MW00932823

Volume 2

MANUAL OF CLINICAL MICROBIOLOGY

12TH EDITION

Volume 2

MANUAL OF CLINICAL MICROBIOLOGY

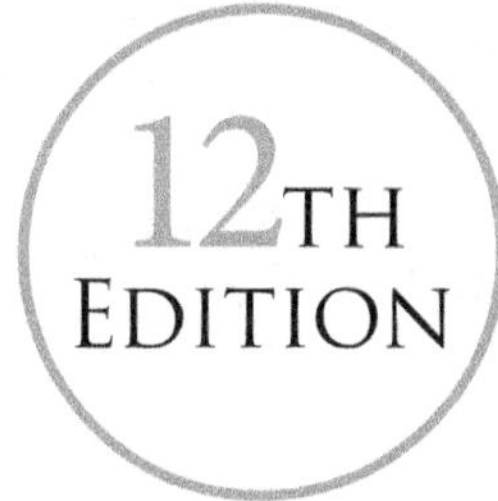

EDITORS-IN-CHIEF

KAREN C. CARROLL
Division of Medical Microbiology,
Department of Pathology, The Johns Hopkins
University School of Medicine,
Baltimore, Maryland

MICHAEL A. PFALLER
Departments of Pathology and Epidemiology
(Emeritus), University of Iowa,
Iowa City, and JMI Laboratories,
North Liberty, Iowa

VOLUME EDITORS

MARIE LOUISE LANDRY
Laboratory Medicine and Internal Medicine,
Yale University, New Haven, Connecticut

ROBIN PATEL
Infectious Diseases Research Laboratory,
Mayo Clinic, Rochester, Minnesota

ALEXANDER J. MCADAM
Department of Laboratory Medicine, Boston
Children's Hospital, Boston, Massachusetts

SANDRA S. RICHTER
Department of Laboratory Medicine,
Cleveland Clinic, Cleveland, Ohio

DAVID W. WARNOCK
Atlanta, Georgia

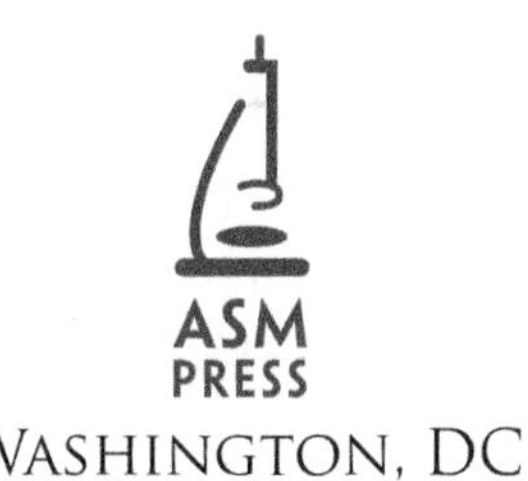

WASHINGTON, DC

Library of Congress Cataloging-in-Publication Data

Names: Carroll, Karen C., editor. | Pfaller, Michael A., editor. | Landry, Marie Louise, editor. | McAdam, Alexander J., editor. | Patel, Robin, M.D., editor. | Richter, Sandra S., editor. | Warnock, D. W., editor.
Title: Manual of clinical microbiology / editors in chief, Karen C. Carroll, Division of Medical Microbiology, Department of Pathology, The Johns Hopkins University School of Medicine, Baltimore, Maryland, Michael A. Pfaller, Departments of Pathology and Epidemiology (emeritus), University of Iowa, Iowa City, and JMI Laboratories, North Liberty, Iowa ; editors, Marie Louise Landry, Laboratory Medicine and Internal Medicine, Yale University, New Haven, Connecticut, Alexander J. McAdam, Department of Laboratory Medicine, Boston Children's Hospital, Boston, Massachusetts, Robin Patel, Infectious Diseases Research Laboratory, Mayo Clinic, Rochester, Minnesota, Sandra S. Richter, Department of Laboratory Medicine, Cleveland Clinic, Cleveland, Ohio, David W. Warnock, Atlanta, Georgia.
Description: 12th edition. | Washington, DC : ASM Press, [2019] | Includes bibliographical references and index.
Identifiers: LCCN 2018057849 | ISBN 9781555819835
Subjects: LCSH: Medical microbiology—Handbooks, manuals, etc. | Diagnostic microbiology—Handbooks, manuals, etc.
Classification: LCC QR46 .M425 2019 | DDC 616.9/041—dc23 LC record available at https://lccn.loc.gov/2018057849

Printed in Canada

SKY14B6885A-5B61-4BA8-A819-9625BDA5F9F8_031521

Address editorial correspondence to: ASM Press, 1752 N St., N.W., Washington, DC 20036-2904, USA.
Send orders to: ASM Press, P.O. Box 605, Herndon, VA 20172, USA.
Phone: 800-546-2416; 703-661-1593. Fax: 703-661-1501.
E-mail: books@asmusa.org
Online: http://estore.asm.org

CONTENTS

Volume 2

section IV

VIROLOGY / 1432

VOLUME EDITOR: MARIE LOUISE LANDRY

SECTION EDITORS: ANGELA M. CALIENDO, CHRISTINE C. GINOCCHIO, RANDALL T. HAYDEN, AND YI-WEI TANG

GENERAL

RNA VIRUSES

DNA VIRUSES

section VII

ANTIFUNGAL AGENTS AND SUSCEPTIBILITY TEST METHODS / 2317

VOLUME EDITOR: DAVID W. WARNOCK
SECTION EDITORS: MARY E. BRANDT AND ELIZABETH M. JOHNSON

section VIII

PARASITOLOGY / 2377

VOLUME EDITOR: DAVID W. WARNOCK
SECTION EDITORS: BOBBI S. PRITT AND GARY W. PROCOP

GENERAL

PARASITES

section IX

ANTIPARASITIC AGENTS AND SUSCEPTIBILITY TEST METHODS / 2643

VOLUME EDITOR: DAVID W. WARNOCK
SECTION EDITORS: GARY W. PROCOP

Editorial Board

Contributors

APRIL N. ABBOTT
Department of Laboratory Medicine, Deaconess Health System, Evansville, Indiana

STEPHAN W. ABERLE
Center for Virology, Medical University of Vienna, Vienna, Austria

SINA M. ADL
University of Saskatchewan, Soil Sciences, College of Agriculture, Saskatoon, Saskatchewan, Canada

MARIA E. AGUERO-ROSENFELD
New York University Langone Health, Pathology, New York, New York

SARAH ABDALLAH AHMED
Westerdijk Fungal Biodiversity Institute, Utrecht, The Netherlands

ALEXANDRE ALANIO
Unité Mycologie Moléculaire, CNRS UMR2000, Centre National de Référence des Mycoses Invasives et Antifongiques, Institut Pasteur, 75724 Paris cedex 15, France

KEVIN ALBY
Department of Pathology and Laboratory Medicine, University of Pennsylvania, Philadelphia, Pennsylvania

DAVID C. ALEXANDER
Cadham Provincial Laboratory and Department of Medical Microbiology & Infectious Diseases, University of Manitoba, Winnipeg, Manitoba, Canada

IBNE M. KARIM ALI
National Center for Emerging and Zoonotic Infectious Diseases, Centers for Disease Control and Prevention, Atlanta, Georgia

GEORGE F. ARAJ
Department of Pathology and Laboratory Medicine, American University of Beirut Medical Center, Beirut, Lebanon

MATTHEW J. ARDUINO
Division of Healthcare Quality Promotion, National Center for Emerging and Zoonotic Infectious Diseases, Centers for Disease Control and Prevention, Atlanta, Georgia

H. RUTH ASHBEE
School of Molecular and Cellular Biology, Faculty of Biological Sciences, University of Leeds, Leeds, United Kingdom

RONALD M. ATLAS
Department of Biology, University of Louisville, Louisville, Kentucky (Retired)

ROBERT L. ATMAR
Departments of Medicine and Molecular Virology & Microbiology, Baylor College of Medicine, Houston, Texas

N. ESTHER BABADY
Department of Laboratory Medicine, Memorial Sloan-Kettering Cancer Center, New York, New York

FAUSTO BALDANTI
Department of Clinical, Surgical, Diagnostics and Pediatric Sciences, University of Pavia, and Molecular Virology Unit, Fondazione IRCCS Policlinico San Matteo, Pavia, Italy

MATTHEW J. BANKOWSKI
Baptist Medical Center Jacksonville, Infectious Diagnostics Laboratory, Jacksonville, Florida

FRÉDÉRIC BARBUT
National Reference Laboratory for Clostridium difficile, Hôpital Saint-Antoine, and EA4065, Université Paris Descartes, Paris, France

JENNIFER DIEN BARD
Department of Pathology and Laboratory Medicine, Children's Hospital Los Angeles, Keck School of Medicine, University of Southern California, Los Angeles, California

CÉCILE BÉBÉAR
USC EA 3671, University of Bordeaux, Department of Bacteriology, French National Reference Center for bacterial STI, Bordeaux University Hospital, Bordeaux, France

KARSTEN BECKER
University Hospital Münster, Institute of Medical Microbiology, Münster, Germany

ELIZABETH L. BERKOW
Centers for Disease Control and Prevention, Mycotic Diseases Branch, Atlanta, Georgia

KATHRYN A. BERNARD
National Microbiology Laboratory-CSCHAH, Public Health Agency of Canada, and Department of Medical Microbiology, University of Manitoba, Winnipeg, Manitoba, Canada

BEVERLEY-ANN BIGGS
Victorian Infectious Diseases Service, Royal Melbourne Hospital, Parkville, Victoria, and Department of Medicine at the Peter Doherty Institute for Infection and Immunity, University of Melbourne, Melbourne, Australia

THOMAS BJARNSHOLT
Department of Clinical Microbiology, Rigshospitalet, and Department of Immunology and Microbiology, Costerton Biofilm Center, Faculty of Health and Medical Sciences, University of Copenhagen, Copenhagen, Denmark

LUCAS S. BLANTON
Department of Internal Medicine – Infectious Diseases, University of Texas Medical Branch, Galveston, Texas

CHANTAL BLEEKER-ROVERS
Radboud University Medical Center, Department of Internal Medicine, and Radboud Expertise Center for Q Fever, Nijmegen, The Netherlands

CHRISTIAN BOGDAN
Mikrobiologisches Institut - Klinische Mikrobiologie, Immunologie und Hygiene, Friedrich-Alexander-Universität (FAU) Erlangen-Nürnberg und Universitätsklinikum Erlangen, Erlangen, Germany

GUY BOIVIN
Department of Microbiology and Infectious Diseases, Laval University, Quebec City, QC, Canada

ANDREW M. BORMAN
United Kingdom National Mycology Reference Laboratory, Public Health England, Bristol, United Kingdom

YAN BOUCHER
University of Alberta, Edmonton, Alberta, Canada

DONALD H. BOUYER
Department of Pathology, University of Texas Medical Branch, Galveston, Texas

PATRICIA A. BRADFORD
Antimicrobial Development Specialists, LLC, Nyack, New York

CLAUDIA BRANDT
Institute for Medical Microbiology and Infection Control, University Hospital, Goethe University, Frankfurt, Germany

MARY E. BRANDT
Office of Laboratory Science and Safety, Centers for Disease Control and Prevention, Atlanta, Georgia

KEVIN E. BROWN
Virus Reference Department, Public Health England, London, United Kingdom

BARBARA A. BROWN-ELLIOTT
Department of Microbiology, The University of Texas Health Science Center at Tyler, Department of Microbiology, Tyler, Texas

DAVID A. BRUCKNER
Department of Pathology & Laboratory Medicine, David Geffen School of Medicine, University of California, Los Angeles, Los Angeles, California

BLAKE W. BUCHAN
Medical College of Wisconsin and Wisconsin Diagnostic Laboratories, Milwaukee, Wisconsin

RICHARD S. BULLER
Department of Pediatrics, Washington University School of Medicine, St. Louis, Missouri

SUSAN M. BUTLER-WU
Department of Pathology and Laboratory Medicine, Keck School of Medicine of USC, Los Angeles, California

ANGELA M. CALIENDO
Alpert Medical School of Brown University, Providence, Rhode Island

VITALIANO CAMA
Division of Parasitic Diseases and Malaria, Centers for Disease Control and Prevention, Atlanta, Georgia

GERALD A. CAPRARO
Carolinas HealthCare System, Clinical Microbiology, Charlotte, North Carolina

DARCIE E. CARPENTER
IHMA, Inc., Schaumburg, Illinois

KAREN C. CARROLL
Division of Medical Microbiology, Department of Pathology, The Johns Hopkins University School of Medicine, Baltimore, Maryland

MARIA DA GLÓRIA SIQUEIRA CARVALHO
Streptococcus Laboratory, Respiratory Diseases Branch, Division of Bacterial Diseases, Centers for Disease Control and Prevention, Atlanta, Georgia

MARIANA CASTANHEIRA
JMI Laboratories, North Liberty, Iowa

ADAM J. CAULFIELD
Spectrum Health Regional Laboratory, Grand Rapids, Michigan

MAIKEN CAVLING-ARENDRUP
Department of Microbiology & Infection Control, Statens Serum Institut; Department of Clinical Microbiology, Rigshospitalet; and Department of Clinical Medicine, University of Copenhagen, Copenhagen, Denmark

ANGELLA CHARNOT-KATSIKAS
Department of Pathology, University of Chicago, Chicago, Illinois

SHARON C.-A. CHEN
Westmead Hospital, Infectious Diseases, Westmead, NSW 2145, Australia

MAX CHERNESKY
Pediatrics, Pathology and Molecular Medicine, McMaster University/St Josephs Healthcare, Hamilton, Ontario, Canada

CHENG-FENG CHIANG
Viral Special Pathogens Branch, Division of High Consequence Pathogens and Pathology, National Center for Emerging and Zoonotic Infectious Diseases, Centers for Disease Control and Prevention, Atlanta, Georgia

SUNWEN CHOU
Department of Medicine, Oregon Health and Sciences University, Portland, Oregon

JENS JØRGEN CHRISTENSEN
Institute of Clinical Medicine, University of Copenhagen, and Department of Clinical Microbiology, Slagelse Hospital, Slagelse, Denmark

OANA CIOFU
Department of Immunology and Microbiology, Costerton Biofilm Center, Faculty of Health and Medical Sciences, University of Copenhagen, Copenhagen, Denmark

JÉRÔME CLAIN
UMR 216 IRD MERIT, Faculty of Pharmacy, Paris Descartes University, 75006 Paris, France

BRYAN R. COBB
Roche Molecular Systems, Pleasanton, California

TOM COENYE
Laboratory of Pharmaceutical Microbiology, Ghent University, Ghent, Belgium

GEORG CONRADS
Division of Oral Microbiology and Immunology, RWTH Aachen University Hospital, Aachen, Germany

PATRICIA S. CONVILLE
Division of Microbiology Devices, Office of In-Vitro Diagnostics and Radiological Health, Center for Devices and Radiological Health, Food and Drug Administration, Silver Spring, Maryland

PIET COOLS
Laboratory Bacteriology Research, Department of Microbiology, Immunology and Clinical Chemistry, Faculty of Medicine and Health Sciences, Ghent University, Ghent, Belgium

JENNIFER R. COPE
National Center for Emerging and Zoonotic Infectious Diseases, Centers for Disease Control and Prevention, Atlanta, Georgia

MARC ROGER COUTURIER
University of Utah/ARUP Laboratories, Pathology/Infectious Disease Microbiology, Salt Lake City, Utah

BART J. CURRIE
Menzies School of Health Research and Northern Territory Medical Program, Royal Darwin Hospital, Darwin, Northern Territory, Australia

KATE CUSCHIERI
Scottish HPV Reference Laboratory, Department of Laboratory Medicine, Royal Infirmary of Edinburgh, Edinburgh, Scotland

MELANIE T. CUSHION
Department of Internal Medicine, Division of Infectious Diseases, University of Cincinnati College of Medicine, and the Cincinnati VA Medical Center, Cincinnati, Ohio

STEVEN D. DALLAS
UT Health San Antonio, Department of Pathology and Laboratory Medicine, San Antonio, Texas

INGER K. DAMON
Centers for Disease Control and Prevention, Division of High Consequence Pathogens and Pathology, Atlanta, Georgia

G. SYBREN DE HOOG
Westerdijk Fungal Biodiversity Institute, Utrecht, The Netherlands

JOHN DEKKER
National Institutes of Health, Bethesda, Maryland

PETER DEPLAZES
Institute of Parasitology, University of Zurich, Zurich, Switzerland

EDWARD P. DESMOND
Mycobacteriology Section, Microbial Diseases Laboratory, California Department of Public Health, Richmond, California

DANIEL J. DIEKEMA
Division of Infectious Diseases, Department of Internal Medicine, and Division of Medical Microbiology, Department of Pathology, University of Iowa College of Medicine, Iowa City, Iowa

ELIZABETH A. DIETRICH
Bacterial Diseases Branch, Division of Vector-Borne Diseases, Centers for Disease Control and Prevention, Fort Collins, Colorado

CHRISTOPHER D. DOERN
Department of Pathology, Virginia Commonwealth University Medical Center, Richmond, Virginia

SHEILA C. DOLLARD
Division of Viral Diseases, Centers for Disease Control and Prevention, Atlanta, Georgia

FRANÇOISE DROMER
Institut Pasteur, Unité de Mycologie Moléculaire, Centre National de Référence des Mycoses Invasives et Antifongiques, CNRS UMR2000, Paris, France

J. STEPHEN DUMLER
Joint Departments of Pathology, Uniformed Services University of the Health Sciences, Walter Reed National Military Medical Center, Joint Pathology Center, Bethesda, Maryland

JAMES J. DUNN
Department of Pathology, Texas Children's Hospital, and Department of Pathology and Immunology, Baylor College of Medicine, Houston, Texas

PAUL H. EDELSTEIN
University of Pennsylvania Perelman School of Medicine, Pathology and Laboratory Medicine, Philadelphia, Pennsylvania

JOHANNES ELIAS
Instiute of Microbiology, DRK Kliniken Berlin, Berlin, Germany

HERMES ESCALANTE
Universidad Nacional de Trujillo, Trujillo, Peru

RICHARD R. FACKLAM
Streptococcus Laboratory, Respiratory Diseases Branch, Division of Bacterial Diseases, Centers for Disease Control and Prevention, Atlanta, Georgia

FERRIC C. FANG
Departments of Laboratory Medicine and Microbiology, University of Washington School of Medicine, Seattle, Washington

JOHN J. FARMER III
United States Public Health Service (Retired), Stone Mountain, Georgia

MATTHEW L. FARON
Medical College of Wisconsin, Milwaukee, Wisconsin

MICHAEL S. FORMAN
Division of Medical Microbiology, Department of Pathology, The Johns Hopkins Medical Institutions, Baltimore, Maryland

STEPHEN J. FORSYTHE
foodmicrobe.com, Nottingham, United Kingdom

KAREN M. FRANK
Department of Laboratory Medicine, National Institutes of Health, Bethesda, Maryland

MATTHIAS FROSCH
Institute of Hygiene and Microbiology, University of Wuerzburg, Wuerzburg, Germany

NAOMI J. GADSBY
Royal Infirmary of Edinburgh, Specialist Virology Centre, Dept. Laboratory Medicine, Edinburgh, Lothian EH16 4SA, United Kingdom

RENEE L. GALLOWAY
Centers for Disease Control and Prevention, Atlanta, Georgia

BHANU P. GANESH
Department of Neurology, The University of Texas Health Science Center at Houston, Houston, Texas

HECTOR H. GARCIA
Universidad Peruana Cayetano Heredia, Center for Global Health, Lima, Peru

LYNNE S. GARCIA
LSG & Associates, Santa Monica, California

DEA GARCIA-HERMOSO
Unité Mycologie Moléculaire, CNRS UMR2000, Centre National de Référence des Mycoses Invasives et Antifongiques, Institut Pasteur, 75724 Paris cedex 15, France

BARBARA C. GÄRTNER
Institute for Microbiology and Hygiene, Saarland University, Faculty of Medicine and Medical Center, Homburg/Saar, Germany

WALTER GEIßDÖRFER
Mikrobiologisches Institut - Klinische Mikrobiologie, Immunologie und Hygiene, Friedrich-Alexander-Universität (FAU) Erlangen-Nürnberg and Universitätsklinikum Erlangen, Erlangen, Germany

PETER GERNER-SMIDT
National Center for Emerging and Zoonotic Infectious Diseases, Centers for Disease Control and Prevention, Atlanta, Georgia

CHRISTINE C. GINOCCHIO
Medical Affairs, bioMérieux/BioFire Diagnostics, Durham, North Carolina

WILLIAM A. GLOVER II
Washington State Public Health Laboratories, Shoreline, Washington

BEATRIZ L. GÓMEZ GIRALDO
School of Medicine and Health Sciences, Translational Microbiology and Emerging Diseases Group (MICROS), Universidad del Rosario, Bogotá, Colombia

MARK D. GONZALEZ
Department of Pathology, Children's Healthcare of Atlanta, Atlanta, Georgia

ALEXANDER L. GRENINGER
Department of Laboratory Medicine, University of Washington, and Vaccine and Infectious Disease Division, Fred Hutchinson Cancer Research Center, Seattle, Washington

JOSEP GUARRO
Universitat Rovira i Virgili, Mycology Unit, Medical School and IISPV, Reus, Spain

CLIFFORD J. GUNTHEL
Infectious Disease Program, Grady Health System, Emory University School of Medicine, Atlanta, Georgia

CATRIONA L. HALLIDAY
Westmead Hospital, Infectious Diseases, Westmead, NSW 2145, Australia

RANDALL T. HAYDEN
Department of Pathology, St. Jude Children's Research Hospital, Memphis, Tennessee

ALBERT HEIM
Hannover Medical School, Virology, Hannover, Germany

WALID HENEINE
Division of HIV/AIDS Prevention, National Center for HIV/AIDS, Viral Hepatitis, STD, and TB Prevention, Centers for Disease Control and Prevention, Atlanta, Georgia

CAROLE J. HICKMAN
Viral Vaccine Preventable Diseases Branch, Division of Viral Diseases, Centers for Disease Control and Prevention, Atlanta, Georgia

SARAH K. HIGHLANDER
Pathogen and Microbiome Division, Translational Genomics Research Institute, Flagstaff, Arizona

RICHARD L. HODINKA
Department of Biomedical Sciences, University of South Carolina School of Medicine Greenville and Greenville Health System, Greenville, South Carolina

NIELS HØIBY
Department of Clinical Microbiology, Rigshospitalet, and Department of Immunology and Microbiology, Costerton Biofilm Center, Faculty of Health and Medical Sciences, University of Copenhagen, Copenhagen, Denmark

MARTIN HOLFELDER
Department of Microbiology, Limbach Laboratory, Heidelberg, Germany

AMY J. HORNEMAN
VA Maryland Health Care System, Pathology and Laboratory Service, Baltimore, Maryland

REBECCA T. HORVAT
Department of Pathology and Laboratory Medicine, University of Kansas School of Medicine, Kansas City, Kansas

DIANA D. HUANG
Department of Microbial Pathogens and Immunity, Rush University Medical Center, Chicago, Illinois

ROMNEY M. HUMPHRIES
Accelerate Diagnostics, Tucson, and Department of Pathology and Laboratory Medicine, University of Arizona, Tucson, Arizona

ELIZABETH A. HUNSPERGER
Diagnostics and Laboratory Systems Program, Centers for Disease Control and Prevention, Centers for Global Health, Division of Global Health Protection, Nairobi, Kenya

JOSEPH P. ICENOGLE
Viral Vaccine Preventable Diseases Branch, Division of Viral Diseases, Centers for Disease Control and Prevention, Atlanta, Georgia

JACQUES IZOPET
Department of Virology, National Reference Center for Hepatitis E virus, CHU Toulouse, and Center for Pathophysiology of Toulouse-Purpan, INSERM UMR1043 / CNRS UMR 5282, CPTP, Toulouse University Paul Sabatier, Toulouse, France

KEITH R. JEROME
Department of Laboratory Medicine, University of Washington, Vaccine and Infectious Disease Division, Fred Hutchinson Cancer Research Center, Seattle, Washington

JUAN A. JIMENEZ
Universidad Nacional Mayor de San Marcos, Laboratorio de Parasitología en Fauna Silvestre y Zoonosis, Lima, Peru

CRYSTAL N. JOHNSON
APC Microbiome Institute and Teagasc Food Research Centre, Moorepark Biosciences Department, Fermoy, Co. Cork, Ireland

ELIZABETH M. JOHNSON
Mycology Reference Laboratory, Public Health England National Infection Service, Bristol, United Kingdom

MALCOLM K. JONES
School of Veterinary Sciences, The University of Queensland, Brisbane, Qld 4072, Australia

JAMES H. JORGENSEN
University of Texas Health Science Center at San Antonio, San Antonio, Texas

NASSIM KAMAR
Center for Pathophysiology of Toulouse-Purpan, INSERM UMR1043 / CNRS UMR 5282, CPTP, Toulouse University Paul Sabatier, and Department of Nephrology and Organ Transplantation, CHU Toulouse, Toulouse, France

PETER KÄMPFER
Institut für Angewandte Mikrobiologie, Universität Giessen, Giessen, Germany

JAMES A. KARLOWSKY
Department of Medical Microbiology and Infectious Diseases, University of Manitoba, Winnipeg, Manitoba, Canada

JENNIFER KEISER
Department of Medical Parasitology and Infection Biology, Swiss Tropical and Public Health Institute, CH-4002 Basel, Switzerland

NANCY P. KELLER
University of Wisconsin-Madison, Medical Microbiology and Immunology and Bacteriology, Madison, Wisconsin

GILBERT J. KERSH
Centers for Disease Control and Prevention, Rickettsial Zoonoses Branch, Atlanta, Georgia

PAUL E. KILGORE
Eugene Applebaum College of Pharmacy and Health Sciences and Department of Family Medicine and Public Health Sciences, School of Medicine, Wayne State University, Detroit, Michigan

LUKE C. KINGRY
Bacterial Diseases Branch, Division of Vector-Borne Diseases, Centers for Disease Control and Prevention, Fort Collins, Colorado

JOHN D. KLENA
Viral Special Pathogens Branch, Division of High Consequence Pathogens and Pathology, National Center for Emerging and Zoonotic Infectious Diseases, Centers for Disease Control and Prevention, Atlanta, Georgia

LAURA M. KOETH
Laboratory Specialists, Inc., Westlake, Ohio

EIJA KÖNÖNEN
Institute of Dentistry, University of Turku, Turku, Finland

THOMAS G. KSIAZEK
Galveston National Laboratory, Department of Pathology, University of Texas Medical Branch, Galveston, Texas

ED KUIJPER
Department of Medical Microbiology, Leiden University Medical Centre, 2333 ZA Leiden, The Netherlands

JAIME LABARCA
Departamento de Enfermedades Infecciosas, Escuela de Medicina, Pontificia Universidad Católica de Chile, Diagonal Paraguay 362, Santiago 8330077, Chile

PHILIPPE LAGACÉ-WIENS
Diagnostic Services, Shared Health, and Department of Medical Microbiology and Infectious Diseases, Max Rady College of Medicine, University of Manitoba, Winnipeg, Manitoba, Canada

DARYL M. LAMSON
Division of Infectious Diseases, Wadsworth Center, New York State Department of Health, Albany, New York

BRIGITTE LAMY
CHU Nice, Université Côte d'Azur and INSERM U1065, Bactériologie, Nice, France

MARIE LOUISE LANDRY
Laboratory Medicine and Internal Medicine, Yale University, New Haven, Connecticut

PAUL A. LAWSON
Department of Microbiology and Plant Biology, University of Oklahoma, Norman, Oklahoma

JACQUES LE BRAS
UMR 216 IRD MERIT, Faculty of Pharmacy, Paris Descartes University, 75006 Paris, France

AMY L. LEBER
Nationwide Children's Hospital, Clinical Microbiology and Immunoserology, Department of Laboratory Medicine, Columbus, Ohio

NATHAN A. LEDEBOER
Department of Pathology, Medical College of Wisconsin, Milwaukee, Wisconsin

KARIN LEDER
Infectious Disease Epidemiology Unit, School of Epidemiology and Preventive Medicine, Monash University, Victorian Infectious Disease Service, Royal Melbourne Hospital, Victoria, Australia

ELLIOT J. LEFKOWITZ
Department of Microbiology, The University of Alabama at Birmingham, Birmingham, Alabama

DIANE S. LELAND
Department of Pathology and Laboratory Medicine, Indiana University School of Medicine, Indianapolis, Indiana

PAUL N. LEVETT
BC Centre for Disease Control Public Health Laboratory, Vancouver, British Columbia, Canada

JAMES S. LEWIS, II
Oregon Health and Science University, Departments of Pharmacy & Infectious Diseases, Portland, Oregon

SHOU-YEAN GRACE LIN
Mycobacteriology Section, Microbial Diseases Laboratory, California Department of Public Health, Richmond, California

DAVID S. LINDSAY
Virginia Tech, Biomedical Sciences and Pathobiology, Blacksburg, Virginia

MARK D. LINDSLEY
Mycotic Diseases Branch, Centers for Disease Control and Prevention, Atlanta, Georgia

ANDREA J. LINSCOTT
Ochsner Medical Center, Department of Pathology and Laboratory Medicine, New Orleans, Louisiana

JOHN J. LiPUMA
Department of Pediatrics and Communicable Diseases, University of Michigan Medical School, Ann Arbor, Michigan

SHAWN R. LOCKHART
Mycotic Diseases Branch, National Center for Emerging and Zoonotic Infectious Diseases, Centers for Disease Control and Prevention, Atlanta, Georgia

MICHAEL LOEFFELHOLZ
Department of Pathology and Clinical Microbiology Laboratory, University of Texas Medical Branch, Galveston, Texas

XIAOYAN LU
Division of Viral Diseases, Centers for Disease Control and Prevention, Atlanta, Georgia

NELL S. LURAIN
Department of Microbial Pathogens and Immunity, Rush University Medical Center, Chicago, Illinois

DUNCAN MacCANNELL
National Center for Emerging and Zoonotic Infectious Diseases, Centers for Disease Control and Prevention, Atlanta, Georgia

HUGO MADRID
Universidad Mayor, Centro de Genómica y Bioinformática, Santiago, Chile

STEVEN D. MAHLEN
Affiliated Laboratory, Inc., Clinical Microbiology, Bangor, Maine

ISABELLA MARTIN
Pathology, Dartmouth-Hitchcock Medical Center, Lebanon, New Hampshire

ALEXANDER MATHIS
Institute of Parasitology, University of Zurich, Zurich, Switzerland

BLAINE MATHISON
ARUP Laboratories, Infectious Disease Division, Salt Lake City, Utah

JAMES B. McAULEY
Rush University Medical Center, Chicago, Illinois

GERALD McDONNELL
DePuy Synthes Companies, Johnson & Johnson, Raritan, New Jersey

ERIN McELVANIA
Pathology, Evanston Hospital/NorthShore University HealthSystem, Evanston, Illinois

KARIN L. McGOWAN
University of Pennsylvania, Department of Pathology and Laboratory Medicine, Perelman School of Medicine, Philadelphia, Pennsylvania (Emeritus)

SARAH L. McGUINNESS
Infectious Disease Epidemiology Unit, School of Epidemiology and Preventive Medicine, Monash University, Department of Infectious Diseases, The Alfred Hospital, Victoria, Australia

DONALD P. McMANUS
QIMR Berghofer Medical Research Institute, Herston, Queensland 4006, Australia

LEONEL MENDOZA
Michigan State University, Microbiology and Molecular Genetics, East Lansing, Michigan

WIELAND MEYER
Westmead Millennium Institute for Medical Research, Infectious Diseases, Westmead, NSW 2145, Australia

LINDA A. FEDERICI MILLER
CMID Pharma Consulting, LLC, Dresher, Pennsylvania

RHODA ASHLEY MORROW
University of Washington and Fred Hutchinson Cancer Research Center, Seattle, Washington

ANNETTE MOTER
Charité-Universitätsmedizin Berlin, Biofilmzentrum des Deutschen Herzzentrums Berlin, Berlin, Germany

IONA MUNJAL
Department of Pediatrics, Montefiore Medical Center and Albert Einstein College of Medicine, and Pfizer Vaccine Clinical Research & Development, Bronx, New York

IRVING NACHAMKIN
Department of Pathology and Laboratory Medicine, Perelman School of Medicine, University of Pennsylvania, Philadelphia, Pennsylvania

ELISABETH NAGY
Institute of Clinical Microbiology, University of Szeged, Szeged, Hungary

RONALD C. NEAFIE
Retired, Former Armed Forces Institute of Pathology, Washington, DC

ALEXANDR NEMEC
Laboratory of Bacterial Genetics, Centre for Epidemiology and Microbiology, National Institute of Public Health, Prague, Czech Republic

TERRY FEI FAN NG
National Center for Immunization and Respiratory Diseases, Centers for Disease Control and Prevention, Atlanta, Georgia

XIAOHUI CHEN NIELSEN
Department of Clinical Microbiology, Slagelse Hospital, Slagelse, Denmark

FREDERICK S. NOLTE
Department of Pathology and Laboratory Medicine, Medical University of South Carolina, Charleston, South Carolina

CARMELLE T. NORICE-TRA
Laboratory of Parasitic Diseases, National Institute of Allergy and Infectious Diseases, National Institutes of Health, Bethesda, Maryland

NIELS NØRSKOV-LAURITSEN
Clinical Microbiology, Aarhus University Hospital, Aarhus, Denmark

SUSAN NOVAK-WEEKLEY
Qvella, Carlsbad, California

THOMAS B. NUTMAN
Laboratory of Parasitic Diseases, National Institute of Allergy and Infectious Diseases, National Institutes of Health, Bethesda, Maryland

KERRY O'DONNELL
Mycotoxin Prevention and Applied Microbiology Research Unit, National Center for Agricultural Utilization Research, ARS-USDA, Peoria, Illinois

VICTORIA A. OLSON
Poxvirus and Rabies Branch, Division of High Consequence Pathogens and Pathologies, Centers for Disease Control and Prevention, Atlanta, Georgia

LILLIAN A. ORCIARI
Poxvirus and Rabies Branch, Division of High Consequence Pathogens and Pathologies, Centers for Disease Control and Prevention, Atlanta, Georgia

OLIVIER ORTHOLARY
Unité Mycologie Moléculaire, CNRS UMR2000, Centre National de Référence des Mycoses Invasives et Antifongiques, Institut Pasteur, 75724 Paris cedex 15, France

BELINDA OSTROWSKY
Department of Medicine, Division of Infectious Disease, Montefiore Medical Center and Albert Einstein College of Medicine, Bronx, New York

S. MICHELE OWEN
National Center for HIV/AIDS, Viral Hepatitis, STD, and TB Prevention, Centers for Disease Control and Prevention, Atlanta, Georgia

GRAEME P. PALTRIDGE
Canterbury Health Laboratories, Microbiology Laboratory, Christchurch 8011, New Zealand

XIAOLI PANG
Provincial Laboratory for Public Health and Department of Laboratory Medicine and Pathology, University of Alberta, Edmonton, Alberta, Canada

NICOLE PARRISH
Pathology, Johns Hopkins University, Baltimore, Maryland

ROBIN PATEL
Infectious Diseases Research Laboratory, Mayo Clinic, Rochester, Minnesota

SHARON J. PEACOCK
Department of Medicine, University of Cambridge, Addenbrooke's Hospital, Cambridge, United Kingdom

MICHAEL PENTELLA
University of Iowa, College of Public Health, Department of Epidemiology, Iowa City, Iowa

DAVID S. PERLIN
Public Health Research Institute, New Jersey Medical School, Rutgers Biomedical and Health Sciences, Newark, New Jersey

JEANNINE M. PETERSEN
Bacterial Diseases Branch, Division of Vector-Borne Diseases, Centers for Disease Control and Prevention, Fort Collins, Colorado

JOSEPH F. PETROSINO
Department of Molecular Virology & Microbiology, Baylor College of Medicine, Houston, Texas

MICHAEL A. PFALLER
Departments of Pathology and Epidemiology (Emeritus), University of Iowa, Iowa City, and JMI Laboratories, North Liberty, Iowa

ALLAN PILLAY
Molecular Surveillance of T. pallidum Unit, Laboratory Reference and Research Branch, Division of STD Prevention, Centers for Disease Control and Prevention, Atlanta, Georgia

BENJAMIN A. PINSKY
Departments of Pathology and Medicine, Stanford University School of Medicine, Stanford, California

JOHANN PITOUT
Department of Pathology and Laboratory Medicine, University of Calgary, and Division of Microbiology, Calgary Laboratory Services, Calgary, Alberta, Canada

BOBBI S. PRITT
Laboratory Medicine and Pathology, Mayo Clinic, Rochester, Minnesota

GARY W. PROCOP
Department of Laboratory Medicine, Pathology and Laboratory Medicine Institute, Cleveland Clinic, Cleveland, Ohio

ELISABETH PUCHHAMMER-STÖCKL
Center for Virology, Medical University of Vienna, Vienna, Austria

JUSTIN D. RADOLF
Departments of Medicine, Pediatrics, Immunology, Molecular Biology and Biophysics, and Genetics and Genome Sciences, UConn Health, Farmington, Connecticut

M. ALI RAI
Cincinnati Veterans Affairs Medical Center, Cincinnati, Ohio

RYAN F. RELICH
Department of Pathology and Laboratory Medicine, Indiana University School of Medicine, Indianapolis, Indiana

L. BARTH RELLER
Departments of Pathology and Medicine, Duke University School of Medicine, Durham, North Carolina

DANIEL D. RHOADS
Case Western Reserve University, Cleveland, Ohio

ELVIRA RICHTER
MVZ Labor Dr. Limbach, TB Laboratory, Heidelberg, Germany

SANDRA S. RICHTER
Clinical Pathology, Cleveland Clinic, Cleveland, Ohio

WINNIE RIDDERBERG
Qiagen Bioinformatics, Aarhus, Denmark

PIERRE E. ROLLIN
Viral Special Pathogens Branch, Centers for Disease Control and Prevention, Atlanta, Georgia

JOSÉ R. ROMERO
Section of Pediatric Infectious Diseases, University of Arkansas for Medical Sciences and Arkansas Children's Hospital, Little Rock, Arkansas

PAUL A. ROTA
National Center for Immunization and Respiratory Diseases, Centers for Disease Control and Prevention, Atlanta, Georgia

KATHRYN L. RUOFF
O'Toole Lab, Department of Microbiology and Immunology, Geisel School of Medicine at Dartmouth, Hanover, New Hampshire

NORBERT RYAN
Bacteriology Laboratory, Victorian Infectious Diseases Reference Laboratory, The Peter Doherty Institute for Infection and Immunity, 792 Elizabeth St., Melbourne 3000, Australia

JIRI G. SAFAR
Case Western Reserve University, Cleveland, Ohio

MAX SALFINGER
Advanced Diagnostic Laboratories, National Jewish Health, Department of Medicine & Mycobacteriology Laboratory, Denver, Colorado

LINOJ SAMUEL
Clinical Microbiology, Henry Ford Health System, Detroit, Michigan

CARLOS A. Q. SANTOS
Division of Infectious Diseases, Rush University Medical Center, Chicago, Illinois

P. S. SATHESHKUMAR
Poxvirus and Rabies Branch, Division of High Consequence Pathogens and Pathologies, Centers for Disease Control and Prevention, Atlanta, Georgia

JULIUS SCHACHTER
Department of Laboratory Medicine, University of California, San Francisco, San Francisco, California

AUDREY N. SCHUETZ
Division of Clinical Microbiology, Department of Laboratory Medicine and Pathology, Mayo Clinic, Rochester, Minnesota

W. EVAN SECOR
Division of Parasitic Diseases and Malaria, Centers for Disease Control and Prevention, Atlanta, Georgia

RUTH HALL SEDLAK
Veterinary Medicine Research and Development, Zoetis, Kalamazoo, Michigan

ARLENE C. SEÑA
Department of Medicine, Division of Infectious Diseases, University of North Carolina at Chapel Hill, Chapel Hill, and Durham County Department of Public Health, Durham, North Carolina

PARHAM SENDI
Institute for Infectious Diseases, University of Bern, Bern, and Department of Infectious Diseases and Hospital Epidemiology, University Hospital Basel, University Basel, Basel, Switzerland

ROBERT W. SHAFER
Departments of Medicine and Pathology, Stanford University, Stanford, California

SUSAN E. SHARP
Kaiser Permanente, Department of Pathology, Portland, Oregon

ROSEMARY C. SHE
Department of Pathology, Keck School of Medicine of the University of Southern California, Los Angeles, California

HARSHA SHEOREY
Department of Microbiology, St Vincent's Hospital Melbourne, Fitzroy, Victoria 3065, Australia

PATRICIA LYNN SHEWMAKER
Streptococcus Laboratory, Respiratory Diseases Branch, Division of Bacterial Diseases, Centers for Disease Control and Prevention, Atlanta, Georgia

WUN-JU SHIEH
Infectious Diseases Pathology Branch, Division of High Consequence Pathogens and Pathology, National Center for Emerging and Zoonotic Infectious Diseases, Centers for Disease Control and Prevention, Atlanta, Georgia

ROBYN Y. SHIMIZU
UCLA HealthSystem, Pathology and Laboratory Medicine, Los Angeles, California

PATRICIA J. SIMNER
John Hopkins University School of Medicine, Pathology, Baltimore, Maryland

KAMALJIT SINGH
NorthShore University HealthSystem, Department of Pathology, Evanston, Illinois

ROBERT L. SKOV
MVZ Synlab Leverkusen GmbH, Leverkusen, Germany, and Statens Serum Institut, Copenhagen, Denmark

MAREK SMIEJA
Department of Pathology and Molecular Medicine, McMaster University, Hamilton, Ontario, Canada

JAMES W. SNYDER
University of Louisville, Department of Pathology and Laboratory Medicine, ULH, Louisville, Kentucky

TANIA C. SORRELL
Westmead Hospital, Infectious Diseases, Westmead, NSW 2145, Australia

BARBARA SPELLERBERG
Institute of Medical Microbiology and Hygiene, University of Ulm, Ulm, Germany

JENNIFER K. SPINLER
Department of Pathology & Immunology, Baylor College of Medicine, and Department of Pathology, Texas Children's Hospital, Houston, Texas

GEROLD STANEK
Medical University of Vienna, Center for Pathophysiology, Infectiology and Immunology, Institute for Hygiene and Applied Immunology, Vienna, Austria

KATHLEEN A. STELLRECHT
Department of Pathology and Laboratory Medicine, Albany Medical College and Albany Medical Center Hospital, Albany, New York

GREGORY A. STORCH
Department of Pediatrics, Washington University School of Medicine, St. Louis, Missouri

RICHARD C. SUMMERBELL
Sporometrics Inc. and Dalla Lana School of Public Health, University of Toronto, Toronto, Ontario, Canada

DEANNA A. SUTTON
Department of Pathology, University of Texas Health Science Center at San Antonio, San Antonio, Texas

WILLIAM M. SWITZER
Division of HIV/AIDS Prevention, National Center for HIV/AIDS, Viral Hepatitis, STD, and TB Prevention, Centers for Disease Control and Prevention, Atlanta, Georgia

WENDY A. SZYMCZAK
Department of Pathology, Montefiore Medical Center and Albert Einstein College of Medicine, Bronx, New York

YI-WEI TANG
Department of Laboratory Medicine, Memorial Sloan Kettering Cancer Center, and Department of Pathology and Laboratory Medicine, Weill Medical College of Cornell University, New York, New York

JOANNA TANNOUS
University of Wisconsin-Madison, Medical Microbiology and Immunology, Madison, Wisconsin

CHERYL L. TARR
Enteric Diseases Laboratory Branch, Division of Foodborne, Waterborne and Environmental Diseases, Centers for Disease Control and Prevention, Atlanta, Georgia

LÚCIA MARTINS TEIXEIRA
Instituto de Microbiologia, Universidade Federal do Rio de Janeiro, Rio de Janeiro, Brazil

SAM R. TELFORD III
Cummings School of Veterinary Medicine, Tufts University, North Grafton, Massachusetts

KATE E. TEMPLETON
Royal Infirmary of Edinburgh, Specialist Virology Centre, Dept. Laboratory Medicine, Edinburgh, Lothian EH16 4SA, United Kingdom

ELITZA S. THEEL
Department of Laboratory Medicine and Pathology, Division of Clinical Microbiology
Mayo Clinic, Rochester, Minnesota

GEORGE R. THOMPSON, III
Department of Internal Medicine, Division of Infectious Diseases, and Department of Medical Microbiology and Immunology, University of California - Davis, Davis, California

JONATHAN S. TOWNER
Viral Special Pathogens Branch, Centers for Disease Control and Prevention, Atlanta, Georgia

EIJA TREES
National Center for Emerging and Zoonotic Infectious Diseases, Centers for Disease Control and Prevention, Atlanta, Georgia

CHRISTINE Y. TURENNE
Clinical Microbiology, Shared Health (Diagnostic Services), and Department of Medical Microbiology & Infectious Diseases, University of Manitoba, Winnipeg, Manitoba, Canada

JOHN D. TURNIDGE
Adelaide Medical School, University of Adelaide, Adelaide, Australia

KERIN TYRRELL
Los Angeles, California

ELIZABETH R. UNGER
Chronic Viral Diseases Branch, National Center for Emerging and Zoonotic Diseases, Centers for Disease Control and Prevention, Atlanta, Georgia

ALEXANDRA VALSAMAKIS
Roche Molecular Systems, Pleasanton, California, and Division of Medical Microbiology, Department of Pathology, The Johns Hopkins Medical Institutions, Baltimore, Maryland

WENDY W. J. VAN DE SANDE
Erasmus MC, Department of Medical Microbiology and Infectious Diseases, Rotterdam, The Netherlands

PETER A. R. VANDAMME
Laboratorium voor Microbiologie, Faculteit Wetenschappen, Universiteit Gent, Ghent, Belgium

MARIO VANEECHOUTTE
Laboratory Bacteriology Research, Department of Microbiology, Immunology and Clinical Chemistry, Faculty of Medicine and Health Sciences, Ghent University, Ghent, Belgium

ALIDA C. M. VELOO
Department of Medical Microbiology and Infection Prevention, University of Groningen, University Medical Center Groningen, Groningen, The Netherlands

JAMES VERSALOVIC
Departments of Pathology & Immunology and Molecular Virology & Microbiology, Baylor College of Medicine, and Department of Pathology, Texas Children's Hospital, Houston, Texas

RAQUEL VILELA
Universidade Federal do Minas Gerais, Faculdade de Farmacia, Campus Pampulha, Belo Horizonte, Minas Gerais CEP: 31.270.901, Brazil

GOVINDA S. VISVESVARA
Centers for Disease Control and Prevention, Atlanta, Georgia (Retired)

ULRICH VOGEL
Institute of Hygiene and Microbiology, University of Wuerzburg, Wuerzburg, Germany

CHRISTOF von EIFF
University Hospital Münster, Institute of Medical Microbiology, Münster, Germany, and Pfizer Pharma GmbH, Berlin, Germany

KEN B. WAITES
Department of Pathology, Diagnostic Mycoplasma Laboratory, University of Alabama at Birmingham, Birmingham, Alabama

DAVID H. WALKER
Department of Pathology, Center for Biodefense and Emerging Infectious Diseases, University of Texas Medical Branch, Galveston, Texas

RICHARD J. WALLACE, JR.
The University of Texas Health Science Center at Tyler, Department of Microbiology, Tyler, Texas

DAVID W. WARNOCK
Atlanta, Georgia

DAVID M. WARSHAUER
Communicable Disease Division, Wisconsin State Laboratory of Hygiene, Madison, Wisconsin

RAINER WEBER
Division of Infectious Diseases and Hospital Epidemiology, University Hospital Zurich, University of Zurich, Zurich, Switzerland

MELVIN P. WEINSTEIN
Departments of Medicine and Pathology & Laboratory Medicine, Rutgers Robert Wood Johnson Medical School, New Brunswick, New Jersey

ANDREJ WEINTRAUB
Karolinska Institutet, Department of Laboratory Medicine, Division of Clinical Microbiology, Stockholm, Sweden

LOUIS M. WEISS
Albert Einstein College of Medicine, Pathology, Bronx, New York

PETER F. WELLER
Harvard Medical School and Division of Infectious Diseases and Allergy and Inflammation Division, Beth Israel Deaconess Medical Center, Boston, Massachusetts

NELE WELLINGHAUSEN
Medical Laboratory Ravensburg, Infection Serology, Ravensburg, Germany

NANCY L. WENGENACK
Division of Clinical Microbiology, Mayo Clinic, Rochester, Minnesota

MICHAEL L. WILSON
Department of Pathology and Laboratory Services, Denver Health Medical Center, Denver, and Department of Pathology, University of Colorado School of Medicine, Aurora, Colorado

FRANK G. WITEBSKY
Microbiology Service, Department of Laboratory Medicine, Warren G. Magnuson Clinical Center, National Institutes of Health, Bethesda, Maryland (Retired)

GAIL L. WOODS
University of Arkansas for Medical Sciences and Arkansas Children's Hospital, Pathology, Little Rock, Arkansas

LIHUA XIAO
College of Veterinary Medicine, South China Agricultural University, Guangzhou, China

PAMELA A. YAGER
Poxvirus and Rabies Branch, Division of High Consequence Pathogens and Pathologies, Centers for Disease Control and Prevention, Atlanta, Georgia

REINHARD ZBINDEN
Institute of Medical Microbiology, University of Zurich, Zurich, Switzerland

SEAN X. ZHANG
Division of Medical Microbiology, Department of Pathology, The Johns Hopkins Hospital, The Johns Hopkins School of Medicine, Baltimore, Maryland

Acknowledgment of Previous Contributors
The *Manual of Clinical Microbiology* is by its nature a continuously revised work which refines and extends the contributions of previous editions. Since its first edition in 1970, many eminent scientists have contributed to this important reference work. The American Society for Microbiology and ASM Press gratefully acknowledge the contributions of all of these generous authors over the life of this *Manual.*

PREFACE

The *Manual of Clinical Microbiology* (MCM) is the most authoritative reference text in the field of clinical microbiology. This edition of the *Manual* benefited from the talents of a team of 22 editors and over 300 authors who were supported by a very capable production team at ASM Press. This, the 12th edition, is presented after the usual 4-year publication cycle following the 11th edition. All of the editorial team are proud members of the American Society for Microbiology and strong supporters of its book publishing arm, ASM Press. We have followed in the footsteps of previous authors and editors of the *Manual* and remain steadfastly committed to the utmost quality and timeliness that the MCM readership has come to expect. It is now clear that the strategy of employing two co-editors in chief of MCM is a good one. The length and scope of the *Manual* now require this division of labor to ensure thoroughness and timeliness of the editing process. We hope that readers of the *Manual* will recognize the commitment to excellence by everyone associated with its production.

We represent the sixth and seventh editors in chief in the 50-year history of the *Manual*. We are grateful for the example set by our predecessors and for the sage advice offered by recent editors in chief Patrick Murray, James Versalovic, and James Jorgensen. We offer our deep appreciation to Ellie Tupper, Senior Production Editor at ASM Press, who provided calm competence in driving the editorial production process.

This is a very dynamic era in clinical microbiology, with new technical tools (MALDI-TOF MS, Sanger and second- and third-generation next-generation sequencing, and other molecular methods) that are profoundly influencing our approaches to organism detection and identification. The *Manual* continues to include classic microbiological techniques such as microscopy and culture as a foundation in addition to the newer methods cited above. Some organisms have become prominent causes of disease recently, e.g., Ebola virus, Zika virus, enterovirus D-68, Gram-negative bacteria that produce carbapenemases, and multi-drug-resistant fungi such as *Candida auris* and *Lomentospora prolificans*. Every effort was made to include up-to-date information on these recently emergent organisms in the *Manual*. Likewise, advances in molecular taxonomy have resulted in major changes in genus and species designations among bacteria, fungi, and protozoan parasites, all of which are reflected in this edition. In addition, the continuing studies of the human microbiome have informed our understanding of normal microbial communities and have posed the possibility of polymicrobial rather than single-agent infections.

In conclusion, we are profoundly grateful for the privilege of guiding the *Manual* through the publication of this 12th edition. We hope that the efforts of the MCM editors and authors will continue to prove useful to the clinical microbiology community.

KAREN C. CARROLL
MICHAEL A. PFALLER

Author and Editor Conflicts of Interest

April N. Abbott (coauthor on chapter 79) has participated in research studies supported by BioFire, Cepheid, ELITech, and Luminex.

Patricia A. Bradford (coauthor on chapter 71) is a consultant for Adenium, Allecra, Antabio, Avego, Aviragen, Bay City, Colgate-Palmolive, Contrafect, Cosmo, Emergent, Entasis, Everest, Genentech, IHMA, Pontifax, Roche, Syndegen, Tetraphase, Theravance, TPG, Wellcome, Zavante, and Zolex.

Gerald A. Capraro (coauthor on chapter 82) has received speaking honoraria from Quidel Diagnostics and is an Advisory Board member for Roche and for DiaSorin Molecular.

Karen C. Carroll (coauthor on chapters 1, 5, and 50; Editor in Chief) has received research funds from Curetis, Inc., GenMark, Inc., and GenePOC, Inc. These funds are paid to Johns Hopkins University School of Medicine. Dr. Carroll also receives travel reimbursement from ASM and IDSA.

Mariana Castanheira (coauthor on chapter 71) holds financial interests or benefits in JMI Laboratories and was contracted to perform services in 2016 for Achaogen, Actelion, Allecra Therapeutics, Allergan, AmpliPhi Biosciences, API, Astellas Pharma, AstraZeneca, Basilea Pharmaceutica, Bayer AG, BD, Biomodels, Cardeas Pharma Corp., CEM-102 Pharma, Cempra, Cidara Therapeutics, Inc., CorMedix, CSA Biotech, Cutanea Life Sciences, Inc., Debiopharm Group, Dipexium Pharmaceuticals, Inc., Duke University, Entasis Therapeutics, Inc., Fortress Biotech, Fox Chase Chemical Diversity Center, Inc., Geom Therapeutics, Inc., GSK Laboratory Specialists, Inc., Medpace, Melinta Therapeutics, Inc., Merck & Co., Inc., Micromyx, MicuRx Pharmaceuticals, Inc., Motif Bio, N8 Medical, Inc., Nabriva Therapeutics, Inc., Nexcida Therapeutics, Inc., Novartis, Paratek Pharmaceuticals, Inc., Pfizer, Polyphor, Rempex, Scynexis, Shionogi, Spero Therapeutics, Symbal Therapeutics, Synlogic, TenNor Therapeutics, TGV Therapeutics, The Medicines Company, Theravance Biopharma, ThermoFisher Scientific, VenatoRx Pharmaceuticals, Inc., Wockhardt, and Zavante Therapeutics, Inc.

Maiken Cavling-Arendrup (coauthor on chapter 134) has received research grants/contract work (paid to Statens Serum Institut) from Amplyx, Basilea, Cidara, F2G, Gilead, Pfizer, and T2Candida, and speaker honoraria from Astellas, Basilea, Gilead, MSD, Novartis, Pfizer, and T2Candida. Dr. Cavling-Arendrup is Chair(wo)man for EUCAST-AFST and has served on past advisory boards for MSD, Pcovery, and Pfizer.

Bryan R. Cobb (coauthor on chapter 94) is an employee of Roche Diagnostics.

Daniel J. Diekema (coauthor on chapter 9) has received research funding from bioMérieux, Inc.

Christopher D. Doern (coauthor on chapter 6) is on a scientific advisory board for ThermoFisher.

Ferric C. Fang (coauthor on chapter 79) has participated in research studies supported by BioFire, Cepheid, ELITech, and Luminex.

Christine C. Ginocchio (coauthor on chapter 82) is an employee of bioMérieux/BioFire Diagnostics.

Walid Heneine (coauthor on chapter 85) has patents for HTLV-3 and HTLV-4 described in the chapter.

Romney M. Humphries (coauthor on chapters 39, 75, and 76) is the Chief Scientific Officer at Accelerate Diagnostics and a member of the CLSI Subcommittee on Antimicrobial Susceptibility Testing.

Amy L. Leber (coauthor on chapter 143) is on the Advisory Board at BioFire Diagnostics.

James S. Lewis, II (chapter 70), is a consultant to Accelerate Diagnostics, Achaogen, Medicines Company, Merck, Paratek, and Tetraphase.

Iona Munjal (coauthor on chapter 10) is the Associate Director of Pfizer Vaccine Clinical Research & Development. Dr. Munjal holds an appointment as an Assistant Professor in the Department of Pediatrics at Montefiore Medical Center/ Albert Einstein College of Medicine.

Susan Novak-Weekley (coauthor on chapter 143) is an employee of Qvella and consultant to GenMark, Asolva, and Copan Diagnostics.

Robin Patel (coauthor on chapters 5 and 50; Volume Editor) reports grants from Accelerate Diagnostics, Allergan, BioFire, CD Diagnostics, Curetis, Hutchison Biofilm Medical Solutions, The Medicines Company, and Merck. Dr. Patel is or has been a consultant to Beckman Coulter, CORMATRIX, Curetis, Diaxonit, Genentech, GenMark Diagnostics, Heraeus Medical GmbH, LBT Innovations Ltd., Morgan Stanley, PathoQuest, Qvella, Selux Dx, St. Jude, and Specific Technologies; monies are paid to Mayo Clinic. In addition, Dr. Patel has a patent on *Bordetella pertussis/parapertussis* PCR issued; a patent on a device/method for sonication, with royalties paid by Samsung to Mayo Clinic; and a patent on an anti-biofilm substance issued. Dr. Patel has served on an Actelion data monitoring board. Dr. Patel receives travel reimbursement from ASM and IDSA, an editor's stipend from ASM and IDSA, and honoraria from the NBME, UpToDate, Inc., and the Infectious Diseases Board Review Course.

David S. Perlin (chapter 133) serves on scientific advisory boards and has received grant support from Amplyx, Astellas, Cidara, Scynexis, Matinas, and Merck. Dr. Perlin holds a U.S. patent for the detection of echinocandin resistance.

Michael A. Pfaller (coauthor on chapters 1 and 9; Editor in Chief) has been an employee of T2 diagnostics and is currently a consultant for JMI Laboratories in North Liberty, Iowa.

Justin D. Radolf (coauthor on chapter 62) receives royalties for syphilis serodiagnostic recombinant proteins from Biokit, SA, through a licensing agreement with UT Southwestern Medical Center, and from Span Diagnostics through a licensing agreement with the University of Connecticut.

Winnie Ridderberg (coauthor on chapter 35) is employed by Qiagen.

Julius Schachter (coauthor on chapter 65) receives research funding from Abbott, Becton Dickinson, and Roche.

Arlene C. Seña (coauthor on chapter 62) receives grant funding from Gilead Sciences and royalties from UpToDate, Inc.

Robert W. Shafer (coauthor on chapter 114) has received research support from Bristol Myers Squibb, Gilead Sciences, Janssen Pharmaceuticals, and Merck Pharmaceuticalss within the past three years.

Patricia J. Simner (coauthor on chapter 75) is an Advisor for the CLSI Subcommittee on Antimicrobial Susceptibility Testing.

Richard C. Summerbell (coauthor on chapter 126) is Research Director at Sporometrics Inc.

William M. Switzer (coauthor on chapter 85) has patents for HTLV-3 and HTLV-4 described in the chapter.

Alexandra Valsamakis (coauthor on chapter 94) has been a consultant for and has had studies funded by Roche Diagnostics.

VIROLOGY

VOLUME EDITOR: MARIE LOUISE LANDRY
SECTION EDITORS: ANGELA M. CALIENDO, CHRISTINE C. GINOCCHIO, RANDALL T. HAYDEN, AND YI-WEI TANG

GENERAL

RNA VIRUSES

section IV

DNA VIRUSES

SUBVIRAL AGENTS

Taxonomy and Classification of Viruses

ELLIOT J. LEFKOWITZ

80

INTRODUCTION

Taxonomy

Taxonomy at its most basic level involves the classification and naming of objects. Living objects have been grouped for hundreds of years according to the Linnaean system (1), a classification scheme that places living things hierarchically into groups of species followed by groupings into higher-level taxa (from genera to families, orders, classes, phyla, kingdoms, and domains, including a number of now-recognized intervening ranks) dependent on common shared characteristics. Taxonomic assignments were originally based on visible structural similarities between organisms. Assignments now also include molecular and genetic information.

Taxonomy functions beyond mere categorization. By having information about and an understanding of a few of the organisms in a group of closely related taxa, it is often possible to extend that knowledge to other organisms in related taxa for which much less biological information may be available. For viruses, this process of comparative analysis plays a critical role in increasing our overall knowledge of the molecular biology, pathogenesis, epidemiology, and evolution of poorly understood or newly isolated viruses. This knowledge enhances our ability to respond to new threats by supporting the development of diagnostics, vaccines, and antiviral therapies.

Viruses

Viruses are not easily placed on the evolutionary tree of life (2–4). They are not accurately represented by side branches sprouting off from the main branches or by their own single branch growing out from the base of the tree. In fact, it is likely that viruses have multiple independent evolutionary origins (5–7) that cannot be easily or completely separated from the evolution of their hosts because they cannot reproduce or evolve separately from their hosts (8, 9). Indeed, the host represents one of the important characteristics of a virus that must be considered when making taxonomic assignments. Therefore, viruses might be better represented as several individual twigs arising from separate branches on the tree of life.

In addition to distinct evolutionary histories, viruses differ from other domains of life in the variety of possible coding molecules they utilize to store their genetic programs (10, 11). Every other domain of life has, as the basic reservoir of its genetic program, double-stranded DNA (dsDNA). Virus genomes may be composed of dsDNA, single-stranded DNA (ssDNA), dsRNA, or ssRNA (which may be positive or negative sense with respect to the mRNA coding strand). In addition, reverse transcription may be a part of their molecular program. Genome topology (linear, circular, single segment, multiple segments) also varies among different viruses. All of these unique features as well as numerous other criteria are taken into account when classifying viruses and making taxonomic assignments.

VIRAL TAXONOMY

ICTV Classification of Viruses

The process of making taxonomic assignments is the responsibility of a number of organizations that have the internationally recognized authority to oversee or contribute to the process by defining the rules, methods, and nomenclature to be used in making assignments for particular domains or subdomains of life (12–14). For viruses, the Virology Division of the International Union of Microbiological Societies has charged the International Committee on Taxonomy of Viruses (ICTV) with the task of developing, refining, and maintaining a universal viral taxonomy (15–17).

The ICTV currently recognizes five hierarchical ranks that are used to define the universal viral taxonomy: order, family, subfamily, genus, and species. The 2016 ICTV viral taxonomy (18) comprises 8 orders, 122 families, 35 subfamilies, 735 genera, and 4,404 species. The official viral taxonomy is published on the ICTV website (http://ictv.global) and in the ICTV report (16). The first report of the ICTV was based on deliberations made at and after the 1968 (Helsinki) International Congress of Virology (19). Subsequent reports have been published at regular intervals, authored by numerous and collaborating virologists, with the last hard-copy report, the ninth, published in 2012. The current (10th) report is now available as an online, open source publication that will release new and updated chapters on each virus family on an ongoing basis (http://ictv.global/report/). These reports provide a history of the efforts and the logic used in forming taxa, term definitions, the official taxonomy, and a description of higher-level taxa.

Initially, the ICTV only recognized and made assignments to ranks at the genus level and above. In 1991, the rank of species was added (20). A virus species is now defined as "the lowest taxonomic level in the hierarchy approved by the ICTV. A species is a monophyletic group of viruses whose properties can be distinguished from those of other species by multiple criteria" (21). In general, every species is a member of a genus, which in turn is a member of a family. A few families are also members of one of the eight orders that are currently recognized, but the majority of viral families do not belong to an order. Some species are not yet assigned to a genus (but may be assigned to a family), and a few genera are not yet assigned to a family; additional biological information must become available before these assignments can be made. Subfamily and order assignments are optional and therefore not necessary to complete a taxonomic hierarchy.

The ICTV is governed by a series of statutes and follows rules and definitions provided by the International Code of Virus Classification and Nomenclature (16, 18, 21, 22) to make taxonomic assignments and name virus taxa. Any modifications or additions to the official ICTV taxonomic classification and names, as well as changes to the statutes or code, must be approved by the voting membership of the ICTV. Any individual can submit proposals to the ICTV for the modification of existing taxa or the creation of new taxa.

In addition to defining the process and rules for virus classification, the ICTV Code also defines the rules to be followed for name assignment. Names for higher-level ranks are composed of a single word ending with a suffix that is dependent on rank. The suffix *-virales* identifies an order. Families are identified by the suffix *-viridae*, subfamilies are identified by the suffix *-virinae*, and genera are identified by the suffix *-virus*. Species names should be as concise as possible, but normally comprise two or more words. It is common for a species name to end with the word "*virus*" or have "*virus*" as a suffix, but this is not required. When written, the names of taxa are italicized, and the first letter of the name is capitalized. (As a part of a species name, the first letter of any proper noun such as a geographic location is also capitalized.) It is often difficult to determine in a particular context if a species name should be written in the formal italicized manner since species names often coincide with the common names used to refer to a virus. Taxa are abstract concepts that do not physically exist. As an example, when referring to the species *Variola virus*, which belongs to the genus *Orthopoxvirus* and the family *Poxviridae*, all names refer to abstract taxa and are therefore written in the formal italicized manner. However, when referring to variola virus, the physical entity that causes smallpox, the name is neither capitalized nor italicized.

The ICTV is only concerned with making taxonomic assignments at the species level and higher, although many viral isolates assigned to one particular species may be further subdivided into categories based on sequence phylogeny, immune reactivity, or other properties. In many cases these subspecies-level assignments are made on an *ad hoc* basis by an individual investigator and reported in a journal article. In other instances, a more organized effort may have been made to subdivide a species into a series of "types" based on a defined set of demarcation criteria. Examples of viruses for which subspecies-level assignments have been made include hepatitis C virus (23), dengue virus (24), and HIV (25).

TABLE 1 Characters used for taxonomic classification

Major categories	Character examples
Name	Virus name, isolate name, synonyms
Isolate information	Location, date, host, tissue, method of isolation, sequence accession number
Virion properties	Morphology (size, envelope, capsid), physicochemical and physical properties, nucleic acid (genome type, size, and configuration), proteins
Genome organization and replication	Attachment, penetration, transcription, translation, protein processing, genome replication, assembly
Biological properties	Host range, transmission, geographical distribution, disease, pathology
Antigenicity	Antigenic determinants, epitopes, serological relationships, immunity, variation, diagnostics, vaccines

CRITERIA FOR TAXONOMIC CLASSIFICATION

Character-Based Descriptors

Taxonomic classification is accomplished by comparing and contrasting sets of characters that can be used to define the properties of any particular taxon. Any aspect of viral biology can be defined by a set of characters. These characters may have values represented by quantitative measures such as the triangulation (T) number used to categorize icosahedral virion capsid structure, or they may be purely qualitative descriptors such as the presence or absence of a host-derived lipid envelope.

Viruses are described by choosing a set of appropriate characters and then assigning values to these characters as necessary (26, 27). Table 1 provides a summary of some of the major categories of characters that might be used for classification along with examples for each category. Many characters have multiple values that might be associated with any one viral taxon or isolate. For example, a particular isolate may be described by the location and date of its isolation, each of which would be associated with the appropriate value (e.g., country and year). Characters describing a particular species may include its host range and a list of diseases associated with viruses belonging to that species.

There is no one master character list utilized by the ICTV for classifying viruses. This is because every taxon is unique, and characters that are useful to describe one taxon may be entirely inappropriate for describing another. The examples provided in Table 1 may be useful as a list of potential characters that might be used for any particular classification, but significant research still needs to be performed to determine the most appropriate set of choices. Character selection and character value assignment can be performed only by investigators with relevant expertise. Therefore, research scientists, who make up the ICTV study groups that are responsible for making taxonomic assignments for each viral family, set the rules of classification for the viruses that fall under their area of expertise (16, 28, 29).

The rules for taxonomic classification are defined by a set of demarcation criteria specific to each rank of every taxonomic hierarchy. Research scientists use these demarcation criteria either to determine that a newly isolated virus belongs to an existing species (and therefore there is no need for it to be further classified) or to submit a proposal to the appropriate study group for the creation of a new species (or higher-level taxa) if the isolate, based on the demarcation criteria, is sufficiently different from other viruses that it warrants the creation of a new taxon. Demarcation criteria are provided in each chapter of the ICTV report describing any particular taxon. Table 2 provides an example of some of the specific criteria utilized

TABLE 2 Criteria for taxonomic classification

Order: *Picornavirales*
- Virion
  - Nonenveloped, icosahedral particles, approximately 30 nm in diameter
  - Capsid proteins composed of three distantly related jelly-roll domains forming particles with pseudo-T=3 symmetry
- Genome
  - Positive-sense ssRNA
  - One or two monocistronic genome segments
  - 5′-bound VPg protein
  - Genome serves as the mRNA
  - Genome typically contains a 3′ polyA tail
- Protein
  - Primary polyprotein translation product proteolytically cleaved into mature proteins by one or more virus-encoded proteinases
  - Functional domains include a superfamily III helicase (Hel), chymotrypsin-like proteinase (Pro); and a superfamily I RNA-dependent RNA polymerase (Pol)
  - The nonstructural proteins are arranged as Hel-VPg-Pro-Pol

Family: *Picornaviridae*
- Genome
  - Single monocistronic genome segment
- Protein
  - Conserved genome organization
  - Conserved set of functional mature proteins
  - Protein sequence conservation (protease-polymerase region)

Genus: *Enterovirus*
- Protein
  - At least 50% amino acid identity over the length of the polyprotein
  - VPg sequence conservation
  - Lacks an L protein
  - Possesses a type-1 internal ribosomal entry site
- Host
  - Virus replication primarily in (but not limited to) the gastrointestinal tract

Species: *Enterovirus C*
- Host
  - Shares a limited range of host cell receptors
  - Shares a limited natural host range (e.g., human)
- Genome
  - Conserved genome map (organization of protein functional domains)
  - Common polyprotein proteolytic processing program
  - Shares a significant degree of compatibility in proteolytic processing, replication, encapsidation, and genetic recombination
- Sequence similarity
  - Amino acid identity: 70% in the polyprotein
  - Amino acid identity: 60% in the P1 structural proteins
  - Amino acid identity: 70% in the 2C + 3CD nonstructural proteins
  - Similar base G+C composition (within 2.5%)
- Phylogeny
  - Monophyletic

to define a species and its upper-level taxa for the species *Enterovirus C* (polioviruses were reclassified as belonging to this species in 2008) (16, 29). Different sets of characters are utilized at each level in the taxonomic hierarchy to describe the viruses that would be assigned to that level and below. The order, family, and genus-level characters are universal and must be present in all viruses assigned to that taxon, while species-level characters do not necessarily need to be present in all members of the species.

Sequence-Based Characters

Characters that describe virus morphology and structure have always been important classification criteria. With the advent of genome sequencing, sequence-based comparison has assumed an increasingly important role in classification. Table 2 provides a number of different sequence-based criteria at each rank that are used to define the important characteristics of that rank. There are conserved functional amino acid domains present in all members of the order *Picornavirales*. Conserved protease and polymerase protein sequences help define the family. A specific level of amino acid conservation across the whole polyprotein is required to place a virus within the *Enterovirus* genus. An even higher level of sequence identity is required for members of a particular species. Classification based on sequence comparison is now one of the major defining characteristics of all viral taxa. How these comparisons are made, how the relationships are measured, and the extent to which they are included in the taxa demarcation criteria vary significantly from taxon to taxon. This is understandable given the inherent differences in mutability between viruses, especially between viruses of different genomic composition. For example, viruses with dsDNA genomes show much less variability at the sequence level in comparison to RNA viruses. This difference is a direct consequence of the error rates of their DNA and RNA polymerases (5). Therefore, the measures used to define specific sequence-based demarcation criteria (as defined by each ICTV study group) will also vary from one taxon to another.

Sequence-based comparisons can be measured using a variety of techniques. The most basic involve pairwise comparisons in which two sequences are aligned and the number of nucleotide or amino acid differences between each aligned position are counted. When comparing multiple sequences, a table of distances is compiled that provides the percent similarity between every possible pairwise comparison in the set. Depending on the particular taxon and hierarchical rank under study, nucleotide or amino acid sequences can be compared, and alignments of complete viral genomes, a portion of the genome, or individual genes can be utilized. By examining these sequence distance tables, a study group can set specific similarity levels that define the demarcation criteria for classification of viruses into different taxa.

More sophisticated analyses based on pairwise sequence comparisons can be utilized to provide alternative methods for visualizing differences, choosing cutoffs, and making assignments. One method used in recent years is the pairwise analysis of sequence conservation (PASC) (30, 31). PASC analysis utilizes pairwise sequence alignments of either whole genomic nucleotide sequences or individual gene nucleotide or amino acid sequences. A pairwise alignment is constructed between every possible pair of available sequences. Once all pairwise alignments had been constructed, the percent identity is calculated for each aligned pair and then plotted against the number of aligned pairs producing similar identities. Figure 1A provides an example of a PASC plot using amino acid alignments of the DNA polymerase gene of virus isolates that belong to the family *Poxviridae* (32). As can be seen, several distinct peaks are produced, each of which corresponds to comparisons between viruses classified into particular ranks of the *Poxviridae* taxonomic hierarchy. The lowest percent identity (20 to 30%) corresponds to comparisons between viruses from different subfamilies. Genus-level comparisons produce multiple peaks from 45 to 75% identity. Peaks for interspecies comparisons vary between 80% and 98%

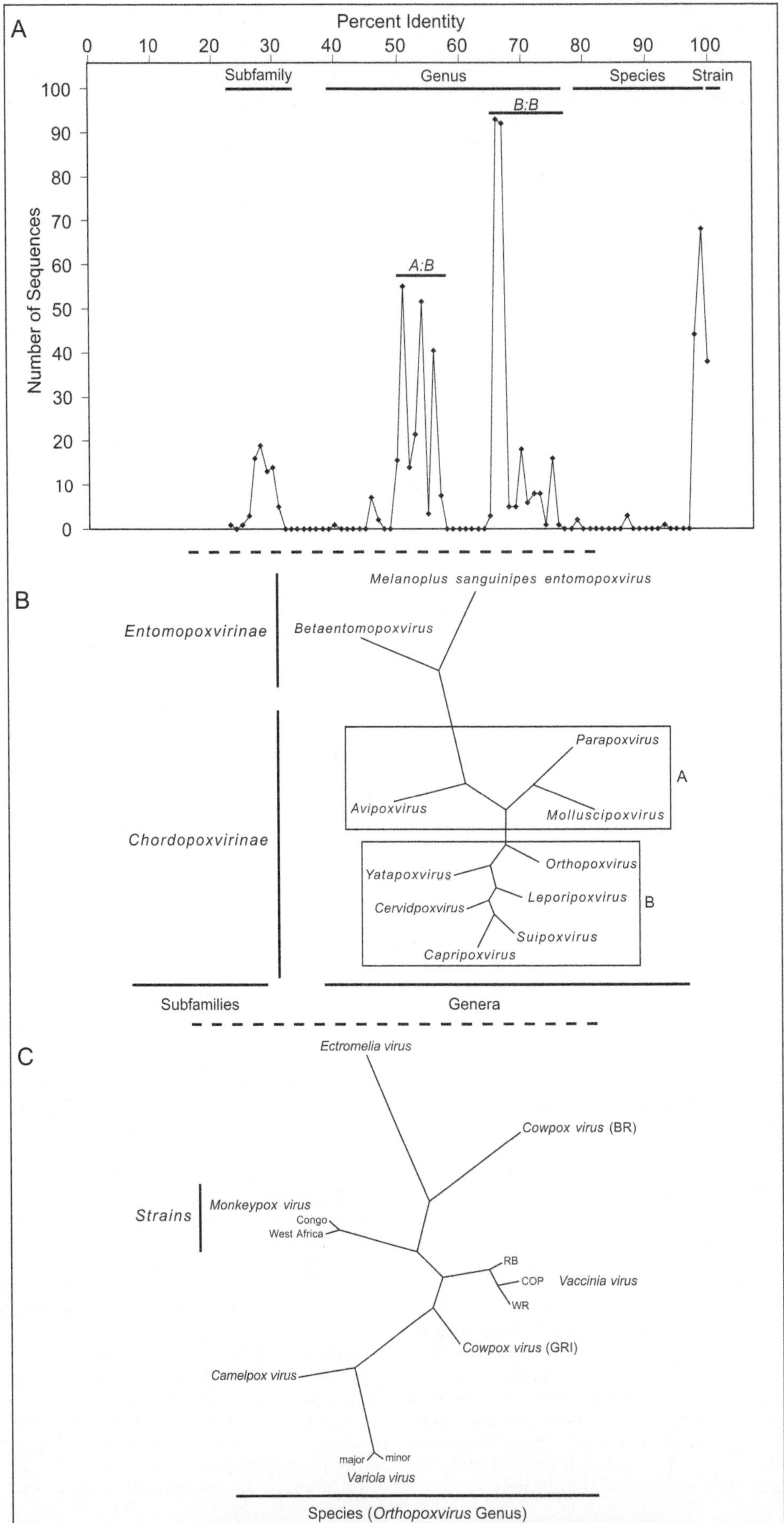
A
Percent Identity
0 10 20 30 40 50 60 70 80 90 100
Subfamily
Genus
Species
Strain
B:B
A:B
Number of Sequences
100 90 80 70 60 50 40 30 20 10 0
B
Entomopoxvirinae
Melanoplus sanguinipes entomopoxvirus
Betaentomopoxvirus
Chordopoxvirinae
Parapoxvirus
Avipoxvirus
Molluscipoxvirus
A
Orthopoxvirus
Yatapoxvirus
Leporipoxvirus
Cervidpoxvirus
B
Suipoxvirus
Capripoxvirus
Subfamilies
Genera
C
Ectromelia virus
Cowpox virus (BR)
Strains
Monkeypox virus
Congo
West Africa
RB
COP
Vaccinia virus
WR
Cowpox virus (GRI)
Camelpox virus
major
minor
Variola virus
Species (Orthopoxvirus Genus)

identity, with the most prominent interspecies peaks occurring at 97% and 98% identity. Intraspecies comparisons (comparisons between strains of the same species) show very high levels of identity of 99% and greater. Figure 1B shows how these taxa are arrayed on the *Poxviridae* phylogenetic tree. By utilizing PASC analysis, a new virus isolate can be compared to all existing isolates, and by plotting its similarity to isolates already assigned to a known taxon, a determination can be made as to whether the new isolate can be assigned to an existing taxon or if a proposal for creation of a new taxon should be considered. It is interesting from a biological point of view that the distinct patterns of conservation exhibited by the peaks present in the PASC graph suggest that the evolutionary history of the protein being analyzed (in this case, poxvirus DNA polymerase) has selected for protein sequences that exhibit distinct peaks of fitness. PASC analysis is utilized by a number of ICTV study groups for making taxonomic assignments (31, 33, 34).

One final sequence-based analysis that is extensively utilized as a demarcation criterion for making taxonomic assignments is phylogenetic analysis (29, 35). Phylogenetic analysis utilizes a multiple sequence alignment constructed from the nucleotide or amino acid sequence of a whole or partial genome or a whole or partial protein sequence (with the exact parameters set for any particular taxon by the appropriate study group). This alignment is then used as the basis for phylogenetic reconstruction in which the evolutionary history of the virus isolates is inferred by applying one of a variety of possible phylogenetic prediction algorithms. The result is a phylogenetic tree showing branching patterns that reflect the evolutionary history of the individual isolates, with branch lengths that are proportional to the number of evolutionary changes that have occurred between each node (both internal and terminal) of the tree. Figure 1B displays a tree that shows the branching topology and distances for subfamilies and genera of the family *Poxviridae*. At this level, it is not possible to discern the species topology for any of the genera, but species-level arrangements can be visualized if, for example, individual species of the genus *Orthopoxvirus* are compared separately (Fig. 1C) (32). The phylogenetic position of a newly described virus can be compared to that of any existing isolate on these trees to determine taxonomic assignment in a manner similar to PASC analysis. Close inspection of Fig. 1C also reveals that the differentiation between species (e.g., *Monkeypox virus* and *Ectromelia virus*) is clearly distinguishable from the differentiation between isolates of the same species (e.g., the Congo and West African monkeypox virus clades).

TAXONOMY OF HUMAN PATHOGENS

Viruses that infect humans fall into five orders: *Bunyavirales*, *Herpesvirales*, *Mononegavirales*, *Nidovirales*, and *Picornavirales* (11, 16, 36). (The other existing orders, the *Caudovirales*, *Ligamenvirales*, and *Tymovirales*, contain only bacteriophage, archaea viruses, and plant viruses, respectively.) Human pathogens are further subdivided into 31 families (not all of which belong to an order), 11 subfamilies, and 81 genera (with each genus usually comprising multiple species). Table 3 provides an overview of the taxa that contain human pathogens, along with representative species for each genus. The information in this table was compiled from the literature (11, 36) and from taxonomic proposals submitted to the ICTV (https://talk.ictvonline.org/files/ictv_official_taxonomy_updates_since_the_8th_report/). Table 4 provides a few of the structural features that define each viral family. Finally, Fig. 2 displays stylized representations of virion morphology for each family.

TAXONOMY DATABASES

ICTV

The ICTV produces an extensive amount of information during the process of classifying and naming viruses that is published regularly in the ICTV report. The ICTV website provides a database of the most recent officially approved viral taxonomy since publication of the last report, as well as historical tables listing the changes in viral taxonomy since the inception of the ICTV. Additional features of the website include a searchable hierarchical list of the current taxonomy, a downloadable spreadsheet, the "Master Species List," that contains a listing of all taxa, access to past and present taxonomy proposals submitted for review to the ICTV Executive Committee, and a forum for discussion of ICTV-related issues. The ICTV also publicizes news and information regarding its efforts in the Virology Division News section of the *Archives of Virology* (15, 37). In addition, following approval of any updates to the taxonomy by the voting membership of the ICTV, an article is published in the *Archives of Virology* that reviews all of the changes and additions (38–41).

NCBI

The National Center for Biotechnology Information (NCBI) provides access to a wide variety of databases containing various types of biological information (42). This includes GenBank, the primary repository of sequence data including viral sequences (43). NCBI also provides RefSeq, a database of reference sequences derived from GenBank records (44). RefSeq contains genomic sequences from representative viruses belonging to each viral species. Viral RefSeq records have been extensively annotated by NCBI curators and in many cases are also reviewed by investigators with expertise on individual viral species. Each viral sequence is linked to the NCBI taxonomic database using a taxonomy ID that is assigned to each taxon at every rank of the viral taxonomic hierarchy. The ICTV and NCBI taxonomies should be completely congruent, but this has not always been the case. The ICTV and NCBI have therefore continued to work to update the NCBI viral taxonomy so that it reflects the official ICTV taxonomy. Unfortunately,

FIGURE 1 Taxonomic demarcation via sequence similarity. (A) PASC analysis was carried out on the viral DNA-dependent DNA polymerase gene (the vaccinia virus E9L gene homolog) for every completely sequenced poxvirus genome. Each protein was aligned to every other protein, and the percent identity of each pairwise comparison was then included in a histogram plot of all possible comparisons. Peaks are identified across the top of the figure according to the taxa represented by particular pairwise sequence comparisons. (B) Phylogenetic reconstruction of the *Poxviridae* family of viruses based on their DNA polymerase protein sequences. Subfamily and genera demarcations are identified. Terminal nodes are labeled according to genus. Sequences belonging to one of the genera labeled either group A or B coincide with the A and B comparison peaks at the top of panel A. (C) Phylogenetic prediction based on the multiple nucleic acid sequence alignment of the core genomic region of each representative orthopoxvirus species or strain. BR, strain Brighton red; GRI, strain GRI-90. Reprinted with modification from *Virus Research* (32) with permission of the publisher.

TABLE 3 Taxonomic classification of viruses infecting humans

Order	Family	Subfamily	Genus	Species (ICTV type species or common examples)
dsDNA, linear[a]				
Herpesvirales	*Herpesviridae*	*Alphaherpesvirinae*	*Simplexvirus*	*Human alphaherpesvirus 1*[b] (herpes simplex virus type 1), *Human alphaherpesvirus 2*[b] (herpes simplex virus type 2), *Macacine alphaherpesvirus 1*[b] (B virus)
			Varicellovirus	*Human alphaherpesvirus 3*[b] (varicella-zoster virus)
		Betaherpesvirinae	*Cytomegalovirus*	*Human betaherpesvirus 5*[b] (human cytomegalovirus)
			Roseolovirus	*Human betaherpesvirus 6A*[b], *6B*[b], *7*[b]
		Gammaherpesvirinae	*Lymphocryptovirus*	*Human gammaherpesvirus 4*[b] (Epstein-Barr virus)
			Rhadinovirus	*Human gammaherpesvirus 8*[b] (Kaposi's sarcoma-associated herpesvirus)
Unassigned	*Adenoviridae*		*Mastadenovirus*	*Human mastadenovirus A*[b]*–G*[b]
Unassigned	*Poxviridae*	*Chordopoxvirinae*	*Molluscipoxvirus*	*Molluscum contagiosum virus*
			Orthopoxvirus	*Cowpox virus, Monkeypox virus, Vaccinia virus, Variola virus*
			Parapoxvirus	*Orf virus*
			Yatapoxvirus	*Yaba monkey tumor virus*
dsDNA, circular				
Unassigned	*Papillomaviridae*[c]		*Alphapapillomavirus*	*Alphapapillomavirus 1* (human papillomavirus 32)
			Betapapillomavirus	*Betapapillomavirus 1* (human papillomavirus 5)
			Gammapapillomavirus	*Gammapapillomavirus 1* (human papillomavirus 4)
			Mupapillomavirus	*Mupapillomavirus 1* (human papillomavirus 1)
			Nupapillomavirus	*Nupapillomavirus 1* (human papillomavirus 41)
Unassigned	*Polyomaviridae*		*Alphapolyomavirus*[b]	*Human polyomavirus 5, 8, 9, 12, 13* (all[d])
			Betapolyomavirus[b]	*Human polyomavirus 1*[b] (BK polyomavirus), *Human polyomavirus 2*[b] (JC polyomavirus), *Human polyomavirus 3*[d], *4*[d]
			Deltapolyomavirus[b]	*Human polyomavirus 6, 7, 10, 11* (all[d])
ssDNA, linear				
Unassigned	*Parvoviridae*	*Parvovirinae*	*Bocaparvovirus*[b]	*Primate bocaparvovirus 1*[d] (human bocavirus 1), *Primate bocaparvovirus 2*[d] (human bocavirus 2a TU)
			Dependoparvovirus[b]	*Adeno-associated dependoparvovirus A*[b] (adeno-associated virus 1–4); *Adeno-associated dependoparvovirus B*[b] (adeno-associated virus 5)
			Erythroparvovirus[b]	*Primate erythroparvovirus 1*[b] (human parvovirus B19)
			Tetraparvovirus[b]	*Primate tetraparvovirus 1*[d] (human parvovirus 4)
ssDNA, circular				
Unassigned	*Anelloviridae*		*Alphatorquevirus*	*Torque teno virus 1* (TTV)
Unassigned	*Circoviridae*[b]		*Circovirus*[b]	*Human associated circovirus 1*[d]
			Cyclovirus[b]	*Human associated cyclovirus 1–11* (all[d])
Unassigned	*Genomoviridae*[b]		*Gemygorvirus*[b]	*Sewage derived gemygorvirus 1*[d]
			Gemykibivirus[b]	*Human associated gemykibivirus 1–5* (all[d])
			Gemyvongvirus[b]	*Human associated gemyvongvirus 1*[d]
dsDNA, reverse transcribing circular				
Unassigned	*Hepadnaviridae*		*Orthohepadnavirus*	*Hepatitis B virus*
ssRNA, linear, positive sense				
Nidovirales	*Coronaviridae*	*Coronavirinae*	*Alphacoronavirus*	*Human coronavirus 229E; Human coronavirus NL63*
			Betacoronavirus	*Betacoronavirus 1, Human coronavirus HKU1, Middle East respiratory syndrome-related coronavirus*[d], *Severe acute respiratory syndrome-related coronavirus*
		Torovirinae	*Torovirus*	*Human torovirus*
Picornavirales	*Picornaviridae*		*Aphthovirus*	*Foot-and-mouth disease virus*
			Cardiovirus[b]	*Cardiovirus B*[d] (saffold virus)
			Cosavirus[b]	*Cosavirus B, D, E, F* (all[d]) (human cosavirus B1, D1, E1, F1)
			Enterovirus	*Enterovirus A* (human coxsackievirus A2; human enterovirus 71) *Enterovirus B* (human coxsackievirus B1; human echovirus) *Enterovirus C* (human poliovirus 1–3; human coxsackievirus A1) *Enterovirus D* (human enterovirus 68, 70, 94) *Rhinovirus A, B, C*
			Hepatovirus	*Hepatovirus A*[b] (hepatitis A virus)
			Kobuvirus[b]	*Aichivirus A*[d] (Aichi virus)
			Parechovirus	*Parechovirus A*[b] (human parechovirus)
			Salivirus[b]	*Salivirus A*[d] (klassevirus)
Unassigned	*Astroviridae*		*Mamastrovirus*	*Mamastrovirus 1, 6, 8, 9* (human astrovirus)
Unassigned	*Caliciviridae*		*Norovirus*	*Norwalk virus*
			Sapovirus	*Sapporo virus*

(Continued on next page)

TABLE 3 Taxonomic classification of viruses infecting humans *(Continued)*

Order	Family	Subfamily	Genus	Species (ICTV type species or common examples)
Unassigned	*Flaviviridae*		*Flavivirus*	*Dengue virus*, *Japanese encephalitis virus*, *Kyasanur Forest disease virus*, *Langat virus*, *Louping ill virus*, *Murray Valley encephalitis virus*, *Omsk hemorrhagic fever virus*, *Powassan virus*, *St. Louis encephalitis virus*, *Tick-borne encephalitis virus*, *Wesselsbron virus*, *West Nile virus*, *Yellow fever virus*, *Zika virus*
			Hepacivirus	*Hepacivirus C* (hepatitis C virus)
			Pegivirus[b]	*Pegivirus A*[d] (GB virus), *Pegivirus H*[d] (human pegivirus 2)
Unassigned	*Hepeviridae*		*Orthohepevirus*[b]	*Orthohepevirus A*[b] (hepatitis E virus)
Unassigned	*Togaviridae*		*Alphavirus*	*Barmah Forest virus*, *Chikungunya virus*, *Eastern equine encephalitis virus*, *Madariaga virus*[d], *Mayaro virus*, *O'nyong-nyong virus*, *Ross River virus*, *Semliki Forest virus*, *Sindbis virus*, *Venezuelan equine encephalitis virus*, *Western equine encephalitis virus*
			Rubivirus	*Rubella virus*
ssRNA, linear, negative sense				
Mononegavirales	*Bornaviridae*		*Bornavirus*	*Mammalian 1 bornavirus*[b] (Borna disease virus), *Mammalian 2 bornavirus*[d] (variegated squirrel bornavirus)
	Filoviridae		*Ebolavirus*	*Bundibugyo ebolavirus*, *Sudan ebolavirus*, *Taï Forest ebolavirus*, *Zaire ebolavirus*
			Marburgvirus	*Marburg marburgvirus*
	Paramyxoviridae		*Henipavirus*	*Hendra henipavirus*[b], *Nipah henipavirus*[b]
			Morbillivirus	*Measles morbillivirus*[b]
			Respirovirus	*Human respirovirus 1*[b], *3*[b] (human parainfluenza virus 1, 3)
			Rubulavirus	*Human rubulavirus 2*[b], *4*[b] (human parainfluenza virus 2, 4), *Mumps rubulavirus*[b]; *Sosuga rubulavirus*[d]
	Pneumoviridae[b]		*Metapneumovirus*	*Human metapneumovirus*
			Orthopneumovirus[b]	*Human orthopneumovirus*[b] (human respiratory syncytial virus)
	Rhabdoviridae		*Ledantevirus*[b]	*Le Dantec ledantevirus*[d], *Nkolbisson ledantevirus*[d]
			Lyssavirus	*Rabies lyssavirus*[b]
			Tibrovirus[b]	*Bas-Congo tibrovirus*[d], *Ekpoma 1 tibrovirus*[d], *Ekpoma 2 tibrovirus*[d]
ssRNA, circular, negative sense				
Unassigned	Unassigned		*Deltavirus*	*Hepatitis delta virus*
ssRNA, linear, negative sense, segmented				
Unassigned	*Orthomyxoviridae*		*Influenzavirus A*	*Influenza A virus*
			Influenzavirus B	*Influenza B virus*
			Influenzavirus C	*Influenza C virus*
ssRNA, linear (noncovalently closed circular), negative sense or ambisense, segmented				
Bunyavirales[b]	*Hantaviridae*[b]		*Orthohantavirus*[b]	*Hantaan orthohantavirus*[b], *Puumala orthohantavirus*[b], *Sin Nombre orthohantavirus*[b], *Thottapalayam orthohantavirus*[b], multiple other species
	Nairoviridae[b]		*Orthonairovirus*[b]	*Crimean-Congo hemorrhagic fever orthonairovirus*[b], *Dugbe orthonairovirus*[b]
	Peribunyaviridae[b]		*Orthobunyavirus*	*Bunyamwera orthobunyavirus*[b], *Bwamba orthobunyavirus*[b], *California encephalitis orthobunyavirus*[b], *Guama orthobunyavirus*[b], *Madrid orthobunyavirus*[b], *Nyando orthobunyavirus*[b], *Oropouche orthobunyavirus*[b], *Tacaiuma orthobunyavirus*[b]
	Phenuiviridae[b]		*Phlebovirus*	*Punta Toro phlebovirus*[b], *Rift Valley fever phlebovirus*[b], *Sandfly fever Naples phlebovirus*[b], *SFTS phlebovirus*[d]
Unassigned	*Arenaviridae*		*Mammarenavirus*[b]	*Chapare mammarenavirus*[b], *Guanarito mammarenavirus*[b], *Junín mammarenavirus*[b], *Lassa mammarenavirus*[b], *Lujo mammarenavirus*[b], *Lymphocytic choriomeningitis mammarenavirus*[b], *Machupo mammarenavirus*[b], *Sabiá mammarenavirus*[b]
dsRNA, linear, segmented				
Unassigned	*Picobirnaviridae*		*Picobirnavirus*	*Human picobirnavirus*
Unassigned	*Reoviridae*	*Sedoreovirinae*	*Orbivirus*	*Changuinola virus*, *Corriparta virus*, *Great Island virus*, *Lebombo virus*, *Orungo virus*
			Rotavirus	*Rotavirus A, B, C*; *Rotavirus H*[d]
			Seadornavirus	*Banna virus*
		Spinareovirinae	*Coltivirus*	*Colorado tick fever virus*
			Orthoreovirus	*Mammalian orthoreovirus*
ssRNA, linear, dimer, reverse transcribing				
Unassigned	*Retroviridae*	*Orthoretrovirinae*	*Deltaretrovirus*	*Primate T-lymphotropic virus 1, 2*
			Lentivirus	*Human immunodeficiency virus 1, 2*
		Spumaretrovirinae	*Spumavirus*	*Simian foamy virus*

[a]dsDNA, double-stranded DNA; ssDNA, single-stranded DNA; dsRNA, double-stranded RNA; ssRNA, single-stranded RNA.
[b]Taxon newly defined or renamed since 2013.
[c]Only one representative human-associated species is provided for each papillomavirus genus.
[d]Species containing newly identified human-associated or human pathogen virus since 2013.

TABLE 4 Summary of important characteristics used to differentiate families of viruses that infect humans

Classification family	Virus properties: Virion				Virus properties: Genome		
	Envelope	Shape	Size (nm)	Nucleocapsid symmetry	Molecule[a]	Structure	Size (kb, kbp)
Adenoviridae	–	Isometric	70–90	Icosahedral	dsDNA, linear	Monopartite, inverted terminal repeats, 5′ ends covalently linked to terminal protein	26–48
Anelloviridae	–	Isometric	30	Icosahedral	ssDNA, (−), circular	Monopartite	2–4
Arenaviridae	+	Spherical	50–300	Helical	ssRNA, (+/−) circular (noncovalently closed)	2 segments (negative or ambisense)	11 (total)
Astroviridae	–	Isometric	28–30	Icosahedral	ssRNA, (+), linear	Monopartite	6–8
Bornaviridae	+	Spherical	90–130	Helical	ssRNA, (−), linear	Monopartite	9
Caliciviridae	–	Isometric	35–40	Icosahedral	ssRNA, (+), linear	Monopartite, 5′-end covalently linked protein (VPg)	7–8
Circoviridae	"–"	Isometric	15–25	Icosahedral	ssDNA, circular	Monopartite	1.7–2.1
Coronaviridae	+	Spherical, pleomorphic	120–160	Helical	ssRNA, (+), linear	Monopartite	26–32
Deltavirus[b]	+	Spherical	36–43	Helical	ssRNA, (−), circular	Monopartite, requires hepatitis B virus for replication	1.7
Filoviridae	+	Filamentous, pleomorphic	80 × 660–800	Helical	ssRNA, (−), linear	Monopartite	19
Flaviviridae	+	Spherical	40–60	Icosahedral	ssRNA, (+), linear	Monopartite	9–13
Genomoviridae	–	Isometric	20–22	Icosahedral	ssDNA, circular	Monopartite	2.2
Hantaviridae	+	Spherical, pleomorphic	80–120	Helical	ssRNA, (−) circular (noncovalently closed)	3 segments	11–13 (total)
Hepadnaviridae	+	Spherical	42–50	Icosahedral	dsDNA, circular	Monopartite, reverse transcribing	3–4
Hepeviridae	–	Isometric	27–34	Icosahedral	ssRNA, (+), linear	Monopartite	7
Herpesviridae	+	Spherical	160–300	Icosahedral	dsDNA, linear	Monopartite, terminal and internal repeats, multiple isomeric forms	125–240
Nairoviridae	+	Spherical, pleomorphic	80–120	Helical	ssRNA, (−) circular (noncovalently closed)	3 segments	19 (total)
Orthomyxoviridae	+	Pleomorphic	80–120	Helical	ssRNA, (−), linear	6–8 segments, depending on genus	10–15 (total)
Papillomaviridae	–	Isometric	55	Icosahedral	dsDNA, circular	Monopartite, supercoiled	7–8
Paramyxoviridae	+	Pleomorphic	150–300	Helical	ssRNA, (−), linear	Monopartite	15–20
Parvoviridae	–	Isometric	21–26	Icosahedral	ssDNA, linear	Monopartite	4–6
Peribunyaviridae	+	Spherical, pleomorphic	80–120	Helical	ssRNA, (−) circular (noncovalently closed)	3 segments	12–13 (total)
Phenuiviridae	+	Spherical, pleomorphic	80–120	Helical	ssRNA, (+/−) circular (noncovalently closed)	3 segments (negative or ambisense)	11–13 (total)
Picobirnaviridae	–	Isometric	33–37	Icosahedral	dsRNA, linear	2 segments	4.2 (total)
Picornaviridae	–	Isometric	30	Icosahedral	ssRNA, (+), linear	Monopartite, 5′-end covalently linked protein (VPg)	7–9
Pneumoviridae	+	Pleomorphic	150–300	Helical	ssRNA, (−), linear	Monopartite	13–15.5
Polyomaviridae	–	Isometric	40–45	Icosahedral	dsDNA, circular	Monopartite, supercoiled	5
Poxviridae	+	Brick shaped or oval	140–260 × 220–450	Complex	dsDNA, linear	Monopartite, inverted terminal repeats, both ends covalently closed	130–375
Reoviridae	–	Isometric	60–85	Icosahedral	dsRNA, linear	10–12 segments, depending on genus	19–32 (total)
Retroviridae	+	Spherical	80–100	Icosahedral	ssRNA, (+), linear	Monopartite, diploid, reverse transcribing	7–13
Rhabdoviridae	+	Bullet shaped	75 × 180	Helical	ssRNA, (−), linear	Monopartite	11–15
Togaviridae	+	Spherical	60–70	Icosahedral	ssRNA, (+), linear	Monopartite	10–12
Prions[c]	NA[d]	Rods	Protein PrP^{SC}	NA	NA	No nucleic acid; self-replicating infectious prion protein (PrP) with a molecular weight of 33,000–35,000	NA

[a]dsDNA, double-stranded DNA; ssDNA, single-stranded DNA; dsRNA, double-stranded RNA; ssRNA, single-stranded RNA; (+), positive sense; (−), negative sense.
[b]Genus (unassigned family).
[c]Not classified by the ICTV.
[d]NA, not applicable.

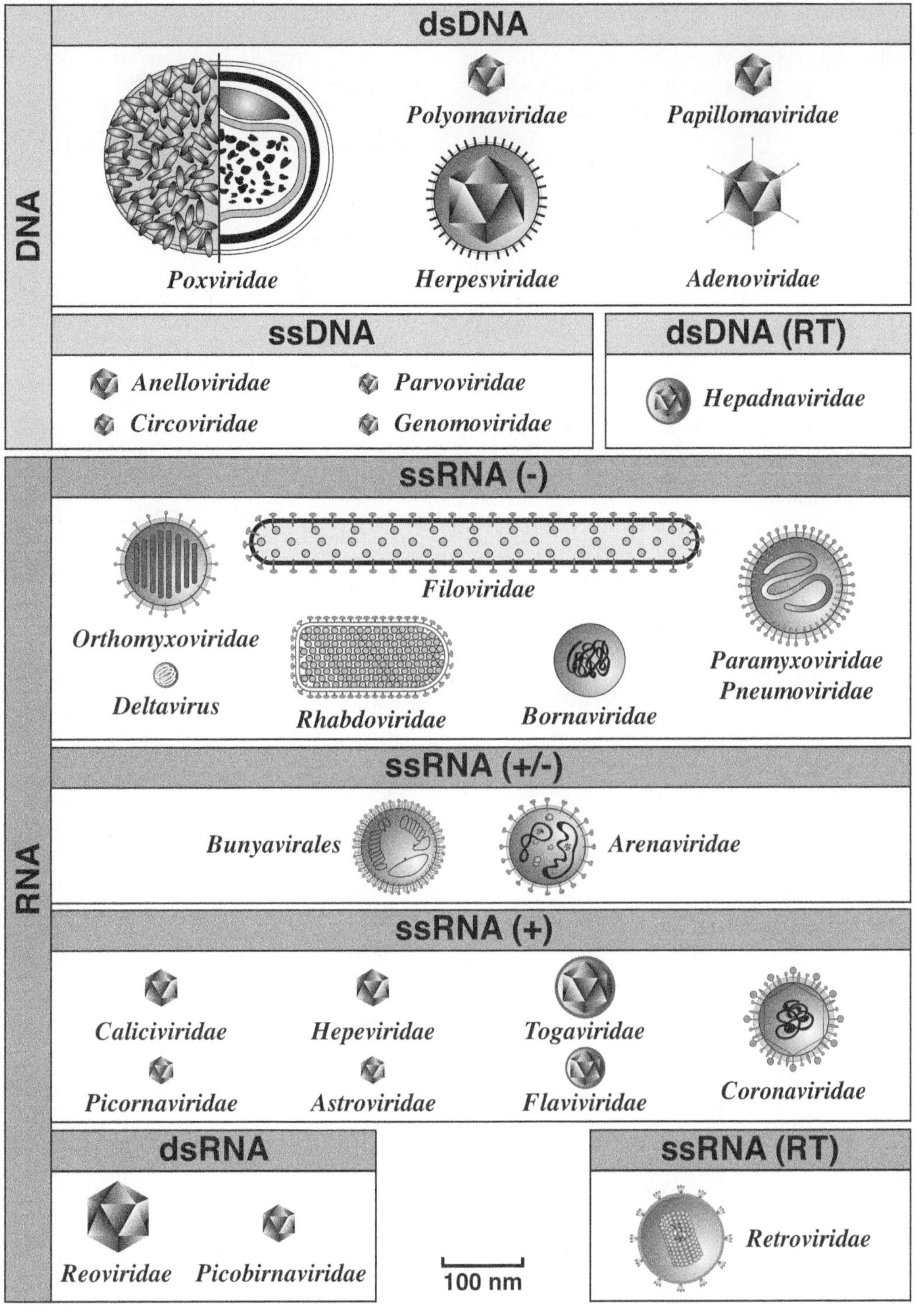

FIGURE 2 Virion morphology. Depiction of the shapes and sizes of viruses of families that include human pathogens. The virions are drawn to scale, but artistic license has been used in representing their structure. In some, the cross-sectional structure of the capsid and envelope is shown with a representation of their genome; for small virions, only their size and symmetry are depicted. RT, reverse transcribing; +, positive sense genome; −, negative sense genome.

the NCBI taxonomy is not automatically updated when new ICTV taxonomy is approved. A lag period of several months usually exists before any official, newly approved ICTV taxonomy is fully represented in the NCBI taxonomy and linked to GenBank and RefSeq sequence records.

FUTURE CHALLENGES

A number of challenges impact viral taxonomic assignment now and in the future. These challenges include discovery of novel, previously unknown viruses (45–47), consideration of the full complement of genetic mechanisms and machinery that viruses use to evolve, including recombination and horizontal gene transfer (48–51), managing vast increases in the amount of available information such as data derived from metagenomic sequencing projects (52–55), determination of new data types (characters) for describing viruses, having only a limited set of characters available for classification (such as only sequence information) (56–58), and creation of additional higher-level taxonomic ranks based on an increase in our knowledge of viral evolution (28, 29).

In 2016 a workshop was organized to discuss metagenomic sequencing and its impact on virus classification (59). A consensus statement published by meeting participants (60) endorsed the taxonomic classification of viruses solely from available metagenomic data and described a set of guidelines for establishing new virus taxa based on metagenomic data. The ICTV Executive Committee endorsed these proposals. Future workshops are planned to discuss some of the other difficult challenges described above. Luckily, new analytical methods, new approaches to classification, and the dedication of investigators worldwide will allow virologists to handle these challenges and deal with future challenges as they arise.

REFERENCES

1. **Linné C, Engel-Ledeboer MSJ, Engel H.** 1964. *Carolus Linnaeus Systema naturae, 1735*. B. de Graff, Nieuwkoop, The Netherlands.
2. **Koonin EV, Senkevich TG, Dolja VV.** 2009. Compelling reasons why viruses are relevant for the origin of cells. *Nat Rev Microbiol* **7:**615.
3. **Mushegian A.** 2008. Gene content of LUCA, the last universal common ancestor. *Front Biosci* **13:**4657–4666.
4. **Villarreal LP.** 2005. *Viruses and the Evolution of Life*. ASM Press, Washington, DC.
5. **Domingo E, Parrish CR, Holland JJ.** 2008. *Origin and Evolution of Viruses*, 2nd ed. Academic Press, San Diego, CA.
6. **Koonin EV, Senkevich TG, Dolja VV.** 2006. The ancient virus world and evolution of cells. *Biol Direct* **1:**29.
7. **Koonin EV, Dolja VV, Krupovic M.** 2015. Origins and evolution of viruses of eukaryotes: the ultimate modularity. *Virology* **479-480:**2–25.
8. **Gibbs AJ, Calisher CH, Garcia-Arenal F.** 1995. *Molecular Basis of Virus Evolution*. Cambridge University Press, Cambridge, United Kingdom.
9. **Koonin EV, Wolf YI, Nagasaki K, Dolja VV.** 2008. The Big Bang of picorna-like virus evolution antedates the radiation of eukaryotic supergroups. *Nat Rev Microbiol* **6:**925–939.
10. **Baltimore D.** 1971. Expression of animal virus genomes. *Bacteriol Rev* **35:**235–241.
11. **Knipe DM, Howley PM.** 2013. *Fields Virology*, 6th ed. Wolters Kluwer/Lippincott Williams & Wilkins Health, Philadelphia, PA.
12. **International Commission on Zoological Nomenclature, International Union of Biological Sciences.** 1999. *International Code of Zoological Nomenclature*, 4th ed. International Trust for Zoological Nomenclature, London, United Kingdom.
13. **Lapage SP, Sneath PHA, Lessel EF, Skerman VBD, Seeliger HPR, Clark WA (ed).** 1992. *International Code of Nomenclature of Bacteria: Bacteriological Code*, 1990 rev ed. ASM Press, Washington, DC.
14. **Polaszek A.** 2005. A universal register for animal names. *Nature* **437:**477.
15. **Adams MJ, Lefkowitz EJ, King AM, Harrach B, Harrison RL, Knowles NJ, Kropinski AM, Krupovic M, Kuhn JH, Mushegian AR, Nibert ML, Sabanadzovic S, Sanfaçon H, Siddell SG, Simmonds P, Varsani A, Zerbini FM, Orton RJ, Smith DB, Gorbalenya AE, Davison AJ.** 2017. 50 years of the International Committee on Taxonomy of Viruses: progress and prospects. *Arch Virol* **162:**1441–1446.
16. **King AMQ, Adams MJ, Carstens EB, Lefkowitz EJ.** 2012. *Virus Taxonomy: Classification and Nomenclature of Viruses: Ninth report of the International Committee on Taxonomy of Viruses*. Academic Press, San Diego, CA.
17. **Schleifer KH.** 2008. The International Union of Microbiological Societies, IUMS. *Res Microbiol* **159:**45–48.
18. **Adams MJ, Lefkowitz EJ, King AMQ, Harrach B, Harrison RL, Knowles NJ, Kropinski AM, Krupovic M, Kuhn JH, Mushegian AR, Nibert M, Sabanadzovic S, Sanfaçon H, Siddell SG, Simmonds P, Varsani A, Zerbini FM, Gorbalenya AE, Davison AJ.** 2017. Changes to taxonomy and the International Code of Virus Classification and Nomenclature ratified by the International Committee on Taxonomy of Viruses (2017). *Arch Virol* **162:**2505–2538.
19. **International Committee on Nomenclature of Viruses, Wildy P.** 1971. *Classification and Nomenclature of Viruses: First Report of the International Committee on Nomenclature of Viruses*. S. Karger, Basel, Switzerland.
20. **Van Regenmortel MHV, Faquet CM, Bishop DHL (ed).** 2000. *Virus Taxonomy: Classification and Nomenclature of viruses: Seventh Report of the International Committee on Taxonomy of Viruses*. Academic Press, San Diego, CA.
21. **Adams MJ, Lefkowitz EJ, King AM, Carstens EB.** 2013. Recently agreed changes to the International Code of Virus Classification and Nomenclature. *Arch Virol* **158:**2633–2639.
22. **Adams MJ, Lefkowitz EJ, King AM, Carstens EB.** 2014. Recently agreed changes to the statutes of the International Committee on Taxonomy of Viruses. *Arch Virol* **159:**175–180.
23. **Smith DB, Bukh J, Kuiken C, Muerhoff AS, Rice CM, Stapleton JT, Simmonds P.** 2014. Expanded classification of hepatitis C virus into 7 genotypes and 67 subtypes: updated criteria and genotype assignment web resource. *Hepatology* **59:**318–327.
24. **Henchal EA, Putnak JR.** 1990. The dengue viruses. *Clin Microbiol Rev* **3:**376–396.
25. **Robertson DL, Anderson JP, Bradac JA, Carr JK, Foley B, Funkhouser RK, Gao F, Hahn BH, Kalish ML, Kuiken C, Learn GH, Leitner T, McCutchan F, Osmanov S, Peeters M, Pieniazek D, Salminen M, Sharp PM, Wolinsky S, Korber B.** 2000. HIV-1 nomenclature proposal. *Science* **288:**55–56.
26. **Büchen-Osmond C.** 1997. Further progress in ICTVdB, a universal virus database. *Arch Virol* **142:**1734–1739.
27. **Buechen-Osmond C, Dallwitz M.** 1996. Towards a universal virus database: progress in the ICTVdB. *Arch Virol* **141:**392–399.
28. **Davison AJ, Eberle R, Ehlers B, Hayward GS, McGeoch DJ, Minson AC, Pellett PE, Roizman B, Studdert MJ, Thiry E.** 2009. The order *Herpesvirales*. *Arch Virol* **154:**171–177.
29. **Le Gall O, Christian P, Fauquet CM, King AM, Knowles NJ, Nakashima N, Stanway G, Gorbalenya AE.** 2008. Picornavirales, a proposed order of positive-sense single-stranded RNA viruses with a pseudo-T = 3 virion architecture. *Arch Virol* **153:**715–727.
30. **Bao Y, Kapustin Y, Tatusova T.** 2008. Virus classification by pairwise sequence comparison (PASC), p 342–348. *In* Mahy BWJ, Van Regenmortel MHV (ed), *Encyclopedia of Virology*, Elsevier, Boston, MA.
31. **Bào Y, Amarasinghe GK, Basler CF, Bavari S, Bukreyev A, Chandran K, Dolnik O, Dye JM, Ebihara H, Formenty P, Hewson R, Kobinger GP, Leroy EM, Mühlberger E, Netesov SV, Patterson JL, Paweska JT, Smither SJ, Takada A, Towner JS, Volchkov VE, Wahl-Jensen V, Kuhn JH.** 2017. Implementation of objective PASC-derived taxon

demarcation criteria for official classification of filoviruses. *Viruses* **9:**106.
32. **Lefkowitz EJ, Wang C, Upton C.** 2006. Poxviruses: past, present and future. *Virus Res* **117:**105–118.
33. **Adams MJ, Antoniw JF, Bar-Joseph M, Brunt AA, Candresse T, Foster GD, Martelli GP, Milne RG, Zavriev SK, Fauquet CM.** 2004. The new plant virus family *Flexiviridae* and assessment of molecular criteria for species demarcation. *Arch Virol* **149:**1045–1060.
34. **Adams MJ, Antoniw JF, Fauquet CM.** 2005. Molecular criteria for genus and species discrimination within the family *Potyviridae*. *Arch Virol* **150:**459–479.
35. **Gorbalenya AE, Enjuanes L, Ziebuhr J, Snijder EJ.** 2006. *Nidovirales*: evolving the largest RNA virus genome. *Virus Res* **117:**17–37.
36. **Loeffelholz MJ, Fenwick BW.** 2017. Taxonomic changes and additions for human and animal viruses, 2012 to 2015. *J Clin Microbiol* **55:**48–52.
37. **Carstens EB.** 2009. Report from the 40th meeting of the Executive Committee of the International Committee of Taxonomy of Viruses. *Arch Virol* **154:**1571–1574.
38. **Adams MJ, King AM, Carstens EB.** 2013. Ratification vote on taxonomic proposals to the International Committee on Taxonomy of Viruses (2013). *Arch Virol* **158:**2023–2030.
39. **Adams MJ, Lefkowitz EJ, King AM, Carstens EB.** 2014. Ratification vote on taxonomic proposals to the International Committee on Taxonomy of Viruses (2014). *Arch Virol* **159:**2831–2841.
40. **Adams MJ, Lefkowitz EJ, King AM, Bamford DH, Breitbart M, Davison AJ, Ghabrial SA, Gorbalenya AE, Knowles NJ, Krell P, Lavigne R, Prangishvili D, Sanfaçon H, Siddell SG, Simmonds P, Carstens EB.** 2015. Ratification vote on taxonomic proposals to the International Committee on Taxonomy of Viruses (2015). *Arch Virol* **160:**1837–1850.
41. **Adams MJ, Lefkowitz EJ, King AM, Harrach B, Harrison RL, Knowles NJ, Kropinski AM, Krupovic M, Kuhn JH, Mushegian AR, Nibert M, Sabanadzovic S, Sanfaçon H, Siddell SG, Simmonds P, Varsani A, Zerbini FM, Gorbalenya AE, Davison AJ.** 2016. Ratification vote on taxonomic proposals to the International Committee on Taxonomy of Viruses (2016). *Arch Virol* **161:**2921–2949.
42. **NCBI Resource Coordinators.** 2017. Database resources of the National Center for Biotechnology Information. *Nucleic Acids Res* **45**(D1)**:**D12–D17.
43. **Benson DA, Cavanaugh M, Clark K, Karsch-Mizrachi I, Lipman DJ, Ostell J, Sayers EW.** 2017. GenBank. *Nucleic Acids Res* **45**(D1)**:**D37–D42.
44. **O'Leary NA, et al.** 2016. Reference sequence (RefSeq) database at NCBI: current status, taxonomic expansion, and functional annotation. *Nucleic Acids Res* **44**(D1)**:**D733–D745.
45. **Assiri A, McGeer A, Perl TM, Price CS, Al Rabeeah AA, Cummings DA, Alabdullatif ZN, Assad M, Almulhim A, Makhdoom H, Madani H, Alhakeem R, Al-Tawfiq JA, Cotten M, Watson SJ, Kellam P, Zumla AI, Memish ZA, KSA MERS-CoV Investigation Team.** 2013. Hospital outbreak of Middle East respiratory syndrome coronavirus. *N Engl J Med* **369:**407–416.
46. **Briese T, Paweska JT, McMullan LK, Hutchison SK, Street C, Palacios G, Khristova ML, Weyer J, Swanepoel R, Egholm M, Nichol ST, Lipkin WI.** 2009. Genetic detection and characterization of Lujo virus, a new hemorrhagic fever-associated arenavirus from southern Africa. *PLoS Pathog* **5:**e1000455.
47. **Lam TT, Zhu H, Guan Y, Holmes EC.** 2016. Genomic analysis of the emergence, evolution, and spread of human respiratory RNA viruses. *Annu Rev Genomics Hum Genet* **17:**193–218.
48. **Lavigne R, Seto D, Mahadevan P, Ackermann HW, Kropinski AM.** 2008. Unifying classical and molecular taxonomic classification: analysis of the *Podoviridae* using BLASTP-based tools. *Res Microbiol* **159:**406–414.
49. **Lima-Mendez G, Van Helden J, Toussaint A, Leplae R.** 2008. Reticulate representation of evolutionary and functional relationships between phage genomes. *Mol Biol Evol* **25:**762–777.
50. **Odom MR, Hendrickson RC, Lefkowitz EJ.** 2009. Poxvirus protein evolution: family wide assessment of possible horizontal gene transfer events. *Virus Res* **144:**233–249.
51. **Walsh DA, Sharma AK.** 2009. Molecular phylogenetics: testing evolutionary hypotheses. *Methods Mol Biol* **502:**131–168.
52. **Delwart EL.** 2007. Viral metagenomics. *Rev Med Virol* **17:**115–131.
53. **Edwards RA, Rohwer F.** 2005. Viral metagenomics. *Nat Rev Microbiol* **3:**504–510.
54. **Monier A, Claverie JM, Ogata H.** 2008. Taxonomic distribution of large DNA viruses in the sea. *Genome Biol* **9:**R106.
55. **Rascovan N, Duraisamy R, Desnues C.** 2016. Metagenomics and the human virome in asymptomatic individuals. *Annu Rev Microbiol* **70:**125–141.
56. **Labonté JM, Reid KE, Suttle CA.** 2009. Phylogenetic analysis indicates evolutionary diversity and environmental segregation of marine podovirus DNA polymerase gene sequences. *Appl Environ Microbiol* **75:**3634–3640.
57. **Schoenfeld T, Patterson M, Richardson PM, Wommack KE, Young M, Mead D.** 2008. Assembly of viral metagenomes from Yellowstone hot springs. *Appl Environ Microbiol* **74:**4164–4174.
58. **Simmonds P.** 2015. Methods for virus classification and the challenge of incorporating metagenomic sequence data. *J Gen Virol* **96:**1193–1206.
59. **Springer Nature.** 2017. A sea change for virology. *Nat Rev Microbiol* **15:**129.
60. **Simmonds P, Adams MJ, Benkő M, Breitbart M, Brister JR, Carstens EB, Davison AJ, Delwart E, Gorbalenya AE, Harrach B, Hull R, King AM, Koonin EV, Krupovic M, Kuhn JH, Lefkowitz EJ, Nibert ML, Orton R, Roossinck MJ, Sabanadzovic S, Sullivan MB, Suttle CA, Tesh RB, van der Vlugt RA, Varsani A, Zerbini FM.** 2017. Consensus statement: virus taxonomy in the age of metagenomics. *Nat Rev Microbiol* **15:**161–168.

Specimen Collection, Transport, and Processing: Virology

JAMES J. DUNN AND BENJAMIN A. PINSKY

81

Given that laboratory data significantly influence medical diagnoses, it is critical that all phases of testing (pre-, intra-, and postanalytical) be approached systematically to ensure the accuracy of results and to detect and correct potential errors. The preanalytical phase is often the most vulnerable part of the testing process and accounts for the majority of errors in laboratory diagnostics (1). Preanalytical steps for viral diagnostics involving specimen selection, collection, transport, and processing are described in this chapter, as well as details for collection of specific sample types. While these recommendations are general guidelines, laboratories must also follow manufacturers' instructions for testing of samples with commercially available kits and reagents.

Preanalytical variables should be controlled to maintain specimen integrity. Therefore, it is important for the laboratory to make available to all specimen-collecting areas within the institution or other locations submitting samples a comprehensive manual of tests available, with indications for appropriate use and specimen collection, which details the appropriate (i) specimen types for specific clinical syndromes (Table 1), (ii) collection devices/containers and transport media when indicated, (iii) collection techniques, (iv) volume of specimen required, (v) specimen labeling, (vi) transport times and storage conditions, and (vii) clinical data, if available (2).

SPECIMEN SELECTION

Viruses infecting humans cause a wide range of diseases. Signs and symptoms of infection largely influence which specimens are collected for virus testing. Additional factors to be considered are epidemiologic details (e.g., travel, exposures, and season) and the patient's immune status. It is important to recognize that viruses differ in their pathogenic mechanisms, their ability to disseminate from the primary site of infection, and the organ systems they infect. Generally, specimen selection is guided by the test best suited to establish a particular diagnosis (synopsized in chapter 83). The diagnosis of certain illnesses requires a basic understanding of viral pathogenesis, organ involvement, and viral epidemiology to determine the appropriate specimen(s) and tests. Specimen selection based on suspicion of a particular virus may be complicated by the fact that similar clinical syndromes can be caused by many different viruses (Table 1). If only the specimens needed to detect a specific virus are collected, other important etiologies may be missed.

Depending on the anatomic site and means of collection, specimens are either nonsterile (i.e., contaminated with bacteria and/or fungi) or sterile. This determines the extent of specimen processing that occurs prior to viral culture, since bacteria and fungi grow rapidly in nutrient-rich cell culture systems. Non-culture-based test methods are less impacted by this distinction. Sterile specimens are obtained from sites that are free of microorganisms in the absence of infection (e.g., blood, cerebrospinal fluid [CSF], and tissue), and there is no contact with nonsterile sites during the collection process. Nonsterile specimens are obtained from sites that contain normal flora (e.g., upper respiratory tract, skin, lower genital tract, and stool), or they are obtained from sterile sites but contact with nonsterile sites is unavoidable during specimen collection (e.g., sputum and voided urine).

SPECIMEN COLLECTION

Since no single diagnostic approach may be optimal for detecting every possible virus in a clinical situation, it may be necessary to utilize a combination of test methods and/or to collect a number of different sample types and/or longitudinal samples for testing to yield the most medically useful information (2). These are particularly important considerations in the era of metagenomic pathogen identification, given that unbiased sequencing methods have not yet been shown to be as sensitive as targeted approaches (3, 4). To optimize viral diagnosis, specimens should be collected as soon as possible after the onset of symptoms. For many viral infections in otherwise healthy and immunocompetent individuals, the likelihood of obtaining positive results is generally greatest within the first 3 days after onset of symptoms and diminishes rapidly as the course of infection proceeds (5). In cases of disseminated disease or in immunocompromised patients, viruses may be identified in clinical samples for prolonged periods (6). Generally, the level and duration of virus shedding depend on the virus, infected organ or organ system, and host factors such as age and immune status (7–9). Specimens with high concentrations of viral particles, viral antigens (Ag), or viral nucleic acids (NA) will improve the laboratory's ability to make an accurate diagnosis. Specimen collection techniques can

TABLE 1 Specimens and methods for detection of viruses

Source and syndrome	Virus(es)[a]	Specimen(s)[b]	Test method(s)[c]
Cardiac			
Myocarditis/pericarditis	Adenoviruses	Blood, respiratory, tissue	Culture, histology, IA, NAAT
	CMV	Blood, tissue, urine	Culture, histology, NAAT
	Enteroviruses	Blood, respiratory, stool, tissue	Culture, NAAT
	Influenza viruses	Respiratory, tissue	Culture, IA, NAAT, serology
Cutaneous			
Exanthematous rash	Adenoviruses	Blood, respiratory	Culture, IA, NAAT
	Chikungunya virus	Blood, urine	NAAT, serology
	Dengue virus	Blood, urine	IA, NAAT, serology
	EBV	Blood	NAAT, serology
	Enteroviruses	Blood, respiratory, stool	Culture, NAAT
	HHV-6	Blood	NAAT, serology
	Measles virus	Blood, respiratory, urine	Culture, NAAT, serology
	Parvovirus B19	Blood	NAAT, serology
	Rubella virus	Blood, respiratory, urine	Culture, serology
	Zika virus	Blood, urine	NAAT, serology
Papillomas/papules	Molluscum contagiosum	Tissue	Cytology, histology
	Human papillomaviruses	Tissue/cells	Cytology, histology, NAAT
Vesicular rash	Enteroviruses	Blood, respiratory, stool, vesicle	Culture, NAAT
	HSV	Lesion	Culture, IA, NAAT
	Poxviruses[d]	Blood, respiratory, tissue, vesicle	Culture, EM, histology, NAAT
	VZV	Respiratory, vesicle	Culture, IA, NAAT
Gastrointestinal			
Diarrhea	Adenoviruses 40 and 41	Stool	IA, NAAT
	Astroviruses	Stool	NAAT
	Caliciviruses	Stool	NAAT
	CMV	Blood, stool, tissue	Culture, histology, NAAT
	Human bocavirus	Stool	NAAT
	Parechoviruses	Stool	Culture, NAAT
	Rotavirus	Stool	IA, NAAT
Hepatitis	Adenoviruses	Blood, tissue	Culture, histology, IA, NAAT
	CMV	Blood, tissue	Culture, histology, NAAT
	EBV	Blood	NAAT, serology
	HAV	Blood	Serology
	HBV	Blood	IA, NAAT, serology
	HCV	Blood	NAAT, serology
	HDV	Blood	IA, serology
	HEV	Blood	NAAT, serology
	HSV	Blood, tissue	Culture, histology, IA, NAAT
Hematologic			
Bone marrow suppression	CMV	Blood, bone marrow	Culture, IA, NAAT
	Dengue virus	Blood, bone marrow	NAAT, serology
	EBV	Blood, bone marrow	Histology, NAAT
	HAV	Blood	NAAT, serology
	HBV	Blood	NAAT, serology
	HCV	Blood	NAAT, serology
	HHV-6	Blood, bone marrow	NAAT
	HHV-8	Blood, bone marrow	Histology, NAAT
	HIV-1	Blood	NAAT, serology
	Parvovirus B19	Blood, bone marrow	NAAT, serology
Hemolytic anemia	CMV	Blood, bone marrow	Culture, IA, NAAT
	EBV	Blood, bone marrow	Histology, NAAT
	HBV	Blood	NAAT, serology
	HCV	Blood	NAAT, serology
Lymphoid (B- and T-cell) disorders	EBV	Blood, bone marrow	Histology, NAAT
	CMV	Blood, bone marrow	Culture, IA, NAAT
	HIV-1	Blood	NAAT, serology
	HHV-8	Blood, bone marrow	IA, NAAT
	HTLV-1	Blood, bone marrow	NAAT, serology

(Continued on next page)

TABLE 1 Specimens and methods for detection of viruses (*Continued*)

Source and syndrome	Virus(es)[a]	Specimen(s)[b]	Test method(s)[c]
Neonatal/fetal	CMV	Amniotic fluid, blood, saliva, urine	Culture, NAAT
	Enteroviruses	Blood, CSF, urine	Culture, NAAT
	HBV	Blood	Serology
	HIV	Blood	NAAT, serology
	HSV	Blood, CSF, vesicle	Culture, IA, NAAT
	Parechoviruses	Blood, CSF, respiratory, urine	Culture, NAAT
	Parvovirus B19	Blood, amniotic fluid	NAAT, serology
	Rubella virus	Blood, urine	Culture, NAAT
	VZV	Amniotic fluid, blood, CSF, vesicle	Culture, IA, NAAT, serology
Neurologic			
Acute flaccid myelitis	Arboviruses	Blood, CSF	NAAT, serology
	Enteroviruses	Blood, CSF, stool, respiratory	Culture, NAAT
Encephalitis	Arboviruses[d]	Blood, CSF	NAAT, serology
	BK virus	CSF, tissue	NAAT
	CMV	CSF	NAAT
	EBV	CSF	NAAT
	Enteroviruses	CSF	Culture, NAAT
	HHV-6	CSF	NAAT
	HSV	CSF	NAAT
	HIV	CSF	NAAT
	Measles virus	Blood, CSF, urine	Culture, NAAT, serology
	Mumps virus	Blood, CSF, saliva, urine	Culture, NAAT, serology
	Parechoviruses	CSF	Culture, NAAT
	Rabies	Blood, CSF, saliva, tissue (nuchal)	IA, NAAT, serology
	VZV	CSF	NAAT
Meningitis	Arboviruses	Blood, CSF	NAAT, serology
	Enteroviruses	CSF	Culture, NAAT
	HSV	CSF	NAAT
	LCMV	Blood, CSF	Serology
	Mumps virus	Blood, CSF, urine	Culture, NAAT, serology
	Parechoviruses	CSF	Culture, NAAT
	VZV	CSF	NAAT
PML[e]	JC virus	CSF, tissue	Histology, NAAT
Ocular			
Conjunctivitis	Adenoviruses	Eye, respiratory	Culture, IA, NAAT
	Enteroviruses	Eye, respiratory	Culture, NAAT
	HSV	Eye	Culture, IA, NAAT
Keratitis	Adenoviruses	Eye, respiratory	Culture, IA, NAAT
	Enteroviruses	Eye, respiratory	Culture, NAAT
	HSV	Eye	Culture, IA, NAAT
	VZV	Eye	Culture, IA, NAAT
Uveitis/retinitis	CMV	Eye	NAAT
	HSV	Eye	NAAT
	VZV	Eye	NAAT
Respiratory			
Bronchiolitis	Adenoviruses	Respiratory	Culture, IA, NAAT
	Enteroviruses	Respiratory	Culture, NAAT
	Human bocavirus	Respiratory	NAAT
	Human coronaviruses	Blood, respiratory	EM, NAAT, serology
	Human metapneumovirus	Respiratory	IA, NAAT
	Influenza viruses	Respiratory	Culture, IA, NAAT
	Parainfluenza viruses	Respiratory	Culture, IA, NAAT
	RSV	Respiratory	Culture, IA, NAAT
	Rhinoviruses	Respiratory	Culture, NAAT
Croup	Human bocavirus	Respiratory	NAAT
	Human coronaviruses	Blood, respiratory	EM, NAAT, serology
	Human metapneumovirus	Respiratory	IA, NAAT
	Influenza viruses	Respiratory	Culture, IA, NAAT
	Parainfluenza viruses	Respiratory	Culture, IA, NAAT
	Rhinoviruses	Respiratory	Culture, NAAT
	RSV	Respiratory	Culture, IA, NAAT

(*Continued on next page*)

TABLE 1 Specimens and methods for detection of viruses (*Continued*)

Source and syndrome	Virus(es)[a]	Specimen(s)[b]	Test method(s)[c]
Parotitis	Adenoviruses	Respiratory	Culture, IA, NAAT
	CMV	Blood, respiratory	Culture, NAAT
	EBV	Blood	NAAT, serology
	Enteroviruses	Blood, respiratory, stool	Culture, NAAT
	HIV-1	Blood	Serology
	Mumps virus	Blood, respiratory, urine	Culture, NAAT, serology
Pharyngitis/URI	Adenoviruses	Respiratory	Culture, IA, NAAT
	EBV	Blood	Serology
	Enteroviruses	Respiratory	Culture, NAAT
	HSV	Respiratory	Culture, NAAT
	Human coronaviruses	Respiratory	NAAT
	Human metapneumovirus	Respiratory	IA, NAAT
	Influenza viruses	Respiratory	Culture, IA, NAAT
	Parainfluenza viruses	Respiratory	Culture, IA, NAAT
	Rhinoviruses	Respiratory	Culture, NAAT
	RSV	Respiratory	Culture, IA, NAAT
Pleurodynia	Enteroviruses	Respiratory	Culture, NAAT
Pneumonia	Adenoviruses	Respiratory	Culture, IA, NAAT
	CMV	Blood, respiratory, tissue	Culture, histology, IA, NAAT
	Hantaviruses	Blood, tissue	NAAT, serology
	HSV	Respiratory, tissue	Culture, histology, NAAT
	Human coronaviruses	Blood, respiratory	NAAT, serology
	Human metapneumovirus	Respiratory	NAAT
	Influenza viruses	Respiratory	Culture, IA, NAAT
	Measles virus	Blood, respiratory, urine	Culture, NAAT, serology
	Parainfluenza viruses	Respiratory	Culture, IA, NAAT
	Rhinoviruses	Respiratory	Culture, NAAT
	RSV	Respiratory	Culture, IA, NAAT
	VZV	Respiratory, tissue	Culture, histology, NAAT
Rhinitis/coryza	Adenoviruses	Respiratory	Culture, IA, NAAT
	Enteroviruses	Respiratory	Culture, NAAT
	Human coronaviruses	Respiratory	NAAT
	Human metapneumovirus	Respiratory	NAAT
	Influenza viruses	Respiratory	Culture, IA, NAAT
	Parainfluenza viruses	Respiratory	Culture, IA, NAAT
	Rhinoviruses	Respiratory	Culture, NAAT
	RSV	Respiratory	Culture, IA, NAAT
Urogenital			
Cervicitis/urethritis	Adenoviruses	Genital	Culture
	CMV	Genital, tissue	Culture, histology, NAAT
	HSV	Genital	Culture, NAAT
Genital warts, carcinoma	HPV	Genital, tissue	Histology, NAAT
Hemorrhagic cystitis	Adenoviruses	Urine	Culture, NAAT
	BK virus	Urine	NAAT
	CMV	Urine	Culture, NAAT
Herpetic lesions	HSV	Lesion	Culture, IA, NAAT
	VZV	Lesion	Culture, IA, NAAT
Orchitis/epididymitis	Mumps virus	Blood	Serology
Papules	Molluscum contagiosum virus	Tissue	Histology
Proctitis	HSV	Rectal	Culture, NAAT

[a]Refer to specific chapters for individual viruses; only common viral pathogens are listed. HHV-6, human herpes virus 6; HAV, hepatitis A virus; HTLV-1, human T-cell lymphotropic virus 1; LCMV, lymphocytic choriomeningitis virus.

[b]Common specimens for viral diagnostics; refer to specific chapters for individual viruses. Respiratory includes throat and nasal swabs, nasal wash, NP aspirate, tracheal, and BAL specimens. Eye includes conjunctiva, cornea, and aqueous and vitreous fluids.

[c]Common detection methods used (listed alphabetically). EM, electron microscopy; IA, immunoassay (such as immunofluorescence-antibody assay, enzyme-linked immunosorbent assay, or immunochromatographic test); NAAT, nucleic acid amplification test.

[d]Smallpox virus as well as hemorrhagic fever viruses (e.g., Ebola virus and Marburg virus) require processing in BSL4 facilities.

[e]PML, progressive multifocal leukoencephalopathy.

greatly affect specimen quality and therefore test results. Collecting an adequate specimen is straightforward when fluids (e.g., CSF, blood, and urine) are sampled, as standard collection procedures are used and are not subject to great variability. However, collection of swab specimens is prone to variability, which can affect the amount of infectious virus, viral nucleic acids, or viral antigens present on the swab.

For serologic diagnosis, the timing of serum collection and type of antibody detected vary for specific viruses. An acute-phase serum specimen should be obtained early in the course of illness for virus-specific IgM testing.

Convalescent-phase serum for IgG testing should be obtained 2 to 4 weeks after the acute-phase specimen or symptom resolution, and both acute and convalescent specimens should be tested concurrently to identify any significant changes in antibody concentration. However, due to the delay in collecting a convalescent-phase specimen, the final result will generally not impact patient treatment, and for this reason, convalescent-phase serologic testing is infrequently performed for clinical purposes. For some viruses (e.g., severe acute respiratory syndrome coronavirus [SARS-CoV]), timing of the collection of the convalescent-phase specimen may extend beyond 4 weeks after the onset of symptoms to reliably rule out infection (10). Additionally, in disease due to reactivation of latent or persistent viruses, there may or may not be a detectable rise in IgM and/or IgG levels. Generally, IgM is more sensitive to freezing and thawing than is IgG, so repetitive freeze/thaw cycles should be avoided.

Health care workers who collect specimens from patients should wear personal protective equipment as appropriate for standard, contact, airborne, or droplet precautions (11, 12). The laboratory should always be notified in advance if rare agents representing a danger to laboratory workers (e.g., hemorrhagic fever viruses and novel influenza viruses) are suspected. Samples in which such viruses are suspected should not be manipulated in laboratories lacking the ability to undertake such handling under the appropriate biosafety level conditions. Some specimens can be handled under enhanced biosafety level 2 (BSL2) or BSL3 conditions for certain viruses (e.g., SARS-CoV). Likewise, laboratories should provide instructions to those collecting and submitting specimens from individuals suspected of harboring a non-BSL2 pathogen. These should generally not be cultured in routine clinical laboratories but rather referred to the relevant state public health laboratory or the Centers for Disease Control and Prevention (CDC; Atlanta, GA). Manipulation of these specimens and tissues, including sera obtained from convalescent patients, may pose a serious biohazard and should be minimized outside a BSL4 laboratory. Use of vacuum tube collection systems is considered safer than use of syringes and needles, which must be disassembled before their contents are transferred to another tube. Procedures that generate aerosols should be minimized. NA extraction procedures, conducted in a biosafety cabinet (BSC), have the advantage of inactivating viruses prior to analysis (13). The appropriate CDC guideline should be consulted for specific information regarding the handling of specimens suspected to contain high-risk pathogens.

TRANSPORT MEDIUM

Depending on the specimen source and type of testing requested, it may be appropriate to place the sample in viral transport medium (VTM). Liquid specimens, such as amniotic fluid, blood, CSF, urine, and bronchoalveolar lavage (BAL) fluid, do not generally require VTM (14). Specimens that are susceptible to drying (e.g., swabs and tissue) must be kept moist in VTM or other buffered solutions designed to maintain the titer of infectious virions for culture, the stability of viral antigens for direct antigen tests, or viral NA for nucleic acid amplification tests (NAATs). However, molecular testing can be an exception, as certain NA have been found to be quite stable in a desiccated state. Dried samples for NAAT have the advantage of (i) relatively long storage capability at room temperature, (ii) reduced biohazard risk to laboratory personnel with no spill risk and reduced infectivity, and (iii) simple and inexpensive ambient-temperature shipping of specimens where maintenance of a cold chain is limited. However, the versatility of a liquid specimen offers obvious advantages (i.e., it can be split and tested by multiple methods). When a complete microbiological workup on a specimen is requested, including viral, bacterial, mycobacterial, and fungal testing, VTM should not be added to the specimen, as this medium contains both antibacterial and antifungal agents. Rather, samples should be collected independently or aliquoted into the appropriate transport media.

The most useful types of transport systems should allow simultaneous detection of viruses by any number of methods, including culture, Ag detection, and NAAT. Although some common viral agents can withstand extended storage in suitable transport media at room temperature, it is generally the case that virus viability decreases over time and, at higher temperatures, this rate of decay is often accelerated. To stabilize the rate of decay, viral transport systems are usually kept on ice until they can be processed for testing. The optimal transport medium should further stabilize virus viability with minimal loss of virus titer, contain components to control potential microbial contamination, have a long shelf life, and be readily available at a reasonable cost (14, 15). Formulations of VTM typically consist of a buffered salt solution, such as Hanks balanced salt solution, buffered with HEPES to maintain a neutral pH, protein-stabilizing agents, such as bovine serum albumin or gelatin, and antimicrobials to prevent bacterial and/or fungal overgrowth. Some laboratories have reported that media designed for collection and transport of bacteriology specimens are also acceptable for collection and transport of viral specimens. Under experimental conditions, bacteriologic swab transport systems allowed NA detection of influenza A virus, echovirus 30, herpes simplex virus 2 (HSV-2), and adenovirus up to 5 days after storage at 4°C or room temperature, albeit with lower sensitivity than swabs in VTM (16).

VTM can be prepared in the laboratory or purchased (Table 2). An advantage of commercially prepared media is that the burden of quality control is shifted from the laboratory to the manufacturer (17). Some transport media also sustain the viability of chlamydiae, mycoplasmas, and ureaplasmas, though culture of these organisms for clinical diagnoses is not commonly performed. The inclusion of sucrose in the media serves as a cryoprotectant to maintain the integrity of viruses if specimens are frozen (−70°C or lower) for prolonged periods. Laboratories should validate the suitability of their selected media for their particular applications, as performances can vary (17, 18).

Manufacturers of commercial assays for NAAT or Ag detection either supply transport media or make recommendations for transport systems that are compatible with their test methods. The manufacturer's package insert should therefore be consulted for information on appropriate collection and transport systems. Most VTM are compatible with NA and Ag detection tests (14, 19). However, note that deviation from the transport media recommended by the manufacturer in the FDA *in vitro* diagnostic package insert requires an in-house validation.

TRANSPORT CONDITIONS

Once a clinical specimen has been collected, it should be transported to the laboratory as soon as possible, since virus viability decreases with time (i.e., some clinically important viruses are more labile than others). The optimal time and temperature for transport, processing, and

TABLE 2 Commercial sources of transport media for viral diagnostics

Medium	Composition	Vol (ml)	Storage temp (°C)
BD Universal VTM[a] (BD Diagnostics)	Basal constituents[b], gelatin, L-cysteine, sucrose, colistin, vancomycin	1 or 3	2–25
Copan Universal transport medium[a] (Copan Diagnostics)	Basal constituents, gelatin, L-cysteine, sucrose, colistin, vancomycin	1, 3, 10	2–25
CVM transport medium[a] (Hardy Diagnostics)	Basal constituents, gelatin, sucrose, colistin, vancomycin	2	2–8
TransPRO CVM transport (Hardy Diagnostics)	Basal constituents, gelatin, L-cysteine, sucrose, colistin, vancomycin	3	2–25
FlexTrans VTM (Trinity Biotech)	Basal constituents, sucrose, gentamicin, streptomycin	2	2–8
Meridian viral transport[a] (Meridian Bioscience)	Tryptose phosphate broth, gelatin, gentamicin	1.5	5–25
MicroTest M4[a] (Remel)	Basal constituents, gelatin, sucrose, colistin, vancomycin	3	2–8
MicroTest M4RT[a] (Remel)	Basal constituents, gelatin, sucrose, gentamicin	3	2–30
MicroTest M5[a] (Remel)	Basal constituents, protein stabilizers, sucrose, colistin, vancomycin	3	2–8
MicroTest M6[a] (Remel)	Basal constituents, gelatin, sucrose, colistin, vancomycin	1.5	2–30
Multitrans medium[a] (Starplex Scientific)	Basal constituents, gelatin, sucrose, sodium bicarbonate, colistin, vancomycin	3	2–25
Puritan UniTranz-RT[a] (Puritan Medical)	Basal constituents, gelatin, sucrose, colistin, vancomycin	1 or 3	2–25
Sigma-VCM medium[a] (Medical Wire & Equipment)	Balanced salt solution, HEPES, disodium hydrogen orthophosphate, sucrose, lactalbumin hydrolysate, colistin, vancomycin, amphotericin B	1, 1.5, 3	5–25
Sigma-Virocult medium[a] (Medical Wire & Equipment)	Balanced salt solution, disodium hydrogen orthophosphate, lactalbumin hydrolysate, chloramphenicol, amphotericin B	1 or 2	5–25
ViraTrans medium (Trinity Biotech)	Basal constituents, gentamicin, penicillin, streptomycin	2	2–8

[a]Product available as swab-transport tube combination.
[b]Basal constituents: Hanks balanced salt solution, bovine serum albumin, L-glutamic acid, HEPES buffer (pH 7.3), phenol red, amphotericin B.

storage (discussed below) of specimens should be adhered to in order to generate accurate and meaningful results. Typically, specimens for viral culture should be transported to the laboratory promptly (ideally, within 2 to 4 hours of collection), since overall diagnostic yield improves when specimens are expeditiously processed for viral culture. The preferred transport temperature for specimens for viral culture is 2 to 8°C. Enzymes present in specimens and capable of inactivating viruses or degrading proteins and nucleic acids are less active at refrigeration temperatures. For longer transport times or submission to reference laboratories, specimens should be stored and shipped under conditions that preserve the integrity of the sample. For example, it may be necessary to transport serum or plasma collected for NA testing frozen. Viability is not a requirement for Ag or NA detection methods; therefore, transport time may be less significant, unless degradation of intact cells, viral proteins, or viral NA is a consideration. However, for timely diagnosis, delay should be avoided during transport of these specimens to the laboratory.

SPECIMEN STORAGE AND PROCESSING

Accredited laboratories are required to specify rejection criteria for specimens that are collected, transported, or stored under improper conditions. Specimens that are unacceptable for testing include those that are (i) unlabeled or improperly labeled, (ii) received in improper or leaking containers, (iii) not appropriate for a particular test, (iv) transported under improper conditions, or (v) received beyond the acceptable transport time limit. At a minimum, the specimen container should be labeled with the patient's full name, a medical record number or unique identifier, the date and time of collection, the specific source, and the name of the collector. Each specimen should be accompanied by a requisition (hard copy or electronic) containing the same information as the specimen container, as well as the patient's location, test(s) requested, source of the specimen, requesting clinician with contact information, and suspected clinical diagnosis (20). Specimens deemed unacceptable that cannot be re-collected (e.g., tissue collected during surgery) may be processed and tested according to the laboratory's clearly defined procedure allowing such exceptions.

Specimens submitted for virus isolation can be held at refrigerated temperature (2 to 8°C) for up to 2 days prior to inoculation onto cell culture. Many viruses lose infectivity at ambient or even refrigeration temperatures. For example, 90% of respiratory syncytial virus (RSV) infectivity is lost after 4 days at 4°C and 24 h at 37°C (21). Freezing of specimens (−70°C or lower) is not recommended for virus isolation, unless specimen processing will not occur within 2 days. The temperature in standard freezers (−20°C) is not low enough to maintain virus infectivity. Certain viruses may also lose infectivity with repeated freeze-thaw cycles, particularly enveloped viruses. Detailed specimen processing protocols for viral culture have been described previously (22, 23). Specimens should be processed using all appropriate biosafety guidelines (24), and a biosafety cabinet should be used when manipulating specimens suspected to contain a virus(es) considered contagious by airborne routes.

Molecular assays are particularly sensitive to substandard preanalytical conditions. For RNA targets such as HIV or HCV, the CLSI recommends that EDTA-treated whole-blood samples be centrifuged and the plasma removed to a secondary tube within 4 hours of phlebotomy, a conservative time frame that may vary depending on the assay manufacturer's requirements (25). However, studies have shown that for HIV-1 viral load testing, whole blood with EDTA and cell-free EDTA-treated plasma can be stored at room temperature for up to 30 hours, at 4°C for up to 14 days, and at −70°C for extended periods of time without significant decreases in viral load signal (26, 27), and HCV RNA is stable in EDTA-treated whole blood for at least 24 hours at room temperature (28). HIV proviral DNA can be detected in acid citrate dextrose (ACD)- or EDTA-treated whole blood for up to 10 days at both 4°C and ambient temperature (29). The preanalytical steps for selected FDA-cleared/approved NAATs are listed in Table 3.

When RNAlater (Qiagen), an RNA stabilization buffer, was used, HCV and HIV plasma viral loads were stable for up to 28 days at 37°C, and HCV viral loads were essentially equivalent after 5 days when samples were transported either frozen or in RNAlater at ambient temperature (30). Under experimental conditions, nonenveloped and enveloped viruses, including HIV-1, retained infectivity after more than 72 h of storage at room temperature in RNAlater (31). Arboviral RNA was stable for at least 35 days when virus-containing samples were stored at 4°C or −20°C in AVL buffer (Buffer A Viral Lysis, Qiagen), a lysis buffer for nucleic acid purification that contains guanidine isothiocyanate and RNase inhibitors (32). AVL buffer has the added property of inactivating viral infectivity. Enterovirus RNA was shown to be stable in CSF specimens stored at 4°C and −80°C for up to 2 weeks, but the half-life in samples stored at room temperature was calculated to be 9 days. In nasopharyngeal (NP) wash specimens, there was a >65% reduction in influenza A virus RNA concentration when samples were maintained at room temperature, 4°C, or −80°C for 2 weeks (33). If no specific RNase inhibitors are used, long-term storage of diagnostic RNA samples should be done preferably at −70°C or lower to inhibit RNase activity, as RNase may limit the stability of RNA even in frozen samples at −20°C (34).

For DNA targets such as cytomegalovirus (CMV), the data on DNA quantification after storage are conflicting, with some studies reporting no decline in CMV DNA levels after 24 h (35), 72 h (36), and 2 weeks (37), while another showed increased levels in blood stored at room temperature or at 4°C prior to plasma separation (38). The increased levels of CMV DNA in plasma separated more than 2 h after collection may be falsely positive or elevated in latently infected patients due to the lysis of leukocytes and release of CMV into plasma during storage. In another study, CMV DNA in EDTA-treated blood was stable for 2 weeks when the samples were stored at room temperature, 4°C, and −80°C, whereas CMV DNA in serum had a half-life of <1, 2, and 3 days when samples were stored at room temperature, 4°C, and −80°C, respectively (33). There was no statistically significant decline in hepatitis B virus (HBV) DNA concentration in plasma stored at both 5°C and 25°C for up to 28 days (27). For HSV, the quantity in oral and genital specimens stored in VTM for 16 months at −20°C was within 1 log of the original concentration for >90% of specimens (39). In CSF specimens, HSV DNA

TABLE 3 Processing and storage conditions for blood specimens with selected FDA-cleared/approved NA tests

Test (manufacturer)	Specimen types	Preseparation conditions	Short-term storage of plasma/serum	Max. no. of freeze/thaw cycles
Aptima HCV RNA Qualitative (Hologic)	EDTA, ACD, citrate, heparin, PPT, or serum	≤24 h, 15–30°C	≤48 h, 2–8°C, or ≤−20°C	3
Aptima HCV Quant Dx (Hologic)	EDTA, ACD, PPT, or serum	≤6 h, 2–30°C	≤24 h, 2–25°C, or ≤5 days, 2–8°C	3
Aptima HIV-1 RNA Qualitative (Hologic)	EDTA, ACD, citrate, PPT, or serum	≤3 days, ≤25°C	≤5 days, 2–8°C, or ≤−20°C	3
Aptima HIV-1 Quant (Hologic)	EDTA, ACD, or PPT	≤24 h, 2–30°C	≤5 days, 2–8°C, or ≤90 days, −20 to −70°C	3
cobas Amplicor HCV Monitor (Roche)	EDTA, ACD, or serum	≤6 h, 2–25°C	≤3 days, 2–8°C or −70°C	2
cobas Amplicor HIV-1 Monitor (Roche)	EDTA or ACD	≤6 h, 2–25°C	≤5 days, 2–8°C, or −70°C	3
cobas AmpliPrep/cobas TaqMan CMV (Roche)	EDTA	≤24 h, ≤25°C	≤7 days, 2–8°C, or ≤6 wk, ≤−20°C	3
cobas AmpliPrep/cobas TaqMan HBV (Roche)	EDTA or serum	≤24 h, 2–25°C	≤3 days, 15–30°C ≤7 days, 2–8°C, or ≤6 wk, −20 to −80°C	5
cobas AmpliPrep/cobas TaqMan HCV (Roche)	EDTA or serum	≤24 h, 2–25°C	≤3 days, 4°C, or ≤6 wk, −20 to −70°C	5
cobas AmpliPrep/cobas TaqMan HIV-1 (Roche)	EDTA	≤24 h, 2–25°C	≤24 h, 15–30°C ≤6 days, 2–8°C, or ≤6 wk −20 to −80°C	5
Qiagen artus CMV RGQ MDx	EDTA	≤24 h, 20–25°C	≤24 h, 20–25°C or ≤8 wk, −15 to −30°C	2
RealTime HBV (Abbott)	EDTA or serum	≤6 h, 2–30°C	≤24 h, 15–30°C ≤3 days, 2–8°C, or ≤−70°C	1[a]
RealTime HCV (Abbott)	EDTA or serum	≤6 h, 2–30°C	≤24 h, 15–30°C ≤3 days, 2–8°C, or ≤60 days, ≤−70°C	1[a]
RealTime HIV-1 (Abbott)	EDTA or ACD	≤6 h, 15–30°C or ≤24 h, 2–8°C	≤24 h, 15–30°C ≤5 days, 2–8°C, or ≤60 days, ≤−20°C	3[a]
RealTime CMV (Abbott)	EDTA	≤24 h, 3–30°C	≤24 h, 15–30°C ≤5 days, 2–8°C, or ≤−70°C	3[a]

[a]Thaw specimens at 15 to 30°C or 2 to 8°C; once thawed, specimens may be stored at 2 to 8°C for ≤6 h.

was detectable by PCR for up to 30 days when samples were stored at temperatures ranging from 23°C to −70°C (40). Human papillomavirus (HPV) DNA stored in two commercial liquid-based cytology media at 2 to 8°C was stable for more than 2 years. However, the reproducibility of results after storage may be affected by the methods of nucleic acid extraction and detection (41). Generally, DNA in tissue is stable for up to 24 h at 4°C, for at least 2 weeks at −20°C, and for at least 2 years at −70°C or lower (25).

Fewer data are available regarding the stability of nucleic acids in stool specimens, although rotavirus RNA has been shown to be stable for up to 2.5 months at ambient temperature (42). Adenovirus DNA in fresh stool collected on sodium dodecyl sulfate (SDS)–EDTA-treated chromatography paper strips was detected after 4 months of storage at −20 to 37°C (43), and under experimental conditions, strips containing various concentrations of norovirus were stable for reverse transcription-PCR detection up to 2 months at temperatures ranging from −80 to 37°C (44).

COLLECTION METHODS AND PROCESSING OF SELECTED SPECIMENS

For commercially available FDA-cleared/approved assays, laboratories must follow manufacturers' instructions for collection and processing of specimens. Assay performance must be verified by the individual laboratory prior to implementing any change in the preanalytical steps described in the manufacturer's package insert (45, 46). For laboratory-developed tests (LDTs), each test site must establish and validate appropriate processing and storage conditions, the extent of which may rely on studies performed by the laboratory or those in published sources. Similarly, if the user changes any aspect of collection or processing for an FDA-cleared/approved assay, the laboratory is then required to perform the necessary validation experiments, as for an LDT.

Amniotic Fluid

Although rare, viral infections during pregnancy may be detrimental to the fetus or newborn. Testing amniotic fluid for viral pathogens is generally based on maternal history or ultrasound-guided indications. Fluid is collected by amniocentesis, and 2 to 5 ml should be submitted to the laboratory in a sterile container. NA detection methods are the most commonly used. NAs should be extracted from samples as soon as possible and stored at 2 to 8°C for up to 48 h or frozen at −70°C or less if testing is delayed beyond 48 h (25). Virus can be isolated in culture, but sensitivity is generally lower than that of NAAT.

For the most accurate diagnosis of prenatal diagnosis of congenital CMV infection, amniotic fluid should be collected between 21 and 23 weeks of fetal gestation (47, 48). If maternal varicella-zoster virus (VZV) infection occurs during the first or second trimester, VZV DNA may be detected in amniotic fluid, but its presence is not necessarily synonymous with the development of congenital varicella syndrome. The presence of parvovirus B19 in amniotic fluid should be correlated with other clinical and prenatal diagnostics, since up to 25% of asymptomatic fetuses may have detectable virus (48).

Blood

Serum, plasma, purified peripheral blood leukocytes, and whole blood have all been used to detect and quantify viral pathogens. The most suitable blood compartment for testing depends on the virus targeted. Quantitative molecular methods performed on blood samples are useful in assessing patient prognosis, treatment response, and antiviral resistance. For viral load monitoring over time, it is particularly important that the sample matrix not be varied. Which blood compartment to test depends on the underlying condition of the patient and whether the viral target dictates that a cellular or cell-free portion be utilized (49–52).

Approximately 3 to 5 ml of blood should be collected in the appropriate anticoagulant vacuum tube. For pediatric specimens, smaller volumes are acceptable, but less than 1 or 2 ml may be inadequate for testing. The most commonly used anticoagulants are EDTA, heparin, and ACD. Anticoagulated blood may be fractionated to allow recovery of leukocytes (see below). EDTA and ACD are the preferred anticoagulants for obtaining plasma for NA testing, since heparin is inhibitory to many NA amplification chemistries (25). In addition, frozen EDTA-treated plasma specimens have improved NA stability compared to those treated with heparin (26).

Whole blood used for NA amplification must be processed to remove inhibitors of DNA and RNA polymerases, such as heme and the metabolic precursors of heme. Many different extraction protocols are used in both commercial and laboratory-developed amplification tests to remove inhibitors and purify nucleic acids (25). Plasma is obtained by centrifuging blood collected in tubes containing spray-dried anticoagulant (EDTA) at 1,500 × g for 20 min at 25°C. Plasma preparation tubes (PPT; Becton-Dickinson [BD], Franklin Lakes, NJ) have spray-dried EDTA and a gel barrier that results in physical separation of plasma and cellular constituents, eliminating the need for decanting plasma. The use of PPT for HIV-1 RNA quantitation has shown falsely elevated viral loads from centrifuged tubes that were stored frozen or for prolonged periods at 2 to 8°C (53–55), likely due to due the presence of cells containing proviral DNA (56, 57). This limitation can be overcome by an additional centrifugation step prior to testing or use of an extraction method that recovers only RNA (58, 59). No decline in hepatitis C virus RNA levels was observed in blood stored in PPT at 4°C for 72 h (60).

When serum is required for serologic or molecular testing, 4 to 8 ml of blood is collected in a serum separator tube (e.g., SST [BD Diagnostics], Corvac [Medtronic], and Vacuette [Greiner Bio-One]) or a tube without anticoagulant. After blood has been allowed to coagulate for 30 min, tubes are centrifuged at 1,000 to 1,300 × g for 10 minutes. The serum fraction, removed to a sterile tube, can be stored at 2 to 8°C for up to 48 hours or frozen at −20°C or lower for longer periods. Whole blood drawn for antibody determination should not be frozen.

For virus isolation, 5 to 10 ml of anticoagulated blood (EDTA or heparin) should be collected by venipuncture and transported to the laboratory at room temperature. Processing of the specimen for leukocyte fractionation should occur within 8 hours. Whole blood should not be used to inoculate cell cultures because of toxicity caused by red blood cells. The buffy coat fraction may also contain erythrocytes. To adequately remove red blood cells and recover both polynuclear and mononuclear cells for inoculation, density gradient methods should be used; a number of density gradient testing kits are commercially available (23). Isolated leukocytes can be cocultured with human diploid fibroblasts, such as MRC-5 cells (tube or shell vial culture) or H&V Mix FreshCells (Diagnostic Hybrids) (shell vial culture) (61), directly stained with fluorescence-labeled monoclonal antibodies (e.g., CMV pp65 antigenemia assay) (62), or extracted to detect viral genomes by molecular techniques. Quantifying leukocyte input is essential for optimizing assay performance and for ensuring inter-run quantitative quality control (63, 64). For recovery of CMV in culture, the shell vial technique is more rapid and sensitive than conventional tube culture (65).

Bone Marrow

Bone marrow can be used to identify viral etiologies of hematologic disorders, including hemophagocytic lymphohistiocytosis, aplastic anemia, and chronic pure red cell aplasia (66, 67) (Table 1). At least 2 ml of bone marrow aspirate should be collected in the appropriate anticoagulant tube. The recommended anticoagulants for NAATs include EDTA and ACD (25). Although the diagnostic yield may be low, bone marrow aspirates for culture should be collected in a syringe or vacuum tube with heparin or EDTA and processed to fractionate the leukocytes as soon as possible after collection (68, 69). Bone marrow specimens should be stored at 2 to 8°C prior to NA extraction. Freezing and thawing of bone marrow lyses red cells, causing release of heme, which may inhibit NA amplification, depending on the extraction procedure and amplification technique (70).

Cerebrospinal Fluid

CSF is an important specimen for diagnosis of viral central nervous system infections (Table 1). CSF is collected using a sterile technique, by inserting a spinal needle into the L4-L5 interspace, located in the midline between the left and right iliac crest. Preferably, 2 to 5 ml should be collected in a sterile, leakproof container. CSF samples should not be centrifuged prior to NA extraction, as many viruses are cell associated. VTM is not added to sterile body fluids such as CSF, since they do not require antimicrobial treatment and dilution in transport media may cause false-negative results. Samples should be transported and stored up to 48 h at 2 to 8°C and frozen at −70°C or lower for longer-term storage. Nucleic acids should typically be extracted prior to testing, since CSF contains globulins, cell-derived proteins, and other uncharacterized substances that inhibit the activity of thermostable polymerases used in PCR (71, 72). However, some studies have demonstrated the suitability of simple methods, such as exposure to high temperature or repetitive freeze-thawing to release nucleic acids (73, 74). For virus isolation, specimens with visible blood may affect recovery of viruses, since antibodies may be present in sufficient concentration to inhibit viral growth. No treatment of CSF is needed before inoculation of cell cultures.

Dried Blood Spots

The use of dried blood spots (DBS) eliminates the need for venipuncture and allows greater flexibility in storage temperature and transport time. DBS samples have been used in NA tests for diagnosis and monitoring of HIV infection, HBV quantification and genotyping, neonatal HSV infection, and detection of congenital CMV infection. Antibodies to viruses such as hepatitis A virus (HAV), HBV, HCV, Epstein-Barr virus (EBV), measles virus, and rubella virus can be detected in DBS, although the performance characteristics vary compared to those of serum testing, depending on the virus. DBS card samples can be prepared from a few drops of blood, typically 15 to 200 μl, obtained from a capillary blood stab, i.e., a finger prick (75). A minimum of 2 hours is needed for air drying of the blood spot. Once dried, DBS should be placed in hermetically sealed bags or containers with sufficient desiccant to minimize moisture exposure, which could allow growth of microorganisms (25). DBS may be transported and stored at room temperature for relatively long periods (depending on the virus) or frozen at −20°C or lower for longer-term storage. Disks punched out from DBS cards normally contain the equivalent of 3.1 to 12.4 μl of blood depending on the punch size (3 to 6 mm) (75). Once dried, HIV-1 RNA in a DBS is stable at ambient temperature or −70°C for at least 1 year, and the virus is typically inactivated (76). Compared to plasma, more than 90% of finger stick DBS samples from solid organ transplant recipients showed less than a 1-$\log_{10}$ deviation in CMV viral load, and the kinetics of CMV viral load during antiviral therapy were comparable (77). In that study, the 95% limit of detection of CMV in DBS was estimated at 2,700 copies/ml (675 IU/ml).

Eye

Eye specimens include swabs or scrapings of the conjunctiva, corneal scrapings, and vitreous and aqueous fluids. Conjunctiva should be cleared of any exudate present with a swab before a specimen is collected. With a second flexible, fine-shafted Dacron or rayon swab premoistened with sterile saline, infected cells from the clean conjunctiva can be obtained and transferred to a vial of VTM or used to prepare a slide for immunofluorescent staining. The AdenoPlus test (Rapid Pathogen Screening, Inc., Sarasota, FL), a lateral-flow immunochromatographic cartridge test for the detection of ocular adenovirus infection, uses a built-in sampling pad to touch the eye and collect fluid from the conjunctiva. The sensitivity of the AdenoPlus test has been reported to be 85%, with a specificity of 98%, compared to PCR (78). Corneal scrapings and swabbing of the cornea are best collected and placed in VTM by a specially trained clinician. Thin smears may be made directly from scrapings or swab specimens for use in immunofluorescent staining. Retinal pathogens are detected in the aqueous and vitreous fluids by NA testing, since they are not easily cultivated from these samples. Direct testing of these surgically obtained fluids has resulted in PCR inhibition (79); therefore, the original specimen may need to be extracted.

Genital

The most common viral causes of genital lesions are HSV-1 and -2, which are easily detected by direct Ag assay (direct fluorescent-antibody assay [DFA]), NAATs, or culture. Cells and fluid from genital ulcers are collected and processed as lesions from skin (discussed below).

Testing of human papillomavirus (HPV) genotypes associated with a high risk of developing cervical cancer (16, 18, 31, 33, 35, 39, 45, 51, 52, 56, 58, 59, 66, 68) is performed using molecular methods on cervical specimens collected with swabs or brushes (detailed in chapter 107). Specimens may be collected in manufacturer-specific systems or FDA-approved/cleared liquid-based cytology solutions used concomitantly for Pap smear preparation. Freshly collected cervical biopsy samples, at least 2 to 5 mm in cross section, may be analyzed in some commercially available NAATs. All specimens should be placed immediately into the specimen transport medium provided by the assay manufacturer and stored, transported, and processed according to their directions. Patient-collected cervicovaginal swab or lavage specimens (80–83) and swabs of penile lesions (84, 85) have also proven reliable for detection of infection with high-risk HPV genotypes. Anal specimens for HPV testing can be collected using a saline-moistened Dacron swab and transported in liquid-based cytology media (86, 87).

Cervical brush specimens in standard transport medium for the HC2 High-Risk HPV DNA Test (Qiagen,

Gaithersburg, MD) may be stored for up to 2 weeks at room temperature, after which they can be stored for an additional week at 2 to 8°C or at −20°C for up to 3 months. Specimens in PreservCyt liquid-based cytology medium (Hologic, Bedford, MA) may be held at 2 to 30°C for up to 3 months for HC2 testing, at 20 to 30°C for up to 18 weeks for Cervista (Hologic, Bedford, MA) testing, and at 2 to 30°C for up to 6 months for cobas HPV (Roche Diagnostics, Indianapolis, IN) testing. For the Aptima HPV assay (Gen-Probe, San Diego, CA), cervical specimens in ThinPrep Pap test vials containing PreservCyt solution should be transported and stored at 2 to 30°C with no more than 30 days at temperatures above 8°C and, for longer storage, at −20°C for up to 24 months. PreservCyt specimens cannot be frozen prior to testing for high-risk HPV genotypes. Specimens collected in SurePath preservative fluid (BD Diagnostics–TriPath, Burlington, NC) may be stored at 2 to 8°C for up to 6 months or at 15 to 30°C for up to 4 weeks after the date of collection for cobas HPV (Roche Diagnostics, Indianapolis, IN) testing. Other methods of testing for high-risk HPV genotypes have not been FDA cleared/approved for use with specimens collected in SurePath preservative fluid.

Oral

An oral specimen provides a noninvasive means of detecting infection, and for some viruses, the onset of salivary shedding can indicate recent acquisition. Different types of oral specimens, including oral mucosal cells (including lesions), whole saliva, glandular duct saliva (from parotid, sublingual, and submandibular glands), and oral mucosal transudates (OMT), can be used for both culture and NA testing methods (88). Oral mucosal cells are dislodged with a swab or plastic spatula; the collection device is then placed in VTM for transport to the laboratory. Saliva is collected by initially tilting the head forward and catching fluid from the lower lip into a collection container and then by catching residual, expectorated fluid after 5 min (88). Parotid gland saliva, useful for diagnosing infectious parotitis, is collected with a swab approximately 30 seconds after massaging the area between the cheek and teeth at the level of the ear (89).

Salivary gland fluid consists primarily of secretory IgA (sIgA), whereas OMT contains a mixture of sIgA, IgG, and IgM. OMT (also called gingival crevicular fluid, crevicular fluid saliva, or crevicular fluid) arise from the capillaries in the buccal mucosa and the base of the pockets between the teeth and gums (gingival crevices) and can be collected with commercially available devices and transported to the laboratory at 2 to 8°C (90). OMT have been used for detection of both IgM and IgG antibodies to measles virus, mumps virus, rubella virus, HIV, and hepatitis viruses (91–93). The performance characteristics of oral fluid for determination of antibodies to HIV and HCV approach those of blood-based specimens (94, 95). However, HIV antibody testing with oral fluid alone is not recommended for patients at high risk of infection, particularly in low-prevalence settings, and should be followed by testing of a blood specimen (95).

Saliva samples are also collected for virus culture and NAAT, primarily for the evaluation of congenital CMV in the neonatal period. In this context, saliva has been shown to be comparable to urine for the diagnosis of congenital CMV using both shell vial culture and NAAT (96).

Respiratory

Viruses causing upper respiratory tract (URT) and lower respiratory tract (LRT) infections can be detected using Ag detection, culture, and NAAT (Table 1). Ideally, diagnostic testing should be completed within a time frame (generally 24 h) that allows the results to be used in patient management (97).

The primary site of replication for many respiratory viruses is the ciliated epithelial cells of the posterior nasopharynx and, to a lesser extent, the anterior nares and oropharynx. Therefore, nasal and throat specimens are traditionally not acceptable for virus detection due to the fact that many viruses are present at low levels in these sites. However, these specimens may be suitable for use in highly sensitive NAATs or when immunocompromised patients may be at risk of bleeding with harsher collection methods.

An NP aspirate is collected by inserting a narrow catheter or tube through the nostril into the posterior nasopharynx. A mucus trap or syringe is connected to the other end, and suction is applied while the tube is slowly withdrawn back through the nostril. Any secretions remaining in the tubing should be flushed into the trap or syringe by aspirating VTM or sterile saline (22, 23). A nasal wash is collected by instilling several milliliters of sterile saline into the nasal cavity using a bulb or syringe with catheter tubing attached. The contents are immediately aspirated by releasing the bulb or pulling the syringe plunger and placed into a tube containing VTM or sterile container. Nasal washes can yield high rates of respiratory virus detection by NA testing with minimal patient discomfort compared to swab, aspirate, and brush sampling (98).

Swabs for respiratory virus testing should be polyester, Dacron, or rayon with plastic or aluminum shafts. Wooden-shaft swabs may contain substances that are toxic to cultured cells. Calcium alginate swabs should not be used, since they may impair recovery of enveloped viruses, interfere with fluorescent-antibody tests, and are inhibitory to some NAATs. Flocked swabs, made from nylon fiber using a proprietary spray-on technology, are designed for optimum specimen absorption and release and have been shown to collect more respiratory epithelial cells than conventional rayon swabs for DFA testing of respiratory viruses (99, 100). Midturbinate flocked swabs are designed with a tapered cone shape, a sampling depth indication gauge, and a greater length and diameter of flocked nylon compared to regular swabs in order to sample a larger surface area of respiratory mucosa, including the inferior and middle turbinate bones. These can be self-collected; they yield numbers of respiratory epithelial cells comparable to those obtained with nasal and NP swabs and, in children, compared favorably with NP aspirates for DFA detection of common respiratory viruses (101, 102). Polyurethane foam-tipped swabs provide an alternative to nylon or Dacron swabs for sampling of the anterior nares in patients that might be at risk for bleeding. Self-collected foam nasal swabs have been shown to be more sensitive than nasal washes for detection of several respiratory viruses by NAAT in immunocompromised patients, and they performed better than flocked nylon swabs for rapid influenza virus antigen testing in children (103, 104).

A swab of the posterior nasopharynx typically yields more virus than a swab of the anterior nares or throat. Here, the flexible, fine-tipped swab is inserted through the nostril along the floor of the nose into the nasopharynx until resistance is felt, then rotated several times, removed, and placed in VTM (23). The swab should be pointed towards the ear rather than towards the top of the head and traverse half the distance between the angles of the nares and pinna. For DFA or NA testing, the sensitivity of flocked NP swabs for detection of respiratory viruses compares favorably to that of nasal wash and NP aspirate specimens (105, 106).

Throat swabs alone are generally inferior specimens for diagnosis of URT infections. However, combined testing of throat swabs with either NP swabs or aspirates can improve the yield of diagnostic etiologies of respiratory infection, as can the testing or pooling of other types of respiratory specimens (105, 107, 108). Throat swabs are collected by depressing the tongue and swabbing the tonsillar area and posterior pharynx thoroughly.

Although the oropharynx and nasopharynx are common portals for the introduction of viruses into the respiratory tract, the presence or absence of a virus in the URT may not be sufficient evidence of LRT disease, as evidenced by cases of severe influenza infection in which URT samples tested negative for the presence of virus, while those from the LRT had detectable virus (109, 110). Similarly, the severe acute respiratory syndrome (SARS) and Middle Eastern respiratory syndrome (MERS) coronaviruses may be detected with greater sensitivity in the LRT than the URT (111). BAL specimens are collected by inserting a fiber-optic bronchoscope into the involved segment of the lung, instilling saline, and applying suction to remove the lavage specimen. BAL specimens for NA testing should be transported and tested within 24 hours of collection, stored at 4°C for up to 72 hours, or frozen at −70°C or lower for future testing (25). Traditionally, sputum has been considered a suboptimal specimen for virus isolation. However, sputum may be a suitable specimen for respiratory virus detection using NAATs (reviewed in reference 112) and has been shown to increase the diagnostic yield over combined nasal and throat specimens in adults with respiratory illness (113). However, in children with radiologic evidence of pneumonia, respiratory pathogen NAAT of induced sputum was shown to have limited diagnostic utility (114). Furthermore, it is possible that viruses identified in sputum may not necessarily represent LRT infection, since they may originate in the oropharynx. Sputum for NAATs should be collected in a sterile container and transported to the laboratory at room temperature within 30 minutes or, if the transportation time is longer, transported at 4°C (25).

Respiratory fluids (e.g., NP aspirates and nasal washes) or swabs in VTM for culture should be vortexed to release cell-associated virus and centrifuged at 500 to 1,000 × *g* for 10 min unless there is a minimal amount of cellular debris. The supernatant can be used directly as the inoculum or further clarified by filtration (0.45-μm pore size) to remove any additional bacterial, fungal, and/or cellular debris. The pelleted cells (washed two or three times in phosphate-buffered saline) may be used for immunofluorescent (IF) staining (22, 23). Application of the concentrated cell suspension to a slide by cytospin preparation can increase the sensitivity of IF staining and reduce the number of inadequate specimens (115). It is not necessary to centrifuge or filter specimens for Ag or NA detection, since these assays should not be affected by microbial contamination. In fact, the loss of host cells may compromise the sensitivity of Ag and NA tests.

Mucus in respiratory specimens can significantly affect Ag detection. In DFA tests, mucus can inhibit adherence of cells to slides and can cause nonspecific fluorescence. It also prevents penetration of the sample into filtration devices. To prevent these complications, mucus threads can be broken by repeated aspiration through a small-bore pipette.

Skin

Viruses can cause rashes with many different appearances, including maculopapular, petechial, and vesicular rashes. Recovery of viruses from maculopapular and petechial rashes requires biopsy of skin, which is not routinely performed. Viral causes of disseminated diseases manifested by maculopapular and petechial rashes are usually identified by their clinical features and laboratory testing of specimen types other than skin, often blood for serologic or NA testing (Table 1), since the virions are not typically found in lesions resulting from the host immune response to infection (116).

Vesicular lesions are commonly caused by HSV, VZV, and enteroviruses. Cells and fluid from fresh vesicles are preferred over other lesion types, such as pustules, ulcers, and crusts, which may not contain sufficient virus for Ag detection, NA testing, or culture. Vesicular fluid can be collected by use of capillary pipettes or syringes or on swabs placed in VTM. Vesicles which have not been opened may have fluid contents withdrawn by means of a sterile tuberculin syringe fitted with a 26- or 27-gauge needle. Prior preparation of the area with disinfectants such as iodophors or alcohol may inactivate the viruses. Therefore, local disinfection should be used after the specimen has been collected. Fluids collected by syringe aspiration should be rinsed promptly into VTM. Alternatively, vesicles may be uncapped using a sterile needle or scalpel and the vesicle fluids adsorbed onto the tip of a sterile swab and placed in VTM. The margins and base of the lesion should be swabbed briskly to obtain infected epithelial cells (22). Cells from ulcers or crusted lesions (after removal of the crust) should be collected by rolling a swab over the same area. Specimens should be collected without causing bleeding, since the presence of neutralizing antibody in blood can impair recovery. Smears for immunofluorescent staining (e.g., for HSV and VZV) can be prepared at the patient's bedside by spreading the material thinly onto a small area in the center of a clean slide. After air drying, slides should be fixed in acetone for 5 to 10 min prior to staining. Swabs or vesicle fluid in VTM can be tested by NAATs, Ag detection, and/or culture. Specimens for viral culture can be inoculated directly after vortexing or first clarified by centrifugation and filtration if debris is present.

Stool and Rectal Swabs

Stool is the optimal specimen for identification of viruses causing gastroenteritis. Many gastroenteritis viruses (e.g., rotavirus) are noncultivable and require Ag or NA tests for detection. Ideally, specimens should be collected within the first 2 to 4 days of illness, since detection rates are reduced in later stages of infection unless the patient's underlying condition allows prolonged shedding. However, most enteroviruses can be recovered in stool for several weeks after onset of symptomatic infection.

Approximately 2 to 5 ml of liquid stool or 2 to 5 g of formed stool should be collected in a clean, dry, leakproof container or in VTM, depending on the type of testing to be performed. Fresh stool specimens can be stored at 4°C for 2 to 3 days if they are not tested immediately after collection. For prolonged storage, specimens should be kept frozen, preferably at −70°C or lower. Specially formulated paper strips have also been used for collection, transport, and storage of stool samples for NA testing of rotavirus, adenovirus types 40 and 41, and norovirus (43, 44, 117). The rectal swab is generally considered an inferior specimen to stool, as it usually collects an insufficient amount of specimen; the utility is directly related to the amount of visible stool collected. For collection, the swab is inserted several centimeters past the anal sphincter, rotated for several seconds, removed, and placed in VTM.

As bacteria comprise a significant proportion of the mass of stool, centrifugation, filtration, or both are often necessary to prevent microbial contamination of cell cultures. For virus isolation, a 10 to 20% (wt/vol) stool suspension is prepared in VTM with antimicrobials and glass beads and vortexed for 1 min, and the suspension is centrifuged at 3,000 × *g* for 15 to 30 min. The clarified supernatant can be filtered through a 0.2- to 0.45-μm pore size filter prior to inoculation of cell cultures (22, 23).

Tissue (Biopsy or Autopsy)

Tissue specimens obtained during surgery or at autopsy can be assessed by several diagnostic methods. Lung, liver, lymph node, kidney, spleen, cardiac, and brain tissue can be used to identify the viral etiology of many clinical syndromes (Table 1). Due to the invasive nature of specimen collection, the laboratory should ensure that a sufficient quantity of tissue is available for all testing requested; otherwise, testing can be prioritized by the clinician. The tissue can be divided in the laboratory in consultation with the pathologist to determine which portions should be submitted for viral diagnostics (118). A small piece of tissue from the leading edge of the affected area should be excised and kept moist in a sterile container, typically with sterile saline if comprehensive microbiologic and histologic testing is requested. Formalin-fixed tissue is unsuitable for viral isolation, and formalin may affect the performance of NAATs, though successful detection of both DNA and RNA viruses in formalin-fixed tissues has been reported (25, 119–121). Touch preparations of cells can be made by pressing tissue against the clean surface of a glass slide multiple times. Once air dried, the slide is fixed in acetone prior to application of staining reagents.

If NA is to be extracted, biopsy samples or large tissue specimens should be kept moist with sterile normal saline or placed in a suitable nucleic acid preservative. While the stability of NAs in tissue specimens varies with tissue type, it is recommended that tissues be transported to the laboratory on wet ice or frozen (25). Fresh tissue specimens for NA detection are minced, treated with proteolytic enzymes, and extracted. Formalin-fixed, paraffin-embedded tissues for NA testing should be stored and transported at ambient temperatures, deparaffinized, and extracted. However, fresh tissue is superior for NA recovery, since formalin treatment induces considerable nucleic acid degradation (25). For viral isolation from tissue, the recommended method is to prepare a 10 to 20% (wt/vol) homogenate, using VTM as a diluent, from small or minced tissue fragments that have been aseptically ground in a tissue grinder (22, 23). The homogenate can be centrifuged (600 to 900 × *g* for 10 min) or allowed to settle by gravity and the supernatant used as the inoculum.

Urine

Urine specimens should be collected as soon as possible after the onset of illness or when congenital or perinatal infection is first suspected. A volume of 5 to 10 ml of urine (midstream or catheter obtained) is collected in a sterile container; no VTM is required. The nature and timing of the collection are not known to have any effect on the reliability of testing methods. For NAATs, ambient storage of fresh unprocessed urine should be minimized, since the low pH and high urea content rapidly denature DNA/RNA (25). Nucleic acids should be extracted before testing, since urine contains substances that can inhibit PCR (122–124). Nucleic acids may be extracted from urine obtained on filter paper disks, or the disks may be used directly in the NAAT as a template without additional purification or elution steps (125–127).

Prior to inoculation of cell culture, urine can be filtered (0.45-μm pore size) or centrifuged (1,000 × *g* for 10 min) to remove bacteria and debris; the pH can be neutralized with sodium bicarbonate (7.5% solution) to reduce toxicity (23). Alternatively, antibiotics can be added directly to the urine, or it can be diluted with VTM to neutralize pH and introduce antimicrobials (22). The mixture should be allowed to stand at room temperature for 15 minutes prior to inoculation of cell cultures.

TRANSPORTATION REGULATIONS

Shipment of specimens to reference or public health laboratories is common practice. All packages that contain infectious substances must meet the shipping regulations of various organizations or agencies. In the United States, the main source for regulations governing specimen and biological shipments is the U.S. Department of Transportation (DOT). The International Air Transport Association (IATA) regulates all shipments on air carriers and provides its own Dangerous Goods Regulations (DGR) (128). Since there is some harmonization between the national and international regulatory bodies, the IATA requirements are usually acceptable under all regulations.

The DGR include specific instructions for packaging and labeling of shipments containing biological or infectious substances, such as patient specimens or cultured microorganisms (128). In the clinical laboratory, materials being shipped generally fall into one of three categories: exempt human specimen, category A, or category B. Category A infectious substances (UN2814 infectious substance, affecting humans) are those transported in a form that, when exposure to it occurs, can cause potentially life-threatening illness (e.g., Ebola virus). The most up-to-date list of category A infectious substances can be found at the International Air Transport Association (IATA) website for Dangerous Goods Regulations (www.iata.org/whatwedo/cargo/dgr/Pages/download.aspx). An infectious substance which does not meet the criteria for inclusion in category A is assigned to category B (UN3373 biological substance, category B) unless it is a patient specimen for which there is minimal likelihood that pathogens are present, in which case it would be labeled an exempt human specimen.

For transportation of any category A infectious substance, packaging must include an inner container, an itemized list of contents, and an outer packaging. The inner packaging must comprise one or more leakproof primary receptacles and leakproof secondary packaging capable of withstanding an internal pressure differential of at least 95 kPa. For liquid specimens, an absorbent material in sufficient quantity to absorb the entire contents must be placed between the primary and secondary packaging. Category B packing instructions are essentially identical to those for category A, although no packing list need be included. Exempt patient specimens are packaged with leakproof primary and secondary receptacles within an outer container of adequate strength. Training of personnel for packaging and shipping dangerous goods must be documented, and recertification is required every 2 years. The DOT may inspect any shipper or receiver of dangerous goods, unannounced, at any time.

SUMMARY

The importance of appropriate specimen collection and handling to ensure accurate laboratory results cannot be overstated, and the laboratory must serve as a resource for clinicians. In some instances, proper collection, transport, and processing of specimens are determined by the manufacturer, whereas laboratories which utilize in-house-developed tests need to verify these preanalytical factors themselves prior to routine clinical testing (45).

The performance characteristics of viral diagnostic tests (sensitivity, specificity, positive predictive value, and negative predictive value) are, to a large extent, dependent on the integrity of viral or host components present in the specimen. For molecular methods, successful testing is based largely on the quality of the nucleic acid purified from the clinical specimen. That quality is directly related to how the specimen is stored and transported to the laboratory after it has been collected from the patient. Detection of viral antigens requires that adequate amounts of intact cellular material from the site of infection be collected and maintained to prevent degradation. Serologic testing is impacted by the timing of collection relative to disease progression. Successful recovery of virus in culture requires maintenance of viability, which can be enhanced by (i) the timing and method of collection to incorporate high titers of virus, (ii) protection from thermal inactivation or drying, and (iii) use of an effective transport system.

REFERENCES

1. **Astion ML, Shojania KG, Hamill TR, Kim S, Ng VL.** 2003. Classifying laboratory incident reports to identify problems that jeopardize patient safety. *Am J Clin Pathol* **120:**18–26.
2. **Grys TE, Smith TF.** 2009. Specimen requirements: selection, collection, transport, and processing, p 18–35. *In* Specter SHR, Young SA, Wiedbrauk DL (ed), *Clinical Virology Manual*, 4th ed. ASM Press, Washington, DC.
3. **Graf EH, Simmon KE, Tardif KD, Hymas W, Flygare S, Eilbeck K, Yandell M, Schlaberg R.** 2016. Unbiased detection of respiratory viruses by use of RNA sequencing-based metagenomics: a systematic comparison to a commercial PCR panel. *J Clin Microbiol* **54:**1000–1007.
4. **Doan T, Acharya NR, Pinsky BA, Sahoo MK, Chow ED, Banaei N, Budvytiene I, Cevallos V, Zhong L, Zhou Z, Lietman TM, DeRisi JL.** 2017. Metagenomic DNA sequencing for the diagnosis of intraocular infections. *Ophthalmology* **124:**1247–1248.
5. **Lau LLH, Cowling BJ, Fang VJ, Chan KH, Lau EHY, Lipsitch M, Cheng CKY, Houck PM, Uyeki TM, Peiris JSM, Leung GM.** 2010. Viral shedding and clinical illness in naturally acquired influenza virus infections. *J Infect Dis* **201:**1509–1516.
6. **Milano F, Campbell AP, Guthrie KA, Kuypers J, Englund JA, Corey L, Boeckh M.** 2010. Human rhinovirus and coronavirus detection among allogeneic hematopoietic stem cell transplantation recipients. *Blood* **115:**2088–2094.
7. **Milbrath MO, Spicknall IH, Zelner JL, Moe CL, Eisenberg JN.** 2013. Heterogeneity in norovirus shedding duration affects community risk. *Epidemiol Infect* **141:**1572–1584.
8. **von Linstow ML, Eugen-Olsen J, Koch A, Winther TN, Westh H, Hogh B.** 2006. Excretion patterns of human metapneumovirus and respiratory syncytial virus among young children. *Eur J Med Res* **11:**329–335.
9. **Walsh EE, Peterson DR, Kalkanoglu AE, Lee FE, Falsey AR.** 2013. Viral shedding and immune responses to respiratory syncytial virus infection in older adults. *J Infect Dis* **207:**1424–1432.
10. **Peiris JSM, Chu CM, Cheng VCC, Chan KS, Hung IFN, Poon LLM, Law KI, Tang BSF, Hon TYW, Chan CS, Chan KH, Ng JSC, Zheng BJ, Ng WL, Lai RWM, Guan Y, Yuen KY, HKU/UCH SARS Study Group.** 2003. Clinical progression and viral load in a community outbreak of coronavirus-associated SARS pneumonia: a prospective study. *Lancet* **361:**1767–1772.
11. **Centers for Disease Control and Prevention.** 2004. *Public Health Guidance for Community-Level Preparedness and Response to Severe Acute Respiratory Syndrome (SARS)*. U.S. Department of Health and Human Services and CDC, Atlanta, GA.
12. **Siegel JD, Rhinehart E, Jackson M, Chiarello L, Health Care Infection Control Practices Advisory Committee.** 2007. 2007 guideline for isolation precautions: preventing transmission of infectious agents in health care settings. *Am J Infect Control* **35**(Suppl 2)**:**S65–S164.
13. **Blow JA, Dohm DJ, Negley DL, Mores CN.** 2004. Virus inactivation by nucleic acid extraction reagents. *J Virol Methods* **119:**195–198.
14. **Josephson SL.** 1997. An update on the collection and transport of specimens for viral culture. *Clin Microbiol Newsl* **19:**57–61.
15. **Johnson FB.** 1990. Transport of viral specimens. *Clin Microbiol Rev* **3:**120–131.
16. **Druce J, Garcia K, Tran T, Papadakis G, Birch C.** 2012. Evaluation of swabs, transport media, and specimen transport conditions for optimal detection of viruses by PCR. *J Clin Microbiol* **50:**1064–1065.
17. **CLSI.** 2013. *Quality Control of Microbiological Transport Systems: Approved Guideline. CLSI document M40-A2.* CLSI, Wayne, PA.
18. **Dunn JJ, Billetdeaux E, Skodack-Jones L, Carroll KC.** 2003. Evaluation of three Copan viral transport systems for the recovery of cultivatable, clinical virus isolates. *Diagn Microbiol Infect Dis* **45:**191–197.
19. **Gleaves CA, Rice DH, Lee CF.** 1990. Evaluation of an enzyme immunoassay for the detection of herpes simplex virus (HSV) antigen from clinical specimens in viral transport media. *J Virol Methods* **28:**133–139.
20. **Hodinka RL.** 2009. Laboratory diagnosis of viral diseases, p 17–35. *In* Shah SS (ed), *Pediatric Practice: Infectious Disease.* McGraw-Hill, New York, NY.
21. **Hambling MH.** 1964. Survival of the respiratory syncytial virus during storage under various conditions. *Br J Exp Pathol* **45:**647–655.
22. **Clarke L.**2010. Specimen collection and processing, p 10.4.1–10.4.11. *In* Garcia LS (ed), *Clinical Microbiology Procedures Handbook*, 3rd ed. ASM Press, Washington, DC.
23. **CLSI.** 2006. Viral culture; approved guideline. CLSI document M41-A. Clinical and Laboratory Standards Institute, Wayne, PA.
24. **Miller JM, Astles R, Baszler T, Chapin K, Carey R, Garcia L, Gray L, Larone D, Pentella M, Pollock A, Shapiro DS, Weirich E, Wiedbrauk D, Biosafety Blue Ribbon Panel, Centers for Disease Control and Prevention.** 2012. Guidelines for safe work practices in human and animal medical diagnostic laboratories. Recommendations of a CDC-convened Biosafety Blue Ribbon Panel. *MMWR Morb Mortal Wkly Rep* **61(Suppl):**1–102.
25. **CLSI.** 2005. Collection, transport, preparation, and storage of specimens for molecular methods; approved guideline. CLSI document MM13-A. Clinical and Laboratory Standards Institute, Wayne, PA.
26. **Ginocchio CC, Wang XP, Kaplan MH, Mulligan G, Witt D, Romano JW, Cronin M, Carroll R.** 1997. Effects of specimen collection, processing, and storage conditions on stability of human immunodeficiency virus type 1 RNA levels in plasma. *J Clin Microbiol* **35:**2886–2893.
27. **José M, Gajardo R, Jorquera JI.** 2005. Stability of HCV, HIV-1 and HBV nucleic acids in plasma samples under long-term storage. *Biologicals* **33:**9–16.
28. **Watson J, Graves S, Ferguson J, D'Este C, Batey R.** 2007. Hepatitis C virus RNA quantitation and degradation studies in whole blood samples in vitro. *Gut* **56:**306–307.
29. **Jennings C, Danilovic A, Scianna S, Brambilla DJ, Bremer JW.** 2005. Stability of human immunodeficiency virus type 1 proviral DNA in whole-blood samples. *J Clin Microbiol* **43:**4249–4250.
30. **Lee DHLL, Li L, Andrus L, Prince AM.** 2002. Stabilized viral nucleic acids in plasma as an alternative shipping method for NAT. *Transfusion* **42:**409–413.
31. **Uhlenhaut C, Kracht M.** 2005. Viral infectivity is maintained by an RNA protection buffer. *J Virol Methods* **128:**189–191.
32. **Blow JA, Mores CN, Dyer J, Dohm DJ.** 2008. Viral nucleic acid stabilization by RNA extraction reagent. *J Virol Methods* **150:**41–44.

33. **Hasan MR, Tan R, Al-Rawahi GN, Thomas E, Tilley P.** 2012. Short-term stability of pathogen-specific nucleic acid targets in clinical samples. *J Clin Microbiol* **50:**4147–4150.
34. **Endler G, Slavka G.** 2010. Stability of the specimen during preanalytics, p 25–34. *In* Kessler HH (ed), *Molecular Diagnostics of Infectious Diseases*. Walter de Gruyter and Co, New York, NY.
35. **Nesbitt SE, Cook L, Jerome KR.** 2004. Cytomegalovirus quantitation by real-time PCR is unaffected by delayed separation of plasma from whole blood. *J Clin Microbiol* **42:**1296–1297.
36. **Roberts TC, Buller RS, Gaudreault-Keener M, Sternhell KE, Garlock K, Singer GG, Brennan DC, Storch GA.** 1997. Effects of storage temperature and time on qualitative and quantitative detection of cytomegalovirus in blood specimens by shell vial culture and PCR. *J Clin Microbiol* **35:**2224–2228.
37. **Abdul-Ali D, Kraft CS, Ingersoll J, Frempong M, Caliendo AM.** 2011. Cytomegalovirus DNA stability in EDTA anticoagulated whole blood and plasma samples. *J Clin Virol* **52:**222–224.
38. **Schäfer P, Tenschert W, Schröter M, Gutensohn K, Laufs R.** 2000. False-positive results of plasma PCR for cytomegalovirus DNA due to delayed sample preparation. *J Clin Microbiol* **38:**3249–3253.
39. **Jerome KR, Huang ML, Wald A, Selke S, Corey L.** 2002. Quantitative stability of DNA after extended storage of clinical specimens as determined by real-time PCR. *J Clin Microbiol* **40:**2609–2611.
40. **Wiedbrauk DL, Cunningham W.** 1996. Stability of herpes simplex virus DNA in cerebrospinal fluid specimens. *Diagn Mol Pathol* **5:**249–252.
41. **Agreda PM, Beitman GH, Gutierrez EC, Harris JM, Koch KR, LaViers WD, Leitch SV, Maus CE, McMillian RA, Nussbaumer WA, Palmer MLR, Porter MJ, Richart GA, Schwab RJ, Vaughan LM.** 2013. Long-term stability of human genomic and human papillomavirus DNA stored in BD SurePath and Hologic PreservCyt liquid-based cytology media. *J Clin Microbiol* **51:**2702–2706.
42. **Fischer TK, Steinsland H, Valentiner-Branth P.** 2002. Rotavirus particles can survive storage in ambient tropical temperatures for more than 2 months. *J Clin Microbiol* **40:**4763–4764.
43. **Zlateva KT, Maes P, Rahman M, Van Ranst M.** 2005. Chromatography paper strip sampling of enteric adenoviruses type 40 and 41 positive stool specimens. *Virol J* **2:**6.
44. **Wollants E, Maes P, Thoelen I, Vanneste F, Rahman M, Van Ranst M.** 2004. Evaluation of a norovirus sampling method using sodium dodecyl sulfate/EDTA-pretreated chromatography paper strips. *J Virol Methods* **122:**45–48.
45. **Burd EM.** 2010. Validation of laboratory-developed molecular assays for infectious diseases. *Clin Microbiol Rev* **23:**550–576.
46. **CLSI.** 2011. Establishing molecular testing in clinical laboratory environments; approved guideline. CLSI document MM19-A. Clinical and Laboratory Standards Institute, Wayne, PA.
47. **Landini MP, Lazzarotto T.** 1999. Prenatal diagnosis of congenital cytomegalovirus infection: light and shade. *Herpes* **6:**45–49.
48. **Mendelson E, Aboudy Y, Smetana Z, Tepperberg M, Grossman Z.** 2006. Laboratory assessment and diagnosis of congenital viral infections: Rubella, cytomegalovirus (CMV), varicella-zoster virus (VZV), herpes simplex virus (HSV), parvovirus B19 and human immunodeficiency virus (HIV). *Reprod Toxicol* **21:**350–382.
49. **Deback C, Fillet AM, Dhedin N, Barrou B, Varnous S, Najioullah F, Bricaire F, Agut H.** 2007. Monitoring of human cytomegalovirus infection in immunosuppressed patients using real-time PCR on whole blood. *J Clin Virol* **40:**173–179.
50. **Hakim H, Gibson C, Pan J, Srivastava K, Gu Z, Bankowski MJ, Hayden RT.** 2007. Comparison of various blood compartments and reporting units for the detection and quantification of Epstein-Barr virus in peripheral blood. *J Clin Microbiol* **45:**2151–2155.
51. **Perlman J, Gibson C, Pounds SB, Gu Z, Bankowski MJ, Hayden RT.** 2007. Quantitative real-time PCR detection of adenovirus in clinical blood specimens: a comparison of plasma, whole blood and peripheral blood mononuclear cells. *J Clin Virol* **40:**295–300.
52. **Ruf S, Behnke-Hall K, Gruhn B, Bauer J, Horn M, Beck J, Reiter A, Wagner HJ.** 2012. Comparison of six different specimen types for Epstein-Barr viral load quantification in peripheral blood of pediatric patients after heart transplantation or after allogeneic hematopoietic stem cell transplantation. *J Clin Virol* **53:**186–194.
53. **Griffith BP, Mayo DR.** 2006. Increased levels of HIV RNA detected in samples with viral loads close to the detection limit collected in Plasma Preparation Tubes (PPT). *J Clin Virol* **35:**197–200.
54. **Rebeiro PF, Kheshti A, Bebawy SS, Stinnette SE, Erdem H, Tang YW, Sterling TR, Raffanti SP, D'Aquila RT.** 2008. Increased detectability of plasma HIV-1 RNA after introduction of a new assay and altered specimen-processing procedures. *Clin Infect Dis* **47:**1354–1357.
55. **Salimnia H, Moore EC, Crane LR, Macarthur RD, Fairfax MR.** 2005. Discordance between viral loads determined by Roche COBAS AMPLICOR human immunodeficiency virus type 1 monitor (version 1.5) standard and ultrasensitive assays caused by freezing patient plasma in centrifuged Becton-Dickinson Vacutainer brand plasma preparation tubes. *J Clin Microbiol* **43:**4635–4639.
56. **Kran AM, Jonassen TO, Sannes M, Jakobsen K, Lind A, Maeland A, Holberg-Petersen M.** 2009. Overestimation of human immunodeficiency virus type 1 load caused by the presence of cells in plasma from plasma preparation tubes. *J Clin Microbiol* **47:**2170–2174.
57. **Wan H, Seth A, Rainen L, Fernandes H.** 2010. Coamplification of HIV-1 proviral DNA and viral RNA in assays used for quantification of HIV-1 RNA. *J Clin Microbiol* **48:**2186–2190.
58. **Fernandes H, Morosyuk S, Abravaya K, Ramanathan M, Rainen L.** 2010. Evaluation of effect of specimen-handling parameters for plasma preparation tubes on viral load measurements obtained by using the Abbott RealTime HIV-1 load assay. *J Clin Microbiol* **48:**2464–2468.
59. **Kraft CS, Binongo JNG, Burd EM, Eaton ME, McCloskey CB, Fernandes H, Hill CE, Caliendo AM.** 2013. Successful use of Plasma Preparation Tubes™ (PPTs) in the COBAS® AmpliPrep/COBAS® TaqMan® HIV-1 test. *J Clin Virol* **57:**77–79.
60. **Grant PR, Kitchen A, Barbara JA, Hewitt P, Sims CM, Garson JA, Tedder RS.** 2000. Effects of handling and storage of blood on the stability of hepatitis C virus RNA: implications for NAT testing in transfusion practice. *Vox Sang* **78:**137–142.
61. **Leland DS, Ginocchio CC.** 2007. Role of cell culture for virus detection in the age of technology. *Clin Microbiol Rev* **20:**49–78 .
62. **St George K, Boyd MJ, Lipson SM, Ferguson D, Cartmell GF, Falk LH, Rinaldo CR, Landry ML.** 2000. A multisite trial comparing two cytomegalovirus (CMV) pp65 antigenemia test kits, Biotest CMV Brite and Bartels/Argene CMV Antigenemia. *J Clin Microbiol* **38:**1430–1433.
63. **Buller RS, Bailey TC, Ettinger NA, Keener M, Langlois T, Miller JP, Storch GA.** 1992. Use of a modified shell vial technique to quantitate cytomegalovirus viremia in a population of solid-organ transplant recipients. *J Clin Microbiol* **30:**2620–2624.
64. **Lipson SM, Falk LH, Lee SH.** 1996. Effect of leukocyte concentration and inoculum volume on the laboratory identification of cytomegalovirus in peripheral blood by the centrifugation culture-antigen detection methodology. *Arch Pathol Lab Med* **120:**53–56.
65. **Buller RS, Gaudreault-Keener M, Rossiter-Fornoff J, Storch GA.** 1995. Direct quantitative comparison of shell vial and conventional culture for detection of CMV viremia. *Clin Diagn Virol* **3:**317–322.
66. **Florea AV, Ionescu DN, Melhem MF.** 2007. Parvovirus B19 infection in the immunocompromised host. *Arch Pathol Lab Med* **131:**799–804.

67. **Maakaroun NR, Moanna A, Jacob JT, Albrecht H.** 2010. Viral infections associated with haemophagocytic syndrome. *Rev Med Virol* **20:**93–105.
68. **Duong S, Dezube BJ, Desai G, Eichelberger K, Qian Q, Kirby JE.** 2009. Limited utility of bone marrow culture: a ten-year retrospective analysis. *Lab Med* **40:**37–38.
69. **Phillips CF, Benyesh-Melnick M, Seidel EH, Fernbach DJ.** 1965. Failure to isolate viral agents from bone marrows of children with acute leukemia. *BMJ* **1:**286–288.
70. **Akane A, Matsubara K, Nakamura H, Takahashi S, Kimura K.** 1994. Identification of the heme compound copurified with deoxyribonucleic acid (DNA) from bloodstains, a major inhibitor of polymerase chain reaction (PCR) amplification. *J Forensic Sci* **39:**362–372.
71. **Greenfield L, White TJ.** 1993. Sample preparation methods, p 122–137. *In* Persing DHST, Tenover FC, White TJ (ed), *Diagnostic Molecular Biology: Principles and Applications*. ASM Press, Washington, DC.
72. **Ratnamohan VM, Cunningham AL, Rawlinson WD.** 1998. Removal of inhibitors of CSF-PCR to improve diagnosis of herpesviral encephalitis. *J Virol Methods* **72:**59–65.
73. **DeBiasi RL, Tyler KL.** 2004. Molecular methods for diagnosis of viral encephalitis. *Clin Microbiol Rev* **17:**903–925.
74. **Lakeman FD, Whitley RJ, National Institute of Allergy and Infectious Diseases Collaborative Antiviral Study Group.** 1995. Diagnosis of herpes simplex encephalitis: application of polymerase chain reaction to cerebrospinal fluid from brain-biopsied patients and correlation with disease. *J Infect Dis* **171:**857–863.
75. **Snijdewind IJ, van Kampen JJ, Fraaij PL, van der Ende ME, Osterhaus AD, Gruters RA.** 2012. Current and future applications of dried blood spots in viral disease management. *Antiviral Res* **93:**309–321.
76. **Brambilla D, Jennings C, Aldrovandi G, Bremer J, Comeau AM, Cassol SA, Dickover R, Jackson JB, Pitt J, Sullivan JL, Butcher A, Grosso L, Reichelderfer P, Fiscus SA.** 2003. Multicenter evaluation of use of dried blood and plasma spot specimens in quantitative assays for human immunodeficiency virus RNA: measurement, precision, and RNA stability. *J Clin Microbiol* **41:**1888–1893.
77. **Limaye AP, Santo Hayes TK, Huang ML, Magaret A, Boeckh M, Jerome KR.** 2013. Quantitation of cytomegalovirus DNA load in dried blood spots correlates well with plasma viral load. *J Clin Microbiol* **51:**2360–2364.
78. **Sambursky R, Trattler W, Tauber S, Starr C, Friedberg M, Boland T, McDonald M, DellaVecchia M, Luchs J.** 2013. Sensitivity and specificity of the AdenoPlus test for diagnosing adenoviral conjunctivitis. *JAMA Ophthalmol* **131:**17–22.
79. **Wiedbrauk DL, Werner JC, Drevon AM.** 1995. Inhibition of PCR by aqueous and vitreous fluids. *J Clin Microbiol* **33:**2643–2646.
80. **Darlin L, Borgfeldt C, Forslund O, Hénic E, Dillner J, Kannisto P.** 2013. Vaginal self-sampling without preservative for human papillomavirus testing shows good sensitivity. *J Clin Virol* **56:**52–56.
81. **Gage JC, Partridge EE, Rausa A, Gravitt PE, Wacholder S, Schiffman M, Scarinci I, Castle PE.** 2011. Comparative performance of human papillomavirus DNA testing using novel sample collection methods. *J Clin Microbiol* **49:**4185–4189.
82. **Gök M, Heideman DA, van Kemenade FJ, Berkhof J, Rozendaal L, Spruyt JWM, Voorhorst F, Beliën JAM, Babovic M, Snijders PJF, Meijer CJ.** 2010. HPV testing on self collected cervicovaginal lavage specimens as screening method for women who do not attend cervical screening: cohort study. *BMJ* **340:**c1040.
83. **Petignat P, Faltin DL, Bruchim I, Tramèr MR, Franco EL, Coutlée F.** 2007. Are self-collected samples comparable to physician-collected cervical specimens for human papillomavirus DNA testing? A systematic review and meta-analysis. *Gynecol Oncol* **105:**530–535.
84. **Hernandez BY, Wilkens LR, Unger ER, Steinau M, Markowitz L, Garvin K, Thompson PJ, Shvetsov YB, O'Dillon K, Dunne EF.** 2013. Evaluation of genital self-sampling methods for HPV detection in males. *J Clin Virol* **58:**168–175.
85. **Ogilvie GS, Taylor DL, Achen M, Cook D, Krajden M.** 2009. Self-collection of genital human papillomavirus specimens in heterosexual men. *Sex Transm Infect* **85:**221–225.
86. **Etienney I, Vuong S, Si-Mohamed A, Fléjou JF, Atienza P, Bauer P, Cytological Diaconesses Group.** 2012. Value of cytologic Papanicolaou smears and polymerase chain reaction screening for human papillomavirus DNA in detecting anal intraepithelial neoplasia: comparison with histology of a surgical sample. *Cancer* **118:**6031–6038.
87. **Goldstone SE, Lowe B, Rothmann T, Nazarenko I.** 2012. Evaluation of the hybrid capture 2 assay for detecting anal high-grade dysplasia. *Int J Cancer* **131:**1641–1648.
88. **Boppana SB, Ross SA, Shimamura M, Palmer AL, Ahmed A, Michaels MG, Sánchez PJ, Bernstein DI, Tolan RW Jr, Novak Z, Chowdhury N, Britt WJ, Fowler KB, National Institute on Deafness and Other Communication Disorders CHIMES Study.** 2011. Saliva polymerase-chain-reaction assay for cytomegalovirus screening in newborns. *N Engl J Med* **364:**2111–2118.
89. **Hindiyeh MY, Aboudy Y, Wohoush M, Shulman LM, Ram D, Levin T, Frank T, Riccardo F, Khalili M, Sawalha ES, Obeidi M, Sabatinelli G, Grossman Z, Mendelson E.** 2009. Characterization of large mumps outbreak among vaccinated Palestinian refugees. *J Clin Microbiol* **47:**560–565.
90. **Holm-Hansen C, Tong G, Davis C, Abrams WR, Malamud D.** 2004. Comparison of oral fluid collectors for use in a rapid point-of-care diagnostic device. *Clin Diagn Lab Immunol* **11:**909–912.
91. **Abernathy E, Cabezas C, Sun H, Zheng Q, Chen MH, Castillo-Solorzano C, Ortiz AC, Osores F, Oliveira L, Whittembury A, Andrus JK, Helfand RF, Icenogle J.** 2009. Confirmation of rubella within 4 days of rash onset: comparison of rubella virus RNA detection in oral fluid with immunoglobulin M detection in serum or oral fluid. *J Clin Microbiol* **47:**182–188.
92. **Hodinka RL, Nagashunmugam T, Malamud D.** 1998. Detection of human immunodeficiency virus antibodies in oral fluids. *Clin Diagn Lab Immunol* **5:**419–426.
93. **Warrener L, Slibinskas R, Chua KB, Nigatu W, Brown KE, Sasnauskas K, Samuel D, Brown D.** 2011. A point-of-care test for measles diagnosis: detection of measles-specific IgM antibodies and viral nucleic acid. *Bull World Health Organ* **89:**675–682.
94. **Lee SR, Kardos KW, Schiff E, Berne CA, Mounzer K, Banks AT, Tatum HA, Friel TJ, Demicco MP, Lee WM, Eder SE, Monto A, Yearwood GD, Guillon GB, Kurtz LA, Fischl M, Unangst JL, Kriebel L, Feiss G, Roehler M.** 2011. Evaluation of a new, rapid test for detecting HCV infection, suitable for use with blood or oral fluid. *J Virol Methods* **172:**27–31.
95. **Pai NP, Balram B, Shivkumar S, Martinez-Cajas JL, Claessens C, Lambert G, Peeling RW, Joseph L.** 2012. Head-to-head comparison of accuracy of a rapid point-of-care HIV test with oral versus whole-blood specimens: a systematic review and meta-analysis. *Lancet Infect Dis* **12:**373–380.
96. **Ross SA, Ahmed A, Palmer AL, Michaels MG, Sánchez PJ, Bernstein DI, Tolan RW Jr, Novak Z, Chowdhury N, Fowler KB, Boppana SB, National Institute on Deafness and Other Communication Disorders CHIMES Study.** 2014. Detection of congenital cytomegalovirus infection by real-time polymerase chain reaction analysis of saliva or urine specimens. *J Infect Dis* **210:**1415–1418.
97. **Ginocchio CC, McAdam AJ.** 2011. Current best practices for respiratory virus testing. *J Clin Microbiol* **49**(Suppl)**:**S44–S48.
98. **Spyridaki IS, Christodoulou I, de Beer L, Hovland V, Kurowski M, Olszewska-Ziaber A, Carlsen KH, Lødrup-Carlsen K, van Drunen CM, Kowalski ML, Molenkamp R, Papadopoulos NG.** 2009. Comparison of four nasal sampling methods for the detection of viral pathogens by RT-PCR-A GA(2)LEN project. *J Virol Methods* **156:**102–106.
99. **Abu-Diab A, Azzeh M, Ghneim R, Ghneim R, Zoughbi M, Turkuman S, Rishmawi N, Issa AE, Siriani I, Dauodi R, Kattan R, Hindiyeh MY.** 2008. Comparison between pernasal flocked swabs and nasopharyngeal aspirates for detection of common respiratory viruses in samples from children. *J Clin Microbiol* **46:**2414–2417.

100. **Daley P, Castriciano S, Chernesky M, Smieja M.** 2006. Comparison of flocked and rayon swabs for collection of respiratory epithelial cells from uninfected volunteers and symptomatic patients. *J Clin Microbiol* **44:**2265–2267.
101. **Faden H.** 2010. Comparison of midturbinate flocked-swab specimens with nasopharyngeal aspirates for detection of respiratory viruses in children by the direct fluorescent antibody technique. *J Clin Microbiol* **48:**3742–3743.
102. **Smieja M, Castriciano S, Carruthers S, So G, Chong S, Luinstra K, Mahony JB, Petrich A, Chernesky M, Savarese M, Triva D.** 2010. Development and evaluation of a flocked nasal midturbinate swab for self-collection in respiratory virus infection diagnostic testing. *J Clin Microbiol* **48:** 3340–3342.
103. **Campbell AP, Kuypers J, Englund JA, Guthrie KA, Corey L, Boeckh M.** 2013. Self-collection of foam nasal swabs for respiratory virus detection by PCR among immunocompetent subjects and hematopoietic cell transplant recipients. *J Clin Microbiol* **51:**324–327.
104. **Scansen KA, Bonsu BK, Stoner E, Mack K, Salamon D, Leber A, Marcon MJ.** 2010. Comparison of polyurethane foam to nylon flocked swabs for collection of secretions from the anterior nares in performance of a rapid influenza virus antigen test in a pediatric emergency department. *J Clin Microbiol* **48:**852–856.
105. **Munywoki PK, Hamid F, Mutunga M, Welch S, Cane P, Nokes DJ.** 2011. Improved detection of respiratory viruses in pediatric outpatients with acute respiratory illness by real-time PCR using nasopharyngeal flocked swabs. *J Clin Microbiol* **49:**3365–3367.
106. **Walsh P, Overmyer CL, Pham K, Michaelson S, Gofman L, DeSalvia L, Tran T, Gonzalez D, Pusavat J, Feola M, Iacono KT, Mordechai E, Adelson ME.** 2008. Comparison of respiratory virus detection rates for infants and toddlers by use of flocked swabs, saline aspirates, and saline aspirates mixed in universal transport medium for room temperature storage and shipping. *J Clin Microbiol* **46:**2374–2376.
107. **Hammitt LL, Kazungu S, Welch S, Bett A, Onyango CO, Gunson RN, Scott JAG, Nokes DJ.** 2011. Added value of an oropharyngeal swab in detection of viruses in children hospitalized with lower respiratory tract infection. *J Clin Microbiol* **49:**2318–2320.
108. **Lieberman D, Lieberman D, Shimoni A, Keren-Naus A, Steinberg R, Shemer-Avni Y.** 2010. Pooled nasopharyngeal and oropharyngeal samples for the identification of respiratory viruses in adults. *Eur J Clin Microbiol Infect Dis* **29:** 733–735.
109. **Mulrennan S, Tempone SS, Ling IT, Williams SH, Gan GC, Murray RJ, Speers DJ.** 2010. Pandemic influenza (H1N1) 2009 pneumonia: CURB-65 score for predicting severity and nasopharyngeal sampling for diagnosis are unreliable. *PLoS One* **5:**e12849.
110. **Yeh E, Luo RF, Dyner L, Hong DK, Banaei N, Baron EJ, Pinsky BA.** 2010. Preferential lower respiratory tract infection in swine-origin 2009 A(H1N1) influenza. *Clin Infect Dis* **50:**391–394.
111. **Chan JF, Lau SK, To KK, Cheng VC, Woo PC, Yuen KY.** 2015. Middle East respiratory syndrome coronavirus: another zoonotic betacoronavirus causing SARS-like disease. *Clin Microbiol Rev* **28:**465–522.
112. **Loens K, Van Heirstraeten L, Malhotra-Kumar S, Goossens H, Ieven M.** 2009. Optimal sampling sites and methods for detection of pathogens possibly causing community-acquired lower respiratory tract infections. *J Clin Microbiol* **47:**21–31.
113. **Falsey AR, Formica MA, Walsh EE.** 2012. Yield of sputum for viral detection by reverse transcriptase PCR in adults hospitalized with respiratory illness. *J Clin Microbiol* **50:**21–24.
114. **Thea DM, Seidenberg P, Park DE, Mwananyanda L, Fu W, Shi Q, Baggett HC, Brooks WA, Feikin DR, Howie SRC, Knoll MD, Kotloff KL, Levine OS, Madhi SA, O'Brien KL, Scott JAG, Antonio M, Awori JO, Baillie VL, DeLuca AN, Driscoll AJ, Higdon MM, Hossain L, Jahan Y, Karron RA, Kazungu S, Li M, Moore DP, Morpeth SC, Ofordile O, Prosperi C, Sangwichian O, Sawatwong P, Sylla M, Tapia MD, Zeger SL, Murdoch DR, Hammitt LL, PERCH Study Group.** 2017. Limited utility of polymerase chain reaction in induced sputum specimens for determining the causes of childhood pneumonia in resource-poor settings: findings from the Pneumonia Etiology for Child Health (PERCH) study. *Clin Infect Dis* **64**(suppl_3)**:**S289–S300.
115. **Landry ML, Ferguson D.** 2010. Cytospin-enhanced immunofluorescence and impact of sample quality on detection of novel swine origin (H1N1) influenza virus. *J Clin Microbiol* **48:**957–959.
116. **Drago F, Rampini P, Rampini E, Rebora A.** 2002. Atypical exanthems: morphology and laboratory investigations may lead to an aetiological diagnosis in about 70% of cases. *Br J Dermatol* **147:**255–260.
117. **Rahman M, Goegebuer T, De Leener K, Maes P, Matthijnssens J, Podder G, Azim T, Van Ranst M.** 2004. Chromatography paper strip method for collection, transportation, and storage of rotavirus RNA in stool samples. *J Clin Microbiol* **42:**1605–1608.
118. **Wilson ML.** 1996. General principles of specimen collection and transport. *Clin Infect Dis* **22:**766–777.
119. **Mills AM, Guo FP, Copland AP, Pai RK, Pinsky BA.** 2013. A comparison of CMV detection in gastrointestinal mucosal biopsies using immunohistochemistry and PCR performed on formalin-fixed, paraffin-embedded tissue. *Am J Surg Pathol* **37:**995–1000.
120. **Folkins AK, Chisholm KM, Guo FP, McDowell M, Aziz N, Pinsky BA.** 2013. Diagnosis of congenital CMV using PCR performed on formalin-fixed, paraffin-embedded placental tissue. *Am J Surg Pathol* **37:**1413–1420.
121. **Reagan-Steiner S, Simeone R, Simon E, Bhatnagar J, Oduyebo T, Free R, Denison AM, Rabeneck DB, Ellington S, Petersen E, Gary J, Hale G, Keating MK, Martines RB, Muehlenbachs A, Ritter J, Lee E, Davidson A, Conners E, Scotland S, Sandhu K, Bingham A, Kassens E, Smith L, St George K, Ahmad N, Tanner M, Beavers S, Miers B, VanMaldeghem K, Khan S, Rabe I, Gould C, Meaney-Delman D, Honein MA, Shieh WJ, Jamieson DJ, Fischer M, Zaki SR, U.S. Zika Pregnancy Registry Collaboration, Zika Virus Response Epidemiology and Surveillance Task Force Pathology Team.** 2017. Evaluation of placental and fetal tissue specimens for Zika virus infection–50 states and District of Columbia, January-December, 2016. *MMWR Morb Mortal Wkly Rep* **66:**636–643.
122. **Behzadbehbahani A, Klapper PE, Vallely PJ, Cleator GM.** 1997. Detection of BK virus in urine by polymerase chain reaction: a comparison of DNA extraction methods. *J Virol Methods* **67:**161–166.
123. **Khan G, Kangro HO, Coates PJ, Heath RB.** 1991. Inhibitory effects of urine on the polymerase chain reaction for cytomegalovirus DNA. *J Clin Pathol* **44:**360–365.
124. **Tang YW, Sefers SE, Li H, Kohn DJ, Procop GW.** 2005. Comparative evaluation of three commercial systems for nucleic acid extraction from urine specimens. *J Clin Microbiol* **43:**4830–4833.
125. **Forman M, Valsamakis A, Arav-Boger R.** 2012. Dried urine spots for detection and quantification of cytomegalovirus in newborns. *Diagn Microbiol Infect Dis* **73:**326–329.
126. **Koyano S, Inoue N, Oka A, Moriuchi H, Asano K, Ito Y, Yamada H, Yoshikawa T, Suzutani T, Japanese Congenital Cytomegalovirus Study Group.** 2011. Screening for congenital cytomegalovirus infection using newborn urine samples collected on filter paper: feasibility and outcomes from a multicentre study. *BMJ Open* **1:**e000118.
127. **Nozawa N, Koyano S, Yamamoto Y, Inami Y, Kurane I, Inoue N.** 2007. Real-time PCR assay using specimens on filter disks as a template for detection of cytomegalovirus in urine. *J Clin Microbiol* **45:**1305–1307.
128. **International Air Transport Association.** 2017. Dangerous Goods Regulations. International Air Transport Association, Montreal, Canada.

Reagents, Stains, Media, and Cell Cultures: Virology

GERALD A. CAPRARO AND CHRISTINE C. GINOCCHIO

82

INTRODUCTION

In 1913, vaccinia virus was first propagated in cell culture for the purpose of vaccine production (1). However, the potential role of cell culture for clinical diagnostics was not highlighted until 1949, when Enders et al. (2) first described the use of cultivated mammalian cells and the observation of cytopathic effect (CPE) for the detection of polioviruses. Today, living cells are used to support the growth of a number of cell-dependent organisms, including viruses and certain bacteria, such as *Chlamydia* spp. and, more rarely, *Mycoplasma* spp. In addition, cultured cells can be used to demonstrate the effects of bacterial toxins excreted from pathogens such as *Shigella* spp., toxigenic *Escherichia coli*, including O157:H7, and toxigenic *Clostridioides difficile* (formerly *Clostridium difficile*), among others. Traditional tube cell culture and rapid cell culture methods (e.g., shell vial) are dependent on the interactions of viruses with a variety of animal, human, and/or insect cells and are utilized in the laboratory setting as substrates for growth, identification, and enumeration of pathogenic viruses (3, 4).

In the era of molecular detection and quantification of viral pathogens, the applicability of viral isolation has been questioned. For many viruses, it is well documented that molecular detection methods are preferred (i) for their greater sensitivity, (ii) for their potential for faster detection and reporting (hours versus overnight or days to weeks), (iii) for their ability to quantify more accurately the amount of virus present in the sample, and (iv) in instances where viral culture may place the laboratory and surrounding environment at risk due to the highly pathogenic nature of the virus (e.g., variola virus, Ebola virus, and avian influenza virus). However, cell culture methods have useful applications (i) when the potential viral agent is not known, (ii) when the cost of other methods of testing is significantly greater than that of cell culture, (iii) for documentation of active infection, (iv) to perform antiviral susceptibility testing, (v) to assess response to antiviral treatment by the detection of viable virus, (vi) for serologic strain typing, (vii) for vaccine and therapeutic clinical trials, and (viii) for laboratories that do not have the ability to perform molecular detection methods. Some molecular assays, for practical reporting purposes, may take as long as overnight cell culture and may not lend themselves to single-specimen testing as well as cell culture does. For these reasons, cell cultures are still an indispensable research and clinical laboratory tool, particularly when combined with the use of highly specific monoclonal antibodies (MAbs) for the detection of common viruses and *Chlamydia* spp. or when cell lines are engineered to produce virus-induced enzymes (5), such as β-galactosidase for the detection of herpes simplex viruses (HSV) (6).

This chapter describes the cell lines, reagents, stains, and media used in association with traditional tube and rapid viral culture techniques. Included are examples of both well-characterized and emerging infectious viral agents that may be encountered in working with viral culture. Sample collection, specimen processing, and culture requirements for individual or classes of viruses are discussed in the appropriate chapters. The reader is referred to a comprehensive review of cell culture (7) and reference document M41-A from the Clinical and Laboratory Standards Institute (Wayne, PA), which provides guidance for viral culture methods, including the applicable biosafety measures required (8). A list of virology services offered by the Centers for Disease Control and Prevention, as well as a downloadable test directory, can be found on the CDC website (https://www.cdc.gov/laboratory/specimen-submission/list.html). The appendix at the end of this chapter lists the manufacturers and suppliers of cell lines, media, and reagents referred to throughout the chapter.

REAGENTS

■ Balanced salt solutions (Hanks' and Earle's)

Hanks' balanced salt solution and Earle's balanced salt solution (EBSS) are the two most commonly used formulations. However, Hanks' balanced salt solution has a better buffering capacity with CO_2, and EBSS has a better buffering capacity with ambient air.

■ Density gradient media

Density gradient media or cell preparation tubes (BD, Franklin Lakes, NJ) are used for the isolation of peripheral blood mononuclear and polymorphonuclear lymphocytes. Separated cells can be used for the direct detection of viruses, such as cytomegalovirus (CMV), using immunostaining methods. Detailed descriptions of the specific uses of the gradient media or tubes and commercial sources are listed in chapter 79.

■ Dulbecco's PBS

Dulbecco's phosphate-buffered saline (PBS) is a maintenance-type medium containing sodium pyruvate and glucose.

■ HEPES

HEPES is a zwitterionic organic chemical buffering agent that maintains physiological pH despite changes in carbon dioxide concentration, in contrast to bicarbonate buffers. HEPES is widely used in culture media.

■ Formalin for cell culture preservation

Formalin can be used to preserve viral CPE in cell culture for both educational and research purposes.

Earle's minimal essential medium .... 81 ml
Formaldehyde (37 to 40% concentration) .... 30 ml

CPE-positive culture tubes should be filled with the solution, sealed, and stored at room temperature.

■ Saline

Normal or physiological saline (0.85%) is commonly used as a diluent.

■ Gentamicin-amphotericin B solution (10×)

Several different combinations of antibiotics and amphotericin B are added to transport media, particularly for pretreatment of specimens such as stool prior to culture inoculation, or are used in refeed medium to reduce both bacterial and fungal contamination. Commercial media containing the appropriate strength of antibiotics and amphotericin B can be purchased. Alternatively, a 10× gentamicin-amphotericin B solution can be added by the laboratory at a ratio of 1:10 (0.1 ml of 10× gentamicin-amphotericin B to every 1.0 ml of specimen). Notably, the effectiveness of antibiotics intended to limit bacterial or fungal contamination of viral culture media may be impacted by the level of antimicrobial resistance patterns for a given community. Laboratories may observe an increase in viral culture contamination, as bacteria and yeast present in patient specimens become resistant. Nonetheless, good quality control (QC) measures necessitate the addition of antimicrobials in transport media. Following receipt by the laboratory of the transport medium containing a specimen, centrifugation may be helpful to reduce cellular artifact overlays or bacterial or fungal contaminants; however, this is not always required. The specimen supernatant is inoculated onto the appropriate cell line(s).

Eagle's minimal essential medium (EMEM) .... 89 ml
Gentamicin (50 mg/ml) .... 1 ml
Amphotericin B (250 μg/ml) .... 10 ml

All ingredients should be combined, and the solution should be stored frozen at −20 to −70°C in working-size aliquots.

■ Trypsin solutions

In lieu of scraping cells from tubes or wells, trypsin solutions are used to disburse cells from the monolayer for repassage and for immunostaining of cell-associated viruses such as adenovirus, CMV, and varicella-zoster virus (VZV). Trypsin solutions made with 2.5% PBS or EDTA solution are commercially available.

■ Tween 20–PBS

Tween 20–PBS, typically used at a working concentration of 0.02% and pH of 7.4, may be used to wash cell monolayers prior to staining with fluorescent MAbs but is not always required. The manufacturers' directions should be followed for specific staining protocols if a commercially available product is used. Tween 20–PBS is stored at room temperature and should be discarded if the solution is turbid or a precipitate develops.

VIROLOGY STAINS

Direct examination of clinical specimens using several methods, such as slide touch preps from unfixed tissue from an excision or biopsy, cytologic examination of tissue scrapings (e.g., Tzanck assay for HSV), smears from mucous membrane scrapings (e.g., HSV or VZV), or sample concentration by cytospin or centrifugation (e.g., respiratory viruses), can provide relatively rapid results. Slides can be prepared at the bedside (e.g., skin scrapings for HSV or VZV) or in the laboratory (e.g., respiratory swabs in transport media) and fixed with 80 to 100% reagent-grade acetone, 95% alcohol, or a cytological fixative, depending on the method.

Traditional staining with hematoxylin and eosin and Wright-Giemsa stains can demonstrate characteristic cell morphologies such as the "owl's eye" nuclear inclusions indicative of CMV or the "smudge cells" that contain large basophilic inclusions consistent with adenovirus. Today, the definitive identification of certain viruses or *Chlamydia* spp. directly in clinical samples is mainly done with MAbs labeled with fluorescein isothiocyanate (FITC), methylrhodamine isothiocyanate, or phycoerythrin with an Evans blue and/or propidium iodide counterstain. Results are available within 15 to 60 min. Additionally, direct fluorescent-antibody (DFA) or indirect fluorescent-antibody (IFA) testing is used for confirmation of viruses isolated in cell culture and for blind staining in centrifugation-enhanced virus isolation methods (discussed below). Minimal equipment (incubator, fluorescent microscope, pipettes, and centrifuge) and moderate technical expertise are required to perform the procedures and interpret the results (reviewed in reference 7).

Commercial reagents, commonly provided at working strength and quality tested to ensure sensitive and specific reactions, cleared by the Food and Drug Administration for *in vitro* diagnostic testing are listed in Table 1. Reagents may be cleared for use with direct specimen testing or for culture confirmation, and in some instances for both applications. Various formats of MAb reagents are available for immunofluorescence testing methods that (i) detect *Chlamydia* spp. (Fig. 1) but do not differentiate, (ii) target a single virus (Fig. 2), (iii) detect and differentiate two or more viruses (Fig. 3), (iv) target a single virus and contain a pool of MAbs that detect multiple additional viruses but do not differentiate (Fig. 4), and (v) detect a family of viruses or multiple viruses using a pool of MAbs but do not differentiate (Fig. 5). Both the location of the fluorescent staining (e.g., cytoplasmic versus nuclear) and the staining pattern (e.g., speckled versus homogeneous) can aid in virus differentiation (Fig. 3).

CELL CULTURES

Good manufacturing practices-regulated commercial vendors (see the appendix) provide tissue culture cells that are sterile, stabilized at the proper pH, thoroughly tested for susceptibility to common pathogens, and carefully screened to be free of potentially harmful endogenous agents, such as foamy viruses and mycoplasmas, that will interfere with the detection of the intended pathogens. Monolayered, ready-to-use cells can be produced at the vendor facility within a day or two of the order, allowing the laboratory flexibility in the quantity and delivery date. Culture cells are provided in a number of ready-to-use formats, including traditional 16- by 125-mm glass round-bottom screw-cap tubes, 1-dram vials (shell vials), flasks, or cluster trays. Ready-to-use cell cultures have a shelf life that is defined by the manufacturer in days or weeks, depending on the cell line or intended pathogen to

TABLE 1 Commercially available DFA and IFA reagents for the detection of chlamydiae and viruses[a]

Target[b]	Use as per manufacturer	Manufacturer and test name
Chlamydia spp.	CC	Trinity Biotech; Bartels *Chlamydia* CC FA kit (not available in the U.S.)
C. trachomatis	CC	Trinity Biotech; MicroTrak *C. trachomatis* culture confirmation
C. trachomatis	DSD	Trinity Biotech; MicroTrak *C. trachomatis* direct specimen kit
Chlamydia spp.	CC	Bio-Rad; Pathfinder *Chlamydia* culture confirmation system
C. trachomatis	DSD	Bio-Rad; Pathfinder *C. trachomatis* DFA kit
Chlamydia spp.	CC	Quidel; D³ DFA *Chlamydia* culture confirmation kit
Chlamydia spp.	CC	Meridian; Merifluor Chlamydia
C. trachomatis	DSD	Remel PathoDX *C. trachomatis* DFA kit
Chlamydia spp.	CC	Remel PathoDX *Chlamydia* culture confirmation kit
CMV	DSD	Millipore; Light Diagnostics CMV pp65 antigenemia IFA kit (RUO)
CMV	CC	Millipore; Light Diagnostics CMV DFA kit
CMV	CC	Millipore; Light Diagnostics CMV IFA kit
CMV	CC	Quidel; D³ DFA CMV immediate early antigen ID kit
CMV	DSD and CC	Trinity Biotech; Bartels CMV fluorescent monoclonal antibody test
CMV	CC	Trinity Biotech; Bartels CMV immediate early antigen (IEA) indirect fluorescent antibody test
Enterovirus	CC	Millipore; Light Diagnostics pan-enterovirus IFA
Enterovirus groups	CC	Millipore; Light Diagnostics enterovirus screening set IFA
Enterovirus	CC	Quidel; D³ IFA enterovirus ID kit
Enterovirus	CC	Remel; Imagen Enterovirus
HSV-1/2 detection	DSD and CC	Millipore; Light Diagnostics SimulFluor HSV 1/2 kit
HSV-1/2 and VZV	DSD and CC	Millipore; Light Diagnostics SimulFluor HSV/VZV kit
HSV species	CC	Quidel; D³ HSV ID
HSV-1/2 typing	CC	Quidel; D³ HSV ID and typing kit
HSV-1/2 typing	CC	Quidel; ELVIS HSV ID and typing
HSV-1/2 detection and typing	CC	Remel; Imagen Herpes Simplex Virus
HSV detection	CC	Trinity Biotech; Bartels HSV fluorescent monoclonal antibody test
HSV-1/2 detection and typing	CC	Trinity Biotech; Bartels HSV type-specific fluorescent antibody test typing kit
HSV-1/2 detection and typing	CC	Trinity Biotech; MicroTrak HSV1/HSV2 culture ID/typing test
HSV-1/2 detection and typing	DSD	Trinity Biotech; MicroTrak HSV1/HSV2 direct specimen ID/typing
VZV	DSD and CC	Meridian; Merifluor VZV
VZV	DSD and CC	Millipore; Light Diagnostics VZV DFA kit
VZV	CC	Quidel; D³ VZV ID kit
Respiratory panel B	DSD and CC	Trinity Biotech; Bartels viral respiratory screening and ID kit
RSV	DSD and CC	Trinity Biotech; Bartels RSV direct fluorescent antibody test
Respiratory panel B	CC	Millipore; Light Diagnostics SimulFluor respiratory screen
Respiratory panel B	CC	Millipore; Light Diagnostics respiratory viral screen and ID DFA kit
Respiratory panel B	CC	Millipore; Light Diagnostics Respiratory Panel I viral screening and ID IFA kit
Influenza viruses A and B	DSD and CC	Millipore; Light Diagnostics SimulFluor Flu A/Flu B IFA
Parainfluenza viruses 1, 2/3	CC	Millipore; Light Diagnostics SimulFluor Para 1, 2, and 3
Parainfluenza viruses 1, 2, 3, adenovirus (dual)	CC	Millipore; Light Diagnostics SimulFluor Para 1, 2, 3/Adeno
RSV/influenza virus A (dual)	CC	Millipore; Light Diagnostics SimulFluor RSV/Flu A
RSV/parainfluenza virus 3 (dual)	CC	Millipore; Light Diagnostics SimulFluor RSV/Para 3
Respiratory panel A/identification	DSD and CC	Quidel; D³ FastPoint L-DFA respiratory virus ID kit
Influenza viruses A and B	DSD and CC	Quidel; D³ FastPoint L-DFA Influenza A/B ID kit
RSV and HMPV	DSD and CC	Quidel; D³ FastPoint L-DFA RSV/MPV ID kit
Respiratory panel B/identification	DSD and CC	Quidel; D³ Ultra screening and ID kit
Respiratory panel C (dual)	DSD and CC	Quidel; D³ Duet Influenza A/Respiratory screening and ID kit
Respiratory panel D (dual)	DSD and CC	Quidel; D³ Duet RSV/respiratory screening and ID kit
HMPV	DSD and CC	Quidel; D³ MPV ID kit
Respiratory panel B pool	DSD and CC	Remel; Imagen Respiratory Screen
Influenza viruses A and B	DSD and CC	Remel; Imagen Influenza A & B
Parainfluenza virus group	DSD and CC	Remel; Imagen Parainfluenza Group
Parainfluenza virus typing	DSD and CC	Remel; Imagen Parainfluenza Typing
RSV	DSD	Remel; Imagen RSV

[a]Refer to manufacturers' websites for Food and Drug Administration and *in vitro* diagnostic status of reagents. Although uses for the reagents may be suggested on manufacturers' websites, all suggested applications may not have been validated by the manufacturer. Abbreviations: adeno, adenovirus; CC, culture confirmation; DSD, direct specimen detection; dual, a two-fluorophore stain; FluA, influenza virus A; ID, identification; IF, immunofluorescence; Para, parainfluenza virus.

[b]Respiratory panel A: adenovirus, influenza viruses A and B, parainfluenza viruses 1, 2, and 3, RSV, HMPV; respiratory panel B: adenovirus, influenza viruses A and B, parainfluenza viruses 1, 2, and 3, RSV; respiratory panel C: adenovirus, influenza virus B, parainfluenza viruses 1, 2, and 3, RSV, and differential detection of influenza virus A; respiratory panel D: adenovirus, influenza viruses A and B, parainfluenza viruses 1, 2, and 3, and differential identification of RSV.

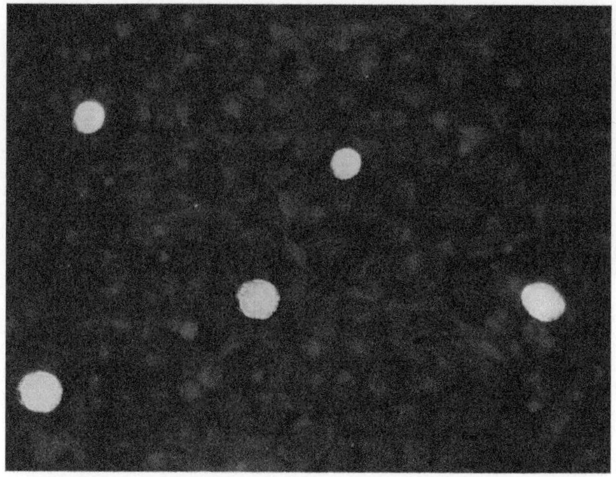

FIGURE 1 Immunofluorescence detection of *C. trachomatis* in McCoy cells. Magnification, ×200. (Courtesy of Quidel.)

be recovered. Some cells are also supplied frozen in shell vials and may be stored for months or years at −70°C or below, ready to use with a simple thaw step and change of medium. Other frozen cells are supplied in cryovials and other containers at a stated density and require the laboratory to subculture them to obtain monolayers in a flask, multiwell plate, shell vial, or tube, depending on the end application (9). Frozen cells can be used as needed and for unexpected situations such as unanticipated increases in the volume of samples, sudden viral outbreaks, or delays in cell shipments.

For laboratories that require special cells not readily available from commercial sources, specific cell types can sometimes be obtained from research laboratories or the American Type Culture Collection (Manassas, VA) and then propagated within the user laboratory. Once the cells are received, the laboratory must confirm sterility, the absence of mycoplasmas and other contaminants, and the appropriate passage or cell duplication number necessary to ensure sensitivity for viral or chlamydial isolation. Cell cultures must be maintained in an environment that allows appropriate cellular replication and proper utility for the tests desired (10). A number of references offer detailed procedures for growing cells from frozen or fresh flasks (4, 8); such procedures are not addressed in this chapter.

To ensure the safety of the technical staff and to prevent cell culture contamination, the laboratory must follow strict procedures for the handling of biohazardous materials throughout the testing process (8, 10). These include (i) the use of class II or higher biological safety cabinets with HEPA filters and, if possible, external venting, certified at least annually; (ii) facilities and procedures that are appropriate to the biohazard level of the viruses tested, as defined by the Centers for Disease Control and Prevention (Atlanta, GA) (11); and (iii) training and annual competency assessment of the laboratory staff. Virology benches and safety cabinets should be disinfected at least daily with a high-level disinfectant, such as 10% sodium hypochlorite (bleach).

■ Traditional cell culture

The common culturable human viral pathogens causing significant infections are readily detected by using a variety of cell types, including the established cell lines listed in Table 2. Cell lines may be primary (e.g., rhesus monkey kidney and rabbit kidney), used for one or two passages; diploid (e.g., human embryonic lung), used for 20 to 50 passages; or heteroploid (e.g., human epidermoid lung carcinoma), which can be passaged indefinitely. The laboratory must maintain sufficient cell types and incubate cell cultures for an optimal length of time and under the appropriate conditions that permit the recovery of the potential range of detectable viruses for all specimen types processed by the laboratory (8, 10, 12). Cell culture systems can be variable and are susceptible to conditions that can adversely affect results, including cell culture source and lineage, age, and condition of the monolayer, number of passages, shipping conditions, and the presence of contaminating agents. For example, in 2012, cultures of rhesus monkey kidney cells distributed to clinical laboratories throughout the United States were found to be contaminated with *Coccidioides immitis* that was endogenous to the harvested monkey kidney (13, 14). As a result of rapid communication of this information and adherence to laboratory safety procedures, there were no adverse effects in terms of personnel infection with this highly infectious fungus (13). Therefore, QC procedures and specific testing guidelines must be followed (8, 10, 15). Shipments of cell culture material

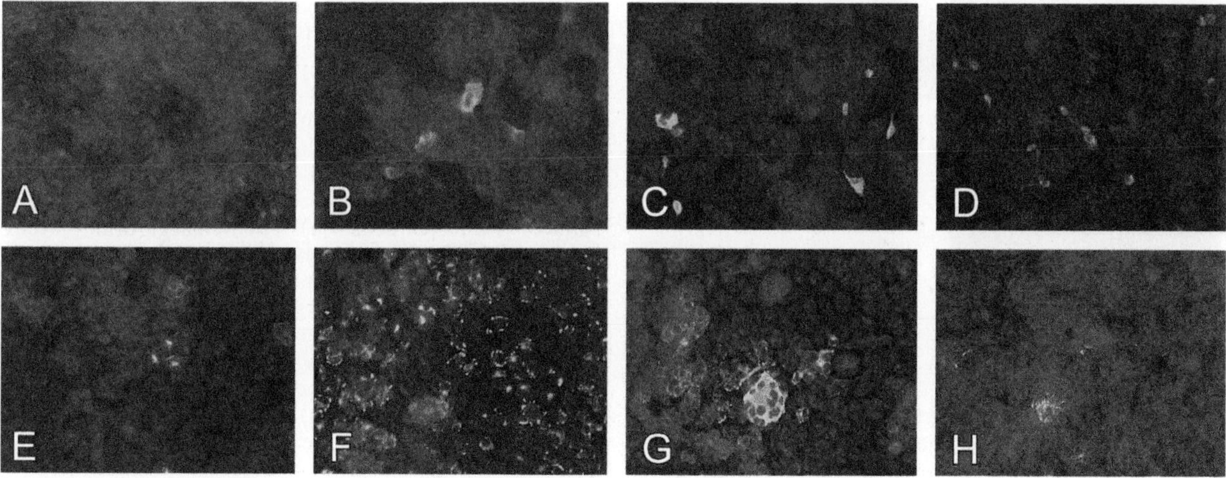

FIGURE 2 Immunofluorescence detection of respiratory pathogens in R-Mix cells using D3 Ultra Kit reagents (Quidel). (A) Uninoculated R-Mix cells; (B) adenovirus; (C) influenza virus A; (D) influenza virus B; (E) parainfluenza virus type 1; (F) parainfluenza virus type 2; (G): parainfluenza virus type 3; (H) RSV. Magnification, ×170. (Courtesy of Quidel.)

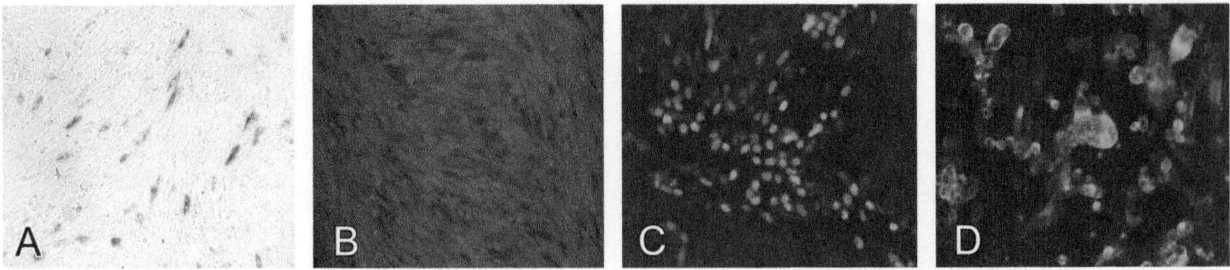

FIGURE 3 Detection of HSV-1 and HSV-2 in ELVIS cells (Quidel). (A) Blue cells positive for HSV with X-Gal stain; (B) immunofluorescence of uninoculated ELVIS cells; (C) HSV-1-positive ELVIS immunofluorescence (note nuclear pattern); (D) HSV-2-positive ELVIS immunofluorescence (note cytoplasmic pattern). Magnification, ×170. (Courtesy of Quidel.)

should be observed microscopically to confirm that the confluency of the monolayer is appropriate (75 to 90%), that the cells are attached to the substratum, that cell appearance is typical, and that no evidence of contaminating viruses, bacteria, or fungi is present, usually signified by cytopathic appearance of the cells before use or turbidity of the cell medium. Cell culture media that will be added to newly shipped cells should also be free of contamination (clear) and near a neutral pH (salmon pink). If the laboratory introduces additives (e.g., L-glutamine or antibiotics) to commercial media, the final solution must be checked for sterility, pH, growth promotion, and the absence of toxicity to cells. The lot number and date of use for all media, buffers, reagents, and additives should also be recorded.

Tubes of cell cultures should be stored in a slanted position with the cell monolayer covered by the medium. Tissue culture cells should ideally be inoculated within 7 days of receipt (8 to 10 days of seeding) for optimal propagation of cell-dependent organisms or demonstration of cytotoxicity. The laboratory should retain all documentation provided by the manufacturer, including cell culture records with cell types, source, passage number, and age of cells. Uninoculated lot-matched tubes, cluster plates, or shell vials that are incubated, maintained, and observed in the same manner as inoculated tissue cells serve as negative controls for CPE, toxicity, exogenous contamination, and procedures such as DFA testing, hemadsorption (HAD), and hemagglutination. Daily inoculation of positive controls to monitor traditional tube culture performance is not routinely performed. However, commonly isolated viruses may be used to perform QC on cell lines when new shipments are received in the laboratory, and they are a source of positive-control material for detection and confirmation methods such as HAD and DFA testing.

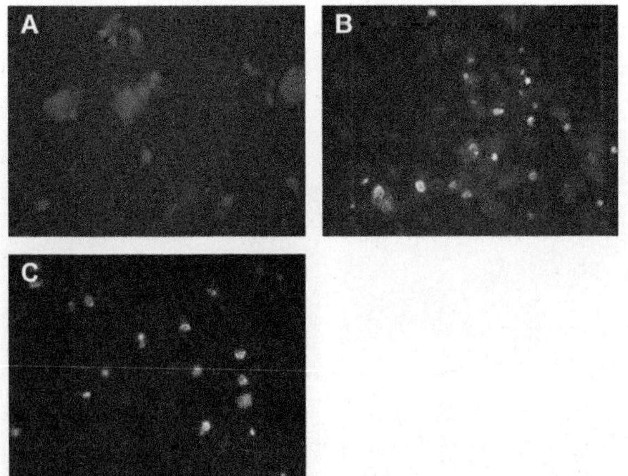

FIGURE 4 Immunofluorescence detection of respiratory pathogens from clinical specimens using Duet stains (Quidel). (A and B) Influenza virus A Duet stain (influenza virus A [gold] and respiratory pool [green] for adenovirus, influenza virus B, parainfluenza virus types 1, 2, and 3, and RSV) on negative cells (A) and influenza virus A-positive cells (B). (C) RSV Duet stain (RSV [gold] and respiratory pool [green] for adenovirus, influenza virus A, influenza virus B, and parainfluenza viruses 1, 2, and 3) on RSV-positive and influenza virus A-positive cells. Magnification, ×170. (Courtesy of Quidel.)

With the exception of a few slower-growing viruses such as CMV, or when viruses are present at very low titers, the time to detection by traditional tube culture methods is generally between 1 and 7 days of inoculation (4). The standard approach for detecting viral proliferation is the microscopic examination of the unstained cell culture monolayer for the presence of CPE. The presence of a virus is indicated by degenerative changes in monolayer cells, including shrinking, swelling, rounding of cells, clustering, and the formation of syncytia, or by complete destruction of the monolayer. Identification of the virus is then based on the CPE characteristics, the cell line involved, the time to detection, specimen type, and confirmation, generally by staining with virus-specific MAbs. Alternatively, for the identification of viruses for which MAbs may not be available, molecular methods or ancillary traditional testing (e.g., acid resistance for rhinoviruses) must be performed. In addition, for certain viruses (influenza, parainfluenza, and mumps viruses) that do not always demonstrate CPE, HAD testing may be done (16).

■ HAD test

HAD refers to the attachment of red blood cells to infected cell culture monolayers. Influenza viruses A and B, parainfluenza viruses 1, 2, 3, and 4, and mumps viruses possess a surface hemagglutinin protein that is expressed on the surfaces of infected cells (16). The hemagglutinin protein binds red blood cells and adsorbs them to the infected-cell membrane. HAD may be performed when there is no visual CPE in culture or as a rapid screen for the presence of an orthomyxovirus or a paramyxovirus in cell culture with a suspicious CPE. HAD testing is usually performed at 3 to 7 days of incubation or at the end of the incubation period (generally 10 to 14 days). A typical HAD procedure involves incubation of guinea pig erythrocytes with viral culture monolayers at 4°C. Microscopic examination of the culture after 30 minutes allows the operator to evaluate for the presence of HAD on the monolayer or hemagglutination in the supernatant. HAD-positive cultures can be further analyzed using MAbs to determine the identity

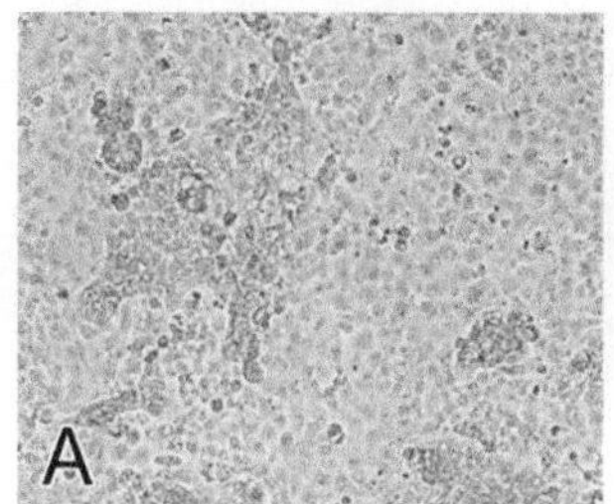

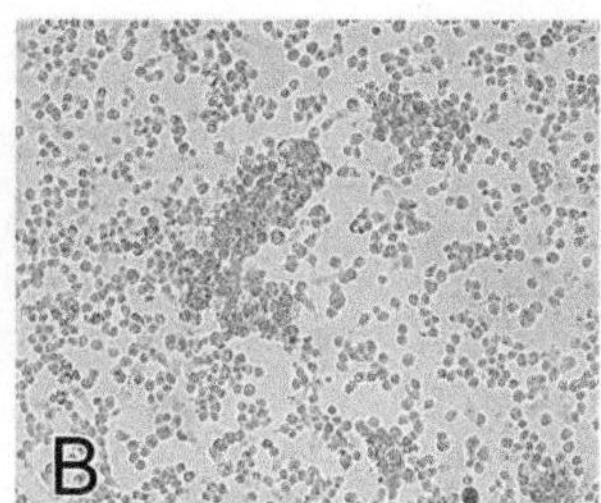

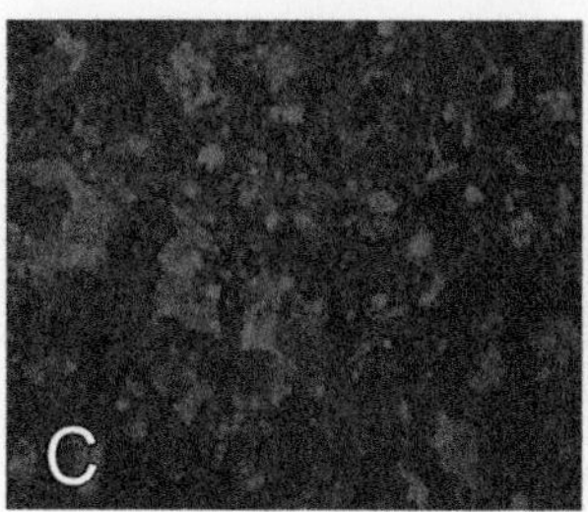

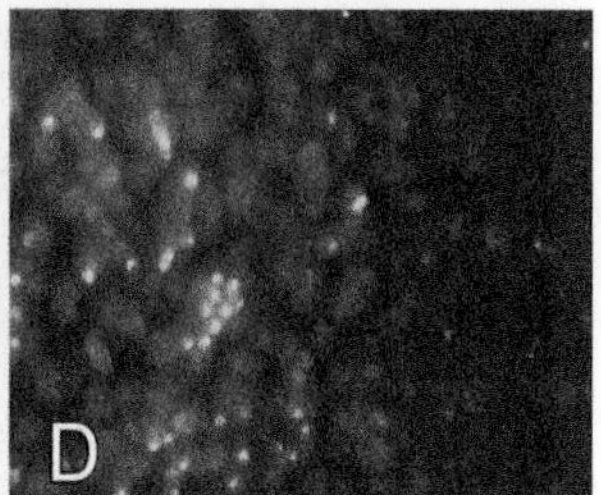

FIGURE 5 Detection of coxsackie B virus in Super E-Mix cells (Quidel). (A) Unstained, uninoculated cells; (B) unstained coxsackie B virus CPE; (C and D) immunofluorescence staining with a pan-enterovirus antibody pool of uninoculated Super E-Mix cells (C) and coxsackie B virus-infected cells (D). Magnification, ×170. (Courtesy of Quidel.)

of the infecting virus. HAD-negative cultures can be reincubated after removal of the erythrocytes and the addition of fresh culture medium. QC using positive and negative control tubes is essential, as variations in HAD testing may occur from laboratory to laboratory and may also occur based on the circulating predominant influenza virus strain (17). Direct MAb staining of the cell monolayer for infectious agents such as influenza and parainfluenza viruses has largely replaced HAD procedures in most clinical laboratories, because staining tends to be more specific and provides more rapid results, which can be critical to patient care.

■ Centrifugation-enhanced rapid cell culture

Centrifugation-enhanced inoculation using cells grown on coverslips in 1-dram shell vials and pre-CPE detection of viral antigen in the monolayer cells by use of MAbs were first described for the detection of *Chlamydia trachomatis* (18). This technique was adapted for the routine detection of CMV using MRC-5 shell vials and staining with MAbs directed against early CMV proteins (19). This pioneering method has reduced the time for virus detection from as long as 10 to 30 days to 16 to 72 h. The important factor in reducing the time to detection is the stressing of the monolayer during centrifugation (20). This process has been shown to increase cell proliferation, decrease cell generation times, alter cell metabolism, increase cell longevity, and activate specific genes.

Rapid cell culture is now commonly used for the detection of *Chlamydia* spp., CMV, enteroviruses, VZV, HSV, mumps viruses, and the main respiratory viruses (adenovirus, human metapneumovirus [HMPV], influenza A and B viruses, parainfluenza viruses 1, 2, and 3, and respiratory syncytial virus [RSV]) (reviewed in reference 7). Centrifugation-enhanced rapid cell culture can be used with standard cell lines (Table 2; Fig. 1) and has been adapted for use with cocultivated cells (Table 3) for the detection of respiratory viruses (R-Mix and R-Mix Too; Quidel Corporation, Athens, OH) (Fig. 2), for the detection of HSV and VZV (H&V-Mix; Quidel) (Fig. 6) (21–23), and with genetically engineered cells such as ELVIS (enzyme-linked virus-inducible system; Quidel) (Table 3) for the detection of HSV (Fig. 3) (24, 25) and Super E-Mix (Quidel) for the detection of enteroviruses (Fig. 5). Identification of the viral pathogen when centrifugation-enhanced rapid cell culture is used is not dependent on the visualization of CPE, allowing technologists not skilled in CPE recognition to perform viral testing. Instead, the virus is detected either by "blind staining" or staining "pre-CPE" with phycoerythrin-, peroxidase-, or FITC-labeled virus-specific MAbs or a combination of phycoerythrin- and FITC-labeled antibodies or by virus-specific induction of enzymes that are detected by the ELVIS HSV system using substrates such as β-galactosidase (6, 24, 25). A significant benefit of using cocultivated cells such as R-Mix, R-Mix Too, H&V-Mix, and Super E-Mix is that they allow the identification of multiple viruses from a single shell vial or cluster tray well, rather than having to use multiple shell vials to cover the range of viruses that the laboratory may wish to detect in a particular sample type. One shell vial can be substituted for up to four different tube cell cultures that require much longer incubation times (10 to 14 days) to identify fewer subspecies of the group.

Since rapid-detection formats are not based on the detection of CPE but use blind staining for either single viruses or multiple viruses, positive- and negative-control slides are required for each day of patient testing. When a single-culture system detects multiple viruses, the detection reagents must be validated for all targets (including any pooled MAb reagents) upon receipt in the laboratory (10, 12). Virus isolate controls can be tested daily and virus types rotated so that during the course of 1 week, the lots of cells and reagents have been tested against all the routinely isolated viruses.

■ ELVIS

ELVIS uses a genetically engineered cell line (BHKICP6LacZ) that was first described by Stabell and Olivo (6). The promoter sequence of the HSV UL97 gene and the *E. coli lacZ* gene were used to stably transform a baby hamster kidney cell line. When the cell line is infected with HSV, the virion-associated transactivator protein VP16 and other transactivating factors such as ICP0 strongly transactivate the UL97 promoter, which in turn activates the *lacZ* gene, resulting in high levels of β-galactosidase activity. Addition of 4-chloro-3-indol-β-D-galactopyranoside (X-Gal) turns a colorless substrate to blue, indicating the presence of HSV-infected cells (Fig. 3A). If HSV typing is required, a fluorescence-labeled MAb that specifically detects HSV-2 (Fig. 3D) and an unlabeled MAb that specifically binds to HSV-1 are incorporated in the staining procedure. If the infected (blue) cells are not detected with the HSV-2 MAb, then the monolayers are stained with anti-mouse immunoglobulin fluorescence-labeled antibody to detect the HSV-1 MAb (Fig. 3C). The ELVIS test is completed within 16 to 24 h for both positive and negative results (24, 25).

■ Cytotoxicity assays

Tissue culture assays using cell types such as human foreskin fibroblasts, MRC-5 cells, and Vero epithelioid cells are commonly used for the detection of toxin-producing strains of *C. difficile* (26–28). Cell culture testing for the presence of *C. difficile* cytotoxin has demonstrated improved sensitivity compared to *C. difficile* toxin A/B enzyme immunoassays. Enteroviruses can cause CPE similar to that caused by *C. difficile* toxin; therefore, the procedure includes the use of a specific antitoxin to *C. difficile* toxin, which creates

TABLE 2 List of cell lines and virus susceptibility profiles

Cell line	Origin	Virus(es)[a]
A-549	Human lung carcinoma	Adenovirus, HSV, influenza virus, HMPV, measles virus, mumps virus, parainfluenza virus, poliovirus, RSV, rotavirus, VZV
AGMK[b]	African green monkey kidney	Enteroviruses, influenza virus, parainfluenza virus
AP61	Mosquito	Arboviruses
B95 or B95a	Epstein-Barr virus-transformed lymphoblastoid	Measles virus, mumps virus
BGMK	Buffalo green monkey kidney	*Chlamydia* spp., coxsackie B virus, HSV, poliovirus
C6/36	Mosquito	Arboviruses
Caco-2	Human epithelial colorectal adenocarcinoma	Astrovirus, HCoV (NL63)
CV-1	African green monkey kidney	Encephalitis viruses (some), HSV, measles virus, mumps virus, rotavirus, SV40, VZV
Graham 293	Human embryonic kidney transformed with adenovirus type 5	Enteric adenoviruses
H292		Adenovirus, coxsackie B virus, echovirus, HSV, mumps virus, parainfluenza virus, poliovirus, RSV, rubella virus
HeLa	Human cervix adenocarcinoma	Adenovirus, CMV, coxsackie B virus, echovirus, HSV, poliovirus, rhinovirus, vesicular stomatitis virus (Indiana strain), VZV
HeLa 229	Human cervix adenocarcinoma	Adenovirus, *Chlamydia* spp., CMV, echovirus, HSV, poliovirus, rhinovirus, vesicular stomatitis virus (Indiana strain), VZV
HEL	Human embryonic lung	Adenovirus, CMV, echovirus, HSV, poliovirus, rhinovirus, vesicular stomatitis virus (Indiana strain), VZV
HEK	Human embryonic kidney	Adenovirus, BK virus, enterovirus, HSV, measles virus, mumps virus, rhinovirus
HEK 293	Human embryonic kidney transformed with adenovirus type 5	Enteric adenoviruses
HEp-2	Human epidermoid carcinoma	Adenovirus, *Chlamydia* spp., coxsackie B virus, HSV, measles virus, parainfluenza virus, poliovirus, RSV
HNK	Human neonatal kidney	Adenovirus, HSV, VZV
Hs27 (HFF[c]; MRHF)	Human foreskin fibroblast	Adenovirus, CMV, echovirus, HSV, mumps virus, poliovirus, rhinovirus, VZV
HuH-7	Human hepatocyte	HCoVs (OC43, 229E)
LLC-MK2	Original, rhesus monkey kidney	Arboviruses (some), enteroviruses (including coxsackie A and B viruses, echoviruses, polioviruses), HMPV (NL-63), influenza virus, MERS-CoV, mumps virus, parainfluenza virus, poxvirus groups, rhinovirus
Mv1Lu	Mink lung	CMV, HSV, influenza virus
McCoy[c]	Mouse fibroblast	*Chlamydia* spp., HSV
MDCK	Madin-Darby canine kidney	Adenovirus (some types), coxsackievirus, influenza virus, reovirus
MNA	Mouse neuroblastoma	Rabies virus
MRC-5	Human fetal lung	Adenovirus, CMV, coxsackie A virus, echovirus, HSV, influenza virus, mumps virus, poliovirus, rhinovirus, RSV, VZV, cytotoxicity for *C. difficile*
NCI-H292	Human pulmonary mucoepidermoid	Adenovirus, BK polyomavirus, enteroviruses (most), HSV, measles virus, reoviruses, rhinoviruses (most), RSV, vaccinia virus
RD	Human rhabdomyosarcoma	Adenovirus, coxsackie A virus, echovirus, HSV, poliovirus
RK[b]	Rabbit kidney	HSV, paramyxoviruses
RhMK[b]	Rhesus monkey kidney	Arboviruses, coxsackie A and B viruses, echoviruses, influenza virus, parainfluenza virus, measles virus, mumps virus, polioviruses
SF	Human foreskin	Adenovirus, CMV, coxsackie A virus, echovirus, HSV, poliovirus, VZV
Vero	African green monkey kidney	Adenovirus, arboviruses (some), *Chlamydia* spp., coxsackie B virus, HMPV, HSV, measles virus, MERS-CoV, mumps virus, poliovirus type 3, rotavirus, rubella virus
Vero E6	African green monkey kidney	Adenovirus, coxsackie B virus, HSV, measles virus, mumps virus, poliovirus type 3, rotavirus, rubella virus, SARS-CoV
Vero 76	African green monkey kidney	Adenovirus, coxsackie B virus, HSV, measles virus, mumps virus, poliovirus type 3, rotavirus, rubella virus, West Nile virus
WI-38	Human lung	Adenovirus, CMV, coxsackie A virus, echovirus, HSV, influenza virus, mumps virus, poliovirus, rhinovirus, RSV, VZV

[a]Abbreviations: HCoV, human coronavirus; MERS-CoV, Middle East respiratory syndrome coronavirus; SARS-CoV, severe acute respiratory syndrome coronavirus.
[b]Primary cell cultures.
[c]Available as fresh and frozen ReadyCells (Quidel).

TABLE 3 List of cocultured cell lines and virus susceptibility profiles[a]

Cell mixture[b]	Cell type	Virus(es)
R-Mix[c]	Mv1Lu (mink lung)	CMV, HSV, influenza virus, SARS-CoV
	A549 (human lung carcinoma)	Adenovirus, HSV, influenza virus, HMPV, measles virus, mumps virus, parainfluenza virus, poliovirus, rotavirus, RSV, VZV
R-Mix Too[c]	MDCK (Madin-Darby canine kidney)	Influenza virus
	A549 (human lung carcinoma)	Adenovirus, HSV, influenza virus, HMPV, measles virus, mumps virus, parainfluenza virus, poliovirus, rotavirus, RSV, VZV
H&V-Mix	CV-1 (African green monkey kidney)	Encephalitis viruses (some), HSV, poliovirus type 1, rotavirus, SV40, VZV
	MRC-5 (human fetal lung)	Adenovirus, CMV, echovirus, HSV, influenza virus, mumps virus, poliovirus, rhinovirus, RSV, VZV
Super E-Mix[c]	sBGMK (Buffalo green monkey kidney) (with degradation activating factor)	*Chlamydia* spp., coxsackie A and B viruses, echovirus, HSV, poliovirus
	A549 (human lung carcinoma)	Adenovirus, HSV, influenza virus, HMPV, measles virus, mumps virus, parainfluenza virus, poliovirus, RSV, rotavirus, VZV
ELVIS	Transfected baby hamster kidney HSV UL97 promoter/*E. coli lacZ* gene	HSV-1, HSV-2

[a]SARS-CoV, severe acute respiratory syndrome coronavirus.
[b]Available from Quidel.
[c]Available as both fresh and frozen cells that do not require propagation but are ready to use.

a more specific assay. The inoculum for this assay can be either liquid stool or a broth culture of a pure *C. difficile* colony recovered in culture. In either scenario, the liquid is diluted, bacteria are removed by membrane filtration, and the tissue culture cells are exposed to the patient material, with and without *C. difficile* antitoxin. Test wells without *C. difficile* antitoxin demonstrating CPE within 12 to 48 h are presumed positive for *C. difficile* toxin if the control well with *C. difficile* antitoxin shows no evidence of CPE. As little as 1 pg of toxin can cause a visible change in cells over a period of hours up to 1 to 2 days.

CELL CULTURE MEDIA

Transport Media and Collection Swabs

An important consideration in using cell culture is ensuring collection of cellular material and maintaining the viability of the organisms from the time of sample collection to inoculation in cell culture. Therefore, time to processing, transport temperature, and the use of transport media need to be evaluated for each sample type. Cell culture media with additives, such as antibiotics and fungicidal agents to inhibit microbial growth, are used to maintain the viability of viruses during sample transport. Transport media may be specific for virus isolation (viral transport media) or also allow the isolation of *Chlamydia*, *Mycoplasma*, and *Ureaplasma* (universal transport media). The types of transport media, uses and components, collection procedures, and swabs are detailed in chapter 81.

■ Growth medium with 10% fetal bovine serum

Cell culture media are an important part of the production and maintenance of cells. Cell culture stocks are generally grown in a richer medium than that which is used for the maintenance of the cells. The higher level of serum or protein in growth medium rapidly enhances cell growth and is used for a day or more before it is replaced by maintenance medium. Standard growth medium consists of EMEM with EBSS and supplemented with 10% heat-inactivated fetal bovine serum (FBS), one or more antimicrobials (gentamicin, penicillin, streptomycin, vancomycin, and/or amphotericin B), and HEPES buffer. Since simian viruses are endogenous to primary monkey kidney cell cultures, media that contain simian virus 5 (SV5) and SV40 antisera are available (Quidel).

■ Maintenance medium

Maintenance medium contains nutrients and buffers that protect the cells during the stage when rapid growth is not desired but healthy monolayers must be controlled for inoculation of specimens and recovery of the etiologic agent. Seeded flasks, tubes, trays, or shell vials may be fed with medium multiple times prior to release from the vendor to ensure that the cells are growing according to specifications and arrive at the user site ready to be used. At the user site, most cells remain stable for a period of a few days without needing changing of the medium with which they were shipped. However, before use, it is common to remove the shipping medium and add a maintenance medium such as 2% FBS EMEM or 10% FBS Hanks' buffer, minimal

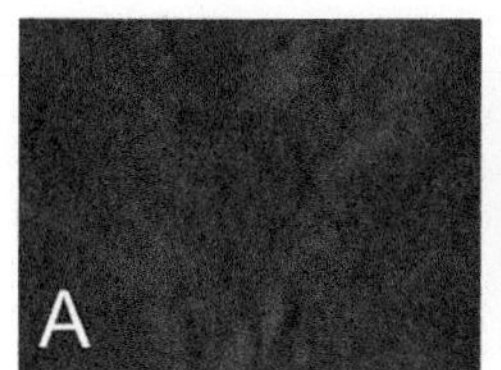

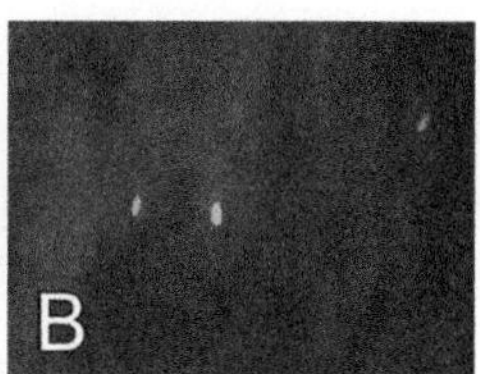

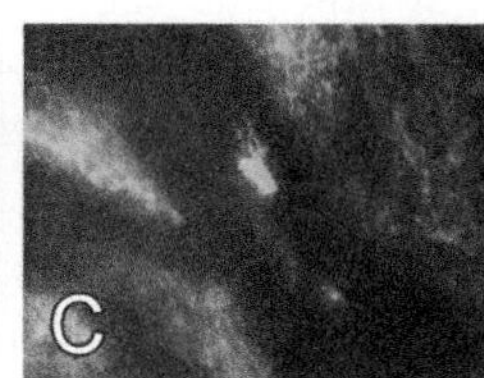

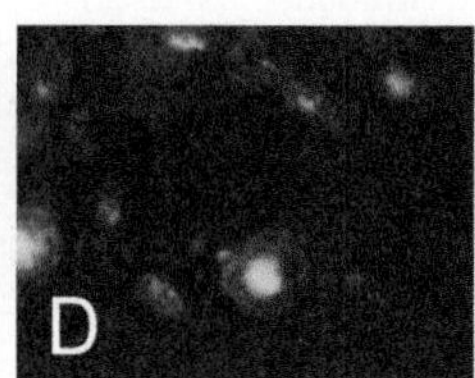

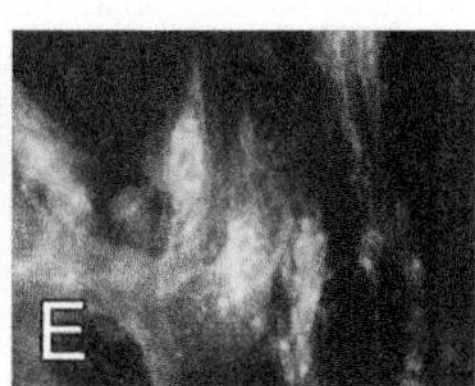

FIGURE 6 Immunofluorescence detection of *Herpesviridae* family viruses in H&V-Mix cells (Quidel). (A) Uninoculated H&V-Mix cells; (B) CMV; (C) VZV; (D) HSV-1; (E) HSV-2. Magnification, ×170. (Courtesy of Quidel.)

essential medium, or, for viruses that would be inhibited by serum proteins (e.g., myxoviruses and paramyxoviruses), R-Mix refeed medium. Trypsin and antimicrobial agents can be added if indicated. Other refeeding media for viruses include E-Mix refeed medium (Quidel) and 5 or 10% FBS growth medium. Tube cell cultures may require refeeding on a weekly or twice-weekly basis; however, the use of shell vial or cluster plate technology usually reduces refeeding to one time just prior to inoculation. Commercial media with and without enrichments, such as PBS, L-glutamine, trypsin, and bactericidal and fungicidal agents, are available.

■ *Chlamydia* isolation medium

Some cell-dependent bacteria, such as *C. trachomatis*, require the cell host to restrict protein synthesis, thus allowing the infecting microbe to replicate more easily. For this reason, media used for propagation of *Chlamydia* spp. in cell culture commonly contain cycloheximide, a protein synthesis inhibitor. Isolation media for *Chlamydia* sp. detection using shell vials generally contain EMEM with EBSS, supplemented with 10% FBS, HEPES, glucose, nonessential amino acids, antibiotics (cycloheximide, gentamicin, or streptomycin), and amphotericin B.

■ EMEM pH 2 to 3

Rhinoviruses require a lower temperature of incubation than many other pathogenic human viruses, and their characteristic CPE can be confused with enterovirus CPE, which has a similar appearance. At this time, MAbs that identify rhinoviruses are not available. For this reason, the acid solutions that can neutralize rhinoviruses, thus reducing viral titers, can be used to differentiate rhinoviruses from enteroviruses, which are not sensitive to low pH. EMEM pH 2 to 3 can be used to test for acid sensitivity.

■ RPMI 1640 medium

RPMI medium consists of glucose, essential amino acids, other amino acids, vitamins, HEPES buffer, antibiotics (such as penicillin and streptomycin), and phenol red as an indicator. This enriched medium is used for lymphocyte cell cultivation and culture of HIV.

Proprietary Media

■ CMV TurboTreat medium

CMV TurboTreat pretreatment medium (Quidel) consists of EMEM with EBSS without phenol red, 10% FBS, HEPES, and gentamicin. Pretreatment of Mv1Lu, R-Mix, and MRC-5 cultures overnight, prior to specimen addition, enhances the recovery of CMV (29).

■ ELVIS replacement medium

ELVIS replacement medium (Quidel) is used with the ELVIS test system and comprises EMEM, FBS, streptomycin, and amphotericin B.

■ R-Mix refeed and rinse medium

R-Mix refeed and rinse medium is used with R-Mix or R-Mix Too fresh and R-Mix or R-Mix Too ReadyCells (frozen shell vial) culture systems (Quidel) and is a defined serum-free medium with trypsin, penicillin, and streptomycin.

QC IN THE DIAGNOSTIC VIROLOGY LABORATORY

The validity of diagnostic test results depends upon the measures employed during each phase of testing—preanalytical, analytical, and postanalytical—as part of an overall quality assurance program. QC in the diagnostic virology laboratory is one component of such a program and refers to the measures included in each assay to verify that the test is working properly and to ensure that a laboratory consistently produces accurate results. Essential to the QC process are the use of internal and external control material and the verification that these controls are performed in accordance with manufacturer criteria for acceptability, adherence to appropriate incubation time and temperatures for the assay, and ensuring that test kits are used prior to expiration. Internal controls demonstrate that each run worked properly, while external controls help to monitor consistent performance of the assay and lot-to-lot variation between kits. Best practice is to establish a QC program for each assay performed by the diagnostic virology laboratory (30, 31). Laboratories must follow the regulations set forth by the College of American Pathologists, CLIA, or other accrediting agency, but at a minimum, controls should be used at the frequency recommended by the assay manufacturer. Several commercial sources provide reliable QC material for purchase, including specific strains, purified nucleic acid, antigens, antibodies, and other biological reagents. Many companies also offer subscription programs for laboratories to participate in external quality assessment and proficiency testing programs. The appendix below lists several manufacturers and suppliers of QC material.

APPENDIX

Sources of Virology Reagents, Stains, Media, Cell Lines, and QC Material (Including Molecular Diagnostics)

American Type Culture Collection
Manassas, VA 20110
http://www.atcc.org

BBI Solutions
Cardiff, Wales, UK
https://www.bbisolutions.com

BD Biosciences
Franklin Lakes, NJ 07417
http://www.bdbiosciences.com

Bio-Rad Laboratories
Hercules, CA 94547
http://www.bio-rad.com

Cambrex Corporation (BioWhittaker Cell Products)
East Rutherford, NJ 07073
http://www.cambrex.com

Lonza, Inc.
Allendale, NJ 07401
http:/www.lonza.com

Maine Molecular Quality Controls, Inc.
Saco, ME 04072
http://mmqci.com

Meridian Bioscience
Cincinnati, OH 45244
http://www.meridianbioscience.com

MilliporeSigma (Chemicon)
Billerica, MA 01821
http://www.millipore.com

Qnostics Ltd
Glasgow, G20 0XA, Scotland, UK and
Shirley, NY 11967
www.qnostics.com

Quality Control for Molecular Diagnostics
Glasgow, Scotland, UK
http://qcmd.org

Quidel (Diagnostic Hybrids)
Athens, OH 45701
http://www.quidel.com

SeraCare Life Sciences
Milford, MA 01757
www.seracare.com

ThermoFisher Scientific (Remel)
Waltham, MA 02451
http://thermofisher.com

Trinity Biotech (Bartels, MicroTrak)
Carlsbad, CA 92008, and
Bray, County Wicklow, Ireland
http://www.trinitybiotech.com

Vircell
Avicena 8, 18016 Granada, Spain
www.en.vircell.com

Zeptometrix Corporation
Buffalo, NY 14202
www.zeptometrix.com

REFERENCES

1. **Stinehardt E, Israeli C, Lambert R.** 1913. Studies on the cultivation of the virus of vaccinia. *J Infect Dis* **13:**204–300.
2. **Enders JF, Weller TH, Robbins FC.** 1949. Cultivation of the Lansing strain of poliomyelitis virus in cultures of various human embryonic tissues. *Science* **109:**85–87.
3. **Landry ML, Leland D.** 2016. Primary isolation of viruses, p 79–94. *In* Loeffelholz MJ, Hodinka RL, Young SA, Pinsky BA (ed), *Clinical Virology Manual*, 5th ed. ASM Press, Washington, DC.
4. **Leland DS.** 1996. *Clinical Virology*. W. B. Saunders, Philadelphia, PA.
5. **Olivo PD.** 1996. Transgenic cell lines for detection of animal viruses. *Clin Microbiol Rev* **9:**321–334.
6. **Stabell EC, Olivo PD.** 1992. Isolation of a cell line for rapid and sensitive histochemical assay for the detection of herpes simplex virus. *J Virol Methods* **38:**195–204.
7. **Leland DS, Ginocchio CC.** 2007. Role of cell culture for virus detection in the age of technology. *Clin Microbiol Rev* **20:**49–78.
8. **Clinical and Laboratory Standards Institute.** 2006. Viral culture. CLSI document M41-A. Clinical and Laboratory Standards Institute, Wayne, PA.
9. **Huang YT, Yan H, Sun Y, Jollick JA, Jr, Baird H.** 2002. Cryopreserved cell monolayers for rapid detection of herpes simplex virus and influenza virus. *J Clin Microbiol* **40:**4301–4303.
10. **Bankowski MJ.** 2016. Quality assurance and quality control in clinical and molecular virology, p 27–34. *In* Loeffelholz MJ, Hodinka RL, Young SA, Pinsky BA (ed), *Clinical Virology Manual*, 5th ed. ASM Press, Washington, DC.
11. **Centers for Disease Control and Prevention.** 2009. Biosafety in microbiological and biomedical laboratories, 5th ed. Centers for Disease Control and Prevention, Atlanta, GA. http://www.cdc.gov/biosafety/publications/bmbl5/BMBL.pdf.
12. **College of American Pathologists.** 2013. *Laboratory Improvement: Laboratory Accreditation Program Checklists*. College of American Pathologists, Chicago, IL.
13. **Ginocchio CC, Lotlikar M, Li X, Elsayed HH, Teng Y, Dougherty P, Kuhles DJ, Chaturvedi S, St George K.** 2013. Identification of endogenous *Coccidioides posadasii* contamination of commercial primary rhesus monkey kidney cells. *J Clin Microbiol* **51:**1288–1290.
14. **Purfield A, Ahmad N, Park BJ, Kuhles D, St George K, Ginocchio C, Harris JR.** 2013. Epidemiology of commercial rhesus monkey kidney cells contaminated with *Coccidioides posadasii*. *J Clin Microbiol* **51:**2005.
15. **Clinical and Laboratory Standards Institute.** 2006. Quality assurance for commercially prepared microbiologic culture media. CLSI document M22-A3. Clinical and Laboratory Standards Institute, Wayne, PA.
16. **Minnich LL, Ray CG.** 1987. Early testing of cell cultures for detection of hemadsorbing viruses. *J Clin Microbiol* **25:**421–422.
17. **Weinberg A, Mettenbrink CJ, Ye D, Yang CF.** 2005. Sensitivity of diagnostic tests for influenza varies with the circulating strains. *J Clin Virol* **33:**172–175.
18. **Johnston SL, Siegel C.** 1992. Comparison of Buffalo green monkey kidney cells and McCoy cells for the isolation of *Chlamydia trachomatis* in shell vial centrifugation culture. *Diagn Microbiol Infect Dis* **15:**355–357.
19. **Gleaves CA, Smith TF, Shuster EA, Pearson GR.** 1984. Rapid detection of cytomegalovirus in MRC-5 cells inoculated with urine specimens by using low-speed centrifugation and monoclonal antibody to an early antigen. *J Clin Microbiol* **19:**917–919.
20. **Hughes JH.** 1993. Physical and chemical methods for enhancing rapid detection of viruses and other agents. *Clin Microbiol Rev* **6:**150–175.
21. **Barenfanger J, Drake C, Mueller T, Troutt T, O'Brien J, Guttman K.** 2001. R-Mix cells are faster, at least as sensitive and marginally more costly than conventional cell lines for the detection of respiratory viruses. *J Clin Virol* **22:**101–110.
22. **Fong CK, Lee MK, Griffith BP.** 2000. Evaluation of R-Mix FreshCells in shell vials for detection of respiratory viruses. *J Clin Microbiol* **38:**4660–4662.
23. **Huang YT, Hite S, Duane V, Yan H.** 2002. CV-1 and MRC-5 mixed cells for simultaneous detection of herpes simplex viruses and varicella zoster virus in skin lesions. *J Clin Virol* **24:**37–43.
24. **LaRocco MT.** 2000. Evaluation of an enzyme-linked viral inducible system for the rapid detection of herpes simplex virus. *Eur J Clin Microbiol Infect Dis* **19:**233–235.
25. **Proffitt MR, Schindler SA.** 1995. Rapid detection of HSV with an enzyme-linked virus inducible system (ELVIS) employing a genetically modified cell line. *Clin Diagn Virol* **4:**175–182.
26. **Donta ST, Shaffer SJ.** 1980. Effects of *Clostridium difficile* toxin on tissue-cultured cells. *J Infect Dis* **141:**218–222.
27. **Ryan RW, Kwasnik I, Tilton RC.** 1980. Rapid detection of *Clostridium difficile* toxin in human feces. *J Clin Microbiol* **12:**776–779.
28. **Thelestam M, Brönnegård M.** 1980. Interaction of cytopathogenic toxin from *Clostridium difficile* with cells in tissue culture. *Scand J Infect Dis Suppl* **12:**(Suppl 22):16–29.
29. **Yang W, Hite S, Huang YT.** 2005. Enhancement of cytomegalovirus detection in mink lung cells using CMV Turbo. *J Clin Virol* **34:**125–128.
30. **Clinical and Laboratory Standards Institute.** 2011. Quality management system: a model for laboratory services. Approved guideline, 4th ed. CLSI document QMS01-A4. Clinical and Laboratory Standards Institute, Wayne, PA.
31. **Clinical and Laboratory Standards Institute.** 2012. ISO 15189: medical laboratories—requirements for quality and competence. Clinical and Laboratory Standards Institute, Wayne, PA.

Algorithms for Detection and Identification of Viruses

MARIE LOUISE LANDRY, ANGELA M. CALIENDO, CHRISTINE C. GINOCCHIO, RANDALL HAYDEN, AND YI-WEI TANG

83

Virology remains a dynamic field. Since the first edition of the *Manual of Clinical Microbiology* in 1970, virology has firmly established itself in the mainstream of clinical laboratory practice. When traditional virologic methods (namely, conventional cell cultures, neutralization tests with antisera for virus identification, manual serologic techniques, and light and electron microscopy) were the mainstay, diagnostic virology was a distinct discipline that was practiced primarily in public health, research, and academic settings. Time to result was slow, and it was often said that the patient was dead or better by the time the result was received.

ADVANCES IN DIAGNOSTICS

Driven by effective antiviral therapies, diagnostic advances have transformed the field, allowing accurate results in a clinically useful time frame. Early technological improvements in the laboratory included enzyme immunoassays, IgM class capture assays, monoclonal antibodies for identification, rapid centrifugation cultures, and direct detection of viral antigens in clinical specimens by immunofluorescence. At the point of care (POC), lateral flow immunochromatography tests were introduced to detect viral antigens or antibodies in 10 to 20 minutes without equipment or reagent additions, allowing immediate impact on clinical decisions. The most transformative, however, has been the introduction of nucleic acid amplification tests (NAATs), which are both rapid and sensitive, can be automated, high-throughput, or random access, and can detect viruses not amenable to routine culture.

Initially, NAAT was confined to a limited number of specialized molecular laboratories, using multistep, technically demanding laboratory-developed methods, and required separate assays optimized for each pathogen. For decades, only a handful of FDA-cleared or -approved commercial NAATs were available. With each new edition of the *Manual*, the transition to molecular methods has accelerated, due to advances in technology, real-time amplification methods, and user-friendly, FDA-approved or -cleared devices.

For years, culture was considered the gold standard because it could detect a variety of pathogens and reveal an unexpected virus. With NAAT syndromic viral panels, first for respiratory viruses and then for meningitis/encephalitis and gastrointestinal pathogens, the relevance of viral culture to clinical management has receded further. Not only are these panels faster, requiring less than 1 hour to a few hours to generate a result, they also detect more viruses than culture and often include nonviral pathogens that can have a similar presentation. They also require less skill than culture. Some require the simple addition of an unprocessed sample into a device and then insertion into the instrument, with approximately 2 minutes of hands-on time. When a more limited diagnosis is sought, another option is a multiplexed minipanel for two or three key pathogens.

For quantitative monitoring of viral load in blood, additional tests have been FDA approved, and substantial effort has been invested in the development and implementation of international quantitative standards that will permit cross-institutional comparisons and interpretive guidelines (e.g., for cytomegalovirus, Epstein-Barr virus, polyomavirus BK, and parvovirus B19). As a result, standardization and commutability have been gradually improved between laboratories. Quantitative NAATs have also required batch testing, often with a limited batch size, and sometimes differing nucleic acid extraction steps for RNA and DNA viruses, as well as separate extraction and amplification instruments. Recent innovations include the ability to accommodate multiple assays in a flexible and automated manner, elimination of the need for separate RNA or DNA extraction, and shorter assay times.

Since the last edition of this *Manual*, rapid influenza virus immunoassays have been reclassified by the FDA as class II (moderate potential harm) and must meet new requirements for minimum performance, including reporting annual reactivity testing of circulating strains. Innovative solutions to improve sensitivity are expected if rapid immunoassays are to remain competitive. If successful, these changes will greatly benefit other POC immunoassays, which, due to their simplicity and low cost, are especially useful in limited-resource settings.

Another paradigm shift occurred in 2015, when the first NAAT was approved for POC use, providing results for influenza virus in 15 min, or in as little as 2 to 5 minutes for some respiratory syncytial virus (RSV) positives. Subsequently, additional CLIA-waived NAATs have been introduced that require the simple addition of a sample to a device, which is then inserted into an instrument. Results are available in 20 to 30 min for influenza virus A and B

TABLE 1 Methods for detection[a] and identification of viruses

Virus	Applicability of detection method[b]					Comments[c]
	Nucleic acid	Antigen	Virus isolation	Antibody	Pathology	
Adenoviruses	A	A	B	B	B	NAAT is most sensitive for detection, but tests vary in ability to detect diverse types. Quantitative NAAT is used to monitor viral load in compromised hosts. Antigen assays are used for ocular, enteric, or respiratory adenoviruses but are less sensitive than culture or NAAT.
Arboviruses	A, C	B	C	A, C	D	NAAT and IgM are useful in acute infection, depending on day of illness and clinical disease. However, NAAT is not commercially available for most neurotropic arboviruses, except WNV. Serologic cross-reactivity is problematic, especially for Zika and dengue viruses; more specific PRNT is available at CDC. Rapid antigen tests are available for dengue virus. Most arboviruses are readily cultured but may require BSL3 or -4 facilities.
Bocaviruses	A	D	D	D	D	NAAT is the only test available for diagnosis. Included in some multiplex respiratory panels. Clinical relevance awaits further investigation.
Coronaviruses OC43, 229E, NL63, HKU1	A	D	D	D	D	NAAT is used for respiratory CoV as part of multiplex panels.
Coronaviruses SARS, MERS	A, C	C	C	C	D	NAAT and antibody tests are available only in public health or research laboratories.
Cytomegalovirus	A	B	B	A	B	NAAT is most sensitive and can determine viral load. pp65 antigenemia is used to determine viral load in blood, but NAAT is much more widely used. Culture can be used for nonblood specimens. IgG antibody is used to determine immune status, and IgM to screen for recent infection. CMV-specific gamma interferon release assay is available to measure cell-mediated immunity.
Enteroviruses and parechoviruses	A	D	B	D	D	NAAT is more sensitive and strongly preferred for CNS infection. Parechovirus requires separate NAAT.
Epstein-Barr virus	A	B	D	A	B	Serology is test of choice for diagnosis of primary infection. NAAT is useful for monitoring viral load in blood. IHC or ISH is used on tissue biopsy specimens.
Filoviruses and arenaviruses	C	C	C	A, C	C	NAAT is key to rapid diagnosis. BSL4 facility is needed for culture, except for LCMV. Patients with severe disease may die without developing antibody. LCMV is diagnosed primarily by serology.
Hantaviruses	C	C	C	A	D	NAAT and serology are equally useful for diagnosis. IHC is used in fatal cases. BSL4 facility is needed for culture. Isolation is difficult.
Hepatitis A virus	D	D	D	A	D	Serology is the standard diagnostic test. False-positive IgM is problematic in low-prevalence areas.
Hepatitis B virus	A	A	D	A	D	Detection of specific viral antigens and antibodies allows diagnosis and monitoring the course of infection. NAAT is used to monitor therapy and determine genotype.
Hepatitis C virus	A	B	D	A	D	Serology is used for diagnosis. NAAT is used to confirm active infection and monitor response to therapy. Genotyping helps determine drug regimen and duration of therapy. Antigen testing is a low-cost POC alternative in low-resource areas.
Hepatitis D virus	A	A	D	A	D	Testing is confined to reference laboratories. Diagnosis is relevant only in the presence of hepatitis B infection. IHC of biopsy tissue is useful for diagnosis.

(Continued on next page)

TABLE 1 Methods for detection[a] and identification of viruses *(Continued)*

Virus	Applicability of detection method[b]					Comments[c]
	Nucleic acid	Antigen	Virus isolation	Antibody	Pathology	
Hepatitis E virus	A, C	D	D	A	D	Serology is the standard diagnostic test, but tests vary in sensitivity and specificity. False-positive IgM is problematic in low-prevalence areas. NAAT is required for accurate diagnosis in transplant patients. Genotyping is performed at CDC for autochthonous cases.
Herpes simplex virus	A	B	B	B	B	NAAT is test of choice, especially for CSF infection. IFA can be used for rapid detection in skin and mucous membrane lesions. Serology is used to determine immune status.
Herpesviruses 6A and 6B	A	D	D	B	D	NAAT is test of choice for diagnosis. Serology can document primary infection in children. Interpretation of HHV-6 NAAT can be complicated by chromosomal integration of virus.
Herpesvirus 7	B	D	D	B	D	NAAT is test of choice but not routinely available.
Herpesvirus 8	A	B	D	A	A	Serology is used to identify infected persons. NAAT of blood may be useful in diagnosis posttransplant and monitoring therapy. IHC is preferred for tissue.
Human immunodeficiency virus	A	A	C	A	D	Serology is primary diagnostic method. Antigen-antibody combination tests reduce seronegative window in acute infection. Quantitative RNA tests are used to guide therapy and monitor response. Proviral DNA tests are useful for diagnosis of neonatal infection.
Human metapneumovirus	A	A	B	D	D	NAAT is the test of choice for diagnosis. IFA and shell vial culture are less sensitive options. Conventional culture is difficult.
Human T-cell lymphotropic virus	B	D	D	A	B	Serology is primary diagnostic method. NAAT is qualitative only; useful if serology is indeterminate.
Influenza viruses	A	A	B	D	D	NAAT is most sensitive and can provide subtype. Rapid antigen tests are lower in sensitivity and specificity. IFA and rapid culture are more accurate. Serology is useful for epidemiological studies or retrospective diagnosis.
Measles viruses	A, C	C	C	A	D	Serology is used for diagnosis and determination of immunity. NAAT is best for acute infection. Isolation can be useful if attempted early (prodromal period to 4 days postrash).
Mumps virus	A, C	C	B	A	D	Serology is used most commonly for diagnosis and determination of immunity. NAAT is useful for diagnosing infection especially among vaccinated individuals.
Noroviruses	A	C	D	D	D	NAAT is test of choice but challenging due to strain variability.
Parainfluenza viruses	A	A	B	D	D	NAAT is more sensitive than isolation. IFA is most common rapid detection method.
Papillomaviruses	A	D	D	D	A	NAAT is test of choice for detection and genotype differentiation. Cytopathology is useful for diagnosis.
Parvovirus B19	A	C	D	A	B	Serology is used to diagnose B19 in immunocompetent individuals. NAAT is test of choice for immunocompromised hosts, early in infection before antibody, and for B19-exposed fetuses.
Polyomaviruses	A	B	D	B	A	NAAT is test of choice, but genetic variability can lead to falsely low or negative results. JC virus DNA detection in CSF is useful for presumptive diagnosis of PML. JC virus antibody is used to predict risk for PML. BK virus DNA quantification in plasma/urine is used for preemptive diagnosis of PVAN. IHC and EM are useful for biopsy tissues.

(Continued on next page)

TABLE 1 Methods for detection[a] and identification of viruses *(Continued)*

Virus	Applicability of detection method[b]					Comments[c]
	Nucleic acid	Antigen	Virus isolation	Antibody	Pathology	
Poxviruses	A, C	C	C	A, C	A	NAAT allows virus inactivation and rapid detection. Electron microscopy is very useful for rapid diagnosis but has limited availability. Smallpox isolation requires BSL3 or -4 and should be attempted only in WHO Collaborating Centers. Vaccinia virus requires BSL2 and grows readily in cell culture.
Rabies virus	C	C	C	A	A, C	For human rabies, testing is done at CDC. NAAT and culture used for saliva, CSF, and tissue; IFA for skin biopsy; serology for CSF and serum. Serology available at commercial laboratories used to monitor antibody titers in vaccinated professionals.
Respiratory syncytial virus	A	A	B	D	D	NAAT is most sensitive. Rapid antigen tests, especially IFA, can be useful in pediatric patients. Serology is useful only for epidemiological studies.
Rhinoviruses	A	D	B	D	D	NAAT is much more sensitive than culture; cross-reaction with enteroviruses can occur.
Rotaviruses	A	A	D	D	D	Antigen detection has been standard test for diagnosis. Rotavirus is now in NAAT gastroenteritis panels. EM is useful if available.
Rubella virus	C	D	C	A	D	Serology is used for diagnosis and immune status. NAAT is used for acute infection. Isolation is useful for postnatal rubella if attempted early (prodromal period to 4 days postrash). In CRS, virus can be isolated for weeks to months after birth.
Transmissible spongiform encephalopathy agents	B	B	D	D	A	Histology is most useful diagnostic test. Surrogate markers popular but lack specificity. Western blot for PrP is performed in specialized laboratories. Real-time quake-induced conversion is used to detect PrP^{Sc}. Human genome sequencing is useful for diagnosis of genetic disorders.
Varicella-zoster virus	A	A	B	B	B	NAAT is most sensitive and increasingly used. IFA on skin lesions is more sensitive than culture. Culture is slow and not sensitive. Serology is most useful for determination of immunity and can be useful in CNS vasculopathy.

[a]Viral nucleic acids (DNA or RNA) can be detected by amplification methods such as PCR. Viral antigens can be detected by a variety of immunoassays. Virus isolation includes conventional cell culture and rapid centrifugation culture with detection of viral antigens by immunostaining. Antibody detection involves measurement of total or class-specific immunoglobulins directed at specific viral antigens. Pathology involves the visualization of virus-induced changes in tissue or cytology smears, including inclusions, multinucleated cells, immunohistochemistry, or *in situ* hybridization, or the visualization of viral particles by electron microscopy.

[b]A, test is generally preferred for routine clinical diagnosis; B, test alternative whose utility may be limited to specific indications, forms of infection, or sample types, as delineated in the rightmost column and in the text of the individual chapters; C, test is limited to public health laboratories, such as CDC, due to specialized testing or biosafety concerns; D, test is not available, is not generally useful, or is used only in research.

[c]Abbreviations: WNV, West Nile virus; PRNT, plaque reduction neutralization test; CDC, Centers for Disease Control and Prevention; BSL, biosafety level; CoV, coronavirus; SARS, severe acute respiratory syndrome; MERS, Middle East respiratory syndrome; CNS, central nervous system; LCMV, lymphocytic choriomeningitis virus; IHC, immunohistochemistry; ISH, *in situ* hybridization; PML, progressive multifocal leukoencephalopathy; PVAN, polyomavirus-associated nephropathy; IFA, immunofluorescence assay; EM, electron microscopy; CRS, congenital rubella syndrome; PrP, prion protein; CMV, cytomegalovirus; HHV, human herpesvirus.

with or without RSV using real-time PCR and in 60 min for 14 respiratory viruses and 3 bacterial pathogens using nested PCR. As an indication of how far the field has come, these POC tests are as sensitive as the best laboratory-performed assays. Thus, any hospital laboratory, emergency department, clinic, or doctor's office can now implement state-of-the-art molecular testing. The main obstacle is no longer lack of technical expertise and laboratory facilities, but cost, of equipment, service contracts, and reagents. Additionally, the expertise of the clinical virologist with regard to interpreting results may be lost, as tests are now performed outside the laboratory setting. For many pathogens, this may not be required, but for some results, such as the detection of latent herpes viruses in cerebrospinal fluid, interpretation can require both clinical and laboratory expertise. Going forward, linking best-practice guidelines to specific test results should be encouraged if the full benefits of an accurate rapid diagnosis are to be realized.

CHALLENGES AND FUTURE PERSPECTIVES

In addition to the advantages of molecular testing, some pitfalls have become apparent as the tests are more widely used. For example, the sensitivities and specificities to detect the same virus often vary for different assays. In addition, despite the fact that the tests target conserved regions of the genome, strain variability and mutations can lead to underquantification of viral load, or even falsely negative results for both qualitative and quantitative assays. Furthermore, as tests become more sensitive, low levels of clinically irrelevant or nonviable viruses may be detected and can be misleading to clinicians. Similarly, interpreting the clinical relevance of multiple viral pathogens in the same sample, especially when relative quantification is not available, is problematic.

Thus, with progress have come new challenges. Laboratories need to choose which platforms and tests to offer. Selecting the appropriate test will depend on the virus(es) sought, sample site, clinical presentation, clinical purpose (e.g., screening, confirmation, diagnosis, or monitoring), patient characteristics, and disease prevalence. Performance characteristics, staff expertise, and cost will also impact that choice. Laboratories must recognize the uses and also the limitations of each test in order to guide clinicians in test selection and in interpreting the results. This *Manual* should serve as a key resource for accomplishing these tasks. The choices available for each virus differ and continue to evolve. Table 1 provides a concise overview for each virus group; however, the reader is referred to the specific chapters for more detailed discussions.

Next-generation sequencing for resistance testing, outbreak management, and characterization and surveillance of pathogens, as well as metagenomics to discover unexpected etiologies of disease, is the next wave of technological advances beginning to move from the research laboratory to the clinical arena. As with other molecular assays, these techniques will provide an impetus to bring virology closer to the rest of clinical microbiology practice. However, there remain a number challenges in the implementation of next-generation sequencing for routine diagnosis, including the technical expertise required, cost of instrumentation, time to results, bioinformatics, and result interpretation. While the pace of change can be daunting for laboratories, it is extremely gratifying to witness the impact of state-of-the-art testing on patient care. As we move forward, it is critical that laboratorians communicate with each other to address problems, including the optimization and standardization of methods, and, in addition, encourage input and feedback from clinicians. Due to the speed of methodological change and the continuing discovery of new viruses and new therapies, keeping abreast of the most recent literature is strongly recommended.

Human Immunodeficiency Viruses*

S. MICHELE OWEN

84

TAXONOMY

Historical Perspective and Origin

The human immunodeficiency virus (HIV) is the etiologic agent of AIDS. The clinical manifestations of AIDS were first recognized in 1981 (1). The search for the cause of this severe cellular immune dysfunction led to isolation of lymphadenopathy-associated virus in 1983 (2). The following year, other researchers isolated cytopathic retroviruses from people with AIDS, which they termed human T-lymphotropic virus type III (3, 4). These viruses were soon confirmed to be identical, and in 1986 the International Committee on the Taxonomy of Viruses designated HIV as the name for the virus that causes AIDS (5).

HIV exists as two major viral species. Both are members of the genus *Lentivirus* within the family *Retroviridae*. HIV type 1 (HIV-1), identified first, is the more virulent of the two and is responsible for the majority of AIDS cases worldwide. HIV-2, first isolated in 1986, has biological and morphologic properties similar to those of HIV-1 but differs in some of its antigenic components (6). HIV-2 is less pathogenic and has a more limited geographic distribution than HIV-1. Both HIV-1 and HIV-2 are related to simian immunodeficiency viruses (SIVs), which are found in 26 species of African primates but do not cause disease in their native hosts (7). Phylogenetic evidence indicates that HIV-1 arose as a consequence of at least three separate zoonotic transmissions of SIV from chimpanzees to humans; four interspecies SIV transmissions from sooty mangabeys are the source of HIV-2 (7, 8). Genetic sequences of HIV have been identified retrospectively in human plasma specimens from as early as 1959 (9).

HIV Classification

HIV viruses are classified based on phylogenetic relatedness of nucleotide sequences. The current classification is hierarchical and consists of types, groups, subtypes, subsubtypes, and recombinant forms (10). Subtypes are often referred to as clades. The most distantly related HIVs are categorized as types: HIV type 1 and HIV type 2. HIV-1 is further characterized into groups: the major (M) group; the more divergent outlier (O) group, the non-M, non-O (N) group, and group P, a new lineage closely related to a gorilla SIV (10–12). Most HIV infections occur with HIV-1 group M, which is differentiated into nine subtypes (A, B, C, D, F, G, H, J, and K). Subtypes A and F are further classified into subsubtypes A1, A2, A3, F1, and F2. The sequences within any one subtype are more similar to each other than to sequences from other subtypes throughout their genomes and represent different lineages of HIV. Eight HIV-2 subtypes (A through H) have been defined; only two, A and B, have been recovered from more than a single individual. When viruses from two or more HIV-1 lineages infect one individual and exchange their genetic material, they are termed recombinant viruses (13). If transmission of the recombinant virus has been documented by whole-genome sequences to three or more people, it is referred to as a circulating recombinant form (CRF), and the CRF is given a numeric designation (13). As of December 2013, CRF01 to CRF55 are recognized (14). Recombinant viruses that have been identified but not documented to have been further transmitted are referred to as unique recombinant forms. The variation in nucleotide sequences can have implications for the biology and transmission of the virus and for patient survival and also helps identify the geographic distribution and epidemiology of HIV infection. From the diagnostic perspective, sequence variation can have significant implications for the reactivity and cross-reactivity of diagnostic tests designed to detect specific viral proteins or peptides.

DESCRIPTION OF THE AGENTS

Structure and Genomic Organization

HIVs are enveloped plus-stranded RNA viruses. The HIV genome is organized similarly to other retroviruses. It contains the *gag*, *pol*, and *env* genes, which encode structural proteins, viral enzymes, and envelope glycoproteins, respectively. These are flanked by long terminal repeats. In addition, the genome comprises open reading frames for *trans*-acting transcriptional activator (Tat), the regulator of viral expression (Rev), and several other proteins such as Vif, Vpr, and Nef.

*This chapter contains significant information presented in chapter 82 by Bernard M. Branson and S. Michele Owen in the 11th edition of this *Manual*.

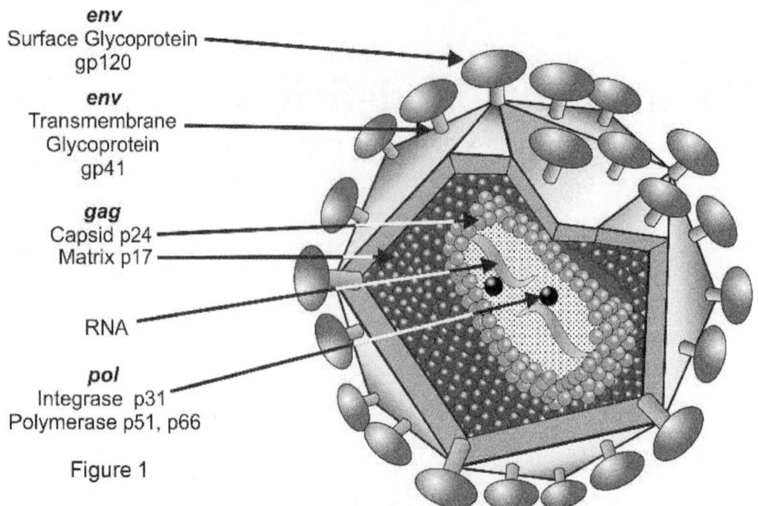

FIGURE 1 Schematic of a viral particle.

Mature viral particles measure 100 to 150 nm in diameter and have a conical core surrounded by a lipid envelope (Fig. 1). The core contains two identical copies of single-stranded RNA, approximately 10 kb in length, which are surrounded by structural proteins that form the nucleocapsid and the matrix shell as well as by-products of the *pol* gene. The lipid envelope is acquired as the virus buds from infected cells. The HIV-1 glycoprotein gp120/41 forms spikes protruding from this envelope. The glycoprotein, a product of the *env* gene, is synthesized as a precursor, gp160, which is cleaved into the heavily glycosylated gp120, forming the majority of the external portion, and the transmembrane gp41 portion, which contains the membrane-spanning domain. The major HIV-1 structural proteins which are encoded by the *gag* gene include p17, p24, p7, and p9. Products of the *pol* gene include the protease, reverse transcriptase (RT), RNase, and integrase.

HIV-2 is structurally analogous to HIV-1, but some of its protein components differ, most notably the outer envelope and transmembrane glycoproteins, gp125 and gp36, as well as the core proteins p16 and p26. The major gene products that are of significance for the diagnosis of HIV-1 and HIV-2 are listed in Table 1.

TABLE 1 Major HIV proteins of diagnostic significance

HIV gene and products	Viral protein/glycoprotein molecular weight	
	HIV-1	HIV-2
env		
Precursor	gp160	gp125
External glycoprotein	gp120	gp105
Transmembrane glycoprotein	gp41	gp36
pol		
Reverse transcriptase	p66	p68
Reverse transcriptase	p51	p53
Endonuclease	p31	p31/34
gag		
Precursor	p55	p56
Core	p24	p27
Matrix	p17	p16

Replication Cycle

The replication cycle of HIV-1 is accomplished *in vivo* in approximately 24 hours (15). Replication begins with the attachment of virus to the target cell via the interaction of gp120 and the cellular receptor CD4. This binding results in gp120 conformational changes which allow the virus to interact with other cellular coreceptor sites, CXCR4 or CCR5. The interaction with CXCR4 occurs primarily with T-cell-tropic, syncytium-inducing viruses (16). In contrast, the β-chemokine receptor CCR5 is involved in macrophage-tropic non-syncytium-inducing HIVs (17).

After fusion with the host cells, HIV enters the cell and RNA is released. HIV particles contain RT, an enzyme that plays a crucial role in the replication process. RT possesses three distinct functions: RNA-dependent DNA polymerase, which serves to synthesize cDNA, RNase H, which degrades RNA from the cDNA-RNA complex, and a DNA-dependent DNA polymerase, which duplicates the cDNA strand. The reverse-transcribed genome is associated with several viral proteins and transported into the nucleus. The DNA copy becomes integrated into the genome of the infected cell by the virally encoded integrase; this integrated retroviral DNA genome is called the provirus. The cDNA then serves as a template for viral RNA. Activation of HIV transcription and gene expression is modulated by cellular transcription factors and by viral regulatory proteins, including Tat, Rev, Nef, and Vrp. The regulatory genes *tat* and *rev* greatly influence the rate of viral replication. The Tat protein increases transcription from the long terminal repeat. The Rev protein facilitates export of unspliced or partially spliced RNAs encoding the viral structural proteins. At the end of the replication cycle, the virion assembles and buds through the plasma membrane.

EPIDEMIOLOGY AND TRANSMISSION

Epidemiology

Approximately 76.1 million people worldwide have become infected with HIV since the start of the pandemic. In 2016, ~1.8 million people became newly infected, and an estimated 36.7 million people were living with

HIV (18). HIV-1 has been reported in virtually every country on earth. Group M viruses are responsible for most HIV-1 infections, with a predominance of subtype C. Subtype B is most prevalent in the United States, Europe, and Australia but is rarely found in Africa, where subtypes A, C, and D predominate. HIV-2 is found predominantly in West African nations, where an estimated 1 to 2 million people are infected with HIV-2. In recent years HIV-2 infections have been reported in countries with historical and socioeconomic ties to West Africa, including Brazil, France, Portugal, and India, and in other countries among immigrants from countries where HIV-2 is endemic (19). In 2017, around 20.9 million people living with HIV had access to antiretroviral therapy, resulting in around 53% (39 to 65%) of all people living with HIV having access to treatment (18).

The CDC estimated that approximately 1.2 million people in the United States were living with HIV at the end of 2014. The demographic characteristics of HIV infection continue to evolve. The CDC now generates annual estimates of the number of new HIV infections, including both those that are diagnosed and those that are undiagnosed. In 2016, 39,782 people received an HIV diagnosis, and the annual number of HIV diagnoses declined 5% between 2011 and 2015.

Men who have sex with men continue to bear the heaviest burden of HIV in the United States. In 2016, gay and bisexual men accounted for 67% (26,570) of all HIV diagnoses and 83% of diagnoses among males. Black/African American gay and bisexual men accounted for the largest number of HIV diagnoses (10,223), followed by Hispanic/Latino (7,425) and white (7,390) gay and bisexual men. In 2016, heterosexual contact accounted for 24% (9,578) of HIV diagnoses. People who inject drugs accounted for 9% (3,425) of HIV diagnoses (which includes 1,201 diagnoses among gay and bisexual men who inject drugs). Overall, from 2011 to 2015, diagnoses among all women declined 16% and among all heterosexuals, diagnoses declined 15%. Similarly, diagnoses in people who inject drugs declined 17% from 2011 to 2015 (20).

Transmission

Both HIV-1 and HIV-2 have the same modes of transmission. The most common mode of transmission is sexual transmission at the genital mucosa through direct contact with infected body fluids, including blood, semen, and vaginal secretions (21). Infection may also occur through inoculation of infected blood, via transfusion of infected blood products, transplantation of infected tissues, from an infected mother to her infant during pregnancy, or by reuse of contaminated needles. The risk of HIV-1 infection from occupational percutaneous exposure to HIV-1-infected blood has been estimated to be 0.3% (22).

The majority of HIV transmissions from mother to child occur in resource-poor countries. The level of maternal HIV-1 DNA in blood and genital fluids has been documented to correlate strongly with mother-to-child transmission (23). HIV transmission can occur *in utero*, during labor and delivery, and during breast-feeding. In the absence of therapeutic intervention, the risk of mother-to-child transmission can range from 15 to 30% and is further increased with breast-feeding. However, the risk can be reduced to less than 2% if antiretroviral therapy is administered to women during pregnancy and labor (24). Antiretroviral treatment of the infant immediately after birth can also significantly decrease the risk of HIV-1 infection in the newborn.

CLINICAL SIGNIFICANCE

Virologic Parameters during the Course of HIV Infection

The natural history of HIV-1 infection can be divided into three phases: a transient acute retroviral syndrome associated with primary infection, an asymptomatic period during which active viral replication continues and disease progresses, and finally, advanced disease resulting in severe immune dysfunction and AIDS. Each of these stages is associated with specific changes in virologic and immunologic parameters. After HIV-1 infection, HIV-1-specific markers appear in the blood in the following chronological order: HIV-1 RNA, p24 antigen, HIV-1 IgM antibody, and HIV-1 IgG antibody (Fig. 2). The exact time at which each of these markers can be detected depends on a number of characteristics of the infecting virus, the type of test used, and individual host immune responses. Immediately after exposure and transmission, HIV-1 replicates in the mucosa, submucosa, and lymphoreticular tissues and the virus cannot be detected in plasma. This period is called the eclipse phase and has been estimated to last 5 to 33 days with an estimated median time of around 11 days (25, 26). Once HIV-1 RNA reaches a concentration of 1 to 5 copies/ ml, it can be detected by sensitive qualitative methods of nucleic acid amplification; at concentrations of 50 copies/ml, it can be detected by quantitative assays used clinically to monitor viral load. HIV-1 p24 antigen is the next analyte that can be detected in the blood (25, 27). However, p24 antigen detection is transient because, as antibodies begin to develop, they bind to the p24 antigen and form immune complexes that interfere with p24 assay detection unless the assay includes steps to disrupt the antigen-antibody complexes. Following the rise of p24 in the blood, IgM-class antibodies are produced (25, 27). Finally, IgG-class antibodies emerge and persist throughout the course of HIV infection. The time period after infection when HIV antibody is not detectable is referred to as the window period. In most infected people, HIV antibody becomes detectable within 1 to 2 months after infection. Figure 2 is a graphic representation of the appearance of viral markers and shows the estimated days postexposure (median, 25th, 75th, and 99th percentiles) at which different tests become reactive when using plasma as the sample type.

Acute Retroviral Syndrome

An estimated 50 to 70% of individuals with HIV infection experience an acute clinical syndrome 3 to 6 weeks after primary infection during which antibodies are often not detectable. Acute HIV-1 infection is a transient symptomatic illness that usually lasts 7 to 14 days and is associated with high levels of HIV-1 replication and a developing virus-specific immune response. Acute HIV-1 infection has been described as a mononucleosis-like syndrome. Clinical symptoms include fever, maculopapular rash, oral ulcers, lymphadenopathy, malaise, weight loss, arthralgia, pharyngitis, and night sweats (28–30). During acute HIV-1 infection, plasma viremia rises, reaching levels of up to 100 million copies of HIV-1 RNA per ml of plasma (31). Destruction of HIV-1-specific CD4+ T lymphocytes and widespread dissemination of the virus, with seeding of lymphoid organs and other tissue reservoirs, occur. During resolution of primary infection, CD4+ T-cell counts rebound and viremia declines before reaching a steady level. This viral set point reflects ongoing viral replication and immune system damage and is an important prognostic indicator (32, 33). In prenatally infected infants, the HIV-1 RNA pattern differs

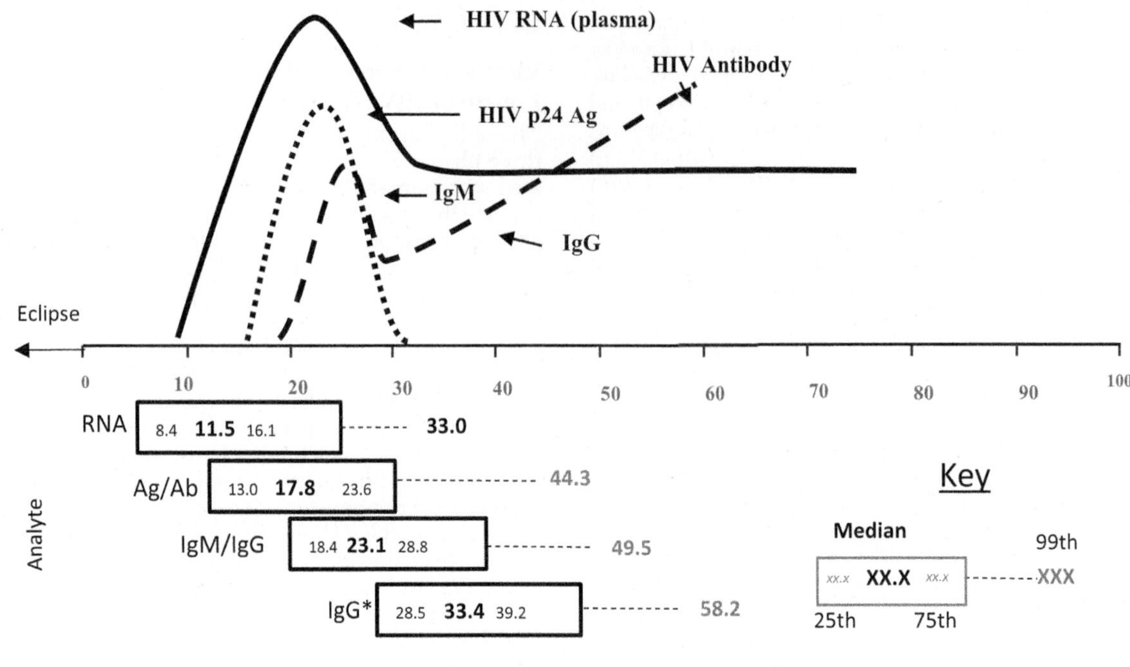

FIGURE 2 Approximate time course (median, 25th, 75th, and 99th percentiles) for appearance of laboratory markers for HIV-1 infection. Units for the vertical axis not noted because their magnitude differs for RNA, p24 antigen, and antibody. From data adapted from reference 84 and updated with data from references 25, 27, 91, and 102.

from that in infected adults: high HIV-1 RNA levels may persist in HIV-infected children for prolonged time periods.

Clinical Latency

In most patients, primary infection with or without the acute syndrome is followed by a prolonged period of clinical latency or smoldering low disease activity. In untreated patients, the length of time from initial infection to the development of clinical immunodeficiency disease varies greatly; the median interval is 10 years. HIV disease with active virus replication is ongoing and progressive during this asymptomatic period. The number of CD4+ lymphocytes declines slowly and the virus continues to replicate. During this asymptomatic period, high titers of virus can be found in lymphoid and other tissue compartments (34). In rapid progressors, AIDS can develop within 1 to 2 years. In contrast, 5 to 10% of HIV-1-infected individuals are long-term nonprogressors and remain symptom-free for longer than 20 years (35). Approximately 0.5% of people with HIV infection, termed elite controllers, are able to spontaneously maintain undetectable levels of virus without antiretroviral therapy.

Disease Progression to AIDS

In the absence of therapy, the continuous replication of HIV-1 in productively infected cells together with the elimination of host cells and chronic immune activation results in deterioration of the immune system. Studies of HIV-1 replication dynamics have shown that, in productively infected lymphocytes, the interval between infection, virus production, and cell death is very short. The half-life of HIV-1 in plasma is thought to be 6 hours, the length of the replication cycle in CD4+ lymphocytes has been estimated at 2.6 days, and 35 million CD4+ cells are thought to be lost daily (36). As the ability of the host to eliminate productively infected cells declines, CD4+ lymphocytes with integrated provirus accumulate. These resting memory CD4+ lymphocytes serve as a long-lived reservoir for HIV-1. This reservoir decays slowly (mean half-life of 44 months) even in treated patients who have had no detectable viremia for as long as 7 years (37). Clinical manifestations of HIV disease can affect nearly every organ system. Destruction of the immune system is clinically manifested by the occurrence of opportunistic infections and tumors. Central nervous system involvement also occurs, most commonly HIV-associated dementia (38). A decline of the CD4+ lymphocyte count below 200 cells/μl marks the onset of immunologic AIDS and predisposition to opportunistic infections caused by viruses, bacteria, fungi, and protozoa; neoplastic disease; HIV encephalopathy; wasting syndrome; and progressive multifocal leukoencephalopathy, which are often the cause of death.

The course of HIV-1 infection and the clinical characteristics of AIDS in children differ from those in adults. The disease progresses rapidly in infants with vertically acquired HIV-1 infection. The most common AIDS-defining conditions in children include *Pneumocystis jirovecii* pneumonia and recurrent bacterial infections.

Public health organizations, including the CDC and the WHO, have published HIV disease classification systems for public health surveillance purposes. All case definitions of HIV infection now require laboratory-confirmed evidence of HIV infection. The current CDC classification system for adults and children categorizes HIV-1 infection into five stages. Stage 0, indicative of early infection, is defined by a negative or indeterminate HIV test result obtained within 180 days of a positive HIV test result. Stage 0 can be established either by testing history (a positive test result

TABLE 2 HIV infection stage, based on age-specific CD4+ T-lymphocyte count or CD4+ T-lymphocyte percentage of total lymphocytes

	Age on date of CD4 T-lymphocyte test					
	<1 year		1–5 years		6 years through adult	
Stage[a]	Cells/μl	%	Cells/μl	%	Cells/μl	%
1	≥1,500	≥34	≥1,000	≥30	≥500	≥26
2	750–1,499	26–33	500–999	22–29	200–499	14–25
3	<750	<26	<500	<22	<200	<14

[a]The stage is based primarily on the CD4+ T-lymphocyte count; the percentage is considered only if the count is missing. Stage 0 is defined by a negative or indeterminate HIV test result obtained within 180 days of a positive HIV test result; cases with no information on CD4+ T-lymphocyte count or percentage are classified as stage unknown.

obtained after a previous negative or indeterminate test result) or by a laboratory testing algorithm that demonstrates the presence of HIV-specific viral markers, such as p24 antigen or nucleic acid (RNA or DNA), in conjunction with a negative or indeterminate antibody test result. Stages 1, 2, and 3 are categorized on the basis of age-specific CD4+ T-lymphocyte counts or percentages indicative of increasing severity (Table 2). Cases with no information on CD4+ T-lymphocyte count or percentage are classified as stage unknown (39).

Therapy and Vaccination

Significant scientific advances in the development of effective antiretroviral therapy have occurred in the past 25 years. The first effective drug against HIV-1, zidovudine, was approved by the FDA in March 1987. Currently, over 30 antiretroviral drugs or combinations of antiviral drugs have been approved by the FDA for the treatment of HIV infections (see the AIDSinfo website, www.aidsinfo.nih.gov, for a list of FDA-approved drugs). Approved antiviral agents used to treat HIV-1 fall into five classes: nucleoside RT inhibitors, nonnucleoside RT inhibitors, protease inhibitors, integrase inhibitors, and entry and fusion inhibitors. Guidelines for the use of antiretroviral agents in adults and in children evolve rapidly. These are updated on a regular basis, and the most recent guidelines can be obtained from the AIDSinfo website.

Several obstacles have hindered the development of effective vaccines against HIV-1, including its inability to induce neutralizing antibodies, the lack of understanding of correlates of protective immunity, the genetic diversity of the virus, and the limitation of animal models (40, 41). However, recent novel engineered bispecific molecules which act as dual-affinity retargeting molecules (DART) and are based on broadly neutralizing antibodies are showing promise with effective antiviral activity in the nanogram range. Future animal and human trials are needed to establish true clinical utility (42).

COLLECTION, STORAGE, AND TRANSPORT OF SPECIMENS

Serum and plasma are the most common specimen types used for routine HIV antibody and antigen determinations in the laboratory. The most common tubes for plasma collection are potassium EDTA, sodium citrate, sodium and lithium heparin, and plasma preparation tubes (PPTs). Prompt separation of serum and plasma from the clot/cellular elements is important to decrease hemolysis and maintain the most viable specimen for testing. Serum or plasma specimens can be transported either at room temperature, refrigerated, or frozen (after removal from cellular components) in screw-cap plastic vials. For antibody immunoassays, serum or plasma specimens may be shipped refrigerated (2 to 8°C) or at ambient temperature (≤37°C) for up to 7 days. For HIV antigen/antibody combination assays, the time that specimens can remain at room temperature is more restrictive. It is necessary to minimize room temperature storage for optimum preservation of p24 antigen. Specimens for the antigen/antibody combination assays available in the United States as of June 2017 can be stored at room temperature for a maximum of 48 to 72 hours or refrigerated at 2 to 8°C for up 7 days. It is important to include specimen transport times as part of the maximum allowable storage times at any given temperature. For long-term storage, serum or plasma specimens should be frozen at −20°C or lower.

Some HIV antibody assays are approved for use with dried blood spots and oral fluid, and some rapid point-of-care HIV assays can be performed with finger-stick whole blood, venipuncture whole blood, or oral fluids. Specific collection devices, procedures, and storage requirements are specified by the test manufacturer for use with these alternative specimen types.

Quantitative HIV-1 RNA viral load assays are most commonly performed on plasma specimens. Plasma for viral load determination is generally collected in potassium EDTA or acid citrate dextrose (ACD) tubes. Heparin anticoagulants inhibit PCR and should not be used for any nucleic acid assay that involves PCR amplification. To ensure accurate HIV-1 RNA quantification in plasma, proper collection, processing, storage, and transport of plasma specimens are essential. For all assays, plasma must be separated from blood cells in a timely manner to prevent RNA degradation. Whole blood can be maintained at room temperature for 6 to 24 hours or stored at 2 to 8°C for up to 24 hours before centrifugation, depending on the specific assay. HIV-1 RNA is generally stable in cell-free plasma refrigerated at 2 to 8°C for 5 to 7 days. For long-term storage, plasma samples should be frozen at −20 to −70°C. HIV-1 RNA remains stable for at least three freeze-thaw cycles.

To simplify the process of collecting and transporting plasma, PPTs (BD Vacutainer PPT, Becton Dickinson), which contain dried EDTA and a gel separator that, after centrifugation, forms a barrier between the plasma and cellular elements, are available and are approved for use with some viral load assays. PPTs provide a closed collection system for the preparation and transport of plasma specimens. Plasma samples do not need to be poured off from PPTs after centrifugation, eliminating plasma transfer and relabeling steps. This improves convenience, decreases risks of error, and improves safety. Initial manufacturer recommendations allowed for either refrigerated or frozen transport of centrifuged PPTs. However, discrepancies in viral loads have been reported to occur in plasma specimens with some assays and with certain handling conditions such as freezing after centrifugation, inadequate storage, and improper centrifugation (43–46). The differences were noted only for samples with viral loads close to the assay limit of detection; a large proportion of samples with undetectable viral load in a standard EDTA aliquot were found to have detectable HIV-1 RNA in the corresponding PPT. As a result, the tube manufacturer has recommended that plasma in PPTs be stored without freezing; plasma from PPTs should be transferred to a secondary tube if plasma specimens need to be stored frozen. The FDA-approved viral load kits have specific volume, collection tube, and specimen storage requirements, so package inserts should be used to determine optimal collection and handling of specimens.

The same collection system and procedures should be used to follow up patients over time because different systems may produce discrepant values. For example, specimens collected in ACD tubes have been shown to yield results that are approximately 15% lower than results obtained with EDTA plasma (45, 47). If a change in collection system or technology is planned, new baseline HIV-1 viral load values should be determined.

Laboratories that test specimens from pediatric patients should investigate flexibility of specimen volume because it may be difficult to obtain the 1 ml of plasma needed for several of the assays. Viral load assays have also been used to measure HIV-1 RNA in specimens other than plasma, including serum, dried blood spots, cerebrospinal fluid, cervical secretions, and seminal plasma (46). The RNA quantity in serum has been found to be lower than that in paired plasma samples, and applications with specimens other than plasma must be validated because they are not included as approved specimen types for the current FDA-approved viral load assays.

Qualitative HIV-1 RNA assays can be conducted with serum and plasma. For the FDA-approved qualitative diagnostic assay, APTIMA (Hologic Incorporated, Marlborough, MA), blood specimens can be collected in glass or plastic tubes. EDTA, ACD, sodium citrate, EDTA PPTs, or serum tubes can be used. For this assay, whole blood can be stored at ≤25°C for up to 72 hours; temperatures not to exceed 30°C are acceptable for not more than 24 hours. Specimens can be stored for an additional 5 days at 2 to 8°C after centrifugation. Plasma separated from cells can be stored for longer periods of time at ≤−20°C.

For HIV-1 resistance assays (genotypic and phenotypic), plasma collected from EDTA, ACD, or EDTA PPTs can be used. Plasma must be separated from the cellular elements within 6 hours of collection and frozen to prevent degradation of RNA. Higher-integrity samples are achieved by minimizing the time before centrifugation and freezing of processed samples. Plasma specimens should be transported frozen and stored at −70°C for optimal results. For HIV-1 DNA and viral culture assays, whole blood is commonly used. Blood should be collected in either EDTA, ACD, or cell preparation tubes. For preparation of the peripheral blood mononuclear cells required for HIV DNA amplification, the blood specimen should not be refrigerated or frozen but instead kept at ambient temperature for no longer than 4 days.

DIRECT DETECTION

p24 Antigen Assays

In the early days of the AIDS epidemic, p24 antigen testing played an important role as a tool for the diagnosis, prognosis, and evaluation of antiretroviral activity and for monitoring of HIV-1-infected cultures. In 1996, the FDA approved the Coulter HIV-1 p24 Ag assay (Coulter Co., Miami, FL) for screening blood products. This test was used for screening blood and plasma donors in the United States for a few years until it was replaced with more sensitive nucleic acid tests (NATs) in 1999 (57). At present, use of individual p24 antigen assays is very limited in the United States. The presence of HIV p24 antigen can be detected in plasma or serum by antigen capture enzyme immunosorbent assay (EIA). Because p24 antigen tests can produce false-positive reactions due to interfering substances and immune complexes, positive samples need to be confirmed by a neutralization procedure (58). p24 antigen is usually not detectable during the first 2 weeks after infection, but during acute infection, it becomes detectable before HIV-1 antibody (Fig. 2). However, detection of p24 antigen is transient because, as HIV-1 antibodies begin to develop, they bind to the p24 antigen and form immune complexes that interfere with p24 assay detection, unless the assay includes steps to disrupt the antigen-antibody complexes (59, 60). Modifications to the HIV-1 antigen test have been made to boost the sensitivity of the assay, including acid or heat treatment for dissociation of antigen-antibody complexes (60–63), and increased sensitivity has been achieved by the addition of signal amplification (62). Heat denaturation combined with tyramide signal amplification has been reported to increase the sensitivity of p24 antigen detection to levels comparable to detection of viral RNA by PCR and can be effective for monitoring of responses to antiretroviral therapy (64–66) and for pediatric diagnosis (67, 68) in resource-limited settings when nucleic acid testing is not feasible.

HIV RNA and DNA Qualitative Assays

The Aptima HIV-1 qualitative RNA assay has clinical utility for identification of acute HIV-1 infection and neonatal HIV-1 infection. The test targets both the long terminal repeat and the *pol* gene of the HIV-1 genome, which allows detection of all HIV-1 group M, N, and O viruses. There are three general steps to the assay: target-specific capture of HIV-1 RNA from the clinical specimen, transcription-mediated amplification, and detection using a hybridization protection assay. The assay has a limit of detection of 30 copies/ml of plasma with a specificity of 99.8%.

Detection of HIV-1 DNA can also be used for HIV diagnosis in special situations such as during the acute phase of infection prior to appearance of antibody, in newborns of infected mothers, or in individuals with suppressed viral replication due to immunologic control or antiretroviral therapy. HIV-1 DNA qualitative assays make use of PCR to amplify conserved regions of the HIV-1 genome to detect proviral HIV-1 DNA in peripheral blood mononuclear cells. There are currently no commercially available FDA-approved proviral DNA tests. However, various laboratory-developed tests based on nested as well as real-time PCR procedures are also used. The limit of detection and ability to detect non-B subtypes vary among these assays. The sensitivity and specificity of previously described HIV-1 DNA PCR assays for the diagnosis of neonatal HIV-1 infection have been reported to be 96% and 99%, respectively, at 1 month of age for HIV-1 subtype B (69). The potential utility of qualitative DNA PCR assays in the diagnosis of vertical HIV-1 transmission has been greatly increased with the development of simple and sensitive procedures for dried blood spots.

HIV RNA Viral Load Assays

Viral load assays, which measure the quantity of HIV-1 RNA present in plasma, are used as prognostic indicators, to monitor response to therapy and to determine infectiousness (33, 70). HIV-1 viral load assays have been used most commonly to guide treatment decisions, but because of the relationship between viral load and potential for virus transmission, they are also used as a tool for guiding treatment as prevention interventions (71). In the United States, four commercial assays are FDA approved and available for the quantification of HIV-1 RNA in plasma. A comparison of the specimen requirements and characteristics of the assays is shown in Table 3. None of the viral load assays detect HIV-2.

The more recent nucleic acid assays offer several advantages over the earlier viral load assays, including very broad linear ranges, extensive automation, and decreased risk of carryover contamination. The RealTime HIV-1 assay uses the automated m2000 system, which has two components: the m2000sp for nucleic acid extraction and loading of sample and master mix into the 96-well optical reaction plate, and the m2000rt for amplification and detection. The assay contains an internal control, which is an unrelated RNA sequence that is added to the sample lysis buffer prior to extraction. RNA is captured by magnetic particles, washed to remove unbound material, and eluted. Once the master mix and sample are combined into the reaction plate, the reaction plate is covered and loaded into the m2000rt; these are the only manual steps of the assay. The amplification and detection utilize TaqMan technology. The HIV-1 oligonucleotide probe is a partially double-stranded complex; the long strand is complementary to the HIV-1 target (integrase) and is labeled at the 5′ end with a fluorophore. The shorter strand is complementary to the 5′ end of the long strand and is labeled with a quencher moiety at its 3′ end. When HIV-1 target is present, the HIV-1-specific strand preferentially hybridizes to the target, allowing emission of fluorescence (72, 73). For calculations of viral load values, two assay calibrators are run in replicates of three to generate a calibration curve; the slope and intercept of the curve are stored on the instrument and used to calculate viral load values. The limit of detection of the assay is 40 copies/ml for a 1.0-ml sample volume, 75 copies/ml for a 0.5-ml sample volume, and 150 copies/ml for a 0.2-ml sample volume. The RealTime assay has been designed to quantify all group M, N, and O viruses and CRFs (72, 74).

The Cobas AmpliPrep/Cobas TaqMan HIV-1 test version 2.0 is also based on real-time TaqMan technology and targets two HIV-1 gene regions, LTR and *gag*. The extraction process is automated on the Cobas AmpliPrep instrument using a generic magnetic silica-based capture method and includes a quantitation standard (QS) that is added to each specimen at a known concentration along with the lysis buffer. The extracted sample and the reaction mix are added to amplification tubes on the AmpliPrep instrument, and the amplification and detection are completed on either the Cobas TaqMan analyzer or the Cobas TaqMan 48 analyzer. Docking the Cobas TaqMan analyzer to the AmpliPrep instrument creates a fully automated system. Alternatively, the amplification tubes can be manually loaded into the Cobas TaqMan 48 analyzer. For calculation of viral load values, the fluorescent readings for the QS and target are checked by the instrument software to ensure that they are valid, crossing threshold values are determined, and the viral load value is calculated from lot-specific calibration constants provided by the manufacturer. The amount of QS added to each sample is constant, so if the critical threshold for the QS has been affected, the HIV-1 target concentration is adjusted accordingly. The Cobas AmpliPrep/Cobas TaqMan HIV-1 test has been designed to quantify all group M viruses including CRFs and can also detect group O and N viruses (74–76).

Recently, Roche received approval for a new platform, Cobas 6800/8800, which offers an integrated workflow and decreases hands-on requirements. These systems also allow for mixed batching, making it possible to perform up to three tests in the same run with no presorting of specimens, so specimens can be tested for comorbid pathogens in addition to HIV. As of 2017, the platform allows for various EDTA plasma volumes including both a 500-μl (650 μl required) and 200-μl (350 μl required) test volume. This platform, like the AmpliPrep/Cobas TaqMan HIV-1, uses a dual target design and has a reported linear range of 20 to 10^7 copies (cp) per ml and a reported limit of detection (LOD) of 13.2 cp/ml when using 500 μl and 50 to 10^7 cp/ml and a LOD of 35.5 cp/ml when using 200 μl of EDTA plasma.

In January 2017, the FDA approved the Aptima HIV-1 Quant assay from Hologic. It is intended for quantitation of HIV-1 RNA in human plasma from HIV-1-infected individuals on the fully automated Panther system. The Aptima assay quantitates HIV-1 RNA groups M, N, and O

TABLE 3 FDA-approved viral load assays and specimen requirements[a]

Test and manufacturer	Amplification method; target	Anticoagulant	Plasma volume	Range (copies/ml)	Standards and controls
Aptima HIV-1 Quant (Hologic Inc., Marlborough, MA)	TMA	EDTA, ACD	240 μl + diluent 700 μl	30 to 10,000,000	3 external controls 1 internal QS 1 internal calibrator
Cobas HIV-1 (Roche Diagnostics, Indianapolis, IN)	Real-time RT-PCR; LTR, *gag* gene	EDTA	200 μl 500 μl	50–10,000,000 20–10,000,000	1 internal QS 3 external controls
Cobas AmpliPrep/Cobas TaqMan HIV-1 version 2.0 (Roche Diagnostics, Indianapolis, IN)	Real-time RT-PCR; LTR, *gag* gene	EDTA	1 ml	20–10,000,000	1 internal QS 3 external controls
RealTime HIV-1 (Abbott Molecular, Des Plaines, IL)	Real-time RT-PCR; integrase gene	EDTA, ACD	200 μl 500 μl 1 ml	40–10,000,000	1 internal control 3 external controls Calibration curve Each new lot or every 6 months

[a]TMA, transcription-mediated amplification.

over the range of 30 to 10,000,000 copies/ml from a 700-µl reaction volume of plasma. The assay utilizes transcription-mediated amplification and includes dual-target amplification and detection systems, targeting two regions of the HIV-1 genome (pol and LTR) independently. An independent signal is generated from amplification of each region to minimize the impact of a mutation in either region. A comparison study conducted with the CE-approved version of the Aptima Quant assay found high concordance of the Aptima assay with the Abbott Real-Time and Roche Cobas AmpliPrep/Cobas TaqMan assays (77). As with previous studies, the greatest variability between assays was at the low end of the dynamic range, near the lower limit of quantitation (72–76). Given the recent approval by the FDA, there are no published studies on the performance of the FDA-approved version of the assay, though based on the package inserts there seems to be little to no difference in the CE-marked and U.S. versions of the assay.

The high cost and complex technical requirements of nucleic acid-based testing strategies have resulted in the development of other types of assays for measuring virus quantity in specimens collected in resource-limited settings. Two such assays are the heat-denatured signal-boosted p24 antigen assays (Perkin Elmer, Wellesley, MA) and the RT assay (ExaVir Load assay; Cavidi AB, Uppsala, Sweden) (78, 79). Although both methods are less sensitive and reproducible than the nucleic acid-based assays, they are affordable alternatives to HIV RNA quantification. Numerous efforts are also under way to develop and market point-of-care quantitative assays for HIV-1 nucleic acids. While there are no FDA-approved assays, such tests are now available outside the United States (80).

ISOLATION PROCEDURES

Because HIV can be isolated from the blood of the majority of HIV-infected individuals, HIV culture was frequently utilized in the early years of the epidemic as a diagnostic or prognostic marker or for assessing the efficacy of antiviral therapy (33, 48). The procedure for HIV culture is elaborate and time-consuming (49). Although a positive culture provides direct evidence of HIV infection, HIV culture is utilized primarily in research laboratories and not for routine diagnosis. To isolate HIV, the patient specimen is first cultured by mixing patient cells with cells from healthy donors stimulated with phytohemagglutinin and interleukin-2; fresh stimulated donor cells must be added weekly because HIV-1 produces cell death. In the second step, the presence of RT or p24 antigen released in the culture supernatants is assayed periodically, generally every 3 to 7 days, for approximately 1 month of culture.

Viral culture assays have been used in phenotypic resistance assays and to determine the viral fitness of HIV-1 (50). However, phenotypic resistance assays based on recombinant DNA technology and amplification of plasma viral RNA have obviated the need for viral isolates (51). A commercially available fitness assay, also referred to as a viral replication capacity (RC) assay, has been developed by Monogram BioSciences (South San Francisco, CA). It measures the ability of HIV-1 from a patient undergoing antiretroviral treatment to replicate *in vitro* compared to a wild-type reference virus. The patient RC value is expressed as a percentage of the RC of the wild-type reference standard. The assay uses a retroviral vector constructed from an infectious clone of HIV-1. The vector contains a luciferase expression cassette inserted within a deleted region of the envelope gene (52). HIV-1 protease and RT sequences are amplified from the patient plasma samples and inserted into the vector. The amount of luciferase produced by patient-derived viruses is then compared to the amount of luciferase produced by well-characterized wild-type reference virus. RC has been suggested as an additional parameter for making decisions regarding antiretroviral therapy. Patients who do not experience increases in viral loads despite the accumulation of multiple resistance mutations have been shown to harbor virus with decreased RC (52, 53). In addition, certain drug resistance mutations have been shown to reduce RC (54, 55); lower RC has also been observed in people who become HIV controllers (56).

SEROLOGIC TESTS

Diagnosis of HIV infection has usually been accomplished via detection of HIV antibody using a sensitive initial immunoassay validated by a subsequent supplemental test (81). Because HIV infection typically lasts for years and the initial infection may be minimally symptomatic, most patients who are identified by antibody detection are in the clinically latent or late phases of the illness. Immunoassays for HIV antibody are rapid and economical, but they suffer an important limitation because of the window period, the time between initial infection and the expression of detectable antibody (27). During the window period, active viral replication and high levels of viremia occur. Different types of antibody immunoassays have different window periods, but all tests based on detection of antibody miss patients during early infection. Recognition that the risk of transmission from people with acute infection is much higher than that from people with established infection (82) and indications of the clinical benefits of antiretroviral treatment during acute HIV infection (83) have served as the impetus to adopt techniques that detect HIV earlier after initial infection. Antigen-antibody combination immunoassays and an HIV-1 nucleic acid test that allow earlier detection of HIV have received FDA approval and play an increasingly important role in HIV diagnosis.

Initial Screening Tests

Considerable progress in the development of HIV immunoassays has been made since the discovery of the virus in 1983. Current methods are summarized in Table 4. HIV immunoassays based on different design principles were generally grouped into generations. Because the generation terminology is becoming somewhat difficult to delineate, assays will be described based on the analytes detected in this chapter. The earliest immunoassays are indirect EIAs that use coated (or immobilized) viral lysate antigens derived from cell culture on a solid phase for antibody capture and an indirect format that detects antibody using an anti-human IgG conjugate. These assays are referred to as IgG-sensitive assays. To increase specificity, significant specimen dilution is required to overcome cross-reactivity with cellular protein contaminants. The next immunoassays were developed to use synthetic peptide or recombinant protein antigens alone or combined with viral lysates to bind HIV antibodies, with an indirect immunoassay format that employs labeled anti-human IgG or protein A, which binds to IgG with high affinity (84). Design of the specific antigenic epitopes in these assays improves sensitivity for HIV-1, HIV-1 group O, and HIV-2, allowing earlier detection of IgG antibodies (85). Eliminating cellular antigens that contaminate viral lysates improves specificity by eliminating cross-reactivity with cellular proteins. To improve detection earlier in the course of infection, immunoassays

TABLE 4 FDA-approved laboratory HIV immunoassays

Test	Markers used for detection	Analytes detected
Conventional EIAs		
Avioq HIV-1 Microelisa system	Viral lysate, native gp160	IgG antibodies
Bio-Rad GS HIV-1/2 PLUS O	Recombinant p24, gp160, HIV-2 gp36, synthetic group O peptide	IgG and IgM antibodies
Bio-Rad GS HIV combo Ag/Ab EIA	Synthetic gp41, recombinant gp160, HIV-2 gp36, synthetic group O peptide, p24 monoclonal antibodies	IgG and IgM antibodies p24 antigen
Chemiluminescent Assays		
Abbott Architect HIV Ag/Ab combo	Synthetic and recombinant gp41 and HIV-2 gp36, group O peptide, p24 monoclonal antibodies	IgG and IgM antibodies p24 antigen
Ortho Vitros Anti-HIV 1+2	Recombinant p24, gp41, gp41/120, HIV-2 gp36	IgG and IgM antibodies
Siemens ADVIA Centaur HIV 1/O/2	Recombinant gp41/120, p24, HIV-2 gp36, synthetic group O peptide	IgG and IgM antibodies
ADVIA Centaur HIV Ag/Ab Combo (CHIV) assay	HIV-1 and HIV-2 recombinant antigens, group O peptide antigen, anti-p24 antibody	IgG and IgM antibodies p24 antigen
Roche Elecsys HIV combi PT assay	Recombinant *env-* and *pol* antigens from HIV-1 and HIV-2 and monoclonal antibodies to p24	IgGM and IgM antibodies p24 antigen
Multiplex Flow Assay		
Bio-Rad BioPlex 2200 HIV Ag/Ab	Recombinant HIV-1 gp160, synthetic group O peptide, HIV-2 gp36 peptide, and p24 monoclonal antibodies	HIV-1 and HIV-2 IgG and IgM antibodies and p24 antigen
Geenius HIV 1/2 confirmatory assay	Recombinant gp36 HIV-2 ENV, gp140 HIV-2 ENV, p31 HIV-1 POL, gp160 HIV-1 ENV, p24 HIV-1 GAG; and synthetic gp41 group M and O HIV-1, envelope peptides	HIV-1 and HIV-2 IgG antibodies

were designed to incorporate synthetic peptide or recombinant antigens to bind HIV antibodies, but in an immunometric antigen sandwich format: HIV antibodies in the specimen bind to HIV antigens on the assay substrate and to antigens conjugated to indicator molecules. This allows detection of both IgM and IgG antibodies. These assays are now being referred to as IgM-sensitive assays. Lower sample dilutions and the ability to detect IgM antibodies (which are expressed before IgG antibodies) further reduce the window period during early seroconversion (25, 86, 87). To further increase detection closer to the time of infection, immunoassays use synthetic peptide or recombinant protein antigens in the same antigen sandwich format to detect IgM and IgG antibodies, and also include monoclonal antibodies to detect p24 antigen. Inclusion of p24 antigen capture allows detection of HIV-1 infection before seroconversion (25, 88–91). Most antigen/antibody immunoassays (termed "combo" assays) do not distinguish antibody reactivity from antigen reactivity. However, one new laboratory antigen/antibody combo assay, BioPlex 2200 HIV Ag-Ab, was FDA approved in July 2015 and is intended for the simultaneous detection and differentiation of the individual analytes related to HIV-1 infection and HIV-2 infection, including HIV-1 p24 antigen, anti-HIV-1 (groups M and O) envelope antibodies, and anti-HIV-2 envelope antibodies.

Analyses of specimens from seroconversion panels have established the approximate time of detection by the different formats of immunoassays. Estimates derived from several data sources are outlined schematically in Fig. 2 (25, 27, 85, 89, 92).

Conventional Immunoassays

Conventional immunoassays for laboratory use consist of EIA and chemiluminescent immunoassay (CIA) methods. Most of the commonly used assays incorporate specific antigens for the detection of HIV-1 groups M and O and HIV-2. HIV antigens (and in fourth-generation assays, anti-p24 antibodies) are adsorbed to a solid phase, usually plates, beads, or tubes, which bind HIV antibodies (or p24 antigen) in the specimens. Antibodies (and with antigen/antibody combo assays, p24 antigen) are conjugated to enzymes (alkaline phosphatase or horseradish peroxidase) or to acridinium esters. The indirect EIA format uses an enzyme-labeled antiglobulin conjugate; the antigen-sandwich EIA and CIA formats use a conjugate with enzyme-labeled HIV antigens (or anti-p24 monoclonal antibodies). With an EIA, the end result is a color change, measured as optical density by a spectrophotometer, proportional to the amount of antibody (or antigen) in the specimen. CIA results are expressed in relative light units, also proportional to the amount of antibody (or antigen) in the specimen. Results are compared to those of a calibrator; a result with a signal to cutoff ratio >1.0 is considered to be reactive. Both EIAs and CIAs are suitable for automation. CIAs, characterized by a shorter processing time and wider dynamic range than EIAs, have been developed for random-access immunochemistry platforms with the potential to make laboratory-based HIV testing simpler and faster. As mentioned above, a recent addition to the HIV test market (BioPlex 2200 HIV Ag-Ab) is an assay that is intended for the simultaneous detection and differentiation of the individual analytes related to HIV-1 and HIV-2 infection and includes the ability to differentiate between antigen and antibody detection. This assay has the potential to improve detection of acute HIV infection. The CDC currently maintains a website that highlights the advantages and disadvantages of currently available FDA-approved HIV diagnostic tests. This information is routinely updated and can be found at https://www.cdc.gov/hiv/pdf/testing/hiv-tests-advantages-disadvantages.pdf.

Rapid Immunoassays

The logistics of conventional laboratory HIV immunoassays require phlebotomy and, typically, a follow-up visit for test results after the specimen has been processed. This complicates HIV testing for many hard-to-reach populations for which phlebotomy is impractical; many people may also fail to return for their test results (93). In addition, an immediate HIV test result is medically desirable in certain circumstances when antiretroviral prophylaxis should be initiated promptly, for example, in assessment of the source patient after an occupational blood or body fluid exposure and for pregnant women in labor whose HIV status is unknown (94, 95). To meet these needs, rapid HIV tests have been developed that are suitable for use at the point of care as well as in clinical laboratories.

Rapid HIV immunoassays are single-use devices that use either immunoconcentration (flow-through) or immunochromatographic (lateral flow) principles (96). Flow-through assays require the sequential addition of specimen, conjugate reagent, and a clarifying buffer through a membrane. Lateral flow assays contain all the necessary reagents and are extremely simple to perform because they require the addition of only specimen or specimen and buffer. Rapid tests differ in their required specimen volumes (range, 3 to 50 μl for whole blood, serum, or plasma) and processing times (range, 1 to 20 minutes). Rapid tests that can use direct, unprocessed specimens (whole blood or oral fluid) have been waived under the Clinical Laboratory Improvement Amendments (CLIA) and are especially well suited for testing outside traditional laboratory settings. Nine rapid HIV antibody tests were FDA-approved in the United States as of December 2017 (Table 5). The disadvantages of rapid assays include their subjective interpretation, possible errors if the reader has vision problems such as color blindness, and potential for procedural errors when performed by less-skilled personnel (97, 98). Accurate specimen volumes must be dispensed and tests read within specified time limits, control lines must be observed, and instructions followed carefully. Rapid tests are useful primarily for small-volume testing. Accurate timing of steps can be adversely affected when multiple specimens are tested simultaneously. Nevertheless, rapid HIV tests have become valuable tools for situations in which rapid results are essential and for outreach settings (99).

Published studies suggest that rapid HIV antibody immunoassays perform similarly to laboratory-based conventional immunoassays in established HIV infection (99, 100). However, most use colloidal gold bound to protein A for detection of antibodies; sensitivity with plasma seroconversion panels is similar to that of IgG-sensitive (second-generation) conventional immunoassays (25, 89, 92). Comparative studies of rapid tests performed on oral fluid, whole blood, and serum demonstrate that rapid tests identified fewer HIV infections than conventional laboratory immunoassays, and sensitivity with oral fluid specimens is lower than that with whole blood or serum in people from populations with increased prevalence of early HIV infection (101, 102). One rapid HIV test that detects and distinguishes HIV antibodies and p24 antigen, the Alere Determine HIV Combo, has received FDA approval (Table 5). Its overall seroconversion sensitivity is similar to that of the IgM-sensitive (third-generation) assays; sensitivity of the antigen component is lower than that of laboratory-based fourth-generation assays (102–104).

Alternative Specimens for Antibody Testing

Alternative specimens to blood, serum, or plasma for HIV antibody testing include oral fluid, urine, and dried blood spots. These may be useful in testing of patients who are reluctant to undergo phlebotomy or who have poor vascular access, in mass-screening settings, in locations in which phlebotomy is impossible, in infants, and for seroprevalence studies. It is essential to employ only specimen collection systems and testing methods designed and validated for the specific specimen type. Oral fluid is a complex mixture of secretions from several different sets of glands, as well as transudated plasma from the capillaries of the gum and mucosa. Glandular secretions of saliva primarily contain secretory IgA, which is not a reliable target for diagnostic testing. Most IgG in the oral cavity derives from the crevicular space between the gums and the teeth, and not from salivary glands, or can be obtained by inducing an oral mucosal transudate. The OraSure specimen collection device is designed to collect oral mucosal transudate for conventional testing (105) with an FDA-approved oral fluid-based HIV-1 EIA. Two rapid tests are FDA approved for use with oral fluid as well as whole blood and plasma specimens. However, false-negative and false-positive immunoassay results and indeterminate Western blot results occur more

TABLE 5 FDA-approved rapid and point-of-care HIV tests

Test	Manufacturer	Specimen types	CLIA category	Antigens represented	FDA approval
OraQuick Advance rapid HIV-1/2 antibody test	Orasure Technologies, Inc.	Oral fluid, whole blood, plasma	Waived; moderate complexity	gp41, gp36	2002
Reveal G3 rapid HIV-1 antibody test	MedMira, Inc.	Serum, plasma	Moderate complexity	gp41, gp120	2003
Uni-Gold Recombigen HIV-1/2	Trinity BioTech	Whole blood, serum, plasma	Waived; moderate complexity	gp41, gp120, gp36	2003
Multispot HIV-1/HIV-2 rapid test	Bio-Rad Laboratories	Serum, plasma	Moderate complexity	gp41, gp36	2004
Alere Clearview HIV 1/2 Stat Pak	Chembio Diagnostics	Whole blood, serum, plasma	Waived; moderate complexity	gp41, gp120, gp36	2006
Alere Clearview Complete HIV 1/2	Chembio Diagnostics	Whole blood, serum, plasma	Waived; moderate complexity	gp41, gp120, gp36	2006
INSTI HIV-1 antibody test kit	Biolytical laboratories	Whole blood, serum, plasma	Waived; moderate complexity	gp41, gp36	2010
Chembio DPP HIV-1/2 assay	Chembio Diagnostics	Oral fluid, whole blood, serum, plasma	Moderate complexity	gp 41, gp120, gp36	2012
Alere Determine HIV 1/2 Ag/Ab combo	Alere Scarborough	Whole blood, serum, plasma	Moderate complexity	gp41, gp120, gp36; p24 antibodies	2013

frequently with oral fluid than with serum specimens (101, 106–108). Dried blood spots, after appropriate elution, can be tested for HIV antibody, p24 antigen, and HIV RNA and produce results comparable to those from matched serum or plasma specimens (67, 109–111). In urine, IgG is found in small quantities relative to serum. Sensitivity and specificity of the FDA-approved EIA and Western blot for urine specimens were lower than with matched serum specimens tested with conventional EIAs (112).

Screening for Atypical and HIV-2 Infections

The prevalence of HIV-1 group M subtypes and CRFs varies geographically. All subtypes and most CRFs are found in sub-Saharan Africa. Subtype B is the predominant strain in the United States, Europe, Canada, and Australia. However, the prevalence of non-B subtypes in these countries is increasing. In the United States, non-B infections account for approximately 3 to 5% of HIV infections (113, 114). Current HIV immunoassays reliably detect the overwhelming majority of HIV-1 group M, B, and non-B subtype infections (115, 116). Only three group O infections have been documented in the United States, all in individuals with a link to West Central Africa. HIV-1 group O infections can be missed by immunoassays that do not contain specific reagents for the detection of antibody to group O (117).

Immunoassays specific for detection of HIV-1 antibodies can detect HIV-2 infections due to cross-reactivity to HIV-1 antigen present in the assay. However, detection of HIV-2 infection by HIV-1-only immunoassays is highly variable: different assays detect 51 to 100% of HIV-2 infections (92). The capability of HIV-1/HIV-2 and HIV-2 assays to detect HIV-2 infections must be demonstrated for the assays to obtain approval by regulatory agencies, and most currently available FDA-approved HIV-1/HIV-2 assays incorporate gp36 antigen for reliable detection of HIV-2 (Table 4, Table 5).

Supplemental Assays for HIV

Initial screening immunoassays for HIV are optimized to provide very high sensitivity, often at the expense of specificity. HIV diagnostic testing therefore relies on a sequence of tests used in combination to improve the accuracy of HIV laboratory diagnosis. Specimens that are nonreactive on the initial immunoassay are generally considered HIV negative. If the initial immunoassay result is reactive, it must be followed by one or more supplemental tests. Four assay methods are FDA-approved as supplemental tests: HIV-1 Western blot, indirect immunofluorescent assay (IFA), qualitative HIV-1 RNA assay, and an HIV-1/HIV-2 antibody differentiation assay. Both the Western blot and IFA are highly specific, but because they rely on viral lysate antigens and anti-human IgG conjugates, they detect HIV-1 later during seroconversion than most currently available conventional initial immunoassays and thus may produce false-negative or indeterminate results (118, 119). In addition, because of cross-reactivity, the HIV-1 Western blot has been interpreted as positive for HIV-1 in 46 to 85% of specimens from people infected with HIV-2 (120, 121). An HIV-1 qualitative RNA assay can be used for the diagnosis of acute HIV-1 infection in serum or plasma from patients without antibodies to HIV-1, and as a supplemental test, when it is reactive, for HIV-1 with specimens repeatedly reactive for HIV antibodies. However, HIV-1 RNA is undetectable in 2 to 5% of HIV-1 Western blot-positive specimens from infected people. Therefore, a specimen with a nonreactive HIV-1 RNA qualitative assay result after repeatedly reactive HIV-1/HIV-2 antibody immunoassay results must undergo supplemental antibody testing to confirm whether HIV-1 or HIV-2 antibodies are present (87, 92). An HIV-1/HIV-2 antibody differentiation assay (Multispot, Bio-Rad Laboratories) was approved by the FDA in 2013 for use as a supplemental test and for differentiation of HIV-1 and HIV-2 antibodies. The production of Multispot was discontinued in July 2016. The Geenius HIV 1/2 Confirmatory Assay (Bio-Rad Laboratories, Redmond, WA), which was FDA approved in 2014, is considered a viable substitute for differentiating antibodies to HIV-1 and HIV-2. The Geenius differentiation assay detects only IgG, so it also detects HIV antibodies later during seroconversion than most currently available conventional initial immunoassays.

Historically, the HIV-1 Western blot has been the "gold standard" for HIV diagnosis (81). The Western blot owes its specificity to separation and concentration of viral components (122). A viral lysate of HIV is applied in a gel under an electric field; the mixture of viral components is separated by their molecular weights into specific "bands." Each viral component becomes relatively pure as it is separated. Components are blotted separately onto a membrane which is cut into strips. The testing laboratory incubates the strips with patient serum, plasma, or dried blood spot eluates and then develops the reaction with an enzyme-labeled anti-human antibody. Antibodies to the following HIV-1-associated antigens can be detected: gp160, gp120, p66, p55, p51, gp41, p31, p24, p17, and p15. Additional viral bands may be described by some manufacturers, and the molecular weight of some antigens might vary slightly between assays produced by different manufacturers. Because Western blot antigens are prepared from HIV grown in cell culture, nonviral cellular proteins may be present on the nitrocellulose strip and lead to nonspecific reactions. The interpretation of HIV-1 Western blots predominantly follows CDC guidelines. A positive result requires detection of at least two of three antigens: p24, gp41, or gp120/160 (81). The absence of all bands is a negative result. The presence of HIV-associated bands not meeting the criteria for positivity or the presence of nonviral bands is interpreted as an indeterminate result. After a reactive initial HIV-1/HIV-2 immunoassay, negative or indeterminate HIV-1 Western blot results should also be followed with additional testing specific for HIV-2 antibodies (123). Western blots that include HIV-2 antigens (e.g., gp36 or gp105) are available outside the United States, but none are FDA approved. Line immunoassays employ a principle similar to that of the Western blot, but recombinant or synthetic antigens are placed on the strip instead of viral lysate antigens from an electrophoretic gel. This approach has the advantage of using only viral antigens in the reaction, eliminating the background from cross-reactivity with nonspecific cellular proteins. The manufacturer also has control over the quantity and type of antigens represented and can include HIV-2 and group O antigens to confirm these infections with a single assay (124). The Inno-LIA HIV I/II Score test (Innogenetics, Gent, Belgium) is a line immunoassay that is widely available outside the United States.

The Fluorognost HIV-1 IFA (Sanochemia) has been used as both an initial screening test and as a supplemental test for HIV-1 infection with serum, plasma, and dried blood spot eluates. HIV-infected and uninfected lymphocytes are fixed on a slide. The slide is incubated first with patient serum and then with a fluorescent-labeled anti-human antibody (125). For interpretation, patterns of fluorescence in infected and uninfected cells are compared for each patient specimen; fluorescence on the infected lymphocytes that exceeds that from nonspecific antibody binding on the uninfected lymphocytes is interpreted as a positive result. Considerable skill is required, and indeterminate results can be produced in patients with autoantibodies and other conditions. In addition to its use as an independent supplemental test, IFA can be used to resolve indeterminate HIV-1 Western blots. An HIV-2-specific IFA has been described, but it is not FDA approved.

The APTIMA HIV-1 qualitative assay is FDA approved for detection of HIV-1. HIV-1 RNA in the test specimen is hybridized to capture nucleotides homologous to highly conserved regions of HIV-1. The hybridized target is then captured onto magnetic microparticles and separated from plasma in a magnetic field. Target amplification occurs via transcription-based nucleic acid amplification. Detection is achieved by chemiluminescent-labeled nucleic acid probes that hybridize specifically to the amplicon. The chemiluminescent signal, measured in a luminometer, is reported as relative light units. Analytical sensitivity is 30 copies/ml of HIV-1 RNA. Quantitative viral HIV-1 and HIV-2 RNA and DNA nucleic acid amplification tests (NAATs) are also available but are not FDA approved for HIV diagnosis.

The Multispot HIV-1/HIV-2 rapid test (Bio-Rad Laboratories, Redmond WA) was a flow-through rapid EIA that differentiated HIV-1 and HIV-2 antibodies in a single-use cartridge. Sensitivity of the Multispot antibody differentiation assay for established HIV infection was comparable to that of the HIV-1 Western blot, but it produced fewer indeterminate results and accurately identified HIV-2 antibodies, including those in specimens misclassified as HIV-1 by the HIV-1 Western blot (118, 119, 126, 127). Because of cross-reactivity, approximately 0.4% of reactive specimens remained dually reactive at the HIV-1 and HIV-2 spots after recommended dilution procedures (119). Although most dually reactive specimens represented HIV-1 infections with cross-reactivity to HIV-2 (128), one U.S. study of five dually reactive specimens found detectable HIV-2 RNA in the one specimen with strong HIV-2 reactivity, suggesting that strong reactivity at the HIV-2 spot indicated the need for further investigation with HIV-2 NAT (126). Testing with Multispot has ended because the manufacturer has ceased production of the test. However, the manufacturer of Multispot introduced a new supplemental test to the market, which according to clinical trials has similar performance characteristics as those described for Multispot. This test, Geenius HIV1/2 supplemental assay (Bio-Rad Laboratories, Redmond, WA), is an immunochromatographic test. The Geenius HIV 1/2 supplemental assay cassette contains antibody-binding protein A, which is conjugated to colloidal gold dye particles, and HIV-1 and HIV-2 antigens (gp36 HIV-2 envelope peptide, gp140 HIV-2 envelope peptides, p31 HIV-1 polymerase peptide, gp160 HIV-1 envelope recombinant protein, gp41 group M and O HIV-1 envelope peptides, and p24 HIV-1 core recombinant protein) which are bound to the membrane solid phase. The sample is applied to the sample plus buffer well. After the sample and buffer have migrated onto the test strip, additional buffer is added to the buffer well. The buffer causes the specimens and reagents to flow laterally and facilitates the binding of antibodies to the antigens. In a reactive sample, the antibodies are captured by the antigens immobilized in the test area. The protein A-colloidal gold binds to the captured antibodies, causing development of pink/purple lines. When there are no HIV antibodies, there are no pink/purple lines in the test area. The sample continues to migrate through the membrane, and a pink/purple line develops in the control (C) area, which contains protein A. In the FDA-approved version, the results are read with a reader that incorporates a standardized algorithm to make a final determination of HIV-1 or HIV-2 reactivity. Several studies have assessed the performance of the Geenius test in the currently recommended laboratory algorithm, and the data indicate comparable performance for detection of HIV-1 and HIV-2 infection compared to the Multispot assay (129–131).

ANTIVIRAL SUSCEPTIBILIES

Resistance testing is an essential element in the management of antiretroviral therapy. It is important for the selection of initial regimens because of the prevalence of transmitted drug resistance in therapy-naive patients and for the selection of the antiretroviral treatment in patients who are failing their current regimen due to the development of antiviral resistance (http://aidsinfo.nih.gov).

The clinical utility of HIV resistance testing has been evaluated in a number of prospective randomized clinical trials (50, 132, 133). Patients whose antiretroviral treatment was based on the results of resistance testing had greater decreases in viral load than patients in whom the antiretroviral regimen was based on prior antiretroviral usage, and the use of resistance testing to guide treatment is cost-effective (134, 135). Two types of methods are available to assay for HIV resistance. Genotyping tests examine the population of viral genomes in the patient sample for the presence of mutations known to confer decreased sensibility to antiretroviral drugs. Phenotypic assays measure viral replication of the patient's virus in the presence of antiretroviral drugs. In addition, HIV tropism assays have become important to evaluate susceptibility to HIV entry inhibitors that target viruses that use CCR5 for cell entry. Table 6 provides a list of the commonly available commercial HIV-1 resistance and tropism assays.

Genotyping Assays

The initial steps of genotypic assays include extraction of viral RNA from plasma and RT-PCR to amplify viral RNA sequences which code for portions of the viral genome that are targeted by antiretroviral drugs. These sequences include genes in the pol region of the virus for RT, protease, and integrase as well as envelope regions related to the entry inhibitors. The nucleotide sequence is determined and examined for the presence of known resistance mutations. This can be accomplished most commonly using automated sequencing technology. The nucleotide sequence of the gene of interest is obtained and compared to the sequence of wild-type virus to identify resistance mutations. The process requires alignment and editing of the sequence, comparison to the wild-type sequence, and final interpretation to identify mutations associated with resistance to specific antiretroviral drugs. FDA-cleared kits containing sequencing reagents and the software programs required for sequence alignment and interpretation are commercially available. The Trugene HIV-1 genotyping kit, which has been discontinued, the OpenGene DNA sequencing system (Siemens Healthcare Diagnostics), and the ViroSeq HIV-1 genotyping system (Abbott Molecular) have been found to perform in an equivalent manner (136). These tests detect mutations in the RT and protease genes but do not detect mutations associated with resistance to the integrase or CCR5 inhibitors. Laboratory-developed tests are available from referral laboratories that detect mutations associated with other classes of drugs such as integrases and entry inhibitors. The databases used for interpretation of resistance mutations require regular updating because the number of new antiretroviral drugs continues to expand.

TABLE 6 Viral RNA HIV-1 resistance and tropism assays

Test	Format	Description[a]
Viroseq HIV-1 genotyping system (Abbott Molecular, Des Plaines, IL)	Genotypic resistance	Detects protease and RT mutations
ViroSeq HIV-1 integrase genotyping kit (RUO) (Abbott Molecular, Des Plaines, IL)	Genotypic resistance	Detects integrase mutations but not FDA approved for clinical use.
GenoSure MG (Monogram Biosciences, South San Francisco, CA)	Genotypic resistance	Detects protease and RT mutations
GenoSure PRIme (Monogram Biosciences, South San Francisco, CA)	Genotypic resistance	Detects protease, RT, and integrase mutations
Trofile (Monogram Biosciences, South San Francisco, CA)	Cell tropism-enotype	Determines virus cell tropism
HIV-1 Genotype (Quest Diagnostics)	Genotypic resistance	Detects protease and RT mutations
HIV-1 Integrase Genotype (Quest Diagnostics)	Genotypic resistance	Detects integrase mutations
HIV-1 Coreceptor Tropism, Ultradeep Sequencing (Quest Diagnostics)	Genotypic resistance and cell tropism	Detect mutations associated with resistance to RTIs and PIs and determines eligibility for therapy with CCR5 antagonist
PhenoSense HIV (RT and protease inhibitors) (Monogram Biosciences, South San Francisco, CA)	Phenotypic resistance	Measures decrease in replication in presence of drug
PhenoSense for entry inhibitor susceptibility (Monogram Biosciences, South San Francisco, CA)	Phenotypic resistance	Measures decrease in replication in presence of drug
PhenoSense integrase (Monogram Biosciences, South San Francisco, CA)	Phenotypic resistance	Measures decrease in replication in presence of drug
PhenoSense Entry (Monogram Biosciences, South San Francisco, CA)	Phenotypic resistance	Assesses resistance to entry inhibitor enfuvirtide
PhenoSense GT (Monogram Biosciences, South San Francisco, CA)	Genotypic and phenotypic resistance	Detects protease and RT mutations and determines decrease in replication in presence of drug
PhenoSense GT Plus Integrase (Monogram Biosciences, South San Francisco, CA)	Genotypic and phenotypic resistance	Detects protease, RT, and integrase mutations and determines decrease in replication in presence of drug

[a]RTIs, reverse transcriptase inhibitors; PIs, protease inhibitors.

One limitation of the FDA-cleared genotypic assays that rely on Sanger sequencing technology is that they are only able to detect mutants that make up major fractions of the patient's virus: resistant variants must constitute at least 25 to 30% of the virus population (137). Although the clinical significance of resistant mutations present at low levels remains to be fully elucidated, there is evidence that minor mutations which are missed by standard genotyping assays can lead to failure of subsequent treatments (138). Because standard genotyping assays lack sensitivity for low-frequency drug resistance mutations, efforts are under way to increase sensitivity by various methods, including PCR-based assays (139) and single-genome analysis (140). These techniques are not FDA cleared. However, given the advantages, next-generation sequencing technologies offer the promise of decreasing the cost of sequencing, and evaluations of this approach for clinical use have been conducted (141). There are laboratory-developed tests that are currently in use by specialty reference labs such as Monogram Biosciences (https://www.monogrambio.com/hiv-tests/genotyping-vs-phenotyping) that are using next-generation sequencing technology.

Phenotyping Assays

Phenotyping assays measure the ability of HIV-1 to grow in the presence of various concentrations of an antiretroviral agent. The amount of drug required to inhibit virus replication by 50% or by 90% is determined and given as a 50% or 90% inhibitory concentration (IC_{50} or IC_{90}). The IC_{50} or IC_{90} obtained with the patient sample is compared to a control wild-type virus, and the result is reported as a relative difference. Early phenotypic resistance assays were labor-intensive because they necessitated the isolation and culture of HIV from the patient's specimen. Currently, commercially available methods use HIV-1 RNA amplified from plasma and are based on recombinant DNA technology. These phenotypic assays are automated but remain labor-intensive and technically complex. They have not been developed in a kit format and are primarily performed by two commercial laboratories: Quest and Monogram Biosciences (South San Francisco, CA). The first step involves extraction of HIV-1 RNA from plasma followed by reverse transcription and PCR amplification of the viral genes. The amplified genes from the patient's specimen are then inserted into vectors that contain a backbone of characterized HIV or are used to make pseudo-viruses containing the patient's viral sequences. Replication of these viruses at different drug concentrations is monitored by expression of a reporter gene and is compared with replication of a reference HIV strain, and recombinants are used in culture to examine resistance. As with genotypic testing, the phenotypic assays can only detect mutant variants that make up at least 25% of the viral population.

In general, genotypic assays are used for recently diagnosed individuals to guide optimal therapy due to reduced cost and shorter turnaround time. In situations of therapy failure, a combination of genotypic and phenotypic assays is often used to guide optimal therapy.

Tropism Assays

The CCR5 inhibitor, maraviroc, has brought about a need for a cell tropism assay, because the drug is only effective against virus that uses CCR5 as a coreceptor for entry. The drug is not active against CXCR4-tropic virus or dual/mixed tropic virus. The tropism assay must be performed prior to initiating maraviroc or any other CCR5 inhibitor to determine whether the virus is CCR5 tropic. Like other drug resistance assays, there are two general approaches in use, and two tropism assays are commercially available. The Trofile assay (Monogram Biosciences) uses the phenotypic approach, and Quest Diagnostics offers an HIV-1 Coreceptor Tropism assay based on Ultradeep Sequencing (Quest Diagnostics), which uses the genotypic approach. For the Trofile assay, the *env* gene from the patient is amplified and used to construct pseudoviruses. Coreceptor tropism is then determined by measuring the ability of the pseudo-viral population to infect CD41/U87 cells that express either CXCR4 or CCR5. Depending on which cells they infect, the viruses are then designated CXCR4 tropic, CCR5 tropic, or dual/mixed tropic (141). Only patients that are solely CCR5 tropic are candidates for a CCR5 inhibitor. Resistance to maraviroc has been reported and results from the development of mutations that allow the virus to use CXCR4 coreceptors or mutations that lead to structural changes in the envelope that prevent the drug from being effective (142, 143).

EVALUATION, INTERPRETATION, AND REPORTING OF RESULTS

Use and Interpretation of Immunoassays

Currently available conventional immunoassays are exquisitely sensitive and specific. False-negative results may occur during early infection, before the appearance of antigen or antibodies (101, 102). Occurrences of delayed seroconversion have also been reported in people taking antiretroviral therapy for pre- and postexposure prophylaxis (144, 145). False-positive results are rare but have been reported to occur transiently after recent immunizations and may also occur in recipients of experimental HIV vaccines (146–148). As with any screening test, positive predictive value may be low in populations with low prevalence. The currently FDA-approved rapid methods have comparable sensitivity to conventional immunoassays for established infection but produce more false-negative results during early infection (149). False-negative and false-positive results occur more frequently with oral fluid than with blood or serum specimens (101, 106).

No single supplemental assay is adequate to confirm the presence of HIV infection in all specimens after a reactive initial immunoassay. The Western blot and IFA are less sensitive than either IgM-sensitive or antigen/antibody combo immunoassays during early infection and may give negative or indeterminate results (86, 150). HIV-1 RNA may be undetectable in 2 to 5% of infected people who are antibody-positive (92, 151). Therefore, the CDC and the Association of Public Health Laboratories published update guidelines for laboratory testing for HIV in 2014 (Fig. 3). These guidelines along with recent technical updates can be found at https://stacks.cdc.gov/view/cdc/23447. The algorithm published in 2014 maximizes the ability to detect acute HIV-1 infections and to correctly classify HIV-2 infections. Testing begins with an initial antigen/antibody combo immunoassay. If reactive, this is followed by an HIV-1/HIV-2 antibody differentiation assay. Reactive results on the initial immunoassay and the antibody differentiation assay confirm the presence of HIV-1 or HIV-2 antibodies; no further testing is necessary. Specimens that are nonreactive or indeterminate on the antibody differentiation assay undergo testing with HIV-1 NAT. A reactive antigen/antibody combo immunoassay result, negative antibody differentiation assay result, and reactive HIV-1 NAT result are consistent with the presence of acute HIV-1 infection; a nonreactive NAT indicates false-positive results from the initial immunoassay. The same sequence of supplemental tests should be performed if an IgM/IgG antibody assay is used as the initial test. Reports of HIV test results should specify all assays that were used, the results of each assay, and an interpretation of the test results. Suggestions for reporting language are available from the New York State Health Department and Clinical and Laboratory Standards Institute and the Association of Public Health Laboratories (152, 153).

Positive results from the testing algorithm indicate the need for HIV medical care and an initial evaluation that includes additional laboratory tests such as HIV-1 viral load, CD4+ determination, and an antiretroviral resistance assay to stage HIV disease and to assist in the selection of

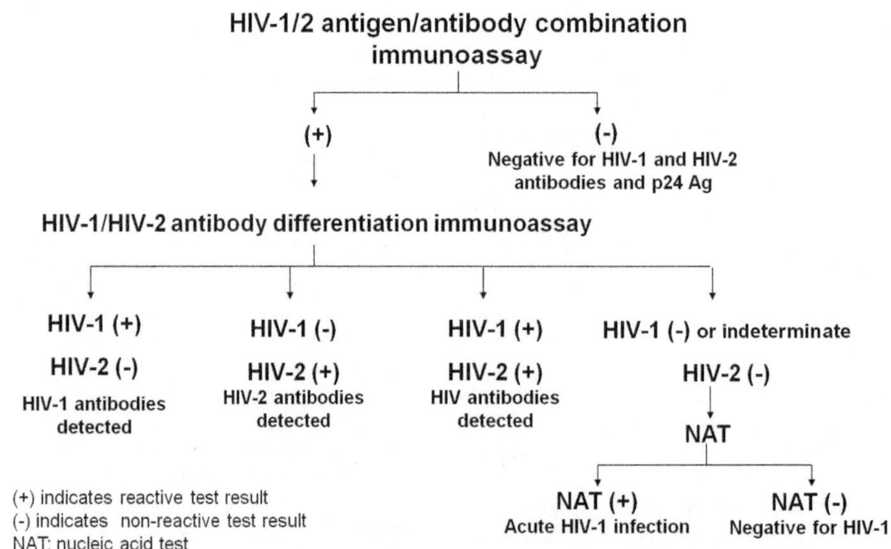

FIGURE 3 Diagnostic HIV testing algorithm showing sequence of follow-up testing.

an initial antiretroviral drug regimen (154). No diagnostic test or algorithm can be completely accurate in all cases of HIV infection. Inconsistent or conflicting test results obtained during the clinical evaluation, or results that are inconsistent with clinical findings, warrant additional testing of follow-up specimens with different assays.

Specimens submitted to a laboratory for testing after a reactive rapid HIV test result that was obtained in an outreach setting should proceed through the same laboratory algorithm as other specimens. This recommendation is based on not having an official record of rapid test results performed in outreach settings. Assays used in the updated CDC laboratory testing algorithm are not suitable for use with oral fluid, dried blood spots, or urine. Testing of these alternative specimens is conducted with the specific immunoassays approved for these types of specimens.

Use and Interpretation of Qualitative HIV RNA and DNA Assays

In adults, HIV-1 RNA tests are primarily used to diagnose acute infection, either as part of the diagnostic algorithm or as part of strategies that conduct pooled testing of specimens that are immunoassay-negative (155, 156). Nucleic acid tests are needed for infant diagnosis because serologic tests are not useful for the detection of HIV infection in infants; maternal antibodies can persist in uninfected, HIV-exposed infants until 18 months of age. Both HIV-1 RNA and DNA tests can be used for the diagnosis of neonatal HIV-1 infection. DNA has often been the preferred method for determining an exposed infant's HIV-1 infection status, but recent studies suggest that HIV-1 RNA is more sensitive at birth and at 4 weeks of age (157). The DNA or RNA assay can be performed on whole blood or dried blood spots, but the specimen collected at birth must be a neonatal and not a cord blood sample: cord blood samples yield a high rate of false-positive results (158). Current recommendations are to test HIV-exposed infants within 14 days of life and at 1 to 2 months and 4 to 6 months after birth, with some experts also recommending testing at birth for improved treatment outcomes and the very recent data related to a functional cure in an infant (159–161). HIV-1 infection in neonates is diagnosed by two positive RNA or DNA tests performed on separate blood samples regardless of age. Qualitative test characteristics vary, and the population tested may influence the optimal test to be used. The Aptima qualitative test may be more sensitive than some HIV-1 DNA tests for the detection of non-B subtypes, CRFs, and group O virus. An advantage of proviral DNA tests is that they generally remain positive even in individuals receiving effective antiretroviral therapy and individuals that naturally suppress virus replication. However, no proviral DNA assays are currently FDA approved.

Use and Interpretation of Viral Load Assays

The clinical utility of HIV-1 viral load testing has been well established. Viral load assays are used widely to monitor changes in plasma viremia during antiretroviral therapy because they are useful for predicting time to progression to AIDS and monitoring responses to therapy. The magnitude of the decrease in viral load is dependent on the effectiveness of the antiretroviral therapy. The goal of optimum therapy is to suppress viral loads below the detection limit of the assay. Baseline testing of HIV-1 RNA viral load should be obtained before initiating therapy, and determinations should be repeated before changing antiretroviral therapy regimens. After initiation of therapy, patients should be tested within 2 to 8 weeks to assess drug efficacy and then every 3 to 4 months to assess durability of response. Updated guidelines on using viral load to guide antiretroviral treatment are maintained at http://aidsinfo.nih.gov/guidelines.

Biological variation of HIV-1 RNA levels among clinically stable patients has been estimated to be approximately 0.3 $\log_{10}$ (162). Reproducibility of commercial assays ranges from 0.1 to 0.3 $\log_{10}$ depending on the region of the assay's dynamic range. The clinical implications of HIV RNA levels in the range of >48 to <200 copies/ml in a patient on antiretroviral therapy are controversial. Persistent HIV RNA levels >200 copies/ml often are associated with evidence of viral evolution and drug resistance mutation accumulation (163); persistent plasma HIV RNA levels in the 200 to 1,000 copies/ml range should therefore be considered as virologic failure. "Blips" of viremia (e.g., viral suppression followed by a detectable HIV RNA level and then subsequent return to undetectable levels) usually are not associated with subsequent virologic failure (164).

Numerous studies comparing the performance of the conventional FDA-approved assays have been conducted showing high correlations between assays and similar net changes in plasma RNA levels after antiretroviral therapy (165–167). Early assays showed larger variations between assays with the same sample, but current-generation assays have been standardized so that the differences between assays are narrowing. Although there is overall good agreement between the different viral load assays, it is still considered optimal for patient care to monitor viral load values over time with the same assay; some variability exists among platforms in immunologically stable patients with very low viral loads near the limits of detection (167).

HIV-1 RNA load testing is sometimes requested to resolve equivocal serologic findings, to facilitate the diagnosis of HIV-1 infection during the acute phase of infection, or for pediatric diagnosis. Viral load tests can be performed for these purposes with a physician's order, but they are not approved by the FDA for the diagnosis of HIV-1 infection, and they should be validated within a laboratory prior to routine use for these purposes. False-positive results can be obtained because of contamination during specimen processing, carryover of amplified products, or by selecting incorrect thresholds for defining positivity.

Use and Interpretation of Resistance Assays

Clinical guidelines for the use of HIV-1 resistance testing in adults are published and updated on a regular basis (168). In general, resistance testing is recommended for patients entering care even if therapy is not immediately initiated, when initiating antiretroviral therapy, for patients failing therapy, for pregnant women, and for patients with acute infection. Genotypic assays are generally more widely available, technically easier to perform, faster, and less expensive than phenotypic assays. In some cases, a resistance mutation may be detectable before a change in the phenotype has occurred, and therefore, genotypic and phenotypic results are not always correlated. One limitation of genotyping assays originates from the complexity of data they generate. In the face of the rapid development of new drugs and new information on HIV-1 resistance, it remains challenging to keep databases updated on which mutations are associated with specific drug combinations. Updated lists of drug-resistant mutations for all classes of drug are available at the International AIDS Society-USA website (http://www.iasusa.org) and the Stanford University website (http://hivdb.stanford.edu/).

Interpretation of HIV-1 genotyping results is complex. It requires knowledge of the identity of mutations associated with each specific drug, the interactions of resistance mutations, and the genetics of cross-resistance. Most systems use a rule-based approach; a group of experts establish interpretation algorithms based on the types of mutations or combination of mutations that are associated with resistance to specific drugs. Depending on the mutations detected, the report indicates, for each drug in each of the antiviral categories, whether HIV in the patient sample shows no evidence of resistance, resistance, or possible resistance, or if evidence is insufficient to categorize the virus in one of the three other categories. These rule-based systems provide easy-to-interpret information to clinicians, but the databases require regular updating. The manufacturer's database update may lag behind the published literature, so clinicians may find it necessary to refer to one of the online databases for the most up-to-date information. For this reason, it is very helpful for laboratories to report both the specific mutations and the interpretation to clinicians so they can easily use online databases.

Phenotyping assays provide results in a format that is more familiar to clinicians. Results are reported as a relative change in IC_{50} compared to wild-type virus. In addition, there is less need for expert interpretation because susceptibility is measured directly. One problem with phenotypic resistance testing is that drugs are used in combination but are not tested in combination. Thus, synergistic effects are not detectable. Cutoffs for a significant change in IC_{50} can also vary greatly depending on the drug. Initially, biological cutoffs were established based on the reproducibility of the assays; however, over time, clinical cutoffs correlated with outcome have been established for most drugs.

Most genotypic and phenotypic assays generally only yield results if the plasma used for testing contains at least 500 HIV-1 RNA copies/ml. Depending on the extraction method used, it may be possible to obtain results on specimens with a lower viral load. Concentration of the virions in plasma by high-speed centrifugation may allow sequencing of specimens with viral loads below 500 copies/ml, but this process may also concentrate inhibitors and interfering substances. Due to the labor and expense involved with genotyping assays, laboratories should establish the lower viral load limit for obtaining reliable sequencing results. In addition, for both types of assays, the resistant viral mutant must constitute at least 20 to 30% of the viral quasi-species to be detected. Cross-contamination can occur with both genotypic and phenotypic resistance assays because both procedures rely on an RT-PCR step to amplify HIV-1 gene sequences. Both methods have clinical utility in managing patients and are widely used in clinical practice. However, given the wider availability, faster turnaround time, and lower cost, most clinicians use genotyping for the initial evaluation of resistance. Phenotyping assays, on the other hand, can help in defining the significance of newly recognized resistance mutations and in elucidating the effects of complex mutation interactions and may be very helpful in determining salvage regimens. The continued improvements in antiretroviral therapy also necessitate continued improvement in drug resistance testing technology. While there are no FDA-cleared tests based on next-generation sequencing technology, there is considerable research and progress toward using this technology for HIV drug resistance monitoring. Potential advantages of such technology are decreased cost and the ability to detect very low levels of resistant virus (169–171). For example, next-generation sequencing has the potential to detect mutations that occur at a frequency as low as 1 to 5% or what is considered to be just above the background of naturally occurring rates of mutation (172).

REFERENCES

1. **Masur H, Michelis MA, Greene JB, Onorato I, Vande Stouwe RA, Holzman RS, Wormser G, Brettman L, Lange M, Murray HW, Cunningham-Rundles S.** 1981. An outbreak of community-acquired *Pneumocystis carinii* pneumonia: initial manifestation of cellular immune dysfunction. *N Engl J Med* **305:**1431–1438.
2. **Barré-Sinoussi F, Chermann JC, Rey F, Nugeyre MT, Chamaret S, Gruest J, Dauguet C, Axler-Blin C, Vézinet-Brun F, Rouzioux C, Rozenbaum W, Montagnier L.** 1983. Isolation of a T-lymphotropic retrovirus from a patient at risk for acquired immune deficiency syndrome (AIDS). *Science* **220:**868–871.
3. **Gallo RC, Salahuddin SZ, Popovic M, Shearer GM, Kaplan M, Haynes BF, Palker TJ, Redfield R, Oleske J, Safai B, White G, Foster P, Markham PD.** 1984. Frequent detection and isolation of cytopathic retroviruses (HTLV-III) from patients with AIDS and at risk for AIDS. *Science* **224:** 500–503.
4. **Levy JA, Hoffman AD, Kramer SM, Landis JA, Shimabukuro JM, Oshiro LS.** 1984. Isolation of lymphocytopathic retroviruses from San Francisco patients with AIDS. *Science* **225:**840–842.
5. **Coffin J, et al.** 1986. What to call the AIDS virus? *Nature* **321:**10.
6. **Clavel F, Guetard D, Brun-Vezinet F, Chamaret S, Rey M, Santos-Ferreira M, Laurent A, Dauguet C, Katlama C, Rouzioux C,** et al. 1986. Isolation of a new human retrovirus from West African patients with AIDS. *Science* **233:**343–346.
7. **Hahn BH, Shaw GM, De Cock KM, Sharp PM.** 2000. AIDS as a zoonosis: scientific and public health implications. *Science* **287:**607–614.
8. **Sharp PM, Bailes E, Robertson DL, Gao F, Hahn BH.** 1999. Origins and evolution of AIDS viruses. *Biol Bull* **196:**338–342.
9. **Zhu T, Korber BT, Nahmias AJ, Hooper E, Sharp PM, Ho DD.** 1998. An African HIV-1 sequence from 1959 and implications for the origin of the epidemic. *Nature* **391:**594–597.
10. **McCutchan FE.** 2006. Global epidemiology of HIV. *J Med Virol* **78**(Suppl 1)**:**S7–S12.
11. **McCutchan FE.** 2000. Understanding the genetic diversity of HIV-1. *AIDS* **14**(Suppl 3)**:**S31–S44.
12. **Plantier JC, Leoz M, Dickerson JE, De Oliveira F, Cordonnier F, Lemée V, Damond F, Robertson DL, Simon F.** 2009. A new human immunodeficiency virus derived from gorillas. *Nat Med* **15:**871–872.
13. **Robertson DL, Anderson JP, Bradac JA, Carr JK, Foley B, Funkhouser RK, Gao F, Hahn BH, Kalish ML, Kuiken C, Learn GH, Leitner T, McCutchan F, Osmanov S, Peeters M, Pieniazek D, Salminen M, Sharp PM, Wolinsky S, Korber B.** 2000. HIV-1 nomenclature proposal. *Science* **288:**55–56.
14. **Los Alamos National Laboratory HIV Sequence Database.** 2 Feb 2012, posting date. HIV and SIV nomenclature. https://www.hiv.lanl.gov/content/sequence/HIV/COMPENDIUM/2012compendium.html.
15. **Perelson AS, Neumann AU, Markowitz M, Leonard JM, Ho DD.** 1996. HIV-1 dynamics *in vivo*: virion clearance rate, infected cell life-span, and viral generation time. *Science* **271:**1582–1586.
16. **Feng Y, Broder CC, Kennedy PE, Berger EA.** 1996. HIV-1 entry cofactor: functional cDNA cloning of a seven-transmembrane, G protein-coupled receptor. *Science* **272:**872–877.
17. **Choe H, Farzan M, Sun Y, Sullivan N, Rollins B, Ponath PD, Wu L, Mackay CR, LaRosa G, Newman W, Gerard N, Gerard C, Sodroski J.** 1996. The beta-chemokine receptors CCR3 and CCR5 facilitate infection by primary HIV-1 isolates. *Cell* **85:**1135–1148.
18. **UNAIDS.** 2017. 2017 global fact sheet. http://www.unaids.org/sites/default/files/media_asset/UNAIDS_FactSheet_en.pdf.
19. **Campbell-Yesufu OT, Gandhi RT.** 2011. Update on human immunodeficiency virus (HIV)-2 infection. *Clin Infect Dis* **52:**780–787.
20. **Centers for Disease Control and Prevention.** 2017. HIV basic statistics. https://www.cdc.gov/hiv/statistics/overview/ataglance.html.

21. **Royce RA, Seña A, Cates W Jr, Cohen MS.** 1997. Sexual transmission of HIV. *N Engl J Med* **336:**1072–1078.
22. **Bell DM.** 1997. Occupational risk of human immunodeficiency virus infection in healthcare workers: an overview. *Am J Med* **102**(5B)**:**9–15.
23. **Montano M, Russell M, Gilbert P, Thior I, Lockman S, Shapiro R, Chang SY, Lee TH, Essex M.** 2003. Comparative prediction of perinatal human immunodeficiency virus type 1 transmission, using multiple virus load markers. *J Infect Dis* **188:**406–413.
24. **Cooper ER, Charurat M, Mofenson L, Hanson IC, Pitt J, Diaz C, Hayani K, Handelsman E, Smeriglio V, Hoff R, Blattner W, Women and Infants' Transmission Study Group.** 2002. Combination antiretroviral strategies for the treatment of pregnant HIV-1-infected women and prevention of perinatal HIV-1 transmission. *J Acquir Immune Defic Syndr* **29:**484–494.
25. **Delaney KP, Hanson DL, Masciotra S, Ethridge SF, Wesolowski L, Owen SM.** 2017. Time until emergence of HIV test reactivity following infection with HIV-1: implications for interpreting test results and retesting after exposure. *Clin Infect Dis* **64:**53–59.
26. **Cohen MS, Shaw GM, McMichael AJ, Haynes BF.** 2011. Acute HIV-1 infection. *N Engl J Med* **364:**1943–1954.
27. **Fiebig EW, Wright DJ, Rawal BD, Garrett PE, Schumacher RT, Peddada L, Heldebrant C, Smith R, Conrad A, Kleinman SH, Busch MP.** 2003. Dynamics of HIV viremia and antibody seroconversion in plasma donors: implications for diagnosis and staging of primary HIV infection. *AIDS* **17:**1871–1879.
28. **Daar ES, Little S, Pitt J, Santangelo J, Ho P, Harawa N, Kerndt P, Giorgi JV, Bai J, Gaut P, Richman DD, Mandel S, Nichols S, Los Angeles County Primary HIV Infection Recruitment Network.** 2001. Diagnosis of primary HIV-1 infection. *Ann Intern Med* **134:**25–29.
29. **Daar ES, Pilcher CD, Hecht FM.** 2008. Clinical presentation and diagnosis of primary HIV-1 infection. *Curr Opin HIV AIDS* **3:**10–15.
30. **Hecht FM, Busch MP, Rawal B, Webb M, Rosenberg E, Swanson M, Chesney M, Anderson J, Levy J, Kahn JO.** 2002. Use of laboratory tests and clinical symptoms for identification of primary HIV infection. *AIDS* **16:**1119–1129.
31. **Kahn JO, Walker BD.** 1998. Acute human immunodeficiency virus type 1 infection. *N Engl J Med* **339:**33–39.
32. **Mellors JW, Muñoz A, Giorgi JV, Margolick JB, Tassoni CJ, Gupta P, Kingsley LA, Todd JA, Saah AJ, Detels R, Phair JP, Rinaldo CR Jr.** 1997. Plasma viral load and CD4+ lymphocytes as prognostic markers of HIV-1 infection. *Ann Intern Med* **126:**946–954.
33. **Mellors JW, Rinaldo CR Jr, Gupta P, White RM, Todd JA, Kingsley LA.** 1996. Prognosis in HIV-1 infection predicted by the quantity of virus in plasma. *Science* **272:**1167–1170.
34. **Pantaleo G, Graziosi C, Demarest JF, Butini L, Montroni M, Fox CH, Orenstein JM, Kotler DP, Fauci AS.** 1993. HIV infection is active and progressive in lymphoid tissue during the clinically latent stage of disease. *Nature* **362:**355–358.
35. **Okulicz JF, Marconi VC, Landrum ML, Wegner S, Weintrob A, Ganesan A, Hale B, Crum-Cianflone N, Delmar J, Barthel V, Quinnan G, Agan BK, Dolan MJ, Infectious Disease Clinical Research Program (IDCRP) HIV Working Group.** 2009. Clinical outcomes of elite controllers, viremic controllers, and long-term nonprogressors in the US Department of Defense HIV natural history study. *J Infect Dis* **200:**1714–1723.
36. **Ho DD, Neumann AU, Perelson AS, Chen W, Leonard JM, Markowitz M.** 1995. Rapid turnover of plasma virions and CD4 lymphocytes in HIV-1 infection. *Nature* **373:**123–126.
37. **Dubravac T, Gahan TF, Pentella MA.** 2013. Use of the Abbott Architect HIV antigen/antibody assay in a low incidence population. *J Clin Virol* **58**(Suppl 1)**:**e76–e78.
38. **Branson BM, Ginocchio CG.** 2013. HIV laboratory diagnosis: new tests and a new algorithm. *J Clin Virol* **58**(Suppl 1)**:**e1–e133.
39. **Selik RM, Mokotoff ED, Branson B, Owen SM, Whitmore S, Hall I.** 2014. Revised surveillance case definition for HIV infection: United States. *MMWR Recommend Rep* **63:**1–10.
40. **Haynes BF, Liao HX, Tomaras GD.** 2010. Is developing an HIV-1 vaccine possible? *Curr Opin HIV AIDS* **5:**362–367.
41. **Taylor BS, Sobieszczyk ME, McCutchan FE, Hammer SM.** 2008. The challenge of HIV-1 subtype diversity. *N Engl J Med* **358:**1590–1602.
42. **Margolis DM, Koup RA, Ferrari G.** 2017. HIV antibodies for treatment of HIV infection. *Immunol Rev* **275:**313–323.
43. **Griffith BP, Mayo DR.** 2006. Increased levels of HIV RNA detected in samples with viral loads close to the detection limit collected in plasma preparation tubes (PPT). *J Clin Virol* **35:**197–200.
44. **Salimnia H, Moore EC, Crane LR, Macarthur RD, Fairfax MR.** 2005. Discordance between viral loads determined by Roche COBAS AMPLICOR human immunodeficiency virus type 1 monitor (version 1.5) standard and ultrasensitive assays caused by freezing patient plasma in centrifuged Becton-Dickinson Vacutainer brand plasma preparation tubes. *J Clin Microbiol* **43:**4635–4639.
45. **Lew J, Reichelderfer P, Fowler M, Bremer J, Carrol R, Cassol S, Chernoff D, Coombs R, Cronin M, Dickover R, Fiscus S, Herman S, Jackson B, Kornegay J, Kovacs A, McIntosh K, Meyer W, Michael N, Mofenson L, Moye J, Quinn T, Robb M, Vahey M, Weiser B, Yeghiazarian T.** 1998. Determinations of levels of human immunodeficiency virus type 1 RNA in plasma: reassessment of parameters affecting assay outcome. TUBE Meeting Workshop Attendees. Technology Utilization for HIV-1 Blood Evaluation and Standardization in Pediatrics. *J Clin Microbiol* **36:**1471–1479.
46. **Griffith BP, Rigsby MO, Garner RB, Gordon MM, Chacko TM.** 1997. Comparison of the Amplicor HIV-1 monitor test and the nucleic acid sequence-based amplification assay for quantitation of human immunodeficiency virus RNA in plasma, serum, and plasma subjected to freeze-thaw cycles. *J Clin Microbiol* **35:**3288–3291.
47. **Ginocchio CC, Wang XP, Kaplan MH, Mulligan G, Witt D, Romano JW, Cronin M, Carroll R.** 1997. Effects of specimen collection, processing, and storage conditions on stability of human immunodeficiency virus type 1 RNA levels in plasma. *J Clin Microbiol* **35:**2886–2893.
48. **Ho DD, Moudgil T, Alam M.** 1989. Quantitation of human immunodeficiency virus type 1 in the blood of infected persons. *N Engl J Med* **321:**1621–1625.
49. **Griffith BP.** 1987. Principles of laboratory isolation and identification of the human immunodeficiency virus (HIV). *Yale J Biol Med* **60:**575–587.
50. **Dykes C, Demeter LM.** 2007. Clinical significance of human immunodeficiency virus type 1 replication fitness. *Clin Microbiol Rev* **20:**550–578.
51. **Hirsch MS, Brun-Vézinet F, D'Aquila RT, Hammer SM, Johnson VA, Kuritzkes DR, Loveday C, Mellors JW, Clotet B, Conway B, Demeter LM, Vella S, Jacobsen DM, Richman DD.** 2000. Antiretroviral drug resistance testing in adult HIV-1 infection: recommendations of an International AIDS Society-USA panel. *JAMA* **283:**2417–2426.
52. **Petropoulos CJ, Parkin NT, Limoli KL, Lie YS, Wrin T, Huang W, Tian H, Smith D, Winslow GA, Capon DJ, Whitcomb JM.** 2000. A novel phenotypic drug susceptibility assay for human immunodeficiency virus type 1. *Antimicrob Agents Chemother* **44:**920–928.
53. **Barbour JD, Wrin T, Grant RM, Martin JN, Segal MR, Petropoulos CJ, Deeks SG.** 2002. Evolution of phenotypic drug susceptibility and viral replication capacity during long-term virologic failure of protease inhibitor therapy in human immunodeficiency virus-infected adults. *J Virol* **76:**11104–11112.
54. **Armstrong KL, Lee TH, Essex M.** 2009. Replicative capacity differences of thymidine analog resistance mutations in subtype B and C human immunodeficiency virus type 1. *J Virol* **83:**4051–4059.
55. **Hsieh SM, Pan SC, Chang SY, Hung CC, Sheng WH, Chen MY, Chang SC.** 2013. Differential impact of resistance-associated mutations to protease inhibitors and nonnucleoside reverse transcriptase inhibitors on HIV-1 replication capacity. *AIDS Res Hum Retroviruses* **29:**1117–1122.

56. **Miura T, Brumme ZL, Brockman MA, Rosato P, Sela J, Brumme CJ, Pereyra F, Kaufmann DE, Trocha A, Block BL, Daar ES, Connick E, Jessen H, Kelleher AD, Rosenberg E, Markowitz M, Schafer K, Vaida F, Iwamoto A, Little S, Walker BD.** 2010. Impaired replication capacity of acute/early viruses in persons who become HIV controllers. *J Virol* **84:**7581–7591.
57. **Stramer SL, Glynn SA, Kleinman SH, Strong DM, Caglioti S, Wright DJ, Dodd RY, Busch MP, National Heart, Lung, and Blood Institute Nucleic Acid Test Study Group.** 2004. Detection of HIV-1 and HCV infections among antibody-negative blood donors by nucleic acid-amplification testing. *N Engl J Med* **351:**760–768.
58. **Fransen K, Mertens G, Stynen D, Goris A, Nys P, Nkengasong J, Heyndrickx L, Janssens W, van der Groen G.** 1997. Evaluation of a newly developed HIV antigen test. *J Med Virol* **53:**31–35.
59. **Goudsmit J, Paul DA, Lange JMA, Speelman H, Van Der Noordaa J, Van Der Helm HJ, De Wolf F, Epstein LG, Krone WJA, Wolters EC, Oleske JM, Coutinho RA.** 1986. Expression of human immunodeficiency virus antigen (HIV-Ag) in serum and cerebrospinal fluid during acute and chronic infection. *Lancet* **328:**177–180.
60. **Bollinger RC Jr, Kline RL, Francis HL, Moss MW, Bartlett JG, Quinn TC.** 1992. Acid dissociation increases the sensitivity of p24 antigen detection for the evaluation of antiviral therapy and disease progression in asymptomatic human immunodeficiency virus-infected persons. *J Infect Dis* **165:** 913–916.
61. **Schüpbach J, Tomasik Z, Knuchel M, Opravil M, Günthard HF, Nadal D, Böni J, Swiss HIV Cohort Study, Swiss HIV Mother + Child Cohort Study.** 2006. Optimized virus disruption improves detection of HIV-1 p24 in particles and uncovers a p24 reactivity in patients with undetectable HIV-1 RNA under long-term HAART. *J Med Virol* **78:**1003–1010.
62. **Pokriefka RA, Manzor O, Markowitz NP, Saravolatz LD, Kvale P, Donovan RM.** 1993. Increased detection of human immunodeficiency virus antigenemia after dissociation of immune complexes at low pH. *J Clin Microbiol* **31:** 1656–1658.
63. **Nadal D, Böni J, Kind C, Varnier OE, Steiner F, Tomasik Z, Schüpbach J.** 1999. Prospective evaluation of amplification-boosted ELISA for heat-denatured p24 antigen for diagnosis and monitoring of pediatric human immunodeficiency virus type 1 infection. *J Infect Dis* **180:**1089–1095.
64. **Pascual A, Cachafeiro A, Funk ML, Fiscus SA.** 2002. Comparison of an assay using signal amplification of the heat-dissociated p24 antigen with the Roche Monitor human immunodeficiency virus RNA assay. *J Clin Microbiol* **40:** 2472–2475.
65. **Schüpbach J.** 2002. Measurement of HIV-1 p24 antigen by signal-amplification-boosted ELISA of heat-denatured plasma is a simple and inexpensive alternative to tests for viral RNA. *AIDS Rev* **4:**83–92.
66. **Respess RA, Cachafeiro A, Withum D, Fiscus SA, Newman D, Branson B, Varnier OE, Lewis K, Dondero TJ.** 2005. Evaluation of an ultrasensitive p24 antigen assay as a potential alternative to human immunodeficiency virus type 1 RNA viral load assay in resource-limited settings. *J Clin Microbiol* **43:**506–508.
67. **Cachafeiro A, Sherman GG, Sohn AH, Beck-Sague C, Fiscus SA.** 2009. Diagnosis of human immunodeficiency virus type 1 infection in infants by use of dried blood spots and an ultrasensitive p24 antigen assay. *J Clin Microbiol* **47:**459–462.
68. **Sherman GG, Stevens G, Stevens WS.** 2004. Affordable diagnosis of human immunodeficiency virus infection in infants by p24 antigen detection. *Pediatr Infect Dis J* **23:** 173–176.
69. **Dunn DT, Brandt CD, Krivinet A, Cassol SA, Roques P, Borkowsky W, De Rossi A, Denamur E, Ehrnst A, Loveday C.** 1995. The sensitivity of HIV-1 DNA polymerase chain reaction in the neonatal period and the relative contributions of intra-uterine and intra-partum transmission. *AIDS* **9:** F7-F11-984.
70. **O'Brien WA, Hartigan PM, Martin D, Esinhart J, Hill A, Benoit S, Rubin M, Simberkoff MS, Hamilton JD, Veterans Affairs Cooperative Study Group on AIDS.** 1996. Changes in plasma HIV-1 RNA and CD4+ lymphocyte counts and the risk of progression to AIDS. *N Engl J Med* **334:**426–431.
71. **Novitsky V, Essex M.** 2012. Using HIV viral load to guide treatment-for-prevention interventions. *Curr Opin HIV AIDS* **7:**117–124.
72. **Swanson P, Holzmayer V, Huang S, Hay P, Adebiyi A, Rice P, Abravaya K, Thamm S, Devare SG, Hackett J Jr.** 2006. Performance of the automated Abbott RealTime HIV-1 assay on a genetically diverse panel of specimens from London: comparison to VERSANT HIV-1 RNA 3.0, AMPLICOR HIV-1 MONITOR v1.5, and LCx HIV RNA quantitative assays. *J Virol Methods* **137:**184–192.
73. **Swanson P, Huang S, Holzmayer V, Bodelle P, Yamaguchi J, Brennan C, Badaro R, Brites C, Abravaya K, Devare SG, Hackett J Jr.** 2006. Performance of the automated Abbott RealTime HIV-1 assay on a genetically diverse panel of specimens from Brazil. *J Virol Methods* **134:**237–243.
74. **Gueudin M, Plantier JC, Lemée V, Schmitt MP, Chartier L, Bourlet T, Ruffault A, Damond F, Vray M, Simon F.** 2007. Evaluation of the Roche Cobas TaqMan and Abbott Real-Time extraction-quantification systems for HIV-1 subtypes. *J Acquir Immune Defic Syndr* **44:**500–505.
75. **Schumacher W, Frick E, Kauselmann M, Maier-Hoyle V, van der Vliet R, Babiel R.** 2007. Fully automated quantification of human immunodeficiency virus (HIV) type 1 RNA in human plasma by the COBAS AmpliPrep/COBAS TaqMan system. *J Clin Virol* **38:**304–312.
76. **Karasi JC, Dziezuk F, Quennery L, Förster S, Reischl U, Colucci G, Schoener D, Seguin-Devaux C, Schmit JC.** 2011. High correlation between the Roche COBAS® AmpliPrep/COBAS® TaqMan® HIV-1, v2.0 and the Abbott m2000 RealTime HIV-1 assays for quantification of viral load in HIV-1 B and non-B subtypes. *J Clin Virol* **52:**181–186.
77. **Hopkins M, Hau S, Tiernan C, Papadimitropoulos A, Chawla A, Beloukas A, Geretti AM.** 2015. Comparative performance of the new Aptima HIV-1 Quant Dx assay with three commercial PCR-based HIV-1 RNA quantitation assays. *J Clin Virol* **69:**56–62.
78. **Braun J, Plantier JC, Hellot MF, Tuaillon E, Gueudin M, Damond F, Malmsten A, Corrigan GE, Simon F.** 2003. A new quantitative HIV load assay based on plasma virion reverse transcriptase activity for the different types, groups and subtypes. *AIDS* **17:**331–336.
79. **Stevens G, Rekhviashvili N, Scott LE, Gonin R, Stevens W.** 2005. Evaluation of two commercially available, inexpensive alternative assays used for assessing viral load in a cohort of human immunodeficiency virus type 1 subtype C-infected patients from South Africa. *J Clin Microbiol* **43:**857–861.
80. **Schito M, Peter TF, Cavanaugh S, Piatek AS, Young GJ, Alexander H, Coggin W, Domingo GJ, Ellenberger D, Ermantraut E, Jani IV, Katamba A, Palamountain KM, Essajee S, Dowdy DW.** 2012. Opportunities and challenges for cost-efficient implementation of new point-of-care diagnostics for HIV and tuberculosis. *J Infect Dis* **205**(Suppl 2)**:**S169–S180.
81. **Centers for Disease Control (CDC).** 1989. Interpretation and use of the Western blot assay for serodiagnosis of human immunodeficiency virus type 1 infections. *MMWR Suppl* **38:** 1–7.
82. **Brenner BG, Roger M, Routy JP, Moisi D, Ntemgwa M, Matte C, Baril JG, Thomas R, Rouleau D, Bruneau J, Leblanc R, Legault M, Tremblay C, Charest H, Wainberg MA, Quebec Primary HIV Infection Study Group.** 2007. High rates of forward transmission events after acute/early HIV-1 infection. *J Infect Dis* **195:**951–959.
83. **Hogan CM, Degruttola V, Sun X, Fiscus SA, Del Rio C, Hare CB, Markowitz M, Connick E, Macatangay B, Tashima KT, Kallungal B, Camp R, Morton T, Daar ES, Little S, A5217 Study Team.** 2012. The setpoint study (ACTG A5217): effect of immediate versus deferred antiretroviral therapy on virologic set point in recently HIV-1-infected individuals. *J Infect Dis* **205:**87–96.

84. **Forsgren A, Nordström K.** 1974. Protein A from *Staphylococcus aureus*: the biological significance of its reaction with IgG. *Ann N Y Acad Sci* **236**(1 Recent Advanc):252–266.
85. **Busch MP, Satten GA.** 1997. Time course of viremia and antibody seroconversion following human immunodeficiency virus exposure. *Am J Med* **102**(5B):117–124, discussion 125–126.
86. **Louie B, Pandori MW, Wong E, Klausner JD, Liska S.** 2006. Use of an acute seroconversion panel to evaluate a third-generation enzyme-linked immunoassay for detection of human immunodeficiency virus-specific antibodies relative to multiple other assays. *J Clin Microbiol* **44**:1856–1858.
87. **Patel P, Mackellar D, Simmons P, Uniyal A, Gallagher K, Bennett B, Sullivan TJ, Kowalski A, Parker MM, LaLota M, Kerndt P, Sullivan PS, Centers for Disease Control and Prevention Acute HIV Infection Study Group.** 2010. Detecting acute human immunodeficiency virus infection using 3 different screening immunoassays and nucleic acid amplification testing for human immunodeficiency virus RNA, 2006-2008. *Arch Intern Med* **170**:66–74.
88. **Ly TD, Ebel A, Faucher V, Fihman V, Laperche S.** 2007. Could the new HIV combined p24 antigen and antibody assays replace p24 antigen specific assays? *J Virol Methods* **143**:86–94.
89. **Masciotra S, McDougal JS, Feldman J, Sprinkle P, Wesolowski L, Owen SM.** 2011. Evaluation of an alternative HIV diagnostic algorithm using specimens from seroconversion panels and persons with established HIV infections. *J Clin Virol* **52**(Suppl 1):S17–S22.
90. **Nasrullah M, Wesolowski LG, Meyer WA III, Owen SM, Masciotra S, Vorwald C, Becker WJ, Branson BM.** 2013. Performance of a fourth-generation HIV screening assay and an alternative HIV diagnostic testing algorithm. *AIDS* **27**:731–737.
91. **Centers for Disease Control and Prevention (CDC).** 2013. Detection of acute HIV infection in two evaluations of a new HIV diagnostic testing algorithm: United States, 2011-2013. *MMWR Morb Mortal Wkly Rep* **62**:489–494.
92. **Owen SM, Yang C, Spira T, Ou CY, Pau CP, Parekh BS, Candal D, Kuehl D, Kennedy MS, Rudolph D, Luo W, Delatorre N, Masciotra S, Kalish ML, Cowart F, Barnett T, Lal R, McDougal JS.** 2008. Alternative algorithms for human immunodeficiency virus infection diagnosis using tests that are licensed in the United States. *J Clin Microbiol* **46**: 1588–1595.
93. **Centers for Disease Control and Prevention (CDC).** 1998. Update: HIV counseling and testing using rapid tests: United States, 1995. *MMWR Morb Mortal Wkly Rep* **47**: 211–215.
94. **Kuhar DT, Henderson DK, Struble KA, Heneine W, Thomas V, Cheever LW, Gomaa A, Panlilio AL.** 2013. Updated US Public Health Service guidelines for the management of occupational exposures to human immunodeficiency virus and recommendations for postexposure prophylaxis. *Infect Control Hosp Epidemiol* **34**:875–892.
95. **Branson BM, Handsfield HH, Lampe MA, Janssen RS, Taylor AW, Lyss SB, Clark JE, Centers for Disease Control and Prevention (CDC).** 2006. Revised recommendations for HIV testing of adults, adolescents, and pregnant women in health-care settings. *MMWR Recomm Rep* **55**(RR-14):1–17, quiz CE1–CE4.
96. **Branson BM.** 2003. Point of care rapid tests for HIV antibodies. *J Lab Med* **27**:288–295.
97. **Granade TC, Parekh BS, Phillips SK, McDougal JS.** 2004. Performance of the OraQuick and Hema-Strip rapid HIV antibody detection assays by non-laboratorians. *J Clin Virol* **30**:229–232.
98. **Gray RH, Makumbi F, Serwadda D, Lutalo T, Nalugoda F, Opendi P, Kigozi G, Reynolds SJ, Sewankambo NK, Wawer MJ.** 2007. Limitations of rapid HIV-1 tests during screening for trials in Uganda: diagnostic test accuracy study. *BMJ* **335**:188.
99. **Campbell S, Fedoriw Y.** 2009. HIV testing near the patient: changing the face of HIV testing. *Clin Lab Med* **29**:491–501.
100. **Delaney KP, Branson BM, Uniyal A, Phillips S, Candal D, Owen SM, Kerndt PR.** 2011. Evaluation of the performance characteristics of 6 rapid HIV antibody tests. *Clin Infect Dis* **52**:257–263.
101. **Stekler JD, O'Neal JD, Lane A, Swanson F, Maenza J, Stevens C, Coombs RW, Dragavon J, Swenson PD, Golden M, Branson BM.** 2013. Relative accuracy of serum, whole blood, and oral fluid HIV tests among Seattle men who have sex with men. *J Clin Virol* **58**(Suppl 1):e119-22.
102. **Pilcher CD, Louie B, Facente S, Keating S, Hackett J Jr, Vallari A, Hall C, Dowling T, Busch MP, Klausner JD, Hecht FM, Liska S, Pandori MW.** 2013. Performance of rapid point-of-care and laboratory tests for acute and established HIV infection in San Francisco. *PLoS One* **8**:e80629.
103. **Masciotra S, Luo W, Youngpairoj AS, Kennedy MS, Wells S, Ambrose K, Sprinkle P, Owen SM.** 2013. Performance of the Alere Determine™ HIV-1/2 Ag/Ab Combo Rapid Test with specimens from HIV-1 seroconverters from the US and HIV-2 infected individuals from Ivory Coast. *J Clin Virol* **58**(Suppl 1):e54–e58.
104. **Laperche S, Leballais L, Ly TD, Plantier JC.** 2012. Failures in the detection of HIV p24 antigen with the Determine HIV-1/2 Ag/Ab Combo rapid test. *J Infect Dis* **206**: 1946–1947; author reply 1949–1950.
105. **Granade TC, Phillips SK, Parekh B, Gomez P, Kitson-Piggott W, Oleander H, Mahabir B, Charles W, Lee-Thomas S.** 1998. Detection of antibodies to human immunodeficiency virus type 1 in oral fluids: a large-scale evaluation of immunoassay performance. *Clin Diagn Lab Immunol* **5**:171–175.
106. **Jafa K, Patel P, Mackellar DA, Sullivan PS, Delaney KP, Sides TL, Newman AP, Paul SM, Cadoff EM, Martin EG, Keenan PA, Branson BM, OraQuick Study Group.** 2007. Investigation of false positive results with an oral fluid rapid HIV-1/2 antibody test. *PLoS One* **2**:e185.
107. **Luo W, Masciotra S, Delaney KP, Charurat M, Croxton T, Constantine N, Blattner W, Wesolowski L, Owen SM.** 2013. Comparison of HIV oral fluid and plasma antibody results during early infection in a longitudinal Nigerian cohort. *J Clin Virol* **58**(Suppl 1):e113–e118.
108. **Wesolowski LG, Sanchez T, MacKellar DA, Branson BM, Ethridge SF, Constantine N, Ketema F, Sullivan PS.** 2009. Evaluation of oral fluid enzyme immunoassay for confirmation of a positive rapid human immunodeficiency virus test result. *Clin Vaccine Immunol* **16**:1091–1092.
109. **Parry JV, Mortimer PP, Nicoll AG.** 1992. Performance assessment of neonatal dried blood spot testing for HIV antibody. *Commun Dis Rep CDR Rev* **2**:R128–R130.
110. **Sullivan TJ, Antonio-Gaddy MS, Richardson-Moore A, Styer LM, Bigelow-Saulsbery D, Parker MM.** 2013. Expansion of HIV screening to non-clinical venues is aided by the use of dried blood spots for Western blot confirmation. *J Clin Virol* **58**(Suppl 1):e123–e126.
111. **Lofgren SM, Morrissey AB, Chevallier CC, Malabeja AI, Edmonds S, Amos B, Sifuna DJ, von Seidlein L, Schimana W, Stevens WS, Bartlett JA, Crump JA.** 2009. Evaluation of a dried blood spot HIV-1 RNA program for early infant diagnosis and viral load monitoring at rural and remote healthcare facilities. *AIDS* **23**:2459–2466.
112. **Urnovitz HB, Sturge JC, Gottfried TD.** 1997. Increased sensitivity of HIV-1 antibody detection. *Nat Med* **3**:1258.
113. **Pyne MT, Hackett J Jr, Holzmayer V, Hillyard DR.** 2013. Large-scale analysis of the prevalence and geographic distribution of HIV-1 non-B variants in the United States. *J Clin Microbiol* **51**:2662–2669.
114. **Brennan CA, Yamaguchi J, Devare SG, Foster GA, Stramer SL.** 2010. Expanded evaluation of blood donors in the United States for human immunodeficiency virus type 1 non-B subtypes and antiretroviral drug-resistant strains: 2005 through 2007. *Transfusion* **50**:2707–2712.
115. **Lee S, Hu J, Tang S, Wood O, Francis K, Machuca A, Rios M, Daniel S, Vockley C, Awazi B, Zekeng L, Hewlett I.** 2006. Evaluation of FDA licensed HIV assays using plasma from Cameroonian blood donors. *J Med Virol* **78**(Suppl 1): S22–S23.

116. **Reynolds SJ, Ndongala LM, Luo CC, Mwandagalirwa K, Losoma AJ, Mwamba KJ, Bazepeyo E, Nzilambi NE, Quinn TC, Bollinger RC.** 2002. Evaluation of a rapid test for the detection of antibodies to human immunodeficiency virus type 1 and 2 in the setting of multiple transmitted viral subtypes. *Int J STD AIDS* **13:**171–173.
117. **Plantier JC, Djemai M, Lemée V, Reggiani A, Leoz M, Burc L, Vessière A, Rousset D, Poveda JD, Henquell C, Gautheret-Dejean A, Barin F.** 2009. Census and analysis of persistent false-negative results in serological diagnosis of human immunodeficiency virus type 1 group O infections. *J Clin Microbiol* **47:**2906–2911.
118. **Styer LM, Sullivan TJ, Parker MM.** 2011. Evaluation of an alternative supplemental testing strategy for HIV diagnosis by retrospective analysis of clinical HIV testing data. *J Clin Virol* **52**(Suppl 1)**:**S35–S40.
119. **Pandori MW, Westheimer E, Gay C, Moss N, Fu J, Hightow-Weidman LB, Craw J, Hall L, Giancotti FR, Mak ML, Madayag C, Tsoi B, Louie B, Patel P, Owen SM, Peters PJ.** 2013. The Multispot rapid HIV-1/HIV-2 differentiation assay is comparable with the Western blot and an immunofluorescence assay at confirming HIV infection in a prospective study in three regions of the United States. *J Clin Virol* **58**(Suppl 1)**:**e92–e96.
120. **Centers for Disease Control and Prevention (CDC).** 2011. HIV-2 Infection Surveillance: United States, 1987-2009. *MMWR Morb Mortal Wkly Rep* **60:**985–988.
121. **Torian LV, Eavey JJ, Punsalang AP, Pirillo RE, Forgione LA, Kent SA, Oleszko WR.** 2010. HIV type 2 in New York City, 2000-2008. *Clin Infect Dis* **51:**1334–1342.
122. **Tsang VC, Peralta JM, Simons AR.** 1983. Enzyme-linked immunoelectrotransfer blot techniques (EITB) for studying the specificities of antigens and antibodies separated by gel electrophoresis. *Methods Enzymol* **92:**377–391.
123. **O'Brien TR, George JR, Epstein JS, Holmberg SD, Schochetman G.** 1992. Testing for antibodies to human immunodeficiency virus type 2 in the United States. *MMWR Recomm Rep* **41**(RR-12)**:**1–9.
124. **Mingle JA.** 1997. Differentiation of dual seropositivity to HIV 1 and HIV 2 in Ghanaian sera using line immunoassay (INNOLIA). *West Afr J Med* **16:**71–74.
125. **Blumberg RS, Sandstrom EG, Paradis TJ, Neumeyer DN, Sarngadharan MG, Hartshorn KL, Byington RE, Hirsch MS, Schooley RT.** 1986. Detection of human T-cell lymphotropic virus type III-related antigens and anti-human T-cell lymphotropic virus type III antibodies by anticomplementary immunofluorescence. *J Clin Microbiol* **23:**1072–1077.
126. **Torian LV, Forgione LA, Punsalang AE, Pirillo RE, Oleszko WR.** 2011. Comparison of Multispot EIA with Western blot for confirmatory serodiagnosis of HIV. *J Clin Virol* **52**(Suppl 1)**:**S41–S44.
127. **Ramos EM, Harb S, Dragavon J, Coombs RW.** 2013. Clinical performance of the Multispot HIV-1/HIV-2 rapid test to correctly differentiate HIV-2 from HIV-1 infection in screening algorithms using third and fourth generation assays and to identify cross reactivity with the HIV-1 Western blot. *J Clin Virol* **58**(Suppl 1)**:**e104–e107.
128. **Gottlieb GS, Sow PS, Hawes SE, Ndoye I, Coll-Seck AM, Curlin ME, Critchlow CW, Kiviat NB, Mullins JI.** 2003. Molecular epidemiology of dual HIV-1/HIV-2 seropositive adults from Senegal, West Africa. *AIDS Res Hum Retroviruses* **19:**575–584.
129. **Fordan S, Bennett B, Lee M, Crowe S.** 2017. Comparative performance of the Geenius™ HIV-1/HIV-2 supplemental test in Florida's public health testing population. *J Clin Virol* **91:**79–83.
130. **Malloch L, Kadivar K, Putz J, Levett PN, Tang J, Hatchette TF, Kadkhoda K, Ng D, Ho J, Kim J.** 2013. Comparative evaluation of the Bio-Rad Geenius HIV-1/2 Confirmatory Assay and the Bio-Rad Multispot HIV-1/2 Rapid Test as an alternative differentiation assay for CLSI M53 algorithm-I. *J Clin Virol* **58**(Suppl 1)**:**e85–e91.
131. **Wesolowski LG, Parker MM, Delaney KP, Owen SM.** 2017. Highlights from the 2016 HIV diagnostics conference: the new landscape of HIV testing in laboratories, public health programs and clinical practice. *J Clin Virol* **91:**63–68.
132. **Cohen CJ, Hunt S, Sension M, Farthing C, Conant M, Jacobson S, Nadler J, Verbiest W, Hertogs K, Ames M, Rinehart AR, Graham NM, VIRA3001 Study Team.** 2002. A randomized trial assessing the impact of phenotypic resistance testing on antiretroviral therapy. *AIDS* **16:**579–588.
133. **Meynard JL, Vray M, Morand-Joubert L, Race E, Descamps D, Peytavin G, Matheron S, Lamotte C, Guiramand S, Costagliola D, Brun-Vézinet F, Clavel F, Girard PM, Narval Trial Group.** 2002. Phenotypic or genotypic resistance testing for choosing antiretroviral therapy after treatment failure: a randomized trial. *AIDS* **16:**727–736.
134. **Weinstein MC, Goldie SJ, Losina E, Cohen CJ, Baxter JD, Zhang H, Kimmel AD, Freedberg KA.** 2001. Use of genotypic resistance testing to guide HIV therapy: clinical impact and cost-effectiveness. *Ann Intern Med* **134:**440–450.
135. **Snedecor SJ, Khachatryan A, Nedrow K, Chambers R, Li C, Haider S, Stephens J.** 2013. The prevalence of transmitted resistance to first-generation non-nucleoside reverse transcriptase inhibitors and its potential economic impact in HIV-infected patients. *PLoS One* **8:**e72784.
136. **Erali M, Page S, Reimer LG, Hillyard DR.** 2001. Human immunodeficiency virus type 1 drug resistance testing: a comparison of three sequence-based methods. *J Clin Microbiol* **39:**2157–2165.
137. **Günthard HF, Wong JK, Ignacio CC, Havlir DV, Richman DD.** 1998. Comparative performance of high-density oligonucleotide sequencing and dideoxynucleotide sequencing of HIV type 1 pol from clinical samples. *AIDS Res Hum Retroviruses* **14:**869–876.
138. **Johnson JA, Li JF, Wei X, Lipscomb J, Irlbeck D, Craig C, Smith A, Bennett DE, Monsour M, Sandstrom P, Lanier ER, Heneine W.** 2008. Minority HIV-1 drug resistance mutations are present in antiretroviral treatment-naïve populations and associate with reduced treatment efficacy. *PLoS Med* **5:**e158.
139. **Johnson JA, Li JF, Wei X, Lipscomb J, Bennett D, Brant A, Cong ME, Spira T, Shafer RW, Heneine W.** 2007. Simple PCR assays improve the sensitivity of HIV-1 subtype B drug resistance testing and allow linking of resistance mutations. *PLoS One* **2:**e638.
140. **Palmer S, Kearney M, Maldarelli F, Halvas EK, Bixby CJ, Bazmi H, Rock D, Falloon J, Davey RT Jr, Dewar RL, Metcalf JA, Hammer S, Mellors JW, Coffin JM.** 2005. Multiple, linked human immunodeficiency virus type 1 drug resistance mutations in treatment-experienced patients are missed by standard genotype analysis. *J Clin Microbiol* **43:**406–413.
141. **Whitcomb JM, Huang W, Fransen S, Limoli K, Toma J, Wrin T, Chappey C, Kiss LD, Paxinos EE, Petropoulos CJ.** 2007. Development and characterization of a novel single-cycle recombinant-virus assay to determine human immunodeficiency virus type 1 coreceptor tropism. *Antimicrob Agents Chemother* **51:**566–575.
142. **MacArthur RD, Novak RM.** 2008. Reviews of anti-infective agents: maraviroc: the first of a new class of antiretroviral agents. *Clin Infect Dis* **47:**236–241.
143. **Tsibris AM, Sagar M, Gulick RM, Su Z, Hughes M, Greaves W, Subramanian M, Flexner C, Giguel F, Leopold KE, Coakley E, Kuritzkes DR.** 2008. *In vivo* emergence of vicriviroc resistance in a human immunodeficiency virus type 1 subtype C-infected subject. *J Virol* **82:**8210–8214.
144. **Prada N, Davis B, Jean-Pierre P, La Roche M, Duh FM, Carrington M, Poles M, Mehandru S, Mohri H, Markowitz M.** 2008. Drug-susceptible HIV-1 infection despite intermittent fixed-dose combination tenofovir/emtricitabine as prophylaxis is associated with low-level viremia, delayed seroconversion, and an attenuated clinical course. *J Acquir Immune Defic Syndr* **49:**117–122.
145. **Terzi R, Niero F, Iemoli E, Capetti A, Coen M, Rizzardini G.** 2007. Late HIV seroconversion after non-occupational post-exposure prophylaxis against HIV with concomitant hepatitis C virus seroconversion. *AIDS* **21:**262–263.
146. **Erickson CP, McNiff T, Klausner JD.** 2006. Influenza vaccination and false positive HIV results. *N Engl J Med* **354:**1422–1423.

147. **Araujo PR, Albertoni G, Arnoni C, Almeida K, Ribeiro J, Rizzo SR, Carvalho FO, Baretto JA, Mangueira C.** 2009. Rubella vaccination and transitory false-positive test results for human immunodeficiency virus type 1 in blood donors. *Transfusion* **49:**2516–2517.
148. **Cooper CJ, Metch B, Dragavon J, Coombs RW, Baden LR, NIAID HIV Vaccine Trials Network (HVTN) Vaccine-Induced Seropositivity (VISP) Task Force.** 2010. Vaccine-induced HIV seropositivity/reactivity in noninfected HIV vaccine recipients. *JAMA* **304:**275–283.
149. **Patel P, Bennett B, Sullivan T, Parker MM, Heffelfinger JD, Sullivan PS, CDC AHI Study Group.** 2012. Rapid HIV screening: missed opportunities for HIV diagnosis and prevention. *J Clin Virol* **54:**42–47.
150. **Styer LM, Sullivan T, Parker MM.** 2012. Validation and clinical use of a HIV-2 viral load assay, p 37. HIV Diagnostics Conference, December 12-14, 2012, Atlanta, GA. http://hivtestingconference.org/2012-2/oral-presentations/
151. **Ren A, Louie B, Rauch L, Castro L, Liska S, Klausner JD, Pandori MW.** 2008. Screening and confirmation of human immunodeficiency virus type 1 infection solely by detection of RNA. *J Med Microbiol* **57:**1228–1233.
152. **Shulman SH, Parker MM.** 2013. Interim guidelines for laboratories on the use of a new diagnostic testing algorithm for human immunodeficiency virus (HIV). *Infection.* https://www.health.ny.gov/diseases/aids/providers/regulations/testing/docs/guidelines_diagnostic_testing.pdf.
153. **CLSI.** 2011. Criteria for laboratory testing and diagnosis of human immunodeficiency virus infection. Approved guideline. Clinical and Laboratory Standards Institute, Wayne, PA.
154. **Panel on Antiretroviral Guidelines for Adults and Adolescents.** 2013. Guidelines for the use of antiretroviral agents in HIV-1-infected adults and adolescents. Department of Health and Human Services.
155. **Long EF.** 2011. HIV screening via fourth-generation immunoassay or nucleic acid amplification test in the United States: a cost-effectiveness analysis. *PLoS One* **6:**e27625.
156. **Stekler J, Swenson PD, Wood RW, Handsfield HH, Golden MR.** 2005. Targeted screening for primary HIV infection through pooled HIV-RNA testing in men who have sex with men. *AIDS* **19:**1323–1325.
157. **Lilian RR, Kalk E, Bhowan K, Berrie L, Carmona S, Technau K, Sherman GG.** 2012. Early diagnosis of *in utero* and intrapartum HIV infection in infants prior to 6 weeks of age. *J Clin Microbiol* **50:**2373–2377.
158. **King SM, American Academy of Pediatrics Committee on Pediatric AIDS, American Academy of Pediatrics Infectious Diseases and Immunization Committee.** 2004. Evaluation and treatment of the human immunodeficiency virus-1-exposed infant. *Pediatrics* **114:**497–505.
159. **López M.** 2013. A multi-step pace towards a cure for HIV: kick, kill, and contain. *AIDS Rev* **15:**190–191.
160. **Lampton LM.** 2013. Functional HIV cure achieved in Mississippi. *J Miss State Med Assoc* **54:**94.
161. **Read JS, Committee on Pediatric AIDS, American Academy of Pediatrics.** 2007. Diagnosis of HIV-1 infection in children younger than 18 months in the United States. *Pediatrics* **120:**e1547–e1562.
162. **Deeks SG, Coleman RL, White R, Pachl C, Schambelan M, Chernoff DN, Feinberg MB.** 1997. Variance of plasma human immunodeficiency virus type 1 RNA levels measured by branched DNA within and between days. *J Infect Dis* **176:**514–517.
163. **Aleman S, Söderbärg K, Visco-Comandini U, Sitbon G, Sönnerborg A.** 2002. Drug resistance at low viraemia in HIV-1-infected patients with antiretroviral combination therapy. *AIDS* **16:**1039–1044.
164. **Nettles RE, Kieffer TL, Kwon P, Monie D, Han Y, Parsons T, Cofrancesco J Jr, Gallant JE, Quinn TC, Jackson B, Flexner C, Carson K, Ray S, Persaud D, Siliciano RF.** 2005. Intermittent HIV-1 viremia (Blips) and drug resistance in patients receiving HAART. *JAMA* **293:**817–829.
165. **Ginocchio CC, Kemper M, Stellrecht KA, Witt DJ.** 2003. Multicenter evaluation of the performance characteristics of the NucliSens HIV-1 QT assay used for quantitation of human immunodeficiency virus type 1 RNA. *J Clin Microbiol* **41:**164–173.
166. **Wojewoda CM, Spahlinger T, Harmon ML, Schnellinger B, Li Q, Dejelo C, Schmotzer C, Zhou L.** 2013. Comparison of Roche Cobas AmpliPrep/Cobas TaqMan HIV-1 test version 2.0 (CAP/CTM v2.0) with other real-time PCR assays in HIV-1 monitoring and follow-up of low-level viral loads. *J Virol Methods* **187:**1–5.
167. **Naeth G, Ehret R, Wiesmann F, Braun P, Knechten H, Berger A.** 2013. Comparison of HIV-1 viral load assay performance in immunological stable patients with low or undetectable viremia. *Med Microbiol Immunol (Berl)* **202:**67–75.
168. **Hirsch MS, Günthard HF, Schapiro JM, Brun-Vézinet F, Clotet B, Hammer SM, Johnson VA, Kuritzkes DR, Mellors JW, Pillay D, Yeni PG, Jacobsen DM, Richman DD.** 2008. Antiretroviral drug resistance testing in adult HIV-1 infection: 2008 recommendations of an International AIDS Society-USA panel. *Clin Infect Dis* **47:**266–285.
169. **Noguera-Julian M, Edgil D, Harrigan PR, Sandstrom P, Godfrey C, Paredes R.** 2017. Next-generation human immunodeficiency virus sequencing for patient management and drug resistance surveillance. *J Infect Dis* **216**(suppl_9):S829–S833.
170. **Moscona R, Ram D, Wax M, Bucris E, Levy I, Mendelson E, Mor O.** 2017. Comparison between next-generation and Sanger-based sequencing for the detection of transmitted drug-resistance mutations among recently infected HIV-1 patients in Israel, 2000-2014. *J Int AIDS Soc* **20:**21846.
171. **Inzaule SC, Hamers RL, Paredes R, Yang C, Schuurman R, Rinke de Wit TF.** 2017. The evolving landscape of HIV drug resistance diagnostics for expanding testing in resource-limited settings. *AIDS Rev* **19:**219–230.
172. **Parikh UM, McCormick K, van Zyl G, Mellors JW.** 2017. Future technologies for monitoring HIV drug resistance and cure. *Curr Opin HIV AIDS* **12:**182–189.

Human T-Cell Lymphotropic Viruses

WILLIAM M. SWITZER, WALID HENEINE, AND S. MICHELE OWEN

85

TAXONOMY

Human T-cell lymphotropic virus types 1 and 2 (HTLV-1 and HTLV-2) are members of the *Deltaretrovirus* genus in the *Retroviridae* family (1). HTLVs likely originated from cross-species transmission of simian T-cell lymphotropic viruses (STLVs); combined, this group of viruses is also referred to as primate T-lymphotropic viruses (PTLVs) (2, 3). While the close phylogenetic relationships of HTLV-1 and STLV-1 indicate a simian origin for HTLV-1, HTLV-2 and STLV-2 are only distantly related, so the exact simian origin of HTLV-2 is unknown. More recently, two novel HTLVs were identified in hunters in Cameroon and were called HTLV-3 and HTLV-4 (2, 4–6). HTLV-3 likely originated from monkeys infected with highly related STLV-3 viruses (2, 4, 5). HTLV-4 is equidistant from all other HTLVs and was recently found to have a gorilla reservoir in Cameroon (7, 8). HTLVs and STLVs are distinct from the *Lentivirus* genus, which includes human immunodeficiency virus types 1 and 2 (HIV-1 and HIV-2) and simian immunodeficiency viruses (1). Classification of HTLV groups using Roman numerals was replaced over a decade ago with Arabic numerals, following the guidelines of the International Committee on Taxonomy of Viruses (1).

DESCRIPTION OF THE AGENT

HTLV-1 and HTLV-2 are enveloped viruses about 80 to 100 nm in diameter; they contain an electron-dense, centrally located nuclear core with less prominent envelope spikes and bud from the cell surface. Electron micrograph studies have not been performed on HTLV-3 and -4, but they likely possess morphologies comparable to HTLV-1 and -2. Within the core are two positive-sense single-stranded RNA genomes. Once a cell is infected, the RNA genome is converted by reverse transcriptase to DNA and integrates into the host genome.

HTLVs are complex retroviruses with regulatory genes in addition to the structural and enzymatic *gag*, *pol*, and *env* genes found in all classical retroviruses. HTLV-1, HTLV-2, HTLV-3, and HTLV-4 all have similar genomic organization: group-specific antigen (*gag*), protease/polymerase (*pro*/*pol*), envelope (*env*), and accessory gene region (*pX*), flanked by long terminal repeats (LTRs) (Fig. 1). Each HTLV group is highly divergent, sharing about 60% nucleotide identity (8–10). The *gag* gene encodes the structural proteins, matrix (p19), capsid (p24), and nucleocapsid (p15) (Fig. 2). The *pro* and *pol* genes encode the protease and the reverse transcriptase enzymes, respectively. The *env* gene encodes the transmembrane and external or surface envelope glycoproteins, gp21 and gp46, respectively.

HTLVs use alternative splicing and internal initiation codons to produce several regulatory and accessory proteins encoded by at least four open reading frames located in the *pX* region of the viral genome between *env* and the 3′ LTR (11, 12). The *pX* region encodes the spliced, regulatory proteins Tax and Rex and several additional open reading frames, some of which are also believed to be involved in viral replication and transport (Fig. 1). Unlike other retroviruses, HTLVs also encode a protein on the antisense strand, called antisense protein of HTLV, that is a repressor of Tax-mediated viral transcription (Fig. 1) (13). Antisense protein of HTLV was first discovered in HTLV-1; it contains a basic leucine zipper (bZIP) motif and was thus originally called HBZ (HTLV-1 bZIP protein) (14, 15). HBZ is also believed to control cellular replication and promote T-lymphocyte proliferation associated with leukemia as seen in some HTLV-1-infected people (13, 16, 17). Antisense proteins of HTLV have now been identified in all primate T-lymphotropic virus groups, suggesting the evolutionary and biological importance of these proteins (8, 10, 13).

HTLV-1 and HTLV-2 use a receptor complex with three different molecules—glucose transporter type 1 (GLUT-1), VEGF-165 receptor neuropilin 1, and heparin sulfate proteoglycans (HSPG)—for cellular entry (18–23). HTLV-1 preferentially infects $CD4^+$ T cells, whereas $CD8^+$ T cells are the primary target for HTLV-2 (18). *In vitro* studies have shown that HTLV-3 can infect both $CD4^+$ and $CD8^+$ T cells and also uses glucose transporter type 1 but does not need heparin sulfate proteoglycans or neuropilin 1 for cellular entry, suggesting that it may use a different complex of receptor molecules (19). Cell receptor studies for HTLV-4 have not been reported yet.

EPIDEMIOLOGY AND TRANSMISSION

Recently, meta-analyses of reliable epidemiologic data from about 1,100 published papers since the discovery of HTLV in 1981 showed that 5 to 10 million people worldwide are

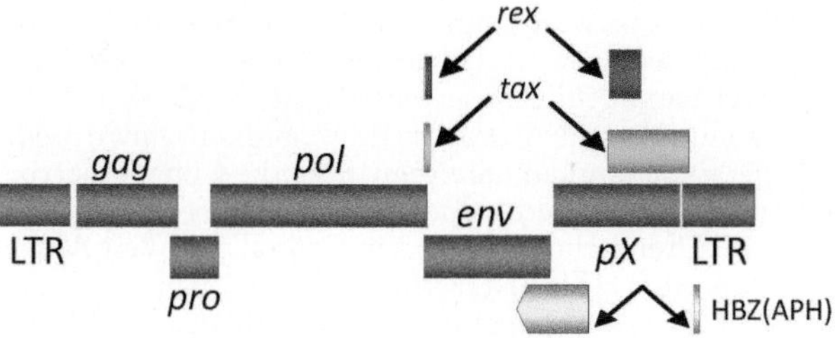

FIGURE 1 Genomic organization of HTLV. LTR, long terminal repeat; Gag, group-specific antigen; *env*, envelope; *pol*, polymerase (including reverse transcriptase and integrase); *pro*, protease; *rex*, regulator of viral expression; *tax*, transcriptional activator; HBZ, HTLV-1 basic leucine zipper-like protein, also known as the antisense protein of HTLV. Miscellaneous accessory genes (not shown) are located in the *pX* region, located between the *env* gene and the 3′ LTR region of HTLV. The Gag and Env proteins are the most immunogenic, and antibodies to these proteins are commonly detected by serological tests (EIA and Western blotting). PCR assays are typically designed to detect regions within the LTR region and *gag*, *pol*, *env*, and/or *tax* genes.

estimated to be infected with HTLV-1, with endemic foci in southwestern Japan, the Caribbean and surrounding islands, large parts of sub-Saharan Africa and Central and South America, some rare areas in Melanesia, the Middle East (northern part of Iran), and Romania (24). The seroprevalence rate in adults ranges from 2 to 17% in the Caribbean islands, and the highest rates (1.7 to 17.4%) are observed in southern Japan (24, 25). While similar meta-analysis estimates of global numbers of HTLV-2 infections have not been reported, it is endemic in Amerindian tribes throughout the Americas, as well as in a few Pygmy tribes in Central Africa, with seroprevalences of about 3% in Pygmies, 1 to 5.8% in South America, 8 to 10% in Central America, and 2 to 13% in North America (26–28). HTLV-3 and HTLV-4 have only been found in a few primate hunters in Cameroon and do not appear to have spread locally or globally, though screening has been limited to only certain non-African populations (2, 4, 5, 29–31). In all areas of endemicity, HTLV-1 and -2 seroprevalence increases with age, especially in women (24, 25, 32). In the United States and Europe, the seroprevalence for both HTLV-1 and HTLV-2 among low-risk populations is less than 1%

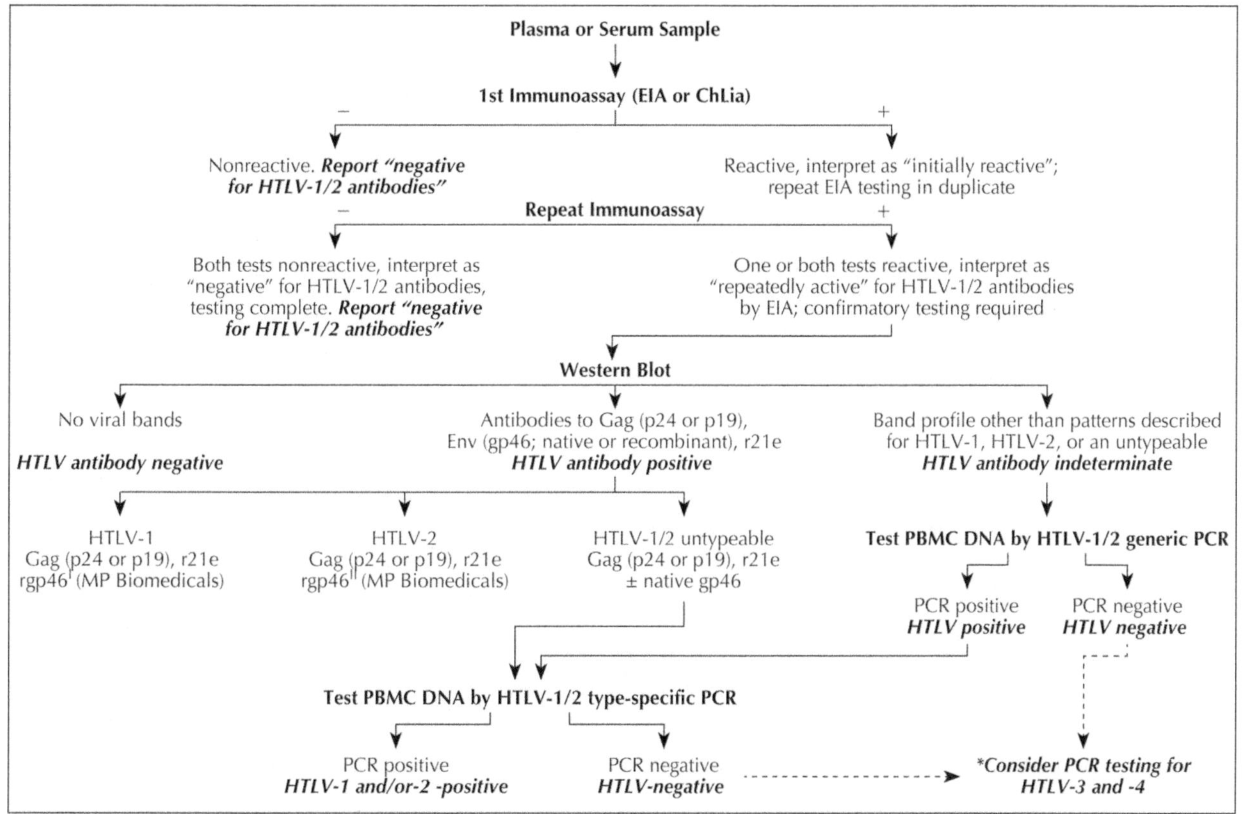

FIGURE 2 Serologic testing algorithm for the detection and confirmation of HTLV-1 and -2 infections. If the initial screening immunoassay (EIA or ChLIA) is reactive, a repeat assay with the same specimen is performed in duplicate. If one or both of the repeat tests are reactive, the specimen is classified as RR (repeat reactive) and supplemental testing is done for confirmation. The WB criteria shown are those used by the manufacturer and not the U.S. Public Health Service Working Group. In some cases, further follow-up is done using HTLV generic and/or type-specific PCR. *, HTLV-3 and -4 PCR are suggested if the patient is linked to Cameroon or West Central Africa. r21e, recombinant p21 envelope (Env) protein; $rgp46^{I}$ and $rgp46^{II}$, recombinant glycoprotein in Env specific for HTLV-1 or HTLV-2, respectively; Gag, group-specific antigen; PBMC, peripheral blood mononuclear cells.

(33, 34). However, high-risk populations such as intravenous drug users (IDUs) in the United States and Europe, in whom HTLV-2 infection predominates over HTLV-1 infection, are reported to have seroprevalences from 0.4 to 20% (24, 25). African-American IDU populations, especially in New Orleans, are at increased risk for HTLV-2 infection (25). IDUs in South Vietnam showed a very high prevalence (>60%) of HTLV-2 infection, which is believed to have been introduced and spread by American military personnel during the Vietnam War (35).

HTLV-1 and HTLV-2 infections are transmitted sexually (mainly male to female), vertically (mother to child, mostly by prolonged breast-feeding), and parenterally (intravenous drug use and blood transfusion) (24, 25, 32). In nonendemic populations, intravenous drug use and sex with IDUs are the most important risk factors for HTLV-2 transmission (24, 25, 32). Both cross-sectional and prospective studies support sexual transmission, and there was a strong concordance of seropositivity between spouses in an area where HTLV-2 is endemic (24, 25, 32). One study showed that transmission mode can affect viral evolution rates, with HTLV-2 strains transmitted between IDUs evolving 150 to 350 times faster than in mother-to-infant transmission (36). The increase in the viral transmission rate between IDUs, which can be many transmissions per year, was proposed to account for the increase in the HTLV-2 evolutionary rate, whereas vertical transmission would be expected to occur just once every 14 to 30 years for a given viral lineage and thus would evolve more slowly (36). This increased rate of transmission and evolution among IDUs may increase the risk for the emergence of HTLV-2 strains with a higher virulence.

Over the past 20 years, highly effective screening programs for volunteer blood donors have been implemented in Japan, Australia, the United States, Canada, and several Caribbean and European countries to reduce the risk of transfusion-related HTLV-1 and HTLV-2 transmission (25, 32–34). For example, in the United States between 1991 to 1996, the incidence rate of seroconversion associated with HTLV in blood donors was estimated to be 1.59 per 100,000 people per year (33), and the residual risk of transmitting HTLV infection by transfusing screened blood was estimated to be 1 in 641,000 (33). From 1998 to 2001, the estimated incidence of new infections among repeat blood donors to the American Red Cross was 0.239 per 100,000 person years, and the estimated risk of collecting blood during the infectious window period was 1:2,993,000 (37). More recently, the American Red Cross found that the HTLV incidence and residual risk of transfusion-transmissible HTLV infection among repeat donors during 2007 to 2008 decreased to 0.21 per 100,000 person years and 1:3,394,086, further demonstrating the success of universal blood screening (38).

Many molecular epidemiologic studies have shown HTLV proviruses to be remarkably stable genetically, which has allowed strong resolution of HTLV phylogenies and molecular dating of these viruses (8, 10, 39–41). The differing evolution rates for HTLV-1 and HIV-1 are due to clonal expansion of HTLV-infected cells versus active replication of HIV-1 (42, 43). While the overall genome of HTLV is highly conserved, nucleotide divergence in the LTR, *tax*, *pol*, and gp21 *env* genes has been exploited to genotype HTLV-1, HTLV-2 and, more recently, HTLV-3 and -4 (29, 44–47). The impact of diversity and emerging variants continues to challenge HTLV serology. An understanding of phylogenetic relationships is therefore useful. There are at least seven major geographic HTLV-1 subtypes which evolved from STLV-1 through several independent interspecies transmissions between simian and human hosts at different geographic locations (2–4): subtype A (cosmopolitan), subtype B (Central African), subtype C (Australo-Melanesian), subtype D (Central African, mainly among Pygmy tribes), subtype E found in an Efe Pygmy from the Congo, subtype F from people in the Democratic Republic of Congo, and subtype G from primate hunters in Central and West Africa (2, 3, 24, 48). HTLV-2 has three subtypes, named 2a, 2b, and 2d (26, 27), whose primate origin has been linked to a single primate, since STLV-2 has only been found in bonobos (3, 49). Subtype 2a is commonly found among IDUs worldwide, whereas subtype 2b is found primarily among Amerindians and in some Pygmies from Cameroon. Subtype 2d has been found in only one Pygmy from the Democratic Republic of Congo. Earlier studies proposed subtype 2c in one Amerindian tribe from Brazil; however, subsequent analysis of complete genomes confirmed this to be a subtype 2a variant (50). HTLV-3 most likely originated from recent cross-species transmission in people exposed to non-human primates in Cameroon (2, 4, 5, 28, 51). Phylogenetic analysis has identified HTLV-3 infection originating from at least four highly divergent STLV-3 subtypes such that there are also four HTLV-3 subtypes (2, 4, 5, 28, 51, 52). Subtypes A and C include the original STLV-3 identified in a baboon from East Africa and STLV-3 in spot-nosed monkeys (*Cercopithecus nictitans*) from Cameroon, but human infection has not been reported yet with either subtype (53–55). Subtype B includes both STLV-3 and HTLV-3 from West-Central Africa, while subtype D has occurred in both monkeys and a human from Cameroon (2–5, 28, 48, 51, 55). A fifth human infection with HTLV-3, another subtype D strain, was reported recently in a farmer in Cameroon who was also infected with HIV-1 (56). HTLV-4 was originally identified in a single hunter from Cameroon (2), but more recently, two additional HTLV-4-infected hunters were identified in Gabon (57). These studies suggest that cross-species transmission of a wide range of STLV lineages to humans is ongoing and not limited to rare historical events. It is currently unknown whether HTLV-3 and -4 represent dead-end infections in humans or have the potential to spread regionally or globally. A new STLV group, STLV-5, has been proposed recently for a macaque STLV originally classified as STLV-1 since detailed phylogenetic analysis showed that it is highly divergent from STLV-1 (58, 59). A human counterpart of STLV-5 has not yet been found. The genetic heterogeneity within HTLV has provided valuable information on geographic clustering, movement of ancient populations, and viral transmission (3, 8, 10, 24, 39, 40, 47, 60, 61).

CLINICAL SIGNIFICANCE

HTLV-1 has been associated with two major diseases: adult T-cell leukemia/lymphoma (ATLL) and HTLV-1-associated myelopathy/tropical spastic paraparesis (HAM/TSP). Disease occurs in less than 5% of infected individuals (24, 25, 32). ATLL exists in four forms: acute, chronic, smoldering, and T-cell non-Hodgkin's lymphoma. The acute form comprises about 75% of all ATLLs and can be rapidly fatal. ATLL is characterized by severe malignant proliferation of $CD4^+$ $CD25^+$ T-lymphocytes diagnosed biologically by seropositivity for HTLV-1, the presence of morphologically distinct $CD3^+/4^+/25^+$ lymphocytes with cleaved nuclei (flower cells), and clonal integration of HTLV-1 proviruses in the tumor cells, as detected by Southern blotting, inverse PCR, or newer technologies such as ultra-deep sequence analysis (17, 62, 63). Both Tax and HBZ are believed to be involved in ATLL development (13, 17, 64).

The clinical features of the chronic neuromyelopathy HAM/TSP are muscle weakness in the legs, hyperreflexia, clonus, extensor plantar responses, sensory disturbances, various urinary manifestations, impotence, and low-back pain (24, 25, 32, 64, 65). Spasticity of the lower legs is the main disability of HAM/TSP, with patients often requiring wheelchairs. The main biological diagnosis includes the presence of high titers of HTLV-specific antibodies in the serum and cerebrospinal fluid. Research studies have shown that levels of HTLV-1-infected cells in the cerebrospinal fluid are over twice those found in the peripheral blood for HAM/TSP patients compared to levels in HTLV-1-infected people with other neurological disorders, and PCR determination of proviral loads in these compartments thus has diagnostic value (64). The estimated lifetime risk of developing HAM/TSP among HTLV-1-infected people is 0.2 to 4% but can vary according to the geographical area, and the disease occurs more frequently in people over 40 years old (24, 25). Other uncommon inflammatory disease associations include infective dermatitis, uveitis, polymyositis, thyroiditis, and pneumonitis and HTLV-associated arthropathy (24, 25, 32, 64, 65). There have also been case reports of increased opportunistic infections in HTLV-1-infected people, such as cytomegalovirus (CMV), *Pneumocystis jirovecii*, herpes zoster, *Cryptococcus*, and *Mycobacterium avium* (25). In research studies, increased viral load has been identified in both ATLL and HAM/TSP patients, compared to asymptomatic infected people, and is one of the best predictors for disease development, though patients with high proviral loads can remain asymptomatic for decades (24, 25, 32, 64).

HTLV-2 has not been definitively associated with malignancy; however, it has shown rare association with a neurological disease resembling HAM/TSP that progresses more slowly and with milder symptoms (25, 66). The estimated lifetime risk of disease development for HTLV-2-infected people is unknown but appears to be less than that estimated for individuals with HTLV-1 infection (25, 26). While the majority of HTLV-2-infected people remain asymptomatic (>95%), recent studies report an increased incidence of infectious diseases (such as bronchitis, pneumonia, tuberculosis, and kidney and/or bladder infections) in HTLV-2-infected people (25, 66). A recent study also found a higher association of all-cause cancer and cancer mortality in a cohort of HTLV-2-infected patients in the United States, suggesting that more research is needed to understand the pathogenic potential of HTLV-2 (67).

HTLV coinfection with HIV can occur in high-risk groups, such as people from endemic HTLV areas and IDUs. To date, a few studies evaluating the impact of HIV-1 coinfection with HTLV have shown that there is an increased frequency of HTLV-1-associated clinical outcomes (lymphoma and neurological disease), especially in individuals with high CD4$^+$ T-cell counts. In contrast, a delayed progression to AIDS is seen in some HTLV-2/HIV-1-coinfected people (68–70). Moreover, HIV therapy that includes highly active antiretroviral therapy in HTLV-2/HIV-1-coinfected people does not affect HTLV-2 proviral burden but has been reported to provide a protective effect from AIDS progression (69, 71). These limited numbers of studies suggest that HIV-1 coinfection may increase the morbidity of HTLV-1-infected patients. A recent study also showed that the Tax proteins of both HTLV-1 and HTLV-2 inhibited HIV-1 replication *in vitro*, suggesting a protective effect of HTLV in HIV-1 infection (68). However, additional studies are needed to determine if coinfection affects the mortality of HTLV-infected patients. The pathogenic potential of HTLV-3 and HTLV-4 is not known and is limited by the small number of infected people identified in surveys of apparently healthy populations (2, 4, 5, 28). In addition, limited studies of patients receiving care at outpatient clinics in Europe or individuals with some cancers in the United States have not identified evidence of HTLV-3 and HTLV-4 infection (29–31, 72).

Treatment options for HTLV-associated diseases are limited (17, 25). Chemotherapy has not proven effective against aggressive forms of ATLL (73–75). Although zidovudine and alpha interferon yield some responses and improve ATLL prognosis, alternative therapies are critically needed (73–75). New drugs such as arsenic trioxide, proteasome inhibitors, retinoids, and angiogenesis inhibitors, as well as cellular immunotherapy, are under investigation (73–75). Allogeneic hematopoietic stem cell transplantation in young people has provided some improvement in survival rates for aggressive ATLL (76). Antiretroviral treatments such as lamivudine and high-dose alpha interferon and beta interferon have been evaluated with HAM/TSP patients and resulted in decreases in proviral loads, alterations in T-cell phenotypes, and anti-*tax* cytotoxic T-cell frequency changes (77). However, results of further follow-up on immunomodulatory therapies have been disappointing, and combination antiretroviral therapies (zidovudine and lamivudine) have been discouraging because of only partial or temporary success in decreasing proviral loads (78, 79). One study using STLV-1-infected baboons treated with zidovudine and sodium valproate showed significant viral load reduction, but clinical trials in HTLV-1-infected humans using both therapeutic agents have not been reported (80). Symptomatic or targeted treatment is still the foundation of HAM/TSP therapy (77, 78). Recently, the integrase inhibitor raltegravir was shown to have potent *in vitro* anti-HTLV-1 activity (81). However, the clinical effects of raltegravir treatment are not clear. In a small study of two people with HAM/TSP and three asymptomatic HTLV-1-infected people, treatment with raltegravir for 12 months did not show any sustained reduction in proviral load (82). For uveitis, topical and systemic corticosteroids appear to improve sight, whereas infective dermatitis responds well to antibiotic treatment (25).

Although animal model studies of various HTLV vaccines have induced neutralizing antibodies (nAb) and strong cytotoxic T-lymphocyte responses using peptides, and synthetic inhibitory peptides and nAb have blocked envelope-mediated viral entry, these vaccines have not yet been used in clinical trials (25). Recently, a subunit vaccine composed of recombinant surface proteins was successful in robustly activating cell-mediated cytotoxic responses and neutralized viral infectivity in mouse models (83). While these studies are promising for the development of potential HTLV vaccines, more research is needed to determine their antiviral and prophylactic efficacy. Recently, studies have shown that the use of Tax or HBZ peptides can infer protective immunity to HTLV-1 infection and development of ATL (76).

COLLECTION AND STORAGE OF SPECIMENS

Serum or plasma is suitable for use in serologic assays for HTLV detection and can be drawn at the time of presentation. Samples should be redrawn at 3 months from seronegative patients who are suspected of having HTLV infection, or those with seroindeterminate Western blot patterns, and should be retested to capture potentially infected people during the seroconversion window period (84). Alternatively, these people can also be tested by qualitative PCR to investigate possible infection, though these assays are not FDA approved but are clinically validated and available at commercial reference laboratories. Serum and plasma specimens can be stored at 4°C or frozen for later use. Package inserts should be consulted for storage limitations and limitations on the number of freeze-thaw cycles permitted. Fresh whole blood collected in EDTA or acid citrate dextrose for the preparation of peripheral blood mononuclear cells (PBMCs), and not plasma or serum, is an appropriate specimen for nucleic acid amplification testing (NAAT) and virus isolation since HTLV-1 and HTLV-2 are cell-associated viruses. PBMCs are typically isolated from fresh whole blood on a Ficoll-Hypaque gradient (discussed in chapter 82). Heparin as a blood anticoagulant is not recommended for NAAT because it interferes with the enzyme used in PCR. DNA is prepared using standard methods and can be stored at −20°C until needed. For virus culture, whole blood is collected in acid citrate dextrose, EDTA, or heparin tubes, and PBMCs are isolated on a Ficoll-Hypaque gradient.

DIRECT EXAMINATION

PCR Detection of Nucleic Acids

Amplification of proviral DNA by PCR is the preferred method for determining infection status, testing the validity of serologic assay results, distinguishing among the four HTLV groups, and studying tissue distribution *in vivo* (84). Qualitative PCR procedures utilizing primers in the *pol*, *env*, or *tax* genes and the LTR have been used to confirm and differentiate between HTLV-1 and -2 (and more recently HTLV-3 and -4) infections (Table 1) (2, 44, 45, 72, 85). These assays utilize HTLV consensus primers that allow amplification of all four viruses, with typing achieved either by hybridizing the product to an HTLV-specific probe or by sequence analysis. A second approach employs type-specific primers and probes in separate amplifications. The PCR products can be detected with labeled internal probes by Southern blot hybridization and with sequencing (44, 85). Most of these assays are performed for research use only, but some are now offered by commercial laboratories. Blood PCR tests offered at commercial reference laboratories are validated to detect only HTLV-1 and -2. Testing of cerebrospinal fluid specimens is not available at commercial laboratories.

Viral detection and quantification of proviral DNA can be performed simultaneously using real-time PCR; RNA viral load estimation from plasma is not feasible in HTLV infection since these viruses are cell associated (29, 44, 46, 47). Noncommercial, quantitative real-time PCR assays have excellent sensitivity and specificity and a broad dynamic range, from 10 to 10^6 copies/reaction, and have been used to define the relationship between proviral load and both pathogenesis and person-to-person transmission risks (25, 86). For example, proviral load is higher among HAM/TSP and ATLL patients than among

TABLE 1 Summary of serological and supplemental confirmatory tests for HTLV infection

Detection method	Description	Reference(s)	Availability in U.S.[a]
Serological screening tests			
EIA	HTLV-1- and HTLV-2-infected cell lysates and/or recombinant antigens used to detect HTLV antibodies by colorimetric readout. Excellent sensitivity and specificity for HTLV-1 and -2. Sensitivity for HTLV-3 and -4 detection is unknown.	25, 45, 82, 91	One FDA-licensed test
ChLIA	Similar to EIA but with chemiluminescent detection	92	One FDA-licensed test
Particle agglutination	Viral lysate coats gelatin or latex particles. Antigen-specific antibodies bind, which results in agglutination of particles. Visual readout by operator.		Research use only
Serological supplementary tests			
Western blot	HTLV-1 viral lysates ± recombinant antigens used to detect HTLV-1- and -2-specific antibodies. May contain recombinant antigens to differentiate antibodies to HTLV-1 and HTLV-2. HTLV-3 and -4 can give variable WB profiles.	45, 91, 97	One FDA-licensed test
LIA	Recombinant or peptide HTLV-1 and HTLV-2 antigens printed onto membrane. Antibodies to individual viral proteins are visualized. HTLV-3 and -4 can give variable results.	45, 91, 98	Research use only
IFA	Antibodies bind to HTLV-1-, HTLV-2-, and STLV-3-infected cells. Detected by secondary anti-human antibody with fluorescent label. Differentiates between antibodies to HTLV-1, HTLV-2, and HTLV-3.	25, 45	Research use only
Nucleic acid detection tests			
Qualitative PCR	Distinguishes between HTLV groups either by using HTLV consensus primers with typing done by HTLV-specific primers and probes in separate tests or by sequence analysis	44, 83	Validated assays available commercially but are not FDA approved or CE marked
Quantitative PCR	Determines proviral DNA copy number by limiting dilution, quantitative competitive PCR, or real-time PCR using HTLV degenerate and/or type-specific primers	25, 29, 46, 47, 84	Research use only

[a]FDA licensed, may be used for blood donor screening and as an aid in clinical diagnosis of HTLV-1 or HTLV-2 infection and related diseases; research use only, not for clinical use.

asymptomatic carriers, suggesting that proviral load may be a prognostic indicator for future disease development (25, 32, 64, 70, 86). Both sexual and mother-to-child transmission are associated with higher HTLV proviral load in the index case (25, 32, 64, 70, 87, 88). Thus, quantification of HTLV proviral load in research studies has provided a better understanding of correlates of transmission and disease progression (25, 32, 64, 70, 87). Since these differences in HTLV proviral loads among asymptomatic and sick patients have been determined in various research studies and a standardized quantitative PCR is currently not available at commercial laboratories, there have been about 5-fold variations in the proviral loads reported across these studies (89). In general, healthy carriers have a proviral load of <3 copies/100 PBMCs compared to 5 to 10 copies/100 PBMCs in people with ATLL (89).

VIRUS ISOLATION AND IDENTIFICATION

Isolation of HTLV has been difficult since these viruses are cell associated (25, 90). Nevertheless, cocultivation of HTLV-infected PBMCs with activated, allogeneic HTLV-negative PBMCs or cord blood cells is used to obtain viral isolates. Tissue culture supernatants are collected weekly for up to 4 to 6 weeks, and the presence of HTLV-1 or HTLV-2 p19 Gag antigen in the supernatant is tested using a research-use-only antigen capture assay (Zeptometrix Corp., Buffalo, NY). Alternatively, PCR methods can be used to monitor for infection in tissue culture cellular DNA. Because of the time required and the labor-intensive nature of this method, virus isolation and tissue culture detection are generally not done for HTLV diagnosis but, rather, serve as research tools to further characterize the viruses. HTLV-3 and HTLV-4 have not yet been isolated *in vitro*.

TYPING SYSTEMS AND SEROLOGIC TESTS

Testing for antibodies to HTLV-1 and HTLV-2 should be performed for all blood donors and patients presenting with relevant clinical signs and symptoms. In the United States, since 1988 all blood donors have been screened for antibodies to both HTLV-1 and HTLV-2 using assays that include both HTLV-1 and HTLV-2 antigens (33, 84, 91). Testing for HTLV-1 and HTLV-2 should also be offered to people who are from areas where HTLV is endemic, who engage in high-risk behaviors such as needle sharing, and who have had sexual contact with persons from either group. Currently, HTLV-1 and HTLV-2 testing is not routinely performed for fertility or pregnancy testing in the United States. This is different from some European countries, as well as some islands in the West Indies, where recommendations have been made to test pregnant and breast-feeding women originating from areas of HTLV-1 endemicity such as Japan (24, 25, 34). In addition, in the United States all donors of viable, leukocyte-rich cells or tissue (e.g., hematopoietic stem/progenitor cells and semen) are screened for HTLV-1 and -2 (92). However, since favorable outcomes for recipients of HTLV-1/2-positive organs in the United States have been reported and given the low prevalence of HTLV-1 in the United States, the Organ Procurement and Transplantation Network/United Network for Organ Sharing Committee in 2009 eliminated the requirement for pretransplant deceased donor HTLV-1/2 testing (92). Organ procurement organization laboratories can continue routine donor screening, including living donors and testing of donors at increased risk of HTLV infection. Organ recipients should also be offered HTLV testing if presenting with any symptoms of HTLV infection. Nonetheless, it may still be prudent to prescreen organ donors from areas with high HTLV endemicity.

The most common screening assays detect antibodies to HTLV in serum or plasma (25, 33, 84). The immunodominant regions of structural and regulatory proteins are well characterized and are used in diagnostic assays that detect and differentiate HTLV-1 and HTLV-2. The major tests for HTLV-1 and HTLV-2 are described in Table 1. The serologic testing algorithm consists of a primary screening assay followed by testing for confirmation and identification of HTLV type (Fig. 2). Assays for the specific detection and discrimination of HTLV-3 and -4 are not currently available (93).

Primary screening assays include enzyme immunoassays (EIA), chemiluminescent immunoassays (ChLIA), particle agglutination (Fujirebio America, Fairfield, NJ), and immunofluorescence assays (IFAs) (Table 1). EIAs are sensitive and simple colorimetric tests that use purified HTLV-infected cell lysates and/or recombinant antigens or synthetic peptides. ChLIA is similar to EIA but uses chemiluminescence for the detection step. The addition of HTLV-2 antigens to screening tests significantly improved the detection of antibodies to HTLV-2 compared with results using tests that contained only HTLV-1 antigens (25, 94). The EIA and ChLIA can be automated and performed on a large scale (94). However, neither EIAs nor ChLIAs can differentiate between HTLV-1 and HTLV-2 infection because of significant sequence identity of the structural proteins between the two viruses; therefore, these screening assays are referred to as tests for HTLV-1/2.

Comparative analysis of various commercial screening assays containing both HTLV-1 and HTLV-2 antigens indicates that sensitivity ranges from 98.9 to 100% for confirmed HTLV-1-positive specimens and 91.5 to 100% for confirmed HTLV-2-positive specimens. Specificity ranges from 90.2 to 100% (25, 95, 96). Currently, one HTLV-1/2 EIA (Avioq HTLV-I/II Microelisa System, Avioq, Inc., Research Triangle Park, NC) and one HTLV-1/2 ChLIA (Abbott Prism HTLV-I/HTLV-II, Abbott Laboratories, Abbott Park, IL) are licensed by the FDA and are available for use in the United States. The Avioq assay was previously called the Vironostika HTLV-I/II Microelisa System and was manufactured by bioMérieux but was not commercially available in the United States for a period of time. Both FDA-approved assays have reported overall sensitivity point estimates of 100% (95% confidence interval [CI] of 99.97 to 100% for Avioq and 99.89 to 99.96% for Abbott). Specificities of 99.93% (95% CI, 99.89 to 99.96%) for Abbott Prism HTLV-I/HTLV-II and 99.95% for Avioq (95% CI, 99.89 to 99.98%) were reported from clinical trial data that supported the licensure of these tests. An independent study by the American Red Cross also showed that the Abbott Prism had a 100% assay sensitivity (95% CI, 99.48 to 100%) (33). Both assays can be used for blood donor screening and as an aid in clinical diagnosis of HTLV-1 and HTLV-2 infection and related diseases. Further attempts have been made to develop a dual EIA algorithm to increase the predictive values of HTLV tests (Fig. 2) (33, 97). Pooling of samples for seroepidemiologic studies has been proposed; however, pooled testing is not recommended for blood donor testing (98).

While most screening assays are highly sensitive, specimens containing low titers of antibodies to HTLV-1 and HTLV-2 from certain areas of HTLV endemicity, or specimens from early seroconverters, may be missed by EIA screening. NAAT can be used to detect infected individuals either with low antibody titers or within their window period prior to the development of an antibody response

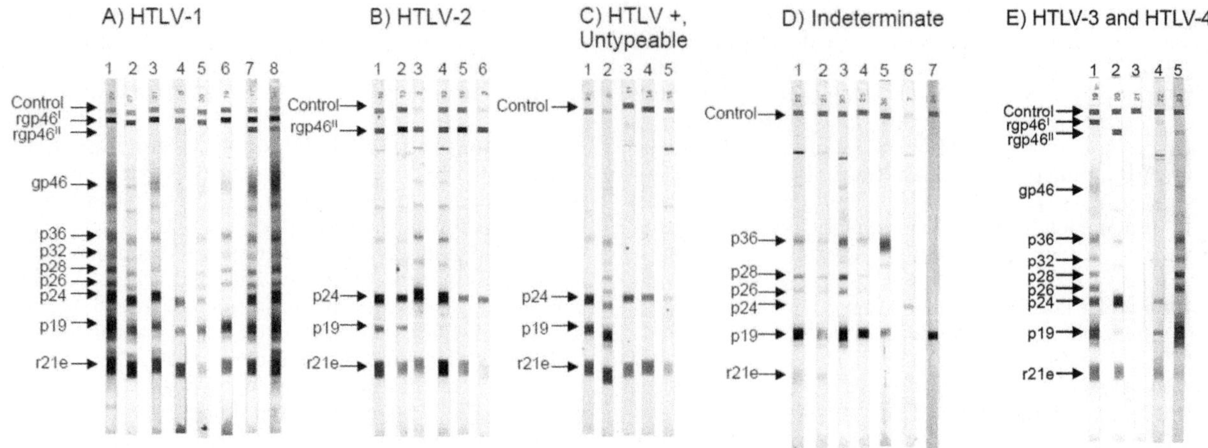

FIGURE 3 WB analysis of representative plasma or serum specimens from people infected with (A) HTLV-1, (B) HTLV-2, (C) HTLV-1/2 untypeable, (D) indeterminate, and (E) HTLV-3 and HTLV-4. Representative seroreactivity patterns are shown for WBs from MP Biomedical (HTLV-2.4 version), which contain HTLV-1 antigens spiked with recombinant r21e (common to HTLV-1 and HTLV-2) and two external envelope recombinant proteins specific for HTLV-1 ($rgp46^{I}$) and HTLV-2 ($rgp46^{II}$). (A) Typical patterns for HTLV-1 reactivity (lanes 1 to 5), atypical reactivity lacking p24 Gag response (lane 6), and specimens with high antibody titers showing dual reactivity to both rgp46 proteins (lanes 7 and 8; titration of sera results in reactivity only to $rgp46^{I}$). (B) Typical patterns for HTLV-2 reactivity (lanes 1 to 6; note that reactivity to the p24 band is stronger than to the p19 band, which is usually absent from sera from HTLV-2-infected people). (C) HTLV-1/2-positive but untypeable specimens, with reactivity to Gag (p24, with or without p19) and r21e but not $gp46^{I}$ or $gp46^{II}$. Lanes 1 and 2: characteristic patterns of specimens that are usually found to contain HTLV-1 after additional testing; lanes 3 to 5: characteristic patterns of specimens that are usually found to contain HTLV-2 after additional testing. (D) Typical patterns from HTLV indeterminate specimens. Shown are typical HTLV Gag indeterminate profiles frequently found in plasma or sera from individuals originating from tropical regions (Central Africa, Papua New Guinea, etc.) (lanes 1 to 4) and those from low-risk populations (lanes 5 to 7). In the great majority of cases, neither HTLV-1 nor HTLV-2 infection could be demonstrated in samples with such seroreactivity using PCR testing. (E) Seroreactivity observed in HTLV-3-infected (lane 4) and HTLV-4-infected (lane 5) people from Cameroon. Plasma from an HTLV-3-infected person was weakly reactive to p24, p19, r21e, and $rgp46^{I}$. Plasma from the HTLV-4-infected person was weakly reactive to p24, r21e, and $rgp46^{II}$ but was strongly reactive to p19, similar to that seen in HTLV-1-infected specimens. Lanes 1 and 2 are from HTLV-1- and -2-infected people, respectively, while lane 3 is reactivity of negative control plasma.

(median window period, 51 days; range, 36 to 72 days) (33). However, while validated NAAT assays may be commercially available, they are not licensed by the FDA nor are they CE-marked for use in Europe.

Supplemental confirmatory or differentiation tests for HTLV-1 and HTLV-2 infection include Western blots (WBs) containing viral lysates supplemented with recombinant proteins, line immunoassays (LIAs; Innogenetics, Ghent, Belgium), and IFAs (Table 1). Although WB assays using purified viral lysates are highly sensitive for detecting p24 and p19 Gag antibodies, they do not always detect antibodies to native Env glycoproteins. An alternative approach used in a second-generation confirmatory assay is a modified WB that contains type-specific gp46 Env recombinant proteins from HTLV-1 and -2 and a truncated form of recombinant p21 Env (r21e) that reduces nonspecific reactivity, improves performance (specificity and sensitivity), and allows differentiation between HTLV-1 and HTLV-2 (MP Diagnostics WB 2.4; MP Biomedicals, Science Park, Singapore) (Fig. 3) (99). The MP Diagnostics WB test was approved by the FDA in December 2014 for detection of antibodies to HTLV-1 and -2 in human serum and plasma.

LIA is another supplementary test consisting of recombinant and synthetic HTLV-1- and HTLV-2-specific antigens printed onto strips (INNO-LIA, Innogenetics) (100); this assay can differentiate between HTLV-1 and HTLV-2 infection. IFAs that detect binding of antibodies from a specimen to HTLV-1- or HTLV-2-infected cells can also be used to discriminate HTLV-1/2 infections and to determine antibody titer (24, 25). WB and LIA confirmatory/supplemental assays have been certified for use in Europe and other areas of endemicity (Brazil, Argentina, West Indies, Iran, and Japan) to confirm any repeatedly EIA-reactive sample (34).

HTLV-3 and HTLV-4 were detected in research studies using commercially available EIAs and WB assays or research-based IFAs that use HTLV-1 and -2 antigens (2, 45, 93). The sensitivity for detecting these new HTLVs with these assays is unknown, and a broad range of WB or LIA profiles is observed which can be confused with those of HTLV-1 or -2. Thus, PCR and sequence analysis are critical for resolving infection with the specific HTLV group.

EVALUATION, INTERPRETATION, AND REPORTING OF RESULTS

A typical algorithm for HTLV testing for diagnostic purposes is outlined in Fig. 2. If the initial screening immunoassay (EIA or ChLIA) is reactive, a repeat assay on the same specimen is performed in duplicate. If one or both of the repeat tests are reactive, the specimen is classified as repeatedly reactive (RR). The RR specimens are subjected to confirmatory supplemental testing that is typically done by WB when available (Fig. 3 and Table 1). Based on the data available in 1992, the U.S. Public Health Service recommended that the diagnostic criteria for confirmation of HTLV-1 or HTLV-2 seropositivity by supplemental tests include demonstration of antibodies to p24 Gag and to native gp46 Env and/or r21e (84). Subsequent data with more sensitive assays suggest that alternative patterns of WB reactivity may be considered. The second-generation modified WB is the most commonly used research-use WB assay worldwide (MP Diagnostics WB 2.4). Specimens with reactivity to p19 Gag (with or without p24 Gag), r21e, and rgp46^{I} are referred to as HTLV-1 positive (Fig. 3A). Sera with reactivity to p24 Gag (with or without p19 Gag), r21e, and rgp46^{II} are referred to as HTLV-2 positive (Fig. 3B). Specimens without immunoreactivity to any WB bands are considered negative for antibodies to HTLV-1 and HTLV-2 (false-positive EIA specimens). Specimens reacting with p24 Gag (with or without p19 Gag) and r21e, but with no reactivity to either rgp46^{I} or rgp46^{II}, are considered HTLV positive but untypeable (Fig. 3C) since PCR analysis of untypeable specimens has identified the presence of HTLV-specific sequences in some cases (2, 44, 85). This type of reactivity could indicate the presence of divergent HTLV such as HTLV-3 and HTLV-4. However, to date, HTLV-3 and -4 have been found only in Cameroon (2, 12–14). Similar interpretive criteria are used for LIA (see manufacturer's instructions).

Both the WB assays and LIA can give indeterminate results (immunoreactivity to a single HTLV gene product or multiple bands not defined as positive above, conditions that do not meet the criteria for seropositivity [Fig. 3D]). Antibody to only Gag proteins (p24, p19) is the most common indeterminate pattern that is observed in EIA-reactive specimens and is an area of intense investigation (101–104). Extensive PCR analyses using primers to detect multiple gene regions have failed to detect HTLV-1 or HTLV-2 proviral sequences in low-risk seroindeterminate people, thus indicating that these individuals are not likely to be infected with HTLV-1 or HTLV-2 (44, 83, 101–104). The possibility that such indeterminate WB results may represent a novel retrovirus with partial homology to HTLV has been explored; however, no DNA amplification was observed using generic PCR primers that would detect HTLV-related viruses (44, 83, 103, 104), with the exception of HTLV-3 and HTLV-4 (2, 4–6, 51). Limited studies have established that individuals with indeterminate WB profiles generally do not have risk factors for HTLV infection (101–104). Indeterminate WB results among low-risk people may represent antibodies to different viral, microbial, and cellular antigens that cross-react with HTLV proteins (101–104) (Fig. 3E). The predictive value of positive WB results is increased in patients with a history of any potential HTLV risk factor, including residence in areas of endemicity, history of a blood transfusion before 1988 or IDU, having multiple sexual partners without condom protection, or having sexual partners or parents from an endemic region (25, 84).

In rare instances, specimens with confirmed HTLV infection have an indeterminate WB pattern of reactivity to p19 Gag (in the absence of p24 Gag) and r21e (25, 101). Likewise, in some instances, antibody to r21e may represent an early antibody response during seroconversion (25, 84). Individuals with such reactivity should be retested in 3 months by EIA and/or PCR (84).

Recent data suggest that a very small number of U.S. patients with chronic progressive neurological disease with HTLV-indeterminate WB patterns may be infected with a defective HTLV or have HTLV-1 in low copy numbers (101). More recently, studies in Japan and Argentina have also reported an association of low proviral loads and HTLV-1 WB indeterminate results (105, 106). Furthermore, both studies also identified genetic mutations that could impact antigen detection, possibly resulting in indeterminate WB patterns. People who have clinical neurological symptoms or are from high-prevalence areas (e.g., African, Asian, South American, and Caribbean countries) with HTLV-1/2-indeterminate reactivity should be further investigated by NAAT and also to exclude HTLV-3 and HTLV-4.

Currently, in the United States decisions to accept blood donations and defer blood donors are based on results of a screening test using ChLIA with reactive specimens tested using a second licensed screening test and the licensed HTLV WB assay. People who are ultimately confirmed to be antibody-positive to HTLV-1 or HTLV-2 will be permanently deferred from donating blood (33, 38). Blood donors with plasma specimens that are RR on screening but not confirmed as seropositive for HTLV-1 or HTLV-2 (including false EIA-reactive and supplemental test indeterminate specimens and specimens for which supplemental testing was not performed) should be notified and deferred if the same test result is obtained on two separate donations (33, 38, 84). Screening tests are weighted toward better sensitivity than specificity because of the public health implications of false-negative results (107). Therefore, in the absence of known risk factors for a given blood donor, RR results from a single-test kit most likely represent false-positive reactions. The positive predictive value of a test result is always a function of the prevalence of disease in the screened population, which for HTLV is extremely low in blood donors following implementation of screening in 1988 (48). The lower the prevalence, the lower the positive predictive value and the lower the specificity of a test. Thus, blood specimens are routinely tested using the dual-screening test algorithm (Fig. 2) to increase the probability of detecting actual infection (33, 38, 97). Since sensitivities are similar in each individual screening test and nonspecific reactivity is not, specimens reactive in both tests are likely true positives (33, 38). Nonetheless, WB-indeterminate results are seen in RR U.S. blood donors but have been shown by PCR to be HTLV negative in nearly all cases (85). Thus, additional testing by PCR or from specimens collected at a later time point is required to resolve infection in these people. Many studies have reported high concordance between WB and PCR results of infected and uninfected U.S. blood donors (33, 107–109). Using NAAT instead of WB has also been suggested for confirmation of RR specimens but requires whole blood or PBMCs and also is not a rapid test (110). A study in 2011 also showed that testing of donors deferred with initially RR results using historic and now discontinued screening EIAs, but without confirmed HTLV infection, could be reconsidered for donation eligibility if a current sample tests negative using the more sensitive and specific ChLIA test (33).

Individuals with HTLV-1- or HTLV-2-positive or indeterminate test results are counseled according to the guidelines established by the U.S. Public Health Service Working Group at the CDC (84). Though published in 1993, the epidemiology of HTLV transmission has not changed, and hence, the guidelines remain effective. These guidelines state that people should be informed that HTLV is not HIV and that their risk of developing HTLV-related diseases is low. HTLV-1- or HTLV-2-infected people are asked not to donate blood, semen, organs, or other tissues and not to share needles or syringes. To prevent transmission of HTLV, the infected person is counseled to use protective measures during sexual activity, and women are counseled to refrain from breast-feeding. People who have indeterminate results on two separate occasions at least 3 months apart should be advised that their specimens were reactive in screening for HTLV-1/2 but that these results could not be confirmed by more specific tests. Further, they should be reassured that indeterminate results are very rarely caused by HTLV-1 or HTLV-2 infection. Repeat serologic and/or PCR testing should be offered to people with indeterminate test results.

Use of trade names is for identification only and does not imply endorsement by the U.S. Department of Health and Human Services, the Public Health Service, or the Centers for Disease Control and Prevention. The findings and conclusions in this report are those of the authors and do not necessarily represent the views of the Centers for Disease Control and Prevention.

REFERENCES

1. **Welkin J, Blomberg J, Boris-Lawrie K, Fan H, Gifford R, Lindemann D, Quackenbush SL, Stoye J.** 2011. Retroviridae, p 477. *In* King AMQ, Lefkowitz E, Adams MJ, Carstens EB (ed), *Virus Taxonomy: Ninth Report of the International Committee on Taxonomy of Viruses*. Elsevier, Waltham, MA.
2. **Wolfe ND, Heneine W, Carr JK, Garcia AD, Shanmugam V, Tamoufe U, Torimiro JN, Prosser AT, Lebreton M, Mpoudi-Ngole E, McCutchan FE, Birx DL, Folks TM, Burke DS, Switzer WM.** 2005. Emergence of unique primate T-lymphotropic viruses among central African bushmeat hunters. *Proc Natl Acad Sci USA* **102:**7994–7999.
3. **Gessain A, Meertens L, Mahieux R.** 2002. *Molecular Epidemiology of Human T Cell Leukemia/Lymphoma Viruses Type 1 and Type 2(HTLV-1/2) and Related Simian Retroviruses (STLV-1, STLV-2, and STLV-L/3)*. Kluwer Academic Publishers, Boston, MA.
4. **Calattini S, Chevalier SA, Duprez R, Bassot S, Froment A, Mahieux R, Gessain A.** 2005. Discovery of a new human T-cell lymphotropic virus (HTLV-3) in Central Africa. *Retrovirology* **2:**30.
5. **Zheng H, Wolfe ND, Sintasath DM, Tamoufe U, Lebreton M, Djoko CF, Diffo JD, Pike BL, Heneine W, Switzer WM.** 2010. Emergence of a novel and highly divergent HTLV-3 in a primate hunter in Cameroon. *Virology* **401:**137–145.
6. **Calattini S, Betsem E, Bassot S, Chevalier SA, Mahieux R, Froment A, Gessain A.** 2009. New strain of human T lymphotropic virus (HTLV) type 3 in a Pygmy from Cameroon with peculiar HTLV serologic results. *J Infect Dis* **199:**561–564.
7. **LeBreton M, Switzer WM, Djoko CF, Gillis A, Jia H, Sturgeon MM, Shankar A, Zheng H, Nkeunen G, Tamoufe U, Nana A, Le Doux Diffo J, Tafon B, Kiyang J, Schneider BS, Burke DS, Wolfe ND.** 2014. A gorilla reservoir for human T-lymphotropic virus type 4. *Emerg Microbes Infect* **3:**e7.
8. **Switzer WM, Salemi M, Qari SH, Jia H, Gray RR, Katzourakis A, Marriott SJ, Pryor KN, Wolfe ND, Burke DS, Folks TM, Heneine W.** 2009. Ancient, independent evolution and distinct molecular features of the novel human T-lymphotropic virus type 4. *Retrovirology* **6:**9.
9. **Calattini S, Chevalier SA, Duprez R, Afonso P, Froment A, Gessain A, Mahieux R.** 2006. Human T-cell lymphotropic virus type 3: complete nucleotide sequence and characterization of the human tax3 protein. *J Virol* **80:**9876–9888.
10. **Switzer WM, Qari SH, Wolfe ND, Burke DS, Folks TM, Heneine W.** 2006. Ancient origin and molecular features of the novel human T-lymphotropic virus type 3 revealed by complete genome analysis. *J Virol* **80:**7427–7438.
11. **Feuer G, Green PL.** 2005. Comparative biology of human T-cell lymphotropic virus type 1 (HTLV-1) and HTLV-2. *Oncogene* **24:**5996–6004.
12. **Bindhu M, Nair A, Lairmore MD.** 2004. Role of accessory proteins of HTLV-1 in viral replication, T cell activation, and cellular gene expression. *Front Biosci* **9:**2556–2576.
13. **Barbeau B, Mesnard JM.** 2011. Making sense out of antisense transcription in human T-cell lymphotropic viruses (HTLVs). *Viruses* **3:**456–468.
14. **Arnold J, Yamamoto B, Li M, Phipps AJ, Younis I, Lairmore MD, Green PL.** 2006. Enhancement of infectivity and persistence *in vivo* by HBZ, a natural antisense coded protein of HTLV-1. *Blood* **107:**3976–3982.
15. **Gaudray G, Gachon F, Basbous J, Biard-Piechaczyk M, Devaux C, Mesnard JM.** 2002. The complementary strand of the human T-cell leukemia virus type 1 RNA genome encodes a bZIP transcription factor that down-regulates viral transcription. *J Virol* **76:**12813–12822.
16. **Satou Y, Yasunaga J, Zhao T, Yoshida M, Miyazato P, Takai K, Shimizu K, Ohshima K, Green PL, Ohkura N, Yamaguchi T, Ono M, Sakaguchi S, Matsuoka M.** 2011. HTLV-1 bZIP factor induces T-cell lymphoma and systemic inflammation *in vivo*. *PLoS Pathog* **7:**e1001274.
17. **Matsuoka M, Jeang KT.** 2011. Human T-cell leukemia virus type 1 (HTLV-1) and leukemic transformation: viral infectivity, Tax, HBZ and therapy. *Oncogene* **30:**1379–1389.
18. **Jones KS, Fugo K, Petrow-Sadowski C, Huang Y, Bertolette DC, Lisinski I, Cushman SW, Jacobson S, Ruscetti FW.** 2006. Human T-cell leukemia virus type 1 (HTLV-1) and HTLV-2 use different receptor complexes to enter T cells. *J Virol* **80:**8291–8302.
19. **Jones KS, Huang YK, Chevalier SA, Afonso PV, Petrow-Sadowski C, Bertolette DC, Gessain A, Ruscetti FW, Mahieux R.** 2009. The receptor complex associated with human T-cell lymphotropic virus type 3 (HTLV-3) Env-mediated binding and entry is distinct from, but overlaps with, the receptor complexes of HTLV-1 and HTLV-2. *J Virol* **83:**5244–5255.
20. **Jones KS, Lambert S, Bouttier M, Bénit L, Ruscetti FW, Hermine O, Pique C.** 2011. Molecular aspects of HTLV-1 entry: functional domains of the HTLV-1 surface subunit (SU) and their relationships to the entry receptors. *Viruses* **3:**794–810.
21. **Jones KS, Petrow-Sadowski C, Huang YK, Bertolette DC, Ruscetti FW.** 2008. Cell-free HTLV-1 infects dendritic cells leading to transmission and transformation of CD4(+) T cells. *Nat Med* **14:**429–436.
22. **Pique C, Jones KS.** 2012. Pathways of cell-cell transmission of HTLV-1. *Front Microbiol* **3:**378.
23. **Lambert S, Bouttier M, Vassy R, Seigneuret M, Petrow-Sadowski C, Janvier S, Heveker N, Ruscetti FW, Perret G, Jones KS, Pique C.** 2009. HTLV-1 uses HSPG and neuropilin-1 for entry by molecular mimicry of VEGF165. *Blood* **113:**5176–5185.
24. **Gessain A, Cassar O.** 2012. Epidemiological aspects and world distribution of HTLV-1 infection. *Front Microbiol* **3:**388.
25. **Beilke MA, Murphy EL.** 2006. The human T-lymphotropic viruses 1 and 2, p 326–358. *In* Wolberding P, Palefsky J (ed), *Viral and Immunological Malignancies*. BC Decker, Inc, Hamilton, Ontario, Canada.
26. **Paiva A, Casseb J.** 2015. Origin and prevalence of human T-lymphotropic virus type 1 (HTLV-1) and type 2 (HTLV-2) among indigenous populations in the Americas. *Rev Inst Med Trop São Paulo* **57:**1–13.
27. **Mauclère P, Afonso PV, Meertens L, Plancoulaine S, Calattini S, Froment A, Van Beveren M, de Thé G, Quintana-Murci L, Mahieux R, Gessain A.** 2011. HTLV-2B strains, similar to those found in several Amerindian tribes, are endemic in central African Bakola Pygmies. *J Infect Dis* **203:**1316–1323.
28. **Calattini S, Betsem E, Bassot S, Chevalier SA, Tortevoye P, Njouom R, Mahieux R, Froment A, Gessain A.** 2011. Multiple retroviral infection by HTLV type 1, 2, 3 and simian foamy virus in a family of Pygmies from Cameroon. *Virology* **410:**48–55.
29. **Duong YT, Jia H, Lust JA, Garcia AD, Tiffany AJ, Heneine W, Switzer WM.** 2008. Short communication: absence of evidence of HTLV-3 and HTLV-4 in patients with

large granular lymphocyte (LGL) leukemia. *AIDS Res Hum Retroviruses* **24:**1503–1505.

30. **Perzova R, Benz P, Abbott L, Welch C, Thomas A, El Ghoul R, Sanghi S, Nara P, Glaser J, Siegal FP, Dosik H, Poiesz BJ.** 2010. Short communication: no evidence of HTLV-3 and HTLV-4 infection in New York State subjects at risk for retroviral infection. *AIDS Res Hum Retroviruses* **26:**1229–1231.
31. **Thomas A, Perzova R, Abbott L, Benz P, Poiesz MJ, Dube S, Loughran T, Ferrer J, Sheremata W, Glaser J, Leon-Ponte M, Poiesz BJ.** 2010. LGL leukemia and HTLV. *AIDS Res Hum Retroviruses* **26:**33–40.
32. **Proietti FA, Carneiro-Proietti AB, Catalan-Soares BC, Murphy EL.** 2005. Global epidemiology of HTLV-I infection and associated diseases. *Oncogene* **24:**6058–6068.
33. **Stramer SL, Notari EP IV, Zou S, Krysztof DE, Brodsky JP, Tegtmeier GE, Dodd RY.** 2011. Human T-lymphotropic virus antibody screening of blood donors: rates of false-positive results and evaluation of a potential donor reentry algorithm. *Transfusion* **51:**692–701.
34. **Taylor GP, Bodéus M, Courtois F, Pauli G, Del Mistro A, Machuca A, Padua E, Andersson S, Goubau P, Chieco-Bianchi L, Soriano V, Coste J, Ades AE, Weber JN.** 2005. The seroepidemiology of human T-lymphotropic viruses: types I and II in Europe: a prospective study of pregnant women. *J Acquir Immune Defic Syndr* **38:**104–109.
35. **Fukushima Y, Takahashi H, Hall WW, Nakasone T, Nakata S, Song P, Duc DD, Hien B, Quang NX, Trinh TN, Nishioka K, Kitamura K, Komuro K, Vahlne A, Honda M.** 1995. Extraordinary high rate of HTLV type II seropositivity in intravenous drug abusers in south Vietnam. *AIDS Res Hum Retroviruses* **11:**637–644.
36. **Salemi M, Lewis M, Egan JF, Hall WW, Desmyter J, Vandamme AM.** 1999. Different population dynamics of human T cell lymphotropic virus type II in intravenous drug users compared with endemically infected tribes. *Proc Natl Acad Sci USA* **96:**13253–13258.
37. **Dodd RY, Notari EP IV, Stramer SL.** 2002. Current prevalence and incidence of infectious disease markers and estimated window-period risk in the American Red Cross blood donor population. *Transfusion* **42:**975–979.
38. **Zou S, Stramer SL, Dodd RY.** 2012. Donor testing and risk: current prevalence, incidence, and residual risk of transfusion-transmissible agents in US allogeneic donations. *Transfus Med Rev* **26:**119–128.
39. **Salemi M, Desmyter J, Vandamme AM.** 2000. Tempo and mode of human and simian T-lymphotropic virus (HTLV/STLV) evolution revealed by analyses of full-genome sequences. *Mol Biol Evol* **17:**374–386.
40. **Van Dooren S, Pybus OG, Salemi M, Liu HF, Goubau P, Remondegui C, Talarmin A, Gotuzzo E, Alcantara LC, Galvão-Castro B, Vandamme AM.** 2004. The low evolutionary rate of human T-cell lymphotropic virus type-1 confirmed by analysis of vertical transmission chains. *Mol Biol Evol* **21:**603–611.
41. **Lemey P, Pybus OG, Van Dooren S, Vandamme AM.** 2005. A Bayesian statistical analysis of human T-cell lymphotropic virus evolutionary rates. *Infect Genet Evol* **5:**291–298.
42. **Asquith B, Zhang Y, Mosley AJ, de Lara CM, Wallace DL, Worth A, Kaftantzi L, Meekings K, Griffin GE, Tanaka Y, Tough DF, Beverley PC, Taylor GP, Macallan DC, Bangham CR.** 2007. *In vivo* T lymphocyte dynamics in humans and the impact of human T-lymphotropic virus 1 infection. *Proc Natl Acad Sci USA* **104:**8035–8040.
43. **Watanabe T.** 2017. Adult T-cell leukemia: molecular basis for clonal expansion and transformation of HTLV-1-infected T cells. *Blood* **129:**1071–1081.
44. **Gallego S, Mangano A, Gastaldello R, Sen L, Medeot S.** 2004. Usefulness of a Nested-polymerase chain reaction for molecular diagnosis of human T-cell lymphotropic virus type I/II. *Mem Inst Oswaldo Cruz* **99:**377–380.
45. **Mahieux R, Gessain A.** 2011. HTLV-3/STLV-3 and HTLV-4 viruses: discovery, epidemiology, serology and molecular aspects. *Viruses* **3:**1074–1090.
46. **Besson G, Kazanji M.** 2009. One-step, multiplex, real-time PCR assay with molecular beacon probes for simultaneous detection, differentiation, and quantification of human T-cell leukemia virus types 1, 2, and 3. *J Clin Microbiol* **47:**1129–1135.
47. **Moens B, López G, Adaui V, González E, Kerremans L, Clark D, Verdonck K, Gotuzzo E, Vanham G, Cassar O, Gessain A, Vandamme AM, Van Dooren S.** 2009. Development and validation of a multiplex real-time PCR assay for simultaneous genotyping and human T-lymphotropic virus type 1, 2, and 3 proviral load determination. *J Clin Microbiol* **47:**3682–3691.
48. **Gessain A, Mahieux R.** 2000. Epidemiology, origin and genetic diversity of HTLV-1 retrovirus and STLV-1 simian affiliated retrovirus. *Bull Soc Pathol Exot* **93:**163–171.
49. **Gessain A, Rua R, Betsem E, Turpin J, Mahieux R.** 2013. HTLV-3/4 and simian foamy retroviruses in humans: discovery, epidemiology, cross-species transmission and molecular virology. *Virology* **435:**187–199.
50. **Vallinoto AC, Ishak MO, Azevedo VN, Vicente AC, Otsuki K, Hall WW, Ishak R.** 2002. Molecular epidemiology of human T-lymphotropic virus type II infection in Amerindian and urban populations of the Amazon region of Brazil. *Hum Biol* **74:**633–644.
51. **Calattini S, Betsem E, Froment A, Bassot S, Chevalier SA, Mahieux R, Gessain A.** 2007. Identification and complete sequence analysis of a new HTLV-3 strain from South Cameroon. 13th International Conference on Human Retrovirology: HTLV and Related Viruses, Hakone, Japan.
52. **Van Dooren S, Salemi M, Pourrut X, Peeters M, Delaporte E, Van Ranst M, Vandamme AM.** 2001. Evidence for a second simian T-cell lymphotropic virus type 3 in *Cercopithecus nictitans* from Cameroon. *J Virol* **75:**11939–11941.
53. **Goubau P, Van Brussel M, Vandamme AM, Liu HF, Desmyter J.** 1994. A primate T-lymphotropic virus, PTLV-L, different from human T-lymphotropic viruses types I and II, in a wild-caught baboon (*Papio hamadryas*). *Proc Natl Acad Sci USA* **91:**2848–2852.
54. **Sintasath DM, Wolfe ND, Lebreton M, Jia H, Garcia AD, Le Doux-Diffo J, Tamoufe U, Carr JK, Folks TM, Mpoudi-Ngole E, Burke DS, Heneine W, Switzer WM.** 2009. Simian T-lymphotropic virus diversity among nonhuman primates, Cameroon. *Emerg Infect Dis* **15:**175–184.
55. **Sintasath DM, Wolfe ND, Zheng HQ, LeBreton M, Peeters M, Tamoufe U, Djoko CF, Diffo JL, Mpoudi-Ngole E, Heneine W, Switzer WM.** 2009. Genetic characterization of the complete genome of a highly divergent simian T-lymphotropic virus (STLV) type 3 from a wild *Cercopithecus mona* monkey. *Retrovirology* **6:**97.
56. **Rodgers MA, Vallari AS, Harris B, Yamaguchi J, Holzmayer V, Forberg K, Berg MG, Kenmenge J, Ngansop C, Awazi B, Mbanya D, Kaptue L, Brennan C, Cloherty G, Ndembi N.** 2017. Identification of rare HIV-1 group N, HBV AE, and HTLV-3 strains in rural South Cameroon. *Virology* **504:**141–151.
57. **Richard L, Mouinga-Ondémé A, Betsem E, Filippone C, Nerrienet E, Kazanji M, Gessain A.** 2016. Zoonotic transmission of two new strains of human T-lymphotropic virus type 4 in hunters bitten by a gorilla in Central Africa. *Clin Infect Dis* **63:**800–803.
58. **Van Dooren S, Meertens L, Lemey P, Gessain A, Vandamme AM.** 2005. Full-genome analysis of a highly divergent simian T-cell lymphotropic virus type 1 strain in *Macaca arctoides*. *J Gen Virol* **86:**1953–1959.
59. **Liégeois F, Lafay B, Switzer WM, Locatelli S, Mpoudi-Ngolé E, Loul S, Heneine W, Delaporte E, Peeters M.** 2008. Identification and molecular characterization of new STLV-1 and STLV-3 strains in wild-caught nonhuman primates in Cameroon. *Virology* **371:**405–417.
60. **Cassar O, Gessain A.** 2017. Serological and molecular methods to study epidemiological aspects of human T-cell lymphotropic virus type 1 infection. *Methods Mol Biol* **1582:**3–24.
61. **Lemey P, Van Dooren S, Vandamme AM.** 2005. Evolutionary dynamics of human retroviruses investigated through full-genome scanning. *Mol Biol Evol* **22:**942–951.

62. **Satou Y, Matsuoka M.** 2013. Virological and immunological mechanisms in the pathogenesis of human T-cell leukemia virus type 1. *Rev Med Virol* **23:**269–280.
63. **Gillet NA, Malani N, Melamed A, Gormley N, Carter R, Bentley D, Berry C, Bushman FD, Taylor GP, Bangham CR.** 2011. The host genomic environment of the provirus determines the abundance of HTLV-1-infected T-cell clones. *Blood* **117:**3113–3122.
64. **Cook LB, Elemans M, Rowan AG, Asquith B.** 2013. HTLV-1: persistence and pathogenesis. *Virology* **435:** 131–140.
65. **Mahieux R, Gessain A.** 2003. HTLV-1 and associated adult T-cell leukemia/lymphoma. *Rev Clin Exp Hematol* **7:**336–361.
66. **Araujo A, Hall WW.** 2004. Human T-lymphotropic virus type II and neurological disease. *Ann Neurol* **56:**10–19.
67. **Biswas HH, Kaidarova Z, Garratty G, Gibble JW, Newman BH, Smith JW, Ziman A, Fridey JL, Sacher RA, Murphy EL, HTLV Outcomes Study.** 2010. Increased all-cause and cancer mortality in HTLV-II infection. *J Acquir Immune Defic Syndr* **54:**290–296.
68. **Barrios CS, Castillo L, Giam CZ, Wu L, Beilke MA.** 2013. Inhibition of HIV type 1 replication by human T lymphotropic virus types 1 and 2 Tax proteins in vitro. *AIDS Res Hum Retroviruses* **29:**1061–1067.
69. **Beilke MA, Theall KP, O'Brien M, Clayton JL, Benjamin SM, Winsor EL, Kissinger PJ.** 2004. Clinical outcomes and disease progression among patients coinfected with HIV and human T lymphotropic virus types 1 and 2. *Clin Infect Dis* **39:**256–263.
70. **Beilke MA, Traina-Dorge VL, Sirois M, Bhuiyan A, Murphy EL, Walls JM, Fagan R, Winsor EL, Kissinger PJ.** 2007. Relationship between human T lymphotropic virus (HTLV) type 1/2 viral burden and clinical and treatment parameters among patients with HIV type 1 and HTLV-1/2 coinfection. *Clin Infect Dis* **44:**1229–1234.
71. **Beilke MA.** 2012. Retroviral coinfections: HIV and HTLV: taking stock of more than a quarter century of research. *AIDS Res Hum Retroviruses* **28:**139–147.
72. **Treviño A, Aguilera A, Caballero E, Benito R, Parra P, Eiros JM, Hernandez A, Calderón E, Rodríguez M, Torres A, García J, Ramos JM, Roc L, Marcaida G, Rodríguez C, Trigo M, Gomez C, de Lejarazu RO, de Mendoza C, Soriano V, HTLV Spanish Study Group.** 2012. Trends in the prevalence and distribution of HTLV-1 and HTLV-2 infections in Spain. *Virol J* **9:**71.
73. **Tsukasaki K, Tobinai K.** 2012. Clinical trials and treatment of ATL. *Leukemia Res Treat* **2012:**101754.
74. **Marçais A, Suarez F, Sibon D, Bazarbachi A, Hermine O.** 2012. Clinical trials of adult T-cell leukaemia/lymphoma treatment. *Leukemia Res Treat* **2012:**932175.
75. **Fields PA, Taylor GP.** 2012. "Antivirals" in the treatment of adult T cell leukaemia- lymphoma (ATLL). *Curr Hematol Malig Rep* **7:**267–275.
76. **Panfil AR, Martinez MP, Ratner L, Green PL.** 2016. Human T-cell leukemia virus-associated malignancy. *Curr Opin Virol* **20:**40–46.
77. **Martin F, Taylor GP.** 2011. Prospects for the management of human T-cell lymphotropic virus type 1-associated myelopathy. *AIDS Rev* **13:**161–170.
78. **Yamano Y, Sato T, Ando H, Araya N, Yagishita N.** 2012. The current and future approaches to the treatment of HTLV-1-associated myelopathy/tropical spastic paraparesis (HAM/TSP). *Nihon Rinsho* **70:**705–713. (In Japanese.)
79. **Yamano Y, Sato T.** 2012. Clinical pathophysiology of human T-lymphotropic virus-type 1-associated myelopathy/tropical spastic paraparesis. *Front Microbiol* **3:**389.
80. **Afonso PV, Mekaouche M, Mortreux F, Toulza F, Moriceau A, Wattel E, Gessain A, Bangham CR, Dubreuil G, Plumelle Y, Hermine O, Estaquier J, Mahieux R.** 2010. Highly active antiretroviral treatment against STLV-1 infection combining reverse transcriptase and HDAC inhibitors. *Blood* **116:**3802–3808.
81. **Seegulam ME, Ratner L.** 2011. Integrase inhibitors effective against human T-cell leukemia virus type 1. *Antimicrob Agents Chemother* **55:**2011–2017.
82. **Treviño A, Parra P, Bar-Magen T, Garrido C, de Mendoza C, Soriano V.** 2012. Antiviral effect of raltegravir on HTLV-1 carriers. *J Antimicrob Chemother* **67:**218–221.
83. **Kuo CW, Mirsaliotis A, Brighty DW.** 2011. Antibodies to the envelope glycoprotein of human T cell leukemia virus type 1 robustly activate cell-mediated cytotoxic responses and directly neutralize viral infectivity at multiple steps of the entry process. *J Immunol* **187:**361–371.
84. **Khabbaz RF, Fukuda K, Kaplan JE.** 1993. Guidelines for counseling human T-lymphotropic virus type I (HTLV-I)- and HTLV type II-infected persons. *Transfusion* **33:**694.
85. **Busch MP, Switzer WM, Murphy EL, Thomson R, Heneine W.** 2000. Absence of evidence of infection with divergent primate T-lymphotropic viruses in United States blood donors who have seroindeterminate HTLV test results. *Transfusion* **40:**443–449.
86. **Kwaan N, Lee TH, Chafets DM, Nass C, Newman B, Smith J, Garratty G, Murphy EL, HTLV Outcomes Study (HOST) Investigators.** 2006. Long-term variations in human T lymphotropic virus (HTLV)-I and HTLV-II proviral loads and association with clinical data. *J Infect Dis* **194:** 1557–1564.
87. **Roucoux DF, Murphy EL.** 2004. The epidemiology and disease outcomes of human T-lymphotropic virus type II. *AIDS Rev* **6:**144–154.
88. **Paiva A, Casseb J.** 2014. Sexual transmission of human T-cell lymphotropic virus type 1. *Rev Soc Bras Med Trop* **47:**265–274.
89. **Kamihira S, Yamano Y, Iwanaga M, Sasaki D, Satake M, Okayama A, Umeki K, Kubota R, Izumo S, Yamaguchi K, Watanabe T.** 2010. Intra- and inter-laboratory variability in human T-cell leukemia virus type-1 proviral load quantification using real-time polymerase chain reaction assays: a multicenter study. *Cancer Sci* **101:**2361–2367.
90. **Derse D, Heidecker G, Mitchell M, Hill S, Lloyd P, Princler G.** 2004. Infectious transmission and replication of human T-cell leukemia virus type 1. *Front Biosci* **9:**2495–2499.
91. **Stramer SL, Hollinger FB, Katz LM, Kleinman S, Metzel PS, Gregory KR, Dodd RY.** 2009. Emerging infectious disease agents and their potential threat to transfusion safety. *Transfusion* **49**(Suppl 2)**:**1S–29S.
92. **Kaul DR, Taranto S, Alexander C, Covington S, Marvin M, Nowicki M, Orlowski J, Pancoska C, Pruett TL, Ison MG, Group HDSA, HTLV Donor Screening Advisory Group.** 2010. Donor screening for human T-cell lymphotrophic virus 1/2: changing paradigms for changing testing capacity. *Am J Transplant* **10:**207–213.
93. **Switzer WM, Hewlett I, Aaron L, Wolfe ND, Burke DS, Heneine W.** 2006. Serologic testing for human T-lymphotropic virus-3 and -4. *Transfusion* **46:**1647–1648.
94. **Qiu X, Hodges S, Lukaszewska T, Hino S, Arai H, Yamaguchi J, Swanson P, Schochetman G, Devare SG.** 2008. Evaluation of a new, fully automated immunoassay for detection of HTLV-I and HTLV-II antibodies. *J Med Virol* **80:** 484–493.
95. **Berini CA, Susana Pascuccio M, Bautista CT, Gendler SA, Eirin ME, Rodriguez C, Pando MA, Biglione MM.** 2008. Comparison of four commercial screening assays for the diagnosis of human T-cell lymphotropic virus types 1 and 2. *J Virol Methods* **147:**322–327.
96. **Jacob F, Magri MC, Costa EA, Santos-Fortuna E, Caterino-de-Araujo A.** 2009. Comparison of signal-to-cutoff values in first, second, and third generation enzyme immunoassays for the diagnosis of HTLV-1/2 infection in "at-risk" individuals from São Paulo, Brazil. *J Virol Methods* **159:** 288–290.
97. **Stramer SL, Foster GA, Dodd RY.** 2006. Effectiveness of human T-lymphotropic virus (HTLV) recipient tracing (lookback) and the current HTLV-I and -II confirmatory algorithm, 1999 to 2004. *Transfusion* **46:**703–707.
98. **Andersson S, Gessain A, Taylor GP.** 2001. Pooling of samples for seroepidemiological surveillance of human T-cell lymphotropic virus types I and II. *Virus Res* **78:** 101–106.

99. **Varma M, Rudolph DL, Knuchel M, Switzer WM, Hadlock KG, Velligan M, Chan L, Foung SK, Lal RB.** 1995. Enhanced specificity of truncated transmembrane protein for serologic confirmation of human T-cell lymphotropic virus type 1 (HTLV-1) and HTLV-2 infections by Western blot (immunoblot) assay containing recombinant envelope glycoproteins. *J Clin Microbiol* **33:**3239–3244.
100. **Sabino EC, Zrein M, Taborda CP, Otani MM, Ribeiro-Dos-Santos G, Sáez-Alquézar A.** 1999. Evaluation of the INNO-LIA HTLV I/II assay for confirmation of human T-cell leukemia virus-reactive sera in blood bank donations. *J Clin Microbiol* **37:**1324–1328.
101. **Abrams A, Akahata Y, Jacobson S.** 2011. The prevalence and significance of HTLV-I/II seroindeterminate Western blot patterns. *Viruses* **3:**1320–1331.
102. **Mahieux R, Horal P, Mauclère P, Mercereau-Puijalon O, Guillotte M, Meertens L, Murphy E, Gessain A.** 2000. Human T-cell lymphotropic virus type 1 gag indeterminate Western blot patterns in Central Africa: relationship to *Plasmodium falciparum* infection. *J Clin Microbiol* **38:** 4049–4057.
103. **Filippone C, Bassot S, Betsem E, Tortevoye P, Guillotte M, Mercereau-Puijalon O, Plancoulaine S, Calattini S, Gessain A.** 2012. A new and frequent human T-cell leukemia virus indeterminate Western blot pattern: epidemiological determinants and PCR results in central African inhabitants. *J Clin Microbiol* **50:**1663–1672.
104. **Rouet F, Meertens L, Courouble G, Herrmann-Storck C, Pabingui R, Chancerel B, Abid A, Strobel M, Mauclere P, Gessain A.** 2001. Serological, epidemiological, and molecular differences between human T-cell lymphotropic virus type 1 (HTLV-1)-seropositive healthy carriers and persons with HTLV-I Gag indeterminate Western blot patterns from the Caribbean. *J Clin Microbiol* **39:**1247–1253.
105. **Kuramitsu M, Sekizuka T, Yamochi T, Firouzi S, Sato T, Umeki K, Sasaki D, Hasegawa H, Kubota R, Sobata R, Matsumoto C, Kaneko N, Momose H, Araki K, Saito M, Nosaka K, Utsunomiya A, Koh KR, Ogata M, Uchimaru K, Iwanaga M, Sagara Y, Yamano Y, Okayama A, Miura K, Satake M, Saito S, Itabashi K, Yamaguchi K, Kuroda M, Watanabe T, Okuma K, Hamaguchi I.** 2017. Proviral features of human T cell leukemia virus Type 1 in carriers with indeterminate Western blot analysis results. *J Clin Microbiol* **55:**2838–2849.
106. **Cánepa C, Salido J, Ruggieri M, Fraile S, Pataccini G, Berini C, Biglione M.** 2015. Low proviral load is associated with indeterminate Western blot patterns in human T-cell lymphotropic virus Type 1 infected individuals: could punctual mutations be related? *Viruses* **7:**5643–5658.
107. **Lal RB, Rudolph DL, Coligan JE, Brodine SK, Roberts CR.** 1992. Failure to detect evidence of human T-lymphotropic virus (HTLV) type I and type II in blood donors with isolated gag antibodies to HTLV-I/II. *Blood* **80:**544–550.
108. **Busch MP, Laycock M, Kleinman SH, Wages JW Jr, Calabro M, Kaplan JE, Khabbaz RF, Hollingsworth CG.** 1994. Accuracy of supplementary serologic testing for human T-lymphotropic virus types I and II in US blood donors. Retrovirus Epidemiology Donor Study. *Blood* **83:**1143–1148.
109. **Kwok S, Lipka JJ, McKinney N, Kellogg DE, Poiesz B, Foung SK, Sninsky JJ.** 1990. Low incidence of HTLV infections in random blood donors with indeterminate Western blot patterns. *Transfusion* **30:**491–494.
110. **Andrade RG, Ribeiro MA, Namen-Lopes MS, Silva SM, Basques FV, Ribas JG, Carneiro-Proietti AB, Martins ML.** 2010. Evaluation of the use of real-time PCR for human T cell lymphotropic virus 1 and 2 as a confirmatory test in screening for blood donors. *Rev Soc Bras Med Trop* **43:** 111–115.

Influenza Viruses*

ROBERT L. ATMAR

86

TAXONOMY

The influenza viruses are members of the family *Orthomyxoviridae*. Antigenic differences in two major structural proteins, the matrix protein (M) and the nucleoprotein (NP), and phylogenetic analyses of the virus genome are used to separate the influenza viruses into four genera within the family: *Influenzavirus A*, *Influenzavirus B*, *Influenzavirus C*, and *Influenzavirus D*. Members of these four genera are also referred to as influenza type A, B, C, and D viruses, respectively. The influenza A viruses are further classified into subtypes based upon characteristics of the two major surface glycoproteins, the hemagglutinin (HA) and neuraminidase (NA). Subtypes are recognized by the lack of cross-reactivity in double immunodiffusion assays with animal hyperimmune sera corresponding to each antigen (1). Currently, 18 HA subtypes and 11 NA subtypes are recognized (2). Within a subtype, strains may be further subclassified into lineages or clades based upon phylogenetic analysis of gene sequences. An example is the classification of the Eurasian lineage of highly pathogenic H5N1 strains into clades and the further subdivision of circulating viruses into second-, third-, fourth- and fifth-order clades (3). Influenza B viruses do not have subtypes, but they are subdivided into two antigenically distinct lineages: B/Victoria and B/Yamagata.

The following information is used in the naming of individual virus strains: type, species of origin (if nonhuman), geographic location of isolation strain, laboratory identification number, year of isolation, and subtype (influenza A viruses only). Thus, an example of a human strain of influenza is A/Texas/50/2012 (H3N2), while A/quail/Vietnam/36/2004 (H5N1) is an example of an avian strain isolated in an epizootic in Asia.

DESCRIPTION OF THE AGENTS

Orthomyxoviruses are enveloped, single-stranded RNA viruses with segmented genomes of negative sense. Influenza A and B viruses have eight RNA segments, while influenza C and D viruses have only seven segments. Gene segments range from ~800 to ~2,500 nucleotides in length, and the entire genome ranges from 10 to 14.6 kb. The segmented genome of influenza viruses allows the exchange of one or more gene segments between two viruses when both infect a single cell. This exchange is called genetic reassortment and results in the generation of new strains containing a mix of genes from both parental viruses. Genetic reassortment between human and avian influenza virus strains led to the generation of the 1957 H2N2 and 1968 H3N2 pandemic strains, and it also played a role in the emergence of the pandemic 2009 H1N1 virus and in H7N9 avian strains from China that are causing infections in people (4).

Influenza viruses are spherical and pleomorphic, with diameters of 80 to 120 nm after serial passage in culture. Filamentous forms also occur and may be up to several micrometers in size. The lipid envelope is derived from the host cell membrane through which maturing virus particles bud, and HA and NA form characteristic rod-like spikes (HA) and spikes with globular heads (NA) on the virus surface. As its name implies, the HA can agglutinate red blood cells from both mammalian (e.g., human [type O], guinea pig, and horse) and avian (e.g., chicken and turkey) species by binding to sialic acid residues. The HA protein is the major antigenic determinant and is used to identify viruses with immune sera. The lipid envelope surrounds the nucleocapsid, which has helical symmetry and consists of the genomic RNA segments, several copies of the polymerase proteins, and the NP. The matrix-1 (M1) protein is present between the nucleocapsid and the envelope, and the matrix-2 (M2) protein forms an ion channel across the envelope in influenza A viruses.

EPIDEMIOLOGY AND TRANSMISSION

Influenza A and B viruses cause annual epidemics in areas with temperate climates, but in tropical climates seasonality is less apparent and influenza viruses can be isolated throughout the year. In the temperate regions of the Northern Hemisphere, epidemics generally occur between December and March, and in the Southern Hemisphere, the epidemic period is usually between May and August. Epidemics are characterized by a sudden increase in febrile respiratory illnesses and absenteeism from school and work, and within a community the epidemic period usually lasts from 3 to 8 weeks. A single subtype (A) or type (B) of influenza virus usually predominates, but epidemics have

*This chapter contains information from chapter 84 by Robert L. Atmar and Stephen E. Lindstrom in the 11th edition of this *Manual*.

occurred in which both A and B viruses or two influenza A virus subtypes were isolated. Global epidemics, or pandemics, occur less frequently and are seen only with influenza A viruses. Pandemics occur following the emergence of an influenza A virus that carries a novel HA and that can be readily transmitted from person to person. The pandemic strain may develop because of genetic reassortment following coinfection of a susceptible host with human and animal influenza viruses or through gradual adaptation of an avian strain to mammalian hosts. Influenza C viruses cause asymptomatic or mild respiratory disease in people. Influenza D viruses infect swine and cattle, but they do not infect people (5).

Influenza viruses are transmitted from person to person primarily via droplets generated by sneezing, coughing, and speaking. Direct or indirect (fomite) contact with contaminated secretions and small-particle aerosols is another potential route of transmission that has been noted. The relative importance of these different routes has not been determined for influenza viruses (6). As for human infections caused by avian strains of influenza virus, direct contact with infected birds has been the most common factor of transmission, and direct inoculation into the pharynx or gastrointestinal tract may lead to infection (7, 8).

The pandemic potential of avian strains of influenza has been a concern since at least 1997, when several human cases of infection with H5N1 viruses occurred in Hong Kong in association with a large poultry outbreak. The outbreak was controlled by slaughtering all poultry in Hong Kong, but H5N1 viruses again caused outbreaks in poultry in China in 2003. By late 2005, the virus had spread to other parts of Asia and to parts of Europe, Africa, and the Middle East. Human cases of H5N1 infection have been directly associated with outbreaks in poultry, and as of 2017 more than 850 human infections have been documented. Most cases have occurred in southeastern Asia, but cases have also been documented in the Middle East and in northern Africa. Most human cases have been due to direct contact with infected birds, but limited human-to-human transmission has also occurred (7). Several mutations in influenza virus genes are required for avian influenza viruses to replicate efficiently in mammalian cells and to transmit by droplet aerosol between ferrets, an animal model of human infection (9, 10). H5N1 viruses continue to evolve and increase diversity, raising the possibility that they may acquire the ability to spread efficiently among humans.

Other avian influenza A virus subtypes are also of concern. An outbreak of H7N7 virus in commercial poultry farms in the Netherlands in 2003 was associated with respiratory illness in >400 persons, although only a single person died (11). Since 2013, H7N9 viruses have emerged in poultry markets in China, with more than 1,200 persons having been infected (12). Sporadic infection of humans with other avian subtypes is occasionally observed. The greatest risk for infection has been exposure to infected poultry, similar to what has been observed with human cases of H5N1.

Swine are another source of novel influenza virus strains that can infect people. In 2009 a novel influenza A/H1N1 virus (pdm09) was initially identified as a cause of significant febrile respiratory illnesses in Mexico and the United States, and it rapidly spread to many countries around the world, which prompted the World Health Organization (WHO) to declare an influenza pandemic. The new strain subsequently replaced previously circulating seasonal H1N1 strains. Other infections with swine virus and antigenically distinct HAs (e.g., variant H3N2) have been identified in the United States (13). Fortunately, most cases are associated with direct or indirect contact with swine, and these variant strains have not spread among the population like the H1N1 pdm09 strain and can be suspected based upon epidemiologic exposures. The transmission of influenza viruses to people from avian and swine species highlights the need for vigilant surveillance for such events.

CLINICAL SIGNIFICANCE

Influenza A and B virus infections typically cause a febrile respiratory illness characterized by fever, cough, upper respiratory tract symptoms (including sore throat, rhinorrhea, and nasal congestion), and systemic symptoms (including headache, myalgia, and malaise). This constellation of symptoms is called influenza, although other clinical presentations, ranging from asymptomatic infection to viral pneumonia, also occur. Illness begins abruptly after a 1- to 5-day incubation period (average, 2 days). Fever generally lasts for 3 to 5 days, but symptoms of dry cough and malaise may persist for several weeks. Complications include otitis media in children, sinusitis, viral pneumonia, secondary bacterial pneumonia, exacerbation of underlying cardiac or pulmonary disease, myositis (including rhabdomyolysis), neurologic problems (seizures, acute encephalitis/encephalopathy, and postinfectious encephalopathy), Reye syndrome (associated with aspirin use), myopericarditis, and death (14–16). In contrast, influenza C viruses cause mild respiratory illnesses that clinically are not distinguishable from common colds.

Influenza A(H5N1) and A(H7N9) viruses also cause a febrile respiratory illness, although lower respiratory tract illness is more prevalent. Upper respiratory tract symptoms may be absent, and gastrointestinal symptoms (watery diarrhea, vomiting, and abdominal pain) occur in some patients (7, 17). Acute encephalitis may occur. H5N1 infection is associated with a high mortality (~60%), with most patients dying of progressive pneumonia. Although overall severity of infection with H7N9 viruses is lower than for H5N1 strains, mortality is still at least 30% (17). Patient age and the presence of underlying diseases have been different among hospitalized patients dying from H5N1 or H7N9 infection (18). Viral replication may be prolonged, and levels of several inflammatory mediators (e.g., interleukin-6, interleukin-8, and interleukin-1beta) in plasma have been higher in fatal cases than in nonfatal cases. Surviving patients develop measurable serum antibody responses 10 to 14 days after symptom onset.

Influenza A and B virus infections spread rapidly through the community, with clinical attack rates having been documented to be as high as 70% following a common source exposure in an enclosed space. Epidemic disease is associated with an increase in hospitalization rates, especially in young children and in the elderly, and an increase in mortality rates in the elderly. Mortality rates have been higher in epidemics caused by influenza A/H3N2 viruses than in those caused by H1N1 or B viruses in the past 20 years. Additional information on the clinical presentation, manifestations, and complications of the diseases can be found in clinical textbooks (14, 15).

There are five licensed antiviral medications available for the treatment of influenza virus infection. Amantadine and rimantadine are adamantanes that block the M2 ion channel. The adamantanes have no activity against influenza B viruses, and unfortunately the currently circulating influenza A viruses have developed resistance so that the adamantanes are not clinically useful as monotherapy for these viruses either. Zanamivir, oseltamivir, and peramivir are NA inhibitors and are active against both influenza A and B viruses. Clinically significant resistance can occur following treatment of immunocompromised patients. Treatment with any of these medications should be initiated within 2 days of symptom onset to have demonstrable clinical benefit, although initiation of treatment of virus-positive hospitalized patients has been recommended at any time during the illness (19). These drugs have also been used for prophylaxis, but annual immunization with a trivalent or quadrivalent influenza vaccine is the primary means of prevention of influenza.

Inactivated influenza vaccines (IIVs), live attenuated influenza virus (LAIV) vaccine, and a recombinant hemagglutinin vaccine (RIV) are licensed in the United States (20). The IIVs are derived from viruses grown in cell culture (ccIIV) or embryonated chicken eggs that are harvested and then inactivated. Viral proteins are partially purified and standardized to contain 15 μg of HA per dose. The IIVs may be trivalent (IIV3), containing influenza A/H1N1, A/H3N2, and B virus strains, or quadrivalent (IIV4), containing influenza B virus strains from two lineages (B/Victoria and B/Yamagata), A/H1N1, and A/H3N2. A high-dose IIV3 containing 60 μg of each HA and an MF59-adjuvanted IIV3 containing 15 μg of each HA are also licensed for adults 65 years of age and older. The RIV3 and RIV4 vaccines contain 45 μg of baculovirus-expressed, recombinant hemagglutinin for an A/H1N1, A/H3N2, and one or two B strains. LAIV4 vaccine is quadrivalent and contains the same strains recommended for IIV4. A reassortant vaccine virus for each strain to be included is derived to contain six internal genes from a parental attenuated influenza (A or B) virus and the HA and NA from the WHO-recommended vaccine strain. It is given topically into the nose, and the virus replicates in the upper respiratory tract (21). The vaccine is licensed in the United States for use in persons 2 to 49 years of age, although 3 years of poor effectiveness against influenza A viruses led the American Committee on Immunization Practices (ACIP) to withdraw its recommendation for its use for 2 years (20). In February 2018, the ACIP recommendation for LAIV use was renewed based upon changes made to correct the poor replicative fitness of the H1N1 component that was identified as the putative cause of LAIV's low effectiveness. The latest guidance for the use of influenza vaccines in the United States can be found online at https://www.cdc.gov/flu/protect/keyfacts.htm.

Due to constant virus evolution causing gradual antigenic changes in the HA protein, viruses included in the influenza vaccines must be updated periodically. The strains to be included in the vaccine are selected twice annually by WHO. Vaccine strains for Northern Hemisphere countries are selected in January and February to make vaccine for use in September. New vaccine alternatives, including those given by other routes and in combination with adjuvants, are undergoing clinical studies.

COLLECTION, TRANSPORT, AND STORAGE OF SPECIMENS

Influenza viruses infect the respiratory epithelium and can be found in respiratory secretions of all types. The level of virus shedding parallels the severity of clinical symptoms in uncomplicated influenza and is maximal in the first several days of illness. Samples should be collected during this time (first 2 to 3 days) to maximize the likelihood of virus detection. A variety of upper respiratory tract samples alone or in combination are routinely used for virus identification, including nasal aspirates, nasal wash fluids, nasal or nasopharyngeal swabs, throat swabs, and throat wash fluids. Virus titers tend to be lower in samples collected from the throat, so assays of these samples alone tend to be less sensitive (22, 23). However, reports of human infection caused by H5N1 and H7N9 strains suggest that throat samples and lower respiratory tract samples may have better diagnostic yields than samples collected from the nose (7, 24). Lower respiratory tract samples, including sputa, tracheal aspirates, and bronchoalveolar lavage fluids, may yield virus and can be assayed when available; some studies have found higher yields with sputum than with upper respiratory samples (25, 26). Virus can occasionally be identified in nonrespiratory clinical samples (7).

Once collected, the clinical samples should be placed in viral transport medium. A number of transport media are suitable for influenza viruses, including veal infusion broth, Hanks balanced salt solution, tryptose phosphate broth, sucrose phosphate buffer, and commercially available cell culture medium. All these media are supplemented with 0.5% bovine serum albumin or 0.1% gelatin to stabilize the virus and antimicrobials (antibiotics and antifungals) to inhibit the growth of other respiratory biota. However, the use of transport medium may interfere with the test performance for certain commercially available virus detection assays; the package inserts of these assays should be consulted if they are to be used for diagnosis (Tables 1 and 2). Influenza virus infectivity is maintained for up to 5 days when samples are placed in transport media and maintained at 4°C (27). Clinical samples should be transported to the diagnostic laboratory as rapidly as possible after collection under these conditions. If a sample cannot be cultured during this time frame, it should be stored immediately at −70°C; storage at higher temperatures (e.g., −20°C) leads to the loss of virus viability. Immediate transport and processing of samples after collection are necessary for immunofluorescence detection of virus antigen in exfoliated epithelial cells.

DIRECT DETECTION

Microscopy

Influenza viruses have been detected in clinical specimens by direct and indirect visualization of their typical morphological appearance by electron microscopy (EM). Immune EM has been the most sensitive EM method and allows differentiation of virus type and subtype when specific hyperimmune sera are used in the assay (28). However, large numbers of viruses (>10^5 to 10^6 per ml) must be present in the clinical sample for successful detection using this diagnostic approach. Because of the need for an experienced microscopist and access to an electron microscope, the relatively high costs of assay performance, and the greater sensitivity of other diagnostic approaches, EM is not routinely used for the diagnosis of influenza virus infection.

Antigen Detection

Antigen detection assays are used in a variety of formats to rapidly detect influenza viruses in clinical specimens and to confirm the identity of isolates grown in culture. These assays are based upon detection of the interaction of viral proteins with specific antibodies. A variety of different formats have been used, including direct and indirect fluorescent antibody (FA) staining, enzyme immunoassay, immunochromatographic assay, and fluoroimmunoassay.

FA assays identify viral antigens present on, or in, infected, exfoliated epithelial cells present in respiratory secretions. Cells are collected on swabs or in aspirates or

TABLE 1 Commercially available kits for detection of influenza A or B viruses by fluorescent antibody staining[a]

Assay format	Kit name (Manufacturer)	Acceptable clinical samples for direct detection; cell culture confirmation	Comments	Influenza virus types detected	Assay sensitivity and specificity for direct detection per mfg. brochure	Assay sensitivity and specificity for isolate identification per mfg. brochure	Other viruses detected
DFA	D^3 Ultra DFA Respiratory Virus Screening & ID kit (Diagnostic Hybrids, Inc.)	NA, NPA, NW; cell culture	Virus-specific MAbs provided mixed for screen and individually for identification	A and B	A: 100%, 100% B: 100%, 98.7–100%	A: 100%, 100% B: 100%, 100%	Ad, P1, P2, P3, RSV
DFA	D^3 Duet DFA Respiratory Virus Screening kit (Diagnostic Hybrids, Inc.)	NA, NPA, NPS, NS; cell culture	Distinguishes influenza A from other respiratory viruses; these viruses (including influenza B) must be identified with reagents from the Ultra kit	A and B	A: 99%, A and B 100% B: 100%, 100%	A: 100%, 100% B: 100%, 100%	Ad, P1, P2, P3, RSV
DFA	D^3 FastPoint DFA Respiratory Virus Screening kit (Diagnostic Hybrids, Inc.)	NA, NPA, NPS, NS, NW	Distinguishes influenza A from influenza B		A: 82.9–100%, 97.5–100% B: 66.7–100%, 99.7–100%	N/A	
DFA	Imagen Influenza Virus A and B (Thermo Fisher Scientific)	NPA; cell culture	Virus-specific MAbs provided mixed for screen and individually for identification	A and B	A: 96.2%, 100% B: 86.7%, 99.5%	A: 100%, 100% B: 100%, 100%	None
DFA	PathoDx Respiratory Virus Panel (Oxoid)	Cell culture only	Not approved for direct use on clinical specimens	A and B	N/A	A: 100%, 100% B: 100%, 100%	Ad, P1, P2, P3, RSV
DFA	Light Diagnostics Simulfluor Viral Diagnostic Screen (Millipore)	Cell culture	Does not distinguish influenza A or influenza B from Ad, P1, P2, or P3	A and B	N/A	A: 95.8–100%, 99.6–100% B: 100%, 100%	Ad, P1, P2, P3, RSV
DFA	Light Diagnostics Simulfluor Flu A/Flu B (Millipore)	BAL, NPA, NPS, NS, NW, TS; cell culture	Distinguishes influenza A from influenza B	A and B	A: 58.8–80%, 98.3–98.6% B: 43.2–50%, 98.3–100%	A: 97.8–100%, 100% B: 100%, 100%	
DFA	Light Diagnostics Simulfluor RSV Flu A (Millipore)	Cell culture	Distinguishes influenza A from RSV	A	N/A	A: 95.8–100%, 99.6–100%	RSV
IFA	Imagen Respiratory Screen (Thermo Fisher Scientific)	NPA; cell culture	Does not distinguish between different viruses in kit	A and B	96.7%, 89.6%[b]	A: 100%, 100% B: 100%, 100%	Ad, P1, P2, P3, RSV
IFA	Light Diagnostics Respiratory Viral Screen IFA (Millipore)	Cell culture	Does not distinguish influenza A or influenza B from Ad, P1, P2, P3, or RSV	A and B	A: 100%, 100% B: 100%, 100%	A: 100%, 100% B: 100%, 100%	Ad, P1, P2, P3, RSV

[a]DFA, direct fluorescent antibody; IFA, indirect fluorescent antibody; NA, nasal aspirate; NPA, nasopharyngeal aspirate; NPS, nasopharyngeal swab; NS, nasal swab; NW, nasal wash; TS, throat swab; N/A, not applicable; Ad, adenovirus; P1, parainfluenza type 1; P2, parainfluenza type 2; P3, parainfluenza type 3; RSV, respiratory syncytial virus.

[b]Sensitivity and specificity for all viruses tested; unable to determine assay parameters for each virus.

TABLE 2 Commercially available, antigen-based RIDT kits for rapid (≤30 minutes) detection of influenza A or B viruses[a,b]

Assay format	Kit name (Manufacturer)	Acceptable clinical samples	Sample collection restrictions	Assay performance time (min)	Assay complexity[c] (510K number)
Dipstick chromatographic immunoassay	Alere Influenza A & B (Alere)	NS	Use the swabs provided in the kit	10	CLIA waived (K092349)
Dipstick chromatographic immunoassay	QuickVue Influenza A+B Test (Quidel Corporation)	NPS, NS	Limited transport media supported	10	CLIA waived (K031899)
Lateral flow chromatographic immunoassay	Biosign Flu A+B (Princeton BioMeditech Corporation); Consult Immunoassay Influenza A&B (McKesson); ImmunoCard STAT! Flu A&B (Meridian Bioscience, Inc.); OraSure Quick Flu Rapid Flu A+B Test (OraSure Technologies, Inc.); OSOM Ultra Flu A&B (Sekisui Diagnostics); Status Flu A&B (Life Sign LLC)	NS, NPS, NPA, NW	Use only swabs supplied with the kit	10–15	CLIA waived (NS, NPS); moderate (NPA, NW) (K083746)[d]
Lateral flow chromatographic immunoassay	Xpect Flu A&B (Thermo Fisher Scientific)	NS, NW, TS	For swab samples, use synthetic-tipped (Dacron or nylon) swabs with aluminum or plastic shafts; cotton tips and wooden shafts not recommended; do not use calcium alginate	15	CLIA moderate (K031565)
Lateral flow chromatographic immunoassay with a reader	Alere BinaxNOW Influenza A&B Card 2 (Alere)[e]	NPS, NS	Swabs included in the kit	15	CLIA waived (K162642)
Lateral flow chromatographic immunoassay with a reader	BD Veritor (Becton Dickinson)[e]	NPS, NS	—	10	CLIA waived (K112277)
Lateral flow chromatographic immunoassay with a reader	BD Veritor (Becton Dickinson)[e]	NA, NW, NPS in transport media	—	10	CLIA moderate (K121797)
Lateral flow fluorescent immunoassay with a reader	Sofia Influenza A+B FIA (Quidel Corporation)[e]	NPA, NPS, NS, NW	Use nylon-flocked swab for NPS and kit swab for NS	15	CLIA waived (K162438)

[a]Additional information on rapid tests can be found at the following website: http://www.cdc.gov/flu/professionals/diagnosis/rapidlab.htm.

[b]NA, nasal aspirate; NPA, nasopharyngeal aspirate; NPS, nasopharyngeal swab; NS, nasal swab; TS, throat swab; NW, nasal wash.

[c]CLIA (Clinical Laboratory Improvement Amendments): CLIA-waived laboratory assays employ methodologies that are so simple and accurate as to render the likelihood of erroneous results negligible. CLIA-moderate complexity assays require some knowledge, training, reagent preparation, processing, proficiency, ability to troubleshoot or interpret, and judgment in the performance of the test. CLIA-waived assays may be used as point-of-care tests; some when used in the laboratory are reclassified as moderate complexity.

[d]Several kits with different names are distributed under the same 510K number.

[e]Requires a reader for assay interpretation.

wash fluids and are washed in cold buffer to remove mucus before being applied and fixed to a microscope slide. Use of cytocentrifugation for application of the cells to slides can improve the number and morphology of cells for evaluation and enhance the accuracy of interpretation. Virus-specific antibodies are applied to the fixed cells; monoclonal antibodies directed against viral proteins that are conserved and expressed in large quantities (e.g., M and NP) are used because of their greater specificity compared to polyclonal sera and are available from a number of manufacturers. A fluorochrome is conjugated to the virus-specific antibody in direct FA (DFA) assays, and it is conjugated to a second antibody that reacts with the virus-specific antibody in indirect FA (IFA) assays. Antibody staining of cells is detected with a fluorescent microscope. Contaminating mucus can cause nonspecific fluorescence that can be reduced by treating the samples with N-acetylcysteine or dithiothreitol and by centrifuging cells through Percoll. DFA and IFA assays take 2 to 4 h to perform, although some diagnostic laboratories batch samples and do not perform tests as soon as the sample is received, delaying the availability of results. In theory, IFA assays should be more sensitive and less specific than DFA assays, but there is significant overlap, noted in published reports, in the sensitivities (50% to 90%) and specificities (generally >90%) of these assays (29). Lower sensitivities may be the result of suboptimal laboratory expertise or malfunctioning equipment (30). An advantage of FA assays is that sample quality can be determined by observing whether an adequate number of epithelial cells are present. In addition, kits are available to screen for other respiratory viruses (e.g., respiratory syncytial virus, parainfluenza viruses, and adenovirus) as well as for influenza A and B viruses (Table 1). These multiplex assays allow for efficient screening for other viral causes of febrile respiratory disease. Disadvantages include the need for specialized equipment (a fluorescent microscope) and the effect of technician expertise on assay performance characteristics (i.e., sensitivity and specificity). Each laboratory should establish its own performance characteristics compared to those of cell culture.

Several immunoassays that use different reporter formats (colorimetric, fluorometric, and chromatographic) have been developed for the detection of influenza virus antigen in clinical specimens. Many of these assays take at least 2 h to perform and have 50% to 80% sensitivity compared to culture methods. RIDT kits that use immunoassay formats for rapid (≤30-min) detection of influenza A and B viruses in clinical specimens are used much more commonly than other antigen detection immunoassay formats (Table 2). The kits use monoclonal antibodies to detect the presence of the influenza A or B nucleoprotein by chromatographic immunoassay. All the kits provide results within 30 min, and some of them can be used as point-of-care tests (i.e., those classified by the Clinical Laboratory Improvement Amendments [CLIA] as waived). The types of specimens that are appropriate for testing vary among the kits, and specific instructions for sample collection and processing must be followed for optimal results. Assay performance characteristics in clinical settings are affected by the age of the patient (generally lower sensitivity in adults), by the amount of virus in the clinical sample, and by the type of specimen analyzed. The sensitivity of antigen detection-based RIDTs for identification of infection was noted to be quite poor in some circumstances during the 2009 H1N1 pandemic (31, 32). The lower sensitivity associated with many of the antigen detection-based RIDTs led the Food and Drug Administration to establish minimum sample sensitivity requirements with appropriate culture or molecular methods as the gold standard (Table 3), to monitor device performance over time to evaluate its ability to identify contemporary strains (available annually from the Centers for Disease Control and Prevention), and to require provisions for evaluating an antigen detection-based RIDT's ability to detect newly emerging influenza virus strains (33). As a result, several previously marketed kits are no longer available, and others have been modified to enhance their performance. Even with these new requirements, a negative RIDT result should not prevent prescription of antiviral treatment for a patient with suspected influenza, especially when influenza is prevalent in the community, and follow-up testing with culture or RT-PCR should be considered (19).

TABLE 3 FDA minimal performance requirements for antigen-based RIDts (28)

	Comparator = molecular assay	Comparator = culture
Sensitivity minimal point estimate		
Influenza A	80%	90%
Influenza B	80%	80%
Sensitivity, 95% CI lower bound		
Influenza A	≥70%	≥80%
Influenza B	≥70%	≥70%
Specificity, minimal point estimate		
Influenza A and B	95%	95%
Specificity, 95% CI lower bound		
Influenza A and B	≥90%	≥90%

Nucleic Acid Analyses

Molecular methods are commonly being used both for the detection and characterization (see below) of influenza viruses. The most commonly used molecular method is reverse transcription (RT)-PCR. Viral nucleic acids are first extracted from clinical samples. The use of guanidinium thiocyanate with silica particles or commercial kits based upon this approach reliably removes inhibitors of the enzymatic amplification that are often present in clinical specimens. Automated extraction instruments decrease the amount of time personnel must spend in sample preparation while increasing the reproducibility of the procedure compared to the use of manual extraction methods, and several commercial assays are licensed to be used in combination with an automated extraction procedure. Reverse transcriptase is used to synthesize cDNA from viral RNA by random hexamers or virus gene-specific oligonucleotides. The cDNA is then amplified by use of virus gene-specific oligonucleotides as primers and a heat-stable DNA polymerase. Resulting amplicons are identified as virus specific by a variety of different methods (e.g., identification by size, hybridization, restriction enzyme mapping, and sequencing).

Many different RT-PCR assays have been developed since the initial description in 1991 of an RT-PCR method to detect and distinguish influenza A, B, and C viruses (34). Assays that identify and distinguish different influenza virus types have targeted conserved genes, such as the matrix gene, and subtype-specific assays have amplified a portion of the HA gene (Table 4). Nested PCR assays have been developed to improve assay sensitivity, but the inherent problem of carryover contamination associated with the use of this assay format limits its utility for most diagnostic laboratories. Real-time RT-PCR assays, which are less vulnerable to cross-contamination, can directly and rapidly detect influenza viruses in clinical specimens with a sensitivity approaching or exceeding that of culture (35). Multiplexed assays able to identify influenza viruses and other respiratory viruses have been developed and have performance characteristics that meet or exceed those of cell culture (36, 37). A variety of methodologies are used to detect amplified products, and different equipment is needed based upon each assay's characteristics. Multiplexed respiratory virus panels may be less sensitive than monoplex molecular assays that target a single virus (36, 37). Genetic drift among circulating viruses can result in mutations in primer and probe target regions, resulting in decreased assay sensitivity, as has been noted for some assays targeting H3N2 viruses in recent years (38). The availability, and FDA clearance, of such assays and their ability to identify multiple other respiratory pathogens (Table 4) has led many diagnostic laboratories to use these assays for respiratory virus diagnosis in place of the more time-consuming cell

TABLE 4 FDA-cleared molecular detection assays for influenza viruses[a,b]

Assay format	Kit name (Manufacturer)	Instrumentation	Acceptable clinical samples	Virus type(s), (subtypes) detected	Influenza target gene(s)	Assay performance time (min)	Assay complexity (510K number)	Other viruses detected	Reference(s)
Isothermal nucleic acid amplification assay—nicking enzyme amplification reaction (NEAR)	Alere i Influenza A&B; Alere i Influenza A&B 2 (Alere)	Alere i	NPS, NS; direct or in VTM	A, B	PB2 (A); PA (B)	<15	CLIA waived (K141520, K171792); Moderate (K163266, K111387)	None	42, 78
Isothermal nucleic acid amplification assay—reverse transcriptase-helicase-dependent amplification (RT-HDA)	Solana Influenza A+B assay (Quidel Corporation)	Solana Instrument	NPS, NS	A, B	Matrix (A, B)	~45	Moderate (K161814)	None	79
Multiplex real-time RT-PCR assay	cobas Liat Influenza A/B (Roche Molecular Diagnostics)	cobas Liat system	NPS	A, B	Matrix (A); NSP (B)	~20	CLIA waived (K111387)	None	78
Multiplex real-time RT-PCR assay	cobas Liat Influenza A/B & RSV (Roche Molecular Diagnostics)	cobas Liat system	NPS	A, B	Matrix (A); NSP (B)	~20	CLIA waived (K153544)	RSV	80
Multiplex real-time RT-PCR assay	Panther Fusion Flu A/B/RSV (Hologic, Inc.)	Panther Fusion system	NPS	A, B	Matrix (A, B)	~150	High (K171963)	RSV	81
Real-time RT-PCR	CDC Human Influenza Virus Real-time RT-PCR Detection and Characterization Panel (CDC)	ABI 7500 Fast DX Real-Time PCR instrument	BAL, BW, NA, NPS, NS, NW, TA, TS, sputum, lung	A (H1, H3, 2009 H1, H5), B (Yamagata lineage [B/Yam], Victoria [B/Vic] lineage)	Matrix (A); NP (A/swine); NSP (B); HA (H1, H3, 2009 H1, H5, B/Yam, B/Vic)	~240	High (K132508)	None	82
Real-time RT-PCR	Joint Biologic Agent Identification Diagnostic System (JBAIDS) Influenza A&B (U.S. Army)	JBAIDS instrument	NPS in VTM, NW	A, B	Matrix (A); NSP (B)	~240	High (K111775)	None	83
Real-time RT-PCR	JBAIDS Influenza A/H5 (Asian lineage) Detection Kit (U.S. Army)	JBAIDS instrument	NPS, TS in VTM	A/H5	HA (H5, Asian lineage)	~240	High (K100287)	None	None

Real-time RT-PCR	JBAIDS Influenza A Subtyping Kit (U.S. Army)	JBAIDS instrument	NPS in VTM, NW	A/H1, A/2009 H1, A/H3, A/swine	HA (H1, 2009 H1, H3); NP (A/swine)	~240	High (K111778)	None	83
Multiplex RT-PCR with colorimetric visualization	Accula Flu A/B Test (Mesa Biotech, Inc.)	Accula Dock instrument	NS	A, B	PB2 (A), Matrix (B)	~30	CLIA waived (K171641)	None	None
Multiplex RT-PCR	artus Influenza A/B RG Kit (Qiagen GmbH)	Rotor-Gene Q MDx instrument	NPS in VTM	A, B	Matrix (A, B)	~240	High (K113323)	None	84
Multiplex real-time RT-PCR	Cepheid Xpert Flu Assay	Cepheid GeneXpert Instrument Systems	NA, NPS, NW in VTM	A, B	Matrix (A); HA (2009 H1); ? for B	75	Moderate (K123191)	None	85, 86
Multiplex real-time RT-PCR	Cepheid Xpert Flu/ RSV XC Assay	Cepheid GeneXpert Instrument Systems	NA, NPS, NW in VTM	A, B	Matrix (A, B), PB2 (A); PA (A); NSP (B)	60	CLIA waived, Moderate (K142045)	RSV	87
Multiplex real-time RT-PCR	Cepheid Xpert Xpress Flu Assay	Cepheid GeneXpert Instrument Systems	NPS in VTM	A, B	Matrix (A, B), PB2 (A), PA (A), NSP (B)	~30	CLIA waived (K171552), Moderate (K162456)	None	None
Multiplex real-time RT-PCR	Cepheid Xpert Xpress Flu/RSV Assay	Cepheid GeneXpert Instrument Systems	NPS in VTM	A, B	Matrix (A, B), PB2 (A), PA (A), NSP (B)	~30	Moderate (K162331)	RSV	88, 89
Multiplex RT-PCR with probe detection using voltammetry	ePlex Respiratory Virus Panel (GenMark Diagnostics, Inc.)	ePlex Instrument	NPS in VTM	A (H1, 2009 H1, H3), B	Matrix (A); PB1 (B); HA (H1, H3, 2009 H1)	~105	Moderate (K163636)	RSVA, RSVB, PIV1, PIV2, PIV3, PIV4, hMPV, Ad, HRV/Ent, CoV	90
Multiplex RT-PCR with probe detection using voltammetry	eSensor Respiratory Virus Panel (GenMark Diagnostics, Inc.)	eSensor XT-8TM System	NPS in VTM	A (H1, 2009 H1, H3), B	Matrix (A); PB1 (B); HA (H1, H3, 2009 H1)	~480	High (K113731)	RSVA, RSVB, PIV1, PIV2, PIV3, hMPV, Ad, HRV/Ent	39, 91
Multiplex RT-PCR with endpoint melt curve analysis	FilmArray Respiratory Panel (BioFire Diagnostics)	FilmArray Instrument, FilmArray System 2.0 or FilmArray Torch System	NPS in VTM	A (H1, 2009 H1, H3), B	Matrix (A); HA (H1, 2009 H1, H3, B)	~60	Moderate (K110764, K160068)	RSV, PIV1, PIV2, PIV3, PIV4, hMPV, HRV/Ent, Ad, OC43, HKU1, 229E, NL63	39, 90
Multiplex RT-PCR with endpoint melt curve analysis	FilmArray Respiratory Panel 2.0 (BioFire Diagnostics)	FilmArray System 2.0 or FilmArray Torch System	NPS in VTM	A (H1, 2009 H1, H3), B	Matrix (A); HA (H1, 2009 H1, H3, B)	~45	Moderate (K170604)	RSV, PIV1, PIV2, PIV3, PIV4, hMPV, HRV/Ent, Ad, OC43, HKU1, 229E, NL63	92

(Continued on next page)

TABLE 4 FDA-cleared molecular detection assays for influenza viruses[a,b] *(Continued)*

Assay format	Kit name (Manufacturer)	Instrumentation	Acceptable clinical samples	Virus type(s), (subtypes) detected	Influenza target gene(s)	Assay performance time (min)	Assay complexity (510K number)	Other viruses detected	Reference(s)
Multiplex RT-PCR with endpoint melt curve analysis	FilmArray Respiratory Panel EZ (BioFire Diagnostics)	FilmArray Instrument	NPS in VTM	A (H1, 2009 H1, H3), B	Matrix (A); HA (H1, 2009 H1, H3, B)	~60	CLIA waived (K152579)	RSV, PIV[c], hMPV, HRV/ Ent, Ad, CoV[c]	None
Multiplex RT-PCR with electrospray ionization-mass spectrometry (ESI-MS)	PLEX-ID Flu (Abbott Laboratories)	PLEX-ID system	NPS	A (H1, H3), B	PB1, NP (A), Matrix (A), PA (A), PB (A), PB2 (B), NS1 (A), HA (2009 H1), NA (2009 H1)	~480	High (K121003)	None	93
Multiplex real-time RT-PCR	ProFast+ Assay (Hologic, Inc.)	Cepheid Smart-Cycler II	NPS in VTM	A (2009 H1, seasonal H1, H3)	HA	~240	High (K101855)	None	93, 94
Multiplex real-time RT-PCR	ProFlu+ Assay (Hologic, Inc.)	Cepheid SmartCycler II	NPS in VTM	A, B	Matrix (A), NSP (B)	~240	High (K110968, K132129, K153219)	RSV	88, 94
Multiplex RT-PCR	Lyra Influenza A+B (Quidel)	ABI 7500 Fast Dx Real-Time PCR Instrument, Quant-Studio Dx Real-Time PCR Instrument, Cepheid SmartCycler II	NS, NPS in VTM	A, B	Matrix (A), NA (B)	<75	Moderate (K112172, K113777, K131728)	None	None
Multiplex real-time RT-PCR	Simplexa Flu A/B & RSV (Focus Diagnostics)	3M Integrated Cycler	NPS in VTM	A, B	Matrix (A, B)	<240	High (K102170)	RSV	95, 96
Multiplex real-time RT-PCR	Simplexa Flu A/B & RSV Direct (Focus Diagnostics)	3M Integrated Cycler	NPS in VTM	A, B	Matrix (A, B)	~60	Moderate (K120413)	RSV	97
Multiplex real-time RT-PCR	Simplexa Influenza A H1N1 (2009) Kit (Focus Diagnostics)	3M Integrated Cycler	NPA, NPS, NS in VTM	A (2009 H1)	Matrix (A), HA (2009 H1)	<240	High (K100148)	None	98
Multiplex real-time RT-PCR with melt curve analysis	ARIES Flu A/B & RSV Assay (Luminex Corporation)	ARIES System, ARIES M1 System	NPS in VTM	A, B	Matrix (A, B)	<120	Moderate (K161220)	RSV	87

Multiplex real-time RT-PCR, target-specific primer extension, fluidic microbead microarray	xTAG Respiratory Virus Panel (Luminex Molecular Diagnostics)	Thermal cycler plus Luminex 100 or 200 system	NPS in VTM	A (H1, H3), B	Matrix (A), HA (H1, H3, B)	~450	High (K063765, K112199)	RSV A, RSV B, PIV1, PIV2, PIV3, hMPV, HRV, Ad	36, 39
Multiplex real-time RT-PCR, target-specific primer extension, fluidic microbead microarray	xTAG Respiratory Virus Panel Fast (Luminex Molecular Diagnostics)	Thermal cycler plus Luminex 100 or 200 system	NPS in VTM	A (H1, H3), B	Matrix (A), HA (H1, H3, B)	~360	High (K103776)	RSV, hMPV, HRV, Ad	96
Multiplex real-time RT-PCR, target-specific primer extension, fluidic microbead microarray	NxTAG Respiratory Virus Panel (Luminex Molecular Diagnostics)	MAGPIX instrument	NPS in VTM	A (seasonal H1, H3), B	Matrix (A, B), HA (H1, H3)	~225	High (K152386)	RSV A, RSV B, PIV1, PIV2, PIV3, PIV4, hMPV, HRV, Ad, OC43, 229E, NL63, HKU1, Boca	99
Multiplex RT-PCR with microarray hybridization	Verigene Respiratory Pathogens Flex Nucleic Acid Test (Luminex Corporation)	Verigene System	NPS in VTM	A (H1, H3, 2009 H1), B	Matrix (A), HA (2009 H1, H3), NSP (B)	~120	Moderate (K143653)	RSV A, RSV B, PIV1, PIV2, PIV3, PIV4, hMPV, HRV, Ad	100

[a]Additional information on rapid tests can be found at the following website: http://www.cdc.gov/flu/professionals/diagnosis/molecular-assays.htm.

[b]BAL, bronchoalveolar lavage; NA, nasal aspirate; NPS, nasopharyngeal swab; NS, nasal swab; TS, throat swab; BW, bronchial wash; NW, nasal wash; TA, tracheal aspirate; VTM, viral transport medium; NP, nucleoprotein; RSV, respiratory syncytial virus; PIV, parainfluenza virus; hMPV, human metapneumovirus; HRV, human rhinovirus; Ent, enterovirus; Ad, adenovirus; Boca, bocavirus; OC43, 229E, NL63, HKU1, human coronavirus (CoV) variants; HA, hemagglutinin; NSP, nonstructural protein; ?, not reported.

[c]Does not differentiate type.

culture methods, and the improved sensitivity of molecular methods is replacing culture methods as the gold standard for influenza virus detection (36, 37, 39).

A number of isothermal molecular amplification assays are undergoing evaluation for direct detection of influenza viruses in clinical samples. These include nucleic acid sequence-based amplification (NASBA), reverse transcription-loop mediated amplification (RT-LAMP), RT-helicase dependent amplification (RT-HDA), and RT-nicking enzyme amplification reaction (RT-NEAR) (40, 41). Nucleic acid amplification occurs at a single temperature without requiring the cycling associated with PCR. All these assays require initial synthesis of complementary DNA with a reverse transcriptase. NASBA uses T7 RNA polymerase to generate RNA amplicons while the other listed methods use a DNA polymerase to produce DNA amplicons. For the DNA-based methods, separation of double-stranded DNA occurs enzymatically rather than as a result of the heat denaturation used in PCR reactions. Successful amplification is detected with a variety of different methods, including molecular beacon probes, turbidity assays (RT-LAMP), and probe hybridization using electrochemical readouts. As with RT-PCR assays, these isothermal amplification methods are more sensitive than culture or immunofluorescent-antibody staining for the diagnosis of influenza virus infection.

The time to a result for molecular assays varies widely depending on the assay used, but it can exceed 4 hours (Table 4). However, some assays provide results in <30 minutes, and there are also several CLIA-waived assays available (Table 4). These assays have improved sensitivity compared to results obtained with rapid antigen detection tests and can be used as point-of-care tests, improving patient care in outpatient settings (32, 42).

ISOLATION PROCEDURES

Influenza virus isolation procedures should be performed under biosafety level 2 (BSL-2) conditions. When the clinical sample comes from a patient suspected to be infected with a highly pathogenic avian influenza (HPAI) virus strain or other avian influenza A viruses with the potential to cause severe human disease, attempts at virus isolation should be performed under BSL-3 or higher conditions (43). Human clinical samples should be processed in separate laboratories and by staff members other than those handling clinical material from swine or birds (44).

Cell Culture

Influenza viruses can be grown in a number of different cell lines, including primary monkey kidney cells, Vero cells, human diploid lung fibroblasts, mink lung epithelial cells, human lung adenocarcinoma (A549) cells, and Madin-Darby canine kidney (MDCK) cells (41, 45, 46). Although some variability can be seen from season to season, MDCK and primary monkey kidney cell lines have similar isolation frequencies (45), and MDCK cells are more sensitive than Vero or diploid lung fibroblast cells (46). Thus, MDCK cells (CCL 34; American Type Culture Collection, Manassas, VA), a continuous polarized cell line, are the most common cell line used for isolation of influenza viruses and will support the growth of type A, B, and C strains. Continuous cell lines do not produce proteases that will cleave the viral HA, a step necessary to produce infectious viral progeny, so exogenous protease must be added to the maintenance medium. L-(Tosylamido-2-phenyl) ethyl chloromethyl ketone (TPCK)-treated trypsin at a concentration of 1 to 2 μg/ml provides the necessary proteolytic activity and is the recommended protease for virus isolation. Chymotrypsin cleavage of the HA prevents the trypsin-mediated enhancement of viral infectivity, and TPCK treatment inactivates chymotrypsin activity, which may contaminate pancreatic extracts of trypsin.

MDCK cells are propagated in growth medium that contains 5% to 10% fetal calf serum (FCS). FCS contains inhibitors that prevent the production of infectious virus, so the FCS must be removed prior to inoculation of the clinical sample (47, 48). The inhibitory effects of FCS can be prevented by washing the cell sheet with Hanks buffer or serum-free medium sufficiently to remove the protein-containing growth medium and then adding serum-free medium to cover the cell sheet. The clinical sample is then inoculated into the medium. After a 2-h incubation, the inoculum-medium mixture is removed and replaced with serum-free medium supplemented with TPCK-treated trypsin. Alternatively, the sample can be inoculated directly onto cells with serum-free medium supplemented with TPCK-treated trypsin and incubated overnight prior to changing of the medium the next day. The cultures are maintained at 33°C to 34°C and monitored for virus growth.

The replication of influenza viruses typically leads to cytopathic effects (CPE) and destruction of the cell sheet within a week after inoculation. CPE may be inapparent or absent in the presence of viral replication, but viral replication can be identified by the ability of the viral HA to bind to sialic residues on the erythrocytes of different animal species. Cultures should be screened every 2 to 3 days by hemadsorption (binding of erythrocytes to the viral HA of infected cells) or hemagglutination (cross-linking of erythrocytes by virus in the culture medium) for evidence of viral replication. To evaluate hemadsorption of cells grown in a tissue culture tube, the monolayer is first examined for CPE (Fig. 1A), and the medium is removed and stored. The cell sheet is rinsed three times with 1 ml of 0.05% guinea pig red blood cells. One milliliter of 0.5% guinea pig red blood cells is then added, and the tube is stored at 4°C for 20 min, with the red blood cell suspension covering the cells. The tube is then shaken, and adherence of red blood cells to the cell sheet is determined microscopically (Fig. 1B). If cytopathic changes are scored as less than 4+ (i.e., less than 75% of cell sheet with CPE), the tissue culture tubes are rinsed with phosphate-buffered saline and re-fed with culture medium. The media collected initially from tubes with 4+ cytopathic changes can be used for further characterization. All procedures are performed in a BSL-2 safety cabinet, and care must be taken to prevent cross-contamination between cultures. Guinea pig red blood cells are more sensitive for detection of influenza virus than are avian cells, but influenza C virus does not agglutinate guinea pig red blood cells. Chicken red blood cells can be used in agglutination assays to identify influenza C viruses. Although most isolates will demonstrate growth within 1 week after inoculation, virus from samples with low infectious titers may require extended culture incubation for 10 to 14 days and additional blind passaging of negative cultures. Presumptive isolates are characterized further, as outlined below.

A disadvantage of traditional cell culture methods is the time needed to obtain a positive result (average, 4 to 5 days). More rapid methods have been developed by inoculating samples onto cell culture monolayers maintained in shell vials or multiwell plates. This approach can use either cell lines employed in traditional cell culture for identification of influenza virus (e.g., MDCK cells) or

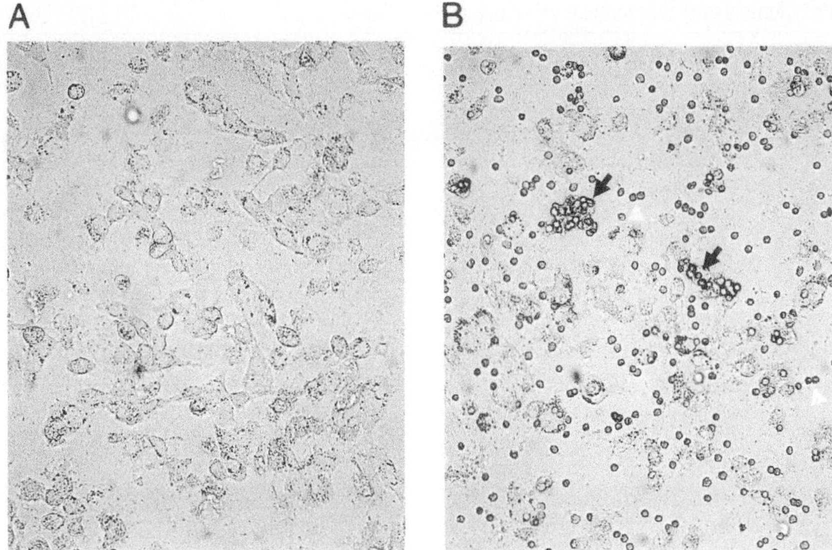

FIGURE 1 Influenza virus-infected MDCK cells. (A) Cytopathic changes. (B) Hemadsorption with guinea pig red blood cells. Red blood cells adsorb to both infected cells (black arrows) and the plastic previously occupied by infected cells and where residual hemagglutinin protein is still present (white arrowheads).

mixed cell cultures (e.g., A549 cells plus mink lung cells) to screen for multiple respiratory viruses (R-Mix Fresh-Cells; Quidel, San Diego, CA), which are reported to detect seasonal influenza virus strains as well as strains with novel hemagglutinins (31, 49). The cells are fixed after 24 to 72 h, and type-specific monoclonal antibodies are used to detect viral antigen. Sensitivity can be lower than that achieved by standard isolation methods, although R-mix cells have been reported to have 82% to 100% sensitivity for detection of influenza A and B viruses (31, 49). Shell vial assays have the disadvantage of not producing virus for additional studies (e.g., antigenic characterization). Screening for viral antigen by immunofluorescence also can be used at the end of the 10- to 14-day incubation period for standard culture prior to discarding of cells (50). This step is usually not necessary if screening by hemadsorption or hemagglutination is being performed, but it may detect virus in the absence of cytopathic changes if other strategies for virus detection are not used.

Isolation from Embryonated Chicken Eggs

The amniotic and allantoic cavities of 10- to 11-day-old embryonated chicken eggs are inoculated with the clinical sample for isolation of influenza A and B viruses. Seven- to 8-day-old eggs are used for isolation of influenza C viruses, although these viruses are also isolated with 10- to 11-day-old eggs. Embryonated eggs have endogenous proteases that can cleave the viral HA to yield infectious virus, so exogenous administration of proteases is not necessary. Inoculated eggs are incubated at 33°C to 34°C for 2 to 3 days (5 days for influenza C viruses), and then both amniotic and allantoic fluids are collected and assayed for hemagglutination activity. Influenza A and B viruses can grow both in cells lining the allantoic cavities and in those lining the amniotic cavities, whereas influenza C virus grows only in cells lining the amniotic cavities of embryonated eggs. If no hemagglutination activity is detected, influenza viruses may still be recovered by performing one or two blind passages. A pool containing equal volumes of the amniotic and allantoic fluids is inoculated into eggs as described above (47).

Isolation and passaging of influenza viruses in eggs can lead to adaptive mutations that include alterations in glycosylation sites in the viral hemagglutinin (51, 52). Such alterations can adversely affect the immunogenicity of egg-passaged viruses used in vaccines, which leads to decreased vaccine effectiveness, as has been observed for egg-passaged inactivated influenza vaccines targeting A/H3N2 viruses (52).

IDENTIFICATION AND TYPING SYSTEMS

A variety of methods are used to identify and characterize influenza virus isolates. The most common are shown in Table 5 and are based upon immunologic or molecular approaches. The initial step is to identify the isolate as an influenza virus and to distinguish it from other respiratory viruses that have the ability to agglutinate or adsorb red blood cells (e.g., parainfluenza viruses and mumps virus). In many instances, it is sufficient to identify the virus by type, and this may be accomplished by immunofluorescent or immunoperoxidase stains or an enzyme-linked immunosorbent assay (ELISA) using commercially available, type-specific antibodies targeting the viral NP or M proteins. These assays are particularly useful for working with cell culture isolates. The rapid immunochromatographic assays described in Table 2 may be able to identify isolates and type them, but there are limited data on the use of these assays for this purpose, and these assays are not approved for this use. Importantly, the immunochromatographic assays may give false-negative results when the quantity of virus in a cell culture harvest is low.

Hemagglutination inhibition (HAI) assays have been performed for more than 75 years and are still used for identification (44, 53). HAI assays can be type, subtype, or strain specific, and they are particularly useful for examining antigenic relationships among strains of the same subtype. HAI is the WHO gold standard for antigenic

TABLE 5 Methods to identify and characterize influenza virus isolates

Assay	Advantages	Limitations
Assays using type- or subtype-specific antisera		
ELISA	Standard assay with known performance characteristics; most labs experienced with assay format	For subtyping of influenza A strains, need to update sera periodically to detect circulating strain
Hemagglutination inhibition	Standard assay with known performance characteristics; no special equipment needed; gold standard for antigenic characterization	For subtyping of influenza A strains, need to update sera periodically to detect circulating strain; many clinical labs not experienced with this method
Immunofluorescence or immunoperoxidase staining of infected cells	Standard assay with known performance characteristics; many labs experienced with assay format; monoclonal antibodies commercially available	For subtyping of influenza A strains, need to update monoclonal antibodies periodically to detect circulating strain
Molecular methods		
RT-PCR	Very sensitive assays	Potential for carryover contamination; need for stringent laboratory controls
Amplicon size	Ease of performance	Potential for false-positive results due to nonspecific amplification
Probe hybridization	Most commonly used approach for confirmation of PCR results; real-time formats eliminate need for post-amplification processes	Depending on hybridization format used, may add time to performance of assay
Restriction analysis	Ease of performance	Need to know specific sequence; requires specific nuclease site; increased handling of post-PCR samples
Genetic sequence	Highest level of identity; sequence data that may be used in other studies	Need for specialized equipment; technically complex; increased cost
Microarray analysis	Potential to analyze multiple genetic sequences simultaneously	Investigational; limited experience

characterization of influenza isolates and vaccine strain selection. Immune sera are usually produced in ferrets, sheep, or chickens. The hemagglutination activity of the virus is quantitated, and a standard amount of viral HA (4 HA units) is mixed with serial 2-fold dilutions of the immune serum and turkey or guinea pig red blood cells. A 4-fold or greater difference in HAI activities between the isolate and the reference strain is an indication that the isolate may be an antigenic variant. Because the HA undergoes antigenic change over time, subtype-specific antisera for interpandemic strains must be prepared and standardized periodically. Thus, subtype identification by HAI is usually performed only as part of surveillance activities or investigation of a case in which there is a strong epidemiologic suspicion of infection with a non-human strain.

Molecular assays can be used for virus identification and characterization. The same RT-PCR assays used for detection of viruses in clinical samples also can be used to identify clinical isolates. An advantage that molecular assays have over immunology-based assays is that the molecular assays can identify influenza A virus subtypes even after significant antigenic variation has occurred because there are well-conserved regions of the HA gene that serve as targets for the primers and probes used for identification. Multiplex assays can also be used to distinguish influenza A and B viruses or to identify HA and NA subtypes (54). Results are determined by identification of amplicon size, by hybridization to type- or subtype-specific probes, and by direct sequencing of the amplicons. If the sequences of different variants are known, it may be possible to identify unique differences by digesting amplified DNA with restriction endonucleases that generate restriction fragment length polymorphisms (RFLP) unique to each strain. For example, this method was used to distinguish two H3N2 variants that cocirculated during a single season (55). Influenza A/Wuhan/359/95 (H3N2) virus-like variants generated amplicons that could be digested with the BstF5I restriction enzyme, whereas amplicons from influenza A/Sydney/05/97 (H3N2) virus-like variants could be digested by HindIII. Given the difficulty to design and perform RFLP analysis and the reduced cost and time required to perform DNA sequencing, direct sequencing of amplicons, or the entire HA gene, has become a more common way to track and characterize specific strains. Electrospray ionization-mass spectrometry is another method that can be used to analyze virus-specific PCR amplicons and to identify novel variants and reassortants when the viral genomic sequence is unknown, as was done with the initial identification of the 2009 H1N1 virus as a likely swine-origin virus (56).

DNA microarrays are being used increasingly in diagnostics for identification of specific pathogens. Oligonucleotide probes are arrayed on a chip or membrane, and hybridization of virus-specific sequences is then detected. The viral sequences can be generated by cDNA synthesis from viral genomic RNA or by amplification of fragments of genomic RNA by RT-PCR. Microarray analysis strategies have been developed that distinguish influenza virus types (A versus B) and subtypes (57, 58) but at the present time they are too costly for most individual laboratories to develop.

Next-generation sequencing methods are being applied to influenza for the analysis of the entire influenza genome (59, 60). The sequence of each segment is determined, which allows a more detailed evaluation of reassortment and evolution of viral genes. This technology has the promise of being able to more fully characterize strains in surveillance studies.

SEROLOGIC TESTS

Influenza virus infections are also identified by serologic methods. Most persons have been infected previously with influenza viruses, so detection of virus-specific immunoglobulin M or other immunoglobulin subclasses has not been particularly useful (61). An exception may be detection of immunoglobulin M responses to novel HAs from avian strains (62). Instead, paired acute- and convalescent-phase serum samples collected at least 10 days apart are needed to detect a significant (4-fold or greater) increase in serum antibody levels. The requirement for paired sera to identify infection makes serology an impractical method for identification of influenza virus infection in the acutely ill individual. Instead, serology is used primarily in surveillance and in epidemiologic studies. The most widely used assay formats include complement fixation, HAI, neutralization, and enzyme immunoassay. Complement fixation identifies type-specific antibodies to the NP, but it is not as sensitive as the other commonly used serologic assays in detecting significant rises in antibody levels. HAI and neutralization antibodies in serum are functionally significant in that higher serum antibody levels correlate with protection from infection and illness, and these antibody levels are used to measure responses to vaccination and to identify infection. HAI antibodies block the binding of the viral HA to sialic acid residues on red blood cells and thus inhibit hemagglutination. Each of the components in the HAI assay may affect the outcome of the test. Human and animal sera may contain nonspecific inhibitors of hemagglutination, but methods to remove these inhibitors have been developed (47). The source of the viral antigen can affect results in that virus initially isolated in cell culture may detect a greater frequency of antibody rises than egg-grown virus (63). The species from which the red blood cells are derived can affect assay results. Chicken and turkey red blood cells are commonly used to measure HAI antibody to human strains of influenza viruses, but they may fail to detect HAI antibodies to avian strains (such as H5N1). Substitution of horse red blood cells can improve HAI assay sensitivity for detection of antibodies to avian influenza virus strains (64). Neutralizing antibodies block viral infectivity and provide a more sensitive assay for detection of antibodies to influenza A and B viruses (65). Neutralization assays are the preferred method for the detection of antibodies to HPAI virus strains (66). Consensus approaches have been developed to allow comparable results to be obtained between laboratories (67). Neutralization assays require the use of live virus, so their use with HPAI virus strains is restricted to those laboratories with BSL-3 or higher facilities. Enzyme immunoassays are also used for detection of antibody responses to whole-virus antigen or to specific viral proteins. The conjugate and the antigen used in the assay are factors that affect the performance characteristics (sensitivity and specificity) of these assays. Enzyme immunoassays are used to measure specific immunoglobulin responses in a variety of clinical specimens (serum samples and respiratory secretions). Serologic assays targeting influenza are not used to manage individual patients clinically, but such tests are useful in vaccine evaluation and in epidemiological and other research studies.

ANTIVIRAL SUSCEPTIBILITIES

Plaque inhibition assays are the "gold standard" for measuring susceptibility to amantadine and rimantadine, but the assays are cumbersome and time-consuming to perform. ELISA methods have also been used to measure decreases in the expression of viral antigens in the presence of these drugs. These assays can be used in combination with genotypic characterization of the M2 gene since *in vitro* and *in vivo* resistance to these drugs is associated with specific M2 gene mutations (68). RT-PCR amplification followed by restriction fragment length polymorphism analysis or direct sequencing of amplicons is a genotypic method used to identify resistant viruses (69). Amplification of the influenza A M2 gene followed by pyrosequencing is a rapid, high-throughput method that allows the rapid and reliable identification of adamantane (amantadine and rimantadine) mutations (70).

Cell culture assays do not reliably identify antiviral susceptibility to the NA inhibitors zanamivir and oseltamivir. Instead, NA enzyme inhibition assays with chemiluminescent or fluorescent substrates are used to identify resistance (71). Several commercially available diagnostic assays (e.g., NA-Star, NA-Fluor, and NA-XTD, Applied Biosystems) are available for *in vitro* screening of influenza virus isolates (72). The results of these assays also correlate with mutations in the NA gene that can be identified by sequencing (73). Molecular approaches can be used to identify known NA gene mutations associated with NAI resistance (e.g., E119V and R292K in A/H3N2, H274Y in A/H1N1, R152K in influenza B) (74). Both traditional terminal deoxynucleotide (Sanger) sequencing and pyrosequencing of the NA gene can successfully identify these mutations. Another strategy to quickly screen a large number of isolates is application of a real-time RT-PCR assay that uses a probe that recognizes wild-type (susceptible) NA sequence. This approach identified all A/H1N1 strains with a H274Y NA gene mutation (75).

Mutations in the HA gene may also lead to a resistance phenotype through decreased binding affinity of HA to cell surface receptors and decreased reliance on NA function to release budding viruses from infected cells. No reliable cell culture system currently exists for identifying HA resistance mutations, so identification relies upon sequencing of the receptor binding site of the HA gene.

EVALUATION, INTERPRETATION, AND REPORTING OF RESULTS

The results of a diagnostic test must be considered in the context of the overall setting in which the test is ordered. Clinicians play a critical role in assessing the plausibility of a test result, but the laboratory also can contribute to this appraisal. Seasonal, epidemiologic, and clinical factors are elements that must be evaluated in addition to the type of assay used. Unexpected laboratory results can be recognized by the laboratory as well as by the clinician. For example, a positive influenza test result when influenza is not recognized to be circulating in the community should prompt an assessment as to whether epidemiologic (e.g., travel history) or clinical (e.g., immunocompromised host) factors support the diagnosis of influenza virus infection. Similarly, a negative result, especially with a less sensitive assay (e.g., a RIDT), should not preclude prescription of antiviral treatment to a patient with signs and symptoms of influenza. Close interactions between the laboratory and clinician are a vital component of a quality control program.

No diagnostic assay has 100% sensitivity and specificity, so false-negative and false-positive results can be expected to occur. Many factors that contribute to lowered sensitivity and specificity are known and can be addressed in ongoing quality control programs. False-negative results may be due to poor quality or inappropriate clinical sample collection, delays in sample transportation or processing, inadequate sample storage (e.g., wrong temperature or transport medium), the time of sample collection during the clinical illness (e.g., later in the illness than recommended, when viral shedding has decreased), the performance characteristics of the diagnostic assay (i.e., lower sensitivity), and the infecting strain (e.g., swine or avian influenza). False-positive results may also be due to other characteristics of the diagnostic assay (i.e., nonspecific reactions), cross-contamination within the laboratory, mislabeling of specimens, and microbial contamination. Standard operating procedures in the collection, transportation, and processing of clinical samples should be established and followed to minimize the occurrence of inaccurate test results. Reagents should be standardized, and periodic assessments of assay performance should be performed with known positive and negative controls. The timing of these assessments will be based upon the type and number of tests being performed and the sources of reagents.

Each laboratory must decide upon the goals of its influenza virus diagnostic program when selecting the diagnostic assays to be performed. Rapid and sensitive assays can favorably affect patient management by allowing the prescription of targeted antiviral therapy and the institution of appropriate infection control isolation procedures. Positive test results may form the basis for offering prophylactic therapy to close contacts of infected patients, especially those contacts with high-risk medical conditions. Early and rapid laboratory diagnosis also can be important for evaluating influenza-like illnesses in the setting of a nosocomial outbreak, at the beginning of the influenza season (before influenza is recognized to be circulating in the community), and in persons with a history of contact with pigs or birds or travel to an area where influenza virus is circulating. Confirmation of swine- or avian-origin virus strains can be accomplished by submission of suspect samples or isolates to a public health laboratory for evaluation. The laboratory's expertise, staffing, and available equipment also will influence test selection. For example, a fluorescent microscope and an experienced technician are necessary for the performance of immunofluorescence assays, and a thermal cycler along with other equipment are needed for RT-PCR assays. If the clinical specimen being tested comes from a patient who may be infected with an HPAI virus strain (e.g., H5N1), nonculture-based assays are currently recommended for laboratories that do not meet the BSL-3 or higher conditions recommended for growth of these strains (43). Commercially available antigen detection assays or the more sensitive H5- and H7-specific RT-PCR assays may be performed with BSL-2 work practices. In the United States, influenza A virus-positive samples from patients meeting the clinical (febrile [>38°C] respiratory illness [cough, sore throat, or dyspnea]) and epidemiologic (contact with poultry or domestic birds or with a patient with known or suspected H5N1 or H7N9 virus infection in a country with endemic transmission of avian influenza) parameters for suspected avian influenza virus infection are referred to the CDC for further evaluation. Selected negative samples may also be sent to the CDC for analysis in consultation with the local public health department (39).

As new strains of influenza virus emerge, the sensitivities of established methods to detect these strains may change. For example, cell lines may have diminished sensitivity to new strains, or the ability to detect influenza virus antigen in infected tissue culture cells (e.g., by hemadsorption) may decrease (50). Thus, it is prudent to reevaluate periodically the performance characteristics of established methods, especially if results do not correlate with those expected based upon clinical and epidemiologic criteria.

Influenza diagnosis is also performed for reasons other than patient management. On the local level, knowledge that influenza is circulating in a community allows diagnosis of influenza based upon clinical symptoms (febrile respiratory illness with cough) with a sensitivity (60% to 80%) similar to that of many rapid antigen tests (76). Influenza viruses isolated in national and global surveillance systems are characterized antigenically and genetically to identify variants. Information gained from these surveillance activities is used in the annual selection of strains for inclusion in updated trivalent influenza vaccines. Surveillance and characterization of isolates also allow the identification of infection with novel subtypes, as has occurred with influenza A/H5N1 and A/H7N9 viruses in Southeast Asia and A/H7N7 strains in the Netherlands (77).

REFERENCES

1. **World Health Organization.** 1980. A revision of the system of nomenclature for influenza viruses: a WHO memorandum. *Bull World Health Organ* **58:**585–591.
2. **Tong S, Zhu X, Li Y, Shi M, Zhang J, Bourgeois M, Yang H, Chen X, Recuenco S, Gomez J, Chen LM, Johnson A, Tao Y, Dreyfus C, Yu W, McBride R, Carney PJ, Gilbert AT, Chang J, Guo Z, Davis CT, Paulson JC, Stevens J, Rupprecht CE, Holmes EC, Wilson IA, Donis RO.** 2013. New world bats harbor diverse influenza A viruses. *PLoS Pathog* **9:**e1003657.
3. **World Health Organization/World Organisation for Animal Health Food Agriculture Organization (WHO/OIE/FAO) H5N1 Evolution Working Group.** 2014. Revised and updated nomenclature for highly pathogenic avian influenza A (H5N1) viruses. *Influenza Other Respir Viruses* **8:**384–388.
4. **Xiang N, Li X, Ren R, Wang D, Zhou S, Greene CM, Song Y, Zhou L, Yang L, Davis CT, Zhang Y, Wang Y, Zhao J, Li X, Iuliano AD, Havers F, Olsen SJ, Uyeki TM, Azziz-Baumgartner E, Trock S, Liu B, Sui H, Huang X, Zhang Y, Ni D, Feng Z, Shu Y, Li Q.** 2016. Assessing change in avian influenza A(H7N9) virus infections during the fourth epidemic—China, September 2015–August 2016. *MMWR Morb Mortal Wkly Rep* **65:**1390–1394.
5. **Ferguson L, Olivier AK, Genova S, Epperson WB, Smith DR, Schneider L, Barton K, McCuan K, Webby RJ, Wan XF.** 2016. Pathogenesis of influenza D virus in cattle. *J Virol* **90:**5636–5642.
6. **Brankston G, Gitterman L, Hirji Z, Lemieux C, Gardam M.** 2007. Transmission of influenza A in human beings. *Lancet Infect Dis* **7:**257–265.
7. **Beigel JH, Farrar J, Han AM, Hayden FG, Hyer R, de Jong MD, Lochindarat S, Nguyen TK, Nguyen TH, Tran TH, Nicoll A, Touch S, Yuen KY, Writing Committee of the World Health Organization (WHO) Consultation on Human Influenza A/H5.** 2005. Avian influenza A (H5N1) infection in humans. *N Engl J Med* **353:**1374–1385.
8. **Li Q, Zhou L, Zhou M, Chen Z, Li F, Wu H, Xiang N, Chen E, Tang F, Wang D, Meng L, Hong Z, Tu W, Cao Y, Li L, Ding F, Liu B, Wang M, Xie R, Gao R, Li X, Bai T, Zou S, He J, Hu J, Xu Y, Chai C, Wang S, Gao Y, Jin L, Zhang Y, Luo H, Yu H, He J, Li Q, Wang X, Gao L, Pang X, Liu G, Yan Y, Yuan H, Shu Y, Yang W, Wang Y, Wu F, Uyeki TM, Feng Z.** 2014. Epidemiology of human infections with avian influenza A(H7N9) virus in China. *N Engl J Med* **370:**520–532.
9. **Herfst S, Schrauwen EJ, Linster M, Chutinimitkul S, de Wit E, Munster VJ, Sorrell EM, Bestebroer TM, Burke DF, Smith DJ, Rimmelzwaan GF, Osterhaus AD, Fouchier RA.** 2012. Airborne transmission of influenza A/H5N1 virus between ferrets. *Science* **336:**1534–1541.
10. **Imai M, Watanabe T, Hatta M, Das SC, Ozawa M, Shinya K, Zhong G, Hanson A, Katsura H, Watanabe S, Li C, Kawakami E, Yamada S, Kiso M, Suzuki Y, Maher EA, Neumann G, Kawaoka Y.** 2012. Experimental adaptation of an influenza H5 HA confers respiratory droplet transmission to a reassortant H5 HA/H1N1 virus in ferrets. *Nature* **486:**420–428.

11. **Koopmans M, Wilbrink B, Conyn M, Natrop G, van der Nat H, Vennema H, Meijer A, van Steenbergen J, Fouchier R, Osterhaus A, Bosman A.** 2004. Transmission of H7N7 avian influenza A virus to human beings during a large outbreak in commercial poultry farms in the Netherlands. *Lancet* **363:**587–593.
12. **Wang X, Jiang H, Wu P, Uyeki TM, Feng L, Lai S, Wang L, Huo X, Xu K, Chen E, Wang X, He J, Kang M, Zhang R, Zhang J, Wu J, Hu S, Zhang H, Liu X, Fu W, Ou J, Wu S, Qin Y, Zhang Z, Shi Y, Zhang J, Artois J, Fang VJ, Zhu H, Guan Y, Gilbert M, Horby PW, Leung GM, Gao GF, Cowling BJ, Yu H.** 2017. Epidemiology of avian influenza A H7N9 virus in human beings across five epidemics in mainland China, 2013–17: an epidemiological study of laboratory-confirmed case series. *Lancet Infect Dis* **17:**822–832.
13. **Nelson MI, Wentworth DE, Das SR, Sreevatsan S, Killian ML, Nolting JM, Slemons RD, Bowman AS.** 2016. Evolutionary dynamics of influenza A viruses in US exhibition swine. *J Infect Dis* **213:**173–182.
14. **Treanor JJ.**2015. Influenza (including avian influenza and swine influenza), p 2000–2024. *In* Bennett JE, Dolin R, Blaser MJ (ed), *Principles and Practice of Infectious Diseases*, 8th ed. Churchill Livingstone, Inc., New York, NY.
15. **Hayden FG, Palese P.** 2017. Influenza virus, p 1009–1058. *In* Richman DD, Whitley RJ, Hayden FG (ed), *Clinical Virology*, 4th ed. ASM Press, Washington, DC.
16. **Sellers SA, Hagan RS, Hayden FG, Fischer WA II.** 2017. The hidden burden of influenza: a review of the extrapulmonary complications of influenza infection. *Influenza Other Respir Viruses* **11:**372–393.
17. **Yu H, Cowling BJ, Feng L, Lau EH, Liao Q, Tsang TK, Peng Z, Wu P, Liu F, Fang VJ, Zhang H, Li M, Zeng L, Xu Z, Li Z, Luo H, Li Q, Feng Z, Cao B, Yang W, Wu JT, Wang Y, Leung GM.** 2013. Human infection with avian influenza A H7N9 virus: an assessment of clinical severity. *Lancet* **382:**138–145.
18. **Wang C, Yu H, Horby PW, Cao B, Wu P, Yang S, Gao H, Li H, Tsang TK, Liao Q, Gao Z, Ip DK, Jia H, Jiang H, Liu B, Ni MY, Dai X, Liu F, Van Kinh N, Liem NT, Hien TT, Li Y, Yang J, Wu JT, Zheng Y, Leung GM, Farrar JJ, Cowling BJ, Uyeki TM, Li L.** 2014. Comparison of patients hospitalized with influenza A subtypes H7N9, H5N1, and 2009 pandemic H1N1. *Clin Infect Dis* **58:**1095–1103.
19. **Harper SA, Bradley JS, Englund JA, File TM, Gravenstein S, Hayden FG, McGeer AJ, Neuzil KM, Pavia AT, Tapper ML, Uyeki TM, Zimmerman RK, Expert Panel of the Infectious Diseases Society of America.** 2009. Seasonal influenza in adults and children—diagnosis, treatment, chemoprophylaxis, and institutional outbreak management: clinical practice guidelines of the Infectious Diseases Society of America. *Clin Infect Dis* **48:**1003–1032.
20. **Grohskopf LA, Sokolow LZ, Broder KR, Olsen SJ, Karron RA, Jernigan DB, Bresee JS.** 2016. Prevention and control of seasonal influenza with vaccines. *MMWR Recomm Rep* **65:**1–54.
21. **Singanayagam A, Zambon M, Lalvani A, Barclay W.** 2018. Urgent challenges in implementing live attenuated influenza vaccine. *Lancet Infect Dis* **18:**e25–e32.
22. **Covalciuc KA, Webb KH, Carlson CA.** 1999. Comparison of four clinical specimen types for detection of influenza A and B viruses by optical immunoassay (FLU OIA test) and cell culture methods. *J Clin Microbiol* **37:**3971–3974.
23. **Kaiser L, Briones MS, Hayden FG.** 1999. Performance of virus isolation and Directigen Flu A to detect influenza A virus in experimental human infection. *J Clin Virol* **14:**191–197.
24. **Yu L, Wang Z, Chen Y, Ding W, Jia H, Chan JF, To KK, Chen H, Yang Y, Liang W, Zheng S, Yao H, Yang S, Cao H, Dai X, Zhao H, Li J, Bao Q, Chen P, Hou X, Li L, Yuen KY.** 2013. Clinical, virological, and histopathological manifestations of fatal human infections by avian influenza A (H7N9) virus. *Clin Infect Dis* **57:**1449–1457.
25. **Falsey AR, Formica MA, Walsh EE.** 2012. Yield of sputum for viral detection by reverse transcriptase PCR in adults hospitalized with respiratory illness. *J Clin Microbiol* **50:**21–24.
26. **Jeong JH, Kim KH, Jeong SH, Park JW, Lee SM, Seo YH.** 2014. Comparison of sputum and nasopharyngeal swabs for detection of respiratory viruses. *J Med Virol* **86:**2122–2127.
27. **Baxter BD, Couch RB, Greenberg SB, Kasel JA.** 1977. Maintenance of viability and comparison of identification methods for influenza and other respiratory viruses of humans. *J Clin Microbiol* **6:**19–22.
28. **Ptáková M, Tůmová B.** 1985. Detection of type A and B influenza viruses in clinical materials by immunoelectronmicroscopy. *Acta Virol* **29:**19–24.
29. **Uyeki TM.** 2003. Influenza diagnosis and treatment in children: a review of studies on clinically useful tests and antiviral treatment for influenza. *Pediatr Infect Dis J* **22:**164–177.
30. **Landry ML.** 2011. Diagnostic tests for influenza infection. *Curr Opin Pediatr* **23:**91–97.
31. **Ginocchio CC, Zhang F, Manji R, Arora S, Bornfreund M, Falk L, Lotlikar M, Kowerska M, Becker G, Korologos D, de Geronimo M, Crawford JM.** 2009. Evaluation of multiple test methods for the detection of the novel 2009 influenza A (H1N1) during the New York City outbreak. *J Clin Virol* **45:**191–195.
32. **Merckx J, Wali R, Schiller I, Caya C, Gore GC, Chartrand C, Dendukuri N, Papenburg J.** 2017. Diagnostic accuracy of novel and traditional rapid tests for influenza infection compared with reverse transcriptase polymerase chain reaction: a systematic review and meta-analysis. *Ann Intern Med* **167:**394–409.
33. **Food and Drug Administration, HHS.** 2017. Microbiology Devices; reclassification of influenza virus antigen detection test systems intended for use directly with clinical specimens. Final order. *Fed Regist* **82:**3609–3619.
34. **Zhang WD, Evans DH.** 1991. Detection and identification of human influenza viruses by the polymerase chain reaction. *J Virol Methods* **33:**165–189.
35. **van Elden LJ, Nijhuis M, Schipper P, Schuurman R, van Loon AM.** 2001. Simultaneous detection of influenza viruses A and B using real-time quantitative PCR. *J Clin Microbiol* **39:**196–200.
36. **Pabbaraju K, Tokaryk KL, Wong S, Fox JD.** 2008. Comparison of the Luminex xTAG respiratory viral panel with in-house nucleic acid amplification tests for diagnosis of respiratory virus infections. *J Clin Microbiol* **46:**3056–3062.
37. **Raymond F, Carbonneau J, Boucher N, Robitaille L, Boisvert S, Wu WK, De Serres G, Boivin G, Corbeil J.** 2009. Comparison of automated microarray detection with real-time PCR assays for detection of respiratory viruses in specimens obtained from children. *J Clin Microbiol* **47:**743–750.
38. **Stellrecht KA.** 2018. The drift in molecular testing for influenza: mutations affecting assay performance. *J Clin Microbiol* **56:**e01531-17.
39. **Popowitch EB, O'Neill SS, Miller MB.** 2013. Comparison of the Biofire FilmArray RP, Genmark eSensor RVP, Luminex xTAG RVPv1, and Luminex xTAG RVP fast multiplex assays for detection of respiratory viruses. *J Clin Microbiol* **51:**1528–1533.
40. **Sidoti F, Bergallo M, Costa C, Cavallo R.** 2013. Alternative molecular tests for virological diagnosis. *Mol Biotechnol* **53:**352–362.
41. **Vemula SV, Zhao J, Liu J, Wang X, Biswas S, Hewlett I.** 2016. Current approaches for diagnosis of influenza virus infections in humans. *Viruses* **8:**96.
42. **Trabattoni E, Le V, Pilmis B, Pean de Ponfilly G, Caisso C, Couzigou C, Vidal B, Mizrahi A, Ganansia O, Le Monnier A, Lina B, Nguyen Van JC.** 2018. Implementation of Alere i Influenza A & B point of care test for the diagnosis of influenza in an ED. *Am J Emerg Med* **36:**916–921.
43. **Centers for Disease Control and Prevention.** 2016. Interim risk assessment and biosafety level recommendations for working with influenza A(H7N9) viruses. https://www.cdc.gov/flu/avianflu/h7n9/risk-assessment.htm (Accessed January 2018).
44. **Webster R, Cox N, Stohr K.** 2004. WHO manual on animal influenza diagnosis and surveillance. http://www.who.int/csr/resources/publications/influenza/en/whocdscsrncs20025.pdf

45. **Frank AL, Couch RB, Griffis CA, Baxter BD.** 1979. Comparison of different tissue cultures for isolation and quantitation of influenza and parainfluenza viruses. *J Clin Microbiol* **10:**32–36.
46. **Reina J, Fernandez-Baca V, Blanco I, Munar M.** 1997. Comparison of Madin-Darby canine kidney cells (MDCK) with a green monkey continuous cell line (Vero) and human lung embryonated cells (MRC-5) in the isolation of influenza A virus from nasopharyngeal aspirates by shell vial culture. *J Clin Microbiol* **35:**1900–1901.
47. **Dowdle WR, Kendal AP, Noble GR.** 1979. Influenza viruses, p 585–609. *In* Lennette EH, Schmidt NJ (ed), *Diagnostic Procedures for Viral, Rickettsial, and Chlamydial Infections*, 5th ed. American Public Health Association, Washington, DC.
48. **Zambon M.** 1998. Laboratory diagnosis of influenza, p 291–313. *In* Nicholson KG, Webster RG, Hay AJ (ed), *Textbook of Influenza*. Blackwell Science, London, England.
49. **Fong CK, Lee MK, Griffith BP.** 2000. Evaluation of R-Mix FreshCells in shell vials for detection of respiratory viruses. *J Clin Microbiol* **38:**4660–4662.
50. **Weinberg A, Mettenbrink CJ, Ye D, Yang CF.** 2005. Sensitivity of diagnostic tests for influenza varies with the circulating strains. *J Clin Virol* **33:**172–175.
51. **Govorkova EA, Kodihalli S, Alymova IV, Fanget B, Webster RG.** 1999. Growth and immunogenicity of influenza viruses cultivated in Vero or MDCK cells and in embryonated chicken eggs. *Dev Biol Stand* **98:**39–51; discussion 73–34.
52. **Zost SJ, Parkhouse K, Gumina ME, Kim K, Diaz Perez S, Wilson PC, Treanor JJ, Sant AJ, Cobey S, Hensley SE.** 2017. Contemporary H3N2 influenza viruses have a glycosylation site that alters binding of antibodies elicited by egg-adapted vaccine strains. *Proc Natl Acad Sci USA* **114:** 12578–12583.
53. **Hirst GK.** 1942. The quantitative determination of influenza virus and antibodies by means of red cell agglutination. *J Exp Med* **75:**49–64.
54. **Zhou B, Deng YM, Barnes JR, Sessions OM, Chou TW, Wilson M, Stark TJ, Volk M, Spirason N, Halpin RA, Kamaraj US, Ding T, Stockwell TB, Salvatore M, Ghedin E, Barr IG, Wentworth DE.** 2017. Multiplex reverse transcription-PCR for simultaneous surveillance of influenza A and B viruses. *J Clin Microbiol* **55:**3492–3501.
55. **O'Donnell FT, Munoz FM, Atmar RL, Hwang LY, Demmler GJ, Glezen WP.** 2003. Epidemiology and molecular characterization of co-circulating influenza A/H3N2 virus variants in children: Houston, Texas, 1997-8. *Epidemiol Infect* **130:**521–531.
56. **Metzgar D, Baynes D, Myers CA, Kammerer P, Unabia M, Faix DJ, Blair PJ.** 2010. Initial identification and characterization of an emerging zoonotic influenza virus prior to pandemic spread. *J Clin Microbiol* **48:**4228–4234.
57. **Townsend MB, Dawson ED, Mehlmann M, Smagala JA, Dankbar DM, Moore CL, Smith CB, Cox NJ, Kuchta RD, Rowlen KL.** 2006. Experimental evaluation of the FluChip diagnostic microarray for influenza virus surveillance. *J Clin Microbiol* **44:**2863–2871.
58. **Sultankulova KT, Chervyakova OV, Kozhabergenov NS, Shorayeva KA, Strochkov VM, Orynbayev MB, Sandybayev NT, Sansyzbay AR, Vasin AV.** 2014. Comparative evaluation of effectiveness of IAVchip DNA microarray in influenza A diagnosis. *Sci World J* **2014:**620580.
59. **Westgeest KB, Russell CA, Lin X, Spronken MI, Bestebroer TM, Bahl J, van Beek R, Skepner E, Halpin RA, de Jong JC, Rimmelzwaan GF, Osterhaus AD, Smith DJ, Wentworth DE, Fouchier RA, de Graaf M, Garcia-Sastre A.** 2014. Genomewide analysis of reassortment and evolution of human influenza A(H3N2) viruses circulating between 1968 and 2011. *J Virol* **88:**2844–2857.
60. **Poon LL, Song T, Rosenfeld R, Lin X, Rogers MB, Zhou B, Sebra R, Halpin RA, Guan Y, Twaddle A, DePasse JV, Stockwell TB, Wentworth DE, Holmes EC, Greenbaum B, Peiris JS, Cowling BJ, Ghedin E.** 2016. Quantifying influenza virus diversity and transmission in humans. *Nat Genet* **48:**195–200.
61. **Rothbarth PH, Groen J, Bohnen AM, de Groot R, Osterhaus AD.** 1999. Influenza virus serology—a comparative study. *J Virol Methods* **78:**163–169.
62. **Katz JM, Lim W, Bridges CB, Rowe T, Hu-Primmer J, Lu X, Abernathy RA, Clarke M, Conn L, Kwong H, Lee M, Au G, Ho YY, Mak KH, Cox NJ, Fukuda K.** 1999. Antibody response in individuals infected with avian influenza A (H5N1) viruses and detection of anti-H5 antibody among household and social contacts. *J Infect Dis* **180:**1763–1770.
63. **Pyhälä R, Pyhälä L, Valle M, Aho K.** 1987. Egg-grown and tissue-culture-grown variants of influenza A (H3N2) virus with special attention to their use as antigens in seroepidemiology. *Epidemiol Infect* **99:**745–753.
64. **Stephenson I, Wood JM, Nicholson KG, Zambon MC.** 2003. Sialic acid receptor specificity on erythrocytes affects detection of antibody to avian influenza haemagglutinin. *J Med Virol* **70:**391–398.
65. **World Health Organization.** 2003. Assays for neutralizing antibody to influenza viruses. Report of an informal scientific workshop, Dresden, 18–19 March 2003. *Wkly Epidemiol Rec* **78:**290–293.
66. **Rowe T, Abernathy RA, Hu-Primmer J, Thompson WW, Lu X, Lim W, Fukuda K, Cox NJ, Katz JM.** 1999. Detection of antibody to avian influenza A (H5N1) virus in human serum by using a combination of serologic assays. *J Clin Microbiol* **37:**937–943.
67. **Laurie KL, Engelhardt OG, Wood J, Heath A, Katz JM, Peiris M, Hoschler K, Hungnes O, Zhang W, Van Kerkhove MD; CONSISE Laboratory Working Group participants.** 2015. International laboratory comparison of influenza microneutralization assays for A(H1N1)pdm09, A(H3N2), and A(H5N1) influenza viruses by CONSISE. *Clin Vaccine Immunol* **22:**957–964.
68. **Belshe RB, Smith MH, Hall CB, Betts R, Hay AJ.** 1988. Genetic basis of resistance to rimantadine emerging during treatment of influenza virus infection. *J Virol* **62:**1508–1512.
69. **Bright RA, Shay DK, Shu B, Cox NJ, Klimov AI.** 2006. Adamantane resistance among influenza A viruses isolated early during the 2005–2006 influenza season in the United States. *JAMA* **295:**891–894.
70. **Deyde VM, Nguyen T, Bright RA, Balish A, Shu B, Lindstrom S, Klimov AI, Gubareva LV.** 2009. Detection of molecular markers of antiviral resistance in influenza A (H5N1) viruses using a pyrosequencing method. *Antimicrob Agents Chemother* **53:**1039–1047.
71. **McKimm-Breschkin J, Trivedi T, Hampson A, Hay A, Klimov A, Tashiro M, Hayden F, Zambon M.** 2003. Neuraminidase sequence analysis and susceptibilities of influenza virus clinical isolates to zanamivir and oseltamivir. *Antimicrob Agents Chemother* **47:**2264–2272.
72. **Murtaugh W, Mahaman L, Healey B, Peters H, Anderson B, Tran M, Ziese M, Carlos MP.** 2013. Evaluation of three influenza neuraminidase inhibition assays for use in a public health laboratory setting during the 2011–2012 influenza season. *Public Health Rep* **128**(Suppl 2)**:**75–87.
73. **Okomo-Adhiambo M, Sheu TG, Gubareva LV.** 2013. Assays for monitoring susceptibility of influenza viruses to neuraminidase inhibitors. *Influenza Other Respir Viruses* **7**(Suppl 1)**:**44–49.
74. **Laplante J, St George K.** 2014. Antiviral resistance in influenza viruses: laboratory testing. *Clin Lab Med* **34:**387–408.
75. **Bolotin S, Robertson AV, Eshaghi A, De Lima C, Lombos E, Chong-King E, Burton L, Mazzulli T, Drews SJ.** 2009. Development of a novel real-time reverse-transcriptase PCR method for the detection of H275Y positive influenza A H1N1 isolates. *J Virol Methods* **158:**190–194.
76. **Monto AS, Gravenstein S, Elliott M, Colopy M, Schweinle J.** 2000. Clinical signs and symptoms predicting influenza infection. *Arch Intern Med* **160:**3243–3247.
77. **Fouchier RA, Schneeberger PM, Rozendaal FW, Broekman JM, Kemink SA, Munster V, Kuiken T, Rimmelzwaan GF, Schutten M, Van Doornum GJ, Koch G, Bosman A, Koopmans M, Osterhaus AD.** 2004. Avian influenza A virus (H7N7) associated with human conjunctivitis and a fatal case of acute respiratory distress syndrome. *Proc Natl Acad Sci USA* **101:**1356–1361.

78. **Nolte FS, Gauld L, Barrett SB.** 2016. Direct comparison of Alere i and cobas Liat Influenza A and B tests for rapid detection of influenza virus infection. *J Clin Microbiol* **54:** 2763–2766.
79. **Mecias-Frias J, Silbert S, Uy D, Widen R.** 2017. *Laboratory Evaluation of the Solana Flu A+B Assay on the Solana Instrument, abstr ASM Microbe, New Orleans, LA, 6/4/2017.* American Society for Microbiology, Washington, DC.
80. **Gibson J, Schechter-Perkins EM, Mitchell P, Mace S, Tian Y, Williams K, Luo R, Yen-Lieberman B.** 2017. Multi-center evaluation of the cobas Liat Influenza A/B & RSV assay for rapid point of care diagnosis. *J Clin Virol* **95:**5–9.
81. **Jost M, Shah A, Douglas P, Hentzen C, Nugent T, Kolk D.** 2016. The modular approach to respiratory syndromic testing with the fully-automated novel Panther Fusion System. *J Clin Virol* **82S:**S32.
82. **Jernigan DB, Lindstrom SL, Johnson JR, Miller JD, Hoelscher M, Humes R, Shively R, Brammer L, Burke SA, Villanueva JM, Balish A, Uyeki T, Mustaquim D, Bishop A, Handsfield JH, Astles R, Xu X, Klimov AI, Cox NJ, Shaw MW.** 2011. Detecting 2009 pandemic influenza A (H1N1) virus infection: availability of diagnostic testing led to rapid pandemic response. *Clin Infect Dis* **52**(Suppl 1): S36–S43.
83. **Thammavong H, Myers C.** 2015. Joint biological agent identification and diagnostic system influenza A and B and influenza A subtyping detection kits. *Open Forum Infect Dis* 2(suppl_1):996.
84. **Gharabaghi F, Tellier R, Cheung R, Collins C, Broukhanski G, Drews SJ, Richardson SE.** 2008. Comparison of a commercial qualitative real-time RT-PCR kit with direct immunofluorescence assay (DFA) and cell culture for detection of influenza A and B in children. *J Clin Virol* **42:**190–193.
85. **Li M, Brenwald N, Bonigal S, Chana K, Osman H, Oppenheim B.** 2012. Rapid diagnosis of influenza: an evaluation of two commercially available RT-PCR assays. *J Infect* **65:**60–63.
86. **Rabaan AA, Bazzi AM, Alshaikh SA.** 2018. Comparison of Cepheid Xpert Flu and Roche RealTime Ready Influenza A/H1N1 Detection Set for detection of influenza A/H1N1. *Diagn Microbiol Infect Dis* **90:**280–285.
87. **McMullen P, Boonlayangoor S, Charnot-Katsikas A, Beavis KG, Tesic V.** 2017. The performance of Luminex ARIES Flu A/B & RSV and Cepheid Xpert Flu/RSV XC for the detection of influenza A, influenza B, and respiratory syncytial virus in prospective patient samples. *J Clin Virol* **95:**84–85.
88. **Cohen DM, Kline J, May LS, Harnett GE, Gibson J, Liang SY, Rafique Z, Rodriguez CA, McGann KM Sr, Gaydos CA, Mayne D, Phillips D, Cohen J.** 2018. Accurate PCR detection of influenza A/B and respiratory syncytial viruses by use of Cepheid Xpert Flu+RSV Xpress Assay in point-of-care settings: comparison to Prodesse ProFlu. *J Clin Microbiol* **56:**e01237-17.
89. **Ling L, Kaplan SE, Lopez JC, Stiles J, Lu X, Tang YW.** 2018. Parallel validation of three molecular devices for simultaneous detection and identification of influenza A and B and respiratory syncytial viruses. *J Clin Microbiol* **56:**e01691-17.
90. **Babady NE, England MR, Jurcic Smith KL, He T, Wijetunge DS, Tang YW, Chamberland RR, Menegus M, Swierkosz EM, Jerris RC, Greene W.** 2018. Multicenter evaluation of the ePlex respiratory pathogen panel for the detection of viral and bacterial respiratory tract pathogens in nasopharyngeal swabs. *J Clin Microbiol* **56:**e01658-17.
91. **Parker J, Fowler N, Walmsley ML, Schmidt T, Scharrer J, Kowaleski J, Grimes T, Hoyos S, Chen J.** 2015. Analytical sensitivity comparison between singleplex real-time PCR and a multiplex PCR platform for detecting respiratory viruses. *PLoS One* **10:**e0143164.
92. **Leber AL, Everhart K, Daly JA, Hopper A, Harrington A, Schreckenberger P, McKinley K, Jones M, Holmberg K, Kensinger B.** 2018. Multicenter evaluation of the Biofire Filmarray respiratory panel 2 for the detection of viruses and bacteria in nasopharyngeal swab samples. *J Clin Microbiol* **56**(6). pii: e01945-17.
93. **Tang YW, Lowery KS, Valsamakis A, Schaefer VC, Chappell JD, White-Abell J, Quinn CD, Li H, Washington CA, Cromwell J, Giamanco CM, Forman M, Holden J, Rothman RE, Parker ML, Ortenberg EV, Zhang L, Lin YL, Gaydos CA.** 2013. Clinical accuracy of a PLEX-ID flu device for simultaneous detection and identification of influenza viruses A and B. *J Clin Microbiol* **51:**40–45.
94. **Van Wesenbeeck L, Meeuws H, Van Immerseel A, Ispas G, Schmidt K, Houspie L, Van Ranst M, Stuyver L.** 2013. Comparison of the FilmArray RP, Verigene RV+, and Prodesse ProFLU+/FAST+ multiplex platforms for detection of influenza viruses in clinical samples from the 2011–2012 influenza season in Belgium. *J Clin Microbiol* **51:** 2977–2985.
95. **Hindiyeh M, Kolet L, Meningher T, Weil M, Mendelson E, Mandelboim M.** 2013. Evaluation of Simplexa Flu A/B & RSV for direct detection of influenza viruses (A and B) and respiratory syncytial virus in patient clinical samples. *J Clin Microbiol* **51:**2421–2424.
96. **Alby K, Popowitch EB, Miller MB.** 2013. Comparative evaluation of the Nanosphere Verigene RV+ assay and the Simplexa Flu A/B & RSV kit for detection of influenza and respiratory syncytial viruses. *J Clin Microbiol* **51:**352–353.
97. **Sutton B, Maggert K, Rowell B, Etter R.** 2014. Comparison of the Focus Diagnostics Simplexa Flu A/B & RSV Direct Assay with the Prodesse ProFlu plus Assay for detection of influenza A virus (IAV), influenza B virus (IBV), and respiratory syncytial virus (RSV) in clinical specimens. *J Mol Diagn* **16:**727–728.
98. **Bogoch II, Andrews JR, Zachary KC, Hohmann EL.** 2013. Diagnosis of influenza from lower respiratory tract sampling after negative upper respiratory tract sampling. *Virulence* **4:**82–84.
99. **Tang YW, Gonsalves S, Sun JY, Stiles J, Gilhuley KA, Mikhlina A, Dunbar SA, Babady NE, Zhang H.** 2016. Clinical evaluation of the Luminex nxTAG respiratory pathogen panel. *J Clin Microbiol* **54:**1912–1914.
100. **Saglik I, Sarınoglu RC, Mutlu D, Cengiz M, Dursun O, Oygur N, Ramazanoglu A, Colak D.** 2016. Respiratory viruses in patients with acute respiratory infections in the pediatric and adults intensive care units. *J Clin Virol* **82S:**S125–S126.

Parainfluenza and Mumps Viruses

RYAN F. RELICH AND DIANE S. LELAND

87

TAXONOMY

The human parainfluenza viruses (HPIVs) and mumps virus (MuV) are taxonomically divided among the genera *Respirovirus* and *Rubulavirus* within the family *Paramyxoviridae*, order *Mononegavirales*. HPIV-1 and HPIV-3 are included in the genus *Respirovirus* and are formally known as *Human respirovirus 1* and *Human respirovirus 3*, respectively. HPIV-2, HPIV-4, and MuV are known formally as *Human rubulavirus 2*, *Human rubulavirus 4*, and *Mumps rubulavirus*, respectively, and also belong to the family *Paramyxoviridae*. These taxonomic revisions are listed in Table 1. Other human-pathogenic paramyxoviruses include members of the genera *Henipavirus* (Hendra and Nipah viruses) and *Morbillivirus* (measles virus). Respiratory syncytial virus (RSV) and human metapneumovirus, once classified as paramyxoviruses, have recently been assigned to the new family *Pneumoviridae* within the order *Mononegavirales*. Paramyxoviruses cause significant human and veterinary diseases whose effects are noted among virus families as "one of the most costly in terms of disease burden and economic impact to our planet" (1).

DESCRIPTION OF THE AGENTS

All of the viruses described in this chapter are enveloped and possess helical nucleocapsids. Particles range in size from ~150 to 350 nm and tend to adopt pleomorphic morphologies that include roughly spherical and filamentous forms; the latter is especially true for HPIV-2 (2). Virions possess monopartite, minus-sense, single-stranded RNA genomes that measure approximately 15 kbp in length and encode 6 to 11 proteins, depending upon the virus. The largest protein, L, is the viral RNA-dependent RNA polymerase. L, along with the phosphoprotein, P, and the nucleocapsid protein, N (or NP), together with the viral RNA, constitutes the viral nucleocapsid. The surface glycoproteins, hemagglutinin-neuraminidase (HN) and fusion protein (F), project from the viral envelope and can be seen by electron microscopy. Rubulaviruses possess a third membrane protein, small hydrophobic protein (SH), which is a 44-amino-acid polypeptide that is believed to inhibit virus-induced host cell apoptosis. The sixth structural protein is a membrane (M) protein. In viral replication, N protein binds to viral RNA, L and P function in transcription and replication, and the HN and F surface glycoproteins interact with the M protein, which attracts assembled nucleocapsids to areas of the plasma membrane that will become the envelopes of the new virions during budding. The HN surface glycoproteins also function in virus-host cell attachment via sialic acid receptors, and the F proteins function in virus-host cell membrane fusion, which allows the viral nucleocapsid to enter and infect a host cell. Diagrams representing the ultrastructure of rubulaviruses and respiroviruses are presented in Fig. 1.

Four species of HPIV have so far been identified. HPIV-4 can be further subdivided into HPIV-4a and HPIV-4b; because these are so closely related, they are referred to as HPIV-4 for the remainder of this discussion. Only one antigenic type of MuV has been identified, although strains show differences in the sequence of the SH protein gene, which constitutes the basis for classification of MuV into 12 genotypes, designated A through L. Among these, genotype G viruses are the most common causes of mumps in the United States. HPIV and MuV are inactivated by temperatures above 50°C, organic solvents, UV irradiation, formalin treatment, low pH (3.0 to 3.4), and desiccation. Preservation by freezing at −70°C or colder is effective, and the addition of 0.5% bovine serum albumin, skim milk, 5% dimethyl sulfoxide, or 2% heat-inactivated serum prior to freezing prolongs infectivity of viral stocks.

Although they are similar in structure and antigenic composition, HPIVs and MuV currently present very different clinical pictures in the United States. The HPIVs are common agents of respiratory infections in children and adults in the United States, and virology laboratories routinely test for HPIV by direct antigen testing, virus isolation, and, most commonly, by molecular methods such as PCR. In contrast, MuV, which was considered one of the common causes of diseases of childhood prior to the introduction of an effective vaccine in 1968, is now relatively uncommon, but mumps outbreaks have become more frequent over the last few years. Despite this, most virology laboratories no longer focus on the isolation and identification of MuV, relegating testing for this agent to reference and public health laboratories. Because of these differences, the HPIVs and MuV are discussed separately below.

TABLE 1 Taxonomy of HPIV and MuV

Virus	Species designation	
	Previous	Current[a]
Human parainfluenza virus type 1	*Human parainfluenza virus 1*	*Human respirovirus 1*
Human parainfluenza virus type 2	*Human parainfluenza virus 2*	*Human rubulavirus 2*
Human parainfluenza virus type 3	*Human parainfluenza virus 3*	*Human respirovirus 3*
Human parainfluenza virus type 4	*Human parainfluenza virus 4*	*Human rubulavirus 4*
Mumps virus	*Mumps virus*	*Mumps rubulavirus*

[a]Current viral species designations according to the International Committee on Taxonomy of Viruses Online (10th) Report on Virus Taxonomy (available at https://talk.ictvonline.org/taxonomy/).

PARAINFLUENZA VIRUSES

Epidemiology and Transmission

HPIVs are thought to be transmitted by large-droplet aerosols and by contact with contaminated surfaces. The viruses have been shown to remain infectious for up to 10 h on porous surfaces; however, HPIV-3 experimentally placed on fingers was shown to lose more than 90% of its infectivity in the first 10 min following application (3). Currently, HPIV-1, -2, -3, and -4 represent approximately 5% of all viruses detected in routine hospital diagnostic laboratories (4). HPIV-1 transmission occurs most often in autumn and biennially. The incidence of HPIV-2 is generally lower than that of HPIV-1 and HPIV-3, occurring biennially with HPIV-1, in alternate years from HPIV-1, or yearly. HPIV-3 occurs yearly, in spring and summer, but can circulate year-round in temperate climates. HPIV-4 is now known to be more prevalent than was previously thought, a result of better and more widely available diagnostic methods, including multiplexed molecular respiratory pathogen detection assays, but it still accounts for many fewer severe infections than other HPIV species. In a study published in 2014, using data obtained by multiplex molecular testing, Frost and colleagues noted that HPIV-4 is a common respiratory pathogen of children, has year-round prevalence, and peaks during the autumn of odd-numbered years (5).

Clinical Significance

HPIVs are associated with upper and lower respiratory tract infections in infants, children, and adults; however, severe disease is generally seen only among those with compromised immune systems. The mean incubation period is estimated to be between 2 and 6 days for HPIV infection (6). These infections are typically fairly mild and self-limited, and mortality is rare in developed countries (7, 8). Reinfection is common, because natural infection does not induce lifelong immunity. HPIV accounts for the majority of cases of viral croup, which is the most common cause of upper airway obstruction in children of 6 months to 6 years of age. Croup is characterized by inspiratory stridor, barking cough, and hoarseness (9).

HPIV-1 is associated with up to 50% of cases of croup reported in the United States, with the majority of cases occurring in children of 7 to 36 months of age. HPIV-2 is associated with croup in immunocompromised or chronically ill children. HPIV-2 also causes typical lower respiratory tract syndromes in otherwise healthy children, with about 60% of infections occurring in children younger than 5 years of age; peak incidence is in children between 1 and

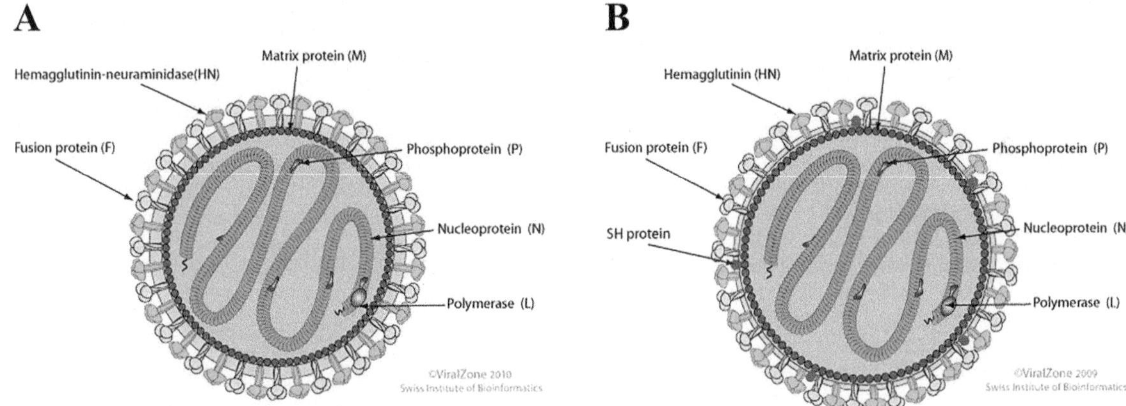

FIGURE 1 Diagrams of respirovirus (A) and rubulavirus (B) ultrastructures. Particles of both types of viruses contain a single strand of minus-sense RNA encapsidated by L, N, and P proteins. The viral genomes are enveloped by a single layer of cellular plasma membrane, below the surface of which is the viral M protein and within which are embedded the viral transmembrane glycoproteins F and HN. In rubulaviruses such as HPIV-2, HPIV-4, and MuV, SH proteins are also present in the viral envelope. (Used with permission from Swiss Institute of Bioinformatics [http://viralzone.expasy.org].)

2 years of age. HPIV-3 is more frequent in infants younger than 6 months of age, with 40% of infections occurring during the first year of life. Only RSV causes more lower respiratory tract infections in neonates and young infants than HPIV-3. HPIV-4 can cause many of the same respiratory symptoms as HPIV-1, -2, and -3; however, it is generally not associated with croup (10). As many as 7% of all hospitalizations for viral acute respiratory illness in children younger than 5 years of age have been shown to be due to HPIV infection (11). HPIV-1, -2, and -3 have also been found in as many as one-third of lower respiratory tract infections in children younger than 5 years of age in the United States and are second only to RSV as a cause of hospitalization for viral lower respiratory tract infections (12).

Although associated with infections in children, HPIVs have the potential for serious pulmonary infections in adults, with HPIV-1 and HPIV-3 being among the four most commonly identified pathogens in adults requiring hospitalization for community-acquired pneumonia (13). HPIVs also cause lower respiratory tract infections in the elderly. Of nine common infections, HPIVs were significantly associated with mortality in those aged ≥75 years; this association was of lower magnitude than that of influenza A virus and RSV—which were significantly associated with mortality in all age groups—but of higher magnitude than that of the other pathogens (14).

HPIV is increasingly recognized as a source of severe morbidity and mortality in immunocompromised patients, especially in those with congenital immunodeficiencies, and is capable of infecting tissues in the gastrointestinal and urinary tracts in these individuals (7). HPIVs replicate productively in respiratory epithelium and generally do not spread systemically unless the host is severely immunocompromised (15). HPIVs cause more than 50% of the respiratory infections in pediatric bone marrow transplant recipients and 19% of those in pediatric solid organ transplant recipients (16). HPIV infection, most commonly HPIV-3 infection, was identified in 3.3% of 5,178 pediatric and adult hematopoietic stem cell transplant recipients, causing both upper and lower respiratory tract infection and resulting in poor outcomes for those with lower respiratory infections (17). HPIVs were detected in 3% of pediatric patients with cystic fibrosis, second only to rhinovirus (18), and, similarly, in 5% of very low birth weight infants, next in frequency behind rhinovirus and RSV (19). In South Korea, HPIVs were the most commonly isolated pathogen among 137 pediatric cancer patients with respiratory viral infections, with 80% of these having been acquired nosocomially (20).

There are currently no U.S. Food and Drug Administration (FDA)-cleared antivirals for treatment of HPIV infections. Ribavirin has been used to treat HPIV infections in immunocompromised patients, but results have varied. Elizaga et al. (21) reported no efficacy for this therapy. In contrast, successful HPIV treatment was reported for intravenous ribavirin therapy (22), oral ribavirin along with methylprednisolone (23), and high ribavirin doses used with early intervention (24). DAS181 (Fludase; Ansun BioPharma), a novel inhaled antiviral agent, offers promise for the treatment of HPIV infections. This agent, a bacterial-human fusion protein with sialidase activity, cleaves α(2,3)- and α(2,6)-linked sialic acids, which are receptors for influenza viruses and HPIVs, from the surfaces of host cells (25). In this way, DAS181 renders the host resistant to infection with these viruses. To date, only a few studies of its efficacy in treating human HPIV infections have been published. In all, participants included either hematopoietic stem cell or solid organ transplant recipients and DAS181 was administered through compassionate-use protocols. In many of the patients, posttreatment viral loads were either undetectable or decreased, and in almost all cases where it was reported, posttreatment pulmonary function improved to some degree (26–32). In addition, DAS181 appeared to be well tolerated by patients and did not appear to have demonstrable side effects in study participants; however, further research is needed to fully evaluate its utility in the treatment of HPIV-associated diseases. To that end, management of HPIV infection symptoms through administration of corticosteroids is recommended (9).

There are currently no FDA-cleared vaccines for the HPIVs. The search continues for an effective HPIV vaccine using live attenuated recombinant HPIVs carrying various mutations and utilizing a bovine PIV-3 strain to express HPIV antigens. All vaccine candidates are still undergoing evaluation for their safety and efficacy: preliminary data for some vaccine candidates are promising (33).

The diagnosis of HPIV infection may be based primarily on clinical signs and symptoms, and laboratory diagnostic studies may not be needed for all patients. However, laboratory assays to confirm HPIV infection, thus differentiating it from the many other viral infections that present with similar respiratory tract signs and symptoms, are widely available, and confirmation of infection may improve patient management and decrease costs (1, 34).

Collection, Transport, and Storage of Specimens

Testing to confirm HPIV infection can include virus isolation, antigen or antibody detection, or, more commonly in modern clinical virology laboratories, detection of viral nucleic acids (Table 2). Viral specimen collection, transport, and storage guidelines are provided earlier in section IV of this *Manual*. For immunofluorescence-based detection, care should be taken to include cellular material in samples collected from respiratory sites. The nasopharynx and oropharynx are primary locations of initial HPIV replication, and children shed virus from 3 to 4 days prior to the onset of clinical symptoms until approximately 10 days past onset. Virus recovery from adults is much more difficult than that from children, although immunocompromised patients and adults with chronic diseases, especially lung disease, have been shown to persistently shed HPIV for many months (12). Throat swabs, nasopharyngeal swabs, nasal washes, and nasal aspirates have all been used successfully to detect HPIV, but specimens from the nasopharynx—which is the primary location of initial HPIV replication—are best. For cultivation-based detection, specimens should be collected, placed in viral transport medium, and kept at 4°C until cell culture inoculation. Inoculation within 24 h of collection is recommended (12). For antigen and molecular tests, refer to the manufacturer's package insert for details regarding specimen collection, handling, and storage prior to testing.

Peripheral blood samples for use in HPIV antibody assays should be collected in tubes without anticoagulant, and serum should be separated from the clot as soon as possible to ensure sample integrity. Serum samples may be stored at 4°C if testing will be performed within 24 to 48 h but should be frozen at −20°C or lower if testing is delayed.

Direct Examination

Microscopy

Fluorescence microscopy remains the most commonly used method for direct microscopic detection of HPIVs in

TABLE 2 Diagnostic methods for HPIV and MuV detection

Virus	Method(s)			
	Isolation	Antigen detection	Molecular testing	Antibody detection
HPIV-1, -2, and -3	Widely available; replicate in PMK cells in 4 to 8 days, little to no CPE; HAD positive	IF[a] only (for direct specimen detection and culture confirmation); widely available as single tests or as part of respiratory virus panel; sensitivity, 70 to 83% compared to culture	Most sensitive method; available at many laboratories as HPIV-1, -2, -3 panel or as part of multitarget respiratory viral panel	May be available at reference laboratories; cross-reactivity with other *Paramyxoviridae*
HPIV-4	Replicates in PMK cells in 4 to 8 days; HAD stronger at room temperature	IF only (for culture confirmation); testing not widely available	Available to many laboratories as part of multitarget respiratory viral panel	Not available at most laboratories
MuV	Widely available; replicates in PMK cells in 6 to 8 days, produces syncytia; HAD positive	IF only (for culture confirmation); testing not widely available	Available at several reference and public health laboratories	Immune status (IgG) testing widely available. Some newer IgM testing methods more effective, not widely available. Cross-reactivity with other *Paramyxoviridae* limits usefulness in confirming acute infection.

[a]IF, immunofluorescence.

clinical specimens: more information concerning this is available in the next section. Histopathologic examination of tissues derived from the lung, pancreas, kidney, and bladder can exhibit syncytia (Fig. 2) that result from the fusion of plasma membranes of neighboring cells, a process mediated by the expression of the viral F protein on the host cell surface (2).

Antigen Detection

HPIV-1, -2, and -3 antigens are routinely detected in clinical specimens through the use of immunofluorescence techniques that employ fluorophore-labeled monoclonal antibodies (MAbs). Cells from nasopharyngeal washes, aspirates, and swabs are fixed on a microscope slide, usually in several cell spots or dots or by cytocentrifugation (35). At least 20 columnar epithelial cells must be present if the assay is to be valid. Many laboratories use pooled MAbs containing antibodies against seven common respiratory pathogens; these are adenovirus, influenza A and B viruses, HPIV-1, -2, and -3, and RSV. These MAbs are applied in either a direct (DFA) or indirect (IFA) fluorescent-antibody staining protocol that detects antigens of all seven viruses. When a positive result is seen, further testing must be done to determine which virus is present. The sensitivity of HPIV antigen detection compared to virus isolation in cell culture varies from laboratory to laboratory and with the various DFA and IFA staining methods and reagents but has been reported to range from 70% (4) to 83% (35). Specificity is very high.

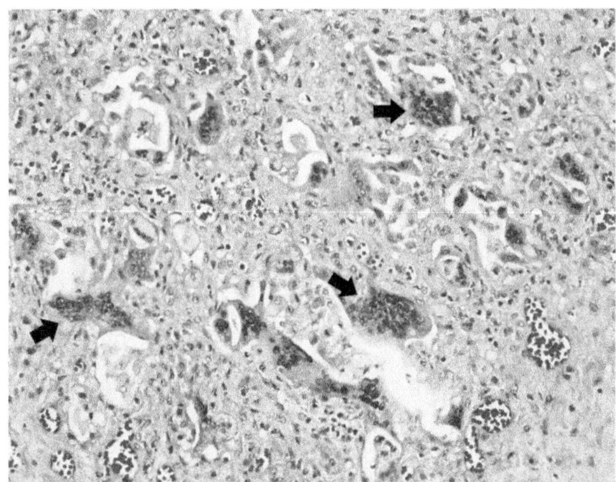

FIGURE 2 Several syncytia (arrows) are demonstrable in this hematoxylin-and-eosin-stained lung tissue section from an infant who died from an HPIV-3 infection. Diffuse alveolar damage, interstitial edema, fibrosis with proteinaceous intra-alveolar exudate, and slit-like, compressed alveolar spaces can be seen.

Pooled and individual MAbs in DFA or IFA formats are commercially marketed in the United States and are FDA cleared for use in detecting HPIV-1, -2, and -3 antigens directly in clinical specimens and for culture confirmation. Distributors of these reagents include, but are not limited to, the following: Diagnostic Hybrids/Quidel (DHI), Athens, OH; Millipore Corporation Light Diagnostics, Temecula, CA; and Trinity Biotech, Carlsbad, CA. FDA-cleared fluorophore-tagged MAbs are available from Millipore Corp. for confirmation of HPIV-4 in cell cultures. HPIV-infected cells demonstrate bright fluorescence that is primarily cytoplasmic and often punctate, with irregular inclusions. A brief overview of the protocol for one HPIV DFA method can be found in reference 36. The principles of DFA and IFA are reviewed in chapter 8 of this *Manual*.

MAb pools that screen for common respiratory viruses are marketed in two DFA formats. In one format, a pool of labeled MAbs is used in initial staining to screen for seven viruses (influenza A virus, influenza B virus, RSV, adenovirus, and HPIV-1 through -3); fresh smears are then prepared and stained with individual MAbs to identify the infecting virus. A second DFA format allows definitive identification of more than one virus simultaneously through the use of two different fluorescent dyes with overlapping spectra (Light Diagnostics SimulFluor reagents [Millipore Corp.] and Duet reagents [DHI]). The reagents are cleared by the FDA for direct specimen testing and for culture confirmation. When stained preparations are examined with a fluorescence microscope with a fluorescein isothiocyanate (FITC) filter set, one antibody produces apple green fluorescence, and the second appears gold or golden orange. The SimulFluor reagents have shown excellent sensitivities and specificities, comparable to those of individual stains, for the respiratory viruses (35).

A rapid format for staining cells in solution is also available (D^3 FastPoint; DHI). This system features three dual-labeled (R-phycoerythrin versus FITC) MAb preparations also containing propidium iodide. HPIV-1, -2, and -3 are detected but not differentiated in this system. In FastPoint testing, after a short incubation of specimen material with the three MAb preparations, the samples are placed on a microscope slide and examined in the wet state with a fluorescence microscope equipped with an FITC filter set. According to the FastPoint package insert (available at https://www.quidel.com/sites/default/files/product/documents/pi-316en_d3_fastpoint_l-dfa_respi_01-120000_v2010jul22_2.pdf), premarket trials showed 85 to 100% sensitivity and 98% to 100% specificity for HPIV-1, -2, and -3 detection by the FastPoint method compared to other HPIV antigen detection methods.

HPIV-4 is not detected by most respiratory virus immunofluorescence screening reagent pools, which screen for only HPIV-1, -2, and -3. Although MAbs are available for immunofluorescence staining of HPIV-4 cell culture isolates, these are not FDA cleared for direct HPIV-4 antigen detection in clinical specimens.

Nucleic Acid Detection Techniques

In the past decade, a number of molecular assays have been developed that permit detection of HPIVs directly from clinical specimens. Initially, these were lab-developed assays that detected individual HPIVs. More recently, multiplexed assays that detect HPIVs, either alone (e.g., Prodesse Pro-Paraflu+; Hologic GenProbe, San Diego, CA) or in combination with other respiratory pathogens (e.g., Luminex NxTAG respiratory pathogen panel [Luminex Corporation, Austin TX]; ePlex respiratory pathogen panel [GenMark DX, Carlsbad, CA]; FilmArray RP [BioFire Diagnostics, Salt Lake City, UT]; and Verigene respiratory pathogens Flex test), have received FDA clearance for *in vitro* diagnostic use. These involve various applications of molecular technology and have unique performance characteristics (Table 3). Of these examples, all but the Prodesse ProParaflu+ detect HPIV-4. These assays have been compared to antigen detection, virus isolation, and other individual and multiplexed molecular methods and have shown excellent sensitivity and specificity and improved analyte detection compared to traditional methods.

The enhanced sensitivity of molecular methods compared to antigen detection and virus isolation is especially important for immunocompromised patients and older patients in whom the viral titer may not be high. Most large virology laboratories employ molecular technologies for detection of all of the common viral respiratory pathogens. Over the past few years, these technologies have been refined and made more "user friendly," (i.e., requiring less technical expertise, exhibiting faster turnaround, and requiring less sophisticated specimen processing, instrumentation, and facilities due to closed systems), allowing smaller laboratories to adopt them and reap their benefits. Experts in viral molecular diagnostics caution users that molecular panels are expensive and should be selected carefully to best fit the needs of the individual laboratory and the patient population it serves. Large multiplexed viral respiratory panels may not be the preferred assay for diagnosis when clinical symptoms are consistent with a particular viral infection already known to be circulating in the community (37).

Isolation and Identification

Many commonly used cell lines support the growth of HPIVs, but the best growth is seen in primary monkey kidney (PMK) cells, including rhesus, cynomolgus, and African green monkey cells (12). LLC-MK2 cells are also acceptable for primary isolation when 2 to 3 μg/ml of *N*-tosyl-L-phenylalanine chloromethyl ketone-treated trypsin is added to the cell culture medium (12). Madin-Darby canine kidney (MDCK), HeLa, Vero, and HEp-2 cells may be used for passaging isolates, but they are not recommended for primary isolation (38). At the time of this writing, commonly used cell lines are available commercially from Quidel/DHI.

In preparing for cell culture inoculation of specimens collected on swabs and transported in a viral transport medium, the transport medium tube should first be vortexed vigorously to dislodge the majority of the clinical specimen from the swab(s) followed by removal and disposal of the swab(s). To minimize sample volume loss during swab removal and disposal, the swab(s) should be pressed against the side of the tube to express as much liquid as possible as it is being removed. The transport medium is then centrifuged at 1,500 × *g* for 10 min. The medium is decanted from cell culture tubes that are to be inoculated, and the supernatant from the centrifuged transport medium, usually 0.2 ml for each tube, is added to each cell culture monolayer. The inoculated tubes are incubated in a horizontal position in a 35 to 37°C incubator for 1 h before excess inoculum is discarded and fresh cell culture maintenance medium (e.g., Eagle's minimal essential medium containing 2% fetal bovine serum) is added. Inoculated cell culture tubes are incubated in rotating racks at 35 to 37°C and examined microscopically on alternate days for 14 days.

In PMK cells, some HPIVs produce a cytopathic effect (CPE) of rounded cells and syncytium formation in 4 to 8 days (Fig. 3B). However, many HPIVs will produce little, if any, CPE in traditional cell culture tubes. Fortunately, HPIVs produce hemagglutinating proteins (e.g., HN) that are inserted into the plasma membranes of infected cells. These proteins bind to erythrocytes and can mediate their adherence to HPIV-infected cells, a phenomenon called hemadsorption (HAD). HAD can be used as another approach for detecting HPIVs in cell cultures. For HAD testing, the culture medium is replaced with a dilute suspension of guinea pig erythrocytes, and the cell culture tubes are refrigerated at 4°C for 30 min; the tubes are then examined microscopically (4). When a hemadsorbing virus is present, erythrocytes adhere to the infected cell monolayer. If a hemadsorbing virus is absent, erythrocytes will not adhere and will float free when the tube is tilted or tapped. Uninfected and infected control tubes should be included in HAD testing. HAD testing may be performed at the end of the typical incubation period of 14 days or earlier, after 3 to 7 days of incubation (38, 39). HPIV-4 hemadsorbs weakly compared to HPIV-1, -2, and -3 at 4°C and more strongly at room temperature. Other members of the family *Paramyxoviridae*, including mumps virus, and other viruses, such as influenza virus, also yield positive HAD test results. Whether the presence of

TABLE 3 FDA-cleared molecular viral respiratory panels that detect HPIVs

Name (manufacturer)[a]	Viruses detected	Method, turnaround time, and complexity
ePlex RP panel (GenMark DX, Carlsbad, CA)	HPIV-1 to -4 (also adenovirus; human coronaviruses 229E, HKU1, NL63, and OC43; human metapneumovirus; human rhinovirus/enterovirus; influenza A [H1, H3, and H1 2009] and B viruses; and RSV [A and B]). Includes the bacterial targets *Chlamydophila pneumoniae* and *Mycoplasma pneumoniae*.	Fully automated closed system with extraction, amplification, and readout in a self-contained plastic cartridge. The cartridge is loaded and placed into the ePlex instrument, which mixes/moves reagents and heats/cools to perform cell lysis, nucleic acid extract/purification, reverse transcription, and PCR. Uses priopnetary eSensor technology. Takes 3–5 min of hands-on time and ~1 h for complete assay. One sample at a time, but scalable testing instrumentation can accommodate up to 24 assays simultaneously; moderately complex.
FilmArray RP[b] (BioFire Diagnostics–formerly Idaho Technologies, Salt Lake City, UT)	HPIV-1 to -4 (also adenovirus, coronaviruses [HKU1, NL63, OC43, and 229E], human metapneumovirus, influenza A [H1, H3, and H1 2009] and B viruses, RSV, and rhinovirus/enterovirus). Includes the bacterial targets *Chlamydophila pneumoniae*, *Mycoplasma pneumoniae*, and *Bordetella pertussis*.	Fully automated closed system with extraction, amplification, and readout in a self-contained plastic pouch. The pouch is placed in a pouch-loading station, rehydrated, and injected with sample. The instrument mixes/moves reagents and heats/cools to perform cell lysis, magnetic bead-based nucleic acid isolation, reverse transcription, and multiple PCRs (1st-stage multiplex and 2nd-stage nested PCRs). Uses endpoint DNA melting curve analysis to automatically generate a result for each target. Takes 3–5 min of hands-on time and ~1 h for complete assay. One sample at a time, but new, scalable testing instrumentation can accommodate up to 12 assays simultaneously (the FilmArray Torch); moderately complex and CLIA-waived systems available.
Luminex NxTAG RP panel (Luminex Corporation, Austin, TX)	HPIV-1 to -4 (also adenovirus; human bocavirus; human coronaviruses 229E, HKU1, NL63, and OC43; human metapneumovirus; human rhinovirus/enterovirus; influenza A [H1 and H3] and B viruses; and RSV [A and B]). Includes the bacterial targets *Chlamydophila pneumoniae*, *Legionella pneumophila*, and *Mycoplasma pneumoniae*.	Open system requires separate extraction and nucleic acid amplification/bead hybridization steps. Amplicons are hybridized to target-specific primers possessing unique DNA tags. DNA polymerase extends perfectly formed complements, at the same time incorporating biotin-dCTP into the extension product. The extension products are added to microwells containing polystyrene microbeads, each of which contains an antitag sequence unique to a specific viral target and all of which are treated with colored dyes to distinguish each bead set. Each tagged primer hybridizes onto its unique antitag complement. Biotinylated extension products hybridizing onto the bead surface are detected with a streptavidin-phycoerythrin reporter molecule. Hybridized and tagged beads are sorted and read on the MAGPIX instrument. Most hands-on time of methods shown, 6–8 h turnaround. Batch testing. Highly complex.
Prodesse ProParaflu+ (Hologic Gen-Probe, San Diego, CA)	HPIV-1 to -3	Open system requires separate extraction. Real-time RT-PCR using multiplex HPIV reagents from Prodesse, 1–2 h turnaround time. Highly complex.
Verigene RP Flex test (Luminex Corporation, Austin, TX)	HPIV-1 to -4 (also adenovirus; human metapneumovirus; influenza A [H1 and H3] and B; RSV [A and B]; and rhinovirus). Includes the bacterial targets *Bordetella pertussis*, *Bordetella parapertussis*/*Bordetella bronchiseptica*, and *Bordetella holmesii*.	Partially open system that combines nucleic acid extraction, target amplification, and hybridization into a test cartridge that is handled by two different instruments: a sample processor and a panel reader, the latter being the central control unit of the system. Four single-use consumables, including an extraction tray, a pipet tip holder assembly, a utility tray, and the test cartridge containing ready-to-use reagents, make up the components of the test system. Samples undergo nucleic acid extraction, amplification, and nanoparticle hybridization within the processing unit, and after ~2 h, the test cartridge is transferred to a reader for interpretation, which takes ~10 s.

[a]RP, respiratory pathogen.
[b]As of this writing, a second-generation FilmArray RP, the RP2, and a FilmArray panel designed for testing lower respiratory tract specimens are in clinical trials.

HPIV is suspected based on the appearance of typical CPE or by a positive HAD test result, confirmatory testing must be done to definitively identify the virus.

Confirmatory testing is routinely completed by immunofluorescence techniques involving the use of HPIV MAbs in DFA or IFA assays, as described for HPIV antigen detection in clinical samples. MAbs against HPIV-1, -2, and -3 are readily available in the various respiratory virus antibody testing kits. However, HPIV-4 antibodies are not included in most testing kits and must be purchased separately. Infected cells are scraped from the cell culture monolayer, concentrated by centrifugation, applied to a microscope slide, fixed, and stained. The presence of apple-green fluorescence when the smear is viewed with a fluorescence microscope confirms the identification of HPIV. Confirmatory testing may also be accomplished by many other methods, including hemagglutination inhibition, complement fixation, neutralization, and molecular assays. These techniques are laborious and time-consuming compared to immunofluorescence methods, so they are seldom used.

Cell cultures grown on coverslips in shell vials or in microwell plates provide an alternative to traditional tube

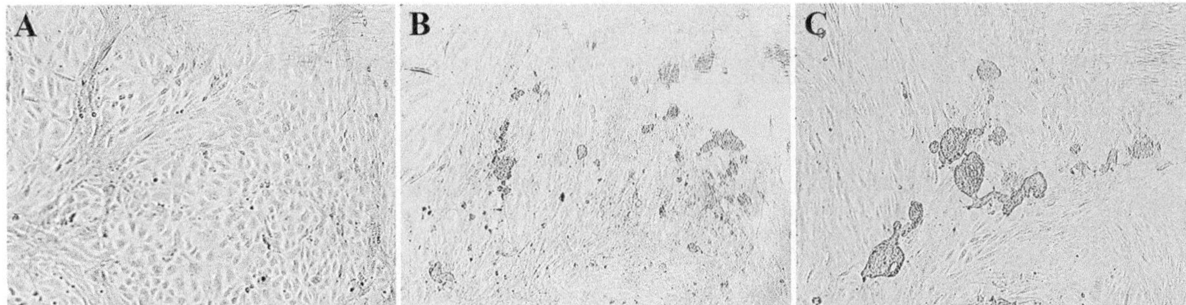

FIGURE 3 CPE of HPIV and MuV in primary rhesus macaque kidney (RhMK) cells. (A) Uninfected RhMK cells; (B) RhMK cells infected with a CPE-producing clinical isolate of HPIV-1 showing some rounded cells and syncytia scattered throughout the field; (C) RhMK cells infected with a clinical isolate of MuV demonstrating syncytia formation. Cell cultures in panels B and C were photographed 6 days postinoculation. Magnification, ×100 (all).

cell cultures for isolation of HPIVs. Centrifugation of the inoculated vials and plates, usually at 700 × g for 1 h, is an important feature of the inoculation process. Inoculated vials or plates are incubated for 24 to 48 h or as long as 5 days. Detection of viral proliferation depends on pre-CPE detection of viral antigens by application of HPIV MAbs to the monolayers in a typical DFA or IFA staining assay. Use of shell vial cultures with centrifugation-enhanced inoculation and pre-CPE detection by immunofluorescence staining has been shown to be very useful in HPIV detection.

Cocultivated mink lung (Mv1Lu) and A549 cells in shell vials, marketed as R-Mix (DHI), are used with centrifugation-enhanced inoculation and pre-CPE detection by a DFA staining technique. Staining involves pooled MAbs to seven respiratory viruses (adenovirus, influenza A and B viruses, HPIV-1, -2, and -3, and RSV). In a comparison of respiratory virus detection in 3,800 clinical samples in R-Mix and in shell vials of PMK, A459, and MRC-5 cells, 33 of 38 (87%) HPIVs were detected after overnight incubation in the R-Mix cells (40). This included 26 of 30 HPIV-1 isolates, 2 of 2 HPIV-2 isolates, and 5 of 6 HPIV-3 isolates. Cocultivated MDCK cells and A549 cells constitute R-Mix Too (DHI). This combination was prepared as an alternative to R-Mix. The HPIVs proliferate very well in R-Mix Too (unpublished data) and are easily detected (Fig. 4A to C).

An overview of the recommended protocol from the manufacturer of R-Mix and R-Mix Too (DHI) is presented here; however, this protocol may be adjusted to meet the needs of the laboratory. Briefly, the processed clinical specimen for respiratory virus detection is inoculated into three vials containing R-Mix or R-Mix Too, and the vials are spun in a centrifuge (700 × g for 1 h). At 16 to 24 h, one vial is stained with respiratory virus screening reagent (which tests for seven respiratory viruses). If fluorescence is observed, the cells are scraped from one of the remaining shell vials, rinsed in phosphate-buffered saline, and spotted onto an eight-well slide; seven of the wells are stained with individual MAbs against the seven respiratory viruses, and the eighth well is used as a control well. If no fluorescence is observed when the first vial is stained, the second vial is stained after an additional 16 to 24 h of incubation. If this vial is positive, the cells are scraped from the remaining vial and stained as described above. If the second vial is negative, the culture may be considered negative for the seven respiratory viruses (i.e., the remaining vial is discarded and the culture is terminated), or the third vial may be observed for CPE for up to 7 days.

Serologic Tests

Most children are born with HPIV-neutralizing antibodies of maternal origin, but these diminish by 6 months of age, allowing more than two-thirds of children to be infected by HPIV during the first year of life. Most children have early serologic evidence of HPIV-3 infection, with HPIV-1 and -2 antibodies developing later, at 2 to 3 years of age. Antibodies to HPIV-4 peak in school-age children (12). Immunoglobulin M (IgM) is produced in most primary HPIV infections of children, so IgM detection in a single sample supports diagnosis of current infection. Likewise, measurement of a

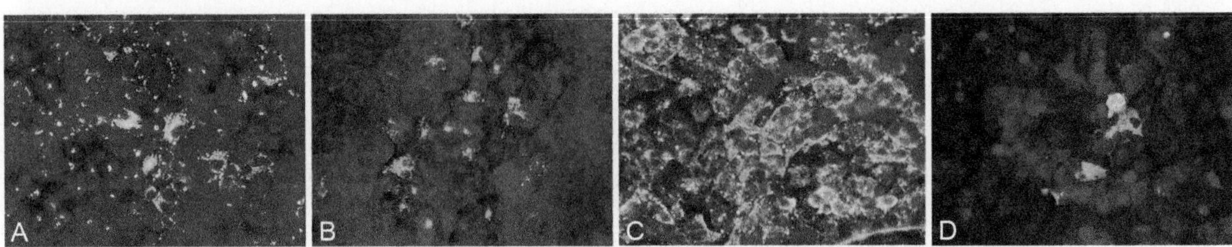

FIGURE 4 Immunofluorescence staining of HPIV-infected R-Mix Too and MuV-infected R-Mix cell cultures. R-Mix Too cells were infected with HPIV-1 (A), HPIV-2 (B), or HPIV-3 (C). (D) R-Mix cells infected with MuV. Magnification, ×200 (all). (A to C) Courtesy of Indiana Pathology Images; (D) courtesy of Quidel/Diagnostic Hybrids, Inc., Athens, OH.

significant increase in the IgG antibody level, which is an increase of 4-fold or more in assays that test serial 2-fold dilutions of serum samples collected 2 weeks apart, supports diagnosis of current infection. Cross-reactivity among the various HPIV types and other paramyxoviruses, such as MuV, makes serologic diagnosis more difficult. Serologic differentiation of the HPIV types is unreliable by all methods; this determination can be made only through virus isolation and antigen typing with MAbs or by molecular methods.

Antibodies to the HN protein may appear early, but antibodies to both HN and F proteins must be present for protection. Immune status determinations are not useful for HPIV. Serology in general is seldom used as a diagnostic approach for HPIV infection because of the wide availability and improved reliability of virus isolation, viral antigen detection, and nucleic acid detection methods.

Principles of various immunoassays are described in detail in chapter 8 of this *Manual*. HPIV antibodies can be detected by many types of assays, including hemagglutination inhibition, complement fixation, and neutralization assays; all of these detect total antibody (IgG and IgM), and most laboratories do not offer these methods due to their cumbersome nature. A detailed procedure for hemagglutination inhibition testing for HPIV antibodies was published previously (38). HPIV antibody detection can be accomplished by enzyme immunoassay (EIA), but commercial kits are not available. Complement fixation is the least sensitive method for antibody detection, and EIA is the most sensitive.

Evaluation, Interpretation, and Reporting of Results

Isolation of HPIV-1, -2, -3, and -4 in traditional, shell vial, or microwell cell cultures and detection of HPIV RNA in clinical samples are the best evidence for current or very recent infection, because HPIV is seldom present in the absence of infection. Rapid reporting of positive results is important (27). As molecular panels that include the HPIVs have become more widely available in formats that produce rapid results, they have become the diagnostic method of choice due to their excellent sensitivity and specificity. Although the sensitivity of HPIV antigen detection by immunofluorescence is lower than that of virus isolation in cell culture or molecular detection, the rapid availability of results and high specificity make such testing useful in patient management. Confirmation of HPIV infection via the serologic route and HPIV immune status determinations is seldom employed due to the difficulties with cross-reactions among the paramyxoviruses.

MUMPS VIRUS

Epidemiology and Transmission

More than 150,000 cases of mumps were expected each year in the United States before aggressive vaccination programs were implemented in the late 1960s. The mumps vaccine was combined with the measles and rubella vaccines to make a trivalent vaccine (MMR). In the United States, the initial dose of MMR is administered to children between 12 and 15 months of age. Vaccination produced a dramatic decline in the incidence of mumps, resulting in fewer than 3,000 cases in the United States by 1985. There was a brief resurgence of mumps in 1986 and 1987 that peaked at 8,000 to 12,000 cases. Following the resurgence, a requirement for a second dose of the MMR vaccine was implemented. This dose is administered to children between ages 4 and 6 or 11 and 13 years (41) but can be given as soon as 28 days following the first dose and has been expected to confer lifelong immunity. The number of mumps cases continued to decline in the United States until the largest U.S. outbreak in 2 decades occurred in the Midwestern states in 2006 (42). More than 6,500 cases were involved in this outbreak. The highest incidence of mumps was in persons aged 18 to 24 years; 83% of these were college students, and 84% of this group, as well as 63% of all those infected in the outbreak, had received two doses of mumps vaccine. The cause of this outbreak is unclear. Potential explanations include waning immunity and incomplete vaccine-induced immunity to circulating wild-type virus (42). In addition, the overall estimate of mumps antibody seroprevalence in the United States in 1999 to 2004 was 90% (43). This is the lower end of the level of immunity (90 to 92%) needed to achieve herd immunity.

During 2009 to 2010, another mumps outbreak occurred in the United States. The outbreak started at a New York summer camp for Orthodox Jewish boys and resulted in 3,502 cases of mumps, 97% of which were in Orthodox Jewish persons, most of whom lived in three neighborhoods in New York (44). As with the 2006 outbreaks, a high percentage of infected individuals had received either one (14%) or two (76%) doses of the MMR vaccine, so waning of vaccine-induced protection against mumps was again suggested as a contributing factor. In addition, it was concluded that the level of immunity required to protect against mumps may depend on the size of the inoculum of virus involved in the exposure, indicating that a particular antibody titer versus protection from infection is not absolute (44). However, in a study of antibody in students prior to the 2006 Kansas outbreak, it was shown that pre-outbreak neutralizing titers were significantly lower among patients who developed mumps than in individuals neither exposed nor infected and in individuals exposed but not infected during the outbreak. However, although those who developed mumps had lower pre-outbreak mumps antibody levels than noninfected individuals, antibody titers overlapped, and no cutoff points clearly separated the groups (45).

At the time of this writing, the incidence of mumps in the United States is higher than prior to the 2006 multistate outbreak. Case counts greater than 1,000 per year have been recorded since 2014. In 2016, there were approximately 5,800 cases of mumps reported to the Centers for Disease Control and Prevention (CDC), and from 1 January to 9 September 2017, the CDC received reports of 4,439 cases, which includes cases from all but three states (46). It remains unclear whether a change in the vaccine itself or in vaccine administration schedules will be needed to prevent future outbreaks in the United States. Studies have suggested that in some vaccinated individuals who later became infected with MuV, susceptibility to the virus could have been associated with either a demonstrably low avidity of vaccine-induced anti-MuV IgG and/or waning concentrations of antibodies over time (47, 48). A recent comparative genomic analysis of contemporary circulating MuV lineages suggests the emergence of strains against which the current vaccine may not provide adequate protection, indicating the need for vaccine reformulation (49). Mumps remains common throughout much of the world, usually infecting 6- to 10-year-old children in the spring in unvaccinated populations.

MuV is transmitted from person to person through respiratory droplets or contaminated fomites and is highly contagious, with approximately 85% of susceptible contacts becoming infected when first exposed. Humans are the only known host and reservoir for the virus. The virus replicates initially in epithelial cells in the upper respiratory tract and in regional lymph nodes. Initial replication is followed by viremia, which results in infection of the salivary glands and other sites. MuV can be isolated from 7 days before through 8 days after the onset of parotitis, but the isolation is more likely and the highest virus loads occur closest to parotitis onset, and virus loads decrease rapidly thereafter. Disease transmission likely occurs before and within 5 days of parotitis onset. Transmission can also occur during the prodromal phase and with subclinical infection (50). The virus is shed in the urine for as long as 14 days after the onset of illness.

Clinical Significance

The average incubation period for mumps is 16 to 18 days. MuV infection is asymptomatic in 25 to 30% of cases and is associated with nonspecific or respiratory symptoms in 50% of cases. Symptoms are typically mild and characterized by slightly elevated temperature and enlargement of one or both parotid glands in 30 to 40% of cases. Complications of mumps include meningoencephalitis (in up to 15% of cases) and, in postpubertal individuals, orchitis in males (in up to 20 to 30% of cases) and oophoritis in females (in up to 7% of cases). Polyarthritis and pancreatitis have also been associated with mumps.

When mumps was a common disease of childhood, the diagnosis was made largely on clinical grounds alone. With the decrease in incidence of mumps, many physicians no longer readily recognize its symptoms. In addition, typical clinical signs and symptoms may be absent in underimmunized or immunocompromised individuals. Parotitis, the hallmark of clinical diagnosis, is now known to be present in other viral and nonviral diseases or conditions, which can complicate the diagnosis of mumps if clinical signs and symptoms alone are used to render a diagnosis. Mumps-like symptoms in acutely ill children who previously received the MMR vaccine have been associated with Epstein-Barr virus, HPIV, adenovirus, and human herpesvirus 6 (51). Therefore, laboratory confirmation of MuV infection is now more important in making the diagnosis.

Collection, Transport, and Storage of Specimens

The accepted laboratory criteria for the diagnosis of MuV infection are isolation of the virus from clinical specimens, detection of MuV RNA via molecular methods, a significant rise between acute- and convalescent-phase antibody titers in serum, or a positive IgM result for mumps. Guidelines for specimen collection, transport, and storage of specimens are presented in chapter 81 in this *Manual*. Specimen collection guidelines differ for diagnosing mumps in unvaccinated and previously vaccinated individuals. Information on sample procurement in both types of host is provided below.

Specimens for MuV isolation in cell culture include saliva or buccal swabs, blood, urine, and cerebrospinal fluid (CSF). Virus can be isolated from saliva and buccal swabs 7 days before and up to 8 days after the onset of parotitis, recovered from the urine for up to 2 weeks after onset of symptoms, isolated from CSF during meningitis, and detected rarely in peripheral blood. Throat swabs and urine samples have been shown to have similar efficacies as sources of MuV (52). It is always advisable to collect samples for virus isolation early in the course of the infection, when the viral titer is the highest. Samples for virus isolation and molecular testing should be collected even sooner in previously vaccinated individuals. In these individuals, neither virus isolation nor molecular methods are likely to yield positive results unless samples are collected within 3 days after onset of parotitis (53). The virus is stable for several days at 4°C, although inoculation of susceptible cell cultures within a few hours of specimen collection is recommended for optimal virus isolation. The virus may survive for months or longer when frozen at −70°C or lower. Information regarding materials and methods for specimen collection (samples for virus detection as well as blood samples for antibody testing), storage, and shipment is available online from the CDC at http://www.cdc.gov/mumps/lab/specimen-collect.html.

An alternative to serum collected by venipuncture is whole blood obtained by finger stick, heel prick, or venipuncture and then spotted on filter paper and dried. Following elution and dilution of the dried blood samples, commercial antibody assays may be used to test the sample for MuV antibody. Results of EIA in testing for MuV IgG and IgM by use of samples collected as blood spots have shown excellent correlation with those obtained in testing of fresh serum. The dried blood spots may be stored for 6 to 24 months without a significant change in antibody testing results (54).

In order to compare IgG or total antibody levels, two samples should be collected, the first (acute phase) as soon as possible after onset of symptoms and the second (convalescent phase) within 2 to 3 weeks following the acute-phase sample. A single serum sample collected within 4 to 10 days of onset is all that is required for IgM-specific antibody testing. If the purpose of the serologic testing is simply to determine the patient's mumps immune status, a single serum sample collected at random is sufficient. Neither comparison of IgG levels in sequential samples nor detection of IgM in a single sample collected early in the infection has been shown to be an effective diagnostic approach for confirming MuV infection in previously vaccinated individuals.

Direct Examination

Microscopy

Diagnosis of mumps does not typically involve direct microscopic examination of clinical specimens, including swab samples and tissues. However, microscopic examination of affected salivary glands reveals an edematous interstitium diffusely infiltrated by macrophages, lymphocytes, and plasma cells, which compress acini and ducts. Neutrophils and necrotic debris may fill the ductal lumen, causing focal damage to the ductal epithelium (36).

Antigen Detection

MuV antigen detection by immunofluorescence in cells from CSF and salivary glands was described in the early 1970s (55, 56). More recent studies of immunofluorescence staining of throat swab specimens for MuV antigen have shown sensitivities as high as 98 to 100% compared to MuV isolation in cell culture (52). Although MuV MAbs are available commercially, most are not FDA cleared for use in direct detection of MuV antigens in tissues and other clinical samples, and most virology laboratories do not offer direct antigen analysis for MuV.

Nucleic Acid Detection

Various molecular approaches have been developed to aid in mumps diagnosis. MuV RNA has been detected by reverse transcriptase PCR (RT-PCR) in oral fluid, CSF (57, 58), saliva or throat, and urine (58) specimens and in MuV isolates from cell culture (57).

Although there are currently no commercially available FDA-cleared molecular assays for mumps detection, two of these assays have been developed and standardized by the CDC, with information available online. Step-by-step procedures are provided and commercial sources of reagents are identified for one standard RT-PCR to detect the SH gene of MuV and for one real-time RT-PCR assay available from the CDC. Molecular assays are more sensitive than virus isolation in culture and can provide sequence information for the coding region of the SH gene that is needed to determine the viral genotype. MuV detection by RT-PCR is offered by many commercial reference laboratories and state public health laboratories; however, most routine virology laboratories rely on MuV isolation as the standard method for diagnosing MuV infection.

Isolation and Identification

MuV proliferates in traditional cell cultures of several cell lines commonly used in viral diagnostic laboratories. These include PMK, human neonatal kidney, HeLa, and Vero cells. A marmoset lymphoblastic cell line, B95a, was shown to be as sensitive for MuV isolation as PMK cells (59). A Vero cell line transfected with a plasmid carrying the gene for human CDw150—a signaling-lymphocytic activation molecule (human SLAM, or hSLAM)—and called Vero/hSLAM has been used for mumps virus isolation (60). Although used originally for isolation of measles virus, these cells have been shown to be effective for MuV isolation as well (53, 61). Directions for cell culture inoculation for swab samples in viral transport medium are the same as those described above in "Parainfluenza Viruses" under "Isolation and Identification."

In cells infected with MuV, CPE characterized by rounded cells and multinucleated giant cells is typical (Fig. 3C), usually appearing after 6 to 8 days of incubation at 35 to 37°C. However, this characteristic CPE may be very subtle, may not appear at all, or may be confused with a similar CPE produced by endogenous contaminant viruses that sometimes infect PMK cells.

MuV infection, like that of the HPIVs, results in the insertion of hemagglutinin proteins into the plasma membranes of infected cells, so MuV-infected cells can be demonstrated through HAD testing. The HAD testing protocol is described above in "Parainfluenza Viruses" under "Isolation and Identification." Whether MuV is detected by CPE production or by a positive HAD result, confirmatory testing must be performed. Confirmatory testing for MuV is routinely performed by fluorescent antibody staining. FDA-cleared mumps MAbs in an IFA format for culture confirmation are available from Millipore Corp.

Many laboratories currently use centrifugation-enhanced inoculation and pre-CPE detection with MAbs to detect MuV within 24 to 48 h after inoculation. Various cell lines can be used in either shell vial or microwell plate formats for this purpose. The recommended centrifugation speeds and times may vary for inoculation, ranging from 700 × *g* for 45 min (52) to 3,000 × *g* for 20 min (40). Up to 66% of MuV-positive samples were identified within 2 days of inoculation in the shell vial system; after 5 days of incubation, the shell vial system was 96% sensitive compared to MuV isolation in traditional cell cultures (62). When various cell lines were compared for efficacy of MuV isolation in shell vials, Vero and LLC-MK2 cells were the most sensitive (100%), followed by MDCK (78%), MRC-5 (44%), and HEp-2 (22%) cells (63). MuV can also be isolated in R-Mix cells (Fig. 4D). An overview of the recommended protocol from the manufacturer of R-Mix (DHI) is presented above in "Parainfluenza Viruses" under "Isolation and Identification."

Because MuV infections in previously vaccinated individuals result in decreased levels of virus shedding into the buccal cavity, virus isolation may be difficult (64). Specimens collected and cultured within 3 days of onset of parotitis may aid in confirming the presence of mumps virus, but negative results do not rule out the infection (42).

Serologic Tests

In MuV infection, IgM is detectable initially within 3 to 5 days of appearance of clinical symptoms and persists for 8 to 12 weeks. IgG is detectable within 7 to 10 days of the onset of symptoms, is maintained at high levels for years, and remains detectable for life. Traditional serologic diagnosis of mumps is based on the detection of virus-specific IgM in a single sample or measurement of a significant increase in the titer of IgG or total antibody, i.e., a 4-fold or greater increase for methods that use serial 2-fold dilutions, between two specimens collected 2 weeks apart. Antibodies produced in MuV infection often cross-react with related viruses, which complicates the interpretation of results. Assays for mumps immune status indicate whether MuV IgG is present at detectable levels or is absent or undetectable. These qualitative results are sufficient, and reporting of titers is unnecessary given that there is no particular antibody level that correlates with protection (44, 45). With the rarity of mumps cases in the United States at present, most laboratories focus MuV serology on immune status testing.

In previously vaccinated persons, serologic diagnosis has very limited use. IgM may be produced weakly or not at all in a secondary immune response. In a recent outbreak, MuV IgM antibodies were detected in fewer than 15% of MuV-infected persons who were previously immunized, and 95% of these patients were positive for MuV IgG (53). False-positive results for MuV IgM are not uncommon and, in addition to being associated with cross-reactivity to a number of other pathogens, have been obtained from pregnant individuals and others without symptoms of MuV infection. Therefore, MuV IgM testing should be limited to patients with illnesses that are clinically compatible with MuV infection, should be performed in conjunction with additional diagnostic tests such as MuV PCR or culture, and should not be used to determine the immune status of individuals.

Basic principles of immunoassays are described in chapter 8 in this *Manual*. MuV antibodies can be detected by many types of assays, including hemagglutination inhibition, complement fixation, and neutralization assays; all of these detect total antibody (IgG and IgM). These methods are usually laborious and are available only at reference or specialty laboratories. A detailed procedure for MuV antibody hemagglutination inhibition testing was published previously (65). The complement fixation technique can be used with two different MuV antigens, V and S. Antibodies against the S antigen appear early, and their levels rise quickly, in contrast to the antibodies to the V antigen, which appear later. The presence of both V and S antibodies is thought to signal a recent past infection, while V antibodies alone signal a long-past infection (38). An IgM capture EIA was used recently for detection of mumps virus IgM (53).

Most diagnostic laboratories use commercially supplied MuV antibody EIA kits, in either manual or automated formats, or IFA testing systems for MuV antibody determinations. Most of these measure only IgG. Antibodies against various MuV proteins are produced, but protection is most closely correlated with antibodies to the MuV HN protein.

Most assays use whole virus or viral extract antigens that detect HN antibody effectively. Written protocols, along with the proper reagents and controls, are included with each commercial product, and each manufacturer's guidelines must be followed if assays are to yield high-quality results. The procedural steps for performance of antibody testing are not published here due to the need for strict adherence to manufacturers' guidelines. None of these MuV antibody assays has been shown to be superior in regard to sensitivity or specificity.

Standard diagnostic tests that detect virus or virus-specific antibody perform inconsistently for individuals with prior immune exposure via either immunization or natural infection. Detection of activated mumps-specific antibody-secreting memory B cells (ASCs) by EIA has been shown to be a more reliable test (66). ASCs are detectable in circulation only following recent activation by antigen. In testing for ASCs, peripheral blood mononuclear cells are cultured in the presence of polyclonal mitogens, and the ASCs are detected by exposure to viral antigen. Trials with this method detected mumps ASCs in recently MMR-vaccinated individuals and in those with clinical mumps during a mumps outbreak. Detection of ASCs appears to be more sensitive for longer periods of time than RT-PCR or IgM EIA and may be useful for diagnosing mumps cases that cannot be confirmed with standard methods and for testing asymptomatic case contacts in an outbreak. Interestingly, mumps ASCs appear to be produced in lower numbers than measles or rubella ASCs, suggesting that mumps infection may not generate robust B-cell memory (66).

Evaluation, Interpretation, and Reporting of Results

Isolation of MuV in traditional or shell vial/microwell cell cultures is evidence of current or very recent infection. The same can be said for the detection of MuV RNA in clinical samples. Rapid antigen detection may also confirm the presence of MuV. However, neither molecular methods nor rapid antigen assays are routinely available in U.S. laboratories, so MuV isolation in culture remains the most sensitive approach. Confirmation of MuV infection via the serologic route is less straightforward. MuV IgM may be detectable, along with significant increases in IgG, in patients infected with related viruses, including the other paramyxoviruses, such as HPIV-1, -2, -3, and -4. In general, cross-reactivity with related viruses can be ruled out by testing for antibodies to the related viruses in parallel with MuV virus antibody testing. The greatest increase in antibody level should identify the true infection. Given the potential lack of serologic test specificity, virus isolation and RNA detection in clinical samples (preferably buccal swabs) remain the most effective ways to confirm infection in unvaccinated individuals.

Virus isolation and RNA detection have also been recommended for mumps diagnosis in individuals with a documented immunization history. Buccal swabs should be procured early (within 3 days of parotitis onset), as the duration of viral replication is likely to be shorter in these hosts. Despite these recommendations, it should be recognized that none of the traditional diagnostic approaches is highly effective for diagnosis of mumps in previously vaccinated individuals. IgM is not consistently observed, so it is not a reliable indicator of recent infection. Virus detection can also be variable, presumably due to low viral loads. Alternative tests may have better diagnostic efficacy. Data from the 2009 outbreak suggest that the IgM capture assay used at the CDC has improved sensitivity compared to commercially available tests in previously vaccinated individuals (~50% for CDC capture versus 9 to 24% for commercial assays) (67). Additionally, use of nucleoprotein RNA as a target enhanced the sensitivity of real-time PCR compared to the historically used SH-based test. The CDC provides guidance online for mumps testing at http://www.cdc.gov/mumps/lab/qa-lab-test-infect.html.

REFERENCES

1. **Henrickson KJ.** 2005. Cost-effective use of rapid diagnostic techniques in the treatment and prevention of viral respiratory infections. *Pediatr Ann* **34:**24–31.
2. **Lamb RA, Parks GD.** 2013. Paramyxoviridae, p 957–995. *In* Knipe DM, Howley PM (ed), *Fields Virology*, 6th ed, vol 1. Lippincott Williams & Wilkins, Philadelphia, PA.
3. **Ansari SA, Springthorpe VS, Sattar SA, Rivard S, Rahman M.** 1991. Potential role of hands in the spread of respiratory viral infections: studies with human parainfluenza virus 3 and rhinovirus 14. *J Clin Microbiol* **29:**2115–2119.
4. **Leland DS.** 1996. *Clinical Virology*. W. B. Saunders Co., Philadelphia, PA.
5. **Frost HM, Robinson CC, Dominguez SR.** 2014. Epidemiology and clinical presentation of parainfluenza type 4 in children: a 3-year comparative study to parainfluenza types 1-3. *J Infect Dis* **209:**695–702.
6. **Lessler J, Reich NG, Brookmeyer R, Perl TM, Nelson KE, Cummings DA.** 2009. Incubation periods of acute respiratory viral infections: a systematic review. *Lancet Infect Dis* **9:** 291–300.
7. **Williams JV, Piedra PA, Englund JA.** 2017. Respiratory syncytial virus, human metapneumovirus, and parainfluenza viruses, p 873–902. *In* Richman DD, Whitley RJ, Hayden FG (ed), *Clinical Virology*, 4th ed. ASM Press, Washington, DC.
8. **Le Bayon JC, Lina B, Rosa-Calatrava M, Boivin G.** 2013. Recent developments with live-attenuated recombinant paramyxovirus vaccines. *Rev Med Virol* **23:**15–34.
9. **Leung AK, Kellner JD, Johnson DW.** 2004. Viral croup: a current perspective. *J Pediatr Health Care* **18:**297–301.
10. **Fairchok MP, Martin ET, Kuypers J, Englund JA.** 2011. A prospective study of parainfluenza virus type 4 infections in children attending daycare. *Pediatr Infect Dis J* **30:**714–716.
11. **Iwane MK, Edwards KM, Szilagyi PG, Walker FJ, Griffin MR, Weinberg GA, Coulen C, Poehling KA, Shone LP, Balter S, Hall CB, Erdman DD, Wooten K, Schwartz B, New Vaccine Surveillance Network.** 2004. Population-based surveillance for hospitalizations associated with respiratory syncytial virus, influenza virus, and parainfluenza viruses among young children. *Pediatrics* **113:**1758–1764.
12. **Henrickson KJ.** 2003. Parainfluenza viruses. *Clin Microbiol Rev* **16:**242–264.
13. **Marx A, Gary HE Jr, Marston BJ, Erdman DD, Breiman RF, Török TJ, Plouffe JF, File TM, Jr, Anderson LJ.** 1999. Parainfluenza virus infection among adults hospitalized for lower respiratory tract infection. *Clin Infect Dis* **29:** 134–140.
14. **van Asten L, van den Wijngaard C, van Pelt W, van de Kassteele J, Meijer A, van der Hoek W, Kretzschmar M, Koopmans M.** 2012. Mortality attributable to 9 common infections: significant effect of influenza A, respiratory syncytial virus, influenza B, norovirus, and parainfluenza in elderly persons. *J Infect Dis* **206:**628–639.
15. **Schomacker H, Schaap-Nutt A, Collins PL, Schmidt AC.** 2012. Pathogenesis of acute respiratory illness caused by human parainfluenza viruses. *Curr Opin Virol* **2:**294–299.
16. **Henrickson KJ, Hoover S, Kehl KS, Hua W.** 2004. National disease burden of respiratory viruses detected in children by polymerase chain reaction. *Pediatr Infect Dis J* **23**(Suppl): S11–S18.
17. **Ustun C, Slabý J, Shanley RM, Vydra J, Smith AR, Wagner JE, Weisdorf DJ, Young JA.** 2012. Human parainfluenza virus infection after hematopoietic stem cell transplantation: risk factors, management, mortality, and changes over time. *Biol Blood Marrow Transplant* **18:**1580–1588.

18. **Burns JL, Emerson J, Kuypers J, Campbell AP, Gibson RL, McNamara S, Worrell K, Englund JA.** 2012. Respiratory viruses in children with cystic fibrosis: viral detection and clinical findings. *Influenza Other Respi Viruses* **6:**218–223.
19. **Miller EK, Bugna J, Libster R, Shepherd BE, Scalzo PM, Acosta PL, Hijano D, Reynoso N, Batalle JP, Coviello S, Klein MI, Bauer G, Benitez A, Kleeberger SR, Polack FP.** 2012. Human rhinoviruses in severe respiratory disease in very low birth weight infants. *Pediatrics* **129:**e60–e67.
20. **Maeng SH, Yoo HS, Choi SH, Yoo KH, Kim YJ, Sung KW, Lee NY, Koo HH.** 2012. Impact of parainfluenza virus infection in pediatric cancer patients. *Pediatr Blood Cancer* **59:**708–710.
21. **Elizaga J, Olavarria E, Apperley J, Goldman J, Ward K.** 2001. Parainfluenza virus 3 infection after stem cell transplant: relevance to outcome of rapid diagnosis and ribavirin treatment. *Clin Infect Dis* **32:**413–418.
22. **Hohenthal U, Nikoskelainen J, Vainionpää R, Peltonen R, Routamaa M, Itälä M, Kotilainen P.** 2001. Parainfluenza virus type 3 infections in a hematology unit. *Bone Marrow Transplant* **27:**295–300.
23. **Shima T, Yoshimoto G, Nonami A, Yoshida S, Kamezaki K, Iwasaki H, Takenaka K, Miyamoto T, Harada N, Teshima T, Akashi K, Nagafuji K.** 2008. Successful treatment of parainfluenza virus 3 pneumonia with oral ribavirin and methylprednisolone in a bone marrow transplant recipient. *Int J Hematol* **88:**336–340.
24. **Chakrabarti S, Collingham KE, Holder K, Oyaide S, Pillay D, Milligan DW.** 2000. Parainfluenza virus type 3 infections in hematopoetic stem cell transplant recipients: response to ribavirin therapy. *Clin Infect Dis* **31:**1516–1518.
25. **Malakhov MP, Aschenbrenner LM, Smee DF, Wandersee MK, Sidwell RW, Gubareva LV, Mishin VP, Hayden FG, Kim DH, Ing A, Campbell ER, Yu M, Fang F.** 2006. Sialidase fusion protein as a novel broad-spectrum inhibitor of influenza virus infection. *Antimicrob Agents Chemother* **50:**1470–1479.
26. **Chen YB, Driscoll JP, McAfee SL, Spitzer TR, Rosenberg ES, Sanders R, Moss RB, Fang F, Marty FM.** 2011. Treatment of parainfluenza 3 infection with DAS181 in a patient after allogeneic stem cell transplantation. *Clin Infect Dis* **53:**e77–e80.
27. **Guzmán-Suarez BB, Buckley MW, Gilmore ET, Vocca E, Moss R, Marty FM, Sanders R, Baden LR, Wurtman D, Issa NC, Fang F, Koo S.** 2012. Clinical potential of DAS181 for treatment of parainfluenza-3 infections in transplant recipients. *Transpl Infect Dis* **14:**427–433.
28. **Drozd DR, Limaye AP, Moss RB, Sanders RL, Hansen C, Edelman JD, Raghu G, Boeckh M, Rakita RM.** 2013. DAS181 treatment of severe parainfluenza type 3 pneumonia in a lung transplant recipient. *Transpl Infect Dis* **15:**E28–E32.
29. **Chalkias S, Mackenzie MR, Gay C, Dooley C, Marty FM, Moss RB, Li T, Routh RL, Walsh SR, Tan CS.** 2014. DAS181 treatment of hematopoietic stem cell transplant patients with parainfluenza virus lung disease requiring mechanical ventilation. *Transpl Infect Dis* **16:**141–144.
30. **Waghmare A, Wagner T, Andrews R, Smith S, Kuypers J, Boeckh M, Moss R, Englund JA.** 2015. Successful treatment of parainfluenza virus respiratory tract infection with DAS181 in 4 immunocompromised children. *J Pediatric Infect Dis Soc* **4:**114–118.
31. **Dhakal B, D'Souza A, Pasquini M, Saber W, Fenske TS, Moss RB, Drobyski WR, Hari P, Abidi MZ.** 2016. DAS181 treatment of severe parainfluenza virus 3 pneumonia in allogeneic hematopoietic stem cell transplant recipients requiring mechanical ventilation. *Case Rep Med* **2016:**8503275.
32. **Salvatore M, Satlin MJ, Jacobs SE, Jenkins SG, Schuetz AN, Moss RB, Van Besien K, Shore T, Soave R.** 2016. DAS181 for treatment of parainfluenza virus infections in hematopoietic stem cell transplant recipients at a single center. *Biol Blood Marrow Transplant* **22:**965–970.
33. **Russell E, Ison MG.** 2017. Parainfluenza virus in the hospitalized adult. *Clin Infect Dis* **65:**1570–1576.
34. **Henrickson KJ.** 2004. Advances in the laboratory diagnosis of viral respiratory disease. *Pediatr Infect Dis J* **23**(Suppl)**:**S6–S10.
35. **Landry ML, Ferguson D.** 2000. SimulFluor respiratory screen for rapid detection of multiple respiratory viruses in clinical specimens by immunofluorescence staining. *J Clin Microbiol* **38:**708–711.
36. **McAdam AJ, Sharpe AH.** 2005. Infectious diseases, p 343–414. *In* Kumar V, Abbas AK, Fausto N (ed), *Robbins and Cotran Pathologic Basis of Disease*, 7th ed. Elsevier Saunders, Philadelphia, PA.
37. **Check W.** April 2012. For respiratory virus detection, a golden age. *CAP Today*. College of American Pathologists, Northfield, IL. http://www.cap.org/apps/cap.portal?_nfpb=true&cntvwrPtlt_actionOverride=%2Fportlets%2FcontentViewer%2Fshow&_windowLabel=cntvwrPtlt&cntvwrPtlt%7BactionForm.contentReference%7D=cap_today%2F0412%2F0412a_respiratory_virus.html&_state=maximized&_pageLabel=cntvwr.
38. **Waner JL, Swierkosz EM.** 2003. Mumps and parainfluenza viruses, p 1368–1377. *In* Murray PR, Baron EJ, Jorgensen JH, Pfaller MA, Yolken RH (ed), *Manual of Clinical Microbiology*, 8th ed, vol 2. ASM Press, Washington, DC.
39. **Minnich LL, Ray CG.** 1987. Early testing of cell cultures for detection of hemadsorbing viruses. *J Clin Microbiol* **25:**421–422.
40. **Dunn JJ, Woolstenhulme RD, Langer J, Carroll KC.** 2004. Sensitivity of respiratory virus culture when screening with R-mix fresh cells. *J Clin Microbiol* **42:**79–82.
41. **Watson JC, Hadler SC, Dykewicz CA, Reef S, Phillips L.** 1998. Measles, mumps, and rubella—vaccine use and strategies for elimination of measles, rubella, and congenital rubella syndrome and control of mumps: recommendations of the Advisory Committee on Immunization Practices (ACIP). *MMWR Recomm Rep* **47**(RR-8)**:**1–57.
42. **Dayan GH, Quinlisk MP, Parker AA, Barskey AE, Harris ML, Schwartz JM, Hunt K, Finley CG, Leschinsky DP, O'Keefe AL, Clayton J, Kightlinger LK, Dietle EG, Berg J, Kenyon CL, Goldstein ST, Stokley SK, Redd SB, Rota PA, Rota J, Bi D, Roush SW, Bridges CB, Santibanez TA, Parashar U, Bellini WJ, Seward JF.** 2008. Recent resurgence of mumps in the United States. *N Engl J Med* **358:**1580–1589.
43. **Kutty PK, Kruszon-Moran DM, Dayan GH, Alexander JP, Williams NJ, Garcia PE, Hickman CJ, McQuillan GM, Bellini WJ.** 2010. Seroprevalence of antibody to mumps virus in the US population, 1999-2004. *J Infect Dis* **202:**667–674.
44. **Barskey AE, Schulte C, Rosen JB, Handschur EF, Rausch-Phung E, Doll MK, Cummings KP, Alleyne EO, High P, Lawler J, Apostolou A, Blog D, Zimmerman CM, Montana B, Harpaz R, Hickman CJ, Rota PA, Rota JS, Bellini WJ, Gallagher KM.** 2012. Mumps outbreak in Orthodox Jewish communities in the United States. *N Engl J Med* **367:**1704–1713.
45. **Cortese MM, Barskey AE, Tegtmeier GE, Zhang C, Ngo L, Kyaw MH, Baughman AL, Menitove JE, Hickman CJ, Bellini WJ, Dayan GH, Hansen GR, Rubin S.** 2011. Mumps antibody levels among students before a mumps outbreak: in search of a correlate of immunity. *J Infect Dis* **204:**1413–1422.
46. **Centers for Disease Control and Prevention.** Mumps cases and outbreaks. https://www.cdc.gov/mumps/outbreaks.html. Last accessed 24 September 2017.
47. **Kontio M, Jokinen S, Paunio M, Peltola H, Davidkin I.** 2012. Waning antibody levels and avidity: implications for MMR vaccine-induced protection. *J Infect Dis* **206:**1542–1548.
48. **Narita M, Matsuzono Y, Takekoshi Y, Yamada S, Itakura O, Kubota M, Kikuta H, Togashi T.** 1998. Analysis of mumps vaccine failure by means of avidity testing for mumps virus-specific immunoglobulin G. *Clin Diagn Lab Immunol* **5:**799–803.
49. **May M, Rieder CA, Rowe RJ.** 2018. Emergent lineages of mumps virus suggest the need for a polyvalent vaccine. *Int J Infect Dis* **66:**1–4.

50. **Kutty PK, Kyaw MH, Dayan GH, Brady MT, Bocchini JA, Reef SE, Bellini WJ, Seward JF.** 2010. Guidance for isolation precautions for mumps in the United States: a review of the scientific basis for policy change. *Clin Infect Dis* **50:** 1619–1628.
51. **Davidkin I, Jokinen S, Paananen A, Leinikki P, Peltola H.** 2005. Etiology of mumps-like illnesses in children and adolescents vaccinated for measles, mumps, and rubella. *J Infect Dis* **191:**719–723.
52. **Reina J, Ballesteros F, Ruiz de Gopegui E, Munar M, Mari M.** 2003. Comparison between indirect immunofluorescence assay and shell vial culture for detection of mumps virus from clinical samples. *J Clin Microbiol* **41:**5186–5187.
53. **Bitsko RH, Cortese MM, Dayan GH, Rota PA, Lowe L, Iversen SC, Bellini WJ.** 2008. Detection of RNA of mumps virus during an outbreak in a population with a high level of measles, mumps, and rubella vaccine coverage. *J Clin Microbiol* **46:**1101–1103.
54. **Condorelli F, Scalia G, Stivala A, Gallo R, Marino A, Battaglini CM, Castro A.** 1994. Detection of immunoglobulin G to measles virus, rubella virus, and mumps virus in serum samples and in microquantities of whole blood dried on filter paper. *J Virol Methods* **49:**25–36.
55. **Boyd JF, Vince-Ribarić V.** 1973. The examination of cerebrospinal fluid cells by fluorescent antibody staining to detect mumps antigen. *Scand J Infect Dis* **5:**7–15.
56. **Lindeman J, Müller WK, Versteeg J, Bots GT, Peters AC.** 1974. Rapid diagnosis of meningoencephalitis, encephalitis. Immunofluorescent examination of fresh and in vitro cultured cerebrospinal fluid cells. *Neurology* **24:**143–148.
57. **Pabbaraju K, Tokaryk KL, Wong S, Fox JD.** 2008. Comparison of the Luminex xTAG respiratory viral panel with in-house nucleic acid amplification tests for diagnosis of respiratory virus infections. *J Clin Microbiol* **46:**3056–3062.
58. **Poggio GP, Rodriguez C, Cisterna D, Freire MC, Cello J.** 2000. Nested PCR for rapid detection of mumps virus in cerebrospinal fluid from patients with neurological diseases. *J Clin Microbiol* **38:**274–278.
59. **Knowles WA, Cohen BJ.** 2001. Efficient isolation of mumps virus from a community outbreak using the marmoset lymphoblastoid cell line B95a. *J Virol Methods* **96:**93–96.
60. **Ono N, Tatsuo H, Hidaka Y, Aoki T, Minagawa H, Yanagi Y.** 2001. Measles viruses on throat swabs from measles patients use signaling lymphocytic activation molecule (CDw150) but not CD46 as a cellular receptor. *J Virol* **75:**4399–4401.
61. **Jin L, Feng Y, Parry R, Cui A, Lu Y.** 2007. Real-time PCR and its application to mumps rapid diagnosis. *J Med Virol* **79:**1761–1767.
62. **Germann D, Gorgievski M, Ströhle A, Matter L.** 1998. Detection of mumps virus in clinical specimens by rapid centrifugation culture and conventional tube cell culture. *J Virol Methods* **73:**59–64.
63. **Reina J, Ballesteros F, Mari M, Munar M.** 2001. Evaluation of different continuous cell lines in the isolation of mumps virus by the shell vial method from clinical samples. *J Clin Pathol* **54:**924–926.
64. **Bellini WJ, Icenogle JP, Hickman CJ.** 2016. Measles, mumps, and rubella viruses, p 293–310. *In* Loeffelholz MJ, Hodinka RL, Young SA, Pinsky BA (ed), *Clinical Virology Manual*, 5th ed. ASM Press, Washington, DC.
65. **Leland DS.** 2002. Measles and mumps, p 683–686. *In* Rose NR, Hamilton RG, Detrick B (ed), *Manual of Clinical Laboratory Immunology*, 6th ed. ASM Press, Washington, DC.
66. **Latner DR, McGrew M, Williams N, Lowe L, Werman R, Warnock E, Gallagher K, Doyle P, Smole S, Lett S, Cocoros N, DeMaria A, Konomi R, Brown CJ, Rota PA, Bellini WJ, Hickman CJ.** 2011. Enzyme-linked immunospot assay detection of mumps-specific antibody-secreting B cells as an alternative method of laboratory diagnosis. *Clin Vaccine Immunol* **18:**35–42.
67. **Rota JS, Rosen JB, Doll MK, McNall RJ, McGrew M, Williams N, Lopareva EN, Barskey AE, Punsalang A Jr, Rota PA, Oleszko WR, Hickman CJ, Zimmerman CM, Bellini WJ.** 2013. Comparison of the sensitivity of laboratory diagnostic methods from a well-characterized outbreak of mumps in New York city in 2009. *Clin Vaccine Immunol* **20:**391–396.

Respiratory Syncytial Virus and Human Metapneumovirus

N. ESTHER BABADY AND YI-WEI TANG

88

RESPIRATORY SYNCYTIAL VIRUS

Taxonomy

Human respiratory syncytial virus (RSV) is a member of the genus *Orthopneumovirus*, family *Pneumoviridae*, order *Mononegavirales* (1, 2). Other members of the genus include morphologically and biologically similar animal viruses, such as the pneumonia virus of mice, bovine RSV, ovine RSV, and caprine RSV. RSV and other pneumoviruses differ from *Paramyxoviridae* viruses in the number and order of genes and the lack of hemagglutinin and neuraminidase activity. RSV was first recovered from humans with pulmonary disease in 1957 by cell culture (3). The virus derives its name from the characteristic formation of multinucleated giant cells (syncytia) in monolayer cell cultures of nonpolarized epithelial cells (4, 5). Only one serotype of RSV has been identified and further subdivided into two major antigenic types, designated RSV A and RSV B (1, 2). These two types are based on variability in the G protein, with only one of six epitopes shared between the two types (1, 6). Studies have suggested that RSV A is more virulent than RSV B, resulting in greater disease severity among hospitalized infants.

Description of the Agent

The enveloped RSV virion consists of a single-stranded, negative-sense, nonsegmented RNA genome with 10 genes that are transcribed into 11 monocistronic polyadenylated messenger RNAs, each of which encodes for a major polypeptide chain (Fig. 1) (1, 2). The virus lipid envelope is derived from the host plasma membrane and contains three structural proteins: the F (fusion) protein, the G (glycosylated) protein, and the SH (short hydrophobic) protein. The F protein initiates viral penetration by fusing viral and cellular membranes and promotes viral spread by fusing the infected cells to adjacent uninfected cells. The G protein mediates attachment of the virus to the host cells, and the SH protein accumulates within lipid-raft structures of the Golgi complex during RSV infection (1, 2). The six other structural proteins include the nucleoprotein (N), the phosphoprotein (P), the polymerase or large protein (L), a matrix protein (M), and two proteins M2-1 and M2-2 (1, 2). The N protein serves as the major structural protein for the nucleocapsid, while the P and L (polymerase or large proteins) are involved in transcription and replication (1, 7). The M protein is present in detergent-solubilized cores and inhibits viral replication in preparation for budding. The M2-1 protein is a transcription regulator that promotes the association of the M and N proteins, and the function of the M2-2 protein is unclear (1, 2, 7). Two nonstructural proteins, NS1 and NS2, are unique to *Pneumovirus*.

During the past decade, there has been significant progress in the understanding of RSV entry, replication, and egress (2, 8). Binding and entry of RSV into the host cell are shown in Fig. 2A. The principal neutralizing determinant on the RSV particle is the RSV-F glycoprotein. The RSV-F protein mediates the fusion reaction that causes mixing of the virus and host cell envelopes, leading to delivery of the virus capsid core contents into the cell (Fig. 2B). The conformation of the RSV-F protein prior to fusion is termed prefusion F, and it exists as a trimer on the surface of the RSV virion. The structures of pre- and postfusion RSV-F were recently elucidated (9). The RSV-F protein undergoes a number of conformational changes during the fusion reaction that bring the virus and host envelopes into close apposition. Disrupting the activity of this protein therefore disrupts viral entry and protects the host against infection (9, 10).

RSV is highly vulnerable to environmental changes. Only 10% of RSV remained infectious after exposure to 55°C for 5 minutes. At room temperature, 10% infectivity was present after 48 hours, and at 4°C, 1% of the infectivity remained after 7 days. The RSV infectivity titer fell by approximately 90% after each freezing and thawing cycle (6, 7). The virus is inactivated quickly by ether, chloroform, and a variety of detergents such as 0.1% sodium deoxycholate, sodium dodecyl sulfate, and Triton X-100. The survival of RSV in the environment depends in part on drying time as well as humidity (6, 7). Long-term storage of RSV can be enhanced by flash freezing in an alcohol and dry ice bath and by adding stabilizing agents such as glycerin or sucrose.

Epidemiology and Transmission

Transmission of RSV occurs via droplets and direct or indirect contact with infected patients and/or contaminated surfaces (6, 7). RSV infections occur year-round worldwide. In the temperate Northern Hemisphere, RSV infections occur in the winter with a peak between December and February. In the temperate Southern Hemisphere, RSV infections peak between May and July, and in a few tropical

Orthopneumovirus - human respiratory syncytial virus A2 (15,222 nt)

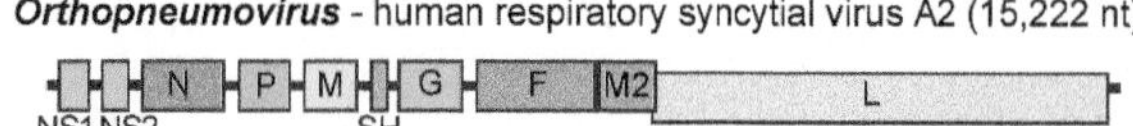

Metapneumovirus - human metapneumovirus NL/00/1 (13,335 nt)

FIGURE 1 *Pneumoviridae*. Genome organization of representative members of the family *Pneumoviridae*. Maps of genomic RNAs in sense (coding) orientation (3′ to 5′) in which each box, drawn approximately to scale, represents a gene encoding a separate mRNA. The M2 mRNA of members of the family *Pneumoviridae* has two overlapping open reading frames, M2-1 and M2-2 (not shown). In the genus *Orthopneumovirus*, human RSV has a gene overlap at M2 and L (staggered boxes). The intergenic sequences are variable (1 to 190 nt long). Reprinted with permission from the International Committee on Taxonomy of Viruses (ICTV): https://talk.ictvonline.org/ictv-reports/ictv_online_report/negative-sense-rna-viruses/w/pneumoviridae#Summary.

locations including Taiwan, Hong Kong, Singapore, Malaysia, and Colombia, semiannual RSV peaks have been identified (11). Epidemiology data have established that both RSV A and RSV B can circulate in the same region in a given respiratory season, with one subtype, commonly RSV A, dominating. The pattern of dominance, however, can shift between seasons, with RSV genotype strains evolving and new strains emerging (12, 13).

In the United States, early reports estimated that 100,000 hospitalizations and 4,500 deaths are related to RSV infection, with excess expenses from $300 million to $600 million for hospitalized infants with RSV in the United States (6). Globally, RSV is a common cause of childhood acute lower respiratory infection and a major cause of hospital admissions in young children, resulting in a substantial burden on health care services (14). The overall increased prevalence of RSV type A over B viruses may be due to a more transient nature of type A-specific immune protection (15). Virtually all children are infected by the time they reach 3 years of age, and repeated infections with RSV are common throughout life. No age group appears to be completely protected against reinfection due to prior exposure (6).

RSV causes hazardous health care-related, or nosocomial, infection and produces outbreaks each year with widespread infection in both children and adults, including medical personnel, who may have a mild enough illness as to not cause absences from work (16, 17). In a classic experiment, volunteers in close physical contact with RSV-infected infants were more readily infected than those who remained 6 feet away, suggesting that small-particle aerosol is less important in the spread of RSV than direct contact with infectious secretions via fomites or large-particle aerosols (6, 7). A targeted infection control intervention has been demonstrated to be cost-effective in reducing the rate of RSV health care-related infections (18, 19). Contact isolation procedures are recommended for RSV-infected patients when they are hospitalized (6, 19).

Clinical Significance

Children

RSV is recognized as the most serious cause of severe acute lower respiratory tract illnesses in young children and infants (14). The incubation period ranges from 2 to 8 days with a median of 4.4 days based on a systematic review (6, 7). Common lower respiratory tract infections include bronchiolitis, tracheobronchitis, and pneumonia (14). Most children with RSV infection are previously healthy children with no underlying conditions and experience recovery from illness after 8 to 15 days (14). Caserta et al. reported the development of a global respiratory severity score based on nine clinical variables as an endpoint for investigation of disease pathogenesis and as an outcome measure for therapeutic interventions (20). Risk factors for acquiring RSV include being under 2 years of age and residential crowding (14). Premature infants and infants with chronic lung disease, major congenital heart diseases, or severe immunodeficiencies are at highest risk of hospital admission for RSV. Based on a recent meta-analysis of the incidence and mortality of severe RSV in children globally, a substantial proportion of RSV-associated morbidity occurs in the first year of life, especially in children born prematurely. These data affirm the importance of RSV disease in the causation of hospitalization and as a significant contributor to pediatric mortality and further demonstrate gestational age as a critical determinant of disease severity. An important limitation of case fatality ratios is the absence of individual patient characteristics of nonsurviving patients. Moreover, case fatality ratios cannot be translated to population-based mortality (21).

Adults

Immunity to RSV is incomplete, and adults are subject to reinfection (15, 22). Adult populations at increased risk for severe RSV infections include nursing home or long-term care residents, adults with underlying heart and lung

FIGURE 2 RSV replication. (Top) Binding and entry of RSV into the host cell. RSV (a) receptors (b) bind to the RSV-G glycoprotein and act to tether the virus particle to the cell surface, initiating the entry process (c) by triggering fusion of the virus and host cell membranes (d). The virion fuses with the cell membrane and enters the cell, one of the last events of virus entry that must take place for successful replication of RSV in the host cell (e). Host cell macropinocytosis of RSV is also a route of entry for RSV (f). It is unclear which receptors are involved in this process (g). Internalization of the virion (h) is dependent on actin rearrangement, phosphatidylinositol 3-kinase activity, and host cell (i) early endosomal Rab5$^+$ vesicles, where proteolytic cleavage of the RSV-F protein triggers delivery of the capsid contents into the host cells by fusion of the virus and endosomal membranes (j). (Bottom) Fusion process between the RSV envelope and cellular membrane. The RSV envelope has multiple protruding RSV-F fusion glycoproteins, anchored via transmembrane domains (a). In the prefusion state, RSV-F exists as a spring-loaded trimer with the major neutralization epitopes shown at the N-terminal region. The major antigenic site Ø exists only on the prefusion trimer and is lost after fusion. Interaction between the RSV-F trimer and a receptor may cause RSV-F to undergo a dramatic conformational shift (b), which leads to insertion of the fusion peptide into the host cell membrane (c) and forcing of the viral and host membranes into close contact (d). Although, for simplicity, only two RSV-F monomers are depicted, the combined force of multiple RSV-F conformational shifts is required to overcome the thermodynamic barrier of mixing membranes and establish a stable fusion pore for viral nucleocapsid delivery (e). Reprinted from Griffiths et al. with permission (2).

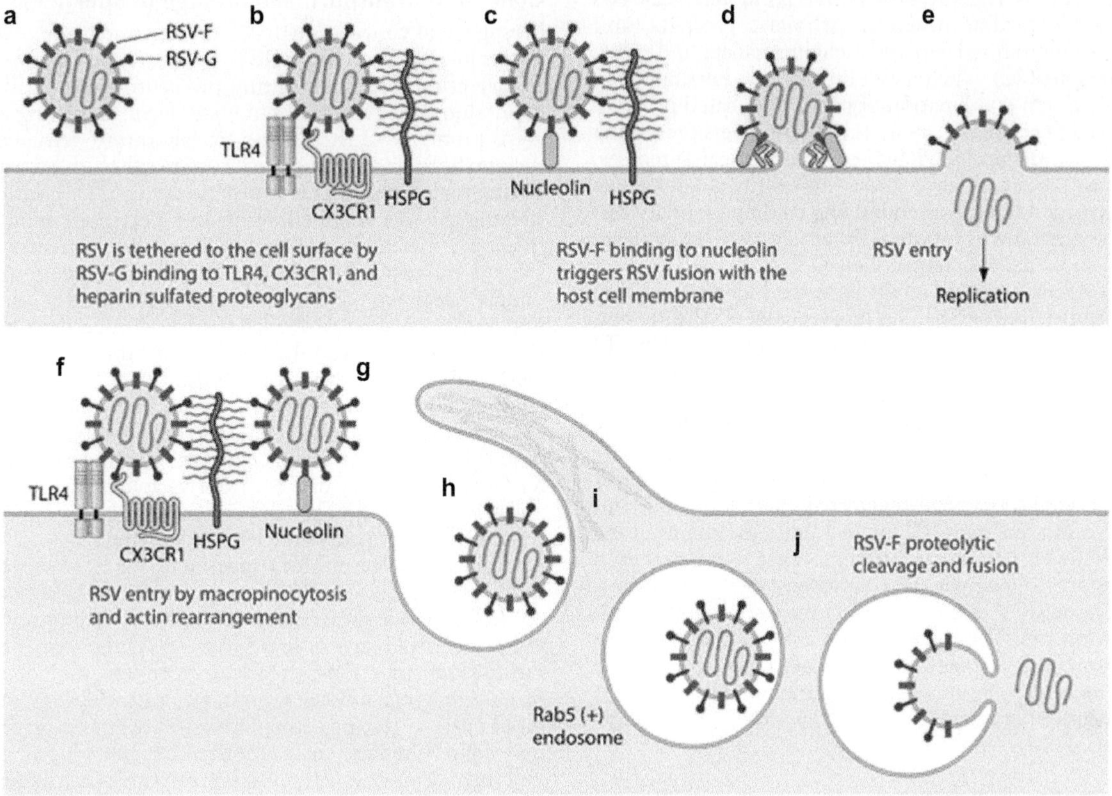

a b c d e

RSV-F
RSV-G

TLR4
CX3CR1
HSPG
Nucleolin
HSPG

RSV is tethered to the cell surface by RSV-G binding to TLR4, CX3CR1, and heparin sulfated proteoglycans

RSV-F binding to nucleolin triggers RSV fusion with the host cell membrane

RSV entry

Replication

f g h i j

TLR4
CX3CR1
HSPG
Nucleolin

RSV entry by macropinocytosis and actin rearrangement

Rab5 (+) endosome

RSV-F proteolytic cleavage and fusion

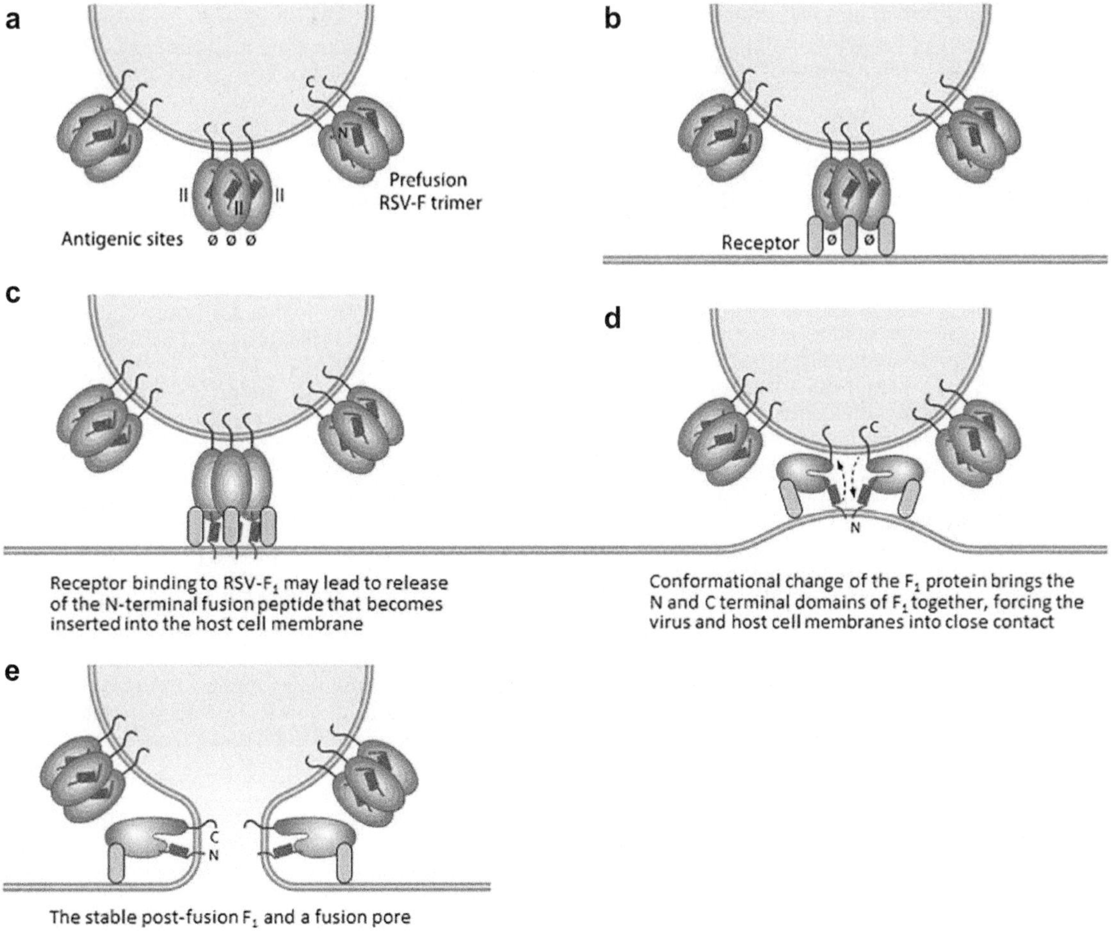

a

C
N
II II II
Prefusion RSV-F trimer
Antigenic sites ø ø ø

b

Receptor ø ø

c

Receptor binding to RSV-F_1 may lead to release of the N-terminal fusion peptide that becomes inserted into the host cell membrane

d

C
N

Conformational change of the F_1 protein brings the N and C terminal domains of F_1 together, forcing the virus and host cell membranes into close contact

e

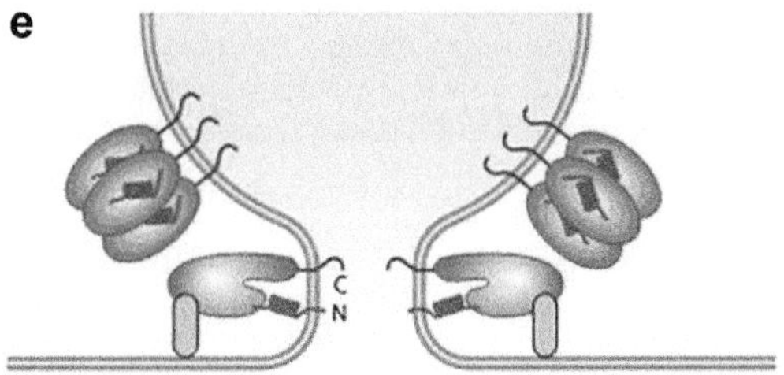

The stable post-fusion F_1 and a fusion pore

diseases such as chronic obstructive pulmonary diseases and chronic cardiac diseases, asthmatic patients, and immune-compromised patients including cancer and transplant patients (22). The burden of RSV in adults has been determined in a combination of population-based prospective surveillance studies, analysis of acute illness presenting for medical care, and modeling of large medical databases. In prospective surveillance studies in healthy elderly adults and high-risk adults with underlying cardiopulmonary disease, the annual wintertime RSV attack rate ranged from 3 to 7% and 2 to 10%, respectively (15, 22).

Immunocompromised adults have the highest morbidity and mortality from RSV. The incidence of RSV infection following hematopoietic stem cell transplantation (HSCT) and solid organ transplantations ranges from 1 to 12%, with 18 to 55% progressing to lower respiratory tract infection (LRTI) and death due to RSV in 7 to 33% (23, 24). Upper respiratory symptoms give way to lower respiratory involvement in 30 to 40% of infected people around day 7 of illness. High-dose total body irradiation and total lymphocyte count less than 100 mm but not serum-neutralizing antibody levels or corticosteroid use were associated with progression from upper-tract to lower-tract disease (24, 25). Data on RSV disease in solid organ transplant recipients are limited. The incidence and risk of RSV infections in solid organ transplant recipients are lower than in the HSCT recipients group, with most common symptoms for RSV infections of fever, cough and dyspnea, and complications (6, 24).

Treatment and Prevention

Treatment of RSV infections can be challenging. Current options include ribavirin and palivizumab (Synagis) for RSV treatment and prophylaxis, respectively (26). Palivizumab is a humanized monoclonal antibody directed at a neutralizing epitope on the postfusion F protein that functions by preventing RSV entry into host cells and is administered as a monthly injection (five-dosage program) in high-risk children during the respiratory season for RSV prophylaxis (26, 27). Palivizumab administration is controversial because of its high cost; several recent abbreviated dosing regimens of palivizumab are confirmed to match the protection for outcomes of RSV infection achieved by the regular five-dosage program (28, 29). Ribavirin is a broad-spectrum nucleoside analogue that targets RNA viruses and can be administered orally, intravenously, or in aerosolized form (30, 31). Data from a large retrospective study of allo-HSCT recipients including both children and adults supported the early initiation of ribavirin therapy for RSV upper respiratory tract infections to prevent progression to LRTI and subsequent mortality from RSV lower respiratory tract infections (32). Over the past 10 years, new antiviral drugs including monoclonal antibodies and nucleoside analogues have shown clinical promise against RSV (2, 30, 31).

Although there is a worldwide need for a preventative vaccine in the pediatric population, an effective and safe RSV vaccine is not yet licensed. The latest and most promising experimental vaccination strategies are based on a conformational analogue of prefusion F, because this form elicits the most potent neutralizing antibodies against RSV, which are reportedly 10- to 100-fold more potent than palivizumab (9, 33). A clinical trial is being conducted (33, 34). A phase II clinical trial by Novavax, using a recombinant RSV-F subunit vaccine, was completed in 2016. The efficacy was reported as a function of circulating neutralizing antibodies (8, 35).

Collection, Transport, and Storage of Specimens

Most general viral specimen collection principles also apply to specimen collection for RSV detection and culture, such as collecting specimens during the acute phase of illness, maintaining recovered cells in intact form, delivering specimens promptly to the diagnostic laboratory, refrigerating specimens if stored temporarily, and sealing them well in O-ring-sealed cryovials if stored on dry ice (7). Heating or freezing the specimen will result in a decreased number of infectious virions in the sample. If a delay of greater than 2 hours is expected between collection and receipt of the sample, specimen containers should be kept at 4°C, including during transport to the laboratory, to effectively isolate RSV. RSV is labile and should ideally be transported to the laboratory and processed for culture within 4 hours of collection because viral titers can significantly decrease with prolonged storage at 4°C. Alternatively, specimens may be snap frozen to prevent viral degradation (36). However, differences in recovery of RSV from various specimen types and transport or storage temperatures are less pronounced with the use of sensitive nucleic acid testing (7).

Appropriate respiratory specimens for RSV detection should reflect the site of infection. RSV infects respiratory epithelial cells and can spread to the lower respiratory tract following 1 to 3 days of incubation (6, 7). For upper respiratory tract infections, the ideal specimens include nasal or nasopharyngeal washes, aspirates, and swabs (6, 7). For rapid antigen testing, nasopharyngeal aspirates or washes had slightly higher sensitivity than nasopharyngeal swabs and nasal aspirates or washes, but no statistical differences were revealed by a systematic review and meta-analysis (37). Nasopharyngeal specimens collected by nylon flocked swabs (e.g., Copan, Brescia, Italy) have more epithelial cells, are easy to elute with the least discomfort, and have been widely used in both rapid antigen and nucleic acid amplification tests (NAATs) (6, 38). Throat swab and saliva specimens are inferior but might be acceptable when it is impractical to obtain nasal or nasopharyngeal specimens. For lower respiratory tract infections, bronchoalveolar lavage fluids, bronchial washings, sputa, and endotracheal aspirates can be used, with bronchoalveolar lavage having the best recovery compared to nasal washes and nose and throat swabs (7, 36). Endotracheal tube aspirate or bronchoalveolar lavage fluid collection is preferred in immune-compromised adults who are being mechanically ventilated (36).

The likelihood of identifying RSV as the etiology of a patient's infection is greatest when a specimen is obtained within the first several days of illness. Viral cultures or antigens usually become negative 1 week after onset of illness in about 50% of patients. However, shedding of live virus in immune-compromised infants has been documented up to 3 weeks after onset of illness (6, 15). The quantity of virus in the upper respiratory tract (nasal aspirates) is nearly equivalent to that found in the lower respiratory tract when tested by quantitative culture or real-time PCR methods (6, 7, 39). In healthy adult volunteers experimentally inoculated with RSV, the mean duration of RSV shedding was 7.4 (±2.5) days, while naturally infected older adults shed the virus on average for 10 to 13 days but for as long as ≥20 days (37, 40, 41).

Direct Examination

Microscopy

Although RSV can be visualized by electron microscopy, its application has been limited to research laboratories.

However, characteristic syncytial cytopathic effects (CPEs) in lung biopsies facilitate the diagnosis.

Antigen Detection

Rapid Antigen Detection Tests

RSV rapid antigen tests (RADTs) can be performed in less than 30 minutes and do not require experienced technologists to perform and interpret test results (37, 42). Results are visualized as a color change or the appearance of a line or sign on a solid membrane as a result of antigen-antibody complex binding. Most RADTs have waived status and can be performed as point-of-care tests (37, 42, 43). However, the sensitivity of these assays is relatively low and highly dependent on the prevalence of RSV in the community (4, 37). Hence, false-positive and false-negative results are a concern depending on the time of the year, and the performance of these tests is considerably reduced during the RSV off-season (44, 45). It is recommended that RADTs be reflexed to culture or NAATs for confirmation (4, 46, 47). A recent systematic review and meta-analysis indicated surprisingly low RSV RADT sensitivity of 29% in adults in comparison to an overall pooled sensitivity of 81% in children (37). Given the observed lack of sensitivity of RSV RADTs in adults, their utility in this population, especially among the elderly and the immunocompromised, is probably very limited (37).

RSV RADTs are commercially available in a variety of platforms and test formats (Table 1). Key factors that influence choice include test accuracy, turnaround time, acceptable specimen types, compatible transport media, and a reliable supply of reagents or kits. BD Veritor RSV (Becton, Dickinson and Company, Franklin Lakes, NJ) and Quidel Sofia RSV (Quidel Corporation, San Diego, CA), the two devices recently cleared by the FDA, employ an instrument-based digital scan of the test strip to improve accuracy (38, 48, 49). Objective result reporting and walk-away testing make the Sofia and the Veritor valuable choices for point-of-care testing. The mariPOC (ArcDia International Oy Ltd., Turku, Finland) is a fully automated, random-access immunoassay method that detects eight respiratory viruses including RSV (50, 51). While test accuracy results were fairly similar between the different rapid tests and the different types of specimens used (37), the lack of objective results by Directigen and the poor sensitivity observed by Quickvue may preclude their value in diagnostic testing (49).

Direct Fluorescent Antibody Tests

Direct fluorescent antibody assays (DFAs) are based on the detection of RSV antigens in respiratory specimens using fluorophore-labeled monoclonal mouse antibodies. The use of monoclonal antibodies in these assays has greatly improved the sensitivity and specificity of the test (Fig. 3). DFA for RSV has reported sensitivities and specificities ranging from 84 to 100% and 86 to 100% when compared to culture or NAATs, respectively (44, 52, 53). RSV DFA reagents are commercially available from a number of companies (Table 2). The sensitivity and specificity of DFA detection are comparable to those of cell culture (54), while test turnaround time is longer than RADT. DFAs offer the advantage of evaluating the specimen quality by visualizing cells on the slide but are fairly labor-intensive and require experienced technologists (4, 37, 42). Multi-analyte DFA reagents to simultaneously detect a panel of common respiratory viruses, including RSV, are also available commercially (54).

Nucleic Acid Detection

Compared with conventional diagnostic tests, NAATs have increased diagnostic yields for RSV detection, with sensitivities ranging from 93.5 to 100% and specificity approaching 100% (Table 3) (39, 55). The RSV N gene has been used as the principal target for developing NAA-based assays because (i) nucleotide sequences in the N gene are highly conserved and (ii) the N gene is preferentially transcribed because it is located nearer the 3′ end of the genome, where transcription and replication initiate (1). Different technical platforms have been described to detect RSV nucleic acids. PCR-based procedures incorporating one-step, nested, random-access, monoplex or multiplex reverse transcriptase PCR (RT-PCR) have been developed and are used for RSV nucleic acid amplification (39, 55–60). Other non-PCR amplification procedures have been described, including nucleic acid sequence-based amplification (39, 55), loop-mediated isothermal amplification (61), multiplex ligation-dependent probe amplification (62), reverse transcription strand invasion-based amplification (63), and nicking enzyme amplification reaction (64). Newer assays provide highly sensitive and specific test results with a considerably shorter test time and have the potential to facilitate RSV detection in point-of-care settings (56, 59, 61, 63, 64).

Numerous multiplex molecular syndromic systems are commercially available (39, 55, 65), and some of them have been cleared by the U.S. FDA for detection of a panel of respiratory viral and bacterial pathogens including RSV (Table 3). The more recent ones include the xTAG respiratory viral panel from Luminex Molecular Diagnostics (Austin, TX), FilmArray respiratory panel from BioFire Diagnostics (Salt Lake City, UT), and eSensor XT-8 respiratory viral panel from GenMark Diagnostics (Pasadena, CA) (66–69). Although the only specimen type that is currently cleared by the FDA for most of these NAATs is nasopharyngeal swabs, most published reports have included analysis of other respiratory specimen types including nasal swabs and bronchoalveolar lavage fluids with sensitivity and specificity similar to those of nasopharyngeal swabs (70, 71). In addition, a wide range of research-use-only tests and analyte-specific reagents (ASRs) are available. Rapid turnaround time, simultaneous detection of an array of pathogens, and superior sensitivity of these multiplex syndromic panels have the potential to decrease emergency department length of stay, reduce diagnostic tests, and shorten the duration of intravenous antibiotic administration (72–75).

Isolation Procedures

Isolation of the virus from respiratory secretions by cell culture remains the "gold standard" method for RSV diagnosis due to its excellent specificity. Furthermore, unlike NAATs, viral culture is not affected by mutations in amplification targets which may result in false-negative results (76), and most specimen types are amenable to culture (47). However, due to the labile nature of RSV, viral culture is no longer the most sensitive and reliable method for diagnosis of RSV infections.

For primary isolation, human heteroploid cells, especially HEp-2, are usually preferred. Other cell lines that may be used but are usually less sensitive include human kidney, amnion, and diploid fibroblastic cells and monkey kidney cells (1, 5, 6). Cell line cultures show characteristic syncytial CPE after 3 to 7 days of incubation (Fig. 3). However, the degree of syncytia formation depends on the type of cell culture, the confluence of the cell monolayer,

TABLE 1 Commercially available RSV and HMPV rapid antigen tests[a]

Virus	Products	Company	Compatible specimens	Assay time	Claimed sensitivity, specificity[b]	Validated sensitivity, specificity[b]	Comments	Reference(s)
RSV	Directigen EZ RSV	BD Diagnostic Systems, Sparks, MD	NPW, NPA, or NPS	15 min	89% 93%	59–86.5% 92.3–98%	Specific antibody used to avoid possible interference with the immunoglobulin therapy	44, 49
	Veritor RSV	BD Diagnostic Systems, Sparks, MD	NPW or NPS	15 min	88–92% 95–98%	59–86.5% 97–99%	Instrument-based digital scan, CLIA-waived test	43, 46, 48, 49
	Alere BinaxNOW RSV	Alere Scarborough, Inc., Scarborough, ME	NW or NPS	15 min	89–93% 93–100%	89–94.6% 88.5–100%	CLIA-waived test	38, 52
	RSVAlert	SA Scientific, San Antonio, TX	NPW, NPA, or NPS	15 min	95.6% 94.1%	57–97% 73–100%	18-month shelf life	
	Tru RSV	Meridian Bioscience, Inc., Cincinnati, OH	NPW, NPA, or NPS	15 min	71.7–92.3% 81.1–96.2%	NA	Pooled monoclonal antibodies detect two RSV antigens	
	Clearview RSV	Alere Scarborough, Inc., Scarborough, ME	NPW, NPA, or NPS	15 min	93.7% 97.7%	NA	CLIA-waived test, for children <6 and adults >60 years old	
	X/pect RSV	Remel, Inc., Kansas City, KS	NPW or NPS	15 min	54.5–100% 94.1–100%	67–78% 96–98%	CLIA-waived test	
	3M Rapid Detection RSV Test	3M Health Care, Saint Paul, MN	NW, NPA, or NPS	15 min	85.3–88.2% 95.1–97.4%	60–87% 96–99%	Automated reader available	
	Sofia RSV	Quidel Corp., San Diego, CA	NW, NPA, or NPS	15 min	86–89% 97–98%	70% 97–100%	Instrument-based digital scan, CLIA-waived test	38, 48, 49
	RSV Respi-Strip/ K-SeT	Coris BioConcept, Gembloux, Belgium	NPW and/ or culture supernatant	10 min	Strip 92.2–96% 98.3–100% K-SeT 92.2–96% 98.3–100%	NA	Rapid in 10 minutes, complete set of sampling devices available	43
	QuickVue RSV	Quidel Corp., San Diego, CA	NW, NPA, or NPS	15 min	83–99% 90–92%	72.5% 97–100%	Negative results do not preclude RSV infection and should be confirmed by culture or NAAT	49
RSV and HMPV	mariPOC test	ArcDia International Oy Ltd., Turku, Finland	NPA or NPS	20 min/ 2 h	100% (RSV), ~100% (HMPV); 100% (both)	89% (RSV), 50% (MPHV); 100.0% (both)	A multianalyte point-of-care antigen system detecting 10 viruses and *Streptococcus pneumoniae*	50, 51

[a]NA, applicable or not available; NW, nasal wash; NPA, nasopharyngeal aspirate; NPS, nasopharyngeal swab; NPW, nasopharyngeal wash.
[b]Compared to cell culture unless specifically noted.

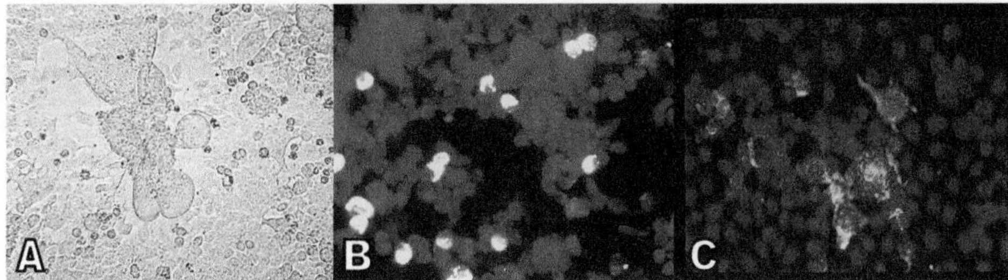

FIGURE 3 Microscopic detection of RSV and HMPV. (A) RSV-infected HEp-2 cells showing that cells have fused, forming large syncytia. (B) Direct immunofluorescence of RSV on a nasopharyngeal swab specimen. (C) Indirect immunofluorescence of HMPV-infected LLC-MK2 centrifugation culture stained with monoclonal antibody MAb-8 (142). Images courtesy of http://www.virology.org/hpphoto3.html (A) and David Ferguson and Marie Landry (B and C).

the medium, the strain and type of virus, the multiplicity of infection, and whether the RSV strain is laboratory adapted. In HEp-2 cells, RSV plaque morphology appears unrelated to disease severity in RSV-infected children (5). The reported sensitivities of conventional tube cell culture have ranged from 57 to 90%, in part due to compromise of virus viability, the technical expertise required, and the cell lines used in the laboratory (1, 6).

The shell vial assay combines centrifugation and immunofluorescence to detect expression of viral antigens on infected cells before development of CPEs, which significantly shorten the length of time needed for detection of the virus to about 16 hours (6, 47). The use of R-Mix cultures (Diagnostic Hybrids/Quidel Corp, Inc., Athens, OH), which contain a mixture of human lung carcinoma A549 and mink lung Mv1Lu cells, has been shown to be a rapid and sensitive method for the detection and identification of respiratory viruses (77, 78). With significantly decreased costs compared to conventional culture, the use of R-Mix was slightly more sensitive than that of RMK, HEp-2, and MRC-5 cell lines used in conventional cultures, and it was several days faster (77). Screening of R-Mix cells after overnight incubation was more sensitive and produced more timely results for RSV and other respiratory viruses and was more reliable than direct antigen testing (78, 79). In addition, R-Mix cell cultures have the major advantage of identifying viruses not detected by direct staining (46, 77).

Identification

The appearance of characteristic syncytial CPEs in cell culture, together with a negative hemadsorption test, may be adequate to establish the presence of RSV during the epidemic season. However, since other respiratory viruses such as parainfluenza virus 3 and measles virus can produce similar CPEs in certain cell lines, clinical virology laboratories confirm RSV detection by performing type-specific immunofluorescence assay (IFA) on infected cells from cell culture vials as a standard practice (47).

Typing Systems

Infections with RSV of type A or B may result in differing clinical manifestations and outcomes; therefore, RSV type information may become useful in clinical patient management if type-specific vaccines or treatments are developed (6, 15). More commonly, RSV type information has been used widely to facilitate epidemiological investigations (80). Several of the molecular commercial assays include concomitant detection and typing of RSV into RSV A and RSV B (Table 3).

Methods commonly used for RSV genotyping include restriction fragment length polymorphisms, Sanger and next-generation sequencing, and heteroduplex mobility assays of the G protein (1, 2, 16, 17). Over 100 genotypes of RSV group A (i.e., GA2, GA5, GA7) and group B (GB3 and GB4) have been identified (1, 81, 82). These highly discriminatory typing techniques have been useful in monitoring possible health care-related RSV infections and facilitating the interruption of RSV outbreaks (16, 17, 81).

Serologic Tests

Serology is primarily useful for epidemiologic studies rather than for clinical diagnosis of RSV infections. Most children have serologic evidence of RSV infection by 2 years of age. A significant proportion (10 to 30%) of young patients with documented RSV infections remain serologically negative, probably due to the immaturity of the infant immune response (6). Assays that detect IgM antibody to RSV show low sensitivity, particularly for infants less than 6 months of age, precluding a definitive diagnosis in a clinically relevant time frame (6, 83). In contrast, serology is most useful in elderly adults, who curiously have the most vigorous antibody responses to RSV (6). Current means of serologic diagnosis for RSV infections include IFA, enzyme immunoassay, complement fixation, and neutralization assays.

Antiviral Susceptibilities

Resistance to ribavirin has not been recognized in the clinical setting. To date, some palivizumab-resistant RSV mutants have been isolated from children receiving monthly administration of palivizumab (84, 85). Palivizumab-resistant strains with mutations of the F protein of K272E and S275F were reported. Mutations leading to amino acid substitutions in the palivizumab binding site of the RSV F protein have been associated with breakthrough RSV infections in patients receiving palivizumab. A recent study reported that palivizumab resistance mutations were identified in 4 (10.2%) of the 39 children studied, of which 1 had documented palivizumab receipt (85). Cell fusion assay by expression of RSV F protein was reported to analyze the mutation of palivizumab-resistant strains (86).

Evaluation, Interpretation, and Reporting of Results

RSV infection among young children is usually diagnosed clinically in the setting of the community's RSV season. Among adults, however, the findings are less specific, and RSV is commonly not suspected. Test results should be interpreted with knowledge of the natural history of

TABLE 2 Commercial RSV and HMPV DFA reagents and their performance

Virus	Products	Company	Manufacturer-claimed performance[a]	Application	Remarks (reference[s])
RSV	Bartels RSV DFA	Trinity Biotech, Jameston, NY	Sensitivity, 88–100%; specificity, 100%	Direct specimen detection and culture confirmation	Single- or dual-reagent DFA available; acquired recently by Trinity Biotech (44)
	Light Diagnostics Respiratory Viral Panel DFA	Millipore, Temecula, CA	Sensitivity, 100%; specificity, 86%	Direct specimen detection and culture confirmation	In either single RSV or panel format; the panel covers RSV, influenza A/B, adenovirus, and parainfluenza viruses 1, 2, and 3
	SimulFluor Respiratory Screen, RSV/flu A or RSV/Para 3	Millipore, Temecula, CA	Sensitivity, 83.3–100%; specificity, 83.8–100%	For screening in clinical specimens and culture	Three formats available; covers RSV, influenza A/B, adenovirus, and parainfluenza 1, 2, and 3 (53, 54)
	D[3] Ultra DFA Respiratory Kit	Quidel, San Diego, CA	Sensitivity, 93%; specificity, 99%	Direct specimen detection and culture confirmation	Covers influenza A and B, RSV, parainfluenza 1, 2, and 3, and adenovirus
	Imagen RSV	Oxoid Ltd., Hampshire, United Kingdom	Sensitivity, 93%; specificity, 98%	Detection or identification in human clinical specimens	Mixture of 3 monoclonal antibodies covering RSV, influenza A, and influenza B (79)
	PathoDx RSV and Respiratory Virus Panel	Remel, Inc., Lenexa, KS	Sensitivity, 77.6–100%; specificity, 98–100%	For clinical specimen detection and culture confirmation	The respiratory panel covers RSV, influenza A/B, adenovirus, and parainfluenza 1, 2, and 3
HMPV	D[3] Ultra DFA HMPV Kit	DHI/Quidel, Athens, OH	Sensitivity, 62.5%; specificity, 99.8%;	Direct specimen detection and culture confirmation	Reference was a combination of culture and NNA assays (44, 157)
	Imagen hMPV DFA test	Thermo Fisher Scientific, Ely, United Kingdom	Sensitivity, 63.2%; specificity, 100.0%	For clinical specimen detection	Sensitivity and specificity were calculated by using culture and NAAT as standards (44)
	Light Diagnostics HMPV Reagent	Millipore, Temecula, CA	ND	Direct specimen detection and culture confirmation	An ASR kit carried by Millipore (134)

[a]Compared to cell culture unless specifically notified. In many cases, the culture used for comparison and validation was suboptimal, making the rapid tests look artificially better. It should be recognized that performance in each laboratory may be different. ND, not done.

TABLE 3 Commercial NAATs for detection and identification of RSV and HMPV

Virus	Test	Manufacturer	Method	Additional targets[a]	Senssitivity (%)	Specificity (%)	Reference(s)
RSV	Alere i RSV[b]	Alere Scarborough, Inc., Scarborough, ME	RNA extraction Isothermal amplification	None	98.0–98.6	97.8–98.6	64
	Xpert Xpress Flu/RSV; Flu/RSV XC	Cepheid, Sunnyvale, CA	RNA extraction Real-time PCR	Flu A, Flu B	97.8–100	100	56, 59, 60
	Prodesse ProFlu+	Hologic, Inc., Marlborough, MA	RNA extraction Real-time PCR	Flu A, Flu B	95–100	97–99	158
	Simplexa Flu A/B & RSV, regular and direct version	Focus Diagnostics, Cypress, CA	RNA extraction (direct: sample heating) Real-time PCR	Flu A, Flu B	91–95	100	158–160
	ARIES Flu A/B and RSV Assay	Luminex Molecular Diagnostics Austin, TX	RNA extraction Real-time PCR	Flu A, Flu B	96.0–98.0	98.4–100	58, 59
	Nanosphere Verigene RV+	Luminex Molecular Diagnostics Austin, TX	Integrated extraction and nanoparticle technology	Flu A, Flu B	100	99	159
	cobas Liat Influenza A/B and RSV Assay[b]	Roche Molecular Diagnostics, Pleasanton, CA	Integrated real-time PCR POCT	Flu A, Flu B	97.8–100	98.4–100	57, 59
HMPV	Pro hMPV	Gen-Probe, San Diego, CA	RNA extraction Real-time PCR	Flu A, Flu B	100	100	161
	Quidel Molecular hMPV Assay	Quidel Molecular, San Diego, CA	RNA extraction Real-time PCR	None	95.2	99.8	
RSV & HMPV	Lyra RSV+hMPV Assay	Quidel Molecular, San Diego, CA	RNA extraction Real-time PCR	None	95.7–96.5	98.0–98.3	
	xTAG Respiratory Viral Panel	Luminex Molecular Diagnostics, Austin, TX	RNA extraction PCR and RT-PCR xMAP suspension array	Flu A, Flu B, PIV1–4, AdV, EnV/RhV, CoV	RSV, 100; HMPH, 96	RSV, 97.4–98.4; HMPV, 98.8	66
	xTAG Respiratory Viral Panel Fast	Luminex Molecular Diagnostics, Austin, TX	RNA extraction PCR and RT-PCR xMAP suspension array	Flu A, Flu B, PIV1–4, AdV, EnV/RhV, CoV, Boca	RSV, 96.6; HMPV, 100	RSV, 100, HMPV, 100	71
	NxTAG Respiratory Pathogen Panel	Luminex Molecular Diagnostics, Austin, TX	RNA extraction PCR and RT-PCR xMAP suspension array	Flu A, Flu B, PIV1–4, AdV, EnV/RhV, CoV, Boca, *Chlamydia pneumoniae*, *Mycoplasma pneumoniae*	RSV, 98.5–100; HMPV, 93.8	RSV, 99.3–99.4; HMPV, 99.1	69

(Continued on next page)

TABLE 3 Commercial NAATs for detection and identification of RSV and HMPV (*Continued*)

Virus	Test	Manufacturer	Method	Additional targets[a]	Senssitivity (%)	Specificity (%)	Reference(s)
	FilmArray Respiratory Panel[c]	BioFire Diagnostics, Salt Lake City, UT	Integrated extraction and nested PCR with melt curve analysis	Flu A, Flu B, PIV1–4, AdV, EnV/RhV, CoV, *C. pneumoniae*, *Bordetella pertussis*, *M. pneumoniae*	RSVA, 86.4; RSVB, 100; HMPV, 96.2	RSVA,100; RSVB, 100; HMPV, 100	68
	FilmArray Respiratory Panel 2	BioFire Diagnostics, Salt Lake City, UT	Integrated extraction and nested PCR with melt curve analysis	Flu A, Flu B, PIV1–4, AdV, EnV/RhV, CoV, *C. pneumoniae*, *B. pertussis*, *Bordetella parapertussis*, *M. pneumoniae*	RSV, 99.4; HMPV, 97.3	RSV, 98.3; HMPV, 99.5	
	eSensor XT-8 Respiratory Viral Panel	GenMark Diagnostics, Pasadena, CA	RNA extraction PCR and RT-PCR Electrochemical detection	Flu A, Flu B, PIV1-3, AdV, RhV	RSVA, 100; RSVB, 95.8; HMPV, 92	RSVA, 100; RSVB, 100; HMPV, 100	67, 73
	ePlex Respiratory Panel	GenMark Diagnostics, Pasadena, CA	Integrated extraction, competitive DNA hybridization and electrochemical detection	Flu A, Flu B, PIV1–4, AdV, EnV/RhV, CoV, *C. pneumoniae*, *M. pneumoniae*	RSV, 92.6–100; HMPV, 71.4–90.0	RSV, 100; HMPV, 100	162, 163
	Nanosphere Verigene RP Flex	Luminex Molecular Diagnostics, Austin, TX	Integrated extraction and nanoparticle technology	Flu A, Flu B, PIV1–4, AdV, RhV, *B. pertussis*, *B. parapertussis/Bordetella bronchiseptica*, *Bordetella holmesii*	RSV, 96–100; HMPV, 97.3	RSV, 98.9–99.8; HMPV, 97.7	62
	Anyplex II	Seegen Inc., Seoul, South Korea	RNA extraction PCR and multiplex real-time PCR	Flu A, Flu B, PIV1–4, AdV, EnV/RhV, CoV, Boca	RSVA, 100; RSVB, 90.6; HMPV, 88.9	RSVA, 100; RSVB, 99.2; HMPV, 99.2	164

[a]AdV, adenovirus; Boca, bocavirus; CoV, coronavirus; EnV/RhV, enterovirus/rhinovirus; PIV, parainfluenza virus; POCT, point-of-care testing.
[b]CLIA waived.
[c]The EZ format is CLIA waived.

RSV infections in the context of the patient's clinical presentation and medical history. Serologic results have little clinical value, and rapid antigen, DFAs, and NAAT-based molecular assays are the tests of choice for laboratory diagnosis. Culture for RSV detection is time-consuming and has a relatively long turnaround time; it is mainly used for specimen types that have not been validated or cleared by NAAT-based molecular assays, as a back-up test for specimens yielding rapid negative antigen results, or when further characterization has been requested.

The availability of rapid antigen assays with a turnaround time as short as 15 minutes makes it possible for clinicians to receive results in a timely fashion. However, due to their relatively low sensitivity, false-negative results can be expected and should not be interpreted as excluding the possibility of RSV infection. To improve detection, DFAs, culture, or RT-PCR assays should be used as back-up tests. NAATs are particularly useful for testing respiratory specimens collected from adults and in the off-season. With the increased number of multiplexed molecular FDA-approved assays, simultaneous detection and identification of common viral pathogens, including RSV, is becoming the main tool for detection and typing of RSV. Rapid near-point-of-care testing has the potential to decrease emergency department stays, reduce diagnostic tests and patient charges, and improve patient care. Notably, three devices including the Alere i RSV, the cobas Liat Influenza A/B & RSV, and the FilmArray Respiratory Panel EZ assays are now CLIA waived. Whereas multiplex NAATs are currently qualitative, real-time NAATs can provide an estimate of viral load. Especially when more than one virus is detected, the viral load information may be helpful in identifying the predominant pathogen. Viral load estimates might also be helpful in determining the rate of RSV clearance, which is especially crucial in immunocompromised patients or pretransplant patients where a positive RSV test result could result in further therapy or a delay in transplant procedures, respectively.

The positive and negative predictive values of these tests vary according to the prevalence of the disease in a particular population during certain seasons. The diagnosis of RSV infection is often made with reasonable accuracy in combination with clinical and epidemiologic findings in infants with lower respiratory tract disease during the epidemic season. Effective exchanges of relevant information between clinicians and the laboratory are essential to good patient care. RSV is extremely labile, and improper specimen collection, transport, and processing, even when sensitive methods such as RT-PCR are used, can lead to false-negative results. The importance of correct specimen collection and prompt specimen transport cannot be overemphasized. Prompt reporting of test results may assist clinicians in discontinuing unnecessary forms of therapy or in implementing infection control precautions, thereby preventing health care-related spread of infection.

HUMAN METAPNEUMOVIRUS

Taxonomy

Human metapneumovirus (HMPV) virus belongs to the order *Mononegavirales*, the family *Pneumoviridae*, and the genus *Metapneumovirus* (87, 88). *Orthopneumovirus*, the other genus in the *Pneumoviridae* family, includes the closely related human RSV. HMPV is the only human pathogen within the *Metapneumovirus* genus, which includes the avian metapneumovirus, also known as turkey rhinotracheitis virus, a cause of respiratory tract infections in turkey, ducks, and chickens (87).

Description of the Agent

HMPV was first isolated in 2001. Viral cultures, in monkey kidney cells, of nasopharyngeal aspirates from symptomatic children under 5 years of age in the Netherlands revealed CPEs that were indistinguishable from CPEs caused by RSV (89). Further analyses showed that the virus was distinct from RSV and most closely related to avian metapneumovirus.

HMPV is an enveloped respiratory virus with a single-stranded nonsegmented negative-sense RNA genome revealing pleomorphic particles measuring 150 to 600 nm (90). The HMPV genome possesses 8 genes ranging in length from 13,280 to 13,278 nucleotides and encoding 9 proteins. HMPV and avian metapneumovirus are distinguished from human RSV and other members of the *Pneumoviridae* family by the absence of genes encoding the nonstructural proteins NS1 and NS2 and by a different gene order in the RNA genome (Fig. 1) (90). Similar to RSV, nucleotide sequences in the nucleoprotein (N) gene are highly conserved. HMPV nucleoprotein (N) and phosphoprotein (P) proteins interact and are recruited to cytoplasmic viral inclusion bodies in HMPV-infected cells. The fusion protein (F) induces virus-cell fusion by binding to heparin sulfate on the host cells and uses multiple Arg-Gly-Asp-binding integrins as attachment and entry receptors (91). The glycosylated protein (G), which is the most variable protein among HMPV isolates, binds to the host cell via cellular glycosaminoglycans including heparin sulfate-like molecules (92).

HMPV strains vary genetically and antigenically and have been classified into two genotypes: genotype A and genotype B, based on the sequence of the F and G genes. Each genotype is further divided into five sublineages (A1, A2a, A2b, B1, and B2) (89, 90), with the A2 sublineage showing the greatest genetic diversity (93–95). A recent study from Malaysia identified a previously unrecognized, novel sublineage of A2, with isolates from other South Asian countries clustering within this novel clade (96).

Epidemiology and Transmission

Since its discovery in 2001, HMPV has been identified worldwide and in all age groups. Most individuals become infected by the age of 5 years as initially demonstrated by serology (89). In a prospective, population-based surveillance for acute respiratory illness or fever among inpatient and outpatient children in three U.S. counties from 2003 through 2009, HMPV infection was found to be associated with a substantial burden of hospitalizations (97). HMPV was detected in 7% of symptomatic children and 1% of asymptomatic control children, with an increase in outpatient visits among children throughout the first 5 years of life, particularly during the first year (97). A Spanish prospective study of symptomatic, hospitalized children under the age of 14 between 2005 and 2014 (98) identified HMPV in 5.5% of cases, a rate similar to a recent U.S. study in which HMPV was identified in 5% of children aged 5 to 13 years presenting with acute respiratory illness as outpatients and in emergency rooms between 2003 and 2009 (99).

Although long-term studies have shown that sporadic infection does occur year-round, HMPV has a seasonal distribution. In temperate countries, most cases occur in winter and spring, often overlapping in part or in whole with the annual RSV epidemic (97). In tropical countries, the peak prevalence occurs in the late summer and early spring between November and April, a period coinciding with the rainy season, with peak prevalence in March (96, 100).

In most longitudinal studies, both antigenic group A and group B were noted to cocirculate in the same location during the epidemic periods and had various patterns of predominance depending on the year (93–96, 100). Antigenic variability is thought to contribute to reinfection throughout the life of the patient and may pose a challenge to vaccine development (93–95).

Formal transmission studies have not been reported, but experts believe that transmission occurs by close or direct contact with contaminated secretions involving large particle aerosols, droplets, or contaminated surfaces (90). Transmission is believed to occur in the first 5 to 6 days when patients are most infectious (101, 102). Using a novel approach that combines bioinformatics and analysis of the F and G gene sequences, the dynamics of HMPV transmission in both pediatric and adult outpatient populations were recently investigated (96). Using this approach, the authors could establish an estimated date of infection between patients belonging to the same cluster of ≥7 days and identify the donor and recipients (96).

Clinical Significance

Humans are the only source of infection. The incubation period of HMPV infection is estimated to range from 4 to 6 days with a median duration of 5 days (101, 102). The signs and symptoms of HMPV are nonspecific and indistinguishable from other viral causes of respiratory tract infections. Detection of HMPV is strongly associated with symptoms in infected patients, with shedding of the virus occurring up to 4 weeks after primary infection (103, 104). HMPV causes a spectrum of diseases ranging from the common cold to lower respiratory tract illnesses including bronchiolitis, pneumonia, croup, and exacerbation of reactive airways disease (105). Studies of patients diagnosed with HPMV revealed that the most common clinical symptoms at presentation include cough, nasal congestion, and rhinorrhea (105, 106). In older adults, dyspnea and wheezing are often present (106, 107), and in pregnant women and immunocompromised hosts, fever is commonly reported (108, 109).

RSV and HMPV coinfections have been reported, which is not surprising given the overlapping seasons. Coinfection with bacteria is not common, except for the complication of otitis media, which is frequent (97). Similar to RSV, HMPV infection can result in significant morbidity in infants and other special populations, including immunocompromised, high-risk patients and elderly adults. About half of the cases of LRTI in children occur in the first 6 months of life, suggesting that young age is a major risk factor for severe disease (97). Progression to LRTI is also a complication of HMPV infections in older adults and immunocompromised patients. In one cohort of immunocompromised pediatric patients, 29% developed LRTI, 23% were admitted to the intensive care unit or required supplemental oxygen, and 5% died from HMPV pneumonia (110). A similar study found that LRTI developed in up to 51% of patients, with respiratory failure and death occurring in 15% and 10%, respectively. Furthermore, coinfection with bacterial or fungal pathogens was identified as the only major risk factor for death (111).

In adult patients with cancer, reports of complications of HMPV vary. In one study, progression to LRTI was independently associated with underlying hematologic malignancies, health care-related infections, and hypoxia at presentation, with a 10% 30-day mortality rate in patients with LRTI compared to 0% in patients who had only upper respiratory tract infections (108). In another study, 55% of cancer patients who were positive for HMPV and had imaging studies done showed evidence of radiographic abnormality, but no fatalities were observed, even in HSCT recipients (112).

In solid organ transplant recipients, upper respiratory tract infections caused by HMPV progressed to LRTI in 50% of patients after a median of 7 days (range, 2 to 31 days). Risk factors identified for progression to LRTI in this cohort included a low lymphocyte count and high C-reactive protein at the time of diagnosis of the upper respiratory tract infection. Coinfection with other viruses and bacteria was common, detected in 39% of patients (113).

Rare complications reported after HMPV infections include encephalitis and meningitis (114, 115) in previously healthy children and adults and cases of myocarditis in adults patients (116, 117). In all cases, patients recovered from the infections without lasting neurological deficits or other sequelae.

There are currently no licensed antiviral agents for the treatment of HMPV (118). Most immunocompetent children and adults infected with HMPV can be managed with supportive care. In immunocompromised hosts, treatment of HMPV infections with ribavirin, a nucleoside analogue approved for the treatment of RSV, intravenous immunoglobulin, or both has been reported, although the exact benefits of these therapeutic approaches remain unclear and will require further evaluation (110, 119).

Several approaches have been used to develop a vaccine for HMPV infection, but to date, all have been unsuccessful (120). In one study, a recombinant HMPV virus, based on wild-type HMPV, elicited an antibody response in 35% of healthy adults inoculated with the virus and was deemed suitable as a parent virus for the development of a live attenuated recombinant HMPV vaccine (121). The vaccine response was overattenuated in a recent phase I clinical trial of an experimental live attenuated recombinant HPMV vaccine administered to adults and HMPV seropositive and seronegative children (122). Thus, further studies are needed to develop an HMPV vaccine.

Shedding can last for a few days to several weeks, raising the potential for HMPV to be a health care-associated infection. In cancer patients, the median range of HMPV shedding was 14 days as detected by PCR, although long-term shedding of up to 80 days was reported from a 1.5-year-old child with pre-B cell acute lymphoblastic leukemia (112, 123). Several health care-associated HMPV infections have been reported in hospitalized children and adults, and contact isolation with excellent handwashing for health care providers is necessary to prevent spread (92, 124–127). There should be increased awareness of HMPV infection in health care settings, particularly when the population that is at risk has a high prevalence of underlying comorbidities (125).

Collection, Transport, and Storage of Specimens

The most frequently used specimens for the recovery and detection of HMPV are nasopharyngeal swabs. Nasopharyngeal flocked swabs have been gradually replacing aspirate specimens without significantly decreasing diagnostic yield (128). Other specimen types used for the diagnosis of upper respiratory tract infection caused by HMPV include nasal washes and nasopharyngeal aspirates, primarily in infants. Typically, nasopharyngeal aspirates are collected from infants using a 10F catheter. Washing the catheter after dispensing, in addition to the collection of material in the collection trap, may enhance yield over use of the trap material alone (129). Diagnosis of HMPV LRTI is accomplished using expectorated or induced sputa, bronchial washings, and bronchoalveolar lavage specimens. Transport is generally performed using standard viral transport media. Specimens should be processed as soon as possible after collection or stored at 4°C for up 72 hours. Incubation at 37°C has been shown to lead to a rapid decrease in HMPV titer (130). For long-term storage of specimens or laboratory stocks, a temperature of −70°C is preferred, with specimens in O-ring-sealed cryovials.

Direct Examination

Microscopy

The virus can be visualized by electron microscopy of the supernatant of HMPV infected cell culture (89, 131). This method was used to describe HMPV when it was first identified (89) but is not sufficiently sensitive, rapid, or reproducible for routine clinical diagnosis use.

Antigen Detection

An automated, multiantigen, point-of-care assay, the mariPOC Respi test (ArcDia Inc., Turku, Finland), is commercially available in Europe for the detection of HMPV antigens from nasopharyngeal aspirate and swab samples (50) (Table 1). In addition to HMPV, the Respi test detects eight other respiratory pathogens—influenza virus A, influenza virus B, RSV, adenovirus, parainfluenza viruses 1 to 3, and *Streptococcus pneumoniae*—with preliminary results reported in 20 minutes. The sensitivity of the mariPOC for HMPV varies across studies from low to high when NAATs are used as the reference method. In one study, the sensitivity and specificity in nasopharyngeal swabs collected from children with respiratory symptoms and/or fever were 50% and 100%, respectively (50), while sensitivity and specificity were higher in another study, at 77.8% and 100%, respectively (132).

Several DFA reagents using mouse monoclonal antibodies specific for HMPV are commercially available for the detection of HMPV antigens in nasopharyngeal samples (Table 2). In one study, the performance characteristics of four HMPV DFA kits on nasopharyngeal aspirate samples were compared (133). Two DFA kits, the Anti-human *Metapneumovirus* (Argene, Verniolle, France) and Imagen hMPV (Oxoid, Thermo Fisher Inc., United Kingdom), gave nonspecific positive signals in samples positive for other viruses (e.g., RSV and adenovirus) and in negative samples. The other two kits that were evaluated, the D^3*Ultra* DFA HMPV (Diagnostic Hybrids Inc./Quidel Corp, Athens, OH) and the Light Diagnostics HMPV DFA Reagent (Millipore, Temecula, CA), were equivalent in their performance with relatively low sensitivity (50%) and great specificity (100%) when compared to RT-PCR. In other reports, the sensitivity of the Light Diagnostics HMPV DFA was higher (85.4%) when evaluated with a larger number of HMPV-positive samples (134), while the sensitivity of the Imagen hMPV was similarly low at 63.2% (44).

Although the sensitivity of antigen tests is generally lower than that of molecular tests, their relative low complexity and cost, high specificity, and rapid turnaround time to results contribute to their continued utility in diagnostic virology. Antigen assays are often used in combination with molecular tests as part of a two-step algorithm where samples are quickly screened using antigen tests and all negative samples are further tested using molecular tests.

Nucleic Acid Detection

The most sensitive test for the identification of HMPV in clinical samples is RT-PCR. Several HMPV NAATs and ASR, including NucliSENS EasyQ HMPV (bioMérieux, Durham, NC), MGB Alert HMPV Detection Reagent ASR (Nanogen, San Diego, CA), Quidel Molecular RSV+HMPV assay (Quidel Corp., San Diego, CA), and Pro HMPV assay (GenProbe Inc, San Diego, CA), are commercially available, and their performance characteristics are contrasted in Table 3.

Recent advances in nucleic acid amplification and identification techniques have allowed for the development of molecular systems that simultaneously detect and differentiate multiple respiratory viruses including HMPV. Most of these devices targeted highly conserved HMPV N or F genes. Currently, several instruments and multiplexed molecular panels are FDA cleared for the detection of respiratory viruses on nasopharyngeal swab samples, with several more panels CE marked in Europe (Table 3). These panels and instruments differ in their degree of multiplexing, complexity, throughput, and turnaround time (135). Given the increased sensitivity of NAATs over viral culture and antigen tests, these assays are now considered the "gold standard" for the detection of viruses including HMPV and are now commonly found in many laboratories. The sensitivity and specificity of each of these panels may vary depending on the reference method used for each or all of the targets, although in general, sensitivities and specificities for HMPV range from 80 to 100% and 95 to 100%, respectively (Table 3).

Syndromic panels that include HMPV offer several advantages. First, given the nonspecific clinical presentation of HMPV infections, syndromic panels allow for each sample tested to be interrogated for multiple pathogens, including in some cases, both viruses and bacteria. Second, syndromic panels allow the detection of coinfections. In one French pediatric cohort, 42.9% of samples positive for HMPV were identified along with another virus (136), while in a Canadian study, 15% of samples positive for HMPV were mixed with another virus, with mixed infections occurring most frequently in specimens from children younger than 6 months and less frequently in older adults (137). However, "coinfections" should be interpreted with caution for several reasons. First, PCR is susceptible to false-positive results due to cross-contamination in some laboratories that perform frequent amplifications. Second, viral genomes can be detected by RT-PCR in respiratory secretions for several weeks or more, even after live virus shedding has ceased. It is difficult to know in this situation if the presence of positive virus-specific nucleic acid signifies active infection or simply a recent acute infection. Although not currently used routinely for diagnosis of HMPV infections, potential future applications of quantitative molecular tests would be to differentiate acute and resolved infections as well as to determine the significance of positive findings (138–141).

Isolation Procedures

HMPV was first isolated in 2001 in the Netherlands using tertiary monkey kidney cells (89). HMPV replicated poorly or not at all in various cell lines commonly used for conventional cell cultures used for respiratory virus diagnosis, such as HEK, HEp-2, and Madin-Darby canine kidney cells. Primary isolation is facilitated by the presence of a low concentration of trypsin, which is not used routinely in diagnostic virology cultures in many laboratories. In one study, rhesus monkey kidney epithelial cells (LLC-MK2 and Vero) and a human airway epithelial cell line (BEAS-2B) were most permissive for HMPV growth. LLC-MK2 cells were tolerant of trypsin and thus remain an ideal cell line for HMPV cultivation (130). In another study, human laryngeal carcinoma (HEp-2) cells were more sensitive than LLC-MK2 cells for isolation of HMPV, detecting HMPV in 88% of samples that tested positive for HMPV by PCR compared to 24% detection using LLC-MK2 cells (131). Centrifugation cultures significantly increased the infectivity of HMPV for cells in monolayer culture (130, 142). HMPV growth in LLC-MK2 cell or Vero cell monolayer cultures is slow, requiring between 10 and 22 days and often several blind passages before CPE appears, especially following primary isolation. The observed CPE is not particularly striking, often appearing only as focal areas of rounding of cells and minor patches of cell-cell fusion (89, 131, 143). A shell vial culture method using R-Mix cells with a mixed monolayer of human adenocarcinoma cells (A549 cells) and mink lung cells (Mv1Lu cells) (Diagnostic Hybrids Inc./Quidel Corp, Athens, OH) and an HMPV-specific monoclonal antibody had a sensitivity of 100% compared with tube culture in one study (144) (Fig. 3C).

Identification

The characteristics of the CPE are not distinct enough that the virus could be identified on this basis, even by trained observers (89, 143). HMPV is suspected when a virus is isolated during the epidemic season in HEp-2, Vero, or LLC-MK2 cells and other possible viruses have been excluded. Specific identification must be made using immunofluorescence with a commercial monoclonal antibody or an RT-PCR test on RNA extracted from cell lysates.

Typing Systems

Sequence analysis of the fusion (F) gene and the glycoprotein (G) gene are the two main targets used to distinguish between the two genotypes, HMPV-A and HMPV-B, with sequence analysis of the nucleocapsid gene additionally used to further delineate the five subtypes, A1, A2a, A2b, B1, and B2 (96, 145, 146). The HMPV G glycoprotein gene exhibits the greatest diversity, with nucleotide and amino acid sequence identities ranging from 52 to 58% and 31 to 35%, respectively, between the two genotypes (90, 147). Reverse transcription nucleic acid amplification followed by bidirectional amplicon sequencing is a common approach used for genotyping of HMPV and has been performed directly from clinical samples (96) or viral culture isolates (145, 146). A few studies investigating the correlation between HMPV genotypes and disease severity have yielded varied results, from no differences in disease severity to either genotype A or B causing more severe diseases (148–151). At present, typing of HMPV isolates is primarily performed for epidemiological investigations. Novel methods such as whole-genome sequencing are currently being investigated and may provide more details of the phylogeny of HMPV species.

Serologic Tests

Serology is generally not useful for clinical diagnosis of HMPV. Diagnosis using serology would require collection of both acute and convalescent titers over a 4- to 8-week period, with diagnosis established by observing a 4-fold increase in titers (152). Several serology methods using both virus-infected cell lysates and recombinant viral proteins in enzyme-linked immunosorbent assays have been reported (89, 153–155). Most of these tests have used reduction of virus plaques or CPE as the readout, but a more objective microneutralization test using a recombinant HMPV expressing green fluorescent protein has been reported (156).

Evaluation, Interpretation, and Reporting of Results

Rapid diagnosis of HMPV infections has greatly improved since its discovery in 2001. Multiple assays are now commercially available, primarily for detection in nasopharyngeal swab specimens. Other specimen types, including lower respiratory tract specimens such as bronchoalveolar lavage fluids, are commonly validated by individual laboratories for use with these assays. The availability of multiplex PCR assays offers laboratories the ability to provide rapid diagnosis in a time frame that allows better management of patients with respiratory tract infections.

A positive test for HMPV must be interpreted in the right clinical context. In general, the diagnosis of HMPV infection is most likely when a positive test, particularly a nucleic acid test, for HMPV infection occurs when testing a respiratory sample during late winter or early spring in temperate climates from a patient with acute respiratory illness. NAAT tests should not be used as tests of cure, because the duration of HMPV shedding is still not well defined. Furthermore, interpretation of a positive nucleic acid test in the presence of nucleic acids from another virus may also be challenging because the clinical impact of coinfections remains unclear. Real-time PCR-based quantitative molecular test results including threshold cycle values may be useful to determine the significance of positive findings as well as to differentiate acute and resolved infections. Inversely correlated to the HMPV loads in clinical specimens, higher threshold cycle values would be more consistent with a resolved infection. However, the value of quantitative HMPV PCR remains to be clearly established. Serology and typing are mostly useful in studies of epidemiology at this time.

REFERENCES

1. **Collins PL, Karron RA.** 2013. Respiratory syncytial virus and metapneumovirus, p 1086–1123. *In* Knipe DM, Howley PM (ed), *Fields Virology*, 6th ed, vol 2. Lippincott Williams & Wilkins, Philadelphia, PA.
2. **Griffiths C, Drews SJ, Marchant DJ.** 2017. Respiratory syncytial virus: infection, detection, and new options for prevention and treatment. *Clin Microbiol Rev* **30:**277–319.
3. **Chanock R, Roizman B, Myers R.** 1957. Recovery from infants with respiratory illness of a virus related to chimpanzee coryza agent (CCA). I. Isolation, properties and characterization. *Am J Hyg* **66:**281–290.
4. **Ginocchio CC.** 2007. Detection of respiratory viruses using non-molecular based methods. *J Clin Virol* **40**(Suppl 1)**:** S11–S14.
5. **Kim YI, Murphy R, Majumdar S, Harrison LG, Aitken J, DeVincenzo JP.** 2015. Relating plaque morphology to respiratory syncytial virus subgroup, viral load, and disease severity in children. *Pediatr Res* **78:**380–388.
6. **Walsh EE, Hall CB.** 2015. Respiratory syncytial virus (RSV), p 1948-1960. *In* Bennett JE, Dolin R, Blaser MJ (ed), *Principles and Practice of Infectious Diseases*, 8th ed, vol 1. Elsevier Saunders, Philadelphia, PA.
7. **Williams JV, Piedra PA, Englund JA.** 2017. Respiratory syncytial virus, human metapneumovirus, and parainfluenza viruses, p 873–902. *In* Richman DD, Whitley RJ, Hayden FG (ed), *Clinical Virology*, vol 4. ASM Press, Washington, DC.

8. **Fearns R, Deval J.** 2016. New antiviral approaches for respiratory syncytial virus and other mononegaviruses: inhibiting the RNA polymerase. *Antiviral Res* **134:**63–76.
9. **McLellan JS, Chen M, Joyce MG, Sastry M, Stewart-Jones GB, Yang Y, Zhang B, Chen L, Srivatsan S, Zheng A, Zhou T, Graepel KW, Kumar A, Moin S, Boyington JC, Chuang GY, Soto C, Baxa U, Bakker AQ, Spits H, Beaumont T, Zheng Z, Xia N, Ko SY, Todd JP, Rao S, Graham BS, Kwong PD.** 2013. Structure-based design of a fusion glycoprotein vaccine for respiratory syncytial virus. *Science* **342:**592–598.
10. **Swanson KA, Settembre EC, Shaw CA, Dey AK, Rappuoli R, Mandl CW, Dormitzer PR, Carfi A.** 2011. Structural basis for immunization with postfusion respiratory syncytial virus fusion F glycoprotein (RSV F) to elicit high neutralizing antibody titers. *Proc Natl Acad Sci USA* **108:**9619–9624.
11. **Bloom-Feshbach K, Alonso WJ, Charu V, Tamerius J, Simonsen L, Miller MA, Viboud C.** 2013. Latitudinal variations in seasonal activity of influenza and respiratory syncytial virus (RSV): a global comparative review. *PLoS One* **8:**e54445.
12. **Jafri HS, Ramilo O, Makari D, Charsha-May D, Romero JR.** 2007. Diagnostic virology practices for respiratory syncytial virus and influenza virus among children in the hospital setting: a national survey. *Pediatr Infect Dis J* **26:**956–958.
13. **Prifert C, Streng A, Krempl CD, Liese J, Weissbrich B.** 2013. Novel respiratory syncytial virus a genotype, Germany, 2011-2012. *Emerg Infect Dis* **19:**1029–1030.
14. **Shi T, et al, RSV Global Epidemiology Network.** 2017. Global, regional, and national disease burden estimates of acute lower respiratory infections due to respiratory syncytial virus in young children in 2015: a systematic review and modelling study. *Lancet* **390:**946–958.
15. **Walsh EE.** 2017. Respiratory syncytial virus infection: an illness for all ages. *Clin Chest Med* **38:**29–36.
16. **Nabeya D, Kinjo T, Parrott GL, Uehara A, Motooka D, Nakamura S, Nahar S, Nakachi S, Nakamatsu M, Maeshiro S, Haranaga S, Tateyama M, Tomoyose T, Masuzaki H, Horii T, Fujita J.** 2017. The clinical and phylogenetic investigation for a nosocomial outbreak of respiratory syncytial virus infection in an adult hemato-oncology unit. *J Med Virol* **89:**1364–1372.
17. **Zhu Y, Zembower TR, Metzger KE, Lei Z, Green SJ, Qi C.** 2017. Investigation of respiratory syncytial virus outbreak on an adult stem cell transplant unit by use of whole-genome sequencing. *J Clin Microbiol* **55:**2956–2963.
18. **Macartney KK, Gorelick MH, Manning ML, Hodinka RL, Bell LM.** 2000. Nosocomial respiratory syncytial virus infections: the cost-effectiveness and cost-benefit of infection control. *Pediatrics* **106:**520–526.
19. **Thorburn K, Kerr S, Taylor N, van Saene HK.** 2004. RSV outbreak in a paediatric intensive care unit. *J Hosp Infect* **57:**194–201.
20. **Caserta MT, Qiu X, Tesini B, Wang L, Murphy A, Corbett A, Topham DJ, Falsey AR, Holden-Wiltse J, Walsh EE.** 2017. Development of a global respiratory severity score for respiratory syncytial virus infection in infants. *J Infect Dis* **215:**750–756.
21. **Stein RT, Bont LJ, Zar H, Polack FP, Park C, Claxton A, Borok G, Butylkova Y, Wegzyn C.** 2017. Respiratory syncytial virus hospitalization and mortality: systematic review and meta-analysis. *Pediatr Pulmonol* **52:**556–569.
22. **Falsey AR, Hennessey PA, Formica MA, Cox C, Walsh EE.** 2005. Respiratory syncytial virus infection in elderly and high-risk adults. *N Engl J Med* **352:**1749–1759.
23. **Chemaly RF, Shah DP, Boeckh MJ.** 2014. Management of respiratory viral infections in hematopoietic cell transplant recipients and patients with hematologic malignancies. *Clin Infect Dis* **59**(Suppl 5)**:**S344–S351.
24. **Pilie P, Werbel WA, Riddell J IV, Shu X, Schaubel D, Gregg KS.** 2015. Adult patients with respiratory syncytial virus infection: impact of solid organ and hematopoietic stem cell transplantation on outcomes. *Transpl Infect Dis* **17:**551–557.
25. **Kim YJ, Guthrie KA, Waghmare A, Walsh EE, Falsey AR, Kuypers J, Cent A, Englund JA, Boeckh M.** 2014. Respiratory syncytial virus in hematopoietic cell transplant recipients: factors determining progression to lower respiratory tract disease. *J Infect Dis* **209:**1195–1204.
26. **Hynicka LM, Ensor CR.** 2012. Prophylaxis and treatment of respiratory syncytial virus in adult immunocompromised patients. *Ann Pharmacother* **46:**558–566.
27. **Sáez-Llorens X, Moreno MT, Ramilo O, Sánchez PJ, Top FH Jr, Connor EM, MEDI-493 Study Group.** 2004. Safety and pharmacokinetics of palivizumab therapy in children hospitalized with respiratory syncytial virus infection. *Pediatr Infect Dis J* **23:**707–712.
28. **Brady MT, Byington CL, Davies HD, American Academy of Pediatrics Committee on Infectious Diseases, American Academy of Pediatrics Bronchiolitis Guidelines Committee.** 2014. Updated guidance for palivizumab prophylaxis among infants and young children at increased risk of hospitalization for respiratory syncytial virus infection. *Pediatrics* **134:**415–420.
29. **Gutfraind A, Galvani AP, Meyers LA.** 2015. Efficacy and optimization of palivizumab injection regimens against respiratory syncytial virus infection. *JAMA Pediatr* **169:**341–348.
30. **Jorquera PA, Tripp RA.** 2017. Respiratory syncytial virus: prospects for new and emerging therapeutics. *Expert Rev Respir Med* **11:**609–615.
31. **DeVincenzo JP, McClure MW, Symons JA, Fathi H, Westland C, Chanda S, Lambkin-Williams R, Smith P, Zhang Q, Beigelman L, Blatt LM, Fry J.** 2015. Activity of oral ALS-008176 in a respiratory syncytial virus challenge study. *N Engl J Med* **373:**2048–2058.
32. **Shah DP, Ghantoji SS, Shah JN, El Taoum KK, Jiang Y, Popat U, Hosing C, Rondon G, Tarrand JJ, Champlin RE, Chemaly RF.** 2013. Impact of aerosolized ribavirin on mortality in 280 allogeneic haematopoietic stem cell transplant recipients with respiratory syncytial virus infections. *J Antimicrob Chemother* **68:**1872–1880.
33. **Liang B, Ngwuta JO, Surman S, Kabatova B, Liu X, Lingemann M, Liu X, Yang L, Herbert R, Swerczek J, Chen M, Moin SM, Kumar A, McLellan JS, Kwong PD, Graham BS, Collins PL, Munir S.** 2017. Improved prefusion stability, optimized codon-usage, and augmented virion packaging enhance the immunogenicity of respiratory syncytial virus (RSV) fusion protein in a vectored vaccine candidate. *J Virol* **91:**e00189-17.
34. **Graham BS.** 2017. Vaccine development for respiratory syncytial virus. *Curr Opin Virol* **23:**107–112.
35. **Glenn GM, Fries LF, Thomas DN, Smith G, Kpamegan E, Lu H, Flyer D, Jani D, Hickman SP, Piedra PA.** 2016. A randomized, blinded, controlled, dose-ranging study of a respiratory syncytial virus recombinant fusion (F) nanoparticle vaccine in healthy women of childbearing age. *J Infect Dis* **213:**411–422.
36. **Englund JA, Piedra PA, Jewell A, Patel K, Baxter BB, Whimbey E.** 1996. Rapid diagnosis of respiratory syncytial virus infections in immunocompromised adults. *J Clin Microbiol* **34:**1649–1653.
37. **Chartrand C, Tremblay N, Renaud C, Papenburg J.** 2015. Diagnostic accuracy of rapid antigen detection tests for respiratory syncytial virus infection: systematic review and meta-analysis. *J Clin Microbiol* **53:**3738–3749.
38. **Rack-Hoch AL, Laniado G, Hübner J.** 2017. Comparison of influenza and RSV diagnostic from nasopharyngeal swabs by rapid fluorescent immunoassay (Sofia system) and rapid bedside testing (BinaxNOW) vs. conventional fluorescent immunoassay in a German university children's hospital. *Infection* **45:**529–532.
39. **Somerville LK, Ratnamohan VM, Dwyer DE, Kok J.** 2015. Molecular diagnosis of respiratory viruses. *Pathology* **47:**243–249.
40. **DeVincenzo JP, Wilkinson T, Vaishnaw A, Cehelsky J, Meyers R, Nochur S, Harrison L, Meeking P, Mann A, Moane E, Oxford J, Pareek R, Moore R, Walsh E, Studholme R, Dorsett P, Alvarez R, Lambkin-Williams R.** 2010. Viral load drives disease in humans experimentally infected with respiratory syncytial virus. *Am J Respir Crit Care Med* **182:**1305–1314.

41. **Walsh EE, Peterson DR, Kalkanoglu AE, Lee FE, Falsey AR.** 2013. Viral shedding and immune responses to respiratory syncytial virus infection in older adults. *J Infect Dis* **207:**1424–1432.
42. **Bruning AHL, Leeflang MMG, Vos JMBW, Spijker R, de Jong MD, Wolthers KC, Pajkrt D.** 2017. Rapid tests for influenza, respiratory syncytial virus, and other respiratory viruses: a systematic review and meta-analysis. *Clin Infect Dis* **65:**1026–1032.
43. **Jonckheere S, Verfaillie C, Boel A, Van Vaerenbergh K, Vanlaere E, Vankeerberghen A, De Beenhouwer H.** 2015. Multicenter evaluation of BD Veritor system and RSV K-SeT for rapid detection of respiratory syncytial virus in a diagnostic laboratory setting. *Diagn Microbiol Infect Dis* **83:**37–40.
44. **Aslanzadeh J, Zheng X, Li H, Tetreault J, Ratkiewicz I, Meng S, Hamilton P, Tang YW.** 2008. Prospective evaluation of rapid antigen tests for diagnosis of respiratory syncytial virus and human metapneumovirus infections. *J Clin Microbiol* **46:**1682–1685.
45. **Elbadawi LI, Haupt T, Reisdorf E, Danz T, Davis JP.** 2015. Use and interpretation of a rapid respiratory syncytial virus antigen detection test among infants hospitalized in a neonatal intensive care unit: Wisconsin, March 2015. *MMWR Morb Mortal Wkly Rep* **64:**857.
46. **Bell JJ, Anderson EJ, Greene WH, Romero JR, Merchant M, Selvarangan R.** 2014. Multicenter clinical performance evaluation of BD Veritor™ system for rapid detection of respiratory syncytial virus. *J Clin Virol* **61:**113–117.
47. **Leland DS, Ginocchio CC.** 2007. Role of cell culture for virus detection in the age of technology. *Clin Microbiol Rev* **20:**49–78.
48. **Kanwar N, Hassan F, Nguyen A, Selvarangan R.** 2015. Head-to-head comparison of the diagnostic accuracies of BD Veritor™ system RSV and Quidel® Sofia® RSV FIA systems for respiratory syncytial virus (RSV) diagnosis. *J Clin Virol* **65:**83–86.
49. **Leonardi GP, Wilson AM, Dauz M, Zuretti AR.** 2015. Evaluation of respiratory syncytial virus (RSV) direct antigen detection assays for use in point-of-care testing. *J Virol Methods* **213:**131–134.
50. **Ivaska L, Niemelä J, Heikkinen T, Vuorinen T, Peltola V.** 2013. Identification of respiratory viruses with a novel point-of-care multianalyte antigen detection test in children with acute respiratory tract infection. *J Clin Virol* **57:** 136–140.
51. **Gunell M, Antikainen P, Porjo N, Irjala K, Vakkila J, Hotakainen K, Kaukoranta SS, Hirvonen JJ, Saha K, Manninen R, Forsblom B, Rantakokko-Jalava K, Peltola V, Koskinen JO, Huovinen P.** 2016. Comprehensive real-time epidemiological data from respiratory infections in Finland between 2010 and 2014 obtained from an automated and multianalyte mariPOC® respiratory pathogen test. *Eur J Clin Microbiol Infect Dis* **35:**405–413.
52. **Moesker FM, van Kampen JJA, Aron G, Schutten M, van de Vijver DAMC, Koopmans MPG, Osterhaus ADME, Fraaij PLA.** 2016. Diagnostic performance of influenza viruses and RSV rapid antigen detection tests in children in tertiary care. *J Clin Virol* **79:**12–17.
53. **Fong CK, Lee MK, Griffith BP.** 2000. Evaluation of R-Mix FreshCells in shell vials for detection of respiratory viruses. *J Clin Microbiol* **38:**4660–4662.
54. **Landry ML, Ferguson D.** 2000. SimulFluor respiratory screen for rapid detection of multiple respiratory viruses in clinical specimens by immunofluorescence staining. *J Clin Microbiol* **38:**708–711.
55. **Yan Y, Zhang S, Tang YW.** 2011. Molecular assays for the detection and characterization of respiratory viruses. *Semin Respir Crit Care Med* **32:**512–526.
56. **Cohen DM, Kline J, May LS, Harnett GE, Gibson J, Liang SY, Rafique Z, Rodriguez CA, McGann KM Sr, Gaydos CA, Mayne D, Phillips D, Cohen J.** 2018. Accurate PCR detection of influenza A/B and RSV using the Cepheid Xpert Flu+RSV Xpress assay in point-of-care settings: comparison to Prodesse ProFlu. *J Clin Microbiol* **56:**e01237-17.
57. **Gibson J, Schechter-Perkins EM, Mitchell P, Mace S, Tian Y, Williams K, Luo R, Yen-Lieberman B.** 2017. Multi-center evaluation of the cobas® Liat® Influenza A/B & RSV assay for rapid point of care diagnosis. *J Clin Virol* **95:**5–9.
58. **Juretschko S, Mahony J, Buller RS, Manji R, Dunbar S, Walker K, Rao A.** 2017. Multicenter clinical evaluation of the Luminex Aries Flu A/B & RSV assay for pediatric and adult respiratory tract specimens. *J Clin Microbiol* **55:** 2431–2438.
59. **Ling L, Kaplan SE, Lopez JC, Stiles J, Lu X, Tang YW.** 2018. Parallel validation of three molecular devices for simultaneous detection and identification of influenza A, B and respiratory syncytial viruses. *J Clin Microbiol* **56:**e01691-17.
60. **Salez N, Nougairede A, Ninove L, Zandotti C, de Lamballerie X, Charrel RN.** 2015. Prospective and retrospective evaluation of the Cepheid Xpert® Flu/RSV XC assay for rapid detection of influenza A, influenza B, and respiratory syncytial virus. *Diagn Microbiol Infect Dis* **81:**256–258.
61. **Hoos J, Peters RM, Tabatabai J, Grulich-Henn J, Schnitzler P, Pfeil J.** 2017. Reverse-transcription loop-mediated isothermal amplification for rapid detection of respiratory syncytial virus directly from nasopharyngeal swabs. *J Virol Methods* **242:**53–57.
62. **Reijans M, Dingemans G, Klaassen CH, Meis JF, Keijdener J, Mulders B, Eadie K, van Leeuwen W, van Belkum A, Horrevorts AM, Simons G.** 2008. RespiFinder: a new multiparameter test to differentially identify fifteen respiratory viruses. *J Clin Microbiol* **46:**1232–1240.
63. **Eboigbodin KE, Moilanen K, Elf S, Hoser M.** 2017. Rapid and sensitive real-time assay for the detection of respiratory syncytial virus using RT-SIBA®. *BMC Infect Dis* **17:**134.
64. **Peters RM, Schnee SV, Tabatabai J, Schnitzler P, Pfeil J.** 2017. Evaluation of Alere i RSV for rapid detection of respiratory syncytial virus in children hospitalized with acute respiratory tract infection. *J Clin Microbiol* **55:**1032–1036.
65. **Caliendo AM.** 2011. Multiplex PCR and emerging technologies for the detection of respiratory pathogens. *Clin Infect Dis* **52**(Suppl 4):S326–S330.
66. **Mahony J, Chong S, Merante F, Yaghoubian S, Sinha T, Lisle C, Janeczko R.** 2007. Development of a respiratory virus panel test for detection of twenty human respiratory viruses by use of multiplex PCR and a fluid microbead-based assay. *J Clin Microbiol* **45:**2965–2970.
67. **Pierce VM, Elkan M, Leet M, McGowan KL, Hodinka RL.** 2012. Comparison of the Idaho Technology FilmArray system to real-time PCR for detection of respiratory pathogens in children. *J Clin Microbiol* **50:**364–371.
68. **Rand KH, Rampersaud H, Houck HJ.** 2011. Comparison of two multiplex methods for detection of respiratory viruses: FilmArray RP and xTAG RVP. *J Clin Microbiol* **49:** 2449–2453.
69. **Tang YW, Gonsalves S, Sun JY, Stiles J, Gilhuley KA, Mikhlina A, Dunbar SA, Babady NE, Zhang H.** 2016. Clinical evaluation of the Luminex NxTAG respiratory pathogen panel. *J Clin Microbiol* **54:**1912–1914.
70. **Azadeh N, Sakata KK, Brighton AM, Vikram HR, Grys TE.** 2015. FilmArray respiratory panel assay: comparison of nasopharyngeal swabs and bronchoalveolar lavage samples. *J Clin Microbiol* **53:**3784–3787.
71. **Babady NE, Mead P, Stiles J, Brennan C, Li H, Shuptar S, Stratton CW, Tang YW, Kamboj M.** 2012. Comparison of the Luminex xTAG RVP Fast assay and the Idaho Technology FilmArray RP assay for detection of respiratory viruses in pediatric patients at a cancer hospital. *J Clin Microbiol* **50:**2282–2288.
72. **Rappo U, Schuetz AN, Jenkins SG, Calfee DP, Walsh TJ, Wells MT, Hollenberg JP, Glesby MJ.** 2016. Impact of early detection of respiratory viruses by multiplex PCR assay on clinical outcomes in adult patients. *J Clin Microbiol* **54:** 2096–2103.
73. **Rogan DT, Kochar MS, Yang S, Quinn JV.** 2017. Impact of rapid molecular respiratory virus testing on real-time decision making in a pediatric emergency department. *J Mol Diagn* **19:**460–467.

74. **Schulert GS, Lu Z, Wingo T, Tang YW, Saville BR, Hain PD.** 2013. Role of a respiratory viral panel in the clinical management of pediatric inpatients. *Pediatr Infect Dis J* **32:**467–472.
75. **Xu M, Qin X, Astion ML, Rutledge JC, Simpson J, Jerome KR, Englund JA, Zerr DM, Migita RT, Rich S, Childs JC, Cent A, Del Beccaro MA.** 2013. Implementation of FilmArray respiratory viral panel in a core laboratory improves testing turnaround time and patient care. *Am J Clin Pathol* **139:**118–123.
76. **Hawkinson D, Abhyankar S, Aljitawi O, Ganguly S, McGuirk JP, Horvat R.** 2013. Delayed RSV diagnosis in a stem cell transplant population due to mutations that result in negative polymerase chain reaction. *Diagn Microbiol Infect Dis* **75:**426–430.
77. **Barenfanger J, Drake C, Mueller T, Troutt T, O'Brien J, Guttman K.** 2001. R-Mix cells are faster, at least as sensitive and marginally more costly than conventional cell lines for the detection of respiratory viruses. *J Clin Virol* **22:**101–110.
78. **St George K, Patel NM, Hartwig RA, Scholl DR, Jollick JA Jr, Kauffmann LM, Evans MR, Rinaldo CR Jr.** 2002. Rapid and sensitive detection of respiratory virus infections for directed antiviral treatment using R-Mix cultures. *J Clin Virol* **24:**107–115.
79. **LaSala PR, Bufton KK, Ismail N, Smith MB.** 2007. Prospective comparison of R-mix shell vial system with direct antigen tests and conventional cell culture for respiratory virus detection. *J Clin Virol* **38:**210–216.
80. **Zlateva KT, Vijgen L, Dekeersmaeker N, Naranjo C, Van Ranst M.** 2007. Subgroup prevalence and genotype circulation patterns of human respiratory syncytial virus in Belgium during ten successive epidemic seasons. *J Clin Microbiol* **45:**3022–3030.
81. **Avadhanula V, Chemaly RF, Shah DP, Ghantoji SS, Azzi JM, Aideyan LO, Mei M, Piedra PA.** 2015. Infection with novel respiratory syncytial virus genotype Ontario (ON1) in adult hematopoietic cell transplant recipients, Texas, 2011-2013. *J Infect Dis* **211:**582–589.
82. **Tran DN, Pham TM, Ha MT, Tran TT, Dang TK, Yoshida LM, Okitsu S, Hayakawa S, Mizuguchi M, Ushijima H.** 2013. Molecular epidemiology and disease severity of human respiratory syncytial virus in Vietnam. *PLoS One* **8:**e45436.
83. **Taggart EW, Hill HR, Martins TB, Litwin CM.** 2006. Comparison of complement fixation with two enzyme-linked immunosorbent assays for the detection of antibodies to respiratory viral antigens. *Am J Clin Pathol* **125:**460–466.
84. **DeVincenzo JP, Hall CB, Kimberlin DW, Sánchez PJ, Rodriguez WJ, Jantausch BA, Corey L, Kahn JS, Englund JA, Suzich JA, Palmer-Hill FJ, Branco L, Johnson S, Patel NK, Piazza FM.** 2004. Surveillance of clinical isolates of respiratory syncytial virus for palivizumab (Synagis)-resistant mutants. *J Infect Dis* **190:**975–978.
85. **Oliveira DB, Iwane MK, Prill MM, Weinberg GA, Williams JV, Griffin MR, Szilagyi PG, Edwards KM, Staat MA, Hall CB, Durigon EL, Erdman DD.** 2015. Molecular characterization of respiratory syncytial viruses infecting children reported to have received palivizumab immunoprophylaxis. *J Clin Virol* **65:**26–31.
86. **Yasui Y, Yamaji Y, Sawada A, Ito T, Nakayama T.** 2016. Cell fusion assay by expression of respiratory syncytial virus (RSV) fusion protein to analyze the mutation of palivizumab-resistant strains. *J Virol Methods* **231:**48–55.
87. **Rima B, Collins P, Easton A, Fouchier R, Kurath G, Lamb RA, Lee B, Maisner A, Rota P, Wang L, Ictv Report Consortium.** 2017. ICTV Virus Taxonomy Profile: *Pneumoviridae*. *J Gen Virol* **98:**2912–2913.
88. **Amarasinghe GK, et al.** 2017. Taxonomy of the order *Mononegavirales*: update 2017. *Arch Virol* **162:**2493–2504.
89. **van den Hoogen BG, de Jong JC, Groen J, Kuiken T, de Groot R, Fouchier RA, Osterhaus AD.** 2001. A newly discovered human pneumovirus isolated from young children with respiratory tract disease. *Nat Med* **7:**719–724.
90. **Schildgen V, van den Hoogen B, Fouchier R, Tripp RA, Alvarez R, Manoha C, Williams J, Schildgen O.** 2011. Human metapneumovirus: lessons learned over the first decade. *Clin Microbiol Rev* **24:**734–754.
91. **Cox RG, Livesay SB, Johnson M, Ohi MD, Williams JV.** 2012. The human metapneumovirus fusion protein mediates entry via an interaction with RGD-binding integrins. *J Virol* **86:**12148–12160.
92. **Chang A, Masante C, Buchholz UJ, Dutch RE.** 2012. Human metapneumovirus (HMPV) binding and infection are mediated by interactions between the HMPV fusion protein and heparan sulfate. *J Virol* **86:**3230–3243.
93. **Aberle JH, Aberle SW, Redlberger-Fritz M, Sandhofer MJ, Popow-Kraupp T.** 2010. Human metapneumovirus subgroup changes and seasonality during epidemics. *Pediatr Infect Dis J* **29:**1016–1018.
94. **Lamson DM, Griesemer S, Fuschino M, St George K.** 2012. Phylogenetic analysis of human metapneumovirus from New York State patients during February through April 2010. *J Clin Virol* **53:**256–258.
95. **Zhang C, Du LN, Zhang ZY, Qin X, Yang X, Liu P, Chen X, Zhao Y, Liu EM, Zhao XD.** 2012. Detection and genetic diversity of human metapneumovirus in hospitalized children with acute respiratory infections in Southwest China. *J Clin Microbiol* **50:**2714–2719.
96. **Chow WZ, Chan YF, Oong XY, Ng LJ, Nor'E SS, Ng KT, Chan KG, Hanafi NS, Pang YK, Kamarulzaman A, Tee KK.** 2016. Genetic diversity, seasonality and transmission network of human metapneumovirus: identification of a unique sub-lineage of the fusion and attachment genes. *Sci Rep* **6:**27730.
97. **Edwards KM, Zhu Y, Griffin MR, Weinberg GA, Hall CB, Szilagyi PG, Staat MA, Iwane M, Prill MM, Williams JV, New Vaccine Surveillance Network.** 2013. Burden of human metapneumovirus infection in young children. *N Engl J Med* **368:**633–643.
98. **García-García ML, Calvo C, Rey C, Díaz B, Molinero MD, Pozo F, Casas I.** 2017. Human metapnuemovirus infections in hospitalized children and comparison with other respiratory viruses. 2005-2014 prospective study. *PLoS One* **12:**e0173504.
99. **Howard LM, Edwards KM, Zhu Y, Griffin MR, Weinberg GA, Szilagyi PG, Staat MA, Payne DC, Williams JV.** 2017. Clinical features of human metapneumovirus infection in ambulatory children aged 5-13 years. *J Pediatric Infect Dis Soc.*
100. **Owor BE, Masankwa GN, Mwango LC, Njeru RW, Agoti CN, Nokes DJ.** 2016. Human metapneumovirus epidemiological and evolutionary patterns in coastal Kenya, 2007-11. *BMC Infect Dis* **16:**301.
101. **Peiris JS, Tang WH, Chan KH, Khong PL, Guan Y, Lau YL, Chiu SS.** 2003. Children with respiratory disease associated with metapneumovirus in Hong Kong. *Emerg Infect Dis* **9:**628–633.
102. **Ebihara T, Endo R, Kikuta H, Ishiguro N, Ishiko H, Hara M, Takahashi Y, Kobayashi K.** 2004. Human metapneumovirus infection in Japanese children. *J Clin Microbiol* **42:**126–132.
103. **Byington CL, Ampofo K, Stockmann C, Adler FR, Herbener A, Miller T, Sheng X, Blaschke AJ, Crisp R, Pavia AT.** 2015. Community surveillance of respiratory viruses among families in the Utah Better Identification of Germs-Longitudinal Viral Epidemiology (BIG-LoVE) Study. *Clin Infect Dis* **61:**1217–1224.
104. **Chonmaitree T, Alvarez-Fernandez P, Jennings K, Trujillo R, Marom T, Loeffelholz MJ, Miller AL, McCormick DP, Patel JA, Pyles RB.** 2015. Symptomatic and asymptomatic respiratory viral infections in the first year of life: association with acute otitis media development. *Clin Infect Dis* **60:**1–9.
105. **Williams JV, Harris PA, Tollefson SJ, Halburnt-Rush LL, Pingsterhaus JM, Edwards KM, Wright PF, Crowe JE Jr.** 2004. Human metapneumovirus and lower respiratory tract disease in otherwise healthy infants and children. *N Engl J Med* **350:**443–450.
106. **Falsey AR, Erdman D, Anderson LJ, Walsh EE.** 2003. Human metapneumovirus infections in young and elderly adults. *J Infect Dis* **187:**785–790.
107. **Walsh EE, Peterson DR, Falsey AR.** 2008. Human metapneumovirus infections in adults: another piece of the puzzle. *Arch Intern Med* **168:**2489–2496.

108. **El Chaer F, Shah DP, Kmeid J, Ariza-Heredia EJ, Hosing CM, Mulanovich VE, Chemaly RF.** 2017. Burden of human metapneumovirus infections in patients with cancer: risk factors and outcomes. *Cancer* **123:**2329–2337.
109. **Lenahan JL, Englund JA, Katz J, Kuypers J, Wald A, Magaret A, Tielsch JM, Khatry SK, LeClerq SC, Shrestha L, Steinhoff MC, Chu HY.** 2017. Human metapneumovirus and other respiratory viral infections during pregnancy and birth, Nepal. *Emerg Infect Dis* **23:**1341–1349.
110. **Chu HY, Renaud C, Ficken E, Thomson B, Kuypers J, Englund JA.** 2014. Respiratory tract infections due to human metapneumovirus in immunocompromised children. *J Pediatric Infect Dis Soc* **3:**286–293.
111. **Scheuerman O, Barkai G, Mandelboim M, Mishali H, Chodick G, Levy I.** 2016. Human metapneumovirus (hMPV) infection in immunocompromised children. *J Clin Virol* **83:**12–16.
112. **Kamboj M, Gerbin M, Huang CK, Brennan C, Stiles J, Balashov S, Park S, Kiehn TE, Perlin DS, Pamer EG, Sepkowitz KA.** 2008. Clinical characterization of human metapneumovirus infection among patients with cancer. *J Infect* **57:**464–471.
113. **Koo HJ, Lee HN, Choi SH, Sung H, Oh SY, Shin SY, Kim HJ, Do KH.** 2018. Human metapneumovirus infection: pneumonia risk factors in solid organ transplantation patients and CT findings. *Transplantation* **102:**699–706.
114. **Fok A, Mateevici C, Lin B, Chandra RV, Chong VH.** 2015. Encephalitis-associated human metapneumovirus pneumonia in adult, Australia. *Emerg Infect Dis* **21:**2074–2076.
115. **Jeannet N, van den Hoogen BG, Schefold JC, Suter-Riniker F, Sommerstein R.** 2017. Cerebrospinal fluid findings in an adult with human metapneumovirus-associated encephalitis. *Emerg Infect Dis* **23:**370.
116. **Choi MJ, Song JY, Yang TU, Jeon JH, Noh JY, Hong KW, Cheong HJ, Kim WJ.** 2016. Acute myopericarditis caused by human metapneumovirus. *Infect Chemother* **48:**36–40.
117. **Weinreich MA, Jabbar AY, Malguria N, Haley RW.** 2015. New-onset myocarditis in an immunocompetent adult with acute metapneumovirus infection. *Case Rep Med* **2015:**814269.
118. **Shahani L, Ariza-Heredia EJ, Chemaly RF.** 2017. Antiviral therapy for respiratory viral infections in immunocompromised patients. *Expert Rev Anti Infect Ther* **15:**401–415.
119. **von Lilienfeld-Toal M, Berger A, Christopeit M, Hentrich M, Heussel CP, Kalkreuth J, Klein M, Kochanek M, Penack O, Hauf E, Rieger C, Silling G, Vehreschild M, Weber T, Wolf HH, Lehners N, Schalk E, Mayer K.** 2016. Community acquired respiratory virus infections in cancer patients: guideline on diagnosis and management by the Infectious Diseases Working Party of the German Society for Haematology and Medical Oncology. *Eur J Cancer* **67:**200–212.
120. **Ren J, Phan T, Bao X.** 2015. Recent vaccine development for human metapneumovirus. *J Gen Virol* **96:**1515–1520.
121. **Talaat KR, Karron RA, Thumar B, McMahon BA, Schmidt AC, Collins PL, Buchholz UJ.** 2013. Experimental infection of adults with recombinant wild-type human metapneumovirus. *J Infect Dis* **208:**1669–1678.
122. **Karron RA, San Mateo J, Wanionek K, Collins PL, Buchholz UJ.** 2017. Evaluation of a live attenuated human metapneumovirus vaccine in adults and children. *J Pediatric Infect Dis Soc*
123. **Richardson L, Brite J, Del Castillo M, Childers T, Sheahan A, Huang YT, Dougherty E, Babady NE, Sepkowitz K, Kamboj M.** 2016. Comparison of respiratory virus shedding by conventional and molecular testing methods in patients with haematological malignancy. *Clin Microbiol Infect* **22:**380e1–380e7.
124. **Kim S, Sung H, Im HJ, Hong SJ, Kim MN.** 2009. Molecular epidemiological investigation of a nosocomial outbreak of human metapneumovirus infection in a pediatric hemato-oncology patient population. *J Clin Microbiol* **47:**1221–1224.
125. **Degail MA, Hughes GJ, Maule C, Holmes C, Lilley M, Pebody R, Bonnet J, Bermingham A, Bracebridge S.** 2012. A human metapneumovirus outbreak at a community hospital in England, July to September 2010. *Euro Surveill* **17:**20145.
126. **Hamada N, Hara K, Matsuo Y, Imamura Y, Kashiwagi T, Nakazono Y, Gotoh K, Ohtsu Y, Ohtaki E, Motohiro T, Watanabe H.** 2014. Performance of a rapid human metapneumovirus antigen test during an outbreak in a long-term care facility. *Epidemiol Infect* **142:**424–427.
127. **Liao RS, Appelgate DM, Pelz RK.** 2012. An outbreak of severe respiratory tract infection due to human metapneumovirus in a long-term care facility for the elderly in Oregon. *J Clin Virol* **53:**171–173.
128. **DeByle C, Bulkow L, Miernyk K, Chikoyak L, Hummel KB, Hennessy T, Singleton R.** 2012. Comparison of nasopharyngeal flocked swabs and nasopharyngeal wash collection methods for respiratory virus detection in hospitalized children using real-time polymerase chain reaction. *J Virol Methods* **185:**89–93.
129. **Semple MG, Booth JA, Ebrahimi B.** 2007. Most human metapneumovirus and human respiratory syncytial virus in infant nasal secretions is cell free. *J Clin Virol* **40:**241–244.
130. **Tollefson SJ, Cox RG, Williams JV.** 2010. Studies of culture conditions and environmental stability of human metapneumovirus. *Virus Res* **151:**54–59.
131. **Chan PK, Tam JS, Lam CW, Chan E, Wu A, Li CK, Buckley TA, Ng KC, Joynt GM, Cheng FW, To KF, Lee N, Hui DS, Cheung JL, Chu I, Liu E, Chung SS, Sung JJ.** 2003. Human metapneumovirus detection in patients with severe acute respiratory syndrome. *Emerg Infect Dis* **9:**1058–1063.
132. **Sanbonmatsu-Gámez S, Pérez-Ruiz M, Lara-Oya A, Pedrosa-Corral I, Riazzo-Damas C, Navarro-Marí JM.** 2015. Analytical performance of the automated multianalyte point-of-care mariPOC® for the detection of respiratory viruses. *Diagn Microbiol Infect Dis* **83:**252–256.
133. **Jokela P, Piiparinen H, Luiro K, Lappalainen M.** 2010. Detection of human metapneumovirus and respiratory syncytial virus by duplex real-time RT-PCR assay in comparison with direct fluorescent assay. *Clin Microbiol Infect* **16:** 1568–1573.
134. **Landry ML, Cohen S, Ferguson D.** 2008. Prospective study of human metapneumovirus detection in clinical samples by use of Light Diagnostics direct immunofluorescence reagent and real-time PCR. *J Clin Microbiol* **46:**1098–1100.
135. **Hanson KE, Couturier MR.** 2016. Multiplexed molecular diagnostics for respiratory, gastrointestinal, and central nervous system infections. *Clin Infect Dis* **63:**1361–1367.
136. **Visseaux B, Collin G, Ichou H, Charpentier C, Bendhafer S, Dumitrescu M, Allal L, Cojocaru B, Desfrère L, Descamps D, Mandelbrot L, Houhou-Fidouh N.** 2017. Usefulness of multiplex PCR methods and respiratory viruses' distribution in children below 15 years old according to age, seasons and clinical units in France: a 3 years retrospective study. *PLoS One* **12:**e0172809.
137. **Fathima S, Lee BE, May-Hadford J, Mukhi S, Drews SJ.** 2012. Use of an innovative web-based laboratory surveillance platform to analyze mixed infections between human metapneumovirus (hMPV) and other respiratory viruses circulating in Alberta (AB), Canada (2009-2012). *Viruses* **4:** 2754–2765.
138. **Scheltinga SA, Templeton KE, Beersma MF, Claas EC.** 2005. Diagnosis of human metapneumovirus and rhinovirus in patients with respiratory tract infections by an internally controlled multiplex real-time RNA PCR. *J Clin Virol* **33:**306–311.
139. **Deng J, Ma Z, Huang W, Li C, Wang H, Zheng Y, Zhou R, Tang YW.** 2013. Respiratory virus multiplex RT-PCR assay sensitivities and influence factors in hospitalized children with lower respiratory tract infections. *Virol Sin* **28:**97–102.
140. **Martin ET, Kuypers J, Wald A, Englund JA.** 2012. Multiple versus single virus respiratory infections: viral load and clinical disease severity in hospitalized children. *Influenza Other Respir Viruses* **6:**71–77.
141. **Utokaparch S, Marchant D, Gosselink JV, McDonough JE, Thomas EE, Hogg JC, Hegele RG.** 2011. The relationship between respiratory viral loads and diagnosis in children presenting to a pediatric hospital emergency department. *Pediatr Infect Dis J* **30:**e18–e23.

142. **Landry ML, Ferguson D, Cohen S, Peret TC, Erdman DD.** 2005. Detection of human metapneumovirus in clinical samples by immunofluorescence staining of shell vial centrifugation cultures prepared from three different cell lines. *J Clin Microbiol* **43:**1950–1952.
143. **Tiwari A, Patnayak DP, Chander Y, Goyal SM.** 2006. Permissibility of different cell types for the growth of avian metapneumovirus. *J Virol Methods* **138:**80–84.
144. **Reina J, Ferres F, Alcoceba E, Mena A, de Gopegui ER, Figuerola J.** 2007. Comparison of different cell lines and incubation times in the isolation by the shell vial culture of human metapneumovirus from pediatric respiratory samples. *J Clin Virol* **40:**46–49.
145. **Huck B, Scharf G, Neumann-Haefelin D, Puppe W, Weigl J, Falcone V.** 2006. Novel human metapneumovirus sublineage. *Emerg Infect Dis* **12:**147–150.
146. **van den Hoogen BG, Herfst S, Sprong L, Cane PA, Forleo-Neto E, de Swart RL, Osterhaus AD, Fouchier RA.** 2004. Antigenic and genetic variability of human metapneumoviruses. *Emerg Infect Dis* **10:**658–666.
147. **Li J, Ren L, Guo L, Xiang Z, Paranhos-Baccalà G, Vernet G, Wang J.** 2012. Evolutionary dynamics analysis of human metapneumovirus subtype A2: genetic evidence for its dominant epidemic. *PLoS One* **7:**e34544.
148. **Moe N, Krokstad S, Stenseng IH, Christensen A, Skanke LH, Risnes KR, Nordbø SA, Døllner H.** 2017. Comparing human metapneumovirus and respiratory syncytial virus: viral co-detections, genotypes and risk factors for severe disease. *PLoS One* **12:**e0170200.
149. **Vicente D, Montes M, Cilla G, Perez-Yarza EG, Perez-Trallero E.** 2006. Differences in clinical severity between genotype A and genotype B human metapneumovirus infection in children. *Clin Infect Dis* **42:**e111–e113.
150. **Schuster JE, Khuri-Bulos N, Faouri S, Shehabi A, Johnson M, Wang L, Fonnesbeck C, Williams JV, Halasa N.** 2015. Human metapneumovirus infection in Jordanian children: epidemiology and risk factors for severe disease. *Pediatr Infect Dis J* **34:**1335–1341.
151. **Papenburg J, Hamelin ME, Ouhoummane N, Carbonneau J, Ouakki M, Raymond F, Robitaille L, Corbeil J, Caouette G, Frenette L, De Serres G, Boivin G.** 2012. Comparison of risk factors for human metapneumovirus and respiratory syncytial virus disease severity in young children. *J Infect Dis* **206:**178–189.
152. **Milder E, Arnold JC.** 2009. Human metapneumovirus and human bocavirus in children. *Pediatr Res* **65:**78R–83R.
153. **Hamelin ME, Boivin G.** 2005. Development and validation of an enzyme-linked immunosorbent assay for human metapneumovirus serology based on a recombinant viral protein. *Clin Diagn Lab Immunol* **12:**249–253.
154. **Sastre P, Ruiz T, Schildgen O, Schildgen V, Vela C, Rueda P.** 2012. Seroprevalence of human respiratory syncytial virus and human metapneumovirus in healthy population analyzed by recombinant fusion protein-based enzyme linked immunosorbent assay. *Virol J* **9:**130.
155. **Te Wierik MJ, Nguyen DT, Beersma MF, Thijsen SF, Heemstra KA.** 2012. An outbreak of severe respiratory tract infection caused by human metapneumovirus in a residential care facility for elderly in Utrecht, the Netherlands, January to March 2010. *Euro Surveill* **17:**20132.
156. **Biacchesi S, Skiadopoulos MH, Yang L, Murphy BR, Collins PL, Buchholz UJ.** 2005. Rapid human metapneumovirus microneutralization assay based on green fluorescent protein expression. *J Virol Methods* **128:**192–197.
157. **Vinh DC, Newby D, Charest H, McDonald J.** 2008. Evaluation of a commercial direct fluorescent-antibody assay for human metapneumovirus in respiratory specimens. *J Clin Microbiol* **46:**1840–1841.
158. **Selvaraju SB, Bambach AV, Leber AL, Patru MM, Patel A, Menegus MA.** 2014. Comparison of the Simplexa™ Flu A/B & RSV kit (nucleic acid extraction-dependent assay) and the Prodessa ProFlu+™ assay for detecting influenza and respiratory syncytial viruses. *Diagn Microbiol Infect Dis* **80:** 50–52.
159. **Alby K, Popowitch EB, Miller MB.** 2013. Comparative evaluation of the Nanosphere Verigene RV+ assay and the Simplexa Flu A/B & RSV kit for detection of influenza and respiratory syncytial viruses. *J Clin Microbiol* **51:**352–353.
160. **Steensels D, Reynders M, Descheemaeker P, Curran MD, Jacobs F, Denis O, Delforge ML, Montesinos I.** 2017. Performance evaluation of direct fluorescent antibody, Focus Diagnostics Simplexa™ Flu A/B & RSV and multi-parameter customized respiratory Taqman® array card in immunocompromised patients. *J Virol Methods* **245:**61–65.
161. **Loeffelholz MJ, Pong DL, Pyles RB, Xiong Y, Miller AL, Bufton KK, Chonmaitree T.** 2011. Comparison of the FilmArray Respiratory Panel and Prodesse real-time PCR assays for detection of respiratory pathogens. *J Clin Microbiol* **49:**4083–4088.
162. **Nijhuis RHT, Guerendiain D, Claas ECJ, Templeton KE.** 2017. Comparison of ePlex respiratory pathogen panel with laboratory-developed real-time PCR assays for detection of respiratory pathogens. *J Clin Microbiol* **55:**1938–1945.
163. **Babady NE, England MR, Jurcic Smith KL, He T, Wijetunge DS, Tang YW, Chamberland RR, Menegus M, Swierkosz EM, Jerris RC, Greene W.** 2017. Multicenter evaluation of the ePlex® respiratory pathogen panel for the detection of viral and bacterial respiratory tract pathogens in nasopharyngeal swabs. *J Clin Microbiol* **6:**01658-17.
164. **Brotons P, Henares D, Latorre I, Cepillo A, Launes C, Muñoz-Almagro C.** 2016. Comparison of NxTAG respiratory pathogen panel and Anyplex II RV16 tests for multiplex detection of respiratory pathogens in hospitalized children. *J Clin Microbiol* **54:**2900–2904.

Measles and Rubella Viruses

CAROLE J. HICKMAN AND JOSEPH P. ICENOGLE

89

MEASLES VIRUS

Taxonomy

Measles is the prototypic member of the genus *Morbillivirus* in the family *Paramyxoviridae*, and it is the only member of the genus that causes human disease (1). The members of this genus generally have restricted host ranges, indicative of long-term association with, and adaptation to, their respective zoonotic hosts. Other genus members include rinderpest virus, canine and phocine distemper viruses, peste des petits ruminants virus, and cetacean morbillivirus.

Description of the Agent

Measles virus is a pleomorphic, enveloped, nonsegmented, single-stranded, negative-sense RNA virus with a virion size ranging from 50 to 510 nm. The measles virus genome is 15,894 nucleotides in length, although occasional variation in genome length has been described (2). The linear genome contains six genes organized on the single strand of RNA in a gene order consistent with most of the paramyxoviruses, i.e., 3′-N, P, M, F, H, and L-5′. Each gene encodes a single protein except the phosphoprotein (P) gene, which also encodes two nonstructural proteins (V and C). The nucleoprotein (N) is produced first and is the most abundant protein. The N protein encapsulates both full-length minus-strand (genome) and full-length plus-strand (antigenome) RNAs.

The protein products of the P and the polymerase (L) genes interact with the full-length viral RNA and form the ribonucleoprotein complex. A membrane derived from the plasma membrane surrounds the viral nucleocapsid structures and includes the gene products from the M, F, and H genes (matrix, fusion, and hemagglutinin proteins, respectively). The F and H envelope proteins are N-linked transmembrane glycoproteins and form a multimeric complex which mediates viral entry (1). The H glycoprotein is the major target for neutralizing antibody. Entry into host cells is initiated by binding of H to one of three host cell receptors: CD46 (3), CD150 (human signaling lymphocyte activation marker [hSLAM]) (4), and nectin-4 (5). CD150 is expressed on many cells of the immune system, including lymphocytes, dendritic cells, and some macrophages (4), while CD46 is expressed on all nucleated human cells. Nectin-4 is present in adherens junctions of the respiratory epithelium (6).

Although measles virus has only a single serotype (monotypic), antigenic and genetic variability has been detected between and among wild-type viruses and vaccine viruses. Thus far, immunity to the vaccine viruses has conferred immunity to clinical disease from other circulating viruses. As an RNA virus, measles virus generates variants during replication due to the lack of proofreading capacity of RNA-dependent polymerases. This has implications for the molecular epidemiological interpretation of nucleotide differences that may be observed in viruses collected during outbreaks. The nucleotide sequence variability among wild-type viruses is most evident in the genes encoding the N and H proteins (7 to 10%), and the maximum sequence variability has been determined to reside in the last 450 nucleotides of the coding region of the N gene (~12%) (7). Based on this sequence region, a standard nomenclature has been established. For molecular epidemiologic purposes, the genotype designations are considered the operational taxonomic unit, while related genotypes are grouped by clades. The World Health Organization (WHO) currently recognizes eight clades, designated A to H. Within these clades, there are 24 recognized genotypes (8), although only seven of the genotypes have been detected during 2010 to 2015 (9). Several recent reviews (10–12) provide an overview of global measles epidemiology and genotype distribution.

Epidemiology and Transmission

Measles virus is an airborne pathogen that is transmitted via inhalation of aerosols, or respiratory droplets. Measles can also be transmitted via direct contact with infected secretions or contaminated fomites. Animal studies indicate that the initial target cells are alveolar macrophages and dendritic cells, which use CD150 for entry (13, 14). Measles virus also spreads to the skin and conjunctiva, replicating in endothelial cells, macrophages, and epithelial cells (15), which results in transportation of measles virus to regional lymph nodes. Infected immune cells then facilitate spread to both lymphoid and nonlymphoid organs. Measles is a highly contagious disease, and following exposure, up to 90% of susceptible persons develop measles (16). In the prevaccine era, more than 90% of individuals acquired measles infections before 10 years of age. The reproduction number (R_0) for measles is estimated to be 9 to 18, higher than that of other viral diseases, such as smallpox or polio.

Based on this measure of transmissibility, the herd immunity threshold necessary to interrupt measles transmission has been estimated to be between 89 and 94% (17).

In unvaccinated populations, measles causes periodic epidemics, with interepidemic periods of 2 to 5 years. These periods decrease as population size and density increase and are directly related to the availability of susceptible individuals for sustained disease transmission. In vaccinated populations, the interval between measles outbreaks increases, and sufficiently high levels of vaccination can interrupt endemic transmission. Among vaccinated populations, the age distribution is determined by which groups lack vaccine- or measles-induced immunity. In the United States, high two-dose measles vaccine coverage has been successful in stopping endemic transmission, and measles was declared to be eliminated in 2000 (18). A panel of experts was convened in 2014 to certify the maintenance of elimination of measles, of rubella, and of congenital rubella syndrome (CRS) from the Western Hemisphere (19). The length of protection afforded by natural infection or vaccination in the absence of circulating wild-type measles virus and subclinical boosting is unclear. While most recent U.S. measles cases have occurred in unvaccinated persons, a small number of cases have been observed among vaccinated and presumptively immune persons (20–25). Cases of measles among adults who received two doses of measles vaccine decades previously are concerning and may indicate that titers of vaccine-induced neutralizing antibodies are waning over time and that immune memory to measles vaccine is more limited than previously believed. Laboratory confirmation of measles in previously vaccinated individuals can be challenging, since IgM assays may give inconclusive results, and although a positive reverse transcription (RT)-PCR assay result from an appropriately timed specimen can provide confirmation, negative results may not rule out a highly suspicious case. Among these individuals, symptoms can range from classic to mild, with reduced intensity and duration of both fever and rash. In fact, laboratory testing indicated that these individuals had a heightened memory response, with high-avidity IgG and an unusually high neutralizing-antibody response (>40,000 mIU) within the first few days of rash (21–23). Suspect measles cases that present with modified symptoms may go unrecognized in the absence of a confirmed measles outbreak. While some reports have indicated that these cases pose a low transmission risk (22, 24, 26, 27), others have indicated that these cases are capable of transmission (23, 25, 28), and good public health practice would dictate that these cases be monitored to assure that contacts, particularly unvaccinated contacts, remain uninfected.

Although measles remains a formidable disease of children in many areas of the world, tremendous strides in global measles control and mortality reduction have occurred (12). Effective use of available live-attenuated measles vaccines and a variety of multidose vaccination strategies (second opportunities for vaccination) have combined to eliminate measles in many large geographic regions, including the Americas, Australia, the Scandinavian countries, and the United Kingdom (29, 30). The current global incidence of measles is 36 cases/million population, reduced from 146 cases/million in 2000 (31, 32). While incidence varies by WHO region and country, in 2015 there were 109 countries with an incidence of <5 cases/million population (31, 32). Recently, financial and logistical difficulties, combined with safety concerns and philosophical objection to vaccination, have resulted in a reemergence of measles cases in some populations with established vaccination programs (33–35). Successful achievement of measles elimination will require redoubling of political and especially financial commitments at a time when such resources are very difficult to secure. Nevertheless, the WHO recommended proceeding to the eventual global eradication of measles, if measurable progress towards reaching the regional measles elimination goals can be achieved (36). In 2012, the Measles and Rubella Initiative initiated a new Global Measles and Rubella Strategic Plan (2012–2020) that offers clear strategies for country immunization managers to achieve the 2015 and 2020 measles and rubella control and elimination goals (37).

Clinical Significance

Uncomplicated Clinical Course

Approximately 1 week to 10 days following infection, the clinical presentation begins with cough, coryza, conjunctivitis, and fever. The prodromal stage then progresses over the next 3 to 4 days, with all symptoms intensifying and the associated fever reaching as high as 105°F. Koplik's spots, pathognomonic for measles, appear on the buccal mucosa in 50 to 90% of cases 2 to 3 days before rash onset and may persist for 1 to 2 days following rash onset. These lesions are small, irregular red spots with a bluish white speck in the center. The erythematous rash appears approximately 2 weeks following infection and is first evident on the forehead or behind the ears. The rash presents as red macules 1 to 2 mm in diameter, becoming maculopapules over the next 3 days. The exanthem is usually most confluent on the face and upper body and initially blanches on pressure. By the end of the second day, the trunk and upper extremities are covered with rash, and by the third day, the lower extremities are affected. The rash resolves in the same sequence, first disappearing from the face and neck. The lesions turn brown, persist for 7 to 10 days, and are followed by a fine desquamation. In most cases, recovery is rapid and complete.

Death resulting from respiratory and neurological causes (see below) occurs in 1 of every 1,000 measles cases. The risk of death is greater for infants and adults than for children and adolescents. However, rates of death from acute measles virus infections in infants and children in developing countries, particularly malnourished populations, can approach 10%, with rates of morbidity being much higher.

Complications

Measles virus infection results in a generalized immunosuppression that may result from the depletion of memory T and B cells (38). This immunosuppression lasts from weeks to months and leads to an increased susceptibility to secondary infections, particularly among children and immunocompromised persons in developing countries (39). The most common complications associated with measles virus infection are otitis media (7 to 9%), pneumonia (1 to 6%), and diarrhea (6%). Notable CNS complications include acute disseminated encephalomyelitis and subacute sclerosing panencephalitis (SSPE). Acute disseminated encephalomyelitis occurs approximately 1 week after rash onset in 1 per 1,000 cases and is manifested clinically by seizures, lethargy, irritability, and/or coma. In the United States in the postelimination era, death resulting from respiratory or neurologic complications has occurred in 1 to 3 of every 1,000 cases.

SSPE is a progressive, inevitably fatal, late neurological complication caused by persistent measles virus infection of the CNS that occurs in approximately 1 to 4 per

10,000 measles cases (15, 40, 41), with higher rates in children <5 years of age. A recent study found even higher rates, reporting that during 1988 to 1991, the incidence of SSPE was 1:1,367 for children <5 years old and 1:609 for children <12 months old at the time of measles disease (42). Only wild-type measles virus nucleic acid sequences have been found in association with this disease, and the use of measles vaccine has largely eliminated SSPE from the United States (41, 43). The average time from natural measles virus infection to manifestations of SSPE is 7 years, and as a result, SSPE may be initially misdiagnosed. The disease characteristically involves personality changes, decreased motor and intellectual capabilities, involuntary movements, and muscular rigidity and ultimately leads to death. The virus is difficult to recover from brain specimens, requiring cocultivation or brain tissue explant techniques, yet measles virus proteins and RNA can readily be detected in brain tissue (44, 45). Patients with SSPE usually have high titers of measles virus-specific IgG antibodies in their sera and cerebrospinal fluid.

Infection during pregnancy is associated with an increased risk of spontaneous termination, fetal and neonatal complications, and prematurity, although there is no convincing evidence that maternal infection with measles virus is associated with congenital malformations.

Atypical measles syndrome occurs only in persons who have previously been vaccinated with multiple doses of formalin-killed measles vaccine and subsequently exposed to wild-type measles virus. An estimated 600,000 to 900,000 persons received the formalin-inactivated vaccine in the United States from 1963 to 1967. The syndrome was believed to result from immunopathological responses due to a combination of the Arthus reaction and delayed hypersensitivity (46). Atypical measles may be prevented by revaccinating with live measles vaccine.

Although some public concern has been raised about a possible relationship between MMR (measles, mumps, and rubella) vaccine and autism, two independent nongovernmental groups, the Institute of Medicine and the American Academy of Pediatrics, have reviewed the evidence and independently concluded that there is no credible evidence that MMR or vaccination causes autism spectrum disorder (47, 48).

In immunocompromised patients, syndromes such as giant-cell pneumonia and measles inclusion body encephalitis (MIBE) have been observed (49, 50). Measles-induced giant-cell pneumonia is usually unrecognized due to the absence of rash. It occurs almost exclusively in patients with T-cell deficiencies, such as leukemia, lymphoma, and HIV infection. Several cases have also been diagnosed following vaccination of children with severe combined-immunodeficiency syndrome (51). MIBE typically occurs within 1 year of infection or vaccination and is generally fatal. There are anecdotal reports of more severe and even fatal measles in HIV-infected patients (52, 53) and recent concern that HIV-infected patients may be at heightened risk for SSPE (54).

Collection, Transport, and Storage of Specimens

Nasopharyngeal (NP) or throat (oropharyngeal) swabs are the preferred samples for detection of measles RNA by RT-PCR or virus isolation. After collection, swabs should be transferred to 1 to 3 ml of viral transport medium and should not be allowed to dry. Measles viruses are sensitive to heat, and infectivity decreases significantly when samples are not kept cold (4 to 8°C). If possible, clinical specimens for RNA detection or virus isolation should be frozen at −70°C to preserve viral viability. If storage at −70°C is not possible, samples can be stored at −20°C. At −20°C, viral viability may be lost, but the integrity of the viral RNA should be maintained, and the RNA can be detected by RT-PCR. If −70°C or −20°C freezers are not available, it is recommended to keep the sample in the refrigerator (4°C). Samples should be transported as soon as possible following collection, and freeze-thaw cycles should be avoided. Specimens for successful molecular detection and virus isolation should be collected as soon after rash onset as possible, since the virus is present in the highest concentrations at that time. Urine samples may also contain virus, and collection of both urine and NP samples can increase the probability of detection. Measles virus is very cell associated, so if possible, the urine (10 to 50 ml) should be centrifuged at 500 × *g* for 10 minutes, preferably at 4°C (55). The sediment can be resuspended in 2 to 3 ml of sterile transport medium, tissue culture medium, or physiological buffered saline. If possible, the resuspended urine sediment should be frozen at −20°C to −70°C and shipped frozen. If facilities for processing the urine are not available, the uncentrifuged urine sample should be kept at 4°C and shipped on cold packs as soon as possible in a leakproof container. Nasal aspirates or bronchial lavage samples may also be used, and under special circumstances, whole blood, serum, brain, and skin biopsy samples may be used. Measles virus is lymphotropic, and macrophages are a known source of infectious virus during natural infection (56). Thus, peripheral blood mononuclear cells (PBMCs) are an excellent source for the isolation of measles virus. PBMCs are obtained from heparinized blood (diluted 1:3 in saline) by sedimentation through density gradients.

A blood specimen (generally 5 ml in a red-top or serum separator tube) should be collected as soon as possible upon suspicion of measles disease. The blood tube should be centrifuged to separate the serum from the clot and the serum aseptically transferred to a sterile tube. Serum specimens should be stored at 4°C and shipped on wet ice packs. A single serum specimen is sufficient in most cases (57). However, measles-specific IgM may not be detectable in serum collected in the first 72 hours after rash onset in approximately 30% of measles cases (58). To assess seroconversion following measles vaccination, paired serum specimens can be tested with IgG enzyme immunoassays or plaque reduction neutralization (PRN) tests (see below). The first specimen should be obtained prior to vaccination and the second approximately 3 to 4 weeks later, so that a rise in measles virus-specific IgG can be measured. Serum samples should be stored at −20°C, but antibody is stable for extended periods at 4°C. Samples for IgM determinations should not be frozen and thawed more than five times. In addition, spinal fluid samples should be obtained if neurological complications are present or suspected. For immunofluorescence assays (IFAs), slides of respiratory specimens should be fixed in cold acetone for 2 minutes and stored at 4°C.

Alternatives to serum specimen collection for the diagnosis of measles include the use of gingival crevicular or oral fluid (OF) and the use of blood spots on filter paper. OF samples have been used both for detection of measles virus-specific IgM and IgG and for detection of hepatitis, rubella, mumps, and other infections (59–61). This specimen collection method is now used almost exclusively for routine measles, rubella, and mumps laboratory surveillance in the United Kingdom (62). The use of OF samples has appeal because the collection method is noninvasive and collection does not require a medical professional. The specimens can also be used for detection of rubella virus, but the lack of a sufficiently sensitive rubella IgM test limits its usage for rubella. OF samples do not require processing in the field and offer the opportunity to detect measles virus-specific IgM for case confirmation and nucleic acids for molecular characterization (63, 64). The overall cost of OF testing is similar to that of traditional serologic testing, but transportation costs tend to be lower, since OF specimens do not generally require a cold chain. Commercial serological assays performed with OF samples can result in heightened background reactivity and decreased sensitivity, and cold chain issues remain a problem with OF specimens in warmer climates. Devices (such as OraSure) containing IgM-stabilizing preservatives should be avoided if molecular testing is to be performed, as these additives inhibit nucleic acid amplification.

Like OF samples, blood spots collected on filter paper do not require processing in the field, and maintaining a cold chain is not necessary. They can be used to test for rubella as well as for measles, and they can be used for molecular characterization of the measles virus genome (65–68). In addition, the eluted serum from blood spots can likely be tested in commercially available measles-specific enzyme-linked immunosorbent assays (ELISAs) without the loss of sensitivity and specificity (65, 69, 70), making this technology very attractive for widespread use. Although still considered an invasive technique, the finger-stick method of sample collection is often more acceptable to parents than phlebotomy (71).

An evaluation and recommendations for the use of dried blood spots (DBS) and OF as diagnostic samples for measles and rubella were published by the WHO in 2008 and endorsed the use of both methods as viable options for measles and rubella surveillance in all regions, especially where patients might resist venipuncture or where special challenges exist with specimen storage or transportation (63). The variations in testing formats and specimen types used in seroprevalence studies on measles and rubella were reviewed recently (72, 73).

Direct Examination

Cytologic Examination

Characteristic cytopathic effects (CPE) of measles virus infection include multinucleated cells and cellular inclusions (intracytoplasmic and intranuclear). Slides can be stained with either Wright stain or hematoxylin and eosin to observe the presence of giant cells with overlapping nuclei (Warthin-Finkeldey giant cells). Tissue samples may be fixed in 10% formalin, embedded in paraffin, sectioned, and then stained with hematoxylin and eosin. Staining of tissue specimens with monoclonal antibodies (see below) to the measles virus N protein can be used for the diagnosis of giant-cell pneumonia and MIBE (74). Verification of isolation of measles virus is typically carried out using immunofluorescence, immunohistochemistry, or RT-PCR.

Immunofluorescence Assay

Measles virus can be detected using an immunofluorescent antibody to examine clinical specimens as well as cell cultures infected with clinical material. The standard assay uses a commercially available monoclonal antibody to the N protein of measles virus and fluorescein-conjugated goat anti-mouse antiserum (see "Confirmation of Measles Virus Isolation" below). Nasopharyngeal aspirates or swabs from the posterior nasopharynx are the specimens of choice and can be diluted in sterile saline solution and centrifuged to pellet the cells. The cell pellets are then washed several times with sterile saline before being applied to a glass slide and fixed in cold acetone for 10 min at −20°C (75, 76). When the measles N monoclonal antibody is used, specific granular or punctate fluorescent staining restricted to the cytoplasm is often observed in multinucleated giant cells.

Nucleic Acid Detection Techniques

Standard RT-PCR and real-time reverse transcriptase quantitative PCR (rRT-qPCR) assays can provide laboratory confirmation of infection in a variety of clinical specimens and infected cells (77, 78). While the collection of both serologic and molecular specimens is recommended to provide the best opportunity of confirming a measles case, molecular detection methods can be more advantageous under certain circumstances. For example, RT-PCR is advantageous for measles case confirmation where IgM testing is compromised by the concurrent or recent use of measles-containing vaccine as part of an outbreak response or in settings of recent vaccine distribution, such as supplemental immunization activities (79). Likewise, molecular detection methods are recommended when genetic characterization of the virus is required to map transmission patterns or link or unlink outbreak cases. Detection of viral RNA can also be useful to classify measles cases from low-prevalence and postelimination settings, since the rate of false positives is lower than that observed for IgM testing. RT-PCR amplification and nucleotide sequencing of the last 450 nucleotides of the coding region of the N protein gene are used for genotype analysis. Genotyping is the only diagnostic method that can distinguish between a vaccine reaction and a wild-type measles virus infection, and a rapid identification method was recently published (80). The use of RT-PCR for case confirmation has increased in recent years and, if specimens are collected early after rash onset, can provide increased sensitivity and specificity compared to serologic testing.

Isolation and Identification of Measles Virus

Measles virus can be isolated from the conjunctiva, nasopharynx, and blood during the latter part of the prodromal period and during the early stages of rash development. Although virus has been isolated from the urine as late as 4 to 7 days after rash onset, viremia generally clears 2 to 3 days after rash onset in parallel with the appearance of antibody. Thus, virus can be most readily isolated within a period from 2 to 4 days prior to rash onset to about 4 days after rash onset. Cell cultures and lines, such as B95a, primary monkey kidney, and Vero cells, can be used for measles virus isolation. However, to improve laboratory safety and efficiency, the Vero/hSLAM cell line is now widely used for measles virus isolation and has been adopted for use in most laboratories in the WHO Global Measles and Rubella Laboratory Network (LabNet). These cells were developed by transfecting the Vero cell line with a plasmid carrying the gene for hSLAM and are permissive for growth of both measles and rubella (81). The hSLAM molecule has been shown to be a cell surface receptor for both wild-type and laboratory-adapted strains of measles. Testing conducted to date indicates that the sensitivity of Vero/hSLAM cells for isolation of measles virus is equivalent to that of B95a cells. Vero/hSLAM cells also express the simian CD46 molecule.

Confirmation of Measles Virus Isolation

Confirmation of isolation is most often achieved by IFA detection using a monoclonal antibody to detect the N protein or other internal antigens in measles virus in infected cells. The infected cells are fixed onto a microscope slide.

Binding of the measles virus-specific antibody is detected using a goat anti-mouse immunoglobulin antibody that is conjugated to fluorescein isothiocyanate. IFA test kits are available from a number of commercial sources. It is also possible to configure an indirect IFA without using a commercial kit. Most monoclonal antibodies to the N protein perform well in the IFA procedure described above. Monoclonal antibodies directed against other viral proteins such as the hemagglutinin and fusion proteins may recognize conformational epitopes that are not stable after acetone fixation. When an in-house IFA is being configured, the appropriate working dilutions of monoclonal antibody and fluorescein isothiocyanate-labeled conjugate have to be determined by experimental titration.

Genotyping

Amplicon sequencing and phylogenetic analysis (genotyping) of the last 450 nucleotides of the measles N gene have proven extremely useful in suggesting the possible source of virus involved in outbreaks, tracking transmission pathways during outbreaks, and differentiating between vaccine and wild-type strains of measles (32, 82, 83). Molecular testing is performed by the CDC and some state public health laboratories, and in 2013, four vaccine-preventable disease (VPD) reference centers (RCs) were created to provide enhanced capacity for VPD testing in a shared service model. Four public health laboratories were chosen through competitive procedures (California Department of Public Health, Minnesota Department of Health, New York State Department of Health [Wadsworth Center], and Wisconsin State Laboratory of Hygiene) and conduct testing, using CDC assays, for four viral and three bacterial diseases, including measles and rubella. The use of these reference centers has increased, and by late 2016, 51 state or county health laboratories had been enrolled and the majority of molecular testing for measles had transitioned from the CDC to RCs. Currently, RCs send test results to CDC by HL7 2.5.1 messaging but report results to the submitter by other methods (phone, fax, or encrypted email) (84), and results are then communicated by the submitting laboratory to the jurisdictional epidemiologists.

Genetic characterization of wild-type measles viruses provides a means to study the transmission pathways of the virus; molecular epidemiology in conjunction with conventional case investigation and epidemiology has permitted the linking of imported cases to their foreign sources. Genotyping is also an essential indicator for establishing and maintaining the elimination status of the United States and the region of the Americas (19). Laboratory-based surveillance for measles and rubella, including genetic characterization of wild-type viruses, is performed throughout the world by the WHO LabNet, which serves 191 of 193 member countries in all WHO regions. In particular, the genetic data can help confirm the sources of virus or suggest a source for unknown-source cases as well as establish links, or the lack thereof, between various cases and outbreaks. Virologic surveillance has helped to document the interruption of transmission of endemic measles in some regions. Thus, molecular characterization of measles viruses has provided a valuable tool for measuring the effectiveness of measles control programs, and virologic surveillance needs to be expanded in all areas of the world and conducted during all phases of measles control (19, 82, 85, 86). It must be emphasized, however, that conventional epidemiology and case investigation must be done hand in hand with the molecular studies to achieve the optimal outcome of this approach.

Serologic Diagnosis

The most widely used laboratory method for the confirmation of clinically diagnosed measles is a serum-based IgM ELISA. Commercial IgM assays are available and in use worldwide by public health, clinical, and commercial laboratories. ELISA was the primary confirmatory test used by the laboratory network of the Pan American Health Organization during the measles control and elimination phases throughout the Americas. The WHO LabNet has also recommended use of the IgM ELISA for laboratory confirmation of measles (87). As regions enter the elimination phase, measles cases become more difficult to diagnose and ELISA results become less reliable. The use of RT-PCR for confirmation has become a routine adjunct for the United States, and in other elimination settings, molecular diagnosis has largely replaced IgM testing due to the lower positive predictive value associated with low disease prevalence. Many regional reference laboratories have also implemented IgG testing and in some cases IgG avidity testing to supplement surveillance and case classification (82, 88). The ELISAs can be done using a single serum specimen, are relatively rapid (2 to 6 h), are simple to perform, and can be used to diagnose acute measles virus infection from the time of rash onset until at least 4 weeks after rash onset. Thus, the ELISA fulfills all of the basic criteria for the accurate, effective, and efficient diagnosis of measles. Both indirect and IgM capture formats have been used (89–91). Though the IgM capture assay format is often regarded as more sensitive than the indirect format, comparative studies of some commercial indirect formatted ELISA kits have demonstrated that the two formats have equivalent sensitivities and specificities (92, 93).

Traditional antibody tests, such as hemagglutination inhibition, PRN, and ELISA, have been used extensively in the serologic confirmation of the clinical diagnosis of measles. However, because of the availability of sensitive and specific commercial kits, ELISA has become the most widely used test format. Commercial IgM and IgG ELISAs are used in confirming clinical diagnosis as well as monitoring measles control programs. Although limited in number, a few available IgG assay kits were found to have sensitivities and specificities that compared favorably with those of PRN (94–96). In general, IgG measurements by ELISA or similar assays have been used for surveillance (antibody prevalence) studies, while PRN has been reserved for studies interested in questions regarding immunity. Most laboratories have trained personnel and are already equipped to run ELISAs.

Commercial laboratories and some large clinical centers performing large-volume testing of measles (and rubella) specimens require high-throughput automated platforms in conjunction with ELISA, chemiluminescent assays, and Luminex immunoassays (97). Although the formats for some of the assays may differ from those of the traditional ELISAs, their performance characteristics and rapid turnaround times make them viable alternatives for large surveillance, seroprevalence, and seroconversion studies (97, 98).

Standard ELISAs

The detection of specific anti-measles virus IgM antibodies by ELISA in serum is the standard method for rapid laboratory confirmation of measles. These microtiter plate assays have various configurations, but in general, serum antibody bound to immobilized antigen is detected with an enzyme-labeled antibody. ELISAs are fast, reliable, and relatively inexpensive and can be adapted for high-throughput use (99, 100). ELISAs using recombinant-expressed

N protein in both capture and indirect formats have high sensitivity and specificity compared to those of other commercial ELISAs (90, 91). Indirect ELISAs are frequently used to detect measles anti-measles virus IgG antibodies to determine immune status but can also be used, when necessary, to detect a 4-fold rise in titer to confirm measles infection.

IgG Avidity Assays

IgG avidity is an indicator of the overall binding strength of IgG antibodies elicited by an antigen. Low-avidity antibodies are synthesized at first exposure to an antigen, and over time (weeks to months), high-avidity antibodies are selected through somatic hypermutation, resulting in high-avidity, antigen-specific IgG. Both in-house and commercial ELISAs to determine the avidity of IgG antibodies to measles virus have been developed (95, 101, 102). These avidity differences can be detected by using protein denaturants, i.e., 6 to 8 M urea or diethylamine (103), in the washing step of the indirect ELISA for measles virus IgG. An avidity index is then calculated by comparing the optical densities obtained with and without the denaturing agent in the wash buffer. These tests can be used to differentiate between primary and secondary responses to vaccination and to natural infection (24, 104). Measles avidity assays are limited in their use and can be used only to rule in a case of measles. Nevertheless, this can be very useful in elimination settings where IgM assays yield indeterminate or questionable results that appear to conflict with clinical presentation and patient history.

PRN

The PRN assay, which measures neutralizing antibodies directed against the surface glycoproteins of measles virus, is more sensitive and specific than hemagglutination inhibition or ELISA (105). Since functional neutralizing antibodies are detected, the PRN assay provides the best serologic correlate for the assessment of immune protection (106, 107). However, the PRN test is not practical for routine serologic diagnosis because it is very labor-intensive, requires paired serum samples, and takes 5 to 7 days to complete. To perform the assay, test serum is diluted (2-fold or 4-fold) in microtiter trays, and a specified number of virus particles are added to each well and incubated to allow the antibody to react with the virus. The serum-virus mixture is then added to tissue culture plates containing confluent Vero cell monolayers and incubated for an hour. The inoculum is removed, and plates are covered with carboxymethyl cellulose to prevent the virus from spreading indiscriminately. Following a 4-day incubation period, plates are stained and plaques are counted. The dilution of serum required to reduce the number of plaques by 50% is the neutralizing antibody titer. A fluorescence-based plaque reduction microneutralization assay for measles virus immunity has been developed and used to evaluate measles immune status among specimens from a large observational study (108). In comparison to standard plaque neutralization assays, these types of assays permit higher-throughput processing of small quantities of serum specimens and are more amenable for use in large serosurveys for assessing immune status.

As mentioned above, laboratory confirmation of measles in vaccinated individuals can be challenging, since IgM may be transient and viral RNA may be less abundant. High concentrations (PRN titer, >40,000) of measles neutralizing antibody have been observed among confirmed measles cases with high-avidity IgG (21–23), and this biomarker can be used to classify clinical measles cases with previous vaccination or disease history. Such cases are infrequent but do occur and were identified during several recent outbreaks of measles (20, 24, 25, 33). In the United States, approximately 8 to 16% of measles cases reported from 2012 to 2015 occurred in vaccinated individuals. IgG avidity testing and PRN testing in combination can be used when case classification requires additional methods to confirm measles infection, usually when the result obtained for IgM is suspected of being a false negative or a false positive and RT-PCR testing was not performed.

Evaluation, Interpretation, and Reporting of Results

Evaluation and interpretation of measles diagnostic results can be complicated, particularly in measles elimination settings. Measles virus infection can be diagnosed by a positive serologic test result for measles IgM antibody, a significant increase in measles IgG antibody concentration in paired acute- and convalescent-phase serum specimens, or isolation of measles virus or identification of measles virus RNA (by RT-PCR assay) from clinical specimens, such as urine, blood, or throat or nasopharyngeal secretions.

Serologic tests can result in false-negative results when serum specimens are collected too early with respect to rash onset. For example, the CDC capture IgM assay, which has a sensitivity and specificity equivalent to those of commercial ELISAs, has been shown to detect IgM in only 77% of true measles cases within the first day of rash onset (109). In addition, measles IgM among previously vaccinated persons suspected of having measles may be muted or fleeting and therefore not detected. Since IgM tests are not 100% specific, false positives will also occur, particularly in elimination settings. Cross-reaction with other agents causing febrile rash illness occurs; parvovirus B19, enteroviruses, or human herpesvirus 6 can give a false-positive result (overall rate of about 4%) when tested in measles IgM ELISAs and vice versa (110, 111). False-positive tests due to the presence of rheumatoid factor (RF) can also occur. Indirect ELISAs appear to be more affected by RF than IgM capture assays. RF is an IgM class immunoglobulin that reacts with IgG and is produced as a result of some viral and autoimmune diseases. Immune complexes may form that contain test antigen-specific IgG and RF IgM. By virtue of the IgG binding to the viral antigen, the IgM component of the RF immune complex is recognized and can result in a falsely positive test. Similar false-positive results can occur in capture assays but appear to be enhanced by the presence of high levels of both antigen-specific antibody and RF (89). Lastly, patients with throat or ear infections occasionally develop a rash following administration of antibiotics. Subsequent serologic specimens sent for measles IgM testing may result in a false-positive test.

The positive predictive values of the ELISAs when disease prevalence is low also become a factor in interpretation. This situation occurs in countries that have eliminated endemic measles but remain vigilant in performing case-based surveillance of rash illnesses. In these geographic regions, both measles IgM and IgG ELISAs are performed on serum specimens from suspected cases due to high vaccine-induced seroprevalence. In this setting, if the IgG test is positive and the IgM test is negative, the case is usually discarded (depending upon the timing of serum collection). In some rare instances, previously vaccinated persons may develop measles, although many of these do have an IgM response (21, 22). There is also evidence that case contacts that have a resident IgG response, due either to a history of natural infection or to vaccination, may develop

TABLE 1 Interpretation of measles ELISA results

ELISA result		Infection history	Current infection	Comment(s)
IgM	IgG			
+	+ or −	Not previously vaccinated, no history of measles	Recent first MCV[a]	Seroconversion,[b] postvaccination; low-avidity IgG, if present
+	+ or −	Not vaccinated, no history of measles	Wild-type measles virus	Seroconversion,[b] classic measles; low-avidity IgG, if present
+	+ or −	Previously vaccinated, primary vaccine failure	Recent second MCV vaccination	Seroconversion,[b] postvaccination; low-avidity IgG confirms primary failure, if present
−	+	Previously vaccinated, IgG positive	Recent second MCV vaccination	IgG level may stay the same or increase; high-avidity IgG
+/−	+	Previously vaccinated, IgG positive	Wild-type measles virus	Symptoms range from classic to mild with modified rash and few symptoms[c]; high-avidity IgG; may have PRN titer of >40,000[b]
+	+	Recently vaccinated	Exposed to wild-type measles virus	Cannot distinguish if vaccine or wild-type virus infection; evaluate on epidemiological grounds[d]
+ or −	+	Distant history of measles	Wild-type measles virus	May have few or no symptoms[d]; if clinically compatible, may have been misdiagnosed initially

[a]MCV, measles virus-containing vaccine.
[b]IgG level depends on timing of specimen collection.
[c]Rare occurrence.
[d]If result is IgM negative, it is helpful to rule out wild-type measles virus infection.

a secondary IgG or an IgM response to currently circulating virus (112, 113). The IgM is generally fleeting and weakly positive and, except for rare instances, should not be a source of diagnostic confusion (79).

Table 1 summarizes the possible interpretations of ELISA results. It should be emphasized that the vast majority of serum specimens submitted for serology yield a test result that is easily interpretable. However, as mentioned earlier, the current CDC *Manual for the Surveillance of Vaccine Preventable Diseases* (114) strongly encourages the collection of both blood and respiratory specimens when persons with suspected measles cases first visit the health care provider. Additionally, laboratorians should be provided with as much clinical and epidemiological information as possible to aid in the final interpretation of the test result(s).

Both rRT-PCR and conventional, endpoint RT-PCR can be used to detect measles virus RNA in a clinical sample to provide laboratory confirmation of infection. Measles rRT-PCR assays are typically more sensitive than the endpoint RT-PCR assays. In general, the endpoint assay is used to amplify the region of the measles genome required to determine the genotype. In elimination settings, it is increasingly important to develop and use molecular tests, because false-positive RT-PCR results rarely occur. Negative RT-PCR results do not rule out a case of measles, since successful detection depends on timing of specimen collection and the quality of the clinical sample. Previously vaccinated persons may have less virus present and therefore shed less virus for a shorter period of time.

Moreover, genomic regions selected for amplification in measles virus RT-qPCR assays do not distinguish between wild-type and vaccine viruses and therefore will be of limited utility in many outbreak settings where vaccine is in use to control the outbreak. The utilization of conventional RT-PCR coupled with nucleotide sequencing and genotyping as confirmatory testing for rRT-PCR is strongly advised. Genotyping will distinguish whether a person has a wild-type measles virus infection or a rash caused by a recent measles vaccination. A rapid identification method has recently been developed (80). Measles virus genotyping can also help establish which foreign country may be the source of an imported U.S. case, since different genotypes circulate in different countries. However, genotyping alone is not sufficient, since each genotype can circulate in multiple countries and even in different regions of the world. Epidemiological information should also be reviewed and considered when investigators are determining which country may be the source of an imported U.S. case.

As with RT-PCR, the interpretation of negative cell culture results should be made with caution, since many factors influence the outcome. Some of the most important considerations include the timing of sample collection, transportation to the laboratory, preparation for culture, and finally, and probably most importantly, the cell culture system used for virus isolation.

RUBELLA VIRUS

Taxonomy

A number of small, enveloped viruses having the same overall genetic organization and replication strategy are grouped into the family *Togaviridae*, which consists of the genus *Rubivirus*, containing only rubella virus, and the genus *Alphavirus*, containing about 25 other viruses, all of which are transmitted by arthropods (e.g., Western equine encephalitis virus). Rubella virus has a restricted host range, and humans appear to be the only species in which rubella virus circulates.

Description of the Agent

Rubella virus virions are particles about 70 nm in diameter that are composed of a core surrounded by a lipid envelope. The core consists of the positive-strand RNA genome (~9,760 nucleotides) and the virus protein C. The viral envelope contains two viral glycoproteins, E1 and E2 (115). The viral RNA replicates in the cytoplasm of infected cells, with nonstructural proteins being translated from the 5′ two-thirds of the genomic RNA and the structural proteins being translated from a subgenomic RNA which is a copy of the 3′ one-third of the genomic RNA. New virions are produced when genomic RNA, the E1 glycoprotein, the E2 glycoprotein, and the C protein assemble at cellular membranes (116, 117).

Rubella viruses currently circulating in the world contain RNAs that differ sufficiently that two clades of rubella viruses, differing by about 10% in the nucleotide sequence, have so far been identified (118, 119). Groups of related viruses within the clades have been classified as genotypes. At present, 12 genotypes and one provisional genotype of rubella viruses have been recognized (120). There is sufficient subgenotype clustering of rubella virus sequences to allow lineages to be defined, although a formal nomenclature for these has not been adopted (121). Only minor immunologic differences exist among circulating viruses. Immunity to one rubella virus has so far proved sufficient to protect against clinical disease caused by other known rubella viruses.

Epidemiology and Transmission

Rubella virus was not isolated until 1962, largely because a specific cell morphology for infected cells is difficult to identify in tissue culture (122, 123). Introduction of rubella vaccine in the United States (licensed in 1969), mostly through childhood immunization, immediately broke the 6- to 9-year epidemic cycle of rubella. The last major U.S. rubella epidemic was in 1964 to 1965, when approximately 20,000 CRS cases and 2,100 neonatal deaths occurred (124). Rubella is less infectious than measles, and a population immunity of 87.5% in the United States is accepted as eliminating significant endemic transmission (125). The combined MMR vaccine was recommended for the United States in 1972. Rubella and CRS have been eliminated in the United States; for example, from 2004 to 2012, only 79 cases of rubella and six cases of CRS were reported in the United States (19, 126). Most mothers of children with CRS were born in countries without rubella immunization programs or with recently organized programs (127). Occasional outbreaks of rubella in some U.S. populations did not spread to undervaccinated populations, suggesting that herd immunity has been protective (128). Indigenous rubella and CRS have been eliminated not only from the United States but also from the Americas. The global Measles and Rubella Strategic Plan (2012–2020) includes goals to eliminate rubella and CRS in at least two WHO regions by 2015 and at least five WHO regions by 2020 (3, 4, 129–131). Despite the possibility of worldwide rubella eradication, rubella remains endemic in many countries, and about 100,000 CRS cases occur annually in the world (132). Infant deaths among CRS cases can be as high as 30% (133, 134). Postnatal transmission of rubella virus is often by close contact with an infected individual, such as occurs in correctional institutions or day care centers.

The safety of the live rubella virus vaccine strains most widely used (RA 27/3) is well documented (135). A recent summary indicated only 1 of 833 infants born to rubella-susceptible mothers who were inadvertently vaccinated after conception was born with abnormalities consistent with CRS (136). However, a small theoretical risk remains. Thus, the Advisory Committee on Immunization Practices recommends avoiding pregnancy after receipt of rubella-containing vaccine for 28 days (16)

Clinical Significance

Rubella (German measles, or 3-day measles) was first described in the 18th century and was accepted as a disease independent of measles and scarlet fever in 1881 (137). Postnatal rubella is characterized by an acute onset and generalized maculopapular rash with mild fever (greater than 99°F) and may include arthritis or arthralgia (mostly in postpubertal females), lymphadenopathy (specifically postauricular and suboccipital nodes), and conjunctivitis. Because disease caused by rubella virus is mild, about 50% of postnatal rubella cases are not diagnosed clinically. In 1941, N. McAlister Gregg first recognized that cataracts in children followed maternal rubella during gestation (138). The association between congenital rubella and a spectrum of significant birth defects, including sensorineural hearing loss, cardiovascular abnormalities, cataracts, congenital glaucoma, and meningoencephalitis, is now accepted. Rubella virus is now recognized as the most potent infectious teratogenic agent yet identified (139).

When rubella occurs in a pregnant woman in the first 11 weeks of gestation, there is a high likelihood of a defect(s) in the infant (about 90%). After 18 weeks, the likelihood of birth defects is much lower, although the infant may still be born with rubella virus infection. Congenital rubella infection (CRI) refers to infants born with rubella virus infection with or without birth defects. Note that by definition, CRS requires a live birth; thus, the full effect of *in utero* rubella infection is underrepresented by CRS; i.e., fetal deaths are not counted as CRS. The current understanding of pathogenesis of CRS is that during viremia, the virus establishes persistent infection in the placenta and then crosses the placenta (in early gestation, this is an ineffective barrier to infection) to infect the differentiating cells of the fetus (140). Since the fetus is incapable of mounting an immune response and transplacental transfer of maternal IgG is blocked during the first trimester, fetal infection often results in viral persistence in multiple organs in the fetus until term and then in infants. Different, multiple cell types can be affected, including endothelial cells, neurons, cardiac and interstitial fibroblasts, and epithelial cells of lungs, kidneys, and ciliary body of the eye. Rubella infection of each cell type is consistent with abnormalities which have been identified in patients with CRS. The congenital abnormalities arise from the direct effects of rubella virus on infected cells as well as from the placenta damage and vascular insufficiency (general growth retardation and neurodegenerative damage). Persistent infection may result in clinical problems presenting later in life, possibly due to direct damage, such as in late-onset deafness, or because of immunopathological mechanisms, such as in pneumonitis. CRI results in both shedding of virus and IgM antibodies in the neonate. Diagnosis is based on detection of rubella virus (RT-PCR or virus culture) or rubella virus-specific IgM in such patients. If congenital defects characteristic of CRS are not present, the infant is diagnosed as having CRI only. The clinical definition of CRS is standardized. Good suspect CRS case identification is crucial to effective CRS surveillance, but laboratory confirmation of rubella virus infection in the newborn by either serologic or virus detection techniques is also critical, especially when only a single defect presents, since the defects characteristic of CRS can occur for other reasons (141).

Collection, Transport, and Storage of Specimens

The measles section of this chapter contains details on sample collection which are not repeated here. Although specimens are collected in the same manner for both diseases, there are important differences in optimal specimen timing, the amount of virus that is present, and storage. Clinical specimens for culture of rubella virus are usually throat swabs or nasopharyngeal secretions diluted into transport medium (e.g., Culturette collection and transport devices).

TABLE 2 Timing of biological markers of rubella virus infection[a]

Diagnostic criterion	Convenient time when many cases are positive (%)	Example of a time when >90% of cases are positive	Approx time for 50% decline[b]
Postnatal rubella			
Virus in throat[c]	Day of rash (90)	2 days before rash	4 days after rash
IgM in serum by ELISA[c]	Day of rash (50)	5 days after rash	6 wk after rash
IgG in serum by ELISA	3 days after rash (50)	8 days after rash	Lifetime
Virus in blood by culture[d]	Day of rash (50)	5 days before rash	1 day after rash
CRS[e]			
Virus in throat[c]	At birth (almost all)	2 wk after birth	3 mo of age
IgM in serum by ELISA	At birth (80)	1 mo of age	6 mo of age
IgG in serum by ELISA[f]			

[a]Times and percentages given are approximate and are meant to guide typical specimen collection. Percentages vary depending on the sensitivity of the assay used. Note that the times listed in the third column were chosen to help guide specimen collection and may not be the earliest time when >90% of cases are positive.

[b]After the maximum number of cases are positive for a given criterion, the approximate time for 50% of cases to become negative.

[c]Alternative specimens, OMT and DBS, have been evaluated for detection of virus (OMT) and IgM (OMT and DBS). See references 63, 64, 143, and 144.

[d]Data taken from reference 164.

[e]Information given is for fetal infection in the first trimester.

[f]Declining levels of maternal IgG and the developing IgG response in a CRS patient lead to high (steady) or increasing IgG levels in the CRS patient through the first year of life.

The virus can also be isolated from a number of other specimens, including cataract tissue and urine (provided that pH is controlled) (112). Specimens for virus detection should be stored at 4°C for short periods (days) or at −70°C for longer periods (weeks); virions lose infectivity at higher temperatures (e.g., 37°C). Virions are rapidly inactivated by mild heat (56°C), detergents, or lipid solvents. Rubella virus-specific IgG can be detected in urine (142). Specimens for serology or culture can be transported by standard methods (e.g., overnight carrier) at 4°C. Alternative specimens such as DBS and oral mucosal transudate (OMT) have been shown to be adequate for surveillance of rubella using IgM detection (DBS and OMT) and virus detection (OMT) (63–65, 143–145). Two caveats should be considered if these alternative specimens are used. First, diagnostic kits are usually not approved by FDA for use with DBS; second, low IgM levels in OMT necessitate the use of highly sensitive detection assays.

The timing of specimen collection is important in postnatal rubella. Rubella virus-specific IgM is the laboratory diagnostic criterion typically used for rubella, but about 50% of rubella cases are IgM negative on the day of rash onset (see Table 2 and related text below). Since postnatal rubella is a mild disease of short duration, special effort may be required to obtain a serum sample 5 to 7 days after the onset of rash, when most rubella patients are strongly IgM positive and before urgency in the patient subsides. Patients with CRS are IgM and virus positive for months; therefore, timing is less critical for these patients.

Direct Examination

Nucleic Acid Detection Techniques

Amplification of rubella virus RNA directly from a clinical specimen using RT-PCR can be used to determine if a patient is infected with rubella virus. Not all RT-PCR protocols are sufficiently sensitive to be used directly with clinical specimens. Assays that can reliably detect 3 to 10 copies of rubella virus RNA are sufficiently sensitive, e.g., most real-time assays. Nested RT-PCR protocols, although difficult to maintain, usually meet this criterion (143, 146, 147).

Many postnatal rubella cases are IgM negative before 4 to 5 days after the onset of rash, and direct detection of viral RNA is the most sensitive test during this time period (143). For example, on the day of rash onset, direct detection of rubella virus RNA by a real-time assay will confirm about twice as many suspected rubella cases as commercial IgM ELISAs. No standard real-time or RT-PCR protocol for detection of viral RNA has been established, and there are currently a number of such tests being used.

Isolation and Identification of the Virus

Growth of rubella virus from clinical specimens can be used to diagnose postnatal rubella, CRS, and CRI (Table 2). Throat swabs taken on the day of rash are usually positive for rubella virus, even though a slightly higher percentage of cases are positive 2 days before rash onset. Virus shedding in the throat declines rapidly, and by 4 days after rash onset, only about 50% of cases are positive. In addition, viral culture is used to monitor virus in CRS and CRI patients for the purpose of determining when isolation of these patients from susceptible contacts can be stopped. The virus will grow in a variety of cell types, including Vero, BHK21, AGMK, and RK-13 cells. The primary problem encountered with tissue culture is the lack of a cell type that produces CPE in a single passage of wild-type viruses. Historically, this problem was overcome by clever assays exploiting the fact that rubella virus growth interferes with the replication of lytic enteroviruses such as coxsackievirus A9. However, such interference assays are quite difficult to maintain (148). Virus growth can now be identified in the absence of CPE using methods such as RT-PCR, IFA, and immunocolorimetric assays (ICA) to detect viral RNA or proteins (147, 149).

The sensitivity of the RT-PCR system used to detect viral RNA from infected tissue culture cells is not critical, since the amount of rubella viral RNA has been amplified by passage in tissue culture (about 10^6-fold) (118, 147). Detection of rubella virus-infected cells in monolayers can also be accomplished by IFA or ICA. It is crucial that IFA and ICA reagents have low background, since rubella virus culture does not produce high levels of progeny virus (about 10^7 PFU/ml for laboratory strains such as f-Therien). Infected cells are easily identified when stained with high-quality reagents. Dilution of specimens may be desirable, since it is useful to have both infected and uninfected cells in the same field. Monoclonal antibodies to the E1, E2, and C proteins, which react with both reduced and nonreduced antigens on Western blots, often work well in the IFA and ICA.

Utility of Sequences Derived from Viral RNA

Sequencing of the nucleic acid amplified directly from specimens or from tissue culture material can provide useful information. Vaccine virus can be differentiated from wild-type viruses (150). Useful information on the origin of imported cases of rubella and CRS can be obtained (127, 151). Documentation of the elimination of rubella can be supported by analysis of sequences obtained over time (152). There are currently two primary limitations to the utility of rubella RNA sequences, limited effort in obtaining rubella virus sequences in many countries (153) and limited standardization of the analysis and nomenclature of clusters of wild-type rubella virus sequences (121). These limitations are not because of the biologic properties of rubella virus and could be overcome by increased effort and/or attention.

Serologic Tests

ELISA

Detection of rubella virus-specific IgM by either IgM capture ELISA or indirect IgM ELISA is the fastest and most cost-effective diagnostic test for recent postnatal infection. Unfortunately, only about 50% of postnatal rubella cases are IgM positive on the day of symptom onset (Table 2) (143). Most postnatal rubella cases have virus-specific IgM detectable by capture ELISA from 5 until 40 days after symptom onset and IgG by indirect ELISA ≥8 days after symptom onset (Fig. 1) (154). A negative IgM serologic result 4 to 5 days after onset should be followed with testing of a serum sample taken as soon as possible thereafter to avoid false-negative results (129). If a serum sample taken at onset and a convalescent-phase serum sample are available, a 4-fold rise in rubella virus-specific IgG is diagnostic for postnatal rubella infection; such sera should be taken as early as possible after disease onset (within 1 week) and about 2 to 3 weeks thereafter. When IgG titers are used for diagnostic purposes, a dilution series of each serum sample should be made and ELISA results for each dilution series compared. A single dilution set is an unreliable measure of the amount of IgG.

The same ELISAs may be used to confirm CRS. Most congenitally infected infants have IgM detectable from birth to 1 month of age (Table 2). The percentage of infants who are IgM positive declines over the first year of life. At 1 year, most infants are negative. In CRS patients, the IgG response increases gradually over the first 9 months, while maternal IgG declines. Thus, high or increasing IgG levels in the first year of life, in the absence of vaccination or significant risk of postnatal rubella, are consistent with CRS. Recommendations for the best times for collection of samples from postnatal rubella and CRS cases have been published (129).

Microbead Assays and Latex Agglutination

A number of commercial microbead assays are available for doing rubella IgM and IgG serology. These tests are the same in principle as ELISAs, but the surface used is a microbead rather than an ELISA plate well. Microbeads are suspended in liquid and can be efficiently and automatically handled as liquids or, if beads are filtered out, as solids. Automated microbead assays often use rapid, sensitive detection methods, such as detection by fluorescent antibodies.

Latex particle agglutination tests consist of latex spheres coated with rubella virus antigen. These particles aggregate in the presence of either rubella virus-specific IgG or IgM.

PRN

PRN is performed when a quantitative assessment of the neutralizing capacity of an antiserum is necessary. A laboratory strain (e.g., f-Therien) should be used, since viruses from clinical specimens do not exhibit CPE. The assay follows a format common to many viruses. The initial step is incubation of 2- or 10-fold dilutions of antiserum and a standard amount of rubella virus (usually about 100 to 200 PFU) in medium or buffer containing protein to inhibit losses on

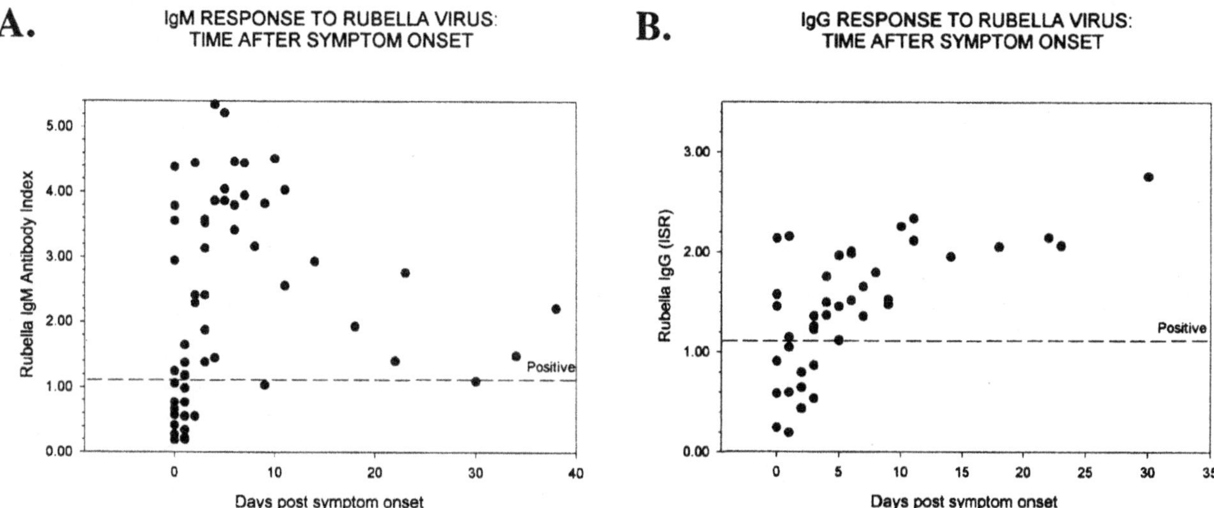

FIGURE 1 Time course of rubella virus-specific IgM and IgG detection by ELISA in sera of rubella patients. Commercial IgM capture ELISA (A) and IgG indirect ELISA (B) were used to detect rubella virus-specific antibodies at the indicated number of days after onset of symptoms (usually rash); antibody index and ISR are the commercial test designations for the ratio of the optical density obtained for the test serum to the optical density obtained for a standard (cutoff) serum. The minimum signal considered positive in each test is indicated by a dashed line. Only results from patients who tested positive for IgM to rubella virus at some time after the onset of symptoms are shown.

surfaces (e.g., 0.1% bovine serum albumin) for 1 h at 35 to 37°C followed by overnight in a refrigerator. A control consisting of virus alone must be included in the assay, since some reduction in the number of plaques is observed during the 1-h incubation. Virus-antiserum specimens are then allowed to attach to confluent Vero cell monolayers for 1 h at 35°C and then overlaid with DEAE dextran (100 μg/ml)-containing medium with agar or carboxymethyl cellulose. Medium in the overlay is typically Dulbecco's modified Eagle's medium; 1% fetal calf serum may also be included to maintain the monolayer. After 6 days, agar/carboxymethyl cellulose is removed and plates are stained with neutral red. Crystal violet can also be used; however, a wash step to remove dead cells should be used prior to crystal violet staining. The ICA for rubella virus can also be used for virus detection (149). The neutralizing capacity of the antiserum is typically reported as the inverse of the antiserum dilution giving a standard reduction in plaques, typically 90% reduction. In both vaccination of nonimmune individuals and postnatal rubella cases, the neutralizing capacity rises at least 100-fold, allowing the easy use of PRN data to confirm past exposure to rubella. However, information on the precise assay used is required to quantitatively compare neutralization capacities of antisera when assays are done in different laboratories (e.g., rubella virus-plaquing efficiency may vary between laboratories). Rubella virus CPE is not even as reproducible as measles virus CPE.

Other Serologic Tests

Avidity tests have been used when IgM detection does not reliably indicate recent infection (e.g., the first serum sample was collected months after clinical symptoms). Low-avidity anti-rubella virus IgG suggests recent infection (111, 155, 156). This test compares the ability of detergents or chaotropic agents to dissociate case IgG and control IgGs from rubella virus proteins. Both high- and low-avidity control sera should be used in each assay. Avidity tests are not widely available and vary in performance (157).

Since the clinical symptoms of postnatal rubella and CRS are dramatically different, it is not surprising that there are significant differences in the immune responses of patients with these diseases. These differences can be observed on Western blots, in which antibodies in sera from CRS patients often demonstrate different reactivity to rubella glycoproteins than those from postnatal rubella patients (158). These tests are not widely used but have been developed in some diagnostic laboratories (128).

Prenatal Screening

The present description of laboratory testing for rubella emphasizes identification of postnatal and congenital rubella cases. However, in the United States, much of the testing is for immunity to rubella, since health care providers should test all pregnant women for immunity by a serum IgG test at the earliest prenatal visit. There are slightly different criteria for rubella immunity that are recommended by various groups (the range is about 10 to 15 IU/ml) (135). Commonly used tests, e.g., ELISA, are standardized to give positive results for 10 IU/ml, the breakpoint defining immunity to rubella in the United States (159). Much of the screening for immunity to rubella virus in the United States is done by automated random-access systems using microparticle immunoassays.

Evaluation, Interpretation, and Reporting of Results

IgM and IgG testing should be done with most sera for both suspected postnatal rubella and CRS cases, since results from both immunoglobulin classes often provide additional information useful for diagnosis. For example, results from a serum sample taken at 8 days after the onset of rash which are positive for IgM but negative for IgG to rubella virus would be inconsistent with the immune response to rubella; usually, the IgM result would be most suspect in this situation (e.g., cross-reaction with antibodies to parvovirus). A serum that tests positive for rubella IgG antibody and negative for IgM is inconsistent with recent postnatal rubella infection in the patient, since the IgM response should precede the IgG response and persist for weeks after rash onset.

A positive result for rubella virus culture is obtained when a positive real-time assay or RT-PCR result is obtained from the culture or at least one cluster of cells is infected, as determined by IFA or ICA. Control cultures must be negative. When an IFA or ICA is used, the expected distribution of viral proteins should be obtained (e.g., E1 glycoprotein distribution when using an E1 monoclonal antibody) (149).

Direct detection of rubella virus RNA by PCR-based protocols requires the laboratory to evaluate the significance of results from such tests. Multiple negative controls and amplified product in more than one specimen from a given patient will increase confidence of a positive diagnosis based on direct RT-PCR. The significance of negative results is usually difficult to determine, since false-negativity rates are usually not available. Sequence variation in wild-type viruses, which can lead to poor primer binding and poor amplification, must be considered when the significance of negative results is evaluated. Nevertheless, when serum from a patient cannot be obtained, or when confirmation of serologic results is desired, direct detection of rubella virus RNA by RT-PCR may be necessary, since it is more rapid than viral culture.

There is often a considerable burden on the laboratory in the diagnosis of rubella. For example, when primary rubella virus infection is suspected for a pregnant woman, false positives and false negatives may lead to incorrect clinical decisions (160). Thus, the laboratorian may be asked to go beyond just communicating false-positivity and false-negativity rates. Testing for recent infection with other viruses that cause clinically similar diseases (e.g., human parvovirus B19) is often prudent. Positive rubella results may be more believable if no other infection is found. Specimen retesting and testing of different specimen types with alternative methods (e.g., serology and viral culture) (Table 2) often yield consistent results and reduce the likelihood of false-positive results. False positives can occur even with IgM capture ELISA. For example, in one study, 1 of 87 sera testing positive for rubella virus-specific IgM by IgM capture ELISA was from a patient whose final diagnosis was primary human parvovirus B19 (111). False negatives can often be identified by testing multiple specimens from a patient (e.g., sera taken 1 week apart). If only a single specimen is available, it may be tested by multiple assays. For example, IgG avidity may resolve the diagnosis from a single serum sample that is IgM positive for both rubella virus and human parvovirus B19 (111, 161).

The significance of decisions resulting from a diagnosis of a CRS-affected pregnancy demands attention by the laboratory to the limitations in interpreting RT-PCR results from prenatal fetal specimens (e.g., from amniotic fluid). Typically, the rate of negative test results from a rubella virus RNA-positive fetus, for example, resulting from a poor specimen, is not known. The percentages of CRS and CRI cases without defects, when positive RT-PCR results from *in utero* specimens at a given gestational age are obtained, are not known. Thus, the possibility of CRI without defects means that a positive test result cannot always conclusively confirm the subsequent birth of a baby with birth defects.

Postnatal rubella can be clinically similar to other diseases, or it can be asymptomatic. Additionally, birth defects characteristic of CRS also occur for other reasons. Thus, the best classification of suspected postnatal rubella and CRS is based on laboratory results rather than clinical presentation. Classification of a postnatal rubella case results in its categorization as suspected, probable, confirmed, or asymptomatic confirmed; for a case of congenital rubella, the categories are suspected CRS, probable CRS, confirmed CRS, and infection only. Positive laboratory results are required to correctly classify asymptomatic confirmed and confirmed cases of postnatal rubella and CRS. Clinical, laboratory, and epidemiological information (e.g., international travel) all may enter into the final clinical decision(s). A full description of classification criteria and recommendations should be consulted (129). One specific diagnostic situation should be noted. A series of tests including a rubella virus IgM test should not be used to determine immunity in a pregnant woman because of the possibility of a false-positive result; immunity should be determined by IgG testing alone. Since standard TORCH (toxoplasmosis, other, rubella, cytomegalovirus, and herpes simplex virus) panels include testing for rubella virus IgM, they should not be used to determine immunity.

Response to Queries about Diseases Recently Associated with Rubella Virus Infection

Rubella virus is not only capable of producing the persistence infections occurring in CRS. Recently, Fuch's uveitis and granulomas in persons with primary immunodeficiency have been associated with the long-term presence of rubella virus nucleic acid or rubella virus (162, 163). Although causal associations with rubella virus and other details of these infections remain to be determined, the full extent of human diseases associated with persistence of rubella infection has clearly not yet been determined.

The findings and conclusions in this chapter are those of the authors and do not necessarily represent the views of the CDC. The use of product names in this chapter does not imply their endorsement by the U.S. Department of Health and Human Services.

REFERENCES

1. **Griffin DE.** 2007. Measles virus, p 1581–1586. *In* Knipe DM, Howley PM, Griffin DE, Lamb RA, Martin MA, Roizman B, Straus SE (ed), *Fields Virology*, 5th ed, vol II. Lippincott Williams &Wilkins, Philadelphia, PA.
2. **Bankamp B, Liu C, Rivailler P, Bera J, Shrivastava S, Kirkness EF, Bellini WJ, Rota PA.** 2014. Wild-type measles viruses with non-standard genome lengths. *PLoS One* **9:**e95470.
3. **Naniche D, Varior-Krishnan G, Cervoni F, Wild TF, Rossi B, Rabourdin-Combe C, Gerlier D.** 1993. Human membrane cofactor protein (CD46) acts as a cellular receptor for measles virus. *J Virol* **67:**6025–6032.
4. **Tatsuo H, Ono N, Tanaka K, Yanagi Y.** 2000. SLAM (CDw150) is a cellular receptor for measles virus. *Nature* **406:**893–897.
5. **Mühlebach MD, Mateo M, Sinn PL, Prüfer S, Uhlig KM, Leonard VH, Navaratnarajah CK, Frenzke M, Wong XX, Sawatsky B, Ramachandran S, McCray PB, Jr, Cichutek K, von Messling V, Lopez M, Cattaneo R.** 2011. Adherens junction protein nectin-4 is the epithelial receptor for measles virus. *Nature* **480:**530–533.
6. **Noyce RS, Bondre DG, Ha MN, Lin LT, Sisson G, Tsao MS, Richardson CD.** 2011. Tumor cell marker PVRL4 (nectin 4) is an epithelial cell receptor for measles virus. *PLoS Pathog* **7:**e1002240.
7. **Rota PA, Featherstone DA, Bellini WJ.** 2008. Molecular epidemiology of measles virus, p 129–150. *In* Oldstone MB, Griffin DE (ed), *Current Topics in Microbiology and Immunology*. Springer Verlag & Co, Berlin, Germany.
8. **World Health Organization.** 2012. Measles virus nomenclature update: 2012. *Wkly Epidemiol Rec* **87:**73–81.
9. **Mulders MN, Rota PA, Icenogle JP, Brown KE, Takeda M, Rey GJ, Ben Mamou MC, Dosseh AR, Byabamazima CR, Ahmed HJ, Pattamadilok S, Zhang Y, Gacic-Dobo M, Strebel PM, Goodson JL.** 2016. Global measles and rubella laboratory network support for elimination goals, 2010-2015. *MMWR Morb Mortal Wkly Rep* **65:**438–442.
10. **Rota PA, Brown K, Mankertz A, Santibanez S, Shulga S, Muller CP, Hübschen JM, Siqueira M, Beirnes J, Ahmed H, Triki H, Al-Busaidy S, Dosseh A, Byabamazima C, Smit S, Akoua-Koffi C, Bwogi J, Bukenya H, Wairagkar N, Ramamurty N, Incomserb P, Pattamadilok S, Jee Y, Lim W, Xu W, Komase K, Takeda M, Tran T, Castillo-Solorzano C, Chenoweth P, Brown D, Mulders MN, Bellini WJ, Featherstone D.** 2011. Global distribution of measles genotypes and measles molecular epidemiology. *J Infect Dis* **204**(Suppl 1)**:** S514–S523.
11. **Coughlin MM, Beck AS, Bankamp B, Rota PA.** 2017. Perspective on global measles epidemiology and control and the role of novel vaccination strategies. *Viruses* **9:**11.
12. **Rota PA, Moss WJ, Takeda M, de Swart RL, Thompson KM, Goodson JL.** 2016. Measles. *Nat Rev Dis Primers* **2:**16049.
13. **Ferreira CS, Frenzke M, Leonard VH, Welstead GG, Richardson CD, Cattaneo R.** 2010. Measles virus infection of alveolar macrophages and dendritic cells precedes spread to lymphatic organs in transgenic mice expressing human signaling lymphocytic activation molecule (SLAM, CD150). *J Virol* **84:**3033–3042.
14. **Lemon K, de Vries R, Mesman A, McQuaid S, van Amerongen G, Yüksel S, Ludlow M, Rennick L, Kuiken T, Rima BK, Geijtenbeek T, Osterhaus AD, Duprex W, de Swart R.** 2011. Early target cells of measles virus after aerosol infection of non-human primates. PLoS Pathog **7:**e1001263.
15. **Ludlow M, McQuaid S, Milner D, de Swart RL, Duprex WP.** 2015. Pathological consequences of systemic measles virus infection. *J Pathol* **235:**253–265.
16. **McLean HQ, Fiebelkorn AP, Temte JL, Wallace GS, Centers for Disease Control and Prevention.** 2013. Prevention of measles, rubella, congenital rubella syndrome, and mumps, 2013: summary recommendations of the Advisory Committee on Immunization Practices (ACIP). *MMWR Recomm Rep* **62**(RR-04)**:**1–34.
17. **Thompson KM.** 2016 Evolution and use of dynamic transmission models for measles and rubella risk and policy analysis. *Risk Anal.* **36:**1383–1403.
18. **Orenstein WA, Papania MJ, Wharton ME.** 2004. Measles elimination in the United States. *J Infect Dis* **189**(Suppl 1)**:**S1–S3.
19. **Papania MJ, Wallace GS, Rota PA, Icenogle JP, Fiebelkorn AP, Armstrong GL, Reef SE, Redd SB, Abernathy ES, Barskey AE, Hao L, McLean HQ, Rota JS, Bellini WJ, Seward JF.** 2014. Elimination of endemic measles, rubella, and congenital rubella syndrome from the Western hemisphere: the US experience. *JAMA Pediatr* **168:**148–155.
20. **Venkat H, Kassem AM, Su CP, Hill C, Timme E, Briggs G, Komatsu K, Robinson S, Sunenshine R, Patel M, Elson D, Gastañaduy P, Brady S, Measles Investigation Team.** 2017. Notes from the field: measles outbreak at a United States immigration and customs enforcement facility—Arizona, May-June 2016. *MMWR Morb Mortal Wkly Rep* **66:**543–544.
21. **Hickman CJ, Hyde TB, Sowers SB, Mercader S, McGrew M, Williams NJ, Beeler JA, Audet S, Kiehl B, Nandy R, Tamin A, Bellini WJ.** 2011. Laboratory characterization of measles virus infection in previously vaccinated and unvaccinated individuals. *J Infect Dis* **204**(Suppl 1)**:**S549–S558.

22. **Rota JS, Hickman CJ, Sowers SB, Rota PA, Mercader S, Bellini WJ.** 2011. Two case studies of modified measles in vaccinated physicians exposed to primary measles cases: high risk of infection but low risk of transmission. *J Infect Dis* **204**(Suppl 1)**:**S559–S563.
23. **Sowers SB, Rota JS, Hickman CJ, Mercader S, Redd S, McNall RJ, Williams N, McGrew M, Walls ML, Rota PA, Bellini WJ.** 2016. High concentrations of measles neutralizing antibodies and high-avidity measles IgG accurately identify measles reinfection cases. *Clin Vaccine Immunol* **23:**707–716.
24. **Hahné SJ, Nic Lochlainn LM, van Burgel ND, Kerkhof J, Sane J, Yap KB, van Binnendijk RS.** 2016. Measles outbreak among previously immunized healthcare workers, the Netherlands, 2014. *J Infect Dis* **214:**1980–1986.
25. **Rosen JB, Rota JS, Hickman CJ, Sowers SB, Mercader S, Rota PA, Bellini WJ, Huang AJ, Doll MK, Zucker JR, Zimmerman CM.** 2014. Outbreak of measles among persons with prior evidence of immunity, New York City, 2011. *Clin Infect Dis* **58:**1205–1210.
26. **Simons E, Ferrari M, Fricks J, Wannemuehler K, Anand A, Burton A, Strebel P.** 2012. Assessment of the 2010 global measles mortality reduction goal: results from a model of surveillance data. *Lancet* **379:**2173–2178.
27. **Jones J, Klein R, Popescu S, Rose K, Kretschmer M, Carrigan A, Trembath F, Koski L, Zabel K, Ostdiek S, Rowell-Kinnard P, Munoz E, Sunenshine R, Sylvester T.** 2015. Lack of measles transmission to susceptible contacts from a health care worker with probable secondary vaccine failure—Maricopa County, Arizona, 2015. *MMWR Morb Mortal Wkly Rep* **64:**832–833.
28. **Ma R, Lu L, Zhangzhu J, Chen M, Yu X, Wang F, Peng X, Wu J.** 2016. A measles outbreak in a middle school with high vaccination coverage and evidence of prior immunity among cases, Beijing, P.R. China. *Vaccine* **34:**1853–1860.
29. **Castillo-Solórzano C, Reef SE, Morice A, Andrus JK, Ruiz Matus C, Tambini G, Gross-Galiano S.** 2011. Guidelines for the documentation and verification of measles, rubella, and congenital rubella syndrome elimination in the region of the Americas. *J Infect Dis* **204**(Suppl 2)**:**S683–S689.
30. **Centers for Disease Control and Prevention.** 2008. Progress in global measles control and mortality reduction, 2000-2007. *MMWR Morb Mortal Wkly Rep* **57:**1303–1306.
31. **Perry RT, Murray JS, Gacic-Dobo M, Dabbagh A, Mulders MN, Strebel PM, Okwo-Bele JM, Rota PA, Goodson JL.** 2015. Progress toward regional measles elimination—worldwide, 2000-2014. *MMWR Morb Mortal Wkly Rep* **64:**1246–1251.
32. **Patel MK, Gacic-Dobo M, Strebel PM, Dabbagh A, Mulders MN, Okwo-Bele JM, Dumolard L, Rota PA, Kretsinger K, Goodson JL.** 2016. Progress toward regional measles elimination—worldwide, 2000-2015. *MMWR Morb Mortal Wkly Rep* **65:**1228–1233.
33. **Breakwell L, Moturi E, Helgenberger L, Gopalani SV, Hales C, Lam E, Sharapov U, Larzelere M, Johnson E, Masao C, Setik E, Barrow L, Dolan S, Chen TH, Patel M, Rota P, Hickman C, Bellini W, Seward J, Wallace G, Papania M.** 2015. Measles outbreak associated with vaccine failure in adults—Federated States of Micronesia, February-August 2014. *MMWR Morb Mortal Wkly Rep* **64:**1088–1092.
34. **De Serres G, Boulianne N, Defay F, Brousseau N, Benoît M, Lacoursière S, Guillemette F, Soto J, Ouakki M, Ward BJ, Skowronski DM.** 2012. Higher risk of measles when the first dose of a 2-dose schedule of measles vaccine is given at 12–14 months versus 15 months of age. *Clin Infect Dis* **55:**394–402.
35. **Hales CM, Johnson E, Helgenberger L, Papania MJ, Larzelere M, Gopalani SV, Lebo E, Wallace G, Moturi E, Hickman CJ, Rota PA, Alexander HS, Marin M.** 2016. Measles outbreak associated with low vaccine effectiveness among adults in Pohnpei State, Federated States of Micronesia, 2014. *Open Forum Infect Dis* **3:**ofw064.
36. **World Health Organization.** 2010. Global eradication of measles: report by the Secretariat. World Health Organization, Geneva, Switzerland. http://apps.who.int/gb/ebwha/pdf_files/WHA63/A63_18-en.pdf
37. **Anonymous.** 2013. Global vaccine action plan. Decade of vaccine collaboration. *Vaccine* **31**(Suppl 2)**:**B5–B31
38. **de Vries RD, McQuaid S, van Amerongen G, Yüksel S, Verburgh RJ, Osterhaus AD, Duprex WP, de Swart RL.** 2012. Measles immune suppression: lessons from the macaque model. *PLoS Pathog* **8:**e1002885.
39. **Griffin DE.** 2010. Measles virus-induced suppression of immune responses. *Immunol Rev* **236:**176–189.
40. **Schönberger K, Ludwig MS, Wildner M, Weissbrich B.** 2013. Epidemiology of subacute sclerosing panencephalitis (SSPE) in Germany from 2003 to 2009: a risk estimation. *PLoS One* **8:**e68909
41. **Bellini WJ, Rota JS, Lowe LE, Katz RS, Dyken PR, Zaki SR, Shieh W-J, Rota PA.** 2005. Subacute sclerosing panencephalitis: more cases of this fatal disease are prevented by measles immunization than was previously recognized. *J Infect Dis* **192:**1686–1693.
42. **Wendorf KA, Winter K, Zipprich J, Schechter R, Hacker JK, Preas C, Cherry JD, Glaser C, Harriman K.** 2017. Subacute sclerosing panencephalitis: the devastating measles complication that might be more common than previously estimated. *Clin Infect Dis* **65:**226–232.
43. **Campbell H, Andrews N, Brown KE, Miller E.** 2007. Review of the effect of measles vaccination on the epidemiology of SSPE. *Int J Epidemiol* **36:**1334–1348.
44. **Katz M, Koprowski H.** 1973. The significance of failure to isolate infectious viruses in cases of subacute sclerosing panencephalitis. Brief report. *Arch Gesamte Virusforsch* **41:** 390–393.
45. **Sidhu MS, Crowley J, Lowenthal A, Karcher D, Menonna J, Cook S, Udem S, Dowling P.** 1994. Defective measles virus in human subacute sclerosing panencephalitis brain. *Virology* **202:**631–641.
46. **Brodsky AL.** 1972. Atypical measles. Severe illness in recipients of killed measles virus vaccine upon exposure to natural infection. *JAMA* **222:**1415–1416.
47. **Taylor LE, Swerdfeger AL, Eslick GD.** 2014. Vaccines are not associated with autism: an evidence-based meta-analysis of case-control and cohort studies. *Vaccine* **32:**3623–3629.
48. **DeStefano F, Price CS, Weintraub ES.** 2013. Increasing exposure to antibody-stimulating proteins and polysaccharides in vaccines is not associated with risk of autism. *J Pediatr* **163:**561–567.
49. **Bitnun A, Shannon P, Durward A, Rota PA, Bellini WJ, Graham C, Wang E, Ford-Jones EL, Cox P, Becker L, Fearon M, Petric M, Tellier R.** 1999. Measles inclusion-body encephalitis caused by the vaccine strain of measles virus. *Clin Infect Dis* **29:**855–861.
50. **Mustafa MM, Weitman SD, Winick NJ, Bellini WJ, Timmons CF, Siegel JD.** 1993. Subacute measles encephalitis in the young immunocompromised host: report of two cases diagnosed by polymerase chain reaction and treated with ribavirin and review of the literature. *Clin Infect Dis* **16:**654–660.
51. **Monafo WJ, Haslam DB, Roberts RL, Zaki SR, Bellini WJ, Coffin CM.** 1994. Disseminated measles infection after vaccination in a child with a congenital immunodeficiency. *J Pediatr* **124:**273–276.
52. **Angel JB, Walpita P, Lerch RA, Sidhu MS, Masurekar M, DeLellis RA, Noble JT, Snydman DR, Udem SA.** 1998. Vaccine-associated measles pneumonitis in an adult with AIDS. *Ann Intern Med* **129:**104–106.
53. **Moss WJ, Monze M, Ryon JJ, Quinn TC, Griffin DE, Cutts F.** 2002. Prospective study of measles in hospitalized, human immunodeficiency virus (HIV)-infected and HIV-uninfected children in Zambia. *Clin Infect Dis* **35:**189–196.
54. **Manesh A, Moorthy M, Bandopadhyay R, Rupali P.** 2017. HIV-associated sub-acute sclerosing panencephalitis—an emerging threat? *Int J STD AIDS* **28:**937–939.
55. **Rota PA, Khan AS, Durigon E, Yuran T, Villamarzo YS, Bellini WJ.** 1995. Detection of measles virus RNA in urine specimens from vaccine recipients. *J Clin Microbiol* **33:** 2485–2488.
56. **Esolen LM, Ward BJ, Moench TR, Griffin DE.** 1993. Infection of monocytes during measles. *J Infect Dis* **168:**47–52.

57. **Tuokko H.** 1984. Comparison of nonspecific reactivity in indirect and reverse immunoassays for measles and mumps immunoglobulin M antibodies. *J Clin Microbiol* **20:**972–976.
58. **Helfand RF, Kebede S, Mercader S, Gary HE, Jr, Beyene H, Bellini WJ.** 1999. The effect of timing of sample collection on the detection of measles-specific IgM in serum and oral fluid samples after primary measles vaccination. *Epidemiol Infect* **123:**451–455.
59. **Helfand RF, Kebede S, Alexander JP, Jr, Alemu W, Heath JL, Gary HE, Jr, Anderson LJ, Beyene H, Bellini WJ.** 1996. Comparative detection of measles-specific IgM in oral fluid and serum from children by an antibody-capture IgM EIA. *J Infect Dis* **173:**1470–1474.
60. **Parry JV, Perry KR, Mortimer PP, Panday S.** 1989. Diagnosis of hepatitis A and B by testing saliva. *J Med Virol* **28:**255–260.
61. **Perry KR, Brown DW, Parry JV, Panday S, Pipkin C, Richards A.** 1993. Detection of measles, mumps, and rubella antibodies in saliva using antibody capture radioimmunoassay. *J Med Virol* **40:**235–240.
62. **Brown DW, Ramsay ME, Richards AF, Miller E.** 1994. Salivary diagnosis of measles: a study of notified cases in the United Kingdom, 1991-3. *BMJ* **308:**1015–1017.
63. **Centers for Disease Control and Prevention.** 2008. Recommendations from an ad hoc meeting of the WHO Measles and Rubella Laboratory Network (LabNet) on use of alternative diagnostic samples for measles and rubella surveillance. *MMWR Morb Mortal Wkly Rep* **57:**657–660.
64. **Jin L, Vyse A, Brown DW.** 2002. The role of RT-PCR assay of oral fluid for diagnosis and surveillance of measles, mumps and rubella. *Bull World Health Organ* **80:**76–77.
65. **Helfand RF, Keyserling HL, Williams I, Murray A, Mei J, Moscatiello C, Icenogle J, Bellini WJ.** 2001. Comparative detection of measles and rubella IgM and IgG derived from filter paper blood and serum samples. *J Med Virol* **65:**751–757.
66. **Punnarugsa V, Mungmee V.** 1991. Detection of rubella virus immunoglobulin G (IgG) and IgM antibodies in whole blood on Whatman paper: comparison with detection in sera. *J Clin Microbiol* **29:**2209–2212.
67. **Sander J, Niehaus C.** 1985. Screening for rubella IgG and IgM using an ELISA test applied to dried blood on filter paper. *J Pediatr* **106:**457–461.
68. **Vejtorp M, Leerhoy J.** 1981. Rubella IgG antibody detection by ELISA using capillary blood samples collected on filter paper and in microtainer tubes. *Acta Pathol Microbiol Scand B* **89:**369–370.
69. **De Swart RL, Nur Y, Abdallah A, Kruining H, El Mubarak HS, Ibrahim SA, Van Den Hoogen B, Groen J, Osterhaus AD.** 2001. Combination of reverse transcriptase PCR analysis and immunoglobulin M detection on filter paper blood samples allows diagnostic and epidemiological studies of measles. *J Clin Microbiol* **39:**270–273.
70. **Mercader S, Featherstone D, Bellini WJ.** 2006. Comparison of available methods to elute serum from dried blood spot samples for measles serology. *J Virol Methods* **137:**140–149.
71. **Wassilak SG, Bernier RH, Herrmann KL, Orenstein WA, Bart KJ, Amler R.** 1984. Measles seroconfirmation using dried capillary blood specimens in filter paper. *Pediatr Infect Dis* **3:**117–121.
72. **Dimech W, Mulders MN.** 2016. A 16-year review of seroprevalence studies on measles and rubella. *Vaccine* **34:**4110–4118.
73. **Dimech W, Mulders MN.** 2016. A review of testing used in seroprevalence studies on measles and rubella. *Vaccine* **34:**4119–4122.
74. **Zaki SR, Bellini WJ.** 1997. Measles, p 233–244. *In* Connor DH, Chandler FW, Schwartz DA, Manz HJ, Lack EE (ed), *Pathology of Infectious Diseases.* Appleton and Lange Publishers, Stamford, CT.
75. **Minnich LL, Goodenough F, Ray CG.** 1991. Use of immunofluorescence to identify measles virus infections. *J Clin Microbiol* **29:**1148–1150.
76. **Smaron MF, Saxon E, Wood L, McCarthy C, Morello JA.** 1991. Diagnosis of measles by fluorescent antibody and culture of nasopharyngeal secretions. *J Virol Methods* **33:**223–229.
77. **Riddell MA, Chibo D, Kelly HA, Catton MG, Birch CJ.** 2001. Investigation of optimal specimen type and sampling time for detection of measles virus RNA during a measles epidemic. *J Clin Microbiol* **39:**375–376.
78. **Fujino M, Yoshida N, Yamaguchi S, Hosaka N, Ota Y, Notomi T, Nakayama T.** 2005. A simple method for the detection of measles virus genome by loop-mediated isothermal amplification (LAMP). *J Med Virol* **76:**406–413.
79. **Hyde TB, Nandy R, Hickman CJ, Langidrik JR, Strebel PM, Papania MJ, Seward JF, Bellini WJ.** 2009. Laboratory confirmation of measles in elimination settings: experience from the Republic of the Marshall Islands, 2003. *Bull World Health Organ* **87:**93–98.
80. **Roy F, Mendoza L, Hiebert J, McNall RJ, Bankamp B, Connolly S, Lüdde A, Friedrich N, Mankertz A, Rota PA, Severini A.** 2017. Rapid identification of measles virus vaccine genotype by real-time PCR. *J Clin Microbiol* **55:**735–743.
81. **Ono N, Tatsuo H, Hidaka Y, Aoki T, Minagawa H, Yanagi Y.** 2001. Measles viruses on throat swabs from measles patients use signaling lymphocytic activation molecule (CDw150) but not CD46 as a cellular receptor. *J Virol* **75:**4399–4401.
82. **Rota PA, Brown KE, Hübschen JM, Muller CP, Icenogle J, Chen MH, Bankamp B, Kessler JR, Brown DW, Bellini WJ, Featherstone D.** 2011. Improving global virologic surveillance for measles and rubella. *J Infect Dis* **204**(Suppl 1)**:**S506–S513.
83. **Bankamp B, Byrd-Leotis LA, Lopareva EN, Woo GK, Liu C, Jee Y, Ahmed H, Lim WW, Ramamurty N, Mulders MN, Featherstone D, Bellini WJ, Rota PA.** 2013. Improving molecular tools for global surveillance of measles virus. *J Clin Virol* **58:**176–182.
84. **Reisdorf E, Bellini WJ, Rota P, Icenogle J, Davis T, Wroblewski K, Hagan CN, Shult P.** 2013. Public health reference laboratories: a model for increasing molecular diagnostic testing and genotyping capacity for measles and rubella, p 41. *Abstr 2013 Association of Public Health Laboratories Meeting.* Association of Public Health Laboratories, Raleigh, NC.
85. **Rota PA, Featherstone DA, Bellini WJ.** 2009. Molecular epidemiology of measles virus. *Curr Top Microbiol Immunol* **330:**129–150.
86. **Bellini WJ, Rota PA.** 2011. Biological feasibility of measles eradication. *Virus Res* **162:**72–79.
87. **World Health Organization.** 2017. Roadmap to elimination standard measles and rubella surveillance. *Wkly Epidemiol Rec* **92:**97–105.
88. **Featherstone DA, Rota PA, Icenogle J, Mulders MN, Jee Y, Ahmed H, de Filippis AM, Ramamurty N, Gavrilin E, Byabamazima C, Dosseh A, Xu W, Komase K, Tashiro M, Brown D, Bellini WJ, Strebel P.** 2011. Expansion of the Global Measles and Rubella Laboratory Network 2005-09. *J Infect Dis* **204**(Suppl 1)**:**S491–S498.
89. **Erdman DD, Anderson LJ, Adams DR, Stewart JA, Markowitz LE, Bellini WJ.** 1991. Evaluation of monoclonal antibody-based capture enzyme immunoassays for detection of specific antibodies to measles virus. *J Clin Microbiol* **29:**1466–1471.
90. **Hummel KB, Erdman DD, Heath J, Bellini WJ.** 1992. Baculovirus expression of the nucleoprotein gene of measles virus and utility of the recombinant protein in diagnostic enzyme immunoassays. *J Clin Microbiol* **30:**2874–2880.
91. **Samuel D, Sasnauskas K, Jin L, Gedvilaite A, Slibinskas R, Beard S, Zvirbliene A, Oliveira SA, Staniulis J, Cohen B, Brown D.** 2003. Development of a measles specific IgM ELISA for use with serum and oral fluid samples using recombinant measles nucleoprotein produced in *Saccharomyces cerevisiae. J Clin Virol* **28:**121–129.
92. **Arista S, Ferraro D, Cascio A, Vizzi E, di Stefano R.** 1995. Detection of IgM antibodies specific for measles virus by capture and indirect enzyme immunoassays. *Res Virol* **146:**225–232.
93. **Ratnam S, Tipples G, Head C, Fauvel M, Fearon M, Ward BJ.** 2000. Performance of indirect immunoglobulin M (IgM) serology tests and IgM capture assays for laboratory diagnosis of measles. *J Clin Microbiol* **38:**99–104.

94. **Cohen BJ, Parry RP, Doblas D, Samuel D, Warrener L, Andrews N, Brown D.** 2006. Measles immunity testing: comparison of two measles IgG ELISAs with plaque reduction neutralisation assay. *J Virol Methods* **131:**209–212.
95. **de Souza VA, Pannuti CS, Sumita LM, Albrecht P.** 1991. Enzyme-linked immunosorbent assay (ELISA) for measles antibody. A comparison with haemagglutination inhibition, immunofluorescence and plaque neutralization tests. *Rev Inst Med Trop São Paulo* **33:**32–36.
96. **Ratnam S, Gadag V, West R, Burris J, Oates E, Stead F, Bouilianne N.** 1995. Comparison of commercial enzyme immunoassay kits with plaque reduction neutralization test for detection of measles virus antibody. *J Clin Microbiol* **33:**811–815.
97. **Haywood B, Patel M, Hurday S, Copping R, Webster D, Irish D, Haque T.** 2014. Comparison of automated chemiluminescence immunoassays with capture enzyme immunoassays for the detection of measles and mumps IgM antibodies in serum. *J Virol Methods* **196:**15–17.
98. **Binnicker MJ, Jespersen DJ, Rollins LO.** 2011. Evaluation of the Bio-Rad BioPlex measles, mumps, rubella, and varicella-zoster virus IgG multiplex bead immunoassay. *Clin Vaccine Immunol* **18:**1524–1526.
99. **Hatchette TF, Scholz H, Bolotin S, Crowcroft NS, Jackson C, McLachlan E, Severini A.** 2017. Calibration and evaluation of quantitative antibody titers for measles virus by using the BioPlex 2200. *Clin Vaccine Immunol* **24:**e00269-16.
100. **Tipples GA, Hamkar R, Mohktari-Azad T, Gray M, Parkyn G, Head C, Ratnam S.** 2003. Assessment of immunoglobulin M enzyme immunoassays for diagnosis of measles. *J Clin Microbiol* **41:**4790–4792.
101. **Tuokko H.** 1995. Detection of acute measles infections by indirect and mu-capture enzyme immunoassays for immunoglobulin M antibodies and measles immunoglobulin G antibody avidity enzyme immunoassay. *J Med Virol* **45:**306–311.
102. **Dina J, Creveuil C, Gouarin S, Viron F, Hebert A, Freymuth F, Vabret A.** 2016. Performance evaluation of the VIDAS(®) measles IgG assay and its diagnostic value for measuring IgG antibody avidity in measles virus infection. *Viruses* **8:**E234.
103. **Mercader S, Garcia P, Bellini WJ.** 2012. Measles virus IgG avidity assay for use in classification of measles vaccine failure in measles elimination settings. *Clin Vaccine Immunol* **19:**1810–1817.
104. **Paunio M, Hedman K, Davidkin I, Peltola H.** 2003. IgG avidity to distinguish secondary from primary measles vaccination failures: prospects for a more effective global measles elimination strategy. *Expert Opin Pharmacother* **4:**1215–1225.
105. **Albrecht P, Herrmann K, Burns GR.** 1981. Role of virus strain in conventional and enhanced measles plaque neutralization test. *J Virol Methods* **3:**251–260.
106. **Chen RT, Markowitz LE, Albrecht P, Stewart JA, Mofenson LM, Preblud SR, Orenstein WA.** 1990. Measles antibody: reevaluation of protective titers. *J Infect Dis* **162:**1036–1042.
107. **Cohen BJ, Audet S, Andrews N, Beeler J, WHO Working Group on Measles Plaque Reduction Neutralization Test.** 2007. Plaque reduction neutralization test for measles antibodies: description of a standardised laboratory method for use in immunogenicity studies of aerosol vaccination. *Vaccine* **26:**59–66.
108. **Haralambieva IH, Ovsyannikova IG, Vierkant RA, Poland GA.** 2008. Development of a novel efficient fluorescence-based plaque reduction microneutralization assay for measles virus immunity. *Clin Vaccine Immunol* **15:**1054–1059.
109. **Helfand RF, Heath JL, Anderson LJ, Maes EF, Guris D, Bellini WJ.** 1997. Diagnosis of measles with an IgM capture EIA: the optimal timing of specimen collection after rash onset. *J Infect Dis* **175:**195–199.
110. **Jenkerson SA, Beller M, Middaugh JP, Erdman DD.** 1995. False positive rubeola IgM tests. *N Engl J Med* **332:**1103–1104.
111. **Thomas HI, Barrett E, Hesketh LM, Wynne A, Morgan-Capner P.** 1999. Simultaneous IgM reactivity by EIA against more than one virus in measles, parvovirus B19 and rubella infection. *J Clin Virol* **14:**107–118.
112. **Bellini WJ, Rota PA.** 1999. Measles (rubeola) virus, p 603–621. *In* Lennette EH, Smith TF (ed), *Laboratory Diagnosis of Viral Infections*, 3rd ed. Marcel Dekker, Inc, New York, NY.
113. **Helfand RF, Kim DK, Gary HE, Jr, Edwards GL, Bisson GP, Papania MJ, Heath JL, Schaff DL, Bellini WJ, Redd SC, Anderson LJ.** 1998. Nonclassic measles infections in an immune population exposed to measles during a college bus trip. *J Med Virol* **56:**337–341.
114. **Centers for Disease Control and Prevention.** 2013. Chapter 7: Measles. *In Manual for the Surveillance of Vaccine-Preventable Diseases*, 6th ed. U.S. Department of Health and Human Services, CDC, Atlanta, GA. http://www.cdc.gov/vaccines/pubs/surv-manual/chpt07-measles.html
115. **DuBois RM, Vaney MC, Tortorici MA, Kurdi RA, Barba-Spaeth G, Krey T, Rey FA.** 2013. Functional and evolutionary insight from the crystal structure of rubella virus protein E1. *Nature* **493:**552–556.
116. **Hobman TC, Chantler JK.** 2007. Rubella virus, p 1069–1100. *In* Knipe DM, Howley PM, Griffin DE, Lamb, Martin MA, Roizman B, Straus SE (ed), *Fields Virology*, 5th ed. Lippincott Williams & Wilkins, Philadelphia, PA.
117. **Battisti AJ, Yoder JD, Plevka P, Winkler DC, Prasad VM, Kuhn RJ, Frey TK, Steven AC, Rossmann MG.** 2012. Cryo-electron tomography of rubella virus. *J Virol* **86:**11078–11085.
118. **Frey TK, Abernathy ES, Bosma TJ, Starkey WG, Corbett KM, Best JM, Katow S, Weaver SC.** 1998. Molecular analysis of rubella virus epidemiology across three continents, North America, Europe, and Asia, 1961-1997. *J Infect Dis* **178:**642–650.
119. **Abernathy E, Chen MH, Bera J, Shrivastava S, Kirkness E, Zheng Q, Bellini W, Icenogle J.** 2013. Analysis of whole genome sequences of 16 strains of rubella virus from the United States, 1961-2009. *Virol J* **10:**32.
120. **World Health Organization.** 2013. Rubella virus nomenclature update: 2013. *Wkly Epidemiol Rec* **88:**337–343.
121. **Rivailler P, Abernathy E, Icenogle J.** 2017. Genetic diversity of currently circulating rubella viruses: a need to define more precise viral groups. *J Gen Virol* **98:**396–404.
122. **Parkman PD, Buescher EL, Artenstein MS.** 1962. Recovery of rubella virus from army recruits. *Proc Soc Exp Biol Med* **111:**225–230.
123. **Weller TH, Neva FA.** 1962. Propagation in tissue culture of cytopathic agents from patients with rubella-like illness. *Proc Soc Exp Biol Med* **111:**215–225.
124. **Reef SE, Cochi SL.** 2006. The evidence for the elimination of rubella and congenital rubella syndrome in the United States: a public health achievement. *Clin Infect Dis* **43**(Suppl 3)**:**S123–S125.
125. **Hyde TB, Kruszon-Moran D, McQuillan GM, Cossen C, Forghani B, Reef SE.** 2006. Rubella immunity levels in the United States population: has the threshold of viral elimination been reached? *Clin Infect Dis* **43**(Suppl 3)**:**S146–S150.
126. **Centers for Disease Control and Prevention.** 2017. Notifiable diseases and mortality tables. https://www.cdc.gov/mmwr/volumes/66/wr/mm6630md.htm?s_cid=mm6630md_w
127. **Centers for Disease Control and Prevention.** 2013. Three cases of congenital rubella syndrome in the postelimination era—Maryland, Alabama, and Illinois, 2012. *MMWR Morb Mortal Wkly Rep* **62:**226–229.
128. **Reef SE, Frey TK, Theall K, Abernathy E, Burnett CL, Icenogle J, McCauley MM, Wharton M.** 2002. The changing epidemiology of rubella in the 1990s: on the verge of elimination and new challenges for control and prevention. *JAMA* **287:**464–472.
129. **Castillo-Solórzano C, Reef SE, Morice A, Vascones N, Chevez AE, Castalia-Soares R, Torres C, Vizzotti C, Ruiz Matus C.** 2011. Rubella vaccination of unknowingly pregnant women during mass campaigns for rubella and congenital rubella syndrome elimination, the Americas 2001–2008. *J Infect Dis* **204**(Suppl 2)**:**S713–S717.
130. **World Health Organization.** 2012. *Surveillance Guidelines for Measles, Rubella and Congenital Rubella Syndrome in the WHO European Region*. World Health Organization, Geneva, Switzerland. http://www.ncbi.nlm.nih.gov/books/NBK143264/

131. **Centers for Disease Control and Prevention.** 2005. Elimination of rubella and congenital rubella syndrome—United States, 1969-2004. *MMWR Morb Mortal Wkly Rep* **54:** 279–282.
132. **Vynnycky E, Adams EJ, Cutts FT, Reef SE, Navar AM, Simons E, Yoshida L-M, Brown DWJ, Jackson C, Peter M. Strebel PM, Dabbagh AJ.** 2016. Using seroprevalence and immunisation coverage data to estimate the global burden of congenital rubella syndrome, 1996-2010: a systematic review. *PLoS One* **11:**e0149160.
133. **Toizumi M, Motomura H, Vo HM, Takahashi K, Pham E, Nguyen HAT, Le TH, Hashizume M, Ariyoshi K, Dang DA, Moriuchi H, Yoshida LM.** 2014. Mortality associated with pulmonary hypertension in congenital rubella syndrome. *Pediatrics* **134:**e519–e526.
134. **Lazar M, Perelygina L, Martines R, Greer P, Paddock CD, Peltecu G, Lupulescu E, Icenogle J, Zaki SR.** 2016. Immunolocalization and distribution of rubella antigen in fatal congenital rubella syndrome. *EBioMedicine* **3:**86–92.
135. **Plotkin SA.** 1999. Rubella vaccine, p 409–439. *In* Plotkin SA, Orenstein WA (ed), *Vaccines*, 3rd ed. W. B. Saunders, Philadelphia, PA.
136. **Minussi L, Mohrdieck R, Bercini M, Ranieri T, Sanseverino MTV, Momino W, Callegari-Jacques SM, Schuler-Faccini L.** 2008. Prospective evaluation of pregnant women vaccinated against rubella in southern Brazil. *Reprod Toxicol* **25:**120–123.
137. **Cooper LZ.** 1985. The history and medical consequences of rubella. *Rev Infect Dis* **7**(Suppl 1):S2–S10.
138. **Gregg NM.** 1941. Congenital cataract following German measles in the mother. *Trans Ophthalmol Soc Aust* **3:**35–46.
139. **Shepard TH.** 1995. *Catalogue of Teratogenic Agents*, 8th ed. Johns Hopkins University Press, Baltimore, MD.
140. **Perelygina L, Icenogle J.** 2018. Togaviruses. *In* Barer M, Irving W (ed), *Medical Microbiology: A Guide to Microbial Infections*, 19th ed. Churchill Livingstone, London, England.
141. **Centers for Disease Control and Prevention.** 2001. Control and prevention of rubella: evaluation and management of suspected outbreaks, rubella in pregnant women, and surveillance for congenital rubella syndrome. *MMWR Recomm Rep* **50**(RR-12)**:**1–23.
142. **Takahashi S, Machikawa F, Noda A, Oda T, Tachikawa T.** 1998. Detection of immunoglobulin G and A antibodies to rubella virus in urine and antibody responses to vaccine-induced infection. *Clin Diagn Lab Immunol* **5:**24–27.
143. **Abernathy E, Cabezas C, Sun H, Zheng Q, Chen MH, Castillo-Solorzano C, Ortiz AC, Osores F, Oliveira L, Whittembury A, Andrus JK, Helfand RF, Icenogle J.** 2009. Confirmation of rubella within 4 days of rash onset: comparison of rubella virus RNA detection in oral fluid with immunoglobulin M detection in serum or oral fluid. *J Clin Microbiol* **47:**182–188.
144. **Helfand RF, Cabezas C, Abernathy E, Castillo-Solorzano C, Ortiz AC, Sun H, Osores F, Oliveira L, Whittembury A, Charles M, Andrus J, Icenogle J.** 2007. Dried blood spots versus sera for detection of rubella virus-specific immunoglobulin M (IgM) and IgG in samples collected during a rubella outbreak in Peru. *Clin Vaccine Immunol* **14:** 1522–1525.
145. **Nokes DJ, Enquselassie F, Nigatu W, Vyse AJ, Cohen BJ, Brown DW, Cutts FT.** 2001. Has oral fluid the potential to replace serum for the evaluation of population immunity levels? A study of measles, rubella and hepatitis B in rural Ethiopia. *Bull World Health Organ* **79:**588–595.
146. **Cooray S, Warrener L, Jin L.** 2006. Improved RT-PCR for diagnosis and epidemiological surveillance of rubella. *J Clin Virol* **35:**73–80.
147. **Zhu Z, Xu W, Abernathy ES, Chen MH, Zheng Q, Wang T, Zhang Z, Li C, Wang C, He W, Zhou S, Icenogle J.** 2007. Comparison of four methods using throat swabs to confirm rubella virus infection. *J Clin Microbiol* **45:**2847–2852.
148. **Chernesky MA, Mahony JB.** 1999. Rubella virus, p 964–969. *In* Murray PR, Baron EJ, Pfaller MA, Tenover FC, Yolken RH (ed), *Manual of Clinical Microbiology*, 7th ed. ASM Press, Washington, DC.
149. **Chen MH, Zhu Z, Zhang Y, Favors S, Xu WB, Featherstone DA, Icenogle JP.** 2007. An indirect immunocolorimetric assay to detect rubella virus infected cells. *J Virol Methods* **146:**414–418.
150. **Frey TK, Abernathy ES.** 1993. Identification of strain-specific nucleotide sequences in the RA 27/3 rubella virus vaccine. *J Infect Dis* **168:**854–864.
151. **Abernathy ES, Hübschen JM, Muller CP, Jin L, Brown D, Komase K, Mori Y, Xu W, Zhu Z, Siqueira MM, Shulga S, Tikhonova N, Pattamadilok S, Incomserb P, Smit SB, Akoua-Koffi C, Bwogi J, Lim WW, Woo GK, Triki H, Jee Y, Mulders MN, de Filippis AM, Ahmed H, Ramamurty N, Featherstone D, Icenogle JP.** 2011. Status of global virologic surveillance for rubella viruses. *J Infect Dis* **204**(Suppl 1)**:**S524–S532.
152. **Icenogle JP, Frey TK, Abernathy E, Reef SE, Schnurr D, Stewart JA.** 2006. Genetic analysis of rubella viruses found in the United States between 1966 and 2004: evidence that indigenous rubella viruses have been eliminated. *Clin Infect Dis* **43**(Suppl 3)**:**S133–S140.
153. **Mulders MN, Serhan F, Goodson JL, Icenogle J, Johnson BW, Rota PA.** 2017. Expansion of surveillance for vaccine-preventable diseases: building on the Global Polio Laboratory Network and the Global Measles and Rubella Laboratory Network platforms. *J Infect Dis* **216**(suppl_1)**:**S324–S330.
154. **Tipples GA, Hamkar R, Mohktari-Azad T, Gray M, Ball J, Head C, Ratnam S.** 2004. Evaluation of rubella IgM enzyme immunoassays. *J Clin Virol* **30:**233–238.
155. **Hofmann J, Kortung M, Pustowoit B, Faber R, Piskazeck U, Liebert UG.** 2000. Persistent fetal rubella vaccine virus infection following inadvertent vaccination during early pregnancy. *J Med Virol* **61:**155–158.
156. **Nedeljkovic J, Jovanovic T, Oker-Blom C.** 2001. Maturation of IgG avidity to individual rubella virus structural proteins. *J Clin Virol* **22:**47–54.
157. **Mubareka S, Richards H, Gray M, Tipples GA.** 2007. Evaluation of commercial rubella immunoglobulin G avidity assays. *J Clin Microbiol* **45:**231–233.
158. **Hyde TB, Sato HK, Hao L, Flannery B, Zheng Q, Wannemuehler K, Ciccone FH, de Sousa Marques H, Weckx LY, Sáfadi MA, de Oliveira Moraes E, Pinhata MM, Olbrich Neto J, Bevilacqua MC, Junior AT, Monteiro TA, Figueiredo CA, Andrus JK, Reef SE, Toscano CM, Castillo-Solorzano C, Icenogle JP, CRS Biomarker Study Group.** 2015. Identification of serologic markers for school-aged children with congenital rubella syndrome. *J Infect Dis* **212:**57–66.
159. **Skendzel LP.** 1996. Rubella immunity. Defining the level of protective antibody. *Am J Clin Pathol* **106:**170–174.
160. **Best JM, O'Shea S, Tipples G, Davies N, Al-Khusaiby SM, Krause A, Hesketh LM, Jin L, Enders G.** 2002. Interpretation of rubella serology in pregnancy—pitfalls and problems. *BMJ* **325:**147–148.
161. **Isaac BM, Zucker JR, Giancotti FR, Abernathy E, Icenogle J, Rakeman JL, Rosen JB.** 2017. Rubella surveillance and diagnostic testing among a low-prevalence population, New York City, 2012-2013. *Clin Vaccine Immunol* **24:**e00102-17.
162. **Abernathy E, Peairs RR, Chen MH, Icenogle J, Namdari H.** 2015. Genomic characterization of a persistent rubella virus from a case of Fuch' uveitis syndrome in a 73 year old man. *J Clin Virol* **69:**104–109.
163. **Perelygina L, Plotkin S, Russo P, Hautala T, Bonilla F, Ochs HD, Joshi A, Routes J, Patel K, Wehr C, Icenogle J, Sullivan KE.** 2016. Rubella persistence in epidermal keratinocytes and granuloma M2 macrophages in patients with primary immunodeficiencies. *J Allergy Clin Immunol* **138:**1436–1439.e11
164. **Davis WJ, Larson HE, Simsarian JP, Parkman PD, Meyer HM, Jr.** 1971. A study of rubella immunity and resistance to infection. *JAMA* **215:**600–608.

Enteroviruses and Parechoviruses

KATHLEEN A. STELLRECHT, DARYL M. LAMSON, AND JOSÉ R. ROMERO

90

TAXONOMY

Enteroviruses (EVs) are members of the *Picornaviridae* family with "pico" meaning very small, "rna" indicating an RNA genome, and "viridae" signifying viruses. Traditional criteria for taxonomy and identification of EVs to subgroups were based on patterns of replication in cell cultures, clinical syndromes or disease, and disease manifestations in suckling mice. The subgroups were poliovirus (PV), coxsackievirus A (CVA), coxsackievirus B (CVB), and echovirus (E). Echoviruses were initially named as the acronym "echo" meaning enteric cytopathic human orphan because they were first isolated from the stool of asymptomatic children and caused a cytopathic effect in cell culture. The criteria classified 67 different human EV serotypes until the designation was dropped in the 1960s, with all subsequent serotypes designated enterovirus (EV) followed by a number beginning with 68 (1, 2).

With the development of molecular sequencing and the limited availability of antisera for characterizing newly identified strains and variant strains, the traditional methods of taxonomy have become challenging. The EV taxonomy was effectively redefined through phylogenetic analysis (3). Currently, EVs predominantly causing disease in humans are divided into seven species: EV A through D and rhinoviruses (RVs) A through C (Table 1) (4). Several EVs originally thought to be distinct serotypes are variants of the same strain (5), and some strains have been reclassified into different groups (6). Furthermore, new EVs have been identified (EV73 to EV121) (http://www.picornaviridae.com/enterovirus/enterovirus.htm) (7). Regarding nomenclature changes, host names have been removed from the EV genus (8), and all classified EVs contain the species in the name (e.g., EV-B111).

Originally identified in 1956 as members of the EV genus based on growth characteristics, echoviruses 22 and 23 are genetically distinct from other EVs and were renamed HPeV1 and HPeV2 (9–11). HPeV3 was identified decades later by molecular methods (12). Analogous to the genotyping of EVs, the use of the *VP1* gene sequence to determine the HPeV genotype is standard (13, 14).

The genus *Parechovirus (PeV)* is now classified into two species, PeV A (previously HPeV) and PeV B [previously Ljungan virus (LV)]; additionally, the host names have been removed from the PeV species. The common names have remained the same to differentiate from the species names (Table 1). PeV A comprises 19 different types, HPeV1 through HPeV19, and PeV B comprises five types, LV1 through LV5 (http://www.picornaviridae.com/parechovirus/parechovirus.htm).

Molecular techniques have led to identification of many additional types of PeV based on the *VP1* gene sequence. Whole-genome sequencing analyses have identified multiple novel intertypic recombinant HPeV strains (15–19). This is not surprising since recombination has been documented to play a role in PeV evolution (20). More whole-genome sequence data are needed to decipher new types versus recombinants, to identify common recombination breakpoints and intertypic recombination events, and to better understand evolutionary relationships between HPeVs.

DESCRIPTION OF THE AGENTS

Like other members of the family *Picornaviridae*, EVs are small (30-nm diameter in the hydrated state), nonenveloped viruses that possess a single-stranded positive (message)-sense RNA genome. Their buoyant density in cesium chloride is 1.30 to 1.34 g/cm^3 (4). Most EVs, from group A to group D, are stable in acid, ether, and chloroform and are insensitive to nonionic detergent. They are inactivated by heat (>56°C), UV light, chlorination, and formaldehyde. In cell culture, most EVs replicate optimally at 36 to 37°C, except for RVs A and B, which replicate optimally at 33°C. RVs are covered more extensively in chapter 91.

The EVs are stable in liquid environments and can survive for many weeks in water, body fluids, and sewage. This is due to several viral properties, including thermostability in the presence of divalent cations, acid stability, and the absence of a lipid envelope.

The EV RNA genome serves as a template for both viral protein translation and RNA replication (Fig. 1) (21). The genome contains a long (approximately 750 bases) 5′-nontranslated region (5′ NTR), which immediately precedes a single open reading frame (ORF) (Fig. 1). The ORF is translated into a single polyprotein that is posttranslationally cleaved into several functional intermediates and the final 11 proteins by virus-encoded proteases. Immediately downstream of the ORF is a short noncoding region of approximately 70 to 100 bases (3′ NTR) and a terminal polyadenylated tail.

TABLE 1 EVs, RVs, and PeVs affecting humans

Virus	Species	Serotypes, types, common name[a]
Enterovirus (EV)	EV A (20 types)	
	Coxsackieviruses (CV)	CV-A2–A8, A10, A12, A14, A16
	Enteroviruses (EV)	EV-A71, A76, A89–A91, A114, A119–A121
	EV B (59 types)	
	Coxsackieviruses (CV)	CV-A9, B1–6
	Echoviruses (E)	E1–7, 9, 11–21, 24–27, 29–33
	Enteroviruses (EV)	EV-B69, B73–B75, B77–B88, B93, B97, B98, B100, B101, B106, B107, B111
	EV C (23 types)	
	Coxsackievirus (CV)	CV-A1, A11, A13, A17, A19–A22, A24
	Poliovirus (PV)	PV1–3
	Enterovirus (EV)	EV-C95, C96, C99, C102, C104, C105, C109, C113, C116–118
	EV D (4 types)	
	Enterovirus (EV)	EV-D68, D70, D94, D111
Rhinovirus (RV)	RV A (80 types)	RV-A1, A2, A7, A9–A13, A15, A16, A18–A25, A28, A30–A34, A36, A38–A41, A43–A47, A49–A51, A53–A68, A71, A73–A78, A80–A82, A85, A88–A90, A94, A96, A98, A100–A109
	RV B (30 serotypes)	RV-B3–6, B14, B17, B26, B27, B35, B37, B42, B48, B52, B69–70, B72, B79, B83–84, B86, B91–93, B97, B99–104
	RV C (55 types)	RV-C1–55
Parechovirus (PeV)	PeV A (19 types)	HPeV A1–19
	PeV B (1 type)	Ljungan (LV) 1

[a]From http://www.picornaviridae.com/enterovirus/enterovirus.htm.
[b]From http://www.picornaviridae.com/parechovirus/parechovirus_a/parechovirus_a.htm.

The EV 5′ and 3′ NTRs play critical roles in the EV life cycle. The 5′ NTR contains multiple regions of predicted higher order structure (i.e., stem loops or domains). A domain located at the extreme 5′ terminus of the 5′ NTR is essential for viral RNA replication. Cap-independent translation of the EV genome is regulated by the internal ribosome entry (IRES) site, which spans a discontinuous region within the 5′ NTR. For PV and several nonpolio enteroviruses (NPEVs), the 5′ NTR has been documented to be a determinant of virulence phenotype and cell type specificity (22, 23). Given the crucial nature of the functions controlled by the 5′ NTR, it is not surprising that nucleotide sequences, with near-absolute conservation among the EVs, exist within this region. These regions of high nucleotide identity have been exploited for the design of primers and probes used for the detection of the EVs. The 3′ NTR has also been demonstrated to play a role in viral RNA replication.

The EV capsid is arranged in 60 repeating protomeric units that confer an icosahedral shape to the virion (Fig. 2) (21). VP1, VP2, and VP3 comprise the surface of the virion and possess an eight-stranded "beta barrel" core structure. The external loops that connect the beta strands are responsible for the differences in surface topography and antigenic diversity among the EVs. Neutralization sites, typically three or four per protomer, are most densely clustered on VP1. VP4 is located internally within the capsid and has no surface-exposed regions.

The resolution of the near-atomic structures of multiple human picornaviruses revealed that the EVs (and RVs) share many conserved structural motifs. Surrounding a conserved protrusion at the 5-fold axis of each pentameric unit (i.e., five protomers) is a narrow deep cleft (25 Å) or canyon. It is into this site that the specific receptors for the EVs bind when the virus encounters a susceptible host cell.

The genomic organization of PeVs is like that of EVs. However, unlike the EVs, PeVs possess only three capsid proteins, VP0, VP3, and VP1, because of the lack of cleavage of VP0. In addition, the PeV IRES is more similar to those of the cardioviruses and aphthoviruses than those of enteroviruses (24). Cryo-electron microscopy has revealed a 28-nm diameter PeV particle similar to other known picornaviruses but with a somewhat smoother surface (25). Sequence similarities between PeVs and the other picornaviruses suggest that the major capsid proteins share the

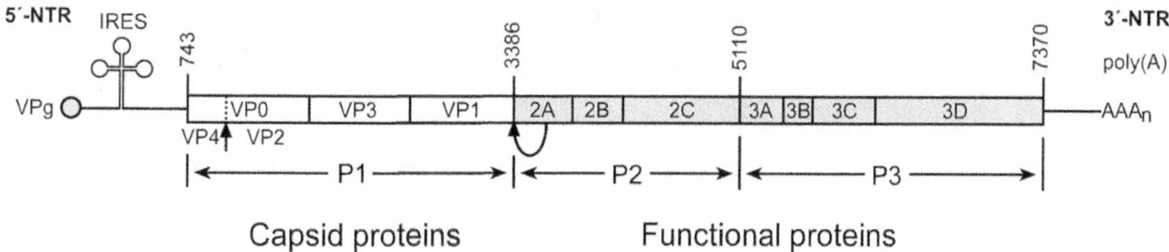

FIGURE 1 Genome organization of PV type 1. The PV genome is a single-stranded positive-sense RNA of approximately 7,500 nucleotides. Nucleotides 743 to 7370 encode the capsid proteins (white boxes in coding regions P1) and functional proteins (gray boxes in coding regions P2 and P3) in a single open reading frame. The 5′ and 3′ NTRs are shown as lines. The IRES is shown schematically with two-dimensional structure. The virus protein VPg is covalently linked to the terminal uracil of the 5′ NTR. Reprinted from reference 21.

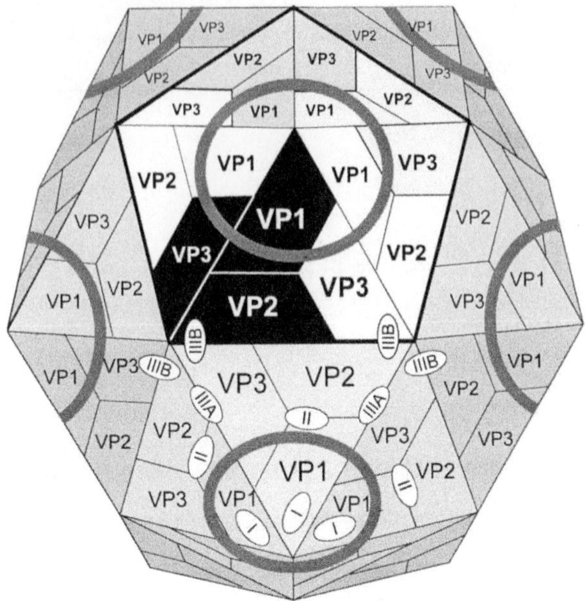

FIGURE 2 Schematic representation of the three-dimensional structure of a PV particle and the four neutralizing antigenetic (N-Ag) sites. The icosahedral capsid structure typical of EVs is composed of 60 protomers, each consisting of the capsid proteins VP1, VP2, and VP3 (black areas). Each of the 12 5-fold symmetry axes is surrounded by five protomers, forming a pentamer (surrounded by a bold black line). The attachment site for the virus-specific receptor is a depression around the 5-fold symmetry axis, also called the canyon (dark gray circles). Each of the three surface-exposed capsid proteins contains immunodominant antigenic sites at which neutralizing antibodies bind. Four N-Ag sites (white ellipses) have been mapped to surface loop extensions. Reprinted from reference 21.

typical beta barrel core structure. Relative to the EVs, the PeVs are predicted to have a flatter surface topography (as shown with cryo-electron microscopy), with antigenic variants determined by the external loops, as for EVs.

EPIDEMIOLOGY AND TRANSMISSION

The EVs and PeVs are ubiquitous agents found worldwide. In regions with temperate climates, most EV infections (70 to 80%) occur in summer and fall. In tropical climates, EV infections occur year-round or with increased incidence during the rainy season. Seasonal differences in incidence have been seen among serotypes of PeV. HPeV3 infections occur mainly during spring and summer, whereas HPeV1 circulates throughout the year, with a nadir in summer months (24, 26, 27)

It is estimated that the EVs infect a billion or more individuals worldwide each year, with 30 to 50 million infections in the United States (28). Except for strictly respiratory strains such as EV-D68 (29), EVs and PeVs are spread mainly by the fecal-oral route and less by respiratory droplets and fomites. Fecal-oral transmission predominates in areas with poor sanitary conditions. Transplacental (i.e., congenital) transmission has been documented (30). These viruses can survive on environmental surfaces for periods long enough to allow transmission from fomites. Hospital nursery and other institutional outbreaks have occurred.

The highest incidence of EV infection is observed in young infants and children of 5 to 10 years of age, with children aged <1 year accounting for almost half of the reported cases in the United States (31). Generally, the incubation period is 3 to 6 days, except for acute hemorrhagic conjunctivitis, which is 24 to 72 hours (32), and secondary infections are observed in >50% of susceptible household members (33). The incidence of PeV infection is highest in children <1 year of age, again with most infections occurring in infants of <6 months of age (34–36). Furthermore, variations in the mean age at which infants had infections with various HPeV types have been documented, with HPeV3 infection occurring at a younger age (24).

Two major patterns of circulating enteroviruses have been observed between 1970 and 2005: epidemic (e.g., E9, E13, E30, and CVB5) and endemic (e.g., CVA9, CVB2, CVB4, and EV71) (31). Epidemic serotypes were characterized by substantial fluctuations in numbers over time with occasional increased incidence. Endemic serotypes had stable and usually low levels of circulation with few changes in incidence. The five most commonly reported serotypes (E9, E11, E30, E6, and CVB5) accounted for 48.1% of the cases. From 2009 to 2013, CVA6 and HPeV3 were the most commonly detected EV and PeV identified, each accounting for 12.3% of cases tested, with most isolates of CVA6 occurring in 2012 (37). A single institution that routinely tested for PeV contributed 94% of all HePV3 isolated in 2012.

In general, mortality is not common with EV infections, with death being reported for 3.3% of cases with known outcomes. Infections with CVB4 and HPeV1 were associated with higher risk for death, and infections with E9 were associated with lower risk for death (31).

The Global Polio Eradication Initiative began in 1988. By 2015, wild poliovirus type 2 infection was certified as having been eradicated by the Global Commission for the Certification of the Eradication of Poliomyelitis (38); by 2016, endemic circulation of wild poliovirus type 1 and 3 had been controlled globally, with the exception of Afghanistan, Nigeria, and Pakistan (39). Efforts toward global polio eradication have resulted in a 99.9% decrease of polio cases, from an estimated 350,000 cases annually to 37 cases in 2016 (39).

CLINICAL SIGNIFICANCE

EVs and PeVs cause a wide array of both localized and systemic infections that affect many organ systems in patients of all ages (Table 2). Generally, no disease is uniquely associated with any specific serotype, and no serotype is uniquely associated with any one disease. This is true even of paralytic poliomyelitis, which has been associated with numerous NPEV serotypes. However, different serotypes of EV have been associated with more-severe disease and/or death in different age groups of children (40). Likewise, HPeV3 is also associated with more-severe disease (13, 24, 34, 41). Encephalitis and a sepsis-like syndrome consisting of high fever, severe irritability, tachycardia, poor perfusion, erythroderma, abdominal distention, and hepatitis have been more frequently associated with PeV3 infection.

The majority of EV and PeV infections are asymptomatic. The most common symptomatic manifestation of infection is acute nonspecific febrile illness, with or without an exanthem. This so-called viral syndrome is one of the most numerically important causes of fever among infants and children. Although this illness itself is benign, it is of great concern because it mimics other more serious illnesses in infants and young children. Distinguishing EV and PeV infections from those due to common bacteria and other viruses is often difficult on clinical grounds alone,

TABLE 2 Clinical syndromes associated with EV and PeV infection

Organ system	Disease
Neurologic	Aseptic meningitis, encephalitis, acute flaccid myelitis
Respiratory	Common cold, stomatitis, hand-foot-and-mouth disease, herpangina, lymphonodular pharyngitis, tonsillitis, rhinitis, bronchiolitis, bronchitis, pneumonia
Cardiovascular	Myocarditis, pericarditis
Miscellaneous	Acute hemorrhagic conjunctivitis (AHC), pleurodynia (Bornholm disease), febrile exanthematous illness, neonatal sepsis

and hence, leads to unnecessary treatment. During summer and fall, the EVs are responsible for 50 to 60% of hospital admissions for the evaluation of acute febrile illness in children and infants (33).

By far the most vexing clinical EV/PeV syndrome that physicians encounter is aseptic meningitis. The EVs are the most common cause of meningitis in the United States and account for over 80% of all viral meningitides (42, 43). More recently, HPeV3 has been recognized to cause a significant number of cases of neonatal sepsis and aseptic meningitis in children <2 years of age (24, 34–36, 44). The onset of symptoms is usually sudden and generally includes fever, headache, occasionally photophobia, vomiting, rash, and myalgias. In young children, symptoms include fever, lethargy, and anorexia, again mimicking bacterial infection. Currently, treatment is supportive with illness generally resolving after a week with no long-term sequelae. An estimated 30,000 to 50,000 hospitalizations for NPEVs meningitis occur each year. The echoviruses and CVBs, particularly E4, E6, E9, E11, E16, and E30 and CVB2 and CVB5, constitute the principal EVs associated with this syndrome.

The term poliomyelitis refers to the inflammatory damage due to infection of the anterior horn cells of the spinal cord. Recognized clinically as acute-onset lower-motor neuron paralysis of one or more muscles, the case fatality rate in the prevaccine era ranged from 5 to 10% (6, 45), and in recent epidemics, as high as 48% (46). Historically, this disease was most commonly associated with the PVs; however, in most countries, this is no longer the case. In regions of the world where the polioviruses have been eradicated, the NPEVs, PeVs, and circulating vaccine-derived PVs (cVDPVs) are now the principal causes of acute flaccid myelitis (AFM). cVDPVs are circulating strains derived from the vaccine (Sabin) strains of PV that have regained the capacity to cause paralytic poliomyelitis, and at least six poliomyelitis outbreaks have been caused by cVDPV (1, 2). It is also important to point out that despite efforts toward polio eradication, these viruses are still endemic in some countries and have served as reservoirs for the reintroduction of polio to other areas.

Multiple NPEV serotypes are also known to cause AFM, in particular EV71. During the fall of 2014, clusters of AFM cases were reported worldwide, concurrent to large outbreaks of EV-D68 severe lower respiratory disease, primarily in children. In the United States, 1,153 identified cases of severe respiratory disease and 107 cases of AFM were reported (47). EV-D68 infection was detected from nasopharyngeal swabs from some of the paralyzed children. To further complicate matters, indications of infections with other organisms were also present in some children, including some coinfections. A similar pattern of increased rates of AFM coinciding with increased rates of EV-D68 respiratory infections occurred again during the fall of 2016, albeit not to the same degree as in 2014. As in previously reported clusters of AFM, no pathogen was consistently isolated from all specimens tested (47). Because the etiology for the AFM has yet to be identified, the CDC emphasizes the importance of expanded AFM testing to include both infectious and noninfectious causes (https://www.cdc.gov/acute-flaccid-myelitis/faqs.html). Studies of the etiology of encephalitis have identified EVs in approximately 3 to 5% of all cases, accounting for 27 to 37% of identified viral etiologies (48, 49). Serotypes from the EV-B and EV-A species are the predominant EV subgroup associated with this syndrome (33, 48–50). PeV has also been shown as a causative agent, particularly among neonates (41). The contribution of PeV to the total number of annual cases of encephalitis is yet unknown. Recently, PeV encephalitis has been linked to significant neurodevelopmental sequelae (51). Rhombencephalitis, a severe and often-fatal form of brainstem encephalitis, has been associated with the EV71 infections in small children from several countries in the Asia-Pacific region (52–54); however, cases in the United States have also been reported (55). Chronic EV meningoencephalitis in agammaglobulinemia occurs and is caused most frequently by the echoviruses, particularly E11.

Myocarditis was once an often-fatal disease associated with EV; however, mortality rates are lower (~10%) with current medical care. Symptoms range from nonspecific (fever, myalgias, palpitations, or exertional dyspnea) to fulminant hemodynamic collapse and sudden death. Myocarditis has been implicated in 8.6 to 12% of cases of sudden cardiac death of young adults (56, 57). CVBs are responsible for one-third to one-half of all cases of acute myocarditis and pericarditis (58), with CVB2 and CVB5 being the most predominant serotypes identified in clinical studies. The echoviruses, PV, and PeVs have also been associated with myopericarditis, but significantly less so than CVB.

Neonatal systemic disease is associated with EV and PeV acquisition *in utero*, perinatally, or within the first 2 weeks of life (24, 30). This syndrome is characterized by multiorgan involvement, with symptoms including lethargy, feeding difficulty, vomiting, tachycardia, dyspnea, cyanosis, jaundice, and diarrhea, with or without fever. Typically, neonatal systemic EV disease is associated with two severe clinical presentations (although infants may present with combinations or organ system involvement): heart failure and hemorrhage-hepatitis syndrome, with hepatic failure and disseminated intravascular coagulation (24, 30, 40). The morbidity and mortality associated with this syndrome are significant, with death occurring rapidly. CVB and echoviruses, particularly serotype 11, are frequently associated with this syndrome. However, other EVs and PeVs are also known to cause this syndrome.

Although originally described for agammaglobulinemic patients, persistent and life-threatening EV infections can also occur in patients with combined variable immunodeficiency, severe combined immunodeficiency, hypogammaglobulinemia, or hyperimmunoglobulin M (hyper-IgM) syndrome, and in those undergoing bone marrow and solid organ transplant. Manifestations almost always include meningoencephalitis. Individuals receiving anti-CD20 monoclonal antibodies (rituximab, obinutuzumab) are at increased risk for severe EV infections (59, 60).

Hand-foot-and-mouth disease (HFMD) has historically been associated with CVA16. However, EV71, which is closely related to polioviruses and CVA16, has been the cause of large outbreaks of HFMD with neurological and systemic complications in the Asia-Pacific region (61). The neurological manifestations range from aseptic meningitis to AFM and brainstem encephalitis, which is associated with systemic features, such as severe pulmonary edema and shock. Although serious disease due to EV71 has been described worldwide, high rates are observed in Asia; the reason for the geographic disparity in presentations is largely unknown but may be related to viral strain differences or to host HLA antigens (61). CVA6, which has been associated with herpangina, has now been linked to outbreaks of atypical HFMD in the United States (62).

Upper respiratory tract signs and symptoms may accompany many of the enteroviral syndromes. The enteroviruses may be causal agents of upper and lower respiratory tract syndromes (e.g., summer cold, pharyngitis, tonsillitis, laryngotracheobronchitis, bronchiolitis, and pneumonia) (55, 63, 64). Enteroviruses have been etiologically linked in up to 15% of cases of upper respiratory tract syndromes (64). The use of nucleic acid amplification methodologies has demonstrated that, depending on the country, the enteroviruses are responsible for up to approximately 19% of lower respiratory tract infections in hospitalized children (65, 66). Several of the EV C types (C104, C109, C117) have been isolated from individuals with pneumonia or respiratory tract disease (67–70).

In recent years, EV-D68 has become recognized as a cause of significant respiratory disease. Originally isolated from four children with pneumonia and bronchiolitis in 1962 (71), the overwhelming majority of reports of its isolation since then (and recently) have been from the respiratory tract as sporadic isolations or as clusters of infections or epidemics (70, 72–77). EV-D68 is phenotypically anomalous among the enteroviruses in that it is acid labile and replicates poorly at 37°C, characteristics commonly found among the RVs (29, 78, 79). Furthermore, EV-D68 was uncommon until recently (70, 75, 77); a 36-year review of nonpolio EV isolates reported to the CDC revealed that only 26 out of 52,812 isolates were EV-D68 (31). Phylogenetic analysis of EV-D68 isolates from around the world has indicated that, over the past 20 years, multiple clades have emerged and spread rapidly (80), possibly accounting for the increase in reported clusters and epidemics worldwide (72–76, 81).

Clinically significant lower respiratory tract disease occurs primarily in young children and infants (72–77, 81) but has been reported in adolescents and adults (70, 72, 75). Underlying conditions such as asthma or wheezing have been reported in approximately 70 to 80% of cases (72, 81). Reported clinical syndromes associated with EV-D68 include pneumonia, bronchiolitis, asthmatic bronchitis, asthma exacerbation, and wheezing (73, 74, 76, 77). Pulmonary signs and symptoms include cough, wheezing, dyspnea, tachycardia, and inter- and subcostal retractions (72, 73, 76, 81). Surprisingly, approximately one-half to three-quarters of children are afebrile. Hypoxia requiring supplemental oxygen is very common and can be severe enough to require admission to intensive care. Some children may require bilevel positive airway pressure ventilation, mechanical ventilation, or even extracorporeal membrane oxygenation. Deaths are uncommon but have been reported. Chest radiographs may show infiltrates and atelectasis.

Other acute clinical EV syndromes of significance include acute hemorrhagic conjunctivitis (predominantly caused by EV70 and a variant CVA24), herpangina, and pleurodynia (Bornholm disease). Data have been presented suggesting a link between EV infections and several chronic illnesses, including amyotrophic lateral sclerosis, chronic fatigue syndrome, polymyositis, congenital hydrocephalus, and attention-deficit/hyperactivity disorder, but definitive proof of causation is lacking (82). However, recent reports strengthen the possible association between enteroviruses and type 1 insulin-dependent diabetes mellitus, although human genetic factors also play an important role (83–85).

In general, the spectrum of diseases caused by PeV is similar to that of EV (24), as are the age groups that are infected. Diarrhea or respiratory symptoms have been described alone or in combination with other syndromes. Evidence linking PeVs as the etiologic cause of epidemic diarrheal disease is lacking, but they may be associated with endemic cases of diarrhea (24). Outbreaks of respiratory disease have been reported, but data for the role of PeV in endemic community respiratory disease are scant. In a cohort of 2,200 persons with respiratory symptoms, PeV was detected in respiratory samples of only 1.2% (86). As with the EV neonatal sepsis, AFM, aseptic meningitis, encephalitis, and myocarditis are seen with PeV infection (particularly type 3). Interestingly, Ljungan virus, a parechovirus previously believed to infect rodents exclusively, has more recently been linked to intrauterine fetal death in humans (87).

COLLECTION, TRANSPORT, AND STORAGE OF SPECIMENS

Specimen selection is important for making a diagnosis of EV infection, as asymptomatic shedding, especially in stool, is common. The specimen collected should correlate with the clinical syndrome (Table 3). Typically, EV infection

TABLE 3 EV and PeV diseases and specimen selection

	Acceptability of specimen[a]					
Disease	Throat[b]	Rectal/Stool[b]	Serum	CSF	Tissue	Conjunctival
Aseptic meningitis			±	+		
Encephalitis	+	+	±	±		
AFM[c]	+	+	±			
Respiratory disease	+					
Myocarditis					+	
AHC[d]						+
Febrile illness			+			
Neonatal sepsis			±			

[a]+, specimen is appropriate for testing; ±, specimen may be appropriate for testing.
[b]Associated with low specificity.
[c]AFM, acute flaccid myelitis.
[d]AHC, acute hemorrhagic conjunctivitis.

begins with viral replication in the epithelial cells of the respiratory or gastrointestinal tract and in the lymphoid follicles of the small intestine followed by viremia, leading to a secondary site of tissue infection. Hence, for patients with aseptic meningitis, cerebrospinal fluid (CSF) is generally the specimen of choice; however, testing serum or plasma can yield better results early in the disease process (88–92) and may be the only option in cases of neonatal sepsis (91). It is important to note that at least in pediatric patients, EV and PeV detection rates are higher in blood and CSF specimens than in nasopharynx specimens (93, 94). Also, if CSF is obtained >2 days after the onset of symptoms, the diagnostic yield may be lower (95).

Prescreening of CSF for pleocytosis (lymphocytosis) is not recommended for pediatric patients because lack of pleocytosis is common, particularly in infants (96–99). The opposite may be true for adults (100). Similarly, in the early stage of the disease, neutrophils may predominate for a few hours. On the other hand, patients with EV encephalitis often have negative CSF PCR results even when they have CSF pleocytosis; in these patients, throat and/or rectal swabs may be the specimen of choice. However, since EV and PeV are associated with prolonged periods of asymptomatic shedding from the throat and gastrointestinal tract (101–105), their presence from these sites is not necessarily proof of cause. Furthermore, viruses detected from sterile sites can differ by 10 to 20% from viruses detected in throat and rectal swabs, because of dual infection (106). It is important to point out that for cases of AFM, it is recommended to collect two stool specimens at least 24 hours apart during the first 14 days following onset of paralysis (1) (https://www.cdc.gov/acute-flaccid-myelitis/hcp/instructions.html).

In cases of myocarditis and pericarditis, myocardial tissue is considered the diagnostic standard (107, 108). Outside of infants less than 1 year old, analyses of blood samples by PCR have been almost uniformly negative (47, 92, 109–111). For cases of herpangina and HFMD, vesicle fluid is an efficient sample for diagnostic testing, with greater yields observed when multiple vesicles are swabbed. For cases of acute hemorrhagic conjunctivitis, the best specimens are conjunctival swabs (1).

Optimal specimens are best transported and stored in viral transport media. But because EVs are stable in liquid environments and can survive for many weeks in water, body fluids, and sewage, rapid transport of specimens to the laboratory is not necessary. In fact, EVs survive at room temperature for 7 days, and at 4°C to −20°C for up to a year (112). Long-term storage at −70°C or colder is recommended to prevent degradation of viral RNA, which also preserves (112) viral infectivity for cell culture for years.

Certain clinical specimens, such as stool, require processing prior to inoculation of cell cultures. Specimen processing procedures for nucleic acid amplification tests (NAAT) should preserve viral capsid integrity so that the EV RNA genome is protected from nucleases that are ubiquitous in body fluids and the environment. Excessive freeze-thaw cycles should be avoided. Residual samples found in clinical laboratory refrigerators may be suitable for nucleic acid-based detection of the EVs because of the inherent environmental stability of the EVs. Specimens that have been handled by automated chemistry or hematology analyzers should be considered compromised because of the potential for cross-contamination with other specimens. Sera for antibody testing are best collected 2 to 4 weeks apart at both acute and convalescent stages. The sera should be frozen at −20°C and tested simultaneously.

DIRECT EXAMINATION

Microscopy

Antigen Detection

Historically, immunofluorescent techniques have not been used for the detection of respiratory infections caused by EVs because these viruses were believed to be associated with self-limited upper respiratory tract infection only.

Nucleic Acid Detection

Currently, NAATs are preferred for the detection of EV and PeV. Cell culture has little clinical utility due to the prolonged time required for viral isolation (up to 10 days for EV and 21 days for PeV). Some serotypes within the EV species C (i.e., CVA1, CVA19, and CVA22), as well as HPeV7-16, either fail to grow in cell culture or their propagation capacity is unknown. Many specimen types (i.e., 25 to 35% of CSF specimens) have titers that are too low to be detected by cell culture (113). Furthermore, studies have demonstrated that the use of EV NAAT testing has a favorable impact on patient care. Outcome studies have demonstrated a correlation between time to result and length of stay (96, 114, 115). Antibiotic usage was reduced, fewer ancillary tests were performed, and hospitalization was shortened and less costly when positive EV results were reported within 24 h (114–118).

NAATs (RT-PCR or nucleic acid sequence-based amplification [NASBA]) are sensitive, specific, rapid, versatile, and clinically useful methods for the detection of EVs (119–121). NAAT of CSF is more sensitive than cell culture, which has a sensitivity of 65 to 75% (121–123). Interestingly, the sensitivity of NAAT for the detection of EV in cases of aseptic meningitis ranges from 70 to 100% despite indications that EVs are the primary causative agent (121, 124–127). One partial reason for this discrepancy is the fact that PeV, which can account for approximately 5% of cases of neonatal sepsis and aseptic meningitis in the United States, is not detected by universal EV RT-PCR assays (9).

A limited number of studies have evaluated the sensitivity and specificity of NAAT with other sample types. For serum, the sensitivity and specificity of RT-PCR range from 81 to 92% and from 98 to 100%, respectively, for the diagnosis of EV infection (122, 128). In contrast, 100- to 1,000-fold greater sensitivity of RT-PCR over culture has been reported for detection of EV and PeV from CSF, throat swabs, or stool specimens (94, 129, 130). In addition to the enhanced sensitivity of NAAT testing, this technology has the added benefit of rapid turnaround times, with results available in as little as 2.5 hours including nucleic acid extraction (131).

Prior to being tested by NAAT, EV RNA must be extracted from specimens to eliminate ubiquitous RNases and to remove potential amplification inhibitors. Only a small sample size, generally 100 to 350 μl of fluid or 1 mg of tissue, is required. The most common methods for RNA extraction are gel membrane or magnetic silica binding. Multiple automated extraction methods have been utilized, including MagNA Pure LC and Compact (Roche Diagnostics System); easyMAG (bioMérieux); and M48, QIAcube, EZ One, and QIAsymphony (Qiagen). An EV RT-PCR assay on the GeneXpert system includes extraction, amplification, and detection all in one cartridge (131). All aspects of NAAT testing, from extraction to detection, are discussed in more detail in chapter 7 of this *Manual*.

Currently, two FDA-approved real-time assays are available for the detection of EV from CSF Cepheid's Xpert

TABLE 4 NAATs for EV and PeV detection from CSF

Assay (Manufacturer)	Method	Target	Regulatory status	Comment	Reference(s)
Xpert EV (Cepheid)	Real-time RT-PCR	5′ NTR	IVD[a]	Extraction, amplification, and detection in a single cartridge	131, 132
Enterovirus R-gene (bioMérieux)	Real-time RT-PCR	5′ NTR	CE-IVD[b]	Used on multiple extraction and real-time PCR platforms	149
MGB Alert Enterovirus (ELITech)	Real-time RT-PCR	5′ NTR	ASR[c]	Uses patented chemistry	
MultiCode Enterovirus Primers (Luminex Corporation)	Real-time RT-PCR	5′ NTR	ASR	Uses labeled primer and proprietary chemistry	
Artus Enterovirus (Qiagen)	Real-time RT-PCR	5′ NTR	RUO[d]		
EV noncommercial reagents	Real-time & conventional RT-PCR	5′ NTR, VP2	LDT[e]		127, 138, 139, 148
Parechovirus R-gene (bioMérieux)	Real-time RT-PCR	5′ NTR	CE-IVD	Used on multiple extraction and real-time PCR platforms	161
HPeV noncommercial reagents	Real-time RT-PCR	5′ NTR	LDT	Detects HPeV 1–16	154–157
Meningitis/Encephalitis (ME) Panel (BioFire)	Real-time RT-PCR	5′ NTR	IVD	Extraction, amplification, and detection of EV, HPeV, and other pathogens in a single pouch	134
FTD Viral Meningitis (Fast Track Diagnostics)	Multiplex real-time RT-PCR	5′ NTR	CE-IVD	Multiplex detection of EV and PeV	162
EV & HPeV Multiplex noncommercial reagents	Multiplex real-time RT-PCR	5′ NTR	LDT	Multiplex detection of EV and PeV	158, 159

[a]IVD, *in vitro* diagnostic (FDA-approved test).
[b]CE-IVD, "Conformité Europèene," which literally means "European Conformity."
[c]ASR, analyte-specific reagent.
[d]RUO, research use only.
[e]LDT, laboratory-developed test.
[f]IC, internal control.

EV and BioFire's Meningitis/Encephalitis (ME) Panel (Table 4). In a multicenter analysis, the Xpert EV had a sensitivity of 95% and specificity of 100% (132). However, in routine clinical practice the sensitivity appeared to be much lower (133). The BioFire ME Panel is a multiplex test system that detects seven viruses, including EV and PeV, six bacteria, and one yeast associated with ME, and demonstrated a sensitivity of 95.7% for EV and 100% for PeV (134). However, more studies with larger numbers of positive PeV and EV samples, as well as a head-to-head comparison with Xpert EV, are needed to better assess the performance of this panel (135).

Additionally, multiplexed respiratory virus assays that include the detection of EV and/or RV are available. In the United States, these systems include xTAG Respiratory Viral Panel, xTAG Respiratory Viral Panel FAST, and VERIGENE Respiratory Tract Infection Test (Luminex Corporation); FilmArray Respiratory Panel, Respiratory Panel EZ, and Respiratory Panel 2 (BioFire Diagnostics); and ePlex Respiratory Pathogen Panel (GenMark Diagnostics). These panels are FDA approved for nasopharyngeal specimens and do not well differentiate EV from RV. Limited data have been reported on direct comparisons of EV/RV components in these assays, but comparisons have been performed on the overall sensitivity and specificity of all the targets, showing varying results (136, 137).

Analyte-specific reagents (ASRs), laboratory-developed tests (LDTs), and CE-IVD (European Conformity)-certified reagents for EV real-time RT-PCR are widely used (Table 4). LDTs routinely target conserved sequences within the 5′ NTR or VP2, for nearly universal amplification of EVs (Table 4); the most frequent 5′ NTR targets are those reported by Rotbart (138) and Chapman et al. (139). While these primers do not detect PeV (discussed below), they do amplify the genomes of several rhinoviruses (140–142) and may miss some strains of EV (143). As with all ASR and LDT, laboratories must develop and validate the assays for themselves.

Despite the increased availability and benefits of real-time PCR, conventional RT-PCR is primarily used for viral typing (144, 145). There is a wide array of detection systems for conventional PCR including agarose gel electrophoresis, reverse transcription loop-mediated isothermal amplification (RT-LAMP) (146, 147), and colorimetric assays using enzyme-linked immunosorbent assay-type formats (127, 148, 149).

With regard to quality control, EV NAATs should include internal controls to detect amplification inhibitors and to assess nucleic acid recovery. EV RNA assay verification experiments and quality assurance performance demonstrate the need for a universal, nominal EV standard; however, none exists. Instead, most laboratories use either quantified EV isolates or transcripts from clones of target regions, both of which must be created and validated in the laboratory. Alternatively, there are commercial sources for EV and PeV viruses for validation and control material. Unfortunately, these viruses are not quantified.

Multicenter proficiency testing programs for LDT EV NAATs indicate that properly designed tests can be equally effective in the detection of EV, regardless of the format used (150). However, other studies have reported marked variation in testing proficiency between centers. In one survey, one-third of participating laboratories were nonproficient in the detection of EV by RT-PCR (112). In another report, 6.8% of participating laboratories recorded false-positive results, pointing to the need for fastidious attention to methods for preventing cross-contamination (150). Overall, these findings underscore the importance of rigorous quality control and periodic proficiency reassessment to ensure uniformly high-quality testing.

Reports detailing the detection of PeVs by RT-PCR have been published (13, 141, 151). Although the original methods were limited to the detection of HPeV 1 and/or 2 (151–153), more recent reports detect at least types 1 through 6 (Table 4) (154–157) and some should detect all 19 (156). To date, only one FDA-approved assay for the detection of PeV is available in the United States, the BioFire ME Panel; as a result, LDTs for single-plex detection or multiplexing of PeV and EV PCR targets are common (158–160). In Europe, two assays are CE-IVD-certified for the detection of PeV, the bioMérieux Parechovirus r-Gene and the Fast Track Diagnostics FTD Viral Meningitis assay (161, 162). The Fast Track assay is a multiplex RT-PCR assay that detects both EV and PeV (Table 4).

ISOLATION PROCEDURES

A combination of human and primate cell lines is typically used for EV and PeV isolation since no single cell line supports the growth of all types. Furthermore, several CVA serotypes do not grow in cell culture (1). The general susceptibilities of commonly used cell lines are summarized in Table 5. Isolation times for EVs from CSF by traditional cell culture techniques range from 4 to 8 days but are shorter (1 to 3 days) from sites with higher viral titers. Recovery time for PeV is variable, dependent upon both virus and cell type, and often are associated with delayed or no cytopathic effect production (163).

Infections of susceptible cell monolayers with EVs result in a characteristic cytopathic effect (CPE), consisting of shrinkage and rounding of individual cells within the monolayers. The nuclei of infected cells exhibit pyknosis. As infection progresses, the cells degenerate and separate from the monolayer. Often the CPE is so characteristic that a presumptive diagnosis of EV infection can be made (Fig. 3). However, experience is necessary, as toxic effects from primary specimens, such as *Clostridioides difficile* toxin, can mimic CPE (164). Although the CPEs for EV and PeV are very similar, differences have long been noted. The CPE for PeV can appear as larger regularly shaped spheres compared to small irregular shapes caused by EVs (Fig. 3) (165).

The relatively low sensitivity of viral culture from CSF (65 to 75%, reviewed in reference 166) is likely due to the presence of neutralizing antibodies, inadequate CSF volume for a comprehensive culture (i.e., inoculate 3 to 5 cell types), low viral load, and resistance of some serotypes to culture. Many serotypes within the EV group C (i.e., CVA1, CVA19, and CVA22) and HPeV7-14 are nonculturable. Historically, stool cultures have been thought to have greater sensitivity for EV/PeV detection than CSF culture (167); however, PCR testing of stool is even more sensitive (130).

TABLE 5 Susceptibilities of cell lines commonly used for isolation of EV and HPeV

	Susceptibility to virus[a]									
		Coxsackie			HPeV					
Cell line	Polio	A[b]	B	Echo	1	2	3	4	5	6
Primary simian (monkey kidney)										
Primary rhesus (pRhMK)	+++	+	+++	+++	+	+	unk	unk	unk	unk
Primary cynomolgus (pCMK)	++++	+	+++	+++	+	+	unk	unk	unk	unk
Buffalo green (BGMK)	+++	+	++++	++	+++	−	++	−	−	−
African green (Vero)	+++	+	+++	++	++++	+	++++[c,d]	++	++	++[d]
Rhesus (LLC-MK2)	+++	+	+++	+++	+++	+++	++[d]	−	−	−
Cynomolgus (tMK)	+++	+	+++	+++	++	++	+	++	+	−
Human										
Human cervix adenocarcinoma (HeLa)	+++	+	+++	+	++	+	−	+	unk	unk
Human colon carcinoma (HT-29)	+++	+	+++	+++	+++	+++	−	+++	+++	+
Human colon carcinoma (CaCo-2)	+++	+	+++	+++	++[d]	±[e]	+[d]	++[e]	−	−
Human embryonic lung fibroblast (HEL)	+++	++	+	+++	−	−	−	−	−	−
Human embryonic lung fibroblast (MRC-5)	+++	+	+	+++	+	+	−	unk	unk	unk
Human embryonic lung fibroblast (WI-38)	++	++	+	+++	+	+	−	unk	unk	unk
Human epidermoid carcinoma (HEp-2)	+++	+	+++	+	++	++	−	unk	unk	unk
Human kidney epithelial (293)	+++	+	++	+++	++	++	−	unk	unk	unk
Human lung carcinoma (A549)	+++	+	+++	+++	++	++	−	++	++	−/+
Human rhabdomyosarcoma (RD)	+++	+++[f]	+	+++	+++[d]	±[d]	+++[d]	+++[d]	++[d]	++[d]
Mouse										
L20B cells[g]	++++	+	−	−	−	−	unk	unk	unk	unk
Super E-mix (combination of BGMK-hDAF[h] and CaCo2)	++	++	++++	++++	++	++	unk	unk	unk	unk

[a]Relative susceptibilities: +, minimally susceptible; ++++, maximally susceptible; −, nonsusceptible; unk, unknown (no published reports). Some EVs are difficult to isolate even on minimally susceptible cell lines.

[b]Some CV-A (A1, A19, and A20) are not readily isolated.

[c]Improved yields after passage.

[d]Delayed CPE.

[e]No CPE.

[f]Many CV-A only grow in RD cells.

[g]L20B cells; L cell line engineered with the PV receptor, CD 155.

[h]BGMK-hDAF, BGMK expressing human decay-accelerating factor.

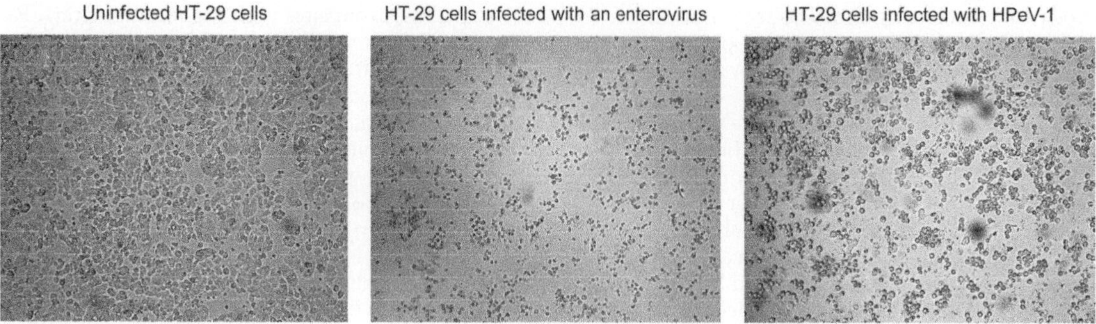

FIGURE 3 Cytopathic effects observed 3 days after infection of HT-29 cells with an EV or HPeV1 isolate after passage on this cell line. Reprinted from reference 165.

Shell vial culture (SVC), in which virus is detected with monoclonal antibodies in the absence of CPE, reduces the time to detection to 2 to 3 days. The sensitivity of SVC may or may not be higher than that of traditional cell culture (168–170) and is probably laboratory and cell line dependent (171). SVC using a mixture of cell lines in a single vial (Super E-Mix containing decay-accelerating factor-expressing BGMK cells and A549 cells, Diagnostic Hybrids Inc., Athens, OH) improves sensitivity (170, 171). Evaluations of the capacity of Super E-Mix to isolate PeV has not been performed; however, it is presumed that at least HPeV1 and 2 would grow in this cell mix because A549 cells are susceptible to infection. The greatest limitation of SVC is the monoclonal antibody used in the detection steps (discussed below).

IDENTIFICATION

Broadly reactive and serotype-specific EV monoclonal antibodies have been developed (172) and applied to cell culture confirmation by immunofluorescence. While preliminary studies suggest that these reagents, used singly and in blends (Dako-Enterovirus 5-D8/1, Dako, Glostrup, Denmark; Pan-Enterovirus blend, Chemicon International Inc.), demonstrated an important role in serotype identifications, further studies have identified several limitations (168, 169, 173). The most notable limitations are cross-reactivity with the Chemicon blend (168) and the lack of EV71 detection with the Dako blend. A pool of anti-EV antibodies has been developed (D3 IFA Enterovirus Identification, Diagnostic Hybrids Inc.), which reportedly has good sensitivity, including the detection of EV71 with little or no cross-reactivity. The concordance of results for identification of clinical EV isolates to the species level with monoclonal blends versus the neutralization assay has demonstrated the latter may be significantly superior for the identification of the EVs (173). These studies appeared to indicate that monoclonal antibodies for EV identification should be used as a preliminary screen for species or serotype identification. With regards to PeV, typing reagents are only available for types 1 and 2, and not all HPeV-2 isolates are neutralized by specific antisera (174).

TYPING SYSTEMS

This virus family exhibits a considerable amount of genetic variability driven by both mutation and recombination (175, 176). However, serotype determination is usually unnecessary for clinical purposes because the diseases caused by the EVs are not serotype specific. Currently, the identification of EV type is most useful for distinguishing between VDPV and NPEVs to facilitate the interpretation of viral culture results in areas where the Sabin PV strains are used for vaccination, as the live vaccine can be shed for 1 to 2 weeks from the throat and can remain in the feces for several weeks to months (32). Identification of NPEV serotypes is useful for epidemiological purposes and for determination of serotypes associated with unusual or novel clinical manifestations, such as flaccid paralysis (1, 2).

Historically, EV serotype determination involved neutralization with the Lim and Benyesh-Melnick (LBM) pools of antisera; however, genetic drift of the EVs over time has given rise to antigenic variants. Furthermore, the procedure is labor-intensive, and the supply of LBM pools available from the World Health Organization is limited (distribution is restricted to reference laboratories).

Sequencing of the *VP1* gene is now the primary method used for typing. Specifically, a 340-bp region that encodes the serotype-specific neutralization epitopes of *VP1* is amplified, sequenced, and analyzed against a sequence database for known EVs (145, 177). A threshold of 25% nucleotide and 12% amino acid divergence in the complete *VP1* gene sequence generally corresponds to the previous serological division of EVs into members of the same or different serotypes (5). A pyrosequencing method based on the assay reported by Nix et al. (145) has also been developed to shorten the time to identify the EV type (178). Molecular typing methods reduce the testing time by weeks (177) over classical serotyping. In addition, these methods of "molecular serotyping" have been extremely useful in characterizing new EV serotypes and identifying "nontypeable" isolates that could not be neutralized by traditional LBM pools (5).

Various molecular methods have been described for either species-specific typing (i.e., PV) or for the detection of multiple EV types. Type-specific real-time assays have been implemented during the recent outbreaks of EV-D68 (179–181), EV-A71, CV-A6, CV-A16 (182), and PV (183). For field deployment and for primary diagnostic settings, isothermal RNA amplification assays have been designed to type CV-A6, CV-A16, EV-A71, and CV-B3. These assays include simultaneous amplification and testing, SAT (184); reverse transcription-isothermal multiple-self-matching-initiated amplification, RT-IMSA (185); and one-step reverse transcription loop-mediated isothermal amplification, RT-LAMP (186–190).

With the lack of available antibodies to perform serotyping and the inability of some PeVs to grow in cell culture, assays were developed that are analogous to the EV VP1 "molecular serotyping" assays (13, 14). These methods have in turn become the standard method to type PeV and have led to the discovery of multiple new PeV types.

SEROLOGIC TEST

In the clinical setting, situations may arise where EV serology is requested; such is the case for myocarditis and determination of congenital infection in pregnant women. However, it has been shown that EV serology has little clinical utility for these patients (191). Complement fixation testing is available from a few commercial laboratories in the United States but is not recommended for the diagnosis of EV infection due to lack of specificity (32). Classically, serologic diagnosis of EV infection involved comparing antibody titers in acute- and convalescent-phase serum in a neutralization assay, with a 4-fold or greater rise in type-specific antibody titer considered as diagnostic of recent infection. However, acute-phase sera are often not obtained because of nonspecific presentations early in EV disease.

Type-specific enzyme-linked immunosorbent assays for the detection of EV serotype-specific IgM antibodies (i.e., CVB- and EV71-specific IgM), as well as heterotypic assays for the detection of IgA, IgM, and IgG antibodies against EVs in general, have been developed (192, 193). Homotypic assays are more relevant to epidemiologic studies than to clinical diagnosis as they appear to be less sensitive than PCR for the diagnosis of EV infection, but they have been successfully applied in such research settings (2, 194). Furthermore, the IgM response to EVs may be nonspecific and can lead to false-positive results (195, 196). Although cross-reactivity with non-EV pathogens has not been studied thoroughly, sera from patients infected with acute hepatitis A virus (a member of the *Picornaviridae* family) have been reported to produce a significant number of false-positive results in an enzyme-linked immunosorbent assay for detection of enterovirus IgM antibodies (193).

Currently there are no commercial reagents for PeV serology testing; hence, testing is limited to epidemiologic studies. Furthermore, the research reagents do not differentiate HPeV types (24).

ANTIVIRAL SUSCEPTIBILITIES

There is no FDA-approved antiviral agent available for the treatment of EV or PeV infections. However, several compounds targeting viral capsid proteins, proteases, polymerase, and other proteins are being developed, including some agents in phase-III clinical trials (197). A promising investigational drug, the WIN compound pleconaril, underwent extensive *in vitro* susceptibility testing against EVs in clinical trials but was not licensed for use by the FDA (198, 199). An antiviral compound with potent activity against the polioviruses, pocapavir, is currently undergoing evaluation and has been used for treatment on a compassionate-use basis (200–202).

EVALUATION, INTERPRETATION, AND REPORTING OF RESULTS

An understanding of the sites where asymptomatic shedding and disease-induced replication occur is critical to the interpretation of EV and PeV test results. Detection of these viruses in the central nervous system, bloodstream, lower respiratory tract, and genitourinary tract implies a true invasive infection and a high-level likelihood of association with current illness. In contrast, they can be shed asymptomatically from the nasopharynx and the gastrointestinal tract for weeks to months. Detection of EVs by virus isolation or NAAT at these sites must be interpreted cautiously because their presence alone does not establish a diagnosis. EV in the feces or nasopharynx of a patient with meningitis may represent residual shedding from an infection from weeks before and may be unrelated to the current illness.

In young children, an additional factor potentially complicating the evaluation of results from these body sites is the administration of live attenuated oral PV in the first years of life. While the vaccine is no longer used in the United States (32), most countries worldwide, including some in Europe, still employ oral PV as part of their vaccination regimes. In such settings it is necessary to test specifically for PV and NPEV.

Another issue with the specificity of NAAT testing from respiratory specimens is that pan-EV assays most likely cross-react with RVs. Many commercial tests do not claim to differentiate between the two. Furthermore, most assays have not been completely evaluated against a large number of EV or RV strains to confirm inclusivity or exclusivity of all strains (203). However, rarely is it necessary clinically to differentiate the viruses, particularly for respiratory infection, and one must remember that RVs are EVs. On the rare occasion differentiation is needed, typing can be performed. But even for viral myocarditis, understanding the etiological agent has more academic than therapeutic benefit.

A further cautionary note is warranted regarding coinfections of the central nervous system with EVs and bacteria (142). In these rare instances, illness was clinically compatible with bacterial meningitis, and EV was later isolated incidentally. Because of the severity of disease, antibiotics would have been used regardless of the sequence of pathogen detection. When the clinical presentation is typical of viral meningitis, coinfection with a clinically "silent" bacterium would be extraordinarily unlikely. Hence, identification of an EV from a sterile site in a patient with a clinically compatible illness is sufficient evidence for establishment of EV causality. PeV NAAT testing should be considered if negative results are obtained for EVs in the setting of clinically compatible disease.

REFERENCES

1. **Oberste MS, Pallansch MA.** 2016. *Enteroviruses and Parechoviruses*, *Clinical Virology Manual*, 5th ed. ASM Press, Washington, DC.
2. **Pallansch MA, Oberste MS.** 2009. Enteroviruses and Parechoviruses, p 249–282. *In* Specter S, Hodinka RL, Young SA, Wiedbrauk DL (ed), *Clinical Virology Manual*, 4th ed. ASM Press, Washington, DC.
3. **Stanway G, Brown F, Christian P, Hovi T, Hyypiä T, King AMQ, Knowles NJ, Lemon SM, Minor PD.** 2005. *Picornaviridae*, p 757–788. *In* Fauquet CM, Mayo MA, Maniloff J, Desselberger U, Ball, LA (ed), *Virus Taxonomy: Eighth Report of the International Committee on the Taxonomy of Viruses*. Elsevier Academic Press, Amsterdam, The Netherlands.
4. **Knowles NJ, Hovi T, Hyypiä T, King AMQ, Lindberg AM, Pallansch MA, Palmenberg AC, Simmonds P, Skern T, Stanway G, Yamashita T, Zell R.** 2012. Picornaviridae, p 855–880. *In* King AMQ, Adams MJ, Carstens EB, Lefkowitz EJ (ed), *Virus Taxonomy: Classification and Nomenclature of Viruses: Ninth Report of the International Committee on Taxonomy of Viruses*. Elsevier, San Diego, CA.
5. **Oberste MS, Maher K, Kilpatrick DR, Pallansch MA.** 1999. Molecular evolution of the human enteroviruses: correlation of serotype with VP1 sequence and application to picornavirus classification. *J Virol* **73:**1941–1948.

6. **Romero JR.** 2017. *Enteroviruses, Clinical Virology*, 4th ed. ASM Press, Washington, DC.
7. **Deshpande JM, Sharma DK, Saxena VK, Shetty SA, Qureshi TH, Nalavade UP.** 2016. Genomic characterization of two new enterovirus types, EV-A114 and EV-A121. *J Med Microbiol* **65:**1465–1471.
8. **Adams MJ, King AM, Carstens EB.** 2013. Ratification vote on taxonomic proposals to the International Committee on Taxonomy of Viruses (2013). *Arch Virol* **158:**2023–2030.
9. **Coller BA, Chapman NM, Beck MA, Pallansch MA, Gauntt CJ, Tracy SM.** 1990. Echovirus 22 is an atypical enterovirus. *J Virol* **64:**2692–2701.
10. **Hyypiä T, Horsnell C, Maaronen M, Khan M, Kalkkinen N, Auvinen P, Kinnunen L, Stanway G.** 1992. A distinct picornavirus group identified by sequence analysis. *Proc Natl Acad Sci USA* **89:**8847–8851.
11. **Stanway G, Kalkkinen N, Roivainen M, Ghazi F, Khan M, Smyth M, Meurman O, Hyypiä T.** 1994. Molecular and biological characteristics of echovirus 22, a representative of a new picornavirus group. *J Virol* **68:**8232–8238.
12. **Ito M, Yamashita T, Tsuzuki H, Takeda N, Sakae K.** 2004. Isolation and identification of a novel human parechovirus. *J Gen Virol* **85:**391–398.
13. **Benschop KS, Schinkel J, Minnaar RP, Pajkrt D, Spanjerberg L, Kraakman HC, Berkhout B, Zaaijer HL, Beld MG, Wolthers KC.** 2006. Human parechovirus infections in Dutch children and the association between serotype and disease severity. *Clin Infect Dis* **42:**204–210.
14. **Nix WA, Maher K, Pallansch MA, Oberste MS.** 2010. Parechovirus typing in clinical specimens by nested or semi-nested PCR coupled with sequencing. *J Clin Virol* **48:** 202–207.
15. **Thoi TC, Than VT, Kim W.** 2014. Whole genomic characterization of a Korean human parechovirus type 1 (HPeV1) identifies recombination events. *J Med Virol* **86:**2084–2091.
16. **Zhao X, Shi Y, Xia Y.** 2016. Genome analysis revealed novel genotypes and recombination of the human parechoviruses prevalent in children in Eastern China. *Gut Pathog* **8:**52.
17. **Alexandersen S, Nelson TM, Hodge J, Druce J.** 2017. Evolutionary and network analysis of virus sequences from infants infected with an Australian recombinant strain of human parechovirus type 3. *Sci Rep* **7:**3861.
18. **Nelson TM, Vuillermin P, Hodge J, Druce J, Williams DT, Jasrotia R, Alexandersen S.** 2017. An outbreak of severe infections among Australian infants caused by a novel recombinant strain of human parechovirus type 3. *Sci Rep* **7:**44423.
19. **Zhao X, Zhou C, Zhang X, Li W, Wan X, Wang Y, Zeng Y, Zhang W.** 2017. The complete genome sequence of a human parechovirus from a child with diarrhea in China revealed intertypic recombination. *Genome Announc* **5:**e00332-17.
20. **Williams CH, Panayiotou M, Girling GD, Peard CI, Oikarinen S, Hyöty H, Stanway G.** 2009. Evolution and conservation in human parechovirus genomes. *J Gen Virol* **90:**1702–1712.
21. **Zeichhardt H, Grunert H-P.** 2000. Enteroviruses, p 252–269. *In* Specter S, Hodinka RL, Young SA (ed), *Clinical Virology Manual*, 3rd ed. ASM Press, Washington, DC.
22. **Bradrick SS, Lieben EA, Carden BM, Romero JR.** 2001. A predicted secondary structural domain within the internal ribosome entry site of echovirus 12 mediates a cell-type-specific block to viral replication. *J Virol* **75:**6472–6481.
23. **Minor PD.** 1996. Poliovirus biology. *Structure* **4:**775–778.
24. **Romero JR, Selvarangan R.** 2011. The human Parechoviruses: an overview. *Adv Pediatr* **58:**65–85.
25. **Seitsonen J, Susi P, Heikkilä O, Sinkovits RS, Laurinmäki P, Hyypiä T, Butcher SJ.** 2010. Interaction of alphaVbeta3 and alphaVbeta6 integrins with human parechovirus 1. *J Virol* **84:**8509–8519.
26. **van der Sanden S, de Bruin E, Vennema H, Swanink C, Koopmans M, van der Avoort H.** 2008. Prevalence of human parechovirus in the Netherlands in 2000 to 2007. *J Clin Microbiol* **46:**2884–2889.
27. **Wolthers KC, Benschop KS, Schinkel J, Molenkamp R, Bergevoet RM, Spijkerman IJ, Kraakman HC, Pajkrt D.** 2008. Human parechoviruses as an important viral cause of sepsis-like illness and meningitis in young children. *Clin Infect Dis* **47:**358–363.
28. **Centers for Disease Control and Prevention (CDC).** 2000. Enterovirus surveillance—United States, 1997–1999. *MMWR Morb Mortal Wkly Rep* **49:**913–916.
29. **Oberste MS, Maher K, Schnurr D, Flemister MR, Lovchik JC, Peters H, Sessions W, Kirk C, Chatterjee N, Fuller S, Hanauer JM, Pallansch MA.** 2004. Enterovirus 68 is associated with respiratory illness and shares biological features with both the enteroviruses and the rhinoviruses. *J Gen Virol* **85:**2577–2584.
30. **Modlin JF.** 1988. Perinatal echovirus and group B coxsackievirus infections. *Clin Perinatol* **15:**233–246.
31. **Khetsuriani N, Lamonte-Fowlkes A, Oberst S, Pallansch MA, Centers for Disease Control and Prevention.** 2006. Enterovirus surveillance—United States, 1970–2005. *MMWR Surveill Summ* **55:**1–20.
32. **American Academy of Pediatrics.** 2015. Enterovirus (Nonpoliovirus), p 333–336. *In* Dw K, Mt B, Ma J, Ss L (ed), *Red Book®: 2015 Report of the Committee on Infectious Diseases*, 28th ed. American Academy of Pediatrics, United States of America. 10.1542/peds.2015-0160.
33. **Modlin JF.** 1996. Update on enterovirus infections in infants and children. *Adv Pediatr Infect Dis* **12:**155–180.
34. **Khatami A, McMullan BJ, Webber M, Stewart P, Francis S, Timmers KJ, Rodas E, Druce J, Mehta B, Sloggett NA, Cumming G, Papadakis G, Kesson AM.** 2015. Sepsis-like disease in infants due to human parechovirus type 3 during an outbreak in Australia. *Clin Infect Dis* **60:**228–236.
35. **Vergnano S, Kadambari S, Whalley K, Menson EN, Martinez-Alier N, Cooper M, Sanchez E, Heath PT, Lyall H.** 2015. Characteristics and outcomes of human parechovirus infection in infants (2008–2012). *Eur J Pediatr* **174:** 919–924.
36. **Midgley CM, Jackson MA, Selvarangan R, Franklin P, Holzschuh EL, Lloyd J, Scaletta J, Straily A, Tubach S, Willingham A, Nix WA, Oberste MS, Harrison CJ, Hunt C, Turabelidze G, Gerber SI, Watson JT.** 2017. Severe parechovirus 3 infections in young infants—Kansas and Missouri, 2014. *J Pediatric Infect Dis Soc.*
37. **Abedi GR, Watson JT, Pham H, Nix WA, Oberste MS, Gerber SI.** 2015. Enterovirus and human parechovirus surveillance—United States, 2009–2013. *MMWR Morb Mortal Wkly Rep* **64:**940–943.
38. **Previsani N, Singh H, St. Pierre J, Boualam L, Fournier-Caruana J, Sutter RW, Zaffran M.** 2017. Global polio eradication: progress towards containment of poliovirus type 2, worldwide 2017. *Wkly Epidemiol Rec* **92:**350–356.
39. **World Health Organization.**2017. Polio Now, *on WHO*. http://polioeradication.org/polio-today/polio-now/this-week/. Accessed July 15, 2017.
40. **Khetsuriani N, Lamonte A, Oberste MS, Pallansch M.** 2006. Neonatal enterovirus infections reported to the national enterovirus surveillance system in the United States, 1983–2003. *Pediatr Infect Dis J* **25:**889–893.
41. **Verboon-Maciolek MA, Groenendaal F, Hahn CD, Hellmann J, van Loon AM, Boivin G, de Vries LS.** 2008. Human parechovirus causes encephalitis with white matter injury in neonates. *Ann Neurol* **64:**266–273.
42. **Strikas RA, Anderson LJ, Parker RA.** 1986. Temporal and geographic patterns of isolates of nonpolio enterovirus in the United States, 1970–1983. *J Infect Dis* **153:**346–351.
43. **Khetsuriani N, Quiroz ES, Holman RC, Anderson LJ.** 2003. Viral meningitis-associated hospitalizations in the United States, 1988–1999. *Neuroepidemiology* **22:**345–352.
44. **Sharp J, Harrison CJ, Puckett K, Selvaraju SB, Penaranda S, Nix WA, Oberste MS, Selvarangan R.** 2013. Characteristics of young infants in whom human parechovirus, enterovirus or neither were detected in cerebrospinal fluid during sepsis evaluations. *Pediatr Infect Dis J* **32:**213–216.
45. **Ferris BG Jr, Auld PA, Cronkhite L, Kaufmann HJ, Kearsley RB, Prizer M, Weinstein L.** 1960. Life-threatening poliomyelitis, Boston, 1955. *N Engl J Med* **262:**371–380.

46. **Patel MK, Konde MK, Didi-Ngossaki BH, Ndinga E, Yogolelo R, Salla M, Shaba K, Everts J, Armstrong GL, Daniels D, Burns C, Wassilak S, Pallansch M, Kretsinger K.** 2012. An outbreak of wild poliovirus in the Republic of Congo, 2010–2011. *Clin Infect Dis* **55:**1291–1298.
47. **Bonwitt J, Poel A, DeBolt C, Gonzales E, Lopez A, Routh J, Rietberg K, Linton N, Reggin J, Sejvar J, Lindquist S, Otten C.** 2017. Acute Flaccid Myelitis Among Children—Washington, September–November 2016. *MMWR Morb Mortal Wkly Rep* **66:**826–829
48. **Huang C, Morse D, Slater B, Anand M, Tobin E, Smith P, Dupuis M, Hull R, Ferrera R, Rosen B, Grady L.** 2004. Multiple-year experience in the diagnosis of viral central nervous system infections with a panel of polymerase chain reaction assays for detection of 11 viruses. *Clin Infect Dis* **39:**630–635.
49. **Fowlkes AL, Honarmand S, Glaser C, Yagi S, Schnurr D, Oberste MS, Anderson L, Pallansch MA, Khetsuriani N.** 2008. Enterovirus-associated encephalitis in the California encephalitis project, 1998–2005. *J Infect Dis* **198:**1685–1691.
50. **Modlin JF, Dagan R, Berlin LE, Virshup DM, Yolken RH, Menegus M.** 1991. Focal encephalitis with enterovirus infections. *Pediatrics* **88:**841–845.
51. **Britton PN, Dale RC, Nissen MD, Crawford N, Elliott E, Macartney K, Khandaker G, Booy R, Jones CA, PAEDS-ACE Investigators.** 2016. Parechovirus encephalitis and neurodevelopmental outcomes. *Pediatrics* **137:**e20152848.
52. **Huang CC, Liu CC, Chang YC, Chen CY, Wang ST, Yeh TF.** 1999. Neurologic complications in children with enterovirus 71 infection. *N Engl J Med* **341:**936–942.
53. **Chan LG, Parashar UD, Lye MS, Ong FG, Zaki SR, Alexander JP, Ho KK, Han LL, Pallansch MA, Suleiman AB, Jegathesan M, Anderson LJ, For the Outbreak Study Group.** 2000. Deaths of children during an outbreak of hand, foot, and mouth disease in Sarawak, Malaysia: clinical and pathological characteristics of the disease. *Clin Infect Dis* **31:**678–683.
54. **Ho M, Chen ER, Hsu KH, Twu SJ, Chen KT, Tsai SF, Wang JR, Shih SR, Taiwan Enterovirus Epidemic Working Group.** 1999. An epidemic of enterovirus 71 infection in Taiwan. *N Engl J Med* **341:**929–935.
55. **Pérez-Vélez CM, Anderson MS, Robinson CC, McFarland EJ, Nix WA, Pallansch MA, Oberste MS, Glodé MP.** 2007. Outbreak of neurologic enterovirus type 71 disease: a diagnostic challenge. *Clin Infect Dis* **45:**950–957.
56. **Fabre A, Sheppard MN.** 2006. Sudden adult death syndrome and other non-ischaemic causes of sudden cardiac death. *Heart* **92:**316–320.
57. **Doolan A, Langlois N, Semsarian C.** 2004. Causes of sudden cardiac death in young Australians. *Med J Aust* **180:**110–112.
58. **Bowles NE, Ni J, Kearney DL, Pauschinger M, Schultheiss HP, McCarthy R, Hare J, Bricker JT, Bowles KR, Towbin JA.** 2003. Detection of viruses in myocardial tissues by polymerase chain reaction: evidence of adenovirus as a common cause of myocarditis in children and adults. *J Am Coll Cardiol* **42:**466–472.
59. **Dendle C, Gilbertson M, Korman TM, Golder V, Morand E, Opat S.** 2015. Disseminated enteroviral infection associated with obinutuzumab. *Emerg Infect Dis* **21:**1661–1663.
60. **Grisariu S, Vaxman I, Gatt M, Elias S, Avni B, Arad A, Pasvolsky O, Raanani P, Paltiel O.** 2016. Enteroviral infection in patients treated with rituximab for non-Hodgkin lymphoma: a case series and review of the literature. *Hematol Oncol* **35:**591–598.
61. **Solomon T, Lewthwaite P, Perera D, Cardosa MJ, McMinn P, Ooi MH.** 2010. Virology, epidemiology, pathogenesis, and control of enterovirus 71. *Lancet Infect Dis* **10:**778–790.
62. **Flett K, Youngster I, Huang J, McAdam A, Sandora TJ, Rennick M, Smole S, Rogers SL, Nix WA, Oberste MS, Gellis S, Ahmed AA.** 2012. Hand, foot, and mouth disease caused by coxsackievirus a6. *Emerg Infect Dis* **18:**1702–1704.
63. **Grist NR, Bell EJ, Assaad F.** 1978. Enteroviruses in human disease. *Prog Med Virol* **24:**114–157.
64. **Chonmaitree T, Mann L.** 1995. *Respiratory Infections, Human Enterovirus Infections*. ASM Press, Washington, DC.
65. **Chung JY, Han TH, Kim SW, Hwang ES.** 2007. Respiratory picornavirus infections in Korean children with lower respiratory tract infections. *Scand J Infect Dis* **39:**250–254.
66. **Renois F, Lévêque N, Deliège PG, Fichel C, Bouin A, Abely M, N'guyen Y, Andréoletti L.** 2013. Enteroviruses as major cause of microbiologically unexplained acute respiratory tract infections in hospitalized pediatric patients. *J Infect* **66:**494–502.
67. **Kaida A, Kubo H, Sekiguchi J, Hase A, Iritani N.** 2012. Enterovirus 104 infection in adult, Japan, 2011. *Emerg Infect Dis* **18:**882–883.
68. **Pankovics P, Boros A, Szabó H, Székely G, Gyurkovits K, Reuter G.** 2012. Human enterovirus 109 (EV109) in acute paediatric respiratory disease in Hungary. *Acta Microbiol Immunol Hung* **59:**285–290.
69. **Piralla A, Rovida F, Baldanti F, Gerna G.** 2010. Enterovirus genotype EV-104 in humans, Italy, 2008–2009. *Emerg Infect Dis* **16:**1018–1021.
70. **Piralla A, Lilleri D, Sarasini A, Marchi A, Zecca M, Stronati M, Baldanti F, Gerna G.** 2012. Human rhinovirus and human respiratory enterovirus (EV68 and EV104) infections in hospitalized patients in Italy, 2008–2009. *Diagn Microbiol Infect Dis* **73:**162–167.
71. **Schieble JH, Fox VL, Lennette EH.** 1967. A probable new human picornavirus associated with respiratory diseases. *Am J Epidemiol* **85:**297–310.
72. **Centers for Disease Control and Prevention (CDC).** 2011. Clusters of acute respiratory illness associated with human enterovirus 68—Asia, Europe, and United States, 2008–2010. *MMWR Morb Mortal Wkly Rep* **60:**1301–1304.
73. **Imamura T, Fuji N, Suzuki A, Tamaki R, Saito M, Aniceto R, Galang H, Sombrero L, Lupisan S, Oshitani H.** 2011. Enterovirus 68 among children with severe acute respiratory infection, the Philippines. *Emerg Infect Dis* **17:**1430–1435.
74. **Kaida A, Kubo H, Sekiguchi J, Kohdera U, Togawa M, Shiomi M, Nishigaki T, Iritani N.** 2011. Enterovirus 68 in children with acute respiratory tract infections, Osaka, Japan. *Emerg Infect Dis* **17:**1494–1497.
75. **Meijer A, van der Sanden S, Snijders BE, Jaramillo-Gutierrez G, Bont L, van der Ent CK, Overduin P, Jenny SL, Jusic E, van der Avoort HG, Smith GJ, Donker GA, Koopmans MP.** 2012. Emergence and epidemic occurrence of enterovirus 68 respiratory infections in The Netherlands in 2010. *Virology* **423:**49–57.
76. **Jacobson LM, Redd JT, Schneider E, Lu X, Chern SW, Oberste MS, Erdman DD, Fischer GE, Armstrong GL, Kodani M, Montoya J, Magri JM, Cheek JE.** 2012. Outbreak of lower respiratory tract illness associated with human enterovirus 68 among American Indian children. *Pediatr Infect Dis J* **31:**309–312.
77. **Renois F, Bouin A, Andreoletti L.** 2013. Enterovirus 68 in pediatric patients hospitalized for acute airway diseases. *J Clin Microbiol* **51:**640–643.
78. **Blomqvist S, Savolainen C, Råman L, Roivainen M, Hovi T.** 2002. Human rhinovirus 87 and enterovirus 68 represent a unique serotype with rhinovirus and enterovirus features. *J Clin Microbiol* **40:**4218–4223.
79. **Ishiko H, Miura R, Shimada Y, Hayashi A, Nakajima H, Yamazaki S, Takeda N.** 2002. Human rhinovirus 87 identified as human enterovirus 68 by VP4-based molecular diagnosis. *Intervirology* **45:**136–141.
80. **Tokarz R, Firth C, Madhi SA, Howie SR, Wu W, Sall AA, Haq S, Briese T, Lipkin WI.** 2012. Worldwide emergence of multiple clades of enterovirus 68. *J Gen Virol* **93:**1952–1958.
81. **Midgley CM, Jackson MA, Selvarangan R, Turabelidze G, Obringer E, Johnson D, Giles BL, Patel A, Echols F, Oberste MS, Nix WA, Watson JT, Gerber SI.** 2014. Severe respiratory illness associated with enterovirus D68—Missouri and Illinois, 2014. *MMWR Morb Mortal Wkly Rep* **63:**798–799.
82. **Abzug MJ.** 2008. The enteroviruses: an emerging infectious disease? The real, the speculative and the really speculative. *Adv Exp Med Biol* **609:**1–15.
83. **Nejentsev S, Walker N, Riches D, Egholm M, Todd JA.** 2009. Rare variants of IFIH1, a gene implicated in antiviral responses, protect against type 1 diabetes. *Science* **324:**387–389.

84. **Redondo MJ, Jeffrey J, Fain PR, Eisenbarth GS, Orban T.** 2008. Concordance for islet autoimmunity among monozygotic twins. *N Engl J Med* **359:**2849–2850.
85. **Yeung WC, Rawlinson WD, Craig ME.** 2011. Enterovirus infection and type 1 diabetes mellitus: systematic review and meta-analysis of observational molecular studies. *BMJ* **342:**d35
86. **Harvala H, Robertson I, McWilliam Leitch EC, Benschop K, Wolthers KC, Templeton K, Simmonds P.** 2008. Epidemiology and clinical associations of human parechovirus respiratory infections. *J Clin Microbiol* **46:**3446–3453.
87. **Niklasson B, Samsioe A, Papadogiannakis N, Kawecki A, Hörnfeldt B, Saade GR, Klitz W.** 2007. Association of zoonotic Ljungan virus with intrauterine fetal deaths. *Birth Defects Res A Clin Mol Teratol* **79:**488–493.
88. **Abzug MJ, Loeffelholz M, Rotbart HA.** 1995. Diagnosis of neonatal enterovirus infection by polymerase chain reaction. *J Pediatr* **126:**447–450.
89. **Nijhuis M, van Maarseveen N, Schuurman R, Verkuijlen S, de Vos M, Hendriksen K, van Loon AM.** 2002. Rapid and sensitive routine detection of all members of the genus enterovirus in different clinical specimens by real-time PCR. *J Clin Microbiol* **40:**3666–3670.
90. **Verboon-Maciolek MA, Nijhuis M, van Loon AM, van Maarssenveen N, van Wieringen H, Pekelharing-Berghuis MA, Krediet TG, Gerards LJ, Fleer A, Diepersloot RJ, Thijsen SF.** 2003. Diagnosis of enterovirus infection in the first 2 months of life by real-time polymerase chain reaction. *Clin Infect Dis* **37:**1–6.
91. **Rittichier KR, Bryan PA, Bassett KE, Taggart EW, Enriquez FR, Hillyard DR, Byington CL.** 2005. Diagnosis and outcomes of enterovirus infections in young infants. *Pediatr Infect Dis J* **24:**546–550.
92. **Harvala H, Griffiths M, Solomon T, Simmonds P.** 2014. Distinct systemic and central nervous system disease patterns in enterovirus and parechovirus infected children. *J Infect* **69:**69–74.
93. **Byington CL, Taggart EW, Carroll KC, Hillyard DR.** 1999. A polymerase chain reaction-based epidemiologic investigation of the incidence of nonpolio enteroviral infections in febrile and afebrile infants 90 days and younger. *Pediatrics* **103:**e27.
94. **de Crom SC, Obihara CC, de Moor RA, Veldkamp EJ, van Furth AM, Rossen JW.** 2013. Prospective comparison of the detection rates of human enterovirus and parechovirus RT-qPCR and viral culture in different pediatric specimens. *J Clin Virol* **58:**449–454.
95. **Kupila L, Vuorinen T, Vainionpää R, Marttila RJ, Kotilainen P.** 2005. Diagnosis of enteroviral meningitis by use of polymerase chain reaction of cerebrospinal fluid, stool, and serum specimens. *Clin Infect Dis* **40:**982–987.
96. **Stellrecht KA, Harding I, Woron AM, Lepow ML, Venezia RA.** 2002. The impact of an enteroviral RT-PCR assay on the diagnosis of aseptic meningitis and patient management. *J Clin Virol* **25**(Suppl 1)**:**S19–26.
97. **Harvala H, Wolthers KC, Simmonds P.** 2010. Parechoviruses in children: understanding a new infection. *Curr Opin Infect Dis* **23:**224–230.
98. **Seiden JA, Zorc JJ, Hodinka RL, Shah SS.** 2010. Lack of cerebrospinal fluid pleocytosis in young infants with enterovirus infections of the central nervous system. *Pediatr Emerg Care* **26:**77–81.
99. **Yun KW, Choi EH, Cheon DS, Lee J, Choi CW, Hwang H, Kim BI, Park KU, Park SS, Lee HJ.** 2012. Enteroviral meningitis without pleocytosis in children. *Arch Dis Child* **97:**874–878.
100. **Wilen CB, Monaco CL, Hoppe-Bauer J, Jackups R Jr, Bucelli RC, Burnham CA.** 2015. Criteria for reducing unnecessary testing for herpes simplex virus, varicella-zoster virus, cytomegalovirus, and enterovirus in cerebrospinal fluid samples from adults. *J Clin Microbiol* **53:**887–895.
101. **Chung PW, Huang YC, Chang LY, Lin TY, Ning HC.** 2001. Duration of enterovirus shedding in stool. *J Microbiol Immunol Infect* **34:**167–170.
102. **Tapia G, Cinek O, Witsø E, Kulich M, Rasmussen T, Grinde B, Rønningen KS.** 2008. Longitudinal observation of parechovirus in stool samples from Norwegian infants. *J Med Virol* **80:**1835–1842.
103. **Witsø E, Palacios G, Cinek O, Stene LC, Grinde B, Janowitz D, Lipkin WI, Rønningen KS.** 2006. High prevalence of human enterovirus a infections in natural circulation of human enteroviruses. *J Clin Microbiol* **44:**4095–4100.
104. **Kolehmainen P, Oikarinen S, Koskiniemi M, Simell O, Ilonen J, Knip M, Hyöty H, Tauriainen S.** 2012. Human parechoviruses are frequently detected in stool of healthy Finnish children. *J Clin Virol* **54:**156–161.
105. **Kapusinszky B, Minor P, Delwart E.** 2012. Nearly constant shedding of diverse enteric viruses by two healthy infants. *J Clin Microbiol* **50:**3427–3434.
106. **Ooi MH, Solomon T, Podin Y, Mohan A, Akin W, Yusuf MA, del Sel S, Kontol KM, Lai BF, Clear D, Chieng CH, Blake E, Perera D, Wong SC, Cardosa J.** 2007. Evaluation of different clinical sample types in diagnosis of human enterovirus 71-associated hand-foot-and-mouth disease. *J Clin Microbiol* **45:**1858–1866.
107. **Magnani JW, Dec GW.** 2006. Myocarditis: current trends in diagnosis and treatment. *Circulation* **113:**876–890.
108. **McManus BM, Seidman M, Klingel K, Luo H.** 2017. *Viral Heart Disease, Clinical Virology*, 4th ed. ASM Press, Washington, DC.
109. **Rogers BB, Alpert LC, Hine EA, Buffone GJ.** 1990. Analysis of DNA in fresh and fixed tissue by the polymerase chain reaction. *Am J Pathol* **136:**541–548.
110. **Simpson KE, Storch GA, Lee CK, Ward KE, Danon S, Simon CM, Delaney JW, Tong A, Canter CE.** 2016. High frequency of detection by PCR of viral nucleic acid in the blood of infants presenting with clinical myocarditis. *Pediatr Cardiol* **37:**399–404.
111. **Akhtar N, Ni J, Stromberg D, Rosenthal GL, Bowles NE, Towbin JA.** 1999. Tracheal aspirate as a substrate for polymerase chain reaction detection of viral genome in childhood pneumonia and myocarditis. *Circulation* **99:**2011–2018.
112. **Van Vliet KE, Muir P, Echevarria JM, Klapper PE, Cleator GM, Van Loon AM.** 2001. Multicenter proficiency testing of nucleic acid amplification methods for the detection of enteroviruses. *J Clin Microbiol* **39:**3390–3392.
113. **Chonmaitree T, Ford C, Sanders C, Lucia HL.** 1988. Comparison of cell cultures for rapid isolation of enteroviruses. *J Clin Microbiol* **26:**2576–2580.
114. **Tattevin P, Minjolle S, Arvieux C, Clayessen V, Colimon R, Bouget J, Michelet C.** 2002. Benefits of management strategy adjustments during an outbreak of enterovirus meningitis in adults. *Scand J Infect Dis* **34:**359–361.
115. **Wallace SS, Lopez MA, Caviness AC.** 2017. Impact of enterovirus testing on resource use in febrile young infants: a systematic review. *Hosp Pediatr* **7:**96–102.
116. **Ramers C, Billman G, Hartin M, Ho S, Sawyer MH.** 2000. Impact of a diagnostic cerebrospinal fluid enterovirus polymerase chain reaction test on patient management. *JAMA* **283:**2680–2685.
117. **Robinson CC, Willis M, Meagher A, Gieseker KE, Rotbart H, Glodé MP.** 2002. Impact of rapid polymerase chain reaction results on management of pediatric patients with enteroviral meningitis. *Pediatr Infect Dis J* **21:**283–286.
118. **Archimbaud C, Chambon M, Bailly JL, Petit I, Henquell C, Mirand A, Aublet-Cuvelier B, Ughetto S, Beytout J, Clavelou P, Labbé A, Philippe P, Schmidt J, Regagnon C, Traore O, Peigue-Lafeuille H.** 2009. Impact of rapid enterovirus molecular diagnosis on the management of infants, children, and adults with aseptic meningitis. *J Med Virol* **81:**42–48.
119. **Fox JD, Han S, Samuelson A, Zhang Y, Neale ML, Westmoreland D.** 2002. Development and evaluation of nucleic acid sequence based amplification (NASBA) for diagnosis of enterovirus infections using the NucliSens Basic Kit. *J Clin Virol* **24:**117–130.
120. **Heim A, Schumann J.** 2002. Development and evaluation of a nucleic acid sequence based amplification (NASBA)

protocol for the detection of enterovirus RNA in cerebrospinal fluid samples. *J Virol Methods* **103:**101–107.

121. **Romero JR.** 1999. Reverse-transcription polymerase chain reaction detection of the enteroviruses. *Arch Pathol Lab Med* **123:**1161–1169.
122. **Rotbart HA, Ahmed A, Hickey S, Dagan R, McCracken GH Jr, Whitley RJ, Modlin JF, Cascino M, O'Connell JF, Menegus MA, Blum D.** 1997. Diagnosis of enterovirus infection by polymerase chain reaction of multiple specimen types. *Pediatr Infect Dis J* **16:**409–411.
123. **Vuorinen T, Vainionpää R, Hyypiä T.** 2003. Five years' experience of reverse-transcriptase polymerase chain reaction in daily diagnosis of enterovirus and rhinovirus infections. *Clin Infect Dis* **37:**452–455.
124. **Olive DM, Al-Mufti S, Al-Mulla W, Khan MA, Pasca A, Stanway G, Al-Nakib W.** 1990. Detection and differentiation of picornaviruses in clinical samples following genomic amplification. *J Gen Virol* **71:**2141–2147.
125. **Rotbart HA.** 1990. Diagnosis of enteroviral meningitis with the polymerase chain reaction. *J Pediatr* **117:**85–89.
126. **Sawyer MH, Holland D, Aintablian N, Connor JD, Keyser EF, Waecker NJ Jr.** 1994. Diagnosis of enteroviral central nervous system infection by polymerase chain reaction during a large community outbreak. *Pediatr Infect Dis J* **13:**177–182.
127. **Stellrecht KA, Harding I, Hussain FM, Mishrik NG, Czap RT, Lepow ML, Venezia RA.** 2000. A one-step RT-PCR assay using an enzyme-linked detection system for the diagnosis of enterovirus meningitis. *J Clin Virol* **17:**143–149.
128. **Abzug MJ, Keyserling HL, Lee ML, Levin MJ, Rotbart HA.** 1995. Neonatal enterovirus infection: virology, serology, and effects of intravenous immune globulin. *Clin Infect Dis* **20:**1201–1206.
129. **Corless CE, Guiver M, Borrow R, Edwards-Jones V, Fox AJ, Kaczmarski EB, Mutton KJ.** 2002. Development and evaluation of a 'real-time' RT-PCR for the detection of enterovirus and parechovirus RNA in CSF and throat swab samples. *J Med Virol* **67:**555–562.
130. **Benschop K, Minnaar R, Koen G, van Eijk H, Dijkman K, Westerhuis B, Molenkamp R, Wolthers K.** 2010. Detection of human enterovirus and human parechovirus (HPeV) genotypes from clinical stool samples: polymerase chain reaction and direct molecular typing, culture characteristics, and serotyping. *Diagn Microbiol Infect Dis* **68:**166–173.
131. **Kost CB, Rogers B, Oberste MS, Robinson C, Eaves BL, Leos K, Danielson S, Satya M, Weir F, Nolte FS.** 2007. Multicenter beta trial of the GeneXpert enterovirus assay. *J Clin Microbiol* **45:**1081–1086.
132. **Nolte FS, Rogers BB, Tang YW, Oberste MS, Robinson CC, Kehl KS, Rand KA, Rotbart HA, Romero JR, Nyquist AC, Persing DH.** 2011. Evaluation of a rapid and completely automated real-time reverse transcriptase PCR assay for diagnosis of enteroviral meningitis. *J Clin Microbiol* **49:**528–533.
133. **de Crom SC, Obihara CC, van Loon AM, Argilagos-Alvarez AA, Peeters MF, van Furth AM, Rossen JW.** 2012. Detection of enterovirus RNA in cerebrospinal fluid: comparison of two molecular assays. *J Virol Methods* **179:**104–107.
134. **Leber AL, Everhart K, Balada-Llasat JM, Cullison J, Daly J, Holt S, Lephart P, Salimnia H, Schreckenberger PC, DesJarlais S, Reed SL, Chapin KC, LeBlanc L, Johnson JK, Soliven NL, Carroll KC, Miller JA, Dien Bard J, Mestas J, Bankowski M, Enomoto T, Hemmert AC, Bourzac KM.** 2016. Multicenter evaluation of BioFire FilmArray Meningitis/Encephalitis Panel for detection of bacteria, viruses, and yeast in cerebrospinal fluid specimens. *J Clin Microbiol* **54:**2251–2261.
135. **Marlowe EM, Novak SM, Dunn JJ, Smith A, Cumpio J, Makalintal E, Barnes D, Burchette RJ.** 2008. Performance of the GeneXpert enterovirus assay for detection of enteroviral RNA in cerebrospinal fluid. *J Clin Virol* **43:**110–113.
136. **Rand KH, Rampersaud H, Houck HJ.** 2011. Comparison of two multiplex methods for detection of respiratory viruses: FilmArray RP and xTAG RVP. *J Clin Microbiol* **49:** 2449–2453.
137. **Popowitch EB, O'Neill SS, Miller MB.** 2013. Comparison of the Biofire FilmArray RP, Genmark eSensor RVP, Luminex xTAG RVPv1, and Luminex xTAG RVP fast multiplex assays for detection of respiratory viruses. *J Clin Microbiol* **51:**1528–1533.
138. **Rotbart HA.** 1990. Enzymatic RNA amplification of the enteroviruses. *J Clin Microbiol* **28:**438–442.
139. **Chapman NM, Tracy S, Gauntt CJ, Fortmueller U.** 1990. Molecular detection and identification of enteroviruses using enzymatic amplification and nucleic acid hybridization. *J Clin Microbiol* **28:**843–850.
140. **Capaul SE, Gorgievski-Hrisoho M.** 2005. Detection of enterovirus RNA in cerebrospinal fluid (CSF) using NucliSens EasyQ Enterovirus assay. *J Clin Virol* **32:**236–240.
141. **Jokela P, Joki-Korpela P, Maaronen M, Glumoff V, Hyypiä T.** 2005. Detection of human picornaviruses by multiplex reverse transcription-PCR and liquid hybridization. *J Clin Microbiol* **43:**1239–1245.
142. **Lai KK, Cook L, Wendt S, Corey L, Jerome KR.** 2003. Evaluation of real-time PCR versus PCR with liquid-phase hybridization for detection of enterovirus RNA in cerebrospinal fluid. *J Clin Microbiol* **41:**3133–3141.
143. **Zoll GJ, Melchers WJ, Kopecka H, Jambroes G, van der Poel HJ, Galama JM.** 1992. General primer-mediated polymerase chain reaction for detection of enteroviruses: application for diagnostic routine and persistent infections. *J Clin Microbiol* **30:**160–165.
144. **Casas I, Palacios GF, Trallero G, Cisterna D, Freire MC, Tenorio A.** 2001. Molecular characterization of human enteroviruses in clinical samples: comparison between VP2, VP1, and RNA polymerase regions using RT nested PCR assays and direct sequencing of products. *J Med Virol* **65:** 138–148.
145. **Nix WA, Oberste MS, Pallansch MA.** 2006. Sensitive, seminested PCR amplification of VP1 sequences for direct identification of all enterovirus serotypes from original clinical specimens. *J Clin Microbiol* **44:**2698–2704.
146. **Wang X, Zhu JP, Zhang Q, Xu ZG, Zhang F, Zhao ZH, Zheng WZ, Zheng LS.** 2012. Detection of enterovirus 71 using reverse transcription loop-mediated isothermal amplification (RT-LAMP). *J Virol Methods* **179:**330–334.
147. **Arita M, Ling H, Yan D, Nishimura Y, Yoshida H, Wakita T, Shimizu H.** 2009. Development of a reverse transcription-loop-mediated isothermal amplification (RT-LAMP) system for a highly sensitive detection of enterovirus in the stool samples of acute flaccid paralysis cases. *BMC Infect Dis* **9:**208.
148. **Smalling TW, Sefers SE, Li H, Tang Y-W.** 2002. Molecular approaches to detecting herpes simplex virus and enteroviruses in the central nervous system. *J Clin Microbiol* **40:** 2317–2322.
149. **Pillet S, Billaud G, Omar S, Lina B, Pozzetto B, Schuffenecker I.** 2010. Multicenter evaluation of the ENTEROVIRUS R-gene real-time RT-PCR assay for the detection of enteroviruses in clinical specimens. *J Clin Virol* **47:**54–59.
150. **Muir P, Ras A, Klapper PE, Cleator GM, Korn K, Aepinus C, Fomsgaard A, Palmer P, Samuelsson A, Tenorio A, Weissbrich B, van Loon AM.** 1999. Multicenter quality assessment of PCR methods for detection of enteroviruses. *J Clin Microbiol* **37:**1409–1414.
151. **Legay V, Chomel JJ, Lina B.** 2002. Specific RT-PCR procedure for the detection of human parechovirus type 1 genome in clinical samples. *J Virol Methods* **102:**157–160.
152. **Joki-Korpela P, Hyypiä T.** 1998. Diagnosis and epidemiology of echovirus 22 infections. *Clin Infect Dis* **27:**129–136.
153. **Oberste MS, Maher K, Pallansch MA.** 1999. Specific detection of echoviruses 22 and 23 in cell culture supernatants by RT-PCR. *J Med Virol* **58:**178–181.
154. **Baumgarte S, de Souza Luna LK, Grywna K, Panning M, Drexler JF, Karsten C, Huppertz HI, Drosten C.** 2008. Prevalence, types, and RNA concentrations of human parechoviruses, including a sixth parechovirus type, in stool samples from patients with acute enteritis. *J Clin Microbiol* **46:**242–248.

155. **Noordhoek GT, Weel JFL, Poelstra E, Hooghiemstra M, Brandenburg AH.** 2008. Clinical validation of a new real-time PCR assay for detection of enteroviruses and parechoviruses, and implications for diagnostic procedures. *J Clin Virol* **41:**75–80.

156. **Nix WA, Maher K, Johansson ES, Niklasson B, Lindberg AM, Pallansch MA, Oberste MS.** 2008. Detection of all known parechoviruses by real-time PCR. *J Clin Microbiol* **46:**2519–2524.

157. **Benschop K, Molenkamp R, van der Ham A, Wolthers K, Beld M.** 2008. Rapid detection of human parechoviruses in clinical samples by real-time PCR. *J Clin Virol* **41:**69–74.

158. **Bennett S, Harvala H, Witteveldt J, McWilliam Leitch EC, McLeish N, Templeton K, Gunson R, Carman WF, Simmonds P.** 2011. Rapid simultaneous detection of enterovirus and parechovirus RNAs in clinical samples by one-step real-time reverse transcription-PCR assay. *J Clin Microbiol* **49:**2620–2624.

159. **Nielsen AC, Böttiger B, Midgley SE, Nielsen LP.** 2013. A novel enterovirus and parechovirus multiplex one-step real-time PCR-validation and clinical experience. *J Virol Methods* **193:**359–363.

160. **Bubba L, Pellegrinelli L, Pariani E, Primache V, Amendola A, Binda S.** 2015. A novel multiplex one-step real-time RT-PCR assay for the simultaneous identification of enterovirus and parechovirus in clinical fecal samples. *J Prev Med Hyg* **56:**E57–E60.

161. **Schuffenecker I, Javouhey E, Gillet Y, Kugener B, Billaud G, Floret D, Lina B, Morfin F.** 2012. Human parechovirus infections, Lyon, France, 2008–10: evidence for severe cases. *J Clin Virol* **54:**337–341.

162. **Walls T, McSweeney A, Anderson T, Jennings LC.** 2017. Multiplex-PCR for the detection of viruses in the CSF of infants and young children. *J Med Virol* **89:**559–561.

163. **Westerhuis BM, Jonker SC, Mattao S, Benschop KS, Wolthers KC.** 2013. Growth characteristics of human parechovirus 1 to 6 on different cell lines and cross-neutralization of human parechovirus antibodies: a comparison of the cytopathic effect and real time PCR. *Virol J* **10:**146.

164. **Faden H, Patel PH, Campagna L.** 2006. Pitfalls in the diagnosis of enteroviral infection in young children. *Pediatr Infect Dis J* **25:**687–690.

165. **Abed Y, Boivin G.** 2006. Human parechovirus types 1, 2 and 3 infections in Canada. *Emerg Infect Dis* **12:**969–975.

166. **DeBiasi RL, Tyler KL.** 2004. Molecular methods for diagnosis of viral encephalitis. *Clin Microbiol Rev* **17:**903–925.

167. **Terletskaia-Ladwig E, Meier S, Hahn R, Leinmüller M, Schneider F, Enders M.** 2008. A convenient rapid culture assay for the detection of enteroviruses in clinical samples: comparison with conventional cell culture and RT-PCR. *J Med Microbiol* **57:**1000–1006.

168. **Klespies SL, Cebula DE, Kelley CL, Galehouse D, Maurer CC.** 1996. Detection of enteroviruses from clinical specimens by spin amplification shell vial culture and monoclonal antibody assay. *J Clin Microbiol* **34:**1465–1467.

169. **Van Doornum GJ, De Jong JC.** 1998. Rapid shell vial culture technique for detection of enteroviruses and adenoviruses in fecal specimens: comparison with conventional virus isolation method. *J Clin Microbiol* **36:**2865–2868.

170. **Buck GE, Wiesemann M, Stewart L.** 2002. Comparison of mixed cell culture containing genetically engineered BGMK and CaCo-2 cells (Super E-Mix) with RT-PCR and conventional cell culture for the diagnosis of enterovirus meningitis. *J Clin Virol* **25**(Suppl 1)**:**S13–S18.

171. **She RC, Crist G, Billetdeaux E, Langer J, Petti CA.** 2006. Comparison of multiple shell vial cell lines for isolation of enteroviruses: a national perspective. *J Clin Virol* **37:**151–155.

172. **Melnick JL, Wenner HA, Phillips CA.** 1979. Enteroviruses, p 471–534. *In* Lennette EH, Schmidt NJ (ed), *Diagnostic Procedures for Viral, Rickettsial and Chlamydia Infections*, 5th ed. American Public Health Association, Washington, DC.

173. **Rigonan AS, Mann L, Chonmaitree T.** 1998. Use of monoclonal antibodies to identify serotypes of enterovirus isolates. *J Clin Microbiol* **36:**1877–1881.

174. **Abed Y, Boivin G.** 2005. Molecular characterization of a Canadian human parechovirus (HPeV)-3 isolate and its relationship to other HPeVs. *J Med Virol* **77:**566–570.

175. **Simmonds P, Welch J.** 2006. Frequency and dynamics of recombination within different species of human enteroviruses. *J Virol* **80:**483–493.

176. **Simmonds P.** 2006. Recombination and selection in the evolution of picornaviruses and other mammalian positive-stranded RNA viruses. *J Virol* **80:**11124–11140.

177. **Oberste MS, Nix WA, Maher K, Pallansch MA.** 2003. Improved molecular identification of enteroviruses by RT-PCR and amplicon sequencing. *J Clin Virol* **26:**375–377.

178. **Silva PA, Diedrich S, de Paula Cardoso D, Schreier E.** 2008. Identification of enterovirus serotypes by pyrosequencing using multiple sequencing primers. *J Virol Methods* **148:**260–264.

179. **Wylie TN, Wylie KM, Buller RS, Cannella M, Storch GA.** 2015. Development and evaluation of an enterovirus D68 real-time reverse transcriptase PCR assay. *J Clin Microbiol* **53:**2641–2647.

180. **Piralla A, Girello A, Premoli M, Baldanti F.** 2015. A new real-time reverse transcription-PCR assay for detection of human enterovirus 68 in respiratory samples. *J Clin Microbiol* **53:**1725–1726.

181. **Ng TF, Montmayeur A, Castro C, Cone M, Stringer J, Lamson DM, Rogers SL, Wang Chern SW, Magaña L, Marine R, Rubino H, Serinaldi D, George KS, Nix WA.** 2016. Detection and genomic characterization of enterovirus D68 in respiratory samples isolated in the United States in 2016. *Genome Announc* **4:**e01350-16.

182. **Puenpa J, Suwannakarn K, Chansaenroj J, Vongpunsawad S, Poovorawan Y.** 2017. Development of single-step multiplex real-time RT-PCR assays for rapid diagnosis of enterovirus 71, coxsackievirus A6, and A16 in patients with hand, foot, and mouth disease. *J Virol Methods* **248:**92–99.

183. **Kilpatrick DR, Ching K, Iber J, Campagnoli R, Freeman CJ, Mishrik N, Liu HM, Pallansch MA, Kew OM.** 2004. Multiplex PCR method for identifying recombinant vaccine-related polioviruses. *J Clin Microbiol* **42:**4313–4315.

184. **Xu J, Cao L, Su L, Dong N, Yu M, Ju J.** 2013. A new accurate assay for Coxsackievirus A 16 by fluorescence detection of isothermal RNA amplification. *J Virol Methods* **193:** 459–462.

185. **Ding X, Nie K, Shi L, Zhang Y, Guan L, Zhang D, Qi S, Ma X.** 2014. Improved detection limit in rapid detection of human enterovirus 71 and coxsackievirus A16 by a novel reverse transcription-isothermal multiple-self-matching-initiated amplification assay. *J Clin Microbiol* **52:**1862–1870.

186. **Lei X, Wen H, Zhao L, Yu X.** 2014. Performance of reversed transcription loop-mediated isothermal amplification technique detecting EV71: a systematic review with meta-analysis. *Biosci Trends* **8:**75–83.

187. **Yan G, Jun L, Kangchen Z, Yiyue G, Yang Y, Xiaoyu Z, Zhiyang S, Lunbiao C.** 2015. Rapid and visual detection of human enterovirus coxsackievirus A16 by reverse transcription loop-mediated isothermal amplification combined with lateral flow device. *Lett Appl Microbiol* **61:**531–537.

188. **Monazah A, Zeinoddini M, Saeeidinia AR.** 2017. Evaluation of a rapid detection for Coxsackievirus B3 using one-step reverse transcription loop-mediated isothermal amplification (RT-LAMP). *J Virol Methods* **246:**27–33.

189. **Zhou F, Kong F, McPhie K, Ratnamohan M, Donovan L, Zeng F, Gilbert GL, Dwyer DE.** 2009. Identification of 20 common human enterovirus serotypes using a RT-PCR-based reverse line blot hybridization assay. *J Clin Microbiol* **47:**2737–2743.

190. **Susi P, Hattara L, Waris M, Luoma-Aho T, Siitari H, Hyypiä T, Saviranta P.** 2009. Typing of enteroviruses by use of microwell oligonucleotide arrays. *J Clin Microbiol* **47:** 1863–1870.

191. **Mahfoud F, Gärtner B, Kindermann M, Ukena C, Gadomski K, Klingel K, Kandolf R, Böhm M, Kindermann I.** 2011. Virus serology in patients with suspected myocarditis: utility or futility? *Eur Heart J* **32:**897–903.

192. **Bell EJ, McCartney RA, Basquill D, Chaudhuri AK.** 1986. Mu-antibody capture ELISA for the rapid diagnosis of enterovirus infections in patients with aseptic meningitis. *J Med Virol* **19:**213–217.
193. **Bendig JW, Molyneaux P.** 1996. Sensitivity and specificity of mu-capture ELISA for detection of enterovirus IgM. *J Virol Methods* **59:**23–32.
194. **Craig ME, Robertson P, Howard NJ, Silink M, Rawlinson WD.** 2003. Diagnosis of enterovirus infection by genus-specific PCR and enzyme-linked immunosorbent assays. *J Clin Microbiol* **41:**841–844.
195. **Pozzetto B, Gaudin OG, Aouni M, Ros A.** 1989. Comparative evaluation of immunoglobulin M neutralizing antibody response in acute-phase sera and virus isolation for the routine diagnosis of enterovirus infection. *J Clin Microbiol* **27:**705–708.
196. **Wang SY, Lin TL, Chen HY, Lin TS.** 2004. Early and rapid detection of enterovirus 71 infection by an IgM-capture ELISA. *J Virol Methods* **119:**37–43.
197. **Chen T-C, Weng K-F, Chang S-C, Lin J-Y, Huang P-N, Shih S-R.** 2008. Development of antiviral agents for enteroviruses. *J Antimicrob Chemother* **62:**1169–1173.
198. **Romero JR.** 2001. Pleconaril: a novel antipicornaviral drug. *Expert Opin Investig Drugs* **10:**369–379.
199. **Webster ADB.** 2005. Pleconaril—an advance in the treatment of enteroviral infection in immuno-compromised patients. *J Clin Virol* **32:**1–6.
200. **McKinlay MA, Collett MS, Hincks JR, Oberste MS, Pallansch MA, Okayasu H, Sutter RW, Modlin JF, Dowdle WR.** 2014. Progress in the development of poliovirus antiviral agents and their essential role in reducing risks that threaten eradication. *J Infect Dis* **210**(Suppl 1)**:** S447–S453.
201. **Torres-Torres S, Myers AL, Klatte JM, Rhoden EE, Oberste MS, Collett MS, McCulloh RJ.** 2015. First use of investigational antiviral drug pocapavir (v-073) for treating neonatal enteroviral sepsis. *Pediatr Infect Dis J* **34:**52–54
202. **Collett MS, Hincks JR, Benschop K, Duizer E, van der Avoort H, Rhoden E, Liu H, Oberste MS, McKinlay MA, Hartford M.** 2017. Antiviral activity of pocapavir in a randomized, blinded, placebo-controlled human oral poliovirus vaccine challenge model. *J Infect Dis* **215:**335–343.
203. **Oberste MS, Pallansch MA.** 2005. Enterovirus molecular detection and typing. *Rev Med Microbiol* **16:**163–171.

Rhinoviruses

MARIE LOUISE LANDRY AND XIAOYAN LU

91

TAXONOMY

Human rhinoviruses (RVs) are members of the family *Picornaviridae*. Previously a separate genus, RVs have been reclassified into three separate species (A, B, C) within the *Enterovirus* genus (1). Other *Picornaviridae* genera that are pathogenic for humans include *Parechovirus*, members of which have been associated with respiratory disease, and *Hepatovirus*. Recently, the *Cardiovirus* genus has been found to contain human pathogens as well (2).

RVs derive their name from the predominant site of their replication and symptomatology, the nose. RV isolates were originally classified into 99 serotypes (RV1 through RV99) based on neutralization with type-specific antisera; subsequent sequencing studies have shown that there are in fact many more types that have not been cultured and typed serologically (see below). While some cross-neutralization occurs, there is no group antigen (3, 4). RV serotypes were further classified into two species: RV-A containing 74 serotypes and RV-B containing 25 serotypes, based on sequence relatedness. The original 99 RV prototype strains isolated in the 1960s and 1970s have been propagated and maintained by the ATCC. One former RV serotype, RV87, has been shown by sequence analysis to be an acid-sensitive strain of enterovirus (EV) D-68 (5, 6).

RV serotypes can be further divided into two groups based on receptor binding (7, 8): (i) a major group (63 RV-A and 25 RV-B serotypes) that binds intercellular adhesion molecule 1 (ICAM-1), a member of the immunoglobulin supergene family that is expressed on the surface of many different cells (9); and (ii) a minor group (11 RV-A serotypes) that binds to members of the low-density lipoprotein receptor family (8).

The wider use of molecular methods in viral diagnostics has led to the discovery (10) of a novel group of RVs identified in patients with lower respiratory tract disease. Classified as a new species "C," these viruses are not new or recently emerging viruses (11), but they have been circulating unnoticed due to their lack of growth in standard cell culture systems used for RV isolation. Recently, RV-C viruses were grown in human sinus epithelium organ cultures (12) and air-liquid interface culture of differentiated airway epithelial cells (13, 14). RV-C was recently discovered to utilize cadherin-related family member 3 receptor (CDHR3) for host cell entry (15). CDHR3 is a transmembrane protein that has been found in human lung, bronchial epithelium, and cultured airway epithelial cells. Interestingly, a coding single nucleotide polymorphism (rs6967330, p.Cys529Tyr) in CDHR3 showed enhanced binding efficiency for RV-C and increased virus production, suggesting that the Cys529Tyr variant could be a risk factor for RV-C-associated childhood wheezing and asthma hospitalization (16).

Sequencing of the complete genomes of the 99 RV-A and RV-B serotypes and available RV-C strains confirmed clustering of all strains into three distinct phylogenetic groups (17). Because serotyping RV-C was not possible due to their refractoriness to cell culture, a genetically based classification system was developed for assigning RV genotypes while retaining the serotype numbering system (18). To date, 55 RV-C genotypes have been assigned using a threshold of ≥13% nucleotide differences in the *VP1* coding region from all RV prototype strains or ≥10% nucleotide difference in the *VP4/VP2* region if the *VP1* sequence is unavailable; thresholds of ≥13% and 12% nucleotide differences in *VP1* for RV-A and RV-B type assignments, respectively, were also proposed (19). By use of the above thresholds, types A44, A95, and A98 have been abolished and combined into types A29, A8, and A54, respectively (19). Designation of an additional 9 RV-A and 6 RV-B genotypes brings the total number of currently recognized RV types to 166.

DESCRIPTION OF THE AGENT

The RV genome is a single-stranded, positive-sense RNA, approximately 7200 nucleotides in length. The genome is composed of a 5′ untranslated region (5′ UTR) coupled with a short peptide (VPg) that serves as a primer for genome replication (20), followed by a single open reading frame that terminates in a 3′ poly (A) tail (Fig. 1). Secondary structures within the 5′ UTR, a cloverleaf domain and an internal ribosomal entry site, are necessary for protein translation. The single polypeptide product of the open reading frame is subsequently proteolytically cleaved into 11 viral proteins (Fig. 1): 4 structural proteins that form the viral capsid (1A through 1D or VP4 through VP1) and 7 nonstructural proteins that are involved with

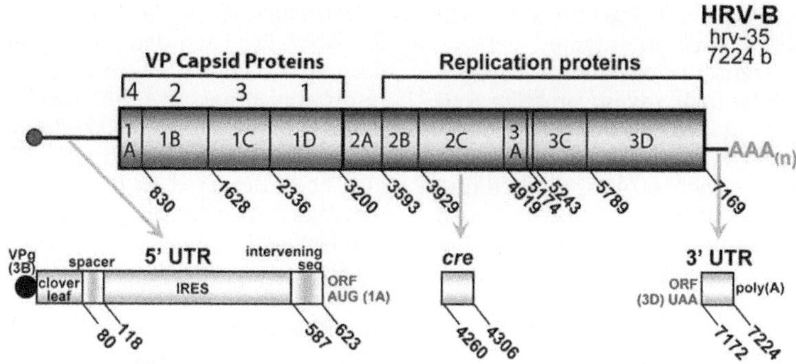

FIGURE 1 Rhinovirus genome structure. The genome consists of a single open reading frame flanked by 5′ and 3′ untranslated regions (UTR). A small viral protein, VPg, is covalently linked to the 5′ UTR. VP, viral protein; IRES, internal ribosome entry site; cre, *cis*-acting replication element. Reproduced with permission from reference 26.

virus replication or polyprotein processing (2A through 2C and 3A through 3D). The 3C protease participates in cleavage of polypeptide and is a target for antiviral drugs.

The RV virion is a small, 20 to 27 nm in diameter, nonenveloped icosahedron comprising 60 protomeric units each consisting of the four structural protein subunits (VP1–VP4). VP1, VP2, and VP3 reside on the exterior of the virion and make up its protein coat. VP1 is the largest, most external, and immunodominant protein of the virus capsid (21). A number of major neutralization sites reside in the VP1 proteins. Located within VP1 is a hydrophobic pocket into which antiviral compounds such as pleconaril bind (22). VP4 resides inside the protein shell. X-ray crystallography and cryoelectron microscopy studies have identified large depressions or "canyons" on each of the 60 protomeric units, which appear to be sites for cell receptor binding and play a critical role in conformational changes that follow attachment (23). Conformational changes in the canyon floor can also be induced by certain antiviral agents, thus inhibiting virus attachment to cells or virus uncoating (22).

RVs replicate in the cytoplasm of infected cells producing infectious virions that sediment at a buoyant density of 1.40 g/liter in cesium chloride. Empty capsids and defective particles lacking one or more structural polypeptides are also produced.

Mutation and recombination are two mechanisms that drive the extensive genetic diversity of RVs and serve as the basis for RV evolution. The 3D RNA-dependent RNA polymerase that facilitates synthesis of new viral genomes has no proofreading capacity and frequently generates mutations. Evidence of recombination between RV-A and RV-C within the 5′ UTR has also been shown: on phylogenetic analysis, the 5′ UTR sequences of some RV-C genotypes cluster within the RV-A clade (24, 25). Although RV-B and RV-C show little evidence of recombination within the genome coding region, recent studies have shown that RV-A sequences have undergone extensive intraspecies recombination during the early stage of diversification into types and several contemporary RV-A strains have been formed by recombination (26, 27).

As they have no lipid envelope, RVs are fairly resistant to inactivation by organic solvents such as ether, chloroform, ethanol, and 5% phenol. Although RVs are relatively thermostable, heating at 50 to 56°C progressively reduces infectivity. RVs are traditionally differentiated from EVs by their loss of infectivity upon exposure to pH 3 for 3 h at room temperature, though this may not be the case with all serotypes and strains.

EPIDEMIOLOGY AND TRANSMISSION

RV infections are widespread and year-round. With use of molecular methods, substantial RV infections have been found in summer and winter (28–30), but transmission typically peaks in autumn and late spring in temperate zones (28).

Seasonal fluctuations have been attributed to improved survival of RV in conditions of high relative indoor humidity and herding together of children when school opens in the fall (31). RV-A and RV-C may co-circulate in equal proportions or may alternate as the predominant species (32–34); RV-B is consistently less frequently detected (34). As the disease burden and diversity of RV infections have become evident, the interest in RV genotyping, molecular epidemiology, and correlating genotype with virulence has intensified (11).

Studies in volunteers have shown that inoculation of virus into the nose or conjunctivae is the most efficient way to initiate infection, although virus can also be transmitted by aerosol inhalation (35, 36). RV is present in highest titers in the nose of infected persons and commonly contaminates their hands and surrounding surfaces. Consequently, investigators have found that RV can be transmitted via hand-to-hand contact (37) or by contaminated fomites, followed by self-inoculation of virus into the nose or conjunctivae (38). Furthermore, transmission can be interrupted by use of tissues impregnated with virucidal agents for nose blowing, by treatment of surfaces with disinfectant, or by application of iodine to the fingers (39). Recent studies have found ethanol hand sanitizers to be more effective than soap and water, and virucidal activity of the sanitizer can be enhanced and prolonged by the addition of organic acids (40). However, a reduction in transmission in a natural setting has not yet been established.

RVs replicate primarily in airway epithelium, but also in the middle ear and sinuses, with an incubation period of 1 to 4 days (41). The peak of virus shedding coincides with the acute rhinitis. Symptoms last 7 days on average, but can persist for 12 to 14 days or more (42, 43); they typically include profuse watery discharge, nasal congestion, sneezing, headache, mild sore throat, cough, and little or no fever. By culture, virus may become undetectable at 4 to 5 days or may be present in low titers for up to

2 to 3 weeks (44). Asymptomatic RV infections are also common, occurring in 20 to 30% of infected persons (28, 45–47). With reverse transcription-PCR (RT-PCR), RV RNA has been detected by some investigators for 4 to 5 weeks after the onset of symptoms, and surprisingly for 2 to 3 weeks prior to onset of symptoms (46, 48). However, genotyping has revealed that such prolonged shedding often represents a series of sequential RV infections with different RV types, some asymptomatic (49). As many as 74 distinct RV types have been found to be co-circulating, including multiple types in the same household (49, 50). Chronic shedding of a single RV type has been documented only in immunocompromised hosts (51).

Symptoms of RV infection parallel the rise and fall of chemical mediators of inflammation (38, 39). Psychological stress and inadequate sleep appear to increase susceptibility and the development of clinical symptoms (52–54). Early studies concluded that immunity is type specific and correlates best with local production of IgA (55, 56).

CLINICAL SIGNIFICANCE

RVs cause approximately two-thirds of cases of the upper respiratory syndrome known as the common cold, and thus they are responsible for more episodes of human illness than any other infectious agent (28, 39). Although considered a trivial illness, the common cold may be acutely disabling, and its cost, in days lost from work, cold remedies, and analgesics, is estimated at $40 billion annually in the United States (57).

With the use of molecular methods, more severe consequences of RV infections have been increasingly recognized. RVs can be the sole etiology of sinusitis and otitis media, as well as facilitating secondary bacterial infections (58–60). RV have been implicated as the major viral cause of exacerbations of asthma, cystic fibrosis, and chronic obstructive pulmonary disease (61–64). Indeed, RV wheezing illness in infancy has been linked to childhood-onset asthma in genetically susceptible children (65, 66). The impact of disease in the elderly is also substantial. In a Canadian study, 59% of outbreaks of respiratory disease in long-term care facilities were due to RVs, and some disease was severe (67)

RV has been increasingly detected in lower respiratory tract infections (68, 69); in patients hospitalized with wheezing or pneumonia (70–73), including school-age children (74); in the elderly (31, 75); and in those with chronic illnesses, cancer, immunosuppressive illnesses, transplants (76–82), or underlying pulmonary disease (64, 83). The clinical manifestations of RV in hospitalized infants are similar to those caused by respiratory syncytial virus; however, the mean age of RV-affected infants tends to be slightly older (72). RVs are commonly found either singly or in combination with other viruses. RVs have been shown to impair the innate immune response (84, 85) and may predispose to invasive pneumococcal disease in children and bacterial superinfections in chronic obstructive pulmonary disease (60, 85–87).

RV-C viruses have been implicated in some studies as the predominant RV species linked to hospitalizations for fever, wheezing, and lower respiratory tract disease, especially in young infants and asthmatic children (32, 88–93). In contrast to classic RV-A and RV-B, RV-C replicates equally well at 37°C and 34°C, facilitating infection in the lower respiratory tract (10). The receptor for EV-C, CDHR3, has been identified as a susceptibility locus for asthma exacerbations (16). However, additional population-based studies are needed before definitive conclusions can be made about the prevalence and virulence of RV species (41).

Although RV viremia has rarely been found by culture, RV RNA has been detected by sensitive molecular methods in the blood of RV-infected young children with severe respiratory illness (14, 94) (including 25% of those with RV-associated asthma exacerbations [47]), and has been predominantly associated with RV-C (14, 94). RVs have also been detected in fecal specimens of children with meningitis, pericarditis, gastroenteritis, and even a healthy child (95–98).

Since RVs have historically been difficult to culture and serotype, there is little information available on the relationships between serotype, clinical manifestations, and virulence (99). With the development of molecular genotyping methods and increased awareness of the disease burden of RV, this currently is an area of intense study (28, 41, 98).

Due to numerous RV types, prospects for a vaccine have been considered negligible. Recently, however, polyvalent inactivated RV vaccines have shown early success in immunizing mice and rhesus macaque monkeys, suggesting that broadly immunogenic response to numerous and diverse RV types is possible (100).

COLLECTION, TRANSPORT, AND STORAGE OF SPECIMENS

In natural infections, RV can generally be isolated in culture from 1 day before to 6 days after onset of cold symptoms, but it is shed in highest concentration on day 1 or 2 of illness. In upper airway disease, RV is excreted in highest titers from the nose, thus nasal rather than throat specimens should be obtained for diagnosis.

Early comparisons of nasal wash, nose swab, throat gargle, and throat swab specimens for the isolation of RV from clinical specimens revealed nasal wash to be the best (56, 101); specimens obtained as follows: tilt the patient's head backward and instill 1 ml of sterile phosphate-buffered saline into one of the nostrils. Then ask the patient to lean forward and allow the washing to drip into a sterile petri dish or other collection container. Repeat with the other nostril until each nostril has been washed with 5 ml of phosphate-buffered saline. The washings are then transferred into a sterile container. However, nasal wash samples are cumbersome to obtain in most clinical settings and may be suboptimal for other respiratory pathogens.

For many years, nasopharyngeal (NP) aspirates have been the standard for infants and young children, but the most convenient and commonly collected sample at present is an NP swab placed in viral transport medium. Well-collected NP swabs can provide detection rates comparable to aspirates and are simpler to obtain (102, 103). A recent study found that while nasal wash detected more RV positives than NP swabs, the difference was not statistically significant when flocked swabs were used (104). Flocked swabs have been shown in some but not all studies to provide superior samples to cotton and some other swab types. However, the small, flexible-shaft, flocked NP swabs are consistently rated as more comfortable for the patient than rigid-shaft, large-tipped collection swabs (104). Midturbinate flocked swabs have provided a yield similar to NP swab results in one report and are amenable to both self-collection and collection of samples from young children by parents (105, 106). Sputum has been reported to be comparable in yield to NP aspirates for respiratory viruses (107).

To diagnose lower respiratory tract infection, endotracheal aspirate, bronchoalveolar lavage (BAL), bronchial wash, or lung biopsy samples should be collected. Sputum, including induced sputum in children, has been recently found to also be useful for diagnosing viral lower respiratory tract disease (103, 108).

All specimens should be transported promptly to the laboratory. For isolation, best results are obtained with prompt inoculation of cell cultures; however, specimens can be held up to 24 h at 4°C in viral transport medium with neutral pH. If longer delays are necessary, specimens should be frozen at −70°C and thawed just prior to inoculation. Freezing does not appear to be detrimental to RV recovery (101). Similar sample handling is recommended for molecular analysis; however, the compatibility of various virus transport media with different extraction reagents must be confirmed in each laboratory, and manufacturers' instructions should be followed for all commercial kits.

DIRECT DETECTION

Antigen

Due to the large number of serotypes and the lack of a common group antigen, antigen detection assays are not used in clinical practice.

Nucleic Acid

Conventional RT-PCR Assays

Wider use of molecular diagnostics has dramatically increased RV detection and greatly enhanced our appreciation of the role of these viruses in respiratory disease. RT-PCR assays have proven more sensitive than culture methods, doubling or even tripling the number of RV infections detected (45, 109–112), and are clearly superior for detection of noncultivable RV strains like RV-C. Nevertheless, culture can occasionally recover some RVs missed by RT-PCR due to variability in techniques and primer or probe mismatches (110, 112, 113).

The first RT-PCR diagnostic assay for RVs was reported by Gama et al. in 1988 (114). Since then, numerous molecular assays have been described. These assays typically target the 5′ UTR of the viral genome that contains highly conserved sequences suitable for molecular assay development. However, most of these assays also detected EVs, because the primer sets used were not able to effectively distinguish between these two virus groups. Earlier strategies to distinguish between RVs and EVs included differential amplicon sizing (115, 116), restriction enzyme digestion of a common-sized amplicon (117), internal probe hybridization (113, 118), and nested PCR using RV-specific primers (93) or annealing and extension times optimized for RV detection (111). Most of these reported methods failed to detect or accurately differentiate all viruses tested, and none evaluated all RV and EV types. RT-PCR and sequencing of amplicons to differentiate RVs from EVs and for identifying virus types (see below) are now commonly used by specialized reference laboratories, but they are still not easily implemented for routine clinical diagnosis (119).

At present, molecular methods are not standardized and those published have differed in types of samples tested, methods of RNA extraction used, primer selection, and amplification and detection conditions. A comparison of the relative sensitivity of 11 published RV primer pairs that used clinical specimens positive for the three recognized RV species demonstrated discordance in performance, especially for the specimens with lower virus loads (120).

Real-Time RT-PCR Assays

Real-time RT-PCR (rRT-PCR) assays for RVs that use SYBR Green, TaqMan hydrolysis probes, or molecular beacons have been developed (43, 79, 96, 119, 121–123). Real-time amplification methods have the advantages of simplicity, reduced risk of amplicon contamination, ability to estimate viral load, and a shortened time to result since detection occurs concurrent with amplification. Though less expensive than probe-based methods, results obtained using SYBR Green and melt-curve analysis can be difficult to interpret (43).

One rRT-PCR assay (14, 43) targeting the 5′ UTR, which was recently modified (14), was shown to detect all recognized RV prototype strains as well as the novel RV-C viruses; it has been used successfully in studies to determine the epidemiology and clinical features of RV infections in different populations (32, 73, 124–126). Although much effort has been devoted to improving the specificity of this assay, it still reacts with some EVs when present at high viral load in the clinical specimen.

Several RV studies have demonstrated a positive correlation between viral load and disease severity, suggesting that virus quantitation may help clarify the clinical relevance of a positive test result (97, 127–130). Although a recent study has shown that rRT-PCR assays can be used to semiquantify RV RNA in clinical material, accurate absolute RV RNA quantification in respiratory specimens is complicated by (i) the lack of an accurately quantified international reference RNA standard, (ii) sequence variation among RV strains that may differentially effect rRT-PCR amplification efficiency, and (iii) variability in sample collection procedures (131).

Multiplexed RT-PCR Assays

Numerous laboratory-developed and commercial multiplex RT-PCR assays based on different amplification platforms and combining multiple respiratory pathogens including RV have been described in recent years. There are currently eight commercial multiplex tests that include RV that have been cleared for *in vitro* diagnostic use in the United States by the FDA: the Luminex xTAG Respiratory Virus Panel (RVP), Luminex xTAG RVP Fast, and Luminex NxTAG Respiratory Pathogen Panel (RPP) (Luminex Molecular Diagnostics, Austin, TX); the FilmArray Respiratory Panel (RP), FilmArray RP2, FilmArray RP EZ (CLIA waived), and FilmArray RP2Plus (BioFire Diagnostics, Salt Lake City, UT); the eSensor RVP and ePlex RPP (GenMark Dx, Carlsbad, CA) (Table 1).

The Luminex xTAG RVPv1, xTAG RVP Fast, and NxTAG RPP utilize multiplex RT-PCR followed by amplicon identification using a fluid-microsphere-based array flow cytometry (132) (133–135) for detection of 12 or 8 viruses and subtypes for the RVPs, respectively, and 18 viruses and subtypes plus 3 bacterial targets for the RPP. The FilmArray RP integrates sample preparation, amplification, and detection into one simple system using a preloaded blister pouch solid array and endpoint melting-curve analysis to detect and identify 20 different respiratory viral and bacterial pathogens in about 1 h. The eSensor RVP uses competitive DNA hybridization and electrochemical detection to identify 14 different respiratory virus types and subtypes, whereas the ePlex RPP detects 15 viral and two bacterial targets. The FilmArray RP, Luminex xTAG RVPv1, xTAG RVP Fast, and ePlex RPP assays do not distinguish between RV and EV, while the eSensor RVP claims to be specific for RV only (136, 137). Most commercial molecular assays require purchase of a dedicated instrument. In contrast, the FTD respiratory pathogens multiplex assay (Fast Track Diagnostics, Luxembourg) uses standard real-time hydrolysis probe chemistries and common real-time PCR

TABLE 1 Commercial multiplex molecular assays for respiratory pathogens, including rhinovirus

Company	Assay	U.S. FDA[a]	Dedicated instrument	RT-PCR	Detection	Post-PCR handling	RV, EV, RV/EV[b]	No. viral and bacterial pathogens identified	Company website	Key reference(s)
AutoGenomics	INFINITI RVP Plus	RUO	Yes	Conventional	Solid array	No	RV (A/B), EV	25	www.autogenomics.com/	159
bioMérieux	FilmArray Respiratory Panel (RP)	IVD	Yes	Real-time	LC green using Cp values and melt-curve analysis	No	RV/EV	20	www.biofiredx.com/	160
	FilmArray RP2	IVD	Yes	Real-time	Same	No	RV/EV	21		
	FilmArray RP EZ (CLIA waived)	IVD	Yes	Real-time	Same	No	RV/EV	14		
	FilmArray RP2Plus	IVD	Yes	Real-time	Same	No	RV/EV	22		
Fast Track Diagnostics	FTD Respiratory pathogens 21	RUO	No	Real-time	Hydrolysis probe	No	RV/EV	21	www.fast-trackdiagnostics.com/	138
GenMark Dx	eSensor Respiratory Viral Panel	IVD	Yes	Conventional	Electrochemical	Yes	RV	14	http://www.genmarkdx.com/	137
	ePlex Respiratory Pathogen Panel	IVD				No	RV/EV	17		161
iCubate	Respiratory-V Cassette	RUO	Yes	Conventional	Solid array	No	RV, Cox/EcV	20	www.icubate.com/	
Luminex	xTag RVP & RVP Fast	IVD	Yes	Conventional	Liquid bead array	Yes	RV (A/B/C)/EV	USA (12 & 8); Europe (18/16)	www.luminexcorp.com/	134, 162–164
	NxTAG Respiratory Pathogen Panel	IVD				No		20		136, 137, 163
	Verigene Respiratory Pathogens	RUO	Yes	Conventional	Solid array	No	RV (A/B/C)/EV	15	www.nanosphere.us/	165
PathoFinder	RespiFinder SMART 22 & SMART 22 Fast	RUO	No	Real-time	Melting-curve analysis	No	RV/EV	21	www.pathofinder.com/	166, 167
Qiagen	ResPLEX II	RUO	Yes	Conventional	Liquid bead array	Yes	RV, Cox/EcV	16	www.qiagen.com/	166
Seegene	Anyplex II RV16	RUO	No	Real-time	Melting-curve analysis	No	RV(A, B, C), EV	16	www.seegene.com/	149
	Seeplex RV15 OneStep ACE Detection	RUO		Conventional	Amplicon size	Yes		15		

[a]RUO, research use only; IVD, FDA-approved for use as *in vitro* diagnostic.
[b]Based on company literature, RV detects rhinovirus (species not indicated); EV detects enterovirus; RV/EV detects both rhinovirus and enterovirus but indistinguishable; CoX/EcV detects coxsackievirus A and B and echovirus.

instrumentation for detection of 21 respiratory pathogens, allowing easy integration into the workflow of laboratories already using standard real-time PCR platforms (138).

At present, few clinical laboratories are either interested in or able to set up homebrew RT-PCR assays for RV, and even if available commercially, these assays may not be used unless they are part of a more comprehensive panel of respiratory pathogens.

These comprehensive multiplex assays have confirmed the frequent detection of RVs in culture-negative clinical samples and have revealed many mixed pathogen infections. However, most are not quantitative and all are costly to implement and maintain. Each commercially available system has its unique advantages and disadvantages, and each user should determine which system is appropriate for their specific diagnostic needs.

Although much effort has been devoted to distinguishing RVs from EVs, in the clinical setting a single assay that detects both virus groups could ultimately prove to be advantageous since some antivirals may be effective against both virus groups (42). Moreover, some EVs (e.g., EV-D68 and coxsackievirus A21 (CV-A21) can also cause respiratory diseases (139–143). Thus, some multiplexed assays have not attempted to separate the two genera, but instead target both (Table 1).

ISOLATION PROCEDURES

Cell Culture

RV species A and B grow only in cells of human or monkey origin. RV species C has not yet been grown in conventional cell culture. Although the original isolation of RVs was in primary monkey kidney cells, these cells have not been consistent in yielding a broad range of isolates. The most commonly used cells in clinical laboratories are the human embryonic lung fibroblast strains WI-38 and MRC-5 (144). WI-38 cells are significantly more sensitive than MRC-5 (101), but MRC-5 cells are more commonly available. Human embryonic kidney (HEK) can also support RV replication. Unfortunately, different lots of normally sensitive cell lines have been found to vary over 100-fold in sensitivity to RV (144); the reasons for this variation are not known. Therefore, for optimal results, simultaneous use of at least two sensitive systems is recommended.

In the research setting, several HeLa cell clones, such as HeLa M or HeLa Ohio cells, HeLa H, HeLa R-19, and HeLa I cells, have been shown to support the replication of RVs to high titers (101). HeLa I cells were found to be more sensitive than WI38, MRC-5, fetal tonsil, HeLa H, or HeLa M cells for recovery of RV from clinical specimens (145). A transduced HeLa-E8 cell line that stably expresses the RV-C CDHR3 receptor has recently been shown to support RV-C propagation (15). These specialized cell lines can be obtained only from research laboratories.

After inoculation, cultures are incubated in standard cell culture medium such as Eagles minimum essential medium with 2% fetal calf serum and antibiotics at a neutral pH. To mimic conditions of the nose, cultures should be incubated at 33 to 35°C with continuous rotation in a roller drum to provide aeration of the monolayer. RV cytopathic effects (CPE) can be observed as early as 24–48 h after inoculation and are often detected by day 4. Passage of infected HeLa cell cultures may be necessary for some isolates before CPE are apparent. In fibroblasts, cellular changes are easier to read and are often detected earlier than in epithelial cell lines. Both large and small rounded, refractile cells with pyknotic nuclei are observed in foci that also contain cellular debris (Fig. 2). RV CPE are similar to EV CPE, but may sometimes be confused with nonspecific changes. The CPE progress over a 2- to 3-day period, with the degree of cellular change

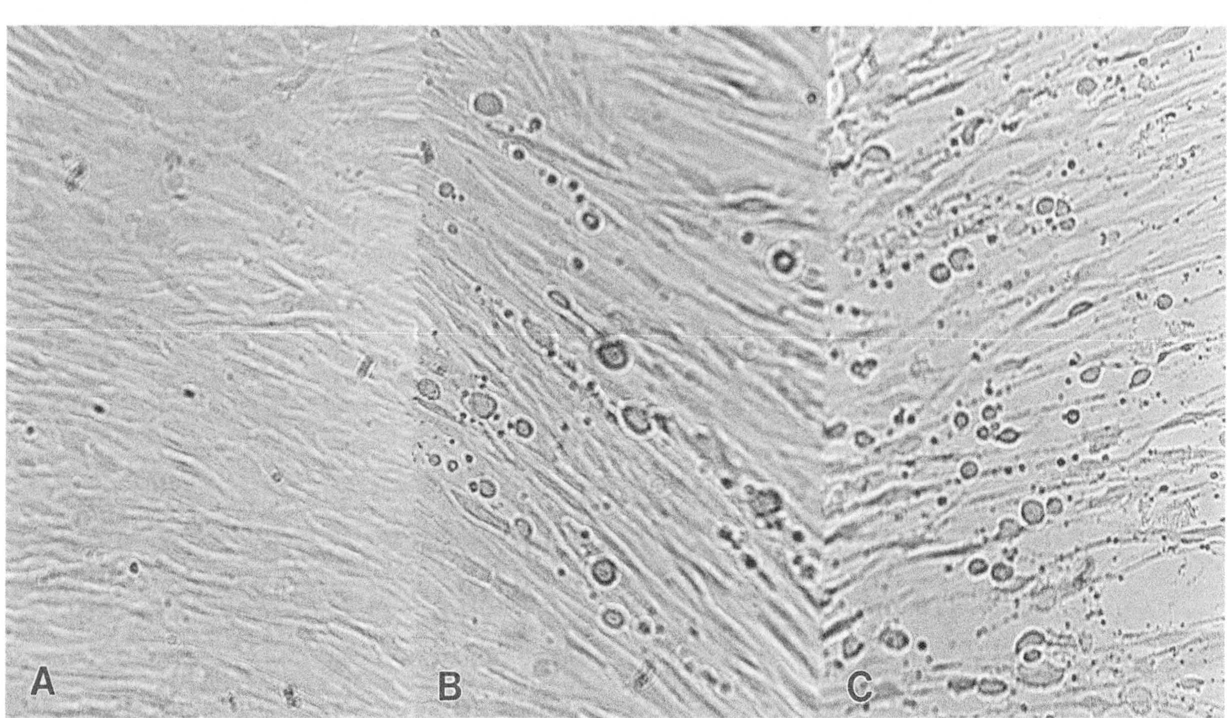

FIGURE 2 Rhinovirus cytopathic effects in human embryonic lung fibroblasts. (A) Uninfected cells. (B) Early focus of rhinovirus CPE. (C) More advanced rhinovirus CPE. Magnification, ×100.

depending on the serotype and the inoculum dose. It should be noted that RV CPE can regress, or virus may inactivate if left too long. Therefore, cultures should be promptly passaged. Passage is also necessary to increase viral titers prior to the performance of identification tests.

Human embryonic lung fibroblast cell cultures should be observed 14 days, with refeeding at 7 days to increase recovery of virus. HeLa cell cultures can be observed for only up to 7 to 8 days, when passage becomes necessary due to nonspecific cell degeneration and rounding.

Rapid centrifugation cultures using HuH7 hepatocellular carcinoma cell line have been reported to detect respiratory viruses, including RV. After 4 days of incubation, RV can be detected in the amplified culture by RT-PCR. While results were faster, HuH7 cells were not as sensitive as MRC-5 conventional cultures incubated for 14 days (109).

Organ and Differentiated Epithelial Cell Culture

Organ cultures of human fetal nasal epithelium or trachea were used in the past to isolate RVs not grown in standard cell cultures, but they are no longer used for this purpose. Recently, however, cultures of nasal, sinus, and tracheal mucosa obtained from biopsy material have been used for research studies of RV pathogenesis (10, 12, 146, 147). Both organ culture and differentiated human airway epithelial cells on air-liquid interface have been used to grow RV-C (13).

IDENTIFICATION

A presumptive diagnosis of RV isolates in cell culture is made by the appearance and progression of characteristic CPE in the appropriate cell lines. In clinical laboratories, further identification of a presumed RV isolate is usually limited to differentiating it from EVs by determining sensitivity to acid pH, although this practice has declined in recent years. Virus neutralization testing with type-specific antisera is time-consuming, costly, and not routinely available. In addition, the recently recognized RV-C strains do not grow in culture and no neutralizing sera are available.

Acid pH Stability

RVs are sensitive to low pH and are inactivated, whereas most EVs remain viable. Thus, a reduction in virus titer of 2 to 3 $\log_{10}$ $TCID_{50}$ can be expected upon exposure of RV to low pH. To perform the test, first passage the isolate to obtain a minimum titer of 10^3 $TCID_{50}$/ml. Then, prepare two solutions of a buffer, such as HEPES, one at pH 3.0 and one at pH 7.0. Add 0.2 ml of unknown virus suspension to 1.8 ml of HEPES pH 3.0, and 0.2 ml of virus to 1.8 ml of HEPES pH 7.0. Keep the mixtures at room temperature for 3 h, adjust the pH to 7.0, make serial dilutions of the mixtures, and inoculate into cell culture. If the unknown virus is an RV, a minimum 2 $\log_{10}$ reduction in viral titer should be evident in the acid-treated sample. For controls, a known RV and a known EV should be treated in a similar fashion.

Temperature Sensitivity

Since RVs often grow best at 33°C, they may be distinguished from EVs by inoculation of parallel serial dilutions of the unknown virus and incubation at 33°C and 37°C. The onset of CPE should be more rapid and the titer of virus obtained should be higher at the lower temperature. Some RV isolates may not show this temperature sensitivity, and this test is no longer used clinically (69).

Immunoassay

Staining of isolates in parallel with both a pan-EV immunofluorescence monoclonal antibody that detects both EV and RV and an EV-specific reagent that detects only EV was shown to rapidly and correctly identify 11 RV isolates in a clinical setting (134).

Virus Identification by RT-PCR and Real-Time RT-PCR

As noted above, RT-PCR and rRT-PCR targeting highly conserved regions of the 5′ UTR can be used for confirmation of RV isolates in cell culture. However, cross-reactions with EV can occur, especially with high-titer EV culture isolates (43, 148).

TYPING SYSTEMS

Serotyping RV by Virus Neutralization

Serotyping of RV isolates by neutralization with type-specific antisera used to be the gold standard for RV identification. However, the neutralization test is expensive and labor-intensive, its results can be delayed for weeks, and few laboratories have the antisera necessary to perform the procedure. Moreover, RV-C strains cannot grow in standard cell culture, and interpreting assay results can be difficult given cross-reactions between some serotypes. Serotyping requires the neutralization of 30 to 100 $TCID_{50}$ of virus-induced CPE by 20 units of antiserum. Hyperimmune antisera for RVs are available through the ATCC. Intersecting serum pools similar to those used for EV identification have been prepared to help narrow the identity of the virus isolate. Identification of the specific serotype is then performed using monospecific antisera. Detailed procedures are described elsewhere (149).

Genotyping RV by Sequencing

Molecular typing based on RT-PCR and amplicon sequencing has essentially replaced serotyping for type-specific identification of RVs. Because the RV VP1 capsid protein contains a number of neutralization domains that correlate with serotype, genotypic identification of RVs based on complete *VP1* sequencing has been proposed using type assignment nucleotide differences thresholds of 13%, 12%, and 13% for RV-A, RV-B, and RV-C, respectively (27). This change has led to only minor revisions of existing serotyping designation (such as reclassification of serotype pairs A8/A95, A29/A44, and A54/A98 as single serotypes). However, because of the high degree of sequence variation in the *VP1* gene and surrounding regions, it has been difficult to design universal primers that will successfully amplify all RV strains, often requiring new primer designs and assay optimization when new RVs are recognized (150). In contrast, genotyping based on sequencing the capsid *VP4/VP2* protein genes has been widely used for RV genotyping in large epidemiological studies (70, 93) due to the availability of conserved regions for primer design that bracket the *VP4/VP2* region. Overall, RV species and type identification based on nucleotide sequences of *VP4/VP2* correlate well with *VP1* genotyping (150).

The RV 5′ UTR contains both highly conserved and variable sequences and has been reported as the most sensitive target for detection and typing of RVs directly from clinical specimens (90, 99). However, sequences from the 5′ UTR cannot unequivocally determine RV species or genotype due to the tendency of some RV-A and RV-C strains to recombine in this region, resulting in incongruent phylogenetic clustering as compared with the capsid coding regions (24, 25, 150).

In a study to determine the relative contribution of the different RV species to hospitalization among young children with acute respiratory illness (125), typing was first performed on all RV RT-PCR-positive specimens by use of primers targeting a partial region of the *VP1* gene (150). *VP1* RT-PCR and sequencing identified an RV genotype in 74% of the specimens. Specimens that were negative by *VP1* RT-PCR were then tested with primers targeting *VP4/VP2*, and an additional 18% were genotyped. The remaining specimens were then tested with primers targeting the 5′ UTR, and an additional 3% were genotyped. The remaining 5% of RT-PCR positive specimens did not yield interpretable sequence data by any method. The presence of multiple RV types in clinical specimens may complicate obtaining unambiguous sequence data when using classical Sanger sequencing methods. Next-generation sequencing methods may prove useful for discriminating among mixed RV infections and studying RV recombination and quasi-species.

SEROLOGIC TESTS

Determination of antibody response is impractical for the diagnosis of RVs in the clinical setting. The number of RV serotypes and the lack of a common antigen make blind serologic testing impractical. Diagnosis by serology is also retrospective since antibody is usually not detectable until 1 to 3 weeks after onset of illness, with IgA predominant in nasal secretions and IgG predominant in serum (149). In research studies, antibody determination by neutralization test is the "gold standard" for serology (151). ELISA using specific serotype antigens has been used to detect serum and nasal IgG and IgA in volunteers inoculated with known RV serotypes, and ELISA was 100 to 10,000 times more sensitive than neutralization (55). Detailed procedures can be found elsewhere (149).

ANTIVIRAL SUSCEPTIBILITIES

Many antivirals show activity against RVs in the laboratory (152). However, inadequate drug delivery to the site of infection has reduced clinical benefit, and treatment remains experimental. Studies have included intranasal administration of soluble ICAM-1 in RV-infected volunteers; use of intranasal ipratropium bromide, an anticholinergic agent, or intranasal imiquimod, an immune response modifier; or administration of antivirals and antimediators in combination (38, 153–155). Efficacy studies in humans of echinacea, an herbal remedy, and zinc tablets have been mixed (156). Although the picornavirus capsid binding agent, pleconaril (Schering-Plough), showed some benefit in clinical trials of natural colds (42), it was not approved for clinical use. A more recent phase II trial of a pleconaril nasal spray remains unpublished (152). Another capsid binding agent, BTA-798 or vapendavir (Aviragen Therapeutics), has had a successful phase II clinical trial in 2010–2011 (98). Although inhibitors of RV 3C protease have shown potent antiviral activity, trials of rupintrivir (Pharmacodia) and PI4KB inhibitor BF738735 (Galapagos, NV) have been halted (152). As an alternative to direct-acting antivirals, such as capsid binding and protease inhibitors, host-targeting inhibitors, such as itraconazole and cyclophilin A, are currently being investigated (157).

EVALUATION, INTERPRETATION, AND REPORTING OF RESULTS

A comparison of RV diagnostic methods is shown in Table 2. Nucleic acid amplification assays have revolutionized RV detection, revealed both the ubiquity of RV infections and the association of RV with serious disease, fostered clinical research, and led to the discovery of RV-C viruses.

In the clinical laboratory, screening for RV is rarely specifically requested. Historically, RVs were isolated in conventional culture when the suspected virus was influenza or respiratory syncytial virus. Following the 2009 influenza pandemic, demand for user-friendly, FDA-approved respiratory virus molecular assays greatly increased, and many of the commercial highly multiplexed RVP and RPP target RV. In clinical laboratories that utilize one of these multiplex tests, RV is often the most commonly identified virus. The frequency of detection can even lead to the impression that RV are "normal flora" and can be ignored.

Thus, the interpretation of a positive RV PCR result can be problematic. RVs are extremely common, occur in asymptomatic persons, are prone to cause serial infections, can be shed for weeks after symptoms resolve, and can occur as coinfections with other viruses or bacteria. Interpretation of a positive RV result in the individual case often relies on risk factors and recovery of other pathogens. While viral load quantification by rRT-PCR may help determine its role in the acute illness, quantitative standards and guidelines are not available and may not correlate in the individual case (97, 128–131, 158). Furthermore, the RVPs and RPPs that include RV detection do not generally provide quantitative results.

Molecular tests also may not accurately distinguish RV from EV (Table 1), and several EVs have been recognized as important respiratory pathogens (139, 141, 143). Although therapy may not differ, more information is needed to determine whether differences in transmission, infection control measures, virus dissemination within the host, samples for diagnostic testing, and presence of extrarespiratory disease merit distinguishing RV from EV.

For laboratories relying on culture methods, though insensitive, isolation of RV-A and -B can be accomplished using commonly available conventional cell systems, such as WI-38, MRC-5, or HEK. Incubation at 33 to 35°C and rotation of cultures provide optimal conditions for virus replication. Differentiation of RV from EV, with which their CPE can be confused, is based on acid-stability testing of isolates or confirmation by RT-PCR.

Specific identification of RV serotypes by neutralization tests or genotypes by sequence-based molecular methods is reserved for epidemiologic and research studies. Serologic testing is also not available outside the research setting.

Molecular techniques are essential for detection of RV-C and to elucidate the role of RVs as lower respiratory tract pathogens and as a significant cause of asthma and chronic obstructive pulmonary disease exacerbations. However, RV detection may not become a high priority for clinical laboratories until the cost-effectiveness and impact of diagnosis on the management of hospitalized patients can be demonstrated or effective therapy becomes available.

TABLE 2 Comparison of diagnostic methods for rhinoviruses

Method	Advantages	Disadvantages/limitations	Clinical applicability	Key reference(s)
RT-PCR or other NAAT[a]	Much more sensitive and rapid than culture methods for RVs. Detects newly recognized RV-C strains. Broadly reactive primers that are most sensitive for detection of RVs in clinical specimens. May also detect EVs. Real-time assays are more rapid, simpler to perform, and less prone to amplicon contamination than conventional or nested PCR assays. Multiplex assays can detect multiple respiratory viruses, and some provide results in 1 h. Instrumentation can automate many steps and may be "sample to answer" format.	Differentiation of RV from EV can be difficult, and it may be reported as picornavirus. EV-D68 may be detected by RV assays. Since the same clinical syndrome may be caused by other viruses, samples must be tested for additional viruses. Assays vary in sensitivity for various RV types. Frequent RV detection by highly multiplexed assays can lead to problems in interpreting clinical relevance.	The standard for detection	See Table 1
Virus isolation	Can recover in culture when RV not specifically requested. RV-A and RV-B replicate in conventional cell cultures used in clinical laboratories (e.g., WI-38, MRC-5, HEK). These cultures may detect other viruses as well as rhinovirus (e.g., CMV, VZV, HSV, adenovirus, EV, RSV).[b]	Optimal recovery of multiple RV serotypes requires use of additional sensitive cell cultures not routinely used in diagnostic laboratories (e.g., HeLa Ohio cells, HeLa I cells, or fetal tonsil). Normally sensitive cells can vary over 100-fold in sensitivity. Differentiation of RV from EV isolates is time-consuming (e.g., quantitative acid sensitivity test). Recently recognized novel RV-C do not grow in standard culture.	For clinical laboratories not using molecular methods	144, 145
Organ culture	Useful in studies of pathogenesis. Biopsy or surgically removed tissues can be used.	Surgically removed and discarded sinus tissues can be used. Fetal nasal or tracheal tissues are not readily available.	Used in pathogenesis research	10
Serology to detect antibody response	May detect some infections not detected by virus isolation. Research tool used after infection of volunteers with a known RV serotype or in epidemiologic studies.	RV antibody testing for clinical diagnosis is impractical due to the large number of RV serotypes, the lack of a common antigen, and the need for acute and convalescent sera.	Used only in research settings	55, 151

[a]RT-PCR, reverse transcription-PCR; NAAT, nucleic acid amplification test.
[b]RV, rhinovirus; EV, enterovirus; CMV, cytomegalovirus; VZV, varicella-zoster virus; HSV, herpes simplex virus; RSV, respiratory syncytial virus.

REFERENCES

1. **Knowles NJ, Hovi T, Hyypiä T, King AMQ, Lindberg AM, Pallansch MA, Palmenberg AC, Simmonds P, Skern T, Stanway G, Yamashita T, Zell R.** 2012. *Picornaviridae*. Elsevier, San Diego, CA.
2. **Zoll J, Erkens Hulshof S, Lanke K, Verduyn Lunel F, Melchers WJG, Schoondermark-van de Ven E, Roivainen M, Galama JMD, van Kuppeveld FJM.** 2009. Saffold virus, a human Theiler's-like cardiovirus, is ubiquitous and causes infection early in life. *PLoS Pathog* **5:**e1000416.
3. **Ledford RM, Patel NR, Demenczuk TM, Watanyar A, Herbertz T, Collett MS, Pevear DC.** 2004. VP1 sequencing of all human rhinovirus serotypes: insights into genus phylogeny and susceptibility to antiviral capsid-binding compounds. *J Virol* **78:**3663–3674.
4. **Laine P, Savolainen C, Blomqvist S, Hovi T.** 2005. Phylogenetic analysis of human rhinovirus capsid protein VP1 and 2A protease coding sequences confirms shared genus-like relationships with human enteroviruses. *J Gen Virol* **86:**697–706.
5. **Savolainen C, Blomqvist S, Mulders MN, Hovi T.** 2002. Genetic clustering of all 102 human rhinovirus prototype strains: serotype 87 is close to human enterovirus 70. *J Gen Virol* **83:**333–340.
6. **Blomqvist S, Savolainen C, Råman L, Roivainen M, Hovi T.** 2002. Human rhinovirus 87 and enterovirus 68 represent a unique serotype with rhinovirus and enterovirus features. *J Clin Microbiol* **40:**4218–4223.
7. **Uncapher CR, DeWitt CM, Colonno RJ.** 1991. The major and minor group receptor families contain all but one human rhinovirus serotype. *Virology* **180:**814–817.
8. **Vlasak M, Roivainen M, Reithmayer M, Goesler I, Laine P, Snyers L, Hovi T, Blaas D.** 2005. The minor receptor group of human rhinovirus (HRV) includes HRV23 and HRV25, but the presence of a lysine in the VP1 HI loop is not sufficient for receptor binding. *J Virol* **79:** 7389–7395.
9. **Rossmann MG, Bella J, Kolatkar PR, He Y, Wimmer E, Kuhn RJ, Baker TS.** 2000. Cell recognition and entry by rhino- and enteroviruses. *Virology* **269:**239–247.
10. **Ashraf S, Brockman-Schneider R, Bochkov YA, Pasic TR, Gern JE.** 2013. Biological characteristics and propagation of human rhinovirus-C in differentiated sinus epithelial cells. *Virology* **436:**143–149.
11. **Arden KE, Mackay IM.** 2010. Newly identified human rhinoviruses: molecular methods heat up the cold viruses. *Rev Med Virol* **20:**156–176.

12. **Bochkov YA, Palmenberg AC, Lee W-M, Rathe JA, Amineva SP, Sun X, Pasic TR, Jarjour NN, Liggett SB, Gern JE.** 2011. Molecular modeling, organ culture and reverse genetics for a newly identified human rhinovirus C. *Nat Med* **17:**627–632.
13. **Ashraf S, Brockman-Schneider R, Gern JE.** 2015. Propagation of rhinovirus-C strains in human airway epithelial cells differentiated at air-liquid interface. *Methods Mol Biol* **1221:**63–70.
14. **Lu X, Schneider E, Jain S, Bramley AM, Hymas W, Stockmann C, Ampofo K, Arnold SR, Williams DJ, Self WH, Patel A, Chappell JD, Grijalva CG, Anderson EJ, Wunderink RG, McCullers JA, Edwards KM, Pavia AT, Erdman DD.** 2017. Rhinovirus viremia in patients hospitalized with community-acquired pneumonia. *J Infect Dis* **216:** 1104–1111.
15. **Bochkov YA, Watters K, Ashraf S, Griggs TF, Devries MK, Jackson DJ, Palmenberg AC, Gern JE.** 2015. Cadherin-related family member 3, a childhood asthma susceptibility gene product, mediates rhinovirus C binding and replication. *Proc Natl Acad Sci USA* **112:**5485–5490.
16. **Bønnelykke K, Sleiman P, Nielsen K, Kreiner-Møller E, Mercader JM, Belgrave D, den Dekker HT, Husby A, Sevelsted A, Faura-Tellez G, Mortensen LJ, Paternoster L, Flaaten R, Mølgaard A, Smart DE, Thomsen PF, Rasmussen MA, Bonàs-Guarch S, Holst C, Nohr EA, Yadav R, March ME, Blicher T, Lackie PM, Jaddoe VW, Simpson A, Holloway JW, Duijts L, Custovic A, Davies DE, Torrents D, Gupta R, Hollegaard MV, Hougaard DM, Hakonarson H, Bisgaard H.** 2014. A genome-wide association study identifies CDHR3 as a susceptibility locus for early childhood asthma with severe exacerbations. *Nat Genet* **46:**51–55.
17. **Palmenberg AC, Spiro D, Kuzmickas R, Wang S, Djikeng A, Rathe JA, Fraser-Liggett CM, Liggett SB.** 2009. Sequencing and analyses of all known human rhinovirus genomes reveal structure and evolution. *Science* **324:**55–59.
18. **Simmonds P, McIntyre C, Savolainen-Kopra C, Tapparel C, Mackay IM, Hovi T.** 2010. Proposals for the classification of human rhinovirus species C into genotypically assigned types. *J Gen Virol* **91:**2409–2419.
19. **McIntyre CL, Knowles NJ, Simmonds P.** 2013. Proposals for the classification of human rhinovirus species A, B and C into genotypically assigned types. *J Gen Virol* **94:**1791–1806.
20. **Paul AV, van Boom JH, Filippov D, Wimmer E.** 1998. Protein-primed RNA synthesis by purified poliovirus RNA polymerase. *Nature* **393:**280–284.
21. **Rossmann MG, Arnold E, Erickson JW, Frankenberger EA, Griffith JP, Hecht H-J, Johnson JE, Kamer G, Luo M, Mosser AG, Rueckert RR, Sherry B, Vriend G.** 1985. Structure of a human common cold virus and functional relationship to other picornaviruses. *Nature* **317:**145–153.
22. **Zhang Y, Simpson AA, Ledford RM, Bator CM, Chakravarty S, Skochko GA, Demenczuk TM, Watanyar A, Pevear DC, Rossmann MG.** 2004. Structural and virological studies of the stages of virus replication that are affected by antirhinovirus compounds. *J Virol* **78:**11061–11069.
23. **Xing L, Casasnovas JM, Cheng RH.** 2003. Structural analysis of human rhinovirus complexed with ICAM-1 reveals the dynamics of receptor-mediated virus uncoating. *J Virol* **77:**6101–6107.
24. **Wisdom A, Kutkowska AE, McWilliam Leitch EC, Gaunt E, Templeton K, Harvala H, Simmonds P.** 2009. Genetics, recombination and clinical features of human rhinovirus species C (HRV-C) infections; interactions of HRV-C with other respiratory viruses. *PLoS One* **4:**e8518.
25. **Huang T, Wang W, Bessaud M, Ren P, Sheng J, Yan H, Zhang J, Lin X, Wang Y, Delpeyroux F, Deubel V.** 2009. Evidence of recombination and genetic diversity in human rhinoviruses in children with acute respiratory infection. *PLoS One* **4:**e6355.
26. **Palmenberg AC, Rathe JA, Liggett SB.** 2010. Analysis of the complete genome sequences of human rhinovirus. *J Allergy Clin Immunol* **125:**1190–1199, quiz 1200–1201.
27. **McIntyre CL, Savolainen-Kopra C, Hovi T, Simmonds P.** 2013. Recombination in the evolution of human rhinovirus genomes. *Arch Virol* **158:**1497–1515.
28. **Brownlee JW, Turner RB.** 2008. New developments in the epidemiology and clinical spectrum of rhinovirus infections. *Curr Opin Pediatr* **20:**67–71.
29. **Linder JE, Kraft DC, Mohamed Y, Lu Z, Heil L, Tollefson S, Saville BR, Wright PF, Williams JV, Miller EK.** 2013. Human rhinovirus C: age, season, and lower respiratory illness over the past 3 decades. *J Allergy Clin Immunol* **131:**69–77.e1–6.
30. **Piotrowska Z, Vázquez M, Shapiro ED, Weibel C, Ferguson D, Landry ML, Kahn JS.** 2009. Rhinoviruses are a major cause of wheezing and hospitalization in children less than 2 years of age. *Pediatr Infect Dis J* **28:**25–29.
31. **Nicholson KG, Kent J, Hammersley V, Cancio E.** 1996. Risk factors for lower respiratory complications of rhinovirus infections in elderly people living in the community: prospective cohort study. *BMJ* **313:**1119–1123.
32. **Miller EK, Edwards KM, Weinberg GA, Iwane MK, Griffin MR, Hall CB, Zhu Y, Szilagyi PG, Morin LL, Heil LH, Lu X, Williams JV.** 2009. A novel group of rhinoviruses is associated with asthma hospitalizations. *J Allergy Clin Immunol* **123:**98–104.e1.
33. **Han TH, Chung JY, Hwang ES, Koo JW.** 2009. Detection of human rhinovirus C in children with acute lower respiratory tract infections in South Korea. *Arch Virol* **154:**987–991.
34. **Onyango CO, Welch SR, Munywoki PK, Agoti CN, Bett A, Ngama M, Myers R, Cane PA, Nokes DJ.** 2012. Molecular epidemiology of human rhinovirus infections in Kilifi, coastal Kenya. *J Med Virol* **84:**823–831.
35. **Dick EC, Jennings LC, Mink KA, Wartgow CD, Inhorn SL.** 1987. Aerosol transmission of rhinovirus colds. *J Infect Dis* **156:**442–448.
36. **Douglas RG Jr.** 1970. Pathogenesis of rhinovirus common colds in human volunteers. *Ann Otol Rhinol Laryngol* **79:** 563–571.
37. **Gwaltney JM Jr, Moskalski PB, Hendley JO.** 1978. Hand-to-hand transmission of rhinovirus colds. *Ann Intern Med* **88:**463–467.
38. **Gwaltney JM Jr.** 1992. Combined antiviral and antimediator treatment of rhinovirus colds. *J Infect Dis* **166:**776–782.
39. **Hendley JO.** 1999. Clinical virology of rhinoviruses. *Adv Virus Res* **54:**453–466.
40. **Turner RB, Fuls JL, Rodgers ND.** 2010. Effectiveness of hand sanitizers with and without organic acids for removal of rhinovirus from hands. *Antimicrob Agents Chemother* **54:**1363–1364.
41. **Bochkov YA, Gern JE.** 2012. Clinical and molecular features of human rhinovirus C. *Microbes Infect* **14:**485–494.
42. **Hayden FG, Herrington DT, Coats TL, Kim K, Cooper EC, Villano SA, Liu S, Hudson S, Pevear DC, Collett M, McKinlay M, Pleconaril Respiratory Infection Study Group.** 2003. Efficacy and safety of oral pleconaril for treatment of colds due to picornaviruses in adults: results of 2 double-blind, randomized, placebo-controlled trials. *Clin Infect Dis* **36:**1523–1532.
43. **Lu X, Holloway B, Dare RK, Kuypers J, Yagi S, Williams JV, Hall CB, Erdman DD.** 2008. Real-time reverse transcription-PCR assay for comprehensive detection of human rhinoviruses. *J Clin Microbiol* **46:**533–539.
44. **Douglas RG Jr, Cate TR, Gerone PJ, Couch RB.** 1966. Quantitative rhinovirus shedding patterns in volunteers. *Am Rev Respir Dis* **94:**159–167.
45. **Johnston SL, Sanderson G, Pattemore PK, Smith S, Bardin PG, Bruce CB, Lambden PR, Tyrrell DA, Holgate ST.** 1993. Use of polymerase chain reaction for diagnosis of picornavirus infection in subjects with and without respiratory symptoms. *J Clin Microbiol* **31:**111–117.
46. **Wright PF, Deatly AM, Karron RA, Belshe RB, Shi JR, Gruber WC, Zhu Y, Randolph VB.** 2007. Comparison of results of detection of rhinovirus by PCR and viral culture in human nasal wash specimens from subjects with and without clinical symptoms of respiratory illness. *J Clin Microbiol* **45:**2126–2129.
47. **Xatzipsalti M, Kyrana S, Tsolia M, Psarras S, Bossios A, Laza-Stanca V, Johnston SL, Papadopoulos NG.** 2005. Rhinovirus viremia in children with respiratory infections. *Am J Respir Crit Care Med* **172:**1037–1040.

48. **Jartti T, Lehtinen P, Vuorinen T, Koskenvuo M, Ruuskanen O.** 2004. Persistence of rhinovirus and enterovirus RNA after acute respiratory illness in children. *J Med Virol* **72:**695–699.
49. **Mackay IM, Lambert SB, Faux CE, Arden KE, Nissen MD, Sloots TP, Nolan TM.** 2013. Community-wide, contemporaneous circulation of a broad spectrum of human rhinoviruses in healthy Australian preschool-aged children during a 12-month period. *J Infect Dis* **207:**1433–1441.
50. **Peltola V, Waris M, Osterback R, Susi P, Hyypiä T, Ruuskanen O.** 2008. Clinical effects of rhinovirus infections. *J Clin Virol* **43:**411–414.
51. **Kaiser L, Aubert JD, Pache JC, Deffernez C, Rochat T, Garbino J, Wunderli W, Meylan P, Yerly S, Perrin L, Letovanec I, Nicod L, Tapparel C, Soccal PM.** 2006. Chronic rhinoviral infection in lung transplant recipients. *Am J Respir Crit Care Med* **174:**1392–1399.
52. **Cohen S, Doyle WJ, Alper CM, Janicki-Deverts D, Turner RB.** 2009. Sleep habits and susceptibility to the common cold. *Arch Intern Med* **169:**62–67.
53. **Cohen S, Janicki-Deverts D, Doyle WJ, Miller GE, Frank E, Rabin BS, Turner RB.** 2012. Chronic stress, glucocorticoid receptor resistance, inflammation, and disease risk. *Proc Natl Acad Sci USA* **109:**5995–5999.
54. **Cohen S, Tyrrell DA, Smith AP.** 1991. Psychological stress and susceptibility to the common cold. *N Engl J Med* **325:**606–612.
55. **Barclay WS, Al-Nakib W.** 1987. An ELISA for the detection of rhinovirus specific antibody in serum and nasal secretion. *J Virol Methods* **15:**53–64.
56. **Cate TR, Couch RB, Johnson KM.** 1964. Studies with rhinoviruses in volunteers: production of illness, effect of naturally acquired antibody, and demonstration of a protective effect not associated with serum antibody. *J Clin Invest* **43:**56–67.
57. **Fendrick AM, Monto AS, Nightengale B, Sarnes M.** 2003. The economic burden of non-influenza-related viral respiratory tract infection in the United States. *Arch Intern Med* **163:**487–494.
58. **Nokso-Koivisto J, Räty R, Blomqvist S, Kleemola M, Syrjänen R, Pitkäranta A, Kilpi T, Hovi T.** 2004. Presence of specific viruses in the middle ear fluids and respiratory secretions of young children with acute otitis media. *J Med Virol* **72:**241–248.
59. **Savolainen-Kopra C, Blomqvist S, Kilpi T, Roivainen M, Hovi T.** 2009. Novel species of human rhinoviruses in acute otitis media. *Pediatr Infect Dis J* **28:**59–61.
60. **Cawcutt K, Kalil AC.** 2017. Pneumonia with bacterial and viral coinfection. *Curr Opin Crit Care* **23:**385–390.
61. **Gern JE.** 2009. Rhinovirus and the initiation of asthma. *Curr Opin Allergy Clin Immunol* **9:**73–78.
62. **Mallia P, Johnston SL.** 2006. How viral infections cause exacerbation of airway diseases. *Chest* **130:**1203–1210.
63. **Burns JL, Emerson J, Kuypers J, Campbell AP, Gibson RL, McNamara S, Worrell K, Englund JA.** 2012. Respiratory viruses in children with cystic fibrosis: viral detection and clinical findings. *Influenza Other Respir Viruses* **6:**218–223.
64. **George SN, Garcha DS, Mackay AJ, Patel AR, Singh R, Sapsford RJ, Donaldson GC, Wedzicha JA.** 2014. Human rhinovirus infection during naturally occurring COPD exacerbations. *Eur Respir J* **44:**87–96.
65. **Calışkan M, Bochkov YA, Kreiner-Møller E, Bønnelykke K, Stein MM, Du G, Bisgaard H, Jackson DJ, Gern JE, Lemanske RF Jr, Nicolae DL, Ober C.** 2013. Rhinovirus wheezing illness and genetic risk of childhood-onset asthma. *N Engl J Med* **368:**1398–1407.
66. **Stone CA Jr, Miller EK.** 2016. Understanding the association of human rhinovirus with asthma. *Clin Vaccine Immunol* **23:**6–10.
67. **Longtin J, Marchand-Austin A, Winter AL, Patel S, Eshaghi A, Jamieson F, Low DE, Gubbay JB.** 2010. Rhinovirus outbreaks in long-term care facilities, Ontario, Canada. *Emerg Infect Dis* **16:**1463–1465.
68. **Hayden FG.** 2004. Rhinovirus and the lower respiratory tract. *Rev Med Virol* **14:**17–31.
69. **Papadopoulos NG, Bates PJ, Bardin PG, Papi A, Leir SH, Fraenkel DJ, Meyer J, Lackie PM, Sanderson G, Holgate ST, Johnston SL.** 2000. Rhinoviruses infect the lower airways. *J Infect Dis* **181:**1875–1884.
70. **Lau SKP, Yip CCY, Lin AWC, Lee RA, So L-Y, Lau Y-L, Chan K-H, Woo PCY, Yuen K-Y.** 2009. Clinical and molecular epidemiology of human rhinovirus C in children and adults in Hong Kong reveals a possible distinct human rhinovirus C subgroup. *J Infect Dis* **200:**1096–1103.
71. **Xiang Z, Gonzalez R, Wang Z, Xiao Y, Chen L, Li T, Vernet G, Paranhos-Baccalà G, Jin Q, Wang J.** 2010. Human rhinoviruses in Chinese adults with acute respiratory tract infection. *J Infect* **61:**289–298.
72. **Korppi M, Kotaniemi-Syrjänen A, Waris M, Vainionpää R, Reijonen TM.** 2004. Rhinovirus-associated wheezing in infancy: comparison with respiratory syncytial virus bronchiolitis. *Pediatr Infect Dis J* **23:**995–999.
73. **Jain S, Williams DJ, Arnold SR, Ampofo K, Bramley AM, Reed C, Stockmann C, Anderson EJ, Grijalva CG, Self WH, Zhu Y, Patel A, Hymas W, Chappell JD, Kaufman RA, Kan JH, Dansie D, Lenny N, Hillyard DR, Haynes LM, Levine M, Lindstrom S, Winchell JM, Katz JM, Erdman D, Schneider E, Hicks LA, Wunderink RG, Edwards KM, Pavia AT, McCullers JA, Finelli L, CDC EPIC Study Team.** 2015. Community-acquired pneumonia requiring hospitalization among U.S. children. *N Engl J Med* **372:**835–845.
74. **Tsolia MN, Psarras S, Bossios A, Audi H, Paldanius M, Gourgiotis D, Kallergi K, Kafetzis DA, Constantopoulos A, Papadopoulos NG.** 2004. Etiology of community-acquired pneumonia in hospitalized school-age children: evidence for high prevalence of viral infections. *Clin Infect Dis* **39:**681–686.
75. **Louie JK, Yagi S, Nelson FA, Kiang D, Glaser CA, Rosenberg J, Cahill CK, Schnurr DP.** 2005. Rhinovirus outbreak in a long term care facility for elderly persons associated with unusually high mortality. *Clin Infect Dis* **41:**262–265.
76. **Christensen MS, Nielsen LP, Hasle H.** 2005. Few but severe viral infections in children with cancer: a prospective RT-PCR and PCR-based 12-month study. *Pediatr Blood Cancer* **45:**945–951.
77. **Gutman JA, Peck AJ, Kuypers J, Boeckh M.** 2007. Rhinovirus as a cause of fatal lower respiratory tract infection in adult stem cell transplantation patients: a report of two cases. *Bone Marrow Transplant* **40:**809–811.
78. **Kumar D, Erdman D, Keshavjee S, Peret T, Tellier R, Hadjiliadis D, Johnson G, Ayers M, Siegal D, Humar A.** 2005. Clinical impact of community-acquired respiratory viruses on bronchiolitis obliterans after lung transplant. *Am J Transplant* **5:**2031–2036.
79. **van Kraaij MG, van Elden LJ, van Loon AM, Hendriksen KA, Laterveer L, Dekker AW, Nijhuis M.** 2005. Frequent detection of respiratory viruses in adult recipients of stem cell transplants with the use of real-time polymerase chain reaction, compared with viral culture. *Clin Infect Dis* **40:**662–669.
80. **Ferguson PE, Gilroy NM, Faux CE, Mackay IM, Sloots TP, Nissen MD, Dwyer DE, Sorrell TC.** 2013. Human rhinovirus C in adult haematopoietic stem cell transplant recipients with respiratory illness. *J Clin Virol* **56:**255–259.
81. **Ison MG, Hayden FG, Kaiser L, Corey L, Boeckh M.** 2003. Rhinovirus infections in hematopoietic stem cell transplant recipients with pneumonia. *Clin Infect Dis* **36:**1139–1143.
82. **Seo S, Waghmare A, Scott EM, Xie H, Kuypers JM, Hackman RC, Campbell AP, Choi SM, Leisenring WM, Jerome KR, Englund JA, Boeckh M.** 2017. Human rhinovirus detection in the lower respiratory tract of hematopoietic cell transplant recipients: association with mortality. *Haematologica* **102:**1120–1130.
83. **Las Heras J, Swanson VL.** 1983. Sudden death of an infant with rhinovirus infection complicating bronchial asthma: case report. *Pediatr Pathol* **1:**319–323.
84. **Proud D, Turner RB, Winther B, Wiehler S, Tiesman JP, Reichling TD, Juhlin KD, Fulmer AW, Ho BY, Walanski AA, Poore CL, Mizoguchi H, Jump L, Moore ML, Zukowski CK, Clymer JW.** 2008. Gene expression profiles during in vivo human rhinovirus infection: insights into the host response. *Am J Respir Crit Care Med* **178:**962–968.

85. **Mallia P, Footitt J, Sotero R, Jepson A, Contoli M, Trujillo-Torralbo MB, Kebadze T, Aniscenko J, Oleszkiewicz G, Gray K, Message SD, Ito K, Barnes PJ, Adcock IM, Papi A, Stanciu LA, Elkin SL, Kon OM, Johnson M, Johnston SL.** 2012. Rhinovirus infection induces degradation of antimicrobial peptides and secondary bacterial infection in chronic obstructive pulmonary disease. *Am J Respir Crit Care Med* **186:**1117–1124.

86. **Peltola V, Heikkinen T, Ruuskanen O, Jartti T, Hovi T, Kilpi T, Vainionpää R.** 2011. Temporal association between rhinovirus circulation in the community and invasive pneumococcal disease in children. *Pediatr Infect Dis J* **30:**456–461.

87. **Walter JM, Wunderink RG.** 2017. Severe respiratory viral infections: new evidence and changing paradigms. *Infect Dis Clin North Am* **31:**455–474.

88. **Khetsuriani N, Lu X, Teague WG, Kazerouni N, Anderson LJ, Erdman DD.** 2008. Novel human rhinoviruses and exacerbation of asthma in children. *Emerg Infect Dis* **14:**1793–1796.

89. **Lamson D, Renwick N, Kapoor V, Liu Z, Palacios G, Ju J, Dean A, St George K, Briese T, Lipkin WI.** 2006. MassTag polymerase-chain-reaction detection of respiratory pathogens, including a new rhinovirus genotype, that caused influenza-like illness in New York State during 2004–2005. *J Infect Dis* **194:**1398–1402.

90. **Lee WM, Kiesner C, Pappas T, Lee I, Grindle K, Jartti T, Jakiela B, Lemanske RF Jr, Shult PA, Gern JE.** 2007. A diverse group of previously unrecognized human rhinoviruses are common causes of respiratory illnesses in infants. *PLoS One* **2:**e966.

91. **Louie JK, Roy-Burman A, Guardia-Labar L, Boston EJ, Kiang D, Padilla T, Yagi S, Messenger S, Petru AM, Glaser CA, Schnurr DP.** 2009. Rhinovirus associated with severe lower respiratory tract infections in children. *Pediatr Infect Dis J* **28:**337–339.

92. **McErlean P, Shackelton LA, Lambert SB, Nissen MD, Sloots TP, Mackay IM.** 2007. Characterisation of a newly identified human rhinovirus, HRV-QPM, discovered in infants with bronchiolitis. *J Clin Virol* **39:**67–75.

93. **Miller EK, Lu X, Erdman DD, Poehling KA, Zhu Y, Griffin MR, Hartert TV, Anderson LJ, Weinberg GA, Hall CB, Iwane MK, Edwards KM, New Vaccine Surveillance Network.** 2007. Rhinovirus-associated hospitalizations in young children. *J Infect Dis* **195:**773–781.

94. **Fuji N, Suzuki A, Lupisan S, Sombrero L, Galang H, Kamigaki T, Tamaki R, Saito M, Aniceto R, Olveda R, Oshitani H.** 2011. Detection of human rhinovirus C viral genome in blood among children with severe respiratory infections in the Philippines. *PLoS One* **6:**e27247.

95. **Lau SK, Yip CC, Lung DC, Lee P, Que TL, Lau YL, Chan KH, Woo PC, Yuen KY.** 2012. Detection of human rhinovirus C in fecal samples of children with gastroenteritis. *J Clin Virol* **53:**290–296.

96. **Tapparel C, Cordey S, Van Belle S, Turin L, Lee W-M, Regamey N, Meylan P, Mühlemann K, Gobbini F, Kaiser L.** 2009. New molecular detection tools adapted to emerging rhinoviruses and enteroviruses. *J Clin Microbiol* **47:**1742–1749.

97. **Harvala H, McIntyre CL, McLeish NJ, Kondracka J, Palmer J, Molyneaux P, Gunson R, Bennett S, Templeton K, Simmonds P.** 2012. High detection frequency and viral loads of human rhinovirus species A to C in fecal samples: diagnostic and clinical implications. *J Med Virol* **84:**536–542.

98. **Miller EK, Mackay IM.** 2013. From sneeze to wheeze: what we know about rhinovirus Cs. *J Clin Virol* **57:**291–299.

99. **Kiang D, Kalra I, Yagi S, Louie JK, Boushey H, Boothby J, Schnurr DP.** 2008. Assay for 5′ noncoding region analysis of all human rhinovirus prototype strains. *J Clin Microbiol* **46:**3736–3745.

100. **Lee S, Nguyen MT, Currier MG, Jenkins JB, Strobert EA, Kajon AE, Madan-Lala R, Bochkov YA, Gern JE, Roy K, Lu X, Erdman DD, Spearman P, Moore ML.** 2016. A polyvalent inactivated rhinovirus vaccine is broadly immunogenic in rhesus macaques. *Nat Commun* **7:**12838.

101. **Arruda E, Crump CE, Rollins BS, Ohlin A, Hayden FG.** 1996. Comparative susceptibilities of human embryonic fibroblasts and HeLa cells for isolation of human rhinoviruses. *J Clin Microbiol* **34:**1277–1279.

102. **Spyridaki IS, Christodoulou I, de Beer L, Hovland V, Kurowski M, Olszewska-Ziaber A, Carlsen K-H, Lødrup-Carlsen K, van Drunen CM, Kowalski ML, Molenkamp R, Papadopoulos NG.** 2009. Comparison of four nasal sampling methods for the detection of viral pathogens by RT-PCR-A GA(2)LEN project. *J Virol Methods* **156:**102–106.

103. **Waris M, Österback R, Lahti E, Vuorinen T, Ruuskanen O, Peltola V.** 2013. Comparison of sampling methods for the detection of human rhinovirus RNA. *J Clin Virol* **58:**200–204.

104. **Debyle C, Bulkow L, Miernyk K, Chikoyak L, Hummel KB, Hennessy T, Singleton R.** 2012. Comparison of nasopharyngeal flocked swabs and nasopharyngeal wash collection methods for respiratory virus detection in hospitalized children using real-time polymerase chain reaction. *J Virol Methods* **185:**89–93.

105. **Larios OE, Coleman BL, Drews SJ, Mazzulli T, Borgundvaag B, Green K, STOP-Flu Study Group, McGeer AJ.** 2011. Self-collected mid-turbinate swabs for the detection of respiratory viruses in adults with acute respiratory illnesses. *PLoS One* **6:**e21335.

106. **Esposito S, Molteni CG, Daleno C, Valzano A, Tagliabue C, Galeone C, Milani G, Fossali E, Marchisio P, Principi N.** 2010. Collection by trained pediatricians or parents of mid-turbinate nasal flocked swabs for the detection of influenza viruses in childhood. *Virol J* **7:**85.

107. **Xiang X, Qiu D, Chan KP, Chan SH, Hegele RG, Tan WC.** 2002. Comparison of three methods for respiratory virus detection between induced sputum and nasopharyngeal aspirate specimens in acute asthma. *J Virol Methods* **101:**127–133.

108. **Falsey AR, Formica MA, Walsh EE.** 2012. Yield of sputum for viral detection by reverse transcriptase PCR in adults hospitalized with respiratory illness. *J Clin Microbiol* **50:**21–24.

109. **Freymuth F, Vabret A, Cuvillon-Nimal D, Simon S, Dina J, Legrand L, Gouarin S, Petitjean J, Eckart P, Brouard J.** 2006. Comparison of multiplex PCR assays and conventional techniques for the diagnostic of respiratory virus infections in children admitted to hospital with an acute respiratory illness. *J Med Virol* **78:**1498–1504.

110. **Hyypiä T, Puhakka T, Ruuskanen O, Mäkelä M, Arola A, Arstila P.** 1998. Molecular diagnosis of human rhinovirus infections: comparison with virus isolation. *J Clin Microbiol* **36:**2081–2083.

111. **Steininger C, Aberle SW, Popow-Kraupp T.** 2001. Early detection of acute rhinovirus infections by a rapid reverse transcription-PCR assay. *J Clin Microbiol* **39:**129–133.

112. **Vuorinen T, Vainionpää R, Hyypiä T.** 2003. Five years' experience of reverse-transcriptase polymerase chain reaction in daily diagnosis of enterovirus and rhinovirus infections. *Clin Infect Dis* **37:**452–455.

113. **Blomqvist S, Skyttä A, Roivainen M, Hovi T.** 1999. Rapid detection of human rhinoviruses in nasopharyngeal aspirates by a microwell reverse transcription-PCR-hybridization assay. *J Clin Microbiol* **37:**2813–2816.

114. **Gama RE, Hughes PJ, Bruce CB, Stanway G.** 1988. Polymerase chain reaction amplification of rhinovirus nucleic acids from clinical material. *Nucleic Acids Res* **16:**9346.

115. **Olive DM, Al-Mufti S, Al-Mulla W, Khan MA, Pasca A, Stanway G, Al-Nakib W.** 1990. Detection and differentiation of picornaviruses in clinical samples following genomic amplification. *J Gen Virol* **71:**2141–2147.

116. **Atmar RL, Georghiou PR.** 1993. Classification of respiratory tract picornavirus isolates as enteroviruses or rhinoviruses by using reverse transcription-polymerase chain reaction. *J Clin Microbiol* **31:**2544–2546.

117. **Papadopoulos NG, Hunter J, Sanderson G, Meyer J, Johnston SL.** 1999. Rhinovirus identification by BglI digestion of picornavirus RT-PCR amplicons. *J Virol Methods* **80:**179–185.

118. **Halonen P, Rocha E, Hierholzer J, Holloway B, Hyypiä T, Hurskainen P, Pallansch M.** 1995. Detection of enteroviruses and rhinoviruses in clinical specimens by PCR and liquid-phase hybridization. *J Clin Microbiol* **33:**648–653.
119. **Deffernez C, Wunderli W, Thomas Y, Yerly S, Perrin L, Kaiser L.** 2004. Amplicon sequencing and improved detection of human rhinovirus in respiratory samples. *J Clin Microbiol* **42:**3212–3218.
120. **Faux CE, Arden KE, Lambert SB, Nissen MD, Nolan TM, Chang AB, Sloots TP, Mackay IM.** 2011. Usefulness of published PCR primers in detecting human rhinovirus infection. *Emerg Infect Dis* **17:**296–298.
121. **Dagher H, Donninger H, Hutchinson P, Ghildyal R, Bardin P.** 2004. Rhinovirus detection: comparison of real-time and conventional PCR. *J Virol Methods* **117:**113–121.
122. **Kares S, Lönnrot M, Vuorinen P, Oikarinen S, Taurianen S, Hyöty H.** 2004. Real-time PCR for rapid diagnosis of entero- and rhinovirus infections using LightCycler. *J Clin Virol* **29:**99–104.
123. **Templeton KE, Forde CB, Loon AM, Claas EC, Niesters HG, Wallace P, Carman WF.** 2006. A multi-centre pilot proficiency programme to assess the quality of molecular detection of respiratory viruses. *J Clin Virol* **35:**51–58.
124. **Jain S, Self WH, Wunderink RG, CDC EPIC Study Team.** 2015. Community-acquired pneumonia requiring hospitalization. *N Engl J Med* **373:**2382.
125. **Iwane MK, Prill MM, Lu X, Miller EK, Edwards KM, Hall CB, Griffin MR, Staat MA, Anderson LJ, Williams JV, Weinberg GA, Ali A, Szilagyi PG, Zhu Y, Erdman DD.** 2011. Human rhinovirus species associated with hospitalizations for acute respiratory illness in young US children. *J Infect Dis* **204:**1702–1710.
126. **Soto-Quiros M, Avila L, Platts-Mills TA, Hunt JF, Erdman DD, Carper H, Murphy DD, Odio S, James HR, Patrie JT, Hunt W, O'Rourke AK, Davis MD, Steinke JW, Lu X, Kennedy J, Heymann PW.** 2012. High titers of IgE antibody to dust mite allergen and risk for wheezing among asthmatic children infected with rhinovirus. *J Allergy Clin Immunol* **129:**1499–1505.e5.
127. **Takeyama A, Hashimoto K, Sato M, Sato T, Kanno S, Takano K, Ito M, Katayose M, Nishimura H, Kawasaki Y, Hosoya M.** 2012. Rhinovirus load and disease severity in children with lower respiratory tract infections. *J Med Virol* **84:**1135–1142.
128. **Utokaparch S, Marchant D, Gosselink JV, McDonough JE, Thomas EE, Hogg JC, Hegele RG.** 2011. The relationship between respiratory viral loads and diagnosis in children presenting to a pediatric hospital emergency department. *Pediatr Infect Dis J* **30:**e18–e23.
129. **Gerna G, Piralla A, Rovida F, Rognoni V, Marchi A, Locatelli F, Meloni F.** 2009. Correlation of rhinovirus load in the respiratory tract and clinical symptoms in hospitalized immunocompetent and immunocompromised patients. *J Med Virol* **81:**1498–1507.
130. **Franz A, Adams O, Willems R, Bonzel L, Neuhausen N, Schweizer-Krantz S, Ruggeberg JU, Willers R, Henrich B, Schroten H, Tenenbaum T.** 2010. Correlation of viral load of respiratory pathogens and co-infections with disease severity in children hospitalized for lower respiratory tract infection. *J Clin Virol* **48:**239–245.
131. **Schibler M, Yerly S, Vieille G, Docquier M, Turin L, Kaiser L, Tapparel C.** 2012. Critical analysis of rhinovirus RNA load quantification by real-time reverse transcription-PCR. *J Clin Microbiol* **50:**2868–2872.
132. **Chandrasekaran A, Manji R, Joseph A, Zhang F, Ginocchio CC.** 2012. Broad reactivity of the Luminex xTAG Respiratory Virus Panel (RVP) assay for the detection of human rhinoviruses. *J Clin Virol* **53:**272–273.
133. **Merante F, Yaghoubian S, Janeczko R.** 2007. Principles of the xTAG respiratory viral panel assay (RVP Assay). *J Clin Virol* **40**(Suppl 1)**:**S31–S35.
134. **Lee CK, Lee HK, Ng CW, Chiu L, Tang JW, Loh TP, Koay ES.** 2017. Comparison of Luminex NxTAG Respiratory Pathogen Panel and xTAG Respiratory Viral Panel FAST Version 2 for the detection of respiratory viruses. *Ann Lab Med* **37:**267–271.
135. **Tang YW, Gonsalves S, Sun JY, Stiles J, Gilhuley KA, Mikhlina A, Dunbar SA, Babady NE, Zhang H.** 2016. Clinical evaluation of the Luminex NxTAG respiratory pathogen panel. *J Clin Microbiol* **54:**1912–1914.
136. **Pierce VM, Hodinka RL.** 2012. Comparison of the GenMark Diagnostics eSensor respiratory viral panel to real-time PCR for detection of respiratory viruses in children. *J Clin Microbiol* **50:**3458–3465.
137. **Popowitch EB, O'Neill SS, Miller MB.** 2013. Comparison of the Biofire FilmArray RP, Genmark eSensor RVP, Luminex xTAG RVPv1, and Luminex xTAG RVP fast multiplex assays for detection of respiratory viruses. *J Clin Microbiol* **51:**1528–1533.
138. **Sakthivel SK, Whitaker B, Lu X, Oliveira DBL, Stockman LJ, Kamili S, Oberste MS, Erdman DD.** 2012. Comparison of fast-track diagnostics respiratory pathogens multiplex real-time RT-PCR assay with in-house singleplex assays for comprehensive detection of human respiratory viruses. *J Virol Methods* **185:**259–266.
139. **Jaramillo-Gutierrez G, Benschop KSM, Claas ECJ, de Jong AS, van Loon AM, Pas SD, Pontesilli O, Rossen JW, Swanink CMA, Thijsen S, van der Zanden AGM, van der Avoort HGAM, Koopmans MPG, Meijer A.** 2013. September through October 2010 multi-centre study in the Netherlands examining laboratory ability to detect enterovirus 68, an emerging respiratory pathogen. *J Virol Methods* **190:**53–62.
140. **Piralla A, Lilleri D, Sarasini A, Marchi A, Zecca M, Stronati M, Baldanti F, Gerna G.** 2012. Human rhinovirus and human respiratory enterovirus (EV68 and EV104) infections in hospitalized patients in Italy, 2008–2009. *Diagn Microbiol Infect Dis* **73:**162–167.
141. **Xiang Z, Gonzalez R, Wang Z, Ren L, Xiao Y, Li J, Li Y, Vernet G, Paranhos-Baccalà G, Jin Q, Wang J.** 2012. Coxsackievirus A21, enterovirus 68, and acute respiratory tract infection, China. *Emerg Infect Dis* **18:**821–824.
142. **Jacobson LM, Redd JT, Schneider E, Lu X, Chern S-WW, Oberste MS, Erdman DD, Fischer GE, Armstrong GL, Kodani M, Montoya J, Magri JM, Cheek JE.** 2012. Outbreak of lower respiratory tract illness associated with human enterovirus 68 among American Indian children. *Pediatr Infect Dis J* **31:**309–312.
143. **Lauinger IL, Bible JM, Halligan EP, Aarons EJ, MacMahon E, Tong CY.** 2012. Lineages, sub-lineages and variants of enterovirus 68 in recent outbreaks. *PLoS One* **7:**e36005.
144. **Brown PK, Tyrrell DA.** 1964. Experiments on the sensitivity of strains of human fibroblasts to infection with rhinoviruses. *Br J Exp Pathol* **45:**571–578.
145. **Geist FC, Hayden FG.** 1985. Comparative susceptibilities of strain MRC-5 human embryonic lung fibroblast cells and the Cooney strain of human fetal tonsil cells for isolation of rhinoviruses from clinical specimens. *J Clin Microbiol* **22:**455–456.
146. **Jang YJ, Lee SH, Kwon HJ, Chung YS, Lee BJ.** 2005. Development of rhinovirus study model using organ culture of turbinate mucosa. *J Virol Methods* **125:**41–47.
147. **Wang JH, Kwon HJ, Chung Y-S, Lee B-J, Jang YJ.** 2008. Infection rate and virus-induced cytokine secretion in experimental rhinovirus infection in mucosal organ culture: comparison between specimens from patients with chronic rhinosinusitis with nasal polyps and those from normal subjects. *Arch Otolaryngol Head Neck Surg* **134:**424–427.
148. **Torgersen H, Skern T, Blaas D.** 1989. Typing of human rhinoviruses based on sequence variations in the 5′ non-coding region. *J Gen Virol* **70:**3111–3116.
149. **Couch RB, Atmar RL.** 1999. *Rhinoviruses*. Marcel Dekker, Inc, New York, NY.
150. **Lu X, Erdman DD.** 2009. Comparison of three typing methods form human rhinoviruses based on sequence analysis of partial 5′NCR, VP4/VP2 and VP1 regions, 25th Annual Clinical Virology Symposium, Daytona Beach, FL.
151. **Douglas RG Jr, Fleet WF, Cate TR, Couch RB.** 1968. Antibody to rhinovirus in human sera. I. Standardization of a neutralization test. *Proc Soc Exp Biol Med* **127:**497–502.

152. **De Palma AM, Vliegen I, De Clercq E, Neyts J.** 2008. Selective inhibitors of picornavirus replication. *Med Res Rev* **28:**823–884.
153. **Clejan S, Mandrea E, Pandrea IV, Dufour J, Japa S, Veazey RS.** 2005. Immune responses induced by intranasal imiquimod and implications for therapeutics in rhinovirus infections. *J Cell Mol Med* **9:**457–461.
154. **Hayden FG, Diamond L, Wood PB, Korts DC, Wecker MT.** 1996. Effectiveness and safety of intranasal ipratropium bromide in common colds: a randomized, double-blind, placebo-controlled trial. *Ann Intern Med* **125:**89–97.
155. **Turner RB, Wecker MT, Pohl G, Witek TJ, McNally E, St George R, Winther B, Hayden FG.** 1999. Efficacy of tremacamra, a soluble intercellular adhesion molecule 1, for experimental rhinovirus infection: a randomized clinical trial. *JAMA* **281:**1797–1804.
156. **Turner RB, Bauer R, Woelkart K, Hulsey TC, Gangemi JD.** 2005. An evaluation of *Echinacea angustifolia* in experimental rhinovirus infections. *N Engl J Med* **353:**341–348.
157. **Bauer L, Lyoo H, van der Schaar HM, Strating JR, van Kuppeveld FJ.** 2017. Direct-acting antivirals and host-targeting strategies to combat enterovirus infections. *Curr Opin Virol* **24:**1–8.
158. **Jansen RR, Wieringa J, Koekkoek SM, Visser CE, Pajkrt D, Molenkamp R, de Jong MD, Schinkel J.** 2011. Frequent detection of respiratory viruses without symptoms: toward defining clinically relevant cutoff values. *J Clin Microbiol* **49:**2631–2636.
159. **Raymond F, Carbonneau J, Boucher N, Robitaille L, Boisvert S, Wu W-K, De Serres G, Boivin G, Corbeil J.** 2009. Comparison of automated microarray detection with real-time PCR assays for detection of respiratory viruses in specimens obtained from children. *J Clin Microbiol* **47:**743–750.
160. **Hayden RT, Gu Z, Rodriguez A, Tanioka L, Ying C, Morgenstern M, Bankowski MJ.** 2012. Comparison of two broadly multiplexed PCR systems for viral detection in clinical respiratory tract specimens from immunocompromised children. *J Clin Virol* **53:**308–313.
161. **Nijhuis RHT, Guerendiain D, Claas ECJ, Templeton KE.** 2017. Comparison of ePlex Respiratory Pathogen Panel with laboratory-developed real-time PCR assays for detection of respiratory pathogens. *J Clin Microbiol* **55:**1938–1945.
162. **Babady NE, Mead P, Stiles J, Brennan C, Li H, Shuptar S, Stratton CW, Tang Y-W, Kamboj M.** 2012. Comparison of the Luminex xTAG RVP Fast assay and the Idaho Technology FilmArray RP assay for detection of respiratory viruses in pediatric patients at a cancer hospital. *J Clin Microbiol* **50:**2282–2288.
163. **Balada-Llasat J-M, LaRue H, Kelly C, Rigali L, Pancholi P.** 2011. Evaluation of commercial ResPlex II v2.0, MultiCode-PLx, and xTAG respiratory viral panels for the diagnosis of respiratory viral infections in adults. *J Clin Virol* **50:** 42–45.
164. **Krunic N, Yager TD, Himsworth D, Merante F, Yaghoubian S, Janeczko R.** 2007. xTAG RVP assay: analytical and clinical performance. *J Clin Virol* **40**(Suppl 1)**:** S39–S46.
165. **Hwang SM, Lim MS, Han M, Hong YJ, Kim TS, Lee HR, Song EY, Park KU, Song J, Kim EC.** 2015. Comparison of xTAG respiratory virus panel and Verigene Respiratory Virus Plus for detecting influenza virus and respiratory syncytial virus. *J Clin Lab Anal* **29:**116–121.
166. **Loens K, van Loon AM, Coenjaerts F, van Aarle Y, Goossens H, Wallace P, Claas EJC, Ieven M, GRACE Study Group.** 2012. Performance of different mono- and multiplex nucleic acid amplification tests on a multipathogen external quality assessment panel. *J Clin Microbiol* **50:**977–987.
167. **Dabisch-Ruthe M, Vollmer T, Adams O, Knabbe C, Dreier J.** 2012. Comparison of three multiplex PCR assays for the detection of respiratory viral infections: evaluation of xTAG respiratory virus panel fast assay, RespiFinder 19 assay and RespiFinder SMART 22 assay. *BMC Infect Dis* **12:**163.

Coronaviruses

NAOMI J. GADSBY AND KATE E. TEMPLETON

92

TAXONOMY

Coronaviruses (CoVs) are so called due to their striking crown of surface projections, reminiscent of the solar corona, which can be seen by electron microscopy (Fig. 1). *Coronaviridae* is one of four families within the order *Nidovirales* and is divided into two subfamilies, *Coronavirinae* and *Torovirinae*. Within *Coronavirinae*, there are four genera, *Alphacoronavirus*, *Betacoronavirus*, *Gammacoronavirus*, and *Deltacoronavirus* (1, 2). Species within the genus *Betacoronavirus* are further differentiated into lineages A, B, C, and D, although these lineages do not have formal taxonomic status. The current phylogenetic relationship of the 30 recognized species within the *Coronavirinae* is illustrated in Fig. 2 (3). To date, six human CoVs (HCoVs) have been described. The genus *Alphacoronavirus* (previously CoV group 1) contains two HCoVs, HCoV-229E and HCoV-NL63, along with a number of other CoVs, including those from bats, pigs, dogs, and cats. The genus *Betacoronavirus* (previously CoV group 2) contains the remaining HCoVs and many other mammalian CoVs. HCoV-OC43 and HCoV-HKU1 are in *Betacoronavirus* lineage A, severe acute respiratory syndrome-related coronavirus (SARS-CoV) is in lineage B, and Middle East respiratory syndrome-related coronavirus (MERS-CoV) is found in lineage C (4). The genera *Gammacoronavirus* (previously CoV group 3) and *Deltacoronavirus* predominantly comprise avian CoV species, with some CoVs found in mammalian species but none thus far in humans (2, 5, 6).

DESCRIPTION OF THE AGENT

Structure

CoVs have very large, linear, positive-stranded RNA genomes approximately 30 kb in size (6). The 5′ two-thirds of the genome is a replicase gene encoding 15 or 16 nonstructural proteins in two overlapping open reading frames, ORF1a and ORF1b. The remaining third of the genome encodes four or five structural proteins, translated from a nested set of subgenomic mRNAs, and contains additional accessory genes specific to particular CoVs. The spherical or pleomorphic virions are enveloped and contain a helical nucleocapsid of nucleoprotein (N) associated with the RNA genome. Embedded in the envelope are 20-nm-long trimers of spike glycoprotein (S), also called peplomers, which have a club-shaped morphology and facilitate attachment to cells. The envelope also contains integral membrane (M) and envelope (E) proteins. CoVs of *Betacoronavirus* lineage A also have 5- to 7-nm spikes of an additional membrane glycoprotein, hemagglutinin-esterase (HE). The molecular biology of CoVs was recently reviewed (7). MERS-CoV is distinct from SARS-CoV in its use of DPP4/CD26 rather than ACE2 as the cellular receptor for entry (8). Work on establishing DPP4 as a receptor has been done in lung cells.

Origin

CoVs have been found in a wide range of domestic and wild mammals and birds; however, the particular diversity of strains found in birds and bats suggests that these animals are the natural reservoirs of CoVs, although this may also be the result of current sampling bias (2, 6). Recent genetic analysis of CoV from bats suggests zoonotic origins for both HCoV-229E and HCoV-NL63 (9–11); specifically, a bat evolutionary origin for HCoV-229E, with camelids as potential intermediate hosts (11, 12). HCoV-OC43 is a subspecies of *Betacoronavirus 1* closely related to other domestic-animal CoVs, particularly bovine CoV, and it is postulated that zoonotic transmission from cattle to humans may have occurred (13). The evolution of HCoV-OC23 in particular is characterized by frequent recombination events, and seven distinct genotypes (A to G) have been described (14). HCoV-HKU1 is distinct from HCoV-OC43 within *Betacoronavirus* lineage A, and its origin is unknown at present (15), although a rodent CoV may be the ancestor of this lineage (16). *Betacoronavirus* lineage B comprises SARS-CoV from humans alongside related CoVs from civets, ferrets, badgers, and bats (2, 17, 18). It is likely that SARS-CoV emerged through recombination of SARS-like CoVs from a natural reservoir in Chinese horseshoe bats and that zoonotic transmission occurred via animals, such as civets, in the exotic-animal markets of southern China (17–20). Although the evolutionary origin of MERS-CoV may be in bats (21, 22), the reservoir for current zoonotic transmission is thought likely to be camelid hosts; several studies have demonstrated high MERS-CoV seroprevalence and viral detection rates particularly in dromedary camels from the Middle East and parts of Africa (23–26). The route of transmission, however, remains unknown, and genomic analyses suggest that

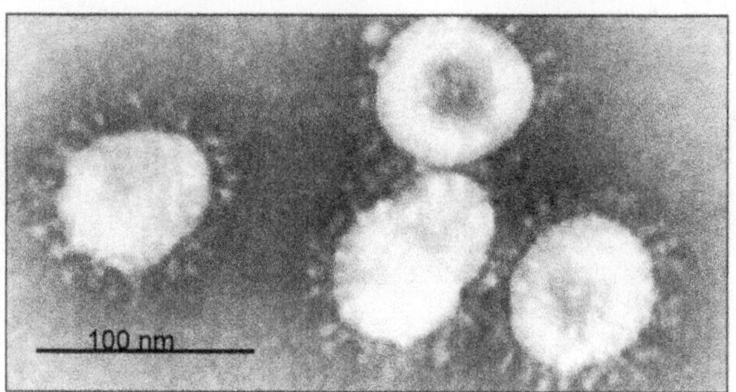

FIGURE 1 Electron micrograph of HCoV-OC43 showing the pleomorphic shape and characteristic coronas made up of surrounding peplomers.

multiple sporadic introductions of MERS-CoV into the human population have occurred, followed by human-to-human transmission (27, 28).

Discovery

In the 1960s, a number of virus strains that had a cytopathic effect, morphology, and biology unlike those of known respiratory viruses were isolated in culture from individuals with respiratory illness in the United States and the United Kingdom (29–31). Isolation of these viruses was difficult and generally required the use of primary organ cultures. They were morphologically and biologically similar and appeared most closely related to infectious bronchitis virus and mouse hepatitis virus. Together, they formed a new group of viruses recognized as coronaviruses in 1968. From this group, HCoV-229E and HCoV-OC43 were subsequently well characterized, owing in part to their existing ability (HCoV-229E) or subsequent adaptation (HCoV-OC43) to propagate *in vitro* (29, 30, 32). In 2003, SARS-CoV was isolated from cell cultures inoculated with respiratory specimens from affected patients; it had CoV-like morphology on electron microscopy and was identified as a novel CoV by sequence analysis (33–38). Experimental infection of cynomolgus macaques demonstrated that it was the etiological agent of SARS (39). Shortly after the SARS epidemic, two further HCoVs were identified; HCoV-NL63 in 2004 (40) and HCoV-HKU1 in 2005 (41). HCoV-NL63 was isolated using a novel cDNA amplified fragment length polymorphism-based technique to identify an unknown virus from culture (40) (Fig. 3). HCoV-HKU1 was identified solely using nucleic acid-based methods because it was refractory to growth in conventional cell lines (41). Retrospective analysis using stored samples has shown that both these "newly discovered" HCoVs have been circulating in the human population for many years (42). MERS-CoV

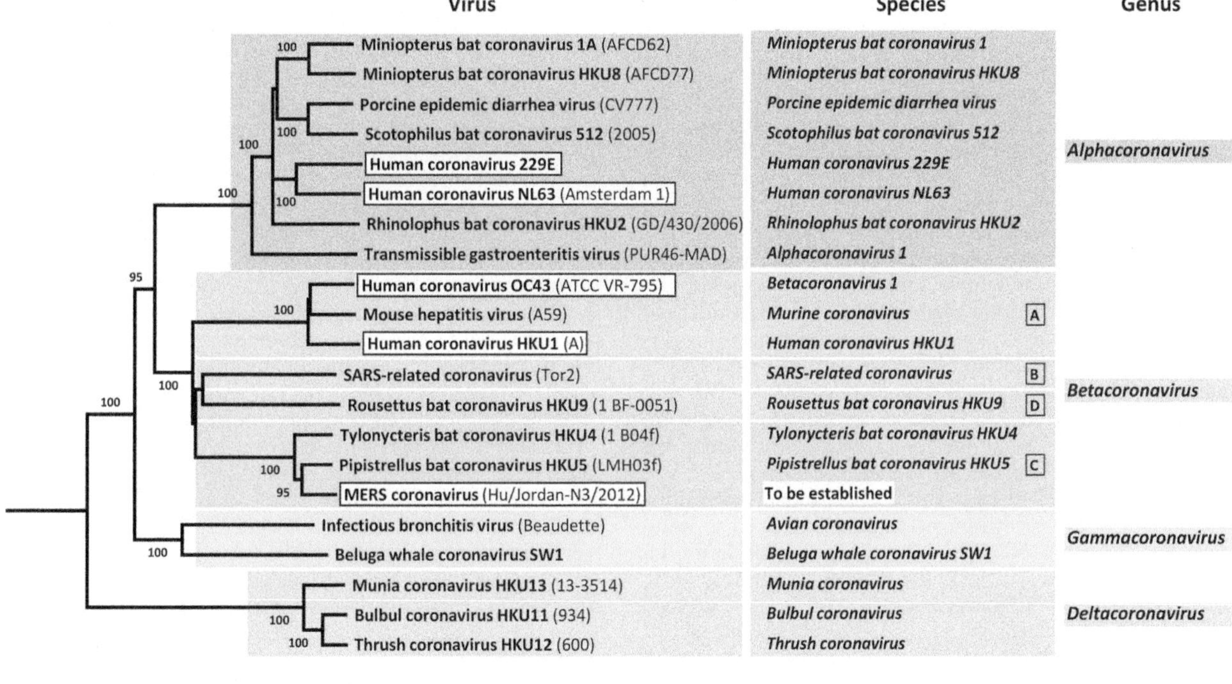

FIGURE 2 Phylogenetic relationships among members of the subfamily *Coronavirinae*. A rooted neighbor-joining tree was generated from amino acid sequence alignments of the replicase proteins encoded by polymerase ORF1b for 20 CoVs, each a representative of a currently recognized CoV species, and for the newly recognized MERS-CoV strain Hu/Jordan-N3/2012; bovine torovirus strain Breda served as an outgroup. Only bootstrap values equal to or larger than 95% are indicated. Virus names are given with strain specifications between parentheses; species and genus names are in italics as per convention. The tree shows the four main monophyletic clusters, corresponding to the genera *Alphacoronavirus*, *Betacoronavirus*, *Gammacoronavirus*, and *Deltacoronavirus*. Also indicated are *Betacoronavirus* lineages A through D (corresponding to former CoV subgroups 2A through D). (Modified from reference 3, kindly provided by R. J. de Groot, and used with permission).

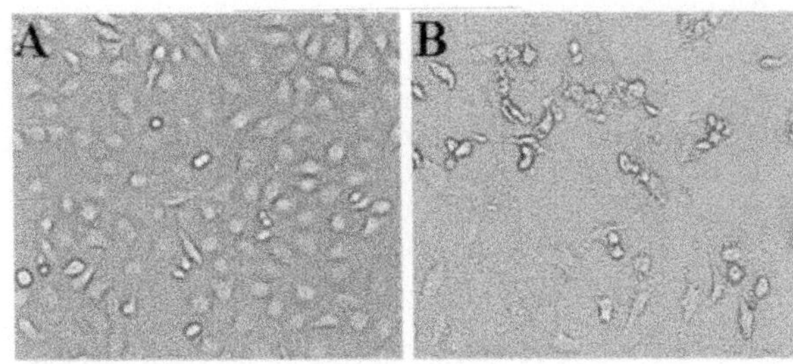

FIGURE 3 HCoV cytopathic effect at 5 days postinfection. (A) Uninfected LLC-MK2 cells. (B) HCoV-NL63-infected LLC-MK2 cells.

was identified in 2012 by pan-CoV reverse transcription-PCR (RT-PCR) and genetic analysis (43). Rhesus macaques experimentally infected with MERS-CoV developed pneumonia, thus establishing a causal relationship between virus and disease (44).

EPIDEMIOLOGY AND TRANSMISSION

HCoV-229E, HCoV-OC43, HCoV-NL63, and HCoV-HKU1 are endemic in humans. In contrast, SARS-CoV has not been reported since early 2004, and MERS-CoV appears to have only recently emerged. The four endemic HCoVs have a worldwide distribution (45–49). Serological surveys carried out several decades ago showed that HCoV infection fluctuated between years, with a higher frequency of serological responses in the winter than in summer months. With the advent of RT-PCR detection, the substantial temporal and geographical variation in HCoV detection and in the predominance of individual HCoVs has been confirmed. This variability makes it hard to draw conclusions about the burden and periodicity of infection from studies describing HCoV epidemiology over only 1 or 2 years. Furthermore, due to their relatively recent discovery, few studies have looked for all four HCoVs simultaneously over long periods of time. From multiyear molecular studies in children and adults, detection by RT-PCR of all four endemic HCoVs typically peaks in the winter and spring months in temperate countries; although HCoV-OC43 and HCoV-NL63 are usually the most commonly detected (42, 45, 46, 50–58) (Fig. 4), other studies have demonstrated higher frequencies of HCoV-229E and HCoV-HKU1 (59). A large Dutch study found that timing and extent of HCoV winter peaks may be related to influenza A epidemics (60), and a 2- to 3-year periodicity has been described for HCoV-NL63, HCoV-229E, and HCoV-OC43 in some RT-PCR and serological studies (57, 61–63) but not in others (42, 45, 53, 58). The combined HCoV detection rate in individuals with acute respiratory illness (ARI) in multiyear studies varies from 1 to 18%, and coinfections with other respiratory viruses are common (45, 46, 51–53, 55, 56, 59). Although HCoVs are detected in all age groups, the highest detection rates are typically seen in young children (Fig. 4) (56).

Historical serological surveys demonstrated that infection with HCoV-229E and HCoV-OC43 could occur on a background of preexisting neutralizing antibody and that apparent reinfection with the same virus species was common (61, 62, 64, 65). Reinfection could also be achieved in experimental inoculations of healthy adults, although it generated subclinical infections under these conditions (66). In longitudinal studies in children, approximately half of the serological responses to HCoV-229E and HCoV-OC43 occurred in the absence of symptoms, suggesting the occurrence of natural subclinical infection (61, 62). Contemporary serological studies have shown that infection with HCoVs is a common event in early childhood, with seropositivity to all four HCoVs generally increasing with age. Seroconversion to at least one HCoV was observed in 24 out of 25 healthy infants by the age of approximately 20 months (51). However, seroconversion was more frequent with HCoV-OC43 and HCoV-NL63 than HCoV-229E and HCoV-HKU1, in line with individual detection frequencies determined by RT-PCR (51). The sequence of HCoV infection in infancy appears to be important, as prior HCoV-OC43 or HCoV-NL63 infection may elicit immunity that protects from subsequent HCoV-HKU1 or HCoV-229E infection, respectively, but not vice versa (51). In two independent cross-sectional seroepidemiologic studies in different populations, the proportion of infants with antibodies to both HCoV-229E and HCoV-NL63 decreased significantly from 0 to 6 months of age but then increased rapidly, so that by the age of 4 years, more than 50% of children were seropositive for both viruses (67, 68). It is likely that this pattern illustrates the waning of maternal antibody and the development of new antibody in response to infection in early childhood. Some studies in adults have reported seroprevalences as high as 90 to 100% for HCoV-229E, HCoV-NL63, and HCoV-OC43, with a lower seroprevalence for HCoV-HKU1 of 59 to 91% (69). However, other studies have found much lower seroprevalences for all four HCoVs (68, 70–72). Differences in study population and geographic location as well as in assay sensitivity and specificity may account for the variation.

The major transmission route of HCoV is likely to be respiratory, although many animal CoVs also have a fecal-oral route of transmission and can replicate in epithelial cells in both the respiratory and gastrointestinal tracts. The isolation of HCoVs from fecal specimens has been described, but it is unclear to what extent HCoVs are transmitted feco-orally. HCoV can be detected by RT-PCR in respiratory secretions for over 3 weeks after the onset of illness, particularly in immunocompromised patients and neonates; however, it is not known if this represents viable virus (73, 74). HCoVs may survive on inanimate surfaces (75), in suspension (76), or as aerosols (77). Therefore, contact-mediated and aerosol-mediated transmission from the environment is a possibility. Nosocomial outbreaks of HCoV have been associated with severe illness in elderly-care facilities and neonatal and pediatric intensive care units (78). The typical incubation period of HCoV-229E, HCoV-OC43, and related strains was shown to be 2 to 5 days in intranasal inoculation experiments in healthy adults; however, it has not been well described for other common HCoVs or in different populations, such as children.

SARS-CoV infection emerged as a zoonosis in Guangdong province, China, in 2002 and then spread globally via human-to-human transmission to cause the SARS pandemic. Mutation in the receptor-binding domain of the S protein may have contributed to adaptation of the virus for human-to-human transmission (79). Global transmission appeared to be largely related to superspreading events involving symptomatic individuals in places such as hospitals, hotels, and residential complexes, and asymptomatic seropositivity in the community was low (36). Initial epidemiological investigations suggested that respiratory droplet secretion or direct or indirect contact were the most likely routes of transmission (37). The generation of aerosols, particularly in hospitals, was also important.

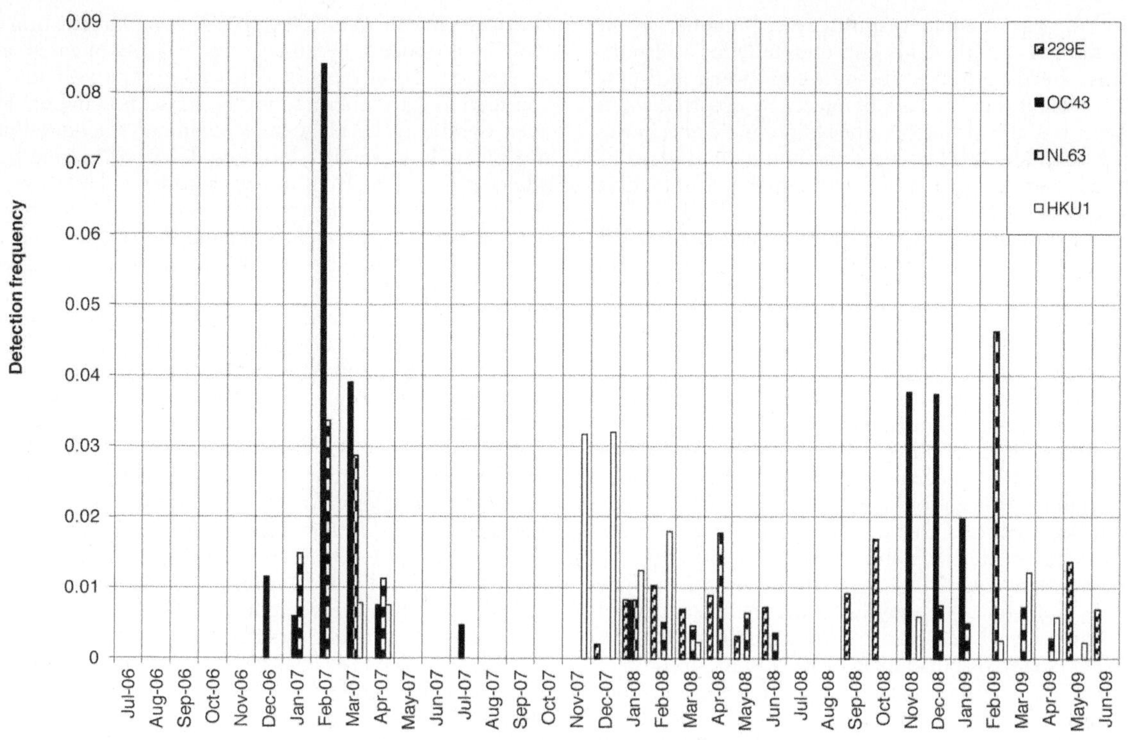

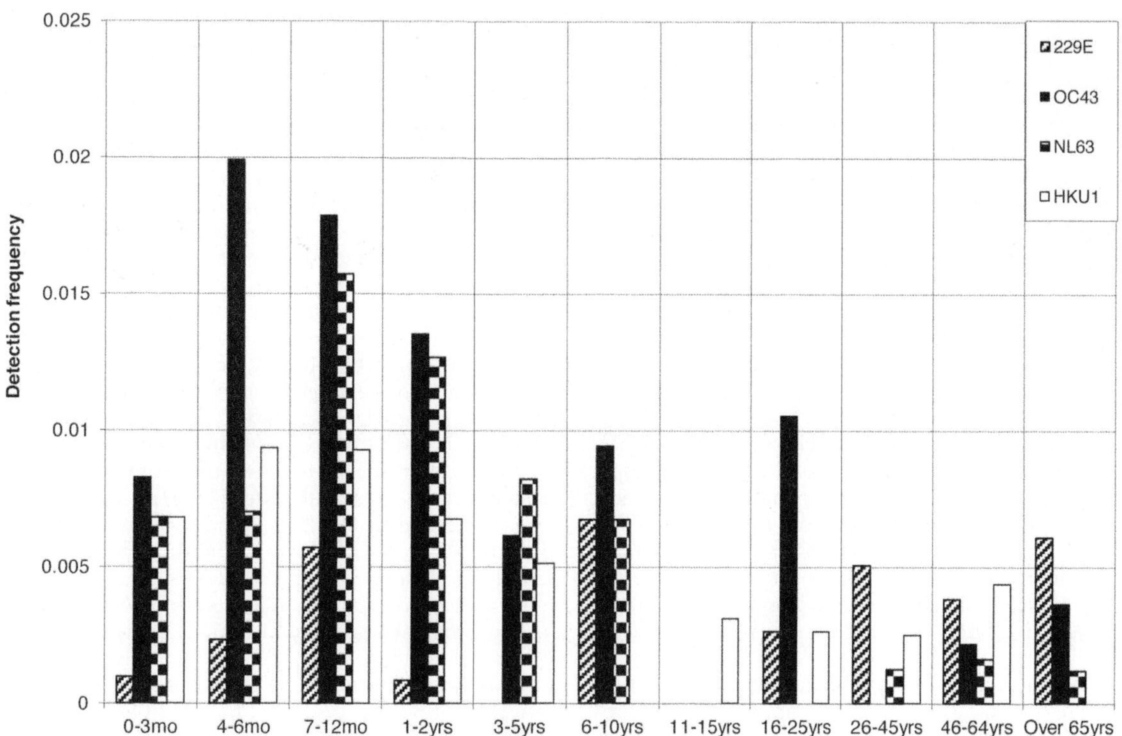

FIGURE 4 HCoV detection frequencies by month and age band over a 3-year period between 2006 and 2009 in Edinburgh, United Kingdom, using multiplex real-time RT-PCR. During this time, 11,661 specimens were tested, with 61 specimens being positive for HCoV-HKU1, 99 for HCoV-OC43, 35 for HCoV-229E, and 75 for HCoV-NL63. (Adapted from reference 46.)

SARS-CoV was shed in respiratory specimens, stool, urine, and other bodily fluids but, unusually for a respiratory virus, shedding peaked in the second week of illness (80). This meant that the peak of infectivity occurred when the patient was already likely to be symptomatic and in the hospital. Public health measures, including rapid identification and quarantine of patients and improved infection control, brought transmission to a halt in mid-2003. SARS-CoV briefly reemerged in Guangdong province in late 2003 from a probable new zoonotic transmission event, and there were also later incidences of laboratory transmission. The incubation period of SARS was typically 2 to 14 days, with a mean of 4 to 5 days, although occasional cases with longer incubation periods were reported (36, 37).

MERS-CoV was first isolated from a patient with severe pneumonia hospitalized in the Kingdom of Saudi Arabia (KSA) in June 2012 (43) but has since been found retrospectively in samples associated with a nosocomial outbreak of severe pneumonia in Jordan in April 2012 (81). Cases have now been reported from 27 countries, mostly linked to travel or residence in the Arabian Peninsula, with approximately 80% cases reported by KSA. Overall seroprevalence in KSA is thought to be very low with the exception of those occupationally exposed to dromedary camels (82). Cases have occurred sporadically or in clusters, and direct contact with dromedary camels has been noted in some but not all cases (83). Raw camel products, such as meat and milk, may also be potentially infectious. Sustained human-to-human transmission has not been observed to date, although limited person-to-person transmission has been identified among close household contacts (84). Significant nosocomial outbreaks have also occurred, the largest being in the Republic of Korea in 2015 (85); as with SARS, transmission has been associated with time to isolation and a small number of superspreading events in hospitals (86). Therefore, contact and droplet transmission-based precautions are recommended in the health care setting, with airborne precautions for aerosol-generating procedures (87). The incubation period for MERS-CoV is estimated at a median of 7 days, with the majority of cases occurring within 2 to 15 days (88). Peak respiratory viral loads and shedding patterns for MERS-CoV appear to be similar to those of SARS-CoV, with the exception of significantly lower levels of detection of MERS-CoV in urine and stool (89).

CLINICAL SIGNIFICANCE

The endemic HCoVs, HCoV-229E, HCoV-OC43, HCoV-NL63, and HCoV-HKU1, are associated with upper respiratory tract infection (URTI) in individuals of all ages and occasionally with lower respiratory-tract infection (LRTI). HCoV-229E and HCoV-OC43 were originally isolated from adults with mild URTI and were demonstrated to cause the symptoms of the "common cold" in human experiments (29, 30, 90, 91). Such experiments have not been carried out with HCoV-NL63 and HCoV-HKU1, so a causal relationship cannot be formally demonstrated. The four endemic HCoVs are associated with similar URTI symptoms such as fever, cough, sore throat, nasal obstruction, and rhinorrhea (47); HCoV-NL63 has been particularly associated with croup in children (49, 63, 92–94). Numerous epidemiological studies have indicated a temporal association with all four of the endemic HCoVs and ARI, and some studies have shown higher rates of HCoV detection in patients with ARI symptoms than in asymptomatic individuals (45). However, other studies have found similar or lower detection rates in hospitalized cases compared to controls, typically 2 to 10% (49, 95, 96). Drawing firm conclusions is difficult, because in the majority of case-control studies, detection rates for HCoV are relatively low, and coinfection with other respiratory viruses is common. However, significant LRTI, such as community-acquired pneumonia and bronchiolitis, has been described in hospitalized adults and children from whom an endemic HCoV was the sole etiologic agent detected (93, 97–99). HCoV has also been associated with significant morbidity due to LRTI in immunocompromised patients, patients with other underlying conditions, and those at the extremes of age (42, 46, 52, 97, 100, 101). Overall, however, it is likely that the burden of severe illness due to endemic HCoVs is relatively minor in comparison to other respiratory viruses, such as adenovirus, influenza virus, and respiratory syncytial virus (102, 103).

Several animal CoVs are known to cause diarrheal disease, but the link between HCoV infection and enteric infection is unclear. At present, HCoVs are thought to play a minor role, if any, in gastrointestinal disease. CoV-like particles have been seen in fecal specimens by electron microscopy, and human "enteric" CoVs, some apparently closely related to the betacoronaviruses bovine CoV and HCoV-OC43, were also isolated from patients with gastrointestinal disease (74, 104, 105). In recent years, work has focused mainly on RT-PCR detection of the four endemic HCoVs; although these have been found occasionally in cases of acute gastroenteritis, they have been equally rarely detected in controls (106–108). Some animal CoVs are also neurotrophic; both HCoV-OC43 and HCoV-229E RNA have been detected in brain tissue, and a fatal case of encephalitis associated with HCoV-OC43 in an immunocompromised child was recently described (109).

SARS-CoV and MERS-CoV cause severe respiratory illness with high mortality rates. During the SARS epidemic, the virus spread to 26 countries, resulting in approximately 8,000 clinical cases and over 700 deaths. The typical SARS clinical presentation was one of initial viral respiratory illness with fever, malaise, and nonproductive cough, followed by an atypical pneumonia with rapid respiratory deterioration. Diarrhea and lymphopenia were also features. Symptoms were milder in children than in adults and the overall crude case fatality rate was 10% (110). MERS-CoV has been predominantly seen in older adults with underlying comorbidities such as diabetes, and, although a spectrum from asymptomatic carriage to severe disease has been reported, most cases to date have been clinically severe (111, 112). MERS-CoV infections have only rarely been detected in children, and these are typically asymptomatic contacts of adult cases (113). At the time of writing, there had been 1,952 laboratory-confirmed cases of infection with MERS-CoV, including 693 deaths, giving a crude case fatality rate of around 35%. The typical clinical course comprises initial viral prodrome with fever, cough, subsequent pneumonia, and respiratory deterioration over several days (111). Severe complications include renal failure, acute respiratory distress syndrome with shock, and, rarely, neurological disease (111, 112, 114). Gastrointestinal symptoms are commonly reported, along with lymphopenia and other hematological abnormalities (111, 112). Adverse maternal and perinatal outcomes have also been noted in MERS-CoV-infected pregnant women (115).

The key to the management of severe HCoV infection is good supportive care, as there is no specific treatment available. Several potential therapeutic agents against SARS-CoV, such as viral protein inhibitors, interferons, and antibodies, have been evaluated *in vitro* and in animal models (116). During the SARS outbreak, several experimental treatments were used in humans, but a retrospective review found no conclusive positive effects of any substance and some potentially harmful effects (117). The biology of MERS-CoV differs in certain important aspects from that of SARS-CoV, and potential treatment options, such as convalescent-phase plasma, interferon with or without ribavirin, and lopinavir/ritonavir, remain, at best, investigational (118).

COLLECTION, TRANSPORT, AND STORAGE OF SPECIMENS

HCoVs can be detected in a range of routine URT and LRT specimens, such as nasopharyngeal swabs, nasopharyngeal aspirates (NPA), nasal washes, and bronchoalveolar lavage fluid. Detection of CoVs in blood, stool, urine, lung biopsy specimens, and postmortem tissue has also been described. In SARS-CoV and MERS-CoV infection, higher viral loads or RT-PCR positivity rates have been found in LRT specimens than in URT specimens and in the second week of illness. Therefore, testing LRT specimens should be the priority where possible, and samples should be taken from multiple sites and at several time points to increase the chances of detection. For MERS-CoV diagnosis specifically, URT samples, LRT samples, and serum are recommended for RT-PCR testing, alongside acute- and convalescent-phase sera for retrospective serological diagnosis (119). Appropriate infection control precautions must be put in place for sample collection, particularly where aerosol-generating procedures are required.

The transport of specimens should be carried out under transport category UN3373 Biological Substance, category B, with packaging complying with instruction P650 (120). Specimens for the direct detection of HCoV can be handled in biosafety level 2 (BSL2) facilities using BSL2 practices, including the use of a biological safety cabinet for potentially aerosol-generating procedures. However, where there is a suspicion of SARS-CoV, MERS-CoV, or other novel CoV infection, the initial handling of infectious samples (respiratory samples, stool, and urine) should be performed in a BSL3 facility; once samples are lysed, BSL2 practices can be followed. Additionally, virus isolation in culture should not be attempted unless laboratories have the relevant expertise, and work with live virus should be carried out only in a BSL3 facility using BSL3 practices. To reduce the risk of laboratory-acquired infection in a novel CoV scenario, nucleic acid-based detection is recommended because it does not require virus propagation and because nucleic acid extraction procedures inactivate the virus. Furthermore, respiratory specimens can be collected, transported, and processed in lysis buffer, thus inactivating the virus at the earliest stage in the diagnostic process.

DIRECT DETECTION

Microscopy

CoVs can be identified by their characteristic morphology on electron microscopy (EM); virions are spherical or pleomorphic, approximately 80 nm in diameter, and with projections around the virus envelope forming a "corona" (Fig. 1). Thin-section EM and negative-stain EM have typically been used for the identification and characterization of HCoVs propagated *in vitro*, rather than for direct detection (29, 30, 34). Cell culture enables amplification of the virus to levels sufficient for detection by EM, so EM is not typically carried out directly on respiratory specimens. However, some laboratories do carry out direct detection of CoVs in fecal specimens by EM, although other direct methods are likely to be more suited to the routine diagnostic setting. EM is most relevant as a complementary method in the search for novel CoVs.

Antigen Detection

Antigen detection assays have the potential to be the most rapid of all detection methods. HCoV antigen is identified directly in clinical specimens by labeled monoclonal antibodies coupled to a detection system such as microscopy. This process may be more convenient than most nucleic acid-based methods for laboratories that lack experience with molecular techniques. However, assays have been developed predominantly in house to detect SARS-CoV, with the majority of assays targeting the abundant nucleocapsid (N) protein in enzyme immunoassay-based formats. Enzyme immunoassays based on chemiluminescent detection and monoclonal antibodies may be particularly effective (121), as SARS-CoV N antigen is detectable in the blood of approximately 60% of patients in the third week of illness (122). Other enzyme-linked immunosorbent assay (ELISA)-based antigen-detection assays have found SARS-CoV N antigen in NPA and stool specimens, particularly after 10 days of illness onset, but rarely in urine (123). The use of immunofluorescence by indirect fluorescent assay (IFA) on cellular preparations from throat washes has also been described (124). The sensitivity of IFA for monoclonal antibody to endemic HCoV or direct fluorescent assays varies depending on the species and is generally lower than that of RT-PCR (125). More recently, ELISA-based methods have been developed for the detection of the N protein from HCoV-229E and HCoV-NL63 (126), along with a rapid antigen test for MERS-CoV N protein (127), but these have not yet been fully clinically evaluated.

Nucleic Acid Detection

Direct detection of nucleic acids in clinical specimens is the most common diagnostic method in use today for HCoV. Detection of nucleic acids is typically more sensitive and specific than other methods. It relies neither on the binding of antigen to potentially cross-reactive antibodies nor on the detection of a timely and specific immune response in individuals. Two strategies have been employed in nucleic acid amplification tests (NAATs) for HCoV. The first is to select a target that is as conserved as possible among all known HCoVs, creating a so-called "pan-CoV" assay; the second is to select a region of the genome that is distinct between the different HCoV species, to generate a series of species-specific assays. Ideally, all four endemic HCoVs should be sought in diagnostic specimens, given our increasing knowledge of their roles as respiratory pathogens. Recent significant advances in our understanding of HCoVs have been made through nucleic acid-based methods, particularly the ability to randomly amplify and sequence nucleic acids from cultures and to compare them to databases to detect novel CoVs (43). Whole-genome sequencing can be carried out directly on respiratory samples (41), although it is not commonplace at this time in most clinical laboratories.

Pan-CoV Assays

Pan-CoV assays enable the detection of CoV infection without anticipation of the species involved. Regions of the conserved polymerase gene within the replicase ORF1a/b have been successfully used in pan-CoV assays, following alignment of known sequences and generation of consensus primers. Some pan-CoV assays use degenerate primers (55), some utilize multiple primer sets (97), and others employ a single set of nondegenerate primers (41). The more degenerate the primers, the lower the sensitivity for known HCoVs, but the higher the likelihood of detecting more distantly related CoVs. Different pan-CoV assays have been shown to vary in their capacity to detect known HCoVs (128), although some have sensitivity equivalent to that of individual species-specific assays (97). Therefore, the choice of approach will depend on the diagnostic objectives. Pan-CoV assays have been used as an initial screening test (97) and also for the detection of unknown viruses growing in cell culture, leading to the discovery of new HCoVs (41). To identify the CoV species, amplicons from pan-CoV assays need to be sequenced and subjected to restriction enzyme digestion or probe hybridization, or positive specimens require further testing with species-specific assays (129).

Species-Specific Assays

Species-specific NAATs are very sensitive and provide species-level identification without sequencing or other postamplification processing. The disadvantage of species-specific assays is that they are likely to miss emerging CoVs that are divergent in sequence, though this may also be the case with pan-CoV NAATs. It is possible to multiplex individual species-specific assays into a single reaction without a loss in sensitivity, thus reducing costs and hands-on time (46). However, some authors using other species-specific NAATs have found that the sensitivity is greater with individual assays (48, 130). Therefore, when HCoV assays are set up, it is wise to assess performance in both formats, in order to find the best arrangement for the individual laboratory. Regions of the N gene have been most commonly used for detection of individual HCoVs; however, assays have been described targeting the membrane protein (M) gene, polymerase gene (replicase ORF1a/1b), spike protein (S) gene, and, most recently, transcriptionally abundant leader sequences in the 5′ UTR (131).

In-House NAATs

NAATs for HCoV mainly utilize PCR technology. As HCoVs have an RNA genome, an initial RT step is required; this can either be carried out separately (two-step RT-PCR) or combined with the PCR assay (one-step RT-PCR). In order to increase sensitivity and specificity, several HCoV RT-PCRs in current diagnostic use are nested, so that the products of an initial round of amplification using outer primers are reamplified with a set of inner primers (46). Detection of amplified products has been traditionally carried out using gel-based electrophoretic systems and UV visualization of DNA bands of the expected size. The use of hybridization probes on a low-density microarray has also been described for a pan-CoV assay (132). However, real-time detection of amplified products, so-called real-time RT-PCR, is now possible. This is achieved through the use of fluorescent dyes that intercalate nonspecifically into double-stranded DNA (93, 133) or fluorescent probes that bind to the nascent DNA in a sequence-specific manner and emit light through a variety of mechanisms, the most common being hydrolysis (46, 131). Real-time RT-PCR has the advantage of a closed-tube format; the reaction vessel is never opened after amplification, thereby reducing the opportunity to contaminate the laboratory environment with DNA template and decreasing the potential for false-positive detection. As it combines amplification and detection in a single step, it is also significantly faster and requires less hands-on time than traditional RT-PCR methods. The sensitivity of real-time RT-PCR for HCoV detection has been shown to be equivalent or superior to that of conventional RT-PCR (134) and nested RT-PCR (46, 135). Examples of real-time RT-PCR assays used for the detection of the four endemic HCoVs are given in Table 1. Real-time RT-PCR can also give a quantitative output; although HCoV viral loads are unlikely to be required in the routine diagnostic setting, viral load profiles are useful in the description of severe disease associated with newly emerging CoVs, where viral load may be a prognostic marker.

Non-PCR-based NAATs are infrequently described, although those using isothermal methods such as loop-mediated isothermal amplification (LAMP) have been successful and may be very suitable in resource-limited settings. A simple, low-cost LAMP assay for HCoV-NL63 has been shown to have sensitivity comparable to that of real-time PCR (136). In most cases, HCoV NAATs have been developed in house by the diagnostic laboratory or adapted from the published method of another laboratory. In either case, this requires a significant initial time commitment from skilled scientific staff in terms of assay development, validation, and evaluation, as well as ongoing support in the routine use of these assays. However, in-house assays are economical to run and can be readily adapted to take into account oligonucleotide binding-site variation in existing HCoVs, or for the detection of emerging HCoVs, such as SARS-CoV and MERS-CoV, as soon as sequence data are available.

Commercial NAATs

The last 5 years have seen a large increase in the number and variety of commercial NAATs for HCoV detection, driven mainly by the development of respiratory virus panels for a syndromic diagnostic approach (Table 2). All respiratory viruses can cause a range of presenting symptoms and complications, and clinical features of ARI caused by different viruses are often indistinguishable. Large commercial panel assays that enable a specimen to be tested for an array of viruses simultaneously may be a viable alternative to the use of multiple in-house real-time PCR assays for routine detection, as well as in outbreak situations, despite their higher unit costs (137). Commercial assays vary significantly in hands-on time, some require more than one reaction tube per sample, and some are particularly suited to high-throughput (e.g., xTAG RVP Fast; Luminex, Austin, TX) or low-throughput (e.g., FilmArray respiratory panel; BioFire, Salt Lake City, UT) settings. Commercial tests are particularly attractive as an alternative to traditional culture and immunofluorescence-based methods in laboratories that require the use of regulatory-body-approved *in vitro* diagnostic tests and/or in laboratories that lack experience with molecular techniques. However, for HCoV detection in particular, although many tests are CE marked (in Europe), few as yet have U.S. Food and Drug Administration (FDA) approval, and not all assays will detect all four endemic HCoVs (Table 2). Direct comparison between commercial and in-house NAATs for HCoV detection has shown a range of performance. However, most comparisons are limited by the overall scarcity of HCoV-positive samples and particularly by the limited number of samples known to contain individual species, making it difficult to draw firm conclusions about sensitivity for individual HCoVs (137–140). This is a rapidly changing field, and it is likely that new commercial tests and modifications to existing ones will continue to come onto the market in the near future.

TABLE 1 Examples of published real-time RT-PCR assays for the detection of endemic HCoVs using different target genes[a]

Reference	Virus	Target gene	Oligonucleotide sequences	Assay format	Reported analytical sensitivity
Gaunt et al., 2010 (46)	HCoV-229E	M	For: CATACTATCAACCCATTCAACAAG Rev: CACGGCAACTGTCATGTATT Probe: ATGAACCTGAACACCTGAAGCCAATCTATG	Multiplex 1-step real-time RT-PCR on ABI7500, hydrolysis probe detection	Detection limit, 66 copies/ reaction
	HCoV-OC43	M	For: CATACYCTGACGGTCACAATAATA Rev: ACCTTAGCAACAGTCATATAAGC Probe: TGCCCAAGAATAGCCAGTACCTAGT		Detection limit, 18 copies/ reaction
	HCoV-NL63	N	For: GTTCTGATAAGGCACCATATAGG Rev: TTTAGGAGGCAAATCAACACG Probe: CGCATACGCCAACGCTCTTGAACA		Detection limit, 69 copies/ reaction
	HCoV-HKU1	N	For: TCCTACTAYTCAAGAAGCTATCC Rev: AATGAACGATTATTGGGTCCAC Probe: TYCGCCTGGTACGATTTTGCCTCA		Detection limit, 9 copies/reaction
Mackay et al., 2012 (48)	HCoV-229E	N	For: ACAACGTGGTCGTCAGGGT Rev: GCAACCCAGACGACACCT Probe: CATCTTTATGGGGTCCTG (MGB)	Individual 1-step real-time RT-PCR on Rotor-Gene 3000/6000/Q, hydrolysis probe detection	Detection limit, ≤10 copies/ reaction
	HCoV-OC43	N	For: GAAGGTCTGCTCCTAATTCCAGAT Rev: TTTGGCAGTATGCTTAGTTACTT Probe: TGCCAAGTTTTGCCAGAACAAGACTAGC		
	HCoV-NL63	N	For: GAGTTCGAGGATCGCTCTAATA Rev: TGAATCCCCCATATTGTGATTAAA Probe: AAAATGTTATTCAGTGCTTTGGTCCTCGTGA		
	HCoV-HKU1	ORF1b (Pol)	For: GTTGGGACGATATGTTACGTCATCTT Rev: TGCTAGTACCACCAGGCTTAACATA Probe: CAACCGCCACACATAA (MGB)		
Kuypers et al., 2007 (97)	HCoV-229E HCoV-OC43 HCoV-NL63 HCoV-HKU1	ORF1b (Pol)	F1: TGGTGGCTGGGACGATATGT F2: TTTATGGTGGTTGGAATAATATGTTG F3: TGGCGGGTGGGATAATATGT F-OC: CCTTATTAAAGATGTTGACAATCCTGTAC R1: GGCATAGCACGATCACACTTAGG R2: GGCAAAGCTCTATCACATTTGG R3: GAGGGCATAGCTCTATCACACTTAGG R-OC: AATACGTAGTAGGTTTGGCATAGCAC P1: ATAATCCCAACCCATRAG P2: ATAGTCCCATCCCATCAA P-OC: CACACTTAGGATAGTCCCA	Individual 1-step real-time RT-PCR, hydrolysis probe detection 229E: F3/P2/R3 NL63: F2/P1/R2 OC43 & HKU1: F1/P1/R1 OC43: F-OC/R-OC/P-OC	10 viral copies/reaction in both consensus and subtype-specific reactions

(Continued on next page)

TABLE 1 Examples of published real-time RT-PCR assays for the detection of endemic HCoVs using different target genes[a] *(Continued)*

Reference	Virus	Target gene	Oligonucleotide sequences	Assay format	Reported analytical sensitivity
Dare et al., 2007 (130); van Elden et al., 2004 (135)	HCoV-229E	N	For: CAGTCAAATGGGCTGATGCA Rev: AAAGGGCTATAAAGAGAATAAGGTATTCT Probe: CCCTGACGACCACGTTGTGGTTCA	Individual 1-step real-time RT-PCR on iCycler iQ, hydrolysis probe detection	100% detection at 50 copies/ reaction, 93% detection at 5 copies/reaction
	HCoV-OC43	N	For: CGATGAGGCTATTCCGACTAGGT Rev: CCTTCCTGAGCCTTCAATATAGTAACC Probe: TCCGCCTGGCACGGTACTCCCT		100% detection at 50 copies/ reaction, 33% detection at 5 copies/reaction
	HCoV-NL63	N	For: GACCAAAGCACTGAATAACATTTTCC Rev: ACCTAATAAGCCTCTTTCTCAACCC Probe: AACACGCT“T”CCAACGAGGTTTCTTCAACTGAG[b]		100% detection at 50 copies/ reaction, 80% detection at 5 copies/reaction
	HCoV-HKU1	ORF1b (Pol)	For: CCTTGCGAATGAATGTGCT Rev: TTGCATCACCACTGCTAGTACCAC Probe: TGTGTGGCGGTTGCTATTATGTTAAGCCTG		100% detection at 50 copies/ reaction, 33% detection at 5 copies/reaction
Esposito et al., 2006 (174)	HCoV-229E	N	For: CGCAAGAATTCAGAACCAGAG Rev: GGGAGTCAGGTTCTTCAACAA Probe: CCACACTTCAATCAAAAGCTCCCAAATG	Individual 2-step real-time RT-PCR on ABI 7700/7500, hydrolysis probe detection	Sensitivity estimated at <500–1,000 copies/ml
	HCoV-OC43	N	For: GCTCAGGAAGGTCTGCTCC Rev: TCCTGCACTAGAGGCTCTGC Probe: TTCCAGATCTACTTCGCGCACATCC		
	HCoV-NL63	N	For: AGGACCTTAAATTCAGACAACGTTCT Rev: GATTACGTTTGCGATTACCAAGACT Probe: TAACAGTTTTAGCACCTTCCTTAGCAACCCAAACA		
	HCoV-HKU1	N	For: AGTTCCCATTGCTTTCGGAGTA Rev: CCGGCTGTGTCTATACCAATATCC Probe: CCCCTTCTGAAGCAA (MGB)		
Chan et al., 2015 (131)	HCoV-229E	5′ UTR leader sequence	For: CTACAGATAGAAAAGTTGCTTT Rev: GGTCGTTTAGTTGAGAAAAGT Probe[c]: AGACT+T+TG+TG+TCT+A+CT	Individual 1-step real-time RT-PCR on LightCycler 96, locked nucleic acid hydrolysis probe detection	Detection limit, 10 RNA copies/ reaction
	HCoV-OC43	5′ UTR leader sequence	For: AAACGTGCGTGCATC Rev: AGATTACAAAAAGATCTAACAAGA Probe[c]: C+TTCA+CTG+ATCT+C+T+TGT		Detection limit, 10 RNA copies/ reaction
	HCoV-NL63	5′ UTR leader sequence	For: GGAGATAGAGAATTTTCTTATTTAGA Rev: GGTTTCGTTTAGTTGAGAAG Probe[c]: TGTGT+C+TAC+T+C+TTCT+CA		Detection limit, 5 RNA copies/ reaction
	HCoV-HKU1	5′ UTR leader sequence	For: CGTACCGTCTATCAGCT Rev: GTTTAGATTTAATGAGATCTGACA Probe[c]: ACGA+T+CT+C+TTG+T+CA		Detection limit, 5 RNA copies/ reaction

[a]Further RT-PCR assays for HCoV-HKU1 have been recently reviewed (15). Abbreviations: For, forward; Rev, reverse; Pol, polymerase; UTR, untranslated region, MGB, minor groove binder.
[b]Internally quenched with BHQ1, indicated by “T.”
[c]The letters following “+” represent locked nucleic acid bases.

TABLE 2 Examples of currently available commercial assays incorporating the detection of endemic HCoVs[a]

Manufacturer	Product	Registration status for endemic-HCoV detection	Method	Platform(s)	Endemic HCoVs detected	Other targets detected	Approved specimen type(s)	Turnaround time
Genmark Dx	ePlex respiratory pathogen panel	CE-IVD, FDA	Single-cartridge combined digital microfluidic extraction and amplification with electrochemical detection	ePlex system (Genmark Dx)	229E, OC43, NL63, HKU1	AdV, hBoV, hMPV, RhV/EV, FA, FA H1, FA H1-2009, FA H3, FB, PIV 1/2/3/4, RSV A/B, MERS-CoV, *Bordetella pertussis*, *Legionella pneumophila*, *Mycoplasma pneumoniae*	NPS	Around 1.5 h, sample to answer
BioFire Diagnostics, bioMérieux[b]	FilmArray respiratory panel	CE-IVD, FDA, TGA	Single-pouch combined extraction and multiplex PCR with endpoint melting curve analysis	FilmArray multiplex PCR system	229E, OC43, NL63, HKU1	AdV, hMPV, RhV/EV, FA, FA H1, FA H1-2009, FA H3, FB, PIV 1/2/3/4, RSV, *B. pertussis*, *Chlamydophila pneumoniae*, *M. pneumoniae*	NPS	About 1 h, sample to answer
	FilmArray RP2plus	CE-IVD				All above plus MERS-CoV, *B. parapertussis*	NPS	Less than 45 min, sample to answer
Luminex Molecular Diagnostics	xTAG RVP Fast v2	CE-IVD	Multiplex PCR with suspension microarray detection	Luminex 100/200 or MAGPIX	229E, OC43, NL63, HKU1	FA, FA H1, FA H3, FA H1N1 2009,[c] FB, RSV A/B, PIV 1/2/3/4, hMPV, hBoV, RhV/EV, AdV	NPS, NPA, BAL	3 h from nucleic acid extraction
	NxTAG	CE-IVD, FDA		Luminex MAGPIX		All above plus *M. pneumoniae*, *C. pneumoniae*, *L. pneumophila*[d]	NPS	<3 h from nucleic acid extraction
PathoFinder	RespiFinder 2SMART	CE-IVD	Multiplex real-time PCR with melting curve analysis	LightCycler 480 (Roche), Rotor-Gene Q (Qiagen)	229E, OC43, NL63/HKU1	FA, FB, FA (H1N1) pdm09, RSV A/B, hMPV, RhV/EV, AdV, PIV 1/2/3/4, hBoV, *L. pneumophila*, *B. pertussis*, *M. pneumoniae*, *C. pneumoniae*	Not stated	2.5 h from nucleic acid extraction
	RespiFinder 22	CE-IVD	Multitube multiplex endpoint PCR with detection by size fragment analysis	ABI 3500 Genetic Analyzer (Applied Biosystems)	229E, OC43, NL63, HKU1	FA, FB, FA (H1N1) pdm09, RSV A/B, hMPV, RhV/EV, AdV, PIV 1/2/3/4, hBoV, *L. pneumophila*, *B. pertussis*, *M. pneumoniae*, *C. pneumoniae*	Not stated	6 h from nucleic acid extraction
	RealAccurate Quadruplex respiratory PCR	CE-IVD	Multitube multiplex real-time PCR	LightCycler 480 (Roche), Rotor-Gene Q (Qiagen)	229E, OC43, NL63/HKU1	FA, FB, FA (H1N1) pdm09, RSV A/B, hMPV A/B, RhV/EV, AdV, PIV 1/2/3/4, hBoV, *L. pneumophila*, *B. pertussis*, *M. pneumoniae*, *C. pneumoniae*	NPS	2 h from nucleic acid extraction

(*Continued on next page*)

TABLE 2 Examples of currently available commercial assays incorporating the detection of endemic HCoVs[a]

Manufacturer	Product	Registration status for endemic-HCoV detection	Method	Platform(s)	Endemic HCoVs detected	Other targets detected	Approved specimen type(s)	Turnaround time
Fast-Track Diagnostics	FTD respiratory pathogens 33/21/21 plus	CE-IVD	Multitube multiplex real-time PCR	AB7500 / 7500 Fast (Life Technologies), Rotor-Gene 3000/6000/Q (Qiagen), CFX96 / DX with CFX software (Bio-Rad), LightCycler 480 (Roche), SmartCycler with Life Science software 2.0d (Cepheid)	229E, OC43, NL63, HKU1	FA, FA H1N1, FB, FC,[e] RhV, PIV 1/2/3/4, hMPV A/B, hBoV, *M. pneumoniae*, RSV A/B, AdV, EV, PeV, *C. pneumoniae*,[f] *Staphylococcus aureus*,[f] *Streptococcus pneumoniae*,[f] *Haemophilus influenzae* type B,[f] *H. influenzae*,[e] *Pneumocystis jirovecii*,[e] *Bordetella* spp.,[e] *Moraxella catarrhalis*,[e] *Klebsiella pneumoniae*,[e] *L. pneumophila*-*L. longbeachae*,[e] *Salmonella* spp.[e]	Nasal/throat swabs, BAL, sputum	Not stated
Seegene	Seeplex RV15 ACE and RV15 one-step ACE	CE-IVD, Health Canada-IVD	Multitube multiplex endpoint PCR with detection by size fragment analysis	MultiNA (Shimadzu), Caliper LabChip Dx (Caliper Life Sciences)	229E/ NL63, OC43	FA, FB, RSV A/B, hMPV, AdV, RhV A/B/C, EV, hBoV 1/2/3/4, PIV 1/2/3/4	NPS, NPA, BAL	Not stated
	Anyplex II RV16 detection	CE-IVD	Multitube multiplex real-time PCR with melting curve analysis	CFX96 (Bio-Rad)	229E, NL63, OC43	FA, FB, RSV A/B, hMPV, AdV, RhV A/B/C, EV, hBoV 1/2/3/4, PIV 1/2/3/4	NPS, NPA, BAL	Not stated
	Allplex respiratory panel assay	CE-IVD	Multitube multiplex real-time PCR	CFX96 (Bio-Rad)	229E, NL63, OC43	FA, FA H1, FA H3, FA H1pdm09, FB, RSV A/B, hMPV, AdV, RhV A/B/C, EV, hBoV, PIV 1/2/3/4, *M. pneumoniae*, *C. pneumoniae*, *L. pneumophila*, *B. pertussis*, *B. parapertussis*, *S. pneumoniae*, *H. influenzae*	NPS, NPA, BAL	4.5 h from nucleic acid extraction
AutoGenomics	Infiniti RVP Plus	CE-IVD	Low-density microarray	Infiniti Plus Analyzer	229E, OC43, NL63, HKU1	FA, FA swine H1N1, FB, PIV 1/2/3/4, RhV A/B, EV A/B/C/D, hMPV A/B, RSV A/B, AdV A/B/C/E	NPA	Not stated
Qiagen	RespiFinder RG panel	CE-IVD	Multiplex real-time PCR with melting curve analysis	Rotor-Gene Q (Qiagen)	229E, OC43, NL63, HKU1	FA, FA H1N1v, FB, RSV A/B, hMPV, AdV, RhV/ EV, hBoV, PIV 1/2/3/4, *M. pneumoniae*, *C. pneumoniae*, *L. pneumophila*, *B. pertussis*	NPS	Not stated
Genomica	CLART PneumoVir 2	CE-IVD	Endpoint multiplex PCR with detection by low-density microarray	Clinical array reader (Genomica)	229E, OC43, NL63	AdV, hMPV A/B, PIV 1/2/3/4a/4b, RhV, RSV A/B, hBoV, EV, FA H1N1, FA H3N2, FA H1N1/2009, FA H7N9, FB, FC	NPW, NPS, BAL	Within a working day

[a]Abbreviations: FA, influenza A virus; FB, influenza B virus; FC, influenza C virus; PIV, parainfluenza virus; RSV, respiratory syncytial virus; AdV, adenovirus; hMPV, human metapneumovirus; RhV, rhinovirus; hBoV, human bocavirus; EV, enterovirus; PeV, parechovirus; CMV, cytomegalovirus; NPS, nasopharyngeal swab; NPW, nasopharyngeal wash; BAL, bronchoalveolar lavage fluid.

[b]Outside the United States, BioFire RP2 has MERS-CoV with no restrictions for testing; in the United States, RP2Plus has MERS-CoV with the limitation that it can be used only for persons with risk factors for MERS-CoV.

[c]RVP Fast v2 only.

[d]CE-IVD only.

[e]FTD 33 only.

[f]FTD 33 and 21 plus only.

SARS-CoV Detection

Both in-house real-time and nested RT-PCR assays targeting the polymerase (replicase ORF1b gene) became available for SARS-CoV soon after the virus was first identified, along with synthetic transcripts to act as positive control material and to enable quantification (33, 34, 36, 37). Later, other NAATs targeting the polymerase and N genes became available, and assays were revised to increase sensitivity of detection, particularly in the first week of illness (141). Isothermal NAATs such as nucleic acid sequence-based amplification and LAMP assays were also described (142), and commercial assays were developed with variable clinical sensitivities and specificities compared to RT-PCR and serology (143, 144). Pan-CoV assays that also detect SARS-CoV are available, but species-specific NAATs are preferred for first-line screening tests (145). A detailed review of NAATs for SARS-CoV, including a comparison of oligonucleotide sequences and assay performance, has been published elsewhere (143).

MERS-CoV Detection

An in-house real-time PCR assay based on a target upstream of the envelope protein (upE) was quickly available for MERS-CoV, along with an alternative but less sensitive real-time PCR assay based on the ORF1b gene and positive control transcripts (146). A real-time RT-PCR assay based on ORF1a was later demonstrated to have higher sensitivity than one based on ORF1b (147). In June 2013, the FDA authorized the emergency use of a real-time RT-PCR assay panel targeting the N and upE genes as an *in vitro* diagnostic test for MERS-CoV (148). Since then, a number of other in-house and commercial real-time RT-PCR assays, along with isothermal methods, have been described, with limited comparative studies (130, 149–153). Currently, the WHO recommends the use of upE assays for initial screening in potential MERS-CoV cases, with confirmation by ORF1a, ORF1b, or N assays (119). If these assays are negative, sequencing of the N or polymerase genes can aid in confirmation (147).

ISOLATION PROCEDURES

Isolation of HCoVs is not effective as a routine diagnostic tool, because many commonly used cell lines are not permissive for growth or do not show obvious cytopathic effect (CPE). CPE is generally nonspecific, and reagents for immunofluorescent detection in culture are not widely available. The use of RT-PCR to detect HCoV in cell culture supernatant has been described, but it may be more efficient in a routine context to carry out NAATs directly on the specimen. HCoV-229E was isolated originally in human embryonic kidney cells but later propagated in a number of human embryonic lung fibroblast cell lines, such as WI-28, L132, and MRC-5 (29, 66, 90, 125, 135, 154). HCoV-OC43 was originally isolated in human embryonic tracheal organ cultures (30) and later adapted to suckling mouse brain and then to cell culture in lines including HRT-18, RD, and HEL (125, 134, 135, 155). HCoV-NL63 was originally isolated in tertiary monkey kidney cells and subsequently propagated in Vero and LLC-MK2 monkey kidney epithelial cell lines (40). Although some reports described HCoV-NL63 CPE by day 4 or 5 of inoculation (Fig. 3), other studies have found low viral titers with slowly developing CPE and with difficulty in sustaining growth (40, 128, 155, 156). HCoV-NL63 growth appears to be more efficient in CaCo-2 cell lines, and this has enabled the development of a cytopathogenic plaque assay (155).

The continuous epithelial cell line HuH7 has been demonstrated to be permissive for HCoV-229E, HCoV-OC43, and HCoV-NL63 (72, 128, 157). However, HCoV-HKU1 has not yet been propagated in any common cell line (41). All four HCoVs, including HCoV-HKU1, were recently successfully propagated on primary human bronchial epithelial cells subpassaged to form pseudostratified human airway epithelial cell cultures (158, 159). In this system, HCoV-NL63 was still difficult to isolate and there was no visible CPE for any of the viruses. HCoV-HKU1 has also now been serially propagated in primary human alveolar type II cells (160). SARS-CoV grows in Vero and fetal rhesus kidney (FRhK-4) cells, and in contrast to other HCoVs, focal CPE occurs and rapidly spreads across the monolayer within 2 to 6 days (33, 34, 37). Human cell lines such as HuH7, HEK-293, and Hep-G2 are also permissive for SARS-CoV infection (161). MERS-CoV was originally isolated in LLC-MK2 and Vero B4 cells (43); however, isolation appears to be more successful in Caco-2 cells (162), and the virus is capable of infecting a wide range of cell lines, including those from primates, pigs, goats, and bats. Inadvertent isolation of a novel CoV in cell culture is therefore a possibility, so where there is a suspicion of SARS-CoV, MERS-CoV, or other novel CoV infection, virus isolation should not be attempted without BSL3 facilities and procedures. NAATs should be used as a first-line test, because they involve virus inactivation. Accidental transmission of SARS-CoV to laboratory workers has been described.

SEROLOGIC TESTS

Serological testing for diagnosis of the endemic HCoVs has largely been replaced by more sensitive and specific NAATs. However, serology is useful in epidemiological studies, enhancing our understanding of HCoV infection and aiding the investigation of outbreaks. It has been particularly important in the diagnosis of cases of novel and emerging HCoVs, such SARS-CoV and MERS-CoV. In these situations, affected patients may not test positive for viral RNA, particularly in the early phase of disease, but retrospectively can be shown to have developed an immune response. The use of viral lysate antigens in ELISA-based serological assays requires propagation of the CoVs to high titers, which is difficult for HCoV-NL63 and not possible for HCoV-HKU1 without primary cultures. Furthermore, serological assays may lack specificity due to the antigenic relatedness among HCoVs, particularly between the alphacoronaviruses HCoV-229E and HCoV-NL63 and between the betacoronaviruses HCoV-OC43 and HCoV-HKU1.

The viral nucleocapsid protein N induces a good immune response, and recombinant N protein has been widely used in ELISA-based assays, as it can be readily expressed and purified without the need for viral culture. Unfortunately, cross-reactivity of serological assays using the full-length or truncated N protein has been reported, particularly between HCoVs of the same genus (68, 71, 163). However, the carboxy-terminal region of the N protein appears to be significantly less homologous between HCoVs, and recombinant N protein-based ELISAs utilizing this region have been successfully developed for all four endemic HCoVs (51, 68, 71). This may be at the expense of some sensitivity, though, as the carboxy-terminal region of the HCoV-OC43 N protein was recently demonstrated to be less immunogenic than the central region (164). The use of recombinant S protein-based ELISAs for HCoV-HKU1 has also been reported (70). The difficulty in culturing some HCoVs is an obstacle to the development of neutralization assays; however, neutralization assays using S-pseudotyped HCoV-HKU1 and HCoV-NL63 viruses can circumvent this problem (70, 72).

As with other HCoVs, most serological assays for SARS-CoV were initially based on antibody detection in acute- and convalescent-phase sera by IFA using fixed infected cells and by ELISA using lysates from cell culture (34, 36). Recombinant N protein-based ELISAs were then developed to remove the requirement for BSL3 containment, with confirmation by Western blots targeting antibodies to both the N and S proteins. Neutralization assays also required cultivation of SARS-CoV and were less practical for routine diagnosis. A number of in-house and commercial serological tests for MERS-CoV have been described, but few have been directly compared; these include protein microarrays, ELISA, whole-virus- and recombinant protein-based IFA, microneutralization, plaque reduction neutralization, and S pseudoparticle neutralization tests, which have the advantage of not requiring live virus (165). However, a recent comparative study showed good correlation between a number of different neutralization tests, including pseudoparticle neutralization tests, and acceptable performance of a commercial S antigen-based ELISA (166). According to current WHO guidance on MERS-CoV, a patient with evidence of seroconversion in at least one screening assay (e.g., ELISA or IFA) and confirmation by a neutralization assay in samples ideally taken at least 14 days apart is considered a confirmed case (119). The use of neutralization tests is advisable to confirm screening results due to cross-reactivity with endemic HCoVs.

EVALUATION, INTERPRETATION, AND REPORTING OF RESULTS

The cornerstone of management of all HCoV infections is the rapid diagnosis of affected individuals, because symptoms may be similar to those caused by other respiratory pathogens. Accurate and timely diagnosis aids surveillance, ensures that appropriate infection control and public health procedures are instigated, and contributes to antibiotic stewardship by providing a viral diagnosis. The generation of a diagnostic test result in which the laboratory and the end user can feel confident requires, among other things, the proper development and validation of HCoV diagnostic tests. Comprehensive guidelines for the development and validation of NAATs are available (167, 168). Participation in internal and external quality assurance (EQA) programs is also essential. Performance in the detection of HCoV by NAATs has been shown to vary between laboratories using Quality Control for Molecular Diagnostics EQA panels (169, 170). EQA enables comparison of proficiency with other diagnostic laboratories and identification of problems with sensitivity and specificity. This is particularly relevant for NAATs, in which ongoing sequence variation in viral RNA genomes, reaction inhibition, and potential contamination are specific challenges. CoV NAATs should be frequently assessed in the light of new sequence information for their ability to detect new viral variants. Furthermore, the use of internal controls added at the specimen extraction stage, which are copurified with viral RNA and are detected by NAAT alongside the HCoV gene target(s), is essential for the detection of RT-PCR inhibition. Finally, the use of good laboratory practice when molecular amplification assays are performed is crucial, and readers are directed to guidance on this subject (168, 171).

It is particularly important in the case of novel or emerging HCoVs, such as SARS-CoV and MERS-CoV, that nationally or internationally agreed-upon protocols for specimen collection, handling, testing, and reporting be followed, including the confirmation of positive diagnostic test results at designated reference laboratories and the involvement of public health specialists (119). Errors in the interpretation and reporting of results can have particularly significant adverse consequences in this context. The rapid reaction of the international diagnostic laboratory community to the emergence of SARS-CoV was mirrored in the recent response to MERS-CoV. In a matter of days after notification of the first case of MERS-CoV, an internationally coordinated effort had produced validated NAATs, which were then widely deployed in specialist laboratories (172). This was a testament to the effectiveness of collaborative international laboratory networks, although standardization and quality control of tests for emerging CoVs are key factors that must be adequately managed in the roll-out process (173). In these situations, the development of commercial tests lags behind because of the regulatory approval process, illustrating the importance of maintaining in-house molecular expertise in diagnostic virology laboratories. The widespread occurrence of CoV in mammals and birds and the potential for interspecies transmission events emphasize the need to be vigilant for the emergence of further human-pathogenic CoVs in the future.

In summary, the four endemic HCoVs make up a small but significant proportion of the viruses found in patients with ARI. Including HCoVs alongside the more common respiratory viruses, such as influenza virus, respiratory syncytial virus, and adenovirus, in diagnostic screening panels will increase the diagnostic pickup rate in ARI, particularly in a pediatric setting. It will also help to further our understanding of the role of HCoVs in respiratory infection.

REFERENCES

1. **Adams MJ, Carstens EB.** 2012. Ratification vote on taxonomic proposals to the International Committee on Taxonomy of Viruses (2012). *Arch Virol* **157:**1411–1422.
2. **de Groot RJ, Baker SC, Baric RS, Enjuanes L, Gorbalenya AE, Holmes KV, Perlman S, Poon L, Rottier PJM, Talbot PJ, Woo PCY, Ziebuhr J.** 2012. Family Coronaviridae, p 806–828. *In* King AMQ, Adams MJ, Carstens EB, Lefkowitz EJ (ed), *Virus Taxonomy: The Ninth Report of the International Committee on Taxonomy of Viruses.* Academic Press, San Diego, CA.
3. **de Groot RJ, Baker SC, Baric RS, Brown CS, Drosten C, Enjuanes L, Fouchier RA, Galiano M, Gorbalenya AE, Memish ZA, Perlman S, Poon LL, Snijder EJ, Stephens GM, Woo PC, Zaki AM, Zambon M, Ziebuhr J.** 2013. Middle East respiratory syndrome coronavirus (MERS-CoV): announcement of the Coronavirus Study Group. *J Virol* **87:**7790–7792.
4. **van Boheemen S, de Graaf M, Lauber C, Bestebroer TM, Raj VS, Zaki AM, Osterhaus AD, Haagmans BL, Gorbalenya AE, Snijder EJ, Fouchier RA.** 2012. Genomic characterization of a newly discovered coronavirus associated with acute respiratory distress syndrome in humans. *mBio* **3:**e00473-12.
5. **Woo PC, Lau SK, Lam CS, Lai KK, Huang Y, Lee P, Luk GS, Dyrting KC, Chan KH, Yuen KY.** 2009. Comparative analysis of complete genome sequences of three avian coronaviruses reveals a novel group 3c coronavirus. *J Virol* **83:**908–917.
6. **Woo PC, Lau SK, Lam CS, Lau CC, Tsang AK, Lau JH, Bai R, Teng JL, Tsang CC, Wang M, Zheng BJ, Chan KH, Yuen KY.** 2012. Discovery of seven novel mammalian and avian coronaviruses in the genus *Deltacoronavirus* supports bat coronaviruses as the gene source of *Alphacoronavirus* and *Betacoronavirus* and avian coronaviruses as the gene source of *Gammacoronavirus* and *Deltacoronavirus*. *J Virol* **86:**3995–4008.

7. **Fehr AR, Perlman S.** 2015. Coronaviruses: an overview of their replication and pathogenesis. *Methods Mol Biol* **1282:** 1–23.
8. **Raj VS, Mou H, Smits SL, Dekkers DH, Müller MA, Dijkman R, Muth D, Demmers JA, Zaki A, Fouchier RA, Thiel V, Drosten C, Rottier PJ, Osterhaus AD, Bosch BJ, Haagmans BL.** 2013. Dipeptidyl peptidase 4 is a functional receptor for the emerging human coronavirus-EMC. *Nature* **495:**251–254.
9. **Dijkman R, van der Hoek L.** 2009. Human coronaviruses 229E and NL63: close yet still so far. *J Formos Med Assoc* **108:**270–279.
10. **Huynh J, Li S, Yount B, Smith A, Sturges L, Olsen JC, Nagel J, Johnson JB, Agnihothram S, Gates JE, Frieman MB, Baric RS, Donaldson EF.** 2012. Evidence supporting a zoonotic origin of human coronavirus strain NL63. *J Virol* **86:** 12816–12825.
11. **Corman VM, Baldwin HJ, Tateno AF, Zerbinati RM, Annan A, Owusu M, Nkrumah EE, Maganga GD, Oppong S, Adu-Sarkodie Y, Vallo P, da Silva Filho LV, Leroy EM, Thiel V, van der Hoek L, Poon LL, Tschapka M, Drosten C, Drexler JF.** 2015. Evidence for an ancestral association of human coronavirus 229E with bats. *J Virol* **89:** 11858–11870.
12. **Corman VM, Eckerle I, Memish ZA, Liljander AM, Dijkman R, Jonsdottir H, Juma Ngeiywa KJ, Kamau E, Younan M, Al Masri M, Assiri A, Gluecks I, Musa BE, Meyer B, Müller MA, Hilali M, Bornstein S, Wernery U, Thiel V, Jores J, Drexler JF, Drosten C.** 2016. Link of a ubiquitous human coronavirus to dromedary camels. *Proc Natl Acad Sci USA* **113:**9864–9869.
13. **Vijgen L, Keyaerts E, Lemey P, Maes P, van Reeth K, Nauwynck H, Pensaert M, van Ranst M.** 2006. Evolutionary history of the closely related group 2 coronaviruses: porcine hemagglutinating encephalomyelitis virus, bovine coronavirus, and human coronavirus OC43. *J Virol* **80:** 7270–7274.
14. **Oong XY, Ng KT, Takebe Y, Ng LJ, Chan KG, Chook JB, Kamarulzaman A, Tee KK.** 2017. Identification and evolutionary dynamics of two novel human coronavirus OC43 genotypes associated with acute respiratory infections: phylogenetic, spatiotemporal and transmission network analyses. *Emerg Microbes Infect* **4:**e3.
15. **Woo PC, Lau SK, Yip CC, Huang Y, Yuen KY.** 2009. More and more coronaviruses: human coronavirus HKU1. *Viruses* **1:** 57–71.
16. **Lau SK, Woo PC, Li KS, Tsang AK, Fan RY, Luk HK, Cai JP, Chan KH, Zheng BJ, Wang M, Yuen KY.** 2015. Discovery of a novel coronavirus, China *Rattus* coronavirus HKU24, from Norway rats supports the murine origin of *Betacoronavirus 1* and has implications for the ancestor of *Betacoronavirus* lineage A. *J Virol* **89:**3076–3092.
17. **Li W, Shi Z, Yu M, Ren W, Smith C, Epstein JH, Wang H, Crameri G, Hu Z, Zhang H, Zhang J, McEachern J, Field H, Daszak P, Eaton BT, Zhang S, Wang LF.** 2005. Bats are natural reservoirs of SARS-like coronaviruses. *Science* **310:** 676–679.
18. **Ge XY, Li JL, Yang XL, Chmura AA, Zhu G, Epstein JH, Mazet JK, Hu B, Zhang W, Peng C, Zhang YJ, Luo CM, Tan B, Wang N, Zhu Y, Crameri G, Zhang SY, Wang LF, Daszak P, Shi ZL.** 2013. Isolation and characterization of a bat SARS-like coronavirus that uses the ACE2 receptor. *Nature* **503:**535–538.
19. **Hu B, Ge X, Wang LF, Shi Z.** 2015. Bat origin of human coronaviruses. *Virol J* **12:**221.
20. **Wu Z, Yang L, Ren X, Zhang J, Yang F, Zhang S, Jin Q.** 2016. ORF8-related genetic evidence for Chinese horseshoe bats as the source of human severe acute respiratory syndrome coronavirus. *J Infect Dis* **213:**579–583.
21. **Corman VM, Ithete NL, Richards LR, Schoeman MC, Preiser W, Drosten C, Drexler JF.** 2014. Rooting the phylogenetic tree of Middle East respiratory syndrome coronavirus by characterization of a conspecific virus from an African bat. *J Virol* **88:**11297–11303.
22. **Anthony SJ, Gilardi K, Menachery VD, Goldstein T, Ssebide B, Mbabazi R, Navarrete-Macias I, Liang E, Wells H, Hicks A, Petrosov A, Byarugaba DK, Debbink K, Dinnon KH, Scobey T, Randell SH, Yount BL, Cranfield M, Johnson CK, Baric RS, Lipkin WI, Mazet JA.** 2017. Further evidence for bats as the evolutionary source of Middle East respiratory syndrome coronavirus. *MBio* **8:**e00373-17.
23. **Reusken CB, Haagmans BL, Müller MA, Gutierrez C, Godeke GJ, Meyer B, Muth D, Raj VS, Smits-De Vries L, Corman VM, Drexler JF, Smits SL, El Tahir YE, De Sousa R, van Beek J, Nowotny N, van Maanen K, Hidalgo-Hermoso E, Bosch BJ, Rottier P, Osterhaus A, Gortázar-Schmidt C, Drosten C, Koopmans MP.** 2013. Middle East respiratory syndrome coronavirus neutralising serum antibodies in dromedary camels: a comparative serological study. *Lancet Infect Dis* **13:**859–866.
24. **Haagmans BL, Al Dhahiry SH, Reusken CB, Raj VS, Galiano M, Myers R, Godeke GJ, Jonges M, Farag E, Diab A, Ghobashy H, Alhajri F, Al-Thani M, Al-Marri SA, Al Romaihi HE, Al Khal A, Bermingham A, Osterhaus AD, AlHajri MM, Koopmans MP.** 2014. Middle East respiratory syndrome coronavirus in dromedary camels: an outbreak investigation. *Lancet Infect Dis* **14:**140–145.
25. **Azhar EI, El-Kafrawy SA, Farraj SA, Hassan AM, Al-Saeed MS, Hashem AM, Madani TA.** 2014. Evidence for camel-to-human transmission of MERS coronavirus. *N Engl J Med* **370:**2499–2505.
26. **Mohd HA, Al-Tawfiq JA, Memish ZA.** 2016. Middle East respiratory syndrome coronavirus (MERS-CoV) origin and animal reservoir. *Virol J* **13:**87.
27. **Cotten M, Watson SJ, Kellam P, Al-Rabeeah AA, Makhdoom HQ, Assiri A, Al-Tawfiq JA, Alhakeem RF, Madani H, AlRabiah FA, Al Hajjar S, Al-nassir WN, Albarrak A, Flemban H, Balkhy HH, Alsubaie S, Palser AL, Gall A, Bashford-Rogers R, Rambaut A, Zumla AI, Memish ZA.** 2013. Transmission and evolution of the Middle East respiratory syndrome coronavirus in Saudi Arabia: a descriptive genomic study. *Lancet* **382:**1993–2002.
28. **Sabir JS, Lam TT, Ahmed MM, Li L, Shen Y, Abo-Aba SE, Qureshi MI, Abu-Zeid M, Zhang Y, Khiyami MA, Alharbi NS, Hajrah NH, Sabir MJ, Mutwakil MH, Kabli SA, Alsulaimany FA, Obaid AY, Zhou B, Smith DK, Holmes EC, Zhu H, Guan Y.** 2016. Co-circulation of three camel coronavirus species and recombination of MERS-CoVs in Saudi Arabia. *Science* **351:**81–84.
29. **Hamre D, Procknow JJ.** 1966. A new virus isolated from the human respiratory tract. *Proc Soc Exp Biol Med* **121:**190–193.
30. **McIntosh K, Dees JH, Becker WB, Kapikian AZ, Chanock RM.** 1967. Recovery in tracheal organ cultures of novel viruses from patients with respiratory disease. *Proc Natl Acad Sci USA* **57:**933–940.
31. **Tyrrell DA, Bynoe ML.** 1965. Cultivation of a novel type of common-cold virus in organ cultures. *BMJ* **1:**1467–1470.
32. **Brucková M, McIntosh K, Kapikian AZ, Chanock RM.** 1970. The adaptation of two human coronavirus strains (OC38 and OC43) to growth in cell monolayers. *Proc Soc Exp Biol Med* **135:**431–435.
33. **Drosten C, Günther S, Preiser W, van der Werf S, Brodt HR, Becker S, Rabenau H, Panning M, Kolesnikova L, Fouchier RA, Berger A, Burguière AM, Cinatl J, Eickmann M, Escriou N, Grywna K, Kramme S, Manuguerra JC, Müller S, Rickerts V, Stürmer M, Vieth S, Klenk HD, Osterhaus AD, Schmitz H, Doerr HW.** 2003. Identification of a novel coronavirus in patients with severe acute respiratory syndrome. *N Engl J Med* **348:**1967–1976.
34. **Ksiazek TG, Erdman D, Goldsmith CS, Zaki SR, Peret T, Emery S, Tong S, Urbani C, Comer JA, Lim W, Rollin PE, Dowell SF, Ling AE, Humphrey CD, Shieh WJ, Guarner J, Paddock CD, Rota P, Fields B, DeRisi J, Yang JY, Cox N, Hughes JM, LeDuc JW, Bellini WJ, Anderson LJ, SARS Working Group.** 2003. A novel coronavirus associated with severe acute respiratory syndrome. *N Engl J Med* **348:** 1953–1966.

35. **Marra MA, et al.** 2003. The genome sequence of the SARS-associated coronavirus. *Science* **300:**1399–1404.
36. **Peiris JS, Lai ST, Poon LL, Guan Y, Yam LY, Lim W, Nicholls J, Yee WK, Yan WW, Cheung MT, Cheng VC, Chan KH, Tsang DN, Yung RW, Ng TK, Yuen KY, SARS Study Group.** 2003. Coronavirus as a possible cause of severe acute respiratory syndrome. *Lancet* **361:**1319–1325.
37. **Poutanen SM, Low DE, Henry B, Finkelstein S, Rose D, Green K, Tellier R, Draker R, Adachi D, Ayers M, Chan AK, Skowronski DM, Salit I, Simor AE, Slutsky AS, Doyle PW, Krajden M, Petric M, Brunham RC, McGeer AJ, National Microbiology Laboratory, Canada; Canadian Severe Acute Respiratory Syndrome Study Team.** 2003. Identification of severe acute respiratory syndrome in Canada. *N Engl J Med* **348:**1995–2005.
38. **Rota PA, Oberste MS, Monroe SS, Nix WA, Campagnoli R, Icenogle JP, Peñaranda S, Bankamp B, Maher K, Chen MH, Tong S, Tamin A, Lowe L, Frace M, DeRisi JL, Chen Q, Wang D, Erdman DD, Peret TC, Burns C, Ksiazek TG, Rollin PE, Sanchez A, Liffick S, Holloway B, Limor J, McCaustland K, Olsen-Rasmussen M, Fouchier R, Günther S, Osterhaus AD, Drosten C, Pallansch MA, Anderson LJ, Bellini WJ.** 2003. Characterization of a novel coronavirus associated with severe acute respiratory syndrome. *Science* **300:**1394–1399.
39. **Fouchier RA, Kuiken T, Schutten M, van Amerongen G, van Doornum GJ, van den Hoogen BG, Peiris M, Lim W, Stöhr K, Osterhaus AD.** 2003. Aetiology: Koch's postulates fulfilled for SARS virus. *Nature* **423:**240.
40. **van der Hoek L, Pyrc K, Jebbink MF, Vermeulen-Oost W, Berkhout RJ, Wolthers KC, Wertheim-van Dillen PM, Kaandorp J, Spaargaren J, Berkhout B.** 2004. Identification of a new human coronavirus. *Nat Med* **10:**368–373.
41. **Woo PC, Lau SK, Chu CM, Chan KH, Tsoi HW, Huang Y, Wong BH, Poon RW, Cai JJ, Luk WK, Poon LL, Wong SS, Guan Y, Peiris JS, Yuen KY.** 2005. Characterization and complete genome sequence of a novel coronavirus, coronavirus HKU1, from patients with pneumonia. *J Virol* **79:**884–895.
42. **Talbot HK, Shepherd BE, Crowe JE Jr, Griffin MR, Edwards KM, Podsiad AB, Tollefson SJ, Wright PF, Williams JV.** 2009. The pediatric burden of human coronaviruses evaluated for twenty years. *Pediatr Infect Dis J* **28:**682–687.
43. **Zaki AM, van Boheemen S, Bestebroer TM, Osterhaus AD, Fouchier RA.** 2012. Isolation of a novel coronavirus from a man with pneumonia in Saudi Arabia. *N Engl J Med* **367:**1814–1820.
44. **Munster VJ, de Wit E, Feldmann H.** 2013. Pneumonia from human coronavirus in a macaque model. *N Engl J Med* **368:**1560–1562.
45. **Cabeça TK, Granato C, Bellei N.** 2013. Epidemiological and clinical features of human coronavirus infections among different subsets of patients. *Influenza Other Respir Viruses* **7:**1040–1047.
46. **Gaunt ER, Hardie A, Claas EC, Simmonds P, Templeton KE.** 2010. Epidemiology and clinical presentations of the four human coronaviruses 229E, HKU1, NL63, and OC43 detected over 3 years using a novel multiplex real-time PCR method. *J Clin Microbiol* **48:**2940–2947.
47. **Lu R, Yu X, Wang W, Duan X, Zhang L, Zhou W, Xu J, Xu L, Hu Q, Lu J, Ruan L, Wang Z, Tan W.** 2012. Characterization of human coronavirus etiology in Chinese adults with acute upper respiratory tract infection by real-time RT-PCR assays. *PLoS One* **7:**e38638.
48. **Mackay IM, Arden KE, Speicher DJ, O'Neil NT, McErlean PK, Greer RM, Nissen MD, Sloots TP.** 2012. Co-circulation of four human coronaviruses (HCoVs) in Queensland children with acute respiratory tract illnesses in 2004. *Viruses* **4:**637–653.
49. **Prill MM, Iwane MK, Edwards KM, Williams JV, Weinberg GA, Staat MA, Willby MJ, Talbot HK, Hall CB, Szilagyi PG, Griffin MR, Curns AT, Erdman DD, New Vaccine Surveillance Network.** 2012. Human coronavirus in young children hospitalized for acute respiratory illness and asymptomatic controls. *Pediatr Infect Dis J* **31:**235–240.
50. **Buecher C, Mardy S, Wang W, Duong V, Vong S, Naughtin M, Vabret A, Freymuth F, Deubel V, Buchy P.** 2010. Use of a multiplex PCR/RT-PCR approach to assess the viral causes of influenza-like illnesses in Cambodia during three consecutive dry seasons. *J Med Virol* **82:**1762–1772.
51. **Dijkman R, Jebbink MF, Gaunt E, Rossen JW, Templeton KE, Kuijpers TW, van der Hoek L.** 2012. The dominance of human coronavirus OC43 and NL63 infections in infants. *J Clin Virol* **53:**135–139.
52. **Regamey N, Kaiser L, Roiha HL, Deffernez C, Kuehni CE, Latzin P, Aebi C, Frey U, Swiss Paediatric Respiratory Research Group.** 2008. Viral etiology of acute respiratory infections with cough in infancy: a community-based birth cohort study. *Pediatr Infect Dis J* **27:**100–105.
53. **Ren L, Gonzalez R, Xu J, Xiao Y, Li Y, Zhou H, Li J, Yang Q, Zhang J, Chen L, Wang W, Vernet G, Paranhos-Baccalà G, Wang Z, Wang J.** 2011. Prevalence of human coronaviruses in adults with acute respiratory tract infections in Beijing, China. *J Med Virol* **83:**291–297.
54. **van der Zalm MM, Uiterwaal CS, Wilbrink B, de Jong BM, Verheij TJ, Kimpen JL, van der Ent CK.** 2009. Respiratory pathogens in respiratory tract illnesses during the first year of life: a birth cohort study. *Pediatr Infect Dis J* **28:**472–476.
55. **Zlateva KT, Coenjaerts FE, Crusio KM, Lammens C, Leus F, Viveen M, Ieven M, Spaan WJ, Claas EC, Gorbalenya AE.** 2013. No novel coronaviruses identified in a large collection of human nasopharyngeal specimens using family-wide CODEHOP-based primers. *Arch Virol* **158:**251–255.
56. **Nickbakhsh S, Thorburn F, Von Wissmann B, McMenamin J, Gunson RN, Murcia PR.** 2016. Extensive multiplex PCR diagnostics reveal new insights into the epidemiology of viral respiratory infections. *Epidemiol Infect* **144:**2064–2076.
57. **Yip CC, Lam CS, Luk HK, Wong EY, Lee RA, So LY, Chan KH, Cheng VC, Yuen KY, Woo PC, Lau SK.** 2016. A six-year descriptive epidemiological study of human coronavirus infections in hospitalized patients in Hong Kong. *Virol Sin* **31:**41–48.
58. **Dominguez SR, Shrivastava S, Berglund A, Qian Z, Góes LG, Halpin RA, Fedorova N, Ransier A, Weston PA, Durigon EL, Jerez JA, Robinson CC, Town CD, Holmes KV.** 2014. Isolation, propagation, genome analysis and epidemiology of HKU1 betacoronaviruses. *J Gen Virol* **95:**836–848.
59. **Lepiller Q, Barth H, Lefebvre F, Herbrecht R, Lutz P, Kessler R, Fafi-Kremer S, Stoll-Keller F.** 2013. High incidence but low burden of coronaviruses and preferential associations between respiratory viruses. *J Clin Microbiol* **51:**3039–3046.
60. **van Asten L, Bijkerk P, Fanoy E, van Ginkel A, Suijkerbuijk A, van der Hoek W, Meijer A, Vennema H.** 2016. Early occurrence of influenza A epidemics coincided with changes in occurrence of other respiratory virus infections. *Influenza Other Respir Viruses* **10:**14–26.
61. **Kaye HS, Dowdle WR.** 1975. Seroepidemiologic survey of coronavirus (strain 229E) infections in a population of children. *Am J Epidemiol* **101:**238–244.
62. **Kaye HS, Marsh HB, Dowdle WR.** 1971. Seroepidemiologic survey of coronavirus (strain OC 43) related infections in a children's population. *Am J Epidemiol* **94:**43–49.
63. **van der Hoek L, Ihorst G, Sure K, Vabret A, Dijkman R, de Vries M, Forster J, Berkhout B, Uberla K.** 2010. Burden of disease due to human coronavirus NL63 infections and periodicity of infection. *J Clin Virol* **48:**104–108.
64. **Monto AS, Lim SK.** 1974. The Tecumseh study of respiratory illness. VI. Frequency of and relationship between outbreaks of coronavirus infection. *J Infect Dis* **129:**271–276.
65. **Schmidt OW, Allan ID, Cooney MK, Foy HM, Fox JP.** 1986. Rises in titers of antibody to human coronaviruses OC43 and 229E in Seattle families during 1975-1979. *Am J Epidemiol* **123:**862–868.
66. **Callow KA, Parry HF, Sergeant M, Tyrrell DA.** 1990. The time course of the immune response to experimental coronavirus infection of man. *Epidemiol Infect* **105:**435–446.
67. **Dijkman R, Jebbink MF, El Idrissi NB, Pyrc K, Müller MA, Kuijpers TW, Zaaijer HL, van der Hoek L.** 2008. Human coronavirus NL63 and 229E seroconversion in children. *J Clin Microbiol* **46:**2368–2373

68. **Shao X, Guo X, Esper F, Weibel C, Kahn JS.** 2007. Seroepidemiology of group I human coronaviruses in children. *J Clin Virol* **40:**207–213.
69. **Gorse GJ, Patel GB, Vitale JN, O'Connor TZ.** 2010. Prevalence of antibodies to four human coronaviruses is lower in nasal secretions than in serum. *Clin Vaccine Immunol* **17:**1875–1880.
70. **Chan CM, Tse H, Wong SS, Woo PC, Lau SK, Chen L, Zheng BJ, Huang JD, Yuen KY.** 2009. Examination of seroprevalence of coronavirus HKU1 infection with S protein-based ELISA and neutralization assay against viral spike pseudotyped virus. *J Clin Virol* **45:**54–60.
71. **Blanchard EG, Miao C, Haupt TE, Anderson LJ, Haynes LM.** 2011. Development of a recombinant truncated nucleocapsid protein based immunoassay for detection of antibodies against human coronavirus OC43. *J Virol Methods* **177:**100–106.
72. **Hofmann H, Pyrc K, van der Hoek L, Geier M, Berkhout B, Pöhlmann S.** 2005. Human coronavirus NL63 employs the severe acute respiratory syndrome coronavirus receptor for cellular entry. *Proc Natl Acad Sci USA* **102:**7988–7993.
73. **Milano F, Campbell AP, Guthrie KA, Kuypers J, Englund JA, Corey L, Boeckh M.** 2010. Human rhinovirus and coronavirus detection among allogeneic hematopoietic stem cell transplantation recipients. *Blood* **115:**2088–2094.
74. **Resta S, Luby JP, Rosenfeld CR, Siegel JD.** 1985. Isolation and propagation of a human enteric coronavirus. *Science* **229:**978–981.
75. **Warnes SL, Little ZR, Keevil CW.** 2015. Human coronavirus 229E remains infectious on common touch surface materials. *mBio* **6:**e01697-15.
76. **Müller A, Tillmann RL, Müller A, Simon A, Schildgen O.** 2008. Stability of human metapneumovirus and human coronavirus NL63 on medical instruments and in the patient environment. *J Hosp Infect* **69:**406–408.
77. **Ijaz MK, Brunner AH, Sattar SA, Nair RC, Johnson-Lussenburg CM.** 1985. Survival characteristics of airborne human coronavirus 229E. *J Gen Virol* **66:**2743–2748.
78. **Birch CJ, Clothier HJ, Seccull A, Tran T, Catton MC, Lambert SB, Druce JD.** 2005. Human coronavirus OC43 causes influenza-like illness in residents and staff of aged-care facilities in Melbourne, Australia. *Epidemiol Infect* **133:**273–277.
79. **Song HD, et al.** 2005. Cross-host evolution of severe acute respiratory syndrome coronavirus in palm civet and human. *Proc Natl Acad Sci USA* **102:**2430–2435.
80. **Cheng PK, Wong DA, Tong LK, Ip SM, Lo AC, Lau CS, Yeung EY, Lim WW.** 2004. Viral shedding patterns of coronavirus in patients with probable severe acute respiratory syndrome. *Lancet* **363:**1699–1700.
81. **Hijawi B, Abdallat M, Sayaydeh A, Alqasrawi S, Haddadin A, Jaarour N, Alsheikh S, Alsanouri T.** 2013. Novel coronavirus infections in Jordan, April 2012: epidemiological findings from a retrospective investigation. *East Mediterr Health J* **19**(Suppl 1)**:**S12–S18.
82. **Müller MA, Meyer B, Corman VM, Al-Masri M, Turkestani A, Ritz D, Sieberg A, Aldabbagh S, Bosch BJ, Lattwein E, Alhakeem RF, Assiri AM, Albarrak AM, Al-Shangiti AM, Al-Tawfiq JA, Wikramaratna P, Alrabeeah AA, Drosten C, Memish ZA.** 2015. Presence of Middle East respiratory syndrome coronavirus antibodies in Saudi Arabia: a nationwide, cross-sectional, serological study. *Lancet Infect Dis* **15:**559–564.
83. **Alraddadi BM, Watson JT, Almarashi A, Abedi GR, Turkistani A, Sadran M, Housa A, Almazroa MA, Alraihan N, Banjar A, Albalawi E, Alhindi H, Choudhry AJ, Meiman JG, Paczkowski M, Curns A, Mounts A, Feikin DR, Marano N, Swerdlow DL, Gerber SI, Hajjeh R, Madani TA.** 2016. Risk factors for primary Middle East respiratory syndrome coronavirus illness in humans, Saudi Arabia, 2014. *Emerg Infect Dis* **22:**49–55.
84. **Memish ZA, Zumla AI, Al-Hakeem RF, Al-Rabeeah AA, Stephens GM.** 2013. Family cluster of Middle East respiratory syndrome coronavirus infections. *N Engl J Med* **368:**2487–2494. CORRECTION *N Engl J Med* **369:**587.
85. **Kim KH, Tandi TE, Choi JW, Moon JM, Kim MS.** 2017. Middle East respiratory syndrome coronavirus (MERS-CoV) outbreak in South Korea, 2015: epidemiology, characteristics and public health implications. *J Hosp Infect* **95:**207–213.
86. **Kim SW, Park JW, Jung HD, Yang JS, Park YS, Lee C, Kim KM, Lee KJ, Kwon D, Hur YJ, Choi BY, Ki M.** 2017. Risk factors for transmission of Middle East respiratory syndrome coronavirus infection during the 2015 outbreak in South Korea. *Clin Infect Dis* **64:**551–557.
87. **World Health Organization.** 2015. Infection prevention and control during health care for probable or confirmed cases of Middle East respiratory syndrome coronavirus (MERS-CoV) infection [WHO/MERS/IPC/15.1]. Interim guidance. Updated 4 June 2015. http://www.who.int/csr/disease/coronavirus_infections/ipc-mers-cov/en/
88. **Park SH, Kim WJ, Yoo JH, Choi JH.** 2016. Epidemiologic parameters of the Middle East respiratory syndrome outbreak in Korea, 2015. *Infect Chemother* **48:**108–117.
89. **Corman VM, Albarrak AM, Omrani AS, Albarrak MM, Farah ME, Almasri M, Muth D, Sieberg A, Meyer B, Assiri AM, Binger T, Steinhagen K, Lattwein E, Al-Tawfiq J, Müller MA, Drosten C, Memish ZA.** 2016. Viral shedding and antibody response in 37 patients with Middle East respiratory syndrome coronavirus infection. *Clin Infect Dis* **62:**477–483.
90. **Bradburne AF, Bynoe ML, Tyrrell DA.** 1967. Effects of a "new" human respiratory virus in volunteers. *BMJ* **3:**767–769.
91. **Bradburne AF, Somerset BA.** 1972. Coronative antibody titres in sera of healthy adults and experimentally infected volunteers. *J Hyg (Lond)* **70:**235–244.
92. **Sung JY, Lee HJ, Eun BW, Kim SH, Lee SY, Lee JY, Park KU, Choi EH.** 2010. Role of human coronavirus NL63 in hospitalized children with croup. *Pediatr Infect Dis J* **29:**822–826.
93. **van der Hoek L, Sure K, Ihorst G, Stang A, Pyrc K, Jebbink MF, Petersen G, Forster J, Berkhout B, Uberla K.** 2005. Croup is associated with the novel coronavirus NL63. *PLoS Med* **2:**e240.
94. **Wu PS, Chang LY, Berkhout B, van der Hoek L, Lu CY, Kao CL, Lee PI, Shao PL, Lee CY, Huang FY, Huang LM.** 2008. Clinical manifestations of human coronavirus NL63 infection in children in Taiwan. *Eur J Pediatr* **167:**75–80.
95. **Singleton RJ, Bulkow LR, Miernyk K, DeByle C, Pruitt L, Hummel KB, Bruden D, Englund JA, Anderson LJ, Lucher L, Holman RC, Hennessy TW.** 2010. Viral respiratory infections in hospitalized and community control children in Alaska. *J Med Virol* **82:**1282–1290.
96. **Rhedin S, Lindstrand A, Hjelmgren A, Ryd-Rinder M, Öhrmalm L, Tolfvenstam T, Örtqvist Å, Rotzén-Östlund M, Zweygberg-Wirgart B, Henriques-Normark B, Broliden K, Naucler P.** 2015. Respiratory viruses associated with community-acquired pneumonia in children: matched case-control study. *Thorax* **70:**847–853.
97. **Kuypers J, Martin ET, Heugel J, Wright N, Morrow R, Englund JA.** 2007. Clinical disease in children associated with newly described coronavirus subtypes. *Pediatrics* **119:**e70–e76.
98. **Templeton KE, Scheltinga SA, van den Eeden WC, Graffelman AW, van den Broek PJ, Claas EC.** 2005. Improved diagnosis of the etiology of community-acquired pneumonia with real-time polymerase chain reaction. *Clin Infect Dis* **41:**345–351.
99. **Jain S, Self WH, Wunderink RG, Fakhran S, Balk R, Bramley AM, Reed C, Grijalva CG, Anderson EJ, Courtney DM, Chappell JD, Qi C, Hart EM, Carroll F, Trabue C, Donnelly HK, Williams DJ, Zhu Y, Arnold SR, Ampofo K, Waterer GW, Levine M, Lindstrom S, Winchell JM, Katz JM, Erdman D, Schneider E, Hicks LA, McCullers JA, Pavia AT, Edwards KM, Finelli L, CDC EPIC Study Team.** 2015. Community-acquired pneumonia requiring hospitalization among U.S. adults. *N Engl J Med* **373:**415–427.
100. **Falsey AR, Walsh EE, Hayden FG.** 2002. Rhinovirus and coronavirus infection-associated hospitalizations among older adults. *J Infect Dis* **185:**1338–1341.

101. **Ogimi C, Waghmare AA, Kuypers JM, Xie H, Yeung CC, Leisenring WM, Seo S, Choi SM, Jerome KR, Englund JA, Boeckh M.** 2017. Clinical significance of human coronavirus in bronchoalveolar lavage samples from hematopoietic cell transplant recipients and patients with hematologic malignancies. *Clin Infect Dis* **64:**1532–1539.
102. **Bosis S, Esposito S, Niesters HG, Zuccotti GV, Marseglia G, Lanari M, Zuin G, Pelucchi C, Osterhaus AD, Principi N.** 2008. Role of respiratory pathogens in infants hospitalized for a first episode of wheezing and their impact on recurrences. *Clin Microbiol Infect* **14:**677–684.
103. **Gaunt ER, Harvala H, McIntyre C, Templeton KE, Simmonds P.** 2011. Disease burden of the most commonly detected respiratory viruses in hospitalized patients calculated using the disability adjusted life year (DALY) model. *J Clin Virol* **52:**215–221.
104. **Gerna G, Passarani N, Battaglia M, Rondanelli EG.** 1985. Human enteric coronaviruses: antigenic relatedness to human coronavirus OC43 and possible etiologic role in viral gastroenteritis. *J Infect Dis* **151:**796–803.
105. **Payne CM, Ray CG, Borduin V, Minnich LL, Lebowitz MD.** 1986. An eight-year study of the viral agents of acute gastroenteritis in humans: ultrastructural observations and seasonal distribution with a major emphasis on coronavirus-like particles. *Diagn Microbiol Infect Dis* **5:**39–54.
106. **Esper F, Ou Z, Huang YT.** 2010. Human coronaviruses are uncommon in patients with gastrointestinal illness. *J Clin Virol* **48:**131–133.
107. **Jevšnik M, Steyer A, Zrim T, Pokorn M, Mrvič T, Grosek Š, Strle F, Lusa L, Petrovec M.** 2013. Detection of human coronaviruses in simultaneously collected stool samples and nasopharyngeal swabs from hospitalized children with acute gastroenteritis. *Virol J* **10:**46.
108. **Paloniemi M, Lappalainen S, Vesikari T.** 2015. Commonly circulating human coronaviruses do not have a significant role in the etiology of gastrointestinal infections in hospitalized children. *J Clin Virol* **62:**114–117.
109. **Morfopoulou S, Brown JR, Davies EG, Anderson G, Virasami A, Qasim W, Chong WK, Hubank M, Plagnol V, Desforges M, Jacques TS, Talbot PJ, Breuer J.** 2016. Human coronavirus OC43 associated with fatal encephalitis. *N Engl J Med* **375:**497–498.
110. **Peiris JS, Guan Y, Yuen KY.** 2004. Severe acute respiratory syndrome. *Nat Med* **10**(Suppl):S88–S97.
111. **Assiri A, Al-Tawfiq JA, Al-Rabeeah AA, Al-Rabiah FA, Al-Hajjar S, Al-Barrak A, Flemban H, Al-Nassir WN, Balkhy HH, Al-Hakeem RF, Makhdoom HQ, Zumla AI, Memish ZA.** 2013. Epidemiological, demographic, and clinical characteristics of 47 cases of Middle East respiratory syndrome coronavirus disease from Saudi Arabia: a descriptive study. *Lancet Infect Dis* **13:**752–761.
112. **Saad M, Omrani AS, Baig K, Bahloul A, Elzein F, Matin MA, Selim MA, Al Mutairi M, Al Nakhli D, Al Aidaroos AY, Al Sherbeeni N, Al-Khashan HI, Memish ZA, Albarrak AM.** 2014. Clinical aspects and outcomes of 70 patients with Middle East respiratory syndrome coronavirus infection: a single-center experience in Saudi Arabia. *Int J Infect Dis* **29:**301–306.
113. **Memish ZA, Al-Tawfiq JA, Assiri A, AlRabiah FA, Al Hajjar S, Albarrak A, Flemban H, Alhakeem RF, Makhdoom HQ, Alsubaie S, Al-Rabeeah AA.** 2014. Middle East respiratory syndrome coronavirus disease in children. *Pediatr Infect Dis J* **33:**904–906.
114. **Arabi YM, Harthi A, Hussein J, Bouchama A, Johani S, Hajeer AH, Saeed BT, Wahbi A, Saedy A, AlDabbagh T, Okaili R, Sadat M, Balkhy H.** 2015. Severe neurologic syndrome associated with Middle East respiratory syndrome corona virus (MERS-CoV). *Infection* **43:**495–501.
115. **Assiri A, Abedi GR, Al Masri M, Bin Saeed A, Gerber SI, Watson JT.** 2016. Middle East respiratory syndrome coronavirus infection during pregnancy: a report of 5 cases from Saudi Arabia. *Clin Infect Dis* **63:**951–953.
116. **Barnard DL, Kumaki Y.** 2011. Recent developments in anti-severe acute respiratory syndrome coronavirus chemotherapy. *Future Virol* **6:**615–631.
117. **Stockman LJ, Bellamy R, Garner P.** 2006. SARS: systematic review of treatment effects. *PLoS Med* **3:**e343.
118. **Mo Y, Fisher D.** 2016. A review of treatment modalities for Middle East respiratory syndrome. *J Antimicrob Chemother* **71:**3340–3350.
119. **World Health Organization.** 2015. Laboratory testing for Middle East respiratory syndrome coronavirus: interim guidance, June 2015. http://www.who.int/csr/disease/coronavirus_infections/mers-laboratory-testing/en/
120. **World Health Organization.** 2015. Guidance on regulations for the transport of infectious substances 2015–2016. http://www.who.int/ihr/publications/who_hse_ihr_2015.2/en/
121. **Fujimoto K, Chan KH, Takeda K, Lo KF, Leung RH, Okamoto T.** 2008. Sensitive and specific enzyme-linked immunosorbent assay using chemiluminescence for detection of severe acute respiratory syndrome viral infection. *J Clin Microbiol* **46:**302–310.
122. **Lau SK, Woo PC, Wong BH, Tsoi HW, Woo GK, Poon RW, Chan KH, Wei WI, Peiris JS, Yuen KY.** 2004. Detection of severe acute respiratory syndrome (SARS) coronavirus nucleocapsid protein in SARS patients by enzyme-linked immunosorbent assay. *J Clin Microbiol* **42:** 2884–2889.
123. **Li YH, Li J, Liu XE, Wang L, Li T, Zhou YH, Zhuang H.** 2005. Detection of the nucleocapsid protein of severe acute respiratory syndrome coronavirus in serum: comparison with results of other viral markers. *J Virol Methods* **130:** 45–50.
124. **Liu IJ, Chen PJ, Yeh SH, Chiang YP, Huang LM, Chang MF, Chen SY, Yang PC, Chang SC, Wang WK, SARS Research Group of the National Taiwan University College of Medicine–National Taiwan University Hospital.** 2005. Immunofluorescence assay for detection of the nucleocapsid antigen of the severe acute respiratory syndrome (SARS)-associated coronavirus in cells derived from throat wash samples of patients with SARS. *J Clin Microbiol* **43:**2444–2448.
125. **Sizun J, Arbour N, Talbot PJ.** 1998. Comparison of immunofluorescence with monoclonal antibodies and RT-PCR for the detection of human coronaviruses 229E and OC43 in cell culture. *J Virol Methods* **72:**145–152.
126. **Sastre P, Dijkman R, Camuñas A, Ruiz T, Jebbink MF, van der Hoek L, Vela C, Rueda P.** 2011. Differentiation between human coronaviruses NL63 and 229E using a novel double-antibody sandwich enzyme-linked immunosorbent assay based on specific monoclonal antibodies. *Clin Vaccine Immunol* **18:**113–118.
127. **Chen Y, Chan KH, Hong C, Kang Y, Ge S, Chen H, Wong EY, Joseph S, Patteril NG, Wernery U, Xia N, Lau SK, Woo PC.** 2016. A highly specific rapid antigen detection assay for on-site diagnosis of MERS. *J Infect* **73:**82–84.
128. **Gerna G, Campanini G, Rovida F, Percivalle E, Sarasini A, Marchi A, Baldanti F.** 2006. Genetic variability of human coronavirus OC43-, 229E-, and NL63-like strains and their association with lower respiratory tract infections of hospitalized infants and immunocompromised patients. *J Med Virol* **78:**938–949.
129. **Silva CS, Mullis LB, Pereira O Jr, Saif LJ, Vlasova A, Zhang X, Owens RJ, Paulson D, Taylor D, Haynes LM, Azevedo MP.** 2014. Human respiratory coronaviruses detected in patients with influenza-like illness in Arkansas, USA. *Virol Mycol* **2014**(Suppl 2):004.
130. **Dare RK, Fry AM, Chittaganpitch M, Sawanpanyalert P, Olsen SJ, Erdman DD.** 2007. Human coronavirus infections in rural Thailand: a comprehensive study using real-time reverse-transcription polymerase chain reaction assays. *J Infect Dis* **196:**1321–1328.
131. **Chan JF, Choi GK, Tsang AK, Tee KM, Lam HY, Yip CC, To KK, Cheng VC, Yeung ML, Lau SK, Woo PC, Chan KH, Tang BS, Yuen KY.** 2015. Development and evaluation of novel real-time reverse transcription-PCR assays with locked nucleic acid probes targeting leader sequences of human-pathogenic coronaviruses. *J Clin Microbiol* **53:** 2722–2726.

132. **de Souza Luna LK, Heiser V, Regamey N, Panning M, Drexler JF, Mulangu S, Poon L, Baumgarte S, Haijema BJ, Kaiser L, Drosten C.** 2007. Generic detection of coronaviruses and differentiation at the prototype strain level by reverse transcription-PCR and nonfluorescent low-density microarray. *J Clin Microbiol* **45:**1049–1052.
133. **Goka EA, Vallely PJ, Mutton KJ, Klapper PE.** 2015. Pan-human coronavirus and human bocavirus SYBR Green and TaqMan PCR assays; use in studying influenza A viruses co-infection and risk of hospitalization. *Infection* **43:**185–192.
134. **Vijgen L, Keyaerts E, Moës E, Maes P, Duson G, Van Ranst M.** 2005. Development of one-step, real-time, quantitative reverse transcriptase PCR assays for absolute quantitation of human coronaviruses OC43 and 229E. *J Clin Microbiol* **43:**5452–5456.
135. **van Elden LJ, van Loon AM, van Alphen F, Hendriksen KA, Hoepelman AI, van Kraaij MG, Oosterheert JJ, Schipper P, Schuurman R, Nijhuis M.** 2004. Frequent detection of human coronaviruses in clinical specimens from patients with respiratory tract infection by use of a novel real-time reverse-transcriptase polymerase chain reaction. *J Infect Dis* **189:**652–657.
136. **Pyrc K, Milewska A, Potempa J.** 2011. Development of loop-mediated isothermal amplification assay for detection of human coronavirus-NL63. *J Virol Methods* **175:**133–136.
137. **Anderson TP, Werno AM, Barratt K, Mahagamasekera P, Murdoch DR, Jennings LC.** 2013. Comparison of four multiplex PCR assays for the detection of viral pathogens in respiratory specimens. *J Virol Methods* **191:**118–121.
138. **Gadsby NJ, Hardie A, Claas EC, Templeton KE.** 2010. Comparison of the Luminex respiratory virus panel fast assay with in-house real-time PCR for respiratory viral infection diagnosis. *J Clin Microbiol* **48:**2213–2216.
139. **Nijhuis RHT, Guerendiain D, Claas ECJ, Templeton KE.** 2017. Comparison of ePlex respiratory pathogen panel with laboratory-developed real-time PCR assays for detection of respiratory pathogens. *J Clin Microbiol* **55:**1938–1945.
140. **Chen JHK, Lam H-Y, Yip CCY, Wong SCY, Chan JFW, Ma ESK, Cheng VCC, Tang BSF, Yuen K-Y.** 2016. Clinical evaluation of the new high-throughput Luminex NxTAG respiratory pathogen panel assay for multiplex respiratory pathogen detection. *J Clin Microbiol* **54:**1820–1825.
141. **Poon LL, Chan KH, Wong OK, Yam WC, Yuen KY, Guan Y, Lo YM, Peiris JS.** 2003. Early diagnosis of SARS coronavirus infection by real time RT-PCR. *J Clin Virol* **28:**233–238.
142. **Poon LL, Wong BW, Chan KH, Ng SS, Yuen KY, Guan Y, Peiris JS.** 2005. Evaluation of real-time reverse transcriptase PCR and real-time loop-mediated amplification assays for severe acute respiratory syndrome coronavirus detection. *J Clin Microbiol* **43:**3457–3459.
143. **Mahony JB, Richardson S.** 2005. Molecular diagnosis of severe acute respiratory syndrome: the state of the art. *J Mol Diagn* **7:**551–559.
144. **Yam WC, Chan KH, Chow KH, Poon LL, Lam HY, Yuen KY, Seto WH, Peiris JS.** 2005. Clinical evaluation of real-time PCR assays for rapid diagnosis of SARS coronavirus during outbreak and post-epidemic periods. *J Clin Virol* **33:**19–24.
145. **Vijgen L, Moës E, Keyaerts E, Li S, Van Ranst M.** 2008. A pancoronavirus RT-PCR assay for detection of all known coronaviruses. *Methods Mol Biol* **454:**3–12.
146. **Corman VM, Eckerle I, Bleicker T, Zaki A, Landt O, Eschbach-Bludau M, van Boheemen S, Gopal R, Ballhause M, Bestebroer TM, Muth D, Müller MA, Drexler JF, Zambon M, Osterhaus AD, Fouchier RM, Drosten C.** 2012. Detection of a novel human coronavirus by real-time reverse-transcription polymerase chain reaction. *Euro Surveill* **17:**20285.
147. **Corman VM, Müller MA, Costabel U, Timm J, Binger T, Meyer B, Kreher P, Lattwein E, Eschbach-Bludau M, Nitsche A, Bleicker T, Landt O, Schweiger B, Drexler JF, Osterhaus AD, Haagmans BL, Dittmer U, Bonin F, Wolff T, Drosten C.** 2012. Assays for laboratory confirmation of novel human coronavirus (hCoV-EMC) infections. *Euro Surveill* **17:**20334.
148. **Lu X, Whitaker B, Sakthivel SK, Kamili S, Rose LE, Lowe L, Mohareb E, Elassal EM, Al-Sanouri T, Haddadin A, Erdman DD.** 2014. Real-time reverse transcription-PCR assay panel for Middle East respiratory syndrome coronavirus. *J Clin Microbiol* **52:**67–75.
149. **Mohamed DH, AlHetheel AF, Mohamud HS, Aldosari K, Alzamil FA, Somily AM.** 2017. Clinical validation of 3 commercial real-time reverse transcriptase polymerase chain reaction assays for the detection of Middle East respiratory syndrome coronavirus from upper respiratory tract specimens. *Diagn Microbiol Infect Dis* **87:**320–324.
150. **Kim MN, Ko YJ, Seong MW, Kim JS, Shin BM, Sung H.** 2016. Analytical and clinical validation of six commercial Middle East respiratory syndrome coronavirus RNA detection kits based on real-time reverse-transcription PCR. *Ann Lab Med* **36:**450–456.
151. **Corman VM, Ölschläger S, Wendtner CM, Drexler JF, Hess M, Drosten C.** 2014. Performance and clinical validation of the RealStar MERS-CoV kit for detection of Middle East respiratory syndrome coronavirus RNA. *J Clin Virol* **60:**168–171.
152. **Shirato K, Yano T, Senba S, Akachi S, Kobayashi T, Nishinaka T, Notomi T, Matsuyama S.** 2014. Detection of Middle East respiratory syndrome coronavirus using reverse transcription loop-mediated isothermal amplification (RT-LAMP). *Virol J* **11:**139.
153. **Douglas CE, Kulesh DA, Jaissle JG, Minogue TD.** 2015. Real-time reverse transcriptase polymerase chain reaction assays for Middle East respiratory syndrome. *Mol Cell Probes* **29:**511–513.
154. **Vabret A, Mouthon F, Mourez T, Gouarin S, Petitjean J, Freymuth F.** 2001. Direct diagnosis of human respiratory coronaviruses 229E and OC43 by the polymerase chain reaction. *J Virol Methods* **97:**59–66.
155. **Herzog P, Drosten C, Müller MA.** 2008. Plaque assay for human coronavirus NL63 using human colon carcinoma cells. *Virol J* **5:**138.
156. **Schildgen O, Jebbink MF, de Vries M, Pyrc K, Dijkman R, Simon A, Müller A, Kupfer B, van der Hoek L.** 2006. Identification of cell lines permissive for human coronavirus NL63. *J Virol Methods* **138:**207–210.
157. **Freymuth F, Vabret A, Rozenberg F, Dina J, Petitjean J, Gouarin S, Legrand L, Corbet S, Brouard J, Lebon P.** 2005. Replication of respiratory viruses, particularly influenza virus, rhinovirus, and coronavirus in HuH7 hepatocarcinoma cell line. *J Med Virol* **77:**295–301.
158. **Dijkman R, Jebbink MF, Koekkoek SM, Deijs M, Jónsdóttir HR, Molenkamp R, Ieven M, Goossens H, Thiel V, van der Hoek L.** 2013. Isolation and characterization of current human coronavirus strains in primary human epithelial cell cultures reveal differences in target cell tropism. *J Virol* **87:**6081–6090.
159. **Pyrc K, Sims AC, Dijkman R, Jebbink M, Long C, Deming D, Donaldson E, Vabret A, Baric R, van der Hoek L, Pickles R.** 2010. Culturing the unculturable: human coronavirus HKU1 infects, replicates, and produces progeny virions in human ciliated airway epithelial cell cultures. *J Virol* **84:**11255–11263.
160. **Dominguez SR, Travanty EA, Qian Z, Mason RJ.** 2013. Human coronavirus HKU1 infection of primary human type II alveolar epithelial cells: cytopathic effects and innate immune response. *PLoS One* **8:**e70129.
161. **Kaye M, Druce J, Tran T, Kostecki R, Chibo D, Morris J, Catton M, Birch C.** 2006. SARS-associated coronavirus replication in cell lines. *Emerg Infect Dis* **12:**128–133.
162. **Muth D, Corman VM, Meyer B, Assiri A, Al-Masri M, Farah M, Steinhagen K, Lattwein E, Al-Tawfiq JA, Albarrak A, Müller MA, Drosten C, Memish ZA.** 2015. Infectious Middle East respiratory syndrome coronavirus excretion and serotype variability based on live virus isolates from patients in Saudi Arabia. *J Clin Microbiol* **53:**2951–2955.
163. **Lehmann C, Wolf H, Xu J, Zhao Q, Shao Y, Motz M, Lindner P.** 2008. A line immunoassay utilizing recombinant nucleocapsid proteins for detection of antibodies to human coronaviruses. *Diagn Microbiol Infect Dis* **61:**40–48.

164. **Liang FY, Lin LC, Ying TH, Yao CW, Tang TK, Chen YW, Hou MH.** 2013. Immunoreactivity characterisation of the three structural regions of the human coronavirus OC43 nucleocapsid protein by Western blot: implications for the diagnosis of coronavirus infection. *J Virol Methods* **187:**413–420.
165. **Chan JF, Sridhar S, Yip CC, Lau SK, Woo PC.** 2017. The role of laboratory diagnostics in emerging viral infections: the example of the Middle East respiratory syndrome epidemic. *J Microbiol* **55:**172–182.
166. **Park SW, Perera RA, Choe PG, Lau EH, Choi SJ, Chun JY, Oh HS, Song KH, Bang JH, Kim ES, Kim HB, Park WB, Kim NJ, Poon LL, Peiris M, Oh MD.** 2015. Comparison of serological assays in human Middle East respiratory syndrome (MERS)-coronavirus infection. *Euro Surveill* **20:**30042.
167. **Saunders N, Zambon M, Sharp I, Siddiqui R, Bermingham A, Ellis J, Vipond B, Sails A, Moran-Gilad J, Marsh P, Guiver M.** 2013. Guidance on the development and validation of diagnostic tests that depend on nucleic acid amplification and detection. *J Clin Virol* **56:**344–354.
168. **Clinical and Laboratory Standards Institute.** 2015. Molecular diagnostic methods for infectious diseases; approved guideline, 3rd ed. CLSI document MM03-Ed3. Clinical and Laboratory Standards Institute, Wayne, PA.
169. **Loens K, van Loon AM, Coenjaerts F, van Aarle Y, Goossens H, Wallace P, Claas EJ, Ieven M, GRACE Study Group.** 2012. Performance of different mono- and multiplex nucleic acid amplification tests on a multipathogen external quality assessment panel. *J Clin Microbiol* **50:** 977–987.
170. **Templeton KE, Forde CB, Loon AM, Claas EC, Niesters HG, Wallace P, Carman WF.** 2006. A multi-centre pilot proficiency programme to assess the quality of molecular detection of respiratory viruses. *J Clin Virol* **35:**51–58.
171. **Standards Unit, Microbiology Services Division, Public Health England.** 2013. UK standards for microbiology investigations: good laboratory practice when performing molecular amplification Assays. Q4:4.4. https://www.gov.uk/government/collections/standards-for-microbiology-investigations-smi
172. **Pereyaslov D, Rosin P, Palm D, Zeller H, Gross D, Brown CS, Struelens MJ, MERS-CoV Working Group.** 2014. Laboratory capability and surveillance testing for Middle East respiratory syndrome coronavirus infection in the WHO European Region, June 2013. *Euro Surveill* **19:**20923.
173. **Pas SD, Patel P, Reusken C, Domingo C, Corman VM, Drosten C, Dijkman R, Thiel V, Nowotny N, Koopmans MP, Niedrig M.** 2015. First international external quality assessment of molecular diagnostics for Mers-CoV. *J Clin Virol* **69:**81–85.
174. **Esposito S, Bosis S, Niesters HG, Tremolati E, Begliatti E, Rognoni A, Tagliabue C, Principi N, Osterhaus AD.** 2006. Impact of human coronavirus infections in otherwise healthy children who attended an emergency department. *J Med Virol* **78:**1609–1615.

Hepatitis A and E Viruses

JACQUES IZOPET AND NASSIM KAMAR

93

TAXONOMY

Hepatitis A Virus

Hepatitis A (HAV) is a species of the genus *Hepatovirus* within the family *Picornaviridae*. HAV is unique in its tropism for the liver, its structure, its physical stability, and its life cycle. HAV has a primitive capsid related to picorna-like viruses (dicistroviruses), which infect insects (1). HAV strains show little variation in nucleotide sequence over time or place. There are six closely related genotypes (I to VI) but only one serotype (2). Genotypes I to III, further divided into subgenotypes A and B, have been associated with infections in humans, while genotypes IV to VI are simian in origin. Evolutionary ancestral forms have been found in small mammals such as bats, rodents, hedgehogs, and shrews (3).

Hepatitis E Virus

Hepatitis E virus (HEV) belongs to the *Hepeviridae* family (4). This family has two genera (*Orthohepevirus* and *Piscihepevirus*) and five species. The species *Orthohepevirus A* includes HEV that infects humans and several other mammals. The other species do not infect humans: *Orthohepevirus B* infects chickens, *Orthohepevirus C* infects rats and ferrets, *Orthohepevirus D* infects bats, and *Piscihepevirus A* infects the cutthroat trout. The species *Orthohepevirus A* consists of at least seven distinct HEV genotypes (4) but only one serotype. Genotypes 1 and 2 infect humans exclusively and are seen in developing countries (5). They are responsible for outbreaks. Genotypes 3 and 4 have an animal reservoir, mainly pigs, and infect humans in developed countries. HEV genotypes 3 and 4 were detected in a large number of animals, such as domestic swine, wild boar, deer, rabbit, and mongoose (5). HEV genotypes 5 and 6 were detected in wild boar in Japan (6) but not yet in humans. HEV genotype 7 was recently detected in camel and was responsible for severe hepatitis E virus infection in an immunosuppressed individual who had regularly consumed milk and meat from camels (7).

DESCRIPTION OF THE AGENTS

Hepatitis A Virus

HAV is a small RNA virus with an icosahedral capsid. There are two forms of fully infectious particles. One form of virion, first identified by Feinstone (8), is nonenveloped and is shed in feces. This form is approximately 27 nm in diameter and has a density of 1.22/cm^3 on iodixanol gradients. The second form, virions circulating in the blood, is cloaked in host cell membranes; the virions' size is 50 to 110 nm and their density is 1.08 g/cm^3 (9). The protein composition of the HAV membrane has been determined by quantitative proteomics analysis (10). While membrane envelopment protects HAV against neutralizing antibody, it also facilitates early but limited detection of HAV infection by plasmacytoid dendritic cells (11). This may account for the minimal type I interferon response observed early in acute HAV infection (12). HAV is resistant to low pH (<3.0) and shows remarkable thermal stability. Cooking or boiling water and food at 85°C for at least 1 minute is necessary to inactivate HAV (13).

The HAV genome is a single-strand positive-sense RNA approximately 7.5 kb long (Fig. 1). It consists of an uncapped 5′ noncoding region including an internal ribosome entry site structure, a single long open reading frame (ORF) encoding a polypeptide of 2,227 amino acids with 3 segments (P1, P2, and P3), and a short 3′ noncoding region that ends in a poly-(A) tail.

The large polyprotein is cleaved into 10 mature proteins (Fig. 1). The P1 segment is processed into the four structural proteins of the viral capsid: VP1, VP2, VP3, and VP4. The largest of the capsid proteins, VP1, is 274 amino acid residues in length in nonenveloped HAV virions and has an 8-kDa carboxyterminal extension (pX, also known as 2A, 71 residues in length) in enveloped HAV virions (9). pX plays a critical role in capsid assembly and HAV envelopment but is cleaved from VP1 by a host proteinase upon loss of the membrane. VP2 contains a YPX3L late domain that binds Alix and vascular protein sorting 4 homolog B (VPS-4B) components of the cellular endosomal sorting complex required for transport (9). VP4, a small polypeptide lacking a terminal myristoylation signal required in the assembly process for the other picornaviruses, is essential for virion formation but is not present in the mature particles. HAV capsid, composed of 12 pentamers, comprises 60 copies of each of the three major proteins, VP1, VP2, and VP3. The remainder of the polyprotein (P2 and P3 segments) is processed into nonstructural proteins required for HAV RNA replication: 2B, 2C, 3A, 3B (also known as VPg, which is covalently linked to the 5′ end of

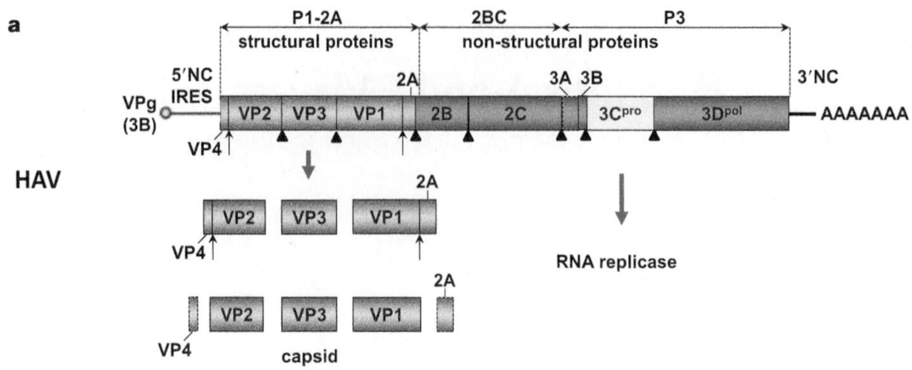

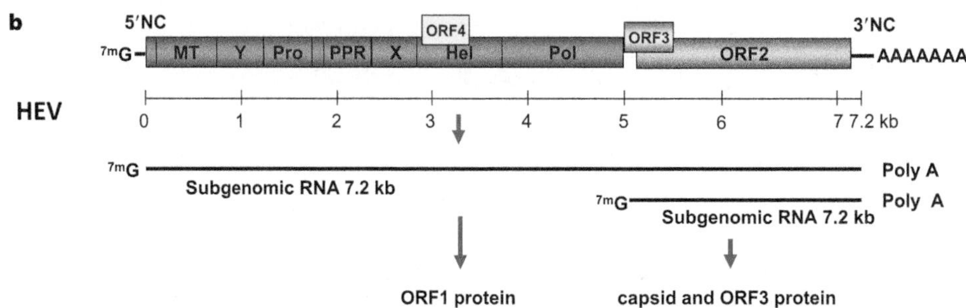

FIGURE 1 Genome organization of HAV and HEV. (A) HAV: The 5′ end of the RNA genome contains an internal ribosome entry site (IRES), and the 3′ end is polyadenylated. The HAV RNA genome contains a single ORF encoding a polyprotein that is processed by the viral protease 3C^{pro} (black triangles). (B) HEV: The 5′ end of the RNA genome is capped with 7-methylguanosine, and the 3′ end is polyadenylated. ORF1 encodes the nonstructural proteins, including a methyltransferase (MT), cysteine protease (P), polyproline region (PPR), macrodomain (X), helicase (Hel), and RNA polymerase (Pol). ORF2 and ORF3 encode the structural proteins from a bi-cistronic subgenomic RNA. ORF4 (genotype 1) interacts with eukaryotic elongation factor 1 isoform-1. NC, noncoding region.

the HAV genome), 3C^{pro} (a cysteine protease responsible for most posttranslational cleavages), and 3D^{pol} (the viral RNA-dependent RNA polymerase).

Non-human primates, especially chimpanzees, were used in the past to investigate the pathogenesis of HAV. A murine model that recapitulates many features of human HAV infection has been developed (14).

Hepatitis E Virus

HEV is a small RNA virus with an icosahedral capsid. Like HAV, there are two forms of infectious particles: the nonenveloped particle and the enveloped particle. Nonenveloped virions, first identified by Balayan (15), are found in the feces. They are 27 to 34 nm in diameter and have a density of 1.22 g/cm^3. Virions circulating in the blood are cloaked in host cell membranes. Their size is 50 to 110 nm and their density is 1.08 g/cm^3 (16–18). HEV is resistant to low pH (<3.0), and cooking time at an internal temperature of 71°C for at least 20 minutes is necessary to inactivate HEV (19, 20).

The HEV genome is a single-strand positive-sense RNA approximately 7.2 kb long (Fig. 1). It consists of a short 5′ noncoding region that is capped with 7-methyl-guanosine, three ORFs (ORF1, ORF2, and ORF3), and a short 3′ noncoding region that ends in a poly-(A) tail.

ORF1 encodes a nonstructural protein about 1,700 amino acids long that is involved in HEV RNA replication. This protein contains several functional domains: a methyltransferase/guanyltransferase, a cysteine protease, a macrodomain (X domain), an RNA helicase that has 5′-nucleoside triphosphatase activity, and an RNA-dependent RNA polymerase (21). A variable region encoding a proline-rich hinge, the polyproline region, is an intrinsically disordered region in which segments of human genes have been identified (22–27). Immunocompromised patients who develop a chronic infection have a highly heterogeneous mixture of polyproline region quasi-species at the acute phase of HEV infection (23). The ORF1 of HEV-1 includes an additional ORF, ORF4 (28). ORF4 is expressed after endoplasmic reticulum stress and interacts with eukaryotic elongation factor 1 isoform-1, thus stimulating virus polymerase activity.

ORF2 encodes the 660-amino-acid virus capsid protein. This protein has three glycosylation sites (Asn 132, Asn 310, and Asn 562) and an N-terminal signal peptide that drives its translocation into the endoplasmic reticulum (29). The capsid protein has been divided into three domains: shell (S), middle (M), and protruding (P). The P domain is the major target for neutralizing antibodies and contains a putative receptor binding domain (30, 31). Capsid monomers self-assemble to form dimers and then the decamers that encapsulate the virus RNA. The capsid consists of 180 copies arranged as an icosahedron with T = 3 symmetry (32). Immunological and structural studies of the capsid protein have contributed to the development of a hepatitis E vaccine (33). Immunocompromised patients with chronic HEV infection are infected with HEV quasi-species whose genome is highly heterogeneous in regions encoding the M and P domains of the capsid protein (34).

ORF3 encodes a small protein (113 residues in HEV-3 and 114 residues in HEV genotypes 1, 2, and 4) that is essential for virus egress. ORF3 protein is associated only with enveloped HEV particles, not with naked HEV particles. The ORF3 protein must be phosphorylated on Ser80 before it can interact with the nonglycosylated form of the capsid protein (35). The ORF3 protein contains a conserved proline-serine-alanine-proline motif that enables it to interact with the endosomal sorting complex required for transport, including the tumor susceptibility gene 101 (Tsg 101) (36–41).

Non-human primates, especially chimpanzees and *Macacus cynomolgus*, were used by different teams to investigate the pathogenesis of HEV. New models for investigating chronic HEV infection based on monkeys or pigs treated with immunosuppressive drugs (42, 43) or human liver chimeric mice (44–47) have been developed.

EPIDEMIOLOGY AND TRANSMISSION

HAV and HEV are both transmitted mainly by the fecal-oral route. However, although the mode of transmission can be quite similar, the epidemiology of HAV and HEV infections is different.

Transmission

Hepatitis A Virus

HAV is highly transmissible and the occurrence of outbreaks is frequently reported, especially from developed countries where herd immunity in the population is low. There is no animal reservoir for human HAV strains.

Water- and Foodborne Transmission

Ingestion of contaminated food or water is a major mode of acquisition of HAV. Swimming in water bodies contaminated by adjacent septic systems or sewage is another mode. A variety of foods have been implicated in hepatitis A outbreaks. Contamination of food products can occur at any point during processing, harvesting, preparation, or distribution. Seafood, vegetables, and fruits are classic vectors (48). The largest hepatitis A outbreak reported was associated with consumption of raw clams in Shanghai in 1988, when around 300,000 individuals were infected (49). Hepatitis A outbreaks through contaminated food and water remain a public health problem in industrialized countries with low or intermediate endemicity.

Person-to-Person Transmission

Close contact between infected and susceptible people is the most common mode of HAV transmission in developing and developed countries. Transmission is facilitated by asymptomatic infections, especially in young children, and the prolonged shedding of HAV in feces before and after the onset of symptoms. This mode of HAV acquisition occurs frequently in closed institutions such as schools, nurseries, and day care centers (50).

Other Modes of Transmission

Outbreaks of HAV infection frequently occur among men who have sex with men (MSM) (51). HAV is not transmitted by the semen but by oral contact with fecally contaminated sites. After initial introduction of HAV into the MSM community, the transmitted variant spreads rapidly and persists for a long period (51).

Outbreaks of HAV infection have been also reported among injecting drug users (52).

Lastly, HAV can be transmitted by transfusion of blood or blood products on rare occasions (53). In some cases, the recipients were anti-HAV IgG positive (53). Due to the sporadic nature of the HAV acute infection among blood donors and the lack of chronic carriers, there is no recommendation for screening blood donors for HAV. However, the plasma industry tests all sources of plasma by HAV nucleic acid testing on mini-pools.

Hepatitis E Virus

The mode of transmission of HEV genotypes 1 and 2 differs from the mode of transmission of genotypes 3 and 4. HEV genotype 1 and 2 infection is observed in developing countries, with severe hepatitis in pregnant women leading to death in up to 25% of cases (5). It can be responsible for outbreaks in high-endemicity areas. Drinking contaminated water is the main route of transmission. Outbreaks are often related to fecal contamination of drinking water supplies (54). Outbreaks have also occurred in refugee camps with limited facilities for water hygiene and sanitation (55, 56). Person-to-person transmission of HEV is uncommon (57, 58). The transmission from infected women to their newborns is well documented (59, 60), and transmission of HEV genotype 1 through blood transfusions has been reported (61, 62).

HEV genotypes 3 and 4 are observed in developed and in high-income countries. Since the reservoir for HEV genotypes 3 and 4 is animals, the main route of transmission of HEV genotypes 3 and 4 is the consumption of HEV-infected animal products, especially undercooked meat. Consumption of infected pork liver, pork products containing liver, and other pork meat consumed raw or undercooked was identified as the main source of HEV infections (63–65). Consumption of infected game meat is another mode of human infection. Strains of rabbit HEV were detected in humans (66, 67). In addition, HEV has been detected in yellow cattle in rural China (68) and in cow milk (69). The shedding of HEV by infected animals can contaminate water sources, leading to the accumulation of HEV in fruits, vegetables, and shellfish. Hence, HEV RNA (HEV genotype 3) was detected on red fruits, strawberries, and salads and in spices (70), as well as in oysters and mussels (71). Recently, it has also been shown in many countries in Europe (72) as well as China (73) and Japan (74) that HEV can be transmitted by transfusion of blood products. Most cases of transfusion-transmitted HEV infection are asymptomatic, and only a small minority of recipients of infected blood products develop symptomatic hepatitis. The frequency of positive HEV RNA blood donors across many countries ranges from 1:600 to 1:14,799 (75). Several developed countries have adopted measures to improve blood safety based on the epidemiology of HEV (76). All blood donations are screened in Ireland (since 2016), the United Kingdom, and the Netherlands (both since 2017). Plasma donations intended for transfusion to patients at risk of severe disease have been selectively screened in France since 2013 (77, 78).

Epidemiology

Hepatitis A Virus

HAV is distributed worldwide. However, the epidemiological patterns vary between populations according to the level of sanitation and socioeconomic status. A classification of HAV endemicity based on age at which 50% seroprevalence is reached in the population has been proposed: very high (<5 years), high (5 to 14 years), intermediate (15 to 34 years), and low (≥35 years) (79) (Fig. 2).

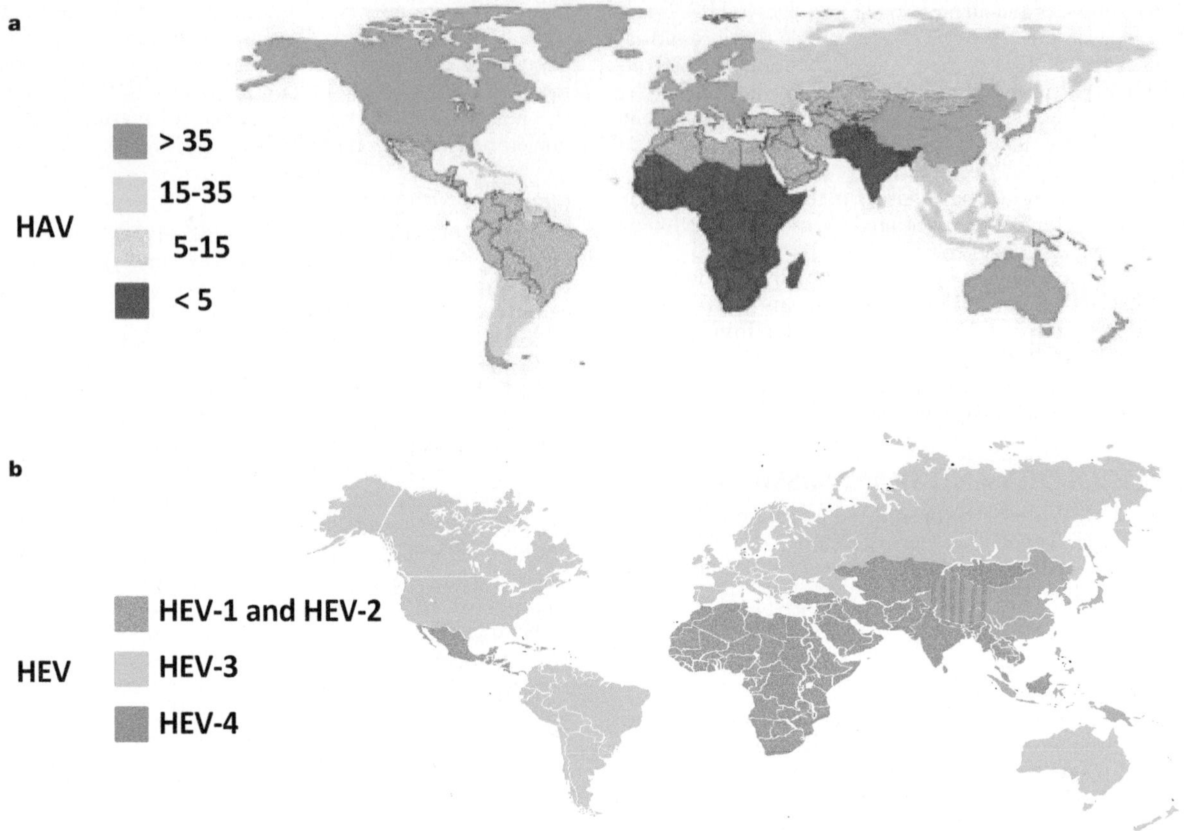

FIGURE 2 Geographic distribution of HAV and HEV infections. (a) HAV: Colors represent different endemicity patterns based on the age in years at which 50% of the population is anti-HAV IgG positive (dark red, very high endemicity [<5 years]; yellow, high endemicity [5 to 15 years]; light green, intermediate endemicity [15 to 35 years]; dark green, low endemicity [>35 years]). (b) HEV: Colors represent the predominant HEV genotypes in the different areas (pink, HEV genotypes 1 and 2; green, HEV genotype 3; blue, HEV genotype 4).

High-Endemicity Pattern

In low-resource countries with poor sanitation, such as most areas in Africa and parts of Asia, rates of HAV transmission are very high and HAV is acquired in early childhood. Infections are asymptomatic and lead to universal protection against HAV subsequently in life. Most people get exposed to HAV and become seropositive before the age of 5 years.

Low-Endemicity Pattern

In high-resource countries with good sanitation and hygienic conditions (North America, Europe, Australia, Japan, etc.), the circulation of HEV is limited and most people in all age groups are susceptible. However, HAV seroprevalence is higher in older age groups due to a cohort effect. In these countries, any introduction of HAV in the population can trigger waves of transmission with symptomatic disease (jaundice), for example, in MSM or through importation of contaminated food.

Intermediate-Endemicity Pattern

In intermediate-resource countries (North Africa, South America, Western Asia, etc.), HAV circulates at a fairly high rate and symptomatic disease occurs in children older than 5 years and young adults. In these countries, socioeconomic development and improved hygiene have led to epidemiologic transition characterized by an increase in the incidence of disease, hospitalizations, and mortality due to hepatitis A despite a reduction in HAV transmission rate (80). This public health problem has led to the introduction of preventive strategies by using universal childhood HAV vaccination (81, 82).

Hepatitis E Virus

HEV Genotypes 1 and 2

HEV genotype 1 is prevalent and highly endemic in South, Central, and Southeast Asia, as well as in Africa and the Middle East (5) (Fig. 2). HEV genotype 2 is prevalent in western Africa and Mexico. In China, over the past decades, the prevalence of HEV genotype 1 that was responsible for frequent outbreaks decreased, while the prevalence of HEV genotype 4 increased. This is likely related to the improvement in sanitation and the increase in income. It is estimated that 20.1 million (95% credible interval = 2.8 to 37.0 million) new infections occur annually in Asia and Africa (83). Determining the real seroprevalence in these areas is difficult due to the use of different serology assays with quite different sensitivities. However, published data show a rate of anti-HEV antibodies in most parts of Asia and Africa ranging from 10 to 40% (84). Most of the cases are adolescents and young adults (5). Infection in children is more often asymptomatic than in adults.

Zoonotic Genotypes

HEV genotype 3 is the main HEV genotype observed in Europe, North America, and South America, while genotype 4 is predominant in Asia (85) (Fig. 2). In Europe, cases of genotype 4 HEV infection are sporadic, and genotype 1 infections are travel-associated. Again, due to the considerable variability in the sensitivity of serology assays, the true seroprevalence is unknown. However, although it varies from one region to another, it seems to be high, i.e., 52% in southwest France (86), above 40% in Germany over the age of 60 years (87), and between 10 and 20% in the United Kingdom, the Benelux, and Germany (85). In the United States, historical data showed a seroprevalence of 21%, while more recent data showed a lower 6% prevalence of anti-HEV IgG (88). However, few data are available for the United States, probably due to the lack of FDA-licensed anti-HEV serology assays.

CLINICAL SIGNIFICANCE

Clinical Presentation and Course

Acute infections with any of the hepatitis viruses cannot be distinguished on clinical characteristics or pathological examinations. Therefore, laboratory markers are one key for diagnosis.

Hepatitis A Virus

Clinical manifestations of HAV infection are varied. Many infections, especially in children less than 5 years old, are asymptomatic. Symptomatic HAV infections include mild anicteric hepatitis, acute hepatitis with jaundice, and acute liver failure. Prolonged acute hepatitis A with relapsing hepatitis has been described, but there is no chronic hepatitis.

Typically, HAV infection begins in symptomatic cases with prodromal symptoms of malaise, vomiting, anorexia, fever, and right upper quadrant abdominal pain after an incubation period of approximately 4 weeks (range, 2 to 6 weeks). Then, patients may develop more severe fever, malaise, loss of appetite, and jaundice that occurs in more than 70% of adults. Dark-colored urine and decolored stools are usually observed. Hepatomegaly and splenomegaly can be present. Peak infectivity occurs 2 weeks before and at least 1 week after the initial symptoms. Acute illness lasts less than 2 months, with a median of 2 weeks. Hepatitis A may cause acute liver failure leading to coagulopathy and encephalopathy. The risk of death increases with age and with underlying liver disease such as chronic hepatitis B or C. Overall, the case-fatality ratio is 0.3%, ranging from 0.1% for children younger than 15 years to 3% for adults older than 50 years. Rarely, pericarditis, renal failure, thrombocytopenia, anemia, Guillain-Barré syndrome, and vasculitis/arthritis may occur in patients with acute HAV infection (89).

Hepatitis E Virus

In the majority of cases, acute HEV infection is asymptomatic whatever the genotype is. Symptoms of acute HEV infection are similar to all acute hepatitis episodes. At the early phase, nonspecific symptoms such as malaise, fever, body aches, nausea, and vomiting are observed. They are followed by the appearance of dark-colored urine and jaundice. Liver enzyme levels rise during the acute phase and return back to the normal range after the resolution of the symptoms. The incubation period is usually 2 to 6 weeks and is followed by an IgM response, which is detected around the time the serum alanine aminotransferase level increases and persists for 6 to 9 months (90). The IgG response can be delayed; it persists for several years, although its exact duration remains uncertain. HEV RNA becomes detectable in the blood and stool during the incubation period and persists for around 4 and 6 weeks, respectively. Capsid antigen persists in the blood for about the same amount of time (91).

Fulminant hepatitis was described in patients with chronic liver disease (acute or chronic hepatitis) who were infected with genotypes 1 or 3 (92, 93), as well as in pregnant women infected by genotype 1 (94, 95). In this last setting, it can lead to death in as high as 15 to 25% of patients. No case of fulminant hepatitis was described in pregnant women infected by genotype 3 or 4 (94, 95). Chronic hepatitis occurs only in immunosuppressed patients infected with genotypes 3 or 4. No case of chronic HEV infection was reported after genotype 1 or 2 infection. In solid organ transplant patients (96–98), stem cell transplant patients (99, 100), HIV-positive patients (101), and patients receiving chemotherapy (102) or immunotherapy (103), spontaneous HEV clearance may not occur and HEV replication can persist beyond 3 or 6 months, leading to chronic hepatitis with progressive fibrosis and cirrhosis (96, 104). After HEV infection, one-third of solid organ transplant patients spontaneously cleared the virus, and the remaining two-thirds developed chronic hepatitis (98, 105). Moreover, nearly 10% of the infected patients developed cirrhosis within a few years after the infection (98, 106). Deep immunosuppression and low specific T-cell response were associated with the evolution to chronic hepatitis (98, 107). The majority of immunosuppressed patients are asymptomatic and present with mild and persistent liver function test abnormalities (98).

In addition to hepatic manifestation, HEV infection can be responsible for extrahepatic manifestations. HEV genotype 1 and 3 infections were associated with neurological manifestations in immunocompetent and immunosuppressed patients (108–110). The most common neurological manifestations associated with HEV infection are Guillain-Barré syndrome (111–114) and neuralgic amyotrophy (115, 116). HEV RNA was detected in the cerebrospinal fluid of patients with neurological manifestations (109, 117). Kidney injuries, such as membranoproliferative glomerulonephritis with and without cryoglobulinemia and membranous glomerulonephritis, were also observed in immunocompetent and immunosuppressed patients infected with HEV genotypes 1 or 3 (118–121). Other extrahepatic manifestations were associated with HEV infection: pancreatitis (only with genotype 1), hematological disorders, myocarditis, thyroiditis, Henoch-Schönlein purpura, and myasthenia gravis.

Vaccines and Antiviral Agents

Hepatitis A Virus

Prophylaxis of HAV infection is effective through passive or active immunization. Passive immunization with human gamma globulin can be used for postexposure prophylaxis (<2 weeks postexposure), especially in immunosuppressed people, in individuals at risk of severe disease, and in infants less than 1 year of age. Postexposure prophylaxis with a single dose of hepatitis A vaccine is the preferred prophylaxis in patients aged between 12 and 40 years (122). Hepatitis A vaccines have supplanted gamma globulin for pre-exposure prophylaxis.

Inactivated hepatitis A vaccines contain viral particles produced in cell culture, purified, inactivated with formalin, and adsorbed to an aluminum hydroxide. Besides hepatitis A monovalent vaccines, combination vaccines including hepatitis A-typhoid vaccine and hepatitis A-hepatitis B vaccine have been licensed. The immunogenicity of the combination vaccines is equivalent to that of the monovalent hepatitis A vaccine. Live-attenuated HAV vaccines are available in China. Traditionally, two doses of inactivated vaccine with an interval of 6 to 12 months are recommended, beginning after 12 months of age. A protective efficacy of nearly 95% has been observed. The protection has been shown to last for at least 10 years, and modeling studies predicted that 88% of individuals who were seronegative prior to vaccination would remain protected for at least 30 years (123).

Optimal strategies regarding the need for HAV vaccination are based on seroprevalence. For high-endemicity countries, vaccination is not routinely recommended. For countries with intermediate endemicity, vaccination of all children may protect the health of adolescents and young adults. In Argentina, a universal immunization of 12-month-old children with a single dose of inactivated HAV vaccine led to marked reduction in the incidence rates of symptomatic hepatitis A, fulminant hepatitis, and liver transplantation (81, 82). For low-endemicity countries, targeted vaccination of high-risk groups (travelers to regions of high HAV endemicity, MSM, injecting drug users, immunosuppressed patients, patients infected with HIV, and patients with chronic liver disease) is generally recommended, but extension to the general population is sometimes an option. In the United States, targeted hepatitis A vaccination began in 1999 for high-risk groups and children living in high-incidence communities. In 2006, the Centers for Disease Control and Prevention recommended that every child be vaccinated between 12 and 23 months.

Individuals with hepatitis A and acute liver failure can be treated with *N*-acetylcysteine. In this setting, liver transplantation is considered for the sickest patients.

Hepatitis E Virus

Two vaccines against HEV have been developed: a 56-kDa subunit antigen (amino acids 112 to 607 of ORF2 expressed in insect cell culture) (124) and a subunit antigen, HEV 239 (amino acids 368 to 606 of ORF2 expressed in *Escherichia coli*) (125). However, only HEV 239 has been licensed for use in humans (125, 126), and it is only licensed in China (125). The Hecolin vaccine demonstrated cross-protection for both genotypes 1 and 4 and was developed to elicit protective antibodies across all HEV genotypes (126). This three-dose vaccine showed a vaccine efficacy of 97% to prevent episodes of symptomatic acute hepatitis (125) and showed long-term efficacy during further follow-up (126). Modeling studies suggest that its protective effect could persist up to 30 years after vaccination (127). The vaccine seems to be safe for pregnant women (128). However, its safety and efficacy have not been tested in patients with chronic hepatitis or in immunosuppressed patients.

In organ transplant patients with chronic hepatitis, the first-line therapeutic option is the reduction of immunosuppression, which allows HEV clearance in one-third of patients (98). In the remaining patients, the use of ribavirin therapy was shown to be efficient for treating HEV infection (129, 130). After 3 months of ribavirin therapy, 78% of patients achieved a sustained virological response (130). A longer duration of therapy, i.e., 6 months instead of 3 months, allowed HEV clearance in relapsers (130). Persistent HEV shedding in stools at the end of therapy was associated with HEV relapse after the end of therapy (131). Ribavirin therapy was also shown to be efficient for treating HEV infection in stem cell transplant patients (132). It has been suggested that ribavirin inhibits HEV replication through the depletion of guanosine triphosphate pools (133). Deep sequencing has identified several HEV RNA mutations, such as G1634R. Recent studies showed that ribavirin increases HEV heterogeneity that seems to be reversible (134–137). However, the role of HEV RNA variants and their impact on HEV treatment outcome are uncertain (134, 135). Pegylated-interferon was also successfully used for treating HEV infection in liver transplant patients (138, 139). However, it cannot be used in other organ transplant patients because it increases the risk of acute rejection (140). Finally, no alternative antiviral therapy to ribavirin or pegylated interferon is available. There are no robust data to recommend the use of ribavirin at the acute HEV phase.

COLLECTION, TRANSPORT, AND STORAGE OF SPECIMENS

Standard methods for the collection, transport, and storage of sera or plasma are adequate. Sera for testing IgM and IgG antibodies to HAV and HEV can be stored at 4°C for weeks but should be frozen (−20°C or −70°C) for long-term conservation. After blood collection in EDTA tubes and centrifugation within 6 hours, plasma can be used immediately for testing for HAV RNA or HEV RNA or be stored at −70°C. HAV RNA and HEV RNA can be detected in stools collected in a sterile container. After dilution in phosphate-buffered saline and filtration, specimens are tested immediately or stored at −70°C.

DIRECT EXAMINATION

Electron Microscopy

Electron microscopy has a historical value for its role in identifying HAV (8) and HEV (15). Recently, electron microscopy was also very useful for identifying the membrane of enveloped forms of HAV and HEV (exosome-like particles) (9, 18). However, it has no diagnostic value due to low sensitivity and the need for specific technical skills.

Antigen Detection

Hepatitis A Virus

HAV antigen can be detected in blood or fecal samples by immunoassays, but this is less sensitive than nucleic acid testing assays. In addition, there are no commercially available tests.

Hepatitis E Virus

Detection of HEV capsid antigen can be used for the diagnosis of HEV infection. A solid-phase antibody sandwich enzyme-linked immunosorbent assay that uses microwell strips coated with anti-HEV antibodies directed against the virus capsid protein has been developed. The sensitivity of this commercial immunoassay (Wantai Biological Pharmacy, China) was 91% (88% in immunocompetent and 94% in immunocompromised patients) (141). The specificity was excellent (100% with no interference from Epstein-Barr virus, cytomegalovirus, or hepatitis C virus infections), but the lowest HEV RNA concentration detected was 800 to 80,000 IU/ml using serial dilutions with HEV RNA-negative anti-HEV antibody-negative plasma (141). This assay could be an alternative for the direct diagnosis of HEV infection for laboratories with no molecular diagnostic facilities.

Nucleic Acid Detection

Hepatitis A Virus

HAV RNA can be detected in blood and stool by RT-PCR before the alanine aminotransferase level increases and clinical illness occurs (53). HAV RNA testing is useful for the detection of very early infections, especially as a safety measure in the plasma industry, and for establishing HAV infection in cases with questionable IgM results. Commercially available tests are listed in Table 1. The limit of detection of current assays is 1 to 46 IU/ml. Laboratory-developed tests must be carefully validated (142). Chemiluminescent fiber-optic genosensor and miniaturized devices are in development (143).

Hepatitis E Virus

Detecting and quantifying HEV RNA in the blood, stools, and other body compartments using nucleic acid amplification technologies with primers targeting regions that are conserved across HEV genotypes is the "gold standard" for the diagnosis of acute HEV infection. Commercially available tests are listed in Table 1. Most real-time PCR assays, including commercial assays, target ORF3 (144, 145). A transcription-mediated amplification assay performed on a fully automated platform is well adapted for high-throughput testing (146) (Table 1). Reverse transcription droplet digital PCR does not require a standard curve and gives absolute quantities of HEV RNA (147). Lastly, the

TABLE 1 Commercial molecular assays for detection and quantification of HAV RNA and HEV RNA

Virus	Manufacturer	Product name	Instrument	Analytical sensitivity	Type of test[a]
HAV	Altona Diagnostics	Real Star HAV RT-PCR	m2000rt (Abbott Diagnostics) Mx3005P QPCR System (Stratagene) Versant kPCR Molecular System AD (Siemens) ABI Prism 7500 SDS (Applied Biosystems) Rotor-Gene 6000 (Corbett Research) Rotor-Gene Q5/6 plex Platform (QIAGEN) CFX96 Real-Time PCR Detection System (Bio-Rad) LightCycler 480 Instrument II (Roche)	46 IU/ml	*In vitro* diagnostics Real-time PCR Qualitative test CE-marked
	Hologic/Grifols	Procleix Parvo/HAV	Tigris, Panther	1 IU/ml	Transfusion, TMA allowing simultaneous detection of HAV and parvovirus B19
	Roche	COBAS Taq Screen DPX	COBAS s201	1 IU/ml	Transfusion, real-time PCR allowing simultaneous detection of HAV and parvovirus B19
HEV	Altona Diagnostics	Real Star HEV RT-PCR	m2000rt (Abbott Diagnostics) Mx3005P QPCR System (Stratagene) Versant kPCR Molecular System AD (Siemens) ABI Prism 7500 SDS (Applied Biosystems) Rotor-Gene 6000 (Corbett Research) Rotor-Gene Q5/6 plex Platform (QIAGEN) CFX96 Real-Time PCR Detection System (Bio-Rad) LightCycler 480 Instrument II (Roche)	20 IU/ml	*In vitro* diagnostics CE-marked Quantitative test Real-time PCR
	Fast-Track Diagnostics	FTD Hepatitis E RNA	ABI 7500 ABI 7500 Fast Bio-Rad CFX96 LightCycler 480 Rotor-Gene 3000/6000/Q SmartCycler	188 IU/ml	*In vitro* diagnostics Quantitative test Real-time PCR CE-marked
	Hologic/Grifols	Procleix HEV	Panther	7 IU/ml	Transfusion, TMA qualitative test
	Roche	COBAS HEV	COBAS 6800	7 IU/ml	Transfusion, real-time PCR qualitative test

[a]TMA, transcription-mediated amplification assay.

loop-mediated isothermal amplification assay provides a one-step, single-tube amplification of HEV RNA without special equipment (148). The limit of detection of current assays is 7 to 188 IU/ml. Quantitative molecular tests are also used to assess the virological response to antiviral therapy (131).

ISOLATION PROCEDURES

Many primary isolates of HAV have been adapted to cell culture. Mutations within the internal ribosome entry site enhance cap-independent viral translation in specific cell lines, while mutations in proteins 2B and 2C promote viral replication in all types of cultured cells (149–151). Standard plaque assays based on cell lines have been developed to determine infectious virus titer. These methods provided data on the survival of HAV in food products and in the environment that can be used in risk-modeling and risk assessment studies (152).

Efficient cell culture systems for HEV are rare and are limited to HEV genotype 3 and 4 strains (153, 154). Insertions of fragments of human genes in the polyproline region of ORF1 seem to play an important role in virus adaptation (22, 27, 155). The main cell systems used for HEV culture are the HepG2/C3A, A549/D3, and PLC/PRF/5 cell lines (18, 155–157). Three-dimensional cell culture for HEV has also been developed (158). Because there are no visible cytopathic effects, viral growth is detected via HEV RNA detection in the supernatant or immunofluorescence straining of HEV-infected cells using polyclonal- or monoclonal-specific antibodies. Regarding HAV, infectivity endpoint methods are used for estimating the stability of HEV in food products or in the environment and the infection risk through specific virus transmission routes. These methods are also used in inactivation/removal studies of different manufacturing steps for plasma-derived medicinal products. Although very useful for research studies, cell culture systems for HAV and HEV have no diagnostic value.

IDENTIFICATION AND TYPING SYSTEMS

The HAV genotype was initially determined by sequencing a 168-nucleotide fragment corresponding to the VP1-2A junction (159, 160). However, current classification of HAV into six genotypes is based on sequences derived from the complete VP1 region (161). Therefore, VP1 is the preferred region for HAV molecular epidemiology studies and outbreak investigations.

HEV genotypes and subgenotypes can be determined by sequencing different regions of the HEV genome such as the ORF2 or ORF1 polymerase regions. This is useful for identifying the source of infection and characterizing the mutations in the polymerase of virus infecting patients in whom ribavirin therapy fails (134, 135).

Thanks to next-generation sequencing technologies, HAV and HEV whole-genome sequences and intrahost spectra of variants provide detailed characterization of viral strains.

SEROLOGIC TESTS

Hepatitis A Virus

Enzyme or chemiluminescent immunoassays for anti-HAV IgM and IgG are commercially available in microplate and multiparametric automated formats (Table 2). No rapid

TABLE 2 Commercial immunoassays available for anti-HAV and anti-HEV antibodies

Virus	Marker	Manufacturer	Product name	Type of test
HAV	Anti-HAV IgM	Abbott	Architect HAVAb-IgM	Automated
		Roche	Cobas Anti-HAV IgM	Automated
		bioMérieux	Vidas HAV IgM	Automated
		Siemens	Advia Centaur Anti-HAV IgM	Automated
		Beckman-Coulter	Access HAV IgM	Automated
		Diasorin	Liaison HAV IgM	Automated
		Ortho	Vitros Anti-HAV IgM	Automated
	Anti-HAV IgG	Abbott	Architect HAVAb-IgG	Automated
	Anti-HAV total antibodies	Roche	Cobas Anti-HAV	Automated
		bioMérieux	Vidas Anti-HAV Total	Automated
		Siemens	Advia Centaur Anti-HAV Total	Automated
		Beckman-Coulter	Access HAV Ab	Automated
		Diasorin	Liaison Anti-HAV	Automated
		Ortho	Vitros Anti-HAV Total	Automated
HEV	Anti-HEV IgM	Wantai	HEV IgM rapid test	Rapid test
		MP Diagnostics	Assure HEV IgM rapid test	Rapid test
		Wantai	HEV ELISA IgM	Microplate
		MP Diagnostics	HEV IgM ELISA	Microplate
		Adaltis	EIAgen HEV M	Microplate
		Mikrogen	recomWELL HEV IgM	Microplate
		Euroimmun	ELISA Anti-Virus HEV IgM	Microplate
		bioMérieux	Vidas Anti-HEV IgM	Automated
	Anti-HEV IgG	Wantai	HEV ELISA IgG	Microplate
		MP Diagnostics	HEV IgG ELISA	Microplate
		Adaltis	EIAgen HEV G	Microplate
		Mikrogen	recomWELL HEV IgG	Microplate
		Euroimmun	ELISA Anti-Virus HEV IgG	Microplate
		bioMérieux	Vidas Anti-HEV IgG	Automated

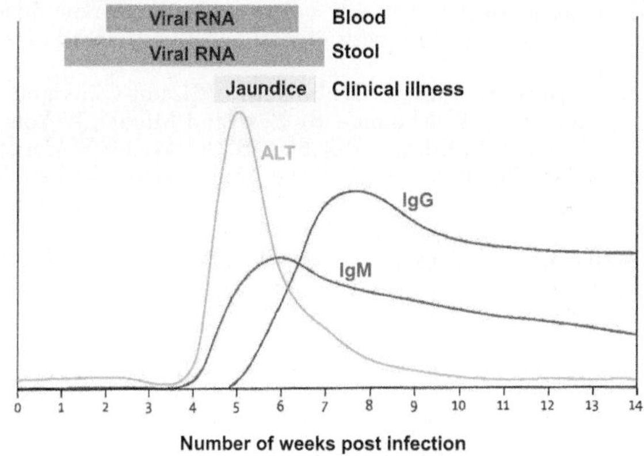

FIGURE 3 Virus detection (HAV RNA or HEV RNA) at different sites and serologic response (IgM and IgG antibodies). ALT, alanine aminotransferase.

immunochromatographic assay is commercially available. The diagnostic performance of HAV immunoassays in terms of sensitivity and specificity is well established (>95%).

The presence of anti-HAV IgM in the serum is a key marker of an acute infection (Fig. 3). Anti-HAV IgM is detectable when the alanine aminotransferase level increases and persists for 3 to 6 months thereafter. False-positive results are possible, especially when the clinical picture is not reflective of HAV infection and in the absence of anti-HAV IgG. IgM can also be detected due to nonspecific polyclonal activation of the immune system (162). In this setting, anti-HAV IgG is detected and IgG avidity for HAV is high (162). Therefore, serologic testing should be limited to people who meet the clinical criteria of hepatitis, particularly in areas where the endemicity pattern is low.

The presence of anti-HAV IgG alone is a marker of past infection or vaccination (Fig. 3). In unvaccinated individuals, testing for anti-HAV IgG can be used for identifying those who require immunization, but the cost-effectiveness of screening depends on age and epidemiologic parameters. Postvaccination tests are not required due to the high efficacy of HAV vaccines.

Hepatitis E Virus

Most enzyme immunoassays for anti-HEV IgM and IgG are commercially available in Europe and Asia in microplate formats (163) (Table 2). Multiparametric automated instruments are in development (164). Several immunochromatographic assays allowing rapid diagnosis are also available in different countries (165, 166). These point-of-care tests that are easy to use and give a result within a few minutes can be very useful in resource-limited countries. The antigens used are usually recombinant ORF2 and/or ORF3 proteins from HEV-1 strains. The diagnostic performance of these immunoassays varies considerably and must be evaluated carefully (163, 167).

The presence of anti-HEV IgM in the serum is a key marker of an acute infection (Fig. 3). Using a validated PCR assay as a reference, studies showed that IgM immunoassays, including rapid tests, had sensitivity of >97% for immunocompetent patients and 80 to 85% for immunosuppressed patients; their specificity was >99.5 % (165, 166, 168). Of note, longitudinal follow-up of patients with proven acute hepatitis E by nucleic acid testing showed a persistence of anti-HEV IgM for 6 to 12 months (91). Several studies using different serum panels have compared the performance of IgM assays (163, 167, 169, 170). In one study, five IgM assays were compared using sera from immunocompetent and immunocompromised individuals with a proven HEV infection (positive HEV RNA) (167). Only 71% of the results from all the assays were concordant. In another study, there were also discrepancies when single samples of 10 seroconversion panels were assayed (163). However, it is difficult to compare the findings of the different studies because differences in assay performance may be related to different versions of the test employed (169).

The presence of anti-HEV IgG alone is a marker of past infection (Fig. 3). Due to large differences in analytical sensitivity between IgG immunoassays, it is difficult to compare seroprevalence rates from different populations obtained by different laboratory methods. Using an international standard (WHO reference reagent established in 2002; National Institute for Biological Standards and Control Code 95/584), the limits of detection of commercial anti-HEV IgG assays vary from 0.25 WHO unit/ml to 2.5 WHO unit/ml. As highlighted in a meta-analysis of studies of HEV seroprevalence in Europe (171), the most sensitive immunoassay (Wantai test) produced the highest estimates of anti-HEV IgG seroprevalence. Several studies showed that in retesting populations initially screened with an insensitive "first-generation" IgG assay, the seroprevalence rose by a factor ranging from 2 to 4 when a more sensitive validated assay was employed (86, 172–175). The determination of anti-HEV IgG concentration could be useful for estimating the risk of reinfection after a natural infection or vaccination (176–178).

EVALUATION, INTERPRETATION, AND REPORTING OF RESULTS

Regarding HAV infection, serologic tests for anti-HAV IgM are essential for identifying new cases and outbreaks. The increasing availability of molecular characterization techniques has made it possible to link apparently sporadic cases and to associate them with slowly evolving multinational outbreaks (51, 179). Hepatitis A is a reportable disease in Europe, the United States, Australia, and many other countries where patient contacts can be managed by hygienic measures and active or passive immunoprophylaxis. At a global level, optimal vaccination policies and recommendations are based on the prevalence of anti-HAV IgG.

Regarding HEV infection, the recent availability of high-performance serologic and molecular tools allowed a significant change in the understanding of global epidemiology (endemicity in many industrialized countries due to zoonotic transmission) and pathology (chronic hepatitis E, neurological manifestations). The good performance of the most recent anti-HEV IgM assays makes them suitable for routine diagnosis. However, HEV RNA testing is necessary in immunocompromised patients because the humoral immune response is frequently impaired in this population. HEV RNA testing is also necessary for identifying chronic infection when the HEV RNA persists for 3 to 6 months and for monitoring interventions based on the reduction of immunosuppression or antiviral therapy. Surveillance systems are in place in most European countries where infections are predominantly caused by HEV genotype 3, the most prevalent virus genotype in the animal reservoirs (180). However, the surveillance strategies and algorithms are quite heterogeneous. Surveillance through reference laboratories exists in France, Germany, the Netherlands, Denmark, and Spain. Hepatitis E is a reportable disease in several countries. Lastly, the recognition of transfusion-transmitted HEV has led to estimations of the recipient risk and the definition of optimal strategies for improving blood safety in several developed countries (76).

REFERENCES

1. **Wang X, Ren J, Gao Q, Hu Z, Sun Y, Li X, Rowlands DJ, Yin W, Wang J, Stuart DI, Rao Z, Fry EE.** 2015. Hepatitis A virus and the origins of picornaviruses. *Nature* **517:**85–88.
2. **Cristina J, Costa-Mattioli M.** 2007. Genetic variability and molecular evolution of hepatitis A virus. *Virus Res* **127:**151–157.
3. **Drexler JF, Corman VM, Lukashev AN, van den Brand JM, Gmyl AP, Brünink S, Rasche A, Seggewiβ N, Feng H, Leijten LM, Vallo P, Kuiken T, Dotzauer A, Ulrich RG, Lemon SM, Drosten C, Hepatovirus Ecology Consortium.** 2015. Evolutionary origins of hepatitis A virus in small mammals. *Proc Natl Acad Sci USA* **112:**15190–15195.
4. **Smith DB, Simmonds P, Jameel S, Emerson SU, Harrison TJ, Meng XJ, Okamoto H, Van der Poel WH, Purdy MA, International Committee on Taxonomy of Viruses Hepeviridae Study Group.** 2014. Consensus proposals for classification of the family *Hepeviridae*. *J Gen Virol* **95:**2223–2232.
5. **Kamar N, Dalton HR, Abravanel F, Izopet J.** 2014. Hepatitis E virus infection. *Clin Microbiol Rev* **27:**116–138.
6. **Li TC, Kataoka M, Takahashi K, Yoshizaki S, Kato T, Ishii K, Takeda N, Mishiro S, Wakita T.** 2015. Generation of hepatitis E virus-like particles of two new genotypes G5 and G6 and comparison of antigenic properties with those of known genotypes. *Vet Microbiol* **178:**150–157.
7. **Lee GH, Tan BH, Teo EC, Lim SG, Dan YY, Wee A, Aw PP, Zhu Y, Hibberd ML, Tan CK, Purdy MA, Teo CG.** 2016. Chronic infection with camelid hepatitis E virus in a liver transplant recipient who regularly consumes camel meat and milk. *Gastroenterology* **150:**355–357.
8. **Feinstone SM, Kapikian AZ, Purcell RH.** 1973. Hepatitis A: detection by immune electron microscopy of a viruslike antigen associated with acute illness. *Science* **182:**1026–1028.
9. **Feng Z, Hensley L, McKnight KL, Hu F, Madden V, Ping L, Jeong SH, Walker C, Lanford RE, Lemon SM.** 2013. A pathogenic picornavirus acquires an envelope by hijacking cellular membranes. *Nature* **496:**367–371.
10. **McKnight KL, Xie L, González-López O, Rivera-Serrano EE, Chen X, Lemon SM.** 2017. Protein composition of the hepatitis A virus quasi-envelope. *Proc Natl Acad Sci USA* **114:**6587–6592.
11. **Feng Z, Li Y, McKnight KL, Hensley L, Lanford RE, Walker CM, Lemon SM.** 2015. Human pDCs preferentially sense enveloped hepatitis A virions. *J Clin Invest* **125:**169–176.
12. **Lanford RE, Feng Z, Chavez D, Guerra B, Brasky KM, Zhou Y, Yamane D, Perelson AS, Walker CM, Lemon SM.** 2011. Acute hepatitis A virus infection is associated with a limited type I interferon response and persistence of intrahepatic viral RNA. *Proc Natl Acad Sci USA* **108:**11223–11228.
13. **Bidawid S, Farber JM, Sattar SA, Hayward S.** 2000. Heat inactivation of hepatitis A virus in dairy foods. *J Food Prot* **63:**522–528.
14. **Hirai-Yuki A, Hensley L, McGivern DR, González-López O, Das A, Feng H, Sun L, Wilson JE, Hu F, Feng Z, Lovell W, Misumi I, Ting JP, Montgomery S, Cullen J, Whitmire JK, Lemon SM.** 2016. MAVS-dependent host species range and pathogenicity of human hepatitis A virus. *Science* **353:**1541–1545.
15. **Balayan MS, Andjaparidze AG, Savinskaya SS, Ketiladze ES, Braginsky DM, Savinov AP, Poleschuk VF.** 1983. Evidence for a virus in non-A, non-B hepatitis transmitted via the fecal-oral route. *Intervirology* **20:**23–31.
16. **Takahashi M, Tanaka T, Takahashi H, Hoshino Y, Nagashima S, Jirintai, Mizuo H, Yazaki Y, Takagi T, Azuma M, Kusano E, Isoda N, Sugano K, Okamoto H.** 2010. Hepatitis E virus (HEV) strains in serum samples can replicate efficiently in cultured cells despite the coexistence of HEV antibodies: characterization of HEV virions in blood circulation. *J Clin Microbiol* **48:**1112–1125.
17. **Feng Z, Lemon SM.** 2014. Peek-a-boo: membrane hijacking and the pathogenesis of viral hepatitis. *Trends Microbiol* **22:**59–64.
18. **Chapuy-Regaud S, Dubois M, Plisson-Chastang C, Bonnefois T, Lhomme S, Bertrand-Michel J, You B, Simoneau S, Gleizes PE, Flan B, Abravanel F, Izopet J.** 2017. Characterization of the lipid envelope of exosome encapsulated HEV particles protected from the immune response. *Biochimie* **141:**70–79.
19. **Barnaud E, Rogée S, Garry P, Rose N, Pavio N.** 2012. Thermal inactivation of infectious hepatitis E virus in experimentally contaminated food. *Appl Environ Microbiol* **78:**5153–5159.
20. **Feagins AR, Opriessnig T, Guenette DK, Halbur PG, Meng XJ.** 2008. Inactivation of infectious hepatitis E virus present in commercial pig livers sold in local grocery stores in the United States. *Int J Food Microbiol* **123:**32–37.
21. **Koonin EV, Gorbalenya AE, Purdy MA, Rozanov MN, Reyes GR, Bradley DW.** 1992. Computer-assisted assignment of functional domains in the nonstructural polyprotein of hepatitis E virus: delineation of an additional group of positive-strand RNA plant and animal viruses. *Proc Natl Acad Sci USA* **89:**8259–8263.
22. **Kenney SP, Meng XJ.** 2015. The lysine residues within the human ribosomal protein S17 sequence naturally inserted into the viral nonstructural protein of a unique strain of hepatitis E virus are important for enhanced virus replication. *J Virol* **89:**3793–3803.
23. **Lhomme S, Garrouste C, Kamar N, Saune K, Abravanel F, Mansuy JM, Dubois M, Rostaing L, Izopet J.** 2014. Influence of polyproline region and macro domain genetic heterogeneity on HEV persistence in immunocompromised patients. *J Infect Dis* **209:**300–303.
24. **Nguyen HT, Torian U, Faulk K, Mather K, Engle RE, Thompson E, Bonkovsky HL, Emerson SU.** 2012. A naturally occurring human/hepatitis E recombinant virus predominates in serum but not in faeces of a chronic hepatitis E patient and has a growth advantage in cell culture. *J Gen Virol* **93:**526–530.
25. **Purdy MA.** 2012. Evolution of the hepatitis E virus polyproline region: order from disorder. *J Virol* **86:**10186–10193.
26. **Shukla P, Nguyen HT, Faulk K, Mather K, Torian U, Engle RE, Emerson SU.** 2012. Adaptation of a genotype 3 hepatitis E virus to efficient growth in cell culture depends on an inserted human gene segment acquired by recombination. *J Virol* **86:**5697–5707.
27. **Shukla P, Nguyen HT, Torian U, Engle RE, Faulk K, Dalton HR, Bendall RP, Keane FE, Purcell RH, Emerson SU.** 2011. Cross-species infections of cultured cells by hepatitis E virus and discovery of an infectious virus-host recombinant. *Proc Natl Acad Sci USA* **108:**2438–2443.
28. **Nair VP, Anang S, Subramani C, Madhvi A, Bakshi K, Srivastava A, Shalimar, Nayak B, Ranjith Kumar CT, Surjit M.** 2016. Endoplasmic reticulum stress induced synthesis of a novel viral factor mediates efficient replication of genotype-1 hepatitis E virus. *PLoS Pathog* **12:**e1005521.
29. **Zafrullah M, Ozdener MH, Kumar R, Panda SK, Jameel S.** 1999. Mutational analysis of glycosylation, membrane translocation, and cell surface expression of the hepatitis E virus ORF2 protein. *J Virol* **73:**4074–4082.
30. **Guu TS, Liu Z, Ye Q, Mata DA, Li K, Yin C, Zhang J, Tao YJ.** 2009. Structure of the hepatitis E virus-like particle suggests mechanisms for virus assembly and receptor binding. *Proc Natl Acad Sci USA* **106:**12992–12997.
31. **Yamashita T, Mori Y, Miyazaki N, Cheng RH, Yoshimura M, Unno H, Shima R, Moriishi K, Tsukihara T, Li TC, Takeda N, Miyamura T, Matsuura Y.** 2009. Biological and immunological characteristics of hepatitis E virus-like particles based on the crystal structure. *Proc Natl Acad Sci USA* **106:**12986–12991.
32. **Xing L, Wang JC, Li TC, Yasutomi Y, Lara J, Khudyakov Y, Schofield D, Emerson SU, Purcell RH, Takeda N, Miyamura T, Cheng RH.** 2011. Spatial configuration of hepatitis E virus antigenic domain. *J Virol* **85:**1117–1124.

33. **Tang X, Yang C, Gu Y, Song C, Zhang X, Wang Y, Zhang J, Hew CL, Li S, Xia N, Sivaraman J.** 2011. Structural basis for the neutralization and genotype specificity of hepatitis E virus. *Proc Natl Acad Sci USA* **108:**10266–10271.
34. **Lhomme S, Abravanel F, Dubois M, Sandres Saune K, Rostaing L, Kamar N, Izopet J.** 2012. Hepatitis E virus quasispecies and the outcome of acute hepatitis E in solid-organ transplant patients. *J Virol* **86:**100006–100014.
35. **Tyagi S, Korkaya H, Zafrullah M, Jameel S, Lal SK.** 2002. The phosphorylated form of the ORF3 protein of hepatitis E virus interacts with its non-glycosylated form of the major capsid protein, ORF2. *J Biol Chem* **277:**22759–22767.
36. **Emerson SU, Nguyen HT, Torian U, Burke D, Engle R, Purcell RH.** 2010. Release of genotype 1 hepatitis E virus from cultured hepatoma and polarized intestinal cells depends on open reading frame 3 protein and requires an intact PXXP motif. *J Virol* **84:**9059–9069.
37. **Kenney SP, Pudupakam RS, Huang YW, Pierson FW, LeRoith T, Meng XJ.** 2012. The PSAP motif within the ORF3 protein of an avian strain of the hepatitis E virus is not critical for viral infectivity *in vivo* but plays a role in virus release. *J Virol* **86:**5637–5646.
38. **Nagashima S, Jirintai S, Takahashi M, Kobayashi T, Tanggis, Nishizawa T, Kouki T, Yashiro T, Okamoto H.** 2014. Hepatitis E virus egress depends on the exosomal pathway, with secretory exosomes derived from multivesicular bodies. *J Gen Virol* **95:**2166–2175.
39. **Nagashima S, Takahashi M, Jirintai, Tanaka T, Yamada K, Nishizawa T, Okamoto H.** 2011. A PSAP motif in the ORF3 protein of hepatitis E virus is necessary for virion release from infected cells. *J Gen Virol* **92:**269–278.
40. **Nagashima S, Takahashi M, Jirintai S, Tanaka T, Nishizawa T, Yasuda J, Okamoto H.** 2011. Tumour susceptibility gene 101 and the vacuolar protein sorting pathway are required for the release of hepatitis E virions. *J Gen Virol* **92:**2838–2848.
41. **Yamada K, Takahashi M, Hoshino Y, Takahashi H, Ichiyama K, Nagashima S, Tanaka T, Okamoto H.** 2009. ORF3 protein of hepatitis E virus is essential for virion release from infected cells. *J Gen Virol* **90:**1880–1891.
42. **Cao D, Cao QM, Subramaniam S, Yugo DM, Heffron CL, Rogers AJ, Kenney SP, Tian D, Matzinger SR, Overend C, Catanzaro N, LeRoith T, Wang H, Piñeyro P, Lindstrom N, Clark-Deener S, Yuan L, Meng XJ.** 2017. Pig model mimicking chronic hepatitis E virus infection in immunocompromised patients to assess immune correlates during chronicity. *Proc Natl Acad Sci USA* **114:**6914–6923.
43. **Gardinali NR, Guimarães JR, Melgaço JG, Kevorkian YB, Bottino FO, Vieira YR, da Silva AC, Pinto DP, da Fonseca LB, Vilhena LS, Uiechi E, da Silva MC, Moran J, Marchevsky RS, Cruz OG, Otonel RA, Alfieri AA, de Oliveira JM, Gaspar AM, Pinto MA.** 2017. Cynomolgus monkeys are successfully and persistently infected with hepatitis E virus genotype 3 (HEV-3) after long-term immunosuppressive therapy. *PLoS One* **12:**e0174070.
44. **Allweiss L, Gass S, Giersch K, Groth A, Kah J, Volz T, Rapp G, Schöbel A, Lohse AW, Polywka S, Pischke S, Herker E, Dandri M, Lütgehetmann M.** 2016. Human liver chimeric mice as a new model of chronic hepatitis E virus infection and preclinical drug evaluation. *J Hepatol* **64:**1033–1040.
45. **Sayed IM, Foquet L, Verhoye L, Abravanel F, Farhoudi A, Leroux-Roels G, Izopet J, Meuleman P.** 2017. Transmission of hepatitis E virus infection to human-liver chimeric FRG mice using patient plasma. *Antiviral Res* **141:**150–154.
46. **Sayed IM, Verhoye L, Cocquerel L, Abravanel F, Foquet L, Montpellier C, Debing Y, Farhoudi A, Wychowski C, Dubuisson J, Leroux-Roels G, Neyts J, Izopet J, Michiels T, Meuleman P.** 2017. Study of hepatitis E virus infection of genotype 1 and 3 in mice with humanised liver. *Gut* **66:** 920–929.
47. **van de Garde MD, Pas SD, van der Net G, de Man RA, Osterhaus AD, Haagmans BL, Boonstra A, Vanwolleghem T.** 2016. Hepatitis E virus (HEV) genotype 3 infection of human liver chimeric mice as a model for chronic HEV infection. *J Virol* **90:**4394–4401
48. **Collier MG, Khudyakov YE, Selvage D, Adams-Cameron M, Epson E, Cronquist A, Jervis RH, Lamba K, Kimura AC, Sowadsky R, Hassan R, Park SY, Garza E, Elliott AJ, Rotstein DS, Beal J, Kuntz T, Lance SE, Dreisch R, Wise ME, Nelson NP, Suryaprasad A, Drobeniuc J, Holmberg SD, Xu F, Hepatitis A Outbreak Investigation Team.** 2014. Outbreak of hepatitis A in the USA associated with frozen pomegranate arils imported from Turkey: an epidemiological case study. *Lancet Infect Dis* **14:**976–981
49. **Halliday ML, Kang LY, Zhou TK, Hu MD, Pan QC, Fu TY, Huang YS, Hu SL.** 1991. An epidemic of hepatitis A attributable to the ingestion of raw clams in Shanghai, China. *J Infect Dis* **164:**852–859
50. **McFarland N, Dryden M, Ramsay M, Tedder RS, Ngui SL, 2008 Winchester HAV Outbreak Team.** 2011. An outbreak of hepatitis A affecting a nursery school and a primary school. *Epidemiol Infect* **139:**336–343
51. **Freidl GS, Sonder GJ, Bovée LP, Friesema IH, van Rijckevorsel GG, Ruijs WL, van Schie F, Siedenburg EC, Yang JY, Vennema H.** 2017. Hepatitis A outbreak among men who have sex with men (MSM) predominantly linked with the EuroPride, the Netherlands, July 2016 to February 2017. *Euro Surveill* **22:**22 http://www.eurosurveillance.org/content/10.2807/1560-7917.ES.2017.22.8.30468.
52. **Spada E, Genovese D, Tosti ME, Mariano A, Cuccuini M, Proietti L, Giuli CD, Lavagna A, Crapa GE, Morace G, Taffon S, Mele A, Rezza G, Rapicetta M.** 2005. An outbreak of hepatitis A virus infection with a high case-fatality rate among injecting drug users. *J Hepatol* **43:**958–964.
53. **da Silva SG, Leon LA, Alves G, Brito SM, Sandes VS, Lima MM, Nogueira MC, Tavares RC, Dobbin J, Apa A, de Paula VS, Oliveira JM, Pinto MA, Ferreira OC Jr, Motta IJ.** 2016. A rare case of transfusion transmission of hepatitis A virus to two patients with haematological disease. *Transfus Med Hemother* **43:**137–141.
54. **Khuroo MS.** 2011. Discovery of hepatitis E: the epidemic non-A, non-B hepatitis 30 years down the memory lane. *Virus Res* **161:**3–14.
55. **Teshale EH, Grytdal SP, Howard C, Barry V, Kamili S, Drobeniuc J, Hill VR, Okware S, Hu DJ, Holmberg SD.** 2010. Evidence of person-to-person transmission of hepatitis E virus during a large outbreak in Northern Uganda. *Clin Infect Dis* **50:**1006–1010.
56. **Centers for Disease Control and Prevention (CDC).** 2013. Investigation of hepatitis E outbreak among refugees: Upper Nile, South Sudan, 2012-2013. *MMWR Morb Mortal Wkly Rep* **62:**581–586.
57. **Aggarwal R, Naik SR.** 1994. Hepatitis E: intrafamilial transmission versus waterborne spread. *J Hepatol* **21:**718–723.
58. **Somani SK, Aggarwal R, Naik SR, Srivastava S, Naik S.** 2003. A serological study of intrafamilial spread from patients with sporadic hepatitis E virus infection. *J Viral Hepat* **10:**446–449.
59. **Khuroo MS, Kamili S, Jameel S.** 1995. Vertical transmission of hepatitis E virus. *Lancet* **345:**1025–1026.
60. **Khuroo MS, Kamili S, Khuroo MS.** 2009. Clinical course and duration of viremia in vertically transmitted hepatitis E virus (HEV) infection in babies born to HEV-infected mothers. *J Viral Hepat* **16:**519–523.
61. **Khuroo MS, Kamili S, Yattoo GN.** 2004. Hepatitis E virus infection may be transmitted through blood transfusions in an endemic area. *J Gastroenterol Hepatol* **19:**778–784.
62. **Arankalle VA, Chobe LP.** 2000. Retrospective analysis of blood transfusion recipients: evidence for post-transfusion hepatitis E. *Vox Sang* **79:**72–74.
63. **Colson P, Borentain P, Queyriaux B, Kaba M, Moal V, Gallian P, Heyries L, Raoult D, Gerolami R.** 2010. Pig liver sausage as a source of hepatitis E virus transmission to humans. *J Infect Dis* **202:**825–834.
64. **Renou C, Roque-Afonso AM, Pavio N.** 2014. Foodborne transmission of hepatitis E virus from raw pork liver sausage, France. *Emerg Infect Dis* **20:**1945–1947 (Erratum, **21:**384.).
65. **Riveiro-Barciela M, Mínguez B, Gironés R, Rodriguez-Frías F, Quer J, Buti M.** 2015. Phylogenetic demonstration

of hepatitis E infection transmitted by pork meat ingestion. *J Clin Gastroenterol* **49:**165–168.

66. **Abravanel F, Lhomme S, El Costa H, Schvartz B, Peron JM, Kamar N, Izopet J.** 2017. Rabbit hepatitis E virus infections in humans, France. *Emerg Infect Dis* **23:**1191–1193.
67. **Izopet J, Dubois M, Bertagnoli S, Lhomme S, Marchandeau S, Boucher S, Kamar N, Abravanel F, Guérin JL.** 2012. Hepatitis E virus strains in rabbits and evidence of a closely related strain in humans, France. *Emerg Infect Dis* **18:**1274–1281.
68. **Yan B, Zhang L, Gong L, Lv J, Feng Y, Liu J, Song L, Xu Q, Jiang M, Xu A.** 2016. Hepatitis E virus in yellow cattle, Shandong, eastern China. *Emerg Infect Dis* **22:**2211–2212.
69. **Huang F, Li Y, Yu W, Jing S, Wang J, Long F, He Z, Yang C, Bi Y, Cao W, Liu C, Hua X, Pan Q.** 2016. Excretion of infectious hepatitis E virus into milk in cows imposes high risks of zoonosis. *Hepatology* **64:**350–359.
70. **Kokkinos P, Kozyra I, Lazic S, Bouwknegt M, Rutjes S, Willems K, Moloney R, de Roda Husman AM, Kaupke A, Legaki E, D'Agostino M, Cook N, Rzez·utka A, Petrovic T, Vantarakis A.** 2012. Harmonised investigation of the occurrence of human enteric viruses in the leafy green vegetable supply chain in three European countries. *Food Environ Virol* **4:**179–191.
71. **Crossan C, Baker PJ, Craft J, Takeuchi Y, Dalton HR, Scobie L.** 2012. Hepatitis E virus genotype 3 in shellfish, United Kingdom. *Emerg Infect Dis* **18:**2085–2087.
72. **Hewitt PE, Ijaz S, Brailsford SR, Brett R, Dicks S, Haywood B, Kennedy IT, Kitchen A, Patel P, Poh J, Russell K, Tettmar KI, Tossell J, Ushiro-Lumb I, Tedder RS.** 2014. Hepatitis E virus in blood components: a prevalence and transmission study in southeast England. *Lancet* **384:**1766–1773.
73. **Zhang L, Jiao S, Yang Z, Xu L, Liu L, Feng Q, Zhang X, Hou Y, He S, Saldanha J, Wang S, Wang B.** 2017. Prevalence of hepatitis E virus infection among blood donors in mainland China: a meta-analysis. *Transfusion* **57:**248–257.
74. **Satake M, Matsubayashi K, Hoshi Y, Taira R, Furui Y, Kokudo N, Akamatsu N, Yoshizumi T, Ohkohchi N, Okamoto H, Miyoshi M, Tamura A, Fuse K, Tadokoro K.** 2017. Unique clinical courses of transfusion-transmitted hepatitis E in patients with immunosuppression. *Transfusion* **57:**280–288.
75. **Izopet J, Lhomme S, Chapuy-Regaud S, Mansuy JM, Kamar N, Abravanel F.** 2017. HEV and transfusion-recipient risk. *Transfus Clin Biol* **24:**176–181.
76. **Domanović D, Tedder R, Blümel J, Zaaijer H, Gallian P, Niederhauser C, Sauleda Oliveras S, O'Riordan J, Boland F, Harritshøj L, Nascimento MSJ, Ciccaglione AR, Politis C, Adlhoch C, Flan B, Oualikene-Gonin W, Rautmann G, Strengers P, Hewitt P.** 2017. Hepatitis E and blood donation safety in selected European countries: a shift to screening? *Euro Surveill* **22:**30514 http://www.eurosurveillance.org/content/10.2807/1560-7917.ES.2017.22.16.30514.
77. **Gallian P, Couchouron A, Dupont I, Fabra C, Piquet Y, Djoudi R, Assal A, Tiberghien P.** 2017. Comparison of hepatitis E virus nucleic acid test screening platforms and RNA prevalence in French blood donors. *Transfusion* **57:**223–224.
78. **Gallian P, Lhomme S, Piquet Y, Sauné K, Abravanel F, Assal A, Tiberghien P, Izopet J.** 2014. Hepatitis E virus infections in blood donors, France. *Emerg Infect Dis* **20:**1914–1917.
79. **Mohd Hanafiah K, Jacobsen KH, Wiersma ST.** 2011. Challenges to mapping the health risk of hepatitis A virus infection. *Int J Health Geogr* **10:**57.
80. **Aggarwal R, Goel A.** 2015. Hepatitis A: epidemiology in resource-poor countries. *Curr Opin Infect Dis* **28:**488–496.
81. **Vizzotti C, González J, Gentile A, Rearte A, Ramonet M, Cañero-Velasco MC, Pérez Carrega ME, Urueña A, Diosque M.** 2014. Impact of the single-dose immunization strategy against hepatitis A in Argentina. *Pediatr Infect Dis J* **33:**84–88.
82. **Vizzotti C, Pippo T, Urueña A, Altuna J, Palópoli G, Hernández ML, Artola MF, Fernández H, Orellano P, Cañero-Velasco MC, Ciocca M, Ramonet M, Diosque M.** 2015. Economic analysis of the single-dose immunization strategy against hepatitis A in Argentina. *Vaccine* **33**(Suppl 1)**:** A227–A232.
83. **Rein DB, Stevens GA, Theaker J, Wittenborn JS, Wiersma ST.** 2012. The global burden of hepatitis E virus genotypes 1 and 2 in 2005. *Hepatology* **55:**988–997.
84. **WHO.** Waterborne Outbreaks of Hepatitis E: Recognition, Investigation and Control. http://www.who.int/hiv/pub/hepatitis/HepE-manual/en/.
85. **Kamar N, Bendall R, Legrand-Abravanel F, Xia NS, Ijaz S, Izopet J, Dalton HR.** 2012. Hepatitis E. *Lancet* **379:** 2477–2488.
86. **Mansuy JM, Bendall R, Legrand-Abravanel F, Sauné K, Miédouge M, Ellis V, Rech H, Destruel F, Kamar N, Dalton HR, Izopet J.** 2011. Hepatitis E virus antibodies in blood donors, France. *Emerg Infect Dis* **17:**2309–2312.
87. **Wenzel JJ, Sichler M, Schemmerer M, Behrens G, Leitzmann MF, Jilg W.** 2014. Decline in hepatitis E virus antibody prevalence in southeastern Germany, 1996-2011. *Hepatology* **60:**1180–1186.
88. **Ditah I, Ditah F, Devaki P, Ditah C, Kamath PS, Charlton M.** 2014. Current epidemiology of hepatitis E virus infection in the United States: low seroprevalence in the National Health and Nutrition Evaluation Survey. *Hepatology* **60:** 815–822.
89. **Vento S, Garofano T, Renzini C, Cainelli F, Casali F, Ghironzi G, Ferraro T, Concia E.** 1998. Fulminant hepatitis associated with hepatitis A virus superinfection in patients with chronic hepatitis C. *N Engl J Med* **338:**286–290.
90. **Huang S, Zhang X, Jiang H, Yan Q, Ai X, Wang Y, Cai J, Jiang L, Wu T, Wang Z, Guan L, Shih JW, Ng MH, Zhu F, Zhang J, Xia N.** 2010. Profile of acute infectious markers in sporadic hepatitis E. *PLoS One* **5:**e13560.
91. **Wen GP, Tang ZM, Yang F, Zhang K, Ji WF, Cai W, Huang SJ, Wu T, Zhang J, Zheng ZZ, Xia NS.** 2015. A valuable antigen detection method for diagnosis of acute hepatitis E. *J Clin Microbiol* **53:**782–788.
92. **Kumar A, Saraswat VA.** 2013. Hepatitis E and acute-on-chronic liver failure. *J Clin Exp Hepatol* **3:**225–230.
93. **Blasco-Perrin H, Madden RG, Stanley A, Crossan C, Hunter JG, Vine L, Lane K, Devooght-Johnson N, Mclaughlin C, Petrik J, Stableforth B, Hussaini H, Phillips M, Mansuy JM, Forrest E, Izopet J, Blatchford O, Scobie L, Peron JM, Dalton HR.** 2015. Hepatitis E virus in patients with decompensated chronic liver disease: a prospective UK/French study. *Aliment Pharmacol Ther* **42:**574–581.
94. **Anty R, Ollier L, Péron JM, Nicand E, Cannavo I, Bongain A, Giordanengo V, Tran A.** 2012. First case report of an acute genotype 3 hepatitis E infected pregnant woman living in South-Eastern France. *J Clin Virol* **54:**76–78.
95. **Renou C, Gobert V, Locher C, Moumen A, Timbely O, Savary J, Roque-Afonso AM, Association Nationale des Hépato-Gastroentérologues des Hôpitaux Généraux (ANGH).** 2014. Prospective study of hepatitis E virus infection among pregnant women in France. *Virol J* **11:**68.
96. **Kamar N, Selves J, Mansuy JM, Ouezzani L, Péron JM, Guitard J, Cointault O, Esposito L, Abravanel F, Danjoux M, Durand D, Vinel JP, Izopet J, Rostaing L.** 2008. Hepatitis E virus and chronic hepatitis in organ-transplant recipients. *N Engl J Med* **358:**811–817.
97. **Gérolami R, Moal V, Colson P.** 2008. Chronic hepatitis E with cirrhosis in a kidney-transplant recipient. *N Engl J Med* **358:**859–860.
98. **Kamar N, Garrouste C, Haagsma EB, Garrigue V, Pischke S, Chauvet C, Dumortier J, Cannesson A, Cassuto-Viguier E, Thervet E, Conti F, Lebray P, Dalton HR, Santella R, Kanaan N, Essig M, Mousson C, Radenne S, Roque-Afonso AM, Izopet J, Rostaing L.** 2011. Factors associated with chronic hepatitis in patients with hepatitis E virus infection who have received solid organ transplants. *Gastroenterology* **140:**1481–1489.
99. **Koenecke C, Pischke S, Beutel G, Ritter U, Ganser A, Wedemeyer H, Eder M.** 2014. Hepatitis E virus infection in a hematopoietic stem cell donor. *Bone Marrow Transplant* **49:**159–160.

100. **Tavitian S, Péron JM, Huynh A, Mansuy JM, Ysebaert L, Huguet F, Vinel JP, Attal M, Izopet J, Récher C.** 2010. Hepatitis E virus excretion can be prolonged in patients with hematological malignancies. *J Clin Virol* **49:**141–144.
101. **Dalton HR, Bendall RP, Keane FE, Tedder RS, Ijaz S.** 2009. Persistent carriage of hepatitis E virus in patients with HIV infection. *N Engl J Med* **361:**1025–1027.
102. **Ollier L, Tieulie N, Sanderson F, Heudier P, Giordanengo V, Fuzibet JG, Nicand E.** 2009. Chronic hepatitis after hepatitis E virus infection in a patient with non-Hodgkin lymphoma taking rituximab. *Ann Intern Med* **150:**430–431.
103. **Bauer H, Luxembourger C, Gottenberg JE, Fournier S, Abravanel F, Cantagrel A, Chatelus E, Claudepierre P, Hudry C, Izopet J, Fabre S, Lefevre G, Marguerie L, Martin A, Messer L, Molto A, Pallot-Prades B, Pers YM, Roque-Afonso AM, Roux C, Sordet C, Soubrier M, Veissier C, Wendling D, Péron JM, Sibilia J, Club Rhumatismes et Inflammation, a section of the French Society of Rheumatology.** 2015. Outcome of hepatitis E virus infection in patients with inflammatory arthritides treated with immunosuppressants: a French retrospective multicenter study. *Medicine (Baltimore)* **94:**e675.
104. **Kamar N, Rostaing L, Legrand-Abravanel F, Izopet J.** 2013. How should hepatitis E virus infection be defined in organ-transplant recipients? *Am J Transplant* **13:**1935–1936.
105. **Kamar N, Abravanel F, Selves J, Garrouste C, Esposito L, Lavayssière L, Cointault O, Ribes D, Cardeau I, Nogier MB, Mansuy JM, Muscari F, Peron JM, Izopet J, Rostaing L.** 2010. Influence of immunosuppressive therapy on the natural history of genotype 3 hepatitis-E virus infection after organ transplantation. *Transplantation* **89:**353–360.
106. **Kamar N, Mansuy JM, Cointault O, Selves J, Abravanel F, Danjoux M, Otal P, Esposito L, Durand D, Izopet J, Rostaing L.** 2008. Hepatitis E virus-related cirrhosis in kidney- and kidney-pancreas-transplant recipients. *Am J Transplant* **8:**1744–1748.
107. **Suneetha PV, Pischke S, Schlaphoff V, Grabowski J, Fytili P, Gronert A, Bremer B, Markova A, Jaroszewicz J, Bara C, Manns MP, Cornberg M, Wedemeyer H.** 2012. Hepatitis E virus (HEV)-specific T-cell responses are associated with control of HEV infection. *Hepatology* **55:**695–708.
108. **Dalton HR, Kamar N, van Eijk JJ, Mclean BN, Cintas P, Bendall RP, Jacobs BC.** 2016. Hepatitis E virus and neurological injury. *Nat Rev Neurol* **12:**77–85.
109. **Kamar N, Bendall RP, Peron JM, Cintas P, Prudhomme L, Mansuy JM, Rostaing L, Keane F, Ijaz S, Izopet J, Dalton HR.** 2011. Hepatitis E virus and neurologic disorders. *Emerg Infect Dis* **17:**173–179.
110. **Woolson KL, Forbes A, Vine L, Beynon L, McElhinney L, Panayi V, Hunter JG, Madden RG, Glasgow T, Kotecha A, Dalton HC, Mihailescu L, Warshow U, Hussaini HS, Palmer J, Mclean BN, Haywood B, Bendall RP, Dalton HR.** 2014. Extra-hepatic manifestations of autochthonous hepatitis E infection. *Aliment Pharmacol Ther* **40:**1282–1291.
111. **van den Berg B, van der Eijk AA, Pas SD, Hunter JG, Madden RG, Tio-Gillen AP, Dalton HR, Jacobs BC.** 2014. Guillain-Barré syndrome associated with preceding hepatitis E virus infection. *Neurology* **82:**491–497.
112. **GeurtsvanKessel CH, Islam Z, Mohammad QD, Jacobs BC, Endtz HP, Osterhaus AD.** 2013. Hepatitis E and Guillain-Barre syndrome. *Clin Infect Dis* **57:**1369–1370.
113. **Fukae J, Tsugawa J, Ouma S, Umezu T, Kusunoki S, Tsuboi Y.** 2016. Guillain-Barré and Miller Fisher syndromes in patients with anti-hepatitis E virus antibody: a hospital-based survey in Japan. *Neurol Sci* **37:**1849–1851.
114. **Stevens O, Claeys KG, Poesen K, Saegeman V, Van Damme P.** 2017. Diagnostic challenges and clinical characteristics of hepatitis E virus-associated Guillain-Barré syndrome. *JAMA Neurol* **74:**26–33.
115. **van Eijk JJ, Madden RG, van der Eijk AA, Hunter JG, Reimerink JH, Bendall RP, Pas SD, Ellis V, van Alfen N, Beynon L, Southwell L, McLean B, Jacobs BC, van Engelen BG, Dalton HR.** 2014. Neuralgic amyotrophy and hepatitis E virus infection. *Neurology* **82:**498–503.
116. **Dalton H, van Eijk JJ, Cintas P, Madden R, Jones C, Webb G, Norton B, Pique J, Lutgens S, Devooght-Johnson N, Woolson KL, Baker J, Saunders M, Househam L, Griffiths J, Abravanel F, Izopet J, Kamar N, van Alfen N, van Engelen BG, Hunter JG, van der Eijk AA, Bendall R, McLean B, Jacobs BC.** 2017. Hepatitis E infection and acute non-traumatic neurological injury: A prospective pilot multicentre study. *J Hepatol* **67:**925–932.
117. **Kamar N, Izopet J, Cintas P, Garrouste C, Uro-Coste E, Cointault O, Rostaing L.** 2010. Hepatitis E virus-induced neurological symptoms in a kidney-transplant patient with chronic hepatitis. *Am J Transplant* **10:**1321–1324.
118. **Kamar N, Weclawiak H, Guilbeau-Frugier C, Legrand-Abravanel F, Cointault O, Ribes D, Esposito L, Cardeau-Desangles I, Guitard J, Sallusto F, Muscari F, Peron JM, Alric L, Izopet J, Rostaing L.** 2012. Hepatitis E virus and the kidney in solid-organ transplant patients. *Transplantation* **93:**617–623.
119. **Ali G, Kumar M, Bali S, Wadhwa W.** 2001. Heptitis E associated immune thrombocytopenia and membranous glomerulonephritis. *Indian J Nephrol* **11:**70–72.
120. **Taton B, Moreau K, Lepreux S, Bachelet T, Trimoulet P, De Ledinghen V, Pommereau A, Ronco P, Kamar N, Merville P, Couzi L.** 2013. Hepatitis E virus infection as a new probable cause of *de novo* membranous nephropathy after kidney transplantation. *Transpl Infect Dis* **15:**E211–E215.
121. **Guinault D, Ribes D, Delas A, Milongo D, Abravanel F, Puissant-Lubrano B, Izopet J, Kamar N.** 2016. Hepatitis E virus-induced cryglobulinemic glomerulonephritis in a non-immunocompromised person. *Am J Kidney Dis* **67:**660–663.
122. **Victor JC, Monto AS, Surdina TY, Suleimenova SZ, Vaughan G, Nainan OV, Favorov MO, Margolis HS, Bell BP.** 2007. Hepatitis A vaccine versus immune globulin for postexposure prophylaxis. *N Engl J Med* **357:**1685–1694.
123. **López EL, Contrini MM, Mistchenko A, Kieffer A, Baggaley RF, Di Tanna GL, Desai K, Rasuli A, Armoni J.** 2015. Modeling the long-term persistence of hepatitis A antibody after a two-dose vaccination schedule in Argentinean children. *Pediatr Infect Dis J* **34:**417–425.
124. **Shrestha MP, Scott RM, Joshi DM, Mammen MP Jr, Thapa GB, Thapa N, Myint KS, Fourneau M, Kuschner RA, Shrestha SK, David MP, Seriwatana J, Vaughn DW, Safary A, Endy TP, Innis BL.** 2007. Safety and efficacy of a recombinant hepatitis E vaccine. *N Engl J Med* **356:**895–903.
125. **Zhu FC, Zhang J, Zhang XF, Zhou C, Wang ZZ, Huang SJ, Wang H, Yang CL, Jiang HM, Cai JP, Wang YJ, Ai X, Hu YM, Tang Q, Yao X, Yan Q, Xian YL, Wu T, Li YM, Miao J, Ng MH, Shih JW, Xia NS.** 2010. Efficacy and safety of a recombinant hepatitis E vaccine in healthy adults: a large-scale, randomised, double-blind placebo-controlled, phase 3 trial. *Lancet* **376:**895–902.
126. **Zhang J, Zhang XF, Huang SJ, Wu T, Hu YM, Wang ZZ, Wang H, Jiang HM, Wang YJ, Yan Q, Guo M, Liu XH, Li JX, Yang CL, Tang Q, Jiang RJ, Pan HR, Li YM, Shih JW, Ng MH, Zhu FC, Xia NS.** 2015. Long-term efficacy of a hepatitis E vaccine. *N Engl J Med* **372:**914–922.
127. **Su YY, Huang SJ, Guo M, Zhao J, Yu H, He WG, Jiang HM, Wang YJ, Zhang XF, Cai JP, Yang CL, Wang ZZ, Zhu FC, Wu T, Zhang J, Xia NS.** 2017. Persistence of antibodies acquired by natural hepatitis E virus infection and effects of vaccination. *Clin Microbiol Infect* **23:**336.e1–336.e4.
128. **Wu T, Zhu FC, Huang SJ, Zhang XF, Wang ZZ, Zhang J, Xia NS.** 2012. Safety of the hepatitis E vaccine for pregnant women: a preliminary analysis. *Hepatology* **55:**2038.
129. **Kamar N, Rostaing L, Abravanel F, Garrouste C, Lhomme S, Esposito L, Basse G, Cointault O, Ribes D, Nogier MB, Alric L, Peron JM, Izopet J.** 2010. Ribavirin therapy inhibits viral replication on patients with chronic hepatitis E virus infection. *Gastroenterology* **139:**1612–1618.
130. **Kamar N, Izopet J, Tripon S, Bismuth M, Hillaire S, Dumortier J, Radenne S, Coilly A, Garrigue V, D'Alteroche L, Buchler M, Couzi L, Lebray P, Dharancy S, Minello A, Hourmant M, Roque-Afonso AM, Abravanel F, Pol S, Rostaing L, Mallet V.** 2014. Ribavirin for chronic

hepatitis E virus infection in transplant recipients. *N Engl J Med* **370:**1111–1120.
131. **Abravanel F, Lhomme S, Rostaing L, Kamar N, Izopet J.** 2015. Protracted fecal shedding of HEV during ribavirin therapy predicts treatment relapse. *Clin Infect Dis* **60:** 96–99.
132. **Tavitian S, Peron JM, Huguet F, Kamar N, Abravanel F, Beyne-Rauzy O, Oberic L, Faguer S, Alric L, Roussel M, Gaudin C, Ysebaert L, Huynh A, Recher C.** 2015. Ribavirin for chronic hepatitis prevention among patients with hematologic malignancies. *Emerg Infect Dis* **21:**1466–1469.
133. **Debing Y, Emerson SU, Wang Y, Pan Q, Balzarini J, Dallmeier K, Neyts J.** 2014. Ribavirin inhibits *in vitro* hepatitis E virus replication through depletion of cellular GTP pools and is moderately synergistic with alpha interferon. *Antimicrob Agents Chemother* **58:**267–273.
134. **Debing Y, Ramière C, Dallmeier K, Piorkowski G, Trabaud MA, Lebossé F, Scholtès C, Roche M, Legras-Lachuer C, de Lamballerie X, André P, Neyts J.** 2016. Hepatitis E virus mutations associated with ribavirin treatment failure result in altered viral fitness and ribavirin sensitivity. *J Hepatol* **65:**499–508.
135. **Lhomme S, Kamar N, Nicot F, Ducos J, Bismuth M, Garrigue V, Petitjean-Lecherbonnier J, Ollivier I, Alessandri-Gradt E, Goria O, Barth H, Perrin P, Saune K, Dubois M, Carcenac R, Lefebvre C, Jeanne N, Abravanel F, Izopet J.** 2016. Mutation in the hepatitis E virus polymerase and outcome of ribavirin therapy. *Antimicrob Agents Chemother* **60:**1608–1614.
136. **Debing Y, Gisa A, Dallmeier K, Pischke S, Bremer B, Manns M, Wedemeyer H, Suneetha PV, Neyts J.** 2014. A mutation in the hepatitis E virus RNA polymerase promotes its replication and associates with ribavirin treatment failure in organ transplant recipients. *Gastroenterology* **147:**1008–1011.e7.
137. **Todt D, François C, Anggakusuma, Behrendt P, Engelmann M, Knegendorf L, Vieyres G, Wedemeyer H, Hartmann R, Pietschmann T, Duverlie G, Steinmann E.** 2016. Antiviral activities of different interferon types and subtypes against hepatitis E virus replication. *Antimicrob Agents Chemother* **60:**2132–2139
138. **Kamar N, Rostaing L, Abravanel F, Garrouste C, Esposito L, Cardeau-Desangles I, Mansuy JM, Selves J, Peron JM, Otal P, Muscari F, Izopet J.** 2010. Pegylated interferon-alpha for treating chronic hepatitis E virus infection after liver transplantation. *Clin Infect Dis* **50:**e30–e33
139. **Haagsma EB, Riezebos-Brilman A, van den Berg AP, Porte RJ, Niesters HG.** 2010. Treatment of chronic hepatitis E in liver transplant recipients with pegylated interferon alpha-2b. *Liver Transpl* **16:**474–477.
140. **Rostaing L, Izopet J, Baron E, Duffaut M, Puel J, Durand D.** 1995. Treatment of chronic hepatitis C with recombinant interferon alpha in kidney transplant recipients. *Transplantation* **59:**1426–1431.
141. **Trémeaux P, Lhomme S, Chapuy-Regaud S, Peron JM, Alric L, Kamar N, Izopet J, Abravanel F.** 2016. Performance of an antigen assay for diagnosing acute hepatitis E virus genotype 3 infection. *J Clin Virol* **79:**1–5.
142. **Costafreda MI, Bosch A, Pintó RM.** 2006. Development, evaluation, and standardization of a real-time TaqMan reverse transcription-PCR assay for quantification of hepatitis A virus in clinical and shellfish samples. *Appl Environ Microbiol* **72:**3846–3855.
143. **Ye K, Manzano M, Muzzi R, Gin KY, Saeidi N, Goh SG, Tok AIY, Marks RS.** 2017. Development of a chemiluminescent DNA fibre optic genosensor to hepatitis A virus (HAV). *Talanta* **174:**401–408.
144. **Abravanel F, Chapuy-Regaud S, Lhomme S, Dubois M, Peron JM, Alric L, Rostaing L, Kamar N, Izopet J.** 2013. Performance of two commercial assays for detecting hepatitis E virus RNA in acute or chronic infections. *J Clin Microbiol* **51:**1913–1916.
145. **Abravanel F, Sandres-Saune K, Lhomme S, Dubois M, Mansuy JM, Izopet J.** 2012. Genotype 3 diversity and quantification of hepatitis E virus RNA. *J Clin Microbiol* **50:**897–902.
146. **Sauleda S, Ong E, Bes M, Janssen A, Cory R, Babizki M, Shin T, Lindquist A, Hoang A, Vang L, Piron M, Casamitjana N, Koppelman M, Danzig L, Linnen JM.** 2015. Seroprevalence of hepatitis E virus (HEV) and detection of HEV RNA with a transcription-mediated amplification assay in blood donors from Catalonia (Spain). *Transfusion* **55:** 972–979.
147. **Nicot F, Cazabat M, Lhomme S, Marion O, Sauné K, Chiabrando J, Dubois M, Kamar N, Abravanel F, Izopet J.** 2016. Quantification of HEV RNA by droplet digital PCR. *Viruses* **8:**233.
148. **Lan X, Yang B, Li BY, Yin XP, Li XR, Liu JX.** 2009. Reverse transcription-loop-mediated isothermal amplification assay for rapid detection of hepatitis E virus. *J Clin Microbiol* **47:**2304–2306.
149. **Day SP, Murphy P, Brown EA, Lemon SM.** 1992. Mutations within the 5′ nontranslated region of hepatitis A virus RNA which enhance replication in BS-C-1 cells. *J Virol* **66:**6533–6540.
150. **Emerson SU, Huang YK, Purcell RH.** 1993. 2B and 2C mutations are essential but mutations throughout the genome of HAV contribute to adaptation to cell culture. *Virology* **194:**475–480.
151. **Yi M, Lemon SM.** 2002. Replication of subgenomic hepatitis A virus RNAs expressing firefly luciferase is enhanced by mutations associated with adaptation of virus to growth in cultured cells. *J Virol* **76:**1171–1180.
152. **Sewlikar S, D'Souza DH.** 2017. Survival of hepatitis A virus and Aichi virus in cranberry-based juices at refrigeration (4 °C). *Food Microbiol* **62:**251–255.
153. **Tanaka T, Takahashi M, Kusano E, Okamoto H.** 2007. Development and evaluation of an efficient cell-culture system for hepatitis E virus. *J Gen Virol* **88:**903–911.
154. **Tanaka T, Takahashi M, Takahashi H, Ichiyama K, Hoshino Y, Nagashima S, Mizuo H, Okamoto H.** 2009. Development and characterization of a genotype 4 hepatitis E virus cell culture system using a HE-JF5/15F strain recovered from a fulminant hepatitis patient. *J Clin Microbiol* **47:**1906–1910.
155. **Lhomme S, Abravanel F, Dubois M, Sandres-Saune K, Mansuy JM, Rostaing L, Kamar N, Izopet J.** 2014. Characterization of the polyproline region of the hepatitis E virus in immunocompromised patients. *J Virol* **88:** 12017–12025.
156. **Johne R, Trojnar E, Filter M, Hofmann J.** 2016. Thermal stability of hepatitis E virus as estimated by a cell culture method. *Appl Environ Microbiol* **82:**4225–4231.
157. **Okamoto H.** 2013. Culture systems for hepatitis E virus. *J Gastroenterol* **48:**147–158.
158. **Berto A, Van der Poel WH, Hakze-van der Honing R, Martelli F, La Ragione RM, Inglese N, Collins J, Grierson S, Johne R, Reetz J, Dastjerdi A, Banks M.** 2013. Replication of hepatitis E virus in three-dimensional cell culture. *J Virol Methods* **187:**327–332.
159. **Brown EA, Jansen RW, Lemon SM.** 1989. Characterization of a simian hepatitis A virus (HAV): antigenic and genetic comparison with human HAV. *J Virol* **63:**4932–4937.
160. **Robertson BH, Jansen RW, Khanna B, Totsuka A, Nainan OV, Siegl G, Widell A, Margolis HS, Isomura S, Ito K, Ishizu T, Moritsugu Y, Lemon SM.** 1992. Genetic relatedness of hepatitis A virus strains recovered from different geographical regions. *J Gen Virol* **73:**1365–1377.
161. **Costa-Mattioli M, Di Napoli A, Ferré V, Billaudel S, Perez-Bercoff R, Cristina J.** 2003. Genetic variability of hepatitis A virus. *J Gen Virol* **84:**3191–3201.
162. **Roque-Afonso AM, Grangeot-Keros L, Roquebert B, Desbois D, Poveda JD, Mackiewicz V, Dussaix E.** 2004. Diagnostic relevance of immunoglobulin G avidity for hepatitis A virus. *J Clin Microbiol* **42:**5121–5124.
163. **Vollmer T, Diekmann J, Eberhardt M, Knabbe C, Dreier J.** 2016. Monitoring of anti-hepatitis E virus antibody seroconversion in asymptomatically infected blood donors: systematic comparison of nine commercial anti-HEV IgM and IgG assays. *Viruses* **8:**232.

164. **Abravanel F, Goutagny N, Perret C, Lhomme S, Vischi F, Averseng A, Chapel A, Dehainault N, Piga N, Dupret-Carruel J, Izopet J.** 2017. Evaluation of two VIDAS ®prototypes for detecting anti-HEV IgG. *J Clin Virol* **89:**46–50.
165. **Abravanel F, Lhomme S, Chapuy-Regaud S, Peron JM, Alric L, Rostaing L, Kamar N, Izopet J.** 2015. Performance of a new rapid test for detecting anti-hepatitis E virus immunoglobulin M in immunocompetent and immunocompromised patients. *J Clin Virol* **70:**101–104.
166. **Legrand-Abravanel F, Thevenet I, Mansuy JM, Saune K, Vischi F, Peron JM, Kamar N, Rostaing L, Izopet J.** 2009. Good performance of immunoglobulin M assays in diagnosing genotype 3 hepatitis E virus infections. *Clin Vaccine Immunol* **16:**772–774.
167. **Norder H, Karlsson M, Mellgren Å, Konar J, Sandberg E, Lasson A, Castedal M, Magnius L, Lagging M.** 2016. Diagnostic performance of five assays for anti-hepatitis E virus IgG and IgM in a large cohort study. *J Clin Microbiol* **54:**549–555.
168. **Abravanel F, Chapuy-Regaud S, Lhomme S, Miedougé M, Peron JM, Alric L, Rostaing L, Kamar N, Izopet J.** 2013. Performance of anti-HEV assays for diagnosing acute hepatitis E in immunocompromised patients. *J Clin Virol* **58:**624–628.
169. **Avellon A, Morago L, Garcia-Galera del Carmen M, Munoz M, Echevarría JM.** 2015. Comparative sensitivity of commercial tests for hepatitis E genotype 3 virus antibody detection. *J Med Virol* **87:**1934–1939.
170. **Drobeniuc J, Meng J, Reuter G, Greene-Montfort T, Khudyakova N, Dimitrova Z, Kamili S, Teo CG.** 2010. Serologic assays specific to immunoglobulin M antibodies against hepatitis E virus: pangenotypic evaluation of performances. *Clin Infect Dis* **51:**e24–e27.
171. **Hartl J, Otto B, Madden RG, Webb G, Woolson KL, Kriston L, Vettorazzi E, Lohse AW, Dalton HR, Pischke S.** 2016. Hepatitis E seroprevalence in Europe: a meta-analysis. *Viruses* **8:**211.
172. **Bendall R, Ellis V, Ijaz S, Thurairajah P, Dalton HR.** 2008. Serological response to hepatitis E virus genotype 3 infection: IgG quantitation, avidity, and IgM response. *J Med Virol* **80:**95–101.
173. **Izopet J, Labrique AB, Basnyat B, Dalton HR, Kmush B, Heaney CD, Nelson KE, Ahmed ZB, Zaman K, Mansuy JM, Bendall R, Sauné K, Kamar N, Arjyal A, Karkey A, Dongol S, Prajapati KG, Adhikary D.** 2015. Hepatitis E virus seroprevalence in three hyperendemic areas: Nepal, Bangladesh and southwest France. *J Clin Virol* **70:**39–42.
174. **Kmush BL, Labrique AB, Dalton HR, Ahmed ZB, Ticehurst JR, Heaney CD, Nelson KE, Zaman K.** 2015. Two generations of "gold standards": the impact of a decade in hepatitis E virus testing innovation on population seroprevalence. *Am J Trop Med Hyg* **93:**714–717.
175. **Wenzel JJ, Preiss J, Schemmerer M, Huber B, Jilg W.** 2013. Test performance characteristics of Anti-HEV IgG assays strongly influence hepatitis E seroprevalence estimates. *J Infect Dis* **207:**497–500.
176. **Abravanel F, Lhomme S, Chapuy-Regaud S, Mansuy JM, Muscari F, Sallusto F, Rostaing L, Kamar N, Izopet J.** 2014. Hepatitis E virus reinfections in solid-organ-transplant recipients can evolve into chronic infections. *J Infect Dis* **209:**1900–1906.
177. **Baylis SA, Crossan C, Corman VM, Blümel J, Scobie L, Dalton HR.** 2015. Unusual serological response to hepatitis E virus in plasma donors consistent with re-infection. *Vox Sang* **109:**406–409.
178. **Schemmerer M, Rauh C, Jilg W, Wenzel JJ.** 2017. Time course of hepatitis E-specific antibodies in adults. *J Viral Hepat* **24:**75–79.
179. **Gossner CM, Severi E, Danielsson N, Hutin Y, Coulombier D.** 2015. Changing hepatitis A epidemiology in the European Union: new challenges and opportunities. *Euro Surveill* **20:**21101 http://www.eurosurveillance.org/content/10.2807/1560-7917.ES2015.20.16.21101.
180. **Adlhoch C, Avellon A, Baylis SA, Ciccaglione AR, Couturier E, de Sousa R, Epštein J, Ethelberg S, Faber M, Fehér Á, Ijaz S, Lange H, Mand'áková Z, Mellou K, Mozalevskis A, Rimhanen-Finne R, Rizzi V, Said B, Sundqvist L, Thornton L, Tosti ME, van Pelt W, Aspinall E, Domanovic D, Severi E, Takkinen J, Dalton HR.** 2016. Hepatitis E virus: assessment of the epidemiological situation in humans in Europe, 2014/15. *J Clin Virol* **82:**9–16.

Hepatitis C Virus

MICHAEL S. FORMAN, BRYAN R. COBB, AND ALEXANDRA VALSAMAKIS

94

TAXONOMY

Hepatitis C virus (HCV) is classified within the family *Flaviviridae* in its own genus *Hepacivirus*. Phylogenetic analysis of helicase sequences has been used to probe its relatedness to other viruses in the family (1). The data suggest that HCV is most closely related to the nonpathogenic human virus GB virus type C. The next closest relatives appear to be the pestiviruses, viruses that infect non-human hosts (bovine viral diarrhea virus and hog cholera virus). HCV is more distantly related to arthropod-borne viruses in the *Flavivirus* genus that infect humans (yellow fever virus, dengue virus, West Nile virus).

DESCRIPTION OF THE AGENT

HCV has an ~9.6-kb positive-sense RNA genome composed of a long open reading frame flanked by terminal 5′ and 3′ untranslated regions (UTRs)(Fig. 1). The 5′ UTR is highly conserved, and the 3′ UTR has a short variable sequence, a poly(U) tract, and a highly conserved element. Structural protein genes include those encoding core (nucleocapsid), p7 (transmembrane protein), and the two glycoproteins, E1 and E2, which are present in the virion envelope. HCV virions exist as lipoviral particles, resulting from the binding of serum lipoproteins (cholesterol, triglycerides, apolipoproteins, and phosphoproteins) to viral glycoproteins (2).

HCV replication in hepatocytes initiates via a multistep entry process (3). Virion-bound lipoproteins engage with the cellular receptor of lipoproteins, SR-B1 (scavenger receptor class B type 1), exposing E2 that then binds the cellular tetraspanin protein CD81, triggering binding of tight junction proteins and clathrin-mediated endocytosis. Within the endosome, E1 and E2 mediate pH-dependent fusion of the virion envelope with the endosomal membrane. In the cytosol, the HCV genome open reading frame is translated into a single polyprotein (approximately 3,000 amino acids) that is subsequently cleaved by host and viral proteases encoded by NS2, NS3, and NS4A genes. The NS3 gene also encodes a helicase. The p7 region encodes a protein that is essential for replication of infectious virus (4); however, its specific function is unknown. The RNA-dependent RNA polymerase (NS5B; Fig. 1) lacks efficient proofreading activity, resulting in extensive genome mutation during replication and quasispecies generation within an infected individual. NS5A is a multifunctional nonstructural phosphoprotein (5). It is a key component of the replication complex and binds other constituents of the complex including RNA-dependent RNA polymerase, RNA, and cyclophilin A, a host protein required for HCV RNA replication. It also appears to play a role in virion assembly. The principal gene targets of current direct-acting antiviral (DAA) regimens are NS3/4 protease, NS5A, and NS5B polymerase (Table 1).

Currently, there are seven major genotypes (Gts) of HCV and more than 50 known subtypes based on genomic sequence heterogeneity (6). Genotypes differ by 30 to 35% of nucleotides, and subtypes by 20 to 25% of nucleotides. Gt1 through Gt3 have a worldwide distribution and account for most HCV infections in Europe and North America. In the United States, the majority of HCV infections in all age groups are Gt1 (75%), followed by Gt2 (13.5%) and Gt3 (5.5%). Gt1subtypes (subtypes 1a and 1b) are now important for appropriate DAA regimen selection (see "Clinical Significance"). In the United States and Asia, Gt1a is more prevalent than Gt1b. Of Gt1 infections in the United States, 75% are Gt1a and 25% are Gt1b; in Asia, 95% are 1a and 5% are 1b (7). In Europe, the prevalence of Gt1a and 1b is comparable (~50% each) (7). Gt4 is most prevalent in the Middle East and North and Central Africa; Gt5 is found primarily in South Africa; Gt6 occurs throughout Asia; Gt7 has been detected in an immigrant from the Congo, and its region of endemicity is unclear (8, 9).

Genetic recombination is an additional source of HCV genetic heterogeneity that was initially thought to be rare but is now increasingly recognized. It likely occurs during coinfection with different HCV strains. Recombination breakpoints occur most commonly in the NS2 to NS3 region, as demonstrated by sequencing (10, 11). Most circulating variants have 5′ sequences derived from genotype 2, with 3′ sequences from other genotypes (Gt2/Gt1, Gt2/Gt5, Gt2/Gt6) (11). The predominance of Gt2 recombinants could have some biologic basis (e.g., increased fitness). Alternatively, these variants may be understudied on a global level, and others may be identified as treatment and associated genotypic testing expand worldwide. Gt2/Gt1 variant strains appear to be most prevalent; of these, the 2k/1b strain is most common (12). This virus was first noted in St. Petersburg and appears to have emerged in the former Soviet Union between 1923 and 1956 (11, 13). It is

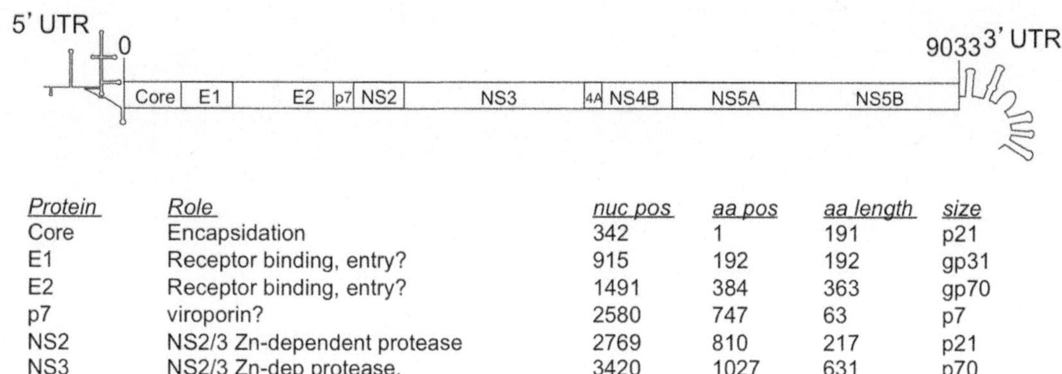

Protein	Role	nuc pos	aa pos	aa length	size
Core	Encapsidation	342	1	191	p21
E1	Receptor binding, entry?	915	192	192	gp31
E2	Receptor binding, entry?	1491	384	363	gp70
p7	viroporin?	2580	747	63	p7
NS2	NS2/3 Zn-dependent protease	2769	810	217	p21
NS3	NS2/3 Zn-dep protease, NS3/4A protease, helicase-NTPase	3420	1027	631	p70
NS4A	cofactor for NS3-4A protease	5313	1658	54	p8
NS4B	membranous web organization	5475	1712	261	p27
NS5A	phosphoprotein	6258	1973	448	p58
NS5B	RNA-dependent RNA polymerase	7602	2421	591	p68

FIGURE 1 HCV genome and protein coding scheme. UTR, untranslated region; E, envelope; NS, nonstructural gene; nuc, nucleotide; pos, position; aa, amino acid; gp, glycoprotein. Numbering according to references 92 and 93.

highly prevalent in former Soviet Republic countries such as Georgia, where prevalence is ~20% among all chronic HCV infections (14). It has also been found in countries with populations that have emigrated from former Soviet bloc countries, such as France, Germany, and Israel. In these countries, 2k/1b has been identified in individuals who were likely infected prior to immigration and in nonimmigrants with high-risk behaviors such as intravenous drug use, suggesting that the variant is now circulating more broadly, along with other endemic strains (11, 12, 15, 16).

Chronic HCV infections with Gt2/1 variants are clinically important because they are not routinely identified and may not be treated with appropriate DAA regimens. HCV genotyping assays that query sequences upstream of the recombination breakpoint (5′ UTR, core, E1) will often identify these variants as Gt2 infections, whereas the DAA target genes (NS3/4, NS5A, NS5B) downstream of the breakpoint are Gt1 sequences. These inaccurately genotyped individuals experience high rates of virologic relapse when treated with Gt2-specific regimens, but they can be cured effectively with Gt1-specific or pan-genotypic regimens (12, 17).

EPIDEMIOLOGY AND TRANSMISSION

HCV is a globally significant pathogen, infecting over 150 million individuals. In the United States, it is the most common blood-borne infection, causing an estimated 3 million chronic infections (18). Acute hepatitis C occurs in the United States at a rate of approximately 0.3 per 100,000, with estimates of 19,000 new infections per year after adjusting for underreporting and asymptomatic infection (19). In the blood-screening era, most transmission occurs after exposure to a low viral inoculum through intravenous drug use, sexual transmission, and occupational exposure to blood such as needlestick (20). Sexual transmission was once thought to be uncommon but is now increasingly recognized, particularly among HIV-infected and HIV-uninfected men who have sex with men (MSM). In HIV-infected MSM, a meta-analysis of studies from 1984 to 2012 demonstrated increasing incidence among individuals who were not injecting drugs; seroconversion was associated with traumatic sex (21). In HIV-uninfected MSM, higher than expected prevalence has been observed in a cohort that was initiating preexposure prophylaxis for HIV; HCV sequencing demonstrated similar strains in HIV-infected and HIV-uninfected individuals in the region, suggesting shared sexual networks play a key role in HCV transmission (22). Injection drug use in the wake of the opioid epidemic is fueling an upsurge in HCV infection in the United States. HCV incidence rates climbed from 2006 to 2012; the greatest increases occurred in young (<30 years of age), nonurban whites (23).

TABLE 1 HCV DAA classes and currently recommended drugs

NS3/4 protease inhibitors	NS5A inhibitors	NS5B polymerase inhibitors
Grazoprevir	Daclatasvir	Dasabuvir
Glecaprevir	Elbasvir	Sofosbuvir
Paritaprevir (dosed with ritonavir)	Ledipasvir	
	Ombitasvir	
Simeprevir	Pibrentasvir	
Voxilaprevir	Velpatasvir	

CLINICAL SIGNIFICANCE

The clinical features of acute infection are depicted in Fig. 2. Most individuals are thought to be asymptomatic. Spontaneous clearance is observed in approximately 25% of acute infections; the remaining individuals become chronically infected. Signs of hepatitis during acute infection are actually positive indicators as they represent early, vigorous antiviral T cell responses associated with spontaneous virus clearance. These responses are minimal or absent in individuals who progress to chronicity (24).

Why some individuals clear their infection while others progress to chronic HCV infection is unknown. To investigate the mechanisms governing clearance, genome-wide association studies have been used to identify genetic determinants that predominate in individuals with spontaneous

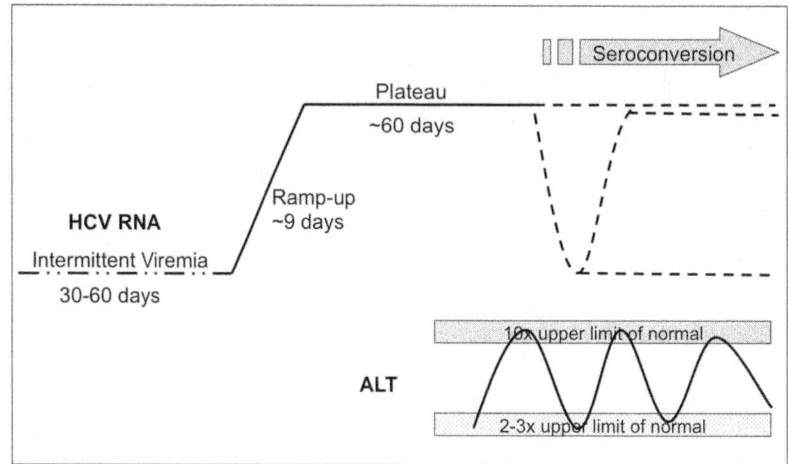

FIGURE 2 Clinical features of acute hepatitis C following exposure to low viral inoculum such as occupational needlestick exposure or community-based exposure (58, 77, 94). Characteristics following higher dose exposure (transfusion with contaminated blood products) may be different. Intermittent viremia phase estimated from needlestick exposure (77). Kinetics of other characteristics derived from seroconversion panels (58). ALT, alanine aminotransferase. Dashed lines indicate potential viremia patterns as defined by HCV RNA levels in peripheral blood. Adapted from reference 58.

clearance versus progression to chronicity. This approach has identified a single nucleotide polymorphism (SNP) in the *DQA1-DQB2 HLA* class II region (25), found on reference SNP (rs)4273729, and multiple SNPs upstream from the *IL28B* gene (26, 27; reviewed in reference 28), of which the most strongly associated are variants on rs12979860 (25) that are independently associated with clearance and additively effective. The homozygous G allele on *HLA* class II rs4273729 and homozygous C allele on *IL28B* rs12979860 are associated with clearance. The homozygous C allele on *HLA* class II rs4273729 and the homozygous T allele on rs12979860 are associated with chronic infection. Heterozygotes tend more toward chronic infection than clearance. *IL28B* encodes interferon λ3, an interferon that stimulates a signaling cascade similar to interferon α and interferon β, but through a distinct receptor. The worldwide geographic distribution of *IL28B* genotypes appears to explain in part the observed racial differences in acute infection outcome (27, 29). Haplotypes associated with resolution are found more commonly in East Asian populations in whom rates of spontaneous clearance are high. Haplotypes associated with progression to chronic infection occur with higher frequency in individuals of African ethnicity, in whom rates of chronic infection are high. How genetic determinants in *HLA* class II and *IL28B* regulate immune responses that mediate HCV clearance is not yet understood.

Disease progression occurs in a relatively small proportion of patients with chronic hepatitis C infection. Over decades, progressive liver damage produces cirrhosis in 10 to 20% of chronic infections and liver failure or hepatocellular carcinoma in approximately 5% of chronic infections (30). However, the overall disease burden is significant due to the number of infected individuals. In fact, liver failure due to chronic hepatitis C infection is the leading cause of liver transplantation in the United States (31). Risk factors for disease progression include diseases or behaviors that induce additional hepatic injury (such as concomitant hepatitis B virus infection and alcohol consumption) or impair antiviral immunity (such as HIV infection). Epidemiologic descriptors such as male gender and older age at infection are also associated with higher risk and faster rate of disease progression.

Unlike other chronic viral infections such as HIV and hepatitis B virus, virologic parameters including viral load and genotype do not predict disease progression or indicate disease severity in chronic hepatitis C (32, 33). Viral load remains fairly constant once chronic hepatitis C infection is established (33), and rates of progression have been found to correlate more with disease severity in the liver, as manifested by the extent of fibrosis on initial liver biopsy (34), than on the level of HCV replication represented by viremia (35).

Therapy for chronic hepatitis C has been revolutionized with the approval of DAA regimens. These drugs have been demonstrated to be highly effective in clinical trials and in general clinical use. Cure rates for Gt1, Gt2, and Gt3 are approximately 90% or greater (36–39). High efficacy has been demonstrated even in individuals with HCV/HIV coinfections, a group that had been considered difficult to treat due to low response rates to interferon-alfa/ribavirin. Response rates to first-line regimens in HIV/HCV coinfection are equivalent to HCV monoinfected individuals; side effect profiles are manageable, and patients on antiretroviral therapy can be safely treated if compatible DAAs are used, greatly simplifying HCV treatment of coinfected individuals (40). Accordingly, guidelines now recommend DAA treatment for all HIV/HCV coinfected patients to prevent the development of significant fibrosis and progression of disease; these complications occur more commonly and more rapidly in coinfected than in HCV monoinfected patients (41–43).

Currently recommended DAAs and their targets are listed in Table 1. Drugs are described in further detail in chapter 113 of this *Manual*. DAA regimens (first line and alternative) are shown in Table 2. Recommendations on all aspects of HCV treatment are updated constantly and are available as Web-based guidelines (http://www.hcvguidelines.org, http://www.easl.eu/_clinical-practice-guideline). Tests that are used currently for the diagnosis and management of chronic hepatitis C are shown in Table 3.

TABLE 2 Current DAA regimens for treatment of chronic hepatitis C

Regimen	Genotype	Drug combination	Treatment duration	Comment
First-line regimens	1a, 1b	ledipasvir/sofosbuvir	8 weeks	Baseline HCV RNA <6 million IU/ml
	1a, 1b, 4, 5, 6	ledipasvir/sofosbuvir	12 weeks	Gt1a and Gt1b: baseline HCV RNA ≥6 million IU/ml
	1a, 1b, 4	elbasvir/grazoprevir	12 weeks	Gt1a: if baseline RAS present, add ribavirin and extend therapy to 16 weeks
	1a, 1b, 2, 3, 4, 5, 6	glecaprevir/pibrentasvir	8 weeks	Pan-genotypic regimen Gt5 and Gt6: extend to 12 weeks in cirrhosis
	1a, 1b, 2, 3, 4, 5, 6	sofosbuvir/velpatasvir	12 weeks	Pan-genotypic regimen
Alternative regimens	1a, 1b, 4	ritonavir-boosted paritaprevir/ ombitasvir/dasabuvir	12 weeks	Gt1a and Gt4: add ribavirin
	1a, 1b	simeprevir/sofosbuvir	12 weeks	
	1a, 1b, 2, 3	daclatasvir/sofosbuvir	12 weeks	

COLLECTION, TRANSPORT, AND STORAGE OF SPECIMENS

Serum and plasma are acceptable for HCV nucleic acid amplification tests (NAATs) and serology tests. Plasma collected in heparin-containing tubes is not acceptable for PCR-based assays since Taq polymerase is inhibited by this anticoagulant. Serum and plasma should be obtained from whole blood as per standard technique, described in chapter 81 of this *Manual*. Requirements for specimen processing and storage, such as recommended intervals between collection/processing, storage conditions, and freeze-thaw cycles, vary by assay; package inserts should be consulted for specific information. Generally, whole blood specimens can be transported at 25°C prior to processing. Dried blood spots (DBSs) have been adapted for use in HCV serology and NAATs with the aim of expanding diagnosis and treatment of chronic hepatitis C into resource-limited settings. With DBSs, accurate results have been obtained with HCV antibody and qualitative HCV RNA assays, but not quantitative HCV RNA tests (44–46), suggesting that DBSs may have utility in identifying individuals with chronic hepatitis C, but they are not suitable for use with tests that are currently recommended for therapeutic monitoring. In HCV core antigen detection tests, DBS sensitivity was inferior to serum (47). DBSs may have limited use for the identification of chronically infected HCV-seropositive individuals with these assays. No HCV diagnostic assays have received regulatory approval for the use of DBSs. Liver tissue is not typically tested, except for histologic assessment of fibrosis in Gt1-infected individuals.

DIRECT DETECTION

Microscopy

By electron microscopy, HCV virions are 55- to 65-nm spheres with 6-nm surface projections. HCV antigens and nucleic acids are detectable in liver sections by immunohistochemistry and *in situ* hybridization, respectively. However, these methods are insensitive and nonspecific; therefore, HCV detection by microscopy has minimal clinical utility.

In the DAA era, histologic assessment to determine liver disease status is used primarily to ensure appropriate treatment of individuals with bridging fibrosis/cirrhosis. Chronic HCV infections in these individuals are more difficult to treat and require more intensive regimens than in patients without cirrhosis (http://www.hcvguidelines.org, http://www.easl.eu/_clinical-practice-guideline). Other uses of histologic assessments include screening for HCV and institution of treatment for cirrhosis-related sequelae.

In response to the disadvantages of liver biopsy (its invasive nature, potential complications, and sampling error), noninvasive tests have been developed, including assessment of liver stiffness through ultrasound (transient elastography) and surrogate markers of fibrosis that can be assessed in peripheral blood. Noninvasive tests are useful for detecting

TABLE 3 Utility of tests for the diagnosis and management of HCV infection

Assay utility	Assay type (accepted specimen)	Indication for use
Diagnosis of acute hepatitis C	HCV RNA detection by qualitative or quantitative NAAT (serum or plasma)	After exposure, for direct detection of HCV after infection (may be sporadic and require serial testing to detect)
	Anti-HCV immunoassay for detection of anti-HCV IgM + IgG (serum or whole blood fingerstick)	After exposure, to document seroconversion
Diagnosis of chronic hepatitis C	Anti-HCV immunoassay for detection of anti-HCV IgM + IgG (serum or whole blood fingerstick)	Screening for infection
	HCV RNA detection by qualitative or quantitative NAAT (serum or plasma)	Confirmation of infection and differentiation between resolution of acute infection and chronic infection
Therapeutic management of chronic hepatitis C	HCV genotype determination (serum or plasma)/ subtype determination for Gt1	Selection of appropriate treatment regimen
	HCV RNA measurement with quantitative NAAT (serum or plasma)	Determine treatment duration for certain therapies (see Table 2 for treatment regimens) Monitoring of therapeutic efficacy
	Antiviral resistance-associated substitution detection (plasma)	Selection of appropriate regimen for treatment of particular HCV genotypes

advanced fibrosis but are poor at distinguishing intermediate fibrosis stages. Biopsy is therefore preferred if this level of accuracy is necessary. Otherwise, noninvasive tests for the detection of advanced fibrosis/cirrhosis have been advocated in the latest treatment guidelines (http://www.hcvguidelines.org, http://www.easl.eu/_clinical-practice-guideline).

Antigen Detection

HCV core antigen detection/quantification tests have been developed as alternatives to HCV RNA assays. The assay that is most widely available and reported in the literature is ARCHITECT HCV Ag (Abbott Diagnostics, Chicago, IL), a chemiluminescent microparticle immunoassay that is marked for use in Europe (Conformité Européene) but has not received regulatory approval in the United States. This test is potentially useful in resource-limited settings due to target stability (eliminating the need for sample storage at ultra-low temperatures), simplified instrumentation, and easier technical protocols that reduce labor/training pressures. The analytical sensitivity ranges from 3 to 13 fmol/liter depending upon genotype, corresponding to approximately 1,000 IU/ml of HCV RNA measured by NAAT. The ARCHITECT HCV Ag assay is linear between 3 and 10,000 fmol/liter, and good quantitative correlation with HCV RNA quantification tests has been observed (48–50).

The utility of these tests in the diagnosis of HCV infections and therapeutic monitoring during DAA treatment has been investigated. Meta-analyses of published data on core antigen assay performance in individuals with known chronic HCV demonstrate sensitivity for the diagnosis of chronic HCV that ranges from 92 to 97% and specificity of ~99% compared to NAAT (51, 52). These data suggest that core antigen assays may be useful as surrogates for NAAT for the diagnosis of chronic HCV in HCV-seropositive individuals, particularly in resource-limited settings where HCV screening is currently limited. In countries that are not resource restricted, where the emphasis is on the identification and treatment of all chronically infected patients, these assays would have limited benefit due to the false-negative rates that are low but significant compared to NAAT. Additionally, studies investigating the utility of core antigen tests for the diagnosis of acute HCV in the seroconversion window (52, 53) and for the documentation of end-of-treatment response after DAA therapy (54) have shown inferior performance compared to NAAT, suggesting they are not optimal in these settings.

Clinical guidelines have taken different approaches regarding core antigen testing. European HCV guidelines recommend the use of these tests in diagnosis and therapeutic monitoring as alternatives if NAATs are not readily available, thereby balancing practical considerations with concerns regarding suboptimal performance compared to NAATs. In contrast, U.S. HCV management guidelines recommend only HCV NAATs with detection limits ≤25 IU/ml for all clinical uses.

Nucleic Acid Detection/Quantification Tests

Clinical Utility

NAAT Usage in the Diagnosis of Acute Hepatitis C

HCV NAATs are useful in establishing the diagnosis of acute HCV infection in seronegative individuals because HCV RNA can be detected as early as 1 week after exposure via needlestick or transfusion (55–57) and at least 4 to 6 weeks prior to seroconversion in a number of transmission settings (58). Testing by sensitive qualitative or quantitative NAATs (Table 4) is recommended (<15 IU/ml in European guidelines [http://www.easl.eu/_clinical-practice-guideline]; ≤25 IU/ml, every 4 to 6 weeks in U.S. guidelines [http://www.hcvguidelines.org]) since HCV RNA levels are low and intermittently detected early after known exposure (58). Treatment of acute infection can be considered for individuals with hepatic dysfunction due to other etiologies, whose disease could be exacerbated by acute hepatitis C. Otherwise, acute infections are managed with a "wait and see" approach, with the rationale that ~25% of

TABLE 4 Commercial HCV NAATs

Test (manufacturer)[a,b]	Extraction chemistry	Amplification method	Measurable range (log10 IU/ml)[c]	Limit of detection (log10 IU/ml)	Reference(s)
Aptima HCV RNA Qualitative Assay (Hologic)[a]	Magnetic microparticle/ target capture	TMA	Not applicable	1.0	
Aptima HCV Quant Dx Assay (Hologic)[a,d]	Magnetic microparticle/ target capture	TMA	1.0–8.0	0.6 plasma 0.5 serum	95
artus HCV RT-PCR QS-RGQ (Qiagen)[b]	Magnetic microparticle/ total nucleic acid	Real-time RT-PCR	1.5–7.4	1.3	96
COBAS AmpliPrep/ COBAS TaqMan v2.0 (Roche)[a,d]	Silica based (total nucleic acid)	Real-time RT-PCR	1.2–8.0	1.2	97
cobas 6800/8800 (Roche)[a,d]	Magnetic microparticle/ total nucleic acid	Real-time RT-PCR	1.2–8.0	1.1	98
RealTime HCV (Abbott)[a,e]	Magnetic microparticle/ total nucleic acid	Real-time RT-PCR	1.1–8.0	1.1	99–101
Versant HCV RNA 1.0 (kPCR) (Siemens Healthineers Global)[b]	Silica based (total nucleic acid)	Real-time RT-PCR	1.2–8.0	1.2	102
Xpert HCV Viral Load Test (Cepheid)[b]	Unreported	Real-time RT-PCR	1.0–8.0	0.6 plasma 0.8 serum	103

[a]FDA approved and Conformité Européenne marked according to European In Vitro Diagnostic Directive 98/79/EC.
[b]Conformité Européenne marked according to European In Vitro Diagnostic Directive 98/79/EC.
[c]Lower limit of quantification/upper limit of quantification of undiluted specimens.
[d]FDA approved in the United States for diagnosis of chronic hepatitis C and for therapeutic monitoring.
[e]FDA approved in the United States for therapeutic monitoring.

patients will spontaneously clear infection. DAA therapy is typically reserved for individuals who progress to chronic infection (HCV RNA detectable twice, at least 12 weeks apart) because they can be cured with short treatment courses (http://www.hcvguidelines.org).

NAAT Usage in the Diagnosis of Chronic Hepatitis C

Given the asymptomatic nature of most acute HCV infections, most patients will be identified in the chronic phase of infection. Chronically infected patients are either asymptomatic and are identified through HCV screening/linkage-to-care efforts or are symptomatic due to disease progression. The diagnosis of chronic HCV is established with antibody screening tests to document infection, followed by HCV RNA NAAT to demonstrate viral replication (Table 3). In immunocompromised individuals who have impaired antibody responses and false-negative serologic test results, documenting the presence of HCV RNA with NAATs is the primary modality for diagnosing chronic HCV infection. Reliance on NAAT as the primary test for HCV infection screening is most important in the setting of HIV. False-negative HCV serology results with second- and third-generation serologic assays have been observed in ~5% of HIV-1-infected individuals. Low CD4 cell counts (<200 cells/μl) have been found to be a risk factor (59, 60). Therefore, NAAT should be performed regardless of serology results to accurately diagnose chronic infection in HIV/HCV coinfected patients whose humoral responses may be impaired.

NAAT Usage in the Management of Chronic Hepatitis C Therapy

In the DAA era, the use of NAATs continues to be critical and is vastly simplified compared to the era of interferon-alfa-based regimens. Their roles in diagnosis and management are summarized in Table 3 and further explained in Fig. 3. Prior to treatment, HCV genotype and RNA levels should be determined in all patients. Genotype is used to determine treatment regimen and duration (see Table 2 for regimens and "Genotyping" section below for further description of these NAATs). In the pegylated interferon-alfa/ribavirin era, genotype was also useful in predicting response to therapy; however, response rates to DAAs are generally uniformly high across genotypes. Testing for the presence of resistance-associated substitutions (RASs) prior to DAA initiation should be performed when considering specific drug regimens for the treatment of particular genotypes (see Table 9 for a summary of RAS testing recommendations and "Antiviral Susceptibility" section below for additional discussion of RAS tests). During treatment, HCV RNA measurement is recommended at week 4 of treatment and 12 weeks after treatment cessation. Additional HCV RNA assessments at end of treatment and 24 weeks after treatment cessation are optional. Testing by sensitive qualitative or quantitative NAATs (Table 4) is recommended (<15 IU/ml in European guidelines [http://www.easl.eu/_clinical-practice-guideline]; ≤25 IU/ml in U.S. guidelines [http://www.hcvguidelines.org]). Baseline HCV RNA quantification is critical as it is the starting point for documentation of cure. On-treatment quantitative HCV RNA testing is limited to week 4; most patients have no detectable HCV RNA at this point. End-of-treatment testing is optional and is used to document treatment efficacy. Cure, defined as continuous absence of detectable HCV RNA (or sustained virologic response, SVR), is ascertained by HCV RNA quantification 12 weeks after treatment cessation (SVR12). In the era of interferon-alfa-based regimens, SVR was conventionally determined 24 weeks after end of treatment. The follow-up period has been shortened to 12 weeks in the DAA era, after an analysis of amassed clinical trial data demonstrated that follow-up periods of 12 and 24 weeks were comparably predictive of SVR (61). Most patients who achieve SVR12 are considered cured. Relapse later than 12 weeks after treatment cessation is rare. One study of clinical trial data demonstrated it occurred in 0.2% of treated patients (62). Recurrence after SVR12 is more commonly due to reinfection in individuals with high-risk behaviors than true relapse (63).

HCV Qualitative and Quantitative NAATs

Commercial HCV NAATs are available in qualitative and quantitative formats (Table 4). Qualitative NAATs are indicated to diagnose chronic hepatitis C in HCV-seropositive individuals. One test (Aptima HCV RNA Qualitative Assay) is currently commercially available; it employs transcription-mediated amplification (TMA)

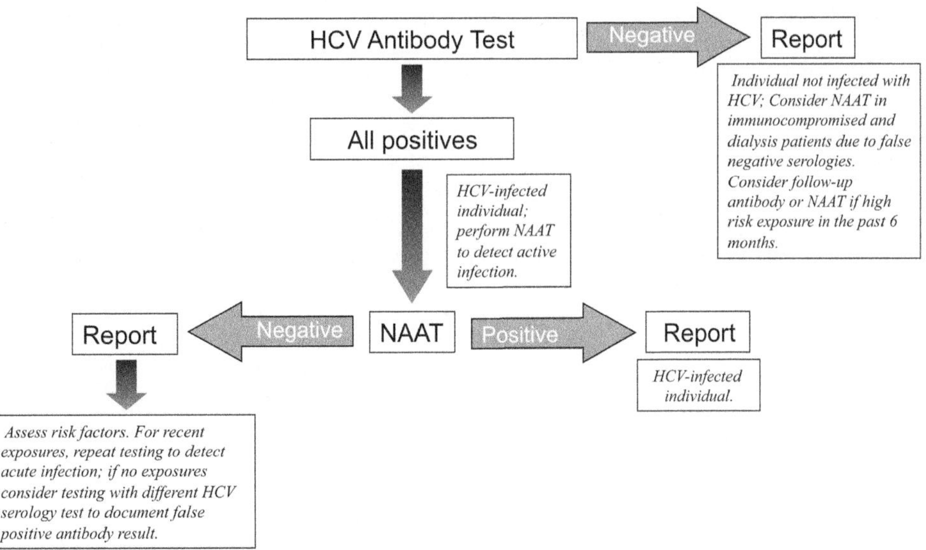

FIGURE 3 Recommended testing algorithm for detection of HCV infection. Derived from reference 85.

chemistry (Table 4; see chapter 7 for description). Quantitative NAATs that employ real-time reverse transcription (RT)-PCR and TMA are available (Table 4). Some quantitative NAATs have received regulatory approval in the United States for chronic hepatitis C diagnosis and therapeutic monitoring indications; others have approval for therapeutic monitoring only (Table 4). All assays amplify and detect highly conserved 5′ UTR sequences. A variety of test platforms for quantitative HCV NAAT have been introduced recently that incorporate new workflows with the aim of improving laboratory efficiency, decreasing labor requirements, and shortening time to result. For example, some instruments (Panther, which performs Aptima HCV Quant Dx, and cobas 6800/8800, which performs cobas HCV) offer features such as random-access testing and complete automation, with testing directly from primary tubes. Others perform testing in individual cartridges (GeneXpert, which performs Xpert HCV Viral Load) that allow for on-demand, random-access testing.

A World Health Organization international calibration standard has been available since 1997; HCV RNA is therefore quantified in international units per milliliter (IU/ml). The Fifth International Standard is currently in use. It consists of plasma from a single Gt1a-infected individual who donated blood prior to seroconversion. This material was then further diluted in HCV seronegative/HCV RNA-negative pooled human plasma. The Fifth International Standard is a biological standard whose concentration was derived by testing at multiple sites (17 laboratories in 11 countries, using five different commercial tests); it has been assigned a value of $5.0\log_{10}$ IU/ml. To permit longitudinal consistency in quantification, the standard was calibrated in parallel with the Second and Fourth International Standards. Whether the current international standard produces harmonization of quantitative results across all available HCV RNA quantitative tests and for all genotypes has not been investigated.

ISOLATION PROCEDURES AND IDENTIFICATION

HCV is a fastidious virus that is not recoverable with mammalian cells (primary or transformed) carried in routine or reference clinical virology laboratories. Virus can be propagated in specialty laboratories using systems for recovery of infectious virus after transfecting permissive cells with HCV molecular clones (64–66) or using a newly reported hepatoma cell line (67). These advances are powerful tools for the development of DAAs and vaccines, but they have not been adopted for diagnostic use.

GENOTYPING

HCV genotyping and subtyping of Gt1 (determination of Gt1a versus Gt1b) are still important. This information is used in clinical management to determine DAA treatment regimen (Table 2) and to guide the need for RAS detection, depending upon the genotype that is present and regimens that are under consideration (see Table 10). Future recommendations on the use of pan-genotypic regimens over genotype-specific regimens will dictate whether these tests will continue to remain clinically useful.

HCV genotypes and subtypes can be determined by commercial (Table 5) and laboratory-developed NAATs (Table 6) based on a variety of biochemical methods

TABLE 5 Commercial HCV RNA genotyping tests[a,b]

Test	Method	Target(s)	Subtyping	Comment	Reference(s)
eSensor HCV Genotyping Test (GenMark)[c]	Amplicon capture with oligonucleotide probes; electrochemical detection with ferrocene-labeled oligonucleotide signal probes	5′ UTR	No	Suitable for use with Roche cobas Ampliprep/cobas TaqMan amplicons. Subtyping unreliable due to 5′ UTR conservation.	104
Versant HCV Genotype (LiPA) 2.0 (Siemens)[d,e]	Reverse hybridization with detection on strips (line probe); automated blot processor and band interpretation instrumentation available.	5′ UTR and core gene	Yes	Some difficulty in reliably distinguishing Gt2 and Gt4 subtypes has been reported. Ghost bands that complicate result interpretation occur less commonly than in version 1.0 (A. Caliendo, personal communication).	105, 106
RealTime HCV Genotype II[d,e] (Abbott)	Real-time RT-PCR	NS5b (Gt1a, 1b), 5′ UTR (Gts1–5)	Yes	96% genotype agreement with LiPA 2.0 and NS5b-based direct sequencing.	107
cobas HCV GT[c] (Roche)	Real-time RT-PCR	5′ UTR, core, NS5B	Gt1a and 1b only		108
Sentosa SQ HCV Genotyping Assay (Vela Diagnostics)[f]	Massively paralleled sequencing (NGS)	NS5B	Yes	Platform combines nucleic acid extraction, library construction, template preparation, sequencing (Ion Torrent technology), and sequence analysis. Has LIS connectivity.	109

[a]Abbreviations: NGS, next-generation sequencing; LIS, laboratory information system.
[b]Genotypes 1–6 can be determined with all assays.
[c]Available globally as a research use only product.
[d]CE marked and approved according to European In Vitro Diagnostic Directive 98/79/EC and approved for use by the U.S. FDA.
[e]In United States, test has been approved by FDA for determination of Gt1–Gt5 but not Gt6. Versions marketed outside the United States can be used for Gt1–Gt6 determination.
[f]CE marked and approved according to European In Vitro Diagnostic Directive 98/79/EC.

TABLE 6 Laboratory-developed HCV RNA genotyping methods

Method	Chemistry	Target(s)	Genotyping	Subtyping	References
Sequencing	Sanger chemistries	NS5B, core, core-E1	1–6	Yes	110–112
Sequencing	Massively parallel sequencing (also referred to as next-generation sequencing and deep sequencing)	Whole genome, NS5B	1–6	Yes	113–116
Subtype-specific PCR	PCR with subtype-specific primers; amplicons of different size detected by gel electrophoresis	Core, NS5B	Gt1a, Gt1b, Gt2a, Gt2b, Gt3a, Gt3b, Gt4, Gt5a, Gt6a	Yes	117, 118

(advantages and disadvantages are summarized in Table 7). Most commercial assays utilize sequence-dependent chemistries that rely on the specificity of test reagents to accurately determine HCV genotype and subtype. For example, real-time RT-PCR utilizes the specificity of primer/probe binding to target HCV RNA in order to determine HCV genotype and subtype, while reverse hybridization is based on hybridization of specimen-derived HCV amplicon sequences to complementary sequences bound onto nylon membranes to determine HCV genotypes and subtypes. Among sequence-dependent tests, assays based on 5′ UTR sequences are generally acceptable for genotype determination but are not suitable for Gt1 subtyping due to the degree of sequence conservation in this region.

TABLE 7 Advantages and disadvantages of HCV genotyping methods[a]

LiPA and real-time PCR

Advantages
- Technically simple
- Utilizes commonly available instrumentation
- Low labor requirement
- Low cost

Disadvantages
- Accuracy issues: genotype miscalls and indeterminate results; cannot identify recombinant strains

Sequencing methods (Sanger, MPS)

Advantages
- Gold standard in accuracy
- WGS: can simultaneously obtain genotype and resistance-associated sequence data
- Can identify recombinant variants
  - WGS: gold standard for recombinant variant identification; genetic breakpoint can be demonstrated
  - Gene-targeted Sanger-based methods: require sequencing of 5′ (5′ UTR, core, E1) and 3′ (NS5A, NS5B) genomic targets to identify recombinant HCV strains
  - Gene-targeted MPS methods: require long-read technologies to identify recombinant HCV strains

Disadvantages
- All methods: infrastructure requirements (instrumentation, informatics), cost
- Metagenomic MPS (unbiased sequencing of all RNAs in plasma): lower depth of coverage (i.e., fewer HCV-specific reads) than methods that include presequencing enrichment steps (HCV RNA capture, HCV-specific PCR) due to high background of human (host) sequence reads (119); requires higher HCV RNA levels than gene-targeted methods (>4.0 $\log_{10}$ IU/ml) (89)

[a]Abbreviations: LiPA, line probe assay; MPS, massively parallel sequencing (also known as next-generation sequencing or deep sequencing.

Analysis of other gene targets such as NS5B, core, and/or core-E1 improves genotype and subtype accuracy. Even with these alternative targets, there are limitations to the accuracy of sequence-directed genotyping methods. With the expansion in HCV diagnosis worldwide, sequence variants are increasing and producing aberrancies in genotype test results. These sequence variants include once-rare genotypes (Gt4, Gt5, and Gt6) and other variants in more common genotypes (Gt1, Gt2, and Gt3). Miscalls of Gt6 as Gt1 or Gt3 by LiPA 2.0 compared to direct sequencing of NS5B or core are particularly problematic as they can lead to inappropriate treatment and therapeutic failure (7, 68). A real-time PCR assay designed to detect only Gt1 and Gt6 in a single reaction and to improve discrimination between these genotypes (Abbott HCV Genotype II PLUS RUO; Abbott Molecular, Des Plaines, IL) has reduced but not eliminated Gt6 miscalls (69, 70). Indeterminate results, demonstrated to be Gt6, Gt2, and Gt3 by Sanger sequencing, have also been observed and must be resolved by an alternative test (68, 71, 72). Considering the tremendous sequence diversity of HCV genomes, tests that rely on sequence binding to make genotype calls may never reach the same level of accuracy as tests based on chemistries that are more sequence agnostic, such as sequencing. A variety of these HCV sequencing methods for genotype determination have been published (Table 6). Advantages and disadvantages of different genotyping methods are listed in Table 7. Of note, recombinant HCV strains can be identified with methods that characterize 5′ regions (5′ UTR, core, E1) and 3′ regions (NS5A and NS5B) such as multitarget sequencing or whole-genome sequencing (WGS) methods; current commercially available tests will not detect these variants (Table 7).

For tests that have received regulatory approval, laboratories must verify accuracy of test performance in-house. More extensive assay verification is required for laboratory-developed tests. From the perspective of accuracy, genotype determination of the more common viruses (Gt1 to Gt3) is fairly straightforward as these samples are readily accessible. Gt4, Gt5, and Gt6 are more problematic as they are found less commonly. Samples containing HCV are available commercially (Gt1 through 3, ProMedDx, Norton, MA; Gt1 through 5, Exact Diagnostics, Fort Worth, TX; Gt1 through 6, BocaBiolistics, Coconut Creek, FL, and SeraCare, Milford, MA) for use in preimplementation accuracy studies. One strategy for samples found to putatively contain these less-common genotypes is to refer them to a reference laboratory for genotype confirmation.

SEROLOGIC TESTS

The diagnosis of HCV infection is usually established with serology assays (Fig. 3). In addition to risk-based testing found in previous hepatitis C screening recommendations

TABLE 8 Recommendations for chronic hepatitis C screening[a]

Serology should be performed in individuals with the following risk factors:
Injection drug use (recent or remote; single or multiple episodes)
Conditions associated with hepatitis C prevalence
  Birth years from 1945 to 1965
  HIV
  Hemophilia with receipt of clotting factors prior to 1987
  Hemodialysis
  Incarceration
  Unexplained aminotransferase elevations
Blood transfusion or organ transplant prior to 1992
Children born to HCV-infected mothers
Needlestick injury or mucosal exposure to HCV-positive blood
Current sexual partners of HCV-infected persons

[a]Synopsized from http://www.hcvguidelines.org.

(listed in Table 8), screening recommendations now also include one-time serology testing for individuals born between 1945 and 1965 (73), the cohort with the projected highest prevalence of chronic hepatitis C. Birth cohort screening has been recommended since previous recommendations were ineffective in identifying what is thought to be the bulk of chronic infections.

Serologic testing for HCV has undergone considerable evolution. The first serologic assay comprised a single NS4 peptide (c-100-3) and was introduced in 1990 shortly after HCV was identified as a major cause of non-A, non-B hepatitis. This assay represented a significant advance, particularly in identifying contaminated blood products and preventing transfusion-transmitted hepatitis C; however, its flaws of low sensitivity and specificity were soon apparent (sensitivity, ~70%; positive predictive values in low- and high-prevalence populations, 30 to 50% and 70 to 85%, respectively) (74). Increased sensitivity and specificity were achieved in second-generation serologic assays. These tests (one of which is still marketed) were better able to detect acute infections due to the incorporation of NS3 and core antigens (Table 9 and Fig. 4), two targets of early antibody responses. The reasons for improved performance of third-generation serologic assays that incorporate NS5 and contain reconfigured NS3 antigen (Fig. 4) are unclear. Improved antigenicity of the alternate NS3 antigen leading to increased detection during early seroconversion has been argued (75). However, the finding of HCV RNA-positive donors who were consistently reactive by third-generation tests but remained unreactive by second-generation versions for over 6 months suggests that more complex immunologic factors may be responsible (76).

With seroconversion panels in which infection has been documented by serology only, the seroconversion window has been documented to decrease from approximately 16 to 10 to 8 weeks with the introduction of first-, second-, and third-generation serology tests, respectively. It is important to note that when infection is documented with NAAT, the seroconversion window with second- and third-generation serology tests is much longer (Fig. 2) (58, 77). Table 9 contains information on HCV serology tests available in the United States; numerous other assays are also available globally (78). A rapid (20- to 40-minute time to result), point-of-care, direct-from-sample cartridge-based immunochromatographic test (CLIA-waived) has been approved by the FDA for use with fingerstick and venipuncture whole blood (OraQuick HCV, Orasure Technologies, Bethlehem, PA). Compared to third-generation serologic tests, reported sensitivity is 94 to 99% and specificity is >99% (79, 80).

Despite improvements in performance characteristics, spurious serology results can still be observed. Second-generation assays are still available (Abbott HCV EIA 2.0; Table 9) and can yield false-negative results due to low sensitivity compared to third-generation assays. Therefore, in the appropriate clinical setting (for example, an individual with sudden onset hepatitis or an occupational exposure such as needlestick from an HCV-infected individual), alternative testing (third-generation serology test or NAAT) should be considered in a patient with a negative second-generation test result. Alternative testing should

TABLE 9 Serologic assays for the detection of anti-HCV antibodies[a]

Test (manufacturer)	Assay type	S/CO threshold[b]	Sensitivity (%)	Specificity (%)	Approved for donor screening	Reference(s)
Abbott HCV EIA 2.0 (Abbott)	Enzyme immunoassay	≥3.8	85.6	98.4	Yes	120
AxSYM Anti-HCV (Abbott)	Microparticle immunoassay	≥10.0	100[c]	94[d]	No	Package insert
ARCHITECT Anti-HCV (Abbott)	Chemiluminescent microparticle	≥5.0	99.7[c]	97.7[d]	No	Package insert
Abbott Prism HCV (Abbott)	Chemiluminescent immunoassay	NA[e]	100	100	Yes	Package insert
Ortho HCV version 3.0 EIA (Ortho)	Enzyme immunoassay	≥3.8	96.9–100	100	Yes	121
VITROS Anti-HCV (Ortho)	Chemiluminescent immunoassay	≥8.0	100	96.5–98.1	No	122, 123
Elecsys Anti-HCV II (Roche)	Electrochemiluminescent immunoassay	≥10	100	99.8	No	124–126
Advia Centaur HCV (Siemens)	Chemiluminescent immunoassay	≥11.0	100	99.9	No	127

[a]All assays approved for diagnostic use by the U.S. Food and Drug Administration.
[b]>95% samples with S/CO ratios above indicated threshold predicted to be confirmed positive.
[c]Expressed in package insert as percent positive agreement.
[d]Expressed in package insert as percent negative agreement.
[e]NA, not available.

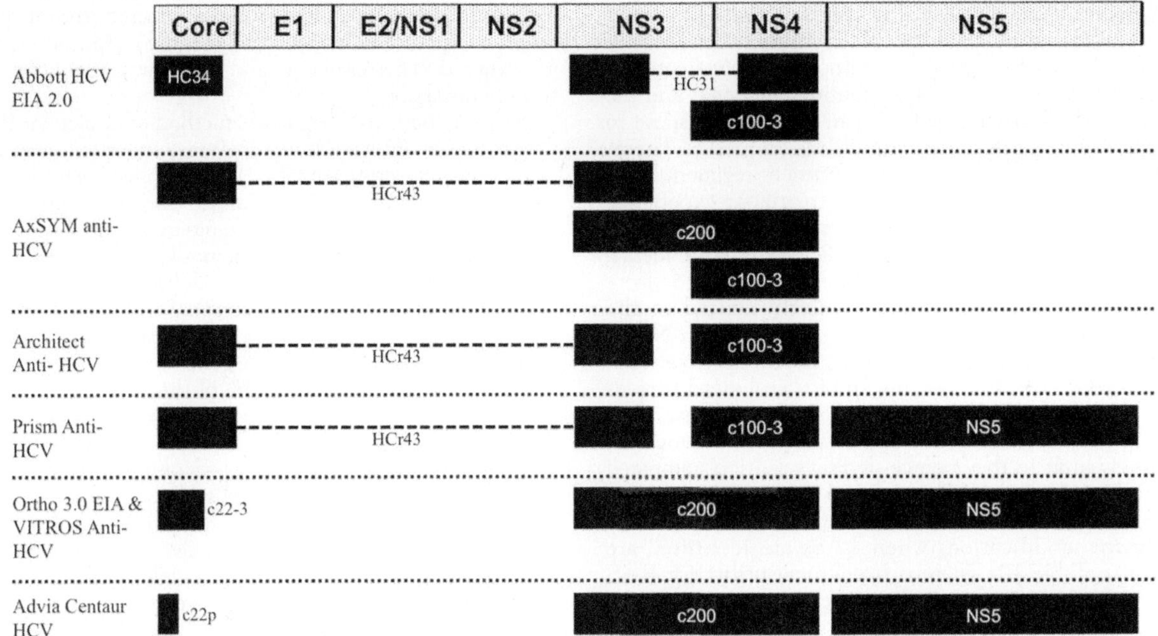

FIGURE 4 Antigens in serology tests currently available commercially in the United States. Abbott HCV EIA 2.0 is the only second-generation screening test currently available. AxSYM, ARCHITECT, Ortho 3.0 EIA, Ortho VITROS, and Advia Centaur are third-generation HCV antibody screening tests. HC34, recombinant antigen containing HCV core protein (amino acids, aa, 1 to 150); HC31, recombinant antigen containing NS3 (aa1192 to 1457) and NS4 (aa1676 to 1931) separated by an 8-aa linker. c100-3, recombinant antigen containing NS3-4 (aa1569 to 1931). HCr43, fusion protein of two noncontiguous antigens, c33c and core protein (aa1 to 150). c200, recombinant antigen containing NS3-4 (aa1192 to 1931). NS5, recombinant antigen (aa2054 to 2995). c22-3, recombinant antigen containing core protein (aa2 to 120). c22p, peptide containing core protein major epitope (aa10 to 53). For Elecsys Anti-HCV II, peptide locations are shown; exact identities are proprietary.

also be considered for any negative serology test result if acute hepatitis C is suspected (see "Evaluation, Interpretation, and Reporting of Results/Interpretation of Results" below for additional discussion). False-negative results have also been observed in immunocompromised patients (HIV with CD4 <100, chemotherapy-treated oncology patients); therefore, NAAT should be performed to definitively exclude infection in these patients (60, 81).

For most antibody screening assays, a positive result is considered initially reactive, and repeat testing in duplicate is required. Results are reported as reactive if two or more replicates are positive. One advantage of certain chemiluminescent and microparticle immunoassays (AxSYM Anti-HCV, Abbott; ARCHITECT Anti-HCV, Abbott; VITROS Anti-HCV, Ortho; Advia Centaur HCV, Siemens) is that initial positive results can be reported as reactive; repeat testing is not required due to the high sensitivities and specificities of these tests.

HCV serologic tests were originally developed as screening assays, with an emphasis on sensitivity and consequent potential for false-positive results. Early recommendations (82) therefore advised confirming all positive results by recombinant immunoblot assay (RIBA) before proceeding to NAAT to avoid erroneous diagnoses. Confirmation of all reactive screening test results was never widely adopted by clinicians or laboratorians outside the blood-screening arena, largely due to the availability of more definitive NAATs and the conviction that RIBA did not represent an adequate confirmatory test as it employed the same antigens as antibody screening tests. Subsequent recommendations included a complex algorithm advising the confirmation of screening results with low signal/cutoff (S/CO) ratios by RIBA, since false positives were most likely to occur in these samples (83). RIBA is no longer being manufactured, and current screening recommendations for chronic HCV (outlined in Fig. 3) have largely jettisoned the concept of confirmatory testing unless a spurious positive result is suspected in an individual with no risk factors. In these instances, S/CO ratios are still useful to guide additional testing although they are not formally mentioned (see Table 9 for assays available in the United States and Europe; S/CO ratios for other assays are described in reference 84); low S/CO ratios typically indicate false-positive serology results. If documentation of a false-positive screening result is required, U.S. guidelines recommend additional testing with an alternative, FDA-approved HCV antibody screening test (85). In other countries, commercial HCV immunoblots are available (INNO-LIA HCV Score, Fujirebio; CE-marked).

ANTIVIRAL SUSCEPTIBILITY

Currently, there is some clinical utility to baseline testing for the presence of RASs that are associated with failure of DAA therapy. HCV exists as a quasispecies in infected individuals, as is true of viruses with RNA genomes that rely on error-prone RNA-dependent RNA polymerases for replication. RASs occur commonly within the quasispecies of untreated individuals.

Unlike other virus infections (HIV), the presence of RAS at baseline is not uniformly predictive of treatment failure.

Rather, certain baseline RASs are associated with treatment failure in the context of specific combinations of HCV genotype and DAA regimens. Additionally, prior treatment failure (with interferon-alfa-containing regimens) and the presence of underlying cirrhosis can further predispose to treatment failure in the setting of baseline RAS. Therefore, a variety of factors including treatment regimen, HCV genotype, underlying cirrhosis, and treatment experience are used to determine the necessity for baseline RAS testing and adjustments to treatment if significant RASs are identified (http://www.hcvguidelines.org) (86).

Baseline RAS detection is currently limited to the NS5A gene. The replicative fitness of HCVs with NS5A RAS is high in the absence of DAAs. These variants have been detected at baseline and for prolonged periods after cessation of DAA treatment (87). In contrast, variant viruses with RASs in NS3/4A and NS5B genes are relatively unfit in the absence of drug selection compared to wild-type HCV. Clinical scenarios that warrant baseline RAS determination, significant RAS, and recommended treatment modifications when RASs are identified are shown in Table 10. There is no clinical utility for RAS detection after treatment failure; therefore, testing in this setting is not recommended.

Most RASs alter the conformation of DAA binding sites and therefore cause an increase in the concentration required for 50% of maximal efficacy (EC50) when tested in HCV replicon systems (86); RASs that are currently clinically actionable cause high-level resistance (≥25-fold increase in EC50 in replicon systems) (http://www.hcvguidelines.org). Interestingly, not all substitutions at RAS positions are equally important. Some are merely polymorphisms while others cause clinically significant resistance. Multiple baseline RASs in a single gene may negatively affect therapeutic response. Preliminary data suggest that three or more RASs in NS5A are associated with ledipasvir/sofosbuvir failure in Gt1b-infected patients with no prior exposure to NS5A inhibitors (88). Additional data are required to better understand the clinical significance of this phenomenon.

Sequencing is the diagnostic method of choice for RAS detection (http://www.hcvguidelines.org, http://www.easl.eu/_clinical-practice-guideline). RASs have been found to be associated with treatment failure only when present at ≥15% of the HCV quasispecies found in plasma; minor variants present at lower frequency do not appear to affect treatment outcome (http://www.hcvguidelines.org, http://www.easl.eu/_clinical-practice-guideline). Consequently, Sanger sequencing chemistry is appropriate for baseline RAS determination because it can identify genetic variants when they are present as at least 10 to 20% of the quasispecies. Massively parallel sequencing (also known as deep sequencing or next-generation sequencing) can also be used for RAS detection. Treatment guidelines recommend that substitutions should only be reported when present in ≥15% of sequence reads (http://www.hcvguidelines.org, http://www.easl.eu/_clinical-practice-guideline). Commercially available assays are limited to a massively parallel sequencing test available for research use only (*Sentosa* SQ HCV Genotyping Assay, Vela Diagnostics) that targets regions in NS3, NS5A, and NS5B for RAS identification.

Many different noncommercial sequencing methods for RAS detection have been reported in the literature. Caution should be taken when implementing target-specific reagents from published Sanger or massively parallel sequencing methods as many primer sets are genotype specific. Efficacy of RAS identification in intended, clinically relevant genotypes should be established during test validation. In theory, WGS would avoid genotype-inclusivity issues of targeted techniques. This approach is impractical as RAS detection is currently a low-volume test in routine clinical laboratories and WGS is cost effective

TABLE 10 Recommendations for RAS testing prior to treatment initiation[a]

Genotype	Drug combination	Treatment: Naïve	Treatment: Experienced	NSB5 testing	Clinically relevant substitutions	Comment
1–6	Glecaprevir/pibrentasvir	X	X	No	—	Treatment duration 8, 12, 16 weeks
1a	Ledipasvir/sofosbuvir	X		No	—	Without cirrhosis, <6M IU/ml before 8-week therapy
			X	Yes	Q30H/R, L31M/V, Y93C/H/N	Without cirrhosis, if >100-fold resistance, treat 12 weeks adding ribavirin (or use different therapy)
1b		X	X	No	L31V	Without cirrhosis, <6M IU/ml before 8-week therapy
1a	Elbasvir/grazoprevir	X	X	Yes	M28A/T, Q30H/R, L31M/V, Y93C/H/N	If present, extend to 16 weeks (or consider different therapy) or 24 weeks with cirrhosis
1b					Y93H	
3	Daclatasvir/sofosbuvir	X		No	—	
			X	Yes		Without cirrhosis before therapy for 12 weeks (or 24 weeks with cirrhosis). With Y93H, add ribavirin
3	Sofosbuvir/velpatasvir				Y93H	Treatment experience (+/− cirrhosis) and treatment naïve with cirrhosis considered for 12 weeks of sofosbuvir/velpatasvir. With Y93H, add ribavirin
1–6	Sofosbuvir/velpatasvir/voxilaprevir	X	X	No	Y93H	Not recommended with 12 weeks of therapy

[a]Synopsized from http://www.hcvguidelines.org.

only in high-volume/high-throughput configurations. A recent meta-analysis that used criteria such as sensitivity (ability to identify RAS in specimens with HCV levels ≥1,000 IU/ml) and genotype inclusivity of published sequencing methods is a useful resource for potential sequencing reagents (89).

IL28B haplotype testing to detect host genetic markers of interferon refractoriness was important before initiating treatment with interferon-alfa-containing regimens to determine probability of response. There is currently no clinical utility for *IL28B* haplotype determination prior to treatment with interferon-free combination DAA regimens. This test had a limited lifespan.

EVALUATION, INTERPRETATION, AND REPORTING OF RESULTS

Interpretation of Results in Acute Hepatitis C

Establishing the diagnosis of acute hepatitis C can be challenging. Most cases of acute hepatitis C are asymptomatic; therefore, serum aminotransferase elevations can be helpful if present but should not be relied upon as the sole indicator of infection. Additionally, seroconversion can be delayed, and HCV RNA detection in plasma can be sporadic. Serology and RNA assessment should therefore both be performed to optimally detect infection. Diagnostic accuracy also requires testing at multiple time points. Single HCV NAAT results do not reliably predict exposure outcome. Transient HCV RNA negativity has been documented early postinfection in individuals who become chronically infected and later at the time of seroconversion (Fig. 2) (90). Transient positive results have been found in those who spontaneously clear virus (58, 91). Testing for infection is recommended for 6 months after a known exposure since the majority of individuals seroconvert by this time (http://www.hcvguidelines.org). Initial testing should be performed as soon as possible after exposure to determine HCV infection status at the time of exposure. Individuals should be tested every 4 to 6 weeks for 6 months with HCV NAAT and serologic assays if they have no prior evidence of HCV infection or with HCV NAAT only if they show evidence of prior resolved HCV infection (HCV seropositive, HCV RNA not detected). In the 6-month period after exposure, HCV RNA detected twice, at least 12 weeks apart, is considered evidence of progression to chronic infection (http://www.hcvguidelines.org).

Interpretation of Results in Chronic Hepatitis C

The lack of potency of interferon-alfa/ribavirin as an antiviral regimen elevated the importance of diagnostic tests (particularly quantitative NAATs) in therapeutic management of chronic hepatitis C, rendering them critical for appropriate decision making with regard to therapeutic duration and determination of response after treatment. Therefore, a full understanding of test performance characteristics (genotype bias, precision, and limit of detection) was required so that results were interpreted accurately and patients were managed appropriately. In the all-oral DAA era, however, tests play a much more limited role in therapeutic management because regimens are so highly potent and efficacious. Essentially, patients will respond to treatment if they are placed on the correct regimen and they take their medicine as prescribed. In this setting, test interpretation issues are subtle or minor. For baseline assessments, laboratories should have a full understanding of the accuracy of their genotyping assays (including accuracy of Gt1a and Gt1b results) and the precision throughout the measuring range of their quantitative NAATs because genotype and HCV RNA levels are used to select optimal treatment regimens. On-treatment testing is limited typically to assessment of HCV RNA level at week 4. Most patients have no detectable HCV RNA by this time; therefore, the impact of factors that can affect quantification and test interpretation during on-treatment monitoring is negligible. Those patients who have detectable HCV RNA at week 4 typically have low or very low levels that are cleared by treatment week 6. The result of "HCV RNA detected, lower than the lower limit of quantification" should be interpreted as a very low level of HCV RNA and not as "HCV RNA not detected." Virtually all patients have no detectable HCV RNA at end of treatment. Most patients who relapse will experience reemergence of HCV RNA 12 weeks after treatment cessation, at levels similar to baseline. Rarely, patients have late relapse, with resurgence of HCV RNA 24 weeks after treatment cessation. This can cause confusion when treatment occurs in the setting of ongoing high-risk behavior because it can be difficult to distinguish between late relapse and new infection. Genotype testing can be performed as a first step in resolving this issue; detection of an HCV genotype different from the original determination indicates reinfection. If the same genotype (or genotype/subtype) is identified in the posttreatment sample, resolution requires sequence determination (typically Sanger sequencing) with comparison of pretreatment and posttreatment HCV sequences. The clinical consequences of sporadic cases of treatment failure or reinfection are minimal, other than health care cost. Given the plethora of DAA regimen options, retreatment is readily undertaken, and cure remains a high probability.

REFERENCES

1. **Ohba K, Mizokami M, Lau JY, Orito E, Ikeo K, Gojobori T.** 1996. Evolutionary relationship of hepatitis C, pesti-, flavi-, plantviruses, and newly discovered GB hepatitis agents. *FEBS Lett* **378:**232–234.
2. **Lavie M, Dubuisson J.** 2017. Interplay between hepatitis C virus and lipid metabolism during virus entry and assembly. *Biochimie* **141:**62–69.
3. **Freedman H, Logan MR, Law JL, Houghton M.** 2016. Structure and function of the Hepatitis C virus envelope glycoproteins E1 and E2: antiviral and vaccine targets. *ACS Infect Dis* **2:**749–762.
4. **Jones CT, Murray CL, Eastman DK, Tassello J, Rice CM.** 2007. Hepatitis C virus p7 and NS2 proteins are essential for production of infectious virus. *J Virol* **81:**8374–8383.
5. **Pawlotsky JM.** 2013. NS5A inhibitors in the treatment of hepatitis C. *J Hepatol* **59:**375–382.
6. **Smith DB, Bukh J, Kuiken C, Muerhoff AS, Rice CM, Stapleton JT, Simmonds P.** 2014. Expanded classification of hepatitis C virus into 7 genotypes and 67 subtypes: updated criteria and genotype assignment web resource. *Hepatology* **59:**318–327.
7. **Welzel TM, Bhardwaj N, Hedskog C, Chodavarapu K, Camus G, McNally J, Brainard D, Miller MD, Mo H, Svarovskaia E, Jacobson I, Zeuzem S, Agarwal K.** 2017. Global epidemiology of HCV subtypes and resistance-associated substitutions evaluated by sequencing-based subtype analyses. *J Hepatol* **67:**224–236.
8. **Gower E, Estes C, Blach S, Razavi-Shearer K, Razavi H.** 2014. Global epidemiology and genotype distribution of the hepatitis C virus infection. *J Hepatol* **61**(Suppl)**:**S45–S57.
9. **Murphy DG, Sablon E, Chamberland J, Fournier E, Dandavino R, Tremblay CL.** 2015. Hepatitis C virus genotype 7, a new genotype originating from central Africa. *J Clin Microbiol* **53:**967–972.

10. **Hedskog C, Doehle B, Chodavarapu K, Gontcharova V, Crespo Garcia J, De Knegt R, Drenth JP, McHutchison JG, Brainard D, Stamm LM, Miller MD, Svarovskaia E, Mo H.** 2015. Characterization of hepatitis C virus intergenotypic recombinant strains and associated virological response to sofosbuvir/ribavirin. *Hepatology* **61:**471–480.
11. **Raghwani J, Thomas XV, Koekkoek SM, Schinkel J, Molenkamp R, van de Laar TJ, Takebe Y, Tanaka Y, Mizokami M, Rambaut A, Pybus OG.** 2012. Origin and evolution of the unique hepatitis C virus circulating recombinant form 2k/1b. *J Virol* **86:**2212–2220.
12. **Susser S, Dietz J, Schlevogt B, Zuckerman E, Barak M, Piazzolla V, Howe A, Hinrichsen H, Passmann S, Daniel R, Cornberg M, Mangia A, Zeuzem S, Sarrazin C.** 2017. Origin, prevalence and response to therapy of hepatitis C virus genotype 2k/1b chimeras. *J Hepatol* **67:**680–686.
13. **Kalinina O, Norder H, Mukomolov S, Magnius LO.** 2002. A natural intergenotypic recombinant of hepatitis C virus identified in St. Petersburg. *J Virol* **76:**4034–4043.
14. **Zakalashvili M, Zarkua J, Weizenegger M, Bartel J, Raabe M, Zangurashvili L, Kankia N, Jashiashvili N, Lomidze M, Telia T, Kerashvili V, Zhamutashvili M, Abramishvili N, Hedskog C, Chodavarapu K, Brainard DM, McHutchison JG, Mo H, Svarovskaia E, Gish RG, Rtskhiladze I, Metreveli D.** 2017. Identification of hepatitis C virus 2k/1b intergenotypic recombinants in Georgia. *Liver Int* **38:**451–457.
15. **Colson P, Borentain P, Dhiver C, Benhaim S, Gerolami R, Tamalet C.** 2016. Recombinant hepatitis C viruses that might hamper accurate genotype classification and choice of treatment with direct-acting agents, southeastern France. *Hepatology* **63:**1400–1402.
16. **Stelzl E, Haas B, Bauer B, Zhang S, Fiss EH, Hillman G, Hamilton AT, Mehta R, Heil ML, Marins EG, Santner BI, Kessler HH.** 2017. First identification of a recombinant form of hepatitis C virus in Austrian patients by full-genome next generation sequencing. *PLoS One* **12:**e0181273.
17. **Karchava M, Chkhartishvili N, Sharvadze L, Abutidze A, Dvali N, Gatserelia L, Dzigua L, Bolokadze N, Dolmazashvili E, Kotorashvili A, Imnadze P, Gamkrelidze A, Tsertsvadze T.** 2018. Impact of hepatitis C virus recombinant form RF1_2k/1b on treatment outcomes within the Georgian national hepatitis C elimination program. *Hepatol Res* **48:**36–44.
18. **Armstrong GL, Wasley A, Simard EP, McQuillan GM, Kuhnert WL, Alter MJ.** 2006. The prevalence of hepatitis C virus infection in the United States, 1999 through 2002. *Ann Intern Med* **144:**705–714.
19. **Wasley A, Grytdal S, Gallagher K, Centers for Disease Control and Prevention (CDC).** 2008. Surveillance for acute viral hepatitis—United States, 2006. *MMWR Surveill Summ* **57:**1–24.
20. **Wang CC, Krantz E, Klarquist J, Krows M, McBride L, Scott EP, Shaw-Stiffel T, Weston SJ, Thiede H, Wald A, Rosen HR.** 2007. Acute hepatitis C in a contemporary US cohort: modes of acquisition and factors influencing viral clearance. *J Infect Dis* **196:**1474–1482.
21. **Hagan H, Jordan AE, Neurer J, Cleland CM.** 2015. Incidence of sexually transmitted hepatitis C virus infection in HIV-positive men who have sex with men. *AIDS* **29:**2335–2345.
22. **Hoornenborg E, Achterbergh RCA, Schim van der Loeff MF, Davidovich U, Hogewoning A, de Vries HJC, Schinkel J, Prins M, van de Laar TJW, Amsterdam PrEP Project team in the HIV Transmission Elimination Amsterdam Initiative, MOSAIC study group.** 2017. MSM starting preexposure prophylaxis are at risk of hepatitis C virus infection. *AIDS* **31:**1603–1610.
23. **Suryaprasad AG, White JZ, Xu F, Eichler BA, Hamilton J, Patel A, Hamdounia SB, Church DR, Barton K, Fisher C, Macomber K, Stanley M, Guilfoyle SM, Sweet K, Liu S, Iqbal K, Tohme R, Sharapov U, Kupronis BA, Ward JW, Holmberg SD.** 2014. Emerging epidemic of hepatitis C virus infections among young nonurban persons who inject drugs in the United States, 2006–2012. *Clin Infect Dis* **59:**1411–1419.
24. **Rehermann B.** 2009. Hepatitis C virus versus innate and adaptive immune responses: a tale of coevolution and coexistence. *J Clin Invest* **119:**1745–1754.
25. **Duggal P, Thio CL, Wojcik GL, Goedert JJ, Mangia A, Latanich R, Kim AY, Lauer GM, Chung RT, Peters MG, Kirk GD, Mehta SH, Cox AL, Khakoo SI, Alric L, Cramp ME, Donfield SM, Edlin BR, Tobler LH, Busch MP, Alexander G, Rosen HR, Gao X, Abdel-Hamid M, Apps R, Carrington M, Thomas DL.** 2013. Genome-wide association study of spontaneous resolution of hepatitis C virus infection: data from multiple cohorts. *Ann Intern Med* **158:**235–245.
26. **Rauch A, Kutalik Z, Descombes P, Cai T, Di Iulio J, Mueller T, Bochud M, Battegay M, Bernasconi E, Borovicka J, Colombo S, Cerny A, Dufour JF, Furrer H, Gunthard HF, Heim M, Hirschel B, Malinverni R, Moradpour D, Mullhaupt B, Witteck A, Beckmann JS, Berg T, Bergmann S, Negro F, Telenti A, Bochud PY.** 2010. Genetic variation in IL28B is associated with chronic hepatitis C and treatment failure: a genome-wide association study. *Gastroenterology* **138:**1338–1345, 1345.e1–7.
27. **Thomas DL, Thio CL, Martin MP, Qi Y, Ge D, O'Huigin C, Kidd J, Kidd K, Khakoo SI, Alexander G, Goedert JJ, Kirk GD, Donfield SM, Rosen HR, Tobler LH, Busch MP, McHutchison JG, Goldstein DB, Carrington M.** 2009. Genetic variation in IL28B and spontaneous clearance of hepatitis C virus. *Nature* **461:**798–801.
28. **Balagopal A, Thomas DL, Thio CL.** 2010. IL28B and the control of hepatitis C virus infection. *Gastroenterology* **139:**1865–1876.
29. **Jiménez-Sousa MA, Fernández-Rodríguez A, Guzmán-Fulgencio M, García-Álvarez M, Resino S.** 2013. Meta-analysis: implications of interleukin-28B polymorphisms in spontaneous and treatment-related clearance for patients with hepatitis C. *BMC Med* **11:**6.
30. **Strader DB, Wright T, Thomas DL, Seeff LB, American Association for the Study of Liver Diseases.** 2004. Diagnosis, management, and treatment of hepatitis C. *Hepatology* **39:**1147–1171.
31. **O'Leary JG, Lepe R, Davis GL.** 2008. Indications for liver transplantation. *Gastroenterology* **134:**1764–1776.
32. **Adinolfi LE, Utili R, Andreana A, Tripodi MF, Rosario P, Mormone G, Ragone E, Pasquale G, Ruggiero G.** 2000. Relationship between genotypes of hepatitis C virus and histopathological manifestations in chronic hepatitis C patients. *Eur J Gastroenterol Hepatol* **12:**299–304.
33. **Yeo AE, Ghany M, Conry-Cantilena C, Melpolder JC, Kleiner DE, Shih JW, Hoofnagle JH, Alter HJ.** 2001. Stability of HCV-RNA level and its lack of correlation with disease severity in asymptomatic chronic hepatitis C virus carriers. *J Viral Hepat* **8:**256–263.
34. **Yano M, Kumada H, Kage M, Ikeda K, Shimamatsu K, Inoue O, Hashimoto E, Lefkowitch JH, Ludwig J, Okuda K.** 1996. The long-term pathological evolution of chronic hepatitis C. *Hepatology* **23:**1334–1340.
35. **Ferreira-Gonzalez A, Shiffman ML.** 2004. Use of diagnostic testing for managing hepatitis C virus infection. *Semin Liver Dis* **24**(Suppl 2)**:**9–18.
36. **Falade-Nwulia O, Suarez-Cuervo C, Nelson DR, Fried MW, Segal JB, Sulkowski MS.** 2017. Oral direct-acting agent therapy for hepatitis C virus infection: a systematic review. *Ann Intern Med* **166:**637–648.
37. **Feld JJ, Maan R, Zeuzem S, Kuo A, Nelson DR, Di Bisceglie AM, Manns MP, Sherman K, Frazier LM, Sterling R, Mailliard M, Schmidt M, Akushevich L, Vainorius M, Fried MW.** 2016. Effectiveness and safety of sofosbuvir-based regimens for chronic HCV genotype 3 infection: results of the HCV-TARGET study. *Clin Infect Dis* **63:**776–783.
38. **Welzel TM, Nelson DR, Morelli G, Di Bisceglie A, Reddy RK, Kuo A, Lim JK, Darling J, Pockros P, Galati JS, Frazier LM, Alqahtani S, Sulkowski MS, Vainorius M, Akushevich L, Fried MW, Zeuzem S, HCV-TARGET Study Group.** 2017. Effectiveness and safety of sofosbuvir plus ribavirin for the treatment of HCV genotype 2 infection: results of the real-world, clinical practice HCV-TARGET study. *Gut* **66:**1844–1852.
39. **Younossi ZM, Park H, Gordon SC, Ferguson JR, Ahmed A, Dieterich D, Saab S.** 2016. Real-world outcomes of ledipasvir/sofosbuvir in treatment-naive patients with hepatitis C. *Am J Manag Care* **22:**SP205–SP211.

40. **Sikavi C, Chen PH, Lee AD, Saab EG, Choi G, Saab S.** 2017. Hepatitis C and human immunodeficiency virus coinfection in the era of direct-acting antiviral agents: no longer a difficult-to-treat population. *Hepatology* **67:**847–857.
41. **Benhamou Y, Bochet M, Di Martino V, Charlotte F, Azria F, Coutellier A, Vidaud M, Bricaire F, Opolon P, Katlama C, Poynard T, The Multivirc Group.** 1999. Liver fibrosis progression in human immunodeficiency virus and hepatitis C virus coinfected patients. *Hepatology* **30:**1054–1058.
42. **Konerman MA, Mehta SH, Sutcliffe CG, Vu T, Higgins Y, Torbenson MS, Moore RD, Thomas DL, Sulkowski MS.** 2014. Fibrosis progression in human immunodeficiency virus/hepatitis C virus coinfected adults: prospective analysis of 435 liver biopsy pairs. *Hepatology* **59:**767–775.
43. **Macías J, Berenguer J, Japón MA, Girón JA, Rivero A, López-Cortés LF, Moreno A, González-Serrano M, Iribarren JA, Ortega E, Miralles P, Mira JA, Pineda JA.** 2009. Fast fibrosis progression between repeated liver biopsies in patients coinfected with human immunodeficiency virus/hepatitis C virus. *Hepatology* **50:**1056–1063.
44. **Dokubo EK, Evans J, Winkelman V, Cyrus S, Tobler LH, Asher A, Briceno A, Page K.** 2014. Comparison of Hepatitis C Virus RNA and antibody detection in dried blood spots and plasma specimens. *J Clin Virol* **59:**223–227.
45. **Greenman J, Roberts T, Cohn J, Messac L.** 2015. Dried blood spot in the genotyping, quantification and storage of HCV RNA: a systematic literature review. *J Viral Hepat* **22:**353–361.
46. **Soulier A, Poiteau L, Rosa I, Hézode C, Roudot-Thoraval F, Pawlotsky JM, Chevaliez S.** 2016. Dried blood spots: a tool to ensure broad access to hepatitis C screening, diagnosis, and treatment monitoring. *J Infect Dis* **213:**1087–1095.
47. **Mohamed Z, Mbwambo J, Shimakawa Y, Poiteau L, Chevaliez S, Pawlotsky JM, Rwegasha J, Bhagani S, Taylor-Robinson SD, Makani J, Thursz MR, Lemoine M.** 2017. Clinical utility of HCV core antigen detection and quantification using serum samples and dried blood spots in people who inject drugs in Dar-es-Salaam, Tanzania. *J Int AIDS Soc* **20:**21856.
48. **Chevaliez S, Soulier A, Poiteau L, Bouvier-Alias M, Pawlotsky JM.** 2014. Clinical utility of hepatitis C virus core antigen quantification in patients with chronic hepatitis C. *J Clin Virol* **61:**145–148.
49. **Ottiger C, Gygli N, Huber AR.** 2013. Detection limit of architect hepatitis C core antigen assay in correlation with HCV RNA, and renewed confirmation algorithm for reactive anti-HCV samples. *J Clin Virol* **58:**535–540.
50. **Ross RS, Viazov S, Salloum S, Hilgard P, Gerken G, Roggendorf M.** 2010. Analytical performance characteristics and clinical utility of a novel assay for total hepatitis C virus core antigen quantification. *J Clin Microbiol* **48:**1161–1168.
51. **Freiman JM, Tran TM, Schumacher SG, White LF, Ongarello S, Cohn J, Easterbrook PJ, Linas BP, Denkinger CM.** 2016. Hepatitis C core antigen testing for diagnosis of hepatitis C virus infection: a systematic review and meta-analysis. *Ann Intern Med* **165:**345–355.
52. **Khan H, Hill A, Main J, Brown A, Cooke G.** 2017. Can hepatitis C virus antigen testing replace ribonucleic acid polymerase chain reaction analysis for detecting hepatitis C virus? A systematic review. *Open Forum Infect Dis* **4:**ofw252.
53. **Laperche S, Nübling CM, Stramer SL, Brojer E, Grabarczyk P, Yoshizawa H, Kalibatas V, El Elkyabi M, Moftah F, Girault A, van Drimmelen H, Busch MP, Lelie N.** 2015. Sensitivity of hepatitis C virus core antigen and antibody combination assays in a global panel of window period samples. *Transfusion* **55:**2489–2498.
54. **Rockstroh JK, Feld JJ, Chevaliez S, Cheng K, Wedemeyer H, Sarrazin C, Maasoumy B, Herman C, Hackett J Jr, Cohen DE, Dawson GJ, Cloherty G, Pawlotsky JM.** 2017. HCV core antigen as an alternate test to HCV RNA for assessment of virologic responses to all-oral, interferon-free treatment in HCV genotype 1 infected patients. *J Virol Methods* **245:**14–18.
55. **Farci P, Alter HJ, Wong D, Miller RH, Shih JW, Jett B, Purcell RH.** 1991. A long-term study of hepatitis C virus replication in non-A, non-B hepatitis. *N Engl J Med* **325:**98–104.
56. **Mosley JW, Operskalski EA, Tobler LH, Buskell ZJ, Andrews WW, Phelps B, Dockter J, Giachetti C, Seeff LB, Busch MP, Transfusion-transmitted Viruses Study and Retrovirus Epidemiology Donor Study Groups.** 2008. The course of hepatitis C viraemia in transfusion recipients prior to availability of antiviral therapy. *J Viral Hepat* **15:**120–128.
57. **Thimme R, Oldach D, Chang KM, Steiger C, Ray SC, Chisari FV.** 2001. Determinants of viral clearance and persistence during acute hepatitis C virus infection. *J Exp Med* **194:**1395–1406.
58. **Glynn SA, Wright DJ, Kleinman SH, Hirschkorn D, Tu Y, Heldebrant C, Smith R, Giachetti C, Gallarda J, Busch MP.** 2005. Dynamics of viremia in early hepatitis C virus infection. *Transfusion* **45:**994–1002.
59. **Chamie G, Bonacini M, Bangsberg DR, Stapleton JT, Hall C, Overton ET, Scherzer R, Tien PC.** 2007. Factors associated with seronegative chronic hepatitis C virus infection in HIV infection. *Clin Infect Dis* **44:**577–583.
60. **Hadlich E, Alvares-Da-Silva MR, Dal Molin RK, Zenker R, Goldani LZ.** 2007. Hepatitis C virus (HCV) viremia in HIV-infected patients without HCV antibodies detectable by third-generation enzyme immunoassay. *J Gastroenterol Hepatol* **22:**1506–1509.
61. **Chen J, Florian J, Carter W, Fleischer RD, Hammerstrom TS, Jadhav PR, Zeng W, Murray J, Birnkrant D.** 2013. Earlier sustained virologic response end points for regulatory approval and dose selection of hepatitis C therapies. *Gastroenterology* **144:**1450–1455.e2.
62. **Sarrazin C, Isakov V, Svarovskaia ES, Hedskog C, Martin R, Chodavarapu K, Brainard DM, Miller MD, Mo H, Molina JM, Sulkowski MS.** 2017. Late relapse versus hepatitis C virus reinfection in patients with sustained virologic response after sofosbuvir-based therapies. *Clin Infect Dis* **64:**44–52.
63. **Simmons B, Saleem J, Hill A, Riley RD, Cooke GS.** 2016. Risk of late relapse or reinfection with hepatitis C virus after achieving a sustained virological response: a systematic review and meta-analysis. *Clin Infect Dis* **62:**683–694.
64. **Lindenbach BD, Evans MJ, Syder AJ, Wölk B, Tellinghuisen TL, Liu CC, Maruyama T, Hynes RO, Burton DR, McKeating JA, Rice CM.** 2005. Complete replication of hepatitis C virus in cell culture. *Science* **309:**623–626.
65. **Wakita T, Pietschmann T, Kato T, Date T, Miyamoto M, Zhao Z, Murthy K, Habermann A, Kräusslich HG, Mizokami M, Bartenschlager R, Liang TJ.** 2005. Production of infectious hepatitis C virus in tissue culture from a cloned viral genome. *Nat Med* **11:**791–796.
66. **Zhong J, Gastaminza P, Cheng G, Kapadia S, Kato T, Burton DR, Wieland SF, Uprichard SL, Wakita T, Chisari FV.** 2005. Robust hepatitis C virus infection in vitro. *Proc Natl Acad Sci USA* **102:**9294–9299.
67. **Yang D, Zuo C, Wang X, Meng X, Xue B, Liu N, Yu R, Qin Y, Gao Y, Wang Q, Hu J, Wang L, Zhou Z, Liu B, Tan D, Guan Y, Zhu H.** 2014. Complete replication of hepatitis B virus and hepatitis C virus in a newly developed hepatoma cell line. *Proc Natl Acad Sci USA* **111:**E1264–E1273.
68. **Yang R, Cong X, Du S, Fei R, Rao H, Wei L.** 2014. Performance comparison of the versant HCV genotype 2.0 assay (LiPA) and the abbott realtime HCV genotype II assay for detecting hepatitis C virus genotype 6. *J Clin Microbiol* **52:**3685–3692.
69. **Mallory MA, Lucic D, Ebbert MT, Cloherty GA, Toolsie D, Hillyard DR.** 2017. Evaluation of the Abbott RealTime HCV genotype II plus RUO (PLUS) assay with reference to core and NS5B sequencing. *J Clin Virol* **90:**26–31.
70. **Mokhtari C, Ebel A, Reinhardt B, Merlin S, Proust S, Roque-Afonso AM.** 2016. Characterization of samples identified as hepatitis C virus genotype 1 without subtype by Abbott RealTime HCV genotype II assay using the new Abbott HCV genotype plus RUO test. *J Clin Microbiol* **54:**296–299.
71. **Benedet M, Adachi D, Wong A, Wong S, Pabbaraju K, Tellier R, Tang JW.** 2014. The need for a sequencing-based assay to supplement the Abbott m2000 RealTime HCV Genotype II assay: a 1 year analysis. *J Clin Virol* **60:**301–304.

72. **González V, Gomes-Fernandes M, Bascuñana E, Casanovas S, Saludes V, Jordana-Lluch E, Matas L, Ausina V, Martró E.** 2013. Accuracy of a commercially available assay for HCV genotyping and subtyping in the clinical practice. *J Clin Virol* **58:**249–253.
73. **Smith BD, Morgan RL, Beckett GA, Falck-Ytter Y, Holtzman D, Teo CG, Jewett A, Baack B, Rein DB, Patel N, Alter M, Yartel A, Ward JW, Centers for Disease Control and Prevention.** 2012. Recommendations for the identification of chronic hepatitis C virus infection among persons born during 1945–1965. *MMWR Recomm Rep* **61**(RR-4)**:**1–32.
74. **Gretch DR.** 1997. Diagnostic tests for hepatitis C. *Hepatology* **26**(Suppl 1)**:**43S–47S.
75. **Uyttendaele S, Claeys H, Mertens W, Verhaert H, Vermylen C.** 1994. Evaluation of third-generation screening and confirmatory assays for HCV antibodies. *Vox Sang* **66:**122–129.
76. **Tobler LH, Stramer SL, Lee SR, Masecar BL, Peterson JE, Davis EA, Andrews WE, Brodsky JP, Kleinman SH, Phelps BH, Busch MP.** 2003. Impact of HCV 3.0 EIA relative to HCV 2.0 EIA on blood-donor screening. *Transfusion* **43:**1452–1459.
77. **Sulkowski MS, Ray SC, Thomas DL.** 2002. Needlestick transmission of hepatitis C. *JAMA* **287:**2406–2413.
78. **Scheiblauer H, El-Nageh M, Nick S, Fields H, Prince A, Diaz S.** 2006. Evaluation of the performance of 44 assays used in countries with limited resources for the detection of antibodies to hepatitis C virus. *Transfusion* **46:**708–718.
79. **Gao F, Talbot EA, Loring CH, Power JJ, Dionne-Odom J, Alroy-Preis S, Jackson P, Bean CL.** 2014. Performance of the OraQuick HCV rapid antibody test for screening exposed patients in a hepatitis C outbreak investigation. *J Clin Microbiol* **52:**2650–2652.
80. **Lee SR, Kardos KW, Schiff E, Berne CA, Mounzer K, Banks AT, Tatum HA, Friel TJ, Demicco MP, Lee WM, Eder SE, Monto A, Yearwood GD, Guillon GB, Kurtz LA, Fischl M, Unangst JL, Kriebel L, Feiss G, Roehler M.** 2011. Evaluation of a new, rapid test for detecting HCV infection, suitable for use with blood or oral fluid. *J Virol Methods* **172:**27–31.
81. **Macedo de Oliveira A, White KL, Beecham BD, Leschinsky DP, Foley BP, Dockter J, Giachetti C, Safranek TJ.** 2006. Sensitivity of second-generation enzyme immunoassay for detection of hepatitis C virus infection among oncology patients. *J Clin Virol* **35:**21–25.
82. **Centers for Disease Control and Prevention.** 1998. Recommendations for prevention and control of hepatitis C virus (HCV) infection and HCV-related chronic disease. *MMWR Recomm Rep* **47**(RR-19)**:**1–39.
83. **Alter MJ, Kuhnert WL, Finelli L.** 2003. Guidelines for laboratory testing and result reporting of antibody to hepatitis C virus. Centers for Disease Control and Prevention. *MMWR Recomm Rep* **52:**1–13, 15; quiz CE11–14.
84. **Ren FR, Lv QS, Zhuang H, Li JJ, Gong XY, Gao GJ, Liu CL, Wang JX, Yao FZ, Zheng YR, Zhu FM, Tiemuer MH, Bai XH, Shan H.** 2005. Significance of the signal-to-cutoff ratios of anti-hepatitis C virus enzyme immunoassays in screening of Chinese blood donors. *Transfusion* **45:**1816–1822.
85. **Centers for Disease Control and Prevention (CDC).** 2013. Testing for HCV infection: an update of guidance for clinicians and laboratorians. *MMWR Morb Mortal Wkly Rep* **62:**362–365.
86. **Weisberg IS, Jacobson IM.** 2017. Primer on hepatitis C virus resistance to direct-acting antiviral treatment: a practical approach for the treating physician. *Clin Liver Dis* **21:**659–672.
87. **Feld JJ.** 2017. Resistance testing: interpretation and incorporation into HCV treatment algorithms. *Clin Liver Dis* **9:** 115–120.
88. **Kozuka R, Hai H, Motoyama H, Hagihara A, Fujii H, Uchida-Kobayashi S, Morikawa H, Enomoto M, Murakami Y, Kawada N, Tamori A.** 2017. The presence of multiple NS5A RASs is associated with the outcome of sofosbuvir and ledipasvir therapy in NS5A inhibitor-naïve patients with chronic HCV genotype 1b infection in a real-world cohort. *J Viral Hepat* 10.1111/jvh.12850.
89. **Bartlett SR, Grebely J, Eltahla AA, Reeves JD, Howe AYM, Miller V, Ceccherini-Silberstein F, Bull RA, Douglas MW, Dore GJ, Harrington P, Lloyd AR, Jacka B, Matthews GV, Wang GP, Pawlotsky JM, Feld JJ, Schinkel J, Garcia F, Lennerstrand J, Applegate TL.** 2017. Sequencing of hepatitis C virus for detection of resistance to direct-acting antiviral therapy: a systematic review. *Hepatol Commun* **1:**379–390.
90. **Busch MP.** 2001. Insights into the epidemiology, natural history and pathogenesis of hepatitis C virus infection from studies of infected donors and blood product recipients. *Transfus Clin Biol* **8:**200–206.
91. **Villano SA, Vlahov D, Nelson KE, Cohn S, Thomas DL.** 1999. Persistence of viremia and the importance of long-term follow-up after acute hepatitis C infection. *Hepatology* **29:**908–914.
92. **Choo QL, Richman KH, Han JH, Berger K, Lee C, Dong C, Gallegos C, Coit D, Medina-Selby R, Barr PJ.** 1991. Genetic organization and diversity of the hepatitis C virus. *Proc Natl Acad Sci USA* **88:**2451–2455.
93. **Major ME, Feinstone SM.** 1997. The molecular virology of hepatitis C. *Hepatology* **25:**1527–1538.
94. **Maheshwari A, Ray S, Thuluvath PJ.** 2008. Acute hepatitis C. *Lancet* **372:**321–332.
95. **Chevaliez S, Dubernet F, Dauvillier C, Hézode C, Pawlotsky JM.** 2017. The new Aptima HCV quant Dx real-time TMA assay accurately quantifies hepatitis C virus genotype 1-6 RNA. *J Clin Virol* **91:**5–11.
96. **Schønning K.** 2014. Comparison of the QIAGEN artus HCV QS-RGQ test with the Roche COBAS Ampliprep/COBAS TaqMan HCV test v2.0 for the quantification of HCV-RNA in plasma samples. *J Clin Virol* **60:**323–327.
97. **Zitzer H, Heilek G, Truchon K, Susser S, Vermehren J, Sizmann D, Cobb B, Sarrazin C.** 2013. Second-generation Cobas AmpliPrep/Cobas TaqMan HCV quantitative test for viral load monitoring: a novel dual-probe assay design. *J Clin Microbiol* **51:**571–577.
98. **Vermehren J, Stelzl E, Maasoumy B, Michel-Treil V, Berkowski C, Marins EG, Paxinos EE, Marino E, Wedemeyer H, Sarrazin C, Kessler HH.** 2017. Multicenter comparison study of both analytical and clinical performance across four Roche hepatitis C virus RNA assays utilizing different platforms. *J Clin Microbiol* **55:**1131–1139.
99. **Chevaliez S, Bouvier-Alias M, Pawlotsky JM.** 2009. Performance of the Abbott real-time PCR assay using m2000sp and m2000rt for hepatitis C virus RNA quantification. *J Clin Microbiol* **47:**1726–1732.
100. **Michelin BD, Muller Z, Stelzl E, Marth E, Kessler HH.** 2007. Evaluation of the Abbott RealTime HCV assay for quantitative detection of hepatitis C virus RNA. *J Clin Virol* **38:**96–100.
101. **Pyne MT, Konnick EQ, Phansalkar A, Hillyard DR.** 2009. Evaluation of the Abbott investigational use only RealTime hepatitis C virus (HCV) assay and comparison to the Roche TaqMan HCV analyte-specific reagent assay. *J Clin Microbiol* **47:**2872–2878.
102. **Kessler HH, Hübner M, Konrad PM, Stelzl E, Stübler MM, Baser MH, Santner BI.** 2013. Genotype impact on HCV RNA levels determined with the VERSANT HCV RNA 1.0 assay (kPCR). *J Clin Virol* **58:**522–527.
103. **McHugh MP, Wu AHB, Chevaliez S, Pawlotsky JM, Hallin M, Templeton KE.** 2017. Multicenter evaluation of the Cepheid Xpert Hepatitis C Virus Viral Load Assay. *J Clin Microbiol* **55:**1550–1556.
104. **Sam SS, Steinmetz HB, Tsongalis GJ, Tafe LJ, Lefferts JA.** 2013. Validation of a solid-phase electrochemical array for genotyping hepatitis C virus. *Exp Mol Pathol* **95:**18–22.
105. **Bouchardeau F, Cantaloube JF, Chevaliez S, Portal C, Razer A, Lefrère JJ, Pawlotsky JM, De Micco P, Laperche S.** 2007. Improvement of hepatitis C virus (HCV) genotype determination with the new version of the INNO-LiPA HCV assay. *J Clin Microbiol* **45:**1140–1145.
106. **Verbeeck J, Stanley MJ, Shieh J, Celis L, Huyck E, Wollants E, Morimoto J, Farrior A, Sablon E, Jankowski-Hennig M, Schaper C, Johnson P, Van Ranst M, Van Brussel M.** 2008. Evaluation of Versant hepatitis C virus genotype assay (LiPA) 2.0. *J Clin Microbiol* **46:**1901–1906.

107. **Colson P, Motte A, Tamalet C.** 2006. Broad differences between the COBAS Ampliprep total nucleic acid isolation-COBAS TaqMan 48 hepatitis C virus (HCV) and COBAS HCV Monitor v2.0 assays for quantification of serum HCV RNA of non-1 genotypes. *J Clin Microbiol* **44:**1602–1603.
108. **Fernández-Caballero JA, Alvarez M, Chueca N, Pérez AB, García F.** 2017. The cobas® HCV GT is a new tool that accurately identifies hepatitis C virus genotypes for clinical practice. *PLoS One* **12:**e0175564.
109. **Dirani G, Paesini E, Mascetra E, Farabegoli P, Dalmo B, Bartolini B, Garbuglia AR, Capobianchi MR, Sambri V.** 2018. A novel next generation sequencing assay as an alternative to currently available methods for hepatitis C virus genotyping. *J Virol Methods* **251:**88–91.
110. **Margraf RL, Page S, Erali M, Wittwer CT.** 2004. Single-tube method for nucleic acid extraction, amplification, purification, and sequencing. *Clin Chem* **50:**1755–1761.
111. **Murphy DG, Willems B, Deschênes M, Hilzenrat N, Mousseau R, Sabbah S.** 2007. Use of sequence analysis of the NS5B region for routine genotyping of hepatitis C virus with reference to C/E1 and 5′ untranslated region sequences. *J Clin Microbiol* **45:**1102–1112.
112. **van Doorn LJ, Kleter B, Pike I, Quint W.** 1996. Analysis of hepatitis C virus isolates by serotyping and genotyping. *J Clin Microbiol* **34:**1784–1787.
113. **Hedskog C, Chodavarapu K, Ku KS, Xu S, Martin R, Miller MD, Mo H, Svarovskaia E.** 2015. Genotype- and subtype-independent full-genome sequencing assay for hepatitis C virus. *J Clin Microbiol* **53:**2049–2059.
114. **Qiu P, Stevens R, Wei B, Lahser F, Howe AY, Klappenbach JA, Marton MJ.** 2015. HCV genotyping from NGS short reads and its application in genotype detection from HCV mixed infected plasma. *PLoS One* **10:**e0122082.
115. **Quer J, Gregori J, Rodríguez-Frias F, Buti M, Madejon A, Perez-del-Pulgar S, Garcia-Cehic D, Casillas R, Blasi M, Homs M, Tabernero D, Alvarez-Tejado M, Muñoz JM, Cubero M, Caballero A, del Campo JA, Domingo E, Belmonte I, Nieto L, Lens S, Muñoz-de-Rueda P, Sanz-Cameno P, Sauleda S, Bes M, Gomez J, Briones C, Perales C, Sheldon J, Castells L, Viladomiu L, Salmeron J, Ruiz-Extremera A, Quiles-Pérez R, Moreno-Otero R, López-Rodríguez R, Allende H, Romero-Gómez M, Guardia J, Esteban R, Garcia-Samaniego J, Forns X, Esteban JI.** 2015. High-resolution hepatitis C virus subtyping using NS5B deep sequencing and phylogeny, an alternative to current methods. *J Clin Microbiol* **53:**219–226.
116. **Trémeaux P, Caporossi A, Thélu MA, Blum M, Leroy V, Morand P, Larrat S.** 2016. Hepatitis C virus whole genome sequencing: current methods/issues and future challenges. *Crit Rev Clin Lab Sci* **53:**341–351.
117. **Ohno O, Mizokami M, Wu RR, Saleh MG, Ohba K, Orito E, Mukaide M, Williams R, Lau JY.** 1997. New hepatitis C virus (HCV) genotyping system that allows for identification of HCV genotypes 1a, 1b, 2a, 2b, 3a, 3b, 4, 5a, and 6a. *J Clin Microbiol* **35:**201–207.
118. **Okamoto H, Kobata S, Tokita H, Inoue T, Woodfield GD, Holland PV, Al-Knawy BA, Uzunalimoglu O, Miyakawa Y, Mayumi M.** 1996. A second-generation method of genotyping hepatitis C virus by the polymerase chain reaction with sense and antisense primers deduced from the core gene. *J Virol Methods* **57:**31–45.
119. **Thomson E, Ip CL, Badhan A, Christiansen MT, Adamson W, Ansari MA, Bibby D, Breuer J, Brown A, Bowden R, Bryant J, Bonsall D, Da Silva Filipe A, Hinds C, Hudson E, Klenerman P, Lythgow K, Mbisa JL, McLauchlan J, Myers R, Piazza P, Roy S, Trebes A, Sreenu VB, Witteveldt J, Barnes E, Simmonds P, STOP-HCV Consortium.** 2016. Comparison of next-generation sequencing technologies for comprehensive assessment of full-length hepatitis C viral genomes. *J Clin Microbiol* **54:**2470–2484.
120. **Abdel-Hamid M, El-Daly M, El-Kafrawy S, Mikhail N, Strickland GT, Fix AD.** 2002. Comparison of second- and third-generation enzyme immunoassays for detecting antibodies to hepatitis C virus. *J Clin Microbiol* **40:**1656–1659.
121. **Colin C, Lanoir D, Touzet S, Meyaud-Kraemer L, Bailly F, Trepo C, HEPATITIS Group.** 2001. Sensitivity and specificity of third-generation hepatitis C virus antibody detection assays: an analysis of the literature. *J Viral Hepat* **8:**87–95.
122. **Ismail N, Fish GE, Smith MB.** 2004. Laboratory evaluation of a fully automated chemiluminescence immunoassay for rapid detection of HBsAg, antibodies to HBsAg, and antibodies to hepatitis C virus. *J Clin Microbiol* **42:**610–617.
123. **Kim S, Kim JH, Yoon S, Park YH, Kim HS.** 2008. Clinical performance evaluation of four automated chemiluminescence immunoassays for hepatitis C virus antibody detection. *J Clin Microbiol* **46:**3919–3923.
124. **Kim B, Ahn HJ, Choi MH, Park Y.** 2018. Retrospective analysis on the diagnostic performances and signal-to-cut-off ratios of the Elecsys Anti-HCV II assay. *J Clin Lab Anal* **32:**e22165.
125. **Pan J, Li X, He G, Yuan S, Feng P, Zhang X, Qiu Y.** 2016. Reflex threshold of signal-to-cut-off ratios of the Elecsys anti-HCV II assay for hepatitis C virus infection. *J Infect Dev Ctries* **10:**1031–1034.
126. **Yang R, Guan W, Wang Q, Liu Y, Wei L.** 2013. Performance evaluation and comparison of the newly developed Elecsys anti-HCV II assay with other widely used assays. *Clin Chim Acta* **426:**95–101.
127. **Denoyel G, van Helden J, Bauer R, Preisel-Simmons B.** 2004. Performance of a new hepatitis C assay on the Bayer ADVIA Centaur Immunoassay System. *Clin Lab* **50:**75–82.

Gastroenteritis Viruses*

XIAOLI PANG AND MAREK SMIEJA

95

TAXONOMY

Rotaviruses

Rotaviruses are classified as members of the *Rotavirus* genus within the family *Reoviridae* (Table 1), which contains 10 other distinct genera. Based on group-specific antigens of the major viral structural protein VP6, rotaviruses are divided into seven groups (A to G) (1). Group-specific epitopes are also found on other structural proteins as well as on some nonstructural proteins. Group A to C rotaviruses infect both humans and animals, with the group A rotaviruses infecting humans most frequently and causing disease mainly in young children. Groups B and C cause infections in swine but have occasionally been associated with foodborne or waterborne outbreaks of human disease in China (group B) and Japan (group C). Group D to G rotaviruses are mainly animal pathogens. Within each group, rotaviruses are further classified into serotypes based on neutralization assays using antibodies against two major outer capsid proteins, VP4 and VP7. VP4 is a spike protein on the capsid surface which is sensitive to protease cleavage; therefore, the types based on the VP4 protein are also called P types (protease sensitive). VP7 is a glycoprotein, and the types based on this protein are also called G types. Both P and G types are also classified as genotypes based on the sequences of the VP4 and VP7 genes. In 2008, a new classification system was recommended, and a Rotavirus Classification Working Group composed of specialists in molecular virology, infectious diseases, epidemiology, and public health was formed to assist in delineation of new genotypes. Scientists discovering a potentially new rotavirus genotype for any of the 11 gene segments are invited to send the novel sequence to the Rotavirus Classification Working Group, where the sequence will be analyzed and a new nomenclature will be recommended as appropriate. To date, 27 G-genotypes and 37 P-genotypes have been reported (2, 3). Genotypes G1P[8], G2P[4], G3P[8], G4P[8], and G12P[8], which was newly merged in 2012, are most common in North America, and genotypes vary from one geographic location to another in different parts of the world.

Caliciviruses

Caliciviruses belong to the family *Caliciviridae* (Table 1) and are a diverse group of human and animal viruses which includes five established genera: *Norovirus* (formerly called Norwalk-like viruses), *Sapovirus* (formerly called Sapporo-like viruses), *Nebovirus*, *Lagovirus*, and *Vesivirus*, as well as four newly proposed genera: *Bavovirus*, *Nacovirus*, *Recovirus*, and *Valovirus* (4, 5). Caliciviruses within the *Norovirus* and *Sapovirus* genera mainly cause gastroenteritis in humans. Within each genus, strains are further grouped into genogroups (G) and genotypes or clusters. Noroviruses are classified into five genogroups (GI to GV) with GI, GII, and GIV found mainly in humans, GII and GIII in pigs and cattle, and GV in mice (6). Based on sequence variations in open reading frame 1 (ORF1) and ORF2, at least 14 genotypes of GI and 29 genotypes of GII have been reported (7). A single genotype of norovirus (genogroup II, genotype 4 [GII.4]) has been found to be predominant in the past decade, causing up to 80% of all norovirus gastroenteritis outbreaks in many countries (8). Norovirus GII.4 has demonstrated a much faster evolution than other strains, and new GII.4 clusters or variants appear to emerge every 2 to 5 years; the latest variant, called the "Sydney strain," caused global epidemic outbreaks in 2012 (9–11). Having dominated for over a decade, however, genotypes of norovirus reveal major changes compared to historical data of its evolution. A gradual reduction in the prevalence of GII.4-associated gastroenteritis outbreaks has been observed since 2012, alongside an increased genetic diversity of norovirus with four novel emerging strains, including GII.17 Kawasaki, first reported in 2014 in China (12), GII.P16/GII.4 Sydney, in 2015 in South Korea (13), GII.P4 New Orleans/GII.4 Sydney strains, in 2016 in Australia (14), and GII.P16/GII.2, in 2016 in Germany (15). These new GII strains have quickly spread globally and have been reported from different continents.

Similar to noroviruses, sapoviruses are grouped into 14 genotypes within 5 genogroups (16, 17). Genogroups GI, GII, GIV, and GV contain human strains of sapovirus, and GIII contains the porcine strains (16).

Enteric Adenoviruses

Human adenoviruses (HAdVs) are members of the family *Adenoviridae* (Table 1) and are divided into seven species (A to G). The species have different tissue tropisms and

*This chapter contains information presented in chapter 93 by Xiaoli Pang and Richard L. Hodinka in the 11th edition of this *Manual*.

TABLE 1 Taxonomy and virological properties of the major gastroenteritis viruses[a]

Virus	Family	Size (nm)	Appearance under EM	Viral genome	Genetic or antigenic types
Rotavirus	*Reoviridae*	70	Wheel-shaped, triple-layered capsid	Segmented dsRNA	7 antigenic groups (A–G) and 27 G and 37 P types
Norovirus	*Caliciviridae*	30–38	SRSV	Linear ss(+)RNA	5 genogroups and 14 types of GI and 29 types of GII
Sapovirus	*Caliciviridae*	30–38	SRSV, with Star of David appearance	Linear ss(+)RNA	5 genogroups and 14 types
Enteric adenoviruses	*Adenoviridae*	70–100	Icosahedral capsid	Linear dsDNA	HAdV40 and HAdV41
Astrovirus	*Astroviridae*	28–30	SRSV, 5- or 6-pointed star shaped	Linear ss(+)RNA	8 serotypes

[a]dsRNA, double-stranded RNA; ss(+)RNA, single-stranded positive-sense RNA; dsDNA, double-stranded DNA; SRSV, small, round, structured virus.

propensities for causing different clinical syndromes; species F is the group most clearly associated with gastroenteritis. Recently, the Human Adenovirus Working Group proposed using whole-genome sequence analyses to characterize and name HAdVs as "type" instead of "serotype" to rectify the misclassification of HAdVs previously characterized by the serological methods of serum neutralization and hemagglutination inhibition that target two small conservative regions on the hexon gene (18, 19). There are now 68 types of HAdVs based on serological assays, whole-genome sequencing, and phylogenomics (18–20). Many adenoviruses are readily isolated from human stools, but their role in the etiology of acute gastroenteritis is unclear. There are two types, however, AdV40 and AdV41 in species F, which are definitively associated with infantile diarrhea and are referred to as enteric adenoviruses (EAdVs). These EAdVs are also known as "fastidious adenoviruses" because they are difficult to grow in cell culture. More recently, other HAdV types, namely, HAdV-52 belonging to species G and HAdV-67 belonging to species D, have been implicated as potentially causing gastroenteritis (20, 21).

Astroviruses

Astroviruses belong to the *Astroviridae* family (Table 1) and are so named because of their characteristic star-like (*astron* = "star" in Greek) surface structure. Two genera of astroviruses, *Mamastrovirus* and *Avastrovirus*, have been described according to their host species; the first group infects mammals and the latter group infects birds (22). Within each genus, there are multiple species of astroviruses named after the hosts in which they replicate. Human astroviruses have been divided into eight types based on antigenic and genetic typing (23). Type 1 appears to be most common, but all eight types have been detected throughout the world.

Other Viruses Causing Gastroenteritis

Other enteric viruses that have been implicated in acute gastroenteritis of humans include coronaviruses and toroviruses, two genera in the *Coronaviridae* family (24), Aichi virus in the genus *Kobuvirus* of the *Picornaviridae* family (25), picobirnaviruses in the *Picobirnaviridae* family (26), and human bocavirus in the genus *Bocavirus* within the *Parvoviridae* family (27). A detailed discussion of these viruses is beyond the scope of this chapter.

DESCRIPTION OF THE AGENTS

Rotaviruses

Rotaviruses are nonenveloped and are among the few human viruses that possess a segmented, double-stranded RNA genome (Table 1). Mature viral particles are approximately 70 nm in diameter with a wheel-like appearance (*rota* = "wheel" in Latin) and possess a triple-layered icosahedral protein capsid composed of an outer layer, an intermediate layer, and an inner core (Fig. 1). The double-stranded RNA genome contains 11 segments ranging in size from ~3,300 (segment 1) to ~660 (segment 11) base pairs (bp), and each segment codes for a single gene product. The gene-coding assignments of the 11 genome segments have been determined; these segments encode six major structural proteins (VP1, VP2, VP3, VP4, VP6, and VP7) that appear on the matured viral particles and six nonstructural proteins (NSP1 to NSP6) that are expressed in infected cells and play important roles in viral genome replication, protein synthesis, capsid assembly, and maturation. The outermost layer of the nucleocapsid contains VP4 and VP7, while the middle layer is composed of VP6, and the innermost core is composed of VP2 and contains a polymerase complex composed of VP1 and VP3. One of the nonstructural proteins, NSP4, is considered to be a viral enterotoxin (28). Similar to influenza viruses, having a segmented genome allows for genetic reassortment of rotavirus strains, resulting in the possible formation of new virus types.

Caliciviruses

Caliciviruses are small (30 to 38 nm), round, nonenveloped viruses possessing a single-stranded, positive-sense RNA genome (Table 1). Sapoviruses have the typical morphology of caliciviruses with the "Star of David" appearance with cup-shaped depressions (*calyx* = "cup" in Latin) on the surface of the virus (Fig. 1). Noroviruses possess a smoother surface structure and therefore also have been called "small round structured viruses" (29). Cryo-electron microscopy and X-ray crystallography analysis of recombinant viral-like particles (VLPs) have revealed that noroviruses possess a T = 3 icosahedral capsid composed of 180 proteins that form 90 dimeric capsomeres. Each capsid protein possesses two major domains, the shell (S) and the protrusion (P) domains. Expression of the P domain in *Escherichia coli* has resulted in self-formation of a subviral particle, the P particle, which maintains the VLP's properties of receptor binding and antigenic recognition (30). This P particle is highly stable and easy to make and has been proposed as a potential subunit vaccine for noroviruses.

The RNA genome of noroviruses is poly(A) tailed and ~7.5 kb in length (31). It is organized into three ORFs, with ORF1 encoding the nonstructural proteins, ORF2 the VP1 capsid protein, and ORF3 a minor structural protein. The sapovirus genome is slightly different in that sequences encoding the nonstructural and capsid proteins are fused into one large ORF.

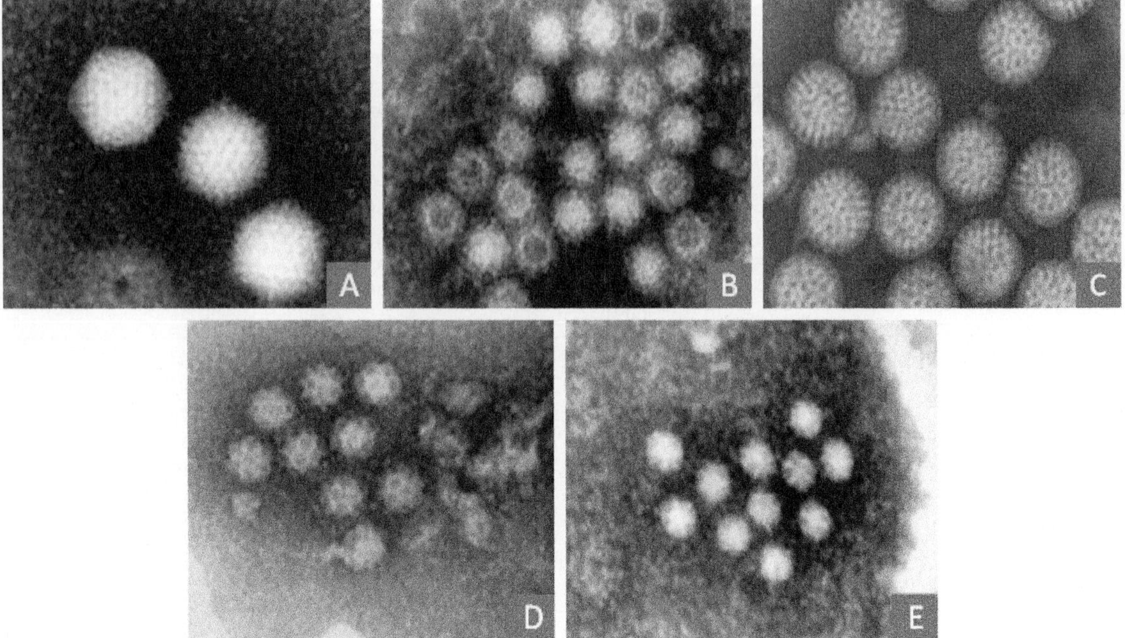

FIGURE 1 Electron micrographs of the major gastroenteritis viruses. (A) Adenovirus, (B) norovirus, (C) rotavirus, (D) sapovirus, (E) astrovirus.

Enteric Adenoviruses

Adenoviruses were named from the Greek word *aden*, meaning "gland" after their original isolation from adenoid tissue and were also called "adenoid-associated viruses." HAdVs have been linked to a number of diseases, including respiratory illness, conjunctivitis, and diarrhea (32). Adenoviruses are nonenveloped, icosahedral particles that are 70 to 100 nm in diameter (Table 1). Mature virions consist of a DNA-containing core surrounded by a capsid composed of hexon, penton, and fiber proteins (Fig. 1). The genome is a linear, nonsegmented double-stranded DNA of 30 to 38 kb, which varies in size from group to group. The capsid is composed of 252 capsomeres, of which 240 are hexons and 12 are pentons. There are a total of 11 viral structural proteins of which the hexons, penton bases, and fibers are of important clinical relevance. These proteins are involved in viral entry (fiber) and intracellular transportation. The fiber proteins extend from the surface of the capsid and interact with primary cellular receptors, which for the majority of adenoviruses, including the EAdVs, is the coxsackievirus B-adenovirus receptor, a transmembrane protein belonging to the immunoglobulin family. The hexon and fiber proteins also contain the major neutralization epitopes.

Astroviruses

Astroviruses are small (28 to 30 nm in diameter), round, nonenveloped viruses with a typical five- or six-pointed star-like appearance (Fig. 1). As determined by X-ray crystallography and computer modeling, the virus has some structural resemblance to the caliciviruses but more strongly resembles the hepatitis E virus. The virions contain a single-stranded, positive-sense RNA genome of about 6.8 kb in length (Table 1). The viral genome contains three ORFs, with ORF1a and ORF1b encoding the nonstructural proteins. ORF1a has a protease motif, transmembrane helices, nuclear localization signals, and a ribosomal frame-shifting signal, whereas ORF1b has an RNA polymerase motif. ORF2 encodes the capsid precursor protein, which is approximately 87 kDa in size and is further cleaved to smaller peptides of 25 to 34 kDa to form mature virions.

EPIDEMIOLOGY AND TRANSMISSION

Viral gastroenteritis occurs in all age groups and socioeconomic classes and in all parts of the world. Important epidemiological features include age, season of the year, duration of symptoms, severity of disease, and exposure and vaccination history (Tables 2 and 3). Severe illness is seen most commonly in children younger than 5 years of age, with the peak incidence observed in children between the ages of 6 months and 2 years. Viruses account for 50 to 90% of acute gastroenteritis requiring hospitalization and 3 to 10% of all pediatric hospital days in this age group. Sporadic illness and outbreaks in healthy adults, elderly populations, and immunosuppressed patients have been described.

Gastroenteritis viruses are transmitted by the fecal-oral route through close contact with infected people or indirectly by contact with contaminated fomites (e.g., shared eating utensils, environmental surfaces, and toys in playrooms). Transmission is highly efficient because of the physical hardiness of gastrointestinal viruses, the high amounts of virus particles concentrated and shed in stools, and resistance of these viruses to various environmental conditions (33). Thus, only a small infectious dose is required. Enteric viruses are stable over wide pH and temperature ranges and even after drying, heating, or freezing, and they are able to survive on human hands and inanimate objects for extended times. Certain viruses, particularly the noroviruses, are readily transmitted by eating or drinking contaminated foods or beverages, which usually results in large outbreaks. Foods may be contaminated by food preparers or handlers who have viral gastroenteritis; water and shellfish may become contaminated by sewage, and eating raw or undercooked shellfish or drinking contaminated water may lead to illness. Enteric viruses are also thought to be

TABLE 2 Transmission and epidemiology of the major gastroenteritis viruses

Virus	Mode(s) of transmission	Target population(s)	Occurrence
Rotavirus	Fecal-oral, respiratory?, food and water?	Children <5 years old (peak activity at 6 months to 2 years of age)	Fall/winter months in temperate climates, year-round in tropical regions
Norovirus	Fecal-oral, foods, water, respiratory?	All age groups	Winter peak, year-round outbreaks common in a variety of settings
Sapovirus	Fecal-oral, respiratory?	Mainly children (primarily infants and toddlers), less so in adults	Sporadic year-round, outbreaks occur
Enteric adenoviruses	Fecal-oral, respiratory?	Mainly infants and young children <5 years old	Sporadic year-round, outbreaks occur
Astrovirus	Fecal-oral, water, respiratory?	Mainly young children	Sporadic year-round, outbreaks occur

transmitted through respiratory secretions, but this has not been fully proven. Most viral diarrheal diseases are endemic, with significant disease burden in both developing and developed countries. Caliciviruses, especially the noroviruses, also cause epidemics of acute gastroenteritis, which is an important public health concern. In countries with temperate climates, viral gastroenteritis does not have the typical summer peak of most bacterium- and parasite-associated gastroenteritis. Instead, viral gastroenteritis is more common in colder seasons, with a typical winter-spring peak. Hospital-associated spread of the enteric viruses, particularly for rotavirus and norovirus, is common without the implementation of appropriate infection prevention and control measures.

Rotaviruses

Prior to widespread vaccination, rotaviruses were the leading cause of severe dehydrating diarrhea in infants and children less than 2 years of age and remain a major cause of childhood deaths in developing countries. The mortality caused by rotavirus infection is now much lower in developed countries, but the disease burden was high in the prevaccine era, representing approximately 2.7 million diarrheal episodes each year in the United States, with significant numbers of physician visits and hospitalizations and substantial medical and societal costs. Infants usually acquire the disease from their siblings or from their parents, who may have subclinical infection. Shedding of rotavirus in stools can occur prior to onset of disease and continue following cessation of diarrhea. Cross-species transmission of rotaviruses has been demonstrated, indicating a potential for zoonotic disease between animals and humans (34).

The histo-blood group antigens (HBGAs) are polymorphic glycans present at the gut mucosa, considered to be attachment ligands used by rotavirus prior to infecting host cells (35–37). The synthesis of HBGAs depends on a group of enzymes that can synthesize the "secretor" antigens and the "Lewis" antigens. The interaction between rotavirus and HBGAs is strain specific and has been observed *in vitro* as well as in population-based studies. For example, P[8] strains can infect individuals that are Lewis positive and secretors but do not infect Lewis-negative and nonsecretor individuals; P[6] strains can infect Lewis-negative individuals regardless of their secretor status (38, 39). Thus, population-based differences in HBGA profiles might explain differences in susceptibility, rotavirus disease burden, genetic diversity of circulating strains, and vaccine effectiveness. More importantly, the proportion of individuals with a specific HBGA profile varies depending on ethnicity. For example, the proportion of individuals who are Lewis-positive secretors accounts for 72%, 55%, and 73% among Caucasians, Africans, and Japanese, respectively, whereas the proportion of individuals who are Lewis negative accounts for 6%, 22%, and 10% in the same ethnic groups (38, 40).

Caliciviruses

Noroviruses are highly contagious and have been recognized as the most important agent of nonbacterial acute

TABLE 3 Selected clinical features of the major gastroenteritis viruses

Virus	Clinical significance	Incubation time (days)	Vomiting (days)	Diarrhea (days)	Virus shedding (days)
Rotavirus	Acute severe dehydrating gastroenteritis, hospital-acquired infections, subclinical infections occur	1–2	2–3	5–8	8–10
Caliciviruses	Noroviruses: moderate to severe acute gastroenteritis, hospital-acquired infections, prolonged shedding and chronic disease in immune-compromised patients; subclinical infections occur Sapoviruses: mild to moderate gastroenteritis; subclinical infections occur	1–2	0.05–1	1–2	1–21
Adenovirus	Moderate to severe gastroenteritis, hospital-acquired infections, persists in immune-compromised patients	8–10	2–3	4–12	8–13
Astrovirus	Mild to moderate gastroenteritis; subclinical infections occur	1–2	1–4	1–4	8–10

gastroenteritis in both developing and developed countries (41). Both common-source outbreaks and sporadic disease can occur. The disease is most common in children, but all ages can be reinfected due to incomplete protective immunity and infected with antigenically different strains. Noroviruses are now recognized as the leading cause of acute gastroenteritis in children in the United States since the numbers of acute gastroenteritis cases associated with rotavirus have declined due to introduction of the rotavirus vaccines (42). Noroviruses commonly cause large outbreaks in closed communities and in a variety of settings, such as hospitals, child care centers, schools, restaurants, nursing homes for the elderly, cruise ships, and military communities or camps. Particular attention has been paid to foodborne outbreaks occurring in nursing homes for the elderly and on cruise ships in the United States and European countries. Chronic diarrhea, increased mortality, and prolonged fecal shedding of noroviruses are often seen in immunocompromised hosts. In recent years, noroviruses have been reported to recognize the ABH (secretor) and Lewis HBGA as receptors (43), and the susceptibility of individuals to norovirus infection is based on the expression of these antigens on the gut epithelium; people devoid of H type 1 epitopes are resistant to infection with noroviruses. Direct evidence of zoonotic transmission of noroviruses remains absent, although noroviruses closely related to human strains have been detected in domestic and wild animals.

Sapoviruses cause disease mainly in children, and sporadic cases and outbreaks in daycare centers and institutional settings have been reported. However, these viruses were recently found to be very common in adult gastroenteritis outbreaks in North America and Europe and are also a common cause of gastroenteritis in solid organ transplantation recipients (44–46).

Enteric Adenoviruses

While the role of EAdVs in acute gastroenteritis is widely accepted, the incidences of adenovirus-related gastroenteritis differ considerably in various studies and locations, with an average of ~5% of cases of pediatric diarrhea being caused by EAdVs. Outbreaks of EAdV-associated diarrhea have been reported in hospitals and child daycare centers. Human EAdV infection does not have the typical winter seasonality of the rotaviruses and caliciviruses, and sporadic cases are reported year-round. Like other enteric pathogens, human EAdVs are frequently detected in stools of children without gastroenteritis. As many as 41% of children acquire EAdV infection during hospitalization for other diseases (47).

Astroviruses

Human astroviruses cause mainly pediatric gastroenteritis. Cases in caregivers of sick children, immunocompromised adults (48), military troops (49), and nursing homes (50) have been reported. Astrovirus infection can be linked to 2 to 10% of cases of pediatric gastroenteritis worldwide, depending on settings and diagnostic tests used. Asymptomatic infections are common in all ages. There is a 70 to 90% seroprevalence of astroviruses among school-age children, indicating frequent infections during childhood.

CLINICAL SIGNIFICANCE

Acute viral gastroenteritis is characterized by a variety of symptoms and signs, including fever, diarrhea, vomiting, abdominal cramps, irritability, lethargy, and dehydration, with rotavirus gastroenteritis considered to be the most severe. Although symptoms of gastroenteritis due to noroviruses, sapoviruses, astroviruses, and the EAdVs are considered to be milder than those of the rotaviruses, increasing data show that noroviruses are frequently detected in hospitalized children and emergency room visitors with acute gastroenteritis, indicating that noroviruses may also cause severe gastroenteritis (42). Headache, anorexia, malaise, myalgia, and nausea may also be observed. Clinical illness is similar for all gastrointestinal viruses, making it difficult, if not impossible, to distinguish which virus is causing the disease based on symptoms alone. The clinical presentation can vary widely: symptoms can appear alone or together and can mimic noninfectious conditions. In general, with the exception of adenoviruses, viral gastroenteritis has a sudden onset following a short incubation period of 1 to 2 days (Table 3). The duration of symptoms is normally less than 7 days, and virus shedding in stools of infected individuals lasts <1 to 2 weeks in most cases but may last longer depending on the virus and host. The stools are usually watery or loose with no mucous or blood, and fecal leukocytes are typically absent or present only in minimal numbers. Viral gastroenteritis is normally self-limited in well-nourished, immunocompetent individuals, and mild disease or asymptomatic infections are common. Severe illness can be seen among infants, younger children, the elderly, and immunocompromised individuals who are unable to effectively rehydrate following loss of fluids due to vomiting and diarrhea and can result in significant morbidity and hospitalizations. For rotaviruses, severe dehydration can be lethal and remains an important cause of infant mortality in developing countries.

Rotaviruses, noroviruses, and adenoviruses can cause acute gastroenteritis and chronic infection in immunocompromised individuals, such as patients who have undergone solid organ or stem cell transplantation or cancer therapy and those infected with human immunodeficiency virus (HIV). In rare cases, the viruses can disseminate systemically and involve other organ systems (51–58). However, viral-associated disease burden in immunocompromised individuals is underestimated due to a lack of routine testing for those viruses in clinical practice. Increasing numbers of studies have shown that immunocompromised individuals are at high risk and susceptible to viral-associated gastroenteritis (54–56, 58, 59). In addition to severe gastroenteritis caused mostly by rotaviruses in healthy young children, immunocompromised adult patients represent another group with much higher prevalence of rotavirus gastroenteritis than that in pediatric patients (55). Norovirus illness can also become debilitating and life-threatening in immunocompromised patients (60). Noroviruses are among the pathogens associated with immunocompromised hosts, causing up to 22% of chronic diarrhea, with prolonged viral shedding in the stools of recipients who underwent allogeneic hematopoietic stem cell and solid organ transplantations (56, 61–65). Noroviruses also can be associated with necrotizing enterocolitis in children (66, 67). Enteric adenovirus infections in immunodeficient individuals, such as hematopoietic stem cell and solid organ transplant recipients, HIV patients, and other individuals with immunosuppressive therapy, are of growing clinical importance (51, 54, 58). Adenovirus infection in these individuals can lead to mild gastroenteritis, asymptomatic infection, and/or severe disease, including gastroenteritis, pneumonitis, hemorrhagic cystitis, hepatitis, and disseminated infection associated with high mortality. Patients can excrete adenoviruses in stool from weeks to months after infection. Potential treatment of adenovirus infection in such clinical settings includes reduction of immunosuppressive drugs, intravenous immunoglobulin, and intravenous antiviral therapy with cidofovir (68).

There are no effective antivirals that can be used for the treatment or prevention of infection and disease caused by gastroenteritis viruses. Treatment involves supportive care including rehydration therapy and restoration of electrolyte balance, which are essential for severe dehydrating cases and for reducing the mortality in developing countries.

Because chronic norovirus diarrhea has been increasingly reported in immunocompromised patients and results in prolonged infection with chronic dehydration that can lead to serious complications, a reduction of immunosuppressive therapy may alleviate the symptoms of gastroenteritis but has an increased risk of graft rejection (69). Recent efforts have used immunoglobulin and nitazoxanide for the treatment of chronic norovirus gastroenteritis in immunocompromised patients through inhibiting viral adherence to the intestinal epithelium and promoting viral clearance from the digestive tract as well as suppressing viral replications (69–71).

The lack of antiviral drugs against rotaviruses and the significant disease burden of rotavirus gastroenteritis were the main driving forces behind the development of rotavirus vaccines. After decades of research and the failure of some earlier vaccine products, two live attenuated rotavirus vaccines were licensed for use in the United States and are now being used worldwide; the pentavalent, three-dose bovine-human reassortant vaccine containing G1-G4 and P[8] types (RotaTeq, Merck & Co., Inc.) was licensed in 2006, and the monovalent, two-dose attenuated human G1P[8] vaccine (Rotarix, GlaxoSmithKline, Inc.) was licensed in 2008. Both vaccines have been shown to be safe and effective in children, providing 80 to 100% protection against severe disease and 70 to 80% protection against rotavirus gastroenteritis of any severity in high- and middle-income countries. Acute gastroenteritis in elderly individuals has also decreased due to increasing herd immunity since introduction of the Rotarix vaccine for children in the United Kingdom in 2013 (72). The Advisory Committee on Immunization Practices recently updated its recommendations for rotavirus vaccination to include the use of Rotarix and RotaTeq for prevention of rotavirus gastroenteritis (73). However, decreased effectiveness (ranging between 39 and 49%) has been reported for both Rotarix and RotaTeq in some low-income countries (74–78). While the decreased effectiveness of rotavirus vaccination might be attributable to factors such as malnutrition, general hygiene, and comorbidities, disparities between prevalent genotypes and those strains covered by vaccines are a major consideration (79, 80). Therefore, it is very important to continually monitor vaccine effectiveness and genotype drifting of rotavirus predominant strains globally, especially in low-income countries.

Since noroviruses cause the great majority of epidemics of viral gastroenteritis, development of vaccines and antivirals against noroviruses is needed. Norovirus vaccines under development are currently focusing on VLPs, which contain the major capsid antigen but lack genetic material for viral replication. VLPs are similar to native viruses morphologically and antigenically, eliciting humoral, mucosal, and cellular immune responses after oral and intranasal administration (81–84). Challenges in norovirus vaccine development include the lack of understanding of herd immunity after infection, particularly the mechanism of the short duration of protective immunity following a natural infection, and the lack of a cell culture and suitable animal model for efficacy studies. The high genetic and antigenic diversity of noroviruses also makes it difficult to select vaccine targets for broad protection. Several norovirus vaccines have been studied in preclinical and clinical trials using VLPs with different routes of administration including intranasal, oral, and intramuscular routes. One of the earlier candidates was a monovalent intranasal GI.1 VLP vaccine that demonstrated a serologic response in 70% of healthy adults who received two doses of the vaccine (81). This candidate vaccine was also efficacious against homologous challenge, reducing the risk of gastroenteritis by 47% and infection by 26%. It was also well tolerated and immunogenic (81). The vaccine was subsequently modified from an intranasal to an intramuscular route of administration and from a monovalent to a bivalent formulation and is now in phase II clinical trials. Modified vaccine contains GI.1 and GII.4 VLPs and is the vaccine furthest along in clinical development (85). Serologic responses were demonstrated for both GI.1 and GII.4, and protection against severe clinical symptoms was observed. However, the vaccine efficacy was only 13.6% against human norovirus infection. Another vaccine in clinical trials is an adenoviral-vector-based norovirus vaccine in a tablet formulation that encodes for a full-length VP1 gene from GI.1. This vaccine recently met the primary and secondary study endpoints for safety and immunogenicity in a phase I trial with adults (85).

At present, preventive and control strategies for gastrointestinal virus infections are aimed at identifying and eliminating the source of infection by promoting standard and contact precautions and good personal hygienic practices (e.g., careful and thorough hand washing with soap and water), performing proper disinfection of environmental surfaces, and identifying and avoiding sick contacts and other potential sources of infection and spread. Certain gastrointestinal viruses (e.g., noroviruses) may be resistant to some common disinfectants and cleaning solutions; sodium hypochlorite is most effective at inactivation of the enteric viruses.

COLLECTION, TRANSPORT, AND STORAGE OF SPECIMENS

Gastroenteritis viruses replicate and cause disease mainly in the intestine, and stool is the foremost specimen of choice for laboratory diagnosis. It is preferable to collect specimens within the first 48 hours of illness since viral shedding is at its maximum at this time and increases the likelihood of virus detection. Specimens collected later in the course of disease have a lower detection rate, although prolonged shedding of some gastroenteritis viruses has been reported after the onset of illness. Stool specimens of a few grams are sufficient for detection by electron microscopy (EM) and antigen or nucleic acid detection methods. The samples can be collected with a bed pan and then transferred into smaller containers or test tubes. Specimens can be recovered from a diaper with a wooden tongue depressor which is then placed in an appropriate container for transport to the laboratory. However, stool collection and transportation are burdensome and may have potential for disease transmission if not handled appropriately. Additionally, waiting for stool to be collected is impractical while patients are on-site in a clinic, and postvisit return rates are poor, leading to delays or missed diagnostic opportunities that can adversely affect outcomes. Anatomically designed sterile flocked rectal swabs (FLOQSwab, Copan Italia, Brescia, Italy) were superior to bulk stool for detection of bacterial pathogens and equivalent for viral pathogens in a study based in Botswana which used commercial multiplex PCR (86). A recent prospective study demonstrated that the flocked rectal swabs described above for stool sampling have an approximately 10% greater chance of identification for enteric pathogen than stool specimens in children with vomiting, diarrhea, or both (87). Thus, when stool is not immediately available and identification for enteric pathogen is urgent, a rectal swab is a suitable alternative sample for diagnostics (87). A standard protocol of rectal swab collection and sample transportation is to be developed. Vomitus material can be used for the detection of gastrointestinal viruses as a supplement to stool specimens (88), but this is not routinely recommended for diagnostic testing. If the patient cannot provide stool or rectal swab samples, the flocked swab is recommended to collect vomitus and to store and ship it by the same method as the rectal swab. In general, stool or rectal swab samples should be stored at 4°C immediately after collection and then promptly transported to the laboratory for processing. If the sample cannot be processed for testing immediately, it should be promptly frozen and stored at −70°C. For research purposes, single-use aliquots of processed specimens should be placed in multiple cryovials for testing and storage. By processing in this manner, specimens are not frozen and thawed repeatedly, thereby avoiding possible degradation of viral particles, proteins, and/or nucleic acids and cross-contamination of specimens. Stool samples can be shipped on wet or dry ice, depending on the storage conditions (e.g., short- or long-term storage). Unnecessary freezing and thawing between shipment and storage should be avoided.

Serum samples can be used for detection of immunoglobulin G (IgG) antibodies against the gastroenteritis viruses. However, such testing is performed mainly in research laboratories and is not suitable for clinical diagnosis of acute infection. The acute-phase serum sample should be collected as soon as possible after onset of illness and tested simultaneously with the convalescent-phase serum sample. Processed serum specimens may be stored at 2 to 8°C for several days pending completion of testing or can be stored frozen at −20°C or colder for prolonged storage. Repeat freezing and thawing should be avoided, and specimens should not be stored in frost-free freezers.

Drinking water, foods and other beverages, and other environmental specimens are normally collected and used to investigate outbreaks of viral gastroenteritis and tracing infectious sources, mainly seen in norovirus infection. If a food item or water is suspected as the source of an outbreak, samples should be obtained as early as possible in the outbreak and stored under appropriate conditions as described above, depending on when the testing will be performed. Since testing of these specimen types is not routinely performed in most diagnostic laboratories and often requires special handling and processing (e.g., filter concentration of 5 to 100 liters of water and processing of food to remove food debris), a laboratory with the capability to test these specimens should be contacted (e.g., a local or regional health department or the Centers for Disease Control and Prevention in Atlanta, GA).

DIRECT DETECTION

Electron Microscopy

EM and immunoelectron microscopy (IEM) have been successfully used for the rapid examination of stool samples for the simultaneous detection and identification of viral agents of gastroenteritis based on the characteristic size and shape of intact viral particles when visualized by negative staining on a support grid (Fig. 1). This offers the main advantages of speed and simplicity. However, due to many disadvantages such as the availability and high cost of the instrument, the requirement for specialized facilities and expertise, and low sensitivity and specificity, EM and IEM have been gradually removed from the clinical diagnostic laboratory for detection of gastroenteritis viruses. Therefore, methods of EM and IEM are not described in this edition of this chapter. Readers can find details of applications of EM and IEM in chapter 93 of 11th edition of this *Manual*.

Antigen Detection Assays

Immunologic assays have been used for the direct detection of gastrointestinal viruses in processed stool samples, and commercial kits are available for some viruses. Common formats of antigen detection assays include conventional 96-well microplate enzyme immunoassays (EIA), latex agglutination tests, and rapid membrane-based immunochromatographic assays. These antigen assays are rapid, inexpensive, simple to perform, and highly suitable for use by most, if not all, clinical laboratories. Stool suspensions of 10 to 20% are normally prepared in phosphate-buffered saline (pH 7.4) or sodium carbonate buffer (pH 9.5) for use in the tests. Overall, the number of available antigen detection assays is limited, and tests remain unavailable for some of the enteric viruses because of the lack of specific antibodies used to capture and detect appropriately conserved viral antigens. In addition, even the performance of existing assays needs to be vastly improved for better sensitivity and specificity. Because of the high degree of genetic and antigenic diversity of enteric viruses, the sensitivity of many antigen detection assays is relatively low to moderate, although still higher than the sensitivity of EM. Monoclonal or hyperimmune antibodies against specific viral capsid proteins, such as the VP6 protein of rotaviruses and the capsid protein or the P domain of the capsid protein of noroviruses, have been used in the development of these antigen detection tests. Due to the lack of a cell culture for human noroviruses, recombinant viral capsid proteins expressed in an *in vitro* system have been used as the source of reagents for assay development.

The more recently developed membrane-based immunochromatographic assays are valuable for small- to moderate-sized laboratories with a demand for diagnosis of sporadic viral gastroenteritis (89). These immunochromatographic kits are designed as dipsticks or self-contained cassettes and usually include built-in positive controls to ensure that the reaction has been performed and interpreted appropriately. The tests require minimal equipment, and the results can be readily visualized. Because of their speed, simplicity, and low cost, immunochromatographic kits are amenable for point-of-care testing. In general, the immunochromatographic assays have a slightly lower sensitivity and specificity than the more conventional EIA-based 96-well microplate systems.

The latex agglutination tests use latex beads coated with virus-specific antibodies and are based on the agglutination of these beads when virus particles or viral antigens present in the specimens bind to the antibody-coated beads. Since some fecal specimens can cause nonspecific agglutination, latex particles coated with nonviral antibodies are also included in the kits. Particulate matter found in some prepared stool suspensions may interfere with the correct reading of the agglutination, and the stools are normally clarified by low-speed centrifugation before the supernatants are mixed with the latex reagent. A positive reaction is indicated by visible clumping (agglutination) occurring within minutes of performing the test. The assays are generally less sensitive than EIAs and immunochromatographic assays but are most useful in small- to moderate-sized diagnostic laboratories (90).

Conventional 96-well microplate EIAs for rotaviruses and adenoviruses have been on the market for years and are still widely used due to their reasonably high sensitivity and specificity with consistent test results. Immunochromatographic tests for rotaviruses and adenoviruses were introduced later and have been readily adopted for diagnostic use. In a comparison of seven commercially available immunochromatographic assays with an EIA for the detection of group A rotaviruses in fecal samples, the results of six immunochromatographic assays were shown to be comparable with those of the EIA, and only one immunochromatographic assay had a significantly lower positive detection rate (91). Immunochromatographic tests for the detection of multiple pathogens such as both rotaviruses and adenoviruses have also been developed. Direct-comparison studies have shown that these assays have sensitivity and specificity comparable to those of the more traditional EIAs and are useful for rapid diagnosis in ambulatory practice (92, 93). Of note, most commercially available adenovirus antigen detection assays are not specific for the EAdV types 40 and 41, with the exception of the Premier Adenoclone-Types 40/41 EIA from Meridian Bioscience (Cincinnati, OH).

Although a number of antigen detection tests are now being developed and commercialized for noroviruses and astroviruses, most of these assays are only CE marked in Europe for *in vitro* diagnostic use and are not available in the United States. Only one norovirus assay (Ridascreen Norovirus 3rd Generation EIA) from R-Biopharm AG (Darmstadt, Germany) has been licensed by the Food and Drug Administration (FDA) for preliminary identification of norovirus when testing multiple specimens during outbreaks. Due to their limited sensitivity and specificity, currently available norovirus antigen assays are used mainly for research and are not recommended for routine clinical diagnosis of individual cases of sporadic disease (94, 95). Several studies evaluating commercial EIA and immunochromatographic kits for detection of norovirus antigens showed much lower sensitivity compared to results obtained using reverse transcription-PCR (RT-PCR), resulting in the detection of significantly lower numbers of GI and GII viruses (94, 95).

Molecular Detection Assays

Diagnosis of viral gastroenteritis based on the identification of viral genomes includes direct detection of viral RNA or DNA by electrophoresis, amplification of viral DNA or RNA by PCR or RT-PCR, and DNA sequencing. Such molecular methods are extremely sensitive and play an increasingly important role in the rapid and accurate detection of the enteric viruses. Nucleic acid amplification tests such as PCR are now the method of choice for the detection of viruses causing gastroenteritis, and a growing literature exists to demonstrate the overall utility of these assays.

Direct Staining of Nucleic Acid Following Electrophoresis

The segmented, double-stranded RNA genome of rotaviruses has traditionally been the target for direct detection and genotyping using electrophoretic methods (96). The viral RNA is extracted from stool specimens and then subjected to separation by polyacrylamide gel electrophoresis followed by silver staining for detection. This technique has been available for many years and is used primarily in research laboratories; the method is as sensitive as EM. It also has been applied to the classification of rotaviruses, in which the appearance of an unusual electropherotype may denote a novel strain or group of rotaviruses. Schematic diagrams of electropherotypes of group A to G rotaviruses have been compiled as a reference. Direct detection and genotyping of viral DNA using this technique has also been applied to the diagnosis of human EAdVs following digestion of the adenoviral genomic DNA with restriction enzymes.

PCR and RT-PCR

Extraction of Nucleic Acids for PCR or RT-PCR

One of the major challenges of viral detection in stool specimens by PCR or RT-PCR is the presence of inhibitors in the samples, which could lead to false-negative results. Such inhibitors can be monitored by adding an internal control to the sample during the nucleic acid extraction and purification process. Approaches to reduce inhibition include dilution of stools and/or extracted nucleic acids; treatment of samples with chelating agents, detergents, or denaturing chemicals during RNA extraction (97); and inclusion of amplification facilitators such as bovine serum albumin and betaines during the PCR (98). Most commercial nucleic acid extraction protocols now use silica- or magnetic bead-based extraction technologies that are simple and efficient and provide appropriate amounts of nucleic acids of high quality that are essentially free of contamination with cellular proteins, carbohydrates, and lipids that may act to inhibit or interfere with downstream amplification.

Nucleic acids extracted from stool specimens usually contain large amounts of nonviral nucleic acids from different microorganisms and host cells that may be nonspecifically amplified by virus-specific primers. These nonspecific PCR products cannot be completely eliminated even under the high-stringency conditions of the reactions. In this case, hybridization with virus-specific probes is usually required as part of the PCR process to confirm the results. Impact of the nonviral nucleic acids present in stool samples on the quality of next-generation sequence (NGS) results has been discerned. Recent studies using NGS for characterization of norovirus demonstrated that the efficiency of NGS can be improved by viral RNA enrichment, including poly(A) tail selection (99), RT-PCR amplification by norovirus-specific primers (100), virus discovery based on cDNA amplified fragment length polymorphism (101), and virus purification (102). Depletion of ribosomal RNA (rRNA) is another possible enrichment approach of eliminating the interrupts (103, 104).

Conventional PCR

Conventional or end-point PCR (cPCR or cRT-PCR) refers to the more traditional amplification process in which amplified product is allowed to accumulate and plateau as the thermal cycling goes to completion or end-point before performing the detection or analysis steps. This type of PCR normally relies on the detection of amplified PCR products by size fractionation using agarose or polyacrylamide gel electrophoresis. By using type-specific primers, cPCR has been widely used to determine the molecular epidemiology of viral gastroenteritis. For example, cRT-PCR is used for genotyping of group A rotaviruses using primers specific to the gene regions that code for the two major viral surface neutralization proteins VP7 (G types) and VP4 (P types) (105). cPCR followed by sequencing of the PCR products also has been commonly used for studies of the molecular epidemiology of noroviruses, the assessment of genetic variation among the various norovirus strains, and the investigation of outbreaks of gastrointestinal disease (6). The major disadvantages of cPCR include the requirement for multiple complex, labor-intensive and time-consuming steps, the low throughput and high variability, and the significant risk of contamination due to the open system and manipulations of amplified products. While cPCR is still commonly used in many research laboratories that study enteric viruses, it does not have wide applicability in diagnostic laboratories.

Real-Time PCR

Currently, monoplex and multiplex real-time PCR is the most common approach for establishing a diagnosis of viral gastroenteritis, and to this end, a number of assays have been developed and implemented by individual laboratories for the detection of the major enteric viruses (Table 4). Simply put, real-time PCR allows for simultaneous detection of specific nucleic acid sequences in real time by using nonspecific intercalating dyes or fluorescent dyes bound to target-specific probes. With real-time PCR, the amplified product is measured at each PCR cycle. Advances in this technology include preoptimized universal reagents and universal conditions for amplification, simplified assay development and design of primers and probes, multiple amplicon detection chemistries and many choices of thermal cyclers, higher throughput capabilities and enhanced reproducibility, flexibility to multiplex assays to detect multiple viruses in a single reaction, a low risk of contamination because of the closed system, increased sensitivity and specificity over the more traditional detection methods, and software-driven operations.

Laboratory-developed real-time PCR assays for the detection of gastroenteritis viruses have been shown to have superior performance characteristics and are much better than any combination of EM and/or antigen detection methods. Antigen testing for rotavirus, while less sensitive than PCR, may be preferred in settings such as developing countries in which low levels of rotavirus may represent recent but not current infection. Antigen is inexpensive and requires less expertise compared with PCR testing. However, in the era of widespread rotavirus vaccination, this higher specificity of antigen testing is much less relevant, and the higher sensitivity of PCR is preferred for clinical laboratory testing in most settings.

PCR-based assays can readily detect coinfections with different enteric viruses and can be coupled with other assays that detect nonviral enteric pathogens. Their sensitivity and specificity are high, with detection limits of 1.5 to 3.6 viral particles per PCR for rotavirus (106) and fewer than 10 RNA copies per PCR reaction for noroviruses (107). The primers of these assays have been selected according to highly conserved regions of the viral genomes, such as those in the VP6, VP2, and NP3 genes of rotaviruses. Primers targeting the rotavirus NP3 gene are particularly useful for broad detection and are capable of detecting most of the common genotypes (G1 to G4 and G9) as well as some rare genotypes, such as G10 and G12

TABLE 4 Selected molecular assays for detection of the major viruses known to cause gastroenteritis

Virus	Primers	Probes	Target gene	Length (bp)	Instrument	Reference
Rotavirus	NSP3F/NSP3R	TaqMan	NSP3	87	ABI:7700/7000/7300/7500	112
	RotaAF1.2/ RotaA R1.2	MGB TaqMan	VP6	145	ABI:7000	113
	VP2F1-5/VP2R1.2	MGB TaqMan	VP2	79	ABI:7900HT	114
Norovirus	COG1F/G1R	TaqMan	ORF1-ORF2 junction region	85-GI	ABI:7700/7000/7300/7500	108
	COG2F/G2R			98-GII		
	Multiplex PCR					
	NV192/193-G1	MGB TaqMan	ORF1-2 junction region	98-GI	ABI PRISM:7700	115
	NV107a,c/NV119-GII			94-GII		
	Multiplex RT-PCR					
	COG1F/G1R-GI	TaqMan	ORF1-2 junction region	85-GI	Roche: LightCycler 1.0	107
	COG2F/G2R-GII			98-GII		
	Mon4F/R-GIV			98-GIV		
	GIF/GIR-GI	MGB TaqMan	ORF1-2 junction region	85-GI	ABI:7000	116
	GIIF and GIVF/GII&IVR			97-GII &IV		
Sapovirus	sapoFa&Fb/sapoR	MGB TaqMan	Polymerase	104	ABI:7000	116
	SaV124F, SaV1F, SaV5F/SaV1245R	MGB TaqMan	Polymerase; capsid junction	104	ABI:7500 Fast	117
	CU-SVF1 and CU-SVF2/Cu-SVR	TaqMan	Polymerase; capsid junction	104	Bio-Rad: iCycler	118
Astrovirus	AstU1-4/AstL1-2	TaqMan	Capsid	218	ABI:7000	119
	HastF/HastR	MGB TaqMan	Capsid	67	ABI:7000	116
Enteric adenovirus	AdenoF/AdenoR	MGB TaqMan	Hexon	130	ABI:7000	113
	EadVF/R	TaqMan	Hexon	135	ABI:7500	120

of rotaviruses (106). However, detection of rotavirus with relatively low sensitivity is still a challenge when the PCR for a double-strand RNA rotavirus is amalgamated with other enteric viruses which are mostly single-strand RNA viruses (such as norovirus, sapovirus, and astrovirus) to form a panel assay. Preheating at 97°C for 5 minutes prior to reverse transcription is an important step to segregate double-strand RNA template, which enhances detection.

The ORF1-ORF2 junction region is the most conserved region of the norovirus genome, with a high level of nucleotide sequence identity across the strains within the genogroups (108). This feature makes the region ideal for designing primers for RT-quantitative PCR (qPCR) assays to achieve high analytical sensitivity as well as a broad range of detection of many norovirus genotypes, including even recent emerging stains of norovirus GII.17 (GII.17 Kawasaki 2014), GII.P16-GII.4 Sydney, and GII.P16-GII.2 (108, 109). However, the primers and probes designed from conserved sequences may not warrant the sensitivity of RT-qPCR because the mutation even with a single nucleotide polymorphism could occur unpredictably (110). Thus, monitoring sequence changes in the primer and probe binding sites should be pursued regularly. With primers specific to individual genogroups (GI and GII), a multiplex real-time PCR which is highly sensitive and useful for typing noroviruses also has been developed (111). The multiplexed assay increases testing efficiency by decreasing test time by 50% and reducing reagent costs compared with those of other real-time PCR methods. A LightCycler real-time RT-PCR assay with additional primers and a probe targeting the GIV norovirus has also been developed (107). Currently, this and the multiplex assays are widely used in clinical and research laboratories worldwide, especially in North America.

Laboratory-developed real-time PCR assays for the detection of sapoviruses, astroviruses, and the EAdVs also have been developed and have been shown to be highly sensitive and specific with increased detection rates over EM and available antigen detection assays (106, 107, 109, 112–120).

Isothermal Amplification Assays

Nucleic acid sequence-based amplification and loop-mediated isothermal amplification (LAMP) assays have been applied to the detection of noroviruses from stool specimens and are categorized as isothermal amplification methods. These assays involve single temperature amplification with no thermal cycling profile. Similar to real-time PCR, the assays have been shown to be extremely sensitive. Nucleic acid sequence-based amplification has been used to detect norovirus RNA, but the detection specificity does not appear to be acceptable for clinical diagnostic use because of the decreased stringency when amplifying viral RNA at relatively low temperatures of ~40°C (121). The LAMP technology has the added advantages of speed and simplicity, with the reaction being performed in a single tube and requiring no more than 1 hour to complete. Reactions normally show a high tolerance to biological products so that extensive nucleic acid extraction is often not necessary and assays require no large equipment and only simple heat blocks or water baths since amplification occurs in low and unchanged temperature conditions, normally at 60 to 65°C. The by-product of LAMP is the production of magnesium pyrophosphate. In positive samples, it precipitates out of solution, causing a turbid reaction that can easily be read using a small turbidity reader. A fluorescent metal indicator can also be added to enhance the readability of the produced turbidity. The simplicity of LAMP assays makes them applicable to laboratories with limited resources and experience in performing molecular methods and which desire rapid turnaround times at the point of care using a robust assay system. Laboratory-developed LAMP assays have been applied to the detection of norovirus GI and GII and have demonstrated compatible results with real-time RT-PCR (122–124). Recently, a commercial LAMP kit for detection of norovirus GI and GII developed by Eiken Chemical Co. (Tokyo, Japan) has improved the detection sensitivity in comparison with laboratory-developed LAMP assays (124). With further development and validation, LAMP assays may prove to be an acceptable alternative to current real-time PCR assays for the detection of enteric viruses.

Multiple NAT Panel Testing for Gastroenteritis Pathogens

Recently, multiplexed and syndrome-specific molecular testing panels using nanotechnology or real-time qPCR platforms for the detection of enteric pathogens have been developed, validated, and implemented in clinical diagnostic laboratories (Table 5). Advances in microelectronics, microfluidics, and microfabrication have paved the way for new and miniature technologies, with the ultimate goal of offering ever simpler, cost-affordable, point-of-care adaptable molecular diagnostic platforms. Nanotechnology is being used to develop sample-in/answer-out testing for laboratories regardless of size, resources, or capacity with the use of the smallest quantities of reagents and samples. It also enables the multiplex diagnostics testing for comprehensive syndrome-specific assessment of the etiology of specific diseases.

To this end, several commercial syndrome-specific multiplex testing platforms have been cleared by the FDA and marketed in recent years, such as the Luminex xTAG Gastrointestinal Pathogen Panel (GPP) (Luminex, Austin, TX), FilmArray gastrointestinal panel (bioMérieux BioFire Diagnostics, Salt Lake City, UT), Verigene Enteric Pathogens Nucleic Acid Test (Nanosphere, U.S.), Allplex Gastrointestinal Panel (Seegene, Seoul, South Korea), and FTD Viral gastroenteritis (Fast Track Diagnostics Ltd., Sliema, Malta). Some of these platforms have been licensed by the FDA, Health Canada, and the European Union. A recent review of the performance of laboratory-developed multiplex PCR assays and two commercial syndrome-specific multiplex testing platforms (the xTAG GPP and FilmArray Gastrointestinal Panel A) demonstrated the superior sensitivity of multiplex PCR assays over conventional methods for detection of most pathogens (125). The xTAG GPP and FilmArray Gastrointestinal Panel A showed comparable results in the detection of multiple enteric pathogens (126). Compared to a laboratory-developed enteric viruses panel based on the multiplex PCR assay, however, a relatively lower sensitivity of the xTAG GPP for detection of norovirus GII.2 has been reported (109). In general, these new technologies with completely automated and closed systems have shown great potential for clinical application to identify enteric pathogens associated with sporadic gastroenteritis and outbreaks, while saving significant time in assay performance (total hands-on time of as little as 2 to 5 minutes) and turn-around-report time (as little as 1 hour). These improvements will provide physicians with prompt clinical intervention and disease control. However, commercial assays generally do not provide Ct (cycle threshold) values, which are available in laboratory-developed tests, thus limiting the ability to identify low-level positives (with high Ct values), which may represent resolved infection or

TABLE 5 Update of commercial molecular assays for the detection of gastroenteritis viruses

Assay	License/ approval information	Principle of the test	Instrument	Vendor	Reference with validation/evaluation data
Luminex xTAG Gastrointestinal Pathogen Panel (GPP)	FDA cleared; IVD[a]	Multiplex RT-PCR and liquid array for 15 pathogens	Luminex system	Luminex, TX	68
BioFire FilmArray GI panel	FDA cleared; IVD	Nested RT-PCR and FilmArray for 24 pathogens	FilmArray platform	bioMérieux	68
Verigene Enteric Pathogens (EP) test	FDA cleared; IVD	Multiplex RT-PCR and array hybridization	Verigene platform	Luminex, TX	https://www.luminexcorp.com/
Allplex Gastrointestinal Full Panel assay	CE; IVD	Multiplex real-time RT-PCR for 25 pathogens in four multiplex qPCR panels	CFX96 real-time PCR detection system (Bio-Rad)	Seegene, Seoul, South Korea	www.seegene.com/neo/en/products/Gastrointestinal/allplex_GI_fp.php
FTD Viral gastroenteritis	CE; IVD	Three multiplex RT-PCRs for 5 gastroenteritis viruses	Applied Biosystems 7500/7500Fast (Thermo Fisher Scientific), CFX96 (Bio-Rad), LightCycler 480 (Roche) and Rotor-Gene 3000, 6000, Q (Qiagen) and SmartCycler (Cepheid)	Fast Track Diagnostics Ltd., Sliema, Malta	http://www.fast-trackdiagnostics.com/human-line/products/ftd-viral-gastroenteritis/

[a]IVD, *In vitro* diagnostic use.

contamination. Furthermore, commercial assays (as well as laboratory-developed tests) require regular verification to ensure that they retain maximal sensitivity for circulating strains. Sequence changes in the virus from mutation, recombination, or new strains could affect test performance. A summary of the current commercial robotic testing platforms is shown in Table 5.

Next-Generation Sequencing

NGS, a fundamentally different approach to classic genetic sequencing, has triggered numerous groundbreaking discoveries and will likely revolutionize genomic science. The principle of NGS is similar to capillary electrophoresis-based Sanger sequencing: the bases of a small DNA fragment are sequentially identified from signals emitted as each fragment is resynthesized from a DNA template strand. NGS extends this process across millions of reactions in a massively parallel manner. Advancement of this technology enables rapid sequencing of large stretches of DNA spanning entire genomes, with the latest instruments being capable of producing hundreds of gigabases of data in a single sequencing run (127). NGS has good features including high-throughput, powerful scalability, tunable resolution, ever-fast speed, and unlimited dynamic range and sensitivity. Since norovirus has a relatively small genome, characterization using direct sequencing can become a new approach to study norovirus. The latest NGS amplicon library preparation kits allow researchers to perform rapid amplification of custom-targeted regions from norovirus genomes. Using this approach, thousands of amplicons spanning multiple samples can be simultaneously prepared and indexed. NGS enables simultaneous analysis of all genomic content of interest in a single experiment (128). With sufficient depth of coverage, NGS sequencing can identify common and rare sequence variations of norovirus in clinical samples (104). NGS is particularly useful for tracking genetic evolution of norovirus and the discovery of emerging variants which may potentially cause outbreaks of norovirus gastroenteritis. It is anticipated that NGS will be adapted for clinical diagnostic workflows with further development of standard reagents and targeting kits in the near future (99, 100, 103, 129, 130).

ISOLATION PROCEDURES

Cell Culture

While growth in cell culture can be used to detect and identify many different viruses from clinical specimens, it is generally time-consuming and not considered sufficient to contribute to meaningful management of a disease like acute gastroenteritis. In addition, most of the enteric viruses that cause human gastroenteritis are fastidious in cell culture and require multiple passages before they can readily grow in cell culture from their primary isolation. Therefore, cell culture is not routinely used in the clinical diagnosis of viral gastroenteritis.

Cell lines for isolation of rotaviruses include MdBK, PK-15, BSC-1, llC-MK2, Ma104, CaCo-2, and HRT-29. To grow the viruses in cell culture, the culture medium must be supplemented with proteases such as trypsin or pancreatin. This approach has been adapted for titration of viruses by plaque assay and serotyping by virus neutralization.

Regardless of the clinical and public health importance of norovirus sporadic and outbreak gastroenteritis, pathogenesis of the virus is still limited because cell cultivability of norovirus remains a key obstacle. Human noroviruses have resisted efforts to establish an *in vitro* culture method for more than 40 years. Several previously reported tentative cell culture systems are not reproducible and support few passages of replication for a single strain of norovirus (131–135). Recently, Ettayebi et al. reported successful cultivation of multiple strains of human norovirus in the human intestinal enteroids, where three-dimensional *in vitro* cultures were derived from proliferating stem cells in crypts isolated from human gastrointestinal tract biopsies or surgical specimens. Bile is required for strain-dependent norovirus replication as a critical factor of the intestinal milieu (136, 137). This culture system recapitulates the human intestinal epithelium and permits human host-pathogen studies of previously noncultivable virus. This preliminary success of norovirus cell culture provides a potential breakthrough for future study of norovirus pathogenesis, immunology, disinfection, and vaccine development, although viral replication and output in the system remain frequently encountered challenges. Norovirus cell culture will have its most significant impact on research and development fields rather than a direct benefit for clinical diagnosis.

EAdV types 40 and 41 grow best in the Graham 293 human embryonic kidney cell line, which has been transformed by adenovirus type 5 DNA. A plaque assay has been developed recently for the detection of EAdV types 40 and 41 (138).

Isolation of astroviruses from clinical samples is difficult, although most of the astrovirus serotypes have been adapted in HEK or llC-MK2 cell culture (139). Propagation of astrovirus cell culture requires the presence of trypsin in the culture medium.

ANTIGENIC AND GENETIC TYPING SYSTEMS

Both antigenic and genetic typing methods are important for understanding the classification and epidemiology of many gastroenteritis viruses and for developing preventive strategies against the diseases caused by these pathogens. Typing of gastroenteritis viruses is used mainly in research laboratories since typing does not affect clinical care and management decisions.

Based on antigenic and genetic variations in the two major surface proteins of rotaviruses, VP7 and VP4, a dual system of antigenic (serotyping) and genetic typing has been used for the classification of human group A rotaviruses. The antigenic typing is accomplished by characterizing the specific interaction of a rotavirus with a panel of monoclonal antibodies representing individual G (VP7) and P (VP4) types of rotaviruses. The genetic typing is performed by RT-PCR using type-specific primers targeting unique regions of the VP7 and VP4 genes. Using this classification system, each strain of rotavirus is dually assigned to a G[P] type by either the antigenic or the genetic typing method. The antigenic typing results are highly correlated with the genetic typing for the G types, while the correlation between antigenic and genetic typing for the P types is low. Due to a limited supply of type-specific antibodies, P genotyping is commonly used. Frequent genetic and antigenic drifting of rotaviruses may result in newly emerging variants which are no longer detectable by the current typing assays (105). It becomes necessary to update the methods and reagents continuously, such as with type-specific monoclonal antibodies for the antigenic typing and primers for the genotyping.

Rotaviruses are also typeable based on the genetic variations in the major structure protein VP6 and the putative viral enterotoxin NSP4 genes. The recently recommended new classification system based on sequence information for all 11 genomic RNA segments is an extension of the previous classification systems. While this new system is challenging due to the requirement of sequencing all 11 genomic segments, it will eventually impact our understanding of the genetic variation, host-pathogen interaction, evolution, and potentially zoonotic nature of human rotaviruses.

Genetic typing provides essential information to further our understanding of norovirus genetic evolution, classification, and molecular epidemiology. The information on the genetic traits of norovirus causing regional gastroenteritis outbreaks in a spatiotemporal manner can be exchanged nationally and internationally to map the trend of norovirus strains that cause endemic, epidemic, or pandemic events. Genetic information on norovirus is also critical for the development of preventive strategies against norovirus infections, such as vaccines. Norovirus is classified into genogroups, subgenogroups, genotypes, and variants based on genotyping results. With the highly diversified genome of norovirus, genotyping may require sequencing of postamplified RT-PCR products. Five regions (designated A, B, C, E, and D) of the genome have been used successfully for genotyping of noroviruses (140–142). In recent years, primers targeting the norovirus viral capsid gene (regions C, E, and D) have been preferred for genotyping use because viral capsid is directly involved in host-receptor interaction and immune response and contains relevant genetic variations. The "gold standard" for genotyping norovirus strains is full capsid sequencing. However, for clinical samples with a high level of norovirus viral load, amplifying partial capsid sequences is more practical and has only slightly less discriminatory power than full capsid sequencing (143). Norovirus has been frequently recombined with ORF1 and ORF2. Use of the capsid gene alone in a current approach of genotyping is not able to identify those recombinant strains. The primers designed in the ORF1/2 junction region were reported to work better for identifying norovirus antigenic drift than recombination events (144).

Genomic DNA restriction enzyme analysis was commonly used before monoclonal antibody-based EIA typing was developed for the detection and typing of EAdVs. In addition, typing PCR or PCR in combination with restriction enzyme analysis has also been developed for the detection and typing of adenoviruses (145, 146). Recently, a real-time qPCR assay was described for detecting HAdVs and identifying EAdVs of types 40 and 41 (147). Field surveillance using various methods suggests that the choice of diagnostic method may influence the epidemiologic picture and disease burden attributed to EAdV infections. There are 68 types of HAdVs grouped into 7 subgroups (A to G) based on serological, whole-genome sequencing, and phylogenomics assays (18–20).

For typing of astroviruses, immunologic assays, such as IEM and a typing enzyme-linked immunosorbent assay, have been described but are not commercially available. The most commonly used RT-PCR typing methods for astroviruses are summarized in a recent review by Guix et al. (148).

SEROLOGIC TESTS

Antibody neutralization tests based on plaque reduction or epitope-blocking assays using type-specific monoclonal antibodies have been described for rotaviruses. There is no neutralization-based serologic test for most other gastroenteritis viruses. However, enzyme-linked immunosorbent assays for antibody detection using specific viral proteins as the capture antigens have been used in epidemiology studies of gastroenteritis viruses. Recombinant viral capsid proteins of caliciviruses and astroviruses generated in a baculovirus vector and other systems are an excellent source of viral antigens for these studies (149). Application of these assays in sero-surveillance against gastroenteritis viruses has played an important role in understanding the importance of these viruses in different populations. Monitoring seroconversion based on a collection of paired acute- and convalescent-phase sera has been used in outbreak investigations.

EVALUATION, INTERPRETATION, AND REPORTING OF RESULTS

There are many issues involved in the laboratory diagnosis of viral gastroenteritis, and detection of gastroenteritis viruses can be quite difficult. As a result, much of viral gastrointestinal disease goes unrecognized. Enteric viruses do not grow well, if at all, in conventional cell culture systems used in clinical laboratories, and there is a definite lack of available reagents and assays for clinical use. Commercial rapid antigen detection tests are available for rotavirus and, to a much lesser extent, for adenovirus types 40 and 41, noroviruses, sapoviruses, and astroviruses; they offer speed in the diagnosis of viral gastrointestinal disease but are not completely sensitive or specific and only detect the pathogen of interest. In recent years, PCR has offered great promise for the diagnosis of viral gastroenteritis and has emerged as the most sensitive and specific method for the detection of viral causes of diarrhea. Real-time PCR is the most widely used molecular method for detecting the viral agents of gastroenteritis.

There are many reasons to attempt a laboratory diagnosis in individuals suspected of having a viral gastrointestinal disease. However, this does not mean that every individual with diarrheal illness has to be tested by a laboratory measure since viral illness is self-limited with short duration, and no specific clinical management is required in most cases. The high cost of many commercial assays is another factor prohibiting such a testing approach. A prompt diagnosis of viral gastroenteritis provides benefit in the management of specific groups of patients by limiting unnecessary antibiotics, laboratory tests, and hospital procedures; reducing hospital stays and sequelae; guiding treatment decisions; and providing earlier informed decision making for better care. Accumulating data have also shown that the major gastroenteritis viruses, such as rotaviruses, noroviruses, and EAdVs, can cause chronic gastroenteritis with prolonged shedding of viruses in the stools of recipients of transplanted organs, HIV patients, and other immunocompromised individuals. Prompt diagnosis in these clinical settings is important to adjust immunosuppressive therapy, to assess prognosis, and to stop the transmission of the disease. Rapid identification and monitoring of the source of infection in outbreaks of acute gastroenteritis, such as water, food, and environmental surfaces, are also important for disease control and prevention in the community. Early identification of food handlers with subclinical infection or chronic shedding of viruses is believed to be important for the prevention of foodborne outbreaks.

The antigen detection methods, although moderate in sensitivity, may be a practical and inexpensive choice for the initial screening of stool samples if tests are available for a specific virus. Commercial antigen detection assays for rotaviruses, EAdVs, and astroviruses can be applied to clinical diagnosis (Table 3). Also, antigenic tests based on type-specific monoclonal antibodies against the G and P types of rotaviruses and various types of astroviruses are widely used in research laboratories. Commercial antigen detection assays for human noroviruses suffer from a lack of sensitivity and specificity and are not recommended for clinical diagnosis, although they may be useful for outbreak investigations.

Nucleic acid-based assays, particularly real-time PCR, are highly sensitive and specific and are increasingly used as the primary method for clinical diagnosis. While less useful in clinical diagnosis, cPCR with type-specific primers and sequencing of the amplified product is appropriate for determining the molecular epidemiology of viral gastroenteritis.

Most gastroenteritis viral families are genetically diverse, which makes clinical diagnosis using PCR and RT-PCR difficult. Human noroviruses have over 40 recognized genetic clusters within three genogroups. Using primers targeting highly conserved regions of the genome, the majority of known human noroviruses can be detected, but there is probably no single primer pair that can detect all strains. In this case, multiple primer sets targeting different regions of the genome can be used to enhance the detection rates. In addition, degenerate primers based on sequence variations of known viral family members have also been used.

Diagnosis of viral gastroenteritis is greatly improving with the availability of commercial multiplex assays for many viral, bacterial, and parasitic pathogens. Despite these advances, noninfectious and toxin-mediated diarrhea may not be diagnosed, and only a minority of presumed infectious diarrhea yields an etiologic diagnosis. To further complicate interpretation, because many viral pathogens may cause subclinical infection or be shed for prolonged periods of time, detecting a virus does not prove it is causally associated with the current diarrheal episode. In some cases, more than one pathogen is detected in the same clinical sample or during the same episode of clinical illness, complicating efforts to determine the true etiology. Thus, care needs to be taken in the interpretation of laboratory results for gastroenteritis viruses. Proper epidemiologic case-control studies are necessary to address these issues.

REFERENCES

1. **Estes MK, Kapikian A.** 2007. Rotaviruses, p 1917–1974. *In* Knipe DM, Howley PM, Griffin DE, Lamb RA, Martin MA, Roizman B, Straus SE (ed), *Fields Virology*, 5th ed. Lippincott Williams & Wilkins, Philadelphia, PA.
2. **Matthijnssens J, Ciarlet M, McDonald SM, Attoui H, Bányai K, Brister JR, Buesa J, Esona MD, Estes MK, Gentsch JR, Iturriza-Gómara M, Johne R, Kirkwood CD, Martella V, Mertens PP, Nakagomi O, Parreño V, Rahman M, Ruggeri FM, Saif LJ, Santos N, Steyer A, Taniguchi K, Patton JT, Desselberger U, Van Ranst M.** 2011. Uniformity of rotavirus strain nomenclature proposed by the Rotavirus Classification Working Group (RCWG). *Arch Virol* **156:**1397–1413.
3. **Trojnar E, Sachsenröder J, Twardziok S, Reetz J, Otto PH, Johne R.** 2013. Identification of an avian group A rotavirus containing a novel VP4 gene with a close relationship to those of mammalian rotaviruses. *J Gen Virol* **94:**136–142.
4. **Green KY, Ando T, Balayan MS, Berke T, Clarke IN, Estes MK, Matson DO, Nakata S, Neill JD, Studdert MJ, Thiel HJ.** 2000. Taxonomy of the caliciviruses. *J Infect Dis* **181**(Suppl 2)**:**S322–S330.
5. **Oliver SL, Asobayire E, Dastjerdi AM, Bridger JC.** 2006. Genomic characterization of the unclassified bovine enteric virus Newbury agent-1 (Newbury1) endorses a new genus in the family *Caliciviridae*. *Virology* **350:**240–250.

6. **Zheng DP, Ando T, Fankhauser RL, Beard RS, Glass RI, Monroe SS.** 2006. Norovirus classification and proposed strain nomenclature. *Virology* **346:**312–323.
7. **Vinjé J.** 2015. Advances in laboratory methods for detection and typing of norovirus. *J Clin Microbiol* **53:**373–381.
8. **Siebenga JJ, Vennema H, Duizer E, Koopmans MP.** 2007. Gastroenteritis caused by norovirus GGII.4, The Netherlands, 1994-2005. *Emerg Infect Dis* **13:**144–146.
9. **Bull RA, Eden JS, Rawlinson WD, White PA.** 2010. Rapid evolution of pandemic noroviruses of the GII.4 lineage. *PLoS Pathog* **6:**e1000831. (Erratum, **6:**10.1371/annotation/19042899-9f1b-4ccc-b13e-2a8faf19421b.)
10. **Hasing ME, Lee BE, Preiksaitis JK, Tellier R, Honish L, Senthilselvan A, Pang XL.** 2013. Emergence of a new norovirus GII.4 variant and changes in the historical biennial pattern of norovirus outbreak activity in Alberta, Canada, from 2008 to 2013. *J Clin Microbiol* **51:**2204–2211.
11. **Zheng DP, Widdowson MA, Glass RI, Vinjé J.** 2010. Molecular epidemiology of genogroup II-genotype 4 noroviruses in the United States between 1994 and 2006. *J Clin Microbiol* **48:**168–177.
12. **Lu J, Sun L, Fang L, Yang F, Mo Y, Lao J, Zheng H, Tan X, Lin H, Rutherford S, Guo L, Ke C, Hui L.** 2015. Gastroenteritis outbreaks caused by norovirus GII.17, Guangdong Province, China, 2014-2015. *Emerg Infect Dis* **21:**1240–1242.
13. **Choi YS, Koo ES, Kim MS, Choi JD, Shin Y, Jeong YS.** 2017. Re-emergence of a GII.4 norovirus Sydney 2012 variant equipped with GII.P16 RdRp and its predominance over novel variants of GII.17 in South Korea in 2016. *Food Environ Virol* **9:**168–178.
14. **Bruggink L, Catton M, Marshall J.** 2016. A norovirus intervariant GII.4 recombinant in Victoria, Australia, June 2016: the next epidemic variant? *Euro Surveill* **21:**30353.
15. **Niendorf S, Jacobsen S, Faber M, Eis-Hübinger AM, Hofmann J, Zimmermann O, Höhne M, Bock CT.** 2017. Steep rise in norovirus cases and emergence of a new recombinant strain GII.P16-GII.2, Germany, winter 2016. *Euro Surveill* **22:**30447.
16. **Farkas T, Zhong WM, Jing Y, Huang PW, Espinosa SM, Martinez N, Morrow AL, Ruiz-Palacios GM, Pickering LK, Jiang X.** 2004. Genetic diversity among sapoviruses. *Arch Virol* **149:**1309–1323.
17. **Hansman GS, Oka T, Katayama K, Takeda N.** 2007. Human sapoviruses: genetic diversity, recombination, and classification. *Rev Med Virol* **17:**133–141.
18. **Seto D, Chodosh J, Brister JR, Jones MS, Members of the Adenovirus Research Community.** 2011. Using the whole-genome sequence to characterize and name human adenoviruses. *J Virol* **85:**5701–5702.
19. **Singh G, Robinson CM, Dehghan S, Schmidt T, Seto D, Jones MS, Dyer DW, Chodosh J.** 2012. Overreliance on the hexon gene, leading to misclassification of human adenoviruses. *J Virol* **86:**4693–4695.
20. **Matsushima Y, Shimizu H, Kano A, Nakajima E, Ishimaru Y, Dey SK, Watanabe Y, Adachi F, Mitani K, Fujimoto T, Phan TG, Ushijima H.** 2013. Genome sequence of a novel virus of the species human adenovirus D associated with acute gastroenteritis. *Genome Announc* **1:**e00068-12.
21. **de Jong JC, Osterhaus AD, Jones MS, Harrach B.** 2008. Human adenovirus type 52: a type 41 in disguise? *J Virol* **82:**3809–3810.
22. **Walter JE, Mitchell DK.** 2003. Astrovirus infection in children. *Curr Opin Infect Dis* **16:**247–253.
23. **Silva PA, Cardoso DD, Schreier E.** 2006. Molecular characterization of human astroviruses isolated in Brazil, including the complete sequences of astrovirus genotypes 4 and 5. *Arch Virol* **151:**1405–1417.
24. **Lai MMC, Perlman S, Anderson LJ.** 2007. Coronaviridae, p 1305–1335. *In* Knipe DM, Howley PM, Griffin DE, Lamb RA, Martin MA, Roizman B, Straus SE (ed), *Fields Virology*, 5th ed. Lippincott Williams & Wilkins, Philadelphia, PA.
25. **Van Regenmortel M, Fauquet CM, Bishop DHL, Carstens E, Estes MK, Lemon S, Maniloff J, Mayo MA, McGeoch DJ, Pringle CR, Wickner R.** 1999. *Virus Taxonomy: Classification and Nomenclature of Viruses. Seventh Report of the International Committee on Taxonomy of Viruses.* Academic Press, New York, NY.
26. **Fregolente MC, de Castro-Dias E, Martins SS, Spilki FR, Allegretti SM, Gatti MS.** 2009. Molecular characterization of picobirnaviruses from new hosts. *Virus Res* **143:**134–136.
27. **Lindner J, Modrow S.** 2008. Human bocavirus: a novel parvovirus to infect humans. *Intervirology* **51:**116–122.
28. **Estes MK, Morris AP.** 1999. A viral enterotoxin. A new mechanism of virus-induced pathogenesis. *Adv Exp Med Biol* **473:**73–82.
29. **Green YK.** 2007. *Caliciviridae*: the noroviruses, p 949–979. *In* Knipe DM, Howley PM, Griffin DE, Lamb RA, Martin MA, Roizman B, Straus SE (ed), *Fields Virology*, 5th ed. Lippincott Williams & Wilkins, Philadelphia, PA.
30. **Tan M, Jiang X.** 2005. The P domain of norovirus capsid protein forms a subviral particle that binds to histo-blood group antigen receptors. *J Virol* **79:**14017–14030.
31. **Jiang X, Wang M, Wang K, Estes MK.** 1993. Sequence and genomic organization of Norwalk virus. *Virology* **195:**51–61.
32. **Wold WSM, Horwitz MS.** 2007. Adenoviruses, p 2395–2436. *In* Knipe DM, Howley PM, Griffin DE, Lamb RA, Martin MA, Roizman B, Straus SE (ed), *Fields Virology*, 5th ed. Lippincott Williams & Wilkins, Philadelphia, PA.
33. **Espinosa AC, Mazari-Hiriart M, Espinosa R, Maruri-Avidal L, Méndez E, Arias CF.** 2008. Infectivity and genome persistence of rotavirus and astrovirus in groundwater and surface water. *Water Res* **42:**2618–2628.
34. **Bányai K, Bogdán A, Domonkos G, Kisfali P, Molnár P, Tóth A, Melegh B, Martella V, Gentsch JR, Szucs G.** 2009. Genetic diversity and zoonotic potential of human rotavirus strains, 2003-2006, Hungary. *J Med Virol* **81:**362–370.
35. **Liu Y, Huang P, Tan M, Liu Y, Biesiada J, Meller J, Castello AA, Jiang B, Jiang X.** 2012. Rotavirus VP8*: phylogeny, host range, and interaction with histo-blood group antigens. *J Virol* **86:**9899–9910.
36. **Hu L, Crawford SE, Czako R, Cortes-Penfield NW, Smith DF, Le Pendu J, Estes MK, Prasad BV.** 2012. Cell attachment protein VP8* of a human rotavirus specifically interacts with A-type histo-blood group antigen. *Nature* **485:**256–259.
37. **Böhm R, Fleming FE, Maggioni A, Dang VT, Holloway G, Coulson BS, von Itzstein M, Haselhorst T.** 2015. Revisiting the role of histo-blood group antigens in rotavirus host-cell invasion. *Nat Commun* **6:**5907.
38. **Nordgren J, Sharma S, Bucardo F, Nasir W, Günaydın G, Ouermi D, Nitiema LW, Becker-Dreps S, Simpore J, Hammarström L, Larson G, Svensson L.** 2014. Both Lewis and secretor status mediate susceptibility to rotavirus infections in a rotavirus genotype-dependent manner. *Clin Infect Dis* **59:**1567–1573.
39. **Van Trang N, Vu HT, Le NT, Huang P, Jiang X, Anh DD.** 2014. Association between norovirus and rotavirus infection and histo-blood group antigen types in Vietnamese children. *J Clin Microbiol* **52:**1366–1374.
40. **Reid ME, Lomas-Francis C, Olsson ML.** 2012. LE Lewis blood group system p. 347–359. *The Blood Group Antigen FactsBook*, 3rd ed. Academic Press, Boston, MA.
41. **Glass RI, Parashar UD, Estes MK.** 2009. Norovirus gastroenteritis. *N Engl J Med* **361:**1776–1785.
42. **Payne DC, Vinjé J, Szilagyi PG, Edwards KM, Staat MA, Weinberg GA, Hall CB, Chappell J, Bernstein DI, Curns AT, Wikswo M, Shirley SH, Hall AJ, Lopman B, Parashar UD.** 2013. Norovirus and medically attended gastroenteritis in U.S. children. *N Engl J Med* **368:**1121–1130.
43. **Huang P, Farkas T, Zhong W, Tan M, Thornton S, Morrow AL, Jiang X.** 2005. Norovirus and histo-blood group antigens: demonstration of a wide spectrum of strain specificities and classification of two major binding groups among multiple binding patterns. *J Virol* **79:**6714–6722.
44. **Hassan-Ríos E, Torres P, Muñoz E, Matos C, Hall AJ, Gregoricus N, Vinjé J.** 2013. Sapovirus gastroenteritis in preschool center, Puerto Rico, 2011. *Emerg Infect Dis* **19:**174–175.

45. **Pang XL, Lee BE, Tyrrell GJ, Preiksaitis JK.** 2009. Epidemiology and genotype analysis of sapovirus associated with gastroenteritis outbreaks in Alberta: 2004–2007. *J Infect Dis* **199:**547–551.
46. **Svraka S, Vennema H, van der Veer B, Hedlund KO, Thorhagen M, Siebenga J, Duizer E, Koopmans M.** 2010. Epidemiology and genotype analysis of emerging sapovirus-associated infections across Europe. *J Clin Microbiol* **48:**2191–2198.
47. **Carraturo A, Catalani V, Tega L.** 2008. Microbiological and epidemiological aspects of rotavirus and enteric adenovirus infections in hospitalized children in Italy. *New Microbiol* **31:**329–336.
48. **Grohmann GS, Glass RI, Pereira HG, Monroe SS, Hightower AW, Weber R, Bryan RT, Enteric Opportunistic Infections Working Group.** 1993. Enteric viruses and diarrhea in HIV-infected patients. *N Engl J Med* **329:**14–20.
49. **Belliot G, Laveran H, Monroe SS.** 1997. Outbreak of gastroenteritis in military recruits associated with serotype 3 astrovirus infection. *J Med Virol* **51:**101–106.
50. **Midthun K, Greenberg HB, Kurtz JB, Gary GWF, Lin FY, Kapikian AZ.** 1993. Characterization and seroepidemiology of a type 5 astrovirus associated with an outbreak of gastroenteritis in Marin County, California. *J Clin Microbiol* **31:**955–962.
51. **Fischer SA.** 2008. Emerging viruses in transplantation: there is more to infection after transplant than CMV and EBV. *Transplantation* **86:**1327–1339.
52. **Kaltsas A, Sepkowitz K.** 2012. Community acquired respiratory and gastrointestinal viral infections: challenges in the immunocompromised host. *Curr Opin Infect Dis* **25:**423–430.
53. **Liakopoulou E, Mutton K, Carrington D, Robinson S, Steward CG, Goulden NJ, Cornish JM, Marks DI.** 2005. Rotavirus as a significant cause of prolonged diarrhoeal illness and morbidity following allogeneic bone marrow transplantation. *Bone Marrow Transplant* **36:**691–694.
54. **Ghosh N, Malik FA, Daver RG, Vanichanan J, Okhuysen PC.** 2017. Viral associated diarrhea in immunocompromised and cancer patients at a large comprehensive cancer center: a 10-year retrospective study. *Infect Dis (Lond)* **49:**113–119.
55. **Bruijning-Verhagen P, Nipshagen MD, de Graaf H, Bonten MJM.** 2017. Rotavirus disease course among immunocompromised patients: 5-year observations from a tertiary care medical centre. *J Infect* **75:**448–454.
56. **Bok K, Prevots DR, Binder AM, Parra GI, Strollo S, Fahle GA, Behrle-Yardley A, Johnson JA, Levenson EA, Sosnovtsev SV, Holland SM, Palmore TN, Green KY.** 2016. Epidemiology of norovirus infection among immunocompromised patients at a tertiary care research hospital, 2010-2013. *Open Forum Infect Dis* **3:**ofw169.
57. **He T, McMillen TA, Qiu Y, Chen LH, Lu X, Pang XL, Kamboj M, Tang YW.** 2017. Norovirus loads in stool specimens of cancer patients with norovirus gastroenteritis. *J Mol Diagn* **19:**836–842.
58. **Portes SAR, Carvalho-Costa FA, Rocha MS, Fumian TM, Maranhão AG, de Assis RM, Xavier MDPTP, Rocha MS, Miagostovich MP, Leite JPG, Volotão EM.** 2017. Enteric viruses in HIV-1 seropositive and HIV-1 seronegative children with diarrheal diseases in Brazil. *PLoS One* **12:**e0183196.
59. **Green KY.** 2014. Norovirus infection in immunocompromised hosts. *Clin Microbiol Infect* **20:**717–723.
60. **Krones E, Högenauer C.** 2012. Diarrhea in the immunocompromised patient. *Gastroenterol Clin North Am* **41:**677–701.
61. **Bok K, Green KY.** 2012. Norovirus gastroenteritis in immunocompromised patients. *N Engl J Med* **367:**2126–2132.
62. **Ye X, Van JN, Munoz FM, Revell PA, Kozinetz CA, Krance RA, Atmar RL, Estes MK, Koo HL.** 2015. Noroviruses as a cause of diarrhea in immunocompromised pediatric hematopoietic stem cell and solid organ transplant recipients. *Am J Transplant* **15:**1874–1881.
63. **Echenique IA, Penugonda S, Stosor V, Ison MG, Angarone MP.** 2015. Diagnostic yields in solid organ transplant recipients admitted with diarrhea. *Clin Infect Dis* **60:**729–737.
64. **Lee LY, Ladner DP, Ison MG.** 2016. Norovirus infection in solid organ transplant recipients: a single-center retrospective study. *Transpl Infect Dis* **18:**932–938.
65. **van Beek J, van der Eijk AA, Fraaij PL, Caliskan K, Cransberg K, Dalinghaus M, Hoek RA, Metselaar HJ, Roodnat J, Vennema H, Koopmans MP.** 2017. Chronic norovirus infection among solid organ recipients in a tertiary care hospital, the Netherlands, 2006-2014. *Clin Microbiol Infect* **23:** 265.e9–265.e13.
66. **Long SS.** 2008. Evidence of norovirus causing necrotizing enterocolitis (NEC) in a NICU. *J Pediatr* **153:**A2.
67. **Turcios-Ruiz RM, Axelrod P, St John K, Bullitt E, Donahue J, Robinson N, Friss HE.** 2008. Outbreak of necrotizing enterocolitis caused by norovirus in a neonatal intensive care unit. *J Pediatr* **153:**339–344.
68. **Matthes-Martin S, Feuchtinger T, Shaw PJ, Engelhard D, Hirsch HH, Cordonnier C, Ljungman P, on behalf of the Fourth European Conference on Infections in Leukemia.** 2012. European guidelines for diagnosis and treatment of adenovirus infection in leukemia and stem cell transplantation: summary of ECIL-4 (2011). *Transpl Infect Dis* **14:**555–563.
69. **Jurgens PT, Allen LA, Ambardekar AV, McIlvennan CK.** 2017. Chronic norovirus infections in cardiac transplant patients. *Prog Transplant* **27:**69–72.
70. **Rossignol JF.** 2014. Nitazoxanide: a first-in-class broad-spectrum antiviral agent. *Antiviral Res* **110:**94–103.
71. **Gairard-Dory AC, Dégot T, Hirschi S, Schuller A, Leclercq A, Renaud-Picard B, Gourieux B, Kessler R.** 2014. Clinical usefulness of oral immunoglobulins in lung transplant recipients with norovirus gastroenteritis: a case series. *Transplant Proc* **46:**3603–3605.
72. **Hungerford D, Vivancos R, Read JM, Iturriza-Gómara M, French N, Cunliffe NA.** 2018. Rotavirus vaccine impact and socioeconomic deprivation: an interrupted time-series analysis of gastrointestinal disease outcomes across primary and secondary care in the UK. *BMC Med* **16:**10.
73. **Cortese MM, Parashar UD, Centers for Disease Control and Prevention (CDC).** 2009. Prevention of rotavirus gastroenteritis among infants and children: recommendations of the Advisory Committee on Immunization Practices (ACIP). *MMWR Recomm Rep* **58**(RR-2)**:**1–25.
74. **Madhi SA, Cunliffe NA, Steele D, Witte D, Kirsten M, Louw C, Ngwira B, Victor JC, Gillard PH, Cheuvart BB, Han HH, Neuzil KM.** 2010. Effect of human rotavirus vaccine on severe diarrhea in African infants. *N Engl J Med* **362:**289–298.
75. **Zaman K, Dang DA, Victor JC, Shin S, Yunus M, Dallas MJ, Podder G, Thiem VD, Mai LTP, Luby SP, Tho LH, Coia ML, Lewis K, Rivers SB, Sack DA, Schödel F, Steele AD, Neuzil KM, Ciarlet M.** 2010. Efficacy of pentavalent rotavirus vaccine against severe rotavirus gastroenteritis in infants in developing countries in Asia: a randomised, double-blind, placebo-controlled trial. *Lancet* **376:**615–623.
76. **Armah GE, Sow SO, Breiman RF, Dallas MJ, Tapia MD, Feikin DR, Binka FN, Steele AD, Laserson KF, Ansah NA, Levine MM, Lewis K, Coia ML, Attah-Poku M, Ojwando J, Rivers SB, Victor JC, Nyambane G, Hodgson A, Schödel F, Ciarlet M, Neuzil KM.** 2010. Efficacy of pentavalent rotavirus vaccine against severe rotavirus gastroenteritis in infants in developing countries in sub-Saharan Africa: a randomised, double-blind, placebo-controlled trial. *Lancet* **376:** 606–614.
77. **Patel M, Pedreira C, De Oliveira LH, Tate J, Orozco M, Mercado J, Gonzalez A, Malespin O, Amador JJ, Umaña J, Balmaseda A, Perez MC, Gentsch J, Kerin T, Hull J, Mijatovic S, Andrus J, Parashar U.** 2009. Association between pentavalent rotavirus vaccine and severe rotavirus diarrhea among children in Nicaragua. *JAMA* **301:** 2243–2251.
78. **Yeung KHT, Tate JE, Chan CC, Chan MCW, Chan PKS, Poon KH, Siu SLY, Fung GPG, Ng KL, Chan IMC, Yu PT, Ng CH, Lau YL, Nelson EAS.** 2016. Rotavirus vaccine effectiveness in Hong Kong children. *Vaccine* **34:**4935–4942.
79. **Patel M, Shane AL, Parashar UD, Jiang B, Gentsch JR, Glass RI.** 2009. Oral rotavirus vaccines: how well will they work where they are needed most? *J Infect Dis* **200**(Suppl 1)**:**S39–S48.

80. **Ramani S, Hu L, Venkataram Prasad BV, Estes MK.** 2016. Diversity in rotavirus-host glycan interactions: a "sweet" spectrum. *Cell Mol Gastroenterol Hepatol* **2:**263–273.
81. **Atmar RL, Bernstein DI, Harro CD, Al-Ibrahim MS, Chen WH, Ferreira J, Estes MK, Graham DY, Opekun AR, Richardson C, Mendelman PM.** 2011. Norovirus vaccine against experimental human Norwalk Virus illness. *N Engl J Med* **365:**2178–2187.
82. **Bernstein DI, Atmar RL, Lyon GM, Treanor JJ, Chen WH, Jiang X, Vinjé J, Gregoricus N, Frenck RW Jr, Moe CL, Al-Ibrahim MS, Barrett J, Ferreira J, Estes MK, Graham DY, Goodwin R, Borkowski A, Clemens R, Mendelman PM.** 2015. Norovirus vaccine against experimental human GII.4 virus illness: a challenge study in healthy adults. *J Infect Dis* **211:**870–878.
83. **Treanor JJ, Atmar RL, Frey SE, Gormley R, Chen WH, Ferreira J, Goodwin R, Borkowski A, Clemens R, Mendelman PM.** 2014. A novel intramuscular bivalent norovirus virus-like particle vaccine candidate: reactogenicity, safety, and immunogenicity in a phase 1 trial in healthy adults. *J Infect Dis* **210:**1763–1771.
84. **Atmar RL, Baehner F, Cramer JP, Song E, Borkowski A, Mendelman PM, NOR-201 Study Group.** 2016. Rapid responses to 2 virus-like particle norovirus vaccine candidate formulations in healthy adults: a randomized controlled trial. *J Infect Dis* **214:**845–853.
85. **Cardemil CV, Parashar UD, Hall AJ.** 2017. Norovirus infection in older adults: epidemiology, risk factors, and opportunities for prevention and control. *Infect Dis Clin North Am* **31:**839–870.
86. **Goldfarb DM, Steenhoff AP, Pernica JM, Chong S, Luinstra K, Mokomane M, Mazhani L, Quaye I, Goercke I, Mahony J, Smieja M.** 2014. Evaluation of anatomically designed flocked rectal swabs for molecular detection of enteric pathogens in children admitted to hospital with severe gastroenteritis in Botswana. *J Clin Microbiol* **52:**3922–3927.
87. **Freedman SB, Xie J, Nettel-Aguirre A, Lee B, Chui L, Pang XL, Zhuo R, Parsons B, Dickinson JA, Vanderkooi OG, Ali S, Osterreicher L, Lowerison K, Tarr PI, Chuck A, Currie G, Eltorki M, Graham T, Jiang J, Johnson D, Kellner J, Lavoie M, Louie M, MacDonald J, MacDonald S, Simmonds K, Svenson L, Tellier R, Drews S, Talbot J, Alberta Provincial Pediatric EnTeric Infection TEam (APPETITE).** 2017. Enteropathogen detection in children with diarrhoea, or vomiting, or both, comparing rectal flocked swabs with stool specimens: an outpatient cohort study. *Lancet Gastroenterol Hepatol* **2:**662–669.
88. **Kirby A, Ashton L, Hart IJ.** 2011. Detection of norovirus infection in the hospital setting using vomit samples. *J Clin Virol* **51:**86–87.
89. **Khamrin P, Tran DN, Chan-it W, Thongprachum A, Okitsu S, Maneekarn N, Ushijima H.** 2011. Comparison of the rapid methods for screening of group a rotavirus in stool samples. *J Trop Pediatr* **57:**375–377.
90. **Lee SY, Hong JH, Lee SW, Lee M.** 2007. Comparisons of latex agglutination, immunochromatography and enzyme immunoassay methods for the detection of rotavirus antigen. *Korean J Lab Med* **27:**437–441. (In Korean.)
91. **Bon F, Kaplon J, Metzger MH, Pothier P.** 2007. Evaluation of seven immunochromatographic assays for the rapid detection of human rotaviruses in fecal specimens. *Pathol Biol (Paris)* **55:**149–153. (In French.)
92. **de Rougemont A, Kaplon J, Billaud G, Lina B, Pinchinat S, Derrough T, Caulin E, Pothier P, Floret D.** 2009. Sensitivity and specificity of the VIKIA Rota-Adeno immunochromatographic test (bioMérieux) and the ELISA IDEIA Rotavirus kit (Dako) compared to genotyping. *Pathol Biol (Paris)* **57:**86–89. (In French.)
93. **Téllez CJ, Montava R, Ribes JM, Tirado MD, Buesa J.** 2008. Evaluation of two immunochromatography kits for rapid diagnosis of rotavirus infections. *Rev Argent Microbiol* **40:**167–170. (In Spanish.)
94. **de Bruin E, Duizer E, Vennema H, Koopmans MP.** 2006. Diagnosis of norovirus outbreaks by commercial ELISA or RT-PCR. *J Virol Methods* **137:**259–264.
95. **Thongprachum A, Khamrin P, Tran DN, Okitsu S, Mizuguchi M, Hayakawa S, Maneekarn N, Ushijima H.** 2012. Evaluation and comparison of the efficiency of immunochromatography methods for norovirus detection. *Clin Lab* **58:**489–493.
96. **Moosai RB, Carter MJ, Madeley CR.** 1984. Rapid detection of enteric adenovirus and rotavirus: a simple method using polyacrylamide gel electrophoresis. *J Clin Pathol* **37:**1404–1408.
97. **Rasool NB, Monroe SS, Glass RI.** 2002. Determination of a universal nucleic acid extraction procedure for PCR detection of gastroenteritis viruses in faecal specimens. *J Virol Methods* **100:**1–16.
98. **Al-Soud WA, Rådström P.** 2001. Purification and characterization of PCR-inhibitory components in blood cells. *J Clin Microbiol* **39:**485–493.
99. **Wong TH, Dearlove BL, Hedge J, Giess AP, Piazza P, Trebes A, Paul J, Smit E, Smith EG, Sutton JK, Wilcox MH, Dingle KE, Peto TE, Crook DW, Wilson DJ, Wyllie DH.** 2013. Whole genome sequencing and *de novo* assembly identifies Sydney-like variant noroviruses and recombinants during the winter 2012/2013 outbreak in England. *J Virol* **10:**335.
100. **Cotten M, Petrova V, Phan MV, Rabaa MA, Watson SJ, Ong SH, Kellam P, Baker S.** 2014. Deep sequencing of norovirus genomes defines evolutionary patterns in an urban tropical setting. *J Virol* **88:**11056–11069.
101. **de Vries M, Oude Munnink BB, Deijs M, Canuti M, Koekkoek SM, Molenkamp R, Bakker M, Jurriaans S, van Schaik BD, Luyf AC, Olabarriaga SD, van Kampen AH, van der Hoek L.** 2012. Performance of VIDISCA-454 in feces-suspensions and serum. *Viruses* **4:**1328–1334.
102. **Vega E, Donaldson E, Huynh J, Barclay L, Lopman B, Baric R, Chen LF, Vinjé J.** 2014. RNA populations in immunocompromised patients as reservoirs for novel norovirus variants. *J Virol* **88:**14184–14196.
103. **Bavelaar HH, Rahamat-Langendoen J, Niesters HG, Zoll J, Melchers WJ.** 2015. Whole genome sequencing of fecal samples as a tool for the diagnosis and genetic characterization of norovirus. *J Clin Virol* **72:**122–125.
104. **Hasing ME, Hazes B, Lee BE, Preiksaitis JK, Pang XL.** 2016. A next generation sequencing-based method to study the intra-host genetic diversity of norovirus in patients with acute and chronic infection. *BMC Genomics* **17:**480.
105. **Iturriza-Gómara M, Kang G, Gray J.** 2004. Rotavirus genotyping: keeping up with an evolving population of human rotaviruses. *J Clin Virol* **31:**259–265.
106. **Jothikumar N, Kang G, Hill VR.** 2009. Broadly reactive TaqMan assay for real-time RT-PCR detection of rotavirus in clinical and environmental samples. *J Virol Methods* **155:**126–131.
107. **Trujillo AA, McCaustland KA, Zheng DP, Hadley LA, Vaughn G, Adams SM, Ando T, Glass RI, Monroe SS.** 2006. Use of TaqMan real-time reverse transcription-PCR for rapid detection, quantification, and typing of norovirus. *J Clin Microbiol* **44:**1405–1412.
108. **Kageyama T, Kojima S, Shinohara M, Uchida K, Fukushi S, Hoshino FB, Takeda N, Katayama K.** 2003. Broadly reactive and highly sensitive assay for Norwalk-like viruses based on real-time quantitative reverse transcription-PCR. *J Clin Microbiol* **41:**1548–1557.
109. **Zhuo R, Cho J, Qiu Y, Parsons BD, Lee BE, Chui L, Freedman SB, Pang X, Alberta Provincial Pediatric EnTeric Infection TEam (APPETITE).** 2017. High genetic variability of norovirus leads to diagnostic test challenges. *J Clin Virol* **96:**94–98.
110. **Zhuo R, Hasing ME, Pang X, Team of Molecular Diagnostics.** 2015. A single nucleotide polymorphism at the TaqMan probe-binding site impedes real-time reverse transcription-PCR-based detection of norovirus GII.4 Sydney. *J Clin Microbiol* **53:**3353–3354.
111. **Pang XL, Preiksaitis JK, Lee B.** 2005. Multiplex real time RT-PCR for the detection and quantitation of norovirus genogroups I and II in patients with acute gastroenteritis. *J Clin Virol* **33:**168–171.

112. **Pang XL, Preiksaitis JK, Lee BE.** 2014. Enhanced enteric virus detection in sporadic gastroenteritis using a multi-target real-time PCR panel: a one-year study. *J Med Virol* **86:**1594–1601.
113. **Logan C, O'Leary JJ, O'Sullivan N.** 2006. Real-time reverse transcription-PCR for detection of rotavirus and adenovirus as causative agents of acute viral gastroenteritis in children. *J Clin Microbiol* **44:**3189–3195.
114. **Gutiérrez-Aguirre I, Steyer A, Boben J, Gruden K, Poljsak-Prijatelj M, Ravnikar M.** 2008. Sensitive detection of multiple rotavirus genotypes with a single reverse transcription-real-time quantitative PCR assay. *J Clin Microbiol* **46:**2547–2554.
115. **Hoehne M, Schreier E.** 2006. Detection of norovirus genogroup I and II by multiplex real-time RT- PCR using a 3′-minor groove binder-DNA probe. *BMC Infect Dis* **6:**69.
116. **Logan C, O'Leary JJ, O'Sullivan N.** 2007. Real-time reverse transcription PCR detection of norovirus, sapovirus and astrovirus as causative agents of acute viral gastroenteritis. *J Virol Methods* **146:**36–44.
117. **Oka T, Katayama K, Hansman GS, Kageyama T, Ogawa S, Wu FT, White PA, Takeda N.** 2006. Detection of human sapovirus by real-time reverse transcription-polymerase chain reaction. *J Med Virol* **78:**1347–1353.
118. **Chan MC, Sung JJ, Lam RK, Chan PK, Lai RW, Leung WK.** 2006. Sapovirus detection by quantitative real-time RT-PCR in clinical stool specimens. *J Virol Methods* **134:**146–153.
119. **Grimm AC, Cashdollar JL, Williams FP, Fout GS.** 2004. Development of an astrovirus RT-PCR detection assay for use with conventional, real-time, and integrated cell culture/RT-PCR. *Can J Microbiol* **50:**269–278.
120. **Ko G, Jothikumar N, Hill VR, Sobsey MD.** 2005. Rapid detection of infectious adenoviruses by mRNA real-time RT-PCR. *J Virol Methods* **127:**148–153.
121. **Moore C, Clark EM, Gallimore CI, Corden SA, Gray JJ, Westmoreland D.** 2004. Evaluation of a broadly reactive nucleic acid sequence based amplification assay for the detection of noroviruses in faecal material. *J Clin Virol* **29:** 290–296.
122. **Iturriza-Gómara M, Xerry J, Gallimore CI, Dockery C, Gray J.** 2008. Evaluation of the Loopamp (loop-mediated isothermal amplification) kit for detecting norovirus RNA in faecal samples. *J Clin Virol* **42:**389–393.
123. **Suzuki Y, Narimatsu S, Furukawa T, Iwakiri A, Miura M, Yamamoto S, Katayama H.** 2011. Comparison of real-time reverse-transcription loop-mediated isothermal amplification and real-time reverse-transcription polymerase chain reaction for detection of noroviruses in municipal wastewater. *J Biosci Bioeng* **112:**369–372.
124. **Yoda T, Suzuki Y, Yamazaki K, Sakon N, Kanki M, Kase T, Takahashi K, Inoue K.** 2009. Application of a modified loop-mediated isothermal amplification kit for detecting norovirus genogroups I and II. *J Med Virol* **81:**2072–2078.
125. **Zhang H, Morrison S, Tang YW.** 2015. Multiplex polymerase chain reaction tests for detection of pathogens associated with gastroenteritis. *Clin Lab Med* **35:**461–486.
126. **Khare R, Espy MJ, Cebelinski E, Boxrud D, Sloan LM, Cunningham SA, Pritt BS, Patel R, Binnicker MJ.** 2014. Comparative evaluation of two commercial multiplex panels for detection of gastrointestinal pathogens by use of clinical stool specimens. *J Clin Microbiol* **52:** 3667–3673.
127. **Srivatsan A, Han Y, Peng J, Tehranchi AK, Gibbs R, Wang JD, Chen R.** 2008. High-precision, whole-genome sequencing of laboratory strains facilitates genetic studies. *PLoS Genet* **4:**e1000139.
128. **Lo YM, Chiu RW.** 2009. Next-generation sequencing of plasma/serum DNA: an emerging research and molecular diagnostic tool. *Clin Chem* **55:**607–608.
129. **Batty EM, Wong TH, Trebes A, Argoud K, Attar M, Buck D, Ip CL, Golubchik T, Cule M, Bowden R, Manganis C, Klenerman P, Barnes E, Walker AS, Wyllie DH, Wilson DJ, Dingle KE, Peto TE, Crook DW, Piazza P.** 2013. A modified RNA-Seq approach for whole genome sequencing of RNA viruses from faecal and blood samples. *PLoS One* **8:**e66129.
130. **Kundu S, Lockwood J, Depledge DP, Chaudhry Y, Aston A, Rao K, Hartley JC, Goodfellow I, Breuer J.** 2013. Next-generation whole genome sequencing identifies the direction of norovirus transmission in linked patients. *Clin Infect Dis* **57:**407–414.
131. **Straub TM, Höner zu Bentrup K, Orosz-Coghlan P, Dohnalkova A, Mayer BK, Bartholomew RA, Valdez CO, Bruckner-Lea CJ, Gerba CP, Abbaszadegan M, Nickerson CA.** 2007. *In vitro* cell culture infectivity assay for human noroviruses. *Emerg Infect Dis* **13:**396–403.
132. **Straub TM, Hutchison JR, Bartholomew RA, Valdez CO, Valentine NB, Dohnalkova A, Ozanich RM, Bruckner-Lea CJ.** 2013. Defining cell culture conditions to improve human norovirus infectivity assays. *Water Sci Technol* **67:**863–868.
133. **Papafragkou E, Hewitt J, Park GW, Greening G, Vinjé J.** 2013. Challenges of culturing human norovirus in three-dimensional organoid intestinal cell culture models. *PLoS One* **8:**e63485.
134. **Herbst-Kralovetz MM, Radtke AL, Lay MK, Hjelm BE, Bolick AN, Sarker SS, Atmar RL, Kingsley DH, Arntzen CJ, Estes MK, Nickerson CA.** 2013. Lack of norovirus replication and histo-blood group antigen expression in 3-dimensional intestinal epithelial cells. *Emerg Infect Dis* **19:**431–438.
135. **Jones MK, Grau KR, Costantini V, Kolawole AO, de Graaf M, Freiden P, Graves CL, Koopmans M, Wallet SM, Tibbetts SA, Schultz-Cherry S, Wobus CE, Vinjé J, Karst SM.** 2015. Human norovirus culture in B cells. *Nat Protoc* **10:**1939–1947.
136. **Ettayebi K, Crawford SE, Murakami K, Broughman JR, Karandikar U, Tenge VR, Neill FH, Blutt SE, Zeng XL, Qu L, Kou B, Opekun AR, Burrin D, Graham DY, Ramani S, Atmar RL, Estes MK.** 2016. Replication of human noroviruses in stem cell-derived human enteroids. *Science* **353:**1387–1393.
137. **Zou WY, Blutt SE, Crawford SE, Ettayebi K, Zeng XL, Saxena K, Ramani S, Karandikar UC, Zachos NC, Estes MK.** 2017. Human intestinal enteroids: new models to study gastrointestinal virus infections. *Methods Mol Biol* Mar 31. doi:10.1007/7651_2017_1. [Epub ahead of print].
138. **Cromeans TL, Lu X, Erdman DD, Humphrey CD, Hill VR.** 2008. Development of plaque assays for adenoviruses 40 and 41. *J Virol Methods* **151:**140–145.
139. **Taylor MB, Grabow WO, Cubitt WD.** 1997. Propagation of human astrovirus in the PLC/PRF/5 hepatoma cell line. *J Virol Methods* **67:**13–18.
140. **Mattison K, Grudeski E, Auk B, Charest H, Drews SJ, Fritzinger A, Gregoricus N, Hayward S, Houde A, Lee BE, Pang XL, Wong J, Booth TF, Vinjé J.** 2009. Multicenter comparison of two norovirus ORF2-based genotyping protocols. *J Clin Microbiol* **47:**3927–3932.
141. **Kojima S, Kageyama T, Fukushi S, Hoshino FB, Shinohara M, Uchida K, Natori K, Takeda N, Katayama K.** 2002. Genogroup-specific PCR primers for detection of Norwalk-like viruses. *J Virol Methods* **100:**107–114.
142. **Pang XL, Preiksaitis JK, Wong S, Li V, Lee BE.** 2010. Influence of novel norovirus GII.4 variants on gastroenteritis outbreak dynamics in Alberta and the Northern Territories, Canada between 2000 and 2008. *PLoS One* **5:**e11599.
143. **Vinjé J, Hamidjaja RA, Sobsey MD.** 2004. Development and application of a capsid VP1 (region D) based reverse transcription PCR assay for genotyping of genogroup I and II noroviruses. *J Virol Methods* **116:**109–117.
144. **Hasing ME, Hazes B, Lee BE, Preiksaitis JK, Pang XL.** 2014. Detection and analysis of recombination in GII.4 norovirus strains causing gastroenteritis outbreaks in Alberta. *Infect Genet Evol* **27:**181–192.
145. **Allard A, Albinsson B, Wadell G.** 2001. Rapid typing of human adenoviruses by a general PCR combined with restriction endonuclease analysis. *J Clin Microbiol* **39:** 498–505.

146. **Xu W, McDonough MC, Erdman DD.** 2000. Species-specific identification of human adenoviruses by a multiplex PCR assay. *J Clin Microbiol* **38:**4114–4120.
147. **Jothikumar N, Cromeans TL, Hill VR, Lu X, Sobsey MD, Erdman DD.** 2005. Quantitative real-time PCR assays for detection of human adenoviruses and identification of serotypes 40 and 41. *Appl Environ Microbiol* **71:** 3131–3136.
148. **Guix S, Bosch A, Pintó RM.** 2005. Human astrovirus diagnosis and typing: current and future prospects. *Lett Appl Microbiol* **41:**103–105.
149. **Jiang X, Wilton N, Zhong WM, Farkas T, Huang PW, Barrett E, Guerrero M, Ruiz-Palacios G, Green KY, Green J, Hale AD, Estes MK, Pickering LK, Matson DO.** 2000. Diagnosis of human caliciviruses by use of enzyme immunoassays. *J Infect Dis* **181**(Suppl 2)**:**S349–S359.

Rabies Lyssavirus*

LILLIAN A. ORCIARI, PAMELA A. YAGER, AND P. S. SATHESHKUMAR

96

TAXONOMY

There are numerous etiologic agents in the genus *Lyssavirus* that result in an acute, fatal viral encephalomyelitis known as rabies in both humans and animals. These agents are single-stranded, bullet-shaped RNA viruses of the order *Mononegavirales* and family *Rhabdoviridae*. The genus includes 14 species, the prototype *Rabies lyssavirus* (RABV) and the less commonly known species of rabies-related lyssaviruses, *Aravan lyssavirus*, *Australian bat lyssavirus*, *Bokeloh bat lyssavirus*, *Duvenhage lyssavirus*, *European bat 1 lyssavirus*, *European bat 2 lyssavirus*, *Ikoma lyssavirus*, *Irkut lyssavirus*, *Khujand lyssavirus*, *Lagos bat lyssavirus*, *Mokola lyssavirus*, *West Caucasian bat lyssavirus*, and *Shimoni bat lyssavirus*; the genus also includes two proposed lyssaviruses, *Lleida bat lyssavirus* and *Gannoruwa bat lyssavirus* (Fig. 1) (1–4). The lyssaviruses were first characterized by serologic neutralization, which was useful in classifying them into related or more distant groups (5). More recently, differences have been defined by nucleotide sequence analysis, and lyssaviruses are grouped as different genotypes or species. Current commercial human and animal vaccines are based on the prototype species, RABV, and provide adequate cross protection against lyssaviruses in phylogroup 1 (*Aravan lyssavirus*, *Australian bat lyssavirus*, *Bokeloh bat lyssavirus*, *Duvenhage lyssavirus*, *European bat 1 lyssavirus*, *European bat 2 lyssavirus*, *Irkut lyssavirus*, *Khujand lyssavirus*, and *Gannoruwa bat lyssavirus*); however, they are less effective against the highly divergent lyssaviruses found in phylogroup 2 (*Lagos bat virus*, *Mokola virus*, and *Shimoni bat lyssavirus*) and phylogroup 3 (*West Caucasian bat virus*, *Ikoma virus*, and *Lleida bat virus*).

DESCRIPTION OF THE AGENT

Lyssavirus virions are bullet-shaped, measure approximately 180 by 75 nm, and consist of five structural proteins: the glycoprotein (G), matrix protein (M), nucleoprotein (N), phosphoprotein (P), and large polymerase protein (L) (Fig. 2). The virus is contained in an envelope bilayer derived from the host cell cytoplasmic membrane during viral budding. Peplomers, G protein trimeric spike inserts of approximately 10 nm, are found within the surface of the virus envelope. The rabies virus G protein binds with host cell surface receptors (adsorption), initiating a cascade in the infectious cycle and replication. Virus-neutralizing antibodies to the G protein produced after vaccination or natural infection may inhibit this process. The inner surface lining of the envelope is formed by the M protein, which binds with the G protein envelope and the viral ribonucleoprotein (RNP) core.

The RNP is composed of tightly wound viral RNA, encapsulated by the phosphorylated N protein and associated with the P and L proteins. All lyssaviruses contain nonsegmented genomes (RNA) of approximately 12 kb. The RNA-nucleoprotein complex is responsible for transcription of genomic RNA into five polyadenylated mRNAs, which are translated into the structural proteins, and for viral replication by providing a template to synthesize complementary full-length (negative-sense) genomic RNA. During assembly, the coiling RNP-M protein binds with the G protein as the completed virus buds from the plasma membrane (6, 7). From a diagnostic viewpoint, the N and G proteins and viral RNA have been the focus of most laboratory research evaluations. Rabies diagnosis in postmortem brain tissues is based on the detection of intracellular viral inclusions, which are collections of RNP. Because the RABV G protein and host cell receptor interactions initiate the infection cycle, the G protein is directly involved in pathogenesis and virulence, induction of immune responses, and binding of neutralizing antibodies. Vaccines prepared from whole virions, purified RABV G proteins, and recombinant viral vaccines encoding RABV G proteins have been used to successfully immunize and protect animals from RABV infections (8–10). In addition, detection of antibody to the G protein has been used as a method to evaluate vaccine potency (10). More detailed reviews of virus replication and virus pathogenesis have been published (11–13). Descriptions of the RABV epidemiology, transmission, clinical signs, and diagnosis are generalizable to the other lyssaviruses.

EPIDEMIOLOGY AND TRANSMISSION

Rabies is a zoonotic disease (primarily an animal disease that may be transmitted to humans). All mammals are susceptible. Although RABV is endemic on five of seven continents, the geographic distributions of the other lyssaviruses are more localized: *Lagos bat virus*, *Shimoni bat virus*, *Mokola virus*, *Duvenhage virus*, and *Ikoma virus* have been

*This chapter contains information presented by Lillian A. Orciari, Cathleen A. Hanlon, and Richard Franka in chapter 94 of the 11th edition of this *Manual*.

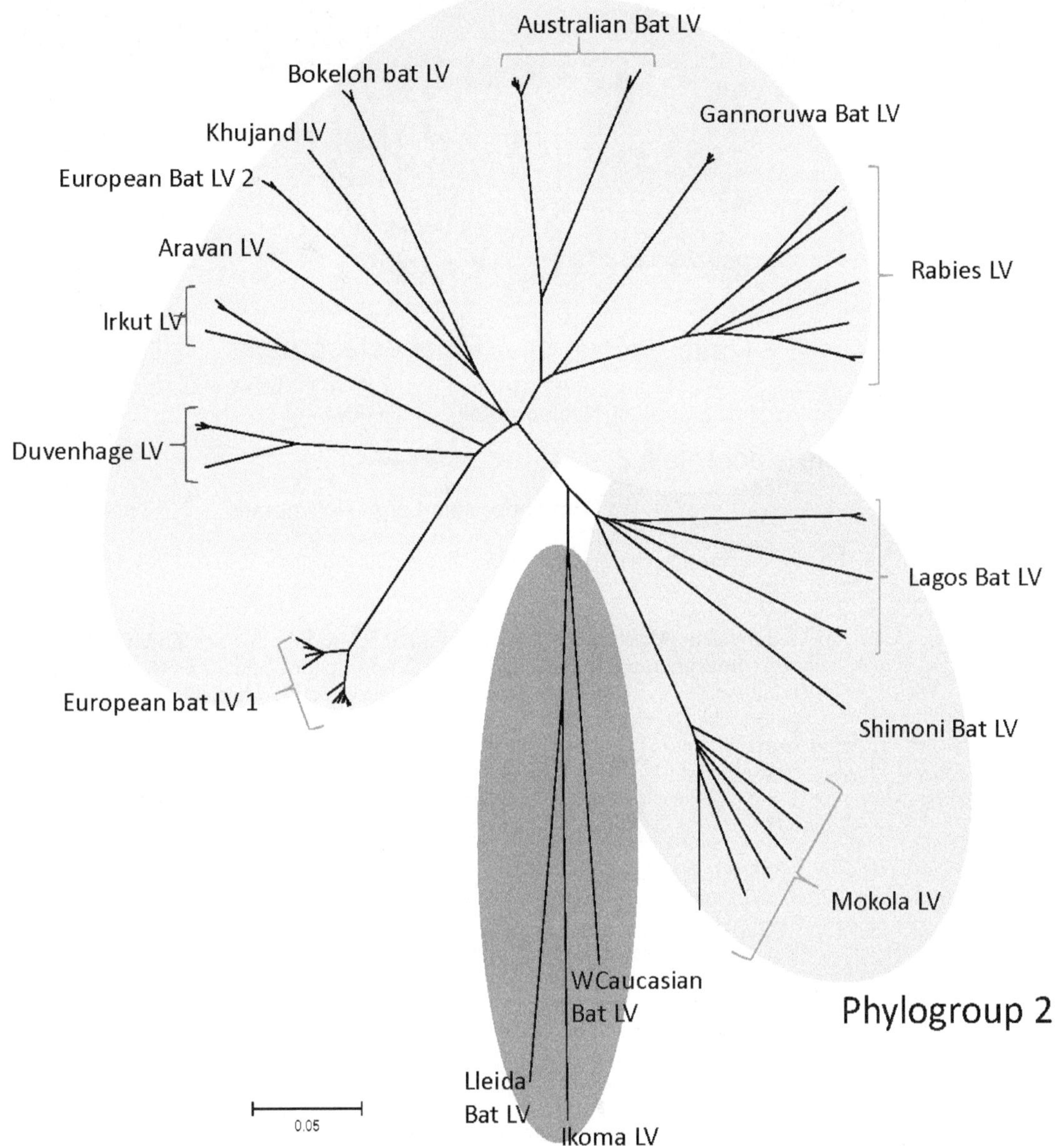

FIGURE 1 Lyssavirus diversity was demonstrated by genome sequence analysis performed using neighbor-joining, maximum-likelihood, and minimum-evolution methods and bootstrap analysis of 500 trees. The consensus tree constructed by the minimum-evolution methods demonstrated topology and lineages consistent with previously published research (1–4). Representative sequences were available for all 14 lyssavirus and 2 proposed lyssaviruses in GenBank. Phylogroup 1 (blue) is composed of RABV and closely related lyssaviruses against which the currently available rabies biologics are effective. These biologics are, however, not effective with the divergent lyssaviruses in phylogroups 2 (yellow) and 3 (pink).

detected only in Africa; *European bat lyssaviruses*, *Bokeloh bat lyssavirus*, and *Lleida bat virus* have been detected only in Europe; *Australian bat lyssavirus* is found exclusively in Australia; and *Aravan bat virus*, *Khujand bat virus*, *Irkut bat virus*, and *West Caucasian bat virus* are restricted to isolations in Eurasia. At present, *Gannoruwa bat lyssavirus (proposed)* has been found only on the island of Sri Lanka. The only lyssavirus detected in the Americas has been RABV. In the United States, more than 6,000 rabies cases are diagnosed annually in animals. The predominant terrestrial reservoir species are raccoons in the Eastern states, skunks in California and the north central and south central states,

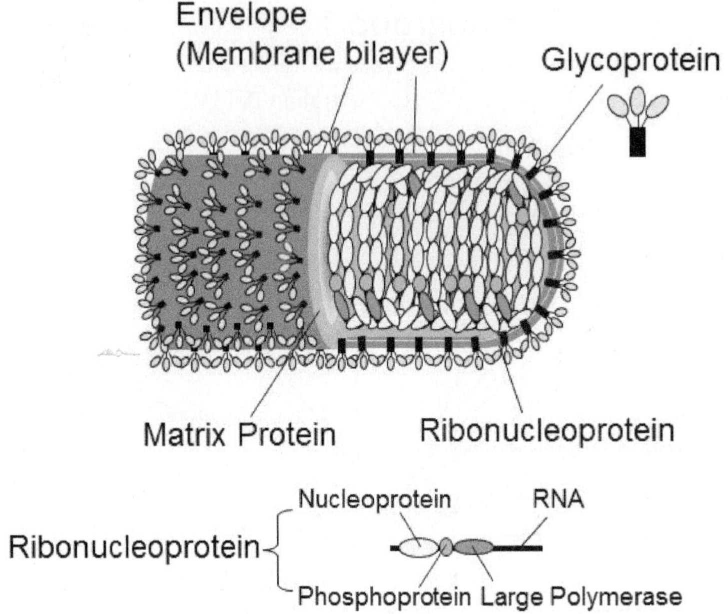

FIGURE 2 Diagram of lyssavirus morphology and structural proteins.

gray foxes in Arizona, Arctic and red foxes in Alaska, and mongooses in Puerto Rico. In addition, there are more than 16 distinct RABVs associated with unique species of insectivorous bats throughout their ranges in North America. Although dogs represent a major reservoir species in most developing nations, enzootic canine rabies virus variants were eradicated in the United States and other developed countries, primarily due to mandatory dog vaccination and stray animal control (14, 15).

Human rabies cases are rare in developed countries where canine rabies is controlled and access to prophylactic biologics is ideal. Fewer than four cases are reported annually in the United States. Despite the relative ease of disease prevention in an exposed human, it is estimated that more than 60,000 preventable human deaths worldwide occur annually. Beyond avoiding contact with wild animals and unvaccinated animals, stray animals, or domestic animals with unknown immunization histories, access to appropriate human rabies postexposure prophylaxis remains an urgent global public health need to avert this preventable human mortality.

The main route of transmission is introduction of saliva containing RABV into a wound via the bite of a rabid animal. Virus may be shed via saliva in high quantities. Human rabies cases due to nonbite exposures are extremely rare. Nonbite exposures include scratches, open wounds, and mucous membranes contaminated with a source of RABV, such as infected saliva or central nervous system (CNS) tissues from a rabid animal. Nosocomial infection (inhalation of accidentally aerosolized RABV) and subsequent mucous membrane contact is a potential source of nonbite exposure. Infection by this route, though rare, has been documented (16, 17). No human rabies cases have been associated with fomite (surface contamination) exposures, most likely because the virus is readily inactivated by drying and by agents such as detergents. In the event of an exposure, immediate wound cleansing with soap and water is essential, followed by appropriate urgent medical care; delays in initiation of human rabies postexposure prophylaxis may result in death.

Lyssaviruses are susceptible to a number of common laboratory disinfectants, such as 1:256 quaternary ammonium compound, 0.5% sodium hypochlorite (10% bleach), iodophors, 70% isopropanol, and 70% ethanol. Chemical disinfectants are less effective when used on items contaminated with brain tissues, heavy suspensions of brain tissue, or even virus suspensions in cell culture media with protein supplements. Decontamination of instruments, laboratory glassware, and disposable waste is best achieved by autoclaving at a minimum of 121°C at 15 lb for 60 minutes (18–20).

CLINICAL SIGNIFICANCE

The initial clinical presentation of rabies in humans and animals may be rather unremarkable and nonspecific. The majority of incubation periods range from several weeks to several months after exposure. Following the prodromal period, an acute neurological phase develops. The majority of rabies cases manifest as an encephalitic form, and less than 20% are observed as a paralytic presentation. Among patients exhibiting classical encephalitic symptoms, generalized arousal or hyperexcitability, including periods of confusion, hallucinations, agitation, or aggressive behavior, may occur, with intermittent lucid periods. Clinical progression may be characterized by difficulty swallowing, hypersalivation, lacrimation, sweating, dilated pupils, and autonomic dysfunction. Cranial nerve dysfunction may include anisocoria and facial or tongue paralysis. Hydrophobic and aerophobic spasms can be severe. In the end stage, multiple systems may be unstable, often leading to coma and invariably death. Rabies continues to have one of the highest case fatality rates of all known illnesses caused by infectious agents.

The paralytic form of presentation includes flaccid muscle weakness, frequently spreading in an ascending pattern to the extremities. In some cases, laryngeal and facial muscle weakness or bilateral deafness occur. These cases may resemble Guillain-Barré syndrome. Other symptoms include urinary incontinence and priapism. Hydrophobia is less common with the paralytic form, but mild inspiratory spasms may be present. Cardiopulmonary complications and instability usually result in cardiac arrest and death (21).

There is no definitive treatment for rabies after clinical signs are apparent. Appropriate management of a patient with rabies is supportive, usually progressing rapidly to respiratory protection through sedation and intubation, as well as complex medical management in attempts to stabilize cardiopulmonary and other major organ system function. Despite the successful outcome of intensive medical management of a high school student from Wisconsin in 2004, specific rabies antiviral treatment does not exist, and the prognosis remains inexorably grim in most cases. The latest information on experimental management of rabies cases may be found on the Medical College of Wisconsin website: http://www.mcw.edu/Pediatrics/InfectiousDiseases/PatientCare/rabies.htm.

Administration of rabies vaccine and human rabies immune globulin (HRIG) to patients with laboratory-confirmed rabies has no proven efficacy, may complicate antemortem testing, and may accelerate the disease process and patient's demise.

All potential RABV exposures need to be evaluated on a case-by-case basis. True human exposures (bite or mucous membrane) to suspect animals or animals proven rabid should receive prompt medical intervention and postexposure prophylaxis as outlined in the Advisory Committee on Immunization Practices (ACIP) guidelines (22), as follows.

Unvaccinated individuals exposed to a rabid animal should receive HRIG at a dose of 20 IU/kg of body weight. The HRIG should be infiltrated around the wound, and any remaining volume should be given at a site distant from where the vaccine was administered. In addition, four doses of a human RABV licensed for use in the United States should be administered on days 0, 3, 7, and 14, and if indicated, a fifth dose should be given at day 28 following exposure. Individuals who previously received immunization against rabies require only two doses of vaccine on days 0 and 3, regardless of the current rabies virus-neutralizing antibody (VNA) titer (22).

Individuals at high risk for RABV exposure (laboratorians, field biologists, and veterinarians) are recommended to receive pre-exposure rabies prophylaxis. According to the current ACIP guidelines for prevention of rabies in humans, a pre-exposure series of three doses of modern cell culture RABV (licensed for use in the United States) should be administered intramuscularly in the deltoid on days 0, 7, and 21 or 28. For all individuals in the high-risk group, determination of rabies VNA titer every 2 years is recommended. Individuals working under higher risk for rabies exposure, such as in research or high-volume diagnostic laboratories, typically have their VNA levels monitored more frequently, such as every 6 months. Pre-exposure vaccination and monitoring of detectable neutralizing antibodies does not ensure protection from a particular exposure. Upon exposure, previously vaccinated individuals require cleansing of the wound and postexposure rabies vaccine doses on days 0 and 3 to prevent clinical disease.

COLLECTION, TRANSPORT, AND STORAGE OF SPECIMENS

A summary of tests, required samples, and shipping and storage conditions is presented in Table 1. Rabies specimen submission guidelines and forms may be found at the Centers for Disease Control and Prevention (CDC) website, https://www.cdc.gov/rabies/resources/specimen-submission-guidelines.html. Diagnosis of rabies in animals requires postmortem examination of the brain. An adequate sample consists of a full cross section of the brain stem (pons, medulla, or midbrain areas) and cerebellum (vermis and right and left lateral lobes inclusive). Removal of CNS tissues should be performed by trained, vaccinated personnel wearing personal protective equipment (at a minimum, a closed-front gown or a lab coat with sleeves, double latex and nitrile or heavy rubber gloves, an N95 respirator, a face shield, safety glasses, and shoe covers). Information on sample collection for postmortem rabies diagnosis in animals may be found at https://www.cdc.gov/rabies/pdf/RabiesDFASPv2.pdf.

Information regarding samples for diagnosis of rabies in humans is available at https://www.cdc.gov/rabies/specific_groups/doctors/ante_mortem.html. The antemortem diagnosis of rabies in humans requires the collection of fresh saliva (no preservatives or transport media), a 5- to 6-mm-diameter full-thickness skin biopsy specimen (nuchal) from the nape of the neck at the hairline, including a minimum of 10 hair follicles (placed on gauze moistened with sterile water with no preservatives or transport media), and serum and cerebrospinal fluid (CSF). The saliva is tested by real-time reverse transcription PCR (RT-PCR). The skin sample is also tested by real-time RT-PCR, and cryostat sections are tested for RABV antigen by a direct fluorescent-antibody (DFA) test. The serum and CSF samples are analyzed by several methods, including rabies virus neutralization using the rapid fluorescent focus inhibition test (RFFIT), and for rabies virus-specific IgG and IgM antibodies that bind to rabies antigens (proteins) in rabies-infected cells by indirect fluorescent antibody (IFA) test. Other samples, such as brain biopsy specimens for RABV antigen detection by the DFA test and real-time RT-PCR and cornea impressions, may be useful in diagnosis of rabies, but these samples are not routinely recommended because of the invasiveness of the collection methods and potential harmful sequelae. For the optimal sensitivity and specificity of antemortem diagnosis, all four samples (serum, CSF, saliva, and skin biopsy samples) should be tested. In some cases, repeated sequential sets of samples may be required to rule out or confirm a diagnosis. Patient specimen and information submission forms may be obtained on https://www.cdc.gov/laboratory/specimen-submission/pdf/form-50-34.pdf and https://www.cdc.gov/rabies/pdf/rorform.pdf. The CDC Rabies Laboratory should be consulted before sample collection and submission (phone, 404-639-1050).

For postmortem diagnosis of rabies in humans, brain samples consisting of a cross section of brain stem and cerebellum, vermis, and right and left lobes are necessary. These samples are tested for RABV antigen, and if it is present, further antigenic and genetic characterization is performed. Formalin-fixed tissues can be analyzed for histopathology and antigen detection. However, these samples are not recommended for primary diagnosis of rabies unless fresh brain tissues are unavailable. Formalin-fixed samples require lengthy preparation time for processing, embedding in paraffin, and sectioning prior to high-complexity experimental diagnostic techniques, which can delay a diagnosis. Postmortem or retained antemortem serum and CSF may be quite useful in confirming a postmortem diagnosis.

The shipment of samples to a testing laboratory for rabies diagnosis should follow the U.S. Department of Transportation's guide to safe transport of infectious substances (https://hazmatonline.phmsa.dot.gov/services/publication_documents/Transporting%20Infectious%20Substances%20Safely.pdf). Packaging of clinical samples for rabies diagnosis should fulfill International Air Transport Association (IATA) regulations for shipment of biological substances, category B, UN 3373. Cell culture isolates and stock virus suspensions carry a higher infection risk, and their packaging should fulfill the IATA regulations for category A, UN 2814 (infectious substance affecting humans)

TABLE 1 Routine tests for rabies diagnosis[a]

Analysis	Test method	Detection	Sample	Source	Requirements	Provider	Results
Microscopic examination	Specialized stains (e.g., H&E and Sellers)	Eosinophilic intracytoplasmic inclusions	Postmortem CNS	Human or animal	Brain stem, cerebellum, hippocampus	Pathology laboratories (hospital, veterinary)	Detects eosinophilic intracytoplasmic inclusions; low sensitivity (60–80%)
Antigen detection by immunofluorescence	DFA	Rabies virus antigen	Postmortem CNS	Human or animal	Full cross section of brain stem and cerebellum	State public health, veterinary laboratories, CDC	Detects rabies virus specific antigen; very high sensitivity (100%)
Antigen detection by immunofluorescence	DFA (cryostat)	Rabies virus antigen	Antemortem nuchal biopsy	Human	Full thickness of skin; 5- to 6-mm cryosections	CDC (some regional or national labs)	Detects rabies virus specific antigen
Antigen detection by immunofluorescence	FF DFA	Rabies virus antigen	FF postmortem CNS	Human or animal	Full cross section of brain stem and cerebellum	CDC (some regional or national labs)	Detects rabies virus specific antigen; very high sensitivity (~100%)
Antigen detection by IHC	IHC	Rabies virus antigen	FF postmortem CNS	Human or animal	Full cross section of brain stem and cerebellum	CDC (some regional or national labs)	Detects rabies virus specific antigen; very high sensitivity (~100%)
Antigen detection by IHC	DRIT	Rabies virus antigen	Postmortem CNS	Human or animal	Full cross section of brain stem and cerebellum	CDC, U.S. Department of Agriculture (some regional or national labs)	Detects rabies virus specific antigen; very high sensitivity (~100%)
Nucleic acid	Real-time RT-PCR	Rabies virus RNA	Postmortem CNS	Human or animal	50 mg of brain stem and cerebellum	CDC (some regional or national labs)	Produces specific RT-PCR amplicons; very sensitive (detects <1 IU) but related to primer specificity
Nucleic acid	Real-time RT-PCR	Rabies virus RNA	Antemortem saliva, throat, skin, other	Human	100 µl of fluid samples or ≤ 50 mg of tissue	CDC (some regional or national labs)	Produces specific RT-PCR amplicons; very sensitive (detects < 1 IU)
Virus isolation	Cell culture (e.g., MNA) and animal inoculation (e.g., MI)	Infectious rabies virus	Postmortem CNS	Human or animal	20% brain homogenate (brain stem and cerebellum)	State public health, veterinary laboratories, CDC	Detects infectious rabies virus
Serology (virus neutralization)	RFFIT, FAVN, MNT	Rabies virus-neutralizing antibodies	Antemortem or postmortem serum or CSF	Human or animal	Serum or CSF	CDC (some commercial, regional or national labs)	Detects neutralizing antibodies. NT are useful in determining immunization status.
Serology by indirect IFA test	IFA	Rabies virus IgG or IgM antibodies	Antemortem or postmortem	Human or animal	Serum or CSF	CDC (some regional or national labs)	Detects specific rabies virus IgM and IgG antibodies from serum or CSF; very sensitive as a diagnostic technique

[a]H&E, hematoxylin and eosin; FF, formalin fixed; NT, neutralization tests; MI, mouse inoculation test; MNT, mouse neutralization test; IU, infectious unit.

and UN 2900 (affecting animals). Fresh-frozen samples for rabies testing should be sent on dry ice (or ice packs for same-day delivery) to the diagnostic laboratory by the most expedient transport or courier method. Paraffin-blocked tissues and tissue sections (slides) should be shipped at ambient temperatures and never frozen.

The validity of laboratory diagnostic tests depends on optimal collection and storage of the samples. The ideal storage temperature for fresh brain tissues for RABV antigen detection, virus isolation, and real-time RT-PCR is −80°C. Storage for short intervals, such as 48 hours or less at 4°C or 4 weeks or less at −20°C, may be adequate for samples that are to be analyzed for RABV antigen. Tissues placed in 10% buffered formalin should remain in the fixative a minimum of 24 to 48 hours at ambient temperature. Formalin-fixed brain tissues should be stored in 70% ethanol at room temperature for long-term storage and never frozen. Paraffin-blocked tissues and tissue sections (slides) should be stored at ambient temperatures and never frozen.

The ideal storage and shipping temperatures for saliva samples for real-time RT-PCR and virus isolation are −80°C or below. Skin biopsy samples for real-time RT-PCR and antigen detection should also be stored at −80°C. Samples for antigen detection may be stored for short intervals at −20°C before testing. Serum and CSF samples for rabies serologic testing should be stored at −20°C or below but may be stored for short intervals prior to testing at 4°C. Whole-blood samples should be centrifuged, and only the serum portion should be submitted for testing. Whole blood should never be shipped in the same container with samples on dry ice, because there is a risk of freezing and hemolysis regardless of packing insulation. Serum samples that demonstrate visible signs of hemolysis or appear chylous are unsatisfactory for testing. Other biological fluids (e.g., vitreous fluids, tracheal washings, and tears) for real-time RT-PCR or virus isolation require storage at −80°C or below.

DIRECT DETECTION METHODS

Direct methods may be used to detect histopathological changes and viral antigen (inclusions) and to observe virion morphology. These methods provide rapid diagnosis within minutes to hours without the need for amplification of virus by isolation, such as in cell culture, or amplification of the viral genome in RT-PCR.

Microscopy

Microscopic examination methods may utilize routine stains (e.g., hematoxylin and eosin) to examine abnormal histopathology consistent with encephalomyelitis, or more specialized stains (e.g., Sellers, Mann's, and Giemsa stains) to observe typical viral eosinophilic intracytoplasmic inclusions, such as classical Negri bodies within neurons (23, 24). Historically, Sellers stain (2:1 methylene blue and basic fuchsin) was most often used for Negri body detection. In contrast with more advanced, sensitive antigen detection methods, this staining procedure is most successfully performed on brain tissues (hippocampi, cerebral cortex pyramidal cells, cerebellum, and Purkinje cells) during the later stages of disease, when inclusions are most abundant and more easily detected. Brain impression slides are stained for 2 to 10 minutes in Sellers stain (the time needed varies depending on the thickness of the impression) and then rinsed with tap water. Typically, intracytoplasmic magenta inclusions that are oval or round with dark blue basophilic granules appear within rabies virus-infected cells of the CNS. Although of historical importance, this method has limitations in specificity and sensitivity. For example, when properly performed, the Sellers staining technique may identify Negri bodies in 50 to 80% of rabid animals.

Observation of virions by electron microscopy allows the examination of their ultrastructure, shape, and size. The technique provides supportive evidence of a rhabdovirus infection but requires careful examination by expertly trained personnel of numerous observational fields of the sample. As such, it is impractical and too costly for routine diagnosis (25).

Antigen Detection

DFA Test

The standard test for RABV antigen detection in CNS tissues is the DFA test. This test is relatively easy to perform by highly trained personnel with specialized equipment, highly specific, approximates 100% sensitivity, and can be completed in 3 or 4 hours. The CDC's protocol for postmortem diagnosis of rabies in animals by DFA testing may be obtained at https://www.cdc.gov/rabies/pdf/RabiesDFASPv2.pdf. In contrast to the nonspecific staining of viral inclusions observed with histologic stains, the RABV diagnostic conjugates consist of antibodies to the whole virion or the RNP, labeled with fluorescein isothiocyanate (FITC). Within infected brain cells, there are abundant collections of RABV proteins (antigen), especially RNP. The conjugates may be hyperimmune polyclonal or monoclonal antibodies directed against highly conserved RABV epitopes.

Impression slides are prepared from a cross section of brain stem and cerebellum (right, left, and vermis) or hippocampi (right and left) if the cerebellum is not available and are fixed in acetone for a minimum of 1 hour at −20°C. The brain impression slides are tested with two different anti-rabies virus conjugates to ensure antigen detection of the diverse RABV variants. When the conjugates are added to impressions of RABV-infected brain tissue and incubated for 30 minutes at 37°C, the labeled antibodies bind with the RABV proteins (antigens) and form specific antigen-antibody-FITC complexes. After the impression slides are washed in phosphate-buffered saline (PBS) twice for 3 to 5 minutes, specific antigen-antibody complexes remain. These complexes fluoresce an intense sparkling apple-green color when observed with a fluorescence microscope equipped with an FITC filter combination. Morphologically, RABV antigen may appear as fluorescing large or small, oval or round inclusions, dust-like particles, or strands (Fig. 3).

DRIT

The direct rapid immunohistochemistry test (DRIT) is an alternative procedure for RABV antigen detection (26). The DRIT uses a cocktail of purified biotinylated anti-rabies virus nucleocapsid monoclonal antibodies (MAbs) to detect RABV antigen. To date, the test has demonstrated sensitivity and specificity equal to that of the DFA test in detecting RABV antigen. The anticipated use for this test method includes confirmatory DFA testing as well as augmentation of passive public health surveillance, since, in contrast with fluorescence microscopy, light microscopy is adaptable to field use. In the United States, the test is currently applied to augment surveillance in samples from animals that have not exposed humans to the virus. However, the DRIT has been accepted by the World Health Organization and World Organization for Animal Health as an alternate test for rabies antigen detection when a fluorescence microscope is not available. Advantages of the procedure include rapidity of the procedure (1 hour to completion), the inactivation of RABV

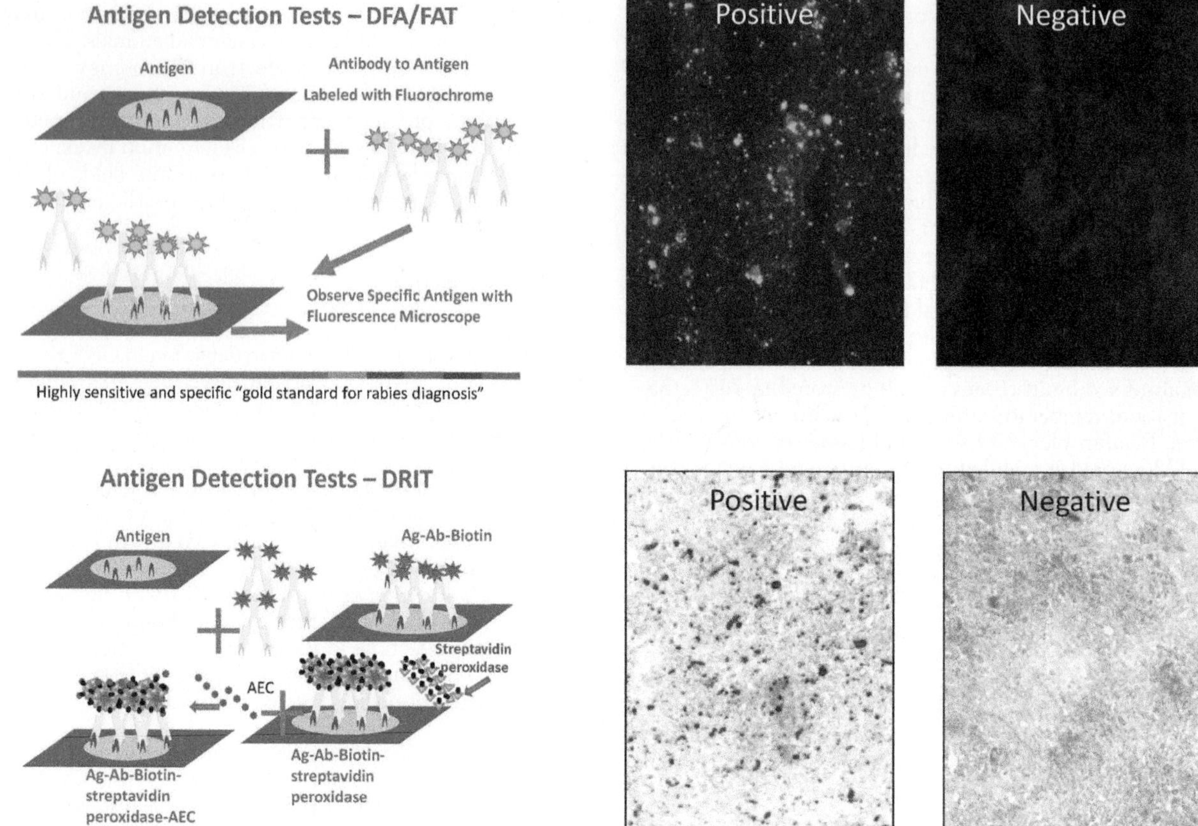

FIGURE 3 Antigen detection by DFA/FAT and DRIT methods. FAT, fluorescent-antibody test.

in test brain impressions by fixation in formalin (in contrast to acetone fixation in the DFA test, which does not completely inactivate RABV), and the minimal equipment requirements (only a standard light microscope). The sample requirements for DRIT are the same as those for the DFA test and other antigen detection methods. (See "Collection, Transport, and Storage of Specimens" above for detailed information.) The DRIT is performed on brain touch impressions prepared as for the DFA test. Slides are fixed in 10% buffered formalin for 10 minutes, rinsed in PBS with 1% Tween 80 (TPBS), and then pretreated with hydrogen peroxide for 10 minutes before primary antibodies are applied. The test is a multistep process involving biotinylated primary antibodies, streptavidin-peroxidase, and 3-amino-9-ethylcarbazole (AEC). First, there is an incubation with biotinylated anti-rabies virus MAbs for 10 minutes, followed by rinsing in TPBS; next is incubation with streptavidin-peroxidase for 10 minutes, followed by rinsing with TPBS; last is incubation with peroxidase substrate (AEC) for 10 minutes to initiate (red) color development, followed by rinsing with distilled water. Slides are counterstained with Gill's hematoxylin for 2 minutes, rinsed with water (and a cover glass is added with water-soluble mounting medium), and observed with a standard light microscope. RABV antigen appears as bright red, large or small, oval or round inclusions, dust-like particles, or strands against a contrasting blue background (Fig. 3).

Formalin-Fixed Tissues

Formalin-fixed CNS tissue samples cannot be tested by the standard DFA test. The fixation process causes chemical cross-linking of proteins. Formalin-fixed tissue samples that have been processed, embedded in paraffin, and sectioned may be tested by a modification of the DFA test for formalin-fixed samples. RABV antigen detection, whether by standard DFA test, DRIT, or modified DFA test on formalin-fixed samples, requires the same tissue sampling of a complete cross section of brain stem and cerebellum. Modifications of the standard DFA test for formalin-fixed samples include heating the slides to 55 to 60°C to melt the paraffin, deparaffinization in xylene, and rehydration of tissue sections in graded alcohols. In addition, a proteinase K digestion for 30 minutes at 37°C is needed for detection of RABV epitopes. Incubation with anti-rabies virus FITC conjugate is longer than the standard DFA test incubation (i.e., 1 hour instead of 30 minutes), and the wash times in PBS (twice at 15 minutes) are longer to clear unbound conjugate from tissue sections (27). The reliability of this method depends on the availability of a high-affinity, highly concentrated polyclonal anti-rabies virus conjugate, because the modified standard DFA test for formalin-fixed tissues may require a working dilution of RABV conjugate as much as 5 to 10 times more concentrated for sensitive and specific detection of RABV antigen in these tissue samples.

An immunohistochemistry (IHC) test for rabies virus antigen detection is an alternative method for formalin-fixed tissue samples that have been processed, embedded in paraffin, and sectioned (28). The IHC protocol also requires heating the slides to 55 to 60°C to melt the paraffin, deparaffinization of tissue sections in xylene, rehydration of tissue sections in graded alcohols, and enzyme digestion but with pronase instead of proteinase K. The remaining IHC test steps are similar to the multistep DRIT: 3% hydrogen peroxide is added for 10 minutes, and the mixture is incubated for 10 minutes to remove endogenous peroxidase activity. Then normal goat serum is added, and slides are incubated for 15 minutes to block nonspecific binding of the primary antibody. The primary anti-rabies virus monoclonal or polyclonal antibodies are added and incubated for 60 minutes. The secondary antispecies biotinylated antibody is added and incubated for 15 minutes, followed by a rinse in TPBS and incubation with streptavidin-peroxidase for 15 minutes. After rinsing with TPBS, slides are incubated with peroxidase substrate, AEC, for 5 to 10 minutes to initiate (red) color development, followed by rinsing with distilled water. Finally, slides are counterstained with Gill's hematoxylin for 2 minutes and rinsed with water, and coverslips are added with water-soluble mounting medium. Slides are observed with a standard light microscope. RABV antigen appears as bright red, large or small, oval or round inclusions or dust-like particles within the cytoplasm of infected neurons against a light blue background of the hematoxylin-stained tissue. Advantages of the IHC test over the standard DFA test modified for formalin-fixed samples include the ability to test for RABV antigen and other etiologies simultaneously by including antibodies to the other agents, the ability to examine the histopathology of tissues, and the ability to observe slides with a standard light microscope rather than fluorescence microscopy. Disadvantages are the time required for the procedure (approximately 6 hours) and the high complexity of the method, requiring optimization of multiple antibodies and reagents.

DFA Test of Nuchal (Neck) Biopsy Specimens

Antemortem DFA tests for RABV antigen are performed on serial 5- to 8-μm tissue cryosections of skin biopsies (from the hairline at the nape of the neck) and provide a rapid method for viral antigen detection in nerves at the base of hair follicles. The DFA test on tissue sections is performed exactly as the standard DFA test on CNS tissues. In its antemortem application, the method has optimized sensitivity but may be negative in early stages of the clinical disease or in later clinical stages if virus-neutralizing antibodies are present. On rare occasions, real-time or nested RT-PCR on a negative DFA test has confirmed a rabies diagnosis when antigen was not present in sufficient quantity to visualize by the DFA test on skin sections.

Nucleic Acid Detection

RT-PCR methods are the most sensitive tests for RABV diagnosis. The sensitivity of RT-PCR depends in part on the sample (type and condition), the integrity of sample handling and storage to preclude contamination and degradation, the particular method of RNA extraction and RT-PCR, the primers selected for amplification, the quality of reagents, individual technical expertise, interpretation of the results, and confirmation methods. The usefulness of traditional RT-PCR as a routine diagnostic test on postmortem (fresh and fixed) CNS tissues is limited. Highly sensitive, broadly reactive, less expensive, and less time-consuming procedures for antigen detection by DFA testing and real-time RT-PCR are more efficient routine tests for rabies diagnosis and confirmatory testing. RT-PCR methods have been essential tools for molecular analysis for decades, but its maximum utility has been the detection of nucleic acid in non-CNS samples (e.g., antemortem saliva, skin, cornea impressions, tears, eye swabs, throat swabs, and postmortem vitreous fluid) when fresh CNS tissues may be unavailable. When all conditions are optimal, traditional RT-PCR can detect as little as 1 infectious unit of RABV. However, real-time or nested RT-PCR increases the sensitivity (10- to 100-fold) to below 1 infectious unit of virus (29, 30). RNA may be limited or degraded in non-CNS samples, and real-time RT-PCR is routinely used on these samples. Until recently, the diversity among lyssaviruses and the lack of specific nondegenerate universal primers have discouraged the use of real-time PCR for detection of rabies virus RNA in non-CNS samples when the rabies virus variant or lyssavirus species is unknown. Recently, broadly reactive rapid real-time RT-PCR assays have been developed for the detection of all lyssaviruses. A newly developed real-time RT-PCR assay named LN34, which uses a combination of degenerate primers and probes has been developed and validated at the CDC for antemortem human and confirmatory postmortem animal testing covered under CLIA (31). The testing has demonstrated sensitivity and specificity equal to that of the DFA test in evaluations to date. The primers and probes of the LN34 assay target the highly conserved noncoding leader region and part of the nucleoprotein coding sequence of the lyssavirus genome and have broad reactivity with all known lyssaviruses.

ISOLATION PROCEDURES

Isolation methods are useful in detecting infectious virus in samples and are sometimes used as confirmatory test alternatives to the standard DFA test. The classical methods include *in vivo* isolation in animals (usually intracerebral inoculation of suckling mice) and *in vitro* virus isolation in cell cultures. For most routine diagnostic needs, the inoculation of cell cultures such as mouse neuroblastoma (MNA; Lonza Inc., Walkersville, MD) or a similar alternative cell culture line, Neuro-2a (CCL 131; ATCC, Rockville, MD), provides the same sensitivity as animal inoculation but with quicker results and without the maintenance required for the use of laboratory animals. For these purposes, 0.4 ml of supernatant from a 20% brain suspension prepared in tissue culture medium with 10% fetal calf serum (MEM10) is inoculated into a suspension of 4×10^6 MNA cells/2 ml and incubated for 1 hour at 37°C. To maximize infection of the cells, gentle mixing of the suspension is performed every 15 minutes. The cell suspension is diluted to a volume of 10 ml with MEM10, 6 ml is transferred to one 25-ml cell culture flask, and the remaining suspension (4 ml) is transferred to 12 Teflon-coated 6-mm slides (or other cell culture slides). At least one slide should be acetone fixed daily and examined by DFA testing for RABV antigen. At least one additional passage of the cell culture (performed in 3 to 5 days) is required to rule out rabies. Ideally, *in vivo* testing use should be reserved for efficacy and safety studies for biologics or virulence and pathogenesis studies. Cell cultures may be useful in the propagation, amplification, and quantification of virus and antibodies; the production of vaccines; determination of the safety of vaccine lots; and the study of rabies virus pathogenesis in particular cells (32, 33).

IDENTIFICATION

As previously described in detail, identification of a *Lyssavirus* infection is made typically by direct examination of brain impressions and demonstration of specific viral inclusions (antigen) by DFA testing. Isolates are also identified in brains of inoculated mice and cell cultures by DFA testing. Electron microscopy may be used to determine the morphologic identification of lyssaviruses by examination of the virion ultrastructure in cell cultures or CNS tissues.

Further secondary characterization of *Lyssavirus* infection may be made by antigenic typing with MAbs, genetic typing with sequence analysis, or investigating patterns of cross-neutralization.

TYPING SYSTEMS

Rabies viruses may be easily identified by antigenic and molecular methods as being associated with the broad groups of carnivore and bat variants. Through antigenic analysis, at least five major reservoirs are detectable among carnivores in the United States. Genetic typing adds resolution and identifies seven distinct virus lineages among the current variants. Antigenic typing is less useful in certain cases involving rabid bats. Nucleotide sequence analysis adds resolution when these bat variant samples and others are being studied. Typing methods are useful under a variety of circumstances, such as determining the RABV variants in human cases with unclear or unknown exposure histories, discovering the emergence of new viruses, monitoring the epidemiologic spread or reemergence of virus in defined geographical areas, detecting spillover or host switching of variants from the predominant host species to another species, and monitoring the success of rabies vaccination programs through characterization of positive samples.

Antigenic Typing

Antigenic typing with MAbs can be performed by an IFA test on acetone-fixed brain impression slides or RABV-infected cell culture grown on slides or by the indirect rapid immunohistochemistry test on formalin-fixed brain impression slides or cell culture slides (34, 35). If direct brain impressions are used, the best results are obtained when 75 to 100% of the microscope fields contain viral antigen. If insufficient antigen is present, it is necessary to amplify the virus by inoculating cell cultures or animals. A panel of seven commercially available murine anti-rabies virus N MAbs may be used to distinguish RABV variants by the different reaction patterns. Antigenic typing methods are less expensive, rapid, and easily performed to determine RABV variants in a few hours. Limitations include the necessity for amplification when antigen amounts are inadequate and a lack of resolution for certain terrestrial and bat rabies virus variants. If antigenic typing results are inconclusive, additional testing can be performed at reference laboratories such as the CDC, which has a more extensive panel of MAbs and resources for sequence analysis (36).

Nucleotide Sequence Analysis

Genetic typing methods for molecular epidemiologic studies have become more routine. The N gene has been the one most frequently used in molecular epidemiology studies. Studies have focused the analyses on short sequences of less than 400 nucleotides; however, current technologies have expanded the focus from partial gene sequences to whole viral genomes (1–4). Currently, there are thousands of N gene sequences (complete and partial) in GenBank for comparison. Lyssavirus researchers typically focus on whole-genome analysis by second-generation sequencing methods and use Sanger sequencing when necessary for resolution of small or difficult regions (4). These data may assist in understanding evolutionary relationships between lyssaviruses (Fig. 1), understanding specific gene functions in host species, and predicting viral pathogenesis, replication, and virion formation.

SEROLOGIC TESTS

The serologic tests for RABV antibody include rabies virus neutralization assays and antibody-binding assay methods. Each varies in sensitivity, specificity, type of antibody detected, and the viral antigen (protein) recognized. These methods are most robust when applied in parallel on sequential samples used to diagnose or monitor rabies in humans (37).

Neutralization Tests

Neutralization tests are essential tools for the prediction of an adequate response to immunization against rabies and for the specific diagnosis of rabies during the later clinical stages. Neutralization of RABV relies on antibodies directed to the outer glycoprotein antigens; these are functional assays measuring performance against active viral infection of cells in culture or, historically, in mice infected with rabies, along with dilutions of test serum. The historic mouse neutralization test has been largely replaced by the RFFIT and a modification of it, the fluorescent antibody virus neutralization test (FAVN) (performed in microtiter 96-well plates). All of these test methods measure the ability of RABV antibodies in serum or CSF samples to neutralize a known standard challenge virus dose. The RFFIT and FAVN are most frequently used to determine the immunization status of vaccinated humans and animals, respectively. When performed in qualified laboratories by qualified personnel, both test methods demonstrate acceptable and similar sensitivity and specificity in determining RABV-neutralizing antibodies; test results are best compared when converted to international units per milliliter on the basis of *a priori* criteria specifying acceptable performance of an international reference standard in each particular run of an assay method (37–40).

IFA Tests

IFA tests are sensitive methods for detection of IgM and IgG antibodies that have bound to rabies virus antigen within infected cells. Binding activity may be present in human serum and CSF and is thus a useful component of the battery of tests applied for antemortem diagnosis (27, 37). It appears that the IFA test may measure antibodies against internal RABV proteins such as RNP rather than rabies G surface protein. Serum or CSF samples are titrated and added to acetone-fixed cell culture slides infected with a RABV challenge virus strain (CVS-11). The endpoint antibody titer is the last dilution demonstrating specific fluorescence. IFA titers are not comparable with levels of *in vivo* virus-neutralizing antibody to the rabies virus G surface proteins.

ANTIMICROBIAL SUSCEPTIBILITIES

As previously described, no specific rabies antiviral biologics are currently licensed, and the prognosis remains inexorably grim. Once clinical signs are present, rabies remains fatal in more than 99% of cases. For the most current information on experimental recommendations and approaches, consult the rabies registry at the Medical College of Wisconsin website: https://www.mcw.edu/Pediatrics/Infectious-Diseases/Patient-Care/Rabies.htm.

EVALUATION, INTERPRETATION, AND REPORTING OF RESULTS

Written protocols, which include quality assurance and quality control measures, are essential for all diagnostic tests.

All reagents for antigen detection should be optimized before use with known positive samples from two or more RABV variants endemic to the geographic region and known negative control samples. The accuracy and limitations of each diagnostic test should be understood before interpretation of the test results (Table 1). The national standard protocol in the United States for rabies diagnosis in postmortem brain tissues is the DFA test. Procedural requirements of the standard DFA test, DRIT, real-time RT-PCR, and isolation methods maximize sensitivity by testing the CNS tissues most likely to be positive in rabid animals (brain stem and cerebellum). The problem of cross-contamination in direct detection and amplification methods can be avoided by processing necropsy samples separately, using separate containers for acetone fixation and rinse steps of DFA tests, and using different dedicated laboratory areas for processing RNA and cDNA samples for RT-PCR. Multiple readers are required to evaluate each of the diagnostic tests and provide quality assurance. Confirmatory DFA testing is required for all rabies diagnostic tests with weak reactions or unusual results (atypical morphology, atypical reactions patterns, and epidemiologic inconsistencies). Samples with nonspecific reactions and inconclusive results should be sent to a reference laboratory for confirmation and alternative testing methods. The incorporation of the CLIA-validated LN34 real-time RT-PCR assay as an additional confirmatory test increases confidence in resolution of indeterminate DFA tests. The timeliness of reporting results directly affects medical intervention in humans and management of exposed animals. Ideally, a primary rabies diagnosis from CNS tissues of suspect animals (or humans) should be made in 24 to 48 hours so that potentially exposed humans and animals may be appropriately managed for the optimal prevention of human and animal rabies.

We thank Michael Niezgoda for providing photomicrographs and Claire E. Hartloge for reviewing the manuscript. We also acknowledge the contributions of other members of the CDC Poxvirus and Rabies Branch.

Use of trade names and commercial sources is for identification only and does not imply endorsement by the U.S. Department of Health and Human Services. The findings and conclusions in this report are those of the authors and do not necessarily represent the views of the funding agency.

REFERENCES

1. **Walker PJ, Blasdell KR, Calisher CH, Dietzgen RG, Kondo H, Kurath G, Longdon B, Stone DM, Tesh RB, Tordo N, Vasilakis N, Whitfield AE, ICTV Report Consortium.** 2018. ICTV Virus Taxonomy Profile: Rhabdoviridae. *J Gen Virol* **99:**447-448.
2. **Marston DA, Ellis RJ, Wise EL, Aréchiga-Ceballos N, Freuling CM, Banyard AC, McElhinney LM, de Lamballerie X, Müller T, Fooks AR, Echevarría JE.** 2017. Complete genome sequence of Lleida bat lyssavirus. *Genome Announc* **5:**e01427-16. 10.1128/genomeA.01427-16.
3. **Gunawardena PS, Marston DA, Ellis RJ, Wise EL, Karawita AC, Breed AC, McElhinney LM, Johnson N, Banyard AC, Fooks AR.** 2016. Lyssavirus in Indian flying foxes, Sri Lanka. *Emerg Infect Dis* **22:**1456–1459.
4. **Horton DL, Banyard AC, Marston DA, Wise E, Selden D, Nunez A, Hicks D, Lembo T, Cleaveland S, Peel AJ, Kuzmin IV, Rupprecht CE, Fooks AR.** 2014. Antigenic and genetic characterization of a divergent African virus, Ikoma lyssavirus. *J Gen Virol* **95:**1025–1032.
5. **Wiktor TJ, Flamand A, Koprowski H.** 1980. Use of monoclonal antibodies in diagnosis of rabies virus infection and differentiation of rabies and rabies-related viruses. *J Virol Methods* **1:**33–46.
6. **Wunner WH.** 2007. Rabies virus, p 23–68. *In* Jackson AC, Wunner WH (ed), *Rabies*, 2nd ed. Academic Press, San Diego, CA.
7. **Mebatsion T, Weiland F, Conzelmann K-K.** 1999. Matrix protein of rabies virus is responsible for the assembly and budding of bullet-shaped particles and interacts with the transmembrane spike glycoprotein G. *J Virol* **73:** 242–250.
8. **Brown CM, Slavinski S, Ettestad P, Sidwa TJ, Sorhage FE, National Association of State Public Health Veterinarians, Compendium of Animal Rabies Prevention and Control Committee.** 2016. Compendium of animal rabies prevention and control, 2016. *J Am Vet Med Assoc* **248:** 505–517.
9. **Maki J, Guiot A-L, Aubert M, Brochier B, Cliquet F, Hanlon CA, King R, Oertli EH, Rupprecht CE, Schumacher C, Slate D, Yakobson B, Wohlers A, Lankau EW.** 2017. Oral vaccination of wildlife using a vaccinia–rabies-glycoprotein recombinant virus vaccine (RABORAL V-RG®): a global review. *Vet Res (Faisalabad)* **48:**57.
10. **Brown LJ, Rosatte RC, Fehlner-Gardiner C, Bachmann P, Ellison JA, Jackson FR, Taylor JS, Davies C, Donovan D.** 2014. Oral vaccination and protection of red foxes (*Vulpes vulpes*) against rabies using ONRAB, an adenovirus-rabies recombinant vaccine. *Vaccine* **32:**984–989.
11. **Albertini AA, Baquero E, Ferlin A, Gaudin Y.** 2012. Molecular and cellular aspects of rhabdovirus entry. *Viruses* **4:** 117–139.
12. **Dietzschold B, Li J, Faber M, Schnell M.** 2008. Concepts in the pathogenesis of rabies. *Future Virol* **3:**481–490
13. **Hooper DC, Roy A, Kean RB, Phares TW, Barkhouse DA.** 2011. Therapeutic immunce clearance of rabies virus from the CNS. *Future Virol* **6:**387–397.
14. **Ma X, Monroe BP, Cleaton JM, Orciari LA, Yager P, Li Y, Kirby JD, Blanton JD, Petersen BW, Wallace RM.** 2018. Rabies surveillance in the United States during 2016. *J Am Vet Med Assoc* **252:**945–957.
15. **World Health Organization.** 2013. World Health Organization Expert Consultation on Rabies, Second Report. WHO Technical Report Series 982. World Health Organization, Geneva, Switzerland.
16. **Center for Disease Control.** 1977. Follow-up on rabies—New York. *MMWR Morb Mortal Wkly Rep* **26:**249–250.
17. **Winkler WG, Fashinell TR, Leffingwell L, Howard P, Conomy P.** 1973. Airborne rabies transmission in a laboratory worker. *JAMA* **226:**1219–1221.
18. **Chosewood LC, Wilson DE (ed).** 2009. *Biosafety in Microbiological and Biomedical Laboratories*, 5th ed. U.S. Department of Health and Human Services publication no. (CDC) 21-111. U.S. Department of Health and Human Services, Washington, D.C. http://www.cdc.gov/biosafety/publications/bmbl5/index.htm/. Accessed 13 September 2017.
19. **Kaplan MM, Wiktor T, Koprowski H.** 1966. An intracerebral assay procedure in mice for chemical inactivation of rabies virus. *Bull World Health Organ* **34:**293–297.
20. **Aiello R, Zecchin B, Tiozzo Caenazzo S, Cattoli G, De Benedictis P.** 2016. Disinfection protocols for necropsy equipment in rabies laboratories: safety of personnel and diagnostic outcome. *J Virol Methods* **234:**75–79.
21. **Jackson AC.** 2007. Human disease, p 309–340. *In* Jackson AC, Wunner WH (ed), *Rabies*, 2nd ed. Academic Press, San Diego, CA.
22. **Centers for Disease Control and Prevention.** 2010. Use of (4-dose) reduced vaccine schedule for post-exposure prophylaxis to prevent human rabies, recommendations of the Advisory Committee on Immunization Practices. *MMWR Recomm Rep* **59**(RR-2)**:**1–9.
23. **Lepine P, Atanasiu P.** 1996. Histopathological diagnosis, p 66–79. *In* Meslin FX, Kaplan MM, Koprowski H (ed), *Laboratory Techniques in Rabies*, 4th ed. World Health Organization, Geneva, Switzerland.
24. **Tierkel ES, Atanasiu P.** 1996. Rapid microscopic examination for Negri bodies and preparation of specimens for biological tests, p 55–65. *In* Meslin FX, Kaplan MM,

Koprowski H (ed), *Laboratory Techniques in Rabies*, 4th ed. World Health Organization, Geneva, Switzerland.

25. **Hummeler K, Atanasiu P.** 1973. Electron microscopy, p 158–164. *In* Kaplan MM, Koprowski H (ed), *Laboratory Techniques in Rabies*, 3rd ed. World Health Organization, Geneva, Switzerland.
26. **Lembo T, Niezgoda M, Velasco-Villa A, Cleaveland S, Ernest E, Rupprecht CE.** 2006. Evaluation of a direct, rapid immunohistochemical test for rabies diagnosis. *Emerg Infect Dis* **12:**310–313.
27. **Whitfield SG, Fekadu M, Shaddock JH, Niezgoda M, Warner CK, Messenger SL, Rabies Working Group.** 2001. A comparative study of the fluorescent antibody test for rabies diagnosis in fresh and formalin-fixed brain tissue specimens. *J Virol Methods* **95:**145–151.
28. **Hamir AN, Moser G, Fu ZF, Dietzschold B, Rupprecht CE.** 1995. Immunohistochemical test for rabies: identification of a diagnostically superior monoclonal antibody. *Vet Rec* **136:**295–296.
29. **Noah DL, Drenzek CL, Smith JS, Krebs JW, Orciari L, Shaddock J, Sanderlin D, Whitfield S, Fekadu M, Olson JG, Rupprecht CE, Childs JE.** 1998. Epidemiology of human rabies in the United States, 1980 to 1996. *Ann Intern Med* **128:**922–930.
30. **Orciari LA, Niezgoda M, Hanlon CA, Shaddock JH, Sanderlin DW, Yager PA, Rupprecht CE.** 2001. Rapid clearance of SAG-2 rabies virus from dogs after oral vaccination. *Vaccine* **19:**4511–4518.
31. **Wadhwa A, Wilkins K, Gao J, Condori Condori RE, Gigante CM, Zhao H, Ma X, Ellison JA, Greenberg L, Velasco-Villa A, Orciari L, Li Y.** 2017. A pan-lyssavirus Taqman real-time RT-PCR assay for the detection of highly variable rabies virus and other lyssaviruses. *PLoS Negl Trop Dis* **11:**e0005258.
32. **Webster LT, Dawson JR.** 1935. Early diagnosis of rabies by mouse inoculation. Measurement of humoral immunity to rabies by mouse protection test. *Proc Soc Exp Biol Med* **32:**570–573.
33. **Webster WA, Casey GA.** 1996. Virus isolation in neuroblastoma cell culture, p 96–104. *In* Meslin FX, Kaplan MM, Koprowski H (ed), *Laboratory Techniques in Rabies*, 4th ed. World Health Organization, Geneva, Switzerland.
34. **Dyer JL, Niezgoda M, Orciari LA, Yager PA, Ellison JA, Rupprecht CE.** 2013. Evaluation of an indirect rapid immunohistochemistry test for the differentiation of rabies virus variants. *J Virol Methods* **190:**29–33.
35. **Smith JS.** 1989. Rabies virus epitopic variation: use in ecologic studies. *Adv Virus Res* **36:**215–253.
36. **Velasco-Villa A, Messenger SL, Orciari LA, Niezgoda M, Blanton JD, Fukagawa C, Rupprecht CE.** 2008. Identification of new rabies virus variant in Mexican immigrant. *Emerg Infect Dis* **14:**1906–1908.
37. **Smith JS, Yager PA, Baer GM.** 1996. A rapid fluorescent focus inhibition test (RFFIT) for determining rabies virus neutralizing antibody, p 181–192. *In* Meslin FX, Kaplan MM, Koprowski H (ed), *Laboratory Techniques in Rabies*, 4th ed. World Health Organization, Geneva, Switzerland.
38. **Vora NM, Basavaraju SV, Feldman KA, Paddock CD, Orciari L, Gitterman S, Griese S, Wallace RM, Said M, Blau DM, Selvaggi G, Velasco-Villa A, Ritter J, Yager P, Kresch A, Niezgoda M, Blanton J, Stosor V, Falta EM, Lyon GM III, Zembower T, Kuzmina N, Rohatgi PK, Recuenco S, Zaki S, Damon I, Franka R, Kuehnert MJ, Transplant-Associated Rabies Virus Transmission Investigation Team.** 2013. Raccoon rabies virus variant transmission through solid organ transplantation. *JAMA* **310:**398–407.
39. **Briggs DJ, Smith JS, Mueller FL, Schwenke J, Davis RD, Gordon CR, Schweitzer K, Orciari LA, Yager PA, Rupprecht CE.** 1998. A comparison of two serological methods for detecting the immune response after rabies vaccination in dogs and cats being exported to rabies-free areas. *Biologicals* **26:**347–355.
40. **Cliquet F, Aubert M, Sagné L.** 1998. Development of a fluorescent antibody virus neutralisation test (FAVN test) for the quantitation of rabies-neutralising antibody. *J Immunol Methods* **212:**79–87.

Arboviruses

ELIZABETH A. HUNSPERGER

97

TAXONOMY

Arthropod-borne viruses (arboviruses) are transmitted to vertebrate hosts through the bites of infected arthropods and cause over 80 diseases in humans. These viruses have been grouped according to their arthropod vectors: mosquitoes, ticks, sand flies, midges, and others (Table 1). There are ~532 taxonomically diverse viruses in seven distinct families: *Togaviridae*, *Flaviviridae*, *Bunyaviridae*, *Reoviridae*, *Rhabdoviridae*, *Orthomyxoviridae*, and *Asfaviridae*. Some of these families are known to infect only arthropods, with no other known host. The medically important arboviruses are found primarily within the families *Togaviridae*, *Flaviviridae*, and *Bunyaviridae*, which are the focus of this chapter. In these three families, there are approximately 312 viruses, of which as many as 70 are medically important. The complete list and characterization of the first discovery and isolation of these viruses can be found in The International Catalog of Arboviruses (https://wwwn.cdc.gov/arbocat/).

DESCRIPTION OF THE AGENT

Arboviruses are RNA viruses of either positive or negative polarity (with the exception of African swine fever virus, in the family *Asfaviridae*). They are enveloped viruses with single-strand and/or segmented RNA genomes and are capable of replication in both insect and mammalian cells. Since most are enveloped viruses, they are not very stable in the environment and cannot survive outside their hosts for very long. Arboviruses range from 40 to 100 nm in size and have an RNA genome of approximately 9 to 22 kb. Many medically important arboviruses have been sequenced (full length or partial, e.g., structural genes), and the sequences are available on GenBank for diagnostic test and vaccine development.

Arbovirus replication takes place in the cytoplasm of susceptible cells following viral entry. For most arboviruses, there are multiple receptors for viral entry that are not well characterized. Some common receptors include heparin sulfate proteoglycans and Dendritic Cell-Specific Intercellular adhesion molecule-3-Grabbing Non-integrin (DC-SIGN) (1, 2). Following viral entry via endosomes, the virus is released into the cytoplasm, typically by a low-pH-induced irreversible conformational change of the structural proteins. For nonsegmented viruses, RNA then circularizes through attachment of the 3′ and 5′ nontranslated regions, forming concatemers that then facilitate replication of the virus (3).

The family *Flaviviridae* has four genera: *Hepacivirus*, *Flavivirus*, *Pegivirus*, and *Pestivirus*. Only the viruses in the genera *Flavivirus* are known to be transmitted through an arthropod vector. These viruses are positive-sense nonsegmented RNA viruses ~40 to 50 nm in diameter whose genome is between 9 and 12 kb. The genome carries three structural genes (encoding envelope [E], capsid [C], and membrane [M] [called "prM" in its immature state] proteins) and seven nonstructural genes (encoding NS1, NS2a, NS2b, NS3, NS4a, NS4b, and NS5), flanked by a 5′ and 3′ untranslated region (Fig. 1A). All genes are essential for viral replication, and some are highly conserved, such as NS3 and NS5. Upon viral entry into a susceptible cell through receptor-mediated endocytosis, pH-induced conformational change of the structural gene product allows the virus to be released into the cytoplasm. The viral RNA is then translated into a single polypeptide. The virus egresses through the secretory pathway.

The family *Togaviridae* is divided into two genera: *Alphavirus* and *Rubivirus*. Only the viruses in the genus *Alphavirus* are transmitted through an arthropod vector. These viruses are positive-sense nonsegmented RNA viruses ~60 to 70 nm in diameter whose genome ranges between 10 and 12 kb. The viruses all contain three structural genes (E1, E2, and C) and four nonstructural genes (nsp1, nsp2, nsp3, and nsp4). These viruses have a 5′ cap and a polyadenylated tail (Fig. 1B). Since these viruses are structurally similar to mRNA in animal cells, the RNA of these viruses is infectious. Like flaviviruses, these viruses infect susceptible cells through receptor-mediated entry, where the viruses are released from the endosome due to conformation change of the E1 protein, inducing acid-dependent fusion. Replication occurs in the cell cytoplasm. Egress of the virus is through preformed nucleocapsids with E1 and E2 glycoproteins on the plasma membrane.

The family *Bunyaviridae* is composed of five genera: *Orthobunyavirus*, *Phlebovirus*, *Nairovirus*, *Hantavirus*, and *Tospovirus* (which infects only plants). Only the viruses in the genera *Orthobunyavirus* and *Phlebovirus* are transmitted through an arthropod vector whose size ranges from ~90 to 100 nm and whose segmented genome is ~10 to 22 kb. These viruses are negative-sense single-stranded RNA viruses composed of three segments (L, M, and S). The L (large) segment primarily encodes the RNA-dependent RNA polymerase (RdRp), and the M (medium) segment encodes the viral glycoproteins; both are negative sense,

TABLE 1 Characteristics of arboviruses affecting humans

Family and genus	Virus common name	Vector	Vaccine	Geographical distribution[a]	Tropism/complication(s)	Other risk factors
Bunyaviridae						
Nairovirus	Crimean-Congo hemorrhagic fever	Tick	None	A	Viscerotropism/hemorrhagic	Potential nosocomial agent
Orthobunyavirus	Bwamba	Mosquito	None	A	Viscerotropism	
	Bunyamwera	Mosquito	None	A	Viscerotropism/encephalitis	
	Guaroa	Mosquito	None	CSA	Viscerotropism	
	Ilesha	Mosquito	None	A	Viscerotropism	
	La Crosse	Mosquito	None	NA	Neurotropism/encephalitis	
	Tahyna	Mosquito	None	E	Viscerotropism	
	Oropouche	Midge	None	CSA	Viscerotropism/hemorrhage, encephalitis	
	Tataguine	Mosquito	None	A	Viscerotropism	
Phlebovirus	Toscana	Sand fly	None	E	Neurotropism/aseptic meningitis	
	Heartland	Tick	None	NA	Possible viscerotropism	
	Bourbon	Tick	None	NA	Possible viscerotropism	
	Severe fever with thrombocytopenia syndrome	Tick	None	SEA	Viscerotropism	
	Sand fly fever (Naples, Sicilian)	Sand fly	None	E, I/SEA	Viscerotropism	
	Rift Valley fever	Mosquito	None	A	Viscerotropism/hemorrhage, encephalitis	
Flaviviridae						
Flavivirus	Bussuquara	Mosquito	None	CSA	Viscerotropism	
	Dengue	Mosquito	DENVAX	A,NA, CSA, I/SEA,O	Viscerotropism/hemorrhage, encephalitis	Transfusion; transplacental transmission; sickle cell anemia
	Japanese encephalitis	Mosquito	SJE-VAX / IXIARO	I/SEA	Neurotropism/encephalitis	
	Kyasanur Forest	Tick	None	I/SEA	Viscerotropism/hemorrhage, encephalitis	
	Tick-borne encephalitis	Tick	Ecepur/ TBE-Immun	E	Neurotropism/encephalitis	Unpasteurized dairy milk
	West Nile/Kunjin	Mosquito	None	NA, CSA, E, I/SEA, O	Neurotropism/encephalitis	Transfusion; organ donation; transplacental transmission
	Powassan	Tick	None	NA	Neurotropism/encephalitis	
	Murray Valley	Mosquito	None	O	Neurotropism/encephalitis	
	Yellow fever	Mosquito	YF-VAX	A, CSA	Viscerotropism/hemorrhage, encephalitis	
	Rocio	Mosquito	None	CSA	Neurotropism/encephalitis	
	Ilheus	Mosquito	None	CSA	Encephalitis	
	Omsk hemorrhagic fever	Tick	None	R	Viscerotropism/hemorrhage	
	St. Louis encephalitis	Mosquito	None	NA, CSA	Neurotropism/encephalitis	
	Zika	Mosquito	None	A/I/SEA/ CSA/NA	Viscerotropism/neurotropism	Transplacental/sexual transmission

Reoviridae						
Coltivirus	Colorado tick fever	Tick	None	NA	Viscerotropism/hemorrhage, encephalitis	
Togaviridae						
Alphavirus	Barmah Forest	Mosquito	None		Viscerotropism	
	Chikungunya	Mosquito	None	A, I/SEA/CSA	Viscerotropism	
	Eastern equine encephalitis	Mosquito	None	NA, CSA	Neurotropism/encephalitis	
	Western equine encephalitis	Mosquito	None	NA	Neurotropism/encephalitis	Transplacental transmission
	Venezuelan equine encephalitis	Mosquito	TC-83	NA, CSA	Neurotropism/encephalitis	
	O'nyong-nyong	Mosquito	None	A	Viscerotropism	
	Mayaro	Mosquito	None	CSA	Viscerotropism	
	Ross River	Mosquito	None	O	Viscerotropism	
	Semliki Forest	Mosquito	None	A	Neurotropism/encephalitis	
	Sindbis	Mosquito	None	A	Viscerotropism	
Rhabdoviridae						
	Vesicular stomatitis	Sand fly	None		Viscerotropism	
	Piry	Mosquito	None	CSA	Viscerotropism	
Orthomyxoviridae						
	Thogotovirus	Tick	None	A	Neurotropism/encephalitis	
	Dhori	Tick	None	I/SEA	Viscerotropism/encephalitis	

[a]A, Africa and Middle East; NA, North America; CSA, Central and/or South America ; E, Europe and/or continental Asia; I/SEA, India and Southeast Asia, including China and Japan; O, Oceania; R, Russia.

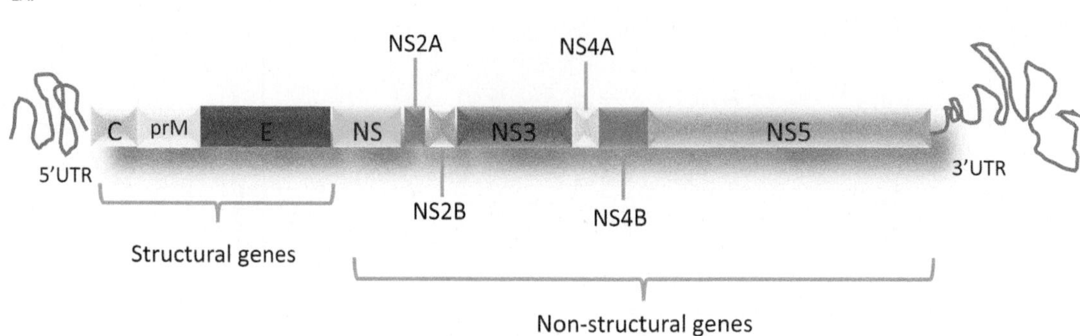

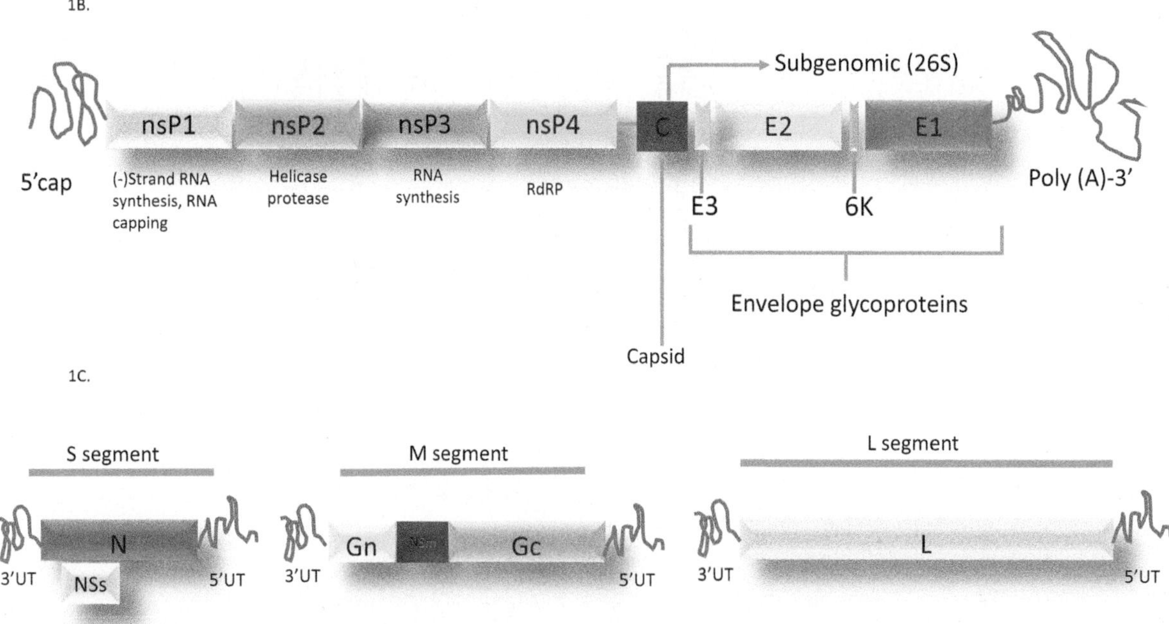

FIGURE 1 (A) Flavivirus genome; (B) alphavirus genome; (C) bunyavirus genome. UTR, untranslated region; RdRP, RNA-dependent RNA polymerase.

whereas the S (small) segment is ambisense and encodes the nucleocapsid proteins in the negative sense and the nonstructural proteins in the positive sense (Fig. 1C). Genetic reassortment can occur between members of the serogroup in the genus *Orthobunyavirus* but not between members of different serogroups in the same genus.

Some arboviruses have developed divergent genomic sequences within species driven by transmission within a specific geographical location, and these viruses are referred to as genotypes, subtypes, or lineages. These genotypes result from the evolution of these virus species within restricted ecological niches, resulting in evolutionary divergence for improved adaptation. Genotypes have been described for virus species in genera in all three families: in *Flavivirus* (*Flaviviridae*), Japanese encephalitis virus (JEV), dengue virus (DENV), yellow fever virus (YFV), and West Nile virus (WNV); in *Alphavirus* (*Togaviridae*), Eastern equine encephalitis virus (EEEV), Western equine encephalitis virus (WEEV), and Venezuelan equine encephalitis virus (VEEV); and in *Bunyavirus* (*Bunyaviridae*), LaCrosse virus (LACV). Within each family of viruses, there is significant nucleic acid homology. The most conserved genes are those corresponding to the RdRp and the nonstructural genes essential for RNA replication. This relatively high level of nucleic acid homology between families of viruses results in gene products that share epitopes targeted by the host for neutralizing antibodies, giving rise to significant cross-reactivity within some arbovirus families. However, these cross-reactive epitopes are often not cross-protective and cause significant challenges in the interpretation of immunodiagnostic tests.

Arboviruses evade the host innate immune response by blocking the interferon response early in the infection. In particular for flaviviruses, type I interferons (alpha/beta interferons) are key mediators of innate antiviral responses which are inhibited by the RdRp NS5 (4). This allows the virus to replicate in the susceptible host to titers sufficient to reinfect an arthropod vector and continue the cycle of transmission. In some instances, the host immune response can further amplify viral titers in the host by facilitating viral entry through Fc receptors. This is often referred to as antibody-dependent enhancement and has been best described for dengue viruses (5).

EPIDEMIOLOGY AND TRANSMISSION

Many mosquito-borne arboviruses are most commonly transmitted in tropical and subtropical regions of the world and are highly dependent on the presence of the vector and an amplifying host. Currently, approximately 40% of the world's population live in tropical regions and are at risk of acquiring an arbovirus infection. The cycle of transmission can be either urban (mosquito to person to mosquito), sylvatic (mosquito to non-human primate to mosquito), or epizootic (mosquito to vertebrate to mosquito, where humans are dead-end incidental hosts). Arbovirus transmission is seasonal, and the highest transmission is commensurate with the abundance of the vector, in the hot and rainy seasons for most mosquito-borne viruses. For arboviruses that are endemic in a population, their transmission can be cyclical; there is sustained annual transmission, with periodic epidemics occurring every 2 to 20 years depending on the host immunity status, vector, virus, and virus reintroduction rates. Often there is no significant difference in infection rate by age or sex; however, in regions of high endemicity, as is observed with dengue viruses, where viral transmission is annual and persistent, the infection rate in younger individuals (<10 years old) tends to be higher than that in adults, because they reflect the susceptible population (6).

The transmission cycle of arboviruses includes an arthropod vector and a vertebrate animal reservoir as the amplifying host, and some have a dead-end or incidental host. Some viruses have evolved an urban and a sylvatic transmission cycle; this has been well documented for chikungunya virus (CHIKV) and YFV. Arboviruses may cause seasonal epidemics, which are often linked to the abundance of the vector, intermediate amplifying hosts, susceptible hosts, and introductions of new genotypes, subtypes, or lineages. Humans have become the principal amplifying host without the need for an intermediate vertebrate amplifying host for arboviruses such as DENV, ZIKV, YFV, and CHIKV. The principal vectors are container-breeding species that require a very small volume of water to lay their eggs; thus, control of larval and adult populations is very difficult. Many factors contribute to the expansion of arboviruses, including travel and urbanization of the human population with uncontrolled urban growth, which contributes to an increase in mosquito breeding sites. In addition, the lack of vector control measures within this environment contributes to this vicious circle of sustained transmission and episodic epidemics.

Most arbovirus infection occurs through the bite of an infected arthropod; however, there are other sources of arbovirus infection, including blood transfusion, organ donations, transplacental transmission, breast milk, laboratory acquisition, and sexual transmission (Table 2). Infection through organ donation was best described for WNV following its emergence in the United States, where transplantation of infected organs caused fatalities in organ recipients (7). These studies prompted the investigation of other arbovirus infections via blood and organ donations, especially DENV, ZIKV, and CHIKV, which cause a high rate of asymptomatic infections (75%) with sufficient viral titers to infect transfusion or organ recipients (8). Other studies have described the presence of CHIKV, WNV, ZIKV, and DENV in breast milk, but vertical transmission through this route is still not well characterized (9–12). Finally, sexual transmission has been described only for ZIKV (13).

Historically, arboviruses were geographically restricted and had limited circulation, being confined to certain continents or specific regions of the world (e.g., tick-borne encephalitis virus [TBEV] circulates in Europe and parts of Asia). However, recent globalization and the spread of competent arbovirus vectors have contributed to the introduction of these viruses in regions of the world where historically they never circulated (e.g., WNV, ZIKV, and CHIKV in the Americas). Environmental factors have also contributed to expansion of arboviruses under conditions which have favored the vector, the virus, or both. Introductions of new arboviruses or their emergence into a new region or continent has become common with the ease of travel and movement of people, animals, and vectors. Also, changes in the vector ecology or number of susceptible hosts in a given population play an important role in arbovirus transmission, particularly where humans are the primary amplifying host. Worldwide globalization has been implicated as the major cause of the introduction of new vectors into regions. This includes increases in travel of infected humans, animals, or vectors, providing a unique environment in which the pathogen adapts and thrives due to the abundance of susceptible hosts (14). For example, WNV commonly circulating in East Africa and in the Middle East was detected and isolated in 1999 in North America. Genetic analysis suggested that the emergence of WNV in the Americas was due to importation of WNV from the Middle East. The method of introduction by either mosquitoes or hosts was not fully determined. Nevertheless, WNV moved across the United States at an alarming speed following its emergence in 1999 in New York. This was due to the increased virus susceptibility of the New World avian amplifying hosts in comparison to the Old World avian host. Hence, the epizootic transmission of WNV in North America caused an alarming number of avian deaths, particularly among corvids, most frequently the American crow (*Corvus brachyrhynchos*) (15). Another example of a rapid geographical expansion of an arbovirus is the transmission of CHIKV primarily by the vector, *Aedes aegypti*. A single point mutation in the membrane fusion glycoprotein of CHIKV increased its adaptation to *Aedes albopictus* and led to large outbreaks in tropical areas of the Indian Ocean (16, 17). Later, in 2014, CHIKV emerged in the Americas, where it was introduced in the small island of St. Martin in the Caribbean. Within 1 year of CHIKV introduction in the Caribbean, the virus had expanded into 26 Caribbean islands and 14 countries, with over 1 million reported cases (reported by the Pan American Health Organization [PAHO]). Although CHIKV has a sylvatic cycle, its transmission is primarily from human to mosquito to human; thus, its expansion into the Americas was believed to be through an infected human traveling from an Asian region of endemicity to the Americas. Sequence analysis determined that the circulating virus was of the Asian genotype (18). Following the chikungunya outbreak, another historical event in arbovirus geographical expansion occurred. The first autochthonous transmission of ZIKV in the Americas was reported in March 2014 in the Easter Island of Chile, and then the virus emerged in Brazil in March of 2015 (19). Previously, ZIKV was thought to circulate mostly in Asia and East Africa regions, causing mild disease with no known outbreaks (20). In the early 2000s, this virus had been expanding in regions of the South Pacific, with the first large outbreak reported in the Federated States of

TABLE 2 Commercial diagnostic tests available for arboviruses

Group	Virus	Name	Manufacturer	Country of origin	Test type
Flavivirus	Dengue	Simplexa Dengue kit	Focus Diagnostics	USA	Molecular
		LightMixKit Dengue Virus	Roche/TIB MOBIOL	Germany	Molecular
		Sentosa SA Dengue I-IV RT-PCR test	Vela Diagnostics	Singapore	Molecular
		Dengue Virus II Real Time RT-PCR kit (CE marked)	Vanunek	Spain	Molecular
		Geno-Sen's Dengue 1-4 Real Time PCR kit	Genome Diagnostics Pvt, Ltd.	Netherlands	Molecular
		Dengue virus (multiplex)	Mikrogen Diagnostik	Germany	Molecular
		Dengue virus	Genesig	United Kingdom	Molecular
		abTES DEN 5 qPCR I kits	AIT Biotech	Singapore	Molecular
		DiaPlexQ Dengue Virus detection kit	SolGent	Korea	Molecular
		Dengue RNA Real Time PCR kit	Co-Diagnostics	USA	Molecular
		RealStar Dengue RT-PCR kit	Altona Diagnostics	Germany	Molecular
		Dengue Virus Real Time RT-PCR kit	Centena Biomed	India	Molecular
		Dengue Virus	TIB MolBiol	Germany	Molecular
		PLATELIA Dengue NS1 Ag	BioRad	France	Antigen
		Dengue NS1 Ag ELISA	Standard Diagnostics, Inc.	Korea	Antigen
		Dengue Early ELISA	Panbio	Australia	Antigen
		DENV Detect IgM MAC ELISA[a]	InBios International, Inc.	USA	Immunodiagnostic
		Dengue Virus IgM Human ELISA kit	Abcam	China	Immunodiagnostic
		Dengue Duo IgM IgG Capture ELISA	Iverness	Australia	Immunodiagnostic
		alphaWell Dengue IgM	Mikrogen Diagnostik	Germany	Immunodiagnostic
		alphaWell Dengue IgG	Mikrogen Diagnostik	Germany	Immunodiagnostic
		NovaLisa Dengue Virus IgM μ-capture	NovaTec Immunodiagnostics GmbH	Germany	Immunodiagnostic
		NovaLisa Dengue IgG	NovaTec Immunodiagnostics GmbH	Germany	Immunodiagnostic
		NovaLisa Dengue IgM	NovaTec Immunodiagnostics GmbH	Germany	Immunodiagnostic
		DENV JE MACE	Venture Technologies Sdn Bhd	Malaysia	Immunodiagnostic
		Focus DENV IgM capture/IgG DxSelect	Focus Diagnostics	USA	Immunodiagnostic
		PATHOZYME-DENGUE IgM/IgG and IgM	Omega	United Kingdom	Immunodiagnostic
		ImmunoComb Dengue IgM & IgG BiSpot	Orgenics	Israel	Immunodiagnostic
		Dengue Virus IgM ELISA	Genway Biotech, Inc.	USA	Immunodiagnostic
		Dengue Virus IgG ELISA	Genway Biotech, Inc.	USA	Immunodiagnostic
		ImmunoLISA Dengue IgM/IgG Capture	Orgenics	Israel	Immunodiagnostic
		ELISA IgM and IgG formats	Panbio	Australia	Immunodiagnostic
		EUROIMMUN DENV Mikrotiter ELISA	Euroimmun	Germany	Immunodiagnostic
		Dengue IgM capture ELISA	Standard Diagnostics, Inc.	Korea	Immunodiagnostic
		Dengue virus IgM ELISA	IBL International	Germany	Immunodiagnostic
		Dengue virus IgG ELISA	IBL International	Germany	Immunodiagnostic
		Dengue virus ELISA kit (HRP)	Novus Biologicals	USA	Immunodiagnostic
		EUROIMMUN DEN 1-4 IIFT Biochip	Euroimmun	Germany	IFA
		Dengue Virus Type 2 Antibody Detection	Progen Biotechnik	Germany	IFA
	West Nile	Geno-Sen's West Nile Virus Real Time PCR kit	Genome Diagnostics Pvt, Ltd.	Netherlands	Molecular
		RealStar WNV RT-PCR kit	Altona Diagnostics	Germany	Molecular
		Artus WNV LC RT-PCR kit and TM kit	Qiagen GmbH	Germany	Molecular
		West Nile Virus	TIB MolBiol	Germany	Molecular
		West Nile Virus Real Time RT-PCR kit	Centena Biomed	India	Molecular
		West Nile Virus (multiplex)	Mikrogen Diagnostik	Germany	Molecular

	West Nile virus IgM Capture ELISA[a] (8/2004)	Panbio	Australia	Immunodiagnostic
	West Nile Detect IgM Capture ELISA[a] (11/2004)	InBios International, Inc.	USA	Immunodiagnostic
	West Nile Virus DxSelect ELISA[a] (6/2004)	Focus Diagnostics	USA	Immunodiagnostic
	EUROIMMUN WNV ELISA (IgM)[a] (8/2016)	Euroimmun	Germany	Immunodiagnostic
	Panbio WNV IFA slides	Panbio	Australia	IFA
St. Louis encephalitis	Arbovirus IFA IgM and IgG	Focus Diagnostics	USA	IFA
Yellow fever	FTD Tropical Fever Africa (YFV multiplex)	Mikrogen Diagnostik	Germany	Molecular
	IFA IgM and IgG	Euroimmun Biochip Technology	Germany	IFA
Japanese encephalitis	Japanese Encephalitis Virus Real Time RT-PCR kit	Vanunek	Spain	Molecular
	Japanese Encephalitis Virus Real Time RT-PCR kit	Centena Biomed	India	Molecular
	Geno-Sen's JEV Real Time PCR kit	Genome Diagnostics Pvt, Ltd.	Netherlands	Molecular
	FTD Tropical Fever Asia (JEV multiplex)	Mikrogen Diagnostik	Germany	Molecular
	JE Detect IgM MAC ELISA	InBios International, Inc.	USA	Immunodiagnostic
	Panbio Japanese Encephalitis - Dengue IgM	Panbio	Australia	Immunodiagnostic
	EUROIMMUN JEV IgG/IgM IIFT	Euroimmun	Germany	Immunodiagnostic
Tick-borne encephalitis	SERION ELISA classic TBE virus IgG/IgM	Virion/serion	Germany	Immunodiagnostic
	IMMUNOZYM FSME IgG All species	Progen Biotechnik	Germany	Immunodiagnostic
	IMMUNOZYM FSME (TBE) IgM	Progen Biotechnik	Germany	Immunodiagnostic
	EUROIMMUN TBEV Mikrotiter ELISA	Euroimmun	Germany	Immunodiagnostic
	EIA TBE Virus IgM / EIA TBEV IgG+avidity	TestLine Clinical Diagnostics	Czech Republic	Immunodiagnostic
	TBEV/FSME IgM ELISA	IBL International	Germany	Immunodiagnostic
	TBEV/FSME IgG ELISA	IBL International	Germany	Immunodiagnostic
	Virotech FSME IgG/IgM ELISA	Sekisui Virotech GmbH	Germany	Immunodiagnostic
	NovaLisa TBEV IgG	NovaTec Immunodiagnostics GmbH	Germany	Immunodiagnostic
	NovaLisa TBEV IgM	NovaTec Immunodiagnostics GmbH	Germany	Immunodiagnostic
	IBL TBE IgG ELISA and IgM ELISA	IBL International	Germany	Immunodiagnostic
Zika	Anti Zika Virus ELISA/IIFT (IgM or IgG)	Euroimmun	Germany	Immunodiagnostic
	ZV IgM ELISA	MyBiosource	Canada	Immunodiagnostic
	anti-Zika virus IgM ELISA kit (μ-capture)	Abcam	China	Immunodiagnostic
	Zika Virus Detect IgM Capture ELISA[b] (8/2016)	InBios International, Inc.	USA	Immunodiagnostic
	anti-Zika virus IgM ELISA kit (μ-capture)	NovaTec	Germany	Immunodiagnostic
	ADVIA Centaur Zika test[b] (9/2017)	Siemen Healthcare Diagnostics, Inc.	USA	Immunodiagnostic
	LIAISON XL Zika Capture IgM assay[b] (4/2017)	DiaSorin Inc.	USA	Immunodiagnostic
	Zika ELITe MGB kit[b] (12/2016)	ELITechGroup, Inc.	USA	Molecular
	RealStar Zika Virus RT-PCR kit[b] (5/2016)	Altona Diagnostics	Germany	Molecular
	Sentosa SA ZIKV RT-PCR test[b] (9/2016)	Vela Diagnostics	Singapore	Molecular
	LightMix Zika rRT-PCR test	Roche	Germany	Molecular
	Zika Virus RNA Qualitative rRT-PCR[b] (4/2016)	Quest Diagnostics	USA	Molecular
	RealStar Zika RT-PCR[b] (5/2016)	Altona Diagnostics	Germany	Molecular
	Aptima Zika assay[b] (6/2016)	Hologic, Inc.	USA	Molecular
	Zika Virus Real-time RT-PCR[b] (7/2016)	Viracor Eurofins	USA	Molecular
	VERSANT Zika RNA 1.0 assay[b] (7/2016)	Siemen Healthcare Diagnostics, Inc.	Germany	Molecular
	xMAP NultiFLEX Zika RNA assay[b] (8-2016)	Luminex Corp	USA	Molecular
	Sentosa SA ZIKV RT-PCR test[b] (9/2016)	Vela Diagnostics	USA	Molecular
	Abbott RealTime ZIKA[b] (11/2016)	Abbott Molecular Inc.	USA	Molecular
	Gene-RADAR Zika Virus test[b] (3/2017)	Nanobiosym Diagnostics, Inc.	USA	Molecular
	TaqPath Zika Virus kit[b] (8/2017)	Thermo Fisher Scientific	USA	Molecular

(Continued on next page)

TABLE 2 Commercial diagnostic tests available for arboviruses *(Continued)*

Group	Virus	Name	Manufacturer	Country of origin	Test type
Alphavirus	Chikungunya	RealStar Chikungunya RT-PCR kit	Altona Diagnostics	Germany	Molecular
		Chik Virus	TIB MolBiol	Germany	Molecular
		abTES CHIKU qPCR I kits	AIT Biotech	Singapore	Molecular
		Sentosa CHIKV RT-PCR test	Vela Diagnostics	Singapore	Molecular
		Chikungunya virus Real Time RT-PCR kit	Centena Biomed	India	Molecular
		Geno-Sen's Chikungunya Virus Real Time PCR kit	Genome Diagnostics Pvt, Ltd.	Netherlands	Molecular
		Chikungunya virus (multiplex)	Mikrogen Diagnostik	Germany	Molecular
		Chikungunya IgG/IgM human ELISA kit	NovaTec Immundiagnostica GmbH	Germany	Immunodiagnostic
		Chikungunya IgM ELISA	Standard Diagnostics, Inc.	Korea	Immunodiagnostic
		Chikungunya virus IgM human ELISA kit	Abcam	China	Immunodiagnostic
		Chikungunya IgM ELISA test kit	Genomix Biotech	India	Immunodiagnostic
		Chikungunya Virus IgG Capture ELISA	Genway Biotech, Inc.	USA	Immunodiagnostic
		Chikungunya IgM u-capture ELISA	IBL International	Germany	Immunodiagnostic
		Chikungunya IgG Capture ELISA	IBL International	Germany	Immunodiagnostic
		Chikungunya Virus IgM u-capture ELISA	Genway Biotech, Inc.	USA	Immunodiagnostic
		EUROIMMUN CHIKV IgG/IgM IIFT	Euroimmun	Germany	IFA
	Ross River	Ross River TAB ELISA	IBL International	Germany	Immunodiagnostic
		Panbio Ross River Virus IgG/IgM	Panbio	Australia	Immunodiagnostic
		Arbovirus IFA IgM and IgG	Focus Diagnostics	USA	IFA
	Eastern encephalitis	Arbovirus IFA IgM and IgG	Focus Diagnostics	USA	IFA
	Western encephalitis	Arbovirus IFA IgM and IgG	Focus Diagnostics	USA	IFA
Bunyavirus	La Crosse	Arbovirus IFA IgM and IgG	Focus Diagnostics	USA	IFA
Phleboviruses	Toscana	TOSCANA VIRUS IgG/IgM	Diesse	Italy	Immunodiagnostic
		Toscana Virus (TOSV) Real Time RT-PCR kit	Vanunek	Spain	Molecular
		EUROIMMUN Sandfly viruses IIFT BIOCHIP	Euroimmun	Germany	IFA
	Naples	EUROIMMUN Sandfly viruses IIFT BIOCHIP	Euroimmun	Germany	IFA
	Rift Valley	Rift Valley Fever Virus PCR kit	Centena Biomed	India	Molecular
		RVF Diagnostics kits IgG, IgM, Antigen	BDLS Diagnostic Test Kits	United Kingdom	Immunodiagnostic
	Crimean-Congo hemorrhagic fever	CCHF IgM, Human	BDLS Diagnostic Test Kits	United Kingdom	Immunodiagnostic

[a]FDA approved (month/year).
[b]FDA emergency use authorization (month/year).

Micronesia island of Yap in 2007 (21). Following its 2015 introduction in Brazil, ZIKV rapidly expanded throughout the Americas and the Caribbean islands, such that within 1 year it had been reported in 11 countries (PAHO website: http://www.paho.org/hq/index.php?option=com_content&view=article&id=11959:timeline-of-emergence-of-zika-virus-in-the-americas&Itemid=41711&lang=en). Previous reports indicated that ZIKV caused a self-limiting mild disease consisting of fever, rash, myalgia, and conjunctivitis; thus, its introduction into the Americas would have not caused high morbidity or mortality in the affected population. However, its association with cases of congenital birth defect of microcephaly reported in newborns infected *in utero* from ZIKV-infected women in Brazil caused a public health emergency and mobilization of global public health agencies (e.g., the World Health Organization [WHO]) (22).

Although the introduction and spread of arboviruses into new regions of the world are alarming, the resurgence of known viruses and the discovery of new viruses are just as important. For example, there have been increasing reports of newly identified cases in the United States of disease caused by Powassan virus, a tick-borne virus discovered in Powassan, Ontario, Canada, in 1958. Climate change favoring the vector abundance has been implicated as the main cause of the detection of these new cases. A vaccine-preventable disease, YF reemerged in Africa and South America in 2016, causing large outbreaks, with a total of 7,509 suspected cases and 171 deaths reported from six different countries (23). This could be due to a shortage in vaccine availability as well as a lack of routine vaccination in countries where the vector and virus are endemic and circulate, especially areas that have the capacity to maintain a sylvatic cycle. Other new viruses have been discovered recently, including Heartland virus (genus *Phlebovirus*), the agent of severe fever with thrombocytopenia syndrome (genus *Phlebovirus*), and Bourbon virus (genus *Thogotovirus*), all of which are transmitted by ticks (24–26). These viruses have caused severe disease and mortality in humans, and there is still much to learn about their natural host and transmission cycle. The most current information on transmission of medically important arboviruses worldwide is available on the Centers for Disease Control and Prevention (CDC) and WHO websites (https://www.cdc.gov/ncezid/dvbd/about.html and www.who.int, listed by disease).

CLINICAL SIGNIFICANCE

Natural infection with an arbovirus occurs when an infected arthropod takes a blood meal from a susceptible person; however, other modes of infection are possible. Many illnesses caused by medically important arboviruses that are human pathogens display broad clinical presentations ranging from mild flu-like symptoms, such as fever, malaise, rash, and headache, to severe disease, with hemorrhage and encephalitis occasionally leading to death. These clinical symptoms can be categorized according to whether the virus is primarily either viscerotropic or neurotropic. Viscerotropic viruses cause febrile illnesses that often present with rash and arthralgia. Additional reported clinical symptoms include myalgia, jaundice, respiratory symptoms, photophobia, and others. A summary of viral tropism and associated complications resulting from severe disease in humans for the commonly reported arboviruses is presented in Table 1. Although most published reports often focus on severe cases, mild forms of disease can cause significant morbidity and sequelae. For example, persons with dengue fever (a mild form of the disease) may be absent from work or school for 7 days or more, with occasional sequelae of fatigue and general malaise that can last for months (27). In more extreme situations, permanent irreversible damage is caused by some arbovirus infections. For example, chikungunya can cause severe arthralgia and loss of function of hands and feet, which may be irreversible (28). Severe WN disease can cause poliomyelitis-like neurological symptoms, including flaccid paralysis, which may lead to permanent damage to the nervous system (29). Similar to poliovirus infection, neurons in the anterior horn of the spinal cord are also vulnerable to WNV. Lastly, as many as 1 out of 10 women who have been infected with ZIKV during their pregnancy could give birth to a baby with congenital defects and particular neurological abnormalities, including microcephaly (30). Zika also causes severe neurological symptoms in adults similar to Guillain-Barré syndrome (31).

Commonly observed clinical symptoms for neurotropic arboviruses include coma, meningitis, flaccid paralysis, encephalitis, microcephaly, and Guillain-Barré syndrome. Neurotropic arboviruses include the genera *Flavivirus* (JEV and TBEV subcomplex), *Alphavirus* (VEEV, EEEV, and WEEV), and *Bunyavirus* (LACV). Neuropathogenesis includes two important yet distinct factors: neuroinvasiveness and neurovirulence. Neuroinvasiveness is the capacity of the virus to invade the central nervous system (CNS) and/or the peripheral nervous system (PNS). Neurovirulence is defined as the replication of the virus within neuron or glial cells in the central nervous system (CNS) and/or peripheral nervous system (PNS). Within the genus *Flavivirus*, JEV and TBEV serocomplex groups have adapted to replicate in the nervous system. Although many non-neurotropic arboviruses are reported to have caused cases of encephalitis, these viruses are not neurotropic, and the reported encephalitis is often observed during multiorgan failure associated with fatal cases (Table 1). The envelope glycoprotein is an important determinant for neurotropism in the genus *Flavivirus* and linked to the glycosylation variants of the envelope gene product. The most important host risk factors for severe flavivirus infection are age, genetics, immunocompromised status, and preexisting flavivirus immunity. Most flavivirus infections cause either an asymptomatic or inapparent infection. The rate of neuroinvasive disease is $\leq$0.1% but varies with the prevalence of the virus in the population. For example, in 2002, during the peak of WNV transmission in the United States, the rate of neuroinvasive disease was 1 in every 150 infections, with a mortality rate of 5 to 10% (32, 33). In nonepidemic years, rates of neuroinvasive disease decreased; however, 2012 was an epidemic year, with rates of neuroinvasive disease comparable to those observed in the 2002 U.S. epidemic (34).

Age is the most common host risk factor documented in both human clinical studies and animal models. Younger individuals have a higher susceptibility to neuroinvasive disease, implying that the developing nervous system is more susceptible to the virus. For example, encephalitis and severe disease in JEV infections are primarily observed in children from 0 to 9 years old. For WNV, neuroinvasive disease increases with age. Younger adults have a higher risk of aseptic meningitis, whereas elderly patients have a higher risk of encephalitis with poor outcome. For the elderly, the risk of neuroinvasive disease is most likely related to a compromised immune system or preexisting medical conditions. Preexisting systemic conditions such as autoimmune diseases, diabetes, and obesity are some of the risk factors associated with WN and dengue severe disease (35, 36). These conditions, which result in a less functional and responsive immune system, are also associated with the reduction in vaccine responsiveness in elderly individuals.

In utero transmission has been poorly studied for most arboviruses; however, the 2015 Zika outbreak in the Americas prompted the first studies that carefully documented *in utero* transmission of an arbovirus (reviewed in reference 37). Cohort studies that monitored pregnant women infected with ZIKV at various stages of their pregnancy documented the infant's developmental abnormalities with specific neurological outcomes. These studies indicated that the fetus or infant had severe cerebral atrophy, ventriculomegaly, and intracranial calcification, seen in *in utero* ultrasound images and after delivery. Although most of the focus has been on the development of microcephaly, there is a wide spectrum of developmental malformations associated with exposure to ZIKV *in utero*, referred to as congenital Zika syndrome (CZS). There are five categories of CZS, including neurological, musculoskeletal, ocular, genitourinary, and others that could not be grouped into specific categories (reviewed in reference 20). Other studies have also shown virus transmission from infected mother to fetus (transplacental transmission), as with DENV and WNV; however, there were no serious outcomes following birth (38, 39).

Viscerotropic arboviruses include but are not limited to DENV, YFV, and Rift Valley fever virus (RVFV) (Table 1). Common clinical symptoms for these viruses are fever, malaise, headache, photophobia, and occasionally rash and arthralgia. Other symptoms include hepatitis and jaundice, which is sometimes misdiagnosed as hepatitis viral infection. A distinct clinical manifestation for these viruses is hemorrhage and shock syndrome. A relatively small percentage (1 to 5%) of symptomatic patients develop hemorrhage during the course of illness, and of those, 0.5 to 5% progress to multiorgan failure and eventually death (40). Disease caused by other viruses that present with viral hemorrhagic syndrome, such as Lassa virus (arenavirus), Ebola virus, and Marburg virus (filoviruses), can be misdiagnosed as hemorrhagic arbovirus syndromes. However, there are sufficient clinical differences between arboviral and other hemorrhagic viral infections as well as geographical constraints to facilitate proper clinical diagnosis.

Since there are few pathognomonic symptoms associated with each arbovirus, there is often misdiagnosis due to nonspecific clinical symptoms during the early acute stage of an infection. Other diseases for which prophylaxis is available or which are vaccine preventable, such as rubella/measles, influenza, leptospirosis, and malaria, have been misdiagnosed as arboviral infections. Clinical misdiagnosis delays appropriate medical treatment and triage of patients. Common misdiagnoses for viscerotropic arboviruses are malaria and leptospirosis. Suspected malaria-infected patients were often treated with antimalaria prophylaxis prior to laboratory confirmation of *Plasmodium* infection. There is no known negative impact of malaria treatment for patients infected with an arbovirus; however, there are no studies to support this observation (41). Encephalitis and hemorrhagic symptoms associated with certain arbovirus infections can aid an accurate clinical diagnosis.

Vaccines and antiviral medications for prophylaxis or treatment are limited for most arboviruses (Table 1). Clinicians principally rely on supportive care, including fluid replacement, analgesics, and transfusion of blood products. When making a diagnosis of arbovirus infection, the clinician should always consider the geographical location where the infection was acquired. Patient information such as vaccine history, travel history, and exposure to vectors should also be considered. While many arboviruses circulate in specific geographical regions, other arboviruses, such as DENV, now circulate in most tropical and subtropical regions of the world due to their rapid geographical expansion. By using known incubation periods, risk of infection by geographical distribution of the virus, and presence of a competent vector, clinical diagnosis can be considerably narrowed. Concurrent infections with either cocirculating arboviruses or other infectious or parasitic diseases (e.g., leptospirosis, influenza, and malaria) can occur (42–44). There is no clear evidence that concurrent infections have higher morbidity or mortality rates, because the small sample size prohibits studies with sufficient statistical power.

COLLECTION, TRANSPORT, AND STORAGE OF SPECIMENS

Serum is the most commonly collected specimen for arbovirus diagnostics; however, other specimens obtained from an acute suspected arbovirus infection in humans may include whole blood, urine, semen, tissues, and saliva, with varying utility. Viscerotropic arboviruses can be detected in sera of infected patients during the first 120 hours (5 days) following symptom or fever onset; however, there are exceptions, including the detection of ZIKV for up to 20 days after onset of illness (days postonset [DPO]) (45). Nucleic acid amplification tests (NAAT) are the most specific and often the most sensitive tests for case confirmation, although for neurotropic viruses, detection of viral nucleic acid in blood is often difficult. Serum specimens are collected in red-top or tiger-top serum separator Vacutainer collection tubes, while whole blood is collected in EDTA-treated Vacutainer blood collection tubes. Other modes of blood collection include obtaining dried blood spots; however, limited studies have validated this technique (46, 47). In order to preserve the nucleic acid integrity, specimens collected during the viremic phase (0 to 5 DPO) should be stored at −80°C. Freeze-thawing of these specimens usually degrades the viral RNA rather quickly and can significantly reduce viral titers, i.e., by as much as 1 log, following a single freeze-thaw cycle. Because humans are the primary amplifying host for several viruses, such as DENV, CHIKV, or YFV, titers of these viruses in blood and tissue are $\sim 10^3$ to 10^9 genome equivalent copies/ml and are readily detected by most molecular diagnostic tests. For neurotropic arboviruses, such as WNV, St. Louis encephalitis virus, and JEV, there exists an intermediate (avian or swine) host; thus, humans are dead-end incidental hosts. For these viruses, identification in blood is less likely due to low viral titers (~10 to 1,000 PFU/ml), which may be below the limit of detection (LOD) of many reverse transcription-PCR (RT-PCR) tests (48). For patients clinically diagnosed with encephalitis or meningitis, a cerebrospinal fluid (CSF) specimen should be tested for the presence of virus-specific antibodies (IgM) (49). However, depending on the immune status of the patient or timing of specimen collection, viral nucleic acid can be detected in CSF by RT-PCR or virus isolation in culture. The sensitivities of these diagnostic tests depend on the infecting virus and the time frame of specimen collection. For cases that are captured prior to neuroinvasion or the onset of encephalitic symptoms, a blood specimen is more likely to yield a positive result than CSF. Recent improvements in PCR technology have shifted the LOD for many of these NAATs so as to detect arboviruses at much lower virus titers. A few studies have shown arboviral persistence, where virus shedding is detected for longer periods of time, such as weeks or months. Studies have reported

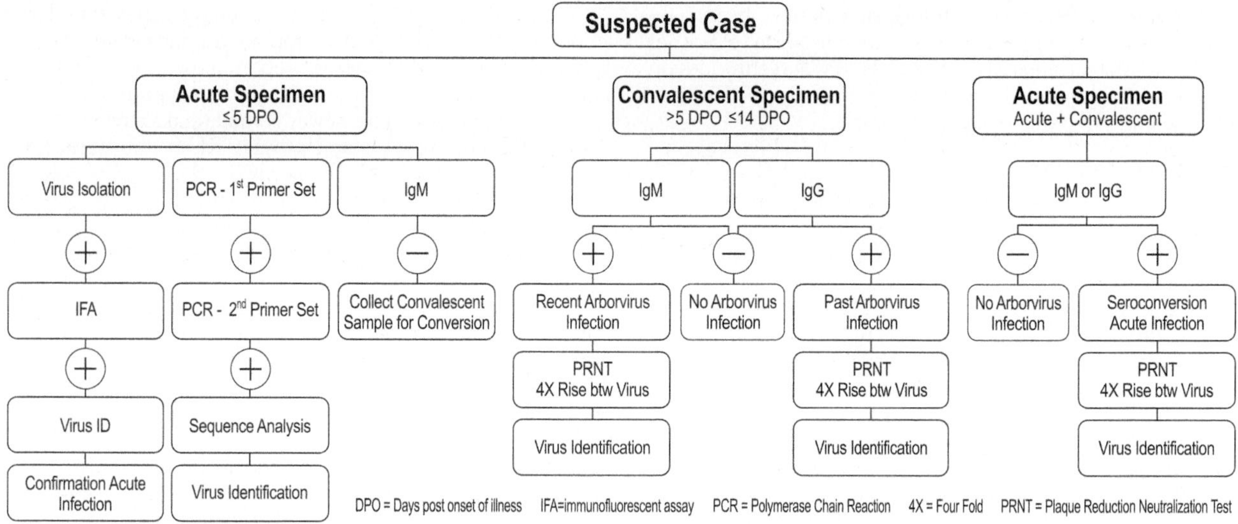

FIGURE 2 Optimal laboratory testing algorithm for human serum specimens for a suspected arbovirus infection. For patients with neuroinvasive disease, IgM is often detectable in CSF when the patient presents with neurological symptoms, and PCR may be negative. The methods depicted may be available only in specialized arbovirus reference laboratories.

virus persistence, particularly for WNV, Colorado tick fever virus, and ZIKV (50). For ZIKV, this viral persistence varied by specimen type, as virus was detected in semen and urine for weeks to months, indicating persistence in tissues such as prostate and kidney (51).

Serum specimens tested for immunodiagnostic tests should be collected during both the acute phase (0 to 5 DPO) and convalescent phase (6 to 14 DPO). Paired specimens provide the highest likelihood of a test result being confirmed by seroconversion by detection of IgM or IgG. For CSF specimens obtained from patients suspected of having a neurotropic arboviral infection, IgM antibodies are detected earlier in the course of infection in CSF than in sera; however, both specimens (serum and CSF) should be obtained for best results. A single IgM-positive serum specimen provides a diagnosis of a recent arbovirus infection; however, acute infection cannot be confirmed due to persistence of the IgM response for some arboviruses (e.g., WNV and ZIKV) (Fig. 2) (52). However, a single IgM-positive CSF specimen is suggestive of an acute arbovirus infection.

Postmortem tissue specimens are collected for direct detection methods from fatal cases. These tissues may include brain, heart, kidney, liver, and placenta. Other specimens collected for diagnostic testing include arthropods, such as ticks, mosquitoes, sand flies, and midges. These specimens are used for virus isolation and/or tested for the presence of viral nucleic acids. Arthropod field tests for virus identification in the vector include rapid tests such as a dipstick test using antibodies directed against a viral antigen (e.g., envelope glycoprotein). These tests are commercially available for WNV, DENV, EEEV, and RFV (53–55).

Ideally, transport of specimens should be rapid, and samples should be frozen and maintained on dry ice. In situations where receipt of specimens is likely to occur within 24 hours of collection, it is best to maintain the specimen at 4°C to avoid a freeze-thaw cycle, and testing should be done immediately upon arrival at the laboratory. Due to the potential infectious nature of the sample, especially for positive-sense RNA viruses, transport of confirmed samples or isolates to the lab should ideally follow International Air Transport Association regulations, which require a triple-packaging method; however, samples from suspected cases can be packaged with the same procedures as any routine diagnostic specimen. Proper personal protective equipment should be used, and specimens should be handled in a biosafety level 2 (BSL2) or BSL3 lab, as specified by the Biosafety and Microbial and Biomedical Laboratories manual (BMBL) (http://www.cdc.gov/biosafety/publications/bmbl5/), and safely manipulated in a type II biological safety cabinet. Specimens that are heat inactivated at 57°C or inactivated via lysis buffer are typically safe to handle outside a biological safety cabinet. Once the specimens are tested, long-term storage should be at −80°C for an indefinite period of time. For specimens that are virus positive or immunopositive, −20°C is best for long-term storage, i.e., up to 20 years.

DIRECT DETECTION

Microscopy

Viral identification via immunohistochemistry testing of biopsy or tissue specimens is primarily performed postmortem. The types of tissue specimens obtained are dependent on the suspected arbovirus infection. Because autopsies are not practiced and/or culturally accepted in some regions of the world where arboviruses circulate, pathology studies for arbovirus-related fatalities are few. The most complete pathology information from fatal cases is primarily from flavivirus-related deaths (JEV, WNV, YFV, and DENV). The specific tissue sampled is determined by viral tropism and varies by arbovirus family and species. For neurotropic viruses that infect the CNS, tissue specimens are collected and tested for the presence of viral antigens or nucleic acid; regions of the CNS tested include the cortex, cerebellum, and brain stem. For JEV, brain autopsies primarily test tissue specimens with NAAT and cell culture virus isolation techniques for confirmation (56, 57). For viscerotropic viruses, such as DENV and YFV, other organs are considered for immunohistochemistry and RT-PCR testing, such as liver, kidney, lymph nodes, spleen, and heart (58, 59). Few pathology studies have been published for the genera *Alphavirus* and *Bunyavirus*. Another method of detection is to use nested RT-PCR techniques on formalin-fixed, paraffin-embedded human tissue to detect viral genome in tissue specimens (60, 61).

Antigen Detection

Viral antigen detection tests have been developed as field tests for rapid identification of viruses in arthropod specimens by targeting the structural proteins (55, 62, 63). Any arthropod specimens that were positive in a rapid diagnostic test were then confirmed by either RT-PCR or virus isolation. Enzyme-linked immunosorbent assays (ELISAs) for viruses such as RVFV and EEEV have been developed for use with mosquito specimens (64, 65). Other antigen tests were developed to detect the nonstructural protein 1 (NS1) antigen of DENV and ZIKV in human sera. The flavivirus NS1 glycoprotein produces a humoral response and is known as a complement-fixing antigen. NS1 is essential for viral replication and is secreted as a hexamer composed of three dimer subunits which is readily detected by ELISA. NS1 tests were developed in a microplate ELISA format for both human and mosquito specimens. Due to their ease of use compared to RT-PCR, these tests have been widely used for diagnostic purposes.

The DENV NS1 ELISA can be implemented in many resource-poor countries for virus surveillance. The sensitivity of the first DENV NS1 antigen capture ELISA ranged from 1 to 4 ng/ml; however, commercial tests have sensitivities of 50 ng/ml of serum (66–68). Results from earlier studies suggested that NS1 levels in blood correlated with disease severity among DENV patients, although these results were not corroborated by later studies (67, 68). DENV NS1 studies suggest that antibodies against DENV NS1 bind to capillary endothelial cells and are responsible for capillary leakage (69). The NS1 glycoprotein has DENV serotype-specific epitopes capable of distinguishing between DENV serotypes in an ELISA (70). However, the NS1 antigen test is less sensitive in secondary DENV infections due to immune complexes formed from multiple DENV exposures (71). The NS1 test is commercially available for DENV, and many investigators have evaluated its sensitivity (60 to 75%) and specificity (71 to 80%) (72–75) (Table 2). Because the specificity of the NS1 test is higher than that of the IgM tests, it may also be useful in differentiating between flaviviruses. However, viruses in the JEV serocomplex group do not develop sufficiently high viral titers, in contrast to what has been observed in DENV infections; therefore, it is unlikely that an NS1 antigen detection test for these flaviviruses will be used for diagnostics.

NS1 antigen detection has been used to detect ZIKV. Homology of ZIKV NS1 to NS1 of other flaviviruses allows differentiation between ZIKV and other flaviviruses, such as DENV. The ZIKV NS1 ELISA has demonstrated a sensitivities of 31.6 and 85.7% for specimens obtained from regions where the virus is nonendemic and endemic, respectively (76). Serum specimens are collected during the viremic phase of the infection to optimize the window of detection where the highest titer of the protein is found.

Nucleic Acid Detection

There are various NAAT methods to detect arbovirus nucleic acid, including conventional and real-time RT-PCR (rRT-PCR), nested PCR, reverse transcription loop-mediated isothermal amplification (RT-LAMP), SYBR green I testing, and use of the TaqMan array. The sensitivity of any NAAT is dependent on the efficiency of the extraction and purification of the target RNA template. Commercial assays for extraction are an improvement over phenol-chloroform extraction techniques, which produced inconsistent results because of RNA degradation during the purification process. The newer commercial assays are often faster and more reliable and provide RNA stabilization to avoid loss of target RNA. The only disadvantage of NAAT is the potential for contamination with target analyte or amplicons; however, separating template-free or clean labs from nucleic acid amplification labs can eliminate potential contamination. Results of NAAT confirm the identity of the infecting virus with a rapid turnaround time. However, these assays are not necessarily available in clinical laboratories and are often found in specialized laboratories, such as CDC, reference, and academic laboratories.

RT-PCR

Conventional RT-PCR uses gel electrophoresis, where the molecular sizes (kilobases) of DNA fragments generated from test samples are compared to those of the amplified DNA fragments of known viral standards. This test cannot be used for nucleic acid quantification, since gel electrophoresis uses ethidium bromide as a method of detection and the sensitivity is dependent on the LOD (1 to 5 ng of nucleic acid) of ethidium bromide. The most sensitive test using conventional RT-PCR is the nested RT-PCR. DENV nested RT-PCR has been shown to have sensitivity almost equivalent to that of rRT-PCR and in some cases better sensitivity when compared by DENV serotypes (77).

rRT-PCR with fluorescently labeled probes has become a routine technique in some laboratories. This is due to its simple format (tubes are not opened after amplification, decreasing the risk of contamination), generally high sensitivity, multiplex capacity, and ability to quantify viral titers. Primers and fluorescent probes are designed to target the conserved regions of the genome for the most specific result. Only when there is uncertainty of the specificity of the primers should a second set of primers and/or sequencing be applied to verify RT-PCR results; however, these additional tests are not required (Fig. 2). Some tests are designed to detect any virus within a particular genus using consensus sequences (e.g., *Flavivirus*, *Alphavirus*, and *Bunyavirus*); these tests are referred to as "pan" or "universal" format tests (78, 79). Universal primers are useful for detecting agents of emerging infectious diseases where an arbovirus is the suspected pathogen. Once the genus of the unknown virus is determined, specific primers for each species within that genus are then used to identify and confirm the infecting pathogen. The fluorescence is measured and captured as cycle threshold values, which are often correlated to either genome equivalent copies or PFU; these values are determined with a standard curve to extrapolate viral load in the specimen.

The recent need for multiplex arbovirus testing has caused researchers to rely on assays that detect DENV (multiplex by serotype), the combination of CHIKV and DENV, or CHIKV, DENV, and ZIKV in a single rRT-PCR (80). These multiplex assays are particularly helpful in regions where multiple arboviruses circulate or for dengue, for which multiple serotypes circulate and physicians are unable to clinically differentiate the infecting pathogen. The only disadvantage with these multiplex assays is that they tend to have lower sensitivities than singleplex formats. Another method of detecting multiple viral targets in singleplex reactions is the use of TaqMan array cards (TAC). As many as 40 pathogens are detected in one card, and multiple arboviruses can be spotted in singleplex rRT-PCR format. Through the use of microfluidics, the specimen migrates into individual wells that have lyophilized primers and probes corresponding to each target pathogen. Due to the lower volume of specimen used in each TAC, the test is less sensitive than most rRT-PCRs or even multiplex rRT-PCRs. The main advantage of this technology is the ability to test for many pathogens with similar etiology in one test (81).

RT-LAMP

The nucleic acid detection technique known as RT-LAMP was developed for various arboviruses. The assay only requires one standard temperature (64°C) and is considered a low-cost alternative to conventional and rRT-PCR, because it does not require thermal cycling. The reaction is a strand displacement reaction using four different primers that recognize six regions of the target gene using *Bst* polymerase instead of *Taq* polymerase. The amplified product can be visually identified either by a white precipitate or by SYBR green, yielding a green or yellow color change. This test has been developed for WNV, JEV, CHIKV, DENV, and RVFV (82–85). A newly developed RT-LAMP using degenerative primers for YFV is highly sensitive; its sensitivity ranges from 83 to 100% during the first 4 days of acute infection, and it has a LOD of 19 PFU/ml (86). The adaptation of the conventional RT-LAMP test using degenerative primers increased the sensitivity to be equivalent to or greater than that of many of the routine molecular diagnostics (e.g., RT-PCR [61.5%], RT-nested PCR [93.8%], quantitative RT-PCR [100%], and conventional RT-LAMP [63.1%]).

ISOLATION PROCEDURES

Arboviruses are generally isolated from serum specimens from infected humans and animals or from extracts from mosquitoes. Virus isolation serves as a confirmatory test for RT-PCR-positive specimens and helps to further characterize circulating strains for molecular epidemiology studies. Most arboviruses can be isolated from blood or tissue if the integrity of the specimen is maintained by appropriate handling and storage. These viruses require various degrees of biological containment (BSL2 or BSL3), and laboratories should consult the BMBL manual for proper biosafety practice. As better sequencing capability becomes available, virus isolation is not always necessary, and it can introduce a bias in sequencing results due to multiple passage of the virus in cell culture. Low-passage-number viruses are preferred for phylogenetic analysis, since these viruses mutate at a rate of 1×10^{-3} substitutions/site/year. Interestingly, arboviruses' mutation rates are 0.21 order of magnitude lower on average, and their rates of synonymous substitutions are lower than those of all other RNA viruses (87). Nevertheless, it is important to obtain viral isolates as reference material for future molecular characterization studies. Virus isolation can identify novel viruses, especially when an RT-PCR-positive sample cannot be categorized by a species-specific RT-PCR assay. For example, a specimen that is positive by universal primers in flavivirus NAAT that cannot then be amplified in a flavivirus species-specific RT-PCR can then be isolated and sequenced to determine whether the virus is a new species within this family or genus.

Arbovirus isolation is performed in either primary cell culture or cell culture lines. Primary cultures typically include primary duck, chicken embryo, monkey, and hamster kidney cells. The common mammalian cell lines used for virus isolation include Vero, LLC-MK2, BHK-21, CER, SW13, and PK cells. Most infecting arboviruses cause characteristic cytopathic effects (CPE) (e.g., plaques, cell fusion, and/or syncytium formation). CPE patterns can assist in determining the genus and possibly the family of virus. Another viral amplification technique includes the intracerebral inoculation of specimen into the brains of 2- to 3-day-old suckling mice (SMB). If virus is present, the mouse will develop paralysis and die within 2 weeks of inoculation. Occasionally, viruses will require multiple passages in SMB for neuroadaptation of the viral isolate. Other organ specimens should also be harvested from infected mice, including liver and kidney. For example, certain orthobunyaviruses replicate at a higher titer in liver than in brain. Adaptation of the viral isolate in cell culture requires inoculation using homogenized infected tissue followed by multiple passages of the virus isolate in cell culture.

Many mosquito-borne arboviruses, including DENV and Sindbis virus, can also be amplified by direct injection into competent mosquitoes, such as *Aedes*, *Culex*, and *Toxorinchites* species (reviewed in reference 88), or in mosquito cell lines (C6/36 and AP61) (89, 90). Occasionally, these viruses can cause persistent infections in mosquito cell lines with no apparent CPE. Careful quality control is required for maintenance of mosquito cell lines to monitor persistent infection by a virus contaminant.

When specimens are submitted for virus identification and isolation to a reference laboratory, multiple cell lines are used, depending on where the specimen is obtained and on known circulating viruses in the region. Typically the specimen is first inoculated into a cell culture using at least one mosquito cell line (C6/36) and various mammalian cell lines, particularly Vero, LLC-MK2, and BHK-21. The inoculated cell culture flask is monitored daily for CPE, and a neutral pH is maintained in the cell culture flasks throughout the virus growth procedure. Acidic environments (pH <6) cause conformational changes in the virus structural proteins, rendering the virus noninfectious. In the absence of CPE, a sample of the culture is tested with virus-specific PCR and/or for the presence of viral antigens using an immunofluorescent assay (IFA) that probes with cross-reactive monoclonal antibodies (MAb) to identify viral family and/or genus. The virus isolate is stored in cell culture medium containing between 10 and 20% fetal bovine serum and at −80°C for future characterization studies. Currently, inoculation in SMB is not permitted in many labs due to Institutional Animal Care and Use Committee rules that prohibit this method of virus amplification. To isolate virus from human or animal serum, susceptible cells are inoculated with undiluted infected serum and two additional serum dilutions of 10^{-1} and 10^{-2} (to avoid viral interference for high-titer virus specimens). If a tissue specimen is received, it is homogenized and diluted on a weight-to-volume basis (10 to 20%).

IDENTIFICATION

IFA is used to identify the virus within infected cells (for either cell culture or tissue specimens) with virus-specific MAbs that target the structural gene products, since they are the most divergent yet conserved within species (Fig. 3). Antigenic characterization using species-specific MAbs cannot differentiate between genotypes or lineages and is useful only for viral species-specific identification. Polyclonal antibodies are also used to determine the virus family, followed by testing with species-specific MAbs. Some of the targeted MAbs cross-react with epitopes identified in all species within a family or genus of viruses.

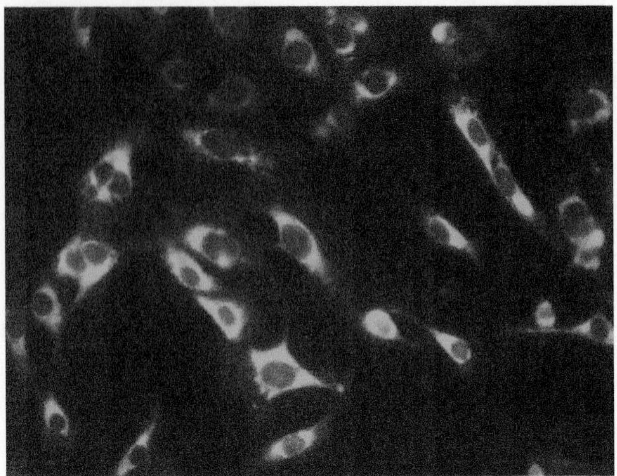

FIGURE 3 IFA for WNV-infected Vero cells using a flavivirus group-specific mouse MAb (6B6C1) and, as the detector, anti-mouse IgG antibody conjugated to fluorescein dye (6-carboxyfluorescein).

These broadly cross-reactive MAbs or polyclonal antibodies identify the family of virus, which can then be tested with specific MAbs that target epitopes within the structural proteins that are conserved between species. Some limitations of IFA are false-positive results due to background and nonspecific antibody reactivity. IFA is a subjective test and highly vulnerable to operator error. Depending on the tissue specimen, the background from the fluorescently tagged antibody can vary significantly. Autofluorescence can occur in certain specimens with high lipid content or an abundance of chitin (protein associated with insect exoskeleton). Sequence analysis provides definitive differentiation between viruses within families and within serocomplex groups that determines the origin and the molecular epidemiology of the virus. Phylogenetic analysis can assist in tracking the virus movement and transmission within a region or throughout the world by spatial and temporal analyses (reviewed in reference 91). This analysis can determine the introduction rate of specific viruses in a region and the rate of evolution. Arbovirus evolution is interdependent on the host and the vector; thus, phylogenetic analysis cannot predict the dominant evolutionary change for increased adaptation to either host or vector (reviewed in reference 14).

Novel methods for virus identification, such as deep sequencing, ultradeep sequencing, and amplicon sequencing (sequencing the same DNA target amplicons many times to find rare mutations), may enhance the identification of new species or families of viruses from tissue, arthropods, or blood. Sequencing provides the advantage of identifying new subtypes of existing viruses or new species in vectors or vertebrate hosts prior to their emergence in the human population. Viruses that may rapidly evolve to infect humans as their amplifying or dead-end incidental host can be rapidly identified for prevention and control measures. For example, Swei et al. reconstructed a newly discovered virus in less than 24 hours, which was significantly faster than conventional sequencing techniques (92). These researchers identified the Lone Star virus, in the genus *Bunyavirus*; this virus is carried by *Amblyomma americanum* ticks and is related to the Heartland virus, which was responsible for an illness reported among farmers in Missouri (25).

SEROLOGICAL TESTS

Hemagglutination

The hemagglutination inhibition assay (HIA) is a classic test used for arbovirus diagnostics and was the basis for virus family classification prior to genome sequencing. The test was first described in 1958 by Clarke and Casals and adapted to a microtiter plate format in 1980 (93). HIA is not antibody isotype specific; thus, it does not differentiate between IgM and IgG. The presence of anti-arbovirus host antibodies in serum specimens inhibits the agglutination of goose erythrocytes, as observed by a button-like appearance of the erythrocyte in the 96-well microtiter plate. Defining a positive HIA titer is influenced by the titer of the positive control used in the test and the infection status (primary or secondary arbovirus infection within the same genus). The results are subjective and vary by the experience of the laboratory technical staff performing the test.

The main advantage of the HIA is that it can be used for surveillance involving multiple hosts, since the test is not species specific. Thus, the HIA is used for vertebrate sentinel surveillance in laboratories that detect multiple cocirculating arboviruses. ELISAs have essentially replaced the HIA in human specimen testing due to the difficulty in standardizing HIA reagents and buffers and the availability of goose erythrocytes. Additionally, the interpretation of the results of HIA is subjective, and cross-reactivity between viruses within the same group or subgroup yields nonspecific results.

Enzyme-Linked Immunosorbent Assay

IgM

The acquired immune response following an arbovirus infection results in the synthesis of IgM antibodies. IgM is detectable in the late acute and the convalescent phases of the infection and is an indication of an acute or recent arbovirus infection. During the acute phase of the infection (the first 5 DPO), a relatively small percentage ($\sim\leq10\%$) of patients have detectable IgM antibodies; however, this varies by DPO, patient, and virus (94). The peak IgM antibody titer occurs in the convalescent phase of the infection (6 to 14 DPO), and ELISA testing during this period yields the most reliable results.

The IgM antibody capture (MAC) ELISA format is preferred by most diagnostic laboratories and commercial diagnostic kits. There are two main reasons for their widespread use. First, the MAC ELISA captures IgM antibodies on a microtiter plate using an anti-human-IgM antibody, thus minimizing the interference of the high-avidity IgG antibodies from binding to the antigen. Second, the MAC ELISA removes nonspecific antibody binding, allowing the use of many different sources of antigen, including unpurified homogeneous protein products composed of a mixture of viral antigens. In the MAC ELISA format, the excess antigen in combination with broadly cross-reactive MAbs that are generally arbovirus group specific increases the sensitivity of the test. Another advantage of the MAC ELISA format is that antigens can be interchanged to compare patient antibody responses to different arboviruses within the same family, mainly due to the use of broadly cross-reactive MAbs conjugated to a detector molecule. The MAC ELISA is highly sensitive but has variable specificity, depending on the cross-reactivity of cocirculating arboviruses. For example, in regions where DENV and JEV cocirculate, there is a high degree of cross-reactivity in the IgM

ELISA results that may require confirmation by neutralization test.

The sensitivity and specificity of the MAC ELISA are dependent on the source of the antigen, the detector antibody, the conjugated chromogen, serum condition (unacceptable serum samples include those that have undergone hemolysis, are lipemic, or are contaminated with bacteria or fungi), and the dilution of the specimen used for the test. The viral antigens used in the MAC ELISA are produced by virus inoculation in SMB or virus-infected cell culture lysate and/or are recombinant antigens produced in bacterial expression vectors. SMB-derived antigens provide the highest sensitivity in the MAC ELISA because they are composed of a high-titer mixture of all viral antigens, yet they provide the least specificity due to their impurity. Conversely, recombinant antigens, developed from immunogenic structural gene products, can be less sensitive yet provide better test specificity. Recombinant antigens may maintain the native conformation or glycosylation of arbovirus structural proteins, which are essential for antibody binding. Those recombinant antigens that maintain the native form of the protein tend to provide the most sensitive and specific results.

IgM kinetics can vary by arbovirus family, genus, and species and by infection status. For example, patients with secondary DENV infections (i.e., those with >1 DENV infection) had lower IgM titers than primary DENV infections (95). In these unique cases where IgM is not detectable, IgG seroconversion can be used to confirm seroconversion (96). In other atypical cases, the IgM response may persist for >3 months or as long as a year, as observed with WNV, ZIKV, and JEV infections (45, 97–99). IgM persistence observed with some arbovirus infections has prompted the development of IgG antibody avidity tests to assess the infection status (acute, recent, or past) (100).

For encephalitic arboviruses, the detection of IgM antibodies in CSF differs from detection in sera. Anti-JEV IgM is detectable in sera approximately 9 to 13 days following the onset of symptoms; however, in the CSF, IgM is detectable as early as 1 day after onset of symptoms (101). Burke et al. determined that, when using only HAI as the diagnostic test to confirm JE in clinical serum specimens, HAI missed 34% of JE cases compared to the MAC ELISA (102). In addition, anti-JEV IgM antibodies can persist in the CSF for as long as a year, suggesting persistent JEV infection of the CNS (103).

IFA has also been used as an indirect IgM test to assess reactivity against arboviruses. Arbovirus-infected cells are fixed and spotted onto a glass microscope slide, and the patient serum specimen is then added. Following incubation, the slides are washed several times to remove excess antibodies from the serum, and a fluorescently labeled anti-human IgM or IgG MAb is then added to the slide. The result is a subjective determination of fluorescently stained cells observed by microscopic analysis (Table 2).

Commercially manufactured IgM ELISAs for some arboviruses with varied sensitivities and specificities are available (Table 2). Reference and public health diagnostic laboratories may use in-house-developed IgM tests; however, many commercial IgM and rapid tests are available for some of the medically important arboviruses, including ZIKV, WNV, JEV, YFV, and DENV (104–106). Some of these commercial tests have very good sensitivity and specificity compared to gold standard or reference tests. Prior to implementing a commercial assay, each diagnostic laboratory should perform a comprehensive independent evaluation (107).

IgG

The presence of anti-arbovirus IgG antibodies in a specimen is an indication of a long-term acquired immunity from a past arbovirus infection. IgG antibodies can be detected for up to 60 years after the initial infection (108). There are two primary methods to measure IgG, direct and indirect ELISA. Direct IgG ELISA is less sensitive than indirect ELISA and requires purified viral antigen. The indirect IgG ELISA is more sensitive and uses a capture antibody to immobilize the viral antigen on a solid surface. This capture step is especially important for unpurified antigens generated from virus infection of SMB, since this antigen is less immunogenic unless it has been captured and concentrated (109). In the indirect assay, the specimen is added to the captured viral antigen and then detected with a secondary anti-human IgG-enzyme-conjugated antibody. The indirect IgG ELISA has essentially replaced the HIA because of its ease of use and improved specificity. The IgG ELISA results are reported as either qualitative or quantitative or as endpoint dilutions (96, 109). However, due to cross-reactivity within families and between species of viruses, the IgG ELISA lacks specificity and may require additional confirmatory testing, such as a neutralization test for virus identification. The IgG ELISA binds all available anti-arbovirus IgG (neutralizing or nonneutralizing antibodies); hence, the test tends to be more sensitive and less specific than the plaque reduction neutralization test (PRNT). Another test for IgG detection in serum specimens is the IFA, as previously described (Table 2).

Some investigators have explored the use of structural antigens other than the envelope protein to increase the specificity of the IgG ELISA for flaviviruses. Cardosa et al. demonstrated that the IgG response to premembrane protein has greater specificity for differentiating between DENV and JEV (110). Other researchers have improved the specificity of the IgG ELISA by using a recombinant polypeptide located in the N-terminal portion of the envelope protein (111). IgG avidity ELISAs have proven useful in differentiating primary versus secondary flavivirus infection (112, 113). The avidity assay uses a stringent 3 to 6 M urea wash buffer to remove nonspecific IgG binding. This stringent wash step has been useful in differentiating acute from past arbovirus infections under unique circumstances in which the IgM response persists (100, 114).

IgG subclasses have been studied as markers of disease severity (115–117). For JEV, subclass IgG1 is the most abundant antibody in the CSF following confirmed cases of clinical encephalitis. Thakare et al. were unable to detect IgG2 in sera or CSF of JE patients and postulated that the IgG1 subclass is more cytophilic than other IgG subclasses and may be more effective in viral clearance (115). For DEN patients, IgG1 and IgG4 subclasses are risk markers for the development of dengue hemorrhagic fever and dengue shock syndrome (the more severe presentation of the disease) (116, 117).

Neutralization

The PRNT is the most specific serological tool for the determination of type-specific antibodies and is most often used to confirm immunodiagnostic test results to determine the infecting arbovirus in convalescent-phase sera (118). This biological assay utilizes the specific interaction of virus and antibody *in vitro*, resulting in the inactivation of the virus such that it is no longer able to infect and replicate in cell culture. PRNT results are presented as the endpoint titer of neutralizing antibodies from serum to a specific virus and may suggest the level of immune protection against the infecting virus. Positive titer results from the PRNT are associated with immune protection in vaccine studies and confirm the infecting virus for IgM- or IgG-positive specimens.

Antibody neutralization has been studied extensively in animal models, natural infections in humans, and *in vitro* cell culture experiments. Neutralizing antibodies are primarily directed against the structural proteins of the virus. The neutralization epitopes for genus *Flavivirus* are located throughout the E glycoprotein, including domain I, domain II, and the surface of domain III (119–121). For the genus *Alphavirus*, the neutralizing epitopes have been mapped primarily to the E2 envelope protein, which is also important for receptor binding and cell entry. Similar E2 epitope clustering in the glycoprotein has been identified for many of the members of the genus *Alphavirus* (e.g., VEEV and Sindbis virus) and Ross River virus (122, 123). Lastly, for the genus *Bunyavirus*, the neutralizing epitopes are found within the G1 glycoprotein (124).

Viral neutralization requires that multiple antibodies occupy the surface of the virion to inhibit the viral infection. This is referred to as the multihit mechanism (125, 126). A homologous antibody response would be more effective in virus neutralization than a heterologous response. A combination of neutralizing, nonneutralizing, and subneutralizing antibodies has a synergistic effect. In other instances, heterologous antibodies are hypothesized to potentiate or enhance viral entry, as observed with DENV and WNV (127–129).

Flaviviruses have both group-specific and type-specific antibody neutralization determinants. The type-specific determinants are cross-reactive in heterologous reactions, causing the cross-reactivity observed in serological IgM and IgG tests. The neutralizing antibody titer required for protective immunity is still not well understood. Vaccine studies have provided information on protective antibody titers for flaviviruses such as YFV, JEV, and DENV; however, many of these studies were of primary infections with attenuated vaccine strains.

The PRNT results are suggestive of the infecting virus; therefore, PRNT is used to differentiate the infecting virus when cross-reactivity is observed in IgM and IgG tests. Because it takes between 5 and 10 days for results (depending on the virus), it is not used for clinical diagnosis. Additionally, this test is not routinely performed in most diagnostic laboratories because it is expensive and requires a tissue culture facility and highly skilled technical staff. To obtain reliable and reproducible PRNT results, laboratories must standardize viral strains and cell lines. Unfortunately, there is no consensus as to the percentage of antibody-induced plaque reduction that constitutes a positive result in the test. Different laboratories set endpoint values of 50%, 70%, or 90% reduction of the total input plaque-forming virus. Each of these endpoint values provides a different level of sensitivity and specificity; thus, although a 90% reduction in plaques provides the highest specificity, it is often less sensitive. In vaccine studies, a 50% reduction in plaques provides the sensitivity needed because of the relatively low neutralization titer produced following vaccination with attenuated strains of viruses in naïve subjects. The challenge of PRNT is the standardization among all end users. As stated previously, three variables account for most of the inconsistent results observed between laboratories: interpretation of the results (using 50, 70, or 90% plaque reduction as the endpoint), the cell lines used in the test, and the laboratory viral strains and growth. In an attempt to standardize the PRNT worldwide for DENV, subject matter experts from around the world published guidelines for PRNT standardization (130). In these guidelines, it was advised that viral growth be standardized such that virus is harvested prior to the plateau of growth between 5 and 7 days postinfection.

EVALUATION, INTERPRETATION, AND REPORTING OF RESULTS

The testing algorithm for diagnosing acute arboviral infection is a matrix divided according to acute-phase and convalescent-phase specimen collection (Fig. 2). The acute-phase serum or CSF specimen (≤5 DPO) is tested for the presence of virus by NAAT, virus isolation, or viral antigen tests or for IgM in CSF for encephalitic viruses. The convalescent-phase serum or CSF specimen (>5 to <14 DPO) is tested for the presence of IgM and IgG antibodies. An acute arbovirus infection is defined as the detection of virus by isolation or NAAT or seroconversion by IgM and/or IgG testing. A single specimen with an IgM-positive test result is suggestive of a recent infection; however, there are several exceptions, especially WNV and ZIKV infections, where there is IgM persistence beyond 120 days (45, 99). There are also cases of viral RNA persistence that have been reported, notably for WNV, ZIKV, and Colorado tick fever virus. The detection of only IgG in a specimen is an indication of a past infection unless there are paired specimens (acute and convalescent phase) indicating a seroconversion. IgM seroconversion in paired specimens is defined as a negative test result in the acute-phase specimen followed by a positive test result in the convalescent-phase specimen. IgG seroconversion is defined the same way as for IgM (negative in acute-phase specimens and positive in convalescent-phase specimens) or as a 4-fold rise in IgG titer from the acute-phase specimen to the convalescent-phase specimen, with a minimum of 5 days between collected specimens. Because of the high degree of cross-reactivity observed within arbovirus genera, serology results are generally confirmed with neutralization tests when definitive diagnosis is required. However, there are certain circumstances where PRNT cannot identify the infecting virus due to multiple exposures to antigenically similar viruses.

The testing algorithm for other specialized epidemiological studies, including seroincidence and/or serosurveys to measure the incidence or prevalence, respectively, in the population, is different from that for diagnostics that define acutely ill patients; thus, diagnostic testing must be modified. Serosurvey studies assess the prevalence and seroincidence of arboviruses measures the rate of infection within the population. Because these epidemiology studies rely on measuring acute, recent, and past infection, the testing algorithm and the interpretation of the test results differ and require other relevant study subject information, such as travel history, vaccination history, age, and other demographics to accurately determine the prevalence or incidence of specific arbovirus infections within a particular population. Thus, decisions regarding the best test to use will be determined by the type of study.

A variety of commercial tests have been developed for the detection of arboviruses (Table 2). These tests include molecular, antibody, antigen, and IFA tests. The formats vary from standard microtiter plate tests to rapid diagnostic tests with variable sensitivity and specificity, as evaluated by the manufacturer or by independent investigators. Advantages of commercial tests include standardization of the ancillary reagents, which allows reproducible results, and manufacturing of the tests using good manufacturing practice. Commercial tests may provide the end user with higher quality assurance, which is often difficult to obtain with in-house laboratory-developed tests (LDT). However, commercial assays can vary in quality (from lot to lot) and in reliability (test availability). Companies may discontinue manufacturing these tests when the market is not profitable, leaving the end user, and reference laboratories in particular, with no other option than to maintain LDTs in their portfolio of tests. Additionally, commercial tests may be cost prohibitive in comparison to LDTs, resulting in a preference for using LDTs despite the fact that LDTs may not be as sensitive as their commercial counterparts. Other aspects of the tests unrelated to their performance that may determine their use in laboratories are the technical time needed to perform the test, storage requirements, reagent stability, and ease of use.

The decision to use commercial assays is country dependent, because regulatory agencies in each country that determine test quality must approve the distribution of these tests. U.S. commercial laboratories prefer to use U.S. Food and Drug Agency (FDA)-approved tests for clinical diagnostics; however, this is not mandatory as long as the tests meet Clinical Laboratory Improvement Amendments and College of American Pathologists standards for validation. In order to reduce duplicative efforts, some countries rely on the FDA regulatory approval process for the use of commercially available tests for clinical diagnosis. Other countries have developed their own internal assessment requirements. There are limited available commercial tests for most arboviruses, with the exception of DENV, JEV, CHIKV, ZIKV, and WNV, and even fewer FDA-approved tests (Table 2). Although many of these tests claim good performance with high sensitivity and specificity, independent evaluations are important corroboration of the company's results. Recent studies involving DENV diagnostics for both IgM tests and NS1 tests determined that the performance of some companies' tests was below the acceptable range for use. These studies also determined that tests that depend on subjective reading of results, such as rapid diagnostic tests, often have large variation due to reader-to-reader variation (104). Thus, diagnostic laboratories must develop a plan to evaluate commercial tests prior to their implementation as routine diagnostics.

REFERENCES

1. **Germi R, Crance JM, Garin D, Guimet J, Lortat-Jacob H, Ruigrok RW, Zarski JP, Drouet E.** 2002. Heparan sulfate-mediated binding of infectious dengue virus type 2 and yellow fever virus. *Virology* **292:**162–168.
2. **Albornoz A, Hoffmann AB, Lozach PY, Tischler ND.** 2016. Early bunyavirus-host cell interactions. *Viruses* **8:**143.
3. **Edgil D, Harris E.** 2006. End-to-end communication in the modulation of translation by mammalian RNA viruses. *Virus Res* **119:**43–51.
4. **Mazzon M, Jones M, Davidson A, Chain B, Jacobs M.** 2009. Dengue virus NS5 inhibits interferon-alpha signaling by blocking signal transducer and activator of transcription 2 phosphorylation. *J Infect Dis* **200:**1261–1270.
5. **Halstead SB.** 2003. Neutralization and antibody-dependent enhancement of dengue viruses. *Adv Virus Res* **60:**421–467.
6. **Tomashek KM, Rivera A, Muñoz-Jordan JL, Hunsperger E, Santiago L, Padro O, Garcia E, Sun W.** 2009. Description of a large island-wide outbreak of dengue in Puerto Rico, 2007. *Am J Trop Med Hyg* **81:**467–474.
7. **Busch MP, Caglioti S, Robertson EF, McAuley JD, Tobler LH, Kamel H, Linnen JM, Shyamala V, Tomasulo P, Kleinman SH.** 2005. Screening the blood supply for West Nile virus RNA by nucleic acid amplification testing. *N Engl J Med* **353:**460–467.
8. **Mohammed H, Linnen JM, Muñoz-Jordán JL, Tomashek K, Foster G, Broulik AS, Petersen L, Stramer SL.** 2008. Dengue virus in blood donations, Puerto Rico, 2005. *Transfusion* **48:**1348–1354.
9. **Arragain L, Dupont-Rouzeyrol M, O'Connor O, Sigur N, Grangeon JP, Huguon E, Dechanet C, Cazorla C, Gourinat AC, Descloux E.** 2017. Vertical transmission of dengue virus in the peripartum period and viral kinetics in newborns and breast milk: new data. *J Pediatric Infect Dis Soc* **6:**324–331.
10. **Gérardin P, Barau G, Michault A, Bintner M, Randrianaivo H, Choker G, Lenglet Y, Touret Y, Bouveret A, Grivard P, Le Roux K, Blanc S, Schuffenecker I, Couderc T, Arenzana-Seisdedos F, Lecuit M, Robillard PY.** 2008. Multidisciplinary prospective study of mother-to-child chikungunya virus infections on the island of La Réunion. *PLoS Med* **5:**e60.
11. **Dupont-Rouzeyrol M, Biron A, O'Connor O, Huguon E, Descloux E.** 2016. Infectious Zika viral particles in breastmilk. *Lancet* **387:**1051.
12. **Hinckley AF, O'Leary DR, Hayes EB.** 2007. Transmission of West Nile virus through human breast milk seems to be rare. *Pediatrics* **119:**e666–e671.
13. **Frank C, Cadar D, Schlaphof A, Neddersen N, Günther S, Schmidt-Chanasit J, Tappe D.** 2016. Sexual transmission of Zika virus in Germany, April 2016. *Euro Surveill* **21:**30252.
14. **Coffey LL, Forrester N, Tsetsarkin K, Vasilakis N, Weaver SC.** 2013. Factors shaping the adaptive landscape for arboviruses: implications for the emergence of disease. *Future Microbiol* **8:**155–176.
15. **Steele KE, Linn MJ, Schoepp RJ, Komar N, Geisbert TW, Manduca RM, Calle PP, Raphael BL, Clippinger TL, Larsen T, Smith J, Lanciotti RS, Panella NA, McNamara TS.** 2000. Pathology of fatal West Nile virus infections in native and exotic birds during the 1999 outbreak in New York City, New York. *Vet Pathol* **37:**208–224.
16. **Schuffenecker I, Iteman I, Michault A, Murri S, Frangeul L, Vaney MC, Lavenir R, Pardigon N, Reynes JM, Pettinelli F, Biscornet L, Diancourt L, Michel S, Duquerroy S, Guigon G, Frenkiel MP, Bréhin AC, Cubito N, Desprès P, Kunst F, Rey FA, Zeller H, Brisse S.** 2006. Genome microevolution of chikungunya viruses causing the Indian Ocean outbreak. *PLoS Med* **3:**e263.
17. **de Lamballerie X, Leroy E, Charrel RN, Ttsetsarkin K, Higgs S, Gould EA.** 2008. Chikungunya virus adapts to tiger mosquito via evolutionary convergence: a sign of things to come? *Virol J* **5:**33.
18. **Stapleford KA, Moratorio G, Henningsson R, Chen R, Matheus S, Enfissi A, Weissglas-Volkov D, Isakov O, Blanc H, Mounce BC, Dupont-Rouzeyrol M, Shomron N, Weaver S, Fontes M, Rousset D, Vignuzzi M.** 2016. Whole-genome sequencing analysis from the chikungunya virus Caribbean outbreak reveals novel evolutionary genomic elements. *PLoS Negl Trop Dis* **10:**e0004402.
19. **Zanluca C, Melo VC, Mosimann AL, Santos GI, Santos CN, Luz K.** 2015. First report of autochthonous transmission of Zika virus in Brazil. *Mem Inst Oswaldo Cruz* **110:**569–572.
20. **Hayes EB.** 2009. Zika virus outside Africa. *Emerg Infect Dis* **15:**1347–1350.
21. **Duffy MR, Chen TH, Hancock WT, Powers AM, Kool JL, Lanciotti RS, Pretrick M, Marfel M, Holzbauer S, Dubray C, Guillaumot L, Griggs A, Bel M, Lambert AJ, Laven J, Kosoy O, Panella A, Biggerstaff BJ, Fischer M, Hayes EB.** 2009. Zika virus outbreak on Yap Island, Federated States of Micronesia. *N Engl J Med* **360:**2536–2543.
22. **Schuler-Faccini L, Ribeiro EM, Feitosa IM, Horovitz DD, Cavalcanti DP, Pessoa A, Doriqui MJ, Neri JI, Neto JM, Wanderley HY, Cernach M, El-Husny AS, Pone MV, Serao CL, Sanseverino MT, Brazilian Medical Genetics Society—Zika Embryopathy Task Force.** 2016. Possible association between Zika virus infection and microcephaly—Brazil, 2015. *MMWR Morb Mortal Wkly Rep* **65:**59–62.

23. **Anonymous.** 2017. Yellow fever in Africa and the Americas, 2016. *Wkly Epidemiol Rec* **92:**442–452.
24. **Kosoy OI, Lambert AJ, Hawkinson DJ, Pastula DM, Goldsmith CS, Hunt DC, Staples JE.** 2015. Novel thogotovirus associated with febrile illness and death, United States, 2014. *Emerg Infect Dis* **21:**760–764.
25. **Pastula DM, Turabelidze G, Yates KF, Jones TF, Lambert AJ, Panella AJ, Kosoy OI, Velez JO, Fisher M, Staples E, Centers for Disease Control and Prevention (CDC).** 2014. Notes from the field: heartland virus disease—United States, 2012-2013. *MMWR Morb Mortal Wkly Rep* **63:**270–271.
26. **Yu XJ, Liang MF, Zhang SY, Liu Y, Li JD, Sun YL, Zhang L, Zhang QF, Popov VL, Li C, Qu J, Li Q, Zhang YP, Hai R, Wu W, Wang Q, Zhan FX, Wang XJ, Kan B, Wang SW, Wan KL, Jing HQ, Lu JX, Yin WW, Zhou H, Guan XH, Liu JF, Bi ZQ, Liu GH, Ren J, Wang H, Zhao Z, Song JD, He JR, Wan T, Zhang JS, Fu XP, Sun LN, Dong XP, Feng ZJ, Yang WZ, Hong T, Zhang Y, Walker DH, Wang Y, Li DX.** 2011. Fever with thrombocytopenia associated with a novel bunyavirus in China. *N Engl J Med* **364:**1523–1532.
27. **Shepard DS, Coudeville L, Halasa YA, Zambrano B, Dayan GH.** 2011. Economic impact of dengue illness in the Americas. *Am J Trop Med Hyg* **84:**200–207.
28. **Borgherini G, Poubeau P, Jossaume A, Gouix A, Cotte L, Michault A, Arvin-Berod C, Paganin F.** 2008. Persistent arthralgia associated with chikungunya virus: a study of 88 adult patients on reunion island. *Clin Infect Dis* **47:**469–475.
29. **Hughes JM, Wilson ME, Sejvar JJ.** 2007. The long-term outcomes of human West Nile virus infection. *Clin Infect Dis* **44:**1617–1624.
30. **Hazin AN, Poretti A, Di Cavalcanti Souza Cruz D, Tenorio M, van der Linden A, Pena LJ, Brito C, Gil LH, de Barros Miranda-Filho D, Marques ET, Turchi Martelli CM, Alves JG, Huisman TA, Microcephaly Epidemic Research Group.** 2016. Computed tomographic findings in microcephaly associated with Zika virus. *N Engl J Med* **374:**2193–2195.
31. **Miller E, Becker Z, Shalev D, Lee CT, Cioroiu C, Thakur K.** 2017. Probable Zika virus-associated Guillain-Barré syndrome: challenges with clinico-laboratory diagnosis. *J Neurol Sci* **375:**367–370.
32. **Sejvar JJ, Haddad MB, Tierney BC, Campbell GL, Marfin AA, Van Gerpen JA, Fleischauer A, Leis AA, Stokic DS, Petersen LR.** 2003. Neurologic manifestations and outcome of West Nile virus infection. *JAMA* **290:**511–515.
33. **Sejvar JJ, Bode AV, Marfin AA, Campbell GL, Pape J, Biggerstaff BJ, Petersen LR.** 2006. West Nile virus-associated flaccid paralysis outcome. *Emerg Infect Dis* **12:**514–516.
34. **Beasley DW, Barrett AD, Tesh RB.** 2013. Resurgence of West Nile neurologic disease in the United States in 2012: what happened? What needs to be done? *Antiviral Res* **99:**1–5.
35. **Murray K, Baraniuk S, Resnick M, Arafat R, Kilborn C, Cain K, Shallenberger R, York TL, Martinez D, Hellums JS, Hellums D, Malkoff M, Elgawley N, McNeely W, Khuwaja SA, Tesh RB.** 2006. Risk factors for encephalitis and death from West Nile virus infection. *Epidemiol Infect* **134:**1325–1332.
36. **Pang J, Hsu JP, Yeo TW, Leo YS, Lye DC.** 2017. Diabetes, cardiac disorders and asthma as risk factors for severe organ involvement among adult dengue patients: a matched case-control study. *Sci Rep* **7:**39872.
37. **Alvarado MG, Schwartz DA.** 2017. Zika virus infection in pregnancy, microcephaly, and maternal and fetal health: what we think, what we know, and what we think we know. *Arch Pathol Lab Med* **141:**26–32.
38. **Nascimento LB, Siqueira CM, Coelho GE, Siqueira JB Jr.** 2017. Symptomatic dengue infection during pregnancy and livebirth outcomes in Brazil, 2007–13: a retrospective observational cohort study. *Lancet Infect Dis* **17:**949–956.
39. **Pridjian G, Sirois PA, McRae S, Hinckley AF, Rasmussen SA, Kissinger P, Buekens P, Hayes EB, O'Leary D, Kuhn S, Swan KF, Xiong X, Wesson DM.** 2016. Prospective study of pregnancy and newborn outcomes in mothers with West Nile illness during pregnancy. *Birth Defects Res A Clin Mol Teratol* **106:**716–723.
40. **Kalayanarooj S.** 2011. Clinical manifestations and management of dengue/DHF/DSS. *Trop Med Health* **39**(Suppl)**:** S83–S87.
41. **Yong LS, Koh KC.** 2013. A case of mixed infections in a patient presenting with acute febrile illness in the tropics. *Case Rep Infect Dis* **2013:**562175.
42. **Sharp TM, Bracero J, Rivera A, Shieh WJ, Bhatnagar J, Rivera-Diez I, Hunsperger E, Munoz-Jordan J, Zaki SR, Tomashek KM.** 2012. Fatal human co-infection with *Leptospira* spp. and dengue virus, Puerto Rico, 2010. *Emerg Infect Dis* **18:**878–880.
43. **Lopez Rodriguez E, Tomashek KM, Gregory CJ, Munoz J, Hunsperger E, Lorenzi OD, Irizarry JG, Garcia-Gubern C.** 2010. Co-infection with dengue virus and pandemic (H1N1) 2009 virus. *Emerg Infect Dis* **16:**882–884.
44. **Epelboin L, Hanf M, Dussart P, Ouar-Epelboin S, Djossou F, Nacher M, Carme B.** 2012. Is dengue and malaria co-infection more severe than single infections? A retrospective matched-pair study in French Guiana. *Malar J* **11:**142.
45. **Paz-Bailey G, Rosenberg ES, Doyle K, Munoz-Jordan J, Santiago GA, Klein L, Perez-Padilla J, Medina FA, Waterman SH, Gubern CG, Alvarado LI, Sharp TM.** 2017. Persistence of Zika virus in body fluids—preliminary report. *N Engl J Med* NEJMoa1613108.
46. **Anders KL, Nguyet NM, Quyen NT, Ngoc TV, Tram TV, Gan TT, Tung NT, Dung NT, Chau NV, Wills B, Simmons CP.** 2012. An evaluation of dried blood spots and oral swabs as alternative specimens for the diagnosis of dengue and screening for past dengue virus exposure. *Am J Trop Med Hyg* **87:**165–170.
47. **Bharucha T, Chanthongthip A, Phuangpanom S, Phonemixay O, Sengvilaipaseuth O, Vongsouvath M, Lee S, Newton PN, Dubot-Pérès A.** 2016. Pre-cut filter paper for detecting anti-Japanese encephalitis virus IgM from dried cerebrospinal fluid spots. *PLoS Negl Trop Dis* **10:**e0004516.
48. **Lanciotti RS, Kerst AJ, Nasci RS, Godsey MS, Mitchell CJ, Savage HM, Komar N, Panella NA, Allen BC, Volpe KE, Davis BS, Roehrig JT.** 2000. Rapid detection of west nile virus from human clinical specimens, field-collected mosquitoes, and avian samples by a TaqMan reverse transcriptase-PCR assay. *J Clin Microbiol* **38:**4066–4071.
49. **Lindsey NP, Fischer M, Neitzel D, Schiffman E, Salas ML, Glaser CA, Sylvester T, Kretschmer M, Bunko A, Staples JE.** 2016. Hospital-based enhanced surveillance for West Nile virus neuroinvasive disease. *Epidemiol Infect* **144:**3170–3175.
50. **Oshiro LS, Dondero DV, Emmons RW, Lennette EH.** 1978. The development of Colorado tick fever virus within cells of the haemopoietic system. *J Gen Virol* **39:**73–79.
51. **Bingham AM, Cone M, Mock V, Heberlein-Larson L, Stanek D, Blackmore C, Likos A.** 2016. Comparison of test results for Zika virus RNA in urine, serum, and saliva specimens from persons with travel-associated Zika virus disease—Florida, 2016. *MMWR Morb Mortal Wkly Rep* **65:**475–478.
52. **Prince HE, Tobler LH, Yeh C, Gefter N, Custer B, Busch MP.** 2007. Persistence of West Nile virus-specific antibodies in viremic blood donors. *Clin Vaccine Immunol* **14:**1228–1230.
53. **Tan CH, Wong PS, Li MZ, Vythilingam I, Ng LC.** 2011. Evaluation of the Dengue NS1 Ag Strip® for detection of dengue virus antigen in *Aedes aegypti* (Diptera: culicidae). *Vector Borne Zoonotic Dis* **11:**789–792.
54. **Sutherland GL, Nasci RS.** 2007. Detection of West Nile virus in large pools of mosquitoes. *J Am Mosq Control Assoc* **23:**389–395.
55. **Wanja E, Parker Z, Rowland T, Turell MJ, Clark JW, Davé K, Davé S, Sang R.** 2011. Field evaluation of a wicking assay for the rapid detection of Rift Valley fever viral antigens in mosquitoes. *J Am Mosq Control Assoc* **27:**370–375.
56. **Johnson RT, Burke DS, Elwell M, Leake CJ, Nisalak A, Hoke CH, Lorsomrudee W.** 1985. Japanese encephalitis: immunocytochemical studies of viral antigen and inflammatory cells in fatal cases. *Ann Neurol* **18:**567–573.
57. **Burke DS, Lorsomrudee W, Leake CJ, Hoke CH, Nisalak A, Chongswasdi V, Laorakpongse T.** 1985. Fatal outcome in Japanese encephalitis. *Am J Trop Med Hyg* **34:**1203–1210.

58. **Basílio-de-Oliveira CA, Aguiar GR, Baldanza MS, Barth OM, Eyer-Silva WA, Paes MV.** 2005. Pathologic study of a fatal case of dengue-3 virus infection in Rio de Janeiro, Brazil. *Braz J Infect Dis* **9:**341–347.
59. **De Brito T, Siqueira SA, Santos RT, Nassar ES, Coimbra TL, Alves VA.** 1992. Human fatal yellow fever. Immunohistochemical detection of viral antigens in the liver, kidney and heart. *Pathol Res Pract* **188:**177–181.
60. **Deubel V, Huerre M, Cathomas G, Drouet MT, Wuscher N, Le Guenno B, Widmer AF.** 1997. Molecular detection and characterization of yellow fever virus in blood and liver specimens of a non-vaccinated fatal human case. *J Med Virol* **53:**212–217.
61. **Bhatnagar J, Guarner J, Paddock CD, Shieh WJ, Lanciotti RS, Marfin AA, Campbell GL, Zaki SR.** 2007. Detection of West Nile virus in formalin-fixed, paraffin-embedded human tissues by RT-PCR: a useful adjunct to conventional tissue-based diagnostic methods. *J Clin Virol* **38:**106–111.
62. **Wanja E, Parker ZF, Odusami O, Rowland T, Davé K, Davé S, Turell MJ.** 2014. Immuno-chromatographic wicking assay for the rapid detection of dengue viral antigens in mosquitoes (Diptera: culicidae). *J Med Entomol* **51:**220–225.
63. **Ryan J, Davé K, Emmerich E, Fernández B, Turell M, Johnson J, Gottfried K, Burkhalter K, Kerst A, Hunt A, Wirtz R, Nasci R.** 2003. Wicking assays for the rapid detection of West Nile and St. Louis encephalitis viral antigens in mosquitoes (Diptera: culicidae). *J Med Entomol* **40:**95–99.
64. **Niklasson BS, Gargan TP II.** 1985. Enzyme-linked immunosorbent assay for detection of Rift Valley fever virus antigen in mosquitoes. *Am J Trop Med Hyg* **34:**400–405.
65. **Brown TM, Mitchell CJ, Nasci RS, Smith GC, Roehrig JT.** 2001. Detection of eastern equine encephalitis virus in infected mosquitoes using a monoclonal antibody-based antigen-capture enzyme-linked immunosorbent assay. *Am J Trop Med Hyg* **65:**208–213.
66. **Young PR, Hilditch PA, Bletchly C, Halloran W.** 2000. An antigen capture enzyme-linked immunosorbent assay reveals high levels of the dengue virus protein NS1 in the sera of infected patients. *J Clin Microbiol* **38:**1053–1057.
67. **Alcon S, Talarmin A, Debruyne M, Falconar A, Deubel V, Flamand M.** 2002. Enzyme-linked immunosorbent assay specific to Dengue virus type 1 nonstructural protein NS1 reveals circulation of the antigen in the blood during the acute phase of disease in patients experiencing primary or secondary infections. *J Clin Microbiol* **40:**376–381.
68. **Libraty DH, Young PR, Pickering D, Endy TP, Kalayanarooj S, Green S, Vaughn DW, Nisalak A, Ennis FA, Rothman AL.** 2002. High circulating levels of the dengue virus nonstructural protein NS1 early in dengue illness correlate with the development of dengue hemorrhagic fever. *J Infect Dis* **186:**1165–1168.
69. **Puerta-Guardo H, Glasner DR, Harris E.** 2016. Dengue virus NS1 disrupts the endothelial glycocalyx, leading to hyperpermeability. *PLoS Pathog* **12:**e1005738.
70. **Xu H, Di B, Pan YX, Qiu LW, Wang YD, Hao W, He LJ, Yuen KY, Che XY.** 2006. Serotype 1-specific monoclonal antibody-based antigen capture immunoassay for detection of circulating nonstructural protein NS1: implications for early diagnosis and serotyping of dengue virus infections. *J Clin Microbiol* **44:**2872–2878.
71. **Buonora SN, Dos Santos FB, Daumas RP, Passos SR, da Silva MH, de Lima MR, Nogueira RM.** 2017. Increased sensitivity of NS1 ELISA by heat dissociation in acute dengue 4 cases. *BMC Infect Dis* **17:**204.
72. **Bessoff K, Delorey M, Sun W, Hunsperger E.** 2008. Comparison of two commercially available dengue virus (DENV) NS1 capture enzyme-linked immunosorbent assays using a single clinical sample for diagnosis of acute DENV infection. *Clin Vaccine Immunol* **15:**1513–1518.
73. **Blacksell SD, Mammen MP, Jr, Thongpaseuth S, Gibbons RV, Jarman RG, Jenjaroen K, Nisalak A, Phetsouvanh R, Newton PN, Day NPJ.** 2008. Evaluation of the Panbio dengue virus nonstructural 1 antigen detection and immunoglobulin M antibody enzyme-linked immunosorbent assays for the diagnosis of acute dengue infections in Laos. *Diagn Microbiol Infect Dis* **60:**43–49.
74. **Dussart P, Labeau B, Lagathu G, Louis P, Nunes MRT, Rodrigues SG, Storck-Herrmann C, Cesaire R, Morvan J, Flamand M, Baril L.** 2006. Evaluation of an enzyme immunoassay for detection of dengue virus NS1 antigen in human serum. *Clin Vaccine Immunol* **13:**1185–1189.
75. **Kumarasamy V, Wahab AHA, Chua SK, Hassan Z, Chem YK, Mohamad M, Chua KB.** 2007. Evaluation of a commercial dengue NS1 antigen-capture ELISA for laboratory diagnosis of acute dengue virus infection. *J Virol Methods* **140:** 75–79.
76. **Steinhagen K, Probst C, Radzimski C, Schmidt-Chanasit J, Emmerich P, van Esbroeck M, Schinkel J, Grobusch MP, Goorhuis A, Warnecke JM, Lattwein E, Komorowski L, Deerberg A, Saschenbrecker S, Stöcker W, Schlumberger W.** 2016. Serodiagnosis of Zika virus (ZIKV) infections by a novel NS1-based ELISA devoid of cross-reactivity with dengue virus antibodies: a multicohort study of assay performance, 2015 to 2016. *Euro Surveill* **21:**30426.
77. **Lanciotti RS, Calisher CH, Gubler DJ, Chang GJ, Vorndam AV.** 1992. Rapid detection and typing of dengue viruses from clinical samples by using reverse transcriptase-polymerase chain reaction. *J Clin Microbiol* **30:**545–551.
78. **Patel P, Landt O, Kaiser M, Faye O, Koppe T, Lass U, Sall AA, Niedrig M.** 2013. Development of one-step quantitative reverse transcription PCR for the rapid detection of flaviviruses. *Virol J* **10:**58.
79. **Lambert AJ, Lanciotti RS.** 2009. Consensus amplification and novel multiplex sequencing method for S segment species identification of 47 viruses of the *Orthobunyavirus*, *Phlebovirus*, and *Nairovirus* genera of the family *Bunyaviridae*. *J Clin Microbiol* **47:**2398–2404.
80. **Pabbaraju K, Wong S, Gill K, Fonseca K, Tipples GA, Tellier R.** 2016. Simultaneous detection of Zika, chikungunya and dengue viruses by a multiplex real-time RT-PCR assay. *J Clin Virol* **83:**66–71.
81. **Liu J, Ochieng C, Wiersma S, Ströher U, Towner JS, Whitmer S, Nichol ST, Moore CC, Kersh GJ, Kato C, Sexton C, Petersen J, Massung R, Hercik C, Crump JA, Kibiki G, Maro A, Mujaga B, Gratz J, Jacob ST, Banura P, Scheld WM, Juma B, Onyango CO, Montgomery JM, Houpt E, Fields B.** 2016. Development of a TaqMan array card for acute-febrile-illness outbreak investigation and surveillance of emerging pathogens, including Ebola virus. *J Clin Microbiol* **54:**49–58.
82. **Toriniwa H, Komiya T.** 2006. Rapid detection and quantification of Japanese encephalitis virus by real-time reverse transcription loop-mediated isothermal amplification. *Microbiol Immunol* **50:**379–387.
83. **Parida M, Horioke K, Ishida H, Dash PK, Saxena P, Jana AM, Islam MA, Inoue S, Hosaka N, Morita K.** 2005. Rapid detection and differentiation of dengue virus serotypes by a real-time reverse transcription-loop-mediated isothermal amplification assay. *J Clin Microbiol* **43:**2895–2903.
84. **Parida MM, Santhosh SR, Dash PK, Tripathi NK, Saxena P, Ambuj S, Sahni AK, Lakshmana Rao PV, Morita K.** 2006. Development and evaluation of reverse transcription-loop-mediated isothermal amplification assay for rapid and real-time detection of Japanese encephalitis virus. *J Clin Microbiol* **44:**4172–4178.
85. **Lu X, Li X, Mo Z, Jin F, Wang B, Zhao H, Shan X, Shi L.** 2012. Rapid identification of chikungunya and dengue virus by a real-time reverse transcription-loop-mediated isothermal amplification method. *Am J Trop Med Hyg* **87:**947–953.
86. **Nunes MR, Vianez JL Jr, Nunes KN, da Silva SP, Lima CP, Guzman H, Martins LC, Carvalho VL, Tesh RB, Vasconcelos PF.** 2015. Analysis of a reverse transcription loop-mediated isothermal amplification (RT-LAMP) for yellow fever diagnostic. *J Virol Methods* **226:**40–51.
87. **Jenkins GM, Rambaut A, Pybus OG, Holmes EC.** 2002. Rates of molecular evolution in RNA viruses: a quantitative phylogenetic analysis. *J Mol Evol* **54:**156–165.
88. **Tabachnick WJ.** 2013. Nature, nurture and evolution of intra-species variation in mosquito arbovirus transmission competence. *Int J Environ Res Public Health* **10:**249–277.

89. **Igarashi A.** 1978. Isolation of a Singh's *Aedes albopictus* cell clone sensitive to dengue and chikungunya viruses. *J Gen Virol* **40:**531–544.
90. **Varma MG, Pudney M, Leake CJ.** 1974. Cell lines from larvae of *Aedes* (*Stegomyia*) *malayensis* Colless and *Aedes* (S) *pseudoscutellaris* (Theobald) and their infection with some arboviruses. *Trans R Soc Trop Med Hyg* **68:**374–382.
91. **Weaver SC, Reisen WK.** 2010. Present and future arboviral threats. *Antiviral Res* **85:**328–345.
92. **Swei A, Russell BJ, Naccache SN, Kabre B, Veeraraghavan N, Pilgard MA, Johnson BJ, Chiu CY.** 2013. The genome sequence of Lone Star virus, a highly divergent bunyavirus found in the *Amblyomma americanum* tick. *PLoS One* **8:**e62083.
93. **Clarke DH, Casals J.** 1958. Techniques for hemagglutination and hemagglutination-inhibition with arthropod-borne viruses. *Am J Trop Med Hyg* **7:**561–573.
94. **Hunsperger EA, Muñoz-Jordán J, Beltran M, Colón C, Carrión J, Vazquez J, Acosta LN, Medina-Izquierdo JF, Horiuchi K, Biggerstaff BJ, Margolis HS.** 2016. Performance of dengue diagnostic tests in a single-specimen diagnostic algorithm. *J Infect Dis* **214:**836–844.
95. **Innis BL, Nisalak A, Nimmannitya S, Kusalerdchariya S, Chongswasdi V, Suntayakorn S, Puttisri P, Hoke CH.** 1989. An enzyme-linked immunosorbent assay to characterize dengue infections where dengue and Japanese encephalitis co-circulate. *Am J Trop Med Hyg* **40:**418–427.
96. **Miagostovich MP, Nogueira RMR, dos Santos FB, Schatzmayr HG, Araújo ESM, Vorndam V.** 1999. Evaluation of an IgG enzyme-linked immunosorbent assay for dengue diagnosis. *J Clin Virol* **14:**183–189.
97. **Prince HE, Tobler LH, Lapé-Nixon M, Foster GA, Stramer SL, Busch MP.** 2005. Development and persistence of West Nile virus-specific immunoglobulin M (IgM), IgA, and IgG in viremic blood donors. *J Clin Microbiol* **43:**4316–4320.
98. **Edelman R, Schneider RJ, Vejjajiva A, Pornpibul R, Voodhikul P.** 1976. Persistence of virus-specific IgM and clinical recovery after Japanese encephalitis. *Am J Trop Med Hyg* **25:**733–738.
99. **Kapoor H, Signs K, Somsel P, Downes FP, Clark PA, Massey JP.** 2004. Persistence of West Nile virus (WNV) IgM antibodies in cerebrospinal fluid from patients with CNS disease. *J Clin Virol* **31:**289–291.
100. **Levett PN, Sonnenberg K, Sidaway F, Shead S, Niedrig M, Steinhagen K, Horsman GB, Drebot MA.** 2005. Use of immunoglobulin G avidity assays for differentiation of primary from previous infections with West Nile virus. *J Clin Microbiol* **43:**5873–5875.
101. **Chanama S, Sukprasert W, Sa-ngasang A, A-nuegoonpipat A, Sangkitporn S, Kurane I, Anantapreecha S.** 2005. Detection of Japanese encephalitis (JE) virus-specific IgM in cerebrospinal fluid and serum samples from JE patients. *Jpn J Infect Dis* **58:**294–296.
102. **Burke DS, Nisalak A, Ussery MA, Laorakpongse T, Chantavibul S.** 1985. Kinetics of IgM and IgG responses to Japanese encephalitis virus in human serum and cerebrospinal fluid. *J Infect Dis* **151:**1093–1099.
103. **Ravi V, Desai AS, Shenoy PK, Satishchandra P, Chandramuki A, Gourie-Devi M.** 1993. Persistence of Japanese encephalitis virus in the human nervous system. *J Med Virol* **40:**326–329.
104. **Hunsperger EA, Yoksan S, Buchy P, Nguyen VC, Sekaran SD, Enria DA, Pelegrino JL, Vázquez S, Artsob H, Drebot M, Gubler DJ, Halstead SB, Guzmán MG, Margolis HS, Nathanson CM, Rizzo Lic NR, Bessoff KE, Kliks S, Peeling RW.** 2009. Evaluation of commercially available anti-dengue virus immunoglobulin M tests. *Emerg Infect Dis* **15:**436–440.
105. **Blacksell SD, Bell D, Kelley J, Mammen MP Jr, Gibbons RV, Jarman RG, Vaughn DW, Jenjaroen K, Nisalak A, Thongpaseuth S, Vongsouvath M, Davong V, Phouminh P, Phetsouvanh R, Day NPJ, Newton PN.** 2007. Prospective study to determine accuracy of rapid serological assays for diagnosis of acute dengue virus infection in Laos. *Clin Vaccine Immunol* **14:**1458–1464.
106. **Ravi V, Robinson JS, Russell BJ, Desai A, Ramamurty N, Featherstone D, Johnson BW.** 2009. Evaluation of IgM antibody capture enzyme-linked immunosorbent assay kits for detection of IgM against Japanese encephalitis virus in cerebrospinal fluid samples. *Am J Trop Med Hyg* **81:**1144–1150.
107. **WHO.** 2009. Evaluation of commercially available anti-dengue virus immunoglobulin M tests. Diagnostics Evaluation Series, no. 3. World Health Organization, Geneva, Switzerland.
108. **Imrie A, Meeks J, Gurary A, Sukhbaatar M, Truong TT, Cropp CB, Effler P.** 2007. Antibody to dengue 1 detected more than 60 years after infection. *Viral Immunol* **20:** 672–675.
109. **Johnson AJ, Martin DA, Karabatsos N, Roehrig JT.** 2000. Detection of anti-arboviral immunoglobulin G by using a monoclonal antibody-based capture enzyme-linked immunosorbent assay. *J Clin Microbiol* **38:**1827–1831.
110. **Cardosa MJ, Wang SM, Sum MSH, Tio PH.** 2002. Antibodies against prM protein distinguish between previous infection with dengue and Japanese encephalitis viruses. *BMC Microbiol* **2:**9.
111. **dos Santos FB, Miagostovich MP, Nogueira RMR, Schatzmayr HG, Riley LW, Harris E.** 2004. Analysis of recombinant dengue virus polypeptides for dengue diagnosis and evaluation of the humoral immune response. *Am J Trop Med Hyg* **71:**144–152.
112. **Matheus S, Deparis X, Labeau B, Lelarge J, Morvan J, Dussart P.** 2005. Discrimination between primary and secondary dengue virus infection by an immunoglobulin G avidity test using a single acute-phase serum sample. *J Clin Microbiol* **43:**2793–2797.
113. **Cordeiro MT, Braga-Neto U, Nogueira RMR, Marques ETA, Jr.** 2009. Reliable classifier to differentiate primary and secondary acute dengue infection based on IgG ELISA. *PLoS One* **4:**e4945.
114. **de Souza VAUF, Fernandes S, Araújo ES, Tateno AF, Oliveira OMNPF, Oliveira RR, Pannuti CS.** 2004. Use of an immunoglobulin G avidity test to discriminate between primary and secondary dengue virus infections. *J Clin Microbiol* **42:**1782–1784.
115. **Thakare JP, Gore MM, Risbud AR, Banerjee K, Ghosh SN.** 1991. Detection of virus specific IgG subclasses in Japanese encephalitis patients. *Indian J Med Res* **93:**271–276.
116. **Koraka P, Suharti C, Setiati TE, Mairuhu ATA, Van Gorp E, Hack CE, Juffrie M, Sutaryo J, Van Der Meer GM, Groen J, Osterhaus ADME.** 2001. Kinetics of dengue virus-specific serum immunoglobulin classes and subclasses correlate with clinical outcome of infection. *J Clin Microbiol* **39:**4332–4338.
117. **Thein S, Aaskov J, Myint TT, Shwe TN, Saw TT, Zaw A.** 1993. Changes in levels of anti-dengue virus IgG subclasses in patients with disease of varying severity. *J Med Virol* **40:** 102–106.
118. **Banoo S, Bell D, Bossuyt P, Herring A, Mabey D, Poole F, Smith PG, Sriram N, Wongsrichanalai C, Linke R, O'Brien R, Perkins M, Cunningham J, Matsoso P, Nathanson CM, Olliaro P, Peeling RW, Ramsay A, TDR Diagnostics Evaluation Expert Panel.** 2010. Evaluation of diagnostic tests for infectious diseases: general principles. *Nat Rev Microbiol* **8(Suppl):**S17–S29.
119. **Modis Y, Ogata S, Clements D, Harrison SC.** 2005. Variable surface epitopes in the crystal structure of dengue virus type 3 envelope glycoprotein. *J Virol* **79:**1223–1231.
120. **Roehrig JT, Bolin RA, Kelly RG.** 1998. Monoclonal antibody mapping of the envelope glycoprotein of the dengue 2 virus, Jamaica. *Virology* **246:**317–328.
121. **Crill WD, Roehrig JT.** 2001. Monoclonal antibodies that bind to domain III of dengue virus E glycoprotein are the most efficient blockers of virus adsorption to Vero cells. *J Virol* **75:**7769–7773.
122. **Roehrig JT, Mathews JH.** 1985. The neutralization site on the E2 glycoprotein of Venezuelan equine encephalomyelitis (TC-83) virus is composed of multiple conformationally stable epitopes. *Virology* **142:**347–356.

123. **Hunt AR, Frederickson S, Maruyama T, Roehrig JT, Blair CD.** 2010. The first human epitope map of the alphaviral E1 and E2 proteins reveals a new E2 epitope with significant virus neutralizing activity. *PLoS Negl Trop Dis* **4:**e739.
124. **Cheng LL, Schultz KT, Yuill TM, Israel BA.** 2000. Identification and localization of conserved antigenic epitopes on the G2 proteins of California serogroup bunyaviruses. *Viral Immunol* **13:**201–213.
125. **Westaway EG.** 1965. The neutralization of arboviruses. II. Neutralization in heterologous virus-serum mixtures with four group B arboviruses. *Virology* **26:**528–537.
126. **Westaway EG.** 1965. The neutralization of arboviruses. I. Neutralization in homologous virus-serum mixtures with two group B arboviruses. *Virology* **26:**517–527.
127. **Halstead SB, O'Rourke EJ.** 1977. Antibody-enhanced dengue virus infection in primate leukocytes. *Nature* **265:** 739–741.
128. **Ferenczi E, Bán E, Abrahám A, Kaposi T, Petrányi G, Berencsi G, Vaheri A.** 2008. Severe tick-borne encephalitis in a patient previously infected by West Nile virus. *Scand J Infect Dis* **40:**759–761.
129. **Pierson TC, Xu Q, Nelson S, Oliphant T, Nybakken GE, Fremont DH, Diamond MS.** 2007. The stoichiometry of antibody-mediated neutralization and enhancement of West Nile virus infection. *Cell Host Microbe* **1:**135–145.
130. **Roehrig JT, Hombach J, Barrett ADT.** 2008. Guidelines for plaque-reduction neutralization testing of human antibodies to dengue viruses. *Viral Immunol* **21:**123–132.

Hantaviruses*

JOHN D. KLENA, CHENG-FENG CHIANG, AND WUN-JU SHIEH

98

Hemorrhagic fever with renal syndrome (HFRS) and hantavirus pulmonary syndrome (HPS; also referred to as hantavirus cardiopulmonary syndrome) are rodent-borne zoonoses caused by several members of the virus family *Hantaviridae*, genus *Orthohantavirus*. A hallmark of HFRS and HPS is a reversible increase in the permeability of small blood vessels. Diagnosis early in the course of disease is critical to the successful management of HFRS and HPS.

TAXONOMY

The International Committee on Taxonomy of Viruses (ICTV) reorganized the order *Bunyavirales* in 2016 and currently recognizes 41 species in the genus *Orthohantavirus* (*Bunyavirales:Hantaviridae*). Unlike other *Bunyavirales* members, hantaviruses are not transmitted by arthropods (1). To be recognized by the ICTV as a species, four mandatory criteria must be met: (i) a hantavirus species is found in a unique ecological niche, i.e., in a different primary rodent reservoir species or subspecies; (ii) a hantavirus species exhibits at least 7% difference in amino acid identity when S and M segment sequences are compared; (iii) a hantavirus species shows at least a 4-fold difference in two-way cross-neutralization tests; and (iv) hantavirus species do not naturally form reassortants with other species (2). Recently, rule 2 was refined to take into account the length and composition of the sequences in addition to amino acid sequence differences ("a 10% difference in S segment similarity and 12% difference in M segment similarity based on complete amino acid sequences") (3, 4). Application of these rules has resulted in the deletion of seven formerly recognized species with the suggestion that they be added as strains of other recognized hantavirus species (5). Pathogenic strains within these species have been identified in the Americas (6–8), Asia (9), and Europe (10); in Africa, only serological evidence of human infection has been presented until now (11, 12) (Table 1).

Hantaviruses were first isolated from Rodentia (e.g., mice, rats, and voles) species; additional reservoirs have been identified in Soricomorpha (e.g., shrews and moles) and Chioptera (e.g., bats) (13) (Table 1). The use of molecular techniques has demonstrated the presence of hantaviruses in new animals and has expanded the list of mammals that appear to be reservoirs (14). However, any given hantavirus species is almost exclusively restricted to a single mammalian reservoir; thus, the geographic distribution of its associated disease is restricted to the range and distribution of its reservoir. In addition, the severity of disease in humans is influenced by the species and strain of hantavirus, with viruses ranging from being noninfectious to having a reported case fatality rate of 50% (14).

Old World hantavirus species are found in Asia and Europe, with Haantan virus being the prototype species of the genus. Pathogenic species of Old World hantavirus are known to cause HFRS. In contrast, pathogenic New World hantavirus species are known to cause HPS. African hantaviruses have yet to be associated with a disease syndrome in humans. It is interesting that the majority of identified African hantaviruses are genetically more diverse than the Old or New World hantaviruses; in part, this has led to their slow discovery and suggests that new diagnostic tools need to be developed to capture potential human pathogenic species.

DESCRIPTION OF THE AGENTS

Hantavirus virions are spherical to pleiomorphic, ranging from 80 to 120 nm in diameter, and possess a lipid bilayer envelope (15). The envelope displays a grid-like pattern that distinguishes them from other *Bunyavirales* (16) (Fig. 1). Spikes, approximately 6 nm in length, are composed of the glycoproteins G1 and G2 (formerly known as Gn and Gc, respectively), and protrude from the envelope of the virion. The virion interior contains ribonucleocapsids—segments of single-stranded genomic RNA complexed with nucleocapsid protein and the RNA-dependent RNA polymerase. The nucleocapsid of hantaviruses has been shown to be a multifunctional protein, interacting with RNA and various viral and cellular proteins, thus participating in genome packaging, RNA chaperoning, intracellular protein transport, DNA degradation, intervention in host translation, and restricting the host immune responses (17).

Organization of the genome of hantaviruses is typical of that of the *Bunyavirales*; each virion consists of a small (S), medium (M), and large (L) segment, all of which are

*This chapter contains material from chapter 96 by Charles F. Fulhorst and Michael D. Bowen in the 11th edition of this *Manual*.

TABLE 1 Hantavirus species associated with human disease

Group and virus[a]	Reservoir	Known geographical distribution	Human disease
Principally associated with members of the rodent family Muridae, subfamily Murinae			
DOBV	*Apodemus agrarius* (striped field mouse), *Apodemus flavicollis* (yellow-necked mouse), *Apodemus ponticus* (Black Sea field mouse)	Central and Eastern Europe	HFRS
HTNV	*Apodemus agrarius*	Asia	HFRS
SAAV	*Apodemus agrarius*	Eastern Europe	HFRS
SANGV	*Hylomyscus simus* (African wood mouse)	Guinea	HFRS
SEOV	*Rattus norvegicus* (brown rat), *Rattus rattus* (black rat)	Asia, worldwide	HFRS
Principally associated with the family Cricetidae, subfamily Arvicolinae			
PUUV	*Myodes glareolus* (bank vole)	Europe	HFRS
Tula virus	*Microtus arvalis* (common vole)	Europe	HFRS
Principally associated with the family Cricetidae, subfamily Neotominae of Sigmodontinae			
ANDV	*Oligoryzomys longicaudatus* (long-tailed colilargo)	South America	HPS
Bayou virus	*Oryzomys palustris* (marsh rice rat)	United States	HPS
Black Creek Canal virus	*Sigmodon hispidus* (hispid cotton rat)	United States	HPS
Choclo virus	*Oligoryzomys fulvescens* (northern pygmy rice rat)	Panama	HPS
Laguna Negra virus	*Calomys laucha* (small vesper mouse), *Calomys callosus* (large vesper mouse)	Argentina, Bolivia, Brazil, Paraguay	HPS
SNV	*Peromyscus maniculatus* (deer mouse), *Peromyscus leucopus* (white-footed mouse)	United States, Canada	HPS
Principally associated with the Eulipoyphla family Soricidae			
Uluguru virus	*Myosorex geata* (Geata mouse shrew)	Tanzania	HFRS

[a]Murinae, Old World rats and mice; Arvicolinae, voles and lemmings; Neotominae and Sigmodontinae, New World rats and mice; Soricidae, shrew.

are unique negative-sense, single-stranded RNA molecules (15). The S segment (1.7 to 2.1 kb) encodes the hantavirus nucleocapsid protein, and in some hantavirus species, an open reading frame overlapping the nucleoprotein and encoding a nonstructural protein has been observed. The M segment (3.6 to 3.7 kb) encodes the glycoprotein precursor, which is cotranslationally cleaved to yield the envelope glycoproteins G1 and G2. The L segment (6.5 to 6.6 kb) encodes an RNA-dependent RNA polymerase and is the most conserved of three genomic segments (3). Consistent with other *Bunyavirales*, ribonucleocapsids display helical symmetry and form circular structures as a result of base pairing by highly conserved, inverse complementary nucleotide sequences at the termini of each genome segment (18).

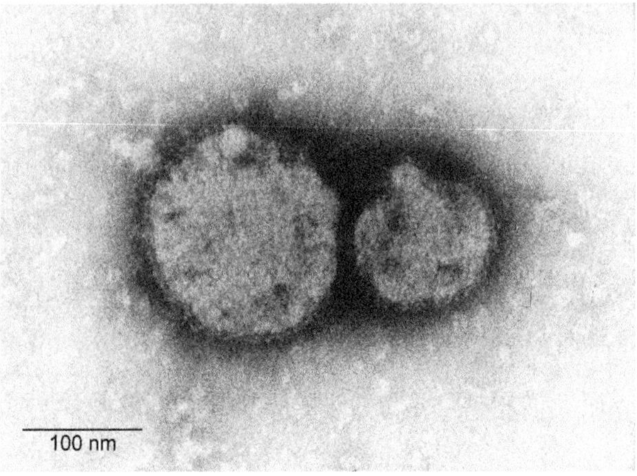

FIGURE 1 Electron micrograph of negatively stained SNV (2% phosphotungstic acid stain, pH 6.5). (Courtesy of Charles Humphrey, Centers for Disease Control and Prevention.)

EPIDEMIOLOGY AND TRANSMISSION

Old World hantaviruses are considered those species that are predominantly found in Asia and Europe. Globally, 150,000 to 200,000 cases of hantavirus infection, and 30,000 HFRS cases, are reported annually, with China experiencing the largest proportion of cases (19, 20). The two most frequently reported hantaviruses in Asia are Hantaan virus (HTNV) and Seoul virus (SEOV). The reservoir for HTNV is *Apodemus agrarius* (striped field mouse), and HTNV causes moderate to severe HFRS in South Korea, China, and eastern Russia. A recent analysis of field and epidemiological data from China (1960 to 2013) supports the idea that Hantaan infections are more pronounced when climactic changes favor rodent population growth and viral transmission (21). The reservoir for SEOV, in contrast, is primarily *Rattus norvegicus* (brown rat), and the virus causes moderate HFRS, though case fatality rates as high as 15% have been reported (22). Because of the widespread distribution of the brown rat, SEOV infections are known to occur globally (23). SEOV in pet rats led to human infections in the United Kingdom in 2012 (24), Sweden in 2013 (25), and the United States in 2017 (26).

Strains of Dobrava-Belgrade virus (DOBV) can cause mild to moderate to severe HFRS in Central and Eastern Europe (22). Three reservoirs are currently recognized for DOBV: *A. agrarius*, *Apodemus flavicollis* (yellow-necked mouse), and *Apodemus ponticus* (Black Sea field mouse). Closely related to but distinct from DOBV is Saaremaa virus (SAAV), which shares the yellow-necked and striped field mouse as reservoirs with DOBV (27). The reservoir for Puumala virus (PUUV) is *Myodes glareolus* (bank vole); PUUV causes nephropathia epidemica, a relatively mild form of HFRS, in Europe and western Russia.

Hantavirus infections in the Americas were unrecognized until 1993, when an outbreak of Sin Nombre virus (SNV), identified in *Peromyscus maniculatus* (deer mouse), occurred in the Four Corners region (New Mexico, Utah, Arizona, and Colorado) of the United States (6). New World hantaviruses have a geographical distribution from Canada through the United States and Latin America to South America. Although New World hantavirus infections do not contribute as significantly to the total hantavirus disease burden as the Old World viruses, SNV and Andes virus (ANDV), found in *Oligoryzomys longicaudatus* (long-tailed colilargo), cause severe disease and are the major causes of HPS in North America and South America, respectively. From 1993 through 2015, 662 HPS cases (230 deaths [35%]) in the United States were reported to the Centers for Disease Control and Prevention; the majority of these cases were attributed to SNV (28). In Buenos Aires province, Argentina, from 2009 through 2014, of 1,386 suspected cases of hantavirus infection, 88 were confirmed as HPS, and the majority of these cases were attributed to ANDV (29). Although there are far fewer HPS cases than HFRS cases each year, outbreaks of HPS usually are highly lethal, with case fatality rates of 20 to 60%.

Since 2006, there have been increasingly successful efforts to identify hantaviruses in Africa (11). Sangassou virus (SANGV) was detected in *Hylomyscus simus* (African wood mouse) (30) and is the first African hantavirus to be cultured (31). Use of a broadly reactive reverse transcription-PCR (RT-PCR) assay based on the most conserved portion of the L segment has led to the discovery of SANGV as well as other African hantaviruses in both western Africa and East Africa (11, 12, 30). New serologic tools designed around the African hantaviruses have been used to perform serosurveys of potential animal reservoirs and humans (12, 32). Evidence is mounting that the African hantaviruses cause disease in humans similar to HFRS (12).

The most common route of transmission by which humans become infected with hantaviruses is through inhalation of aerosolized droplets of urine, saliva, or respiratory secretions from infected rodents or by inhalation of aerosolized particles of feces, dust, or other organic matter contaminated with secretions or excretions from infected rodents or reservoir species (33). Other means of infection, such as infection after the bite of a rodent or other reservoir species, are rare, and human-to-human transmission has been documented only for ANDV during the acute phase of illness (7).

The risk of infection in humans is dependent upon the frequency and intensity of human exposure to infected rodents and their secretions or excretions. The cleaning of closed quarters occupied by infected rodents has been repeatedly associated with an increased risk of infection (34–37). Given the relative ease of modern travel and the time lag from symptom onset to diagnosis, epidemiological challenges remain with respect to identifying and locating individuals that have potentially been exposed to hantavirus-infected rodents during an HPS outbreak investigation (38).

CLINICAL SIGNIFICANCE

The clinical and pathological features of severe HFRS and HPS are associated with acute thrombocytopenia and a reversible increase in microvascular (capillary) permeability. A major difference between the two syndromes is that the retroperitoneum is the major site of the vascular leak in HFRS, whereas the lungs and thoracic cavity are the major sites of the vascular leak in HPS.

The length of the incubation period in HFRS and HPS is usually 2 to 4 weeks but can range from a few days to 2 months. The clinical course of HFRS can be divided into five phases: prodrome (typically 3 to 7 days), hypotensive (several hours to 4 days), oliguric (4 to 5 days), diuretic (7 to 11 days), and convalescent (weeks to months). Similarly, the clinical course of HPS can be divided into four phases: prodrome (3 to 6 days), cardiopulmonary (7 to 10 days), diuretic (1 to 3 days), and convalescent (weeks to months). Death in HFRS is usually due to shock in the hypotensive or diuretic phase. Death in HPS is usually attributed to hypoxia (pulmonary edema) or shock in the cardiopulmonary phase.

In severe HFRS caused by HTNV or DOBV, the prodrome usually begins with an abrupt onset of high fever, chills, headache, blurred vision, malaise, and anorexia and then includes severe abdominal or lumbar pain, gastrointestinal symptoms, facial flushing, petechiae, and an erythematous rash or conjunctival hemorrhage. The hypotensive phase begins with a characteristic decrease in platelet number followed by defervescence and abrupt onset of hypotension, which may progress to shock and more apparent hemorrhagic manifestations. Other abnormalities may include elevated serum levels of aspartate transaminase (39). In the oliguric phase, blood pressure returns to normal or becomes high, urinary output falls dramatically, concentrations of serum creatinine and blood urea nitrogen increase, and severe hemorrhage may occur. Spontaneous diuresis, with polyuria greater than 3 liters per day, heralds the onset of recovery. Distinct clinical phases are less obvious in HFRS caused by SEOV and nephropathia epidemica, and visible superficial hemorrhages usually do not occur in nephropathia epidemica (40). Pathological findings in HFRS at autopsy include effusions in body cavities, retroperitoneal edema, and enlarged, congested, hemorrhagic kidneys (41).

HPS was first recognized in 1993 as a highly fatal disease in the southwestern United States (6). The original description of HPS (42) was subsequently modified to include mild infections that do not result in radiographic evidence of pulmonary disease (43). It is now recognized that HPS sometimes includes renal impairment and, at least in South America, bleeding manifestations (44–46). The prodrome in HPS is characterized by fever, myalgia, and malaise. Other symptoms that may occur during the prodrome include headache, dizziness, anorexia, abdominal pain, nausea, vomiting, and diarrhea. Nonproductive cough and tachypnea usually mark the onset of pulmonary edema. Fully developed HPS is characterized by rapidly progressive (time span of 4 to 24 hours) noncardiogenic pulmonary edema, hypoxemia, large volumes of pleural effusion, and cardiogenic shock. Hypotension and oliguria are the result of shock. Myocardial depression may occur and contribute to shock (47). The diuretic phase is characterized by rapid clearance of pulmonary edema and resolution of fever and shock. Hematologic abnormalities in HPS at hospitalization include thrombocytopenia, hemoconcentration with elevated hematocrit, and leukocytosis with the presence of large, reactive (immunoblastic) lymphocytes (48, 49). Other laboratory abnormalities may include elevated levels of hepatic enzymes, hypoalbuminemia, metabolic acidosis, and, in severe cases, lactic acidosis. The gross abnormalities in fatal HPS seen at autopsy include copious amounts of frothy fluid in bronchi and other airways; heavy, edematous lungs; and large volumes of pleural fluid (49, 50).

Therapy

Treatment of HFRS and HPS starts with addressing the clinical symptoms after the patient is hospitalized. In HFRS patients, shock symptoms may be managed with vasopressors and intravenous fluids. Hemodialysis is also provided when patients show signs of acute kidney failure (51). HPS patients should be oxygenated by mechanical ventilation and/or extracorporeal membrane oxygenation, since the disease can rapidly progress to respiratory failure or cardiogenic shock (52). When given early after disease onset, ribavirin has shown beneficial effects in HFRS patients in studies conducted in China and Korea (53, 54). In contrast, ribavirin did not appreciably affect outcome in HPS patients in two U.S. trials (55, 56).

Animal Models

To date, rodents, shrews, voles, and bats have been identified as natural hosts of hantaviruses (11). These small mammals are asymptomatic after infection and consequently become the reservoir for transmitting hantavirus horizontally through their excreta (57). Because these animals do not recapitulate human disease, they are not viable models for hantavirus research. No evidence of vertical hantavirus transmission has been documented (58, 59). Newborn mice infected with HTNV develop neurological disorders and succumb to death (60, 61), but this disease does not mimic HFRS seen in humans, and thus, no rodent models of HFRS caused by Old World hantaviruses exist. However, limited successes have been reported with using cynomolgus macaques as a disease model for PUUV; these animals develop a less severe form of HFRS upon infection than that in humans (62, 63).

Among New World hantaviruses, ANDV has been shown to cause a lethal disease course similar to HPS in Syrian golden hamsters (64–66). Maporal and Laguna Negra viruses induce deaths and elicit HPS-like diseases in hamsters (67, 68). A recent study showed that rhesus macaques receiving lung homogenates from SNV-infected deer mice develop a clinical disease resembling HPS in humans (69).

Antivirals

Currently, no antiviral compounds have been approved by the U.S. Food and Drug Administration for preventing or treating HFRS or HPS. However, in addition to ribavirin, favipiravir (T-705; 6-fluoro-3-hydroxy-2-pyrazinecarboxamide) is a nucleoside analog reported to inhibit Maporal virus, DOBV, and ANDV in rodent disease models (70–72). Another nucleoside analog, ETAR (1-β-D-ribofuranosyl-3-ethynyl-[1,2,4] triazole), was also found to suppress HTNV infection in newborn mice (73).

Nucleoprotein (N) of hantaviruses plays an important role in viral genome packaging, viral RNA synthesis, and translation. Salim and colleagues have demonstrated that several chemical inhibitors interrupt the interaction between ANDV N and viral RNA, abolish viral RNA synthesis and translation, and inhibit ANDV replication in cell culture (74). Another virus-targeting antiviral, lactoferrin, binds viral glycoprotein (G), inhibits viral adsorption to cells, and increases the survival of infected newborn mice (75, 76). In addition, hantavirus G2 envelope protein is a class II fusion protein and part of the G protein complex (77, 78). When triggered, it fuses the viral membrane with the endosomal membrane under acidic conditions (79, 80). A study has shown that hantavirus membrane fusion and cell entry are inhibited by protein fragments spanning domain III and the stem region of ANDV G2 protein. The results suggested that these fragments blocked up to 60% of ANDV infection in Vero-E6 cells (81).

Several studies performed in rodents have demonstrated that passive transfer of neutralizing antibodies to HTNV or ANDV can protect animals from challenge with the same virus (82–84). Furthermore, light-chain portions of antibodies (Fab) from a PUUV-immune patient were cloned into a phage display library, and Fab fragments were screened for viral G protein binding activity and for neutralizing activity against PUUV in cell culture (85). Four of 13 Fab clones showed a 44 to 54% reduction in the number of PUUV foci (85). In another study, antibodies produced in geese treated with a DNA vaccine encoding ANDV G protein effectively protected hamsters when administered 5 days after ANDV challenge (86). Due to the absence of mammalian Fc, the Fab fragment and IgY from geese did not elicit undesired immune responses, making these antibodies attractive potential candidates for vaccine development.

RNA interference is a posttranscriptional, sequence-specific RNA degradation process observed in eukaryotic cells and is considered a defense mechanism against viral infection (87). Small interfering RNA (siRNA) pools targeting each of the ANDV genome segments (S, M, and L) have been tested for efficacy in reducing viral replication in Vero-E6 and human primary lung endothelial cells (HMVEC-L), a primary target of ANDV infection in humans (88). Interestingly, the siRNA pool targeting the S segment inhibited ANDV replication in Vero-E6 cells more effectively than did siRNA pools targeting the L or M segment. In contrast, the siRNA pool targeting M segment reduced ANDV titers in HMVEC-L cells (88). Moreover, in a recent study, a single-chain antibody that recognized HTNV G protein (scFv) was fused to a cationic peptide from protamine, which was in turn complexed with the siRNA against the M segment. This chimeric protein recognized HTNV G protein in the infected cells (61). The bound fusion protein was internalized, delivering the siRNA cargo into the cytosol of infected cells (89). The results suggest that the siRNA complexes not only were able to inhibit HTNV replication in the infected Vero-E6 cells but also targeted the brain cells of the infected newborn mice and effectively protected them from death (61).

In addition to antivirals directly targeting hantaviruses, several antivirals targeting host proteins have been explored. Cellular entry of pathogenic hantaviruses is mediated by β_3 integrin on the host cells (90, 91). Hall and colleagues used multiple cyclic peptides to block the attachment of SNV and ANDV to β_3 integrin receptor, inhibiting *in vitro* replication of these viruses by 50% (92–94). However, other receptors and cellular entry pathways have also been implicated in hantavirus infection (95–97). Combinations of several antivirals may be necessary to effectively combat hantavirus infection.

Hantavirus infection causes increased capillary permeability and vascular leakage. Infection of endothelial cells activates the kinin-kallikrein system and releases bradykinin (98). The binding of bradykinin to bradykinin B2 receptor in turn triggers an inflammatory response, resulting in blood vessel dilation and decreased blood pressure. Icatibant is a peptidomimetic antagonist of bradykinin B2 receptor that blocks the binding of bradykinin to its receptor and prevents the subsequent inflammatory response. Taylor et al. have shown that icatibant blocks the openings in human umbilical vein endothelial cell monolayers after infection with ANDV or HTNV (98). In addition, another report documented that a patient infected with PUUV recovered from the illness after icatibant treatment (99).

Vaccines

No vaccines have been approved by the U.S. Food and Drug Administration for preventing hantavirus infection. Vaccines based on viruses inactivated by formalin or β-propiolactone have been developed and used in South Korea and China to combat HFRS in humans (100, 101). These vaccines are based on virus particles harvested from the brains of suckling mice or from cell cultures infected with HTNV or SEOV. In China, vaccines based on HTNV and/or SEOV have been used in regions of high endemicity since 1995 (101). Hantavax from South Korea was tested with a three-dose schedule. Recipients generated sufficient levels of neutralizing antibodies against HTNV after the last vaccine dose, and the protective immunity lasted 2 years (102). In Russia, inactivated PUUV and DOBV were combined to create a bivalent vaccine. Combined with an aluminum hydroxide adjuvant, this vaccine induced production of neutralizing antibodies against both PUUV and DOBV in BALB/c mice (103).

Chimeric viruses have been made from nonreplicating adenovirus vectors. Adenoviruses expressing ANDV N, G1, or G2 protein protect hamsters from ANDV challenge (104). An alternative approach using replication-competent canine adenovirus expressing SEOV G1 or G2 was also shown to elicit neutralizing antibodies against SEOV infection in mice (105, 106).

Virus-like particles (VLPs) containing virus core particles have often been used as platforms to accommodate self or foreign viral proteins. Li and colleagues generated VLPs by coexpressing HTNV N, G1, and G2 proteins in Chinese hamster ovary cells. Immune responses induced by inoculating mice with these VLPs were compared with responses produced by Chinese bivalent inactivated vaccines (based on HTNV and SEOV) (107). VLP vaccination resulted in higher levels of cellular immune response to N protein than the inactivated vaccine did (107). Furthermore, ANDV or PUUV G1 and G2 proteins have been shown to self-assemble into VLPs, which reacted with patient sera (108).

Compared with the vaccines mentioned above, DNA vaccines are easier to construct and have the advantage of eliciting long-term humoral and cellular immune responses. DNA vaccines containing the M or S gene (encoding G or N protein, respectively) have been made using HTNV, SEOV, PUUV, ANDV, and SNV sequences. Various model animals given these vaccines were subsequently challenged with the corresponding hantavirus. In general, better immune responses and protection were seen in nonhuman primates and rabbits than in hamsters, and G protein constructs induced stronger immune responses than did N protein constructs (64, 84, 109–111). Finally, volunteers receiving gene-gun-delivered DNA vaccines encoding G protein of HTNV or PUUV developed neutralizing antibody titers toward respective virus. Most of the volunteers (seven of nine) receiving both HTNV and PUUV DNA vaccines developed neutralizing antibodies against PUUV; the three who responded most strongly to the PUUV vaccine also had strong neutralizing antibody responses to HTNV (112).

COLLECTION, TRANSPORT, AND STORAGE OF SPECIMENS

As the rules regarding shipment of potentially pathogenic specimens are subject to change, the clinician should consult with local health authorities and/or national (or international) reference laboratories that maintain diagnostic capability for hantaviruses before shipping clinical specimens to a diagnostic laboratory for current guidance.

Infectious hantavirus has been isolated from blood, serum, urine and cerebral spinal fluid collected during the acute phase of clinical disease (33), and therefore, these and other biological materials should be considered potentially infectious to humans. The U.S. Department of Health and Human Services has recommended the following precautions for the handling of hantavirus clinical specimens: (i) sera from potential HFRS or HPS cases should be handled at biosafety level 2 (BSL2), (ii) potentially infectious tissue specimens should be handled at BSL2 using BSL3 practices, (iii) all procedures that could result in splatter or aerosolization of human body fluids should be done inside a certified biological safety cabinet, and (iv) propagation of virus in cell culture and virus purification should be carried out in a BSL3 facility using BSL3 practices (113). Because hantaviruses are thermolabile (114), they can be inactivated by agents that disrupt lipid membranes; these include many commercial products as well as acids, alcohols, sodium hypochlorite, paraformaldehyde, and UV irradiation (115–117). Laboratory-acquired infections have been reported previously (118, 119), and although the survival of hantaviruses in the environment in liquids, aerosols, or a dried state is not well understood, infectious virions in dried cell culture medium and in liquids maintained at low temperatures have been reported to persist for 2 or more days (33).

As previously reported (37), blood, serum, and plasma samples for serology may be stored at 4°C and shipped to the diagnostic laboratory on cold packs if there is no significant delay between collection and testing. If this is not possible, specimens should be stored at −20°C or lower and shipped on dry ice. Any biological material to be used for RNA extraction and/or viral isolation (e.g., blood, blood clots, and solid tissues) should be stored continuously (without freeze-thawing) at −70°C or lower and shipped on dry ice in order to preserve the integrity of the viral RNA and viral infectivity. Samples shipped by air should be packaged, documented, and shipped in accordance with International Air Transport Association Dangerous Goods Regulations (https://www.iata.org/pages/default.aspx). In the United States, ground shipping must comply with regulations issued by the U.S. Department of Transportation (49 CFR, parts 171 to 178).

DIRECT EXAMINATION

As previously reported, none of the laboratory assays used for diagnosis of hantaviral infections in humans have been standardized (37); no hantavirus diagnostic assays have received approval from the U.S. Food and Drug Administration. Commercially produced European diagnostic test kits are sold for research use only in the United States, if available at all.

Microscopy

The major histopathologic change in HPS is massive intra-alveolar edema and capillaritis in the lung (Fig. 2). Prominent immunoblasts may be observed in the spleen (Fig. 3).

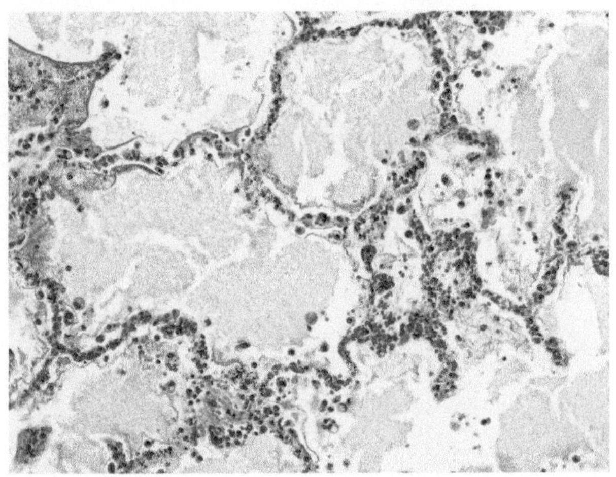

FIGURE 2 Photomicrograph of human lung tissue from a fatal case of HPS showing massive intra-alveolar edema and inflammation in pulmonary microvasculature (capillaritis).

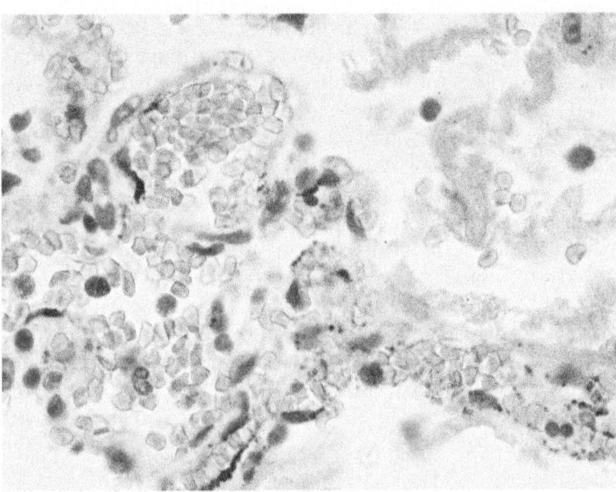

FIGURE 4 Photomicrograph of human lung tissue from a fatal case of HPS showing hantaviral antigen in pulmonary microvasculature, with hantaviral antigen stained red by using immunohistochemistry.

However, these histopathologic changes are nonspecific and need further ancillary tests, such as immunohistochemical or molecular assays for confirmation of diagnosis. Direct electron-microscopic examination of tissues is of limited diagnostic value but has been used to detect virions and viral replicative structures in autopsy samples. Electron-microscopic examination of autopsy tissues from HFRS and HPS patients found that mature virions are infrequent in tissues and can be difficult to identify due to considerable polymorphism in size and shape. Structures determined to be hantaviral inclusion bodies were seen more often than intact virions (50, 120).

Antigen Detection

Immunohistochemistry has been used to detect hantaviral antigens in tissues from fatal HFRS cases, biopsy materials from nephropathia epidemica cases, and tissues from fatal HPS cases (Fig. 4) (50). Polyclonal antibodies (e.g., immune sera from humans, experimentally infected rabbits, and experimentally or naturally infected rodents) and murine monoclonal antibodies have been used as primary antibodies in immunohistochemical assays. Fatal HPS is associated with widespread distribution of hantaviral antigen in lung, spleen, kidney, and heart tissues, with antigen primarily localized within endothelial cells of capillaries and other small blood vessels (50). Immunohistochemical assays for diagnosis of hantaviral infections in humans are limited to the few institutions that have access to the appropriate primary antibodies and control tissues.

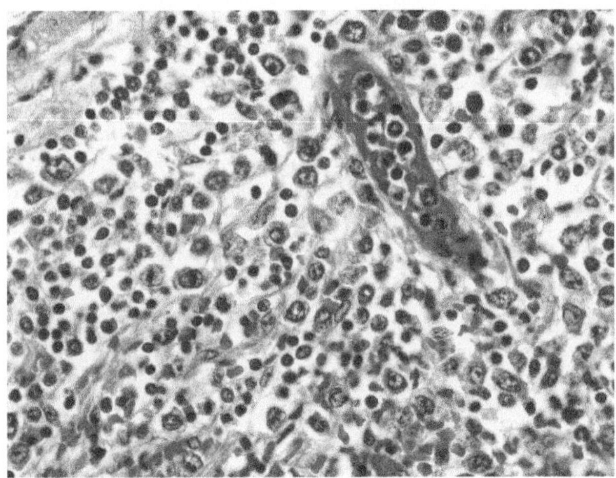

FIGURE 3 Photomicrograph of human spleen tissue from a fatal case of HPS showing prominent immunoblasts.

IDENTIFICATION

Nucleic Acid Detection

RT-PCR is a widely used molecular diagnostic method for hantavirus detection. Samples like serum, whole blood, bronchoalveolar lavage fluid, and organ fragments from suspected cases (or, occasionally, rodents) have been received for hantavirus testing at the CDC (26, 121). In addition to confirming hantavirus infection by detecting viral RNA, the resulting PCR product may be sequenced to identify the virus through phylogenetic analysis. Hantavirus RNA can be detected by RT-PCR in human samples from 3 to 10 days after symptom onset. Prior knowledge of the circulating species of hantavirus in a geographic location supports the use of primers specific for hantavirus S and M segments targeting that species (8, 122). Concurrent circulation of several hantavirus types in a region complicates such identification. For example, both New World hantaviruses and the Old World hantavirus SEOV are present in wild rodent populations in the United States (23, 123, 124). To detect currently known hantaviruses in such samples, a set of four pan-hantavirus primers against the highly conserved L segment was designed, and a protocol of nested RT-PCR was developed at the CDC (23). A similar nested RT-PCR targeting the L segment was also used to discover a novel hantavirus in an African wood mouse sample (30). Additionally, researchers used primers against conserved regions of the M segment of HTNV/SEOV or PUUV/Prospect Hill virus in nested RT-PCR and sequenced the products to identify what is now known as SNV (6, 125).

Real-time RT-PCR is another sensitive test for diagnosing hantavirus infection. It has advantages, such as the ability to quantify viral loads in the samples and shorter detection times due to smaller amplicons (126, 127).

However, high sequence diversity among the known hantaviruses has prevented the design of a robust set of primers and probes for an efficient pan-hantavirus real-time RT-PCR. Therefore, application of real-time RT-PCR is restricted to detection of genetically closely related hantaviruses cocirculating in a region and following up contacts of a known case of hantavirus infection (26, 121, 127, 128).

RT-PCR can detect the presence of viral RNA only when the patient is in the acute phase of the infection, when viremia is still ongoing. Often, viral RNA is undetectable by PCR by the time the patient is hospitalized. PCR should be considered a complementary method, along with serologic assays, such as IgM/IgG enzyme-linked immunosorbent assay (ELISA), to create a complete diagnostic panel to conclusively detect or rule out hantavirus infection.

Serologic Tests

Diagnosis of hantavirus infection usually begins with clinical and epidemiological information gathered from patients, e.g., history of fever, myalgia, thrombocytopenia, renal failure, or respiratory distress, and whether the individuals had a recent exposure to rodent excreta. Laboratory testing is then conducted after samples have been received from a suspected case. In addition to nucleic acid detection methods such as RT-PCR (discussed above), several serologic tests are used for hantavirus diagnosis.

The immunofluorescence assay (IFA) is considered one of the earliest serologic tests developed for hantavirus diagnosis (129). IFA uses hantavirus-infected cells fixed as an antigen on glass plates. Diluted serum samples are added to the plates to detect the viral antigens. However, low virus yield in preparations of certain hantavirus antigens and high levels of background signal from nonspecific antibody binding can affect the quality and interpretation of IFA results. Multiparametric IFAs have been developed and are commercially available in Europe. Matrices on biochips are coated with HTNV-, PUUV-, SEOV-, SAAV-, DOBV-, SNV-, and ANDV-infected cells to react with serum samples. A report suggested that the performance of such multiparametric IFAs is comparable to many in-house-developed IFAs and ELISAs (130).

However, the most commonly used serologic tests for hantavirus detection are ELISAs. In general, significant levels of hantavirus-specific IgM can be found in the serum of HFRS and HPS patients after the onset of clinical symptoms (125, 131). As the disease progresses into the acute phase, IgG responses against hantaviruses become detectable (132, 133). In patients with HFRS, anti-hantavirus IgM may last for 6 months after the acute phase ends, and IgG can be detected up to 10 years later in some cases (133, 134). In contrast, in HPS patients, anti-hantavirus IgM levels decline after 2 to 3 months postinfection, though IgG levels may be maintained for up to 3 years (132, 135).

To detect hantavirus-specific IgM antibodies, an IgM capture ELISA has been developed and is routinely performed by the CDC, many state public health laboratories, and some commercial reference laboratories (125). The assay uses goat anti-μ captured IgM from samples to bind viral antigens in infected cell lysates, instead of immobilizing viral antigens to a solid substrate as in some commercially available indirect IgM assays (136, 137). The results appear to be significantly more accurate, with fewer false-positive results than in indirect assays (138). However, the entire process of performing IgM-capture ELISA takes over 4 hours, which is longer than the time required for an indirect ELISA.

In contrast to IgM assays, IgG titers in samples are measured by an indirect ELISA. A study of B cell maturation processes has suggested that the majority of epitopes recognized by IgG are continuous, specific, and less abundant than those recognized by IgM (139). Therefore, the short, linear peptides on the surface of coated viral antigens represent the predominant epitopes recognized by IgG. Lysates of hantavirus-infected Vero-E6 cells are the source of viral antigens to be used if BSL3 laboratories are available (125). Otherwise, recombinant N protein has been produced as the antigen for IgM and IgG ELISAs (137, 138, 140, 141). However, caution must be taken in interpreting data based on the detection of antibodies against a single protein's epitopes, which may increase the chances of false-negative results.

It is important to note that the specific hantavirus antigens used in an ELISA can detect other hantaviruses. A phylogenetic analysis suggests that SNV is a prototype of New World hantaviruses (142). SNV antigens can be used to detect IgM or IgG against all known New World hantaviruses (143–145). IgG from sera of patients infected with PUUV cross-reacts with recombinant N protein of HTNV, SEOV, DOBV, or SNV (146).

Immunoblotting is another serological test for hantavirus detection that has been made commercially available in Europe (137, 147). In the commercially available assay, nitrocellulose test strips are coated with electrophoretically separated, full-length N proteins of PUUV and HTNV or with recombinant N terminus of N proteins from PUUV, HTNV, SEOV, DOBV, and SNV. The strip also contains a control band for isotype differentiation (IgG or IgM). These immunoblots have been shown to be highly sensitive for IgG detection in acute HFRS, but immunoblotting for IgM has only 76% specificity (137).

Of all the serologic tests described so far, only neutralization assays can allow the determination of which hantavirus serotype is responsible for an infection. Neutralization (or reduction) of virus infectivity is measured by counting viral plaques or foci in monolayers of Vero-E6 cells overlaid with agarose or methylcellulose. The focus reduction neutralization test (FRNT) has been used to identify hantavirus serotypes by comparing the titers in serum samples with those of related hantaviruses (148, 149). A 4-fold difference in neutralizing antibody titers between tested hantaviruses is indicated as a criterion to determine hantavirus serotype (148). However, FRNT requires culturing cells in BSL3 laboratories, which are not readily available. In addition, this assay is time-consuming and laborious. In summary, FRNT can be used to determine specific hantavirus infection when next-generation sequencing, an expensive alternative, is not available.

Virus Isolation

Isolation of hantavirus from natural hosts is difficult yet necessary for analyzing biological properties of these viruses. It is most common to use blood, serum, urine, or tissue homogenate samples from infected individuals or animals to inoculate cultured cells. Vero-E6 cells are the cell line of choice for virus isolation due to their genetic defect in interferon production. About 2 weeks after inoculation, hantavirus-infected cells can be identified by immunofluorescence assays (150–153). Repeated passaging of inoculated cells may be needed to achieve successful virus isolation (150). However, hantaviruses passaged in cell culture often adapt to the cells, altering their properties. Reports have shown that PUUV isolated from Vero-E6 cells contains mutations in S and L segments compared to the wild-type virus isolated from bank voles, the virus's natural host; moreover, the cell culture isolate could no longer infect bank voles (154, 155). In addition, some hantaviruses have been shown to infect cultured cells more efficiently than others do (156).

Several studies have shown that hantaviruses can be successfully isolated from laboratory animals. The choice of laboratory animal is typically based on the relationship of its genetic background to those of the natural virus hosts (157, 158). However, PUUV has been isolated from hamsters, which are only distantly related to bank voles (159). Other factors, such as the age of the animals and the route of inoculation, may also play a role in the success of virus isolation from laboratory animals (158).

EVALUATION, INTERPRETATION, AND REPORTING OF RESULTS

Currently there is no specific treatment for hantavirus infections, and diagnosis during the prodromal phase is critical to the successful management of HFRS and HPS. However, early diagnosis is challenging, because the prodromal phase of hantavirus infection is nonspecific, with thrombocytopenia being the only abnormal and significant laboratory finding during this phase (160). If health care providers in regions where hantaviral disease is endemic are presented with patients who develop thrombocytopenia combined with additional symptoms, including fever, tachycardia and tachypnea, hantavirus infection should be suspected. As previously mentioned, ANDV can be transmitted from person to person; therefore, the importance of a rapid diagnosis not only increases the likelihood of successful patient management but also is necessary for implementation of appropriate isolation procedures to prevent virus transmission to health care providers and limit possible spread to other persons who may have been in contact with the case patient (161).

The laboratory criteria for diagnosis of HPS (and HFRS) established by the CDC (see https://www.cdc.gov/hantavirus/health-care-workers/hps-case-definition.html) are as follows:

- Presence of orthohantavirus-specific IgM in persons who meet the case definition for HPS (see http://www.cdc.gov/hantavirus/health-care-workers/hps-case-definition.html) or a 4-fold or greater increase in titers of orthohantavirus-specific IgG in paired acute- and convalescent-phase serum samples
- Positive RT-PCR assay for orthohantavirus-specific RNA in plasma or other types of biological specimens
- Positive immunohistochemistry assay for orthohantaviral antigen in lung, spleen, kidney, or other solid tissues

The gold standard for hantavirus diagnosis is serology, and in the majority of cases, antibodies of IgM and IgG classes can be detected during the prodrome phase (14, 162, 163). Controls for IgM capture ELISA and IgG ELISA (e.g., sera from laboratory-confirmed HPS cases) and immunohistochemistry assays are essential for correct interpretation of the assay results. Most local laboratories do not have direct access to these materials. Thus, diagnostic testing is often limited to federal laboratories, research institutions that have a specific interest in HFRS or HPS, and a small number of commercial laboratories. In addition, because of the lack of standardized methods, overall quality of laboratory testing is highly variable. For example, a 2010 external quality control study for serological diagnosis of hantavirus infections involving 18 laboratories in Europe and Canada revealed that only 53% and 76% of IgM- and IgG-positive samples, respectively, were diagnosed correctly (164).

RT-PCR assays can be used to provide additional information, and subsequent sequence analysis of amplified orthohantavirus segments can be used to speciate the virus responsible for infection. Similar to the serologic methods, assays must be properly controlled using known positive reference and negative controls.

As previously stated by Fulhorst and Bowen (37), the "requirement for reporting HFRS and HPS varies among local health agencies and from country to country. In the United States, reporting of HPS cases is mandated at the state level, and HPS is listed as a notifiable disease in the National Notifiable Diseases Surveillance System maintained by the Centers for Disease Control and Prevention, although reporting is not compulsory." The CDC has the capacity to perform diagnostic and confirmatory laboratory tests (including the μ-capture ELISA for anti-hantavirus IgM, ELISA for anti-hantavirus IgG, RT-PCR and real-time RT-PCR assays for hantavirus-specific RNA, and next-generation sequencing). Confirmatory ELISA and RT-PCR assays are normally completed within 24 to 48 hours after receipt of diagnostic specimens at the Viral Special Pathogens Branch [Centers for Disease Control and Prevention, Mail Stop-070, 1600 Clifton Rd., Atlanta, GA 30333; phone, 404-639-0114; fax, 404-718-2175].

The findings and conclusions in this chapter are those of the authors and do not necessarily represent the views of the CDC. The use of product names does not imply their endorsement by the U.S. Department of Health and Human Services.

REFERENCES

1. **Vaheri A, Strandin T, Hepojoki J, Sironen T, Henttonen H, Mäkelä S, Mustonen J.** 2013. Uncovering the mysteries of hantavirus infections. *Nat Rev Microbiol* **11**:539–550.
2. **Nichol ST, Beaty BJ, Elliott RM, Goldbach R, Plyusnin A, Schmaljohn CS, Tesh RB.** 2005. Family Bunyaviridae, p 695-716. *In* Fauquet CM, Mayo MA, Maniloff J, Desselberger U, Ball LA (ed), *Viral Taxonomy: VIIIth Report of the International Committee of Taxonomy of Viruses*. Elsevier, London, United Kingdom.
3. **Maes P, Klempa B, Clement J, Matthijnssens J, Gajdusek DC, Krüger DH, Van Ranst M.** 2009. A proposal for new criteria for the classification of hantaviruses, based on S and M segment protein sequences. *Infect Genet Evol* **9**:813–820.
4. **Klempa B, Avsic-Zupanc T, Clement J, Dzagurova TK, Henttonen H, Heyman P, Jakab F, Kruger DH, Maes P, Papa A, Tkachenko EA, Ulrich RG, Vapalahti O, Vaheri A.** 2013. Complex evolution and epidemiology of Dobrava-Belgrade hantavirus: definition of genotypes and their characteristics. *Arch Virol* **158**:521–529.
5. **Adams MJ, Lefkowitz EJ, King AMQ, Harrach B, Harrison RL, Knowles NJ, Kropinski AM, Krupovic M, Kuhn JH, Mushegian AR, Nibert M, Sabanadzovic S, Sanfaçon H, Siddell SG, Simmonds P, Varsani A, Zerbini FM, Gorbalenya AE, Davison AJ.** 2017. Changes to taxonomy and the International Code of Virus Classification and Nomenclature ratified by the International Committee on Taxonomy of Viruses (2017). *Arch Virol* **162**:2505–2538.
6. **Nichol ST, Spiropoulou CF, Morzunov S, Rollin PE, Ksiazek TG, Feldmann H, Sanchez A, Childs J, Zaki S, Peters CJ.** 1993. Genetic identification of a hantavirus associated with an outbreak of acute respiratory illness. *Science* **262**:914–917.
7. **Padula PJ, Edelstein A, Miguel SDL, López NM, Rossi CM, Rabinovich RD.** 1998. Hantavirus pulmonary syndrome outbreak in Argentina: molecular evidence for person-to-person transmission of Andes virus. *Virology* **241**:323–330.

8. **Johnson AM, Bowen MD, Ksiazek TG, Williams RJ, Bryan RT, Mills JN, Peters CJ, Nichol ST.** 1997. Laguna Negra virus associated with HPS in western Paraguay and Bolivia. *Virology* **238:**115–127.
9. **Lee HW, Lee PW, Johnson KM.** 1978. Isolation of the etiologic agent of Korean hemorrhagic fever. *J Infect Dis* **137:**298–308.
10. **Gligic A, Dimkovic N, Xiao SY, Buckle GJ, Jovanovic D, Velimirovic D, Stojanovic R, Obradovic M, Diglisic G, Micic J, Asher DM, LeDuc JW, Yanagihara R, Gajdusek DC.** 1992. Belgrade virus: a new hantavirus causing severe hemorrhagic fever with renal syndrome in Yugoslavia. *J Infect Dis* **166:**113–120.
11. **Witkowski PT, Klempa B, Ithete NL, Auste B, Mfune JKE, Hoveka J, Matthee S, Preiser W, Kruger DH.** 2014. Hantaviruses in Africa. *Virus Res* **187:**34–42.
12. **Heinemann P, Tia M, Alabi A, Anon J-C, Auste B, Essbauer S, Gnionsahe A, Kigninlman H, Klempa B, Kraef C, Kruger N, Leendertz FH, Ndhatz-Sanogo M, Schaumburg F, Witkowski PT, Akoua-Koffi CG, Kruger DH.** 2016. Human infections by non-rodent-associated hantaviruses in Africa. *J Infect Dis* **214:**1507–1511.
13. **Yanagihara R, Gu SH, Arai S, Kang HJ, Song J-W.** 2014. Hantaviruses: rediscovery and new beginnings. *Virus Res* **187:**6–14.
14. **Kruger DH, Figueiredo LTM, Song J-W, Klempa B.** 2015. Hantaviruses—globally emerging pathogens. *J Clin Virol* **64:**128–136.
15. **Plyusnin A, Beaty BJ, Elliott RM, Goldbach R, Kormelink R, Lundkvist A, Schmaljohn CS, Tesh RB.** 2012. Family *Bunyaviridae*, p 725–741. *In* King AMQ, Lefkowitz EJ, Adams MJ, Carstens EB (ed), *Virus Taxonomy: Ninth Report of the International Committee on Taxonomy of Viruses (ICTV)*. Elsevier Academic Press, San Diego, CA.
16. **Martin ML, Lindsey-Regnery H, Sasso DR, McCormick JB, Palmer E.** 1985. Distinction between Bunyaviridae genera by surface structure and comparison with Hantaan virus using negative stain electron microscopy. *Arch Virol* **86:** 17–28.
17. **Reuter M, Krüger DH.** 2018. The nucleocapsid protein of hantaviruses: much more than a genome-wrapping protein. *Virus Genes* **54:**5–16.
18. **Blasdell K, Hentonnen H, Buchy P.** 2012. Hantavirus genetic diversity, p 179–216. *In* Morand S (ed), *New Frontiers of Molecular Epidemiology of Infectious Diseases*. Springer Science+Business Media, New York, NY.
19. **Bi Z, Formenty PB, Roth CE.** 2008. Hantavirus infection: a review and global update. *J Infect Dev Ctries* **2:**3–23.
20. **Watson DC, Sargianou M, Papa A, Chra P, Starakis I, Panos G.** 2014. Epidemiology of Hantavirus infections in humans: a comprehensive, global overview. *Crit Rev Microbiol* **40:**261–272.
21. **Tian H, Yu P, Cazelles B, Xu L, Tan H, Yang J, Huang S, Xu B, Cai J, Ma C, Wei J, Li S, Qu J, Laine M, Wang J, Tong S, Stenseth NC, Xu B.** 2017. Interannual cycles of Hantaan virus outbreaks at the human-animal interface in central China are controlled by temperature and rainfall. *Proc Natl Acad Sci USA* **114:**8041–8046.
22. **Ermonval M, Baychelier F, Tordo N.** 2016. What do we know about how hantaviruses interact with their different hosts? *Viruses* **8:**223.
23. **Woods C, Palekar R, Kim P, Blythe D, de Senarclens O, Feldman K, Farnon EC, Rollin PE, Albariño CG, Nichol ST, Smith M.** 2009. Domestically acquired Seoul virus causing hemorrhagic fever with renal syndrome—Maryland, 2008. *Clin Infect Dis* **49:**e109–e112.
24. **Jameson LJ, Taori SK, Atkinson B, Levick P, Featherstone CA, van der Burgt G, McCarthy N, Hart J, Osborne JC, Walsh AL, Brooks TJ, Hewson R.** 2013. Pet rats as a source of hantavirus in England and Wales, 2013. *Euro Surveill* **18:**20415
25. **Lundkvist A, Verner-Carlsson J, Plyusnina A, Forslund L, Feinstein R, Plyusnin A.** 2013. Pet rat harbouring Seoul hantavirus in Sweden, June 2013. *Euro Surveill* **18:**20521.
26. **Fill MA, Mullins H, May AS, Henderson H, Brown SM, Chiang CF, Patel NR, Klena JD, de St Maurice A, Knust B, Nichol ST, Dunn JR, Schaffner W, Jones TF.** 2017. Notes from the field: multiple cases of Seoul virus Infection in a household with infected pet rats—Tennessee, December 2016–April 2017. *MMWR Morb Mortal Wkly Rep* **66:**1081–1082.
27. **Klempa B, Schmidt HA, Ulrich R, Kaluz S, Labuda M, Meisel H, Hjelle B, Krüger DH.** 2003. Genetic interaction between distinct Dobrava hantavirus subtypes in *Apodemus agrarius* and *A. flavicollis* in nature. *J Virol* **77:**804–809.
28. **de St Maurice A, Ervin E, Schumacher M, Yaglom H, VinHatton E, Melman S, Komatsu K, House J, Peterson D, Buttke D, Ryan A, Yazzie D, Manning C, Ettestad P, Rollin P, Knust B.** 2017. Exposure characteristics of hantavirus pulmonary syndrome patients, United States, 1993-2015. *Emerg Infect Dis* **23:**733–739.
29. **Iglesias AA, Bellomo CM, Martinez VP.** 2016. Sindrome pulmonar por hantavirus en Buenos Aires, 2009-2014. *Medicina (Buenos Aires)* **76:**1–9.
30. **Klempa B, Fichet-Calvet E, Lecompte E, Auste B, Aniskin V, Meisel H, Denys C, Koivogui L, ter Meulen J, Krüger DH.** 2006. Hantavirus in African wood mouse, Guinea. *Emerg Infect Dis* **12:**838–840.
31. **Klempa B, Witkowski PT, Popugaeva E, Auste B, Koivogui L, Fichet-Calvet E, Strecker T, Ter Meulen J, Krüger DH.** 2012. Sangassou virus, the first hantavirus isolate from Africa, displays genetic and functional properties distinct from those of other *Murinae*-associated hantaviruses. *J Virol* **86:**3819–3827.
32. **Klempa B, Koivogui L, Sylla O, Koulemou K, Auste B, Krüger DH, ter Meulen J.** 2010. Serological evidence of human hantavirus infections in Guinea, West Africa. *J Infect Dis* **201:**1031–1034.
33. **Centers for Disease Control and Prevention.** 1994. Laboratory management of agents associated with hantavirus pulmonary syndrome: interim biosafety guidelines. *MMWR Recomm Rep* **43**(RR-7)**:**1–7
34. **Armstrong LR, Zaki SR, Goldoft MJ, Todd RL, Khan AS, Khabbaz RF, Ksiazek TG, Peters CJ.** 1995. Hantavirus pulmonary syndrome associated with entering or cleaning rarely used, rodent-infested structures. *J Infect Dis* **172:**1166.
35. **Crowcroft NS, Infuso A, Ilef D, Le Guenno B, Desenclos JC, Van Loock F, Clement J.** 1999. Risk factors for human hantavirus infection: Franco-Belgian collaborative case-control study during 1995-6 epidemic. *BMJ* **318:**1737–1738.
36. **Mills JN, Corneli A, Young JC, Garrison LE, Khan AS, Ksiazek TG, Centers for Disease Control and Prevention.** 2002. Hantavirus pulmonary syndrome—United States: updated recommendations for risk reduction. *MMWR Recomm Rep* **51**(RR-9)**:**1–12
37. **Fulhorst CF, Bowen MD.** 2015. Hantaviruses, p 1660–1668. *In* Jorgensen JH, Pfaller MA, Carroll KC, Funke G, Landry ML, Richter SS, Warnock DW (ed), *Manual of Clinical Microbiology*, 11th ed. ASM Press, Washington, DC..
38. **Roehr B.** 2012. US officials warn 39 countries about risk of hantavirus among travellers to Yosemite. *BMJ* **345:**e6054.
39. **Park SC, Pyo HJ, Soe JB, Lee MS, Kim YH, Byun KS, Kang KH, Kim MJ, Kim JS, Lee HW, Lee YJ, Seong IW, Baek LJ.** 1989. A clinical study of hemorrhagic fever with renal syndrome caused by Seoul virus infection. *Korean J Intern Med* **4:**130–135.
40. **Lee HW, van der Groen G.** 1989. Hemorrhagic fever with renal syndrome. *Prog Med Virol* **36:**62–102
41. **Lukes RJ.** 1954. The pathology of thirty-nine fatal cases of epidemic hemorrhagic fever. *Am J Med* **16:**639–650.
42. **Duchin JS, Koster FT, Peters CJ, Simpson GL, Tempest B, Zaki SR, Ksiazek TG, Rollin PE, Nichol S, Umland ET, Moolenaar RL, Reef SE, Nolte KB, Gallaher MM, Butler JC, Breiman RF, The Hantavirus Study Group.** 1994. Hantavirus pulmonary syndrome: a clinical description of 17 patients with a newly recognized disease. *N Engl J Med* **330:**949–955.
43. **Kitsutani PT, Denton RW, Fritz CL, Murray RA, Todd RL, Pape WJ, Frampton JW, Young JC, Khan AS, Peters CJ, Ksiazek TG.** 1999. Acute Sin Nombre hantavirus infection without pulmonary syndrome, United States. *Emerg Infect Dis* **5:**701–705.

44. **Castillo C, Naranjo J, Sepúlveda A, Ossa G, Levy H.** 2001. Hantavirus pulmonary syndrome due to Andes virus in Temuco, Chile: clinical experience with 16 adults. *Chest* **120:**548–554.
45. **Riquelme R, Rioseco ML, Bastidas L, Trincado D, Riquelme M, Loyola H, Valdivieso F.** 2015. Hantavirus pulmonary syndrome, southern Chile, 1995-2012. *Emerg Infect Dis* **21:**562–568.
46. **Riquelme R, Riquelme M, Torres A, Rioseco ML, Vergara JA, Scholz L, Carriel A.** 2003. Hantavirus pulmonary syndrome, southern Chile. *Emerg Infect Dis* **9:**1438–1443.
47. **Hallin GW, Simpson SQ, Crowell RE, James DS, Koster FT, Mertz GJ, Levy H.** 1996. Cardiopulmonary manifestations of hantavirus pulmonary syndrome. *Crit Care Med* **24:**252–258.
48. **Koster F, Foucar K, Hjelle B, Scott A, Chong YY, Larson R, McCabe M.** 2001. Rapid presumptive diagnosis of hantavirus cardiopulmonary syndrome by peripheral blood smear review. *Am J Clin Pathol* **116:**665–672.
49. **Nolte KB, Feddersen RM, Foucar K, Zaki SR, Koster FT, Madar D, Merlin TL, McFeeley PJ, Umland ET, Zumwalt RE.** 1995. Hantavirus pulmonary syndrome in the United States: a pathological description of a disease caused by a new agent. *Hum Pathol* **26:**110–120.
50. **Zaki SR, et al.** 1995. Hantavirus pulmonary syndrome. Pathogenesis of an emerging infectious disease. *Am J Pathol* **146:**552–579
51. **Rista E, Pilaca A, Akshija I, Rama A, Harja E, Puca E, Bino S, Cadri V, Kota M, Nestor T, Arjan H.** 2017. Hemorrhagic fever with renal syndrome in Albania. Focus on predictors of acute kidney injury in HFRS. *J Clin Virol* **91:**25–30.
52. **Jonsson CB, Hooper J, Mertz G.** 2008. Treatment of hantavirus pulmonary syndrome. *Antiviral Res* **78:**162–169.
53. **Huggins JW, Hsiang CM, Cosgriff TM, Guang MY, Smith JI, Wu ZO, LeDuc JW, Zheng ZM, Meegan JM, Wang QN, Oland DD, Gui XE, Gibbs PH, Yuan GH, Zhang TM.** 1991. Prospective, double-blind, concurrent, placebo-controlled clinical trial of intravenous ribavirin therapy of hemorrhagic fever with renal syndrome. *J Infect Dis* **164:**1119–1127.
54. **Rusnak JM, Byrne WR, Chung KN, Gibbs PH, Kim TT, Boudreau EF, Cosgriff T, Pittman P, Kim KY, Erlichman MS, Rezvani DF, Huggins JW.** 2009. Experience with intravenous ribavirin in the treatment of hemorrhagic fever with renal syndrome in Korea. *Antiviral Res* **81:**68–76.
55. **Chapman LE, Mertz GJ, Peters CJ, Jolson HM, Khan AS, Ksiazek TG, Koster FT, Baum KF, Rollin PE, Pavia AT, Holman RC, Christenson JC, Rubin PJ, Behrman RE, Bell LJ, Simpson GL, Sadek RF, Ribavirin Study Group.** 1999. Intravenous ribavirin for hantavirus pulmonary syndrome: safety and tolerance during 1 year of open-label experience. *Antivir Ther* **4:**211–219
56. **Mertz GJ, Miedzinski L, Goade D, Pavia AT, Hjelle B, Hansbarger CO, Levy H, Koster FT, Baum K, Lindemulder A, Wang W, Riser L, Fernandez H, Whitley RJ, Collaborative Antiviral Study Group.** 2004. Placebo-controlled, double-blind trial of intravenous ribavirin for the treatment of hantavirus cardiopulmonary syndrome in North America. *Clin Infect Dis* **39:**1307–1313.
57. **Meyer BJ, Schmaljohn CS.** 2000. Persistent hantavirus infections: characteristics and mechanisms. *Trends Microbiol* **8:**61–67.
58. **Taruishi M, Yoshimatsu K, Hatsuse R, Okumura M, Nakamura I, Arikawa J.** 2008. Lack of vertical transmission of Hantaan virus from persistently infected dam to progeny in laboratory mice. *Arch Virol* **153:**1605–1609.
59. **Childs JE, Korch GW, Glass GE, LeDuc JW, Shah KV.** 1987. Epizootiology of Hantavirus infections in Baltimore: isolation of a virus from Norway rats, and characteristics of infected rat populations. *Am J Epidemiol* **126:**55–68.
60. **McKee KT, Jr, Kim GR, Green DE, Peters CJ.** 1985. Hantaan virus infection in suckling mice: virologic and pathologic correlates. *J Med Virol* **17:**107–117.
61. **Yang J, Sun JF, Wang TT, Guo XH, Wei JX, Jia LT, Yang AG.** 2017. Targeted inhibition of hantavirus replication and intracranial pathogenesis by a chimeric protein-delivered siRNA. *Antiviral Res* **147:**107–115.
62. **Groen J, Gerding M, Koeman JP, Roholl PJ, van Amerongen G, Jordans HG, Niesters HG, Osterhaus AD.** 1995. A macaque model for hantavirus infection. *J Infect Dis* **172:** 38–44.
63. **Klingström J, Stoltz M, Hardestam J, Ahlm C, Lundkvist A.** 2008. Passive immunization protects cynomolgus macaques against Puumala hantavirus challenge. *Antivir Ther* **13:** 125–133
64. **Hooper JW, Larsen T, Custer DM, Schmaljohn CS.** 2001. A lethal disease model for hantavirus pulmonary syndrome. *Virology* **289:**6–14.
65. **Campen MJ, Milazzo ML, Fulhorst CF, Obot Akata CJ, Koster F.** 2006. Characterization of shock in a hamster model of hantavirus infection. *Virology* **356:**45–49.
66. **Wahl-Jensen V, Chapman J, Asher L, Fisher R, Zimmerman M, Larsen T, Hooper JW.** 2007. Temporal analysis of Andes virus and Sin Nombre virus infections of Syrian hamsters. *J Virol* **81:**7449–7462.
67. **Milazzo ML, Eyzaguirre EJ, Molina CP, Fulhorst CF.** 2002. Maporal viral infection in the Syrian golden hamster: a model of hantavirus pulmonary syndrome. *J Infect Dis* **186:**1390–1395.
68. **Hardcastle K, Scott D, Safronetz D, Brining DL, Ebihara H, Feldmann H, LaCasse RA.** 2016. Laguna Negra virus infection causes hantavirus pulmonary syndrome in Turkish hamsters (*Mesocricetus brandti*). *Vet Pathol* **53:**182–189.
69. **Safronetz D, Prescott J, Feldmann F, Haddock E, Rosenke R, Okumura A, Brining D, Dahlstrom E, Porcella SF, Ebihara H, Scott DP, Hjelle B, Feldmann H.** 2014. Pathophysiology of hantavirus pulmonary syndrome in rhesus macaques. *Proc Natl Acad Sci USA* **111:**7114–7119.
70. **Gowen BB, Wong MH, Jung KH, Smee DF, Morrey JD, Furuta Y.** 2010. Efficacy of favipiravir (T-705) and T-1106 pyrazine derivatives in phlebovirus disease models. *Antiviral Res* **86:**121–127.
71. **Gowen BB, Wong MH, Jung KH, Sanders AB, Mendenhall M, Bailey KW, Furuta Y, Sidwell RW.** 2007. In vitro and in vivo activities of T-705 against arenavirus and bunyavirus infections. *Antimicrob Agents Chemother* **51:**3168–3176.
72. **Safronetz D, Falzarano D, Scott DP, Furuta Y, Feldmann H, Gowen BB.** 2013. Antiviral efficacy of favipiravir against two prominent etiological agents of hantavirus pulmonary syndrome. *Antimicrob Agents Chemother* **57:**4673–4680.
73. **Chung DH, Kumarapperuma SC, Sun Y, Li Q, Chu YK, Arterburn JB, Parker WB, Smith J, Spik K, Ramanathan HN, Schmaljohn CS, Jonsson CB.** 2008. Synthesis of 1-beta-D-ribofuranosyl-3-ethynyl-[1,2,4]triazole and its in vitro and in vivo efficacy against Hantavirus. *Antiviral Res* **79:**19–27.
74. **Salim NN, Ganaie SS, Roy A, Jeeva S, Mir MA.** 2016. Targeting a novel RNA-protein interaction for therapeutic intervention of hantavirus disease. *J Biol Chem* **291:**24702–24714.
75. **Murphy ME, Kariwa H, Mizutani T, Yoshimatsu K, Arikawa J, Takashima I.** 2000. In vitro antiviral activity of lactoferrin and ribavirin upon hantavirus. *Arch Virol* **145:**1571–1582.
76. **Murphy ME, Kariwa H, Mizutani T, Tanabe H, Yoshimatsu K, Arikawa J, Takashima I.** 2001. Characterization of in vitro and in vivo antiviral activity of lactoferrin and ribavirin upon hantavirus. *J Vet Med Sci* **63:**637–645.
77. **Löber C, Anheier B, Lindow S, Klenk HD, Feldmann H.** 2001. The Hantaan virus glycoprotein precursor is cleaved at the conserved pentapeptide WAASA. *Virology* **289:**224–229.
78. **Tischler ND, Gonzalez A, Perez-Acle T, Rosemblatt M, Valenzuela PD.** 2005. Hantavirus Gc glycoprotein: evidence for a class II fusion protein. *J Gen Virol* **86:**2937–2947.
79. **Higa MM, Petersen J, Hooper J, Doms RW.** 2012. Efficient production of Hantaan and Puumala pseudovirions for viral tropism and neutralization studies. *Virology* **423:**134–142.
80. **Ray N, Whidby J, Stewart S, Hooper JW, Bertolotti-Ciarlet A.** 2010. Study of Andes virus entry and neutralization using a pseudovirion system. *J Virol Methods* **163:**416–423.
81. **Barriga GP, Villalón-Letelier F, Márquez CL, Bignon EA, Acuña R, Ross BH, Monasterio O, Mardones GA, Vidal SE, Tischler ND.** 2016. Inhibition of the hantavirus fusion process by predicted domain III and stem peptides from glycoprotein Gc. *PLoS Negl Trop Dis* **10:**e0004799.

82. **Xu Z, Wei L, Wang L, Wang H, Jiang S.** 2002. The in vitro and in vivo protective activity of monoclonal antibodies directed against Hantaan virus: potential application for immunotherapy and passive immunization. *Biochem Biophys Res Commun* **298:**552–558.
83. **Zhang XK, Takashima I, Hashimoto N.** 1989. Characteristics of passive immunity against hantavirus infection in rats. *Arch Virol* **105:**235–246.
84. **Custer DM, Thompson E, Schmaljohn CS, Ksiazek TG, Hooper JW.** 2003. Active and passive vaccination against hantavirus pulmonary syndrome with Andes virus M genome segment-based DNA vaccine. *J Virol* **77:**9894–9905.
85. **de Carvalho Nicacio C, Lundkvist A, Sjölander KB, Plyusnin A, Salonen EM, Björling E.** 2000. A neutralizing recombinant human antibody Fab fragment against Puumala hantavirus. *J Med Virol* **60:**446–454.
86. **Haese N, Brocato RL, Henderson T, Nilles ML, Kwilas SA, Josleyn MD, Hammerbeck CD, Schiltz J, Royals M, Ballantyne J, Hooper JW, Bradley DS.** 2015. Antiviral biologic produced in DNA vaccine/goose platform protects hamsters against hantavirus pulmonary syndrome when administered post-exposure. *PLoS Negl Trop Dis* **9:**e0003803.
87. **Umbach JL, Cullen BR.** 2009. The role of RNAi and microRNAs in animal virus replication and antiviral immunity. *Genes Dev* **23:**1151–1164.
88. **Chiang CF, Albariño CG, Lo MK, Spiropoulou CF.** 2014. Small interfering RNA inhibition of Andes virus replication. *PLoS One* **9:**e99764.
89. **Rowe RK, Suszko JW, Pekosz A.** 2008. Roles for the recycling endosome, Rab8, and Rab11 in hantavirus release from epithelial cells. *Virology* **382:**239–249.
90. **Gavrilovskaya IN, Shepley M, Shaw R, Ginsberg MH, Mackow ER.** 1998. β_3 integrins mediate the cellular entry of hantaviruses that cause respiratory failure. *Proc Natl Acad Sci USA* **95:**7074–7079.
91. **Gavrilovskaya IN, Brown EJ, Ginsberg MH, Mackow ER.** 1999. Cellular entry of hantaviruses which cause hemorrhagic fever with renal syndrome is mediated by beta3 integrins. *J Virol* **73:**3951–3959
92. **Hall PR, Leitão A, Ye C, Kilpatrick K, Hjelle B, Oprea TI, Larson RS.** 2010. Small molecule inhibitors of hantavirus infection. *Bioorg Med Chem Lett* **20:**7085–7091.
93. **Hall PR, Hjelle B, Njus H, Ye C, Bondu-Hawkins V, Brown DC, Kilpatrick KA, Larson RS.** 2009. Phage display selection of cyclic peptides that inhibit Andes virus infection. *J Virol* **83:**8965–8969.
94. **Hall PR, Hjelle B, Brown DC, Ye C, Bondu-Hawkins V, Kilpatrick KA, Larson RS.** 2008. Multivalent presentation of antihantavirus peptides on nanoparticles enhances infection blockade. *Antimicrob Agents Chemother* **52:**2079–2088.
95. **Choi Y, Kwon YC, Kim SI, Park JM, Lee KH, Ahn BY.** 2008. A hantavirus causing hemorrhagic fever with renal syndrome requires gC1qR/p32 for efficient cell binding and infection. *Virology* **381:**178–183.
96. **Raftery MJ, Lalwani P, Krautkrämer E, Peters T, Scharffetter-Kochanek K, Krüger R, Hofmann J, Seeger K, Krüger DH, Schönrich G.** 2014. β2 integrin mediates hantavirus-induced release of neutrophil extracellular traps. *J Exp Med* **211:**1485–1497.
97. **Chiang CF, Flint M, Lin JS, Spiropoulou CF.** 2016. Endocytic pathways used by Andes virus to enter primary human lung endothelial cells. *PLoS One* **11:**e0164768.
98. **Taylor SL, Wahl-Jensen V, Copeland AM, Jahrling PB, Schmaljohn CS.** 2013. Endothelial cell permeability during hantavirus infection involves factor XII-dependent increased activation of the kallikrein-kinin system. *PLoS Pathog* **9:**e1003470.
99. **Vaheri A, Strandin T, Jääskeläinen AJ, Vapalahti O, Jarva H, Lokki ML, Antonen J, Leppänen I, Mäkelä S, Meri S, Mustonen J.** 2014. Pathophysiology of a severe case of Puumala hantavirus infection successfully treated with bradykinin receptor antagonist icatibant. *Antiviral Res* **111:**23–25.
100. **Maes P, Clement J, Van Ranst M.** 2009. Recent approaches in hantavirus vaccine development. *Expert Rev Vaccines* **8:**67–76.
101. **Zhang YZ, Zou Y, Fu ZF, Plyusnin A.** 2010. Hantavirus infections in humans and animals, China. *Emerg Infect Dis* **16:**1195–1203.
102. **Song JY, Woo HJ, Cheong HJ, Noh JY, Baek LJ, Kim WJ.** 2016. Long-term immunogenicity and safety of inactivated Hantaan virus vaccine (Hantavax™) in healthy adults. *Vaccine* **34:**1289–1295.
103. **Krüger DH, Schönrich G, Klempa B.** 2011. Human pathogenic hantaviruses and prevention of infection. *Hum Vaccin* **7:**685–693.
104. **Safronetz D, Hegde NR, Ebihara H, Denton M, Kobinger GP, St Jeor S, Feldmann H, Johnson DC.** 2009. Adenovirus vectors expressing hantavirus proteins protect hamsters against lethal challenge with andes virus. *J Virol* **83:**7285–7295.
105. **Yuan ZG, Li XM, Mahmmod YS, Wang XH, Xu HJ, Zhang XX.** 2009. A single immunization with a recombinant canine adenovirus type 2 expressing the seoul virus Gn glycoprotein confers protective immunity against Seoul virus in mice. *Vaccine* **27:**5247–5251.
106. **Yuan ZG, Luo SJ, Xu HJ, Wang XH, Li J, Yuan LG, He LT, Zhang XX.** 2010. Generation of E3-deleted canine adenovirus type 2 expressing the Gc glycoprotein of Seoul virus by gene insertion or deletion of related terminal region sequences. *J Gen Virol* **91:**1764–1771.
107. **Li C, Liu F, Liang M, Zhang Q, Wang X, Wang T, Li J, Li D.** 2010. Hantavirus-like particles generated in CHO cells induce specific immune responses in C57BL/6 mice. *Vaccine* **28:**4294–4300.
108. **Acuña R, Cifuentes-Muñoz N, Márquez CL, Bulling M, Klingström J, Mancini R, Lozach PY, Tischler ND.** 2014. Hantavirus Gn and Gc glycoproteins self-assemble into virus-like particles. *J Virol* **88:**2344–2348.
109. **Hooper JW, Kamrud KI, Elgh F, Custer D, Schmaljohn CS.** 1999. DNA vaccination with hantavirus M segment elicits neutralizing antibodies and protects against seoul virus infection. *Virology* **255:**269–278.
110. **Hooper JW, Custer DM, Thompson E, Schmaljohn CS.** 2001. DNA vaccination with the Hantaan virus M gene protects Hamsters against three of four HFRS hantaviruses and elicits a high-titer neutralizing antibody response in rhesus monkeys. *J Virol* **75:**8469–8477.
111. **Hooper JW, Custer DM, Smith J, Wahl-Jensen V.** 2006. Hantaan/Andes virus DNA vaccine elicits a broadly cross-reactive neutralizing antibody response in nonhuman primates. *Virology* **347:**208–216.
112. **Hooper JW, Moon JE, Paolino KM, Newcomer R, McLain DE, Josleyn M, Hannaman D, Schmaljohn C.** 2014. A phase 1 clinical trial of Hantaan virus and Puumala virus M-segment DNA vaccines for haemorrhagic fever with renal syndrome delivered by intramuscular electroporation. *Clin Microbiol Infect* **20**(Suppl 5)**:**110–117.
113. **U.S. Department of Health and Human Services.** 2009. Viral agents, p 200–232. *In* Chosewood LC, Wilson DE (ed), *Biosafety in Microbiological and Biomedical Laboratories*, 5th ed. Centers for Disease Control and Prevention, Atlanta, GA.
114. **Saluzzo JF, Leguenno B, Van der Groen G.** 1988. Use of heat inactivated viral haemorrhagic fever antigens in serological assays. *J Virol Methods* **22:**165–172.
115. **Vapalahti O, Mustonen J, Lundkvist A, Henttonen H, Plyusnin A, Vaheri A.** 2003. Hantavirus infections in Europe. *Lancet Infect Dis* **3:**653–661.
116. **Kraus AA, Priemer C, Heider H, Kruger DH, Ulrich R.** 2005. Inactivation of Hantaan virus-containing samples for subsequent investigations outside biosafety level 3 facilities. *Intervirology* **48:**255–261.
117. **Maes P, Li S, Verbeeck J, Keyaerts E, Clement J, Van Ranst M.** 2007. Evaluation of the efficacy of disinfectants against Puumala hantavirus by real-time RT-PCR. *J Virol Methods* **141:**111–115.
118. **Lloyd G, Jones N.** 1986. Infection of laboratory workers with hantavirus acquired from immunocytomas propagated in laboratory rats. *J Infect* **12:**117–125.
119. **Lee HW, Johnson KM.** 1982. Laboratory-acquired infections with Hantaan virus, the etiologic agent of Korean hemorrhagic fever. *J Infect Dis* **146:**645–651.

120. **Hung T, Zhou JY, Tang YM, Zhao TX, Baek LJ, Lee HW.** 1992. Identification of Hantaan virus-related structures in kidneys of cadavers with haemorrhagic fever with renal syndrome. *Arch Virol* **122:**187–199.
121. **Kerins JL, Koske SE, Kazmierczak J, Austin C, Gowdy K, Dibernardo A, Seoul Virus Working Group, Canadian Seoul Virus Investigation Group (Federal), Canadian Seoul Virus Investigation Group (Provincial).** 2018. Outbreak of Seoul virus among rats and rat owners—United States and Canada, 2017. *MMWR Morb Mortal Wkly Rep* **67:**131–134.
122. **Mattar S, Guzmán C, Figueiredo LT.** 2015. Diagnosis of hantavirus infection in humans. *Expert Rev Anti Infect Ther* **13:**939–946.
123. **Childs JE, Glass GE, Ksiazek TG, Rossi CA, Oro JG, Leduc JW.** 1991. Human-rodent contact and infection with lymphocytic choriomeningitis and Seoul viruses in an inner-city population. *Am J Trop Med Hyg* **44:**117–121.
124. **Easterbrook JD, Kaplan JB, Vanasco NB, Reeves WK, Purcell RH, Kosoy MY, Glass GE, Watson J, Klein SL.** 2007. A survey of zoonotic pathogens carried by Norway rats in Baltimore, Maryland, USA. *Epidemiol Infect* **135:**1192–1199.
125. **Ksiazek TG, Peters CJ, Rollin PE, Zaki S, Nichol S, Spiropoulou C, Morzunov S, Feldmann H, Sanchez A, Khan AS, Mahy BWJ, Wachsmuth K, Butler JC.** 1995. Identification of a new North American hantavirus that causes acute pulmonary insufficiency. *Am J Trop Med Hyg* **52:**117–123.
126. **Saksida A, Duh D, Korva M, Avsic-Zupanc T.** 2008. Dobrava virus RNA load in patients who have hemorrhagic fever with renal syndrome. *J Infect Dis* **197:**681–685.
127. **Kramski M, Meisel H, Klempa B, Krüger DH, Pauli G, Nitsche A.** 2007. Detection and typing of human pathogenic hantaviruses by real-time reverse transcription-PCR and pyrosequencing. *Clin Chem* **53:**1899–1905.
128. **Aitichou M, Saleh SS, McElroy AK, Schmaljohn C, Ibrahim MS.** 2005. Identification of Dobrava, Hantaan, Seoul, and Puumala viruses by one-step real-time RT-PCR. *J Virol Methods* **124:**21–26.
129. **Engler O, Klingstrom J, Aliyev E, Niederhauser C, Fontana S, Strasser M, Portmann J, Signer J, Bankoul S, Frey F, Hatz C, Stutz A, Tschaggelar A, Mutsch M.** 2013. Seroprevalence of hantavirus infections in Switzerland in 2009: difficulties in determining prevalence in a country with low endemicity. *Euro Surveill* **18:**20660.
130. **Lederer S, Lattwein E, Hanke M, Sonnenberg K, Stoecker W, Lundkvist Å, Vaheri A, Vapalahti O, Chan PK, Feldmann H, Dick D, Schmidt-Chanasit J, Padula P, Vial PA, Panculescu-Gatej R, Ceianu C, Heyman P, Avšič-Županc T, Niedrig M.** 2013. Indirect immunofluorescence assay for the simultaneous detection of antibodies against clinically important old and new world hantaviruses. *PLoS Negl Trop Dis* **7:**e2157.
131. **Clement J, McKenna P, Groen J, Osterhaus A, Colson P, Vervoort T, van der Groen G, Lee HW.** 1995. Epidemiology and laboratory diagnosis of hantavirus (HTV) infections. *Acta Clin Belg* **50:**9–19.
132. **Bostik P, Winter J, Ksiazek TG, Rollin PE, Villinger F, Zaki SR, Peters CJ, Ansari AA.** 2000. Sin nombre virus (SNV) Ig isotype antibody response during acute and convalescent phases of hantavirus pulmonary syndrome. *Emerg Infect Dis* **6:**184–188.
133. **Elgh F, Wadell G, Juto P.** 1995. Comparison of the kinetics of Puumala virus specific IgM and IgG antibody responses in nephropathia epidemica as measured by a recombinant antigen-based enzyme-linked immunosorbent assay and an immunofluorescence test. *J Med Virol* **45:**146–150.
134. **Lundkvist A, Björsten S, Niklasson B.** 1993. Immunoglobulin G subclass responses against the structural components of Puumala virus. *J Clin Microbiol* **31:**368–372
135. **Ye C, Prescott J, Nofchissey R, Goade D, Hjelle B.** 2004. Neutralizing antibodies and Sin Nombre virus RNA after recovery from hantavirus cardiopulmonary syndrome. *Emerg Infect Dis* **10:**478–482
136. **Goeijenbier M, Hartskeerl RA, Reimerink J, Verner-Carlsson J, Wagenaar JF, Goris MG, Martina BE, Lundkvist Å, Koopmans M, Osterhaus AD, van Gorp EC, Reusken CB.** 2014. The hanta hunting study: underdiagnosis of Puumala hantavirus infections in symptomatic non-travelling leptospirosis-suspected patients in the Netherlands, in 2010 and April to November 2011. *Euro Surveill* **19:**20878.
137. **Schubert J, Tollmann F, Weissbrich B.** 2001. Evaluation of a pan-reactive hantavirus enzyme immunoassay and of a hantavirus immunoblot for the diagnosis of nephropathia epidemica. *J Clin Virol* **21:**63–74.
138. **Prince HE, Su X, Hogrefe WR.** 2007. Utilization of hantavirus antibody results generated over a five-year period to develop an improved serologic algorithm for detecting acute Sin Nombre hantavirus infection. *J Clin Lab Anal* **21:**7–13.
139. **Tuteja R, Agarwal A, Vijayakrishnan L, Nayak BP, Gupta SK, Kumar V, Rao KV.** 1997. B cell responses to a peptide epitope. II: multiple levels of selection during maturation of primary responses. *Immunol Cell Biol* **75:**245–252.
140. **Padula PJ, Rossi CM, Della Valle MO, Martínez PV, Colavecchia SB, Edelstein A, Miguel SD, Rabinovich RD, Segura EL.** 2000. Development and evaluation of a solid-phase enzyme immunoassay based on Andes hantavirus recombinant nucleoprotein. *J Med Microbiol* **49:**149–155.
141. **Figueiredo LT, Moreli ML, Borges AA, de Figueiredo GG, Badra SJ, Bisordi I, Suzuki A, Capria S, Padula P.** 2009. Evaluation of an enzyme-linked immunosorbent assay based on Araraquara virus recombinant nucleocapsid protein. *Am J Trop Med Hyg* **81:**273–276
142. **Montoya-Ruiz C, Diaz FJ, Rodas JD.** 2014. Recent evidence of hantavirus circulation in the American tropic. *Viruses* **6:**1274–1293.
143. **Iversson LB, da Rosa AP, Rosa MD, Lomar AV, Sasaki Mda G, LeDuc JW.** 1992. 1994. Human infection by Hantavirus in southern and southeastern Brazil. *Rev Assoc Med Bras* **40:**85–92. [In Portuguese.]
144. **Khan AS, Spiropoulou CF, Morzunov S, Zaki SR, Kohn MA, Nawas SR, McFarland L, Nichol ST.** 1995. Fatal illness associated with a new hantavirus in Louisiana. *J Med Virol* **46:**281–286.
145. **López N, Padula P, Rossi C, Lázaro ME, Franze-Fernández MT.** 1996. Genetic identification of a new hantavirus causing severe pulmonary syndrome in Argentina. *Virology* **220:**223–226.
146. **Elgh F, Linderholm M, Wadell G, Tärnvik A, Juto P.** 1998. Development of humoral cross-reactivity to the nucleocapsid protein of heterologous hantaviruses in nephropathia epidemica. *FEMS Immunol Med Microbiol* **22:**309–315.
147. **Zöller L, Scholz J, Stohwasser R, Giebel LB, Sethi KK, Bautz EK, Darai G.** 1989. Immunoblot analysis of the serological response in Hantavirus infections. *J Med Virol* **27:**231–237.
148. **Valdivieso F, Vial P, Ferres M, Ye C, Goade D, Cuiza A, Hjelle B.** 2006. Neutralizing antibodies in survivors of Sin Nombre and Andes hantavirus infection. *Emerg Infect Dis* **12:**166–168.
149. **Bharadwaj M, Nofchissey R, Goade D, Koster F, Hjelle B.** 2000. Humoral immune responses in the hantavirus cardiopulmonary syndrome. *J Infect Dis* **182:**43–48.
150. **Galeno H, Mora J, Villagra E, Fernandez J, Hernandez J, Mertz GJ, Ramirez E.** 2002. First human isolate of Hantavirus (Andes virus) in the Americas. *Emerg Infect Dis* **8:**657–661.
151. **Godoy P, Marsac D, Stefas E, Ferrer P, Tischler ND, Pino K, Ramdohr P, Vial P, Valenzuela PD, Ferrés M, Veas F, López-Lastra M.** 2009. Andes virus antigens are shed in urine of patients with acute hantavirus cardiopulmonary syndrome. *J Virol* **83:**5046–5055.
152. **Song JW, Kang HJ, Gu SH, Moon SS, Bennett SN, Song KJ, Baek LJ, Kim HC, O'Guinn ML, Chong ST, Klein TA, Yanagihara R.** 2009. Characterization of Imjin virus, a newly isolated hantavirus from the Ussuri white-toothed shrew (Crocidura lasiura). *J Virol* **83:**6184–6191.

153. **Jameson LJ, Logue CH, Atkinson B, Baker N, Galbraith SE, Carroll MW, Brooks T, Hewson R.** 2013. The continued emergence of hantaviruses: isolation of a Seoul virus implicated in human disease, United Kingdom, October 2012. *Euro Surveill* **18:**4–7
154. **Lundkvist A, Cheng Y, Sjölander KB, Niklasson B, Vaheri A, Plyusnin A.** 1997. Cell culture adaptation of Puumala hantavirus changes the infectivity for its natural reservoir, *Clethrionomys glareolus*, and leads to accumulation of mutants with altered genomic RNA S segment. *J Virol* **71:**9515–9523
155. **Nemirov K, Lundkvist A, Vaheri A, Plyusnin A.** 2003. Adaptation of Puumala hantavirus to cell culture is associated with point mutations in the coding region of the L segment and in the noncoding regions of the S segment. *J Virol* **77:**8793–8800.
156. **Kariwa H, Arikawa J, Takashima I, Isegawa Y, Yamanishi K, Hashimoto N.** 1994. Enhancement of infectivity of hantavirus in cell culture by centrifugation. *J Virol Methods* **49:**235–244.
157. **Klingström J, Heyman P, Escutenaire S, Sjölander KB, De Jaegere F, Henttonen H, Lundkvist A.** 2002. Rodent host specificity of European hantaviruses: evidence of Puumala virus interspecific spillover. *J Med Virol* **68:**581–588.
158. **Li JL, Ling JX, Chen LJ, Wei F, Luo F, Liu YY, Xiong HR, How W, Yang ZQ.** 2013. An efficient method for isolation of Hantaan virus through serial passages in suckling mice. *Intervirology* **56:**172–177.
159. **Seto T, Tkachenko EA, Morozov VG, Tanikawa Y, Kolominov SI, Belov SN, Nakamura I, Hashimoto N, Kon Y, Balakiev AE, Dzagurnova TK, Medvedkina OA, Nakauchi M, Ishizuka M, Yoshii K, Yoshimatsu K, Ivanov LV, Arikawa J, Takashima I, Kariwa H.** 2011. An efficient in vivo method for the isolation of Puumala virus in Syrian hamsters and the characterization of the isolates from Russia. *J Virol Methods* **173:**17–23.
160. **Llah ST, Mir S, Sharif S, Khan S, Mir MA.** 2018. Hantavirus induced cardiopulmonary syndrome: a public health concern. *J Med Virol* **90:**1003–1009.
161. **Martinez VP, Bellomo C, San Juan J, Pinna D, Forlenza R, Elder M, Padula PJ.** 2005. Person-to-person transmission of Andes virus. *Emerg Infect Dis* **11:**1848–1853.
162. **Krüger DH, Ulrich R, Lundkvist A.** 2001. Hantavirus infections and their prevention. *Microbes Infect* **3:**1129–1144.
163. **Khan AS, Gaviria M, Rollin PE, Hlady WG, Ksiazek TG, Armstrong LR, Greenman R, Ravkov E, Kolber M, Anapol H, Sfakianaki ED, Nichol ST, Peters CJ, Khabbaz RF.** 1996. Hantavirus pulmonary syndrome in Florida: association with the newly identified Black Creek Canal virus. *Am J Med* **100:**46–48.
164. **Richter MH, Hanson JD, Cajimat MNB, Milazzo ML, Fulhorst CF.** 2010. Geographical range of Rio Mamoré virus (family *Bunyaviridae*, genus *Hantavirus*) in association with the small-eared pygmy rice rat (*Oligoryzomys microtis*). *Vector Borne Zoonotic Dis* **10:**613–620.

Arenaviruses and Filoviruses

JONATHAN S. TOWNER, PIERRE E. ROLLIN, YI-WEI TANG, AND THOMAS G. KSIAZEK

99

This chapter focuses on the viral hemorrhagic fever (VHF) viruses from two taxa, the families *Arenaviridae* (1) and *Filoviridae* (2). Some, but not all, members of these virus families cause severe, frequently fatal VHF in localized areas of the world. Although exotic in North America, these viruses are important public health problems in Africa and South America and have the potential of being introduced into the United States by travelers returning from these areas. The arenaviruses and, particularly, the filoviruses have been associated with serious health care-related outbreaks involving health care workers and laboratory personnel. However, more recent outbreaks have generally been in settings where infection control has been lax. The lack of health care-related transmission associated with Lassa or Marburg hemorrhagic fever cases imported into the United States or Europe would suggest that the implementation of standard infection control practices is sufficient to prevent virus spread within the medical care setting. During the West African Ebola outbreak, several infected health care workers were evacuated to the United States and Europe. The U.S. guidelines for patient evaluation and management and sample collection, shipping, and processing have been updated (http://www.cdc.gov/vhf/ebola/index.html). Unfortunately, such practices are not always possible in resource-poor regions in Africa or South America (http://www.cdc.gov/vhf/ebola/hcp/limiting-heat-burden.html).

Continuing detection and isolation of new arenavirus and filovirus species from new geographic locations remain important for public health. The similarity of initial isolation, clinical management, and viral diagnostic procedures for patients with suspected arenavirus or filovirus infections is the rationale for grouping these taxonomically distinct viruses in this chapter. Viruses from other taxonomic families, including *Bunyaviridae* and *Flaviviridae* (chapters 97 and 98), have also been associated with VHF (3).

TAXONOMY AND DESCRIPTION OF THE AGENTS

Arenaviridae

The family *Arenaviridae* comprises 43 named viruses which have unique morphologic and physiochemical characteristics. Antigenic relationships are established mainly on the basis of broadly reactive antibody binding assays, including complement fixation, indirect fluorescent-antibody (IFA), and enzyme-linked immunosorbent assays (ELISA) (1). Both serologic and phylogenetic analyses of the viruses divide the arenaviruses into two complexes. The lymphocytic choriomeningitis (LCM), or Old World, complex contains LCM virus and the Lassa viruses, including a number of apparently benign Lassa-like but unique viruses, Mopeia from Mozambique and Zimbabwe and Mobala and Ippy from the Central African Republic. All have been isolated from rodents of the family *Muridae*. Other arenaviruses have been isolated, or identified through molecular detection and sequencing, either from rodents (Merino Walk [4], Menekre and Gbagroube [5], Kodoko [6], and Morogoro [7] viruses; Lemniscomys and Mus minutoides viruses [8]; and Luna virus [9]) or from humans (Lujo virus, from an outbreak of human fatal hemorrhagic fever patients with person-to-person transmission [3, 10]; Lunk [9], Gairo [11], Mariental and Okahandja [12], Wenzhou [13], and Cardamones and Loei River [14] viruses). The Tacaribe or New World complex includes Tacaribe, Junin, Machupo, Amapari, Cupixi, Parana, Latino, Pichinde, Tamiami, Flexal, Guanarito, Sabia, Oliveros, Whitewater Arroyo, Pirital, Bear Canyon (15), Ocozocoaula de Espinosa (16), Allpahuayo (17), Tonto Creek and Big Brushy Tank (18), Real de Catorce (19), Catarina (16), Pampa (20), Skinner Tank (16), Chapare (21), Middle Pease River (22), Patawa (23), and Pinhal (24) viruses. Some of the viruses have not yet been isolated and are known only from molecular sequence data. All the rodent isolates of New World complex viruses have been from rodents of the family *Muridae* subfamily *Sigmodontinae*, while Tacaribe virus was originally isolated from bats. Highly divergent arenaviruses have been identified in boas and boid snakes with snake inclusion body disease (25, 26) and the Boa Av NL B3 virus (25). The Old and New World arenavirus complexes are distantly related; only when very high-titer antisera are used can cross-reactions be observed. Monoclonal antibodies with specificities for structural proteins of arenaviruses suggest that the N protein is the group-reactive determinant, whereas the envelope glycoproteins (G1 and G2) are responsible for type specificity (1, 27).

The morphology of arenaviruses is distinctive in thin-section electron microscopy (28) and was the basis for first associating LCM virus with Machupo virus and ultimately associating these viruses with all the viruses in the present family. Three major virion structural proteins are usually found (27). The virus glycoprotein precursor is processed into two glycoproteins, G1 (50,000 to 72,000 Da) and G2 (31,000 to 41,000 Da), which constitute the virion envelope and spikes and which both serve as highly type-specific neutralization targets. In addition, a stable signal peptide is retained as an essential subunit in the mature glycoprotein complex (29). The third major protein is the N protein (63,000 to 72,000 Da), which is clearly associated with the virion RNA and is considered the nucleocapsid protein. Four RNA species can be isolated from intact arenavirus virions. Two are virus specific and are ambisense in coding strategy: the small (S) RNA (22S) (encoding the N protein and virus glycoprotein precursor) and the large (L) RNA (31S) (encoding the viral L polymerase and the Z protein, a regulatory element) (1). In addition, ribosomal 28S and 18S species are isolated in virions in different proportions depending on external conditions.

Arenaviruses mature by budding at the cytoplasmic membrane, and host proteins are incorporated into the virion envelope. Vero cells infected with each of the viruses contain distinctive intracytoplasmic inclusion bodies, immunoreactive with anti-N but not anti-G1 or anti-G2 antibody. All arenaviruses are readily inactivated by ethyl ether, chloroform, sodium deoxycholate, and acidic media (pH less than 5). β-Propiolactone (30) and gamma irradiation (31) are both reported to inactivate arenavirus infectivity while preserving reactivity in standard serologic tests.

Filoviridae

The filoviruses, including both ebolaviruses and marburgviruses, have a common morphology and similar genomic organization and complement of structural proteins (2). Marburgvirus and ebolavirus virion RNAs are nonsegmented, negative-sense, single-stranded RNAs, approximately 19 kb long and 4.0×10^6 to 4.5×10^6 Da. The viral genomes are linearly arranged in a manner consistent with other nonsegmented, negative-sense, and single-stranded RNA viruses. Some sequence similarity to the paramyxoviruses, especially in the nucleocapsid and polymerase proteins, was noted. However, comparison with other filovirus protein sequences confirms that filoviruses are highly distinct. Furthermore, filoviruses are sufficiently distinct by ultrastructural and serologic criteria to warrant separate taxonomic status as members of the family *Filoviridae* (2, 28, 32).

Marburgviruses and ebolaviruses have at least seven virus-specific structural proteins, expressed from seven genes (2). For ebolaviruses, the ribonucleoprotein complex contains L (180 kDa), N (104 kDa), VP30 (30 kDa), and VP35 (35 kDa) in loose association. L is an RNA-dependent RNA polymerase, and VP35 may play a role similar to the P protein of paramyxoviruses and rhabdoviruses. GP (125 kDa) is the major spike protein; VP40 (a matrix protein) plus VP24 make up the remaining protein content of the multilayered envelope (2, 32). The GP of ebolaviruses and marburgviruses can be differentiated by the presence or absence of *N*- and O-linked glycans and by the lack, in marburgviruses, of the second open reading frame coding for the small/soluble glycoprotein expressed during ebolavirus infection *in vitro* and *in vivo* (2). When grown in Vero (or Vero E6) or MA-104 cells, the GP of marburgviruses is totally devoid of terminal sialic acid, whereas that of ebolaviruses has abundant (2-3)-linked sialic acid. Phylogenetic analysis of filovirus genomes clearly separates these viruses into three genera: *Ebolavirus*, *Marburgvirus*, and the newly identified *Cuevavirus*. The genus *Ebolavirus* contains five species: *Zaire ebolavirus*, *Sudan ebolavirus*, *Reston ebolavirus*, *Taï Forest ebolavirus* (formerly known as *Ivory Coast ebolavirus*), and *Bundibugyo ebolavirus* (33), and each contains one virus (Ebola virus [EBOV], Sudan virus [SUDV], Reston virus [RESTV], Taï Forest (TAFV) virus, and Bundibugyo virus [BDBV], respectively). The genus *Marburgvirus* has just a single virus species, *Marburg marburgvirus*, which contains two viruses, Marburg virus (MARV) and Ravn virus (RAVV) (34). Though not known to be clinically relevant for humans, the genus *Cuevavirus* has just a single virus species, *Lloviu cuevavirus*, which contains a single virus, Lloviu virus (LLOV). Lloviu virus has not been cultured, but full-length genomes were detected in several dead *Miniopterus schreibersii* bats in Europe (35).

Despite their unusual long rod-like morphologic properties, filoviruses resemble the other lipid-enveloped viruses, including the arenaviruses, in being susceptible to heat, lipid solvents, β-propiolactone (30), formaldehyde, UV light, and gamma radiation (31). These viruses are stable at room temperature for several hours but are destabilized by incubation at 60°C for 1 h.

EPIDEMIOLOGY AND TRANSMISSION

Arenaviridae

Arenaviruses are maintained in nature by association with specific mammalian hosts (Table 1), in which they produce chronic viremia and/or viruria. The viruses are routinely isolated from blood and urine samples of their specific rodent host. Naturally occurring human disease can usually be traced to direct or indirect contact with infected rodents. Aerosol infectivity is thought to be an important natural route of infection as well. Attempts to implicate arthropod vectors have been unsuccessful, but ectoparasites taken from viremic mammalian hosts have occasionally yielded arenavirus isolates. Of the 39 named mammalian members of the family *Arenaviridae*, 9 are known to be human pathogens. Health care-related transmission is well described for Lassa and Machupo viruses. Lujo virus was identified during a health care-related outbreak involving five people, four of whom died (36). Because of the high level of virus circulation in West Africa (mostly Nigeria, Sierra Leone, Guinea, and Liberia), Lassa fever is the VHF most frequently exported to areas of nonendemicity, including multiple instances in the United States and Europe.

Filoviridae

Marburg and Ebola hemorrhagic fevers are now referred to as Marburg virus disease (MVD) and Ebola virus disease (EVD) because less than 50% of confirmed patients present with any kind of hemorrhage. Marburg virus was first recognized in 1967, when 32 people in Germany and Yugoslavia became infected following contact with monkey kidneys, primary tissue cultures derived from monkeys imported from Uganda, or sick patients (2, 32). Ebolaviruses first emerged in two major disease outbreaks, which occurred almost simultaneously in Zaire (now Democratic Republic of the Congo) and Sudan (now South Sudan) in 1976. Despite their simultaneous emergence, these viruses were later shown to be two distinct viruses (now known as EBOV and SUDV), based on serologic and sequence analysis criteria (2). In 1989 and 1990, RESTV was isolated from cynomolgus monkeys being held in quarantine in Reston, VA, and Perkasie, PA, following their importation

TABLE 1 Currently recognized arenaviruses and filoviruses and associated human diseases

Virus, date isolated	Natural host	Geographic distribution	Naturally occurring human disease	Human laboratory infections
Old World arenaviruses				
Lymphocytic choriomeningitis, 1933	*Mus musculus* (house mouse)	Americas, Europe	Undifferentiated febrile illness, aseptic meningitis; rarely serious	Common; usually mild, but 5 were fatal
Lassa, 1969	*Mastomys* sp. (multimammate rat)	West Africa, imported cases in Europe, Japan, USA	Lassa fever; mild to severe and fatal disease	Common; often severe
Mopeia, 1977	*Mastomys natalensis* (multimammate rat)	Mozambique, Zimbabwe, Tanzania	Unknown	None; little experience
Mobala, 1983	*Praomys* sp. (soft-furred mouse)	Central African Republic	Unknown	None; little experience
Ippy, 1984	*Arvicanthis* sp. (grass rats)	Central African Republic	Unknown	None
Merino Walk, 1985	*Myotomys unisulcatus* (Busk Karoo rat)	Republic of South Africa	Unknown	None
Menekre, 2005 (only sequence available)	*Hylomyscus* sp. (African wood mouse)	Ivory Coast	Unknown	None
Gbagroube, 2005 (only sequence available)	*Mus (Nannomys) setulosus* (African pigmy mouse)	Ivory Coast	Unknown	None
Morogoro, 2007 (only sequence available)	*Mastomys natalensis* (multimammate rat)	Tanzania	Unknown	None
Kodoko, 2007	*Mus (Nannomys) minutoides* (savannah pygmy mouse)	Guinea	Unknown	None
Lujo, 2008	Unknown	Zambia, Republic of South Africa	Fatal hemorrhagic fever	None
Luna, 2009	*Mastomys natalensis* (multimammate rat)	Zambia	Unknown	None
Lemniscomys, 2010 (only sequence available)	*Lemniscomys rosalia* (multimammate rat)	Tanzania	Unknown	None
Mus minutoides, 2010 (only sequence available)	*Mus minutoides* (savannah pygmy mouse)	Tanzania	Unknown	None
Lunk, 2012 (only sequence available)	*Mus minutoides* (savannah pygmy mouse)	Zambia	Unknown	None
Gairo, 2015	*Mastomys natalensis* (multimammate rat)	Tanzania	Unknown	None
Mariental, 2015	*Micaelamys [Aethomys] namaquensis* (Namaqua rock mice)	Namibia	Unknown	None
Okahandja, 2015	*Micaelamys [Aethomys] namaquensis* (Namaqua rock mice)	Namibia	Unknown	None
Wenzhou, 2015	*Rattus norvegicus* (brown rat), *R. flavipectus* (yellow breasted rat), *R. losea* (lesser ricefield rat), *R. rattus* (black rat), *Suncus murinus* (house shrew)	China	Unknown	None detected
Wenzhou, Cardamones variant, 2016	*Rattus norvegicus* (brown rat), *R. exulans* (Pacific rat)	Cambodia	Fever and respiratory syndrome	None detected
Loei River, 2016	*Bandicota indica* (bandicoot rat), *B. savilei* (Savile's bandicoot rat), *Niviventer fulvescens* (Indomalayan niviventer)	Thailand	Unknown	None detected
New World arenaviruses				
Tacaribe, 1956	*Artibeus* sp. bats	Trinidad, West Indies	Unknown	One suspected; moderately symptomatic
Junin, 1958	*Calomys musculinus* (drylands vesper mouse)	Argentina	Argentinian hemorrhagic fever	Common; often severe
Machupo, 1963	*Calomys callosus* (large vesper mouse)	Bolivia	Bolivian hemorrhagic fever	Common; often severe
Cupixi, 1965	*Oryzomys gaeldi* (rice rat)	Brazil	Unknown	None detected
Amapari,1965	*Neacomys guianae* (Guiana bristly mouse)	Brazil	Unknown	None detected

(Continued on next page)

TABLE 1 Currently recognized arenaviruses and filoviruses and associated human diseases *(Continued)*

Virus, date isolated	Natural host	Geographic distribution	Naturally occurring human disease	Human laboratory infections
New World arenaviruses *(Continued)*				
Parana, 1970	*Oryzomys buccinatus* (Paraguayan rice rat)	Paraguay	Unknown	None detected
Tamiami, 1970	*Sigmodon hispidus* (hispid cotton rat)	Florida, USA	Antibodies detected	None detected
Pichinde, 1971	*Oryzomys albigularis* (Tomes's rice rat)	Colombia	Unknown	Occasional; mild to asymptomatic
Latino, 1973	*Calomys callosus* (large vesper mouse)	Bolivia	Unknown	None detected
Flexal, 1977	*Oryzomys* spp. (rice rats)	Brazil	None detected	One recognized (severe)
Guanarito, 1989	*Zygodontomys brevicauda* (short-tailed cane mouse)	Venezuela	Venezuelan hemorrhagic fever	None detected
Sabia, 1993	Unknown	Brazil	Viral hemorrhagic fever	Two recognized (both severe)
Oliveros, 1996	*Bolomys obscuris* (dark bolo mouse)	Argentina	Unknown	None detected
Whitewater Arroyo, 1997	*Neotoma* spp. (wood rats)	USA: New Mexico, Oklahoma, Utah, California, Colorado	Unknown	None detected
Pirital, 1997	*Sigmodon alstoni* (Alston's cotton rat)	Venezuela	Unknown	None detected
Pampa, 1997	*Bolomys* sp.	Argentina	Unknown	None detected
Bear Canyon, 1998	*Peromyscus californicus* (California mouse), *Neotoma macrotis* (large-eared woodrat)	USA: California	Unknown	None detected
Ocozocoautla de Espinosa, 2000 (only sequence available)	*Peromyscus mexicanus* (Mexican deer mouse)	Mexico	Unknown	None detected
Allpahuayo, 2001	*Oecomys bicolor*, (bicolored arboreal rice rat), *Oecomys paricola* (Brazilian arboreal rice rat	Peru	Unknown	None detected
Tonto Creek, 2001	*Neotoma albigula* (white-throated woodrat)	USA: Arizona	Unknown	None detected
Big Brushy Tank, 2002	*Neotoma albigula* (white-throated woodrat)	USA: Arizona	Unknown	None detected
Real de Catorce, 2005 (only sequence available)	*Neotoma leucodon* (white-toothed woodrat)	Mexico	Unknown	None detected
Catarina, 2007	*Neotoma micropus* (southern plains woodrat)	USA: Texas	Unknown	None detected
Skinner Tank, 2008	*Neotoma mexicana* (Mexican woodrat)	USA: Arizona	Unknown	None detected
Chapare, 2008	Unknown	Bolivia	Single fatal hemorrhagic fever case	None detected
Middle Pease River, 2015	*Neotoma micropus* (southern plain woodrat)	USA: Texas	Unknown	None detected
Patawa, 2015 (only sequence available)	*Oecomys rutilus* (red arboreal rice rat), *Oecomys auyantepui* (North Amazonian arboreal rice rat)	French Guiana	Unknown	None detected
Pinhal, 2015 (only sequence available)	*Calomys tener* (delicate vester mouse)	Brazil	Unknown	None detected
Unclassified arenaviruses				
Golden Gate, 2009	*Boa constrictor* (boa constrictor)	USA: California	Unknown	None detected
Collierville, 2009 (only sequence available)	*Boa constrictor* (boa constrictor)	USA: California	Unknown	None detected
CAS, 2009 (only sequence available)	*Corallus annulatus* (annulated tree boa)	USA: California	Unknown	None detected
Boa Av NL B3, 2013 (only sequence available)	*Boa constrictor* (boa constrictor)	Netherlands	Unknown	None detected

(Continued on next page)

TABLE 1 Currently recognized arenaviruses and filoviruses and associated human diseases (*Continued*)

Virus, date isolated	Natural host	Geographic distribution	Naturally occurring human disease	Human laboratory infections
Filoviruses				
Marburg, 1967	Bats, *Rousettus aegyptiacus*	Imported in Germany and Yugoslavia; Kenya, Zimbabwe, Democratic Republic of Congo, Angola, Uganda; imported single cases in Netherlands and USA	Fatal cases	Yes
Ebola, 1976	Bats?	Democratic Republic of Congo, Gabon, Republic of Congo, Guinea with spread to Sierra Leone and Liberia	Fatal cases	Yes
Sudan, 1976	Bats?	Sudan, Uganda	Fatal cases	None detected
Reston, 1989	Bats?	Philippines, imported infected primates in USA and Italy	No symptoms reported	Seroconversion in non-human primate handlers, pig farmers, and slaughterhouse workers
Taï Forest, 1994	Bats?	Ivory Coast	Febrile illness, survived	None detected
Bundibugyo, 2007	Bats?	Uganda, Democratic Republic of Congo	Fatal cases	None detected

from the Philippines (37), while in 1994, the only known human infection with TAFV occurred in a veterinarian investigating deaths among chimpanzees in the Ivory Coast (Côte d'Ivoire) (38). From 1995 to 2005, EBOV emerged sporadically in Zaire (now Democratic Republic of Congo), Gabon, and Republic of Congo, with some human cases associated with exposure to infected non-human primates (3, 39). The emergence of SUDV has thus far been restricted to Uganda and southern Sudan (now South Sudan), causing outbreaks in 2000 (425 cases), 2004 (17 cases), and in a series of small clusters, in 2011, 2012, and 2013 (40, 41). An outbreak due to marburgviruses, both MARV and RAVV, involving gold miners and secondary contacts, started in 1998 and continued into 2000 in eastern Democratic Republic of Congo (2) and was linked to bats found in that mine based on reverse transcription PCR (RT-PCR) and serology (42). The highest seroprevalence was found in the cave-dwelling Egyptian rousette bat (species *Rousettus aegyptiacus*). The largest known outbreak of MVD occurred in 2005 in Uige, northern Angola, causing 252 cases with 227 deaths (2, 43). The source of the outbreak was not determined.

In 2005, Ebola virus RT-PCR-positive fruit bats were found in Gabon (44), the first time genetic material for any ebolavirus was found in a bat. In 2007 and 2008, EBOV was responsible for two small outbreaks in Kasai-Occidental (Democratic Republic of the Congo) (http://www.who.int/csr/don/2009_02_17/en/index.html). Also in 2007, a new distinct ebolavirus, BDBV, was isolated during an outbreak, centered in and around Bundibugyo in western Uganda (33), where 131 suspected, probable, or confirmed cases were reported from August to December 2007. In 2008, RESTV was isolated from swine tissues during the laboratory investigation of samples from a 2007 outbreak of high-mortality disease in swine in farms in the Philippines, which was thought to be atypical porcine reproductive and respiratory syndrome (PRRS) (45). PRRS and Circo 2 viruses were also isolated from the swine, leaving it unclear to what extent RESTV contributed to the disease symptoms. The exact role of RESTV in the clinical process is still unclear. In 2011, RESTV was detected by RT-PCR in piglets in Shanghai, China, as part of routine screening efforts for PRRS virus (46). This finding may be indicative of continued maintenance of RESTV in pigs, with possible distribution to other countries through trade. Experimental infections of swine with RESTV isolated from Philippine pigs did not cause clinically notable disease, although the virus was shed, and detectable antibodies developed in experimental infections in the laboratory (18). This virus species appears to be less virulent for humans than are other filovirus species, since in 1990, four workers at the U.S. quarantine facility were found to have antibody to RESTV without having experienced disease, and several slaughterhouse and pig farm workers from the outbreak in the Philippines were also found with antibody without associated clinical disease (http://www.who.int/csr/resources/publicationsHSE_EPR_2009_2.pdf).

In 2007, four workers from a lead ore mine near Ibanda, Uganda, were infected with marburgviruses, three with MARV and one with RAVV. Two patients died, and the subsequent investigations led to the detection of marburgvirus RT-PCR-positive Egyptian rousette fruit bats and, for the first time, the isolation of both marburgviruses from this potential reservoir (47, 48). In 2008, MVD was diagnosed in two tourists infected with MARV who independently visited the same Egyptian rousette bat-inhabited cave (Python Cave, Queen Elizabeth National Park) in western Uganda. The first case was a Dutch woman who subsequently died of MVD in the Netherlands (49). The second patient was an American woman from Colorado who, following hospitalization in the United States, recovered and was diagnosed retrospectively.

Through 2018, a total of 21 marburgvirus isolates have been obtained directly from Egyptian rousette bats caught in Uganda. A single case of EVD associated with SUDV was reported in 2011 in Uganda (50), but in 2012, four unrelated outbreaks occurred: SUDV in Kibaale (Uganda) in July and August, BDBV in Isiro (Democratic Republic of Congo) from August to October, MARV in Kabale (Uganda) in October and November, and SUDV in Luwero (Uganda) in November (51). In early 2014, the Guinean Ministry of Health reported an outbreak of EVD in the forest region of the country. This outbreak, caused by EBOV, quickly became the biggest outbreak ever, causing more than 28,000 confirmed and probable cases primarily in Guinea, Sierra Leone, and Liberia. For the first time, multiple public health institutions and research laboratories deployed and supported mobile laboratories (up to 32) for rapid diagnostic detection of EVD in all the affected countries. Most of these field labs used molecular assays which were recently FDA/WHO emergency use approved. There were multiple medical evacuations of infected medical responders to Europe and the United States as well as infected travelers sometimes causing secondary cases in Senegal, Mali, Nigeria, and the United States (52). An update can be found at http://www.who.int/csr/disease/ebola/en/. Multiple health care workers in developed countries, including the United States, became infected. In response, the CDC defined multiple tiers of hospital readiness, consisting of (i) frontline health care facilities, (ii) Ebola assessment hospitals, and (iii) Ebola treatment centers. Ultimately, 81 facilities in the United States were evaluated for their readiness to care for EVD patients, resulting in the certification of 55 hospitals by state health departments as Ebola treatment centers. In 2017 and 2018, EVD (caused by EBOV) reemerged three times in separate outbreaks in Democratic Republic of the Congo in the Bas-Uele, Equateur, and Nord-Kivu provinces, respectively. This last outbreak caused more than 211 cases and 135 deaths as of the time of this writing (14 October 2018).

CLINICAL SIGNIFICANCE

Patients with VHF frequently present with similar, nonspecific clinical signs resembling malaria, typhoid fever, and pharyngitis. A detailed travel history, coupled with a high index of suspicion and availability of definitive virologic tools, should facilitate rapid diagnosis and the timely implementation of appropriate patient isolation, clinical management procedures, and public health measures. For EVD, U.S. guidance documents are available online (http://www.cdc.gov/vhf/ebola/hcp/ed-management-patients-possible-ebola.html and http://www.cdc.gov/vhf/ebola/hcp/patient-management-us-hospitals.html).

Arenaviridae

Among the known arenavirus human pathogens, LCM virus produces the least severe infection (53). A modest proportion of LCM infections are subclinical. A "typical" LCM case is usually heralded by fever, myalgia, retro-orbital headache, weakness, and anorexia. Especially during the first week, prominent symptoms include sore throat, chills, vomiting, cough, retrosternal pain, and arthralgia. Rash occurs but is infrequent. In about one-third of the patients, fever recurs, coinciding with the onset of frank neurologic involvement, usually aseptic meningitis but less frequently, meningoencephalitis. Complete recovery is almost always the rule. Thus, LCM infections are temporarily debilitating but rarely fatal, even when neurologic complications arise. *In utero* infections with LCM virus are a cause of significant birth defects of the central nervous and ocular systems (54). Fatal forms of LCM infections have been reported in several clusters following transplantation of organs from LCM virus-infected donors to immunosuppressed recipients (55–57).

Lassa, Junin, and Machupo virus infections are much more severe. Lassa fever patients usually present at the hospital within 5 to 7 days of onset and complain of sore throat, severe lower back pain, and conjunctivitis. These signs and symptoms usually increase in severity during the following week and are accompanied by nausea, vomiting, diarrhea, chest and abdominal pain, headache, cough, dizziness, and tinnitus. Later, pneumonitis and pleural and pericardial effusions with friction rub frequently occur. A maculopapular rash may develop, but frank hemorrhage is seen in only a proportion of the more severe cases. Bleeding from puncture sites and mucous membranes and melena are more common. Although mild or unapparent infections occur, approximately 15 to 20% of hospitalized patients die, usually as a result of sudden cardiovascular collapse resulting from hepatic, pulmonary, and myocardial failure. Few Lassa fever patients develop central nervous system signs, although tinnitus or deafness may develop as recovery begins. Lassa fever is a particularly severe disease among pregnant women, for whom mortality rates are somewhat higher. The disease course in children is similar to that in adults, but in infants a condition described as swollen-baby syndrome, characterized by anasarca, abdominal distension, and bleeding, is typical. Clinical laboratory studies are not usually helpful for Lassa fever; specific virologic testing is required, especially in a setting where Lassa fever is less common or where mild, atypical cases are occurring.

The clinical pictures for Argentinian hemorrhagic fever due to Junin virus and Bolivian hemorrhagic fever due to Machupo virus are well characterized; for Venezuelan hemorrhagic fever due to Guanarito virus, Sabia virus in Brazil, and Chapare virus with a single confirmed case in Bolivia, less information is available (3). However, all these infections are sufficiently similar to each other to be discussed as a single entity, South American or New World arenavirus hemorrhagic fevers. Incubation periods range from 7 to 14 days, and very few subclinical cases are thought to occur. Following gradual onset of fever, anorexia, and malaise over several days, constitutional signs involving the gastrointestinal, cardiovascular, and central nervous systems become apparent by the time patients present to the hospital. On initial examination, Argentinian hemorrhagic fever and Bolivian hemorrhagic fever patients are febrile, acutely ill, and mildly hypotensive. They frequently complain of back pain, epigastric pain, headache, retro-orbital pain, photophobia, dizziness, constipation or diarrhea, and coughing. Flushing of the face, neck, and chest and bleeding from the gums are common. Enanthem is almost invariably present; petechiae or tiny vesicles spread over the erythematous palate and fauces. Neurologic involvement, ranging from mild irritability and lethargy to abnormalities in gait, tremors of the upper extremities, and in severely ill patients, coma, delirium, and convulsions, occurs in more than half of the patients. During the second week of illness, clinical improvement may begin or complications may develop. Complications include extensive petechial hemorrhages, blood oozing from puncture wounds, melena, and hematemesis. These manifestations of capillary damage and thrombocytopenia do not result in life-threatening blood loss. However, hypotension and shock may develop, often in combination with serious neurologic signs, among

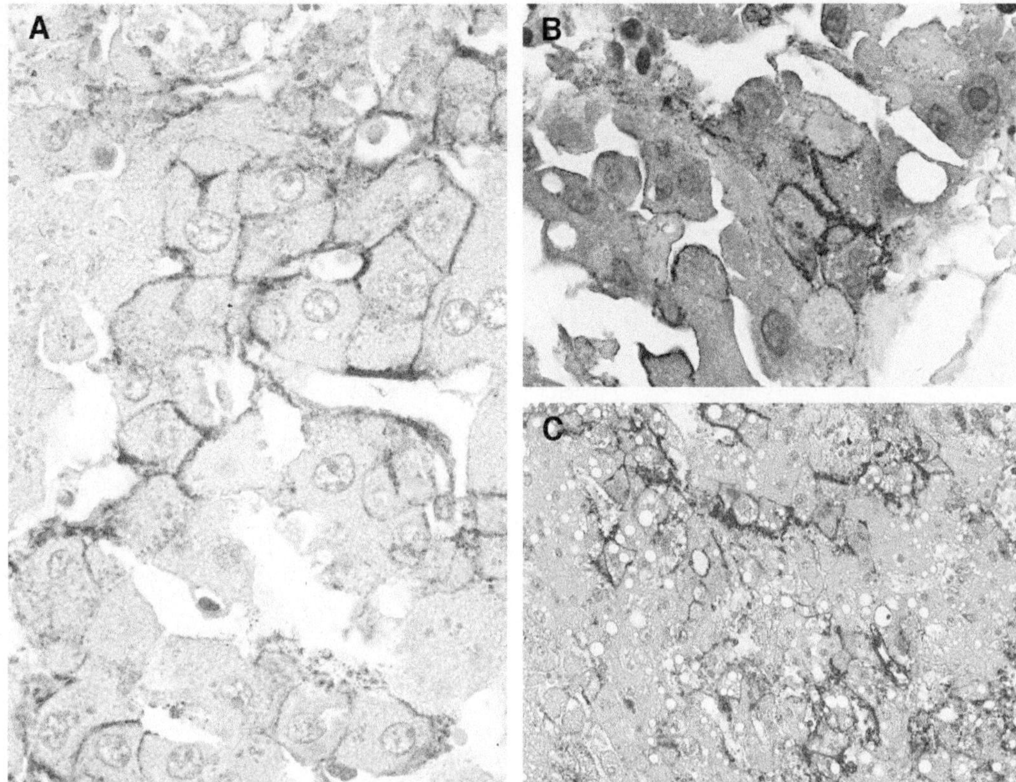

FIGURE 1 By immunohistochemistry, abundant virus antigens are seen within the cytoplasm of hepatocytes and sinusoidal lining cells in the liver of patients infected by (A) Lassa virus, original magnification ×158; (B) Lujo virus, original magnification ×158; (C) LCM virus (transplant patient), original magnification ×50 (immunoalkaline phosphatase staining, naphthol fast red substrate with light hematoxylin counterstain).

the 15% of patients who die. Survivors begin to show improvement by the third week. Recovery is slow; weakness, fatigue, and mental difficulties may last for weeks, and a significant proportion of patients relapse with a "late neurologic syndrome," which includes headache, cerebellar tremor, and cranial nerve palsies. In contrast to Lassa fever, clinical laboratory studies are frequently useful. Total leukocyte counts usually fall to 1,000 to 2,000 cells/mm^3, although the differential remains normal. Platelet counts fall precipitously, usually to between 25,000 and 100,000/mm^3. Routine clotting parameters are usually normal or slightly abnormal; however, patients with severe cases may show evidence of disseminated intravascular coagulation.

In the single Lujo virus outbreak in southern Africa, involving five confirmed cases, the patients presented with nonspecific febrile illness with headache and myalgia following an incubation ranging from 7 to 13 days (36). A morbilliform rash was evident in three Caucasian patients on days 6 to 8 of illness, but not in two African patients. In the four fatal cases, the disease course was biphasic. The second phase, starting around 1 week post onset was characterized by a rapid deterioration with respiratory distress, neurological signs, and circulatory collapse. All patients had thrombocytopenia on admission to hospital (platelet count range 20 to 104 × 10^9/liter). Three patients had normal white cell counts, and two had leukopenia on admission, while four developed leucocytosis during the illness. The last patient (the only one surviving) was treated with the antiviral drug ribavirin.

In fatal arenavirus infections histopathologic findings include multifocal hepatocellular necrosis with minimal inflammatory response, interstitial pneumonitis, myocarditis, and lymphoid depletion. Extensive arenavirus antigens are seen in parenchymal cells as well as cells of the mononuclear phagocytic system, much more than morphologic lesions would suggest (Fig. 1).

Filoviridae

EVD and MVD cases are clinically similar, although the frequencies of reported signs and symptoms vary among individuals. Clinical features of EVD and clinical management in high-resource and low-resource settings were recently reviewed (58–60). Following incubation periods of 4 to 16 days, onset is sudden and is marked by fever, chills, headache, anorexia, and myalgia. These signs are soon followed by nausea, vomiting, sore throat, abdominal pain, and diarrhea. When first examined, patients are usually overtly ill, dehydrated, apathetic, and disoriented. Pharyngeal and conjunctival injection is usual. Within several days, a characteristic maculopapular rash over the trunk, petechiae, and mucous membrane hemorrhages can appear. Gastrointestinal bleeding, accompanied by intense epigastric pain, is common, as are petechiae and bleeding from puncture wounds and mucous membranes. In the West Africa EVD outbreak, hemorrhages were less frequent, but profuse diarrhea was frequently observed and was responsible for severe dehydration (60) (http://www.cdc.gov/vhf/ebolahcp/clinician-information-us-healthcare-settings.html). High titers of EBOV are found in bodily fluids, including blood,

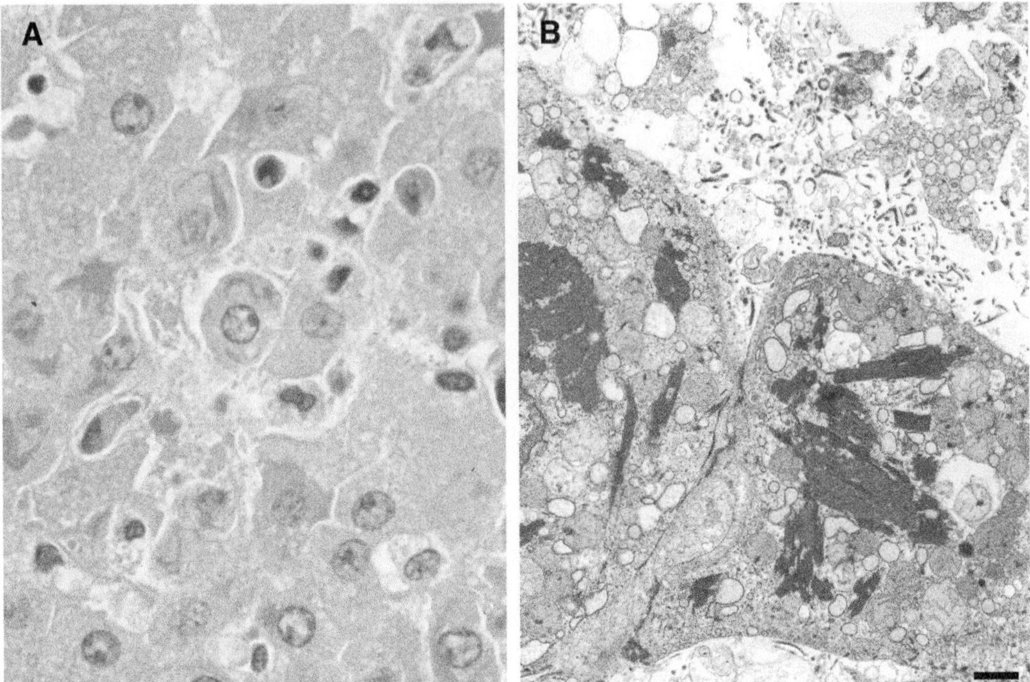

FIGURE 2 Ebola virus hemorrhagic fever. (A) Section of liver showing hepatocellular necrosis, numerous intracytoplasmic, eosinophilic Ebola viral inclusions, and sinusoidal dilatation and congestion. Hematoxylin and eosin stain; original magnification ×250. (B) Several Ebola viral inclusions are seen in a thin-section electron micrograph of liver. The inclusions consist of viral nucleocapsids mostly seen in a longitudinal section. Numerous viral particles are also seen in sinusoidal spaces; scale bar, 100 nm. (Courtesy of C. S. Goldsmith.).

and present a major risk factor for those caring for EVD patients. Shock develops shortly before death, often 6 to 16 days after the onset of illness. Abnormalities in coagulation parameters include fibrin split products and prolonged prothrombin and partial thromboplastin times, suggesting that disseminated intravascular coagulation is typically a terminal event and is usually associated with multiorgan failure (61). Clinical laboratory studies usually reveal profound leukopenia early, and sometimes moderately elevated at a later stage. Platelet counts decline to 50,000 to 100,000/mm^3 during the hemorrhagic phase. Severe hypokalemia can be seen when profuse vomiting and diarrhea are seen. Liver enzymes and creatinine levels parallel the liver and kidney failure encountered in the latter stages of the disease.

In fatal filovirus infections, disseminated infection and necrosis in major organs such as liver, spleen, lung, kidney, skin, and gonads are extensive. Extensive hepatocellular necrosis associated with the formation of characteristic viral inclusion is seen in fatal Ebola virus infections. Lymphoid depletion, microvascular infection, and injury are seen in all filovirus infections. Abundant antigens and nucleic acids can be seen in all major organs by using immunohistochemistry and *in situ* hybridization (Fig. 2 and 3). For patients that recover, virus can persist for many months in seminal fluid, a feature first observed in patients infected with MARV in 1967 but found frequently in convalescent men infected with EBOV in West Africa (62, 63). On rare occasions this leads to sexual transmission of virus, in one instance over 470 days after symptom onset (64). Other rare instances of EBOV residing in immune-privileged sites include the eye, causing uveitis, and cerebrospinal fluid, detected 9 months after clearing viremia (64, 65).

Therapy of VHF follows general principles: symptomatic treatment with careful maintenance of fluid balance and management of bleeding diathesis. The antiviral drug ribavirin, if used early in the course of the disease, is effective in Lassa hemorrhagic fever in reducing mortality and duration of disease (3, 66). Ribavirin is also effective in Junin hemorrhagic fever and has been used to treat Bolivian hemorrhagic fever, Lujo infection, and LCM infection in immune-compromised patients (3, 36, 56). It was recently reported that the compound KP-146 [(5-(5-(2,3-dihydrobenzo[b][1,4] dioxin-6-yl)-4′-methoxy-[1,1′-biphenyl]-3-yl)thiophene-2-carboxamide] had strong anti-LCM virus activity in cultured cells (67). Major challenges of developing a vaccine against Lassa virus include the very high genetic diversity and lack of a profitable commercial market for major vaccine manufacturers. No antiviral drugs are yet commercially available against filovirus, but some postexposure treatment has showed some efficacy in non-human primate models such as recombinant human activated protein C, small-interfering RNA, and immunotherapy using cocktails of monoclonal antibody (68, 69). During the West Africa Ebola outbreak, convalescent immune plasma, cocktails of monoclonal antibody, and antiviral were administrated through compassionate use in patients, with mixed results (69–71). There are no licensed vaccines for arenaviruses and filoviruses. Several vaccine candidates against Ebola virus infections have been developed and have shown promising results in human clinical trials (72–77).

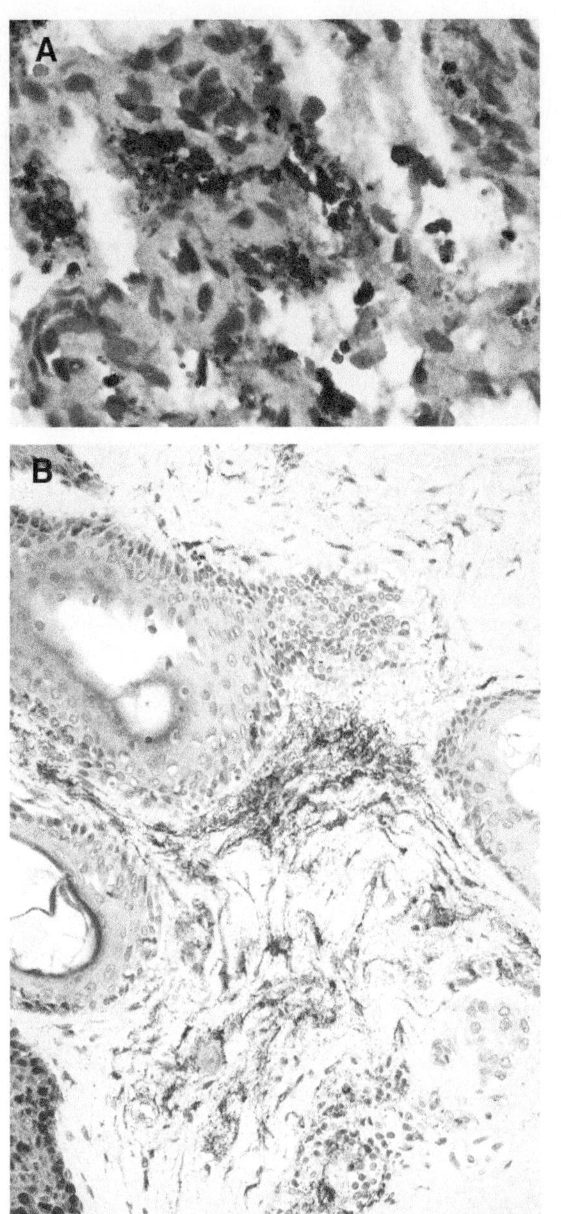

FIGURE 3 (A) Using immunohistochemistry, abundant Ebola virus antigens (in red) are seen in the lymph node of a pig infected by Ebola Reston virus. Original magnification ×158. (B) Skin showing massive viral burden as seen in this section immunostained for Ebola antigens. Original magnification ×50 (immunoalkaline phosphatase staining, naphthol fast red substrate with light hematoxylin counterstain).

COLLECTION, TRANSPORT, AND STORAGE OF SPECIMENS

Safety and Security

Some arenaviruses (Lassa, Junin, Machupo, Sabia, Guanarito, Chapare, and Lujo) and all filoviruses are classified as biosafety level 4 (BSL4) agents, because there is a high risk of infection of laboratory personnel, and appropriate precautions must be taken (78) (http://www.cdc.gov/vhf/ebola/hcp/interim-guidance-specimen-collection-submission-patients-suspected-infection-ebola.html#update1). For laboratories, basic guidance written for EBOV but applicable to other high-consequence pathogens can be found at https://www.cdc.gov/vhf/ebola/healthcare-us/laboratories/index.html. Most are also classified in the United States as select agents by the Department of Health and Human Services and should be handled as such (http://www.selectagents.gov/ and http://www.cdc.gov/vhf/ebola/hcp/select-agent-regulations.html). However, for the arenavirus LCM virus, diagnostic specimens and cell culture manipulations are performed at BSL2, while procedures that might generate aerosols of concentrated virus are performed at BSL3. Ebolaviruses and marburgviruses have been classified as tier 1 select agents, and additional regulations exist for possessing, using, or transferring tier 1 select agents and toxins (http://www.selectagents.gov/Regulations.html). At a minimum, barrier nursing procedures should be implemented, and personnel caring for the patient and handling diagnostic specimens should wear disposable caps, gowns, shoe covers, surgical gloves, and face masks (preferably full-face respirators equipped with high-efficiency particulate air filters) (79). Gloves should be disinfected immediately if they come in direct contact with infected blood or secretions. Manipulation of these specimens and tissues, including sera obtained from convalescent patients, may pose a serious biohazard and should be minimized outside a BSL4 laboratory (78, 79). Use of vacutainer tubes (e.g., BD Vacutainer) is considered safer than use of syringes and needles, which must be disassembled before their contents are transferred to another tube. Procedures which generate aerosols (e.g., centrifugation) should be minimized and performed only if additional protective measures, such as keeping the equipment in a class I or II laminar flow hood, are taken. For specialized procedures, the infectivity of samples may be greatly reduced, if not totally inactivated, by the addition of Triton X-100 and heating. Heating to 60°C for 1 h may reduce infectivity in diagnostic specimens (80) and is acceptable for measurement of heat-stable substances such as electrolytes, blood urea nitrogen, and creatinine. When the equipment is available, sterilization by ^{60}Co γ-irradiation is the preferred method of inactivation. Extraction of RNA from infectious samples by using guanidinium thiocyanate (with a proper ratio, at least 1 to 5 or 1 to 10 of lysis reagents) should be conducted in a laminar-flow hood. Note that some lysis buffers do not completely inactivate high-titer specimens without certain conditions (80, 81). After this step, the extracted RNAs are no longer infectious.

Specimen Collection

For virus isolation, antigen detection, and RT-PCR, serum, heparinized plasma, or whole blood should be collected during the acute, febrile stages of illness and frozen on dry ice or in liquid nitrogen vapor. In the United States, the guidance for Ebola sample collection and submission has been updated (http://www.cdc.gov/vhf/ebola/hcp/interim-guidance-specimen-collection-submission-patients-suspected-infection-ebola.html). Storage at higher temperatures (above −70°C) leads to losses in infectivity. Blood obtained in early convalescence for diagnostic purposes may be infectious despite the presence of antibodies, and it should be handled accordingly (78, 79). In addition to blood samples, throat wash specimens have also been used for virus isolation during infections with arenaviruses (Lassa, Junin, and Machupo). LCM virus may be recovered from acute-phase serum samples obtained during the first week after onset but more likely from cerebrospinal fluid during the period of meningeal involvement and from the brain at autopsy but is rarely, if ever, recovered from throat washings or urine specimens. LCM virus has been easily isolated from the blood of immunocompromised organ transplant recipients. Chapare and Lujo viruses were isolated from blood during the acute phase of the disease. Filoviruses are usually recovered from acute-phase serum samples; various specimens including throat washings, oropharyngeal secretions, urine, soft tissue effusions, semen, and anterior eye fluid have yielded filovirus isolates, even occasionally when the specimens were obtained late in convalescence.

Postmortem Specimens

Lassa, Machupo, and Junin viruses; marburgviruses; and ebolaviruses are all readily isolated from specimens of spleen, lymph nodes, liver, and kidney obtained at autopsy but rarely, if ever, from brain or other central nervous system tissues. Autopsies may be attempted on a limited basis but only by highly trained personnel such as those in the Infectious Diseases Pathology Branch at the CDC. Notably, Lassa virus is usually isolated from the placentas of infected pregnant women. In the severe and fatal clinical forms observed after organ transplant, LCM virus was isolated from several organs by biopsies taken before death or at autopsy. Lujo virus was isolated from liver at autopsy. Formaldehyde-fixed tissues and paraffin-embedded blocks are also suitable for histopathology and immunohistochemical identification of viral antigens and should be conserved and shipped at room temperature.

Shipping

If an arenavirus or filovirus infection is suspected based on clinical and epidemiological evidence, and before sending the specimens, the clinicians should consult with the local health authorities and the relevant laboratories listed below that maintain BSL4 facilities and a diagnostic capability for these agents. For all testing of infectious material, samples should be packaged in accordance with current recommendations (International Air Transport Association: http://www.iata.org/index.htm). Packages should be sent by rapid courier, and preliminary results could be expected within 24 to 48 hours after receipt of the specimens.

1. Centers for Disease Control and Prevention, Viral Special Pathogens Branch, 1600 Clifton Rd., Atlanta, GA 30333. Phone: (404) 639-1115. Fax: (404) 639-1118. URL: http://www.cdc.gov/vhf/ebola/hcp/interim-guidance-specimen-collection-submission-patients-suspected-infection-ebola.html.
2. U.S. Army Medical Research Institute of Infectious Diseases, Headquarters, Fort Detrick, 1425 Porter St., Frederick, MD 21702-5011. Phone: (301) 619-2833. Fax: (301) 610-4625.
3. Center for Applied Microbiology and Research, Novel and Dangerous Pathogens, Manor Farm Rd., Porton Down, Salisbury, Wiltshire SP4 0JG, United Kingdom. Phone: 0980-612224. Fax: 0980-611310.
4. National Institute for Communicable Diseases, Special Viral Pathogens Laboratory, 1 Modderfontein Rd., Private Bag X4, Sandringham, Johannesburg, South Africa. Phone: 27 (11) 386 6376 or 082 903 9131. Fax: 27 (11) 882 3741.
5. Bernhard-Nocht-Institute for Tropical Medicine, Department of Virology, Bernhard-Nocht-Str 74, 20359 Hamburg, Germany. Phone: 49 (40) 42818 421.
6. Special Pathogens Program, National Microbiology Laboratory, Public Health Agency of Canada, 1015 Arlington St., Winnipeg, Manitoba R3E 3R2, Canada. Phone: (204) 789-6019.
7. Unite de Biologie des Infections Virales Emergentes CNR des Fievres Hemorragiques Virales, Institute Pasteur, 21 avenue Tony Garnier, 69365 Lyon cedex 07, France. Phone: 33 043728244340.

Several BSL4 laboratories are available in Europe (http://www.enivd.de/index.htm), and in the United States, other BSL4 laboratories with diagnostic capability may be available in the near future.

DIRECT EXAMINATION

Electron Microscopy

Individual arenavirus virions are pleomorphic and range in size from 60 to 280 nm (mean, 110 to 130 nm) (Fig. 4, top). A unit membrane envelops the structure and is covered with club-shaped, 10-nm projections. No symmetry has been discerned. The most prominent and distinctive feature of these virions is the presence of different numbers of electron-dense particles (usually 2 to 10), which may be connected by fine filaments. These particles, 20 to 25 nm in diameter, are identical to host cell ribosomes by biochemical and oligonucleotide analysis (28). Immunoelectron microscopy techniques also work well for diagnosis of

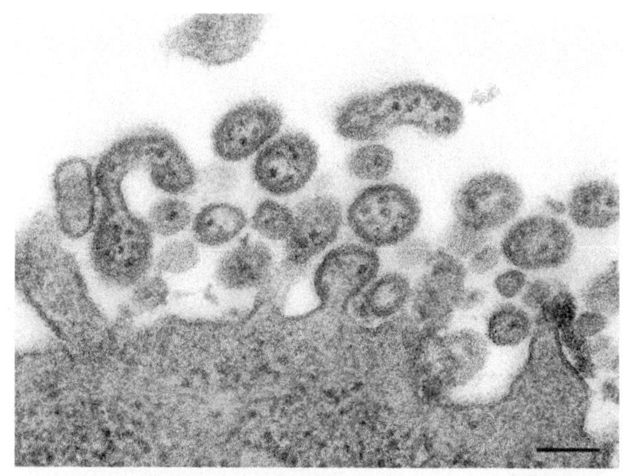

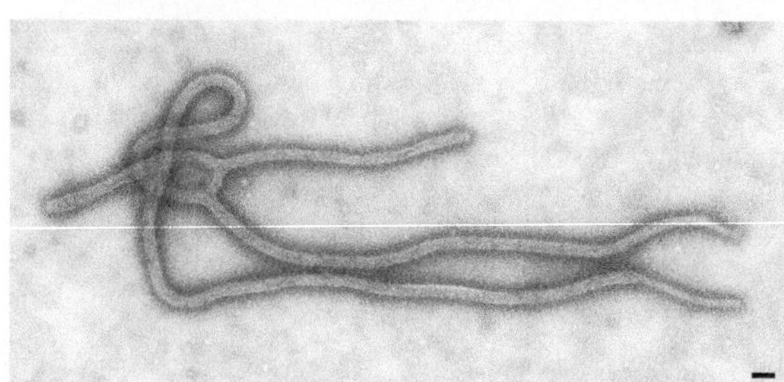

FIGURE 4 Ultrastructural characteristics of LCM virus and Ebola virus as seen in tissue culture cells. (Top) Lymphocytic choriomeningitis virus, an arenavirus, showing pleomorphic enveloped particles with internal ribosome-like granules; scale bar, 100 nm. (Courtesy of C. S. Goldsmith.) (Bottom) Ebola virus isolate, a filovirus, showing enveloped filamentous particles around 80 nm wide. Some filaments can occasionally measure up to 15,000 nm in length; scale bar, 100 nm. (Courtesy of C. S. Goldsmith.).

arenavirus infections, although the morphology of the virions is less striking for arenaviruses than filoviruses.

Marburgviruses and ebolaviruses have been successfully visualized directly by electron microscopy of both heparinized blood and urine obtained during the febrile period as well as in tissue culture supernatant fluids. The combination of the size and shape of the virions is sufficiently characteristic to allow a morphologic diagnosis of filovirus (28, 37, 82). The virus particles are very large, typically 790 to 970 nm long and consistently 80 nm in diameter. Bizarre structures of widely different lengths are frequently found in negatively stained preparations, sometimes exceeding 14,000 nm, as well as branching, circular, or "6" shapes, probably resulting from coenvelopment of multiple nucleocapsids during budding (Fig. 4, bottom) (28, 82, 83).

Ebolavirus inclusions are often seen in thin-section electron micrographs of liver. The inclusions consist of viral nucleocapsids mostly seen in longitudinal sections. Numerous viral particles are also seen in sinusoidal spaces (Fig. 2B). These virions can be differentiated and identified as marburgviruses or ebolaviruses by immunoelectron microscopy techniques (82, 83).

Antigen Detection

IFA staining of impression smears or air-dried suspensions of the liver, spleen, or kidney have been used successfully to detect cytoplasmic inclusion bodies associated with marburgvirus infection; clumps of marburgvirus antigen have also been observed by IFA examination of infected, dried, citrated blood smears. This approach was successfully adapted to the diagnosis of RESTV in impression smears from blood, tissues, and nasal turbinates, as it was to the detection of Junin virus-infected cells in peripheral blood and urinary sediment. Hematoxylin and eosin staining of the liver reveals hepatocellular necrosis, numerous intracytoplasmic, eosinophilic ebolavirus inclusions, as well as sinusoidal dilatation and congestion (Fig. 2A). Immunohistochemical techniques for detection of filovirus and arenavirus antigens in formalin-fixed tissues provide more satisfactory results than those of IFA examination of frozen, acetone-fixed sections (84–87). Obtaining frozen sections for diagnosis is rarely worth the biohazard incurred, especially since the threshold sensitivity for detection exceeds 6 $\log_{10}$ PFU/g. For filoviruses, paraffin blocks of tissues are sectioned. Sections are deparaffinized, hydrated, digested with protease, and stained for the presence of viral antigens with immune rabbit serum or cocktails of murine monoclonal antibodies (37, 86, 87). Biotinylated secondary antibody is then reacted, and the product is developed with a streptavidin-alkaline phosphatase system. Substitution of other chromogens can further increase sensitivity while reducing background (84). In the 2007–2008 epizootic of Reston virus in swine in the Philippines (45), ebolavirus antigens were detected in different tissues, including lymph nodes (Fig. 3A). Remarkable success was reported in the application of immunohistochemistry to the demonstration of Ebola virus antigens in formalin-fixed skin biopsy specimens obtained from deceased Ebola hemorrhagic fever patients in Zaire in 1995 (3, 87) (Fig. 3B). Immunohistochemistry was used to confirm the diagnosis of a fatal Lassa fever case in a New Jersey patient returning from West Africa (Fig. 1A). It was the immunohistochemistry assays on a liver biopsy (Fig. 1B) which first indicated the arenavirus etiology of a disease observed in South Africa, leading to the description of Lujo virus (36). In the cluster of LCM cases occurring through organ transplants (55, 56), very abundant LCM virus antigen could be found in a number of organs (Fig. 1C).

An antigen capture ELISA for quantitative detection of arenavirus and filovirus antigens in viremic sera and tissue culture supernatants can be used for early detection and identification of these agents (88–91). These tests reliably detect antigens in samples inactivated by heat-detergent treatment, β-propiolactone, or irradiation; therefore, they can be conducted safely without elaborate containment facilities. The threshold sensitivities for these assays are approximately 2.1 to 2.5 $\log_{10}$ PFU/ml, so they are sufficiently sensitive to detect antigen in most acute-phase VHF viremias and to detect viruses at the concentrations present in throat wash and urine samples. Further, antigen capture ELISAs are much more tolerant of genetic variation than RT-PCR-based detection methods and consequently are more likely to be successful at detecting new viruses (16, 33). Substitution of one or several monoclonal antibodies of high avidity and appropriate specificities for polyclonal sera (mostly against nucleoprotein and VP40) generally increases the sensitivities and specificities of these rapid antigen enzyme immunoassays (91–93). During the EVD outbreak in West Africa, multiple lateral flow assays were successfully developed for use with whole blood and plasma (94–97). Although FDA emergency use authorization (EUA) was granted, they reportedly suffered from lower sensitivity relative to RT-PCR-based methods and from false positives and negatives (98, 99).

Nucleic Acid Detection

For rapid acute case identification, RT-PCR followed by genome analysis has generally replaced antigen-antibody methods, primarily due to its ease of use, lower detection limits, and complete inactivation of the samples in the first extraction step (81, 100). However because RT-PCR-based methods are more prone to cross-contamination problems, we would still encourage its use in combination with traditional methods (virus isolation and/or serology) when possible. Real-time RT-PCR assays are common because of their automation potential, machine reporting capabilities, and ability to rapidly quantitate virus loads, features that are useful for measuring convalescence and potential effects of antiviral therapies (100, 101).

Arenaviridae

The considerable genetic variation among Lassa viruses requires caution in primer design if diagnosis of infections originating in more than one geographic area is being considered (102–106). To remediate this problem, primers targeting the 5′ region of the S RNA have been developed (107) and are used on a routine basis on a very large set of patients presenting at Irrua Specialist Teaching Hospital in Nigeria (108). In limited-resource settings, real-time PCR assays would reduce the reported low rate (13/1,650, 0.8% in Irrua) of PCR contamination but still lack field validation (100). Likewise, various strategies for RT-PCR have been devised to detect Junin virus RNA in clinical materials (20, 103, 104, 109). Some of these are reputed to be far more sensitive than conventional isolation procedures, especially in the presence of antibody. Any method which promises to be a reliable substitute for procedures that entail the manipulation of infectious BSL4 virus deserves attention. However, the ability to isolate and retain the virus has obvious advantages and should not be abandoned. Even in instances in which the etiological agent has been identified, the shipment of clinical material to an appropriate reference laboratory should be highly encouraged.

Filoviridae
Protocols which maximize detection are usually based on conserved sequences within the N, VP40, VP35, or L genes, while fine discrimination and phylogeny are based on the more variable GP region (2, 34, 110, 111). The sensitivity of RT-PCR for various ebolavirus species is similar to that of conventional isolation. During the SUDV outbreak in Gulu, Uganda, a nested RT-PCR-based assay was very valuable because of its ability to identify early patients prior to identification by any other available tests and for early convalescent specimens, which had already cleared detectable antigen. Using NP-based real-time quantitative RT-PCR, the viral load was found to correlate with disease outcome (40, 112). During the 2005 Marburg hemorrhagic fever outbreak in Angola and the 2012 outbreak in Uganda, Marburg virus real-time PCR assays were developed and effectively applied, respectively, in laboratories (Luanda and Entebbe) and in the field (Uige and Kabale) (43, 51, 113). Other platforms are available (111, 114, 115), and reverse-transcription loop-mediated isothermal amplification has been reported (116–118). During the West Africa Ebola outbreak, numerous nucleic acid amplification assays targeting NP, VP40, and GP genes were used in the field and in Europe and the United States (119–121). The U.S. FDA granted Ebola virus EUAs for over 10 nucleic acid amplification-based assays, including the BioFire and GeneXpert systems (Table 2) (119, 120, 122–125). However, the vast majority of clinical specimens in West Africa were tested using real-time RT-PCR, including the CDC lab in Bo, Sierra Leone, which tested over 27,000 samples during 15 months of operation (126).

ISOLATION PROCEDURES

Cell Culture

Most arenavirus and filovirus species grow well in cell culture. However, due to facility requirements (virus culture should not be attempted in BSL2 laboratories), cell culture is not recommended for routine clinical diagnostic use. Clinical specimens and clarified tissue homogenates are diluted in a suitable maintenance medium and adsorbed in small volumes to cell monolayers grown in suitable vessels, such as T-25 tissue culture flasks. If no antigen is detected by IFA by 14 days, the sample is considered negative, but supernatant fluids should be blind-passaged to confirm the absence of virus. To confirm the presence and identity of the virus, scraped cells are tested by immunofluorescence assay, and supernatant fluids are tested by antigen capture ELISA or RT-PCR techniques.

Arenaviridae
Cocultivation of Hypaque-Ficoll-separated peripheral blood leukocytes with susceptible cells has increased the isolation frequency of Junin virus. Cocultivation of lymphocytes from spleens of experimentally infected animals has yielded Lassa virus late in convalescence, even after neutralizing antibody has appeared. The technique merits systematic development for the remaining arenavirus and filovirus pathogens. Adequate cell culture systems such as Vero E6 exist for the isolation of LCM virus. LCM virus can grow to high titers in cell culture but cause little or no cytopathic effect.

Although historically, Machupo and Junin viruses were isolated by inoculation of newborn hamsters and mice, respectively, Vero E6 cells are approximately as sensitive and are far less cumbersome to manage in BSL4 containment. Furthermore, Vero cells usually permit isolation and identification within 1 to 5 days, a significant advantage over the use of animals, since 7 to 20 days of incubation are required for illness to develop in the animals (1).

Filoviridae
The best general method currently available for isolation of filoviruses is the inoculation of appropriate cell cultures (usually Vero cells) followed by IFA or other immunologically or nucleic acid-specific testing of the inoculated cells for the presence of viral antigens or genomic RNA at intervals. Other cell lines, including human diploid lung (MRC-5) and BHK-21 cells, also work; MA-104 cells (a fetal rhesus monkey kidney cell line) may be more sensitive than Vero cells for some strains (2).

Animal Inoculation

Arenaviridae
Intracranial inoculation of weanling mice is still regarded by some as the most sensitive established indicator of LCM virus (127). Care must be taken to use mice from a colony known to be free of LCM virus. Many LCM virus isolates produce a characteristic convulsive disease within 5 to 7 days, which is nearly pathognomonic. Brains from dead mice may be used to prepare ELISA antigens or may be subjected to IFA or IHC staining to obtain presumptive identification. Clarified mouse brain may also be used as the antigen for confirmatory testing by neutralization or RT-PCR.

Most LCM virus strains are also lethal for guinea pigs. The pathogenicity of virulent Lassa virus strains for outbred Swiss albino mice inoculated intracranially seems to vary with different sources; mice should not be seriously considered for Lassa virus isolations. Strain 13/N guinea pigs develop hemorrhagic disease after Lujo virus inoculation (128). For the New World arenaviruses, particularly Junin virus, young adult guinea pigs inoculated either intracranially or peripherally have been used. Guinea pigs die 7 to 18 days after Junin virus inoculation. Strain 13 guinea pigs are exquisitely sensitive to most Lassa virus strains and uniformly die 12 to 18 days after inoculation; outbred Hartley strain guinea pigs are somewhat less susceptible. Newborn mice (1 to 3 days old) are highly susceptible to Junin virus inoculated intracranially; newborn hamsters are believed to be more sensitive to Machupo virus.

Filoviridae
Marburgviruses and the EBOV and SUDV viruses produce febrile responses in guinea pigs 4 to 10 days after inoculation; however, none of these viruses kill guinea pigs consistently on primary inoculation, and only EBOV and Marburg virus have been adapted to uniform lethality by sequential guinea pig passages. EBOV is usually pathogenic for newborn mice inoculated intracranially, but SUDV, RESTV, and marburgviruses are not. Recently SCID mice were successfully used to isolate EBOV from clinical material, including semen, from the West Africa Ebola outbreak (129).

IDENTIFICATION OF VIRUS

Typing Antisera

Detection of viral antigens in infected tissue culture cells (usually Vero or MA-104) permits a presumptive diagnosis, provided that the serologic reagents have been tested against all the reference arenaviruses and filoviruses expected in a given laboratory, thus permitting an

TABLE 2 Nucleic acid amplification-based devices with EUA for detection of Ebola viruses[a]

Device name	Laboratory	Date EUA granted	Specimen types	Principle and method	Instrument	Targets	Applications
EZ1 real-time RT-PCR assay	U.S. Department of Defense	5 August 2014	Inactivated whole blood or plasma	Real-time PCR (TaqMan)	ABI 7500 FAST DX, JBAIDS or Roche LightCycler	Ebola Zaire virus	Individuals in affected areas with signs and symptoms of Ebola virus infection or who are at risk for exposure or may have been exposed to the Ebola Zaire virus in conjunction with epidemiological risk factors
Ebola virus NP/ VP40 real-time RT-PCR assay (119, 122)	Centers for Disease Control and Prevention	10 October 2014	Whole blood, serum, and plasma	Real-time RT-PCR, NP, or VP40 targets	ABI 7500 FAST DX, later on extended to BioRad CFX96 Touch real-time PCR	Ebola Zaire virus	Individuals in affected areas with signs and symptoms of Ebola virus infection and/or epidemiological risk factors
FilmArray Biothreat-E/ NGDS BT-E (120, 123, 124)	BioFire Defense	25 October 2014	Whole blood, urine	Nested PCR followed by solid microarray	FilmArray instrument	Ebola Zaire virus	Individuals with signs and symptoms of Ebola virus infection in conjunction with epidemiological risk factors
RealStar Ebolavirus RT-PCR kit 1.0 (125)	Altona Diagnostics	10 November 2014	EDTA plasma	Real-time PCR (TaqMan)	ABI 7500 SDS, ABI 7500 Fast SDS, LightCycler 480 II, or CFX96 system/ Dx real-time system	Ebolaviruses including the Zaire	Individuals with signs and symptoms of Ebola virus infection in conjunction with epidemiological risk factors
LightMix Ebola Zaire rRT-PCR test	Roche Molecular Systems, Inc.	23 December 2014	Whole blood	Real-time PCR (dual-hybridization)	LightCycler and Cobas z 480 analyzer	Ebola Zaire virus	Individuals with signs and symptoms of Ebola virus disease
Xpert Ebola assay (119, 122)	Cepheid	23 March 2015	EDTA venous whole blood	Real-time PCR (TaqMan)	GeneXpert instrument	Ebola Zaire virus	Individuals with signs and symptoms of Ebola virus infection in conjunction with epidemiological risk factors
Idylla Ebola virus triage test	Biocartis NV, Belgium	26 May 201	EDTA venous whole blood	Real-time PCR (TaqMan)	Idylla system	Ebola Zaire virus	Individuals with signs and symptoms of Ebola virus infection in conjunction with epidemiological risk factors

[a]Modified from https://www.fda.gov/MedicalDevices/Safety/EmergencySituations/ucm161496.htm.

interpretation of virus cross-reactions. Virus isolates in cell culture supernatant fluids or tissue homogenates are presumptively or specifically identified by their reactivity with diagnostic antisera in various serologic tests (see below). Specific polyclonal antisera are prepared in adult guinea pigs, hamsters, rabbits, rats, or mice inoculated intraperitoneally with infectious virus. Rhesus and cynomolgus monkeys that are convalescent from experimental infections are also reasonable sources for larger quantities of immune sera. Polyvalent polyclonal "typing" sera or ascitic fluids made by immunization with a number of viruses within the families have also been useful in early identification of virus isolates and in immunohistochemistry on unknown patient materials. Diagnostic antisera produced by single injection of infectious virus are less cross-reactive and usually have higher titers than those produced by multiple injections of inactivated antigens. To further reduce the induction of extraneous antibodies, input virus should be derived from tissues or cells homologous to the species being immunized; likewise, the virus suspension should be stabilized with homologous serum or serum proteins. Sera produced for use in the IFA tests and ELISA should be collected 30 to 60 days after inoculation; sera for neutralization tests should be collected later. All sera must be inactivated and rigorously tested for the presence of live virus before being removed from a BSL4 environment.

Specific murine monoclonal antibodies with high specificities for N and GP epitopes of LCM virus, Lassa virus, Junin virus (130, 131), and other arenaviruses are frequently used, as well as monoclonal antibodies against the different proteins of the filoviruses. Reference reagents for all of these viruses are not generally available outside of the appropriately equipped specialized laboratories.

Immunofluorescence

To process infected cells for IFA examination and presumptive identification, inoculated cell monolayers are dispersed by using glass beads or a rubber policeman or trypsinization, washed, and placed onto circular areas of specially prepared Teflon-coated slides. These "spot slides" are air dried, fixed in acetone at room temperature for 10 min, and either stained quickly or stored frozen at −70°C. Although acetone fixation greatly reduces the number of infectious intracellular viruses, spot slides prepared in this manner should still be considered infectious and handled accordingly. Gamma irradiation has been used to render spot slides noninfectious (31), with no diminution in fluorescent-antigen intensity. Alternatively, infected cells may be biologically inactivated with β-propiolactone (30). Gamma irradiation is recommended if the appropriate equipment is available.

For direct FA tests, specific immune globulins conjugated to fluorescein are used with Evans blue counterstain. Specific viral fluorescence is characterized by intense, punctate to granular aggregates confined to the cytoplasm of infected cells. Specific marburgvirus and ebolavirus fluorescence may include large, bizarrely shaped aggregates up to 10 μm across. Nonspecific fluorescence is rarely a problem in IFA procedures for these viruses. Detection of marburgviruses, ebolaviruses, Lassa virus, and LCM virus antigens by the IFA test is usually considered sufficient for a definitive diagnosis, although Lassa and LCM viruses cross-react at low levels in this test (132). Detection of Junin or Machupo virus antigens by the IFA test constitutes a presumptive diagnosis, since these viruses can be reliably distinguished from each other only by neutralization tests or sequencing. IFA formats for viral detection are more cumbersome and cross-reactive but can be used if direct conjugates are unavailable. Immunohistochemical techniques for detecting arenaviruses (84) and filoviruses (85, 86) with a variety of chromogens can also be applied. A multiplex nucleic acid suspension bead array was reported for detection and subtyping of filoviruses (133).

SEROLOGIC DIAGNOSIS

IFA Test

Until the early 1990s, the IFA test was widely regarded as the most practical single method for documenting recent infections with filoviruses or for large prevalence studies (134). Preparation of spot slides with infected Vero cells is identical to the procedure described above. Some refinements to enhance reproducibility and quality between spot slide lots have been suggested (135). Although monovalent spot slides are usually desired and are prepared with cells optimally infected with a single virus, polyvalent spot slides can also be prepared by mixing cells infected with different viruses selected from these or other taxonomic groups which have similar geographic distributions (136). The requirement for a BSL4 facility to produce the spot slides could be avoided by using recombinant antigen-expressing cells (137). Discrepancies in titers determined by different laboratories, or even different investigators, are common. In addition, in most of the severe and fatal forms of these diseases, the patients may not develop a humoral response and may die without detectable antibodies. This technique is not recommended for acute diagnosis of hemorrhagic fevers.

ELISA for Detection of IgG and IgM Antibodies

For all intents and purposes, the IgG and IgM ELISAs have replaced the more subjective IFA tests and remain the serologic tests of choice (90, 132). ELISA procedures for Lassa virus-specific IgG and IgM have been developed and successfully used on field-collected human sera (88, 92). When this ELISA is used in combination with the Lassa antigen capture ELISA described above, virtually all Lassa fever patients can be specifically diagnosed within hours of hospital admission. A simplification of this procedure, which entails the use of infected Vero cell detergent lysate as the antigen, diluted in phosphate-buffered saline and adsorbed directly to the microtiter plate wells, has been developed for ebolaviruses (89, 90, 138) and adapted to marburgviruses and LCM virus. Test sera are serially diluted, with a 1:100 initial dilution, and incubated with antigen in a format analogous to the antigen capture ELISA described above. Following incubation, washing, and addition of horseradish peroxidase-conjugated anti-human antibodies, 2,2′-azinobis(3-ethylbenzthiazolinesulfonic acid) (ABTS) substrate is added for color development. Species-specific conjugates allow testing of other animal species during epidemiological studies. To avoid the use of several conjugates during epidemiological studies, protein A-protein G conjugate can be used. Samples are considered positive if the optical density at 410 nm exceeds the mean plus 3 standard deviations for the normal-serum controls. This procedure can be further modified to detect virus-specific IgM by coating the plates with anti-human IgM followed by test serum dilutions and cell slurry antigens and then using the antigen capture protocol. These IgG and IgM ELISA procedures have worked well with specimens obtained from humans during natural infection and from animals experimentally infected with Lassa, Machupo, Junin, and filoviruses. Several assays based on recombinant proteins were developed during the EVD outbreak in West Africa but suffered from nonspecific reactivity. A simplification of the ELISA plate procedure, substituting filter paper disks, has been reported for RESTV (139); it appears to sacrifice some sensitivity and precision in comparison with the more established procedures but may find application in a field setting. All of these developmental assays are sufficiently robust to warrant field testing. Recombinant full or truncated proteins have also been proposed and used as antigen for ELISAs (140–142).

Neutralization Tests

For the arenaviruses, plaque reduction tests with Vero cells are generally used. For measuring the levels of neutralizing antibody to Lassa and LCM viruses, which are both difficult to neutralize and are poor inducers of this antibody, test sera are diluted, usually 1:10, in medium containing 10% guinea pig serum as a complement source, and mixed with serial dilutions of challenge virus. Titers are expressed as a $\log_{10}$ neutralization index, defined as $\log_{10}$ PFU in control minus $\log_{10}$ PFU in test serum. For Junin and Machupo viruses, the more conventional serum dilution-constant virus format is normally used, although the constant serum-virus dilution format is equally useful for distinguishing among virus strains. Neutralizing-antibody responses require weeks to months to evolve but persist for years. Performance of these tests is restricted to laboratories equipped to handle the infectious viruses.

In survivors, neutralizing antibodies to Lassa virus first appear very late in convalescence (6 weeks or later), long after the viremia has disappeared. This pattern of early IFA and delayed neutralizing-antibody response is similar for LCM virus infections. Neutralizing antibodies against Junin and Machupo viruses become detectable 3 to 4 weeks after onset, soon after the termination of viremia. While these antibodies are thought to be important in protection against reinfection, their role in resolution of acute infections is less firmly established (68, 143).

As described above, reliable tests for measuring the levels of neutralizing antibody to filoviruses are not currently available.

Western Blotting

Western blotting is feasible for demonstrating antibodies to arenaviruses and filoviruses. However, it has never been applied systematically or routinely to diagnosis, although it was proposed as a confirmatory test to supplement the IFA test for filovirus antibodies (135). Detection of the nucleocapsid (N) band plus either VP30 or VP24 was taken as diagnostic. The Western blotting procedure was further refined by miniaturization, using the Phast system sodium dodecyl sulfate-polyacrylamide gel electrophoresis and transblot apparatus (Phast Western blot system). This test has not been routinely used for antibody detection.

Other Serologic Tests

Other serologic tests have been applied to diagnosis but have largely been abandoned: the gel diffusion precipitation test for arenaviruses, the CF test, the reverse passive-hemagglutination (and inhibition) test utilizing Lassa virus antibody-coated erythrocytes, a radioimmunoassay, using ^{125}I-labeled staphylococcal protein A for Ebola. Western blotting and radioimmunoassay procedures are used in specialized laboratories to determine the fine specificities of monoclonal antibodies and occasionally to confirm the results of individual sera found positive by the ELISA test (142).

ANTIVIRAL SUSCEPTIBILITIES

Current antiarenavirus therapy is limited to an off-label use of ribavirin, and no viral resistance mutants to ribavirin have been reported. LCM virus variants with increased resistance to KP-146 did not emerge after serial passages in the presence of KP-146 (67). No antiviral drugs are yet commercially available against filovirus, and no viral mutants in relation to increased drug resistance have been reported in the clinical trials (69–71).

EVALUATION AND INTERPRETATION OF RESULTS

Early diagnosis of arenavirus and filovirus infections is desirable since specific immune plasma and appropriately selected antiviral drugs are, in certain cases, effective when treatment is initiated soon after onset. Early recognition of these infections should also trigger strict isolation procedures to prevent the spread of disease to patient contacts. In areas where specific viruses are endemic, the index of suspicion is often high, and experienced clinicians may be remarkably accurate in rendering an accurate diagnosis of fully developed cases on clinical grounds alone. However, even in these areas, specific virologic and serologic tests are required to confirm clinical impressions, since many other diseases, including malaria, typhoid, rickettsial infections, idiopathic thrombocytopenia, and viral hepatitis, may masquerade as an arenavirus or filovirus infection. In other countries, where evacuated suspected (or confirmed) patients or recent travelers showing symptoms are evaluated, a rapid confirmation is needed, and RT-PCR or real-time PCR-based tests are preferred (106, 107, 119–121).

Since patients with most of the severe and fatal forms of these diseases can die without developing detectable levels of antibody, timely diagnosis requires a means of detecting RNA, infectious virus, or antigen in the field. The RT-PCR-based assays targeting viral RNA are without question the most sensitive assays and are widely used for the reasons previously discussed (100). The rapid antigen lateral flow assays used at the point of care hold promise for use in detecting clinically relevant concentrations of virus in plasma, sera, body fluids, and tissues (37, 88–90, 94–96, 144). However, the sensitivity of these assays needs improvement to avoid false negatives.

RT-PCR assays lessen the need to isolate infectious virus to establish a definitive diagnosis, but virus isolation remains important for subsequent genetic and pathogenesis studies. The ability to amplify viral genomes from infected tissues, and even from formalin-fixed tissues, and to sequence the reaction products has eclipsed serologic methods of identification and classification of arenaviruses (103–105) and filoviruses (33, 40). With the exception of LCM virus, which may be handled at a lower containment level, isolation attempts of these viruses should not be done outside a BSL4 laboratory (78). A combination of several laboratory techniques should be used to confirm any clinical suspicion of hemorrhagic fevers.

Among arenavirus infections, Lassa virus is usually able to be detected (virus isolation, antigen detection, RT-PCR) from acute-phase sera of hospitalized patients soon after admission, frequently in the presence of specific IgM antibody, and a detectable antibody response does not necessarily signal imminent recovery; viremia frequently persists, and some patients die despite an antibody response. Junin, Machupo, and LCM viruses are recovered less frequently, and diagnosis is usually based on the detection of specific antibodies later in the course of the disease. The presence of specific IgM ELISA-detectable antibodies in the cerebrospinal fluid of LCM patients constitutes a definitive diagnosis, and for all arenavirus infections, the presence of specific IgM antibodies is indicative of recent infection. The extent to which heterologous arenavirus infection and/or reinfection broadens antibody specificity has not been systematically evaluated for any of the available serologic tests. Neutralizing antibodies against arenaviruses persist for long periods, perhaps for life, and thus provide the most reliable basis for determining the minimum resistance of a population to reinfection. The role of neutralizing antibody in acute recovery is less clear. The protective efficacy of passively administered immune plasma is believed to be a direct function of neutralizing-antibody titers, and plasma should be selected on this basis, especially for Junin and Lassa fever (68, 143).

For filoviruses, the combination of RT-PCR, antigen detection, and IgM are the more valuable techniques for acute case diagnosis. The FDA issued over 10 EUAs to authorize the emergency use of both nucleic acid amplification and rapid antigen assays (94–96, 119, 120, 122–125). Because of the time required for culture and the biohazard, virus isolation data for these viruses are usually available only retrospectively. Marburgviruses and ebolaviruses are usually easily isolated from acute-phase serum samples. A rising IgM or IgG ELISA titer constitutes a strong presumptive diagnosis. Since IgM titers do not persist for long, a decreasing titer suggests a recent infection which occurred perhaps only within the several months. In general, IgG and IgM antibodies show a stronger reactivity to homologous ebolavirus antigens. Because of the low sensitivity of the IgM ELISA to heterologous antigen, there are some limitations in using the IgM ELISA prior to identification of the virus species. In contrast, IgG antibodies are relatively cross-reactive to heterologous antigens (145).

The highest priority for future development is refinement of the available diagnostic tools to permit definitive diagnosis and virus identification in the field, at the bedside, or in the frontline clinic. PCR-based assays enable field laboratories to diagnose acute disease almost in real time. Proper tailoring of primers should permit the design of tests with the proper degree of specificity. However, the emergence of new arenaviruses, as well as BDBV, in the past decade, serves as a reminder that broadly reactive, grouping reagents are still required to augment the newly evolving tools of conventional and real-time PCR and capture ELISAs based on extremely specific monoclonal antibodies and gene sequences.

An investment in rapid diagnosis should result in more timely intervention with effective implementation of appropriate public health measures and use of evolving treatment regimens. The implementation of appropriate infection control measures has been demonstrated to greatly reduce the transmission and dissemination of these highly virulent viral pathogens.

ACKNOWLEDGMENTS

We thank Bobbie Rae Erickson and Deborah Cannon of the Diagnostics Team within the Viral Special Pathogens Branch for many helpful discussions. The findings and conclusions in this chapter are those of the authors and do not represent the official position of their funding agencies.

REFERENCES

1. **Buchmeier MJ, de la Torre JC, Peters CJ.** 2013. Arenaviridae, p 1283–1303. *In* Knipe DM, Howley PM (ed), *Fields Virology*, 6th ed. Lippincott Williams & Wilkins, Philadelphia, PA.
2. **Feldmann H, Sanchez A, Geisbert TW.** 2013. Filoviridae: Marburg and Ebola viruses, p 923–956. *In* Knipe DM, Howley PM (ed), *Fields Virology*, 6th ed. Lippincott Williams & Wilkins, Philadelphia, PA.
3. **Peters CJ.** 2006. Emerging infections: lessons from the viral hemorrhagic fevers. *Trans Am Clin Climatol Assoc* **117:** 189–196; discussion 196-187.
4. **Palacios G, Savji N, Hui J, Travassos da Rosa A, Popov V, Briese T, Tesh R, Lipkin WI.** 2010. Genomic and phylogenetic characterization of Merino Walk virus, a novel arenavirus isolated in South Africa. *J Gen Virol* **91:**1315–1324.
5. **Coulibaly-N'Golo D, Allali B, Kouassi SK, Fichet-Calvet E, Becker-Ziaja B, Rieger T, Olschläger S, Dosso H, Denys C, Ter Meulen J, Akoua-Koffi C, Günther S.** 2011. Novel arenavirus sequences in *Hylomyscus* sp. and *Mus* (*Nannomys*) *setulosus* from Côte d'Ivoire: implications for evolution of arenaviruses in Africa. *PLoS One* **6:**e20893.
6. **Lecompte E, ter Meulen J, Emonet S, Daffis S, Charrel RN.** 2007. Genetic identification of Kodoko virus, a novel arenavirus of the African pigmy mouse (*Mus Nannomys minutoides*) in West Africa. *Virology* **364:**178–183.
7. **Günther S, Hoofd G, Charrel R, Röser C, Becker-Ziaja B, Lloyd G, Sabuni C, Verhagen R, van der Groen G, Kennis J, Katakweba A, Machang'u R, Makundi R, Leirs H.** 2009. Mopeia virus-related arenavirus in natal multimammate mice, Morogoro, Tanzania. *Emerg Infect Dis* **15:** 2008–2012.
8. **de Bellocq JG, Borremans B, Katakweba A, Makundi R, Baird SJ, Becker-Ziaja B, Günther S, Leirs H.** 2010. Sympatric occurrence of 3 arenaviruses, Tanzania. *Emerg Infect Dis* **16:**692–695.
9. **Ishii A, Thomas Y, Moonga L, Nakamura I, Ohnuma A, Hang'ombe B, Takada A, Mweene A, Sawa H.** 2011. Novel arenavirus, Zambia. *Emerg Infect Dis* **17:**1921–1924.
10. **Briese T, Paweska JT, McMullan LK, Hutchison SK, Street C, Palacios G, Khristova ML, Weyer J, Swanepoel R, Egholm M, Nichol ST, Lipkin WI.** 2009. Genetic detection and characterization of Lujo virus, a new hemorrhagic fever-associated arenavirus from southern Africa. *PLoS Pathog* **5:**e1000455.
11. **Gryseels S, Rieger T, Oestereich L, Cuypers B, Borremans B, Makundi R, Leirs H, Günther S, Goüy de Bellocq J.** 2015. Gairo virus, a novel arenavirus of the widespread *Mastomys natalensis*: genetically divergent, but ecologically similar to Lassa and Morogoro viruses. *Virology* **476:**249–256.
12. **Witkowski PT, Kallies R, Hoveka J, Auste B, Ithete NL, Šoltys K, Szemes T, Drosten C, Preiser W, Klempa B, Mfune JK, Kruger DH.** 2015. Novel arenavirus isolates from Namaqua rock mice, Namibia, southern Africa. *Emerg Infect Dis* **21:**1213–1216.
13. **Li K, Lin XD, Wang W, Shi M, Guo WP, Zhang XH, Xing JG, He JR, Wang K, Li MH, Cao JH, Jiang ML, Holmes EC, Zhang YZ.** 2015. Isolation and characterization of a novel arenavirus harbored by rodents and shrews in Zhejiang province, China. *Virology* **476:**37–42.
14. **Blasdell KR, Becker SD, Hurst J, Begon M, Bennett M.** 2008. Host range and genetic diversity of arenaviruses in rodents, United Kingdom. *Emerg Infect Dis* **14:**1455–1458.
15. **Fulhorst CF, Bennett SG, Milazzo ML, Murray HL Jr, Webb JP Jr, Cajimat MN, Bradley RD.** 2002. Bear Canyon virus: an arenavirus naturally associated with the California mouse (*Peromyscus californicus*). *Emerg Infect Dis* **8:** 717–721.
16. **Cajimat MN, Milazzo ML, Bradley RD, Fulhorst CF.** 2012. Ocozocoautla de Espinosa virus and hemorrhagic fever, Mexico. *Emerg Infect Dis* **18:**401–405.
17. **Moncayo AC, Hice CL, Watts DM, Travassos de Rosa AP, Guzman H, Russell KL, Calampa C, Gozalo A, Popov VL, Weaver SC, Tesh RB.** 2001. Allpahuayo virus: a newly recognized arenavirus (Arenaviridae) from arboreal rice rats (*Oecomys bicolor* and *Oecomys paricola*) in northeastern Peru. *Virology* **284:**277–286.
18. **Milazzo ML, Amman BR, Cajimat MN, Méndez-Harclerode FM, Suchecki JR, Hanson JD, Haynie ML, Baxter BD, Milazzo C Jr, Carroll SA, Carroll DS, Ruthven DC III, Bradley RD, Fulhorst CF.** 2013. Ecology of Catarina virus (family Arenaviridae) in southern Texas, 2001-2004. *Vector Borne Zoonotic Dis* **13:**50–59.

19. **Inizan CC, Cajimat MN, Milazzo ML, Barragán-Gomez A, Bradley RD, Fulhorst CF.** 2010. Genetic evidence for a Tacaribe serocomplex virus, Mexico. *Emerg Infect Dis* **16:**1007–1010.
20. **Lozano ME, Posik DM, Albariño CG, Schujman G, Ghiringhelli PD, Calderón G, Sabattini M, Romanowski V.** 1997. Characterization of arenaviruses using a family-specific primer set for RT-PCR amplification and RFLP analysis. Its potential use for detection of uncharacterized arenaviruses. *Virus Res* **49:**79–89.
21. **Delgado S, Erickson BR, Agudo R, Blair PJ, Vallejo E, Albariño CG, Vargas J, Comer JA, Rollin PE, Ksiazek TG, Olson JG, Nichol ST.** 2008. Chapare virus, a newly discovered arenavirus isolated from a fatal hemorrhagic fever case in Bolivia. *PLoS Pathog* **4:**e1000047.
22. **Cajimat MN, Milazzo ML, Mauldin MR, Bradley RD, Fulhorst CF.** 2013. Diversity among Tacaribe serocomplex viruses (family Arenaviridae) associated with the southern plains woodrat (*Neotoma micropus*). *Virus Res* **178:**486–494.
23. **Lavergne A, de Thoisy B, Donato D, Guidez A, Matheus S, Catzeflis F, Lacoste V.** 2015. Patawa virus, a new arenavirus hosted by forest rodents in French Guiana. *EcoHealth* **12:**339–346.
24. **Bisordi I, Levis S, Maeda AY, Suzuki A, Nagasse-Sugahara TK, de Souza RP, Pereira LE, Garcia JB, Cerroni MP, de A e Silva F, dos Santos CL, da Fonseca BA.** 2015. Pinhal virus, a new arenavirus isolated from *Calomys tener* in Brazil. *Vector Borne Zoonotic Dis* **15:**694–700.
25. **Bodewes R, Kik MJ, Raj VS, Schapendonk CM, Haagmans BL, Smits SL, Osterhaus AD.** 2013. Detection of novel divergent arenaviruses in boid snakes with inclusion body disease in The Netherlands. *J Gen Virol* **94:**1206–1210.
26. **Stenglein MD, Sanders C, Kistler AL, Ruby JG, Franco JY, Reavill DR, Dunker F, Derisi JL.** 2012. Identification, characterization, and *in vitro* culture of highly divergent arenaviruses from boa constrictors and annulated tree boas: candidate etiological agents for snake inclusion body disease. *MBio* **3:**e00180-12.
27. **Buchmeier MJ, Parekh BS.** 1987. Protein structure and expression among arenaviruses. *Curr Top Microbiol Immunol* **133:**41–57.
28. **Murphy FA, Whitfield SG.** 1975. Morphology and morphogenesis of arenaviruses. *Bull World Health Organ* **52:**409–419.
29. **Burri DJ, Pasquato A, da Palma JR, Igonet S, Oldstone MB, Kunz S.** 2013. The role of proteolytic processing and the stable signal peptide in expression of the Old World arenavirus envelope glycoprotein ectodomain. *Virology* **436:**127–133.
30. **Van der Groen G, Elliot LH.** 1982. Use of betapropionolactone inactivated Ebola, Marburg and Lassa intracellular antigens in immunofluorescent antibody assay. *Ann Soc Belg Med Trop* **62:**49–54.
31. **Elliott LH, McCormick JB, Johnson KM.** 1982. Inactivation of Lassa, Marburg, and Ebola viruses by gamma irradiation. *J Clin Microbiol* **16:**704–708.
32. **Kiley MP, Cox NJ, Elliott LH, Sanchez A, DeFries R, Buchmeier MJ, Richman DD, McCormick JB.** 1988. Physicochemical properties of Marburg virus: evidence for three distinct virus strains and their relationship to Ebola virus. *J Gen Virol* **69:**1957–1967.
33. **Towner JS, Sealy TK, Khristova ML, Albariño CG, Conlan S, Reeder SA, Quan PL, Lipkin WI, Downing R, Tappero JW, Okware S, Lutwama J, Bakamutumaho B, Kayiwa J, Comer JA, Rollin PE, Ksiazek TG, Nichol ST.** 2008. Newly discovered Ebola virus associated with hemorrhagic fever outbreak in Uganda. *PLoS Pathog* **4:**e1000212.
34. **Sanchez A, Trappier SG, Ströher U, Nichol ST, Bowen MD, Feldmann H.** 1998. Variation in the glycoprotein and VP35 genes of Marburg virus strains. *Virology* **240:**138–146.
35. **Negredo A, Palacios G, Vázquez-Morón S, González F, Dopazo H, Molero F, Juste J, Quetglas J, Savji N, de la Cruz Martínez M, Herrera JE, Pizarro M, Hutchison SK, Echevarría JE, Lipkin WI, Tenorio A.** 2011. Discovery of an Ebolavirus-like filovirus in Europe. *PLoS Pathog* **7:** e1002304.
36. **Paweska JT, Sewlall NH, Ksiazek TG, Blumberg LH, Hale MJ, Lipkin WI, Weyer J, Nichol ST, Rollin PE, McMullan LK, Paddock CD, Briese T, Mnyaluza J, Dinh TH, Mukonka V, Ching P, Duse A, Richards G, de Jong G, Cohen C, Ikalafeng B, Mugero C, Asomugha C, Malotle MM, Nteo DM, Misiani E, Swanepoel R, Zaki SR, Outbreak Control and Investigation Teams.** 2009. Nosocomial outbreak of novel arenavirus infection, southern Africa. *Emerg Infect Dis* **15:**1598–1602.
37. **Jahrling PB, Geisbert TW, Johnson ED, Peters CJ, Dalgard DW, Hall WC.** 1990. Preliminary report: isolation of Ebola virus from monkeys imported to USA. *Lancet* **335:**502–505.
38. **Le Guenno B, Formenty P, Wyers M, Gounon P, Walker F, Boesch C.** 1995. Isolation and partial characterisation of a new strain of Ebola virus. *Lancet* **345:**1271–1274.
39. **Georges-Courbot MC, Sanchez A, Lu CY, Baize S, Leroy E, Lansout-Soukate J, Tévi-Bénissan C, Georges AJ, Trappier SG, Zaki SR, Swanepoel R, Leman PA, Rollin PE, Peters CJ, Nichol ST, Ksiazek TG.** 1997. Isolation and phylogenetic characterization of Ebola viruses causing different outbreaks in Gabon. *Emerg Infect Dis* **3:**59–62.
40. **Towner JS, Rollin PE, Bausch DG, Sanchez A, Crary SM, Vincent M, Lee WF, Spiropoulou CF, Ksiazek TG, Lukwiya M, Kaducu F, Downing R, Nichol ST.** 2004. Rapid diagnosis of Ebola hemorrhagic fever by reverse transcription-PCR in an outbreak setting and assessment of patient viral load as a predictor of outcome. *J Virol* **78:**4330–4341.
41. **Onyango CO, Opoka ML, Ksiazek TG, Formenty P, Ahmed A, Tukei PM, Sang RC, Ofula VO, Konongoi SL, Coldren RL, Grein T, Legros D, Bell M, De Cock KM, Bellini WJ, Towner JS, Nichol ST, Rollin PE.** 2007. Laboratory diagnosis of Ebola hemorrhagic fever during an outbreak in Yambio, Sudan, 2004. *J Infect Dis* **196**(Suppl 2):S193–S198 .
42. **Swanepoel R, Smit SB, Rollin PE, Formenty P, Leman PA, Kemp A, Burt FJ, Grobbelaar AA, Croft J, Bausch DG, Zeller H, Leirs H, Braack LE, Libande ML, Zaki S, Nichol ST, Ksiazek TG, Paweska JT, International Scientific and Technical Committee for Marburg Hemorrhagic Fever Control in the Democratic Republic of Congo.** 2007. Studies of reservoir hosts for Marburg virus. *Emerg Infect Dis* **13:**1847–1851.
43. **Towner JS, Khristova ML, Sealy TK, Vincent MJ, Erickson BR, Bawiec DA, Hartman AL, Comer JA, Zaki SR, Ströher U, Gomes da Silva F, del Castillo F, Rollin PE, Ksiazek TG, Nichol ST.** 2006. Marburgvirus genomics and association with a large hemorrhagic fever outbreak in Angola. *J Virol* **80:**6497–6516.
44. **Leroy EM, Kumulungui B, Pourrut X, Rouquet P, Hassanin A, Yaba P, Délicat A, Paweska JT, Gonzalez JP, Swanepoel R.** 2005. Fruit bats as reservoirs of Ebola virus. *Nature* **438:**575–576.
45. **Barrette RW, Metwally SA, Rowland JM, Xu L, Zaki SR, Nichol ST, Rollin PE, Towner JS, Shieh WJ, Batten B, Sealy TK, Carrillo C, Moran KE, Bracht AJ, Mayr GA, Sirios-Cruz M, Catbagan DP, Lautner EA, Ksiazek TG, White WR, McIntosh MT.** 2009. Discovery of swine as a host for the Reston Ebolavirus. *Science* **325:**204–206.
46. **Pan Y, Zhang W, Cui L, Hua X, Wang M, Zeng Q.** 2014. Reston virus in domestic pigs in China. *Arch Virol* **159:**1129–1132.
47. **Amman BR, Carroll SA, Reed ZD, Sealy TK, Balinandi S, Swanepoel R, Kemp A, Erickson BR, Comer JA, Campbell S, Cannon DL, Khristova ML, Atimnedi P, Paddock CD, Kent Crockett RJ, Flietstra TD, Warfield KL, Unfer R, Katongole-Mbidde E, Downing R, Tappero JW, Zaki SR, Rollin PE, Ksiazek TG, Nichol ST, Towner JS.** 2012. Seasonal pulses of Marburg virus circulation in juvenile Rousettus aegyptiacus bats coincide with periods of increased risk of human infection. *PLoS Pathog* **8:**e1002877.
48. **Towner JS, Amman BR, Sealy TK, Carroll SA, Comer JA, Kemp A, Swanepoel R, Paddock CD, Balinandi S, Khristova ML, Formenty PB, Albarino CG, Miller DM, Reed ZD, Kayiwa JT, Mills JN, Cannon DL, Greer PW, Byaruhanga E, Farnon EC, Atimnedi P, Okware S, Katongole-Mbidde E, Downing R, Tappero JW, Zaki SR, Ksiazek TG, Nichol ST, Rollin PE.** 2009. Isolation of genetically diverse Marburg viruses from Egyptian fruit bats. *PLoS Pathog* **5:**e1000536.

49. **Timen A, Koopmans MP, Vossen AC, van Doornum GJ, Günther S, van den Berkmortel F, Verduin KM, Dittrich S, Emmerich P, Osterhaus AD, van Dissel JT, Coutinho RA.** 2009. Response to imported case of Marburg hemorrhagic fever, the Netherlands. *Emerg Infect Dis* **15:** 1171–1175.
50. **Shoemaker T, MacNeil A, Balinandi S, Campbell S, Wamala JF, McMullan LK, Downing R, Lutwama J, Mbidde E, Ströher U, Rollin PE, Nichol ST.** 2012. Reemerging Sudan Ebola virus disease in Uganda, 2011. *Emerg Infect Dis* **18:**1480–1483.
51. **Albariño CG, Shoemaker T, Khristova ML, Wamala JF, Muyembe JJ, Balinandi S, Tumusiime A, Campbell S, Cannon D, Gibbons A, Bergeron E, Bird B, Dodd K, Spiropoulou C, Erickson BR, Guerrero L, Knust B, Nichol ST, Rollin PE, Ströher U.** 2013. Genomic analysis of filoviruses associated with four viral hemorrhagic fever outbreaks in Uganda and the Democratic Republic of the Congo in 2012. *Virology* **442:**97–100.
52. **Carroll MW, et al.** 2015. Temporal and spatial analysis of the 2014-2015 Ebola virus outbreak in West Africa. *Nature* **524:**97–101.
53. **Lehmann-Grube F.** 1972. Persistent infection of the mouse with the virus of lymphocytic choriomeningitis. *J Clin Pathol Suppl (R Coll Pathol)* **6:**8–21.
54. **Mets MB, Barton LL, Khan AS, Ksiazek TG.** 2000. Lymphocytic choriomeningitis virus: an underdiagnosed cause of congenital chorioretinitis. *Am J Ophthalmol* **130:** 209–215.
55. **Centers for Disease Control and Prevention (CDC).** 2008. Brief report: lymphocytic choriomeningitis virus transmitted through solid organ transplantation—Massachusetts, 2008. *MMWR Morb Mortal Wkly Rep* **57:**799–801.
56. **Fischer SA, Graham MB, Kuehnert MJ, Kotton CN, Srinivasan A, Marty FM, Comer JA, Guarner J, Paddock CD, DeMeo DL, Shieh WJ, Erickson BR, Bandy U, DeMaria A Jr, Davis JP, Delmonico FL, Pavlin B, Likos A, Vincent MJ, Sealy TK, Goldsmith CS, Jernigan DB, Rollin PE, Packard MM, Patel M, Rowland C, Helfand RF, Nichol ST, Fishman JA, Ksiazek T, Zaki SR, LCMV in Transplant Recipients Investigation Team.** 2006. Transmission of lymphocytic choriomeningitis virus by organ transplantation. *N Engl J Med* **354:**2235–2249.
57. **MacNeil A, Ströher U, Farnon E, Campbell S, Cannon D, Paddock CD, Drew CP, Kuehnert M, Knust B, Gruenenfelder R, Zaki SR, Rollin PE, Nichol ST, LCMV Transplant Investigation Team.** 2012. Solid organ transplant-associated lymphocytic choriomeningitis, United States, 2011. *Emerg Infect Dis* **18:**1256–1262.
58. **Marshall Lyon G, Mehta AK, Ribner BS.** 2017. Clinical management of patients with Ebola virus disease in high-resource settings. *Curr Top Microbiol Immunol* **411:** 115–137.
59. **Muñoz-Fontela C, McElroy AK.** 2017. Ebola virus disease in humans: pathophysiology and immunity. *Curr Top Microbiol Immunol* **411:**141–169.
60. **Sprecher A, Van Herp M, Rollin PE.** 2017. Clinical management of Ebola virus disease patients in low-resource settings. *Curr Top Microbiol Immunol* **411:**93–113.
61. **Rollin PE, Bausch DG, Sanchez A.** 2007. Blood chemistry measurements and D-dimer levels associated with fatal and nonfatal outcomes in humans infected with Sudan Ebola virus. *J Infect Dis* **196**(Suppl 2): S364–S371.
62. **Lyon GM, Mehta AK, Varkey JB, Brantly K, Plyler L, McElroy AK, Kraft CS, Towner JS, Spiropoulou C, Ströher U, Uyeki TM, Ribner BS, Emory Serious Communicable Diseases Unit.** 2014. Clinical care of two patients with Ebola virus disease in the United States. *N Engl J Med* **371:** 2402–2409.
63. **Vetter P, Fischer WA II, Schibler M, Jacobs M, Bausch DG, Kaiser L.** 2016. Ebola virus shedding and transmission: review of current evidence. *J Infect Dis* **214**(suppl 3): S177–S184.
64. **Diallo B, Sissoko D, Loman NJ, Bah HA, Bah H, Worrell MC, Conde LS, Sacko R, Mesfin S, Loua A, Kalonda JK, Erondu NA, Dahl BA, Handrick S, Goodfellow I, Meredith LW, Cotten M, Jah U, Guetiya Wadoum RE, Rollin P, Magassouba N, Malvy D, Anglaret X, Carroll MW, Aylward RB, Djingarey MH, Diarra A, Formenty P, Keïta S, Günther S, Rambaut A, Duraffour S.** 2016. Resurgence of Ebola virus disease in Guinea linked to a survivor with virus persistence in seminal fluid for more than 500 days. *Clin Infect Dis* **63:**1353–1356.
65. **Varkey JB, Shantha JG, Crozier I, Kraft CS, Lyon GM, Mehta AK, Kumar G, Smith JR, Kainulainen MH, Whitmer S, Ströher U, Uyeki TM, Ribner BS, Yeh S.** 2015. Persistence of Ebola virus in ocular fluid during convalescence. *N Engl J Med* **372:**2423–2427.
66. **McCormick JB, King IJ, Webb PA, Scribner CL, Craven RB, Johnson KM, Elliott LH, Belmont-Williams R.** 1986. Lassa fever. Effective therapy with ribavirin. *N Engl J Med* **314:**20–26.
67. **Miranda PO, Cubitt B, Jacob NT, Janda KD, de la Torre JC.** 2018. Mining a Kröhnke pyridine library for anti-arenavirus activity. *ACS Infect Dis* **4:**815–824.
68. **Jahrling PB, Geisbert TW, Geisbert JB, Swearengen JR, Bray M, Jaax NK, Huggins JW, LeDuc JW, Peters CJ.** 1999. Evaluation of immune globulin and recombinant interferon-alpha2b for treatment of experimental Ebola virus infections. *J Infect Dis* **179**(Suppl 1):S224–S234.
69. **Connor J, Kobinger G, Olinger G.** 2017. Therapeutics against filovirus infection. *Curr Top Microbiol Immunol* **411:**263–290.
70. **Davey RT Jr, Dodd L, Proschan MA, Neaton J, Neuhaus Nordwall J, Koopmeiners JS, Beigel J, Tierney J, Lane HC, Fauci AS, Massaquoi MBF, Sahr F, Malvy D, PREVAIL II Writing Group, Multi-National PREVAIL II Study Team.** 2016. A randomized, controlled trial of ZMapp for Ebola virus infection. *N Engl J Med* **375:**1448–1456.
71. **van Griensven J, Edwards T, Baize S, Ebola-Tx Consortium.** 2016. Efficacy of convalescent plasma in relation to dose of Ebola virus antibodies. *N Engl J Med* **375:**2307–2309.
72. **Ewer K, et al.** 2016. A monovalent chimpanzee adenovirus Ebola vaccine boosted with MVA. *N Engl J Med* **374:** 1635–1646.
73. **Henao-Restrepo AM, Camacho A, Longini IM, Watson CH, Edmunds WJ, Egger M, Carroll MW, Dean NE, Diatta I, Doumbia M, Draguez B, Duraffour S, Enwere G, Grais R, Gunther S, Gsell PS, Hossmann S, Watle SV, Kondé MK, Kéïta S, Kone S, Kuisma E, Levine MM, Mandal S, Mauget T, Norheim G, Riveros X, Soumah A, Trelle S, Vicari AS, Røttingen JA, Kieny MP.** 2017. Efficacy and effectiveness of an rVSV-vectored vaccine in preventing Ebola virus disease: final results from the Guinea ring vaccination, open-label, cluster-randomised trial (Ebola Ça Suffit!). *Lancet* **389:**505–518.
74. **Kennedy SB, Bolay F, Kieh M, Grandits G, Badio M, Ballou R, Eckes R, Feinberg M, Follmann D, Grund B, Gupta S, Hensley L, Higgs E, Janosko K, Johnson M, Kateh F, Logue J, Marchand J, Monath T, Nason M, Nyenswah T, Roman F, Stavale E, Wolfson J, Neaton JD, Lane HC, PREVAIL I Study Group.** 2017. Phase 2 placebo-controlled trial of two vaccines to prevent Ebola in Liberia. *N Engl J Med* **377:** 1438–1447.
75. **Ledgerwood JE, DeZure AD, Stanley DA, Coates EE, Novik L, Enama ME, Berkowitz NM, Hu Z, Joshi G, Ploquin A, Sitar S, Gordon IJ, Plummer SA, Holman LA, Hendel CS, Yamshchikov G, Roman F, Nicosia A, Colloca S, Cortese R, Bailer RT, Schwartz RM, Roederer M, Mascola JR, Koup RA, Sullivan NJ, Graham BS, VRC 207 Study Team.** 2017. Chimpanzee adenovirus vector Ebola vaccine. *N Engl J Med* **376:**928–938.
76. **Marzi A, Robertson SJ, Haddock E, Feldmann F, Hanley PW, Scott DP, Strong JE, Kobinger G, Best SM, Feldmann H.** 2015. VSV-EBOV rapidly protects macaques against infection with the 2014/15 Ebola virus outbreak strain. *Science* **349:**739–742.

77. **Regules JA, Beigel JH, Paolino KM, Voell J, Castellano AR, Hu Z, Muñoz P, Moon JE, Ruck RC, Bennett JW, Twomey PS, Gutiérrez RL, Remich SA, Hack HR, Wisniewski ML, Josleyn MD, Kwilas SA, Van Deusen N, Mbaya OT, Zhou Y, Stanley DA, Jing W, Smith KS, Shi M, Ledgerwood JE, Graham BS, Sullivan NJ, Jagodzinski LL, Peel SA, Alimonti JB, Hooper JW, Silvera PM, Martin BK, Monath TP, Ramsey WJ, Link CJ, Lane HC, Michael NL, Davey RT Jr, Thomas SJ, rVSVΔG-ZEBOV-GP Study Group.** 2017. A recombinant vesicular stomatitis virus Ebola vaccine. *N Engl J Med* **376:**330–341.
78. **CDC-NIH.** 2009. *Biosafety in Microbiological and Biomedical Laboratories*, 5th ed. U.S. Department of Health and Human Services, Washington, DC. https://www.cdc.gov/biosafety/publications/bmbl5/bmbl.pdf.
79. **Centers for Disease Control and Prevention (CDC).** 1995. Update: management of patients with suspected viral hemorrhagic fever—United States. *MMWR Morb Mortal Wkly Rep* **44:**475–479.
80. **Haddock E, Feldmann F, Feldmann H.** 2016. Effective chemical inactivation of Ebola virus. *Emerg Infect Dis* **22:** 1292–1294.
81. **Towner JS, Sealy TK, Ksiazek TG, Nichol ST.** 2007. High-throughput molecular detection of hemorrhagic fever virus threats with applications for outbreak settings. *J Infect Dis* **196**(Suppl 2)**:**S205–S212.
82. **Geisbert TW, Jahrling PB.** 1995. Differentiation of filoviruses by electron microscopy. *Virus Res* **39:**129–150.
83. **Geisbert TW, Jaax NK.** 1998. Marburg hemorrhagic fever: report of a case studied by immunohistochemistry and electron microscopy. *Ultrastruct Pathol* **22:**3–17.
84. **Connolly BM, Jenson AB, Peters CJ, Geyer SJ, Barth JF, McPherson RA.** 1993. Pathogenesis of Pichinde virus infection in strain 13 guinea pigs: an immunocytochemical, virologic, and clinical chemistry study. *Am J Trop Med Hyg* **49:**10–24.
85. **Connolly BM, Steele KE, Davis KJ, Geisbert TW, Kell WM, Jaax NK, Jahrling PB.** 1999. Pathogenesis of experimental Ebola virus infection in guinea pigs. *J Infect Dis* **179**(Suppl 1)**:**S203–S217.
86. **Jaax NK, Davis KJ, Geisbert TJ, Vogel P, Jaax GP, Topper M, Jahrling PB.** 1996. Lethal experimental infection of rhesus monkeys with Ebola-Zaire (Mayinga) virus by the oral and conjunctival route of exposure. *Arch Pathol Lab Med* **120:**140–155.
87. **Zaki SR, Shieh WJ, Greer PW, Goldsmith CS, Ferebee T, Katshitshi J, Tshioko FK, Bwaka MA, Swanepoel R, Calain P, Khan AS, Lloyd E, Rollin PE, Ksiazek TG, Peters CJ.** 1999. A novel immunohistochemical assay for the detection of Ebola virus in skin: implications for diagnosis, spread, and surveillance of Ebola hemorrhagic fever. Commission de Lutte contre les Epidémies à Kikwit. *J Infect Dis* **179**(Suppl 1)**:** S36–S47.
88. **Bausch DG, Rollin PE, Demby AH, Coulibaly M, Kanu J, Conteh AS, Wagoner KD, McMullan LK, Bowen MD, Peters CJ, Ksiazek TG.** 2000. Diagnosis and clinical virology of Lassa fever as evaluated by enzyme-linked immunosorbent assay, indirect fluorescent-antibody test, and virus isolation. *J Clin Microbiol* **38:**2670–2677.
89. **Ksiazek TG, Rollin PE, Jahrling PB, Johnson E, Dalgard DW, Peters CJ.** 1992. Enzyme immunosorbent assay for Ebola virus antigens in tissues of infected primates. *J Clin Microbiol* **30:**947–950.
90. **Ksiazek TG, Rollin PE, Williams AJ, Bressler DS, Martin ML, Swanepoel R, Burt FJ, Leman PA, Khan AS, Rowe AK, Mukunu R, Sanchez A, Peters CJ.** 1999. Clinical virology of Ebola hemorrhagic fever (EHF): virus, virus antigen, and IgG and IgM antibody findings among EHF patients in Kikwit, Democratic Republic of the Congo, 1995. *J Infect Dis* **179**(Suppl 1)**:**S177–S187.
91. **Niikura M, Ikegami T, Saijo M, Kurane I, Miranda ME, Morikawa S.** 2001. Detection of Ebola viral antigen by enzyme-linked immunosorbent assay using a novel monoclonal antibody to nucleoprotein. *J Clin Microbiol* **39:**3267–3271.
92. **Niklasson BS, Jahrling PB, Peters CJ.** 1984. Detection of Lassa virus antigens and Lassa virus-specific immunoglobulins G and M by enzyme-linked immunosorbent assay. *J Clin Microbiol* **20:**239–244.
93. **Saijo M, Georges-Courbot MC, Fukushi S, Mizutani T, Philippe M, Georges AJ, Kurane I, Morikawa S.** 2006. Marburgvirus nucleoprotein-capture enzyme-linked immunosorbent assay using monoclonal antibodies to recombinant nucleoprotein: detection of authentic Marburgvirus. *Jpn J Infect Dis* **59:**323–325.
94. **Boisen ML, Cross RW, Hartnett JN, Goba A, Momoh M, Fullah M, Gbakie M, Safa S, Fonnie M, Baimba F, Koroma VJ, Geisbert JB, McCormick S, Nelson DK, Millett MM, Oottamasathien D, Jones AB, Pham H, Brown BL, Shaffer JG, Schieffelin JS, Kargbo B, Gbetuwa M, Gevao SM, Wilson RB, Pitts KR, Geisbert TW, Branco LM, Khan SH, Grant DS, Garry RF.** 2016. Field validation of the ReEBOV antigen rapid test for point-of-care diagnosis of Ebola virus infection. *J Infect Dis* **214**(suppl 3)**:**S203–S209.
95. **Broadhurst MJ, Kelly JD, Miller A, Semper A, Bailey D, Groppelli E, Simpson A, Brooks T, Hula S, Nyoni W, Sankoh AB, Kanu S, Jalloh A, Ton Q, Sarchet N, George P, Perkins MD, Wonderly B, Murray M, Pollock NR.** 2015. ReEBOV antigen rapid test kit for point-of-care and laboratory-based testing for Ebola virus disease: a field validation study. *Lancet* **386:**867–874.
96. **Cross RW, Boisen ML, Millett MM, Nelson DS, Oottamasathien D, Hartnett JN, Jones AB, Goba A, Momoh M, Fullah M, Bornholdt ZA, Fusco ML, Abelson DM, Oda S, Brown BL, Pham H, Rowland MM, Agans KN, Geisbert JB, Heinrich ML, Kulakosky PC, Shaffer JG, Schieffelin JS, Kargbo B, Gbetuwa M, Gevao SM, Wilson RB, Saphire EO, Pitts KR, Khan SH, Grant DS, Geisbert TW, Branco LM, Garry RF.** 2016. Analytical validation of the ReEBOV antigen rapid test for point-of-care diagnosis of Ebola virus infection. *J Infect Dis* **214**(suppl 3)**:** S210–S217.
97. **Jean Louis F, Huang JY, Nebie YK, Koivogui L, Jayaraman G, Abiola N, Vansteelandt A, Worrel MC, Shang J, Murphy LB, Fitter DL, Marston BJ, Martel L.** 2017. Implementation of broad screening with Ebola rapid diagnostic tests in Forécariah, Guinea. *Afr J Lab Med* **6:**484.
98. **Phan JC, Pettitt J, George JS, Fakoli LS III, Taweh FM, Bateman SL, Bennett RS, Norris SL, Spinnler DA, Pimentel G, Sahr PK, Bolay FK, Schoepp RJ.** 2016. Lateral flow immunoassays for Ebola virus disease detection in Liberia. *J Infect Dis* **214**(suppl 3)**:**S222–S228.
99. **VanSteelandt A, Aho J, Franklin K, Likofata J, Kamgang JB, Keita S, Koivogui L, Magassouba N, Martel LD, Dahourou AG.** 2017. Operational evaluation of rapid diagnostic testing for Ebola virus disease in Guinean laboratories. *PLoS One* **12:**e0188047.
100. **Drosten C, Kümmerer BM, Schmitz H, Günther S.** 2003. Molecular diagnostics of viral hemorrhagic fevers. *Antiviral Res* **57:**61–87.
101. **Günther S, Asper M, Röser C, Luna LK, Drosten C, Becker-Ziaja B, Borowski P, Chen HM, Hosmane RS.** 2004. Application of real-time PCR for testing antiviral compounds against Lassa virus, SARS coronavirus and Ebola virus *in vitro*. *Antiviral Res* **63:**209–215.
102. **Andersen KG, et al, Viral Hemorrhagic Fever Consortium.** 2015. Clinical sequencing uncovers origins and evolution of Lassa virus. *Cell* **162:**738–750.
103. **Bowen MD, Peters CJ, Nichol ST.** 1996. The phylogeny of New World (Tacaribe complex) arenaviruses. *Virology* **219:**285–290.
104. **Bowen MD, Peters CJ, Nichol ST.** 1997. Phylogenetic analysis of the Arenaviridae: patterns of virus evolution and evidence for cospeciation between arenaviruses and their rodent hosts. *Mol Phylogenet Evol* **8:**301–316.
105. **Bowen MD, Rollin PE, Ksiazek TG, Hustad HL, Bausch DG, Demby AH, Bajani MD, Peters CJ, Nichol ST.** 2000. Genetic diversity among Lassa virus strains. *J Virol* **74:** 6992–7004.

106. **Drosten C, Göttig S, Schilling S, Asper M, Panning M, Schmitz H, Günther S.** 2002. Rapid detection and quantification of RNA of Ebola and Marburg viruses, Lassa virus, Crimean-Congo hemorrhagic fever virus, Rift Valley fever virus, dengue virus, and yellow fever virus by real-time reverse transcription-PCR. *J Clin Microbiol* **40:**2323–2330.
107. **Olschläger S, Lelke M, Emmerich P, Panning M, Drosten C, Hass M, Asogun D, Ehichioya D, Omilabu S, Günther S.** 2010. Improved detection of Lassa virus by reverse transcription-PCR targeting the 5′ region of S RNA. *J Clin Microbiol* **48:**2009–2013.
108. **Asogun DA, Adomeh DI, Ehimuan J, Odia I, Hass M, Gabriel M, Olschläger S, Becker-Ziaja B, Folarin O, Phelan E, Ehiane PE, Ifeh VE, Uyigue EA, Oladapo YT, Muoebonam EB, Osunde O, Dongo A, Okokhere PO, Okogbenin SA, Momoh M, Alikah SO, Akhuemokhan OC, Imomeh P, Odike MA, Gire S, Andersen K, Sabeti PC, Happi CT, Akpede GO, Günther S.** 2012. Molecular diagnostics for Lassa fever at Irrua specialist teaching hospital, Nigeria: lessons learnt from two years of laboratory operation. *PLoS Negl Trop Dis* **6:**e1839.
109. **Lozano ME, Enría D, Maiztegui JI, Grau O, Romanowski V.** 1995. Rapid diagnosis of Argentine hemorrhagic fever by reverse transcriptase PCR-based assay. *J Clin Microbiol* **33:**1327–1332.
110. **Sanchez A, Ksiazek TG, Rollin PE, Miranda ME, Trappier SG, Khan AS, Peters CJ, Nichol ST.** 1999. Detection and molecular characterization of Ebola viruses causing disease in human and nonhuman primates. *J Infect Dis* **179**(Suppl 1)**:**S164–S169.
111. **Vieth S, Drosten C, Lenz O, Vincent M, Omilabu S, Hass M, Becker-Ziaja B, ter Meulen J, Nichol ST, Schmitz H, Günther S.** 2007. RT-PCR assay for detection of Lassa virus and related Old World arenaviruses targeting the L gene. *Trans R Soc Trop Med Hyg* **101:**1253–1264.
112. **Trappier SG, Conaty AL, Farrar BB, Auperin DD, McCormick JB, Fisher-Hoch SP.** 1993. Evaluation of the polymerase chain reaction for diagnosis of Lassa virus infection. *Am J Trop Med Hyg* **49:**214–221.
113. **Grolla A, Lucht A, Dick D, Strong JE, Feldmann H.** 2005. Laboratory diagnosis of Ebola and Marburg hemorrhagic fever. *Bull Soc Pathol Exot* **98:**205–209.
114. **Panning M, Laue T, Olschlager S, Eickmann M, Becker S, Raith S, Courbot MC, Nilsson M, Gopal R, Lundkvist A, di Caro A, Brown D, Meyer H, Lloyd G, Kummerer BM, Gunther S, Drosten C.** 2007. Diagnostic reverse-transcription polymerase chain reaction kit for filoviruses based on the strain collections of all European biosafety level 4 laboratories. *J Infect Dis* **196**(Suppl 2)**:**S199–S204.
115. **Weidmann M, Mühlberger E, Hufert FT.** 2004. Rapid detection protocol for filoviruses. *J Clin Virol* **30:**94–99.
116. **Kurosaki Y, Takada A, Ebihara H, Grolla A, Kamo N, Feldmann H, Kawaoka Y, Yasuda J.** 2007. Rapid and simple detection of Ebola virus by reverse transcription-loop-mediated isothermal amplification. *J Virol Methods* **141:** 78–83.
117. **Kurosaki Y, Magassouba N, Oloniniyi OK, Cherif MS, Sakabe S, Takada A, Hirayama K, Yasuda J.** 2016. Development and evaluation of reverse transcription-loop-mediated isothermal amplification (RT-LAMP) assay coupled with a portable device for rapid diagnosis of Ebola virus disease in Guinea. *PLoS Negl Trop Dis* **10:**e0004472.
118. **Oloniniyi OK, Kurosaki Y, Miyamoto H, Takada A, Yasuda J.** 2017. Rapid detection of all known Ebolavirus species by reverse transcription-loop-mediated isothermal amplification (RT-LAMP). *J Virol Methods* **246:**8–14.
119. **Jansen van Vuren P, Grobbelaar A, Storm N, Conteh O, Konneh K, Kamara A, Sanne I, Paweska JT.** 2016. Comparative evaluation of the diagnostic performance of the prototype Cepheid GeneXpert Ebola assay. *J Clin Microbiol* **54:**359–367.
120. **Southern TR, Racsa LD, Albariño CG, Fey PD, Hinrichs SH, Murphy CN, Herrera VL, Sambol AR, Hill CE, Ryan EL, Kraft CS, Campbell S, Sealy TK, Schuh A, Ritchie JC, Lyon GM III, Mehta AK, Varkey JB, Ribner BS, Brantly KP, Ströher U, Iwen PC, Burd EM.** 2015. Comparison of FilmArray and quantitative real-time reverse transcriptase PCR for detection of Zaire Ebolavirus from contrived and clinical specimens. *J Clin Microbiol* **53:**2956–2960.
121. **Weller SA, Bailey D, Matthews S, Lumley S, Sweed A, Ready D, Eltringham G, Richards J, Vipond R, Lukaszewski R, Payne PM, Aarons E, Simpson AJ, Hutley EJ, Brooks T.** 2016. Evaluation of the Biofire FilmArray BioThreat-E test (v2.5) for rapid identification of Ebola virus disease in heat-treated blood samples obtained in Sierra Leone and the United Kingdom. *J Clin Microbiol* **54:** 114–119.
122. **Semper AE, Broadhurst MJ, Richards J, Foster GM, Simpson AJ, Logue CH, Kelly JD, Miller A, Brooks TJ, Murray M, Pollock NR.** 2016. Performance of the GeneXpert Ebola assay for diagnosis of Ebola virus disease in Sierra Leone: a field evaluation study. *PLoS Med* **13:**e1001980.
123. **Gay-Andrieu F, Magassouba N, Picot V, Phillips CL, Peyrefitte CN, Dacosta B, Dore A, Kourouma F, Ligeon-Ligeonnet V, Gauby C, Longuet C, Scullion M, Faye O, Machuron JL, Miller M.** 2017. Clinical evaluation of the BioFire FilmArray((R)) BioThreat-E test for the diagnosis of Ebola virus disease in Guinea. *J Clin Virol* **92:**20–24.
124. **Leski TA, Ansumana R, Taitt CR, Lamin JM, Bangura U, Lahai J, Mbayo G, Kanneh MB, Bawo B, Bockarie AS, Scullion M, Phillips CL, Horner CP, Jacobsen KH, Stenger DA.** 2015. Use of the FilmArray system for detection of Zaire Ebolavirus in a small hospital in Bo, Sierra Leone. *J Clin Microbiol* **53:**2368–2370.
125. **Rieger T, Kerber R, El Halas H, Pallasch E, Duraffour S, Günther S, Ölschläger S.** 2016. Evaluation of RealStar reverse transcription-polymerase chain reaction kits for filovirus detection in the laboratory and field. *J Infect Dis* **214**(suppl 3)**:**S243–S249.
126. **Flint M, Goodman CH, Bearden S, Blau DM, Amman BR, Basile AJ, Belser JA, Bergeron É, Bowen MD, Brault AC, Campbell S, Chakrabarti AK, Dodd KA, Erickson BR, Freeman MM, Gibbons A, Guerrero LW, Klena JD, Lash RR, Lo MK, McMullan LK, Momoh G, Massally JL, Goba A, Paddock CD, Priestley RA, Pyle M, Rayfield M, Russell BJ, Salzer JS, Sanchez AJ, Schuh AJ, Sealy TK, Steinau M, Stoddard RA, Taboy C, Turnsek M, Wang D, Zemtsova GE, Zivcec M, Spiropoulou CF, Ströher U, Towner JS, Nichol ST, Bird BH.** 2015. Ebola virus diagnostics: the US Centers for Disease Control and Prevention Laboratory in Sierra Leone, August 2014 to March 2015. *J Infect Dis* **212**(Suppl 2)**:**S350–S358.
127. **Hotchin J, Sikora E.** 1975. Laboratory diagnosis of lymphocytic choriomeningitis. *Bull World Health Organ* **52:** 555–559.
128. **Bird BH, Dodd KA, Erickson BR, Albariño CG, Chakrabarti AK, McMullan LK, Bergeron E, Ströeher U, Cannon D, Martin B, Coleman-McCray JD, Nichol ST, Spiropoulou CF.** 2012. Severe hemorrhagic fever in strain 13/N guinea pigs infected with Lujo virus. *PLoS Negl Trop Dis* **6:**e1801.
129. **Sissoko D, Duraffour S, Kerber R, Kolie JS, Beavogui AH, Camara AM, Colin G, Rieger T, Oestereich L, Pályi B, Wurr S, Guedj J, Nguyen THT, Eggo RM, Watson CH, Edmunds WJ, Bore JA, Koundouno FR, Cabeza-Cabrerizo M, Carter LL, Kafetzopoulou LE, Kuisma E, Michel J, Patrono LV, Rickett NY, Singethan K, Rudolf M, Lander A, Pallasch E, Bockholt S, Rodríguez E, Di Caro A, Wölfel R, Gabriel M, Gurry C, Formenty P, Keïta S, Malvy D, Carroll MW, Anglaret X, Günther S.** 2017. Persistence and clearance of Ebola virus RNA from seminal fluid of Ebola virus disease survivors: a longitudinal analysis and modelling study. *Lancet Glob Health* **5:**e80–e88.
130. **Buchmeier MJ, Lewicki HA, Tomori O, Oldstone MB.** 1981. Monoclonal antibodies to lymphocytic choriomeningitis and pichinde viruses: generation, characterization, and cross-reactivity with other arenaviruses. *Virology* **113:** 73–85.

131. **Sanchez A, Pifat DY, Kenyon RH, Peters CJ, McCormick JB, Kiley MP.** 1989. Junin virus monoclonal antibodies: characterization and cross-reactivity with other arenaviruses. *J Gen Virol* **70:**1125–1132.
132. **Wulff H, Johnson KM.** 1979. Immunoglobulin M and G responses measured by immunofluorescence in patients with Lassa or Marburg virus infections. *Bull World Health Organ* **57:**631–635.
133. **Bergqvist C, Holmström P, Lindegren G, Lagerqvist N, Leijon M, Falk KI.** 2015. Multiplex nucleic acid suspension bead arrays for detection and subtyping of filoviruses. *J Clin Microbiol* **53:**1368–1370.
134. **Ambrosio AM, Feuillade MR, Gamboa GS, Maiztegui JI.** 1994. Prevalence of lymphocytic choriomeningitis virus infection in a human population of Argentina. *Am J Trop Med Hyg* **50:**381–386.
135. **Elliott LH, Bauer SP, Perez-Oronoz G, Lloyd ES.** 1993. Improved specificity of testing methods for filovirus antibodies. *J Virol Methods* **43:**85–99.
136. **Johnson KM, Elliott LH, Heymann DL.** 1981. Preparation of polyvalent viral immunofluorescent intracellular antigens and use in human serosurveys. *J Clin Microbiol* **14:**527–529.
137. **Ikegami T, Saijo M, Niikura M, Miranda ME, Calaor AB, Hernandez M, Manalo DL, Kurane I, Yoshikawa Y, Morikawa S.** 2002. Development of an immunofluorescence method for the detection of antibodies to Ebola virus subtype Reston by the use of recombinant nucleoprotein-expressing HeLa cells. *Microbiol Immunol* **46:**633–638.
138. **Ksiazek TG, West CP, Rollin PE, Jahrling PB, Peters CJ.** 1999. ELISA for the detection of antibodies to Ebola viruses. *J Infect Dis* **179**(Suppl 1)**:**S192–S198.
139. **Kalter SS, Heberling RL, Barry JD, Tian PY.** 1995. Detection of Ebola-Reston (Filoviridae) virus antibody by dot-immunobinding assay. *Lab Anim Sci* **45:**523–525.
140. **Ikegami T, Saijo M, Niikura M, Miranda ME, Calaor AB, Hernandez M, Manalo DL, Kurane I, Yoshikawa Y, Morikawa S.** 2003. Immunoglobulin G enzyme-linked immunosorbent assay using truncated nucleoproteins of Reston Ebola virus. *Epidemiol Infect* **130:**533–539.
141. **Saijo M, Niikura M, Morikawa S, Ksiazek TG, Meyer RF, Peters CJ, Kurane I.** 2001. Enzyme-linked immunosorbent assays for detection of antibodies to Ebola and Marburg viruses using recombinant nucleoproteins. *J Clin Microbiol* **39:**1–7.
142. **Fukushi S, Tani H, Yoshikawa T, Saijo M, Morikawa S.** 2012. Serological assays based on recombinant viral proteins for the diagnosis of arenavirus hemorrhagic fevers. *Viruses* **4:**2097–2114.
143. **Jahrling PB, Peters CJ.** 1984. Passive antibody therapy of Lassa fever in cynomolgus monkeys: importance of neutralizing antibody and Lassa virus strain. *Infect Immun* **44:**528–533.
144. **Rollin PE, Williams RJ, Bressler DS, Pearson S, Cottingham M, Pucak G, Sanchez A, Trappier SG, Peters RL, Greer PW, Zaki S, Demarcus T, Hendricks K, Kelley M, Simpson D, Geisbert TW, Jahrling PB, Peters CJ, Ksiazek TG.** 1999. Ebola (subtype Reston) virus among quarantined nonhuman primates recently imported from the Philippines to the United States. *J Infect Dis* **179**(Suppl 1)**:** S108–S114.
145. **MacNeil A, Reed Z, Rollin PE.** 2011. Serologic cross-reactivity of human IgM and IgG antibodies to five species of Ebola virus. *PLoS Negl Trop Dis* **5:**e1175.

Herpes Simplex Viruses and Herpes B Virus

ALEXANDER L. GRENINGER, RHODA ASHLEY MORROW, AND KEITH R. JEROME

100

TAXONOMY

Herpes simplex virus (HSV) types 1 and 2, formally designated human herpesvirus 1 and human herpesvirus 2, respectively, are members of the family *Herpesviridae*. Along with varicella-zoster virus (VZV) (human herpesvirus 3), and a number of viruses primarily affecting non-human hosts, they comprise the subfamily *Alphaherpesvirinae*.

DESCRIPTION OF THE AGENT

The herpesviruses are thought to have coevolved with their hosts (1, 2), and thus the earliest documentation of presumptive herpes simplex infection appears shortly after the development of writing and clinical observation. The infectious nature of HSV was demonstrated in 1919 (3). The concepts of seropositivity and recurrence developed in the 1930s (4, 5). In the 1960s, antigenically distinct strains (HSV-1 and HSV-2) were identified. HSV-1 and HSV-2 are two of nine known human herpesviruses. In addition, herpes B virus ("Herpesvirus simiae"), a herpesvirus infecting macaques, is a rare but important zoonotic pathogen in humans.

The linear, double-stranded genome is 152 kilobase pairs for HSV-1 and 155 kilobase pairs for HSV-2. HSV-1 and HSV-2 share 83% nucleotide identity within their protein-coding regions. The genome is organized into a unique long and a unique short region, each of which is flanked by inverted-repeat regions. Although significant stretches of sequence are conserved between unrelated clinical isolates, identification of isolates can be achieved by sequencing, PCR, or restriction endonuclease digestion.

The HSV virion is 120 to 300 nm in diameter, with a central electron-dense core containing the DNA, an icosahedral capsid consisting of 162 capsomeres surrounding the core, and a tegument layer surrounded by a spiked envelope containing viral glycoproteins that aid in attachment, penetration, and immune evasion. The envelope is a trilaminar, lipid-rich layer derived largely from the nuclear membrane of the infected cell. Because the viral envelope is lipid rich, the virus is readily inactivated. Lipid solvents such as 70% ethanol or isopropanol (but not alcohol >95%), Lysol, bleach, exposure to pH of <5 or >11, or temperatures of >56°C for 30 minutes will all eliminate infectivity (6, 7).

Viral replication begins with attachment to the target cell via cell type-dependent host receptors (8, 9). After attachment, the viral envelope and cell membrane fuse, releasing the capsid into the cell. The capsid is translocated to the nuclear pores (10, 11), and DNA is released into the nucleus. The tegument protein VP16 induces expression of the immediate early, or alpha, proteins, which in turn transactivate the expression of the early, or beta, genes. The early genes are maximally expressed 5 to 7 hours after infection and are involved in the synthesis of progeny viral DNA. DNA replication is required for optimal synthesis of the late, or gamma, genes, which are mainly structural proteins. Progeny DNA is processed and assembled into preformed capsids within the cell nucleus. The DNA-containing capsids attach to patches of the nuclear membrane that contain viral tegument proteins and viral glycoproteins. In sensory ganglia neurons, the virus establishes latency, and episomal HSV DNA is maintained for the lifetime of the infected individual. Upon reactivation, nucleocapsids are transported anterograde to the axon terminus, where the final assembly of enveloped virus occurs (12), typically with infection of surrounding epithelial cells. The replication cycle is complete within about 20 hours in epithelial cells.

Innate immune mechanisms such as activation of macrophages, NK cells, and interferon production play a predominant role in the control of primary infection, while both innate and adaptive immunity are important in the control of recurrences. Although both cellular and humoral immunity are thought to be important, people with defective cellular immunity often show severe HSV infections, while those with agammaglobulinemia do not (13). $CD4^+$ T cells infiltrate mucocutaneous lesions early in lesion development (14), followed by cytotoxic T lymphocytes (15). HSV-specific T cells can be detected early in lesion development and persist at the lesion site after healing (16, 17). T cells also play an important role in controlling viral reactivation from the dorsal root ganglia, via noncytotoxic mechanisms that do not result in neuronal death (18).

Functional antibody responses include complement-independent and complement-dependent viral neutralization (19). IgG, IgM, and IgA responses to individual viral proteins arise within the first weeks after infection (13). IgM wanes after 2 to 3 months, appearing sporadically thereafter, and in about a third of patients after recurrent genital herpes episodes. Antibody titer may or may not rise after recurrences (20). However, IgG titers are maintained for years after primary infection.

Most epitopes are shared between HSV-1 and HSV-2. As a result, it is difficult to distinguish antibodies to HSV-1 from those to HSV-2 (21). In particular, in HSV-1-seropositive patients, seroconversion to HSV-2 is accompanied by brisk anamnestic responses to HSV-1, resulting in the predominant antibody response being directed toward HSV-1 rather than to HSV-2 for prolonged periods (21). While type-specific epitopes have been demonstrated on the major viral proteins, only glycoprotein G (gG) elicits predominantly type-specific responses.

EPIDEMIOLOGY AND TRANSMISSION

HSV infections occur worldwide with no seasonal distribution. The virus is spread by direct contact with virus in secretions. Incubation periods range from 1 to 26 days. The prevalence of HSV-1 infection increases gradually from childhood, reaching 80% or more in later years (22). In contrast, the seroprevalence of HSV-2 remains low until adolescence and the onset of sexual activity. The incidence of antibodies to HSV-2 in the United States reached 21% in the period of 1988 to 1994; however, in more recent years seropositivity rates declined to 16% for the period of 2005 to 2008 (23) and 12% for 2015 to 2016 (24). The rate of seropositivity varies widely, reaching more than 50% in some demographic groups (25, 26). In general, the seroprevalence of HSV-2 is higher in the United States than in other developed countries (27, 28).

A large percentage of individuals who are seropositive for HSV-1 and/or HSV-2 are unaware of the infection (26, 29). Such people make up an important reservoir of infection. The risk of genital HSV transmission has been reported to be reduced by 30 to 50% through the use of condoms (30, 31), and a more recent case-crossover analysis of previous study data suggests that the reduction of transmission may be substantially more than previously estimated (32). Transmission is also reduced approximately 50% by disclosure of HSV infection status to sexual partners (33) and by approximately 50% with suppressive antiviral therapy in the source partner (34). It is likely that combining these approaches further reduces risk.

Future studies of epidemiology and transmission of HSV-1 and HSV-2 will be informed by the growing availability of genomic sequence data for these viruses. As of mid-2017, approximately 150 genomes are available in NCBI for each of HSV-1 and HSV-2—an increase of more than 10-fold over the previous 4 years. Genomic sequencing of HSV-1 and HSV-2 is difficult owing to the extraordinarily high GC content (70%), the presence of many repeats, and the need to enrich from human DNA. Early studies of HSV genomic evolution and diversity highlighted the overall limited diversity among the sequenced viruses as well as the role played by both intertypic (HSV-1 × HSV-2) and intratypic (HSV-1 × HSV-1) recombination and the high burden of homopolymeric frameshift mutations (35, 36). Indeed, the majority of HSV-2 sequences deposited to date contain HSV-1 sequences (37, 38). New methods allow direct sequencing from clinical specimens rather than cultured isolates as was required previously (38). Many unanswered questions remain concerning the evolution of HSV-1 and HSV-2 genomes in transmission chains and global diversity, especially in sub-Saharan Africa.

CLINICAL SIGNIFICANCE

Primary Infection

Most HSV-1 infections are acquired early in childhood as subclinical or unrecognized infections. Young children may present with classic primary HSV-1 infection characterized by gingivostomatitis, fever, and marked submandibular lymphadenopathy. Oral lesions progress to ulceration and heal without scarring over 2 to 3 weeks. Adolescents may present with pharyngitis and mononucleosis.

Primary infection with HSV-2 classically presents as herpes genitalis with extensive, bilateral vesicles, fever, inguinal lymphadenopathy, and dysuria. Lesions ulcerate and heal without scarring within 3 weeks. Secondary lesions may develop in the second to third week. Subclinical or unrecognized primary infection with HSV-2 is common.

The proportion of primary genital infections due to HSV-1 is increasing (39), from about 10% in 1983 to 32% in 1995 (40, 41), and it is now the major cause of first-episode anogenital infections in at least some populations (42–44). In a large study of young women age 18 to 30, primary infection with HSV-1 was more than twice as common as infection with HSV-2 (44), and of clinically recognized primary HSV-1 infections, more than 75% were genital rather than oral. This trend is thought to result from changing sexual practices, including increased oral-genital exposure (42). The clinical presentation of primary genital HSV-1 cannot be distinguished from that of HSV-2. However, recurrent disease (see below) is less common with genital HSV-1 than HSV-2 (40, 45), and thus determining the infecting virus type is useful for prognostic purposes.

Latency and Recurrent Disease

Primary infection with HSV-1 or HSV-2 is followed by the establishment of latency in sensory ganglia, typically the trigeminal ganglia for orolabial disease and the lumbosacral dorsal root ganglia for genital disease. Periodically, the virus reactivates and travels via the nerve axon to oral or genital sites, resulting in release of infectious virus and, in some cases, lesion formation. Recurrent disease has milder symptoms and a shorter time to lesion healing than primary episodes (40, 46). The frequency of HSV-2 genital recurrences varies widely among individuals, ranging from none to 12 or more per year (47), with a mean rate of 0.33 recurrences/month. Orolabial HSV-1 recurrence rates are lower, with a mean of 0.12 episodes/month, while genital HSV-1 infection recurs even less frequently (mean 0.02 episodes/month) (48). While HSV-2 may be isolated from the pharynx during primary genital herpes episodes, orolabial HSV-2 recurrences are extremely infrequent (48).

Asymptomatic or Subclinical Infection

Approximately 70 to 90% of individuals with HSV-2 antibodies have not been diagnosed with genital herpes (26, 29). Over half of such people recognize and present with symptoms after education regarding manifestations of HSV disease (49, 50). In addition, about 20% of patients presenting with first episodes of genital herpes have serologic evidence of having been infected for some time (51). These episodes most closely resemble recurrent disease, with relatively mild symptoms. The risk of recurrence is similar between patients presenting with true primary and first recognized recurrent episodes (20). Most patients with genital herpes have episodes of subclinical virus excretion from anogenital sites; these constitute an important source of transmission. The copy number of HSV DNA can sometimes be as high during subclinical episodes as when symptoms occur (52). In general, oral shedding of HSV-1 occurs somewhat less frequently than genital shedding of HSV-2 (53). Oral shedding of HSV-2 and genital shedding of HSV-1 are comparatively rare, particularly outside the setting of newly acquired disease (48, 53, 54).

Neonatal Herpes

The most serious consequence of genital HSV infection is neonatal herpes. Infection usually occurs during vaginal delivery when the infant is exposed to HSV in maternal secretions. The risk of maternal-to-infant transmission is 10-fold higher in mothers experiencing unrecognized primary infection during the time of labor than in those shedding HSV as a result of recurrent, subclinical reactivation. This conclusion was drawn in part from the finding that the neonatal infection rate is 54 per 100,000 among HSV-seronegative mothers, 26 per 100,000 among mothers with only HSV-1 antibody, and 22 per 100,000 among all mothers with HSV-2 antibody (55, 56). Transmission of HSV-1 occurs at a significantly higher rate than that of HSV-2 (56, 57). The high rate of transmission during primary disease means that 50 to 80% of all cases of neonatal herpes occur in children of women who acquire genital HSV infection near term (58, 59). Pregnant women who present with HSV infection should undergo both a type-specific serologic assay and viral typing, to identify infants at highest risk for infection (60).

Infected neonates can present with HSV disease localized to the skin, eyes, and mucosa or with more serious central nervous system (CNS) or disseminated disease but often have nonspecific presentation (61, 62). The mortality rate for untreated neonates with disseminated disease exceeds 70%. Early diagnosis and antiviral therapy while disease is localized to the skin can substantially reduce the morbidity and mortality associated with neonatal infections (63, 64). PCR should be used to test samples from lesions, other mucosal sites, cerebrospinal fluid (CSF), and blood (61, 65–67). Although culture has continued to be advocated for surface specimens (68), the superior sensitivity of PCR for surface specimens is well established (52). Specimen swabs from body sites may be combined prior to HSV testing, according to established guidelines (68).

Herpes CNS Disease in the Immunocompetent Host

HSV is the most common cause of fatal sporadic encephalitis in the United States (69). HSV-1 is associated with more focal encephalitis in the temporal lobe, while HSV-2 has been associated with meningitis and milder neurological disease (70). HSV encephalitis presents as fever, behavioral changes, and altered consciousness, resulting from localized temporal lobe involvement. Without treatment, mortality exceeds 70%, and few survivors recover normal neurologic function. Early treatment with acyclovir reduces morbidity and mortality; however, residual neurologic impairment is common (71). HSV PCR of CSF is the test of choice but should not be used as a test of cure (72, 73). Culture of CSF is not acceptable for diagnosis of HSV encephalitis.

Genital HSV may be followed by sporadic meningitis or recurrent meningitis (Mollaret's syndrome) characterized by headache, fever, photophobia, and lymphocytic pleocytosis (74, 75). The condition is self-limiting and typically resolves within 1 week. HSV also can be associated with myelitis, radiculitis, ascending paralysis, autonomic nerve dysfunction, and possibly Bell's palsy.

Systemic HSV Infection in Hospitalized Adults

HSV can sometimes be detected by PCR in the blood during primary HSV disease (76) and in recurrent herpes labialis (77). It can also occasionally be detected in the blood of hospitalized adults, either immunocompetent or immunocompromised (78, 79). Hospitalized patients with detectable HSV viremia frequently have clinical symptoms, including hepatitis, fever, CNS alterations, skin lesions, abdominal pain, or sepsis, although it has not been established that HSV is the cause of these symptoms. Nevertheless, hospitalized patients with detectable HSV viremia do have a high rate of mortality, suggesting a role for testing. Patients with HSV hepatitis can have high viral loads in the plasma, which can be the first indication of HSV as the etiology of an often fatal, though treatable, hepatitis (80).

Ocular Herpes Infections

HSV is the most common viral cause of corneal infection in the United States, affecting 400,000 to 500,000 people (81, 82). Most corneal HSV infections are limited to the epithelial layer, causing characteristic branching ulcerations, pain, photophobia, and blurred vision. HSV epithelial keratitis responds well to oral or topical therapy (see below). Such superficial infections heal without loss of vision. HSV infection may extend to the corneal stroma, leading to scarring and opacification of the cornea. Stromal HSV infections respond favorably to a combination of corticosteroids and topical or oral antivirals (83, 84). Ocular HSV infection is significantly more likely to be due to HSV-1 than HSV-2 (85).

Herpes in the Immunocompromised Host

Immunosuppressed individuals with defective cell-mediated immunity frequently develop symptomatic HSV disease. HSV infections in such individuals can be severe, with extensive mucocutaneous necrosis and involvement of contiguous tissues leading to esophagitis or proctitis. Disseminated HSV, which can lead to meningoencephalitis, pneumonitis, hepatitis, and coagulopathy, may be more common in immunocompromised and hospitalized patients than is generally recognized (78, 86). Disseminated infections require intravenous antiviral therapy and monitoring for development of antiviral resistance.

Antiviral Therapy

Several antiviral drugs including acyclovir, valacyclovir, penciclovir, and famciclovir are now widely used to treat mucocutaneous and genital herpes (87, 88) and for long-term suppression of recurrent episodes. These drugs are selectively activated by the viral thymidine kinase and have minimal side effects. Suppressive therapy reduces the risk of viral transmission between HSV-discordant partners (34). *N*-Docosanol, a nonprescription topical medication that inhibits viral-host membrane fusion, and topical acyclovir are used for the treatment of herpes labialis. HSV conjunctivitis, blepharitis, and dendritic keratitis are treated either topically with trifluridine, idoxuridine, or vidarabine or orally with acyclovir, valacyclovir, or famciclovir (83). In cases with stromal involvement, the addition of topical corticosteroids reduces the persistence of inflammation (83). Neonatal herpes, herpes encephalitis, and severe infections in immunocompromised patients require prompt intravenous antiviral therapy (89). The alternative agents foscarnet, cidofovir, and vidarabine are generally reserved for acyclovir-resistant herpes infections (88, 90). A new compound, pritelivir, targeting the HSV helicase/primase complex, has shown efficacy in clinical trials (91–93), with reduced genital HSV shedding, and is likely to provide an additional therapeutic option in the future.

COLLECTION, TRANSPORT, AND STORAGE OF SPECIMENS

Samples for DNA amplification (PCR) require careful collection and handling, which are essential to ensure adequate specimen and avoid contamination of the sample with exogenous viral DNA. For lesions or mucocutaneous sites, a dedicated specimen should be collected with a Dacron swab in viral transport medium (VTM) or digestion buffer (94). Serum, plasma, and CSF do not require special handling. Heparin can inhibit PCR and therefore is not an acceptable anticoagulant. Specimens for PCR can be maintained at 4°C for up to 72 hours, but longer storage should be at −20°C (95, 96).

For culture, specimens from lesions or mucocutaneous sites should be placed in VTM and kept at a controlled temperature to retain optimal infectivity. VTM is made of balanced salt solutions such as Hanks balanced salt solution, Stuart's medium, Leibovitz-Emory medium, veal infusion broth, or tryptose phosphate broth buffered to maintain a neutral pH. Protein-stabilizing agents such as gelatin or bovine serum albumin are added as well as antibiotics to prevent bacterial overgrowth (97). Most VTM are inappropriate for bacterial or chlamydial transport. However, Multi-Microbe M4 media from Remel (Lenexa, KS) and Universal Transport Medium from Copan (Murrieta, CA) are suitable for viruses, *Chlamydia*, *Mycoplasma*, and *Ureaplasma*. It is important that laboratories validate the suitability of the selected media for their particular applications, because performance can vary.

Necrotic debris or exudate should be removed from mucosal sites (endocervix, anogenital areas, conjunctiva, and throat) or lesions with a cotton swab prior to sampling. The lesion base must be vigorously rubbed with Dacron, rayon, or cotton swabs on aluminum shafts to ensure that infected cells at the base of the lesion are collected. Calcium alginate swabs and swabs with wooden shafts inhibit infectivity and enzyme-mediated DNA amplification (97, 98). Swabs are then placed into VTM for transport. Several manufacturers offer combined swab/media packaging, such as the Copan Universal Transport Medium system and the Remel Multi-microbe M4 system.

Samples should be shipped cold (on ample ice packs) but not frozen. Prolonged (>48 hours) storage should be at −70°C. HSV stability is reduced significantly at 22°C compared with 4°C; in one study, median half-lives of virus in Copan CVM were 6.8 days (HSV-1) and 4.9 days (HSV-2) at 4°C but only 1.9 days (HSV-1) and 3.8 days (HSV-2) at 22°C (99). With other transport media, reported half-lives of HSV-1 have ranged from 0.5 to 4 days at 22°C and from 1 to 180 days at 4°C (100).

A single transport vial may provide specimen for both viral culture and direct antigen detection tests. Alternatively, slides for direct fluorescent antibody detection can be prepared immediately after collection by gently spreading the material on a swab in a thin layer over a clean microscope slide. The slide is air-dried and fixed in cold acetone before transport.

Fluids such as tracheal aspirates should be collected aseptically and transported without VTM. Urine should be collected by clean catch and refrigerated before transport. Once in the laboratory, urine is diluted 1:1 with culture medium prior to cell culture. Corneal samples are obtained with a scalpel blade, and cells are suspended in VTM. Tissue is placed in VTM in a sterile container. Prolonged storage of tissue requires immersion in sterile 50% neutral glycerol in saline or, alternatively, in culture medium with 5% fetal bovine serum. Fresh tissue samples can also be frozen, sectioned, applied to slides, and fixed in acetone.

DIRECT DETECTION

Detection of virus in patient samples without an intervening culture amplification step provides the most rapid diagnosis. PCR or other DNA amplification techniques provide the best sensitivity of the direct detection approaches and have become the method of choice for most laboratories. Immunostaining methods to detect antigen require less expertise than cytopathic effect (CPE)-based culture methods and are usually less expensive than culture or DNA amplification.

DNA Amplification

PCR or other amplification approaches are the most sensitive methods for direct detection of HSV (101). This is especially important in situations where sensitivity is critical, such as CSF, but recently PCR has been increasingly adopted for anogenital and other specimen types as well. For many years, DNA amplification for HSV was available in the United States only through laboratory-developed tests. In 2010, however, the FDA granted the first of several clearances to DNA-based HSV tests, and the availability of FDA-cleared assays has accelerated the trend from culture toward DNA testing. Several FDA-cleared direct-from-specimen assays have gained popularity due to limited hands-on time and high sensitivity (95 to 100%) and specificity (95 to 100%) (102–107). These assays do not require DNA extraction, and results are available in approximately 1 hour, with a hands-on time of 2 to 5 minutes, and show excellent reproducibility (108). Not all FDA-cleared direct-from-sample assays provide quantitative results like those that are typically provided by laboratory-developed or FDA-cleared *in vitro* diagnostic real-time PCR assays. Quantification of virus may be useful in monitoring the response to antiviral therapy, particularly in HSV encephalitis or neonatal herpes infections (109).

Whether testing is done in an FDA-cleared or laboratory-developed test format, precautions to prevent contamination of the sample and the inclusion of frequent negative controls within the assay are critical (110, 111). Some laboratories include isopsoralens or uracil-*N*-glycosylase in their PCR amplifications, preventing the amplification of PCR products in subsequent reactions. The likelihood of laboratory contamination by amplicon is reduced by using real-time PCR detection systems that eliminate the need for postamplification manipulation of the PCR product. Laboratories performing PCR testing should participate in a regular proficiency testing program, such as those provided by the College of American Pathologists (www.cap.org) or Quality Control for Molecular Diagnostics (www.qcmd.org).

Depending on the gene targets and detection methods, PCR can be set up to detect both HSV-1 and HSV-2 (94, 112) or to allow distinction of HSV-1 from HSV-2 (94, 113). PCR primers have been described amplifying portions of HSV genes encoding thymidine kinase (U_L23); DNA polymerase (U_L30); DNA binding protein (U_L42); glycoproteins B, C, D, and G (U_L27, U_L44, U_s6, U_s4, respectively); and many others. The choice of target gene is probably not a critical factor for HSV PCR, and efficient and sensitive assays have been developed using a variety of target genes. Instead, laboratories should ensure that the primers and probes in any contemplated assay follow the principles of efficient PCR assay design (114). Distinction of HSV-1 and HSV-2 can be achieved using type-specific primers or probes, melting curve analysis, restriction enzyme analysis, or direct sequencing. Ideally, typing information should be provided at the time of initial HSV detection, to avoid delays in providing appropriate prognosis, counseling, and medical management.

PCR is the gold standard for detection of HSV in CSF, neonatal, and ocular specimens and is increasingly used in other sample types as well. Substantial differences in performance have been reported in interlaboratory comparisons, particularly in sensitivity for detection of low-positive specimens (115). Published analytical sensitivities for detection of HSV in CSF for sample-to-answer platforms range from 50 to 250 copies per ml, although most package inserts report analytical sensitivity in terms of 50% tissue culture infective dose/ml (116, 117). There is no consensus on the required sensitivity for CSF testing, and interlaboratory differences are exacerbated by the current lack of an international reference standard for HSV. Thus, it is important to carefully consider the laboratory's or manufacturer's reputation, performance data, and test turnaround times before selecting a provider of DNA amplification testing.

As stated above, FDA-approved commercial molecular assays for HSV are a recent and growing phenomenon (Table 1) and were generally preceded by CE-marked assays that have been available in Europe for many years. The EraGen Multi-Code-RTx HSV 1&2 kit was FDA-cleared in 2010 for qualitative detection and typing of HSV in vaginal lesion swabs from symptomatic female patients only and is now available from Luminex Corp. (Austin, TX). The assay is based on PCR amplification using a synthetic isoC:isoG DNA base pair. It was initially cleared for use on samples extracted using the Roche MagNA Pure LC instrument and amplified on the Roche LightCycler real-time PCR instrument (Basel, Switzerland). FDA clearance was subsequently obtained for specimens extracted using the bioMérieux NucliSens easyMag extraction system as well. Luminex now markets this as an FDA-cleared qualitative HSV-1 and HSV-2 direct-from-sample assay on the ARIES platform; however, the assay is not FDA-cleared for CSF.

The ProbeTec herpes simplex viruses (HSV 1 & 2) Q^X amplified DNA assays (BD, Franklin Lakes, NJ) use strand displacement amplification for the qualitative detection and differentiation of HSV-1 and HSV-2. The assays

TABLE 1 FDA-cleared molecular amplification tests for HSV

Test	Manufacturer	Amplification technology	Approved specimen types	Qualitative vs quantitative	HSV typing?	Instrumentation
Multi-Code-RTx HSV 1&2 kit	Luminex, Austin, TX	PCR	Vaginal lesion swabs from symptomatic female patients	Qualitative	Yes	Extraction using Roche MagNA Pure LC or bioMérieux NucliSens easyMag; amplification on Roche LightCycler
ProbeTec herpes simplex viruses (HSV 1 & 2) Q^X amplified DNA assays	BD, Franklin Lakes, NJ	Strand displacement amplification	Clinician-collected external anogenital lesion specimens	Qualitative	Yes	BD Viper system in extracted mode
AmpliVue HSV 1+2 assay	Quidel, San Diego, CA	Helicase-dependent amplification	Cutaneous and mucocutaneous lesion specimens from symptomatic patients	Qualitative	Yes	Single-use handheld disposable detection device
FilmArray meningitis/ encephalitis	BioFire, Salt Lake City, UT	Nested real-time PCR	CSF	Qualitative	Yes	Sample to answer, single-use pouch
Simplexa HSV1&2 direct kit	Focus	PCR	CSF/swab	Qualitative	Yes	Sample to answer, single-use disc
Aries HSV1&2 assay	Luminex, Austin, TX	Real-time PCR	Swab	Qualitative	Yes	Sample to answer, single-use assay
Lyra Direct HSV1+2/VZV assay	Quidel, San Diego, CA	Real-time PCR	Swab	Qualitative	Yes	Extraction; amplification on variety of real-time thermocyclers
Solana HSV 1+2/ VZV assay	Quidel, San Diego, CA	Helicase-dependent amplification	Cutaneous and mucocutaneous lesion specimens from symptomatic patients	Qualitative	Yes	Dedicated amplification/ detection instrument
artus HSV-1/2 QS-RGQ MDx kit	Qiagen	Real-time PCR	Swab	Qualitative	Yes	Qiasymphony extraction, Rotor-Gene Q MDx amplification
Cobas HSV1 and 2 test	Roche, Switzerland	Real-time PCR	Swab	Qualitative	Yes	Cobas 4800 extraction
Anyplex II HSV-1/2 assay	Seegene, South Korea	Real-time PCR	Swab, female	Qualitative	Yes	Qiagen extraction, Cepheid SmartCycler II Dx amplification
Sentosa SA201 HSV-1/2 PCR test	Vela, Fairfield, NJ	Real-time PCR	Male or female skin lesions from anogenital or oral sites	Qualitative	Yes	Rotor-Gene Q MDx 5plex HRM instrument

are performed on the fully automated BD Viper system in extracted mode and were FDA cleared in 2011 for testing of clinician-collected external anogenital lesion specimens. In a large head-to-head comparison, the assay proved to be far more sensitive than culture and had specificity and sensitivity of 95.1 to 100% compared to the University of Washington PCR assay (118).

The IsoAmp HSV assay (BioHelix, Beverly, MA) is FDA cleared for detection of HSV-1 and -2 in genital and oral lesion specimens from symptomatic patients. The IsoAmp HSV assay was based on a helicase-dependent amplification technology and a unique single-use handheld disposable detection device, allowing rapid (1.5 hour) turnaround time. The assay did not differentiate between HSV-1 and -2. In a comparison with viral culture, the IsoAmp HSV assay had a sensitivity of 100% and a specificity of 96.3%; the analytical sensitivities for HSV-1 and HSV-2 were 5.5 and 34.1 copies per reaction, respectively (119). After the acquisition of BioHelix by Quidel (San Diego, CA), the isothermal helicase-dependent amplification technology was incorporated into the FDA-cleared Quidel AmpliVue HSV 1+2 assay, which provides differentiation of HSV-1 from HSV-2. Quidel also offers the FDA-cleared Lyra Direct HSV 1+2/VZV assay, which is a multiplex PCR assay that detects and differentiates HSV-1, HSV-2, and varicella-zoster virus, and the Solana HSV 1+2/VZV assay, a multiplex helicase-dependent amplification-based test for the detection and differentiation of HSV-1, HSV-2, and VZV.

Other rapid sample-to-answer FDA-cleared tests include the BioFire FilmArray meningitis/encephalitis panel and the Focus Simplexa HSV-1 and HSV-2. Of these, only the Simplexa is cleared for both CSF and swabs. The FilmArray detects 14 pathogens directly from CSF, in addition to HSV1/2, and had a sensitivity of 100% on 16 HSV1/2-positive specimens across 1,560 prospectively collected CSF specimens (117). Notably, three false-positive HSV1/2 results were found during the study; these and similar false-positive HSV results have been ascribed to preanalytical contamination (120). The Simplexa assay also showed 96.2% (50/52) sensitivity and 97.9% (47/48) specificity on 100 CSF specimens, and further testing of discrepant samples suggested that sensitivity could be 100% (105).

Other Nucleic Acid-Based Tests

In situ hybridization or solution hybridization methods are not as widely used as DNA amplification, indirect fluorescent antigen, or direct fluorescent antibody assay (DFA). These tests use DNA or RNA probes, some of which are type specific. The sensitivity of direct hybridization methods is limited (approximately 1×10^5 copies/ml), and thus these approaches have been largely replaced by PCR or other amplification methods.

Microscopy

Changes that are characteristic for HSV are sometimes visible in fixed, stained cells from lesions (Tzanck preparations) or cervical scrapings (Papanicalou stains) or hematoxylin and eosin stains of fixed tissue (121). Enlarged or degenerating cells, syncytium formation, chromatin margination, a "ground glass" appearance of the cytoplasm, and nuclear inclusions are typical of HSV-infected cells. These methods are widely available but lack sensitivity and specificity (122). Virus-specific methods are preferred.

Antigen

Slides are prepared with cells from the patient's specimen, fixed, and coated with antibody preparations against HSV-1 and HSV-2 or against type-common epitopes. Some manufacturers offer dual anti-HSV and anti-VZV reagent combinations. If the antibodies are linked to a fluorophore such as fluorescein isothiocyanate, the test is a DFA. If bound anti-HSV antibodies are detected with secondary antibodies conjugated to fluorophore, the test is an indirect fluorescent antibody assay. Same-well testing can be performed using antibody conjugates with different fluorophores for HSV-1 and HSV-2 (123). DFA is 10 to 87% as sensitive as culture, with higher sensitivity from vesicular lesions and poor sensitivity from healing lesions (48). DFA is far less sensitive than PCR (124), and validated commercial kits for DFA are not readily available. The reported sensitivity of cytospin DFA has varied widely; in one study it was higher than culture for detecting HSV from swab specimens (125), while another study, using different DFA antibody and cell culture systems, reported sensitivity of 31% versus culture (126). Different sample types such as ocular or mucosal swabs may vary widely in providing adequate cells for accurate DFA results. The Light Diagnostics Simulfluor assay (Millipore, Billerica, MA) has been reported to have a sensitivity of 80.0% and a specificity of 98.8% compared to culture (123) and a sensitivity of 86.2% in a multimethod comparison including two PCR-based assays (127). Immunohistochemistry has been described for the detection of HSV in tissue but suffers from the same reduced sensitivities compared to culture and molecular methods (128).

ISOLATION PROCEDURES

Although molecular testing is increasingly preferred, virus detection methods including culture and modified culture are used to diagnose mucocutaneous, genital, and ocular lesions (Table 2). Conventional culture uses cells that are permissive for HSV-1 and HSV-2 as well as other viruses that may be of diagnostic importance. Inoculated cells are examined frequently for CPE (see below). In our laboratory, 95% of HSV isolates produce CPE by day 5; only 5% require 5 to 14 days. Mink lung cells, rhabdomyosarcoma cells, human diploid fibroblasts such as MRC-5 and WI-38, and human epidermoid carcinoma lines such as HEp-2 and A549 are commercially available. Direct comparisons suggest that test sensitivity can be markedly affected by the cells used, particularly with a low-titer HSV inoculum (129).

Infected cells develop cytoplasmic granulation and then become large, round, and refractile. Clusters or "foci" of infected cells appear early after inoculation in diploid fibroblast or epidermoid carcinoma lines (Fig. 1). CPE in A549 cells is characterized by syncytium formation; particularly with HSV-2 (130). Cells then lyse and detach from the substrate with eventual destruction of the monolayer. Other readouts from cell culture such as the shell vial culture with indirect fluorescent antigen or engineered beta-galactosidase reporters with DFA (ELVIS system) allow for more sensitive and rapid culture-based typing of HSV, with turnaround times as short as 1 day (131). Culture remains helpful when testing for acyclovir resistance is required, and it can be less expensive than molecular methods, but the increased sensitivity and limited hands-on time of PCR relative to culture limit its overall utility.

IDENTIFICATION AND TYPING

Other viruses, as well as toxic factors in specimens, can mimic the CPE of HSV (Fig. 2A). Confirmation of putative HSV CPE is accomplished using commercially available polyclonal or monoclonal antibodies against type-common

TABLE 2 Selected diagnostic tests for HSV

Syndrome	Sample	Lab tests	Comment
Oral or genital lesion	Swab in VTM	Culture, shell vial	Viability must be preserved.
		DFA, cytospin DFA	Cell architecture must be maintained.
		PCR	Better stability than culture.
Recurrent genital symptoms; culture-negative	Serum	Western blot	Limited availability. Good confirmatory test.
	Serum	gG-specific ELISA	FDA approved
	Capillary blood	gG-based point-of-care tests	FDA approved
	Swab in VTM	PCR	Better sensitivity than culture
Neonatal herpes	CSF; blood in EDTA	PCR	Collect separate CSF for PCR.
	Eye, mouth, nasal, and rectal swabs	Culture, DFA, PCR	Blood in EDTA (purple top)
Ocular herpes	Swab in VTM	PCR, culture, DFA	Clinical presentation may be sufficient for diagnosis.
Conjunctivitis	Corneal scraping	PCR, culture, DFA	
Dendritic corneal ulcers			
Encephalitis	CSF, brain tissue	PCR	Culture of CSF should not be performed.
Recurrent lymphocytic meningitis	CSF	PCR	Culture is far less sensitive than PCR and is not recommended.

or type-specific epitopes. The most widely used reagents are fluorescein conjugated for use in fluorescent antibody tests (Table 3). Spin amplification methods reduce the time required to detect HSV in culture by detecting viral proteins before CPE develops (129). The most widely used technique involves centrifuging the sample onto monolayers of cells on cover slips that are placed in the bottom of small vials ("shell vials") or in the wells of flat-bottomed plates. After 16 to 48 hours' incubation, the cover slips or plates are subjected to antigen detection tests for HSV (123). Increasingly, typing and identification are performed by molecular methods. All of the direct-from-sample tests described above (Luminex Aries, BioFire meningitis/encephalitis, Focus Simplexa) differentiate between HSV-1 and HSV-2 during the initial PCR and do not require additional tests for identification.

SEROLOGIC TESTS

Because nearly all HSV structural proteins have extensive antigenic cross-reactivity, only IgG tests based on the type-specific HSV gG accurately distinguish HSV-1 and HSV-2 antibodies (21, 132, 133). Tests based on crude antigen mixtures are still marketed but have unacceptably low sensitivity and specificity, especially for detecting new HSV-2 infections in those with prior HSV-1 (21, 132, 134, 135). FDA-approved IgM tests decrease the time to detecting seroconversion in new infections but cannot accurately distinguish new from established infections (136). IgM-based tests can also be prone to false-positive results (137, 138) and thus should be confirmed by other approaches. Tests for HSV-2 antibody avidity can discriminate accurately between first episodes (low avidity) and recurrent episodes (high avidity) in most cases (139). However, these tests are not commercially available.

Western Blot

The HSV Western blot used by the University of Washington laboratory uses nitrocellulose blots prepared with human diploid fibroblast-infected cell proteins. Western blot detects antibodies to multiple viral proteins, including those to the type-specific glycoproteins gG-1 and gG-2 (140). About 20% of sera must be preabsorbed against sepharose beads coated with HSV-1 or HSV-2 proteins and retested to give definitive results. This combination of tests gives a very accurate determination of HSV-1 versus HSV-2 antibody status (140) and is considered the "gold standard" for comparison of other serologic assays.

Commercial Type-Specific gG-Based Assays

A number of manufacturers now offer FDA-approved assays using gG as the target antigen. As noted above, gG-based assays are preferred over those based on crude antigen mixtures, due to their ability to distinguish antibodies to HSV-1 versus HSV-2. Microplate format enzyme immunoassays (EIAs) include the HerpeSelect ELISA (enzyme-linked immunosorbent assay) from Focus Diagnostics (Cypress, CA), the Captia HSV 1 and HSV 2 IgG type-specific ELISA test kits (Trinity Biotech, Bray, Ireland), the anti-HSV-1 and anti-HSV-2 ELISA IgG kits from Euroimmun (Lubeck, Germany), the HSV-1 IgG ELISA test from Gold Standard Diagnostics (Davis, CA), the SeraQuest HSV-1- and HSV-2-specific IgG assays (Miami, FL), and the Zeus ELISA HSV-1 and -2 test systems (Raritan, NJ). The Roche Elecsys HSV-1 IgG and HSV-2 IgG assays are FDA cleared for use on several automated immunoassay instruments. Some newer assays utilize microparticle-based detection technology, which provides the possibility of multiplexing and offers potential advantages in assay throughput and reproducibility. The Plexus HerpeSelect 1 and 2 IgG test kit (Focus, Cypress, CA), the BioPlex 2200 HSV-1 and -2 kit (Bio-Rad), and the AtheNA Multi-lyte HSV1&2 (Zeus Scientific, Raritan, NJ) utilize Luminex detection technology (Luminex, Austin, TX). The Liaison HSV-1 and HSV-2 type-specific IgG tests are bead-based chemiluminescent immunoassays requiring the use of the Liaison Analyzer (Diasorin, Saluggia, Italy). Finally, simple gG-based lateral flow assays are available that are designed for point-of-care testing. These include the HerpeSelect Express IgG (Focus Diagnostics), which distinguishes antibodies to HSV-1 and HSV-2, and the BiokitHSV-2 Rapid Test (Biokit, Barcelona, Spain).

The commercial gG-based tests perform well in clinical use in North America. When compared with the University of Washington Western blot, HerpeSelect ELISA had 91 to 96% sensitivity with 92 to 95% specificity for HSV-1, and 96 to 100% sensitivity with 96 to 97% specificity for HSV-2. HerpeSelect Immunoblot had 99 to 100% sensitivity with 93 to 96% specificity for HSV-1, and 97 to 100% sensitivity and 94 to 98% specificity for HSV-2 (133). The BioPlex assay had sensitivity and specificity for HSV-1 of 85% and 98% and for HSV-2 of 100% and 95%,

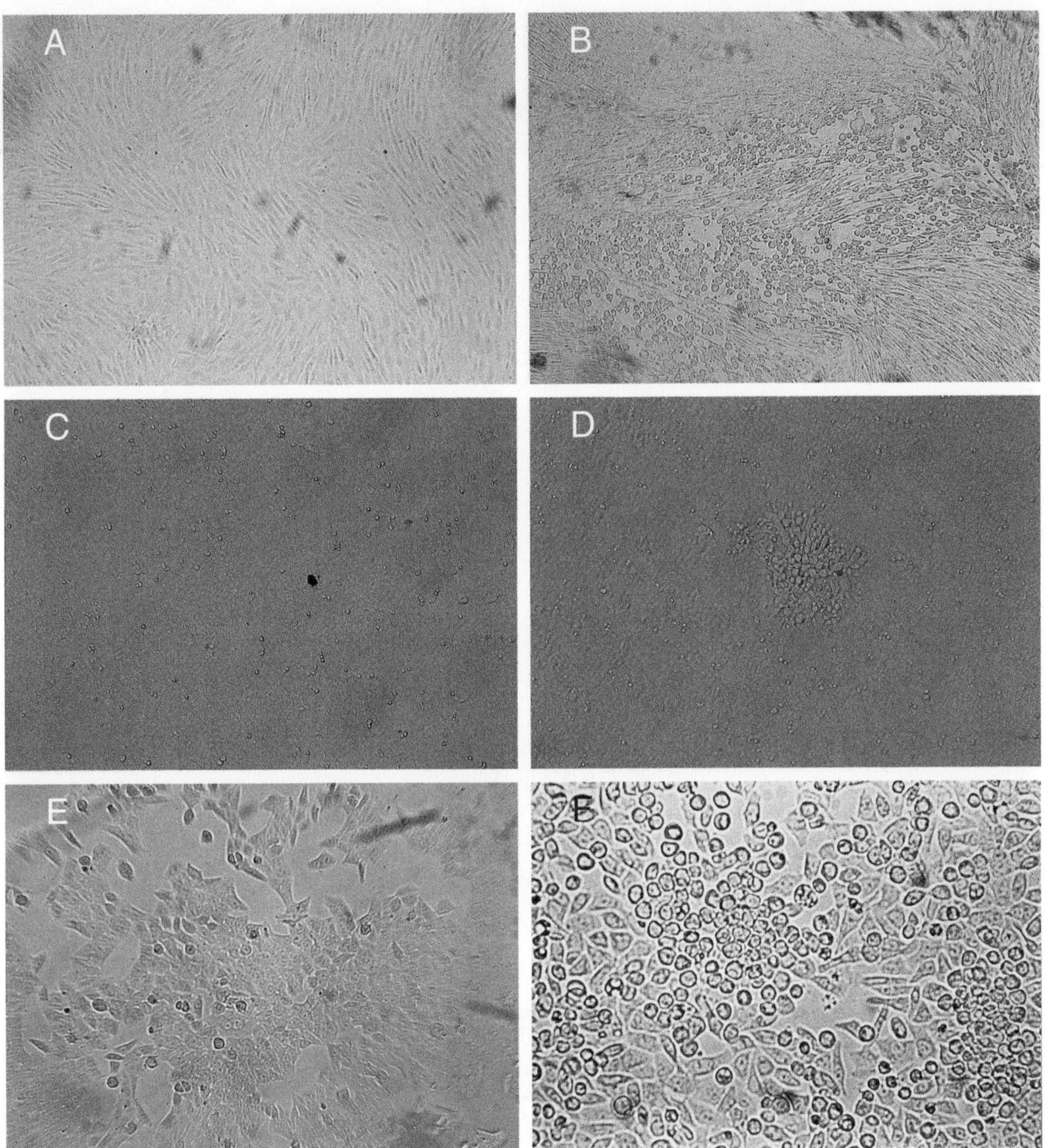

FIGURE 1 (A) Normal human diploid fibroblasts. Magnification, ×400. (B) HSV-1 in human diploid fibroblasts. Magnification, ×400. (C) Normal mink lung. Magnification, ×100. (D) HSV-2 in mink lung cells. Magnification, ×100. (E) Normal Hep-2 cells. Magnification, ×400. (F) HSV-2 in Hep-2 cells. Magnification, ×400.

respectively, when compared to Western blot (136). The Luminex-based assays show good agreement with the Focus HerpeSelect EIA: 94.9% for the AtheNA Multi-lyte HSV1&2, 97.8% for the BioPlex 2200 HSV-1 and -2 kit, and 97.4% for the Plexus HerpeSelect 1 and 2 IgG test kit (141). For point-of-care tests, the POCkit-HSV-2 test (now BiokitHSV-2 Rapid Test) had 93 to 96% sensitivity with 95 to 98% specificity in comparison tests (133). While performance characteristics against Western blot are not available, the HerpeSelect Express IgG assay had 100% sensitivity and 97.3% specificity when compared to the HerpeSelect ELISA (142). The median time to seroconversion is approximately 2 to 3 weeks for HerpeSelect-HSV ELISA and the BiokitHSV-2 Rapid Test (143, 144).

ANTIVIRAL SUSCEPTIBILITIES

Acyclovir-resistant strains of HSV typically result from mutation of the gene encoding the viral thymidine kinase and more rarely from mutations in the HSV polymerase,

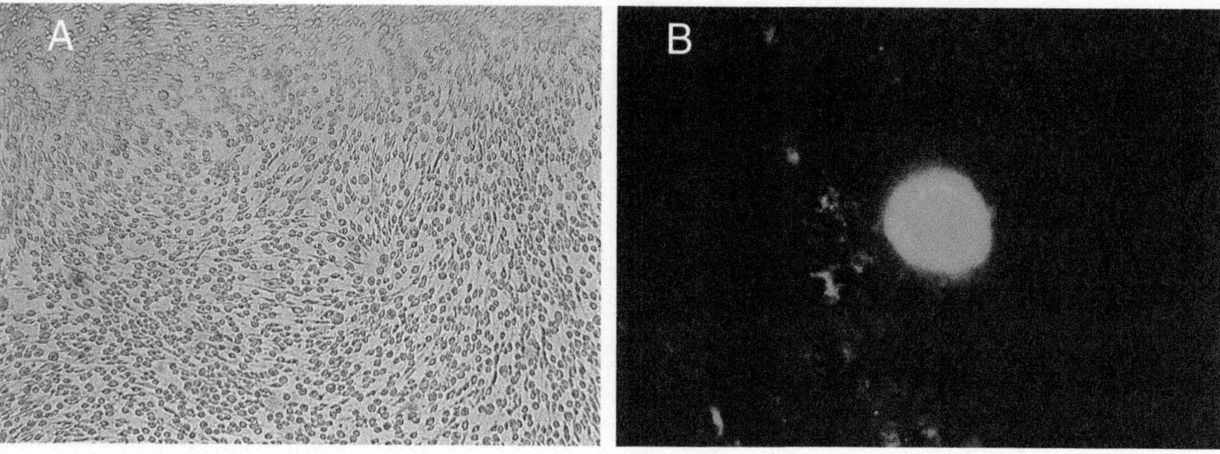

FIGURE 2 (A) Toxicity in human diploid fibroblasts. Magnification, ×100. (B) HSV-2 direct fluorescent antibody confirmatory test.

while foscarnet resistance arises due to mutations in the HSV polymerase only. Resistance to pritelivir, a newer antiviral for HSV, is associated with mutations in the HSV helicase and primase genes but has not been seen *in vivo* (145). Prolonged use of antivirals can lead to selection of resistant strains, especially in immunocompromised individuals and neonates (146). Strains with detectable *in vitro* resistance can also be isolated from patients who have never received acyclovir (147). Such isolates are rarely of clinical significance in immunocompetent individuals, and these people generally respond well to acyclovir (148). However, resistance can occasionally be observed in immune-privileged sites even in immunocompetent individuals (149). Acyclovir-resistant HSV can lead to treatment failure (148), and thus laboratory confirmation of resistance can inform patient management decisions. Some patients with suspected acyclovir-resistant virus respond to increased dosage of drug. For most patients, second-line therapy requires the use of less desirable drugs such as foscarnet or cidofovir. However, since some mutations in the HSV polymerase cause acyclovir resistance but do not affect sensitivity to penciclovir, testing for susceptibility to individual antivirals may be warranted in certain circumstances (146), because it may allow the use of a less toxic drug.

Susceptibility testing can be performed by phenotypic assays, because genotypic tests are currently for research use only. Among the phenotypic assays, plaque reduction is considered the gold standard (146, 148). Alternative phenotypic assays include antigen reduction by EIA and genome reduction by DNA hybridization (146). In general, a 50% inhibitory concentration of <2 μg/ml is used as the threshold for susceptibility and correlates relatively well with clinical response (150). However, false determinations of resistance are common in the various phenotypic assays, and interlaboratory variability is significant (146). Thus, clinical correlation of testing results is essential. Given the long turnaround time of phenotypic testing for antiviral resistance and improvements in sequencing, there is likely a future role for genotypic antiviral susceptibility testing. Currently, a major drawback of genotypic assays is that frameshift or nonsense mutations are possible throughout the relevant gene, requiring complete sequencing of the

TABLE 3 Monoclonal antibodies for HSV-1 and HSV-2 detection, confirmation, and typing by immunofluorescence

Reagent	Source	Intended use	Comments
Light Diagnostics SimulFluor HSV 1/2	Millipore, Billerica, MA	Confirmation of CPE in cell culture Direct examination of clinical specimens prepared by cytospin	HSV-1: whole-cell stain (apple green) HSV-2: cytoplasmic or membrane stain (yellow) Simultaneous testing for both HSV-1, HSV-2
Light Diagnostics SimulFluor HSV/VZV	Millipore, Billerica, MA	Confirmation of CPE in cell culture Direct examination of clinical specimens prepared by cytospin	Simultaneous testing for both HSV-1, HSV-2, and VZV
Light Diagnostics HSV1 and HSV2 DFA typing kit	Millipore, Billerica, MA	Differentiation of HSV-1 and HSV-2 in direct specimens and cell culture	Requires separate spots for HSV-1 and HSV-2
D3 DFA identification and typing kit	Diagnostic Hybrids, Athens, OH	Confirmation of CPE and typing in cell culture	HSV-1: strong focal nuclear staining HSV-2: strong nuclear and perinuclear staining
MicroTrak HSV 1 & 2 culture ID/typing test	Trinity Biotech, Jamestown, NY	Confirmation of CPE and typing in cell culture Antigen detection prior to CPE by shell vial	HSV-1: nuclear staining HSV-2: strong nuclear stain, with speckled cytoplasmic staining

gene for definitive results (146). More complete databases of mutations associated with antiviral resistance will be required to definitively link genotype to resistance.

EVALUATION, INTERPRETATION, AND REPORTING OF RESULTS

Laboratory results are best interpreted in the context of the patient's presentation and history and with the knowledge of the natural history of HSV infection.

Interpretation of Virus Detection Tests

Interpretation of positive test results depends on the specificity of the test. Specificity of culture is extremely high if confirmatory tests are performed. With its excellent sensitivity and specificity, PCR is the test of choice in most situations. PCR is most reliable when closed system methods are used and lab practices are strictly followed to avoid contamination of specimens with exogenous HSV DNA. Even when using a closed system, preanalytical contamination of HSV PCR assays may occur, either at the ordering site or in the laboratory. Despite these caveats, in practice, positive culture or PCR results are highly diagnostic in patients with lesions due to gingivostomatitis, genital herpes, or ocular infections. Positive fluorescent antibody tests from lesions or ocular swabs are considered reliable. HSV found in the CNS, in tissues, in blood, or in the eye by culture or PCR is diagnostic. Positive cultures or positive PCR tests in symptomatic infants at 1 to 3 weeks of life are highly diagnostic (151).

For other patients, interpretation of a positive viral detection test requires caution. One potential confounding issue is the simultaneous presence of multiple potential pathogens. For example, respiratory secretions from immunocompromised patients may contain HSV in addition to the presumably causative agent such as respiratory syncytial, influenza, parainfluenza, or adenovirus (152, 153). HSV may also be shed concurrently with other pathogens from oral or anogenital sites or may not be the cause of the episodic syndrome that triggered testing. Syphilis and chancroid are the most likely alternative causes of genital ulcers in the United States. In a series of patients with genital ulcers other than those typical of herpes (vesiculopustular lesions), 65% had only herpes detected, while 20% had both syphilis and herpes detected (154). HSV results from such patients need to be interpreted in the context of laboratory testing for other pathogens in the differential diagnosis. Symptoms of HSV gingivostomatitis or genital infection can be mimicked by noninfectious causes, such as Stevens-Johnson syndrome, or by other infectious agents. Because of the sporadic nature of asymptomatic HSV shedding (155), swabs of oral or anogenital sites can also yield positive HSV culture, PCR, or antigen tests when the underlying cause of disease is not herpes. Even in meningitis, an HSV-positive result may not mean that clinicians should not consider additional causes; clinical correlation is always required (120). The increasing availability of syndromic multiplex testing will likely help increase our understanding of the role of multiple pathogens in infection.

Positive cultures or PCR results from skin, conjunctival, mouth, or nasal swabs from neonates less than 24 hours old may reflect maternal virus rather than neonatal infection. Neonates born to mothers shedding HSV from the genital tract at labor and delivery may be tested 24 to 72 hours after birth, the likely time frame for receiving maternal culture or PCR results. Most babies developing neonatal herpes present between 9 and 14 days of life (156), well beyond the time frame where maternal viral contamination would be a problem. However, early initiation of therapy is strongly associated with a favorable outcome (157), and thus current opinion favors aggressive monitoring and treatment (61).

PCR has adequate sensitivity to detect shedding of HSV in individuals with asymptomatic infection or negative cultures (158–160) and also to detect HSV in CSF, a specimen with a low yield of HSV by culture. The sensitivity of HSV PCR for HSV encephalitis has been reported to be about 96%, and the specificity 99% (105, 117, 161). Since the viral load in CSF can be quite low in HSV encephalitis, it is critical that PCR assays are optimized to provide the best possible limit of detection. PCR has much greater sensitivity than culture for detection of genital HSV-2 both from lesions and during periods of subclinical shedding (52). PCR can detect virus early in lesion development before culture positivity and can remain positive for several days after HSV lesions become negative by culture (158, 162). PCR positivity in such cases probably represents infectious virus below the limit of detection by culture, and PCR positivity is quickly lost in the absence of active shedding (159). False negatives can occur in PCR, due to reaction failure or the presence of inhibitors in clinical specimens. It is therefore critical that only negative reactions accompanied by positive internal controls be accepted as true negatives (163). In addition, PCR false negatives can occur due to sequence variation in the primer- or probe-binding regions (127). Importantly, a negative PCR result for HSV does not rule out HSV disease, since specimens taken very early or late in the course of disease may not have viral DNA (164). This is especially true in pediatric populations; for example, in one series, nearly 25% of infants with CNS HSV infections had negative CSF PCR results (151). The specificity of PCR for detection of HSV encephalitis has been reported to be greater than 98% (165); thus, all HSV-positive PCR results demand immediate attention. In patients with CNS HSV infections, HSV PCR may become negative after about 7 days of antiviral therapy (161). The persistence or reemergence of virus after antiviral therapy has been associated with a poor clinical outcome (166).

Quantitative PCR may be useful in monitoring the response to antiviral therapy. Successful therapy is associated with a decline in viral load in the CSF (109, 167–169), and a long duration of viral detectability is associated with poor outcome (170). Quantification of HSV may also have prognostic value. Patients with higher viral loads have been reported to have worse clinical outcomes (171); in one study, those with >100 copies/μl (100,000 copies/ml) of CSF had worse outcomes than patients with lower levels (169). However, other groups have reported no association between CSF viral load and clinical outcome (167, 168, 170, 172).

Interpretation of Type-Specific Serology

Type-specific serology is useful when culture or other virus detection methods are not available, when specimen collection or transport is inadequate, or for evaluation of serostatus in the absence of clinical disease. Serology based on gG-1 and gG-2 is vital for diagnosing subclinical and unrecognized HSV infections. Many experts believe that better recognition of genital HSV-2 infections by increased use of accurate gG-based serologic tests could help slow the spread of genital herpes (173–175). However, the U.S. Preventive Services Task Force, after review of potential benefit and harm, recently recommended against serologic screening for genital HSV infection in asymptomatic people (176).

As with other herpes laboratory tests, serology tests based on gG must be ordered and interpreted with care. First, due to the low specificity of non-gG-based commercial tests, it is important to ensure that a gG-based test is used. If so, a positive test for HSV-2 antibodies in a patient with genital lesions is highly likely to be a true positive. A positive HSV-2 antibody test in a patient without a history compatible with genital herpes may be a false positive and should be confirmed by testing with a different type-specific test (177). Negative HSV-2 test results in a patient with symptomatic genital disease may indicate genital HSV-1; no test can distinguish between antibodies elicited by oral versus genital HSV-1, and definitive diagnosis in such cases rests on direct detection of virus. False-negative tests may also occur during seroconversion; sera drawn 4 to 6 weeks later should also be tested. While "index values" in HSV-2 EIAs have been shown to rise during seroconversion, index values alone are not reliable indicators of early versus established infection (178). IgM tests based on gG-1 and gG-2 are not available commercially. The available IgM tests cannot distinguish new from established symptomatic episodes with sufficient accuracy and are not recommended (136).

As noted above, type-specific serology is critical for identifying pregnant women with new HSV infections, who are at high risk for transmitting virus to their neonates (61, 175). Determining HSV-2 serostatus early in pregnancy has been recommended so that treatment options can be considered (175). If a herpes culture from the anogenital region is positive at labor or delivery, a negative maternal type-specific serology indicates high risk (30 to 50%) for neonatal herpes. A positive maternal serology by Western blot or equivalent test indicates a lower risk of transmission (1 to 3%).

HERPES B VIRUS

Description of the Agent

Herpes B virus, also known as Macacine (formerly Cercopithecine) herpesvirus 1 or monkey B virus, is similar to HSV in terms of genome size and structure and in terms of virion morphology. Herpes B virus DNA has 161 ± 12 kilobase pairs (179) and is extremely (approximately 75%) G+C rich.

The replication cycle of herpes B virus is very similar to HSV. Herpes B virus is detectable as soon as 6 hours postinfection, and titers of virus stabilize by 24 to 36 hours (180). At least nine herpes B virus glycoproteins have been identified, and at least two of these share antigenic determinants with glycoproteins B and D of HSV (181). As an enveloped virus, herpes B virus can be inactivated by lipid solvents, UV light, or heat, and thus, cell-free virus is inactivated rapidly in the environment.

Clinical Significance

Herpes B virus is the simian counterpart to HSV in Old World monkeys of the genus *Macaca*, including the rhesus, cynomolgus, Japanese, Taiwan, and stumptail macaques. The virus can affect the oropharynx or genital areas and is spread between animals via biting, sexual activity, or other close contact (182, 183). The seroprevalence of herpes B virus among adult macaques in the wild is nearly 75% (184). Among animals housed in outdoor breeding corrals, the seroprevalence is approximately 22% before 2.5 years of age, rising to more than 97% among animals 2.5 years or older (185). Primary infection in the macaque is often asymptomatic, but the virus establishes latency and can reactivate. Reactivation can be triggered by stress, such as the transition of animals from freedom to captivity, or crowded conditions. Recurrent disease in macaques is typically characterized by vesicular lesions of the tongue and buccal mucosa, progressing to ulceration. Encephalitis is rare but can occur. Asymptomatic shedding of virus can occur.

In 1932 a researcher was bitten by a macaque and developed ascending myelitis and encephalitis, culminating in death. Herpes B virus was subsequently described (186). Sporadic cases of herpes B virus infection in humans have subsequently been described in the literature. Humans can be infected via animal bites, mucosal or eye exposure (187), inoculation of broken skin, needlesticks, or potentially, via aerosols. The possibility of herpes B virus transmission makes macaques unsuitable as pets (188). Safety precautions for workers with close contact with macaques and recommendations for postexposure management have been published (189). Primary cell cultures from macaques also represent a potential source of virus (189).

Herpes B virus disease is severe in humans, with a mortality rate of 70% or higher without treatment. The first symptoms usually appear 3 to 5 days after exposure (although they can appear up to several weeks later) and include a localized vesicular lesion at the site of inoculation, erythema, and edema. Lymphangitis and lymphadenopathy follow, with fever, myalgia, vomiting, and cramping. Neurologic signs develop quickly, starting with meningeal irritation, diplopia, and altered sensation, progressing to paralysis, altered mentation, respiratory depression, seizures, and death within 10 days to 6 weeks. Human-to-human transmission appears to be extremely rare (190). Asymptomatic infection in humans also appears to be rare. In one study of over 300 primate handlers (of whom more than 150 had a history of exposures), none had antibody to herpes B virus (191).

Acyclovir is effective against herpes B virus, although the 50% effective dose is 10-fold higher than for HSV. Ganciclovir is somewhat more effective than acyclovir (192), although clinical experience with ganciclovir is limited. Foscarnet has also been used in some cases (187). Postexposure therapy can often prevent the development of acute disease (193). The preferred drug for postexposure prophylaxis is oral valacyclovir (189), due to its improved bioavailability (189). Clinical disease necessitates intravenous antiviral therapy. Intravenous therapy should be continued until symptoms resolve and two or more viral cultures are negative after having been held for 10 to 14 days, at which time therapy can be switched to oral antivirals (189). Reactivation and relapse have occurred in some patients upon cessation of antiviral therapy. Many clinicians therefore recommend continuing oral antiviral therapy indefinitely.

Collection, Transport, and Storage of Specimens

Because herpes B virus should be propagated only under biosafety level 4 conditions, diagnostic specimens are best handled by specialized reference laboratories (see below). Other laboratories should take precautions to ensure that herpes B virus specimens are not confused with HSV specimens and thus cultured under lower biosafety conditions, since amplification of virus in culture increases the risk to laboratory personnel. Lesion swabs should be taken from each collection site using separate, sterile Dacron or cotton swabs with wooden or plastic shafts. Swabs or biopsy tissue should be placed into separate tubes containing 1 to 2 ml of viral transport media. Specimens can be stored in the refrigerator for up to 1 week or at $<-60°$ C indefinitely.

Reference Laboratories for Herpes B

Advice regarding proper specimen collection and submission of specimens for herpes B diagnosis can be obtained from the CDC (http://www.cdc.gov/herpesbvirus/index.html) or from the National B Virus Resource Laboratory, Atlanta, GA (404-413-6550; http://www.gsu.edu/bvirus).

Identification of Virus and Serodiagnosis

Herpes B virus can be cultured in monkey kidney and chick embryo cells. A characteristic cytopathic effect similar to that of HSV is seen, with polykaryon formation and intranuclear Cowdry type A inclusion bodies. Confirmation of herpes B virus in culture can be done using monoclonal antibodies or molecular techniques. PCR for herpes B virus (194–196) is generally preferred over culture for diagnostic purposes, since it is comparatively rapid, highly sensitive and specific, and avoids the need to amplify infectious virus to high titers.

Serodiagnosis of herpes B virus infections has been complicated by extensive cross-reactivity with HSV-1 and HSV-2. However, careful ELISA and Western blot tests have been developed that allow discrimination of antibodies to herpes B virus, HSV-1, and HSV-2 (197–199). Serologic testing can be useful for evaluation of potentially infected animals involved in human exposures and for screening research animals. Serial determinations of serostatus from potentially exposed individuals are also useful adjuncts for diagnosis (187, 189).

REFERENCES

1. **Gentry GA, Rana S, Hutchinson M, Starr P.** 1988. Evolution of herpes and pox viruses and their hosts: a problem with the molecular clock. *Intervirology* **29:**277–280.
2. **Gentry GA, Lowe M, Alford G, Nevins R.** 1988. Sequence analyses of herpesviral enzymes suggest an ancient origin for human sexual behavior. *Proc Natl Acad Sci USA* **85:** 2658–2661.
3. **Lowenstein.** 1919. Aetiologische untersuchungen uber den fieberhaften, herpes. *Meunch Med Wochenschr* **66:**769–770.
4. **Burnet FM, Williams SW.** 1939. Herpes simplex: a new point of view. *Med J Aust* **1:**637–642.
5. **Brain RT.** 1932. The demonstration of herpetic antibody in human sera by complement fixation, and the correlation between its presence and infection with herpes virus. *Br J Exp Pathol* **13:**166–167.
6. **Croughan WS, Behbehani AM.** 1988. Comparative study of inactivation of herpes simplex virus types 1 and 2 by commonly used antiseptic agents. *J Clin Microbiol* **26:**213–215.
7. **Tyler R, Ayliffe GA.** 1987. A surface test for virucidal activity of disinfectants: preliminary study with herpes virus. *J Hosp Infect* **9:**22–29.
8. **Spear PG.** 2004. Herpes simplex virus: receptors and ligands for cell entry. *Cell Microbiol* **6:**401–410.
9. **Heldwein EE, Krummenacher C.** 2008. Entry of herpesviruses into mammalian cells. *Cell Mol Life Sci* **65:**1653–1668.
10. **Tognon M, Furlong D, Conley AJ, Roizman B.** 1981. Molecular genetics of herpes simplex virus. V. Characterization of a mutant defective in ability to form plaques at low temperatures and in a viral fraction which prevents accumulation of coreless capsids at nuclear pores late in infection. *J Virol* **40:** 870–880.
11. **Batterson W, Furlong D, Roizman B.** 1983. Molecular genetics of herpes simplex virus. VII. Further characterization of a temperature-sensitive mutant defective in release of viral DNA and in other stages of viral reproductive cycle. *J Virol* **45:** 397–407.
12. **Diefenbach RJ, Miranda-Saksena M, Douglas MW, Cunningham AL.** 2008. Transport and egress of herpes simplex virus in neurons. *Rev Med Virol* **18:**35–51.
13. **Ashley R, Koelle DM.** 1992. Immune responses to genital herpes infection, p 201–238. *In* Quinn TC (ed), *Advances in Host Defense Mechanisms: Sexually Transmitted Diseases*, vol 8. Raven Press, New York, NY.
14. **Cunningham AL, Turner RR, Miller AC, Para MF, Merigan TC.** 1985. Evolution of recurrent herpes simplex lesions. An immunohistologic study. *J Clin Invest* **75:**226–233.
15. **Koelle DM, Posavad CM, Barnum GR, Johnson ML, Frank JM, Corey L.** 1998. Clearance of HSV-2 from recurrent genital lesions correlates with infiltration of HSV-specific cytotoxic T lymphocytes. *J Clin Invest* **101:**1500–1508.
16. **Zhu J, Koelle DM, Cao J, Vazquez J, Huang ML, Hladik F, Wald A, Corey L.** 2007. Virus-specific CD8+ T cells accumulate near sensory nerve endings in genital skin during subclinical HSV-2 reactivation. *J Exp Med* **204:**595–603.
17. **Zhu J, Peng T, Johnston C, Phasouk K, Kask AS, Klock A, Jin L, Diem K, Koelle DM, Wald A, Robins H, Corey L.** 2013. Immune surveillance by CD8αα+ skin-resident T cells in human herpes virus infection. *Nature* **497:**494–497.
18. **Knickelbein JE, Khanna KM, Yee MB, Baty CJ, Kinchington PR, Hendricks RL.** 2008. Noncytotoxic lytic granule-mediated CD8+ T cell inhibition of HSV-1 reactivation from neuronal latency. *Science* **322:**268–271.
19. **Dix RD, Pereira L, Baringer JR.** 1981. Use of monoclonal antibody directed against herpes simplex virus glycoproteins to protect mice against acute virus-induced neurological disease. *Infect Immun* **34:**192–199.
20. **Reeves WC, Corey L, Adams HG, Vontver LA, Holmes KK.** 1981. Risk of recurrence after first episodes of genital herpes. Relation to HSV type and antibody response. *N Engl J Med* **305:**315–319.
21. **Ashley R, Cent A, Maggs V, Nahmias A, Corey L.** 1991. Inability of enzyme immunoassays to discriminate between infections with herpes simplex virus types 1 and 2. *Ann Intern Med* **115:**520–526.
22. **Nahmias AJ, Lee FK, Beckman-Nahmias S.** 1990. Sero-epidemiological and -sociological patterns of herpes simplex virus infection in the world. *Scand J Infect Dis Suppl* **69**(Suppl):19–36.
23. **Centers for Disease Control and Prevention (CDC).** 2010. Seroprevalence of herpes simplex virus type 2 among persons aged 14-49 years: United States, 2005-2008. *MMWR Morb Mortal Wkly Rep* **59:**456–459.
24. **McQuillan G, Kruszon-Moran D, Flagg EW,** Paulose-Ram R. 2018. Prevalence of herpes simplex virus type 1 and type 2 in persons aged 14-49: United States, 2015-2016. *NCHS Data Brief* no. 304.
25. **Johnson RE, Nahmias AJ, Magder LS, Lee FK, Brooks CA, Snowden CB.** 1989. A seroepidemiologic survey of the prevalence of herpes simplex virus type 2 infection in the United States. *N Engl J Med* **321:**7–12.
26. **Xu F, Sternberg MR, Kottiri BJ, McQuillan GM, Lee FK, Nahmias AJ, Berman SM, Markowitz LE.** 2006. Trends in herpes simplex virus type 1 and type 2 seroprevalence in the United States. *JAMA* **296:**964–973.
27. **Smith JS, Robinson NJ.** 2002. Age-specific prevalence of infection with herpes simplex virus types 2 and 1: a global review. *J Infect Dis* **186**(Suppl 1):S3–S28.
28. **Malkin JE.** 2004. Epidemiology of genital herpes simplex virus infection in developed countries. *Herpes* **11**(Suppl 1): 2A–23A.
29. **Fleming DT, McQuillan GM, Johnson RE, Nahmias AJ, Aral SO, Lee FK, St Louis ME.** 1997. Herpes simplex virus type 2 in the United States, 1976 to 1994. *N Engl J Med* **337:** 1105–1111.
30. **Wald A, Langenberg AG, Krantz E, Douglas JM Jr, Handsfield HH, DiCarlo RP, Adimora AA, Izu AE, Morrow RA, Corey L.** 2005. The relationship between condom use and herpes simplex virus acquisition. *Ann Intern Med* **143:** 707–713.
31. **Martin ET, Krantz E, Gottlieb SL, Magaret AS, Langenberg A, Stanberry L, Kamb M, Wald A.** 2009. A pooled analysis of the effect of condoms in preventing HSV-2 acquisition. *Arch Intern Med* **169:**1233–1240.

32. **Stanaway JD, Wald A, Martin ET, Gottlieb SL, Magaret AS.** 2012. Case-crossover analysis of condom use and herpes simplex virus type 2 acquisition. *Sex Transm Dis* **39:** 388–393.
33. **Wald A, Krantz E, Selke S, Lairson E, Morrow RA, Zeh J.** 2006. Knowledge of partners' genital herpes protects against herpes simplex virus type 2 acquisition. *J Infect Dis* **194:** 42–52.
34. **Corey L, Wald A, Patel R, Sacks SL, Tyring SK, Warren T, Douglas JM Jr, Paavonen J, Morrow RA, Beutner KR, Stratchounsky LS, Mertz G, Keene ON, Watson HA, Tait D, Vargas-Cortes M, Valacyclovir HSV Transmission Study Group.** 2004. Once-daily valacyclovir to reduce the risk of transmission of genital herpes. *N Engl J Med* **350:**11–20.
35. **Szpara ML, Gatherer D, Ochoa A, Greenbaum B, Dolan A, Bowden RJ, Enquist LW, Legendre M, Davison AJ.** 2014. Evolution and diversity in human herpes simplex virus genomes. *J Virol* **88:**1209–1227.
36. **Newman RM, Lamers SL, Weiner B, Ray SC, Colgrove RC, Diaz F, Jing L, Wang K, Saif S, Young S, Henn M, Laeyendecker O, Tobian AA, Cohen JI, Koelle DM, Quinn TC, Knipe DM.** 2015. Genome sequencing and analysis of geographically diverse clinical isolates of herpes simplex virus 2. *J Virol* **89:**8219–8232.
37. **Burrel S, Boutolleau D, Ryu D, Agut H, Merkel K, Leendertz FH, Calvignac-Spencer S.** 2017. Ancient recombination events between human herpes simplex viruses. *Mol Biol Evol* **34:**1713–1721.
38. **Koelle DM, Norberg P, Fitzgibbon MP, Russell RM, Greninger AL, Huang ML, Stensland L, Jing L, Magaret AS, Diem K, Selke S, Xie H, Celum C, Lingappa JR, Jerome KR, Wald A, Johnston C.** 2017. Worldwide circulation of HSV-2 × HSV-1 recombinant strains. *Sci Rep* **7:**44084.
39. **Brugha R, Keersmaekers K, Renton A, Meheus A.** 1997. Genital herpes infection: a review. *Int J Epidemiol* **26:** 698–709.
40. **Corey L, Adams HG, Brown ZA, Holmes KK.** 1983. Genital herpes simplex virus infections: clinical manifestations, course, and complications. *Ann Intern Med* **98:**958–972.
41. **Wald A, Zeh J, Selke S, Ashley RL, Corey L.** 1995. Virologic characteristics of subclinical and symptomatic genital herpes infections. *N Engl J Med* **333:**770–775.
42. **Roberts C.** 2005. Genital herpes in young adults: changing sexual behaviours, epidemiology and management. *Herpes* **12:**10–14.
43. **Ryder N, Jin F, McNulty AM, Grulich AE, Donovan B.** 2009. Increasing role of herpes simplex virus type 1 in first-episode anogenital herpes in heterosexual women and younger men who have sex with men, 1992-2006. *Sex Transm Infect* **85:**416–419.
44. **Bernstein DI, Bellamy AR, Hook EW III, Levin MJ, Wald A, Ewell MG, Wolff PA, Deal CD, Heineman TC, Dubin G, Belshe RB.** 2013. Epidemiology, clinical presentation, and antibody response to primary infection with herpes simplex virus type 1 and type 2 in young women. *Clin Infect Dis* **56:**344–351.
45. **Engelberg R, Carrell D, Krantz E, Corey L, Wald A.** 2003. Natural history of genital herpes simplex virus type 1 infection. *Sex Transm Dis* **30:**174–177.
46. **Spruance SL.** 1992. The natural history of recurrent oral-facial herpes simplex virus infection. *Semin Dermatol* **11:** 200–206.
47. **Benedetti J, Corey L, Ashley R.** 1994. Recurrence rates in genital herpes after symptomatic first-episode infection. *Ann Intern Med* **121:**847–854.
48. **Lafferty WE, Coombs RW, Benedetti J, Critchlow C, Corey L.** 1987. Recurrences after oral and genital herpes simplex virus infection. Influence of site of infection and viral type. *N Engl J Med* **316:**1444–1449.
49. **Langenberg A, Benedetti J, Jenkins J, Ashley R, Winter C, Corey L.** 1989. Development of clinically recognizable genital lesions among women previously identified as having "asymptomatic" herpes simplex virus type 2 infection. *Ann Intern Med* **110:**882–887.
50. **Frenkel LM, Garratty EM, Shen JP, Wheeler N, Clark O, Bryson YJ.** 1993. Clinical reactivation of herpes simplex virus type 2 infection in seropositive pregnant women with no history of genital herpes. *Ann Intern Med* **118:**414–418.
51. **Diamond C, Selke S, Ashley R, Benedetti J, Corey L.** 1999. Clinical course of patients with serologic evidence of recurrent genital herpes presenting with signs and symptoms of first episode disease. *Sex Transm Dis* **26:**221–225.
52. **Wald A, Huang ML, Carrell D, Selke S, Corey L.** 2003. Polymerase chain reaction for detection of herpes simplex virus (HSV) DNA on mucosal surfaces: comparison with HSV isolation in cell culture. *J Infect Dis* **188:** 1345–1351.
53. **Leone P, Warren T, Hamed K, Fife K, Wald A.** 2007. Famciclovir reduces viral mucosal shedding in HSV-seropositive persons. *Sex Transm Dis* **34:**900–907.
54. **Wald A, Ericsson M, Krantz E, Selke S, Corey L.** 2004. Oral shedding of herpes simplex virus type 2. *Sex Transm Infect* **80:**272–276.
55. **Prober CG, Sollender WM, Yasukawa LL, Au DS, Yeager AS, Arvin AM.** 1987. Low risk of herpes simplex virus infections in neonates exposed to the virus at the time of vaginal delivery to mothers with recurrent genital herpes simplex virus infections. *N Engl J Med* **316:**240–244.
56. **Brown ZA, Wald A, Morrow RA, Selke S, Zeh J, Corey L.** 2003. Effect of serologic status and cesarean delivery on transmission rates of herpes simplex virus from mother to infant. *JAMA* **289:**203–209.
57. **Kropp RY, Wong T, Cormier L, Ringrose A, Burton S, Embree JE, Steben M.** 2006. Neonatal herpes simplex virus infections in Canada: results of a 3-year national prospective study. *Pediatrics* **117:**1955–1962.
58. **Brown ZA, Selke S, Zeh J, Kopelman J, Maslow A, Ashley RL, Watts DH, Berry S, Herd M, Corey L.** 1997. The acquisition of herpes simplex virus during pregnancy. *N Engl J Med* **337:**509–516.
59. **Sullender WM, Yasukawa LL, Schwartz M, Pereira L, Hensleigh PA, Prober CG, Arvin AM.** 1988. Type-specific antibodies to herpes simplex virus type 2 (HSV-2) glycoprotein G in pregnant women, infants exposed to maternal HSV-2 infection at delivery, and infants with neonatal herpes. *J Infect Dis* **157:**164–165.
60. **ACOG Committee on Practice Bulletins.** 2007. ACOG Practice Bulletin. Clinical management guidelines for obstetrician-gynecologists. No. 82 June 2007. Management of herpes in pregnancy. *Obstet Gynecol* **109:**1489–1498.
61. **Corey L, Wald A.** 2009. Maternal and neonatal herpes simplex virus infections. *N Engl J Med* **361:**1376–1385.
62. **Kohl S.** 2002. The diagnosis and treatment of neonatal herpes simplex virus infection. *Pediatr Ann* **31:**726–732.
63. **Whitley R, Arvin A, Prober C, Burchett S, Corey L, Powell D, Plotkin S, Starr S, Alford C, Connor J, Jacobs R, Nahmias A, Soong S-J, Infectious Diseases Collaborative Antiviral Study Group.** 1991. A controlled trial comparing vidarabine with acyclovir in neonatal herpes simplex virus infection. *N Engl J Med* **324:**444–449.
64. **Whitley RJ, Arvin AM.** 1995. Herpes simplex virus infection, p 354–376. *In* Remingon J, Klein J (ed), *Infectious Diseases of the Fetus and Newborn*, 4th ed. The W.B. Saunders Co., Philadelphia, PA.
65. **Diamond C, Mohan K, Hobson A, Frenkel L, Corey L.** 1999. Viremia in neonatal herpes simplex virus infections. *Pediatr Infect Dis J* **18:**487–489.
66. **Pinninti SG, Kimberlin DW.** 2013. Neonatal herpes simplex virus infections. *Pediatr Clin North Am* **60:**351–365.
67. American Academy of **Pediatrics.** 2012. Herpes simplex, p 398–408. *In* Pickering LK, Baker CJ, Kimberlin DW, Long SS (ed), *Red Book: 2012 Report of the Committee on Infectious Diseases*, 29th ed. American Academy of Pediatrics, Elk Grove Village, IL.
68. **Kimberlin DW, Baley J, Committee on Infectious Diseases, Committee on Fetus and Newborn.** 2013. Guidance on management of asymptomatic neonates born to women with active genital herpes lesions. *Pediatrics* **131:**e635–e646.

69. **Olson LC, Buescher EL, Artenstein MS, Parkman PD.** 1967. Herpesvirus infections of the human central nervous system. *N Engl J Med* **277:**1271–1277.
70. **Tang YW, Mitchell PS, Espy MJ, Smith TF, Persing DH.** 1999. Molecular diagnosis of herpes simplex virus infections in the central nervous system. *J Clin Microbiol* **37:**2127–2136.
71. **Gordon B, Selnes OA, Hart J Jr, Hanley DF, Whitley RJ.** 1990. Long-term cognitive sequelae of acyclovir-treated herpes simplex encephalitis. *Arch Neurol* **47:**646–647.
72. **Domingues RB, Tsanaclis AM, Pannuti CS, Mayo MS, Lakeman FD.** 1997. Evaluation of the range of clinical presentations of herpes simplex encephalitis by using polymerase chain reaction assay of cerebrospinal fluid samples. *Clin Infect Dis* **25:**86–91.
73. **Cinque P, Cleator GM, Weber T, Monteyne P, Sindic CJ, van Loon AM.** 1996. The role of laboratory investigation in the diagnosis and management of patients with suspected herpes simplex encephalitis: a consensus report. The EU Concerted Action on Virus Meningitis and Encephalitis. *J Neurol Neurosurg Psychiatry* **61:**339–345.
74. **Yamamoto LJ, Tedder DG, Ashley R, Levin MJ.** 1991. Herpes simplex virus type 1 DNA in cerebrospinal fluid of a patient with Mollaret's meningitis. *N Engl J Med* **325:** 1082–1085.
75. **Schmutzhard E.** 2001. Viral infections of the CNS with special emphasis on herpes simplex infections. *J Neurol* **248:** 469–477.
76. **Juhl D, Mosel C, Nawroth F, Funke AM, Dadgar SM, Hagenström H, Kirchner H, Hennig H.** 2010. Detection of herpes simplex virus DNA in plasma of patients with primary but not with recurrent infection: implications for transfusion medicine? *Transfus Med* **20:**38–47.
77. **Youssef R, Shaker O, Sobeih S, Mashaly H, Mostafa WZ.** 2002. Detection of herpes simplex virus DNA in serum and oral secretions during acute recurrent herpes labialis. *J Dermatol* **29:**404–410.
78. **Berrington WR, Jerome KR, Cook L, Wald A, Corey L, Casper C.** 2009. Clinical correlates of herpes simplex virus viremia among hospitalized adults. *Clin Infect Dis* **49:** 1295–1301.
79. **Beersma MF, Verjans GM, Metselaar HJ, Osterhaus AD, Berrington WR, van Doornum GJ.** 2011. Quantification of viral DNA and liver enzymes in plasma improves early diagnosis and management of herpes simplex virus hepatitis. *J Viral Hepat* **18:**e160–e166.
80. **Levitsky J, Duddempudi AT, Lakeman FD, Whitley RJ, Luby JP, Lee WM, Fontana RJ, Blei AT, Ison MG, US Acute Liver Failure Study Group.** 2008. Detection and diagnosis of herpes simplex virus infection in adults with acute liver failure. *Liver Transpl* **14:**1498–1504.
81. **Pepose JD.** 1996. Herpes simplex virus diseases: anterior segment of the eye, p 905–932. *In* Pepose JD, Holland GN, Wilhelmus KR (ed), *Ocular Infection and Immunity*. Mosby, St. Louis, MO.
82. **Dawson C.** 1995. Management of herpes simplex eye diseases, p 127–136. *In* Griffiths PD (ed), *Clinical Management of Herpes Viruses*. IOS Press, Washington, DC.
83. **Khan BF, Pavan-Langston D.** 2004. Clinical manifestations and treatment modalities in herpes simplex virus of the ocular anterior segment. *Int Ophthalmol Clin* **44:**103–133.
84. **Knickelbein JE, Hendricks RL, Charukamnoetkanok P.** 2009. Management of herpes simplex virus stromal keratitis: an evidence-based review. *Surv Ophthalmol* **54:**226–234.
85. **Al-Dujaili LJ, Clerkin PP, Clement C, McFerrin HE, Bhattacharjee PS, Varnell ED, Kaufman HE, Hill JM.** 2011. Ocular herpes simplex virus: how are latency, reactivation, recurrent disease and therapy interrelated? *Future Microbiol* **6:**877–907.
86. **Zahariadis G, Jerome KR, Corey L.** 2003. Herpes simplex virus-associated sepsis in a previously infected immunocompetent adult. *Ann Intern Med* **139:**153–154.
87. **Centers for Disease Control and Prevention.** 2002. Guidelines for treatment of sexually transmitted diseases. *MMWR Morb Mortal Wkly Rep* **51:**12–17.
88. **Superti F, Ammendolia MG, Marchetti M.** 2008. New advances in anti-HSV chemotherapy. *Curr Med Chem* **15:**900–911.
89. **Diamond C, Corey L.** 1999. Antiviral drugs and therapy, p 349–364. *In* Root RK, Stamm W, Waldvogel F, Corey L (ed), *Clinical Infectious Diseases: a Practical Approach*. University Press, Oxford, United Kingdom.
90. **Kimberlin DW, Coen DM, Biron KK, Cohen JI, Lamb RA, McKinlay M, Emini EA, Whitley RJ.** 1995. Molecular mechanisms of antiviral resistance. *Antiviral Res* **26:** 369–401.
91. **Tyring S, Wald A, Zadeikis N, Dhadda S, Takenouchi K, Rorig R.** 2012. ASP2151 for the treatment of genital herpes: a randomized, double-blind, placebo- and valacyclovir-controlled, dose-finding study. *J Infect Dis* **205:**1100–1110.
92. **Wald A, Corey L, Timmler B, Magaret A, Warren T, Tyring S, Johnston C, Kriesel J, Fife K, Galitz L, Stoelben S, Huang ML, Selke S, Stobernack HP, Ruebsamen-Schaeff H, Birkmann A.** 2014. Helicase-primase inhibitor pritelivir for HSV-2 infection. *N Engl J Med* **370:**201–210.
93. **Wald A, Timmler B, Magaret A, Warren T, Tyring S, Johnston C, Fife K, Selke S, Huang ML, Stobernack HP, Zimmermann H, Corey L, Birkmann A, Ruebsamen-Schaeff H.** 2016. Effect of pritelivir compared with valacyclovir on genital HSV-2 shedding in patients with frequent recurrences: a randomized clinical trial. *JAMA* **316:** 2495–2503.
94. **Ryncarz AJ, Goddard J, Wald A, Huang M-L, Roizman B, Corey L.** 1999. Development of a high-throughput quantitative assay for detecting herpes simplex virus DNA in clinical samples. *J Clin Microbiol* **37:**1941–1947.
95. **Waldhuber MG, Denham I, Wadey C, Leong-Shaw W, Cross GF.** 1999. Detection of herpes simplex virus in genital specimens by type-specific polymerase chain reaction. *Int J STD AIDS* **10:**89–92.
96. **Jerome KR, Huang ML, Wald A, Selke S, Corey L.** 2002. Quantitative stability of DNA after extended storage of clinical specimens as determined by real-time PCR. *J Clin Microbiol* **40:**2609–2611.
97. **Specter S, Jeffries D.** 1996. Detection of virus and viral antigens, p 309–322. *In* Mahy BW, Kangro HL (ed), *Virology Methods Manual*. Harcourt, New York, NY.
98. **Crane LR, Gutterman PA, Chapel T, Lerner AM.** 1980. Incubation of swab materials with herpes simplex virus. *J Infect Dis* **141:**531.
99. **Dunn JJ, Billetdeaux E, Skodack-Jones L, Carroll KC.** 2003. Evaluation of three Copan viral transport systems for the recovery of cultivatable, clinical virus isolates. *Diagn Microbiol Infect Dis* **45:**191–197.
100. **Jensen C, Johnson FB.** 1994. Comparison of various transport media for viability maintenance of herpes simplex virus, respiratory syncytial virus, and adenovirus. *Diagn Microbiol Infect Dis* **19:**137–142.
101. **Slomka MJ.** 2000. Current diagnostic techniques in genital herpes: their role in controlling the epidemic. *Clin Lab* **46:**591–607.
102. **Young S, Body B, Moore F, Dunbar S.** 2016. Multicenter evaluation of the Luminex® ARIES® HSV 1&2 Assay for the detection of herpes simplex virus types 1 and 2 in cutaneous and mucocutaneous lesion specimens. *Expert Rev Mol Diagn* **16:**1241–1249.
103. **Heaton PR, Espy MJ, Binnicker MJ.** 2015. Evaluation of 2 multiplex real-time PCR assays for the detection of HSV-1/2 and Varicella zoster virus directly from clinical samples. *Diagn Microbiol Infect Dis* **81:**169–170.
104. **Kuypers J, Boughton G, Chung J, Hussey L, Huang ML, Cook L, Jerome KR.** 2015. Comparison of the Simplexa HSV1 & 2 Direct kit and laboratory-developed real-time PCR assays for herpes simplex virus detection. *J Clin Virol* **62:**103–105.
105. **Binnicker MJ, Espy MJ, Irish CL.** 2014. Rapid and direct detection of herpes simplex virus in cerebrospinal fluid by use of a commercial real-time PCR assay. *J Clin Microbiol* **52:**4361–4362.

106. **Faron ML, Ledeboer NA, Patel A, Beqa SH, Yen-Lieberman B, Kohn D, Leber AL, Mayne D, Northern WI, Buchan BW.** 2016. Multicenter evaluation of Meridian Bioscience HSV 1&2 molecular assay for detection of herpes simplex virus 1 and 2 from clinical cutaneous and mucocutaneous specimens. *J Clin Microbiol* **54:**2008–2013.
107. **Teo JW, Chiang D, Jureen R, Lin RT.** 2015. Clinical evaluation of a helicase-dependant amplification (HDA)-based commercial assay for the simultaneous detection of HSV-1 and HSV-2. *Diagn Microbiol Infect Dis* **83:**261–262.
108. **Binnicker MJ, Espy MJ, Duresko B, Irish C, Mandrekar J.** 2017. Automated processing, extraction and detection of herpes simplex virus types 1 and 2: a comparative evaluation of three commercial platforms using clinical specimens. *J Clin Virol* **89:**30–33.
109. **Ando Y, Kimura H, Miwata H, Kudo T, Shibata M, Morishima T.** 1993. Quantitative analysis of herpes simplex virus DNA in cerebrospinal fluid of children with herpes simplex encephalitis. *J Med Virol* **41:**170–173.
110. **Landry ML.** 1995. False-positive polymerase chain reaction results in the diagnosis of herpes simplex encephalitis. *J Infect Dis* **172:**1641–1643.
111. **Kwok S, Higuchi R.** 1989. Avoiding false positives with PCR. *Nature* **339:**237–238.
112. **Kúdelová M, Murányiová M, Kúdela O, Rajcáni J, Lehtinen M, Stankovic J, Arvaja M, Bálint O.** 1995. Detection of herpes simplex virus DNA by polymerase chain reaction in the cerebrospinal fluid of patients with viral meningoencephalitis using primers for the glycoprotein D gene. *Acta Virol* **39:**11–17.
113. **Kimura H, Shibata M, Kuzushima K, Nishikawa K, Nishiyama Y, Morishima T.** 1990. Detection and direct typing of herpes simplex virus by polymerase chain reaction. *Med Microbiol Immunol (Berl)* **179:**177–184.
114. **Kramer MF, Coen DM.** 2001. Enzymatic amplification of DNA by PCR: standard procedures and optimization. *Curr Protoc Immunol* **Chapter 10:**Unit 10 20.
115. **Schloss L, van Loon AM, Cinque P, Cleator G, Echevarria JM, Falk KI, Klapper P, Schirm J, Vestergaard BF, Niesters H, Popow-Kraupp T, Quint W, Linde A.** 2003. An international external quality assessment of nucleic acid amplification of herpes simplex virus. *J Clin Virol* **28:** 175–185.
116. **Köller T, Kurze D, Lange M, Scherdin M, Podbielski A, Warnke P.** 2016. Implementation and evaluation of a fully automated multiplex real-time PCR assay on the BD Max platform to detect and differentiate *Herpesviridae* from cerebrospinal fluids. *PLoS One* **11:**e0153991.
117. **Leber AL, Everhart K, Balada-Llasat JM, Cullison J, Daly J, Holt S, Lephart P, Salimnia H, Schreckenberger PC, DesJarlais S, Reed SL, Chapin KC, LeBlanc L, Johnson JK, Soliven NL, Carroll KC, Miller JA, Dien Bard J, Mestas J, Bankowski M, Enomoto T, Hemmert AC, Bourzac KM.** 2016. Multicenter evaluation of BioFire FilmArray meningitis/encephalitis panel for detection of bacteria, viruses, and yeast in cerebrospinal fluid specimens. *J Clin Microbiol* **54:**2251–2261.
118. **Van Der Pol B, Warren T, Taylor SN, Martens M, Jerome KR, Mena L, Lebed J, Ginde S, Fine P, Hook EW III.** 2012. Type-specific identification of anogenital herpes simplex virus infections by use of a commercially available nucleic acid amplification test. *J Clin Microbiol* **50:** 3466–3471.
119. **Kim HJ, Tong Y, Tang W, Quimson L, Cope VA, Pan X, Motre A, Kong R, Hong J, Kohn D, Miller NS, Poulter MD, Kong H, Tang YW, Yen-Lieberman B.** 2011. A rapid and simple isothermal nucleic acid amplification test for detection of herpes simplex virus types 1 and 2. *J Clin Virol* **50:**26–30.
120. **Gomez CA, Pinsky BA, Liu A, Banaei N.** 2016. Delayed diagnosis of tuberculous meningitis misdiagnosed as herpes simplex virus-1 encephalitis with the FilmArray syndromic polymerase chain reaction panel. *Open Forum Infect Dis* **4:**ofw245.
121. **Nahass GT, Goldstein BA, Zhu WY, Serfling U, Penneys NS, Leonardi CL.** 1992. Comparison of Tzanck smear, viral culture, and DNA diagnostic methods in detection of herpes simplex and varicella-zoster infection. *JAMA* **268:** 2541–2544.
122. **Corey L, Spear PG.** 1986. Infections with herpes simplex viruses (1). *N Engl J Med* **314:**686–691.
123. **Chan EL, Brandt K, Horsman GB.** 2001. Comparison of Chemicon SimulFluor direct fluorescent antibody staining with cell culture and shell vial direct immunoperoxidase staining for detection of herpes simplex virus and with cytospin direct immunofluorescence staining for detection of varicella-zoster virus. *Clin Diagn Lab Immunol* **8:**909–912.
124. **Coyle PV, Desai A, Wyatt D, McCaughey C, O'Neill HJ.** 1999. A comparison of virus isolation, indirect immunofluorescence and nested multiplex polymerase chain reaction for the diagnosis of primary and recurrent herpes simplex type 1 and type 2 infections. *J Virol Methods* **83:**75–82.
125. **Landry ML, Ferguson D, Wlochowski J.** 1997. Detection of herpes simplex virus in clinical specimens by cytospin-enhanced direct immunofluorescence. *J Clin Microbiol* **35:**302–304.
126. **Sanders C, Nelson C, Hove M, Woods GL.** 1998. Cytospin-enhanced direct immunofluorescence assay versus cell culture for detection of herpes simplex virus in clinical specimens. *Diagn Microbiol Infect Dis* **32:**111–113.
127. **Gitman MR, Ferguson D, Landry ML.** 2013. Comparison of Simplexa HSV 1 & 2 PCR with culture, immunofluorescence, and laboratory-developed TaqMan PCR for detection of herpes simplex virus in swab specimens. *J Clin Microbiol* **51:**3765–3769.
128. **Strickler JG, Manivel JC, Copenhaver CM, Kubic VL.** 1990. Comparison of *in situ* hybridization and immunohistochemistry for detection of cytomegalovirus and herpes simplex virus. *Hum Pathol* **21:**443–448.
129. **Zhao LS, Landry ML, Balkovic ES, Hsiung GD.** 1987. Impact of cell culture sensitivity and virus concentration on rapid detection of herpes simplex virus by cytopathic effects and immunoperoxidase staining. *J Clin Microbiol* **25:** 1401–1405.
130. **Landry ML, Hsiung GD.** 1994. *Herpesviridae*, p 238–268. *In* Hsiung GD, Fong CKY, Landry ML (ed), *Hsiung's Diagnostic Virology*. Yale University Press, New Haven, CT.
131. **Crist GA, Langer JM, Woods GL, Procter M, Hillyard DR.** 2004. Evaluation of the ELVIS plate method for the detection and typing of herpes simplex virus in clinical specimens. *Diagn Microbiol Infect Dis* **49:**173–177.
132. **Martins TB, Woolstenhulme RD, Jaskowski TD, Hill HR, Litwin CM.** 2001. Comparison of four enzyme immunoassays with a Western blot assay for the determination of type-specific antibodies to herpes simplex virus. *Am J Clin Pathol* **115:**272–277.
133. **Ashley RL.** 2001. Sorting out the new HSV type specific antibody tests. *Sex Transm Infect* **77:**232–237.
134. **Morrow RA, Brown ZA.** 2005. Common use of inaccurate antibody assays to identify infection status with herpes simplex virus type 2. *Am J Obstet Gynecol* **193:**361–362.
135. **Morrow RA, Friedrich D.** 2003. Inaccuracy of certain commercial enzyme immunoassays in diagnosing genital infections with herpes simplex virus types 1 or 2. *Am J Clin Pathol* **120:**839–844.
136. **Morrow R, Friedrich D.** 2006. Performance of a novel test for IgM and IgG antibodies in subjects with culture-documented genital herpes simplex virus-1 or -2 infection. *Clin Microbiol Infect* **12:**463–469.
137. **Torfason EG, Diderholm H.** 1982. False RIA IgM titres to herpes simplex virus and cytomegalovirus: factors causing them, and their absorption by protein A-Sepharose/ IgG-protein A-Sepharose. *J Med Virol* **10:**157–170.
138. **Berth M, Bosmans E.** 2009. Acute parvovirus B19 infection frequently causes false-positive results in Epstein-Barr virus- and herpes simplex virus-specific immunoglobulin M determinations done on the Liaison platform. *Clin Vaccine Immunol* **16:**372–375.

139. **Morrow RA, Friedrich D, Krantz E, Wald A.** 2004. Development and use of a type-specific antibody avidity test based on herpes simplex virus type 2 glycoprotein G. *Sex Transm Dis* **31:**508–515.
140. **Ashley RL, Militoni J, Lee F, Nahmias A, Corey L.** 1988. Comparison of Western blot (immunoblot) and glycoprotein G-specific immunodot enzyme assay for detecting antibodies to herpes simplex virus types 1 and 2 in human sera. *J Clin Microbiol* **26:**662–667.
141. **Binnicker MJ, Jespersen DJ, Harring JA.** 2010. Evaluation of three multiplex flow immunoassays compared to an enzyme immunoassay for the detection and differentiation of IgG class antibodies to herpes simplex virus types 1 and 2. *Clin Vaccine Immunol* **17:**253–257.
142. **Laderman EI, Whitworth E, Dumaual E, Jones M, Hudak A, Hogrefe W, Carney J, Groen J.** 2008. Rapid, sensitive, and specific lateral-flow immunochromatographic point-of-care device for detection of herpes simplex virus type 2-specific immunoglobulin G antibodies in serum and whole blood. *Clin Vaccine Immunol* **15:**159–163.
143. **Ashley-Morrow R, Krantz E, Wald A.** 2003. Time course of seroconversion by HerpeSelect ELISA after acquisition of genital herpes simplex virus type 1 (HSV-1) or HSV-2. *Sex Transm Dis* **30:**310–314.
144. **Ashley RL, Eagleton M, Pfeiffer N.** 1999. Ability of a rapid serology test to detect seroconversion to herpes simplex virus type 2 glycoprotein G soon after infection. *J Clin Microbiol* **37:**1632–1633.
145. **Edlefsen PT, Birkmann A, Huang ML, Magaret CA, Kee JJ, Diem K, Goldner T, Timmler B, Stoelben S, Ruebsamen-Schaeff H, Zimmermann H, Warren T, Wald A, Corey L.** 2016. No evidence of pritelivir resistance among herpes simplex virus type 2 isolates after 4 weeks of daily therapy. *J Infect Dis* **214:**258–264.
146. **Weinberg A, Leary JJ, Sarisky RT, Levin MJ.** 2007. Factors that affect *in vitro* measurement of the susceptibility of herpes simplex virus to nucleoside analogues. *J Clin Virol* **38:** 139–145.
147. **Parris DS, Harrington JE.** 1982. Herpes simplex virus variants restraint to high concentrations of acyclovir exist in clinical isolates. *Antimicrob Agents Chemother* **22:**71–77.
148. **Moellering RC Jr, Graybill JR, McGowan JE Jr, Corey L.** 2007. Antimicrobial resistance prevention initiative–an update: proceedings of an expert panel on resistance. *Am J Infect Control* **35:**S1–S23; quiz S24–S26.
149. **Andrei G, Snoeck R.** 2013. Herpes simplex virus drug-resistance: new mutations and insights. *Curr Opin Infect Dis* **26:**551–560.
150. **Safrin S, Elbeik T, Phan L, Robinson D, Rush J, Elbaggari A, Mills J.** 1994. Correlation between response to acyclovir and foscarnet therapy and *in vitro* susceptibility result for isolates of herpes simplex virus from human immunodeficiency virus-infected patients. *Antimicrob Agents Chemother* **38:**1246–1250.
151. **Kimberlin DW, Lakeman FD, Arvin AM, Prober CG, Corey L, Powell DA, Burchett SK, Jacobs RF, Starr SE, Whitley RJ, National Institute of Allergy and Infectious Diseases Collaborative Antiviral Study Group.** 1996. Application of the polymerase chain reaction to the diagnosis and management of neonatal herpes simplex virus disease. *J Infect Dis* **174:**1162–1167.
152. **De Vos N, Van Hoovels L, Vankeerberghen A, Van Vaerenbergh K, Boel A, Demeyer I, Creemers L, De Beenhouwer H.** 2009. Monitoring of herpes simplex virus in the lower respiratory tract of critically ill patients using real-time PCR: a prospective study. *Clin Microbiol Infect* **15:** 358–363.
153. **Daubin C, Vincent S, Vabret A, du Cheyron D, Parienti JJ, Ramakers M, Freymuth F, Charbonneau P.** 2005. Nosocomial viral ventilator-associated pneumonia in the intensive care unit: a prospective cohort study. *Intensive Care Med* **31:**1116–1122.
154. **Mertz KJ, Trees D, Levine WC, Lewis JS, Litchfield B, Pettus KS, Morse SA, St Louis ME, Weiss JB, Schwebke J, Dickes J, Kee R, Reynolds J, Hutcheson D, Green D, Dyer I, Richwald GA, Novotny J, Weisfuse I, Goldberg M, O'Donnell JA, Knaup R, The Genital Ulcer Disease Surveillance Group.** 1998. Etiology of genital ulcers and prevalence of human immunodeficiency virus coinfection in 10 US cities. *J Infect Dis* **178:**1795–1798.
155. **Mark KE, Wald A, Magaret AS, Selke S, Olin L, Huang ML, Corey L.** 2008. Rapidly cleared episodes of herpes simplex virus reactivation in immunocompetent adults. *J Infect Dis* **198:**1141–1149.
156. **Whitley RJ, Kimberlin DW.** 1997. Treatment of viral infections during pregnancy and the neonatal period. *Clin Perinatol* **24:**267–283.
157. **Kimberlin DW, Lin CY, Jacobs RF, Powell DA, Corey L, Gruber WC, Rathore M, Bradley JS, Diaz PS, Kumar M, Arvin AM, Gutierrez K, Shelton M, Weiner LB, Sleasman JW, de Sierra TM, Weller S, Soong SJ, Kiell J, Lakeman FD, Whitley RJ, National Institute of Allergy and Infectious Diseases Collaborative Antiviral Study Group.** 2001. Safety and efficacy of high-dose intravenous acyclovir in the management of neonatal herpes simplex virus infections. *Pediatrics* **108:**230–238.
158. **Boggess KA, Watts DH, Hobson AC, Ashley RL, Brown ZA, Corey L.** 1997. Herpes simplex virus type 2 detection by culture and polymerase chain reaction and relationship to genital symptoms and cervical antibody status during the third trimester of pregnancy. *Am J Obstet Gynecol* **176:** 443–451.
159. **Wald A, Corey L, Cone R, Hobson A, Davis G, Zeh J.** 1997. Frequent genital herpes simplex virus 2 shedding in immunocompetent women. Effect of acyclovir treatment. *J Clin Invest* **99:**1092–1097.
160. **Wald A, Zeh J, Selke S, Warren T, Ryncarz AJ, Ashley R, Krieger JN, Corey L.** 2000. Reactivation of genital herpes simplex virus type 2 infection in asymptomatic seropositive persons. *N Engl J Med* **342:**844–850.
161. **Boivin G.** 2004. Diagnosis of herpesvirus infections of the central nervous system. *Herpes* **11**(Suppl 2)**:**48A–56A.
162. **Ramaswamy M, McDonald C, Smith M, Thomas D, Maxwell S, Tenant-Flowers M, Geretti AM.** 2004. Diagnosis of genital herpes by real time PCR in routine clinical practice. *Sex Transm Infect* **80:**406–410.
163. **Cone RW, Hobson AC, Huang ML.** 1992. Coamplified positive control detects inhibition of polymerase chain reactions. *J Clin Microbiol* **30:**3185–3189.
164. **Puchhammer-Stöckl E, Presterl E, Croÿ C, Aberle S, Popow-Kraupp T, Kundi M, Hofmann H, Wenninger U, Gödl I.** 2001. Screening for possible failure of herpes simplex virus PCR in cerebrospinal fluid for the diagnosis of herpes simplex encephalitis. *J Med Virol* **64:**531–536.
165. **Whitley RJ.** 2006. Herpes simplex encephalitis: adolescents and adults. *Antiviral Res* **71:**141–148.
166. **Kimura H, Aso K, Kuzushima K, Hanada N, Shibata M, Morishima T.** 1992. Relapse of herpes simplex encephalitis in children. *Pediatrics* **89:**891–894.
167. **Wildemann B, Ehrhart K, Storch-Hagenlocher B, Meyding-Lamadé U, Steinvorth S, Hacke W, Haas J.** 1997. Quantitation of herpes simplex virus type 1 DNA in cells of cerebrospinal fluid of patients with herpes simplex virus encephalitis. *Neurology* **48:**1341–1346.
168. **Revello MG, Baldanti F, Sarasini A, Zella D, Zavattoni M, Gerna G.** 1997. Quantitation of herpes simplex virus DNA in cerebrospinal fluid of patients with herpes simplex encephalitis by the polymerase chain reaction. *Clin Diagn Virol* **7:**183–191.
169. **Domingues RB, Lakeman FD, Mayo MS, Whitley RJ.** 1998. Application of competitive PCR to cerebrospinal fluid samples from patients with herpes simplex encephalitis. *J Clin Microbiol* **36:**2229–2234.
170. **Schloss L, Falk KI, Skoog E, Brytting M, Linde A, Aurelius E.** 2009. Monitoring of herpes simplex virus DNA types 1 and 2 viral load in cerebrospinal fluid by real-time PCR in patients with herpes simplex encephalitis. *J Med Virol* **81:**1432–1437.

171. **Bhullar SS, Chandak NH, Purohit HJ, Taori GM, Daginawala HF, Kashyap RS.** 2014. Determination of viral load by quantitative real-time PCR in herpes simplex encephalitis patients. *Intervirology* **57:**1–7.
172. **Hjalmarsson A, Granath F, Forsgren M, Brytting M, Blomqvist P, Sköldenberg B.** 2009. Prognostic value of intrathecal antibody production and DNA viral load in cerebrospinal fluid of patients with herpes simplex encephalitis. *J Neurol* **256:**1243–1251.
173. **Handsfield HH.** 2000. Public health strategies to prevent genital herpes: where do we stand? *Curr Infect Dis Rep* **2:** 25–30.
174. **Corey L, Handsfield HH.** 2000. Genital herpes and public health: addressing a global problem. *JAMA* **283:**791–794.
175. **Brown ZA.** 2000. HSV-2 specific serology should be offered routinely to antenatal patients. *Rev Med Virol* **10:**141–144.
176. **Bibbins-Domingo K, Grossman DC, Curry SJ, Davidson KW, Epling JW Jr, García FA, Kemper AR, Krist AH, Kurth AE, Landefeld CS, Mangione CM, Phillips WR, Phipps MG, Pignone MP, Silverstein M, Tseng CW, US Preventive Services Task Force.** 2016. Serologic screening for genital herpes infection: US Preventive Services Task Force recommendation statement. *JAMA* **316:**2525–2530.
177. **Morrow RA, Friedrich D, Meier A, Corey L.** 2005. Use of "Biokit HSV-2 Rapid Assay" to improve the positive predictive value of Focus HerpeSelect HSV-2 ELISA. *BMC Infect Dis* **5:**84.
178. **Ashley Morrow R, Krantz E, Friedrich D, Wald A.** 2006. Clinical correlates of index values in the focus HerpeSelect ELISA for antibodies to herpes simplex virus type 2 (HSV-2). *J Clin Virol* **36:**141–145.
179. **Ludwig H.** 1972. Genetic material of herpesviruses. I. Biophysical-chemical characterization of herpesvirus DNAs. *Med Microbiol Immunol (Berl)* **157:**186–211.
180. **Hilliard JK, Eberle R, Lipper SL, Munoz RM, Weiss SA.** 1987. Herpesvirus simiae (B virus): replication of the virus and identification of viral polypeptides in infected cells. *Arch Virol* **93:**185–198.
181. **Norrild B, Ludwig H, Rott R.** 1978. Identification of a common antigen of herpes simplex virus bovine herpes mammillitis virus, and B virus. *J Virol* **26:**712–717.
182. **Weigler BJ, Hird DW, Hilliard JK, Lerche NW, Roberts JA, Scott LM.** 1993. Epidemiology of cercopithecine herpesvirus 1 (B virus) infection and shedding in a large breeding cohort of rhesus macaques. *J Infect Dis* **167:**257–263.
183. **Weigler BJ, Scinicariello F, Hilliard JK.** 1995. Risk of venereal B virus (cercopithecine herpesvirus 1) transmission in rhesus monkeys using molecular epidemiology. *J Infect Dis* **171:**1139–1143.
184. **Orcutt RP, Pucak GJ, Foster HL, Kilcourse JT, Ferrell T.** 1976. Multiple testing for the detection of B virus antibody in specially handled rhesus monkeys after capture from virgin trapping grounds. *Lab Anim Sci* **26:**70–74.
185. **Weigler BJ, Roberts JA, Hird DW, Lerche NW, Hilliard JK.** 1990. A cross sectional survey for B virus antibody in a colony of group housed rhesus macaques. *Lab Anim Sci* **40:**257–261.
186. **Gay FP, Holden M.** 1933. The herpes encephalitis problem. *J Infect Dis* **53:**287–303.
187. **CDC.** 1998. Fatal cercopithecine herpesvirus 1 (B virus) infection following mucocutaneous exposure and interim recommendations for worker protection. *MMWR* **47:**1073–1076.
188. **Ostrowski SR, Leslie MJ, Parrott T, Abelt S, Piercy PE.** 1998. B-virus from pet macaque monkeys: an emerging threat in the United States? *Emerg Infect Dis* **4:**117–121.
189. **Cohen JI, Davenport DS, Stewart JA, Deitchman S, Hilliard JK, Chapman LE, B Virus Working Group.** 2002. Recommendations for prevention of and therapy for exposure to B virus (cercopithecine herpesvirus 1). *Clin Infect Dis* **35:**1191–1203.
190. **Centers for Disease Control and Prevension.** 1987. B virus infection in humans—Pensacola, Florida. *MMWR* **36:** 289–290.
191. **Freifeld AG, Hilliard J, Southers J, Murray M, Savarese B, Schmitt JM, Straus SE.** 1995. A controlled seroprevalence survey of primate handlers for evidence of asymptomatic herpes B virus infection. *J Infect Dis* **171:**1031–1034.
192. **Zwartouw HT, Humphreys CR, Collins P.** 1989. Oral chemotherapy of fatal B virus (herpesvirus simiae) infection. *Antiviral Res* **11:**275–283.
193. **Holmes GP, Chapman LE, Stewart JA, Straus SE, Hilliard JK, Davenport DS.** 1995. Guidelines for the prevention and treatment of B-virus infections in exposed persons. The B Virus Working Group. *Clin Infect Dis* **20:**421–439.
194. **Scinicariello F, English WJ, Hilliard J.** 1993. Identification by PCR of meningitis caused by herpes B virus. *Lancet* **341:**1660–1661.
195. **Scinicariello F, Eberle R, Hilliard JK.** 1993. Rapid detection of B virus (herpesvirus simiae) DNA by polymerase chain reaction. *J Infect Dis* **168:**747–750.
196. **Slomka MJ, Brown DW, Clewley JP, Bennett AM, Harrington L, Kelly DC.** 1993. Polymerase chain reaction for detection of herpesvirus simiae (B virus) in clinical specimens. *Arch Virol* **131:**89–99.
197. **Katz D, Hilliard JK, Eberle R, Lipper SL.** 1986. ELISA for detection of group-common and virus-specific antibodies in human and simian sera induced by herpes simplex and related simian viruses. *J Virol Methods* **14:**99–109.
198. **Fujima A, Ochiai Y, Saito A, Omori Y, Noda A, Kazuyama Y, Shoji H, Tanabayashi K, Ueda F, Yoshikawa Y, Hondo R.** 2008. Discrimination of antibody to herpes B virus from antibody to herpes simplex virus types 1 and 2 in human and macaque sera. *J Clin Microbiol* **46:**56–61.
199. **Katz D, Shi W, Wildes MJ, Krug PW, Hilliard JK.** 2012. Reassessing the detection of B-virus-specific serum antibodies. *Comp Med* **62:**516–526.

Varicella-Zoster Virus

ELISABETH PUCHHAMMER-STÖCKL AND STEPHAN W. ABERLE

101

TAXONOMY

Varicella-zoster virus (VZV) belongs to the family *Herpesviridae*, based on morphological criteria, and is one of the eight human pathogenic herpesviruses identified so far. On the basis of its biological properties, it is classified, together with herpes simplex virus (HSV), as a member of the subfamily *Alphaherpesvirinae* (genus *Varicellovirus*, species *Human Herpesvirus 3* [HHV-3]).

DESCRIPTION OF THE AGENT

VZV is an enveloped virus with a diameter of about 180 to 200 nm (Fig. 1). It contains an icosahedral nucleocapsid surrounded by a tegument structure, a lipid envelope that allows the virus to be degraded by lipid solvents, and a linear double-stranded DNA genome (1). The viral genome has an approximate length of 125,000 bp and contains at least 70 viral genes (2). The VZV genome consists of a unique long region, a unique short region, and flanking internal and terminating repeat regions, and it can exist in four isomeric forms (Fig. 2).

VZV may infect susceptible cells either by fusion at the cell surface or by endocytosis. Virus replication takes place in the nucleus of the infected cell, and similar to what occurs in other herpesviruses, the progression of viral gene expression is highly regulated. Not all VZV gene functions are yet known. The especially well-characterized ones include some transcription regulator proteins (IE 61 to IE 63), viral enzymes such as thymidine kinase (TK; encoded by open reading frame [ORF] 36), the DNA polymerase (ORF 28), and various VZV glycoproteins, such as gB (ORF 31), gE (ORF 68), and gH (ORF 37), which are required for virus attachment and for inducing a host immune response.

VZV exhibits low genomic diversity among isolates in comparison to other herpesviruses (3). From full genome sequencing, five major VZV clades and two provisional genotypes have been established (4, 5). There is no evidence that naturally circulating VZV strains differ significantly in virulence.

EPIDEMIOLOGY AND TRANSMISSION

VZV is ubiquitous and highly contagious, and primary infection with VZV therefore usually occurs in early childhood. Prevaccination seroepidemiological studies in 11 European countries have shown that in most areas, more than 90% of 10- to 15-year-olds were seropositive for VZV (6). In the United States, the incidence of varicella has declined significantly since 1995, when the VZV vaccine was generally introduced (7).

Primary infection with VZV is most likely acquired by virus transmission through aerosols. Cell-free virus is also produced at high levels in the skin vesicles, and thus the fluid from these vesicles is also highly infectious. Infection occurs by inoculation of the respiratory tract mucosa and replication in tonsillar lymphoid tissue, from which the virus is then disseminated, most likely by T cells (1). The incubation period is 10 to 21 days. During this incubation time, the virus is spread by viremia, may also replicate in reticuloendothelial organs, and finally infects cutaneous epithelial cells, which are the major sites of virus replication (1). Eventually, the infected host begins to shed virus by the respiratory route. New vesicles containing infectious fluid may appear for several days after rash onset. Individuals are no longer infectious once the last set of vesicles has dried and crusted.

After primary VZV infection, the virus remains latent in ganglia. Upon reactivation, herpes zoster may develop. Herpes zoster rash vesicles are filled with virus-containing fluid and may be also a source of primary infection for susceptible, VZV-seronegative individuals. Virus can also be transmitted from mother to child during pregnancy (8).

CLINICAL SIGNIFICANCE

Varicella (chickenpox) is the manifestation of primary infection with VZV. The clinical appearance of chickenpox is usually dominated by a generalized vesicular rash. Sometimes, symptoms such as fever, malaise, and abdominal pain are seen as prodromal symptoms 24 to 48 hours before and during the first days after the onset of the rash. New vesicles develop during the first 3 to 6 days of varicella. Due to its characteristic clinical appearance, the diagnosis of varicella is often a clinical one and does not require laboratory confirmation. Clinical reinfection with VZV has been described for immunocompetent and immunosuppressed individuals (9, 10).

Complications associated with chickenpox can occur (11), and older age, immunosuppression, and pregnancy are considered to be generally associated with a higher

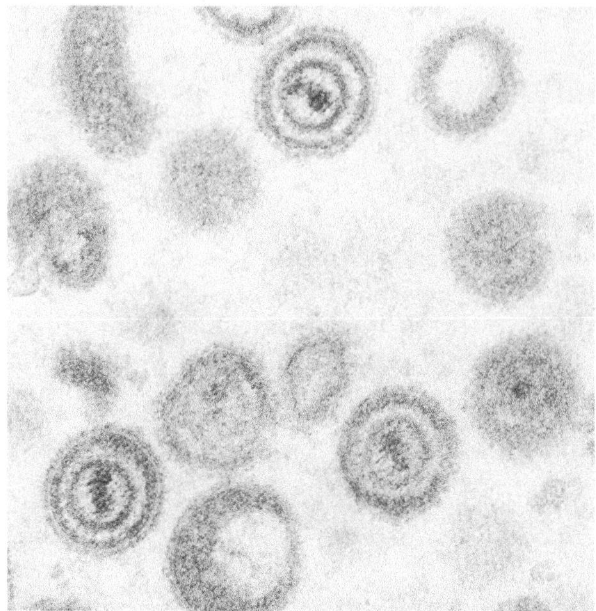

FIGURE 1 Electron micrograph of VZV in skin vesicle fluid from a patient with varicella. Magnification, ×100,000. (Reprinted from reference 125.)

complication rate. The most frequent complications seen with chickenpox are secondary bacterial infections of the skin lesions, which can lead to abscesses, lymphadenitis, and, rarely, bacteremia and sepsis. In healthy adults especially, varicella may be complicated by VZV pneumonia, which is 25 times more frequent in these patients than in children and has been described to be especially severe in pregnant women (12). The hospitalization rate among adults with varicella is about 32 per 1,000 reported cases, which is more than 6 times higher than in children (13).

VZV encephalitis can occur during chickenpox, due to primary infection or to postinfection processes, and often presents with symptoms of acute cerebellar ataxia (14). Other varicella complications include hepatitis, nephritis, and acute thrombocytopenia. In immunosuppressed patients, extensive general dissemination can occur, leading to multiorgan infection and death if not treated early.

Primary infection with VZV during the first 21 weeks of gestation may lead to congenital varicella syndrome in the fetus, characterized by cutaneous scarifications, atrophy of the extremities, and in rare cases, seizures, microcephaly, and other sequelae. The association between the clinical syndrome and VZV has been confirmed by detection of viral DNA by PCR in fetal tissue (15). The incidence is low, <1% in the first 2 trimesters (16). Neonatal varicella can result in severe disseminated infection in babies born within 4 days before to 2 days after the maternal varicella rash appears.

After primary infection, VZV persists in the host in a latent state in sensory trigeminal and dorsal root ganglia. VZV reaches the sensory ganglia, most likely by retrograde axonal transport from skin lesions, and eventually also by hematogenous spread (1). Variable amounts of virus, ranging from about 500 to 55,000 viral genome copies per 100,000 ganglion cells, have been detected in latently infected hosts (17). During VZV latency, transcription and translation of different genes are observed (18). The virus is kept under control mostly by the host's VZV-specific T-cell immunity. When this immunity decreases due to immunosuppression or older age, reactivation of the virus may occur.

Reactivation of VZV can lead to limited subclinical local infection, or the virus may spread via neurons to the skin, resulting in the clinical syndrome herpes zoster. Herpes zoster is mostly characterized as a vesicular rash, typically limited in immunocompetent hosts to the dermatome innervated by a single sensory nerve (1). It is often preceded and accompanied by intense neuropathic pain due to sensory neuron involvement. The eye may be affected, resulting in zoster ophthalmicus. An increase in the VZV-specific T-cell response limits viral spread. The most frequent complication of herpes zoster is postherpetic neuralgia, which presents as severe pain and may last for up to several months after herpes zoster.

In immunocompetent hosts, the most severe complications of herpes zoster are associated with VZV infections of the central nervous system (CNS). Viral meningitis, myelitis, or encephalitis may be observed, with encephalitis probably occurring due to neuronal spread. Cases of facial palsy syndrome are also seen. In most cases, the diagnosis of herpes zoster is a clinical one, based on its characteristic appearance and the distribution of vesicles. In some cases, however, reactivation may also result in zoster sine herpete, a syndrome of undefined local pain that is sometimes also associated with CNS infection that occurs in the absence of a vesicular rash. The diagnosis of zoster sine herpete can be provided only by virological investigation. It may occur more commonly than previously thought. Approximately 25% of cases with CNS complications due to virologically confirmed VZV reactivation occurred in the context of zoster sine herpete (19). Furthermore, VZV reactivation can cause intra- and extracranial vasculopathy.

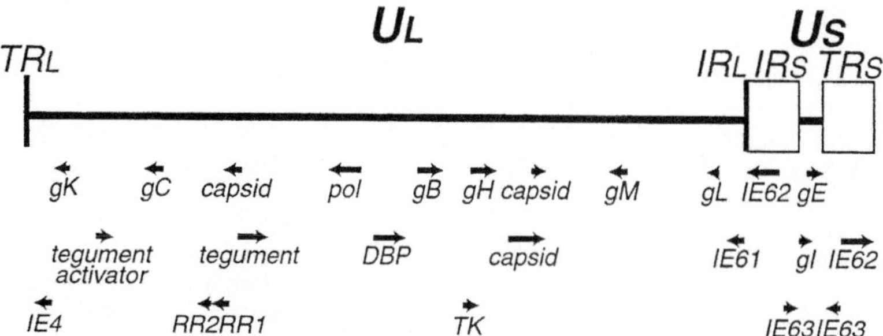

FIGURE 2 Schematic of the VZV linear double-stranded DNA genome. UL, unique long segment (100 kbp); US, unique short segment (5.4 kbp); TRS and TRL, terminal repeats; IRS and IRL, internal repeats. The arrows indicate the direction of the transcription of the viral genes indicated. RR, ribonucleotide reductase; DBP, DNA-binding protein. (Reprinted from reference 126.)

TABLE 1 Diagnostic tests for VZV-induced disease

Method	Target(s)	Suitable specimens (disease)	Comment
PCR	ORF 17, 29, 31, 62, and 69	Fluid, cells, or crust from lesions (varicella, herpes zoster) Blood (disseminated infection, zoster sine herpete) CSF (encephalitis, meningitis, myelitis, facial palsy, zoster sine herpete) Tissue (autopsy)	Most sensitive method. Faster time to result than culture. Quantification possible.
DFA	gE	Cells from lesions (varicella, herpes zoster) Tissue (autopsy)	More sensitive than culture. Rapid time to results (<2 h); random access.
Culture	Infectious virus	Lesion fluid or cells (varicella, herpes zoster) Blood (disseminated infection, zoster sine herpete) Tissue (autopsy)	Positive early in disease (<2 days after rash onset). Recovery can be difficult, as virus is very labile. Traditional diagnostic standard now largely replaced by PCR due to lack of sensitivity and slow time to result (7–10 days for CPE).
Serology	Anti-VZV IgM, IgG	Serum (primarily to assess immunity)	Not recommended for use in disease diagnosis; false-positive and false-negative IgM results may arise. To test IgG levels, 7–10 days required between acute- and convalescent-phase samples.

VZV infection of arteries should be considered in patients with transient ischemic attacks, stroke, or giant cell arteritis, in particular if it follows zoster or varicella (20, 21).

In the immunosuppressed host, primary infection and reactivation can lead to severe and possibly life-threatening generalized infection. In the prevaccine era, severe disseminated primary infection associated with high mortality was a particular concern in immunosuppressed children. This remains an important entity in undervaccinated populations. After bone marrow or solid-organ transplantation, patients frequently exhibit episodes of VZV reactivation, which sometimes proceed to severe disseminated infection and to the development of visceral zoster, a clinical picture characterized by severe abdominal pain and associated with the involvement of internal organs, such as the liver, colon, or lung (22–26). Among solid-organ transplant recipients, lung transplant patients especially have an increased risk for VZV complications (27), but VZV can also cause substantial problems in patients with hematological malignancies or after hematopoietic stem cell transplantation (28). HIV-infected individuals may also undergo severe episodes of VZV reactivation and dissemination, especially during AIDS, and they may exhibit an unusual clinical presentation (29–31). VZV can also play a role in the development of immune reconstitution inflammatory syndrome, and mucocutaneous zoster may occur within 4 weeks after the initiation of highly active antiretroviral therapy (HAART) (32).

Disease caused by VZV can be prevented by vaccination. A live attenuated varicella vaccine derived from the Japanese Oka strain was developed in the early 1970s. It was approved in the United States in 1995 for persons who are susceptible to chickenpox and is currently also recommended in various European countries (33). The childhood vaccination policy in the United States has led to a substantial decrease in varicella incidence (34), disease severity, and associated complications (35). An Oka-derived and a nonlive recombinant vaccine have also been developed to boost immunity against VZV in older patients in order to prevent zoster reactivation (36, 37).

Varicella zoster immune globulin may prevent severe varicella and is thus given to high-risk patient populations to avoid the development of disease. Seronegative women during the first 21 weeks of pregnancy receive the commercially available VZV immune globulin up to 72 hours after VZV exposure, to avoid the development of congenital varicella syndrome in the fetus (8). In immunosuppressed VZV-seronegative patients, such as hematopoietic cell transplant patients, application of VZV immune globulin has been recommended up to 96 hours postexposure to inhibit the development of severe generalized infections (38).

Early and rapid diagnosis of VZV infection is important. Different detection methods are available (summarized in Table 1). Due to its sensitivity, PCR has largely supplanted culture and become the preferred method in many instances. Antigen detection is still useful, as it can be performed rapidly and in a random-access format. Serology is most useful to ascertain immunity.

Specific antiviral treatment of VZV infection and reactivation is possible. If treatment is necessary, it is usually performed with nucleoside analogues, such as acyclovir or penciclovir, or with the better orally bioavailable prodrugs valacyclovir and famciclovir. Brivudine is another nucleoside analogue that has proven effective against VZV (39). Anti-VZV treatment is applied in immunosuppressed hosts and in immunocompetent patients when clinical complications arise. In addition, herpes zoster reactivation is also treated to limit the development of postherpetic neuralgia and to prevent ocular involvement.

COLLECTION, TRANSPORT, AND STORAGE OF SPECIMENS

Various specimens can be used for diagnosis (Table 1), depending on the clinical presentation and test method. Vesicular fluid contains cell-free virus, mostly at high concentrations. Since nearly all patients with varicella and many patients with herpes zoster show a vesicular rash, and because collection of vesicular fluid is very convenient, laboratory diagnosis from vesicular fluid is a major diagnostic tool for detection or confirmation of VZV infection or reactivation. The vesicular fluid can be collected using capillary pipettes or syringes. For PCR analysis, vesicular fluid can also be collected on swabs and submitted to the laboratory in physiological saline or in viral transport medium. If further virus culture is planned, it should be kept in mind that virus collected on swabs is less stable and is also further diluted in the medium, which may decrease the efficiency of virus culture.

VZV DNA is detectable by PCR in plasma, serum, whole blood, and peripheral blood mononuclear cells (PBMCs). Plasma or serum is conventionally used due to ease of preparation. Whole-blood specimens should be submitted in anticoagulants other than heparin if PCR testing is to be performed, as heparin can inhibit *Taq* polymerases. Virus can be recovered from PBMCs early in disease; however, this method is used primarily in research. Cerebrospinal fluid (CSF) should be submitted in a sterile container. Usually, uncentrifuged CSF is used for detection of VZV DNA, but virus can also be detected in the cellular fraction or in supernatant.

Tissue is tested primarily at autopsy. In disseminated disease, tissue testing has now largely been replaced by PCR of blood specimens due to test sensitivity and ease of specimen procurement. Cells from tissue can be stained by immunofluorescence. Touch preparations of cells are prepared by pressing tissue (typically 10 to 15 mm) against the clean surface of a glass slide multiple times, over a length of 30 to 40 mm. Slides are air dried, fixed in cold acetone, and stained with reagents used in antigen detection (see below). Tissue homogenates can be prepared as described in chapter 81 and tested by culture or PCR.

Generally, VZV DNA, which is ultimately amplified by PCR methods, is quite stable during collection, transport, and storage. VZV virions, however, are quite labile; therefore, specimens should be placed into culture as quickly as possible after collection if isolation is required. Samples for PCR can be stored at −20°C. Virus isolation from frozen samples is largely ineffective unless cellular fractions are stored in cryoprotectant medium at −80°C.

DIRECT EXAMINATION

Microscopy

One of the oldest direct detection methods is the Tzanck test. In this assay, cellular material is scraped from the base of vesicular lesions and put onto glass slides. These smears are then stained, examined under a microscope, and screened for multinucleated giant cells, which contain multiple eosinophilic intranuclear inclusions representing viral capsids (Fig. 3). However, since the presence of these cells is characteristic both of HSV and VZV infections, a specific diagnosis of VZV cannot be made with this test. VZV can be visualized by electron microscopy, but this method also does not allow a clear differentiation between the different herpesviruses (Fig. 1).

Antigen Detection

VZV antigen detection from cell-containing vesicle material by direct fluorescent-antibody assay (DFA) is sometimes still used for rapid detection of VZV infection in hospitalized patients. Cell suspensions obtained by skin scrapings from the base of the vesicle are applied to glass slides, fixed with cold acetone, and dried. Then cells are stained with fluorescently labeled monoclonal antibodies (MAbs) for 30 min at 37°C in a humidified chamber. After a washing step, cells are covered with a coverslip, and staining is visualized by fluorescence microscopy (Fig. 4) (40). VZV-specific monoclonal antibodies are commercially available (Merifluor; Meridian Diagnostics, Meridian Bioscience Inc., Cincinnati, OH; Light Diagnostics, Chemicon/Merck) as well as dual HSV/VZV monoclonal antibody pools (SimulFlor HSV/VZV; Light Diagnostics, Chemicon/Merck). Antigen detection is clearly less sensitive than PCR-based methods for direct detection of virus from clinical material and can be performed only from samples containing intact cells, which limits its general applicability (41).

Nucleic Acid Detection

Over the last decade, nucleic acid (NA) amplification-based techniques, especially PCR assays, have become standard tools for the diagnosis of VZV disease. These techniques have revolutionized the diagnosis of VZV disease of the CNS, of disseminated VZV infection in immunocompromised patients, and the identification of herpes zoster in patients who do not develop the typical rash. The advantages of these molecular techniques are that they require only small volumes of input material and are highly sensitive and rapid.

Since the description of the first detection of VZV DNA in CSF by conventional PCR (42), the PCR techniques used have changed substantially. Real-time PCR methods (reviewed in chapter 5) that are more sensitive and can be quantitative have replaced older PCR techniques and are now routinely performed in many diagnostic laboratories.

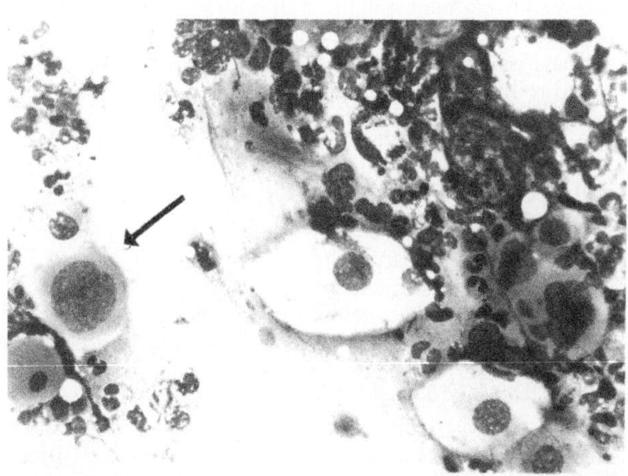

FIGURE 3 Giemsa-stained preparation of material from the base of a vesicular lesion. Magnification, ×102. The arrow indicates a giant cell with a folded nucleus characteristic of VZV or HSV.

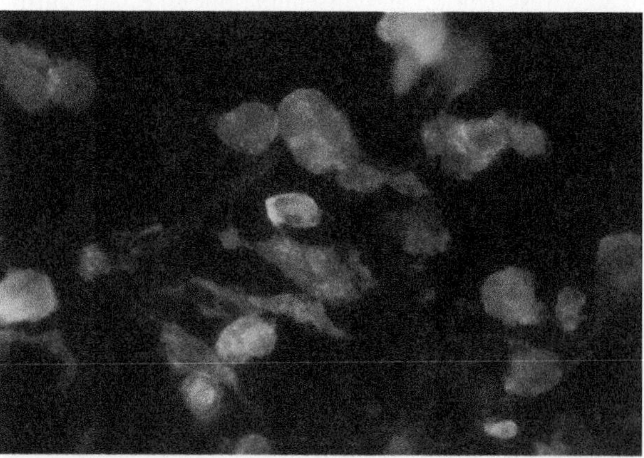

FIGURE 4 Immunofluorescence assay for the detection of VZV-positive cells from a patient with zoster. A smear of a skin vesicle was fixed and stained with monoclonal antibody to VZV gE. Magnification, ×200.

Numerous in-house PCR tests have been published for amplifying various gene segments of the VZV genome (Table 1). There is no generally preferred target sequence, and the genetic variability between virus strains is low. An increasing number of commercially available VZV nucleic acid test kits are being developed, such as VZV tracer (Affigene; Cepheid), the VZV PCR kit (Abbott Laboratories), and Artus VZV PCR kits (Qiagen). Protocols have also been designed for simultaneous amplification of VZV together with various other viruses causing similar clinical pictures. Commercially available tests include Artus Herpes Virus LC-PCR kits (Qiagen; CE marked for *in vitro* diagnostic use in Europe, available for research use only in Canada, and not available in the United States), HSV1 HSV2 VZV R-gene (Argene Inc.; CE marked for *in vitro* diagnostic use in Europe and available for research use only in the United States), and the Lyra Direct HSV 1+2/VZV assay (Quidel Corp.; FDA approved), and the Biofire Film Array meningitis/encephalitis panel (bioMérieux; FDA cleared and CE marked). These multiplex PCRs are able to identify a variety of diagnostically important viruses simultaneously, either within one tube or by parallel detection in a single PCR run (43, 44). VZV detection and quantification by PCR can be performed in various clinical materials (for an overview, see Table 2). Quantified VZV DNA for use as nucleic acid detection and quantification test controls is

TABLE 2 Quantitative VZV DNA results with different clinical materials from patients with different VZV-associated diseases[a]

Material	Clinical syndrome	No. investigated	% PCR positive	Viral load: Median, mean, or geometric mean	Viral load: Range	Reference
Vesicle	Varicella	3		1.0×10^8 co/ml		69
	Zoster	3		7.4×10^8 co/ml		69
CSF	Meningitis	17		4.110^3 co/ml	$50–1.710^6$ co/ml	19
	Meningitis	25		2.7×10^4 co/ml	$2 \times 10^3–5.2 \times 10^5$ co/ml	54
	Meningitis	25		2.9×10^4 co/ml	$4 \times 10^2–2.7 \times 10^5$ co/ml	55
	Encephalitis	13		7.4×10^4 co/ml	$1 \times 10^3–2.6 \times 10^8$ co/ml	19
	Encephalitis	19		8.6×10^4 co/ml	$3 \times 10^2–2.1 \times 10^8$ co/ml	54
	Encephalitis	20		1.1×10^5 co/ml	$4.3 \times 10^3–2.4 \times 10^7$ co/ml	55
	CNS infection	16		3.1×10^3 co/ml	$1.1 \times 10^2–4 \times 10^4$ co/ml	56
Saliva	Ramsay Hunt syndrome	25	52		$30–1.410^6$ co/50 μl	127
	Facial palsy without rash	31	55		$10–1 \times 10^5$ co/50 μl	127
	Zoster	54	100		$8–2.7 \times 10^7$ co/ml	66
Whole blood	Varicella in adults	34	100	5×10^2 co/ml	$20–10^5$ co/ml	73
	Varicella	8	87.5	1.6×10^3 co/ml	$2 \times 10^2–1.1 \times 10^4$ co/ml	72
	Zoster dermatomal	9	90	2×10^2 co/ml	$10^2–9 \times 10^2$ co/ml	72
	Zoster multidermatomal	5	100	2.7×10^3 co/ml	$9 \times 10^2–3 \times 10^5$ co/ml	72
	Healthy control	20	0			72
	Blood donors	100	0			82
PBMCs	Varicella	9	100	12 co/10^5 cells		68
	Varicella	19	73	4.9×10^2 co/10^5 cells	$5–5 \times 10^3$ co/10^5 cells	69
	Varicella	21	48		$1.4 \times 10^2–3.4 \times 10^3$ co/10^5 cells	70
	Zoster	10	20	10 co/10^5 cells		69
	Zoster	71	16		$10–10^2$ co/10^5 cells	70
	Zoster	130	78	9×10^2 co/10^5 cells	$40–2.9 \times 10^4$ co/10^5 cells	74
	Healthy controls	28	0			69
	Healthy controls (50 ml blood)	53	5	1.3×10^3 co/10^5 cells	$6 \times 10^2–5 \times 10^3$ co/10^5 cells	74
Serum/plasma	Varicella	18	89	2.0×10^3 co/ml	$100–2 \times 10^5$ co/ml	72
	Varicella	5	100	10^4 co/ml		68
	Disseminated varicella	1		1.2×10^7 co/ml		80
	Zoster dermatomal	9	67	100 co/ml		72
	Zoster multidermatomal	6	100	2.7×10^3 co/ml		72
	Zoster	9	100	1.7×10^3 co/ml	$1.8 \times 10^2–10^4$ co/ml	77
	Zoster	12		7×10^3 co/ml	$4 \times 10^2–2 \times 10^5$ co/ml	76
	Zoster	36	78	4.3×10^2 co/ml	$<10^2–2 \times 10^6$ co/ml	78
	Zoster disseminated	4	100	2.1×10^5 co/ml	$2.5 \times 10^3–7.4 \times 10^5$ co/ml	77
	Zoster visceral disseminated	1		2×10^5 co/ml		81
	Meningitis	35	31		$<10^2–6.7 \times 10^4$ co/ml	78
	Encephalitis	18	72	3.3×10^2 co/ml	$<10^2–1.2 \times 10^6$ co/ml	78
	Healthy control	10	0			72
Aqueous humor	Acute retinal necrosis	2			9×10^2 and 5.5×10^6 co/ml	128
	Anterior uveitis	8		2.5×10^5 co/ml	$3.8 \times 10^2–1.2 \times 10^7$ co/ml	85
Tissue	Postmortem	17	100	9×10^3 co/10^5 GC	$5.8 \times 10^2–5.5 \times 10^4$ co/10^5 GC	17

[a]Abbreviations: co, copies; GC, ganglion cells.

provided by various manufacturers, such as Advanced Biotechnologies, Inc. (Columbia, MD), and Zeptometrix Corp. (Buffalo, NY), and by the National Institute for Biological Standards and Control (South Mimms, Hertfordshire, United Kingdom).

VZV DNA from vesicular fluid and skin scrapings can be detected easily by PCR. This helps to discriminate quickly between vesicular lesions caused by VZV and those due to various other causes, especially HSV-1 or HSV-2 infection. The benefit of VZV PCR was also shown for the diagnosis of vaccine-modified varicella disease (41). VZV DNA can be detected by PCR in crusting lesions (45) and in skin scrapings in VZV-associated facial palsy even in the absence of visible vesicular lesions (46). The easy access and the high virus detection rates make dermal lesions an ideal material to be used not only for diagnosis but also for further genotyping of vaccine and wild-type (WT) strains using genotype-specific PCR strategies (47, 48).

Analysis of CSF using nucleic acid amplification has become the method of choice for diagnosis of neurological disease associated with VZV, such as cerebellitis, aseptic meningitis, and encephalitis. Using PCR, it was found that neurological disease is an important and not infrequent complication in immunocompetent as well as immunosuppressed patients. VZV DNA was detected in CSF of up to 10% of patients presenting with clinical symptoms of aseptic meningitis and (meningo)encephalitis (49–51). PCR analysis is also useful for the diagnosis of VZV-induced neurological symptoms in cases where the characteristic vesicular rash appears only after the start of CNS infection, or even in cases of zoster sine herpete (19, 52–54). No rash was observed in about a quarter of all cases of patients suffering from VZV-associated neurological symptoms (19, 53, 54). Higher mean VZV DNA loads were found in CSF of patients with herpes zoster-associated encephalitis than with meningitis (Fig. 5A) (19, 55) and in patients requiring intensive-care treatment than in those who did not, although overlap was observed among individual patients in each of the compared groups (Fig. 5B) (19). Virus is predominantly detected within 1 week after the onset of clinical symptoms, but in cases of VZV-induced neurological symptoms without rash, virus can be detected in the second week of disease (19, 53).

In cases of varicella-induced cerebellar ataxia, the amount of viral DNA has been shown to be generally low (42, 56, 57), supporting the theory that these symptoms might be mediated by the antiviral immune response. After initiation of antiviral therapy, CSF usually becomes negative for VZV DNA in the follow-up in uncomplicated cases (42). In contrast, the continuous presence of viral DNA has been found in individual HIV-infected patients in spite of therapy, and this was associated with the death of these patients (58).

PCR testing plays an important role in the diagnosis of acute VZV-associated peripheral facial palsy occurring as a neurological complication in the course of VZV reactivation. In cases of Ramsay Hunt syndrome, virus can be detected not only in vesicles of the auricles and the oral cavity but also in the facial nerve sheath, middle ear mucosa, and CSF (59). As the rash is mostly hidden in the ear or mouth and may be faint or delayed, only sensitive testing for the presence of VZV by PCR has shown that a considerable number of idiopathic peripheral facial palsy or Bell's palsy cases are due to VZV reactivation. Using PCR methods, VZV was detected in saliva samples of 58% of patients with VZV-induced facial palsy, with 64% of those cases presenting without characteristic rash (60). Virus was shown to be present in oropharyngeal swabs until day 12 in patients with acute peripheral facial palsy (61). VZV DNA levels in saliva were about 10^4 copies higher and recovery of facial function was worse in patients with facial palsy and oropharyngeal lesions than in those with facial palsy alone (61). VZV can be detected rarely in CSF samples of patients with facial palsy (59, 62), and smaller amounts of virus are found in these patients than in those presenting with meningitis and encephalitis (Fig. 5C) (19, 54, 63).

In saliva, VZV DNA was detectable in 30% of healthy astronauts, indicating that subclinical reactivation is frequent (64, 65). In patients with herpes zoster, VZV DNA was found in saliva of 54 out of 54 patients, including those with thoracic or vertebral zoster. The VZV loads ranged from 8×10^0 to 2.7×10^7 copies/ml (66).

VZV DNA is also detectable in PBMCs (67–70) and in whole blood (71–74), and although the viremia is assumed to be cell associated, viral DNA can also be detected in serum or plasma (68, 72, 75–77). Viremia is detected by PCR in up to 100% of cases of acute varicella, but virus can also be detected in the blood compartment in cases of herpes zoster. VZV DNA was detected in 47 to 93% of serum samples obtained within the first 8 days after the start of herpes zoster from otherwise healthy patients (75, 78). In a small cohort of nine immunocompetent patients with herpes zoster, all were found to be VZV DNA positive when the amount of plasma analyzed was increased to

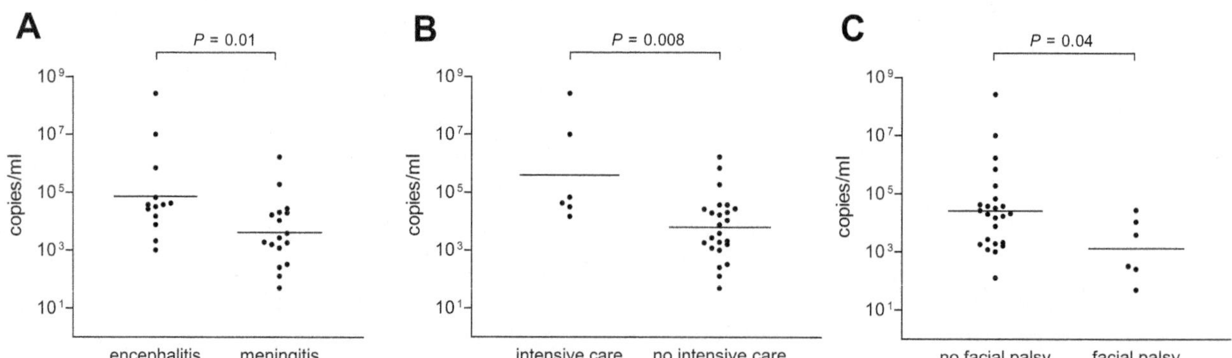

FIGURE 5 Comparison of the amount of VZV DNA in CSF according to the neurological diagnosis (A), the severity of disease (B), and the presence of acute peripheral facial palsy with meningeal signs (C). The geometric mean values are shown by horizontal lines. The *P* values were calculated using the Mann-Whitney *U* test. (Modified from reference 19, with permission.)

1 ml (77). Quantitative analysis showed that viral loads may range from 5 to 5 × 10^3 copies/10^5 cells in PBMCs, from 20 to 10^5 copies/ml in whole blood, and from 100 to 2 × 10^6 copies/ml in plasma or serum. The virus load is higher in patients with acute varicella than in those with herpes zoster (72). A higher viral load correlates with a larger number of skin lesions and more severe disease (73), as well as with the presence of multidermatomal zoster (72). The viral load was lower in samples taken only a few days after the start of varicella symptoms (69) and was found to be negative in convalescent-phase sera of patients with shingles (75). When a highly sensitive nested PCR assay was used, VZV DNA was also detected in PBMCs of patients with facial palsy without dermal lesions (79). VZV DNA in serum with viral loads ranging from 50 to 1.2 × 10^6 copies/ml was also found in patients with meningitis and encephalitis, including 6 cases out of 32 without rash (78).

Virus detection in blood is important for the diagnosis of complicated or clinically unclear courses of varicella or herpes zoster, especially in cases in which the appearance of a rash is delayed or completely lacking, and also in cases of visceral dissemination (77, 80, 81). In immunocompromised patients, quantitative PCR analysis proved to be an important tool for monitoring the clinical course of disease and assessing therapeutic success (76, 77, 80, 81).

VZV is not detectable in the blood in the majority of healthy control patients, even with sensitive PCR methods (82), unless a very large volume of blood (50 ml) is used (74). In other studies, VZV was detectable in 2 to 3% of PBMC samples taken from immunocompetent individuals without clinical signs of VZV illness (70, 83). These findings support the assumption that asymptomatic reactivation of latent virus may occur and may be important for boosting host immunity to the virus (84).

VZV PCR can be performed from aqueous humor and has been found to be helpful in confirming VZV-associated ocular disease. Viral load in the aqueous humor of patients with anterior uveitis corresponds to the extent of iris atrophy (85).

Identification of VZV by PCR in bronchoalveolar lavage specimens has been reported and seems to be useful for the successful early diagnosis of severe VZV pneumonitis (86). The detection of VZV DNA in tissue samples by PCR is also possible and has been used to confirm the association between VZV and congenital varicella syndrome (15, 87). Generally, the use of highly sensitive PCR techniques may be especially important for confirming the diagnosis of VZV-related disease in cases of less disseminated or milder disease associated with lower viral loads (46, 70) or for samples obtained later in the course of disease after the initiation of antiviral therapy.

ISOLATION AND IDENTIFICATION

Cell Culture Methods

Virus isolation provides the basis for phenotypic characterization of individual VZV strains, for generating VZV-infected cells for serological tests, such as the fluorescent-antibody-to-membrane-antibody (FAMA) test, and for the phenotypic analysis of VZV drug resistance. Many laboratories use human foreskin fibroblasts for isolation of VZV from clinical samples. Other sensitive host cells include diploid human cell lines, preferably derived from fetal kidney, fetal lung, human lung carcinoma (A549), or human melanoma cell lines, and non-human cell lines, such as primary monkey kidney cells (40, 88). A cell mixture (CV-1 and MRC-5) is commercially available for the recovery of herpesviruses including VZV (H&V Mix; Diagnostic Hybrids, A Quidel Company). VZV maintains a high level of genetic stability during the culturing procedure. Cell cultures are performed at 37°C under sterile conditions, and the medium used is usually Eagle's minimal essential medium, prepared in Hanks' or Earle's balanced salt solution containing neomycin and glutamine and supplemented with 10% fetal bovine serum for the growth medium and 1 to 2% fetal bovine serum for maintenance. The medium is heat inactivated at 56°C for 30 min. The need for a medium change is indicated by a drop in pH, and this change is required at least once weekly. When virus culture is done for diagnostic purposes, the clinical material is adsorbed onto the cell monolayer or inoculated directly into the medium, and the cells are then incubated at 37°C and evaluated daily by microscopy. The development of a cytopathic effect (CPE) is variable, but a CPE is usually visible from 4 days up to maximally 2 weeks. The CPE consists of small foci of rounded and swollen cells. Confirmation of VZV infection is done by PCR or by staining monolayer cells with VZV-specific monoclonal antibodies (described below). Shell vial centrifugation cultures can provide results in 2 to 5 days and are more sensitive than conventional cultures for VZV but less sensitive than PCR.

Virus Identification from Cell Culture

Specific identification of VZV from clinical material in cell culture after the emergence of a CPE is necessary because it may be difficult to distinguish VZV from other herpesviruses. For identification by VZV-specific PCR, supernatant is taken from the culture, and DNA is extracted and subjected to PCR. Monolayers can also be stained with VZV-specific MAbs when approximately 50% of the monolayer demonstrates CPE suggestive of VZV. For this purpose, cell monolayers are washed with phosphate-buffered saline (PBS). Then monolayer cells are scraped into 0.5 ml PBS. Slides are prepared by directly applying the suspension to a glass slide using a cytocentrifuge. Slides are air dried and then fixed in cold acetone for 10 minutes. Following a washing with PBS, cells are stained with VZV-specific MAbs. Commercial reagents approved for use in culture confirmation include the D^3 DFA VZV detection kit (Quidel) as well as the MAbs listed in "Antigen Detection" above. After a 30-min incubation at 37°C, monolayers are washed in PBS and rinsed in distilled water. Excess moisture is removed by blotting around wells. Stained cells should not be allowed to dry, as this produces artifactual fluorescence. Mounting medium and a coverslip are applied, and the staining is visualized by fluorescence microscopy.

Genetic VZV Strain Characterization

Genetic identification of VZV is performed by different molecular methods, directly from clinical specimens, but primarily on a research basis. Characterization of VZV strains is usually done by PCR assays followed by restriction fragment length polymorphism analysis or by sequencing of characteristic fragments and determination of single-nucleotide polymorphisms (89). Genetic analysis of virus strains has proven that the VZV strains identified during varicella are identical within an outbreak and are also identical to those present in subsequent herpes zoster (90). It has been shown that VZV strains vary between geographic areas (3, 89).

Characterization of VZV strains may be especially important for differentiating between WT strains and Oka vaccine strains after vaccination, for determining the etiology of a postvaccination rash, for analyzing the association between vaccination and the development of herpes zoster, and also for assessing whether transmission of vaccine virus to susceptible persons has occurred. Different methods for discrimination between WT and vaccine strains have been published, and in this regard, much attention has been focused on VZV ORF 62 because most nonsynonymous VZV vaccine mutations occur in this ORF. In particular, SmaI and NaeI sites in ORF 62 have been shown to allow the discrimination of vaccine strains from WT strains and also from the Oka parental strain (91).

In addition, real-time PCR assays based on sequence polymorphisms, especially in ORF 62, have also been established (48, 92).

The analysis of the Oka vaccine itself has shown that it contains a mixture of different strains that also differ in the R2 repeat region (93). The development of rash after vaccination seems to be associated with the emergence of certain strains that are closely related to the Oka parental strain (94).

SEROLOGIC TESTS

Antibodies against VZV develop in the course of primary infection, are directed against various proteins of the virus, and can be detected in most cases within 3 days after the appearance of the rash. Serological testing can be used for confirmation of primary infections, where it is applied especially in clinically atypical cases. Detection of VZV-specific antibodies (Abs) is also routinely used for determining the immune status. This may be required in patients who cannot remember their varicella history and is especially important in pretransplantation evaluations as well as after virus exposure to guide prophylaxis with varicella immune globulin in high-risk individuals, such as solid-organ or bone marrow transplant patients, pregnant women, and health care workers. In addition, it may be used for monitoring a patient's immune status after vaccination, although assessment of vaccine efficacy is not routinely performed. A variety of serological methods that differ in specificity, sensitivity, and utility are available for detecting VZV-specific Abs.

Specialized IgG Detection Tests

A number of different serologic assays are performed in specialized or referral laboratories, often for research purposes. One such test is the FAMA test, which is considered the gold standard for serological testing (95) and which correlates best with protection against varicella (96). A flow cytometry-adapted version of the FAMA assay has also been developed (97). The FAMA titer, however, is not predictive of long-term protection after vaccination. Although high seroconversion rates have been described after vaccination, a loss of FAMA-detectable Abs is generally observed over time (98). The FAMA test is labor-intensive and nonautomated. A noncommercial and apparently very sensitive enzyme immunoassay (EIA) developed by Merck, based on the detection of VZV glycoprotein preparations, has been used for extended postvaccination serostudies. EIA titers of 5 glycoprotein EIA units/ml or more at 6 weeks after vaccination have been associated with a high degree of protection against breakthrough for the following 7 years (99). However, the fact that breakthroughs have also been observed after this Ab level has been achieved suggests that glycoprotein EIA levels correlating with long-term protection have not been adequately defined. Other IgG detection assays that are used in specialized settings include the anticomplement immunofluorescence test, the time-resolved fluorescence immunoassay (100), and plaque reduction assays that detect neutralizing Abs against varicella; these tests are important tools for confirming that vaccine-induced Abs are in fact neutralizing circulating WT VZV strains (101).

IgG Detection Tests in Routine Diagnostic Laboratories

Clinical laboratories typically use commercial immunoassays, and a variety of different formats are available, including EIA (colorimetric and fluorescence detection), chemoluminescence, and immunoassays. These tests have the advantage of being less laborious than the FAMA test, do not require any additional VZV cell culture procedures, and can be interpreted objectively; many are automated, and some instruments are random access. The different tests use either whole VZV-infected-cell lysate as the specific antigen or, in some cases, purified glycoprotein, and the test procedure is done according to the manufacturer's protocol. In some laboratories, noncommercial, in-house EIAs have been established for routine detection of VZV-specific Abs, mostly with whole viral lysates as the test antigen (100, 102–104).

Validation of commercial tests is usually done by comparison to the FAMA test, and the results obtained show that these assays are generally less sensitive than the FAMA test. Commercial immunoassays have been shown to detect Abs in 43 to 92% of naturally infected individuals identified as seropositive by the FAMA test or an adapted FAMA protocol (105). In their specificity, commercial immunoassays are more similar to the FAMA test (102). Considering that one aim of an Ab test is usually to determine if a person is susceptible to infection and thus a candidate for vaccination, the lower sensitivity of the commercial immunoassays leads to more unnecessary vaccinations. The risks associated with this, however, are low compared to the risk of infection of a person who has been falsely declared immune. Immunoassays are typically used to detect VZV-specific Abs in blood, but they may also serve to detect Abs in CSF.

IgG Avidity Assays

To discriminate recent from past infections or to assess the impairment of Ab development in immunosuppressed patients, VZV IgG antibodies may be further tested for their avidity (106–108). For this purpose, an EIA is run in duplicate, and one of the runs is treated with dilutions of sodium thiocyanate or with diethylamine (106, 107). The avidity index is calculated as the ratio of the optical density of the treated sample to that of the untreated sample. The lower the optical density of the treated sample relative to that of the untreated sample, the more Abs of low avidity are present in the sample, which is a sign of a recent infection.

IgM Assays

Testing for IgM antibodies is usually performed by commercially available EIAs and may be used as an additional tool to identify primary VZV infection when the clinical picture is not typical for varicella. Detection of VZV-specific IgM Abs in CSF is sometimes performed retrospectively to confirm intrathecal VZV Ab production after VZV infection of the CNS. VZV IgM was also identified in 37% of patients with herpes zoster, for up to 4 to 5 weeks after onset of lesions (109).

Cellular Immunity

It has been shown that VZV-specific cellular immunity is the key factor in keeping VZV in a latent state. T-cell-mediated immunity consists of CD4 and CD8 effector and memory cells and is detected up to 2 weeks after the rash appears (110). A decrease in cellular immunity, which is observed with increasing age or during immunosuppression, facilitates VZV reactivation and development of herpes zoster (111). Cellular immunity against VZV can be measured with a gamma interferon enzyme-linked immunospot assay or intracellular cytokine staining followed by fluorescence-activated cell sorting analysis (112–114). The identification of VZV-stimulated cytokines may be used to assess the VZV-specific immunocompetence in transplant recipients (108, 115) or to identify protection against VZV after vaccination, in patients negative for VZV-specific Abs (107). However, these methods are so far mainly investigational.

ANTIVIRAL THERAPY AND SUSCEPTIBILITY

Most VZV strains are fully susceptible to antiviral drugs. Resistance against acyclovir or penciclovir has been observed primarily in HIV-infected individuals in the pre-HAART era, in transplant recipients, and in hemato-oncological patients.

Development of drug resistance may lead to uncontrolled viral dissemination, visceral complication, and death of the patient (116, 117). Data from *in vitro* studies and investigation of resistant WT isolates have shown that acyclovir resistance is mostly associated with mutations in the VZV TK gene and is only rarely due to mutations in the VZV DNA polymerase (118). Foscarnet and cidofovir can be used for treatment of acyclovir-resistant strains. Resistant VZV strains may be detected only in specific compartments, and therefore, when screening for drug-resistant VZV strains is performed, samples from all affected body sites should be investigated (119). Antiviral susceptibility of VZV strains can be determined phenotypically. Changes in virus replication in the presence of different concentrations of various drugs are measured in most cases by plaque reduction assay in human diploid lung cells. The 50% effective doses of acyclovir have been shown to range from 2.06 μM to 6.28 μM (120). Other methods that have been described include the late-antigen synthesis reduction assay (121) and phenotypic characterization of the TK gene without the need for virus isolation (122). Phenotypic analysis has several disadvantages that limit its clinical utility: time to result typically is prolonged, limiting its use in clinical decision-making; it cannot easily be performed from all clinical materials; and it may be not sensitive enough for detection of minor resistant VZV populations. Therefore, genotypic resistance testing is preferred for clinical use, as it is rapid and can be performed from different clinical materials. Genotypic resistance testing is mostly done by sequencing of certain regions of the VZV TK gene that are associated with resistance to acyclovir (123) and of parts of the polymerase gene. A number of defined VZV mutations have been described so far, and their influence on resistance against different drugs has been proven by phenotypic data (124). Resistance testing is so far performed only in research settings and is not applied in routine diagnostics.

EVALUATION, INTERPRETATION, AND REPORTING OF RESULTS

For appropriate evaluation and interpretation of test results, knowledge about the clinical background of the individual patient is of the utmost importance. The interpretation of the results is dependent on whether a primary infection with VZV is suspected or whether the patient has already had chickenpox. In addition, it is important to know whether a patient is immunosuppressed.

Primary infection is usually diagnosed based on clinical presentation. Virus can be detected from vesicles by PCR and antigen detection assays and from pustules and even crusts by PCR. The results of serologic tests can be suggestive but are not definitively diagnostic of primary infection. For example, IgM (alone or in the presence of low IgG) or a 4-fold increase in IgG in convalescent-phase serum can be observed during primary infection; however, these seroresponses can also be detected during reactivation.

Herpes zoster can also be diagnosed clinically; however, confirmation may be necessary if vesicles are limited or otherwise indistinct in appearance from those seen in other types of infection. Detection of virus in vesicle fluid is preferred.

The presence of VZV in blood can be observed by PCR assays during chickenpox and sometimes during VZV reactivation. In most immunocompromised hosts, detection of VZV in blood by PCR is generally indicative of severe disease. It should be noted, however, that VZV DNA can also be detected in the blood of HIV patients with localized zoster. The same holds true for the detection of VZV DNA in CSF, which is generally considered a pathological finding. Both clinical situations usually require immediate antiviral treatment.

However, highly sensitive detection of virus DNA does not always prove the causality of disease. VZV DNA may also be found due to secondary and/or subclinical reactivation, but then it will be observed mostly at clearly lower levels than during VZV disease. In this context, the quantitative evaluation and reporting of VZV DNA levels is gaining significance. Within immunocompromised patients, so far no defined VZV-DNA thresholds in blood exist for distinguishing subclinical reactivation from clinically relevant and potentially fatal disease. However, severe visceral infections are clearly associated with higher virus load levels in blood (Table 2). Studies have also shown that high VZV DNA levels in CSF may be associated with the expression and severity of CNS disease (Fig. 5). It may therefore be useful to assess and report quantitative results in the setting of VZV CNS disease. In the pre-PCR era, Ab detection in CSF and quantitation in comparison to blood Ab levels were used for diagnosis of VZV infections of the CNS. The detection of IgM Abs is considered a proof for intrathecal Ab production, as is an increase of the IgG Ab CSF/serum ratio in relation to a test of the blood-brain barrier function, i.e., the albumin CSF/serum ratio. The clinical significance of these tests in VZV infections of the CNS and their value for therapeutic decisions are limited, as they allow a diagnosis only late in the course of disease, in contrast to PCR tests of CSF, which identify virus replication already at an earlier stage of disease. Serology from CSF was, however, described to be of certain value for detection of VZV vasculopathy (20, 21).

The major importance of Ab assays, of which commercial immunoassays are currently the most commonly used, lies in their ability to identify previously infected individuals, as indicated by anti-VZV IgG Abs in the absence of IgM. This information can be used to guide further vaccination decisions. However, this may result in the vaccination of seropositive individuals, since these tests are not as sensitive as other gold standard formats.

REFERENCES

1. **Cohen J, Straus SE, Arvin AM.** 2007. Varicella zoster virus, replication, pathogenesis and management, p 2773–2818. *In* Knipe DM, Howley PM (ed), *Fields Virology*, 5th ed. Lippincott, Williams and Wilkins, Philadelphia, PA.
2. **Davison AJ, Scott JE.** 1986. The complete DNA sequence of varicella-zoster virus. *J Gen Virol* **67:**1759–1816.
3. **Quinlivan M, Breuer J.** 2006. Molecular studies of Varicella zoster virus. *Rev Med Virol* **16:**225–250.
4. **Loparev VN, Rubtcova EN, Bostik V, Govil D, Birch CJ, Druce JD, Schmid DS, Croxson MC.** 2007. Identification of five major and two minor genotypes of varicella-zoster virus strains: a practical two-amplicon approach used to genotype clinical isolates in Australia and New Zealand. *J Virol* **81:**12758–12765.
5. **Breuer J, Grose C, Norberg P, Tipples G, Schmid DS.** 2010. A proposal for a common nomenclature for viral clades that form the species varicella-zoster virus: summary of VZV Nomenclature Meeting 2008, Barts and the London School of Medicine and Dentistry, 24-25 July 2008. *J Gen Virol* **91:**821–828.
6. **Nardone A, de Ory F, Carton M, Cohen D, van Damme P, Davidkin I, Rota MC, de Melker H, Mossong J, Slacikova M, Tischer A, Andrews N, Berbers G, Gabutti G, Gay N, Jones L, Jokinen S, Kafatos G, de Aragón MV, Schneider F, Smetana Z, Vargova B, Vranckx R, Miller E.** 2007. The comparative sero-epidemiology of varicella zoster virus in 11 countries in the European region. *Vaccine* **25:**7866–7872.
7. **Papaloukas O, Giannouli G, Papaevangelou V.** 2014. Successes and challenges in varicella vaccine. *Ther Adv Vaccines* **2:**39–55.
8. **Enders G, Bolley I, Miller E, Cradock-Watson J, Ridehalgh M.** 1994. Consequences of varicella and herpes zoster in pregnancy: prospective study of 1739 cases. *Lancet* **343:**1548–1551.
9. **Gershon AA, Steinberg SP, Gelb L.** 1984. Clinical reinfection with varicella-zoster virus. *J Infect Dis* **149:**137–142.
10. **Hall S, Maupin T, Seward J, Jumaan AO, Peterson C, Goldman G, Mascola L, Wharton M.** 2002. Second varicella infections: are they more common than previously thought? *Pediatrics* **109:**1068–1073.
11. **Galil K, Brown C, Lin F, Seward J.** 2002. Hospitalizations for varicella in the United States, 1988 to 1999. *Pediatr Infect Dis J* **21:**931–934.
12. **Kaneko T, Ishigatsubo Y.** 2004. Varicella pneumonia in adults. *Intern Med* **43:**1105–1106.
13. **Marin M, Watson TL, Chaves SS, Civen R, Watson BM, Zhang JX, Perella D, Mascola L, Seward JF.** 2008. Varicella among adults: data from an active surveillance project, 1995–2005. *J Infect Dis* **197**(Suppl 2)**:**S94–S100.
14. **van der Maas NA, Bondt PE, de Melker H, Kemmeren JM.** 2009. Acute cerebellar ataxia in the Netherlands: a study on the association with vaccinations and varicella zoster infection. *Vaccine* **27:**1970–1973.
15. **Puchhammer-Stöckl E, Kunz C, Wagner G, Enders G.** 1994. Detection of varicella zoster virus (VZV) DNA in fetal tissue by polymerase chain reaction. *J Perinat Med* **22:**65–69.
16. **Smith CK, Arvin AM.** 2009. Varicella in the fetus and newborn. *Semin Fetal Neonatal Med* **14:**209–217.
17. **Cohrs RJ, Randall J, Smith J, Gilden DH, Dabrowski C, van Der Keyl H, Tal-Singer R.** 2000. Analysis of individual human trigeminal ganglia for latent herpes simplex virus type 1 and varicella-zoster virus nucleic acids using real-time PCR. *J Virol* **74:**11464–11471.
18. **Kennedy PG, Grinfeld E, Bell JE.** 2000. Varicella-zoster virus gene expression in latently infected and explanted human ganglia. *J Virol* **74:**11893–11898.
19. **Aberle SW, Aberle JH, Steininger C, Puchhammer-Stöckl E.** 2005. Quantitative real time PCR detection of Varicella-zoster virus DNA in cerebrospinal fluid in patients with neurological disease. *Med Microbiol Immunol (Berl)* **194:**7–12.
20. **Nagel MA, Jones D, Wyborny A.** 2017. Varicella zoster virus vasculopathy: the expanding clinical spectrum and pathogenesis. *J Neuroimmunol* **308:**112–117.
21. **Nagel MA, Cohrs RJ, Mahalingam R, Wellish MC, Forghani B, Schiller A, Safdieh JE, Kamenkovich E, Ostrow LW, Levy M, Greenberg B, Russman AN, Katzan I, Gardner CJ, Häusler M, Nau R, Saraya T, Wada H, Goto H, de Martino M, Ueno M, Brown WD, Terborg C, Gilden DH.** 2008. The varicella zoster virus vasculopathies: clinical, CSF, imaging, and virologic features. *Neurology* **70:**853–860.
22. **Gourishankar S, McDermid JC, Jhangri GS, Preiksaitis JK.** 2004. Herpes zoster infection following solid organ transplantation: incidence, risk factors and outcomes in the current immunosuppressive era. *Am J Transplant* **4:**108–115.
23. **Miller GG, Dummer JS.** 2007. Herpes simplex and varicella zoster viruses: forgotten but not gone. *Am J Transplant* **7:**741–747.
24. **Pergam SA, Limaye AP, AST Infectious Diseases Community of Practice.** 2009. Varicella zoster virus (VZV) in solid organ transplant recipients. *Am J Transplant* **9**(Suppl 4)**:**S108–S115.
25. **Zuckerman RA, Limaye AP.** 2013. Varicella zoster virus (VZV) and herpes simplex virus (HSV) in solid organ transplant patients. *Am J Transplant* **13**(Suppl 3)**:**55–66.
26. **Okuma HS, Kobayashi Y, Makita S, Kitahara H, Fukuhara S, Munakata W, Suzuki T, Maruyama D, Tobinai K.** 2016. Disseminated herpes zoster infection initially presenting with abdominal pain in patients with lymphoma undergoing conventional chemotherapy: a report of three cases. *Oncol Lett* **12:**809–814.
27. **Carby M, Jones A, Burke M, Hall A, Banner N.** 2007. Varicella infection after heart and lung transplantation: a single-center experience. *J Heart Lung Transplant* **26:**399–402.
28. **Styczynski J, Reusser P, Einsele H, de la Camara R, Cordonnier C, Ward KN, Ljungman P, Engelhard D, Second European Conference on Infections in Leukemia.** 2009. Management of HSV, VZV and EBV infections in patients with hematological malignancies and after SCT: guidelines from the Second European Conference on Infections in Leukemia. *Bone Marrow Transplant* **43:**757–770.
29. **Franco-Paredes C, Bellehemeur T, Merchant A, Sanghi P, DiazGranados C, Rimland D.** 2002. Aseptic meningitis and optic neuritis preceding varicella-zoster progressive outer retinal necrosis in a patient with AIDS. *AIDS* **16:**1045–1049.
30. **Gnann JW Jr.** 2002. Varicella-zoster virus: atypical presentations and unusual complications. *J Infect Dis* **186**(Suppl 1)**:**S91–S98.
31. **Vafai A, Berger M.** 2001. Zoster in patients infected with HIV: a review. *Am J Med Sci* **321:**372–380.
32. **Feller L, Wood NH, Lemmer J.** 2007. Herpes zoster infection as an immune reconstitution inflammatory syndrome in HIV-seropositive subjects: a review. *Oral Surg Oral Med Oral Pathol Oral Radiol Endod* **104:**455–460.
33. **Sengupta N, Booy R, Schmitt HJ, Peltola H, Van-Damme P, Schumacher RF, Campins M, Rodrigo C, Heikkinen T, Seward J, Jumaan A, Finn A, Olcén P, Thiry N, Weil-Olivier C, Breuer J.** 2008. Varicella vaccination in Europe: are we ready for a universal childhood programme? *Eur J Pediatr* **167:**47–55.
34. **Seward JF, Watson BM, Peterson CL, Mascola L, Pelosi JW, Zhang JX, Maupin TJ, Goldman GS, Tabony LJ, Brodovicz KG, Jumaan AO, Wharton M.** 2002. Varicella disease after introduction of varicella vaccine in the United States, 1995–2000. *JAMA* **287:**606–611.
35. **Vázquez M, LaRussa PS, Gershon AA, Steinberg SP, Freudigman K, Shapiro ED.** 2001. The effectiveness of the varicella vaccine in clinical practice. *N Engl J Med* **344:** 955–960.
36. **Harpaz R, Ortega-Sanchez IR, Seward JF.** 2008. Prevention of herpes zoster: recommendations of the Advisory Committee on Immunization Practices (ACIP). *MMWR Recomm Rep* **57:**1–30.
37. **Cunningham AL, Lal H, Kovac M, Chlibek R, Hwang SJ, Díez-Domingo J, Godeaux O, Levin MJ, McElhaney JE, Puig-Barberà J, Vanden Abeele C, Vesikari T, Watanabe D, Zahaf T, Ahonen A, Athan E, Barba-Gomez JF, Campora L, de Looze F, Downey HJ, Ghesquiere W, Gorfinkel I, Korhonen T, Leung E, McNeil SA, Oostvogels L, Rombo L, Smetana J, Weckx L, Yeo W, Heineman TC, ZOE-70 Study Group.** 2016. Efficacy of the herpes zoster subunit vaccine in adults 70 years of age or older. *N Engl J Med* **375:**1019–1032.

38. **Zaia J, Baden L, Boeckh MJ, Chakrabarti S, Einsele H, Ljungman P, McDonald GB, Hirsch H, Center for International Blood and Marrow Transplant Research, National Marrow Donor Program, European Blood and Marrow Transplant Group, American Society of Blood and Marrow Transplantation, Canadian Blood and Marrow Transplant Group, Infectious Disease Society of America, Society for Healthcare Epidemiology of America, Association of Medical Microbiology and Infectious Diseases Canada, Centers for Disease Control and Prevention.** 2009. Viral disease prevention after hematopoietic cell transplantation. *Bone Marrow Transplant* **44:**471–482.
39. **Andrei G, Snoeck R.** 2013. Advances in the treatment of varicella-zoster virus infections. *Adv Pharmacol* **67:**107–168.
40. **Coffin SE, Hodinka RL.** 1995. Utility of direct immunofluorescence and virus culture for detection of varicella-zoster virus in skin lesions. *J Clin Microbiol* **33:**2792–2795.
41. **Leung J, Harpaz R, Baughman AL, Heath K, Loparev V, Vázquez M, Watson BM, Schmid DS.** 2010. Evaluation of laboratory methods for diagnosis of varicella. *Clin Infect Dis* **51:**23–32.
42. **Puchhammer-Stöckl E, Popow-Kraupp T, Heinz FX, Mandl CW, Kunz C.** 1991. Detection of varicella-zoster virus DNA by polymerase chain reaction in the cerebrospinal fluid of patients suffering from neurological complications associated with chickenpox or herpes zoster. *J Clin Microbiol* **29:**1513–1516.
43. **Weidmann M, Armbruster K, Hufert FT.** 2008. Challenges in designing a Taqman-based multiplex assay for the simultaneous detection of Herpes simplex virus types 1 and 2 and Varicella-zoster virus. *J Clin Virol* **42:**326–334.
44. **Stöcher M, Leb V, Bozic M, Kessler HH, Halwachs-Baumann G, Landt O, Stekel H, Berg J.** 2003. Parallel detection of five human herpes virus DNAs by a set of real-time polymerase chain reactions in a single run. *J Clin Virol* **26:**85–93.
45. **Mols JF, Ledent E, Heineman TC.** 2013. Sampling of herpes zoster skin lesion types and the impact on viral DNA detection. *J Virol Methods* **188:**145–147.
46. **Yamakawa K, Hamada M, Takeda T.** 2007. Different real-time PCR assays could lead to a different result of detection of varicella-zoster virus in facial palsy. *J Virol Methods* **139:**227–229.
47. **Sauerbrei A, Eichhorn U, Gawellek S, Egerer R, Schacke M, Wutzler P.** 2003. Molecular characterisation of varicella-zoster virus strains in Germany and differentiation from the Oka vaccine strain. *J Med Virol* **71:**313–319.
48. **Parker SP, Quinlivan M, Taha Y, Breuer J.** 2006. Genotyping of varicella-zoster virus and the discrimination of Oka vaccine strains by TaqMan real-time PCR. *J Clin Microbiol* **44:**3911–3914.
49. **Kupila L, Vuorinen T, Vainionpää R, Hukkanen V, Marttila RJ, Kotilainen P.** 2006. Etiology of aseptic meningitis and encephalitis in an adult population. *Neurology* **66:**75–80.
50. **Dupuis M, Hull R, Wang H, Nattanmai S, Glasheen B, Fusco H, Dzigua L, Markey K, Tavakoli NP.** 2011. Molecular detection of viral causes of encephalitis and meningitis in New York State. *J Med Virol* **83:**2172–2181.
51. **de Ory F, Avellón A, Echevarría JE, Sánchez-Seco MP, Trallero G, Cabrerizo M, Casas I, Pozo F, Fedele G, Vicente D, Pena MJ, Moreno A, Niubo J, Rabella N, Rubio G, Pérez-Ruiz M, Rodríguez-Iglesias M, Gimeno C, Eiros JM, Melón S, Blasco M, López-Miragaya I, Varela E, Martinez-Sapiña A, Rodríguez G, Marcos MA, Gegúndez MI, Cilla G, Gabilondo I, Navarro JM, Torres J, Aznar C, Castellanos A, Guisasola ME, Negredo AI, Tenorio A, Vázquez-Morón S.** 2013. Viral infections of the central nervous system in Spain: a prospective study. *J Med Virol* **85:**554–562.
52. **Echevarría JM, Casas I, Tenorio A, de Ory F, Martínez-Martín P.** 1994. Detection of varicella-zoster virus-specific DNA sequences in cerebrospinal fluid from patients with acute aseptic meningitis and no cutaneous lesions. *J Med Virol* **43:**331–335.
53. **Koskiniemi M, Piiparinen H, Rantalaiho T, Eränkö P, Färkkilä M, Räihä K, Salonen EM, Ukkonen P, Vaheri A.** 2002. Acute central nervous system complications in varicella zoster virus infections. *J Clin Virol* **25:**293–301.
54. **Persson A, Bergström T, Lindh M, Namvar L, Studahl M.** 2009. Varicella-zoster virus CNS disease—viral load, clinical manifestations and sequels. *J Clin Virol* **46:**249–253.
55. **Rottenstreich A, Oz ZK, Oren I.** 2014. Association between viral load of varicella zoster virus in cerebrospinal fluid and the clinical course of central nervous system infection. *Diagn Microbiol Infect Dis* **79:**174–177.
56. **Růžek D, Piskunova N, Žampachová E.** 2007. High variability in viral load in cerebrospinal fluid from patients with herpes simplex and varicella-zoster infections of the central nervous system. *Clin Microbiol Infect* **13:**1217–1219.
57. **Aberle SW, Puchhammer-Stöckl E.** 2002. Diagnosis of herpesvirus infections of the central nervous system. *J Clin Virol* **25**(Suppl 1)**:**79–85.
58. **Cinque P, Bossolasco S, Vago L, Fornara C, Lipari S, Racca S, Lazzarin A, Linde A.** 1997. Varicella-zoster virus (VZV) DNA in cerebrospinal fluid of patients infected with human immunodeficiency virus: VZV disease of the central nervous system or subclinical reactivation of VZV infection? *Clin Infect Dis* **25:**634–639.
59. **Murakami S, Nakashiro Y, Mizobuchi M, Hato N, Honda N, Gyo K.** 1998. Varicella-zoster virus distribution in Ramsay Hunt syndrome revealed by polymerase chain reaction. *Acta Otolaryngol* **118:**145–149.
60. **Furuta Y, Ohtani F, Kawabata H, Fukuda S, Bergström T.** 2000. High prevalence of varicella-zoster virus reactivation in herpes simplex virus-seronegative patients with acute peripheral facial palsy. *Clin Infect Dis* **30:**529–533.
61. **Furuta Y, Fukuda S, Suzuki S, Takasu T, Inuyama Y, Nagashima K.** 1997. Detection of varicella-zoster virus DNA in patients with acute peripheral facial palsy by the polymerase chain reaction, and its use for early diagnosis of zoster sine herpete. *J Med Virol* **52:**316–319.
62. **Stjernquist-Desatnik A, Skoog E, Aurelius E.** 2006. Detection of herpes simplex and varicella-zoster viruses in patients with Bell's palsy by the polymerase chain reaction technique. *Ann Otol Rhinol Laryngol* **115:**306–311.
63. **Grahn A, Hagberg L, Nilsson S, Blennow K, Zetterberg H, Studahl M.** 2013. Cerebrospinal fluid biomarkers in patients with varicella-zoster virus CNS infections. *J Neurol* **260:**1813–1821.
64. **Mehta SK, Cohrs RJ, Forghani B, Zerbe G, Gilden DH, Pierson DL.** 2004. Stress-induced subclinical reactivation of varicella zoster virus in astronauts. *J Med Virol* **72:**174–179.
65. **Gershon AA.** 2011. The history and mystery of VZV in saliva. *J Infect Dis* **204:**815–816.
66. **Mehta SK, Tyring SK, Gilden DH, Cohrs RJ, Leal MJ, Castro VA, Feiveson AH, Ott CM, Pierson DL.** 2008. Varicella-zoster virus in the saliva of patients with herpes zoster. *J Infect Dis* **197:**654–657.
67. **Gilden DH, Devlin M, Wellish M, Mahalingham R, Huff C, Hayward A, Vafai A.** 1989. Persistence of varicella-zoster virus DNA in blood mononuclear cells of patients with varicella or zoster. *Virus Genes* **2:**299–305.
68. **Ito Y, Kimura H, Hara S, Kido S, Ozaki T, Nishiyama Y, Morishima T.** 2001. Investigation of varicella-zoster virus DNA in lymphocyte subpopulations by quantitative PCR assay. *Microbiol Immunol* **45:**267–269.
69. **Kimura H, Kido S, Ozaki T, Tanaka N, Ito Y, Williams RK, Morishima T.** 2000. Comparison of quantitations of viral load in varicella and zoster. *J Clin Microbiol* **38:**2447–2449.
70. **Mainka C, Fuss B, Geiger H, Höfelmayr H, Wolff MH.** 1998. Characterization of viremia at different stages of varicella-zoster virus infection. *J Med Virol* **56:**91–98.
71. **Bezold G, Lange M, Pillekamp H, Peter RU.** 2002. Varicella zoster viraemia during herpes zoster is not associated with neoplasia. *J Eur Acad Dermatol Venereol* **16:**357–360.
72. **de Jong MD, Weel JF, Schuurman T, Wertheim-van Dillen PM, Boom R.** 2000. Quantitation of varicella-zoster virus DNA in whole blood, plasma, and serum by PCR and electrochemiluminescence. *J Clin Microbiol* **38:**2568–2573.
73. **Malavige GN, Jones L, Kamaladasa SD, Wijewickrama A, Seneviratne SL, Black AP, Ogg GS.** 2008. Viral load, clinical disease severity and cellular immune responses in primary varicella zoster virus infection in Sri Lanka. *PLoS One* **3:**e3789.

74. **Quinlivan ML, Ayres K, Ran H, McElwaine S, Leedham-Green M, Scott FT, Johnson RW, Breuer J.** 2007. Effect of viral load on the outcome of herpes zoster. *J Clin Microbiol* **45:**3909–3914.
75. **Dobec M, Bossart W, Kaeppeli F, Mueller-Schoop J.** 2008. Serology and serum DNA detection in shingles. *Swiss Med Wkly* **138:**47–51.
76. **Kalpoe JS, Kroes AC, Verkerk S, Claas EC, Barge RM, Beersma MF.** 2006. Clinical relevance of quantitative varicella-zoster virus (VZV) DNA detection in plasma after stem cell transplantation. *Bone Marrow Transplant* **38:**41–46.
77. **Kronenberg A, Bossart W, Wuthrich RP, Cao C, Lautenschlager S, Wiegand ND, Mullhaupt B, Noll G, Mueller NJ, Speck RF.** 2005. Retrospective analysis of varicella zoster virus (VZV) copy DNA numbers in plasma of immunocompetent patients with herpes zoster, of immunocompromised patients with disseminated VZV disease, and of asymptomatic solid organ transplant recipients. *Transpl Infect Dis* **7:**116–121.
78. **Grahn A, Bergström T, Runesson J, Studahl M.** 2016. Varicella-zoster virus (VZV) DNA in serum of patients with VZV central nervous system infections. *J Infect* **73:**254–260.
79. **Terada K, Niizuma T, Kawano S, Kataoka N, Akisada T, Orita Y.** 1998. Detection of varicella-zoster virus DNA in peripheral mononuclear cells from patients with Ramsay Hunt syndrome or zoster sine herpete. *J Med Virol* **56:** 359–363.
80. **Beby-Defaux A, Brabant S, Chatellier D, Bourgoin A, Robert R, Ruckes T, Agius G.** 2009. Disseminated varicella with multiorgan failure in an immunocompetent adult. *J Med Virol* **81:**747–749.
81. **Rau R, Fitzhugh CD, Baird K, Cortez KJ, Li L, Fischer SH, Cowen EW, Balow JE, Walsh TJ, Cohen JI, Wayne AS.** 2008. Triad of severe abdominal pain, inappropriate antidiuretic hormone secretion, and disseminated varicella-zoster virus infection preceding cutaneous manifestations after hematopoietic stem cell transplantation: utility of PCR for early recognition and therapy. *Pediatr Infect Dis J* **27:**265–268.
82. **Hudnall SD, Chen T, Allison P, Tyring SK, Heath A.** 2008. Herpesvirus prevalence and viral load in healthy blood donors by quantitative real-time polymerase chain reaction. *Transfusion* **48:**1180–1187.
83. **Schünemann S, Mainka C, Wolff MH.** 1998. Subclinical reactivation of varicella-zoster virus in immunocompromised and immunocompetent individuals. *Intervirology* **41:**98–102.
84. **Arvin A.** 2005. Aging, immunity, and the varicella-zoster virus. *N Engl J Med* **352:**2266–2267.
85. **Kido S, Sugita S, Horie S, Miyanaga M, Miyata K, Shimizu N, Morio T, Mochizuki M.** 2008. Association of varicella zoster virus load in the aqueous humor with clinical manifestations of anterior uveitis in herpes zoster ophthalmicus and zoster sine herpete. *Br J Ophthalmol* **92:**505–508.
86. **Cowl CT, Prakash UB, Shawn Mitchell P, Migden MR.** 2000. Varicella-zoster virus detection by polymerase chain reaction using bronchoalveolar lavage specimens. *Am J Respir Crit Care Med* **162:**753–754.
87. **Nikkels AF, Delbecque K, Pierard GE, Wienkotter B, Schalasta G, Enders M.** 2005. Distribution of varicella-zoster virus DNA and gene products in tissues of a first-trimester varicella-infected fetus. *J Infect Dis* **191:**540–545.
88. **Grose C, Brunel PA.** 1978. Varicella-zoster virus: isolation and propagation in human melanoma cells at 36 and 32 degrees C. *Infect Immun* **19:**199–203.
89. **Breuer J.** 2010. VZV molecular epidemiology. *Curr Top Microbiol Immunol* **342:**15–42.
90. **Straus SE, Hay J, Smith H, Owens J.** 1983. Genome differences among varicella-zoster virus isolates. *J Gen Virol* **64:**1031–1041.
91. **Quinlivan M, Hawrami K, Barrett-Muir W, Aaby P, Arvin A, Chow VT, John TJ, Matondo P, Peiris M, Poulsen A, Siqueira M, Takahashi M, Talukder Y, Yamanishi K, Leedham-Green M, Scott FT, Thomas SL, Breuer J.** 2002. The molecular epidemiology of varicella-zoster virus: evidence for geographic segregation. *J Infect Dis* **186:**888–894.
92. **Harbecke R, Oxman MN, Arnold BA, Ip C, Johnson GR, Levin MJ, Gelb LD, Schmader KE, Straus SE, Wang H, Wright PF, Pachucki CT, Gershon AA, Arbeit RD, Davis LE, Simberkoff MS, Weinberg A, Williams HM, Cheney C, Petrukhin L, Abraham KG, Shaw A, Manoff S, Antonello JM, Green T, Wang Y, Tan C, Keller PM, Shingles Prevention Study Group.** 2009. A real-time PCR assay to identify and discriminate among wild-type and vaccine strains of varicella-zoster virus and herpes simplex virus in clinical specimens, and comparison with the clinical diagnoses. *J Med Virol* **81:**1310–1322.
93. **Sauerbrei A, Zell R, Wutzler P.** 2007. Analysis of repeat units in the R2 region among different Oka varicella-zoster virus vaccine strains and wild-type strains in Germany. *Intervirology* **50:**40–44.
94. **Quinlivan M, Gershon AA, Steinberg SP, Breuer J.** 2005. An evaluation of single nucleotide polymorphisms used to differentiate vaccine and wild type strains of varicella-zoster virus. *J Med Virol* **75:**174–180.
95. **Breuer J, Schmid DS, Gershon AA.** 2008. Use and limitations of varicella-zoster virus-specific serological testing to evaluate breakthrough disease in vaccinees and to screen for susceptibility to varicella. *J Infect Dis* **197**(Suppl 2)**:** S147–S151.
96. **Williams V, Gershon A, Brunell PA.** 1974. Serologic response to varicella-zoster membrane antigens measured by direct immunofluorescence. *J Infect Dis* **130:**669–672.
97. **Lafer MM, Weckx LY, de Moraes-Pinto MI, Garretson A, Steinberg SP, Gershon AA, LaRussa PS.** 2011. Comparative study of the standard fluorescent antibody to membrane antigen (FAMA) assay and a flow cytometry-adapted FAMA assay to assess immunity to varicella-zoster virus. *Clin Vaccine Immunol* **18:**1194–1197.
98. **Saiman L, LaRussa P, Steinberg SP, Zhou J, Baron K, Whittier S, Della-Latta P, Gershon AA.** 2001. Persistence of immunity to varicella-zoster virus after vaccination of healthcare workers. *Infect Control Hosp Epidemiol* **22:**279–283.
99. **Li S, Chan IS IV, Matthews H, Heyse JF, Chan CY, Kuter BJ, Kaplan KM, Vessey SJ, Sadoff JC.** 2002. Inverse relationship between six week postvaccination varicella antibody response to vaccine and likelihood of long term breakthrough infection. *Pediatr Infect Dis J* **21:**337–342.
100. **Maple PA, Gray J, Breuer J, Kafatos G, Parker S, Brown D.** 2006. Performance of a time-resolved fluorescence immunoassay for measuring varicella-zoster virus immunoglobulin G levels in adults and comparison with commercial enzyme immunoassays and Merck glycoprotein enzyme immunoassay. *Clin Vaccine Immunol* **13:**214–218.
101. **Sauerbrei A, Stefanski J, Gruhn B, Wutzler P.** 2011. Immune response of varicella vaccinees to different varicella-zoster virus genotypes. *Vaccine* **29:**3873–3877.
102. **de Ory F, Echevarría JM, Kafatos G, Anastassopoulou C, Andrews N, Backhouse J, Berbers G, Bruckova B, Cohen DI, de Melker H, Davidkin I, Gabutti G, Hesketh LM, Johansen K, Jokinen S, Jones L, Linde A, Miller E, Mossong J, Nardone A, Rota MC, Sauerbrei A, Schneider F, Smetana Z, Tischer A, Tsakris A, Vranckx R.** 2006. European seroepidemiology network 2: standardisation of assays for seroepidemiology of varicella zoster virus. *J Clin Virol* **36:** 111–118.
103. **Chris Maple PA, Gunn A, Sellwood J, Brown DW, Gray JJ.** 2009. Comparison of fifteen commercial assays for detecting varicella zoster virus IgG with reference to a time resolved fluorescence immunoassay (TRFIA) and the performance of two commercial assays for screening sera from immunocompromised individuals. *J Virol Methods* **155:**143–149.
104. **Sauerbrei A, Wutzler P.** 2006. Serological detection of varicella-zoster virus-specific immunoglobulin G by an enzyme-linked immunosorbent assay using glycoprotein antigen. *J Clin Microbiol* **44:**3094–3097.
105. **Larussa P, Steinberg S, Waithe E, Hanna B, Holzman R.** 1987. Comparison of five assays for antibody to varicella-zoster virus and the fluorescent-antibody-to-membrane-antigen test. *J Clin Microbiol* **25:**2059–2062.

106. **L'Huillier AG, Ferry T, Courvoisier DS, Aebi C, Cheseaux JJ, Kind C, Rudin C, Nadal D, Hirschel B, Sottas C, Siegrist CA, Posfay-Barbe KM, Pediatric Infectious Diseases Group of Switzerland, Group of Switzerland (PIGS), Swiss HIV Cohort Study (SHCS), Swiss Mother & Child HIV Cohort Study (MoCHiV).** 2012. Impaired antibody memory to varicella zoster virus in HIV-infected children: low antibody levels and avidity. *HIV Med* **13:**54–61.
107. **Behrman A, Lopez AS, Chaves SS, Watson BM, Schmid DS.** 2013. Varicella immunity in vaccinated healthcare workers. *J Clin Virol* **57:**109–114.
108. **Prelog M, Schönlaub J, Jeller V, Almanzar G, Höfner K, Gruber S, Eiwegger T, Würzner R.** 2013. Reduced varicella-zoster-virus (VZV)-specific lymphocytes and IgG antibody avidity in solid organ transplant recipients. *Vaccine* **31:**2420–2426.
109. **Min SW, Kim YS, Nahm FS, Yoo H, Choi E, Lee PB, Choo H, Park ZY, Yang CS.** 2016. The positive duration of varicella zoster immunoglobulin M antibody test in herpes zoster. *Medicine (Baltimore)* **95:**e4616.
110. **Weinberg A, Levin MJ.** 2010. VZV T cell-mediated immunity. *Curr Top Microbiol Immunol* **342:**341–357.
111. **Arvin AM.** 2008. Humoral and cellular immunity to varicella-zoster virus: an overview. *J Infect Dis* **197**(Suppl 2)**:**S58–S60.
112. **Frey CR, Sharp MA, Min AS, Schmid DS, Loparev V, Arvin AM.** 2003. Identification of CD8+ T cell epitopes in the immediate early 62 protein (IE62) of varicella-zoster virus, and evaluation of frequency of CD8+ T cell response to IE62, by use of IE62 peptides after varicella vaccination. *J Infect Dis* **188:**40–52.
113. **Vossen MT, Gent MR, Weel JF, de Jong MD, van Lier RA, Kuijpers TW.** 2004. Development of virus-specific CD4+ T cells on reexposure to varicella-zoster virus. *J Infect Dis* **190:**72–82.
114. **Sadaoka K, Okamoto S, Gomi Y, Tanimoto T, Ishikawa T, Yoshikawa T, Asano Y, Yamanishi K, Mori Y.** 2008. Measurement of varicella-zoster virus (VZV)-specific cell-mediated immunity: comparison between VZV skin test and interferon-gamma enzyme-linked immunospot assay. *J Infect Dis* **198:**1327–1333.
115. **Merindol N, Salem Fourati I, Brito RM, Grenier AJ, Charrier E, Cordeiro P, Caty M, Mezziani S, Malette B, Duval M, Alfieri C, Ovetchkine P, Le Deist F, Soudeyns H.** 2012. Reconstitution of protective immune responses against cytomegalovirus and varicella zoster virus does not require disease development in pediatric recipients of umbilical cord blood transplantation. *J Immunol* **189:**5016–5028.
116. **Breton G, Fillet AM, Katlama C, Bricaire F, Caumes E.** 1998. Acyclovir-resistant herpes zoster in human immunodeficiency virus-infected patients: results of foscarnet therapy. *Clin Infect Dis* **27:**1525–1527.
117. **van der Beek MT, Vermont CL, Bredius RG, Marijt EW, van der Blij-de Brouwer CS, Kroes AC, Claas EC, Vossen AC.** 2013. Persistence and antiviral resistance of varicella zoster virus in hematological patients. *Clin Infect Dis* **56:**335–343.
118. **Coen DM, Richman DD.** 2007. Antiviral agents, p 447–486. *In* Knipe DM, Howley PM (ed), *Fields Virology*, 5th ed. Lippincott, Williams and Wilkins, Philadelphia, PA.
119. **Brink AA, van Gelder M, Wolffs PF, Bruggeman CA, van Loo IH.** 2011. Compartmentalization of acyclovir-resistant varicella zoster virus: implications for sampling in molecular diagnostics. *Clin Infect Dis* **52:**982–987.
120. **Biron KK, Elion GB.** 1980. In vitro susceptibility of varicella-zoster virus to acyclovir. *Antimicrob Agents Chemother* **18:**443–447.
121. **Fillet AM, Dumont B, Caumes E, Visse B, Agut H, Bricaire F, Huraux JM.** 1998. Acyclovir-resistant varicella-zoster virus: phenotypic and genetic characterization. *J Med Virol* **55:**250–254.
122. **Suzutani T, Saijo M, Nagamine M, Ogasawara M, Azuma M.** 2000. Rapid phenotypic characterization method for herpes simplex virus and varicella-zoster virus thymidine kinases to screen for acyclovir-resistant viral infection. *J Clin Microbiol* **38:**1839–1844.
123. **Talarico CL, Phelps WC, Biron KK.** 1993. Analysis of the thymidine kinase genes from acyclovir-resistant mutants of varicella-zoster virus isolated from patients with AIDS. *J Virol* **67:**1024–1033.
124. **Andrei G, Topalis D, Fiten P, McGuigan C, Balzarini J, Opdenakker G, Snoeck R.** 2012. In vitro-selected drug-resistant varicella-zoster virus mutants in the thymidine kinase and DNA polymerase genes yield novel phenotype-genotype associations and highlight differences between antiherpesvirus drugs. *J Virol* **86:**2641–2652.
125. **Chen JJ, Zhu Z, Gershon AA, Gershon MD.** 2004. Mannose 6-phosphate receptor dependence of varicella zoster virus infection in vitro and in the epidermis during varicella and zoster. *Cell* **119:**915–926.
126. **Gershon AA, Silverstein SJ.** 2002. Varicella-zoster virus, p 413–432. *In* Richman DD, Whitley RJ, Hayden FG (ed), *Clinical Virology*, 2nd ed. ASM Press, Washington, DC.
127. **Furuta Y, Ohtani F, Sawa H, Fukuda S, Inuyama Y.** 2001. Quantitation of varicella-zoster virus DNA in patients with Ramsay Hunt syndrome and zoster sine herpete. *J Clin Microbiol* **39:**2856–2859.
128. **Asano S, Yoshikawa T, Kimura H, Enomoto Y, Ohashi M, Terasaki H, Nishiyama Y.** 2004. Monitoring herpesvirus DNA in three cases of acute retinal necrosis by real-time PCR. *J Clin Virol* **29:**207–210.

Human Cytomegalovirus

RICHARD L. HODINKA

102

TAXONOMY

Human cytomegalovirus (CMV), formally designated human herpesvirus 5 (HHV-5) by the International Committee on Taxonomy of Viruses, is a member of the family *Herpesviridae*, which includes herpes simplex virus types 1 (HHV-1) and 2 (HHV-2), varicella-zoster virus (HHV-3), Epstein-Barr virus (HHV-4), and HHV-6, -7, and -8. It is classified in the subfamily *Betaherpesvirinae* with cytomegaloviruses of other animal species based on its tropism for salivary glands, slow growth in cell culture, and strict species specificity. Human CMV is the type species of the genus *Cytomegalovirus*, and its name is derived from the enlargement of cells ("cyto" = cell, "mega" = large) infected by the virus. Regions of genome sequence homology between CMV and herpesviruses 6 and 7 have been identified, and HHV-6 and HHV-7 are now classified with CMV among the betaherpesviruses.

DESCRIPTION OF THE AGENT

Complete CMV particles have a diameter of 120 to 200 nm and consist of a core containing a large (220- to 240-kb) linear double-stranded DNA genome, an icosahedral capsid with 162 capsomeres, an amorphous tegument or matrix, and a surrounding phospholipid-rich envelope. The CMV genome is the largest of the herpesviruses and consists of more than 170 nonoverlapping open reading frames that encode structural and regulatory proteins and proteins that function to modulate the immune system of the host. Electron-microscopic features of CMV include virions morphologically indistinguishable from those of other herpesviruses, a high ratio of defective viral particles, and the presence of spherical particles called dense bodies. Viral replication occurs in the nucleus of the host cell and involves the expression of immediate early (α), early (β), and late (γ) classes of genes. The viral envelope is formed as assembled nucleocapsids bud from the inner surface of the nuclear membrane.

Molecular and immunologic techniques, including whole-genome sequencing directly from clinical specimens (1), have been used to study variation among CMV strains. Although it has been shown that different strains of CMV are 95% homologous to the standard laboratory reference strains AD-169 and Towne, genetically distinct CMV genotypes that display polymorphisms in multiple coding and noncoding regions of the virus genome have been identified in various human hosts, including healthy adults and children, congenitally infected infants, transplant recipients, and AIDS patients (1–3). Strain diversity has been observed within a single individual and between individuals and has been associated with specific differences in geographic distribution, transmission, tissue tropism, immunopathogenesis, and clinical manifestations of disease, but the exact role and importance of CMV genotypes in infection and disease are not well understood and remain largely unknown.

CMV is inactivated by a number of physical and chemical treatments, including heat (56°C for 30 min), low pH, lipid solvents, UV light, and cycles of freezing and thawing.

EPIDEMIOLOGY AND TRANSMISSION

CMV has a worldwide distribution and infects humans of all ages, with no seasonal or epidemic patterns of transmission. The seroprevalence of CMV increases with age in all populations and ranges from 40 to 100%; the virus is acquired earlier in life and the prevalence is highest among lower socioeconomic groups in crowded living conditions. CMV can be transmitted vertically and horizontally, and infections are classified as being acquired before birth (congenital), at the time of delivery (perinatal), or later in life (postnatal). Groups at increased risk for CMV infection include child care workers, pregnant women, infants infected *in utero*, very low-birth-weight and premature infants (born at <1,500 g and <30 weeks gestational age), and individuals whose immune systems are compromised.

Most infections are acquired by direct close personal contact with individuals who are shedding virus. Since CMV has been detected in many body fluids, including saliva, urine, breast milk, tears, stool, vaginal and cervical secretions, blood, and semen, it is clear that transmission can occur in a variety of ways. Prolonged shedding of virus after congenital or acquired CMV infection contributes to the ease of virus spread; virus may be excreted for weeks, months, or even years following a primary infection.

Transplacental infection of the fetus can occur following primary or recurrent infection of a pregnant woman, but the risk of CMV transmission to the fetus and the rate of symptomatic fetal infection are much higher with primary maternal infection. The incidence of fetal damage is highest if infection occurs during the first 12 to 16 weeks of pregnancy. Maternal illness may be mild, with fever and nonspecific symptoms, but is not clinically apparent in most pregnant women. Newborns can also acquire infection at the time of delivery by contact with virus in the birth canal. Nearly 10% of women shed CMV in the genital tract at or near the time of delivery, and virus is transmitted to approximately 50% of the newborns. Such infants begin to excrete virus at 3 to 12 weeks of age but usually remain asymptomatic. Mother-to-infant transmission of CMV through breast milk is very common; very low-birth-weight preterm infants are at greatest risk for developing disease. Of children who attend child care centers and enter as toddlers, 20 to 70% experience CMV infection over a 1- to 2-year period. Infection is usually asymptomatic, but the children may transmit CMV to their parents and other caregivers, posing a risk to an unborn fetus if a woman is pregnant at the time. Susceptible health care workers and employees of child care centers are at risk of occupational exposure. In adolescents and adults, sexual transmission of CMV may occur and is an important route of CMV spread.

Similar to infections with other herpesviruses, primary infection with CMV results in the establishment of a lifelong persistent or latent infection. Reactivation of the virus can occur in response to different stimuli, particularly immunosuppression. The sites of latent infection are thought to include various tissues, endothelial cells, and leukocytes. Therefore, CMV can be transmitted through transfusion of blood products and by exposure to tissue and hematopoietic stem cells during transplantation and may lead to severe disease in infants with very low birth weights, pregnant women, transplant recipients and other immunocompromised hosts, and critically ill immunocompetent patients.

CLINICAL SIGNIFICANCE

CMV infections are common and usually asymptomatic in otherwise healthy children and adults; however, the incidence and spectrum of disease in newborns and in immunocompromised hosts establish this virus as an important human pathogen (4, 5).

Immunocompetent Host

The vast majority of immunocompetent children and adults who acquire CMV infection postnatally remain asymptomatic. Cell-mediated immunity is most important in controlling infection, and CMV-specific $CD4^+$ and $CD8^+$ lymphocytes play a critical role.

Symptoms in young adults can mimic the infectious mononucleosis syndrome caused by Epstein-Barr virus and include prolonged fever (persisting for 2 to 3 weeks), malaise, an atypical lymphocytosis, and mild hepatitis without the production of heterophile antibody. Exudative pharyngitis is frequently absent, and lymphadenopathy and splenomegaly are less common with CMV-associated infectious mononucleosis. Organ-specific diseases, including colitis, hepatitis, encephalitis, pneumonia, anterior uveitis, and multisystem involvement with fever of unknown origin, have also been observed in the immunocompetent host but are rare.

A link between CMV infection in the immunocompetent host and other clinical conditions has been suggested, including for atherosclerosis, hypertension, malignancies such as glioblastoma and breast cancer, new-onset diabetes, inflammatory and autoimmune diseases, Alzheimer's disease, and immunosenescence in the elderly. It is unclear whether CMV truly contributes to these diseases or is an innocent bystander. More recently, there has been an increase in the number of reports of severe CMV infection associated with poor outcomes in hospitalized, critically ill immunocompetent patients (6, 7). Reactivation of CMV is common in these patients and is linked to increased length of stay in the hospital and/or intensive care unit, prolonged duration of mechanical ventilation, severe sepsis, high disease severity, and mortality (8).

Fetus and Newborn Infant

CMV infection has been detected in 0.2 to 2.5% of newborn infants and is the most common identified infectious cause of congenital disease. Approximately 10 to 15% of congenitally infected infants develop symptoms during the newborn period; possible manifestations range from severe disease, with any combination of intrauterine growth retardation, jaundice, hepatosplenomegaly, petechiae, thrombocytopenic purpura, myocarditis, pneumonitis, microcephaly, periventricular calcifications, deafness, and chorioretinitis, to more limited involvement. Symptomatic infants may die of complications within the first months of life; more commonly, they survive but are neurologically damaged and will have long-term health problems, such as sensorineural hearing loss (the most common chronic condition following congenital CMV infection), visual impairment, seizures, or psychomotor and/or intellectual disabilities. It is now recognized that even congenitally infected infants who are asymptomatic at birth may develop progressive hearing loss later in life.

Perinatal or postnatal infection with CMV may occur in term and preterm infants as a result of exposure to maternal cervicovaginal secretions during delivery, ingestion of breast milk after delivery, and blood transfusions. In high-risk preterm newborns, morbidity and mortality can be significant, and hepatosplenomegaly, neutropenia, thrombocytopenia, atypical lymphocytosis, hemolytic anemia, pneumonitis, and necrotizing enterocolitis have been described.

Although a large proportion of congenital CMV infections are attributed to primary maternal infection in the developed world, studies in resource-poor settings have shown similar rates of sequelae, especially hearing loss, following primary or reactivated maternal infection (5). Therefore, contrary to past beliefs, preexisting infection and development of CMV antibody in the mother may not eliminate the risk for significant infection in the infant. Thus far, it appears that perinatally and postnatally infected infants do not develop late neurologic sequelae of infection.

Immunocompromised Host

CMV infections are frequent and occasionally severe in children or adults with congenital or acquired defects of cellular immunity, such as patients with AIDS, cancer patients (particularly those with leukemia and lymphoma receiving chemotherapy), and recipients of solid organ and hematopoietic stem cell transplants. Infections in these patients may be due to reactivation of latent virus or primary infection or reinfection with exogenous virus, which may be introduced by blood transfusions or by the grafted organ. Symptoms tend to be most severe after primary infection; however, reactivation infection or reinfection in a severely immunocompromised host may also cause serious illness.

CMV is the most common viral infection in the setting of transplantation, with symptomatic infection developing in 20 to 60% of transplant recipients within the first year posttransplantation. The frequency and severity of CMV infection in organ transplant recipients are variable and depend on the type of transplant, the source of the donated organ, the immune status of the recipient, and the duration of the immunosuppressive therapy (9, 10). The highest occurrence of CMV disease is seen in CMV-seronegative recipients receiving a transplanted organ from a CMV-seropositive donor. Active infection usually occurs between 1 and 4 months after transplantation, when patients are at the height of their immunosuppression. The widespread use of antiviral drugs for prophylaxis or preemptive therapy following transplantation has resulted in the emergence of late-onset (>90 days posttransplant) CMV disease (11). The major symptoms in these patients represent a nonspecific "viral syndrome" and usually include fever, malaise, lethargy, myalgia or arthralgia, leukopenia, thrombocytopenia, and hepatitis. Specific organ damage may lead to pneumonitis in recipients of lung or heart-lung transplants; the development of myocarditis, retinitis, or accelerated vascular damage and atherosclerosis after cardiac transplantation; hepatitis and pancreatitis in liver and pancreas transplant recipients, respectively; and gastrointestinal disease. CMV infection in transplant recipients has also been associated with delayed or failed bone marrow engraftment, an increased incidence or severity of graft-versus-host disease, and an increased risk of graft rejection in solid organ transplants. Death may occur as a result of various complications, including bacterial and fungal superinfections. CMV infection, particularly when associated with pneumonitis, is an important cause of morbidity and mortality after hematopoietic stem cell transplantation.

In patients infected with HIV, active CMV infection usually occurs with advanced immunosuppression (e.g., $CD4^+$ lymphocyte counts drop below 50 to 100 cells/μl) and is primarily the result of reactivation of latent infection. Retinitis is the most common clinical presentation, with destruction of the retina and damage to the optic nerve without treatment or improvement in the immune system. CMV is also an important cause of fever, gastrointestinal infections including esophagitis, gastritis, enteritis, and ulcerative colitis, encephalitis, and polyradiculomyelopathy. CMV pneumonia is uncommon in the setting of HIV infection. There has been a significant decline in severe CMV disease in AIDS patients with the introduction of highly active antiretroviral therapy (12).

Treatment and Prevention

Over the years, four antiviral drugs have been licensed by the U.S. Food and Drug Administration (FDA) for treatment and prevention of CMV infections; these include ganciclovir, its prodrug valganciclovir, foscarnet, and cidofovir (9, 10, 13). These drugs target the viral DNA polymerase and affect viral DNA replication. The initial drug of choice is ganciclovir, although valganciclovir is now also widely used as preemptive, curative, and maintenance therapy or for prophylaxis in transplant recipients due to its better bioavailability compared to ganciclovir. Both drugs can be administered orally or intravenously. Foscarnet and cidofovir are considered second-line therapeutic drugs used primarily in AIDS patients with CMV retinitis; foscarnet is also used for treating ganciclovir-resistant CMV. All four drugs are associated with significant drug-related toxicities, and drug resistance has emerged over time. Newborns with congenital or perinatal CMV disease may benefit from treatment with ganciclovir or valganciclovir, but experience is limited, and additional clinical trials are warranted. The use of antiviral drugs to treat CMV infections in immunocompetent adults is seldom indicated, and further studies are needed in hospitalized, critically ill immunocompetent patients with CMV to determine if treatment is beneficial. CMV immune globulin is approved by the FDA and has been used in combination with antiviral drugs to treat and prevent disease after organ transplant.

Novel therapies have been developed, including letermovir (a CMV UL56 terminase inhibitor), maribavir (an oral inhibitor of the CMV UL97 kinase), and brincidofovir (an oral derivative of cidofovir), which have been shown to be more potent than current antiviral drugs against CMV with lesser toxicity (14, 15). Letermovir was recently FDA approved as an oral drug for the prophylaxis of CMV infection and disease in adult CMV-seropositive recipients of an allogeneic hematopoietic stem cell transplant; it has no reported major adverse effects (16, 17). Maribavir and brincidofovir have been successfully used to treat ganciclovir-resistant CMV infection, while neither drug has shown efficacy in phase III trials for prophylactic use in allogeneic hematopoietic stem cell transplant recipients. Several drugs with activity against CMV have been repurposed as adjunct therapy for the treatment of multidrug-resistant or refractory CMV infections, including leflunomide, approved for treatment of rheumatoid arthritis; artesunate, an antimalarial drug; and sirolimus and everolimus, rapamycin drugs used to prevent transplant rejection. The efficacy of these drugs remains to be determined in clinical trials.

More recently, cellular adoptive immunotherapy involving the transfer of CMV-seropositive transplant donor-derived CMV-reactive cytotoxic T lymphocytes has matured as a novel therapeutic approach to restore immune competence and treat CMV infections that are unresponsive to therapy following solid organ or hematopoietic stem cell transplants (18–22). Adoptive transfer of CMV-specific T cells from third-party donors also has showed promise, resulting in the establishment of cryopreserved third-party donor T-cell banks for off-the-shelf treatment of refractory infections (23). The efficacy of this treatment modality awaits clinical trials.

There are currently no licensed vaccines available for prevention of CMV disease. A number of candidate vaccines have been developed and are in various stages of preclinical and clinical evaluation (24–26). These include preparations derived from attenuated or replication-defective viruses or noninfectious particles, recombinant subunit vaccines, and DNA/RNA or viral-vector gene-based vaccines. The safety and immunogenicity of these vaccines have been demonstrated in phase I clinical trials, and phase II trials have shown promise for an adjuvanted recombinant surface glycoprotein B vaccine, gB/MF59, and a DNA vaccine, ASP0113, consisting of plasmids encoding phosphoprotein 65 and glycoprotein B. Phase III trials are now under way for the ASP0113 vaccine.

Asymptomatic excretion with CMV is common, and standard precautions and good personal hygienic practices (e.g., careful handwashing) can help decrease the possibility of transmission. Common disinfectants containing alcohol, detergents, and chlorine are effective in inactivating the virus. Transmission of CMV by blood transfusion or through breast milk can be minimized by using leukoreduced and/or CMV-seronegative blood products or treating breast milk by pasteurization, freezing and thawing, or ultraviolet-C irradiation.

COLLECTION, TRANSPORT, AND STORAGE OF SPECIMENS

At present, a variety of methods are available for use in the diagnosis and management of patients infected with CMV (Table 1). These include isolation of the virus in cell

TABLE 1 Laboratory methods for diagnosis and monitoring of CMV infections

Method	Principle	Specimen	Test time	Sensitivity	Specificity	Clinical usefulness
Virus isolation						
Conventional tube culture	Viral growth in cell culture with CPE	Various body fluids and tissues	2–4 wk	Low–moderate	High	Slow and involves considerable time, labor, and resources; currently has limited diagnostic utility; viral isolates used for phenotypic susceptibility testing
Spin amplification shell vial culture	Viral growth in cell culture with pre-CPE antigen detection	Various body fluids and tissues	16–24 h	Low–moderate	High	More rapid and more sensitive than tube cultures for diagnosis of CMV infection; limited use in some laboratories; molecular testing generally preferred
Direct examination						
Histopathology/ immunohistochemistry	Histologic detection of CMV-infected cells	Tissues	24–48 h	Low–moderate	Moderate–high	Most useful for definitive diagnosis of tissue-invasive disease; perform CMV-specific immunohistochemical staining in conjunction with histopathology for increased sensitivity
Antigen detection (antigenemia assay)	Immunocytochemical detection of pp65 protein in leukocytes	Peripheral whole-blood leukocytes	2–5 h	Moderate–high	Moderate–high	Rapid and relatively simple to perform; subjective interpretation and lack of standardization; semiquantitative test useful for diagnosis of clinical disease, initiating preemptive therapy and monitoring responses to therapy
Nucleic acid detection	Qualitative and quantitative real-time PCR; digital PCR	Qualitative PCR: various body fluids and tissues Quantitative PCR: plasma, whole blood Digital PCR: plasma	1–3 h	High	High	Superior performance characteristics and standardized materials; qualitative assays are highly sensitive but may not differentiate active disease from infection or latency; quantitative tests now considered to be best method to provide rapid and accurate diagnosis of CMV disease, identify patients at risk of developing disease, assess disease progression and risk of relapse, direct initiation of preemptive therapy, monitor response to therapy, and predict viral resistance and treatment failure; digital PCR offers quantification without need for standards and a calibration curve
Serology	Detection of IgM and IgG antibodies and IgG avidity	Serum	1–2 h	Moderate–high	Moderate–high	Rapid and simple to perform; detection of CMV-specific IgM or seroconversion from negative to positive IgG antibody useful in diagnosis of recent or active primary CMV infection; screening of blood and organ donors and recipients for IgG against CMV is important in preventing transmission of CMV to high-risk individuals; measurements of CMV IgG avidity are useful to distinguish primary from nonprimary CMV infections in pregnant women
Cell-mediated immunity assays	Measurements of interferon gamma release from T lymphocytes exposed to CMV-specific proteins and/or peptide epitopes	Peripheral whole-blood lymphocytes	16–24 h	Moderate	Moderate–high	Assessment of CMV-specific immune responses and reconstitution; may be useful for risk stratification of viremia and disease and in guiding treatment and other management decisions in immunocompromised hosts such as transplant recipients; several assays are commercially available

(continued)

TABLE 1 Laboratory methods for diagnosis and monitoring of CMV infections (*continued*)

Method	Principle	Specimen	Test time	Sensitivity	Specificity	Clinical usefulness
Antiviral susceptibility tests						
Phenotypic assays	Measure inhibition or suppression of viral replication in cell culture in presence of varied concentrations of antiviral drug	Virus isolates	2–6 wk	Moderate–high	High	Direct measure of effect a drug has on growth of virus; can identify novel drug-resistant mutations and can determine amount of drug needed to inhibit virus; cumbersome and labor-intensive and assays do not provide results in a clinically relevant time frame; not practical to use
Genotypic assays	PCR and sequencing of amplified products or direct sequencing alone	Plasma, whole blood, other body fluids and tissues	24–48 h	High	High	Rapid detection of known genetic mutations that confer resistance to one or more of the currently available antiviral drugs active against CMV; can greatly impact choices of initial and alternative therapy and can predict treatment failure and identify potential cross-resistance to multiple drugs; drug-resistant virus below 20–30% of total population may not be detected unless next-generation deep sequencing techniques are used; available mainly in reference and commercial laboratories
Genotype determination	PCR and sequencing of amplified products or direct sequencing alone	Various body fluids, tissues	24–48 h	High	High	Characterization of genetic diversity among CMV strains and identification of multiple and mixed genotypes within immunocompromised hosts may be beneficial for predicting disease severity and the kinetics of viral clearance during treatment of active CMV infection; method is mainly investigational

culture, histologic and cytologic techniques, assays for the direct detection and/or quantification of viral proteins or nucleic acids, serologic tests, phenotypic and genotypic assays to screen for antiviral drug resistance, and tests to measure cellular immune function of the host and control of CMV infection. The selection of assays to perform and the choice of specimen(s) to be tested depend on the patient population and clinical situation and the intended use of the individual tests. The details of specimen collection and processing are given in chapter 79.

Specimens for Direct Detection

Tissue specimens, respiratory secretions (e.g., saliva and bronchoalveolar lavage fluid), urine sediment, cerebrospinal fluid (CSF), peripheral whole blood, plasma, umbilical cord blood, amniotic fluid, aqueous humor and vitreous fluid, and peripheral blood leukocytes have been used for the direct detection of CMV antigens or nucleic acids from various patient populations.

Blood specimens have proven most useful for identification and monitoring of CMV disease in immunocompromised hosts. Purified blood leukocytes are used in the CMV antigenemia assay, while whole blood, plasma obtained from anticoagulated whole blood, serum obtained from clotted blood, and purified peripheral blood leukocytes have all been used to quantitate CMV DNA in molecular amplification assays. EDTA is currently the preferred anticoagulant for molecular testing, since it is considered the most effective stabilizer of nucleic acids in blood. The optimal frequency of blood collection remains to be established for surveillance of different patient groups, although it is common practice to submit blood specimens once a week while monitoring viral loads during preemptive antiviral therapy (9, 10). The first specimen should be collected at the start of therapy to establish a baseline viral load (27).

There is considerable debate about which blood compartment is best suited for the detection of CMV DNA (28–30). Although peripheral blood leukocytes were commonly used in the past, whole blood and plasma are now considered the specimens of choice (31). Whole blood has been shown to yield the highest levels and most frequent and earliest detection of CMV DNA of all blood compartments examined (28) and may represent the most practical specimen for laboratories to process for use in the diagnosis and monitoring of CMV disease, since it requires little processing prior to extraction of the DNA and both cell-associated and extracellular viruses can be detected. The choice of extraction platforms and chemistries should be considered when whole blood is processed, as CMV DNA yields may vary depending on the protocols used for isolation of nucleic acids. Also, delays in sample preparation can result in lysis of leukocytes after blood collection, which may result in inaccurate quantitation of CMV DNA if either purified leukocytes or plasma is used as a specimen source (32). A potential limitation for the use of whole blood is the possibility of variation in leukocyte counts from patient to patient; this may lead to erroneous quantitative measurements if fluctuations in cell numbers are not taken into consideration. Also, detection of low levels of CMV DNA in whole blood may not always correlate with active CMV disease, and persistent DNA-emia in whole blood may lead to overtreatment until results are negative or below a defined threshold predictive of a clinical response. Plasma may be preferable in neutropenic patients, who may have inadequate numbers of leukocytes for testing, and it may be a better specimen source for predicting CMV disease. Plasma DNA-emia also may be a better predictor of relapse at day 21 of treatment than DNA-emia in whole blood (31). When patients are monitored over time, the same specimen type should be used to minimize the variations observed between different blood compartments.

For the CMV antigenemia assay, a total of 4 to 7 ml of whole blood is usually recommended for collection, but at least 10 ml of blood may be required for patients with severe neutropenia (e.g., absolute neutrophil counts of less than 200/mm^3). Any type of anticoagulated blood can be used, including blood collected in heparin, EDTA, sodium citrate, or acid citrate dextrose, although the most extensive experience has been with using heparin or EDTA. The blood should be kept at 4°C during storage and transport and should be processed within 6 to 8 h of collection for accurate and reliable quantitation of the viral load and within 24 h and no later than 48 h for qualitative testing (33). A decrease in quantitative antigenemia levels after storage of blood specimens for 24 h to 48 h has been described, although most positive specimens remain positive after this time when held at 4°C (33–35). As a general rule, specimens for molecular amplification should be stored at 4°C immediately after collection and then promptly transported to the laboratory for processing. CMV DNA has been shown to be stable in whole blood when stored for 14 days at 4°C and for up to 21 days at 4°C when plasma is separated from whole blood (35, 36). These findings were consistent over a wide range of CMV DNA concentrations. Single-use aliquots of processed specimens should be placed in multiple cryovials for testing and storage. When they are processed in this manner, specimens are not frozen and thawed repeatedly and are never returned to the original specimen cryovial, thereby avoiding possible degradation of the DNA and cross-contamination of specimens, respectively. If not tested immediately, specimens should be promptly frozen and stored at −70°C or colder.

For prenatal diagnosis of congenital CMV infection, collection of amniotic fluid has largely replaced chorionic villus sampling or cordocentesis to collect fetal blood. Amniotic fluid should be collected after 21 to 23 weeks of fetal gestation and at least 6 to 8 weeks from the estimated onset of maternal infection for best sensitivity (37, 38). Neonatal blood collected at birth and dried on paper (e.g., Guthrie cards) as blood spots has been described for neonatal screening and for retrospective diagnosis in patients beyond the neonatal period with a clinical suspicion of congenital CMV infection (39). However, dried blood spots and blood in general are not as sensitive as urine or saliva for newborn screening. Dried blood spots have also been used for rapid genotyping of CMV strains in congenitally infected newborns (40) and for quantification of CMV DNA in solid organ transplant recipients (41). Both liquid- and dried-saliva specimens have proven useful for sensitive and specific detection of CMV DNA in newborns (42). For diagnosis of congenital infection in the neonate, samples of saliva, urine, or both collected within the first 3 weeks of life should be used (38). Saliva specimens (rather than urine) are now considered the most convenient sample type to collect and have been shown to be as reliable as urine for detection of CMV DNA for effective screening of neonates for congenital CMV infection and sensorineural hearing loss.

Impression smears, frozen sections, or formaldehyde-fixed and paraffin-embedded material can be used for *in situ* hybridization, immunohistochemical staining, or histopathologic examination of tissue specimens obtained from patients with pneumonia, gastrointestinal disease, hepatitis, myocarditis, retinitis, pancreatitis, nephritis, cystitis, or central nervous system disease.

More recently, measurements of CMV DNA viral load in bronchoalveolar lavage fluid have proven useful in the diagnosis of CMV pneumonia in solid organ and hematopoietic stem cell transplant recipients and infants suspected of CMV infection and disease without the need for performing more invasive procedures to obtain lung tissue (43–45).

Specimens for Virus Isolation

CMV can be isolated from a variety of body fluids and tissues; however, urine, respiratory secretions (e.g., saliva, throat washings, and bronchoalveolar lavage fluid), and anticoagulated whole blood (leukocytes) are most commonly used for diagnostic purposes.

Urine specimens should be clean-voided specimens. Because excretion of CMV in urine is intermittent, increased recovery of the virus is possible by processing more than one specimen. Adjustment of urine specimens to pH 7.0 with 0.1 N NaOH or 0.1 N HCl is recommended to reduce toxicity to cell cultures. Centrifuging urine specimens to obtain sediment-enriched samples has been advocated but is usually unnecessary and may produce toxicity more frequently than do uncentrifuged urine samples.

Blood leukocyte cultures have been used in the evaluation of immunocompromised patients. Detection of CMV in leukocytes is often a better indicator of symptomatic CMV infection than is shedding of virus in urine or respiratory secretions, although the sensitivity of cultures from blood is inadequate in comparison to that of molecular methods or the antigenemia assay. Fresh blood collected in the presence of heparin, sodium citrate, acid citrate dextrose, or EDTA may be used. A number of procedures for obtaining peripheral blood leukocytes have been described. However, density gradient centrifugation with either Ficoll-Hypaque or a mixture of sodium metrizoate and dextran 500 is most suitable for a clinical laboratory. Both mononuclear cells and granulocytes are efficiently separated from erythrocytes in a single step. The procedure is rapid and easy to perform, and the reagents are commercially available. Compared with traditional sedimentation methods, the technique results in a greater number of virus isolates and an increased yield of infectious foci or plaques. Alternatively, the direct lysis procedure described below may be used, although a reduced ability to culture CMV following direct erythrocyte lysis has been observed.

Bronchial washings and tissue biopsy and autopsy specimens, particularly of lungs, kidneys, spleen, liver, brain, the gastrointestinal tract, and retinas, also can be processed for virus isolation. Recovery of CMV from tissues is strong evidence for organ involvement. All tissue specimens should be placed in a suitable viral transport medium immediately after collection.

Since CMV loses infectivity when subjected to freezing and thawing, specimens for virus isolation should be kept at 4°C in an ice-water bath or refrigerator until they can be used to inoculate cultures, preferably within a few hours after collection. When prolonged transport times are unavoidable, infectivity is reasonably well preserved for at least 48 h at 4°C. In general, it is never a good idea to hold specimens for CMV isolation at room temperature, and specimens should be transported to the laboratory as quickly as possible after collection to maintain viability of the virus. If freezing the specimen is necessary, an equal volume of 0.4 M sucrose-phosphate added to the specimen helps preserve viral infectivity. All frozen specimens should be stored at −70°C or colder or in liquid nitrogen. Loss of virus infectivity occurs if specimens are stored at −20°C.

All specimens are treated with antibiotics before inoculation of cell cultures.

Specimens for Serologic Testing

Single serum specimens for immunoglobulin G (IgG) antibody testing are useful in screening for evidence of past infection with CMV and for identifying individuals at risk for CMV infection. This approach is especially helpful in testing sera from organ transplant donors and recipients before transplantation and from donors of blood products that are to be administered to premature infants or hematopoietic stem cell transplant patients. Also, knowing the immune status of women prior to conception may be helpful in identifying individuals who may be most susceptible to primary CMV infection following pregnancy.

For serologic diagnosis of recent CMV infection, detection of IgM in a single serum specimen may be beneficial, or paired sera should be obtained at least 2 weeks apart for testing for IgG antibody. The acute-phase serum sample should be collected as soon as possible after onset of illness and tested simultaneously with the convalescent-phase serum sample. If congenital infection is suspected, specimens from mother, fetus, and newborn can be submitted for the evaluation of IgG and IgM antibodies for the detection of prenatal, natal, and postnatal CMV infections. When testing for IgM in the fetus, blood should be collected after 22 weeks of gestation, since fetal synthesis of antibodies starts at 20 weeks of gestation and may not reach detectable levels for 1 to 2 more weeks.

Processed serum specimens may be stored at 2 to 8°C for several days pending the completion of testing or can be stored frozen at −20°C or colder for more extended periods of time. Repeat freezing and thawing should be avoided, and specimens should not be stored in frost-free freezers.

Testing saliva or oral fluids for CMV-specific antibodies has been previously suggested as a noninvasive alternative to the collection of blood from children, although neither specimen is routinely used in this setting. In patients with CMV neurologic disease, CSF may be tested for viral antibody if paired with a serum specimen collected on or close to the same date. However, the yield of such testing is low and limited by delays in intrathecal production of virus-specific antibody and passive transfer of serum antibodies across a damaged blood-brain barrier. As a general rule, screening for CMV-specific IgG and/or IgM antibodies to diagnose congenital CMV infection and antibody testing of CSF for the diagnosis of CMV neurologic disease have limited utility and have been largely replaced by more direct methods, like PCR.

Specimens for Measurement of Cell-Mediated Immunity

Whole blood in lithium or sodium heparin as the anticoagulant is collected for assays that measure cell-mediated immune responses to CMV infection (46–48). For enzyme-linked immunosorbent spot (ELISPOT) tests, a total of 7.5 to 12 ml of whole blood is typically used to purify peripheral blood mononuclear cells (PBMCs) according to established procedures and then stimulate the cells at 37°C for 16 to 20 h using defined CMV antigens. The number of cells is adjusted to 2.0 to 2.5 × 10^5/reaction for use in the assay. For the QuantiFERON-CMV assay, a total of 1.0 ml of whole blood is collected into each of three tubes containing either CMV antigens, phytohemagglutinin (a mitogen) as the positive control, or only heparin as the negative control dried on the inner wall of the individual tubes. The blood is vigorously mixed by shaking for 5 seconds to ensure that the entire inner surface of each tube has been coated with blood and then immediately stored at 37°C for 16 to 24 h to stimulate cells before processing by centrifugation to obtain plasma for testing. Plasma samples can be stored for up to 4 weeks at 2 to 8°C or for extended times at −20°C or below prior to testing. For assays that use flow cytometry to measure functional analysis of immune cells using intracellular cytokine staining or staining of antigen-specific receptor-carrying T lymphocytes, either whole blood or purified PBMCs can be used. A total of 2 to 3 ml of whole blood is used for assays that measure intracellular synthesis of ATP in stimulated $CD4^+$ T cells.

DIRECT EXAMINATION

Histopathologic testing, antigenemia assays, and qualitative and quantitative molecular methods have been routinely used for the direct detection of CMV from clinical samples. Histologic or immunohistochemical staining of tissue biopsy specimens is most useful in the diagnosis of localized CMV tissue-invasive disease, while antigenemia assays and molecular amplification tests are now the standard of care for testing and monitoring patients at increased risk for severe CMV disease, diagnosing active CMV disease, and monitoring response to therapy (10, 49, 50).

Histopathologic Testing

Characteristic large cells (cytomegalic cells) with basophilic intranuclear inclusions and, on occasion, eosinophilic cytoplasmic inclusions can be seen in routine sections of CMV-infected biopsy or autopsy material following staining with Wright-Giemsa, hematoxylin and eosin, or Papanicolaou stain (Fig. 1). The nuclear inclusion has the appearance of an "owl's eye" because it has marginated chromatin that is typically surrounded by a clear halo that extends to the nuclear membrane. The presence of characteristic cytologic changes seen by histopathologic testing suggests CMV infection and, while less sensitive than molecular methods like PCR, is more predictive of disease, especially in the gastrointestinal tract, and correlates with active disease in most cases. Overall, histopathologic diagnosis of CMV disease involves time and labor and is relatively insensitive, and since CMV can infect tissues without producing morphologic changes, failure to find typical cytomegalic cells does not exclude the possibility of CMV infection; additional virologic or serologic confirmation is suggested.

The sensitivity and specificity of histopathologic testing can be increased by using immunohistochemical staining with CMV-specific monoclonal or polyclonal antibody to detect CMV antigens or *in situ* hybridization with CMV-specific DNA probes to detect CMV nucleic acids. For years, the detection of CMV in intestinal mucosal epithelium or lung tissue by immunohistochemistry has been considered an important part of the evaluation of solid organ and hematopoietic stem cell transplant recipients with gastrointestinal symptoms or pneumonia, particularly given that viral loads in blood may be undetectable or low in these clinical settings. A major obstacle to tissue diagnosis of CMV is the need to perform invasive procedures to obtain biopsy specimens for testing. Consequently, tissue biopsy samples are not always obtained, and finding CMV in blood by antigen or nucleic acid detection is often used as a substitute to support the clinical suspicion of tissue-invasive disease.

Antigen Detection

The CMV antigenemia assay is a sensitive, specific, and rapid method for the early diagnosis of CMV infection and

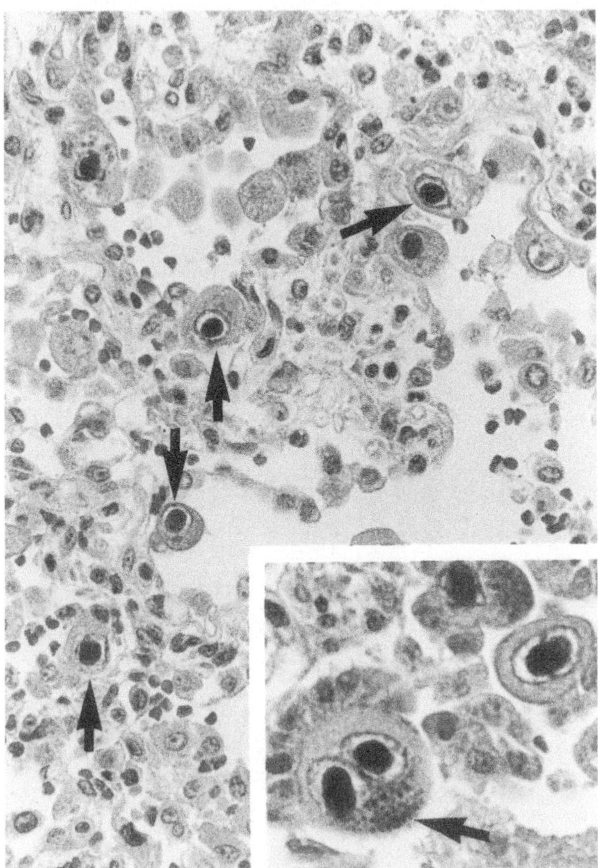

FIGURE 1 Fixed hematoxylin-and-eosin-stained lung tissue from a patient with interstitial pneumonia. Note the numerous giant cells that possess large intranuclear inclusions surrounded by characteristically clear halos (arrows). Less pronounced granular inclusions may also be present in the cytoplasm (inset). (Courtesy of Eduardo Ruchelli.)

can be used for routine monitoring of patients at high risk for severe CMV disease, including recipients of solid organ and hematopoietic stem cell transplants, HIV-infected patients, and patients treated with immunomodulating drugs. The test is relatively simple to perform and is based on immunocytochemical detection of the 65-kDa lower-matrix phosphoprotein (pp65) in the nuclei of peripheral blood leukocytes. By using this assay, CMV can be detected before the onset of symptoms and the viral load can be quantified to assist in predicting and differentiating CMV disease from asymptomatic infection (51, 52). The procedure has also been used to evaluate the efficacy of antiviral therapy and to predict treatment failure and the development of viral resistance (53, 54), to prompt the institution of preemptive therapy (55, 56), to detect CMV in leukocytes of CSF from AIDS patients with infections of the central nervous system, and for diagnosis of congenital CMV infection, CMV gastrointestinal disease, pneumonia, and liver disease, and CMV infection in the immunocompetent host. Positive antigenemia results are of value when one is attempting to diagnose tissue-invasive disease, whereas negative results are not helpful due to the relatively low sensitivity of the assay in this setting. The pp65 protein has also been found in endothelial cells circulating in the blood of immunocompromised patients, and some investigators have suggested that infection of these cells is associated with organ involvement and more advanced disease (57, 58). The results of the antigenemia assay correlate well with the quantitative detection of CMV DNA in whole blood, leukocytes, or plasma in molecular amplification assays (29, 59–63).

In the antigenemia assay, leukocytes (mainly polymorphonuclear leukocytes) are enriched from freshly collected whole blood by sedimentation with dextran. A method for direct lysis of erythrocytes and subsequent isolation of leukocytes from whole blood has been described (64) and is routinely used by laboratories performing this test. This modification allows a shorter total assay time and the capability of processing more specimens. Following sedimentation, the remaining erythrocytes are lysed with ammonium chloride, the granulocytes are counted in a hemocytometer or automated cell-counting instrument, and a known number of cells (usually 2×10^5, although variations of 5×10^4 to 1×10^6 cells have been used) are cytocentrifuged onto microscope slides. The cells are fixed with formaldehyde or paraformaldehyde, permeabilized with the nonionic detergent Nonidet P-40, and stained with suitable monoclonal antibodies directed against CMV pp65. These processes are followed by incubation of the cells with a fluorescein isothiocyanate-labeled secondary antibody diluted in a counterstain. Slides are read by microscopy at magnification of ×200 to ×400. Positive results are viewed as homogeneous yellow to apple-green fluorescence within the nuclei of infected cells (Fig. 2).

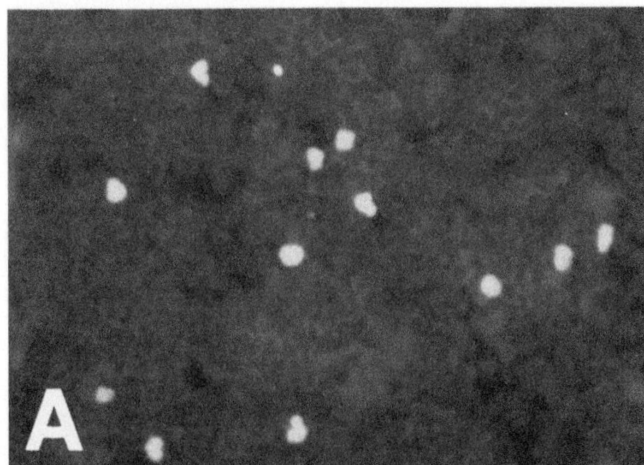

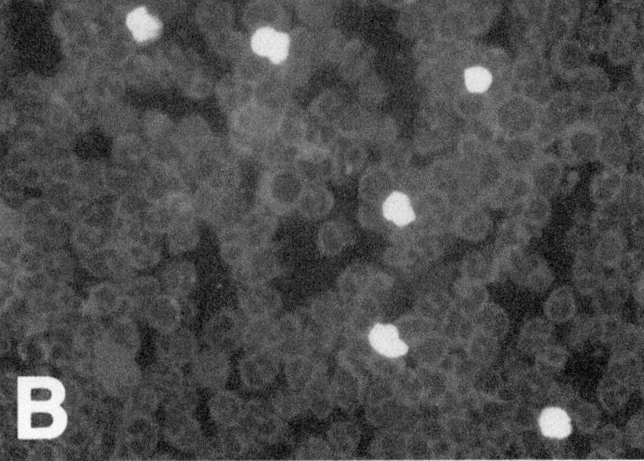

FIGURE 2 CMV antigen-positive polymorphonuclear leukocytes. Note the nuclear staining when a monoclonal antibody directed against pp65 is used. Magnification, ×100 (A) and ×400 (B).

Quantitative results are usually expressed as the number of antigen-positive cells per total number of leukocytes evaluated. Absolute CMV antigenemia values or specific thresholds to predict symptomatic disease or prompt administration of preemptive antiviral therapy have not been fully established for interpretation of quantitative testing, and they appear to be different between patient populations. Therefore, it is more important to monitor patients and trend relative rises and/or falls in the level of antigen-positive cells in multiple blood specimens collected over time than it is to rely on a single test result. The presence of small numbers of antigen-positive cells generally indicates asymptomatic infection, whereas increasingly larger numbers are more strongly associated with clinically significant disease. In patients with severe immunosuppression (e.g., after allogeneic hematopoietic stem cell transplantation), however, even very small numbers of antigen-positive cells may be significant. For transplant recipients, the frequency and extent of monitoring vary with the institution and from one transplant population to another and depend on the medical approach taken to manage CMV infection and disease (10, 49, 50).

The major advantages of the antigenemia assay are that it is more sensitive than either conventional tube or shell vial cultures for the detection of CMV from blood; it can be completed in 2 to 4 h, providing same-day turnaround of results; and the procedure can be readily modified for quantitative measure of the viral load. The assay has the disadvantages of being labor-intensive and time-consuming, particularly when large numbers of specimens are being processed; the blood must be processed in a timely manner for accurate results; and the test should be performed by personnel with experience in immunocytochemical techniques due to the subjective nature of the interpretation. Considerable time, effort, and expertise are needed in isolating and counting cells, adjusting the cell concentration to 10^6/ml before preparing the slides for staining, and then reading the stained slides. Also, interlaboratory variability exists with regard to the exact procedures used to perform the antigenemia assay (65–67), although it is not likely that the assay will undergo further standardization, since most laboratories now perform quantitative molecular tests for monitoring CMV infections. Commercial kits containing monoclonal antibodies and other reagents needed to perform the antigenemia assay are available (Table 2). Several of these assays have been licensed by the FDA, and comparative studies have demonstrated equivalent performance. Because of the low throughput, the antigenemia assay is best suited for laboratories processing small numbers of specimens.

Nucleic Acid Detection

Over the years, molecular amplification assays have progressively replaced the antigenemia assay and other nonmolecular direct detection tests for the diagnosis and monitoring of CMV infections. PCR is the most preferred and widely used molecular method for the detection of CMV DNA and mRNAs, and the sensitivity and specificity of PCR for diagnosis of active CMV infection have been evaluated (68–72). Amplification has been performed with a variety of primer pairs from regions of genes encoding the immediate early antigen (UL122-123 locus), the major immediate early antigen (UL122-123 locus), the DNA polymerase (UL54), glycoproteins B (UL55) and H (UL75), pp65 (UL83), pp67 (UL65), US17, HXFL4, the EcoRI D fragment, the HindIII X fragment, the pp150 tegument protein (UL32), and the major capsid protein (UL86) and the

TABLE 2 Available commercial CMV antigenemia assays

Manufacturer	Product[a]	Recommended blood collection and processing				No. of cells per slide	Monoclonal antibody used	Total assay time (h)	Selected reference(s)
		Amt (ml)	Anticoagulant used	Storage conditions	Cell separation technique				
Bio-Rad (IQ Products)	CMV Brite	5–10	Heparin or EDTA	20–25°C for 6–8 h	Dextran sedimentation	1.5×10^5	C10/C11	4–5	166, 167
	CMV Brite Turbo	3–5	EDTA	20–25°C for 6–8 h	Direct erythrocyte lysis with NH_4Cl	2.0×10^5	C10/C11	2	167–169
bioMérieux, Inc.	Argene CINAkit HCMV ppUL83 rapid antigenemia	7	Heparin or EDTA	2–8°C for up to 24 h	Dextran sedimentation or direct erythrocyte lysis with NH_4Cl	2.0×10^5	1C3 + AYM-1	4–5 or 2	167, 170
Millipore Sigma	Light Diagnostics CMV pp65 antigenemia	5–10	Heparin or EDTA	20–25°C for up to 24 h	Dextran sedimentation or direct erythrocyte lysis with NH_4Cl	2.0×10^5	Proprietary	4–5 or 2	171

[a]CMV Brite, CMV Brite Turbo, and CINAkit are FDA approved for qualitative testing only; the Light Diagnostics kit is not FDA approved; all kits are CE marked.

junction between the glycoprotein B and major immediate early antigen genes. Based on published literature, the most common targets for CMV PCR include glycoprotein B, the immediate early antigen, the major immediate early antigen, and US17 genes followed by the pp65 and polymerase genes. Not all primers are equally sensitive in amplifying CMV DNA, and in several studies, the sensitivity of the assay was increased by amplifying genomic regions from both the immediate early and the late CMV genes or by using nested primers specific to a single gene fragment. The use of both gene fragments enabled the detection of a variety of clinical isolates, indicating that strain variability is not a limiting factor for PCR diagnosis of CMV. PCR has been used successfully to detect CMV DNA in a variety of clinical specimens from transplant recipients, patients with AIDS, and infants with congenital infection. It also has been used for the continued surveillance of immunocompromised patients and for evaluation of the therapeutic efficacy of antiviral drugs.

Of concern with PCR for CMV diagnosis is whether the test can distinguish between active disease and asymptomatic infection or latency. CMV DNA-emia is considered to be the best predictor of CMV disease, and CMV DNA has been successfully detected in whole blood, purified peripheral blood leukocytes, plasma, and serum by PCR. However, PCR is extremely sensitive, and the qualitative detection of CMV DNA in these specimens has limited value in predicting symptomatic disease and in monitoring the success of antiviral therapy in immunocompromised patients. CMV DNA can be detected in blood by PCR in the absence of disease and can be found for weeks or months after successful therapy of symptomatic patients (53, 73, 74). However, there are clinical settings in which qualitative PCR appears to be useful, including in the use of saliva, urine, tissue, amniotic fluid, or fetal blood for diagnosis of congenital CMV infection and the aqueous or vitreous humor in patients with CMV retinitis. Also, a negative result from qualitative PCR of blood has a high negative predictive value for excluding systemic CMV disease and has been used over the years as an initial screen of blood specimens before quantifying CMV DNA from only those samples that are positive. However, the recent commercial availability of highly sensitive quantitative molecular assays most likely eliminates any need for qualitative testing of blood specimens.

Qualitative PCR can also be used on fresh, unfixed tissue specimens from immunocompromised patients with suspected localized or compartmentalized tissue-invasive disease. However, careful consideration should be given to whether detection of CMV by highly sensitive molecular methods truly represents infection of the organ or possible contamination with the virus from infected extracellular fluids that bathe the tissue. While negative PCR results would suggest absence of CMV tissue-invasive infection, positive results may not be significant and should be correlated with clinical and histopathologic findings and detection of CMV viremia, DNA-emia, or antigenemia in blood. In this regard, *in situ* hybridization or immunohistochemical staining may be helpful in localizing the virus within the tissue. More recently, CMV PCR on formalin-fixed, paraffin-embedded tissues was shown to be a useful adjunct to immunohistochemistry for the diagnosis of tissue-invasive disease (75, 76) and can provide a more specific diagnosis than performing CMV PCR on fresh, unfixed tissue.

Similar to the antigenemia assay, measuring the level of CMV DNA in blood appears to be necessary to predict and diagnose CMV disease in immunocompromised hosts (10, 49, 50). Consequently, a number of quantitative and semiquantitative molecular assays have been developed over the years and have included target and signal amplification methods. Most laboratories now use quantitative real-time PCR (77–83) because it allows detection of amplified nucleic acids as they accumulate, and technological advances have provided rapid and accurate quantification over a dynamic range of orders of magnitude, using a variety of different chemistries and platforms. Also, assays for CMV can be multiplexed with tests for other herpesviruses for simultaneous monitoring following transplantation (84, 85). The performances of individual PCR assays have been compared to those of the antigenemia assay and culture as well as to each other (59, 61, 62, 86–91). Overall, these molecular methods provide quantitative results comparable to those obtained by the antigenemia assay; they are also more sensitive than culture for detecting CMV infection and can detect CMV before the onset of clinical symptoms. It has been shown that transplant recipients and AIDS patients with active CMV disease have higher levels of CMV DNA and that a rapid rise in the CMV DNA copy number correlates with the presence of symptoms and drug failure during treatment (60, 92–94). Also, Rasmussen et al. (95) have determined that quantitation of CMV DNA from peripheral blood leukocytes can be used to identify HIV-infected patients at risk for development of symptomatic CMV retinitis. It has also been determined that immunocompromised patients with CMV disease have more CMV DNA in either whole blood, plasma, or leukocyte fractions than do patients without disease but that the level of CMV DNA in whole blood or leukocytes is higher than that in plasma (60, 96). Quantitation of CMV in plasma, therefore, may be less sensitive for monitoring CMV infection, although a positive result may correlate better with active disease.

Although there is general agreement between PCR and antigenemia assays, the quantitative numerical relationship is not exact, and differences should be expected, since these assays measure different biological features of CMV replication and infection. PCR is extremely sensitive; it may detect CMV earlier than the antigenemia assay and may continue to be positive after antigen testing is negative. Conversely, negative PCR results have been reported for patients with low numbers of positive cells in the antigenemia assay (62). Therefore, depending on the test and parameters used, these assays may be more or less sensitive compared to one another and may have higher or lower positive predictive values for CMV disease. As in the antigenemia assay, absolute CMV DNA levels or threshold values for predicting symptomatic disease and initiating preemptive therapy have not been fully elucidated and may differ by specimen type and testing platform selected and from one laboratory and patient population to another. It is currently more important to monitor the relative changes in DNA levels from serial blood specimens collected over time and tested using the same assay and specimen type. If desired, specific cutoff levels should be prospectively determined based on the assay and specimen used and the type of patients being monitored. Because of the high sensitivity of PCR and depending upon the cutoff value selected, the positive predictive value for symptomatic CMV disease may vary and may affect clinical decision-making and the initiation and length of antiviral therapy.

Quantitative PCR methods have been used for the estimation of CMV DNA levels in urine, saliva, amniotic fluid, dried blood spots, and CSF of CMV-infected patients (37, 38, 41, 42, 97, 98), but more research is needed to assess the clinical relevance of quantitating CMV DNA from these specimens. It has been shown that the prognosis of congenital CMV infection may be directly related to the amount of CMV in the urine and/or saliva of an infected neonate, that measurements of CMV DNA in the blood and urine of a pregnant woman may be predictive of transmission to the fetus, that quantitating CMV DNA in the CSF of AIDS patients may help determine if disorders of the central nervous system are attributable more to CMV than to the direct effects of HIV or other opportunistic pathogens, and that measuring the CMV viral load in bronchoalveolar lavage specimens may be an appropriate and less invasive way to diagnose CMV pneumonia in immunocompromised patients (43–45).

In general, real-time PCR assays for the detection and quantification of CMV DNA are sensitive, specific, and reproducible and significantly reduce the time necessary to report results that may have an impact on the care and management of patients. The method offers the distinct advantages of being less technically demanding and less expensive to perform than more conventional assays, and quality reagents and automated instruments for nucleic acid extraction and amplification and detection are readily available and greatly improve the potential for standardization and increased accuracy of results. The assays also require a lower specimen volume for testing and can be easily performed on neutropenic patients with low leukocyte counts. The DNA is stable during extended specimen transport and storage times, and large numbers of specimens can be efficiently processed. Furthermore, the overall risk of amplicon contamination has been greatly minimized, as real-time platforms are closed systems.

Various commercial real-time qualitative and quantitative PCR assays are now available as either analyte-specific reagents or packaged as complete kits (Table 3). However, many real-time PCR assays for CMV have been developed in the laboratory by the end user and differ in many parameters, including the types and volumes of specimens used; the collection, transport, processing, and storage of the specimens; the nucleic acid target selected; the choice and design of suitable oligonucleotide primers and probes; optimization of specimen extraction and PCR amplification conditions; the controls and calibration standards used; the method chosen to detect and/or quantify the amplified product; the upper and lower limits of detection and quantification; the accuracy and precision; and the quantitative units of measure and viral loads reported from one laboratory and method to another. Many of the assays require additional validation, and there is a definite need for traceable and commutable international reference materials that include both standards and controls for institutional comparison of results, since significant variability in CMV quantification has been observed between laboratories (99–102). To this end, the first international CMV standard was developed by the World Health Organization (WHO) in 2010 and is available from the National Institute of Biological Standards and Controls in the United Kingdom as NIBSC code 09/162. The standard is whole virus prepared from the CMV Merlin strain, and the material was initially evaluated in a worldwide collaborative study involving 32 laboratories performing a range of molecular amplification assays for CMV (103). Secondary material calibrated against this standard now can be purchased from commercial manufacturers, and a second standard reference material (SRM 2366a) has been made available from the National Institute of Standards and Technology in the United States (104). This reference standard comprises a bacterial artificial chromosome carrying the complete virus genome of the Towne strain of CMV. Use of these standard reference materials and the recommended reporting of viral loads in international units per milliliter have allowed improved interassay agreement among different laboratories using different quantitative molecular assays (105–108) and should facilitate the establishment of defined testing algorithms and cutoff values that predict clinical disease and improve management and outcomes in CMV-infected patients (109–112).

Several commercial quantitative assays have been developed using this international standard and have been licensed by the FDA, including the Abbott RealTime CMV assay, Qiagen artus CMV RGQ MDx kit, Roche cobas AmpliPrep/cobas TaqMan CMV test, and Roche cobas CMV test for use on the cobas 4800 and 6800/8800 automated systems (Table 3). The tests are performed on automated platforms, and results are expressed in international units per milliliter. The level of agreement between assays has been shown to be high across different laboratories during evaluations of these systems. Although the development of international standards and the greater availability of commercial assays have definitely helped harmonize CMV viral load testing and reporting, the intra- and interlaboratory variability has not been completely eliminated and is thought to be due to assay design and a variety of analytical factors apart from universal standards that are traceable and commutable (102, 105, 113–117).

More recently, digital PCR has been developed as a quantitative method, and the clinical utility of this assay for the accurate quantification of CMV from plasma specimens has been demonstrated in several studies (118–120). Digital PCR is similar to quantitative real-time PCR in that the same reaction components and amplification conditions are used, but they differ in how the amplified target is measured. The assay is performed by partitioning a sample reaction mixture into thousands of smaller picoliter- or nanoliter-scale individual PCRs and is based on the assumption that partitioning of the sample will follow a Poisson distribution, resulting in individual reactions with either a single target molecule or no target at all. Reaction mixtures that contain a target molecule will amplify and show positive fluorescence during PCR, while reactions with no target will be negative. Following PCR, the negative and positive reactions are counted, and the results are used to calculate the number of copies of target in the sample based on Poisson statistical analysis. Digital PCR has the major advantages of offering absolute quantification of CMV DNA without the requirement for reference standards or the need for a calibration curve to facilitate measurements of viral load. The assay has improved inter- and intralaboratory precision over that of current quantitative methods (121) and is less affected by poor amplification efficiency and interfering substances that may be present in clinical specimens (119, 122). However, digital PCR does not appear to be as sensitive as real-time PCR for quantitative detection of CMV, and further optimization is required (119).

Several digital PCR platforms are commercially availably and differ primarily in how individual reactions are partitioned, using either water-oil emulsion droplets or microchip-based arrays. They include the RainDrop Plus Digital PCR system (RainDance Technologies), QX200 Droplet digital PCR system (Bio-Rad), BioMark HD system (Fluidigm Corporation), and QuantStudio 3D digital PCR system (Life Technologies). None of the commercial systems have been approved by the FDA to date. Limited data currently exist in support of digital PCR for CMV

TABLE 3 Selected commercial real-time PCR molecular assays available for qualitative and quantitative detection of CMV[a]

Manufacturer	Product	Specimen (ml)	Gene target(s)	Measurement	Regulatory status	Selected reference(s)
Abbott Molecular	Abbott RealTime CMV	Plasma in U.S.; whole blood and plasma outside U.S.	UL34 and UL80.5	Quantitative; calibrated against 1st WHO International Standard for Human CMV; linear range is 50 IU/ml to 156 million IU/ml for plasma in U.S.; 31.2 IU/ml to 156 million IU/ml for plasma and 62.4 IU/ml to 156 million IU/ml for whole blood outside the U.S.	FDA approved; CE marked	172–175
Altona Diagnostics	RealStar CMV PCR kits 1.0 and 1.2	Plasma	Proprietary	Qualitative and quantitative; calibrated against 1st WHO International Standard for Human CMV; validated with different extraction and real-time PCR instruments; linear range varies by which instruments are used	CE marked only	176
bioMérieux, Inc.	Argene CMV R-gene	Whole blood, plasma, serum, urine, CSF, amniotic fluid, BAL, tissue	UL83 pp65	Qualitative and quantitative; validated with different extraction and real-time PCR instruments; linear range varies by which instruments and sample types are used	CE marked only	177
	Argene CMV HHV6,7,8 R-gene	Whole blood, plasma, serum, urine, CSF, amniotic fluid, BAL, tissue	CMV UL83 pp65; HHV-6 U57; HHV-7 U42; HHV-8 ORF26	Qualitative and quantitative; validated with different extraction and real-time PCR instruments; linear range varies by which instruments and sample types are used	CE marked only	30, 178
ELITechGroup	CMV ELITe MGB kit	Whole blood, plasma, urine, saliva, CSF, amniotic fluid	UL123 MIEA	Qualitative and quantitative; validated with different extraction and real-time PCR instruments; linear range varies by which instruments and sample types are used	CE marked only	179, 180
	Alert Q-CMV Real Time Complete kit	Whole blood, plasma, amniotic fluid, leukocyte and granulocyte suspensions	UL123 MIEA	Qualitative and quantitative; validated with different extraction and real-time PCR instruments; linear range varies by which instruments and sample types are used	CE marked only	181
Focus Diagnostics	Simplexa CMV	Whole blood or plasma	UL83 pp65	Quantitative; calibrated against 1st WHO International Standard for Human CMV; linear range is 713 IU/ml to 396 million IU/ml	CE marked only	179
	CMV primers	Various	UL 83 pp65	Qualitative and quantitative; analytical and performance characteristics must be established by the end user	ASR for laboratory-developed assays	
Luminex Corp.	Multicode CMV primers	Various	UL54 pol	Qualitative and quantitative; analytical and performance characteristics must be established by the end user	ASR for laboratory-developed assays	179
Qiagen, Inc.	artus CMV RGQ MDx kit	Plasma	UL123 MIEA	Quantitative; calibrated against 1st WHO International Standard for Human CMV; linear range is 159 IU/ml to 79.4 million IU/ml	FDA approved; CE marked	182, 183
	artus CMV RG, TM, LC, and QS-RGQ PCR kits	Plasma	UL123 MIEA	Quantitative; validated with different extraction and real-time PCR instruments; linear range varies by which instruments are used	CE marked only	178, 184
Roche Diagnostics	cobas AmpliPrep/cobas TaqMan CMV test	Plasma	UL54 pol	Quantitative; calibrated against 1st WHO International Standard for Human CMV; linear range is 137 IU/ml to 9.1 million IU/ml	FDA approved; CE marked	172, 180, 185–190
	cobas CMV for cobas 4800 and 6800/8800 systems	Plasma	UL54 pol (smaller amplicon)	Quantitative; calibrated against 1st WHO International Standard for Human CMV; linear range is 34.5 IU/ml to 10 million IU/ml	FDA approved; CE marked	

[a]Abbreviations: BAL, bronchoalveolar lavage; pol, polymerase; MIEA, major immediate early antigen; ASR, analyte-specific reagent.

viral load testing, and studies comparing digital PCR to the existing FDA-approved quantitative real-time PCR systems for measurements of CMV viral load are needed to better understand the applicability and use of this newer technology in clinical laboratories.

Ultimately, the clinical utility of these assays depends on their accuracy, reproducibility, precision, ease of use, cost, availability, and predictive value. Molecular methods, however, are now considered invaluable additions to the analytical tools already being used to provide a rapid diagnosis of established CMV disease, identify patients at risk of developing disease, assess the progression of disease and the risk of relapse, direct the initiation of preemptive therapy, monitor the response to therapy, predict viral resistance and treatment failure, and define when antiviral susceptibility testing should be performed to identify emerging CMV resistance.

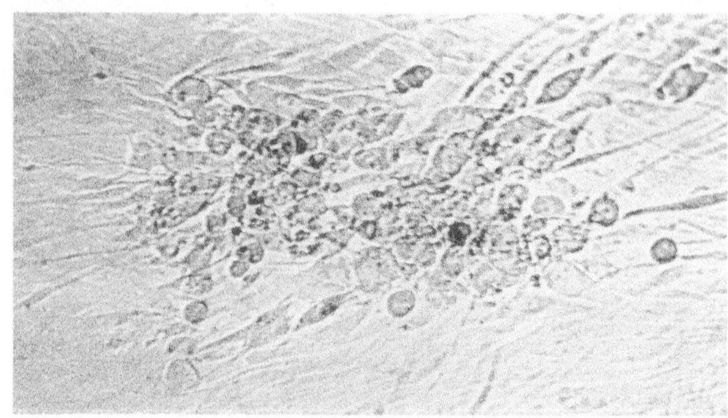

FIGURE 3 CPE produced by a CMV isolate in human skin fibroblasts 10 days postinoculation. Unstained preparation; magnification, ×100. (Courtesy of Sergio Stagno.)

ISOLATION PROCEDURES

Cell Cultures

Human fibroblasts best support the growth of CMV and therefore are used for diagnostic purposes. Acceptable fibroblast cultures include those prepared from human embryonic tissues or foreskins and serially passaged diploid human fetal lung strains, such as WI-38, MRC-5, and IMR-90. Diploid fibroblast cells should be used at a low passage number, since they may become less susceptible to CMV infection with increasing cell generations. Several of these fibroblast cell lines are commercially available. Culture systems for the detection of CMV in clinical specimens include conventional tube cultures and spin amplification shell vial assays. Although cultures are still performed in some laboratories, their use and clinical utility for CMV have diminished, owing to the much better overall performance and ease of use of newer and more efficient non-culture-based detection methods.

Conventional Tube Culture

Specimens to be tested are added in a volume of 0.2 ml to tubes of confluent fibroblasts maintained in Eagle minimal essential medium with 2% fetal bovine serum. Alternatively, the tubes are drained of medium, the inocula are absorbed for 1 h in a stationary position or by centrifugation at 700 × *g* for 45 min at 30 to 33°C, and then fresh medium is added. After inoculation, the tubes can be rolled or kept stationary at 37°C. Twenty-four hours later, the medium is changed in tubes inoculated with urine or leukocyte specimens. Thereafter, and for other types of specimens, the medium is changed once a week or more frequently as the pH of the culture medium changes or if toxicity appears. When toxicity necessitates passage of the culture, cells rather than culture medium should be passaged, since CMV remains mostly cell associated. Cells are removed by addition of 0.25% trypsin–0.1% EDTA to the monolayers and incubation at 37°C for approximately 1 min. When the cells detach, Eagle minimal essential medium with 2% fetal bovine serum is added, and the cells are used to inoculate fresh tubes. Tubes are examined for cytopathic effect (CPE) for at least 4 weeks for most specimens (6 weeks for leukocyte specimens). Control, uninoculated cultures are handled in the same manner as those inoculated with clinical specimens.

CMV isolates are normally identified solely on the basis of characteristic CPE and host cell range. The time of appearance and the extent of CPE depend on the amounts of virus present in specimens. In cultures inoculated with urine from a congenitally infected newborn, CPE may develop by 24 h and progress rapidly to involve most of the monolayer if the virus titer in the urine is extremely high. More commonly, foci of CPE, consisting of enlarged, rounded, refractile cells, appear during the first week, and progression of CPE to surrounding cells proceeds slowly (Fig. 3). In cultures inoculated with urine or respiratory specimens from older individuals, CPE usually appears within 2 weeks. Leukocyte cultures may not become positive until after 3 to 6 weeks. The usual slow progression of CPE in tube cultures inoculated with clinical specimens is due, at least in part, to limited release of virus into extracellular fluid. With strains of CMV that have been serially passaged, including laboratory-adapted strains, greater amounts of extracellular virus are released and CPE progresses more rapidly. Viruses such as adenovirus and varicella-zoster virus occasionally produce CPE indistinguishable from that of CMV, so suspected CMV isolates are best confirmed by an immunofluorescence assay (IFA) using monoclonal or polyclonal antibodies that are available from various commercial sources. The appearance of typical nuclear fluorescence of infected cells indicates the presence of CMV. PCR or other molecular amplification methods also can be used for confirmation of suspected isolates.

For storage of fresh isolates, monolayers exhibiting CPE are treated with trypsin-EDTA, and the cells obtained are suspended in Eagle minimal essential medium with 10% fetal bovine serum and 10% dimethyl sulfoxide and then frozen at −70°C. Infectivity can be better maintained for long periods by storage in liquid nitrogen.

Spin Amplification Shell Vial Assay

The spin amplification shell vial assay has been used extensively as a rapid culture method for the detection of CMV in clinical specimens and has largely replaced the slower conventional tube cultures in most laboratories. The technique is based on the amplification of virus in cell cultures after low-speed centrifugation and detects viral antigens produced early in the replication of CMV, before the development of CPE. Even low titers of virus present in specimens are easily amplified and rapidly detected within 24 h. Monoclonal antibodies are commercially available and are used for the detection of CMV early antigens.

MRC-5 fibroblast cells are grown to confluency on 12-mm-diameter round coverslips in 3.7-ml (1-dram) shell vials and inoculated with 0.2 ml of specimen. Shell vials of MRC-5 cells can be obtained commercially or prepared in the laboratory. Monolayers should be inoculated within

1 week after preparation, since older monolayers demonstrate decreased sensitivity to CMV and increased toxicity. Two vials should be inoculated for urine, tissue, and bronchoalveolar lavage fluid specimens, and three vials should be inoculated for blood specimens. Alternatively, disruption of purified leukocytes by sonication before their use in the shell vial assay may increase the sensitivity of CMV detection from blood. Increasing the frequency of blood collection and the volume of blood obtained also may enhance the diagnostic yield of the shell vial assay from this specimen. After inoculation, the vials are centrifuged at 700 × *g* for 40 min at 25°C, and then 2.0 ml of Eagle minimum essential medium containing 2% fetal bovine serum and antibiotics is added. The cultures are incubated at 37°C for 16 to 24 h, fixed with acetone, and stained. A longer incubation time may be used, but the time should be determined by each laboratory on the basis of individual experience, the reagents and staining technique used, and whether monolayers are purchased or prepared in the laboratory. Uninfected and CMV-infected monolayers are included as negative and positive controls, respectively. Mink lung (ML) cells, a non-human continuous cell line, are comparable to MRC-5 fibroblasts for the detection of CMV in clinical specimens by shell vial culture. A distinct advantage of using ML cells is that this cell line can be propagated and passaged in the laboratory for a long time without a decrease in susceptibility to CMV. Significantly less toxicity and an increase in the number of CMV-positive nuclei were also observed with ML cells. Coverslips are scanned at a magnification of ×200 to ×250, and specific staining is confirmed at ×400 to ×630. Positive cells contain yellow to apple-green fluorescent nuclei against a red cytoplasmic background. Staining of immediate early antigen appears as an even matte yellow to green fluorescence with specks of brighter yellow or green (Fig. 4A). Viral inclusions (owl's eyes) may be visible in the nuclei (Fig. 4B).

The spin amplification shell vial assay has the important features of being rapid, sensitive, and specific, but skilled technical personnel and close attention to the quality of specimens, monolayers, and reagents are required for optimum performance.

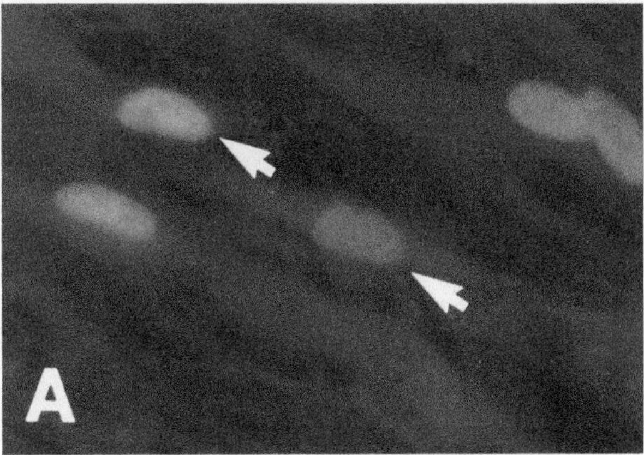

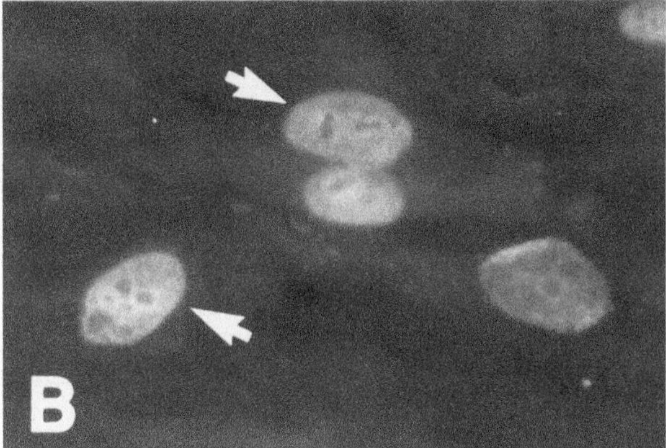

FIGURE 4 Demonstration of CMV early antigens in the nuclei (arrows) of infected MRC-5 cells following shell vial culture and IFA staining. (A) Staining of immediate early antigen appears as an even matte yellow to green fluorescence with specks of brighter yellow to green. (B) Viral inclusions (owl's eyes) may be visible in the nuclei. Magnification, ×400.

SEROLOGIC TESTS

A variety of tests with high sensitivities and specificities are available for the detection of either IgM or IgG antibodies to CMV (123). In deciding which test to perform, one should consider such factors as the number of specimens to be tested, the patient population, cost, turnaround time, equipment needs, and ease of performance. The method that is chosen depends on the needs of individual laboratories. For small-volume laboratories, IFA may be more cost-effective and practical, while enzyme immunoassays (EIAs) may be more suitable for laboratories with higher volumes of specimens. Overall, detection of CMV-specific IgM or determination of a seroconversion from a negative to a positive IgG antibody response can be useful for the diagnosis of primary CMV infection in certain clinical settings, and the screening of blood and organ donors and recipients plays an important role in preventing the transmission of latent CMV to patients at high risk for severe CMV disease.

Enzyme Immunoassays

Over the years, solid-phase EIAs have largely replaced other traditional methods for detecting antibodies to CMV. The assay format is versatile, as the solid phase may include microwell plates, polystyrene beads, microparticles, or paramagnetic particles, and detection of antibody can occur using fluorochrome, chemiluminescent, and electrochemiluminescent molecules to generate an accurate signal. The main advantages of the EIA are that it is rapid, sensitive, and specific. In addition, multiple specimens can be handled daily at a relatively low cost. Kits that detect CMV IgG are available from a number of commercial sources (Table 4). The kits are easy to use, and the manufacturers have provided detailed instructions. All the materials necessary to perform the assay are included, and the reagents are stable with time. Some companies also provide a spectrophotometer and automated plate washer, which otherwise must be purchased separately at additional expense. The development of robotics technology has led to the commercial availability of both fully automated and semiautomated EIA instruments that include sample dispensers, diluters, washers, and spectrophotometers with complete computer programming and generation of electronic and written reports. Some automated instruments also have random-access capability, which is a major advance that allows continuous loading and management of multiple specimens as they are received in the laboratory and permits individualized testing profiles to be applied to each sample. Random-access systems are also commonly associated with reagent and waste monitoring and automated calibrations and maintenance routines.

TABLE 4 Selected commercial immunoassay systems for CMV IgM, IgG, and IgG avidity antibody detection

Manufacturer	System(s)	CMV test availability	
		In U.S.	Outside U.S.
Abbott Diagnostics	Architect i1000SR, i2000SR, i4000SR	None	IgM, IgG, and IgG avidity
Beckman Coulter, Inc.	Access/Access 2	None	IgM and IgG
	Unicel DxI 600, DxI 800, DxC 600i, DxC 660i, DxC 680i, DxC 860i, DxC 880i	None	IgM and IgG
bioMérieux, Inc.	VIDAS/Mini-VIDAS	IgM and IgG	IgM, IgG, and IgG avidity
Bio-Rad Laboratories	BioPlex 2200	IgM and IgG	IgM and IgG
	EVOLIS Premium/EVOLIS Twin Plus	IgM and IgG	IgM and IgG
DiaSorin, Inc.	ETI-MAX 3000	IgM capture and IgG	None
	LIAISON	IgM and IgG	IgM, IgG, and IgG avidity
Diesse Diagnostica	Reagent kits	IgM capture, IgG and IgG avidity	IgM capture, IgG and IgG avidity
Euroimmun	Reagent kits	IgM, IgG, and IgG avidity	IgM, IgG, and IgG avidity
Mikrogen Diagnostik	Reagent kits	IgM, IgG, and IgG avidity	IgM, IgG, and IgG avidity
Ortho Clinical Diagnostics	VITROS ECi	None	IgM and IgG
	VITROS 3600/5600	None	IgM and IgG
Radim Diagnostics	Reagent kits	IgM capture, IgG and IgG avidity	IgM capture, IgG and IgG avidity
Roche Diagnostics	cobas 8000 (e602 module)	IgM and IgG; IgG avidity under development	IgM, IgG, and IgG avidity
	cobas 6000 (e601 module)	IgM and IgG; IgG avidity under development	IgM, IgG, and IgG avidity
	cobas 4000 (e411 module)	IgM and IgG; IgG avidity under development	IgM, IgG, and IgG avidity
Siemens Healthcare Diagnostics	ADVIA Centaur CP, XP, XPT	IgM and IgG under development	IgM and IgG under development
	IMMULITE 2000/2000 XPi	IgM and IgG	IgM and IgG
	IMMULITE 1000	IgM and IgG	IgM and IgG
Technogenetics	Reagent kits	None	IgM, IgG, and IgG avidity
Trinity Biotech	Use of semiautomated washers and readers, Trinity Biotech DSX/DS2 automated open systems, or other open platforms that can be programmed to perform all analytical steps for Trinity Biotech immunoassays (e.g., Awareness Technology Chem Well 2910, Bio-Rad PhD/PhD Ix and EVOLIS Premium/EVOLIS Twin Plus, Diamedix MAGO 4S/MAGO Plus, Dynex Technologies Agility, GRIFOLS Triturus, Inova Diagnostics Quanta-Lyser 240/160/2 and DSX/DS2)	IgM capture and IgG	IgM capture and IgG
Vidia	Reagent kits	IgM capture, IgG and IgG avidity	IgM capture, IgG and IgG avidity
Virion/Serion	Reagent kits	IgM and IgG	IgM and IgG
Wampole (Alere)	Use of semiautomated washers and readers, Alere DSX/DS2 automated open systems, or other open platforms that can be programmed to perform all analytical steps for Alere immunoassays (e.g., Awareness Technology Chem Well 2910, Bio-Rad PhD/PhD Ix and EVOLIS Premium/EVOLIS Twin Plus, Diamedix MAGO 4S and MAGO Plus, Dynex Technologies Agility, GRIFOLS Triturus, Inova Diagnostics Quanta-Lyser 240/160/2 and DSX/DS2)	IgM and IgG	IgM and IgG
Zeus Scientific	AtheNA Multi-Lyte	IgG	IgG

More recently, an EIA that uses the envelope glycoproteins B and H to distinguish CMV strain-specific antibody responses was developed (124). This assay may be useful for identifying strain diversity in different patient populations and may provide a better understanding of the implications of infection with multiple CMV strains and the role of strain-specific antibody in the protective immune response against CMV.

Immunofluorescence Assays

Indirect and anticomplement IFAs are commonly used methods for detecting CMV antibodies. In the indirect IFA, dilutions of test serum are incubated with virus-infected cells that have been fixed to a glass microscope slide. Specific antibody-antigen complexes are detected using an anti-human immunoglobulin antibody conjugated with fluorescein isothiocyanate and fluorescence microscopy. Anticomplement immunofluorescence is similar to the indirect IFA. It differs, however, in that the test serum is first heat inactivated to remove endogenous complement activity and then incubated with virus-infected cells on glass slides. An exogenous source of complement is added and bound by any specific antigen-antibody complexes that have formed. A fluorescein-labeled anticomplement antibody is then added; it binds to the C3 component of complement, and the slides are read using a fluorescence microscope. Anticomplement IFA amplifies the fluorescent signal above what can be seen using an indirect IFA, allowing the detection of small amounts of antibody or antibodies of low avidity. IFAs are useful and inexpensive methods that offer the advantages of speed and simplicity for the qualitative and quantitative detection of CMV antibodies. Commercial kits are readily available, or antigen-coated slides and labeled secondary antibodies can be purchased separately. The major disadvantages of IFA systems are that they require a fluorescence microscope and darkroom for examining slides and that extensive training is needed to read and interpret the test results.

CMV IgM Antibody Measurements

Commercial reagents and complete EIA and IFA diagnostic kits are available for measuring CMV IgM antibodies (Table 4) and are most useful in the diagnosis of CMV infection in newborns. The procedures are essentially the same as those used to detect IgG antibodies, except that anti-human IgM antibodies labeled with suitable markers are used to detect CMV-specific IgM bound to viral antigens on the solid phase. A recognized pitfall of CMV IgM assays is the occurrence of false-positive and false-negative reactions. False-positive reactions occur when sera contain unusually high levels of rheumatoid factor in the presence of specific CMV IgG. Rheumatoid factor is an immunoglobulin, usually of the IgM class, that reacts with IgG. It is produced in some rheumatologic, vasculitic, and viral diseases, including CMV infection. IgM rheumatoid factor forms a complex with IgG that may contain CMV-specific IgG. The CMV IgG binds to CMV antigen, carrying nonviral IgM with it; in this setting, a test designed to detect IgM will produce a false-positive result. False-negative reactions occur if high levels of specific IgG antibodies competitively block the binding of IgM to CMV antigen. Therefore, it is highly recommended to separate IgM and IgG fractions before testing to decrease the incidence of both false-positive and false-negative IgM test results.

Rapid and simple methods for the removal of interfering rheumatoid factor and IgG molecules from serum have been developed. These include selective absorption of IgM to a solid phase and removal of IgG by using hyperimmune anti-human IgG antibody, staphylococcal protein A, or recombinant protein G from group G streptococci. Serum pretreatment methods are now readily available and are incorporated into the procedures of commercially available IFA and EIA kits, which have resulted in more reliable IgM tests. More recently, reverse capture solid-phase IgM assays have been used as an alternative approach to avoiding false-positive or false-negative results. This method uses a solid phase coated with an anti-human IgM antibody to capture the IgM from a serum specimen, after which competing IgG antibody and immune complexes are removed by washing. The bound IgM antibody is then exposed to specific CMV antigen, and an enzyme-conjugated second antibody and substrate are added. The development and use of recombinantly derived CMV proteins as a source of antigenic substrate also have greatly improved the performance of IgM assays.

Although the detection of CMV-specific IgM may be beneficial in the determination of recent or active infection, the results should be interpreted with caution. Because IgM does not cross the placenta, a positive result from a single serum specimen from an infected newborn is diagnostic. However, there may be a lack of or delay in production of IgM in the newborn. Testing for the presence of CMV-specific IgM antibody beyond the newborn period is usually not recommended, since IgM antibody can appear in both primary and reactivated CMV infections and can persist for extended periods after a primary infection. This complicates the interpretation of test results, particularly for pregnant women or immunocompromised patients, and may not be indicative of recent or active infection. The detection of CMV-specific IgM in maternal serum is not indicative of virus transmission to the fetus, since fewer than 10% of pregnant women who are positive for CMV IgM actually give birth to a congenitally infected infant. Like newborns, immunocompromised individuals also may have a delay in IgM production or may be unable to mount a significant IgM antibody response. Lastly, patients with Epstein-Barr virus-induced infectious mononucleosis or chicken pox due to varicella-zoster virus may produce heterotypic IgM responses, resulting in false-positive CMV IgM test results.

IgG Avidity Assay

Given the described limitations of CMV IgM testing, measurements of CMV-specific IgG avidity have proven useful for distinguishing primary from nonprimary infections, particularly in women suspected of having CMV during pregnancy (37, 38, 125). CMV-specific IgG of low avidity is produced during the first weeks to months following primary infection, while IgG antibody of increasingly higher avidity is produced with past or nonprimary infections.

Commercial CMV-specific IgG avidity assays are available (Table 4), and the tests are performed primarily by making simple modifications to conventional EIA protocols (125). In the assays, separate aliquots of a serum sample are reacted in parallel with CMV-specific antigens bound to a solid phase, and either urea (preferred), potassium thiocyanate, or guanidine chloride is used as a denaturant on one of the sample aliquots to preferentially dissociate and differentiate the weaker binding strength of low-avidity antibody-antigen reactions from the more strongly bound high-avidity antibody-antigen reactions. The avidity of CMV-specific IgG in the sample is determined based on the differences in optical density values measured between the two sample aliquots tested and is expressed as an avidity index. Most of the available IgG avidity kits are formatted as EIAs, whereas one has been designed as an immunoblot assay (Mikrogen Diagnostik, Neuried, Germany). Some of the reagent kits can be purchased in the United States, but none are FDA approved for clinical use, and none of the IgG avidity assays on automated platforms are available in the United States.

Various studies (37, 125–127) have provided convincing evidence that in a pregnant woman suspected of having a CMV infection, finding low-avidity CMV-specific IgG antibody in combination with a positive CMV IgM result is reliable evidence for primary infection and an increased risk of *in utero* transmission to the fetus, whereas detection of high-avidity CMV IgG in the presence of a positive CMV IgM result most likely indicates reactivation or a past infection (Table 5). The maturation of IgG avidity has been shown to progress gradually from low avidity for the first 3 to 4 months following infection to high avidity by 5 to 6 months after infection, with a transition period of 1 to 2 months between, in which intermediate avidity index values may be observed. Therefore, finding high-avidity CMV IgG in a pregnant woman during the first trimester would strongly indicate infection prior to conception and a low risk of giving birth to a CMV-infected infant, whereas detection of low-avidity CMV IgG at any time during pregnancy would indicate infection after conception and the possible need for invasive procedures to determine if the fetus is infected. Although an intermediate CMV IgG avidity is concerning for result interpretation, intermediate results have been shown to be more comparable to high-avidity results and most suggestive of reactivation or past infection. With respect to the kinetics of maturation of CMV-specific IgG avidity, it has been shown that pregnant women with positive CMV IgM results and low IgG avidity indexes who display a rapid increase in IgG avidity over time have a higher risk of transmitting the virus to the unborn fetus (128).

TABLE 5 Interpretation of CMV-specific IgM, IgG, and IgG avidity assays in women suspected of having CMV infection during pregnancy

IgM	IgG	IgG avidity	Interpretation
Negative	Negative	Not applicable	No infection; at risk for primary CMV infection
Positive	Negative	Not applicable	Very recent CMV infection; increased risk of vertical transmission to fetus; also document seroconversion from negative to positive CMV IgG antibody
Positive	Positive	Low	Possible acute infection; IgM positive results in combination with low IgG avidity results are considered reliable evidence for primary CMV infection in a pregnant woman and an increased risk of vertical transmission to the fetus; additional procedures can be performed to detect CMV infection in the fetus
Positive	Positive	High or Intermediate	Reactivation of previously acquired latent infection or past infection; low risk of vertical transmission to the fetus
Negative	Positive	Not applicable	Normally indicates past infection; IgG avidity testing may be warranted if heightened clinical suspicion of CMV infection

Routinely, CMV-specific IgG avidity testing is performed reflexively only on CMV IgG-positive samples that are also positive for CMV IgM antibody. However, it has been shown that this algorithm may miss roughly 1 to 3% of primary CMV infections in which CMV IgG-positive specimens are negative for CMV IgM antibody (125).

Measurement of CMV-Specific Cell-Mediated Immunity

CMV-specific $CD4^+$ and $CD8^+$ T-cell responses are critical to the control of CMV replication and the onset of symptomatic infections. Over the years, a number of methods have been developed to assess the CMV-specific cell-mediated immune response (46–48, 129–131). These include enzyme-linked immunosorbent assay (ELISA) (132–136) and ELISPOT assays (137–141), multicolored flow cytometry (142–146), and the use of major histocompatibility (MHC) class I and II tetramers (147–149). The assays are procedurally different, but the basic principle is essentially the same. ELISA and ELISPOT assays measure the release of gamma interferon following stimulation of whole blood or PBMCs with CMV-specific antigens or peptides. Multicolored flow cytometry is used to stain for the intracellular accumulation of gamma interferon and other cytokines (e.g., tumor necrosis factor alpha, interleukin 2, and interleukin 6) in response to CMV-specific antigen stimulation. Lastly, CMV-specific antigen-associated MHC class I and II tetramers are used to bind to T-cell receptors on the surface of $CD8^+$ and $CD4^+$ T cells, respectively, to quantify the T cells that are specific for given CMV antigens and their matched MHC alleles (147–149). Assays like the QuantiFERON-CMV (Qiagen, Hilden, Germany), T-SPOT.CMV ELISPOT (Oxford Immunotec Ltd., Milton, United Kingdom), and T-Track CMV ELISPOT (Lophius Biosciences, Regensburg, Germany) have been commercialized and formulated into complete kits and have received CE marking in Europe (Table 6). Also, individual CMV-specific proteins and peptides (primarily pp65 and IE-1 antigens) and individual reagents and ready-to-use reagent kits are available from a number of manufacturers for the development of user-defined gamma interferon release assays and flow-cytometric T-cell enumeration tests. The ImmuKnow assay (Eurofins Viracor-IBT Laboratories, Lee's Summit, MO), which measures the intracellular concentration of ATP from stimulated $CD4^+$ T cells, is the only FDA-approved test and detects overall immune function rather than specific cell-mediated immune responses against CMV; testing is available only through Eurofins Viracor-IBT Laboratories (Table 6).

A number of studies have demonstrated the clinical application of these assays to assess immune reconstitution and identify transplant recipients at increased risk for CMV viremia and a higher incidence of disease following transplantation, to guide decision-making regarding prophylaxis and preemptive therapies, and for risk stratification

TABLE 6 Selected immunologic assays available for CMV-specific immune monitoring[a]

Assay (manufacturer)	Principle	Specimen	Test time (h)	Important features	References
QuantiFERON-CMV (Qiagen)	Uses a cocktail of 22 CMV-specific peptides to stimulate T cells in whole blood; then measures release of IFN-γ into plasma by ELISA	3 ml whole blood; 1 ml/tube	19–27	Performed on small volume of blood; uses specialized blood collection tubes; measures only $CD8^+$ T-cell responses; restricted to certain HLA class I types; high rate of indeterminate (uninterpretable) results; commercial kit; CE marked only	132–136, 138, 139
T-SPOT.CMV (Oxford Immunotec Ltd)	Uses CMV-specific IE-1 and pp65 proteins to stimulate isolated PBMCs; then measures release of antibody-captured and membrane-bound IFN-γ by ELISPOT	2–12 ml whole blood depending on age	21–25	Measurement performed at single-cell level; measures responses of $CD4^+$ and $CD8^+$ T cells, NK cells, and NKT cells; independent of HLA types; commercial kit; CE marked only	
T-TRACK CMV (Lophius Biosciences)	Uses CMV-specific IE-1 and pp65 proteins to stimulate isolated PBMCs; then measures release of antibody-captured and membrane-bound IFN-γ by ELISPOT	7.5 ml whole blood	20–24	Measurement performed at single-cell level; measures responses of $CD4^+$ and $CD8^+$ T cells, NK cells, and NKT cells; independent of HLA types; commercial kit; CE marked only	191–193
FastImmune Intracellular Cytokine Detection (BD Biosciences)	Uses a CMV-specific pp65 peptide mixture to stimulate T cells in whole blood or isolated PBMCs; then measures intracellular accumulation of IFN-γ and other cytokines using flow cytometry	1–7 ml whole blood	8–24	Stimulated cells are stained with monoclonal antibodies directed against IFN-γ and other cytokines (e.g., IL-2, IL-6, TNF-α); measures responses of $CD4^+$ and $CD8^+$ T cells; independent of HLA types; commercial antibodies available	194, 195
iTAg MHC Tetramers (Beckman Coulter)	Uses CMV-specific peptide-conjugated MHC class I and II tetramers to enumerate T cells in whole blood (preferred) or PBMCs; then analysis by flow cytometry	0.5–1 ml of whole blood	1–2	Performed on small volume of blood; procedure is fast and relatively simple; measures responses of CD4+ and/or CD8+ T cells; reagents are commercially available	147–149
ImmuKnow (Eurofins Viracor-IBT Laboratories)	Uses phytohemagglutinin to stimulate T cells; then captures CD4+ cells and measures concentration of synthesized ATP released from lysed cells	2–3 ml whole blood	24	Broadly measures degree of immune function; not specific for CMV; testing available through Viracor Eurofins Clinical Diagnostics; commercial kit; FDA approved only	196–198

[a]Abbreviations: IFN-γ, gamma interferon; IE-1, immediate early protein-1; HLA, human leukocyte antigen; NK, natural killer cells; NKT, natural killer T cells; IL, interleukin; TNF, tumor necrosis factor.

of patients before transplantation (46–48, 129). Therefore, in combination with quantitative monitoring of viral load in blood, the use of tests for immune monitoring has been recommended in the most recent updated international CMV consensus guidelines on the management of CMV in transplant patients (10). A low or declining viral load in the presence of a robust or increasing CMV-specific cell-mediated immune response in a transplant recipient may indicate a low risk for disease and a possible opportunity to stop antiviral therapy and adjust immunosuppressive treatment. This would be in contrast to detecting high or increasing viral loads with low or declining CMV-specific cellular immune function, which may indicate a high risk for CMV complications and the need to start or continue antiviral therapy, begin cellular adoptive immunotherapy, or adjust the immunosuppressive drugs. Recently, CMV-specific cell-mediated immune responses also have been assessed in pregnant women, and studies have revealed that the maternal CMV-specific cell-mediated immune response is a predictor of CMV transmission to the fetus (138, 139).

ANTIVIRAL SUSCEPTIBILITY TESTING

The resistance of CMV to antiviral drugs used to treat and prevent CMV infection and disease has emerged as a growing problem in immunocompromised hosts (150–152). Prolonged and repeated use of these drugs in transplant recipients and patients with AIDS has been associated with the development of antiviral resistance and progressive or recurrent CMV disease. CMV resistance is the result of specific genetic mutations in the catalytic domain of the UL97 phosphotransferase gene, leading to a deficiency in drug phosphorylation, and alterations in the UL54 viral DNA polymerase gene (15, 150, 151). Mutations in the UL97 gene confer resistance to ganciclovir and valganciclovir, whereas mutations in the UL54 gene confer resistance to ganciclovir, valganciclovir, cidofovir, and foscarnet. Resistance to the newer antiviral agents also has been described and is mediated by alterations in the UL56 gene for letermovir, the UL54 gene for brincidofovir and the UL97 gene for maribavir (15). CMV isolates resistant to ganciclovir remain susceptible to maribavir and vice versa, since the resistance mutation for maribavir is in a different location on the UL97 gene.

The described emergence of antiviral drug resistance has led to a definite need for *in vitro* antiviral susceptibility testing. Laboratory confirmation of drug resistance in the setting of rising, rebounding, or persistently high viral loads during prolonged therapy (median of 5 months) is essential for defining the mechanisms of antiviral resistance, for determining the frequency with which drug-resistant CMV mutants emerge in clinical practice, for predicting treatment failure and identifying cross-resistance to other antiviral agents, for instituting the most appropriate alternative therapy, and for the evaluation of new antiviral agents. Testing for suspected drug resistance generally should be considered when there is new or worsening CMV disease following a minimum of 6 or more weeks of cumulative antiviral drug exposure, including more than 2 weeks of ongoing therapy that has been appropriately dosed and delivered (10, 15). A number of phenotypic and genotypic assays have been described for testing the susceptibility of CMV to antiviral agents (150, 153).

Phenotypic assays, and more specifically plaque reduction assays, have been considered the reference methods for many years. These assays measure the ability of CMV to grow in cell culture in the presence of various concentrations of antiviral drug. They offer the distinct advantage of being a direct measure of CMV susceptibility to any antiviral drug and can provide data on the concentration of drug needed to inhibit viral replication. The effective dose is normally defined as the dose resulting in a 50% reduction in plaque formation. Phenotypic assays generally require isolation and passage of the virus to high titer in cell culture before testing begins, which can be quite difficult to do for wild-type CMV isolates, and are rarely used in clinical practice today, as they are cumbersome, labor-intensive, and expensive and have turnaround times that are far too long to permit the results to be clinically relevant, owing to the very slow growth of CMV in culture. Also, the assays are subjective and not well standardized, which may result in significant variability within and between different laboratories.

Genotypic assays are currently the method of choice for measuring susceptibility of CMV to antiviral drugs and offer speed, objectivity, sensitivity, and efficiency in direct screening and analysis of clinical specimens, including whole blood, plasma, other body fluids, and tissue, or of CMV isolates, and they allow earlier detection of the emergence of drug resistance than phenotypic assays. They are designed to identify mutations that are known to confer resistance, and current genotypic testing typically includes identification of mutations in the CMV UL97 phosphotransferase gene and the UL54 DNA polymerase gene that confer resistance to ganciclovir, valganciclovir, foscarnet, and/or cidofovir. These assays normally involve using PCR for amplification of specific viral genes and sequencing of the amplified products to identify polymorphisms; some assays use specific probes to detect selected mutations or use restriction endonuclease digestion of amplified products to identify alterations in the viral genome known to be associated with viral resistance to a given viral agent. Information on the phenotypes associated with specific resistance gene mutations has been published and can be beneficial to support the use of specific treatment options where drug resistance is suspected or proven (150). This is particularly true in the management of refractory or resistant CMV infections with defined UL97 or UL54 mutations (15).

Newer genotypic assays have been developed and involve automated sequencing methods performed directly from specimens without the need for PCR amplification (154, 155); they usually require a minimum quantity of 1,000 copies/ml of CMV DNA for the most reliable results, and mutant strains that comprise $<$20 to 30% of the viral population may not be detected. Next-generation sequencing and deep sequencing methods are now being used to overcome these limitations and offer more sensitive detection of minor variants and emerging mutant subpopulations (156, 157). For fast interpretation of sequence data from CMV genotypic resistance testing, a Web-based search tool called Mutation Resistance Analyzer has been developed; this tool links the sequence to a database containing all published mutations in the UL97 and UL54 genes and the corresponding antiviral drug susceptibility phenotypes (158). The major disadvantage of current genotypic assays is that they detect only known drug-resistant mutations, and the results may be confounded by the presence of mutations that have no bearing on drug resistance. In this regard, phenotypic assays are still required to identify drug-resistant viruses with novel mutations for antiviral resistance but now involve genetic transfer of the mutation sequences to a laboratory-adapted reference CMV strain or artificial cloning system for rapid recombinant phenotyping (153).

The overall complexities of phenotypic and genotypic assays make both methods less than routine for most clinical laboratories, and these assays are primarily available in specialized reference laboratories. Also, the continued development of novel antiviral agents with efficacy against CMV and the emergence of resistance to these drugs when used clinically will make it necessary to continuously update antiviral susceptibility assays.

EVALUATION, INTERPRETATION, AND REPORTING OF RESULTS

There are a number of points to consider when choosing which tests to perform for the detection of CMV. Conventional tube cultures are highly specific and can detect unexpected viruses but are generally too slow and insensitive to have an impact on clinical decision-making when CMV is being considered as the primary pathogen. Shell vial cultures decrease the time required for detecting CMV in culture, but the sensitivity varies by specimen type and from laboratory to laboratory. Cultures also are often positive in the absence of true CMV disease; this is particularly true when urine or respiratory specimens are screened for CMV, in which shedding of CMV is common during asymptomatic infection and is usually not suggestive of more-severe illness. Isolation of CMV in culture may be useful for postpartum and *in utero* diagnosis of congenital CMV infection and tissue invasive disease, and CMV isolates may be needed for certain phenotypic antiviral susceptibility assays.

In the immunocompromised host, the use of direct detection methods to diagnose CMV disease is most beneficial for patient care. However, virologic or serologic detection of CMV indicates infection but does not establish whether the infection is responsible for symptomatic illness. CMV is ubiquitous, and asymptomatic excretion is high in patients who never progress to disease. Reactivation of latent virus is also common, and other pathogens may be simultaneously present in patients with overt disease. To implicate CMV as the cause of an illness, laboratory confirmation of active disease in an appropriate clinical setting is required. In this regard, most clinical virology laboratories have largely replaced their conventional tube and shell vial culture systems with CMV pp65 antigen assays or, to a much greater extent, with molecular methods for accurate CMV detection and/or quantification from blood. Quantitative measures of CMV antigenemia or CMV DNA-emia can provide a rapid diagnosis of established disease, identify patients at risk of developing new or relapsing disease, and assess the progression of disease and the resolution of symptoms. They are also useful for directing the initiation of preemptive therapy, monitoring the response to antiviral drugs during prophylaxis and preemptive therapy, and predicting treatment failure and the emergence of drug-resistant virus.

Evaluating trends in viral loads and measuring the rate of elevation in the viral load over time are currently more useful than interpreting a single test result in relation to a defined cutoff value, since the initial viral load, the rate at which it rises, and its persistence with time may predict the risk of CMV disease and possible relapse and aid in establishing treatment failure. Serial monitoring of high-risk patients also may be beneficial with respect to aiding in the decreased use of and exposure to antivirals, leading to a more cost-effective and focused use of such agents. However, significant variations in approaches to measuring viral loads and using the results among transplant centers that monitor and manage CMV infections have been reported (159), and practices need further optimization among institutions. The availability of licensed commercial quantitative molecular CMV tests calibrated to the WHO international CMV standard has improved the agreement of viral load values and has allowed comparisons across laboratories using these assays.

Interpretation should be done with caution, as not all changes in quantitative CMV DNA levels may reflect a substantial biological or clinical difference, especially if the changes are small and fall within the expected range of variability for the assay used. Threefold changes ($>0.5 \log_{10}$) usually cannot be explained by inherent biological or assay variability and likely reflect a biologically and clinically relevant change in the level of CMV DNA-emia. However, molecular quantitative CMV DNA assays can have greater variability at the lower limit of sensitivity, and 5-fold ($>0.7 \log_{10}$) differences between measurements nearer the lower limit may be more reflective of a substantial biological or clinical change. Also, an isolated positive result for CMV DNA-emia may not be indicative of disease and the need for immediate antiviral treatment, particularly in asymptomatic patients. Lastly, negative viral load results do not always exclude CMV disease in symptomatic patients; end-organ involvement, particularly in the gastrointestinal tract and lungs, may occur in the absence of detectable levels of CMV DNA-emia. Histopathologic examination and/or PCR can be useful in immunocompromised hosts for the diagnosis of specific organ invasive diseases. However, detection of CMV in tissue specimens must be interpreted with caution, particularly when infections with more than one organism are documented, as the relative importance of each pathogen in producing clinical illness may be difficult to determine. The degree of histological involvement may help in determining the role and severity of CMV in causing disease. There is a particular need to differentiate CMV infection from graft rejection in transplant patients, since the administration of potent immunosuppressive antirejection drugs during active CMV infection can result in life-threatening disease.

The isolation of CMV from urine, respiratory secretions, or other body fluids within the first 3 weeks of life is the traditional means of confirming the diagnosis of congenital infection in newborns. Urine is the preferred specimen because it contains greater amounts of virus, and the virus therefore grows quickly in culture. PCR has also been used effectively to find CMV DNA in urine and saliva of congenitally infected infants (42, 160), and CMV has been detected in blood of infants with congenital infection by the antigenemia assay and PCR. Real-time PCR of saliva obtained at birth is now considered a highly sensitive and specific approach for detection of CMV-associated sensorineural hearing loss in asymptomatic infants who fail a newborn hearing test prior to hospital discharge (160). Similar to urine specimens, high titers of CMV are shed in saliva of infected newborns, and saliva is an easier sample to collect for newborn screening by PCR. Attempts to isolate or detect virus from maternal blood leukocytes and from amniotic fluid and fetal blood and tissue by molecular and/or antigen-based tests may provide useful information for prenatal diagnosis of congenital CMV infection (5, 37, 38, 161). While such prenatal testing is a sensitive indicator of maternal or fetal CMV infection, positive results do not predict which infants will have disease. In this regard, quantitative measures of viral load in congenital CMV infection may prove beneficial for predicting symptomatic outcome and for guiding patient management. It has been demonstrated that elevated levels of CMV DNA in blood during early infancy are associated with hearing loss in newborns with symptomatic and asymptomatic congenital CMV infection (162, 163). Also, quantitative real-time PCR has been used to quantify CMV DNA from amniotic fluid samples to predict fetal and neonatal outcomes (164) and to test umbilical cord blood to screen for neonatal CMV infection at delivery (165). Infants not previously tested but found to be excreting virus after 3 weeks of age may have either congenital or acquired infection. Standard serologic and virologic tests do not differentiate between these possibilities.

In general, serologic tests for CMV-specific IgG antibody have limited value for the diagnosis of acute infection, since the results are obtained retrospectively and are not predictive of disease. Also, the transplacental passage of maternal IgG antibody begins at 18 weeks of gestation and confounds the diagnosis of CMV infection in the neonate, and immunocompromised hosts may not mount a normal immune response or may have been given blood transfusions or intravenous immunoglobulins that contain detectable CMV IgG antibodies. Nonetheless, a history of seroconversion from a negative to a positive IgG antibody response to CMV is diagnostic of primary infection and may be beneficial in evaluating a pregnant woman with symptoms of viral disease. For pregnant women with preexisting CMV-specific IgG and/or IgM antibody, however, IgG avidity testing may be more helpful in distinguishing primary from nonprimary infections and for predicting CMV transmission to the fetus. Whenever possible, serologic diagnoses of CMV infection should be confirmed by other virologic methods. CMV-specific IgG serologic assays play a more important role as a screening tool in the determination of an individual's immune status to CMV. Detection of CMV-specific IgG in a single serum specimen indicates exposure to CMV at some time in the past. Negative serum antibody titers may exclude CMV infection. In the evaluation of an organ donor and recipient, a seronegative recipient who receives an organ or blood products from a seropositive donor is at increased risk for developing primary CMV infection and serious disease. Knowing the serostatus of the donor and recipient is therefore important in determining the treatment or prophylaxis to be used and in considering the type of donor to be selected and blood products to be given.

Immune-based tests that monitor CMV-specific T-cell responses and measure immune reconstitution in immunocompromised hosts may have value in identifying those at highest risk for CMV viremia and disease, in instituting preemptive, prophylactic, and/or adoptive immune-based therapies, and in altering treatment and management decisions. With the commercial development and continued standardization of immune monitoring assays, clinical laboratories should be poised to broadly adopt this technology.

The application of virologic methods, including conventional and shell vial culture, rapid direct-detection assays, and immunologic testing, should be combined with clinical assessment of the patient to provide an accurate, reliable diagnosis of CMV infection and disease and to allow subsequent prompt, appropriate patient management and timely intervention with specific antiviral therapy. It is imperative that health care providers and laboratorians alike know which tests for CMV are most appropriate for different patient populations and to have a complete understanding of the advantages and limitations of each test and the meaning of the test results.

REFERENCES

1. **Hage E, Wilkie GS, Linnenweber-Held S, Dhingra A, Suárez NM, Schmidt JJ, Kay-Fedorov PC, Mischak-Weissinger E, Heim A, Schwarz A, Schulz TF, Davison AJ, Ganzenmueller T.** 2017. Characterization of human cytomegalovirus genome diversity in immunocompromised hosts by whole-genome sequencing directly from clinical specimens. *J Infect Dis* **215:**1673–1683.
2. **Renzette N, Gibson L, Jensen JD, Kowalik TF.** 2014. Human cytomegalovirus intrahost evolution—a new avenue for understanding and controlling herpesvirus infections. *Curr Opin Virol* **8:**109–115.
3. **Renzette N, Pokalyuk C, Gibson L, Bhattacharjee B, Schleiss MR, Hamprecht K, Yamamoto AY, Mussi-Pinhata MM, Britt WJ, Jensen JD, Kowalik TF.** 2015. Limits and patterns of cytomegalovirus genomic diversity in humans. *Proc Natl Acad Sci USA* **112:**E4120–E4128.
4. **Boeckh M, Geballe AP.** 2011. Cytomegalovirus: pathogen, paradigm, and puzzle. *J Clin Invest* **121:**1673–1680.
5. **Manicklal S, Emery VC, Lazzarotto T, Boppana SB, Gupta RK.** 2013. The "silent" global burden of congenital cytomegalovirus. *Clin Microbiol Rev* **26:**86–102.
6. **Osawa R, Singh N.** 2009. Cytomegalovirus infection in critically ill patients: a systematic review. *Crit Care* **13:**R68
7. **Rafailidis PI, Mourtzoukou EG, Varbobitis IC, Falagas ME.** 2008. Severe cytomegalovirus infection in apparently immunocompetent patients: a systematic review. *Virol J* **5:**47.
8. **Limaye AP, Boeckh M.** 2010. CMV in critically ill patients: pathogen or bystander? *Rev Med Virol* **20:**372–379
9. **Razonable RR.** 2013. Management strategies for cytomegalovirus infection and disease in solid organ transplant recipients. *Infect Dis Clin North Am* **27:**317–342.
10. **Kotton CN, Kumar D, Caliendo AM, Asberg A, Chou S, Danziger-Isakov L, Humar A, Transplantation Society International CMV Consensus Group.** 2013. Updated international consensus guidelines on the management of cytomegalovirus in solid-organ transplantation. *Transplantation* **96:**333–360.
11. **Husain S, Pietrangeli CE, Zeevi A.** 2009. Delayed onset CMV disease in solid organ transplant recipients. *Transpl Immunol* **21:**1–9.
12. **Steininger C, Puchhammer-Stöckl E, Popow-Kraupp T.** 2006. Cytomegalovirus disease in the era of highly active antiretroviral therapy (HAART). *J Clin Virol* **37:**1–9.
13. **Ahmed A.** 2011. Antiviral treatment of cytomegalovirus infection. *Infect Disord Drug Targets* **11:**475–503.
14. **Boeckh M, Murphy WJ, Peggs KS.** 2015. Recent advances in cytomegalovirus: an update on pharmacologic and cellular therapies. *Biol Blood Marrow Transplant* **21:**24–29.
15. **El Chaer F, Shah DP, Chemaly RF.** 2016. How I treat resistant cytomegalovirus infection in hematopoietic cell transplantation recipients. *Blood* **128:**2624–2636.
16. **Marty FM, Ljungman P, Chemaly RF, Maertens J, Dadwal SS, Duarte RF, Haider S, Ullmann AJ, Katayama Y, Brown J, Mullane KM, Boeckh M, Blumberg EA, Einsele H, Snydman DR, Kanda Y, DiNubile MJ, Teal VL, Wan H, Murata Y, Kartsonis NA, Leavitt RY, Badshah C.** 2017. Letermovir prophylaxis for cytomegalovirus in hematopoietic-cell transplantation. *N Engl J Med* **377:**2433–2444.
17. **Chemaly RF, Ullmann AJ, Stoelben S, Richard MP, Bornhäuser M, Groth C, Einsele H, Silverman M, Mullane KM, Brown J, Nowak H, Kölling K, Stobernack HP, Lischka P, Zimmermann H, Rübsamen-Schaeff H, Champlin RE, Ehninger G, AIC246 Study Team.** 2014. Letermovir for cytomegalovirus prophylaxis in hematopoietic-cell transplantation. *N Engl J Med* **370:**1781–1789.
18. **Roddie C, Peggs KS.** 2017. Immunotherapy for transplantation-associated viral infections. *J Clin Invest* **127:**2513–2522.
19. **Blyth E, Withers B, Clancy L, Gottlieb D.** 2016. CMV-specific immune reconstitution following allogeneic stem cell transplantation. *Virulence* **7:**967–980.
20. **Roemhild A, Reinke P.** 2016. Virus-specific T-cell therapy in solid organ transplantation. *Transpl Int* **29:**515–526.
21. **Pei XY, Zhao XY, Chang YJ, Liu J, Xu LP, Wang Y, Zhang XH, Han W, Chen YH, Huang XJ.** 2017. Cytomegalovirus-specific T-cell transfer for refractory cytomegalovirus infection after haploidentical stem cell transplantation: the quantitative and qualitative immune recovery for cytomegalovirus. *J Infect Dis* **216:**945–956.
22. **Boeckh M, Corey L.** 2017. Adoptive immunotherapy of viral infections: should infectious disease embrace cellular immunotherapy? *J Infect Dis* **216:**926–928.
23. **O'Reilly RJ, Prockop S, Hasan AN, Koehne G, Doubrovina E.** 2016. Virus-specific T-cell banks for 'off the shelf' adoptive therapy of refractory infections. *Bone Marrow Transplant* **51:** 1163–1172.
24. **Schleiss MR, Permar SR, Plotkin SA.** 2017. Progress toward development of a vaccine against congenital cytomegalovirus infection. *Clin Vaccine Immunol* **24:**e00268-17.
25. **Anderholm KM, Bierle CJ, Schleiss MR.** 2016. Cytomegalovirus vaccines: current status and future prospects. *Drugs* **76:**1625–1645.
26. **Griffiths P, Plotkin S, Mocarski E, Pass R, Schleiss M, Krause P, Bialek S.** 2013. Desirability and feasibility of a vaccine against cytomegalovirus. *Vaccine* **31**(Suppl 2)**:** 197–203.
27. **Kraft CS, Armstrong WS, Caliendo AM.** 2012. Interpreting quantitative cytomegalovirus DNA testing: understanding the laboratory perspective. *Clin Infect Dis* **54:**1793–1797.
28. **Razonable RR, Brown RA, Wilson J, Groettum C, Kremers W, Espy M, Smith TF, Paya CV.** 2002. The clinical use of various blood compartments for cytomegalovirus (CMV) DNA quantitation in transplant recipients with CMV disease. *Transplantation* **73:**968–973.
29. **Garrigue I, Boucher S, Couzi L, Caumont A, Dromer C, Neau-Cransac M, Tabrizi R, Schrive M-H, Fleury H, Lafon M-E.** 2006. Whole blood real-time quantitative PCR for cytomegalovirus infection follow-up in transplant recipients. *J Clin Virol* **36:**72–75.
30. **Koidl C, Bozic M, Marth E, Kessler HH.** 2008. Detection of CMV DNA: is EDTA whole blood superior to EDTA plasma? *J Virol Methods* **154:**210–212.

31. **Lisboa LF, Asberg A, Kumar D, Pang X, Hartmann A, Preiksaitis JK, Pescovitz MD, Rollag H, Jardine AG, Humar A.** 2011. The clinical utility of whole blood versus plasma cytomegalovirus viral load assays for monitoring therapeutic response. *Transplantation* **91:**231–236.
32. **Sanchez JL, Storch GA.** 2002. Multiplex, quantitative, real-time PCR assay for cytomegalovirus and human DNA. *J Clin Microbiol* **40:**2381–2386.
33. **Landry ML, Ferguson D, Cohen S, Huber K, Wetherill P.** 1995. Effect of delayed specimen processing on cytomegalovirus antigenemia test results. *J Clin Microbiol* **33:**257–259.
34. **Boeckh M, Woogerd PM, Stevens-Ayers T, Ray CG, Bowden RA.** 1994. Factors influencing detection of quantitative cytomegalovirus antigenemia. *J Clin Microbiol* **32:**832–834.
35. **Abdul-Ali D, Kraft CS, Ingersoll J, Frempong M, Caliendo AM.** 2011. Cytomegalovirus DNA stability in EDTA anti-coagulated whole blood and plasma samples. *J Clin Virol* **52:**222–224.
36. **Xie L, Liang X-N, Deng Y, Wang J, He Y, Li T-J, Huang S, Qin X, Li S.** 2014. Effects of storage time on cytomegalovirus DNA stability in plasma determined by quantitative real-time PCR. *J Virol Methods* **207:**196–199.
37. **Saldan A, Forner G, Mengoli C, Gussetti N, Palù G, Abate D.** 2017. Testing for cytomegalovirus in pregnancy. *J Clin Microbiol* **55:**693–702.
38. **Rawlinson WD, Boppana SB, Fowler KB, Kimberlin DW, Lazzarotto T, Alain S, Daly K, Doutré S, Gibson L, Giles ML, Greenlee J, Hamilton ST, Harrison GJ, Hui L, Jones CA, Palasanthiran P, Schleiss MR, Shand AW, van Zuylen WJ.** 2017. Congenital cytomegalovirus infection in pregnancy and the neonate: consensus recommendations for prevention, diagnosis, and therapy. *Lancet Infect Dis* **17:**e177–e188.
39. **Boppana SB, Ross SA, Novak Z, Shimamura M, Tolan RW Jr, Palmer AL, Ahmed A, Michaels MG, Sánchez PJ, Bernstein DI, Britt WJ, Fowler KB, National Institute on Deafness and Other Communication Disorders CMV and Hearing Multicenter Screening (CHIMES) Study.** 2010. Dried blood spot real-time polymerase chain reaction assays to screen newborns for congenital cytomegalovirus infection. *JAMA* **303:**1375–1382.
40. **de Vries JJC, Wessels E, Korver AMH, van der Eijk AA, Rusman LG, Kroes ACM, Vossen ACTM.** 2012. Rapid genotyping of cytomegalovirus in dried blood spots by multiplex real-time PCR assays targeting the envelope glycoprotein gB and gH genes. *J Clin Microbiol* **50:**232–237.
41. **Limaye AP, Santo Hayes TK, Huang ML, Magaret A, Boeckh M, Jerome KR.** 2013. Quantitation of cytomegalovirus DNA load in dried blood spots correlates well with plasma viral load. *J Clin Microbiol* **51:**2360–2364.
42. **Boppana SB, Ross SA, Shimamura M, Palmer AL, Ahmed A, Michaels MG, Sánchez PJ, Bernstein DI, Tolan RW, Jr, Novak Z, Chowdhury N, Britt WJ, Fowler KB, National Institute on Deafness and Other Communication Disorders CHIMES Study.** 2011. Saliva polymerase-chain-reaction assay for cytomegalovirus screening in newborns. *N Engl J Med* **364:**2111–2118.
43. **Beam E, Germer JJ, Lahr B, Yao JDC, Limper AH, Binnicker MJ, Razonable RR.** 2018. Cytomegalovirus (CMV) DNA quantification in bronchoalveolar lavage fluid of immunocompromised patients with CMV pneumonia. *Clin Transplant* **32:**e13149.
44. **Boeckh M, Stevens-Ayers T, Travi G, Huang ML, Cheng GS, Xie H, Leisenring W, Erard V, Seo S, Kimball L, Corey L, Pergam SA, Jerome KR.** 2017. Cytomegalovirus (CMV) DNA quantitation in bronchoalveolar lavage fluid from hematopoietic stem cell transplant recipients with CMV pneumonia. *J Infect Dis* **215:**1514–1522.
45. **Govender K, Jeena P, Parboosing R.** 2017. Clinical utility of bronchoalveolar lavage cytomegalovirus viral loads in the diagnosis of cytomegalovirus pneumonitis in infants. *J Med Virol* **89:**1080–1087.
46. **Egli A, Humar A, Kumar D.** 2012. State-of-the-art monitoring of cytomegalovirus-specific cell-mediated immunity after organ transplant: a primer for the clinician. *Clin Infect Dis* **55:**1678–1689.
47. **Calarota SA, Aberle JH, Puchhammer-Stöckl E, Baldanti F.** 2015. Approaches for monitoring of non virus-specific and virus-specific T-cell response in solid organ transplantation and their clinical applications. *J Clin Virol* **70:**109–119.
48. **Fernández-Ruiz M, Kumar D, Humar A.** 2014. Clinical immune-monitoring strategies for predicting infection risk in solid organ transplantation. *Clin Transl Immunology* **3:**e12.
49. **Razonable RR, Hayden RT.** 2013. Clinical utility of viral load in management of cytomegalovirus infection after solid organ transplantation. *Clin Microbiol Rev* **26:**703–727.
50. **Natori Y, Alghamdi A, Tazari M, Miller V, Husain S, Komatsu T, Griffiths P, Ljungman P, Orchanian-Cheff A, Kumar D, Humar A, CMV Consensus Forum.** 2017. Use of viral load as a surrogate marker in clinical studies of cytomegalovirus in solid organ transplantation: a systematic review and meta-analysis. *Clin Infect Dis* **66:**617–631 10.1093/cid/cix793.
51. **Gerna G, Revello MG, Percivalle E, Zavattoni M, Parea M, Battaglia M.** 1990. Quantification of human cytomegalovirus viremia by using monoclonal antibodies to different viral proteins. *J Clin Microbiol* **28:**2681–2688.
52. **Landry ML, Ferguson D.** 1993. Comparison of quantitative cytomegalovirus antigenemia assay with culture methods and correlation with clinical disease. *J Clin Microbiol* **31:** 2851–2856.
53. **Gerna G, Zipeto D, Parea M, Revello MG, Silini E, Percivalle E, Zavattoni M, Grossi P, Milanesi G.** 1991. Monitoring of human cytomegalovirus infections and ganciclovir treatment in heart transplant recipients by determination of viremia, antigenemia, and DNAemia. *J Infect Dis* **164:** 488–498.
54. **van den Berg AP, Tegzess AM, Scholten-Sampson A, Schirm J, van der Giessen M, The TH, van Son WJ.** 1992. Monitoring antigenemia is useful in guiding treatment of severe cytomegalovirus disease after organ transplantation. *Transpl Int* **5:**101–107.
55. **Baldanti F, Lilleri D, Gerna G.** 2008. Human cytomegalovirus load measurement and its applications for pre-emptive therapy in patients undergoing hematopoietic stem cell transplantation. *Hematol Oncol* **26:**123–130.
56. **Tan BH, Chlebicka NL, Hong Low JG, Chong TYR, Chan KP, Goh YT.** 2008. Use of the cytomegalovirus pp65 antigenemia assay for preemptive therapy in allogeneic hematopoietic stem cell transplantation: a real-world review. *Transpl Infect Dis* **10:**325–332.
57. **Gerna G, Zavattoni M, Baldanti F, Furione M, Chezzi L, Revello MG, Percivalle E.** 1998. Circulating cytomegalic endothelial cells are associated with high human cytomegalovirus (HCMV) load in AIDS patients with late-stage disseminated HCMV disease. *J Med Virol* **55:**64–74.
58. **Salzberger B, Myerson D, Boeckh M.** 1997. Circulating cytomegalovirus (CMV)-infected endothelial cells in marrow transplant patients with CMV disease and CMV infection. *J Infect Dis* **176:**778–781.
59. **Cariani E, Pollara CP, Valloncini B, Perandin F, Bonfanti C, Manca N.** 2007. Relationship between pp65 antigenemia levels and real-time quantitative DNA PCR for Human Cytomegalovirus (HCMV) management in immunocompromised patients. *BMC Infect Dis* **7:**138.
60. **Gerna G, Furione M, Baldanti F, Sarasini A.** 1994. Comparative quantitation of human cytomegalovirus DNA in blood leukocytes and plasma of transplant and AIDS patients. *J Clin Microbiol* **32:**2709–2717.
61. **Mengoli C, Cusinato R, Biasolo MA, Cesaro S, Parolin C, Palù G.** 2004. Assessment of CMV load in solid organ transplant recipients by pp65 antigenemia and real-time quantitative DNA PCR assay: correlation with pp67 RNA detection. *J Med Virol* **74:**78–84.
62. **Sanghavi SK, Abu-Elmagd K, Keightley MC, St George K, Lewandowski K, Boes SS, Bullotta A, Dare R, Lassak M, Husain S, Kwak EJ, Paterson DL, Rinaldo CR.** 2008. Relationship of cytomegalovirus load assessed by real-time PCR to pp65 antigenemia in organ transplant recipients. *J Clin Virol* **42:**335–342.

63. **The TH, van der Ploeg M, van den Berg AP, Vlieger AM, van der Giessen M, van Son WJ.** 1992. Direct detection of cytomegalovirus in peripheral blood leukocytes—a review of the antigenemia assay and polymerase chain reaction. *Transplantation* **54:**193–198.
64. **Ho SKN, Lo C-Y, Cheng IKP, Chan T-M.** 1998. Rapid cytomegalovirus pp65 antigenemia assay by direct erythrocyte lysis and immunofluorescence staining. *J Clin Microbiol* **36:**638–640.
65. **Gerna G, Percivalle E, Torsellini M, Revello MG.** 1998. Standardization of the human cytomegalovirus antigenemia assay by means of in vitro-generated pp65-positive peripheral blood polymorphonuclear leukocytes. *J Clin Microbiol* **36:**3585–3589.
66. **The TH, van den Berg AP, Harmsen MC, van der Bij W, van Son WJ.** 1995. The cytomegalovirus antigenemia assay: a plea for standardization. *Scand J Infect Dis Suppl* **99**(Suppl)**:**25–29.
67. **Verschuuren EA, Harmsen MC, Limburg PC, van Der Bij W, van Den Berg AP, Kas-Deelen AM, Meedendorp B, van Son WJ, The TH.** 1999. Towards standardization of the human cytomegalovirus antigenemia assay. *Intervirology* **42:**382–389.
68. **Demmler GJ, Buffone GJ, Schimbor CM, May RA.** 1988. Detection of cytomegalovirus in urine from newborns by using polymerase chain reaction DNA amplification. *J Infect Dis* **158:**1177–1184.
69. **Hsia K, Spector DH, Lawrie J, Spector SA.** 1989. Enzymatic amplification of human cytomegalovirus sequences by polymerase chain reaction. *J Clin Microbiol* **27:**1802–1809.
70. **Olive DM, Simsek M, Al-Mufti S.** 1989. Polymerase chain reaction assay for detection of human cytomegalovirus. *J Clin Microbiol* **27:**1238–1242.
71. **Shibata D, Martin WJ, Appleman MD, Causey DM, Leedom JM, Arnheim N.** 1988. Detection of cytomegalovirus DNA in peripheral blood of patients infected with human immunodeficiency virus. *J Infect Dis* **158:**1185–1192.
72. **Wolf DG, Spector SA.** 1992. Diagnosis of human cytomegalovirus central nervous system disease in AIDS patients by DNA amplification from cerebrospinal fluid. *J Infect Dis* **166:**1412–1415.
73. **Bitsch A, Kirchner H, Dennin R, Hoyer J, Fricke L, Steinhoff J, Sack K, Bein G.** 1993. The long persistence of CMV DNA in the blood of renal transplant patients after recovery from CMV infection. *Transplantation* **56:**108–112.
74. **Stanier P, Taylor DL, Kitchen AD, Wales N, Tryhorn Y, Tyms AS.** 1989. Persistence of cytomegalovirus in mononuclear cells in peripheral blood from blood donors. *BMJ* **299:**897–898.
75. **Mills AM, Guo FP, Copland AP, Pai RK, Pinsky BA.** 2013. A comparison of CMV detection in gastrointestinal mucosal biopsies using immunohistochemistry and PCR performed on formalin-fixed, paraffin-embedded tissue. *Am J Surg Pathol* **37:**995–1000.
76. **Folkins AK, Chisholm KM, Guo FP, McDowell M, Aziz N, Pinsky BA.** 2013. Diagnosis of congenital CMV using PCR performed on formalin-fixed, paraffin-embedded placental tissue. *Am J Surg Pathol* **37:**1413–1420.
77. **Gault E, Michel Y, Dehée A, Belabani C, Nicolas JC, Garbarg-Chenon A.** 2001. Quantification of human cytomegalovirus DNA by real-time PCR. *J Clin Microbiol* **39:**772–775.
78. **Gourlain K, Salmon D, Gault E, Leport C, Katlama C, Matheron S, Costagliola D, Mazeron MC, Fillet AM, Predivir Study Group, CMV AC11 Study Group.** 2003. Quantitation of cytomegalovirus (CMV) DNA by real-time PCR for occurrence of CMV disease in HIV-infected patients receiving highly active antiretroviral therapy. *J Med Virol* **69:**401–407.
79. **Griscelli F, Barrois M, Chauvin S, Lastere S, Bellet D, Bourhis J-H.** 2001. Quantification of human cytomegalovirus DNA in bone marrow transplant recipients by real-time PCR. *J Clin Microbiol* **39:**4362–4369.
80. **Guiver M, Fox AJ, Mutton K, Mogulkoc N, Egan J.** 2001. Evaluation of CMV viral load using TaqMan CMV quantitative PCR and comparison with CMV antigenemia in heart and lung transplant recipients. *Transplantation* **71:**1609–1615.
81. **Leruez-Ville M, Ouachée M, Delarue R, Sauget A-S, Blanche S, Buzyn A, Rouzioux C.** 2003. Monitoring cytomegalovirus infection in adult and pediatric bone marrow transplant recipients by a real-time PCR assay performed with blood plasma. *J Clin Microbiol* **41:**2040–2046.
82. **Machida U, Kami M, Fukui T, Kazuyama Y, Kinoshita M, Tanaka Y, Kanda Y, Ogawa S, Honda H, Chiba S, Mitani K, Muto Y, Osumi K, Kimura S, Hirai H.** 2000. Real-time automated PCR for early diagnosis and monitoring of cytomegalovirus infection after bone marrow transplantation. *J Clin Microbiol* **38:**2536–2542.
83. **Mengelle C, Pasquier C, Rostaing L, Sandres-Sauné K, Puel J, Berges L, Righi L, Bouquies C, Izopet J.** 2003. Quantitation of human cytomegalovirus in recipients of solid organ transplants by real-time quantitative PCR and pp65 antigenemia. *J Med Virol* **69:**225–231.
84. **Ono Y, Ito Y, Kaneko K, Shibata-Watanabe Y, Tainaka T, Sumida W, Nakamura T, Kamei H, Kiuchi T, Ando H, Kimura H.** 2008. Simultaneous monitoring by real-time polymerase chain reaction of Epstein-Barr virus, human cytomegalovirus, and human herpesvirus-6 in juvenile and adult liver transplant recipients. *Transplant Proc* **40:**3578–3582.
85. **Wada K, Kubota N, Ito Y, Yagasaki H, Kato K, Yoshikawa T, Ono Y, Ando H, Fujimoto Y, Kiuchi T, Kojima S, Nishiyama Y, Kimura H.** 2007. Simultaneous quantification of Epstein-Barr virus, cytomegalovirus, and human herpesvirus 6 DNA in samples from transplant recipients by multiplex real-time PCR assay. *J Clin Microbiol* **45:**1426–1432.
86. **Bestetti A, Pierotti C, Terreni M, Zappa A, Vago L, Lazzarin A, Cinque P.** 2001. Comparison of three nucleic acid amplification assays of cerebrospinal fluid for diagnosis of cytomegalovirus encephalitis. *J Clin Microbiol* **39:**1148–1151.
87. **Blank BS, Meenhorst PL, Mulder JW, Weverling GJ, Putter H, Pauw W, van Dijk WC, Smits P, Lie-A-Ling S, Reiss P, Lange JM.** 2000. Value of different assays for detection of human cytomegalovirus (HCMV) in predicting the development of HCMV disease in human immunodeficiency virus-infected patients. *J Clin Microbiol* **38:**563–569.
88. **Pellegrin I, Garrigue I, Ekouevi D, Couzi L, Merville P, Merel P, Chene G, Schrive MH, Trimoulet P, Lafon ME, Fleury H.** 2000. New molecular assays to predict occurrence of cytomegalovirus disease in renal transplant recipients. *J Infect Dis* **182:**36–42.
89. **Razonable RR, Brown RA, Espy MJ, Rivero A, Kremers W, Wilson J, Groettum C, Smith TF, Paya CV.** 2001. Comparative quantitation of cytomegalovirus (CMV) DNA in solid organ transplant recipients with CMV infection by using two high-throughput automated systems. *J Clin Microbiol* **39:**4472–4476.
90. **Tong CY, Cuevas LE, Williams H, Bakran A.** 2000. Comparison of two commercial methods for measurement of cytomegalovirus load in blood samples after renal transplantation. *J Clin Microbiol* **38:**1209–1213.
91. **Wattanamano P, Clayton JL, Kopicko JJ, Kissinger P, Elliot S, Jarrott C, Rangan S, Beilke MA.** 2000. Comparison of three assays for cytomegalovirus detection in AIDS patients at risk for retinitis. *J Clin Microbiol* **38:**727–732.
92. **Drouet E, Colimon R, Michelson S, Fourcade N, Niveleau A, Ducerf C, Boibieux A, Chevallier M, Denoyel G.** 1995. Monitoring levels of human cytomegalovirus DNA in blood after liver transplantation. *J Clin Microbiol* **33:**389–394.
93. **Gerdes JC, Spees EK, Fitting K, Hiraki J, Sheehan M, Duda D, Jarvi T, Roehl C, Robertson AD.** 1993. Prospective study utilizing a quantitative polymerase chain reaction for detection of cytomegalovirus DNA in the blood of renal transplant patients. *Transplant Proc* **25:**1411–1413.
94. **Zipeto D, Baldanti F, Zella D, Furione M, Cavicchini A, Milanesi G, Gerna G.** 1993. Quantification of human cytomegalovirus DNA in peripheral blood polymorphonuclear leukocytes of immunocompromised patients by the polymerase chain reaction. *J Virol Methods* **44:**45–55.
95. **Rasmussen L, Morris S, Zipeto D, Fessel J, Wolitz R, Dowling A, Merigan TC.** 1995. Quantitation of human cytomegalovirus DNA from peripheral blood cells of human immunodeficiency virus-infected patients could predict cytomegalovirus retinitis. *J Infect Dis* **171:**177–182.

96. **Zipeto D, Morris S, Hong C, Dowling A, Wolitz R, Merigan TC, Rasmussen L.** 1995. Human cytomegalovirus (CMV) DNA in plasma reflects quantity of CMV DNA present in leukocytes. *J Clin Microbiol* **33:**2607–2611.
97. **Revello MG, Gerna G.** 2002. Diagnosis and management of human cytomegalovirus infection in the mother, fetus, and newborn infant. *Clin Microbiol Rev* **15:**680–715.
98. **Shinkai M, Spector SA.** 1995. Quantitation of human cytomegalovirus (HCMV) DNA in cerebrospinal fluid by competitive PCR in AIDS patients with different HCMV central nervous system diseases. *Scand J Infect Dis* **27:**559–561.
99. **Caliendo AM, Shahbazian MD, Schaper C, Ingersoll J, Abdul-Ali D, Boonyaratanakornkit J, Pang X-L, Fox J, Preiksaitis J, Schönbrunner ER.** 2009. A commutable cytomegalovirus calibrator is required to improve the agreement of viral load values between laboratories. *Clin Chem* **55:** 1701–1710.
100. **Pang XL, Fox JD, Fenton JM, Miller GG, Caliendo AM, Preiksaitis JK, American Society of Transplantation Infectious Diseases Community of Practice, Canadian Society of Transplantation.** 2009. Interlaboratory comparison of cytomegalovirus viral load assays. *Am J Transplant* **9:** 258–268.
101. **Wolff DJ, Heaney DL, Neuwald PD, Stellrecht KA, Press RD.** 2009. Multi-site PCR-based CMV viral load assessment-assays demonstrate linearity and precision, but lack numeric standardization: a report of the association for molecular pathology. *J Mol Diagn* **11:**87–92.
102. **Hayden RT, Yan X, Wick MT, Rodriguez AB, Xiong X, Ginocchio CC, Mitchell MJ, Caliendo AM, College of American Pathologists Microbiology Resource Committee.** 2012. Factors contributing to variability of quantitative viral PCR results in proficiency testing samples: a multivariate analysis. *J Clin Microbiol* **50:**337–345.
103. **Fryer JF, Heath AB, Minor PD, Kessler H, Rawlinson W, Boivin G, Preiksaitis J, Pang X-L, Barranger C, Alain S, Bressollette-Bodin C, Hamprecht K, Grewing T, Constantoulakis P, Ghisetti V, Capobianchi MR, Abbate I, Olivo C, Lazzarotto T, Baldanti F, Inoue N, Müller F, Corcoran C, Hardie D, Prieto J, Schuurman R, van Loon A, Ho S, Hillyard D, Hodinka R, Louise Landry M, Caliendo A, Lurain N, Sung L, Gulley M, Atkinson C, Bible J, Guiver M, Collaborative Study Group.** 2016. A collaborative study to establish the 1st WHO International Standard for human cytomegalovirus for nucleic acid amplification technology. *Biologicals* **44:**242–251.
104. **Haynes RJ, Kline MC, Toman B, Scott C, Wallace P, Butler JM, Holden MJ.** 2013. Standard reference material 2366 for measurement of human cytomegalovirus DNA. *J Mol Diagn* **15:**177–185.
105. **Hayden RT, Shahbazian MD, Valsamakis A, Boonyaratanakornkit J, Cook L, Pang XL, Preiksaitis JK, Schönbrunner ER, Caliendo AM.** 2013. Multicenter evaluation of a commercial cytomegalovirus quantitative standard: effects of commutability on interlaboratory concordance. *J Clin Microbiol* **51:**3811–3817.
106. **Rychert J, Danziger-Isakov L, Yen-Lieberman B, Storch G, Buller R, Sweet SC, Mehta AK, Cheeseman JA, Heeger P, Rosenberg ES, Fishman JA.** 2014. Multicenter comparison of laboratory performance in cytomegalovirus and Epstein-Barr virus viral load testing using international standards. *Clin Transplant* **28:**1416–1423.
107. **Abbate I, Piralla A, Calvario A, Callegaro A, Giraldi C, Lunghi G, Gennari W, Sodano G, Ravanini P, Conaldi PG, Vatteroni M, Gaeta A, Paba P, Cavallo R, Baldanti F, Lazzarotto T, AMCLI – Infections in Transplant Working Group GLaIT.** 2016. Nation-wide measure of variability in HCMV, EBV and BKV DNA quantification among centers involved in monitoring transplanted patients. *J Clin Virol* **82:**76–83.
108. **Hirsch HH, Lautenschlager I, Pinsky BA, Cardeñoso L, Aslam S, Cobb B, Vilchez RA, Valsamakis A.** 2013. An international multicenter performance analysis of cytomegalovirus load tests. *Clin Infect Dis* **56:**367–373.
109. **Dioverti MV, Lahr BD, Germer JJ, Yao JD, Gartner ML, Razonable RR.** 2017. Comparison of standardized cytomegalovirus (CMV) viral load thresholds in whole blood and plasma of solid organ and hematopoietic stem cell transplant recipients with CMV infection and disease. *Open Forum Infect Dis* **4:**ofx143.
110. **Griffiths PD, Rothwell E, Raza M, Wilmore S, Doyle T, Harber M, O'Beirne J, Mackinnon S, Jones G, Thorburn D, Mattes F, Nebbia G, Atabani S, Smith C, Stanton A, Emery VC.** 2016. Randomized controlled trials to define viral load thresholds for cytomegalovirus pre-emptive therapy. *PLoS One* **11:**e0163722.
111. **Martín-Gandul C, Pérez-Romero P, Sánchez M, Bernal G, Suárez G, Sobrino M, Merino L, Cisneros JM, Cordero E, Spanish Network for Research in Infectious Diseases.** 2013. Determination, validation and standardization of a CMV DNA cut-off value in plasma for preemptive treatment of CMV infection in solid organ transplant recipients at lower risk for CMV infection. *J Clin Virol* **56:**13–18.
112. **Razonable RR, Åsberg A, Rollag H, Duncan J, Boisvert D, Yao JD, Caliendo AM, Humar A, Do TD.** 2013. Virologic suppression measured by a cytomegalovirus (CMV) DNA test calibrated to the World Health Organization international standard is predictive of CMV disease resolution in transplant recipients. *Clin Infect Dis* **56:**1546–1553.
113. **Hayden RT, Sun Y, Tang L, Procop GW, Hillyard DR, Pinsky BA, Young SA, Caliendo AM.** 2017. Progress in quantitative viral load testing: variability and impact of the WHO quantitative international standards. *J Clin Microbiol* **55:** 423–430.
114. **Preiksaitis JK, Hayden RT, Tong Y, Pang XL, Fryer JF, Heath AB, Cook L, Petrich AK, Yu B, Caliendo AM.** 2016. Are we there yet? Impact of the first international standard for cytomegalovirus DNA on the harmonization of results reported on plasma samples. *Clin Infect Dis* **63:** 583–589.
115. **Hayden RT, Preiksaitis J, Tong Y, Pang X, Sun Y, Tang L, Cook L, Pounds S, Fryer J, Caliendo AM.** 2015. Commutability of the first world health organization international standard for human cytomegalovirus. *J Clin Microbiol* **53:**3325–3333.
116. **Hayden RT, Gu Z, Sam SS, Sun Y, Tang L, Pounds S, Caliendo AM.** 2015. Comparative evaluation of three commercial quantitative cytomegalovirus standards by use of digital and real-time PCR. *J Clin Microbiol* **53:**1500–1505.
117. **Jones S, Webb EM, Barry CP, Choi WS, Abravaya KB, Schneider GJ, Ho SY.** 2016. Commutability of cytomegalovirus WHO international standard in different matrices. *J Clin Microbiol* **54:**1512–1519.
118. **Hayden RT, Gu Z, Sam SS, Sun Y, Tang L, Pounds S, Caliendo AM.** 2016. Comparative performance of reagents and platforms for quantitation of cytomegalovirus DNA by digital PCR. *J Clin Microbiol* **54:**2602–2608.
119. **Hayden RT, Gu Z, Ingersoll J, Abdul-Ali D, Shi L, Pounds S, Caliendo AM.** 2013. Comparison of droplet digital PCR to real-time PCR for quantitative detection of cytomegalovirus. *J Clin Microbiol* **51:**540–546.
120. **Sedlak RH, Cook L, Cheng A, Magaret A, Jerome KR.** 2014. Clinical utility of droplet digital PCR for human cytomegalovirus. *J Clin Microbiol* **52:**2844–2848.
121. **Kuypers J, Jerome KR.** 2017. Applications of digital PCR for clinical microbiology. *J Clin Microbiol* **55:**1621–1628.
122. **Dingle TC, Sedlak RH, Cook L, Jerome KR.** 2013. Tolerance of droplet-digital PCR vs real-time quantitative PCR to inhibitory substances. *Clin Chem* **59:**1670–1672.
123. **Hodinka RL.** 2010. Serological tests in clinical virology, p 133–150. *In* Jerome KR (ed), *Lennette's Laboratory Diagnosis of Viral Infections*, 4th ed. Informa Healthcare USA, Inc., New York, NY.
124. **Novak Z, Ross SA, Patro RK, Pati SK, Reddy MK, Purser M, Britt WJ, Boppana SB.** 2009. Enzyme-linked immunosorbent assay method for detection of cytomegalovirus strain-specific antibody responses. *Clin Vaccine Immunol* **16:**288–290.

125. **Prince HE, Lapé-Nixon M.** 2014. Role of cytomegalovirus (CMV) IgG avidity testing in diagnosing primary CMV infection during pregnancy. *Clin Vaccine Immunol* **21:** 1377–1384.
126. **Grangeot-Keros L, Mayaux MJ, Lebon P, Freymuth F, Eugene G, Stricker R, Dussaix E.** 1997. Value of cytomegalovirus (CMV) IgG avidity index for the diagnosis of primary CMV infection in pregnant women. *J Infect Dis* **175:** 944–946.
127. **Lazzarotto T, Spezzacatena P, Pradelli P, Abate DA, Varani S, Landini MP.** 1997. Avidity of immunoglobulin G directed against human cytomegalovirus during primary and secondary infections in immunocompetent and immunocompromised subjects. *Clin Diagn Lab Immunol* **4:**469–473.
128. **Ebina Y, Minematsu T, Morioka I, Deguchi M, Tairaku S, Tanimura K, Sonoyama A, Nagamata S, Morizane M, Yamada H.** 2015. Rapid increase in the serum cytomegalovirus IgG avidity index in women with a congenitally infected fetus. *J Clin Virol* **66:**44–47.
129. **Han SH.** 2017. Immunological prediction of cytomegalovirus (CMV) replication risk in solid organ transplantation recipients: approaches for regulating the targeted anti-CMV prevention strategies. *Infect Chemother* **49:**161–175.
130. **Costa C, Saldan A, Cavallo R.** 2012. Evaluation of virus-specific cellular immune response in transplant patients. *World J Virol* **1:**150–153.
131. **Lacey SF, Diamond DJ, Zaia JA.** 2004. Assessment of cellular immunity to human cytomegalovirus in recipients of allogeneic stem cell transplants. *Biol Blood Marrow Transplant* **10:**433–447.
132. **Tey SK, Kennedy GA, Cromer D, Davenport MP, Walker S, Jones LI, Crough T, Durrant ST, Morton JA, Butler JP, Misra AK, Hill GR, Khanna R.** 2013. Clinical assessment of anti-viral CD8+ T cell immune monitoring using QuantiFERON-CMV® assay to identify high risk allogeneic hematopoietic stem cell transplant patients with CMV infection complications. *PLoS One* **8:**e74744.
133. **Yong MK, Cameron PU, Slavin M, Morrissey CO, Bergin K, Spencer A, Ritchie D, Cheng AC, Samri A, Carcelain G, Autran B, Lewin SR.** 2017. Identifying cytomegalovirus complications using the Quantiferon-CMV assay after allogeneic hematopoietic stem cell transplantation. *J Infect Dis* **215:**1684–1694.
134. **Sood S, Haifer C, Yu L, Pavlovic J, Gow PJ, Jones RM, Visvanathan K, Angus PW, Testro AG.** 2015. Targeted individual prophylaxis offers superior risk stratification for cytomegalovirus reactivation after liver transplantation. *Liver Transpl* **21:**1478–1485.
135. **Abate D, Saldan A, Mengoli C, Fiscon M, Silvestre C, Fallico L, Peracchi M, Furian L, Cusinato R, Bonfante L, Rossi B, Marchini F, Sgarabotto D, Rigotti P, Palù G.** 2013. Comparison of cytomegalovirus (CMV) enzyme-linked immunosorbent spot and CMV quantiferon gamma interferon-releasing assays in assessing risk of CMV infection in kidney transplant recipients. *J Clin Microbiol* **51:**2501–2507.
136. **Clari MÁ, Muñoz-Cobo B, Solano C, Benet I, Costa E, Remigia MJ, Bravo D, Amat P, Navarro D.** 2012. Performance of the QuantiFERON-cytomegalovirus (CMV) assay for detection and estimation of the magnitude and functionality of the CMV-specific gamma interferon-producing CD8(+) T-cell response in allogeneic stem cell transplant recipients. *Clin Vaccine Immunol* **19:**791–796.
137. **Abate D, Saldan A, Forner G, Tinto D, Bianchin A, Palù G.** 2014. Optimization of interferon gamma ELISPOT assay to detect human cytomegalovirus specific T-cell responses in solid organ transplants. *J Virol Methods* **196:**157–162
138. **Saldan A, Forner G, Mengoli C, Tinto D, Fallico L, Peracchi M, Gussetti N, Palù G, Abate D.** 2016. Comparison of the cytomegalovirus (CMV) enzyme-linked immunosorbent spot and CMV QuantiFERON cell-mediated immune assays in CMV-seropositive and -seronegative pregnant and nonpregnant women. *J Clin Microbiol* **54:**1352–1356.
139. **Forner G, Saldan A, Mengoli C, Gussetti N, Palù G, Abate D.** 2016. Cytomegalovirus (CMV) enzyme-linked immunosorbent spot assay but not CMV QuantiFERON assay is a novel biomarker to determine risk of congenital CMV infection in pregnant women. *J Clin Microbiol* **54:**2149–2154.
140. **Costa C, Balloco C, Sidoti F, Mantovani S, Rittà M, Piceghello A, Fop F, Messina M, Cavallo R.** 2014. Evaluation of CMV-specific cellular immune response by EliSPOT assay in kidney transplant patients. *J Clin Virol* **61:**523–528.
141. **Rittà M, Costa C, Sidoti F, Ballocco C, Ranghino A, Messina M, Biancone L, Cavallo R.** 2015. Pre-transplant assessment of CMV-specific immune response by Elispot assay in kidney transplant recipients. *New Microbiol* **38:** 329–335.
142. **Muñoz-Cobo B, Solano C, Benet I, Costa E, Remigia MJ, de la Cámara R, Nieto J, López J, Amat P, Garcia-Noblejas A, Bravo D, Clari MÁ, Navarro D.** 2012. Functional profile of cytomegalovirus (CMV)-specific CD8+ T cells and kinetics of NKG2C+ NK cells associated with the resolution of CMV DNAemia in allogeneic stem cell transplant recipients. *J Med Virol* **84:**259–267.
143. **Giménez E, Blanco-Lobo P, Muñoz-Cobo B, Solano C, Amat P, Pérez-Romero P, Navarro D.** 2015. Role of cytomegalovirus (CMV)-specific polyfunctional CD8+ T-cells and antibodies neutralizing virus epithelial infection in the control of CMV infection in an allogeneic stem-cell transplantation setting. *J Gen Virol* **96:**2822–2831.
144. **Giménez E, Muñoz-Cobo B, Solano C, Amat P, de la Cámara R, Nieto J, López J, Remigia MJ, Garcia-Noblejas A, Navarro D.** 2015. Functional patterns of cytomegalovirus (CMV) pp65 and immediate early-1-specific CD8(+) T cells that are associated with protection from and control of CMV DNAemia after allogeneic stem cell transplantation. *Transpl Infect Dis* **17:**361–370.
145. **Mena-Romo JD, Pérez Romero P, Martín-Gandul C, Gentil MÁ, Suárez-Artacho G, Lage E, Sánchez M, Cordero E.** 2017. CMV-specific T-cell immunity in solid organ transplant recipients at low risk of CMV infection. Chronology and applicability in preemptive therapy. *J Infect* **75:**336–345.
146. **Ciáurriz M, Beloki L, Zabalza A, Bandrés E, Mansilla C, Pérez-Valderrama E, Lachén M, Rodríguez-Calvillo M, Ramírez N, Olavarría E.** 2017. Functional specific-T-cell expansion after first cytomegalovirus reactivation predicts viremia control in allogeneic hematopoietic stem cell transplant recipients. *Transpl Infect Dis* **19:**e12778.
147. **Borchers S, Luther S, Lips U, Hahn N, Kontsendorn J, Stadler M, Buchholz S, Diedrich H, Eder M, Koehl U, Ganser A, Mischak-Weissinger E.** 2011. Tetramer monitoring to assess risk factors for recurrent cytomegalovirus reactivation and reconstitution of antiviral immunity post allogeneic hematopoietic stem cell transplantation. *Transpl Infect Dis* **13:**222–236.
148. **Gratama JW, Boeckh M, Nakamura R, Cornelissen JJ, Brooimans RA, Zaia JA, Forman SJ, Gaal K, Bray KR, Gasior GH, Boyce CS, Sullivan LA, Southwick PC.** 2010. Immune monitoring with iTAg MHC tetramers for prediction of recurrent or persistent cytomegalovirus infection or disease in allogeneic hematopoietic stem cell transplant recipients: a prospective multicenter study. *Blood* **116:** 1655–1662.
149. **Brooimans RA, Boyce CS, Popma J, Broyles DA, Gratama JW, Southwick PC, Keeney M.** 2008. Analytical performance of a standardized single-platform MHC tetramer assay for the identification and enumeration of CMV-specific CD8+ T lymphocytes. *Cytometry A* **73A:**992–1000.
150. **Lurain NS, Chou S.** 2010. Antiviral drug resistance of human cytomegalovirus. *Clin Microbiol Rev* **23:**689–712
151. **Campos AB, Ribeiro J, Boutolleau D, Sousa H.** 2016. Human cytomegalovirus antiviral drug resistance in hematopoietic stem cell transplantation: current state of the art. *Rev Med Virol* **26:**161–182.
152. **Le Page AK, Jager MM, Iwasenko JM, Scott GM, Alain S, Rawlinson WD.** 2013. Clinical aspects of cytomegalovirus antiviral resistance in solid organ transplant recipients. *Clin Infect Dis* **56:**1018–1029.

153. **Huang DD, Bankowski MJ.** 2015. Susceptibility test methods: viruses, p 1913–1931. *In* Jorgensen JH, Pfaller MA, Carroll KC, Funke G, Landry ML, Richter SS, Warnock DW (ed), *Manual of Clinical Microbiology*, 11th ed. ASM Press, Washington, DC.
154. **Daikoku T, Saito K, Aihara T, Ikeda M, Takahashi Y, Hosoi H, Nishida T, Takemoto M, Shiraki K.** 2013. Rapid detection of human cytomegalovirus UL97 and UL54 mutations for antiviral resistance in clinical specimens. *Microbiol Immunol* **57:**396–399.
155. **Hall Sedlak R, Castor J, Butler-Wu SM, Chan E, Cook L, Limaye AP, Jerome KR.** 2013. Rapid detection of human cytomegalovirus UL97 and UL54 mutations directly from patient samples. *J Clin Microbiol* **51:**2354–2359.
156. **Sahoo MK, Lefterova MI, Yamamoto F, Waggoner JJ, Chou S, Holmes SP, Anderson MW, Pinsky BA.** 2013. Detection of cytomegalovirus drug resistance mutations by next-generation sequencing. *J Clin Microbiol* **51:**3700–3710.
157. **Chou S, Ercolani RJ, Sahoo MK, Lefterova MI, Strasfeld LM, Pinsky BA.** 2014. Improved detection of emerging drug-resistant mutant cytomegalovirus subpopulations by deep sequencing. *Antimicrob Agents Chemother* **58:** 4697–4702.
158. **Chevillotte M, von Einem J, Meier BM, Lin FM, Kestler HA, Mertens T.** 2010. A new tool linking human cytomegalovirus drug resistance mutations to resistance phenotypes. *Antiviral Res* **85:**318–327.
159. **Navarro D, San-Juan R, Manuel O, Giménez E, Fernández-Ruiz M, Hirsch HH, Grossi PA, Aguado JM, ESGICH CMV Survey Study Group, European Study Group of Infections in Compromised Hosts (ESGICH), Society of Clinical Microbiology and Infectious Diseases (ESCMID).** 2017. Cytomegalovirus infection management in solid organ transplant recipients across European centers in the time of molecular diagnostics: an ESGICH survey. *Transpl Infect Dis* **19:**e12773.
160. **de Vries JJC, van der Eijk AA, Wolthers KC, Rusman LG, Pas SD, Molenkamp R, Claas EC, Kroes ACM, Vossen ACTM.** 2012. Real-time PCR versus viral culture on urine as a gold standard in the diagnosis of congenital cytomegalovirus infection. *J Clin Virol* **53:**167–170.
161. **Lazzarotto T, Guerra B, Lanari M, Gabrielli L, Landini MP.** 2008. New advances in the diagnosis of congenital cytomegalovirus infection. *J Clin Virol* **41:**192–197.
162. **Boppana SB, Fowler KB, Pass RF, Rivera LB, Bradford RD, Lakeman FD, Britt WJ.** 2005. Congenital cytomegalovirus infection: association between virus burden in infancy and hearing loss. *J Pediatr* **146:**817–823.
163. **Bradford RD, Cloud G, Lakeman AD, Boppana S, Kimberlin DW, Jacobs R, Demmler G, Sanchez P, Britt W, Soong S-J, Whitley RJ, National Institute of Allergy and Infectious Diseases Collaborative Antiviral Study Group.** 2005. Detection of cytomegalovirus (CMV) DNA by polymerase chain reaction is associated with hearing loss in newborns with symptomatic congenital CMV infection involving the central nervous system. *J Infect Dis* **191:**227–233.
164. **Goegebuer T, Van Meensel B, Beuselinck K, Cossey V, Van Ranst M, Hanssens M, Lagrou K.** 2009. Clinical predictive value of real-time PCR quantification of human cytomegalovirus DNA in amniotic fluid samples. *J Clin Microbiol* **47:**660–665.
165. **Theiler RN, Caliendo AM, Pargman S, Raynor BD, Berga S, McPheeters M, Jamieson DJ.** 2006. Umbilical cord blood screening for cytomegalovirus DNA by quantitative PCR. *J Clin Virol* **37:**313–316.
166. **Landry MLD, Ferguson D, Stevens-Ayers T, de Jonge MWA, Boeckh M.** 1996. Evaluation of CMV Brite kit for detection of cytomegalovirus pp65 antigenemia in peripheral blood leukocytes by immunofluorescence. *J Clin Microbiol* **34:**1337–1339.
167. **St George K, Boyd MJ, Lipson SM, Ferguson D, Cartmell GF, Falk LH, Rinaldo CR, Landry ML.** 2000. A multisite trial comparing two cytomegalovirus (CMV) pp65 antigenemia test kits, biotest CMV brite and Bartels/Argene CMV antigenemia. *J Clin Microbiol* **38:**1430–1433.
168. **Landry ML, Ferguson D.** 2000. 2-Hour cytomegalovirus pp65 antigenemia assay for rapid quantitation of cytomegalovirus in blood samples. *J Clin Microbiol* **38:**427–428.
169. **Visser CE, van Zeijl CJ, de Klerk EP, Schillizi BM, Beersma MF, Kroes AC.** 2000. First experiences with an accelerated CMV antigenemia test: CMV Brite Turbo assay. *J Clin Virol* **17:**65–68.
170. **May G, Kuhn JE, Eing BR.** 2006. Comparison of two commercially available pp65 antigenemia tests and COBAS Amplicor CMV Monitor for early detection and quantification of episodes of human CMV-viremia in transplant recipients. *Intervirology* **49:**261–265.
171. **Percivalle E, Genini E, Chiesa A, Gerna G.** 2008. Comparison of a new Light Diagnostics and the CMV Brite to an in-house developed human cytomegalovirus antigenemia assay. *J Clin Virol* **43:**13–17.
172. **Tsai HP, Tsai YY, Lin IT, Kuo PH, Chen TY, Chang KC, Wang JR.** 2016. Comparison of two commercial automated nucleic acid extraction and integrated quantitation real-time PCR platforms for the detection of cytomegalovirus in plasma. *PLoS One* **11:**e0160493.
173. **Tremblay MA, Rodrigue MA, Deschênes L, Boivin G, Longtin J.** 2015. Cytomegalovirus quantification in plasma with Abbott RealTime CMV and Roche Cobas Amplicor CMV assays. *J Virol Methods* **225:**1–3.
174. **Schnepf N, Scieux C, Resche-Riggon M, Feghoul L, Xhaard A, Gallien S, Molina JM, Socié G, Viglietti D, Simon F, Mazeron MC, Legoff J.** 2013. Fully automated quantification of cytomegalovirus (CMV) in whole blood with the new sensitive Abbott RealTime CMV assay in the era of the CMV international standard. *J Clin Microbiol* **51:**2096–2102.
175. **Clari MÁ, Bravo D, Costa E, Muñoz-Cobo B, Solano C, Remigia MJ, Giménez E, Benmarzouk-Hidalgo OJ, Pérez-Romero P, Navarro D.** 2013. Comparison of the new Abbott Real Time CMV assay and the Abbott CMV PCR kit for the quantitation of plasma cytomegalovirus DNAemia. *Diagn Microbiol Infect Dis* **75:**207–209.
176. **Berth M, Benoy I, Christensen N.** 2016. Evaluation of a standardised real-time PCR based DNA-detection method (Realstar®) in whole blood for the diagnosis of primary human cytomegalovirus (CMV) infections in immunocompetent patients. *Eur J Clin Microbiol Infect Dis* **35:**245–249
177. **Gouarin S, Vabret A, Scieux C, Agbalika F, Cherot J, Mengelle C, Deback C, Petitjean J, Dina J, Freymuth F.** 2007. Multicentric evaluation of a new commercial cytomegalovirus real-time PCR quantitation assay. *J Virol Methods* **146:**147–154.
178. **Michelin BD, Hadzisejdic I, Bozic M, Grahovac M, Hess M, Grahovac B, Marth E, Kessler HH.** 2008. Detection of cytomegalovirus (CMV) DNA in EDTA whole-blood samples: evaluation of the quantitative *artus* CMV LightCycler PCR kit in conjunction with automated sample preparation. *J Clin Microbiol* **46:**1241–1245.
179. **Binnicker MJ, Espy ME.** 2013. Comparison of six real-time PCR assays for qualitative detection of cytomegalovirus in clinical specimens. *J Clin Microbiol* **51:**3749–3752.
180. **Costa C, Sidoti F, Mantovani S, Gregori G, Proietti A, Ghisetti V, Cavallo R.** 2016. Comparison of two molecular assays for detection of cytomegalovirus DNA in whole blood and plasma samples from transplant recipients. *New Microbiol* **39:**186–191.
181. **Allice T, Cerutti F, Pittaluga F, Varetto S, Franchello A, Salizzoni M, Ghisetti V.** 2008. Evaluation of a novel real-time PCR system for cytomegalovirus DNA quantitation on whole blood and correlation with pp65-antigen test in guiding pre-emptive antiviral treatment. *J Virol Methods* **148:**9–16.
182. **Costa C, Mantovani S, Balloco C, Sidoti F, Fop F, Cavallo R.** 2013. Comparison of two nucleic acid extraction and testing systems for HCMV-DNA detection and quantitation on whole blood specimens from transplant patients. *J Virol Methods* **193:**579–582.
183. **Forman M, Wilson A, Valsamakis A.** 2011. Cytomegalovirus DNA quantification using an automated platform for

nucleic acid extraction and real-time PCR assay setup. *J Clin Microbiol* **49:**2703–2705.

184. **Hanson KE, Reller LB, Kurtzberg J, Horwitz M, Long G, Alexander BD.** 2007. Comparison of the Digene Hybrid Capture system cytomegalovirus (CMV) DNA (version 2.0), Roche CMV UL54 analyte-specific reagent, and QIAGEN RealArt CMV LightCycler PCR reagent tests using AcroMetrix OptiQuant CMV DNA quantification panels and specimens from allogeneic-stem-cell transplant recipients. *J Clin Microbiol* **45:**1972–1973.
185. **Kerschner H, Bauer C, Schlag P, Lee S, Goedel S, Popow-Kraupp T.** 2011. Clinical evaluation of a fully automated CMV PCR assay. *J Clin Virol* **50:**281–286.
186. **Pritt BS, Germer JJ, Gomez-Urena E, Bishop CJ, Mandrekar JN, Irish CL, Yao JD.** 2013. Conversion to the COBAS AmpliPrep/COBAS TaqMan CMV test for management of CMV disease in transplant recipients. *Diagn Microbiol Infect Dis* **75:**440–442.
187. **Boaretti M, Sorrentino A, Zantedeschi C, Forni A, Boschiero L, Fontana R.** 2013. Quantification of cytomegalovirus DNA by a fully automated real-time PCR for early diagnosis and monitoring of active viral infection in solid organ transplant recipients. *J Clin Virol* **56:**124–128.
188. **Cardeñoso L, Pinsky BA, Lautenschlager I, Aslam S, Cobb B, Vilchez RA, Hirsch HH.** 2013. CMV antigenemia and quantitative viral load assessments in hematopoietic stem cell transplant recipients. *J Clin Virol* **56:**108–112.
189. **Mannonen L, Loginov R, Helanterä I, Dumoulin A, Vilchez RA, Cobb B, Hirsch HH, Lautenschlager I.** 2014. Comparison of two quantitative real-time CMV-PCR tests calibrated against the 1st WHO international standard for viral load monitoring of renal transplant patients. *J Med Virol* **86:**576–584.
190. **Babady NE, Cheng C, Cumberbatch E, Stiles J, Papanicolaou G, Tang YW.** 2015. Monitoring of cytomegalovirus viral loads by two molecular assays in whole-blood and plasma samples from hematopoietic stem cell transplant recipients. *J Clin Microbiol* **53:**1252–1257.
191. **Banas B, Böger CA, Lückhoff G, Krüger B, Barabas S, Batzilla J, Schemmerer M, Köstler J, Bendfeldt H, Rascle A, Wagner R, Deml L, Leicht J, Krämer BK.** 2017. Validation of T-Track® CMV to assess the functionality of cytomegalovirus-reactive cell-mediated immunity in hemodialysis patients. *BMC Immunol* **18:**15.
192. **Kim SH, Lee HJ, Kim SM, Jung JH, Shin S, Kim YH, Sung H, Lee SO, Choi SH, Kim YS, Woo JH, Han DJ.** 2015. Diagnostic usefulness of cytomegalovirus (CMV)-specific T cell immunity in predicting CMV infection after kidney transplantation: a pilot proof-of-concept study. *Infect Chemother* **47:**105–110.
193. **Jung J, Lee HJ, Kim SM, Kang YA, Lee YS, Chong YP, Sung H, Lee SO, Choi SH, Kim YS, Woo JH, Lee JH, Lee JH, Lee KH, Kim SH.** 2017. Diagnostic usefulness of dynamic changes of CMV-specific T-cell responses in predicting CMV infections in HCT recipients. *J Clin Virol* **87:**5–11.
194. **San-Juan R, Navarro D, García-Reyne A, Montejo M, Muñoz P, Carratala J, Len O, Fortun J, Muñoz-Cobo B, Gimenez E, Eworo A, Sabe N, Meije Y, Martín-Davila P, Andres A, Delgado J, Jimenez C, Amat P, Fernández-Ruiz M, López-Medrano F, Lumbreras C, Aguado JM, REIPI Network.** 2015. Effect of long-term prophylaxis in the development of cytomegalovirus-specific T-cell immunity in D+/R– solid organ transplant recipients. *Transpl Infect Dis* **17:**637–646.
195. **Clari MA, Aguilar G, Benet I, Belda J, Giménez E, Bravo D, Carbonell JA, Henao L, Navarro D.** 2013. Evaluation of cytomegalovirus (CMV)-specific T-cell immunity for the assessment of the risk of active CMV infection in non-immunosuppressed surgical and trauma intensive care unit patients. *J Med Virol* **85:**1802–1810.
196. **Andrikopoulou E, Mather PJ.** 2014. Current insights: use of Immuknow in heart transplant recipients. *Prog Transplant* **24:**44–50.
197. **Quaglia M, Cena T, Fenoglio R, Musetti C, Cagna D, Radin E, Roggero S, Amoroso A, Magnani C, Stratta P.** 2014. Immune function assay (Immunknow) drop over first 6 months after renal transplant: a predictor of opportunistic viral infections? *Transplant Proc* **46:**2220–2223.
198. **Pérez-Jacoiste Asín MA, Fernández-Ruiz M, López-Medrano F, Aquilino C, González E, Ruiz-Merlo T, Gutiérrez E, San Juan R, Paz-Artal E, Andrés A, Aguado JM.** 2016. Monitoring of intracellular adenosine triphosphate in CD4(+) T cells to predict the occurrence of cytomegalovirus disease in kidney transplant recipients. *Transpl Int* **29:**1094–1105.

Epstein-Barr Virus

BARBARA C. GÄRTNER AND FAUSTO BALDANTI

103

Epstein-Barr virus (EBV) is associated with a wide variety of disease states ranging from infectious mononucleosis (IM) to malignant disorders. Antibody assays are used primarily for patients with suspected IM. A variety of immunoassays, blotting assays, and flow cytometry tests have been used. Assays targeting viral capsid antigen (VCA) IgG, VCA IgM, and EBV nuclear antigen 1 (EBNA 1) IgG are favored. Additional assays, such as avidity testing or viral load measurement, are only rarely necessary to establish the diagnosis of IM. The detection of heterophile antibodies is sometimes useful for diagnosing young adults with typical IM symptoms, but it often lacks sensitivity and specificity, particularly in young children and when symptoms are atypical. Antibody assays detecting early antigen (EA) are rarely useful because of their heterogeneity and poor specificity. Assays that measure EBV in peripheral blood using quantitative nucleic acid amplification testing (QNAAT) are being used mainly for transplant recipients and for patients with EBV-associated malignant disorders. The best evidence exists for EBV DNA monitoring to trigger preemptive therapy to prevent posttransplant lymphoproliferative disorders (PTLD) in high-risk transplant recipients, as well as for the diagnosis and treatment monitoring of nasopharyngeal carcinoma (NPC). An international reference standard for EBV DNA significantly reduced variability for viral load measurement. QNAAT values that could be used as trigger points for intervention are under investigation but may vary by specimen type, clinical setting, and patient group. Dynamic changes in viral load, rather than absolute QNAAT values alone, may be important in patient management.

TAXONOMY

EBV is a member of the *Herpesviridae* and belongs to the subfamily *Gammaherpesvirinae* (1). EBV is closely related to another human pathogen, human herpesvirus 8, which also replicates in epithelial cells and establishes long-term latency in lymphocytes. However, EBV is the only human pathogen in the genus *Lymphocryptovirus*; human herpesvirus 8 belongs to the genus *Rhadinovirus*.

DESCRIPTION OF THE AGENT

Morphologically, EBV is a typical herpesvirus with 162 capsomeres in an icosahedral arrangement surrounded by a lipid-rich envelope. The virus has a double-stranded, 172-kbp DNA genome which exists in a linear form in the mature virion and in a circular episomal form in latently infected cells. The genome consists of a series of unique sequences alternating with internal repeats, all sandwiched between two terminal repeat elements which are joined during circularization. Integration of viral DNA into host chromosomal DNA occurs rarely and has been documented primarily for lymphoblastoid cell lines.

EBV primarily infects naïve B cells. This requires the binding of the major EBV outer envelope glycoprotein gp350/220 with the cellular complement receptor C3d (also known as CD21 or CR2) and gp42 with the major histocompatibility complex class II molecule. *In vivo*, EBV uses the highly regulated, sequentially expressed proteins described below to persist in the host and transmit infection. It is believed to do this by usurping normal B cell physiologic processes. EBV replaces antigen, T cell help, the B cell receptor, and other signals that result in cellular activation, proliferation, differentiation, and survival, mimicking pathways followed when naïve B cells encounter antigen with the end result of establishing latency in memory B cells (2). *In vitro*, EBV transforms B cells into lymphoblastoid cell lines. Although CD21-negative epithelial cells of the oropharynx are the most important site of viral replication and amplification (3), monocytes may also be productively infected by EBV (4, 5). In some clinical settings, T and NK (natural killer) cells also demonstrate evidence of infection (6). EBV nuclear antigens—EBNA 1, EBNA 2, EBNA 3 (also referred to as EBNA 3a), EBNA 4 (EBNA 3b), EBNA 5 (EBNA LP), and EBNA 6 (EBNA 3c)—and latent membrane proteins (LMP 1, 2A, and 2B) may be expressed in B cells. Four types of B cell latency have been defined, based on various levels of expression of the latency-associated proteins (7, 8). In latency type 0, only EBV-encoded RNAs (EBERs) and rightward transcripts from the BamHIA gene are expressed. EBER 1 and EBER 2 are nonpolyadenylated RNAs, are therefore not translated to a protein, and act to inhibit antiviral effects by interferon as well as apoptosis. EBERs are present in high copy numbers (10^6 to 10^7 copies) in virtually all EBV-infected cells. This expression profile is seen in memory B cells of healthy carriers. In latency type I, in addition to the type 0 expression profile, EBNA 1 is detectable; this is observed in Burkitt's lymphoma. In latency type II, LMP 1 and 2 are expressed in addition to gene products of latency type I; this is observed in germinal center and memory B cells in the tonsil and malignancies, including Hodgkin's lymphoma, NPC, nasal NK cell lymphoma, chronic active EBV infection, and nasopharyngeal lymphoma. Finally, in latency type III, all EBNA proteins are detectable; this is observed in naïve B cells of the tonsil during acute infection and in immunodeficiency-related lymphoproliferative disorders (2).

EBV has a highly restricted host range. Although during acute EBV infection, as many as 10% of all circulating B cells, representing 50% or more of all memory B cells, may be infected, in a healthy individual remote from infection, only in about 1 to 50 B cells per million EBV genomes may be found (9). During lytic replication, more than 70 proteins are expressed, including the VCAs and the EAs used in diagnostics. This occurs primarily in epithelial cells and in B cells as they undergo plasmacytoid differentiation.

EPIDEMIOLOGY AND TRANSMISSION

Virtually everyone becomes infected with EBV at some time during his or her life. In lower socioeconomic strata and developing countries, EBV infection occurs mainly during the first years of life and is usually subclinical. However, in developed countries, particularly in upper socioeconomic strata, only about 60% are infected before puberty. In these settings, infection often occurs in adolescence and early adult life, resulting in an IM syndrome or atypical symptomatic infection in 23 to 89% of cases (10). As a result, by the age of 20 years, ~90% of individuals are seropositive, and by the age of 40, almost 99% of the population have seroconverted.

Transmission of EBV occurs primary through saliva exchange in adolescents and adults, mainly through deep kissing (10). EBV shedding in saliva is continuous, persistent, and rapid in all previously infected subjects (3, 11). Therefore, the use of saliva for the diagnosis of acute infections is discouraged. Although infection via blood products is possible, the importance of blood products as a source of EBV infection is uncertain, particularly in settings where blood products are universally leukodepleted.

Among transplant recipients, latently EBV-infected cells transmitted with the donor organ or hematopoietic stem cells from seropositive donors to seronegative recipients are the most important source of infection in the early posttransplantation period.

EBV strains may be classified into types 1 and 2 (sometimes referred to as types A and B, respectively) based on the polymorphism of their EBNA 2 genes. Both EBV types have a worldwide distribution, though they predominate in different geographical areas. Dual infections with the two types are not uncommon. In immunosuppressed individuals, coinfection with multiple strains of EBV has also been demonstrated (12).

CLINICAL SIGNIFICANCE

EBV is associated with a variety of disease states in immunocompetent and immunosuppressed individuals. Longitudinal studies with African children with acute EBV infection suggest that asymptomatic infection at a very early age (before 6 months) may be related to higher and more persistent viral loads in peripheral blood because of age-related immune immaturity; a relationship of early infection to risk for Burkitt's lymphoma has been postulated (13). Passive maternal antibody may provide protection against infection very early in life, although the duration of that protection is uncertain (14).

IM is believed to be an immunopathologic disease with symptoms resulting from an uncontrolled T cell response of a more mature immune system to a self-limited lymphoproliferative process and perhaps high viral loads. In this model, EBV DNA positivity in blood precedes clinical symptoms (15). In young adults with acute symptomatic EBV infection, EBV DNA (possibly representing virions) is rapidly cleared from plasma within a week of symptom onset, but EBV DNA in whole blood (perhaps representing episomal DNA in latently infected B cells) takes up to 200 days or more to clear to levels seen in healthy carriers (10, 15, 16).

Symptoms vary from mild to severe, and data suggest that the initial viral inoculum, viral type (type 1 versus 2), and human leukocyte antigen class 1 polymorphisms may be risk factors for symptomatic disease (17–19). The classical symptom triad of IM is fever, sore throat, and lymphadenopathy; symptoms and signs such as pharyngitis, tonsillitis, hepatitis, splenomegaly, and lymphocytosis with atypical lymphocytes are often present. Rash in a variety of forms is seen in up to 15% of IM patients (20). Earlier, it was believed that using antibiotics, especially ampicillin or amoxicillin, might cause antibiotic-associated rash in over 80% of patients with IM (21). However, a recent study indicated that this number is far too high and that rash occurs with antibiotic treatment in an only slightly higher percentage than without (22). This antibiotic-associated rash is not predictive of future drug intolerance.

The time span between infection and symptoms is relatively long, ranging from 30 to 50 days (15, 23), and clinical disease generally persists for 1 to 4 weeks or longer. However, protracted illness and postinfectious fatigue and/or depression for up to a year are not uncommon (24). Atypical presentations in which hematologic features such as anemia, including autoimmune hemolytic anemia thrombocytopenia, or neurologic conditions such as meningoencephalitis, radiculitis, or mononeuritis predominate can occur. When visceral organs are affected, almost any symptom resulting from inflammation of the affected organ may be seen (25). Death due to IM is rare but has been described; it occurs most often as a result of splenic rupture (26), airway obstruction, or neurologic complications (25). A severe and sometimes fatal complication of primary infection is hemophagocytic lymphohistiocytosis, a hemophagocytic syndrome characterized by an uncontrolled macrophage activation and phagocytosis caused by virally driven T cell response. Extremely high levels of EBV DNA are observed in both peripheral blood mononuclear cells (PBMC) and sera of patients with this complication (6, 27, 28). Atypical presentations, including acute cholestatic hepatitis sometimes misdiagnosed as acute cholecystitis, are common in older subjects (>40 years) with acute EBV infection (29). EBV is often reactivated in healthy individuals, but reactivation has not been clearly associated with symptoms.

It should also be noted that primary EBV infections cause only approximately 50 to 90% of mononucleosis syndromes (29). Other infectious agents, such as acute cytomegalovirus, adenovirus, *Toxoplasma gondii*, and human immunodeficiency virus (HIV), as well as lymphoma and autoimmune diseases can cause symptoms and signs similar to those seen in EBV-associated IM.

In vitro, acyclovir, ganciclovir, and foscarnet inhibit EBV replication through blockade of viral DNA polymerase. However, the *in vivo* efficacy of these antivirals is unclear.

In addition, since pathogenesis of IM appears to be (at least in part) immune mediated, treatment with antivirals blocking viral shedding proved to have no or only small effects on IM symptoms. Indeed, a meta-analysis showed only minor benefits associated with acyclovir use for IM treatment (30). Antiviral therapy is therefore not recommended for treatment of nonsevere IM. Meta-analysis of steroid use in nonsevere IM showed no relevant effects as well (31). However, steroids may be useful in complicated or severe disease (25). Uncomplicated IM is generally treated with supportive treatment only. Importantly, trauma to the spleen has to be avoided.

Chronic active EBV infection is a rare, severe (often fatal) EBV-associated condition most often described to occur in Asian children; it is believed to be a precursor state for T/NK lymphoma (32). It is characterized by a clonal expansion of EBV-infected T cells and NK cells and a high EBV DNA load in both PBMC and serum or plasma. The EBV DNA in serum and plasma is believed to be free DNA rather than virion associated. Patients often show atypical patterns of EA antibodies (6, 33). Although chemotherapy and immunomodulatory therapy have been attempted as treatment, most cases are chemotherapy resistant. Hematopoietic stem cell transplantation (HSCT) is currently the preferred treatment option (6, 34).

EBV is highly oncogenic and is associated with a variety of tumors affecting multiple embryologic layers (meso- and endoderm) (Table 1). The oncogenic potential of EBV relies on the ability of its latency genes to mimic several growth factors, transcription factors, and factors interfering with cell apoptosis (Table 2). In addition, EBV-transformed cells are able to avoid T cell recognition through inhibition of major histocompatibility complex signaling and exploitation of the PD-1/PDL1 pathway (Table 2). EBV-associated neoplasms are primarily of lymphoid and epithelial origin, not related to obvious immunosuppression. On the other hand, immune impairment associated with HIV infection and anti-rejection treatments in transplant patients strongly promotes development of EBV-induced lymphoproliferation (PTLD), lymphomas, and leiomyosarcomas. Increased incidence of NPC has also been observed in immunocompromised patients. Finally, EBV and the closely related Kaposi sarcoma herpes virus (human herpesvirus 8) are often copresent in rare lymphomas in immunocompromised individuals (e.g., those with multicentric Castleman disease or primary effusion lymphoma).

TABLE 1 EBV-associated tumors and expression of EBV latency genes[a]

EBV latency type	EBV latency gene expression	Malignancy	Embryologic layer origin
I	EBNA-1	Burkitt's lymphoma	Mesoderm
	EBERs	Gastric carcinoma	Endoderm
II	EBNA 1	NPC	Endoderm
	LMP 1, 2A, 2B	Hodgkin's disease	Mesoderm
	EBERs	Nasal T/NK lymphoma	Mesoderm
III	EBNA 1, 2, 3A, 3B, 3C, LP	AIDS-associated non-Hodgkin's disease lymphoma	Mesoderm
	LMP 1, 2A, 2B, EBERs	PTLD	Mesoderm
Other	EBNA 1, 2, EBERs	Leiomyosarcoma	Mesoderm

[a]Modified from reference 180.

TABLE 2 EBV gene products and their role in oncogenesis[a]

EBV gene product	Function
EBNA 1	Sequence-specific DNA-binding protein essential for orienting EBV genome replication by viral polymerase during the lytic cycle and by cell polymerases during latency; essential for segregation of EBV episomes in dividing cells at mitosis; proteasome interference; immune evasion
EBNA 2	Upregulation of CD23 and c-*myc*, interaction with Notch signaling pathway; cell immortalization
EBNA 3A	Interaction with CBF1 (Notch signaling pathway); cell immortalization
EBNA 3B	Interaction with CBF1; dispensable for cell immortalization
EBNA 3C	Interaction with CBF1, interference with pRB, upregulation of LMP-1; cell immortalization
EBNA LP	Interaction with EBNA-2 to interfere with pRB and p53, interaction with Notch signaling pathway; cell immortalization
LMP 1	Mimics a constitutively active CD40 receptor, upregulation of Bcl-2; cell immortalization; upregulation of PDL1; immune evasion
LMP 2A and LMP 2B	Maintenance of latency
EBERs 1 and 2	Latency-associated transcripts
BCRF1 (vIL10)	Mimics interleukin 10 functions; immune evasion
BNLF2a	Interference with TAP1; immune evasion
BARFs	Interaction with Notch signaling pathway; dispensable for immortalization

[a]Data from references 35 and 181–183.

The EBV genome has been found in tumor cells in >95% of endemic Burkitt's lymphomas and NPC, <5 to 70% of cases of Hodgkin's disease (depending on the subtype), 2 to 16% of gastric adenocarcinomas, 40 to >90% of T/NK lymphomas (depending on the subtype), and 40 to 95% of lymphoepithelioma-like carcinomas (35).

In a recent review article, Thorley-Lawson elegantly described how the EBV latency genetic program(s) mirrors the normal B lymphocyte programming and how superimposed EBV genetic reprogramming of B lymphocytes at different maturation stages might lead to the emergence of the various B lymphomas on the basis of costimuli (malaria infection for Burkitt's lymphoma) and the crossing of specific cell checkpoints (36).

Due to the limited impact of the EBV lytic cycle in the pathogenesis of EBV-associated tumors, there is no proven role for current antiviral agents (which target the viral DNA polymerase, which is actually inactive during latency) in the management of these malignancies; standard cancer treatment is used for management. EBV can persist asymptomatically in the vast majority of infected individuals on the basis of an efficient innate and adaptive cellular immune control (37). Adoptive immunotherapy targeting specific EBV proteins expressed in some EBV-associated malignancies has been successfully used for some patients and is being explored further in clinical trials (38–42).

Initial anecdotal reports suggesting a role for EBV during exacerbations of chronic inflammatory bowel diseases (43) have recently been backed up in the context of new immunosuppressive regimens also involving the use of biologicals (44–47).

Primary immunodeficiencies and, as their prototype, X-linked lymphoproliferative syndrome are rare hereditary immunodeficiencies primarily involving the inability of T cells and NK cells to engage EBV-infected B cells (48, 49). Affected patients become symptomatic after exposure to EBV because of EBV's exquisite tropism for B cells, developing acute fatal IM or lymphoproliferative disorders and/or dysgammaglobulinemia. For some of these immunodeficiencies, the genetic defects have been identified. Untreated, these diseases are often lethal, and patients benefit from stem cell transplantation (50). The role of antiviral therapy early during acute EBV infection in these patients is uncertain; treatment with anti-CD20 antibody has been advocated by some investigators.

In immunocompromised patients, both primary infection and EBV reactivation can result in lymphoproliferative disorders. PTLD represents a spectrum of disorders varying from benign polyclonal proliferations to true malignancies containing clonal chromosomal abnormalities. PTLD is often extranodal, can be restricted to the allograft after solid-organ transplantation (SOT), and, unlike lymphoma in immunocompetent patients, can involve the brain in isolation or as part of multisystem disease. Principal risk factors are (i) EBV primary infection after transplantation in the setting of SOT and (ii) severe T cell depletion (e.g., after administration of T cell antibodies or following infusion of a manipulated graft) in both SOT and HSCT settings (51–53). Although >90% of early (first posttransplant year) PTLD lesions after SOT have demonstrable EBV, >50% of late PTLD is EBV negative at presentation (54). It is believed that loss of EBV in late PTLDs might reflect the cell replication-promoting nature of the virus in early polyclonal phases, while chromosomal abnormalities in oligo- and monoclonal lymphoproliferations might *per se* sustain uncontrolled cell proliferation. Adoptive immunity strategies for controlling EBV-induced PTLDs target virus antigens in proliferating cells; thus, they might be ineffective in advanced PTLDs. Incidence of PTLD (especially EBV-positive PTLD) has declined over the years, probably reflecting progress in optimizing immunosuppression and the use of prophylactic measures as a result of EBV DNA monitoring (55).

EBV-related lymphomas are also common malignancies seen in HIV-infected and AIDS patients. Burkitt's lymphoma, lymphomas of the central nervous system (CNS), and smooth muscle tumors are strongly associated with EBV (~90%) (56, 57); the latter are also observed in transplant recipients (58). Oral hairy leukoplakia, a white nonmalignant lesion of the lateral borders of the tongue observed mainly in HIV patients but also in patients using steroid inhalers for respiratory disorders, is associated with lytic EBV infection and is responsive to antiviral therapy (59, 60).

Some SOT recipients experiencing primary EBV infection or PTLD have sustained elevation of EBV DNA load in blood after asymptomatic infection or resolution of EBV disease or PTLD (61, 62). These patients show a chronic high EBV DNA load phenotype. Although a study of pediatric thoracic SOT suggests that 45% of patients with this phenotype developed late-onset EBV-positive PTLD at a median follow-up of 7 years (63), risk appears, in part, to be organ specific, with intermediate risk having been observed after intestinal SOT (64) and low risk after liver SOT at the same center (62). The persistence of EBV DNA in blood has also been observed in children and adults with HIV infection as well. EBV DNA thresholds in blood of individual patients as well as in EBV infection of NK and T cells have been observed in this setting (65). The pathogenesis of this EBV infection state is unknown. A chronic high EBV DNA load without progression to an EBV-associated disorder might indicate that the immune system is still able to control EBV-driven proliferation, although at a lower level than in immunocompetent individuals (61).

The prevention and management of PTLD are complex, requiring a multidisciplinary team that includes transplant physicians, infectious disease specialists, virologists, and hematologists/oncologists, and this is reviewed elsewhere (66–69). Approaches used include immune reconstitution by lowering immunosuppression (only to prevent PTLD) and adoptive immunotherapy, the reduction of tumor burden by surgery or radiotherapy, and the use of chemotherapeutic and biological agents, particularly anti-CD20 therapy and cytotoxic chemotherapy (54, 70).

Although antiviral drugs with or without intravenous immunoglobulins have been used to treat PTLD, there is no evidence to suggest that these agents impact clinical outcome. PTLD lesions, when clinically apparent, contain almost exclusively latently infected cells. The strategy of combining antiviral agents targeting the lytic EBV cycle with drugs, such as arginine butyrate and bortezomib, that induce EBV lytic replication in latently infected PTLD cells was used previously but is not used any longer due to the wide spectrum of other therapeutic options (71). On theoretical grounds, antiviral drugs and intravenous immunoglobulins might have greater efficacy in preventing or modifying the course of primary or reactivation EBV infection early after SOT and HSCT in patients at high risk of transplant- or community-acquired EBV infection. However, a recent meta-analysis did not show a significant benefit, and thus, the use of prophylactic antiviral agents in these settings remains controversial (72). Reconstitution of the EBV-specific immune response is key to the management of PTLD and often initially involves reduction of immunosuppression (73). Adoptive immunotherapy using EBV-specific cytotoxic T cell therapies (autologous or allogeneic T cells) has demonstrated efficacy in both disease prevention and treatment (69, 74). This resulted in third-party T cell banks, such as that in Aberdeen, which collected T cells from healthy blood donors to provide T cells for SOT (75–77).

There is no approved vaccine against EBV. Vaccines for prophylactic and therapeutic use are under development. For prophylactic use, prototype vaccines failed to prevent EBV infection but were effective in partly preventing symptomatic disease (78, 79). Studies addressing the use of an EBV vaccine in treatment of NPC are under way (80).

COLLECTION, TRANSPORT, AND STORAGE OF SPECIMENS

For the rare circumstances in which oropharyngeal viral excretion is studied, 5 to 10 ml of throat gargle, collected in serum-free tissue culture medium or Hanks' balanced salt solution, can be used. Approximately 5 to 10 ml of heparinized or EDTA-treated blood is required either for cell culture and detection of EBV-transformed B cells or for antigen detection in B cells by immunostaining or immunofluorescent *in situ* hybridization studies (see below). Blood specimens should be processed as soon as possible, although refrigeration for up to 24 h is acceptable for antigen detection. Fresh biopsy samples or thin cryosections (5 μm) are preferable to formalin-fixed material for antigen detection in tissues.

TABLE 3 Materials and methods for prevention, diagnosis, and monitoring of EBV disease and EBV-associated malignancies[a]

Suspected EBV-associated condition and clinical setting	Validated method(s)	Suitable specimen	Approx value for clinical significance[b]
IM	Serology	Serum	
Chronic active EBV infection	QNAAT	Mononuclear cells	$10^{2.0}$ IU/μg DNA (vs. patients with past infection); $10^{3.2}$ IU/μg DNA (vs. patients with IM)[c]
EBV-positive CNS lymphoma	QNAAT	CSF	~10^4 EBV DNA copies/ml[d]
Prevention of PTLD using preemptive therapy in high-risk patients	QNAAT	Plasma	~10^2–10^4 EBV DNA copies/ml
		Whole blood	10^3–10^5 EBV DNA copies/ml
Screening for NPC in high-risk populations	QNAAT	Plasma/serum	~20 EBV DNA copies/ml (repeated testing)
		Nasopharyngeal brushings	~200 EBV DNA copies/ng DNA
	Serology[e]	EBV-specific IgA	Not defined
Monitoring NPC response to therapy	QNAAT	Plasma/serum	Not defined
Diagnosis of primary immunodeficiencies, such as XLP[f]	Genetic analysis	Host cells	Specific associated gene mutations

[a]EBV-associated tumors are diagnosed by detecting EBV antigens or EBER in the respective biopsy.

[b]Approximate levels of EBV viral load for clinical significance are based on data reported, most often from single centers, using a variety of often nonstandardized assays. Only in a few studies were assays calibrated to the international reference standard.

[c]Mononuclear cells showed higher sensitivity and specificity compared to plasma, since disease is most often due to clonal expansion of EBV-infected T or NK cells (70).

[d]A parallel quantification in blood is highly advised, especially in transplanted patients, in case of leaking blood-brain barrier or blood-stained CSF sampling, in order to estimate potential CSF contamination by circulating EBV DNA.

[e]Less useful than NAAT.

[f]XLP, X-linked lymphoproliferative syndrome.

Nucleic acid amplification testing (NAAT) is currently most frequently used to detect EBV in blood, cerebrospinal fluid (CSF), and biopsy samples. The choice of sample matrix depends on the EBV-associated disease of interest and the clinical setting in which the test is being used (Table 3). For example, investigators have proposed sampling of PBMC in chronic active EBV infection (81), tumor cells from CSF in AIDS-related primary CNS lymphoma (82), and whole blood or plasma after transplantation (83, 84). Plasma but not whole blood has been recommended as the preferred sampling matrix in IM (11, 85) and in diseases in which malignant cells do not necessarily circulate in blood, such as NPC (86), nasal T/NK cell lymphoma (87), and Hodgkin's lymphoma (88).

The optimal sample matrix for monitoring transplant recipients and patients under immunosuppression has not been definitely determined. However, EBV DNA in cell-free samples might better correlate with an active infection, whereas whole blood or PBMC are more sensitive but similarly less specific (89). Indeed, in patients with malignancies, EBV DNA in plasma was shown to derive from degrading cells rather than replicating virus (90). For serial monitoring of individual patients, it is particularly important that the sample matrix not be varied. The sample quantity required varies, but it is advisable to provide at least 1 ml of plasma or whole blood. Source blood specimens for serum, plasma, or PBMC should be processed as soon as possible. If the transport time is less than 24 h, samples may be kept at room temperature until separated. Separated materials can thereafter be stored at 4 to 7°C for a few days or frozen. Whole blood can be stored for a few days at room temperature or frozen without further processing. For long-term storage, freezing at −70°C is recommended. For detection of EBV in peripheral blood lymphocytes by DNA hybridization, 5 to 10 ml of heparinized or EDTA-treated blood is required.

QNAAT of CSF hatts been used for the diagnosis of EBV-associated CNS disease, particularly lymphoma. CSF without additives should be sent, processed, and stored as described above for blood specimens being tested for EBV DNA by NAAT; at least 0.5 ml should be submitted for testing when possible. EBV DNA quantification in a paired blood sample is advised, especially for immunocompromised individuals, to distinguish intrathecal DNA synthesis versus blood contamination.

Tissues (e.g., nasopharyngeal brushings for NPC) and biopsy samples to be examined for viral nucleic acids or antigens should be collected and refrigerated in saline or balanced salt solutions. Fresh-frozen samples are preferred. For patients with NPC, endoscope-guided nasopharyngeal brushings are an important sample matrix. A brush covered by a plastic catheter should be used to prevent contamination by cells from nonnasopharyngeal sites. The brush tip can be placed in transport medium and transferred immediately to the laboratory or stored at −80°C.

For antibody assays detecting heterophile antibody, whole blood, serum, or capillary fingertip blood may be used for most point-of-care tests. For EBV-specific tests, 50 μl or even less, acute-phase serum may be sufficient; however, it is advisable to provide 1 to 2 ml. Plasma can be used, but serum is preferable. Serum can be stored at 5°C for several months. For long-term storage, freezing at −20°C or −70°C is recommended.

DIRECT EXAMINATION

Electron microscopy, virus isolation, and antigen detection by immunohistochemistry are primarily research tools. EBV DNA detection by molecular methods, mainly NAAT, is the most common and often the only method used for routine direct detection.

Microscopy

Electron microscopy is not an appropriate diagnostic technique for EBV diagnosis, since most EBV-associated disease is associated with latent infection and virions are rarely present in sufficient quantity to be detected.

EBV Antigen Detection by Immunohistochemistry and EBER Detection by *In Situ* Hybridization

Antibodies specific to a wide range of EBV antigens have been used to detect EBV in tissue biopsy samples using immunohistochemical techniques. Studies using antibodies targeting EBNA 1, EBNA 2, LMP 1, LMP 2, BamHI H right-frame 1 protein (BHRF 1), BamHI Z left-frame 1 protein (BZLF 1), BamHI M right-frame 1 protein (BMRF 1), and others have been described previously (7, 91–93). EBNA 1 is the only antigen expressed in all EBV-infected cells expressing EBV proteins (cells with latency states other than latency state 0). However, the sensitivity of immunohistochemistry techniques for the detection of EBV-infected cells using currently available EBNA 1 antibodies is lower than that observed using *in situ* hybridization targeting EBER (7). EBER is present in high copy numbers in EBV-infected cells regardless of latency state. This has made its detection using *in situ* hybridization techniques ideal and the gold standard for detecting EBV-infected cells in tissues and tumors (94). Despite this, some authors report having documented EBER-negative EBV-infected cells (95).

The cellular tropism of EBV in the peripheral blood of patients with high persistent EBV viral loads is also being studied using assays that combine immunofluorescent staining for cell surface proteins (cell phenotyping) with fluorescent or *in situ* hybridization using nucleic acid probes for EBER (96, 97) or other targets (98). Detection can be performed on slides by microscopy or in suspension by flow cytometry. These assays are not yet available in routine diagnostic laboratories.

Nucleic Acid Amplification Techniques

Molecular techniques are important tools for the detection of EBV in clinical specimens. The choice of method and sample matrix is dependent upon the clinical question being addressed (Table 1).

Clinical diagnostic assays for direct detection of EBV DNA can be performed on a wide range of clinical specimens following DNA extraction. A variety of primers, probes, and techniques have been used. In general, quantitative viral load assessment is superior to qualitative detection, and a wide variety of commercial assays are available (99, 100). Quantitative real-time PCR is the most popular currently used technology for measuring EBV viral load in patients at risk for EBV-associated disorders. Earlier studies demonstrated significant variability (4 $\log_{10}$) among laboratories, limiting the validity of interinstitutional result comparison (101). In October 2011, the WHO approved the first international standard for EBV (a whole-virus preparation of EBV B95-8 with a potency of 5×10^6 IU/ml) created by the National Institute for Biological Standards and Controls (United Kingdom) (102).

Assessment of viral load can be broken down into two basic strategies, based upon the genomic region being targeted. (i) The conserved BamHI W region, coding for a long internal repeat sequence of EBNA 1, is present in multiple copies (7 to 11 copies) in EBV-infected cells. NAAT targeting this region has maximal sensitivity in clinical samples (103). (ii) The genes for LMP 1 or thymidine kinase or other parts of the EBNA 1 gene are often targeted in quantitative PCRs, since these are single-copy regions (104). Recently, it was shown that the two concepts differ in viral load by around 0.5 $\log_{10}$ (103) when they are calibrated against the international standard. It must be kept in mind that the international standard uses B95-8 cells with 11 copies of the BamHI W region (103), but clinical strains might have fewer copies. However, even between NAATs using single-copy genes, target-specific quantitative differences in results were obtained (105–108). Gene targets that result in small amplicons may be more useful when viral DNA is measured in plasma samples, since EBV DNA in plasma is often free DNA, i.e., not encapsidated, and so may be highly fragmented (90, 109).

For accurate quantitation, the standards should be extracted together with the clinical samples in a matrix resembling the clinical sample. They should not be diluted in buffer, although the international reference standard is reconstituted in nuclease-free water. To date, most of the commercially available NAATs are calibrated using the international standard, significantly reducing variability between assays (110–112). However, these studies also suggest that calibrators are not the only issue preventing result harmonization. Commercial reagents and gene targets used also contribute to result variability (111). Indeed, a standardization strategy based upon the WHO international standard and taking into account all technical variables proved to be of help in reducing result variability among centers to 0.5 $\log_{10}$ (113).

Results should be reported in international units per milliliter. Normalization of viral load by using cell number or micrograms of DNA is generally unnecessary in routine diagnostics when samples of whole blood or CSF are tested. Studies showed a close correlation between results reported in copies per milliliter and those reported as copies per microgram of DNA when whole blood was tested. Similar dynamic trending in patients using both reporting formats was also observed, suggesting that normalization to cell number or genomic DNA in cellular specimens may also be unnecessary (114, 115). There is a strong correlation among viral loads measured in cell-containing samples, such as PBMC, B cells, and whole blood (116), but a weaker correlation between these results and those obtained with plasma or serum. Results from biopsy samples should be reported in international units per microgram of DNA; when coamplification of a cellular single-copy gene is performed, results should be reported in international units per number of cells.

The precision of EBV NAAT is such that changes in values should be at least 3-fold (0.5 $\log_{10}$ IU/ml) to be considered to represent biologically important changes in viral replication. QNAAT variability is greatest for low viral loads. Thus, for viral load values at or near the limit of quantification, QNAAT viral load changes may need to be greater than 5-fold (0.7 $\log_{10}$ IU/ml) to be considered significant.

Appropriate controls for extraction, contamination, and inhibition should always be included in the assays. Participation in external quality control programs is mandatory for all clinical diagnostic laboratories. Proficiency panels are available in both Europe (e.g., Quality Control for Molecular Diagnostics; http://www.QCMD.org) and North America (College of American Pathologists; http://www.cap.org).

ISOLATION, IDENTIFICATION, AND TYPING PROCEDURES

EBV isolation is currently not routinely performed in diagnostic laboratories. Freshly fractionated human cord blood lymphocytes are inoculated with cell-free, filtered saliva or throat gargle specimens and monitored for 4 weeks. Direct sequencing of EBV isolates using next-generation deep-sequencing techniques is also being explored for strain typing directly from clinical samples (117). However, since there are currently no data to allow clear prediction of a patient's clinical course or treatment outcome based on EBV strain polymorphisms, EBV genotyping is not useful in clinical practice.

SEROLOGIC TESTS

Heterophile Antibodies

Heterophile antibodies are not EBV specific. The test for them relies on the detection of antibodies reacting with erythrocytes of non-human animals that develop as a result of polyclonal B cell stimulation occurring in the setting of IM. Historically, sheep erythrocytes were used (Paul-Bunnell test) as assay targets, but the assays using them lacked sensitivity (118). Later, horse erythrocytes were used, and to improve specificity, the Davidsohn differential test was added. This test discriminates between the EBV heterophile response and the heterophile response seen in serum sickness and rheumatic diseases (i.e., it targets the Forssman antigen). To exclude agglutination resulting from heterophile antibodies against the non-EBV Forssman antigen, in the Davidsohn differential test, these non-EBV-related heterophile antibodies are first removed by adsorption of serum with guinea pig kidney cells that express the Forssman antigen. As an additional control, serum is also adsorbed with bovine erythrocytes not expressing the IM antigen. When the two adsorbed sera are then mixed with sheep or horse erythrocytes, stronger agglutination in the guinea pig-adsorbed serum indicates a positive result.

Latex agglutination tests using erythrocyte antigens are currently used for heterophile antibody detection and show a high degree of specificity (118). Although they are all intended for laboratory and point-of-care use, the agglutination assays may not be suitable for use by persons without laboratory training. Evaluation of a true positive agglutination result requires experience, since spontaneous agglutination will inevitably develop after some time. Immunochromatographic methods may therefore be easier to read and perform better than agglutination assays in point-of-care settings (118).

EBV-Specific Antibodies

Serologic testing using EBV-specific assays remains the method of choice for the diagnosis or exclusion of EBV infection (Table 4) (119, 120). The tests differ in methods, antigens, and antibody isotypes tested for. Although immunofluorescence assays (IFAs) and blotting techniques are more reliable, enzyme immunoassays (EIAs) and chemiluminescence assays (CLIAs) are used most frequently.

TABLE 4 Overview of commercial products for EBV diagnosis[a]

Method	No. of products	Differences between kits	Advantages	Limitations
Heterophile antibodies				
Slide agglutination tests	~40 kits	Mostly latex particles; rarely bovine, horse, or sheep erythrocytes	Very rapid (<15 min), inexpensive	Measures heterophile antibodies; can be positive for 1 year after IM; not specific for EBV; can be positive with lymphoma, acute HIV, or other infectious agents
Immunochromatographic strip tests			Very rapid (<15 min), inexpensive, easier to read than agglutination tests	
EBV-specific antibodies				
Immunochromatographic strip or paddle tests	~2 kits	Different antigens	Rapid (<25 min)	Depending on the kit, the spectrum of antigens may not be sufficient
EIA				
ELISA	~15 kits	Different antigens and antigen preparations	Might be combined with avidity testing for atypical results	Turnaround time of ~2–3 h, interpretation schema of some manufacturers include diagnoses that are not clinically relevant
Dot technique	1 kit		Combined with CMV, *T. gondii*	Turnaround time of ~2–3 h
CLIA	~2 kits	Different antigens and antigen preparations	Rapid (<1 h); random access; avidity testing commercially available	Specific instruments needed
Flow cytometry based, with microparticles	~3 kits	Combined with CMV, or combined with heterophile antibodies	Rapid (<1 h); reaction to specific antigens similar to blot assay	Specific instruments needed; variable quality of antigens
Immunofluorescence	3 kits	With EBNA (ACIF) or without	Gold standard, high specificity, might be combined with avidity testing	EBNA ACIF detects not only IgG against EBNA 1 but also against EBNA 2; must be combined with a non-IFA method to detect only EBNA 1 IgG; labor-intensive; turnaround time of ~2–3 h
Immunoblotting	~10 kits	Western blot or line blots	Line blots are easier to read; excellent as confirmation for atypical results; can be combined with avidity testing	Expensive, labor-intensive; turnaround time of ~2–3 h
EBV viral load				
Real-time PCR	~10 kits	Different gene targets; different amplicon lengths	High sensitivity and specificity	Different kits are not always comparable; calibration to the international standard is important

[a]ELISA, enzyme-linked immunosorbent assay; CMV, cytomegalovirus.

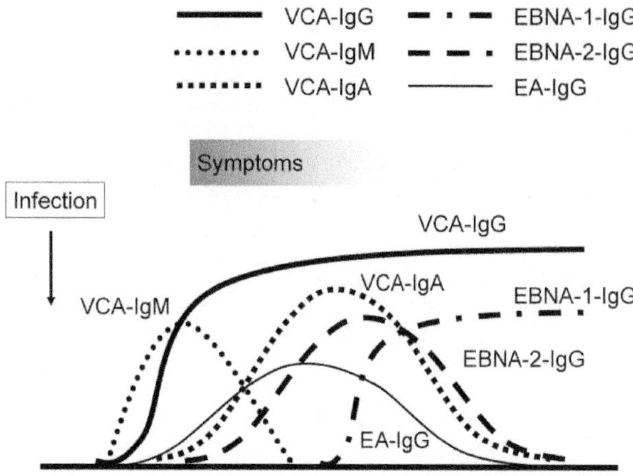

FIGURE 1 Development of antibodies to EBV antigens following primary infection. While there is marked interpatient and interlaboratory variation in titers, the typical relative development of titers by antibody class and antigen specificity is given.

At present, flow cytometry-based assays are used in some laboratories to detect EBV antibodies to different antigens at the same time, in a multiplex approach (multiplex flow immunoassays). In the case of unclear results, any of these methods may be supplemented by avidity testing. Traditionally, antibodies to three antigen complexes have been measured, including VCA, EA, and EBNA. In addition, different immunoglobulin isotypes (IgG, IgM, and sometimes IgA) can be detected. The large numbers of assays can lead to complex antibody patterns, making results difficult to interpret. When possible, kits from the same manufacturer should be used for detecting different markers in an individual patient. The antibody profile for a patient with suspected mononucleosis is presented in Fig. 1.

Immunofluorescence together with immunoblotting is the gold standard for EBV serology at present. IFAs have fairly uniform performance characteristics, principally because suppliers use the same cell substrates. Their sensitivity is similar to or even lower than that of EIA (121). The performance of EIAs and blotting assays is much more variable, due to the plethora of antigen preparations used in the different kits. These range from cell extracts to recombinant or fusion proteins and synthetic peptides (121). This means that reference criteria established for interpretation of IFAs may not apply to all EIAs, even when the antigens are referred to by the same name. For example, EBNA is a complex of several large, native proteins detected in Raji cells by anticomplement immunofluorescence (ACIF); in EIAs, the same designation may be given to a single oligopeptide derived from EBNA 1 or an EBNA 1 recombinant protein. Recombinant proteins and peptides, however, are easier to standardize than cell-grown antigens and assays using synthetic antigens.

Multiplex flow immunoassays, also called flow cytometry-based microparticle assays, have become more popular, since they allow parallel detection of different antigens. In theory, up to 100 uniquely identifiable fluorescently labeled microspheres can be detected with this technique, each particle coated with a different antigen (122–125). This approach combines the advantages of a complete antibody profile, like that of a blot, with a turnaround time of 1 to 2 h as well as a random-access feature. In addition to EBV-specific antigens, some assays also include heterophile antibodies or non-EBV antigens. However, specialized instruments are necessary for signal detection.

Moreover, rapid tests using immunochromatography (e.g., on strips) have been developed for EBV, enabling a fast diagnosis (from less than 5 min up to ~20 min) from a single sample. These tests are particularly suited to point-of-care use.

Avidity testing, measuring the strength of antibody-antigen binding, is available for all methods, not only for EIA. It can be used to differentiate between a primary infection (low avidity) and a past infection (high avidity). Avidity is calculated as the percentage of signal loss resulting from pretreatment of the serum with urea compared with a regular assay (119). These assays are used more often in Europe than in North America.

VCA is a complex of different proteins (e.g., p18, p23, and p150), and antibodies to these antigens are not detectable at the same time, explaining differences in test performances.

Anti-EA/D (diffuse distribution in cells) and anti-EA/R (restricted to cytoplasm) are antibodies traditionally measured with Raji cells activated to enter the lytic phase by phorbol ester or sodium butyrate. Ethanol fixation eliminates the EA/R complex; cells fixed in ethanol are used for studies of EA/D antibodies. Tests using cell-derived and recombinant EA proteins are available but often lack both specificity and sensitivity (118, 124, 126). Because of their high heterogeneity with respect to the specific protein targeted and consequently their low comparability, EA assays are only rarely useful for the diagnosis of acute EBV infection. Furthermore, EA antibodies are present in a significant proportion of healthy blood donors and may thus be more problematic than helpful for diagnosis of acute EBV infection (120). Only in NPC do EA antibodies play a diagnostic role (127).

ACIF detecting not only EBNA 1 but also EBNA 2 is no longer used in routine diagnostics, since commercial EIAs containing cell-derived EBNA or, even better, recombinant EBNA 1 (p72) are available and demonstrate high sensitivity (≥95%).

For the serologic diagnosis of EBV infection in the United States, EBV antibody panels of two, three, or four markers are commonly performed using EIA; IFA is less frequently used. Antibody panels can include VCA IgG and VCA IgM only; VCA IgG, VCA IgM, and EBNA IgG; or the last three antibodies plus antibody to EA. If an atypical pattern is observed (Table 5), retesting options include repeating the EIA, testing by other methods (such as IFA, blotting, or CLIA), or repeat testing of a second follow-up blood sample in 1 to 2 weeks.

An alternative algorithm frequently used in Europe for serologic diagnosis is provided in Fig. 2. In this cost-effective approach, stepwise analysis and data interpretation feature testing for EBNA-1 IgG in serum as the key initial step. This schema is feasible for assays with short turnaround times and random access (e.g., CLIA). EBNA 1 IgG antibodies normally appear between 6 weeks and 7 months after onset of IM and should be negative in acute IM. They are maintained for life and are therefore a good marker of prior infection. However, in about 5 to 10% of patients, EBNA 1 IgG may be present in low titers or even undetectable (128). Increasing age, severe immunosuppression, and rheumatic disorders are often reasons for reduced or absent EBNA 1 IgG titers. Diagnosis of primary EBV infections should not rely solely on the detection of VCA IgM, since both false-positive and false-negative results are possible. False positives result mainly from the

TABLE 5 Typical EBV serological profiles using the most frequently employed antigens and Ig isotypes[a]

Condition	Antigen, Ig isotype					
	VCA, IgG	VCA, IgM	VCA, IgA	EA/D, IgG	EA/R, IgG	EBNA, Ig
Susceptible/no previous exposure	–	–	–	–	–	–
Primary infection	++	+++	+	+	+/–	–
Past infection	+	–	+/–	–	+/–	+
Inconclusive: primary or past infection[b]	+	+	+/–	+/–	+/–	+
Inconclusive: primary or past infection[c]	+	–	+/–	+/–	+/–	–
Chronic active EBV infection	+++	+	++	++	+	+/–
Nasopharyngeal carcinoma	+++	–	+++	+++	+	+++
X-linked lymphoproliferative syndrome	+/–	–	–	–	–	–

[a]+/–, Antibodies absent or present; +, antibodies present; ++, antibodies present in elevated titers; +++, antibodies present in strongly elevated titers. EA/D, early antigen/diffuse; EA/R, early antigen/restricted; EBNA, EBV nuclear antigen; EBV, Epstein-Barr virus; VCA, virus capsid antigens. Atypical patterns include VCA IgM positive only, EBNA positive only, or VCA IgM and EBNA positive but VCA IgG negative. Atypical patterns merit repeat testing, testing of a follow-up sample, or testing by alternate methods.

[b]Primary infection with early detection of EBNA1 IgG, or past infection with a prolonged detection of VCA IgM. The antibody titer might help to distinguish primary from past infection; e.g., a high IgM titer combined with a very low EBNA1 IgG might indicate a primary infection, whereas a past infection might be more likely if EBNA1 IgG is present at a high titer and VCA IgM has a low positive value. Additional methods are available to distinguish both infections (see text).

[c]Primary infection without VCA IgM, or past infection with loss of EBNA1 IgG. Depending on the time since exposure, VCA IgM may no longer be detectable in patients with symptoms of infectious mononucleosis. Some patients with past infection lose EBNA1 IgG over time.

presence of rheumatoid factor cross-reacting with other herpesvirus infections and antinuclear factors (129). False negatives may result from insufficiently sensitive assays or when the specimen is collected late, during a period after IgM has disappeared.

In rare cases, immunoblotting including VCA p23, VCA p18, and EBNA 1 p72 may be performed (128). VCA p18 may be important, since antibodies of the IgM class are detectable quite early during infection, whereas IgG antibodies are produced late (similar to EBNA 1 IgG).

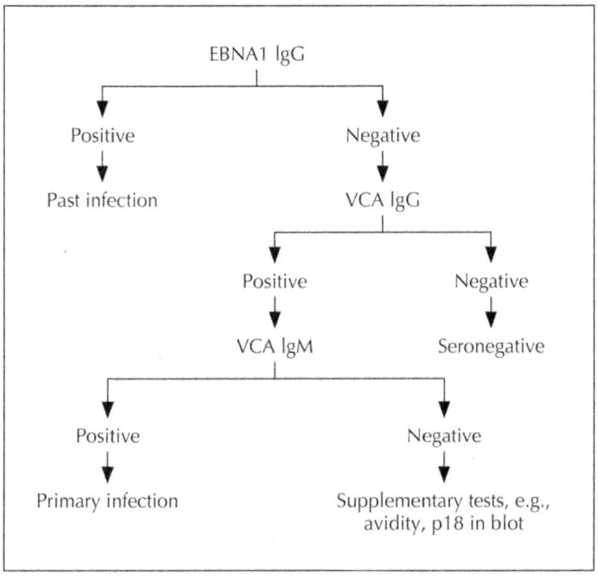

FIGURE 2 Diagnostic algorithm and interpretation scheme based on EBNA 1 used with microparticle multiplex assays or rapid tests with random access in Europe. Diagnostic procedures and interpretation may start with EBNA 1 IgG. If this parameter is positive, a past infection is proven; if EBNA 1 IgG is negative, a negative VCA IgG results in the diagnosis of seronegative and a positive VCA IgM in the diagnosis of a primary infection. If VCA IgG is positive and the other parameters are negative, supplementary tests should be applied, e.g., avidity testing or blotting using p18 antigen.

Thus, a VCA IgG using p18 might be used as substitute for EBNA 1 IgG (124) or as an additional test. If EBNA 1 IgG and p18 IgG are negative, an avidity test for VCA IgG can be informative (128).

In the setting of NPC, different antibody isotypes (mainly IgA but also IgG) targeting a wide variety of antigens (LMP 2, LMP 1, thymidine kinase, BamHI Z-encoded EBV replication activator, EBNA 1, and Zta) have been studied for disease diagnosis. However, for routine diagnostics, VCA and EA have turned out to be the most important ones (130).

EVALUATION, INTERPRETATION, AND REPORTING OF RESULTS

Infectious Mononucleosis

Antibody assays are the method of choice for diagnosing acute EBV infection in immunocompetent hosts. NAAT might be an option for some patients but is usually discouraged in this setting, since EBV DNA may also be detected in healthy seropositive individuals (85, 131, 132). Studies suggest that EBV DNA is cleared rapidly from plasma (within 15 days of IM) (11) but persists significantly longer in whole blood, with clearance from this matrix occurring in most subjects within 200 days (133). Detection of infection in young children (<12 months) in the presence of maternal antibody using serologic techniques is problematic. The use of NAAT to document infection in this setting may be useful and requires further study (13, 85).

Heterophile antibodies are a marker of IM but not necessarily of acute EBV infection. High levels of heterophile antibodies are seen during the first month of IM, normally followed by a rapid decrease. Low but persisting heterophile antibody titers can be found after primary EBV for up to 1 year (119), which can be misleading, and more importantly, heterophile antibodies can sometimes be found in an acute HIV infection, lymphoma, or infection with other infectious agents (e.g., cytomegalovirus, rubella virus, or *T. gondii*) (134, 135). EBV-specific serology should always be performed in settings where the interpretation of a positive heterophile result is uncertain. False-negative heterophile antibody results (15 to 20%) are the rule among young children (118, 136, 137) but also occur for adolescents and adults, particularly when atypical clinical presentations are present. Thus, a negative heterophile antibody test should be supplemented with EBV-specific serology when EBV infection is suspected.

Almost all IM patients have high titers of IgG to various lytic-phase EBV antigens (VCA and EA) but lack antibodies to the EBNA antigens (for details, see Fig. 1). The patient's EBV status can generally be ascertained from a single serum sample by measuring VCA IgG, VCA IgM, and EBNA 1 IgG. In upwards of 90 to 95% of cases, the antibody profile is sufficiently distinct to determine whether the patient (i) is still susceptible to EBV, (ii) has a current primary infection, or (iii) has a past infection (Table 3). The use of terminology such as "recent," "convalescent," or "reactivated" infection, as suggested by some manufacturers in result reporting, is discouraged, since as these diagnoses correspond to infection states in healthy individuals, they are of limited clinical relevance when testing is performed for symptomatic patients. The exact antibody titers and the time needed to develop the complete antibody profile of past infection vary widely between individuals and do not correlate with severity of disease (133, 138). Thus, quantitative measurement of antibodies is of limited usefulness in routine diagnostics.

Nasopharyngeal Carcinoma

In the past, NPC serology—specifically, testing for VCA IgA and EA IgA—has been used as a tumor marker. However, tests for EBV DNA and EBV microRNAs (miRNAs) are superior to serology, since viral load follows a faster kinetics than antibody production and half-life (139–141). For example, EBV DNA becomes rapidly undetectable within a few hours of tumor surgery (142). In a recent screening study, repeated positive EBV DNA in plasma (detection limit, 20 copies/ml) had a sensitivity of 97.1% and a specificity of 98.6% for NPC (143). EBV DNA at different time points prior to, during, and after treatment, as well as its clearance rate, acts as a tumor marker (144–147). DNA is present in plasma and exists as free nonencapsidated DNA in NPC (148). Moreover, EBV DNA load in nasopharyngeal brushings is an important tool to establish diagnosis, especially for early stage disease. In a recent study, a cutoff of 225 copies/ng of DNA had a sensitivity of 96% and a specificity of 97% (149).

Transplantation

In the setting of transplantation, EBV serostatus determination is required for risk stratification. Serostatus determination is problematic with young children and recently transfused patients because of passive antibody. In these settings, donors are considered seropositive and recipients seronegative for risk stratification purposes.

High EBV DNA loads often predict symptoms and signs of EBV-associated PTLD occurring early after transplantation. Routine posttransplantation monitoring of EBV viral load has been recommended for PTLD prevention in high-risk settings (66, 69). Monitoring is combined with preemptive interventions that include mainly reduction in immunosuppression after SOT (69) and rituximab (anti-CD20) therapy after HSCT (84). Reductions in the incidence of early EBV-positive PTLD have been reported by centers using this approach (55). Alternatively, in HSCT recipients, a preemptive adoptive immunotherapy approach (using previously primed donor cells) has been proposed in some centers (69). However, EBV DNA thresholds that could be used as trigger points for intervention remain undefined at a global level. Along with the absolute EBV DNA level, its kinetics may play an important role in defining risk.

In high-risk asymptomatic SOT recipients being serially monitored, the use of EBV DNA load determination as a diagnostic test (i.e., levels above a specific quantitative threshold being diagnostic of PTLD) usually has good sensitivity for detecting EBV-positive PTLD but misses EBV-negative PTLD and some cases of localized PTLD (68). However, it has poor specificity, resulting in good negative predictive values (greater than 90%) but poor positive predictive values (as low as 28% and not greater than 65%) in these populations. Monitoring over the first year after transplantation after SOT and for the first 6 months after HSCT in high-risk populations is recommended in international guidelines (69, 84). In patients with posttransplant primary EBV infection, screening intervals for up to 2 to 3 years are suggested (69). At present, routine monitoring is not recommended in patients at low risk for PTLD or after the individual high-risk period for PTLD (69, 84).

EBV DNA-emia is frequently detected in EBV-seropositive patients after transplantation, and quantitative EBV levels have been proposed as a marker of global immunosuppression that might guide immunosuppressive treatment in this setting (150–153). However, recent studies using Torque teno virus load for the same purpose showed promising results, with the advantage that it could be applied for almost all patients and not only for EBV-positive individuals (154–156).

Without a history of recent or past monitoring, a one-time EBV DNA load in patients presenting with symptoms or signs (usually mass lesions) is difficult to interpret.

Data on the use of EBV NAAT with peripheral blood to monitor PTLD treatment response and predict PTLD relapse are limited. A short-term fall and clearance of EBV DNA in blood coincident with clinical and histologic regression in response to interventions, such as reduction of immunosuppression (157) and adoptive immunotherapy (76), have been observed in PTLD patients and patients with high viral loads receiving preemptive therapy. In contrast, when rituximab was used, EBV DNA levels in cellular blood components often fell dramatically and remained low even when disease progressed and relapsed (158, 159). In pediatric SOT patients, particularly those experiencing primary infection, asymptomatic intermittent or persistent EBV DNA rebound occurs frequently with no short-term consequences (157). Adult PTLD patients have been observed to relapse in the presence of a persistently low viral load (158).

Chronic Active EBV Infection

In patients with chronic active EBV infection, DNA load testing in plasma and in PBMC has been evaluated, and cutoffs using the international standard as reference are established. In PBMC, a cutoff of $10^{2.0}$ IU/μg of DNA can be used with excellent sensitivity and specificity (99.0% and 97.4%) when values are compared to those for patients with past infection. However, when values are compared to those for patients with IM, the cutoff increases to $10^{3.2}$ IU/μg of DNA, and sensitivity and specificity decrease to 81.6% and 86.5% (81).

EBV DNA Load in CSF

Testing of viral load in the CNS is often used to assist in the diagnosis of CNS lymphoma, particularly in immunodeficient patients, based on the observation that CSF EBV

DNA loads in patients with CNS lymphoma are higher than those seen in peripheral blood or may be detectable only in CSF (160). However, the detection of EBV DNA in CSF has a limited positive predictive value for CNS lymphoma, since it is has poor specificity. The prevalence and quantitative levels of CSF EBV DNA observed in non-EBV-related disorders are rather high (160–163). Use of quantitative levels of EBV DNA in CSF in parallel with blood may improve diagnostic specificity (160, 162, 163). Tissue diagnosis remains the gold standard for the diagnosis of CNS lymphoma, with the presence of EBV being documented using immunohistochemistry or *in situ* hybridization in biopsy tissue.

Patients with EBV infections and a background of primary immunodeficiencies, such as X-linked lymphoproliferative syndrome, typically have high EBV DNA loads and do not develop EBNA antibodies. The definitive diagnosis of these conditions requires genetic studies to detect specific associated hereditary mutations (48).

EBV DNA Load in Critically Ill Patients

Elevated EBV DNA load can be found as an epiphenomenon in various disorders, and in critically ill immunocompetent individuals as well. However, it does not seem to negatively influence the outcome (164). Moreover, EBV DNA is detectable to a high percentage in bronchoalveolar fluid mainly without an underlying EBV-related disorder, calling the use of EBV detection in this sample matrix into question (165).

FUTURE PERSPECTIVES

Adjunctive laboratory testing may improve the specificity of high viral load as a predictor of PTLD. The best-studied and most promising tests are assays measuring EBV-specific T cell responses. Different methods have been used for this purpose, such as intracellular cytokine staining, enzyme-linked immunospot assay, and peptide major histocompatibility complex multimer staining (166–169). Although these assays are still not widely utilized in routine laboratory practice, data suggest that the specificity and positive predictive value of EBV DNA load can be significantly improved when it is analyzed in the context of EBV-specific T cell response. In particular, the level of virus-specific $CD4^+$ and $CD8^+$ T cell response appears to be a promising predictive marker for development of PTLD in transplant recipients (166–169).

A particularly interesting source of new EBV diagnostics involves the study of host and viral miRNAs, a class of small noncoding RNAs that are involved in gene regulation by inhibition of protein translation or mRNA degradation (170). Different EBV-associated disorders seem to exhibit a specific miRNA profile. Research with miRNAs has been particularly groundbreaking in hematologic malignancies. Several studies have confirmed that miRNAs play important roles in B cell differentiation and lymphoma pathogenesis and are prognostic for clinical outcome (170, 171). EBV itself encodes 44 mature miRNAs in two gene clusters, BHRF 1 and BART (BamHI A rightward transcripts), and viral and human miRNAs interact with each other in host gene regulation (172–175). An advantage of the study of miRNAs is that due to their small size and molecular stability, they can be studied in formalin-fixed paraffin-embedded tissue used for diagnostic purposes and have been detected in plasma samples (176). Human and EBV miRNA profiles are being extensively studied in a number of EBV-associated malignancies to understand pathogenesis, develop new therapeutic targets, and tailor therapy, as well as being studied as prognostic markers (144, 146, 172, 173, 177–179).

REFERENCES

1. **Longnecker R, Kieff E, Cohen JL.** 2013. Epstein-Barr virus, p 1898–1959. *In* Knipe DM, Howley PM, Cohen JL, Griffin DE, Lamb RA, Martin MA, Racaniello VR, Roizman B (ed), *Fields Virology*, 6th ed. Lippincott Williams &Wilkins, Philadelphia, PA.
2. **Thorley-Lawson DA, Gross A.** 2004. Persistence of the Epstein-Barr virus and the origins of associated lymphomas. *N Engl J Med* **350:**1328–1337.
3. **Hadinoto V, Shapiro M, Sun CC, Thorley-Lawson DA.** 2009. The dynamics of EBV shedding implicate a central role for epithelial cells in amplifying viral output. *PLoS Pathog* **5:**e1000496.
4. **Guerreiro-Cacais AO, Li L, Donati D, Bejarano MT, Morgan A, Masucci MG, Hutt-Fletcher L, Levitsky V.** 2004. Capacity of Epstein-Barr virus to infect monocytes and inhibit their development into dendritic cells is affected by the cell type supporting virus replication. *J Gen Virol* **85:**2767–2778.
5. **Savard M, Bélanger C, Tremblay MJ, Dumais N, Flamand L, Borgeat P, Gosselin J.** 2000. EBV suppresses prostaglandin E2 biosynthesis in human monocytes. *J Immunol* **164:** 6467–6473.
6. **Kimura H, Ito Y, Kawabe S, Gotoh K, Takahashi Y, Kojima S, Naoe T, Esaki S, Kikuta A, Sawada A, Kawa K, Ohshima K, Nakamura S.** 2012. EBV-associated T/NK-cell lymphoproliferative diseases in nonimmunocompromised hosts: prospective analysis of 108 cases. *Blood* **119:**673–686.
7. **Gulley ML, Tang W.** 2008. Laboratory assays for Epstein-Barr virus-related disease. *J Mol Diagn* **10:**279–292.
8. **Middeldorp JM, Brink AA, van den Brule AJ, Meijer CJ.** 2003. Pathogenic roles for Epstein-Barr virus (EBV) gene products in EBV-associated proliferative disorders. *Crit Rev Oncol Hematol* **45:**1–36.
9. **Wagner HJ, Bein G, Bitsch A, Kirchner H.** 1992. Detection and quantification of latently infected B lymphocytes in Epstein-Barr virus-seropositive, healthy individuals by polymerase chain reaction. *J Clin Microbiol* **30:**2826–2829.
10. **Balfour HH, Jr, Odumade OA, Schmeling DO, Mullan BD, Ed JA, Knight JA, Vezina HE, Thomas W, Hogquist KA.** 2013. Behavioral, virologic, and immunologic factors associated with acquisition and severity of primary Epstein-Barr virus infection in university students. *J Infect Dis* **207:** 80–88.
11. **Fafi-Kremer S, Morand P, Germi R, Ballout M, Brion JP, Genoulaz O, Nicod S, Stahl JP, Ruigrok RW, Seigneurin JM.** 2005. A prospective follow-up of Epstein-Barr virus LMP1 genotypes in saliva and blood during infectious mononucleosis. *J Infect Dis* **192:**2108–2111.
12. **Gratama JW, Oosterveer MA, Weimar W, Sintnicolaas K, Sizoo W, Bolhuis RL, Ernberg I.** 1994. Detection of multiple 'Ebnotypes' in individual Epstein-Barr virus carriers following lymphocyte transformation by virus derived from peripheral blood and oropharynx. *J Gen Virol* **75:**85–94.
13. **Piriou E, Asito AS, Sumba PO, Fiore N, Middeldorp JM, Moormann AM, Ploutz-Snyder R, Rochford R.** 2012. Early age at time of primary Epstein-Barr virus infection results in poorly controlled viral infection in infants from Western Kenya: clues to the etiology of endemic Burkitt lymphoma. *J Infect Dis* **205:**906–913.
14. **Piriou ER, van Dort K, Nanlohy NM, Miedema F, van Oers MH, van Baarle D.** 2004. Altered EBV viral load setpoint after HIV seroconversion is in accordance with lack of predictive value of EBV load for the occurrence of AIDS-related non-Hodgkin lymphoma. *J Immunol* **172:** 6931–6937.
15. **Dunmire SK, Grimm JM, Schmeling DO, Balfour HH, Jr, Hogquist KA.** 2015. The incubation period of primary Epstein-Barr virus infection: viral dynamics and immunologic events. *PLoS Pathog* **11:**e1005286.

16. **Fafi-Kremer S, Morand P, Brion JP, Pavese P, Baccard M, Germi R, Genoulaz O, Nicod S, Jolivet M, Ruigrok RW, Stahl JP, Seigneurin JM.** 2005. Long-term shedding of infectious Epstein-Barr virus after infectious mononucleosis. *J Infect Dis* **191:**985–989.
17. **Crawford DH, Macsween KF, Higgins CD, Thomas R, McAulay K, Williams H, Harrison N, Reid S, Conacher M, Douglas J, Swerdlow AJ.** 2006. A cohort study among university students: identification of risk factors for Epstein-Barr virus seroconversion and infectious mononucleosis. *Clin Infect Dis* **43:**276–282.
18. **McAulay KA, Higgins CD, Macsween KF, Lake A, Jarrett RF, Robertson FL, Williams H, Crawford DH.** 2007. HLA class I polymorphisms are associated with development of infectious mononucleosis upon primary EBV infection. *J Clin Invest* **117:**3042–3048.
19. **Johannsen EC, Kaya KM.** 2014. Epstein-Barr virus, p 1754–1771. *In* Bennett JE, Dolin R, Blaser MJ (ed), *Mandell, Douglas, and Bennett's Principles and Practice of Infectious Diseases*, 8th ed. Elsevier Saunders, Philadelphia, PA.
20. **Pullen H, Wright N, Murdoch JM.** 1967. Hypersensitivity reactions to antibacterial drugs in infectious mononucleosis. *Lancet* **ii:**1176–1178.
21. **Patel BM.** 1967. Skin rash with infectious mononucleosis and ampicillin. *Pediatrics* **40:**910–911.
22. **Chovel-Sella A, Ben Tov A, Lahav E, Mor O, Rudich H, Paret G, Reif S.** 2013. Incidence of rash after amoxicillin treatment in children with infectious mononucleosis. *Pediatrics* **131:**e1424–e1427.
23. **Hoagland RJ.** 1964. The incubation period of infectious mononucleosis. *Am J Public Health Nations Health* **54:** 1699–1705.
24. **Petersen I, Thomas JM, Hamilton WT, White PD.** 2006. Risk and predictors of fatigue after infectious mononucleosis in a large primary-care cohort. *QJM* **99:**49–55.
25. **Rafailidis PI, Mavros MN, Kapaskelis A, Falagas ME.** 2010. Antiviral treatment for severe EBV infections in apparently immunocompetent patients. *J Clin Virol* **49:**151–157.
26. **Bartlett A, Williams R, Hilton M.** 2016. Splenic rupture in infectious mononucleosis: a systematic review of published case reports. *Injury* **47:**531–538.
27. **Kimura H, Ito Y, Suzuki R, Nishiyama Y.** 2008. Measuring Epstein-Barr virus (EBV) load: the significance and application for each EBV-associated disease. *Rev Med Virol* **18:** 305–319.
28. **Maakaroun NR, Moanna A, Jacob JT, Albrecht H.** 2010. Viral infections associated with haemophagocytic syndrome. *Rev Med Virol* **20:**93–105.
29. **Hurt C, Tammaro D.** 2007. Diagnostic evaluation of mononucleosis-like illnesses. *Am J Med* **120:**911.e1–911.e8.
30. **De Paor M, O'Brien K, Fahey T, Smith SM.** 2016. Antiviral agents for infectious mononucleosis (glandular fever). *Cochrane Database Syst Rev* **12:**CD011487.
31. **Rezk E, Nofal YH, Hamzeh A, Aboujaib MF, AlKheder MA, Al Hammad MF.** 2015. Steroids for symptom control in infectious mononucleosis. *Cochrane Database Syst Rev* (11):CD004402.
32. **Fujiwara S, Kimura H, Imadome K, Arai A, Kodama E, Morio T, Shimizu N, Wakiguchi H.** 2014. Current research on chronic active Epstein-Barr virus infection in Japan. *Pediatr Int* **56:**159–166.
33. **Kimura H, Morishima T, Kanegane H, Ohga S, Hoshino Y, Maeda A, Imai S, Okano M, Morio T, Yokota S, Tsuchiya S, Yachie A, Imashuku S, Kawa K, Wakiguchi H, Japanese Association for Research on Epstein-Barr Virus and Related Diseases.** 2003. Prognostic factors for chronic active Epstein-Barr virus infection. *J Infect Dis* **187:**527–533.
34. **Sawada A, Inoue M, Kawa K.** 2017. How we treat chronic active Epstein-Barr virus infection. *Int J Hematol* **105:** 406–418.
35. **Thompson MP, Kurzrock R.** 2004. Epstein-Barr virus and cancer. *Clin Cancer Res* **10:**803–821.
36. **Thorley-Lawson DA.** 2015. EBV persistence—introducing the virus. *Curr Top Microbiol Immunol* **390:**151–209.
37. **Münz C.** 2016. Epstein Barr virus—a tumor virus that needs cytotoxic lymphocytes to persist asymptomatically. *Curr Opin Virol* **20:**34–39.
38. **Roskrow MA, Suzuki N, Gan Y, Sixbey JW, Ng CY, Kimbrough S, Hudson M, Brenner MK, Heslop HE, Rooney CM.** 1998. Epstein-Barr virus (EBV)-specific cytotoxic T lymphocytes for the treatment of patients with EBV-positive relapsed Hodgkin's disease. *Blood* **91:**2925–2934.
39. **Chia WK, Teo M, Wang WW, Lee B, Ang SF, Tai WM, Chee CL, Ng J, Kan R, Lim WT, Tan SH, Ong WS, Cheung YB, Tan EH, Connolly JE, Gottschalk S, Toh HC.** 2014. Adoptive T-cell transfer and chemotherapy in the first-line treatment of metastatic and/or locally recurrent nasopharyngeal carcinoma. *Mol Ther* **22:**132–139.
40. **Bollard CM, Rooney CM, Heslop HE.** 2012. T-cell therapy in the treatment of post-transplant lymphoproliferative disease. *Nat Rev Clin Oncol* **9:**510–519.
41. **Secondino S, Zecca M, Licitra L, Gurrado A, Schiavetto I, Bossi P, Locati L, Schiavo R, Basso S, Baldanti F, Maccario R, Locatelli F, Siena S, Pedrazzoli P, Comoli P.** 2012. T-cell therapy for EBV-associated nasopharyngeal carcinoma: preparative lymphodepleting chemotherapy does not improve clinical results. *Ann Oncol* **23:**435–441.
42. **Comoli P, Basso S, Zecca M, Pagliara D, Baldanti F, Bernardo ME, Barberi W, Moretta A, Labirio M, Paulli M, Furione M, Maccario R, Locatelli F.** 2007. Preemptive therapy of EBV-related lymphoproliferative disease after pediatric haploidentical stem cell transplantation. *Am J Transplant* **7:** 1648–1655.
43. **Spieker T, Herbst H.** 2000. Distribution and phenotype of Epstein-Barr virus-infected cells in inflammatory bowel disease. *Am J Pathol* **157:**51–57.
44. **Ciccocioppo R, Racca F, Paolucci S, Campanini G, Pozzi L, Betti E, Riboni R, Vanoli A, Baldanti F, Corazza GR.** 2015. Human cytomegalovirus and Epstein-Barr virus infection in inflammatory bowel disease: need for mucosal viral load measurement. *World J Gastroenterol* **21:**1915–1926.
45. **Magro F, Santos-Antunes J, Albuquerque A, Vilas-Boas F, Macedo GN, Nazareth N, Lopes S, Sobrinho-Simões J, Teixeira S, Dias CC, Cabral J, Sarmento A, Macedo G.** 2013. Epstein-Barr virus in inflammatory bowel disease-correlation with different therapeutic regimens. *Inflamm Bowel Dis* **19:**1710–1716.
46. **Sankaran-Walters S, Ransibrahmanakul K, Grishina I, Hung J, Martinez E, Prindiville T, Dandekar S.** 2011. Epstein-Barr virus replication linked to B cell proliferation in inflamed areas of colonic mucosa of patients with inflammatory bowel disease. *J Clin Virol* **50:**31–36.
47. **Perfetti V, Baldanti F, Lenti MV, Vanoli A, Biagi F, Gatti M, Riboni R, Dallera E, Paulli M, Pedrazzoli P, Corazza GR.** 2016. Detection of active Epstein-Barr virus infection in duodenal mucosa of patients with refractory celiac disease. *Clin Gastroenterol Hepatol* **14:**1216–1220.
48. **Tangye SG, Palendira U, Edwards ES.** 2017. Human immunity against EBV-lessons from the clinic. *J Exp Med* **214:** 269–283.
49. **Lu KT, Schwartzberg PL.** 2010. To B or not to B. *Blood* **116:** 3120–3121.
50. **Booth C, Gilmour KC, Veys P, Gennery AR, Slatter MA, Chapel H, Heath PT, Steward CG, Smith O, O'Meara A, Kerrigan H, Mahlaoui N, Cavazzana-Calvo M, Fischer A, Moshous D, Blanche S, Pachlopnik Schmid J, Latour S, de Saint-Basile G, Albert M, Notheis G, Rieber N, Strahm B, Ritterbusch H, Lankester A, Hartwig NG, Meyts I, Plebani A, Soresina A, Finocchi A, Pignata C, Cirillo E, Bonanomi S, Peters C, Kalwak K, Pasic S, Sedlacek P, Jazbec J, Kanegane H, Nichols KE, Hanson IC, Kapoor N, Haddad E, Cowan M, Choo S, Smart J, Arkwright PD, Gaspar HB.** 2011. X-linked lymphoproliferative disease due to SAP/SH2D1A deficiency: a multicenter study on the manifestations, management and outcome of the disease. *Blood* **117:**53–62 *ERRATUM Blood* **118:**5060.
51. **Cherikh WS, Kauffman HM, McBride MA, Maghirang J, Swinnen LJ, Hanto DW.** 2003. Association of the type of

induction immunosuppression with posttransplant lymphoproliferative disorder, graft survival, and patient survival after primary kidney transplantation. *Transplantation* **76:** 1289–1293.

52. **Landgren O, Gilbert ES, Rizzo JD, Socié G, Banks PM, Sobocinski KA, Horowitz MM, Jaffe ES, Kingma DW, Travis LB, Flowers ME, Martin PJ, Deeg HJ, Curtis RE.** 2009. Risk factors for lymphoproliferative disorders after allogeneic hematopoietic cell transplantation. *Blood* **113:** 4992–5001.
53. **Walker RC.** 1995. Pretransplant assessment of the risk for posttransplant lymphoproliferative disorder. *Transplant Proc* **27**(Suppl 1)**:**41.
54. **Trappe R, Oertel S, Leblond V, Mollee P, Sender M, Reinke P, Neuhaus R, Lehmkuhl H, Horst HA, Salles G, Morschhauser F, Jaccard A, Lamy T, Leithäuser M, Zimmermann H, Anagnostopoulos I, Raphael M, Riess H, Choquet S, German PTLD Study Group, European PTLD Network.** 2012. Sequential treatment with rituximab followed by CHOP chemotherapy in adult B-cell post-transplant lymphoproliferative disorder (PTLD): the prospective international multicentre phase 2 PTLD-1 trial. *Lancet Oncol* **13:**196–206.
55. **Caillard S, Lamy FX, Quelen C, Dantal J, Lebranchu Y, Lang P, Velten M, Moulin B, French Transplant Centers.** 2012. Epidemiology of posttransplant lymphoproliferative disorders in adult kidney and kidney pancreas recipients: report of the French registry and analysis of subgroups of lymphomas. *Am J Transplant* **12:**682–693.
56. **Purgina B, Rao UN, Miettinen M, Pantanowitz L.** 2011. AIDS-related EBV-associated smooth muscle tumors: a review of 64 published cases. *Pathol Res Int* **2011:**561548.
57. **Jonigk D, Laenger F, Maegel L, Izykowski N, Rische J, Tiede C, Klein C, Maecker-Kolhoff B, Kreipe H, Hussein K.** 2012. Molecular and clinicopathological analysis of Epstein-Barr virus-associated posttransplant smooth muscle tumors. *Am J Transplant* **12:**1908–1917.
58. **Conrad A, Brunet AS, Hervieu V, Chauvet C, Buron F, Collardeau-Frachon S, Rivet C, Cassier P, Testelin S, Lachaux A, Morelon E, Thaunat O.** 2013. Epstein-Barr virus-associated smooth muscle tumors in a composite tissue allograft and a pediatric liver transplant recipient. *Transpl Infect Dis* **15:**E182–E186.
59. **Triantos D, Porter SR, Scully C, Teo CG.** 1997. Oral hairy leukoplakia: clinicopathologic features, pathogenesis, diagnosis, and clinical significance. *Clin Infect Dis* **25:**1392–1396.
60. **Chambers AE, Conn B, Pemberton M, Robinson M, Banks R, Sloan P.** 2015. Twenty-first-century oral hairy leukoplakia—a non-HIV-associated entity. *Oral Surg Oral Med Oral Pathol Oral Radiol* **119:**326–332.
61. **Gotoh K, Ito Y, Ohta R, Iwata S, Nishiyama Y, Nakamura T, Kaneko K, Kiuchi T, Ando H, Kimura H.** 2010. Immunologic and virologic analyses in pediatric liver transplant recipients with chronic high Epstein-Barr virus loads. *J Infect Dis* **202:**461–469.
62. **Green M, Soltys K, Rowe DT, Webber SA, Mazareigos G.** 2009. Chronic high Epstein-Barr viral load carriage in pediatric liver transplant recipients. *Pediatr Transplant* **13:**319–323.
63. **Bingler MA, Feingold B, Miller SA, Quivers E, Michaels MG, Green M, Wadowsky RM, Rowe DT, Webber SA.** 2008. Chronic high Epstein-Barr viral load state and risk for late-onset posttransplant lymphoproliferative disease/lymphoma in children. *Am J Transplant* **8:**442–445.
64. **Lau AH, Soltys K, Sindhi RK, Bond G, Mazariegos GV, Green M.** 2010. Chronic high Epstein-Barr viral load carriage in pediatric small bowel transplant recipients. *Pediatr Transplant* **14:**549–553.
65. **Bekker V, Scherpbier H, Beld M, Piriou E, van Breda A, Lange J, van Leth F, Jurriaans S, Alders S, Wertheim-van Dillen P, van Baarle D, Kuijpers T.** 2006. Epstein-Barr virus infects B and non-B lymphocytes in HIV-1-infected children and adolescents. *J Infect Dis* **194:**1323–1330.
66. **Allen UD, Preiksaitis JK, AST Infectious Diseases Community of Practice.** 2013. Epstein-Barr virus and posttransplant lymphoproliferative disorder in solid organ transplantation. *Am J Transplant* **13**(Suppl 4)**:**107–120.
67. **Zimmermann H, Trappe RU.** 2011. Therapeutic options in post-transplant lymphoproliferative disorders. *Ther Adv Hematol* **2:**393–407.
68. **Baldanti F, Rognoni V, Cascina A, Oggionni T, Tinelli C, Meloni F.** 2011. Post-transplant lymphoproliferative disorders and Epstein-Barr virus DNAemia in a cohort of lung transplant recipients. *Virol J* **8:**421.
69. **San-Juan R, Comoli P, Caillard S, Moulin B, Hirsch HH, Meylan P, ESCMID Study Group of Infection in Compromised Hosts.** 2014. Epstein-Barr virus-related post-transplant lymphoproliferative disorder in solid organ transplant recipients. *Clin Microbiol Infect* **20**(Suppl 7)**:**109–118.
70. **Styczynski J, Gil L, Tridello G, Ljungman P, Donnelly JP, van der Velden W, Omar H, Martino R, Halkes C, Faraci M, Theunissen K, Kalwak K, Hubacek P, Sica S, Nozzoli C, Fagioli F, Matthes S, Diaz MA, Migliavacca M, Balduzzi A, Tomaszewska A, Camara RL, van Biezen A, Hoek J, Iacobelli S, Einsele H, Cesaro S, Infectious Diseases Working Party of the European Group for Blood and Marrow Transplantation.** 2013. Response to rituximab-based therapy and risk factor analysis in Epstein Barr virus-related lymphoproliferative disorder after hematopoietic stem cell transplant in children and adults: a study from the Infectious Diseases Working Party of the European Group for Blood and Marrow Transplantation. *Clin Infect Dis* **57:**794–802.
71. **Mentzer SJ, Perrine SP, Faller DV.** 2001. Epstein-Barr virus post-transplant lymphoproliferative disease and virus-specific therapy: pharmacological re-activation of viral target genes with arginine butyrate. *Transpl Infect Dis* **3:**177–185.
72. **AlDabbagh MA, Gitman MR, Kumar D, Humar A, Rotstein C, Husain S.** 2017. The role of antiviral prophylaxis for the prevention of Epstein-Barr virus-associated posttransplant lymphoproliferative disease in solid organ transplant recipients: a systematic review. *Am J Transplant* **17:**770–781.
73. **Reshef R, Vardhanabhuti S, Luskin MR, Heitjan DF, Hadjiliadis D, Goral S, Krok KL, Goldberg LR, Porter DL, Stadtmauer EA, Tsai DE.** 2011. Reduction of immunosuppression as initial therapy for posttransplantation lymphoproliferative disorder. *Am J Transplant* **11:**336–347.
74. **Gottschalk S, Rooney CM.** 2015. Adoptive T-cell immunotherapy. *Curr Top Microbiol Immunol* **391:**427–454.
75. **Vickers MA, Wilkie GM, Robinson N, Rivera N, Haque T, Crawford DH, Barry J, Fraser N, Turner DM, Robertson V, Dyer P, Flanagan P, Newlands HR, Campbell J, Turner ML.** 2014. Establishment and operation of a Good Manufacturing Practice-compliant allogeneic Epstein-Barr virus (EBV)-specific cytotoxic cell bank for the treatment of EBV-associated lymphoproliferative disease. *Br J Haematol* **167:**402–410.
76. **Haque T, Wilkie GM, Jones MM, Higgins CD, Urquhart G, Wingate P, Burns D, McAulay K, Turner M, Bellamy C, Amlot PL, Kelly D, MacGilchrist A, Gandhi MK, Swerdlow AJ, Crawford DH.** 2007. Allogeneic cytotoxic T-cell therapy for EBV-positive posttransplantation lymphoproliferative disease: results of a phase 2 multicenter clinical trial. *Blood* **110:**1123–1131.
77. **Haque T, McAulay KA, Kelly D, Crawford DH.** 2010. Allogeneic T-cell therapy for Epstein-Barr virus-positive posttransplant lymphoproliferative disease: long-term follow-up. *Transplantation* **90:**93–94.
78. **Sokal EM, Hoppenbrouwers K, Vandermeulen C, Moutschen M, Léonard P, Moreels A, Haumont M, Bollen A, Smets F, Denis M.** 2007. Recombinant gp350 vaccine for infectious mononucleosis: a phase 2, randomized, double-blind, placebo-controlled trial to evaluate the safety, immunogenicity, and efficacy of an Epstein-Barr virus vaccine in healthy young adults. *J Infect Dis* **196:**1749–1753.
79. **Elliott SL, Suhrbier A, Miles JJ, Lawrence G, Pye SJ, Le TT, Rosenstengel A, Nguyen T, Allworth A, Burrows SR, Cox J, Pye D, Moss DJ, Bharadwaj M.** 2008. Phase I trial of a CD8+ T-cell peptide epitope-based vaccine for infectious mononucleosis. *J Virol* **82:**1448–1457.

80. **Hui EP, Taylor GS, Jia H, Ma BB, Chan SL, Ho R, Wong WL, Wilson S, Johnson BF, Edwards C, Stocken DD, Rickinson AB, Steven NM, Chan AT.** 2013. Phase I trial of recombinant modified vaccinia ankara encoding Epstein-Barr viral tumor antigens in nasopharyngeal carcinoma patients. *Cancer Res* **73:**1676–1688.
81. **Ito Y, Suzuki M, Kawada J, Kimura H.** 2016. Diagnostic values for the viral load in peripheral blood mononuclear cells of patients with chronic active Epstein-Barr virus disease. *J Infect Chemother* **22:**268–271.
82. **Bower M, Palfreeman A, Alfa-Wali M, Bunker C, Burns F, Churchill D, Collins S, Cwynarski K, Edwards S, Fields P, Fife K, Gallop-Evans E, Kassam S, Kulasegaram R, Lacey C, Marcus R, Montoto S, Nelson M, Newsom-Davis T, Orkin C, Shaw K, Tenant-Flowers M, Webb A, Westwell S, Williams M, British HIV Association.** 2014. British HIV Association guidelines for HIV-associated malignancies 2014. *HIV Med* **15**(Suppl 2)**:**1–92.
83. **Humar A, Michaels M, AST ID Working Group on Infectious Disease Monitoring.** 2006. American Society of Transplantation recommendations for screening, monitoring and reporting of infectious complications in immunosuppression trials in recipients of organ transplantation. *Am J Transplant* **6:**262–274.
84. **Styczynski J, Reusser P, Einsele H, de la Camara R, Cordonnier C, Ward KN, Ljungman P, Engelhard D.** 2009. Management of HSV, VZV and EBV infections in patients with hematological malignancies and after SCT: guidelines from the Second European Conference on Infections in Leukemia. *Bone Marrow Transplant* **43:**757–770.
85. **Jiang SY, Yang JW, Shao JB, Liao XL, Lu ZH, Jiang H.** 2016. Real-time polymerase chain reaction for diagnosing infectious mononucleosis in pediatric patients: a systematic review and meta-analysis. *J Med Virol* **88:**871–876.
86. **Liu TB, Zheng ZH, Pan J, Pan LL, Chen LH.** 2017. Prognostic role of plasma Epstein-Barr virus DNA load for nasopharyngeal carcinoma: a meta-analysis. *Clin Invest Med* **40:**E1–E12.
87. **Tse E, Kwong YL.** 2014. Management of advanced NK/T-cell lymphoma. *Curr Hematol Malig Rep* **9:**233–242.
88. **Gandhi MK, Lambley E, Burrows J, Dua U, Elliott S, Shaw PJ, Prince HM, Wolf M, Clarke K, Underhill C, Mills T, Mollee P, Gill D, Marlton P, Seymour JF, Khanna R.** 2006. Plasma Epstein-Barr virus (EBV) DNA is a biomarker for EBV-positive Hodgkin's lymphoma. *Clin Cancer Res* **12:**460–464.
89. **Kanakry JA, Hegde AM, Durand CM, Massie AB, Greer AE, Ambinder RF, Valsamakis A.** 2016. The clinical significance of EBV DNA in the plasma and peripheral blood mononuclear cells of patients with or without EBV diseases. *Blood* **127:**2007–2017.
90. **Ryan JL, Fan H, Swinnen LJ, Schichman SA, Raab-Traub N, Covington M, Elmore S, Gulley ML.** 2004. Epstein-Barr virus (EBV) DNA in plasma is not encapsidated in patients with EBV-related malignancies. *Diagn Mol Pathol* **13:**61–68.
91. **Connolly Y, Littler E, Sun N, Chen X, Huang PC, Stacey SN, Arrand JR.** 2001. Antibodies to Epstein-Barr virus thymidine kinase: a characteristic marker for the serological detection of nasopharyngeal carcinoma. *Int J Cancer* **91:**692–697.
92. **Grässer FA, Murray PG, Kremmer E, Klein K, Remberger K, Feiden W, Reynolds G, Niedobitek G, Young LS, Mueller-Lantzsch N.** 1994. Monoclonal antibodies directed against the Epstein-Barr virus-encoded nuclear antigen 1 (EBNA1): immunohistologic detection of EBNA1 in the malignant cells of Hodgkin's disease. *Blood* **84:**3792–3798.
93. **Niedobitek G, Herbst H.** 2006. In situ detection of Epstein-Barr virus and phenotype determination of EBV-infected cells. *Methods Mol Biol* **326:**115–137.
94. **Weiss LM, Chen YY.** 2013. EBER in situ hybridization for Epstein-Barr virus. *Methods Mol Biol* **999:**223–230.
95. **Junying J, Herrmann K, Davies G, Lissauer D, Bell A, Timms J, Reynolds GM, Hubscher SG, Young LS, Niedobitek G, Murray PG.** 2003. Absence of Epstein-Barr virus DNA in the tumor cells of European hepatocellular carcinoma. *Virology* **306:**236–243.
96. **Kimura H, Miyake K, Yamauchi Y, Nishiyama K, Iwata S, Iwatsuki K, Gotoh K, Kojima S, Ito Y, Nishiyama Y.** 2009. Identification of Epstein-Barr virus (EBV)-infected lymphocyte subtypes by flow cytometric in situ hybridization in EBV-associated lymphoproliferative diseases. *J Infect Dis* **200:**1078–1087.
97. **Kawabe S, Ito Y, Gotoh K, Kojima S, Matsumoto K, Kinoshita T, Iwata S, Nishiyama Y, Kimura H.** 2012. Application of flow cytometric in situ hybridization assay to Epstein-Barr virus-associated T/natural killer cell lymphoproliferative diseases. *Cancer Sci* **103:**1481–1488.
98. **Calattini S, Sereti I, Scheinberg P, Kimura H, Childs RW, Cohen JI.** 2010. Detection of EBV genomes in plasmablasts/plasma cells and non-B cells in the blood of most patients with EBV lymphoproliferative disorders by using immuno-FISH. *Blood* **116:**4546–4559.
99. **Gulley ML, Tang W.** 2010. Using Epstein-Barr viral load assays to diagnose, monitor, and prevent posttransplant lymphoproliferative disorder. *Clin Microbiol Rev* **23:**350–366.
100. **Gärtner B, Preiksaitis JK.** 2010. EBV viral load detection in clinical virology. *J Clin Virol* **48:**82–90.
101. **Preiksaitis JK, Pang XL, Fox JD, Fenton JM, Caliendo AM, Miller GG, American Society of Transplantation Infectious Diseases Community of Practice.** 2009. Interlaboratory comparison of Epstein-Barr virus viral load assays. *Am J Transplant* **9:**269–279.
102. **Fryer JF, Heath AB, Wilkinson DE, Minor PD, Collaborative Study Group.** 2016. A collaborative study to establish the 1st WHO international standard for Epstein-Barr virus for nucleic acid amplification techniques. *Biologicals* **44:**423–433.
103. **Sanosyan A, Fayd'herbe de Maudave A, Bollore K, Zimmermann V, Foulongne V, Van de Perre P, Tuaillon E.** 2017. The impact of targeting repetitive BamHI-W sequences on the sensitivity and precision of EBV DNA quantification. *PLoS One* **12:**e0183856.
104. **Ruf S, Wagner HJ.** 2013. Determining EBV load: current best practice and future requirements. *Expert Rev Clin Immunol* **9:**139–151.
105. **Ryan JL, Fan H, Glaser SL, Schichman SA, Raab-Traub N, Gulley ML.** 2004. Epstein-Barr virus quantitation by real-time PCR targeting multiple gene segments: a novel approach to screen for the virus in paraffin-embedded tissue and plasma. *J Mol Diagn* **6:**378–385.
106. **Tsai DE, Douglas L, Andreadis C, Vogl DT, Arnoldi S, Kotloff R, Svoboda J, Bloom RD, Olthoff KM, Brozena SC, Schuster SJ, Stadtmauer EA, Robertson ES, Wasik MA, Ahya VN.** 2008. EBV PCR in the diagnosis and monitoring of posttransplant lymphoproliferative disorder: results of a two-arm prospective trial. *Am J Transplant* **8:**1016–1024.
107. **Ishii H, Ogino T, Berger C, Köchli-Schmitz N, Nagato T, Takahara M, Nadal D, Harabuchi Y.** 2007. Clinical usefulness of serum EBV DNA levels of BamHI W and LMP1 for nasal NK/T-cell lymphoma. *J Med Virol* **79:**562–572.
108. **Le QT, Jones CD, Yau TK, Shirazi HA, Wong PH, Thomas EN, Patterson BK, Lee AW, Zehnder JL.** 2005. A comparison study of different PCR assays in measuring circulating plasma Epstein-Barr virus DNA levels in patients with nasopharyngeal carcinoma. *Clin Cancer Res* **11:**5700–5707.
109. **Stevens SJ, Verkuijlen SA, Hariwiyanto B, Harijadi, Fachiroh J, Paramita DK, Tan IB, Haryana SM, Middeldorp JM.** 2005. Diagnostic value of measuring Epstein-Barr virus (EBV) DNA load and carcinoma-specific viral mRNA in relation to anti-EBV immunoglobulin A (IgA) and IgG antibody levels in blood of nasopharyngeal carcinoma patients from Indonesia. *J Clin Microbiol* **43:**3066–3073.
110. **Semenova T, Lupo J, Alain S, Perrin-Confort G, Grossi L, Dimier J, Epaulard O, Morand P, Germi R.** 2016. Multicenter evaluation of whole-blood Epstein-Barr viral load standardization using the WHO international standard. *J Clin Microbiol* **54:**1746–1750.
111. **Hayden RT, Sun Y, Tang L, Procop GW, Hillyard DR, Pinsky BA, Young SA, Caliendo AM.** 2017. Progress in quantitative viral load testing: variability and impact of the WHO quantitative international standards. *J Clin Microbiol* **55:**423–430.

112. **Rychert J, Danziger-Isakov L, Yen-Lieberman B, Storch G, Buller R, Sweet SC, Mehta AK, Cheeseman JA, Heeger P, Rosenberg ES, Fishman JA.** 2014. Multicenter comparison of laboratory performance in cytomegalovirus and Epstein-Barr virus viral load testing using international standards. *Clin Transplant* **28:**1416–1423.
113. **Abbate I, Piralla A, Calvario A, Callegaro A, Giraldi C, Lunghi G, Gennari W, Sodano G, Ravanini P, Conaldi PG, Vatteroni M, Gaeta A, Paba P, Cavallo R, Baldanti F, Lazzarotto T, AMCLI–Infections in Transplant Working Group GLaIT.** 2016. Nation-wide measure of variability in HCMV, EBV and BKV DNA quantification among centers involved in monitoring transplanted patients. *J Clin Virol* **82:**76–83.
114. **Hakim H, Gibson C, Pan J, Srivastava K, Gu Z, Bankowski MJ, Hayden RT.** 2007. Comparison of various blood compartments and reporting units for the detection and quantification of Epstein-Barr virus in peripheral blood. *J Clin Microbiol* **45:**2151–2155.
115. **Ruf S, Behnke-Hall K, Gruhn B, Bauer J, Horn M, Beck J, Reiter A, Wagner HJ.** 2012. Comparison of six different specimen types for Epstein-Barr viral load quantification in peripheral blood of pediatric patients after heart transplantation or after allogeneic hematopoietic stem cell transplantation. *J Clin Virol* **53:**186–194.
116. **Baldanti F, Gatti M, Furione M, Paolucci S, Tinelli C, Comoli P, Merli P, Locatelli F.** 2008. Kinetics of Epstein-Barr virus DNA load in different blood compartments of pediatric recipients of T-cell-depleted HLA-haploidentical stem cell transplantation. *J Clin Microbiol* **46:**3672–3677.
117. **Kwok H, Chiang AK.** 2016. From conventional to next generation sequencing of Epstein-Barr virus genomes. *Viruses* **8:**60.
118. **Bruu AL, Hjetland R, Holter E, Mortensen L, Natås O, Petterson W, Skar AG, Skarpaas T, Tjade T, Asjø B.** 2000. Evaluation of 12 commercial tests for detection of Epstein-Barr virus-specific and heterophile antibodies. *Clin Diagn Lab Immunol* **7:**451–456.
119. **De Paschale M, Clerici P.** 2012. Serological diagnosis of Epstein-Barr virus infection: problems and solutions. *World J Virol* **1:**31–43.
120. **Odumade OA, Hogquist KA, Balfour HH, Jr.** 2011. Progress and problems in understanding and managing primary Epstein-Barr virus infections. *Clin Microbiol Rev* **24:**193–209.
121. **Hess RD.** 2004. Routine Epstein-Barr virus diagnostics from the laboratory perspective: still challenging after 35 years. *J Clin Microbiol* **42:**3381–3387.
122. **Gu AD, Mo HY, Xie YB, Peng RJ, Bei JX, Peng J, Li MY, Chen LZ, Feng QS, Jia WH, Zeng YX.** 2008. Evaluation of a multianalyte profiling assay and an enzyme-linked immunosorbent assay for serological examination of Epstein-Barr virus-specific antibody responses in diagnosis of nasopharyngeal carcinoma. *Clin Vaccine Immunol* **15:**1684–1688.
123. **Wong J, Sibani S, Lokko NN, LaBaer J, Anderson KS.** 2009. Rapid detection of antibodies in sera using multiplexed self-assembling bead arrays. *J Immunol Methods* **350:** 171–182.
124. **Klutts JS, Ford BA, Perez NR, Gronowski AM.** 2009. Evidence-based approach for interpretation of Epstein-Barr virus serological patterns. *J Clin Microbiol* **47:**3204–3210.
125. **Binnicker MJ, Jespersen DJ, Harring JA, Rollins LO, Beito EM.** 2008. Evaluation of a multiplex flow immunoassay for detection of epstein-barr virus-specific antibodies. *Clin Vaccine Immunol* **15:**1410–1413.
126. **Gärtner BC, Kortmann K, Schäfer M, Mueller-Lantzsch N, Sester U, Kaul H, Pees H.** 2000. No correlation in Epstein-Barr virus reactivation between serological parameters and viral load. *J Clin Microbiol* **38:**2458.
127. **Tay JK, Chan SH, Lim CM, Siow CH, Goh HL, Loh KS.** 2016. The role of Epstein-Barr virus DNA load and serology as screening tools for nasopharyngeal carcinoma. *Otolaryngol Head Neck Surg* **155:**274–280.
128. **Bauer G.** 2001. Simplicity through complexity: immunoblot with recombinant antigens as the new gold standard in Epstein-Barr virus serology. *Clin Lab* **47:**223–230.
129. **Linde A, Kallin B, Dillner J, Andersson J, Jägdahl L, Lindvall A, Wahren B.** 1990. Evaluation of enzyme-linked immunosorbent assays with two synthetic peptides of Epstein-Barr virus for diagnosis of infectious mononucleosis. *J Infect Dis* **161:**903–909.
130. **Chen Y, Xin X, Cui Z, Zheng Y, Guo J, Chen Y, Lin Y, Su G.** 2016. Diagnostic value of serum Epstein-Barr virus capsid antigen-IgA for nasopharyngeal carcinoma: a meta-analysis based on 21 studies. *Clin Lab* **62:**1155–1166.
131. **Ling PD, Lednicky JA, Keitel WA, Poston DG, White ZS, Peng R, Liu Z, Mehta SK, Pierson DL, Rooney CM, Vilchez RA, Smith EO, Butel JS.** 2003. The dynamics of herpesvirus and polyomavirus reactivation and shedding in healthy adults: a 14-month longitudinal study. *J Infect Dis* **187:**1571–1580.
132. **Maurmann S, Fricke L, Wagner HJ, Schlenke P, Hennig H, Steinhoff J, Jabs WJ.** 2003. Molecular parameters for precise diagnosis of asymptomatic Epstein-Barr virus reactivation in healthy carriers. *J Clin Microbiol* **41:**5419–5428.
133. **Balfour HH, Jr, Verghese P.** 2013. Primary Epstein-Barr virus infection: impact of age at acquisition, coinfection, and viral load. *J Infect Dis* **207:**1787–1789.
134. **Vidrih JA, Walensky RP, Sax PE, Freedberg KA.** 2001. Positive Epstein-Barr virus heterophile antibody tests in patients with primary human immunodeficiency virus infection. *Am J Med* **111:**192–194.
135. **Walensky RP, Rosenberg ES, Ferraro MJ, Losina E, Walker BD, Freedberg KA.** 2001. Investigation of primary human immunodeficiency virus infection in patients who test positive for heterophile antibody. *Clin Infect Dis* **33:**570–572.
136. **Sumaya CV, Ench Y.** 1985. Epstein-Barr virus infectious mononucleosis in children. II. Heterophil antibody and viral-specific responses. *Pediatrics* **75:**1011–1019.
137. **Linderholm M, Boman J, Juto P, Linde A.** 1994. Comparative evaluation of nine kits for rapid diagnosis of infectious mononucleosis and Epstein-Barr virus-specific serology. *J Clin Microbiol* **32:**259–261.
138. **Balfour HH, Jr, Dunmire SK, Hogquist KA.** 2015. Infectious mononucleosis. *Clin Transl Immunology* **4:**e33.
139. **Fan H, Nicholls J, Chua D, Chan KH, Sham J, Lee S, Gulley ML.** 2004. Laboratory markers of tumor burden in nasopharyngeal carcinoma: a comparison of viral load and serologic tests for Epstein-Barr virus. *Int J Cancer* **112:** 1036–1041.
140. **Lin JC, Wang WY, Liang WM, Chou HY, Jan JS, Jiang RS, Wang JY, Twu CW, Liang KL, Chao J, Shen WC.** 2007. Long-term prognostic effects of plasma Epstein-Barr virus DNA by minor groove binder-probe real-time quantitative PCR on nasopharyngeal carcinoma patients receiving concurrent chemoradiotherapy. *Int J Radiat Oncol Biol Phys* **68:** 1342–1348.
141. **Adham M, Greijer AE, Verkuijlen SA, Juwana H, Fleig S, Rachmadi L, Malik O, Kurniawan AN, Roezin A, Gondhowiardjo S, Atmakusumah D, Stevens SJ, Hermani B, Tan IB, Middeldorp JM.** 2013. Epstein-Barr virus DNA load in nasopharyngeal brushings and whole blood in nasopharyngeal carcinoma patients before and after treatment. *Clin Cancer Res* **19:**2175–2186.
142. **To EW, Chan KC, Leung SF, Chan LY, To KF, Chan AT, Johnson PJ, Lo YM.** 2003. Rapid clearance of plasma Epstein-Barr virus DNA after surgical treatment of nasopharyngeal carcinoma. *Clin Cancer Res* **9:**3254–3259.
143. **Chan KCA, Woo JKS, King A, Zee BCY, Lam WKJ, Chan SL, Chu SWI, Mak C, Tse IOL, Leung SYM, Chan G, Hui EP, Ma BBY, Chiu RWK, Leung SF, van Hasselt AC, Chan ATC, Lo YMD.** 2017. Analysis of plasma Epstein-Barr virus DNA to screen for nasopharyngeal cancer. *N Engl J Med* **377:**513–522.
144. **He ML, Luo MX, Lin MC, Kung HF.** 2012. MicroRNAs: potential diagnostic markers and therapeutic targets for EBV-associated nasopharyngeal carcinoma. *Biochim Biophys Acta* **1825:**1–10.
145. **Wong AM, Kong KL, Tsang JW, Kwong DL, Guan XY.** 2012. Profiling of Epstein-Barr virus-encoded microRNAs in

nasopharyngeal carcinoma reveals potential biomarkers and oncomirs. *Cancer* **118:**698–710.

146. **Zhang G, Zong J, Lin S, Verhoeven RJ, Tong S, Chen Y, Ji M, Cheng W, Tsao SW, Lung M, Pan J, Chen H.** 2015. Circulating Epstein-Barr virus microRNAs miR-BART7 and miR-BART13 as biomarkers for nasopharyngeal carcinoma diagnosis and treatment. *Int J Cancer* **136:** E301–E312.
147. **Wang WY, Twu CW, Chen HH, Jiang RS, Wu CT, Liang KL, Shih YT, Chen CC, Lin PJ, Liu YC, Lin JC.** 2013. Long-term survival analysis of nasopharyngeal carcinoma by plasma Epstein-Barr virus DNA levels. *Cancer* **119:**963–970.
148. **Chan KC, Zhang J, Chan AT, Lei KI, Leung SF, Chan LY, Chow KC, Lo YM.** 2003. Molecular characterization of circulating EBV DNA in the plasma of nasopharyngeal carcinoma and lymphoma patients. *Cancer Res* **63:**2028–2032.
149. **Zheng XH, Lu LX, Li XZ, Jia WH.** 2015. Quantification of Epstein-Barr virus DNA load in nasopharyngeal brushing samples in the diagnosis of nasopharyngeal carcinoma in southern China. *Cancer Sci* **106:**1196–1201.
150. **Lee TC, Savoldo B, Rooney CM, Heslop HE, Gee AP, Caldwell Y, Barshes NR, Scott JD, Bristow LJ, O'Mahony CA, Goss JA.** 2005. Quantitative EBV viral loads and immunosuppression alterations can decrease PTLD incidence in pediatric liver transplant recipients. *Am J Transplant* **5:**2222–2228.
151. **Bakker NA, Verschuuren EA, Erasmus ME, Hepkema BG, Veeger NJ, Kallenberg CG, van der Bij W.** 2007. Epstein-Barr virus-DNA load monitoring late after lung transplantation: a surrogate marker of the degree of immunosuppression and a safe guide to reduce immunosuppression. *Transplantation* **83:**433–438.
152. **Doesch AO, Konstandin M, Celik S, Kristen A, Frankenstein L, Sack FU, Schnabel P, Schnitzler P, Katus HA, Dengler TJ.** 2008. Epstein-Barr virus load in whole blood is associated with immunosuppression, but not with post-transplant lymphoproliferative disease in stable adult heart transplant patients. *Transpl Int* **21:**963–971.
153. **Ahya VN, Douglas LP, Andreadis C, Arnoldi S, Svoboda J, Kotloff RM, Hadjiliadis D, Sager JS, Woo YJ, Pochettino A, Schuster SJ, Stadtmauer EA, Tsai DE.** 2007. Association between elevated whole blood Epstein-Barr virus (EBV)-encoded RNA EBV polymerase chain reaction and reduced incidence of acute lung allograft rejection. *J Heart Lung Transplant* **26:**839–844.
154. **Görzer I, Jaksch P, Strassl R, Klepetko W, Puchhammer-Stöckl E.** 2017. Association between plasma Torque teno virus level and chronic lung allograft dysfunction after lung transplantation. *J Heart Lung Transplant* **36:**366–368.
155. **Schiemann M, Puchhammer-Stöckl E, Eskandary F, Kohlbeck P, Rasoul-Rockenschaub S, Heilos A, Kozakowski N, Görzer I, Kikić Ž, Herkner H, Böhmig GA, Bond G.** 2017. Torque teno virus load—inverse association with antibody-mediated rejection after kidney transplantation. *Transplantation* **101:**360–367.
156. **Focosi D, Macera L, Pistello M, Maggi F.** 2014. Torque Teno virus viremia correlates with intensity of maintenance immunosuppression in adult orthotopic liver transplant. *J Infect Dis* **210:**667–668.
157. **Green M, Cacciarelli TV, Mazariegos GV, Sigurdsson L, Qu L, Rowe DT, Reyes J.** 1998. Serial measurement of Epstein-Barr viral load in peripheral blood in pediatric liver transplant recipients during treatment for posttransplant lymphoproliferative disease. *Transplantation* **66:** 1641–1644.
158. **Oertel S, Trappe RU, Zeidler K, Babel N, Reinke P, Hummel M, Jonas S, Papp-Vary M, Subklewe M, Dörken B, Riess H, Gärtner B.** 2006. Epstein-Barr viral load in whole blood of adults with posttransplant lymphoproliferative disorder after solid organ transplantation does not correlate with clinical course. *Ann Hematol* **85:**478–484.
159. **Yang J, Tao Q, Flinn IW, Murray PG, Post LE, Ma H, Piantadosi S, Caligiuri MA, Ambinder RF.** 2000. Characterization of Epstein-Barr virus-infected B cells in patients with posttransplantation lymphoproliferative disease: disappearance after rituximab therapy does not predict clinical response. *Blood* **96:**4055–4063.
160. **Yanagisawa K, Tanuma J, Hagiwara S, Gatanaga H, Kikuchi Y, Oka S.** 2013. Epstein-Barr viral load in cerebrospinal fluid as a diagnostic marker of central nervous system involvement of AIDS-related lymphoma. *Intern Med* **52:**955–959.
161. **Cocuzza CE, Piazza F, Musumeci R, Oggioni D, Andreoni S, Gardinetti M, Fusco L, Frigo M, Banfi P, Rottoli MR, Confalonieri P, Rezzonico M, Ferrò MT, Cavaletti G, EBV-MS Italian Study Group.** 2014. Quantitative detection of Epstein-Barr virus DNA in cerebrospinal fluid and blood samples of patients with relapsing-remitting multiple sclerosis. *PLoS One* **9:**e94497 *ERRATUM PLoS One* **9:**e103890.
162. **Corcoran C, Rebe K, van der Plas H, Myer L, Hardie DR.** 2008. The predictive value of cerebrospinal fluid Epstein-Barr viral load as a marker of primary central nervous system lymphoma in HIV-infected persons. *J Clin Virol* **42:** 433–436.
163. **Weinberg A, Li S, Palmer M, Tyler KL.** 2002. Quantitative CSF PCR in Epstein-Barr virus infections of the central nervous system. *Ann Neurol* **52:**543–548.
164. **Walton AH, Muenzer JT, Rasche D, Boomer JS, Sato B, Brownstein BH, Pachot A, Brooks TL, Deych E, Shannon WD, Green JM, Storch GA, Hotchkiss RS.** 2014. Reactivation of multiple viruses in patients with sepsis. *PLoS One* **9:**e98819.
165. **Friedrichs I, Bingold T, Keppler OT, Pullmann B, Reinheimer C, Berger A.** 2013. Detection of herpesvirus EBV DNA in the lower respiratory tract of ICU patients: a marker of infection of the lower respiratory tract? *Med Microbiol Immunol (Berl)* **202:**431–436.
166. **Calarota SA, Chiesa A, Zelini P, Comolli G, Minoli L, Baldanti F.** 2013. Detection of Epstein-Barr virus-specific memory CD4+ T cells using a peptide-based cultured enzyme-linked immunospot assay. *Immunology* **139:**533–544.
167. **Sebelin-Wulf K, Nguyen TD, Oertel S, Papp-Vary M, Trappe RU, Schulzki A, Pezzutto A, Riess H, Subklewe M.** 2007. Quantitative analysis of EBV-specific CD4/CD8 T cell numbers, absolute CD4/CD8 T cell numbers and EBV load in solid organ transplant recipients with PLTD. *Transpl Immunol* **17:**203–210.
168. **Smets F, Latinne D, Bazin H, Reding R, Otte JB, Buts JP, Sokal EM.** 2002. Ratio between Epstein-Barr viral load and anti-Epstein-Barr virus specific T-cell response as a predictive marker of posttransplant lymphoproliferative disease. *Transplantation* **73:**1603–1610.
169. **Meij P, van Esser JW, Niesters HG, van Baarle D, Miedema F, Blake N, Rickinson AB, Leiner I, Pamer E, Lowenberg B, Cornelissen JJ, Gratama JW.** 2003. Impaired recovery of Epstein-Barr virus (EBV)-specific CD8+ T lymphocytes after partially T-depleted allogeneic stem cell transplantation may identify patients at very high risk for progressive EBV reactivation and lymphoproliferative disease. *Blood* **101:**4290–4297.
170. **Di Lisio L, Martinez N, Montes-Moreno S, Piris-Villaespesa M, Sanchez-Beato M, Piris MA.** 2012. The role of miRNAs in the pathogenesis and diagnosis of B-cell lymphomas. *Blood* **120:**1782–1790.
171. **Alencar AJ, Malumbres R, Kozloski GA, Advani R, Talreja N, Chinichian S, Briones J, Natkunam Y, Sehn LH, Gascoyne RD, Tibshirani R, Lossos IS.** 2011. MicroRNAs are independent predictors of outcome in diffuse large B-cell lymphoma patients treated with R-CHOP. *Clin Cancer Res* **17:**4125–4135.
172. **Fink SE, Gandhi MK, Nourse JP, Keane C, Jones K, Crooks P, Jöhrens K, Korfel A, Schmidt H, Neumann S, Tiede A, Jäger U, Dührsen U, Neuhaus R, Dreyling M, Borchert K, Südhoff T, Riess H, Anagnostopoulos I, Trappe RU.** 2014. A comprehensive analysis of the cellular and EBV-specific microRNAome in primary CNS PTLD identifies different patterns among EBV-associated tumors. *Am J Transplant* **14:**2577–2587.
173. **Kim DN, Lee SK.** 2012. Biogenesis of Epstein-Barr virus microRNAs. *Mol Cell Biochem* **365:**203–210.

174. **Martín-Pérez D, Vargiu P, Montes-Moreno S, León EA, Rodríguez-Pinilla SM, Lisio LD, Martínez N, Rodríguez R, Mollejo M, Castellvi J, Pisano DG, Sánchez-Beato M, Piris MA.** 2012. Epstein-Barr virus microRNAs repress BCL6 expression in diffuse large B-cell lymphoma. *Leukemia* **26:**180–183.
175. **Riley KJ, Rabinowitz GS, Yario TA, Luna JM, Darnell RB, Steitz JA.** 2012. EBV and human microRNAs co-target oncogenic and apoptotic viral and human genes during latency. *EMBO J* **31:**2207–2221.
176. **Nourse JP, Crooks P, Keane C, Nguyen-Van D, Mujaj S, Ross N, Jones K, Vari F, Han E, Trappe R, Fink S, Gandhi MK.** 2012. Expression profiling of Epstein-Barr virus-encoded microRNAs from paraffin-embedded formalin-fixed primary Epstein-Barr virus-positive B-cell lymphoma samples. *J Virol Methods* **184:**46–54.
177. **Imig J, Motsch N, Zhu JY, Barth S, Okoniewski M, Reineke T, Tinguely M, Faggioni A, Trivedi P, Meister G, Renner C, Grässer FA.** 2011. microRNA profiling in Epstein-Barr virus-associated B-cell lymphoma. *Nucleic Acids Res* **39:**1880–1893.
178. **Jun SM, Hong YS, Seo JS, Ko YH, Yang CW, Lee SK.** 2008. Viral microRNA profile in Epstein-Barr virus-associated peripheral T cell lymphoma. *Br J Haematol* **142:**320–323.
179. **Kim DN, Chae HS, Oh ST, Kang JH, Park CH, Park WS, Takada K, Lee JM, Lee WK, Lee SK.** 2007. Expression of viral microRNAs in Epstein-Barr virus-associated gastric carcinoma. *J Virol* **81:**1033–1036.
180. **Hsu JL, Glaser SL.** 2000. Epstein-barr virus-associated malignancies: epidemiologic patterns and etiologic implications. *Crit Rev Oncol Hematol* **34:**27–53.
181. **Rowe M, Zuo J.** 2010. Immune responses to Epstein-Barr virus: molecular interactions in the virus evasion of CD8+ T cell immunity. *Microbes Infect* **12:**173–181.
182. **Hansen TH, Bouvier M.** 2009. MHC class I antigen presentation: learning from viral evasion strategies. *Nat Rev Immunol* **9:**503–513.
183. **Grywalska E, Rolinski J.** 2015. Epstein-Barr virus-associated lymphomas. *Semin Oncol* **42:**291–303.

Human Herpesviruses 6A, 6B, and 7*

ALEXANDER L. GRENINGER, RUTH HALL SEDLAK, AND KEITH R. JEROME

104

HUMAN HERPESVIRUS 6

Taxonomy

Human herpesvirus (HHV) 6A, HHV-6B, and HHV-7 are three distinct virus species that make up the *Roseolovirus* genus (1). Although HHV-6A and HHV-6B were originally considered subtypes of the same viral species, they were officially classified as distinct viral species in 2012 (2). Together with cytomegalovirus (CMV), which is discussed in a separate chapter, the roseoloviruses represent the four human viruses of the *Betaherpesvirus* subfamily. Roseoloviruses share many features of their genomic architecture and genetic content, the ability to replicate and establish latent infections in lymphocytes, associations with febrile rash in young children and with a variety of neurologic disorders, and the ability to act as opportunistic pathogens in immunocompromised patients. HHV-6A and HHV-6B have the ability to genetically recombine with each other in the laboratory (3). For convenience, we sometimes refer to HHV-6A and HHV-6B collectively as HHV-6 when there are no discriminating data.

Description of the Agent

HHV-6 virions are about 200 nm in diameter and consist of four major components: a double-stranded DNA genome (160 to 170 kb) within the core of an icosahedral capsid surrounded by a proteinaceous tegument, all of which is surrounded by a lipid bilayer envelope containing a variety of viral and cellular proteins. The viral genomes carry approximately 100 unique genes. HHV-6A and HHV-6B share approximately 95% nucleotide identity with each other, which is by far the highest similarity of any two species of human herpesvirus. By comparison, HHV-6A and B share approximately 60% nucleotide identity in alignable regions with HHV-7 and are essentially unalignable in nucleotide space with CMV (<45% nucleotide identity in housekeeping genes).

A recent genomic study of HHV-6B showed that actively replicating HHV-6B strains cluster by geographical origin and are highly similar to each other, with an average pairwise nucleotide identity of >99.9% (4). Comparatively few genome sequences from acute infections of HHV-6A are available, although the pairwise sequencing identity among HHV-6A strains suggests similar conservation to that seen in HHV-6B.

Epidemiology and Transmission

Epidemiology

The seroprevalence of HHV-6A and HHV-6B together is high (>90%) (5), but as discussed later, extensive cross-reactivity has hindered large-scale assessment of the specific seroprevalence of each virus. Transmission is thought to occur mainly via saliva (6). Most individuals become infected by the age of 2 or 3 years (7). In the United States, Japan, and Europe, HHV-6B is typically acquired in early childhood and infects nearly all individuals, and HHV-6A prevalence in these areas may exceed 50% by adulthood. In Zambia, HHV-6A was reported in >85% of asymptomatic infants, suggesting possible international differences in the epidemiology of the HHV-6 variants (8). However, in Uganda, over 90% of newly acquired HHV-6 infections by infants were HHV-6B (9). Further studies will be required to develop a full understanding of regional differences.

Tissue Distribution

The cell surface receptor for HHV-6A is CD46, while the receptor for HHV-6B is CD134 (10). As such, the tissue distribution of the two viruses appears to be distinct, although the differential detection of the two viruses is confounded by their differing prevalence. HHV-6B DNA has been detected in as many as 90% of peripheral blood mononuclear cell (PBMC) specimens, >80% of brains, >90% of tonsils (in epithelial cells of tonsillar crypts), and 40 to 90% of oral fluid and nasal mucus specimens; it has been detected less frequently in skin, lungs, endomyocardial biopsy specimens, goblet cells and histiocytes of the large intestine, cervical fluids, and ocular aqueous humor. HHV-6B is commonly detected in the gastrointestinal tract of transplant patients (11). The receptor tropism may be associated with delayed T-cell reconstitution in transplant patients with reactivated HHV-6 (12). During primary infection in young children in the United States, HHV-6A was found by PCR in 2.5% of PBMC and 17% of cerebrospinal fluid (CSF) specimens, while HHV-6B was

*This chapter contains information presented by Philip E. Pellett and Graham Tipples in chapter 102 of the 11th edition of this *Manual*.

found in 99% of PBMC and 86% of CSF specimens (13). The median salivary viral level of HHV-6B increases from approximately 10^3 copies of HHV-6/ml at 1 week postinfection to 10^5 copies of HHV-6/ml by 8 weeks postinfection (7). Shedding may persist at substantial levels into adulthood (14, 15). HHV-6A DNA was reported to be present in over half of lung specimens, mostly in conjunction with HHV-6B (16). In a study of adult brains from 40 consecutive autopsies, 28% were positive for HHV-6A and 75% for HHV-6B (17). For bone marrow transplant recipients, HHV-6A and HHV-6B have both been detected in plasma, but HHV-6B was the species overwhelmingly detected in PBMC (18, 19).

Latency, Persistence, and Transmission

Other than during the acute phase of roseola, HHV-6 can seldom be detected by culture. However, HHV-6 DNA can be detected in PBMC from 90% of children by PCR, and transcripts can occasionally be detected in asymptomatic children (~1% of specimens) (20). This suggests that latent infection is established in PBMC. Latent HHV-6B has been detected in monocytes, PBMC-derived dendritic cells, and their CD34+ bone marrow progenitors (21). Unlike other human herpesviruses, HHV-6A and -6B appear to establish latency via integration into subtelomeric regions of host cells, rather than as episomes (22). The cell tropism of HHV-6A latency is less well understood, although latency has been established in oligodendrocytes *in vitro* (23). Both HHV-6B and HHV-7 are detected in high proportions of salivary glands, suggesting that it is a critical reservoir of persistent infection and shedding (24, 25). Primary infection with HHV-6 typically occurs with the waning of maternal antibody, with transmission likely occurring via saliva (6). HHV-6 was not detected in breast milk, suggesting that it is not a significant vehicle for transmission (26). Little is known of HHV-6A transmission.

Unique among the human herpesviruses, approximately 1% of the population harbors inherited chromosomally integrated HHV-6 (iciHHV-6) genomes at a chromosomal telomere. This occurs via vertical transmission through the germ line, and as such, all cells in these individuals harbor viral DNA (22, 27). iciHHV-6 can result in persistence of high levels of HHV-6 DNA in CSF and blood, which is most commonly observed in posttransplant patients (28). It is still unclear how frequently iciHHV-6 reactivates, although recent reports suggest it is possible (29, 30) and may explain some cases of congenital infection (31, 32). While some iciHHV-6B strains genomically cluster with acute HHV-6B strains, many unrelated iciHHV-6 cases share identical iciHHV-6 sequences, suggesting a founder effect in inheritance of HHV-6 (4, 33).

Clinical Significance

While infections with HHV-6 are generally subclinical or mild in immunocompetent individuals, they can be severe in immunocompromised persons.

Primary Infection

HHV-6 primary infection causes roseola (also called roseola infantum, sixth disease, and exanthem subitum) and accounts for 10 to 20% of febrile illness presenting to the emergency department in the 6- to 12-month-old population (34). While HHV-6B is the predominant etiologic agent of roseola, rare cases of HHV-6A-associated roseola or febrile illness have been reported. About 94% of children are symptomatic at the time of primary infection, with specifically associated symptoms including fever (58%), fussiness (70%), rhinorrhea (66%), diarrhea (26%), rash (31%), and roseola (24%) (7).

Classic roseola symptoms include an abrupt rise in temperature (39 to 40°C), which persists for 3 to 5 days. Fever abatement coincides with onset of a blanching maculopapular rash (Fig. 1), which resolves within 3 days. Initial appearance of the rash is on the neck, behind the ears, and on the back, followed by spread to the rest of the body. The illness lasts 2 to 7 days, usually with no sequelae. Other clinical symptoms of roseola may include lymphadenopathy, erythematous tympanic membranes, and uvulopalatoglossal junctional papules (Nagayama spots) prior to rash onset.

Primary HHV-6 infection may also present as fever without rash or rash without fever, because three-quarters of cases do not meet clinical definitions of roseola. Less common but more severe forms of primary HHV-6 infection may include fever of >40°C, respiratory tract distress, diarrhea, and convulsions. Although seizures are rare for HHV-6 primary infections, primary HHV-6 infections account for a significant portion of febrile seizures in young children (35, 36). Recent studies have also suggested a relationship between HHV-6, febrile seizures, and the subsequent development of mesial temporal lobe epilepsy (37, 38). Other serious but rare complications reported with HHV-6 primary infections include hepatosplenomegaly, Gianatti syndrome (an acrodermatitis of childhood that has been associated with hepatitis B virus and Epstein-Barr

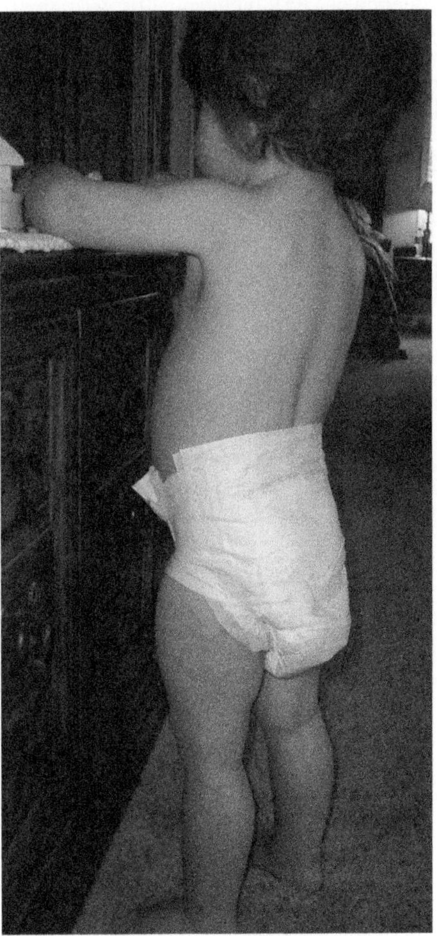

FIGURE 1 Child with roseola during primary HHV-6B infection. Public domain photo from M. Davis.

virus infections), bulging fontanels, aseptic meningitis, encephalitis (perhaps 1% of meningitis and encephalitis cases) (35), poor neurologic outcomes following congenital infection, and disseminated fatal infection.

Primary HHV-6 infection in adults is rare but can be severe. Clinical presentation in these cases may include a mononucleosis-like illness, prolonged lymphadenopathy, and fulminant hepatitis.

Transplant Recipients and Immunosuppressed Populations

HHV-6 reactivation generally occurs in the context of immune suppression. For example, HHV-6 can reactivate in AIDS patients and lead to disseminated infection (39). The most common clinical setting for HHV-6 reactivation is transplantation. Most cases are due to HHV-6B; less than 3% are thought to result from HHV-6A. In contrast, HHV-6B can be detected in plasma or serum in 30 to 50% of transplant recipients (40–42). Reactivation typically occurs within the first 2 to 4 weeks posttransplant; the median time to HHV-6 reactivation was reported to be 20 days for HHV-6, compared to 27 days for HHV-7 and 36 days for CMV (5).

Multiple disease manifestations have been associated with HHV-6 reactivation in transplant recipients. Of these, encephalitis is the best documented. HHV-6 associated encephalitis occurs in approximately 1% of hematopoietic cell transplants and can lead to damage of the limbic system, brain stem, and hippocampus, manifesting in seizures, cognitive problems, and abnormal electroencephalogram. The frequency of HHV-6 encephalitis varies by transplant type; it reaches approximately 10% in cord blood transplant recipients (42), while it appears to be much less frequent in solid organ transplantation (41, 43). Interestingly, levels of HHV-6 DNA found in CSF during reactivation tend to be higher than during primary disease (44). HHV-6 also appears to have effects on the central nervous system that are subtler than frank encephalitis, including delirium and cognitive decline after hematopoietic cell transplantation (45).

HHV-6 reactivation after transplant has also been associated with other clinical manifestations. Myelosuppression and delayed engraftment have been reported (46, 47). Several studies have also associated HHV-6 with the development of acute graft-versus-host disease (40, 46, 48, 49). Interestingly, one study suggests that either HHV-6 reactivation or acute graft-versus-host disease predisposes to the subsequent development of the other (50); future studies should clarify the mechanisms and causality of this relationship. HHV-6 may contribute to allograft dysfunction and rejection; in one study of liver transplantation, some patients with graft hepatitis responded favorably to antiviral therapy (51). Beyond allografts, HHV-6 has also been reported to affect organs in the context of hematopoietic cell transplantation, including liver (52) and lung (53). Detection of HHV-6 in bronchoalveolar lavage has been associated with idiopathic pneumonia syndrome (53). Finally, HHV-6 has been associated with an increased risk of CMV reactivation, both in hematopoietic (40, 54) and solid organ transplants (55, 56). Coreactivation of HHV-6 and CMV is associated with a worse outcome in intensive care unit patients than either virus alone (57). Similarly, several studies have demonstrated that HHV-6 reactivation is a predictor of increased mortality after hematopoietic cell transplantation (40, 46, 58). Whether these relationships indicate a causal relationship or instead merely reflect the underlying immunosuppression remains to be established. Despite these associations, a randomized clinical trial of patients after liver transplant demonstrated no clinical benefit from routine monitoring for HHV-6 (59).

iciHHV-6 may affect clinical outcomes in immunocompromised patients, but further study is required (60, 61). Acute graft-versus-host disease grades 2 to 4 have been shown to be more frequent when recipients or donors had iciHHV-6. CMV viremia is also more frequent among recipients with iciHHV-6 (62).

Other

Drug-Induced Hypersensitivity Syndromes

Exposure to certain drugs occasionally results in a severe and sometimes fatal reaction variously known as drug-induced hypersensitivity syndrome, drug rash with eosinophilia and systemic symptoms, and anticonvulsant hypersensitivity syndrome (63). HHV-6 reactivations have been identified specifically in the acute phases of drug rash with eosinophilia and systemic symptoms cases but not in toxic epidermal necrolysis or Stevens-Johnson syndrome (64). It remains to be seen whether HHV-6 contributes to either initiation or exacerbation of the events or instead represents a biomarker of immune activation (65).

Hashimoto's Thyroiditis

Hashimoto's thyroiditis (HT) is an autoimmune condition in which the thyroid gland is gradually destroyed. The disease is more common in women and is thought to result from a combination of genetic and environmental factors. Two studies have reported a higher prevalence and viral load of HHV-6 in thyroid fine-needle aspirates or thyroid tissue from HT/autoimmune thyroid disease patients compared to controls (66, 67). Immunohistochemistry revealed expression of HHV-6 antigens on thyroid tissue from HT patients. Higher natural killer cell activity and T-cell responses to HHV-6-infected thyroid cells were observed in HT patients compared to controls, suggesting a possible role in pathogenesis.

Cardiomyopathy and Cardiovascular Disease

HHV-6B antigens and DNA have been detected in damaged cardiac tissues of patients with acute and chronic cardiomyopathies (68, 69). A study of 19,597 participants, with a 0.58% prevalence of iciHHV-6, found a 3.3 times greater prevalence of angina pectoris in iciHHV-6-positive individuals compared to non-iciHHV-6-positive individuals but no association with myocardial infarction (70).

Other Diseases

There is no conclusive evidence for causal associations between HHV-6 and multiple sclerosis, malignancy, or chronic fatigue syndrome. A population-based case-control study of 1,090 women with incident breast cancer and 1,053 controls from British Columbia and Ontario (Canada) found no statistically significant associations between inherited chromosomally integrated HHV-6 and breast cancer in women (odds ratio 0.87). HHV-6 has been suggested to be a biomarker for physiological fatigue associated with military training but is not associated with chronic fatigue syndrome or other pathological fatigue syndromes (71). For many of these associations, proof of causality will require randomized clinical trials using an efficacious antiviral drug (72).

Therapy

Antiviral treatment of HHV-6 has been reviewed in depth (5). No antivirals are licensed for treatment of HHV-6. Therapeutic approaches are similar to those for human

CMV, including ganciclovir, cidofovir, and foscarnet, which show *in vitro* activity against HHV-6. Artesunate has anti-HHV-6 activity *in vitro* and was reported to effectively treat a case of HHV-6B-associated myocarditis (68). The few trials completed to date on the use of antivirals for HHV-6 have not demonstrated statistically significant improvements in outcomes (73–75). Nevertheless, it is considered prudent to use antiviral therapy in the setting of HHV-6 reactivation in immunocompromised individuals (76). It is important to distinguish iciHHV-6 from HHV-6 reactivation when considering antiviral therapy for patients with detectable HHV-6, and clinical symptoms should weigh heavily in treatment decisions (27). Indeed, testing for iciHHV-6 is often used to justify stopping antiviral therapy in the setting of a positive HHV-6 PCR without clear symptoms. Nevertheless, it is important to recognize that HHV-6 reactivation and disease can occur in the setting of iciHHV-6, and thus the presence of iciHHV-6 is by itself not enough to justify halting treatment if symptoms are compatible with HHV-6 disease.

Collection, Transport, and Storage of Specimens

Saliva specimens can be collected for virus detection by various methods, including filter paper strips (77), oral swabs, throat swabs, and expectorated saliva collection. Plasma should be separated from cells shortly after collection to avoid false-positive results for individuals with iciHHV-6 due to release of cellular DNA. Serum, plasma, CSF, bronchoalveolar lavage fluid, and cells or tissues intended for PCR can be shipped frozen. A single freeze-thaw cycle was associated with a 10-fold decrease in HHV-6 quantitation in one study (14). CSF specimens for testing by the FilmArray Meningitis/Encephalitis panel (BioFire/bioMérieux, Salt Lake City, UT) can be stored for up to 1 day at room temperature, or up to 7 days under refrigeration. Whole blood is the specimen of choice for iciHHV-6 testing using droplet digital PCR (78).

Direct Examination

Direct detection of HHV-6 can be done by immunohistochemistry (79, 80), *in situ* hybridization, and *in situ* or other PCR (81, 82). The most common method of detection by far is PCR. The sensitivity of PCR is of particular value for the detection of HHV-6, given that even during periods of viral activity, viral DNA can be at relatively low concentrations. A multitude of PCR strategies have been published that utilize numerous HHV-6 genomic targets and, in some instances, inclusion in multiplex assays (83, 84). HHV-6A and HHV-6B can readily be distinguished by appropriate choice of PCR primers and probes. Reverse transcription PCR for detection of HHV-6 mRNA can be useful for specific detection of active HHV6 replication and may be useful to discriminate between latent virus and reactivation (85), which may be particularly relevant in the setting of iciHHV-6.

Quantitative PCR (from whole blood or PBMC) is useful for the determination of baseline viral load levels in transplant patients, with significant increases above baseline indicating active infection and increased risk of clinical disease. Testing can be performed on plasma, serum, whole blood, or PBMC. We recommend the use of plasma for HHV-6 PCR. Detection of HHV-6 DNA in serum or plasma appears to correlate well with indicators of active replication (86); in contrast, detection of HHV-6 in other sample types can result from the presence of latently infected cells or DNA released from them.

As is the case for all quantitative real-time PCR assays, testing for HHV-6 should incorporate a coamplified internal positive control, and ideally the two HHV-6 species should be distinguished. Important variables that need to be carefully standardized and incorporated into the sensitivity calculation and interpretation are the amount of material initially lysed to prepare the template (e.g., volume of fluid or number of cells) and the amount of this material that is included in each reaction mixture (87, 88).

Selected reference laboratories performing HHV-6 testing are summarized in Table 1. Thorough evaluations of HHV-6 PCR assays are essential (83), as are ongoing comparisons and proficiency testing to improve the standardization of quantitative assays (89). Interlaboratory quantitative agreement for HHV-6 viral load is poor (89, 90). To address this, the World Health Organization has recently made a provisional international standard available for HHV-6, which consists of cultured Z29 type strain for HHV-6B and the GS type strain for HHV-6A. Both of these standards have been noted to have large tandem repeats in the origin of replication and the potential for large genomic rearrangements, similar to that seen in the JC and BK polyomaviruses (3, 91–93), and as such, diagnostic PCR assays should avoid these regions. HHV-6 has recently been included in an FDA-cleared multiplex PCR panel for meningitis/encephalitis, and it is likely that HHV-6 detection in the context of encephalitis will increase as more labs perform HHV-6 testing (Table 2) (94).

Digital PCR quantitation is especially attractive for HHV-6 given the ability to accurately count copies of human and viral DNA. In digital PCR, a sample is divided into thousands of individual partitions, each of which undergoes PCR amplification to the endpoint. The proportion of partitions with positive amplification allows calculation of the starting concentration of analyte. Digital PCR is substantially more accurate and precise than traditional quantitative PCR (qPCR). The accuracy of digital PCR may also provide a solution to the poor commutability of quantitative testing discussed above.

Isolation Procedures

HHV-6 can be isolated from patient PBMC by cocultivation with stimulated human umbilical cord blood lymphocytes (95–97), but virus culture is not used for routine clinical diagnostics.

Identification

HHV-6 virions have typical herpesvirus morphology by electron microscopy, i.e., approximately 200-nm spherical enveloped virions containing a 90- to 110-nm icosahedral capsid with an electron-dense core surrounded by an amorphous tegument (1). Numerous monoclonal antibodies are available (both commercially and from research laboratories) that react with HHV-6A and/or HHV-6B (98).

Typing Systems

HHV-6A and HHV-6B can be typed through the use of species-specific monoclonal antibodies and species-specific PCR assays. In many cases, differentiation of HHV-6A and HHV-6B is not essential for patient management, but assays that discriminate between HHV-6A and HHV-6B may be useful in the setting of coinfection or the presence of iciHHV-6 (99) and may lead to a better understanding of the clinical manifestations of these viruses. Typing systems have typically been based on primer binding regions that are highly conserved between HHV-6A and HHV-6B, with an intervening region that can be targeted by probes specific for one or the other virus. However, the recent expansion of

TABLE 1 Selected reference laboratories offering HHV-6 and HHV-7 testing

Laboratory	Website	HHV-6 PCR	HHV-6 Serology	iciHHV-6	HHV-7 PCR	HHV-7 Serology
ARUP Laboratories	www.aruplab.com	qPCR (serum, plasma, CSF)	IgM, IgG			
Coppe Labs	http://www.coppelabs.com/	qPCR, reverse transcription PCR (plasma, whole blood, CSF, bone marrow, tissue)		PCR (hair follicles, nail clippings)		
Labcorp	www.labcorp.com	PCR, qPCR (serum, plasma, whole blood, CSF)	IgM, IgG			
Mayo Medical Labs	www.mayomedicallaboratories.com	PCR, qPCR (serum, plasma, whole blood, CSF, BAL, bone marrow)				
Quest Diagnostics	www.questdiagnostics.com	qPCR (serum, plasma, whole blood, CSF, BAL, bone marrow, urine)	IgM, IgG		qPCR (serum, plasma, whole blood)	IgM, IgG
University of Washington	www.depts.washington.edu/uwviro	PCR, qPCR (serum, plasma, whole blood, CSF, BAL, bone marrow, tissue)		ddPCR (whole blood)		
Viracor	www.viracor-eurofins.com	PCR, qPCR (serum, plasma, whole blood, CSF, BAL, bone marrow, urine, stool, tissue)	IgM, IgG		PCR, qPCR (serum, plasma, whole blood, CSF, BAL, bone marrow, urine, stool, tissue)	

[a]BAL, bronchoalveolar lavage fluid; ddPCR, droplet digital PCR.

whole HHV-6 genomes available in GenBank allows other approaches to PCR assay design as well.

Serologic Tests

Numerous serologic methods for detecting HHV-6 antibodies have been described, and commercial reagents are available. These serologic methods have limited utility for diagnosis of primary infections and are unable to reliably identify HHV-6 reactivations. Recent versus past infections have been discriminated through the use of immunofluorescence-based antibody avidity tests, though these are not available clinically (100). Maturation from low- to high-avidity HHV-6 antibody following primary HHV-6 infection takes approximately 5 months.

TABLE 2 FDA-cleared and CE-IVD marked assays for HHV-6 detection

Regulatory status	Name	Manufacturer	LoD[a]	Gene target	Sensitivity	Specificity
FDA cleared						
	FilmArray Meningitis/Encephalitis panel	BioFire/bioMérieux	10,000 copies/ml	Unknown	85.7%	99.7%
CE/IVD marked						
	HHV-6 ELITe MGB kit	ELITechGroup	132 copies/ml	ORF13R, U67	100%	100%
	RealStar HHV-6 PCR kit	Altona	50 copies/ml	Unknown	100%	100%
	artus HHV-6 RG PCR kit	Qiagen	2 copies/μl DNA extract	Unknown	100%	100%
	Herpes virus type 6 (HHV6) PCR Kit CE/IVD	Emelca	5 copies/μl DNA extract	U67		
	Human herpes virus 6/7 (HHV-6/7) PCR kit	GeneProof	500 copies/ml	U57		
	CMV HHV6,7,8 R-Gene	bioMérieux	555 copies/ml whole blood	U57	100%	96.40%
	RealLine HHV-6	Bioron	100 copies/sample	U72	100%	100%

[a]LOD, limit of detection.

Antibody avidity testing can also be used to differentiate between HHV-6 and HHV-7 primary infections. Neutralizing antibodies typically become detectable 3 to 8 days following the onset of fever during primary infection.

Due to their protein sequence homology, there is extensive serologic cross-reactivity between HHV-6A and HHV-6B and also substantial cross-reactivity with HHV-7 and CMV (100, 101). The simultaneous rise in antibodies to both HHV-6 and human CMV seen in some patients may be due to the combination of simultaneous activity of both viruses together with responses to cross-reactive antigens. One assay has been reported to distinguish between antibodies to HHV-6A and HHV-6B (102), but this assay has not found widespread use. Despite some serologic cross-reactivity between HHV-6 and HHV-7, adsorption methods and antibody avidity tests can be used for differentiation (100).

Antiviral Susceptibilities

The highest *in vitro* antiviral sensitivities and selectivities have consistently been seen for foscarnet, cidofovir, and ganciclovir. Similar to human CMV, mutations in the HHV-6 U69-encoded protein kinase or the HHV-6 U38-encoded DNA polymerase gene can cause HHV-6 resistance to these drugs (103, 104). HHV-6 antiviral susceptibility testing is not available clinically, but a rapid PCR-based genotyping assay for U69-associated mutations for ganciclovir resistance has been developed (105). Ganciclovir-resistant HHV-6 has been reported in post-transplantation cases, but it is extraordinarily rare (106).

Evaluation, Interpretation, and Reporting of Results

The diagnosis of HHV-6 infection is complicated by the varying clinical manifestations, the ability of the virus to establish and later reactivate from latency, and the entity of iciHHV-6. As such, the testing ordered and the interpretation of results should rely heavily on the clinical presentation.

The most common presentation of HHV-6 is primary infection in young children. As described previously in this chapter, such presentation is usually quite typical; while the rash of exanthem subitum (roseola) can be visually dramatic, systemic symptoms and fever are comparatively mild. While primary infection with roseoloviruses leads to significant health care utilization (7), in uncomplicated cases clinical diagnosis without confirmatory lab testing may suffice. On the other hand, testing in such circumstances may be justified if it is likely to provide other benefits such as preventing unnecessary hospitalization or excessive use of antibiotics. As a more severe presentation, roseoloviruses account for approximately one-third of cases of febrile status epilepticus (36), and inclusion of HHV-6 in the differential diagnosis is warranted, along with PCR testing of CSF and plasma.

The most usual setting for HHV-6 testing is in the context of immunosuppression, especially hematopoietic cell or solid organ transplantation. Again, HHV-6 can present with a variety of end-organ complications, but the most common is central nervous system alteration. The mainstay of laboratory diagnosis is PCR testing. While there are currently no FDA-cleared quantitative assays available for HHV-6, a wide variety of validated HHV-6 DNA load assays are available from reference and other laboratories (Tables 1 and 2). It is important to recognize that interlaboratory agreement for quantitative HHV-6 PCR testing is poor; as such, there are no widely accepted quantitative thresholds for therapy, and clinicians should avoid comparing viral load measurements from different labs. This situation may improve with the recent introduction of a WHO international standard, although previous experience with the CMV international standard suggests that this will not completely solve the issue of interlaboratory commutability (107).

For most clinical presentations, we recommend PCR testing on plasma or serum, along with another specimen based on the clinical symptoms present (CSF, bronchoalveolar lavage fluid, or tissue). Most laboratories interpret the detection of virus in such samples as suggestive of a pathogenic role for HHV-6; however, with improved standardization of assays it may be possible in the future to define viral load thresholds that can better guide clinical treatment decisions. The lack of detection of HHV-6 in plasma does not rule out localized active infection in a specific organ or tissue. On the other hand, it is important to recognize that detection of low-level HHV-6 in cellular specimens such as tissue or whole blood can also reflect the presence of latent virus rather than active viral replication. Finally, as with all PCR assays for a single analyte, it is important to note that the presence of HHV-6 does not rule out the possible presence of other copathogens. The recent development of simple-to-perform and highly multiplexed assays that include HHV-6, such as the BioFire FilmArray (bioMérieux), may be helpful in this regard; as always, the clinical context should drive test selection and result interpretation.

The detection of HHV-6 DNA by PCR can be especially difficult to interpret in the context of iciHHV-6. Cellular specimens from such patients have high HHV-6 levels, but plasma from such patients is also typically PCR positive due to the release of cellular DNA (which by definition includes viral DNA in cases of iciHHV-6). Thus, it is often useful to rule out iciHHV-6 in patients with high-level HHV-6 in plasma, especially if such levels are not consistent with the clinical presentation. Previously, testing for iciHHV-6 required fluorescence *in situ* hybridization or quantitative PCR analysis of hair follicles or fingernail clippings, but the introduction of digital PCR has allowed the development of rapid and accessible testing for iciHHV-6. In the context of iciHHV-6, the precision of digital PCR is more important in that it allows the simultaneous quantitation of HHV-6 and a human reference gene (RPP30). Because people with iciHHV-6 have one copy of HHV-6 in each cell, iciHHV-6 is ruled out if the ratio of HHV-6 to cellular genome equivalents (two RPP30/cell) falls outside a range of 1 ± 0.07 (78), with the exception of rare individuals with two or more copies of iciHHV-6, in whom the virus/genome ratio will still fall close to 2.0, 3.0, or higher integers. Some experts have suggested that testing for iciHHV-6 should be routine in the management of transplant patients (108).

Although iciHHV-6 can explain high viral loads in plasma, it is important to recognize that patients with iciHHV-6 can still have active HHV-6 replication with associated pathology. For patients with underlying iciHHV-6A, HHV-6B reactivation can be identified by a multiplexed type-specific digital PCR assay (99); presumably the converse, although rare, would be true as well. For patients with iciHHV-6B, active replication cannot be diagnosed by qPCR or digital PCR because of the background reactivity. In this case, the detection of viral RNA transcripts by reverse transcription real-time qPCR appears very promising for distinguishing latent from active infections, although such assays are not yet widely available.

Beyond PCR and its variants, other testing modalities for HHV-6 have extremely limited roles in clinical management. Culture has been considered the "gold standard" approach for direct detection, but it is labor-intensive, slow, and insensitive and thus is not suited for clinical use. Serologic testing is more valuable in population-based studies of viral acquisition and prevalence; the use of paired sera in primary infection is too slow to be clinically useful, and IgM testing is unable to reliably detect primary versus recurrent infection (109).

HHV-7

Taxonomy and Description of the Agent

HHV-7 is one of three distinct viral species (along with HHV-6A and HHV-6B) that compose the *Roseolovirus* genus (1). Together with CMV, the roseoloviruses represent the four human viruses of the *Betaherpesvirus* subfamily. Roseoloviruses share many features of their genomic architecture and genetic content, the ability to replicate and establish latent infections in lymphocytes, associations with febrile rash in young children and with a variety of neurologic disorders, and the ability to act as opportunistic pathogens in immunocompromised patients. HHV-7 virions are approximately 170 nm in diameter and consist of four major components: a double-stranded DNA genome (145 kb) within the core of an icosahedral capsid surrounded by a proteinaceous tegument, all of which is surrounded by a lipid bilayer envelope that is studded with a variety of viral and cellular proteins. Less sequence data is available for HHV-7 compared to the other roseoloviruses, but HHV-7 genomes carry approximately 100 unique genes and share approximately 60% nucleotide identity in alignable regions with HHV-6A and HHV-6B.

Epidemiology and Transmission

Epidemiology

Like HHV-6, HHV-7 infection is highly prevalent (110) and infects most individuals during childhood. The typical age for primary infection with HHV-7 may be somewhat older (median 26 months) than for HHV-6 (111).

Tissue Distribution

HHV-7 mainly infects CD4+ lymphocytes, although the virus can likely infect other cell types as well (112, 113). The major cellular receptor is CD4, most likely in conjunction with cellular glycoproteins (114). HHV-7 antigens have been detected in salivary gland acini, lungs, skin, and mammary glands, and more sporadically, in the liver, kidneys, and tonsils (115). HHV-7 DNA has been detected by PCR in PBMC, salivary glands, gastric mucosa, skin, cervical swabs, bronchoalveolar lavage samples, and brain (116), although in some cases DNA detection may reflect the presence of infected CD4+ T cells. Infectious HHV-7 is easily isolated from the saliva of healthy adults. The ability to detect HHV-7 DNA in uncultured lymphocytes by PCR, along with the inability to detect infectious virus in the absence of T-cell activation, suggests that the virus establishes latency in CD4+ cells. A recent report suggests that, like HHV-6, HHV-7 may occasionally integrate into the germ line, resulting in iciHHV-7 (117).

Transmission

HHV-7 is frequently detectable by PCR in saliva from healthy adults. It has been suggested that salivary levels of HHV-7 and/or HHV-6 may represent a biomarker for physiological as opposed to pathological fatigue (71). While the most plausible route of transmission is via saliva, HHV-7 has also been detected in breast milk, urine, and cervical secretions. In contrast to HHV-6, congenital transmission of HHV-7 appears to occur rarely if at all (118).

Clinical Significance

Primary Infection

Like HHV-6, HHV-7 can cause exanthema subitum (roseola), although it may cause this condition less frequently than does HHV-6. As noted above, the typical age for primary infection with HHV-7 may be somewhat older (median 26 months) than for HHV-6 (111). Among children with symptomatic primary disease there appears to be no difference between HHV-6 and HHV-7 in terms of degree of fever, rash, or gastrointestinal symptoms. However, children with primary HHV-7 infection may be at higher risk for seizures compared to those with primary HHV-6 infection (35, 111).

Immunocompromised Patients

Like all herpesviruses, HHV-7 establishes latency after primary infection, and thus reactivation can later occur, particularly in the setting of immunodeficiency. The frequency of recurrence after solid organ transplantation has been estimated to be 0 to 45%, with most cases occurring in the first 2 to 4 weeks posttransplant (119). In general, symptomatic disease associated with HHV-7 has not been well documented, although scattered case reports have been published. A randomized clinical trial of patients after liver transplant demonstrated no clinical benefit from routine monitoring for HHV-7 (59).

Other

HHV-7 DNA has been detected more frequently and at higher loads in affected tissues from nonimmunocompromised patients with interstitial pneumonia (120, 121). HHV-7 DNA has been found in 20 to 50% of bronchoalveolar lavage and transbronchial biopsy specimens from lung transplant patients (122), but assignment of a causative role is difficult because of the frequent codetection of CMV and the fact that common antivirals have activity against both viruses. An association between HHV-7 and pityriasis rosea has been suggested, but the data are inconclusive (123, 124). HHV-7 DNA has been detected in various tissues in individual cases, with uncertain clinical significance.

Therapy

In general, HHV-7 is inhibited by the same drugs used for HHV6 and CMV (ganciclovir, foscarnet, and cidofovir) (125), although the inhibitory concentrations may be higher for HHV-7 (126). Drug-resistant HHV-7 has not been reported clinically, but there would appear to be no biological reason that it could not emerge. Specific therapeutic regimens for HHV-7 have not been defined; given the tenuous clinical associations for HHV-7, frequent coinfection with other betaherpesviruses, and similar drug susceptibility profiles, this is likely to remain the case indefinitely.

Collection, Transport, and Storage of Specimens

Specimens for HHV-7 testing should be handled as described above for HHV-6.

Direct Examination

By electron microscopy, HHV-7 virions have appearances typical of herpesviruses. Monoclonal antibodies are available commercially, from some research laboratories

(127), and from the NIH AIDS reagent program. Real-time PCR methods for HHV-7 have been described (84, 128), including multiplex assays for detection of multiple herpesviruses (83, 84). A reference laboratory performing HHV-7 testing is noted in Table 1. HHV-7 is currently not included in the BioFire FilmArray Meningitis/Encephalitis panel.

Isolation Procedures

HHV-7 can be cultured using methods similar to those for HHV-6. HHV-7 isolates initially propagated in primary cell culture or previously adapted HHV-7 strains (e.g., strain SB) can be grown in SupT1 cells. Although culture of primary isolate HHV-7 is possible, it is not of practical utility for clinical diagnostics (95).

Identification

The PCR methods described above provide sensitive, specific, and rapid ways to unambiguously identify the virus. Monoclonal antibodies can be useful for immunohistochemistry on tissue specimens, but this does not have a role in clinical diagnosis.

Typing Systems

Biologically meaningful subtypes of HHV-7 have not been identified.

Serologic Tests

Serologic testing for HHV-7 does not have a substantial role in clinical management. No FDA-cleared reagents are available. Previously reported HHV-7 serologic assays include neutralization tests, immunoblotting, immunoprecipitation, immunofluorescence assay, and enzyme-linked immunosorbent assay (ELISA) (reviewed in reference 127). In one comparison of immunofluorescence assay, immunoblots, and ELISA, the overall performances of the three assays were quite similar, with a small sensitivity advantage for the ELISA and a specificity advantage for the immunoblot assay (129). As described above for HHV-6, antibody avidity testing may distinguish primary from recurrent HHV-7 infections (100).

Antiviral Susceptibilities

Antiviral susceptibility testing does not have a role in clinical management of HHV-7 infection. As noted above, inhibition of HHV-7 may require higher concentrations of antivirals than other betaherpesviruses.

Evaluation, Interpretation, and Reporting of Results

Given the generally mild nature of HHV-7 infections and the tenuous associations with more severe clinical disease, specific testing for HHV-7 is rarely indicated. PCR and serologic testing for HHV-7 is available from certain large reference laboratories. HHV-7 is not included in most meningitis/encephalitis panels available from reference laboratories or in the BioFire FilmArray Meningitis/Encephalitis panel. Given the frequent codetection of other pathogens in the context of HHV-7, it is important to recognize that the detection of HHV-7 does not rule out the presence of other viruses or nonviral infectious agents, many of which have clearer roles in disease pathogenesis.

FUTURE DIRECTIONS

HHV-6A, HHV6B, and HHV-7 can cause clinically relevant infections that require accurate clinical and laboratory diagnosis. However, the need for testing is generally limited to defined groups, especially the immunocompromised and pediatric populations. Future work should focus on clarifying the roles of these viruses in disease pathogenesis and on distinguishing normal carriage of these viruses from virally induced pathogenesis. With the growing availability of rapid multiplex PCR testing and the inclusion of HHV-6 in these licensed panels, we expect a significant rise in the number of new HHV-6 detections and increased interest and insight into clinical disease associations with the roseoloviruses.

REFERENCES

1. **Yamanishi K, Mori Y, Pellett PE.** 2013. Human herpesvirus 6 and 7, p 2058–2079, *Fields Virology*, 6th ed, vol 2. Lippincott Williams & Wilkins, Philadelphia, PA.
2. **Ablashi D, Agut H, Alvarez-Lafuente R, Clark DA, Dewhurst S, DiLuca D, Flamand L, Frenkel N, Gallo R, Gompels UA, Höllsberg P, Jacobson S, Luppi M, Lusso P, Malnati M, Medveczky P, Mori Y, Pellett PE, Pritchett JC, Yamanishi K, Yoshikawa T.** 2014. Classification of HHV-6A and HHV-6B as distinct viruses. *Arch Virol* **159:**863–870.
3. **Greninger A, Roychoudhury P, Makhsous N, Hanson D, Chase J, Krueger G, Xie H, Huang M-L, Saunders L, Ablashi D, Koelle DM, Cook L, Jerome KR.** 2017. Copy number heterogeneity, large origin tandem repeats, and interspecies recombination in HHV-6A and HHV-6B reference strains. *bioRxiv* **92:e00135-18.** 10.1101/193805.
4. **Greninger A, Knudsen G, Roychoudhury P, Hanson D, Sedlak RAH, Xie H, Guan J, Nguyen T, Peddu V, Boeckh M, Huang M-L, Cook L, Depledge D, Zerr D, Koelle D, Gantt S, Yoshikawa T, Caserta M, Hill J, Jerome K.** 2017. Genomic and proteomic analysis of human herpesvirus 6 reveals distinct clustering of acute versus inherited forms and reannotation of reference strain. *bioRxiv* 10.1101/181248:181248.
5. **De Bolle L, Naesens L, De Clercq E.** 2005. Update on human herpesvirus 6 biology, clinical features, and therapy. *Clin Microbiol Rev* **18:**217–245.
6. **Rhoads MP, Magaret AS, Zerr DM.** 2007. Family saliva sharing behaviors and age of human herpesvirus-6B infection. *J Infect* **54:**623–626.
7. **Zerr DM, Meier AS, Selke SS, Frenkel LM, Huang M-L, Wald A, Rhoads MP, Nguy L, Bornemann R, Morrow RA, Corey L.** 2005. A population-based study of primary human herpesvirus 6 infection. *N Engl J Med* **352:**768–776.
8. **Bates M, Monze M, Bima H, Kapambwe M, Clark D, Kasolo FC, Gompels UA.** 2009. Predominant human herpesvirus 6 variant A infant infections in an HIV-1 endemic region of sub-Saharan Africa. *J Med Virol* **81:**779–789.
9. **Gantt S, Orem J, Krantz EM, Morrow RA, Selke S, Huang M-L, Schiffer JT, Jerome KR, Nakaganda A, Wald A, Casper C, Corey L.** 2016. Prospective characterization of the risk factors for transmission and symptoms of primary human herpesvirus infections among Ugandan infants. *J Infect Dis* **214:**36–44.
10. **Tang H, Serada S, Kawabata A, Ota M, Hayashi E, Naka T, Yamanishi K, Mori Y.** 2013. CD134 is a cellular receptor specific for human herpesvirus-6B entry. *Proc Natl Acad Sci USA* **110:**9096–9099.
11. **Lempinen M, Halme L, Arola J, Honkanen E, Salmela K, Lautenschlager I.** 2012. HHV-6B is frequently found in the gastrointestinal tract in kidney transplantation patients. *Transpl Int* **25:**776–782.
12. **Quintela A, et al, Lyon HEMINF Study Group.** 2016. HHV-6 infection after allogeneic hematopoietic stem cell transplantation: from chromosomal integration to viral co-infections and T-cell reconstitution patterns. *J Infect* **72:**214–222.
13. **Hall CB, Caserta MT, Schnabel KC, Long C, Epstein LG, Insel RA, Dewhurst S.** 1998. Persistence of human herpesvirus 6 according to site and variant: possible greater neurotropism of variant A. *Clin Infect Dis* **26:**132–137.

14. **Collot S, Petit B, Bordessoule D, Alain S, Touati M, Denis F, Ranger-Rogez S.** 2002. Real-time PCR for quantification of human herpesvirus 6 DNA from lymph nodes and saliva. *J Clin Microbiol* **40:**2445–2451.
15. **Matrajt L, Gantt S, Mayer BT, Krantz EM, Orem J, Wald A, Corey L, Schiffer JT, Casper C.** 2017. Virus and host-specific differences in oral human herpesvirus shedding kinetics among Ugandan women and children. *Sci Rep* **7:**13105.
16. **Cone RW, Huang ML, Hackman RC, Corey L.** 1996. Coinfection with human herpesvirus 6 variants A and B in lung tissue. *J Clin Microbiol* **34:**877–881.
17. **Chan PK, Ng HK, Hui M, Cheng AF.** 2001. Prevalence and distribution of human herpesvirus 6 variants A and B in adult human brain. *J Med Virol* **64:**42–46.
18. **Nitsche A, Müller CW, Radonic A, Landt O, Ellerbrok H, Pauli G, Siegert W.** 2001. Human herpesvirus 6A DNA is detected frequently in plasma but rarely in peripheral blood leukocytes of patients after bone marrow transplantation. *J Infect Dis* **183:**130–133.
19. **Secchiero P, Carrigan DR, Asano Y, Benedetti L, Crowley RW, Komaroff AL, Gallo RC, Lusso P.** 1995. Detection of human herpesvirus 6 in plasma of children with primary infection and immunosuppressed patients by polymerase chain reaction. *J Infect Dis* **171:**273–280.
20. **Caserta MT, McDermott MP, Dewhurst S, Schnabel K, Carnahan JA, Gilbert L, Lathan G, Lofthus GK, Hall CB.** 2004. Human herpesvirus 6 (HHV6) DNA persistence and reactivation in healthy children. *J Pediatr* **145:**478–484.
21. **Luppi M, Barozzi P, Morris C, Maiorana A, Garber R, Bonacorsi G, Donelli A, Marasca R, Tabilio A, Torelli G.** 1999. Human herpesvirus 6 latently infects early bone marrow progenitors *in vivo*. *J Virol* **73:**754–759.
22. **Arbuckle JH, Medveczky MM, Luka J, Hadley SH, Luegmayr A, Ablashi D, Lund TC, Tolar J, De Meirleir K, Montoya JG, Komaroff AL, Ambros PF, Medveczky PG.** 2010. The latent human herpesvirus-6A genome specifically integrates in telomeres of human chromosomes *in vivo* and *in vitro*. *Proc Natl Acad Sci U S A* **107:**5563–5568.
23. **Ahlqvist J, Fotheringham J, Akhyani N, Yao K, Fogdell-Hahn A, Jacobson S.** 2005. Differential tropism of human herpesvirus 6 (HHV-6) variants and induction of latency by HHV-6A in oligodendrocytes. *J Neurovirol* **11:**384–394.
24. **Sada E, Yasukawa M, Ito C, Takeda A, Shiosaka T, Tanioka H, Fujita S.** 1996. Detection of human herpesvirus 6 and human herpesvirus 7 in the submandibular gland, parotid gland, and lip salivary gland by PCR. *J Clin Microbiol* **34:**2320–2321.
25. **Di Luca D, Mirandola P, Ravaioli T, Frigatti A, Monini P, Cassai E, Sighinolfi L, Dolcetti R.** 1995. Human herpesviruses 6 and 7 in salivary glands and shedding in saliva of healthy and human immunodeficiency virus positive individuals. *J Med Virol* **45:**462–468.
26. **Fujisaki H, Tanaka-Taya K, Tanabe H, Hara T, Miyoshi H, Okada S, Yamanishi K.** 1998. Detection of human herpesvirus 7 (HHV-7) DNA in breast milk by polymerase chain reaction and prevalence of HHV-7 antibody in breast-fed and bottle-fed children. *J Med Virol* **56:**275–279.
27. **Pellett PE, Ablashi DV, Ambros PF, Agut H, Caserta MT, Descamps V, Flamand L, Gautheret-Dejean A, Hall CB, Kamble RT, Kuehl U, Lassner D, Lautenschlager I, Loomis KS, Luppi M, Lusso P, Medveczky PG, Montoya JG, Mori Y, Ogata M, Pritchett JC, Rogez S, Seto E, Ward KN, Yoshikawa T, Razonable RR.** 2012. Chromosomally integrated human herpesvirus 6: questions and answers. *Rev Med Virol* **22:**144–155.
28. **Ward KN, Thiruchelvam AD, Couto-Parada X.** 2005. Unexpected occasional persistence of high levels of HHV-6 DNA in sera: detection of variants A and B. *J Med Virol* **76:**563–570.
29. **Pantry SN, Medveczky PG.** 2017. Latency, integration, and reactivation of human herpesvirus-6. *Viruses* **9:**194.
30. **Hill JA, Sedlak RH, Zerr DM, Huang ML, Yeung C, Myerson D, Jerome KR, Boeckh MJ.** 2015. Prevalence of chromosomally integrated human herpesvirus 6 in patients with human herpesvirus 6-central nervous system dysfunction. *Biol Blood Marrow Transplant* **21:**371–373.
31. **Leong HN, Tuke PW, Tedder RS, Khanom AB, Eglin RP, Atkinson CE, Ward KN, Griffiths PD, Clark DA.** 2007. The prevalence of chromosomally integrated human herpesvirus 6 genomes in the blood of UK blood donors. *J Med Virol* **79:**45–51.
32. **Hall CB, Caserta MT, Schnabel K, Shelley LM, Marino AS, Carnahan JA, Yoo C, Lofthus GK, McDermott MP.** 2008. Chromosomal integration of human herpesvirus 6 is the major mode of congenital human herpesvirus 6 infection. *Pediatrics* **122:**513–520.
33. **Zhang E, Bell AJ, Wilkie GS, Suárez NM, Batini C, Veal CD, Armendáriz-Castillo I, Neumann R, Cotton VE, Huang Y, Porteous DJ, Jarrett RF, Davison AJ, Royle NJ.** 2017. Inherited chromosomally integrated human herpesvirus 6 genomes are ancient, intact and potentially able to reactivate from telomeres. *J Virol* **91:**e01137-17.
34. **Hall CB, Long CE, Schnabel KC, Caserta MT, McIntyre KM, Costanzo MA, Knott A, Dewhurst S, Insel RA, Epstein LG.** 1994. Human herpesvirus-6 infection in children. A prospective study of complications and reactivation. *N Engl J Med* **331:**432–438.
35. **Ward KN, Andrews NJ, Verity CM, Miller E, Ross EM.** 2005. Human herpesviruses-6 and -7 each cause significant neurological morbidity in Britain and Ireland. *Arch Dis Child* **90:**619–623.
36. **Epstein LG, Shinnar S, Hesdorffer DC, Nordli DR, Hamidullah A, Benn EKT, Pellock JM, Frank LM, Lewis DV, Moshe SL, Shinnar RC, Sun S, FEBSTAT Study Team.** 2012. Human herpesvirus 6 and 7 in febrile status epilepticus: the FEBSTAT study. *Epilepsia* **53:**1481–1488.
37. **Kawamura Y, Nakayama A, Kato T, Miura H, Ishihara N, Ihira M, Takahashi Y, Matsuda K, Yoshikawa T.** 2015. Pathogenic role of human herpesvirus 6B infection in mesial temporal lobe epilepsy. *J Infect Dis* **212:**1014–1021.
38. **Leibovitch EC, Jacobson S.** 2015. Human herpesvirus 6 as a viral trigger in mesial temporal lobe epilepsy. *J Infect Dis* **212:**1011–1013.
39. **Knox KK, Carrigan DR.** 1994. Disseminated active HHV-6 infections in patients with AIDS. *Lancet* **343:**577–578.
40. **Zerr DM, Boeckh M, Delaney C, Martin PJ, Xie H, Adler AL, Huang ML, Corey L, Leisenring WM.** 2012. HHV-6 reactivation and associated sequelae after hematopoietic cell transplantation. *Biol Blood Marrow Transplant* **18:**1700–1708.
41. **Razonable RR.** 2013. Human herpesviruses 6, 7 and 8 in solid organ transplant recipients. *Am J Transplant* **13**(Suppl 3)**:**67–77.
42. **Scheurer ME, Pritchett JC, Amirian ES, Zemke NR, Lusso P, Ljungman P.** 2013. HHV-6 encephalitis in umbilical cord blood transplantation: a systematic review and meta-analysis. *Bone Marrow Transplant* **48:**574–580.
43. **Vinnard C, Barton T, Jerud E, Blumberg E.** 2009. A report of human herpesvirus 6-associated encephalitis in a solid organ transplant recipient and a review of previously published cases. *Liver Transpl* **15:**1242–1246.
44. **Kawamura Y, Sugata K, Ihira M, Mihara T, Mutoh T, Asano Y, Yoshikawa T.** 2011. Different characteristics of human herpesvirus 6 encephalitis between primary infection and viral reactivation. *J Clin Virol* **51:**12–19.
45. **Zerr DM, Fann JR, Breiger D, Boeckh M, Adler AL, Xie H, Delaney C, Huang ML, Corey L, Leisenring WM.** 2011. HHV-6 reactivation and its effect on delirium and cognitive functioning in hematopoietic cell transplantation recipients. *Blood* **117:**5243–5249.
46. **Dulery R, Salleron J, Dewilde A, Rossignol J, Boyle EM, Gay J, de Berranger E, Coiteux V, Jouet JP, Duhamel A, Yakoub-Agha I.** 2012. Early human herpesvirus type 6 reactivation after allogeneic stem cell transplantation: a large-scale clinical study. *Biol Blood Marrow Transplant* **18:**1080–1089.
47. **Zerr DM, Corey L, Kim HW, Huang ML, Nguy L, Boeckh M.** 2005. Clinical outcomes of human herpesvirus 6 reactivation after hematopoietic stem cell transplantation. *Clin Infect Dis* **40:**932–940.

48. **Hill JA, Koo S, Guzman Suarez BB, Ho VT, Cutler C, Koreth J, Armand P, Alyea EP III, Baden LR, Antin JH, Soiffer RJ, Marty FM.** 2012. Cord-blood hematopoietic stem cell transplant confers an increased risk for human herpesvirus-6-associated acute limbic encephalitis: a cohort analysis. *Biol Blood Marrow Transplant* **18:**1638–1648.
49. **Gotoh M, Yoshizawa S, Katagiri S, Suguro T, Asano M, Kitahara T, Akahane D, Okabe S, Tauchi T, Ito Y, Ohyashiki K.** 2014. Human herpesvirus 6 reactivation on the 30th day after allogeneic hematopoietic stem cell transplantation can predict grade 2–4 acute graft-versus-host disease. *Transpl Infect Dis* **16:**440–449.
50. **Pichereau C, Desseaux K, Janin A, Scieux C, Peffault de Latour R, Xhaard A, Robin M, Ribaud P, Agbalika F, Chevret S, Socié G.** 2012. The complex relationship between human herpesvirus 6 and acute graft-versus-host disease. *Biol Blood Marrow Transplant* **18:**141–144.
51. **Buyse S, Roque-Afonso AM, Vaghefi P, Gigou M, Dussaix E, Duclos-Vallée JC, Samuel D, Guettier C.** 2013. Acute hepatitis with periportal confluent necrosis associated with human herpesvirus 6 infection in liver transplant patients. *Am J Clin Pathol* **140:**403–409.
52. **Hill JA, Myerson D, Sedlak RH, Jerome KR, Zerr DM.** 2014. Hepatitis due to human herpesvirus 6B after hematopoietic cell transplantation and a review of the literature. *Transpl Infect Dis* **16:**477–483.
53. **Seo S, Renaud C, Kuypers JM, Chiu CY, Huang ML, Samayoa E, Xie H, Yu G, Fisher CE, Gooley TA, Miller S, Hackman RC, Myerson D, Sedlak RH, Kim YJ, Fukuda T, Fredricks DN, Madtes DK, Jerome KR, Boeckh M.** 2015. Idiopathic pneumonia syndrome after hematopoietic cell transplantation: evidence of occult infectious etiologies. *Blood* **125:**3789–3797.
54. **Tormo N, Solano C, de la Cámara R, Garcia-Noblejas A, Cardeñoso L, Clari MA, Nieto J, López J, Hernández-Boluda JC, Remigia MJ, Benet I, Navarro D.** 2010. An assessment of the effect of human herpesvirus-6 replication on active cytomegalovirus infection after allogeneic stem cell transplantation. *Biol Blood Marrow Transplant* **16:**653–661.
55. **Razonable RR, Brown RA, Humar A, Covington E, Alecock E, Paya CV, Group PVS, PV16000 Study Group.** 2005. Herpesvirus infections in solid organ transplant patients at high risk of primary cytomegalovirus disease. *J Infect Dis* **192:**1331–1339.
56. **Humar A, Malkan G, Moussa G, Greig P, Levy G, Mazzulli T.** 2000. Human herpesvirus-6 is associated with cytomegalovirus reactivation in liver transplant recipients. *J Infect Dis* **181:**1450–1453.
57. **Lopez Roa P, Hill JA, Kirby KA, Leisenring WM, Huang ML, Santo TK, Jerome KR, Boeckh M, Limaye AP.** 2015. Coreactivation of human herpesvirus 6 and cytomegalovirus is associated with worse clinical outcome in critically ill adults. *Crit Care Med* **43:**1415–1422.
58. **de Pagter PJ, Schuurman R, Visscher H, de Vos M, Bierings M, van Loon AM, Uiterwaal CS, van Baarle D, Sanders EA, Boelens J.** 2008. Human herpes virus 6 plasma DNA positivity after hematopoietic stem cell transplantation in children: an important risk factor for clinical outcome. *Biol Blood Marrow Transplant* **14:**831–839.
59. **Fernández-Ruiz M, Kumar D, Husain S, Lilly L, Renner E, Mazzulli T, Moussa G, Humar A.** 2015. Utility of a monitoring strategy for human herpesviruses 6 and 7 viremia after liver transplantation: a randomized clinical trial. *Transplantation* **99:**106–113.
60. **Lee SO, Brown RA, Razonable RR.** 2012. Chromosomally integrated human herpesvirus-6 in transplant recipients. *Transpl Infect Dis* **14:**346–354.
61. **Clark DA.** 2016. Clinical and laboratory features of human herpesvirus 6 chromosomal integration. *Clin Microbiol Infect* **22:**333–339.
62. **Hill JA, Magaret AS, Hall-Sedlak R, Mikhaylova A, Huang M-L, Sandmaier BM, Hansen JA, Jerome KR, Zerr DM, Boeckh M.** 2017. Outcomes of hematopoietic cell transplantation using donors or recipients with inherited chromosomally integrated HHV-6. *Blood* **130:**1062–1069.
63. **Descamps V, Ranger-Rogez S.** 2014. DRESS syndrome. *Joint Bone Spine* **81:**15–21.
64. **Ishida T, Kano Y, Mizukawa Y, Shiohara T.** 2014. The dynamics of herpesvirus reactivations during and after severe drug eruptions: their relation to the clinical phenotype and therapeutic outcome. *Allergy* **69:**798–805.
65. **Cho YT, Yang CW, Chu CY.** 2017. Drug reaction with eosinophilia and systemic symptoms (DRESS): an interplay among drugs, viruses, and immune system. *Int J Mol Sci* **18:**E1243.
66. **Caselli E, Zatelli MC, Rizzo R, Benedetti S, Martorelli D, Trasforini G, Cassai E, degli Uberti EC, Di Luca D, Dolcetti R.** 2012. Virologic and immunologic evidence supporting an association between HHV-6 and Hashimoto's thyroiditis. *PLoS Pathog* **8:**e1002951.
67. **Sultanova A, Cistjakovs M, Gravelsina S, Chapenko S, Roga S, Cunskis E, Nora-Krukle Z, Groma V, Ventina I, Murovska M.** 2017. Association of active human herpesvirus-6 (HHV-6) infection with autoimmune thyroid gland diseases. *Clin Microbiol Infect* **23:**50.e1–50.e5.
68. **Hakacova N, Klingel K, Kandolf R, Engdahl E, Fogdell-Hahn A, Higgins T.** 2013. First therapeutic use of Artesunate in treatment of human herpesvirus 6B myocarditis in a child. *J Clin Virol* **57:**157–160.
69. **Bigalke B, Klingel K, May AE, Kandolf R, Gawaz MG.** 2007. Human herpesvirus 6 subtype A-associated myocarditis with 'apical ballooning'. *Can J Cardiol* **23:**393–395.
70. **Gravel A, Dubuc I, Morissette G, Sedlak RH, Jerome KR, Flamand L.** 2015. Inherited chromosomally integrated human herpesvirus 6 as a predisposing risk factor for the development of angina pectoris. *Proc Natl Acad Sci USA* **112:**8058–8063.
71. **Aoki R, Kobayashi N, Suzuki G, Kuratsune H, Shimada K, Oka N, Takahashi M, Yamadera W, Iwashita M, Tokuno S, Nibuya M, Tanichi M, Mukai Y, Mitani K, Kondo K, Ito H, Nakayama K.** 2016. Human herpesvirus 6 and 7 are biomarkers for fatigue, which distinguish between physiological fatigue and pathological fatigue. *Biochem Biophys Res Commun* **478:**424–430.
72. **Leibovitch EC, Jacobson S.** 2014. Evidence linking HHV-6 with multiple sclerosis: an update. *Curr Opin Virol* **9:**127–133.
73. **Ogata M, Satou T, Inoue Y, Takano K, Ikebe T, Ando T, Ikewaki J, Kohno K, Nishida A, Saburi M, Miyazaki Y, Ohtsuka E, Saburi Y, Fukuda T, Kadota J.** 2013. Foscarnet against human herpesvirus (HHV)-6 reactivation after allo-SCT: breakthrough HHV-6 encephalitis following antiviral prophylaxis. *Bone Marrow Transplant* **48:**257–264.
74. **Ishiyama K, Katagiri T, Hoshino T, Yoshida T, Yamaguchi M, Nakao S.** 2011. Preemptive therapy of human herpesvirus-6 encephalitis with foscarnet sodium for high-risk patients after hematopoietic SCT. *Bone Marrow Transplant* **46:**863–869.
75. **Ogata M, Satou T, Kawano R, Goto K, Ikewaki J, Kohno K, Ando T, Miyazaki Y, Ohtsuka E, Saburi Y, Saikawa T, Kadota JI.** 2008. Plasma HHV-6 viral load-guided preemptive therapy against HHV-6 encephalopathy after allogeneic stem cell transplantation: a prospective evaluation. *Bone Marrow Transplant* **41:**279–285.
76. **Zerr DM.** 2012. Human herpesvirus 6 (HHV-6) disease in the setting of transplantation. *Curr Opin Infect Dis* **25:**438–444.
77. **Zerr DM, Huang ML, Corey L, Erickson M, Parker HL, Frenkel LM.** 2000. Sensitive method for detection of human herpesviruses 6 and 7 in saliva collected in field studies. *J Clin Microbiol* **38:**1981–1983.
78. **Sedlak RH, Cook L, Huang M-L, Magaret A, Zerr DM, Boeckh M, Jerome KR.** 2014. Identification of chromosomally integrated human herpesvirus 6 by droplet digital PCR. *Clin Chem* **60:**765–772.
79. **Lautenschlager I, Linnavuori K, Höckerstedt K.** 2000. Human herpesvirus-6 antigenemia after liver transplantation. *Transplantation* **69:**2561–2566.
80. **Nishimura N, Yoshikawa T, Ozaki T, Sun H, Goshima F, Nishiyama Y, Asano Y, Kurata T, Iwasaki T.** 2005. *In vitro* and *in vivo* analysis of human herpesvirus-6 U90 protein expression. *J Med Virol* **75:**86–92.

81. **Blumberg BM, Mock DJ, Powers JM, Ito M, Assouline JG, Baker JV, Chen B, Goodman AD.** 2000. The HHV6 paradox: ubiquitous commensal or insidious pathogen? A two-step *in situ* PCR approach. *J Clin Virol* **16:**159–178.
82. **Opsahl ML, Kennedy PGE.** 2005. Early and late HHV-6 gene transcripts in multiple sclerosis lesions and normal appearing white matter. *Brain* **128:**516–527.
83. **Deback C, Agbalika F, Scieux C, Marcelin AG, Gautheret-Dejean A, Cherot J, Hermet L, Roger O, Agut H.** 2008. Detection of human herpesviruses HHV-6, HHV-7 and HHV-8 in whole blood by real-time PCR using the new CMV, HHV-6, 7, 8 R-gene kit. *J Virol Methods* **149:**285–291.
84. **Wada K, Mizoguchi S, Ito Y, Kawada J, Yamauchi Y, Morishima T, Nishiyama Y, Kimura H.** 2009. Multiplex real-time PCR for the simultaneous detection of herpes simplex virus, human herpesvirus 6, and human herpesvirus 7. *Microbiol Immunol* **53:**22–29.
85. **Caserta MT, Hall CB, Schnabel K, Lofthus G, Marino A, Shelley L, Yoo C, Carnahan J, Anderson L, Wang H.** 2010. Diagnostic assays for active infection with human herpesvirus 6 (HHV-6). *J Clin Virol* **48:**55–57.
86. **Boutolleau D, Fernandez C, André E, Imbert-Marcille BM, Milpied N, Agut H, Gautheret-Dejean A.** 2003. Human herpesvirus (HHV)-6 and HHV-7: two closely related viruses with different infection profiles in stem cell transplantation recipients. *J Infect Dis* **187:**179–186.
87. **Martró E, Cannon MJ, Dollard SC, Spira TJ, Laney AS, Ou C-Y, Pellett PE.** 2004. Evidence for both lytic replication and tightly regulated human herpesvirus 8 latency in circulating mononuclear cells, with virus loads frequently below common thresholds of detection. *J Virol* **78:**11707–11714.
88. **Gautheret-Dejean A, Henquell C, Mousnier F, Boutolleau D, Bonnafous P, Dhédin N, Settegrana C, Agut H.** 2009. Different expression of human herpesvirus-6 (HHV-6) load in whole blood may have a significant impact on the diagnosis of active infection. *J Clin Virol* **46:**33–36.
89. **Flamand L, Gravel A, Boutolleau D, Alvarez-Lafuente R, Jacobson S, Malnati MS, Kohn D, Tang Y-W, Yoshikawa T, Ablashi D.** 2008. Multicenter comparison of PCR assays for detection of human herpesvirus 6 DNA in serum. *J Clin Microbiol* **46:**2700–2706.
90. **de Pagter PJ, Schuurman R, de Vos NM, Mackay W, van Loon AM.** 2010. Multicenter external quality assessment of molecular methods for detection of human herpesvirus 6. *J Clin Microbiol* **48:**2536–2540.
91. **Greninger AL, Bateman AC, Atienza EE, Wendt S, Makhsous N, Jerome KR, Cook L.** 2017. Copy number heterogeneity of JC virus standards. *J Clin Microbiol* **55:**824–831.
92. **Bateman AC, Greninger AL, Atienza EE, Limaye AP, Jerome KR, Cook L.** 2017. Quantification of BK virus standards by quantitative real-time PCR and droplet digital PCR is confounded by multiple virus populations in the WHO BKV international standard. *Clin Chem* **63:**761–769.
93. **Stamey FR, Dominguez G, Black JB, Dambaugh TR, Pellett PE.** 1995. Intragenomic linear amplification of human herpesvirus 6B oriLyt suggests acquisition of oriLyt by transposition. *J Virol* **69:**589–596.
94. **Leber AL, Everhart K, Balada-Llasat J-M, Cullison J, Daly J, Holt S, Lephart P, Salimnia H, Schreckenberger PC, DesJarlais S, Reed SL, Chapin KC, LeBlanc L, Johnson JK, Soliven NL, Carroll KC, Miller J-A, Dien Bard J, Mestas J, Bankowski M, Enomoto T, Hemmert AC, Bourzac KM.** 2016. Multicenter evaluation of BioFire FilmArray meningitis/encephalitis panel for detection of bacteria, viruses, and yeast in cerebrospinal fluid specimens. *J Clin Microbiol* **54:**2251–2261.
95. **Black JB, Pellett PE.** 2000. Antiviral screening assays for human herpesviruses 6 and 7. *Methods Mol Med* **24:**129–138.
96. **De Bolle L, Van Loon J, De Clercq E, Naesens L.** 2005. Quantitative analysis of human herpesvirus 6 cell tropism. *J Med Virol* **75:**76–85
97. **Osman HK, Wells C, Baboonian C, Kangro HO.** 1993. Growth characteristics of human herpesvirus-6: comparison of antigen production in two cell lines. *J Med Virol* **39:**303–311.
98. **Arsenault S, Gravel A, Gosselin J, Flamand L.** 2003. Generation and characterization of a monoclonal antibody specific for human herpesvirus 6 variant A immediate-early 2 protein. *J Clin Virol* **28:**284–290.
99. **Sedlak RH, Hill JA, Nguyen T, Cho M, Levin G, Cook L, Huang ML, Flamand L, Zerr DM, Boeckh M, Jerome KR.** 2016. Detection of human herpesvirus 6B (HHV-6B) reactivation in hematopoietic cell transplant recipients with inherited chromosomally integrated HHV-6A by droplet digital PCR. *J Clin Microbiol* **54:**1223–1227.
100. **Ward KN.** 2005. The natural history and laboratory diagnosis of human herpesviruses-6 and -7 infections in the immunocompetent. *J Clin Virol* **32:**183–193.
101. **Braun DK, Dominguez G, Pellett PE.** 1997. Human herpesvirus 6. *Clin Microbiol Rev* **10:**521–567.
102. **Burbelo PD, Bayat A, Wagner J, Nutman TB, Baraniuk JN, Iadarola MJ.** 2012. No serological evidence for a role of HHV-6 infection in chronic fatigue syndrome. *Am J Transl Res* **4:**443–451.
103. **Bonnafous P, Naesens L, Petrella S, Gautheret-Dejean A, Boutolleau D, Sougakoff W, Agut H.** 2007. Different mutations in the HHV-6 DNA polymerase gene accounting for resistance to foscarnet. *Antivir Ther* **12:**877–888.
104. **Bonnafous P, Boutolleau D, Naesens L, Deback C, Gautheret-Dejean A, Agut H.** 2008. Characterization of a cidofovir-resistant HHV-6 mutant obtained by *in vitro* selection. *Antiviral Res* **77:**237–240.
105. **Isegawa Y, Matsumoto C, Nishinaka K, Nakano K, Tanaka T, Sugimoto N, Ohshima A.** 2010. PCR with quenching probes enables the rapid detection and identification of ganciclovir-resistance-causing U69 gene mutations in human herpesvirus 6. *Mol Cell Probes* **24:**167–177.
106. **Bounaadja L, Piret J, Goyette N, Boivin G.** 2013. Analysis of HHV-6 mutations in solid organ transplant recipients at the onset of cytomegalovirus disease and following treatment with intravenous ganciclovir or oral valganciclovir. *J Clin Virol* **58:**279–282.
107. **Hayden RT, Preiksaitis J, Tong Y, Pang X, Sun Y, Tang L, Cook L, Pounds S, Fryer J, Caliendo AM.** 2015. Commutability of the First World Health Organization International Standard for Human Cytomegalovirus. *J Clin Microbiol* **53:** 3325–3333.
108. **Kaufer BB, Flamand L.** 2014. Chromosomally integrated HHV-6: impact on virus, cell and organismal biology. *Curr Opin Virol* **9:**111–118.
109. **de Oliveira Vianna RA, Siqueira MM, Camacho LA, Setúbal S, Knowles W, Brown DW, de Oliveira SA.** 2008. The accuracy of anti-human herpesvirus 6 IgM detection in children with recent primary infection. *J Virol Methods* **153:**273–275.
110. **Clark DA, Freeland ML, Mackie LK, Jarrett RF, Onions DE.** 1993. Prevalence of antibody to human herpesvirus 7 by age. *J Infect Dis* **168:**251–252.
111. **Caserta MT, Hall CB, Schnabel K, Long CE, D'Heron N.** 1998. Primary human herpesvirus 7 infection: a comparison of human herpesvirus 7 and human herpesvirus 6 infections in children. *J Pediatr* **133:**386–389.
112. **Katsafanas GC, Schirmer EC, Wyatt LS, Frenkel N.** 1996. *In vitro* activation of human herpesviruses 6 and 7 from latency. *Proc Natl Acad Sci USA* **93:**9788–9792.
113. **Berneman ZN, Ablashi DV, Li G, Eger-Fletcher M, Reitz MS Jr, Hung CL, Brus I, Komaroff AL, Gallo RC.** 1992. Human herpesvirus 7 is a T-lymphotropic virus and is related to, but significantly different from, human herpesvirus 6 and human cytomegalovirus. *Proc Natl Acad Sci USA* **89:**10552–10556.
114. **Secchiero P, Sun D, De Vico AL, Crowley RW, Reitz MS Jr, Zauli G, Lusso P, Gallo RC.** 1997. Role of the extracellular domain of human herpesvirus 7 glycoprotein B in virus binding to cell surface heparan sulfate proteoglycans. *J Virol* **71:**4571–4580.
115. **Kempf W, Adams V, Mirandola P, Menotti L, Di Luca D, Wey N, Müller B, Campadelli-Fiume G.** 1998. Persistence of human herpesvirus 7 in normal tissues detected by expression of a structural antigen. *J Infect Dis* **178:**841–845.

116. **Chapenko S, Roga S, Skuja S, Rasa S, Cistjakovs M, Svirskis S, Zaserska Z, Groma V, Murovska M.** 2016. Detection frequency of human herpesviruses-6A, -6B, and -7 genomic sequences in central nervous system DNA samples from post-mortem individuals with unspecified encephalopathy. *J Neurovirol* **22:**488–497.
117. **Prusty BK, Gulve N, Rasa S, Murovska M, Hernandez PC, Ablashi DV.** 2017. Possible chromosomal and germline integration of human herpesvirus 7. *J Gen Virol* **98:**266–274.
118. **Hall CB, Caserta MT, Schnabel KC, Boettrich C, McDermott MP, Lofthus GK, Carnahan JA, Dewhurst S.** 2004. Congenital infections with human herpesvirus 6 (HHV6) and human herpesvirus 7 (HHV7). *J Pediatr* **145:**472–477.
119. **Razonable RR, Paya CV.** 2002. The impact of human herpesvirus-6 and -7 infection on the outcome of liver transplantation. *Liver Transpl* **8:**651–658.
120. **Yamamoto K, Yoshikawa T, Okamoto S, Yamaki K, Shimokata K, Nishiyama Y.** 2005. HHV-6 and 7 DNA loads in lung tissues collected from patients with interstitial pneumonia. *J Med Virol* **75:**70–75.
121. **Costa C, Bergallo M, Delsedime L, Solidoro P, Donadio P, Cavallo R.** 2009. Acute respiratory distress syndrome associated with HHV-7 infection in an immunocompetent patient: a case report. *New Microbiol* **32:**315–316.
122. **Costa C, Delsedime L, Solidoro P, Curtoni A, Bergallo M, Libertucci D, Baldi S, Rinaldi M, Cavallo R.** 2010. Herpesviruses detection by quantitative real-time polymerase chain reaction in bronchoalveolar lavage and transbronchial biopsy in lung transplant: viral infections and histopathological correlation. *Transplant Proc* **42:**1270–1274.
123. **Chuh AAT, Chan HHL, Zawar V.** 2004. Is human herpesvirus 7 the causative agent of pityriasis rosea? A critical review. *Int J Dermatol* **43:**870–875.
124. **Broccolo F, Drago F, Careddu AM, Foglieni C, Turbino L, Cocuzza CE, Gelmetti C, Lusso P, Rebora AE, Malnati MS.** 2005. Additional evidence that pityriasis rosea is associated with reactivation of human herpesvirus-6 and -7. *J Invest Dermatol* **124:**1234–1240.
125. **De Clercq E, Naesens L, De Bolle L, Schols D, Zhang Y, Neyts J.** 2001. Antiviral agents active against human herpesviruses HHV-6, HHV-7 and HHV-8. *Rev Med Virol* **11:**381–395.
126. **Yoshida M, Yamada M, Tsukazaki T, Chatterjee S, Lakeman FD, Nii S, Whitley RJ.** 1998. Comparison of antiviral compounds against human herpesvirus 6 and 7. *Antiviral Res* **40:**73–84.
127. **Black JB, Pellett PE.** 1999. Human herpesvirus 7. *Rev Med Virol* **9:**245–262.
128. **Bergallo M, Costa C, Terlizzi ME, Sidoti F, Margio S, Astegiano S, Ponti R, Cavallo R.** 2009. Development of a LUX real-time PCR for the detection and quantification of human herpesvirus 7. *Can J Microbiol* **55:**319–325
129. **Black JB, Schwarz TF, Patton JL, Kite-Powell K, Pellett PE, Wiersbitzky S, Bruns R, Müller C, Jäger G, Stewart JA.** 1996. Evaluation of immunoassays for detection of antibodies to human herpesvirus 7. *Clin Diagn Lab Immunol* **3:**79–83.

Human Herpesvirus 8

SHEILA C. DOLLARD AND CLIFFORD J. GUNTHEL

105

TAXONOMY

Human herpesvirus 8 (HHV-8) is classified in the genus *Rhadinovirus* of the subfamily *Gammaherpesvirinae* based on sequence and biological properties. Its closest human herpesvirus relative is Epstein-Barr virus (EBV), which is also a member of the subfamily *Gammaherpesvirinae*. The other known human herpesviruses are herpes simplex virus 1 and 2, varicella-zoster virus, cytomegalovirus, human herpesvirus 6A and 6B, and human herpesvirus 7.

DESCRIPTION OF THE AGENT

The HHV-8 genome is double-stranded DNA approximately 160 kb long and contains over 85 genes, including several genes of host derivation (1, 2). All herpesviruses consist of an icosahedral capsid surrounded by a membrane envelope. The capsid contains the viral DNA. HHV-8 is the most recently discovered human herpesvirus. In the 1960s, virus-like particles were cultured from biopsy material from Kaposi's sarcoma (KS) (3). Subsequently, investigators analyzed genetic material from lesions to identify what they termed Kaposi's sarcoma-associated herpesvirus (KSHV) (4), also referred to as HHV-8 because of its association with diseases other than KS. As with all herpesviruses, HHV-8 infection is lifelong. Following primary infection, herpesviruses enter a state of viral latency with minimal gene expression, an effective adaptation to escape the host antiviral response which presents diagnostic challenges.

EPIDEMIOLOGY AND TRANSMISSION

The most common disease associated with HHV-8 infection is KS, for which there are four recognized epidemiologic categories: (i) epidemic KS, associated with human immunodeficiency virus (HIV) disease, the predominant form of KS in the United States and Europe; (ii) classical KS, seen in older Mediterranean men; (iii) endemic KS, which occurs in sub-Saharan Africa; and (iv) iatrogenic KS, which occurs in organ transplant recipients. HHV-8 infection alone is not sufficient to cause KS. The main cofactor appears to be immunosuppression, which can be caused by immune senescence, malnutrition, intercurrent illnesses, antirejection agents, or AIDS (5). HHV-8 stands out as the only human herpesvirus with low prevalence in most of the world. Low HHV-8 seroprevalence (<5%) is seen in North America and Northern and Western Europe, where the occurrence of KS is almost entirely limited to men who have sex with men (MSM) with AIDS, and in a portion of organ transplant recipients (6).

Transmission of HHV-8 appears to be via saliva for both casual and sexual transmission. In regions of Africa where HHV-8 is endemic, transmission is horizontal and casual, beginning early in childhood. In countries where the virus is not endemic, including the United States, HHV-8 transmission is primarily sexual and concentrated among MSM. Heterosexual transmission appears to be rare, for reasons that are not understood (7). HHV-8 can be transmitted by injection drug use (8). Transmission by blood transfusion has been documented only in countries where HHV-8 seroprevalence is high and blood is not leukoreduced, such as Uganda (9). The frequency of HHV-8 transmission by organ transplantation increases with the HHV-8 prevalence in a region (10), which is a growing area of interest in the field of HHV-8 diagnostics due to an increase in the number of HIV-positive patients receiving transplants and, in some cases, serving as donors (11).

CLINICAL SIGNIFICANCE

Kaposi's Sarcoma

HHV-8 is in the small group of DNA viruses that cause cancer in humans, along with EBV, human papillomavirus, and hepatitis B virus. HHV-8 causes KS, which commonly manifests as red-purple to brown-black lesions on the skin or mucous membranes. Lesions vary in appearance from substantially raised and nodular (Fig. 1) to flat and plaque-like (Fig. 2). The lower extremities tend to be a preferred area of cutaneous involvement, often with associated lymphedema; the result can be painful and disfiguring. Lymph nodes as well as visceral organs (lung, gastrointestinal tract, liver, and bone) can also be affected; pulmonary KS is associated with significant morbidity and mortality. Increased KS disease activity has been associated with concurrent infections, such as pneumocystis pneumonia (5, 12).

Pathologically, KS lesions are characterized by the presence of spindle cells, an irregular blood vessel network, and a cellular inflammatory infiltrate. The associated extravasated red blood cells are the source of the hyperpigmentation that

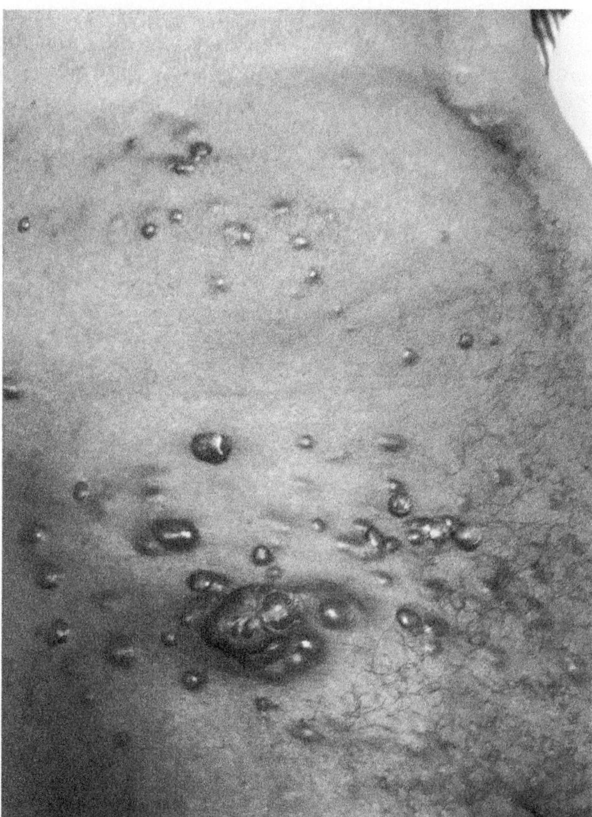

FIGURE 1 Typical cutaneous KS nodules on the torso of a man with AIDS.

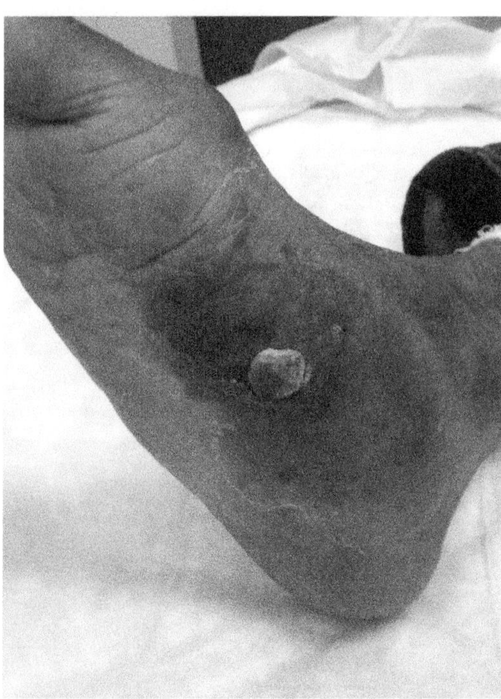

FIGURE 2 Exophytic KS tumor arising from a background of a KS plaque on the foot.

the clinician recognizes as KS (13). Long-term remissions from KS can be achieved with immune reconstitution. The incidence of KS among persons living with AIDS (PLWA) in North America and Europe has declined substantially with the introduction of combined antiretroviral therapy (cART) (14). Although herpesvirus-specific antiviral therapy, mainly ganciclovir, can prevent the development of KS, serious side effects preclude its use for this indication, since cART is effective for both prevention and management of KS (15). Posttransplant KS can be managed in most cases by modifying the level of immunosuppressive therapy and not treating the KS directly.

PEL, MCD, and KICS

Three less common HHV-8-associated diseases are primary effusion lymphoma (PEL), multicentric Castleman disease (MCD), and KSHV inflammatory cytokine syndrome (KICS). PEL is a rare, aggressive, non-Hodgkin lymphoma that arises in body cavities but usually does not present with distinct tumor masses. Typically occurring in PLWA, PEL has also been observed in other immunodeficiency states. PEL comprises only about 4% of all AIDS-associated non-Hodgkin lymphomas (16). Virtually all cases of PEL harbor HHV-8, and half are coinfected with EBV (16, 17). MCD is characterized by constitutional symptoms and diffuse lymphadenopathy. HHV-8 is associated with the plasmablastic variant of MCD, more commonly seen in HIV-infected individuals. MCD is diagnosed by histopathology, and KS is often codiagnosed on lymph node biopsies (17). Abnormal laboratory results include anemia, pancytopenia, hypoalbuminemia, hypergammaglobulinemia, and elevated inflammatory markers (17). KICS is another HHV-8-associated inflammatory syndrome that presents similarly to MCD but lacks the histopathology diagnostic features of MCD. KS is often clinically present with KICS. HHV-8 and inflammatory cytokines levels are elevated (18).

COLLECTION, TRANSPORT, AND STORAGE OF SPECIMENS

Serology is the preferred method to identify HHV-8 infection because of low, usually undetectable, viral load. Serum and plasma can be used interchangeably in most HHV-8 serologic tests, and standard procedures for collection and storage of serum and plasma apply. PCR is mainly used for measurement of HHV-8 viral load in blood, as it can predict disease risk and measure response to therapy (discussed further under "Nucleic Acid Detection" below). Preferred specimens for viral load measurements are whole blood or peripheral blood mononuclear cells and not plasma, since HHV-8 is primarily cell associated. Viral DNA is often present in the saliva (more often than blood) and is used for many research studies on transmission and epidemiology. All fluids and tissues for PCR testing should be stored at −60°C to −80°C after collection, prior to testing.

DIRECT EXAMINATION

Antigen Detection

Immunohistochemistry (IHC) and *in situ* hybridization (ISH) allow the direct identification of viral transcripts and proteins in infected tissues. IHC and ISH have proven useful for confirming the diagnosis of KS in lesions with non-typical pathologies and ruling out KS in the case of other spindle cell lesions. IHC and ISH can more closely link viral expression to a given disease process, which results in better understanding of viral pathogenesis and allows more precisely targeted therapy (26–28).

Nucleic Acid Detection

Most HHV-8-infected individuals do not have detectable viral DNA in their blood; therefore, PCR is not a useful screen test to establish HHV-8 infection. HHV-8 DNA is detected by PCR in the blood of 30 to 50% of AIDS patients with KS and in 5 to 20% of HIV-infected, HHV-8-seropositive individuals without KS and is rarely detected at all in HHV-8-seropositive, HIV-negative individuals (19–21). The clinical value of PCR testing is to provide information on disease risk, transmission, and response to antiviral therapy (21, 22). Engels and colleagues performed HHV-8 PCR testing on blood collected from 132 HIV-infected MSM without KS, 31 of whom developed KS later (22). They showed that men with HHV-8 viremia one year prior to KS diagnosis had 10 times the risk for developing KS than men without viremia had (22). Laney and colleagues monitored 96 HIV-infected, HHV-8-infected MSM for 2 years at 4-month intervals; 47 of the men had KS. They found a significant association between changes in KS disease severity and HHV-8 viral load. The data were insufficient to confirm a threshold viral load for disease risk; however, patients with progressing disease were eight times more likely to have viral loads greater than 10,000 genome copies per million cells than patients with regressing disease (21). Several smaller studies cited in the Engels and Laney papers reported similar associations between HHV-8 viremia and KS disease severity.

Numerous PCR primer sets specific for the viral genes ORF (open reading frame) 26 (4), ORF 25 (23), K6 (24), and ORF 73 (25) have been described, and PCR tests are available commercially (Table 1). HHV-8 DNA is present in high concentrations in KS lesions, but collection of biopsy material is painful for the patient and is not standard for diagnosis.

ISOLATION PROCEDURES

There are currently no cell culture systems for isolation of HHV-8 virus from clinical specimens. Although HHV-8 can infect and establish latency in a broad range of host cells, efficient replication and serial passage of clinical isolates in cell lines have not been demonstrated. Human B-cell lines naturally infected with HHV-8 are in wide use as serodiagnostic reagents. The virus is latent in most cells and can be induced with stimulants such as phorbol ester (tetradecanoyl phorbol acetate) and sodium butyrate.

IDENTIFICATION AND TYPING SYSTEMS

HHV-8 DNA is identified with PCR testing and through direct detection of viral proteins and transcripts with IHC/ISH staining. Targeted sequencing of viral DNA is performed to identify genome subtypes in the study of transmission and epidemiology but is not routine practice in the clinical setting.

SEROLOGIC TESTS

KS is normally a clinical diagnosis that does not involve laboratory testing other than possible histological examination of a lesion biopsy. The main application of HHV-8 serologic testing has been to establish the presence of HHV-8 infection for

TABLE 1 Commercial diagnostic tests for HHV-8

Test type and company	Test format	Product no.	Contact information[a]	Approval (FDA[b]/CE)
IgG antibody				
LabCorp	IFA (whole cell)	841155	800-762-4344	No/No
Quest Diagnostics, Inc.	IFA (whole cell)	37959	866-697-8378; https://www.questdiagnostics.com/testcenter/TestDetail.action?ntc=37959	No/No
Advanced Biotechnologies	ELISA (whole cell)	15-501-000	https://abionline.com/product/kshvhhv-8-igg-antibody-elisa-kit/	No/No
Advanced Biotechnologies	IFA (whole cell)	Discontinued in 2014	Discontinued in 2014	Discontinued in 2014
DiaSorin	IFA (whole cell); unavailable in U.S.	V18 HHV-8	800-328-1482; https://www.diasorin.com/en	No/No
PCR				
LabCorp	Quantitative	009985/45700	800-762-4344	No/No
Quest Diagnostics	Quantitative	19798	866-697-8378; https://www.questdiagnostics.com/testcenter/TestDetail.action?ntc=19798	No/No
ARUP Laboratories	Quantitative	2013089	800-522-2787; http://ltd.aruplab.com/Tests/Pub/2013089	No/No
bioMérieux, Inc.	Multiplex for HHV-6, -7, and -8, CMV	69-100B-01 R-Gene	http://www.biomerieux.co.uk/product/cmv-hhv678-r-gene	Yes/Yes
Bioron	Quantitative	Discontinued in 2015	Discontinued in 2015	Discontinued in 2015

[a]HHV-8 tests are not listed on all company websites, and a phone call may be required.
[b]FDA, Food and Drug Administration.

epidemiologic or clinical research. PCR is not used to establish HHV-8 infection due to extremely low levels of viremia that are undetectable by PCR in most people without disease.

Most published serologic tests for HHV-8 have been developed by research laboratories and are not commercially available. The two main test formats are immunofluorescence assays (IFA) based on human B-cell lines, naturally infected with HHV-8 that express either lytic or latent viral antigens, and enzyme-linked immunosorbent assays (ELISA) based on individual viral proteins or peptides. Several studies have compared the performance of HHV-8 serologic tests, and the majority of them show 80 to 95% concordance and sensitivity with sera from patients with AIDS-associated KS but show considerable discordance (<50% agreement) with sera from various risk groups without KS or from blood donors (20, 29, 30). The biological challenge with HHV-8 serology is the weak antibody response in immunocompetent people, which can involve different subsets of antigens between individuals (31). Another challenge is identifying truly negative serum panels to establish assay specificity, when most HHV-8 infection is asymptomatic without detectable viremia.

Assay comparison studies have consistently shown that the lytic antigen IFA is the most sensitive HHV-8 test (>95%), with reasonable specificity (>95%) when used by experienced laboratories (20, 32). However, the IFA is labor-intensive and subject to variable interpretation and is therefore not suitable for clinical use or high-throughput testing. Numerous HHV-8 epidemiologic studies have been conducted using two ELISAs developed by the National Cancer Institute; however, the combined estimated sensitivity on samples from the U.S. population was 80 to 90% (29); thus, clinical use would require improved performance. To address the shortcomings of individual tests, most research labs use combinations of HHV-8 assays to achieve higher sensitivity and specificity (20, 29, 30), but multiple test algorithms are not practical for clinical use.

Commercial serologic tests for HHV-8 are listed in Table 1, none of which is approved by the Food and Drug Administration or has received the CE marking. The only commercial tests currently available in the United States are the lytic antigen IFA (LabCorp and Quest) and an ELISA (ABI); however, two large multicenter studies found that the ABI ELISA showed poor sensitivity (<50%) in patients with KS (20, 32). The very limited options for HHV-8 serologic testing underscore the need for a convenient and validated test.

HHV-8 serologic testing in the setting of organ transplantation is a growing area of interest despite the lack of a suitable test. Serologic screening of donors and recipients in regions where HHV-8 is endemic and possibly of high-risk individuals (MSM and intravenous-drug users) in regions where the virus is not endemic may be warranted (10, 33, 34). The transplant community has seen the gradual acceptance of liver and kidney transplantation in HIV-positive patients (11), who are at higher risk for HHV-8 infection and therefore for posttransplant KS.

ANTIMICROBIAL SUSCEPTIBILITIES

There have not been reports of development of antimicrobial resistance with herpesvirus-specific antiviral therapies for KS, which is mainly ganciclovir, because they are rarely used in the management of KS. Cost and toxicity prohibit these agents from being utilized as preventative chemotherapy options, especially since cART has been effective in preventing KS. There is no evidence that the addition of an antiherpesvirus therapy would have additional efficacy beyond cART alone (35).

EVALUATION, INTERPRETATION, AND REPORTING OF RESULTS

Diagnosis of HHV-8-associated disease is usually clinical, without the use of HHV-8-specific diagnostic tests. Diagnosis of HHV-8 infection is done mainly with serologic testing due to the low detectability of viral DNA in most infections. Most serologic tests have been developed in-house by research laboratories and are used for research purposes only. There is currently no consensus on which serologic tests are the most accurate. HHV-8 PCR testing is generally more straightforward, but its applications are limited to studies on transmission, disease risk, and response to therapy.

The findings and conclusions in this document are those of the authors and do not necessarily represent the official position of the Centers for Disease Control and Prevention or Emory University.

The authors thank Phili Wong at CDC for thoroughly exploring the availability of commercial diagnostic tests for Table 1.

REFERENCES

1. **Neipel F, Fleckenstein B.** 1999. The role of HHV-8 in Kaposi's sarcoma. *Semin Cancer Biol* **9:**151–164.
2. **Moore PS, Chang Y.** 2003. Kaposi's sarcoma-associated herpesvirus immunoevasion and tumorigenesis: two sides of the same coin? *Annu Rev Microbiol* **57:**609–639.
3. **Giraldo G, Beth E, Haguenau F.** 1972. Herpes-type virus particles in tissue culture of Kaposi's sarcoma from different geographic regions. *J Natl Cancer Inst* **49:**1509–1526.
4. **Chang Y, Cesarman E, Pessin MS, Lee F, Culpepper J, Knowles DM, Moore PS.** 1994. Identification of herpesvirus-like DNA sequences in AIDS-associated Kaposi's sarcoma. *Science* **266:**1865–1869.
5. **Antman K, Chang Y.** 2000. Kaposi's sarcoma. *N Engl J Med* **342:**1027–1038.
6. **Cohen A, Wolf DG, Guttman-Yassky E, Sarid R.** 2005. Kaposi's sarcoma-associated herpesvirus: clinical, diagnostic, and epidemiological aspects. *Crit Rev Clin Lab Sci* **42:**101–153.
7. **Engels EA, Atkinson JO, Graubard BI, McQuillan GM, Gamache C, Mbisa G, Cohn S, Whitby D, Goedert JJ.** 2007. Risk factors for human herpesvirus 8 infection among adults in the United States and evidence for sexual transmission. *J Infect Dis* **196:**199–207.
8. **Cannon MJ, Dollard SC, Smith DK, Klein RS, Schuman P, Rich JD, Vlahov D, Pellett PE, HIV Epidemiology Research Study Group.** 2001. Blood-borne and sexual transmission of human herpesvirus 8 in women with or at risk for human immunodeficiency virus infection. *N Engl J Med* **344:**637–643.
9. **Hladik W, Dollard SC, Mermin J, Fowlkes AL, Downing R, Amin MM, Banage F, Nzaro E, Kataaha P, Dondero TJ, Pellett PE, Lackritz EM.** 2006. Transmission of human herpesvirus 8 by blood transfusion. *N Engl J Med* **355:**1331–1338.
10. **Lebbé C, Legendre C, Francès C.** 2008. Kaposi sarcoma in transplantation. *Transplant Rev (Orlando)* **22:**252–261.
11. **Stock PG, Barin B, Murphy B, Hanto D, Diego JM, Light J, Davis C, Blumberg E, Simon D, Subramanian A, Millis JM, Lyon GM, Brayman K, Slakey D, Shapiro R, Melancon J, Jacobson JM, Stosor V, Olson JL, Stablein DM, Roland ME.** 2010. Outcomes of kidney transplantation in HIV-infected recipients. *N Engl J Med* **363:**2004–2014.
12. **Douglas JL, Gustin JK, Moses AV, Dezube BJ, Pantanowitz L.** 2010. Kaposi sarcoma pathogenesis: a triad of viral infection, oncogenesis and chronic inflammation. *Transl Biomed* **1:**172.

13. **Hong Y-K, Foreman K, Shin JW, Hirakawa S, Curry CL, Sage DR, Libermann T, Dezube BJ, Fingeroth JD, Detmar M.** 2004. Lymphatic reprogramming of blood vascular endothelium by Kaposi sarcoma-associated herpesvirus. *Nat Genet* **36:**683–685.
14. **Engels EA, Pfeiffer RM, Goedert JJ, Virgo P, McNeel TS, Scoppa SM, Biggar RJ, HIV/AIDS Cancer Match Study.** 2006. Trends in cancer risk among people with AIDS in the United States 1980-2002. *AIDS* **20:**1645–1654.
15. **Martin RW III, Hood AF, Farmer ER.** 1993. Kaposi sarcoma. *Medicine (Baltimore)* **72:**245–261.
16. **Cesarman E.** 2011. Gammaherpesvirus and lymphoproliferative disorders in immunocompromised patients. *Cancer Lett* **305:**163–174.
17. **Bhutani M, Polizzotto MN, Uldrick TS, Yarchoan R.** 2015. Kaposi sarcoma-associated herpesvirus-associated malignancies: epidemiology, pathogenesis, and advances in treatment. *Semin Oncol* **42:**223–246.
18. **Polizzotto MN, Uldrick TS, Wyvill KM, Aleman K, Marshall V, Wang V, Whitby D, Pittaluga S, Jaffe ES, Millo C, Tosato G, Little RF, Steinberg SM, Sereti I, Yarchoan R.** 2016. Clinical features and outcomes of patients with symptomatic Kaposi sarcoma herpesvirus (KSHV)-associated inflammation: prospective characterization of KSHV inflammatory cytokine syndrome (KICS). *Clin Infect Dis* **62:**730–738.
19. **Boivin G, Côté S, Cloutier N, Abed Y, Maguigad M, Routy JP.** 2002. Quantification of human herpesvirus 8 by real-time PCR in blood fractions of AIDS patients with Kaposi's sarcoma and multicentric Castleman's disease. *J Med Virol* **68:**399–403.
20. **Pellett PE, Wright DJ, Engels EA, Ablashi DV, Dollard SC, Forghani B, Glynn SA, Goedert JJ, Jenkins FJ, Lee TH, Neipel F, Todd DS, Whitby D, Nemo GJ, Busch MP, Retrovirus Epidemiology Donor Study.** 2003. Multicenter comparison of serologic assays and estimation of human herpesvirus 8 seroprevalence among US blood donors. *Transfusion* **43:**1260–1268.
21. **Laney AS, Cannon MJ, Jaffe HW, Offermann MK, Ou CY, Radford KW, Patel MM, Spira TJ, Gunthel CJ, Pellett PE, Dollard SC.** 2007. Human herpesvirus 8 presence and viral load are associated with the progression of AIDS-associated Kaposi's sarcoma. *AIDS* **21:**1541–1545.
22. **Engels EA, Biggar RJ, Marshall VA, Walters MA, Gamache CJ, Whitby D, Goedert JJ.** 2003. Detection and quantification of Kaposi's sarcoma-associated herpesvirus to predict AIDS-associated Kaposi's sarcoma. *AIDS* **17:**1847–1851.
23. **Stamey FR, Patel MM, Holloway BP, Pellett PE.** 2001. Quantitative, fluorogenic probe PCR assay for detection of human herpesvirus 8 DNA in clinical specimens. *J Clin Microbiol* **39:**3537–3540.
24. **de Sanjosé S, Marshall V, Solà J, Palacio V, Almirall R, Goedert JJ, Bosch FX, Whitby D.** 2002. Prevalence of Kaposi's sarcoma-associated herpesvirus infection in sex workers and women from the general population in Spain. *Int J Cancer* **98:**155–158.
25. **Pauk J, Huang ML, Brodie SJ, Wald A, Koelle DM, Schacker T, Celum C, Selke S, Corey L.** 2000. Mucosal shedding of human herpesvirus 8 in men. *N Engl J Med* **343:** 1369–1377.
26. **Katano H, Sato Y, Kurata T, Mori S, Sata T.** 2000. Expression and localization of human herpesvirus 8-encoded proteins in primary effusion lymphoma, Kaposi's sarcoma, and multicentric Castleman's disease. *Virology* **269:**335–344.
27. **Chadburn A, Wilson J, Wang YL.** 2013. Molecular and immunohistochemical detection of Kaposi sarcoma herpesvirus/human herpesvirus-8. *Methods Mol Biol* **999:** 245–256.
28. **Benevenuto de Andrade BA, Ramírez-Amador V, Anaya-Saavedra G, Martínez-Mata G, Fonseca FP, Graner E, Paes de Almeida O.** 2014. Expression of PROX-1 in oral Kaposi's sarcoma spindle cells. *J Oral Pathol Med* **43:** 132–136.
29. **Engels EA, Whitby D, Goebel PB, Stossel A, Waters D, Pintus A, Contu L, Biggar RJ, Goedert JJ.** 2000. Identifying human herpesvirus 8 infection: performance characteristics of serologic assays. *J Acquir Immune Defic Syndr* **23:** 346–354.
30. **Schatz O, Monini P, Bugarini R, Neipel F, Schulz TF, Andreoni M, Erb P, Eggers M, Haas J, Buttò S, Lukwiya M, Bogner JR, Yaguboglu S, Sheldon J, Sarmati L, Goebel FD, Hintermaier R, Enders G, Regamey N, Wernli M, Stürzl M, Rezza G, Ensoli B.** 2001. Kaposi's sarcoma-associated herpesvirus serology in Europe and Uganda: multicentre study with multiple and novel assays. *J Med Virol* **65:**123–132.
31. **Chandran B, Smith MS, Koelle DM, Corey L, Horvat R, Goldstein E.** 1998. Reactivities of human sera with human herpesvirus-8-infected BCBL-1 cells and identification of HHV-8-specific proteins and glycoproteins and the encoding cDNAs. *Virology* **243:**208–217.
32. **Chiereghin A, Barozzi P, Petrisli E, Piccirilli G, Gabrielli L, Riva G, Potenza L, Cappelli G, De Ruvo N, Libri I, Maggiore U, Morelli MC, Potena L, Todeschini P, Gibertoni D, Labanti M, Sangiorgi G, La Manna G, Pinna AD, Luppi M, Lazzarotto T.** 2017. Multicenter prospective study for laboratory diagnosis of HHV8 infection in solid organ donors and transplant recipients and evaluation of the clinical impact after transplantation. *Transplantation* **101:** 1935–1944.
33. **Riva G, Luppi M, Barozzi P, Forghieri F, Potenza L.** 2012. How I treat HHV8/KSHV-related diseases in posttransplant patients. *Blood* **120:**4150–4159.
34. **Le J, Gantt S, AST Infectious Diseases Community of Practice.** 2013. Human herpesvirus 6, 7 and 8 in solid organ transplantation. *Am J Transplant* **13**(Suppl 4)**:**128–137.
35. **Martin DF, Kuppermann BD, Wolitz RA, Palestine AG, Li H, Robinson CA, Roche Ganciclovir Study Group.** 1999. Oral ganciclovir for patients with cytomegalovirus retinitis treated with a ganciclovir implant. *N Engl J Med* **340:** 1063–1070.

Adenoviruses

ALBERT HEIM AND RANDALL T. HAYDEN

106

In 1953, Rowe and colleagues described an "adenoid degeneration agent" that induced spontaneous deterioration of tissue cultures prepared from adenoids of children (1). In 1954, Hilleman and Werner cultivated a similar agent from military recruits with respiratory illnesses and called it RI-67 (2). The two viruses were subsequently shown to be related, and in 1956 the term "adenovirus" was proposed to acknowledge their initial source. Epidemiologic studies soon identified the virus as a major cause of acute respiratory, ocular, and gastrointestinal disease. In the mid-1960s, human adenoviruses were found to cause tumors in rodents, prompting studies that revealed fundamental processes of molecular biology but failed to link the virus convincingly to human cancer. More recently, adenoviruses have generated considerable interest as vectors for gene delivery, as opportunistic pathogens affecting immunocompromised patients, and even as emerging human pathogens.

TAXONOMY

Human adenoviruses belong to the *Adenoviridae* family, *Mastadenovirus* genus. Seven species of human mastadenoviruses (A through G) have been recognized by the International Committee on Taxonomy of Viruses (ICTV) based on immunologic, biologic, and genetic properties (Table 1). However, the term "human mastadenovirus" is not commonly used in the field of medical microbiology, and therefore the widely accepted but vernacular term "human adenovirus" (HAdV) will be used in this chapter.

Within each HAdV species, there are many types, which were defined by serology (cross-neutralization) up to (sero) type 51. Complete genomic sequences of all these types are available on GenBank. Subsequently, a type 22 strain isolated from a disease (epidemic keratoconjunctivitis) not associated with this type was sequenced and found to have a multiple recombinant genome. Most of it originated from epidemic keratoconjunctivitis-associated types 8 and 37 and only the neutralization epitope sequence originating from type 22 (3, 4). Therefore, an alternative means of classifying new strains as novel (geno-)types by phylogenetic analysis of complete genomic sequences was proposed, and the above-mentioned strain was labeled type 53. This option to define genotypes with recombinant genomes provoked an intensive taxonomic discussion among adenovirologists (5–9). Previously, recombinant isolates with a hexon sequence of one serotype (e.g., 7) and a fiber sequence of another serotype (e.g., 3) were sometimes detected by serological typing but were designated "intermediate strains" (e.g., 7H3) because they give contradictory typing results in serological typing assays (neutralization and hemagglutination inhibition [HAI]). Contemporary isolates will likely be typed by genomic sequencing and, if novel, labeled as new genotypes according to the genotype definition (e.g., type 66). Eventually, the Human Adenovirus Working Group (http://hadvwg.gmu.edu/) was established to coordinate and standardize the process of assigning type numbers to novel HAdV strains. To date, 85 types have been accepted. All newer types (52 to 85) are defined as genotypes, but there is still the option to define new adenovirus serotypes (by serological criteria). Compared to the serotype definition, the definition of adenovirus genotypes has the advantage of a better association of types with virulence and clinical symptoms.

Because it is usually not significant in diagnostics to indicate how a certain adenovirus type was defined, it is advisable to use the term "type" (as in this chapter) except when it should be stressed that a certain adenovirus type has serotype or genotype properties (e.g., in studies of immunity or molecular evolution). Many of the new genotypes are recombinants of older serotypes of the same HAdV species and cross-neutralize with one of these, but a few of the new genotypes (e.g., type 54) also have novel neutralization epitopes and thus could also fulfill the definition of a new serotype (10, 11).

Within a given type, molecular variants can be defined by full-length genomic sequencing or by restriction enzyme analysis. These variants are called subtypes or "genome types" (not to be confused with genotypes) and result from variations in DNA that can be detected by restriction enzyme analysis (and, of course, by full-length sequencing) but do not result in different serologic properties (12). Genome types are designated with lowercase letters after the numbered type, with the reference prototype denoted by the letter "p" (e.g., adenovirus genome type 21p or 21a). A few previously published genome types, subtypes, and intermediate strains, which are more virulent or cause a different disease than the prototype, have already been relabeled recently as new types according to the genotype definition, e.g., genome type 19a as type 64 (13).

TABLE 1 Properties of the 51 human adenovirus serotypes by species characteristics[a]

HAdV species	Serotype(s)	Oncogenic potential[b]	% G+C	HA[c]		Fiber length (nm)
				Rhesus	Rat	
A	12, 18, 31	High	47–49	−	±	28–31
B1	3, 7, 16, 21, 50	Weak	50–52	+	−	9–11
B2	11, 14, 34, 35	Weak	50–52	+	−	9–11
C	1, 2, 5, 6	None	57–59	−	±	23–31
D	8–10, 13, 15, 17, 19, 20, 22–30, 32, 33, 36–39, 42–49, 51	None	57–60	±	+	12–13
E	4	None	58	−	±	17
F	40, 41	None	52	−	±	18, 29

[a]Modified from reference 121 with permission of the publisher.
[b]In rodents.
[c]−, Absent HA; ±, partial HA; +, complete HA.

DESCRIPTION OF THE AGENT

Adenoviruses are large, nonenveloped, icosahedral viruses 70 to 90 nm in diameter (Fig. 1). Each particle consists of a single, linear, double-stranded DNA molecule of about 36 kb that encodes approximately 40 genes. The DNA is covalently attached to a terminal protein at both 5′ ends and encased by core proteins. A viral protease is also present. Seven structural proteins form the capsid.

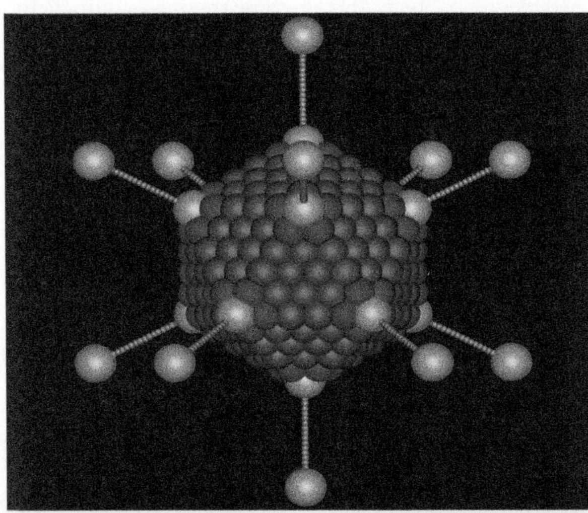

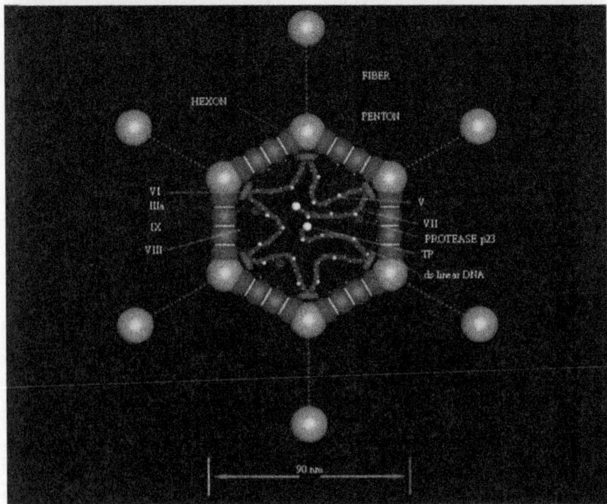

FIGURE 1 Model of an adenovirus particle. (Top) Exterior. (Bottom) Interior.

The major capsid proteins are the hexon, penton base, and fiber. The capsid is formed primarily by 252 capsomeres consisting of the 240 trimeric hexons that form 20 triangular faces and 12 pentons, one at each of the 12 vertices. Each penton consists of a pentameric base and a trimeric fiber, a rod-like projection of variable length with a terminal knob which interacts with cellular receptors. The hexon has antigenic sites common to all HAdVs, but these sites reside within the capsid, so neutralizing antibodies are not induced. The hexon also contains on its outer surface the ε determinant, which induces serotype-specific neutralizing antibodies. The fiber has mostly serotype-specific antigenic determinants and some species specificity. The knob region of the fiber includes the γ determinant, which is responsible for hemagglutination *in vitro*.

Productive infection begins by attachment of the viral fiber knobs to cell surface molecules, such as the coxsackie adenovirus receptor, although most types of species B and certain types of species D use CD46 or sialic acid, respectively. The specificity of this interaction is an important determinant of tissue tropism. Following secondary interaction of capsids with integrins, particles are internalized by endocytosis and are transported to the nucleus, where viral transcription and DNA replication initiate. Viral structural proteins synthesized in the cytoplasm likewise migrate to the nucleus, where the particles assemble and aggregate, forming large crystalline arrays (Fig. 2A). Productive infection results in 10,000 to over a million viral particles per cell, only 1 to 5% of which are infectious.

Latent infection can follow acute adenovirus infection, but latent infection is not well understood. Early studies showed latency mostly associated with species C adenoviruses in the mucosal T lymphocytes of tonsils and adenoids of asymptomatic young children. More-recent work has shown a wider spectrum of viral species and has demonstrated viral genomic material in gastrointestinal-associated lymphoid cells (14–16). Similar reservoirs may exist elsewhere in the body. The highest quantities of viral DNA are detectable in the tissues of young children, suggesting that virus stores may decline with age (17). Low levels of viral DNA (<1,000 copies/ml) are occasionally detectable in peripheral blood (circulating white blood cells) of healthy individuals (18–20).

EPIDEMIOLOGY AND TRANSMISSION

Adenovirus infections are common and ubiquitous. Adenoviruses are responsible for 1 to 5% of respiratory infections overall but induce 2 to 24% of all respiratory infections and 5 to 15% of all acute diarrheal illnesses in children and 30 to 70% of all respiratory illnesses in unvaccinated new

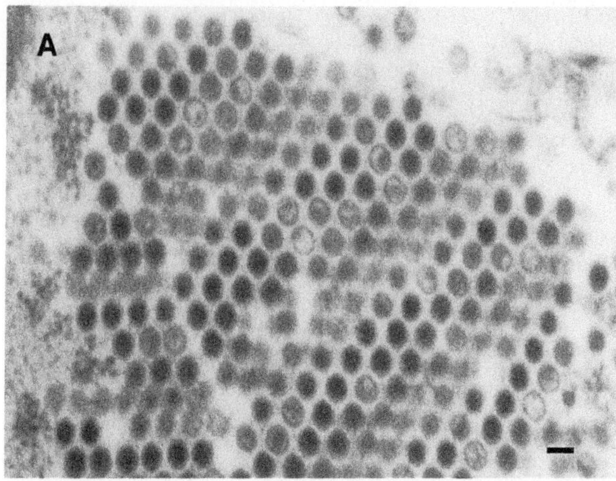

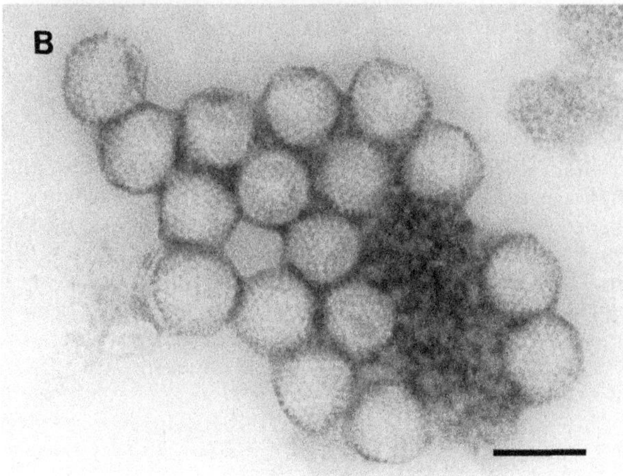

FIGURE 2 Ultrastructure of adenovirus particles. (A) Transmission EM of a hepatocyte nucleus containing complete (dark) and empty (clear) adenovirus particles. (B) Direct EM of a cluster of adenovirus particles in stool from a child with diarrhea. Bar = 100 nm.

military recruits. Most infections occur in the first few years of life, and about half are asymptomatic. By the age of 10, most children have been infected with one or more types. Coinfection with different types and different species is documented, especially when different body sites are sampled (21). The incidence of infection is highest in crowded closed settings, such as day care centers, boarding schools, geriatric facilities, military training camps, and hospitals. Intrafamilial transmissions are common. There is no obvious difference in susceptibility by gender or ethnic group. Infections occur worldwide, with some differences in types associated with various syndromes in other parts of the world.

Adenovirus infections can be epidemic, endemic, or sporadic, with the pattern of circulation, specific syndrome, and severity varying by type, population, and route of exposure. Sporadic infections occur year-round.

Respiratory infections are most often associated with species HAdV-B, HAdV-C, and HAdV-E, with types 1, 2, 5, and 6 causing endemic infections and subsequent latency (most frequently in young children) and types 4, 7, 14, and 21 causing small epidemics mostly in winter to early summer. A survey of U.S. isolates conducted in 2004 to 2006 identified the most common types in civilians as 3, 2, 1, and 5, with an increasing amount of type 21, which can cause serious lower respiratory tract illness (LRTI) (22–24). Epidemics of severe respiratory disease in U.S. military recruits typically occur in the winter and spring. Historically, types 4 and 7 were the most common causes and were controlled by a vaccination program. After termination of the vaccination program in 1999, type 4 predominated, with lesser amounts of species B types 7 and 21 detected. Reintroduction of vaccination in 2011 reduced the incidence of type 4 infections in the military and the clinical severity of respiratory infections (25). An emerging variant of type 14 (14p1, previously labeled 14a) was also identified in the military (22, 26), but it has also caused clusters of severe LRTI and fatalities among civilians in several states (27).

Large epidemics of keratoconjunctivitis are caused mostly by species HAdV-D types 8, 37, and 64 (previously subtype 19a) and less frequently by types 53 and 54; the latter seems to predominate in Asia. Smaller outbreaks of conjunctivitis caused by types 3, 4, and 7 (of species HAdV-B and -E) occur in the summertime and are associated with contaminated swimming pool water. In contrast to epidemic keratoconjunctivitis, these infections hardly ever affect the cornea.

Adenovirus-associated gastroenteritis is caused primarily by types 40 and 41 of species HAdV-F, which are also known as the "enteric adenoviruses." These infections are endemic globally and occur year-round. Types 12, 18, 31, and 61 of species HAdV-A can cause small gastroenteritis outbreaks, and gastroenteritis can also be observed during respiratory infections with types 1, 2, and 5.

Adenovirus infections in people with primary or acquired immunodeficiencies are frequently reported (28). Infections are most frequent and severe in pediatric recipients of hematopoietic stem cell transplantation (HSCT), with an incidence of infection up to 30%. Risk factors for disease in this population include young age, allogeneic transplantation, T-cell depletion, graft mismatch, cord blood transplantation, and severe graft-versus-host disease (29). Many infections in pediatric HSCT recipients are endogenous reactivations of latent infections with adenovirus types of species HAdV-C and perhaps other species, for example, HAdV-A (28, 30, 31), but *de novo* infections can also be observed. Infections with types of species HAdV-C clearly predominate in all HSCT age groups. Type 31 of species HAdV-A is frequently found in pediatric HSCT recipients but not in adult recipients, where types of species HAdV-B and -D can be found occasionally (32, 33). Mixed or sequential infections with different types are also common (34).

Data for solid organ transplantation recipients are more limited (35), but this group generally experiences fewer and milder infections than HSCT recipients. Adenovirus infections are frequently associated with increased immunosuppression for the treatment of organ rejection. The lowest incidence is for renal transplant patients, who tend to suffer from species HAdV-B adenoviruses (types 7, 11, 34, and 35), which usually cause hemorrhagic cystitis and occasionally transplant nephritis. Adenovirus infections can be observed more frequently in lung, small bowel, or liver transplant recipients and lead to graft dysfunction (or loss) and fatalities. Infections with species C viruses (types 1, 2, and 5) are the most common. Transplant patients can acquire adenovirus as a result of endogenous reactivation of the virus from recipient or donor tissue, as well as from the community or hospital.

Adenoviruses once caused many serious infections in human immunodeficiency virus/AIDS patients, mostly with species D types rarely identified in other settings (36). The introduction of highly active antiretroviral therapy has dramatically reduced the incidence of such infections in this population.

Transmission occurs primarily by the respiratory or fecal-oral route. Airborne transmission occurs by small droplets and, to a lesser extent, large-droplet aerosols. Fecal-oral spread probably accounts for the majority of enteric adenovirus infections. Adenoviruses are also spread by contaminated fomites, fingers, and liquids, such as ophthalmic solutions and sewage. Eye trauma facilitates infection and the spread of keratoconjunctivitis in environments with high levels of airborne particulates. The infection's spread among new military recruits may involve direct contact as well as aerosol exposure via ventilation systems. Physical stress and fatigue may be contributory host factors in this setting for infection and severe disease affecting the lower respiratory tract. The mean incubation period for most respiratory tract infections is 5.6 days, for eye infections about 1 week, and for gastroenteritis 3 to 10 days (37).

Transmission is facilitated by adenoviral resistance to many disinfectants and physical treatments. The stability of particles in gastric secretions, bile, and pancreatic proteases also permits passage through the stomach, followed by replication in the intestine. The prolonged period of virus shedding from various body sites aids transmission as well. The duration of shedding varies by type, body site, patient age, and immune status. In general, nonenteric adenoviruses are shed for several days by adults with upper respiratory tract infections, for a few weeks in ocular infections, and for 3 to 6 weeks from the throat or stool of children with respiratory or generalized illness. Infected children may excrete the virus initially from the respiratory tract and later from the gastrointestinal tract. Excretion in stool can be intermittent and prolonged for 18 months or longer after recovery (38). Although the possibility of serial reinfection cannot be ruled out in all cases, a recent study of adenovirus DNA detection in intestinal biopsies of children clearly supports the concept of adenovirus latency and persistent infections (15, 16). In contrast, enteric adenoviruses of species HAdV-F are shed for only a few days after recovery. Immunocompromised individuals shed adenovirus longer than immunocompetent individuals.

CLINICAL SIGNIFICANCE

The spectrum of adenovirus-associated disease is broad due to the many types and their different tissue tropisms (Table 2). Clinical manifestations also depend on the age and immune status of the infected person. Most infections affect the respiratory tract, eye, and gastrointestinal tract, with less involvement of the urinary tract, heart, central nervous system, liver, pancreas, and genital tract. Solid-organ involvement and disseminated disease are seen primarily in immunocompromised patients.

Most respiratory tract infections occur early in life and are self-limited and mild. Usual signs and symptoms are fever, nasal congestion, coryza, pharyngitis, cervical adenopathy, and cough, with or without otitis media. An exudative tonsillitis clinically indistinguishable from infection with group A streptococcus has been described. A pertussis-like syndrome has been reported, although adenoviruses are more likely to be copathogens or to reactivate in this syndrome than to be a significant cause. The role of adenoviruses in asthma remains controversial (39). Adenoviral lower respiratory tract infections, such as croup, bronchitis, bronchiolitis, and pneumonia, can be severe and sometimes fatal, particularly in young children less than 2 years of age. Long-term sequelae (bronchitis obliterans, bronchiectasis, and chronic atelectasis) of these lower respiratory tract infections are frequent in some populations, but additional studies on this topic are needed (40). Higher mortality is reported for types 4 (genome type 4a), 5, 14 (genome type 14p1), 21 (subtype 21a), and 66 (previously labeled genome type 7h or intermediate strain 7H3) and when extrapulmonary manifestations occur (22, 23, 41–43).

TABLE 2 Adenovirus diseases, associated types, hosts, and suitable specimens[a]

Disease	Associated type(s)		Frequent hosts	Specimen(s)
	Frequent	Infrequent		
URTI	1–3, 5, 7	4, 6, 11, 14, 15, 18, 21, 29, 31	Infants, children	NP aspirate or swab, throat swab
LRTI	3, 4, 7, 14, 21, 55	1, 2, 5, 7, 8, 11, 35, 66	Infants, children, IP	NP aspirate or swab, BAL fluid, lung tissue
Pertussis syndrome	5	1–3, 12, 19	Children	Throat swab
Acute respiratory disease	4, 7	2, 3, 5, 8, 11, 14, 21, 35	Military recruits	Throat swab, BAL fluid, lung tissue, NP aspirate or swab
Acute conjunctivitis	1–4, 7	6, 9–11, 15–17, 19, 20, 22, 37	Children	Conjunctival swab or scraping
Acute hemorrhagic conjunctivitis	11	2–8, 14, 15, 19, 37	Children	Conjunctival swab or scraping
Pharyngoconjunctival fever	3, 4, 7	1, 2, 5, 6, 8, 11–17, 19–21, 29, 37	Children	NP aspirate or swab, throat swab, conjunctival swab or scraping
Epidemic keratoconjunctivitis	8, 37, 53, 54, 64 (=19a)	2–5, 7, 10, 11, 13–17, 21, 23, 29, 56	Individuals of any age	Conjunctival swab or scraping
Gastroenteritis	40, 41	1–3, 5, 7, 12–18, 21, 25, 26, 29, 31, 52	Children	Stool
Hemorrhagic cystitis	11	7, 21, 34, 35	Children, IP	Urine
Hepatitis	1–3, 5, 7	4, 31	Infants, children, IP	Liver tissue, blood
Myocarditis	7, 21		Children	Heart tissue, blood
Meningoencephalitis	7	1–3, 5, 6, 11, 12, 26, 32	Children, IP	Brain tissue, cerebrospinal fluid
Sexually transmitted disease	2, 37	1, 4, 5, 7, 9, 11, 18, 19, 31, 49	Teens, adults	Lesion swab
Disseminated disease	1, 2, 5, 11, 31, 34, 35	3, 6, 7, 14, 21, 29, 32, 37–39, 43, 45	IP, newborns	Blood, BAL fluid, urine, involved tissue

[a]Modified from reference 121 with permission of the publisher. ARDS, acute respiratory distress syndrome; BAL, bronchoalveolar lavage; IP, immunocompromised people; NP, nasopharyngeal; LRTI, lower respiratory tract illness; URTI, upper respiratory tract illness.

Frequent outbreaks of adenovirus-associated acute respiratory disease in young military recruits were noted beginning in 1953. Symptoms included febrile cold-like illness, pharyngitis with tonsillitis, bronchitis, and pneumonia. Hospitalization rates were as high as 50%, and some fatalities occurred due to severe LRTI, which resulted in acute respiratory distress syndrome. Vaccines directed against serotypes 4 and 7, the most common serotypes involved at the time, were introduced for this population in 1980 and significantly reduced disease. In 1996, vaccine production lapsed, and the problem recurred until reintroduction of the vaccine (again to serotypes 4 and 7) to the military in 2011. Although the current outbreaks in military facilities are not as severe as in the prevaccine era, they continue to be problematic and involve a broader array of serotypes (22, 25). In particular, type 14 has been associated with numerous outbreaks in recent years among both military recruits and the general population (42, 43). Interestingly, type 4 has been an uncommon cause of respiratory disease in civilians.

Ocular adenovirus infections are common. Acute follicular conjunctivitis is usually superficial and resolves without consequence in a few weeks. Epidemics of acute hemorrhagic conjunctivitis similar to those caused by enterovirus are also described. Pharyngoconjunctival fever is a follicular conjunctivitis accompanied by upper respiratory tract symptoms, fever, and occasionally lymphadenopathy, pharyngitis, and malaise. All these infections do not affect the cornea and are frequently caused by types 3, 4, and 7 of species HAdV-B and HAdV-E but also by many other types. Epidemic keratoconjunctivitis is a more serious infection that starts with conjunctivitis but progresses with corneal erosions and infiltrates, which impair vision, and painful edema of the eyelids. Inflammatory symptoms may resolve in 2 weeks, although reduced vision due to chronic infiltrates of the cornea ("numuli"), photophobia, and foreign-body sensation may persist for months to years. Most cases of epidemic conjunctivitis are caused by types 8, 37, 53, 54, and 64, which are all members of species HAdV-D.

The enteric adenovirus types 40 and 41 are a common cause of viral gastroenteritis in children less than 2 years old (Table 2). Diarrhea is usually watery and nonbloody, lacks fecal leukocytosis, and lasts a mean of 10 days, which is somewhat longer than diarrhea due to rotavirus (44). Mild fever, vomiting, and abdominal pain can occur, and respiratory symptoms are sometimes present. Most immunocompetent patients recover uneventfully, although infants with ileostomies or colostomies can have prolonged symptoms, and rare fatalities have been reported for immunocompetent patients. Gastrointestinal syndromes infrequently associated with nonenteric adenovirus infections include intussusception, acute mesenteric lymphadenitis, and appendicitis.

Clinical manifestations of adenovirus in immunocompromised patients depend on the individual's underlying disease or transplanted organ, patient age, and type involved (31, 45, 46). Presentations in HSCT patients most often start with endogenous reactivation in the gastrointestinal tract (asymptomatic or symptomatic adenovirus shedding with the feces) or less frequently with *de novo* infections of, e.g., the respiratory or gastrointestinal tract. Disease can affect single organs (e.g., hemorrhagic cystitis, pneumonia, hepatitis, enteritis), but disseminated disease is frequently observed. This includes high-level viremia (usually detected as DNA-emia by quantitative PCR) associated with sepsis-like symptoms and infection of multiple organs (e.g., hepatitis and pneumonia) resulting in high mortality rates (exceeding 80% in some studies) (47, 48).

Infections in solid organ transplantation patients can involve the graft or other organ systems. In liver transplant patients, infections are most often associated with diarrhea, graft hepatitis, and pneumonia (49, 50). Enterocolitis, with occasional spread to the liver, occurs in intestinal transplant recipients. The major clinical presentation in renal transplant patients is acute hemorrhagic cystitis and, to a lesser extent, graft nephritis and pneumonia (51). Without adenovirus diagnostics, graft nephritis can be mixed up with rejection, and increased immunosuppression may result in graft loss. Recent work has also reported systemic involvement of other organs (52). Infections of the graft in lung transplant recipients can result in necrotizing pneumonitis, leading to respiratory failure and progressive graft loss. Bronchiolitis obliterans can be a late consequence.

In the post-highly active antiretroviral therapy era, clinical manifestations in patients with human immunodeficiency virus infections are uncommon. AIDS patients have presented with adenovirus-associated pneumonia, meningoencephalitis, and hepatitis as well as disseminated disease.

Less common clinical manifestations include exanthems, neonatal disease, which can be severe and frequently fatal, neurologic manifestations, such as meningoencephalitis and encephalitis, acute myocarditis in otherwise healthy people or associated with graft rejection in cardiac transplant patients, macrophage activation syndrome, and genitourinary disease, including genital lesions and urethritis. The role of adenoviruses in fetal demise remains unclear. Adenovirus type 36 has recently been linked to obesity (53), although this association remains controversial. Some adenovirus infections resemble Kawasaki disease, but adenovirus has also been described concomitantly with Kawasaki disease, so one should be cautious when making these diagnoses (54). In general, detection of adenovirus DNA by highly sensitive PCR can be misleading because latent adenovirus infections can result in positive PCR results coincidental with any disease of another etiology. Quantification of adenovirus DNA can be helpful to discern disease-associated adenovirus replication from latent adenovirus infections.

COLLECTION, TRANSPORT, AND STORAGE OF SPECIMENS

Adenoviruses are best detected from affected sites early in the course of illness. Suitable specimens vary with the clinical syndrome and test requirements (Table 2). Collection of cell-rich specimens usually results in the highest sensitivity. Flocked nylon swabs (Copan Diagnostics, Murrieta, CA) have shown excellent yield compared to that from cotton swabs or nasopharyngeal aspirates for the detection of respiratory viruses, including adenovirus (55–57). When a deep-seated or disseminated infection is suspected and tissue from the affected sites is unavailable, collection from multiple sites (e.g., respiratory, stool, and urine) or blood is recommended.

Recovery is best if specimens are kept cold (2 to 8°C), transported, and processed as described in earlier chapters. Suitable viral transport media can be laboratory prepared or purchased from commercial sources. Some commercial formulations, such as MicroTest multimicrobe medium M4RT (Remel, Lenexa, KS) or universal transport medium UTM (Copan), preserve infectivity for prolonged periods at room temperature and are also suitable for detection of viral antigen or DNA (58). If plasma or serum samples are being tested, they should be separated within several hours of collection. Specimens, virus isolates, or DNA extracts can be frozen at −70°C indefinitely, with minimal loss of activity. Storage of specimens for adenovirus DNA detection by PCR is also feasible in –20°C freezers. Long-term storage in self-defrosting freezers and repeated freeze-thaw cycles ultimately reduce infectivity and degrade adenovirus DNA. Such conditions are not recommended for storage of any clinical specimens.

Adenoviruses are highly resistant to inactivation by chemical and physical treatment. Most types are stable for a week at 36°C, for several weeks at room temperature, and for several months at 4°C. Infectivity is retained for several weeks on paper or in saline and for over a month on nonporous surfaces. Strict adherence to conventional safety practices, such as the use of personal protective equipment and biologic safety cabinets, disinfection of work surfaces, and handwashing, minimizes laboratory infections. Avoid hand-to-eye or hand-to-mouth contact due to the affinity of adenoviruses for mucosal and ocular tissue. Treatments that eliminate infectivity include a 1:10 dilution of household bleach (0.5% sodium hypochlorite) for 30 min, heating to 56°C for 30 min or 60°C for 2 min, and autoclaving. Type 4 is especially heat resistant. Alcohol-based hand gels can destroy infectivity, although several minutes of contact may be required for some products. Variable disinfection is achieved with povidone-iodine, formaldehyde, and UV light. Viral DNA can be detected long after loss of infectivity.

DIRECT DETECTION

Microscopy

Adenovirus-infected cells can be visualized by light microscopy as "smudge cells" in hematoxylin-and-eosin-stained or Wright-Giemsa-stained tissues, fluid sediments, or cultures. Smudge cells are large late-stage-infected cells containing solitary, central, basophilic nuclear inclusions composed of adenoviral particles (Fig. 2A). Other types of inclusions have been described as well (59). Adenoviral inclusions can be mistaken for those of cytomegalovirus, herpes simplex virus, or polyomavirus. Further identification by immunohistochemistry or *in situ* hybridization is recommended to avoid misdiagnosis (60, 61). The characteristic morphology of adenovirus particles permits their detection by electron microscopy (EM) without the need for further identification. Particles, often in large crystalline arrays, can be visualized in the infected cells by transmission EM (Fig. 2A). The large quantity of virus (10^6 to 10^9 particles/ml) in the stools of children with acute diarrhea (Fig. 2B) also permits detection by direct EM (62). The sensitivity of direct EM can be increased by ultracentrifugation, by immunoelectron microscopy using antihexon antibodies, or by a special ultracentrifuge rotor (Airfuge; Beckman Coulter, Inc., Fullerton, CA) that permits concentration of virus onto grids prior to examination (63). Few clinical laboratories have access to EM facilities, so other methods are typically used.

Antigen Detection

Antigen detection can be used for the rapid detection of adenoviruses in respiratory, ocular, and gastrointestinal tract specimens. Sensitivity is often poor, particularly when adults or immunocompromised patients are tested, and particularly compared to the sensitivities of molecular methods (64, 65). Most antigen assays target conserved regions of the adenovirus hexon protein and utilize monoclonal antibodies (MAbs). Immunofluorescence (IF), enzyme immunoassay (EIA), and lateral-flow immunochromatography (IC) are the most common formats.

IF can be used for definitive identification of culture isolates and for primary detection of respiratory tract infections. Suitable specimens for direct detection are washes, aspirates, and swabs containing exfoliated ciliated columnar epithelial cells from the posterior nasopharynx or midturbinate. Touch preparations of fresh tissue or frozen or formalin-fixed tissue sections can be tested as well. However, these may not be approved applications for a given commercial reagent and as such would require further validation prior to routine clinical use. General techniques for IF are described in chapter 82. Positive cells usually display condensed nuclear or granular cytoplasmic staining (Fig. 3). Although indirect IF is highly sensitive and specific, direct IF can also provide satisfactory and more rapid results (66). Labeled MAbs directed solely against adenovirus or pools of MAbs labeled with different fluorochromes directed against adenoviruses and other respiratory viruses can be used. Pools may be most economical for laboratories with a low prevalence of adenovirus. The reported sensitivity of IF for adenovirus detection in respiratory specimens is 40 to 60% of that of culture, which is lower than the detection rate of most other respiratory viruses. A sensitivity higher (60 to 80%) than that of culture is achievable using cytocentrifugation (66) and specimens from pediatric patients. The specificity of IF for adenovirus is excellent (>99%) in most studies.

Antigen detection can also be performed by EIA, IC, or latex agglutination. These technologies are fully described in other chapters. Two types of EIA are available, a type 40- and 41-specific EIA and a generic EIA to detect all types (67, 68). Both assays utilize microtiter plates and adenovirus-specific MAbs as capture and detector reagents. This format is most economical for large laboratories which usually test in batch mode. The sensitivity of the type 40/41 assay compared to that of Graham 293 cell culture or EM is >90% in most studies, although sensitivity can be lower with some variants (69). Specificity is >97%. The generic EIA detects species F and other species in a single reaction.

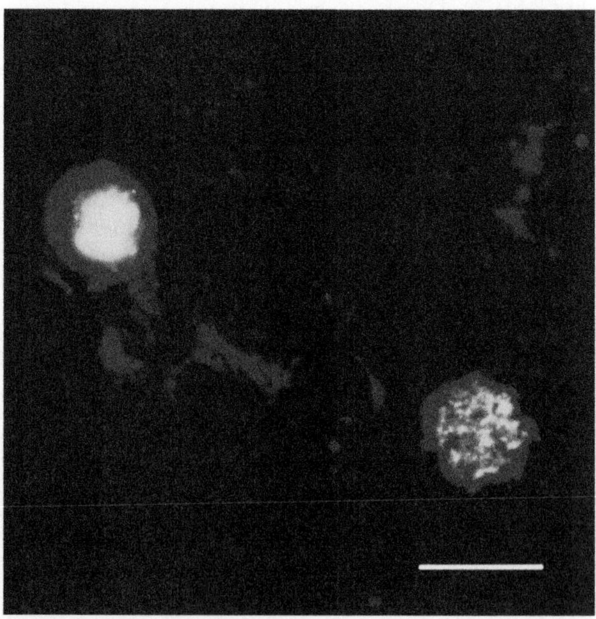

FIGURE 3 Adenovirus antigen demonstrated in two cells of a nasopharyngeal aspirate by direct IF using a rhodamine-conjugated antibody (yellow). Bar = 40 μm.

Some have shown high sensitivity (>95%) when stool is tested, but the sensitivity is only 65 to 75% when other specimen types are tested. Urine may give the lowest value, and occasional false-positive reactions occur (67, 70).

The IC format is attractive for smaller laboratories because tests can be run individually, and results are usually available in less than 30 min. The SAS rapid adenovirus test (SA Scientific, San Antonio, TX) is a membrane-based immunogold assay for testing eye swabs, nasopharyngeal secretions, and fecal material. Initial reports suggested good sensitivity (84 to 95%) compared to that of culture and PCR on nasopharyngeal specimens, but sensitivity was only 55% when a broader array of specimen types was evaluated (64, 71). Performance is best with specimens from young children. The AdenoPlus (Quidel, San Diego, CA) is a lateral flow immunoassay for testing eye swabs and is marketed as a point-of-care test. Reports on its sensitivity compared to PCR were contradictory in two studies, with 85% and 39.5%, but both studies reported a high specificity, 98% and 95.5%, respectively (72, 73).

Nucleic Acid Detection

Nucleic acid detection has become commonplace for sensitive and rapid viral detection and quantification. In fact, adenovirus has been detected by PCR or similar amplification methods in virtually all specimen types, so the appropriate specimen depends largely on the associated disease (Table 2). In almost all reports, irrespective of the specific method used, the sensitivity of PCR has usually exceeded that of antigen detection or culture (74). Direct detection of viral DNA (without amplification) is feasible in stool specimens by gel electrophoresis after restriction enzyme digestion and in tissues specimens by *in situ* hybridization but has become almost obsolete as a diagnostic procedure since highly sensitive PCR protocols have become available.

Detection of all adenoviral types by PCR represents a tremendous challenge in test design. It is therefore incumbent on both the developer and the user of such tests to verify the sensitivity of a given assay for the whole range of adenoviral types of clinical importance in the population being tested. Where quantitative tests are used, colinearity should be assessed across detectable viral types to ensure accuracy when a non-type-specific calibration curve is used. Calculation of amplification efficiencies for different types can be helpful to estimate colinearity. Clinical specificity should also be determined whenever possible because adenovirus DNA can be found in healthy control subjects due to persistence of adenovirus DNA after symptomatic infections or due to asymptomatic adenovirus infections. On average, fewer than 2% of specimens from healthy individuals contain low concentrations of adenovirus DNA, although values can vary significantly depending on the patient population and the specimen type (e.g., whole blood versus plasma/serum) (18–20, 75). Somewhat higher detection rates have been reported for chronic conditions (such as asthma), for tonsil and adenoid tissue, and for gastrointestinal biopsy specimens with negative pathology (17, 39, 76). Each laboratory should therefore define the clinical significance of positive PCR results in its patient population and sample types. For quantitative tests, threshold values can be established which indicate the clinical significance of a positive result. In the case of qualitative real-time PCRs, threshold cycle values may be helpful to discern clinically significant acute infections from persistence of adenovirus DNA, but threshold cycle values have to be validated carefully.

Both endpoint PCR and real-time amplification methods are in current use. Degenerate or nondegenerate primers and probes for the hexon or fiber gene or for the viral-associated RNA I and II regions are usually selected due to the extensive homology of these regions among types. Many assays utilize multiple primer and probe sets for uniform detection or quantification of all types, but this is also feasible with a single primer and probe set (19, 77–81). Over the years, a variety of laboratory-developed tests have been described in the literature. More recently, commercial tests that are cleared or approved for *in vitro* diagnostics (Table 3) have

TABLE 3 Commercial PCR assays (FDA cleared or approved[a]) available in the United States for the detection of adenovirus infections either as singleplex PCRs or as part of multiplex PCRs

Manufacturer	Test name	Specimen types/DNA extracted from[a]	Adenovirus types detected	Format
Luminex Molecular Diagnostics	xTAG respiratory viral panel (xTAG RVP and xTAG RVP FAST)	Nasopharyngeal swabs	Not specified (probably all respiratory types)	Broad respiratory panel/ endpoint detection
Luminex Molecular Diagnostics	xTAG gastrointestinal pathogen panel	Stool	Types 40 and 41	Broad gastrointestinal panel/ endpoint detection
bioMérieux (BioFire)	FilmArray respiratory panel 2 (RP2)	Nasopharyngeal swabs	23 types of species HAdV-A, -B, -C, -D, -E, and -F (probably generic)	Broad respiratory panel/ endpoint detection
bioMérieux (BioFire)	FilmArray respiratory panel (RP)	Nasopharyngeal swabs	Types of species HAdV-B, -C, and -E (85)	Broad respiratory panel/ endpoint detection
bioMérieux (BioFire)	FilmArray gastrointesinal panel	Stool	Types 40 and 41	Broad gastrointestinal panel/ endpoint detection
GenMark Diagnostics	ePlex respiratory pathogen panel	Nasopharyngeal swabs	(Probably all respiratory types)	Broad respiratory panel/ endpoint detection
Hologic Gen-Probe	Prodesse ProAdeno+ assay	Nasopharyngeal swabs	Types 1–51 (probably generic)	Adenovirus-only testing/ real-time detection
bioMérieux	Adenovirus r-gene (U.S.)	Nasopharyngeal swab, wash, and aspirate[a]	Types 1–60 (probably generic)	Adenovirus-only testing/ real-time detection
Quidel	Lyra adenovirus assay	Nasal and nasopharyngeal swabs[a]	Types 1–52 (probably generic)	Adenovirus-only testing/ real-time detection

[a]According to https://www.fda.gov/MedicalDevices/ProductsandMedicalProcedures/InVitroDiagnostics/ucm330711.htm#microbial. Accessed 13 June 2017.

been marketed (82–85). While many of these have largely been approved only for detection of respiratory tract or gastrointestinal tract infections, their availability represents a marked advance in our ability to rapidly and accurately detect adenoviral infections.

Detection formats described for endpoint PCR methods have included gel electrophoresis, Southern blotting or liquid hybridization and capture onto microtiter plates, and fluidic or solid-phase microarrays (86). Conventional assays that detect all adenoviruses as well as multiplex PCRs for adenoviruses, herpesviruses, and other respiratory viruses have been reported (21, 87, 88). Increasingly, highly multiplexed methods that detect a full range of respiratory viruses have been developed and marketed (82–85). The sensitivities of such systems for adenovirus and the spectra of adenovirus types detected are widely varied among platforms and test versions. Early versions of some systems have shown marked weakness in the detection of adenovirus compared to other respiratory pathogens. While the trend has been for manufacturers to ameliorate such issues in subsequent test versions (85), the sensitivity of such tests for all diagnostically relevant types should be critically assessed prior to implementation. Real-time PCR is most often used when targeting adenovirus alone, rather than in a panel approach, because it is more rapid and less prone to contamination than endpoint PCR and can provide quantitative results. Many real-time laboratory-developed tests have been described (19, 63, 77–79, 81), and commercial real-time PCRs are available, but all of those on the U.S. market claim only qualitative detection of adenovirus DNA. Quantification with the help of these assays may be feasible but needs to be thoroughly validated by the laboratory with the help of external standards. A European (CE-marked) version of the bioMérieux R-Gene assay permits quantitative adenovirus DNA detection.

The major application of quantitative real-time PCR is the detection and quantification of DNA-emia to predict current or incipient disseminated adenovirus disease in immunocompromised patients (89, 90). Detection and quantification of DNA-emia can be performed using plasma, peripheral blood mononuclear cells, or whole blood. No significant differences in qualitative sensitivity have been observed among these specimen types, although viral load values were slightly higher for whole blood and plasma than for peripheral blood mononuclear cells in one recent report (91). Quantitative tests have increasingly been applied to other sample types, such as stool, in an effort to improve the clinically predictive value of positive results (92) or to achieve early diagnosis of reactivation in pediatric HSCT patients (46). High virus loads are clearly associated with acute infections and clinically significant reactivations in HSCT patients.

Many transplant centers now assess DNA-emia with such quantitative tests on a weekly basis for several months after transplantation and subsequently when symptoms appear. Routine screening has become especially commonplace for pediatric HSCT patients. Screening of asymptomatic patients can be used to trigger preemptive therapy (29). A threshold value of 1×10^4 copies/ml was proposed for starting preemptive therapy because lower virus loads did not influence mortality (33, 93). However, there is no single threshold value of DNA-emia that can be recommended in general due to differences in assay characteristics and patient populations and the lack of universal calibration standards. Some experts follow *in vivo* dynamic changes by repeat testing 2 or 3 days after a single low viral load to identify patients with a rapid increase before initiating treatment. In patients with diagnosed adenoviral infection, changing viral load values can be used to assess the clinical response to antivirals and predict outcomes (94).

ISOLATION PROCEDURES

Although historically considered the reference standard, viral isolation is now used with decreasing frequency. Viral culture is slower than antigen or DNA assays and, with some specimen types, can be less sensitive than PCR, yet it remains useful to detect types that might be missed by direct methods and yields infectious progeny for further identification and typing. Most specimens are suitable for culture (Table 2). Exceptions are blood and cerebrospinal fluid, which may contain insufficient virus to be cultivated or may contain virus neutralized by antibodies. For these specimens, DNA amplification is typically preferred.

Adenoviruses grow best in human epithelial cells. Primary human embryonic or neonatal kidney cells are the most sensitive but are rarely available, so human epithelial cell lines, such as A549, Hep2, or sometimes HeLa or KB, are used. Human fibroblasts and non-human cells, such as Vero and primary monkey kidney cells that contain endogenous simian virus 40, may support adenovirus replication, but the yield is low. Enteric adenoviruses (species HAdV-F) are often termed "fastidious" because they are noncultivable or grow slowly in routine cell lines. Cultivation of enteric adenoviruses is most successful in Graham 293 cells (44).

Adenoviruses can be isolated by conventional tube culture or shell vial centrifugation culture (SVCC). These methods are detailed in earlier chapters. Although SVCC is popular because it produces rapid results, tube culture remains useful to detect low concentrations of virus or slow-growing types, particularly of species A or D, which may not be evident for 3 or 4 weeks. Holding tubes for 2 weeks is customary for routine diagnostic work. If tubes are held for longer periods, cells should be subpassaged at least once to maintain the health of the monolayer. Typical cytopathic effects (CPEs) consist of grape-like aggregates of swollen, refractile cells (Fig. 4B). Aggregates may not develop with species D, and a web-like flattening is described for serotypes 3 and 7 (95). CPE is usually evident in 2 to 7 days in A549 cells but may be less characteristic and slower to appear in other cell types. As infection progresses, cells can become highly granular and detach completely from the surface. Most infectious virus remains cell associated so that high-titer preparations can be produced by several freeze-thaw cycles of harvested cells. CPE that develops within hours after inoculation with concentrated preparations is known as "lysis from without" or "early CPE" and is a toxic effect due to free penton base proteins in the inoculum. It can be prevented by using a lower concentration of the inoculum.

A significant proportion of culture-positive specimens can be detected in A549 or Hep2 SVCC after 1 to 5 days of incubation and should be confirmed using fluorophore-conjugated MAbs directed against the adenovirus hexon protein. Often the MAb preparations used to identify viral antigen in direct specimens can be used in SVCC. Maximum detection of fluorescent foci requires at least 30 min of centrifugation at $700 \times g$ (20). The sensitivity of SVCC compared to that of tube culture under these conditions is approximately 50% at 24 h, increases somewhat at 2 days, and can approach 100% by 5 days (67, 96–99). Similar results can be achieved using 24-well microtiter plates. Lower detection rates are reported if human fibroblast or monkey cells are used (100). Dexamethasone, which

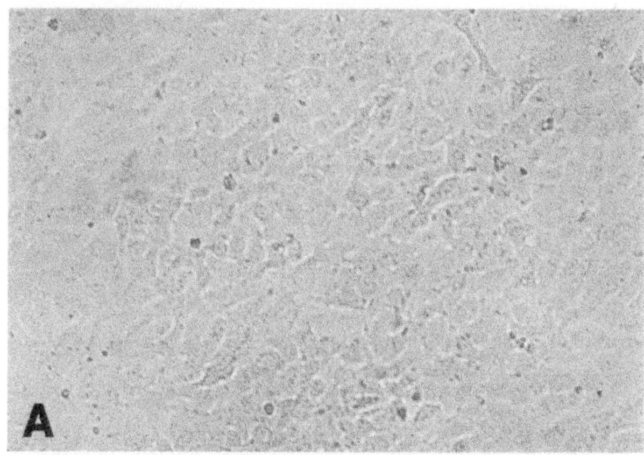

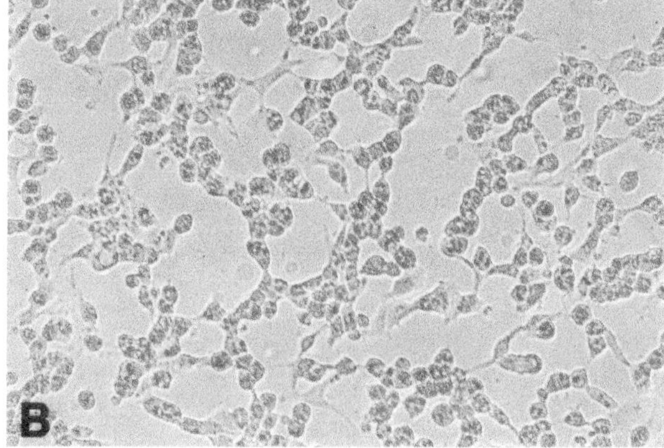

FIGURE 4 Adenovirus CPE in A549 cells. (A) Uninfected cells. (B) Advanced adenovirus CPE. Magnification, ×100.

enhances the identification of some viruses in SVCC, does not improve adenovirus detection in SVCC (101). Recovery of adenoviruses from respiratory sources in R-Mix (Diagnostic Hybrids Inc., Athens, OH), a mixture of A549 and mink lung cells, is lower than that for parainfluenza or influenza viruses (102). Enteric adenoviruses can be detected in SVCC if appropriate cells lines are used (103), but other approaches are more sensitive and convenient.

IDENTIFICATION

Culture isolates should be definitively identified before a report is generated. For diagnostic work, genus-specific identification is usually sufficient. Most immunologic or molecular methods for direct detection of adenoviruses are suitable for this purpose. Identification by IF is most often used for culture isolates because the technique is simple and rapid. For IF, cells that appear to contain adenovirus should be harvested when at least 20% of the monolayer shows CPE. Other methods that can be used for identification are latex agglutination, IC, or PCR. On occasion, CPE-positive variants or new types that cannot be identified by these methods emerge. Under these circumstances, EM of infected cells or DNA sequence-based methods may aid in identification.

TYPING SYSTEMS

Typing of adenoviruses into species or types is used primarily for epidemiology or studies of pathogenesis or to reveal the cause of an unusual or especially severe infection. Traditional and molecular typing methods are available. Traditional typing requires a viral isolate and detects serologically recognized differences in fiber and hexon epitopes. Molecular typing can be performed with isolates or directly on PCR-positive specimens. Typing by serology and molecular methods is usually in agreement for serotypes, but discrepant results can be obtained with many of the new genotypes. These require molecular typing if they share common neutralization epitopes with older serotypes.

Molecular typing has increasingly replaced serology as the method of choice for routine strain typing and epidemiologic studies. Sequence-based typing is rapid and highly accurate. Some assays can be performed directly with clinical material if amplification is performed by generic or multiplex PCR, or sometimes by nested PCR, to obtain sufficient DNA for sequencing (104). Alternative methods of analysis can include measurement of product length, restriction endonuclease analysis (REA), REA followed by DNA sequencing, mass spectrometry (79, 105–107) or probe-based methods including reverse line blotting, in-well hybridization, type- or species-specific real-time PCR, and solid-phase microarrays (108–110). Many of these alternative methods cannot identify all adenovirus types or are limited to typing on a species level, whereas nucleic acid sequencing methods are more comprehensive (86, 104, 111). Sequence analysis of polymorphisms in long nucleotide repeats (microsatellites) is proposed to track strains (112). Sequencing of hypervariable regions 1 to 6 or 7 of the hexon gene (which code for the main neutralization epitope ε) yields results identical to the classical serotyping by neutralization testing ("imputed serology") (104, 113, 114). However, genotypes which share neutralization epitopes with other types cannot be identified by sequencing of the hexon gene, and additional sequencing of the fiber gene and the penton gene may be required (115). This and even sequencing of the complete genome is also advisable if an unusual disease association is observed with the typing result based on the hexon gene sequence because an already described or novel genotype can be suspected (4, 6, 116, 117).

Sequencing of complete adenovirus genomes by next-generation sequencing is required for definite identification of multiple recombinant genotypes, identification of novel genotypes, and sometimes for tracing of infection chains and other epidemiological questions (7, 23, 24, 117–119). Results of all other methods (REA, partial sequencing of hexon gene) can be deduced from complete genomic sequencing, so it can be regarded as the reference method for molecular typing.

Restriction endonuclease analysis does not require amplification of adenovirus DNA by PCR (120), but highly positive specimens or culture isolates and interpretation of cleavage patterns can be challenging and sometimes even misleading (23, 24). REA is still used, however, in addition to classical serotyping, for identification of new genome types (not to be confused with genotypes) associated with severe disease. Single-stranded confirmation polymorphism and heteroduplex mobility assays are other direct approaches.

Traditional serotyping is performed by provisionally determining the species of an isolate by hemagglutination (Table 1) or, if the isolate is from stools, by a species F (serotype 40/41)-specific EIA. Serotyping by hemagglutination inhibition (HAI) or serum neutralization (SN) is then performed, utilizing specific antisera that define the serotypes of that species. HAI is the easier assay, but SN is the primary arbiter of serotype. However, it may give misleading results with the novel genotypes. Modified SN procedures are preferred for speed and simplicity over the conventional 7-day test with human epithelial cells (or 293 cells for stool isolates). Intersecting pools of antibody mixtures reduce the number of individual reactions. Modified SN tests include a 3-day test with monkey kidney cells and a 5-day microneutralization test with Vero cells (121). If HAI and SN give contradictory typing results on isolates, these were previously labeled as intermediate types, but nowadays complete genomic sequencing is advisable to identify the precise genotype. However, SN remains the "gold standard" to classify novel serotypes.

SEROLOGIC TESTS

Most primary adenovirus infections (in immunocompetent patients) are accompanied by a diagnostic rise in virus-specific immunoglobulin G (IgG), a less-predictable IgA response, and an IgM response in 20 to 50% of cases. Neutralizing antibodies can persist a decade or more in a relatively undiminished titer, probably maintained by periodic reinfection, reactivation, and heterotypic anamnestic antibody responses. The IgG response can be delayed in many children for months after infection and may not appear in immunocompromised individuals. An IgM response occasionally occurs when virus reactivates.

In recent years, serodiagnosis of adenovirus infections has largely been superseded by other methods of virus detection. Its current use is for epidemiologic investigations, to confirm associations between virus detection and unusual clinical outcome, and to study the immune response. The value of serology for patient care is limited due to the retrospective nature of demonstrating seroconversion, false-negative results due to the delay of the IgG response in children, the insensitivity of IgM assays, persistent infections, and the lack of antibody responses in immunocompromised individuals. False positives also occur due to heterotypic responses or late antibody increases in children unrelated to their current problem.

Serology is typically performed by documenting at least a 4-fold rise in virus-specific IgG (seroconversion) or by detecting an IgM response in the right setting. For clinical work, it is usually sufficient to know that adenovirus caused the infection, so a genus-specific EIA to detect IgG or IgM antibodies against the hexon protein is adequate. Formats with a viral antigen preparation or a "capture" immunoglobulin on the solid phase are commercially available and sensitive. Serotype-specific antibody tests are infrequently used for diagnosis but can pinpoint serotypes responsible for a cluster of infections when other specimens are unavailable. HAI and SN are the serotype-specific assays of choice. SN is the standard, with the 3-day monkey kidney test or microneutralization preferred and may be required prior to gene therapy studies with adenovirus vectors. Complement fixation, indirect IF, latex agglutination, and radioimmunoassay are rarely used. Assays utilizing genetically modified cells and fluorescent reporter molecules as surrogates for SN activity are increasingly used for serosurveys (122).

Treatment and Prevention

Most adenovirus infections of immunocompetent patients are mild and self-limiting and do not require antiviral treatment, but LRTI can be severe and even fatal. A reduction of immunosuppressive therapy, if feasible, is essential in immunosuppressed patients because severe manifestations of adenovirus infections, e.g., disseminated disease, are clearly associated with immunosuppression.

Several antivirals, including ganciclovir, ribavirin, and cidofovir, an acyclic nucleoside phosphonate analogue and broad-spectrum antiviral agent, as well as the antiretroviral drugs zalcitabine, alovudine, and stavudine have *in vitro* activities against adenovirus. Ribavirin was initially reported to have *in vitro* activity only against species C types but is now said to be active against most isolates of species A, B, and D and all isolates of species C (123). All adenovirus types are susceptible to cidofovir *in vitro*, including the emerging adenovirus type 14p1, which is associated with severe lower respiratory tract infection, whereas this type is not susceptible to ribavirin (124). Although cidofovir resistance can develop with serial passage *in vitro*, little resistance has so far been detected in isolates from cidofovir-treated patients (123).

Cidofovir is frequently used to treat a variety of clinical presentations, mostly in immunocompromised patients. Despite the significant side effects of cidofovir (nephrotoxicity, myelosuppression, and uveitis), regimens with acceptable levels of toxicity have been developed (125). Prospective controlled clinical trials have never been published, but retrospective studies reported efficacies of up to 98% in HSCT patients and a reduction of mortality in comparison to previously published studies (33, 125). However, several cases of treatment failure were also reported, and these may be associated with a late start of therapy when symptoms and high virus loads ($>1 \times 10^6$ copies/ml) in peripheral blood are already present (94, 126). Therefore, guidelines from the European Conference on Infections in Leukemia include recommendations for preemptive therapy with cidofovir in high-risk patients (as defined by host factors, transplant type, and viremia, which is usually detected as DNA-emia by quantitative PCR) (29). Weekly surveillance of DNA-emia for high-risk patients in the first few months posttransplantation is recommended, followed by preemptive cidofovir treatment if results are positive or rising. This strategy still does not completely eliminate adenovirus disease, however, and some pediatric patients clear their DNA-emia spontaneously without treatment (125). The use of a threshold value of virus loads (e.g., 1×10^4 copies/ml) for triggering cidofovir treatment is discussed to avoid overtreatment and thus unnecessary side effects because low virus loads do not influence mortality of HSCT patients (29, 33, 93). However, quantification of adenovirus loads may differ significantly between laboratories because an international standard is not available. Quantitative detection of adenovirus shedding ($>10^6$ copies/ml) by additional weekly monitoring of stool specimens is helpful for early detection of patients at a high risk for significant DNA-emias (33, 46, 127). However, gastrointestinal panel PCRs which only detect types 40 and 41 of species HAdV-F are not appropriate for this purpose because detection of shedding of species HAdV-A, -B, and C is essential because these, but not species HAdV-F, are associated with significant mortality in HSCT patients (31). Highly multiplexed PCR panels for respiratory viruses are also not appropriate because they can fail to detect types (e.g., 31) of nonrespiratory adenovirus species (e.g., A), which are significant pathogens in HSCT patients (85).

A lipid conjugate of cidofovir, brincidofovir (CMX001; hexadecyloxypropyl cidifovir) has shown promise in early studies for the treatment of adenoviral infections (128). Brincidofovir can be administered orally, with good absorption, and reaches higher intracellular concentrations than cidofovir, with lower toxicity. It has shown potent *in vitro* antiviral activity against a wide range of double-stranded DNA viruses, and evidence points to less toxicity than that of cidofovir (129). In a multicenter retrospective study comparing brincidofovir with cidofovir for preemptive treatment of HSCT patients, significantly more virological responses were observed with brincidofovir (130). Diarrhea is the main side effect of brincidofovir. A randomized placebo-controlled clinical trial of brincidofovir for the preemptive treatment of asymptomatic HAdV DNA-emia in HSCT patients did not show a significant effect on the primary endpoint, defined as the proportion of subjects experiencing treatment failure, either progression to probable or definitive adenovirus disease or confirmed increasing adenovirus DNA-emia (131). However, a positive trend was observed for brincidofovir 100 mg (2 mg/kg if <50 kg) twice weekly, but not for 200 mg once weekly. Perhaps the study was underpowered because of the three-arm design.

Ganciclovir has only a moderate effect *in vivo* and is no longer recommended for clinical use. Ribavirin has been used with somewhat greater success, but many failures and fatalities were reported (28). Ribavirin may be somewhat effective against hemorrhagic cystitis, probably due to the high drug concentrations achievable in urine.

Another promising strategy is immunotherapy using donor lymphocyte infusion or the adoptive transfer of adenovirus virus-specific cytotoxic T lymphocytes (132, 133). Both approaches, with or without concomitantly administered antivirals, have improved outcomes for HSCT patients in some studies. To avoid inducing graft-versus-host disease with donor lymphocyte infusion, adenovirus-specific cytotoxic lymphocytes have been produced *in vitro*. A strategy to expand naive cord blood T cells *in vitro* with efficacy against adenovirus, Epstein-Barr virus, and cytomegalovirus infections has shown promise (134).

A vaccine against HAdV types 4 and 7 is available to prevent respiratory infections, which can even present as acute respiratory distress syndrome in military recruits (Table 2). The vaccine consists of nonattenuated live virus which is applied in enteric coated tablets. An enteric infection with these types induces immunity and thus protects against subsequent respiratory infections with these types. This vaccine is safe and highly effective for use in young and healthy adults (135), and it also reduces HAdV contamination on building surfaces of military bases (136). However, this vaccine is only available for the U.S. military, and the safety of the vaccine is questionable in groups (for example, immunosuppressed patients) at high risk for severe respiratory infections.

EVALUATION, INTERPRETATION, AND REPORTING OF RESULTS

The clinical spectrum of adenoviral disease is broad, so laboratory testing is usually required for accurate diagnosis. Selection of tests should be guided by the patient's symptoms and immune status, the interval between disease onset and specimen collection, and laboratory expertise. In the past few years, testing has shifted primarily toward molecular methods, such that most adenovirus infections can now be detected within hours when automated "sample-to-answer" systems are used or within 1 to 2 days when quantitative laboratory-developed test-based assays are used. The use of culture (centrifugation or tube culture) continues to diminish. Antigen testing has found limited application, and serologic testing rarely provides clinically actionable data. Testing can be aimed at systemic detection in blood samples (primarily in immunocompromised patients) or at detection in sites of end-organ involvement. In the latter instance, histopathology and adjunctive immunohistochemical and *in situ* hybridization continue to play an important role.

Interpretation of positive results can be challenging since many adenovirus infections are asymptomatic or are due to adenovirus latency. Accurate interpretation should consider patient and specimen characteristics, test method, and under some circumstances, the adenovirus type or quantity detected (137). This requires close communication between the laboratory and the clinician. In general, detection of virus from the involved organ or in large quantities in a patient with an illness that is epidemiologically associated with adenovirus is evidence that adenovirus is the actual cause of the disease.

PCR-based methodology has now displaced culture and antigen detection as the method of choice for rapid detection of adenoviral respiratory tract infection. These assays typically have a high degree of sensitivity. Higher rates of detection can be expected in samples from children, because virus is typically shed at higher titers and for longer periods in children than in adults. This can also coincide with a more recently acquired, clinically relevant infection with another respiratory pathogen. Caution is advised in the selection of test methods, because the complex phylogeny of adenoviruses can present a daunting assay design challenge. A given test, though claiming broad detection capabilities, may have significantly reduced sensitivity for specific adenoviral types or species. Nonetheless, both sensitivity and speed of detection have markedly improved over time, and the rapid reporting of such results can have a positive impact on patient and fiscal outcomes (138, 139). The sensitivity advantage of PCR over other methods is such that confirmatory reflex testing by PCR for samples testing negative by other methods should be considered in critically ill or high-risk populations. Although typically utilized for immunocompromised patients, assessment of DNA-emia may be a useful adjunct for the diagnosis of severe adenoviral disease in immunocompetent children (76). The exquisite sensitivity of PCR can also present challenges, however. Low viral DNA loads can be detected in specimens from asymptomatic subjects. Results of tissue PCR may be particularly hard to interpret in the absence of correlative viral inclusions that are positive by immunohistochemistry or *in situ* hybridization. Furthermore, the clinical significance of continued shedding of adenovirus after resolution of symptomatology is an unresolved issue (137).

In contrast, ocular adenoviral detection by EIA, IC, culture, or PCR may be considered diagnostic. Adenovirus encephalitis and meningitis occur infrequently, so studies comparing traditional and newer methods of detection are lacking, although PCR of cerebrospinal fluid is likely to be the optimum approach.

Adenovirus gastroenteritis in immunocompetent patients is best detected by a type 40/41-specific immunoassay or gastrointestinal panel PCRs of stools. Interpretation is usually straightforward, because viral shedding is infrequent past the symptomatic period. In contrast, nonenteric adenoviruses can be detected in stools of asymptomatic immunocompetent and immunocompromised patients for prolonged periods. In the latter group, severe gastrointestinal disease can result, and detection in the stool can presage potentially fatal disseminated infection. High viral loads in excess of 10^6 genome copies/ml of stool have been shown to be predictive of subsequent DNA-emia in allogeneic stem cell transplant recipients. Detection and quantification of nonenteric adenoviruses in stools of immunocompromised patients can be achieved by generic real-time PCR protocols but not by gastrointestinal panel PCRs designed to detect only enteric adenovirus (types 40/41). Detection of adenovirus in the stools of transplant recipients does not rule out graft-versus-host disease.

Detection of adenovirus in urine has also been associated with hemorrhagic cystitis. Among immunocompetent patients, this picture is typically seen in pediatric patients, with a male predominance, in association with adenovirus types 11, 34, and 35. In HSCT patients, hemorrhagic cystitis may be severe and might be the initial site of severe disease or dissemination (48). However, as in other organ systems, adenovirus may be shed asymptomatically in the urine, and the predictive value of routine testing for this sample type is unclear, with some investigators failing to show an association between adenoviruria and hemorrhagic cystitis in HSCT patients.

Diagnosis of adenovirus disease in immunocompromised patients is challenging due to the many copathogens, the high rates of asymptomatic virus shedding, and the protean manifestations of adenovirus infections in this population. HSCT and solid organ transplantation recipients are at highest risk of severe disease and are the usual focus of testing. Some centers utilize surveillance cultures or PCR studies of multiple body sites to detect virus in temporal association with the onset of new symptoms. Involvement is then classified as infection, probable disease, or definite disease, depending on the number of virus-positive sites, symptoms, or histologic confirmation. DNA-emia testing by quantitative PCR is an alternative strategy and is more frequently used nowadays. DNA-emia is usually present during severe or fatal adenovirus infection and often precedes the development of disease, although not all PCR-positive patients become symptomatic. Therefore, many centers now monitor weekly DNA-emia quantitatively in high-risk transplant patients, treat preemptively based on single high-positivity results or dynamic increases from low baselines, and reevaluate DNA-emia to assess response to treatment. Similar approaches may be useful to assess the clinical effectiveness of new treatment modalities for adenoviral disease. However, caution is warranted in adapting universal or consensus breakpoints for institution of therapy. The lack of international quantitative standards, together with wide variations in methodology, and the potential for inaccuracies in quantification across different types for individual assays mean that treatment thresholds must continue to be verified based on the test in use and the population being assessed in any given institution.

REFERENCES

1. **Rowe WP, Huebner RJ, Gilmore LK, Parrott RH, Ward TG.** 1953. Isolation of a cytopathogenic agent from human adenoids undergoing spontaneous degeneration in tissue culture. *Proc Soc Exp Biol Med* **84:**570–573.
2. **Hilleman MR, Werner JH.** 1954. Recovery of new agent from patients with acute respiratory illness. *Proc Soc Exp Biol Med* **85:**183–188.
3. **Engelmann I, Madisch I, Pommer H, Heim A.** 2006. An outbreak of epidemic keratoconjunctivitis caused by a new intermediate adenovirus 22/H8 identified by molecular typing. *Clin Infect Dis* **43:**e64–e66.
4. **Walsh MP, Chintakuntlawar A, Robinson CM, Madisch I, Harrach B, Hudson NR, Schnurr D, Heim A, Chodosh J, Seto D, Jones MS.** 2009. Evidence of molecular evolution driven by recombination events influencing tropism in a novel human adenovirus that causes epidemic keratoconjunctivitis. *PLoS One* **4:**e5635.
5. **de Jong JC, Osterhaus AD, Jones MS, Harrach B.** 2008. Human adenovirus type 52: a type 41 in disguise? *J Virol* **82:**3809, author reply 3809–3810.
6. **Walsh MP, Seto J, Jones MS, Chodosh J, Xu W, Seto D.** 2010. Computational analysis identifies human adenovirus type 55 as a re-emergent acute respiratory disease pathogen. *J Clin Microbiol* **48:**991–993.
7. **Seto D, Chodosh J, Brister JR, Jones MS, Members of the Adenovirus Research Community.** 2011. Using the whole-genome sequence to characterize and name human adenoviruses. *J Virol* **85:**5701–5702.
8. **Kajon AE, Echavarria M, de Jong JC.** 2013. Designation of human adenovirus types based on sequence data: an unfinished debate. *J Clin Virol* **58:**743–744.
9. **Seto D, Jones MS, Dyer DW, Chodosh J.** 2013. Characterizing, typing, and naming human adenovirus type 55 in the era of whole genome data. *J Clin Virol* **58:**741–742.
10. **Akiyoshi K, Suga T, Fukui K, Taniguchi K, Okabe N, Fujimoto T.** 2011. Outbreak of epidemic keratoconjunctivitis caused by adenovirus type 54 in a nursery school in Kobe City, Japan in 2008. *Jpn J Infect Dis* **64:**353–355.
11. **Ishiko H, Shimada Y, Konno T, Hayashi A, Ohguchi T, Tagawa Y, Aoki K, Ohno S, Yamazaki S.** 2008. Novel human adenovirus causing nosocomial epidemic keratoconjunctivitis. *J Clin Microbiol* **46:**2002–2008.
12. **Crawford-Miksza LK, Schnurr DP.** 1996. Adenovirus serotype evolution is driven by illegitimate recombination in the hypervariable regions of the hexon protein. *Virology* **224:** 357–367.
13. **Zhou X, Robinson CM, Rajaiya J, Dehghan S, Seto D, Jones MS, Dyer DW, Chodosh J.** 2012. Analysis of human adenovirus type 19 associated with epidemic keratoconjunctivitis and its reclassification as adenovirus type 64. *Invest Ophthalmol Vis Sci* **53:**2804–2811.
14. **Garnett CT, Erdman D, Xu W, Gooding LR.** 2002. Prevalence and quantitation of species C adenovirus DNA in human mucosal lymphocytes. *J Virol* **76:**10608–10616.
15. **Roy S, Calcedo R, Medina-Jaszek A, Keough M, Peng H, Wilson JM.** 2011. Adenoviruses in lymphocytes of the human gastro-intestinal tract. *PLoS One* **6:**e24859.
16. **Kosulin K, Geiger E, Vecsei A, Huber WD, Rauch M, Brenner E, Wrba F, Hammer K, Innerhofer A, Potschger U, Lawitschka A, Matthes-Leodolter S, Fritsch G, Lion T.** 2016. Persistence and reactivation of human adenoviruses in the gastrointestinal tract. *Clin Microbiol Infect* **22:** 381. e1–381.e8.
17. **Garnett CT, Talekar G, Mahr JA, Huang W, Zhang Y, Ornelles DA, Gooding LR.** 2009. Latent species C adenoviruses in human tonsil tissues. *J Virol* **83:**2417–2428.
18. **Flomenberg P, Gutierrez E, Piaskowski V, Casper JT.** 1997. Detection of adenovirus DNA in peripheral blood mononuclear cells by polymerase chain reaction assay. *J Med Virol* **51:**182–188.
19. **Heim A, Ebnet C, Harste G, Pring-Akerblom P.** 2003. Rapid and quantitative detection of human adenovirus DNA by real-time PCR. *J Med Virol* **70:**228–239.
20. **Shike H, Shimizu C, Kanegaye J, Foley JL, Burns JC.** 2005. Quantitation of adenovirus genome during acute infection in normal children. *Pediatr Infect Dis J* **24:**29–33.
21. **Echavarria M, Maldonado D, Elbert G, Videla C, Rappaport R, Carballal G.** 2006. Use of PCR to demonstrate presence of adenovirus species B, C, or F as well as coinfection with two adenovirus species in children with flu-like symptoms. *J Clin Microbiol* **44:**625–627.
22. **Gray GC, McCarthy T, Lebeck MG, Schnurr DP, Russell KL, Kajon AE, Landry ML, Leland DS, Storch GA, Ginocchio CC, Robinson CC, Demmler GJ, Saubolle MA, Kehl SC, Selvarangan R, Miller MB, Chappell JD, Zerr DM, Kiska DL, Halstead DC, Capuano AW, Setterquist SF, Chorazy ML, Dawson JD, Erdman DD.** 2007. Genotype prevalence and risk factors for severe clinical adenovirus infection, United States 2004-2006. *Clin Infect Dis* **45:** 1120–1131.
23. **Hage E, Huzly D, Ganzenmueller T, Beck R, Schulz TF, Heim A.** 2014. A human adenovirus species B subtype 21a associated with severe pneumonia. *J Infect* **69:** 490–499.

24. **Kajon AE, Hang J, Hawksworth A, Metzgar D, Hage E, Hansen CJ, Kuschner RA, Blair P, Russell KL, Jarman RG.** 2015. Molecular epidemiology of adenovirus type 21 respiratory strains isolated from US military trainees (1996-2014). *J Infect Dis* **212:**871–880.
25. **Yun HC, Young AN, Caballero MY, Lott L, Cropper TL, Murray CK.** 2015. Changes in clinical presentation and epidemiology of respiratory pathogens associated with acute respiratory illness in military trainees after reintroduction of adenovirus vaccine. *Open Forum Infect Dis* **2:**ofv120.
26. **Metzgar D, Osuna M, Kajon AE, Hawksworth AW, Irvine M, Russell KL.** 2007. Abrupt emergence of diverse species B adenoviruses at US military recruit training centers. *J Infect Dis* **196:**1465–1473.
27. **Louie JK, Kajon AE, Holodniy M, Guardia-LaBar L, Lee B, Petru AM, Hacker JK, Schnurr DP.** 2008. Severe pneumonia due to adenovirus serotype 14: a new respiratory threat? *Clin Infect Dis* **46:**421–425.
28. **Lion T.** 2014. Adenovirus infections in immunocompetent and immunocompromised patients. *Clin Microbiol Rev* **27:**441–462.
29. **Matthes-Martin S, Feuchtinger T, Shaw PJ, Engelhard D, Hirsch HH, Cordonnier C, Ljungman P, Fourth European Conference on Infections in L.** 2012. European guidelines for diagnosis and treatment of adenovirus infection in leukemia and stem cell transplantation: summary of ECIL-4 (2011). *Transpl Infect Dis* **14:**555–563.
30. **Veltrop-Duits LA, van Vreeswijk T, Heemskerk B, Thijssen JC, El Seady R, Jol-van der Zijde EM, Claas EC, Lankester AC, van Tol MJ, Schilham MW.** 2011. High titers of pre-existing adenovirus serotype-specific neutralizing antibodies in the host predict viral reactivation after allogeneic stem cell transplantation in children. *Clin Infect Dis* **52:** 1405–1413.
31. **Ganzenmueller T, Heim A.** 2012. Adenoviral load diagnostics by quantitative polymerase chain reaction: techniques and application. *Rev Med Virol* **22:**194–208.
32. **Ganzenmueller T, Buchholz S, Harste G, Dammann E, Trenschel R, Heim A.** 2011. High lethality of human adenovirus disease in adult allogeneic stem cell transplant recipients with high adenoviral blood load. *J Clin Virol* **52:**55–59.
33. **Mynarek M, Ganzenmueller T, Mueller-Heine A, Mielke C, Gonnermann A, Beier R, Sauer M, Eiz-Vesper B, Kohstall U, Sykora KW, Heim A, Maecker-Kolhoff B.** 2014. Patient, virus, and treatment-related risk factors in pediatric adenovirus infection after stem cell transplantation: results of a routine monitoring program. *Biol Blood Marrow Transplant* **20:**250–256.
34. **Kroes AC, de Klerk EP, Lankester AC, Malipaard C, de Brouwer CS, Claas EC, Jol-van der Zijde EC, van Tol MJ.** 2007. Sequential emergence of multiple adenovirus serotypes after pediatric stem cell transplantation. *J Clin Virol* **38:** 341–347.
35. **Ison MG, Green M, AST Infectious Diseases Community of Practice.** 2009. Adenovirus in solid organ transplant recipients. *Am J Transplant* **9**(Suppl 4)**:**S161–S165.
36. **De Jong JC, Wermenbol AG, Verweij-Uijterwaal MW, Slaterus KW, Wertheim-Van Dillen P, Van Doornum GJ, Khoo SH, Hierholzer JC.** 1999. Adenoviruses from human immunodeficiency virus-infected individuals, including two strains that represent new candidate serotypes Ad50 and Ad51 of species B1 and D, respectively. *J Clin Microbiol* **37:**3940–3945.
37. **Lessler J, Reich NG, Brookmeyer R, Perl TM, Nelson KE, Cummings DA.** 2009. Incubation periods of acute respiratory viral infections: a systematic review. *Lancet Infect Dis* **9:** 291–300.
38. **Fox JP, Brandt CD, Wassermann FE, Hall CE, Spigland I, Kogon A, Elveback LR.** 1969. The virus watch program: a continuing surveillance of viral infections in metropolitan New York families. VI. Observations of adenovirus infections: virus excretion patterns, antibody response, efficiency of surveillance, patterns of infections, and relation to illness. *Am J Epidemiol* **89:**25–50.
39. **Thavagnanam S, Christie SN, Doherty GM, Coyle PV, Shields MD, Heaney LG.** 2010. Respiratory viral infection in lower airways of asymptomatic children. *Acta Paediatr* **99:**394–398.
40. **Murtagh P, Giubergia V, Viale D, Bauer G, Pena HG.** 2009. Lower respiratory infections by adenovirus in children. Clinical features and risk factors for bronchiolitis obliterans and mortality. *Pediatr Pulmonol* **44:**450–456.
41. **Carballal G, Videla C, Misirlian A, Requeijo PV, Aguilar MC.** 2002. Adenovirus type 7 associated with severe and fatal acute lower respiratory infections in Argentine children. *BMC Pediatr* **2:**6.
42. **Esposito DH, Gardner TJ, Schneider E, Stockman LJ, Tate JE, Panozzo CA, Robbins CL, Jenkerson SA, Thomas L, Watson CM, Curns AT, Erdman DD, Lu X, Cromeans T, Westcott M, Humphries C, Ballantyne J, Fischer GE, McLaughlin JB, Armstrong G, Anderson LJ.** 2010. Outbreak of pneumonia associated with emergent human adenovirus serotype 14: Southeast Alaska, 2008. *J Infect Dis* **202:**214–222.
43. **Tate JE, Bunning ML, Lott L, Lu X, Su J, Metzgar D, Brosch L, Panozzo CA, Marconi VC, Faix DJ, Prill M, Johnson B, Erdman DD, Fonseca V, Anderson LJ, Widdowson MA.** 2009. Outbreak of severe respiratory disease associated with emergent human adenovirus serotype 14 at a US Air Force training facility in 2007. *J Infect Dis* **199:** 1419–1426.
44. **Uhnoo I, Svensson L, Wadell G.** 1990. Enteric adenoviruses. *Baillieres Clin Gastroenterol* **4:**627–642.
45. **Echavarría M.** 2008. Adenoviruses in immunocompromised hosts. *Clin Microbiol Rev* **21:**704–715.
46. **Lion T, Kosulin K, Landlinger C, Rauch M, Preuner S, Jugovic D, Pötschger U, Lawitschka A, Peters C, Fritsch G, Matthes-Martin S.** 2010. Monitoring of adenovirus load in stool by real-time PCR permits early detection of impending invasive infection in patients after allogeneic stem cell transplantation. *Leukemia* **24:**706–714.
47. **Heim A.** 2011. Advances in the management of disseminated adenovirus disease in stem cell transplant recipients: impact of adenovirus load (DNAemia) testing. *Expert Rev Anti Infect Ther* **9:**943–945.
48. **Echavarria MS, Ray SC, Ambinder R, Dumler JS, Charache P.** 1999. PCR detection of adenovirus in a bone marrow transplant recipient: hemorrhagic cystitis as a presenting manifestation of disseminated disease. *J Clin Microbiol* **37:** 686–689.
49. **McGrath D, Falagas ME, Freeman R, Rohrer R, Fairchild R, Colbach C, Snydman DR.** 1998. Adenovirus infection in adult orthotopic liver transplant recipients: incidence and clinical significance. *J Infect Dis* **177:**459–462.
50. **Ronan BA, Agrwal N, Carey EJ, De Petris G, Kusne S, Seville MT, Blair JE, Vikram HR.** 2014. Fulminant hepatitis due to human adenovirus. *Infection* **42:**105–111.
51. **Florescu MC, Miles CD, Florescu DF.** 2013. What do we know about adenovirus in renal transplantation? *Nephrol Dial Transplant* **28:**2003–2010.
52. **Watcharananan SP, Avery R, Ingsathit A, Malathum K, Chantratita W, Mavichak V, Chalermsanyakorn P, Jirasiritham S, Sumethkul V.** 2011. Adenovirus disease after kidney transplantation: course of infection and outcome in relation to blood viral load and immune recovery. *Am J Transplant* **11:**1308–1314.
53. **Almgren M, Atkinson R, He J, Hilding A, Hagman E, Wolk A, Thorell A, Marcus C, Näslund E, Östenson CG, Schalling M, Lavebratt C.** 2012. Adenovirus-36 is associated with obesity in children and adults in Sweden as determined by rapid ELISA. *PLoS One* **7:**e41652.
54. **Jaggi P, Kajon AE, Mejias A, Ramilo O, Leber A.** 2013. Human adenovirus infection in Kawasaki disease: a confounding bystander? *Clin Infect Dis* **56:**58–64.
55. **Walsh P, Overmyer CL, Pham K, Michaelson S, Gofman L, DeSalvia L, Tran T, Gonzalez D, Pusavat J, Feola M, Iacono KT, Mordechai E, Adelson ME.** 2008. Comparison of respiratory virus detection rates for infants and toddlers by use

of flocked swabs, saline aspirates, and saline aspirates mixed in universal transport medium for room temperature storage and shipping. *J Clin Microbiol* **46:**2374–2376.

56. **Abu-Diab A, Azzeh M, Ghneim R, Ghneim R, Zoughbi M, Turkuman S, Rishmawi N, Issa AE, Siriani I, Dauodi R, Kattan R, Hindiyeh MY.** 2008. Comparison between pernasal flocked swabs and nasopharyngeal aspirates for detection of common respiratory viruses in samples from children. *J Clin Microbiol* **46:**2414–2417.
57. **Fujimoto T, Enomoto M, Konagaya M, Taniguchi K.** 2009. Usefulness of flocked swabs for sample collection of adenovirus. *Kansenshogaku Zasshi* **83:**398–400. (In Japanese.)
58. **Romanowski EG, Bartels SP, Vogel R, Wetherall NT, Hodges-Savola C, Kowalski RP, Yates KA, Kinchington PR, Gordon YJ.** 2004. Feasibility of an antiviral clinical trial requiring cross-country shipment of conjunctival adenovirus cultures and recovery of infectious virus. *Curr Eye Res* **29:**195–199.
59. **Bayón MN, Drut R.** 1991. Cytologic diagnosis of adenovirus bronchopneumonia. *Acta Cytol* **35:**181–182.
60. **Landry ML, Fong CK, Neddermann K, Solomon L, Hsiung GD.** 1987. Disseminated adenovirus infection in an immunocompromised host. Pitfalls in diagnosis. *Am J Med* **83:** 555–559.
61. **Matsuse T, Matsui H, Shu CY, Nagase T, Wakabayashi T, Mori S, Inoue S, Fukuchi Y, Orimo H.** 1994. Adenovirus pulmonary infections identified by PCR and *in situ* hybridisation in bone marrow transplant recipients. *J Clin Pathol* **47:**973–977.
62. **Brown M.** 1990. Laboratory identification of adenoviruses associated with gastroenteritis in Canada from 1983 to 1986. *J Clin Microbiol* **28:**1525–1529.
63. **Hammond GW, Hazelton PR, Chuang I, Klisko B.** 1981. Improved detection of viruses by electron microscopy after direct ultracentrifuge preparation of specimens. *J Clin Microbiol* **14:**210–221.
64. **Levent F, Greer JM, Snider M, Demmler-Harrison GJ.** 2009. Performance of a new immunochromatographic assay for detection of adenoviruses in children. *J Clin Virol* **44:** 173–175.
65. **Ivaska L, Niemelä J, Heikkinen T, Vuorinen T, Peltola V.** 2013. Identification of respiratory viruses with a novel point-of-care multianalyte antigen detection test in children with acute respiratory tract infection. *J Clin Virol* **57:**136–140.
66. **Landry ML, Ferguson D.** 2000. SimulFluor respiratory screen for rapid detection of multiple respiratory viruses in clinical specimens by immunofluorescence staining. *J Clin Microbiol* **38:**708–711.
67. **August MJ, Warford AL.** 1987. Evaluation of a commercial monoclonal antibody for detection of adenovirus antigen. *J Clin Microbiol* **25:**2233–2235.
68. **Herrmann JE, Perron-Henry DM, Blacklow NR.** 1987. Antigen detection with monoclonal antibodies for the diagnosis of adenovirus gastroenteritis. *J Infect Dis* **155:**1167–1171.
69. **Moore P, Steele AD, Lecatsas G, Alexander JJ.** 1998. Characterisation of gastro-enteritis-associated adenoviruses in South Africa. *S Afr Med J* **88:**1587–1592.
70. **Gleaves CA, Militoni J, Ashley RL.** 1993. An enzyme immunoassay for the direct detection of adenovirus in clinical specimens. *Diagn Microbiol Infect Dis* **17:**57–59.
71. **Fujimoto T, Okafuji T, Okafuji T, Ito M, Nukuzuma S, Chikahira M, Nishio O.** 2004. Evaluation of a bedside immunochromatographic test for detection of adenovirus in respiratory samples, by comparison to virus isolation, PCR, and real-time PCR. *J Clin Microbiol* **42:**5489–5492.
72. **Sambursky R, Trattler W, Tauber S, Starr C, Friedberg M, Boland T, McDonald M, DellaVecchia M, Luchs J.** 2013. Sensitivity and specificity of the AdenoPlus test for diagnosing adenoviral conjunctivitis. *JAMA Ophthalmol* **131:**17–22.
73. **Kam KY, Ong HS, Bunce C, Ogunbowale L, Verma S.** 2015. Sensitivity and specificity of the AdenoPlus point-of-care system in detecting adenovirus in conjunctivitis patients at an ophthalmic emergency department: a diagnostic accuracy study. *Br J Ophthalmol* **99:**1186–1189.
74. **Kuypers J, Campbell AP, Cent A, Corey L, Boeckh M.** 2009. Comparison of conventional and molecular detection of respiratory viruses in hematopoietic cell transplant recipients. *Transpl Infect Dis* **11:**298–303.
75. **Jartti T, Jartti L, Peltola V, Waris M, Ruuskanen O.** 2008. Identification of respiratory viruses in asymptomatic subjects: asymptomatic respiratory viral infections. *Pediatr Infect Dis J* **27:**1103–1107.
76. **Landry ML, Ferguson D.** 2009. Polymerase chain reaction and the diagnosis of viral gastrointestinal disease due to cytomegalovirus, herpes simplex virus and adenovirus. *J Clin Virol* **45:**83–84.
77. **Claas EC, Schilham MW, de Brouwer CS, Hubacek P, Echavarria M, Lankester AC, van Tol MJ, Kroes AC.** 2005. Internally controlled real-time PCR monitoring of adenovirus DNA load in serum or plasma of transplant recipients. *J Clin Microbiol* **43:**1738–1744.
78. **Damen M, Minnaar R, Glasius P, van der Ham A, Koen G, Wertheim P, Beld M.** 2008. Real-time PCR with an internal control for detection of all known human adenovirus serotypes. *J Clin Microbiol* **46:**3997–4003.
79. **Ebner K, Suda M, Watzinger F, Lion T.** 2005. Molecular detection and quantitative analysis of the entire spectrum of human adenoviruses by a two-reaction real-time PCR assay. *J Clin Microbiol* **43:**3049–3053.
80. **Gu Z, Belzer SW, Gibson CS, Bankowski MJ, Hayden RT.** 2003. Multiplexed, real-time PCR for quantitative detection of human adenovirus. *J Clin Microbiol* **41:**4636–4641.
81. **Huang ML, Nguy L, Ferrenberg J, Boeckh M, Cent A, Corey L.** 2008. Development of multiplexed real-time quantitative polymerase chain reaction assay for detecting human adenoviruses. *Diagn Microbiol Infect Dis* **62:**263–271.
82. **Gadsby NJ, Hardie A, Claas EC, Templeton KE.** 2010. Comparison of the Luminex respiratory virus panel fast assay with in-house real-time PCR for respiratory viral infection diagnosis. *J Clin Microbiol* **48:**2213–2216.
83. **Pierce VM, Elkan M, Leet M, McGowan KL, Hodinka RL.** 2012. Comparison of the Idaho Technology FilmArray system to real-time PCR for detection of respiratory pathogens in children. *J Clin Microbiol* **50:**364–371.
84. **Pierce VM, Hodinka RL.** 2012. Comparison of the GenMark Diagnostics eSensor respiratory viral panel to real-time PCR for detection of respiratory viruses in children. *J Clin Microbiol* **50:**3458–3465.
85. **Song E, Wang H, Salamon D, Jaggi P, Leber A.** 2016. Performance characteristics of FilmArray respiratory panel v1.7 for detection of adenovirus in a large cohort of pediatric nasopharyngeal samples: one test may not fit all. *J Clin Microbiol* **54:**1479–1486 .
86. **Pehler-Harrington K, Khanna M, Waters CR, Henrickson KJ.** 2004. Rapid detection and identification of human adenovirus species by adenoplex, a multiplex PCR-enzyme hybridization assay. *J Clin Microbiol* **42:**4072–4076.
87. **Kim SR, Ki CS, Lee NY.** 2009. Rapid detection and identification of 12 respiratory viruses using a dual priming oligonucleotide system-based multiplex PCR assay. *J Virol Methods* **156:**111–116.
88. **Müller R, Ditzen A, Hille K, Stichling M, Ehricht R, Illmer T, Ehninger G, Rohayem J.** 2009. Detection of herpesvirus and adenovirus co-infections with diagnostic DNA-microarrays. *J Virol Methods* **155:**161–166.
89. **Echavarria M, Forman M, van Tol MJ, Vossen JM, Charache P, Kroes AC.** 2001. Prediction of severe disseminated adenovirus infection by serum PCR. *Lancet* **358:**384–385.
90. **Lion T, Baumgartinger R, Watzinger F, Matthes-Martin S, Suda M, Preuner S, Futterknecht B, Lawitschka A, Peters C, Potschger U, Gadner H.** 2003. Molecular monitoring of adenovirus in peripheral blood after allogeneic bone marrow transplantation permits early diagnosis of disseminated disease. *Blood* **102:**1114–1120.
91. **Perlman J, Gibson C, Pounds SB, Gu Z, Bankowski MJ, Hayden RT.** 2007. Quantitative real-time PCR detection of adenovirus in clinical blood specimens: a comparison of plasma, whole blood and peripheral blood mononuclear cells. *J Clin Virol* **40:**295–300.

92. **Jeulin H, Salmon A, Bordigoni P, Venard V.** 2011. Diagnostic value of quantitative PCR for adenovirus detection in stool samples as compared with antigen detection and cell culture in haematopoietic stem cell transplant recipients. *Clin Microbiol Infect* **17:**1674–1680.
93. **Lee YJ, Chung D, Xiao K, Papadopoulos EB, Barker JN, Small TN, Giralt SA, Zheng J, Jakubowski AA, Papanicolaou GA.** 2013. Adenovirus viremia and disease: comparison of T cell-depleted and conventional hematopoietic stem cell transplantation recipients from a single institution. *Biol Blood Marrow Transplant* **19:**387–392.
94. **Leruez-Ville M, Minard V, Lacaille F, Buzyn A, Abachin E, Blanche S, Freymuth F, Rouzioux C.** 2004. Real-time blood plasma polymerase chain reaction for management of disseminated adenovirus infection. *Clin Infect Dis* **38:**45–52.
95. **Lipson SM, Poshni IA, Ashley RL, Grady LJ, Ciamician Z, Teichberg S.** 1993. Presumptive identification of common adenovirus serotypes by the development of differential cytopathic effects in the human lung carcinoma (A549) cell culture. *FEMS Microbiol Lett* **113:**175–182.
96. **Espy MJ, Hierholzer JC, Smith TF.** 1987. The effect of centrifugation on the rapid detection of adenovirus in shell vials. *Am J Clin Pathol* **88:**358–360.
97. **Mahafzah AM, Landry ML.** 1989. Evaluation of immunofluorescent reagents, centrifugation, and conventional cultures for the diagnosis of adenovirus infection. *Diagn Microbiol Infect Dis* **12:**407–411.
98. **Olsen MA, Shuck KM, Sambol AR, Flor SM, O'Brien J, Cabrera BJ.** 1993. Isolation of seven respiratory viruses in shell vials: a practical and highly sensitive method. *J Clin Microbiol* **31:**422–425.
99. **Rabalais GP, Stout GG, Ladd KL, Cost KM.** 1992. Rapid diagnosis of respiratory viral infections by using a shell vial assay and monoclonal antibody pool. *J Clin Microbiol* **30:**1505–1508.
100. **Van Doornum GJ, De Jong JC.** 1998. Rapid shell vial culture technique for detection of enteroviruses and adenoviruses in fecal specimens: comparison with conventional virus isolation method. *J Clin Microbiol* **36:**2865–2868.
101. **Woods GL, Yamamoto M, Young A.** 1988. Detection of adenovirus by rapid 24-well plate centrifugation and conventional cell culture with dexamethasone. *J Virol Methods* **20:**109–114 .
102. **LaSala PR, Bufton KK, Ismail N, Smith MB.** 2007. Prospective comparison of R-mix shell vial system with direct antigen tests and conventional cell culture for respiratory virus detection. *J Clin Virol* **38:**210–216.
103. **Durepaire N, Ranger-Rogez S, Denis F.** 1996. Evaluation of rapid culture centrifugation method for adenovirus detection in stools. *Diagn Microbiol Infect Dis* **24:**25–29.
104. **Sarantis H, Johnson G, Brown M, Petric M, Tellier R.** 2004. Comprehensive detection and serotyping of human adenoviruses by PCR and sequencing. *J Clin Microbiol* **42:**3963–3969.
105. **Blyn LB, Hall TA, Libby B, Ranken R, Sampath R, Rudnick K, Moradi E, Desai A, Metzgar D, Russell KL, Freed NE, Balansay M, Broderick MP, Osuna MA, Hofstadler SA, Ecker DJ.** 2008. Rapid detection and molecular serotyping of adenovirus by use of PCR followed by electrospray ionization mass spectrometry. *J Clin Microbiol* **46:**644–651.
106. **Lu X, Erdman DD.** 2006. Molecular typing of human adenoviruses by PCR and sequencing of a partial region of the hexon gene. *Arch Virol* **151:**1587–1602.
107. **Okada M, Ogawa T, Kubonoya H, Yoshizumi H, Shinozaki K.** 2007. Detection and sequence-based typing of human adenoviruses using sensitive universal primer sets for the hexon gene. *Arch Virol* **152:**1–9.
108. **Cao Y, Kong F, Zhou F, Xiao M, Wang Q, Duan Y, Kesson AM, McPhie K, Gilbert GL, Dwyer DE.** 2011. Genotyping of human adenoviruses using a PCR-based reverse line blot hybridisation assay. *Pathology* **43:**488–494.
109. **López-Campos G, Coiras M, Sánchez-Merino JP, López-Huertas MR, Spiteri I, Martín-Sánchez F, Pérez-Breña P.** 2007. Oligonucleotide microarray design for detection and serotyping of human respiratory adenoviruses by using a virtual amplicon retrieval software. *J Virol Methods* **145:**127–136.
110. **Ylihärsilä M, Harju E, Arppe R, Hattara L, Hölsä J, Saviranta P, Soukka T, Waris M.** 2013. Genotyping of clinically relevant human adenoviruses by array-in-well hybridization assay. *Clin Microbiol Infect* **19:**551–557.
111. **Banik U, Adhikary AK, Suzuki E, Inada T, Okabe N.** 2005. Multiplex PCR assay for rapid identification of oculopathogenic adenoviruses by amplification of the fiber and hexon genes. *J Clin Microbiol* **43:**1064–1068.
112. **Houng HS, Lott L, Gong H, Kuschner RA, Lynch JA, Metzgar D.** 2009. Adenovirus microsatellite reveals dynamics of transmission during a recent epidemic of human adenovirus serotype 14 infection. *J Clin Microbiol* **47:**2243–2248.
113. **Madisch I, Harste G, Pommer H, Heim A.** 2005. Phylogenetic analysis of the main neutralization and hemagglutination determinants of all human adenovirus prototypes as a basis for molecular classification and taxonomy. *J Virol* **79:**15265–15276.
114. **Madisch I, Wölfel R, Harste G, Pommer H, Heim A.** 2006. Molecular identification of adenovirus sequences: a rapid scheme for early typing of human adenoviruses in diagnostic samples of immunocompetent and immunodeficient patients. *J Med Virol* **78:**1210–1217.
115. **McCarthy T, Lebeck MG, Capuano AW, Schnurr DP, Gray GC.** 2009. Molecular typing of clinical adenovirus specimens by an algorithm which permits detection of adenovirus coinfections and intermediate adenovirus strains. *J Clin Virol* **46:**80–84.
116. **Kaneko H, Aoki K, Ohno S, Ishiko H, Fujimoto T, Kikuchi M, Harada S, Gonzalez G, Koyanagi KO, Watanabe H, Suzutani T.** 2011. Complete genome analysis of a novel intertypic recombinant human adenovirus causing epidemic keratoconjunctivitis in Japan. *J Clin Microbiol* **49:**484–490.
117. **Robinson CM, Singh G, Henquell C, Walsh MP, Peigue-Lafeuille H, Seto D, Jones MS, Dyer DW, Chodosh J.** 2011. Computational analysis and identification of an emergent human adenovirus pathogen implicated in a respiratory fatality. *Virology* **409:**141–147.
118. **Hage E, Espelage W, Eckmanns T, Lamson DM, Pantó L, Ganzenmueller T, Heim A.** 2017. Molecular phylogeny of a novel human adenovirus type 8 strain causing a prolonged, multi-state keratoconjunctivitis epidemic in Germany. *Sci Rep* **7:**40680.
119. **Robinson CM, Singh G, Lee JY, Dehghan S, Rajaiya J, Liu EB, Yousuf MA, Betensky RA, Jones MS, Dyer DW, Seto D, Chodosh J.** 2013. Molecular evolution of human adenoviruses. *Sci Rep* **3:**1812.
120. **Adrian T, Wadell G, Hierholzer JC, Wigand R.** 1986. DNA restriction analysis of adenovirus prototypes 1 to 41. *Arch Virol* **91:**277–290.
121. **Hierholzer JC.** 1995. Adenoviruses, p 169–188. *In* Lenette EH, Lenette DA, Lenette ET (ed), *Diagnostic Procedures for Viral, Rickettsial, and Chlamydial Infections*. American Public Health Association, Washington, DC.
122. **Sprangers MC, Lakhai W, Koudstaal W, Verhoeven M, Koel BF, Vogels R, Goudsmit J, Havenga MJ, Kostense S.** 2003. Quantifying adenovirus-neutralizing antibodies by luciferase transgene detection: addressing preexisting immunity to vaccine and gene therapy vectors. *J Clin Microbiol* **41:**5046–5052.
123. **Morfin F, Dupuis-Girod S, Frobert E, Mundweiler S, Carrington D, Sedlacek P, Bierings M, Cetkovsky P, Kroes AC, van Tol MJ, Thouvenot D.** 2009. Differential susceptibility of adenovirus clinical isolates to cidofovir and ribavirin is not related to species alone. *Antivir Ther* **14:**55–61.
124. **Darr S, Madisch I, Heim A.** 2008. Antiviral activity of cidofovir and ribavirin against the new human adenovirus subtype 14a that is associated with severe pneumonia. *Clin Infect Dis* **47:**731–732 .
125. **Yusuf U, Hale GA, Carr J, Gu Z, Benaim E, Woodard P, Kasow KA, Horwitz EM, Leung W, Srivastava DK, Handgretinger R, Hayden RT.** 2006. Cidofovir for the treatment of adenoviral infection in pediatric hematopoietic stem cell transplant patients. *Transplantation* **81:**1398–1404 .

126. **Caruso Brown AE, Cohen MN, Tong S, Braverman RS, Rooney JF, Giller R, Levin MJ.** 2015. Pharmacokinetics and safety of intravenous cidofovir for life-threatening viral infections in pediatric hematopoietic stem cell transplant recipients. *Antimicrob Agents Chemother* **59:**3718–3725.
127. **Srinivasan A, Klepper C, Sunkara A, Kang G, Carr J, Gu Z, Leung W, Hayden RT.** 2015. Impact of adenoviral stool load on adenoviremia in pediatric hematopoietic stem cell transplant recipients. *Pediatr Infect Dis J* **34:**562–565.
128. **Florescu DF, Pergam SA, Neely MN, Qiu F, Johnston C, Way S, Sande J, Lewinsohn DA, Guzman-Cottrill JA, Graham ML, Papanicolaou G, Kurtzberg J, Rigdon J, Painter W, Mommeja-Marin H, Lanier R, Anderson M, van der Horst C.** 2012. Safety and efficacy of CMX001 as salvage therapy for severe adenovirus infections in immunocompromised patients. *Biol Blood Marrow Transplant* **18:** 731–738 .
129. **Florescu DF, Keck MA.** 2014. Development of CMX001 (Brincidofovir) for the treatment of serious diseases or conditions caused by dsDNA viruses. *Expert Rev Anti Infect Ther* **12:**1171–1178 .
130. **Hiwarkar P, Amrolia P, Sivaprakasam P, Lum SH, Doss H, O'Rafferty C, Petterson T, Patrick K, Silva J, Slatter M, Lawson S, Rao K, Steward C, Gassas A, Veys P, Wynn R, United Kingdom Paediatric Bone Marrow Transplant Group.** 2017. Brincidofovir is highly efficacious in controlling adenoviremia in pediatric recipients of hematopoietic cell transplant. *Blood* **129:**2033–2037.
131. **Grimley MS, Chemaly RF, Englund JA, Kurtzberg J, Chittick G, Brundage TM, Bae A, Morrison ME, Prasad VK.** 2017. Brincidofovir for asymptomatic adenovirus viremia in pediatric and adult allogeneic hematopoietic cell transplant recipients: a randomized placebo-controlled phase II trial. *Biol Blood Marrow Transplant* **23:**512–521.
132. **Leen AM, Christin A, Myers GD, Liu H, Cruz CR, Hanley PJ, Kennedy-Nasser AA, Leung KS, Gee AP, Krance RA, Brenner MK, Heslop HE, Rooney CM, Bollard CM.** 2009. Cytotoxic T lymphocyte therapy with donor T cells prevents and treats adenovirus and Epstein-Barr virus infections after haploidentical and matched unrelated stem cell transplantation. *Blood* **114:**4283–4292.
133. **Qian C, Campidelli A, Wang Y, Cai H, Venard V, Jeulin H, Dalle JH, Pochon C, D'aveni M, Bruno B, Paillard C, Vigouroux S, Jubert C, Ceballos P, Marie-Cardine A, Galambrun C, Cholle C, Clerc Urmes I, Petitpain N, De Carvalho Bittencourt M, Decot V, Reppel L, Salmon A, Clement L, Bensoussan D.** 2017. Curative or pre-emptive adenovirus-specific T cell transfer from matched unrelated or third party haploidentical donors after HSCT, including UCB transplantations: a successful phase I/II multicenter clinical trial. *J Hematol Oncol* **10:**102 .
134. **Childs RW, Zerbe CS.** 2009. Expanding multiviral reactive T cells from cord blood. *Blood* **114:**1725–1726 .
135. **Kuschner RA, Russell KL, Abuja M, Bauer KM, Faix DJ, Hait H, Henrick J, Jacobs M, Liss A, Lynch JA, Liu Q, Lyons AG, Malik M, Moon JE, Stubbs J, Sun W, Tang D, Towle AC, Walsh DS, Wilkerson D, Adenovirus Vaccine Efficacy Trial Consortium.** 2013. A phase 3, randomized, double-blind, placebo-controlled study of the safety and efficacy of the live, oral adenovirus type 4 and type 7 vaccine, in U.S. military recruits. *Vaccine* **31:**2963–2971 .
136. **Broderick M, Myers C, Balansay M, Vo S, Osuna A, Russell K.** 2017. Adenovirus 4/7 vaccine's effect on disease rates is associated with disappearance of adenovirus on building surfaces at a military recruit base. *Mil Med* **182:** e2069–e2072.
137. **Kalu SU, Loeffelholz M, Beck E, Patel JA, Revai K, Fan J, Henrickson KJ, Chonmaitree T.** 2010. Persistence of adenovirus nucleic acids in nasopharyngeal secretions: a diagnostic conundrum. *Pediatr Infect Dis J* **29:**746–750 .
138. **Rocholl C, Gerber K, Daly J, Pavia AT, Byington CL.** 2004. Adenoviral infections in children: the impact of rapid diagnosis. *Pediatrics* **113:**e51–e56 .
139. **Udeh BL, Schneider JE, Ohsfeldt RL.** 2008. Cost effectiveness of a point-of-care test for adenoviral conjunctivitis. *Am J Med Sci* **336:**254–264 .

Human Papillomaviruses

KATE CUSCHIERI AND ELIZABETH R. UNGER

107

TAXONOMY

Papillomaviruses (PVs) are in the family *Papillomaviridae*. PV virions (~55-nm diameter) are nonenveloped with an icosahedral capsid composed of 72 capsomers enclosing a single double-stranded DNA circular genome (~8 kb). The genome is organized into early and late genes with an upstream (noncoding) regulatory region. The two late genes code for the structural capsid proteins (L1, major; L2, minor). Systematic classification of PVs is based on the nucleic acid sequence of the L1 open reading frame (ORF). The International Committee on Taxonomy of Viruses (ICTV) recognizes 49 genera within the family, each designated by a Greek letter (e.g., *Alphapapillomavirus*, *Betapapillomavirus*). Human papillomaviruses (HPVs), PVs that infect humans, are found in five of these genera (Fig. 1). The genus name with a number (e.g., *Alphapapillomavirus* 9) is used to designate a species, and within species "strains" are designated as types, numbered in order of their recognition, and, particularly in the epidemiological and clinical context, HPVs are generally described at the level of "type" or genotype. Designation of a new type requires a full genome sequence and a >10% difference in the L1 ORF sequence compared to the closest known type. Sequence variation less than 10% is recognized, but there is currently no agreement on a systematic nomenclature. Commonly, differences between 10 and 2% are called subtypes, and those less than 2% are called variants. Currently, more than 200 HPV types are recognized. The International HPV Reference Center at the Karolinska Institute confirms sequences of novel types and assigns HPV type numbers. The Papillomavirus Episteme (PaVE) is a curated database of PV genomic sequences along with sequence analysis tools (1).

DESCRIPTION OF THE GROUP OF ORGANISMS

The large, closely related PV family are host species restricted and are restricted to infecting epithelial surfaces. Replication occurs in the host cell nucleus, and both replication and transcription rely on host cell machinery. Transcription occurs from only one strand and in one direction, using different promoters for early and late proteins. ORFs of proteins frequently overlap, and transcriptional regulation is complex and regulated by poorly understood methods of processing and splicing polycistronic messages. The productive viral infection is completed as fully differentiated cells are shed from the epithelial surface; thus, infection is nonlytic. Viral restriction to the epithelial compartment and the lack of host cell necrosis contribute to the evasion of the host immune response. All known HPVs require terminal epithelial differentiation for completion of the viral life cycle, and therefore conventional cell culture methods cannot be used to isolate or propagate HPV (see reviews of the biology of HPV in references 1 and 2).

The genomic organization of HPV 16 is shown as an example, because all HPVs share some homology (Fig. 2). The noncoding upstream regulatory region (also called the long control region) includes binding sites for cellular transcription factors and viral proteins that regulate replication and gene expression. The core genes (E1, E2, E4, E5, L1, L2) have important functions in genome replication and packaging in all HPV types. E1 is an essential origin recognition protein for replication. E2 interacts with E1 to enhance the specificity of E1 binding and exerts a key influence on the regulation of other early proteins. E4 plays a role in late phases of the viral life cycle, binding to cytokeratin and helping to disrupt cell structure and release virions as cells are shed. The major capsid protein, L1, generally forms into pentameric capsids forming the viral protein shell. When produced in protein expression systems *in vitro*, recombinant L1 proteins self-assemble into viral-like particles (VLPs) that retain type-specific neutralizing epitopes and have an electron microscopic appearance very similar to native virions. The minor capsid protein, L2, plays key roles in encapsidating the viral genome and in viral uncoating during infection. It may also facilitate viral entry.

The other genes (E5, E6, E7) also are essential for replication and completion of the productive life cycle, but their properties differ between genera, and for the genus *Alphapapillomavirus* also by species. The properties of E5, E6, and E7 influence the propensity of the virus to persist, transition into a deregulated or abortive life cycle, and introduce oncogenesis (see section on clinical significance below). The functions of these proteins also influence the particular epithelial environment characteristic of viral types. For example, *Alphapapillomavirus* favors nonkeratinizing

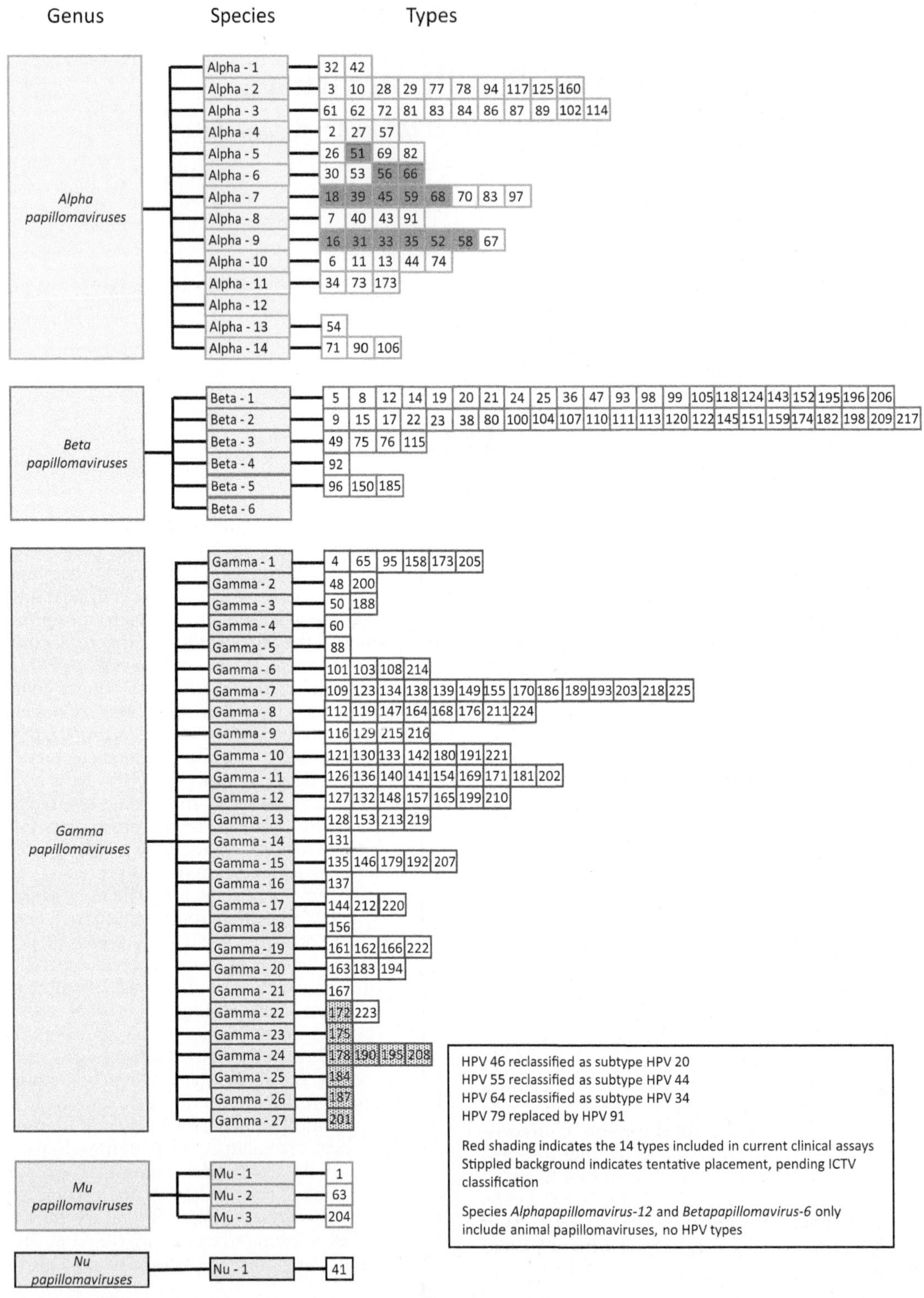

FIGURE 1 The family *Papillomaviridae* based on nucleotide sequence of the L1 gene. Only HPV types are included. *Alphapapillomavirus* species include HPV types with tropism for cutaneous and mucosal epithelia. The mucosal high-risk types found in anogenital precancers and cancers (red shading) are in this genus, as are low-risk types found in genital warts, recurrent respiratory papillomatosis, and focal epithelial hyperplasia. Cutaneous types in this genus are associated with benign common warts, flat warts, plantar warts, and filiform warts. Hand warts are particularly common, often near the nail. The other genera include HPV types with tropism for cutaneous epithelia. *Betapapillomavirus* species are usually subclinical but can cause cutaneous lesions in those with immune disorders, such as epidermodysplasia verruciformis, or with immune suppression. They have been implicated in nonmelanoma skin cancer in patients with epidermodysplasia verruciformis, particularly in association with sunlight. HPV types in the *Gamma-*, *Mu-*, and *Nupapillomavirus* species are usually subclinical but have been associated with skin lesions, most notably *Mupapillomavirus* types HPV 1 and 63 in hand and foot warts. *Mupapillomavirus* species have not been reported in cancers, while types in the *Gamma-* and *Nupapillomavirus* genera have been occasionally detected in skin cancer.

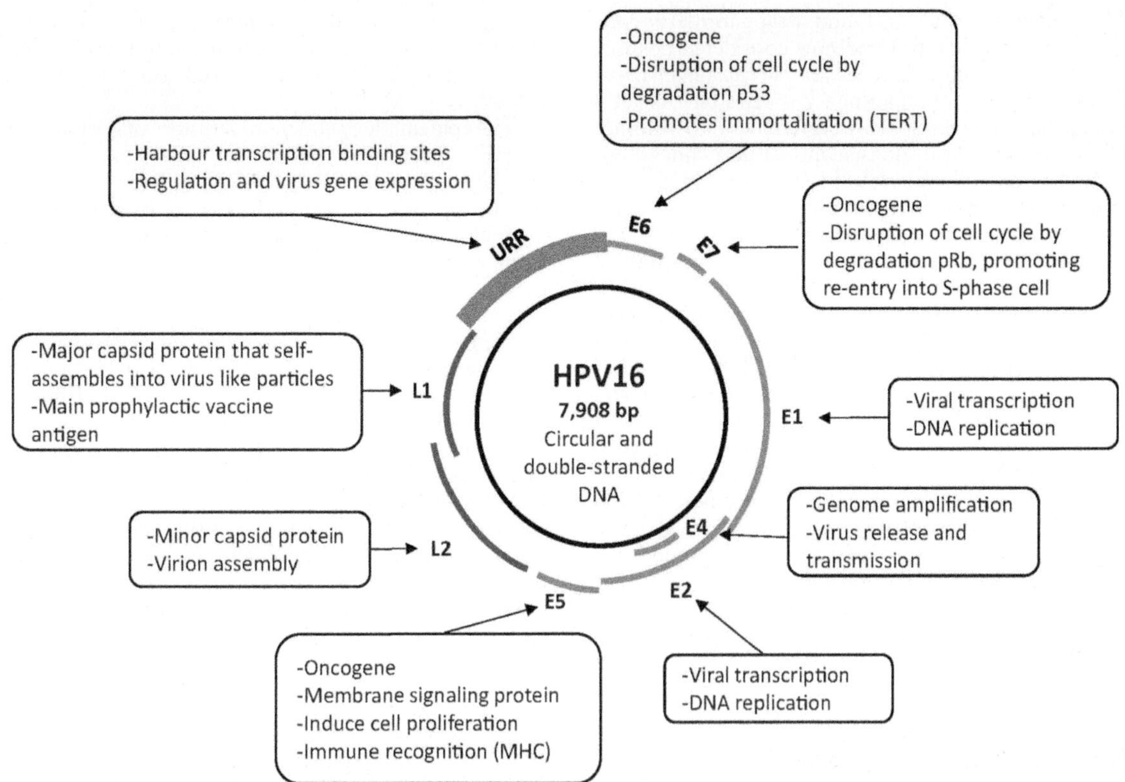

FIGURE 2 Genomic organization of HPV as exemplified by HPV 16. From reference 78, with permission.

mucosa, whereas *Beta-*, *Gamma-*, *Mu-*, and *Nupapillomavirus* favor keratinizing or cutaneous epithelia.

HPV infection requires the viral particle to move from the cell surface through the cytoplasm to the nucleus, where the viral genome is replicated. The details of the steps in this process are still being characterized and appear to differ between *in vitro* studies using quasivirions (i.e., VLPs encapsidating HPV genomes expressed from packaging plasmids) and *in vivo* native HPV virions. The current model (see reference 3) is that *in vivo* virions bind to the basement membrane and then secondarily to the cell surface, largely mediated by L1 interactions. Neutralizing antibodies to L1 can block this binding. While binding may occur through a variety of extracellular matrix proteins, heparan sulfate appears to be required for transfer to the cell surface. Coreceptors may be involved in binding and entry steps that involve conformation changes in the viral protein surface exposing L2 to furin cleavage. This step appears to be essential, because antibodies to L2 block viral entry (4). The virus is internalized through endocytosis, a slow process that occurs over several hours.

HPV initiates infection in primitive basal-like epithelial cells, accessed through minor trauma or at specialized sites of epithelial transition. Many infections are completely asymptomatic. Productive infection commonly results in expansion of the infected basal and differentiating cells, recognized as a wart or papilloma. Most infections are transient and clear spontaneously or are no longer detectable (are latent). Latent infection in basal epithelial cells is well documented in animal PVs and is suspected to occur in humans (5).

HPV infections that are not cleared may persist as a productive or latent infection, and some types (see below) may eventually be involved in oncogenesis. The interval between acquisition and development of cancer is generally quite long, at least 10 years. The HPV oncogenic pathway can be considered a nonproductive infection or abortive infection, i.e., one in which daughter viruses are not produced, which is consistent with other viruses that cause cancer (see references 5–7). The E6 and E7 proteins that are essential for promoting viral production by extending the cellular replication cycle can contribute to genomic instability and the accumulation of cellular mutations within proliferating cells. Integration of HPV may occur, most often disrupting E1 and E2 expression and contributing to further overexpression of E6 and E7 and adding to stepwise neoplastic progression. Integration is not part of the normal life cycle but can be detected in some precancers. The episomal viral genome may integrate as either a single copy or multitandem copies. HPV integration is frequent in HPV-associated cancers but is not absolutely required. HPV-associated cancers may have integrated HPV DNA, extrachromosomal episomal HPV, or a mixture of these. In most cancers with only extrachromosomal HPV, the viral genome has been methylated or mutated to allow overexpression of HPV E6 and E7.

Of the approximately 40 *Alphapapillomavirus* types frequently detected in anogenital samples, the International Agency for Research on Cancer (IARC) has designated 12 HPV types as oncogenic or high-risk based on their association with cancers (8). The 14 high-risk types detected in all clinical HPV assays to date (either directly or through cross-reactivity) include the 12 types considered oncogenic by the IARC (HPV 16, 18, 31, 33, 35, 39, 45, 51, 52, 56, 58, and 59), an additional type designated by the IARC as probably oncogenic (HPV 68), and a type formerly considered oncogenic (HPV 66) and now considered possibly oncogenic. These high-risk types are *Alphapapillomavirus* types, mostly in alpha-9 and alpha-7 species (see Fig. 1). Some *Betapapillomavirus* species are thought to interact with UV light to result in nonmelanoma skin cancer, but the biology is not well understood (9). Currently, there is no justification or indication for clinical testing of types other than a subset of *Alphapapillomavirus*.

A host antibody response occurs in less than half of those infected. The lack of a consistent humoral immune response explains the need to rely on genomic differences for taxonomy (i.e., HPV genotypes not serotypes), as well as the limitation of serology in natural history studies and the inappropriateness of HPV serology for diagnostic testing. Serum antibodies have been detected to a variety of HPV proteins, but those directed against type-specific conformational epitopes in L1 VLPs have been most studied in response to natural infection and HPV vaccines. Animal and *in vitro* systems demonstrate that these antibodies are neutralizing, i.e., protect from infection (see reference 10). The immune response to natural infection is stronger in females than males; there is evidence for modest protection against type-specific reinfection in females but not males (see reference 11). The immune response to HPV vaccines is equally strong in males and females (12).

EPIDEMIOLOGY AND TRANSMISSION

Due to the strong species specificity, there are no animal reservoirs or vectors for HPV. In most situations, transmission requires close epithelial contact. The epidemiology and transmission of genital and nongenital infections differ significantly. Nongenital infections manifesting as hand and foot warts are most common in children and adolescents. Spread is by direct contact, although environmental transmission is suggested by the increased risk among those who walk barefoot in pool or shower areas and for hand warts as an occupational risk for butchers and meat handlers (see section on cutaneous warts below).

The epidemiology and natural history of genital or mucosal HPV differ by anatomic site, by sex, and by age (13). In addition, the method of sampling and assay (discussed in subsequent sections) also influences study results. As an overview, sexual contact, not confined to penetrative sex, is the dominant mode of transmission, with incidence and prevalence closely following age of sexual debut and numbers of sexual partners. HPV is the most common sexually transmitted infection, and estimates suggest that nearly every sexually active person is likely exposed over their lifetime. Vertical transmission and nonsexual horizontal transmission are rare but can occur particularly in the first 2 years of life, with the former thought to be the mechanism for juvenile onset recurrent respiratory papillomatosis (see "Clinical Significance" below). Fomite transmission is considered a possibility because of the stability of the virus, but the frequency and likelihood of nonsexual transmission are unclear (14).

The natural history of cervical HPV infection has been studied most intensively. Cervical cancer was the first malignancy linked to HPV (15). Cervical cancer screening on the basis of exfoliated cervical cytology (the Pap test) resulted in a good understanding of the progression of cervical neoplasia, established the importance of sampling the cervical transformation zone, and provided reliable methods for sampling the relatively accessible cervix. It is now clear that cervical HPV is usually acquired around the time of sexual debut, and the peak population prevalence is in late adolescence/early adulthood (Fig. 3). Infection with one of the oncogenic types is required but not sufficient for neoplastic progression. The peak population prevalence of high-grade cervical precancers follows 5 to 10 years after HPV acquisition, indicating the need for persistent

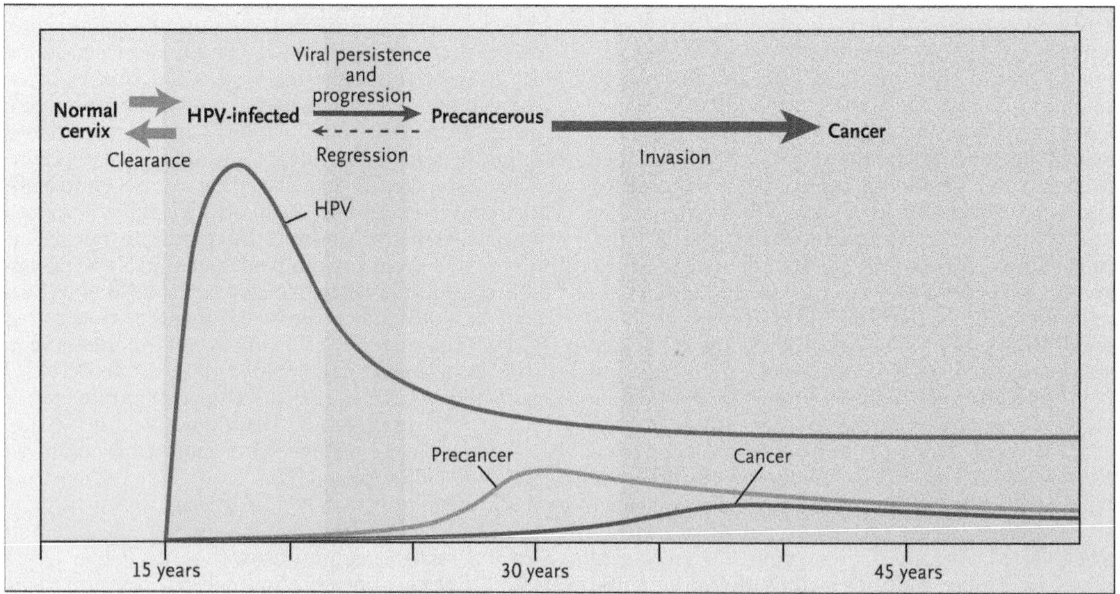

FIGURE 3 The natural history of cervical HPV. The peak prevalence of transient infections with high-risk types of HPV (blue line) occurs among women during their teens and 20s, after the initiation of sexual activity. The peak prevalence of cervical precancerous conditions occurs approximately 10 years later (green line), and the peak prevalence of invasive cancers occurs at 40 to 50 years of age (red line). (The peaks of the curves are not drawn to scale.) From reference 79, with permission.

infection and additional behavioral and environmental factors such as smoking and chronic inflammation. If precancers do not regress and are not detected and removed, invasion may occur with time, generally several years. Thus, the rare invasive cancer arises slowly, decades after initial infection.

As noted previously, most HPV infections, even those with oncogenic types, clear spontaneously. However, persistent infection with one of the oncogenic types is associated with risk for cervical cancer, and high-risk HPV is necessary but not sufficient for cervical cancer. The natural history of cervical HPV is summarized in Fig. 3. The long delay between infection and cancer made cervical cancer screening with cytology feasible. The requirement of HPV for cervical cancer means that preventing infection can prevent cancer, thus providing the basis of the prophylactic HPV vaccines (see section on prophylactic HPV vaccines below). Further, detection of HPV nucleic acid can be used as a risk marker for cervical disease either as an adjunct to cytology or as a primary screening test (see genotyping section below).

CLINICAL SIGNIFICANCE

HPV infections can induce proliferation beyond that which would be naturally programmed by the cell, and this can have subclinical or clinical consequences—and, with regard to the latter, a benign or a malignant trajectory. HPV types that reside in the *Alpha-*, *Beta-*, *Gamma-*, *Mu-*, and *Nupapillomavirus* genera can give rise to infections that have clinical sequelae (16). Species groups which unite a group of phylogenetically related types often confer similar risks/manifestations, although there are exceptions, so a clinical "phenotype" cannot be reliably predicted given knowledge of a species group. Interestingly, advances in the resolving power of sequencing technologies have revealed that differential clinical risks and tropisms can exist even at the level of variant. For example, certain variants of HPV 16 are more likely to be associated with glandular abnormalities, and HPV 16 variants which have a high degree of E7 conservation (compared to canonical type) confer a worse prognosis compared to variants with a greater number of nucleotide polymorphisms (17). Given that the substantial fraction of clinical morbidity is associated with types within the *Alphapapillomavirus* genus, particular focus is given to the clinical implications of these types in the sections below.

Cutaneous Warts

Cutaneous warts are the most common manifestations of HPV infection, with an estimated prevalence of around 7 to 12% in the general population. The common wart (verruca vulgaris) is frequently caused by HPV types 2 and 4 and appears as individual lesions or clusters, most frequently on the hands, particularly near the nail-beds. Common warts are particularly prevalent in childhood. Inherently benign lesions, they represent a cosmetic issue and are rarely painful. Plantar warts (verruca plantaris) are caused most frequently by HPV 1; these are often referred to in lay terms as "veruccas" and frequently appear as hyperkeratotic lesions on the soles of the feet, which may be painful, particularly with pressure. Acquisition of plantar warts is associated with swimming pools, where wet skin is more vulnerable to microabrasions, allowing entry of the viral particle to the basement epithelium. Other types of cutaneous warts include periungual warts, associated with nail biting, and the flat wart (verruca plana), which can occur as multiple flesh-colored protrusions often on the face but also on the neck, hands, wrists, and knees. The rarer filoform warts present as elongated lesions on the outer edge of lips or the rims of eyelids. Histologically, warts are associated with hypertrophy of all dermal layers and hyperkeratosis of the horny layer. Regression of warts can occur without intervention, although the key immune drivers of resolution are not well known and recurrence is, unfortunately, common.

Anogenital Warts (AGWs)

These warts are generally noticed by the patient as visible cauliflower-like growths that may be pink, tan, or hyperpigmented. They can be found anywhere on the anogenital epithelium, including vulva, perineum, penile, and perianal areas. The majority of AGWs are caused by HPV types 6 and 11. The management and treatment of AGWs represent a significant clinical burden. In a large UK-based assessment, AGWs accounted for 16 out of 100 referrals to genitourinary medicine clinics (18). Recurrence of AGWs is common, and another episode is experienced within a year of clearance in about 50% of patients. Symptoms include burning sensation, pruritis, discharge, and bleeding. Genital warts are straightforward to diagnose clinically, so HPV testing to confirm clinical suspicion of warts is not recommended, particularly as knowledge of the HPV type would not inform any management or treatment decisions. Anogenital warts rarely develop into cancer. The rare Buschke-Löwenstein tumor, sometimes referred to as the giant condyloma acuminatum of Buschke and Löwenstein, is a slow-progressing tumor that is locally aggressive, similar to verrucous carcinoma. The most common location is on the glans penis, and these lesions are more common in males than females.

Warts in Immunocompromised Populations

Warts are more common in immunocompromised individuals, including organ transplant recipients, those infected with HIV, and pregnant women. For example, it is estimated that around 40% of renal transplant recipients develop cutaneous warts within a year of transplantation. Iatrogenic immunosuppression in organ transplant recipients is also associated with increased replication of beta-PVs in the skin, and it is notable that there is a 250-fold risk of actinic keratoses and skin cancers in transplant recipients (19). The rare, autosomal recessive hereditary skin disorder epidermodysplasia verruciformis is a chronic immune disorder that results in high susceptibility to HPV infection at least partially due to impairment of T cell cytotoxicity against HPV-infected cells. Extensive flat and papillomatous warts appearing on the hands, face, trunk, and extremities are characteristic, and malignancies arise in 30 to 70% of patients, particularly in sun-exposed skin. Many HPV types are found in epidermodysplasia verruciformis lesions, including types 4, 5, 8, 9, 12, and 15, and concurrent infection with multiple types is common.

Oral and Upper Respiratory Tract Warts

Recurrent Respiratory Papillomatosis (RRP)

RRP is a rare condition characterized by benign papillomatous lesions of the larynx and other parts of the upper respiratory tract that are characteristically resistant to treatment. The onset may be in childhood (juvenile onset) or in adulthood. Patients usually present with hoarseness, voice changes, or other airway dysfunction such as chronic shortness of breath. Definitive diagnosis of RRP is made based on characteristic appearance on endoscopy and histopathology of biopsy. Nearly all RRP lesions are caused by HPV types 6 and 11, and HPV testing does not have a role in diagnosis or management. Despite the benign histology, significant morbidity occurs due to the frequent need for surgeries, potential damage to vocal cords, and possibility of respiratory obstruction. Malignant progression rarely occurs but has been reported, particularly in lesions that extend into the lower respiratory tract (20, 21).

Oral Papillomatosis

A variety of benign lesions may arise in the oral mucosa, and the occurrence of multiple lesions on the buccal mucosa is known as oral florid papillomatosis. HPV types associated with oral papillomatosis are those more commonly found in the genital tract.

HPV and Cancer

Globally, 570,000 cancers per year in women and 60,000 cases in men are attributable to HPV, representing, respectively, 8.6% and 0.8% of all cancers (22). Anogenital cancers with an evidence-based HPV etiology are cervical, vulvar, vaginal, anal, and penile cancer, although the attributable fraction of high-risk HPV (HR-HPV)-driven disease varies according to anatomical site (as described below). In addition, certain squamous cell cancers of the oropharynx (the area of the pharynx between the soft-palate and the epiglottis) are associated with HR-HPV, most notably the tonsil and the base of the tongue.

A precursor or preinvasive phase to anogenital squamous cancers exists, called intraepithelial neoplasia, graded 1 to 3 via histopathology, where 3 indicates the greatest degree of abnormality. An alternative terminology for squamous precancers similar to that used for cytology is being introduced in the United States: low- or high-grade squamous intraepithelial lesions (23). Cancer precursors of glandular lesions are rarer than squamous precancers and are designated as adenocarcinoma *in situ* without grading. The natural history of HPV infection, preinvasive lesions, and cancer is understood most fully for the cervix, and this has informed comprehensive screening options. The natural history of other anogenital cancers is less well understood, and no preinvasive phase for oropharyngeal cancer is reliably detected.

Cervical Cancer and Precancer

Cervical cancer is the most common HPV-driven cancer, with around 530,000 incident cases per year (22). Around 80% of cancers arise in low- and middle-income countries where the provision of primary and secondary prevention strategies via vaccination and screening are scarce, as are treatment options. The most common histologic type of cervical cancer is squamous cell carcinoma, arising in the squamous or metaplastic epithelium (70 to 75%). Adenocarcinomas, of glandular origin, are rarer (~20%), and other rare types account for around 5% of cervical cancer. Persistent infection with HR-HPV is the principal risk factor for the development of cervical cancer, and around 95% are HR-HPV positive, with HPV 16 and 18 accounting for 70%. Explanations for the absence of HR-HPV in cervical cancer include technical challenges in detecting highly fragmented viral genomes and/or a "hit and run" theory where, in some tumors, the virus exerts a malignant phenotype in the earlier stages of lesion development but is no longer present in the cancer. Certainly, there are rare cervical histological subtypes (such as clear cell adenocarcinoma) that are associated with a low prevalence of HPV (<30%) (24). With respect to preinvasive lesions, cervical intraepithelial neoplasia 1 (CIN 1) is considered a low-grade lesion, characteristic of a productive HPV infection, and is often managed conservatively given the high rate of natural clearance. CIN 2 and CIN 3 are considered high-grade lesions (high-grade squamous intraepithelial lesions). While CIN 3 is less heterogeneous and is a more robust diagnostic entity for significant precancerous disease, CIN 2 is usually the threshold for treatment in countries that have screening programs. Treatment of CIN is via surgical or ablative techniques to remove the affected area, and women who have had high-grade cervical lesions are at a significantly greater risk of recurrence of cervical disease than the general population (25). While clearance of CIN without intervention does occur, precise data on the rates of clearance, particularly high-grade CIN, are imperfect given the ethical issues pertaining to observational natural history studies. However, as noted earlier, the process from HPV infection to invasive cancer usually takes decades.

Anal and Penile Cancer

The second most common HPV-associated anogenital cancer is anal cancer, with around 40,000 incident cases per year globally. Similar to cervical cancer, most anal cancers have an HPV etiology, with the majority caused by HPV 16. The incidence of anal cancer is rising in both women and men for reasons that are not well understood but may be influenced by changing sexual practices. In addition, men who have sex with men are at significantly greater risk of anal cancer, as are people infected with HIV, and this has informed recommendations for targeted vaccination in these groups (26). Knowledge gaps exist with respect to the natural history and progression rate of preinvasive anal disease to cancer and, while anal cancer screening options (using cytology and high-resolution anoscopy) exist in certain settings, the traction and success of these approaches are behind those for cervical cancer, particularly because interventions to remove anal intraepithelial neoplasia (AIN) can result in significant morbidity (27). Penile cancer is relatively rare, at around 26,000 incident cases per year, of which ~50% are HPV positive (nearly all HPV 16). Warty/basoloid histology is more associated with HPV positivity than other histologic types.

Vulvar and Vaginal Cancer

Global estimates of incident cases of vulvar cancer are 34,000, with 8,500 attributable to HPV. The dominant type in HPV-associated vulvar cancer is HPV 16. Vulvar intraepithelial neoplasia (VIN) may be histologically classified as "usual type" (uVIN) or "differentiated type" (dVIN). The importance of this subtyping is that uVIN is more associated with HPV and more likely to be found in younger women, whereas dVIN is generally HPV negative and most often found in older, postmenopausal women.

Vaginal cancer is a rare cancer, with 15,000 incident cases globally, of which approximately 75% are associated with HPV (largely HPV 16). Vaginal cancer is found more frequently in postmenopausal women. Organized screening programs do not exist for vulvar and vaginal cancers, although cervical screening (and associated follow-up) provides an opportunity for identifying lesions clinically to some extent.

Oropharyngeal Cancer

The number of incident cases of oropharyngeal squamous cell carcinoma (OPSCC) is estimated at 96,000 globally. The attributable fraction of HPV-associated OPSCC varies significantly depending on country, ranging from 15 to 65% (28). However, a consistent observation is that 90% of HR-HPV-positive OPSCC is HPV-16. The incidence of OPSCC has risen dramatically in the last 2 decades, and in some countries, particularly those with cervical screening programs, the incidence of OPSCC may exceed that of cervical cancer. The reasons for the increase in OPSCC have included temporal changes in sexual behaviors, particularly around oral sex practices, although a rise in non-HPV-associated OPSCC—associated with alcohol consumption and tobacco—has also been observed. HR-HPV-positive OPSCC has a better prognosis than its HPV-negative counterpart in terms of disease progression and survival, and trials to determine whether knowledge of HPV status can influence/inform therapeutic options in OPSCC patients are under way. To this end, HPV annotation and testing may play an increasing role in the management of this disease (29, 30).

Prophylactic HPV Vaccines: Primary Cancer Prevention

As noted above, preventing HPV infection should prevent the development of cancer. This is the basis for the three currently licensed prophylactic HPV vaccines. These formulations all are protein based, composed of HPV L1 VLPs, and are noninfectious. They differ in the protein expression system used for production, the adjuvant, and the number of types targeted. All target HPV 16 and 18. Cervarix (GlaxoSmith Kline) targets those two types (2vHPV); Gardasil (Merck) also targets HPV 6 and 11, the types that cause genital warts (4vHPV); Gardasil 9 (Merck) additionally targets HPV 31, 33, 45, 52, and 58 (9vHPV) (31). These vaccines were approved on the basis of large multinational phase 3 clinical trials that demonstrated their safety and effectiveness for disease outcomes. More recently, the population-level impact on HPV prevalence, genital warts, and cervical disease has been noted in countries that have implemented national immunization programs (32).

The vaccines work by eliciting a largely type-specific neutralizing antibody response to conformationally intact VLPs in the vaccine, although significant cross-protection for HPV types 31, 33, and 45 has been demonstrated for 2vHPV as well as to some extent for 4vHPV vaccines (33). All three vaccines were originally approved with a three-dose schedule, following a prime-boost system (i.e., an initial dose to prime antibodies, with titers further raised by subsequent doses). Dosing regimens vary somewhat according to country-specific settings, but the WHO recommends two doses for 15-year-old girls and three doses for those who are older than 15 and those who are HIV positive (with doses to be a minimum of 6 months apart) (34). Reduced doses reduce the cost of the vaccine as well as the challenges of administration, factors that could remove barriers to vaccine introduction in low- and middle-income countries where cancer rates are high. *Post hoc* analysis of randomized controlled trial data indicates that one dose of vaccine may be effective, and prospective trials to investigate the efficacy of one dose are now under way (35).

The vaccine is efficacious in females and males; as a result, some countries have opted for gender-neutral vaccination programs. In situations where vaccine coverage of females is high, the cost effectiveness of gender-neutral programs is reduced due to "herd protection" (the overall reduced risk to nonvaccinated individuals due to decreased pathogen prevalence in the population caused by vaccination). Decisions on vaccinating males may not be entirely predicated on cost-effectiveness and vary by country (36, 37). Targeted programs for men who have sex with men have also been implemented given that they are not conferred herd protection from female-only programs and are at excess risk of HPV-associated disease compared to men who have sex with women exclusively (38).

COLLECTION, TRANSPORT, AND STORAGE OF SPECIMENS

This section focuses on specimen collection issues related to HPV detection and typing assays. As noted above, HPV serology has limited applications. The evaluation of HPV antibodies requires no specialized handling of blood and is usually performed on serum, although plasma can be used.

Because HPV cannot be cultured and is cell associated, HPV infection is studied indirectly based on detection and typing of nucleic acid extracts from a particular cellular sample. Samples from one anatomic site give no information about the possibility of infection at a different site. Tissue samples can be used, but for screening and natural history/epidemiology studies, samples collected noninvasively are required. The sample collection methods need to match requirements of the molecular assay, which may vary based on assay format and sensitivity. Requirements for transport and storage depend on collection media and the time interval to testing. The main requirement is sufficient preservation of the nucleic acids to allow the HPV assay to be valid.

Cervical sampling methods were established following approaches that had been used to optimize collection of exfoliated cells for the Pap test. After visualization of the cervix at the time of speculum examination, cells are collected from the epithelial surface of the transformation zone and endocervix using a variety of collection devices, such as swabs, brushes, or brooms. The collection device is turned a specified number of turns to ensure cellular yield. The cellular sample can be placed in a variety of collections fluids such as STM (Qiagen), PreservCyt (Hologic), or SurePath (Becton Dickinson). This approach remains preferred for samples used in cervical cancer screening, but vaginal self-collection methods developed for epidemiologic studies are being optimized to reach nonparticipants in cervical screening (39, 40). In most formats, women collect the sample by inserting the collection device into the vagina, similar to the method of inserting a tampon. The collection device can be a simple swab or more complicated specialized devices. Sampling by washing or lavage, similar to the use of a vaginal douche has also been used (41).

First-void urine samples also collect cells from the vaginal pool that represent the cervix, and this approach is being used in epidemiologic studies as well as being explored for screening (42, 43). While not used in clinical management, anal sampling follows methods similar to those for the cervix to collect cells for cytology or HPV testing. The anorectal junction is the area where most lesions occur, and swabs or brushes are positioned to exfoliate cells in the area, either by turning or rubbing. Self-collection methods have been successfully used in epidemiologic studies.

Epidemiological studies of HPV in male genital samples were originally hindered by difficulties in sampling the keratinized penile and scrotal areas. Methods using fine-grained emery papers to dislodge cells were used, but firm rubbing of the genital surface with Dacron or foam swabs can be used. Self-sampling can be as effective as samples collected by health care providers.

The oropharynx is difficult to sample noninvasively. Oral rinse and gargle using mouthwash or saline are the best options for collecting cells for epidemiological work. If lesions are visible, the surface may be sampled using a swab or brush.

The type-specific prevalence of HPV in precancers and cancers has relied largely on studies of formalin-fixed paraffin-embedded samples stored in pathology archives. The formalin cross-links limit the size of the DNA, and tissue preservation varies when routine processing is used. Methods of extraction need to be optimized (44). Histologic sectioning must be adapted to avoid PCR contamination (use of disposable fresh blade for each block, gloves, no water bath). A "sandwich" method of sectioning is recommended which involves cutting the first and last sections for hematoxylin and eosin staining, permitting verification of the lesion in the intervening section used for testing.

Because research has consistently indicated that detection of HR-HPV has prognostic importance in oropharyngeal cancers, sampling methods appropriate for clinical testing are being explored. A variety of material has been used, including fresh or formalin-fixed samples of the primary tumor or lymph node metastasis, as well as cellular material from fine-needle aspirates. Guidelines are still in development, and methods require standardization to improve reliability (30, 45).

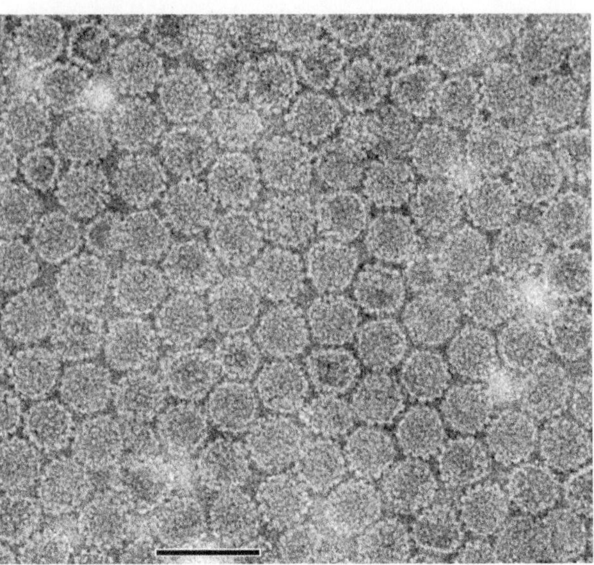

FIGURE 5 Negative-stain electron micrograph of HPV 18 recombinant L1 VLPs packed into a hexagonal array. Bar represents 100 nm. (Image courtesy of Charles Humphrey, Centers for Disease Control and Prevention.)

DIRECT EXAMINATION

Microscopy

Conventional light microscopy on histology specimens is the basis for diagnosis of the HPV-associated diseases described in the section on clinical significance above. In addition, microscopy of cervical cytology specimens, the Pap test, has been effective in cervical cancer screening. A well-defined perinuclear halo, referred to as koilocytosis, is a characteristic feature of cells from a low-grade cervical lesion (Fig. 4). Koilocytosis may also be seen in histology of warts and low-grade cervical biopsies. While histology and cytology changes are suggestive of HPV, specific detection of HPV requires molecular methods (see section on nucleic acid detection).

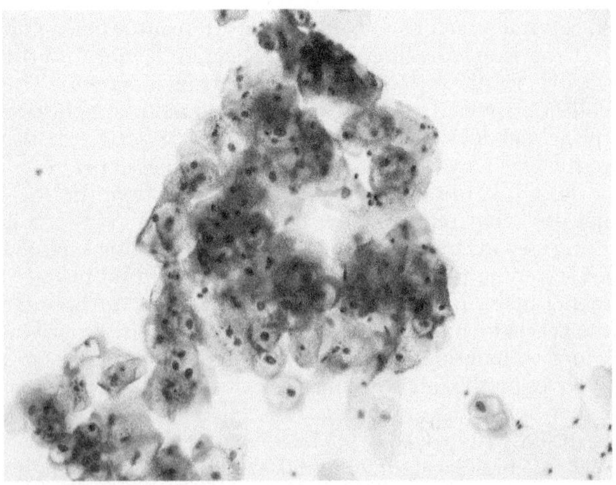

FIGURE 4 Koilocytosis. Exfoliated cervical cells showing a sharply demarcated large halo around nuclei known as koilocytosis. This is characteristic of productive HPV infection and would be given a cytology diagnosis of low-grade intraepithelial neoplasia. ThinPrep slide, Papanicolaou stain, original magnification 200×. (Image courtesy of Sue Mehew, Royal Infirmary of Edinburgh, United Kingdom.)

HPV viral particles may be visible by electron microscopy (EM) in lesions associated with high viral production. In general, EM is not used for HPV detection and diagnosis. The EM of complete viral particles and VLPs is very similar, and type-specific changes are difficult to discern. The EM appearance of VLPs is one method used in quality control of reagents used for HPV serology (Fig. 5).

Antigen Detection

Antigen detection is not used to identify or type HPV. For clinical applications relying on HPV as an indicator of disease, direct detection of HPV proteins, particularly the E6/E7 oncoproteins overexpressed in precancer and cancer, has been investigated. Simple assays for protein detection would simplify cervical cancer screening methods. A lateral flow assay for E6 oncoproteins was developed for point-of-care testing in low- and middle-income countries) (46). This has been commercialized as the OncoE6 cervical test (Arbor Vitae Corporation, Fremont, CA), which currently targets HPV 16 and 18 E6 proteins. Use has shown some promise in low-resource settings (47, 48).

Nucleic Acid Detection

In clinical applications, HPV serves as a biomarker for detection of underlying disease (as in cervical cancer) or as a guide to prognosis (as in oropharyngeal cancer). HPV detection is important in epidemiologic research studies and monitoring of the impact of HPV vaccines, but there is no treatment for HPV *per se*. While many assays could be used for either application, the focus for research is often analytic sensitivity and specificity, the numbers of copies of the virus that can be accurately detected. By contrast, clinical assays need to evaluate sensitivity and specificity with respect to disease detection (discussed further in the section on validation metrics). This chapter focuses on HPV tests that are used clinically. Current indications for clinical HPV testing are summarized in Table 1.

Nucleic acid amplification technologies (NAATs) are the mainstay of clinical HPV tests, particularly those aimed

TABLE 1 Summary of indications for clinical HPV testing for cervical screening and disease management[a]

Indication	Advantages	Limitations
Primary screening	Sensitive for the detection of CIN 2+; longer screening intervals possible after an HPV-negative result Opportunities for self-sampling in hard-to-reach populations Less affected by the impact of vaccination compared to cytology (?) Objective; more practical for countries that do not have the infrastructure for cytology-based screening	Although sensitive, will not detect all CIN 2+ Prevalence of "screen" HR-HPV positives higher than screen cytology positives Low positive predictive value of HR-HPV test for significant disease requires additional triage
Triage of low-grade cytologic abnormalities	Sensitive for the detection of CIN 2+ Reduced intensity of follow-up in those who test HPV negative and minimization of unnecessary colposcopy referrals	Low PPV, particularly in LSIL where prevalence of HR-HPV can be 70–80%
Posttreatment monitoring (test of cure)	Sensitive for the detection of residual CIN 2+ Reduced intensity of follow-up for the majority who test HPV negative	Low PPV of those who test HR-HPV positive after treatment (~20% at 6 months)
Prognosis	Oropharyngeal squamous cell carcinomas that are positive for HPV may be managed less aggressively	Standards for sampling and testing are still under development

[a]LSIL, low-grade squamous intraepithelial lesions; PPV, positive predictive value.

to inform screening and management of cervical disease. In this regard, HPV is no different from other targets within clinical virology laboratories inasmuch as culture and *in situ* technologies have made way for molecular approach(es) due to advantages in sensitivity, consistency, and automation. The rise in commercially available HPV tests in the last 10 years has been dramatic, and there is an almost overwhelming choice of assays which vary in their chemistry, level of automation, platform, genotype range, and importantly, the amount of performance data associated with their application.

The most recent review of HPV assays that were commercially available in 2015 detailed 193 separate assays (and 127 variants/derivatives thereof) (49). The majority of those assays lacked peer-reviewed publications on analytical and/or clinical performance relative to cervical disease. Given the high prevalence of subclinical HPV infection relative to cervical disease, high analytical sensitivity, while prized for other viruses and in research, is not necessarily an advantage for HPV tests used for cervical screening. The strength of HR-HPV assays for cervical cancer screening rests on their high sensitivity and negative predictive value. Increasing analytic sensitivity can erode clinical specificity, resulting in too many unnecessary referrals for further evaluation. To mitigate against the use of assays that are not fit for purpose, validation metrics for assays used in cervical screening have been proposed. Described in the validation metrics section below, these require that assays meet a minimum level of technical and clinical performance before they can be endorsed for clinical use. The importance of ongoing validation and verification of HPV assays must be emphasized.

Broadly speaking, HPV NAATs may be separated by (i) the method of amplification (signal or target), (ii) whether they are DNA or RNA based, and (iii) the level of genotyping they offer (limited, extended, or broad spectrum). Table 2 shows some examples of assays and their key characteristics, including those listed above. Another conceptual but important category is whether assays have been clinically validated and have regulatory approval for use in cervical screening. Decisions on test selection include considerations similar to those for other analytes (Table 3).

In contrast to assays for many other viruses, there are currently no commercial assays which offer strict viral load (VL) quantification for HPV. It is difficult to accurately and reproducibly normalize HPV copy number because it is unevenly distributed within lesional and nonlesional tissue. Observed copy numbers could change depending on how well the exfoliated cellular sample represents the lesion. In addition, infections with multiple HPV types are common, and it is not clear whether the cumulative viral copy number or type-specific copy number is most important. Finally, while most studies support an association between increasing HPV 16 VL and the likelihood of CIN 3, it has not been possible to establish a clinically meaningful threshold for risk, for example (50). Productive infections can actually have higher copy numbers than nonproductive infections when HPV may integrate. Recent work indicates that VL at a single time point is less helpful than sequential VL measurement where the crucial output is not an absolute value but rather the slope between two points (with an exponential, log-type increase associated with an adverse outcome) (51). Certainly, most commercially available assays, particularly those used for cervical screening, are validated at the qualitative level, and any semiquantitative measure that can be derived from the data is used according to the particular interest/objective of the user rather than the behest of the manufacturer.

Amplification Strategies and Targets

The majority of NAATs are based on target amplification, frequently PCR but also including transcription-mediated amplification or nucleic acid sequence-based amplification for RNA targets. While a variety of HPV genomic regions may be targeted, assays which amplify L1 are the most common, followed by those that target E6. Furthermore, primer/probe selection may be generic for multiple *Alphapapillomavirus* species encompassing multiple types or be type specific.

Assay-reporting strategies vary greatly. They range from visual interpretation of colorimetric hybridization of amplicons to an immobilized array of probes on a strip, to entirely automated real-time PCR systems which automatically convert a Ct (cycle threshold) value to a "positive" or "negative" result. Ideally, assays also include concurrent

TABLE 2 Approaches to molecular HPV testing according to target, underlying technology, and extent of genotyping capability

Category	Detection technology, examples	Commercially available assay, examples	Comments	Applications
HR-HPV DNA screening tests[a,b]	Target-based amplification using consensus primers (e.g., real-time PCR) or signal-based amplification	Hybrid Capture 2 (HC2) HPV DNA test (Qiagen Inc., Gaithersburg, MD) Amplicor HPV test (Roche Molecular Systems Inc., Alameda, CA) 13 High-risk HPV real-time PCR kit (Hybridibio, Beijing, China) CareHPV test (Qiagen Inc., Gaithersburg, MD)	HC2 was the first HPV test to be FDA approved. It is a signal-based amplification assay. HC2 has often been used as a comparator assay on which the technical and clinical performance of emerging assays are based, given the amount of data associated with its application. The CareHPV test is a test designed with low- and middle-income countries in mind.	HPV primary screening Triage of low-grade abnormalities Test of cure of treatment
HR-HPV DNA screening tests with concurrent or reflex typing[c]	Usually target-based amplification Genotyping element can involve type-specific primers/probes or a consensus approach where the amplicon is then subjected to a "secondary" type-specific detection	Cobas 4800 HPV test (Roche Molecular Systems Inc., Alameda, CA) Xpert HPV (Cepheid, Sunnyvale, CA) BD Onclarity HPV Assay (BD Diagnostics, Sparks, MD) RealTime High Risk HPV test (Abbott Molecular, Des Plaines, IL)	The level of genotyping ranges from HPV 16 and 18 (with HPV 18 sometimes indistinguishable from HPV 45) to delineation of 6 genotypes with a further 8 genotypes detected as 3 groups (as is the case for the Onclarity assay). An increasing number have FDA approval, including all those listed as examples in the adjacent cell.	As above and triage of women who are HR-HPV positive on primary screen
HPV DNA full genotyping tests	Various, including but not confined to target amplification prior to reverse line blot hybridization, Luminex-based detection, capillary electrophoresis, multiplex real-time PCR, PCR coupled with sequencing, and mass spectrometry; for details please refer to reference 32	Linear Array HPV Genotyping Test (Roche Molecular Systems Inc., Alameda, CA) Papillocheck high-risk test (Greiner Bio-One, Frickenhausen, Germany) Clart HPV 2 – papillomavirus clinical arrays (Genomica, Coslada, Spain) Anyplex II HPV HR Detection (Seegene, Seoul, Korea)	Largest group of commercially available HPV tests with a number of underlying and detection technologies. Extent and range of types detected vary significantly between assays. Generally less automated than the above two categories. Not generally applied for cervical screening/disease management.	Research and development Epidemiology Vaccine monitoring
HR-HPV E6/E7 mRNA tests (including those with typing capability)	Includes NASBA, real-time PCR, target-mediated amplification	APTIMA HPV assay (Hologic, Madison, WI) NucliSENS Easy Q HPV (bioMérieux, Marcy l'Etoile, France) PreTect SEE (Norchip, Klokkarstua, Norway) QuantiVirus HPV E6/E7 mRNA for cervical cancer (DiaCarta LLC, Hayward, CA)	Fewer RNA- than DNA-based tests. Argument that mRNA approaches may be more specific (compared to DNA approaches) for the detection of clinically significant HPV infection given that E6/E7 transcript is detected, which may be a better indicator of oncogenic activity compared to DNA amplification of a structural gene. The APTIMA HPV assay is currently the only mRNA-based test to have FDA approval for use in cervical screening and disease management.	Dependent on assay. However, for FDA-approved assay (APTIMA): HPV primary screening Triage of low-grade abnormalities Test of cure of treatment

[a]Screening tests target 12 HPV types considered high-risk according to the International Agency of Research on Cancer in addition to HPV 66 and HPV 68.

[b]There are a group of tests which target a subset of types within the 12 HR-HPV types defined by the IARC. These are not included in this table because the above categories are generally applied for clinical, screening, and epidemiological applications.

[c]Reflex typing: a secondary test must be performed after an initial positive result has been generated in order to determine the type-specific content. Concurrent typing: genotyping information is provided as a function of a single assay.

TABLE 3 Considerations for selection of HPV assay

What is the context/driver for testing?

Epidemiological: Requires assay with genotyping capability, ideally amenable to diverse biospecimens. If the result will not affect the screening/patient pathway, regulatory approval is not a priority.

Research: Depends on the nature of the research, i.e., basic or applied. High analytical sensitivity may be a priority for the former. If the result will not affect the screening/patient pathway, regulatory approval is not required.

Clinical: What is the evidence base for the particular application? Does it fulfill recognized minimum criteria for performance? Regulatory approval is important (mandatory in certain countries). Is genotyping used for the screening/patient pathway? If so, does the platform offer this as a concurrent or reflex facility?

Location of the testing site

Low- and middle-income countries (LMICs): Costly tests/platforms which require sophisticated machinery and a high level of supportive laboratory infrastructure may be inappropriate. Ease of use and portability are clearly important. Logistical barriers to patient follow-up in LMICs may favor near-to-patient or point-of-care testing.

High income: What is the nature of the program? Nationally organized and monitored screening programs generally rely on centralized laboratories, resulting in standardized methods. A greater variability of laboratory services is associated with opportunistic programs where individualized practice is more common.

Throughput demands

For high-throughput testing (e.g., primary screening), robust automation is essential in addition to technical support from commercial provider to minimize impact on turnaround/service. What are the contingencies for platform downtime? What are the options/solutions for automation of preanalytical steps (i.e., sample preparation prior to extraction)?

Technical demands and cost

What equipment/instruments are required? Is specialized equipment needed that will have no other applications in the laboratory? What technical experience and skill are required? What are reagent/supply costs per assay? What is the cost of equipment maintenance?

amplification of a human housekeeping or endogenous gene, produced in every cell (such as glyceraldehyde-3-phosphate dehydrogenase or beta-globin) as a control for sample "adequacy." This endogenous control also gives an indication that inhibitors of the reaction are not present. For both indications, the positive control probe is not a substitute for careful standardized sample collection, and it cannot fully exclude problems.

Compared to target amplification assays, fewer tests use signal amplification. However, of note, the first HPV test to receive FDA approval for use in cervical screening—the Digene Hybrid Capture 2 HPV DNA test (HC2, Qiagen)—is based on signal amplification. The HC2 assay is associated with significant longitudinal data on clinical performance and has been used as a comparator against which emerging assays are assessed (52). As with any assay developed and validated for clinician-collected samples, performance on self-collected samples requires reestablishing clinical performance. There is evidence suggesting that self-collected samples (see section on sampling) require target-based amplification tests to achieve clinical sensitivity comparable to that obtained with a clinician-taken sample (39).

Because HPV is a double-stranded DNA virus, most molecular tests focus on the direct amplification of DNA. RNA-based tests are rarer, although the FDA-approved Aptima HPV assay (Hologic), which relies on detection of E6/E7 mRNA via transcription-mediated amplification, is relatively well established for cervical screening (53). There is some evidence to indicate that detection of mRNA of oncogenes as opposed to detection of DNA of a structural gene (L1) may reduce detection of transient HPV infection, conferring greater clinical specificity. However, many who test positive for HPV E6/E7 mRNA have transient infection.

Genotyping

As described earlier, even within the group of HR-HPV types, natural history studies confirm the absolute risk for CIN 2+ to be stratified by type, with HPV 16 having the highest risk (54). Additionally, type-specific persistent infection poses a significantly greater risk for lesion development than sequential infection with different HPV types over the same time. As a consequence, genotyping provides value and insight to longitudinal epidemiological and research studies following type-specific trends. HPV genotyping has generated important data on the impact of the prophylactic HPV vaccines in both trial settings and at the population/program level (33, 55). Furthermore, given the gradations of risk even within the high-risk category, HPV genotyping can exert a role in screening and clinical management.

HPV screening is now a reality in many settings, either as a primary screen or as a cotest with cervical cytology. The high negative predictive value of an HPV test allows screening intervals to be extended, but the high sensitivity comes with a lower specificity, risking overreferral of women for follow-up. Because HPV prevalence is highest in young women (below age 25 to 30 years), in whom the risk for cervical disease is low, primary screening with HPV testing is generally reserved for women over age 25. This avoids detection of clinically insignificant HPV and improves the specificity for detection of cervical disease. Even with age restriction, additional testing is needed to improve the efficiency of clinical management. Between countries, there is some heterogeneity of practice with regard to how HPV-positive women are triaged (56). Specific identification of HPV 16 and 18 is one of the more evidence-based indications for referral to colposcopy because of the established higher risk of cervical disease in women with HPV 16/18 (57). There is also some evidence that the HR-HPV group could be further divided into additional categories with discrete risk and associated management guidelines. This would warrant the use of assays with more extensive genotyping. One such proposal identified five groups to guide management (from greatest to least 3-year risk of CIN 3+): (i) HPV 16, (ii) HPV 18/45, (iii) HPV 31/33/58/52, (iv) HPV 51/35/39/56/59/66/68, and (v) HPV negative. Management ranged from immediate colposcopy and biopsy even if colposcopic impression is negative (ii) to a return to routine screening (v) (58).

Most of the clinically validated, high-throughput HPV assays that have appeared on the market in the last 5 years incorporate a level of genotyping that includes HPV 16 and 18, with HPV 18 sometimes indistinguishable from HPV 45 (59). There is between-assay variation as to whether the genotyping element is provided concurrently or as a reflex after a positive result. Assays that provide broad-spectrum typing capability (whether confined to high-risk types or not) tend to be less automated/high throughput. Although this is a rapidly evolving field, FDA-approved assays that offer extended genotyping beyond HPV 16/18, which reconcile with service-laboratory demands on throughput, now exist. For example, one such assay, the Onclarity HPV test (Becton Dickinson), provides an output that delineates six HPV types individually (16, 18, 31, 45, 51, and 52) and three groups of HPV types: 33/58, 56/59/66, and 35/39/68.

With respect to resolution of types other than the high-risk types, there is no evidence to indicate that this is justified for patient management (60). Identification of types that are considered "possibly carcinogenic" does not inform a clear clinical management strategy. Although possibly carcinogenic types may, by definition, be associated with cancer, the frequency of this is so low that they are excluded from the scope of assays approved by regulatory agencies (such as the FDA) for HPV primary cervical cancer screening. The incremental increase in sensitivity achieved by including these additional types does not offset a substantial loss in specificity (61). This is not meant to criticize the existence of broad-spectrum genotyping assays, because these are important for research and surveillance endeavors. However, as with all HPV testing in the screening and clinical context, HPV genotyping should be confined to evidence-based application(s).

Level of Automation and Technical Complexity

The variety of available assays and throughput requirements is reflected in the variety of equipment platforms created to accommodate them. These range from large analyzers which can process hundreds of samples per day and incorporate preanalytic solutions for uncapping primary vials to near-patient (point-of-care) tests that can be performed in primary care or the field. Physical separation of high-throughput analyzers into an extraction and amplification platform is increasingly being replaced by single units that incorporate both. In addition, batch processing/testing in a classic 96-well format is making way for random access options with continual loading. Moreover, a number of the higher-throughput assays are delivered on platforms that accommodate other molecular microbial targets such as *Chlamydia trachomatis* and blood-borne viruses.

In terms of technical complexity, again, there is considerable variation across platforms and with respect to what is demanded in terms of supportive infrastructure, including both the physical environment and staff skill sets. These are important elements when considering what may be applicable in low- and middle-income countries. Indeed, certain assays lend themselves to this context more readily, including an assay based on the chemical principles of HC2 but with lower complexity and demands on electricity (Care HPV, Qiagen) and an assay which requires simple addition of 1 ml of sample to a cartridge (Xpert HPV, Cepheid). Xpert HPV was the first test accepted for the WHO list of prequalified *in vitro* diagnostics for cervical cancer screening (http://www.who.int/diagnostics_laboratory/evaluations/pq-list/hiv-vrl/171221_final_pq_report_pqdx_0268_070_00.pdf).

Next-Generation Sequencing Assays

Next-generation sequencing (NGS) methods are rapidly transitioning into clinical laboratories, and while none of the HPV NGS methods are ready for clinical applications, many research applications are already reported (e.g., 62–64). NGS methods have the potential to broaden the spectrum of HPV types that can be studied, relying, for example, on broad-coverage target enrichment (65). In addition, these methods can provide detailed information on HPV variants and integration status. Methods that bar code and sequence consensus amplicons of the L1 region provide less information on the virus, but the shorter reads allow for increased multiplexing. Improved methods and refinements in bioinformatics pipelines could significantly increase the reliability and decrease the cost of such methods for epidemiologic studies.

Adjunctive/Triage Tests

There is a clear demand to develop assays that can risk-stratify, or "triage," clinically significant HPV infections from trivial ones that will clear. With the increasing move to molecular HPV testing as a primary screen, this demand becomes particularly apposite. Triage tests are clearly important because they inform whether a female requires examination at a colposcopy clinic or can be managed more conservatively (66). Arguably, the triage tests that are the most evidence based for the risk stratification of HPV infection are cytology and limited genotyping (using HPV 16/18 typing as described above in the genotyping section). The greater risk of cancer associated with HPV 16 and 18 infection (compared to other HR-HPV types) has justified this triage approach; however, because not all cancers are associated with types 16/18, women who are HPV positive/HPV 16-18 negative still require a level of monitoring. In a similar fashion, while HPV positive/cytology abnormal women are generally referred to colposcopy, the level of risk in HPV-positive, cytology-normal women is not so low as to recommend discharge to routine recall (67). So far, the identification of a triage test which offers a binary outcome of referral to colposcopy versus return to routine screening has proved elusive, and this is evidenced in the internationally varied approaches to triage (56).

The performance of cytology can be further enhanced by the use of adjunctive biomarker staining using immunocytochemistry. Protein markers indicative of abnormal proliferation, known to be overexpressed in high-grade disease such as p16INK4a (alone or in combination with another proliferation marker, Ki67), have been used to this end. Proponents suggest that addition of these biomarkers removes a level of subjectivity from morphological interpretation, with a red nucleus within a brown cytoplasm serving as an easily found marker of disease. Detractors suggest that because a level of subjective interpretation is still required, it does not satisfy the demands of a complete molecular solution to cervical screening that molecular HR-HPV testing may presage.

One area of growing research is the development and application of assays which detect methylation. Methylation is the transfer of CH_3 groups to GC-rich areas of the genome in a manner which can affect gene regulation. The development of tools which target methylation signatures builds on the longstanding evidence base that certain "abnormal" methylation patterns are a hallmark of aberrant cell proliferation and cancer development, including in cervical cancer. Developments in sequencing technologies such as pyrosequencing and NGS have facilitated the transition of basic knowledge to laboratory tests.

Hypermethylation of L1 confers a risk for development of lesions, particularly for HPV 16, and hypermethylation of host genes including *CADM1*, *EPB41L3*, *FAM19A4*, *MAL*, *miR-124*, *PAX1*, and *SOX1* is also associated with cancer risk. While methylation assays are currently less established/applied than HPV NAATs, development of these assays is increasing, as is their application to cervical screening contexts (68).

ISOLATION PROCEDURES

HPV cannot be isolated from lesional tissues or cells by conventional methods. Propagation of HPV by any method has been challenging because the viral life cycle is tightly linked to differentiation of the host cell. The first successful method to passage HPV *in vitro* grafted samples under the renal capsule of athymic mice (69). Subsequently, a variety of systems were developed to study PV infection (recently reviewed in reference 70). Organotypic raft cultures provide a fully differentiating environment, and human keratinocytes with episomal HPV can reproduce the full viral life cycle. HPV can be introduced to monolayer cultures using packaging cell lines and methods similar to those used to produce VLPs and quasi-virions (71, 72). These are important research methods but play no role in clinical identification of HPV.

SEROLOGIC TESTS

As noted in earlier sections, HPV types are not based on serology, because of the weak and inconsistent immune response to natural infection. Therefore, HPV serology is not used clinically, and there are no commercially available assays for detecting HPV antibodies. However, HPV serology is an important research tool and is increasingly important, such as in HPV vaccine trials. The approval of reduced dosing schedules and next-generation biosimilar vaccines may need to rely on the noninferiority of antibody titers (73). The efficacy of current vaccines makes placebo-controlled trials unethical and is reducing the population burden of targeted types, making disease endpoints and even HPV DNA endpoints infeasible.

HPV antibody tests used in HPV vaccinology have been reviewed (74). Neutralization assays are considered the best correlate of antibody function. These use pseudovirions, L1 VLPs with signaling plasmid, as a model for infection and require *in vitro* mammalian cell culture. Neutralizing antibodies block pseudovirions from binding and releasing their signaling plasmid into the cells. After washing and evaluating signal, the extent of signal reduction induced by the sample compared with a blank provides a semiquantitative measure of neutralizing antibodies. However, neutralizing assays are time-consuming, and enzyme-linked immunosorbent assays (ELISAs) of some form are more often used. Prior to using an ELISA, verification of the correlation between ELISA and neutralization assay results is required. ELISAs can be direct binding assays (generally targeting IgG) or can be competitive, in which case a type-specific monoclonal antibody directed against one neutralizing epitope competes with serum immunoglobulins of any class. Increasingly, immunoassays need to be multiplexed (using multianalyte wells or bead-based methods) to allow monitoring of a response to the nine types targeted by Gardasil 9. Interassay variation can be expected because of differences in the assay design (75). Use of the parallel-line method of assay interpretation improves interlaboratory comparability. International standards allow results to be reported in international units, the only approach that allows direct comparison between assay formats. Standards are available from the National Institute for Biological Standards and Controls for HPV 16 and 18 antibodies, with others under development.

EVALUATION, INTERPRETATION, AND REPORTING OF RESULTS

Validation Metrics and Quality Monitoring

The nature of assay validation depends on the application. If the goal is investigative and relies on the discrimination of very low levels of viral target in the sample, then assays with a high analytical sensitivity are required. When the investigative focus relies on longitudinal trends in type-specific prevalence in the population, such as monitoring HPV vaccine impact, long-term assay stability is another important consideration. Use of the same assay with strict monitoring of quality control is required to avoid assay-driven differences confounding real-life changes.

Regarding assays that are suitable for cervical screening contexts, it is essential that their performance is calibrated to disease endpoints to minimize detection of clinically irrelevant infection. A framework devised in 2009 by Meijer and colleagues set out a pathway for the validation of HPV assays for primary cervical screening in women aged 30 and above, and this process has been adopted widely in the HPV community (52). In this framework, performance of the candidate assay is assessed relative to that of a "gold-standard" assay with a well-established, acceptable detection capability for CIN 2+. With this framework, which also incorporates a minimum requirement for inter- and intralab reproducibility, samples used for the validation should be derived from a cervical screening context. This is an important element because although the initial clinical performance data of emerging assays are frequently derived from colposcopy referral populations (given their disease-enriched nature), such referral populations do not resemble primary screening populations with respect to the amount and nature of disease and the relevant demands of the tests thereof. HPV assays that have FDA approval have, so far, particular applications (which include primary screening and triage of low-grade abnormality) paired with particular sample collection and processing methods. As with any assay used for patient management, ongoing validation is multifaceted and dynamic, and while demonstration and verification of performance via FDA approval and/or Certificate of European standards are important, so is independent evaluation using the validation frameworks described above.

Demonstration of technical competence in the setting where the assay will be delivered, as well as ongoing quality monitoring and assessment—which include, but are by no means confined to, participation in external quality assessment schemes—are essential (76). Furthermore, laboratories which perform diagnostic testing are obliged to meet the standards of their external accreditation body; such standards include a sizable component for verification and ongoing quality monitoring, and HPV testing is no exception to such scrutiny. Proficiency testing programs are available for some assays through accrediting groups such as the College of American Pathologists. Usually, these programs use defined samples (cloned DNA) and do not fully evaluate all steps of the assay. The International HPV Center offers a proficiency panel for HPV DNA typing that is appropriate for laboratories involved in epidemiology and

HPV vaccine monitoring (77). Interlaboratory exchange of samples and QC repeats are also methods to help laboratories ensure the reliability of their results. International standards for HPV DNA and HPV antibodies are available from the National Institute for Biological Standards and Controls. In addition, plasmid constructs are available from the International HPV Reference Center.

The findings in this chapter are those of the authors and do not represent the official position of the Centers for Disease Control and Prevention.

REFERENCES

1. **Van Doorslaer K, Li Z, Xirasagar S, Maes P, Kaminsky D, Liou D, Sun Q, Kaur R, Huyen Y, McBride AA.** 2017. The Papillomavirus Episteme: a major update to the papillomavirus sequence database. *Nucleic Acids Res* **45**(D1):D499–D506.
2. **Doorbar J, Egawa N, Griffin H, Kranjec C, Murakami I.** 2015. Human papillomavirus molecular biology and disease association. *Rev Med Virol* **25**(Suppl 1):2–23.
3. **DiGiuseppe S, Bienkowska-Haba M, Guion LG, Sapp M.** 2017. Cruising the cellular highways: how human papillomavirus travels from the surface to the nucleus. *Virus Res* **231:**1–9.
4. **Kwak K, Jiang R, Wang JW, Jagu S, Kirnbauer R, Roden RB.** 2014. Impact of inhibitors and L2 antibodies upon the infectivity of diverse alpha and beta human papillomavirus types. *PLoS One* **9:**e97232.
5. **Doorbar J.** 2006. Molecular biology of human papillomavirus infection and cervical cancer. *Clin Sci (Lond)* **110:**525–541.
6. **Doorbar J, Quint W, Banks L, Bravo IG, Stoler M, Broker TR, Stanley MA.** 2012. The biology and life-cycle of human papillomaviruses. *Vaccine* **30**(Suppl 5):F55–F70.
7. **McBride AA, Warburton A.** 2017. The role of integration in oncogenic progression of HPV-associated cancers. *PLoS Pathog* **13:**e1006211.
8. **IARC.** 2012. Human Papillomaviruses, p 255–314, *IARC Mongraphs on the Evaluation of Carcinogenic Risks to Humans*, vol 100B, *Biological Agents*. IARC, Lyons, France.
9. **Tommasino M.** 2017. The biology of beta human papillomaviruses. *Virus Res* **231:**128–138.
10. **Stanley M, Pinto LA, Trimble C.** 2012. Human papillomavirus vaccines: immune responses. *Vaccine* **30**(Suppl 5):F83–F87.
11. **Beachler DC, Jenkins G, Safaeian M, Kreimer AR, Wentzensen N.** 2016. Natural acquired immunity against subsequent genital human papillomavirus infection: a systematic review and meta-analysis. *J Infect Dis* **213:**1444–1454.
12. **Iversen OE, Miranda MJ, Ulied A, Soerdal T, Lazarus E, Chokephaibulkit K, Block SL, Skrivanek A, Nur Azurah AG, Fong SM, Dvorak V, Kim KH, Cestero RM, Berkovitch M, Ceyhan M, Ellison MC, Ritter MA, Yuan SS, DiNubile MJ, Saah AJ, Luxembourg A.** 2016. Immunogenicity of the 9-valent HPV vaccine using 2-dose regimens in girls and boys vs a 3-dose regimen in women. *JAMA* **316:**2411–2421.
13. **Giuliano AR, Nyitray AG, Kreimer AR, Pierce Campbell CM, Goodman MT, Sudenga SL, Monsonego J, Franceschi S.** 2015. EUROGIN 2014 roadmap: differences in human papillomavirus infection natural history, transmission and human papillomavirus-related cancer incidence by gender and anatomic site of infection. *Int J Cancer* **136:**2752–2760.
14. **Ryndock EJ, Meyers C.** 2014. A risk for non-sexual transmission of human papillomavirus? *Expert Rev Anti Infect Ther* **12:**1165–1170.
15. **zur Hausen H, Meinhof W, Scheiber W, Bornkamm GW.** 1974. Attempts to detect virus-specific DNA in human tumors. I. Nucleic acid hybridizations with complementary RNA of human wart virus. *Int J Cancer* **13:**650–656.
16. **Egawa N, Doorbar J.** 2017. The low-risk papillomaviruses. *Virus Res* **231:**119–127.
17. **Mirabello L, Yeager M, Cullen M, Boland JF, Chen Z, Wentzensen N, Zhang X, Yu K, Yang Q, Mitchell J, Roberson D, Bass S, Xiao Y, Burdett L, Raine-Bennett T, Lorey T, Castle PE, Burk RD, Schiffman M.** 2016. HPV16 sublineage associations with histology-specific cancer risk using HPV whole-genome sequences in 3200 women. *J Natl Cancer Inst* **108:**djw100.
18. **Thurgar E, Barton S, Karner C, Edwards SJ.** 2016. Clinical effectiveness and cost-effectiveness of interventions for the treatment of anogenital warts: systematic review and economic evaluation. *Health Technol Assess* **20:**v–vi, 1–486.
19. **Wieland U, Kreuter A, Pfister H.** 2014. Human papillomavirus and immunosuppression. *Curr Probl Dermatol* **45:**154–165.
20. **Derkay CS, Wiatrak B.** 2008. Recurrent respiratory papillomatosis: a review. *Laryngoscope* **118:**1236–1247.
21. **Fortes HR, von Ranke FM, Escuissato DL, Araujo Neto CA, Zanetti G, Hochhegger B, Souza CA, Marchiori E.** 2017. Recurrent respiratory papillomatosis: a state-of-the-art review. *Respir Med* **126:**116–121.
22. **de Martel C, Plummer M, Vignat J, Franceschi S.** 2017. Worldwide burden of cancer attributable to HPV by site, country and HPV type. *Int J Cancer* **141:**664–670.
23. **Darragh TM, Colgan TJ, Thomas Cox J, Heller DS, Henry MR, Luff RD, McCalmont T, Nayar R, Palefsky JM, Stoler MH, Wilkinson EJ, Zaino RJ, Wilbur DC, Members of the LAST Project Work Groups.** 2013. The Lower Anogenital Squamous Terminology Standardization project for HPV-associated lesions: background and consensus recommendations from the College of American Pathologists and the American Society for Colposcopy and Cervical Pathology. *Int J Gynecol Pathol* **32:**76–115.
24. **Chen W, Molijn A, Enqi W, Zhang X, Jenkins D, Yu X, Quint W, Schmidt JE, Li J, Pirog E, Liu B, Li Q, Liu X, Li L, Qiao Y, Chinese HPV Typing Group.** 2016. The variable clinicopathological categories and role of human papillomavirus in cervical adenocarcinoma: a hospital based nation-wide multi-center retrospective study across China. *Int J Cancer* **139:**2687–2697.
25. **Strander B, Andersson-Ellström A, Milsom I, Sparén P.** 2007. Long term risk of invasive cancer after treatment for cervical intraepithelial neoplasia grade 3: population based cohort study. *BMJ* **335:**1077.
26. **Kirby T.** 2018. MSM in England to be offered free HPV vaccination. *Lancet Oncol* **19:**e148.
27. **Martin D, Balermpas P, Winkelmann R, Rödel F, Rödel C, Fokas E.** 2018. Anal squamous cell carcinoma: state of the art management and future perspectives. *Cancer Treat Rev* **65:**11–21.
28. **Hussein AA, Helder MN, de Visscher JG, Leemans CR, Braakhuis BJ, de Vet HCW, Forouzanfar T.** 2017. Global incidence of oral and oropharynx cancer in patients younger than 45 years versus older patients: a systematic review. *Eur J Cancer* **82:**115–127.
29. **Gillison ML, Chaturvedi AK, Anderson WF, Fakhry C.** 2015. Epidemiology of human papillomavirus-positive head and neck squamous cell carcinoma. *J Clin Oncol* **33:**3235–3242.
30. **Lewis JS Jr, Beadle B, Bishop JA, Chernock RD, Colasacco C, Lacchetti C, Moncur JT, Rocco JW, Schwartz MR, Seethala RR, Thomas NE, Westra WH, Faquin WC.** 2018. Human papillomavirus testing in head and neck carcinomas: guideline from the College of American Pathologists. *Arch Pathol Lab Med* **142:**559–597.
31. **Roden RBS, Stern PL.** 2018. Opportunities and challenges for human papillomavirus vaccination in cancer. *Nat Rev Cancer* **18:**240–254.
32. **Brisson M, Bénard É, Drolet M, Bogaards JA, Baussano I, Vänskä S, Jit M, Boily MC, Smith MA, Berkhof J, Canfell K, Chesson HW, Burger EA, Choi YH, De Blasio BF, De Vlas SJ, Guzzetta G, Hontelez JAC, Horn J, Jepsen MR, Kim JJ, Lazzarato F, Matthijsse SM, Mikolajczyk R, Pavelyev A, Pillsbury M, Shafer LA, Tully SP, Turner HC, Usher C, Walsh C.** 2016. Population-level impact, herd immunity, and elimination after human papillomavirus vaccination: a systematic review and meta-analysis of predictions from transmission-dynamic models. *Lancet Public Health* **1:**e8–e17.

33. **Kavanagh K, Pollock KG, Cuschieri K, Palmer T, Cameron RL, Watt C, Bhatia R, Moore C, Cubie H, Cruickshank M, Robertson C.** 2017. Changes in the prevalence of human papillomavirus following a national bivalent human papillomavirus vaccination programme in Scotland: a 7-year cross-sectional study. *Lancet Infect Dis* **17:**1293–1302.
34. **WHO.** 2017. Human papillomavirus vaccines: WHO position paper, May 2017. *Wkly Epidemiol Rec* **92:**241–268.
35. **Kreimer AR, Herrero R, Sampson JN, Porras C, Lowy DR, Schiller JT, Schiffman M, Rodriguez AC, Chanock S, Jimenez S, Schussler J, Gail MH, Safaeian M, Kemp TJ, Cortes B, Pinto LA, Hildesheim A, Gonzalez P, Costa Rica HPV Vaccine Trial (CVT) Group.** 2018. Evidence for single-dose protection by the bivalent HPV vaccine: review of the Costa Rica HPV vaccine trial and future research studies. *Vaccine* **36:**4774–4782.
36. **Sabeena S, Bhat PV, Kamath V, Arunkumar G.** 2018. Global human papilloma virus vaccine implementation: an update. *J Obstet Gynaecol Res* **44:**989–997.
37. **Malagón T, Laurie C, Franco EL.** 2018. Human papillomavirus vaccination and the role of herd effects in future cancer control planning: a review. *Expert Rev Vaccines* **17:**395–409.
38. **Zhang L, Regan DG, Ong JJ, Gambhir M, Chow EPF, Zou H, Law M, Hocking J, Fairley CK.** 2017. Targeted human papillomavirus vaccination for young men who have sex with men in Australia yields significant population benefits and is cost-effective. *Vaccine* **35:**4923–4929.
39. **Arbyn M, Verdoodt F, Snijders PJ, Verhoef VM, Suonio E, Dillner L, Minozzi S, Bellisario C, Banzi R, Zhao FH, Hillemanns P, Anttila A.** 2014. Accuracy of human papillomavirus testing on self-collected versus clinician-collected samples: a meta-analysis. *Lancet Oncol* **15:**172–183.
40. **Ogilvie G, Nakisige C, Huh WK, Mehrotra R, Franco EL, Jeronimo J.** 2017. Optimizing secondary prevention of cervical cancer: recent advances and future challenges. *Int J Gynaecol Obstet* **138**(Suppl 1)**:**15–19.
41. **Trevitt SSS, Wood A.** 2014. *New and Emerging Self-Sampling Technologies for Human Papillomavirus (HPV) Testing.* Horizon Scanning Research & Intelligence Centre, Birminghan, UK.
42. **Vorsters A, Micalessi I, Bilcke J, Ieven M, Bogers J, Van Damme P.** 2012. Detection of human papillomavirus DNA in urine: a review of the literature. *Eur J Clin Microbiol Infect Dis* **31:**627–640.
43. **Leeman A, Del Pino M, Molijn A, Rodriguez A, Torné A, de Koning M, Ordi J, van Kemenade F, Jenkins D, Quint W.** 2017. HPV testing in first-void urine provides sensitivity for CIN2+ detection comparable with a smear taken by a clinician or a brush-based self-sample: cross-sectional data from a triage population. *BJOG* **124:**1356–1363.
44. **Lagheden C, Eklund C, Kleppe SN, Unger ER, Dillner J, Sundström K.** 2016. Validation of a standardized extraction method for formalin-fixed paraffin-embedded tissue samples. *J Clin Virol* **80:**36–39.
45. **Schache AG, Liloglou T, Risk JM, Filia A, Jones TM, Sheard J, Woolgar JA, Helliwell TR, Triantafyllou A, Robinson M, Sloan P, Harvey-Woodworth C, Sisson D, Shaw RJ.** 2011. Evaluation of human papilloma virus diagnostic testing in oropharyngeal squamous cell carcinoma: sensitivity, specificity, and prognostic discrimination. *Clin Cancer Res* **17:**6262–6271.
46. **Schweizer J, Lu PS, Mahoney CW, Berard-Bergery M, Ho M, Ramasamy V, Silver JE, Bisht A, Labiad Y, Peck RB, Lim J, Jeronimo J, Howard R, Gravitt PE, Castle PE.** 2010. Feasibility study of a human papillomavirus E6 oncoprotein test for diagnosis of cervical precancer and cancer. *J Clin Microbiol* **48:**4646–4648.
47. **Mariano VS, Lorenzi AT, Scapulatempo-Neto C, Stein MD, Resende JC, Antoniazzi M, Villa LL, Levi JE, Longatto-Filho A, Fregnani JH.** 2016. A low-cost HPV immunochromatographic assay to detect high-grade cervical intraepithelial neoplasia. *PLoS One* **11:**e0164892.
48. **Zhao FH, Jeronimo J, Qiao YL, Schweizer J, Chen W, Valdez M, Lu P, Zhang X, Kang LN, Bansil P, Paul P, Mahoney C, Berard-Bergery M, Bai P, Peck R, Li J, Chen F, Stoler MH, Castle PE.** 2013. An evaluation of novel, lower-cost molecular screening tests for human papillomavirus in rural China. *Cancer Prev Res (Phila)* **6:**938–948.
49. **Poljak M, Kocjan BJ, Oštrbenk A, Seme K.** 2016. Commercially available molecular tests for human papillomaviruses (HPV): 2015 update. *J Clin Virol* **76**(Suppl 1)**:**S3–S13.
50. **Rajeevan MS, Swan DC, Nisenbaum R, Lee DR, Vernon SD, Ruffin MT, Horowitz IR, Flowers LC, Kmak D, Tadros T, Birdsong G, Husain M, Srivastava S, Unger ER.** 2005. Epidemiologic and viral factors associated with cervical neoplasia in HPV-16-positive women. *Int J Cancer* **115:**114–120.
51. **Depuydt CE, Thys S, Beert J, Jonckheere J, Salembier G, Bogers JJ.** 2016. Linear viral load increase of a single HPV-type in women with multiple HPV infections predicts progression to cervical cancer. *Int J Cancer* **139:**2021–2032.
52. **Meijer CJ, Berkhof J, Castle PE, Hesselink AT, Franco EL, Ronco G, Arbyn M, Bosch FX, Cuzick J, Dillner J, Heideman DA, Snijders PJ.** 2009. Guidelines for human papillomavirus DNA test requirements for primary cervical cancer screening in women 30 years and older. *Int J Cancer* **124:**516–520.
53. **Cook DA, Smith LW, Law J, Mei W, van Niekerk DJ, Ceballos K, Gondara L, Franco EL, Coldman AJ, Ogilvie GS, Jang D, Chernesky M, Krajden M.** 2017. Aptima HPV assay versus Hybrid Capture® 2 HPV test for primary cervical cancer screening in the HPV FOCAL trial. *J Clin Virol* **87:**23–29.
54. **Schiffman M, Burk RD, Boyle S, Raine-Bennett T, Katki HA, Gage JC, Wentzensen N, Kornegay JR, Aldrich C, Tam T, Erlich H, Apple R, Befano B, Castle PE.** 2015. A study of genotyping for management of human papillomavirus-positive, cytology-negative cervical screening results. *J Clin Microbiol* **53:**52–59.
55. **Kreimer AR, Struyf F, Del Rosario-Raymundo MR, Hildesheim A, Skinner SR, Wacholder S, Garland SM, Herrero R, David MP, Wheeler CM, González P, Jiménez S, Lowy DR, Pinto LA, Porras C, Rodriguez AC, Safaeian M, Schiffman M, Schiller JT, Schussler J, Sherman ME, Bosch FX, Castellsague X, Chatterjee A, Chow SN, Descamps D, Diaz-Mitoma F, Dubin G, Germar MJ, Harper DM, Lewis DJ, Limson G, Naud P, Peters K, Poppe WA, Ramjattan B, Romanowski B, Salmeron J, Schwarz TF, Teixeira JC, Tjalma WA, Costa Rica Vaccine Trial Group, PATRICIA Study Group.** 2015. Efficacy of fewer than three doses of an HPV-16/18 AS04-adjuvanted vaccine: combined analysis of data from the Costa Rica Vaccine and PATRICIA Trials. *Lancet Oncol* **16:**775–786.
56. **Wentzensen N, Schiffman M, Palmer T, Arbyn M.** 2016. Triage of HPV positive women in cervical cancer screening. *J Clin Virol* **76**(Suppl 1)**:**S49–S55.
57. **Huh WK, Ault KA, Chelmow D, Davey DD, Goulart RA, Garcia FA, Kinney WK, Massad LS, Mayeaux EJ, Saslow D, Schiffman M, Wentzensen N, Lawson HW, Einstein MH.** 2015. Use of primary high-risk human papillomavirus testing for cervical cancer screening: interim clinical guidance. *J Low Genit Tract Dis* **19:**91–96.
58. **Schiffman M, Hyun N, Raine-Bennett TR, Katki H, Fetterman B, Gage JC, Cheung LC, Befano B, Poitras N, Lorey T, Castle PE, Wentzensen N.** 2016. A cohort study of cervical screening using partial HPV typing and cytology triage. *Int J Cancer* **139:**2606–2615.
59. **Castle PE, Smith KM, Davis TE, Schmeler KM, Ferris DG, Savage AH, Gray JE, Stoler MH, Wright TC Jr, Ferenczy A, Einstein MH.** 2015. Reliability of the Xpert HPV assay to detect high-risk human papillomavirus DNA in a colposcopy referral population. *Am J Clin Pathol* **143:**126–133.
60. **Ronco G, Giorgi Rossi P.** 2018. Role of HPV DNA testing in modern gynaecological practice. *Best Pract Res Clin Obstet Gynaecol* **47:**107–118.
61. **Arbyn M, Snijders PJ, Meijer CJ, Berkhof J, Cuschieri K, Kocjan BJ, Poljak M.** 2015. Which high-risk HPV assays fulfil criteria for use in primary cervical cancer screening? *Clin Microbiol Infect* **21:**817–826.
62. **Yi X, Zou J, Xu J, Liu T, Liu T, Hua S, Xi F, Nie X, Ye L, Luo Y, Xu L, Du H, Wu R, Yang L, Liu R, Yang B, Wang J, Belinson JL.** 2014. Development and validation of a new

HPV genotyping assay based on next-generation sequencing. *Am J Clin Pathol* **141:**796–804.
63. **Cullen M, Boland JF, Schiffman M, Zhang X, Wentzensen N, Yang Q, Chen Z, Yu K, Mitchell J, Roberson D, Bass S, Burdette L, Machado M, Ravichandran S, Luke B, Machiela MJ, Andersen M, Osentoski M, Laptewicz M, Wacholder S, Feldman A, Raine-Bennett T, Lorey T, Castle PE, Yeager M, Burk RD, Mirabello L.** 2015. Deep sequencing of HPV16 genomes: a new high-throughput tool for exploring the carcinogenicity and natural history of HPV16 infection. *Papillomavirus Res* **1:**3–11.
64. **Ambulos NP Jr, Schumaker LM, Mathias TJ, White R, Troyer J, Wells D, Cullen KJ.** 2016. Next-generation sequencing-based HPV genotyping assay validated in formalin-fixed, paraffin-embedded oropharyngeal and cervical cancer specimens. *J Biomol Tech* **27:**46–52.
65. **Li T, Unger ER, Batra D, Sheth M, Steinau M, Jasinski J, Jones J, Rajeevan MS.** 2017. Universal human papillomavirus typing assay: whole-genome sequencing following target enrichment. *J Clin Microbiol* **55:**811–823.
66. **Cuschieri K, Ronco G, Lorincz A, Smith L, Ogilvie G, Mirabello L, Carozzi F, Cubie H, Wentzensen N, Snijders P, Arbyn M, Monsonego J, Franceschi S.** 2018. Eurogin roadmap 2017: triage strategies for the management of HPV-positive women in cervical screening programs. *Int J Cancer* **143:**735–745.
67. **Katki HA, Schiffman M, Castle PE, Fetterman B, Poitras NE, Lorey T, Cheung LC, Raine-Bennett T, Gage JC, Kinney WK.** 2013. Benchmarking CIN 3+ risk as the basis for incorporating HPV and Pap cotesting into cervical screening and management guidelines. *J Low Genit Tract Dis* **17**(Suppl 1): S28–S35.
68. **Verlaat W, Snijders PJF, Novianti PW, Wilting SM, De Strooper LMA, Trooskens G, Vandersmissen J, Van Criekinge W, Wisman GBA, Meijer CJLM, Heideman DAM, Steenbergen RDM.** 2017. Genome-wide DNA methylation profiling reveals methylation markers associated with 3q gain for detection of cervical precancer and cancer. *Clin Cancer Res* **23:**3813–3822.
69. **Kreider JW, Howett MK, Wolfe SA, Bartlett GL, Zaino RJ, Sedlacek T, Mortel R.** 1985. Morphological transformation *in vivo* of human uterine cervix with papillomavirus from condylomata acuminata. *Nature* **317:**639–641.
70. **Biryukov J, Meyers C.** 2015. Papillomavirus infectious pathways: a comparison of systems. *Viruses* **7:**4303–4325.
71. **Wang HK, Duffy AA, Broker TR, Chow LT.** 2009. Robust production and passaging of infectious HPV in squamous epithelium of primary human keratinocytes. *Genes Dev* **23:** 181–194.
72. **Bienkowska-Haba M, Luszczek W, Myers JE, Keiffer TR, DiGiuseppe S, Polk P, Bodily JM, Scott RS, Sapp M.** 2018. A new cell culture model to genetically dissect the complete human papillomavirus life cycle. *PLoS Pathog* **14:**e1006846.
73. **Lowy DR, Herrero R, Hildesheim A, Participants in the IARC/NCI Workshop on Primary Endpoints for Prophylactic HPV Vaccine Trials.** 2015. Primary endpoints for future prophylactic human papillomavirus vaccine trials: towards infection and immunobridging. *Lancet Oncol* **16:**e226–e233.
74. **Pinto LA, Dillner J, Beddows S, Unger ER.** 2018. Immunogenicity of HPV prophylactic vaccines: serology assays and their use in HPV vaccine evaluation and development. *Vaccine* **36:**4792–4799.
75. **Schiller JT, Lowy DR.** 2009. Immunogenicity testing in human papillomavirus virus-like-particle vaccine trials. *J Infect Dis* **200:**166–171.
76. **Carozzi FM, Del Mistro A, Cuschieri K, Frayle H, Sani C, Burroni E.** 2016. HPV testing for primary cervical screening: laboratory issues and evolving requirements for robust quality assurance. *J Clin Virol* **76**(Suppl 1):S22–S28.
77. **Eklund C, Forslund O, Wallin KL, Dillner J, Loeffelholz MJ.** 2014. Global improvement in genotyping of human papillomavirus DNA: the 2011 HPV LabNet International Proficiency Study. *J Clin Microbiol* **52:**449–459.
78. **Taberna M, Mena M, Pavón MA, Alemany L, Gillison ML, Mesía R.** 2017. Human papillomavirus-related oropharyngeal cancer. *Ann Oncol* **28:**2386–2398.
79. **Schiffman M, Castle PE.** 2005. The promise of global cervical-cancer prevention. *N Engl J Med* **353:**2101–2104.

Human Polyomaviruses

GREGORY A. STORCH AND RICHARD S. BULLER

108

TAXONOMY

Since the last edition of this *Manual*, the pace of identification of new human polyomaviruses (HPyVs) has slowed; with two new HPyVs identified, the total number of HPyVs is now 14. The polyomaviruses were formerly members of the *Papovaviridae* family but have been reclassified into the family *Polyomaviridae*. A recent updated, sequence-based revision of polyomavirus taxonomy was accepted by the International Committee on Taxonomy of Viruses in December 2015 (1). The updated taxonomy divides the *Polyomaviridae* family into four genera: *Alpha-*, *Beta-*, *Gamma-*, and *Deltapolyomavirus*. Polyomavirus species will be named with the host species followed by *polyomavirus* and a number indicating the temporal sequence of their identification. Note that, as with other virus families, this taxonomy results in some HPyVs having an official taxonomic designation and a common name. For example, the human species has the common name BK polyomavirus (BKPyV), but the official taxonomic name is now *Human polyomavirus 1* (*HPyV 1*). For the remainder of this chapter, where there is a choice between a common and taxonomic name, the common name will be employed. The *Alphapolyomavirus* genus contains the following human viruses: Merkel cell polyomavirus (MCPyV, *HPyV 5*), trichodysplasia spinulosa polyomavirus (TSPyV, *HPyV 8*), *HPyV 9*, *HPyV 12*, and the recently identified New Jersey polyomavirus (NJPyV, *HPyV 13*) (2). HPyVs in the *Betapolyomavirus* genus include BK polyomavirus (BKPyV, *HPyV 1*), JC polyomavirus (JCPyV, *HPyV 2*), Karolinska Institute (KI) polyomavirus (KIPyV, *HPyV 3*), and Washington University (WU) polyomavirus (WUPyV, *HPyV 4*). Currently, there are no HPyVs in the *Gammapolyomavirus* genus, while the *Deltapolyomavirus* genus contains *HPyV 6*, *HPyV 7*, Malawi (MW) polyomavirus (MWPyV, *HPyV 10*), and Saint Louis (STL) polyomavirus (STLPyV, *HPyV 11*). The most recently identified HPyV is Lyon IARC polyomavirus (LIPyV, *HPyV 14*). LIPyV is most closely related to raccoon polyomavirus, which tentatively places it in the *Alphapolyomavirus* genus (3). Table 1 displays the current taxonomy of the human polyomaviruses.

Because some of the novel HPyVs were discovered nearly simultaneously in more than one laboratory, different names for what appear to be the same virus, or strains of the same virus, can be found in the literature. For example, the virus MxPyV (4, 5) appears to be the same species as MWPyV (*HPyV 10*) (6). In a previous edition of this *Manual*, lymphocytic polyomavirus (LPyV), a strain of African green monkey polyomavirus, was listed here because antibodies to that virus were reported in humans, suggesting infection by LPyV or a closely related virus. It now appears that *HPyV 9* is likely the closely related virus responsible for those findings (7).

From a diagnostic perspective, further subclassification of polyomaviruses is primarily important for BKPyV and JCPyV. BKPyV was originally divided into six subtypes based on VP1 gene sequences. However, whole-genome sequence data now support the existence of four subtypes (I to IV), with two subtypes reclassified as subgroups of subtype I (8). Subtypes vary in prevalence and geographic distribution (9). Subtype I is most prevalent and is found worldwide; subtype IV is second most prevalent and is found mostly in Asia and Europe. Subtypes II and III are uncommon and are found throughout the world. JCPyV has seven genotypes that, like BKPyV, are associated with different geographic areas and human populations and have multiple subtypes (10). Subtype-dependent quantification and detection bias has been observed and can contribute to interassay differences in quantification and detection (see Nucleic Acid Amplification Methods below).

DESCRIPTION OF THE AGENTS

The polyomaviruses are small (40- to 45-nm diameter), icosahedral, nonenveloped viruses with circular, double-stranded DNA genomes. The size of the genome is relatively small, with all the human viruses, including the newly identified members and SV40, falling within the range of ~4,800 to ~5,400 bp. JCPyV, BKPyV, and SV40 have been extensively characterized. The newly identified viruses have been less well studied.

The genome is organized into an early region that is transcribed prior to DNA replication and a late region transcribed after DNA replication. The noncoding control region (NCCR) separates the early and late regions and includes the origin of replication (11).

Early region transcripts code for the large and small T antigens, nonstructural proteins that regulate viral replication, control of viral transcription, induction of host cell division, and transformation. Late gene transcripts code for viral capsid proteins VP1, VP2, and VP3. VP1 is the major

TABLE 1 Taxonomy of human polyomaviruses (family *Polyomaviridae*)

Species	Common name (abbreviation)
Genus *Alphapolyomavirus*	
Human polyomavirus 5	Merkel cell polyomavirus (MCPyV)
Human polyomavirus 8	Trichodysplasia spinulosa polyomavirus (TSPyV)
Human polyomavirus 9	(HPyV9)
Human polyomavirus 12	(HPyV12)
Human polyomavirus 13	New Jersey polyomavirus (NJPyV)
Human polyomavirus 14[a]	Lyon IARC polyomavirus (LIPyV)
Genus *Betapolyomavirus*	
Human polyomavirus 1	BK virus (BKPyV)
Human polyomavirus 2	JC virus (JCPyV)
Human polyomavirus 3	KI (Karolinska Institute) virus (KIPyV)
Human polyomavirus 4	WU (Washington University) virus (WUPyV)
Genus *Deltapolyomavirus*	
Human polyomavirus 6	(HPyV6)
Human polyomavirus 7	(HPyV7)
Human polyomavirus 10	Malawi polyomavirus (MWPyV)
Human polyomavirus 11	Saint Louis polyomavirus (STLPyV)

[a]Putative human polyomavirus. The virus has not been formally named or classified.

capsid protein that comprises ~80% of the capsid and is the only surface-exposed protein (11). The late regions of JCPyV, BKPyV, and SV40 also code for a fourth late protein termed the agnoprotein, the function of which is incompletely understood, but which appears to be a nonstructural protein involved in viral assembly and release from infected cells (11).

The genomic organization of the newly identified polyomaviruses appears to be similar to those previously described, with open reading frames identified for the T antigens, VP1, VP2, and VP3 (2, 3, 6, 12–14). These viruses appear to differ from JCPyV and BKPyV in that there is no agnoprotein open reading frame (6, 12–14).

The NCCRs of the human viruses BK and JCPyV are hypervariable sequences of ~300 to 500 bp in length. In addition to the origin of replication, the NCCR contains the promoters for early and late gene transcription. The variable nature of the NCCR is apparent when sequences of this region are compared between viruses obtained from different anatomical sites. The NCCR sequence from kidney and urine isolates is referred to as the archetype. Viruses with archetype NCCR sequences do not replicate well in cell cultures and may be the infectious form of the virus. Rearrangements of the archetype NCCR may be found in the brain at the site of disease.

One little-understood characteristic of polyomaviruses is their ability to establish persistent infections. For the two most clinically significant HPyVs, BKPyV and JCPyV, studies using molecular methods, such as PCR and *in situ* hybridization, have suggested the genitourinary tract, the central nervous system, and the hematopoietic system as potential sites of persistence (15). The molecular mechanism responsible for establishing and maintaining persistence is not known, however.

Lastly, studies have demonstrated that MCPyV can integrate into host cell chromosomes, a step that appears to be important in the development of at least some Merkel cell carcinomas (16). A case report describing the integration of a novel strain of BKyPV in chromosome 12 in a case of urothelial carcinoma suggests that HPyVs may be a factor in some human cancers (17).

EPIDEMIOLOGY AND TRANSMISSION

The two most important HPyVs, BKPyV and JCPyV, appear to infect most humans by adulthood. Seroepidemiologic studies reveal that 50% of children acquire anti-BKPyV antibodies by the age of 3 years and anti-JCPyV antibodies by 6 years of age (18). For all older age groups, the seroprevalence for both viruses ranges from 55% to 85%, although there is more variability in the age of seroconversion for JCPyV (19). The route of BKPyV and JCPyV transmission is largely speculative, in part because primary infection does not appear to cause clinical illness, although there are reports of signs and symptoms such as fever or respiratory illness accompanying seroconversion (19). Respiratory and oral transmission has been hypothesized because JCPyV can infect tonsillar cells (20) and has been detected in tonsillar tissue (21). Using a multiplex PCR assay capable of detecting HPyVs 1 to 13 to test tonsillar tissue specimens, Sadeghi et al. reported detection of JCPyV, WUPyV, MCPyV, *HPyV* 6, and TSPyV, suggesting this tissue as a possible site of infection and/or persistence for these viruses (22). Studies of oral and respiratory specimens, however, have failed to detect BKPyV and JCPyV (23, 24). Uro-oral transmission has been hypothesized, and circumstantial evidence consists of intermittent BKPyV and JCPyV excretion in urine of immunocompetent and immunocompromised individuals (19, 25), detection of BKPyV and JCPyV in sewage samples (26–28), and the stability of these non-enveloped viruses. A study of stool specimens obtained from Mexican infants found BKPyV in 18% of specimens from 64% of the infants; these findings suggest that the gastrointestinal tract may also be a site of infection and persistence (29).

Less is known about the epidemiology and transmission of other HPyVs. WUPyV and KIPyV are found in respiratory secretions and have been widely detected around the globe (30–38). WUPyV has been detected in respiratory secretions of a 1-day-old infant, raising the possibility of *in utero* or intrapartum infection (36). Studies have also detected WUPyV in small numbers of serum and stool specimens (39, 40). MCPyV is also found in respiratory specimens, and seroprevalences of 50% and 80% in children and adults have been documented, suggesting that infection is common (16, 41–43). Likewise, seroprevalence for TSPyV infection is 74% in adults, and evidence exists that the respiratory tract is the site of infection (44, 45).

Epidemiological studies of the more recently identified HPyVs are in their infancy, with initial seroepidemiological studies suggesting that infection with these viruses is also common. Those studies show low seroprevalence in children, rising in adulthood to 25% to 90%, depending on the virus (46, 47). Caution must be exercised in the interpretation of these findings as cross-reactions are possible among the polyomaviruses and it is likely that unidentified HPyVs could further confound the results (47). A recent seroepidemiologic study of 450 sera from age- and sex-matched controls from a U.S. skin cancer study reported that for *HPyV 1* to *10*, seroprevalences ranged from 17.6% for *HPyV* 9 to 99.1% for *HPyV 10* (48). The same study indicated that individual sera had demonstrable antibodies against from 1 to 10 different HPyVs, with a mean of ~7 HPyVs.

It appears that infection with HPyVs is common in the human population, with variations in the age of acquisition of a particular virus and the likely route of infection.

In addition to the HPyVs, humans were also exposed to the non-human primate polyomavirus SV40 between 1955 and 1963, when some incompletely formalin-inactivated lots of polio vaccine were found to be contaminated. Monkey kidney cell cultures used to prepare the vaccine were found to be the source of the SV40 contamination. About 200 cases of paralytic polio occurred because of the presence of infectious poliovirus in the vaccine. Although ~100 million Americans were vaccinated during this period, it is not known how many of the lots contained infectious SV40 or how many people became infected with SV40 as the result of this accident (49). Some studies have suggested ongoing transmission of SV40 in the human population (29), but rigorous confirmation is lacking.

CLINICAL SIGNIFICANCE

Polyomaviruses cause a number of diseases in different patient populations (Table 2). Current understanding is that with the possible exception of respiratory infection and disease due to WUPyV or KIPyV, diseases due to HPyVs appear to occur primarily in immunocompromised patients. Progressive multifocal leukoencephalopathy (PML) is a rare disease of the central nervous system (CNS) that occurs in certain groups of immunocompromised patients and is characterized by destruction of myelin-producing oligodendrocytes by JCPyV. Focal demyelination in white

TABLE 2 Diseases associated with HPyV

Virus(es)	Disease association	Comment(s) (reference[s])
BKPyV	Polyomavirus-associated nephropathy (PVAN)	Seen primarily in kidney transplant recipients (58); occurs rarely in other immunocompromised hosts (HIV, hematologic malignancy, hematopoietic stem cell transplant, transplant of organs other than kidney, and congenital immunodeficiency).
	Hemorrhagic cystitis	Observed primarily in BMT recipients with a prevalence of 10–25% in this population (70).
	Rare associations	CNS and pneumonia have been reported (59).
JCPyV	Progressive multifocal leukoencephalopathy (PML)	Observed in patients with compromised cellular immunity (HIV/AIDS, malignancy, and immunomodulatory therapies used to treat multiple sclerosis and psoriasis) (51, 190–193).
	PVAN	Associated with rare cases of BKPyV-negative PVAN (68, 69, 128).
	Rare associations	Other central nervous system diseases such as cerebral atrophy and granule cell neuronopathy have been reported (55–57).
WUPyV and KIPyV	No firm disease association	Detected in respiratory secretions, stool specimens, and blood (31, 32, 35, 36, 74–79, 143) and tissues of immunocompromised patients (80–82).
MCPyV	Merkel cell carcinoma	Associated with 75%–88% of Merkel cell carcinoma tumors (16, 83, 194, 195); MCPyV has also been detected in respiratory specimens, suggesting a mode of acquisition (41, 42, 86).
HPyV6 and HPyV7	No firm disease association	Detected on the skin of 11–14% of the healthy individuals tested (85) and patients with a variety of dermatologic conditions such rashes, pruritic and dyskeratotic dermatoses, and keratoacanthomas (93–95).
TSPyV	Trichodysplasia spinulosa	TSPyV has been associated with trichodysplasia spinulosa from various geographic locations (89, 91, 196–198), although viral DNA has also been rarely detected in normal tissues (89). Also, there has been a report of detecting TSPyV in tissues of a fatal case of myocarditis (92).
HPyV9	No firm disease association	Initially identified in the serum of a kidney transplant patient and subsequently found in rare specimens from other immunocompromised patients. The close relationship of HPyV9 to the non-human primate virus LPyV may explain the occurrence of anti-LPyV antibodies in human sera (7).
MWPyV	No firm disease association	Initially identified in the stool from a Malawian child with diarrhea and subsequently in stools from the United States (6). May be the same viral species as those initially reported as MxPyV from stool (5) and as HPyV10 from warts from an immunocompromised patient (4). The virus has also been detected in respiratory specimens, but there is no clear evidence for its causing either respiratory or gastrointestinal disease (97, 98).
STLPyV	No firm disease association	Initially identified in the stool from a Malawian child and subsequently in ~1% of stools tested from the United States and Gambia (13). The virus has been reported as a coinfecting agent with known GI pathogens as well as being more common in asymptomatic patients (96).
HPyV12	No firm disease association	Initially identified in liver tissue from a cancer patient and subsequently in other liver specimens and rare colon, rectum, and stool specimens from similar patients (12).
NJPyV	No firm disease association	Identified in endothelial cells at locations with myositis in a pancreatic transplant recipient (2).
LIPyV	No firm disease association	Identified in ~2% of skin and oral gargle specimens tested (3).
SV40	No firm disease association	Primate virus found to contaminate polio vaccine (49, 99–101).

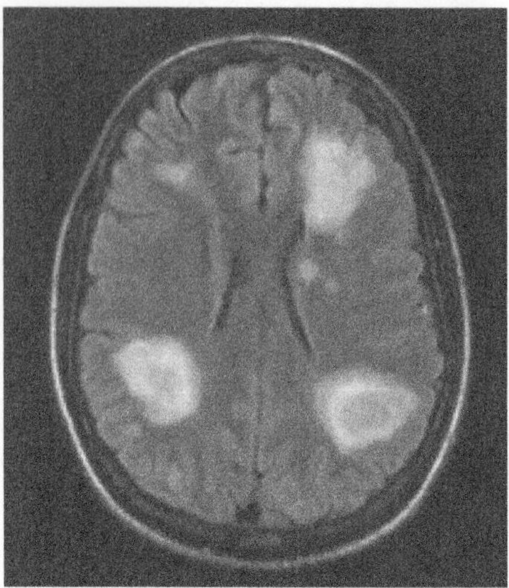

FIGURE 1 MR image showing the brain of a patient with lesions of advanced PML. Lesions are seen bilaterally in frontal lobes and in parietooccipital subcortical regions. Note that the cortex is spared, with lesions primarily in white matter, consistent with the pathology of demyelination of white matter tracts (fluid-attenuated inversion recovery T2-weighted MR). Reprinted with permission of the publisher, Lippincott Williams & Wilkins, from reference 189.

matter can be visualized by neuroimaging studies such as magnetic resonance (MR) imaging (Fig. 1). Neurological signs and symptoms include gait or other motor disturbances and cognitive abnormalities (50). Prognosis is poor, with long-term survival usually <12 months unless underlying immunosuppression can be reduced (11). Prior to the development of highly active antiretroviral therapy (HAART), PML occurred primarily in severely immunocompromised HIV-infected individuals. With the advent of HAART, PML has become less common in the HIV-infected patient population but has now appeared in patients treated with immunomodulatory monoclonal antibodies, including natalizumab (Tysabri), used to treat multiple sclerosis; efalizumab (Raptiva, since removed from the market), used to treat psoriasis; rituximab (Maptera), used to treat systemic lupus erythematosus and lymphoproliferative diseases; and infliximab (Remicade), used to treat Crohn's disease and psoriasis (51). PML risk appears to be highest and has been studied most thoroughly for natalizumab as a treatment for multiple sclerosis. In this group, PML had an early incidence of ~3/1,000 patients treated, with three risk factors recognized: duration of natalizumab treatment, prior use of immunosuppressive medication, and positive JCPyV antibody status (52, 53). However, a recent study reported much higher incidences of PML in JCPyV-seropositive patients treated with natalizumab, in particular, an incidence of 19.5/1,000 during treatment months 25 through 48 for patients with prior immunosuppressive treatment (54). Prior to effective anti-HIV therapy, mortality from PML was nearly 100%, but it has now fallen to about 50%. Mortality for PML induced by immunomodulatory agents is lower, although it can produce severe neurological sequelae (55). Other CNS diseases such as cerebral atrophy and granule cell neuronopathy appear to be rare forms of JCPyV infection (55, 56). A case report of an atypical case of JCPyV encephalopathy in a kidney transplant recipient whose illness responded to allograft removal and cessation of immunosuppressive therapy demonstrated the importance of looking for JCPyV as a cause of CNS disease in other groups of immunocompromised individuals (57).

BKPyV has tropism for uroepithelial cells and can cause a spectrum of illness. Asymptomatic shedding can occur in urine of normal individuals (especially during pregnancy and in the elderly) and of immunocompromised patients. Polyomavirus-associated nephropathy (PVAN) occurs in immunocompromised patients and is the result of BKPyV replication in renal tubular epithelial cells with destruction of those cells. It is most common in renal transplant recipients (58) but has also been described as a rare cause of nephropathy in other groups of immunocompromised individuals, including those with HIV, hematologic malignancy, hematopoietic stem cell transplant, transplant of organs other than kidney, and congenital immunodeficiency (59).

In PVAN, disease is typically preceded by increasing levels of virus that are initially found in urine, followed by viremia (60, 61). Without clinical intervention, PVAN can result in renal graft dysfunction and, ultimately, graft loss (62). In a prospective study of 78 renal transplant recipients, the probability of developing PVAN was 8% (61). Renal transplant patients may have a propensity to develop PVAN because of the use of more aggressive immunosuppression regimens (62), BKPyV acquisition from the donor kidney, or HLA-mediated predisposition (63, 64). PVAN is treated by reducing immunosuppression; certain antiviral compounds, including cidofovir and the investigational drug brincidofovir, have also been used (60, 65–67). JCPyV has also been reported to rarely cause PVAN (68, 69).

Other pathological conditions associated with BKPyV include hematuria, ureteral stenosis, and hemorrhagic cystitis. Hemorrhagic cystitis is due to BKPyV infection of the bladder epithelium. It occurs most commonly in the setting of hematopoietic stem cell transplantation and is seen less frequently in other immunocompromised states including HIV infection. Allogeneic stem cell recipients are at particular risk, with disease occurring several weeks after transplant, differentiating it from chemotherapy-associated disease, which generally occurs immediately after receipt of the drug. Hemorrhagic cystitis is associated with significant morbidity but is rarely fatal (70). The risk of developing hemorrhagic cystitis has been shown to correlate with increased levels of BKPyV viruria (71) and viremia (72). Treatment is supportive, although the use of select antiviral drugs has been attempted (70). Rarer examples of other BKPyV diseases in immunocompromised patients, including those with HIV infection and posttransplant immunosuppression, include disseminated disease, CNS infection, retinitis, colitis, vasculitis, and pneumonia (59, 73). There have also been concerns that BKPyV may be involved in the development of certain human cancers, in particular, prostate cancer. Currently, however, more evidence is needed to answer the question of whether BKPyV is a significant cause of any human cancers (73).

Attempts to link the more newly identified HPyV with specific human diseases are ongoing. KIPyV and WUPyV have frequently been detected in respiratory specimens but have not been firmly associated with human disease because of the frequent presence of other coinfecting respiratory viruses and their detection in asymptomatic patients (10, 74). However, some recent reports have shown that WUPyV or KIPyV can be detected as a sole agent from normal patients with respiratory disease, suggesting that these viruses may cause respiratory disease in some instances (75–79). Case reports of WUPyV being detected in respiratory tissues of immunosuppressed patients with different conditions have also been reported, but a definitive link between virus infection and disease in these patients was not proven (80–82).

Merkel cell carcinoma is a rare, highly aggressive human neuroepithelial tumor of the skin noted for its high mortality. In 2008, MCPyV was discovered in specimens from this tumor by use of molecular viral discovery techniques (83) (Table 2). Subsequent studies have demonstrated MCPyV to be clonally integrated in the genomes of ~80% of Merkel cell carcinomas (16). MCPyV has also been detected in skin samples from healthy individuals (84), with one report indicating that MCPyV is chronically shed from the skin of healthy individuals as intact virions, suggesting a possible mode of transmission (85). MCPyV is also found in respiratory tract specimens, including from patients with acute respiratory tract disease (41, 42, 86), although whether MCPyV is a cause of respiratory disease is not clear. The fact that MCPyV infection appears to be ubiquitous and Merkel cell carcinoma is uncommon suggests that factors other than the virus are also important in the development of this cancer. Identified risk factors include immune suppression, sun exposure, female sex, and age >69 years (16, 84).

Trichodysplasia spinulosa is a rare skin disease that occurs only in immunocompromised individuals (84). In 2010, TSPyV was identified in specimens from a heart transplant recipient with the disease (87); this finding confirmed an earlier report of polyomavirus-like particles seen in electron micrographs (88). High viral loads and the presence of viral proteins in trichodysplasia spinulosa lesions suggest active TSPyV replication in diseased tissues (89). As with some of the other HPyVs, TSPyV infection appears to be ubiquitous, with seroepidemiological studies indicating low seroprevalence in children that rises to ~70% in adults (90, 91). Despite the high rate of seropositivity to TSPyV, the number of cases of trichodysplasia spinulosa is very low. More frequent occurrence of the disease with primary infection rather than with reactivation has been suggested (45). High levels of the virus in blood and cerebrospinal fluid, suggesting dissemination, have also been described (45). A case report from Japan described a fatal case of myocarditis in an apparently immunologically normal 7-month-old girl. TSPyV was the only pathogen detected in heart tissue, but a causal role was not proven (92).

HPyV 6 and 7 have been shown to be shed from skin (85), with recent reports suggesting an association of these viruses with certain dermatological diseases (93, 94). A study of nonmelanoma skin lesions reported presence of HPyV 6 in 42% of keratoacanthomas. *HPyV* 6 was also detected in several other skin cancers but not at rates significantly different from detection on normal skin (95). While interesting, these results require further work to prove a causal role for *HPyV* 6 and 7 in these diseases.

STLPyV and MWPyV have been detected in respiratory and stool specimens from symptomatic patients, but proof of a pathogenic role is lacking since they are frequently detected in the presence of coinfecting pathogens and the prevalence of detection is frequently higher in asymptomatic than symptomatic individuals (96–98). Evidence is also lacking to date for the pathogenicity of the remaining HPyVs, NJPyV, and LIPyV.

Lastly, because of the known ability of polyomaviruses to cause cancer, there have long been concerns that these viruses could be a cause of some human cancers. Over the years there have been many attempts to link SV40 with human cancers, with some of the attempts being reported as successful. However, there has been an inability to reproduce the results of some studies because of factors such as contamination with plasmids and serological cross-reactions between BKPyV and JCPyV (49). Although debatable, the general consensus today is that apart from MCPyV, there is currently no convincing evidence that either human or animal polyomaviruses are a significant cause of human cancers. Readers interested in this subject are referred to several excellent reviews on this topic (49, 99–101).

COLLECTION, TRANSPORT, AND STORAGE OF SPECIMENS

Although systematic studies of clinical specimens have not been reported for polyomaviruses, they appear to be quite stable, as would be expected for nonenveloped DNA viruses. A study of JCPyV stability in sewage at 20°C found a t_{90} value (time required for a reduction of 90% of the viral concentration, as measured by quantitative PCR) of 64 days and a t_{99} of 127 days with a greater t_{90} value obtained when the virus was suspended in phosphate-buffered saline (111 days) (102). These data suggest that standard guidelines for the collection, transport, and storage of specimens for viral diagnostics (see chapter 81 of this *Manual*) should be appropriate for polyomaviruses.

Specimens commonly submitted for the detection of polyomaviruses include blood, cerebrospinal fluid (CSF), urine, respiratory specimens, and tissue. Polyomaviruses can be recovered from peripheral blood mononuclear cells, usually for research purposes. Because detection of HPyVs in the clinical laboratory generally relies on molecular methods, guidelines for collection and transport of specimens are those that apply to molecular testing (see chapter 81 and reference 103). When available, manufacturers' directions for collection, transport, and storage of specimens should be followed. Since nucleic acid detection methods are the primary means by which polyomaviruses are detected in clinical specimens, extracted DNA should be stored in tightly sealed low-binding plastic tubes to prevent evaporation and binding of DNA to the walls of the tubes (103). DNA can be stored in Tris-EDTA buffer for up to 1 year at 2 to 8°C, −20°C for up to 7 years, or at −70°C or lower for at least 7 years (103). Others have shown that quantification of viral nucleic acids is not affected by frozen storage of patient specimens at −20°C or refrigeration at 4°C of nucleic acid extracts (104).

DIRECT EXAMINATION

Microscopy

Histologic assessment of renal biopsy material is the gold standard for the diagnosis of PVAN (60). PVAN is a tubulointerstitial nephritis that can resemble allograft rejection on histopathologic examination (58, 105–107). However, in contrast to rejection, characteristic basophilic, intranuclear viral inclusions may be observed in PVAN (Fig. 2) (58, 105, 107). Due to its patchy nature, at least two tissue biopsy specimens should be examined prior to ruling out PVAN (60, 106). Papanicolaou stain of urine sediment from patients with PVAN reveals abnormal inclusion-bearing cells referred to as "decoy cells" because of their resemblance to malignant cancer cells (Fig. 2) (108).

Antemortem direct microscopic examination of tissue is performed less commonly for PML than for PVAN due to the risks involved in obtaining brain biopsy material. In brain biopsy specimens, PML appears as foci of

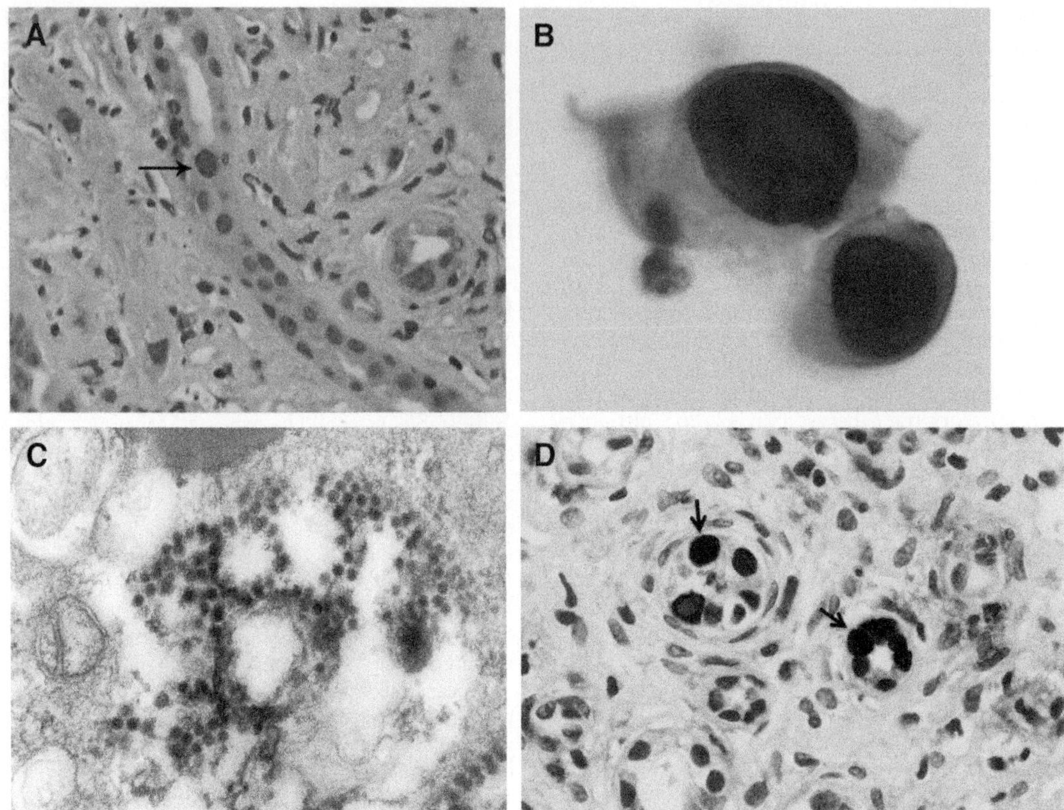

FIGURE 2 PVAN pathology. (A) Photomicrograph of hematoxylin- and eosin-stained renal biopsy specimen, showing nuclear inclusion (arrow) in epithelial cell in collecting duct (magnification, ×200). (B) Photomicrograph of Papanicolaou-stained decoy cells from the urine of a patient with PVAN, demonstrating the typical enlarged basophilic nuclei (magnification, ×400). (C) Electron micrograph of a renal biopsy specimen, showing arrays of typical 40- to 45-nm diameter polyomavirus virions (magnification, ×12,000). (D) Photomicrograph of an immunostained renal biopsy specimen, showing staining of homogeneous type one nuclear inclusions (arrows) in epithelial cells of distal tubes. (Images courtesy of Helen Liapis, Washington University.)

demyelination-containing macrophages, enlarged oligodendrocytes with basophilic or eosinophilic nuclear inclusions, and enlarged bizarre astrocytes with pleomorphic nuclei, typically in the subcortical white matter (Fig. 3) (109–111). The so-called "classic histopathologic triad" of demyelination, bizarre astrocytes, and enlarged oligodendroglial nuclei has been incorporated into a consensus statement for the diagnosis of PML (112).

Electron microscopy (EM) can be used in the diagnosis of PVAN and PML. Intracellularly, polyomaviruses appear as 40-nm-diameter virions packed in paracrystalline arrays or so-called "stick and ball" or "spaghetti and meatballs" structures (Fig. 2 and 3)(113–115). Extracellular BKPyV virions are found by EM in aggregates called "Haufen" in urine of hematopoietic stem cell transplant patients (116, 117) and PVAN patients (118). EM may be useful in the diagnosis of Merkel cell carcinoma because polyomavirus particles have been observed in some cases (119). EM has also been used to demonstrate typical polyomavirus virions in tissue from patients with trichodysplasia spinulosa (89).

Antigen Detection

Immunohistochemical staining of tissue sections by use of antibodies reactive with polyomavirus antigens has been employed as an adjunct to histopathological examination of tissue for the diagnosis of PVAN (58, 114, 120, 121) and PML (115, 122) (Fig. 2 and 3). In the case of PVAN, the demonstration of polyomavirus antigen can help in determining whether PVAN or rejection is the cause of renal pathology. Commercially available antibodies raised against the SV40 large T antigen are most commonly used for this purpose (see http://www.biocompare.com for suppliers). These antibodies are cross-reactive with JCPyV and BKPyV antigens and can be used to detect polyomaviruses but cannot be used to definitively identify which virus is present. JCPyV- and BKPyV-specific monoclonal antibodies against respective VP1 proteins are available and can be used for this purpose. For trichodysplasia spinulosa, a lab-developed, noncommercial immunofluorescence assay has been used to detect VP1 proteins of TSPyV in affected tissues (89).

Nucleic Acid Detection

ISH

In situ hybridization (ISH) using probes specific for BKPyV or JCPyV is an adjunct histopathologic method sometimes employed for the laboratory diagnosis of PVAN and PML (Fig. 3) (65, 120, 123–125). Addition of a PCR step may increase sensitivity (124). In the case of PVAN, as is also true for immunohistochemical staining, ISH can aid in discriminating PVAN from rejection by localizing the presence of BKPyV nucleic acid to the site of pathology.

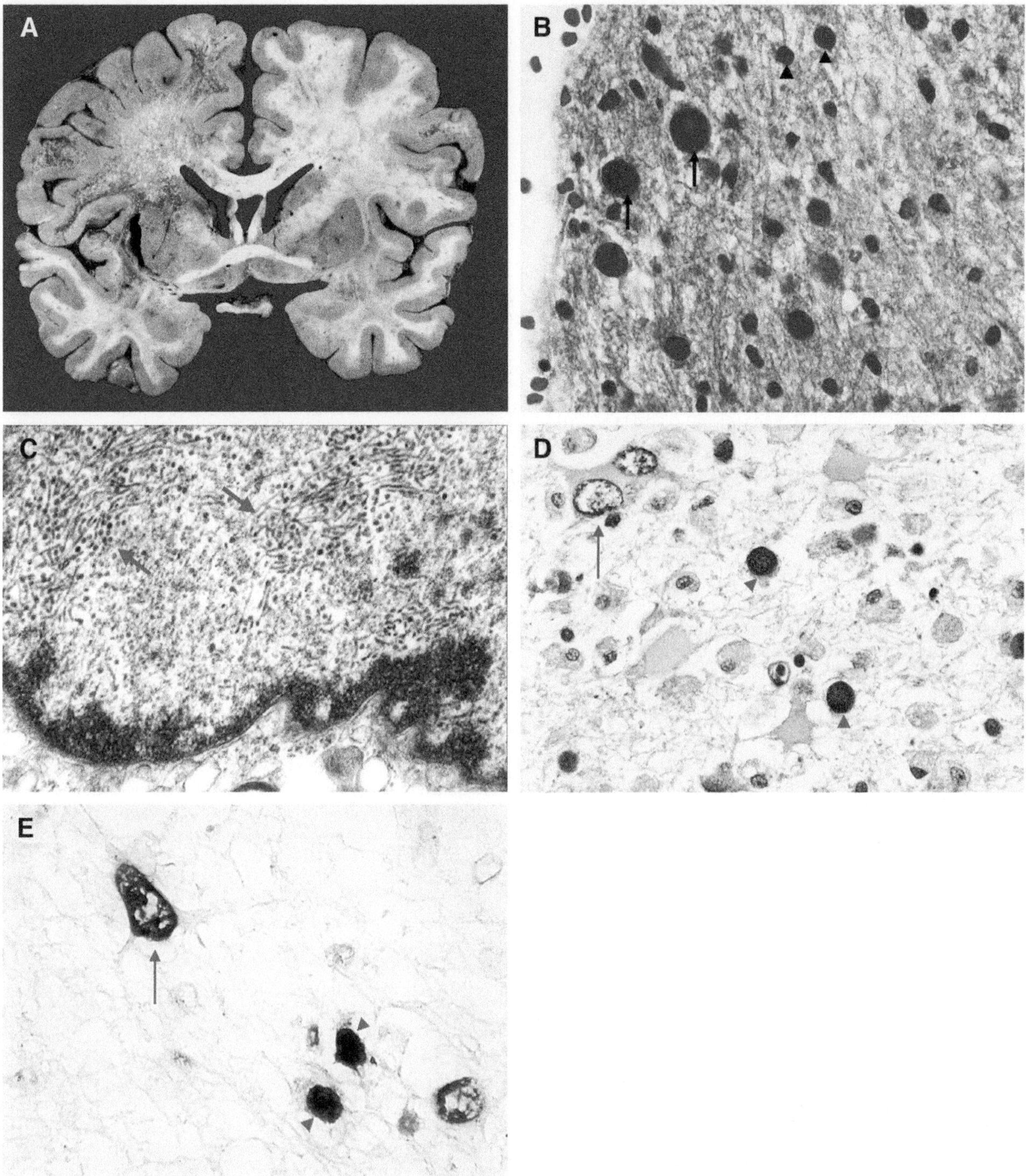

FIGURE 3 PML pathology. (A) Gross section of the brain from a patient with PML, demonstrating asymmetric focal patches of involvement mostly confined to the white matter. (B) Photomicrograph of hematoxylin- and eosin-stained section of brain from a patient with PML, showing "plum colored" oligodendroglial nuclei (arrows), some with marginated chromatin and inclusions. Infected oligodendrocytes are markedly enlarged compared to more normal sized oligodendroglia (arrowheads) (magnification, ×400). (C) Electron micrograph of brain from a patient with PML, showing the "stick and ball" or "spaghetti and meatballs" (arrows) appearance of JCPyV in an oligodendrocyte (magnification, ×58,000). (D) Photomicrograph of an immunostained brain section, demonstrating JCPyV proteins in enlarged immunoreactive oligodendroglial nuclei (arrowhead) but little involvement of atypical astrocytes (arrow) (magnification, ×600). (E) Photomicrograph of ISH with a labeled JCPyV probe, showing a positive signal in oligodendrocytes (arrowheads) and an atypical labeled astrocyte (arrow) (magnification, ×1000). (Images courtesy of Robert Schmidt, Washington University.)

Biotin- and digoxigenin-labeled BKPyV and JCPyV probes suitable for ISH are commercially available (Enzo Life Sciences, Farmingdale, NY).

NAATs

Although analyte-specific reagents and research-use-only reagents are available, there are currently no Food and Drug Administration (FDA) approved or cleared assays for the detection or quantification of polyomaviruses. Laboratories are therefore left to develop their own tests and confront various issues including selecting suitable extraction methods, controlling for various biochemical steps in testing, and choosing an amplification method and reagents. Information specific to polyomavirus nucleic acid amplification tests (NAATs) addressing these issues is provided below.

Template Extraction

The ideal performance characteristics for BKPyV and JCPyV NAATs are different. Monitoring for PVAN is usually performed with quantitative NAATs for BKPyV that must be reproducible (yielding results with low coefficients of variation), but not necessarily exquisitely sensitive, as low virus concentrations are not considered significant in most instances. In contrast, extremely sensitive assays for the detection of JCPyV are desirable for use in the diagnosis of PML because levels of JCPyV DNA in CSF may be low. The nucleic acid extraction method should be selected to help meet these different performance criteria. For BKPyV the few published studies of extraction methods suggest that standard manual and automated extraction methods are sufficient (see below). Similar studies of extraction methods for JCPyV are not available. Because sensitivity is important for the detection of JCPyV, laboratories may choose to investigate the efficiency of different extraction methods for JCPyV. However, such an evaluation would be complicated by the lack of an available source for JCPyV virions, thus requiring the use of patient-derived CSF known to contain the virus. Alternatively, laboratories could study the efficiency of different extraction methods with other nonenveloped viruses such as adenoviruses.

Several evaluations that examine the ability of different methods to extract and purify BKPyV DNA from clinical specimens have been published (126–130). In general, there were minimal differences between the automated and manual methods examined, although one study noted a difference in the ability to remove PCR inhibitors from urine between two automated platforms (131), and differences were observed in the relative amounts of hands-on or turnaround times for the different methods.

Cross-contamination between specimens due to the extremely high levels of viruria that are present in some specimens is a major concern in BKPyV DNA extraction. No evidence of cross-contamination was observed with an automated extractor, suggesting that instrumentation is a viable option (132). Extraction may not be necessary if small sample volumes can be used in NAATs. Two microliters of unprocessed urine added to a 20-μl PCR reaction produced qualitative and quantitative BKPyV results that were not significantly different from those with samples extracted with a manual spin column method (133). A larger sample volume (5 μl) resulted in inhibition.

Internal Controls

Internal positive controls are particularly important when testing urine specimens for polyomaviruses. Such controls can be used to detect, but cannot distinguish between, problems that arise during extraction, such as incomplete elimination of amplification inhibitors (the primary concern with urine specimens) or poor nucleic acid extraction efficiency. Chemically modified, noninfectious BKPyV virions that can be used as extraction controls are commercially available (ZeptoMetrix, Buffalo, NY). A seven-member inhibition panel consisting of quantified substances recognized as being inhibitors of NAAT reactions is also available (AcroMetrix, Benicia, CA) and can be used during test validation to assess assay robustness in the presence of known inhibitors.

Positive Controls and Standards

All NAAT reactions require the use of positive and negative controls while quantitative NAATs require an additional set of quantitated standards for use in construction of a standard curve. There are several options available for laboratories seeking controls and standards for use in NAATs for polyomaviruses. BKPyV and JCPyV control materials are commercially available (whole virus and plasmids encoding entire virus genomes [American Type Culture Collection, Manassas, VA], quantified viral DNA [Advanced Biotechnologies Inc., Columbia, MD], and quantitated inactivated BKPyV virions [Zeptometrix]). A WHO international standard for BKPyV became available in 2016 from the National Institute for Biological Standards and Controls in the United Kingdom (www.nibsc.org). There are no commercially available materials for the newly identified polyomaviruses. For these viruses, laboratories can either identify positive specimens that can be used to clone viral DNA and produce controls and standards or contact researchers in the field for materials.

Nucleic Acid Amplification Methods

Conventional laboratory methods for viral diagnosis such as cell culture, rapid antigen detection, and serology have significant drawbacks for the laboratory diagnosis of HPyVs, while other methods such as immunohistochemical stains, EM, and ISH are traditionally not performed in microbiology laboratories. Therefore, for most diagnostic microbiology laboratories, nucleic acid amplification is the method of choice for the detection and/or quantitation of HPyVs in clinical specimens. For BKPyV, quantitative methods are required (134).

NAATs for BKPyV and JCPyV are challenging to design because of species-specific sequence variation. Sequence differences among BKPyV subtypes can affect detection by PCR. A recent study of seven different BKPyV assays employing two different calibrators reported significant variability in quantification related to the calibrators employed and, more importantly, to primer and probe designs. The most important cause of error was nucleotide mismatch between viruses and amplification/detection oligonucleotides, particularly in the case of BKPyV subtypes III and IV (135). Assays biased toward subtype I failed to detect some samples containing subtype III or IV virus. An assay using two modified primer/probe sets was better able to accurately quantify all subtypes detected in the study. Another study found significant nucleotide mismatches in up to 31% of the BKPyV strains when primers and probes from five published real-time PCR assays were aligned against 716 sequences, with subtypes IVa, IVb, and IVc being most problematic (136). Another report detailed the use of primers and probes with degenerate bases to improve detection of BKPyV sequence variants (137). Laboratories should be alert to flattened amplification curves, which may indicate nucleotide polymorphisms in the primer or probe binding sequences that could affect the accuracy of viral load determination.

TABLE 3 Commercial nucleic acid amplification products available in the United States for the detection of JCPyV and BKPyV

Virus(es)	Product (manufacturer)	Comment(s) (regulatory status)[a]
BKPyV	BK Virus R-gene Primers/Probe (bioMérieux, Durham, NC)	Primer and probes for 5′ nuclease real-time assay targeting a sequence in the large T antigen (RUO)
	BK Virus R-gene Quantification Kit (bioMérieux)	Kit for the quantification of BKPyV, using 5′ nuclease real-time assay. Includes extraction, inhibition, sensitivity, and negative controls (RUO)
	BKV Primer Pair (Focus Diagnostics, Cypress, CA)	Primers for a real-time assay using a FAM-labeled forward primer amplifying a segment of the VP2 gene (ASR)
	MGB Alert BK virus primers and probe (ELITechGroup, Princeton, NJ)	Separate set of primers and MGB probe, capable of performing a melt curve analysis, targeting a sequence in the VP1 region (ASR)
	MultiCode BK Virus Primers (Luminex, Madison, WI)	Set of primers targeting VP3; combined with use of synthetic bases, allows for amplification and real-time detection (ASR)
JCPyV	JC Virus R-gene Primers and Probe (bioMérieux)	Primer and probes for 5′ nuclease real-time assay targeting a sequence in the large T antigen (RUO)
	MultiCode JC Virus Primers (Luminex)	Set of primers targeting VP3; combined with use of synthetic bases, allows for amplification and real-time detection (ASR)
JCPyV/BKPyV	JC/BK Consensus (bioMérieux)	Amplification and differentiation of JCPyV and BKPyV through PCR and product hybridization to probes in a microwell plate (RUO)

[a]ASR, analyte-specific reagent; FAM, 6-carboxyfluorescein amidite; MGB, minor groove binder; RUO, research use only.

The availability of the WHO international standard is an important development that should allow interlaboratory standardization, with reporting of results in international units rather than copy number. A caveat in using this standard is based on a recent report indicating that the WHO standard consists of multiple viral populations, including some with deletions of portions of the BKPyV large T antigen, a region that is targeted by some PCR assays. The deletions can potentially result in overestimation of BKPyV levels by quantitative assays using the standard (138).

Sequence variability may also affect JCPyV NAATs. False-negative NAAT results (proved by amplification of an alternate target) have been reported in an individual with progressive CNS illness and polyomavirus-like particles by EM in brain biopsy material (139). Attention to this issue in the assay design phase is important; broadly reactive real-time PCR reagents and less variable target sequences have been described (135–137, 140, 141). Additionally, laboratories should align their primers and probes against new sequences at regular intervals to ensure detection of these viruses. At the time of writing, studies of the comparative sensitivity of assays for JCPyV have not been published.

PCR methods have also been published for the newly identified HPyVs, although because of the novelty of these agents, much less information is available regarding sequence variation. Conventional PCR methods are available (32, 35, 142), and real-time PCR assays employing TaqMan probes (36, 39, 143, 144) have been reported for WUPyV and KIPyV. Conventional PCR assays (83) and real-time PCR assays employing TaqMan probes have also been published (41, 42) for MCPyV. PCR assays for the more recently discovered HPyVs are also available, including HPyV6 and HPyV7 (85), TSPyV (87, 89), MWPyV (5, 6), STLPyV (13), HPyV9 (7, 145), and HPyV12 (12).

ISOLATION AND CULTURE PROCEDURES

JCPyV and BKPyV can be isolated and propagated in cell culture (146–148), although currently there is no role for these methods in the laboratory diagnosis of HPyV infections. JCPyV demonstrates restricted host range (human cells only) and can be grown in primary embryonic cells, human brain-derived cells (particularly astrocytes and oligodendrocyte precursors), and the permanent cell line SVG. BKPyV has an expanded host range compared to JCPyV and can grow in similar primary cell cultures, primary human embryonic kidney and lung cells, human foreskin fibroblasts, and continuous cell lines (HeLa and monkey cell lines such as CV-1 and Vero). The cytopathic effect of both viruses includes cellular translucency, nuclear enlargement, and gradual loss of the monolayer. Successful propagation often requires weeks and multiple rounds of blind passage. Most virus remains cell associated.

SEROLOGIC TESTS

Serologic tests for HPyV are primarily used for risk assessment in specific clinical settings (see below) and otherwise are investigational tools used for seroepidemiologic studies. The majority of assays are laboratory developed. For JCPyV and BKPyV, two types of serological tests have been described: hemagglutination inhibition (HAI) and enzyme immunoassays (EIAs) employing either crude antigens or virus-like particles (VLPs). Detection of an antibody response by HAI is based on the capacity of specific antiviral antibodies to inhibit the agglutination of human erythrocytes mediated by the viral structural VP1 proteins of JCPyV and BKPyV (148). The development of EIAs for the detection of antibodies to both BKPyV and JCPyV was made possible when engineered cell lines capable of producing adequate amounts of JCPyV antigen were developed (149). A comparison of EIA and HAI demonstrated that antibody titers measured by the two assay formats were statistically significantly correlated, although EIA titers were higher (150). VLPs have also been used as antigens in EIAs for the detection of antibodies. VLPs are empty particles that retain the full antigenicity of intact virions. They form spontaneously when viral capsid proteins are expressed in certain systems and are preferred as antigen sources for EIAs because they contain native conformational epitopes that may be missing when other forms of viral antigens are employed (151). An assay that simultaneously detects antibodies to 13 different human polyomaviruses has been described (152).

Even though JCPyV and BKPyV are closely related, it appears that the antigenic epitopes responsible for the human antibody response are not cross-reactive and antibody tests can discriminate between infection by these two viruses (150). In contrast, it appears that seroreactivity to SV40 is due largely to cross-reactivity with BKPyV (151, 153, 154). The identification of novel HPyVs in recent years has complicated polyomavirus serology and highlighted issues associated with the interpretation of some polyomavirus serologic assays. Further complicating matters, it appears that human sera contain antibodies that can react with animal polyomaviruses, suggesting possible transmission from animal to human. This finding and the likelihood that more HPyVs will be discovered suggest that caution should be employed when interpreting the results of some HPyV assays. These and other issues concerning HPyV serology are covered in depth in a recent review (47).

For BKPyV, studies have demonstrated a positive correlation between kidney donor BKPyV antibody titers and infection in the transplant recipient (62). While this observation is striking, it is not currently used in clinical practice. Antibody testing for JCPyV is used to assess the risk of PML in patients for whom treatment with natalizumab or other immunosuppressive monoclonal antibodies is under consideration (155–157). At the time of writing, commercial availability was limited to the Stratify JCV antibody test produced by Focus Diagnostics (Cypress, CA), which is cleared by the FDA. This test is an ELISA that uses VLPs as the antigen and expresses the result as an index, with results >0.4 considered positive.

ANTIVIRAL SUSCEPTIBILITIES

For PML, a number of antiviral agents have been considered, including cidofovir, an acyclic nucleoside phosphonate; brincidofovir (CMX-001), a lipidated prodrug of cidofovir; topotecan, an inhibitor of DNA topoisomerase I; leflunomide, an immunosuppressive agent with antiviral properties; vidarabine (ARA-A) and cytarabine (ARA-C), synthetic nucleosides that inhibit viral DNA polymerases; and alpha interferon (158). Following evidence that JCPyV uses the serotonin 2A receptor to infect cells in the CNS, interest has been shown in investigating drugs such as risperidone that bind to this receptor and are approved for treatment of certain neuropsychiatric diseases (159), although another study reported that infection of cells by JCPyV was independent of the serotonin receptor (160). A study that examined a collection of 2,000 currently approved drugs found evidence that the antimalarial drug mefloquine had activity against JCPyV *in vitro* (161). Unfortunately, a clinical trial of mefloquine treatment for PML was stopped early when interim data indicated that the drug offered no benefit (162). For some of these agents, antiviral activity against JCPyV has been demonstrated *in vitro*, and encouraging results have been reported in case reports. However, the ability to carry out systematic studies has been hampered by the fact that PML is a rare disease and the majority of patients are HIV infected and receiving potentially confounding anti-HIV therapy, making it difficult to evaluate the effect of the drug being studied. Unfortunately, most clinical studies of antiviral treatments for PML have failed to demonstrate a consistent benefit (163–167), and there are no currently FDA-approved drugs for the treatment of this devastating disease. Current approaches to therapy include optimal HAART for HIV-infected patients, with the aim of increasing CD4 cell counts and decreasing HIV RNA level (50). For non-HIV-infected individuals, reversal or amelioration of the immunosuppressed state ultimately responsible for the disease is recommended (163). While not an antiviral therapy, removal of immunomodulatory agents such as natalizumab can be achieved with plasma exchange. This in turn can trigger an immune reconstitution inflammatory syndrome, a condition that while dangerous can improve survival, although sequelae are common (55).

Many of the same agents studied as possible antiviral treatments for PML have also been investigated for the treatment of BKPyV PVAN and, less commonly, hemorrhagic cystitis. In addition to these compounds, fluoroquinolone antibiotics and intravenous immunoglobulin have also been studied. Similar to the situation with the development of antiviral drugs for the treatment of PML, there are currently no FDA-approved agents for the treatment of BKPyV diseases. The lack of antivirals can be attributed to several factors, including the need for prospective, randomized, controlled studies, the nephrotoxicity exhibited by a number of the drugs, and the confounding variable of the near-universal approach of improving immune function in transplant recipients showing signs of BKPyV disease by some form of reduction in the level of immunosuppression. A review of the literature on antiviral treatment of PVAN found a total of only 184 patients in 27 published studies examining the use of cidofovir, 189 patients in 18 studies of the use of leflunomide, and 14 patients in 2 studies of the use of fluoroquinolones, with the authors concluding that there was no consensus on the use of antivirals for PVAN (168). Currently, there is an ongoing phase 1/2 study of the use of nucleoside analogs for treating BKPyV infection (169), but until this or potential future studies can demonstrate a benefit for a particular antiviral, the mainstay of current therapy for PVAN is the reduction of immunosuppression, although in cases where a patient is in danger of losing a graft to PVAN, a course of an antiviral may be of use (170–172).

EVALUATION, INTERPRETATION, AND REPORTING OF RESULTS

The current recommendation for laboratory testing for PVAN is to monitor levels of the BKPyV in urine and blood after renal transplantation and to reduce immunosuppression when viruria or viremia reaches levels that predict progression to disease (134). Testing for BKPyV viruria has a high negative predictive value and a variable positive predictive value for the development of PVAN, with sustained high levels of viruria (>10^7 copies/ml) having a positive predictive value of up to 67% (172). Sustained high levels of BKPyV viruria are frequently followed by the appearance of viremia. The majority of individuals with PVAN have been found to have BKPyV viremia, with the positive predictive value for viremia being ~60% for the development of PVAN (172). A management algorithm published in 2013 for management of BKPyV infection after solid organ transplantation in adults recommended regular monitoring for BKPyV replication by testing urine or plasma every 1 to 3 months for the first 2 years after the transplant and annually until the fifth year posttransplant. Urine screening could be done by PCR or by cytologic examination looking for decoy cells. A positive test by either method should be followed by testing plasma by PCR. An alternative approach is to screen plasma directly. Detection of plasma viremia at a level of >10,000 DNA copies/ml has been recommended as an indication for renal biopsy and/or reduction of immunosuppressive medication (134). However, because this recommendation was made before the availability of an international standard, it may be difficult to apply because of interassay variability.

These recommendations are helpful in directing NAAT use and interpretation of NAAT results. However, implementing them is complicated by interlaboratory variability in BKPyV quantification because of the previous lack of internationally recognized standards that can serve as calibrators and by the use of assays that may not optimally detect and quantify all BKPyV strains. For example, in 2008, the College of American Pathologists sent four proficiency samples to laboratories performing quantitative BKPyV assays to compare results among the different assays. All 48 laboratories (38 using user-developed assays and 10 using commercial tests) that tested a sample that did not contain BKPyV DNA reported a negative result. When BKPyV-positive specimens were tested, the results were less encouraging. The sample producing the most variation was tested by 41 laboratories with the following results: mean, 700,946 copies/ml; standard deviation (SD), 1,729,692 copies/ml; coefficient of variation (CV), 246.8%; range, 129 to 10,400,000 copies/ml. For 35 laboratories that also reported log-transformed data on this specimen, the results were as follows: mean, 4.806; SD, 1.231; and range, 1.02 to 6.51. The BKPyV-positive specimen with the lowest CV produced the following results: mean, 277,288 copies/ml; SD, 284,990; CV, 102.8%; and range, 7,800 to 945,000 copies/ml. (All data used with the permission of the College of American Pathologists.) Obviously, there is a significant amount of interlaboratory variation in quantitative BKPyV results. It is hoped that the current availability of a WHO quantitative standard will improve interlaboratory variability for BKPyV as has occurred for other viruses when international standards became available (173).

Laboratories are encouraged to calibrate their BKPyV assays with the international standard to achieve better interlaboratory standardization. Other general principles are also encouraged, including minimizing intralaboratory variability with careful coordination between physicians and the laboratory to establish in-house viruria and viremia thresholds for adjusting immunosuppression regimens, at least until reliable general recommendations based on the international standard become available. The additional effort this requires is clearly worthwhile, since successful implementation of testing algorithms has been shown to significantly reduce PVAN incidence (170, 174).

To draw accurate conclusions regarding the course of infection, patients should be monitored at one site if possible. Sequential measurements by different laboratories are difficult to interpret given the likelihood of interlaboratory differences in BKPyV quantification. The laboratory should educate physicians and transplant coordinators about this issue.

In cases where PVAN is suspected and BKPyV titers are negative or low, the possibility of a false negative should be considered, due potentially to sequence mismatches between the virus and real-time PCR primers or probe. Alternatively, it may be possible that JCPyV is responsible, in which case it may be best to try to identify this virus either in biopsy material by histological methods or in plasma. Shedding of this virus is common in the urine and may not indicate the presence of a causative organism. Unfortunately, guidelines for interpreting JCPyV levels in peripheral blood are not available.

Quantitative NAATs of urine from BMT recipients to either predict the development of or diagnose hemorrhagic cystitis may also be useful. High levels of viruria ($>1 \times 10^9$/ml) can be seen in hemorrhagic cystitis due to BKPyV (71, 175); a negative result suggests another cause of this condition. The interpretation of BKPyV viruria is complicated by the fact that BMT recipients frequently excrete BKPyV in their urine and by the lack of guidelines for thresholds that can be applied to predicting or diagnosing disease. Studies have yielded variable data. One report suggested that viruria of 10^9 to 10^{10} or more copies/ml, an increase of $\geq 3 \log_{10}$ relative to baseline levels, may help implicate BKPyV as the cause (70). Another found that levels of BKPyV viremia of $>10^4$ copies/ml were associated with hemorrhagic cystitis (70); however, this relationship was not observed in a similar study (71). The applicability of any recommendations for quantitative thresholds that are not referenced to the international standard is limited.

Serology and culture have little role in the diagnosis of PML. Most individuals are seropositive for JCPyV by adulthood; culture requires special cells and prolonged incubation and is insensitive. Therefore, the preferred diagnostic test for PML is a JCPyV-specific NAAT. The detection of JCPyV DNA in CSF is distinctly abnormal. In combination with appropriate imaging studies and patient history, it is strongly suggestive of PML. JCPyV NAAT sensitivities in CSF range from 42% to 100%, with most reports between 70% and 80%; specificities range from 92% to 100% (176). False-negative JCPyV PCR results in patients with PML, possibly due to mismatches between primers and/or probe sequences and the corresponding viral sequences (139, 177), have been observed. Additionally, decreased PCR sensitivity has been reported in the HAART era (89.5% pre-HAART versus 57.5% HAART, with the negative predictive value falling from 98% to 89%) (178). These findings underscore the fact that a negative JCPyV result cannot rule out the presence of PML. It may be advantageous to retest CSF with a different NAAT if the initial result is negative in a presumptive case of PML. It should be noted that in patients with natalizumab-induced PML who are treated with plasma exchange to remove the drug, JCPyV DNA has been reported to persist in the CSF for periods ranging from months to years (179).

Because of the devastating nature of PML, NAATs have been evaluated for their ability to identify patients at increased risk for developing PML or to provide a prognosis for those patients who have already been diagnosed. A single qualitative test for JCPyV DNA in urine and blood does not appear to be useful for the identification of patients at risk of PML, as demonstrated by studies of individuals with HIV and those with immunosuppression unrelated to HIV (including immunomodulatory therapy with natalizumab) (180, 181), and is therefore not recommended. Persistent viruria and rising urine viral loads have been found to be associated with the development of PML in HIV-positive patients (182). However, a large study that tested >12,000 urine and blood specimens from 1,397 natalizumab-treated multiple sclerosis patients for the presence of JCPyV DNA reported the following: (i) the prevalence of JCPyV viremia was very low in treated patients (<1%) and similar to that seen in untreated healthy controls; (ii) the detection of JCPyV viremia did not correlate with the development of PML; and (iii) the prevalence of JCPyV viruria was high (~25%) at both baseline and after 48 weeks of treatment, leading the authors to conclude that detection of viremia or viruria was not useful in determining the risk of development of PML in this population (183).

Quantitative PCR for the determination of the JCPyV load in the CSF of PML patients has been reported to be potentially useful as a prognostic measure for disease progression. However, because of small study sizes and the lack of standardized quantitative JCPyV NAATs, it has been difficult to formulate guidelines for threshold CSF viral loads. Different reports have indicated, roughly, that JCPyV CSF viral loads of between 10^4 and 10^5 copies/ml separate those PML patients whose disease progresses quickly from those whose illness is stable or progressing more slowly (181, 184–186).

The commercial Stratify JCV offered by Focus Diagnostics is used to determine the JCPyV serostatus of multiple sclerosis patients undergoing natalizumab therapy. Data supporting use of this test to determine risk for development of PML come from a study that revealed that 54% of 831 multiple sclerosis patients were seropositive for JCPyV and that the 17 patients who subsequently developed PML were all JCPyV seropositive (155). In the same study it was reported that the JCPyV false-seronegative rate was 2.5%, as determined by the detection of viruria in 5 of 204 seronegative patients. However, another study of natalizumab-treated patients found a much higher false-seronegative rate of 35% in 17 patients with JCPyV viremia, suggesting that while the determination of JCPyV serostatus may be useful in helping to evaluate the risk of development of PML, other measures of risk need to be developed and employed to supplement serology and that JCPyV serology needs to be interpreted with caution (187).

Current recommendations call for use of the Stratify assay for risk assessment in patients being considered for treatment with natalizumab. In this assay, index values less than 0.2 are considered negative and values >0.4 are considered positive. Values between 0.2 and 0.4 are considered intermediate and are followed up with a confirmatory inhibition assay. Patients who are negative for JC antibodies or are positive with an antibody index <1.5 should be retested every 6 months during treatment with natalizumab. Those who are positive with an antibody index >1.5 either at baseline or on repeat testing are at increased risk for PML with recommendations for increased frequency of brain MRI scans and consideration of discontinuation of natalizumab therapy (188).

Laboratory testing for the newly identified HPyVs is considered investigational at this time, so it is not possible to offer meaningful interpretations for test results for these agents.

REFERENCES

1. **Calvignac-Spencer S, Feltkamp MC, Daugherty MD, Moens U, Ramqvist T, Johne R, Ehlers B, *Polyomaviridae* Study Group of the International Committee on Taxonomy of Viruses.** 2016. A taxonomy update for the family *Polyomaviridae*. *Arch Virol* **161:**1739–1750.
2. **Mishra N, Pereira M, Rhodes RH, An P, Pipas JM, Jain K, Kapoor A, Briese T, Faust PL, Lipkin WI.** 2014. Identification of a novel polyomavirus in a pancreatic transplant recipient with retinal blindness and vasculitic myopathy. *J Infect Dis* **210:**1595–1599.
3. **Gheit T, Dutta S, Oliver J, Robitaille A, Hampras S, Combes JD, McKay-Chopin S, Le Calvez-Kelm F, Fenske N, Cherpelis B, Giuliano AR, Franceschi S, McKay J, Rollison DE, Tommasino M.** 2017. Isolation and characterization of a novel putative human polyomavirus. *Virology* **506:**45–54.
4. **Buck CB, Phan GQ, Raiji MT, Murphy PM, McDermott DH, McBride AA.** 2012. Complete genome sequence of a tenth human polyomavirus. *J Virol* **86:**10887.
5. **Yu G, Greninger AL, Isa P, Phan TG, Martínez MA, de la Luz Sanchez M, Contreras JF, Santos-Preciado JI, Parsonnet J, Miller S, DeRisi JL, Delwart E, Arias CF, Chiu CY.** 2012. Discovery of a novel polyomavirus in acute diarrheal samples from children. *PLoS One* **7:**e49449.
6. **Siebrasse EA, Reyes A, Lim ES, Zhao G, Mkakosya RS, Manary MJ, Gordon JI, Wang D.** 2012. Identification of MW polyomavirus, a novel polyomavirus in human stool. *J Virol* **86:**10321–10326.
7. **Scuda N, Hofmann J, Calvignac-Spencer S, Ruprecht K, Liman P, Kühn J, Hengel H, Ehlers B.** 2011. A novel human polyomavirus closely related to the African green monkey-derived lymphotropic polyomavirus. *J Virol* **85:**4586–4590.
8. **Luo C, Bueno M, Kant J, Martinson J, Randhawa P.** 2009. Genotyping schemes for polyomavirus BK, using gene-specific phylogenetic trees and single nucleotide polymorphism analysis. *J Virol* **83:**2285–2297.
9. **Zhong S, Randhawa PS, Ikegaya H, Chen Q, Zheng HY, Suzuki M, Takeuchi T, Shibuya A, Kitamura T, Yogo Y.** 2009. Distribution patterns of BK polyomavirus (BKV) subtypes and subgroups in American, European and Asian populations suggest co-migration of BKV and the human race. *J Gen Virol* **90:**144–152.
10. **Cook L.** 2016. Polyomaviruses. *Microbiol Spectr* **4(4):** doi:10.1128/microbiolspec.DMIH2-0010-2015.
11. **Imperiale MJ, Major EO.** 2007. Polyomaviruses, p 2263–2298. *In* Knipe DM, Howley PM, Griffin DE, Martin MA, Lamb RA, Roizman B, Straus SE (ed), *Fields Virology*, 5th ed, vol 2. Lippincott Williams & Wilkins, Philadelphia, PA.
12. **Korup S, Rietscher J, Calvignac-Spencer S, Trusch F, Hofmann J, Moens U, Sauer I, Voigt S, Schmuck R, Ehlers B.** 2013. Identification of a novel human polyomavirus in organs of the gastrointestinal tract. *PLoS One* **8:**e58021.
13. **Lim ES, Reyes A, Antonio M, Saha D, Ikumapayi UN, Adeyemi M, Stine OC, Skelton R, Brennan DC, Mkakosya RS, Manary MJ, Gordon JI, Wang D.** 2013. Discovery of STL polyomavirus, a polyomavirus of ancestral recombinant origin that encodes a unique T antigen by alternative splicing. *Virology* **436:**295–303.
14. **Van Ghelue M, Khan MT, Ehlers B, Moens U.** 2012. Genome analysis of the new human polyomaviruses. *Rev Med Virol* **22:**354–377.
15. **Imperiale MJ, Jiang M.** 2016. Polyomavirus persistence. *Annu Rev Virol* **3:**517–532.
16. **DeCaprio JA.** 2017. Merkel cell polyomavirus and Merkel cell carcinoma. *Philos Trans R Soc Lond B Biol Sci* **372:**372.
17. **Kenan DJ, Mieczkowski PA, Burger-Calderon R, Singh HK, Nickeleit V.** 2015. The oncogenic potential of BK-polyomavirus is linked to viral integration into the human genome. *J Pathol* **237:**379–389.
18. **Taguchi F, Kajioka J, Miyamura T.** 1982. Prevalence rate and age of acquisition of antibodies against JC virus and BK virus in human sera. *Microbiol Immunol* **26:**1057–1064.
19. **Knowles WA.** 2006. Discovery and epidemiology of the human polyomaviruses BK virus (BKV) and JC virus (JCV). *Adv Exp Med Biol* **577:**19–45.
20. **Monaco MC, Atwood WJ, Gravell M, Tornatore CS, Major EO.** 1996. JC virus infection of hematopoietic progenitor cells, primary B lymphocytes, and tonsillar stromal cells: implications for viral latency. *J Virol* **70:**7004–7012.
21. **Monaco MC, Jensen PN, Hou J, Durham LC, Major EO.** 1998. Detection of JC virus DNA in human tonsil tissue: evidence for site of initial viral infection. *J Virol* **72:**9918–9923.
22. **Sadeghi M, Wang Y, Ramqvist T, Aaltonen LM, Pyöriä L, Toppinen M, Söderlund-Venermo M, Hedman K.** 2017. Multiplex detection in tonsillar tissue of all known human polyomaviruses. *BMC Infect Dis* **17:**409.
23. **Berger JR, Miller CS, Mootoor Y, Avdiushko SA, Kryscio RJ, Zhu H.** 2006. JC virus detection in bodily fluids: clues to transmission. *Clin Infect Dis* **43:**e9–e12.
24. **Sundsfjord A, Spein AR, Lucht E, Flaegstad T, Seternes OM, Traavik T.** 1994. Detection of BK virus DNA in nasopharyngeal aspirates from children with respiratory infections but not in saliva from immunodeficient and immunocompetent adult patients. *J Clin Microbiol* **32:**1390–1394.
25. **Zhong S, Zheng HY, Suzuki M, Chen Q, Ikegaya H, Aoki N, Usuku S, Kobayashi N, Nukuzuma S, Yasuda Y, Kuniyoshi N, Yogo Y, Kitamura T.** 2007. Age-related urinary excretion of BK polyomavirus by nonimmunocompromised individuals. *J Clin Microbiol* **45:**193–198.
26. **Bofill-Mas S, Formiga-Cruz M, Clemente-Casares P, Calafell F, Girones R.** 2001. Potential transmission of human polyomaviruses through the gastrointestinal tract after exposure to virions or viral DNA. *J Virol* **75:**10290–10299.

27. **Bofill-Mas S, Girones R.** 2003. Role of the environment in the transmission of JC virus. *J Neurovirol* **9**(Suppl 1)**:**54–58.
28. **Bofill-Mas S, Pina S, Girones R.** 2000. Documenting the epidemiologic patterns of polyomaviruses in human populations by studying their presence in urban sewage. *Appl Environ Microbiol* **66:**238–245.
29. **Vanchiere JA, Carillo B, Morrow AL, Jiang X, Ruiz-Palacios GM, Butel JS.** 2016. Fecal polyomavirus excretion in infancy. *J Pediatric Infect Dis Soc* **5:**210–213.
30. **Abed Y, Wang D, Boivin G.** 2007. WU polyomavirus in children, Canada. *Emerg Infect Dis* **13:**1939–1941.
31. **Abedi Kiasari B, Vallely PJ, Corless CE, Al-Hammadi M, Klapper PE.** 2008. Age-related pattern of KI and WU polyomavirus infection. *J Clin Virol* **43:**123–125.
32. **Allander T, Andreasson K, Gupta S, Bjerkner A, Bogdanovic G, Persson MA, Dalianis T, Ramqvist T, Andersson B.** 2007. Identification of a third human polyomavirus. *J Virol* **81:** 4130–4136.
33. **Bialasiewicz S, Whiley DM, Lambert SB, Jacob K, Bletchly C, Wang D, Nissen MD, Sloots TP.** 2008. Presence of the newly discovered human polyomaviruses KI and WU in Australian patients with acute respiratory tract infection. *J Clin Virol* **41:**63–68.
34. **Bialasiewicz S, Whiley DM, Lambert SB, Wang D, Nissen MD, Sloots TP.** 2007. A newly reported human polyomavirus, KI virus, is present in the respiratory tract of Australian children. *J Clin Virol* **40:**15–18.
35. **Gaynor AM, Nissen MD, Whiley DM, Mackay IM, Lambert SB, Wu G, Brennan DC, Storch GA, Sloots TP, Wang D.** 2007. Identification of a novel polyomavirus from patients with acute respiratory tract infections. *PLoS Pathog* **3:**e64.
36. **Le BM, Demertzis LM, Wu G, Tibbets RJ, Buller R, Arens MQ, Gaynor AM, Storch GA, Wang D.** 2007. Clinical and epidemiologic characterization of WU polyomavirus infection, St. Louis, Missouri. *Emerg Infect Dis* **13:**1936–1938.
37. **Lin F, Zheng M, Li H, Zheng C, Li X, Rao G, Zheng M, Wu F, Zeng A.** 2008. WU polyomavirus in children with acute lower respiratory tract infections, China. *J Clin Virol* **42:** 94–102.
38. **Payungporn S, Chieochansin T, Thongmee C, Samransamruajkit R, Theamboolers A, Poovorawan Y.** 2008. Prevalence and molecular characterization of WU/KI polyomaviruses isolated from pediatric patients with respiratory disease in Thailand. *Virus Res* **135:**230–236.
39. **Neske F, Blessing K, Pröttel A, Ullrich F, Kreth HW, Weissbrich B.** 2009. Detection of WU polyomavirus DNA by real-time PCR in nasopharyngeal aspirates, serum, and stool samples. *J Clin Virol* **44:**115–118.
40. **Ren L, Gonzalez R, Xu X, Li J, Zhang J, Vernet G, Paranhos-Baccalà G, Jin Q, Wang J.** 2009. WU polyomavirus in fecal specimens of children with acute gastroenteritis, China. *Emerg Infect Dis* **15:**134–135.
41. **Bialasiewicz S, Lambert SB, Whiley DM, Nissen MD, Sloots TP.** 2009. Merkel cell polyomavirus DNA in respiratory specimens from children and adults. *Emerg Infect Dis* **15:**492–494.
42. **Goh S, Lindau C, Tiveljung-Lindell A, Allander T.** 2009. Merkel cell polyomavirus in respiratory tract secretions. *Emerg Infect Dis* **15:**489–491.
43. **Tolstov YL, Pastrana DV, Feng H, Becker JC, Jenkins FJ, Moschos S, Chang Y, Buck CB, Moore PS.** 2009. Human Merkel cell polyomavirus infection II. MCV is a common human infection that can be detected by conformational capsid epitope immunoassays. *Int J Cancer* **125:**1250–1256.
44. **Bialasiewicz S, Byrom L, Fraser C, Clark J.** 2017. Potential route of transmission for trichodysplasia spinulosa polyomavirus. *J Infect Dis* **215:**1175–1176.
45. **van der Meijden E, Horváth B, Nijland M, de Vries K, Rácz EK, Diercks GF, de Weerd AE, Clahsen-van Groningen MC, van der Blij-de Brouwer CS, van der Zon AJ, Kroes ACM, Hedman K, van Kampen JJA, Riezebos-Brilman A, Feltkamp MCW.** 2017. Primary polyomavirus infection, not reactivation, as the cause of trichodysplasia spinulosa in immunocompromised patients. *J Infect Dis* **215:**1080–1084.
46. **DeCaprio JA, Garcea RL.** 2013. A cornucopia of human polyomaviruses. *Nat Rev Microbiol* **11:**264–276.
47. **Moens U, Van Ghelue M, Song X, Ehlers B.** 2013. Serological cross-reactivity between human polyomaviruses. *Rev Med Virol* **23:**250–264.
48. **Gossai A, Waterboer T, Nelson HH, Michel A, Willhauck-Fleckenstein M, Farzan SF, Hoen AG, Christensen BC, Kelsey KT, Marsit CJ, Pawlita M, Karagas MR.** 2016. Seroepidemiology of human polyomaviruses in a US population. *Am J Epidemiol* **183:**61–69.
49. **Shah KV.** 2007. SV40 and human cancer: a review of recent data. *Int J Cancer* **120:**215–223.
50. **Weber T.** 2008. Progressive multifocal leukoencephalopathy. *Neurol Clin* **26:**833–854, x–xi.
51. **Assetta B, Atwood WJ.** 2017. The biology of JC polyomavirus. *Biol Chem* **398:**839–855.
52. **Bloomgren G, Richman S, Hotermans C, Subramanyam M, Goelz S, Natarajan A, Lee S, Plavina T, Scanlon JV, Sandrock A, Bozic C.** 2012. Risk of natalizumab-associated progressive multifocal leukoencephalopathy. *N Engl J Med* **366:**1870–1880.
53. **Sørensen PS, Bertolotto A, Edan G, Giovannoni G, Gold R, Havrdova E, Kappos L, Kieseier BC, Montalban X, Olsson T.** 2012. Risk stratification for progressive multifocal leukoencephalopathy in patients treated with natalizumab. *Mult Scler* **18:**143–152.
54. **Borchardt J, Berger JR.** 2016. Re-evaluating the incidence of natalizumab-associated progressive multifocal leukoencephalopathy. *Mult Scler Relat Disord* **8:**145–150.
55. **Ferenczy MW, Marshall LJ, Nelson CD, Atwood WJ, Nath A, Khalili K, Major EO.** 2012. Molecular biology, epidemiology, and pathogenesis of progressive multifocal leukoencephalopathy, the JC virus-induced demyelinating disease of the human brain. *Clin Microbiol Rev* **25:**471–506.
56. **Tan CS, Koralnik IJ.** 2010. Progressive multifocal leukoencephalopathy and other disorders caused by JC virus: clinical features and pathogenesis. *Lancet Neurol* **9:**425–437.
57. **Bialasiewicz S, Hart G, Oliver K, Agnihotri SP, Koralnik IJ, Viscidi R, Nissen MD, Sloots TP, Burke MT, Isbel NM, Burke J.** 2017. A difficult decision: atypical JC polyomavirus encephalopathy in a kidney transplant recipient. *Transplantation* **101:**1461–1467.
58. **Nickeleit V, Singh HK, Mihatsch MJ.** 2003. Polyomavirus nephropathy: morphology, pathophysiology, and clinical management. *Curr Opin Nephrol Hypertens* **12:**599–605.
59. **Siguier M, Sellier P, Bergmann JF.** 2012. BK-virus infections: a literature review. *Med Mal Infect* **42:**181–187.
60. **Bohl DL, Brennan DC.** 2007. BK virus nephropathy and kidney transplantation. *Clin J Am Soc Nephrol* **2**(Suppl 1)**:** S36–S46.
61. **Hirsch HH, Knowles W, Dickenmann M, Passweg J, Klimkait T, Mihatsch MJ, Steiger J.** 2002. Prospective study of polyomavirus type BK replication and nephropathy in renal-transplant recipients. *N Engl J Med* **347:** 488–496.
62. **Ramos E, Drachenberg CB, Papadimitriou JC, Hamze O, Fink JC, Klassen DK, Drachenberg RC, Wiland A, Wali R, Cangro CB, Schweitzer E, Bartlett ST, Weir MR.** 2002. Clinical course of polyoma virus nephropathy in 67 renal transplant patients. *J Am Soc Nephrol* **13:**2145–2151.
63. **Bohl DL, Storch GA, Ryschkewitsch C, Gaudreault-Keener M, Schnitzler MA, Major EO, Brennan DC.** 2005. Donor origin of BK virus in renal transplantation and role of HLA C7 in susceptibility to sustained BK viremia. *Am J Transplant* **5:**2213–2221.
64. **Vera-Sempere FJ, Rubio L, Felipe-Ponce V, Garcia A, Sanahuja MJ, Zamora I, Ramos D, Beneyto I, Sánchez-Plumed J.** 2006. Renal donor implication in the origin of BK infection: analysis of genomic viral subtypes. *Transplant Proc* **38:**2378–2381.
65. **Bonvoisin C, Weekers L, Xhignesse P, Grosch S, Milicevic M, Krzesinski JM.** 2008. Polyomavirus in renal transplantation: a hot problem. *Transplantation* **85**(Suppl)**:**S42–S48.
66. **Dall A, Hariharan S.** 2008. BK virus nephritis after renal transplantation. *Clin J Am Soc Nephrol* **3**(Suppl 2)**:**S68–S75.

67. **Reisman L, Habib S, McClure GB, Latiolais LS, Vanchiere JA.** 2014. Treatment of BK virus-associated nephropathy with CMX001 after kidney transplantation in a young child. *Pediatr Transplant* **18:**E227–E231.
68. **Kazory A, Ducloux D, Chalopin JM, Angonin R, Fontanière B, Moret H.** 2003. The first case of JC virus allograft nephropathy. *Transplantation* **76:**1653–1655.
69. **Wen MC, Wang CL, Wang M, Cheng CH, Wu MJ, Chen CH, Shu KH, Chang D.** 2004. Association of JC virus with tubulointerstitial nephritis in a renal allograft recipient. *J Med Virol* **72:**675–678.
70. **Dropulic LK, Jones RJ.** 2008. Polyomavirus BK infection in blood and marrow transplant recipients. *Bone Marrow Transplant* **41:**11–18.
71. **Leung AY, Suen CK, Lie AK, Liang RH, Yuen KY, Kwong YL.** 2001. Quantification of polyoma BK viruria in hemorrhagic cystitis complicating bone marrow transplantation. *Blood* **98:**1971–1978.
72. **Erard V, Kim HW, Corey L, Limaye A, Huang ML, Myerson D, Davis C, Boeckh M.** 2005. BK DNA viral load in plasma: evidence for an association with hemorrhagic cystitis in allogeneic hematopoietic cell transplant recipients. *Blood* **106:**1130–1132.
73. **Ambalathingal GR, Francis RS, Smyth MJ, Smith C, Khanna R.** 2017. BK polyomavirus: clinical aspects, immune regulation, and emerging therapies. *Clin Microbiol Rev* **30:**503–528.
74. **Babakir-Mina M, Ciccozzi M, Perno CF, Ciotti M.** 2011. The novel KI, WU, MC polyomaviruses: possible human pathogens? *New Microbiol* **34:**1–8.
75. **Bialasiewicz S, Rockett RJ, Barraclough KA, Leary D, Dudley KJ, Isbel NM, Sloots TP.** 2016. Detection of recently discovered human polyomaviruses in a longitudinal kidney transplant cohort. *Am J Transplant* **16:**2734–2740.
76. **Dehority WN, Eickman MM, Schwalm KC, Gross SM, Schroth GP, Young SA, Dinwiddie DL.** 2017. Complete genome sequence of a KI polyomavirus isolated from an otherwise healthy child with severe lower respiratory tract infection. *J Med Virol* **89:**926–930.
77. **Kennedy JL, Denson JL, Schwalm KS, Stoner AN, Kincaid JC, Abramo TJ, Thompson TM, Ulloa EM, Burchiel SW, Dinwiddie DL.** 2017. Complete genome sequence of a novel WU polyomavirus isolate from Arkansas, USA, associated with acute respiratory infection. *Genome Announc* **5:**e01452-16.
78. **Rao S, Lucero MG, Nohynek H, Tallo V, Lupisan SP, Garcea RL, Simões EAF, ARIVAC Consortium.** 2016. WU and KI polyomavirus infections in Filipino children with lower respiratory tract disease. *J Clin Virol* **82:**112–118.
79. **Rockett RJ, Bialasiewicz S, Mhango L, Gaydon J, Holding R, Whiley DM, Lambert SB, Ware RS, Nissen MD, Grimwood K, Sloots TP.** 2015. Acquisition of human polyomaviruses in the first 18 months of life. *Emerg Infect Dis* **21:**365–367.
80. **Bijol V, Willby M, Erdman D, Paddock C, Zaki S, Goldsmith C, DeLeon-Carnes M, Batten B, Jones T, Shieh W-J, Menegus M.** 2009. WU polyomavirus infection in an immunocompromised host: histological, ultrastructural and molecular evidence of multi-organ involvement. Twenty-Fifth Annual Clinical Virology Symposium, Daytona Beach, FL.
81. **Siebrasse EA, Nguyen NL, Willby MJ, Erdman DD, Menegus MA, Wang D.** 2016. Multiorgan WU polyomavirus infection in bone marrow transplant recipient. *Emerg Infect Dis* **22:**24–31.
82. **Siebrasse EA, Pastrana DV, Nguyen NL, Wang A, Roth MJ, Holland SM, Freeman AF, McDyer J, Buck CB, Wang D.** 2015. WU polyomavirus in respiratory epithelial cells from lung transplant patient with Job syndrome. *Emerg Infect Dis* **21:**103–106.
83. **Feng H, Shuda M, Chang Y, Moore PS.** 2008. Clonal integration of a polyomavirus in human Merkel cell carcinoma. *Science* **319:**1096–1100.
84. **Moens U, Ludvigsen M, Van Ghelue M.** 2011. Human polyomaviruses in skin diseases. *Pathol Res Int* **2011:**123491.
85. **Schowalter RM, Pastrana DV, Pumphrey KA, Moyer AL, Buck CB.** 2010. Merkel cell polyomavirus and two previously unknown polyomaviruses are chronically shed from human skin. *Cell Host Microbe* **7:**509–515.
86. **Shikova E, Emin D, Alexandrova D, Shindov M, Kumanova A, Lekov A, Moens U.** 2017. Detection of Merkel cell polyomavirus in respiratory tract specimens. *Intervirology* **60:**28–32.
87. **van der Meijden E, Janssens RW, Lauber C, Bouwes Bavinck JN, Gorbalenya AE, Feltkamp MC.** 2010. Discovery of a new human polyomavirus associated with trichodysplasia spinulosa in an immunocompromized patient. *PLoS Pathog* **6:**e1001024.
88. **Haycox CL, Kim S, Fleckman P, Smith LT, Piepkorn M, Sundberg JP, Howell DN, Miller SE.** 1999. Trichodysplasia spinulosa—a newly described folliculocentric viral infection in an immunocompromised host. *J Investig Dermatol Symp Proc* **4:**268–271.
89. **Kazem S, van der Meijden E, Kooijman S, Rosenberg AS, Hughey LC, Browning JC, Sadler G, Busam K, Pope E, Benoit T, Fleckman P, de Vries E, Eekhof JA, Feltkamp MC.** 2012. Trichodysplasia spinulosa is characterized by active polyomavirus infection. *J Clin Virol* **53:**225–230.
90. **Chen T, Mattila PS, Jartti T, Ruuskanen O, Söderlund-Venermo M, Hedman K.** 2011. Seroepidemiology of the newly found trichodysplasia spinulosa-associated polyomavirus. *J Infect Dis* **204:**1523–1526.
91. **van der Meijden E, Kazem S, Burgers MM, Janssens R, Bouwes Bavinck JN, de Melker H, Feltkamp MC.** 2011. Seroprevalence of trichodysplasia spinulosa-associated polyomavirus. *Emerg Infect Dis* **17:**1355–1363.
92. **Tsuzuki S, Fukumoto H, Mine S, Sato N, Mochizuki M, Hasegawa H, Sekizuka T, Kuroda M, Matsushita T, Katano H.** 2014. Detection of trichodysplasia spinulosa-associated polyomavirus in a fatal case of myocarditis in a seven-month-old girl. *Int J Clin Exp Pathol* **7:**5308–5312.
93. **Ho J, Jedrych JJ, Feng H, Natalie AA, Grandinetti L, Mirvish E, Crespo MM, Yadav D, Fasanella KE, Proksell S, Kuan SF, Pastrana DV, Buck CB, Shuda Y, Moore PS, Chang Y.** 2015. Human polyomavirus 7-associated pruritic rash and viremia in transplant recipients. *J Infect Dis* **211:**1560–1565.
94. **Nguyen KD, Lee EE, Yue Y, Stork J, Pock L, North JP, Vandergriff T, Cockerell C, Hosler GA, Pastrana DV, Buck CB, Wang RC.** 2017. Human polyomavirus 6 and 7 are associated with pruritic and dyskeratotic dermatoses. *J Am Acad Dermatol* **76:**932–940.e3.
95. **Beckervordersandforth J, Pujari S, Rennspiess D, Speel EJ, Winnepenninckx V, Diaz C, Weyers W, Haugg AM, Kurz AK, Zur Hausen A.** 2016. Frequent detection of human polyomavirus 6 in keratoacanthomas. *Diagn Pathol* **11:**58.
96. **Li K, Zhang C, Zhao R, Xue Y, Yang J, Peng J, Jin Q.** 2015. The prevalence of STL polyomavirus in stool samples from Chinese children. *J Clin Virol* **66:**19–23.
97. **Ma FL, Li DD, Wei TL, Li JS, Zheng LS.** 2017. Quantitative detection of human Malawi polyomavirus in nasopharyngeal aspirates, sera, and feces in Beijing, China, using real-time TaqMan-based PCR. *Virol J* **14:**152.
98. **Rockett RJ, Sloots TP, Bowes S, O'Neill N, Ye S, Robson J, Whiley DM, Lambert SB, Wang D, Nissen MD, Bialasiewicz S.** 2013. Detection of novel polyomaviruses, TSPyV, HPyV6, HPyV7, HPyV9 and MWPyV in feces, urine, blood, respiratory swabs and cerebrospinal fluid. *PLoS One* **8:**e62764.
99. **Poulin DL, DeCaprio JA.** 2006. Is there a role for SV40 in human cancer? *J Clin Oncol* **24:**4356–4365.
100. **Rollison DE.** 2006. Epidemiologic studies of polyomaviruses and cancer: previous findings, methodologic challenges and future directions. *Adv Exp Med Biol* **577:**342–356.
101. **Vilchez RA, Butel JS.** 2004. Emergent human pathogen simian virus 40 and its role in cancer. *Clin Microbiol Rev* **17:**495–508.
102. **Bofill-Mas S, Albinana-Gimenez N, Clemente-Casares P, Hundesa A, Rodriguez-Manzano J, Allard A, Calvo M, Girones R.** 2006. Quantification and stability of human adenoviruses and polyomavirus JCPyV in wastewater matrices. *Appl Environ Microbiol* **72:**7894–7896.

103. **Subcommittee on Sample Collection and Handling for Molecular Test Methods.** 2005. Collection, transport, preparation, and storage of specimens for molecular methods; Approved Guideline, CLSI document MM13-A, vol 25. Clinical and Laboratory Standards Institute, Wayne, PA.
104. **Khare R, Grys TE.** 2016. Specimen requirements selection, collection, transport, and processing, p 59–77. *In* Loeffelholz MJ (ed), *Cinical Virology Manual*, 5th ed. ASM Press, Washington, DC.
105. **Drachenberg CB, Beskow CO, Cangro CB, Bourquin PM, Simsir A, Fink J, Weir MR, Klassen DK, Bartlett ST, Papadimitriou JC.** 1999. Human polyoma virus in renal allograft biopsies: morphological findings and correlation with urine cytology. *Hum Pathol* **30:**970–977.
106. **Drachenberg CB, Papadimitriou JC, Hirsch HH, Wali R, Crowder C, Nogueira J, Cangro CB, Mendley S, Mian A, Ramos E.** 2004. Histological patterns of polyomavirus nephropathy: correlation with graft outcome and viral load. *Am J Transplant* **4:**2082–2092.
107. **Randhawa PS, Finkelstein S, Scantlebury V, Shapiro R, Vivas C, Jordan M, Picken MM, Demetris AJ.** 1999. Human polyoma virus-associated interstitial nephritis in the allograft kidney. *Transplantation* **67:**103–109.
108. **Singh HK, Bubendorf L, Mihatsch MJ, Drachenberg CB, Nickeleit V.** 2006. Urine cytology findings of polyomavirus infections. *Adv Exp Med Biol* **577:**201–212.
109. **Ahsan N, Shah KV.** 2006. Polyomaviruses and human diseases. *Adv Exp Med Biol* **577:**1–18.
110. **Khalili K, Gordon J, White MK.** 2006. The polyomavirus, JCV and its involvement in human disease. *Adv Exp Med Biol* **577:**274–287.
111. **White MK, Sariyer IK, Gordon J, Delbue S, Pietropaolo V, Berger JR, Khalili K.** 2016. Diagnostic assays for polyomavirus JC and progressive multifocal leukoencephalopathy. *Rev Med Virol* **26:**102–114.
112. **Berger JR, Aksamit AJ, Clifford DB, Davis L, Koralnik IJ, Sejvar JJ, Bartt R, Major EO, Nath A.** 2013. PML diagnostic criteria: consensus statement from the AAN Neuroinfectious Disease Section. *Neurology* **80:**1430–1438.
113. **Herrera GA, Veeramachaneni R, Turbat-Herrera EA.** 2005. Electron microscopy in the diagnosis of BK-polyoma virus infection in the transplanted kidney. *Ultrastruct Pathol* **29:**469–474.
114. **Latif S, Zaman F, Veeramachaneni R, Jones L, Uribe-Uribe N, Turbat-Herrera EA, Herrera GA.** 2007. BK polyomavirus in renal transplants: role of electron microscopy and immunostaining in detecting early infection. *Ultrastruct Pathol* **31:**199–207.
115. **Mesquita R, Björkholm M, Ekman M, Bogdanovic G, Biberfeld P.** 1996. Polyomavirus-infected oligodendrocytes and macrophages within astrocytes in progressive multifocal leukoencephalopathy (PML). *APMIS* **104:**153–160.
116. **Biel SS, Nitsche A, Kurth A, Siegert W, Ozel M, Gelderblom HR.** 2004. Detection of human polyomaviruses in urine from bone marrow transplant patients: comparison of electron microscopy with PCR. *Clin Chem* **50:**306–312.
117. **Laskin BL, Singh HK, Beier UH, Moatz T, Furth SL, Bunin N, Witte D, Goebel J, Davies SM, Dandoy C, Jodele S, Nickeleit V.** 2016. The noninvasive urinary polyomavirus Haufen test predicts BK virus nephropathy in children after hematopoietic cell transplantation: a pilot study. *Transplantation* **100:**e81–e87.
118. **Singh HK, Andreoni KA, Madden V, True K, Detwiler R, Weck K, Nickeleit V.** 2009. Presence of urinary Haufen accurately predicts polyomavirus nephropathy. *J Am Soc Nephrol* **20:**416–427.
119. **Wetzels CT, Hoefnagel JG, Bakkers JM, Dijkman HB, Blokx WA, Melchers WJ.** 2009. Ultrastructural proof of polyomavirus in Merkel cell carcinoma tumour cells and its absence in small cell carcinoma of the lung. *PLoS One* **4:**e4958.
120. **Hirsch HH, Brennan DC, Drachenberg CB, Ginevri F, Gordon J, Limaye AP, Mihatsch MJ, Nickeleit V, Ramos E, Randhawa P, Shapiro R, Steiger J, Suthanthiran M, Trofe J.** 2005. Polyomavirus-associated nephropathy in renal transplantation: interdisciplinary analyses and recommendations. *Transplantation* **79:**1277–1286.
121. **Liptak P, Kemeny E, Ivanyi B.** 2006. Primer: histopathology of polyomavirus-associated nephropathy in renal allografts. *Nat Clin Pract Nephrol* **2:**631–636.
122. **Jochum W, Weber T, Frye S, Hunsmann G, Lüke W, Aguzzi A.** 1997. Detection of JC virus by anti-VP1 immunohistochemistry in brains with progressive multifocal leukoencephalopathy. *Acta Neuropathol* **94:**226–231.
123. **Procop GW, Beck RC, Pettay JD, Kohn DJ, Tuohy MJ, Yen-Lieberman B, Prayson RA, Tubbs RR.** 2006. JC virus chromogenic in situ hybridization in brain biopsies from patients with and without PML. *Diagn Mol Pathol* **15:**70–73.
124. **von Einsiedel RW, Samorei IW, Pawlita M, Zwissler B, Deubel M, Vinters HV.** 2004. New JC virus infection patterns by in situ polymerase chain reaction in brains of acquired immunodeficiency syndrome patients with progressive multifocal leukoencephalopathy. *J Neurovirol* **10:**1–11.
125. **Zheng H, Murai Y, Hong M, Nakanishi Y, Nomoto K, Masuda S, Tsuneyama K, Takano Y.** 2007. JC [corrected] virus detection in human tissue specimens. *J Clin Pathol* **60:**787–793.
126. **Bergallo M, Costa C, Gribaudo G, Tarallo S, Baro S, Negro Ponzi A, Cavallo R.** 2006. Evaluation of six methods for extraction and purification of viral DNA from urine and serum samples. *New Microbiol* **29:**111–119.
127. **Cook L, Atienza EE, Bagabag A, Obrigewitch RM, Jerome KR.** 2009. Comparison of methods for extraction of viral DNA from cellular specimens. *Diagn Microbiol Infect Dis* **64:**37–42.
128. **Dundas N, Leos NK, Mitui M, Revell P, Rogers BB.** 2008. Comparison of automated nucleic acid extraction methods with manual extraction. *J Mol Diagn* **10:**311–316.
129. **Mengelle C, Mansuy JM, Sauné K, Barthe C, Boineau J, Izopet J.** 2012. A new highly automated extraction system for quantitative real-time PCRs from whole blood samples: routine monitoring of opportunistic infections in immunosuppressed patients. *J Clin Virol* **53:**314–319.
130. **Tang YW, Sefers SE, Li H, Kohn DJ, Procop GW.** 2005. Comparative evaluation of three commercial systems for nucleic acid extraction from urine specimens. *J Clin Microbiol* **43:**4830–4833.
131. **Kim S, Park SJ, Namgoong S, Sung H, Kim MN.** 2009. Comparative evaluation of two automated systems for nucleic acid extraction of BK virus: NucliSens easyMAG versus BioRobot MDx. *J Virol Methods* **162:**208–212.
132. **Beuselinck K, van Ranst M, van Eldere J.** 2005. Automated extraction of viral-pathogen RNA and DNA for high-throughput quantitative real-time PCR. *J Clin Microbiol* **43:**5541–5546.
133. **Pang XL, Martin K, Preiksaitis JK.** 2008. The use of unprocessed urine samples for detecting and monitoring BK viruses in renal transplant recipients by a quantitative real-time PCR assay. *J Virol Methods* **149:**118–122.
134. **Hirsch HH, Randhawa P, AST Infectious Diseases Community of Practice.** 2013. BK polyomavirus in solid organ transplantation. *Am J Transplant* **13**(Suppl 4)**:**179–188.
135. **Hoffman NG, Cook L, Atienza EE, Limaye AP, Jerome KR.** 2008. Marked variability of BK virus load measurement using quantitative real-time PCR among commonly used assays. *J Clin Microbiol* **46:**2671–2680.
136. **Luo C, Bueno M, Kant J, Randhawa P.** 2008. Biologic diversity of polyomavirus BK genomic sequences: implications for molecular diagnostic laboratories. *J Med Virol* **80:**1850–1857.
137. **Dumoulin A, Hirsch HH.** 2011. Reevaluating and optimizing polyomavirus BK and JC real-time PCR assays to detect rare sequence polymorphisms. *J Clin Microbiol* **49:** 1382–1388.
138. **Bateman AC, Greninger AL, Atienza EE, Limaye AP, Jerome KR, Cook L.** 2017. Quantification of BK virus standards by quantitative real-time PCR and droplet digital PCR is confounded by multiple virus populations in the WHO BKV international standard. *Clin Chem* **63:**761–769.
139. **Landry ML, Eid T, Bannykh S, Major E.** 2008. False negative PCR despite high levels of JC virus DNA in spinal fluid: implications for diagnostic testing. *J Clin Virol* **43:**247–249.

140. **Pang XL, Doucette K, LeBlanc B, Cockfield SM, Preiksaitis JK.** 2007. Monitoring of polyomavirus BK virus viruria and viremia in renal allograft recipients by use of a quantitative real-time PCR assay: one-year prospective study. *J Clin Microbiol* **45:**3568–3573.
141. **Ryschkewitsch CF, Jensen PN, Major EO.** 2013. Multiplex qPCR assay for ultra sensitive detection of JCV DNA with simultaneous identification of genotypes that discriminates non-virulent from virulent variants. *J Clin Virol* **57:**243–248.
142. **Norja P, Ubillos I, Templeton K, Simmonds P.** 2007. No evidence for an association between infections with WU and KI polyomaviruses and respiratory disease. *J Clin Virol* **40:**307–311.
143. **Bialasiewicz S, Whiley DM, Lambert SB, Gould A, Nissen MD, Sloots TP.** 2007. Development and evaluation of real-time PCR assays for the detection of the newly identified KI and WU polyomaviruses. *J Clin Virol* **40:**9–14.
144. **Mourez T, Bergeron A, Ribaud P, Scieux C, de Latour RP, Tazi A, Socié G, Simon F, LeGoff J.** 2009. Polyomaviruses KI and WU in immunocompromised patients with respiratory disease. *Emerg Infect Dis* **15:**107–109.
145. **Sauvage V, Foulongne V, Cheval J, Ar Gouilh M, Pariente K, Dereure O, Manuguerra JC, Richardson J, Lecuit M, Burguière A, Caro V, Eloit M.** 2011. Human polyomavirus related to African green monkey lymphotropic polyomavirus. *Emerg Infect Dis* **17:**1364–1370.
146. **Beckmann AM, Shah KV.** 1983. Propagation and primary isolation of JCV and BKV in urinary epithelial cell cultures. *Prog Clin Biol Res* **105:**3–14.
147. **Sack GH, Felix JS, Lanahan AA.** 1980. Plaque formation and purification of BK virus in cultured human urinary cells. *J Gen Virol* **50:**185–190.
148. **Shah KV.** 1995. Polyomaviruses, p 505-510. *In* Lennette EH, Lennette DA, Lennette ET (ed), *Diagnostic Procedures for Viral, Rickettsial, and Chlamydial Infections*, 7th ed. American Public Health Association, Washington, DC.
149. **Frye S, Trebst C, Dittmer U, Petry H, Bodemer M, Hunsmann G, Weber T, Lüke W.** 1997. Efficient production of JC virus in SVG cells and the use of purified viral antigens for analysis of specific humoral and cellular immune response. *J Virol Methods* **63:**81–92.
150. **Hamilton RS, Gravell M, Major EO.** 2000. Comparison of antibody titers determined by hemagglutination inhibition and enzyme immunoassay for JC virus and BK virus. *J Clin Microbiol* **38:**105–109.
151. **Viscidi RP, Clayman B.** 2006. Serological cross reactivity between polyomavirus capsids. *Adv Exp Med Biol* **577:**73–84.
152. **Kamminga S, van der Meijden E, Wunderink HF, Touzé A, Zaaijer HL, Feltkamp MCW.** 2018. Development and evaluation of a broad bead-based multiplex immunoassay to measure IgG seroreactivity against human polyomaviruses. *J Clin Microbiol* **56:**e01566-17.
153. **Knowles WA, Pipkin P, Andrews N, Vyse A, Minor P, Brown DW, Miller E.** 2003. Population-based study of antibody to the human polyomaviruses BKV and JCV and the simian polyomavirus SV40. *J Med Virol* **71:**115–123.
154. **Viscidi RP, Rollison DE, Viscidi E, Clayman B, Rubalcaba E, Daniel R, Major EO, Shah KV.** 2003. Serological cross-reactivities between antibodies to simian virus 40, BK virus, and JC virus assessed by virus-like-particle-based enzyme immunoassays. *Clin Diagn Lab Immunol* **10:**278–285.
155. **Gorelik L, Lerner M, Bixler S, Crossman M, Schlain B, Simon K, Pace A, Cheung A, Chen LL, Berman M, Zein F, Wilson E, Yednock T, Sandrock A, Goelz SE, Subramanyam M.** 2010. Anti-JC virus antibodies: implications for PML risk stratification. *Ann Neurol* **68:**295–303.
156. **Lee P, Plavina T, Castro A, Berman M, Jaiswal D, Rivas S, Schlain B, Subramanyam M.** 2013. A second-generation ELISA (STRATIFY JCV™ DxSelect™) for detection of JC virus antibodies in human serum and plasma to support progressive multifocal leukoencephalopathy risk stratification. *J Clin Virol* **57:**141–146.
157. **Plavina T, Berman M, Njenga M, Crossman M, Lerner M, Gorelik L, Simon K, Schlain B, Subramanyam M.** 2012. Multi-site analytical validation of an assay to detect anti-JCV antibodies in human serum and plasma. *J Clin Virol* **53:**65–71.
158. **Roskopf J, Trofe J, Stratta RJ, Ahsan N.** 2006. Pharmacotherapeutic options for the management of human polyomaviruses. *Adv Exp Med Biol* **577:**228–254.
159. **Focosi D, Fazzi R, Montanaro D, Emdin M, Petrini M.** 2007. Progressive multifocal leukoencephalopathy in a haploidentical stem cell transplant recipient: a clinical, neuroradiological and virological response after treatment with risperidone. *Antiviral Res* **74:**156–158. h
160. **Chapagain ML, Verma S, Mercier F, Yanagihara R, Nerurkar VR.** 2007. Polyomavirus JC infects human brain microvascular endothelial cells independent of serotonin receptor 2A. *Virology* **364:**55–63.
161. **Brickelmaier M, Lugovskoy A, Kartikeyan R, Reviriego-Mendoza MM, Allaire N, Simon K, Frisque RJ, Gorelik L.** 2009. Identification and characterization of mefloquine efficacy against JC virus in vitro. *Antimicrob Agents Chemother* **53:**1840–1849.
162. **Clifford DB, Nath A, Cinque P, Brew BJ, Zivadinov R, Gorelik L, Zhao Z, Duda P.** 2013. A study of mefloquine treatment for progressive multifocal leukoencephalopathy: results and exploration of predictors of PML outcomes. *J Neurovirol* **19:**351–358.
163. **Berger JR.** 2000. Progressive multifocal leukoencephalopathy. *Curr Treat Options Neurol* **2:**361–368.
164. **De Luca A, Ammassari A, Pezzotti P, Cinque P, Gasnault J, Berenguer J, Di Giambenedetto S, Cingolani A, Taoufik Y, Miralles P, Marra CM, Antinori A, Gesida 9/99, IRINA, ACTG 363 Study Groups.** 2008. Cidofovir in addition to antiretroviral treatment is not effective for AIDS-associated progressive multifocal leukoencephalopathy: a multicohort analysis. *AIDS* **22:**1759–1767.
165. **Gasnault J, Taoufik Y, Goujard C, Kousignian P, Abbed K, Boue F, Dussaix E, Delfraissy JF.** 1999. Prolonged survival without neurological improvement in patients with AIDS-related progressive multifocal leukoencephalopathy on potent combined antiretroviral therapy. *J Neurovirol* **5:**421–429.
166. **Hall CD, Dafni U, Simpson D, Clifford D, Wetherill PE, Cohen B, McArthur J, Hollander H, Yainnoutsos C, Major E, Millar L, Timpone J.** 1998. Failure of cytarabine in progressive multifocal leukoencephalopathy associated with human immunodeficiency virus infection. AIDS Clinical Trials Group 243 Team. *N Engl J Med* **338:**1345–1351.
167. **Marra CM, Rajicic N, Barker DE, Cohen BA, Clifford D, Donovan Post MJ, Ruiz A, Bowen BC, Huang ML, Queen-Baker J, Andersen J, Kelly S, Shriver S, Adult AIDS Clinical Trials Group 363 Team.** 2002. A pilot study of cidofovir for progressive multifocal leukoencephalopathy in AIDS. *AIDS* **16:**1791–1797.
168. **Hilton R, Tong CY.** 2008. Antiviral therapy for polyomavirus-associated nephropathy after renal transplantation. *J Antimicrob Chemother* **62:**855–859.
169. **Kuypers DR.** 2012. Management of polyomavirus-associated nephropathy in renal transplant recipients. *Nat Rev Nephrol* **8:**390–402.
170. **Ramos E, Drachenberg CB, Wali R, Hirsch HH.** 2009. The decade of polyomavirus BK-associated nephropathy: state of affairs. *Transplantation* **87:**621–630.
171. **Rinaldo CH, Hirsch HH.** 2007. Antivirals for the treatment of polyomavirus BK replication. *Expert Rev Anti Infect Ther* **5:**105–115.
172. **Wiseman AC.** 2009. Polyomavirus nephropathy: a current perspective and clinical considerations. *Am J Kidney Dis* **54:**131–142.
173. **Hayden RT, Sun Y, Tang L, Procop GW, Hillyard DR, Pinsky BA, Young SA, Caliendo AM.** 2017. Progress in quantitative viral load testing: variability and impact of the WHO quantitative international standards. *J Clin Microbiol* **55:**423–430.
174. **Brennan DC, Agha I, Bohl DL, Schnitzler MA, Hardinger KL, Lockwood M, Torrence S, Schuessler R, Roby T, Gaudreault-Keener M, Storch GA.** 2005. Incidence of BK with tacrolimus versus cyclosporine and impact of preemptive immunosuppression reduction. *Am J Transplant* **5:** 582–594.

175. **Bogdanovic G, Priftakis P, Giraud G, Kuzniar M, Ferraldeschi R, Kokhaei P, Mellstedt H, Remberger M, Ljungman P, Winiarski J, Dalianis T.** 2004. Association between a high BK virus load in urine samples of patients with graft-versus-host disease and development of hemorrhagic cystitis after hematopoietic stem cell transplantation. *J Clin Microbiol* **42:**5394–5396.
176. **Cinque P, Scarpellini P, Vago L, Linde A, Lazzarin A.** 1997. Diagnosis of central nervous system complications in HIV-infected patients: cerebrospinal fluid analysis by the polymerase chain reaction. *AIDS* **11:**1–17.
177. **Sheikh SI, Stemmer-Rachamimov A, Attar EC.** 2009. Autopsy diagnosis of progressive multifocal leukoencephalopathy with JC virus-negative CSF after cord blood stem-cell transplantation. *J Clin Oncol* **27:**e46–e47.
178. **Marzocchetti A, Di Giambenedetto S, Cingolani A, Ammassari A, Cauda R, De Luca A.** 2005. Reduced rate of diagnostic positive detection of JC virus DNA in cerebrospinal fluid in cases of suspected progressive multifocal leukoencephalopathy in the era of potent antiretroviral therapy. *J Clin Microbiol* **43:**4175–4177.
179. **Ryschkewitsch CF, Jensen PN, Monaco MC, Major EO.** 2010. JC virus persistence following progressive multifocal leukoencephalopathy in multiple sclerosis patients treated with natalizumab. *Ann Neurol* **68:**384–391.
180. **Clifford DB.** 2008. Natalizumab and PML: a risky business? *Gut* **57:**1347–1349.
181. **Koralnik IJ, Boden D, Mai VX, Lord CI, Letvin NL.** 1999. JC virus DNA load in patients with and without progressive multifocal leukoencephalopathy. *Neurology* **52:**253–260.
182. **Grabowski MK, Viscidi RP, Margolick JB, Jacobson LP, Shah KV.** 2009. Investigation of pre-diagnostic virological markers for progressive multifocal leukoencephalopathy in human immunodeficiency virus-infected patients. *J Med Virol* **81:**1140–1150.
183. **Rudick RA, O'Connor PW, Polman CH, Goodman AD, Ray SS, Griffith NM, Jurgensen SA, Gorelik L, Forrestal F, Sandrock AW, Goelz SE.** 2010. Assessment of JC virus DNA in blood and urine from natalizumab-treated patients. *Ann Neurol* **68:**304–310.
184. **Bossolasco S, Calori G, Moretti F, Boschini A, Bertelli D, Mena M, Gerevini S, Bestetti A, Pedale R, Sala S, Sala S, Lazzarin A, Cinque P.** 2005. Prognostic significance of JC virus DNA levels in cerebrospinal fluid of patients with HIV-associated progressive multifocal leukoencephalopathy. *Clin Infect Dis* **40:**738–744.
185. **Delbue S, Tremolada S, Ferrante P.** 2008. Application of molecular tools for the diagnosis of central nervous system infections. *Neurol Sci* **29**(Suppl 2)**:**S283–S285.
186. **Yiannoutsos CT, Major EO, Curfman B, Jensen PN, Gravell M, Hou J, Clifford DB, Hall CD.** 1999. Relation of JC virus DNA in the cerebrospinal fluid to survival in acquired immunodeficiency syndrome patients with biopsy-proven progressive multifocal leukoencephalopathy. *Ann Neurol* **45:**816–821.
187. **Major EO, Frohman E, Douek D.** 2013. JC viremia in natalizumab-treated patients with multiple sclerosis. *N Engl J Med* **368:**2240–2241.
188. **McGuigan C, Craner M, Guadagno J, Kapoor R, Mazibrada G, Molyneux P, Nicholas R, Palace J, Pearson OR, Rog D, Young CA.** 2016. Stratification and monitoring of natalizumab-associated progressive multifocal leukoencephalopathy risk: recommendations from an expert group. *J Neurol Neurosurg Psychiatry* **87:**117–125.
189. **Snyder MD, Storch GA, Clifford DB.** 2005. Atypical PML leading to a diagnosis of common variable immunodeficiency. *Neurology* **64:**1661.
190. **Eng PM, Turnbull BR, Cook SF, Davidson JE, Kurth T, Seeger JD.** 2006. Characteristics and antecedents of progressive multifocal leukoencephalopathy in an insured population. *Neurology* **67:**884–886.
191. **Kleinschmidt-DeMasters BK, Tyler KL.** 2005. Progressive multifocal leukoencephalopathy complicating treatment with natalizumab and interferon beta-1a for multiple sclerosis. *N Engl J Med* **353:**369–374.
192. **Langer-Gould A, Atlas SW, Green AJ, Bollen AW, Pelletier D.** 2005. Progressive multifocal leukoencephalopathy in a patient treated with natalizumab. *N Engl J Med* **353:**375–381.
193. **Van Assche G, Van Ranst M, Sciot R, Dubois B, Vermeire S, Noman M, Verbeeck J, Geboes K, Robberecht W, Rutgeerts P.** 2005. Progressive multifocal leukoencephalopathy after natalizumab therapy for Crohn's disease. *N Engl J Med* **353:**362–368.
194. **Becker JC, Houben R, Ugurel S, Trefzer U, Pföhler C, Schrama D.** 2009. MC polyomavirus is frequently present in Merkel cell carcinoma of European patients. *J Invest Dermatol* **129:**248–250.
195. **Foulongne V, Kluger N, Dereure O, Brieu N, Guillot B, Segondy M.** 2008. Merkel cell polyomavirus and Merkel cell carcinoma, France. *Emerg Infect Dis* **14:**1491–1493.
196. **Fischer MK, Kao GF, Nguyen HP, Drachenberg CB, Rady PL, Tyring SK, Gaspari AA.** 2012. Specific detection of trichodysplasia spinulosa–associated polyomavirus DNA in skin and renal allograft tissues in a patient with trichodysplasia spinulosa. *Arch Dermatol* **148:**726–733.
197. **Matthews MR, Wang RC, Reddick RL, Saldivar VA, Browning JC.** 2011. Viral-associated trichodysplasia spinulosa: a case with electron microscopic and molecular detection of the trichodysplasia spinulosa-associated human polyomavirus. *J Cutan Pathol* **38:**420–431.
198. **Wanat KA, Holler PD, Dentchev T, Simbiri K, Robertson E, Seykora JT, Rosenbach M.** 2012. Viral-associated trichodysplasia: characterization of a novel polyomavirus infection with therapeutic insights. *Arch Dermatol* **148:**219–223.

Parvovirus B19 and Bocaviruses

KEVIN E. BROWN

109

TAXONOMY

Parvoviruses are small (~22-nm-diameter), nonenveloped icosahedral viruses with a linear single-stranded DNA genome. They take their name from *parvum*, the Latin for "small," and *Parvoviridae* are among the smallest known DNA-containing viruses that infect mammalian cells. The *Parvoviridae* are divided into two subfamilies, *Parvovirinae* and *Densovirinae*, on the basis of their ability to infect vertebrate or invertebrate cells, respectively. The viruses of vertebrates (*Parvovirinae*) are currently subdivided into eight genera on the basis of their number of open reading frames, their transcription map, their ability to replicate efficiently either autonomously or with helper virus, and their sequence homology. The eight genera are *Amdoparvovirus*, *Aveparvovirus*, *Bocaparvovirus*, *Copiparvovirus*, *Dependoparvovirus*, *Erythroparvovirus*, *Protoparvovirus*, and *Tetraparvovirus* (1).

At least five different parvoviruses are known to infect humans. Parvovirus B19 (B19V) is the best characterized and is classified as the type member of the *Erythroparvovirus* genus. The other viruses are the human bocaviruses (*Bocaparvovirus*), PARV4 (*Tetraparvovirus*), human bufavirus (*Protoparvovirus*), and the nonpathogenic adeno-associated viruses (*Dependoparvoviruses*). Tusavirus (*Protoparvovirus*) has also been found in human fecal material, but it is not known if it really is a human virus.

PARVOVIRUS B19

Description of the Agent

B19V has the typical features of a member of the *Parvoviridae*: the virions are nonenveloped, are 15 to 28 nm in diameter, and show icosahedral symmetry (Fig. 1). The virions hemagglutinate through the primary viral receptor, blood group P, also known as globoside (2–4).

The genome consists of a single strand of DNA of 5,596 nucleotides, with long inverted terminal repeat sequences at each end. The genome has two large open reading frames (ORFs), with the left ORF encoding the nonstructural protein (NS) and the right ORF encoding the two capsid proteins, VP1 and VP2, by alternative splicing.

The B19V virion is an icosahedron consisting of 60 copies of the capsid proteins, of which 95% is VP2, with 5% or less being the larger VP1 protein (5). VP2 capsid proteins self-assemble to form virus-like particles (VLPs) in the absence of B19V DNA; VP1 is not required for capsid formation (6, 7). Although three different genotypes have been described, there is serological cross-reactivity, and thus only one serotype.

In 1985, the virus was officially recognized as a member of the *Parvoviridae*, and the International Committee on Taxonomy of Viruses recommended the name B19V to prevent confusion with other viruses (i.e., human papillomavirus). It is classified as a member of the *Erythroparvovirus* genus with the name parvovirus B19 (official abbreviation, B19V) (1).

Epidemiology and Transmission

B19V is a common cause of infection in humans, and although there is some variation in different countries (8), 50% of 15-year-olds and 80% of the elderly have detectable IgG (9, 10). Infections in temperate climates are more common in late winter, spring, and early summer months. Rates of infection may also increase every 3 to 5 years, and this is reflected by corresponding increases in the major clinical manifestations of B19V infection, mainly transient aplastic crisis (TAC) and erythema infectiosum (11).

The virus can be readily transmitted by close contact through the respiratory route. In one study, the secondary attack rate from symptomatic patients to susceptible (IgG-negative) household contacts was approximately 50% (11). The highest secondary attack rates and also seroprevalence and annual seroconversion rates are seen among workers with close contact with young children, e.g., day care providers and school personnel (10, 12).

Infectious virus can also be found in serum, and infection can be transmitted by blood and blood products. Although ~1% of blood donations have low-level B19V DNA detectable (13), reports of transmission of B19V infection by individual units of blood or platelets are rare. However, transmission from pooled products is more common, and recommendations in Europe and America now require all plasma pools for fractionation to be screened for high-titer parvovirus DNA to try to minimize the transmission of B19V by blood products.

Currently there is no vaccine for B19V, although B19V VLPs expressed in either insect or yeast cells are highly immunogenic (14, 15), and the results of phase 1 trials looked promising. However, a more recent, larger trial was

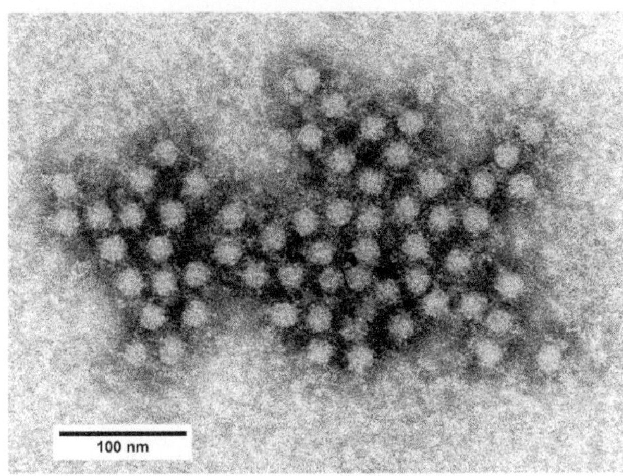

FIGURE 1 Immunoelectron microscopy of parvovirus B19, showing typical 22-nm particles clumped together with a polyclonal human serum. Image courtesy of Hazel Appleton.

stopped due to the development of unexplained skin rashes in three recipients (16).

Clinical Significance

B19V primarily infects erythroid progenitor cells, inducing cell death through apoptosis and cessation of red cell production. Thus, the presentation of infection depends on the significance of the drop in red cell production and/or the immune response to infection, and unlike many virus infections, the disease manifestation of infection with B19V varies widely with the immunologic and hematologic status of the host (Table 1).

Healthy Individuals—Normal Immune Response

Although a significant number of infections are asymptomatic, the major manifestation of B19V infection is erythema infectiosum, also known as fifth disease or slapped-cheek disease, due to the characteristic facial rash After a 2- to 5-day nonspecific prodromal illness (fever, chills, and myalgia) (Fig. 2A), the classic slapped-cheek rash appears, followed 1 to 4 days later by erythematous maculopapular exanthem on the trunk and limbs. This rash is almost certainly immune-mediated, and the timing correlates to detection of an antibody response. As the rash on the trunk and limbs fades, it takes on a typical lacy appearance. There may be great variation in the dermatological appearance, and rarely, it may present as papulo-purpuric "glove and sock" syndrome (17). The classic slapped-cheek appearance is more common in children than adults, and the second-stage eruption may vary from a very faint erythema that is easily missed to a florid exanthema and may be transient or recurrent over 1 to 3 weeks.

In children, B19V infection is usually mild and of short duration. However, in adults and especially in women, there is a symmetrical arthropathy primarily affecting the small joints of the hands and feet in approximately 50% of patients (18). Joint symptoms often last 1 to 3 weeks, although in 20% of affected women, arthralgia or frank arthritis may persist or recur for >2 months or even years. In the absence of a history of rash, the symptoms may be mistaken for acute rheumatoid arthritis, especially as B19V infection can be associated with transient rheumatoid factor production (19). It has been postulated that B19V is involved in the initiation and perpetuation of rheumatoid arthritis leading to joint lesions (20), but these results have not been reproducible by other groups. In contrast, parvoviral B19V DNA is frequently found in synovial tissue of patients with rheumatoid arthritis, chronic arthropathy, and control subjects, and it seems unlikely that B19V plays a role in classic erosive rheumatoid arthritis. The association of B19V and juvenile rheumatic disease is more convincing (21), but whether it is the cause of the disease or one of many potential triggers is less clear.

Patients with Increased Erythropoiesis

TAC, the abrupt cessation of red cell production (Fig. 2B) due to B19V, has been described in a wide range of patients with underlying hemolytic disorders, including hereditary spherocytosis, thalassemia, and red cell enzymopathies such as pyruvate kinase deficiency and autoimmune hemolytic anemia (22). Even in hematologically normal individuals, acute anemia or a drop in red cell count has been observed (23, 24). Other blood lineages may also be affected, and there may be varying degrees of neutropenia, thrombocytopenia, and transient pancytopenia (22). Rarely, the patient may present with a petechial or purpuric rash, and some cases of idiopathic thrombocytopenia purpura (25) and Henoch–Schönlein purpura (26) have also been linked to B19V infection.

Although it is a self-limiting disease, patients with aplastic crisis can be severely ill, with dyspnea, lassitude, and even confusion due to the worsening anemia. Congestive heart failure and severe bone marrow necrosis may develop (27, 28), and the illness can be fatal (29). TAC is readily treated by blood transfusion.

Infection during Pregnancy and Congenital Infection

B19V is a known cause of fetal hydrops and miscarriage. Studies have estimated an increased fetal loss of

TABLE 1 Clinical diseases associated with parvovirus B19 infection, and methods of diagnosis

Host(s)	Disease presentation	IgM	IgG	PCR	Quantitative PCR[a]
Healthy children	Fifth disease	Positive	Positive	Positive	>10^4 IU/ml
Healthy adults (often women)	Polyarthropathy syndrome	Positive within 3 months of onset	Positive	Positive	>10^4 IU/ml
Patients with increased erythropoiesis	Transient aplastic crisis	Negative/positive	Negative/ positive	Positive	Often >10^{12} IU/ml, but rapidly decreases
Immunodeficient or immunocompetent patients	Persistent anemia/ pure-red-cell aplasia	Negative/weakly positive	Negative/weakly positive	Positive	Often >10^{12} IU/ml, but should be >10^6 in the absence of treatment
Fetus (<20 weeks)	Hydrops fetalis/ congenital anemia	Negative/positive	Positive	Positive amniotic fluid or tissue	NA

[a]Abbreviations: IU, international units (1 IU equals ~1 genome); NA, not applicable.

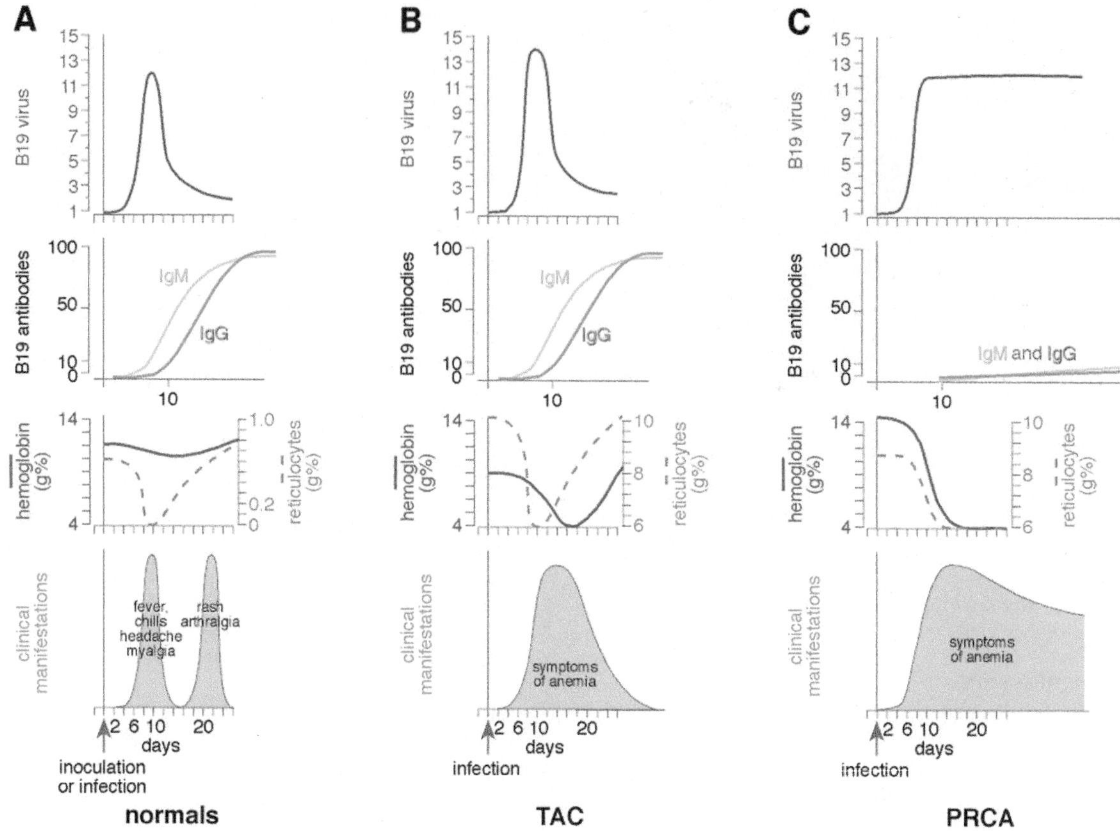

FIGURE 2 Time course of B19 infections in healthy individuals (A), patients with TAC (B), and immunosuppressed patients (C). PRCA, pure-red-cell aplasia. Figure reprinted with permission from *New England Journal* (**350**:586–597, 2004).

9% in women with confirmed B19V infection in the first 20 weeks of pregnancy (30–32). Many cases of parvovirus B19-induced hydrops fetalis are now treated with intrauterine blood transfusion.

Rare cases of congenital anemia after a history of maternal B19V exposure have been reported (33). In these cases, the virus load is generally low and the anemia does not respond to immunoglobulin therapy. The B19V infection may mimic Diamond-Blackfan anemia (34), and the role of *in utero* B19V infection in inducing constitutional bone marrow failure such as that in Diamond-Blackfan anemia is still not clear.

Immunosuppressed and Immunocompromised Patients

In patients with a compromised immune system, there may be a failure to induce a neutralizing antibody response, leading to chronic infection of erythroid progenitors and, as a consequence, prolonged failure of red cell production and development of a chronic anemia (Fig. 2C). Persistent B19 infection resulting in pure-red-cell aplasia has been reported in a wide variety of immunosuppressed patients, ranging from patients with congenital immunodeficiency, AIDS, and lymphoproliferative disorders to transplant patients (35). The stereotypical presentation is with persistent anemia rather than the immune-mediated symptoms of rash or arthropathy. Often there is a pure-red-cell aplasia, but other lineages may also be affected. Treatment is by reduction of the immunosuppression, if this is feasible, or, more often, administration of immunoglobulin (36, 37).

Other Presentations

B19V infection has been associated with a wide range of other manifestations, including vasculitis, hepatitis, myocarditis (and cardiomyopathies), glomerulonephritis, Kawasaki disease, and virus-associated hemophagocytic syndrome (38).

Treatment

Treatment for all presentations of B19V infection is for symptoms only. B19V does not encode either a DNA polymerase or viral proteases, so targets for antivirals are limited. Although cidofovir has been shown to have some antiparvovirus activity *in vivo* (39), this has not been demonstrated *in vitro*.

Collection, Transport, and Storage of Specimens

Due to its small DNA genome and lack of a lipid envelope, B19V is resistant to most types of physical inactivation and is relatively heat stable. Therefore, no special precautions are needed for transportation and storage of most clinical specimens, although repeated freeze-thaw cycles should be prevented where possible. Serum (or plasma) samples should be obtained, if possible, and should permit measurement of both viral load and B19V-specific IgM and IgG levels. Additional samples may include cerebrospinal fluid (for investigation of neurologic infection), amniotic fluid (for investigations in pregnancy), and bone marrow samples (hematologic disease), but these should always be in addition to serum samples where possible, as interpretation may be difficult without a concurrent serum sample.

For investigation of fetal deaths, fetal tissue can be used, either frozen or fixed, although frozen material is preferable for DNA analysis. Samples can usually be transported at room temperature, with the exception of tissue samples (and especially fetal liver samples), which, if not fixed, should be frozen as soon as possible after collection and kept frozen if possible until processed (due to the large amount of proteases and DNase activity often present in such samples).

Direct Examination

Microscopy

Infected cells are characterized both *in vivo* and *in vitro* by the presence of giant pronormoblasts, or lantern cells (40). These are early erythroid cells, 25 to 32 μm in diameter, with cytoplasmic vacuolization, immature chromatin, and large eosinophilic nuclear inclusion bodies (Fig. 3). Electron microscopy of such cells shows that the inclusion is made up of large viral arrays, which can be confirmed by monoclonal antibody staining. These cells can be found in bone marrow of infected individuals at the time of their peak viremia and occasionally in the peripheral circulation (41). Although they have been said to be pathognomonic of B19V infection, similar cells can be seen in bone marrows of patients with other infections, including HIV, and so should not be used for diagnosis of parvovirus B19 infection without other confirmation.

When seen as a large viral array within a cell, parvovirus B19 can be readily identified. However, often the infected cells do not have inclusions, and in these cases, electron microscopy cannot always distinguish intracellular virus from ribosomes, limiting its practicalities except as a research tool.

High viral loads (>10^9 IU/ml) can be detected in serum samples (after concentration) by election microscopy, in which the characteristic 22-nm icosahedral virions can be seen (Fig. 1). Immuno-electron microscopy using polyclonal serum to clump the virions together can increase the sensitivity and makes the virions easier to identify.

Antigen Detection

Antigen detection, generally done using monoclonal antibodies, can be used with standard histochemistry (Fig. 4) to identify infected cells in tissues or in cell culture. It is relatively insensitive and can be useful for identifying infected cells in cases where the significance of low levels of B19V DNA is unknown. Its role in clinical microbiology is limited.

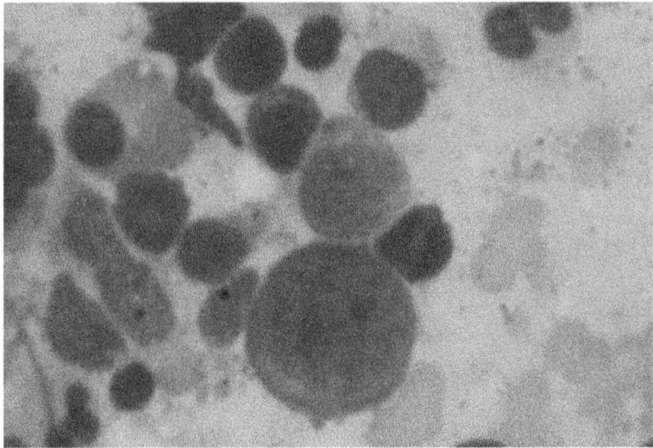

FIGURE 3 Lantern cell, or giant pronormoblast, typical of parvovirus B19 infection.

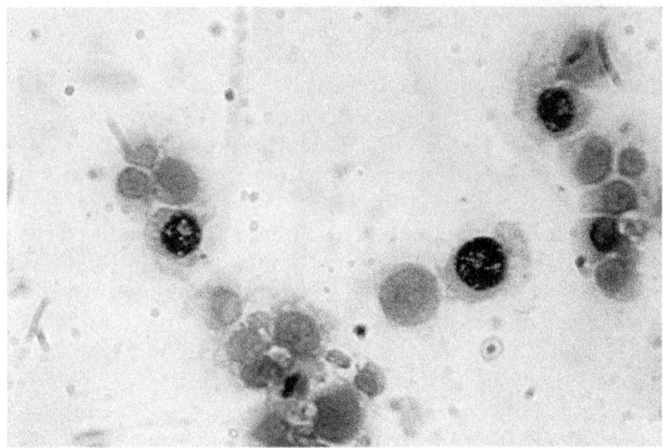

FIGURE 4 Immunohistochemistry of infected erythroid progenitor cells from human fetal liver, stained with anticapsid antibody. Note the typical intranuclear localization of capsid protein.

B19V antigen-based assays are relatively insensitive (>10^6 virus particles/ml), but antigen detection can be used for detecting high concentrations of virus in serum or plasma settings, and it has been suggested as a screening method for detecting high-titer virus in blood and plasma samples (42).

Nucleic Acid Detection

Detection of B19V DNA is the preferred method for identifying B19V in samples. Although *in situ* hybridization can been used to identify B19V DNA within specific cells, and direct hybridization was used for many years to detect B19V DNA in serum samples, DNA detection is now more commonly done by PCR. Due to the exquisite sensitivity of PCR, B19V DNA can then remain detectable for months or even years at low levels, even following complete recovery, and thus, quantitative PCR is required to distinguish recent infection from previous infection with the virus. All assays should be calibrated against the WHO B19V nucleic acid amplification technology standard (43) and the results reported as international units per milliliter.

A large number of different PCR primers (and probes) have been described in the literature (44–47), and commercial assays are available from a number of different companies, including Abbott, Altona, Argene, Artus, Fast-track, Focus, Ingenetix, and Roche, but there are few studies comparing the different assays, and none are currently FDA approved for diagnostic testing. When an assay is being chosen, primers should be designed from the more conserved parts of the virus genome, such as the region in the NS gene where there is a second ORF (48, 49), and should be chosen to specifically detect all three genotypes. Although the genome is relatively conserved, a single nucleotide difference may markedly alter the sensitivity of the assay (50). There is now a first WHO International Reference Panel available comprising the different genotypes so that assays can be checked to make sure that all three genotypes will be detectable in an assay (49).

Detection of viral RNA can be very useful for confirming the presence of replicating virus and active infection. Often, this is achieved through amplification across a spliced junction, so that there is distinction between the spliced RNA and viral DNA (51). This is generally used only as a research tool.

Isolation Procedures

B19V, like all autonomous parvoviruses, is dependent on mitotically active cells for its own replication. B19V also has a very narrow target cell range and can be efficiently propagated only in human erythroid progenitor cells. For erythroid progenitors from bone marrow, susceptibility to parvovirus B19 increases with differentiation; the pluripotent stem cell appears to be spared, and the main target cells are CD36-positive erythroid colony-forming cells and erythroblasts (52). Thus, B19V cannot be grown in standard tissue culture.

A number of semipermissive cell lines have been described, including UT7/Epo (53, 54) and KU812Ep6 (55) cells. However, more efficient replication is obtained using primary cultures from bone marrow or fetal liver (40, 56). Methods for enhancing erythroid differentiation have been developed, so that efficient B19 replication can now be achieved in the research laboratory (57).

Typing Systems

Parvovirus B19 is now recognized to have three different genotypes, with ~10% variability at the DNA level between genotypes (48, 58, 59). Most of the B19V identified is genotype 1 (58), the original B19V genotype, which is distributed worldwide. Genotype 3 seems to be the predominant B19V genotype in Ghana, representing more than 90% of the sequences identified (60). Genotype 2 has been primarily identified in tissues of older patients (born before 1973), suggesting that it may have circulated more frequently prior to the 1970s (61). However, blood samples or donations containing high-titer genotype 2 are occasionally identified (62, 63), and genotype 2 and 3 sequences have been identified in blood and tissues from many different parts of the world (64–66), suggesting a more widespread distribution than originally assumed. Although rare, patients with low levels of more than one genotype have been described (67).

Despite the differences in the DNA sequences, the capsid protein sequence is conserved between the different genotypes, and there is evidence for both serological cross-reactivity and cross-neutralization (68). There is no evidence of significant differences in virological or disease characteristics among genotypes (69, 70).

Serological Tests

Serological surveys were originally performed using counterimmunoelectrophoresis, which is relatively insensitive, but this was superseded by radioimmunoassays and now almost universally by enzyme immunoassays. Due to the inability to grow B19V in standard cell culture systems, early serology assays were based on the use of synthetic peptides (71) or fusion proteins in *Escherichia coli* (72) as the antigen. However, the epitopes presented by these products do not accurately reproduce the epitopes of the native capsids, and the sensitivity and specificity were disappointing. The production of B19V capsid proteins as VLPs using baculovirus (7, 73) or yeast (74) expression systems appears to have overcome these problems, with results based on these antigens showing good correlation with assays based on native virus. The antigens are relatively easy to mass produce and are noninfectious.

Immunoassays using VLPs as antigens are generally both sensitive and specific. Although B19V IgM can be detected by both IgM capture assays and indirect assays, capture assays appear to be more sensitive assays and less prone to false-positive results due to rheumatoid factor. In contrast, IgG assays are probably more sensitive in an indirect (or sandwich) format, especially for seroprevalence studies. Commercial immunoassays for both B19V IgM and IgG are available from a number of different companies, including BioELISA, Diasorin (previously Biotrin), DRG, EurImmune, IBL, Focus, Mikrogen, MyBiosource, and Serion, but several of these are designated for research use only, and in the United States, only the Diasorin assay is FDA approved for diagnostic use.

Antibody to virus is usually present by the seventh day of illness (aplastic crisis) or the day after the onset of rash and is probably detectable lifelong thereafter, although some waning of antibody has been suggested (75). In immunocompetent individuals, the early antibody response is to the major capsid protein VP2, but as the immune response matures, reactivity to the minor capsid protein, VP1, dominates (76, 77). Sera from patients with persistent B19V infection typically have antibody to VP2 but not to VP1 (78). Thus, a number of other formats for assays have been described, including epitope-specific assays and avidity tests for B19 infection (76, 79). Apart from a commercial immunoblot assay (Mikrogen), these assays are all laboratory-developed assays and are not available outside research laboratories. In specialist settings and in combination with B19V DNA viral load, these assays may be useful, especially for confirming the timing of recent infection, e.g., during pregnancy (80).

Although assays to detect neutralizing antibodies have been described (46), they are very time-consuming and not used outside the research setting.

Evaluation, Interpretation, and Reporting of Results

The diagnosis of parvovirus B19 infection is very dependent on the host characteristics and the presentation of the illness, with either serology or quantitative PCR being the most appropriate assay depending on the circumstances (Table 1; Fig. 2).

For otherwise healthy children or adults presenting with the immune-mediated rash illness consistent with B19V (i.e., slapped-cheek rash or rash of erythema infectiosum), appropriate testing is for the detection of parvovirus B19 IgM, as the high-titer viremic stage correlates with the time of the prodrome (Fig. 2A). The IgM remains detectable for several months following infection. B19V IgG is also detectable within a day of onset of the rash and then remains detectable lifelong. Patients with fifth disease do have detectable B19V DNA in blood, with titers of $>10^4$ IU/ml. At 2 to 3 months following infection, B19V DNA levels fall to $<10^4$ IU/ml, and low-level B19V DNA may remain detectable in blood and tissues for the rest of the patient's life. False-positive B19 IgM serology can occur with other acute rash infections, including measles and rubella, and may mislead clinicians. In addition, B19V infection may be associated with production of rheumatoid factor (81) and has produced false-positive serology results in other assays (82). Measurement of the B19 viral load can then be useful in determining the specificity of the IgM result.

Patients with increased red cell turnover, and presenting with TAC, often have 10^8 to 10^{14} IU/ml of virus DNA detectable in their blood (Fig. 2B), and diagnosis should be by quantitative PCR. IgM and IgG are not initially detectable, and the diagnosis can be missed if these assays are not combined with detection of B19V DNA. Assays for detection of B19V antigen in serum or plasma are not recommended, as they can give false-negative results due to immune complex formation.

Similar high viral loads and undetectable IgM (and IgG) in the serum at the time of presentation are also seen in the rare patients who present with a petechial or purpuric rash. In these patients, parvovirus B19 infection cannot be excluded on the basis of a negative IgM test alone.

Immunosuppressed or immunocompromised patients with persistent parvovirus infection often have low or absent antibody response but high titers (>10^6 IU/ml) of B19V DNA in blood or serum (Fig. 2C). Diagnosis should be made using quantitative PCR.

B19V infection in the fetus is usually suspected following confirmation of maternal infection. However, infection of the fetus follows maternal infection, and it can be that the mother's B19 IgM response is negative at the time of the fetal hydrops. In these cases, B19V IgG avidity and/or B19V DNA viral load may be useful in determining the time of maternal infection (80, 83).

As low levels of B19V DNA remain detectable in serum or tissues of otherwise healthy immunocompetent individuals following an acute infection, the finding of low-titer B19V DNA alone should not be interpreted as an indicator of recent infection or the causal agent of pathology.

HUMAN BOCAVIRUSES

Human bocavirus (HBoV) was discovered in 2005 as part of a virus discovery program to identify the causes of lower respiratory tract infections in children (84). This respiratory human bocavirus is now classified as HBoV1. The related viruses HBoV2, HBoV3, and HBoV4 have been detected in fecal samples (85–87).

Description of the Agent

HBoV1 has the typical structure of a member of the *Parvoviridae*. The full-length genome of HBoV1 is 5,543 nucleotides, with dissimilar hairpin sequences at the 5′ and 3′ ends. The genome has three large ORFs (as seen in other members of the genus *Bocaparvovirus*) encoding the nonstructural protein (NS1), the capsid proteins (VP1 and VP2), and a second nonstructural protein (NP1) (88).

The major capsid protein, VP2, has been expressed in insect cells and self-assembles to form VLPs (Fig. 5) that are the basis of most serology assays. The coding sequences for the other human bocaviruses have also been determined (HBoV2 [85], HBoV3 [89], and HBoV4 [87]). The different human bocavirus species show between 10% and 30% divergence, with increased genetic variation and evidence for recombination between HBoV2 and HBoV4 (87).

Epidemiology and Transmission

HBoVs have a worldwide distribution and have been identified in all countries that have looked for them. HBoV1 is predominantly found in respiratory secretions and is found in 2 to 20% of samples from children with upper or lower respiratory tract disease (90). Although HBoV1 DNA can be detected throughout the year, primary infection is predominantly in the winter and spring months (84, 91, 92), as for other respiratory infections. Based on serological studies using HBoV1 as the antigen, most, if not all, individuals are infected in early childhood before the age of 6 (93).

HBoV2, HBoV3, and HBoV4 are identified predominantly in fecal samples, both in patients (children and adults) with gastroenteritis and in healthy controls (87, 90). HBoV2 appears to be the most commonly identified species, followed by HBoV3 and then HBoV4 (90, 93). This is also reflected in the seroepidemiology, with seroprevalence being reported as follows: HBoV1 > HboV2 > HBoV3 > HBoV4.

HBoV1 appears to be transmitted predominantly by the respiratory route, although HBoV1 DNA has been detected in urine and fecal samples (94, 95), suggesting that it may also be spread by the fecal-oral route.

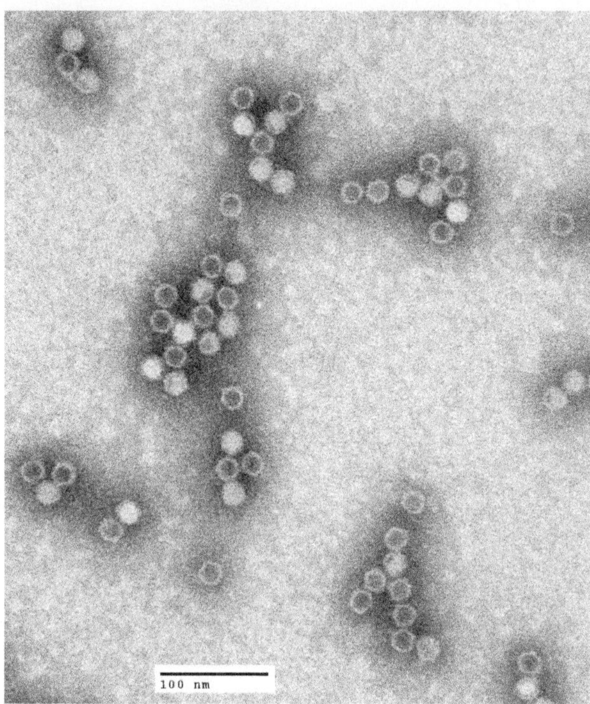

FIGURE 5 Bocavirus VLPs expressed in insect cells.

HBoV2 to -4 are found mainly in fecal samples and appear to be spread by the fecal route.

Clinical Significance

Although HBoV1 DNA is commonly found in respiratory secretions of hospitalized children with respiratory symptoms, in many cases HBoV1 is found with other pathogens, raising questions as to whether it is the main cause of symptoms (90). It is now clear that there can be prolonged persistence of bocavirus DNA in respiratory tract (and fecal) samples, and several groups have shown that if a tighter definition for diagnosing HBoV1 infection is used (high viral load in respiratory secretions, DNA in serum, and/or a serological response), HBoV1 infection is associated with both upper and lower respiratory tract infection, and specifically with wheezing (96–98).

Similar criteria for the diagnosis of infection due to the fecal bocaviruses have not been identified, and although HBoV2 to -4 can be found in patients with acute gastroenteritis, in controlled studies they are found in healthy controls at similar rates (99, 100).

Direct Examination

Microscopy and Antigen Detection

Although parvovirus-like particles had been observed in fecal samples by electron microscopy, it is only with the identification of the nucleic acid sequence that their true identity has been confirmed. Microscopy and antigen detection do not have a role in diagnosis and management of bocavirus infection.

Nucleic Acid Detection

The mainstay of bocavirus diagnosis is nucleic acid detection by PCR. A number of different primers and probes have been described (90–111), but there have been virtually no studies comparing the relative specificity or sensitivity of the different assays. The NS1 and NP1 regions are the most conserved region of the virus and therefore the preferred target area. Commercial assays have also been produced (e.g., Argene, Fast-track Diagnostics, and Gentaur), often as part of a multiplex combined with other respiratory targets.

Isolation Procedures

HBoV1 can be grown in human airway epithelia (112), and cells in the respiratory tract are presumed to be the main site of replication during infection. Although HBoV1 can be grown *in vitro* in well-differentiated airway epithelial cells (113), replication is inefficient, and for most cases, virus detection is generally done by detection of viral DNA by PCR.

Typing Systems

At least four different human bocaviruses have been described, and they can be readily distinguished based on their DNA sequence using specific primers The viruses are also serologically distinct, although antigenic differences are used more to characterize the serological response than to identify the viruses (114).

Serologic Tests

As with B19V, several groups have expressed the major capsid protein of human bocavirus capsids in insect cells (Fig. 5) and developed serological assays to detect both IgM and IgG (115). In addition, bocavirus IgG avidity assays have been described (116). However, most assays probably measure cross-reacting antibodies to any of the four different human bocaviruses, and there have been only a few studies to try to distinguish between the antibody responses (114). None of these assays are widely commercially available, although SinoeGeneclon advertises a human bocavirus IgM assay.

Evaluation, Interpretation, and Reporting of Results

It is now recognized that diagnosis of human bocavirus infection should not be based on detection of bocavirus DNA in respiratory or fecal samples alone, because of the persistence of DNA at these sites. For HBoV1, detection should be based on the detection of viral DNA in the serum and on evidence by serology of recent infection. This is generally indicated by evidence of IgG seroconversion or by detection of IgM or low-avidity antibody. If serum is not available for serology and PCR, then high-titer ($>10^4$ genome copies/ml) HBoV1 DNA in respiratory secretions should be used (90).

Similar criteria have not been developed for HBoV2 to -4 infections.

HUMAN PARVOVIRUS 4

Human parvovirus 4 (PARV4) was also discovered in 2005 as part of a virus discovery program looking for new viruses in plasma samples using sequence-independent single-primer amplification. The initial sample was from a daily-injecting intravenous-drug user with signs of acute viral infection (117).

So far, 5,268 nucleotides of the sequence have been identified, and although this represents the full-length genome, the terminal inverted repeat sequences are incomplete (117). The genome has two large ORFs but a very different transcription profile from other parvoviruses; it is now classified in the new genus *Tetraparvovirus*.

The PARV4 sequences can be divided into three main groups or genotypes. Genotypes 1 and 2 are predominantly found in America and Europe, and genotype 3 is found in Africa. Although there may be differences in transmission (this has not been confirmed), it is not known if there are any other differences in virology or pathogenicity between the genotypes.

Testing of pooled plasma products from Europe and North America showed that PARV4 DNA can be readily detected in plasma pools (4 to 5%), with viral loads varying from <100 copies/ml to 4×10^6 copies/ml (118). The prevalence may be significantly higher in other parts of the world.

PARV4 has not been grown in culture, but several groups have expressed capsid protein in insect cells. Serological studies suggest that infection is unusual in the general population (119), but seroprevalence is higher in those with needle-sharing activities and those who receive blood products (120), as well as in some parts of Africa (121). Although the main route of transmission in Europe and North America appears to be parenteral, transmission through the fecal-oral route cannot be dismissed.

Very little information is available on the clinical features of acute infection with PARV4, with only very limited studies on cohorts of groups at high risk of acquiring infection through parenteral exposure (122, 123).

Diagnosis is generally by the detection of PARV4 viral DNA by PCR. Patients with acute infection appear to have transient high levels of PARV4 DNA in serum. However, the duration of the high-level viremia before the development of an IgM and IgG response is not known. No commercial assays are available for PARV4, and testing for PARV4 is a research tool only.

HUMAN BUFAVIRUS AND TUSIVIRUS

Human bufavirus (BuV) was also discovered by a metagenomic analysis, this time of fecal material from children with diarrhea in Burkina Faso in 2012 (124). A range of different viruses were discovered, including human bufavirus, a novel member of the genus *Protoparvovirus*. As with other novel parvoviruses, the full coding region was obtained but with incomplete terminal hairpin sequences. Three distinct BuV genotypes have been described (125); all were obtained from fecal samples of children or adults with gastroenteritis, albeit with low viral loads, and these viruses were often associated with other pathogens (126–129). Antibody assays are in development and suggest that in Finland, 5% of adults have had previous infection (130). Seroepidemiology studies from other countries have not been reported.

Another *Protoparvovirus*, tusivirus, was also detected in fecal samples from a Tunisian child with diarrhea in 2014, but whether this virus is a true human pathogen is still unclear (131).

REFERENCES

1. **Tijssen P, Agbandje-McKenna M, Almendral JM, Bergoin M, Flegel TW, Hedman K, Kleinschmidt JA, Pintel D, Tattersall P.** 2011. Parvoviridae, p 405–425. *In* King AMQ, Adams MJ, Carstens EB, Lefkowitz EJ (ed), *Virus Taxonomy: IXth Report of the International Committee on Taxonomy of Viruses*, 9th ed. Elsevier, San Diego, CA.
2. **Brown KE, Anderson SM, Young NS.** 1993. Erythrocyte P antigen: cellular receptor for B19 parvovirus. *Science* **262:**114–117.
3. **Brown KE, Cohen BJ.** 1992. Haemagglutination by parvovirus B19. *J Gen Virol* **73:**2147–2149.

4. **Brown KE, Hibbs JR, Gallinella G, Anderson SM, Lehman ED, McCarthy P, Young NS.** 1994. Resistance to parvovirus B19 infection due to lack of virus receptor (erythrocyte P antigen). *N Engl J Med* **330:**1192–1196.
5. **Kajigaya S, Shimada T, Fujita S, Young NS.** 1989. A genetically engineered cell line that produces empty capsids of B19 (human) parvovirus. *Proc Natl Acad Sci USA* **86:**7601–7605.
6. **Brown CS, DiSumma FM, Rommelaere J, Dege AY, Cornelis JJ, Dinsart C, Spaan WJ.** 2002. Production of recombinant H1 parvovirus stocks devoid of replication-competent viruses. *Hum Gene Ther* **13:**2135–2145.
7. **Kajigaya S, Fujii H, Field A, Anderson S, Rosenfeld S, Anderson LJ, Shimada T, Young NS.** 1991. Self-assembled B19 parvovirus capsids, produced in a baculovirus system, are antigenically and immunogenically similar to native virions. *Proc Natl Acad Sci USA* **88:**4646–4650.
8. **Kelly HA, Siebert D, Hammond R, Leydon J, Kiely P, Maskill W.** 2000. The age-specific prevalence of human parvovirus immunity in Victoria, Australia compared with other parts of the world. *Epidemiol Infect* **124:**449–457.
9. **Mossong J, Hens N, Friederichs V, Davidkin I, Broman M, Litwinska B, Siennicka J, Trzcinska A, Van Damme P, Beutels P, Vyse A, Shkedy Z, Aerts M, Massari M, Gabutti G.** 2008. Parvovirus B19 infection in five European countries: seroepidemiology, force of infection and maternal risk of infection. *Epidemiol Infect* **136:**1059–1068.
10. **Röhrer C, Gärtner B, Sauerbrei A, Böhm S, Hottenträger B, Raab U, Thierfelder W, Wutzler P, Modrow S.** 2008. Seroprevalence of parvovirus B19 in the German population. *Epidemiol Infect* **136:**1564–1575.
11. **Chorba T, Coccia P, Holman RC, Tattersall P, Anderson LJ, Sudman J, Young NS, Kurczynski E, Saarinen UM, Moir R, Lawrence DN, Jason JM, Evatt B.** 1986. The role of parvovirus B19 in aplastic crisis and erythema infectiosum (fifth disease). *J Infect Dis* **154:**383–393.
12. **van Rijckevorsel, GG, Bovee LP, Damen M, Sonder GJ, Schim van der Loeff MF, van den Hoek A.** 2012. Increased seroprevalence of IgG-class antibodies against cytomegalovirus, parvovirus B19, and varicella-zoster virus in women working in child day care. *BMC Public Health* **12:**475.
13. **Kleinman SH, Glynn SA, Lee TH, Tobler L, Montalvo L, Todd D, Kiss JE, Shyamala V, Busch MP, National Heart, Lung, Blood Institute Retrovirus Epidemiology Donor Study (REDS-II).** 2007. Prevalence and quantitation of parvovirus B19 DNA levels in blood donors with a sensitive polymerase chain reaction screening assay. *Transfusion* **47:**1756–1764.
14. **Bansal GP, Hatfield JA, Dunn FE, Kramer AA, Brady F, Riggin CH, Collett MS, Yoshimoto K, Kajigaya S, Young NS.** 1993. Candidate recombinant vaccine for human B19 parvovirus. *J Infect Dis* **167:**1034–1044.
15. **Chandramouli S, Medina-Selby A, Coit D, Schaefer M, Spencer T, Brito LA, Zhang P, Otten G, Mandl CW, Mason PW, Dormitzer PR, Settembre EC.** 2013. Generation of a parvovirus B19 vaccine candidate. *Vaccine* **31:** 3872–3878.
16. **Bernstein DI, El Sahly HM, Keitel WA, Wolff M, Simone G, Segawa C, Wong S, Shelly D, Young NS, Dempsey W.** 2011. Safety and immunogenicity of a candidate parvovirus B19 vaccine. *Vaccine* **29:**7357–7363.
17. **Parez N, Dehée A, Michel Y, Veinberg F, Garbarg-Chenon A.** 2009. Papular-purpuric gloves and socks syndrome associated with B19V infection in a 6-year-old child. *J Clin Virol* **44:**167–169.
18. **Woolf AD, Campion GV, Chishick A, Wise S, Cohen BJ, Klouda PT, Caul O, Dieppe PA.** 1989. Clinical manifestations of human parvovirus B19 in adults. *Arch Intern Med* **149:**1153–1156.
19. **Naides SJ, Field EH.** 1988. Transient rheumatoid factor positivity in acute human parvovirus B19 infection. *Arch Intern Med* **148:**2587–2589.
20. **Takahashi Y, Murai C, Shibata S, Munakata Y, Ishii T, Ishii K, Saitoh T, Sawai T, Sugamura K, Sasaki T.** 1998. Human parvovirus B19 as a causative agent for rheumatoid arthritis. *Proc Natl Acad Sci USA* **95:**8227–8232.
21. **Lehmann HW, Knöll A, Küster RM, Modrow S.** 2003. Frequent infection with a viral pathogen, parvovirus B19, in rheumatic diseases of childhood. *Arthritis Rheum* **48:** 1631–1638.
22. **Young N.** 1988. Hematologic and hematopoietic consequences of B19 parvovirus infection. *Semin Hematol* **25:**159–172.
23. **Hamon MD, Newland AC, Anderson MJ.** 1988. Severe aplastic anaemia after parvovirus infection in the absence of underlying haemolytic anaemia. *J Clin Pathol* **41:**1242.
24. **Anderson MJ, Higgins PG, Davis LR, Willman JS, Jones SE, Kidd IM, Pattison JR, Tyrrell DA.** 1985. Experimental parvoviral infection in humans. *J Infect Dis* **152:**257–265.
25. **Foreman NK, Oakhill A, Caul EO.** 1988. Parvovirus-associated thrombocytopenic purpura. *Lancet* **332:** 1426–1427.
26. **Lefrère JJ, Courouc‌é AM, Muller JY, Clark M, Soulier JP, Mortimer PP, Cohen BJ, Rossiter MA, Fairhead SM, Rahman AFMS.** 1985. Human parvovirus and purpura. *Lancet* **326:**730–731.
27. **Conrad ME, Studdard H, Anderson LJ.** 1988. Aplastic crisis in sickle cell disorders: bone marrow necrosis and human parvovirus infection. *Am J Med Sci* **295:**212–215.
28. **Godeau B, Galacteros F, Schaeffer A, Morinet F, Bachir D, Rosa J, Portos JL.** 1991. Aplastic crisis due to extensive bone marrow necrosis and human parvovirus infection in sickle cell disease. *Am J Med* **91:**557–558.
29. **Serjeant GR, Serjeant BE, Thomas PW, Anderson MJ, Patou G, Pattison JR.** 1993. Human parvovirus infection in homozygous sickle cell disease. *Lancet* **341:**1237–1240.
30. **Miller E, Fairley CK, Cohen BJ, Seng C.** 1998. Immediate and long term outcome of human parvovirus B19 infection in pregnancy. *Br J Obstet Gynaecol* **105:**174–178.
31. **Enders M, Klingel K, Weidner A, Baisch C, Kandolf R, Schalasta G, Enders G.** 2010. Risk of fetal hydrops and non-hydropic late intrauterine fetal death after gestational parvovirus B19 infection. *J Clin Virol* **49:**163–168.
32. **Yaegashi N.** 2000. Pathogenesis of nonimmune hydrops fetalis caused by intrauterine B19 infection. *Tohoku J Exp Med* **190:**65–82.
33. **Brown KE, Green SW, Antunez de Mayolo J, Young NS, Bellanti JA, Smith SD, Smith TJ.** 1994. Congenital anaemia after transplacental B19 parvovirus infection. *Lancet* **343:**895–896.
34. **Heegaard ED, Hasle H, Skibsted L, Bock J, Brown KE.** 2000. Congenital anemia caused by parvovirus B19 infection. *Pediatr Infect Dis J* **19:**1216–1218.
35. **Frickhofen N, Young NS.** 1989. Persistent parvovirus B19 infections in humans. *Microb Pathog* **7:**319–327.
36. **Kurtzman GJ, Meyers P, Cohen B, Amunullah A, Young NS.** 1988. Persistent B19 parvovirus infection as a cause of severe chronic anaemia in children with acute lymphocytic leukaemia. *Lancet* **332:**1159–1162.
37. **Crabol Y, et al.** 2013. Intravenous immunoglobulin therapy for pure red cell aplasia related to human parvovirus B19 infection: a retrospective study of 10 patients and review of the literature. *Clin Infect Dis* **56:**968–977.
38. **Qiu J, Söderlund-Venermo M, Young NS.** 2017. Human parvoviruses. *Clin Microbiol Rev* **30:**43–113.
39. **Bonvicini, F, Bua G, Manaresi E, Gallinella G.** 2016. Enhanced inhibition of parvovirus B19 replication by cidofovir in extendedly exposed erythroid progenitor cells. *Virus Res* **220:**47–51.
40. **Ozawa K, Kurtzman G, Young N.** 1987. Productive infection by B19 parvovirus of human erythroid bone marrow cells in vitro. *Blood* **70:**384–391.
41. **Van Horn DK, Mortimer PP, Young N, Hanson GR.** 1986. Human parvovirus-associated red cell aplasia in the absence of underlying hemolytic anemia. *Am J Pediatr Hematol Oncol* **8:**235–239.
42. **Sakata H, Matsubayashi K, Ihara H, Sato S, Kato T, Wakisaka A, Tadokoro K, Yu MY, Baylis SA, Ikeda H, Takamoto S.** 2012. Impact of chemiluminescent enzyme immunoassay screening for human parvovirus B19 antigen in Japanese blood donors. *Transfusion* **53:**2556–2566.

43. **Baylis SA, Chudy M, Blümel J, Pisani G, Candotti D, José M, Heath AB.** 2010. Collaborative study to establish a replacement World Health Organization International Standard for parvovirus B19 DNA nucleic acid amplification technology (NAT)-based assays. *Vox Sang* **98**(3p2)**:**441–446.
44. **Manaresi E, Gallinella G, Zuffi E, Bonvicini F, Zerbini M, Musiani M.** 2002. Diagnosis and quantitative evaluation of parvovirus B19 infections by real-time PCR in the clinical laboratory. *J Med Virol* **67:**275–281.
45. **Hokynar K, Norja P, Laitinen H, Palomäki P, Garbarg-Chenon A, Ranki A, Hedman K, Söderlund-Venermo M.** 2004. Detection and differentiation of human parvovirus variants by commercial quantitative real-time PCR tests. *J Clin Microbiol* **42:**2013–2019.
46. **Wong S, Brown KE.** 2006. Development of an improved method of detection of infectious parvovirus B19. *J Clin Virol* **35:**407–413.
47. **Toppinen, M, Norja P, Aaltonen LM, Wessberg S, Hedman L, Soderlund-Venermo M, Hedman K.** 2015. A new quantitative PCR for human parvovirus B19 genotypes. *J Virol Methods* **218:**40–45.
48. **Nguyen QT, Wong S, Heegaard ED, Brown KE.** 2002. Identification and characterization of a second novel human erythrovirus variant, A6. *Virology* **301:**374–380.
49. **Baylis SA, Ma L, Padley DJ, Heath AB, Yu MW, Collaborative Study Group.** 2012. Collaborative study to establish a World Health Organization International genotype panel for parvovirus B19 DNA nucleic acid amplification technology (NAT)-based assays. *Vox Sang* **102:**204–211.
50. **Baylis SA, Fryer JF, Grabarczyk P.** 2007. Effects of probe binding mutations in an assay designed to detect parvovirus B19: implications for the quantitation of different virus genotypes. *J Virol Methods* **139:**97–99.
51. **Bostic JR, Brown KE, Young NS, Koenig S.** 1999. Quantitative analysis of neutralizing immune responses to human parvovirus B19 using a novel reverse transcriptase-polymerase chain reaction-based assay. *J Infect Dis* **179:**619–626.
52. **Takahashi T, Ozawa K, Takahashi K, Asano S, Takaku F.** 1990. Susceptibility of human erythropoietic cells to B19 parvovirus in vitro increases with differentiation. *Blood* **75:**603–610.
53. **Komatsu N, Yamamoto M, Fujita H, Miwa A, Hatake K, Endo T, Okano H, Katsube T, Fukumaki Y, Sassa S, Miura Y.** 1993. Establishment and characterization of an erythropoietin-dependent subline, UT-7/Epo, derived from human leukemia cell line, UT-7. *Blood* **82:**456–464.
54. **Shimomura S, Komatsu N, Frickhofen N, Anderson S, Kajigaya S, Young NS.** 1992. First continuous propagation of B19 parvovirus in a cell line. *Blood* **79:**18–24.
55. **Miyagawa E, Yoshida T, Takahashi H, Yamaguchi K, Nagano T, Kiriyama Y, Okochi K, Sato H.** 1999. Infection of the erythroid cell line, KU812Ep6 with human parvovirus B19 and its application to titration of B19 infectivity. *J Virol Methods* **83:**45–54.
56. **Yaegashi N, Shiraishi H, Takeshita T, Nakamura M, Yajima A, Sugamura K.** 1989. Propagation of human parvovirus B19 in primary culture of erythroid lineage cells derived from fetal liver. *J Virol* **63:**2422–2426.
57. **Wong S, Zhi N, Filippone C, Keyvanfar K, Kajigaya S, Brown KE, Young NS.** 2008. Ex vivo-generated CD36+ erythroid progenitors are highly permissive to human parvovirus B19 replication. *J Virol* **82:**2470–2476.
58. **Servant A, Laperche S, Lallemand F, Marinho V, De Saint Maur G, Meritet JF, Garbarg-Chenon A.** 2002. Genetic diversity within human erythroviruses: identification of three genotypes. *J Virol* **76:**9124–9134.
59. **Nguyen QT, Sifer C, Schneider V, Allaume X, Servant A, Bernaudin F, Auguste V, Garbarg-Chenon A.** 1999. Novel human erythrovirus associated with transient aplastic anemia. *J Clin Microbiol* **37:**2483–2487.
60. **Candotti D, Etiz N, Parsyan A, Allain JP.** 2004. Identification and characterization of persistent human erythrovirus infection in blood donor samples. *J Virol* **78:**12169–12178.
61. **Norja P, Hokynar K, Aaltonen LM, Chen R, Ranki A, Partio EK, Kiviluoto O, Davidkin I, Leivo T, Eis-Hübinger AM, Schneider B, Fischer HP, Tolba R, Vapalahti O, Vaheri A, Söderlund-Venermo M, Hedman K.** 2006. Bioportfolio: lifelong persistence of variant and prototypic erythrovirus DNA genomes in human tissue. *Proc Natl Acad Sci USA* **103:**7450–7453.
62. **Blümel J, Eis-Hübinger AM, Stühler A, Bönsch C, Gessner M, Löwer J.** 2005. Characterization of parvovirus B19 genotype 2 in KU812Ep6 cells. *J Virol* **79:**14197–14206.
63. **Cohen BJ, Gandhi J, Clewley JP.** 2006. Genetic variants of parvovirus B19 identified in the United Kingdom: implications for diagnostic testing. *J Clin Virol* **36:**152–155.
64. **Wong S, Young NS, Brown KE.** 2003. Prevalence of parvovirus B19 in liver tissue: no association with fulminant hepatitis or hepatitis-associated aplastic anemia. *J Infect Dis* **187:**1581–1586.
65. **Sanabani S, Neto WK, Pereira J, Sabino EC.** 2006. Sequence variability of human erythroviruses present in bone marrow of Brazilian patients with various parvovirus B19-related hematological symptoms. *J Clin Microbiol* **44:**604–606.
66. **Corcoran C, Hardie D, Yeats J, Smuts H.** 2010. Genetic variants of human parvovirus B19 in South Africa: cocirculation of three genotypes and identification of a novel subtype of genotype 1. *J Clin Microbiol* **48:**137–142.
67. **Schneider, B, Fryer JF, Oldenburg J, Brackmann HH, Baylis SA, Eis-Hubinger AM.** 2008. Frequency of contamination of coagulation factor concentrates with novel human parvovirus PARV4. *Haemophilia* **14:**978–986.
68. **Corcoran A, Doyle S, Allain JP, Candotti D, Parsyan A.** 2005. Evidence of serological cross-reactivity between genotype 1 and genotype 3 erythrovirus infections. *J Virol* **79:**5238–5239, author reply 5239.
69. **Ekman A, Hokynar K, Kakkola L, Kantola K, Hedman L, Bondén H, Gessner M, Aberham C, Norja P, Miettinen S, Hedman K, Söderlund-Venermo M.** 2007. Biological and immunological relations among human parvovirus B19 genotypes 1 to 3. *J Virol* **81:**6927–6935.
70. **Blümel J, Rinckel LA, Lee DC, Roth NJ, Baylis SA.** 2012. Inactivation and neutralization of parvovirus B19 Genotype 3. *Transfusion* **52:**1490–1497.
71. **Fridell E, Trojnar J, Wahren B.** 1989. A new peptide for human parvovirus B19 antibody detection. *Scand J Infect Dis* **21:**597–603.
72. **Morinet F, D'Auriol L, Tratschin JD, Galibert F.** 1989. Expression of the human parvovirus B19 protein fused to protein A in *Escherichia coli*: recognition by IgM and IgG antibodies in human sera. *J Gen Virol* **70:**3091–3097.
73. **Brown CS, Salimans MM, Noteborn MH, Weiland HT.** 1990. Antigenic parvovirus B19 coat proteins VP1 and VP2 produced in large quantities in a baculovirus expression system. *Virus Res* **15:**197–211.
74. **Lowin T, Raab U, Schroeder J, Franssila R, Modrow S.** 2005. Parvovirus B19 VP2-proteins produced in *Saccharomyces cerevisiae*: comparison with VP2-particles produced by baculovirus-derived vectors. *J Vet Med B Infect Dis Vet Public Health* **52:**348–352.
75. **Goeyvaerts N, Hens N, Aerts M, Beutels P.** 2011. Model structure analysis to estimate basic immunological processes and maternal risk for parvovirus B19. *Biostatistics* **12:**283–302.
76. **Söderlund M, Brown CS, Spaan WJ, Hedman L, Hedman K.** 1995. Epitope type-specific IgG responses to capsid proteins VP1 and VP2 of human parvovirus B19. *J Infect Dis* **172:**1431–1436.
77. **Musiani M, Manaresi E, Gallinella G, Venturoli S, Zuffi E, Zerbini M.** 2000. Immunoreactivity against linear epitopes of parvovirus B19 structural proteins. Immunodominance of the amino-terminal half of the unique region of VP1. *J Med Virol* **60:**347–352.
78. **Kurtzman GJ, Cohen BJ, Field AM, Oseas R, Blaese RM, Young NS.** 1989. Immune response to B19 parvovirus and an antibody defect in persistent viral infection. *J Clin Invest* **84:**1114–1123.

79. **Söderlund M, Brown CS, Cohen BJ, Hedman K.** 1995. Accurate serodiagnosis of B19 parvovirus infections by measurement of IgG avidity. *J Infect Dis* **171:**710–713.
80. **Enders M, Weidner A, Rosenthal T, Baisch C, Hedman L, Söderlund-Venermo M, Hedman K.** 2008. Improved diagnosis of gestational parvovirus B19 infection at the time of nonimmune fetal hydrops. *J Infect Dis* **197:**58–62.
81. **Page, C, Francois C, Goeb V, Duverlie G.** 2015. Human parvovirus B19 and autoimmune diseases. Review of the literature and pathophysiological hypotheses. *J Clin Virol* **72:**69–74.
82. **Thomas HI, Barrett E, Hesketh LM, Wynne A, Morgan-Capner P.** 1999. Simultaneous IgM reactivity by EIA against more than one virus in measles, parvovirus B19 and rubella infection. *J Clin Virol* **14:**107–118.
83. **Maple PA, Hedman L, Dhanilall P, Kantola K, Nurmi V, Söderlund-Venermo M, Brown KE, Hedman K.** 2014. Identification of past and recent parvovirus B19 infection in immunocompetent individuals by quantitative PCR and enzyme immunoassays: a dual-laboratory study. *J Clin Microbiol* **52:**947–956.
84. **Allander T, Tammi MT, Eriksson M, Bjerkner A, Tiveljung-Lindell A, Andersson B.** 2005. Cloning of a human parvovirus by molecular screening of respiratory tract samples. *Proc Natl Acad Sci USA* **102:**12891–12896.
85. **Arthur JL, Higgins GD, Davidson GP, Givney RC, Ratcliff RM.** 2009. A novel bocavirus associated with acute gastroenteritis in Australian children. *PLoS Pathog* **5:**e1000391.
86. **Kapoor A, Slikas E, Simmonds P, Chieochansin T, Naeem A, Shaukat S, Alam MM, Sharif S, Angez M, Zaidi S, Delwart E.** 2009. A newly identified bocavirus species in human stool. *J Infect Dis* **199:**196–200.
87. **Kapoor A, Simmonds P, Slikas E, Li L, Bodhidatta L, Sethabutr O, Triki H, Bahri O, Oderinde BS, Baba MM, Bukbuk DN, Besser J, Bartkus J, Delwart E.** 2010. Human bocaviruses are highly diverse, dispersed, recombination prone, and prevalent in enteric infections. *J Infect Dis* **201:**1633–1643.
88. **Chen AY, Cheng F, Lou S, Luo Y, Liu Z, Delwart E, Pintel D, Qiu J.** 2010. Characterization of the gene expression profile of human bocavirus. *Virology* **403:**145–154.
89. **Kapoor A, Hornig M, Asokan A, Williams B, Henriquez JA, Lipkin WI.** 2011. Bocavirus episome in infected human tissue contains non-identical termini. *PLoS One* **6:**e21362.
90. **Jartti T, Hedman K, Jartti L, Ruuskanen O, Allander T, Söderlund-Venermo M.** 2012. Human bocavirus-the first 5 years. *Rev Med Virol* **22:**46–64.
91. **Schildgen O, Müller A, Allander T, Mackay IM, Völz S, Kupfer B, Simon A.** 2008. Human bocavirus: passenger or pathogen in acute respiratory tract infections? *Clin Microbiol Rev* **21:**291–304.
92. **Manning A, Russell V, Eastick K, Leadbetter GH, Hallam N, Templeton K, Simmonds P.** 2006. Epidemiological profile and clinical associations of human bocavirus and other human parvoviruses. *J Infect Dis* **194:**1283–1290.
93. **Kantola K, Hedman L, Allander T, Jartti T, Lehtinen P, Ruuskanen O, Hedman K, Söderlund-Venermo M.** 2008. Serodiagnosis of human bocavirus infection. *Clin Infect Dis* **46:**540–546.
94. **Khamrin P, Malasao R, Chaimongkol N, Ukarapol N, Kongsricharoern T, Okitsu S, Hayakawa S, Ushijima H, Maneekarn N.** 2012. Circulating of human bocavirus 1, 2, 3, and 4 in pediatric patients with acute gastroenteritis in Thailand. *Infect Genet Evol* **12:**565–569.
95. **Vicente D, Cilla G, Montes M, Pérez-Yarza EG, Pérez-Trallero E.** 2007. Human bocavirus, a respiratory and enteric virus. *Emerg Infect Dis* **13:**636–637.
96. **Don M, Söderlund-Venermo M, Valent F, Lahtinen A, Hedman L, Canciani M, Hedman K, Korppi M.** 2010. Serologically verified human bocavirus pneumonia in children. *Pediatr Pulmonol* **45:**120–126.
97. **Söderlund-Venermo M, Lahtinen A, Jartti T, Hedman L, Kemppainen K, Lehtinen P, Allander T, Ruuskanen O, Hedman K.** 2009. Clinical assessment and improved diagnosis of bocavirus-induced wheezing in children, Finland. *Emerg Infect Dis* **15:**1423–1430.
98. **Christensen A, Nordbø SA, Krokstad S, Rognlien AG, Døllner H.** 2010. Human bocavirus in children: monodetection, high viral load and viraemia are associated with respiratory tract infection. *J Clin Virol* **49:**158–162.
99. **Nawaz S, Allen DJ, Aladin F, Gallimore C, Iturriza-Gómara M.** 2012. Human bocaviruses are not significantly associated with gastroenteritis: results of retesting archive DNA from a case control study in the UK. *PLoS One* **7:**e41346.
100. **Risku M, Kätkä M, Lappalainen S, Räsänen S, Vesikari T.** 2012. Human bocavirus types 1, 2 and 3 in acute gastroenteritis of childhood. *Acta Paediatr* **101:**e405–e410.
101. **Abdel-Moneim, AS, Kamel MM, Hamed DH, Hassan SS, Soliman MS, Al-Quraishy SA, El Kholy AA.** 2016. A novel primer set for improved direct gene sequencing of human bocavirus genotype-1 from clinical samples. *J Virol Methods* **228:**108–113.
102. **Allander T, Jartti T, Gupta S, Niesters HG, Lehtinen P, üsterback R, Vuorinen T, Waris M, Bjerkner A, Tiveljung-Lindell A, van den Hoogen BG, Hyypiä T, Ruuskanen O.** 2007. Human bocavirus and acute wheezing in children. *Clin Infect Dis* **44:**904–910.
103. **Kantola K, Sadeghi M, Antikainen J, Kirveskari J, Delwart E, Hedman K, Söderlund-Venermo M.** 2010. Real-time quantitative PCR detection of four human bocaviruses. *J Clin Microbiol* **48:**4044–4050.
104. **Foulongne V, Rodière M, Segondy M.** 2006. Human bocavirus in children. *Emerg Infect Dis* **12:**862–863.
105. **Lin, F, Zeng A, Yang N, Lin H, Yang E, Wang S, Pintel D, Qiu J.** 2007. Quantification of human bocavirus in lower respiratory tract infections in China. *Infect Agents Cancer* **2:**3.
106. **Lu X, Chittaganpitch M, Olsen SJ, Mackay IM, Sloots TP, Fry AM, Erdman DD.** 2006. Real-time PCR assays for detection of bocavirus in human specimens. *J Clin Microbiol* **44:**3231–3235.
107. **Niang MN, Diop OM, Sarr FD, Goudiaby D, Malou-Sompy H, Ndiaye K, Vabret A, Baril L.** 2010. Viral etiology of respiratory infections in children under 5 years old living in tropical rural areas of Senegal: the EVIRA project. *J Med Virol* **82:**866–872.
108. **Qu XW, Duan ZJ, Qi ZY, Xie ZP, Gao HC, Liu WP, Huang CP, Peng FW, Zheng LS, Hou YD.** 2007. Human bocavirus infection, People's Republic of China. *Emerg Infect Dis* **13:**165–168.
109. **Regamey N, Kaiser L, Roiha HL, Deffernez C, Kuehni CE, Latzin P, Aebi C, Frey U, Swiss Paediatric Respiratory Research Group.** 2008. Viral etiology of acute respiratory infections with cough in infancy: a community-based birth cohort study. *Pediatr Infect Dis J* **27:**100–105.
110. **Schenk T, Huck B, Forster J, Berner R, Neumann-Haefelin D, Falcone V.** 2007. Human bocavirus DNA detected by quantitative real-time PCR in two children hospitalized for lower respiratory tract infection. *Eur J Clin Microbiol Infect Dis* **26:**147–149.
111. **Tozer SJ, Lambert SB, Whiley DM, Bialasiewicz S, Lyon MJ, Nissen MD, Sloots TP.** 2009. Detection of human bocavirus in respiratory, fecal, and blood samples by real-time PCR. *J Med Virol* **81:**488–493.
112. **Huang Q, Deng X, Yan Z, Cheng F, Luo Y, Shen W, Lei-Butters DC, Chen AY, Li Y, Tang L, Söderlund-Venermo M, Engelhardt JF, Qiu J.** 2012. Establishment of a reverse genetics system for studying human bocavirus in human airway epithelia. *PLoS Pathog* **8:**e1002899.
113. **Dijkman R, Koekkoek SM, Molenkamp R, Schildgen O, van der Hoek L.** 2009. Human bocavirus can be cultured in differentiated human airway epithelial cells. *J Virol* **83:**7739–7748.
114. **Kantola K, Hedman L, Arthur J, Alibeto A, Delwart E, Jartti T, Ruuskanen O, Hedman K, Söderlund-Venermo M.** 2011. Seroepidemiology of human bocaviruses 1-4. *J Infect Dis* **204:**1403–1412.
115. **Lindner J, Karalar L, Zehentmeier S, Plentz A, Pfister H, Struff W, Kertai M, Segerer H, Modrow S.** 2008. Humoral immune response against human bocavirus VP2 virus-like particles. *Viral Immunol* **21:**443–449.

116. **Hedman L, Söderlund-Venermo M, Jartti T, Ruuskanen O, Hedman K.** 2010. Dating of human bocavirus infection with protein-denaturing IgG-avidity assays—secondary immune activations are ubiquitous in immunocompetent adults. *J Clin Virol* **48:**44–48
117. **Jones MS, Kapoor A, Lukashov VV, Simmonds P, Hecht F, Delwart E.** 2005. New DNA viruses identified in patients with acute viral infection syndrome. *J Virol* **79:**8230–8236.
118. **Fryer JF, Kapoor A, Minor PD, Delwart E, Baylis SA.** 2006. Novel parvovirus and related variant in human plasma. *Emerg Infect Dis* **12:**151–154.
119. **Maple PA, Beard S, Parry RP, Brown KE.** 2013. Testing UK blood donors for exposure to human parvovirus 4 using a time-resolved fluorescence immunoassay to screen sera and Western blot to confirm reactive samples. *Transfusion* **53:**2575-2584.
120. **Sharp CP, Lail A, Donfield S, Simmons R, Leen C, Klenerman P, Delwart E, Gomperts ED, Simmonds P.** 2009. High frequencies of exposure to the novel human parvovirus PARV4 in hemophiliacs and injection drug users, as detected by a serological assay for PARV4 antibodies. *J Infect Dis* **200:**1119–1125.
121. **Drexler JF, Reber U, Muth D, Herzog P, Annan A, Ebach F, Sarpong N, Acquah S, Adlkofer J, Adu-Sarkodie Y, Panning M, Tannich E, May J, Drosten C, Eis-Hübinger AM.** 2012. Human parvovirus 4 in nasal and fecal specimens from children, Ghana. *Emerg Infect Dis* **18:**1650–1653.
122. **Sharp CP, Lail A, Donfield S, Gomperts ED, Simmonds P.** 2012. Virologic and clinical features of primary infection with human parvovirus 4 in subjects with hemophilia: frequent transmission by virally inactivated clotting factor concentrates. *Transfusion* **52:**1482–1489.
123. **Matthews PC, Malik A, Simmons R, Sharp C, Simmonds P, Klenerman P.** 2014. PARV4: an emerging tetraparvovirus. *PLoS Pathog* **10:**e1004036.
124. **Phan TG, Vo NP, Bonkoungou IJ, Kapoor A, Barro N, O'Ryan M, Kapusinszky B, Wang C, Delwart E.** 2012. Acute diarrhea in West African children: diverse enteric viruses and a novel parvovirus genus. *J Virol* **86:** 11024–11030.
125. **Yahiro T, Wangchuk S, Tshering K, Bandhari P, Zangmo S, Dorji T, Tshering K, Matsumoto T, Nishizono A, Söderlund-Venermo M, Ahmed K.** 2014. Novel human bufavirus genotype 3 in children with severe diarrhea, Bhutan. *Emerg Infect Dis* **20:**1037–1039.
126. **Altay A, Yahiro T, Bozdayi G, Matsumoto T, Sahin F, Ozkan S, Nishizono A, Söderlund-Venermo M, Ahmed K.** 2015. Bufavirus genotype 3 in Turkish children with severe diarrhoea. *Clin Microbiol Infect* **21:**965.e1–965.e4.
127. **Ayouni S, Estienney M, Hammami S, Guediche MN, Pothier P, Aouni M, Belliot G, de Rougemont A.** 2016. Cosavirus, salivirus and bufavirus in diarrheal Tunisian infants. *PLoS One* **11:**e0162255.
128. **Chieochansin T, Vutithanachot V, Theamboonlers A, Poovorawan Y.** 2015. Bufavirus in fecal specimens of patients with and without diarrhea in Thailand. *Arch Virol* **160:**1781–1784.
129. **Huang DD, Wang W, Lu QB, Zhao J, Guo CT, Wang HY, Zhang XA, Tong YG, Liu W, Cao WC.** 2015. Identification of bufavirus-1 and bufavirus-3 in feces of patients with acute diarrhea, China. *Sci Rep* **5:**13272.
130. **Väisänen E, Paloniemi M, Kuisma I, Lithovius V, Kumar A, Franssila R, Ahmed K, Delwart E, Vesikari T, Hedman K, Söderlund-Venermo M.** 2016. Epidemiology of two human protoparvoviruses, bufavirus and tusavirus. *Sci Rep* **6:**39267.
131. **Phan TG, Sdiri-Loulizi K, Aouni M, Ambert-Balay K, Pothier P, Deng X, Delwart E.** 2014. New parvovirus in child with unexplained diarrhea, Tunisia. *Emerg Infect Dis* **20:**1911–1913.

Poxviruses

VICTORIA A. OLSON, P. S. SATHESHKUMAR, AND INGER K. DAMON

110

TAXONOMY

All poxviruses described in this chapter belong to the family *Poxviridae* and subfamily *Chordopoxviridae* (see chapter 80 of this volume). The genera and species of the viruses discussed in this chapter are shown in Table 1. DNA-based assays, including DNA sequencing, are the most precise methods for poxvirus genus, species, strain, and variant identification and differentiation. The G+C contents of orthopoxviruses (OPXVs), yatapoxviruses, *Molluscum contagiosum virus* (MCV), and parapoxviruses are ~33, ~32, ~60, and ~63%, respectively.

DESCRIPTION OF THE AGENTS

Virions are large and brick shaped (OPXVs, yatapoxviruses, and molluscipoxvirus) or ovoid (parapoxviruses). Virions range in length from 220 to 450 nm and in width and depth from 140 to 260 nm. The appearances of virions under an electron microscope vary somewhat with sample preparation. By cryo-electron microscopy, in unstained, unfixed vitrified specimens, vaccinia virus (VACV) appears as smooth, rounded rectangles and has a uniform core surrounded by a 30-nm-thick membrane. In conventional negatively stained thin sections, the core appears dumbbell shaped and is surrounded by a complex series of membranes. Lateral bodies occupy the space between the outer membrane and the bar of the dumbbell and may play a role in immunomodulation (1).

Virus particles contain about half of the approximately 200 proteins encoded by the viral genome. Virions consist of structural proteins and enzymes, including a virtually complete RNA polymerase system for primary transcription of viral genes (2). The genome is a 130- to 375-kbp (depending upon the genus) double-stranded DNA molecule that is encapsidated in a nucleoprotein complex inside the core. The genome is covalently closed at each end, and its ends are hairpin-like telomeres. Complete genome DNA sequences have been reported for several different poxviruses. GenBank entries are compiled at a dedicated website (https://virology.uvic.ca/).

During virus replication (2), virion morphogenesis begins in the cytoplasm in areas known as cytoplasmic viral factories, where cellular organelles are largely absent. Thin-section electron microscopy observations of cells early after infection show crescent-shaped membrane structures, which progress to ovoid structures, called immature virions, which enclose a dense nucleoprotein complex. Primary transcription precedes the production of the crescents (cup shaped in three dimensions) and the immature virions. Brick-shaped, membrane-covered mature virions (MVs; also known as intracellular MVs) form as the viral core condenses. These features aid the electron microscopist in the identification of poxviruses in clinical materials (3).

A small portion of MVs may be further transported on microtubules from the viral factory and processed to acquire a bilayer tegument (envelope) of Golgi or endosomal membrane that contains specific viral proteins. The intracellular enveloped MV then moves along cellular microtubules to the cell surface, where the outermost membrane fuses with the cellular membrane to reveal a cell-associated enveloped virus (EV) on the cell surface. The cell-associated EV can prompt actin polymerization behind the virion, which may facilitate cell-to-cell infection with virus. EVs can also exit the cell to spread more distantly.

To date, cellular proteins that function as a poxvirus receptor have not been identified. EV and MV forms of VACV attach to cells differently; however, the MV membrane possesses an entry-fusion complex required for entry into the host cell. The common result of entry is uncoating of the particle, release of viral contents into the cell, and initiation of virus-controlled transcription of early-class proteins. Reviews of virion entry, morphogenesis, and exiting processes have been published (4–7).

EPIDEMIOLOGY AND TRANSMISSION

All current, naturally occurring poxviruses that infect humans are sporadic zoonotic agents except the *Molluscipoxvirus* MCV, which is transmitted strictly between humans. The zoonotic poxviruses include members of the genera OPXV (monkeypox virus [MPXV], cowpox virus [CPXV], and VACV subspecies, including buffalopox virus [BPXV]), *Parapoxvirus* (orf, pseudocowpox, sealpox, and papular stomatitis viruses), and *Yatapoxvirus* (tanapox virus [TPV], Yaba monkey tumor virus [YMTV], and Yaba-like disease virus [YLDV]). Orf virus and MCV infections are the most common poxvirus infections worldwide. These dermatologic lesions often can be readily identified, and laboratory confirmation of clinical diagnosis is often not utilized (8–10).

TABLE 1 Taxonomy of poxviruses that infect humans

Genus	Species
Orthopoxvirus	*Variola virus, Vaccinia virus, Cowpox virus, Monkeypox virus*
Parapoxvirus	*Orf virus, Pseudocowpox virus,*[a] *Bovine papular stomatitis virus, Sealpox virus*
Yatapoxvirus	*Tanapox virus, Yaba-like disease virus, Yaba monkey tumor virus*
Molluscipoxvirus	*Molluscum contagiosum virus*

[a]Causes milker's nodule in humans.

Orthopoxviruses

VARV

Variola virus (VARV), the cause of smallpox, had a strict human host range and no known animal reservoir. The virus was most often transmitted between humans by large-droplet respiratory particles inhaled by susceptible persons who had close, face-to-face contact with an infectious person. It was spread less commonly by aerosol, by direct contact with the rash lesion, or by sloughed crust material from the scab (11). Smallpox is no longer found in nature after a coordinated global vaccination campaign, and the known stocks of VARV are held at two World Health Organization (WHO) Collaborating Centers.

MPXV

Human monkeypox was first reported in 1970 in the Democratic Republic of Congo (DRC). Since 1970, the disease has been seen in Liberia, the Ivory Coast, Sierra Leone, Nigeria, Benin, Cameroon, Republic of Congo, Central African Republic, and Gabon, but most cases have been in the DRC. In the 1980s, serosurveys and virologic investigations in the DRC by the WHO indicated that (i) monkeys are sporadically infected, as are humans; (ii) three-fourths of cases, mainly those in children under 15 years of age, were from animal contact; (iii) the protective efficacy of smallpox vaccination is about 85%; (iv) MPXV has a broad host range, including squirrels (*Funisciurus* spp. and *Heliosciurus* spp.); and (v) human monkeypox has a secondary attack rate of 8% among unvaccinated contacts within households (i.e., it is much less transmissible than smallpox). In an outbreak in the DRC, about 250 serosubstantiated cases of monkeypox occurred among 0.5 million people in 78 villages from February 1996 to October 1997. Unlike those in the earlier investigations, about three-fourths of the cases appeared to result from secondary human-to-human transmission; within households, the transmission rate appeared to be about the same as that found in the 1981 to 1986 surveillance (12–15). More recent case series have been reported from the DRC (16, 17), and disease with a sustained chain of human-to-human transmission was reported in the Republic of Congo in 2003 (18).

The emergence of monkeypox in the United States during an outbreak in 2003 provides another example of the ability of this zoonotic disease to exploit new ecologic niches. North American prairie dogs, which became diseased after exposure to infected West African rodent(s), subsequently infected and caused illness in the U.S. human population (19). The characterization of human disease in the United States caused by this imported West African MPXV variant, and its comparison with disease classically described in the Congo Basin in the 1980s, enabled clinical and epidemiologic descriptions of distinct monkeypox diseases (20, 21).

VACV

Certain strains of VACV were used for human vaccination to globally eradicate smallpox (11, 22). Since the early 1980s, vaccinia and certain other poxviruses have served as recombinant vectors for the expression of a variety of proteins, including vaccine immunogens. Infection can be transmitted to laboratory workers by accidental exposure, and significant pathology has been observed in unvaccinated individuals (23). Vaccination is therefore currently recommended for personnel working with live, replicative OPXVs, including VACV.

The origin and natural host of VACV are uncertain (24). VACV infections are not generally regarded as naturally occurring, although vaccinee-to-cattle and cattle-to-human transmissions occurred on farms during the smallpox eradication campaign. Sporadic outbreaks of infection caused by the VACV subspecies BPXV that involve transmission between milking buffalo, cattle, and people have been reported, mainly in India but also in Egypt, Bangladesh, Pakistan, and Indonesia. Vaccinia-like lesions have been observed on the animals' teats and the milkers' hands. Biological data and limited DNA analyses of isolates from an outbreak in India in 1985 suggest that BPXV may be derived from VACV strains transmitted from humans to livestock during the smallpox vaccination era (25).

Quite interestingly, multiple distinct VACVs, possibly related to the vaccine strain used during smallpox eradication in Brazil, were described in cattle and their farm worker handlers in rural Rio de Janeiro (26, 27) as well as various locales within the state of Minas Gerais (26, 28–30). Historic collections, when reevaluated with additional techniques, suggest that vaccinia-like viruses were previously isolated in the 1960s and 1970s (31). Inadvertent exposure to a VACV-vectored recombinant rabies virus vaccine dispersed to control rabies in wildlife has resulted in at least two instances of human infection; in both cases, the bait was encountered via the family dog (32, 33).

CPXV

Cowpox, a rare occupational infection of humans, can be acquired by contact with infected cows. Other animals (e.g., infected rats, pet cats, and zoo and circus elephants) have more often been sources of the disease in contemporary settings. CPXV is a rather diverse species and has been isolated from humans and a variety of animals in Europe and adjoining regions of Asia (34, 35). An outbreak in Europe associated human disease to contact with pet rats (36). A serosurvey of wild animals in Great Britain found OPXV antibodies in a portion of bank and field voles and wood mice, which is consistent with small rodents being reservoir hosts (37).

Yatapoxviruses

The epidemiology and natural history of yatapoxviruses are poorly understood. YMTV and YLDV infections have occurred in animal handlers (38); however, TPV is the main naturally occurring human pathogen in the genus *Yatapoxvirus* (39). Tanapox is an endemic zoonosis of equatorial Africa that is thought to be transmitted mechanically to humans by biting insects, especially during the rainy season (50). Reports have demonstrated that travelers to regions where the disease is endemic can be infected (41, 42).

Parapoxviruses

Many different parapoxvirus diseases occur in humans (39, 43), generally as occupational infections: milker's nodule (in dairy cattle, the disease is termed pseudocowpox or paravaccinia), orf (in sheep and goats, the disease has been referred to as orf, contagious ecthyma, contagious pustular dermatitis, contagious pustular stomatitis, and sore mouth), and papular stomatitis (in calves and beef cattle, the disease is termed bovine papular stomatitis). Parapoxvirus infections are transmitted to humans by direct contact with infected livestock through abraded skin on the hands and fingers, and ocular autoinoculation sometimes occurs (39, 43). Sealpox virus infections have been transmitted to humans from pinnipeds (44).

Molluscipoxvirus

MCV is the sole member of the genus *Molluscipoxvirus*. MCV appears to have a human-restricted host range, and it does not grow readily in culture. Molluscum contagiosum occurs worldwide. In children it is transmitted by direct skin contact, and sexual transmission occurs in adults (39).

CLINICAL SIGNIFICANCE

Orthopoxviruses

A global commission of the WHO declared smallpox eradicated in December 1979, and the declaration was sanctioned by the World Health Assembly in May 1980 (11). Human monkeypox, an emerging zoonotic smallpox-like disease caused by MPXV, with recurrent (and likely endemic) disease in the Congo Basin countries of Africa, is now regarded as the most serious naturally occurring human poxvirus infection (12, 16, 20, 45). The emergence of MPXV as a human pathogen in the United States in 2003 is a classic example of a pathogen's exploitation of new ecologic niches and hosts.

VARV

VARV major strains produced "variola major," a syndrome consisting of a severe prodrome, fever, prostration, and a rash. Toxemia or other forms of systemic shock led to case fatality rates of up to 30%, with secondary attack rates of 30 to 80% among unvaccinated contacts within households. VARV minor strains (alastrim, amass, and kaffir viruses) produced "variola minor," a less severe infection with case fatality rates of less than 1%, although secondary attack rates among unvaccinated contacts were as high as rates of VARV major infections. DNA and biological data have indicated that alastrim viruses (VARV minor) obtained from Europe and South America are similar to each other but distinct from the so-called African VARV minor viruses, which appear to be variants of VARV major (8). Epidemiologically, the disease syndromes were discriminated by case fatality rates; current sequence data indicate that the genetic distinctions between strains causing major or minor disease manifestations are multiple and varied. The last naturally occurring smallpox case occurred in Somalia in October 1977, although a fatal laboratory-associated infection with VARV major occurred at the University of Birmingham, Birmingham, England, in August 1978 (11).

Naturally acquired VARV infection caused a systemic febrile rash illness. For ordinary smallpox, the most common clinical presentation, after an asymptomatic incubation period of 10 to 14 days (range, 7 to 17 days), was fever, quickly rising to about 103°F, sometimes with dermal petechiae. Associated constitutional symptoms included backache, headache, vomiting, and prostration. Within a day or two after the incubation period, a systemic rash appeared that was characteristically centrifugally distributed (i.e., lesions were present in greater numbers on the oral mucosa, face, and extremities than on the trunk). Initially, the rash lesions appeared macular, then papular, enlarging and progressing to a vesicle by day 4 to 5 and a pustule by day 7; lesions were encrusted and scabby by day 14 and sloughed off. Skin lesions were deep seated and were in the same stage of development on any one area of the body. Milder and more severe forms of the rash were also documented. Less severe manifestations (modified smallpox, or variola sine eruptione) occurred in some vaccinated individuals, whereas hemorrhagic or flat-pox types of smallpox occurred in patients with impaired immune responses.

VARV major smallpox was differentiated into four main clinical types: (i) ordinary smallpox (~90% of cases) produced viremia, fever, prostration, and rash; (ii) modified smallpox (5% of cases) produced a mild prodrome with few skin lesions in previously vaccinated people; (iii) flat smallpox (5% of cases) produced slowly developing focal lesions with generalized infection and an ~50% fatality rate; and (iv) hemorrhagic smallpox (<1% of cases) induced bleeding into the skin and the mucous membranes and was invariably fatal within a week of onset. A discrete type of the ordinary form resulted from alastrim VARV minor infection (11).

Prior to its eradication, smallpox as a clinical entity was relatively easy to recognize, but other exanthematous illnesses were mistaken for this disease (11). For example, the rash of severe chicken pox, caused by varicella-zoster virus, was often misdiagnosed as that of smallpox. However, chicken pox produces a centripetally distributed rash and rarely appears on the palms and soles. In addition, in the case of chicken pox, prodromal fever and systemic manifestations are mild, if present at all. Chicken pox lesions are superficial, and lesions in different developmental stages may be present on the same area of the body. Other diseases confused with vesicular-stage smallpox included monkeypox, generalized vaccinia, disseminated herpes zoster, disseminated herpes simplex virus infection, drug reactions (eruptions), erythema multiforme, enteroviral infections, scabies, insect bites, impetigo, and molluscum contagiosum. Diseases confused with hemorrhagic smallpox included acute leukemia, meningococcemia, and idiopathic thrombocytopenic purpura. The Centers for Disease Control and Prevention (CDC), in collaboration with numerous professional organizations, has developed an algorithm for evaluating patients for smallpox. The algorithm and additional information are available at https://www.cdc.gov/smallpox/clinicians/diagnosis-evaluation.html. Experience with the algorithm was summarized previously (46).

MPXV

Reviews of human monkeypox infection are available (12, 45). Monkeypox was first recognized by P. von Magnus in Copenhagen, Denmark, in 1958 as an exanthem of primates in captivity. Later, the disease was seen in other captive animals, including primates in zoos and animal import centers.

The clinical appearance of human monkeypox, typified by the Congo Basin variant, is much like that of smallpox, with fever, a centrifugally distributed vesiculopustular rash (appearing also on the palms and soles), respiratory distress, and in some cases, death from systemic shock. Like VARV, MPXV appears to enter through skin abrasions or the mucosa of the upper respiratory tract, where it produces an exanthem and cough. During the primary viremia, the virus migrates to regional lymph nodes, and during secondary viremia, it disseminates throughout the body and the skin rash appears. During the prodrome, lymphadenopathy (generally inguinal) with fever and headache is common. Individual skin lesions develop through stages of macule, papule, vesicle, and pustule. Sequelae involve secondary infections, permanent scarring and pitting at the sites of the lesions, and sometimes alopecia and corneal opacities. Acute illness in the United States in 2003, caused by the West African variant, appeared generally more mild (20, 21); genomic sequence analyses, comparative epidemiologic data, and clinical data support the existence of two distinct clades of MPXV. Additional information on clinical manifestations of disease (47) is also available.

VACV

Humans have historically encountered VACV most commonly in the form of smallpox vaccine (now called vaccinia vaccine), a live-virus preparation that is cross-protective against other OPXV infections. The most recent recommendations of the Advisory Committee on Immunization Practices (ACIP) on vaccinia vaccination are available at https://www.cdc.gov/mmwr/volumes/65/wr/mm6510a2.htm (48). The ACIP recommends vaccination as a safeguard for laboratory and health care workers who are at high risk of OPXV infection. In the United States, the CDC Drug Service provides the vaccine after CDC approval of a formal request for this purpose by the administering physician. Vaccinia immunoglobulin is available to treat possible postvaccination complications, which can be severe.

Vaccination is performed by using a multiple puncture technique that causes a local lesion, which develops and recedes in a distinctive manner in primary vaccinees during a 3-week period. At the site of percutaneous vaccination, a papule forms within 2 to 5 days, and the lesion reaches maximum size (about 1 cm in diameter) by 8 to 10 days postvaccination after evolving through vesicle and pustule stages; an areola may encircle the site. The pustule dries into a scab, which usually separates by 14 to 21 days after vaccination. In some vaccinated children, fevers with temperatures as high as about 100°F have occurred but have been uncommon in adults, and a regional lymphadenopathy has been observed.

Because of an increased risk for serious adverse events, such as eczema vaccinatum or vaccinia necrosum, the ACIP has stated that the vaccine is contraindicated for persons with eczema or immunocompromising conditions. The contraindications of vaccinia vaccination are described in the ACIP report (48). Despite attempts to prescreen potential vaccinees for contraindications, instances of generalized vaccinia rash, which may arise 10 to 14 days postvaccination, continue to be reported (49). On a clinical basis alone, it is often difficult to distinguish between generalized vaccinia, which represents virus presumably spread hematogenously, and a form of erythema multiforme, which may be immunologically mediated. Laboratory identification of virus within the disseminated rash may differentiate these conditions (49). Alternatively, nonreplicating modified vaccinia Ankara-based vaccine is currently being considered for contraindicated individuals.

CPXV

In humans, cowpox lesions occur mainly on the fingers, with reddening and swelling. Autoinoculation of other parts of the body may occur, and severe systemic infections have been reported in those with immune-compromising conditions. Skin lesions are likened to those from a primary vaccinia vaccination. The site becomes papular, and a vesicle develops in 4 to 5 days. Healing takes about 3 weeks (34).

Yatapoxviruses

The three members of the genus *Yatapoxvirus* (TPV, YLDV, and YMTV) are serologically related (38). DNA maps of TPV and YLDV are extremely similar, suggesting that they are the same agent. However, these DNA maps are markedly different from YMTV DNA maps, even though the DNA from the three viruses cross-hybridizes extensively (50).

TPV and YLDV infections in humans consist of a brief fever, followed by development of firm, elevated, round, maculopapular nodules which become necrotic and are distinct from the vesiculopustular lesions of OPXV infections. Generally, few lesions develop, and these occur primarily on the skin of the upper arms, face, neck, or trunk (51). Symptoms that occur prior to the appearance of lesions include fever, backache, and headache. Lesions become umbilicate without pustulation during recovery from infection. They usually heal in 2 to 4 weeks. YMTV produces epidermal histiocytomas, tumor-like masses of histiocytic polygonal mononuclear cell infiltrates that advance to suppurative inflammation.

Parapoxviruses

Human parapoxvirus infection is normally associated with an exposure to sheep, goats, and/or cattle. Milker's nodule occurs as a reddened hemispheric papule that matures into a purplish, smooth, firm nodule varying up to 2 cm in diameter. The lesions usually are not painful and can persist for about 6 weeks. Human orf virus infection is usually found on the fingers, hands, and arms but may also be found on the face and neck. Fever and swelling of draining lymph nodes may be present, and the lesions often ulcerate and are painful. Autoinoculation of the eye may lead to serious sequelae (9). Contact with (e.g., skinning of) certain wild animals, including deer, reindeer, chamois, and Japanese serow, has also been a source of human parapoxvirus infection. Technicians handling gray seals have contracted sealpox virus (43, 44).

Molluscipoxvirus

In children and teenagers, molluscum contagiosum lesions generally appear on the trunk, limbs (except the palms and soles), and face, where there may be ocular involvement. Infection is usually transmitted by direct skin contact. When MCV infection is transmitted sexually among teenagers and adults, the lesions are mostly on the lower abdomen, pubis, inner thighs, and genitalia. Lesions are pearly, flesh-colored, raised, firm, umbilicated nodules, about 5 mm in diameter. The lesions tend to disseminate by autoinoculation. Prior to highly active antiretroviral therapy, MCV was an opportunistic pathogen in approximately 15% of patients with AIDS in the United States. Restriction endonuclease mapping of isolates suggests that there are at least three MCV subtypes (10). Two predominant MCV subtypes, MCV I and MCV II, have been detected in a limited number of samples examined by restriction pattern and base sequence analyses, but no correlation of subtype with disease syndrome or geographic distribution has been confirmed (9, 10). A rapid PCR and restriction fragment length polymorphism analysis using skin lesion material for differentiating the MCV subtypes has been described (52).

Antiviral Therapy

Currently there are no drugs approved for use in the treatment of poxvirus infections; this is an area of active research and development (53). The experimental drug ST-246 (TPOXX), an inhibitor of poxvirus egress, appears to be effective against OPXV diseases, including VARV and MPXV infections of non-human primates (54), and has been used investigationally in the treatment of human smallpox (vaccinia) vaccine adverse events (55). The DNA polymerase inhibitor cidofovir and its orally bioavailable derivative, CMX-001 (brincidofovir), similarly have *in vitro* and *in vivo* data to support anti-OPXV activity and have been used as investigational agents in the treatment of smallpox (vaccinia) vaccine adverse events (56). Vaccinia immunoglobulin is licensed for use as a treatment for severe adverse events associated with vaccination and can be obtained from the CDC.

COLLECTION, HANDLING, AND STORAGE OF SPECIMENS

A suspected case of smallpox should be immediately reported to the appropriate local or state health department. After review by the health department, the case should be immediately reported to the CDC if the diagnosis of smallpox is still suspected. Current international recommendations advise that work with VARV be done using WHO-sanctioned biosafety level 4 (BSL4) laboratories. Two WHO collaborating centers (WHOCC) currently have the capability to handle smallpox specimens: one at the CDC in Atlanta, the other at the State Center for Virology and Biotechnology, Koltsovo, Russia. The WHOCC at the CDC also has containment facilities appropriate to work with MPXV and other exotic poxviruses (e.g., TPV). Generally, clinical specimens suspected of containing other poxviruses (e.g., parapoxviruses and MCV) can be tested by experienced staff using BSL2 containment facilities and equipment. Additionally, laboratories testing samples from laboratory workers with potential occupational exposures to VACV may wish to consider vaccination of staff, in addition to the use of BSL3 containment facilities, equipment, and work practices.

Suitable specimens for laboratory testing of most suspected poxvirus infections are at least two to four scabs and/or material from vesicular lesions. Scabs can be separated from the underlying intact skin with a scalpel or a 26-gauge needle, and each specimen should be stored in separate containers to avoid cross-contamination. Coexistent infectious rash illnesses, including simultaneous chicken pox and monkeypox infections, have been noted (15).

Lesions should be sampled so that both the vesicle fluid and the overlying skin are collected. Once the overlying skin is lifted off and placed in a specimen container, the base of the vesicle should be vigorously swabbed with a wooden applicator or polyester or cotton swab. The viscous material can be submitted on the swab or applied onto a clean glass microscope slide and air dried. A "touch prep" can be prepared by pressing a clean slide onto the opened lesion by using a gradual pressing motion. If available, three electron microscope grids can be applied in succession (shiny side to the unroofed vesicle) to the lesion by using minimal, moderate, and moderate pressure. The glass slides and electron microscope grids should be allowed to air dry for about 10 min and then placed in a slide holder or a grid carrier box for transport to a laboratory.

Alternative lesion sampling processes, including storing material on appropriate filter paper types, are being evaluated. Sample storage in transport medium (as done, for example, with herpesviruses) is discouraged, since specimen dilution decreases the sensitivity of direct evaluation by electron microscopy. Specific recommendations for electron microscopy sampling and specimen processing can be found on the Internet (https://www.cdc.gov/smallpox/lab-personnel/specimen-collection/negative-stain.html). Biopsy of lesions may also provide material suitable for direct viral evaluation or immunohistochemistry. A 3- to 4-mm punch biopsy specimen can be obtained, and the specimen can be bisected, with half placed in formalin for immunohistochemical testing and the remainder placed in a specimen collection container. Blood and throat swabs obtained from patients with suspected smallpox during the prodromal febrile phase and early in the rash phase were also a potential source of virus during the smallpox era (11).

Patient serum can also be obtained for serology to substantiate viral infection diagnoses or to infer a retrospective diagnosis. Paired acute- and convalescent-phase serum specimens can be of great value for diagnosis of infection. In this case, serum should be obtained as early as possible in the disease course and then 3 to 4 weeks later.

Most virus-containing specimens should be stored frozen at −20°C or on dry ice until samples reach their transport destination. Storage at standard refrigerator temperatures is acceptable for less than 7 days. Electron microscopy grids and formalin-fixed tissues should be kept at room temperature.

CLINICAL UTILITY OF LABORATORY TESTS FOR POXVIRUS DIAGNOSIS

Poxvirus infections can often be distinguished by the appearances of rashes and associated dermatopathologies (58). In addition, multiple different clinical laboratory tests can be useful for identifying and differentiating poxviruses, including electron microscopy, antigenic testing, nucleic acid detection, determination of virus growth features, and serology. The utility of these test methods for the diagnosis of poxvirus infections is shown in Table 2.

DIRECT DETECTION

Microscopy

Electron microscopy is a first-line method for laboratory diagnosis of poxvirus infections. Negative-stain electron microscopy of lesion samples was widely used during the smallpox eradication era. Because the clinical diagnosis of

TABLE 2 Diagnostic tests for poxviruses[a]

Virus(es)	HP	EM	HA	NAAT	Isolation	Serology
Orthopoxviruses	X	X	X	X	X[b]	X
Parapoxviruses	X	X		X	X[c]	X
Yatapoxviruses	X	X		X	X[c]	X
Molluscum contagiosum virus	X	X		X		

[a]Abbreviations: HP, histopathology; EM, electron microscopy; HA, hemagglutination; NAAT, nucleic acid test. An X indicates the utility of the test for the specified virus(es).

[b]Pock formation on CAM and tissue culture isolation are useful.

[c]Isolation in tissue culture only; viruses do not produce pocks on CAM.

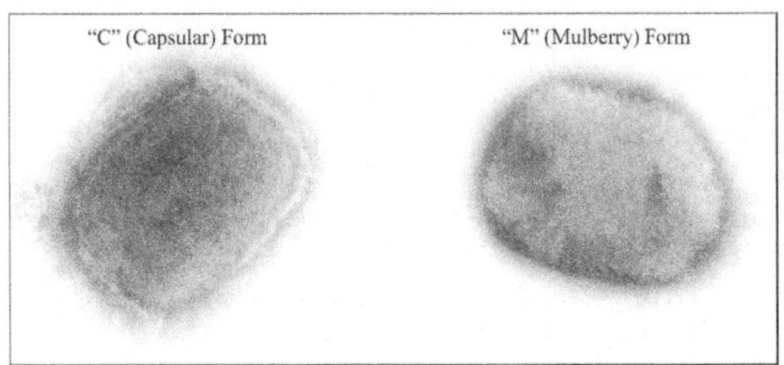

FIGURE 1 A negative-stain electron micrograph demonstrates the two forms of the brick-shaped MPXV from a cell culture. The surfaces of M (mulberry) virions are covered with short, whorled filaments, while C (capsular)-form virions penetrated by stain present as a sharply defined, dense core surrounded by several laminated zones of differing densities. (Image 3945 from the CDC Public Health Image Library; courtesy of C. Goldsmith, I. Damon, and S. Zaki.)

poxvirus infection is now infrequent, electron microscopy observations may provide one of the first clues to the cause of an unidentified rash illness. Although electron microscopy can distinguish between OPXV and parapoxvirus morphologies, it cannot differentiate between species. OPXVs have a distinctive brick-shaped, knobby morphology when examined with sodium phosphotungstate or other heavy-metal negative stains (Fig. 1). Parapoxviruses appear ovoid with a spiraling crisscross surface. The relative sensitivity of the negative-stain method was about 95% for detecting VARVs in smallpox lesions and about 75% for detecting VACV (59, 60). Sensitivity may be improved by directly pressing a prepared grid into the base of an unroofed skin lesion, as described above (61). Descriptions of methods for negative-stain evaluation and pictures of negative-stained particles are available on the Internet (https://www.cdc.gov/smallpox/lab-personnel/specimen-collection/negative-stain.html) and elsewhere (60, 62).

Poxviruses produce inclusions that have characteristic appearances when stained with May-Grunwald Giemsa and hematoxylin-eosin. Perinuclear basophilic or B-type cytoplasmic inclusions (virus factories or viroplasm) are observed in cells infected with any of the poxviruses and represent sites of virus replication. Certain species of OPXVs (e.g., CPXV) produce acidophilic inclusions or A-type inclusions. Depending on the strain, A-type inclusions may or may not contain virions.

Antigen Detection

OPXV is the only genus whose members produce a hemagglutinin antigen, which is detectable by hemadsorption or hemagglutination assays using chicken erythrocytes that are pretested and found to be suitable for such tests. OPXV antigen can also be rapidly detected by the Tetracore Orthopox BioThreat assay, which uses a lateral flow system to rapidly detect the presence of virus in clinical specimens. It has been shown to recognize VACV and MPXV at levels that may be found in rash lesions (63). Direct detection of poxvirus antigens in clinical specimens is not routinely performed in many laboratories as a diagnostic assay.

Nucleic Acid Detection

PCR analysis is used by the WHOCC at the CDC to detect poxvirus DNA in samples. A recent development is the validation of a "pan-poxvirus" PCR assay, which can screen specimens for the presence of poxviruses other than avipoxviruses (64). Multiple single-gene PCR assays, followed by restriction fragment length polymorphism analysis or sequence analysis of the amplicon, permit species identification of OPXVs. A number of different targets are used, including the hemagglutinin gene, which is unique to the genus OPXV, the gene for the B cytokine response modifier (CrmB, one of several different tumor necrosis factor receptor homologs produced by OPXVs), and the gene for the A-type inclusion protein. In these assays, DNA that is present in any OPXV is amplified (Table 3). The amplicon is digested with the appropriate restriction endonuclease, and digested fragments are electrophoresed. Fragment sizes are compared to reference restriction fragment length polymorphism profiles to discriminate species. Conventional PCR tests for other poxvirus genera have also been reported (65). Other nucleic acid diagnostic approaches include random amplified polymorphic DNA fragment length polymorphism for OPXV species and strain discrimination (66, 67). Microchips have also been utilized to identify the poxvirus species by discernment of PCR-amplified, fluorescence-labeled DNA fragment hybridization to OPXV species-specific immobilized DNA.

The high sensitivity of and rapid results from real-time PCR assays make them attractive for laboratory clinical diagnostic use (68). In the United States, many national reference laboratories, as well as the Laboratory Response Network laboratories, use this format of nucleic acid testing for rapid response to diagnose suspected OPXV infections and/or to rule out smallpox infections. The use of a probe or probes in this type of assay allows for the specificity; however, the extreme sensitivity of the assays can lead to false-positive contaminants from specimen carryover. Many of these methods for detection of OPXVs and other poxviruses are summarized in Table 4. These types of assays are performed primarily at specific reference centers, including the CDC Poxvirus Program/WHOCC for Smallpox and Other Poxvirus Infections and certain Laboratory Response Network laboratories proficient in OPXV diagnostics. Several real-time PCR assays for the detection of OPXV or VARV have gained regulatory approval by the Food and Drug Administration.

TABLE 3 Conventional PCR assays for OPXV detection

Target	Primers (amplicon size, bp)	Detection method[a]	Reference(s)
Hemagglutinin	EACP1/EACP2 (Old World viruses) (900)	*Taq*I	83
	NACP1/NACP2 (New World viruses) (600)	RsaI	
CrmB	VL2N/VL33 (vaccinia virus, 1,200; monkeypox, variola, cowpox viruses, 1,300)	NlaIII[b]	84
A-type inclusion body protein	ATI-low-1/ATI-up-1 (1,500–1,700)	BglII or XbaI	85, 86

[a]Amplicons are digested with specified restriction enzymes to distinguish different viruses.
[b]To distinguish monkeypox, variola, and cowpox viruses.

TABLE 4 Real-time PCR assays for poxvirus detection[a]

Genus (genera); species[b]	Genetic target[c]	Platform and method	Comments	Limitations	Limit of detection (no. of genomic copies)	Reference
Orthopoxvirus*, *Parapoxvirus*, *Molluscipoxvirus	Assay 1: E_ORF_C (OPXV) (FAM) Assay 2: orf envelope protein (parapoxvirus) (VIC) Assay 3: MC001R (molluscipoxvirus) (FAM and VIC)	TaqMan	Multiplex assay that detects which genus of poxvirus is causing the infection based on multicolor profile and includes a control for cellular DNA		<10	87
Orthopoxvirus	Hemagglutinin/ A56R	LightCycler with hybridization probes	Melting curve analysis differentiates VARV from other OPXVs	Several cowpox and camelpox virus strains have the same melting temperature as VARV	5–10	88
***Orthopoxvirus*;** *Variola virus*, *Monkeypox virus*, *Cowpox virus*, and *Vaccinia virus*	Assay 1: A38R (VAR) (FAM) Assay 2: B7R (MPXV) (TAMRA) Assay 3: D11L (CWXV) (JOE) Assay 4: B10R (VACV) (Cy5)	TaqMan	Multiplex assay that detects which species of *Orthopoxvirus* is causing the infection based on multicolor profile		NA	66
***Orthopoxvirus*;** *Variola virus* and *Monkeypox virus*	Assay 1: B12R (VARV) (FAM) Assay 2: F13L (MPXV) (JOE)	TaqMan	Multiplex assay with differently labeled probes allows for simultaneous detection and differentiation of viruses		NA	89
***Orthopoxvirus*;** *Variola virus*	Hemagglutinin/ A56R	TaqMan	VARV specific probe cleavage		25	90
***Orthopoxvirus*;** *Variola virus*	Hemagglutinin/ A56R	LightCycler with hybridization probes	Melting curve analysis differentiates VARV from other OPXVs	Several CPXV strains have the same melting temperature as VARV	2.74–9.88	91
***Orthopoxvirus*;** *Variola virus*	Assay 1: Rpo 18 Assay 2: VETF Assay 3: A13L (VARV) Assay 4: A13L (nVAR-OPXV)	LightCycler with hybridization probes	Melting curve analysis differentiates VARV		NA	92
***Orthopoxvirus*;** *Variola virus*	Assay 1: B10R Assay 2: B9R Assay 3: hemagglutinin/A56R	TaqMan		Assay 1 and 2: some CPXV strains are amplified. Assay 3: identical with the assay described in reference 37 with a slightly shortened probe	12–25	93
***Orthopoxvirus*;** *Variola virus*	14 kDa/A27L	LightCycler with hybridization probes	Melting curve analysis differentiates VARV from other OPXVs		>12	94
***Orthopoxvirus*;** *Variola virus*	CrmB	LightCycler with hybridization probes	Melting curve analysis differentiates VARV from other OPXVs	Specific identification of VARV has to be performed by restriction enzyme analysis of PCR amplicons	5	95

(Continued on next page)

TABLE 4 Real-time PCR assays for poxvirus detection[a] *(Continued)*

Genus (genera); species[b]	Genetic target[c]	Platform and method	Comments	Limitations	Limit of detection (no. of genomic copies)	Reference
Orthopoxvirus; *Variola virus*	CrmB	Two TaqMan probes	One probe is VARV specific		10–100	96
Orthopoxvirus; *Variola virus*	Assay 1: A4L Assay 2: A36R Assay 3: A13L Assay 4: E9L	TaqMan	Probes designed to be specific for VARV detection	Certain strains of CPXV were found to cross react with A13L and E9L assays	250	97
Orthopoxvirus; *Variola virus*	14 kDa/A27L	TaqMan	Two probes; one probe is VARV-specific		25	98
Orthopoxvirus; *Variola virus*	Hemagglutinin/A56R	TaqMan	Two probes; one probe is VARV specific		50–100	99
Orthopoxvirus; *Variola virus*	Hemagglutinin/A56R	LightCycler with hybridization probes	Melting curve analysis differentiates VARV from other OPXVs		13–1,300	100
Orthopoxvirus; *Monkeypox virus*	Assay 1: B5R (MPXV) Assay 2: E9L (nVAR-OPXV)		MPXV-specific assay (MGB probe) Nonvariola OPXV detection assay (TaqMan)	MGB probe performs optimally only in the iCycler iQ and SmartCycler platforms	Assay 1: 10 ng Assay 2: 2 pg–20 fg	101
Orthopoxvirus; *Monkeypox virus*	Assay 1: G2R (MPX) Assay 2: G2R (MPXV, West African) Assay 3: C3L (MPXV, Congo Basin)	TaqMan			3.5	102
Orthopoxvirus; *Vaccinia virus*	E9L	TaqMan with MGB probe			NA	103
Orthopoxvirus; *Vaccinia virus*	B8R	TaqMan			10–10^6	104
Orthopoxvirus; *Cowpox virus*	D11L	TaqMan			20	105
Orthopoxvirus; *Cowpox virus*	A55R	TaqMan		Certain CPXVs have this target deleted	NA	106
Orthopoxvirus; *Cowpox virus*	D8L	TaqMan			20	107
Yatapoxvirus	101 nt of PstIL fragment	TaqMan		Detects YLDV, TPV, not YMTV	8	108
Parapoxvirus; *Orf virus*	B2L	TaqMan			10–10^6	109
Parapoxvirus; *Orf virus*	RNA polymerase	TaqMan	Two different primer-probe sets, one specific for parapoxviruses and one specific for orf virus		NA	110
Parapoxvirus; *Orf virus*	DNA polymerase	TaqMan		Not tested for specificity against other parapoxviruses	15	111
Parapoxvirus; *Orf virus*	ORFVO24 (NF-κB inhibitor)	TaqMan		Not tested for specificity against other parapoxviruses	15	112
Parapoxvirus; *Orf virus*	DNA polymerase	TaqMan	Duplex assay using two differently labeled probes, one for orf virus and one for capripoxvirus	Not tested for specificity against other parapoxviruses	175	113

(Continued on next page)

TABLE 4 Real-time PCR assays for poxvirus detection[a] *(Continued)*

Genus (genera); species[b]	Genetic target[c]	Platform and method	Comments	Limitations	Limit of detection (no. of genomic copies)	Reference
Parapoxvirus; *Orf virus*, *Pseudocowpox virus*, and *Bovine papular stomatitis virus*	RNA polymerase gene	TaqMan	Four different primer-probe sets, one generic for parapoxviruses and one each specific for orf, pseudocowpox virus, and bovine papular stomatitis virus		10	114
Parapoxvirus	B2L	TaqMan			4.7	57
Molluscipoxvirus; *Molluscum contagiosum virus*	P43K, MC080R	TaqMan	Pyrosequencing of the p43K product differentiates MCV1 and MCV2		10	115

[a]Abbreviations: FAM, 6-carboxyfluorescein; JOE, 6-carboxy-4′,5′-dichloro-2′,7′-dimethoxyfluorescein; MGB, minor groove binder; NA, not reported; n-VAR-OPXV, non-variola OPXV; TAMRA, 6-carboxytetramethylrhodamine; VETF, virus early transcription factor.

[b]Boldface indicates the genus name.

[c]OPXV assays use the target's vaccinia virus Copenhagen nomenclature.

ISOLATION AND IDENTIFICATION

OPXVs can be grown in a variety of established cell culture lines, including Vero, BS-C-1, CV-1, LLCMK-2 monkey kidney cells, human embryonic lung fibroblasts, HeLa cells, chicken embryo fibroblasts, and MRC-5 human diploid fibroblast cells, as well as in fetal rhesus monkey kidney FHRK-4 cells. Propagation of samples at high risk for smallpox should not be attempted except at a WHOCC for smallpox. Cytopathic effects (CPE) appear as cell rounding with long cytoplasmic extensions (Fig. 2 and 3). In some cases, syncytium formation can also be seen; in Fig. 3B, this is seen in the MPXV-induced CPE. The timing of CPE is dependent on infectious inoculum. Most laboratories will confirm the presence of a specific OPXV via PCR (see above). Methods for growing and discriminating the morphologies of OPXVs on the chorioallantoic membranes (CAMs) of 12-day-old chicken embryos have been described (59, 60, 69, 70). OPXVs are the only human poxviruses that produce pocks (69, 70) on the CAMs of fertile chicken eggs; pock morphology is useful for biologic species and variant differentiation. Parapoxviruses, yatapoxviruses, and MCV do not form pocks on the CAM, in contrast to avipoxviruses, leporipoxviruses, and capripoxviruses. Poxvirus genera can usually be identified and differentiated by virus neutralization testing with hyperimmune reference sera (25, 39, 59, 60, 71). However, it can be difficult to identify the infecting species, since poxviruses are antigenically closely related within a given genus.

SEROLOGIC TESTS

Orthopoxviruses

When virus-containing clinical specimens are not available, antibody detection may be the only way to define the etiology of the disease. Serologic methods currently used to detect antibodies against human OPXVs include enzyme-linked immunosorbent assays (ELISAs), the virus neutralization test, Western blotting, and hemagglutination inhibition. Various protocols for poxvirus serologic testing used at the CDC are detailed elsewhere (40).

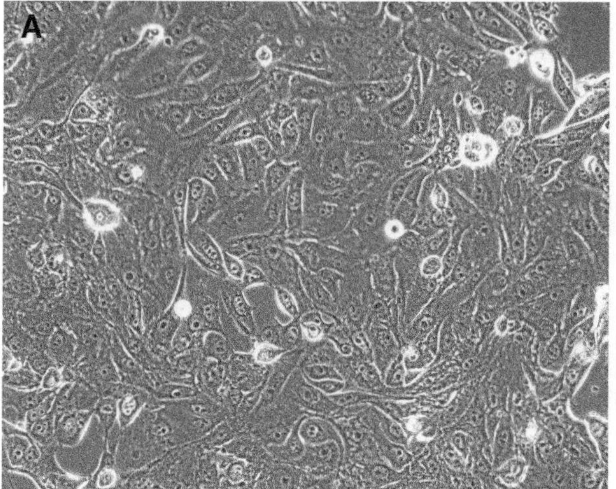

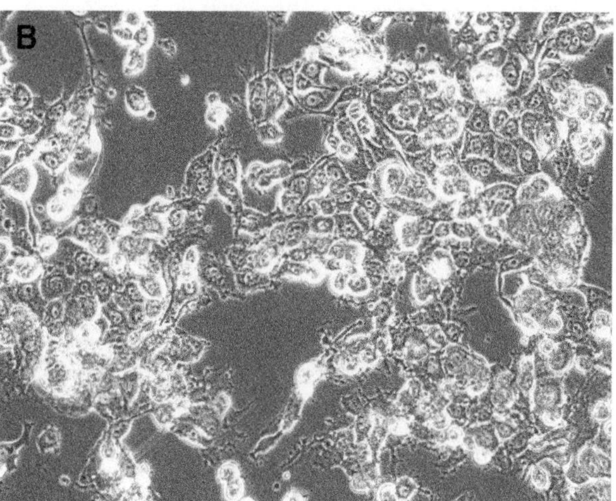

FIGURE 2 VACV (Dryvax) CPE in FHRK-4 cells. (A) Early CPE; (B) mature CPE. (Images courtesy of V. Olson.)

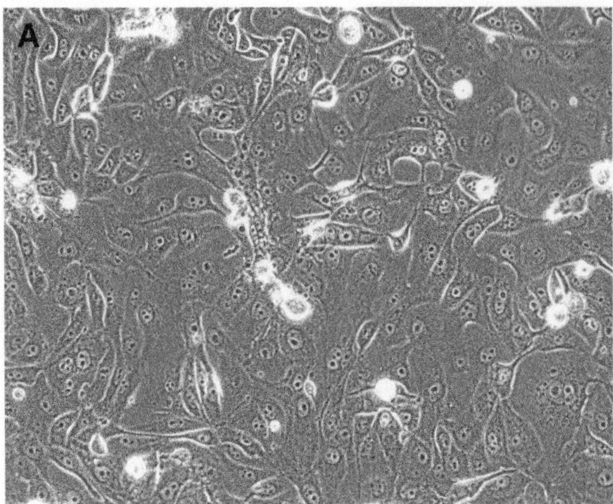

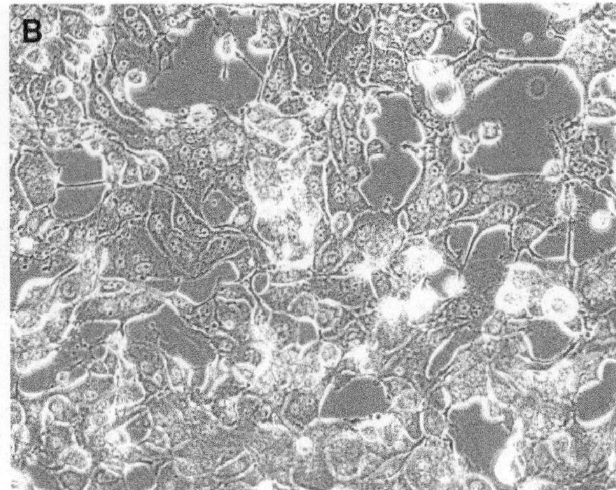

FIGURE 3 Monkeypox (Congo Basin clade, v79-I-005) CPE in FRHK-4 cells. (A) Early CPE; (B) mature CPE with syncytia. (Images courtesy of V. Olson.)

The description of an OPXV immunoglobulin M (IgM) assay indicates great promise to enhance investigations of OPXV infection outbreaks, often semiretrospective in nature (40). This technique offers the advantage of measuring recent infection or illness with an OPXV. It is useful for evaluating disease incidence in epidemiologic surveillance studies. For example, during the 2003 U.S. monkeypox outbreak, the IgM capture assay demonstrated ~95% sensitivity and ~95% specificity for epidemiologically linked and laboratory test-confirmed patients when sera were obtained between days 4 and 56 after rash onset. A low-grade response, termed "equivocal," awaits further research. This assay was also used to detect anti-OPXV IgM in the cerebrospinal fluid of an encephalitic patient with monkeypox (72). A peptide-based ELISA for the identification of MPXV-specific antibodies has been reported (73, 74). The peptide-based ELISA was capable of differentiating between MPXV and VACV. However, this ELISA is known to cross-react with VARV and, due to sequence conservation across the OPXVs, is also likely to cross-react with many strains of CPXVs. It remains an investigational tool rather than a clinical test, since its clinical utility has not been further established. An MPXV-specific antibody has been isolated, and characterization of the epitope has provided insight into the design of peptides to be used in a monkeypox-specific serological assay (75, 76).

In the current state of bioterrorism response awareness, tests to evaluate residual protection from previous vaccination are being requested. It is important to note that there is not one routine immunologic test that defines a person's degree of protection against a poxvirus infection, and determination of protection requires a concert of cell-mediated and humoral immune responses. Studies (77) suggest that humoral responses may be the critical component of recovery from and survival of a systemic OPXV infection. The presence of neutralizing antibodies generally indicates recovery from an infection but not always protracted protection against future infection. Neutralizing antibodies against OPXVs may be detectable as early as 6 days after infection or vaccination. Neutralizing antibodies have been detected as long as 20 years after vaccinia vaccination or natural infection with other human OPXVs.

The OPXV neutralization test has been traditionally performed by looking for a reduction in plaque number. This was improved upon using a green fluorescent protein-tagged VACV and measuring viral entry into tissue culture cells (78, 79). In the virus neutralization assay, a 4-fold rise in antibody titer between serum samples drawn during the acute and convalescent phases is usually considered diagnostic of poxvirus infection. When only one serum specimen is available from one phase of infection, confirmation of a clinical diagnosis may be difficult or impossible. Because OPXVs are closely related, serum cross-absorption tests, such as those performed in immunofluorescent-antibody or immunodiffusion methods, have been used with variable success with patient and animal sera. OPXV antigen cross-absorption assays have been performed using hyperimmune animal sera and have been utilized in serosurveys for animal and human monkeypox infection (59, 60). False-positive results should be ruled out by using appropriate control sets of sera of known provenance.

The Western blot assay is performed essentially as described by Towbin et al. (80) and uses various antigens, including purified virus and sometimes the concentrate of culture fluid from infected cells maintained under medium that contains 1% or no serum supplement. Few laboratories are using this method, as reliable standardization has not been achieved.

Pseudocowpox, Orf, Tanapox, and Molluscum Contagiosum Viruses

Serologic methods used to help confirm parapoxvirus infections (milker's nodule and orf) have included ELISAs (81) and Western blot assays that use various antigen preparations. Serologic testing for TPV infection by standard ELISA (81) with antigens obtained from concentrates of infected cell culture, by an indirect immunofluorescent antibody test, and by neutralizing test has been moderately effective. Optimally, sera should be collected at the time of actual disease and 3 to 5 weeks or later after the presumed onset date. Because MCV cannot be readily grown in culture, no routine serologic test is available. Molluscum contagiosum is readily diagnosed clinically, often with the aid of electron microscopy and histopathologic testing performed by a diagnostic facility.

EVALUATION, INTERPRETATION, AND REPORTING OF RESULTS

For confirmation of an infectious agent, cell culture or another mechanism for demonstrating viable virus should be regarded as the gold standard. Propagation of samples at high risk for smallpox should not be attempted except at a WHOCC for smallpox. Given the lack of readily available or feasible tissue culture methods, the use of multiple diagnostic assays or techniques improves the specificity of a diagnosis. Nucleic acid amplification tests, while sensitive, can result in false-positive results. A proficiency survey of nucleic acid amplification tests performed by 33 labs spanning three geographic areas (Europe, Australasia, and the United States) found a substantial rate of false-positive results (<12%), highlighting the need for sound molecular practices, which becomes even more critical when tests for potential biothreat agents are carried out (82). The use of multiple nucleic acid tests, with different detection targets, can improve the specificity of a diagnosis. Electron microscopy can be used to evaluate generically for the presence of a poxvirus and to infer the presence of infectious mature form if multiple virus forms are present, but it cannot be used to make a specific genus diagnosis except in the case of parapoxvirus infections. Serologic assays are available at a few reference laboratories worldwide but can only rarely be used to make a specific species diagnosis. Histochemistry combined with immunologic analysis can be used to identify poxvirus genera in a few reference centers worldwide. A combination of nucleic acid amplification, growth of agent in culture, serology, electron microscopy, and/or immunohistochemistry techniques improves the sensitivity and specificity of a diagnosis.

The findings and conclusions in this chapter are those of the authors and do not necessarily represent the views of the CDC. The use of product names in this manuscript does not imply their endorsement by the U.S. Department of Health and Human Services.

REFERENCES

1. **Schmidt FI, Bleck CK, Reh L, Novy K, Wollscheid B, Helenius A, Stahlberg H, Mercer J.** 2013. Vaccinia virus entry is followed by core activation and proteasome-mediated release of the immunomodulatory effector VH1 from lateral bodies. *Cell Rep* **4:**464–476.
2. **Moss B.** 2013. Poxviridae, p 2129–2159. *In* Knipe D, Howley P, Cohen JI, Griffin DE, Lamb RA, Martin MA, Racaniello VR, Roizman B (ed), *Fields Virology*, 6th ed. Lippincott Williams and Wilkins, New York, NY.
3. **Reed KD, Melski JW, Graham MB, Regnery RL, Sotir MJ, Wegner MV, Kazmierczak JJ, Stratman EJ, Li Y, Fairley JA, Swain GR, Olson VA, Sargent EK, Kehl SC, Frace MA, Kline R, Foldy SL, Davis JP, Damon IK.** 2004. The detection of monkeypox in humans in the Western Hemisphere. *N Engl J Med* **350:**342–350.
4. **Moss B.** 2006. Poxvirus entry and membrane fusion. *Virology* **344:**48–54.
5. **Smith GL, Law M.** 2004. The exit of vaccinia virus from infected cells. *Virus Res* **106:**189–197.
6. **Smith GL, Murphy BJ, Law M.** 2003. Vaccinia virus motility. *Annu Rev Microbiol* **57:**323–342.
7. **Smith GL, Vanderplasschen A, Law M.** 2002. The formation and function of extracellular enveloped vaccinia virus. *J Gen Virol* **83:**2915–2931.
8. **Damon IK.** 2007. Poxviruses, p 2947–2977. *In* Knipe DM, Howley PM, Griffin DE, Lamb RA, Martin MA, Roizman B, Straus SE (ed), *Fields Virology*, vol 5. Lippincott Williams and Wilkins, New York, NY.
9. **Pepose JS, Esposito JJ.** 1996. Molluscum contagiosum, orf, and vaccinia virus ocular infections in humans, p 846–856. *In* Pepose JS, Holland GN, Wilhelmus KR (ed), *Ocular Infections and Immunity*. Mosby Year Book, Inc., St. Louis, MO.
10. **Porter CD, Blake NW, Cream JJ, Archard LC.** 1992. Molluscum contagiosum virus, p 233–257. *In* Wright D, Archard LC (ed), *Molecular and Cellular Biology of Sexually Transmitted Diseases*. Chapman and Hall, London, England.
11. **Fenner FD, Henderson DA, Arita I, Jezek Z, Ladnyi I.** 1988. Smallpox and its eradication. World Health Organization, Geneva, Switzerland.
12. **Breman JG.** 2000. Monkeypox: an emerging infection for humans? p 45–67. *In* Scheld WM, Craig WA, Hughes JM (ed), *Emerging Infections 4*. ASM Press, Washington, DC.
13. **Centers for Disease Control and Prevention.** 1997. Human monkeypox—Kasai Oriental, Democratic Republic of Congo, February 1996-October 1997. *Morb Mortal Wkly Rep* **46:**1168–1171.
14. **Centers for Disease Control and Prevention.** 1997. Human monkeypox—Kasai Oriental, Zaire 1996-1997. *Morb Mortal Wkly Rep* **46:**304–307.
15. **Hutin YJ, Williams RJ, Malfait P, Pebody R, Loparev VN, Ropp SL, Rodriguez M, Knight JC, Tshioko FK, Khan AS, Szczeniowski MV, Esposito JJ.** 2001. Outbreak of human monkeypox, Democratic Republic of Congo, 1996 to 1997. *Emerg Infect Dis* **7:**434–438.
16. **Weinstein RA, Nalca A, Rimoin AW, Bavari S, Whitehouse CA.** 2005. Reemergence of monkeypox: prevalence, diagnostics, and countermeasures. *Clin Infect Dis* **41:** 1765–1771.
17. **Meyer H, Perrichot M, Stemmler M, Emmerich P, Schmitz H, Varaine F, Shungu R, Tshioko F, Formenty P.** 2002. Outbreaks of disease suspected of being due to human monkeypox virus infection in the Democratic Republic of Congo in 2001. *J Clin Microbiol* **40:**2919–2921.
18. **Learned LA, Reynolds MG, Wassa DW, Li Y, Olson VA, Karem K, Stempora LL, Braden ZH, Kline R, Likos A, Libama F, Moudzeo H, Bolanda JD, Tarangonia P, Boumandoki P, Formenty P, Harvey JM, Damon IK.** 2005. Extended interhuman transmission of monkeypox in a hospital community in the Republic of the Congo, 2003. *Am J Trop Med Hyg* **73:**428–434.
19. **Centers for Disease Control and Prevention.** 2003. Update: multistate outbreak of monkeypox—Illinois, Indiana, Kansas, Missouri, Ohio, and Wisconsin, 2003. *Morb Mortal Wkly Rep* **52:**642–646.
20. **Likos AM, Sammons SA, Olson VA, Frace AM, Li Y, Olsen-Rasmussen M, Davidson W, Galloway R, Khristova ML, Reynolds MG, Zhao H, Carroll DS, Curns A, Formenty P, Esposito JJ, Regnery RL, Damon IK.** 2005. A tale of two clades: monkeypox viruses. *J Gen Virol* **86:** 2661–2672.
21. **Chen N, Li G, Liszewski MK, Atkinson JP, Jahrling PB, Feng Z, Schriewer J, Buck C, Wang C, Lefkowitz EJ, Esposito JJ, Harms T, Damon IK, Roper RL, Upton C, Buller RM.** 2005. Virulence differences between monkeypox virus isolates from West Africa and the Congo basin. *Virology* **340:**46–63.
22. **Fenner F, Wittek R, Dumbell KR.** 1989. *The Orthopoxviruses*. Academic Press, New York, NY.
23. **Lewis FM, Chernak E, Goldman E, Li Y, Karem K, Damon IK, Henkel R, Newbern EC, Ross P, Johnson CC.** 2006. Ocular vaccinia infection in laboratory worker, Philadelphia, 2004. *Emerg Infect Dis* **12:**134–137.
24. **Carroll DS, Emerson GL, Li Y, Sammons S, Olson V, Frace M, Nakazawa Y, Czerny CP, Tryland M, Kolodziejek J, Nowotny N, Olsen-Rasmussen M, Khristova M, Govil D, Karem K, Damon IK, Meyer H.** 2011. Chasing Jenner's vaccine: revisiting *Cowpox virus* classification. *PLoS One* **6:**e23086.
25. **Dumbell K, Richardson M.** 1993. Virological investigations of specimens from buffaloes affected by buffalopox in Maharashtra State, India between 1985 and 1987. *Arch Virol* **128:**257–267.
26. **Damaso CR, Esposito JJ, Condit RC, Moussatché N.** 2000. An emergent poxvirus from humans and cattle in Rio de Janeiro State: Cantagalo virus may derive from Brazilian smallpox vaccine. *Virology* **277:**439–449.
27. **Schatzmayr HG, Lemos ER, Mazur C, Schubach A, Majerowicz S, Rozental T, Schubach TM, Bustamante MC, Barth OM.** 2000. Detection of poxvirus in cattle associated with human cases in the State of Rio de Janeiro: preliminary report. *Mem Inst Oswaldo Cruz* **95:**625–627.

28. **Marques JT, Trindade GD, da Fonseca FG, Dos Santos JR, Bonjardim CA, Ferreira PC, Kroon EG.** 2001. Characterization of ATI, TK and IFN-α/βR genes in the genome of the BeAn 58058 virus, a naturally attenuated wild Orthopoxvirus. *Virus Genes* **23:**291–301.
29. **Nagasse-Sugahara TK, Kisielius JJ, Ueda-Ito M, Curti SP, Figueiredo CA, Cruz AS, Silva MM, Ramos CH, Silva MC, Sakurai T, Salles-Gomes LF.** 2004. Human vaccinia-like virus outbreaks in São Paulo and Goiás States, Brazil: virus detection, isolation and identification. *Rev Inst Med Trop São Paulo* **46:**315–322.
30. **Trindade GS, da Fonseca FG, Marques JT, Diniz S, Leite JA, De Bodt S, Van der Peer Y, Bonjardim CA, Ferreira PC, Kroon EG.** 2004. Belo Horizonte virus: a vaccinia-like virus lacking the A-type inclusion body gene isolated from infected mice. *J Gen Virol* **85:**2015–2021.
31. **da Fonseca FG, Trindade GS, Silva RL, Bonjardim CA, Ferreira PC, Kroon EG.** 2002. Characterization of a vaccinia-like virus isolated in a Brazilian forest. *J Gen Virol* **83:**223–228.
32. **Centers for Disease Control and Prevention.** 2009. Human vaccinia infection after contact with a raccoon rabies vaccine bait—Pennsylvania, 2009. *Morb Mortal Wkly Rep* **58:** 1204–1207.
33. **Rupprecht CE, Blass L, Smith K, Orciari LA, Niezgoda M, Whitfield SG, Gibbons RV, Guerra M, Hanlon CA.** 2001. Human infection due to recombinant vaccinia-rabies glycoprotein virus. *N Engl J Med* **345:**582–586.
34. **Baxby D, Bennett M, Getty B.** 1994. Human cowpox 1969-93: a review based on 54 cases. *Br J Dermatol* **131:**598–607.
35. **Bennett M, Gaskell CJ, Baxby D, Gaskell RM, Kelly DF, Naidoot J.** 1990. Feline cowpox virus infection. *J Small Anim Pract* **31:**167–173.
36. **Campe H, Zimmermann P, Glos K, Bayer M, Bergemann H, Dreweck C, Graf P, Weber BK, Meyer H, Büttner M, Busch U, Sing A.** 2009. Cowpox virus transmission from pet rats to humans, Germany. *Emerg Infect Dis* **15:**777–780.
37. **Bennett M, Crouch AJ, Begon M, Duffy B, Feore S, Gaskell RM, Kelly DF, McCracken CM, Vicary L, Baxby D.** 1997. Cowpox in British voles and mice. *J Comp Pathol* **116:**35–44.
38. **Rouhandeh H.** 1988. Yaba virus, p 1–15. *In* Darai G (ed), *Virus Diseases in Laboratory and Captive Animals.* Martinus Nijhoff, Boston, MA.
39. **Fenner F, Nakano JH.** 1988. Poxviridae: the poxviruses, p 177–207. *In* Lennette EH, Halonen P, Murphy FA (ed), *Laboratory Diagnosis of Infectious Diseases: Principles and Practice*, vol 2. *Viral, Rickettsial, and Chlamydial Diseases.* Springer-Verlag, New York, NY.
40. **Karem KL, Reynolds M, Braden Z, Lou G, Bernard N, Patton J, Damon IK.** 2005. Characterization of acute-phase humoral immunity to monkeypox: use of immunoglobulin M enzyme-linked immunosorbent assay for detection of monkeypox infection during the 2003 North American outbreak. *Clin Diagn Lab Immunol* **12:**867–872.
41. **Dhar AD, Werchniak AE, Li Y, Brennick JB, Goldsmith CS, Kline R, Damon I, Klaus SN.** 2004. Tanapox infection in a college student. *N Engl J Med* **350:**361–366.
42. **Stich A, Meyer H, Köhler B, Fleischer K.** 2002. Tanapox: first report in a European traveller and identification by PCR. *Trans R Soc Trop Med Hyg* **96:**178–179.
43. **Robinson AJ, Lyttle DJ.** 1992. Parapoxviruses: their biology and potential as recombinant vaccine vectors, p 285–327. *In* Binns MM, Smith GL (ed), *Recombinant Poxviruses.* CRC Press, Inc., Boca Raton, FL.
44. **Clark C, McIntyre PG, Evans A, McInnes CJ, Lewis-Jones S.** 2005. Human sealpox resulting from a seal bite: confirmation that sealpox virus is zoonotic. *Br J Dermatol* **152:**791–793.
45. **Jezek Z, Fenner F.** 1988. Human monkeypox. *Monogr Virol* **17:** 1–140.
46. **Seward JF, Galil K, Damon I, Norton SA, Rotz L, Schmid S, Harpaz R, Cono J, Marin M, Hutchins S, Chaves SS, McCauley MM.** 2004. Development and experience with an algorithm to evaluate suspected smallpox cases in the United States, 2002-2004. *Clin Infect Dis* **39:**1477–1483.
47. **Huhn GD, Bauer AM, Yorita K, Graham MB, Sejvar J, Likos A, Damon IK, Reynolds MG, Kuehnert MJ.** 2005. Clinical characteristics of human monkeypox, and risk factors for severe disease. *Clin Infect Dis* **41:**1742–1751.
48. **Petersen, BW, Harms TJ, Reynolds MG, Harrison LH.** 2016. Use of vaccinia virus smallpox vaccine in laboratory and health care personnel at risk for occupational exposure to orthopoxviruses—recommendations of the Advisory Committee on Immunization Practices (ACIP), 2015. *Morb Mortal Wkly Rep* **65:**257–262.
49. **Kelly CD, Egan C, Davis SW, Samsonoff WA, Musser KA, Drabkin P, Miller JR, Taylor J, Cirino NM.** 2004. Laboratory confirmation of generalized vaccinia following smallpox vaccination. *J Clin Microbiol* **42:**1373–1375.
50. **Knight JC, Novembre FJ, Brown DR, Goldsmith CS, Esposito JJ.** 1989. Studies on Tanapox virus. *Virology* **172:**116–124.
51. **Jezek Z, Arita I, Szczeniowski M, Paluku KM, Ruti K, Nakano JH.** 1985. Human tanapox in Zaire: clinical and epidemiological observations on cases confirmed by laboratory studies. *Bull World Health Organ* **63:**1027–1035.
52. **Nuñez A, Funes JM, Agromayor M, Moratilla M, Varas AJ, Lopez-Estebaranz JL, Esteban M, Martin-Gallardo A.** 1996. Detection and typing of molluscum contagiosum virus in skin lesions by using a simple lysis method and polymerase chain reaction. *J Med Virol* **50:**342–349.
53. **Smee DF.** 2008. Progress in the discovery of compounds inhibiting orthopoxviruses in animal models. *Antivir Chem Chemother* **19:**115–124.
54. **Huggins J, Goff A, Hensley L, Mucker E, Shamblin J, Wlazlowski C, Johnson W, Chapman J, Larsen T, Twenhafel N, Karem K, Damon IK, Byrd CM, Bolken TC, Jordan R, Hruby D.** 2009. Nonhuman primates are protected from smallpox virus or monkeypox virus challenges by the antiviral drug ST-246. *Antimicrob Agents Chemother* **53:** 2620–2625.
55. **Vora S, Damon I, Fulginiti V, Weber SG, Kahana M, Stein SL, Gerber SI, Garcia-Houchins S, Lederman E, Hruby D, Collins L, Scott D, Thompson K, Barson JV, Regnery R, Hughes C, Daum RS, Li Y, Zhao H, Smith S, Braden Z, Karem K, Olson V, Davidson W, Trindade G, Bolken T, Jordan R, Tien D, Marcinak J.** 2008. Severe eczema vaccinatum in a household contact of a smallpox vaccinee. *Clin Infect Dis* **46:**1555–1561.
56. **Centers for Disease Control and Prevention.** 2009. Progressive vaccinia in a military smallpox vaccinee—United States, 2009. *Morb Mortal Wkly Rep* **58:**532–536.
57. **Nitsche A, Büttner M, Wilhelm S, Pauli G, Meyer H.** 2006. Real-time PCR detection of parapoxvirus DNA. *Clin Chem* **52:**316–319.
58. **Moriello KA, Cooley J.** 2001. Difficult dermatologic diagnosis. Contagious viral pustular dermatitis (orf), goatpox, dermatophilosis, dermatophytosis, bacterial pyoderma, and mange. *J Am Vet Med Assoc* **218:**19–20.
59. **Nakano JH.** 1978. Comparative diagnosis of poxvirus diseases, p 267–339. *In* Kurstak E, Kurstak C (ed), *Comparative Diagnosis of Viral Diseases.* Academic Press, New York, NY.
60. **Nakano JH.** 1979. Poxviruses, p 257–308. *In* Lennette EH, Schmidt NJ (ed), *Diagnostic Procedures for Viral, Rickettsial, and Chlamydial Infections.* American Public Health Association, Inc., Washington, DC.
61. **Gelderblom HR, Hazelton PR.** 2000. Specimen collection for electron microscopy. *Emerg Infect Dis* **6:**433–434.
62. **Long GW, Nobel J, Jr, Murphy FA, Herrmann KL, Lourie B.** 1970. Experience with electron microscopy in the differential diagnosis of smallpox. *Appl Microbiol* **20:**497–504.
63. **Townsend MB, MacNeil A, Reynolds MG, Hughes CM, Olson VA, Damon IK, Karem KL.** 2013. Evaluation of the Tetracore Orthopox BioThreat® antigen detection assay using laboratory grown orthopoxviruses and rash illness clinical specimens. *J Virol Methods* **187:**37–42.
64. **Li Y, Meyer H, Zhao H, Damon IK.** 2010. GC content-based pan-pox universal PCR assays for poxvirus detection. *J Clin Microbiol* **48:**268–276.

65. **Torfason EG, Guðnadóttir S.** 2002. Polymerase chain reaction for laboratory diagnosis of orf virus infections. *J Clin Virol* **24:**79–84.
66. **Shchelkunov SN, Gavrilova EV, Babkin IV.** 2005. Multiplex PCR detection and species differentiation of orthopoxviruses pathogenic to humans. *Mol Cell Probes* **19:**1–8.
67. **Stemmler M, Neubauer H, Meyer H.** 2001. Comparison of closely related orthopoxvirus isolates by random amplified polymorphic DNA and restriction fragment length polymorphism analysis. *J Vet Med B Infect Dis Vet Public Health* **48:**647–654.
68. **Fedorko DP, Preuss JC, Fahle GA, Li L, Fischer SH, Hohman P, Cohen JI.** 2005. Comparison of methods for detection of vaccinia virus in patient specimens. *J Clin Microbiol* **43:**4602–4606.
69. **Westwood JC, Phipps PH, Boulter EA.** 1957. The titration of vaccinia virus on the chorioallantoic membrane of the developing chick embryo. *J Hyg (Lond)* **55:**123–139.
70. **World Health Organization.** 1960. Guide to the laboratory diagnosis of smallpox for smallpox eradication programmes. World Health Organization, Geneva, Switzerland.
71. **Cole GA, Blanden RV.** 1982. Immunology of poxviruses, p 1–19. *In* Nahmias AJ, O'Reilly RJ (ed), *Comprehensive Immunology*, vol 9. Plenum Press, New York, NY.
72. **Sejvar JJ, Chowdary Y, Schomogyi M, Stevens J, Patel J, Karem K, Fischer M, Kuehnert MJ, Zaki SR, Paddock CD, Guarner J, Shieh WJ, Patton JL, Bernard N, Li Y, Olson VA, Kline RL, Loparev VN, Schmid DS, Beard B, Regnery RR, Damon IK.** 2004. Human monkeypox infection: a family cluster in the midwestern United States. *J Infect Dis* **190:**1833–1840.
73. **Hammarlund E, Lewis MW, Carter SV, Amanna I, Hansen SG, Strelow LI, Wong SW, Yoshihara P, Hanifin JM, Slifka MK.** 2005. Multiple diagnostic techniques identify previously vaccinated individuals with protective immunity against monkeypox. *Nat Med* **11:**1005–1011.
74. **Dubois ME, Hammarlund E, Slifka MK.** 2012. Optimization of peptide-based ELISA for serological diagnostics: a retrospective study of human monkeypox infection. *Vector Borne Zoonotic Dis* **12:**400–409.
75. **Roumillat LF, Patton JL, Davis ML.** 1984. Monoclonal antibodies to a monkeypox virus polypeptide determinant. *J Virol* **52:**290–292.
76. **Hughes LJ, Goldstein J, Pohl J, Hooper JW, Lee Pitts R, Townsend MB, Bagarozzi D, Damon IK, Karem KL.** 2014. A highly specific monoclonal antibody against monkeypox virus detects the heparin binding domain of A27. *Virology* **464-465:**264–273.
77. **Edghill-Smith Y, Golding H, Manischewitz J, King LR, Scott D, Bray M, Nalca A, Hooper JW, Whitehouse CA, Schmitz JE, Reimann KA, Franchini G.** 2005. Smallpox vaccine-induced antibodies are necessary and sufficient for protection against monkeypox virus. *Nat Med* **11:** 740–747.
78. **Earl PL, Americo JL, Moss B.** 2003. Development and use of a vaccinia virus neutralization assay based on flow cytometric detection of green fluorescent protein. *J Virol* **77:** 10684–10688.
79. **Johnson MC, Damon IK, Karem KL.** 2008. A rapid, high-throughput vaccinia virus neutralization assay for testing smallpox vaccine efficacy based on detection of green fluorescent protein. *J Virol Methods* **150:**14–20.
80. **Towbin H, Staehelin T, Gordon J.** 1979. Electrophoretic transfer of proteins from polyacrylamide gels to nitrocellulose sheets: procedure and some applications. *Proc Natl Acad Sci USA* **76:**4350–4354.
81. **Conroy JM, Stevens RW, Hechemy KE.** 1991. Enzyme immunoassays, p 87–92. *In* Balows A, Hausler WJ, Herman KI, Isenberg HD, Shadomy HJ (ed), *Manual of Clinical Microbiology*, vol 5. American Society for Microbiology, Washington, DC.
82. **Niedrig M, Meyer H, Panning M, Drosten C.** 2006. Follow-up on diagnostic proficiency of laboratories equipped to perform orthopoxvirus detection and quantification by PCR: the second international external quality assurance study. *J Clin Microbiol* **44:**1283–1287.
83. **Ropp SL, Jin Q, Knight JC, Massung RF, Esposito JJ.** 1995. PCR strategy for identification and differentiation of small pox and other orthopoxviruses. *J Clin Microbiol* **33:** 2069–2076.
84. **Loparev VN, Massung RF, Esposito JJ, Meyer H.** 2001. Detection and differentiation of Old World orthopoxviruses: restriction fragment length polymorphism of the *crmB* gene region. *J Clin Microbiol* **39:**94–100.
85. **Meyer H, Ropp SL, Esposito JJ.** 1997. Gene for A-type inclusion body protein is useful for a polymerase chain reaction assay to differentiate orthopoxviruses. *J Virol Methods* **64:**217–221.
86. **Meyer H, Ropp SL, Esposito JJ.** 1998. Poxviruses, p 199–211. *In* Warnes A, Stephenson J (ed), *Methods in Molecular Medicine: Diagnostic Virology Protocols*. Humana Press, Totowa, NJ.
87. **Schroeder K, Nitsche A.** 2010. Multicolour, multiplex real-time PCR assay for the detection of human-pathogenic poxviruses. *Mol Cell Probes* **24:**110–113.
88. **Espy MJ, Cockerill FR, III, Meyer RF, Bowen MD, Poland GA, Hadfield TL, Smith TF.** 2002. Detection of smallpox virus DNA by LightCycler PCR. *J Clin Microbiol* **40:** 1985–1988.
89. **Maksyutov, RA, Gavrilova EV, Shchelkunov SN.** 2016. Species-specific differentiation of variola, monkeypox, and varicella-zoster viruses by multiplex real-time PCR assay. *J Virol Methods* **236:**215–220.
90. **Sofi Ibrahim M, Kulesh DA, Saleh SS, Damon IK, Esposito JJ, Schmaljohn AL, Jahrling PB.** 2003. Real-time PCR assay to detect smallpox virus. *J Clin Microbiol* **41:**3835–3839.
91. **Panning M, Asper M, Kramme S, Schmitz H, Drosten C.** 2004. Rapid detection and differentiation of human pathogenic orthopox viruses by a fluorescence resonance energy transfer real-time PCR assay. *Clin Chem* **50:**702–708.
92. **Nitsche A, Ellerbrok H, Pauli G.** 2004. Detection of orthopoxvirus DNA by real-time PCR and identification of variola virus DNA by melting analysis. *J Clin Microbiol* **42:** 1207–1213.
93. **Kulesh DA, Baker RO, Loveless BM, Norwood D, Zwiers SH, Mucker E, Hartmann C, Herrera R, Miller D, Christensen D, Wasieloski LP, Jr, Huggins J, Jahrling PB.** 2004. Smallpox and *pan*-orthopox virus detection by real-time 3′-minor groove binder TaqMan assays on the Roche LightCycler and the Cepheid Smart Cycler platforms. *J Clin Microbiol* **42:**601–609.
94. **Olson VA, Laue T, Laker MT, Babkin IV, Drosten C, Shchelkunov SN, Niedrig M, Damon IK, Meyer H.** 2004. Real-time PCR system for detection of orthopoxviruses and simultaneous identification of smallpox virus. *J Clin Microbiol* **42:**1940–1946.
95. **Carletti F, Di Caro A, Calcaterra S, Grolla A, Czub M, Ippolito G, Capobianchi MR, Horejsh D.** 2005. Rapid, differential diagnosis of orthopox- and herpesviruses based upon real-time PCR product melting temperature and restriction enzyme analysis of amplicons. *J Virol Methods* **129:** 97–100.
96. **Fedele CG, Negredo A, Molero F, Sánchez-Seco MP, Tenorio A.** 2006. Use of internally controlled real-time genome amplification for detection of variola virus and other orthopoxviruses infecting humans. *J Clin Microbiol* **44:** 4464–4470.
97. **Kondas AV, Olson VA, Li Y, Abel J, Laker M, Rose L, Wilkins K, Turner J, Kline R, Damon IK.** 2015. Variola virus-specific diagnostic assays: characterization, sensitivity, and specificity. *J Clin Microbiol* **53:**1406–1410.
98. **Scaramozzino N, Ferrier-Rembert A, Favier AL, Rothlisberger C, Richard S, Crance JM, Meyer H, Garin D.** 2007. Real-time PCR to identify variola virus or other human pathogenic orthopox viruses. *Clin Chem* **53:**606–613.
99. **Aitichou M, Javorschi S, Ibrahim MS.** 2005. Two-color multiplex assay for the identification of orthopox viruses with real-time LUX- PCR. *Mol Cell Probes* **19:**323–328.

100. **Putkuri N, Piiparinen H, Vaheri A, Vapalahti O.** 2009. Detection of human orthopoxvirus infections and differentiation of smallpox virus with real-time PCR. *J Med Virol* **81:** 146–152.
101. **Li Y, Olson VA, Laue T, Laker MT, Damon IK.** 2006. Detection of monkeypox virus with real-time PCR assays. *J Clin Virol* **36:**194–203.
102. **Li Y, Zhao H, Wilkins K, Hughes C, Damon IK.** 2010. Real-time PCR assays for the specific detection of monkeypox virus West African and Congo Basin strain DNA. *J Virol Methods* **169:**223–227.
103. **Baker JL, Ward BM.** 2014. Development and comparison of a quantitative TaqMan-MGB real-time PCR assays to three other methods of quantifying vaccinia virions. *J Virol Methods* **196:**126–132.
104. **Nitsche A, Steger B, Ellerbrok H, Pauli G.** 2005. Detection of vaccinia virus DNA on the LightCycler by fluorescence melting curve analysis. *J Virol Methods* **126:**187–195.
105. **Gavrilova EV, Shcherbakov DN, Maksyutov RA, Shchelkunov SN.** 2010. Development of real-time PCR assay for specific detection of cowpox virus. *J Clin Virol* **49:** 37–40.
106. **McCollum AM, Austin C, Nawrocki J, Howland J, Pryde J, Vaid A, Holmes D, Weil MR, Li Y, Wilkins K, Zhao H, Smith SK, Karem K, Reynolds MG, Damon IK.** 2012. Investigation of the first laboratory-acquired human cowpox virus infection in the United States. *J Infect Dis* **206:**63–68.
107. **Maksyutov RA, Gavrilova EV, Meyer H, Shchelkunov SN.** 2015. Real-time PCR assay for specific detection of cowpox virus. *J Virol Methods* **211:**8–11.
108. **Zimmermann P, Thordsen I, Frangoulidis D, Meyer H.** 2005. Real-time PCR assay for the detection of tanapox virus and yaba-like disease virus. *J Virol Methods* **130:**149–153.
109. **Gallina L, Dal Pozzo F, Mc Innes CJ, Cardeti G, Guercio A, Battilani M, Ciulli S, Scagliarini A.** 2006. A real time PCR assay for the detection and quantification of orf virus. *J Virol Methods* **134:**140–145.
110. **Lederman ER, Green GM, DeGroot HE, Dahl P, Goldman E, Greer PW, Li Y, Zhao H, Paddock CD, Damon IK.** 2007. Progressive ORF virus infection in a patient with lymphoma: successful treatment using imiquimod. *Clin Infect Dis* **44:**e100–e103.
111. **Bora DP, Venkatesan G, Bhanuprakash V, Balamurugan V, Prabhu M, Siva Sankar MS, Yogisharadhya R.** 2011. TaqMan real-time PCR assay based on DNA polymerase gene for rapid detection of Orf infection. *J Virol Methods* **178:**249–252.
112. **Du, H, Li W, Hao W, Liao X, Li M, Luo S.** 2013. Taqman real-time PCR assay based on ORFV024 gene for rapid detection of orf infection. *Toxicol Mech Methods* **23:**308–314.
113. **Venkatesan, G, Balamurugan V, Bhanuprakash V.** 2014. TaqMan based real-time duplex PCR for simultaneous detection and quantitation of capripox and orf virus genomes in clinical samples. *J Virol Methods* **201:**44–50
114. **Zhao, H, Wilkins K, Damon IK, Li Y.** 2013. Specific qPCR assays for the detection of orf virus, pseudocowpox virus and bovine papular stomatitis virus. *J Virol Methods* **194:**229–234.
115. **Trama JP, Adelson ME, Mordechai E.** 2007. Identification and genotyping of molluscum contagiosum virus from genital swab samples by real-time PCR and pyrosequencing. *J Clin Virol* **40:**325–329.

Hepatitis B and D Viruses*

YI-WEI TANG, REBECCA T. HORVAT, AND MARIE-LOUISE LANDRY

111

HEPATITIS B VIRUS

Taxonomy

Hepatitis B virus (HBV), which was discovered in blood specimens from Australian aborigines in 1965 (1), is an enveloped DNA virus in the genus *Orthohepadnavirus* of the *Hepadnaviridae* family. HBV has a narrow host range and infects only species closely related to humans, such as gibbons and several monkey species (2). As with other viruses in this family, the HBV genome is partially double stranded. It has a circular DNA molecule that replicates via an RNA intermediate. The replication of HBV DNA by reverse transcription is unique for human DNA viruses (2).

Description of the Agent

HBV is a 42-nm, partially double-stranded DNA virus that replicates in the nucleus of the host cell. HBV-infected cells have no cytopathic features because the virus causes little damage to the host cell (2). The virion is composed of HBsAg embedded in a lipid membrane surrounding a viral nucleocapsid core. The complete virus particle is known as the Dane particle, after its discoverer (3). The viral nucleocapsid core is surrounded by a specific viral core protein (HBcAg) and encloses a single molecule of partially double-stranded DNA, hepatitis B e antigen (HBeAg), and a DNA-dependent polymerase (Fig. 1A). The terminology used to describe the various antigens and antibodies associated with HBV as they appear at different stages of infection is given in Table 1.

HBV particles found in the sera of patients with active HBV infection reveal three distinct morphologic entities in varying proportions (Fig. 1A and B). The most abundant forms (by a factor of 10^4 to 10^6) are the small, pleomorphic, spherical, noninfectious particles (17 to 25 nm in diameter). These noninfectious particles have a low buoyant density, reflecting the presence of lipids from the host cell membrane (2). Less numerous are the tubular or filamentous forms, which have diameters similar to those of the small particles. The third and least numerous particle is the complete HBV virion, with a diameter of approximately 42 to 47 nm (3). At present, there is no native cell culture system that supports the growth of HBV (4).

The HBV genome is approximately 3,200 bases and contains overlapping genes (Fig. 1C). There are four open reading frames in the complete minus strand. These genes encode the structural proteins (HBsAg and HBcAg), replicative proteins (polymerase and X protein), and regulatory proteins. The genome is compact, and most sequences are essential for productive infection (2).

As shown in Fig. 2, HBV infection of hepatocytes is initiated by low-affinity attachment to heparin sulfate proteoglycan. Subsequent specific binding to the sodium taurocholate cotransporting polypeptide (NTCP), a heptocyte-specific receptor (5, 6), induces entry of the viral particle into its target cells (4, 7). The HBV virion is then taken up and uncoated. The partially double-stranded, relaxed circular DNA is converted by the host polymerase to a covalently closed circular DNA (cccDNA) template in the cell nucleus. The cccDNA form is used as a template for transcription of the pregenomic RNA (pgRNA) and mRNA (2). The pgRNA is transcribed from the cccDNA in the nucleus and then moves into the cytoplasm of the host cell. In the cytoplasm, the pgRNA serves as the template for the HBV reverse transcriptase enzyme as well as the core protein. At the same time, the polymerase converts the pgRNA to a new circular DNA molecule (4). Early in infection, some newly synthesized genomes from the cytoplasm circulate back to the nucleus to build up and maintain the pool of cccDNA (2).

The HBV genome is highly efficient in that every nucleotide in the genome is in at least one coding region. More than half of the genome is transcribed in more than one open reading frame. Four viral mRNA transcripts are translated into HBV proteins. These viral mRNAs are transcribed from different promoter regions on the cccDNA template (Fig. 1C). The longest mRNA acts as the template for genome replication (pgRNA) and also the translation of precore, core (HBcAg), and polymerase proteins (2). The second transcript encodes the pre-S1 protein (39 kb), pre-S2 protein (33 kDa), and S protein (24 kDa; also known as HBsAg). A third transcript encodes the pre-S2 protein and the S protein. The smallest mRNA codes for the X protein, which is responsible for transactivating transcription. Mature virions are produced by transcription of RNA into a circular DNA molecule. The long RNA transcript and the polymerase protein are packaged into mature core particles, and the reverse transcriptase enzyme synthesizes a new viral DNA genome. These particles are then transported to the

*This chapter contains information presented by Rebecca T. Horvat and Ryan Taylor in chapter 108 of the 11th edition of this *Manual*.

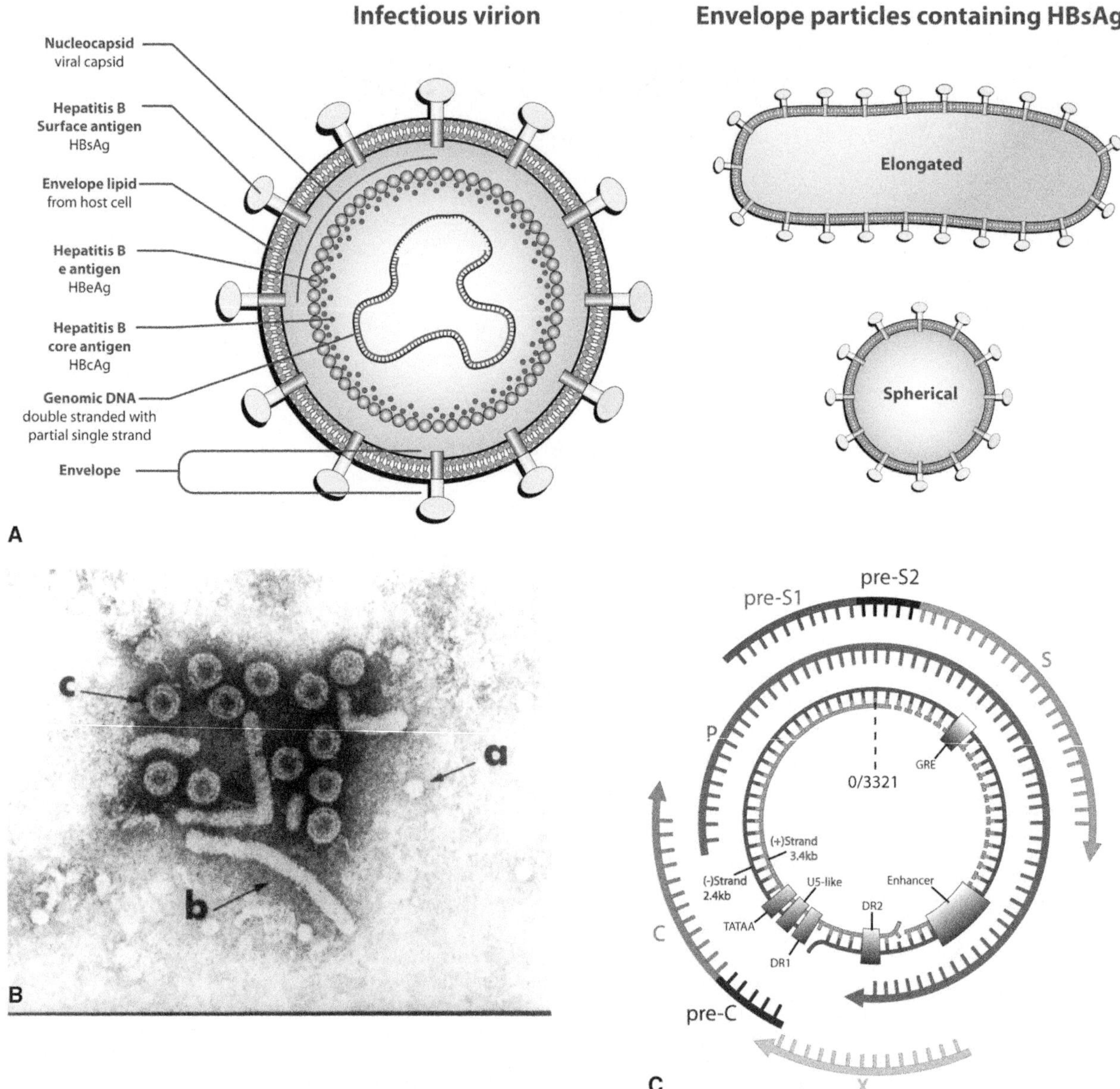

FIGURE 1 (A) The intact infectious HBV virion and the empty particles are shown. The two HBV particles (right) composed of HBsAg are shown as an elongated or tubular particle and as a spherical particle. These particles vastly outnumber the virions. (Designed by the University of Kansas Graphic Design Department, 2009.) (B) Electron micrograph of serum showing the presence of three distinct morphologic entities: 17- to 25-nm-diameter pleomorphic, spherical particles (a), tubular or filamentous forms with diameters similar to those of the small particles (b), and 42- to 47-nm-diameter double-shelled spherical particles representing the HBV virion (Dane particle) (c). Magnification, $\times 10^5$. (C) Diagrammatic representation of HBV coding regions. The functioning genome is a double-stranded circular DNA molecule, shown in the middle. RNA transcripts (arrows) are generated using both the plus-strand [(+) Strand] and minus-strand [(−)Strand] DNA templates. The largest transcript codes for the viral polymerase shown around the genome as the P transcript. The transcript for surface antigen (S) is produced as three separate transcripts, pre-S1, pre-S2, and S. The core protein is translated from the C transcript. HBeAg is encoded within the HB core gene. The transactivating protein is coded by the X transcript. (Designed by the University of Kansas Graphic Design Department, 2009.)

HBsAg in the endoplasmic reticulum of the host cell and exported from the cell. The unused HBsAg is also released from infected cells as spherical and filamentous particles devoid of HBV genomes or core proteins. Thus, these HBsAg particles are used as a diagnostic marker in serum to detect active viral replication (8–10).

The envelope proteins of HBsAg are made up of three polypeptides encoded by the S/pre-S region of the HBV genome (Fig. 1C). The major protein is the smallest peptide. It is encoded by the S region and is a glycosylated polypeptide. The middle protein, encoded by the S and the pre-S2 regions, has an additional glycosylation site.

TABLE 1 HBV markers in different stages of infection and convalescence[a]

Stage of infection	Molecular marker: HBV DNA	Protein antigen markers		HBV-specific antibody markers			
				Anti-HBc			
		HBsAg	HBeAg	IgM	Total	Anti-HBe	Anti-HBs
Susceptible	–	–	–	–	–	–	–
Early incubation	+	–	–	–	–	–	–
Late incubation	+	+	–/+	–	–	–	–
Acute infection	+	+	+	+	+	–	–
HBsAg-negative window in acute infection	– (<10^3 IU/ml)	–	–	+	+	–	–
Recent infection[b]	–/+	–	–	++	+	+	+++
Remote resolved infection[c]	–	–	–	–	+	+/–	+
Immune tolerant carrier	+++	+	+	–	+	–	–
Immune active carrier	++ (>10^5 IU/ml)	+	–/+	–/+	+++	–	–
Inactive carrier	– (<10^3 IU/ml)	+	–	–	+	+	–
HBeAg negative chronic infection[d]	++	+	–	+/–	+	+/–	–
HBsAg variant infection[e]	++/+	–	+/–	+/–	+	+/–	–
Chronic low-level infection[c]	–/+	–	–	–	+	+/–	–
Vaccination response	–	–	–	–	–	–	+
Recent vaccination[f]	–	+	–	–	–	–	–

[a]–, not detected; +, detected; –/+, sometimes detected; ++, detected at high levels; +++, detected at very high levels; HBsAg, complex antigen found on surface of HBV and on 20-nm-diameter particles and tubular forms; HBcAg, antigen associated with 27-nm-diameter core of HBV; HBeAg, protein that results from the proteolytic cleavage of the precore/core protein by cellular proteases and secreted as soluble protein in serum.

[b]This description can be applied to early convalescence and to individuals that remain HBV DNA positive for prolonged periods in the absence of HBsAg.

[c]The term "remote infection" can be applied to individuals with anti-HBc in the absence of other serologic markers, including DNA. These patients may or may not have anti-HBs. There is evidence that these patients may reactivate HBV during immunosuppression or treatment for hepatitis C virus.

[d]Precore or core promoter region mutations may result in HBeAg-negative results despite high HBV DNA levels.

[e]HBsAg variants or escape mutants may not be detected by immunoassays.

[f]HBsAg can be detected in serum for 18 days after vaccination, and up to 52 days in dialysis patients.

The large S protein consists of 389 to 400 amino acids encoded by the pre-S1, pre-S2, and S regions of the genome. The production of HBsAg exceeds what is needed for virion production, and this excess antigen circulates in the blood of infected individuals as spherical and tubular particles and can be detected in clinical assays to detect active HBV infection (Fig. 1A,B) (11). This antigen may persist in the serum for variable periods after initial infection and in some patients can be as high as 10^{13} per ml.

Two additional HBV-specific proteins play a key role in diagnostic testing. HBcAg and HBeAg have different antigenic specificities, and both can be distinguished from HBsAg. HBcAg is a polypeptide encoded by the C gene of HBV and is translated from the pregenomic mRNA (Fig. 1C). The precore sequence within the C gene contains the start codon for HBeAg translation (11). Because of the different start codons, the two proteins, HBcAg and HBeAg, are antigenically unrelated. HBeAg lacks the viral DNA-binding domain found on HBcAg. The first 29 amino acid residues of the HBeAg are encoded in the precore region of the C gene. This part of HBeAg directs the protein to the host endoplasmic reticulum. In the endoplasmic reticulum this "homing" portion of the protein is cleaved off, and HBeAg is released from the host cell to the blood. In the blood HBeAg is a soluble protein or is bound to albumin, α-1-antitrypsin, or immunoglobulin. It is a dependable marker for the presence of intact virions, indicating high infectivity. In some HBV strains, a mutation at the end of the precore region of the C gene results in a stop codon which prevents the translation of HBeAg. These precore mutants contribute to the pathogenesis of chronic HBV disease, leading to acute exacerbation of disease (11, 12). Other HBV gene mutations have been observed in the core, core promoter, envelope, and polymerase regions. The envelope protein variants become relevant, because some of them lead to antigenic changes that are not recognized by HBs antibody. These viruses are called escape HBV mutants and are resistant to HBsAg vaccine-induced neutralizing antibody and do not respond to hepatitis B immunoglobulin (HBIG) therapy (11, 13, 14).

Epidemiology and Transmission

HBV infections are prevalent around the world and represent a global public health problem. Roughly 30% of the world's population shows serological evidence of current or past HBV infection. The WHO estimates that approximately 600,000 people die each year as a result of acute or chronic HBV (10). About half the total hepatocellular carcinoma (HCC) mortality in 2010 was attributed to HBV infection, and from 1990 to 2010, the worldwide mortality associated with cancer increased by 62%, and that associated with cirrhosis increased by 29% (15).

The majority of these HBV-infected individuals live in Asia or Africa (Fig. 3). Approximately one-fourth of adults who were infected with HBV as children experience serious complications from liver cirrhosis and/or HCC linked to chronic HBV (10). In 2015, it was estimated that 21,900 new cases occurred, and approximately 850,000 individuals live with HBV infection in the United States (https://www.cdc.gov/hepatitis/statistics/2015surveillance/commentary.htm). In the United States, most infections are in adults, in whom the risk of chronic infection is lower. In contrast, outside the United States, perinatal exposure is more common and leads to chronic HBV infections (10, 16).

The most common modes of HBV transmission are vertical transmission (mother to child perinatally), early childhood infections from close contact with infected individuals, sexual activity (both heterosexual and male

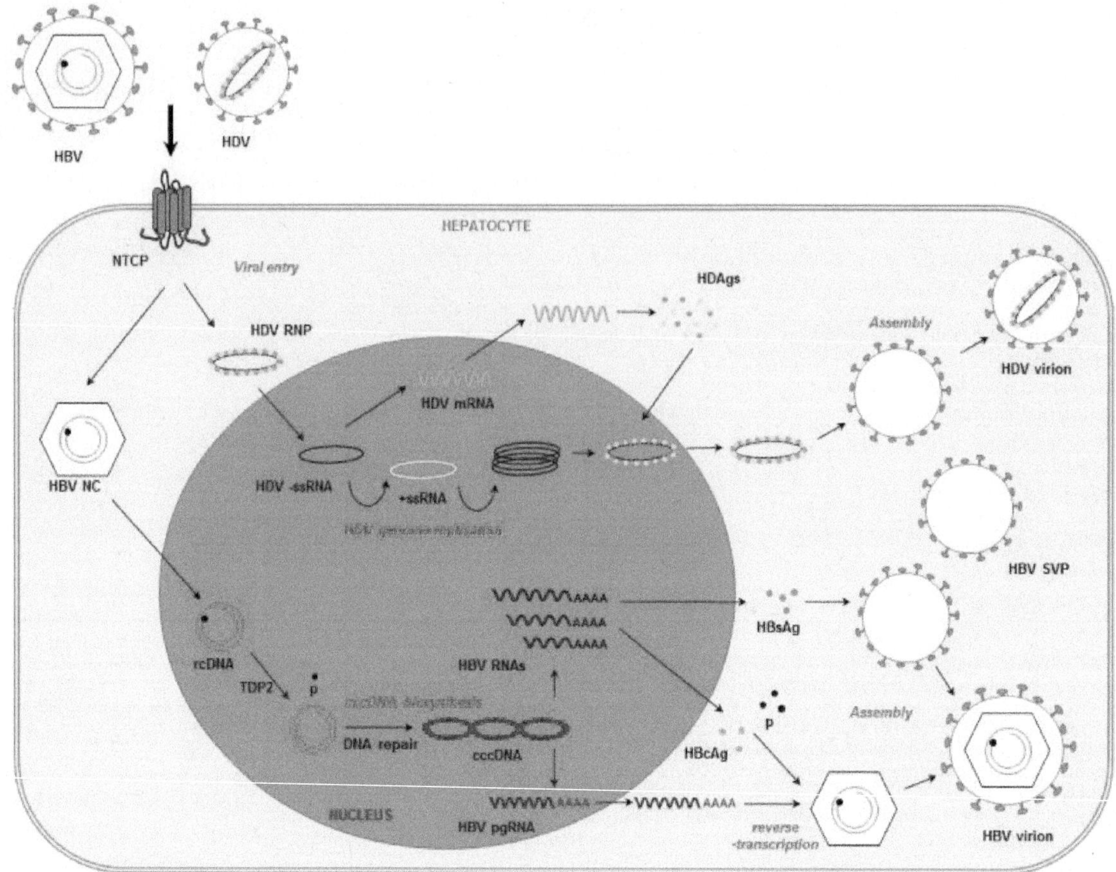

FIGURE 2 Schematic representation of the HBV and HDV life cycles in hepatocytes. HDV RNP, HDV ribonucleoprotein; HBV NC, HBV nucleocapsid; rcDNA, relaxed circular DNA; −/+ssRNA, negative/positive single-stranded RNA; cccDNA, covalently closed circular DNA; HBV pgRNA, HBV pregenomic RNA; HDAgs, hepatitis D antigens; HBcAg, HBV core antigen; HBsAg, HBV surface antigen; p, HBV polymerase; HBV SVP, HBV subviral particle; TDP2, tyrosyl-DNA phosphodiesterase 2. Reprinted from reference 4 with permission.

homosexual), and injection drug use or other physical contact with infected body fluids (occupational exposure, contaminated blood products, etc.) (2, 10). HBV is not transmitted by casual activities such as talking, hand holding, or hugging, by ingestion of food or water, or from a cough or sneeze.

Clinical Significance

HBV infects hepatocytes, leading to either an acute infection that resolves or a chronic infection that lasts for years. In infected individuals, subclinical hepatitis presents as a mild disease without symptoms or jaundice. It is not uncommon for many HBV-infected people to be asymptomatic early in disease. Nevertheless, some patients may have vague symptoms such as abdominal pain, nausea without jaundice (anicteric hepatitis), or nausea with jaundice (icteric hepatitis). HBV infections can result in the complete recovery of the patient, fulminant hepatitis with mortality, or a chronic viral infection. Progression from acute to chronic HBV varies with age, occurring in approximately 90% of perinatal, 20% of childhood, and <5% of adult infections (17). Though terminology has varied over time and between international societies, four phases of chronic HBV disease are commonly recognized: (i) immune tolerant, (ii) immune active, (iii) immune inactive, and (iv) reactivation (https://www.cdc.gov/mmwr/volumes/67/rr/pdfs/rr6701-H.pdf) (10, 18, 19).

The incubation period of acute HBV infection ranges from 6 weeks to 6 months. During this time the infection can be symptomatic or asymptomatic. Newborns infected with HBV usually have chronic, asymptomatic infections, while older children and adults are typically symptomatic during a primary infection (2, 10).

The symptoms of acute HBV infection are often mild but sometimes include physical signs such as jaundice, dark urine, clay-colored stools, and hepatomegaly (2, 10, 19). Some patients experience weight loss, right upper quadrant pain, and a tender, enlarged liver. Acute HBV infections are usually self-limited, and most patients recover completely after specific antibodies (anti-HBs) clear the virus (10, 19).

The disease outcome of acute HBV is age dependent, and most patients with acute disease are adults. Acute liver damage is caused by the host immune response to HBV-infected hepatocytes (10). This results in massive necrosis, which can lead to permanent damage to the liver. Mortality associated with fulminant hepatic failure is high without liver transplantation. After transplantation, HBV reinfection of the "new" liver is common, resulting in injury to the new liver in some patients. HBIG and/or antiviral therapy

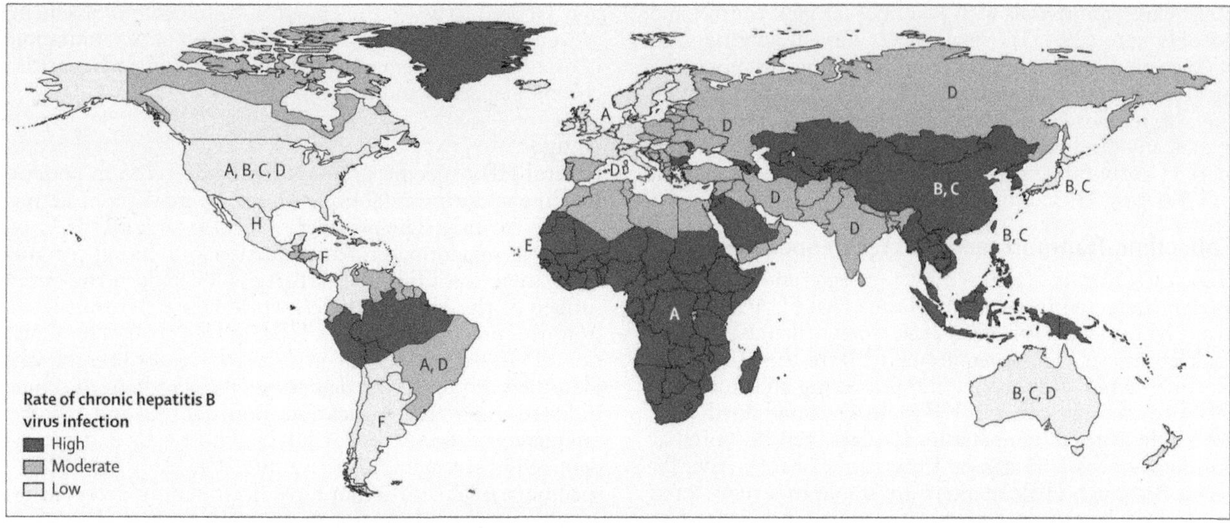

FIGURE 3 Worldwide distribution of major HBV genotypes and frequency of chronic infection. HBV prevalence in the population is defined as high, >8%; intermediate, 2 to 7%; low, <2%. Reprinted from reference 10 with permission.

can prevent this outcome (19, 20). Pathologic features of acute HBV include both degenerative and regenerative liver parenchymal changes that lead to lobular disarray. Patients with perinatally acquired HBV are usually immune tolerant to HBV antigens. This explains the absence of severe liver disease despite high levels of virus (10). Patients who continue to have detectable HBsAg or detectable HBV DNA in serum for at least 6 months after infection are considered to have chronic HBV infections (19). Chronic carriers can remain positive for HBsAg indefinitely, although some HBsAg-positive patients spontaneously convert to HBsAg negative after the appearance of anti-HBs. Many of these patients continue to have detectable HBV DNA (2, 10, 18). Symptoms of chronic HBV are generally nonspecific and may be unrecognized for years.

Most HBV-infected individuals progress to the immune active phase, in which a liver biopsy shows inflammation with fibrosis, thus the term "active." This pathology results from a persistent immune response to the HBV proteins on infected hepatocytes. The last phase of chronic HBV infection is the inactive carrier phase, characterized by less inflammation as determined by liver biopsy and normal liver enzyme levels. These patients have a lower risk for HCC (18).

Chronic HBV infection is associated with an increased risk for HCC (15, 18, 21). During HBV infection, the viral DNA randomly integrates into the hepatocyte genome. Over time this results in high levels of integrated viral DNA in host cells that can persist for years. Since the viral DNA integrates randomly, the number of integration sites also increases over time (19). Some of this randomly integrated viral DNA can activate cellular proto-oncogenes or suppress the regulation of gene expression (21). In addition, some HBV proteins, such as the X protein and the truncated pre-S/S protein, are potent transactivators of cellular genes (22, 23). Likewise, several other factors have been associated with the development of HCC, such as smoking, alcohol consumption, infections with other hepatotropic viruses (hepatitis C), and mycotoxins (aflatoxin) (15).

Safe and effective vaccines against HBV have been available since 1981. The complete HBV vaccination series is protective in >95% of infants, children, and young adults (10, 16). Vaccine-induced protection lasts at least 20 years and may be lifelong. Universal vaccination is recommended at birth, in childhood, and for adults in high-risk settings. Nonimmune individuals with a known or suspected exposure to HBV should be given HBV vaccine as soon as possible after the exposure, in addition to HBIG. In January 2018, updated recommendations for the prevention of HBV infection in the United States from the Advisory Committee on Immunization Practices were released by the Centers for Disease Control and Prevention (CDC) (https://www.cdc.gov/mmwr/volumes/67/rr/pdfs/rr6701-H.pdf). Two single-antigen vaccines (HBsAg only) and two combination vaccines (HBsAg in combination with other vaccines) were included. These vaccines require three spaced doses, at 0, 1, and 6 months. In March 2018, a more immunogenic adjuvanted HBV vaccine was approved for use in adults, which requires only two doses, 4 weeks apart, and may be more immunogenic for patients with compromised immune systems. Information on the Heplisav-B vaccine is available on the CDC website (https://www.cdc.gov/vaccines/schedules/vacc-updates/heplisav-b.html) (24, 25).

Chronic HBV infections should be treated with lifelong antiviral drugs. Historically, the goals of treating chronic HBV are to suppress viral replication and slow the progression of liver damage (2, 10, 26, 27). With the advent of new, curative therapies for patients with hepatitis C, a discussion has taken place to define what it means to be "cured" of chronic HBV (26, 28, 29). At present, drugs to treat HBV are classified into two categories, the pegylated interferons and the nucleoside/nucleotide analogs. The FDA has approved the nucleoside/nucleotide analogs adefovir, entecavir, tenofovir, emtricitabine, and telbivudine for use in the United States (19, 26, 27, 30). In late 2016, the FDA approved tenofovir alafenamide, a tenofovir prodrug, for treatment of adults with chronic HBV infection with compensated liver disease. Since tenofovir alafenamide has greater plasma stability and more efficiently delivers tenofovir to hepatocytes, it can be given at a lower dose once a day, improving renal and bone laboratory safety parameters (31, 32).

With the discovery of NTCP as an HBV receptor (4–7), HBV entry inhibitors are now under investigation as a novel class of antivirals with potential for viral control and possibly cure (29, 33). Small molecules interacting with NTCP exhibit antiviral activity, including the immunosuppressive drug cyclosporin A (33, 34). A pre-S1 peptide (i.e., Myrcludex B) derived from the HBV envelope, and specifically binding to the receptor, was shown to exhibit marked antiviral activity in cell culture, animal models, and patients (33, 35, 36).

Collection, Transport, and Storage of Specimens

HBV infection is diagnosed by serologic and molecular markers detected in serum or plasma. All FDA-approved assays have specific specimen requirements defined in their package inserts. These requirements state the acceptable specimen types and describe the processing and storage of the specimen. In general, HBV antigens and antibodies are stable at room temperature for days, can be stored at 4°C for months, and can be frozen at −20 to −70°C for years. Although HBV markers are stable in serum stored at −70°C, repetitive freezing and thawing can lead to their degradation. The use of hemolyzed samples should be avoided due to the potential of these specimens to interfere with the detection signals used in immunoassays.

Both serum and plasma (EDTA or acid-citrate-dextrose [ACD]) can be used for nucleic acid analysis (37). However, for consistent results, serial testing should be performed using the same sample type and the same kit whenever possible. Depending on the manufacturer's instructions for the kit employed, serum or plasma should be separated from cells within 6 to 24 h and stored at 4°C for 3 to 7 days until tested. For long-term storage, serum or plasma should be kept at −70°C. Heparinized plasma is unacceptable for most nucleic acid analysis because heparin interferes with *Taq* polymerase-mediated PCR. There is evidence that HBV DNA is stable and detectable without a loss of sensitivity after multiple freeze-thaw cycles (38). Dried blood spots on filter paper and dried specimen storage transportation systems have been successfully used for HBV serology and nucleic acid testing (39–41). Useful information about many diagnostic tests can be found by consulting the FDA website and the specific year of test approval (http://www.fda.gov/MedicalDevices/ProductsandMedicalProcedures/DeviceApprovalsandClearances/Recently-ApprovedDevices/default.htm).

The HBV virion is very hardy and remains infectious for at least 7 days outside the host (37). Thus, spills or splashes should be cleaned using absorbent material and disinfected with an appropriate disinfectant. Decontamination should be carried out while wearing gloves. Laboratory personnel should regard all specimens as potentially infectious (42). The Occupational Safety and Health Administration (OSHA) standards for occupational exposure to blood-borne pathogens are designed to protect employees exposed to blood and other potentially infectious materials. OSHA mandates that all employees whose job requirements put them at risk for blood-borne pathogens be offered HBV vaccine at no cost. OSHA standards and additional safety recommendations can be found in the literature.

Direct Detection

The diagnosis of HBV uses a combination of tests (43, 44). These assays detect specific HBV proteins, nucleic acid, and specific antibodies in plasma or serum (Table 2).

Microscopy

Electron microscopy for detection of HBV does not play a role in the diagnosis of disease. However, a liver biopsy may be used to assess the extent of histologic involvement as well as the response to therapy. Histologic examination is useful for distinguishing among acute viral hepatitis, chronic hepatitis, and cirrhosis.

Antigen

Several HBV-specific proteins can be detected in patient specimens during infection. These are markers of active viral replication. The presence of HBsAg and/or HBeAg in serum occurs during primary infection and during chronic HBV infection (Table 1). HBsAg is located on the outer surface of the HBV particles, while HBeAg is translated from the precore mRNA of HBcAg (Fig. 1C). The function of HBeAg and its role in disease have not been clearly identified; however, the detection of this protein in serum indicates high viral replication. Both HBsAg and HBeAg are made in large excess by infected host cells and can be detected in serum during active infection (2, 10, 45). HBV-specific antigens in serum have been mainly detected by enzyme or chemiluminescence immunoassays. The presence of viral antigens in tissue can be determined through the use of immunohistochemistry.

Diagnostic assays with high sensitivity and specificity are available to detect these HBV antigens. Table 1 lists the biomarkers used to determine the stage of HBV disease. HBV antigens are detected by using solid-phase assays based on capture with a monoclonal antibody and then detected with a second antibody attached to a signal. These assays commonly use microparticles with different compositions and sizes and are usually performed on automated instruments (9, 46). Antigen capture and detection reagents are specific for the major immunodominant region of HBsAg. Current detection methods use enzyme or chemiluminescence immunoassays to detect specific antigens (Table 2). Hepatitis B core-related antigen is considered an emerging marker for chronic HBV in some studies but currently remains a research tool (47).

HBsAg

The detection of HBsAg in serum plays a central role in establishing the diagnosis of HBV infection. Each HBsAg assay is approved by the FDA for diagnostic use only; for testing donors of blood, organs, and tissue only; or for both applications. The package insert should be consulted to determine what sample types have been approved for use with each HBsAg test (Table 2).

The presence of HBsAg in the serum indicates that the patient is considered infectious. Patients who resolve an acute infection eventually produce anti-HBs (see "Serologic Tests" below). However, when HBsAg is present, anti-HBs can be negative in diagnostic tests because the antibody is bound to the HBsAg.

For all commercially available diagnostic assays, any specimens that are nonreactive for HBsAg are considered negative and do not require further testing. In contrast, specimens reactive for HBsAg are often repeated to verify positive results. These repeatedly HBsAg-positive results are usually confirmed by a neutralization assay provided by the manufacturer consistent with FDA approval protocols. If the HBsAg-reactive serum is neutralized by the anti-HBs, then the specimen is considered positive for HBsAg. Conversely, if the anti-HBs does not neutralize the HBsAg, then the HBsAg test must be considered nonconfirmed. A new specimen should be requested and/or the patient should be tested for other markers of HBV infection such as IgM anti-HBc or total anti-HBc.

All HBsAg assays are capable of detecting subnanogram amounts of protein with no loss of specificity (46, 48).

TABLE 2 Commercial systems for serologic testing of HBV antigens and antibodies available in the United States

Manufacturer	Test	Method[a]	Analytes	Acceptable specimens[b]	Reportable range[c,d] (level for immunity; range)	Approved uses[e]
Abbott Laboratories	Architect	CLIA	HBsAg[f], anti-HBc total, anti-HBc IgM	Serum, plasma (no citrate)	Qualitative	A
			Anti-HBs	Serum, plasma (no citrate)	Qualitative or quantitative (≥12 mIU/ml immune; range, 4.23 to >1,000 mIU/ml)	A, D
	Prism	CLIA	HBsAg	Serum, plasma	Qualitative	C
			Anti-HBc total	Serum, plasma (no heparin)	Qualitative	C
Bio-Rad Laboratories	Genetic Systems	EIA	HBsAg 3.0	Serum, plasma, and cadaveric serum	Qualitative	B
	Monolisa	EIA	Anti-HBc total, anti-HBc IgM	Serum, plasma	Qualitative	A
			Anti-HBs PLUS	Serum, plasma (citrate may give lower values)	Qualitative or quantitative (≥10 mIU/ml immune; range, 2 to 1,000 mIU/ml)	A, D
DiaSorin	ETI	EIA	HBsAg, anti-HBc total, anti-HBc IgM	Serum, plasma	Qualitative	A
			HBeAg, anti-HBe	Serum, plasma	Qualitative	A
			Anti-HBs	Serum, plasma	Qualitative only (>10 mIU/ml positive)	A, D
Ortho Clinical Diagnostics	Vitros	CLIA	HBsAg, anti-HBc total, anti-HBc IgM	Serum, plasma (heparin and/or citrate can lower sample/cutoff ratio in some HBsAg or anti-HBc IgM reactive samples)	Qualitative	A
			HBeAg, anti-HBe	Serum	Qualitative	A
			Anti-HBs	Serum	Qualitative or quantitative (≥12 mIU/ml positive; range, 4.23 to 1,000 mIU/ml)	A, D
Roche Diagnostics	Elecsys	ECLIA	HBsAg II[g], anti-HBc total, anti-HBc IgM	Serum, plasma	Qualitative	A
			HBeAg	Serum, plasma		A
			Anti-HBs	Serum, plasma (EDTA only)	Qualitative or quantitative (≥11.5 mIU/ml positive; range, 3.5 to 1,000 mIU/ml)	A, D
Siemens Healthcare Diagnostics	Advia Centaur	CLIA	HBsAg, HBsAg II[g], anti-HBc total, anti-HBc IgM	Serum, plasma (no citrate, except for HBsAg II)	Qualitative	A
			HBeAg, anti-HBe 1, anti-HBe 2	Serum, plasma (no citrate)	Qualitative	A
			Anti-HBs2	Serum, plasma (no citrate)	Qualitative or quantitative (≥12 mIU/ml immune; range, 3.1 to 1,000 mIU/ml)	A, D
	Immulite	CLIA	HBsAg, anti-HBc total, anti-HBc IgM	Serum, plasma[e]	Qualitative	A
			Anti-HBs	Serum, plasma (heparin only)	Qualitative or quantitative (≥12 mIU/ml immune; range, 3.0 to 1,000 mIU/ml)	A, D

[a]CLIA, chemiluminescent immunoassay; EIA, enzyme immunoassay; ECLIA, electrochemiluminescence.
[b]Serum includes specimens collected in serum separator tubes; plasma includes collections in potassium EDTA, sodium citrate, sodium heparin, lithium heparin, and/or plasma separator tubes unless otherwise stated for a specific test.
[c]All information on methods is derived from FDA submissions and manufacturers' information when available.
[d]All samples with reactive and/or gray zone/indeterminate results are retested in duplicate before reporting results. See package insert for specific instructions.
[e]A, diagnostic use only; not for use in evaluation of blood, blood products, or tissue or blood donors; B, diagnostic use and screening of blood, blood products, and/or tissue or blood donors; C, screening of blood, blood products, and/or tissue or blood donors only; D, evaluation of postvaccination response.
[f]All assays require positive HBsAg results to be repeated and confirmed with a separate confirmation assay specific for each kit.
[g]Detects HBsAg wild type and escape mutants.

For diagnostic applications, this level of sensitivity is sufficient to detect the HBsAg in the sera of individuals with actively replicating HBV. However, a recent concern is that some assays cannot detect variants of HBsAg that have mutations within the major antigenic region of the protein. These mutant HBsAg proteins can be missed by some diagnostic assays (9, 13), so initial testing should include the detection of antibodies to both HBsAg and HB core, and if needed, molecular assays should be used for confirmation (9).

The major antigenic determinant on the HBsAg is designated the "a" determinant. This antigenic site is formed by a conformational structure containing a disulfide bond that results in a specific three-dimensional epitope. The region between amino acids 124 and 147 is found within the major hydrophilic loop of the protein (8, 48–50). There is a concern that current diagnostic assays do not detect HBsAg with alterations within this major antigenic epitope, since some HBsAg assays use monoclonal antibodies that capture the HBsAg using this immunodominant epitope. These HBV strains are known as "escape mutants." The first escape mutant that was described occurred in a child born to an HBV-positive mother who transmitted HBV to the child despite vaccination and HBIG (45). This virus had a substitution of arginine for glycine in HBsAg at amino acid position 145. A single amino acid change altered the antigenic portion of the protein such that vaccine-induced antibody no longer recognized the antigen. This allowed the altered virus to persist in the infant. Subsequently, the patient remained positive for HBV DNA and HBsAg (with mutation) for longer than 12 years. Since that time, a number of other substitution mutants within the "a" determinant region of HBsAg have been recognized. Recent studies have evaluated HBsAg assays to determine their ability to detect well-defined HBsAg mutants and have found that some mutations in the HBsAg may be missed by diagnostic assays (45, 48). Many assays have been updated to better detect mutants (e.g., HBsAg II [Table 2]) (9). Nevertheless, the CDC recently reported a hemodialysis patient who was HBsAg negative as determined by several commercial assays yet had an HBV DNA level of 14,200,000 IU/ml (51).

In response to the concern that blood donors with an HBsAg mutant may not be identified by HBV antigen assays, most countries screen blood donors for anti-HBc in addition to screening for HBsAg. Blood donors in the United States are also tested for HBV DNA (48). Individuals with positive tests for HBV DNA and anti-HBc and/or patients with positive results for HBeAg and/or HBV DNA but negative for HBsAg could be infected with an escape mutant (49).

Serum HBsAg quantification has been recently reported as a useful marker to predict disease activity and monitor treatment response in chronic hepatitis B and is widely used in Europe and Asia but not yet in the United States (8, 9). The HBsAg level is considered a surrogate for transcriptional activity of cccDNA, independent of HBV DNA replication and viral load. It can assist in the differentiation of immune tolerance and immune clearance in HBeAg-positive patients, predict inactive disease and spontaneous HBsAg seroclearance in HBeAg-negative patients, and identify HBV-positive mothers at highest risk for maternofetal transmission (52). The determination of HBsAg level is pivotal to individualize pegylated interferon treatment (8). Due to the development of new antiviral treatments aiming at HBsAg seroclearance as a functional cure, the HBsAg quantification in serum may become a mandatory measurement. The third international standard for HBsAg is available from the WHO (53, 54). Devices which measure HBsAg levels in IU/milliliter include the Abbott Architect HBsAg, DiaSorin LiaisonXL Murex HBsAg Quant, and Roche Elecsys HBsAg II. A head-to-head comparison of three assays indicated a good correlation between them but clearly showed an influence of both the genotype and the presence of "a" determinant variants in HBsAg quantification (9). Quantitative commercial assays are available in Europe but are not yet FDA approved in the United States. However, at the time of this writing, Quest Diagnostics reference laboratory offers a quantitative HBsAg using the Vitros assay.

HBeAg

The detection of HBeAg in serum is a sign of rapid viral replication usually associated with high HBV DNA levels. HBeAg-positive patients are highly infectious. However, some HBV strains do not make HBeAg due to a precore mutation. Patients infected with these mutant strains may have high HBV DNA levels in the absence of detectable HBeAg (49). Several commercial assays are available for the detection of HBeAg in serum. HBeAg-positive samples should be HBsAg and HBV DNA positive. If not, the result should be questioned and investigated further to ensure validity prior to reporting (Table 2).

Nucleic Acid Detection

Molecular assays to quantitate HBV DNA are used for the initial evaluation of HBV infections and the monitoring of patients with chronic infections during treatment (43, 44). In addition, as mentioned above, blood donors are routinely screened for HBV DNA using qualitative tests to identify donors in the early stage of HBV infection.

A number of quantitative assays, most using real-time PCR, have been developed to detect and monitor HBV DNA levels in infected patients (50, 55–59). In addition, loop-mediated isothermal amplification has been reported as a rapid and sensitive qualitative test option for use in resource-limited areas (60). Monitoring of HBV DNA levels provides information on the effectiveness of antiviral treatment and can indicate when a change in the antiviral regimen is needed. Most of the available assays have a lower limit of detection, between 5 and 50 copies/ml, and can quantify levels up to 1 billion copies/ml. This wide range of quantitation allows for monitoring HBV DNA early after infection and identifying HBV infections resistant to antiviral therapy (Table 3) (56). Recent studies have shown that the persistent suppression of HBV DNA is a primary measure of therapeutic success (19). A high level of HBV DNA following resolution of clinical hepatitis indicates a failure to control viral replication (26, 44).

Commercially available HBV DNA assays differ in their limits of detection, dynamic ranges, and methods used to measure DNA levels (Table 3). An international HBV DNA standard was established in 2001 by the WHO in response to the need to standardize HBV DNA quantification (38, 61). The current third WHO standard virus preparation is a high-titer genotype A2 preparation (code 10/264) which has been assigned a potency of $10^{5.93}$ IU/ml when constituted in 0.5 ml of nuclease-free water (62). The WHO standard has allowed results for different HBV DNA assays to be reported in IU per milliliter.

However, despite the availability of this standard, the various quantitative assays usually have different IU to copy number conversion factors, demonstrating their variability. Thus, the best practice is the consistent monitoring of patients using the same manufacturer's assay in the same laboratory (43, 44, 56).

TABLE 3 Molecular assays used to detect HBV nucleic acid

Manufacturer	Assay	Method	Platform	Specimens	Quantitative range	Sensitivity[a]	Approved uses[b]
Abbott Molecular	Abbott RealTime HBV	Real-time PCR	M2000	Serum, plasma (EDTA)	10–10^9 IU/ml	6.4 IU/ml for plasma 3.82 IU/ml for serum	A
Hologic	Aptima HBV Quant	TMA	Panther system	Serum, plasma (EDTA, ACD)	10–10^9 IU/ml	4.8 IU/ml for plasma 5.9 IU/ml for serum	A
Qiagen	*artus* HBV PCR	Real-time PCR	Roto-Gene	Plasma (EDTA, ACD)	10–10^9 IU/ml	3.8 IU/ml	A
			Lightcycler		10–10^{10} IU/ml	5.8 IU/ml	A
Roche Molecular Systems	COBAS AmpliPrep/ COBAS TaqMan v.2.0	Real-time PCR	Ampliprep/TaqMan Analyzer	Serum, plasma (EDTA)	20–1.7×10^8 IU/ml	20 IU/ml	A
	cobas HBV	Real-time PCR	Cobas 4800 Cobas 6800/8800	Serum, plasma (EDTA)	10–10^9 IU/ml	2.4 serum–2.7 plasma IU/ml; lower if sample input is <0.5 ml	A
	cobas AmpliScreen HBV	PCR followed by hybridization	Cobas Amplicor Analyzer	Serum, plasma (EDTA, ACD), cadaveric serum or plasma	Qualitative	4.41 (multiprep); 15.99 (standard prep) IU/ml	B
	cobas TaqScreen MPX	Real-time PCR (multiplex)	Cobas 6800/8800		Qualitative	1.3–1.4 IU/ml	B
Grifols USA	Procleix Ultrio	TMA[c] (multiplex)	Tigris		Qualitative	8.5 IU/ml	B
	Procleix Ultrio Plus	TMA (multiplex)	Tigris		Qualitative	4.1 IU/ml	B

[a]All assays claim to detect genotypes A to H; Qiagen and Roche assays claim ability to detect precore mutations.
[b]A, Monitor response to antiviral therapy; B, screen donor blood or blood products for presence of HBV DNA.
[c]TMA, transcription mediate amplification.

Some of the variability of HBV DNA quantification may occur during collection and processing of the specimen. Most assays use serum or plasma (EDTA or ACD) as the specimen of choice. In general, the tube should be centrifuged and the serum or plasma separated from the cells within 6 to 24 h after collection, as specified in the package insert for the kit employed. The manufacturer's instructions should be followed for approved specimen types and collection tubes, as well as processing and storage conditions and temperature. Repeated freezing and thawing should be avoided, because this may reduce assay sensitivity.

Most commercial assays quantitate HBV DNA and cover an 8- to 9-$\log_{10}$ range, which permits the accurate evaluation of HBV levels above a million down to very low levels that occur during treatment or in inactive carriers. Several studies have shown that a reduction of 2 $\log_{10}$ in HBV DNA levels in the first 6 months of antiviral therapy indicates treatment efficacy (38, 51, 53).

Isolation Procedures

Although HBV can infect hepatocytes *in vitro*, culture of HBV is not used as a diagnostic test. Recently, the discovery of NTCP as a key HBV/HDV cell entry factor (5, 6) has opened the door to a new era of investigation, because NTCP-overexpressing hepatoma cells acquire susceptibility to HBV and HDV infections (4). These advances should result in the development of cell culture models to improve our knowledge of virus-host interactions, and potentially of virus characterization.

Identification

The methods for identification of HBV infection use a combination of molecular, antigenic, and serologic methods described in "Direct Detection" above and "Serologic Tests" below.

Typing Systems

Antigenic variation occurs naturally in HBV due to genetic heterogeneity. These various genetic differences are used to classify HBV into 10 distinct genotypes, with over 40 subgenotypes (63). Genotypes A through H are presented in Table 4. Two more genotypes, I and J, are pending ratification by the International Committee on Taxonomy of Viruses. HBV genotypes are distinguished by a genetic divergence of 8% or more within the complete nucleotide sequence (2, 10, 16). There are substantial data that have correlated HBV genotypes with disease outcome. The most common genotypes associated with chronic HBV infections are B and C. Patients with genotype B are more likely to spontaneously convert to anti-HBeAg and thus have less severe liver damage. Genotype C is more common in Asia and has been associated with a high risk of progression to cirrhosis. However, in European studies, genotype D has been shown to be more likely to be associated with active liver disease than other genotypes (49). It is noted that most of these patients acquired these infections in childhood and had more exposure to HBV than other patients evaluated. It is not clear yet how the variances in HBV genotypes affect clinical outcomes. It is possible that the differences are associated with the viral expression of immune epitopes or the loss of critical control over viral replication such as precore and core promoter mutations. Thus, in spite of the intriguing studies of HBV genotypes, the role of HBV genotyping in predicting clinical and therapeutic outcomes has not been firmly established. However, with additional studies, the value of HBV genotyping to determine specific treatment will likely become apparent (10, 14, 26).

TABLE 4 HBV genotypes and major geographic circulation

Genotype[a]	Subtypes and serotypes	Genome size (nucleotides)	Geographic connection	Disease relationship
A	Subtypes A1–A3; serotypes adw2, ayw1	3,221	Northwestern Europe, Spain, Poland, USA, Central Africa, India, Brazil	HCC and cirrhosis in older patients; core promoter mutations (A1762T, G1764A) detected
B	Subtypes B1–B6; serotypes adw2, ayw1	3,215	Southeast Asia, Taiwan, Japan, Indonesia, China, Australia	HCC and cirrhosis in both younger and older patients; precore mutations (G1896A) detected
C	Subtypes C1–C4; serotypes adw2, adrq+, adrq−, ayr	3,215	Asia, Indonesia, India, Australia, USA, Brazil	Higher risk of HCC and cirrhosis than with genotype B; precore mutations (G1896A) and core promoter mutations (A1762T, G1764A) detected
D	Subtypes D1–D4; serotypes ayw2, ayw3	3,182	Mediterranean area, Middle East, India, Spain, USA, Brazil (generally found worldwide)	Chronic HBV, cirrhosis in older patients; precore mutations (G1896A) and core promoter mutations (A1762T, G1764A) detected
E	Subtypes unknown; serotype ayw4	3,212	West Africa	Unknown
F	Subtypes D1–D4; serotypes adw4q−, adw2, ayw4	3,215	Central and South America, Bolivia, Venezuela, Polynesia, Alaska	HCC in young children and adults
G	Subtypes unknown; serotype adw2	3,248	Australia, France, Germany, USA	Almost always is a coinfection with other HBV types
H	Subtypes unknown; serotype adw4	3,215	Central and South America, USA	Unknown

[a]Two additional genotypes, I and J, are pending ratification by the International Committee on Taxonomy of Viruses.

Serologic Tests

Serologic tests for HBV-specific antibodies are used to determine the stage of HBV disease and to establish immunity after HBV vaccination. As the host mounts an immune response, the first antibodies to appear are IgM specific for HBc (IgM anti-HBc); this is followed by the appearance of total anti-HBc, anti-HBe, and finally anti-HBs (20) (Fig. 4). A number of commercial assays are available for HBV serologic testing (Table 2).

IgM Anti-HBc

IgM anti-HBc persists for several weeks to months after an initial infection. The detection of IgM anti-HBc indicates an infection of less than 6 months' duration (Table 1). During this stage of disease, the patient's liver enzymes may be elevated. A negative IgM anti-HBc result excludes a recent, acute infection but does not rule out chronic infection (43, 44, 64). The presence of IgM anti-HBc identifies patients who are acutely infected; such patients often have high levels of HBV DNA (64). IgM anti-HBc is also the only serologic marker that is positive during the seronegative window of acute HBV, when HBsAg has declined to an undetectable level but before anti-HBs appears. During this period, HBsAg is bound in immune complexes to anti-HBs, thus rendering both undetectable by immunoassay.

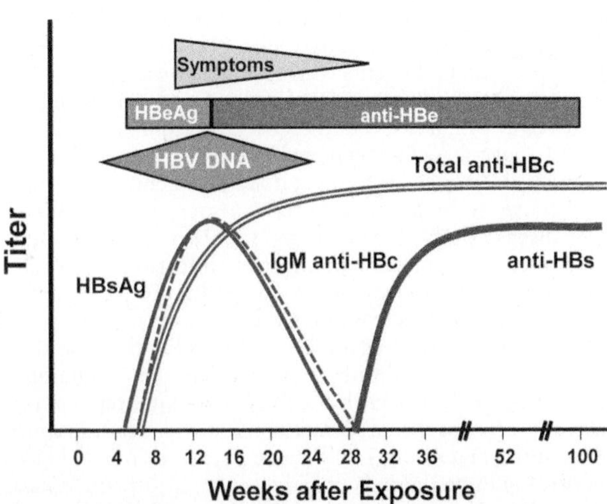

FIGURE 4 Typical sequence of serologic markers in patients with acute HBV infection with resolution of symptoms.

Total Anti-HBc

A negative anti-HBc test indicates that a person does not have a history of infection with HBV. A positive total anti-HBc result can indicate an acute infection, in which the patient is also HBsAg positive and IgM anti-HBc positive, a resolved (HBsAg-negative) infection, or a chronic (HBsAg-positive) HBV infection (Table 1) (26, 64). Total anti-HBc antibodies remain after IgM anti-HBc disappears and can be detected for many years. These antibodies persist longer than anti-HBs. Thus, total anti-HBc is the best marker for documenting prior exposure to HBV infection. Vaccines do not include HBcAg; thus, vaccination induces only anti-HBs. Therefore, anti-HBc is not present in vaccinated individuals unless they were infected with HBV prior to vaccination (65). Individuals positive for anti-HBc without any other serologic evidence of HBV infection (i.e., isolated anti-HBc) should be considered exposed to HBV (64). This serologic pattern is consistent with a remote, past HBV infection that has resolved or with an occult HBV infection with very low viral DNA levels (10). Thus, HBV DNA testing should be performed in all patients with isolated anti-HBc. Many patients with isolated anti-HBc may be coinfected with hepatitis C virus and/or human immunodeficiency virus (HIV) (66). Rarely, isolated anti-HBc could be a nonspecific result.

Commercial kits for detection of total anti-HBc are available and use a variety of methods and instrumentation (Table 2). All assays use recombinant HBc antigen for capture of antibody.

Anti-HBs

A negative result for anti-HBs in the absence of any other HBV-specific antigen or antibody indicates that a person has not been infected with HBV and has not been vaccinated with HBV. A positive result is consistent with immunity to HBV due to an infection or from effective vaccination (Table 1). Anti-HBs quantitation panels are commercially available and should be used when validating anti-HBs assays.

Anti-HBs is a key serologic marker for both vaccine-induced immunity and immunity due to infection. As HBV vaccination has become more widespread, this serologic marker is used to monitor vaccine success. Both the WHO and CDC recognize a level of >10 mIU/ml of anti-HBs as an indication of protective immunity. However, it has been demonstrated that levels of anti-HBs determined by one commercial assay system cannot be compared with those detected with a different system despite the use of international standards (67). Thus, levels designated positive by different test kits may vary (Table 2).

Postvaccination testing for the presence of anti-HBs is not recommended for infants, children, or most adults. The CDC lists exceptions to this rule, which are infants born to mothers who are HBsAg positive, immunocompromised patients, dialysis patients, and to confirm successful vaccination in health care workers to prevent the transmission of HBV in the health care setting (68).

HBV escape mutants in which the HBsAg has mutated can result in HBV infections despite vaccine-induced anti-HBs antibody (49). In these situations, both HBsAg and anti-HBs may be detected simultaneously in the patient's blood (51).

Anti-HBe

A positive test for anti-HBe is associated with a decrease in viral replication and thus viral titer (Table 1). During acute infection, these antibodies are bound to HBeAg; the antibody is not detected until the HBeAg levels decrease.

Patients who have recovered from acute HBV infection have detectable anti-HBe, anti-HBc, and anti-HBs. Interestingly, patients infected with HBeAg-negative strains of HBV still have anti-HBe (26).

Test algorithms for HBeAg and anti-HBe kits vary. Generally, immunoassays have indeterminate or gray zones. If a sample repeatedly yields indeterminate values, additional testing should be performed with a new specimen.

Antiviral Susceptibility Testing

Therapy for HBV usually requires long-term treatment with nucleoside or nucleotide analogs. A disadvantage of long-term therapy is the subsequent development of antiviral resistance. As noted above, HBV replicates through an RNA intermediate. The HBV RNA-dependent DNA polymerase is not precise during rapid replication cycles and does not correctly proofread the final copies, leading to frequent errors. Some of these errors create resistant mutants, which are selected in the presence of antiviral agents (26, 69). Over time, the HBV strains with antiviral resistance become the major viral species. The current recommendation is that a patient who has a 1-$\log_{10}$ increase from the lowest HBV DNA level should be evaluated for the development of antiviral resistance (26, 69).

Recently, the nomenclature of HBV antiviral resistance was standardized to track nucleotide changes associated with drug resistance and to recognize new mutations (69, 70). Antiviral resistance mutations can be detected by molecular methods that recognize known mutations associated with resistance (12). Methods used to detect these mutations are available; however, the interpretation of results is not always straightforward. Some mutations predict resistance to multiple drugs. A single mutation at A181T is associated with resistance to lamivudine, adefovir, tenofovir, and telbivudine (12, 71). In other situations genetic sequence changes may not confer resistance when present alone but do contribute to resistance when additional mutations are present. Many of these single nucleotide changes have no recognized phenotype and may represent the random genetic changes found in viruses that use a reverse transcriptase during replication (69, 70). For more information on HBV antiviral resistance mutations, see chapters 114 and 115 of this *Manual*.

There are currently no FDA-approved commercial IVD kits for resistance genotyping, but testing for antiviral resistance mutations by genetic sequencing is available at reference laboratories (72). The INNO-LIPA HBV Multi-DR (Fujirebio Diagnostics, Malvern, PA) is a line probe assay available for diagnostic use in Europe and for research use only in the United States. It employs biotinylated amplicons that hybridize to membrane-bound oligonucleotides that represent a mutation sequence. The second-generation line probe assay allows for simultaneous detection of HBV wild-type motif, lamivudine, telbivudine, emtricitabine, adefovir, and entecavir resistance-associated mutations (73–76). Some disadvantages of line probe assays are that the reading of the reaction lines on each strip can be difficult (up to 34 lines per strip), faint bands can be problematic to interpret, and at times the test results show no bands in viral preparations with known mutations (74–76).

A second assay (Trugene HBV genotyping kit; Siemens Medical Solutions Diagnostics) is only available as a research-use-only assay. This system detects antiviral mutations by direct sequencing from specimens, including specimens with low HBV levels (72, 77, 78). Comparison between the sequence assay and the line probe hybridization assay shows a high concordance (77).

A number of individual laboratory-developed assays have been used to detect antiviral mutations in HBV. Sanger DNA sequencing can be used to detect such mutations directly. The advantage of DNA sequencing is that it is accurate and mutations can be identified in any part of the HBV genome (64, 74). However, a serious disadvantage is that these methods lack sensitivity and detect mutants present in 10 to 30% of the viral population. This level of detection does not always consistently identify resistance mutants, which make up at least 10% of the virus population (74). Next-generation sequencing is now being used to detect minor viral populations that could emerge during antiviral treatment (76, 79). These HBV variants are present in the patient in low numbers and can have random genetic changes that lead to antiviral drug resistance. During treatment, the HBV variants can be monitored to determine when the patient needs a change in therapy (79–85).

Phenotypic testing is used to detect HBV antiviral resistance in research and development laboratories. These methods detect drug resistance based on the use of molecular or cellular techniques or using animal models and are not available for clinical use. Recently, NTCP-overexpressing hepatoma cell lines have been used to screen for antivirals targeting cell entry (86, 87). These novel cell culture systems should provide useful tools not only to improve our understanding of the HBV life cycles, but also in antiviral susceptibility testing.

Evaluation, Interpretation, and Reporting of Results

HBV infection leads to several disease presentations, from acute hepatitis with fulminant hepatic failure to chronic hepatitis leading to cirrhosis and/or HCC. The initial assessment for suspected viral hepatitis should include laboratory tests that measure serum transaminases, direct and total bilirubin, albumin and total protein, a complete blood count, coagulation tests, and alpha fetoprotein. The specific laboratory tests to detect and monitor HBV infection are a mix of viral antigen detection, molecular measurements of HBV DNA, and serologic markers (Table 1). Patients who are negative for HBsAg, anti-HBc, and HBV DNA are not infected with HBV.

In a typical acute HBV infection, HBsAg can be detected by immunoassay 2 to 4 weeks before the liver enzyme levels become abnormal and before symptoms appear. Using molecular amplification methods, HBV DNA can be detected before HBsAg and long before the onset of symptoms. During acute HBV disease, once symptoms appear and serum transaminases are elevated, IgM anti-HBc and total anti-HBc are also detectable as liver damage is associated with the immune response. At this phase, a period of peak viral replication, HBeAg may also be detectable. Most patients with an active HBV infection that resolves have anti-HBs that are detectable shortly after the disappearance of HBsAg. The levels of IgM anti-HBc eventually decline over several months as the disease either resolves or becomes chronic. Figure 4 illustrates a typical serologic pattern that occurs in patients with an acute HBV infection.

Note that if HBsAg alone is detected in a blood sample without anti-HBc, rather than early HBV infection, the explanation is usually recent vaccination, since HBsAg can be routinely detectable in blood for 18 days after vaccination, and even up to 52 days in dialysis patients (https://www.cdc.gov/mmwr/volumes/67/rr/pdfs/rr6701-H.pdf). Thus, a history of recent vaccination should be sought and interpretive comments should include this possibility.

Chronic HBV stages can be distinguished using a combination of laboratory tests and clinical signs (Table 1; Fig. 5). The immune tolerant phase usually occurs when the patient acquires HBV infection at birth or during early childhood. Infection in this case is associated with a high level of viral production and the presence of HBeAg. There is an absence of liver disease despite high levels of HBV replication as a consequence of immune tolerance; however, the underlying pathology is poorly understood.

As the host's immune response matures, the patient often moves to the immune active phase (also referred to as the HBeAg-positive chronic hepatitis phase), during which HBV-specific epitopes are recognized by the host immune system, leading to immune-mediated injury in the liver. Individuals who acquire HBV perinatally often transition from the immune tolerant phase to the HBeAg-positive chronic hepatitis phase between 20 and 30 years of age. The liver biopsy in this stage shows active inflammation accompanied by fibrosis. Patients who remain HBeAg positive have a higher risk of progressing to liver disease due to the induction of a chronically active immune response by high rates of HBV replication. Such patients have high HBV DNA levels and increased levels of serum transaminases. While HBsAg-positive patients can transmit HBV sexually, percutaneously, or perinatally, individuals with detectable HBeAg pose the highest risk of transmitting HBV to others.

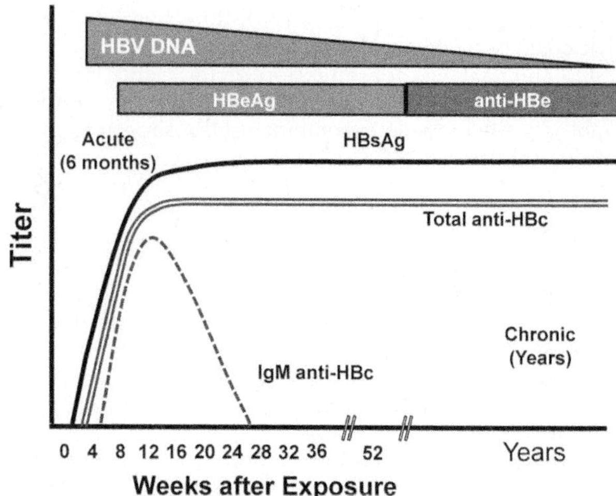

FIGURE 5 Typical sequence of serologic markers in patients with HBV infection that progresses to chronicity. In patients with chronic HBV infection, both HBsAg and IgG anti-HBc remain persistently detectable, generally for life. HBeAg is variably present in these patients.

However, if these individuals develop anti-HBe and HBeAg negativity, they move to the inactive carrier phase (Table 1). The transition from the immune tolerant phase to the inactive carrier phase is often not recognized, since patients are often asymptomatic. While the inactive carrier phase is characterized by the seroconversion to anti-HBe, patients can alternate between low and undetectable levels of HBV DNA. The seroconversion to anti-HBe is associated with a decrease in liver damage and the normalization of serum transaminase levels. Mild hepatitis may be noted on biopsy. Many patients remain in this phase for years.

A portion of inactive HBsAg carriers (about one-third) develop chronic hepatitis which recurs in the absence of HBeAg in their sera (HBeAg-negative chronic hepatitis). These patients are infected with an HBV variant that cannot express HBeAg due to mutations in the precore or core promoter regions of the HBV core gene. Patients with chronic hepatitis that are HBeAg negative are more likely to have more advanced liver disease in spite of lower serum HBV DNA levels.

Patients infected with an HBsAg escape mutant can test negative for HBsAg but are positive when tested for anti-HBc and HBV DNA. In some individuals the presence of anti-HBc alone may be the only evidence of an active, occult HBV infection of remote origin. These patients, especially those on dialysis, should have HBV DNA testing to exclude a low-level carrier state.

In a new development, quantitative HBsAg has been proposed as a surrogate marker for transcriptional activity of intrahepatic cccDNA, independent of HBV DNA replication, and thus is increasingly recognized as a useful marker to differentiate phases of chronic HBV (8, 9). Consequently, diagnostic assays are becoming available to inform HBV prognosis and therapy.

Passive transfer of anti-HBs or anti-HBc may be observed in neonates of mothers with current or past HBV infections. However, passive-antibody levels decline gradually over 3 to 6 months, while levels of antibody induced by infection are stable over many years. Since blood donations are tested for HBsAg and total anti-HBc, passive transfer of these HBV markers following blood transfusions is unlikely.

Anti-HBs without anti-HBc develops in individuals who receive hepatitis B vaccine (which contains only HBsAg), and anti-HBs levels of ≥10 mIU/ml are considered protective. Most individuals vaccinated for HBV have detectable levels of anti-HBs; however, some vaccinated people test negative due to waning levels of anti-HBs. They usually respond to a challenge dose of HBsAg vaccine with an anamnestic response in approximately 2 weeks. Studies of vaccinated individuals who no longer have detectable anti-HBs show that infection can occur but is blunted by the anamnestic anti-HBs response such that liver damage is minimal and symptoms do not occur. In contrast, an HBsAg-negative carrier may fail to produce detectable levels of anti-HBs after vaccination. Individuals who do not have a detectable response to the first series of HBV vaccine should be given a second vaccine series. Individuals who do not respond to the second vaccination series should be considered susceptible to HBV infection and should be given HBV immunoglobulin prophylaxis after any known exposure to HBV-positive body fluid. It is important to note that some HBV vaccine nonresponders are chronically infected with HBV. Thus, individuals who do not have detectable anti-HBs after two vaccine series should be tested for HBsAg and anti-HBc.

Testing for the HBV genotype is currently not required except for selected patients from regions around the world that have variability in HBV genotypes (Table 4). While the "gold standard" for assessing inflammatory activity (grade) and degree of fibrosis (stage) is the liver biopsy, noninvasive assessments of liver fibrosis are increasingly used in lieu of biopsy (http://www.who.int/hepatitis/publications/guidelines-hepatitis-c-b-testing/en/).

Molecular assays are used to determine HBV DNA levels and contribute to establishing the stage of disease in newly diagnosed patients. They are also used to monitor patients on antiviral therapy. The reduction of HBV DNA during antiviral therapy is a measure of treatment response and predicts histologic improvement. Increasing HBV DNA levels are associated with chronic liver disease, cirrhosis, and possibly death. The WHO standard for HBV DNA has helped standardization of HBV DNA assays, and results are now reported in international units per milliliter.

Antiviral therapy is given to patients to prevent progression of liver disease. The decision to begin therapy is generally based on the presence or absence of cirrhosis, the alanine aminotransferase level, and the HBV DNA level (http://www.who.int/hepatitis/publications/guidelines-hepatitis-c-b-testing/en/). During the course of therapy, treatment response is monitored using biochemical, virologic, serologic, and histologic results. Currently, the most accurate monitor of virologic activity is the HBV DNA level using an assay with a wide dynamic range. The loss of HBsAg, seroconversion to anti-HBs, and long-lasting suppression of HBV DNA indicate a successful response to therapy. Patients who appear to have suppressed HBV DNA levels are monitored periodically because relapse due to antiviral resistance is possible. The most reliable measure of a successful long-term treatment response is the sustained suppression of HBV DNA.

In addition, treatment of pregnant women with HBV viral loads >200,000 IU/ml is recommended beginning in the third trimester regardless of alanine aminotransferase levels to reduce the risk of perinatal transmission (https://www.cdc.gov/mmwr/volumes/67/rr/pdfs/rr6701-H.pdf). All patients with HCC should be treated, and patients with chronic HBV starting immunosuppressive drugs should be given prophylactic therapy to prevent HBV reactivation (https://www.cdc.gov/mmwr/volumes/67/rr/pdfs/rr6701-H.pdf; http://www.who.int/hepatitis/publications/guidelines-hepatitis-c-b-testing/en/). Treatment of hepatitis C virus with direct-acting antivirals can lead to HBV reactivation in coinfected patients (88), and thus patients should be either treated for HBV or monitored for reactivation at regular intervals if treatment criteria are not met (https://www.cdc.gov/mmwr/volumes/67/rr/pdfs/rr6701-H.pdf; http://www.who.int/hepatitis/publications/guidelines-hepatitis-c-b-testing/en/).

When HBV DNA levels increase by 1 $\log_{10}$ in a patient taking antiviral treatment, it may indicate antiviral resistance. It is not recommended that resistance testing be performed before starting therapy, even if the patient has a very high viral level. Resistance detection is useful only after a patient has been treated for several months and fails to show an HBV DNA reduction of at least 1 $\log_{10}$. Such patients are classified as primary nonresponders. They should be tested for the presence of resistant mutants to assist in selecting a new treatment regimen. For successfully treated patients who have a virologic breakthrough, antiviral resistance testing should also be performed to determine selection of resistant viral strains.

In summary, diagnostic testing is essential for HBV prevention and treatment. Thus, increasing the accessibility and uptake of diagnostic testing in all resource settings is essential in reducing the disease burden worldwide. Strategies include using dried blood spots for testing and implementing rapid antigen and molecular testing, including at the point of care (39–41, 43) (http://www.who.int/hepatitis/publications/guidelines-hepatitis-c-b-testing/en/). Most important, however, is linking patients to care.

HEPATITIS D VIRUS

Taxonomy

Hepatitis D virus (HDV) is the only virus in the genus *Deltaviridae*. HDV is not classified into a viral family because it is a unique virus that is unable to replicate without the presence of HBV. Thus, it is a subviral particle rather than a true virus (89, 90). HDV was first described in 1977 in Italian patients with chronic HBV who developed episodes of serious acute disease (91). The HDV particle is similar to those of plant subviral agents (92). However, there are some major differences between the plant viroids and HDV. The plant viroids do not encode a specific protein and do not utilize a host or helper virus as HDV does with HBV (90, 92, 93).

Description of the Agent

HDV is generally spherical, with an average diameter ranging from 36 to 43 nm, which is slightly smaller than that of the HBV particle. The circular, single-stranded, negative-sense 1.7-kb RNA genome of HDV encodes only a single protein, the HDV nucleocapsid protein, known as the hepatitis delta antigen (HDAg). It is nonglycosylated and is produced in two forms: a short peptide consisting of a 195-amino-acid 24-kDa protein and a larger peptide consisting of a 214-amino-acid 27-kDa protein (90, 93, 94). The protein cannot assemble into viral particles without the presence of HBsAg. The HDV RNA genome is surrounded by HDAg, which is surrounded by HBsAg. Consequently, HDAg is undetectable on the complete HDV particle. In spite of this, infected individuals produce antibody to the HDV antigen (anti-HDV). However, anti-HDV does not neutralize this particle, whereas anti-HBs does have neutralizing activity (93).

HDV relies on host cell machinery for replication, and the viral genome (and antigenome) serves as a ribozyme for self-ligation and cleavage (89, 90). Similar to HBV, HDV binds to hepatocytes via the heptocyte-specific receptor NTCP (7, 89) (Fig. 2). The replication of the HDV genome uses the host RNA polymerase II rather than an HDV- or HBV-encoded RNA polymerase (93). The only enzymatic activity inherent to HDV is mediated by RNA elements termed ribozymes which cleave the newly synthesized, circular RNA genomes, producing linear molecules (95). After that cleavage, replication of the HDV genome occurs via a rolling-circle mechanism with self-cleavage (89, 93).

Epidemiology and Transmission

Worldwide, it is estimated that approximately 15 to 20 million people are HDV carriers (94, 96). Several areas of the world have a high prevalence of HDV-infected individuals, including countries bordering the Mediterranean, the Middle East, Central Asia, West Africa, the Amazon Basin, and the South Pacific Islands (96). In these areas of endemicity, HDV appears to be transmitted by close person-to-person spread, such as household contact. Additionally, many individuals have acquired HDV through exposure to blood-contaminated needles and blood products. Persistent epidemics of severe acute HDV have been observed in these populations, which have high HBV carrier rates (94, 96). Eight genotypes of HDV have been identified, each with its own distinct geographic distributions and outcomes (90, 94). HDV isolates of genotype I have been reported in every part of the world, while the milder HDV II genotype is found primarily in Asia, including Japan, Taiwan, and Russia. HDV genotype III has been isolated only in northern South America (Peru, Venezuela, and Colombia) and is associated with severe acute hepatitis. Mixed infections of genotypes I and II, or II and IIb, have been reported in Taiwan (97).

Clinical Significance

HDV can be transmitted only to individuals who are infected with HBV already or when both viral agents are transmitted together. A coinfection occurs when a naive individual is infected simultaneously with both viruses; coinfection occurs in only 2% of cases (Fig. 6) (93). A superinfection occurs when an individual chronically infected with HBV is infected with HDV (Fig. 7) (93). Superinfection occurs in more than 90% of infected patients (96). Acute HDV superinfection has a greater risk of fulminant hepatitis and liver failure than HBV infection alone. Likewise, chronic HDV infection is the most severe form of viral hepatitis, which is associated with more rapidly progressing liver damage than infection with HBV alone (94).

Rates of fulminant hepatitis can be as high as 5% in patients with HBV and HDV coinfection (93, 96). A biphasic clinical course is sometimes observed during coinfection. HDV infection does not increase the rate of chronicity of acute HBV but may convert an asymptomatic or mild, chronic HBV infection into a rapidly progressive, fulminant or severe disease (94, 98). Limited success has been achieved in treating chronic HDV patients with gamma interferon. High-dose, long-term therapy is required, and relapses are common after therapy is stopped (93, 94, 98). Patients with HDV who have hepatic decompensation are candidates for liver transplantation and in general have had favorable outcomes (94).

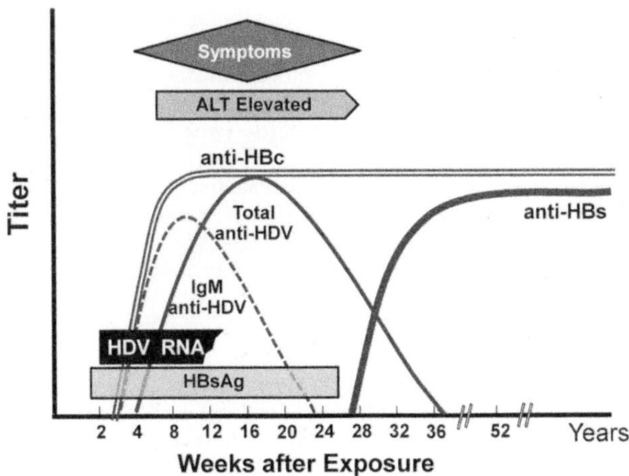

FIGURE 6 Serologic course of HDV infection, with resolution when the virus is acquired as a coinfection with HBV.

The failure of HBV-specific nucleoside analogues to suppress the HBV helper function, and the limitations of experimental systems to study the HDV life cycle, have impeded the development of HDV-specific drugs (94, 99). It appears that therapy with alpha interferon in combination with either ribavirin or lamivudine is not useful in treating chronic HDV infections (98). However, interference with entry through blockade of the HBV/HDV-specific receptor NTCP by Myrcludex B (35, 98, 100, 101), and inhibition of assembly by blockade of farnesyltransferase using either lonafarnib (102, 103) or nucleic acid polymers such as REP 2139-Ca (94, 104), have shown promising results in phase II studies. Successful vaccination for HBV also prevents HDV infection, since HDV cannot replicate in the absence of a concurrent HBV infection.

Collection, Transport, and Storage of Specimens

HDV infection is diagnosed by serologic and molecular markers using serum or plasma and is suspected for HBV-infected patients from countries in which HDV is prevalent. Patients with chronic hepatitis B not responding to

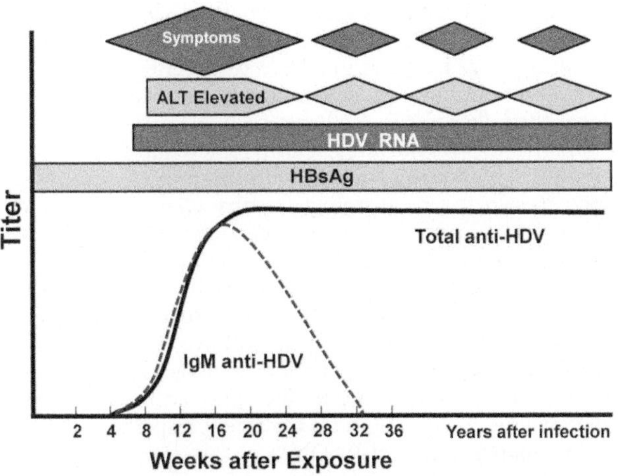

FIGURE 7 Serologic course of HDV infection when the virus is acquired as a superinfection with HBV. Symptoms and alanine aminotransferase (ALT) levels are shown to indicate the intermittent nature of symptoms and liver involvement.

antiviral treatment, or with liver damage despite a low viral load (HBV DNA <2,000 IU/ml), should also be tested.

Direct Detection

HDV infections can be diagnosed by detecting HDAg or, more recently, HDV RNA in serum and in liver tissue (93, 105). Currently, the most common method for HDV RNA detection is reverse transcription real-time PCR (106–109). While liver ultrasounds, elastrography and fibroscans remain the effective ways of monitoring chronic HDV progression, a declining HDV RNA level usually indicates a response to treatment (94, 99, 105). Qualitative and quantitative HDV RNA tests are now available in major reference laboratories.

Typing

Sequencing has been the sole technique used for HDV genotype determination. Although it is unclear if differences in the HDV genome play a role in disease presentation, this genomic diversity is likely related to discrepant results in HDV IgM antibodies and HDV viral loads between clinical laboratories, as reported in a recent French national quality control study (105, 110).

Serologic Tests

The first test used for the diagnosis of HDV infection is often HDV antibody using commercial or laboratory-developed enzyme immunoassay (106, 110, 111). Two kits, the DiaSorin (Saluggia, Piedmont, Italy) and the Cusabio (Wuhan, Hubei, China), were recently evaluated and are commercially available (111). A positive result for anti-HDV may indicate either acute or chronic HDV infection and should be followed with an HDV RNA test, which determines whether the infection is active. IgM anti-HDV can be detected during either a coinfection or a superinfection. Anti-HDV IgM testing can help to determine disease activity and to predict treatment response (112, 113).

Evaluation, Interpretation, and Reporting of Results

Recently, there has been a resurgence of interest in HDV infections, due to improvements in diagnostic testing and emerging new therapies. HDV infections lead to more serious liver diseases than HBV infection alone, such as faster progression to liver fibrosis, increased risk of liver cancer, and earlier decompensated cirrhosis and liver failure. It is important that people with HBV/HDV coinfection are diagnosed early. The first step in the diagnosis of HDV infection is testing HBsAg-positive individuals for anti-HDV antibody using commercially available kits. In anti-HDV-positive patients, HDV RNA in serum is tested to determine whether the antibody reflects an ongoing active HDV infection or represents a past HDV infection. In the HDV-positive individual with liver disease, it is critical to distinguish acute HDV/HBV coinfection from chronic HDV superinfection in HBsAg carriers; the course, prognosis, and management of the two conditions are different.

The differential diagnosis can be achieved through testing a battery of HDV and HBV markers, which combine in patterns characteristic for each condition. Standardized commercial assays are available to determine IgG and IgM antibodies to HDV. Several laboratory-developed tests to qualitatively and quantitatively detect HDV RNA in plasma or serum are available in major reference laboratories. These molecular results should be interpreted with caution because they are not yet standardized and the sensitivities and the results from different laboratories can vary (105).

REFERENCES

1. **Blumberg BS, Alter HJ, Visnich S.** 1965. A "new" antigen in leukemia sera. *JAMA* **191:**541–546.
2. **Seeger CFZ, Mason WS.** 2013. Hepadnaviruses, p 2185–2221. *In* Knipe DM, Howley PM (ed), *Fields Virology*, 6th ed. Lippincott Williams & Wilkins, Philadelphia, PA.
3. **Dane DS, Cameron CH, Briggs M.** 1970. Virus-like particles in serum of patients with Australia-antigen-associated hepatitis. *Lancet* **1:**695–698.
4. **Verrier ER, Colpitts CC, Schuster C, Zeisel MB, Baumert TF.** 2016. Cell culture models for the investigation of hepatitis B and D virus infection. *Viruses* **8:**261.
5. **Ni Y, Lempp FA, Mehrle S, Nkongolo S, Kaufman C, Fälth M, Stindt J, Königer C, Nassal M, Kubitz R, Sültmann H, Urban S.** 2014. Hepatitis B and D viruses exploit sodium taurocholate co-transporting polypeptide for species-specific entry into hepatocytes. *Gastroenterology* **146:**1070–1083.
6. **Yan H, Zhong G, Xu G, He W, Jing Z, Gao Z, Huang Y, Qi Y, Peng B, Wang H, Fu L, Song M, Chen P, Gao W, Ren B, Sun Y, Cai T, Feng X, Sui J, Li W.** 2012. Sodium taurocholate cotransporting polypeptide is a functional receptor for human hepatitis B and D virus. *eLife* **3:**10.7554/eLife.00049.
7. **Li W.** 2015. The hepatitis B virus receptor. *Annu Rev Cell Dev Biol* **31:**125–147.
8. **Cornberg M, Wong VW, Locarnini S, Brunetto M, Janssen HLA, Chan HL.** 2017. The role of quantitative hepatitis B surface antigen revisited. *J Hepatol* **66:**398–411.
9. **Thibault V, Servant-Delmas A, Ly TD, Roque-Afonso AM, Laperche S.** 2017. Performance of HBsAg quantification assays for detection of hepatitis B virus genotypes and diagnostic escape-variants in clinical samples. *J Clin Virol* **89:** 14–21.
10. **Trépo C, Chan HL, Lok A.** 2014. Hepatitis B virus infection. *Lancet* **384:**2053–2063.
11. **Tong S, Revill P.** 2016. Overview of hepatitis B viral replication and genetic variability. *J Hepatol* **64**(Suppl):S4–S16.
12. **Łapiński TW, Pogorzelska J, Flisiak R.** 2012. HBV mutations and their clinical significance. *Adv Med Sci* **57:**18–22.
13. **Kajiwara E, Tanaka Y, Ohashi T, Uchimura K, Sadoshima S, Kinjo M, Mizokami M.** 2008. Hepatitis B caused by a hepatitis B surface antigen escape mutant. *J Gastroenterol* **43:**243–247.
14. **Rajoriya N, Combet C, Zoulim F, Janssen HLA.** 2017. How viral genetic variants and genotypes influence disease and treatment outcome of chronic hepatitis B. Time for an individualised approach? *J Hepatol* **67:**1281–1297.
15. **Lozano R, et al.** 2012. Global and regional mortality from 235 causes of death for 20 age groups in 1990 and 2010: a systematic analysis for the Global Burden of Disease Study 2010. *Lancet* **380:**2095–2128. (Erratum, **381:**628.)
16. **Nelson NP, Easterbrook PJ, McMahon BJ.** 2016. Epidemiology of hepatitis B virus infection and impact of vaccination on disease. *Clin Liver Dis* **20:**607–628. (Erratum, **21:**xiii.)
17. **Croagh CM, Lubel JS.** 2014. Natural history of chronic hepatitis B: phases in a complex relationship. *World J Gastroenterol* **20:**10395–10404.
18. **Lok AS, McMahon BJ, Brown RS Jr, Wong JB, Ahmed AT, Farah W, Almasri J, Alahdab F, Benkhadra K, Mouchli MA, Singh S, Mohamed EA, Abu Dabrh AM, Prokop LJ, Wang Z, Murad MH, Mohammed K.** 2016. Antiviral therapy for chronic hepatitis B viral infection in adults: a systematic review and meta-analysis. *Hepatology* **63:**284–306.
19. **Sorrell MF, Belongia EA, Costa J, Gareen IF, Grem JL, Inadomi JM, Kern ER, McHugh JA, Petersen GM, Rein MF, Strader DB, Trotter HT.** 2009. National Institutes of Health consensus development conference statement: management of hepatitis B. *Hepatology* **49**(Suppl):S4–S12.
20. **Bauer T, Sprinzl M, Protzer U.** 2011. Immune control of hepatitis B virus. *Dig Dis* **29:**423–433.
21. **Dandri M, Petersen J.** 2016. Mechanism of hepatitis B virus persistence in hepatocytes and its carcinogenic potential. *Clin Infect Dis* **62**(Suppl 4):S281–S288.
22. **Chen BF.** 2018. Hepatitis B virus pre-S/S variants in liver diseases. *World J Gastroenterol* **24:**1507–1520.

23. **Geng M, Xin X, Bi LQ, Zhou LT, Liu XH.** 2015. Molecular mechanism of hepatitis B virus X protein function in hepatocarcinogenesis. *World J Gastroenterol* **21:**10732–10738.
24. **Jackson S, Lentino J, Kopp J, Murray L, Ellison W, Rhee M, Shockey G, Akella L, Erby K, Heyward WL, Janssen RS, Adams M, Bolshoun D, Bruce T, Chuang R, DeSantis D, Fiel T, Fitzgibbons W, Francyk D, Geisberg H, Giep S, Godbole N, Haas T, Halpern S, Inzerello A, Jennings W, Kaiser S, Kay J, Kirby W, Lending R, Levins P, Molin C, Noss M, Kotek L, Reynolds M, Riffer E, Schumacher D, Severance R, Solano R, Tejada A, Tharenos L, Throne M, Turner M, Wolf T, Woodruff M, HBV-23 Study Group.** 2018. Immunogenicity of a two-dose investigational hepatitis B vaccine, HBsAg-1018, using a Toll-like receptor 9 agonist adjuvant compared with a licensed hepatitis B vaccine in adults. *Vaccine* **36:**668–674.
25. **Blumberg EA.** 2018. Prevention of hepatitis B virus infection in the United States: recommendations of the Advisory Committee on Immunization Practices: a summary of the MMWR report. *Am J Transplant* **18:**1285–1286.
26. **Gish RG, Given BD, Lai CL, Locarnini SA, Lau JY, Lewis DL, Schluep T.** 2015. Chronic hepatitis B: virology, natural history, current management and a glimpse at future opportunities. *Antiviral Res* **121:**47–58.
27. **Tang LSY, Covert E, Wilson E, Kottilil S.** 2018. Chronic hepatitis B infection: a review. *JAMA* **319:**1802–1813.
28. **Block TM, Locarnini S, McMahon BJ, Rehermann B, Peters MG.** 2017. Use of current and new endpoints in the evaluation of experimental hepatitis B therapeutics. *Clin Infect Dis* **64:**1283–1288.
29. **Zeisel MB, Lucifora J, Mason WS, Sureau C, Beck J, Levrero M, Kann M, Knolle PA, Benkirane M, Durantel D, Michel ML, Autran B, Cosset FL, Strick-Marchand H, Trépo C, Kao JH, Carrat F, Lacombe K, Schinazi RF, Barré-Sinoussi F, Delfraissy JF, Zoulim F.** 2015. Towards an HBV cure: state-of-the-art and unresolved questions—report of the ANRS workshop on HBV cure. *Gut* **64:**1314–1326.
30. **Shamliyan TA, MacDonald R, Shaukat A, Taylor BC, Yuan JM, Johnson JR, Tacklind J, Rutks I, Kane RL, Wilt TJ.** 2009. Antiviral therapy for adults with chronic hepatitis B: a systematic review for a National Institutes of Health Consensus Development Conference. *Ann Intern Med* **150:**111–124.
31. **Buti M, Gane E, Seto WK, Chan HL, Chuang WL, Stepanova T, Hui AJ, Lim YS, Mehta R, Janssen HL, Acharya SK, Flaherty JF, Massetto B, Cathcart AL, Kim K, Gaggar A, Subramanian GM, McHutchison JG, Pan CQ, Brunetto M, Izumi N, Marcellin P, GS-US-320-0108 Investigators.** 2016. Tenofovir alafenamide versus tenofovir disoproxil fumarate for the treatment of patients with HBeAg-negative chronic hepatitis B virus infection: a randomised, double-blind, phase 3, non-inferiority trial. *Lancet Gastroenterol Hepatol* **1:**196–206.
32. **Chan HL, Fung S, Seto WK, Chuang WL, Chen CY, Kim HJ, Hui AJ, Janssen HL, Chowdhury A, Tsang TY, Mehta R, Gane E, Flaherty JF, Massetto B, Gaggar A, Kitrinos KM, Lin L, Subramanian GM, McHutchison JG, Lim YS, Acharya SK, Agarwal K, GS-US-320-0110 Investigators.** 2016. Tenofovir alafenamide versus tenofovir disoproxil fumarate for the treatment of HBeAg-positive chronic hepatitis B virus infection: a randomised, double-blind, phase 3, non-inferiority trial. *Lancet Gastroenterol Hepatol* **1:**185–195.
33. **Urban S, Bartenschlager R, Kubitz R, Zoulim F.** 2014. Strategies to inhibit entry of HBV and HDV into hepatocytes. *Gastroenterology* **147:**48–64.
34. **Shimura S, Watashi K, Fukano K, Peel M, Sluder A, Kawai F, Iwamoto M, Tsukuda S, Takeuchi JS, Miyake T, Sugiyama M, Ogasawara Y, Park SY, Tanaka Y, Kusuhara H, Mizokami M, Sureau C, Wakita T.** 2017. Cyclosporin derivatives inhibit hepatitis B virus entry without interfering with NTCP transporter activity. *J Hepatol* **66:**685–692.
35. **Donkers JM, Zehnder B, van Westen GJP, Kwakkenbos MJ, IJzerman AP, Oude Elferink RPJ, Beuers U, Urban S, van de Graaf SFJ.** 2017. Reduced hepatitis B and D viral entry using clinically applied drugs as novel inhibitors of the bile acid transporter NTCP. *Sci Rep* **7:**15307.
36. **Ye X, Zhou M, He Y, Wan Y, Bai W, Tao S, Ren Y, Zhang X, Xu J, Liu J, Zhang J, Hu K, Xie Y.** 2016. Efficient inhibition of hepatitis B virus infection by a preS1-binding peptide. *Sci Rep* **6:**29391.
37. **Baleriola C, Johal H, Jacka B, Chaverot S, Bowden S, Lacey S, Rawlinson W.** 2011. Stability of hepatitis C virus, HIV, and hepatitis B virus nucleic acids in plasma samples after long-term storage at -20°C and -70°C. *J Clin Microbiol* **49:**3163–3167.
38. **Saldanha J, Gerlich W, Lelie N, Dawson P, Heermann K, Heath A, WHO Collaborative Study Group.** 2001. An international collaborative study to establish a World Health Organization international standard for hepatitis B virus DNA nucleic acid amplification techniques. *Vox Sang* **80:**63–71.
39. **Jardi R, Rodriguez-Frias F, Buti M, Schaper M, Valdes A, Martinez M, Esteban R, Guardia J.** 2004. Usefulness of dried blood samples for quantification and molecular characterization of HBV-DNA. *Hepatology* **40:**133–139.
40. **Villar LM, de Oliveira JC, Cruz HM, Yoshida CF, Lampe E, Lewis-Ximenez LL.** 2011. Assessment of dried blood spot samples as a simple method for detection of hepatitis B virus markers. *J Med Virol* **83:**1522–1529.
41. **Zanoni M, Giron LB, Vilhena C, Sucupira MC, Lloyd RM Jr, Diaz RS.** 2012. Comparative effectiveness of dried-plasma hepatitis B virus viral load (VL) testing in three different VL commercial platforms using ViveST for sample collection. *J Clin Microbiol* **50:**145–147.
42. **Bhat M, Ghali P, Deschenes M, Wong P.** 2012. Hepatitis B and the infected health care worker: public safety at what cost? *Can J Gastroenterol* **26:**257–260.
43. **Peeling RW, Boeras DI, Marinucci F, Easterbrook P.** 2017. The future of viral hepatitis testing: innovations in testing technologies and approaches. *BMC Infect Dis* **17**(Suppl 1)**:**699.
44. **Song JE, Kim DY.** 2016. Diagnosis of hepatitis B. *Ann Transl Med* **4:**338.
45. **Gerlich WH, Bremer C, Saniewski M, Schüttler CG, Wend UC, Willems WR, Glebe D.** 2010. Occult hepatitis B virus infection: detection and significance. *Dig Dis* **28:**116–125.
46. **Amini A, Varsaneux O, Kelly H, Tang W, Chen W, Boeras DI, Falconer J, Tucker JD, Chou R, Ishizaki A, Easterbrook P, Peeling RW.** 2017. Diagnostic accuracy of tests to detect hepatitis B surface antigen: a systematic review of the literature and meta-analysis. *BMC Infect Dis* **17**(Suppl 1)**:**698.
47. **Mak LY, Wong DK, Cheung KS, Seto WK, Lai CL, Yuen MF.** 2018. Review article: hepatitis B core-related antigen (HBcrAg): an emerging marker for chronic hepatitis B virus infection. *Aliment Pharmacol Ther* **47:**43–54.
48. **Servant-Delmas A, Mercier-Darty M, Ly TD, Wind F, Alloui C, Sureau C, Laperche S.** 2012. Variable capacity of 13 hepatitis B virus surface antigen assays for the detection of HBsAg mutants in blood samples. *J Clin Virol* **53:**338–345.
49. **Chotiyaputta W, Lok AS.** 2009. Hepatitis B virus variants. *Nat Rev Gastroenterol Hepatol* **6:**453–462.
50. **Thibault V, Pichoud C, Mullen C, Rhoads J, Smith JB, Bitbol A, Thamm S, Zoulim F.** 2007. Characterization of a new sensitive PCR assay for quantification of viral DNA isolated from patients with hepatitis B virus infections. *J Clin Microbiol* **45:**3948–3953.
51. **Hendrickson B, Kamili S, Timmons T, Iwen PC, Pedati C, Safranek T.** 2018. Notes from the field: false-negative hepatitis B surface antigen test results in a hemodialysis patient: Nebraska, 2017. *MMWR Morb Mortal Wkly Rep* **67:**311–312.
52. **Wang CC, Tseng KC, Hsieh TY, Tseng TC, Lin HH, Kao JH.** 2016. Assessing the durability of entecavir-treated hepatitis B using quantitative HBsAg. *Am J Gastroenterol* **111:**1286–1294.
53. **Seiz PL, Mohr C, Wilkinson DE, Ziebuhr J, Schüttler CG, Gerlich WH, Glebe D.** 2016. Characterization of the 3rd International Standard for hepatitis B virus surface antigen (HBsAg). *J Clin Virol* **82:**166–172.
54. **Wilkinson DE, Seiz PL, Schüttler CG, Gerlich WH, Glebe D, Scheiblauer H, Nick S, Chudy M, Dougall T, Stone L, Heath AB, Collaborative Study Group.** 2016. International collaborative study on the 3rd WHO international standard for hepatitis B surface antigen. *J Clin Virol* **82:**173–180.

55. **Allice T, Cerutti F, Pittaluga F, Varetto S, Gabella S, Marzano A, Franchello A, Colucci G, Ghisetti V.** 2007. COBAS AmpliPrep-COBAS TaqMan hepatitis B virus (HBV) test: a novel automated real-time PCR assay for quantification of HBV DNA in plasma. *J Clin Microbiol* **45:**828–834.
56. **Caliendo AM, Valsamakis A, Bremer JW, Ferreira-Gonzalez A, Granger S, Sabatini L, Tsongalis GJ, Wang YF, Yen-Lieberman B, Young S, Lurain NS.** 2011. Multilaboratory evaluation of real-time PCR tests for hepatitis B virus DNA quantification. *J Clin Microbiol* **49:**2854–2858.
57. **Chevaliez S, Bouvier-Alias M, Laperche S, Pawlotsky JM.** 2008. Performance of the Cobas AmpliPrep/Cobas TaqMan real-time PCR assay for hepatitis B virus DNA quantification. *J Clin Microbiol* **46:**1716–1723.
58. **Pyne MT, Vest L, Clement J, Lee J, Rosvall JR, Luk K, Rossi M, Cobb B, Hillyard DR.** 2012. Comparison of three Roche hepatitis B virus viral load assay formats. *J Clin Microbiol* **50:**2337–2342.
59. **Chevaliez S, Dauvillier C, Dubernet F, Poveda JD, Laperche S, Hézode C, Pawlotsky JM.** 2017. The New Aptima HBV Quant real-time TMA assay accurately quantifies hepatitis B virus DNA from genotypes A to F. *J Clin Microbiol* **55:**1211–1219.
60. **Nyan DC, Ulitzky LE, Cehan N, Williamson P, Winkelman V, Rios M, Taylor DR.** 2014. Rapid detection of hepatitis B virus in blood plasma by a specific and sensitive loop-mediated isothermal amplification assay. *Clin Infect Dis* **59:**16–23.
61. **Heermann KH, Gerlich WH, Chudy M, Schaefer S, Thomssen R, Eurohep Pathobiology Group.** 1999. Quantitative detection of hepatitis B virus DNA in two international reference plasma preparations. *J Clin Microbiol* **37:**68–73.
62. **Fryer JF, Heath AB, Wilkinson DE, Minor PD, Collaborative Study Group.** 2017. A collaborative study to establish the 3rd WHO international standard for hepatitis B virus for nucleic acid amplification techniques. *Biologicals* **46:**57–63.
63. **Locarnini S, Hatzakis A, Chen DS, Lok A.** 2015. Strategies to control hepatitis B: public policy, epidemiology, vaccine and drugs. *J Hepatol* **62**(Suppl)**:**S76–S86.
64. **Rotman Y, Brown TA, Hoofnagle JH.** 2009. Evaluation of the patient with hepatitis B. *Hepatology* **49**(Suppl)**:**S22–S27.
65. **Gerlich WH, Caspari G.** 1999. Hepatitis viruses and the safety of blood donations. *J Viral Hepat* **6**(Suppl 1)**:**6–15.
66. **Wu T, Kwok RM, Tran TT.** 2017. Isolated anti-HBc: the relevance of hepatitis B core antibody: a review of new issues. *Am J Gastroenterol* **112:**1780–1788.
67. **Huzly D, Schenk T, Jilg W, Neumann-Haefelin D.** 2008. Comparison of nine commercially available assays for quantification of antibody response to hepatitis B virus surface antigen. *J Clin Microbiol* **46:**1298–1306.
68. **Centers for Disease Control and Prevention (CDC).** 2012. Updated CDC recommendations for the management of hepatitis B virus-infected health-care providers and students. *MMWR Recomm Rep* **61**(RR-3)**:**1–12.
69. **Liu SH, Seto WK, Lai CL, Yuen MF.** 2016. Hepatitis B: treatment choice and monitoring for response and resistance. *Expert Rev Gastroenterol Hepatol* **10:**697–707.
70. **Caligiuri P, Cerruti R, Icardi G, Bruzzone B.** 2016. Overview of hepatitis B virus mutations and their implications in the management of infection. *World J Gastroenterol* **22:**145–154.
71. **Tatti KM, Korba BE, Stang HL, Peek S, Gerin JL, Tennant BC, Schinazi RF.** 2002. Mutations in the conserved woodchuck hepatitis virus polymerase FLLA and YMDD regions conferring resistance to lamivudine. *Antiviral Res* **55:**141–150.
72. **Neumann-Fraune M, Beggel B, Kaiser R, Obermeier M.** 2014. Hepatitis B virus drug resistance tools: one sequence, two predictions. *Intervirology* **57:**232–236.
73. **Guirgis BS, Abbas RO, Azzazy HM.** 2010. Hepatitis B virus genotyping: current methods and clinical implications. *Int J Infect Dis* **14:**e941–e953.
74. **Alidjinou EK, Bocket L, Pigot V, Lambert V, Hallaert C, Canva V, Hober D.** 2018. Sanger sequencing versus INNO-LiPA® HBV PreCore assay for routine detection of precore and basal core promoter mutations in hepatitis virus B chronically infected patients. *Diagn Microbiol Infect Dis* **90:**277–279.
75. **Doutreloigne J, Van Hecke E.** 2011. Revision of interpretation criteria of the INNO-LiPA HBV genotyping assay. *J Clin Microbiol* **49:**3446.
76. **Mese S, Arikan M, Cakiris A, Abaci N, Gumus E, Kursun O, Onel D, Ustek D, Kaymakoglu S, Badur S, Yenen OS, Bozkaya E.** 2013. Role of the line probe assay INNO-LiPA HBV DR and ultradeep pyrosequencing in detecting resistance mutations to nucleoside/nucleotide analogues in viral samples isolated from chronic hepatitis B patients. *J Gen Virol* **94:**2729–2738.
77. **Basaras M, Arrese E, Blanco S, Arroyo LS, Ruiz P, Cisterna R.** 2013. Comparison of INNO-LIPA and TRUGENE assays for genotyping and drug-resistance mutations in chronic hepatitis B virus infection. *Intervirology* **56:**190–194.
78. **Gintowt AA, Germer JJ, Mitchell PS, Yao JD.** 2005. Evaluation of the MagNA Pure LC used with the TRUGENE HBV genotyping kit. *J Clin Virol* **34:**155–157.
79. **Lowe CF, Merrick L, Harrigan PR, Mazzulli T, Sherlock CH, Ritchie G.** 2016. Implementation of next-generation sequencing for hepatitis B virus resistance testing and genotyping in a clinical microbiology laboratory. *J Clin Microbiol* **54:**127–133.
80. **Bayliss J, Yuen L, Rosenberg G, Wong D, Littlejohn M, Jackson K, Gaggar A, Kitrinos KM, Subramanian GM, Marcellin P, Buti M, Janssen HLA, Gane E, Sozzi V, Colledge D, Hammond R, Edwards R, Locarnini S, Thompson A, Revill PA.** 2017. Deep sequencing shows that HBV basal core promoter and precore variants reduce the likelihood of HBsAg loss following tenofovir disoproxil fumarate therapy in HBeAg-positive chronic hepatitis B. *Gut* **66:**2013–2023.
81. **Gong L, Han Y, Chen L, Liu F, Hao P, Sheng J, Li XH, Yu DM, Gong QM, Tian F, Guo XK, Zhang XX.** 2013. Comparison of next-generation sequencing and clone-based sequencing in analysis of hepatitis B virus reverse transcriptase quasispecies heterogeneity. *J Clin Microbiol* **51:**4087–4094.
82. **Margeridon-Thermet S, Svarovskaia ES, Babrzadeh F, Martin R, Liu TF, Pacold M, Reuman EC, Holmes SP, Borroto-Esoda K, Shafer RW.** 2013. Low-level persistence of drug resistance mutations in hepatitis B virus-infected subjects with a past history of lamivudine treatment. *Antimicrob Agents Chemother* **57:**343–349.
83. **Quer J, Rodríguez-Frias F, Gregori J, Tabernero D, Soria ME, García-Cehic D, Homs M, Bosch A, Pintó RM, Esteban JI, Domingo E, Perales C.** 2017. Deep sequencing in the management of hepatitis virus infections. *Virus Res* **239:**115–125.
84. **Rodriguez-Frías F, Tabernero D, Quer J, Esteban JI, Ortega I, Domingo E, Cubero M, Camós S, Ferrer-Costa C, Sánchez A, Jardí R, Schaper M, Homs M, Garcia-Cehic D, Guardia J, Esteban R, Buti M.** 2012. Ultra-deep pyrosequencing detects conserved genomic sites and quantifies linkage of drug-resistant amino acid changes in the hepatitis B virus genome. *PLoS One* **7:**e37874.
85. **Yamani LN, Yano Y, Utsumi T, Juniastuti, Wandono H, Widjanarko D, Triantanoe A, Wasityastuti W, Liang Y, Okada R, Tanahashi T, Murakami Y, Azuma T, Soetjipto, Lusida MI, Hayashi Y.** 2015. Ultradeep sequencing for detection of quasispecies variants in the major hydrophilic region of hepatitis B virus in Indonesian patients. *J Clin Microbiol* **53:**3165–3175.
86. **Iwamoto M, Watashi K, Tsukuda S, Aly HH, Fukasawa M, Fujimoto A, Suzuki R, Aizaki H, Ito T, Koiwai O, Kusuhara H, Wakita T.** 2014. Evaluation and identification of hepatitis B virus entry inhibitors using HepG2 cells overexpressing a membrane transporter NTCP. *Biochem Biophys Res Commun* **443:**808–813.
87. **Kaneko M, Futamura Y, Tsukuda S, Kondoh Y, Sekine T, Hirano H, Fukano K, Ohashi H, Saso W, Morishita R, Matsunaga S, Kawai F, Ryo A, Park SY, Suzuki R, Aizaki H, Ohtani N, Sureau C, Wakita T, Osada H, Watashi K.** 2018. Chemical array system, a platform to identify novel hepatitis B virus entry inhibitors targeting sodium taurocholate cotransporting polypeptide. *Sci Rep* **8:**2769.

88. **Wang C, Ji D, Chen J, Shao Q, Li B, Liu J, Wu V, Wong A, Wang Y, Zhang X, Lu L, Wong C, Tsang S, Zhang Z, Sun J, Hou J, Chen G, Lau G.** 2017. Hepatitis due to reactivation of hepatitis B virus in endemic areas among patients with hepatitis C treated with direct-acting antiviral agents. *Clin Gastroenterol Hepatol* **15:**132–136.
89. **Sureau C, Negro F.** 2016. The hepatitis delta virus: replication and pathogenesis. *J Hepatol* **64**(Suppl)**:**S102–S116.
90. **Taylor JM, Purcell RH, Farci P.** 2013. Hepatitis D (delta) virus, p 2222–2241. *In* Knipe DM, Howley PM (ed), *Fields Virology*, 6th ed. Lippincott Williams & Wilkins, Philadelphia, PA.
91. **Rizzetto M, Canese MG, Aricò S, Crivelli O, Trepo C, Bonino F, Verme G.** 1977. Immunofluorescence detection of new antigen-antibody system (delta/anti-delta) associated to hepatitis B virus in liver and in serum of HBsAg carriers. *Gut* **18:**997–1003.
92. **Flores R, Grubb D, Elleuch A, Nohales MA, Delgado S, Gago S.** 2011. Rolling-circle replication of viroids, viroid-like satellite RNAs and hepatitis delta virus: variations on a theme. *RNA Biol* **8:**200–206.
93. **Taylor JM.** 2012. Virology of hepatitis D virus. *Semin Liver Dis* **32:**195–200.
94. **Lempp FA, Ni Y, Urban S.** 2016. Hepatitis delta virus: insights into a peculiar pathogen and novel treatment options. *Nat Rev Gastroenterol Hepatol* **13:**580–589.
95. **Been MD.** 2006. HDV ribozymes. *Curr Top Microbiol Immunol* **307:**47–65.
96. **Rizzetto M, Ciancio A.** 2012. Epidemiology of hepatitis D. *Semin Liver Dis* **32:**211–219.
97. **Lin HH, Lee SS, Yu ML, Chang TT, Su CW, Hu BS, Chen YS, Huang CK, Lai CH, Lin JN, Wu JC.** 2015. Changing hepatitis D virus epidemiology in a hepatitis B virus endemic area with a national vaccination program. *Hepatology* **61:**1870–1879.
98. **Niro GA, Smedile A, Ippolito AM, Ciancio A, Fontana R, Olivero A, Valvano MR, Abate ML, Gioffreda D, Caviglia GP, Rizzetto M, Andriulli A.** 2010. Outcome of chronic delta hepatitis in Italy: a long-term cohort study. *J Hepatol* **53:**834–840.
99. **Yurdaydin C.** 2017. Recent advances in managing hepatitis D. *F1000Res* 6:1596. doi:10.12688/f1000research.11796.1.
100. **Blank A, Markert C, Hohmann N, Carls A, Mikus G, Lehr T, Alexandrov A, Haag M, Schwab M, Urban S, Haefeli WE.** 2016. First-in-human application of the novel hepatitis B and hepatitis D virus entry inhibitor myrcludex B. *J Hepatol* **65:**483–489.
101. **Bogomolov P, Alexandrov A, Voronkova N, Macievich M, Kokina K, Petrachenkova M, Lehr T, Lempp FA, Wedemeyer H, Haag M, Schwab M, Haefeli WE, Blank A, Urban S.** 2016. Treatment of chronic hepatitis D with the entry inhibitor myrcludex B: first results of a phase Ib/IIa study. *J Hepatol* **65:**490–498.
102. **Koh C, Canini L, Dahari H, Zhao X, Uprichard SL, Haynes-Williams V, Winters MA, Subramanya G, Cooper SL, Pinto P, Wolff EF, Bishop R, Ai Thanda Han M, Cotler SJ, Kleiner DE, Keskin O, Idilman R, Yurdaydin C, Glenn JS, Heller T.** 2015. Oral prenylation inhibition with lonafarnib in chronic hepatitis D infection: a proof-of-concept randomised, double-blind, placebo-controlled phase 2A trial. *Lancet Infect Dis* **15:**1167–1174.
103. **Yurdaydin C, Keskin O, Kalkan Ç, Karakaya F, Çalişkan A, Karatayli E, Karatayli S, Bozdayi AM, Koh C, Heller T, Idilman R, Glenn JS.** 2018. Optimizing lonafarnib treatment for the management of chronic delta hepatitis: the LOWR HDV-1 study. *Hepatology* **67:**1224–1236.
104. **Beilstein F, Blanchet M, Vaillant A, Sureau C.** 2018. Nucleic acid polymers are active against hepatitis delta virus infection *in vitro*. *J Virol* **92:**e01416-17.
105. **Olivero A, Smedile A.** 2012. Hepatitis delta virus diagnosis. *Semin Liver Dis* **32:**220–227.
106. **Coller KE, Butler EK, Luk KC, Rodgers MA, Cassidy M, Gersch J, McNamara AL, Kuhns MC, Dawson GJ, Kaptue L, Bremer B, Wedemeyer H, Cloherty GA.** 2018. Development and performance of prototype serologic and molecular tests for hepatitis delta infection. *Sci Rep* **8:**2095.
107. **Kodani M, Martin A, Mixson-Hayden T, Drobeniuc J, Gish RR, Kamili S.** 2013. One-step real-time PCR assay for detection and quantitation of hepatitis D virus RNA. *J Virol Methods* **193:**531–535.
108. **Mederacke I, Bremer B, Heidrich B, Kirschner J, Deterding K, Bock T, Wursthorn K, Manns MP, Wedemeyer H.** 2010. Establishment of a novel quantitative hepatitis D virus (HDV) RNA assay using the Cobas TaqMan platform to study HDV RNA kinetics. *J Clin Microbiol* **48:**2022–2029.
109. **Scholtes C, Icard V, Amiri M, Chevallier-Queyron P, Trabaud MA, Ramière C, Zoulim F, André P, Dény P.** 2012. Standardized one-step real-time reverse transcription-PCR assay for universal detection and quantification of hepatitis delta virus from clinical samples in the presence of a heterologous internal-control RNA. *J Clin Microbiol* **50:**2126–2128.
110. **Brichler S, Le Gal F, Neri-Pinto F, Mansour W, Roulot D, Laperche S, Gordien E.** 2014. Serological and molecular diagnosis of hepatitis delta virus infection: results of a French national quality control study. *J Clin Microbiol* **52:**1694–1697.
111. **Chow SK, Atienza EE, Cook L, Prince H, Slev P, Lape-Nixon M, Jerome KR.** 2016. Comparison of enzyme immunoassays for detection of antibodies to hepatitis D virus in serum. *Clin Vaccine Immunol* **23:**732–734.
112. **Mederacke I, Yurdaydin C, Dalekos GN, Bremer B, Erhardt A, Cakaloglu Y, Yalcin K, Gurel S, Zeuzem S, Zachou K, Bozkaya H, Dienes HP, Manns MP, Wedemeyer H, Hep-Net/International Delta Hepatitis Study Group.** 2012. Anti-HDV immunoglobulin M testing in hepatitis delta revisited: correlations with disease activity and response to pegylated interferon-α2a treatment. *Antivir Ther* **17:**305–312.
113. **Wranke A, Heidrich B, Ernst S, Calle Serrano B, Caruntu FA, Curescu MG, Yalcin K, Gurel S, Zeuzem S, Erhardt A, Luth S, Papatheodoridis GV, Bremer B, Stift J, Grabowski J, Kirschner J, Port K, Cornberg M, Falk CS, Dienes HP, Hardtke S, Manns MP, Yurdaydin C, Wedemeyer H.** 2014. Anti-HDV IgM as a marker of disease activity in hepatitis delta. *PLoS One* **9:**e101002.

Prion Diseases

DANIEL D. RHOADS AND JIRI G. SAFAR

112

TAXONOMY

Prion diseases (1), originally called transmissible spongiform encephalopathies (2), are invariably fatal neurodegenerative diseases that affect humans and animals. The unusual biological and biochemical properties of the infectious agent causing the disease were first recognized in studies of scrapie in sheep, which is the prototypic prion disease (3). Specifically, the resistance of the scrapie agent to inactivation by formalin and heat treatments, which were commonly used to produce vaccines against viral illnesses, suggested that the scrapie agent might be different from viruses. Two decades later, the scrapie agent's extreme resistance to inactivation by radiation was documented (4–6). The partial purification of the transmissible agent in rodent-adapted disease led to the discovery that a protein is required for transmission (7–10), and procedures that eliminate or damage nucleic acids do not alter scrapie infectivity (1, 5, 6, 11). On the basis of these seminal findings, Stanley Prusiner proposed the term "prion" to distinguish these proteinaceous infectious particles from both viroids and viruses, and he was awarded a Nobel prize for this work (1, 12). The currently accepted model of prion disease posits that the infectious pathogen is a misfolded protein, designated PrP^{Sc}, where "Sc" is an abbreviation for "scrapie." This protein is a pathogenic conformational isoform of the normal cellular prion protein, PrP^{C}, which is encoded by the host's prion protein (*PRNP*) gene (13) and which is expressed in variable amounts in all healthy mammalian cells. The discovery that misfolded proteins may be infectious represented a new biological paradigm, and although originally deemed heretical, this protein-only model is now supported by a wealth of biochemical, genetic, and animal studies (14–19), including recent success in generating infectious prions *in vitro* from recombinant protein (20–23). Most human prion disease is described as sporadic because no epidemiological link has been identified, but genetics and environmental exposure can play a role in the development of prion disease. Prions cause scrapie in sheep; bovine spongiform encephalopathy (BSE) in cattle; chronic wasting disease (CWD) in cervids; and Gerstmann-Sträussler-Scheinker disease (GSS), fatal familial insomnia (FFI), kuru, variably protease-sensitive prionopathy (VPSPR), and several types of Creutzfeldt-Jakob disease (CJD) in humans.

DESCRIPTION OF THE AGENT

The remarkable progress in the past decade provided new insights into the biology and pathophysiology of prion diseases and indicated that the pathogenic and infectious PrP^{Sc} conformer is largely composed of beta-sheets. PrP^{Sc} self-replicates by binding to alpha-helical monomers of PrP^{C}, which causes a conformational change to convert PrP^{C} to PrP^{Sc}. This conformational change has a domino-like cascade with more protein converting to the oligomeric, amyloid-forming PrP^{Sc} state with a predominantly beta-sheet secondary structure (24–28). Although the exact structural intermediate steps remain poorly understood, many lines of evidence show that multiple diseases and clinical presentations are attributed to the variations in the conformational structure of PrP^{Sc} (29–33) (see "Epidemiology and Transmission," below).

The human *PRNP* gene, which codes for normal PrP^{C}, is composed of two exons, the second of which contains the single open reading frame encoding a 253-amino-acid preprotein (34). Both N-terminal and C-terminal signal peptides are cleaved in the endoplasmic reticulum. The C-terminal signal peptide is replaced with the glycosylphosphatidylinositol cell membrane anchor, and two complex sugar chains are linked to asparagine 181 and 197 (29–31). In normal PrP^{C}, five glycine-rich octapeptide repeats are coded for by *PRNP* codons 51 through 90. Codon 129 encodes either a methionine (M) or a valine (V), and this polymorphism plays a significant role in the susceptibility to disease and in disease phenotypes (see Epidemiology and Transmission section).

Monomeric PrP^{C} in the alpha helical conformation is susceptible to proteolytic degradation. The predominantly beta-sheet conformation that is present in PrP^{Sc} results in resistance to degradation by proteinase K treatment. PrP^{Sc} typically forms large insoluble aggregates. These characteristics of PrP^{C} and PrP^{Sc} have been used to aid in the diagnosis of prion disease (see Identification section). The conformational transition that underlies these pronounced changes is believed to involve refolding of the C-terminal region whereby the α-helical structures of PrP^{C} are replaced by beta-sheets with variable particle assembly patterns (35). Although insolubility and protease resistance were the original defining features of PrP^{Sc}, the finding of protease-sensitive small oligomers of pathogenic

PrP^{Sc} (36, 37) significantly broadened our knowledge of the spectrum of pathogenic conformers, and this finding has led to the discoveries of new animal and human prion diseases, such as atypical scrapie in sheep (38) and VPSPR in humans (39).

In healthy individuals, PrP^{C} is a membrane-associated glycoprotein, evolutionarily similar to the ZIP family of metal ion transport proteins (40). The flexibility and structure of octapeptide repeats coordinating zinc and copper transport are able to impact diverse biological endpoints (41). Although data accumulated in the past indicate that the PrP^{C} serves as an essential receptor for cytotoxicity of PrP^{Sc} as well as a substrate for the conversion to PrP^{Sc} (42, 43), the exact physiological function of PrP^{C} remains elusive (44). The variable neurotoxicity and specific infectivity of PrP^{Sc}, and the absence of amyloid fibrillar forms in a growing number of newly recognized prion diseases (39, 45), led some researchers to question the causative link with PrP^{Sc} and to predict a hypothetical lethal (PrPL) subform, presumably responsible for the toxicity and symptomatic stage of the disease (46, 47). The PrPL protein remains to be found, and recent experiments demonstrated that the high replication potency of CJD prions correlates with the brain levels of oligomeric PrP^{Sc} and the progression rate of human prion diseases *in vivo* (31, 32), and rising levels of these small oligomeric species of PrP^{Sc} convert the asymptomatic plateau of prion infectivity into a symptomatic stage (48). Cumulatively, these recent data argue that small PrP^{Sc} particles control the prion conversion as well as the cytotoxic effect mediated by PrP^{C} and that they represent the previously proposed PrPL species.

EPIDEMIOLOGY AND TRANSMISSION

Most prion disease in humans arises sporadically, but some are attributed to *PRNP* mutations, and still others are caused by zoonotic or iatrogenic transmission (Table 1) (30). Prion diseases include variant CJD (vCJD), GSS, FFI, kuru, VPSPR, and clinically and histologically diverse forms of sporadic CJD (sCJD). Human prion diseases—for which there is no therapy or cure—are characterized by deposits of pathogenic prion protein (PrP^{Sc}) in the brain and multifocal neuropathologic features with neuronal loss, spongiform changes, and astrocytic proliferation (30, 49). CJD generally occurs with an incidence between 0.5 and 2 cases per million annually. In the aging population of the United States, recent national mortality surveillance indicates an annual CJD incidence of between 4 and 6 cases per million among those 65 years of age and older (50). However, the rising age-adjusted incidence of CJD observed independently in the United Kingdom (http://www.cjd.ed.ac.uk/sites/default/files/report24.pdf) and in the United States (https://www.cdc.gov/prions/cjd/occurrence-transmission.html) in the past 10 years suggests that factors other than age, but as of yet unidentified, may be contributing to this trend.

TABLE 1 Types of human prion disease

Etiology	Phenotype
Acquired	Variant Creutzfeldt-Jakob disease
	Iatrogenic Creutzfeldt-Jakob disease
	Kuru
Sporadic	Creutzfeldt-Jakob disease (sCJD)[a]
	sCJD subtype 129 M/M (or M/V) 1
	sCJD subtype 129 V/V 1
	sCJD subtype 129 M/M 2
	sCJD subtype 129 M/V 2
	sCJD subtype 129 V/V 2
	Fatal insomnia
	Variably protease-sensitive prionopathy
Genetic	Genetic Creutzfeldt-Jakob disease
	Fatal familial insomnia
	Gerstmann-Sträussler-Scheinker disease

[a]sCJD subtypes are classified by their *PRNP* codon 129 amino acid(s) (i.e., methionine [M] and/or valine [V]) and by the type of migration seen in the proteinase K-resistant prion protein (see Fig. 1) (108).

Sporadic CJD

Several explanations have been proposed for the etiology of sporadic forms of CJD, which account for approximately 85% of all prion disease in humans. One hypothesis is that spontaneous somatic mutations in the *PRNP* gene may occur, which would lead to production of PrP^{C} that can easily convert to PrP^{Sc}, and this pathophysiology would be analogous to the pathophysiology of genetic CJD (gCJD). A second hypothesis is that rare stochastic conformational changes in the structure of PrP^{C} occur, which can result in spontaneous creation of the PrP^{Sc} conformer, which can then propagate (51). A third hypothesis is that at least some cases of apparent sCJD are actually acquired forms of CJD that have resulted from covert, low-level exposure to a "common external factor," which has not been identified (52). These three explanations presuppose that the PrP^{Sc} would have to be capable of recruiting wild-type PrP^{C}; this process might occur with some mutations or conformations but is unlikely to occur with others (53). A fourth hypothesis suggests that small amounts of PrP^{Sc}-like isoforms are normally present in the brain but are bound to other proteins (e.g., heat shock proteins), which prevent PrP^{Sc} from causing disease. However, this protective mechanism fails with aging (54, 55).

A number of *PRNP* polymorphisms have been described (56, 57). One of the most commonly studied risk modifiers in developing CJD is the *PRNP* codon 129. Homozygosity of methionine at codon 129 is a risk factor for developing sCJD, whereas valine at codon 129 is somewhat protective (49, 58, 59). Worldwide, the prevalence of this polymorphism is varied. In individuals of Asian descent, the 129M allele has a frequency of up to 0.97 (60), and in Europeans the 129M allele frequency is about 0.65 (57). In those from kuru-endemic areas, the valine variant is slightly more prevalent than the methionine allele (57, 58).

Genetic Prion Disease

Several genetic prion diseases have been described: gCJD, GSS, and FFI. Various mutations in *PRNP* have been identified and linked to these genetic prion diseases. The *PRNP* mutations are missense or nonsense point mutations, or the mutations result in an increase in the number of glycine-rich octapeptide repeats present in PrP (see Description of the Agent section) (57, 61, 62). Some of these diseases have unique histological features and clinical presentations. Allele counts in 16,025 definite and probable prion disease cases in 9 countries reported 59 rare *PRNP* variants, but many of these variants have unknown or low penetrance and exist also in the general population (56). The most common mutation associated with gCJD is the E200K *PRNP* mutation, which has a clinical presentation that is indistinguishable from sCJD (57). FFI and GSS are well described (63). The *PRNP* mutation associated with FFI is D178N (64). Some fatal insomnia cases are not FFI and have not been linked to a *PRNP* mutation, and this prion disease is described as sporadic fatal insomnia (64). A number of *PRNP* mutations have been associated with GSS, but the classic mutation is P102L. Symptoms in genetic prion disease typically begin sometime after 50 years of age.

Acquired Prion Disease

Kuru is a well-studied form of acquired prion disease. In the recent past, the Fore people of Papua New Guinea practiced endocanabalism as part of their death and mourning ritual (65, 66). Through these ritualistic feasts, the prions that cause kuru were spread within the tribe, mainly to the women and children who were the predominant participants in the feasts. The Fore have an increased frequency of the 129V PRNP allele when compared to other groups. The Fore individuals with methionine-valine heterozygosity at PRNP codon 129 who developed kuru did so later in life, and the progression of symptoms after onset was slower than for other homozygous genotypes (67, 68). Additionally, a novel PrP variant, G127V, with strong protection against the disease in the heterozygous state, was likely under positive evolutionary selection during the epidemic of kuru (69). The cessation of endocanabalism within the tribe brought an end to the kuru epidemic, but the study of kuru and the Fore people revealed that the incubation period for prion disease from transmission to symptomatology can be as long as 50 years (70).

vCJD is acquired by humans by exposure to BSE. BSE is sometimes referred to as "mad cow disease" and is a prion disease of cattle, which is analogous to scrapie in sheep and CJD in humans. Prions from cattle with BSE can be transmitted to humans, which can result in human prion disease; this human disease is termed "new variant CJD" or "variant CJD" (71–73). vCJD was first identified in 1996 in the United Kingdom where, as of April 2017, 178 probable and definite cases have been reported. An additional 53 cases have been identified in residents of 11 countries outside the United Kingdom, including 4 cases in the United States. Epidemiologic evidence from the four vCJD cases in U.S. residents indicated that they were infected in the United Kingdom (two cases), in Saudi Arabia (one case), and in either Kuwait or Russia (one case) (74).

An outbreak of BSE in the 1980s in the United Kingdom is thought to have originated from feeding protein-rich by-products from animal carcasses (including neural tissue remnants containing prions) to cattle (71). Subsequently, an outbreak of vCJD in the United Kingdom began in the late 1990s (71–73, 75). The individuals who developed vCJD have been typically younger than those affected with sCJD. Additionally, three individuals who have developed vCJD likely acquired the disease via therapeutic transfusion of human blood products that were donated from individuals with preclinical vCJD (76, 77).

Animal studies have demonstrated that all codon 129 genotypes are susceptible to developing vCJD (78), but until 2016, vCJD had exclusively been described in individuals who are homozygous for methionine at *PRNP* codon 129 (79). Because of the potential for developing transmitted prion disease decades after exposure, it is still uncertain if individuals with M129V PrP who were exposed to BSE are completely resistant to developing vCJD or if they simply have a longer incubation time before onset of symptoms, similar to those exposed to kuru. There is concern that heterozygous individuals may have a longer incubation period for vCJD than those individuals homozygous for methionine. In 2017, a single case report was published that described the first case of vCJD in an individual who was heterozygous at *PRNP* codon 129 (80). At this time, it is not known if this case represents the first case in a "second wave" of vCJD that will occur in *PRNP* M129V individuals or if the case is an atypical isolated occurrence.

The recently recognized atypical (H and L) forms of BSE are being reported with comparable frequency worldwide but are observed mainly in older cattle, thus making these atypical forms difficult to detect (81). The origin of this disease is unknown, but extrapolation from experimental humanized transgenic data suggests that L-BSE may propagate in humans as an unrecognized form of sCJD (82).

In addition to BSE, another prion disease of potential public health concern in the United States is CWD of deer and elk. The CWD in these farmed and free-ranging cervids has been endemic for decades in areas of Colorado and Wyoming, but since 2000 the disease has been detected in 19 additional states, two Canadian provinces, South Korea, and Norway (83). Unlike the BSE outbreak in cattle, CWD prions are highly infectious among cervids, and the disease is readily transmissible animal-to-animal through contact and through exposure to CWD prions in the environment (e.g., via cervid feces) (84). No reports have suggested that exposure of humans to CWD prions can cause disease (85–87). The experimental evidence suggests the existence of a species barrier against CWD transmission to humans, but it is unclear how protective this species barrier may be, because other primates are not protected. As many as 100% of intracerebrally and 92% of orally inoculated squirrel monkeys developed prion disease after CWD prion exposure (88, 89). The potential transmission of animal prion diseases, such as BSE and CWD, to humans directly or via an intermediate animal host has resulted in ongoing public health surveillance. These public health efforts are proactive and precautionary given the current high level of uncertainty (83).

Iatrogenic CJD (iCJD) is the result of transmission of prion disease via the therapeutic use of prion-contaminated human products or prion-contaminated reusable devices. More than 200 cases of iatrogenic transmission of sCJD have been attributed to the use of growth hormone derived from cadaveric pituitary glands, and more than 200 cases have been attributed to contaminated dura mater grafts (77, 90). Since the discovery of prion transmission via cadaveric growth hormone and dura mater grafts, measures have been implemented to prevent further exposure of individuals to prions via therapeutic products derived from humans. Although vCJD appears to have been transmitted via therapeutic blood transfusions, transmission of sCJD via blood transfusion has not been identified as a means of transmission (76). About a dozen cases of iCJD have been attributed to uncommon transmission events including neurosurgical instruments, electroencephalogram needles, and corneal transplants (77). Because of the potential for transmitting prions via reusable instrumentation exposed to neural tissue, guidelines recommend quarantine and/or more extensive decontamination and/or destruction of these instruments if it is suspected that they may have been exposed to prions (see Decontamination section).

Transmission of Prions in the Health Care Setting

Potential prion transmission causes concern for several reasons. First, prion disease is infrequently encountered, so many individuals only have a cursory working knowledge of prion transmission. Second, laboratory studies indicate that standard decontamination and sterilization procedures may be insufficient to completely remove infectivity from prion-contaminated instruments. Third, uncertainty still remains regarding how prions can and cannot be transmitted.

For example, vCJD appears to be potentially transmitted via blood transfusions or ingestion of contaminated beef products, but sCJD appears to be potentially transmissible only through more invasive exposures (e.g., neurosurgery or exposure to cadaver-derived therapeutics derived from neural tissue). Fourth, the incubation period between prion exposure/transmission and symptomatology can be decades, so it is difficult to definitively conclude that certain exposures (or potential exposures) to prions do not result in the transmission of the disease. Fifth, there is no prophylaxis or cure for prion disease.

Although a large epidemiological study of health care professionals concluded that the data did not support any overall increased occupational risk for health care workers (91), increased caution should be taken in the health care setting, specifically regarding neurosurgical patients. While the Centers for Disease Control and Prevention (CDC) and the World Health Organization (WHO) have devised risk assessment and decontamination protocols for the prevention of iatrogenic transmission of prion diseases (see Decontamination section), incidents of possible exposure to prions have unfortunately occurred in the United States (57, 92). The experience of vCJD after BSE exposure and the experience of kuru indicate that a delay of 10 years or longer between exposure and detectable human prion disease is likely, so short-term human outcomes cannot be used to gauge the efficacy of prion infection control practices. These characteristics of prion disease and the methodological limitations of retrospective epidemiological studies support a conservative approach in maintaining current precautionary measures (92).

CLINICAL SIGNIFICANCE

Human prion diseases often arise sporadically but have been transmitted to humans both iatrogenically and zoonotically, can have decades-long incubation periods, and are universally fatal. This combination of characteristics makes prion diseases an important entity for public health monitoring. The variability in clinical presentation can make prion diseases difficult to differentiate from other age-related brain neurodegenerative disorders, and postmortem brain analysis is currently the "gold standard" for diagnosing prion diseases (93–95). However, recent advances in radiological imaging and clinical laboratory testing have significantly improved the predictive value of antemortem testing (see Identification section).

The incubation period for CJD can be months to decades, but once symptoms emerge and a diagnosis is achieved, its course typically involves rapid neuropsychiatric decline, which is classically described as "rapidly progressive dementia," and death within months (49). No means of preventing sCJD or genetic prion disease (in individuals with a *PRNP* mutation) are currently known. Beyond supportive care, no specific medical therapy for CJD is currently available.

sCJD can present with various clinical manifestations including rapid cognitive deterioration, movement disorders, sleep disturbances, visual symptoms, behavioral changes, and psychiatric changes (96). The disease often progresses to myoclonus and akinetic mutism before death, which typically occurs within 6 months after diagnosis (97).

Genetic prion diseases can present in different ways depending on the underlying genetic mutation, and the symptomatic course is often months to years longer and more slowly progressive than sCJD. FFI classically presents with sleep disturbances including insomnia. GSS classically presents with signs and symptoms of cerebellar dysfunction, such as ataxia.

iCJD can present months to years after exposure. In iCJD, shorter incubation periods are observed when prions are directly transmitted to the brain, and longer incubation periods are observed when prions are transmitted via peripheral inoculation.

vCJD has been described as affecting a younger cohort than sCJD; individuals diagnosed with vCJD are often around 30 years of age, but the age range is broad. vCJD often manifests with psychiatric symptoms and progresses to death over the course of 12 to 18 months (49, 92).

The differential diagnosis of prion disease includes rapidly progressive variants of dementias that are usually chronic and slowly progressive, autoimmune diseases, vascular disease, metabolic diseases, vitamin deficiency, malignancy, and infection (98).

COLLECTION, TRANSPORT, AND STORAGE OF SPECIMENS

Standard precautions are necessary when collecting and handling specimens that may contain prions. Surgical instruments used to collect specimens for prion testing should ideally be disposed of after use. Alternatively, instruments and devices should be decontaminated using methods known to inactivate prions (99) (see Decontamination section). The CDC's *Biosafety in Microbiological and Biomedical Laboratories*, 5th ed., recommends that "unfixed samples of brain, spinal cord, and other tissues containing human prions should be processed with extreme care in a BSL-2 [biosafety level 2] facility utilizing BSL-3 practices" (100). Specimens such as blood for genetic testing, cerebrospinal fluid (CSF) and biopsies for diagnostic testing, and brains for autopsy should be stored and transported according to the reference laboratory's protocols. Neurologic tissue to be sectioned for histopathologic analysis should be handled and processed in accordance with College of American Pathologists recommendations, which ideally involves formic acid decontamination of the tissue before paraffin embedding (101). Shipping of specimens should be performed by trained individuals in accordance with government regulations. The National Prion Disease Pathology Surveillance Center recommends shipping all specimens as UN 3373, Category B material (102).

Decontamination

Prions are not inactivated using routine decontamination methods commonly employed in the clinical microbiology laboratory. For example, prions can maintain infectivity after alcohol fixation, formalin fixation, autoclaving, and even dry heat incineration, reducing specimens to ash (103). Although prions can maintain their infectivity after harsh treatment, no iatrogenic transmission of prions via contaminated surgical equipment has been identified since the 1970s, and human transmission of prions from potentially contaminated surfaces has never been identified (99).

Central nervous system (CNS) tissues are known to harbor the highest titer of transmissible prions, but detectable prions have also been identified from other body sites, even blood (104). Individuals with vCJD have been noted to have infectivity in reticuloendothelial tissues, albeit lower than in CNS (105). The current WHO guidelines, published in 1999, recommend handling blood and body fluids other than CSF using routine handling precautions (106). These WHO guidelines recommend against testing prion-contaminated CSF on automated instruments, but this guideline is difficult to practically implement because the diagnosis of CJD is often obtained days, weeks, or months after CSF has been tested in clinical laboratories.

Several infection control guidelines for prion diseases are available online:

- The United Kingdom (https://www.gov.uk/government/publications/guidance-from-the-acdp-tse-risk-management-subgroup-formerly-tse-working-group)
- The WHO (http://www.who.int/csr/resources/publications/bse/WHO_CDS_CSR_APH_2000_3/en/)
- The CDC *Biosafety in Microbiological and Biomedical Laboratories*, 5th edition, section VIII, part H (https://www.cdc.gov/biosafety/publications/bmbl5/BMBL5_sect_VIII_h.pdf)

Generally, if materials to be decontaminated can withstand the harsh treatment, the rule of thumb for decontamination of possible prion-contaminated material is to immerse the material or cover the contaminated surface with 1N sodium hydroxide (or 20,000 ppm of sodium hypochlorite) for 1 hour before neutralizing the chemical decontaminant and then proceeding with routine disinfection procedures (107).

The CDC recommends that laboratories handling prions from human tissue should use biosafety level 2 (BSL-2) laboratory practices (100). Although prions have been identified from many sites in individuals with CJD, CNS tissue typically contains prions at much higher titers than other tissues, blood, or CSF. The CDC recommends that CNS tissues from autopsy specimens containing prions should be processed "with extreme care in a BSL-2 facility utilizing BSL-3 practices" during autopsy. In the United States, the National Prion Disease Pathology Surveillance Center, which is sponsored by the CDC, has expertise in performing CJD autopsies and can be consulted. For those laboratories that are accredited by the College of American Pathologists (CAP), the CAP Anatomic Pathology Checklist explicitly describes special handling instructions for histology tissue specimens suspected of containing prions (101).

IDENTIFICATION

Autopsy is currently the gold standard for the diagnosis and classification of prion diseases and the determination of disease origin (49). However, antemortem studies have diagnostic value, and a confident diagnosis of CJD can often be made before death. Clinical presentation (see Clinical Significance section), family history, brain tissue studies, CSF analyses, genetic testing, magnetic resonance imaging (MRI) of the brain, and electroencephalogram can all contribute to the diagnosis of prion disease (49, 95, 108).

Classification of Prions

Human prion diseases are phenotypically heterogeneous (29–31, 49), and premortem clinical diagnosis has poor specificity. Although improved laboratory testing methods for CSF and brain MRI studies are helping to improve the reliability of clinical diagnosis, examination of brain tissue specimens remains the gold standard for determining disease origin. Two major determinants of prion disease phenotype and origin are the conformational structure of the pathogenic prion protein (PrP^{Sc}), which generates higher (type 1) or lower (type 2) molecular weight fragments after proteolysis on Western blot (Fig. 1), and the *PRNP* codon 129 polymorphism with methionine (M) or valine (V). In combination with neuropathological characteristics,

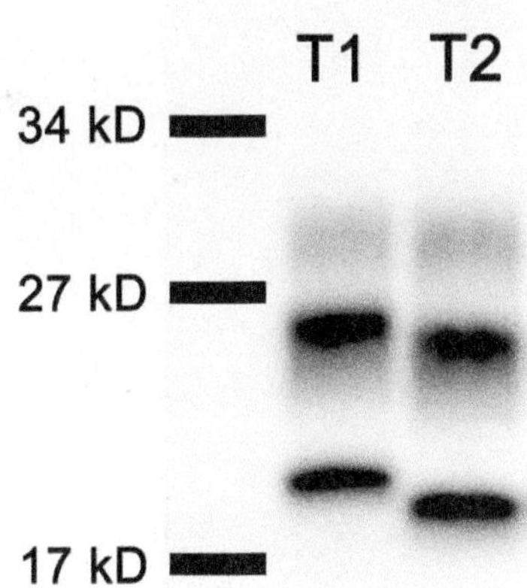

FIGURE 1 A Western blot of proteinase K-treated brain tissue specimens is depicted. PrP^{Sc} that is resistant to proteinase degradation is seen as bands. A specimen with type 1 prion protein is in the T1 lane, and a specimen with type 2 prion protein is in the T2 lane. Three bands are visible in each lane, with the lowest-molecular-weight bands (approximately 21 kDa [kD] in the T1 lane and approximately 19 to 20 kDa in the T2 lane) representing the unglycosylated PrP^{Sc}, the bands near 26 kDa representing mono-glycosylated PrP^{Sc}, and the faint bands near 29 kDa representing di-glycosylated PrP^{Sc}.

these factors are now used to classify sporadic human prion diseases and have been adopted by prion surveillance centers worldwide (30, 49, 95). This classification scheme describes six subtypes of sCJD: MM1, MV1, VV1, MM2, MV2, and VV2 (108, 109). sCJD subtypes MM1 and MV1 are often considered a single subtype due to their similar phenotypic findings. Over half of sCJD cases can be classified as subtype MM1, but mixed subtypes can be found in one-fifth of individuals (108–110). Notably, these subtypes correlate strongly with unique histopathological findings of the brain at autopsy to the extent that neuropathological findings often are predictive of the prion subtype (111). Different prion subtypes are associated with different clinical courses of disease (94) and represent different prion strains with distinctly different conformational structures of prion particles (29, 31–33, 112).

Western Blot

PrP^{Sc} is typically proteinase K resistant, and brain tissue can be treated with proteinase K, which digests proteins other than PrP^{Sc}. Any PrP^{Sc} that remains after proteinase K treatment can be detected and classified by electrophoretic migration pattern (93, 108–110). Three bands of PrP^{Sc} with increasing molecular weight are visible by Western blot: an unglycosylated band, a mono-glycoslyated band, and a di-glycoslyated band. Unglycosylated PrP^{Sc} with a molecular weight of 20 to 21 kDa is classified as type 1, and unglycosylated PrP^{Sc} with a molecular weight of 19 kDa is classified as type 2 (Fig. 1) (108). Notably, VPSPR has been reported in which the PrP^{Sc} can be digested with proteinase K (39, 78).

Histopathology

Brain tissue obtained by biopsy or autopsy can be used for histology studies (Fig. 2). Classic histological findings of the brain in individuals with CJD include spongiform degeneration, neuron loss, and astrogliosis (95). Specific neuropathological findings can be used to predict the prion subtype (111). Key histological findings can guide the diagnosis. Immunohistochemical staining of PrP is used to

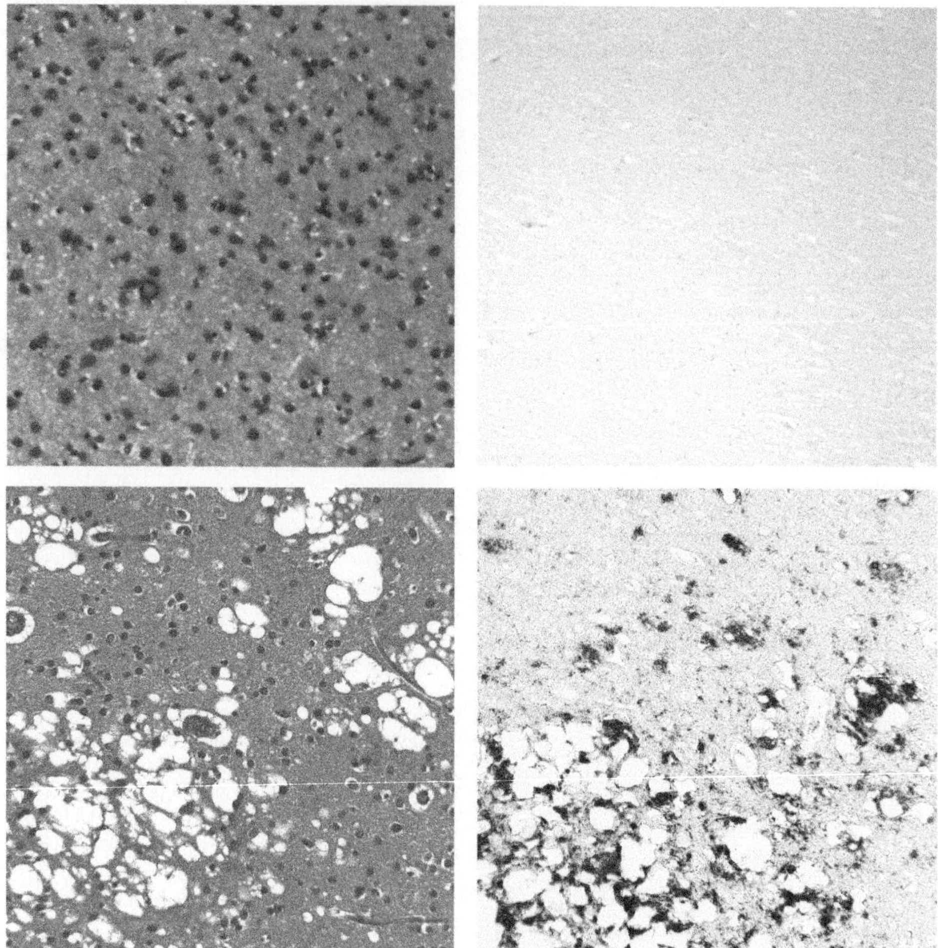

FIGURE 2 Micrographs of tissue sections of human brain occipital cortex are depicted. The top panels depict normal tissue; the bottom panels depict findings seen in sCJD. The left panels are stained with hematoxylin and eosin, and coarse fused vacuolization (spongiform changes) is present in the lower-left panel, which is a diagnostic feature of prion disease. The tissue sections in the right panels have been treated with proteinase, which degrades normal cellular prion protein. After proteinase treatment, the tissue was stained with an immunohistochemical stain to detect any prion protein that resisted proteinase treatment. These remaining prion protein deposits are evidenced as brown aggregates, and this finding is a diagnostic feature of prion disease.

characterize the disease; for example, florid plaques of PrP^{Sc} deposited in the cortex are a key feature of vCJD. Other histological features and the location within the brain where those feature are identified can be used to suggest one of the six subtypes of sCJD (94, 110, 111). PrP^{Sc} has been reliably identified in lymphoid tonsils in individuals with vCJD but is absent in individuals with sCJD (113).

Magnetic Resonance Imaging (MRI)

Diffusion-weighted MRI is estimated to have a sensitivity of about 90% in identifying prion disease, and a key sign is restricted diffusion in the gray matter (Fig. 3) that has been associated with spongiform changes (114). Hyperintensity using fluid-attenuated inversion recovery or T2 imaging has been associated with the astrocytosis present in prion disease. Areas that are commonly involved include the cortex, basal ganglia, striatum (caudate and putamen), and thalamus (including the pulivnar).

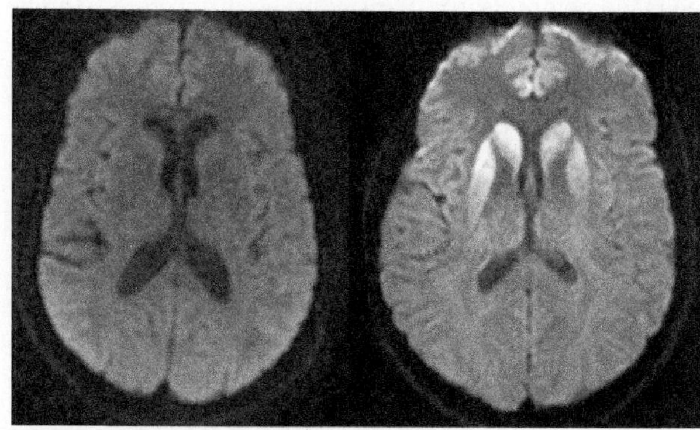

FIGURE 3 Diffusion-weighted MRIs of two brains. The image on the left does not demonstrate signs of prion disease. The image on the right demonstrates hyperintensity in the basal ganglia, which is associated with prion disease.

There may be value in positron emission tomography or single photon emission computed tomography in diagnosing prion disease, but MRI remains the mainstay in the radiological evaluation of suspected CJD (115, 116). Some radiological findings are suggestive of certain types (e.g., sCJD, vCJD, gCJD) or subtypes (e.g., MM1, MV2, etc.) of prion disease (114, 116).

Electroencephalography

A classic finding in an individual with prion disease is bilateral periodic discharges in the electroencephalogram, which are described as periodic sharp wave complexes (114). However, this method of identifying prion disease has low sensitivity (~50%) and may only be evident late in the disease course (114).

Blood, Urine, and Nasal Brushings

Research is being conducted to try to detect prions in peripheral blood, urine, nasal brushings, skin, and internal organs in individuals who may have prion disease, but this testing is not currently available for clinical use (117–120). Research studies have demonstrated that these specimen types may have adequate sensitivity and specificity for clinical testing or blood product screening, but these studies have generally only been performed at single centers. The studies that detected PRP^{Sc} from urine and blood have focused on detecting vCJD (117, 120), so the potential applicability to detecting sCJD has not been established.

Cerebrospinal Fluid

Several diagnostic tests can be performed on CSF, which can be helpful in diagnosing or ruling out prion disease. Two types of tests are typically performed. The first type examines the CSF for nonspecific markers of neurodegeneration. The second type examines the CSF for PrP^{Sc}, which is the causative agent of disease.

Multiple assays can be used to identify brain tissue breakdown products in the CSF, including 14-3-3, tau, neuron-specific enolase, and α-synuclein. A 14-3-3 assay is the classic test used to detect prion disease, and it is often still used despite the availability of more sensitive and specific assays (121). Either a Western blot or an enzyme-linked immunosorbent assay can be used to identify elevated 14-3-3. Another important nonspecific marker is total tau, which is commonly identified by enzyme-linked immunosorbent assay (49, 122). Because prion disease causes rapid deterioration of the brain tissue, these markers are sensitive in detecting prion disease. However, many other diagnoses can cause elevated levels, so these markers lack specificity. More slowly progressive forms of prion disease, such as some genetic prion diseases, may have levels of markers of neurodegeneration that are lower than more rapidly progressive prion diseases.

Real-time quaking-induced conversion (RT-QuIC) was recently developed as a novel assay to detect PrP^{Sc} (123, 124). This assay does not identify surrogate markers of disease, but it detects replication (seeding) activity of prions. The assay uses recombinant PrP^{C} as a reagent substrate, and the assay is seeded with CSF from a patient that is suspected of having prion disease. If PrP^{Sc} is present in the CSF, the PrP^{Sc} template induces misfolding of the PrP^{C} substrate *in vitro*. These misfolded proteins are detected by an increase in relative fluorescence of the reporter reagent, thioflavin T (Fig. 4). The second generation of CSF RT-QuIC reached a sensitivity of 92 to 95% and specificity of 98.5% in the detection of human prion diseases (125).

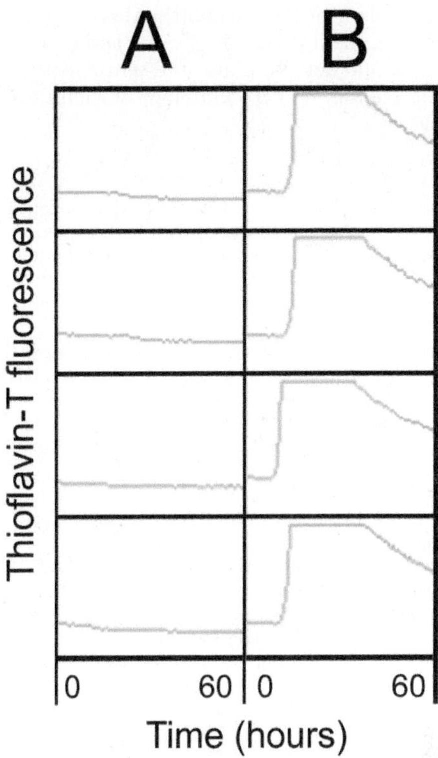

FIGURE 4 RT-QuIC curves are depicted for CSF specimens from two patients tested in quadruplicate (125). Specimen A demonstrates negative RT-QuIC results with no increase in fluorescence above the baseline. Specimen B demonstrates positive RT-QuIC results with a sharp increase in relative fluorescence and gradual degradation of signal.

Genetic Testing of *PRNP*

As with any genetic testing, a genetic counselor should be consulted before a living individual is tested. *PRNP* sequence analysis can be performed to determine the codon 129 genotype and to interrogate the gene for mutations which can cause genetic prion diseases (13, 57). Genetic testing can be performed using peripheral blood collected from living individuals or from tissue collected during autopsy. The most common mutation associated with gCJD is E200K, but many other *PRNP* mutations have also been described (57, 96, 126).

EVALUATION, INTERPRETATION, AND REPORTING OF RESULTS

Ideally, laboratories should be informed when the possibility of prion disease is being considered by the ordering provider. Laboratories should be informed of this consideration before receiving CSF or CNS tissue specimens for testing, so appropriate laboratory precautions and subsequent decontamination can be undertaken. Laboratory evaluation of CSF or CNS tissue from individuals suspected of having prion disease should follow their institutional policies and procedures for handling, testing, and decontamination (see Decontamination section). The diagnosis or exclusion of prion disease should be based on the whole clinical picture including clinical and family history, symptomatology, neurological signs, radiographic findings, and laboratory results. MRI and CSF testing can play an especially important role in evaluating the likelihood of prion disease in living patients (see Identification section). Autopsy remains the gold standard in definitively diagnosing and characterizing prion disease, and autopsy plays an essential role in investigating the etiology and epidemiology of each individual's prion disease.

REFERENCES

1. **Prusiner SB.** 1982. Novel proteinaceous infectious particles cause scrapie. *Science* **216:**136–144.
2. **Gajdusek DC.** 1967. Slow-virus infections of the nervous system. *N Engl J Med* **276:**392–400.
3. **Gordon WS.** 1946. Advances in veterinary research. *Vet Rec* **58:**516–525.
4. **Latarjet R, Muel B, Haig DA, Clarke MC, Alper T.** 1970. Inactivation of the scrapie agent by near monochromatic ultraviolet light. *Nature* **227:**1341–1343.
5. **Alper T, Cramp WA, Haig DA, Clarke MC.** 1967. Does the agent of scrapie replicate without nucleic acid? *Nature* **214:**764–766.
6. **Alper T, Haig DA, Clarke MC.** 1966. The exceptionally small size of the scrapie agent. *Biochem Biophys Res Commun* **22:**278–284.
7. **Prusiner SB, McKinley MP, Groth DF, Bowman KA, Mock NI, Cochran SP, Masiarz FR.** 1981. Scrapie agent contains a hydrophobic protein. *Proc Natl Acad Sci USA* **78:**6675–6679.
8. **Bolton DC, McKinley MP, Prusiner SB.** 1982. Identification of a protein that purifies with the scrapie prion. *Science* **218:**1309–1311.
9. **Safar J, Ceroni M, Piccardo P, Liberski PP, Miyazaki M, Gajdusek DC, Gibbs CJ Jr.** 1990. Subcellular distribution and physicochemical properties of scrapie-associated precursor protein and relationship with scrapie agent. *Neurology* **40:**503–508.
10. **Ceroni M, Piccardo P, Safar J, Gajdusek DC, Gibbs CJ Jr.** 1990. Scrapie infectivity and prion protein are distributed in the same pH range in agarose isoelectric focusing. *Neurology* **40:**508–513.
11. **Alper T, Haig DA, Clarke MC.** 1978. The scrapie agent: evidence against its dependence for replication on intrinsic nucleic acid. *J Gen Virol* **41:**503–516.
12. **Anonymous.** 2014. Stanley B. Prusiner: biographical. Nobel prize.org. http://www.nobelprize.org/nobel_prizes/medicine/laureates/1997/prusiner-bio.html. Accessed 21 June 2017.
13. **Anonymous.** 2017. Online Mendelian Inheritance in Man, OMIM®, McKusick-Nathans Institute of Genetic Medicine, Johns Hopkins University (Baltimore, MD). http://www.omim.org/entry/176640. Accessed 20 June 2017.
14. **Prusiner SB, Scott MR, DeArmond SJ, Cohen FE.** 1998. Prion protein biology. *Cell* **93:**337–348.
15. **Prusiner SB (ed).** 2004. *Prion Biology and Diseases*. Cold Spring Harbor Laboratory Press, Cold Spring Harbor, NY.
16. **Caughey B, Baron GS, Chesebro B, Jeffrey M.** 2009. Getting a grip on prions: oligomers, amyloids, and pathological membrane interactions. *Annu Rev Biochem* **78:**177–204.
17. **Cobb NJ, Surewicz WK.** 2009. Prion diseases and their biochemical mechanisms. *Biochemistry* **48:**2574–2585.
18. **Collinge J, Clarke AR.** 2007. A general model of prion strains and their pathogenicity. *Science* **318:**930–936.
19. **Morales R, Abid K, Soto C.** 2007. The prion strain phenomenon: molecular basis and unprecedented features. *Biochim Biophys Acta* **1772:**681–691.
20. **Legname G, Baskakov IV, Nguyen H-OB, Riesner D, Cohen FE, DeArmond SJ, Prusiner SB.** 2004. Synthetic mammalian prions. *Science* **305:**673–676.
21. **Wang F, Wang X, Yuan CG, Ma J.** 2010. Generating a prion with bacterially expressed recombinant prion protein. *Science* **327:**1132–1135.
22. **Deleault NR, Harris BT, Rees JR, Supattapone S.** 2007. Formation of native prions from minimal components *in vitro*. *Proc Natl Acad Sci USA* **104:**9741–9746.
23. **Kim JI, Cali I, Surewicz K, Kong Q, Raymond GJ, Atarashi R, Race B, Qing L, Gambetti P, Caughey B, Surewicz WK.** 2010. Mammalian prions generated from bacterially expressed prion protein in the absence of any mammalian cofactors. *J Biol Chem* **285:**14083–14087.
24. **Safar J.** 1996. Spectroscopic conformational studies of prion protein isoforms and the mechanism of transformation. *Semin Virol* **7:**207–214.
25. **Safar J, Roller PP, Gajdusek DC, Gibbs CJ Jr.** 1994. Scrapie amyloid (prion) protein has the conformational characteristics of an aggregated molten globule folding intermediate. *Biochemistry* **33:**8375–8383.
26. **Safar J, Roller PP, Gajdusek DC, Gibbs CJ Jr.** 1993. Conformational transitions, dissociation, and unfolding of scrapie amyloid (prion) protein. *J Biol Chem* **268:**20276–20284.
27. **Caughey BW, Dong A, Bhat KS, Ernst D, Hayes SF, Caughey WS.** 1991. Secondary structure analysis of the scrapie-associated protein PrP 27–30 in water by infrared spectroscopy. *Biochemistry* **30:**7672–7680.
28. **Pan K-M, Baldwin M, Nguyen J, Gasset M, Serban A, Groth D, Mehlhorn I, Huang Z, Fletterick RJ, Cohen FE, Prusiner SB.** 1993. Conversion of α-helices into β-sheets features in the formation of the scrapie prion proteins. *Proc Natl Acad Sci USA* **90:**10962–10966.
29. **Safar JG, Xiao X, Kabir ME, Chen S, Kim C, Haldiman T, Cohen Y, Chen W, Cohen ML, Surewicz WK.** 2015. Structural determinants of phenotypic diversity and replication rate of human prions. *PLoS Pathog* **11:**e1004832.
30. **Safar JG.** 2012. Molecular pathogenesis of sporadic prion diseases in man. *Prion* **6:**108–115.
31. **Safar JG.** 2012. Molecular mechanisms encoding quantitative and qualitative traits of prion strains, p 161–179. *In* Gambetti P (ed), *Prions and Diseases*, vol 1. Springer Verlag, New York, NY.
32. **Kim C, Haldiman T, Surewicz K, Cohen Y, Chen W, Blevins J, Sy MS, Cohen M, Kong Q, Telling GC, Surewicz WK, Safar JG.** 2012. Small protease sensitive oligomers of PrPSc in distinct human prions determine conversion rate of PrP(C). *PLoS Pathog* **8:**e1002835.
33. **Kim C, Haldiman T, Cohen Y, Chen W, Blevins J, Sy MS, Cohen M, Safar JG.** 2011. Protease-sensitive conformers in broad spectrum of distinct PrPSc structures in sporadic Creutzfeldt-Jakob disease are indicator of progression rate. *PLoS Pathog* **7:**e1002242.
34. **Anonymous.** Homo sapiens prion protein (PRNP), transcript variant 1, mRNA. NCBI Nucleotide Database. https://goo.gl/68HGr2. Accessed 20 June 2017.
35. **Smirnovas V, Kim JI, Lu X, Atarashi R, Caughey B, Surewicz WK.** 2009. Distinct structures of scrapie prion protein (PrPSc)-seeded versus spontaneous recombinant prion protein fibrils revealed by hydrogen/deuterium exchange. *J Biol Chem* **284:**24233–24241.
36. **Safar J, Wille H, Itri V, Groth D, Serban H, Torchia M, Cohen FE, Prusiner SB.** 1998. Eight prion strains have PrP(^{Sc}) molecules with different conformations. *Nat Med* **4:**1157–1165.
37. **Tzaban S, Friedlander G, Schonberger O, Horonchik L, Yedidia Y, Shaked G, Gabizon R, Taraboulos A.** 2002. Protease-sensitive scrapie prion protein in aggregates of heterogeneous sizes. *Biochemistry* **41:**12868–12875.
38. **Benestad SL, Sarradin P, Thu B, Schönheit J, Tranulis MA, Bratberg B.** 2003. Cases of scrapie with unusual features in Norway and designation of a new type, Nor98. *Vet Rec* **153:**202–208.
39. **Gambetti P, Dong Z, Yuan J, Xiao X, Zheng M, Alshekhlee A, Castellani R, Cohen M, Barria MA, Gonzalez-Romero D, Belay ED, Schonberger LB, Marder K, Harris C, Burke JR, Montine T, Wisniewski T, Dickson DW, Soto C, Hulette CM, Mastrianni JA, Kong Q, Zou WQ.** 2008. A novel human disease with abnormal prion protein sensitive to protease. *Ann Neurol* **63:**697–708.
40. **Watts JC, Huo H, Bai Y, Ehsani S, Won Jeon AH, Shi T, Daude N, Lau A, Young R, Xu L, Carlson GA, Williams D, Westaway D, Schmitt-Ulms G.** 2009. Interactome analyses identify ties of PrP and its mammalian paralogs to oligomannosidic N-glycans and endoplasmic reticulum-derived chaperones. *PLoS Pathog* **5:**e1000608. (Erratum, doi:10.1371/annotation/9eb11869-6acb-49b0-978e-abedc3cc545a.)
41. **Mays CE, Kim C, Haldiman T, van der Merwe J, Lau A, Yang J, Grams J, Di Bari MA, Nonno R, Telling GC, Kong Q, Langeveld J, McKenzie D, Westaway D, Safar JG.** 2014. Prion disease tempo determined by host-dependent substrate reduction. *J Clin Invest* **124:**847–858.

42. **Aguzzi A, Blättler T, Klein MA, Räber AJ, Hegyi I, Frigg R, Brandner S, Weissmann C.** 1997. Tracking prions: the neurografting approach. *Cell Mol Life Sci* **53:**485–495.
43. **Sailer A, Büeler H, Fischer M, Aguzzi A, Weissmann C.** 1994. No propagation of prions in mice devoid of PrP. *Cell* **77:**967–968.
44. **Aguzzi A, Falsig J.** 2012. Prion propagation, toxicity and degradation. *Nat Neurosci* **15:**936–939.
45. **Colby DW, Wain R, Baskakov IV, Legname G, Palmer CG, Nguyen HO, Lemus A, Cohen FE, DeArmond SJ, Prusiner SB.** 2010. Protease-sensitive synthetic prions. *PLoS Pathog* **6:**e1000736.
46. **Sandberg MK, Al-Doujaily H, Sharps B, De Oliveira MW, Schmidt C, Richard-Londt A, Lyall S, Linehan JM, Brandner S, Wadsworth JD, Clarke AR, Collinge J.** 2014. Prion neuropathology follows the accumulation of alternate prion protein isoforms after infective titre has peaked. *Nat Commun* **5:**4347.
47. **Sandberg MK, Al-Doujaily H, Sharps B, Clarke AR, Collinge J.** 2011. Prion propagation and toxicity *in vivo* occur in two distinct mechanistic phases. *Nature* **470:**540–542.
48. **Mays CE, van der Merwe J, Kim C, Haldiman T, McKenzie D, Safar JG, Westaway D.** 2015. Prion infectivity plateaus and conversion to symptomatic disease originate from falling precursor levels and increased levels of oligomeric PrPSc species. *J Virol* **89:**12418–12426.
49. **Puoti G, Bizzi A, Forloni G, Safar JG, Tagliavini F, Gambetti P.** 2012. Sporadic human prion diseases: molecular insights and diagnosis. *Lancet Neurol* **11:**618–628.
50. **Holman RC, Belay ED, Christensen KY, Maddox RA, Minino AM, Folkema AM, Haberling DL, Hammett TA, Kochanek KD, Sejvar JJ, Schonberger LB.** 2010. Human prion diseases in the United States. *PLoS One* **5:**e8521.
51. **Prusiner SB.** 2001. Shattuck lecture: neurodegenerative diseases and prions. *N Engl J Med* **344:**1516–1526.
52. **Linsell L, Cousens SN, Smith PG, Knight RS, Zeidler M, Stewart G, de Silva R, Esmonde TF, Ward HJ, Will RG.** 2004. A case-control study of sporadic Creutzfeldt-Jakob disease in the United Kingdom: analysis of clustering. *Neurology* **63:**2077–2083.
53. **Tremblay P, Ball HL, Kaneko K, Groth D, Hegde RS, Cohen FE, DeArmond SJ, Prusiner SB, Safar JG.** 2004. Mutant PrP^{Sc} conformers induced by a synthetic peptide and several prion strains. *J Virol* **78:**2088–2099.
54. **Safar JG, DeArmond SJ, Kociuba K, Deering C, Didorenko S, Bouzamondo-Bernstein E, Prusiner SB, Tremblay P.** 2005. Prion clearance in bigenic mice. *J Gen Virol* **86:**2913–2923.
55. **Yuan J, Xiao X, McGeehan J, Dong Z, Cali I, Fujioka H, Kong Q, Kneale G, Gambetti P, Zou WQ.** 2006. Insoluble aggregates and protease-resistant conformers of prion protein in uninfected human brains. *J Biol Chem* **281:**34848–34858.
56. **Minikel EV, et al, Exome Aggregation Consortium (ExAC).** 2016. Quantifying prion disease penetrance using large population control cohorts. *Sci Transl Med* **8:**322ra9.
57. **Collinge J, Whitfield J, McKintosh E, Beck J, Mead S, Thomas DJ, Alpers MP.** 2006. Kuru in the 21st century: an acquired human prion disease with very long incubation periods. *Lancet* **367:**2068–2074.
58. **Lee KS, Magalhães AC, Zanata SM, Brentani RR, Martins VR, Prado MA.** 2001. Internalization of mammalian fluorescent cellular prion protein and N-terminal deletion mutants in living cells. *J Neurochem* **79:**79–87.
59. **Palmer MS, Dryden AJ, Hughes JT, Collinge J.** 1991. Homozygous prion protein genotype predisposes to sporadic Creutzfeldt-Jakob disease. *Nature* **352:**340–342.
60. **Jeong BH, Nam JH, Lee YJ, Lee KH, Jang MK, Carp RI, Lee HD, Ju YR, Ahn Jo S, Park KY, Kim YS.** 2004. Polymorphisms of the prion protein gene (PRNP) in a Korean population. *J Hum Genet* **49:**319–324.
61. **Mastrianni JA.** 1993. Genetic prion diseases. *In* Pagon RA, Adam MP, Ardinger HH, Wallace SE, Amemiya A, Bean LJH, Bird TD, Ledbetter N, Mefford HC, Smith RJH, Stephens K (ed), *GeneReviews*. https://www.ncbi.nlm.nih.gov/books/NBK1229/.
62. **Takada LT, Kim MO, Cleveland RW, Wong K, Forner SA, Gala II, Fong JC, Geschwind MD.** 2017. Genetic prion disease: experience of a rapidly progressive dementia center in the United States and a review of the literature. *Am J Med Genet B Neuropsychiatr Genet* **174:**36–69.
63. **Llorens F, Zarranz JJ, Fischer A, Zerr I, Ferrer I.** 2017. Fatal familial insomnia: clinical aspects and molecular alterations. *Curr Neurol Neurosci Rep* **17:**30.
64. **Montagna P, Gambetti P, Cortelli P, Lugaresi E.** 2003. Familial and sporadic fatal insomnia. *Lancet Neurol* **2:**167–176.
65. **Mead S, Stumpf MP, Whitfield J, Beck JA, Poulter M, Campbell T, Uphill JB, Goldstein D, Alpers M, Fisher EM, Collinge J.** 2003. Balancing selection at the prion protein gene consistent with prehistoric kurulike epidemics. *Science* **300:**640–643.
66. **Wadsworth JD, Joiner S, Linehan JM, Desbruslais M, Fox K, Cooper S, Cronier S, Asante EA, Mead S, Brandner S, Hill AF, Collinge J.** 2008. Kuru prions and sporadic Creutzfeldt-Jakob disease prions have equivalent transmission properties in transgenic and wild-type mice. *Proc Natl Acad Sci USA* **105:**3885–3890.
67. **Cervenáková L, Goldfarb LG, Garruto R, Lee HS, Gajdusek DC, Brown P.** 1998. Phenotype-genotype studies in kuru: implications for new variant Creutzfeldt-Jakob disease. *Proc Natl Acad Sci USA* **95:**13239–13241.
68. **Lee HS, Brown P, Cervenáková L, Garruto RM, Alpers MP, Gajdusek DC, Goldfarb LG.** 2001. Increased susceptibility to Kuru of carriers of the PRNP 129 methionine/methionine genotype. *J Infect Dis* **183:**192–196.
69. **Asante EA, Smidak M, Grimshaw A, Houghton R, Tomlinson A, Jeelani A, Jakubcova T, Hamdan S, Richard-Londt A, Linehan JM, Brandner S, Alpers M, Whitfield J, Mead S, Wadsworth JD, Collinge J.** 2015. A naturally occurring variant of the human prion protein completely prevents prion disease. *Nature* **522:**478–481.
70. **Wadsworth JD, Joiner S, Linehan JM, Asante EA, Brandner S, Collinge J.** 2008. The origin of the prion agent of kuru: molecular and biological strain typing. *Philos Trans R Soc Lond B Biol Sci* **363:**3747–3753.
71. **Brown P, Will RG, Bradley R, Asher DM, Detwiler L.** 2001. Bovine spongiform encephalopathy and variant Creutzfeldt-Jakob disease: background, evolution, and current concerns. *Emerg Infect Dis* **7:**6–16.
72. **Hill AF, Desbruslais M, Joiner S, Sidle KCL, Gowland I, Collinge J, Doey LJ, Lantos P.** 1997. The same prion strain causes vCJD and BSE. *Nature* **389:**448–450, 526.
73. **Will RG, Ironside JW, Zeidler M, Cousens SN, Estibeiro K, Alperovitch A, Poser S, Pocchiari M, Hofman A, Smith PG.** 1996. A new variant of Creutzfeldt-Jakob disease in the UK. *Lancet* **347:**921–925.
74. **CDC.** 2017. vCJD cases reported in the US. https://www.cdc.gov/prions/vcjd/vcjd-reported.html. Accessed 21 June 2017.
75. **Spencer MD, Knight RS, Will RG.** 2002. First hundred cases of variant Creutzfeldt-Jakob disease: retrospective case note review of early psychiatric and neurological features. *BMJ* **324:**1479–1482.
76. **Urwin PJ, Mackenzie JM, Llewelyn CA, Will RG, Hewitt PE.** 2016. Creutzfeldt-Jakob disease and blood transfusion: updated results of the UK Transfusion Medicine Epidemiology Review Study. *Vox Sang* **110:**310–316.
77. **Brown P, Brandel JP, Sato T, Nakamura Y, MacKenzie J, Will RG, Ladogana A, Pocchiari M, Leschek EW, Schonberger LB.** 2012. Iatrogenic Creutzfeldt-Jakob disease, final assessment. *Emerg Infect Dis* **18:**901–907.
78. **Diack AB, Ritchie DL, Peden AH, Brown D, Boyle A, Morabito L, Maclennan D, Burgoyne P, Jansen C, Knight RS, Piccardo P, Ironside JW, Manson JC.** 2014. Variably protease-sensitive prionopathy, a unique prion variant with inefficient transmission properties. *Emerg Infect Dis* **20:**1969–1979.
79. **Ironside JW, McCardle L, Horsburgh A, Lim Z, Head MW.** 2002. Pathological diagnosis of variant Creutzfeldt-Jakob disease. *APMIS* **110:**79–87.
80. **Mok T, Jaunmuktane Z, Joiner S, Campbell T, Morgan C, Wakerley B, Golestani F, Rudge P, Mead S, Jäger HR, Wadsworth JD, Brandner S, Collinge J.** 2017. Variant Creutzfeldt-Jakob disease in a patient with heterozygosity at PRNP codon 129. *N Engl J Med* **376:**292–294.

81. **Masujin K, Orrú CD, Miyazawa K, Groveman BR, Raymond LD, Hughson AG, Caughey B.** 2016. Detection of atypical H-type bovine spongiform encephalopathy and discrimination of bovine prion strains by real-time quaking-induced conversion. *J Clin Microbiol* **54:**676–686. (Erratum, **54:**1407. doi:10.1128/JCM.00472-16.)
82. **Jaumain E, Quadrio I, Herzog L, Reine F, Rezaei H, Andréoletti O, Laude H, Perret-Liaudet A, Haïk S, Béringue V.** 2016. Absence of evidence for a causal link between bovine spongiform encephalopathy strain variant L-BSE and known forms of sporadic Creutzfeldt-Jakob disease in human PrP transgenic mice. *J Virol* **90:**10867–10874.
83. **Waddell L, Greig J, Mascarenhas M, Otten A, Corrin T, Hierlihy K.** 2018. Current evidence on the transmissibility of chronic wasting disease prions to humans-A systematic review. *Transbound Emerg Dis* 10.1111/tbed.12612.
84. **Hoover CE, Davenport KA, Henderson DM, Denkers ND, Mathiason CK, Soto C, Zabel MD, Hoover EA.** 2017. Pathways of prion spread during early chronic wasting disease in deer. *J Virol* **91:** e00077-17.
85. **Kurt TD, Sigurdson CJ.** 2016. Cross-species transmission of CWD prions. *Prion* **10:**83–91.
86. **Barria MA, Balachandran A, Morita M, Kitamoto T, Barron R, Manson J, Knight R, Ironside JW, Head MW.** 2014. Molecular barriers to zoonotic transmission of prions. *Emerg Infect Dis* **20:**88–97.
87. **CDC.** 2015. Chronic Wasting Disease (CWD) Transmission. https://www.cdc.gov/prions/cwd/transmission.html. Accessed 21 June 2017.
88. **Race B, Meade-White KD, Phillips K, Striebel J, Race R, Chesebro B.** 2014. Chronic wasting disease agents in nonhuman primates. *Emerg Infect Dis* **20:**833–837.
89. **Race B, Meade-White KD, Miller MW, Barbian KD, Rubenstein R, LaFauci G, Cervenakova L, Favara C, Gardner D, Long D, Parnell M, Striebel J, Priola SA, Ward A, Williams ES, Race R, Chesebro B.** 2009. Susceptibilities of nonhuman primates to chronic wasting disease. *Emerg Infect Dis* **15:**1366–1376.
90. **Rudge P, Jaunmuktane Z, Adlard P, Bjurstrom N, Caine D, Lowe J, Norsworthy P, Hummerich H, Druyeh R, Wadsworth JD, Brandner S, Hyare H, Mead S, Collinge J.** 2015. Iatrogenic CJD due to pituitary-derived growth hormone with genetically determined incubation times of up to 40 years. *Brain* **138:**3386–3399.
91. **Alcalde-Cabero E, Almazan-Isla J, Brandel JP, Breithaupt M, Catarino J, Collins S, Hayback J, Hoftberger R, Kahana E, Kovacs GG, Ladogana A, Mitrova E, Molesworth A, Nakamura Y, Pocchiari M, Popovic M, Ruiz-Tovar M, Taratuto A, van Duijn C, Yamada M, Will RG, Zerr I, de Pedro Cuesta J.** 2012. Health professions and risk of sporadic Creutzfeldt-Jakob disease, 1965 to 2010. *Euro Surveill* **17:**20144. http://www.eurosurveillance.org/content/10.2807/ese.17.15.20144-en.
92. **Bonda DJ, Manjila S, Mehndiratta P, Khan F, Miller BR, Onwuzulike K, Puoti G, Cohen ML, Schonberger LB, Cali I.** 2016. Human prion diseases: surgical lessons learned from iatrogenic prion transmission. *Neurosurg Focus* **41:**E10.
93. **Monari L, Chen SG, Brown P, Parchi P, Petersen RB, Mikol J, Gray F, Cortelli P, Montagna P, Ghetti B, Goldfarb LG, Gajdusek DC, Lugaresi E, Gambetti P, Autilio-Gambetti L.** 1994. Fatal familial insomnia and familial Creutzfeldt-Jakob disease: different prion proteins determined by a DNA polymorphism. *Proc Natl Acad Sci USA* **91:**2839–2842.
94. **Parchi P, Giese A, Capellari S, Brown P, Schulz-Schaeffer W, Windl O, Zerr I, Budka H, Kopp N, Piccardo P, Poser S, Rojiani A, Streichemberger N, Julien J, Vital C, Ghetti B, Gambetti P, Kretzschmar H.** 1999. Classification of sporadic Creutzfeldt-Jakob disease based on molecular and phenotypic analysis of 300 subjects. *Ann Neurol* **46:**224–233.
95. **Gambetti P, Kong Q, Zou W, Parchi P, Chen SG.** 2003. Sporadic and familial CJD: classification and characterisation. *Br Med Bull* **66:**213–239.
96. **Owen J, Beck J, Campbell T, Adamson G, Gorham M, Thompson A, Smithson S, Rosser E, Rudge P, Collinge J, Mead S.** 2014. Predictive testing for inherited prion disease: report of 22 years experience. *Eur J Hum Genet* **22:**1351–1356.
97. **Geissen M, Krasemann S, Matschke J, Glatzel M.** 2007. Understanding the natural variability of prion diseases. *Vaccine* **25:**5631–5636.
98. **Geschwind MD, Haman A, Miller BL.** 2007. Rapidly progressive dementia. *Neurol Clin* **25:**783–807, vii.
99. **CDC.** 2015. Creutzfeldt-Jakob disease, classic (CJD) infection control. https://www.cdc.gov/prions/cjd/infection-control.html. Accessed 21 June 2017.
100. **CDC.** 2009. Section VIII-H: prion diseases. *In* Chosewood LC, Wilson DE (ed), *Biosafety in Microbiological and Biomedical Laboratories (BMBL)*, 5th ed. U.S. Department of Health and Human Services. https://www.cdc.gov/biosafety/publications/bmbl5/BMBL5_sect_VIII_h.pdf.
101. **Anonymous.** 2015. *Anatomic Pathology Checklist.* College of American Pathologists, Northfield, IL.
102. **Anonymous.** Contact and shipping information. National Prion Disease Pathology Surveillance Center, Case Western Reserve University. https://case.edu/medicine/pathology/divisions/prion-center/resources-for-professionals/contact-and-shipping-information/. Accessed 27 June 2017.
103. **Brown P, Liberski PP, Wolff A, Gajdusek DC.** 1990. Resistance of scrapie infectivity to steam autoclaving after formaldehyde fixation and limited survival after ashing at 360 degrees C: practical and theoretical implications. *J Infect Dis* **161:**467–472.
104. **Concha-Marambio L, Pritzkow S, Moda F, Tagliavini F, Ironside JW, Schulz PE, Soto C.** 2016. Detection of prions in blood from patients with variant Creutzfeldt-Jakob disease. *Sci Transl Med* **8:**370ra183.
105. **WHO.** 2010. WHO tables on tissue infectivity distribution in transmissible spongiform encephalopathies. World Health Organization, Geneva, Switzerland. http://www.who.int/bloodproducts/tablestissueinfectivity.pdf.
106. **WHO.** 1999. WHO infection control guidelines for transmissible spongiform encephalopathies. Report of WHO consultation in Geneva, Switzerland, 23–26 March 1999. World Health Organization, Geneva, Switzerland. http://www.who.int/csr/resources/publications/bse/whocdscsraph2003.pdf.
107. **Belay ED, Blase J, Sehulster LM, Maddox RA, Schonberger LB.** 2013. Management of neurosurgical instruments and patients exposed to Creutzfeldt-Jakob disease. *Infect Control Hosp Epidemiol* **34:**1272–1280.
108. **Parchi P, Castellani R, Capellari S, Ghetti B, Young K, Chen SG, Farlow M, Dickson DW, Sima AA, Trojanowski JQ, Petersen RB, Gambetti P.** 1996. Molecular basis of phenotypic variability in sporadic Creutzfeldt-Jakob disease. *Ann Neurol* **39:**767–778.
109. **Gambetti P, Cali I, Notari S, Kong Q, Zou WQ, Surewicz WK.** 2011. Molecular biology and pathology of prion strains in sporadic human prion diseases. *Acta Neuropathol* **121:**79–90.
110. **Schoch G, Seeger H, Bogousslavsky J, Tolnay M, Janzer RC, Aguzzi A, Glatzel M.** 2006. Analysis of prion strains by PrPSc profiling in sporadic Creutzfeldt-Jakob disease. *PLoS Med* **3:**e14.
111. **Parchi P, de Boni L, Saverioni D, Cohen ML, Ferrer I, Gambetti P, Gelpi E, Giaccone G, Hauw JJ, Höftberger R, Ironside JW, Jansen C, Kovacs GG, Rozemuller A, Seilhean D, Tagliavini F, Giese A, Kretzschmar HA.** 2012. Consensus classification of human prion disease histotypes allows reliable identification of molecular subtypes: an inter-rater study among surveillance centres in Europe and USA. *Acta Neuropathol* **124:**517–529.
112. **Haldiman T, Kim C, Cohen Y, Chen W, Blevins J, Qing L, Cohen ML, Langeveld J, Telling GC, Kong Q, Safar JG.** 2013. Co-existence of distinct prion types enables conformational evolution of human PrPSc by competitive selection. *J Biol Chem* **288:**29846–29861.
113. **Hill AF, Antoniou M, Collinge J.** 1999. Protease-resistant prion protein produced *in vitro* lacks detectable infectivity. *J Gen Virol* **80:**11–14.
114. **Letourneau-Guillon L, Wada R, Kucharczyk W.** 2012. Imaging of prion diseases. *J Magn Reson Imaging* **35:**998–1012.
115. **Caobelli F, Cobelli M, Pizzocaro C, Pavia M, Magnaldi S, Guerra UP.** 2015. The role of neuroimaging in evaluating patients affected by Creutzfeldt-Jakob disease: a systematic review of the literature. *J Neuroimaging* **25:**2–13.

116. **Risacher SL, Saykin AJ.** 2013. Neuroimaging biomarkers of neurodegenerative diseases and dementia. *Semin Neurol* **33:**386–416.

117. **Sawyer EB, Edgeworth JA, Thomas C, Collinge J, Jackson GS.** 2015. Preclinical detection of infectivity and disease-specific PrP in blood throughout the incubation period of prion disease. *Sci Rep* **5:**17742.

118. **Orrú CD, Bongianni M, Tonoli G, Ferrari S, Hughson AG, Groveman BR, Fiorini M, Pocchiari M, Monaco S, Caughey B, Zanusso G.** 2014. A test for Creutzfeldt-Jakob disease using nasal brushings. *N Engl J Med* **371:** 519–529.

119. **Notari S, Moleres FJ, Hunter SB, Belay ED, Schonberger LB, Cali I, Parchi P, Shieh WJ, Brown P, Zaki S, Zou WQ, Gambetti P.** 2010. Multiorgan detection and characterization of protease-resistant prion protein in a case of variant CJD examined in the United States. *PLoS One* **5:**e8765.

120. **Moda F, Gambetti P, Notari S, Concha-Marambio L, Catania M, Park KW, Maderna E, Suardi S, Haïk S, Brandel JP, Ironside J, Knight R, Tagliavini F, Soto C.** 2014. Prions in the urine of patients with variant Creutzfeldt-Jakob disease. *N Engl J Med* **371:**530–539.

121. **Weber T, Aguzzi A.** 1997. The spectrum of transmissible spongiform encephalopathies. *Intervirology* **40:**198–212.

122. **Leitão MJ, Baldeiras I, Almeida MR, Ribeiro MH, Santos AC, Ribeiro M, Tomás J, Rocha S, Santana I, Oliveira CR.** 2016. CSF Tau proteins reduce misdiagnosis of sporadic Creutzfeldt-Jakob disease suspected cases with inconclusive 14-3-3 result. *J Neurol* **263:**1847–1861.

123. **Atarashi R, Satoh K, Sano K, Fuse T, Yamaguchi N, Ishibashi D, Matsubara T, Nakagaki T, Yamanaka H, Shirabe S, Yamada M, Mizusawa H, Kitamoto T, Klug G, McGlade A, Collins SJ, Nishida N.** 2011. Ultrasensitive human prion detection in cerebrospinal fluid by real-time quaking-induced conversion. *Nat Med* **17:**175–178.

124. **Wilham JM, Orrú CD, Bessen RA, Atarashi R, Sano K, Race B, Meade-White KD, Taubner LM, Timmes A, Caughey B.** 2010. Rapid end-point quantitation of prion seeding activity with sensitivity comparable to bioassays. *PLoS Pathog* **6:**e1001217.

125. **Foutz A, Appleby BS, Hamlin C, Liu X, Yang S, Cohen Y, Chen W, Blevins J, Fausett C, Wang H, Gambetti P, Zhang S, Hughson A, Tatsuoka C, Schonberger LB, Cohen ML, Caughey B, Safar JG.** 2017. Diagnostic and prognostic value of human prion detection in cerebrospinal fluid. *Ann Neurol* **81:**79–92.

126. **van der Kamp MW, Daggett V.** 2009. The consequences of pathogenic mutations to the human prion protein. *Protein Eng Des Sel* **22:**461–468.

ANTIVIRAL AGENTS AND SUSCEPTIBILITY TEST METHODS

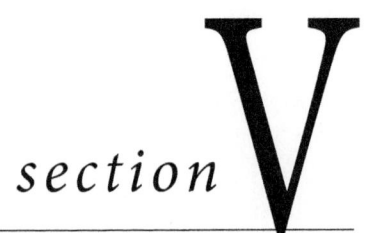

VOLUME EDITOR: MARIE LOUISE LANDRY

SECTION EDITORS: ANGELA M. CALIENDO, CHRISTINE C. GINOCCHIO, RANDALL T. HAYDEN, AND YI-WEI TANG

Antiviral Agents*

CARLOS A. Q. SANTOS AND NELL S. LURAIN

113

The use of antiviral agents for the treatment of viral diseases continues to expand. Most of the agents currently approved by the Food and Drug Administration (FDA) are active against one or more of the following viruses: human immunodeficiency virus types 1 and 2 (HIV-1 and HIV-2), hepatitis viruses B and C (HBV and HCV), the human herpesviruses, and influenza A and B viruses. This chapter is organized according to these virus groups with cross-referencing for agents with activity against more than one group of viruses. The major targets of these agents are viral replication enzymes, proteases, and entry/exit pathways (1–4). In a few cases, approved drugs for the above families of viruses have also been used to treat viruses in other families. The expanded spectrum of drug usage is discussed in the individual drug sections.

AGENTS AGAINST HIV-1 AND HIV-2

There are now five classes of antiviral agents for the treatment of HIV-1: (i) nucleoside/nucleotide reverse transcriptase inhibitors (NRTIs/NtRTIs), (ii) nonnnucleoside reverse transcriptase inhibitors (NNRTIs), (iii) protease inhibitors (PIs), (iv) entry/fusion inhibitors, and (v) integrase strand transfer inhibitors (INSTIs). Current information on each drug is available through the AIDSinfo website (http://AIDSinfo.nih.gov), which has separate guidelines for the use of approved antiretroviral agents in adolescents and adults, children, and pregnant HIV-1-infected women (5–7). These guidelines describe the agents along with dosage, adverse effects, and drug interactions. Working groups for each of these patient populations regularly update the guidelines. Additional information can be obtained from the package inserts available from the pharmaceutical company websites. Changes in recommended drug doses as well as observed adverse effects and drug interactions occur frequently, making it necessary to consult the most up-to-date sources.

Antiretroviral agents are administered in combinations of different drug classes termed combined antiretroviral therapy (cART) to maximize efficacy and to minimize the induction of drug resistance. cART is now generally regarded as any combination regimen designed to achieve the goal of complete virus suppression. These regimens comprise a minimum of three drugs, which are usually NNRTI based (two NRTIs and/or NtRTIs plus one NNRTI), PI based (two NRTIs and/or NtRTIs plus one or more PIs), or more recently, INSTI based (two NRTIs and/or NtRTIs plus an INSTI) (5).

There are currently 25 approved antiretroviral drugs (1) with numerous possible combinations for treatment regimens. Recommended regimens for adults and adolescents are given in the guidelines (5) for treatment-naive and treatment-experienced patients. The large number of drugs creates a tremendous potential for drug interactions among the different classes as well as interactions with other types of drugs prescribed for conditions associated with HIV infection. Close monitoring of these complex interactions is required to avoid detrimental changes in drug levels and/or toxicity.

Table 1 summarizes the structure, mechanism of action, and major adverse effects of the individual drugs and drug combinations approved by the FDA. The drug interactions described below for each drug are only highlights of potential interactions. Frequent updates and more-comprehensive information can be obtained from the AIDSinfo website listed above.

Nucleoside and/or Nucleotide Reverse Transcriptase Inhibitors

The NRTI-NtRTI class of drugs is not active as administered but must be phosphorylated by cellular kinases to the nucleoside triphosphate form, which may lack a 3′hydroxyl group for DNA chain elongation. The NRTIs require triphosphorylation, while the NtRTIs require only diphosphorylation (1). These antiviral agents act as competitive inhibitors of the viral reverse transcriptase (RT), which results in chain termination. They are active against both the HIV-1 and HIV-2 RTs, and they are used as dual-combination backbones in regimens with NNRTIs, PIs, and INSTIs (5). Several of them also are active against the HBV DNA polymerase, which has RT activity (see "Agents against Hepatitis B Virus" below) (3). Lactic acidosis with hepatic steatosis is a rare but very serious adverse effect associated with all members of this class. These toxic effects of NRTIs and NtRTIs appear to be the result of inhibition of the mitochondrial DNA polymerase γ (8).

*This chapter contains information presented by Aimee C. Hodowanec, Kenneth D. Thompson, and Nell S. Lurain in chapter 110 of the 11th edition of this *Manual*.

TABLE 1 Antiviral agents for HIV therapy[a]

Antiviral agent (abbreviation)	Trade name (pharmaceutical company[b])	Mechanism of action/ route of administration	Major adverse effects[c]
Nucleoside or nucleotide reverse transcriptase inhibitors (NRTI-NtRTIs)			
Abacavir (ABC)	Ziagen (GSK)	Converted to triphosphate analogue of dGTP by cellular kinases, competitive inhibitor of RT, viral DNA chain terminator; administered orally	Hypersensitivity reaction associated with HLA-B*5701
Didanosine (ddI)	Videx (BMS)	Converted to dideoxy triphosphate analogue of dATP by cellular kinases Activity and administration similar to ABC	Pancreatitis, peripheral neuropathy, nausea, diarrhea
Emtricitabine (FTC)	Emtriva (Gilead)	Converted to triphosphate analogue of dCTP by cellular kinases Activity and administration similar to ABC	Minimal toxicity, skin hyperpigmentation, posttreatment exacerbation of hepatitis B coinfection
Lamivudine (3TC)	Epivir (GSK)	Converted to triphosphate analogue of dCTP by cellular kinases Activity and administration similar to ABC	Minimal toxicity, posttreatment exacerbation of hepatitis B coinfection
Stavudine (d4T)	Zerit (BMS)	Converted to triphosphate analogue of dTTP by cellular kinases Activity and administration similar to ABC	Peripheral neuropathy, lipodystrophy; motor weakness
Tenofovir alafenamide (TAF)	Vemlidy (Gilead)	Diester hydrolysis required for conversion to tenofovir, monophosphate analogue requires diphosphorylation by cellular kinases Activity and administration similar to ABC	Asthenia, headache, GI symptoms, cough, posttreatment exacerbation of hepatitis B coinfection
Tenofovir disoproxil fumarate (TDF)	Viread (Gilead)	Same as TAF	Asthenia, headache, GI symptoms, cough, decrease in bone mineral density, lipodystrophy, posttreatment exacerbation of hepatitis B coinfection
Zidovudine (AZT or ZDV)	Retrovir (GSK)	Converted to triphosphate analogue of dTTP by cellular kinases Activity and administration similar to ABC	Bone marrow suppression, GI symptoms, headache, insomnia
Nucleoside or nucleotide reverse transcriptase inhibitors (NRTI-NtRTI) combined formulations			
Abacavir (ABC) + lamivudine (3TC)	Epzicom (GSK)	See individual NRTIs above	See individual NRTIs above
Abacavir (ABC) + zidovudine (AZT) + lamivudine (3TC)	Trizivir (GSK)	See individual NRTIs above	See individual NRTIs above
Emtricitabine (FTC) + tenofovir (TDF) + efavirenz (EFV)	Atripla (Gilead and BMS)	See individual NTRIs-NtRTIs above	See individual NTRIs-NtRTIs above
Tenofovir (TDF) + emtricitabine (FTC)	Truvada (Gilead)	See individual NTRIs-NtRTIs above	See individual NTRIs-NtRTIs above
Nonnucleoside reverse transcriptase inhibitors (NNRTIs)			
Efavirenz (EFV)	Sustiva (BMS)	Noncompetitive inhibitor binds to HIV-1 RT close to catalytic site, disrupts normal polymerization function Administered orally	Skin rash (Stevens-Johnson syndrome), psychiatric symptoms, CNS symptoms (e.g., dizziness, insomnia, confusion), elevated transaminases, teratogenic
Etravirine (ETR)	Intelence (Tibotec)	Activity and administration similar to EFV	Skin rash (Stevens-Johnson syndrome), GI symptoms
Nevirapine (NVP)	Viramune (BI)	Activity and administration similar to EFV	Severe hepatotoxicity, skin rashes (Stevens-Johnson syndrome)
Rilpivirine (RPV)	Edurant (Tibotec)	Activity and administration similar to EFV	Rash, depression, headache, insomnia, hepatotoxicity

(Continued on next page)

TABLE 1 Antiviral agents for HIV therapy[a] *(Continued)*

Antiviral agent (abbreviation)	Trade name (pharmaceutical company[b])	Mechanism of action/ route of administration	Major adverse effects[c]
Protease inhibitors			
Atazanavir (ATV)	Reyataz (BMS)	Peptidomimetic protease. Binds competitively to active site of HIV protease, prevents cleavage of viral polyprotein precursors, produces immature, noninfectious viral particles Administered orally	Indirect hyperbilirubinemia, prolonged PR interval, hyperglycemia; fat redistribution; increased bleeding episodes with hemophilia, nephrolithiasis
Darunavir (DRV)	Prezista (Tibotec)	Nonpeptidic protease Inhibits protease dimerization Prevents cleavage of viral polyprotein Administered orally	Skin rash (Stevens-Johnson syndrome), hepatotoxicity, hyperglycemia, fat redistribution, GI symptoms, elevated transaminase, increased bleeding episodes with hemophilia, nephrolithiasis
Fosamprenavir (FPV)	Lexiva (GSK)	Converted to amprenavir by cellular phosphatases Activity and administration similar to ATV	Skin rash, GI symptoms, headache, hyperlipidemia, fat redistribution, elevated transaminases, hyperglycemia, increased bleeding episodes with hemophilia
Indinavir (IDV)	Crixivan (Merck)	Activity and administration similar to ATV	Nephrolithiasis/urolithiasis, GI symptoms, indirect hyperbilirubinemia, hyperlipidemia, hemolytic anemia, headache, hyperglycemia, fat redistribution, increased bleeding episodes with hemophilia
Lopinavir (LPV) + ritonavir (RTV)	Kaletra (Abbott)	Activity and administration similar to ATV	GI symptoms, asthenia, hyperlipidemia, elevated transaminase, hyperglycemia, hyperlipidemia, fat redistribution, elevated transaminases, increased bleeding episodes with hemophilia
Nelfinavir (NFV)	Viracept (Pfizer)	Activity and administration similar to ATV	Diarrhea, hyperlipidemia, hyperglycemia, fat redistribution, elevated transaminases, increased bleeding episodes with hemophilia
Ritonavir (RTV)	Norvir (Abbott)	Activity and administration similar to ATV	Severe GI symptoms, circumoral paresthesias, hyperlipidemia, hepatitis, asthenia, taste disturbance, hyperglycemia, fat redistribution, increased bleeding episodes with hemophilia
Saquinavir (SQV)	Invirase (Roche)	Activity and administration similar to ATV	GI symptoms, hyperlipidemia, elevated transaminase, headache, hyperglycemia, hyperlipidemia, fat redistribution, increased bleeding episodes with hemophilia
Tipranavir (TPV)	Aptivus (BI)	Nonpeptidic protease Activity and administration similar to DRV	Hepatotoxicity, hyperglycemia, sulfa allergy skin rash, hyperlipidemia, fat redistribution, increased bleeding episodes with hemophilia, rare intracranial hemorrhage
Entry inhibitors			
Enfuvirtide (T20)	Fuzeon (Roche)	Binds to first heptad repeat in gp41, prevents conformational changes required for fusion of viral and cellular membranes Administered by injection	Local injection site reactions, pneumonia, hypersensitivity reactions
Maraviroc (MVC)	Selzentry (Pfizer)	CCR5 coreceptor antagonist Allosteric binding to CCR5 alters conformation, prevents gp120 binding Administered orally	Upper respiratory infections, cough, pyrexia, rash, dizziness

(Continued on next page)

TABLE 1 Antiviral agents for HIV therapy[a] *(Continued)*

Antiviral agent (abbreviation)	Trade name (pharmaceutical company[b])	Mechanism of action/ route of administration	Major adverse effects[c]
Integrase strand transfer inhibitors			
Dolutegravir (DTG)	Tivicay (Viiv/GSK)	Prevents formation of covalent bond between unintegrated HIV DNA and host DNA, preventing formation of provirus Administered orally	Headache, insomnia, fatigue, elevated AST/ALT, elevated CPK
Elvitegravir (EVG) + cobicistat (COBI) + TDF + FTC	Stribild (Gilead)	EVG: prevents formation of covalent bond between unintegrated HIV DNA and host DNA, preventing formation of provirus Requires pharmacologic boosting Administered orally Cobicistat: pharmacokinetic enhancer, inhibits CYP3A4. TDF and FTC: see protease inhibitors above	Coformulation EG-COBI-TDF-FTC: GI symptoms, renal impairment, decreased bone density
Raltegravir (RAL)	Isentress (Merck)	Prevents formation of covalent bond between unintegrated HIV DNA and host DNA, preventing formation of provirus. Administered orally	Headache, GI symptoms, asthenia, fatigue, pyrexia, CPK elevation

[a]Note: all NRTI/NtRTIs carry the warning of lactic acidosis and severe hepatomegaly with steatosis.

[b]Pharmaceutical companies: Abbott Laboratories, North Chicago, IL; BI, Boehringer Ingelheim Pharmaceuticals, Ridgefield, CT; BMS, Bristol-Meyers Squibb, Princeton, NJ; Gilead Sciences, Foster City, CA; GSK, GlaxoSmithKline, Research Triangle Park, NC; Merck & Co., Whitehouse Station, NJ; Pfizer, New York, NY; Roche Pharmaceuticals, Nutley, NJ; Tibotec Therapeutics, Division of Ortho Biotech Products, L.P., Raritan, NJ.

[c]Abbreviations: GI, gastrointestinal (symptoms include nausea, vomiting, and diarrhea); AST, aspartate aminotransferase; ALT, alanine aminotransferase; CPK, creatine phosphokinase.

Abacavir

Pharmacology

The oral bioavailability of abacavir (ABC) is 83%. The plasma half-life is 1.5 h, and the intracellular half-life is 12 to 26 h. ABC can be administered with or without food. It is metabolized by alcohol dehydrogenase and glucuronyltransferase, and 82% of the metabolites are excreted by the kidneys. Placental passage has been demonstrated in animal studies (7). ABC penetration of the central nervous system (CNS) is adequate to inhibit HIV replication (9). ABC is recommended for therapy in combination with dolutegravir (DTG) and lamivudine (3TC). The guidelines recommend using caution when prescribing ABC in patients with high risk for cardiovascular disease, because studies have shown both a lack of association as well as increased risk of cardiovascular disease (10–12). ABC is contraindicated in patients who are positive for the HLA-B*5701 major histocompatibility complex class I allele, which is associated with a hypersensitivity reaction to the drug (5, 13). Combination formulations of two and three NRTIs and/or NtRTIs containing ABC are commercially available (Table 1).

Drug Interactions

ABC decreases the level of methadone. Ethanol increases the concentration of ABC in plasma through common metabolic pathways (5).

Didanosine

Pharmacology

The oral bioavailability of didanosine (ddI) is 30 to 40%. The serum half-life is 1.5 h, and the intracellular half-life is >20 h. It should be administered without food. One-half of the drug is excreted by the kidney. There is low penetration of the CNS, but ddI has been shown to cross the human placenta (7). ddI is no longer recommended for use in treatment-naive patients (7).

Drug Interactions

Administration of ddI with either d4T or tenofovir disoproxil fumarate (TDF) can increase the rate and severity of toxicities associated with each individual drug. Ganciclovir (GCV), valganciclovir (val-GCV), ribavirin (RBV), and allopurinol also increase ddI exposure, leading to increased ddI toxicity (5, 14, 15).

Emtricitabine

Pharmacology

The oral bioavailability of emtricitabine (FTC) is 93%. The plasma half-life is 10 h, and the intracellular half-life is >20 h. FTC can be administered with or without food. It is excreted mostly unchanged (86%) by the kidneys, and the remainder is eliminated in the feces. It has intermediate penetration of cells of the CNS (16) and has been shown to cross the placenta (7). FTC is recommended as a preferred drug in combination with tenofovir (TDF) in NNRTI-based, PI-based, or INSTI-based regimens for treatment-naive patients. Coadministration with 3TC is not recommended, because both drugs have similar resistance patterns and there is no therapeutic advantage for the combination (5).

Drug Interactions

No significant interactions with other antiretroviral agents have been reported (5, 17).

Lamivudine

Pharmacology

The oral bioavailability of lamivudine (3TC) is 86%. The serum half-life is 5 to 7 h, and the intracellular half-life is 18 to 22 h. The drug can be administered with or without food, and 71% is excreted by the kidney. 3TC crosses the human placenta (7) and has intermediate penetration of the CNS (16). 3TC is recommended in alternative dual-NRTI regimens with tenofovir (TDF or tenofovir alafenamide [TAF]), combined with either an NNRTI, PI, or INSTI for treatment-naive patients (5). Coadministration of 3TC with FTC is not recommended (see " Emtricitabine" above).

Drug Interactions

3TC is actively excreted by the kidney by the organic cationic transport system; therefore, possible interactions should be considered with other drugs that use the same pathway, such as trimethoprim-sulfamethoxazole (5).

Stavudine

Pharmacology

The oral bioavailability of stavudine (d4T) is 86%. The serum half-life is 1.0 h, and the intracellular half-life is 7.5 h. d4T can be administered with or without food. Half of the drug is excreted by the kidneys. Placental passage occurs in animals, and d4T has intermediate penetrance of the CNS (7, 18). d4T is no longer recommended for use in treatment-naive patients because of toxicity (5). It has been replaced by ABC or zidovudine (ZDV) in first-line pediatric regimens (19).

Drug Interactions

d4T combined with ddI can increase the rate and severity of toxicities associated with each individual drug. ZDV and RBV inhibit the phosphorylation of d4T (20, 21).

Tenofovir Disoproxil Fumarate and Tenofovir Alafenamide

Pharmacology

The oral bioavailability of the prodrug tenofovir disoproxil fumarate (TDF) metabolized to tenofovir is 25% without food and 39% with a high-fat meal, although the drug is administered without regard to meals. The serum half-life is 17 h, and the intracellular half-life is >60 h. The drug is excreted mostly unchanged (70 to 80%) by the kidneys. TDF has been shown to cross the placenta in animal studies, but it has low penetrance of the CNS (7, 16). It is less likely than other NRTIs-NtRTIs to be associated with mitochondrial toxicity; however, renal dysfunction and decreased bone mineral density have been reported with TDF use. TDF is recommended in initial regimens with dual NRTI-NtRTI combinations including FTC with elvitegravir (EVG) and cobicistat (COBI) (5, 22).

Tenofovir alafenamide (TAF) is another prodrug of tenofovir, which appears to be equally effective as an antiretroviral agent as TDF, but at a much lower dose (23). Consequently, TAF is associated with lower bone density loss and nephrotoxicity compared to TDF (22). TAF is approved in combined formulations such as EVG-COBI-FTC or darunavir (DRV)-ritonavir (RTV)/FTC for initial antiretroviral therapy (5).

Drug Interactions

TDF increases the concentration of ddI in plasma, leading to increased toxicity (14). There may be increased toxicity associated with coadministration of GCV, val-GCV, acyclovir (ACV), or cidofovir (CDV) (5).

TAF is a substrate for P-glycoprotein. Drugs that decrease TAF through this pathway include anticonvulsants, antimycobacterials, and St. John's wort (5).

Zidovudine

Pharmacology

The oral bioavailability of zidovudine (ZDV) is 60%, with a serum half-life of 1.1 h and intracellular half-life of 7 h. ZDV can be administered without regard to meals. It is metabolized to the glucuronide form, which is excreted by the kidneys.

ZDV crosses the blood-brain barrier to achieve effective concentrations in the CNS (16) and also crosses the placenta. ZDV with 3TC is an alternative dual-NRTI backbone for combination regimens in pregnant women (7). It can be given intravenously to pregnant women during labor to prevent maternal-fetal transmission if the mother has ≥400 copies/ml of HIV or if the HIV viral load is unknown near the time of delivery. Intrapartum ZDV is no longer recommended for HIV-infected mothers who achieve virologic control on cART. ZDV can be administered orally to the child at birth either alone or in combination with nevirapine (NVP) and/or 3TC (7, 24). For adults and adolescents, ZDV can be given with 3TC as a dual-NRTI backbone with NNRTI-based and PI-based regimens. However, this is no longer considered a preferred or alternative regimen, because it requires twice-daily dosing and has greater associated toxicity than TDF-FTC or ABC-3TC (5).

Drug Interactions

ZDV inhibits the phosphorylation of d4T by thymidine kinase (24). RBV inhibits phosphorylation of ZDV (21). GCV and alpha-interferon may enhance the hematologic toxicity associated with ZDV (25, 26).

NRTI/NtRTI Combination Formulations

There are multiple fixed-dose combinations involving NRTIs and NtRTIs, which are available as commercial formulations for convenience of administration: ABC-3TC-ZDV (Trizivir), ABC-3TC (Epzicom), FTC-TDF (Truvada), 3TC-ZDV (Combivir), FTC-TDF-efavirenz (EFV) (Atripla), FTC-rilpivirine (RPV)-TDF (Complera), FTC-EVG-COBI-TDF (Stribild), FTC/RPV/TAF (Odefsey), FTC/TAF (Descovy), and EVG-COBI-FTC-TAF (Genvoya). Clinical trials have shown the triple combination ABC-3TC-ZDV to be equivalent to PI-based regimens but inferior to NNRTI-based regimens (5). Therefore, ABC-3TC-ZDV is no longer recommended for initial therapy. The dual combinations are used as NRTI-NtRTI backbones in combination with an NNRTI, PI, or INSTI in triple- or quadruple-drug therapy. The triple coformulation FTC-TAF (or TAF)-EFV is a preferred initial regimen, while FTC-RPV-TAF and FTC-RPV-TDF (or TAF) are considered alternative regimens (7).

Nonnucleoside Reverse Transcriptase Inhibitors

Drugs in the NNRTI class do not require intracellular anabolism for activation. There is no common structure; however, they bind noncompetitively to the HIV-1 RT close to the catalytic site. Disruption of DNA polymerization activity leads to premature DNA chain termination. The HIV-2 RT is resistant to this class of drugs (1).

There are currently four available NNRTIs: NVP, EFV, etravirine, and RPV. All are metabolized by the cytochrome P450 (CYP450) system, which also metabolizes the PIs (see below) and other drugs used to treat conditions associated with HIV infection. The common pathway can lead to serious interactions, which either induce or inhibit individual drug metabolism.

In the past NNRTIs were preferred for first-line therapeutic regimens with two NRTIs and/or NtRTIs for the following reasons: (i) there is a low incidence of gastrointestinal symptoms; (ii) NNRTIs have a long half-life that tolerates missed doses; and (iii) use of NNRTIs saves PIs for future regimens. The disadvantages of the NNRTIs are (i) the relatively low number of mutations required to confer cross-resistance to many of the drugs in this class and (ii) side effects related to the CNS (7). As a result, NNRTIs are now components of recommended alternative regimens, with INSTIs replacing them in the preferred initial regimens.

Efavirenz

Pharmacology

The oral bioavailability of efavirenz (EFV) is <1%. The serum half-life is 52 to 76 h. The drug should be administered without food. EFV is 99.5% protein bound in the plasma, mainly to albumin. CNS penetration is intermediate (16), but EFV has been shown to cross the placenta in animals (7). EFV is metabolized by CYP3A4 and CYP2B6 and is an inducer and inhibitor of CYP3A4. Glucuronidated metabolites are excreted in the urine (14 to 34%) and eliminated in the feces (16 to 61%). EFV-FTC-TDF (or TAF) is recommended as an alternative regimen except in pregnant women, because teratogenic effects have been observed in cynomolgus monkeys during the first trimester of pregnancy (7).

Drug Interactions

Dose modifications may be necessary for potential drug interactions between EFV and the following: indinavir (IDV), lopinavir-RTV (LPV-r), fosamprenavir (FPV), nelfinavir (NFV), saquinavir (SQV), clarithromycin, rifabutin, rifampin, simvastatin, lovastatin, methadone, itraconazole, anticonvulsants, and oral contraceptives (5). Contraindicated drugs are rifapentine, cisapride, midazolam, triazolam, ergot derivatives, St. John's wort, voriconazole, HCV PIs, and in treatment-experienced patients, atazanavir (ATV).

Etravirine

Pharmacology

The oral bioavailability of etravirine (ETR) is unknown. The serum half-life is 41 h ± 21 h. Drug levels are reduced under fasting conditions; therefore, ETR should be taken with meals. ETR is 99.9% protein bound in plasma, mainly to albumin. It is not known whether ETR penetrates the CNS or crosses the placenta. ETR is metabolized by CYP3A4, CYP2C9, and CYP2C19. It induces CYP3A4 and inhibits CYP2C9 and CYP2C19. It is also an inducer of P-glycoprotein (5). ETR is eliminated in the feces (93.7%) and excreted in the urine (1.2%) (27). It has not been studied in large trials of treatment-naive patients and therefore is not recommended for treatment in this population. ETR is reported to be active against HIV-1 strains that are resistant to other NNRTIs, including HIV-1 group O (28); therefore, it is currently used in regimens for treatment-experienced patients who have failed therapy (1, 27, 29).

Drug Interactions

Dose modifications may be required for the following: LPV-r, SQV, antiarrhythmics, dexamethasone, erectile dysfunction drugs, warfarin, lipid-lowering drugs, diazepam, and antifungal agents. ETR should not be coadministered with the following drugs: EFV, NVP, ATV, FPV, tipranavir (TPV), hormonal contraceptives, St. John's wort, clarithromycin, antimycobacterials (if coadministered with RTV-boosted PI), and phenobarbital (5, 27).

Nevirapine

Pharmacology

The oral bioavailability of nevirapine (NVP) is >90%, and the serum half-life is 25 to 30 h. NVP is 60% protein bound. Penetration into the CNS is high; the concentration in the cerebrospinal fluid is 45% of the concentration in plasma (16). NVP can be administered with or without food. It is both a substrate and an inducer of CYP3A4 and CYP2B6 (5). Glucuronidated metabolites are excreted in the urine (80%) and feces (10%). NVP is known to cross the human placenta (7). It has been used in resource-limited regions as a single oral agent in an intrapartum/newborn prophylaxis regimen to prevent mother-to-child transmission (7, 30). It is also under study as part of three-drug regimens to prevent perinatal transmission (7, 31). However, NVP has been associated with serious hepatic events and has a low barrier to resistance, and therefore, it is no longer considered a preferred or alternative agent for initial therapy. In certain circumstances NVP may be considered in women with $CD4^+$ T cell counts of ≤250 cells/mm^3 or in males with counts of ≤400 cells/mm^3 in the absence of moderate to severe hepatic impairment (Child-Pugh class B or C) (5).

Drug Interactions

NVP reduces the concentrations in plasma of IDV, SQV, oral contraceptives, fluconazole, ketoconazole, clarithromycin, and methadone (21). Coadministration of ATV, ETR, rifampin, rifapentine, St. John's wort, or HCV PIs with NVP is contraindicated (5).

Rilpivirine

Pharmacology

The oral bioavailability of rilpivirine (RPV) is unknown, and the serum half-life is 50 h. It is not known whether RPV penetrates the CNS or crosses the placenta. RPV should be administered with food. It is a CYP3A4 substrate (5). RPV in combination with TDF-FTC or ABC-3TC is an alternative regimen for treatment-naive patients. However, RPV use is not recommended in patients with a pretreatment HIV viral load of >100,000 copies/ml, because it has been associated with virologic failure in these patients. In addition, patients with $CD4^+$ T cell counts of <200 cells/mm^3 are more likely to experience virologic failure when treated with an RPV-based regimen (5). RPV is metabolized by CYP3A4 and eliminated in urine and feces.

Drug Interactions

Drugs that are contraindicated are antimycobacterials, anticonvulsants, proton pump inhibitors, HCV PIs, dexamethasone, and St. John's wort (5).

Protease Inhibitors

PIs, like the NNRTIs, require no intracellular anabolism for antiviral activity. The target is the HIV-encoded protease, which is required for posttranslational processing of the precursor gag polyprotein (32). Most PIs are peptidomimetic, because they contain the peptide bond normally cleaved by the protease (1). TPV and DRV are nonpeptidic molecules that are reported to inhibit protease dimerization as well as normal enzymatic activity (33). The relative activity of PIs against the HIV-1 versus HIV-2 protease varies among the drugs and is dependent on the amino acid sequences of the target binding sites (34).

PIs are commonly used in cART regimens in combination with NRTI and/or NtRTIs for maximum antiretroviral activity and to minimize the development of resistance. PI-based regimens introduced initially led to treatment failure related to their limited bioavailability, frequent dosing, and toxicity. There are several characteristics of these drugs that lead to these treatment-related problems. They are highly bound to plasma protein, mainly alpha-1 acid glycoprotein (AAG) (35). The low concentration of unbound drug is responsible for the therapeutic activity as well as toxicity. PIs are substrates for P-glycoprotein and multidrug resistance-associated protein. These are efflux transporters, which enhance elimination of the drugs from cells in the intestine, liver, and kidneys and reduce intracellular drug concentrations (36). All of the PIs are metabolized in the intestine and liver by enzymes of the CYP450 system (37), mainly by CYP3A4, CYP2C9, and CYP2C19. An individual PI can induce and/or inhibit specific CYP450 isoenzymes, which can enhance or reduce its own metabolism or that of other PIs. As noted above, the CYP450 system metabolizes the NNRTIs and numerous other drugs that may be used for conditions associated with HIV infection. Thus, the choice of treatment regimens is complicated by multiple potential drug-drug interactions, which may enhance toxicity and/or require dose modifications of coadministered drugs (5).

Although most PIs are inhibitors of CYP3A4, RTV is the most inhibitory. For this reason, RTV is used in boosting regimens to improve the pharmacokinetic profile of a second PI (38). Subtherapeutic concentrations of RTV increase the systemic exposure of a second PI by reducing the rate of metabolism and increasing the half-life (37), which lowers dosing requirements and food effects for the second drug. An example is LPV, which alone has very little bioavailability and a very short half-life but in combination with RTV is used therapeutically in alternative regimens for treatment-naive patients and in salvage therapy (5, 38, 39). The effect of RTV on the pharmacokinetics of other PIs varies as a result of differences in interaction with components of the CYP450 system that determine bioavailability. Specific recommendations are described below for each drug.

Atazanavir

Pharmacology

Atazanavir (ATV) is an azapeptide PI that differs structurally from other peptidomimetic PIs. The bioavailability is undetermined, and the serum half-life is 7 h. The bioavailability, however, is increased by administration with food. ATV is 86% protein bound and penetrates the CNS (40). It is metabolized in the liver by CYP3A4, and it is also an inhibitor of this enzyme. The metabolites are eliminated in the feces (79%) and urine (13%). ATV crosses the placenta at minimal levels. It is an inhibitor, inducer, and substrate for P-glycoprotein (7).

ATV has the advantage of once-daily dosing as well as a high genetic barrier to resistance. ATV boosted with RTV or COBI is a recommended alternative PI in regimens with TDF (or TAF)-FTC (5, 41).

Drug Interactions

Drugs that may require dose modifications or cautious use with ATV include antifungal agents, antiarrhythmics, clarithromycin, colchicine, oral contraceptives, anticonvulsants, rifabutin, erectile dysfunction agents, H2 receptor antagonists, antacids, and buffered medications. Drugs that are contraindicated for coadministration with ATV include IDV, NVP, ETR, EFV (in treatment-experienced patients), HCV PIs, antihistamines, bepridil, simvastatin, lovastatin, antimycobacterials, cisapride, proton pump inhibitors, neurologic agents, ergot derivatives, St. John's wort, and irinotecan (5).

Cobicistat

Pharmacology

Cobicistat (COBI) is a structural analogue of RTV, but it has no direct antiviral activity for HIV or HCV. Like RTV it serves as a pharmacoenhancer for other antiviral agents. It is a component of several fixed-dose antiretroviral regimens: ATV-COBI, DRV-COBI, EVG-COBI-FTC-TDF (or TAF) (42, 43). It is not interchangeable with RTV for boosting FPV, SQV, or TPV. COBI should be given with food. COBI is 97 to 98% protein bound. The half-life is 3 to 4 h (higher with ATZ than DRV), and it is excreted in feces and urine. COBI is a substrate and a very strong inhibitor of CYP3A4 as well as an inhibitor of CYP2D6 and P-glycoprotein.

Drug Interactions

As an analogue of an HIV PI, COBI has a similar profile of drug interactions. It should not be administered with any PIs coformulated with RTV (FPV, SQV, TPV, LPV). Other contraindicated drugs include EFV, ETV, NVP, antiarrhythmics, macrolide/ketolide antibiotics, antifungals, antimycobacterials, HCV antivirals, neurologic agents, erectile dysfunction drugs, and anticonvulsants.

Darunavir

Pharmacology

The bioavailability of darunavir (DRV) is 37% alone and 82% when boosted with RTV, and the serum half-life is 15 h when boosted. It should be administered with food. The plasma protein binding is 95%, mainly to AAG. DRV is metabolized in the liver by CYP3A4, for which it is an inhibitor, and it is an inducer of CYP2C9 and P-glycoprotein. It is eliminated in the feces (79.5%) and the urine (13.9%). DRV boosted with RTV is a preferred PI in regimens with two NRTIs or NtRTIs for treatment-naive patients and pregnant women (7).

Drug Interactions

Drugs that may require dose modifications are the antidepressants paroxetine and sertraline, erectile dysfunction drugs, antifungals, atorvastatin, and rosuvastatin. Drugs that are contraindicated are EFV, ETR, NVP, HCV PIs, neurologic agents, lovastatin, simvastatin, antimycobacterials, ergot derivatives, St. John's wort, cisapride, anticonvulsants, and fluticasone.

Fosamprenavir

Pharmacology

Fosamprenavir (FPV) is a prodrug with no antiviral activity which must be converted to amprenavir (APV) by cellular phosphatases (44). The bioavailability of APV is undetermined, and the serum half-life is 7.7 h. It can be administered with or without food. The plasma protein binding is 90%. APV is metabolized in the liver by CYP3A4, for which it is an inhibitor and inducer (45). It is eliminated in the feces (75%) and urine (14%). It is not known whether APV crosses the placenta (7). FPV boosted with RTV has high penetrance in the CNS (16). However, it is not recommended for treatment-naive patients (5).

Drug Interactions

Drugs that may require dose modifications or cautious use with FPV include erectile dysfunction drugs, antifungals,

EFV, NVP, LPV/r, SQV, RTV, rifabutin atorvastatin, and methadone. Drugs that are contraindicated for coadministration with FPV include ETR, DLV, HCV protease and NS5A inhibitors, simvastatin, lovastatin, antimycobacterials, cardiac agents, cisapride, neurologic agents, antihistamines, ergot derivatives, St. John's wort, and oral contraceptives (5, 21).

Indinavir

Pharmacology

The bioavailability of indinavir (IDV) is 65%, and the serum half-life is 1.5 to 2.0 h. IDV should be administered with low-caloric, low-fat food. It is 60% plasma protein bound, mainly to AAG (46). IDV is a substrate and an inhibitor of CYP3A4. The majority of the drug (83%) is eliminated as metabolites in the feces. There is minimal passage of IDV across the placenta (7), but RTV-boosted IDV penetrates the CNS (16, 47).

RTV-boosted or -unboosted IDV is not recommended as a component of PI-based regimens for treatment-naive patients, because of inconvenient dosing (unboosted) and the adverse complication of nephrolithiasis (RTV boosted) (5).

Drug Interactions

Coadministered drugs that may require dose modifications or cautious use include DLV, ddI, EFV, NFV, NVP, RTV, SQV, antiarrhymics, antifungal agents, anticonvulsants, calcium channel blockers, atorvastatin, methadone, colchicine, and vitamin C, especially in grapefruit juice. Drugs that are contraindicated for coadministration with IDV include ATV, TPV, amiodarone, simvastatin, lovastatin, antimycobacterials, ergot derivatives, neurologic agents, cisapride, erectile dysfunction drugs, and St. John's wort (5, 21).

Lopinavir-Ritonavir

Pharmacology

LPV is administered only in combination with low-dose RTV (LPV-r), and the combined formulation (Kaletra) is commercially available. The bioavailability of LPV-r is undetermined, and the half-life is 5 to 6 h. The oral tablet formulation can be taken with or without food; the oral solution should be taken with food of moderate fat content. The plasma protein binding is 99%, mainly to AAG. LPV-r is an inhibitor and a substrate of CYP3A4 and to a lesser extent CYP2D6. It is eliminated mainly in the feces (82.6%) and urine (10.4%) as metabolites. LPV crosses the placenta (7). LPV-r has high penetration of the CNS (16) and is a component of recommended alternative PI-based regimens with two NRTIs/NtRTIs for treatment-naive patients (5).

Drug Interactions

Drugs that may require dose modifications when coadministered with LPV-r include erectile dysfunction drugs, rosuvastatin, atorvastatin, calcium channel blockers, and methadone. Drugs that are contraindicated for coadministration include DRV, FPV, TPV, simvastatin, lovastatin, oral contraceptives, neurologic agents, anticonvulsants, antiarrhythmics, antimycobacterials, antihistamines, cisapride, cardiac agents, HCV antivirals, ergot derivatives, fluticasone, and St. John's wort (5, 21).

Nelfinavir

Pharmacology

The bioavailability of nelfinavir (NFV) is 20 to 80%, and the serum half-life is 3.5 to 5 h. NFV shows the greatest accumulation in cells of all the PIs; however, the protein binding is >98% (35). It should be administered with food. NFV is both an inhibitor and inducer of CYP3A4 (45). The majority of the drug (87%) is eliminated in the feces. There is minimal placental passage (7) and low penetration of the CNS (16). NFV is not recommended in PI-based regimens with two NRTIs and/or NtRTIs for treatment-naive patients because of lower antiretroviral efficacy (5). Boosting with RTV does not affect exposure.

Drug Interactions

Drugs that require dose modifications or cautious use include rifabutin, atorvastatin, anticonvulsants, methadone, and erectile dysfunction agents. Drugs that are contraindicated for coadministration with NFV include TPV, antiarrhythmics, simvastatin, lovastatin, antimycobacterials, cisapride, neurologic agents, antihistamines, ergot derivatives, St. John's wort, proton pump inhibitors, and oral contraceptives (5, 21).

Ritonavir

Pharmacology

The oral bioavailability of ritonavir (RTV) is undetermined, and the serum half-life is 3 to 5 h. RTV should be administered with food. It is 98% plasma protein bound and is metabolized by CYP3A. The major metabolite is isopropylthiazole, which has the same antiviral activity as the parent drug. RTV is eliminated in the feces (86.4%) and urine (11.3%) (5). Passage across the placenta is minimal (7).

The main role of RTV in current HIV therapeutics is to enhance the pharmacokinetics of a second PI (38), because RTV is a very strong inhibitor of CYP3A4. Low-dose RTV is a pharmacoenhancer of IDV, FPV, SQV, LPV, ATV, TPV, and DRV. RTV alone in PI-based regimens is not recommended because of gastrointestinal intolerance (5). RTV-boosted PIs are recommended in combination with two NRTIs and/or NtRTIs in PI-based regimens for treatment-naive and treatment-experienced patients (5, 38).

Drug Interactions

As a very strong inhibitor of CYP3A4, RTV has numerous potential drug interactions requiring close monitoring (5, 21). Coadministered drugs that may require dose modifications or cautious use include antifungals, clarithromycin, atorvastatin, pravastatin, rosuvastatin, anticonvulsants, methadone, erectile dysfunction drugs, atovaquone, quinine, antidepressants, and theophylline. Drugs that are contraindicated for coadministration with RTV include ETR, antiarrhythmics, simvastatin, lovastatin, antimycobacterials, cisapride, neurologic agents, ergot derivatives, oral contraceptives, and St. John's wort.

Saquinavir

Pharmacology

The oral bioavailability of saquinavir (SQV) is approximately 4%. The serum half-life is 1 to 2 h. SQV is both a substrate and inhibitor of CYP3A4 and P-glycoprotein. It should be administered with food. SQV is 97% bound to plasma proteins and is eliminated mainly in the feces (81%) (5). There is minimal passage of SQV across the placenta (7) and very low penetrance of the CNS (16). SQV RTV-boosted and unboosted regimens with two NRTIs and/or NtRTIs are not recommended for treatment-naive patients (5).

Drug Interactions

Coadministered drugs or foods that require dose modifications or cautious use include antifungal agents, antiarrhythmics, atorvastatin, rosuvastatin, anticonvulsants, methadone, erectile dysfunction agents, proton pump inhibitors, and grapefruit juice. Drugs that are contraindicated for coadministration with SQV include TPV, DRV, antihistamines, fluticasone, simvastatin, lovastatin, antimycobacterials, cisapride, neurologic agents, oral contraceptives, ergot derivatives, HCV antivirals, St. John's wort, garlic supplements, and dexamethasone (5, 21).

Tipranavir

Pharmacology

Tipranavir (TPV) is a nonpeptidic PI (48). The oral bioavailability is undetermined, and the half-life is 6 h. It can be administered with or without food. TPV is >99.9% protein bound in plasma to both albumin and AAG. It is metabolized mainly through CYP3A4, and it is also a CYP3A4 and CYP2C19 inducer. TPV is eliminated in the feces (82.3%) and urine (4.4%). It is not known whether TPV crosses the placenta (7), and penetration of the CNS is low (16). TPV requires coadministration with RTV to reach effective levels in plasma (37, 49). TPV is not recommended for use in PI-based regimens for treatment-naive patients. The current indicated use is in patients who are highly treatment experienced or who are infected with virus strains resistant to multiple PIs.

Drug Interactions

Coadministration of TPV with the following drugs may require dose modification: colchicine, rosuvastatin, methadone, antifungals, and anticonvulsants. Coadministration of the following drugs is contraindicated: ATV, ETR, FPV, LPN, NFV, SQV, cardiac agents, antimycobacterials, lovastatin, simvastatin, neurologic agents, ergot derivatives, cisapride, antihistamines, HCV antivirals, oral contraceptives, erectile dysfunction agents, St. John's wort, and fluticasone (5, 37, 49).

Entry Inhibitors

Antiretroviral agents that target the entry of HIV into the host cell have been developed. Enfuvirtide (T20), a fusion inhibitor, was the first of these drugs to be approved. It is a linear synthetic peptide of 36 L-amino acids that binds to the first heptad repeat in the gp41 subunit of the HIV-1 envelope glycoprotein. The sequence of the peptide was derived from that of HIV-1_{LAI}, a subtype B strain (50). The binding prevents conformational changes that are required for fusion between the virus envelope and the cell membrane (51). Entry is inhibited, thereby preventing infection of the target cell.

Maraviroc (MVC), a CCR5 antagonist, is a second drug that targets viral entry. The use of this drug is dependent on the prior determination of the viral tropism, because only virus strains utilizing the CCR5 coreceptor (R5) are susceptible. The rationale for this antiviral target is that coreceptor tropism of primary HIV-1 infection is most commonly CCR5, and the switch to CXCR4 or dual tropism occurs much later in the course of infection. Allosteric binding of MVC to the CCR5 coreceptor results in a conformational change, which inhibits HIV-1 gp120 binding and viral entry into the target cell (52).

Enfuvirtide

Pharmacology

The bioavailability of enfuvirtide (T20) by subcutaneous injection is 84% (51), and the serum half-life is 3.8 h. T20 is 92% protein bound in plasma. It is assumed that the metabolism of the drug produces the constituent amino acids, which enter the amino acid pool in the body and are recycled. It is not active against HIV-2, but there are recent data suggesting that it is active against HIV-1 non-B subtypes and possibly group O as well (53). Limited data indicate that T20 does not cross the placenta (7) and that it does not penetrate the CNS (54). T20 is not recommended for use in NNRTI- or PI-based regimens in treatment-naive patients, because of its low barrier to resistance, and it requires injection for delivery. T20 is currently used in salvage therapy regimens for treatment-experienced patients who have not responded to their current antiretroviral therapy (7, 55).

Drug Interactions

There is no evidence that T20 induces or inhibits any of the CYP450 isoenzymes; therefore, it is unlikely to interact with any of the drugs that are metabolized by the CYP450 system. No significant interactions with other antiretroviral drugs have been identified (51).

Maraviroc

Pharmacology

Maraviroc (MVC) prevents HIV-1 binding of CCR5 (R5) strains to the CCR5 coreceptor but has no activity against CXCR4 (X4) strains. The bioavailability is 33%, and the serum half-life is 14 to 18 h. It is 76% protein bound in the plasma to both albumin and AAG. It can be administered with or without food. MVC is a substrate for CYP3A4 and P-glycoprotein and is eliminated in the feces (76%) and urine (20%). It is not known whether MVC crosses the placenta (7). Although MVC may be used in combination with two NRTIs and/or NtRTIs in treatment-naive patients known to have R5-tropic virus, it is not considered a preferred or alternative agent because of its twice-daily dosing schedule and need for tropism testing (7, 56).

Drug Interactions

Coadministration of MVC with the following drugs may require dose modification: antifungals, anticonvulsants, rifabutin, EFV, EVG boosted with COBI (EVG/c), raltegravir (RAL), ETR, and all PIs except TPV. Coadministration with antimycobacterials, HCV antivirals, and St. John's wort is contraindicated.

Integrase Strand Transfer Inhibitors

INSTIs, a class of antiretroviral drugs, target the HIV-1 integrase enzyme that mediates transfer of the reverse-transcribed HIV-1 DNA into the host chromosome. The activity of this enzyme includes 3′ processing of the reverse transcribed DNA to generate hydroxyls at the 3′ ends of both strands followed by strand transfer that joins viral and host DNA. The approved integrase inhibitors are recommended with two NRTI/NtRTIs for first-line therapy regimens for treatment-naive patients (1, 7).

Raltegravir

Pharmacology

Raltegravir (RAL) is active against HIV-1 group O isolates (28) as well as HIV-1 group M and HIV-2 (57). Its bioavailability has not been established, and its serum half-life is 7 to 12 h. It is 83% protein bound in plasma. RAL crosses the placenta (7). It can be administered with or without food. It is eliminated in the feces (51%) and urine (32%).

Clearance is by UDP-glucuronosyltransferase glucuronidation. It is not metabolized by the CYP450 enzymes. RAL with FTC-TDF or TAF is now an INSTI-based recommended regimen for treatment-naive patients (5, 58, 59).

Drug Interactions

Because RAL is not an inducer, inhibitor, or substrate of CYP450 enzymes, it does not affect the pharmacokinetics of most of the drugs that interact with the other classes of antiretroviral agents (5, 57, 59). Coadministration of the following drugs may require dose modification: antacids, antimycobacterials, anticonvulsants, ETR, and TPV boosted with RTV (TPV/r).

Elvitegravir

Pharmacology

Currently, elvitegravir (EVG) is approved only in coformulation with other antivirals plus the pharmacoenhancer COBI (EVG-COBI-TDF or TAF-FTC; Stribild). It achieves therapeutic concentrations only when combined with COBI. EVG has a serum half-life of 13 h. It is 99% protein bound in plasma (60). EVG should be taken with food. Cerebrospinal fluid and placental penetration levels are unknown. The combination pill EVG-COBI-TDF-FTC is a recommended option for treatment-naive patients (5).

EVG is a CYP3A4 substrate and CYP2C9 inducer. COBI was developed for use with EVG, because COBI has no anti-HIV activity, but like RTV, it is a strong inhibitor of CYP3A4. The result is higher concentrations of EVG at lower doses (61). COBI also interacts with intestinal transport proteins to increase absorption of other anti-HIV drugs, including ATZ/c and DRV/c (42, 43, 59).

Drug Interactions

EVG is primarily metabolized by the CYP450 pathway and therefore interacts with other drugs that utilize this pathway. Because EVG is available only as a coformulated tablet, data regarding interactions of EVG alone are lacking. EVG-COBI-TDF-FTC administration should be separated from antacid administration by more than 2 hours. Coadministration of NVP, RPV, ATV boosted with COBI (ATV/c) (or with RTV [ATV/r]), DRV/c (or r), FPV/r, LPV/r, SQV/r, TPV/r, antimycobacterials, anticonvulsants, antidepressants, antifungal agents, neurologic agents, HCV antivirals, ergot derivatives, lovastatin, simvastatin, and St. John's wort is contraindicated (5).

Dolutegravir

Pharmacology

DTG is approved for use in both HIV treatment-naive and treatment-experienced patients. It has been shown to have little cross-resistance with the other INSTIs, RAL, and EVG (62). DTG has a 14-hour half-life and can therefore be administered once a day in select patients. Twice-daily dosing is recommended in patients with known or suspected INSTI resistance and when coadministered with EFV, FPV/r, TPV/r, or rifampin (63). DTG can be administered with or without food (64). It is a P-glycoprotein substrate and is eliminated in the feces (53%) and urine (31%). DTG does not inhibit CYP450 enzymes, and therefore, like RAL, it does not interact with drugs that are metabolized by these enzymes.

Drug Interactions

Coadministration with the following drugs may require dose modification: anticonvulsants, EFV, FPV/r, TPV/r, and mycobacterials. The following drugs should not be coadministered with DTG: carbamazepine, phenytoin, NVP, phenobarbital, and St. John's wort.

AGENTS AGAINST HEPATITIS C VIRUS

Increased understanding of the genome and virology of hepatitis C virus (HCV) has led to advances in the efficacy and tolerability of HCV treatment. Multiple direct-acting antivirals (DAAs) which interfere with specific steps in HCV replication have been developed. This has led to combination treatment regimens that are interferon free, pangenotypic, and administered in single daily doses. The four classes of DAAs defined according to their mechanism of action and therapeutic target are the nonstructural proteins 3/4A (NS3/4A) PIs, NS5B nucleoside polymerase inhibitors, NS5B nonnucleoside polymerase inhibitors, and NS5A inhibitors (65). DAAs are available in multiple fixed-dose combinations (summarized in Table 2). While RBV is still used in combination with DAAs, interferon-based regimens are no longer used because of their poor tolerability. Given the rapidly changing landscape of HCV treatment, please visit www.hcvguidelines.org for the most current information (66).

NS3/4A Protease Inhibitors

NS3/4A PIs inhibit a serine protease involved in posttranslational processing of HCV by blocking the NS3 catalytic site or the NS3/NS4A interaction. In addition, NS3/NS4A PIs prevent blockage of TIR domain-containing adaptor protein-inducing interferon beta (TRIF)-mediated Toll-like receptor and Cardif-mediated retinoic acid inducible gene 1 signaling, which results in induction of interferons and promotion of viral elimination (67). The first-generation PIs telaprevir and bocepravir have been replaced by more potent and better-tolerated antivirals. Grazoprevir, paritaprevir, simeprevir, voxilaprevir, and glecaprevir are PIs available in the United States.

Grazoprevir

Pharmacology

Grazoprevir is a pangenotypic PI that is only available in combination with the NS5A inhibitor elbasvir (68). Its absorption is not affected by meals and is 27% bioavailable. It has a predominantly hepatic distribution and is highly protein bound. It is metabolized hepatically, has a half-life of 31 hours, and is predominantly excreted in the feces. It can be used in patients with any degree of renal impairment, including those on dialysis, without the need for dose modifications. It is contraindicated in patients with Child-Pugh class B or C cirrhosis.

Drug Interactions

Grazoprevir is metabolized by CYP3A enzymes and should not be given with moderate and strong inducers or strong inhibitors of this system (69). It is also a substrate of OATP1B1/3 and should not be coadministered with drugs that inhibit this enzyme. Coadministration is contraindicated with rifampin, phenytoin, carbamazepine, St. John's wort, cyclosporine, and some antiretroviral agents such as PIs and EFV. Coadministration is not recommended with nafcillin, ketoconazole, etravirine, COBI, or modafinil.

Paritaprevir

Pharmacology

Paritaprevir is coadministered with low-dose RTV for a pharmacologic boosting effect, and these drugs are available as a fixed-dose combination with ombitasvir, which is an

TABLE 2 Antiviral agents for HCV therapy[a]

Antiviral agents and approved fixed combinations	Trade name (pharmaceutical company[b])	Mechanism of action/ route of administration	Major adverse effects
Ribavirin	Copegus (Genentech) Rebetol (Merck)	Mechanism not established Administered orally only in combination with another DAA	Anemia[c], myocardial infarction, teratogenic, hypersensitivity, impairment of pulmonary function, GI symptoms[d]
Sofosbuvir	Sovaldi (Gilead)	A nucleotide analogue inhibitor of HCV NS5B polymerase Inhibits viral RNA synthesis Administered orally	Fatigue, insomnia, headache, GI symptoms, bradycardia with amiodorone
Simeprevir	Olysio (Janssen)	Binds to NS34A protease active site, preventing viral replication Administered orally	Photosensitivity, rash, bradycardia with amiodorone
Sofosbuvir + ledipasvir	Harvoni (Gilead)	NS5A inhibitor (ledipasvir) and nucleotide analogue inhibitor of HCV NS5B polymerase (sofosbuvir) Administered orally	Fatigue, insomnia, headache, GI symptoms
Ombitasvir + paritaprevir + ritonavir + dasabuvir	Viekira Pak (AbbVie)	NS5A inhibitor (ombitasvir), NS3/4A protease inhibitor (paritaprevir), and NS5B RNA polymerase inhibitor (dasabuvir) Ritonavir is an HIV protease inhibitor with no anti-HCV activity	Fatigue, rash, GI symptoms, insomnia, pruritus
Ombitasvir + paritaprevir + ritonavir	Technivie (AbbVie)	Same combination of antiviral agents as above, without dasabuvir	Same as above
Grazoprevir + elbasvir	Zepatier (Merck)	NS5A inhibitor (elbasvir), NS3/4A protease inhibitor (elbasvir)	Fatigue, headache, GI symptoms
Daclatasvir	Daklinza (Bristol-Meyers Squibb)	NS5A inhibitor for use with sofosbuvir	Fatigue, headache
Velpatasvir + sofosbuvir	Epclusa (Gilead)	NS5A inhibitor (velpatasvir), NS5B inhibitor (sofosbuvir)	Fatigue, headache
Voxilaprevir + velpatasvir + voxilaprevir	Vosevi (Gilead)	Protease inhibitor (voxilaprevir), NS5A inhibitor (velpatasvir), NS5B inhibitor (sofosbuvir)	Headache, fatigue, GI symptoms
Glecaprevir + pibrentasvir	Mavyret (Gilead)	Protease inhibitor (glecaprevir), NS5A inhibitor (pibrentasvir)	Headache, fatigue

[a]Note: all DAA HCV antiviral agents carry the warning that HBV reactivation has been reported in coinfected patients being treated for HCV but not HBV and can lead to fulminant hepatitis.
[b]Pharmaceutical companies: AbbVie, North Chicago, IL; Bristol-Meyers Squibb, Princeton, NJ; Genentech, San Francisco, CA; Gilead, Foster City, CA; Janssen Pharmaceutica, Beerse, Belgium; Merck & Co., Inc., Whitehouse Station, NJ; Roche Pharmaceuticals, Nutley, NJ.
[c]Ribavirin can cause anemia via hemolysis or decreased red cell production.
[d]GI (gastrointestinal) symptoms include nausea, vomiting, and diarrhea.

NS5A inhibitor (70). Ombitasvir, paritaprevir, and RTV are typically given with the nonnucleoside NS5B inhibitor dasabuvir. Paritaprevir is well absorbed when administered with food, has a 53% bioavailability, and is very highly protein bound. Its half-life is 5.5 hours, and it is primarily excreted in the feces. Renal insufficiency is not expected to clinically affect levels of paritaprevir, and no dose adjustment is warranted by mild hepatic impairment. Its use is contraindicated in moderate to severe (Child-Pugh classes B and C) hepatic impairment.

Drug Interactions

Paritaprevir is metabolized by CYP3A4 and to a lesser extent by CYP3A5 (71). Common drugs that should not be coadministered are anticonvulsants, rifampin, St. John's wort, certain oral contraceptives, and salmeterol. Close monitoring with statins, cyclosporine, tacrolimus, and antiarrhythmics is warranted.

Simeprevir

Pharmacology

Simeprevir was the first available second-generation PI, and it has been used in combination with sofosbuvir with or without RBV for chronic genotype 1 infection (72). It has a bioavailability of 62% with food and is very highly protein bound. Its half-life is 41 hours, and it is primarily excreted in the feces. No dose adjustment is necessary with renal insufficiency, and its use is not recommended in patients with moderate or severe (Child-Pugh classes B and C) hepatic impairment.

Drug Interactions

Simeprevir undergoes oxidative metabolism by CYP3A4 and possibly CYP2C8 and CYP2C19 (72). Significant inducers or inhibitors of these enzymes will lead to alterations in simeprevir concentrations. Simeprevir in turn can affect the levels of other drugs by inhibiting OATP1B1/3.

Coadministration with RTV, HIV PIs, EFV, NVP, statins, St. John's wort, and cyclosporine among many others is not recommended. Simeprevir can be safely administered with tacrolimus or sirolimus.

Voxilaprevir

Pharmacology

Voxilaprevir is a pangenotypic inhibitor of the NS3/4A protease that has been studied in combination with sofosbuvir and velpatasvir for previously treated patients without sustained virologic response (73). It is well absorbed and highly protein bound and is primarily excreted in the feces. No dosage adjustment is required for mild or moderate renal impairment, and use is not recommended in patients with moderate or severe hepatic impairment.

Drug Interactions

Voxilaprevir is metabolized through CYP3A4. Coadministration with phenytoin, phenobarbital, oxcarbazepine, rifabutin, rifapentine, ATV, LPV, TPV, EFV, and cyclosporine is not recommended (74).

Glecaprevir

Pharmacology

Glecaprevir is a pangenotypic inhibitor of the NS3/4A protease that has been formulated in combination with the NS5A inhibitor pibrentasvir for previously treated patients without sustained virologic response (75). It is highly protein bound and is primarily excreted in feces. No dosage adjustment is required with mild, moderate, or severe renal impairment, including those on dialysis. It is not recommended in patients with moderate or severe hepatic impairment.

Drug Interactions

Glecaprevir is metabolized by CYP3A. Coadministration with digoxin, carbamazepine, rifampin, ethinyl estradiol-containing medications such as combined oral contraceptives, St. John's wort, ATV, DRV, LPV, RTV, HMG-CoA reductase inhibitors, and cyclosporine is not recommended (75).

NS5A Inhibitors

The NS5A protein plays a role in hepatitis C viral replication and assembly (76, 77). However, the precise molecular mechanisms by which it accomplishes these functions remain poorly characterized. While NS5A inhibitors are effective across all genotypes, they have a low barrier to resistance and variable toxicity profiles. They have been shown to have very high SVR rates among patients with genotype 1 infection when given in combination with other direct-acting antivirals with or without RBV (78, 79). Available NS5A inhibitors are ledipasvir, ombitasvir, elbasvir, velpatasvir, and pibrentasvir, each available in fixed-dose combinations with other direct-acting antivirals, and daclatasvir.

Ledipasvir

Pharmacology

Ledipasvir is coformulated with sofosbuvir and is administered with or without RBV depending on the patient population (78). It is well absorbed and is highly protein bound. Its half-life is 47 h, and it is primarily excreted in the feces. While ledipasvir needs no dose adjustment for severe renal insufficiency, its coformulated drug sofosbuvir accumulates with severe renal impairment. No dose adjustment is needed for mild or moderate renal insufficiency or in the setting of moderate or severe (Child Pugh class B or C) hepatic impairment.

Drug Interactions

Ledipasvir undergoes slow oxidative metabolism via an unknown mechanism and is a substrate of the P-glycoprotein drug transporter (78). Coadministration is not recommended with rifampin, St. John's wort, carbamazepine, phenytoin, phenobarbital, or TPV. Increased gastric pH levels may decrease its absorption. Acid-suppressing agents can be coadministered if needed, but low doses should be used.

Ombitasvir

Pharmacology

Ombitasvir is only available as a fixed-dose coformulation with the PIs paritaprevir and RTV, which is typically given with the NS5B inhibitor dasabuvir (70). These drugs are administered with or without RBV depending on the patient population, for the treatment of chronic genotype 1 infection (80). Ombitasvir-paritaprevir-RTV coadministered with RBV but without dasabuvir is used for genotype 4 infections (81). Ombitasvir is well absorbed when administered with food and has a bioavailability of 48%. Its half-life is 21 to 25 h, and it is primarily excreted in the feces. Renal impairment is not expected to significantly alter its levels, but it has not been studied in patients with severe renal insufficiency. Its use is contraindicated for patients with moderate to severe (Child Pugh classes B and C) hepatic impairment.

Drug Interactions

Ombitasvir is metabolized by amide hydrolysis and oxidative metabolism (70). Because it is coformulated with paritaprevir and RTV, which are metabolized by CYP3A4 and CYP3A5, the fixed-dose combination has considerable drug interactions and should not be administered with anticonvulsants, rifampin, St. John's wort, certain oral contraceptives, or salmeterol.

Elbasvir

Pharmacology

Elbasvir is only available as a fixed-dose combination with the PI grazoprevir (69). It is administered with or without RBV depending on certain patient characteristics (82). Prior to administration of this drug, patients with genotype 1a infection should be tested for the presence of NS5A resistance-associated substitutions. Elbasvir has a bioavailability of 32% and is highly protein bound. Its half-life is 24 h, and it is primarily excreted in the feces. It can be used in patients with any degree of renal impairment without the need for dose modifications. It is contraindicated in patients with Child-Pugh class B or C cirrhosis.

Drug Interactions

Elbasvir undergoes partial oxidative metabolism via CYP3A, just like its coformulated drug grazoprevir (69). Coadministration is contraindicated with rifampin, phenytoin, carbamazepine, St. John's wort, cyclosporine, and some antiretroviral agents such as PIs and EFV. Coadministration is not recommended with nafcillin, ketoconazole, etravirine, COBI, or modafinil.

Velpatasvir

Pharmacology

Velpatasvir is a pangenotypic NS5A inhibitor that is only available as a fixed-dose combination with the

NS5B inhibitor sofosbuvir (83). It is highly protein bound and has a half-life of 15 h. It is primarily excreted in the feces. No dose adjustment is necessary for mild or moderate renal insufficiency or Child Pugh class B or C hepatic impairment. Preliminary studies suggest that severe renal impairment does not affect levels of velpatasvir. However, its coformulated drug sofosbuvir accumulates with renal impairment.

Drug Interactions

Velpatasvir is a substrate of the P-glycoprotein drug transporter and should not be coadministered with rifampin, rifabutin, rifapentine, St. John's wort, carbamazepine, phenytoin, phenobarbital, oxcarbazepine, or TPV (83). Increased gastric pH levels may decrease its absorption. If acid-suppressing agents need to be used, only low doses of proton pump inhibitors should be given, and velpatasvir should be administered without food.

Pibrentasvir

Pharmacology

Pibrentasvir is an NS5A inhibitor that is formulated in combination with glecaprevir for previously treated patients without sustained virologic response (75). It is highly protein bound and is primarily excreted in the feces. No dosage adjustment is required with mild, moderate, or severe renal impairment, including those on dialysis. It is not recommended in patients with moderate or severe hepatic impairment.

Drug Interactions

Pibrentasvir is not extensively metabolized and is excreted unchanged in the feces (75). Since it is coformulated with glecaprevir, which is metabolized by CYP3A, coadministration with digoxin, carbamazepine, rifampin, ethinyl estradiol-containing medications such as combined oral contraceptives, St. John's wort, ATV, DRV, LPV, RTV, HMG-CoA reductase inhibitors, and cyclosporine is not recommended.

Daclatasvir

Pharmacology

Daclatasvir is typically used in combination with sofosbuvir (79). It is 67% bioavailable and is highly protein bound. Its half-life is 12 to 15 h, and it is primarily excreted in the feces. No dosage adjustments are required for renal or hepatic impairment.

Drug Interactions

Daclatasvir is primarily metabolized by CYP3A4 and should not be given with strong inducers or inhibitors of this enzyme (84). Coadministration is not recommended with rifampin, phenytoin, carbamazepine, or St. John's wort. Daclatasvir is also an inhibitor of P-glycoprotein transporter and organic anion transporting polypeptide 1B1 and 1B3. Dose adjustments of digoxin may be warranted when it is coadministered with daclatasvir.

NS5B RNA-Dependent RNA Polymerase Inhibitors

NS5B is an RNA-dependent RNA polymerase that is also involved in posttranslational processing. Its structure is highly conserved across all hepatitis C virus genotypes, giving NS5B inhibitors activity against all six genotypes (67). There are two kinds of polymerase inhibitors: nucleoside/nucleotide analogues such as sofosbuvir and nonnucleoside analogues such as dasabuvir. Nucleoside/nucleotide analogues are activated within the hepatocyte through phosphorylation which competes with nucleotides, resulting in chain termination during RNA replication. As a class, nucleoside polymerase inhibitors have moderate to high efficacy against all six genotypes and a very high barrier to resistance. In contrast, nonnucleoside polymerase inhibitors are less potent and more genotype specific, with all drugs from this class having been optimized for genotype 1.

Sofosbuvir

Pharmacology

Sofosbuvir is the first NS5B nucleoside polymerase inhibitor to have been developed, and it is used in various combinations with other direct-acting antivirals against hepatitis C (85, 86). It can be taken without regard to food and has a half-life of 0.4 h. It is primarily excreted in the urine. No dose adjustment is necessary for patients with a glomerular filtration rate greater than 30 ml/minute. Sofosbuvir exposure is increased in patients with severe renal impairment, including patients on dialysis. It can be used without regard to hepatic impairment.

Drug Interactions

Sofosbuvir is a substrate of the P-glycoprotein drug transporter, so inducers of these enzymes may decrease sofosbuvir levels (85). Coadministration is not recommended with rifampin, rifabutin, rifapentine, St. John's wort, carbamazepine, phenytoin, phenobarbital, oxcarbazepine, or TPV. Coadministering sofosbuvir and amiodarone is also not recommended, because of reports of symptomatic bradycardia and fatal cardiac arrest.

Dasabuvir

Pharmacology

Dasabuvir is packaged with ombitasvir-paritaprevir-RTV (70, 71). It is 70% bioavailable and very highly protein bound. Its half-life is 6 hours, and it is excreted primarily in the feces. Because of its lower potency and higher threshold for resistance, it is used as an adjunct to more potent direct-acting antivirals.

Drug Interactions

Dasabuvir is metabolized by CYP2C8 and CYP3A. It should not be coadministered with anticonvulsants, rifampin, St. John's wort, ethinyl estradiol-containing products, or salmeterol.

Ribavirin

Pharmacology

The bioavailability of ribavirin (RBV) is reported to be 52% (87) and is increased by a high-fat meal; therefore, RBV should be administered with food. The half-life in plasma is 120 to 170 h, and the drug may persist in other body compartments for up to 6 months. The pathway for elimination has not been determined. RBV appears not to be a substrate for the CYP450 isoenzymes. It is used as a standard therapy, always in combination with other antiviral agents, for the treatment of HCV. RBV monotherapy is not effective against HCV infection.

RBV has been used as a monotherapy to treat other RNA viruses, including respiratory syncytial virus, Lassa fever virus, influenza virus, parainfluenza virus, and hantavirus; however, there are no conclusive data demonstrating RBV treatment efficacy (88–95). An aerosolized formulation of RBV (Virazole; Valeant Pharmaceuticals, Costa

Mesa, CA) has been approved for the treatment of hospitalized infants and young children with severe respiratory syncytial virus lower respiratory tract infections.

Drug Interactions

Coadministration of ddI or d4T with RBV is contraindicated. ZDV plus RBV is linked to higher rates of anemia (5, 96).

AGENTS AGAINST HEPATITIS B VIRUS

Because a large percentage of patients are coinfected with HIV, agents with activity against HBV are categorized according to whether they have activity against both viruses or only HBV. Of the drugs that are specifically approved for HBV, only telbivudine (LdT) is active against HBV, while 3TC, TDF, TAF, adefovir (ADV), and entecavir (ETV) are active against both HBV and HIV (Table 3). Though neither ADV nor ETV is currently recommended for the treatment of HIV, use of these agents should be avoided in HIV/HBV-coinfected patients who are not on a suppressive antiretroviral regimen in order to prevent the development of HIV resistance. FTC is approved only for HIV, but it has been shown to have activity against HBV (97, 98). The common target for antiviral drugs active against both viruses is the RT function of the HIV and HBV replication enzymes (99–101).

Chronic HBV infection plays an important role in the morbidity and mortality of HIV-infected patients (102). The strategy for selecting antiviral therapy regimens for coinfected patients is based on the need to treat one or both viruses. If only HIV requires treatment, drugs with activity against both HIV and HBV, such as 3TC or TDF, should be withheld. If only HBV needs to be treated, drugs without HIV activity, such as LdT, can be used. However, it is recommended that all patients with HIV and HBV coinfection be started on cART regardless of CD4 count, because this may slow the progression of liver disease (98). cART regimens with dual NRTIs and/or NtRTIs, such as TDF with 3TC or FTC, that suppress replication of both viruses are preferred (98, 102). 3TC monotherapy rapidly selects for HBV resistance (103); therefore, combination therapy with one NRTI (3TC or FTC) and one NtRTI (TDF or ADV) is required. Of note, there are eight HBV genotypes (A to H), each with certain geographic predilections (104). There is evidence that the genotype impacts interferon responsiveness. In particular, in the treatment of hepatitis B e antigen-positive chronic hepatitis B, greater rates of hepatitis B e antigen seroconversion have been observed for genotype A than for genotype D and for genotype B than for genotype C (105). A correlation between genotype and treatment response to other anti-HBV therapies has not been established.

Nucleoside/Nucleotide Analogues

Adefovir Dipivoxil

Pharmacology

Adefovir (ADV)-dipivoxil is a diester prodrug that is converted to the active drug ADV. ADV-dipivoxil is administered without regard to food, and the bioavailability is 59%. The half-life of ADV is 7.5 h, and it is excreted by the kidneys. There are no data for placental passage of the drug.

ADV was originally developed as an antiretroviral drug; however, the high dose required for HIV therapy is associated with nephrotoxicity (101). A much lower dosage is effective against HBV (99, 102). ADV is effective for treatment of chronic HBV infection. The rate of viral load decline is slower, but development of drug resistance is delayed compared to that seen with other NRTIs and NtRTIs (106) that are active against HBV. The primary

TABLE 3 Antiviral agents for HBV therapy[a]

Antiviral agent (abbreviation)	Trade name (pharmaceutical company[b])	Mechanism of action/route of administration	Major adverse effects
Adefovir dipovoxil (ADV)	Hepsera (Gilead)	Prodrug converted to the nucleotide monophosphate analogue of adenosine Inhibitor of HBV RT DNA polymerase, viral DNA chain terminator Administered orally	Headache, asthenia, GI symptoms, nephrotoxicity
Entecavir (ETV)	Baraclude (BMS)	Guanosine analogue inhibitor of HBV RT DNA polymerase functions: priming, reverse transcription, positive-strand DNA synthesis Administered orally	Headache, fatigue, dizziness
Lamivudine (3TC)	See HIV antivirals, Table 1	Cytidine analogue inhibitor of HBV RT DNA polymerase	Minimal toxicity (see HIV antivirals)
Telbivudine (LdT)	Tyzeka (Novartis)	Thymidine analogue inhibitor of HBV RT DNA polymerase	Fatigue, increased creatine kinase, headache, myopathy, cough, GI symptoms
Tenofovir (TDF/TAF)	See HIV antivirals, Table 1	Inhibitor of HBV DNA polymerase	Asthenia, headache, GI symptoms (see HIV antivirals)

[a]Note: Except for interferon, all HBV antiviral agents are N(t)RTIs, some of which have anti-HIV activity (see Table 1), and all carry the warning of lactic acidosis and severe hepatomegaly with steatosis. All agents also carry a warning of severe acute exacerbations (flares) of HBV in patients who have discontinued anti-HBV therapy.

[b]Pharmaceutical companies: BMS, Bristol-Meyers Squibb, Princeton, NJ; Gilead Sciences, Foster City, CA; Novartis Pharmaceuticals Corporation, East Hanover, NJ.

role of ADV is in the treatment of 3TC-resistant HBV infection (107). However, TDF and entecavir have largely replaced ADV for this indication.

Drug Interactions

ADV is not a substrate, inhibitor, or inducer of any of the CYP450 isoenzymes. There is no interaction with 3TC, ETV, or TDF. It is possible that drugs that reduce renal function or compete for active tubular secretion could increase the concentration of ADV and/or the coadministered drug in serum.

Emtricitabine

Pharmacology

See the discussion on HIV antiviral agents above and Table 1. Emtricitabine (FTC) is approved for antiviral therapy in HIV-infected patients. It has activity against HBV but is not licensed for HBV antiviral therapy. FTC and 3TC are biochemically similar and appear to be interchangeable for potential use in treatment of HIV-HBV-coinfected patients. However, they also share the same HBV resistance mutations; therefore, combined therapy with these two drugs is not recommended (101, 102). In addition, as with 3TC, severe acute exacerbations of HBV can occur once therapy is discontinued (98).

Drug Interactions

See the discussion on HIV antiviral agents above.

Entecavir

Pharmacology

The bioavailability of entecavir (ETV) is approximately 100%, and the half-life is 24 h. ETV should be administered without food. It is excreted by the kidney (62 to 73%) mainly as unmetabolized drug. ETV maintains activity against 3TC-resistant HBV, but a higher dose is recommended for patients with 3TC-resistant HBV infection (102). ETV has shown low activity against HIV; however, there is evidence that resistance mutations are selected. For this reason, it is recommended that ETV be used in HIV-coinfected patients only if they are receiving effective antiretroviral therapy (99, 102, 108).

Drug Interactions

ETV is not a substrate, inhibitor, or inducer of any of the CYP450 isoenzymes. There is no interaction with 3TC, ADV, or TDF. It is possible that drugs that reduce renal function or compete for active tubular secretion could increase the concentration of ETV and/or the coadministered drug in serum.

Lamivudine

Pharmacology

See the discussion on HIV antiviral agents above as well as Table 1. Lamivudine (3TC) was the first nucleoside analogue that was approved for chronic HBV infection. Because it has activity against both HIV and HBV, it has been effective in reducing loads of both viruses in plasma as part of cART regimens. However, HBV-specific drug resistance mutations are selected over long-term therapy at a higher rate (20% per year) in coinfected patients than in those that are HIV negative (90). Selection of HBV drug resistance mutations eventually decreases efficacy for treatment of chronic hepatitis. Discontinuation of 3TC in HBV-infected patients can produce severe flare-ups of hepatitis, which are usually self-limited but have been fatal in a few cases. Another common problem is the rebound viremia that occurs when therapy is terminated (98). This is thought to be derived from the viral covalently closed circular DNA (cccDNA), which is not affected by nucleoside or nucleotide therapy and remains in the infected hepatocytes (101). For coinfected patients, recent recommendations suggest using combination dual NTRI-NtRTI therapy that includes TDF to reduce the rate of selection of HBV 3TC-resistant strains (109).

Drug Interactions

See the discussion on HIV antiviral agents above.

Telbivudine

Pharmacology

The bioavailability of telbivudine (LdT) is 68%, and it can be administered with or without food. The half-life is 40 to 50 h, and the drug is excreted mainly by the kidneys. LdT has a relatively low genetic barrier to resistance; therefore, it is not recommended as a first-line drug for treatment of chronic HBV (110). Hepatitis exacerbations have been reported upon discontinuation of LdT.

Drug Interactions

LdT does not alter the pharmacokinetics of other nucleoside or nucleotide analogues used in the treatment of HBV (e.g., 3TC, ADV, or TDF). Coadministration with PEG-IFN 2a may be associated with increased risk of peripheral neuropathy (99).

Tenofovir Disoproxil Fumarate and Tenofovir Alafenamide

Pharmacology

See the discussion on HIV antiviral agents above as well as Table 1. Tenofovir disoproxil fumarate (TDF) is approved for treatment of both HBV- and HIV-infected patients. It does not show cross-resistance with HBV 3TC-resistant mutants, and it appears to have a lower potential for selection of resistance mutations. For this reason, TDF and FTC or TDF and 3TC are recommended as dual-nucleoside backbones in therapeutic regimens to reduce the possibility of selection of HBV drug-resistant strains in coinfected patients who are on antiretroviral therapy (98, 99, 102, 109). TAF is another prodrug of tenofovir, which appears to be effective as TDF in treating hepatitis B but at a much lower dose (111).

Drug Interactions

See the discussion on HIV antiviral drugs above.

AGENTS AGAINST HERPESVIRUSES

Most of the antiviral compounds that are approved to treat the eight human herpesviruses are nucleoside or nucleotide analogues, which inhibit DNA replication. Several of these compounds require phosphorylation by a virus-encoded enzyme as well as cellular kinases for activation. The ultimate target of most of these drugs is the viral DNA polymerase, although other enzymatic steps in DNA synthesis also may be inhibited (1). In addition to the nucleoside and nucleotide analogues, the antiherpesvirus compounds include a pyrophosphate analogue (foscarnet [FOS]) that targets the viral DNA polymerase directly and an entry inhibitor (docosanol). The structure, mode of action, route of administration, and adverse effects of each drug are summarized in Table 4.

TABLE 4 Antiviral agents for herpesviruses

Antiviral agent (abbreviation)	Trade name (pharmaceutical company[a])	Mechanism of action/route of administration	Major adverse effects	Antiviral activity
Acyclovir (ACV)	Zovirax (GSK)	Converted to guanosine monophosphate by viral kinase Converted to triphosphate by cellular kinases DNA chain terminator Oral or intravenous formulations	Minimal toxicity GI symptoms,[b] headache, nephrotoxicity Precipitation in renal tubules if maximum solubility exceeded	HSV-1, HSV-2, VZV
Valacyclovir (Val-ACV)	Valtrex (GSK)	L-Valyl ester prodrug of ACV with increased bioavailability Activity same as ACV	GI symptoms, headache, dizziness, abdominal pain, nephrotoxicity, thrombotic thrombocytopenia, hemolytic uremic syndrome (high dosage)	HSV-1, HSV-2, VZV, HCMV[c]
Cidofovir (CDV)	Vistide (Gilead)	Cytidine nucleotide analogue Converted to di- and triphosphate by cellular kinases DNA chain terminator (2 successive molecules required); intravenous administration with probenecid	CDV: renal toxicity, decreased intraocular pressure, neutropenia, fever Probenecid: headache, GI symptoms, rash	HCMV,[d] HSV-1, HSV-2, VZV
Foscarnet (FOS)	Foscavir (AstraZeneca)	Pyrophosphate analogue Noncompetitive inhibitor of DNA polymerase pyrophosphate binding site Intravenous formulation only	Renal impairment, fever, nausea, anemia, diarrhea, vomiting, headache, seizures, altered serum electrolytes	HCMV, HSV-1, HSV-2, EBV
Ganciclovir (GCV)	Cytovene (Roche)	Guanosine analogue Converted to monophosphate by HCMV UL97 kinase or HSV or VZV TK DNA chain terminator Oral and intravenous formulations	Fever, neutropenia, anemia, thrombocytopenia, impaired renal function, diarrhea	HCMV,[e] HSV-1, HSV-2
Valganciclovir (Val-GCV)	Valcyte (Roche)	Oral prodrug of GCV with increased bioavailability Activity same as GCV	Diarrhea, neutropenia, nausea, headache, and anemia	HCMV[e]
Letermovir	Prevymis (Merck)	Inhibitor of HCMV terminase complex	Nausea, diarrhea, vomiting, peripheral edema, cough, headache, fatigue, abdominal pain	HCMV
Penciclovir (PCV)	Denavir (Novartis)	Guanosine analogue Mode of action similar to ACV Limited DNA chain elongation Topical formulation only	Headache and application site reaction no different from placebo	HSV-1[f]
Famciclovir	Famvir (Novartis)	Oral prodrug of PCV Mode of action same as PCV	Headache, GI symptoms, anorexia	HSV-1, HSV-2, VZV
Trifluridine	Viroptic (Monarch)	Mode of action not established, may inhibit viral DNA synthesis Ophthalmic aqueous solution for topical use	Burning on instillation and palpebral edema, punctate keratopathy, hypersensitivity reaction, stromal edema, keratitis sicca, hyperemia, increased ocular pressure	HSV-1[g]
Docosanol	Abreva (GSK)	Prevents HSV entry into cells by inhibition of fusion between HSV envelope and cell membrane Nonprescription topical cream formulation	Headache and skin rash	Oral HSV

[a]Pharmaceutical companies: AstraZeneca, Wilmington, DE; BMS, Gilead Sciences, Foster City, CA; GSK, GlaxoSmithKline, Research Triangle Park, NC; Monarch Pharmaceutical, Bristol, TN; Novartis, East Hanover, NJ; Roche Pharmaceuticals, Nutley, NJ.

[b]GI (gastrointestinal) symptoms include nausea, vomiting, and diarrhea.

[c]Valacyclovir is used in some transplant settings for HCMV prophylaxis.

[d]Cidofovir also has reported activity against human papillomavirus, polyomavirus, adenovirus, and poxvirus.

[e]Ganciclovir and valganciclovir also have *in vitro* activity against EBV, HHV-6, HHV-7, and HHV-8.

[f]Penciclovir is used to treat herpes labialis but also has activity against HSV2 and VZV.

[g]Trifluridine is used to treat herpes keratitis but also has activity against HSV2 and VZV.

Acyclovir and Valacyclovir

Pharmacology

The pharmacokinetics of acyclovir (ACV) after oral administration has been evaluated in healthy volunteers and in immunocompromised patients with herpes simplex virus (HSV) and varicella-zoster virus (VZV) infection. The plasma protein binding for valganciclovir (val-ACV) is 13.5 to 17.9% and for ACV is 22 to 33%. The bioavailability of ACV administered as val-ACV is 54%, while the bioavailability resulting from oral ACV is 12 to 20%. The ACV half-life is 2.5 to 3.3 h in patients with normal renal function but increases to 14 h in patients with end-stage renal disease (112). ACV may be administered with or without food. Valacyclovir (val-ACV), the L-valyl ester prodrug, is rapidly converted to ACV after oral administration (112). ACV is phosphorylated by the viral thymidine kinases of HSV-1, HSV-2, and VZV and by the UL97 kinase of human cytomegalovirus (HCMV) (113).

ACV is excreted by the kidney with inactive metabolites 9-[(carboxymethoxy) methyl] guanine and 8-hydroxy-9-[2-(hydroxyethoxy)methyl] guanine. A dosage adjustment is recommended for patients with reduced renal function (112).

Spectrum of Activity

ACV and val-ACV are active against HSV-1, HSV-2, VZV, and Epstein-Barr virus (EBV) (4). Of note, ACV and val-ACV are active only against replicating virus. Therefore, their role in the treatment of EBV-associated disease processes, which are primarily driven by latent virus, is limited (114). In addition, both drugs have some activity against HCMV. Although ACV and val-ACV are not recommended for HCMV treatment, they have been used prophylactically to prevent HCMV disease in some patients following transplantation (115, 116).

Drug Interactions

There are no clinically significant drug-drug interactions in patients with normal renal function.

Cidofovir

Pharmacology

Cidofovir (CDV) is a nucleotide analogue of deoxycytidine monophosphate, which does not require a virus-encoded enzyme for activation. After phosphorylation by cellular kinases, CDV diphosphate becomes the active nucleotide triphosphate, which inhibits the HCMV DNA polymerase. In HCMV, two successive CDV molecules must be incorporated for complete chain termination (117).

CDV must be administered with probenecid (118, 119). Approximately 90% of the CDV dose administered is recovered unchanged in the urine within 24 hours. The half-life is 2.4 to 3.2 h. When CDV is administered with probenecid, the renal clearance of CDV is reduced to a level consistent with creatinine clearance, suggesting that probenecid blocks active renal tubular secretion of CDV (118). *In vitro*, CDV is less than 6% bound to plasma or serum proteins.

Spectrum of Activity

CDV is active against several herpesviruses, including HCMV, HSV, and VZV (4). CDV also has antiviral activity against poxviruses (120), adenovirus (121), polyomaviruses (122), and human papillomavirus (123, 124).

Drug Interactions

No clinically significant interactions have been identified for CDV. However, the required administration of probenecid with CDV may produce drug-drug interactions resulting from the potential block of acidic drug transport in the kidney (118).

Foscarnet

Pharmacology

Pharmacokinetic data indicate that foscarnet (FOS) undergoes negligible metabolism, appears to be distributed widely by the circulation, and is eliminated via the renal route. The available data, however, indicate that the pharmacokinetics of the drug varies among patients and within the individual patient, particularly with regard to plasma FOS levels (125). The FOS terminal half-life determined by urinary excretion is 87.5 ± 41.8 h, possibly due to release of FOS from bone (126). Approximately 90% of FOS is excreted as unchanged drug in urine. Systemic clearance of FOS decreases and half-life increases with diminishing renal function, which may require FOS dosage modification (127).

Spectrum of Activity

Although FOS is active against several herpesviruses, including HSV, HCMV, VZV, and EBV, it is most commonly used to treat drug-resistant HSV and HCMV.

Drug Interactions

Because FOS is reported to decrease calcium concentrations in serum, caution is advised for patients receiving agents known to affect calcium levels in serum such as intravenous pentamidine. Renal impairment is a major adverse effect of FOS; therefore, the use of FOS in combination with other potentially nephrotoxic drugs such as aminoglycosides and amphotericin B (128) should be avoided.

Ganciclovir and Valganciclovir

Pharmacology

Ganciclovir (GCV) is an acyclic nucleoside analogue of 2′-deoxyguanosine, which requires phosphorylation by a viral kinase to become active. GCV monophosphate is subsequently phosphorylated to the di- and triphosphate forms by cellular kinases (1, 4).

val-GCV, the L-valyl ester prodrug of GCV, is rapidly converted to GCV after oral administration (129). Val-GCV should be administered with food. The bioavailability of val-GCV is 60.9% compared to 5.6% for the oral formulation of GCV. The half-life of GCV is 4 h in healthy volunteers and 6.5 h in transplant recipients (130, 131). GCV is only 1 to 2% protein bound. Renal excretion of unchanged drug by glomerular filtration and active tubular secretion is the major route of elimination (91%).

Spectrum of Activity

GCV is active against HCMV as well as HSV-1, HSV-2, VZV, EBV, HHV-6, HHV-7, and HHV-8 (132–135).

Drug Interactions

Coadministration of GCV with ddI results in significantly increased levels of ddI (133). Coadministration of GCV with ZDV requires dose modifications of both drugs because of their common adverse hematological effects of neutropenia and anemia. Dosage modifications may also be required with drugs that inhibit renal tubular secretion, such as probenecid. Imipenem-cilastatin should not be administered with GCV (133).

Letermovir

Pharmacology

Letermovir prevents HCMV replication by inhibiting the terminase complex (pUL51, pUL56, pUL89), resulting in an inability to cleave concatemeric genomic viral DNA and package genomes into preformed virus capsids. It is orally bioavailable and has a half-life of 12 hours. It is primarily excreted in the feces. In a phase 3, double-blind trial of HCMV-seropositive hematopoietic stem cell transplant recipients, the efficacy of letermovir in preventing active HCMV infection was compared to placebo through week 24 after transplant (152). The trial found that 37.5% of patients on letermovir developed active CMV infection versus 60.6% of patients on placebo. Most cases of active HCMV infection were asymptomatic DNAemia. HCMV disease was rare. Adverse events were similar in the two groups, and myelotoxic and nephrotoxic events were similar. The results of this study led to FDA approval for letermovir in 2017.

Spectrum of Activity

Letermovir is active only against HCMV and does not have activity against other herpesviruses, including HSV and VZV.

Drug Interactions

Letermovir is highly protein bound and metabolized in the liver. It is a P-glycoprotein and CYP3A4 inhibitor and can increase serum concentrations of amlodipine, atorvastatin, cilostazol, cyclosporine, and ibrutinib, among others.

Penciclovir and Famciclovir

Pharmacology

Famciclovir is the oral prodrug diacetyl 6-deoxy analogue of penciclovir (PCV) (136), which undergoes rapid conversion to the active compound, PCV. Famciclovir was developed to improve the bioavailability of the parent compound (137). PCV is available only as a 1% cream for the topical treatment of herpes labialis (138). The bioavailability of PCV is 77%, and the half-life is 2 h. It can be given with or without food. PCV is <20% protein bound and is eliminated in the urine (73%) and feces (27%) (139). Although PCV is structurally related to ACV, it has a higher affinity for the HSV thymidine kinases than ACV. However, ACV triphosphate has a higher affinity for the HSV DNA polymerase than does PCV triphosphate. As a result, the two compounds have similar anti-HSV potencies (140).

Spectrum of Activity

PCV and famciclovir are active against HSV-1, HSV-2, and VZV (141). Neither of these compounds is active against other human herpesviruses.

Drug Interactions

No clinically significant drug interactions have been identified for PCV.

Trifluridine

Pharmacology

Trifluridine is a fluorinated pyrimidine nucleoside approved for the topical treatment of epithelial keratitis caused by HSV (142). It has activity against HSV-1, HSV-2, and vaccinia virus (143). Intraocular penetration of trifluridine occurs after topical instillation into the eye. Decreased corneal integrity or stromal or uveal inflammation may enhance the penetration of trifluridine into the aqueous humor. Systemic absorption following therapeutic dosing with trifluridine appears to be negligible (144).

Drug Interactions

There are no reported drug interactions by the topical route of administration.

n-Docosanol

Pharmacology

n-Docosanol exhibits *in vitro* antiviral activity against several lipid-enveloped viruses including HSV-1, HSV-2, and respiratory syncytial virus (145). A topical preparation of *n*-docosanol is available without prescription as a 10% cream for the treatment of herpes labialis.

Drug Interactions

There are no reported drug interactions with topical administration.

Other Drugs against Herpesviruses

There are several antiviral agents that are undergoing clinical trials or that are approved for conditions other than antiviral therapy. Maribavir is an antiviral agent in the benzimidazole drug class (146). Maribavir is not phosphorylated by the UL97 kinase but inhibits UL97 kinase activity directly. It has been found to be effective *in vitro* against GCV-resistant strains of HCMV, with taste disturbances as the only adverse side effect (147). Unfortunately, phase 3 clinical trials in stem cell and liver transplant recipients found maribavir to be inadequate for prevention of CMV disease (148, 149). However, new clinical trials have been launched to address speculation that the lack of demonstrable efficacy may be due to inadequate dosing (https://clinicaltrials.gov; NCT02927067 and NCT02931539).

Brincidofovir is an orally administered lipid conjugate of CDV (150). It has *in vitro* activity against all of the herpesviruses, including GCV-resistant CMV and ACV-resistant HSV, as well as polyomaviruses, poxviruses, and adenovirus (151). However, severe diarrhea and increased mortality led to the failure of a phase III trial (https://clinicaltrials.gov; NCT01769170). New formulations may lead to future trials to pursue the treatment of targeted patients.

Two helicase/primase inhibitors, pritelivir and amenamevir, have shown efficacy in phase II studies (153, 154). Pritelivir and amenamevir show *in vitro* activity against HSV-1 and HSV-2, while amenamevir also shows activity against VZV.

Two additional drugs that are approved for other medical conditions have been reported to have antiviral activity against HCMV, although no clinical trials have been conducted. These are leflunomide, which is approved for treatment of rheumatoid arthritis (155, 156), and artesunate, which is an antimalarial agent (157, 158).

AGENTS AGAINST INFLUENZA VIRUSES

The two classes of antiviral agents for the treatment of influenza are M2 protein inhibitors and neuraminidase inhibitors (159–161). The structure, mode of action, route of administration, and adverse effects of each drug are summarized in Table 5. Recommendations for the use of these antivirals for influenza prevention and therapy are available from the Centers for Disease Control and Prevention website (http://www.cdc.gov/flu).

TABLE 5 Antiviral agents for influenza virus

Antiviral agent	Trade name (pharmaceutical company[a])	Mechanism of action/ route of administration	Major adverse effects
Amantadine/ rimantadine	Symmetrel/Flumadine (Endo/Forrest)	Prevents release of nucleic acid by interfering with viral M2 protein Administered orally	CNS symptoms,[b] GI symptoms[c]
Oseltamivir	Tamiflu (Genentech) (Gilead [licensor])	Sialic acid analogue Competitive inhibitor of neuraminidase affecting release of influenza virus particles from host cells Administered orally	GI symptoms[c] (usually mild), transient neuropsychiatric symptoms[d]
Peramivir	Rapivab (Biocryst)	Same as oseltamivir Administered intravenously	GI symptoms[c], leukopenia/ neutropenia
Zanamivir	Relenza (GSK)	Same as oseltamivir Administered by oral inhalation	Respiratory function deterioration after inhalation

[a]Pharmaceutical companies: Biocryst Pharmaceuticals, Durham, NC; Endo Pharmaceuticals, Inc., Chadds Ford, PA; Forrest Laboratories, Inc., St. Louis, MO; Licensor: Gilead Sciences, Inc., Foster City, CA; GSK, GlaxoSmithKline, Research Triangle Park, NC.
[b]CNS symptoms include confusion, anxiety, insomnia, difficulty concentrating, dizziness, hallucinations, and seizures.
[c]GI (gastrointestinal) symptoms include nausea, vomiting, and anorexia.
[d]Neuropsychiatric symptoms include self-injury and delirium.

M2 Protein Inhibitors

The virus-encoded M2 protein facilitates the hydrogen ion-mediated dissociation of the matrix protein-ribonucleoprotein complex within the endosome and the release of the viral ribonucleoprotein into the cytoplasm of the host cell. The M2 inhibitors block the passage of H^+ ions through the M2 ion channel, which prevents uncoating of the virus (1, 162, 163).

Amantadine and Rimantadine

The adamantanes differ in their metabolism and adverse effects, but they have similar antiviral activity against influenza A viruses. Neither drug has activity against influenza B viruses. Recent reports indicate that both the seasonal influenza virus, H3N2, and the current pandemic virus, H1N1, have a high incidence of resistance to both drugs (1, 164, 165); therefore, the adamantanes are no longer recommended for influenza prophylaxis and empiric therapy.

Neuraminidase Inhibitors

The influenza virus neuraminidase is an envelope glycoprotein that cleaves the terminal sialic residues, releasing the virion from the infected cell. The virus-encoded neuraminidase allows the influenza virus to spread from cell to cell. Three neuraminidase inhibitors are approved for the treatment of influenza A and B viruses: oseltamivir, zanamivir, and peramivir (166, 167). Of these, oseltamivir is the most widely used. In 2007 to 2008, a high percentage of seasonal H1N1 influenza virus isolates were resistant to oseltamivir as the result of a single amino acid substitution, but they remained sensitive to zanamivir (164, 168). However, for the 2013–2014 season the CDC reported that 98.2% of the 2009 H1N1 pandemic virus strains were susceptible to oseltamivir and 100% were susceptible to zanamivir (https://www.cdc.gov/flu/about/qa/antiviralresistance.htm).

Oseltamivir

Pharmacology

Oseltamivir phosphate is an ethyl ester prodrug that requires ester hydrolysis for conversion to the active form, oseltamivir carboxylate. After oral administration, oseltamivir phosphate is readily absorbed from the gastrointestinal tract and is extensively converted to oseltamivir carboxylate, predominantly by hepatic esterases (169). At least 75% of an oral dose reaches the systemic circulation as oseltamivir carboxylate. The binding of oseltamivir carboxylate to plasma protein is low. The plasma half-life is 6 to 10 h. There are fewer side effects if administered with food. Oseltamivir carboxylate is not further metabolized and is eliminated in the urine (170). The efficacy of oseltamivir in preventing naturally occurring influenza illness has been demonstrated in treatment and prophylaxis studies (171–173).

Drug Interactions

Studies of oseltamivir suggest that clinically significant drug interactions are unlikely, because neither the drug nor the metabolite oseltamivir carboxylate is a substrate for the CYP450 isoenzymes or for glucuronyltransferases. The potential exists for interaction with other agents such as probenecid that are excreted in the urine by the same pathways (170). Oseltamivir should not be administered in a time period 2 weeks before and 48 h after administration of live influenza vaccine.

Peramivir

Pharmacology

Peramivir was approved in late 2014 for the treatment of uncomplicated influenza. Peramivir has poor oral bioavailability and is therefore only available as an intravenous formulation that is administered as a single dose. It is primarily eliminated by the kidneys (174).

Drug Interactions

There are no significant drug interactions (174).

Zanamivir

Zanamivir treatment has been shown to reduce the severity and duration of naturally occurring, uncomplicated influenza illness in adults (175). Zanamivir is administered only to the respiratory tract by oral inhalation using a blister pack (176). The contents of each blister are inhaled using a specially designed breath-activated plastic device for the inhaling powder. This route rapidly provides high local concentrations at the site of delivery. Because of the respiratory route of administration, zanamivir is contraindicated in patients with underlying airway disease such as asthma. As noted above, the H1N1 strains that have become resistant to oseltamivir remain sensitive to zanamivir.

Pharmacology

The absolute oral bioavailability of zanamivir is low, averaging 2%. After intranasal or oral inhaled administration, a median of 10 to 20% of the dose is systemically absorbed, with maximum concentrations in serum generally reached within 1 to 2 hours. The remaining 70 to 80% is left in the oropharynx and is eliminated in the feces. The median serum half-life ranges between 2.5 and 5.5 hours, and the systemically absorbed drug is excreted unchanged in the urine. The low level of absorption of the drug after inhalation produces low concentrations in serum with only modest systemic zanamivir exposure (170).

Drug Interactions

Zanamivir is not metabolized; therefore, there is a very low potential for drug-drug interaction (177).

REFERENCES

1. **De Clercq E, Li G.** 2016. Approved antiviral drugs over the past 50 years. *Clin Microbiol Rev* **29:**695–747.
2. **Li G, De Clercq E.** 2017. Current therapy for chronic hepatitis C: the role of direct-acting antivirals. *Antiviral Res* **142:**83–122.
3. **Fung J, Lai CL, Seto WK, Yuen MF.** 2011. Nucleoside/nucleotide analogues in the treatment of chronic hepatitis B. *J Antimicrob Chemother* **66:**2715–2725.
4. **Field HJ, Vere Hodge RA.** 2013. Recent developments in anti-herpesvirus drugs. *Br Med Bull* **106:**213–249.
5. **Panel on Antiretroviral Guidelines for Adults and Adolescents.** 2017. Guidelines for the use of antiretroviral agents in HIV-1-infected adults and adolescents. http://www.aidsinfo.nih.gov/ContentFiles/AdultandAdolescentGL.pdf. Accessed 18 August 2017.
6. **Panel on Antiretroviral Therapy and Medical Management of HIV-Infected Children.** 2017. Guidelines for Use of Antiretroviral Agents in Pediatric HIV Infection. http://aidsinfo.nih.gov/contentfiles/lvguidelines/pediatricguidelines.pdf. Accessed 18 August 2017.
7. **Panel on Treatment of HIV-Infected Pregnant Women and Prevention of Perinatal Transmission.** 2017. Recommendation for use of antiretroviral drugs in pregnanat HIV-infected women for maternal health and interventions to reduce perinatal HIV transmission in the United States. http://aidsinfo.nih.gov/contentfiles/lvguidelines/PerinatalGL.pdf. Accessed 18 August 2017.
8. **Côté HC, Brumme ZL, Craib KJ, Alexander CS, Wynhoven B, Ting L, Wong H, Harris M, Harrigan PR, O'Shaughnessy MV, Montaner JS.** 2002. Changes in mitochondrial DNA as a marker of nucleoside toxicity in HIV-infected patients. *N Engl J Med* **346:**811–820.
9. **Capparelli EV, Letendre SL, Ellis RJ, Patel P, Holland D, McCutchan JA.** 2005. Population pharmacokinetics of abacavir in plasma and cerebrospinal fluid. *Antimicrob Agents Chemother* **49:**2504–2506.
10. **Hsue PY, Hunt PW, Wu Y, Schnell A, Ho JE, Hatano H, Xie Y, Martin JN, Ganz P, Deeks SG.** 2009. Association of abacavir and impaired endothelial function in treated and suppressed HIV-infected patients. *AIDS* **23:**2021–2027.
11. **Marcus JL, Neugebauer RS, Leyden WA, Chao CR, Xu L, Quesenberry CP Jr, Klein DB, Towner WJ, Horberg MA, Silverberg MJ.** 2016. Use of abacavir and risk of cardiovascular disease among HIV-infected individuals. *J Acquir Immune Defic Syndr* **71:**413–419.
12. **Ribaudo HJ, Benson CA, Zheng Y, Koletar SL, Collier AC, Lok JJ, Smurzynski M, Bosch RJ, Bastow B, Schouten JT, ACTG A5001/ALLRT Protocol Team.** 2011. No risk of myocardial infarction associated with initial antiretroviral treatment containing abacavir: short and long-term results from ACTG A5001/ALLRT. *Clin Infect Dis* **52:**929–940.
13. **Mallal S, Phillips E, Carosi G, Molina JM, Workman C, Tomazic J, Jägel-Guedes E, Rugina S, Kozyrev O, Cid JF, Hay P, Nolan D, Hughes S, Hughes A, Ryan S, Fitch N, Thorborn D, Benbow A, PREDICT-1 Study Team.** 2008. HLA-B*5701 screening for hypersensitivity to abacavir. *N Engl J Med* **358:**568–579.
14. **Pruvost A, Negredo E, Benech H, Theodoro F, Puig J, Grau E, García E, Moltó J, Grassi J, Clotet B.** 2005. Measurement of intracellular didanosine and tenofovir phosphorylated metabolites and possible interaction of the two drugs in human immunodeficiency virus-infected patients. *Antimicrob Agents Chemother* **49:**1907–1914.
15. **Ray AS, Olson L, Fridland A.** 2004. Role of purine nucleoside phosphorylase in interactions between 2′,3′-dideoxyinosine and allopurinol, ganciclovir, or tenofovir. *Antimicrob Agents Chemother* **48:**1089–1095.
16. **Tozzi V, Balestra P, Salvatori MF, Vlassi C, Liuzzi G, Giancola ML, Giulianelli M, Narciso P, Antinori A.** 2009. Changes in cognition during antiretroviral therapy: comparison of 2 different ranking systems to measure antiretroviral drug efficacy on HIV-associated neurocognitive disorders. *J Acquir Immune Defic Syndr* **52:**56–63.
17. **Perry CM.** 2009. Emtricitabine/tenofovir disoproxil fumarate: in combination with a protease inhibitor in HIV-1 infection. *Drugs* **69:**843–857.
18. **Foudraine NA, Hoetelmans RM, Lange JM, de Wolf F, van Benthem BH, Maas JJ, Keet IP, Portegies P.** 1998. Cerebrospinal-fluid HIV-1 RNA and drug concentrations after treatment with lamivudine plus zidovudine or stavudine. *Lancet* **351:**1547–1551.
19. **Fortuin-de Smidt M, de Waal R, Cohen K, Technau KG, Stinson K, Maartens G, Boulle A, Igumbor EU, Davies MA.** 2017. First-line antiretroviral drug discontinuations in children. *PLoS One* **12:**e0169762.
20. **Havlir DV, Tierney C, Friedland GH, Pollard RB, Smeaton L, Sommadossi JP, Fox L, Kessler H, Fife KH, Richman DD.** 2000. *In vivo* antagonism with zidovudine plus stavudine combination therapy. *J Infect Dis* **182:**321–325.
21. **Piscitelli SC, Gallicano KD.** 2001. Interactions among drugs for HIV and opportunistic infections. *N Engl J Med* **344:**984–996.
22. **Raffi F, Orkin C, Clarke A, Slama L, Gallant J, Daar E, Henry K, Santana-Bagur J, Stein DK, Bellos N, Scarsella A, Yan M, Abram ME, Cheng A, Rhee MS.** 2017. Brief report: long-term (96-week) efficacy and safety after switching from tenofovir disoproxil fumarate to tenofovir alafenamide in HIV-infected, virologically suppressed adults. *J Acquir Immune Defic Syndr* **75:**226–231.
23. **Ruane PJ, DeJesus E, Berger D, Markowitz M, Bredeek UF, Callebaut C, Zhong L, Ramanathan S, Rhee MS, Fordyce MW, Yale K.** 2013. Antiviral activity, safety, and pharmacokinetics/pharmacodynamics of tenofovir alafenamide as 10-day monotherapy in HIV-1-positive adults. *J Acquir Immune Defic Syndr* **63:**449–455.
24. **Durand-Gasselin L, Pruvost A, Dehée A, Vaudre G, Tabone MD, Grassi J, Leverger G, Garbarg-Chenon A, Bénech H, Dollfus C.** 2008. High levels of zidovudine (AZT) and its intracellular phosphate metabolites in AZT- and AZT-lamivudine-treated newborns of human immunodeficiency virus-infected mothers. *Antimicrob Agents Chemother* **52:**2555–2563.
25. **Castello G, Mela G, Cerruti A, Mencoboni M, Lerza R.** 1995. Azidothymidine and interferon-alpha *in vitro* effects on hematopoiesis: protective *in vitro* activity of IL-1 and GM-CSF. *Exp Hematol* **23:**1367–1371
26. **Cimoch PJ, Lavelle J, Pollard R, Griffy KG, Wong R, Tarnowski TL, Casserella S, Jung D.** 1998. Pharmacokinetics of oral ganciclovir alone and in combination with zidovudine, didanosine, and probenecid in HIV-infected subjects. *J Acquir Immune Defic Syndr Hum Retrovirol* **17:**227–234.

27. **Johnson LB, Saravolatz LD.** 2009. Etravirine, a next-generation nonnucleoside reverse-transcriptase inhibitor. *Clin Infect Dis* **48:**1123–1128.
28. **Briz V, Garrido C, Poveda E, Morello J, Barreiro P, de Mendoza C, Soriano V.** 2009. Raltegravir and etravirine are active against HIV type 1 group O. *AIDS Res Hum Retroviruses* **25:**225–227.
29. **Häggblom A, Lindbäck S, Gisslén M, Flamholc L, Hejdeman B, Palmborg A, Leval A, Herweijer E, Valgardsson S, Svedhem V.** 2017. HIV drug therapy duration; a Swedish real world nationwide cohort study on InfCareHIV 2009-2014. *PLoS One* **12:**e0171227.
30. **Mmiro FA, Aizire J, Mwatha AK, Eshleman SH, Donnell D, Fowler MG, Nakabiito C, Musoke PM, Jackson JB, Guay LA.** 2009. Predictors of early and late mother-to-child transmission of HIV in a breastfeeding population: HIV Network for Prevention Trials 012 experience, Kampala, Uganda. *J Acquir Immune Defic Syndr* **52:**32–39.
31. **Samuel R, Julian MN, Paredes R, Parboosing R, Moodley P, Singh L, Naidoo A, Gordon M.** 2016. HIV-1 drug resistance by ultra-deep sequencing following short course zidovudine, single-dose nevirapine, and single-dose tenofovir with emtricitabine for prevention of mother-to-child transmission. *J Acquir Immune Defic Syndr* **73:**384–389.
32. **Eron JJ Jr.** 2000. HIV-1 protease inhibitors. *Clin Infect Dis* **30**(Suppl 2)**:**S160–S170.
33. **Koh Y, Matsumi S, Das D, Amano M, Davis DA, Li J, Leschenko S, Baldridge A, Shioda T, Yarchoan R, Ghosh AK, Mitsuya H.** 2007. Potent inhibition of HIV-1 replication by novel non-peptidyl small molecule inhibitors of protease dimerization. *J Biol Chem* **282:**28709–28720.
34. **Menéndez-Arias L, Tözsér J.** 2008. HIV-1 protease inhibitors: effects on HIV-2 replication and resistance. *Trends Pharmacol Sci* **29:**42–49.
35. **Ford J, Khoo SH, Back DJ.** 2004. The intracellular pharmacology of antiretroviral protease inhibitors. *J Antimicrob Chemother* **54:**982–990.
36. **Zeldin RK, Petruschke RA.** 2004. Pharmacological and therapeutic properties of ritonavir-boosted protease inhibitor therapy in HIV-infected patients. *J Antimicrob Chemother* **53:**4–9.
37. **Boffito M, Maitland D, Samarasinghe Y, Pozniak A.** 2005. The pharmacokinetics of HIV protease inhibitor combinations. *Curr Opin Infect Dis* **18:**1–7.
38. **Youle M.** 2007. Overview of boosted protease inhibitors in treatment-experienced HIV-infected patients. *J Antimicrob Chemother* **60:**1195–1205.
39. **Cooper CL, van Heeswijk RP, Gallicano K, Cameron DW.** 2003. A review of low-dose ritonavir in protease inhibitor combination therapy. *Clin Infect Dis* **36:**1585–1592.
40. **Orrick JJ, Steinhart CR.** 2004. Atazanavir. *Ann Pharmacother* **38:**1664–1674.
41. **Havlir DV, O'Marro SD.** 2004. Atazanavir: new option for treatment of HIV infection. *Clin Infect Dis* **38:**1599–1604.
42. **Elliot ER, Amara A, Pagani N, Else L, Moyle G, Schoolmeesters A, Higgs C, Khoo S, Boffito M.** 2017. Once-daily atazanavir/cobicistat and darunavir/cobicistat exposure over 72 h post-dose in plasma, urine and saliva: contribution to drug pharmacokinetic knowledge. *J Antimicrob Chemother* **72:**2035–2041.
43. **Lepist EI, Phan TK, Roy A, Tong L, Maclennan K, Murray B, Ray AS.** 2012. Cobicistat boosts the intestinal absorption of transport substrates, including HIV protease inhibitors and GS-7340, *in vitro*. *Antimicrob Agents Chemother* **56:**5409–5413.
44. **Wire MB, Shelton MJ, Studenberg S.** 2006. Fosamprenavir : clinical pharmacokinetics and drug interactions of the amprenavir prodrug. *Clin Pharmacokinet* **45:**137–168.
45. **Fellay J, Marzolini C, Decosterd L, Golay KP, Baumann P, Buclin T, Telenti A, Eap CB.** 2005. Variations of CYP3A activity induced by antiretroviral treatment in HIV-1 infected patients. *Eur J Clin Pharmacol* **60:**865–873.
46. **Sudhakaran S, Rayner CR, Li J, Kong DC, Gude NM, Nation RL.** 2007. Differential protein binding of indinavir and saquinavir in matched maternal and umbilical cord plasma. *Br J Clin Pharmacol* **63:**315–321.
47. **Isaac A, Taylor S, Cane P, Smit E, Gibbons SE, White DJ, Drake SM, Khoo S, Back DJ.** 2004. Lopinavir/ritonavir combined with twice-daily 400 mg indinavir: pharmacokinetics and pharmacodynamics in blood, CSF and semen. *J Antimicrob Chemother* **54:**498–502.
48. **Yeni P.** 2003. Tipranavir: a protease inhibitor from a new class with distinct antiviral activity. *J Acquir Immune Defic Syndr* **34**(Suppl 1)**:**S91–S94.
49. **Kiser JJ.** 2008. Pharmacologic characteristics of investigational and recently approved agents for the treatment of HIV. *Curr Opin HIV AIDS* **3:**330–341.
50. **Covens K, Kabeya K, Schrooten Y, Dekeersmaeker N, Van Wijngaerden E, Vandamme AM, De Wit S, Van Laethem K.** 2009. Evolution of genotypic resistance to enfuvirtide in HIV-1 isolates from different group M subtypes. *J Clin Virol* **44:**325–328.
51. **Mould DR, Zhang X, Nieforth K, Salgo M, Buss N, Patel IH.** 2005. Population pharmacokinetics and exposure-response relationship of enfuvirtide in treatment-experienced human immunodeficiency virus type 1-infected patients. *Clin Pharmacol Ther* **77:**515–528.
52. **Vandekerckhove L, Verhofstede C, Vogelaers D.** 2009. Maraviroc: perspectives for use in antiretroviral-naive HIV-1-infected patients. *J Antimicrob Chemother* **63:**1087–1096.
53. **Depatureaux A, Charpentier C, Collin G, Leoz M, Descamps D, Vessière A, Damond F, Rousset D, Brun-Vézinet F, Plantier JC.** 2010. Baseline genotypic and phenotypic susceptibilities of HIV-1 group O to enfuvirtide. *Antimicrob Agents Chemother* **54:**4016–4019.
54. **Price RW, Parham R, Kroll JL, Wring SA, Baker B, Sailstad J, Hoh R, Liegler T, Spudich S, Kuritzkes DR, Deeks SG.** 2008. Enfuvirtide cerebrospinal fluid (CSF) pharmacokinetics and potential use in defining CSF HIV-1 origin. *Antivir Ther* **13:**369–374
55. **Xiong S, Borrego P, Ding X, Zhu Y, Martins A, Chong H, Taveira N, He Y.** 2016. A helical short-peptide fusion inhibitor with highly potent activity against human immunodeficiency virus type 1 (HIV-1), HIV-2, and simian immunodeficiency virus. *J Virol* **91:**e01839-16
56. **MacArthur RD, Novak RM.** 2008. Reviews of anti-infective agents: maraviroc: the first of a new class of antiretroviral agents. *Clin Infect Dis* **47:**236–241.
57. **Podany AT, Scarsi KK, Fletcher CV.** 2017. Comparative clinical pharmacokinetics and pharmacodynamics of HIV-1 integrase strand transfer inhibitors. *Clin Pharmacokinet* **56:** 25–40.
58. **Lennox JL, DeJesus E, Lazzarin A, Pollard RB, Madruga JV, Berger DS, Zhao J, Xu X, Williams-Diaz A, Rodgers AJ, Barnard RJ, Miller MD, DiNubile MJ, Nguyen BY, Leavitt R, Sklar P, STARTMRK investigators.** 2009. Safety and efficacy of raltegravir-based versus efavirenz-based combination therapy in treatment-naive patients with HIV-1 infection: a multicentre, double-blind randomised controlled trial. *Lancet* **374:**796–806.
59. **Elliot E, Chirwa M, Boffito M.** 2017. How recent findings on the pharmacokinetics and pharmacodynamics of integrase inhibitors can inform clinical use. *Curr Opin Infect Dis* **30:** 58–73
60. **Ramanathan S, Mathias AA, German P, Kearney BP.** 2011. Clinical pharmacokinetic and pharmacodynamic profile of the HIV integrase inhibitor elvitegravir. *Clin Pharmacokinet* **50:**229–244.
61. **Arribas JR, Eron J.** 2013. Advances in antiretroviral therapy. *Curr Opin HIV AIDS* **8:**341–349
62. **Eron JJ, Clotet B, Durant J, Katlama C, Kumar P, Lazzarin A, Poizot-Martin I, Richmond G, Soriano V, Ait-Khaled M, Fujiwara T, Huang J, Min S, Vavro C, Yeo J, Walmsley SL, Cox J, Reynes J, Morlat P, Vittecoq D, Livrozet J-M, Fernandez PV, Gatell JM, DeJesus E, DeVente J, Lalezari JP, McCurdy LH, Sloan LA, Young B, LaMarca A, Hawkins T, VIKING Study Group.** 2013. Safety and efficacy of dolutegravir in treatment-experienced subjects with raltegravir-resistant HIV type 1 infection: 24-week results of the VIKING Study. *J Infect Dis* **207:**740–748.

63. **Min S, Song I, Borland J, Chen S, Lou Y, Fujiwara T, Piscitelli SC.** 2010. Pharmacokinetics and safety of S/GSK1349572, a next-generation HIV integrase inhibitor, in healthy volunteers. *Antimicrob Agents Chemother* **54:** 254–258.
64. **Cahn P, Pozniak AL, Mingrone H, Shuldyakov A, Brites C, Andrade-Villanueva JF, Richmond G, Buendia CB, Fourie J, Ramgopal M, Hagins D, Felizarta F, Madruga J, Reuter T, Newman T, Small CB, Lombaard J, Grinsztejn B, Dorey D, Underwood M, Griffith S, Min S, extended SAILING Study Team.** 2013. Dolutegravir versus raltegravir in antiretroviral-experienced, integrase-inhibitor-naive adults with HIV: week 48 results from the randomised, double-blind, non-inferiority SAILING study. *Lancet* **382:**700–708.
65. **Poordad F, Dieterich D.** 2012. Treating hepatitis C: current standard of care and emerging direct-acting antiviral agents. *J Viral Hepat* **19:**449–464.
66. **AASLD-IDSA.** 2017. Recommendations for testing, managing, and treating hepatitis C. http://www.hcvguidelines.org. Accessed 18 August 2017.
67. **Pockros PJ.** 2010. New direct-acting antivirals in the development for hepatitis C virus infection. *Therap Adv Gastroenterol* **3:**191–202.
68. **Lahser FC, Bystol K, Curry S, McMonagle P, Xia E, Ingravallo P, Chase R, Liu R, Black T, Hazuda D, Howe AY, Asante-Appiah E.** 2016. The Combination of grazoprevir, a hepatitis C virus (HCV) NS3/4A protease inhibitor, and elbasvir, an HCV NS5A inhibitor, demonstrates a high genetic barrier to resistance in HCV genotype 1a replicons. *Antimicrob Agents Chemother* **60:**2954–2964.
69. **Zeuzem S, Ghalib R, Reddy KR, Pockros PJ, Ben Ari Z, Zhao Y, Brown DD, Wan S, DiNubile MJ, Nguyen BY, Robertson MN, Wahl J, Barr E, Butterton JR.** 2015. Grazoprevir-elbasvir combination therapy for treatment-naive cirrhotic and noncirrhotic patients with chronic hepatitis C virus genotype 1, 4, or 6 infection: a randomized trial. *Ann Intern Med* **163:**1–13.
70. **Feld JJ, Kowdley KV, Coakley E, Sigal S, Nelson DR, Crawford D, Weiland O, Aguilar H, Xiong J, Pilot-Matias T, DaSilva-Tillmann B, Larsen L, Podsadecki T, Bernstein B.** 2014. Treatment of HCV with ABT-450/r-ombitasvir and dasabuvir with ribavirin. *N Engl J Med* **370:**1594–1603.
71. **Zeuzem S, Jacobson IM, Baykal T, Marinho RT, Poordad F, Bourlière M, Sulkowski MS, Wedemeyer H, Tam E, Desmond P, Jensen DM, Di Bisceglie AM, Varunok P, Hassanein T, Xiong J, Pilot-Matias T, DaSilva-Tillmann B, Larsen L, Podsadecki T, Bernstein B.** 2014. Retreatment of HCV with ABT-450/r-ombitasvir and dasabuvir with ribavirin. *N Engl J Med* **370:**1604–1614.
72. **Lawitz E, Sulkowski MS, Ghalib R, Rodriguez-Torres M, Younossi ZM, Corregidor A, DeJesus E, Pearlman B, Rabinovitz M, Gitlin N, Lim JK, Pockros PJ, Scott JD, Fevery B, Lambrecht T, Ouwerkerk-Mahadevan S, Callewaert K, Symonds WT, Picchio G, Lindsay KL, Beumont M, Jacobson IM.** 2014. Simeprevir plus sofosbuvir, with or without ribavirin, to treat chronic infection with hepatitis C virus genotype 1 in non-responders to pegylated interferon and ribavirin and treatment-naive patients: the COSMOS randomised study. *Lancet* **384:**1756–1765.
73. **Bourlière M, Gordon SC, Flamm SL, Cooper CL, Ramji A, Tong M, Ravendhran N, Vierling JM, Tran TT, Pianko S, Bansal MB, de Lédinghen V, Hyland RH, Stamm LM, Dvory-Sobol H, Svarovskaia E, Zhang J, Huang KC, Subramanian GM, Brainard DM, McHutchison JG, Verna EC, Buggisch P, Landis CS, Younes ZH, Curry MP, Strasser SI, Schiff ER, Reddy KR, Manns MP, Kowdley KV, Zeuzem S, POLARIS-1 and POLARIS-4 Investigators.** 2017. Sofosbuvir, velpatasvir, and voxilaprevir for previously treated HCV infection. *N Engl J Med* **376:**2134–2146.
74. **Gane EJ, Shiffman ML, Etzkorn K, Morelli G, Stedman C, Davis MN, Hinestrosa F, Dvory-Sobol H, Huang KC, Osinusi A, McNally J, Brainard DM, McHutchison JG, Thompson AJ, Sulkowski MS, GS-US-342-1553 Investigators.** 2017. Sofosbuvir-velpatasvir with ribavirin for 24 weeks in HCV patients previously treated with a direct-acting antiviral regimen. *Hepatology* **66:**1083–1089.
75. **Poordad F, Felizarta F, Asatryan A, Sulkowski MS, Reindollar RW, Landis CS, Gordon SC, Flamm SL, Fried MW, Bernstein DE, Lin CW, Liu R, Lovell SS, Ng TI, Kort J, Mensa FJ.** 2017. Glecaprevir and pibrentasvir for 12 weeks for hepatitis C virus genotype 1 infection and prior direct-acting antiviral treatment. *Hepatology* **66:**389–397.
76. **Evans MJ, Rice CM, Goff SP.** 2004. Phosphorylation of hepatitis C virus nonstructural protein 5A modulates its protein interactions and viral RNA replication. *Proc Natl Acad Sci USA* **101:**13038–13043.
77. **Tellinghuisen TL, Foss KL, Treadaway J.** 2008. Regulation of hepatitis C virion production via phosphorylation of the NS5A protein. *PLoS Pathog* **4:**e1000032.
78. **Kowdley KV, Gordon SC, Reddy KR, Rossaro L, Bernstein DE, Lawitz E, Shiffman ML, Schiff E, Ghalib R, Ryan M, Rustgi V, Chojkier M, Herring R, Di Bisceglie AM, Pockros PJ, Subramanian GM, An D, Svarovskaia E, Hyland RH, Pang PS, Symonds WT, McHutchison JG, Muir AJ, Pound D, Fried MW, ION-3 Investigators.** 2014. Ledipasvir and sofosbuvir for 8 or 12 weeks for chronic HCV without cirrhosis. *N Engl J Med* **370:**1879–1888.
79. **Sulkowski MS, Gardiner DF, Rodriguez-Torres M, Reddy KR, Hassanein T, Jacobson I, Lawitz E, Lok AS, Hinestrosa F, Thuluvath PJ, Schwartz H, Nelson DR, Everson GT, Eley T, Wind-Rotolo M, Huang SP, Gao M, Hernandez D, McPhee F, Sherman D, Hindes R, Symonds W, Pasquinelli C, Grasela DM, AI444040 Study Group.** 2014. Daclatasvir plus sofosbuvir for previously treated or untreated chronic HCV infection. *N Engl J Med* **370:**211–221.
80. **Ferenci P, Bernstein D, Lalezari J, Cohen D, Luo Y, Cooper C, Tam E, Marinho RT, Tsai N, Nyberg A, Box TD, Younes Z, Enayati P, Green S, Baruch Y, Bhandari BR, Caruntu FA, Sepe T, Chulanov V, Janczewska E, Rizzardini G, Gervain J, Planas R, Moreno C, Hassanein T, Xie W, King M, Podsadecki T, Reddy KR, PEARL-III Study, PEARL-IV Study.** 2014. ABT-450/r-ombitasvir and dasabuvir with or without ribavirin for HCV. *N Engl J Med* **370:**1983–1992.
81. **Hézode C, Asselah T, Reddy KR, Hassanein T, Berenguer M, Fleischer-Stepniewska K, Marcellin P, Hall C, Schnell G, Pilot-Matias T, Mobashery N, Redman R, Vilchez RA, Pol S.** 2015. Ombitasvir plus paritaprevir plus ritonavir with or without ribavirin in treatment-naive and treatment-experienced patients with genotype 4 chronic hepatitis C virus infection (PEARL-I): a randomised, open-label trial. *Lancet* **385:**2502–2509.
82. **Lawitz E, Gane E, Pearlman B, Tam E, Ghesquiere W, Guyader D, Alric L, Bronowicki JP, Lester L, Sievert W, Ghalib R, Balart L, Sund F, Lagging M, Dutko F, Shaughnessy M, Hwang P, Howe AY, Wahl J, Robertson M, Barr E, Haber B.** 2015. Efficacy and safety of 12 weeks versus 18 weeks of treatment with grazoprevir (MK-5172) and elbasvir (MK-8742) with or without ribavirin for hepatitis C virus genotype 1 infection in previously untreated patients with cirrhosis and patients with previous null response with or without cirrhosis (C-WORTHY): a randomised, open-label phase 2 trial. *Lancet* **385:**1075–1086.
83. **Feld JJ, Jacobson IM, Hézode C, Asselah T, Ruane PJ, Gruener N, Abergel A, Mangia A, Lai CL, Chan HL, Mazzotta F, Moreno C, Yoshida E, Shafran SD, Towner WJ, Tran TT, McNally J, Osinusi A, Svarovskaia E, Zhu Y, Brainard DM, McHutchison JG, Agarwal K, Zeuzem S, ASTRAL-1 Investigators.** 2015. Sofosbuvir and velpatasvir for HCV genotype 1, 2, 4, 5, and 6 infection. *N Engl J Med* **373:**2599–2607.
84. **Nelson DR, Cooper JN, Lalezari JP, Lawitz E, Pockros PJ, Gitlin N, Freilich BF, Younes ZH, Harlan W, Ghalib R, Oguchi G, Thuluvath PJ, Ortiz-Lasanta G, Rabinovitz M, Bernstein D, Bennett M, Hawkins T, Ravendhran N, Sheikh AM, Varunok P, Kowdley KV, Hennicken D, McPhee F, Rana K, Hughes EA, ALLY-3 Study Team.** 2015. All-oral 12-week treatment with daclatasvir plus sofosbuvir in patients with hepatitis C virus genotype 3 infection: ALLY-3 phase III study. *Hepatology* **61:**1127–1135.

85. **Afdhal N, Zeuzem S, Kwo P, Chojkier M, Gitlin N, Puoti M, Romero-Gomez M, Zarski JP, Agarwal K, Buggisch P, Foster GR, Bräu N, Buti M, Jacobson IM, Subramanian GM, Ding X, Mo H, Yang JC, Pang PS, Symonds WT, McHutchison JG, Muir AJ, Mangia A, Marcellin P, ION-1 Investigators.** 2014. Ledipasvir and sofosbuvir for untreated HCV genotype 1 infection. *N Engl J Med* **370:**1889–1898.
86. **Foster GR, Afdhal N, Roberts SK, Bräu N, Gane EJ, Pianko S, Lawitz E, Thompson A, Shiffman ML, Cooper C, Towner WJ, Conway B, Ruane P, Bourlière M, Asselah T, Berg T, Zeuzem S, Rosenberg W, Agarwal K, Stedman CA, Mo H, Dvory-Sobol H, Han L, Wang J, McNally J, Osinusi A, Brainard DM, McHutchison JG, Mazzotta F, Tran TT, Gordon SC, Patel K, Reau N, Mangia A, Sulkowski M, ASTRAL-2 Investigators, ASTRAL-3 Investigators.** 2015. Sofosbuvir and velpatasvir for HCV genotype 2 and 3 infection. *N Engl J Med* **373:**2608–2617.
87. **Preston SL, Drusano GL, Glue P, Nash J, Gupta SK, McNamara P.** 1999. Pharmacokinetics and absolute bioavailability of ribavirin in healthy volunteers as determined by stable-isotope methodology. *Antimicrob Agents Chemother* **43:**2451–2456
88. **Bonney D, Razali H, Turner A, Will A.** 2009. Successful treatment of human metapneumovirus pneumonia using combination therapy with intravenous ribavirin and immune globulin. *Br J Haematol* **145:**667–669.
89. **Crotty S, Maag D, Arnold JJ, Zhong W, Lau JY, Hong Z, Andino R, Cameron CE.** 2000. The broad-spectrum antiviral ribonucleoside ribavirin is an RNA virus mutagen. *Nat Med* **6:**1375–1379.
90. **Leyssen P, Balzarini J, De Clercq E, Neyts J.** 2005. The predominant mechanism by which ribavirin exerts its antiviral activity *in vitro* against flaviviruses and paramyxoviruses is mediated by inhibition of IMP dehydrogenase. *J Virol* **79:**1943–1947.
91. **Liu V, Dhillon GS, Weill D.** 2010. A multi-drug regimen for respiratory syncytial virus and parainfluenza virus infections in adult lung and heart-lung transplant recipients. *Transpl Infect Dis* **12:**38–44.
92. **Mertz GJ, Miedzinski L, Goade D, Pavia AT, Hjelle B, Hansbarger CO, Levy H, Koster FT, Baum K, Lindemulder A, Wang W, Riser L, Fernandez H, Whitley RJ, Collaborative Antiviral Study Group.** 2004. Placebo-controlled, double-blind trial of intravenous ribavirin for the treatment of hantavirus cardiopulmonary syndrome in North America. *Clin Infect Dis* **39:**1307–1313.
93. **Nguyen JT, Hoopes JD, Smee DF, Prichard MN, Driebe EM, Engelthaler DM, Le MH, Keim PS, Spence RP, Went GT.** 2009. Triple combination of oseltamivir, amantadine, and ribavirin displays synergistic activity against multiple influenza virus strains *in vitro*. *Antimicrob Agents Chemother* **53:**4115–4126.
94. **Patterson JL, Fernandez-Larsson R.** 1990. Molecular mechanisms of action of ribavirin. *Rev Infect Dis* **12:**1139–1146.
95. **Smee DF, Hurst BL, Wong MH, Bailey KW, Morrey JD.** 2009. Effects of double combinations of amantadine, oseltamivir, and ribavirin on influenza A (H5N1) virus infections in cell culture and in mice. *Antimicrob Agents Chemother* **53:**2120–2128.
96. **Perronne C.** 2006. Antiviral hepatitis and antiretroviral drug interactions. *J Hepatol* **44**(Suppl)**:**S119–S125.
97. **Gish RG, Trinh H, Leung N, Chan FK, Fried MW, Wright TL, Wang C, Anderson J, Mondou E, Snow A, Sorbel J, Rousseau F, Corey L.** 2005. Safety and antiviral activity of emtricitabine (FTC) for the treatment of chronic hepatitis B infection: a two-year study. *J Hepatol* **43:**60–66.
98. **Panel on Antiretroviral Guidelines for Adults and Adolescents.** 2013. Guidelines for the use of antiretroviral agents in HIV-1-infected adults and adolescents. Department of Health and Human Services, Washington, DC.
99. **Fontana RJ.** 2009. Side effects of long-term oral antiviral therapy for hepatitis B. *Hepatology* **49**(Suppl)**:**S185–S195.
100. **Soriano V, Puoti M, Bonacini M, Brook G, Cargnel A, Rockstroh J, Thio C, Benhamou Y.** 2005. Care of patients with chronic hepatitis B and HIV co-infection: recommendations from an HIV-HBV International Panel. *AIDS* **19:**221–240.
101. **Younger HM, Bathgate AJ, Hayes PC.** 2004. Review article: nucleoside analogues for the treatment of chronic hepatitis B. *Aliment Pharmacol Ther* **20:**1211–1230.
102. **Soriano V, Puoti M, Peters M, Benhamou Y, Sulkowski M, Zoulim F, Mauss S, Rockstroh J.** 2008. Care of HIV patients with chronic hepatitis B: updated recommendations from the HIV-Hepatitis B Virus International Panel. *AIDS* **22:**1399–1410.
103. **Mohanty SR, Cotler SJ.** 2005. Management of hepatitis B in liver transplant patients. *J Clin Gastroenterol* **39:**58–63
104. **Erhardt A, Blondin D, Hauck K, Sagir A, Kohnle T, Heintges T, Häussinger D.** 2005. Response to interferon alfa is hepatitis B virus genotype dependent: genotype A is more sensitive to interferon than genotype D. *Gut* **54:**1009–1013.
105. **Wai CT, Chu CJ, Hussain M, Lok AS.** 2002. HBV genotype B is associated with better response to interferon therapy in HBeAg(+) chronic hepatitis than genotype C. *Hepatology* **36:**1425–1430
106. **Kaplan JE, Benson C, Holmes KH, Brooks JT, Pau A, Masur H.** 2009. Guidelines for prevention and treatment of opportunistic infections in HIV-infected adults and adolescents: recommendations from CDC, the National Institutes of Health, and the HIV Medicine Association of the Infectious Diseases Society of America. *MMWR Recomm Rep* **58:**1–207; quiz CE201–204.
107. **van Bömmel F, Zöllner B, Sarrazin C, Spengler U, Hüppe D, Möller B, Feucht HH, Wiedenmann B, Berg T.** 2006. Tenofovir for patients with lamivudine-resistant hepatitis B virus (HBV) infection and high HBV DNA level during adefovir therapy. *Hepatology* **44:**318–325.
108. **McMahon MA, Jilek BL, Brennan TP, Shen L, Zhou Y, Wind-Rotolo M, Xing S, Bhat S, Hale B, Hegarty R, Chong CR, Liu JO, Siliciano RF, Thio CL.** 2007. The HBV drug entecavir: effects on HIV-1 replication and resistance. *N Engl J Med* **356:**2614–2621.
109. **Jain MK, Comanor L, White C, Kipnis P, Elkin C, Leung K, Ocampo A, Attar N, Keiser P, Lee WM.** 2007. Treatment of hepatitis B with lamivudine and tenofovir in HIV/HBV-coinfected patients: factors associated with response. *J Viral Hepat* **14:**176–182.
110. **Nash K.** 2009. Telbivudine in the treatment of chronic hepatitis B. *Adv Ther* **26:**155–169.
111. **Chan HL, Fung S, Seto WK, Chuang WL, Chen CY, Kim HJ, Hui AJ, Janssen HL, Chowdhury A, Tsang TY, Mehta R, Gane E, Flaherty JF, Massetto B, Gaggar A, Kitrinos KM, Lin L, Subramanian GM, McHutchison JG, Lim YS, Acharya SK, Agarwal K, GS-US-320-0110 Investigators.** 2016. Tenofovir alafenamide versus tenofovir disoproxil fumarate for the treatment of HBeAg-positive chronic hepatitis B virus infection: a randomised, double-blind, phase 3, non-inferiority trial. *Lancet Gastroenterol Hepatol* **1:**185–195.
112. **Ormrod D, Scott LJ, Perry CM.** 2000. Valaciclovir: a review of its long term utility in the management of genital herpes simplex virus and cytomegalovirus infections. *Drugs* **59:**839–863.
113. **Talarico CL, Burnette TC, Miller WH, Smith SL, Davis MG, Stanat SC, Ng TI, He Z, Coen DM, Roizman B, Biron KK.** 1999. Acyclovir is phosphorylated by the human cytomegalovirus UL97 protein. *Antimicrob Agents Chemother* **43:**1941–1946
114. **Whitley RJ, Gnann JW Jr.** 1992. Acyclovir: a decade later. *N Engl J Med* **327:**782–789.
115. **Hazar V, Kansoy S, Küpesiz A, Aksoylar S, Kantar M, Yeşilipek A.** 2004. High-dose acyclovir and pre-emptive ganciclovir in prevention of cytomegalovirus disease in pediatric patients following peripheral blood stem cell transplantation. *Bone Marrow Transplant* **33:**931–935.
116. **Reischig T, Jindra P, Mares J, Cechura M, Svecová M, Hes O, Opatrný K Jr, Treska V.** 2005. Valacyclovir for cytomegalovirus prophylaxis reduces the risk of acute renal allograft rejection. *Transplantation* **79:**317–324.

117. **Xiong X, Smith JL, Chen MS.** 1997. Effect of incorporation of cidofovir into DNA by human cytomegalovirus DNA polymerase on DNA elongation. *Antimicrob Agents Chemother* **41:**594–599
118. **Cundy KC, Petty BG, Flaherty J, Fisher PE, Polis MA, Wachsman M, Lietman PS, Lalezari JP, Hitchcock MJ, Jaffe HS.** 1995. Clinical pharmacokinetics of cidofovir in human immunodeficiency virus-infected patients. *Antimicrob Agents Chemother* **39:**1247–1252.
119. **Wolf DL, Rodríguez CA, Mucci M, Ingrosso A, Duncan BA, Nickens DJ.** 2003. Pharmacokinetics and renal effects of cidofovir with a reduced dose of probenecid in HIV-infected patients with cytomegalovirus retinitis. *J Clin Pharmacol* **43:** 43–51.
120. **Duraffour S, Mertens B, Meyer H, van den Oord JJ, Mitera T, Matthys P, Snoeck R, Andrei G.** 2013. Emergence of cowpox: study of the virulence of clinical strains and evaluation of antivirals. *PLoS One* **8:**e55808.
121. **Matthes-Martin S, Feuchtinger T, Shaw PJ, Engelhard D, Hirsch HH, Cordonnier C, Ljungman P, Fourth European Conference on Infections in Leukemia.** 2012. European guidelines for diagnosis and treatment of adenovirus infection in leukemia and stem cell transplantation: summary of ECIL-4 (2011). *Transpl Infect Dis* **14:**555–563.
122. **Kuten SA, Patel SJ, Knight RJ, Gaber LW, DeVos JM, Gaber AO.** 2014. Observations on the use of cidofovir for BK virus infection in renal transplantation. *Transpl Infect Dis* **16:**975–983.
123. **Shehab N, Sweet BV, Hogikyan ND.** 2005. Cidofovir for the treatment of recurrent respiratory papillomatosis: a review of the literature. *Pharmacotherapy* **25:**977–989.
124. **Fusconi M, Grasso M, Greco A, Gallo A, Campo F, Remacle M, Turchetta R, Pagliuca G, De Vincentiis M.** 2014. Recurrent respiratory papillomatosis by HPV: review of the literature and update on the use of cidofovir. *Acta Otorhinolaryngol Ital* **34:**375–381
125. **Lietman PS.** 1992. Clinical pharmacology: foscarnet. *Am J Med* **92(2A):**S8–S11.
126. **Chrisp P, Clissold SP.** 1991. Foscarnet: a review of its antiviral activity, pharmacokinetic properties and therapeutic use in immunocompromised patients with cytomegalovirus retinitis. *Drugs* **41:**104–129.
127. **Aweeka F, Gambertoglio J, Mills J, Jacobson MA.** 1989. Pharmacokinetics of intermittently administered intravenous foscarnet in the treatment of acquired immunodeficiency syndrome patients with serious cytomegalovirus retinitis. *Antimicrob Agents Chemother* **33:**742–745.
128. **Schwarz A, Perez-Canto A.** 1998. Nephrotoxicity of antiinfective drugs. *Int J Clin Pharmacol Ther* **36:**164–167
129. **Curran M, Noble S.** 2001. Valganciclovir. *Drugs* **61:** 1145–1150; discussion 1151–1152.
130. **Pescovitz MD, Rabkin J, Merion RM, Paya CV, Pirsch J, Freeman RB, O'Grady J, Robinson C, To Z, Wren K, Banken L, Buhles W, Brown F.** 2000. Valganciclovir results in improved oral absorption of ganciclovir in liver transplant recipients. *Antimicrob Agents Chemother* **44:**2811–2815.
131. **Wiltshire H, Paya CV, Pescovitz MD, Humar A, Dominguez E, Washburn K, Blumberg E, Alexander B, Freeman R, Heaton N, Zuideveld KP, Valganciclovir Solid Organ Transplant Study Group.** 2005. Pharmacodynamics of oral ganciclovir and valganciclovir in solid organ transplant recipients. *Transplantation* **79:**1477–1483.
132. **Casper C, Krantz EM, Corey L, Kuntz SR, Wang J, Selke S, Hamilton S, Huang ML, Wald A.** 2008. Valganciclovir for suppression of human herpesvirus-8 replication: a randomized, double-blind, placebo-controlled, crossover trial. *J Infect Dis* **198:**23–30.
133. **Cvetković RS, Wellington K.** 2005. Valganciclovir: a review of its use in the management of CMV infection and disease in immunocompromised patients. *Drugs* **65:**859–878.
134. **Sun HY, Wagener MM, Singh N.** 2008. Prevention of posttransplant cytomegalovirus disease and related outcomes with valganciclovir: a systematic review. *Am J Transplant* **8:**2111–2118.
135. **Torres-Madriz G, Boucher HW.** 2008. Immunocompromised hosts: perspectives in the treatment and prophylaxis of cytomegalovirus disease in solid-organ transplant recipients. *Clin Infect Dis* **47:**702–711.
136. **Vere Hodge RA, Sutton D, Boyd MR, Harnden MR, Jarvest RL.** 1989. Selection of an oral prodrug (BRL 42810; famciclovir) for the antiherpesvirus agent BRL 39123 [9-(4-hydroxy-3-hydroxymethylbut-l-yl)guanine; penciclovir]. *Antimicrob Agents Chemother* **33:**1765–1773.
137. **Luber AD, Flaherty JF Jr.** 1996. Famciclovir for treatment of herpesvirus infections. *Ann Pharmacother* **30:**978–985.
138. **Schmid-Wendtner MH, Korting HC.** 2004. Penciclovir cream: improved topical treatment for herpes simplex infections. *Skin Pharmacol Physiol* **17:**214–218.
139. **Simpson D, Lyseng-Williamson KA.** 2006. Famciclovir: a review of its use in herpes zoster and genital and orolabial herpes. *Drugs* **66:**2397–2416.
140. **Bacon TH, Levin MJ, Leary JJ, Sarisky RT, Sutton D.** 2003. Herpes simplex virus resistance to acyclovir and penciclovir after two decades of antiviral therapy. *Clin Microbiol Rev* **16:**114–128.
141. **Earnshaw DL, Bacon TH, Darlison SJ, Edmonds K, Perkins RM, Vere Hodge RA.** 1992. Mode of antiviral action of penciclovir in MRC-5 cells infected with herpes simplex virus type 1 (HSV-1), HSV-2, and varicella-zoster virus. *Antimicrob Agents Chemother* **36:**2747–2757.
142. **Chilukuri S, Rosen T.** 2003. Management of acyclovir-resistant herpes simplex virus. *Dermatol Clin* **21:**311–320.
143. **Pepose JS, Margolis TP, LaRussa P, Pavan-Langston D.** 2003. Ocular complications of smallpox vaccination. *Am J Ophthalmol* **136:**343–352.
144. **Carmine AA, Brogden RN, Heel RC, Speight TM, Avery GS.** 1982. Trifluridine: a review of its antiviral activity and therapeutic use in the topical treatment of viral eye infections. *Drugs* **23:**329–353.
145. **Katz DH, Marcelletti JF, Khalil MH, Pope LE, Katz LR.** 1991. Antiviral activity of 1-docosanol, an inhibitor of lipid-enveloped viruses including herpes simplex. *Proc Natl Acad Sci USA* **88:**10825–10829.
146. **Trofe J, Pote L, Wade E, Blumberg E, Bloom RD.** 2008. Maribavir: a novel antiviral agent with activity against cytomegalovirus. *Ann Pharmacother* **42:**1447–1457.
147. **Ma JD, Nafziger AN, Villano SA, Gaedigk A, Bertino JS Jr.** 2006. Maribavir pharmacokinetics and the effects of multiple-dose maribavir on cytochrome P450 (CYP) 1A2, CYP 2C9, CYP 2C19, CYP 2D6, CYP 3A, N-acetyltransferase-2, and xanthine oxidase activities in healthy adults. *Antimicrob Agents Chemother* **50:**1130–1135.
148. **Marty FM, Ljungman P, Papanicolaou GA, Winston DJ, Chemaly RF, Strasfeld L, Young JA, Rodriguez T, Maertens J, Schmitt M, Einsele H, Ferrant A, Lipton JH, Villano SA, Chen H, Boeckh M, Maribavir 1263-300 Clinical Study Group.** 2011. Maribavir prophylaxis for prevention of cytomegalovirus disease in recipients of allogeneic stem-cell transplants: a phase 3, double-blind, placebo-controlled, randomised trial. *Lancet Infect Dis* **11:**284–292.
149. **Winston DJ, Saliba F, Blumberg E, Abouljoud M, Garcia-Diaz JB, Goss JA, Clough L, Avery R, Limaye AP, Ericzon BG, Navasa M, Troisi RI, Chen H, Villano SA, Uknis ME, 1263-301 Clinical Study Group.** 2012. Efficacy and safety of maribavir dosed at 100 mg orally twice daily for the prevention of cytomegalovirus disease in liver transplant recipients: a randomized, double-blind, multicenter controlled trial. *Am J Transplant* **12:**3021–3030.
150. **Price NB, Prichard MN.** 2011. Progress in the development of new therapies for herpesvirus infections. *Curr Opin Virol* **1:**548–554.
151. **Florescu DF, Pergam SA, Neely MN, Qiu F, Johnston C, Way S, Sande J, Lewinsohn DA, Guzman-Cottrill JA, Graham ML, Papanicolaou G, Kurtzberg J, Rigdon J, Painter W, Mommeja-Marin H, Lanier R, Anderson M, van der Horst C.** 2012. Safety and efficacy of CMX001 as salvage therapy for severe adenovirus infections in immunocompromised patients. *Biol Blood Marrow Transplant* **18:**731–738.

152. **Marty FM, Ljungman P, Chemaly RF, Maertens J, Dadwal SS, Duarte RF, Haider S, Ullmann AJ, Katayama Y, Brown J, Mullane KM, Boeckh M, Blumberg EA, Einsele H, Snydman DR, Kanda Y, DiNubile MJ, Teal VL, Wan H, Murata Y, Kartsonis NA, Leavitt RY, Badshah C.** 2017. Letermovir prophylaxis for cytomegalovirus in hematopoietic-cell transplantation. *N Engl J Med* **377:**2433–2444.
153. **Tyring S, Wald A, Zadeikis N, Dhadda S, Takenouchi K, Rorig R.** 2012. ASP2151 for the treatment of genital herpes: a randomized, double-blind, placebo- and valacyclovir-controlled, dose-finding study. *J Infect Dis* **205:**1100–1110.
154. **Wald A, Corey L, Timmler B, Magaret A, Warren T, Tyring S, Johnston C, Kriesel J, Fife K, Galitz L, Stoelben S, Huang ML, Selke S, Stobernack HP, Ruebsamen-Schaeff H, Birkmann A.** 2014. Helicase-primase inhibitor pritelivir for HSV-2 infection. *N Engl J Med* **370:**201–210.
155. **Avery RK, Bolwell BJ, Yen-Lieberman B, Lurain N, Waldman WJ, Longworth DL, Taege AJ, Mossad SB, Kohn D, Long JR, Curtis J, Kalaycio M, Pohlman B, Williams JW.** 2004. Use of leflunomide in an allogeneic bone marrow transplant recipient with refractory cytomegalovirus infection. *Bone Marrow Transplant* **34:**1071–1075.
156. **Levi ME, Mandava N, Chan LK, Weinberg A, Olson JL.** 2006. Treatment of multidrug-resistant cytomegalovirus retinitis with systemically administered leflunomide. *Transpl Infect Dis* **8:**38–43.
157. **Efferth T, Romero MR, Wolf DG, Stamminger T, Marin JJ, Marschall M.** 2008. The antiviral activities of artemisinin and artesunate. *Clin Infect Dis* **47:**804–811.
158. **Shapira MY, Resnick IB, Chou S, Neumann AU, Lurain NS, Stamminger T, Caplan O, Saleh N, Efferth T, Marschall M, Wolf DG.** 2008. Artesunate as a potent antiviral agent in a patient with late drug-resistant cytomegalovirus infection after hematopoietic stem cell transplantation. *Clin Infect Dis* **46:**1455–1457.
159. **American Academy of Pediatrics Committee on Infectious Diseases.** 2007. Antiviral therapy and prophylaxis for influenza in children. *Pediatrics* **119:**852–860.
160. **Monto AS.** 2003. The role of antivirals in the control of influenza. *Vaccine* **21:**1796–1800.
161. **Oxford JS.** 2007. Antivirals for the treatment and prevention of epidemic and pandemic influenza. *Influenza Other Respir Viruses* **1:**27–34.
162. **Jing X, Ma C, Ohigashi Y, Oliveira FA, Jardetzky TS, Pinto LH, Lamb RA.** 2008. Functional studies indicate amantadine binds to the pore of the influenza A virus M2 proton-selective ion channel. *Proc Natl Acad Sci USA* **105:**10967–10972.
163. **van der Vries E, Schutten M, Boucher CA.** 2011. The potential for multidrug-resistant influenza. *Curr Opin Infect Dis* **24:**599–604.
164. **Hurt AC, Holien JK, Parker MW, Barr IG.** 2009. Oseltamivir resistance and the H274Y neuraminidase mutation in seasonal, pandemic and highly pathogenic influenza viruses. *Drugs* **69:**2523–2531.
165. **Suzuki Y, Saito R, Zaraket H, Dapat C, Caperig-Dapat I, Suzuki H.** 2010. Rapid and specific detection of amantadine-resistant influenza A viruses with a Ser31Asn mutation by the cycling probe method. *J Clin Microbiol* **48:**57–63.
166. **Dobson J, Whitley RJ, Pocock S, Monto AS.** 2015. Oseltamivir treatment for influenza in adults: a meta-analysis of randomised controlled trials. *Lancet* **385:**1729–1737.
167. **McLaughlin MM, Skoglund EW, Ison MG.** 2015. Peramivir: an intravenous neuraminidase inhibitor. *Expert Opin Pharmacother* **16:**1889–1900.
168. **Cheng PK, To AP, Leung TW, Leung PC, Lee CW, Lim WW.** 2010. Oseltamivir- and amantadine-resistant influenza virus A (H1N1). *Emerg Infect Dis* **16:**155–156.
169. **Hill G, Cihlar T, Oo C, Ho ES, Prior K, Wiltshire H, Barrett J, Liu B, Ward P.** 2002. The anti-influenza drug oseltamivir exhibits low potential to induce pharmacokinetic drug interactions via renal secretion-correlation of *in vivo* and *in vitro* studies. *Drug Metab Dispos* **30:**13–19.
170. **Fiore AE, Fry A, Shay D, Gubareva L, Bresee JS, Uyeki TM, Centers for Disease Control and Prevention (CDC).** 2011. Antiviral agents for the treatment and chemoprophylaxis of influenza: recommendations of the Advisory Committee on Immunization Practices (ACIP). *MMWR Recomm Rep* **60:**1–24
171. **Bowles SK, Lee W, Simor AE, Vearncombe M, Loeb M, Tamblyn S, Fearon M, Li Y, McGeer A, Oseltamivir Compassionate Use Program Group.** 2002. Use of oseltamivir during influenza outbreaks in Ontario nursing homes, 1999–2000. *J Am Geriatr Soc* **50:**608–616.
172. **Hayden FG, Belshe R, Villanueva C, Lanno R, Hughes C, Small I, Dutkowski R, Ward P, Carr J.** 2004. Management of influenza in households: a prospective, randomized comparison of oseltamivir treatment with or without postexposure prophylaxis. *J Infect Dis* **189:**440–449.
173. **Whitley RJ.** 2007. The role of oseltamivir in the treatment and prevention of influenza in children. *Expert Opin Drug Metab Toxicol* **3:**755–767.
174. **Wester A, Shetty AK.** 2016. Peramivir injection in the treatment of acute influenza: a review of the literature. *Infect Drug Resist* **9:**201–214.
175. **Moscona A.** 2005. Neuraminidase inhibitors for influenza. *N Engl J Med* **353:**1363–1373.
176. **Ison MG, Gnann JW Jr, Nagy-Agren S, Treannor J, Paya C, Steigbigel R, Elliott M, Weiss HL, Hayden FG, NIAID Collaborative Antiviral Study Group.** 2003. Safety and efficacy of nebulized zanamivir in hospitalized patients with serious influenza. *Antivir Ther* **8:**183–190
177. **Cass LM, Efthymiopoulos C, Bye A.** 1999. Pharmacokinetics of zanamivir after intravenous, oral, inhaled or intranasal administration to healthy volunteers. *Clin Pharmacokinet* **36**(Suppl 1)**:**1–11.

Mechanisms of Resistance to Antiviral Agents

ROBERT W. SHAFER, GUY BOIVIN, AND SUNWEN CHOU

114

Understanding the mechanisms of viral drug resistance is critical for clinical management of individuals receiving antiviral therapy, for developing new antiviral drugs, and for drug resistance surveillance. This chapter reviews the mechanisms of resistance to antiviral drugs used to treat seven common viral infections: herpes simplex (HSV), cytomegalovirus (CMV), varicella-zoster virus (VZV), human immunodeficiency virus type 1 (HIV-1), influenza A and B, hepatitis B (HBV), and hepatitis C (HCV).

Antiviral drug resistance is mediated most often by mutations in the molecular targets of drug therapy, and the development of drug resistance is the most compelling evidence that an antiviral drug acts specifically by inhibiting the virus rather than its cellular host. Drug-resistant virus subpopulations may exist at low levels in clinical isolates or may arise only during drug exposure. The error-prone polymerase enzymes in RNA viruses render the development of resistance more frequent than in DNA viruses.

Drug-resistant viruses are identified by *in vitro* passage experiments in which wild-type viruses are cultured in increasing concentrations of an inhibitory drug and by *ex vivo* analysis of virus isolates obtained from individuals receiving antiviral therapy. Measuring drug susceptibility involves culturing a fixed inoculum of virus in serial dilutions of an inhibitory drug. The drug concentration required to inhibit virus replication by 50% (EC_{50}) is the most commonly used measure of susceptibility. Drug susceptibility assays are not designed to determine the drug concentration required to inhibit virus replication *in vivo*. They are instead designed to identify viruses with reduced drug susceptibility relative to wild-type viruses. The clinical significance of reductions in drug susceptibility is determined by studying the treatment response of individuals harboring viruses with reduced susceptibility.

One of the fundamental paradigms of viral drug resistance to emerge in the past 2 decades is that antiviral drug resistance mutations often consist of major mutations that reduce drug susceptibility by themselves and accessory mutations that generally compensate for the decreased fitness associated with many of the major mutations. With a few notable exceptions, major drug resistance mutations do not occur in previously untreated patients, whereas accessory mutations are often polymorphic.

The success in developing antivirals for the treatment of chronic viral infections and the increased recognition of the threat posed by a range of acute viral infections has led to the recent identification of multiple new investigational antiviral compounds. A few of these are entering phase II and III clinical trials and may eventually be approved for treating human influenza viruses, severe respiratory syncytial virus infections, and several endemic viruses with high morbidity and/or mortality (1–4). Of interest, several of the compounds in development differ from most currently approved antivirals in that they appear to have broad-spectrum antiviral activity. For example, nitazoxanide is a repurposed antiparasitic compound which appears to have both broad-spectrum antiviral and immunomodulatory activities and has demonstrated anti-influenza activity in a phase II clinical trial (5, 6). Favipiravir and GS-5734 are inhibitors of RNA-dependent RNA polymerase, which also appear to have activity against several RNA viruses (7, 8). However, because most of these investigational antivirals are at least several years from potential FDA approval and because little is currently known about their mechanisms of resistance, they will not be reviewed in this chapter.

HERPES VIRUSES

All current FDA-approved drugs for treatment of herpesvirus infections target the viral DNA polymerase (Table 1). Nucleoside analogs that are selectively phosphorylated by viral enzymes are preferred as the initial therapy. Oral bioavailability is improved by the use of prodrugs that are metabolized to the parent drug. Acyclovir (ACV), its prodrug valacyclovir, and famciclovir, the prodrug of penciclovir (PCV), have been used successfully for genital HSV infections, VZV infections, and mucocutaneous HSV infections in immunocompromised hosts. Ganciclovir (GCV) and its prodrug valganciclovir are used to treat CMV infection. These guanosine analog antivirals are supplemented by foscarnet (phosphonoformate, FOS), a pyrophosphate analog, and cidofovir (CDV), a cytosine nucleotide analog, which do not depend on prior activation by viral enzymes. FOS and CDV are generally used as second- and third-line drugs when there is a lack of response to initial therapy. Letermovir is an orally bioavailable CMV terminase inhibitor, which recently underwent successful phase III testing for prevention of clinically significant CMV infection after hematopoietic cell transplantation (ClinicalTrials.gov identifier NCT02137772). Maribavir is an orally dosed

TABLE 1 Mechanisms and mutations associated with herpesvirus antiviral drug resistance

Virus	Antiviral agent(s)	Mechanism of resistance	Drug resistance mutations
HSV	Acyclovir, valacyclovir, penciclovir, famciclovir	TK (UL23) and/or DNA polymerase (UL30) mutations	TK frameshift (commonly at strings of multiple G or C bases) or substitution mutations causing a TK-deficient phenotype and cross-resistance among the four drugs; less commonly, TK mutations conferring altered substrate specificity, or DNA polymerase mutations clustered in palm and finger domains
	Foscarnet	DNA polymerase (UL30) mutations	Mutations clustering in palm and finger domains (including probable pyrophosphate binding regions)
	Cidofovir	DNA polymerase (UL30) mutations	Mutations in exonuclease, palm and finger domains (based on limited data from laboratory strains)
VZV	Acyclovir, valacyclovir, penciclovir, famciclovir	TK (ORF36) and/or DNA polymerase (ORF28) mutations	TK frameshift or substitution mutations causing a TK-deficient phenotype and cross-resistance among the four drugs; less commonly, TK-altered or DNA polymerase mutations
	Foscarnet	DNA polymerase (ORF28) mutations	Mutations clustering in palm and finger domains (including probable pyrophosphate binding regions)
	Cidofovir	DNA polymerase (ORF28) mutations	No VZV-specific data are available
CMV	Ganciclovir	UL97 kinase and/or DNA polymerase (UL54) mutations	Usually UL97 mutations at codons 460, 520, and 590 to 607 with M460V/I, H520Q, C592G, A594V, L595S, and C603W being most common; DNA polymerase mutations less common, mainly at exonuclease and thumb domains, e.g., at residues 408, 412, 522, 545, and 987, usually adding to preexisting UL97 mutations
	Foscarnet	DNA polymerase (UL54) mutations	Mutations in amino terminal, palm and finger domains (including probable pyrophosphate binding regions), e.g., at residues 700, 715, 756, 781, 802, and 809; some may also decrease ganciclovir ± cidofovir susceptibility
	Cidofovir	DNA polymerase (UL54) mutations	Exonuclease and thumb domains with cross-resistance to ganciclovir; low-grade cross-resistance from some foscarnet-associated mutations.
	Letermovir	Terminase gene (UL56, UL89, UL51) mutations	Usually at UL56 codons 231 to 261, 325, or 369; mutation at C325 confers absolute resistance; rare mutations in UL89 and UL51 genes observed in cell culture
	Maribavir	UL97 kinase and/ or UL27 gene mutations	UL97 mutations in ATP-binding region (codons 335 to 480), commonly T409M and H411Y/N; diverse UL27 mutations confer borderline or low-grade decreased susceptibility

inhibitor of the CMV UL97 kinase that was unsuccessful in a similar phase III clinical trial for prevention of CMV infection (NCT00411645) but at higher doses was reported to be active in subsequent phase II trials for treatment of resistant or refractory CMV infections in transplant recipients (NCT01611974), and phase III treatment trials have been initiated (NCT02931539).

Herpes Simplex Virus

ACV and PCV are initially monophosphorylated by the HSV thymidine kinase (TK), and then converted to triphosphates by cellular enzymes. ACV triphosphate causes chain termination of replicating DNA and formation of a dead-end complex that strongly inhibits the viral DNA polymerase (9). As compared with ACV, PCV triphosphate is formed at a higher concentration and persists longer in infected cells but is a less potent inhibitor of the viral DNA polymerase (10). Because the viral TK enzyme is not essential for HSV replication, a wide variety of TK mutations may decrease the phosphorylation of nucleoside analogs, and this is by far the most common mechanism of ACV and PCV resistance (11, 12). TK mutations confer no cross-resistance to drugs that act independently of virally mediated phosphorylation, including FOS and CDV.

Drug-resistant TK mutants are classified as TK negative, usually arising from frameshift or stop mutations that delete important functional domains, or TK low, where the mutation reduces the phosphorylation of both natural nucleosides and antiviral drugs (11–14). TK-altered mutants that selectively reduce the phosphorylation of antiviral nucleosides occur less commonly. Although TK mutations selected by PCV may differ from those selected by ACV, cross-resistance is expected (12, 15). Among clinical isolates, frameshifting nucleotide insertion or deletion mutations at homopolymeric TK loci (e.g., runs of G bases) are among the most common (14). TK amino acid substitutions that confer drug resistance cluster at conserved regions such as ATP and nucleoside binding sites (residues 51 to 63 and 168 to 176), while many other substitutions represent baseline polymorphism and tend to involve nonconserved residues (12). The effect of specific mutations on TK activity and drug susceptibility can be defined by site-directed mutagenesis of control strains, contributing to an increasing database (12). Mixed heterogeneous populations of resistant genotypes evolve in individual subjects (16, 17). Because of remaining uncertainties in genotypic diagnosis, phenotypic resistance assays remain in common use (11, 12).

TK-negative HSV mutants are attenuated in mouse models with respect to virulence, latency, and reactivation potential (18). However, animal studies (19) and clinical case reports (20, 21) show that resistant viruses cause overt disease and recurrent infection. Even isolates with frameshift mutations that are predicted to be TK negative may in fact express some TK activity that enables reactivation from latency (19), through such mechanisms as ribosomal frameshifting (22). Although drug-resistant HSV TK mutants can easily be selected in cell culture, the frequency of isolation of ACV-resistant HSV in clinical practice is typically <1% in immunocompetent hosts and 7 to 16% in immunocompromised hosts (23, 24). Hematopoietic cell transplant recipients are a high-risk population (24), with 28% of those with viral breakthrough during ACV prophylaxis having resistant virus in a recent prospective study (25). ACV-resistant corneal HSV isolates were found in 11 (6.4%) of 173 immunocompetent patients with keratitis (26); this may result from persistence and reactivation of virus, including resistant strains, at sanctuary sites evading normal host immune defenses (13, 17).

DNA polymerase (pol) mutations are occasionally responsible for HSV resistance to ACV, PCV, FOS, and CDV (12, 14, 27). Because the viral DNA polymerase is an essential gene for replication, mutations are more selective and usually consist of single amino acid changes in functional domains of the enzyme. Mutations conferring ACV resistance are distributed among several conserved pol regions, with clustering of mutations in palm and finger structure domains (12, 27) and frequent cross-resistance to FOS. Unlike the situation with GCV and CMV, there is no clustering of resistance mutations in the exonuclease domains of pol. Little is known about the range of CDV-resistance mutations in clinical isolates, but available information suggests that there is limited cross-resistance with ACV or FOS (11–13).

Varicella-Zoster Virus

VZV infections are generally treated with the oral prodrugs valacyclovir or famciclovir or with intravenous ACV. Drug resistance is rarely a concern in normal hosts, but immunocompromised subjects may develop prolonged and recurrent infection, increasing the risk of emergence of resistant strains after extensive antiviral treatment (11, 28, 29).

Mechanisms of VZV drug resistance are analogous to those of HSV. Most ACV-resistant VZV contains TK gene mutations that result in TK deficiency or altered substrate specificity, including stop, frameshift, and substitution mutations (11). Detection of such mutations may be used for genotypic resistance assays, since the phenotypic resistance testing of VZV clinical isolates is more limited than for HSV. Although VZV TK has less sequence polymorphism than the HSV TK (30), uncharacterized amino acid substitutions may prevent clear interpretation. Alternative drugs used for ACV-resistant VZV are usually FOS and CDV, since their antiviral activity is not TK dependent. Less commonly, ACV resistance may result from mutations clustering in the palm and finger structure domains of the VZV DNA polymerase, with some mutations conferring FOS cross-resistance (27).

Cytomegalovirus

CMV lacks a TK but does have another kinase encoded by the UL97 gene, which is essential for the production of normal amounts of infectious virus in cell culture and is a potential antiviral drug target (31). GCV, the standard initial therapy for CMV disease, is monophosphorylated by the UL97 kinase and subsequently converted to the active triphosphate form in infected cells (32). Risk factors for CMV drug resistance are prolonged viral replication as seen in immunocompromised hosts coupled with a cumulative antiviral drug exposure of several months (33). Genotypic resistance testing for CMV is standard clinical practice because of the unavailability of timely phenotypic testing on clinical isolates. An extensive database of resistance mutations validated by recombinant phenotyping (34–36) provides a basis for practice guidelines (37).

More than 90% of GCV-resistant CMV isolates contain UL97 mutations that are proven or presumed to impair GCV phosphorylation with relative preservation of biological kinase function (32). UL97 mutations in GCV-resistant CMV isolates are preferentially localized to codons 460, 520, and 590 to 607, with the seven most common mutations being M460V/I, H520Q, C592G, A594V, L595S, and C603W (36). These specific mutations confer a 5- to 10-fold increased resistance to GCV (drug EC_{50}), except for C592G, which confers a 3-fold increase. Various other point mutations and in-frame deletion mutations conferring varying degrees of GCV resistance have been observed, mainly at codons 590 to 607 (38). UL97 mutation is not known or expected to be involved in resistance to FOS or CDV.

After prolonged exposure to GCV, mutations in the UL54 DNA polymerase (pol) gene may be selected, usually adding to pre-existing UL97 mutations and contributing to an increased overall level of resistance to the drug (39, 40), although the pol mutations by themselves typically confer low-grade (2- to 5-fold) GCV resistance. Uncommonly, mutation in the pol gene may be the initial marker of GCV resistance (36). Cross-resistance to other drugs is expected for GCV-resistant pol mutants. Mutations conferring GCV and significant (up to 20-fold) CDV resistance have been reported at pol codons 301, 408 to 413, and 501 to 545, which correspond to exonuclease regions, and at codons 978 to 988 (thumb structure domain), notably A987G (36). Exonuclease mutants may bypass the usual stalling of the polymerase enzyme that occurs after the incorporation of GCV triphosphate and one additional nucleotide (41).

FOS resistance mutations are mostly located in the amino-terminal, palm, and finger structure domains of the CMV DNA polymerase, ranging from codons 552 to 982 (34–36). FOS resistance mutations generally confer 2- to 5-fold increased EC_{50} values and often a reduction in viral growth fitness. FOS resistance mutations, especially in the finger domain, may confer low-grade GCV ± CDV cross-resistance (36), likely involving polymerase residues with roles in recognition of the incoming nucleotide triphosphate and in pyrophosphate exchange. Uncommonly, single pol mutations (e.g., A834P or 981-2del) are sufficient to confer significant resistance to all three drugs—GCV, CDV, and FOS (34–36). Despite a large database of baseline sequence polymorphisms and phenotyped mutants, there remain a number of pol sequence variants of unclear relevance for drug resistance that require characterization by recombinant phenotyping (42).

Letermovir resistance mutations primarily map to the UL56 component of the CMV terminase complex. Most of the current information derives from *in vitro* selection experiments (43, 44), where numerous mutations in the UL56 codon range of 229 to 369 readily emerge to confer varying degrees of resistance. Absolute resistance (EC_{50} increased by >3,000-fold, approaching cytotoxic concentrations) commonly results from a single step mutation at codon 325 causing amino acid substitutions such as C325F/R/Y (43, 44) but can also arise from a combination of other mutations. The C325 mutants retain near normal growth fitness *in vitro* (43, 44). The frequency and distribution of mutations in clinical use of letermovir have not yet been defined. The first one to be reported from a clinical trial is UL56 V236M (45), which confers 30- to 45-fold increased EC_{50}.

Mutations arising after maribavir exposure to confer substantial drug resistance map to the ATP binding site of the UL97 kinase drug target (46). Among the most commonly encountered *in vitro* and in treated subjects are T409M, which confers ~80-fold increased EC_{50}, and H411N/Y, which confer 9- to 12-fold increased EC_{50} (46–48). These UL97 mutations do not confer GCV cross-resistance (46), but mutation at codon 342 within the p-loop has been reported to confer dual maribavir-GCV resistance without knocking out UL97 kinase activity (49). Diverse mutations in a separate gene, UL27, may confer low-grade maribavir resistance (50), probably by modulating host cell metabolism in a way that affects the antiviral activity of maribavir (51).

HUMAN IMMUNODEFICIENCY VIRUS

Of the approximately 30 FDA-approved antiretroviral (ARV) drugs, the most commonly used include (i) six nucleoside reverse transcriptase (RT) inhibitors (NRTIs): the cytosine analogs lamivudine and emtricitabine, the tenofovir prodrugs tenofovir disoproxil fumarate and tenofovir alafenamide, and abacavir and zidovudine; (ii) three nonnucleoside RT inhibitors (NNRTIs): efavirenz, rilpivirine, and etravirine; (iii) three pharmacologically boosted protease inhibitors (PIs): ritonavir-boosted lopinavir and ritonavir- or cobicistat (a CYP4503A inhibitor)-boosted atazanavir, and ritonavir- or cobicistat-boosted darunavir; and (iv) four integrase inhibitors (INIs), also referred to as integrase strand transfer inhibitors (INSTIs): raltegravir, elvitegravir, dolutegravir, and bictegravir. In addition, two approved entry inhibitors, the fusion inhibitor enfuvirtide and the CCR5 inhibitor maraviroc, are used in a number of limited clinical situations (Table 2). Because tenofovir

TABLE 2 Genetic mechanisms of resistance to ARV agents

Drug class	Mechanism(s)	DRMs[a]
NRTIs[b]	(i) Mutations that allow RT to discriminate between NRTIs and cellular nucleoside triphosphates (ii) Mutations that promote ATP-dependent hydrolytic removal of chain-terminating nucleotide monophosphates; also called TAMs	Abacavir (ABC): K65R/N, K70E/Q/G, L74V/I, Y115F, M184V/I; multiple TAMs including T215Y/F; MDR mutations Emtricitabine (FTC) and lamivudine (3TC): M184V/I >> K65R/N >> MDR mutations Tenofovir (TDF) and tenofovir alafenamide (TAF): K65R/N, K70E/Q/G, Y115F; multiple TAMs, including T215Y/F; MDR mutations Zidovudine (AZT, ZDV): TAMs; MDR mutations
NNRTIs	Mutations in the NNRTI-binding pocket of RT that interfere with inhibitor binding	Nevirapine (NVP): K101E/P, K103N/S, V106A/M, Y181C/I/V, Y188L/C/H, G190A/S/E/Q, F227L/C, and M230L Efavirenz (EFV): L100I, K101E/P, K103N/S, V106A/M, Y188L/C/H, G190A/S/E/Q, P225H, F227C, and M230L Etravirine (ETR): L100I, K101E/P, Y181C/I/V, G190E/Q, F227C, and M230L Rilpivirine (RPV): L100I, K101E/P, E138A/G/K/Q/R, Y181C/I/V, Y188L, G190E/Q, F227C, and M230L Accessory DRMs: A98G, K101H, V108I, V179D/E/F, and K238T
PIs[c]	Protease mutations in or near the substrate cleft that interfere with inhibitor binding or compensate for the decreased replication associated with substrate cleft mutations	Atazanavir (ATV/r): V32I, M46I/L, I47V, G48V/M, I50L, I54V/T/A/S/L/M, V82A/C/F/M/S/T, I84V/A/C, N88S, and L90M Darunavir (DRV/r): V32I, I47V/A, I50V, I54L/M, L76V, and I84/V/A/C Lopinavir (LPV/r): L24I, V32I, M46I/L, I47V/A, G48V/M, I50V, I54V/T/A/S/L/M, L76V, V82A/C/F/M/S/T, I84A/C/V, and L90M Accessory DRMs: L10F, V11I/L, K20T, L33F, G73/S/T/C/A, T74P, and L89V
INIs	Mutations in residues surrounding the enzyme's active site	Raltegravir (RAL): T66K, E92Q, G118R, F121Y, Y143C/R/H/A/G/K/S, Q148H/R/K, and N155H Elvitegravir (EVG): T66A/I/K, E92Q, G118R, F121Y, P145S, Q146P, S147G, Q148H/R/K, N155H, and R263K Dolutegravir (DTG): T66K, E92Q, G118R, Q148H/R/K, N155H, and R263K Bictegravir (BIC): Preliminary data suggest a profile similar to DTG Accessory mutations: H51Y, L74F/M, Q95K, T97A, E138A/K/T, G140S/A/C, S153F/Y, E157Q, G163R/K, and S230R
Fusion inhibitor (enfuvirtide)	Mutations in the first heptad repeat region (HR1) of the gp41 transmembrane protein that interfere with inhibitor binding	Gp41 mutations: G36D/E/S/V, I37V, V38A/E/G/M, Q48H, N42T, N43D/K/S, L44M, and L45M
CCR5 inhibitor (maraviroc)	Expansion of preexisting CXCR4-tropic variants that were not detected before therapy gp120 mutations that facilitate gp120 binding to an inhibitor-bound CCR5 molecule	CXCR4-tropic gp120 variants: Positively charged residues at positions 11 and 25 of the V3 loop of gp120 and several other combinations of mutations primarily but not exclusively within the V3 loop are associated with CXCR4 tropism There is no consistent pattern of gp120 mutations associated with virus binding to an inhibitor-bound CCR5 receptor

[a]TAMs (thymidine analog mutations): M41L, D67N, K70R, L210W, T215F/Y, K219Q/E. Multidrug-resistance (MDR) mutations: (i) Q151M ± A62V, V75I, F77L, F116Y; (ii) T69S_SS (insertion) ± ≥1 TAMs.

[b]Because of their toxicities, the NRTIs didanosine (ddI) and stavudine (d4T) are no longer routinely recommended for ARV therapy and are in fact usually contraindicated. The susceptibility of both ARVs is reduced by most discriminatory DRMs and combinations of TAMs, although M184V/I increase stavudine susceptibility (https://hivdb.stanford.edu/dr-summary/resistance-notes/NRTI/).

[c]There are few, if any, remaining indications for the PIs fosamprenavir, indinavir, nelfinavir, saquinavir, and tipranavir (73). The nelfinavir-associated DRMs D30N and N88D were once among the most commonly observed DRMs when nelfinavir was in widespread use. These two DRMs are still occasionally observed in cases of transmitted drug resistance. N88D is associated with potential low-level atazanavir resistance. There are several scenarios in which viruses that are resistant to atazanavir, darunavir, and lopinavir retain susceptibility to tipranavir. Specifically, the DRMs I50V, I54L, and L76V are darunavir-resistance mutations that increase tipranavir susceptibility (https://hivdb.stanford.edu/dr-summary/resistance-notes/PI/).

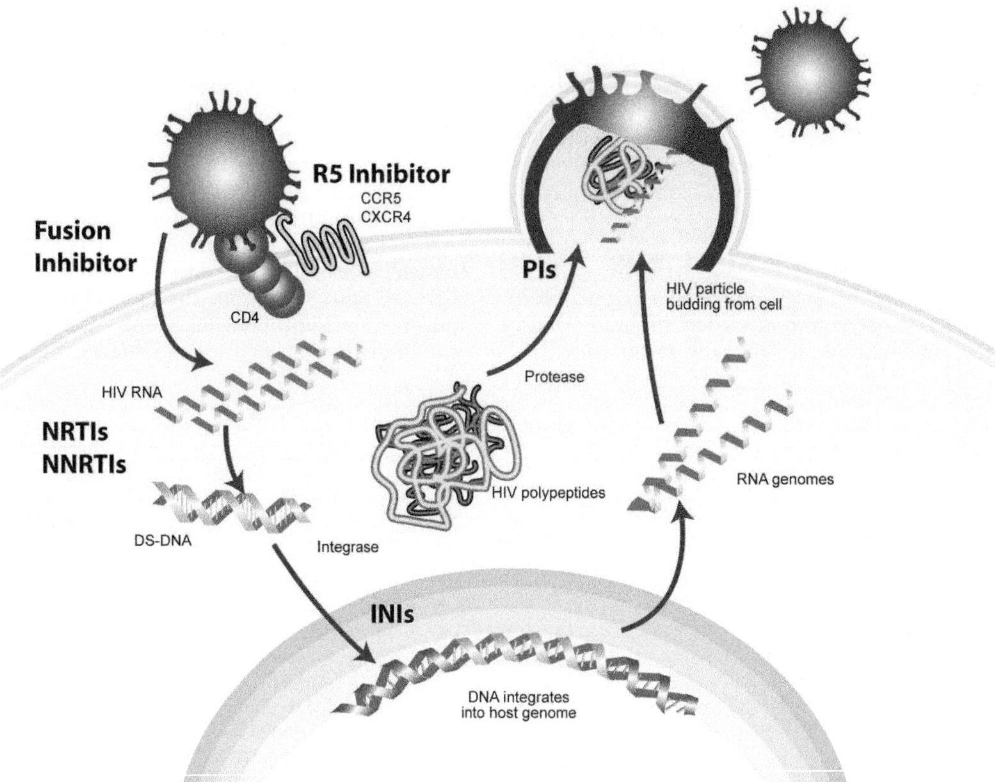

FIGURE 1 Simplified version of the HIV-1 replication cycle showing the steps at which the six approved classes of antiretroviral drugs act: fusion inhibitor, CCR5 (chemokine receptor) inhibitor, NRTIs (nucleoside reverse transcriptase inhibitors), NNRTIs (nonnucleoside reverse transcriptase inhibitors), INIs (integrase inhibitors), and PIs (protease inhibitors).

disoproxil fumarate and tenofovir alafenamide have similar resistance profiles, they will henceforth both be referred to as tenofovir. Although tenofovir alafenamide achieves higher intracellular levels than tenofovir disoproxil fumarate, it has not been shown to have greater activity against tenofovir-resistant strains. Figure 1 depicts the steps in the HIV-1 replication cycle at which each of the ARV classes act.

HIV-1 genetic variability results from the high rate of RT enzyme errors, the high rate of virus replication *in vivo*, recombination when viruses with different sequences infect the same cell, and the accumulation of proviral variants during the course of infection. The virus population within an individual consists of an ensemble of innumerable related genotypes often called a quasispecies. The selection of drug-resistant variants depends on the extent to which virus replication continues during incompletely suppressive therapy, the ease of acquisition of a particular mutation, and the effect of drug-resistance mutations on drug susceptibility and virus replication (52).

In previously untreated individuals with drug-susceptible HIV-1, a number of different drug combinations lead to prolonged virus suppression and, in most patients, immune reconstitution. Once complete HIV-1 suppression is achieved, it usually persists indefinitely if therapy is not interrupted. However, because ARV therapy does not inhibit proviral HIV-1 DNA, viral eradication is not possible. Recurrent viremia and immunological decline ensue whenever therapy is discontinued, regardless of the previous duration of virological suppression.

HIV-1 drug resistance may be acquired or transmitted. Drug resistance is acquired in patients in whom ongoing virus replication occurs in the presence of incompletely suppressive therapy. Whereas incompletely suppressive therapy was once a consequence of an insufficient number of active drugs, it is now usually a consequence of incomplete adherence. The proportion of HIV-1-infected people with transmitted NRTI or NNRTI resistance is about 15% in North America and up to 10% or higher in many other regions including Europe, Australia, parts of South and Central America, the Caribbean, and several countries in sub-Saharan Africa (53, 54). The presence of either acquired or transmitted drug resistance before starting a new ARV treatment regimen is associated with reduced virological response to that regimen (55).

NRTI Resistance

NRTIs must be triphosphorylated (or diphosphorylated in the case of the nucleotide analog tenofovir) to their active form. The dependence of NRTIs on intracellular phosphorylation complicates the *in vitro* assessment of their activity because phosphorylation occurs at different rates in the highly activated lymphocytes used for susceptibility testing and the wider variety of cells infected *in vivo*, explaining why NRTI resistance levels differ in their dynamic ranges (56). Specifically, clinical isolates from people failing NRTI therapy may have several hundred-fold reductions in susceptibility to zidovudine, lamivudine, and emtricitabine but rarely have more than 5- to 10-fold reductions in susceptibility to abacavir and tenofovir. Slight reductions in susceptibility to this second category of drugs, however, are clinically significant.

There are two biochemical mechanisms of NRTI resistance. One mechanism is mediated by discriminatory mutations that reduce RT affinity for an NRTI, preventing its addition to the growing DNA chain (57). Another mechanism is mediated by mutations that facilitate primer unblocking through the phosphorolytic removal of NRTIs incorporated into the HIV-1 primer chain (58). Primer unblocking mutations, because they are selected by the thymidine analog inhibitors zidovudine and stavudine, are also referred to as thymidine analog mutations (TAMs). The most common TAMs include M41L, D67N, K70R, L210W, T215Y/F, and K219Q/E. A subset of these mutations—M41L, L210W, and T215Y—is associated with greater cross-resistance to abacavir and tenofovir (59, 60). Although thymidine analogs are now used infrequently, particularly in high-income countries, TAMs remain common because they often persist in individuals who have been treated for many years and because many are readily transmissible.

Lamivudine and emtricitabine have a low genetic barrier to resistance in that a single mutation—the discriminatory mutation M184V (or less commonly, M184I)—confers >200-fold reduced susceptibility to these drugs. Indeed, M184V is the most common mutation to emerge in patients developing virological failure on a first-line regimen. Although M184V limits the antiviral activity of lamivudine and emtricitabine, they retain efficacy because M184V reduces HIV-1 fitness and increases susceptibility to zidovudine and tenofovir (56, 61).

In patients receiving regimens without thymidine analogs, K65R, K70E/Q/G, L74V/I, and Y115F are the mutations that occur most commonly in combination with M184V (62). K65R reduces susceptibility to tenofovir, abacavir, lamivudine, and emtricitabine and increases susceptibility to zidovudine (63). L74V/I reduces abacavir susceptibility. Y115F reduces abacavir and tenofovir susceptibility. K65N and K70E/Q/G reduce susceptibility to tenofovir and abacavir.

T69SSS and Q151M are multi-NRTI resistance mutations. T69SSS is a double amino insertion at HIV-1 RT position 69, which usually occurs with multiple TAMs, and in this setting, it causes intermediate resistance to lamivudine and emtricitabine and high-level resistance to the remaining NRTIs (64). Q151M usually occurs in combination with several otherwise uncommon mutations (A62V, V75I, F77L, and F116Y). It causes intermediate resistance to tenofovir, lamivudine, and emtricitabine and high-level resistance to the remaining NRTIs (65, 66). Amino acid deletions between codons 67 and 70 are also associated with multi-NRTI resistance. Deletions at codon 67 generally occur with multiple TAMs or Q151M (67). Deletions at codon 69 generally occur with K65R or Q151M (67).

NNRTI Resistance

The NNRTIs inhibit HIV-1 RT allosterically by binding to a hydrophobic pocket about 10 angstroms from its active site (57). This hydrophobic NNRTI-binding pocket is less well conserved than the enzyme's dNTP-binding active site. Indeed, HIV-2 and many HIV-1 group O viruses are intrinsically resistant to most NNRTIs, and HIV-1 group M viruses have greater interisolate variability in their susceptibility to NNRTIs than to NRTIs (68).

Resistance emerges rapidly when NNRTIs are administered as monotherapy, suggesting that NNRTI resistance can be caused by the selection of preexisting low-abundance populations of mutant viruses. For example, a single dose of nevirapine used to prevent mother-to-child HIV transmission often selected for NNRTI-resistant mutants that were detected by standard sequencing for several months and that interfered with the subsequent response to an NNRTI-containing treatment regimen (69).

Nevirapine and efavirenz have low genetic barriers to resistance in that a single mutation in the NNRTI-binding pocket may result in high-level resistance. Etravirine has a higher genetic barrier to resistance in that two or more mutations are usually required to cause high-level resistance (70). Etravirine's higher genetic barrier to resistance is a result of its ability to rearrange itself, thereby adopting multiple binding modes within the NNRTI-binding pocket (71). Although rilpivirine has a similar structure to etravirine, its genetic barrier to clinically significant resistance is lower than that of etravirine because it is administered at a much lower dose.

The most common major NNRTI mutations are L100I, K101E/P, K103N/S, V106A/M, Y181C/I/V, Y188C/H/L, G190A/S/E/Q, and M230L (72, 73). With the exception of Y181C/I/V, each confers intermediate- or high-level reductions in susceptibility to efavirenz. L100I, K101E/P, Y181C/I/V, G190E, and M230L reduce susceptibility to etravirine and rilpivirine, and Y188L reduces susceptibility to rilpivirine but not etravirine. In addition, the previously unrecognized mutations E138K/G/Q/A are among the most common mutations to emerge in patients receiving rilpivirine (74). Although these mutations reduce rilpivirine susceptibility only minimally, they are among the most common mutations to emerge in patients with virological failure on a rilpivirine-containing regimen.

PI Resistance

Of the nine FDA-approved PIs, ritonavir is administered solely at subtherapeutic doses to increase the tissue concentrations of other PIs via its inhibition of the cytochrome P4503A pathway. Of the remaining eight PIs, lopinavir (which is coformulated with ritonavir) and ritonavir- or cobicistat-boosted atazanavir and darunavir are used most frequently.

More than 80 nonpolymorphic PI-selected mutations have been reported (75). Most of these reduce susceptibility to one or more PIs (76). Mutations in the substrate cleft, including D30N, V32I, I47V/A, G48V/M, I50V/L, V82A/T/L/F/S, and I84V, reduce PI binding affinity. Several mutations in the enzyme flap, including M46I/L and I54V/M/L/T/S/A, and in the enzyme core, including L76V and N88S, also markedly reduce susceptibility. These and other accessory mutations indirectly reshape the substrate cleft or compensate for the decreased kinetics of enzymes with substrate cleft mutations (77). Compensatory mutations at several Gag cleavage sites are also selected during PI treatment (78).

Ritonavir-boosted lopinavir and, in particular, ritonavir- or cobicistat-boosted darunavir have high genetic barriers to resistance, with multiple mutations required before antiviral activity is compromised (79, 80). Lopinavir/r alone and darunavir/r alone are each effective at fully suppressing the HIV-1 RNA level below detectable levels for 48 weeks in most patients, and monotherapy with these PIs is a highly effective simplification regimen (81). Viruses from patients with virological failure on an initial boosted-PI-containing regimen rarely contain PI-resistance mutations, suggesting that such virological failure may often result from nonadherence rather than PI resistance (82, 83). Indeed, a high proportion of such patients often experience resuppression of virus levels without a change in therapy (84, 85).

INI Resistance

Following reverse transcription and the generation of double-stranded viral DNA, HIV-1 IN catalyzes the cleavage of the conserved 3′ dinucleotide CA (3′ processing) and the ligation of the viral 3′-OH ends to the 5′-DNA of host chromosomal DNA (strand transfer). HIV-1 IN is composed of three functional domains: the N-terminal domain encompassing amino acids 1 to 50; the catalytic core domain (CCD), which encompasses amino acids 51 to 212 and contains the catalytic triad D64, D116, and E152; and the C-terminal domain, which encompasses amino acids 213 to 288 and binds host DNA nonspecifically. IN strand transfer inhibitors bind the CCD active site and chelate the divalent metal ions critical for enzymatic function. Raltegravir was licensed in 2008. Elvitegravir was licensed in 2012 as a fixed-dose combination (FDC) with the CYP3A4 inhibitor cobicistat and the NRTIs tenofovir and emtricitabine. Dolutegravir was licensed in 2013 by itself and as an FDC with abacavir and lamivudine. Bictegravir was licensed in 2018 as a fixed-dose combination with tenofovir alafenamide and emtricitabine.

There are crystal structures of the CCD plus C-terminal domain, the CCD plus N-terminal domain, and the CCD bound to the prototype diketo acid inhibitor 5CITEP (86–88). But the relative conformation of the CCD, N-terminal domain, and C-terminal domain and the tetrameric functional form of HIV-1 IN have been inferred primarily from crystallographic studies of the homologous IN of the prototype foamy virus (89) and more recently of a cryo-electron microscopic structure showing the catalytically active HIV-1 IN strand-transfer complex catalytically joined to viral and target DNA (90).

Many of the mutations with the greatest effect on reducing INI susceptibility are highly conserved residues in the INI binding site and residues 140 to 149, which form a flexible loop that is important for catalysis following IN-DNA binding. Q148 interacts with a 5′ terminal cytosine of viral DNA and likely forms a hydrogen bond with most INIs (88, 91). N155 points into the active site and forms a hydrogen bond with D116, one of the three catalytic aspartate residues (92). Y143 is part of the highly flexible active site loop that participates in DNA and INI binding.

There are three main overlapping genetic pathways to raltegravir resistance: (i) Q148H/R/K ± G140S/A/C ± E138A/K, (ii) N155H ± E92Q, and (iii) Y143C/R ± T97A (93, 94). Elvitegravir resistance is caused primarily by the first two mutational pathways and by T66A/I/K and S147G (95). Dolutegravir has a high genetic barrier to resistance. Most reports of clinically significant phenotypic resistance to dolutegravir were in patients with previous virological failure on a raltegravir-containing regimen. In these patients, the most common mutations associated with resistance included Q148H/R/K in combination with E138A/K/T ± G140A/C/S (96). However, as dolutegravir use has expanded, there has been a gradually increasing number of reports of dolutegravir resistance associated with other INI resistance mutations including N155H as well as with two uncommon mutations, G118R and R263K, that have been selected by dolutegravir *in vitro* and in a small number of patients receiving dolutegravir monotherapy (97–101). The clinical significance of these mutations is not well understood because they cause a minimal 2-fold or less reduction in dolutegravir susceptibility, are associated with reduced viral replication, and rarely occur in combination with other dolutegravir resistance mutations. Preliminary studies suggest that there is a high correlation between the phenotypic effects of INI drug-resistance mutations on dolutegravir and the recently approved INI bictegravir (102).

Fusion Inhibitor Resistance

The HIV-1 envelope consists of surface (gp120) and transmembrane (gp41) glycoproteins. gp120 binds to the CD4 receptor and to one of the chemokine coreceptors (CCR5 or CXCR4) on target cells. After gp120-CD4-coreceptor binding, gp41 undergoes a conformational change that promotes fusion of viral and cellular membranes. Two heptad repeat regions (HR1 and HR2) of gp41 form a helical bundle that contains trimers belonging to HR1 and HR2. Enfuvirtide is a highly active synthetic peptide that inhibits fusion by binding to HR1 and preventing its bundling with HR2.

Enfuvirtide-resistant isolates contain either single or double mutations between positions 36 and 45 of gp41 HR1 (103, 104). Single mutants typically have on the order of 10-fold reduced enfuvirtide susceptibility, whereas double mutants typically have on the order of 100-fold reduced susceptibility. Despite being one of the most potent inhibitors, the genetic barrier to enfuvirtide resistance is low, with virological rebound emerging rapidly when enfuvirtide is not administered with a sufficient number of other active inhibitors (105).

CCR5 Inhibitor Resistance

Maraviroc allosterically inhibits gp120 *env* of CCR5-tropic HIV-1 strains from binding to the seven-transmembrane G protein-coupled CCR5 receptor (106). Whereas HIV-1 gp120 binds to the N terminus and second extracellular loop region of CCR5, maraviroc binds to a pocket formed by the transmembrane helices (106). In patients receiving CCR5 inhibitors, the most common mechanism of virological failure is the expansion of preexisting CXCR4 tropic viruses that are intrinsically resistant to CCR5 inhibitors (107). Positively charged residues at positions 11 and 25 of the V3 loop of gp120 and several less common combinations of mutations primarily but not exclusively within the V3 loop are associated with CXCR4 tropism (108).

During *in vitro* passage experiments, CCR5 inhibitor resistance develops by a different mechanism—gp120 mutations that enable HIV-1 to bind to the CCR5/CCR5-inhibitor complex, resulting in a plateau in the maximal percent inhibition at maximal CCR5 inhibitor concentrations (109). This mechanism of resistance occurs rarely in patients, and when it does, it is not associated with a consistent pattern of responsible mutations (110).

Intersubtype Variation

During its spread among humans, group M HIV-1 has evolved into multiple subtypes that differ from one another by 10 to 30% along their genomes (111). HIV-1 protease and RT of different subtypes differ by 10 to 12% of their nucleotides and 5 to 6% of their amino acids. Naturally occurring polymorphisms differ among subtypes, but these polymorphisms do not appear to be responsible for clinically significant effects on drug susceptibility.

Subtype B viruses comprise 95% of HIV-1 strains in the United States and 60% of strains in Europe but only about 10% of strains worldwide. Subtype B viruses played an outsized role in the earliest ARV development efforts and in the earliest studies of ARV resistance. Nonetheless, existing ARVs appear equally effective at treating subtype B and nonsubtype B viruses. Moreover, with several notable exceptions, most HIV-1 drug-resistance mutations occur in similar proportions in different subtypes (76). For example, subtype C viruses have a unique polyadenine stretch between codons 63 and 65, which predisposes them to substitute a guanosine triphosphate (G) for an adenosine trisphosphate (A) at the second position of codon 65 after tenofovir exposure, resulting in the drug-resistance mutation K65R (112, 113). Most other examples of preferentially selected drug-resistance mutations result from intersubtype differences in codon usage. For example, in efavirenz-treated individuals, the NNRTI-resistance mutation V106M occurs much more often in subtype C viruses than in other subtypes because V106M requires a single-base-pair change in subtype C viruses, GTG (V) → ATG (M), but a two-base-pair change in all other subtypes, GTA (V) → ATG (M) (114).

HEPATITIS B VIRUS

HBV is a partially double-stranded DNA virus of about 3.2 kb. Following infection, its genome localizes to the nucleus, where it is converted to the covalently closed circular DNA (cccDNA) form that serves as a template for transcription of mRNA and genomic RNA. Genomic RNA is then reverse-transcribed to viral DNA, and the resulting viral cores either bud into the endoplasmic reticulum and are exported from the cell or return to the nucleus for conversion back to cccDNA. HBV cccDNA can be eliminated by cell turnover but not by drug therapy, and therefore eradication of infection occurs infrequently (115–117).

HBV replicates at a high rate, producing about 10^{11} virions per day (118). In the absence of therapy, HBV DNA levels are often as high as 10^8 to 10^{10} copies/ml. HBV polymerase, because it has RT activity, is functionally and structurally similar to HIV-1 RT and has an error rate similar to that of other retroviruses (119). However, the overlapping arrangement of open reading frames in the HBV genome limits the viability of many spontaneous mutants (120). For example, the nucleotides encoding the HBV polymerase also encode the HBV envelope in a different reading frame. Therefore, the rate at which mutations become fixed is considerably lower than that for HIV-1 (121).

HBV is classified into at least eight genotypes differing from one another by about 10% of their nucleotides. Several small studies suggest that viruses belonging to different genotypes may respond differently to interferon or differ in their predilection for certain drug-resistance mutations, but there is no evidence that genotype influences the likelihood of responding virologically to drug therapy (122–126).

Anti-HBV Drug Therapy

There are two forms of interferon and six nucleoside analogs approved for the treatment of chronic HBV infection (Table 3). Alpha interferon was approved in 1992, and pegylated alpha interferon 2a was approved in 2005. Pegylated interferon remains an important treatment option because 1 year of therapy offers the possibility of sustained virological remission (127). Lamivudine (in 1998), adefovir (in 2002), entecavir (in 2005), telbivudine (in 2006), tenofovir (in 2008), and tenofovir alafenamide (in 2015) have also been approved. Tenofovir and tenofovir alafenamide have similar indications and drug-resistance profiles. The ARV drug emtricitabine, which is similar to lamivudine in its chemical structure and antiviral activity, is also used for HBV treatment because it is coformulated with tenofovir and tenofovir alafenamide for treating HIV-1.

The preferred treatment regimens are monotherapy with entecavir, tenofovir, or tenofovir alafenamide. Each of these drugs is a potent HBV inhibitor. Drug resistance has never developed in patients receiving tenofovir or tenofovir alafenamide for initial therapy and has only very rarely developed in patients receiving entecavir for initial therapy (127–130). The recently approved inhibitor tenofovir alafenamide has demonstrated efficacy similar to tenofovir and is associated with reduced evidence of renal dysfunction and osteopenia (127, 131).

The use of lamivudine, adefovir, and telbivudine has diminished greatly because of the high incidence of virological failure and drug resistance associated with long-term therapy with these drugs. Lamivudine resistance develops in 15 to 30% of patients treated for 3 years, 40 to 50% of patients treated for 3 years, and 70% of patients treated for 5 years (132). Telbivudine resistance develops in 25% of patients treated for 2 years (133). Adefovir resistance develops in 10% and 30% of patients after 2 and 5 years, respectively (134).

HBV RT and NRTI Resistance

Homology modeling suggests that HBV polymerase shares regions similar to the fingers, palm, and thumb

TABLE 3 Genetic mechanisms of resistance to inhibitors of HBV[a]

Drug class	Mechanism(s)	DRMs
Interferon	Unknown	Unknown
NRTIs	Mutations that allow RT to discriminate between NRTIs and naturally occurring nucleoside triphosphates; whether some of these mutations also cause primer unblocking is not known	L-nucleosides: Lamivudine (LAM, 3TC): M204I/V, L180M + M204V, and A181T/V Telbivudine (LDT): M204I, L180M + M204V, and A181T/V Accessory DRMs: L80I, I169T, V173L, T184G, S202G/I, and M250V
		Deoxyguanosine analog: Entecavir (ETV): M204I/V + L180M Accessory DRMs: L80I, I169T, V173L, T184G, S202G/I, and M250V
		Acyclic nucleotides: Adefovir (ADV): A181T/V and N236T Tenofovir (TDF): A181T/V and N236T Tenofovir alafenamide (TAF): A181T/V and N236T

[a]Emtricitabine (FTC) is not FDA approved for the treatment of HBV. Its activity and cross-resistance profile are similar to those of lamivudine. It is frequently used in combination with tenofovir to treat HIV coinfected patients.

configuration of HIV-1 (135, 136). High-level (>1,000-fold) lamivudine resistance is caused by a mutation, M204V/I, which is in the YMDD motif, characteristic of all RTs, and which is analogous to M184V/I, the HIV-1 lamivudine-resistance mutations (137, 138). M204V/I mutations are also frequently accompanied by compensatory mutations, particularly L180M (126). M204V/I mutations cause high-level cross-resistance to emtricitabine and telbivudine but do not reduce susceptibility to the acyclic nucleotides, adefovir and tenofovir (137, 138). Although viruses with M204V/I replicate less well than wild-type viruses, the development of M204V/I is associated with virological and clinical progression (139, 140).

Adefovir and tenofovir retain complete *in vitro* susceptibility to viruses with M204V/I and their associated mutations (141, 142). However, because tenofovir and tenofovir alafenamide are more potent than adefovir and have a higher genetic barrier to resistance, they are recommended for treating patients with lamivudine resistance (137). Adefovir resistance is caused by the mutations N236T and A181V/T (143–145). Although the levels of reduced susceptibility associated with these mutations—3- to 10-fold—are much lower than the levels of M204V/I-associated lamivudine resistance, these reductions are associated with virological breakthrough in patients receiving adefovir (143). N236T confers low-level cross-resistance to tenofovir and tenofovir alafenamide but not to lamivudine, entecavir, or telbivudine (146, 147).

A181V and A181T emerge with lamivudine and more commonly with adefovir (144, 148, 149). A181T causes a stop codon in the S protein reading frame, potentially allowing for ongoing hepatocellular replication without accompanying viral load rebound (150). Isolates with these mutations remain susceptible to entecavir but have minimally reduced *in vitro* cross-resistance to tenofovir and tenofovir alafenamide (137, 147, 151).

High-level etravirine resistance results from the combination of M204V/I plus L180I and one or more of the following mutations: I169T, T184G, S202I, and M250V (137, 147, 152). Although entecavir retains considerable antiviral activity against lamivudine-resistant variants, the risk of virological failure and emergence of high-level entecavir resistance is significant when entecavir is used to treat patients with lamivudine-resistance mutations (125, 153–156).

Although tenofovir retains considerable antiviral activity in patients with adefovir-resistance mutations, the virological response to tenofovir monotherapy is slower than in patients without such mutations (157, 158). Therefore, in patients with adefovir-resistance mutations but without a history of lamivudine or lamivudine-resistance mutations, entecavir alone is usually recommended. However, in patients with multidrug resistance, tenofovir (or tenofovir alafenamide) plus either lamivudine, emtricitabine, or entecavir is recommended (147, 156, 159). However, once viral suppression occurs, tenofovir or tenofovir alafenamide alone may be sufficient for long-term therapy (160).

HEPATITIS C

HCV is a positive-sense, single-stranded enveloped virus with a genome of about 9.5 kb. HCV replication occurs in a membrane-associated cytoplasmic replicase complex, consisting of the nonstructural proteins NS3 protease, NS4A protease cofactor, NS5B RNA-dependent RNA polymerase (RdRp), and two membrane-associated proteins, NS4B and NS5A. NS4B is a membrane anchor protein, and NS5A plays an essential role in modulating RdRp function and has multiple interactions with host proteins (161). After synthesizing a negative-sense RNA intermediate, multiple positive-sense progeny RNAs are generated for either RNA translation or incorporation into virus particles (161).

There are six main human HCV genotypes, differing from one another by >30% of their genomes, and two recently described but extremely rare genotypes (162, 163). Each of these six main genotypes can be subdivided into subtypes that differ from one another by >15% of their genomes (162). HCV genotypes 1 and 3 (GT1 and GT3) account for an estimated 46% and 30% of worldwide infections, respectively (163). Like other RdRps, HCV polymerase has a high error rate, estimated at 10^{-4} substitutions per nucleotide per round of replication (164). HCV exists *in vivo* as an ensemble of viral genomes differing from one another by up to 5 to 10%, referred to as quasispecies (165).

HCV plasma levels typically range from $10^{4.5}$ to $10^{6.5}$ IU/ml. HCV has an estimated half-life of less than 3 hours, and in the absence of antiviral therapy, up to 10^{12} virions are produced daily (166). HCV persists in up to 70 to 80% of untreated infected people. The absence of a stable intracellular reservoir, however, makes viral eradication possible. Indeed, the absence of detectable plasma virus at 12 and/or 24 weeks following a treatment regimen constitutes a sustained virological response (SVR) and usually a virological cure (167).

HCV has been studied *in vitro* using stably transfected replicons capable of autonomous replication but unable to produce infectious HCV particles and using chimeric versions of the unique JFH-1 infectious clone (168–170). These assays have been essential for discovering antiviral agents, quantifying their inhibitory activity, selecting drug resistance mutations, and assessing the phenotypic effects of various mutations (168–170).

Anti-HCV Therapy

Prior to 2011, pegylated interferon plus ribavirin for 6 to 12 months was the only recommended treatment for HCV. In 2011, the first-generation PIs telaprevir and boceprevir became the first FDA-approved directly acting agents (DAAs) approved for use in combination with pegylated interferon plus ribavirin for treating GT1 HCV. Combinations of these PIs with interferon and ribavirin increased the cure rate for GT1 to about 70% but were associated with a high frequency of toxicity and PI resistance. Interferon and the first-generation PIs have since been replaced by newer DAAs that when used in FDCs achieve SVR rates that are usually >95%.

Between 2013 and 2017, 13 DAAs were approved by the FDA: the nucleotide analog RdRp inhibitor (NI; sofosbuvir), five PIs (simeprevir, paritaprevir, grazoprevir, glecaprevir, and voxilaprevir), six NS5A inhibitors (daclatasvir, ledipasvir, ombitasvir, elbasvir, velpatasvir, and pibrentasvir), and the nonnucleoside RdRp inhibitor dasabuvir (Table 4). Sofosbuvir is available alone and as part of three FDCs. The PI simeprevir (171) and the NS5A inhibitor daclatasvir (172) are available only alone. The remaining DAAs are available in FDCs or, in the case of dasabuvir, used with an FDC.

Current FDCs recommended for initial therapy include (i) sofosbuvir/ledipasvir for GT1 and GT4 viruses (173), (ii) ritonavir-boosted paritaprevir (paritaprevir/r)/ombitasvir plus dasabuvir for GT1 viruses and paritaprevir/r/ombitasvir for GT4 viruses (174), (iii) grazoprevir/elbasvir for GT1 and GT4 viruses (175); (iv) sofosbuvir/velpatasvir for all genotypes (176), and (v) glecaprevir/pibrentasvir for all genotypes (177). Sofosbuvir/velpatasvir/voxilaprevir is

TABLE 4 Genetic mechanisms of resistance to HCV inhibitors

Drug class	Mechanism(s)	RASs[a]
Interferon	Viral and host genotypic factors	None
Ribavirin	None known	None
Nucleos(t)ide inhibitors	NS5B mutations near the active site that inhibit nucleoside analog incorporation	Sofosbuvir (SOF): L159F, S282T, and V321A Accessory RASs: C316N and L320F
NNIs	NS5B mutations that prevent binding to the NNI binding pockets	Dasabuvir: C316Y, M414I/T, C451R, A553T, G554S, S556G, G558R (174, 200)
PIs[b]	Mutations in or near the NS3 protease substrate binding cleft	Simeprevir: F43I/S/V, Q80K/R, R155K/T, A156G/S/T/V, D168A/E/H/I/T/V/Y (204) Paritaprevir: F43L, Y56H, R155G/K/S/T A156T, D168A/E/F/H/N/V/Y (174, 185, 200, 206) Grazoprevir: Y56F/H, R155K/Q, A156G/T/V, V158A, D168A/E/G/N/S/V/Y (35, 175, 185) Glecaprevir: Y56H, Q80K/R, R155K/T, A156G/T/V, D168A/L/R/T (177) Voxilaprevir: A156L/T/V; RASs at positions 41 and 168 were also selected *in vitro* and contributed to reduced susceptibility (179)
NS5A inhibitors[c]	NS5A N-terminal domain mutations that interfere with binding to NS5A inhibitors	Daclatasvir: M28T, Q30E/H/K/R/S, L31F/M/V, H58D, Y93C/H/N (172, 214) Ombitasvir: M28A/T/V, Q30E/K/R, L31V, H58D, Y93C/H/L/N (174, 200) Ledipasvir: K24R, M28A/G/T, Q30E/G/H/K/L/R/Y, L31M/V, P32L/S, H58D, A92K, Y93C/H/N/S (173, 187, 217) Elbasvir: M28A/G/S/T, Q30D/E/G/H/K/L/R/S/Y, L31F/M/V, H58D, Y93C/H/N/S (167, 175) Velpatasvir: Y93H/N; additional RASs including Q30R and L31I/M/V in GT1b and M28T, A30K, L31V, and E92K in GT3 contribute to reduced susceptibility (176, 211) Pibrentasvir: All single RASs reduce susceptibility <10-fold; several combinations of RASs reduce susceptibility >100-fold (177, 212)

[a]The term "resistance-associated substitutions" (RASs) is preferred to "drug resistance mutations" in the HCV field because the consensus amino acids, the amino acids selected by DAA therapy, and the phenotypic effects of DAA-selected amino acids are highly genotype and subtype dependent. This table lists amino acid variants selected *in vitro* or in patients and shown to reduce drug susceptibility in one or more HCV genotypes. The amino acid preceding the position is the consensus for GT1A. RASs are listed in order of position and, at each position, in alphabetical order. RAS positions are underlined if one or more amino acids at that position are selected commonly during therapy or associated with markedly reduced *in vitro* susceptibility. Most of the data in this table are from GT1a and GT1b viruses. Comprehensive data on naturally occurring RASs in different genotypes in DAA-naive individuals have also been published (203). Comprehensive data on the RASs selected in different genotypes during therapy and on the phenotypes of RASs in different genotypes are generally found in the package insert for each DAA as well as in two recent reviews (183, 217).

[b]Telaprevir and boceprevir are no longer recommended under any circumstances. The most common telaprevir and boceprevir RASs included V36A/C/L/M, T54A/S, R155K/T, and A156S/V/T for both PIs and V170A for boceprevir. Simeprevir is no longer routinely recommended, although it may have a role in several restricted circumstances in regions where it is the most affordable option.

[c]Preexisting NS5A inhibitor RASs are common because many exist as the consensus or as common polymorphisms in one or more genotype. M28L occurs in a high proportion of GT1, GT2, and GT4 viruses; Q30A/K/L/R occur in a high proportion of GT1 to GT4 viruses; and L31M occurs in a high proportion of GT2 and GT4 viruses (203). Y93H occurs in about 10% of GT1b viruses and 5 to 10% of GT3 viruses (187).

available for pan-genotypic treatment of patients who have experienced previous virological failure on DAA therapy, especially those exposed to an NS5A inhibitor-containing regimen (178, 179).

Treatment guidelines are complicated because treatment efficacy is influenced by HCV genotype, the presence of cirrhosis, previous virological failure on an interferon-containing regimen, previous virological failure on an interferon-free DAA treatment regimen, and the duration of therapy (167, 180). Moreover, ribavirin remains an important adjunct to many interferon-free DAA-containing regimens, particularly for treating GT1 and GT3 patients with cirrhosis, previous treatment failures, or known or likely DAA resistance (181, 182).

Principles of HCV Drug Resistance

Many studies have identified HCV mutations that emerge during *in vitro* passage experiments and in patients with virological failure. The term "resistance-associated substitutions" (RASs) is preferred to "drug-resistance mutations" in the HCV field because the consensus amino acids, the amino acids selected by DAAs, and their phenotypic effects are highly genotype dependent. The phenotypic effect of RASs has been assessed primarily in GT1 subtype a (GT1a) and subtype b (GT1b) replicons and infectious clones. Because an increasing number of studies are being performed in GT2 to GT6 replicons and clones, it has become apparent that the same DAA often selects for different RASs in different genotypes and that the same RASs often have different effects in different genotypes. Drug-resistance profiles may also differ between different subtypes within the same genotype, though only differences between GT1a and GT1b have been well studied. Although there is extensive cross-resistance within the PI and NS5A classes, the newer DAAs in these classes generally have pan-genotypic activity and substantially higher genetic barriers to resistance.

Analyses linking specific RASs to SVR rates have also been complicated by the complex interplay between RASs, DAA regimens, HCV genotype and subtype, the extent of liver disease, and duration of therapy. To make these analyses tractable, most studies have focused on those

RASs with the greatest reductions in susceptibility, which is >100-fold reduced susceptibility for the NS5A inhibitors and >10-fold reduced susceptibility for the PIs (183–186). A consensus is also emerging that RASs detectable by Sanger sequencing or at levels ≥15% by next-generation sequencing are more clinically significant than RASs present at lower levels (167, 187).

The effects of the detection of baseline RASs on SVR rates have been studied in multiple clinical trials. Most of these studies evaluated the clinical significance of polymorphic RASs in DAA-naive patients. In this population, there are several clinical scenarios in which the presence of a major NS5A inhibitor RAS has been shown to reduce SVR rates (167, 188–191). Indications for genotypic resistance testing, however, have been slow to evolve because sequencing assays are not widely available or standardized and because the effect of baseline RASs on the success of therapy is often not large (167, 190, 192). Nonetheless, indications for genotypic resistance testing will continue to evolve and may eventually play an increased role, particularly in the management of patients with previous virological failure on a DAA-containing regimen.

Nucleotide and Nonnucleoside RdRp Inhibitor Resistance

HCV RdRp is encoded by the 530 N-terminal amino acids of the NS5B gene. A C-terminal extension of NS5B anchors the catalytic domain to the endoplasmic reticulum as part of a larger viral replication complex. HCV RdRp, like other polymerases, contains palm, thumb, and finger subdomains that enclose the RNA template groove and glycine-aspartate-aspartate (GDD) catalytic triad (193). Approved HCV RdRp inhibitors include the chain-terminating nucleotide analog sofosbuvir and the nonnucleoside RdRp inhibitor (NNI) dasabuvir.

The catalytic site of RdRp is highly conserved across genotypes, accounting for the pan-genotypic activity of sofosbuvir. The active site mutation S282T is the main RAS selected *in vitro* by sofosbuvir in all HCV genotypes (194, 195). S282T is associated with 3- to 20-fold reduced sofosbuvir susceptibility depending on genotype and is associated with markedly reduced virus replication fitness (194, 195). In clinical trials, it has been observed transiently in just one patient receiving sofosbuvir (196).

L159F occurs in 7% of genotype 1b sequences from DAA-naive patients but is otherwise nonpolymorphic (197). As determined by Sanger sequencing, it develops in about 5% of patients receiving sofosbuvir, often in combination with the compensatory mutation C316N or L320F (196, 198). L159F confers a minimal 1.2- to 2.0-fold reduction in sofosbuvir susceptibility depending on genotype. V321A is a nonpolymorphic mutation selected by sofosbuvir in fewer than 5% of patients with virological failure (197). It confers a minimal 1.2- to 1.4-fold reduction in sofosbuvir susceptibility and is associated with reduced replication capacity (197). Despite their minimal effects on *in vitro* susceptibility, L159F and V321A may be associated with an increased risk of not attaining SVR in those patients at greatest risk for virological failure (197, 198).

Dasabuvir is the only FDA-approved NNI. It binds allosterically to a pocket between the RdRp palm and thumb subdomains. It is active against GT1a and GT1b virus variants and is used in combination with the FDC paritaprevir/r/ombitasvir (199). The most common treatment-emergent dasabuvir RASs include C316Y, M414T, S556G, and several additional RASs between positions 553 and 561 (174, 200). Although S556G occurs in 10 to 35% of GT1b viruses from DAA-naive patients and is associated with about 10-fold reduced susceptibility, it has not been shown to reduce the response to paritaprevir/r/ombitasvir plus dasabuvir (200, 201).

Protease Inhibitors

The NS3 serine protease comprises the 189 N-terminal amino acids of NS3. NS3 protease forms a heterodimer with the 54-amino acid NS4A, and together they function to cleave four sites in the HCV polypeptide precursor to generate the N termini of NS4A, NS4B, NS5A, and NS5B. HCV protease also appears to take part in host immune evasion by cleaving several critical intracellular immune mediators (161). Multiple structures of protease with and without inhibitors have been solved by X-ray crystallography (202). HCV protease contains an H57, D81, and S139 catalytic triad characteristic of other members of the trypsin family of serine proteases.

As new PIs have been approved, their genotypic spectrum of activity has broadened and their genetic barrier to resistance has increased. The first-wave first-generation PIs, telaprevir and boceprevir, were active against GT1 strains but vulnerable to many RASs. The second-wave first-generation PIs simeprevir, paritaprevir, and grazoprevir were approved for treating GT1 and GT4 strains. However, simeprevir was less active against GT1 strains compared with the four subsequently approved PIs (171, 185). The second-generation PIs glecaprevir and voxilaprevir were approved in 2017 as part of FDCs for treating all HCV genotypes (177, 179).

The most common RASs for the PI class occur in or near the protease substrate cleft at positions 36, 43, 54, 55, 56, 80, 155, 156, 168, and 170 (183, 201). With the exception of Q80K, these RASs are nonpolymorphic in GT1 strains. Q80K is a polymorphism that occurs in about 30% of DAA-naive GT1b-infected patients in North America. It seems to be less frequent in European GT1b patients. It reduces simeprevir susceptibility about 10-fold (203, 204), and in several clinical scenarios, it reduces SVR rates to simeprevir-containing regimens (183, 189).

The most relevant RASs for the four most recently approved PIs are substitutions at positions 155, 156, and 168. Depending on the PI, the genotype, and the amino acid substitution, RASs at these positions may reduce susceptibility up to 100-fold (185, 186, 202). Most emergent RASs at these positions reduce viral fitness and are gradually replaced by wild-type variants in the weeks to months following treatment discontinuation (190, 205). Of these RASs, paritaprevir selects for R155G/K/S, A156T, and D168A/E/F/H/N/V/Y *in vitro* and primarily for R155K and D168V *in vivo* (174, 200, 206), and grazoprevir selects for R155K, A156G/T/V, and D168A/E/G/N/S/V/Y *in vitro* and primarily for D168 mutations *in vivo* (35, 175). Although Q168 is the consensus GT3 amino acid (203), this residue does not appear to explain the markedly reduced activity of paritaprevir and grazoprevir against GT3 viruses (207). Few data are available on the RASs selected in patients receiving the FDCs containing the second-generation PIs, glecaprevir and voxilaprevir (177, 179).

NS5A Inhibitors

NS5A is an ~450-amino-acid membrane-associated phosphoprotein that is an essential part of the HCV replicase complex. It is anchored to the endoplasmic reticulum through an N-terminal amphipathic α-helix and contains a structured N-terminal domain that in a dimeric form likely binds HCV RNA (161, 208). NS5A inhibitors bind to the NS5A N-terminal domain (domain I) and appear to prevent NS5A from binding viral RNA and thus interfering with the formation of the HCV replicase complex and inhibiting viral particle assembly and release (208–210). Each of the NS5A inhibitors has picomolar potencies, and as new NS5A inhibitors have been approved, their spectrum of activity has broadened and their genetic barrier to resistance has increased (211, 212).

The NS5A inhibitor RASs occur in the N terminus of NS5A between positions 24 and 93 and develop in most patients with virological failure on an NS5A inhibitor-containing regimen (200, 213). They often occur in synergistic combinations that can counteract the extraordinary potency of many NS5A inhibitors (190, 208, 214). Most NS5A inhibitor RASs are associated with a minimal fitness cost, and when they emerge during therapy, they are likely to persist for many months to years, even in the absence of selective drug pressure (190, 213, 214).

The most commonly occurring GT1 RASs selected *in vitro* and in patients receiving an NS5A inhibitor occur at positions 28, 30, 31, and 93, sites at which NS5A inhibitors bind to the NS5A N-terminal domain (208). The most common clinically significant RASs are M28A/G/T, Q30D/E/G/H/K/L/R/T, L31I/M/V, and Y93C/H/N/S in GT1a and L31V and Y93H/N in GT1b (167, 187, 215).

In GT1a viruses, the following RASs confer >100-fold reductions in susceptibility to one or more inhibitors: M28T for daclatasvir and ombitasvir; Q30R for daclatasvir, ombitasvir, ledipasvir, and elbasvir; L31M or L31V for daclatasvir, ombitasvir, ledipasvir, and elbasvir; and Y93H/N for daclatasvir, ombitasvir, ledipasvir, elbasvir, and velpatasvir (190). Y93H/N may be the most significant RAS because it confers >1,000-fold reduced susceptibility to each NS5A inhibitor except pibrentasvir. Additional, less commonly occurring RASs include K24G/N/R, P32L/S, H58DL//R, and A92K/T (183, 208).

Many NS5A inhibitor RASs are highly polymorphic. For example, M28L occurs in a high proportion of GT1, GT2, and GT4 viruses from NS5A inhibitor-naive patients; Q30A/K/L/R occur in a high proportion of GT1, GT2, GT3, and GT4 viruses; and L31M occurs in a high proportion of GT2 and GT4 strains (203, 208). Y93H occurs in about 10% of GT1b strains and 5% of GT3 strains (203, 216). Overall, one or more RASs are likely to be detectable by Sanger sequencing prior to therapy in 10% of GT1 and 20% of GT3 viruses (189, 203, 217).

As of 2107, the American Association for the Study of Liver Diseases/Infectious Diseases Society of America guidelines recommend that NS5A genotypic resistance testing be performed for GT1a-infected patients in whom elbasvir/grazoprevir is being considered (188), GT1a-infected interferon-experienced patients in whom ledipasvir/sofosbuvir is being considered (187, 217), and GT3 treatment-naive cirrhotic patients or interferon-experienced patients in whom daclatasvir/sofosbuvir or velpatasvir/sofosbuvir is being considered (190, 218). In these patients, the detection of pretherapy RASs associated with >100-fold reduced susceptibility would lead to a recommendation to add ribavirin and/or prolong therapy or to consider the use of a different DAA-containing regimen (190).

Ribavirin

Ribavirin will likely remain an important component of many regimens because it is active against viruses of all genotypes, does not select for resistance, and increases the SVR rate of many regimens (181, 182). Ribavirin's most likely mechanism of action is to increase viral mutagenesis. This mechanism is most consistent with its observed clinical effects and with deep-sequencing studies (219, 220). Ribavirin has also been proposed to weakly directly inhibit HCV RNA polymerase (182). No mechanism for ribavirin resistance has been identified.

INFLUENZA

Influenza A and B viruses have segmented minus-strand RNA genomes, each associated with many copies of the nucleoprotein as well as the three polymerase (PA, PB1, and PB2) proteins in the ribonucleoprotein complex. Embedded in the membrane of influenza A and B viruses are two spiked glycoproteins, hemagglutinin (HA) and neuraminidase (NA), and a matrix (M)-2 channel protein.

Sixteen HA and nine NA influenza A antigenic subtypes have been reported, predominantly in avian species. A subset of these has infected humans. In particular, influenza A viruses of the H1N1, H2N2, and H3N2 subtypes have been responsible for human epidemics and pandemics over the last century. In 2009, a swine-origin influenza A(H1N1) variant [A(H1N1)pdm09] emerged in Mexico and spread worldwide, causing the first pandemic of the 21st century (221). Influenza B viruses are also responsible for annual epidemics. Since 1983, influenza B isolates have been divided into two genetically distinct lineages (i.e., B/Yamagata/16/1988- and B/Victoria/2/87-like viruses). Besides human influenza strains, two highly pathogenic avian influenza species are responsible for several human infections: A(H5N1), which has been widely disseminated in water fowl since at least 1997 and has infected people in China, Southeast Asia, the Middle East, Africa, and Europe (222), and A(H7N9), which has infected more than 1,400 people in China since March 2013 (223).

There are two classes of licensed anti-influenza drugs in the United States: M2 channel blockers (the adamantane derivatives amantadine and rimantadine) and NA inhibitors (zanamivir, oseltamivir, and peramivir) (Table 5). M2 channel blockers are currently inactive against circulating influenza A viruses and are intrinsically inactive against influenza B viruses (224). On the other hand, NA inhibitors are active against most influenza A and B viruses. Zanamivir, which is approved for inhaled use, is also available as an investigational intravenous preparation for emergency use (225). Peramivir, an intravenous NA inhibitor which was licensed in Japan and Korea in 2010, has been recently approved in other countries, including the United States and Canada (226).

M2 Channel Blockers

M2 is a tetrameric pH-activated proton-selective channel that plays a role in virus uncoating (227). Passage of hydrogen ions through the M2 channel into the virion following endocytosis promotes M1 dissociation from the ribonucleoprotein complexes. Amantadine and rimantadine interfere with the penetration of hydrogen ions through the M2 channel, thereby preventing transport of the ribonucleoprotein complex to the nucleus (228).

Adamantane resistance used to develop in about 30% of people receiving amantadine or rimantadine after a few days of therapy (229, 230). Amantadine- and rimantadine-resistant variants cause typical disease and are transmissible in humans (229). Natural resistance to the adamantanes has emerged since 2004 in A/H3N2 viruses and since 2009 in A(H1N1)pdm09 viruses, so this class of antivirals is not currently recommended. Resistance is due to substitutions

TABLE 5 Genetic mechanisms of resistance to influenza virus inhibitors

Drug class	Mechanism(s)	Drug resistance mutations
M2 channel blockers: Amantadine Rimantadine	M2 transmembrane mutations that block hydrogen ion transfer	Mutations at residues 26, 27, 30, 31, and 34, particularly S31N Most circulating lineages of A(H3N2), A(H1N1)pdm09, and the pathogenic avian influenza strains A(H5N1) and A(H7N9) are resistant as a result of S31N Influenza B viruses do not possess the M2 ion channel and are naturally resistant to adamantanes
Neuraminidase inhibitors: Oseltamivir Zanamivir Peramivir	Framework or catalytic neuraminidase mutations associated with decreased inhibitor binding	A(H1N1) and A(H1N1)pdm09: Oseltamivir: H274Y, E119G/D, Y155H, I222M/R/K, S246N/G, N294S Zanamivir: Q136K, E119G/D, Y155H, I222R Peramivir: H274Y, Q136K, E119G/D A(H3N2): Oseltamivir: E119V/I, R292K, N294S, Del245-248 Zanamivir: D151A, R292K, E119I, N294S Peramivir: R292K, E119I A(H5N1): Oseltamivir: H274Y, N294S Peramivir: H274Y A(H7N9): Oseltamivir: R292K, E119V, I222R/K Zanamivir: R292K, I222R Peramivir: R292K, I222R Influenza B: Oseltamivir: R152K, R371K, D198N/E, I222T Zanamivir: R152K, R371K, D198N/E, I222T Peramivir: D198N, R152K

at one of five codons (26, 27, 30, 31, and 34) of the M2 protein (231) (Table 5).

Neuraminidase Inhibitors (NAIs)

The HA and NA proteins play a major role during the influenza virus life cycle. While HA is responsible for virus attachment to the sialic acid receptors on the host cell, the enzymatic activity of the NA cleaves off the terminal *N*-acetyl neuraminic acid (Neu5Ac) on these α2,3 and α2,6 sialic acid moieties. Such NA activity is important for virion release from the host cell and for facilitating viral spread throughout the respiratory tract (232).

The three-dimensional structures of NA from influenza B and from several influenza A subtypes have been solved by X-ray crystallography (232–234). NA is a homotetramer containing monomers of about 470 amino acids depending on the type and subtype. NA has a hydrophobic stalk peptide at its N terminus, which is responsible for membrane anchoring. A globular head contains its active site—a pocket into which sialic acid and substrate analogs bind. The most commonly used numbering system is based on alignment to the influenza A N2 subtype.

Influenza NAs of different A subtypes differ from one another at about 50% of their amino acids, and influenza A differs from influenza B at about 70% of its amino acids. Nonetheless, the folded structure of the polypeptide brings into proximity a number of amino acids that are nearly invariant in all influenza strains. Eight of these strain-invariant amino acids directly contact sialic acid: R118, D151, R152, R224, E276, R292, R371, and Y406. Eleven provide the framework that supports these catalytic residues: E119, R156, W178, S179, D198, I222, E227, H274, E277, N294, and E425 (235, 236).

NA inhibitors are sialic acid analogs that competitively inhibit NA. They are active against a wide range of human and avian strains, including influenza B and each of the nine identified avian influenza A NA subtypes (224, 236, 237). Although they are intrinsically less active against influenza B than A, NA inhibitors have nonetheless demonstrated clinical efficacy at treating influenza B at the doses used in clinical trials (224). Oseltamivir, which is administered orally, is a carbocyclic analog of sialic acid with a bulky side chain necessitating a conformation change in NA to allow binding (234). Because zanamivir is administered as an aerosol and because its structure is more similar to the natural sialic acid than oseltamivir, zanamivir resistance occurs much less frequently than oseltamivir resistance (237). The intravenous formulation of peramivir enables it to be a suitable antiviral option for severe influenza cases (226), although it is not approved for this specific indication in the United States.

The NA mutations responsible for NAI resistance depend on the influenza type (A or B) and subtype (e.g., N1 or N2) for influenza A (Table 5). In addition, specific genetic lineages within an influenza A subtype may differ in their levels of NAI susceptibility and in their predisposition to specific NAI-resistance mutations. Therefore, ongoing genotypic and phenotypic surveillance is required to identify changes in the intrinsic susceptibility and replicative capacity of circulating NA variants and the spectrum of mutations selected in patients receiving NAIs.

NAI susceptibility is monitored primarily by genotypic and enzymatic NA inhibition assays (238, 239). Genotypic assays are useful for clinical management and surveillance (239). Enzymatic assays are useful for surveillance and for characterizing novel NA variants. Cell culture assays are possible but must be interpreted cautiously because the cells used for culture have variable concentrations of glycoconjugate receptors, and different influenza viruses vary in their dependence on NA activity (240, 241).

During the first few years of its use, oseltamivir resistance was reported to occur in about 1 to 4% of treated adults and in a higher proportion of treated children (242, 243). There was no evidence of naturally occurring oseltamivir resistance, and there were no reports of transmitted resistance (244). In the 2007–2008 season, a significant proportion of worldwide H1N1 infections were caused by a strain containing the oseltamivir-resistant framework mutation H274Y (245, 246). By the 2008–2009 season, >95% of seasonal H1N1 strains in the United States and Europe were oseltamivir resistant (245, 247). This strain disappeared with the advent of the 2009 pandemic virus, and resistance levels returned to 1 to 2% in immunocompetent subjects (248).

H274Y reduces oseltamivir susceptibility by several hundred- to several thousand-fold and causes high-level cross-resistance to peramivir but not zanamivir (244). Although *in vitro* cell culture and ferret model experiments showed that old viruses with H274Y had greatly diminished replication (249), the H274Y-containing H1N1 viruses that emerged after 2006 to 2007 retained their *in vitro* replicative capacity, transmissibility, and pathogenicity (250). Indeed, epidemiologic and molecular phylogenetic data suggest that the fixation of H274Y in 2007–2008 H1N1 strains was not a result of selective drug pressure (251). Rather, H274Y evolved in the dominant circulating strain in seasonal 2007–2008 H1N1 viruses, probably due to the presence of permissive NA substitutions such as R221Q, V233M, and D343N (234, 252). Reverse genetics and mutagenesis experiments further confirmed the major permissive effect of the R221Q change in the A/Brisbane/579/2007 (H1N1) background in restoring the attenuating impact of the H274Y mutation (253, 254).

H274Y is the most frequently occurring NAI-resistance mutation in patients receiving oseltamivir (255) and has been more recently reported in community clusters of A (H1N1)pdm09 viruses in Australia in 2011 (256) and in Japan in 2014 (257). Although H5N1 viruses are intrinsically susceptible to oseltamivir and zanamivir (258, 259), virological failure resulting from H274Y appears to occur at a higher frequency among patients receiving oseltamivir than in pre-2007 seasonal H1N1 and in A(H1N1)pdm09 strains (260).

Additional NAI-resistance mutations in A(H1N1) or A(H1N1)pdm09 include Q136K, Y155H, I222M/K/R/V, S246N/G, and N294S (237, 261, 262). I222 and S246 mutations appear to increase the replication fitness of viruses with H274Y and to cause low-level resistance (5- to 30-fold reduced susceptibility) to oseltamivir and zanamivir when they occur alone (261, 262). Q136K and Y155H are uncommon naturally occurring N1 mutations which reduce zanamivir (Q136K) and oseltamivir and zanamivir (Y155H) susceptibility >30-fold (241, 263). Q136K was present at low proportions in primary clinical specimens but rose during cell culture, raising questions about its clinical significance (263, 264). Recent clinical studies reported the emergence of E119G/D mutants responsible for cross-resistance to all tested NA inhibitors (265, 266).

Among H3N2 viruses, the catalytic and framework substitutions R292K, E119I/V, and N294S and the deletion Del245-248 have been reported in patients receiving oseltamivir (237, 243, 255, 267, 268). E119I and E119V reduce oseltamivir susceptibility by more than 30-fold and cause low-level cross-resistance to zanamivir (E119I) (Table 5). R292K and N294S cause high-level oseltamivir resistance and lower levels of zanamivir cross-resistance. R292K, E119V, and I222K/R have also been reported in H7N9 viruses from patients receiving oseltamivir (269, 270).

Among influenza B viruses, the most commonly reported NAI-resistance mutations include D198E/N, I222T, R152K, and R371K. D198N and I222T reduce oseltamivir and zanamivir susceptibility by less than 10-fold (224). R371K, which was identified in a 2004 to 2008 surveillance study, was associated with >100-fold reduced susceptibility to oseltamivir and about 30-fold reduced susceptibility to zanamivir (246). R152K, which causes high-level resistance to both oseltamivir and zanamivir, has been reported in an immunocompromised patient receiving prolonged therapy with inhaled zanamivir (271). A WHO committee has recently established levels of NAI resistance by virus type. For influenza A virus, reduced and highly reduced inhibitions are defined by 10- to 100-fold and >100-fold increases, respectively, in IC_{50} levels by the NA assay. For influenza B viruses, reduced inhibition and highly reduced inhibition are defined by 5- to 50-fold and >50-fold increases, respectively, in IC_{50} levels (272). It is noteworthy that only the H274Y in H1N1 viruses has been unequivocally associated with clinical drug failure (273).

REFERENCES

1. **Koszalka P, Tilmanis D, Hurt AC.** 2017. Influenza antivirals currently in late-phase clinical trial. *Influenza Other Respir Viruses* **11:**240–246.
2. **Brendish NJ, Clark TW.** 2017. Antiviral treatment of severe non-influenza respiratory virus infection. *Curr Opin Infect Dis* **30:**573–578.
3. **Boldescu V, Behnam MAM, Vasilakis N, Klein CD.** 2017. Broad-spectrum agents for flaviviral infections: dengue, Zika and beyond. *Nat Rev Drug Discov* **16:**565–586.
4. **Bixler SL, Duplantier AJ, Bavari S.** 2017. Discovering drugs for the treatment of Ebola virus. *Curr Treat Options Infect Dis* **9:**299–317.
5. **Haffizulla J, Hartman A, Hoppers M, Resnick H, Samudrala S, Ginocchio C, Bardin M, Rossignol JF, US Nitazoxanide Influenza Clinical Study Group.** 2014. Effect of nitazoxanide in adults and adolescents with acute uncomplicated influenza: a double-blind, randomised, placebo-controlled, phase 2b/3 trial. *Lancet Infect Dis* **14:**609–618.
6. **Rossignol JF.** 2014. Nitazoxanide: a first-in-class broad-spectrum antiviral agent. *Antiviral Res* **110:**94–103.
7. **Zhang T, Zhai M, Ji J, Zhang J, Tian Y, Liu X.** 2017. Recent progress on the treatment of Ebola virus disease with favipiravir and other related strategies. *Bioorg Med Chem Lett* **27:**2364–2368.
8. **Sheahan TP, Sims AC, Graham RL, Menachery VD, Gralinski LE, Case JB, Leist SR, Pyrc K, Feng JY, Trantcheva I, Bannister R, Park Y, Babusis D, Clarke MO, Mackman RL, Spahn JE, Palmiotti CA, Siegel D, Ray AS, Cihlar T, Jordan R, Denison MR, Baric RS.** 2017. Broad-spectrum antiviral GS-5734 inhibits both epidemic and zoonotic coronaviruses. *Sci Transl Med* **9:**eaal3653.
9. **Reardon JE, Spector T.** 1989. Herpes simplex virus type 1 DNA polymerase. Mechanism of inhibition by acyclovir triphosphate. *J Biol Chem* **264:**7405–7411.
10. **Earnshaw DL, Bacon TH, Darlison SJ, Edmonds K, Perkins RM, Vere Hodge RA.** 1992. Mode of antiviral action of penciclovir in MRC-5 cells infected with herpes simplex virus type 1 (HSV-1), HSV-2, and varicella-zoster virus. *Antimicrob Agents Chemother* **36:**2747–2757.
11. **Piret J, Boivin G.** 2014. Antiviral drug resistance in herpesviruses other than cytomegalovirus. *Rev Med Virol* **24:**186–218.
12. **Sauerbrei A, Bohn-Wippert K, Kaspar M, Krumbholz A, Karrasch M, Zell R.** 2016. Database on natural polymorphisms and resistance-related non-synonymous mutations in thymidine kinase and DNA polymerase genes of herpes simplex virus types 1 and 2. *J Antimicrob Chemother* **71:**6–16.
13. **Andrei G, Snoeck R.** 2013. Herpes simplex virus drug-resistance: new mutations and insights. *Curr Opin Infect Dis* **26:**551–560.
14. **Burrel S, Aime C, Hermet L, Ait-Arkoub Z, Agut H, Boutolleau D.** 2013. Surveillance of herpes simplex virus resistance to antivirals: a 4-year survey. *Antiviral Res* **100:**365–372.

15. **Sarisky RT, Quail MR, Clark PE, Nguyen TT, Halsey WS, Wittrock RJ, O'Leary Bartus J, Van Horn MM, Sathe GM, Van Horn S, Kelly MD, Bacon TH, Leary JJ.** 2001. Characterization of herpes simplex viruses selected in culture for resistance to penciclovir or acyclovir. *J Virol* **75:**1761–1769.
16. **Andrei G, Georgala A, Topalis D, Fiten P, Aoun M, Opdenakker G, Snoeck R.** 2013. Heterogeneity and evolution of thymidine kinase and DNA polymerase mutants of herpes simplex virus type 1: implications for antiviral therapy. *J Infect Dis* **207:**1295–1305.
17. **Pan D, Kaye SB, Hopkins M, Kirwan R, Hart IJ, Coen DM.** 2014. Common and new acyclovir resistant herpes simplex virus-1 mutants causing bilateral recurrent herpetic keratitis in an immunocompetent patient. *J Infect Dis* **209:**345–349.
18. **Chen SH, Pearson A, Coen DM, Chen SH.** 2004. Failure of thymidine kinase-negative herpes simplex virus to reactivate from latency following efficient establishment. *J Virol* **78:** 520–523.
19. **Grey F, Sowa M, Collins P, Fenton RJ, Harris W, Snowden W, Efstathiou S, Darby G.** 2003. Characterization of a neurovirulent aciclovir-resistant variant of herpes simplex virus. *J Gen Virol* **84:**1403–1410.
20. **Morfin F, Thouvenot D, Aymard M, Souillet G.** 2000. Reactivation of acyclovir-resistant thymidine kinase-deficient herpes simplex virus harbouring single base insertion within a 7 Gs homopolymer repeat of the thymidine kinase gene. *J Med Virol* **62:**247–250.
21. **Saijo M, Suzutani T, Itoh K, Hirano Y, Murono K, Nagamine M, Mizuta K, Niikura M, Morikawa S.** 1999. Nucleotide sequence of thymidine kinase gene of sequential acyclovir-resistant herpes simplex virus type 1 isolates recovered from a child with Wiskott-Aldrich syndrome: evidence for reactivation of acyclovir-resistant herpes simplex virus. *J Med Virol* **58:**387–393.
22. **Pan D, Coen DM.** 2012. Quantification and analysis of thymidine kinase expression from acyclovir-resistant G-string insertion and deletion mutants in herpes simplex virus-infected cells. *J Virol* **86:**4518–4526.
23. **Stránská R, Schuurman R, Nienhuis E, Goedegebuure IW, Polman M, Weel JF, Wertheim-Van Dillen PM, Berkhout RJ, van Loon AM.** 2005. Survey of acyclovir-resistant herpes simplex virus in the Netherlands: prevalence and characterization. *J Clin Virol* **32:**7–18.
24. **Frobert E, Burrel S, Ducastelle-Lepretre S, Billaud G, Ader F, Casalegno JS, Nave V, Boutolleau D, Michallet M, Lina B, Morfin F.** 2014. Resistance of herpes simplex viruses to acyclovir: an update from a ten-year survey in France. *Antiviral Res* **111:**36–41.
25. **Kakiuchi S, Tsuji M, Nishimura H, Yoshikawa T, Wang L, Takayama-Ito M, Kinoshita H, Lim CK, Fujii H, Yamada S, Harada S, Oka A, Mizuguchi M, Taniguchi S, Saijo M.** 2017. Association of the emergence of acyclovir-resistant herpes simplex virus type 1 with prognosis in hematopoietic stem cell transplantation patients. *J Infect Dis* **215:**865–873.
26. **Duan R, de Vries RD, Osterhaus AD, Remeijer L, Verjans GM.** 2008. Acyclovir-resistant corneal HSV-1 isolates from patients with herpetic keratitis. *J Infect Dis* **198:**659–663.
27. **Topalis D, Gillemot S, Snoeck R, Andrei G.** 2016. Distribution and effects of amino acid changes in drug-resistant α and β herpesviruses DNA polymerase. *Nucleic Acids Res* **44:** 9530–9554.
28. **Nikkels AF, Snoeck R, Rentier B, Pierard GE.** 1999. Chronic verrucous varicella zoster virus skin lesions: clinical, histological, molecular and therapeutic aspects. *Clin Exp Dermatol* **24:**346–353.
29. **van der Beek MT, Vermont CL, Bredius RG, Marijt EW, van der Blij-de Brouwer CS, Kroes AC, Claas EC, Vossen AC.** 2013. Persistence and antiviral resistance of varicella zoster virus in hematological patients. *Clin Infect Dis* **56:**335–343.
30. **Hoffmann A, Döring K, Seeger NT, Bühler M, Schacke M, Krumbholz A, Sauerbrei A.** 2017. Genetic polymorphism of thymidine kinase (TK) and DNA polymerase (pol) of clinical varicella-zoster virus (VZV) isolates collected over three decades. *J Clin Virol* **95:**61–65.
31. **Prichard MN.** 2009. Function of human cytomegalovirus UL97 kinase in viral infection and its inhibition by maribavir. *Rev Med Virol* **19:**215–229.
32. **Sullivan V, Talarico CL, Stanat SC, Davis M, Coen DM, Biron KK.** 1992. A protein kinase homologue controls phosphorylation of ganciclovir in human cytomegalovirus-infected cells. *Nature* **358:**162–164. (Erratum, **366:**756.)
33. **Fisher CE, Knudsen JL, Lease ED, Jerome KR, Rakita RM, Boeckh M, Limaye AP.** 2017. Risk factors and outcomes of ganciclovir-resistant cytomegalovirus infection in solid organ transplant recipients. *Clin Infect Dis* **65:**57–63.
34. **Campos AB, Ribeiro J, Boutolleau D, Sousa H.** 2016. Human cytomegalovirus antiviral drug resistance in hematopoietic stem cell transplantation: current state of the art. *Rev Med Virol* **26:**161–182.
35. **Komatsu TE, Pikis A, Naeger LK, Harrington PR.** 2014. Resistance of human cytomegalovirus to ganciclovir/valganciclovir: a comprehensive review of putative resistance pathways. *Antiviral Res* **101:**12–25.
36. **Lurain NS, Chou S.** 2010. Antiviral drug resistance of human cytomegalovirus. *Clin Microbiol Rev* **23:**689–712.
37. **Kotton CN, Kumar D, Caliendo AM, Asberg A, Chou S, Danziger-Isakov L, Humar A, Transplantation Society International CMV Consensus Group.** 2013. Updated international consensus guidelines on the management of cytomegalovirus in solid-organ transplantation. *Transplantation* **96:**333–360.
38. **Chou S, Ercolani RJ, Vanarsdall AL.** 2017. Differentiated levels of ganciclovir resistance conferred by mutations at codons 591 to 603 of the cytomegalovirus UL97 kinase gene. *J Clin Microbiol* **55:**2098–2104.
39. **Chou S, Van Wechel LC, Lichy HM, Marousek GI.** 2005. Phenotyping of cytomegalovirus drug resistance mutations by using recombinant viruses incorporating a reporter gene. *Antimicrob Agents Chemother* **49:**2710–2715.
40. **Smith IL, Cherrington JM, Jiles RE, Fuller MD, Freeman WR, Spector SA.** 1997. High-level resistance of cytomegalovirus to ganciclovir is associated with alterations in both the UL97 and DNA polymerase genes. *J Infect Dis* **176:**69–77.
41. **Chen H, Beardsley GP, Coen DM.** 2014. Mechanism of ganciclovir-induced chain termination revealed by resistant viral polymerase mutants with reduced exonuclease activity. *Proc Natl Acad Sci USA* **111:**17462–17467.
42. **Chou S, Boivin G, Ives J, Elston R.** 2014. Phenotypic evaluation of previously uncharacterized cytomegalovirus DNA polymerase sequence variants detected in a valganciclovir treatment trial. *J Infect Dis* **209:**1219–1226.
43. **Chou S.** 2015. Rapid *in vitro* evolution of human cytomegalovirus UL56 mutations that confer letermovir resistance. *Antimicrob Agents Chemother* **59:**6588–6593.
44. **Goldner T, Hempel C, Ruebsamen-Schaeff H, Zimmermann H, Lischka P.** 2014. Geno- and phenotypic characterization of human cytomegalovirus mutants selected *in vitro* after letermovir (AIC246) exposure. *Antimicrob Agents Chemother* **58:**610–613.
45. **Lischka P, Michel D, Zimmermann H.** 2016. Characterization of Cytomegalovirus breakthrough events in a phase 2 prophylaxis trial of letermovir (AIC246, MK 8228). *J Infect Dis* **213:**23–30.
46. **Chou S.** 2008. Cytomegalovirus UL97 mutations in the era of ganciclovir and maribavir. *Rev Med Virol* **18:**233–246.
47. **Schubert A, Ehlert K, Schuler-Luettmann S, Gentner E, Mertens T, Michel D.** 2013. Fast selection of maribavir resistant cytomegalovirus in a bone marrow transplant recipient. *BMC Infect Dis* **13:**330.
48. **Strasfeld L, Lee I, Tatarowicz W, Villano S, Chou S.** 2010. Virologic characterization of multidrug-resistant cytomegalovirus infection in 2 transplant recipients treated with maribavir. *J Infect Dis* **202:**104–108.
49. **Chou S, Ercolani RJ, Marousek G, Bowlin TL.** 2013. Cytomegalovirus UL97 kinase catalytic domain mutations that confer multidrug resistance. *Antimicrob Agents Chemother* **57:**3375–3379.

50. **Chou S.** 2009. Diverse cytomegalovirus UL27 mutations adapt to loss of viral UL97 kinase activity under maribavir. *Antimicrob Agents Chemother* **53:**81–85.
51. **Bigley TM, Reitsma JM, Terhune SS.** 2015. Antagonistic relationship between human cytomegalovirus pUL27 and pUL97 activities during infection. *J Virol* **89:**10230–10246.
52. **Coffin JM.** 1995. HIV population dynamics *in vivo*: implications for genetic variation, pathogenesis, and therapy. *Science* **267:**483–489.
53. **Rhee SY, et al.** 2015. Geographic and temporal trends in the molecular epidemiology and genetic mechanisms of transmitted HIV-1 drug resistance: an individual-patient- and sequence-level meta-analysis. *PLoS Med* **12:**e1001810.
54. **Gupta RK, Gregson J, Parkin N, Haile-Selassie H, Tanuri A, Andrade Forero L, Kaleebu P, Watera C, Aghokeng A, Mutenda N, Dzangare J, Hone S, Hang ZZ, Garcia J, Garcia Z, Marchorro P, Beteta E, Giron A, Hamers R, Inzaule S, Frenkel LM, Chung MH, de Oliveira T, Pillay D, Naidoo K, Kharsany A, Kugathasan R, Cutino T, Hunt G, Avila Rios S, Doherty M, Jordan MR, Bertagnolio S.** 2018. HIV-1 drug resistance before initiation or re-initiation of first-line antiretroviral therapy in low-income and middle-income countries: a systematic review and meta-regression analysis. *Lancet Infect Dis* **18:**346–355.
55. **World Health Organization.** 2017. HIVDR global report 2017. http://www.who.int/hiv/topics/drugresistance/en.
56. **Whitcomb JM, Parkin NT, Chappey C, Hellmann NS, Petropoulos CJ.** 2003. Broad nucleoside reverse-transcriptase inhibitor cross-resistance in human immunodeficiency virus type 1 clinical isolates. *J Infect Dis* **188:**992–1000.
57. **Singh K, Marchand B, Kirby KA, Michailidis E, Sarafianos SG.** 2010. Structural aspects of drug resistance and inhibition of HIV-1 reverse transcriptase. *Viruses* **2:**606–638.
58. **Menéndez-Arias L.** 2008. Mechanisms of resistance to nucleoside analogue inhibitors of HIV-1 reverse transcriptase. *Virus Res* **134:**124–146.
59. **Lanier ER, Ait-Khaled M, Scott J, Stone C, Melby T, Sturge G, St Clair M, Steel H, Hetherington S, Pearce G, Spreen W, Lafon S.** 2004. Antiviral efficacy of abacavir in antiretroviral therapy-experienced adults harbouring HIV-1 with specific patterns of resistance to nucleoside reverse transcriptase inhibitors. *Antivir Ther* **9:**37–45.
60. **Miller MD, Margot N, Lu B, Zhong L, Chen SS, Cheng A, Wulfsohn M.** 2004. Genotypic and phenotypic predictors of the magnitude of response to tenofovir disoproxil fumarate treatment in antiretroviral-experienced patients. *J Infect Dis* **189:**837–846.
61. **Melikian GL, Rhee SY, Taylor J, Fessel WJ, Kaufman D, Towner W, Troia-Cancio PV, Zolopa A, Robbins GK, Kagan R, Israelski D, Shafer RW.** 2012. Standardized comparison of the relative impacts of HIV-1 reverse transcriptase (RT) mutations on nucleoside RT inhibitor susceptibility. *Antimicrob Agents Chemother* **56:**2305–2313.
62. **Rhee SY, Varghese V, Holmes SP, Van Zyl GU, Steegen K, Boyd MA, Cooper DA, Nsanzimana S, Saravanan S, Charpentier C, de Oliveira T, Etiebet MA, Garcia F, Goedhals D, Gomes P, Günthard HF, Hamers RL, Hoffmann CJ, Hunt G, Jiamsakul A, Kaleebu P, Kanki P, Kantor R, Kerschberger B, Marconi VC, D'amour Ndahimana J, Ndembi N, Ngo-Giang-Huong N, Rokx C, Santoro MM, Schapiro JM, Schmidt D, Seu L, Sigaloff KCE, Sirivichayakul S, Skhosana L, Sunpath H, Tang M, Yang C, Carmona S, Gupta RK, Shafer RW.** 2017. Mutational correlates of virological failure in individuals receiving a WHO-recommended tenofovir-containing first-line regimen: an international collaboration. *EBioMedicine* **18:**225–235.
63. **Parikh UM, Bacheler L, Koontz D, Mellors JW.** 2006. The K65R mutation in human immunodeficiency virus type 1 reverse transcriptase exhibits bidirectional phenotypic antagonism with thymidine analog mutations. *J Virol* **80:**4971–4977.
64. **Winters MA, Coolley KL, Girard YA, Levee DJ, Hamdan H, Shafer RW, Katzenstein DA, Merigan TC.** 1998. A 6-basepair insert in the reverse transcriptase gene of human immunodeficiency virus type 1 confers resistance to multiple nucleoside inhibitors. *J Clin Invest* **102:**1769–1775.
65. **Shirasaka T, Kavlick MF, Ueno T, Gao WY, Kojima E, Alcaide ML, Chokekijchai S, Roy BM, Arnold E, Yarchoan R.** 1995. Emergence of human immunodeficiency virus type 1 variants with resistance to multiple dideoxynucleosides in patients receiving therapy with dideoxynucleosides. *Proc Natl Acad Sci USA* **92:**2398–2402.
66. **Shafer RW, Kozal MJ, Winters MA, Iversen AK, Katzenstein DA, Ragni MV, Meyer WA III, Gupta P, Rasheed S, Coombs R, Katzman M, Fiscus S, Merigan TC.** 1994. Combination therapy with zidovudine and didanosine selects for drug-resistant human immunodeficiency virus type 1 strains with unique patterns of pol gene mutations. *J Infect Dis* **169:**722–729.
67. **Menéndez-Arias L.** 2013. Molecular basis of human immunodeficiency virus type 1 drug resistance: overview and recent developments. *Antiviral Res* **98:**93–120.
68. **Parkin NT, Hellmann NS, Whitcomb JM, Kiss L, Chappey C, Petropoulos CJ.** 2004. Natural variation of drug susceptibility in wild-type Human Immunodeficiency Virus Type 1. *Antimicrob Agents Chemother* **48:**437–443.
69. **Jourdain G, Ngo-Giang-Huong N, Le Coeur S, Bowonwatanuwong C, Kantipong P, Leechanachai P, Ariyadej S, Leenasirimakul P, Hammer S, Lallemant M, Perinatal HIV Prevention Trial Group.** 2004. Intrapartum exposure to nevirapine and subsequent maternal responses to nevirapine-based antiretroviral therapy. *N Engl J Med* **351:**229–240.
70. **Vingerhoets J, Tambuyzer L, Azijn H, Hoogstoel A, Nijs S, Peeters M, de Béthune MP, De Smedt G, Woodfall B, Picchio G.** 2010. Resistance profile of etravirine: combined analysis of baseline genotypic and phenotypic data from the randomized, controlled phase III clinical studies. *AIDS* **24:**503–514.
71. **Das K, Clark AD Jr, Lewi PJ, Heeres J, De Jonge MR, Koymans LM, Vinkers HM, Daeyaert F, Ludovici DW, Kukla MJ, De Corte B, Kavash RW, Ho CY, Ye H, Lichtenstein MA, Andries K, Pauwels R, De Béthune MP, Boyer PL, Clark P, Hughes SH, Janssen PA, Arnold E.** 2004. Roles of conformational and positional adaptability in structure-based design of TMC125-R165335 (etravirine) and related non-nucleoside reverse transcriptase inhibitors that are highly potent and effective against wild-type and drug-resistant HIV-1 variants. *J Med Chem* **47:**2550–2560.
72. **Wensing AM, Calvez V, Günthard HF, Johnson VA, Paredes R, Pillay D, Shafer RW, Richman DD.** 2017. 2017 Update of the drug resistance mutations in HIV-1. *Top Antivir Med* **24:**132–133.
73. **Paredes R, Tzou PL, van Zyl G, Barrow G, Camacho R, Carmona S, Grant PM, Gupta RK, Hamers RL, Harrigan PR, Jordan MR, Kantor R, Katzenstein DA, Kuritzkes DR, Maldarelli F, Otelea D, Wallis CL, Schapiro JM, Shafer RW.** 2017. Collaborative update of a rule-based expert system for HIV-1 genotypic resistance test interpretation. *PLoS One* **12:**e0181357.
74. **Rimsky L, Vingerhoets J, Van Eygen V, Eron J, Clotet B, Hoogstoel A, Boven K, Picchio G.** 2012. Genotypic and phenotypic characterization of HIV-1 isolates obtained from patients on rilpivirine therapy experiencing virologic failure in the phase 3 ECHO and THRIVE studies: 48-week analysis. *J Acquir Immune Defic Syndr* **59:**39–46.
75. **Shahriar R, Rhee SY, Liu TF, Fessel WJ, Scarsella A, Towner W, Holmes SP, Zolopa AR, Shafer RW.** 2009. Nonpolymorphic human immunodeficiency virus type 1 protease and reverse transcriptase treatment-selected mutations. *Antimicrob Agents Chemother* **53:**4869–4878.
76. **Rhee SY, Sankaran K, Varghese V, Winters MA, Hurt CB, Eron JJ, Parkin N, Holmes SP, Holodniy M, Shafer RW.** 2016. HIV-1 protease, reverse transcriptase, and integrase variation. *J Virol* **90:**6058–6070.
77. **Ali A, Bandaranayake RM, Cai Y, King NM, Kolli M, Mittal S, Murzycki JF, Nalam MN, Nalivaika EA, Ozen A, Prabu-Jeyabalan MM, Thayer K, Schiffer CA.** 2010. Molecular basis for drug resistance in HIV-1 protease. *Viruses* **2:**2509–2535.

78. **Fun A, Wensing AM, Verheyen J, Nijhuis M.** 2012. Human immunodeficiency virus Gag and protease: partners in resistance. *Retrovirology* **9:**63.
79. **King MS, Rode R, Cohen-Codar I, Calvez V, Marcelin AG, Hanna GJ, Kempf DJ.** 2007. Predictive genotypic algorithm for virologic response to lopinavir-ritonavir in protease inhibitor-experienced patients. *Antimicrob Agents Chemother* **51:**3067–3074.
80. **de Meyer S, Vangeneugden T, van Baelen B, de Paepe E, van Marck H, Picchio G, Lefebvre E, de Béthune MP.** 2008. Resistance profile of darunavir: combined 24-week results from the POWER trials. *AIDS Res Hum Retroviruses* **24:** 379–388.
81. **Arribas JR, Girard PM, Paton N, Winston A, Marcelin AG, Elbirt D, Hill A, Hadacek MB.** 2016. Efficacy of protease inhibitor monotherapy vs. triple therapy: meta-analysis of data from 2303 patients in 13 randomized trials. *HIV Med* **17:**358–367.
82. **Dolling DI, Dunn DT, Sutherland KA, Pillay D, Mbisa JL, Parry CM, Post FA, Sabin CA, Cane PA, UK HIV Drug Resistance Database (UKHDRD), UK Collaborative HIV Cohort Study (UK CHIC).** 2013. Low frequency of genotypic resistance in HIV-1-infected patients failing an atazanavir-containing regimen: a clinical cohort study. *J Antimicrob Chemother* **68:**2339–2343.
83. **El Bouzidi K, White E, Mbisa JL, Sabin CA, Phillips AN, Mackie N, Pozniak AL, Tostevin A, Pillay D, Dunn DT, UK HIV Drug Resistance Database (UKHDRD) and the UK Collaborative HIV Cohort (UK CHIC) Study Steering Committees.** 2016. HIV-1 drug resistance mutations emerging on darunavir therapy in PI-naive and -experienced patients in the UK. *J Antimicrob Chemother* **71:**3487–3494.
84. **Zheng Y, Hughes MD, Lockman S, Benson CA, Hosseinipour MC, Campbell TB, Gulick RM, Daar ES, Sax PE, Riddler SA, Haubrich R, Salata RA, Currier JS.** 2014. Antiretroviral therapy and efficacy after virologic failure on first-line boosted protease inhibitor regimens. *Clin Infect Dis* **59:**888–896.
85. **López-Cortés LF, Castaño MA, López-Ruz MA, Rios-Villegas MJ, Hernández-Quero J, Merino D, Jiménez-Aguilar P, Marquez-Solero M, Terrón-Pernía A, Tellez-Pérez F, Viciana P, Orihuela-Cañadas F, Palacios-Baena Z, Vinuesa-Garcia D, Fajardo-Pico JM, Romero-Palacios A, Ojeda-Burgos G, Pasquau-Liaño J.** 2016. Effectiveness of ritonavir-boosted protease inhibitor monotherapy in clinical practice even with previous virological failures to protease inhibitor-based regimens. *PLoS One* **11:**e0148924.
86. **Goldgur Y, Craigie R, Cohen GH, Fujiwara T, Yoshinaga T, Fujishita T, Sugimoto H, Endo T, Murai H, Davies DR.** 1999. Structure of the HIV-1 integrase catalytic domain complexed with an inhibitor: a platform for antiviral drug design. *Proc Natl Acad Sci USA* **96:**13040–13043.
87. **Wang JY, Ling H, Yang W, Craigie R.** 2001. Structure of a two-domain fragment of HIV-1 integrase: implications for domain organization in the intact protein. *EMBO J* **20:** 7333–7343.
88. **Chen X, Tsiang M, Yu F, Hung M, Jones GS, Zeynalzadegan A, Qi X, Jin H, Kim CU, Swaminathan S, Chen JM.** 2008. Modeling, analysis, and validation of a novel HIV integrase structure provide insights into the binding modes of potent integrase inhibitors. *J Mol Biol* **380:**504–519.
89. **Hare S, Gupta SS, Valkov E, Engelman A, Cherepanov P.** 2010. Retroviral intasome assembly and inhibition of DNA strand transfer. *Nature* **464:**232–236.
90. **Passos DO, Li M, Yang R, Rebensburg SV, Ghirlando R, Jeon Y, Shkriabai N, Kvaratskhelia M, Craigie R, Lyumkis D.** 2017. Cryo-EM structures and atomic model of the HIV-1 strand transfer complex intasome. *Science* **355:** 89–92.
91. **Johnson AA, Santos W, Pais GC, Marchand C, Amin R, Burke TR Jr, Verdine G, Pommier Y.** 2006. Integration requires a specific interaction of the donor DNA terminal 5′-cytosine with glutamine 148 of the HIV-1 integrase flexible loop. *J Biol Chem* **281:**461–467.
92. **McColl DJ, Chen X.** 2010. Strand transfer inhibitors of HIV-1 integrase: bringing IN a new era of antiretroviral therapy. *Antiviral Res* **85:**101–118.
93. **Fransen S, Gupta S, Frantzell A, Petropoulos CJ, Huang W.** 2012. Substitutions at amino acid positions 143, 148, and 155 of HIV-1 integrase define distinct genetic barriers to raltegravir resistance *in vivo*. *J Virol* **86:**7249–7255.
94. **Hurt CB, Sebastian J, Hicks CB, Eron JJ.** 2014. Resistance to HIV integrase strand transfer inhibitors among clinical specimens in the United States, 2009-2012. *Clin Infect Dis* **58:**423–431.
95. **Abram ME, Hluhanich RM, Goodman DD, Andreatta KN, Margot NA, Ye L, Niedziela-Majka A, Barnes TL, Novikov N, Chen X, Svarovskaia ES, McColl DJ, White KL, Miller MD.** 2013. Impact of primary elvitegravir resistance-associated mutations in HIV-1 integrase on drug susceptibility and viral replication fitness. *Antimicrob Agents Chemother* **57:**2654–2663.
96. **Eron JJ, Clotet B, Durant J, Katlama C, Kumar P, Lazzarin A, Poizot-Martin I, Richmond G, Soriano V, Ait-Khaled M, Fujiwara T, Huang J, Min S, Vavro C, Yeo J, VIKING Study Group.** 2013. Safety and efficacy of dolutegravir in treatment-experienced subjects with raltegravir-resistant HIV type 1 infection: 24-week results of the VIKING Study. *J Infect Dis* **207:**740–748.
97. **Anstett K, Brenner B, Mesplede T, Wainberg MA.** 2017. HIV drug resistance against strand transfer integrase inhibitors. *Retrovirology* **14:**36.
98. **Oldenbuettel C, Wolf E, Ritter A, Noe S, Heldwein S, Pascucci R, Wiese C, Von Krosigk A, Jaegel-Guedes E, Jaeger H, Balogh A, Koegl C, Spinner CD.** 2017. Dolutegravir monotherapy as treatment de-escalation in HIV-infected adults with virological control: DoluMono cohort results. *Antivir Ther* **22:**169–172.
99. **Quashie PK, Mesplède T, Han YS, Oliveira M, Singhroy DN, Fujiwara T, Underwood MR, Wainberg MA.** 2012. Characterization of the R263K mutation in HIV-1 integrase that confers low-level resistance to the second-generation integrase strand transfer inhibitor dolutegravir. *J Virol* **86:**2696–2705.
100. **Brenner BG, Thomas R, Blanco JL, Ibanescu RI, Oliveira M, Mesplède T, Golubkov O, Roger M, Garcia F, Martinez E, Wainberg MA.** 2016. Development of a G118R mutation in HIV-1 integrase following a switch to dolutegravir monotherapy leading to cross-resistance to integrase inhibitors. *J Antimicrob Chemother* **71:**1948–1953.
101. **Wijting I, Rokx C, Boucher C, van Kampen J, Pas S, de Vries-Sluijs T, Schurink C, Bax H, Derksen M, Andrinopoulou ER, van der Ende M, van Gorp E, Nouwen J, Verbon A, Bierman W, Rijnders B.** 2017. Dolutegravir as maintenance monotherapy for HIV (DOMONO): a phase 2, randomised non-inferiority trial. *Lancet HIV* **4:**e547–e554.
102. **Tsiang M, Jones GS, Goldsmith J, Mulato A, Hansen D, Kan E, Tsai L, Bam RA, Stepan G, Stray KM, Niedziela-Majka A, Yant SR, Yu H, Kukolj G, Cihlar T, Lazerwith SE, White KL, Jin H.** 2016. Antiviral activity of bictegravir (GS-9883), a novel potent HIV-1 integrase strand transfer inhibitor with an improved resistance profile. *Antimicrob Agents Chemother* **60:**7086–7097.
103. **Sista PR, Melby T, Davison D, Jin L, Mosier S, Mink M, Nelson EL, DeMasi R, Cammack N, Salgo MP, Matthews TJ, Greenberg ML.** 2004. Characterization of determinants of genotypic and phenotypic resistance to enfuvirtide in baseline and on-treatment HIV-1 isolates. *AIDS* **18:**1787–1794.
104. **Mink M, Mosier SM, Janumpalli S, Davison D, Jin L, Melby T, Sista P, Erickson J, Lambert D, Stanfield-Oakley SA, Salgo M, Cammack N, Matthews T, Greenberg ML.** 2005. Impact of human immunodeficiency virus type 1 gp41 amino acid substitutions selected during enfuvirtide treatment on gp41 binding and antiviral potency of enfuvirtide *in vitro*. *J Virol* **79:**12447–12454.
105. **Lu J, Deeks SG, Hoh R, Beatty G, Kuritzkes BA, Martin JN, Kuritzkes DR.** 2006. Rapid emergence of enfuvirtide resistance in HIV-1-infected patients: results of a clonal analysis. *J Acquir Immune Defic Syndr* **43:**60–64.

106. **Tan Q, Zhu Y, Li J, Chen Z, Han GW, Kufareva I, Li T, Ma L, Fenalti G, Li J, Zhang W, Xie X, Yang H, Jiang H, Cherezov V, Liu H, Stevens RC, Zhao Q, Wu B.** 2013. Structure of the CCR5 chemokine receptor-HIV entry inhibitor maraviroc complex. *Science* **341:**1387–1390.
107. **Westby M, Lewis M, Whitcomb J, Youle M, Pozniak AL, James IT, Jenkins TM, Perros M, van der Ryst E.** 2006. Emergence of CXCR4-using human immunodeficiency virus type 1 (HIV-1) variants in a minority of HIV-1-infected patients following treatment with the CCR5 antagonist maraviroc is from a pretreatment CXCR4-using virus reservoir. *J Virol* **80:**4909–4920.
108. **Hartley O, Klasse PJ, Sattentau QJ, Moore JP.** 2005. V3: HIV's switch-hitter. *AIDS Res Hum Retroviruses* **21:**171–189.
109. **Westby M, Smith-Burchnell C, Mori J, Lewis M, Mosley M, Stockdale M, Dorr P, Ciaramella G, Perros M.** 2007. Reduced maximal inhibition in phenotypic susceptibility assays indicates that viral strains resistant to the CCR5 antagonist maraviroc utilize inhibitor-bound receptor for entry. *J Virol* **81:**2359–2371.
110. **Jiang X, Feyertag F, Meehan CJ, McCormack GP, Travers SA, Craig C, Westby M, Lewis M, Robertson DL.** 2015. Characterizing the diverse mutational pathways associated with R5-tropic maraviroc resistance: HIV-1 that uses the drug-bound CCR5 coreceptor. *J Virol* **89:**11457–11472.
111. **Tebit DM, Arts EJ.** 2011. Tracking a century of global expansion and evolution of HIV to drive understanding and to combat disease. *Lancet Infect Dis* **11:**45–56.
112. **Coutsinos D, Invernizzi CF, Xu H, Moisi D, Oliveira M, Brenner BG, Wainberg MA.** 2009. Template usage is responsible for the preferential acquisition of the K65R reverse transcriptase mutation in subtype C variants of human immunodeficiency virus type 1. *J Virol* **83:**2029–2033.
113. **Gregson J, et al, TenoRes Study Group.** 2016. Global epidemiology of drug resistance after failure of WHO recommended first-line regimens for adult HIV-1 infection: a multicentre retrospective cohort study. *Lancet Infect Dis* **16:** 565–575.
114. **Brenner B, Turner D, Oliveira M, Moisi D, Detorio M, Carobene M, Marlink RG, Schapiro J, Roger M, Wainberg MA.** 2003. A V106M mutation in HIV-1 clade C viruses exposed to efavirenz confers cross-resistance to non-nucleoside reverse transcriptase inhibitors. *AIDS* **17:**F1–F5.
115. **Werle-Lapostolle B, Bowden S, Locarnini S, Wursthorn K, Petersen J, Lau G, Trepo C, Marcellin P, Goodman Z, Delaney WE IV, Xiong S, Brosgart CL, Chen SS, Gibbs CS, Zoulim F.** 2004. Persistence of cccDNA during the natural history of chronic hepatitis B and decline during adefovir dipivoxil therapy. *Gastroenterology* **126:**1750–1758.
116. **Wong DK, Seto WK, Fung J, Ip P, Huang FY, Lai CL, Yuen MF.** 2013. Reduction of hepatitis B surface antigen and covalently closed circular DNA by nucleos(t)ide analogues of different potency. *Clin Gastroenterol Hepatol* **11:** 1004-10e1.
117. **Lucifora J, Protzer U.** 2016. Attacking hepatitis B virus cccDNA: the holy grail to hepatitis B cure. *J Hepatol* **64**(Suppl)**:**S41–S48.
118. **Nowak MA, Bonhoeffer S, Hill AM, Boehme R, Thomas HC, McDade H.** 1996. Viral dynamics in hepatitis B virus infection. *Proc Natl Acad Sci USA* **93:**4398–4402.
119. **Hollinger FB.** 2007. Hepatitis B virus genetic diversity and its impact on diagnostic assays. *J Viral Hepat* **14**(Suppl 1)**:** 11–15.
120. **Zaaijer HL, van Hemert FJ, Koppelman MH, Lukashov VV.** 2007. Independent evolution of overlapping polymerase and surface protein genes of hepatitis B virus. *J Gen Virol* **88:**2137–2143.
121. **Soriano V, Perelson AS, Zoulim F.** 2008. Why are there different dynamics in the selection of drug resistance in HIV and hepatitis B and C viruses? *J Antimicrob Chemother* **62:** 1–4.
122. **Fung SK, Lok AS.** 2004. Hepatitis B virus genotypes: do they play a role in the outcome of HBV infection? *Hepatology* **40:**790–792.
123. **Moucari R, Martinot-Peignoux M, Mackiewicz V, Boyer N, Ripault MP, Castelnau C, Leclere L, Dauvergne A, Valla D, Vidaud M, Nicolas-Chanoine MH, Marcellin P.** 2009. Influence of genotype on hepatitis B surface antigen kinetics in hepatitis B e antigen-negative patients treated with pegylated interferon-alpha2a. *Antivir Ther* **14:** 1183–1188.
124. **Tong S, Revill P.** 2016. Overview of hepatitis B viral replication and genetic variability. *J Hepatol* **64**(Suppl)**:** S4–S16.
125. **Li X, Liu Y, Xin S, Ji D, You S, Hu J, Zhao J, Wu J, Liao H, Zhang XX, Xu D.** 2017. Comparison of detection rate and mutational pattern of drug-resistant mutations between a large cohort of genotype B and genotype C hepatitis B virus-infected patients in north China. *Microb Drug Resist* **23:**516–522.
126. **Zhang HY, Liu LG, Ye CY, Chen CH, Hang SX, Zhu Z, Shen HY, Huang ZY, Chen WY, Xue Y.** 2018. Evolution of drug-resistant mutations in HBV genomes in patients with treatment failure during the past seven years (2010-2016). *Virus Genes* **54:**41–47.
127. **Lampertico P, Agarwal K, Berg T, Buti M, Janssen HLA, Papatheodoridis G, Zoulim F, Tacke F, European Association for the Study of the Liver.** 2017. EASL 2017 clinical practice guidelines on the management of hepatitis B virus infection. *J Hepatol* **67:**370–398.
128. **Tenney DJ, Rose RE, Baldick CJ, Pokornowski KA, Eggers BJ, Fang J, Wichroski MJ, Xu D, Yang J, Wilber RB, Colonno RJ.** 2009. Long-term monitoring shows hepatitis B virus resistance to entecavir in nucleoside-naïve patients is rare through 5 years of therapy. *Hepatology* **49:**1503–1514.
129. **Kitrinos KM, Corsa A, Liu Y, Flaherty J, Snow-Lampart A, Marcellin P, Borroto-Esoda K, Miller MD.** 2014. No detectable resistance to tenofovir disoproxil fumarate after 6 years of therapy in patients with chronic hepatitis B. *Hepatology* **59:**434–442.
130. **Liu Y, Corsa AC, Buti M, Cathcart AL, Flaherty JF, Miller MD, Kitrinos KM, Marcellin P, Gane EJ.** 2017. No detectable resistance to tenofovir disoproxil fumarate in HBeAg+ and HBeAg- patients with chronic hepatitis B after 8 years of treatment. *J Viral Hepat* **24:**68–74.
131. **Scott LJ, Chan HLY.** 2017. Tenofovir alafenamide: a review in chronic hepatitis B. *Drugs* **77:**1017–1028.
132. **Lai CL, Dienstag J, Schiff E, Leung NW, Atkins M, Hunt C, Brown N, Woessner M, Boehme R, Condreay L.** 2003. Prevalence and clinical correlates of YMDD variants during lamivudine therapy for patients with chronic hepatitis B. *Clin Infect Dis* **36:**687–696.
133. **Liaw YF, Gane E, Leung N, Zeuzem S, Wang Y, Lai CL, Heathcote EJ, Manns M, Bzowej N, Niu J, Han SH, Hwang SG, Cakaloglu Y, Tong MJ, Papatheodoridis G, Chen Y, Brown NA, Albanis E, Galil K, Naoumov NV, GLOBE Study Group.** 2009. 2-Year GLOBE trial results: telbivudine is superior to lamivudine in patients with chronic hepatitis B. *Gastroenterology* **136:**486–495.
134. **Hadziyannis SJ, Tassopoulos NC, Heathcote EJ, Chang TT, Kitis G, Rizzetto M, Marcellin P, Lim SG, Goodman Z, Ma J, Brosgart CL, Borroto-Esoda K, Arterburn S, Chuck SL, Adefovir Dipivoxil 438 Study Group.** 2006. Long-term therapy with adefovir dipivoxil for HBeAg-negative chronic hepatitis B for up to 5 years. *Gastroenterology* **131:** 1743–1751.
135. **Das K, Xiong X, Yang H, Westland CE, Gibbs CS, Sarafianos SG, Arnold E.** 2001. Molecular modeling and biochemical characterization reveal the mechanism of hepatitis B virus polymerase resistance to lamivudine (3TC) and emtricitabine (FTC). *J Virol* **75:**4771–4779.
136. **Bartholomeusz A, Tehan BG, Chalmers DK.** 2004. Comparisons of the HBV and HIV polymerase, and antiviral resistance mutations. *Antivir Ther* **9:**149–160.
137. **Lok AS, Zoulim F, Locarnini S, Bartholomeusz A, Ghany MG, Pawlotsky JM, Liaw YF, Mizokami M, Kuiken C, Hepatitis B Virus Drug Resistance Working Group.**

2007. Antiviral drug-resistant HBV: standardization of nomenclature and assays and recommendations for management. *Hepatology* **46:**254–265.

138. **Devi U, Locarnini S.** 2013. Hepatitis B antivirals and resistance. *Curr Opin Virol* **3:**495–500.
139. **Liaw YF, Chien RN, Yeh CT.** 2004. No benefit to continue lamivudine therapy after emergence of YMDD mutations. *Antivir Ther* **9:**257–262.
140. **Di Marco V, Di Stefano R, Ferraro D, Almasio PL, Bonura C, Giglio M, Parisi P, Cappello M, Alaimo G, Craxì A.** 2005. HBV-DNA suppression and disease course in HBV cirrhosis patients on long-term lamivudine therapy. *Antivir Ther* **10:**431–439.
141. **Peters MG, Hann HW, Martin P, Heathcote EJ, Buggisch P, Rubin R, Bourliere M, Kowdley K, Trepo C, Gray DF, Sullivan M, Kleber K, Ebrahimi R, Xiong S, Brosgart CL.** 2004. Adefovir dipivoxil alone or in combination with lamivudine in patients with lamivudine-resistant chronic hepatitis B. *Gastroenterology* **126:**91–101.
142. **Westland CE, Yang H, Delaney WE IV, Wulfsohn M, Lama N, Gibbs CS, Miller MD, Fry J, Brosgart CL, Schiff ER, Xiong S.** 2005. Activity of adefovir dipivoxil against all patterns of lamivudine-resistant hepatitis B viruses in patients. *J Viral Hepat* **12:**67–73.
143. **Fung SK, Chae HB, Fontana RJ, Conjeevaram H, Marrero J, Oberhelman K, Hussain M, Lok AS.** 2006. Virologic response and resistance to adefovir in patients with chronic hepatitis B. *J Hepatol* **44:**283–290.
144. **Borroto-Esoda K, Miller MD, Arterburn S.** 2007. Pooled analysis of amino acid changes in the HBV polymerase in patients from four major adefovir dipivoxil clinical trials. *J Hepatol* **47:**492–498.
145. **Santantonio T, Fasano M, Durantel S, Barraud L, Heichen M, Guastadisegni A, Pastore G, Zoulim F.** 2009. Adefovir dipivoxil resistance patterns in patients with lamivudine-resistant chronic hepatitis B. *Antivir Ther* **14:**557–565.
146. **Marcellin P, Lau GK, Bonino F, Farci P, Hadziyannis S, Jin R, Lu ZM, Piratvisuth T, Germanidis G, Yurdaydin C, Diago M, Gurel S, Lai MY, Button P, Pluck N, Peginterferon Alfa-2a HBeAg-Negative Chronic Hepatitis B Study Group.** 2004. Peginterferon alfa-2a alone, lamivudine alone, and the two in combination in patients with HBeAg-negative chronic hepatitis B. *N Engl J Med* **351:**1206–1217.
147. **Zoulim F, Locarnini S.** 2013. Optimal management of chronic hepatitis B patients with treatment failure and antiviral drug resistance. *Liver Int* 33(Suppl 1)**:**116–124.
148. **Yatsuji H, Noguchi C, Hiraga N, Mori N, Tsuge M, Imamura M, Takahashi S, Iwao E, Fujimoto Y, Ochi H, Abe H, Maekawa T, Tateno C, Yoshizato K, Suzuki F, Kumada H, Chayama K.** 2006. Emergence of a novel lamivudine-resistant hepatitis B virus variant with a substitution outside the YMDD motif. *Antimicrob Agents Chemother* **50:**3867–3874.
149. **Villet S, Pichoud C, Billioud G, Barraud L, Durantel S, Trépo C, Zoulim F.** 2008. Impact of hepatitis B virus rtA181V/T mutants on hepatitis B treatment failure. *J Hepatol* **48:**747–755.
150. **Warner N, Locarnini S.** 2008. The antiviral drug selected hepatitis B virus rtA181T/sW172* mutant has a dominant negative secretion defect and alters the typical profile of viral rebound. *Hepatology* **48:**88–98.
151. **Liu Y, Miller MD, Kitrinos KM.** 2017. Tenofovir alafenamide demonstrates broad cross-genotype activity against wild-type HBV clinical isolates and maintains susceptibility to drug-resistant HBV isolates *in vitro*. *Antiviral Res* **139:** 25–31.
152. **Tenney DJ, Levine SM, Rose RE, Walsh AW, Weinheimer SP, Discotto L, Plym M, Pokornowski K, Yu CF, Angus P, Ayres A, Bartholomeusz A, Sievert W, Thompson G, Warner N, Locarnini S, Colonno RJ.** 2004. Clinical emergence of entecavir-resistant hepatitis B virus requires additional substitutions in virus already resistant to lamivudine. *Antimicrob Agents Chemother* **48:**3498–3507.
153. **Tenney DJ, Rose RE, Baldick CJ, Levine SM, Pokornowski KA, Walsh AW, Fang J, Yu CF, Zhang S, Mazzucco CE, Eggers B, Hsu M, Plym MJ, Poundstone P, Yang J, Colonno RJ.** 2007. Two-year assessment of entecavir resistance in lamivudine-refractory hepatitis B virus patients reveals different clinical outcomes depending on the resistance substitutions present. *Antimicrob Agents Chemother* **51:**902–911.
154. **Sherman M, Yurdaydin C, Simsek H, Silva M, Liaw YF, Rustgi VK, Sette H, Tsai N, Tenney DJ, Vaughan J, Kreter B, Hindes R, AI463026 Benefits of Entecavir for Hepatitis B Liver Disease (BEHoLD) Study Group.** 2008. Entecavir therapy for lamivudine-refractory chronic hepatitis B: improved virologic, biochemical, and serology outcomes through 96 weeks. *Hepatology* **48:**99–108.
155. **Koffi J, Egounlety R, Pradat P, Lebosse F, Si-Ahmed SN, Lussier V, Chevallier P, Bailly F, Zoulim F.** 2014. Impact of lamivudine-resistance mutations on entecavir treatment outcome in hepatitis B. *Eur J Gastroenterol Hepatol* **26:**146–154.
156. **Lim YS.** 2017. Management of antiviral resistance in chronic hepatitis B. *Gut Liver* **11:**189–195.
157. **van Bömmel F, de Man RA, Wedemeyer H, Deterding K, Petersen J, Buggisch P, Erhardt A, Hüppe D, Stein K, Trojan J, Sarrazin C, Böcher WO, Spengler U, Wasmuth HE, Reinders JG, Möller B, Rhode P, Feucht HH, Wiedenmann B, Berg T.** 2010. Long-term efficacy of tenofovir monotherapy for hepatitis B virus-monoinfected patients after failure of nucleoside/nucleotide analogues. *Hepatology* **51:**73–80.
158. **Berg T, Zoulim F, Moeller B, Trinh H, Marcellin P, Chan S, Kitrinos KM, Dinh P, Flaherty JF Jr, McHutchison JG, Manns M.** 2014. Long-term efficacy and safety of emtricitabine plus tenofovir DF vs. tenofovir DF monotherapy in adefovir-experienced chronic hepatitis B patients. *J Hepatol* **60:**715–722.
159. **Zoulim F, Białkowska-Warzecha J, Diculescu MM, Goldis AE, Heyne R, Mach T, Marcellin P, Petersen J, Simon K, Bendahmane S, Klauck I, Wasiak W, Janssen HL.** 2016. Entecavir plus tenofovir combination therapy for chronic hepatitis B in patients with previous nucleos(t)ide treatment failure. *Hepatol Int* **10:**779–788.
160. **Kim DY, Lee HW, Song JE, Kim BK, Kim SU, Kim DY, Ahn SH, Han KH, Park JY.** 2018. Switching from tenofovir and nucleoside analogue therapy to tenofovir monotherapy in virologically suppressed chronic hepatitis B patients with antiviral resistance. *J Med Virol* **90:**497–502.
161. **Bartenschlager R, Lohmann V, Penin F.** 2013. The molecular and structural basis of advanced antiviral therapy for hepatitis C virus infection. *Nat Rev Microbiol* **11:** 482–496.
162. **Smith DB, Bukh J, Kuiken C, Muerhoff AS, Rice CM, Stapleton JT, Simmonds P.** 2014. Expanded classification of hepatitis C virus into 7 genotypes and 67 subtypes: updated criteria and assignment web resource. *Hepatology* **59:** 318–327.
163. **Messina JP, Humphreys I, Flaxman A, Brown A, Cooke GS, Pybus OG, Barnes E.** 2015. Global distribution and prevalence of hepatitis C virus genotypes. *Hepatology* **61:** 77–87.
164. **Powdrill MH, Tchesnokov EP, Kozak RA, Russell RS, Martin R, Svarovskaia ES, Mo H, Kouyos RD, Götte M.** 2011. Contribution of a mutational bias in hepatitis C virus replication to the genetic barrier in the development of drug resistance. *Proc Natl Acad Sci USA* **108:**20509–20513.
165. **Fan X, Mao Q, Zhou D, Lu Y, Xing J, Xu Y, Ray SC, Di Bisceglie AM.** 2009. High diversity of hepatitis C viral quasispecies is associated with early virological response in patients undergoing antiviral therapy. *Hepatology* **50:** 1765–1772.
166. **Herrmann E, Neumann AU, Schmidt JM, Zeuzem S.** 2000. Hepatitis C virus kinetics. *Antivir Ther* **5:**85–90.
167. **European Association for the Study of the Liver.** 2017. EASL recommendations on treatment of hepatitis C 2016. *J Hepatol* **66:**153–194.

168. **Kwong AD, Najera I, Bechtel J, Bowden S, Fitzgibbon J, Harrington P, Kempf D, Kieffer TL, Koletzki D, Kukolj G, Lim S, Pilot-Matias T, Lin K, Mani N, Mo H, O'Rear J, Otto M, Parkin N, Pawlotsky JM, Petropoulos C, Picchio G, Ralston R, Reeves JD, Schooley RT, Seiwert S, Standring D, Stuyver L, Sullivan J, Miller V, Forum for Collaborative Human Immunodeficiency Virus Research, HCV Drug Development Advisory Group (HCV DRAG), Sequence Analysis Working Group (SAWG), Phenotype Analysis Working Group (PAWG).** 2011. Sequence and phenotypic analysis for resistance monitoring in hepatitis C virus drug development: recommendations from the HCV DRAG. *Gastroenterology* **140:**755–760.
169. **Lohmann V, Bartenschlager R.** 2014. On the history of hepatitis C virus cell culture systems. *J Med Chem* **57:** 1627–1642.
170. **Fourati S, Pawlotsky JM.** 2015. Virologic tools for HCV drug resistance testing. *Viruses* **7:**6346–6359.
171. **Johnson & Johnson.** 2017. Olysio (simeprevir) capsules, for oral use. Initial U.S. approval: 2013. https://www.olysio.com/shared/product/olysio/prescribing-information.pdf.
172. **Bristol-Myers Squibb.** 2017. Daklinza (daclastavir) tablets, for oral use. Initial U.S. approval: 2015. https://packageinserts.bms.com/pi/pi_daklinza.pdf.
173. **Gilead Sciences.** 2017. Harvoni (ledipasvir and sofosbuvir) tablets, for oral use. Initial U.S. approval: 2014. https://www.gilead.com/~/media/Files/pdfs/medicines/liver-disease/harvoni/harvoni_pi.pdf.
174. **Abbvie Inc.** 2015. Viekira Pak (ombitasvir, paritaprevir, and ritonavir tablets; dasabuvir tablets): U.S. prescribing information. https://www.rxabbvie/viekirapak/viekirapak_pi.html.
175. **Merck.** 2017. Zepatier (elbasvir and grazoprevir tablets, for oral use: U.S. prescribing information 2016. https://www.merck.com/product/usa/pi_circulars/z/zepatier/zepatier_pi.pdf.
176. **Gilead Sciences.** 2017. Epclusa (sofosbuvir and velpatasvir) tablets, for oral use. Initial U.S. approval: 2016. http://www.gilead.com/~/media/Files/pdfs/medicines/liver-disease/epclusa/epclusa_pi.pdf.
177. **Abbvie Inc.** 2017. Mavyret (glecaprevir and pibrentasvir) tablets, for oral use. Initial U.S. Approval 2017. http://www.rxabbvie.com/pdf/mavyret_pi.pdf.
178. **Bourlière M, Gordon SC, Flamm SL, Cooper CL, Ramji A, Tong M, Ravendhran N, Vierling JM, Tran TT, Pianko S, Bansal MB, de Lédinghen V, Hyland RH, Stamm LM, Dvory-Sobol H, Svarovskaia E, Zhang J, Huang KC, Subramanian GM, Brainard DM, McHutchison JG, Verna EC, Buggisch P, Landis CS, Younes ZH, Curry MP, Strasser SI, Schiff ER, Reddy KR, Manns MP, Kowdley KV, Zeuzem S, POLARIS-1 and POLARIS-4 Investigators.** 2017. Sofosbuvir, velpatasvir, and voxilaprevir for previously treated HCV infection. *N Engl J Med* **376:**2134–2146.
179. **Gilead Sciences.** 2017. Vosevi (sofosbuvir, velpatasvir, and voxilaprevir) tablets for oral use. Initial U.S. approval: 2017. https://www.accessdata.fda.gov/drugsatfda_docs/label/2017/209195s000lbl.pdf.
180. **American Association for the Study of Liver Diseases.** 2017. Initial treatment of HCV infection. http://www.hcvguidelines.org/treatment-naive.
181. **Feld JJ, Jacobson IM, Sulkowski MS, Poordad F, Tatsch F, Pawlotsky JM.** 2017. Ribavirin revisited in the era of direct-acting antiviral therapy for hepatitis C virus infection. *Liver Int* **37:**5–18.
182. **Loustaud-Ratti V, Debette-Gratien M, Jacques J, Alain S, Marquet P, Sautereau D, Rousseau A, Carrier P.** 2016. Ribavirin: past, present and future. *World J Hepatol* **8:** 123–130.
183. **Pawlotsky JM.** 2016. Hepatitis C virus resistance to direct-acting antiviral drugs in interferon-free regimens. *Gastroenterology* **151:**70–86.
184. **Wyles DL, Luetkemeyer AF.** 2017. Understanding hepatitis C virus drug resistance: clinical implications for current and future regimens. *Top Antivir Med* **25:**103–109.
185. **Jensen SB, Serre SB, Humes DG, Ramirez S, Li YP, Bukh J, Gottwein JM.** 2015. Substitutions at NS3 residue 155, 156, or 168 of hepatitis C virus genotypes 2 to 6 induce complex patterns of protease inhibitor resistance. *Antimicrob Agents Chemother* **59:**7426–7436.
186. **Serre SB, Jensen SB, Ghanem L, Humes DG, Ramirez S, Li YP, Krarup H, Bukh J, Gottwein JM.** 2016. Hepatitis C virus genotype 1 to 6 protease inhibitor escape variants: *in vitro* selection, fitness, and resistance patterns in the context of the infectious viral life cycle. *Antimicrob Agents Chemother* **60:**3563–3578.
187. **Zeuzem S, Mizokami M, Pianko S, Mangia A, Han KH, Martin R, Svarovskaia E, Dvory-Sobol H, Doehle B, Hedskog C, Yun C, Brainard DM, Knox S, McHutchison JG, Miller MD, Mo H, Chuang WL, Jacobson I, Dore GJ, Sulkowski M.** 2017. NS5A resistance-associated substitutions in patients with genotype 1 hepatitis C virus: prevalence and effect on treatment outcome. *J Hepatol* **66:** 910–918.
188. **Boyd SD, Tracy L, Komatsu TE, Harrington PR, Viswanathan P, Murray J, Sherwat A.** 2017. US FDA perspective on elbasvir/grazoprevir treatment for patients with chronic hepatitis C virus genotype 1 or 4 infection. *Clin Drug Investig* **37:**317–326.
189. **Carter W, Connelly S, Struble K.** 2017. Reinventing HCV treatment: past and future perspectives. *J Clin Pharmacol* **57:**287–296.
190. **American Association for the Study of Liver Diseases / Infectious Diseases Society of America.** 2017. HCV resistance primer. http://www.hcvguidelines.org/evaluate/resistance.
191. **Harrington PR, Komatsu TE, Deming DJ, Donaldson EF, O'Rear JJ, Naeger LK.** 2017. Impact of hepatitis C virus polymorphisms on direct-acting antiviral treatment efficacy: regulatory analyses and perspectives. *Hepatology*.
192. **Molino S, Martin MT.** 2017. Hepatitis C virus resistance testing in genotype 1: the changing role in clinical utility. *Ann Pharmacother* **51:**811–816.
193. **Appleby TC, Perry JK, Murakami E, Barauskas O, Feng J, Cho A, Fox D III, Wetmore DR, McGrath ME, Ray AS, Sofia MJ, Swaminathan S, Edwards TE.** 2015. Structural basis for RNA replication by the hepatitis C virus polymerase. *Science* **347:**771–775.
194. **Lam AM, Espiritu C, Bansal S, Micolochick Steuer HM, Niu C, Zennou V, Keilman M, Zhu Y, Lan S, Otto MJ, Furman PA.** 2012. Genotype and subtype profiling of PSI-7977 as a nucleotide inhibitor of hepatitis C virus. *Antimicrob Agents Chemother* **56:**3359–3368.
195. **Xu S, Doehle B, Rajyaguru S, Han B, Barauskas O, Feng J, Perry J, Dvory-Sobol H, Svarovskaia ES, Miller MD, Mo H.** 2017. *In vitro* selection of resistance to sofosbuvir in HCV replicons of genotype-1 to -6. *Antivir Ther* **22:**587–597.
196. **Svarovskaia ES, Dvory-Sobol H, Parkin N, Hebner C, Gontcharova V, Martin R, Ouyang W, Han B, Xu S, Ku K, Chiu S, Gane E, Jacobson IM, Nelson DR, Lawitz E, Wyles DL, Bekele N, Brainard D, Symonds WT, McHutchison JG, Miller MD, Mo H.** 2014. Infrequent development of resistance in genotype 1-6 hepatitis C virus-infected subjects treated with sofosbuvir in phase 2 and 3 clinical trials. *Clin Infect Dis* **59:**1666–1674.
197. **Svarovskaia ES, Gane E, Dvory-Sobol H, Martin R, Doehle B, Hedskog C, Jacobson IM, Nelson DR, Lawitz E, Brainard DM, McHutchison JG, Miller MD, Mo H.** 2016. L159F and V321A sofosbuvir-associated hepatitis C virus NS5B substitutions. *J Infect Dis* **213:**1240–1247.
198. **Donaldson EF, Harrington PR, O'Rear JJ, Naeger LK.** 2015. Clinical evidence and bioinformatics characterization of potential hepatitis C virus resistance pathways for sofosbuvir. *Hepatology* **61:**56–65.
199. **Kati W, Koev G, Irvin M, Beyer J, Liu Y, Krishnan P, Reisch T, Mondal R, Wagner R, Molla A, Maring C, Collins C.** 2015. *In vitro* activity and resistance profile of dasabuvir, a nonnucleoside hepatitis C virus polymerase inhibitor. *Antimicrob Agents Chemother* **59:**1505–1511.

200. **Krishnan P, Tripathi R, Schnell G, Reisch T, Beyer J, Irvin M, Xie W, Larsen L, Cohen D, Podsadecki T, Pilot-Matias T, Collins C.** 2015. Resistance analysis of baseline and treatment-emergent variants in hepatitis C virus genotype 1 in the AVIATOR study with paritaprevir-ritonavir, ombitasvir, and dasabuvir. *Antimicrob Agents Chemother* **59:**5445–5454.

201. **Sarrazin C.** 2016. The importance of resistance to direct antiviral drugs in HCV infection in clinical practice. *J Hepatol* **64:**486–504.

202. **Romano KP, Ali A, Aydin C, Soumana D, Ozen A, Deveau LM, Silver C, Cao H, Newton A, Petropoulos CJ, Huang W, Schiffer CA.** 2012. The molecular basis of drug resistance against hepatitis C virus NS3/4A protease inhibitors. *PLoS Pathog* **8:**e1002832.

203. **Welzel TM, Bhardwaj N, Hedskog C, Chodavarapu K, Camus G, McNally J, Brainard D, Miller MD, Mo H, Svarovskaia E, Jacobson I, Zeuzem S, Agarwal K.** 2017. Global epidemiology of HCV subtypes and resistance-associated substitutions evaluated by sequencing-based subtype analyses. *J Hepatol* **67:**224–236.

204. **Lenz O, Verbinnen T, Lin TI, Vijgen L, Cummings MD, Lindberg J, Berke JM, Dehertogh P, Fransen E, Scholliers A, Vermeiren K, Ivens T, Raboisson P, Edlund M, Storm S, Vrang L, de Kock H, Fanning GC, Simmen KA.** 2010. *In vitro* resistance profile of the hepatitis C virus NS3/4A protease inhibitor TMC435. *Antimicrob Agents Chemother* **54:**1878–1887.

205. **Bagaglio S, Uberti-Foppa C, Morsica G.** 2017. Resistance mechanisms in hepatitis C virus: implications for direct-acting antiviral use. *Drugs* **77:**1043–1055.

206. **Pilot-Matias T, Tripathi R, Cohen D, Gaultier I, Dekhtyar T, Lu L, Reisch T, Irvin M, Hopkins T, Pithawalla R, Middleton T, Ng T, McDaniel K, Or YS, Menon R, Kempf D, Molla A, Collins C.** 2015. *In vitro* and *in vivo* antiviral activity and resistance profile of the hepatitis C virus NS3/4A protease inhibitor ABT-450. *Antimicrob Agents Chemother* **59:**988–997.

207. **Soumana DI, Kurt Yilmaz N, Ali A, Prachanronarong KL, Schiffer CA.** 2016. Molecular and dynamic mechanism underlying drug resistance in genotype 3 hepatitis C NS3/4A protease. *J Am Chem Soc* **138:**11850–11859.

208. **Issur M, Götte M.** 2014. Resistance patterns associated with HCV NS5A inhibitors provide limited insight into drug binding. *Viruses* **6:**4227–4241.

209. **Ascher DB, Wielens J, Nero TL, Doughty L, Morton CJ, Parker MW.** 2014. Potent hepatitis C inhibitors bind directly to NS5A and reduce its affinity for RNA. *Sci Rep* **4:**4765.

210. **Kwon HJ, Xing W, Chan K, Niedziela-Majka A, Brendza KM, Kirschberg T, Kato D, Link JO, Cheng G, Liu X, Sakowicz R.** 2015. Direct binding of ledipasvir to HCV NS5A: mechanism of resistance to an HCV antiviral agent. *PLoS One* **10:**e0122844.

211. **Lawitz EJ, Dvory-Sobol H, Doehle BP, Worth AS, McNally J, Brainard DM, Link JO, Miller MD, Mo H.** 2016. Clinical resistance to velpatasvir (GS-5816), a novel pan-genotypic inhibitor of the hepatitis C virus NS5A protein. *Antimicrob Agents Chemother* **60:**5368–5378.

212. **Ng TI, Krishnan P, Pilot-Matias T, Kati W, Schnell G, Beyer J, Reisch T, Lu L, Dekhtyar T, Irvin M, Tripathi R, Maring C, Randolph JT, Wagner R, Collins C.** 2017. *In vitro* antiviral activity and resistance profile of the next-generation hepatitis C virus NS5A inhibitor pibrentasvir. *Antimicrob Agents Chemother* **61:** e02558-16.

213. **Wyles D, Mangia A, Cheng W, Shafran S, Schwabe C, Ouyang W, Hedskog C, McNally J, Brainard DM, Doehle BP, Svarovskaia E, Miller MD, Mo H, Dvory-Sobol H.** 2018. Long-term persistence of HCV NS5A resistance associated substitutions after treatment with the HCV NS5A inhibitor, ledipasvir, without sofosbuvir. *Antivir Ther* **23:**229–238.

214. **Wang C, Sun JH, O'Boyle DR II, Nower P, Valera L, Roberts S, Fridell RA, Gao M.** 2013. Persistence of resistant variants in hepatitis C virus-infected patients treated with the NS5A replication complex inhibitor daclatasvir. *Antimicrob Agents Chemother* **57:**2054–2065.

215. **Wang C, Valera L, Jia L, Kirk MJ, Gao M, Fridell RA.** 2013. *In vitro* activity of daclatasvir on hepatitis C virus genotype 3 NS5A. *Antimicrob Agents Chemother* **57:**611–613.

216. **Hernandez D, Zhou N, Ueland J, Monikowski A, McPhee F.** 2013. Natural prevalence of NS5A polymorphisms in subjects infected with hepatitis C virus genotype 3 and their effects on the antiviral activity of NS5A inhibitors. *J Clin Virol* **57:**13–18.

217. **Sarrazin C, Dvory-Sobol H, Svarovskaia ES, Doehle BP, Pang PS, Chuang SM, Ma J, Ding X, Afdhal NH, Kowdley KV, Gane EJ, Lawitz E, Brainard DM, McHutchison JG, Miller MD, Mo H.** 2016. Prevalence of resistance-associated substitutions in HCV NS5A, NS5B, or NS3 and outcomes of treatment with ledipasvir and sofosbuvir. *Gastroenterology* **151:**501–512.e1.

218. **Foster GR, Afdhal N, Roberts SK, Bräu N, Gane EJ, Pianko S, Lawitz E, Thompson A, Shiffman ML, Cooper C, Towner WJ, Conway B, Ruane P, Bourlière M, Asselah T, Berg T, Zeuzem S, Rosenberg W, Agarwal K, Stedman CA, Mo H, Dvory-Sobol H, Han L, Wang J, McNally J, Osinusi A, Brainard DM, McHutchison JG, Mazzotta F, Tran TT, Gordon SC, Patel K, Reau N, Mangia A, Sulkowski M, ASTRAL-2 Investigators, ASTRAL-3 Investigators.** 2015. Sofosbuvir and velpatasvir for HCV genotype 2 and 3 infection. *N Engl J Med* **373:**2608–2617.

219. **Cuevas JM, Torres-Puente M, Jiménez-Hernández N, Bracho MA, García-Robles I, Wrobel B, Carnicer F, del Olmo J, Ortega E, Moya A, González-Candelas F.** 2008. Genetic variability of hepatitis C virus before and after combined therapy of interferon plus ribavirin. *PLoS One* **3:**e3058.

220. **Dietz J, Schelhorn SE, Fitting D, Mihm U, Susser S, Welker MW, Füller C, Däumer M, Teuber G, Wedemeyer H, Berg T, Lengauer T, Zeuzem S, Herrmann E, Sarrazin C.** 2013. Deep sequencing reveals mutagenic effects of ribavirin during monotherapy of hepatitis C virus genotype 1-infected patients. *J Virol* **87:**6172–6181.

221. **Novel Swine-Origin Influenza A (H1N1) Virus Investigation Team.** 2009. Emergence of a novel swine-origin influenza A (H1N1) virus in humans. *N Engl J Med* **360:**2605–2615.

222. **Writing Committee of the Second World Health Organization Consultation on Clinical Aspects of Human Infection with Avian Influenza A (H5N1) Virus.** 2008. Update on avian influenza A (H5N1) virus infection in humans. *N Engl J Med* **358:**261–273.

223. **WHO.** 2017. Human infection with avian influenza A(H7N9) virus: China. http://www.who.int/csr/don/13-september-2017-ah7n9-china/en/.

224. **Burnham AJ, Baranovich T, Govorkova EA.** 2013. Neuraminidase inhibitors for influenza B virus infection: efficacy and resistance. *Antiviral Res* **100:**520–534.

225. **Härter G, Zimmermann O, Maier L, Schubert A, Mertens T, Kern P, Wöhrle J.** 2010. Intravenous zanamivir for patients with pneumonitis due to pandemic (H1N1) 2009 influenza virus. *Clin Infect Dis* **50:**1249–1251.

226. **Alame MM, Massaad E, Zaraket H.** 2016. Peramivir: a novel intravenous neuraminidase inhibitor for treatment of acute influenza infections. *Front Microbiol* **7:**450.

227. **Cady SD, Luo W, Hu F, Hong M.** 2009. Structure and function of the influenza A M2 proton channel. *Biochemistry* **48:**7356–7364.

228. **Pielak RM, Schnell JR, Chou JJ.** 2009. Mechanism of drug inhibition and drug resistance of influenza A M2 channel. *Proc Natl Acad Sci USA* **106:**7379–7384. (Erratum, **106:**11425.)

229. **Hayden FG, Hay AJ.** 1992. Emergence and transmission of influenza A viruses resistant to amantadine and rimantadine. *Curr Top Microbiol Immunol* **176:**119–130.

230. **Shiraishi K, Mitamura K, Sakai-Tagawa Y, Goto H, Sugaya N, Kawaoka Y.** 2003. High frequency of resistant viruses harboring different mutations in amantadine-treated children with influenza. *J Infect Dis* **188:**57–61.

231. **Hussain M, Galvin HD, Haw TY, Nutsford AN, Husain M.** 2017. Drug resistance in influenza A virus: the epidemiology and management. *Infect Drug Resist* **10:**121–134.

232. **Smith BJ, McKimm-Breshkin JL, McDonald M, Fernley RT, Varghese JN, Colman PM.** 2002. Structural studies of the resistance of influenza virus neuramindase to inhibitors. *J Med Chem* **45:**2207–2212.
233. **Russell RJ, Haire LF, Stevens DJ, Collins PJ, Lin YP, Blackburn GM, Hay AJ, Gamblin SJ, Skehel JJ.** 2006. The structure of H5N1 avian influenza neuraminidase suggests new opportunities for drug design. *Nature* **443:**45–49.
234. **Collins PJ, Haire LF, Lin YP, Liu J, Russell RJ, Walker PA, Martin SR, Daniels RS, Gregory V, Skehel JJ, Gamblin SJ, Hay AJ.** 2009. Structural basis for oseltamivir resistance of influenza viruses. *Vaccine* **27:**6317–6323.
235. **Colman PM, Hoyne PA, Lawrence MC.** 1993. Sequence and structure alignment of paramyxovirus hemagglutinin-neuraminidase with influenza virus neuraminidase. *J Virol* **67:**2972–2980.
236. **von Itzstein M.** 2007. The war against influenza: discovery and development of sialidase inhibitors. *Nat Rev Drug Discov* **6:**967–974.
237. **Nguyen HT, Fry AM, Gubareva LV.** 2012. Neuraminidase inhibitor resistance in influenza viruses and laboratory testing methods. *Antivir Ther* **17**(1 Pt B)**:**159–173.
238. **Zambon MC.** 2013. Surveillance for antiviral resistance. *Influenza Other Respir Viruses* **7**(Suppl 1)**:**37–43.
239. **Okomo-Adhiambo M, Sleeman K, Lysén C, Nguyen HT, Xu X, Li Y, Klimov AI, Gubareva LV.** 2013. Neuraminidase inhibitor susceptibility surveillance of influenza viruses circulating worldwide during the 2011 Southern Hemisphere season. *Influenza Other Respir Viruses* **7:**645–658.
240. **Zambon M, Hayden FG, Global Neuraminidase Inhibitor Susceptibility Network.** 2001. Position statement: global neuraminidase inhibitor susceptibility network. *Antiviral Res* **49:**147–156.
241. **McKimm-Breschkin JL, Williams J, Barrett S, Jachno K, McDonald M, Mohr PG, Saito T, Tashiro M.** 2013. Reduced susceptibility to all neuraminidase inhibitors of influenza H1N1 viruses with haemagglutinin mutations and mutations in non-conserved residues of the neuraminidase. *J Antimicrob Chemother* **68:**2210–2221.
242. **Whitley RJ, Hayden FG, Reisinger KS, Young N, Dutkowski R, Ipe D, Mills RG, Ward P.** 2001. Oral oseltamivir treatment of influenza in children. *Pediatr Infect Dis J* **20:**127–133.
243. **Kiso M, Mitamura K, Sakai-Tagawa Y, Shiraishi K, Kawakami C, Kimura K, Hayden FG, Sugaya N, Kawaoka Y.** 2004. Resistant influenza A viruses in children treated with oseltamivir: descriptive study. *Lancet* **364:** 759–765.
244. **McKimm-Breschkin J, Trivedi T, Hampson A, Hay A, Klimov A, Tashiro M, Hayden F, Zambon M.** 2003. Neuraminidase sequence analysis and susceptibilities of influenza virus clinical isolates to zanamivir and oseltamivir. *Antimicrob Agents Chemother* **47:**2264–2272.
245. **Dharan NJ, Gubareva LV, Meyer JJ, Okomo-Adhiambo M, McClinton RC, Marshall SA, St George K, Epperson S, Brammer L, Klimov AI, Bresee JS, Fry AM, Oseltamivir-Resistance Working Group.** 2009. Infections with oseltamivir-resistant influenza A(H1N1) virus in the United States. *JAMA* **301:**1034–1041.
246. **Sheu TG, Deyde VM, Okomo-Adhiambo M, Garten RJ, Xu X, Bright RA, Butler EN, Wallis TR, Klimov AI, Gubareva LV.** 2008. Surveillance for neuraminidase inhibitor resistance among human influenza A and B viruses circulating worldwide from 2004 to 2008. *Antimicrob Agents Chemother* **52:**3284–3292.
247. **Lackenby A, Hungnes O, Dudman SG, Meijer A, Paget WJ, Hay AJ, Zambon MC.** 2008. Emergence of resistance to oseltamivir among influenza A(H1N1) viruses in Europe. *Euro Surveill* **13:**8026.
248. **Gubareva LV, Trujillo AA, Okomo-Adhiambo M, Mishin VP, Deyde VM, Sleeman K, Nguyen HT, Sheu TG, Garten RJ, Shaw MW, Fry AM, Klimov AI.** 2010. Comprehensive assessment of 2009 pandemic influenza A (H1N1) virus drug susceptibility *in vitro*. *Antivir Ther* **15:**1151–1159.
249. **Ives JA, Carr JA, Mendel DB, Tai CY, Lambkin R, Kelly L, Oxford JS, Hayden FG, Roberts NA.** 2002. The H274Y mutation in the influenza A/H1N1 neuraminidase active site following oseltamivir phosphate treatment leave virus severely compromised both *in vitro* and *in vivo*. *Antiviral Res* **55:**307–317.
250. **Baz M, Abed Y, Simon P, Hamelin ME, Boivin G.** 2010. Effect of the neuraminidase mutation H274Y conferring resistance to oseltamivir on the replicative capacity and virulence of old and recent human influenza A(H1N1) viruses. *J Infect Dis* **201:**740–745.
251. **Chao DL.** 2013. Modeling the global transmission of antiviral-resistant influenza viruses. *Influenza Other Respir Viruses* **7**(Suppl 1)**:**58–62.
252. **Bloom JD, Gong LI, Baltimore D.** 2010. Permissive secondary mutations enable the evolution of influenza oseltamivir resistance. *Science* **328:**1272–1275.
253. **Abed Y, Pizzorno A, Bouhy X, Boivin G.** 2011. Role of permissive neuraminidase mutations in influenza A/Brisbane/59/2007-like (H1N1) viruses. *PLoS Pathog* **7:**e1002431.
254. **Abed Y, Pizzorno A, Bouhy X, Boivin G.** 2015. Permissive changes in the neuraminidase play a dominant role in improving the viral fitness of oseltamivir-resistant seasonal influenza A(H1N1) strains. *Antiviral Res* **114:**57–61.
255. **Whitley RJ, Boucher CA, Lina B, Nguyen-Van-Tam JS, Osterhaus A, Schutten M, Monto AS.** 2013. Global assessment of resistance to neuraminidase inhibitors, 2008–2011: the Influenza Resistance Information Study (IRIS). *Clin Infect Dis* **56:**1197–1205.
256. **Hurt AC, Hardie K, Wilson NJ, Deng YM, Osbourn M, Leang SK, Lee RT, Iannello P, Gehrig N, Shaw R, Wark P, Caldwell N, Givney RC, Xue L, Maurer-Stroh S, Dwyer DE, Wang B, Smith DW, Levy A, Booy R, Dixit R, Merritt T, Kelso A, Dalton C, Durrheim D, Barr IG.** 2012. Characteristics of a widespread community cluster of H275Y oseltamivir-resistant A(H1N1)pdm09 influenza in Australia. *J Infect Dis* **206:**148–157.
257. **Takashita E, Kiso M, Fujisaki S, Yokoyama M, Nakamura K, Shirakura M, Sato H, Odagiri T, Kawaoka Y, Tashiro M.** 2015. Characterization of a large cluster of influenza A(H1N1)pdm09 viruses cross-resistant to oseltamivir and peramivir during the 2013-2014 influenza season in Japan. *Antimicrob Agents Chemother* **59:**2607–2617.
258. **Leneva IA, Goloubeva O, Fenton RJ, Tisdale M, Webster RG.** 2001. Efficacy of zanamivir against avian influenza A viruses that possess genes encoding H5N1 internal proteins and are pathogenic in mammals. *Antimicrob Agents Chemother* **45:**1216–1224.
259. **Leneva IA, Roberts N, Govorkova EA, Goloubeva OG, Webster RG.** 2000. The neuraminidase inhibitor GS4104 (oseltamivir phosphate) is efficacious against A/Hong Kong/156/97 (H5N1) and A/Hong Kong/1074/99 (H9N2) influenza viruses. *Antiviral Res* **48:**101–115.
260. **de Jong MD, Tran TT, Truong HK, Vo MH, Smith GJ, Nguyen VC, Bach VC, Phan TQ, Do QH, Guan Y, Peiris JS, Tran TH, Farrar J.** 2005. Oseltamivir resistance during treatment of influenza A (H5N1) infection. *N Engl J Med* **353:**2667–2672.
261. **Pizzorno A, Abed Y, Bouhy X, Beaulieu E, Mallett C, Russell R, Boivin G.** 2012. Impact of mutations at residue I223 of the neuraminidase protein on the resistance profile, replication level, and virulence of the 2009 pandemic influenza virus. *Antimicrob Agents Chemother* **56:**1208–1214.
262. **Hurt AC, Lee RT, Leang SK, Cui L, Deng YM, Phuah SP, Caldwell N, Freeman K, Komadina N, Smith D, Speers D, Kelso A, Lin RT, Maurer-Stroh S, Barr IG.** 2011. Increased detection in Australia and Singapore of a novel influenza A(H1N1)2009 variant with reduced oseltamivir and zanamivir sensitivity due to a S247N neuraminidase mutation. *Euro Surveill* **16:**19909.
263. **Hurt AC, Holien JK, Parker M, Kelso A, Barr IG.** 2009. Zanamivir-resistant influenza viruses with a novel neuraminidase mutation. *J Virol* **83:**10366–10373.

264. **Okomo-Adhiambo M, Nguyen HT, Abd Elal A, Sleeman K, Fry AM, Gubareva LV.** 2014. Drug susceptibility surveillance of influenza viruses circulating in the United States in 2011-2012: application of the WHO antiviral working group criteria. *Influenza Other Respir Viruses* **8:**258–265.
265. **L'Huillier AG, Abed Y, Petty TJ, Cordey S, Thomas Y, Bouhy X, Schibler M, Simon A, Chalandon Y, van Delden C, Zdobnov E, Boquete-Suter P, Boivin G, Kaiser L.** 2015. E119D neuraminidase mutation conferring pan-resistance to neuraminidase inhibitors in an A(H1N1)pdm09 isolate from a stem-cell transplant recipient. *J Infect Dis* **212:**1726–1734.
266. **Tamura D, DeBiasi RL, Okomo-Adhiambo M, Mishin VP, Campbell AP, Loechelt B, Wiedermann BL, Fry AM, Gubareva LV.** 2015. Emergence of multidrug-resistant influenza A(H1N1)pdm09 virus variants in an immunocompromised child treated with oseltamivir and zanamivir. *J Infect Dis* **212:**1209–1213.
267. **Ison MG, Gubareva LV, Atmar RL, Treanor J, Hayden FG.** 2006. Recovery of drug-resistant influenza virus from immunocompromised patients: a case series. *J Infect Dis* **193:** 760–764.
268. **Abed Y, Baz M, Boivin G.** 2009. A novel neuraminidase deletion mutation conferring resistance to oseltamivir in clinical influenza A/H3N2 virus. *J Infect Dis* **199:**180–183.
269. **Hu Y, Lu S, Song Z, Wang W, Hao P, Li J, Zhang X, Yen HL, Shi B, Li T, Guan W, Xu L, Liu Y, Wang S, Zhang X, Tian D, Zhu Z, He J, Huang K, Chen H, Zheng L, Li X, Ping J, Kang B, Xi X, Zha L, Li Y, Zhang Z, Peiris M, Yuan Z.** 2013. Association between adverse clinical outcome in human disease caused by novel influenza A H7N9 virus and sustained viral shedding and emergence of antiviral resistance. *Lancet* **381:**2273–2279.
270. **Marjuki H, Mishin VP, Chesnokov AP, Jones J, De La Cruz JA, Sleeman K, Tamura D, Nguyen HT, Wu HS, Chang FY, Liu MT, Fry AM, Cox NJ, Villanueva JM, Davis CT, Gubareva LV.** 2015. Characterization of drug-resistant influenza A(H7N9) variants isolated from an oseltamivir-treated patient in Taiwan. *J Infect Dis* **211:**249–257.
271. **Gubareva LV, Matrosovich MN, Brenner MK, Bethell RC, Webster RG.** 1998. Evidence for zanamivir resistance in an immunocompromised child infected with influenza B virus. *J Infect Dis* **178:**1257–1262.
272. **WHO.** 2012. Meetings of the WHO working group on surveillance of influenza antiviral susceptibility: Geneva, November 2011 and June 2012. *Wkly Epidemiol Rec* **87:** 369–374.
273. **Monto AS.** 2009. Implications of antiviral resistance of influenza viruses. *Clin Infect Dis* **48:**397–399.

Susceptibility Test Methods: Viruses

DIANA D. HUANG, BENJAMIN A. PINSKY, AND MATTHEW J. BANKOWSKI

115

FDA-approved antiviral drugs are available and used for the treatment and management of herpes simplex virus types 1 and 2 (HSV-1 and HSV-2), human cytomegalovirus (HCMV), varicella-zoster virus (VZV), human immunodeficiency virus (HIV-1) (1), hepatitis B virus (HBV), hepatitis C virus (HCV) (2, 3), and influenza virus. When the drugs are used over long periods of time and/or inconsistently, variants may be selected which may become drug resistant and are no longer susceptible to therapy (4–11). Since these variants are transmissible, learning whether the virus may be drug resistant is a critical step in the treatment strategy (12).

Testing for viral susceptibility is now standard practice for the management of viral infections for optimum patient care. The only FDA-cleared assays available for viral susceptibility testing over the past decade target the HIV-1 protease (Pro) and reverse transcriptase (RT) genes. However, interest in testing for susceptibility has increased for other viruses, such as HBV, HCV, and HIV-1, for which there are newly approved antiviral drugs; this testing is done using research-use-only (RUO) test kits or analyte-specific reagents in laboratory-developed tests (LDTs) (13).

ANTIVIRAL RESISTANCE AND CAUSES OF DRUG FAILURE

Failure to respond to drug therapy can occur for different reasons. More commonly, the virus population being treated is inherently resistant to the drug(s) being given. Alternatively, host biological and sociobehavioral factors (e.g., therapeutic nonadherence) may influence therapeutic success. Viral susceptibility testing can identify resistant populations and guide patient management strategies.

True Antiviral Resistance

Antiviral resistance is expressed as a drop in the efficacy of a drug to inhibit viral replication. Resistance is demonstrated clinically by an increase or no change in amounts of circulating virus in the infected individual despite active treatment. The loss of susceptibility can be measured by *in vitro* testing, which evaluates the phenotypic activity of drug-virus combinations. If the decrease in drug effect is related to specific mutations in the virus genome, affecting function of the protein which the drug targets, then the resistance to that drug may be an inherently transmissible feature of the virus. This genotypic and phenotypic expression provides combined evidence for the loss of drug activity against the virus and is documented during drug development. Independent confirmation of these correlations is made by antiviral testing of viral isolates obtained from participants in clinical drug trials. Diagnostic assays may then be developed that measure the change in response of the virus to a drug and/or identify the presence of the specific viral mutations associated with the observed loss of susceptibility. Interpretations of the data from these assays are used to clinically manage viral infections.

Host Factors

The failure to respond to therapy may occur even if the infecting virus does not harbor any mutations associated with antiviral susceptibility. Host physiologic factors can interfere with a successful clinical response. The genetic background of the host may lessen the effect of the drug, as host polymorphisms, such as those identified for the IL28b gene, may affect the activity or bioavailability of pegylated interferon (peg-IFN)–ribavirin in HCV treatment (14–16). Another nonviral factor is the potential for drug-drug interactions. For example, in early clinical trials of the newer protease inhibitors to treat chronic HCV infection, pharmacokinetic influences and drug-drug interactions occurred with some HIV-1 protease treatments in HIV-HCV-coinfected individuals (17). Coadministration of the HCV and HIV protease inhibitors could then cause the viral loads of either virus to increase (18). In this scenario, there were no identified mutations associated with antiviral resistance present in the viral genomes.

Patient Sociobehavioral Influence

Individuals undergoing drug treatment may not adhere to their prescribed antiviral regimen for a variety of reasons. For instance, physiologic and psychological side effects associated with antiretroviral drugs and IFN treatment may occur, fueling patient intolerance for the drug. The acute and long-term symptoms, as well as complexities of the treatment, such as pill burden and timing, may initiate problems with adherence (19). Consequently, the patient may choose to suspend treatment on his or her own. In addition, consistent access to and follow-through of therapy may be difficult for some individuals due to socioeconomic concerns (20). This results in treatment gaps which foster the selection or generation of an underlying genetically resistant viral population. In this type of patient, the class of drug to which the virus has become resistant is no longer effective for future use (21). Clinical trials and studies are now being conducted that study adherence outcomes (22–24) and include genotypic resistance testing.

CLINICAL INDICATIONS FOR ANTIVIRAL SUSCEPTIBILITY TESTING

It is important to distinguish when the lack of effective response to treatment with an antiviral drug results from true antiviral resistance, i.e., genetic changes in the patient's virus. Clinical resistance to a particular antiviral drug can be misinterpreted as viral resistance. The failure to recognize this difference could result in the inappropriate use of more toxic drugs, leading to higher morbidity and mortality with much higher test costs. For example, a transplant patient who is immunosuppressed may show an increasing CMV viral load for the first few weeks of therapy in the presence of antiviral drug. This rise is less likely to be evidence of development of drug resistance, as it is unusual for CMV to acquire resistance within the initial six weeks of treatment (25).

The clinical category and status of the patient are important in determining whether antiviral resistance testing is indicated. Table 1 presents instances for both immunocompetent and immunocompromised patients for whom resistance testing should be considered. In general, sustained or increasing viral load with a worsening clinical condition is a reliable indicator for the presence of emerging drug resistance. If these markers of resistance are present, it may be prudent to test the virus directly for drug resistance. Antiviral susceptibility test methods can be phenotypic or genotypic. The choice will often rely on the specific virus being tested. Interpretation of the testing data may be more complex for individuals on combination therapy.

TESTING METHODS: PHENOTYPIC ASSAYS

Plaque Reduction Assay and Dye Uptake

The standard method of antiviral susceptibility testing is the plaque reduction assay (PRA) (Fig. 1). The PRA test principle relies on the ability of the antiviral agent to inhibit the production of viral plaques at a predetermined drug concentration. A 50% inhibitory concentration (IC_{50}) is then calculated and subsequently reported in micrograms per milliliter or micromolar units. A higher IC_{50} for the sample virus than for a wild-type control strain denotes resistance. Depending on the virus, this value may vary for the drug. This method is especially useful for the herpesviruses (e.g., HSV, CMV, and VZV) but is time-consuming and exhibits an extended turnaround time of about 2 to 3 days for HSV, approximately 7 days for VZV, and at least a month for CMV (26–29).

The PRA involves two testing phases. The first entails growing the clinical isolate in susceptible cells to obtain a viral stock whose titer can be determined for infectivity. For a slowly growing virus such as CMV, generation of the stock could take 3 to 4 weeks. The titration of the stock is performed by plaquing serial dilutions to quantitate the relative numbers of infectious virus particles, which for CMV takes about 10 days.

The second testing phase determines the susceptibility of the virus stock to an antiviral drug using the PRA. Here, an inoculum containing a defined number of infectious virus particles from the stock (for instance, 100) is incubated in the presence of serial dilutions of the antiviral drug of interest. If the virus is susceptible to that drug, there will be a reduction in the number of plaques as the concentration of the drug increases. Resistance will be evident by minimal plaque reduction compared to growth in the absence of drug. The PRA for CMV could add another 10 days to the protocol, so that the total time to assess drug resistance could be 4 to 6 weeks (25). Results for a faster-growing virus, such as HSV, may take less time to obtain.

There is also the question of method standardization, for which an approved standard document from the Clinical and Laboratory Standards Institute (CLSI) for HSV has been published (M33A). The use of a phenotypic method such as PRA is still recommended, because of the presence of uncharacterized mutations among the herpesviruses that can contribute to antiviral resistance. Table 2 lists the proposed guidelines for interpreting antiviral susceptibility results for PRA of herpes group and influenza A viruses.

TABLE 1 Clinical situation where antiviral resistance testing may be indicated

Clinical category	Clinical status	Indicator(s) of resistance
Immunocompetent host (e.g., influenza virus or genital HSV infection)	Culture or molecular testing evidence of viral infection and disease with clinical indications for short-term antiviral therapy	Sustained culture positivity with known therapeutic drug adherence Sustained or increasing viral load by quantitative molecular testing Worsening clinical condition without evidence of infection by other agents Epidemiological evidence of emerging antiviral resistance (e.g., oseltamivir resistance for influenza virus A)
Immunocompromised host (e.g., immunosuppression due to cancer, transplantation, or AIDS)	Prolonged antiviral drug therapy or combination therapy used for prophylaxis or treatment	Increasing viremia or viral load while on long-term antiviral therapy, a history of failed antiviral therapy Unexplained worsening of clinical disease condition Documented cross-resistance known from the use of specific antiviral drugs (e.g., HIV-1 antiretroviral therapy) Suboptimal viral load reductions achieved (e.g., lack of success with a change of HIV-1 therapy even with baseline retesting)

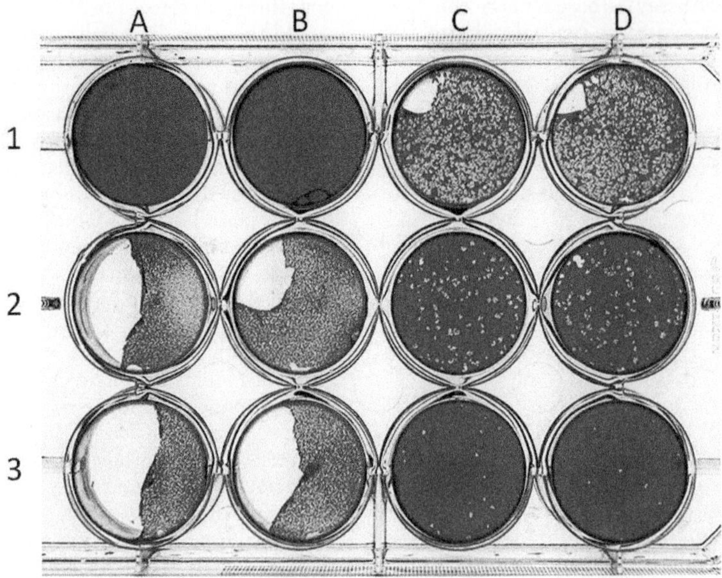

FIGURE 1 An example of a PRA (i.e., phenotypic test) used for determining acyclovir resistance in HSV-1. The reduction in the number of plaques is shown for an acyclovir-sensitive HSV-1 isolate tested in duplicate starting with uninfected cells in the first two wells (1A and 1B). Increasing acyclovir concentrations are added downward to duplicate wells beginning with 2A and 2B, continuing to 3A and 3B, and moving from the top right downward (1C/1D to 3C/3D) of the 12-well microtiter plate. The lowest number of plaques appears in wells 3C and 3D, where the highest concentration of acyclovir is added.

TABLE 2 Proposed guidelines for phenotypic antiviral susceptibility results of herpes group viruses and influenza virus A

Virus	Antiviral agent	Method	IC_{50} denoting resistance	Reference(s)
HSV	Acyclovir	PRA	≥2 μg/ml	29
		DNA hybridization DU	≥2 μg/ml	9, 143
		PRA	≥3 μg/ml	29, 144
	Famciclovir (active metabolite 5 penciclovir)	PRA and DNA hybridization	Definitive breakpoints cannot be established	145, 166
	Foscarnet	PRA	>100 μg/ml	147
	Vidarabine	PRA	≥2-fold increase of IC_{50} compared to control or pretherapy isolate	148
HCMV	Cidofovir	PRA and DNA hybridization	>2 μM	62–64
	Foscarnet	PRA and DNA hybridization	>400 μM	63, 149
			>324 μM	64
	Ganciclovir	PRA and DNA hybridization	≥3–4-fold increase of IC_{50} compared to pretherapy isolate or control strain (~3 μg/ml)	70, 150, 151
			>6 μM	62, 63
			>8 μM	64
Influenza virus A	Amantadine-rimantadine	EIA	>0.1 μg/ml	5, 6
Influenza virus A and B	Oseltamivir and zanamivir	NI assay	>8-fold decrease in NA activity	128, 152
VZV	Acyclovir	PRA and DNA hybridization	≥3–4-fold increase of IC_{50} compared to pretherapy isolate or to control strain	26, 153, 154
	Famciclovir	PRA and DNA hybridization	Definitive breakpoints cannot be established	166
	Foscarnet	Late antigen reduction assay	300 μM	154

The dye uptake (DU) assay is based upon the ability of viable cells to incorporate the neutral red vital dye (29). It is used for antiviral susceptibility testing of HSV. An IC_{50} is calculated similarly to the PRA but measured colorimetrically.

Enzyme Immunoassays

Enzyme immunoassays (EIAs) have also been developed for antiviral susceptibility testing (5–7, 30–32). These methods have been used successfully for both the herpesviruses and influenza virus A. They compare favorably with the PRA method but are less labor-intensive and allow a quantitative measurement. This method measures absorbance as related to viral antigen detection in viral infected cells and results in the determination of an IC_{50}.

Neuraminidase Inhibition Assay

Three neuraminidase (NA or N) inhibitors (NIs)—oseltamivir, zanamivir, and peramivir—have been FDA approved for the treatment of both influenza virus A and B infection (33). A fluorogenic assay resulting in the generation of an IC_{50} was developed and has been used successfully to detect antiviral resistance to the three NI drugs (34, 35). It was subsequently commercialized and is available under the name NA-Star or NA-XTD (Applied Biosystems, Foster City, CA). A rapid bioluminescence-based assay, the QFlu Combo test (Cellex, Inc., Rockville, MD), detects influenza virus A and B and the sensitivity of their neuraminidases to oseltamivir and zanamivir in a single test (36). This assay kit is CE marked and also available as an RUO kit in the United States.

Recombinant Viral Assays

Recombinant viral assays (RVA) for drug susceptibility have been developed for clinical use. These assays monitor phenotypic behavior in the presence of an antiviral drug that can be attributed to specific genes on the virus genome, which may contain mutations known to correlate with antiviral resistance. The first clinically useful RVA was used to measure the phenotypic resistance of HIV-1 to protease and RT inhibitors.

In the RVA protocol strategy, the gene of interest (e.g., the HIV-1 protease or RT gene) is PCR amplified directly from virus in the patient specimen. Afterwards, the PCR product is ligated into a retroviral vector from which the protease or RT gene was removed. The concept is that the ligation adds back the protease or RT activity associated with the gene from the patient's virus. The vector also has the *env* gene, which codes for the receptor binding protein, replaced with a reporter gene coding for a light-emitting protein, such as luciferase. This vector, which now contains the HIV-1 gene of interest, is then cotransfected into a susceptible cell line along with a different plasmid. However, this plasmid contains a gene to provide a non-HIV receptor-binding protein able to attach to and infect the chosen test cells. After transfection, the newly assembled chimeric virus, called a pseudotype, incorporates the gene for the non-HIV receptor-binding protein, the genome from the retroviral vector containing the added HIV-1 protease or RT gene from the patient virus, and the reporter gene. The pseudotype virus can now infect the cells of choice to start replication for a single round. This RVA strategy allows the activity of the protease or RT derived from patient HIV to be tested in cells in the presence of antiretroviral drugs. Measurements of the replication efficiency of the engineered virus can be monitored by light emission of the luciferase expressed in the cells only during successful replication of the virus. Chimeric virus containing a protease or RT sensitive to the antiviral drug would then not emit light from infected cells, while virus containing a protease or RT resistant to the antiviral drug would emit measurable light.

The RVA is labor-intensive and time-consuming and requires a long turnaround time. RVA utilizes cell culture. However, the use of a standard cell line also provides assay consistency that is not possible with the use of primary cells, such as peripheral blood mononuclear cells. An advantage of a recombinant assay over conventional culture is that it provides direct evidence of the antiviral activity associated with a specific gene derived from the virus population in a patient specimen. Also, if an RVA is linked with genotyping of the patient's virus to show the presence of known resistance mutations, a direct correlation between the levels of phenotypic resistance and the mutations observed could be made, especially in patients on a complex treatment regimen. This information would allow a more accurate snapshot of HIV-1 resistance and could offer the clinician a more accurate choice of antiretroviral drugs available if a change in treatment is contemplated.

Modifications of the RVA have been made to allow fusion, integrase, and coreceptor usage to be monitored in instances where inhibitors of these HIV-1 activities are candidates for a patient's antiviral therapy. Currently, HIV-1 RVA testing is provided from commercial reference labs. Available RVAs measure HIV-1 protease-RT, fusion, integrase, and coreceptor activities. There is also an LDT variation of this strategy that has been developed for CMV resistance testing in which a linkage between phenotypic and genotypic data has been made (37).

GENOTYPIC ASSAYS

The gene targets for antiviral genotypic testing and their respective mutations are shown in Table 3 and Table 4. There are 43 drugs currently available for treatment of HIV-1, targeting the protease, RT, integrase, viral fusion, and entry (38, 39). The list of mutations associated with resistance to these and newly approved inhibitors is updated every 2 years. The current list can be downloaded from the International Antiviral Society-USA website (http://www.iasusa.org/sites/default/files/tam/24-4-132.pdf) or from the Stanford HIV Drug Resistance Database (http://hivdb.stanford.edu). Knowledge of the mutations is the basis for genotyping assays used to identify antiviral resistance. Analysis of raw genotyping sequence data using Sanger sequencing protocols involves subjective input from an operator for final processing and interpretation. This expertise requires specific training and experience in order to correctly identify relevant mutations in the template. The basic flow of a Sanger genotypic assay is shown in Fig. 2. Commercial reference laboratories and large medical centers offer these highly complex FDA-approved or -cleared tests or LDTs. A basic report often consists of a section showing the relevant mutations associated with drug resistance, followed by an interpretation of the mutations. Smaller diagnostic laboratories with the proper training and equipment can also perform antiviral genotypic assays. However, there is a need for strict control of the generation of results and accurate and correct interpretation of the data for laboratories of any size. Newer platforms represented by next-generation sequencing (NGS) are commonly protocols that are LDT. No FDA-cleared or -approved assays are currently available for analysis of antiviral drug resistance mutations. Since assay strategies are not standardized, guidelines for consistent performance and analysis of these assays have not yet been developed.

TABLE 3 Gene targets used for antiviral resistance testing with genotypic methods

Virus group	Virus	Antiviral agent(s)	Gene target(s)	Gene mutation(s)	References
Herpesviruses	CMV	Cidofovir	UL54	See Table 4	See Table 4
		Foscarnet	UL54		
		Ganciclovir	UL54, UL97		
		Maribavir	UL97		
		Valganciclovir	UL54, UL97		
	HSV	Acyclovir Valacyclovir Penciclovir Famciclovir	TK and/or DNA polymerase	P57H, D59P, K62N, R51W, E83K, A175V, indels, nucleotide substitutions	145, 155–166
		Foscarnet	DNA polymerase	Regions II, III, and VI	
		Cidofovir	DNA polymerase	Regions δC and II	
	VZV	Acyclovir, valacyclovir Penciclovir Famciclovir	TK and/or DNA polymerase	Frameshift and substitution mutations	164, 167, 168
		Foscarnet	DNA polymerase	Regions II, III, and VI	
		Cidofovir	DNA polymerase	Not specific	
Influenza viruses	Type A	Amantadine	M2 protein	26, 27, 30, 31, 34	5, 6, 152, 169–174
		Rimantadine	M2 protein	26, 27, 30, 31, 34	
		Oseltamivir	NA	H275Y, E119V, R292K, N294S	
		Zanamivir	NA	T198I, R152K	
	Type B	Oseltamivir	NA	R152K	
		Zanamivir	NA	R152K	
Hepatitis viruses	HBV	Adefovir	Pol-RT (B, D)	rtA181TV, rtN236T	175–194
		Entecavir	Pol-RT (A, B, C, E)	rtI169T, rtV173L, rtL180M, rtT184G/S/A/I/L, rtM204V/I, rtS202G/C/I, rtM250I/V	
		Lamivudine	Pol-RT (A, B, C)	rtL80V/I, rtL180M, rtM204V/I/S/A	
		Telbivudine	Pol-RT (A, B, C)	rtL80V/I, rtL180M, rtM204V/I/S/A	
		Tenofovir	Pol RT (B, C, D)	rtL180M, rtM204V, rtN236T	
	HCV	Daclatasvir, sofosbuvir	NS5A/NS5B	NS5A GT1a M28A/G/T, Q30D/E/H/G/K/L/R, L31F/M/V, Y93C/H/N/S	109
		Grazoprevir, elbasvir Ledipasvir, sofosbuvir Paritaprevir, ombitasvir, ritonovir Paritaprevir, ombitasvir, dasabuvir, ritonovir	NS3/4A/NS5A NS5A/NS5B NS3/4A/NS5A/CYP3A NS3/4A/NS5A/NS5B/CYP3A	NS5A GT1a M28A/G/T, Q30D/E/H/G/K/L/R, L31F/M/V, Y93C/H/N/S	
		Simeprevir, sofosbuvir	NS3/4A/NS5B	Q80K	
		Telaprevir, peg-IFN, ribavirin	NS3/4A	V36C, R155K, A156T/V	
		Velpatasvir, sofosbuvir	NS5A/NS5B		
		Voxilaprevir, velpatasvir, sofosbuvir	NS3/4A/NS5A/NS5B		

Genotypic Platforms

Genotypic platforms used for antiviral susceptibility testing may include Sanger sequencing, pyrosequencing, NGS, *in vitro* reverse hybridization line probe assay (LiPA), and single nucleotide polymorphism (SNP) analysis. Real-time RT-PCR allelic discrimination is also being evaluated as an LDT targeting single mutations (40, 41). In general, these assays analyze data and yield results more quickly than phenotypic testing, often at a lower cost. Currently, sequencing assays are more frequently used to detect well-characterized mutations associated with antiviral resistance. They are also capable of identifying novel mutations associated with antiviral resistance. However, most sequencing platforms will require the use of bioinformatics software for accurate and reproducible data interpretation.

Viral genomes with multiple, clustered resistance mutations are mostly analyzed by the use of assays based on Sanger dideoxynucleotide sequencing (42). For example, in the case of HIV-1 or HCV chronic infection, the viral population consists of multiple variants referred to as "quasispecies" (43). Raw data from Sanger sequencing are displayed in chromatograms, which can show the presence of minor populations in the total virus population. The operator should evaluate the chromatograms and proofread the data manually to determine that the quality of the sequence chromatogram produced is of acceptable resolution (44) (Fig, 2). Every consensus sequence

TABLE 4 CMV UL54 and UL97 gene targets and the associated mutations conferring antiviral resistance[a]

Gene region	Mutation[b]	CMV susceptibility[c]		
		Cidofovir	Foscarnet	Ganciclovir
UL97 (phosphotransferase)	M460V, M460I, H520Q, Del 591–594, A594V, L595S, L595F, Del 595, C603W, C607Y	NA	NA	R
Other mutations at or next to UL97 codons involved in ganciclovir resistance	L595T, L595W, E596G, E596G, N597I, G598V, K599M, Del 600, C603Y, C606D	NA	NA	R
UL54 (DNA Pol)[d]	N408D, D413E, **L501F**, L501I, T503I, P522S, L545S, G678S, I722V, Y751H, **A809V**, A987G	R	S	R
	F412V, **F412C**, K805Q, K513R, K513E	R	S or R	R
	P522A, G841A	ND	S	R
	D588E, **L802M**	S or R	R	S or R
	T700A	S	R (S)[e]	S
	V715M	S	R	S
	V781I	S	R	R
	T821I	R	R	R

[a]References 25, 60, 149, and 195–204.
[b]Boldface indicates resistance confirmed by recombinant virus data.
[c]S, sensitive; R, resistant; NA, UL97 is not a target for this drug; ND, phenotype is not determined or known at this time.
[d]Most of the UL54 mutants also have UL97 mutations.
[e]A single foscarnet-sensitive strain was found with this mutation.

developed should include sequencing of the PCR-derived template in both the forward and reverse directions in order to ensure sequence accuracy by verifying the presence of the identical mutation(s) in both strands of the sequencing template. This process will validate true nucleotide change as opposed to an artifact generated during the sequencing protocol (i.e., a breach in the enzyme proofreading or inconsistencies during the preparation of the sequencing sample). Sanger sequencing is useful in monitoring longer contiguous regions of the genome. Good-quality sequencing reactions can yield 600 to 700 readable nucleotides per sequencing primer, assuming that the template is generated from a clean PCR product. However, Sanger sequencing does not detect a variant in a mixed virus population reproducibly if the minor population is less than ~20%.

Pyrosequencing is another sequencing method used for identifying mutations associated with antiviral drug resistance. Pyrosequencing is fundamentally different from Sanger sequencing in several ways and is described thoroughly by Metzker (45). Pyrosequencing methods are not FDA approved or cleared for use in antiviral susceptibility testing at this time.

NGS methods also have been applied to genotypic antiviral drug resistance testing and are capable of detecting minor populations typically between 1 and 5%, or in some cases less than 1% (46). These technologies, also referred to as ultradeep, high-throughput, or massively parallel sequencing, can detect much lower levels of variants in mixed samples because of the number of genomic reads which are obtained by parallel sequencing of amplified clones or single molecules. These valuable sequence data provide a snapshot of the population of the infectious agent in the patient. NGS also allows accurate verification of variants that might otherwise be misinterpreted using Sanger sequencing. Though NGS technology is rapidly evolving, current NGS methods for genotypic antiviral resistance testing commonly use targeted PCR amplification to enrich for the resistance gene sequences of interest. In addition, sequencing library preparation involves the addition of platform-specific adapter sequences and sequence barcodes for multiplexing, as well as the generation of fragments or amplicons of the appropriate size to be sequenced. At this point in time, NGS yields sequence data ranging from approximately 150 to 300 bases in length. Interpreting the large volume of raw sequence data is challenging and requires laboratories to place the data into a bioinformatics pipeline for analysis and alignment in order to identify the sequence variants present in a clinical sample (47). Once the variants are identified, a database of drug resistance mutations that takes into account their association with phenotype, treatment, and clinical outcomes, as well as their interactions with one another, if known, should be used to render an interpretation. As library preparation techniques, sequencing methods, bioinformatics approaches, and resistance databases improve and automation of the entire process becomes more common, NGS is likely to serve as an important tool for the diagnosis and management of viral resistance (47). As laboratories consider the implementation of NGS technology, many outstanding questions remain, including those concerning the clinical impact of low-level drug resistance mutations and the threshold at which mutations should be reported.

LiPA testing for antiviral susceptibility testing involves PCR-generated biotin-tagged oligonucleotides from the genetic region of interest of the patient's virus. The amplified product is then hybridized to oligonucleotide probes bound to nitrocellulose strips, spatially embedded on this solid matrix. The probes are derived from a reference virus genome and contain single mutations, which correlate to antiviral drug resistance. Both the probes for the reference and the mutation sequences are on the membrane. Each single mutation to be identified is represented by a different probe. The pattern of probe reactivity on the strip (i.e., a color reaction produced by an EIA-type process) indicates the mutations present in the patient's viral population. The LiPA assay will detect only known, previously identified mutations specific for the probes included in the

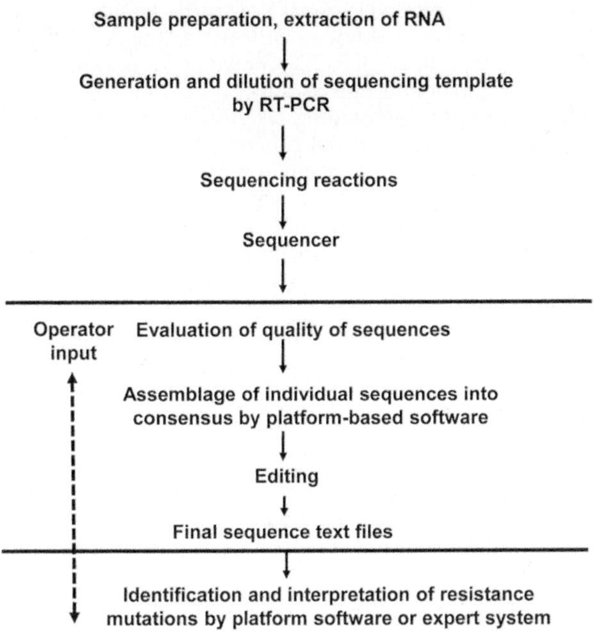

FIGURE 2 General protocol for Sanger sequence-based genotypic assays of plasma samples. The individual steps that are performed in sequence-based genotypic assays are shown. Above the first line are components that are accomplished as a result of specified protocol instructions and instruments. After completion of the block, the subsequent steps are performed with subjective input from the operator within a software program that will accept the chromatograms generated by the sequencer. The operator then chooses the portion of the reference sequence containing the unknown mutations for use in the software of his or her choice. This is followed by alignment and editing of the sequences to identify these mutations in the patient samples. The most commonly used consensus sequences of HIV-1 strains are HIV-1 strain HXB2 and HIV-1 Consensus B. If the operator is using an in-house genotyping assay for other viruses, the reference sequence used should be based upon the literature or common practice.

test kit (48). LiPA is also not FDA approved or cleared for use in antiviral susceptibility testing at this time.

Real-time PCR and SNP assays have also been developed for antiviral susceptibility testing. They are especially useful for detecting antiviral resistance in influenza virus A infection with the introduction of anti-neuraminidase inhibitor drugs (49, 50). SNP assays are multiplexed, so that more than one primer-probe pair is added to each reaction. The probes will distinguish, for example, a wild-type virus from one that carries a resistance mutation. The probes for each are labeled with a different fluorescent dye, and detection of the bound dye indicates the presence or absence of the mutation. These assays are mostly LDTs (using analyte-specific reagents) and are more likely to be performed by large commercial reference laboratories.

Applications (Genotyping)

Herpesviruses

HCMV

There are currently no FDA-approved or -cleared kits or systems or RUO kits to screen for HCMV antiviral drug resistance mutations. Sanger sequencing is currently used to screen for mutations in HCMV isolates associated with ganciclovir resistance, as well as to screen for resistance to newer drugs for HCMV treatment, such as letermovir (51–53). Direct sequencing of HCMV from blood, cerebrospinal fluid, and culture isolates has also been successful in determining drug resistance (54–56). NGS methods have also been applied to the diagnosis of HCMV drug resistance and have demonstrated improved sensitivity for the detection of low-level variants compared to Sanger sequencing (57, 58). Genotyping offers a much faster turnaround than phenotyping and is now the test of choice for HCMV antiviral drug resistance for patient samples with a minimum virus load (VL) of 1,000 copies/ml (59).

The UL97 (phosphotransferase) and UL54 (DNA polymerase) genes are well-documented targets for numerous mutations associated with HCMV antiviral drug resistance (Tables 3 and 4) (60). Mutations associated with ganciclovir resistance may be identified by sequencing the entire UL97 gene, including the region covering the conserved domains linked to phosphotransferase activity (25, 61–64). However, newly discovered mutations associated with antiviral susceptibility are still being documented, especially in immunocompromised populations (e.g., transplant recipients) (53, 65, 66). UL97 mutations have long been known to be associated with ganciclovir resistance (64, 67, 68). Mutations in UL54 are also known to be linked to resistance in ganciclovir, foscarnet, and cidofovir (codons 300 to 1000) (60, 69). Sequencing of both the UL54 and UL97 genes requires multiple primers to generate multiple PCR products, factors that will increase the cost and complexity of this assay. It is for these reasons, as well as the limited number of tests from individual institutions, that the assay is usually performed by large academic medical centers or commercial reference laboratories.

HCMV genotyping sequence data from antiviral resistance testing must be carefully interpreted, because some common mutations observed in genotypic assays may not be responsible for phenotypic resistance. For example, a moderate number of the codon changes identified in UL97 are not associated with antiviral drug resistance (63). The laboratory should confirm such mutations with those identified by "recombinant phenotyping" (25) if the literature is not supportive or if clinical drug efficacy has not been achieved (60, 62, 70). The ratio of IC_{50}s for mutants versus wild type can fluctuate up to ~30% in replicate assays for a given mutation, but a ratio usually of at least 2 has been associated with resistance in UL97 (25). In these instances, the aforementioned recombinant assays (37) which have been developed for HCMV may be considered.

HSV-1 and -2

Currently available antiviral drugs for HSV infection are acyclovir (ACV), penciclovir (PCV), and their prodrugs, valacyclovir and famiciclovir (Table 3). These drugs target the HSV viral thymidine kinase (TK) and DNA polymerase (Pol). Drug-resistant isolates frequently develop in HSV-infected immunocompromised patients. The use of antiviral susceptibility testing is especially useful for this patient population (Table 1).

Common target genes for genotypic sequencing assays are the HSV TK gene (UL23) and the DNA Pol gene (UL30), which are associated with ACV and PCV drug resistance (71). Many cases of ACV resistance correlate with observed mutations in UL23, especially in areas of homopolymer repeats consisting of guanines or cytosines where hypermutation occurs (72, 73). In contrast, the mutations found in clinical isolates observed in UL30 are scattered over structural regions II, III, VI, and VII (71).

Phenotypic antiviral susceptibility testing should be considered when ACV and PCV treatment fails and other reasons for drug failure are ruled out. HSV genotyping is not commonly requested, and there are no specific guidelines available to aid in the interpretation of the mutations for drug resistance. Therefore, the resulting mutations are usually compared to the published literature in order to distinguish true antiviral resistance from viral polymorphisms (70).

VZV

In cases of VZV infection, treatment is usually initiated if the patient is immunocompromised (e.g., HIV-infected, transplant, and cancer patients). Some of the antiviral drugs used for HSV infection are used for VZV infection and target similar genes (i.e., the TK and DNA Pol genes) (Table 3). There are fewer studies in the literature on antiviral drug resistance in VZV than in HSV. However, there are supportive data for genotypic testing from a phenotypic study (74), which examined cross-reactivity patterns associated with mutations in the VZV TK and DNA Pol genes. Mutations correlating with drug resistance were mapped for both genes, and this information could be used as a source reference for evaluation of mutations found in genotypic assays. However, the phenotypic method has been mostly offered as a commercial reference laboratory test, though as of this writing, no clinical laboratories in the United States currently offer VZV susceptibility testing.

HIV

Genotypic testing for antiretroviral resistance mutations is used for monitoring treatment failures (11, 75, 76) and is recommended for baseline screening of newly diagnosed patients (http://www.aidsinfo.nih.gov/Guidelines). Regularly updated algorithms released by expert panels are used to interpret mutations detected in genotypic assays. There is currently one FDA-cleared test kit for HIV-1 genotyping, the ViroSeq HIV-1 genotyping system (Abbott Diagnostics) (21, 77–81). This assay employs RT-nonnested PCR amplification of the HIV-1 protease (codons 1 to 99) and RT (codons 1 to 335) genes followed by Sanger sequencing. The assay was validated for HIV-1 subtype B strains, but it has been used successfully for genotyping non-subtype B strains, including HIV-1 recombinants (78, 80, 82–84) which show mutations similar to those observed for subtype B (85). A second FDA-cleared test, the TrueGene HIV-1 genotyping assay (Siemens Healthcare Diagnostics, Deerfield, IL), was discontinued in 2014. In recent years, a growing number of clinical laboratories, including academic, commercial, and government-supported laboratories, have also developed LDT genotyping assays, several of which utilize NGS methods (86).

The drugs currently available to treat HIV-1 infection target the protease, RT, integrase, viral fusion, and entry (http://aidsinfo.nih.gov/drugs; https://www.fda.gov/forpatients/illness/hivaids/treatment/ucm118915.htm). In the past 10 or more years, new HIV-1 drugs for non-protease, non-RT targets have been FDA approved. For example, enfuvirtide targets the fusion peptide in gp41 coded for in the *env* gene and is used as an option in heavily treatment-experienced individuals. Resistance mutations for enfuvirtide have been mapped to the *env* first heptad repeat sequence in gp41 (codons 35 to 43) (87). Raltegravir, elvitegravir, and dolutegravir are integrase strand-transfer inhibitors targeting the integrase protein coded for in the Pol gene (88). Maraviroc is an entry inhibitor based on CCR5 usage and is associated with the V3 loop in the *env* gene (39).

Currently, genotypic assays to identify known antiviral mutations for these drugs are primarily being developed as LDTs. One commercial RUO genotyping kit is available for the detection of integrase resistance mutations, the ViroSeq HIV-1 integrase genotyping system (Abbott). There are no RUO or FDA-approved commercially available kits to screen for resistance to maraviroc or other CCR5 inhibitors. The expanded use of maraviroc as a first-line treatment option in drug-naïve individuals carrying virus with a CCR5 tropism requires determination of the baseline coreceptor usage of the virus. A phenotypic assay, Trofile (Monogram Biosciences/LabCorp, South San Francisco, CA), is commercially available to determine if the virus employs the CCR5 or CXCR4 coreceptor. Because this phenotypic testing requires cloning of patient-derived HIV-1 envelope protein genes to generate recombinant pseudoviruses for evaluation, a virus load of ≥1,000 copies/ml of plasma is necessary to ensure reliable target amplification. In patients with undetectable plasma virus loads for whom substitution of a CCR5 inhibitor is being considered, whole blood may be used to determine the tropism of the HIV-1 reservoir (Trofile DNA).

Molecular phenotypic assays are costly, and the turnaround time is lengthy. An alternative strategy to determine coreceptor usage is to sequence the V3 loop. Here, the genotypic determination of resistance to maraviroc entails the observation of a coreceptor switch from a CCR5 sequence profile to a mixed-coreceptor profile or solely a CXCR4 profile in the V3 loop. The consensus sequences generated are subsequently submitted to interactive websites employing databases correlating genotype with phenotypic outcome. The analysis infers coreceptor usage using different algorithms to determine the amino acid patterns and net charges of the entire V3 loop or only positions 11 and 25, which predict CCR5 and CXCR4 usage (89–91). Two algorithms frequently used to predict coreceptor tropism are the position-specific scoring matrix (92) and the Geno2pheno coreceptor algorithm (93). The successful use of this strategy as a clinical tool has been evaluated and reported by several groups (90, 94, 95). Although protocols for sequencing the V3 loop have been circulating for years, development of the various algorithms for analysis, some of which are free web-based services, has made this an approach feasible for LDT users.

NGS-based genotypic assays to determine HIV coreceptor tropism are available clinically, including the HIV-1 CCR5 tropism test (V3), offered by the British Columbia Centre for Excellence in HIV/AIDS (Vancouver, Canada) (95), the HIV-1 Coreceptor Tropism, Ultradeep Sequencing, offered by a major U.S. reference laboratory (96), and DEEPGEN HIV (developed by University Hospitals Case Medical Center, Cleveland, OH), which also assesses resistance mutations in the protease, RT, and integrase genes (86).

Hepatitis Virus

HBV. The 5′ nucleoside/nucleotide analogs approved for the management of chronic HBV infection targeting the HBV DNA polymerase and RT coding regions are listed in Table 3 (97, 98). IFN-α2b and peg-IFN–ribavirin have been the recommended treatment. However, treatment efficacy is dependent upon the HBV subtype (99, 100), and interferon does not directly target HBV. Since HBV is difficult to culture, genotyping methods are the tests of choice to monitor resistance. HBV genotypic assays detect known mutations (Table 3) in the polymerase and RT genes. The most common genotypic method for HBV genotyping is to directly sequence the polymerase and RT genes in HBV from plasma and determine the resistance-associated mutations. Alternatively, the generation of a PCR product from the specimen can be interrogated using specific probes in a reverse hybridization assay (98).

There are no FDA-approved or -cleared sequencing assay systems for HBV antiviral susceptibility testing. There is at least one RUO kit available for HBV genotyping (Abbott Diagnostics). This assay utilizes Sanger sequencing and targets an area of the HBV Pol-RT gene between bases 130 and 1161, where known antiviral resistance mutations reside. There is no software associated with this assay to generate a consensus sequence from the chromatograms, but the use of SeqScape v2.5 or later is recommended for the analysis. The parameters used in the analysis of the HBV sequence in SeqScape are provided with the test kit protocol. The RUO TruGene HBV genotyping kit (Siemens Healthcare Diagnostics) was discontinued in 2014.

There are also LDT sequencing assays to detect the HBV genotype and/or to detect antiviral drug resistance (101). The ability to consistently detect variants in the HBV population using Sanger sequencing-based genotyping assays is usually not achievable unless the minority population is greater than 25% (97, 101). However, this method is capable of detecting all mutations that are known or compensatory, as well as novel mutations that might be associated with antiviral resistance (98). Interpretation of the associated mutations requires a virtual phenotype and the consensus data must be analyzed further by other relational databases such as SeqHepB (Evivar) (102, 103). NGS methods are beginning to be applied to HBV (104), though tests are not widely available for clinical purposes.

A commercial (CE-marked) reverse hybridization assay, INNO-LiPA HBV DR, version 2 (Innogenetics N.V., Ghent, Belgium), which is capable of detecting known HBV mutations in the Pol-RT gene, is also available outside the United States. These mutations are associated with resistance to lamivudine, adefovir, emtricitabine, and telbivudine (48, 105) (Table 3). This assay is more sensitive for the detection of minority HBV populations compared to Sanger sequencing. It is also less labor-intensive than the population sequencing method (97). However, the sensitivity can be affected by neighboring polymorphisms within the sequence (105, 106). The RUO INNO-LiPA HBV genotyping kit (Innogenetics), based on the HBsAg (HBV surface antigen) sequence, can also be used for HBV genotyping (107).

HCV. Treatment of chronic HCV infection was historically limited to peg-IFN–ribavirin therapy. Success of this treatment varied and was affected by the virus genotype. Genotype 1 is the least responsive to IFN therapy, and infection with this genotype is the most likely to evolve into a chronic infection (108). Therefore, management of HCV infection required virus genotyping to predict the efficacy of peg-IFN–ribavirin. Over the past several years, there has been a revolution in the development of antiviral therapies for HCV. These direct-acting antiviral agents include drugs targeting the nonstructural protein 3/4A (NS3/4A) serine protease, the NS5A replication complex, and the NS5B polymerase (Table 3). The current recommendations comprise combination therapies targeting at least two of these proteins, and all first-line regimens are now IFN free (www.hcvguidelines.org). These regimens are extremely effective, with sustained virological responses obtained in more than 90% of cases, even in patients who have already developed cirrhosis. Genotyping remains an important component of regimen selection, though several drug combinations now provide pangenotypic coverage (sofosbuvir-velpatasvir; sofosbuvir-velpatasvir-voxilaprevir).

According to the guidelines of the American Association for the Study of Liver Disease and the Infectious Disease Society of America (AASLD/IDSA), the clinical utility of HCV genotypic susceptibility testing is currently limited to two specific conditions: (i) infection with HCV genotype 1a, both with and without cirrhosis, when treatment with elbasvir-grazoprevir is initiated; and (ii) infection with HCV genotype 1a with cirrhosis when simeprevir-sofosbuvir is initiated (Table 3) (109). Though not part of the IDSA guidelines, genotypic susceptibility testing is also recommended in the daclatasvir package insert for patients infected with HCV genotype 1a with cirrhosis when daclatasvir-sofosbuvir is initiated. The identification of these NS5A and NS3/4a resistance-associated amino acid substitutions (RASs) may also be useful to tailor therapy in genotype 1 infected patients that have failed NS5A containing regimens or simeprevir-sofosbuvir.

There are currently no FDA-approved/cleared assays available to identify NS3/4A or NS5A RASs. A number of laboratory-developed HCV sequencing assays have been evaluated for RAS detection (110, 111), and an NGS-based combined genotyping and NS3/4a/NS5A RAS assay received CE marking in 2016 (Sentosa SQ HCV genotyping assay; Vela Diagnostics, Singapore). In the United States, sequence-based HCV RAS testing is commercially available at several reference laboratories. Additional HCV regimens are expected to be approved in the near term (112), so close monitoring of the HCV resistance literature and professional society guidelines will be necessary to remain up to date with the rapidly evolving indications for RAS testing.

Influenza Virus

Mutations responsible for influenza virus A resistance to amantidine and rimantidine have been mapped to the gene encoding the M2 protein (6) (Table 3). However, these drugs are no longer recommended, because current circulating influenza virus A strains show heightened resistance. Current guidelines for the treatment of influenza recommend the use of the neuraminidase inhibitors oseltamivir, zanamivir, and peramivir (113–115) as the drugs of choice against influenza virus A (116). Mutations conferring resistance to the neuraminidase inhibitor drugs are located on the neuraminidase (NA) gene, including the most common neuraminidase inhibitor resistance mutation in the 2009 influenza virus A H1N1, NA H275Y. Numerous genotypic assays for the determination of anti-neuraminidase resistance have been developed as LDTs. These include real-time assays (49, 117), RT-PCR with high-resolution melt (118), a SNP analysis method performed by capillary electrophoresis (50), and a real-time allelic discrimination assay (41), which was adopted by WHO for screening influenza virus A H1N1. These assays primarily target H275Y of the seasonal virus (H1N1) and some 2009 H1N1 viruses (119); however, sequencing assays are also performed to detect other resistance mutations in the NA gene, and both Sanger and pyrosequencing protocols have been reported in the literature (120–123). It should be noted in review of the mutations in Table 3 that the exact numbering may vary depending upon the viral subtype. NGS methods are also being developed for influenza virus typing, subtyping, and genotypic drug resistance (124–127). Detection of mutations is more likely to be performed for infected high-risk immunocompromised individuals and for surveillance purposes (127).

INTERPRETATION OF GENOTYPIC ANTIVIRAL SUSCEPTIBILITY TESTING

The FDA-cleared genotypic assay for HIV susceptibility, ViroSeq (Abbott), which was cleared in 2002, includes kit-associated software to analyze the raw data sequences generated from each sample to produce a consensus sequence. In turn, the assay provides guideline-based interpretations of the mutations found in the consensus sequence and generate a formal report. The report helps the physician in choosing the regimen for the patient by indicating the likelihood of antiretroviral drug efficacy. FDA clearance included the software validation and periodic updates of the guidelines for use and interpretation. This system is considered the model protocol for diagnostic genotype testing used for antiviral susceptibility drug testing formats. The ViroSeq HIV-1 integrase genotyping kit (RUO; Abbott) has associated software that allows analysis of the sequences generated to form a consensus sequence. A drug resistance report can also be created for the sample.

Bioinformatics: Virtual Phenotypes

Results generated using RUO assays or LDTs are dependent upon bioinformatics sources for providing an interpretation. The laboratory has the option of analyzing the data following Sanger sequencing at various steps in the protocol (Fig. 2). The clinician has the task of determining the significance of the mutations observed based upon the interpretation provided by the laboratory. These assays are mostly represented by the antiviral susceptibility testing for HBV, HCV, and HIV-1 infections.

The clinical laboratory wishing to perform their own sequence-based antiviral susceptibility assays with either an RUO assay or an LDT will need access to analysis software to examine raw sequence data. Software for general sequence analysis and for the formation of consensus sequences can be purchased. Access to specialized "expert systems," as explained by Shafer (11), will also be needed to complete the interpretation. These systems are interactive, complex databases that use rules-based algorithms for individual drugs and associated mutations to infer the significance of the data (Table 5). The algorithms are guided by knowledge-based systems, which associate primary and secondary mutations, phenotypic data, and clinical outcomes.

Another consideration that should be addressed is access to adequate secured computer space or servers for storage of the raw data, software, and analysis results. These cumulative files of sample data analysis can be very extensive for Sanger sequencing and especially NGS. If the laboratories or their institutions are in a position to allocate this computer storage space, it can be very useful for comparison purposes when a patient is being monitored over time. There are also commercial entities available that can provide this service at a cost.

Models for knowledge-based expert systems originated from commercial entities. A system developed early in the era of highly active antiretroviral therapy was the Virtual Phenotype system based on the Antivirogram (Virco; acquired by Jannsen Diagnostics). Genotypic sequence data, obtained from a clinical sample sent to this company, were analyzed and interpreted by an algorithm by comparison against a private database in order to infer a phenotype (11, 128). Their extensive database contained known genotypes which were correlated with phenotypes and/or clinical outcomes. The Virtual Phenotype system is not available as of December 31, 2013. The Monogram Biosciences GenoSure MG and GenoSure PRIme tests compare an HIV genotype, derived from a submitted specimen, to their own expansive database of linked genotypes and phenotypes. A newer offering, GenoSure Archive, uses NGS analysis to examine archived DNA in infected cells from patients with good suppression of their HIV viral load. The objective is to identify resistance mutations and predict phenotypic resistance using a proprietary algorithm

Consensus sequences can also be submitted through noncommercial interactive websites where interpretative data providing a virtual phenotype are returned to the submitting laboratory (Table 5). These sites are useful but are not regulated or standardized at this time. They employ different algorithms for different virus-drug combinations and allow different levels of operator input (91–93, 102, 103, 129–132). The databases linked with their algorithms connecting genotype and phenotype are also public. The reliability and consistency of the sites have been compared by several investigators (90, 91, 94). Most of these sites can examine consensus sequences to detect relevant mutations linked to resistance, and some can provide interpretations of the significance of the observed mutations with regard to drug efficacy. Some of the sites also provide additional tools for further analyses. All of these sites analyze data derived by Sanger sequencing or consensus sequences derived from NGS methods. Though Geno2pheno offers a module that accepts data directly from ultradeep pyrosequencing (95, 133–137), this method (454 Genome Sequencer; Roche Molecular Diagnostics) is not supported by the manufacturer, as of mid-2016.

Test Interpretation

There is often minimal or no standardization among the various antiviral testing methods at a technical level, but required proficiency testing provides some assurance of quality. Sequencing assays can be affected by several factors. Assuming that the laboratory follows good laboratory practices, adhering to the stringency of defined use and separation of space to control the possibility of contamination is critical. This is especially important when the VL of the patient sample is low. The commercial kits for HIV-1 were optimized for a minimum VL of 1,000 to 2,000 copies/ml of virus in the patient sample, and additional safeguards to reduce the effects of contamination were added within the protocol by using nonnested PCR to produce the sequencing template. Initial required volumes for extraction were ~200 to 500 μl of specimen, usually plasma. In situations where the initial starting volumes are much lower, such as genotyping from dried blood spots or when the VL is reduced to near undetectable, many LDTs incorporate nested PCR into the protocols, an approach which is vulnerable to contamination. Generation of quality data in these circumstances can still occur if the assay is performed under rigorous conditions.

The analysis software provided with FDA-cleared diagnostic sequencing assays incorporates algorithms to accurately provide interpretations generated from test results. Updates to the algorithms are also FDA cleared before they are released. Alternatively, non-FDA-cleared Sanger genotyping assays developed as LDTs rely upon the individual laboratory to establish test performance and to provide useful interpretations. The sources for such interpretations may be the literature, testing by the laboratory, established online databases (e.g., http://hivdb.stanford.edu), or other sources. Though there is no standardization or oversight of the interpretation algorithms used, the inferred clinical significance of the data may be very similar regardless of the algorithm used. Ultimately, the use of these results

TABLE 5 Bioinformatics-based sites for analysis of resistance from genotyped samples

Sites	User fee	Virus	Genotyped target area	Interactive	Sample submitted	Information provided	Other comments/features
Stanford University HIV-1 Drug Resistance Database (Stanford University, Palo Alto)	No	HIV	Protease-RT Integrase	Yes	FASTA file of multiple sequences; Test file ok for a single sequence	Resistance mutations Polymorphisms Clinical interpretations Subtype Genotype/phenotype correlations	New Web-based link allows individuals and institutions to use site database tools. Interactive tools for epidemiologic and treatment observations
Geno2pheno (Max Planck Institute, part of GENAFOR, Bonn, Germany)	No	HIV	Protease-RT Integrase GAG Coreceptor use	Yes	FASTA file of consensus sequence Clinical data from patient	Resistance mutations Polymorphisms Clinical interpretations Subtype	Most established modules
		HCV	Protease - NS3	Yes	Plain or FASTA file of consensus sequence	Resistance mutations Clinical phenotypic interpretations	Data include interpreted phenotype based on genotype Should not be sole basis for clinical decisions
			NS5B NS5A		FASTA file of consensus sequence	Genotype, subgenotype	
		HBV	Pol gene/Surface gene	Yes	FASTA file of consensus sequence	Pol gene mutations SHB gene mutations Predicted phenotype for 5 antiretroviral drugs	Interpretations require substantial RT sequence to be submitted. Should not be sole basis for clinical decisions
PSSM (position specific scoring matrices) (University of Washington, Seattle, WA)	No	HIV	Coreceptor	No	FASTA of V3 amino acids	Predicts coreceptor usage based on charged V3 loop amino acids	Developed for subtypes B and C Does not predict subtype

(*Continued on next page*)

TABLE 5 Bioinformatics-based sites for analysis of resistance from genotyped samples *(Continued)*

Sites	User fee	Virus	Genotyped target area	Interactive	Sample submitted	Information provided	Other comments/features
SmartGene integrated database network system (IDNS)	Yes	HIV	Protease-RT Integrase GAG gp41-gp120 (V3)	Yes	Sequence chromatogram files FASTA files FAST Q files Sff files	Resistance mutations Polymorphisms Clinical interpretations Subtype Quantitation of minority variants	Provides user capability to work with and edit chromatograms within module Network links to sites with different databases and algorithms for clinical interpretation allowing comparisons. Site acts as a secured application and data management center with storage of cumulative data able to be recalled for analysis.
	Yes	HCV	NS3, NS4 HCV 5′ UTR NS5B NS5A	Yes	Sequence chromatogram files FASTA files FAST Q files Sff files	Resistance mutations Subtype Quantitation of minority variants	Same as above
	Yes	Influenza virus	HA NA		Sequence chromatogram files FASTA files	Resistance mutations Subtype	Same as above
	Yes	HSV TK Pol			Sequence chromatogram files FASTA files	Resistance mutations Subtype	Same as above
SeqHepB (ABL SA, Luxembourg)	Yes	HBV	Pol gene (RT)	Yes	Sequence chromatogram files FASTA files FAST Q files BAM/SAM Patient blood	Resistance mutations Polymorphisms Clinical interpretations Genotype Serotype	Linked to *in vitro* phenotypic database

and the interpretations provided by the laboratory in care of the patient are the responsibility of the laboratory medical director and primary health care provider.

For LDTs that are based on NGS, test performance should be optimized prior to actual sequencing on the instrument. In light of the ability of the assay to identify mutations down to a 1%-of-population level, there are some artificial parameters that could affect the accuracy of low-level detection, especially since there is less opportunity to evaluate and edit the raw sequence data. These include potential errors made during reverse transcription or PCR to generate the single-molecule sequencing templates (138). Further analysis of the sequence data in an established bioinformatics pipeline program will also be essential to accurate interpretation of the mutations identified (47). The pipelines available are in various stages of development; some are more user-friendly, and many do not charge for use. A good description of the pipelines is presented by Noguera-Julian et al. (47).

FUTURE DIRECTIONS AND EMERGING TECHNOLOGIES

Methods for antiviral susceptibility testing have dramatically evolved over recent years in parallel with emerging molecular technologies. Genotypic testing methods utilizing nucleic acid amplification and sequencing have become invaluable tools for detecting resistance in viruses that are difficult to culture or are noncultivatable (e.g., HBV and HCV) and are now performed routinely for the clinical management of viral infections. Genotypic resistance testing is possible because the genes and nucleotide positions of the variants responsible for antiviral resistance to many antiviral therapies have been identified and characterized. As virus culture-based methods are phased out in clinical virology laboratories, clinical phenotypic resistance assays are primarily limited to rapidly replicating viruses (e.g., HSV) and cases in which resistance is suspected but the genotypic testing is inconclusive (e.g., HIV-1). From a research perspective, phenotypic assays remain critical for the detection of emerging resistance and confirmation of newly identified resistance-associated mutations.

An area of ongoing improvement for both phenotypic and genotypic assays is efforts to improve assay harmonization and standardization. Examples include a CLSI approach reported for HSV plaque assays (139) and approaches for CMV genotypic testing using the UL97 gene target (67, 140). In addition, proficiency testing materials are available from several suppliers for HIV-1 genotypic antiviral susceptibility testing.

The pharmaceutical industry is actively investigating and developing new antiviral drugs, especially for chronic viral disease agents (e.g., HCV, HBV, and HIV-1). Concurrently, antiviral resistance assays must be developed for detecting and monitoring resistance to these novel therapeutics. This is particularly important due to the high cost of such new antivirals and the potential for long-term use, which is conducive to the development of resistance. An important goal is to develop assays that predict the likelihood of emerging resistance. Such assays may be possible using NGS technologies, which can detect variants at levels of <5%. However, the clinical significance of the presence of such small populations will have to be determined. Also, as previously mentioned, there are logistical concerns with data management and storage, as well as with proficiency and consistency in expertise which should be addressed in parallel with assay development.

In addition, there is an increasing interest in the use of alternative specimen types, such as dried blood spots, whose ease of collection and transport may facilitate the availability of viral genotyping, particularly for HIV-1, in remote, underserved populations (141). While many genotypic assays utilize sequencing technologies for their broad coverage of drug resistance mutations, simpler, less costly screening tests for a limited number of well-characterized mutations may also be used to guide treatment strategies when sequencing is unavailable and the treatment regimens in use result in a narrow spectrum of mutations. For example, recent work evaluating HIV-1 antiviral resistance indicates that a panel of just six mutations would capture nearly 99% of individuals in low- and middle-income countries failing a first-line regimen containing nucleoside reverse transcriptase inhibitors and/or nonnucleoside reverse transcriptase inhibitors (142). Such targeted allele-specific point mutation assays could be used in the clinical laboratory setting or adapted for use in sample-to-answer systems for near-care or point-of-care testing.

It is very likely that antiviral susceptibility testing applications will evolve quickly as new technology is introduced and the characteristics of viral infection and treatment change. Evaluation of the clinical significance of the data acquired from these new technologies will need to keep pace.

REFERENCES

1. **Arts EJ, Hazuda DJ**. 2012. HIV-1 antiretroviral drug therapy. *Cold Spring Harb Perspect Med* **2:**a007161.
2. **Wyles DL**. 2013. Antiviral resistance and the future landscape of hepatitis C virus infection therapy. *J Infect Dis* **207**(Suppl 1)**:**S33–S39.
3. **Fox AN, Jacobson IM**. 2012. Recent successes and noteworthy future prospects in the treatment of chronic hepatitis C. *Clin Infect Dis* **55**(Suppl 1)**:**S16–S24.
4. **Bean B, Fletcher C, Englund J, Lehrman SN, Ellis MN**. 1987. Progressive mucocutaneous herpes simplex infection due to acyclovir-resistant virus in an immunocompromised patient: correlation of viral susceptibilities and plasma levels with response to therapy. *Diagn Microbiol Infect Dis* **7:**199–204.
5. **Belshe RB, Burk B, Newman F, Cerruti RL, Sim IS**. 1989. Resistance of influenza A virus to amantadine and rimantadine: results of one decade of surveillance. *J Infect Dis* **159:**430–435.
6. **Belshe RB, Smith MH, Hall CB, Betts R, Hay AJ**. 1988. Genetic basis of resistance to rimantadine emerging during treatment of influenza virus infection. *J Virol* **62:**1508–1512.
7. **Berkowitz FE, Levin MJ**. 1985. Use of an enzyme-linked immunosorbent assay performed directly on fixed infected cell monolayers for evaluating drugs against varicella-zoster virus. *Antimicrob Agents Chemother* **28:**207–210.
8. **Biron KK**. 1991. Ganciclovir-resistant human cytomegalovirus clinical isolates; resistance mechanisms and in vitro susceptibility to antiviral agents. *Transplant Proc* **23**(Suppl 3)**:**162–167.
9. **Englund JA, Zimmerman ME, Swierkosz EM, Goodman JL, Scholl DR, Balfour HH, Jr**. 1990. Herpes simplex virus resistant to acyclovir. A study in a tertiary care center. *Ann Intern Med* **112:**416–422.
10. **Lok AS**. 2007. Navigating the maze of hepatitis B treatments. *Gastroenterology* **132:**1586–1594.
11. **Shafer RW**. 2002. Genotypic testing for human immunodeficiency virus type 1 drug resistance. *Clin Microbiol Rev* **15:**247–277.
12. **DeGruttola V, Dix L, D'Aquila R, Holder D, Phillips A, Ait-Khaled M, Baxter J, Clevenbergh P, Hammer S, Harrigan R, Katzenstein D, Lanier R, Miller M, Para M, Yerly S, Zolopa A, Murray J, Patick A, Miller V, Castillo S, Pedneault L, Mellors J**. 2000. The relation between baseline HIV drug resistance and response to antiretroviral therapy: re-analysis of retrospective and prospective studies using a standardized data analysis plan. *Antivir Ther* **5:**41–48.

13. **Burd EM.** 2010. Validation of laboratory-developed molecular assays for infectious diseases. *Clin Microbiol Rev* **23:**550–576.
14. **Thursz M, Yee L, Khakoo S.** 2011. Understanding the host genetics of chronic hepatitis B and C. *Semin Liver Dis* **31:**115–127.
15. **Lampertico P, Viganò M, Cheroni C, Facchetti F, Invernizzi F, Valveri V, Soffredini R, Abrignani S, De Francesco R, Colombo M.** 2013. IL28B polymorphisms predict interferon-related hepatitis B surface antigen seroclearance in genotype D hepatitis B e antigen-negative patients with chronic hepatitis B. *Hepatology* **57:**890–896.
16. **Holzinger ER, Ritchie MD.** 2012. Integrating heterogeneous high-throughput data for meta-dimensional pharmacogenomics and disease-related studies. *Pharmacogenomics* **13:**213–222.
17. **Rodríguez-Torres M.** 2013. Focus on drug interactions: the challenge of treating hepatitis C virus infection with direct-acting antiviral drugs in the HIV-positive patient. *Curr Opin Infect Dis* **26:**50–57.
18. **Taylor LE, Swan T, Mayer KH.** 2012. HIV coinfection with hepatitis C virus: evolving epidemiology and treatment paradigms. *Clin Infect Dis* **55**(Suppl 1)**:**S33–S42.
19. **Yee HS, Chang MF, Pocha C, Lim J, Ross D, Morgan TR, Monto A, Department of Veterans Affairs Hepatitis C Resource Center Program, National Hepatitis C Program Office.** 2012. Update on the management and treatment of hepatitis C virus infection: recommendations from the Department of Veterans Affairs Hepatitis C Resource Center Program and the National Hepatitis C Program Office. *Am J Gastroenterol* **107:**669–689, quiz 690.
20. **Bangsberg DR, Hecht FM, Charlebois ED, Zolopa AR, Holodniy M, Sheiner L, Bamberger JD, Chesney MA, Moss A.** 2000. Adherence to protease inhibitors, HIV-1 viral load, and development of drug resistance in an indigent population. *AIDS* **14:**357–366.
21. **Cingolani A, Antinori A, Rizzo MG, Murri R, Ammassari A, Baldini F, Di Giambenedetto S, Cauda R, De Luca A.** 2002. Usefulness of monitoring HIV drug resistance and adherence in individuals failing highly active antiretroviral therapy: a randomized study (ARGENTA). *AIDS* **16:**369–379.
22. **Genberg BL, Wilson IB, Bangsberg DR, Arnsten J, Goggin K, Remien RH, Simoni J, Gross R, Reynolds N, Rosen M, Liu H, MACH14 Investigators.** 2012. Patterns of antiretroviral therapy adherence and impact on HIV RNA among patients in North America. *AIDS* **26:**1415–1423.
23. **Sivay MV, Li M, Piwowar-Manning E, Zhang Y, Hudelson SE, Marzinke MA, Amico RK, Redd A, Hendrix CW, Anderson PL, Bokoch K, Bekker LG, van Griensven F, Mannheimer S, Hughes JP, Grant R, Eshleman SH, HPTN 067/ADAPT Study Team.** 2017. Characterization of HIV seroconverters in a TDF/FTC PrEP study: HPTN 067/ADAPT. *J Acquir Immune Defic Syndr* **75:**271–279.
24. **Zhang Y, Clarke W, Marzinke MA, Piwowar-Manning E, Beauchamp G, Breaud A, Hendrix CW, Cloherty GA, Emel L, Rose S, Hightow-Weidman L, Siegel M, Shoptaw S, Fields SD, Wheeler D, Eshleman SH.** 2017. Evaluation of a multidrug assay for monitoring adherence to a regimen for HIV pre-exposure prophylaxis in a clinical study, HIV Prevention Trials Network 073. *Antimicrob Agents Chemother* **61:**e02743-16.
25. **Lurain NS, Chou S.** 2010. Antiviral drug resistance of human cytomegalovirus. *Clin Microbiol Rev* **23:**689–712.
26. **Biron KK, Elion GB.** 1980. In vitro susceptibility of varicella-zoster virus to acyclovir. *Antimicrob Agents Chemother* **18:**443–447.
27. **Biron KK, Stanat SC, Sorrell JB, Fyfe JA, Keller PM, Lambe CU, Nelson DJ.** 1985. Metabolic activation of the nucleoside analog 9-[(2-hydroxy-1-(hydroxymethyl)ethoxy]methyl)guanine in human diploid fibroblasts infected with human cytomegalovirus. *Proc Natl Acad Sci USA* **82:**2473–2477.
28. **Hayden FG, Cote KM, Douglas RG, Jr.** 1980. Plaque inhibition assay for drug susceptibility testing of influenza viruses. *Antimicrob Agents Chemother* **17:**865–870.
29. **McLaren C, Ellis MN, Hunter GA.** 1983. A colorimetric assay for the measurement of the sensitivity of herpes simplex viruses to antiviral agents. *Antiviral Res* **3:**223–234.
30. **Rabalais GP, Levin MJ, Berkowitz FE.** 1987. Rapid herpes simplex virus susceptibility testing using an enzyme-linked immunosorbent assay performed in situ on fixed virus-infected monolayers. *Antimicrob Agents Chemother* **31:**946–948.
31. **Safrin S, Palacios E, Leahy BJ.** 1996. Comparative evaluation of microplate enzyme-linked immunosorbent assay versus plaque reduction assay for antiviral susceptibility testing of herpes simplex virus isolates. *Antimicrob Agents Chemother* **40:**1017–1019.
32. **Safrin S, Phan L, Elbeik T.** 1995. A comparative evaluation of three methods of antiviral susceptibility testing of clinical herpes simplex virus isolates. *Clin Diagn Virol* **4:**81–91.
33. **Winquist AG, Fukuda K, Bridges CB, Cox NJ.** 1999. Neuraminidase inhibitors for treatment of influenza A and B infections. *Morb Mortal Wkly Rep* **48**(RR14)**:**1–9.
34. **Wetherall NT, Trivedi T, Zeller J, Hodges-Savola C, McKimm-Breschkin JL, Zambon M, Hayden FG.** 2003. Evaluation of neuraminidase enzyme assays using different substrates to measure susceptibility of influenza virus clinical isolates to neuraminidase inhibitors: report of the neuraminidase inhibitor susceptibility network. *J Clin Microbiol* **41:**742–750.
35. **Murtaugh W, Mahaman L, Healey B, Peters H, Anderson B, Tran M, Ziese M, Carlos MP.** 2013. Evaluation of three influenza neuraminidase inhibition assays for use in a public health laboratory setting during the 2011–2012 influenza season. *Public Health Rep* **128**(Suppl 2)**:**75–87.
36. **Marjuki H, Mishin VP, Sleeman K, Okomo-Adhiambo M, Sheu TG, Guo L, Xu X, Gubareva LV.** 2013. Bioluminescence-based neuraminidase inhibition assay for monitoring influenza virus drug susceptibility in clinical specimens. *Antimicrob Agents Chemother* **57:**5209–5215.
37. **Chou S.** 2010. Recombinant phenotyping of cytomegalovirus UL97 kinase sequence variants for ganciclovir resistance. *Antimicrob Agents Chemother* **54:**2371–2378.
38. **Blanco JL, Whitlock G, Milinkovic A, Moyle G.** 2015. HIV integrase inhibitors: a new era in the treatment of HIV. *Expert Opin Pharmacother* **16:**1313–1324.
39. **DHHS Panel on Antiretroviral Guidelines for Adults and Adolescents.** Guidelines for the use of antiretroviral agents in HIV-1-infected adults and adolescents living with HIV. https://aidsinfo.nih.gov/contentfiles/lvguidelines/adultandadolescentgl.pdf.
40. **Wainberg MA, Zaharatos GJ, Brenner BG.** 2011. Development of antiretroviral drug resistance. *N Engl J Med* **365:**637–646.
41. **Nakauchi M, Ujike M, Obuchi M, Takashita E, Takayama I, Ejima M, Oba K, Konomi N, Odagiri T, Tashiro M, Kageyama T, influenza virus surveillance group of Japan.** 2011. Rapid discrimination of oseltamivir-resistant 275Y and -susceptible 275H substitutions in the neuraminidase gene of pandemic influenza A/H1N1 2009 virus by duplex one-step RT-PCR assay. *J Med Virol* **83:**1121–1127.
42. **Sanger F, Nicklen S, Coulson AR.** 1977. DNA sequencing with chain-terminating inhibitors. *Proc Natl Acad Sci USA* **74:**5463–5467.
43. **Delwart EL, Pan H, Sheppard HW, Wolpert D, Neumann AU, Korber B, Mullins JI.** 1997. Slower evolution of human immunodeficiency virus type 1 quasispecies during progression to AIDS. *J Virol* **71:**7498–7508.
44. **Huang DD, Eshleman SH, Brambilla DJ, Palumbo PE, Bremer JW.** 2003. Evaluation of the editing process in human immunodeficiency virus type 1 genotyping. *J Clin Microbiol* **41:**3265–3272.
45. **Metzker ML.** 2010. Sequencing technologies—the next generation. *Nat Rev Genet* **11:**31–46.
46. **Lefterova MI, Suarez CJ, Banaei N, Pinsky BA.** 2015. Next-generation sequencing for infectious disease diagnosis and management: a report of the Association for Molecular Pathology. *J Mol Diagn* **17:**623–634.
47. **Noguera-Julian M, Edgil D, Harrigan PR, Sandstrom P, Godfrey C, Paredes R.** 2017. Next-generation human immunodeficiency virus sequencing for patient management and drug resistance surveillance. *J Infect Dis* **216**(Suppl 9)**:**S829–S833.

48. **Hussain M, Fung S, Libbrecht E, Sablon E, Cursaro C, Andreone P, Lok AS.** 2006. Sensitive line probe assay that simultaneously detects mutations conveying resistance to lamivudine and adefovir. *J Clin Microbiol* **44:**1094–1097.
49. **Hindiyeh M, Ram D, Mandelboim M, Meningher T, Hirsh S, Robinov J, Levy V, Orzitzer S, Azar R, Grossman Z, Mendelson E.** 2010. Rapid detection of influenza A pandemic (H1N1) 2009 virus neuraminidase resistance mutation H275Y by real-time reverse transcriptase PCR. *J Clin Microbiol* **48:**1884–1887.
50. **Duan S, Boltz DA, Li J, Oshansky CM, Marjuki H, Barman S, Webby RJ, Webster RG, Govorkova EA.** 2011. Novel genotyping and quantitative analysis of neuraminidase inhibitor resistance-associated mutations in influenza a viruses by single-nucleotide polymorphism analysis. *Antimicrob Agents Chemother* **55:**4718–4727.
51. **Goldner T, Hempel C, Ruebsamen-Schaeff H, Zimmermann H, Lischka P.** 2014. Geno- and phenotypic characterization of human cytomegalovirus mutants selected in vitro after letermovir (AIC246) exposure. *Antimicrob Agents Chemother* **58:**610–613.
52. **Chou S.** 2015. Rapid in vitro evolution of human cytomegalovirus UL56 mutations that confer letermovir resistance. *Antimicrob Agents Chemother* **59:**6588–6593.
53. **Bowman LJ, Melaragno JI, Brennan DC.** 2017. Letermovir for the management of cytomegalovirus infection. *Expert Opin Investig Drugs* **26:**235–241.
54. **Boivin G, Chou S, Quirk MR, Erice A, Jordan MC.** 1996. Detection of ganciclovir resistance mutations quantitation of cytomegalovirus (CMV) DNA in leukocytes of patients with fatal disseminated CMV disease. *J Infect Dis* **173:**523–528.
55. **Spector SA, Hsia K, Wolf D, Shinkai M, Smith I.** 1995. Molecular detection of human cytomegalovirus and determination of genotypic ganciclovir resistance in clinical specimens. *Clin Infect Dis* **21**(Suppl 2)**:**S170–S173.
56. **Wolf DG, Smith IL, Lee DJ, Freeman WR, Flores-Aguilar M, Spector SA.** 1995. Mutations in human cytomegalovirus UL97 gene confer clinical resistance to ganciclovir and can be detected directly in patient plasma. *J Clin Invest* **95:**257–263.
57. **Sahoo MK, Lefterova MI, Yamamoto F, Waggoner JJ, Chou S, Holmes SP, Anderson MW, Pinsky BA.** 2013. Detection of cytomegalovirus drug resistance mutations by next-generation sequencing. *J Clin Microbiol* **51:**3700–3710.
58. **Chou S, Ercolani RJ, Sahoo MK, Lefterova MI, Strasfeld LM, Pinsky BA.** 2014. Improved detection of emerging drug-resistant mutant cytomegalovirus subpopulations by deep sequencing. *Antimicrob Agents Chemother* **58:**4697–4702.
59. **Kotton CN, Kumar D, Caliendo AM, Asberg A, Chou S, Danziger-Isakov L, Humar A, Transplantation Society International CMV Consensus Group.** 2013. Updated international consensus guidelines on the management of cytomegalovirus in solid-organ transplantation. *Transplantation* **96:**333–360.
60. **Erice A.** 1999. Resistance of human cytomegalovirus to antiviral drugs. *Clin Microbiol Rev* **12:**286–297.
61. **Baldanti F, Underwood MR, Stanat SC, Biron KK, Chou S, Sarasini A, Silini E, Gerna G.** 1996. Single amino acid changes in the DNA polymerase confer foscarnet resistance and slow-growth phenotype, while mutations in the UL97-encoded phosphotransferase confer ganciclovir resistance in three double-resistant human cytomegalovirus strains recovered from patients with AIDS. *J Virol* **70:**1390–1395.
62. **Chou S, Guentzel S, Michels KR, Miner RC, Drew WL.** 1995. Frequency of UL97 phosphotransferase mutations related to ganciclovir resistance in clinical cytomegalovirus isolates. *J Infect Dis* **172:**239–242.
63. **Erice A, Gil-Roda C, Pérez JL, Balfour HH, Jr, Sannerud KJ, Hanson MN, Boivin G, Chou S.** 1997. Antiviral susceptibilities and analysis of UL97 and DNA polymerase sequences of clinical cytomegalovirus isolates from immunocompromised patients. *J Infect Dis* **175:**1087–1092.
64. **Smith IL, Cherrington JM, Jiles RE, Fuller MD, Freeman WR, Spector SA.** 1997. High-level resistance of cytomegalovirus to ganciclovir is associated with alterations in both the UL97 and DNA polymerase genes. *J Infect Dis* **176:**69–77.
65. **Hantz S, Michel D, Fillet AM, Guigonis V, Champier G, Mazeron MC, Bensman A, Denis F, Mertens T, Dehee A, Alain S.** 2005. Early selection of a new UL97 mutant with a severe defect of ganciclovir phosphorylation after valaciclovir prophylaxis and short-term ganciclovir therapy in a renal transplant recipient. *Antimicrob Agents Chemother* **49:**1580–1583.
66. **Iwasenko JM, Scott GM, Naing Z, Glanville AR, Rawlinson WD.** 2011. Diversity of antiviral-resistant human cytomegalovirus in heart and lung transplant recipients. *Transpl Infect Dis* **13:**145–153.
67. **Lurain NS, Weinberg A, Crumpacker CS, Chou S, Adult AIDS Clinical Trials Group—CMV Laboratories.** 2001. Sequencing of cytomegalovirus UL97 gene for genotypic antiviral resistance testing. *Antimicrob Agents Chemother* **45:**2775–2780.
68. **Chou S, Ercolani RJ, Marousek G, Bowlin TL.** 2013. Cytomegalovirus UL97 kinase catalytic domain mutations that confer multidrug resistance. *Antimicrob Agents Chemother* **57:**3375–3379.
69. **Lurain NS, Thompson KD, Holmes EW, Read GS.** 1992. Point mutations in the DNA polymerase gene of human cytomegalovirus that result in resistance to antiviral agents. *J Virol* **66:**7146–7152.
70. **Storch GA.** 2000. *Essentials of Diagnostic Virology*. Churchill Livingstone, New York, NY.
71. **Piret J, Boivin G.** 2011. Resistance of herpes simplex viruses to nucleoside analogues: mechanisms, prevalence, and management. *Antimicrob Agents Chemother* **55:**459–472.
72. **Gaudreau A, Hill E, Balfour HH, Jr, Erice A, Boivin G.** 1998. Phenotypic and genotypic characterization of acyclovir-resistant herpes simplex viruses from immunocompromised patients. *J Infect Dis* **178:**297–303.
73. **Morfin F, Souillet G, Bilger K, Ooka T, Aymard M, Thouvenot D.** 2000. Genetic characterization of thymidine kinase from acyclovir-resistant and -susceptible herpes simplex virus type 1 isolated from bone marrow transplant recipients. *J Infect Dis* **182:**290–293.
74. **Andrei G, Topalis D, Fiten P, McGuigan C, Balzarini J, Opdenakker G, Snoeck R.** 2012. In vitro-selected drug-resistant varicella-zoster virus mutants in the thymidine kinase and DNA polymerase genes yield novel phenotype-genotype associations and highlight differences between antiherpesvirus drugs. *J Virol* **86:**2641–2652.
75. **Hirsch MS, Brun-Vézinet F, D'Aquila RT, Hammer SM, Johnson VA, Kuritzkes DR, Loveday C, Mellors JW, Clotet B, Conway B, Demeter LM, Vella S, Jacobsen DM, Richman DD.** 2000. Antiretroviral drug resistance testing in adult HIV-1 infection: recommendations of an International AIDS Society—USA panel. *JAMA* **283:**2417–2426.
76. **Hirsch MS, Conway B, D'Aquila RT, Johnson VA, Brun-Vézinet F, Clotet B, Demeter LM, Hammer SM, Jacobsen DM, Kuritzkes DR, Loveday C, Mellors JW, Vella S, Richman DD, International AIDS Society—USA Panel.** 1998. Antiretroviral drug resistance testing in adults with HIV infection: implications for clinical management. International AIDS Society—USA Panel. *JAMA* **279:**1984–1991.
77. **Grant RM, Kuritzkes DR, Johnson VA, Mellors JW, Sullivan JL, Swanstrom R, D'Aquila RT, Van Gorder M, Holodniy M, Lloyd RM, Jr, Reid C, Morgan GF, Winslow DL.** 2003. Accuracy of the TRUGENE HIV-1 genotyping kit. *J Clin Microbiol* **41:**1586–1593.
78. **Cunningham S, Ank B, Lewis D, Lu W, Wantman M, Dileanis JA, Jackson JB, Palumbo P, Krogstad P, Eshleman SH.** 2001. Performance of the applied biosystems ViroSeq human immunodeficiency virus type 1 (HIV-1) genotyping system for sequence-based analysis of HIV-1 in pediatric plasma samples. *J Clin Microbiol* **39:**1254–1257.
79. **Erali M, Page S, Reimer LG, Hillyard DR.** 2001. Human immunodeficiency virus type 1 drug resistance testing: a comparison of three sequence-based methods. *J Clin Microbiol* **39:**2157–2165.
80. **Mracna M, Becker-Pergola G, Dileanis J, Guay LA, Cunningham S, Jackson JB, Eshleman SH.** 2001. Performance of Applied Biosystems ViroSeq HIV-1 Genotyping System for sequence-based analysis of non-subtype B human immunodeficiency virus type 1 from Uganda. *J Clin Microbiol* **39:**4323–4327.

81. **Tural C, Ruiz L, Holtzer C, Schapiro J, Viciana P, González J, Domingo P, Boucher C, Rey-Joly C, Clotet B, Havana Study Group.** 2002. Clinical utility of HIV-1 genotyping and expert advice: the Havana trial. *AIDS* **16:**209–218.
82. **Jagodzinski LL, Cooley JD, Weber M, Michael NL.** 2003. Performance characteristics of human immunodeficiency virus type 1 (HIV-1) genotyping systems in sequence-based analysis of subtypes other than HIV-1 subtype B. *J Clin Microbiol* **41:**998–1003.
83. **Beddows S, Galpin S, Kazmi SH, Ashraf A, Johargy A, Frater AJ, White N, Braganza R, Clarke J, McClure M, Weber JN.** 2003. Performance of two commercially available sequence-based HIV-1 genotyping systems for the detection of drug resistance against HIV type 1 group M subtypes. *J Med Virol* **70:**337–342.
84. **Eshleman SH, Hackett J Jr, Swanson P, Cunningham SP, Drews B, Brennan C, Devare SG, Zekeng L, Kaptué L, Marlowe N.** 2004. Performance of the Celera Diagnostics ViroSeq HIV-1 Genotyping System for sequence-based analysis of diverse human immunodeficiency virus type 1 strains. *J Clin Microbiol* **42:**2711–2717.
85. **Kantor R, Katzenstein DA, Efron B, Carvalho AP, Wynhoven B, Cane P, Clarke J, Sirivichayakul S, Soares MA, Snoeck J, Pillay C, Rudich H, Rodrigues R, Holguin A, Ariyoshi K, Bouzas MB, Cahn P, Sugiura W, Soriano V, Brigido LF, Grossman Z, Morris L, Vandamme AM, Tanuri A, Phanuphak P, Weber JN, Pillay D, Harrigan PR, Camacho R, Schapiro JM, Shafer RW.** 2005. Impact of HIV-1 subtype and antiretroviral therapy on protease and reverse transcriptase genotype: results of a global collaboration. *PLoS Med* **2:**e112.
86. **Gibson RM, Meyer AM, Winner D, Archer J, Feyertag F, Ruiz-Mateos E, Leal M, Robertson DL, Schmotzer CL, Quiñones-Mateu ME.** 2014. Sensitive deep-sequencing-based HIV-1 genotyping assay to simultaneously determine susceptibility to protease, reverse transcriptase, integrase, and maturation inhibitors, as well as HIV-1 coreceptor tropism. *Antimicrob Agents Chemother* **58:**2167–2185.
87. **Lu J, Deeks SG, Hoh R, Beatty G, Kuritzkes BA, Martin JN, Kuritzkes DR.** 2006. Rapid emergence of enfuvirtide resistance in HIV-1-infected patients: results of a clonal analysis. *J Acquir Immune Defic Syndr* **43:**60–64.
88. **Thierry E, Deprez E, Delelis O.** 2017. Different pathways leading to integrase inhibitors resistance. *Front Microbiol* **7:**2165.
89. **Lin NH, Kuritzkes DR.** 2009. Tropism testing in the clinical management of HIV-1 infection. *Curr Opin HIV AIDS* **4:**481–487.
90. **Garrido C, Roulet V, Chueca N, Poveda E, Aguilera A, Skrabal K, Zahonero N, Carlos S, García F, Faudon JL, Soriano V, de Mendoza C.** 2008. Evaluation of eight different bioinformatics tools to predict viral tropism in different human immunodeficiency virus type 1 subtypes. *J Clin Microbiol* **46:**887–891.
91. **Seclén E, Garrido C, González MM, González-Lahoz J, de Mendoza C, Soriano V, Poveda E.** 2010. High sensitivity of specific genotypic tools for detection of X4 variants in antiretroviral-experienced patients suitable to be treated with CCR5 antagonists. *J Antimicrob Chemother* **65:**1486–1492.
92. **Jensen MA, Coetzer M, van 't Wout AB, Morris L, Mullins JI.** 2006. A reliable phenotype predictor for human immunodeficiency virus type 1 subtype C based on envelope V3 sequences. *J Virol* **80:**4698–4704.
93. **Lengauer T, Sander O, Sierra S, Thielen A, Kaiser R.** 2007. Bioinformatics prediction of HIV coreceptor usage. *Nat Biotechnol* **25:**1407–1410.
94. **Sánchez V, Masiá M, Robledano C, Padilla S, Lumbreras B, Poveda E, De Mendoza C, Soriano V, Gutiérrez F.** 2011. A highly sensitive and specific model for predicting HIV-1 tropism in treatment-experienced patients combining interpretation of V3 loop sequences and clinical parameters. *J Acquir Immune Defic Syndr* **56:**51–58.
95. **Swenson LC, Mo T, Dong WW, Zhong X, Woods CK, Jensen MA, Thielen A, Chapman D, Lewis M, James I, Heera J, Valdez H, Harrigan PR.** 2011. Deep sequencing to infer HIV-1 co-receptor usage: application to three clinical trials of maraviroc in treatment-experienced patients. *J Infect Dis* **203:**237–245.
96. **Kagan RM, Johnson EP, Siaw M, Biswas P, Chapman DS, Su Z, Platt JL, Pesano RL.** 2012. A genotypic test for HIV-1 tropism combining Sanger sequencing with ultradeep sequencing predicts virologic response in treatment-experienced patients. *PLoS One* **7:**e46334.
97. **Valsamakis A.** 2007. Molecular testing in the diagnosis and management of chronic hepatitis B. *Clin Microbiol Rev* **20:**426–439.
98. **Lok AS, Zoulim F, Locarnini S, Bartholomeusz A, Ghany MG, Pawlotsky JM, Liaw YF, Mizokami M, Kuiken C, Hepatitis B Virus Drug Resistance Working Group.** 2007. Antiviral drug-resistant HBV: standardization of nomenclature and assays and recommendations for management. *Hepatology* **46:**254–265.
99. **Janssen HL, van Zonneveld M, Senturk H, Zeuzem S, Akarca US, Cakaloglu Y, Simon C, So TM, Gerken G, de Man RA, Niesters HG, Zondervan P, Hansen B, Schalm SW, HBV 99-01 Study Group, Rotterdam Foundation for Liver Research.** 2005. Pegylated interferon alfa-2b alone or in combination with lamivudine for HBeAg-positive chronic hepatitis B: a randomised trial. *Lancet* **365:**123–129.
100. **Sonneveld MJ, Janssen HL.** 2011. Chronic hepatitis B: peginterferon or nucleos(t)ide analogues? *Liver Int* **31**(Suppl 1)**:** 78–84.
101. **Bartholomeusz A, Schaefer S.** 2004. Hepatitis B virus genotypes: comparison of genotyping methods. *Rev Med Virol* **14:**3–16.
102. **Shaw T, Bartholomeusz A, Locarnini S.** 2006. HBV drug resistance: mechanisms, detection and interpretation. *J Hepatol* **44:**593–606.
103. **Yuen LK, Ayres A, Littlejohn M, Colledge D, Edgely A, Maskill WJ, Locarnini SA, Bartholomeusz A.** 2007. SeqHepB: a sequence analysis program and relational database system for chronic hepatitis B. *Antiviral Res* **75:**64–74.
104. **Lowe CF, Merrick L, Harrigan PR, Mazzulli T, Sherlock CH, Ritchie G.** 2016. Implementation of next-generation sequencing for hepatitis B virus resistance testing and genotyping in a clinical microbiology laboratory. *J Clin Microbiol* **54:** 127–133.
105. **Niesters HG, Zoulim F, Pichoud C, Buti M, Shapiro F, D'Heuvaert N, Celis L, Doutreloigne J, Sablon E.** 2010. Validation of the INNO-LiPA HBV DR assay (version 2) in monitoring hepatitis B virus-infected patients receiving nucleoside analog treatment. *Antimicrob Agents Chemother* **54:**1283–1289.
106. **Lok AS, Zoulim F, Locarnini S, Mangia A, Niro G, Decraemer H, Maertens G, Hulstaert F, De Vreese K, Sablon E.** 2002. Monitoring drug resistance in chronic hepatitis B virus (HBV)-infected patients during lamivudine therapy: evaluation of performance of INNO-LiPA HBV DR assay. *J Clin Microbiol* **40:**3729–3734.
107. **Osiowy C, Giles E.** 2003. Evaluation of the INNO-LiPA HBV genotyping assay for determination of hepatitis B virus genotype. *J Clin Microbiol* **41:**5473–5477.
108. **Ghany MG, Kim HY, Stoddard A, Wright EC, Seeff LB, Lok AS, HALT-C Trial Group.** 2011. Predicting clinical outcomes using baseline and follow-up laboratory data from the hepatitis C long-term treatment against cirrhosis trial. *Hepatology* **54:**1527–1537.
109. **Bagaglio S, Uberti-Foppa C, Morsica G.** 2017. Resistance mechanisms in hepatitis C virus: implications for direct-acting antiviral use. *Drugs* **77:**1043–1055.
110. **Andre-Garnier E, Besse B, Rodallec A, Ribeyrol O, Ferre V, Luco C, Le Guen L, Bourgeois N, Gournay J, Billaud E, Raffi F, Coste-Burel M, Imbert-Marcille BM.** 2017. An NS5A single optimized method to determine genotype, subtype and resistance profiles of hepatitis C strains. *PLoS One* **12:**e0179562.
111. **Welzel TM, Bhardwaj N, Hedskog C, Chodavarapu K, Camus G, McNally J, Brainard D, Miller MD, Mo H, Svarovskaia E, Jacobson I, Zeuzem S, Agarwal K.** 2017. Global epidemiology of HCV subtypes and resistance-associated substitutions evaluated by sequencing-based subtype analyses. *J Hepatol* **67:**224–236.

112. **Kardashian AA, Pockros PJ.** 2017. Novel emerging treatments for hepatitis C infection: a fast-moving pipeline. *Therap Adv Gastroenterol* **10:**277–282.
113. **McLaughlin MM, Skoglund EW, Ison MG.** 2015. Peramivir: an intravenous neuraminidase inhibitor. *Expert Opin Pharmacother* **16:**1889–1900.
114. **Sato M, Ito M, Suzuki S, Sakuma H, Takeyama A, Oda S, Watanabe M, Hashimoto K, Miyazaki K, Kawasaki Y, Hosoya M.** 2015. Influenza viral load and peramivir kinetics after single administration and proposal of regimens for peramivir administration against resistant variants. *Antimicrob Agents Chemother* **59:**1643–1649.
115. **Yoo JW, Choi SH, Huh JW, Lim CM, Koh Y, Hong SB.** 2015. Peramivir is as effective as oral oseltamivir in the treatment of severe seasonal influenza. *J Med Virol* **87:**1649–1655.
116. **Fiore AE, Fry A, Shay D, Gubareva L, Bresee JS, Uyeki TM, Centers for Disease Control and Prevention (CDC).** 2011. Antiviral agents for the treatment and chemoprophylaxis of influenza—ecommendations of the Advisory Committee on Immunization Practices (ACIP). *MMWR Recomm Rep* **60:**1–24.
117. **Trevino C, Bihon S, Pinsky BA.** 2011. A synonymous change in the influenza A virus neuraminidase gene interferes with PCR-based subtyping and oseltamivir resistance mutation detection. *J Clin Microbiol* **49:**3101–3102.
118. **Chen N, Pinsky BA, Lee BP, Lin M, Schrijver I.** 2011. Ultrasensitive detection of drug-resistant pandemic 2009 (H1N1) influenza A virus by rare-variant-sensitive high-resolution melting-curve analysis. *J Clin Microbiol* **49:** 2602–2609.
119. **Renaud C, Boudreault AA, Kuypers J, Lofy KH, Corey L, Boeckh MJ, Englund JA.** 2011. H275Y mutant pandemic (H1N1) 2009 virus in immunocompromised patients. *Emerg Infect Dis* **17:**653–660, quiz 765.
120. **Bright RA, Medina MJ, Xu X, Perez-Oronoz G, Wallis TR, Davis XM, Povinelli L, Cox NJ, Klimov AI.** 2005. Incidence of adamantane resistance among influenza A (H3N2) viruses isolated worldwide from 1994 to 2005: a cause for concern. *Lancet* **366:**1175–1181.
121. **Centers for Disease Control and Prevention (CDC).** 2009. Update: drug susceptibility of swine-origin influenza A (H1N1) viruses, April 2009. *MMWR Morb Mortal Wkly Rep* **58:**433–435.
122. **Deyde VM, Okomo-Adhiambo M, Sheu TG, Wallis TR, Fry A, Dharan N, Klimov AI, Gubareva LV.** 2009. Pyrosequencing as a tool to detect molecular markers of resistance to neuraminidase inhibitors in seasonal influenza A viruses. *Antiviral Res* **81:**16–24.
123. **Deyde VM, Xu X, Bright RA, Shaw M, Smith CB, Zhang Y, Shu Y, Gubareva LV, Cox NJ, Klimov AI.** 2007. Surveillance of resistance to adamantanes among influenza A(H3N2) and A(H1N1) viruses isolated worldwide. *J Infect Dis* **196:**249–257.
124. **Ghedin E, Laplante J, DePasse J, Wentworth DE, Santos RP, Lepow ML, Porter J, Stellrecht K, Lin X, Operario D, Griesemer S, Fitch A, Halpin RA, Stockwell TB, Spiro DJ, Holmes EC, St George K.** 2011. Deep sequencing reveals mixed infection with 2009 pandemic influenza A (H1N1) virus strains and the emergence of oseltamivir resistance. *J Infect Dis* **203:**168–174.
125. **McGinnis J, Laplante J, Shudt M, George KS.** 2016. Next generation sequencing for whole genome analysis and surveillance of influenza A viruses. *J Clin Virol* **79:**44–50.
126. **Zhao J, Liu J, Vemula SV, Lin C, Tan J, Ragupathy V, Wang X, Mbondji-Wonje C, Ye Z, Landry ML, Hewlett I.** 2016. Sensitive detection and simultaneous discrimination of influenza A and B viruses in nasopharyngeal swabs in a single assay using next-generation sequencing-based diagnostics. *PLoS One* **11:**e0163175.
127. **Tamura D, DeBiasi RL, Okomo-Adhiambo M, Mishin VP, Campbell AP, Loechelt B, Wiedermann BL, Fry AM, Gubareva LV.** 2015. Emergence of multidrug-resistant influenza A(H1N1)pdm09 virus variants in an immunocompromised child treated with oseltamivir and zanamivir. *J Infect Dis* **212:**1209–1213.
128. **Mayer KH, Hanna GJ, D'Aquila RT.** 2001. Clinical use of genotypic and phenotypic drug resistance testing to monitor antiretroviral chemotherapy. *Clin Infect Dis* **32:**774–782.
129. **Sing T, Low AJ, Beerenwinkel N, Sander O, Cheung PK, Domingues FS, Büch J, Däumer M, Kaiser R, Lengauer T, Harrigan PR.** 2007. Predicting HIV coreceptor usage on the basis of genetic and clinical covariates. *Antivir Ther* **12:**1097–1106.
130. **Shafer RW, Jung DR, Betts BJ.** 2000. Human immunodeficiency virus type 1 reverse transcriptase and protease mutation search engine for queries. *Nat Med* **6:**1290–1292.
131. **Shafer RW.** 2006. Rationale and uses of a public HIV drug-resistance database. *J Infect Dis* **194**(Suppl 1)**:**S51–S58.
132. **Rhee SY, Gonzales MJ, Kantor R, Betts BJ, Ravela J, Shafer RW.** 2003. Human immunodeficiency virus reverse transcriptase and protease sequence database. *Nucleic Acids Res* **31:**298–303.
133. **Vandenbroucke I, Van Marck H, Mostmans W, Van Eygen V, Rondelez E, Thys K, Van Baelen K, Fransen K, Vaira D, Kabeya K, De Wit S, Florence E, Moutschen M, Vandekerckhove L, Verhofstede C, Stuyver LJ.** 2010. HIV-1 V3 envelope deep sequencing for clinical plasma specimens failing in phenotypic tropism assays. *AIDS Res Ther* **7:**4.
134. **Bunnik EM, Swenson LC, Edo-Matas D, Huang W, Dong W, Frantzell A, Petropoulos CJ, Coakley E, Schuitemaker H, Harrigan PR, van 't Wout AB.** 2011. Detection of inferred CCR5- and CXCR4-using HIV-1 variants and evolutionary intermediates using ultra-deep pyrosequencing. *PLoS Pathog* **7:**e1002106.
135. **Gonzalez-Serna A, McGovern RA, Harrigan PR, Vidal F, Poon AF, Ferrando-Martinez S, Abad MA, Genebat M, Leal M, Ruiz-Mateos E.** 2012. Correlation of the virological response to short-term maraviroc monotherapy with standard and deep-sequencing-based genotypic tropism prediction methods. *Antimicrob Agents Chemother* **56:**1202–1207.
136. **Besse B, Coste-Burel M, Bourgeois N, Feray C, Imbert-Marcille BM, André-Garnier E.** 2012. Genotyping and resistance profile of hepatitis C (HCV) genotypes 1–6 by sequencing the NS3 protease region using a single optimized sensitive method. *J Virol Methods* **185:**94–100.
137. **Rodriguez C, Soulié C, Marcelin AG, Calvez V, Descamps D, Charpentier C, Flandre P, Recordon-Pinson P, Bellecave P, Pawlotsky JM, Masquelier B, ANRS AC11 Study Group.** 2015. HIV-1 coreceptor usage assessment by ultra-deep pyrosequencing and response to maraviroc. *PLoS One* **10:**e0127816.
138. **Smit E.** 2014. Antiviral resistance testing. *Curr Opin Infect Dis* **27:**566–572.
139. **NCCLS.** 2004. Antiviral susceptibility testing: herpes simplex virus by plaque reduction assay. Approved standard M33. National Committee for Clinical Laboratory Standards, Wayne, PA.
140. **Landry ML, Stanat S, Biron K, Brambilla D, Britt W, Jokela J, Chou S, Drew WL, Erice A, Gilliam B, Lurain N, Manischewitz J, Miner R, Nokta M, Reichelderfer P, Spector S, Weinberg A, Yen-Lieberman B, Crumpacker C.** 2000. A standardized plaque reduction assay for determination of drug susceptibilities of cytomegalovirus clinical isolates. *Antimicrob Agents Chemother* **44:**688–692.
141. **Singh D, Dhummakupt A, Siems L, Persaud D.** 2017. Alternative sample types for HIV-1 antiretroviral drug resistance testing. *J Infect Dis* **216**(Suppl 9)**:**S834–S837.
142. **Rhee SY, Jordan MR, Raizes E, Chua A, Parkin N, Kantor R, Van Zyl GU, Mukui I, Hosseinipour MC, Frenkel LM, Ndembi N, Hamers RL, Rinke de Wit TF, Wallis CL, Gupta RK, Fokam J, Zeh C, Schapiro JM, Carmona S, Katzenstein D, Tang M, Aghokeng AF, De Oliveira T, Wensing AM, Gallant JE, Wainberg MA, Richman DD, Fitzgibbon JE, Schito M, Bertagnolio S, Yang C, Shafer RW.** 2015. HIV-1 drug resistance mutations: potential applications for point-of-care genotypic resistance testing. *PLoS One* **10:**e0145772.
143. **Swierkosz EM, Scholl DR, Brown JL, Jollick JD, Gleaves CA.** 1987. Improved DNA hybridization method for detection of acyclovir-resistant herpes simplex virus. *Antimicrob Agents Chemother* **31:**1465–1469.

144. **Balows A (ed).** 1991. *Manual of Clinical Microbiology*, 5th ed. American Society for Microbiology, Washington, DC.
145. **Leary JJ, Wittrock R, Sarisky RT, Weinberg A, Levin MJ.** 2002. Susceptibilities of herpes simplex viruses to penciclovir and acyclovir in eight cell lines. *Antimicrob Agents Chemother* **46:**762–768.
146. **Sarisky RT, Quail MR, Clark PE, Nguyen TT, Halsey WS, Wittrock RJ, O'Leary Bartus J, Van Horn MM, Sathe GM, Van Horn S, Kelly MD, Bacon TH, Leary JJ.** 2001. Characterization of herpes simplex viruses selected in culture for resistance to penciclovir or acyclovir. *J Virol* **75:** 1761–1769.
147. **Safrin S, Assaykeen T, Follansbee S, Mills J.** 1990. Foscarnet therapy for acyclovir-resistant mucocutaneous herpes simplex virus infection in 26 AIDS patients: preliminary data. *J Infect Dis* **161:**1078–1084.
148. **Safrin S, Crumpacker C, Chatis P, Davis R, Hafner R, Rush J, Kessler HA, Landry B, Mills J, The AIDS Clinical Trials Group.** 1991. A controlled trial comparing foscarnet with vidarabine for acyclovir-resistant mucocutaneous herpes simplex in the acquired immunodeficiency syndrome. *N Engl J Med* **325:**551–555.
149. **Chou S, Marousek G, Guentzel S, Follansbee SE, Poscher ME, Lalezari JP, Miner RC, Drew WL.** 1997. Evolution of mutations conferring multidrug resistance during prophylaxis and therapy for cytomegalovirus disease. *J Infect Dis* **176:**786–789.
150. **Drew WL, Miner RC, Busch DF, Follansbee SE, Gullett J, Mehalko SG, Gordon SM, Owen WF, Matthews TR, Buhles WC, DeArmond B.** 1991. Prevalence of resistance in patients receiving ganciclovir for serious cytomegalovirus infection. *J Infect Dis* **163:**716–719.
151. **Pépin JM, Simon F, Dazza MC, Brun-Vézinet F.** 1992. The clinical significance of in vitro cytomegalovirus susceptibility to antiviral drugs. *Res Virol* **143:**126–128.
152. **Gubareva LV, Matrosovich MN, Brenner MK, Bethell RC, Webster RG.** 1998. Evidence for zanamivir resistance in an immunocompromised child infected with influenza B virus. *J Infect Dis* **178:**1257–1262.
153. **Jacobson MA, Berger TG, Fikrig S, Becherer P, Moohr JW, Stanat SC, Biron KK.** 1990. Acyclovir-resistant varicella zoster virus infection after chronic oral acyclovir therapy in patients with the acquired immunodeficiency syndrome (AIDS). *Ann Intern Med* **112:**187–191.
154. **Safrin S, Berger TG, Gilson I, Wolfe PR, Wofsy CB, Mills J, Biron KK.** 1991. Foscarnet therapy in five patients with AIDS and acyclovir-resistant varicella-zoster virus infection. *Ann Intern Med* **115:**19–21.
155. **Bacon TH, Levin MJ, Leary JJ, Sarisky RT, Sutton D.** 2003. Herpes simplex virus resistance to acyclovir and penciclovir after two decades of antiviral therapy. *Clin Microbiol Rev* **16:**114–128.
156. **Coen DM.** 1996. Antiviral drug resistance in herpes simplex virus. *Adv Exp Med Biol* **394:**49–57.
157. **Frobert E, Ooka T, Cortay JC, Lina B, Thouvenot D, Morfin F.** 2005. Herpes simplex virus thymidine kinase mutations associated with resistance to acyclovir: a site-directed mutagenesis study. *Antimicrob Agents Chemother* **49:** 1055–1059.
158. **Morfin F, Thouvenot D.** 2003. Herpes simplex virus resistance to antiviral drugs. *J Clin Virol* **26:**29–37.
159. **Reyes M, Shaik NS, Graber JM, Nisenbaum R, Wetherall NT, Fukuda K, Reeves WC, Task Force on Herpes Simplex Virus Resistance.** 2003. Acyclovir-resistant genital herpes among persons attending sexually transmitted disease and human immunodeficiency virus clinics. *Arch Intern Med* **163:**76–80.
160. **Safrin S, Phan L.** 1993. In vitro activity of penciclovir against clinical isolates of acyclovir-resistant and foscarnet-resistant herpes simplex virus. *Antimicrob Agents Chemother* **37:**2241–2243.
161. **Sauerbrei A, Deinhardt S, Zell R, Wutzler P.** 2010. Testing of herpes simplex virus for resistance to antiviral drugs. *Virulence* **1:**555–557.
162. **Sauerbrei A, Vödisch S, Bohn K, Schacke M, Gronowitz S.** 2013. Screening of herpes simplex virus type 1 isolates for acyclovir resistance using DiviTum® assay. *J Virol Methods* **188:**70–72.
163. **Bestman-Smith J, Boivin G.** 2003. Drug resistance patterns of recombinant herpes simplex virus DNA polymerase mutants generated with a set of overlapping cosmids and plasmids. *J Virol* **77:**7820–7829.
164. **Gilbert C, Bestman-Smith J, Boivin G.** 2002. Resistance of herpesviruses to antiviral drugs: clinical impacts and molecular mechanisms. *Drug Resist Updat* **5:**88–114.
165. **Frobert E, Cortay JC, Ooka T, Najioullah F, Thouvenot D, Lina B, Morfin F.** 2008. Genotypic detection of acyclovir-resistant HSV-1: characterization of 67 ACV-sensitive and 14 ACV-resistant viruses. *Antiviral Res* **79:**28–36.
166. **Morfin F, Thouvenot D, De Turenne-Tessier M, Lina B, Aymard M, Ooka T.** 1999. Phenotypic and genetic characterization of thymidine kinase from clinical strains of varicella-zoster virus resistant to acyclovir. *Antimicrob Agents Chemother* **43:**2412–2416.
167. **Hatchette T, Tipples GA, Peters G, Alsuwaidi A, Zhou J, Mailman TL.** 2008. Foscarnet salvage therapy for acyclovir-resistant varicella zoster: report of a novel thymidine kinase mutation and review of the literature. *Pediatr Infect Dis J* **27:**75–77.
168. **Abed Y, Baz M, Boivin G.** 2006. Impact of neuraminidase mutations conferring influenza resistance to neuraminidase inhibitors in the N1 and N2 genetic backgrounds. *Antivir Ther* **11:**971–976.
169. **Collins PJ, Haire LF, Lin YP, Liu J, Russell RJ, Walker PA, Martin SR, Daniels RS, Gregory V, Skehel JJ, Gamblin SJ, Hay AJ.** 2009. Structural basis for oseltamivir resistance of influenza viruses. *Vaccine* **27:**6317–6323.
170. **Hurt AC, Holien JK, Barr IG.** 2009. In vitro generation of neuraminidase inhibitor resistance in A(H5N1) influenza viruses. *Antimicrob Agents Chemother* **53:**4433–4440.
171. **Kiso M, Mitamura K, Sakai-Tagawa Y, Shiraishi K, Kawakami C, Kimura K, Hayden FG, Sugaya N, Kawaoka Y.** 2004. Resistant influenza A viruses in children treated with oseltamivir: descriptive study. *Lancet* **364:**759–765.
172. **Le QM, Kiso M, Someya K, Sakai YT, Nguyen TH, Nguyen KH, Pham ND, Ngyen HH, Yamada S, Muramoto Y, Horimoto T, Takada A, Goto H, Suzuki T, Suzuki Y, Kawaoka Y.** 2005. Avian flu: isolation of drug-resistant H5N1 virus. *Nature* **437:**1108.
173. **McKimm-Breschkin J, Trivedi T, Hampson A, Hay A, Klimov A, Tashiro M, Hayden F, Zambon M.** 2003. Neuraminidase sequence analysis and susceptibilities of influenza virus clinical isolates to zanamivir and oseltamivir. *Antimicrob Agents Chemother* **47:**2264–2272.
174. **Allen MI, Deslauriers M, Andrews CW, Tipples GA, Walters KA, Tyrrell DL, Brown N, Condreay LD, Lamivudine Clinical Investigation Group.** 1998. Identification and characterization of mutations in hepatitis B virus resistant to lamivudine. *Hepatology* **27:**1670–1677.
175. **Choe WH, Hong SP, Kim BK, Ko SY, Jung YK, Kim JH, Yeon JE, Byun KS, Kim KH, Ji SI, Kim SO, Lee CH, Kwon SY.** 2009. Evolution of hepatitis B virus mutation during entecavir rescue therapy in patients with antiviral resistance to lamivudine and adefovir. *Antivir Ther* **14:**985–993.
176. **Das K, Xiong X, Yang H, Westland CE, Gibbs CS, Sarafianos SG, Arnold E.** 2001. Molecular modeling and biochemical characterization reveal the mechanism of hepatitis B virus polymerase resistance to lamivudine (3TC) and emtricitabine (FTC). *J Virol* **75:**4771–4779.
177. **Delaney WE, IV, Yang H, Westland CE, Das K, Arnold E, Gibbs CS, Miller MD, Xiong S.** 2003. The hepatitis B virus polymerase mutation rtV173L is selected during lamivudine therapy and enhances viral replication in vitro. *J Virol* **77:**11833–11841.
178. **Ono SK, Kato N, Shiratori Y, Kato J, Goto T, Schinazi RF, Carrilho FJ, Omata M.** 2001. The polymerase L528M mutation cooperates with nucleotide binding-site mutations, increasing hepatitis B virus replication and drug resistance. *J Clin Invest* **107:**449–455.

179. **Warner N, Locarnini S.** 2008. The antiviral drug selected hepatitis B virus rtA181T/sW172* mutant has a dominant negative secretion defect and alters the typical profile of viral rebound. *Hepatology* **48:**88–98.
180. **Warner N, Locarnini S, Kuiper M, Bartholomeusz A, Ayres A, Yuen L, Shaw T.** 2007. The L80I substitution in the reverse transcriptase domain of the hepatitis B virus polymerase is associated with lamivudine resistance and enhanced viral replication in vitro. *Antimicrob Agents Chemother* **51:**2285–2292.
181. **Santantonio T, Fasano M, Durantel S, Barraud L, Heichen M, Guastadisegni A, Pastore G, Zoulim F.** 2009. Adefovir dipivoxil resistance patterns in patients with lamivudine-resistant chronic hepatitis B. *Antivir Ther* **14:**557–565.
182. **Tenney DJ, Levine SM, Rose RE, Walsh AW, Weinheimer SP, Discotto L, Plym M, Pokornowski K, Yu CF, Angus P, Ayres A, Bartholomeusz A, Sievert W, Thompson G, Warner N, Locarnini S, Colonno RJ.** 2004. Clinical emergence of entecavir-resistant hepatitis B virus requires additional substitutions in virus already resistant to lamivudine. *Antimicrob Agents Chemother* **48:**3498–3507.
183. **Tenney DJ, Rose RE, Baldick CJ, Levine SM, Pokornowski KA, Walsh AW, Fang J, Yu CF, Zhang S, Mazzucco CE, Eggers B, Hsu M, Plym MJ, Poundstone P, Yang J, Colonno RJ.** 2007. Two-year assessment of entecavir resistance in lamivudine-refractory hepatitis B virus patients reveals different clinical outcomes depending on the resistance substitutions present. *Antimicrob Agents Chemother* **51:**902–911.
184. **Tenney DJ, Rose RE, Baldick CJ, Pokornowski KA, Eggers BJ, Fang J, Wichroski MJ, Xu D, Yang J, Wilber RB, Colonno RJ.** 2009. Long-term monitoring shows hepatitis B virus resistance to entecavir in nucleoside-naïve patients is rare through 5 years of therapy. *Hepatology* **49:**1503–1514.
185. **Westland CE, Yang H, Delaney WE, IV, Wulfsohn M, Lama N, Gibbs CS, Miller MD, Fry J, Brosgart CL, Schiff ER, Xiong S.** 2005. Activity of adefovir dipivoxil against all patterns of lamivudine-resistant hepatitis B viruses in patients. *J Viral Hepat* **12:**67–73.
186. **Angus P, Vaughan R, Xiong S, Yang H, Delaney W, Gibbs C, Brosgart C, Colledge D, Edwards R, Ayres A, Bartholomeusz A, Locarnini S.** 2003. Resistance to adefovir dipivoxil therapy associated with the selection of a novel mutation in the HBV polymerase. *Gastroenterology* **125:**292–297.
187. **Borroto-Esoda K, Miller MD, Arterburn S.** 2007. Pooled analysis of amino acid changes in the HBV polymerase in patients from four major adefovir dipivoxil clinical trials. *J Hepatol* **47:**492–498.
188. **Fung SK, Chae HB, Fontana RJ, Conjeevaram H, Marrero J, Oberhelman K, Hussain M, Lok AS.** 2006. Virologic response and resistance to adefovir in patients with chronic hepatitis B. *J Hepatol* **44:**283–290.
189. **Hadziyannis SJ, Tassopoulos NC, Heathcote EJ, Chang TT, Kitis G, Rizzetto M, Marcellin P, Lim SG, Goodman Z, Ma J, Brosgart CL, Borroto-Esoda K, Arterburn S, Chuck SL, Adefovir Dipivoxil 438 Study Group.** 2006. Long-term therapy with adefovir dipivoxil for HBeAg-negative chronic hepatitis B for up to 5 years. *Gastroenterology* **131:**1743–1751.
190. **Villet S, Pichoud C, Billioud G, Barraud L, Durantel S, Trépo C, Zoulim F.** 2008. Impact of hepatitis B virus rtA181V/T mutants on hepatitis B treatment failure. *J Hepatol* **48:**747–755.
191. **Yang H, Westland C, Xiong S, Delaney WE, IV.** 2004. In vitro antiviral susceptibility of full-length clinical hepatitis B virus isolates cloned with a novel expression vector. *Antiviral Res* **61:**27–36.
192. **Yeh CT, Chien RN, Chu CM, Liaw YF.** 2000. Clearance of the original hepatitis B virus YMDD-motif mutants with emergence of distinct lamivudine-resistant mutants during prolonged lamivudine therapy. *Hepatology* **31:**1318–1326.
193. **Zoulim F, Locarnini S.** 2009. Hepatitis B virus resistance to nucleos(t)ide analogues. *Gastroenterology* **137:**1593-1608.e2.
194. **Abraham B, Lastere S, Reynes J, Bibollet-Ruche F, Vidal N, Segondy M.** 1999. Ganciclovir resistance and UL97 gene mutations in cytomegalovirus blood isolates from patients with AIDS treated with ganciclovir. *J Clin Virol* **13:**141–148.
195. **Baldanti F, Sarasini A, Silini E, Barbi M, Lazzarin A, Biron KK, Gerna G.** 1995. Four dually resistant human cytomegalovirus strains from AIDS patients: single mutations in UL97 and UL54 open reading frames are responsible for ganciclovir- and foscarnet-specific resistance, respectively. *Scand J Infect Dis Suppl* **99:**103–104.
196. **Baldanti F, Silini E, Sarasini A, Talarico CL, Stanat SC, Biron KK, Furione M, Bono F, Palù G, Gerna G.** 1995. A three-nucleotide deletion in the UL97 open reading frame is responsible for the ganciclovir resistance of a human cytomegalovirus clinical isolate. *J Virol* **69:**796–800.
197. **Bowen EF, Cherrington JM, Lamy PD, Griffiths PD, Johnson MA, Emery VC.** 1999. Quantitative changes in cytomegalovirus DNAemia and genetic analysis of the UL97 and UL54 genes in AIDS patients receiving cidofovir following ganciclovir therapy. *J Med Virol* **58:**402–407.
198. **Bowen EF, Johnson MA, Griffiths PD, Emery VC.** 1997. Development of a point mutation assay for the detection of human cytomegalovirus UL97 mutations associated with ganciclovir resistance. *J Virol Methods* **68:**225–234.
199. **Chou S, Meichsner CL.** 2000. A nine-codon deletion mutation in the cytomegalovirus UL97 phosphotransferase gene confers resistance to ganciclovir. *Antimicrob Agents Chemother* **44:**183–185.
200. **Cihlar T, Fuller MD, Mulato AS, Cherrington JM.** 1998. A point mutation in the human cytomegalovirus DNA polymerase gene selected in vitro by cidofovir confers a slow replication phenotype in cell culture. *Virology* **248:**382–393.
201. **Erice A, Borrell N, Li W, Miller WJ, Balfour HH, Jr.** 1998. Ganciclovir susceptibilities and analysis of UL97 region in cytomegalovirus (CMV) isolates from bone marrow recipients with CMV disease after antiviral prophylaxis. *J Infect Dis* **178:**531–534.
202. **Cihlar T, Fuller MD, Cherrington JM.** 1998. Characterization of drug resistance-associated mutations in the human cytomegalovirus DNA polymerase gene by using recombinant mutant viruses generated from overlapping DNA fragments. *J Virol* **72:**5927–5936.
203. **Hanson MN, Preheim LC, Chou S, Talarico CL, Biron KK, Erice A.** 1995. Novel mutation in the UL97 gene of a clinical cytomegalovirus strain conferring resistance to ganciclovir. *Antimicrob Agents Chemother* **39:**1204–1205.

MYCOLOGY

section 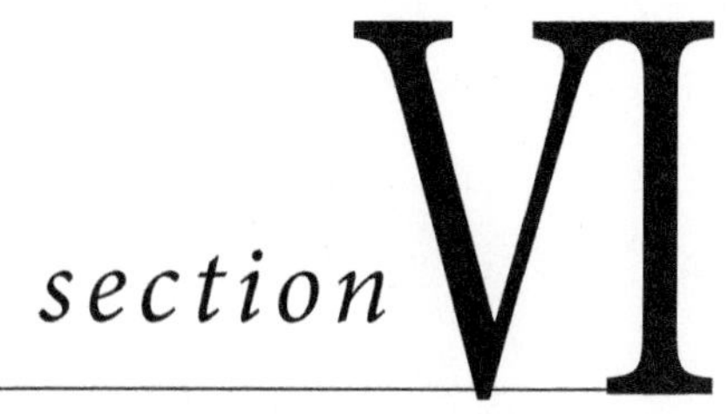

VOLUME EDITOR: DAVID W. WARNOCK

SECTION EDITORS: MARY E. BRANDT AND ELIZABETH M. JOHNSON

GENERAL

FUNGI

Taxonomy, Classification, and Nomenclature of Fungi

MARY E. BRANDT AND DAVID W. WARNOCK

116

There are at least 135,000 named species of fungi. However, it has been estimated that the number of undescribed species ranges from 1 million to more than 10 million, and it has been calculated that about 1,000 to 1,500 new species are described each year (1). Of the named species of fungi, fewer than 500 have commonly been associated with human or animal disease, and no more than 50 are capable of causing infection in otherwise normal individuals (2). On the other hand, an increasing number of ubiquitous environmental molds are now being implicated as opportunistic pathogens capable of producing serious or lethal disease in hosts that are immunocompromised or debilitated. These molds are organisms whose natural habitats are in the soil or on plants, wood, compost heaps, or decomposing food. Many are familiar to mycologists, plant pathologists, and food microbiologists, but they present problems for the clinical microbiologist who often has had no formal training in the identification of fungi. Fungal identification can be challenging and sometimes frustrating because of the importance placed on the morphological characteristics of the organisms and the need to become familiar with a range of different structures and terms. Indeed, it is fair to state that obscure mycological terms have been one of the major factors that discourage many microbiologists from mastering fungal identification. However, the advent of rapid DNA sequencing has transformed this process, facilitating the accurate identification of clinical isolates. Molecular analysis has had a substantial impact on the taxonomy, classification, and nomenclature of fungi, including many species of medical importance.

MORPHOLOGICAL CHARACTERISTICS OF THE FUNGI

Fungi form a separate clade of eukaryotic organisms which differ from other groups in several major respects. Fungal cells are encased within a rigid cell wall, mostly composed of chitin, glucan, chitosan, mannan, and glycoproteins in various combinations. These features contrast with the animals, which have no cell walls, and the plants, which have cellulose as the major cell wall component. As in other eukaryotic organisms, fungal cells have a true nucleus with a surrounding membrane, and cell division is accompanied by meiosis or mitosis.

Fungi are heterotrophic (lacking in chlorophyll) and therefore require preformed organic carbon compounds for their nutrition. Fungi live embedded in a food source or medium and obtain their nourishment by secreting enzymes into the external substrate and by absorbing the released nutrients through their cell wall. Fungi are found throughout nature, performing an essential service in returning to the soil nutrients removed by plants.

Fungi can be multicellular or unicellular. In multicellular organisms, the basic structural unit is a chain of multinucleate, tubular, filament-like cells (termed a hypha). In most multicellular fungi the vegetative stage consists of a mass of branching hyphae, termed a mycelium or thallus. Each individual hypha has a rigid cell wall and increases in length as a result of apical growth with mitotic cell division. In the more primitive fungi, the hyphae remain aseptate (without cross-walls). In the more advanced groups, however, the hyphae are divided into compartments or cells by the development of more or less frequent cross-walls, termed septa. Such hyphae are referred to as being septate. Fungi that exist in the form of microscopic multicellular mycelium are commonly called molds.

Many fungi that exist in the form of independent single cells propagate by budding out similar cells from their surface. The bud may become detached from the parent cell, or it may remain attached and itself produce another bud. In this way, a chain of cells may be produced. Fungi that do not produce hyphae, but just consist of a loose arrangement of budding cells are called yeasts. Under certain conditions, continued elongation of the parent cell before it buds results in a chain of elongated cells, termed a pseudohypha. Unlike a true hypha, the connection between adjacent pseudohyphal cells shows a marked constriction. Yeasts are neither a natural nor a formal taxonomic group but are a growth form seen in a wide range of unrelated fungi.

Many medically important fungi change their growth form as part of the process of tissue invasion. These so-called dimorphic pathogens usually change from a multicellular mold form in the natural environment to a budding, single-celled yeast form in tissue under the influence of temperature as they exhibit thermal dimorphism. *Histoplasma capsulatum*, *Blastomyces dermatitidis*, *Paracoccidioides brasiliensis*, and *Sporothrix schenckii* are the best-known examples of this dimorphic change, but many other fungal pathogens show subtle morphological differences between forms found in tissue and in culture.

Fungi reproduce by means of microscopic propagules called spores or conidia. The term "conidium" (plural, conidia) is used to describe propagules that result from an asexual process (involving mitosis only). Except for the occasional mutation, asexual conidia are identical to the parent. They are generally short-lived propagules that are produced in enormous numbers to ensure dispersion to new habitats. Many fungi are also capable of sexual reproduction (involving meiosis, preceded by fusion of the nuclei of two cells). Some species are self-fertile (homothallic) and able to form sexual structures between different cells within an individual thallus. Most, however, are heterothallic and do not form their sexual structures unless two compatible isolates come into contact. Once two compatible haploid nuclei have fused, meiosis can occur, and this leads to the production of the sexual spores. In some species the haploid sexual spores are borne singly on specialized generative cells, and the whole structure is microscopic in size. In other cases, however, the spores are produced in millions in macroscopic "fruiting bodies" such as mushrooms. Sexual reproduction and its accompanying structures form one scheme for the classification of the fungi.

NOMENCLATURE OF FUNGI

The scientific names of fungi are subject to the International Code of Nomenclature for algae, fungi, and plants (ICN) that was adopted in 2011 (http://www.iapt-taxon.org/nomen/main.php). The ICN rules must be followed when proposing the name for a new fungal species; otherwise the name being proposed can be rejected as invalid (3). The main requirements for valid publication are that the name must be in Latin binomial form, that the proposal is accompanied by an English or Latin description, that a living culture of the specimen on which the author based the description of the species has been deposited in a recognized culture collection, and that the name has been registered with the online taxonomy database MycoBank (http://www.mycobank.org/) and has been assigned a MycoBank registration number.

Names of fungi may have to be changed for a number of reasons. Many common and widely distributed species of fungi have been described as new many times and thus have come to have more than one name. In general, the correct name for any species is the earliest name published in line with the requirements of the code of nomenclature. The later names are termed synonyms. To avoid confusion, however, the ICN permits certain exceptions. The most significant of these is when an earlier generic name has been overlooked, a later name is in common use, and a reversion to the earlier name would cause problems (3).

Another reason for changing the name of a fungus is when new research necessitates the transfer of a species from one genus to another or establishes it as the type of a new genus. Such changes are quite in order, but with the provision that the specific epithet should remain unchanged, except for inflection according to the rules of Latin grammar. However often a species is transferred to a new genus, the correct species epithet is always the first one that was applied to that particular organism. As an example, when *Phialophora parasitica* was moved to a new genus, it became *Phaeoacremonium parasiticum*.

If there is one complication of fungal nomenclature that is confusing to many microbiologists, it is the fact that a large number of fungi appear to bear more than one name. This is an apparent departure from the basic principle of biological classification, in which an organism can only have one correct name. As described in the previous section of this chapter, many fungi have an asexual stage (or anamorph), characterized by the production of asexual conidia, and a sexual stage (or teleomorph) characterized by sexual spores (e.g., ascospores, basidiospores). Many fungi propagate asexually and the teleomorph is unknown or only rarely encountered. Because of this, mycologists have often given separate names to the asexual and sexual stages. Often this is because the anamorph and teleomorph were described and named at different times without the connection between them being recognized. With the widespread application of molecular methods, it is now possible to confirm that these separate forms constitute a single species. As a consequence, there are numerous instances where the different names that have been applied to the asexual and sexual forms of the same species are now redundant (4).

These developments are reflected in the most recent code of nomenclature. As of 1 January 2013, the system of permitting separate anamorph and teleomorph names ended; the dual-naming system is no longer permitted, and mycologists have begun the process of choosing one name from several existing names for many fungal species. All legitimate names proposed for a species, whether for the sexual or asexual form, can in the future serve as the correct name for that species. Working groups and committees have been established under the auspices of the International Commission on the Taxonomy of Fungi (ICTF) (http://www.fungaltaxonomy.org/subcommissions), and these will propose lists of accepted and rejected names for ratification.

TAXONOMY AND CLASSIFICATION OF THE FUNGI

The advent of molecular phylogenetics has led to a revolution in the classification of fungi. In the past, this was largely based on their morphological characteristics, rather than on the physiological and biochemical differences that were of such importance in bacterial classification. In recent years, however, comparative DNA sequence analysis has led to a radical and ongoing revision of the fungal tree of life based on a phylogenetic approach to species recognition (5, 6). With phylogenetic species recognition, a species is defined as a group of organisms that share concordance of multiple gene genealogies (DNA sequences at different genetic loci), rather than organisms that share a common morphology or organisms that can mate with one another. Portions of genes are often used to construct the genealogies. Concordant branches among the gene trees are used to connect species. Many different genes and gene fragments have been explored, but the most widely used remain the conserved regions encoding the ribosomal RNA genes, in particular the two internal transcribed spacer regions of ribosomal DNA.

Advances in molecular phylogenetic analysis have led to major revisions in the classification of eukaryotic organisms, including the fungi. One proposal from Adl et al. (7) divided the eukaryotes into five monophyletic lineages or supergroups: the SAR (derived from the acronym of three groups united in this clade: Stramenopiles, Alveolata, and Rhizaria), Archaeplastida, Excavata, Amoebozoa, and Opisthokonta (see chapter 135). In this phylogenetic classification, these supergroups replace the previous kingdoms that encompassed the eukaryotes. The true fungi make up a monophyletic clade and are classified in the supergroup Opisthokonta. This also includes the single-celled animals and several protist clades (7). Molecular analysis has also led to a number of organisms being reassigned to the fungi, most notably *Pneumocystis jirovecii*, now placed in the phylum Ascomycota, and the microsporidia (see chapters 121 and 131).

In addition to the true fungi, there are a number of human and animal pathogens, including *Pythium insidiosum* and *Rhinosporidium seeberi*, that have long been studied by mycologists (see chapter 130). These organisms, while not fungi *sensu strictu*, are "parafungi" or "pseudofungi," protists sharing fungal-like morphological features with the true fungi. *Lagenidium* spp. and *P. insidiosum* were formerly classified in the kingdom Straminopila, phylum Oomycota. These slime-fungal-like organisms develop sparsely septate mycelioid structures similar to those seen in filamentous fungi. They are closely related to some algal groups and for this reason are now placed in the SAR supergroup (7). *R. seeberi* is a nonculturable organism that produces large spherical sporangia filled with endospores in tissue. It is now placed in the supergroup Opisthokonta, Ichthyosporea (Mesomycetozoea), clade Holozoa (7).

One of the consequences of the widespread employment of molecular analysis for fungal identification and classification has been the discovery of genetically distinct populations that deserve species status. These newly recognized cryptic species, which can only be distinguished by DNA sequencing, have been found within many medically important species. For example, *Coccidioides posadasii* has been separated from *Coccidioides immitis* (8), while *Blastomyces gilchristii* and *Paracoccidioides lutzii* are genetically distinct from *B. dermatitidis* and *P. brasiliensis* (9, 10). It is unclear at present whether the detection of these particular cryptic species contributes to patient management. However, this may change, and there are examples where cryptic species have been found to possess distinct phenotypic characteristics of potential clinical relevance. For instance, it is now accepted that *Aspergillus fumigatus* is a species complex that comprises in excess of 40 cryptic species, several of which are less susceptible to azole and echinocandin antifungal agents (11).

The sexual spores and their mode of production have historically formed the main basis for the classification of fungi into the Zygomycota, Ascomycota, and Basidiomycota. In some fungi, however, the asexual stage, or anamorph, has proved so successful as a means of rapid dispersal to new habitats that the sexual stage, or teleomorph, has disappeared, or at least has not been discovered. Even in the absence of the teleomorph, it is now often possible to assign these fungi to the Ascomycota or Basidiomycota on the basis of DNA sequences of the anamorphs (12). In the past, these asexual fungi were classified in an artificial group, the "Fungi Imperfecti" (also termed the "form-division Deuteromycota") and were divided into artificial form-classes according to the morphological characteristics of their asexual reproductive structures. There is no longer any separate formal grouping for those fungi that appear to be strictly anamorphic, or for which no teleomorph has been discovered. Nonetheless, mycologists continue to employ the asexual reproductive characteristics of molds, at least for routine identification purposes (see below).

Kingdom Fungi

Traditionally, the kingdom Fungi has been organized in a hierarchical manner, each rank being named with, and recognizable by, a particular ending: phylum, -mycota; subphylum, -mycotina; class, -mycetes; order, -ales; family: -aceae (13). Each family is composed of a number of genera, and these are divided into species. With the advent of molecular phylogenetics, there has been particular instability in the use of higher taxonomic ranks because of the comparative nature of the data and also because no "gold standard" exists to define boundaries between different groups at any level (4). In their comprehensive phylogenetic classification of the kingdom Fungi, Hibbett et al. (14) accepted 7 phyla, 10 subphyla, 35 classes, 12 subclasses, and 129 orders. While these familiar grouping names are no longer used in the latest revision to eukaryote classification (7), this rank-based approach has been retained for this discussion.

The seven phyla that constitute the true fungi are the Ascomycota, Basidiomycota, Blastocladiomycota, Chytridiomycota, Glomeromycota, Microsporidia, and Neocallimastigomycota. The clade containing the Ascomycota and Basidiomycota is classified as the subkingdom Dikarya (14). The phylum Zygomycota is no longer accepted due to its polyphyletic nature (14). Because of remaining doubts about relationships between the groups that were formerly placed in this phylum, these organisms have been divided among the phylum Glomeromycota and four subphyla *incertae sedis* (Latin for "of uncertain position," not assigned to any phylum). The subphylum Mucoromycotina has been proposed to accommodate the Mucorales, while the subphylum Entomophthoromycotina has been created for the Entomophthorales (14).

A simplified taxonomic scheme illustrating the major groups of medically important fungi is presented in Table 1. These groups are described in the following sections. A simplified key to their identification is provided in Table 2.

Subphyla Mucoromycotina and Entomophthoromycotina (formerly Phylum Zygomycota)

The traditional Zygomycota have been divided among the phylum Glomeromycota and four subphyla, pending resolution of further taxonomic questions (14). In these groups of lower fungi, the thallus is pauciseptate and consists of wide, hyaline (colorless) branched hyphal elements. The asexual spores (termed sporangiospores) are nonmotile and are often produced inside a closed sac, termed a sporangium, the wall of which ruptures to release them, although in some genera the spores are formed around a vesicle at the tip of the sporangiophore. Sexual reproduction leads to the formation of a single large zygospore with a thickened wall. Most of the medically important species are heterothallic and do not form their sexual structures unless two compatible isolates come into contact.

The subphylum Mucoromycotina contains the order Mucorales, which is the most clinically important and includes the genera *Lichtheimia* (formerly *Absidia*), *Mucor*, *Rhizomucor*, and *Rhizopus*. The subphylum Entomophthoromycotina contains one order of medical importance, the Entomophthorales. The Entomophthorales group includes the genera *Basidiobolus* and *Conidiobolus*, agents of subcutaneous infections.

Phylum Basidiomycota

Most members of this group of higher fungi have a septate, filamentous thallus, but some are typical yeasts. Sexual reproduction leads to the formation of haploid basidiospores on the outside of a generative cell, termed a basidium. Three subphyla (Agaricomycotina, Pucciniomycotina, and Ustilagomycotina) and 15 classes are recognized (14), but only a few members of this large phylum are of medical

TABLE 1 Simplified taxonomic scheme illustrating major groups of the kingdom Fungi in which medically important fungi are classified[a]

Phylum or subphylum	Class	Order	Representative genera
Mucoromycotina		Mucorales	*Lichtheimia, Rhizopus*
Entomophthoromycotina		Entomophthorales	*Basidiobolus, Conidiobolus*
Basidiomycota	Tremellomycetes	Filobasidiales and Tremellales	*Cryptococcus*
	Agaricomycetes	Agaricales	*Schizophyllum*
Ascomycota	Pneumocystidomycetes	Pneumocystidales	*Pneumocystis*
	Saccharomycetes	Saccharomycetales	*Issatchenkia, Kluyveromyces* (teleomorphs of *Candida* spp.); *Saccharomyces*
	Eurotiomycetes	Onygenales	*Arthroderma* (teleomorphs of *Microsporum* and *Trichophyton* spp); *Ajellomyces* (teleomorphs of *Blastomyces* and *Histoplasma* spp.)
		Eurotiales	*Emericella, Eurotium, Neosartorya* (teleomorphs of *Aspergillus* spp.)
	Sordariomycetes	Hypocreales	*Gibberella, Nectria* (teleomorphs of *Fusarium* spp.)
		Microascales	*Pseudallescheria* (teleomorph of *Scedosporium* spp.)

[a]Modified from reference 14.

importance. The most prominent are the basidiomycetous yeasts with anamorphic stages belonging to the genera *Cryptococcus*, *Malassezia*, and *Trichosporon* (see chapter 120). The genus *Cryptococcus* belongs to the subphylum Agaricomycotina. Within this subphylum, molecular analysis has demonstrated that *Cryptococcus* is polyphyletic, with species distributed among five major lineages within the class Tremellomycetes. Most cluster in in the orders Tremellales and Filobasidiales (15).

In culture, filamentous basidiomycetes often produce fast-growing, nonsporulating (sterile) white colonies with clamp connections. These are hyphal outgrowths which, at cell division, make a connection between the two cells, forming a bypass around the septum to allow the migration of a nucleus. The basidia are often produced in macroscopic structures, termed basidiomata or basidiocarps, and the basidiospores are often forcibly discharged. Asexual reproduction is variable, with some species producing spores like those of the Ascomycota (see below), but many others are not known to produce spores at all. Most filamentous basidiomycetes are wood-rotting fungi or obligate plant pathogens. Historically, the most frequently reported clinically important filamentous basidiomycete has been *Schizophyllum commune* (16, 17). With the advent of DNA sequencing, many of these sterile or nonculturable fungi, including *Ceriporia lacerata* and *Hormographiella aspergillata* (16, 17), can now be identified in clinical laboratories.

Phylum Ascomycota

This large phylum contains almost 50% of all named fungal species and accounts for around 80% of fungi of medical importance (2). Three subphyla (Pezizomycotina, Saccharomycotina, and Taphrinomycotina) are recognized (14). Sexual reproduction leads to the development of haploid spores, termed ascospores, which are produced in a saclike structure termed an ascus. The Ascomycota show a gradual transition from primitive forms that produce single asci to species that produce large structures, termed ascocarps or ascomata, containing numerous asci. Variations in ascus structure are of major importance in the classification of these fungi. Asexual reproduction consists of the

TABLE 2 Simplified key to the main groups of medically important fungi

1a Fungus not culturable on routine media, occurs as cyst-like cells in tissue	Pneumocystidomycetes
1b Fungus cultivable	2
2a Colonies consist of budding cells at 30°C.	3
2b Colonies consist of hyphae at 30°C	5
3a Colonies black.	Black yeast
3b Colonies white, cream, pink, or red	4
4a Urease test positive	Basidiomycetous yeasts
4b Urease test negative	Ascomycetous yeasts
5a Hyphae septate	6
5b Hyphae nearly aseptate (pauciseptate).	9
6a Clamp connections present	Filamentous basidiomycetes
6b Clamp connections absent	7
7a Fruiting bodies absent	Hyphomycetes
7b Fruiting bodies present	8
8a Fruiting bodies containing ascospores in asci	Eurotiomycetes
8b Fruiting bodies containing conidia.	Coelomycetes
9a Sporulation abundant	Mucormycetes, Entomophthoromycetes
9b Sporulation absent; zoospores formed in water cultures.	Oomycota

production of conidia (singular, conidium), from a generative or conidiogenous cell. In some species the conidiogenous cell cannot be distinguished from the rest of the mycelium. In others, a special structure is produced which bears one or more conidiogenous cells. Many genetically unrelated species among the Ascomycota have very similar conidial structures, while other genetically similar species differ vastly in their morphological characteristics.

The subphylum Taphrinomycotina contains only one medically important genus, *Pneumocystis*, formerly classified as a member of the kingdom Protozoa, but now reassigned to the class Pneumocystidiomycetes on the basis of small-subunit rDNA and other gene sequence comparisons (18). The subphylum Saccharomycotina contains a single class of medical importance, the Saccharomycetes, to which belong most pathogenic ascomycetous yeasts. The subphylum Pezizomycotina contains two classes of medical importance: the Eurotiomycetes and the Sordariomycetes, which encompass the filamentous ascomycetes.

The order Saccharomycetales, which belongs to the class Saccharomycetes, is characterized by vegetative yeast cells which proliferate by budding or fission. These fungi do not produce ascomata, the ascus being formed by direct transformation of a budding vegetative cell, by "mother-bud" conjugation, or by conjugation between two independent single cells. Many members of this order have an anamorphic stage belonging to the genus *Candida*. This genus, which consists of around 200 anamorphic species, has teleomorphs in more than 10 different genera, including *Clavispora*, *Debaryomyces*, *Issatchenkia*, *Kluyveromyces*, and *Pichia* (19). Many of these will be renamed as the "one fungus one name" concept is applied.

In the class Eurotiomycetes sexual reproduction leads to the formation of ascomata containing asci with ascospores. This class has seven orders that include species pathogenic to humans. Among the more important are the Onygenales, which contains the teleomorphs of the dermatophytes and a number of dimorphic systemic pathogens (including *H. capsulatum* and *B. dermatitidis*), and the Eurotiales, which includes the teleomorphs of the anamorphic genera *Aspergillus* and *Penicillium*. In the class Sordariomycetes, the order Hypocreales contains many of the teleomorphs of the anamorphic genus *Fusarium*. In addition, the teleomorphs of numerous melanized fungi of medical importance belong to a number of orders in the classes Eurotiomycetes or Sordariomycetes. These include the Capnodiales, Chaetothyriales, Microascales, Pleosporales, Hypocreales, and Ophiostomatales.

Although most of the septate molds that are isolated in clinical laboratories belong to one of the classes described above, it is unusual to encounter their sexual reproductive structures in routine cultures. The few species which do produce ascomata in relative abundance include *Pseudallescheria boydii* (anamorph: *Scedosporium boydii*) and *Emericella nidulans* (anamorph: *Aspergillus nidulans*). For the most part, however, routine identification of these molds is based on the form and arrangement of the asexual spore-bearing structures and the manner in which the spores are produced (see below).

Phylum Microsporidia

Microsporidians, some of which are obligate parasites of humans, have long been classified with the protozoa. However, molecular phylogenetic analysis has indicated that these organisms belong among the fungi (20), and the phylum Microsporidia within the kingdom Fungi has been created to accommodate them (14) (see chapter 131).

IDENTIFICATION OF YEASTS

Yeasts are neither a natural nor a formal taxonomic group but are a growth form found in a wide range of unrelated ascomycetous and basidiomycetous fungi. Their identification relies on a combination of morphological, physiological, and biochemical characteristics. Useful morphological characteristics include the color of the colonies; the size and shape of the cells; the presence of a capsule around the cells; the production of hyphae, pseudohyphae, or arthroconidia; and the production of chlamydospores. Useful biochemical tests include the assimilation and fermentation of sugars and the assimilation of nitrate. Most yeasts of medical importance can be identified using one of the commercial test systems that are based on sugar assimilation of isolates. However, it is important to remember that microscopic examination of cultures on cornmeal agar is essential to avoid confusion between organisms with identical biochemical profiles (see chapter 118). In many laboratories, biochemical methods have been supplanted with DNA sequencing or matrix-assisted laser desorption ionization–time of flight mass spectrometry (MALDI-TOF) (21). These approaches have shortened the turnaround time for identification and have obviated the need for additional biochemical confirmatory testing.

The so-called black yeasts are not a formal taxonomic group, but the description is applied to a wide range of unrelated ascomycetous and basidiomycetous fungi that are able to produce melanized budding cells at some stage in their life cycle (22). Because most of these fungi are also able to produce true mycelium, their routine identification has traditionally been based on the morphological characteristics of the asexual spore-bearing structures and the manner in which the spores are produced. Molecular methods and MALDI-TOF are now being used to identify these organisms (23).

CLASSIFICATION AND IDENTIFICATION OF ANAMORPHIC MOLDS

Most of the septate molds that are isolated in clinical laboratories do not produce their sexual reproductive structures in routine cultures. While these organisms can now be sequenced and their correct positions in the fungal kingdom determined, in the past their classification and identification were based on the manner in which the asexual spores are produced. Two artificial form-classes of anamorphic or "mitosporic" molds were informally recognized, based on the mode of conidium formation. The Hyphomycetes produce their conidia directly on the hyphae or on specialized conidiophores, while the Coelomycetes have more elaborate reproductive structures, termed conidiomata. Although these form-classes are no longer formally recognized, they continue to offer a useful framework for identification based on morphology.

Form-Class Coelomycetes

Three artificial orders are recognized: the Sphaeropsidales, Melanconiales, and Pycnothyriales. In the Sphaeropsidales, the conidia are produced in conidiomata that are either spherical with an apical opening and with conidiogenous cells lining the inner cavity wall (termed pycnidia) or are open and cup-shaped, in which case the conidiogenous cells cover the conidiomatal surface (termed acervuli). A few members of this form-class are common pathogens of humans. One of the more frequently encountered species is *Neoscytalidium dimidiatum*, a plant pathogen which can also cause infections of the skin and nails. Until recently, this species was known by the synanamorph name *Scytalidium dimidiatum*.

Form-Class Hyphomycetes

The Hyphomycetes contains a large number of septate anamorphic molds of medical importance, including the genera *Aspergillus*, *Blastomyces*, *Cladophialophora*, *Fusarium*, *Histoplasma*, *Microsporum*, *Penicillium*, *Phialophora*, *Scedosporium*, and *Trichophyton*. In addition, numerous Hyphomycetes have been reported as occasional opportunistic pathogens of humans. For this reason, it is important for clinical microbiologists to be able to recognize and correctly identify this group of fungi.

As mentioned earlier, the process of conidiogenesis is of major importance in the identification of these molds. Two basic methods of conidiogenesis can be distinguished: thallic conidiogenesis, in which an existing hyphal cell is converted into one or more conidia, and blastic conidiogenesis, in which conidia are produced as a result of some form of budding process (for a detailed discussion of this topic, see reference 22).

Thallic Conidiogenesis

In this form of conidiogenesis the conidia are produced from an existing hyphal cell. Arthroconidia, which are derived from the fragmentation of an existing hypha, represent the simplest form of thallic conidiogenesis and have evolved in many different groups of fungi. The first step in the examination of cultures of these molds should be to ascertain whether another spore form is present. If so, identification should be based on that form. The few molds of medical importance which produce arthroconidia as their sole means of conidiogenesis include *Coccidioides* species.

Aleurioconidia are formed from the side or tip of an existing hypha and, during the initial stage before a septum is laid down, can resemble short hyphal branches. This form of thallic conidiogenesis is characteristic of the dermatophytes (*Epidermophyton*, *Microsporum*, and *Trichophyton* spp.), as well as a number of dimorphic systemic pathogens, including *B. dermatitidis*, *H. capsulatum*, and *P. brasiliensis*.

Blastic Conidiogenesis

Many fungi have evolved some form of repeated budding that allows them to produce large numbers of asexual spores from a single conidiogenous cell. There are two basic forms of blastic conidiogenesis: holoblastic development, in which all layers of the wall of the conidiogenous cell swell out to form the conidium, and enteroblastic development, in which the conidium is produced from within the conidiogenous cell, the outer layers of the cell wall breaking open and an inner layer extending through the opening to become the new spore wall. These two forms of blastic conidiogenesis can be further subdivided according to the details of spore development.

Almost all the molds that produce holoblastic conidia have melanized cell walls and thus are similar in colonial appearance. The morphological characteristics of their conidia and the manner in which the spores are produced serve as the main distinguishing features. Holoblastic conidia range in size from minute unicellular to large thick-walled multicelled conidia. In some species, the first-formed conidium buds to produce a second, and the second produces a third, and so on until a chain of conidia is produced, with the youngest at its tip (acropetal). Because each spore can produce more than one bud, a branching chain becomes possible (e.g., *Cladophialophora* species). In another group, the conidiogenous cell that produced the first spore then grows past it to produce a second. If this process is repeated, it will result in an elongated conidiogenous cell with numerous lateral single spores along its sides. This is termed sympodial development and is typical of species of *Bipolaris* and *Exserohilum*.

In molds that produce enteroblastic conidia, the wall of the conidium is derived from the inner layer of the wall of the conidiogenous cell. This permits a succession of conidia to be produced from the same point. There are two main forms of enteroblastic conidiogenesis: phialidic, in which the specialized conidiogenous cell from which the conidia are produced is termed a phialide, and annellidic, in which the conidiogenous cell is termed an annellide.

In phialidic conidiogenesis, the first blown-out cell breaks open at its tip and remains as a collarette, from the inside of which conidia are produced in succession. In some species, the collarette is distinct (e.g., *Phialophora* species), but in others it is almost invisible at the tip of the phialide. In some phialidic molds, such as species of *Fusarium* and *Acremonium*, the conidia are not firmly attached to each other and often move aside to accumulate in a wet mass around the phialide. In other phialidic molds, such as species of *Aspergillus* and *Penicillium*, continuous replenishment of the inner wall of the tip of the phialide results in the formation of an unbranched chain of connected conidia, with the youngest at the base (basipetal).

Annellides, like phialides, are conidiogenous cells which produce conidia at their tips in unbranched chains (e.g., *Scopulariopsis* species) or in wet masses (e.g., *Scedosporium* species). In annellidic conidiogenesis the first blown-out cell becomes a conidium, and subsequent conidia are formed by blowing out through the scar of the previous one. Unlike phialides, annellides increase in length each time a new spore is produced. An old annellide that has produced many conidia will have a number of apical scars or annellations at its tip.

IDENTIFICATION OF MOLDS

Most molds can be identified after growth in culture, but the criteria for recognition often differ from the fundamental characteristics that are used as a basis for classification. Macroscopic characteristics, such as colonial form, surface color, pigmentation, and growth rate, are often helpful in mold identification. Although the culture medium, incubation temperature, age of the culture, and amount of inoculum can influence colonial appearance and growth rate, these characteristics remain sufficiently constant to be useful in the process of identification. Molds that fail to sporulate in culture may be impossible to speciate using morphology, and it is therefore important to select culture conditions which favor sporulation. Although molds often grow best on rich media, such as Sabouraud's dextrose agar, overproduction of mycelium often results in loss of sporulation. In such cases subculture to a low-nutrient medium may help to stimulate sporulation.

POLYPHASIC IDENTIFICATION

A frequent problem with the traditional morphological approach to fungal identification is that nonsporulating organisms cannot be identified or given a taxonomic placement. With comparative DNA sequence analysis, most such isolates can now be identified and classified by applying phylogenetic species recognition concepts.

Interpretive criteria for the identification of fungi using DNA sequencing have been published (24).

Many clinical laboratories today employ DNA sequencing and/or MALDI-TOF as part of their routine protocol for fungal identification. In circumstances where morphology-based identification is not helpful, an isolate may be a candidate for these methods of identification. This approach may be useful when an isolate displays atypical morphology, fails to sporulate, requires lengthy incubation or incubation on specialized media to sporulate, or if the phenotypic results are nonspecific or confusing. Precise identification of particular isolates may also be necessary as part of outbreak investigations or during other studies of the epidemiologic significance of particular groups of organisms. In these cases, DNA sequencing may be required. A polyphasic approach to fungal identification that combines both morphologic and genotypic approaches may be the most useful, practical, and cost-effective way forward for fungal identification at this time (25).

COMMON MYCOLOGICAL TERMS

Acervulus (plural, acervuli): an open or cup-shaped structure on which conidia are formed.

Acropetal: describes a chain of conidia in which new spores are formed at the tip of the chain.

Aleurioconidium (plural, aleurioconidia): a thallic conidium that is formed from the end of an undifferentiated hypha or from a short side-branch.

Aleuriospore: *see* Aleurioconidium.

Anamorph: the asexual form of a fungus.

Annellide: a specialized conidiogenous cell from which a succession of spores is produced and which has a column of apical scars at its tip.

Annelloconidium (plural, annelloconidia): a blastic conidium that is formed from an annellide.

Annellospore: *see* Annelloconidium.

Apophysis: the enlargement of a sporangium just below the columella.

Appressorium (plural, appressoria): a swelling on a germ-tube or hypha, typical of *Colletotrichum* spp.

Arthroconidium (plural, arthroconidia): a thallic conidium produced as the result of fragmentation of an existing hypha into separate cells.

Arthrospore: *see* Arthroconidium.

Ascocarp: a structure that contains asci.

Ascoma (plural, ascomata): *see* Ascocarp.

Ascospore: a haploid spore produced within an ascus following meiosis.

Ascus (plural, asci): a thin-walled sac containing ascospores, characteristic of the Ascomycota.

Aseptate: without cross-walls or septa.

Ballistoconidium: a conidium that is forcibly discharged.

Ballistospore: *see* Ballistoconidium.

Basidiocarp: a structure that produces basidia.

Basidioma (plural, basidiomata): *see* Basidiocarp.

Basidiospore: a haploid spore produced on a basidium following meiosis.

Basidium: a cell upon which basidiospores are produced, characteristic of the Basidiomycota.

Basipetal: describes a chain of conidia in which new spores are formed at the base of the chain.

Blastic: one of the two basic forms of conidiogenesis in which enlargement of the conidial initial occurs before a delimiting septum is laid down.

Blastoconidium (plural, blastoconidia): a blastic conidium produced by the enlargement of a part of a conidiogenous cell before a septum is laid down.

Blastospore: *see* Blastoconidium.

Catenate: in chains.

Cerebriform: term used to describe colonies with a convoluted surface.

Chlamydospore: a resting conidium, formed as a result of the enlargement of an existing hyphal cell.

Clade: a phylogenetic group consisting of an ancestral species and all its descendants. Clades (and subclades) can be recognized at any given taxonomic level.

Clavate: club-like in shape, narrowing toward the base.

Cleistothecium (plural, cleistothecia): a form of closed ascocarp with no predefined opening, which splits open to release the ascospores.

Coelomycete: an artificial taxonomic grouping referring to anamorphic molds that form conidia within a specialized multihyphal structure, such as an acervulus or pycnidium.

Collarette: a cup-shaped structure at the tip of a conidiogenous cell.

Columella (plural, columellae): the swollen tip of the sporangiophore projecting into the sporangium in some Mucorales.

Conidiogenesis: the process of conidium formation.

Conidiogenous cell: any cell that produces or becomes a conidium.

Conidioma (plural, conidiomata): a specialized conidia-bearing structure.

Conidiophore: a specialized hypha or cell on which, or as part of which, conidia are produced.

Conidium (plural, conidia): an asexual spore.

Cruciate: term used to describe spores with septa in the form of a cross.

Cryptic species: a species recognized by nucleic acid variation that had not been recognized as distinct on the basis of its morphological characteristics.

Cuneiform: term used to describe spores that are thinner at one end than the other.

Dematiaceous: darkly pigmented.

Denticle: a small tooth-like projection on which a spore is borne.

Distoseptate: term used to describe spores in which the individual cells are each surrounded by a sac-like wall distinct from the outer wall.

Echinulate: term used to describe spores with small pointed spines.

Endoconidium (plural, endoconidia): a conidium formed inside a hypha.

Enteroblastic: a form of conidiogenesis in which conidia are produced from within a conidiogenous cell.

Euseptate: term used to describe spores in which the outer and inner wall of the septum are continuous.

Floccose: term used to describe colonies with a cotton-like texture.

Fusiform: term used to describe spores with a spindle-like shape.

Geniculate: an irregular conidiogenous cell formed by some holoblastic molds.

Glabrous: term used to describe colonies with a wax-like texture.

Gymnothecium (plural, gymnothecia): an ascocarp in which the asci are distributed within a loose network of hyphae.

Heterothallic: a self-sterile fungus; sexual reproduction cannot take place unless two compatible mating strains are present.

Hilum: a slightly prominent scar at the base of a conidium.

Holoblastic: a form of conidiogenesis in which both the inner and outer walls of the conidiogenous cell swell out to form the conidium.

Homothallic: a self-compatible fungus; sexual reproduction can take place within an individual strain.

Hülle cell: a large, thick-walled, sterile cell found in some *Aspergillus* spp.

Hyaline: colorless, transparent, translucent.

Hypha (plural, hyphae): one of the individual filaments that make up the mycelium of a fungus. Hyphomycete: an artificial taxonomic grouping referring to anamorphic molds that form conidia directly on the hyphae or on specialized conidiophores.

Macroconidium (plural, macroconidia): the larger of two different sizes of conidia produced by a fungus in the same manner.

Merosporangium (plural, merosporangia): a cylindrical outgrowth from the end of a sporangiophore in which a chain-like series of sporangiospores is produced, characteristic of *Syncephalastrum* spp.

Meristematic: perpetual increase in biomass in all directions with concordant septum formation.

Metula (plural, metulae): a conidiophore branch that bears phialides, characteristic of *Aspergillus* and *Penicillium* spp.

Microconidium (plural, microconidia): the smaller of two different sizes of conidia produced by a fungus in the same manner.

Mitosporic: term used to describe an anamorphic fungus.

Mold: a filamentous fungus.

Moniliaceous: hyaline or lightly colored.

Muriform cell: a thick-walled, darkly pigmented cell found in tissues affected by chromoblastomycosis.

Mycelium: a mass of branching filaments which make up the vegetative growth of a fungus.

Oligokaryotic cell: a cell with several nuclei.

Oospore: a sexual spore produced in the Oomycota.

Ostiole: the opening through which spores are released from an ascocarp or pycnidium.

Pauciseptate: having few septa

Perithecium (plural, perithecia): a flask-shaped ascocarp with an apical opening (ostiole) through which the ascospores are released.

Phialide: a specialized conidiogenous cell from which a succession of spores is produced.

Pleoanamorphism: term used to describe a fungus that has more than one anamorph.

Pleomorphic: term used to describe a nonsporing strain of a fungus.

Pseudohypha (plural, pseudohyphae): a chain of yeast cells which have arisen as a result of budding and have elongated without becoming detached from each other, forming a hypha-like filament.

Punctate: term used to describe colonies marked with small spots.

Pycnidiospore: a conidium formed within a pycnidium.

Pycnidium (plural, pycnidia): a flask-shaped structure with an apical opening (ostiole) inside of which conidia are produced.

Pyriform: pear-like in shape.

Rhizoid: a short branching hypha that resembles a root.

Sclerotic body: *see* Muriform cell.

Sclerotium (plural, sclerotia): a firm mass of hyphae, normally having no spores in or on it.

Septate: having cross-walls or septa.

Septum (plural, septa): a cross-wall in a fungal hypha or spore.

Sessile: not having a stem.

Sibling species: species that share the same, most recent common ancestor.

Species complex: a monophyletic clade of species with equivalent clinical relevance.

Sporangiole: *see* Sporangiolum.

Sporangiolum (plural, sporangiolia): a small sporangium containing a small number of asexual spores, characteristic of the Mucorales.

Sporangiophore: a specialized hypha upon which a sporangium develops.

Sporangiospore: asexual spore produced in a sporangium, characteristic of the Glomeromycota.

Sporangium (plural, sporangia): a closed sac-like structure containing asexual spores, characteristic of the Glomeromycota. This term has also been used in the members of kingdom Straminipila to denominate the segmented hyphal structures (and not to the vesicles containing zoospores) giving origin to a germ tube developing terminal vesicles in which biflagellate zoospores are cleaved.

Sporodochium (plural, sporodochia): a specialized structure in which conidia are borne on a compact mass of short conidiophores.

Stroma (plural, stromata): a solid mass of hyphae, sometimes bearing spores on short conidiophores or having ascocarps or pycnidia embedded in it.

Sympodial: term used to describe the development of a single conidium at successive sites along a lengthening conidiogenous cell.

Synanamorph: term applied to any one of two or more anamorphs which have the same teleomorph.

Synnema (plural, synnemata): a compact group of erect and sometimes fused conidiophores bearing conidia at the tip, along the upper portion of the sides, or both.

Teleomorph: the sexual form of a fungus.

Thallic: one of the two basic forms of conidiogenesis in which enlargement of the conidial initial occurs after a delimiting septum has been laid down.

Thallus: the vegetative growth of a fungus.

Vesicle: the swollen tip of the conidiophore in *Aspergillus* spp. or the swollen part of a sporogenous cell in other fungi.

Villose: term used to describe spores covered with long hairs.

Yeast: a unicellular, budding fungus.

Zoospore: a motile asexual spore.

Zygospore: a thick-walled, sexual spore, produced in the Glomeromycota.

REFERENCES

1. **Blackwell M.** 2011. The fungi: 1, 2, 3 . . . 5.1 million species? *Am J Bot* **98:**426–438.
2. **Guarro J, Gené J, Stchigel AM.** 1999. Developments in fungal taxonomy. *Clin Microbiol Rev* **12:**454–500.
3. **Hawksworth DL.** 2011. A new dawn for the naming of fungi: impacts of decisions made in Melbourne in July 2011 on the future publication and regulation of fungal names. *IMA Fungus* **2:**155–162.
4. **de Hoog GS, Chaturvedi V, Denning DW, Dyer PS, Frisvad JC, Geiser D, Gräser Y, Guarro J, Haase G, Kwon-Chung K-J, Meis JF, Meyer W, Pitt JI, Samson RA, Taylor JW, Tintelnot K, Vitale RG, Walsh TJ, Lackner M, ISHAM Working Group on Nomenclature of Medical Fungi.** 2015. Name changes in medically important fungi and their implications for clinical practice. *J Clin Microbiol* **53:**1056–1062.
5. **Taylor JW, Jacobson DJ, Kroken S, Kasuga T, Geiser DM, Hibbett DS, Fisher MC.** 2000. Phylogenetic species recognition and species concepts in fungi. *Fungal Genet Biol* **31:**21–32.
6. **Hawksworth DL.** 2006. Pandora's mycological box: molecular sequences vs. morphology in understanding fungal relationships and biodiversity. *Rev Iberoam Micol* **23:**127–133.
7. **Adl SM, Simpson AG, Lane CE, Lukeš J, Bass D, Bowser SS, Brown MW, Burki F, Dunthorn M, Hampl V, Heiss A, Hoppenrath M, Lara E, Le Gall L, Lynn DH, McManus H, Mitchell EA, Mozley-Stanridge SE, Parfrey LW, Pawlowski J, Rueckert S, Shadwick L, Schoch CL, Smirnov A, Spiegel FW.** 2012. The revised classification of eukaryotes. *J Eukaryot Microbiol* **59:**429–514. (Erratum, **60:**321.)
8. **Fisher MC, Koenig GL, White TJ, Taylor JW.** 2002. Molecular and phenotypic description of *Coccidioides posadasii* sp. nov., previously recognized as the non-California population of *Coccidioides immitis*. *Mycologia* **94:**73–84.
9. **Brown EM, McTaggart LR, Zhang SX, Low DE, Stevens DA, Richardson SE.** 2013. Phylogenetic analysis reveals a cryptic species *Blastomyces gilchristii*, sp. nov. within the human pathogenic fungus *Blastomyces dermatitidis*. *PLoS One* **8:**e59237. (Erratum, **11:**e0168018.)
10. **Teixeira MM, Theodoro RC, Oliveira FF, Machado GC, Hahn RC, Bagagli E, San-Blas G, Soares Felipe MS.** 2014. *Paracoccidioides lutzii* sp. nov.: biological and clinical implications. *Med Mycol* **52:**19–28.
11. **Balajee SA, Gribskov JL, Hanley E, Nickle D, Marr KA.** 2005. *Aspergillus lentulus* sp. nov., a new sibling species of *A. fumigatus*. *Eukaryot Cell* **4:**625–632.
12. **Blackwell M.** 1993. Phylogenetic systematics and ascomycetes, p 93–103. *In* Reynolds DR, Taylor JW (ed), *The Fungal Holomorph: Mitotic, Meiotic and Pleomorphic Speciation in Fungal Systematics*. CABI Publishing, Wallingford, United Kingdom.
13. **Kirk PM, Cannon PF, Minter DW, Stalpers JA.** 2008. *Dictionary of the Fungi*, 10th ed. CABI Publishing, Wallingford, United Kingdom.
14. **Hibbett DS, et al.** 2007. A higher-level phylogenetic classification of the *Fungi*. *Mycol Res* **111:**509–547.
15. **Kwon-Chung KJ, Boekhout T, Wickes BL, Fell JW.** 2011. Systematics of the genus *Cryptococcus* and its type species *C. neoformans*, p 3–16. *In* Heitman J, Kozel TR, Kwon-Chung KJ, Perfect JR, Casadevall A (ed), *Cryptococcus: from Human Pathogen to Model Yeast*. ASM Press, Washington, DC.
16. **Brandt ME.** 2013. Filamentous basidiomycetes in the clinical laboratory. *Curr Fungal Infect Rep* **7:**219–223.
17. **Chowdhary A, Kathuria S, Agarwal K, Meis JF.** 2014. Recognizing filamentous basidiomycetes as agents of human disease: a review. *Med Mycol* **52:**782–797.
18. **Alexopoulos CJ, Mims CW, Blackwell M.** 1996. *Introductory Mycology*, 4th ed. John Wiley and Sons, Inc, New York, NY.
19. **Kurtzman CP, Fell JW, Boekhout T (ed).** 1998. *The Yeasts, a Taxonomic Study*, 5th ed. Elsevier, Amsterdam, The Netherlands.
20. **Thomarat F, Vivarès CP, Gouy M.** 2004. Phylogenetic analysis of the complete genome sequence of *Encephalitozoon cuniculi* supports the fungal origin of microsporidia and reveals a high frequency of fast-evolving genes. *J Mol Evol* **59:**780–791.
21. **Cassagne C, Normand AC, L'Ollivier C, Ranque S, Piarroux R.** 2016. Performance of MALDI-TOF MS platforms for fungal identification. *Mycoses* **59:**678–690.
22. **de Hoog GS, Guarro J, Gené J, Figueras MJ.** 2000. *Atlas of Clinical Fungi*, 2nd ed. Centraalbureau voor Schimmelcultures, Baarn, The Netherlands.
23. **Singh A, Singh PK, Kumar A, Chander J, Khanna G, Roy P, Meis JF, Chowdhary A.** 2017. Molecular and matrix-assisted laser desorption ionization-time of flight mass spectrometry-based characterization of clinically significant melanized fungi in India. *J Clin Microbiol* **55:**1090–1103.
24. **Clinical and Laboratory Standards Institute.** 2007. *Interpretive Criteria for Identification of Bacteria and Fungi by DNA Target Sequencing; Approved Guideline*, MM18-A. Clinical and Laboratory Standards Institute, Wayne, PA.
25. **Balajee SA, Sigler L, Brandt ME.** 2007. DNA and the classical way: identification of medically important molds in the 21st century. *Med Mycol* **45:**475–490.

Specimen Collection, Transport, and Processing: Mycology

ELIZABETH L. BERKOW AND KARIN L. MCGOWAN

117

SPECIMEN COLLECTION AND TRANSPORT

As in bacteriology, the goals of a good mycology laboratory are to accurately isolate and identify fungi suspected of causing infection. It is our responsibility to provide the guidelines for proper specimen selection, collection, and transport to the laboratory. Table 1 is a listing of the types of specimens most commonly submitted for fungal culture (1–3) (Fig. 1). Once collected properly, all specimens should be transported in leakproof sterile containers and processed as soon as possible. Anaerobic transport media or anaerobic containers should never be used for fungi. Fungi are quite resilient, but because some fungi can be affected by temperatures above 37°C and below 10°C, transport at room temperature is recommended. Dermatophytes are particularly sensitive to cold temperatures. With the exception of skin, hair, and nails, specimens that contain normal bacterial biota should be transported as rapidly as possible because bacterial overgrowth can inhibit slower-growing fungi as well as reduce fungal viability. If such specimens cannot be transported to the laboratory within 2 h, they should be stored at 4°C.

As with other infectious diseases, the best specimen for determining the causative agent comes from the site of active infection (e.g., cerebrospinal fluid [CSF] for meningitis). For a number of fungal diseases, however, peripheral specimens as well as specimens from the active site may also be useful. Table 2 is a listing of the clinical sites associated with recovery of different pathogenic fungi. Laboratories should not hesitate to suggest that peripheral specimens be taken when specific fungal diseases are suspected. Prostate fluid, for example, is an excellent high-yield specimen when endemic mycoses are suspected, but it is a specimen not often submitted to clinical laboratories (4–8).

Fortunately, many of the specimen collection and transport guidelines for mycology are similar to those used in bacteriology. In instances where they differ, it is critical to convey that information to physicians and nurses. One such difference is in specimen volume. The volume of material required for fungal cultures usually exceeds that used in bacteriology, because several types of specimens (body fluids, respiratory secretions, etc.) need to be concentrated or pretreated prior to plating to maximize recovery of fungi. In general, except for a few specific sites noted in Table 1, specimens submitted on swabs are not optimal for recovering fungi, and this practice should be discouraged.

Mycology laboratories should be encouraged to offer physicians different types of fungal cultures. The choice of medium used for primary isolation as well as the length and temperature of incubation can vary with the culture request. For example, fungal culture choices can include a dermatophyte culture for hair, skin, and nail specimens; a rule-out *Candida* culture for vaginal, urine, skin, and throat specimens; a fungal blood culture (lysis-centrifugation culture); and a complete fungal culture. By choosing the culture type, physicians can signal the laboratory when they suspect a specific pathogen, which can often reduce the time that cultures need to be kept in the laboratory.

SPECIMEN HANDLING, PRETREATMENT, AND SAFETY

If specimens that are unacceptable for any reason are received in the laboratory, they should be rejected and the appropriate physicians should be notified. Poor-quality specimens can result in incorrect information, including false-negative results. As required by the Joint Commission (an independent organization which accredits and certifies health care programs in the United States, formerly called JCAHO), a requisition must accompany each specimen and must include the following: patient name, age, sex, and location or address, physician name, specific culture site, date and time of specimen collection, name of the person who collected the specimen, clinical diagnosis, and any special culture request. In addition, each specimen must have a firmly attached label indicating the patient name, location, physician, and date and time of collection (9).

Pretreatment of several specimen types is necessary to maximize the recovery of fungi (2, 3). While this takes additional time and effort, it allows the laboratory to make the most of every specimen submitted, particularly for those that are difficult to obtain from patients. Pretreatment procedures are listed in Table 3 and include centrifugation of urine and sterile body fluids, mincing of nail and tissue specimens, lysis and centrifugation of blood or bone marrow received in Isolator tubes (Wampole Laboratories, Alere, Inc., Orlando, FL), and lysis by mucolytic agents, followed by centrifugation, for respiratory secretions. Such procedures release fungi enclosed within cells, concentrate fungal material in the specimen, and help to reduce or eliminate bacteria present in contaminated specimens because of the

TABLE 1 Specimen collection and transport guidelines[a]

Specimen type	Collection procedure	Processing procedure	Transport time and temperature	Comments
Abscess (drainage, exudate, pus, wound)	Clean surface with 70% alcohol. Collect from active peripheral edge with sterile needle and syringe. If open, use swab system or aspirate.	If thick, pretreat similar to sputum specimen.	If ≤2 h, RT	Examine for grains or granules and note color if present.
Blood	Disinfect skin with iodine tincture or chlorhexidine prior to obtaining (2). Use maximum volume of blood recommended for the system used.	Manual	If ≤2 h, RT; if longer, RT	All systems for bacteria will recover all yeast except for *Malassezia* spp. but will not recover molds. Special fungal media for automated systems are best for molds.
		Biphasic (Septi-Chek)	If ≤2 h, RT; if longer, RT	
		Automated (BACTEC [BD Diagnostics, Sparks, MD], BacT/ALERT [bioMérieux, Durham, NC], VersaTREK [TREK Diagnostic Systems, Cleveland, OH])	If ≤2 h, RT; if longer, RT	
		Lysis-centrifugation (manual or Isolator)	If ≤2 h, RT; if longer, RT but process in ≤16 h	Lysis-centrifugation systems are good for recovery of molds, especially those causing endemic mycoses. They give high contamination and false-positive rates.
Bone marrow	Collect aseptically in a heparinized syringe or lysis-centrifugation tube.	Clotted bone marrow is an unacceptable specimen.	If ≤15 min, RT; if longer, RT	Pediatric Isolator tubes are best.
Catheter tip (intravascular)	Remove distal 3–5 cm of line tip and place in sterile container.	Method of Maki et al. (39); used for catheter tips but not validated for fungi.	If ≤15 min, RT; if longer, 4°C	Avoid media containing cycloheximide.
Cutaneous (hair, skin nails)	Disinfect all types with 70% alcohol. Hair: hair root is most important, plucking is best; submit 10–12 hairs in sterile dry container or envelope. Skin: scrape with dull edge of a scalpel or glass slide, or vigorously brush in a circular motion with a soft-bristle toothbrush. Nails: clip or scrape with a scalpel. Material under nail should also be scraped. Submit in sterile container or clean, dry paper envelope.	Only the leading edge of a lesion should be sampled, as centers are often nonviable. All specimens should be pressed gently into the agar with a sterile swab, do not streak agar plates. If used, toothbrushes should be pressed gently into agar as well.	If ≤72 h, RT (very stable) Never refrigerate, as dermatophytes are sensitive to cold.	Select hairs which fluoresce under a Wood's light. Hair and skin can be collected with soft-bristle toothbrush. For pityriasis versicolor (*M. furfur*), olive oil or a paper disc saturated with olive oil should be placed on the first quadrant of agar plate.
Eye (corneal scraping, vitreous humor)	Corneal scraping: taken by physicians and media/slides inoculated directly. Vitreous humor: needle aspiration.	Corneal: inoculate non-inhibitory media in X- or C-shape motion. Vitreous humor: concentrate by centrifugation, use sediment for media and smears.	If ≤15 min, RT; if longer, RT If ≤15 min, RT; if longer, RT	Very little material usually available. Avoid media with cycloheximide.
Medical devices	Collected surgically. Transport in sterile container.	Use sterile scalpel to collect (by scraping) biofilm or vegetative growth.	If ≤15 min, RT; if longer, 4°C	Avoid media containing cycloheximide. Device material recovered best by using liquid medium.

(Continued on next page)

TABLE 1 Specimen collection and transport guidelines[a] (*Continued*)

Specimen type	Collection procedure	Processing procedure	Transport time and temperature	Comments
Prostate fluid	Have patient empty bladder and then massage prostate gland to yield fluid.	Inoculate media directly or transport in sterile wide-mouth container.	If ≤15 min, RT; if longer, RT	Fluid should always be examined microscopically. The first urine following massage has a high yield. This fluid is excellent for detection of endemic mycoses.
Respiratory tract, lower (sputum, bronchial aspirate, BAL fluid)	Use first morning sputum collected after brushing teeth. Collect brushings and BAL fluid surgically. Place all samples in sterile containers. Inoculate media containing antimicrobial agents with and without cycloheximide.	Viscous lower respiratory specimens should be pretreated and centrifuged to concentrate their contents.	If ≤2 h, RT; if longer, 4°C	Saliva and 24-h sputum are unacceptable specimens. Methods for mycobacterial decontamination are not acceptable.
Respiratory, upper (oral, oropharyngeal, and sinus samples)	Swab oral lesions, avoiding tongue. Use thin wire or flexible swab for oropharynx. Collect sinus contents surgically.	Use swab transport system for oral and oropharyngeal samples. Place sinus contents in sterile container.	Oral: if ≤2 h, RT; if longer, RT Sinus: if ≤15 min, RT; if longer, RT	Selective and chromogenic media are best for recovery of *Candida*.
Sterile body fluids (CSF and pericardial, peritoneal, and synovial fluids)	Collect as for bacteriology. Concentrate by centrifugation, and use sediment for inoculation. Clots should be ground.	Except CSF, put sterile body fluids in sterile Vacutainer tubes with heparin or lysis-centrifugation tube to prevent blood clotting. Except for CSF, blood culture bottles can be used for recovery of yeast.	If ≤15 min, RT; if longer, RT; never refrigerate.	Sterile fluid sediment should always be examined microscopically. With specimen volumes ≤2 ml, fluid should be plated directly using as much fluid on each plate as possible.
Stool	Specimen use should be discouraged.			
Tissue	Collected surgically. A larger volume is needed than for bacteriology.	Use a sterile container, keep moist (saline drops) to prevent drying. Except with *H. capsulatum*, mincing (not grinding) is critical. Tissue pieces should be pressed into the agar so they are partially embedded. Grind tissue for recovery of *H. capsulatum*.	If ≤15 min, RT; if longer, RT	Tissue biopsy recommended for invasive disease. Examine subcutaneous tissue for granules (see information for abscesses).
Urine	First morning clean catch, suprapubic, or catheterized specimens; 24-h specimens are unacceptable.	Use a sterile container or urine transport system. Concentrate specimens by centrifugation, and use sediment for inoculation.	If ≤2 h, RT; if longer, 4°C; urine transport systems can stay at RT for up to 72 h.	Chromogenic media best for *Candida*. Use sediment for microscopic examination.
Vaginal	Collect as for bacteriology.	Swab transport system or sterile container for washings.	If ≤2 h, RT; if longer, RT	Antibacterial media or chromogenic agars are best for recovery of *Candida*.

[a]Abbreviations: BAL, bronchoalveolar lavage fluid; RT, room temperature.

action of mucolytic agents, such as *N*-acetyl-L-cysteine, 5% oxalic acid, or dithiothreitol (Sputolysin; Millipore Sigma, Burlington, MA).

All work in mycology should be carried out in a certified type 2 laminar-airflow biosafety cabinet whenever possible. Biosafety level 2 procedures are recommended for personnel working with clinical specimens that may contain dimorphic fungi as well as other potential pathogenic fungi. Gloves should be worn for processing specimens and cultures. A number of techniques are available for examining clinical specimens microscopically, and these are discussed in a later chapter of this *Manual*. There are different biosafety regulations in Europe and other countries, and for this reason, practices may differ.

SPECIMEN PROCESSING AND CULTURE GUIDELINES

Abscess (Drainage, Exudate, Pus, and Wound Material)

Abscess specimens should be collected from the active peripheral edge of open abscesses or aspirated from closed abscesses by use of a syringe. Abscess, pus, or drainage

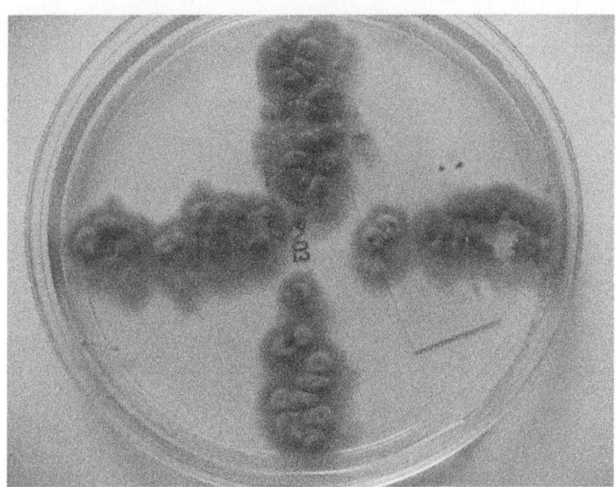

FIGURE 1 Growth of a dermatophyte (*Trichophyton soudanense*) after 4 days of aerobic incubation at 30°C following toothbrush inoculation of Mycosel agar. (Courtesy of Marilyn A. Leet, Children's Hospital of Philadelphia, Philadelphia, PA.)

material should be examined for grains or granules by use of a dissecting microscope. The presence of grains or granules is indicative of a mycetoma, which is discussed at greater length in chapter 128 of this *Manual*. If none are present, the material can be inoculated directly onto medium. If the specimen is thick, it should be pretreated similarly to a sputum specimen. If present, grains and granules should be teased out of the specimen and washed in sterile distilled water, sterile saline, or either solution plus antibiotics. The color of the granules should be noted and recorded. A portion should be crushed between two glass slides and examined microscopically for the presence of hyphae. Both true fungal hyphae and bacteria (branching Gram-positive rods) can be observed with grains. If branching Gram-positive rods are seen, a modified acid-fast stain should be performed to look for *Nocardia*. Another portion of the grains and granules should be crushed by using a sterile technique (sterile glass rod or mortar and pestle) and then inoculated directly onto medium (10).

Blood

Fungemia is a major cause of morbidity and mortality in hospitalized patients, with *Candida* species being the major cause (11, 12). Early detection of organisms in the bloodstream is incredibly important because it is an indicator of disseminated disease. As in bacteriology, the volume of blood, the blood-to-broth ratio, and the number of blood cultures are all critical factors, with the volume of blood being the most important variable. For adults, 20 to 30 ml per culture, divided between two bottles, is recommended for the highest recovery rate and the shortest time to detection (13–16). Studies recommend a 5- to 10-fold dilution of blood in broth, and dilutions of <1:5 may result in reduced recovery of organisms (11, 17). For infants and children, total blood volumes based on the weight of the patient are currently recommended (17–19). Fungemia is almost always continuous, so the timing of obtaining a blood culture for fungi is not critical (14, 20). Both iodine tincture and chlorhexidine are effective for skin decontamination prior to obtaining the blood culture (21).

There are presently a wide variety of manual, biphasic, automated, and continuously monitoring systems for blood cultures, but no single commercial system or culture medium

TABLE 2 Common clinical sites for laboratory recovery of pathogenic fungi

Disease	Recovery from specimen[a]														
	Blood	Bone	Bone marrow	Brain	CSF	Eye	Hair	Nails	Joint fluid	Prostate fluid	Lower respiratory tract	Sinus/nasal cavity	Skin[b]	Tissue	Urine
Aspergillosis		X		X		X		X			X	X	X	X	X
Blastomycosis		X		X	X				X	X	X	X	X	X	X
Candidiasis	X	X	X	X	X	X		X	X	X	X	X	X	X	X
Chromoblastomycosis				X								X	X	X	
Coccidioidomycosis	X	X	X	X	X				X	X	X	X	X	X	X
Cryptococcosis	X	X	X	X	X	X					X		X	X	X
Fusariosis (hyalohyphomycosis)	X		X	X		X		X	X		X	X	X	X	
Histoplasmosis	X	X	X	X	X	X					X		X	X	X
Mucormycosis/ entomophthoromycosis		X		X		X					X	X	X	X	
Paracoccidioidomycosis	X		X	X	X					X	X	X	X	X	
Penicilliosis/*Talaromyces marneffei* infection	X	X	X	X					X				X	X	X
Pneumocystosis		X	X								X			X	
Pseudoallescheriosis/scedosporiosis	X		X		X	X					X		X	X	
Sporotrichosis	X	X			X						X		X	X	
Trichosporonosis	X	X	X	X	X	X			X	X	X	X	X	X	X

[a]X, recovery of fungus from indicated specimen.
[b]Includes skin and mucous membranes.

TABLE 3 Pretreatment of clinical specimens prior to plating

Specimen	Pretreatment	Comments
Abscess, drainage, pus, granules	Granules should be washed and crushed; other materials should be centrifuged at 2,000 × *g* for 10 min.	Essential for best recovery
Blood, bone marrow	Lysis in Isolator tubes and then centrifugation for 30 min at 3,000 × *g*, using a 35° fixed-angle rotor or swinging bucket	Critical for detection of *H. capsulatum* and other dimorphic fungi
Body fluids	Centrifugation at 2,000 × *g* for 10 min or membrane filtration	Essential for best recovery with volumes ≥1 ml; blood clots should be teased apart
Nails	Mince; gently push pieces down into agar	Essential for maximum recovery of dermatophytes
Respiratory secretions (bronchoalveolar lavage fluid, sputum)	Lysis with mucolytic agents,[a] followed by centrifugation at 2,000 × *g* for 10 min	Critical for *Pneumocystis jirovecii* as very difficult to isolate in culture; improves recovery for other mycoses
Tissue	Mince or grind in a mortar; push pieces down into agar	Essential for best recovery; for zygomycetes and other molds, mincing is best; for *H. capsulatum*, grinding is best
Urine	Centrifugation at 2,000 × *g* for 10 min	Essential for best recovery, particularly with deep mycoses

[a]N-Acetyl-L-cysteine, 5% oxalic acid, or dithiothreitol (Sputolysin; Millipore Sigma, Burlington, MA).

can detect all potential blood pathogens. If manual blood cultures are used, a biphasic system is best for fungi (Septi-Chek; Becton Dickinson Diagnostic Systems, Sparks, MD), and the agar slant should be rewashed with the broth-blood mixture each time the bottles are examined. Many automated and continuously monitoring systems are available, and several have medium modifications to enhance fungal growth. These include the BACTEC (BD Diagnostics, Sparks, MD), BacT/ALERT 3D (bioMérieux, Durham, NC), and VersaTREK (Thermo Scientific, Oakwood Village, OH) blood culture systems. Use of these mycosis bottles ensures the highest sensitivity for detecting fungemia (22). Studies evaluating all of these systems have shown that they can recover all pathogenic yeast species except non-*pachydermatis Malassezia* spp. (23). Even without specific fungal media, automated and continuously monitoring systems are able to recover *Candida*, *Cryptococcus*, *Rhodotorula*, and *Trichosporon* spp., with sensitivities equal to or higher than those of manual or lysis-centrifugation methods (13, 14, 24–31). Automated systems with routine bacteriology media are not, however, satisfactory for molds and *Nocardia* spp. (31).

Lysis-centrifugation performed either manually or by using the commercially available Isolator collection system is a more sensitive method for recovery of molds and dimorphic fungi such as *Histoplasma capsulatum* (14, 31, 32). Several studies, however, have argued against the routine use of lysis-centrifugation for all fungal blood cultures because of high contamination rates, high false-positivity rates, and times to detection of yeasts equivalent to or shorter than those of automated systems (25, 26, 33). If molds are suspected, either a special fungal medium for an automated system, such as BACTEC MYCO/F lytic medium or BacT/ALERT MB, or a lysis-centrifugation system should be considered (34). Blood placed in either adult or pediatric Isolator tubes should be kept at room temperature until it is processed, ideally within 16 h of collection. Sediment from lysis-centrifugation should be streaked onto a variety of enriched media not containing cycloheximide and onto a chocolate agar plate (35). The only yeast species requiring special processing are the lipophilic *Malassezia* species, such as *Malassezia furfur*, which require lipids for growth (23). This can be achieved by overlaying solid medium with a thin layer of olive oil or adding a paper disk saturated with olive oil to a subculture plate or plates containing sediment from a lysis-centrifugation tube (10, 17, 36). Specialized media such as modified Dixon's, Leeming's, and Ushijima's media can also be used to isolate *Malassezia* species, if available.

Bone Marrow

Bone marrow is most useful for the diagnosis of disseminated candidiasis, cryptococcosis, and histoplasmosis. Approximately 0.5 ml (pediatrics) to 3 ml (adults) should be collected aseptically in a heparinized syringe or pediatric Isolator tube. Because lysis-centrifugation enhances the recovery of *H. capsulatum* and other molds, the use of Isolator tubes is the method of choice for these organisms. Clotted bone marrow is an unacceptable specimen. With the exception of *H. capsulatum*, fungi are rarely seen in bone marrow aspirates from immunocompetent hosts. For immunocompromised patients, however, bone marrow is an excellent specimen, and *Aspergillus* spp., *Candida* spp., *Cryptococcus* spp., *H. capsulatum*, and *Talaromyces marneffei* can all be observed (37). While it is quite clear that microscopic examination of Giemsa-stained bone marrow can be diagnostic, recent data show that compared with other, less-invasive methods, such as blood cultures, bone marrow aspirate cultures are of limited value and should be performed only selectively (38). Bone marrow should not be placed in blood culture bottles, because with many continuously monitoring systems, the specimen will quickly register a false-positive result due to CO_2 from massive numbers of white blood cells.

Catheter Tips (Intravascular)

If performed simultaneously with blood cultures, quantitative bacterial and fungal cultures have been advocated to demonstrate catheter tip colonization. Acceptable specimens are intravenous or intra-arterial catheter tips, with the distal 3 to 5 cm of the line tip being submitted to the laboratory for culture. Specimens should be placed in a sterile container and transported and stored at room temperature (39). The semiquantitative method of Maki et al. is the most common method used in clinical laboratories, where the catheter tip is rolled across the surface of an agar plate four times and cultures yielding ≥15 CFU are considered positive, although quantitative culture techniques (sonication) may also be used (40). The semiquantitative method distinguishes infection (≥15 colonies) from contamination and is considered a more specific method to diagnose catheter-related septicemia than culturing the catheter tip in broth.

Cutaneous Specimens (Hair, Skin, and Nails)

Hair

The hair root is the most important part to culture for detection of fungi, so plucking or pulling rather than cutting hair is recommended. The area should be cleaned with 70% alcohol and allowed to dry. Infected hairs can appear dull, broken, and faded. Hairs which fluoresce under Wood's light should also be selected for culture. Hair should be submitted in a sterile container or clean, dry paper envelope. Hair can also be collected by using a soft-bristle toothbrush and rubbing in a circular motion over margins or patches of alopecia (hair loss) (41).

Skin

The area should be cleaned with 70% alcohol and allowed to dry. The skin should then be scraped with the dull edge of a scalpel or glass slide or vigorously brushed in a circular motion with a soft-bristle toothbrush (41). Only the leading edge of a skin lesion should be sampled, because the centers of lesions are frequently nonviable. Skin can be submitted in a sterile container or clean, dry paper envelope or on a toothbrush.

Nails

Nails should be cleaned with 70% alcohol and then clipped or scraped with a scalpel. If material is present under the leading edge of the nail, it should also be scraped and submitted in a sterile container or paper envelope designed specifically for this purpose. Prior to being plated, nail pieces should be pulverized or minced by use of a scalpel.

All cutaneous specimens should be inoculated into the agar medium by gently pressing them onto the agar with a sterile swab or scalpel. The pieces should be distributed evenly over the agar surface; the plate should not be streaked with a sterile loop. If a toothbrush is used to collect skin and/or hair specimens, the brush should be pressed gently onto the surface of the agar in four or five places on the plate, leaving an imprint. If organisms are present, growth will occur within the bristle imprint. By nature, cutaneous specimens are usually contaminated with bacteria. For this reason, a plate of inhibitory medium with chloramphenicol and cycloheximide, such as Mycosel, should be used for dermatophytes. As *Trichosporon* spp., the cause of white piedra, *Piedraia hortae*, the cause of black piedra, *Hortaea werneckii*, the cause of tinea nigra, and *Neoscytalidium dimidiatum*, a cause of both nail and skin infections, are sensitive to both chloramphenicol and cycloheximide, samples of hair and skin from patients suspected of having these infections should also be inoculated onto a noninhibitory medium such as Sabouraud dextrose agar. More common nondermatophyte causes of nail infection such as *Scopulariopsis* and *Fusarium* species are also sensitive to cycloheximide, so all nail samples should be cultured on both inhibitory and noninhibitory media. For patients suspected of having pityriasis versicolor, caused by *Malassezia furfur*, direct microscopy is normally diagnostic, but a noninhibitory medium such as Sabouraud dextrose agar can be inoculated, and then olive oil or a paper disk saturated with olive oil should be placed on the first quadrant of the plate. *M. furfur* grows best at ≥35°C but can grow at 30°C. Cutaneous specimens should never be refrigerated, because dermatophytes are sensitive to low temperatures.

Eye Specimens (Corneal Scrapings and Vitreous Humor)

Several types of eye infections require that corneal scrapings and/or vitreous humor be obtained by an ophthalmologist. These include mycotic or fungal keratitis, fungal endophthalmitis, and extension oculomycosis. Mycotic or fungal keratitis is an infection of the cornea. The most common causes are *Acremonium* spp., *Aspergillus* spp., *Candida albicans*, *Candida parapsilosis*, *Candida tropicalis*, *Curvularia* spp., and *Fusarium* spp. (42, 43). Fungal endophthalmitis is usually a late-stage result of hematogenous dissemination of a systemic fungal infection. It can involve many areas of the eye and surrounding tissues. The most common causes are *Aspergillus* spp., *Blastomyces dermatitidis*, *Candida* spp., *Cryptococcus neoformans*, *Coccidioides* spp., *H. capsulatum*, *Paracoccidioides brasiliensis*, and *Sporothrix schenckii* (42, 43). Extension oculomycosis is a result of rhinocerebral mucormycosis, and like fungal endophthalmitis, it may involve many areas of the eye and surrounding tissues. The diagnosis of these infections requires attempting to demonstrate the organism on a microscopic examination plus positive culture. Corneal scrapings are taken by physicians, and media are inoculated directly by use of a heat-sterilized platinum spatula (44). Very little material is usually obtained because of the risks of corneal thinning or perforation. Physicians should be instructed to first inoculate the specimen directly onto a noninhibitory medium, such as Sabouraud dextrose agar, and then to place some material on a sterile glass slide (in the center) for staining. The scraping should be placed in two or three places on the plate, using an X- or C-shaped motion (3). The inoculated plate should be kept at room temperature and transported immediately to the laboratory. Vitreous, or vitreous humor, is the clear, gelatinous material that fills the space between the lens of the eye and the retina. When taken by physicians, vitreous is often diluted with irrigation fluid. For this reason, it should be concentrated by centrifugation, and the sediment should be used to inoculate media and to make smears. Specimens should be placed onto Sabouraud dextrose agar, inhibitory mold agar, and/or brain heart infusion (BHI) agar with 10% sheep blood and incubated at 30°C. Media containing cycloheximide should be avoided (42, 43, 45).

Medical Devices

A wide variety of medical devices (contact lenses, stents, wound-healing dressings, contraceptives, surgical implants, replacement joints, etc.) may be submitted for fungal culture. Most are collected surgically and should be submitted in a sterile container and transported and stored at room temperature. Each should be examined for vegetative growth and biofilms, and if these are present, they should be scraped from the device by use of a sterile scalpel for direct inoculation of agar media and broth (3). Specimens should be placed onto Sabouraud dextrose agar, inhibitory mold agar, and/or BHI agar with 10% sheep blood and incubated at 30°C. Media containing cycloheximide should be avoided. If biofilm or vegetative growth areas are not obvious, portions of the device should be placed in a broth medium such as BHI broth and incubated at 30°C. Quantitative (sonication) broth culture may also be performed.

Prostate Fluid

Prostate fluid consists of secretions of the testes, seminal vesicles, prostate, and bulbourethral glands. After the bladder is emptied, the prostate gland is massaged to yield pure prostatic fluid. The prostate is frequently seeded when organisms are present in the bloodstream. A key clinical sign in males with endemic mycoses is the complaint of a history of chronic urinary tract infections but negative urine cultures. Prostatic fluid from such patients is frequently positive when cultured for fungi. The secretions should also be examined microscopically. After the prostate fluid is obtained, the next urine specimen should also be obtained and submitted for culture, because this urine has a high yield (4–8).

Lower Respiratory Tract Specimens (Sputum, Bronchial Aspirate, and Bronchoalveolar Lavage Fluid)

After a patient's teeth have been brushed, sputum should be collected as a first morning specimen. Neither saliva nor 24-h sputum specimens are acceptable for fungal culture. Viscous lower respiratory tract specimens should be pretreated before being processed. Lysis with mucolytic agents, such as *N*-acetyl-L-cysteine, 5% oxalic acid, or dithiothreitol (Sputolysin, Millipore Sigma, Burlington, MA), followed by centrifugation at 2,000 × *g* for 10 min and then plating of the sediment, greatly increases the yield and improves the recovery of many fungi. Sodium hydroxide, which is used to concentrate specimens for detection of mycobacteria, should not be used because it inhibits the growth of many fungi (e.g., *Aspergillus* spp.). Unfortunately, centrifugation also increases the number of bacteria in the sediment, and for this reason, media containing antimicrobial agents, with and without cycloheximide, should be used. As in bacteriology, lower respiratory tract specimens should be examined for the presence of blood, pus, or necrotic portions, since these have the highest yields (46, 47). Because *Candida* spp. are the most common yeasts isolated from respiratory specimens of patients with cystic fibrosis, use of a chromogenic medium that is selective and differential for *Candida* is recommended (48). *Scedosporium* is now the second most common mold associated with cystic fibrosis, and use of a *Scedosporium*-selective medium containing the antifungal agents dichloran and benomyl has been proposed to improve isolation of this mold in this patient population (49).

Upper Respiratory Tract Specimens (Oral and Oropharyngeal Specimens)

The mucosal surfaces of gums, oral lesions, and oropharyngeal specimens submitted for fungal culture are usually screened for candidiasis. When thrush is suspected, lesions should be scraped gently with moist swabs and submitted for microscopy and a rule-out yeast culture. Antibacterial media or chromogenic agars for *Candida* spp. should be inoculated. While culture is not required to make the diagnosis of candidiasis, it can be useful if microscopy is not available in an outpatient setting or if species other than *C. albicans* are suspected. On rare occasions, oral lesions can be seen with histoplasmosis or paracoccidioidomycosis, but they do not resemble those seen with *Candida* spp. If these are suspected, a full fungal culture and microscopic smear should be performed. The use of nasal swabs should be discouraged because of contamination from environmental spores in the nasal cavity, making interpretation of culture results difficult. Nasal tissue and sinus washings are better specimens and should be plated on a variety of media containing antibiotics, but not cycloheximide, since significant pathogens recovered from these sites (*Aspergillus* spp.) are sensitive to cycloheximide (50).

Sterile Body Fluids (CSF and Pericardial, Peritoneal, and Synovial Fluids)

With the exception of CSF, sterile body fluids are often placed in sterile Vacutainer tubes with heparin to prevent blood clotting. Lysis-centrifugation Isolator tubes can also be used for this purpose. With specimen volumes of ≥2 ml, these tubes plus CSF lumbar puncture tubes should be centrifuged at 2,000 × *g* for 10 min, and the sediment should be used to inoculate media. The supernatant fluid can be used for serologic tests (45). With specimen volumes of ≤2 ml, the specimen should be plated directly, using as much fluid on each plate as possible. Use of a Cytospin centrifuge to prepare microscopic smears is recommended (51, 52). Because sterile fluids are rarely culture positive for fungi, many laboratories inoculate medium slants with screw-cap lids rather than plates to avoid questions concerning possible contamination. In some countries, a purity plate is placed in the biosafety cabinet when sterile body fluids or tissues are being processed. Growth on the purity plate would signal a contamination event during processing.

Stool

Submission of stool specimens for routine fungal culture should be discouraged. Many *Candida* spp. are part of the normal stool biota, and anything that disrupts the normal gastrointestinal tract biota, such as diet or use of antibiotics, can yield a predominance of yeast when stool is cultured. Neither colonization with yeast nor a predominance of yeast indicates invasive disease with *Candida*. If invasive disease of the gastrointestinal tract is suspected, a colonoscopy and tissue biopsy should be performed (53, 54).

Tissue

With one exception (*H. capsulatum*), fungi present in tissue are best recovered when the tissue is minced, not ground. For the mucoraceous molds, in particular, mincing is critical for the recovery of organisms. Tissues should be minced by use of a scalpel, and the pieces of tissue should be pressed into the agar so they are partially embedded (55) (Fig. 2). Two to four pieces should be placed onto each culture plate being inoculated. Further streaking of the plate with sterile

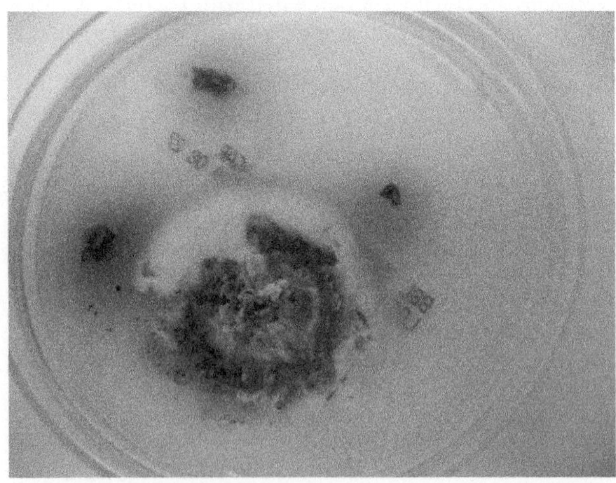

FIGURE 2 Early growth of *Talaromyces marneffei* from a tissue piece embedded in Sabouraud dextrose agar with gentamicin incubated aerobically at 30°C. (Courtesy of Marilyn A. Leet, Children's Hospital of Philadelphia, Philadelphia, PA.)

loops should not be done. When the medium is inoculated this way, fungi grow out directly from the piece of tissue. Laboratories often question if growth on agar plates is contamination. When growth comes directly from the tissue piece, it is unquestionably significant growth. A portion of the specimen can be ground for microscopic examination and/or smears.

When *H. capsulatum* is suspected, the tissue should be ground or homogenized. Because this pathogen is intracellular, organisms need to be released from the cells to be available to grow on media. If needed, a small amount of sterile broth or distilled water can be added to smooth the process of grinding. Subcutaneous tissue should be examined for the presence of granules (as described above, for abscesses). Homogenate or tissue pieces should be inoculated onto enriched media containing antibacterial agents, and for systemic mycoses, enriched media containing both blood and antibacterial agents are best.

Urine

Clean-catch, suprapubic, or catheterized urine specimens should all be obtained as first morning specimens. Large volumes (10 to 50 ml) give the best results and should be centrifuged for maximum recovery, particularly for agents of deep mycoses. Urine should be centrifuged at 2,000 × *g* for 10 min. The sediment should be used for microscopic smears and inoculation of media. Quantification of organisms, as performed in bacteriology, is not useful (36). Twenty-four-hour urine specimens are not acceptable.

Vaginal Specimens

Vaginal specimens submitted for fungal culture are frequently screened just for vaginal candidiasis. For this reason, having a rule-out *Candida* culture as a culture choice is helpful for clinicians and laboratorians. *Candida* spp. are part of the normal vaginal biota, and their presence alone is not significant. Appropriate clinical symptoms plus a positive microscopic examination or culture are sufficient to diagnose vaginal candidiasis. Culture is not required to confirm vaginal candidiasis, but microscopic examinations are not available in all settings, while culture is available. Antibacterial media or chromogenic agars for *Candida* spp. should be inoculated. On rare occasions, vaginal lesions can be seen with histoplasmosis or paracoccidioidomycosis. These lesions do not resemble those seen with *Candida* spp. If these are suspected, a full fungal culture and microscopic smear should be performed.

REFERENCES

1. **Hazen KC.** 1998. Mycology and aerobic actinomycetes, p 255–283. *In* Isenberg HD (ed), *Essential Procedures for Clinical Microbiology*. American Society for Microbiology, Washington, DC.
2. **Merz WG, Roberts GD.** 1999. Detection and recovery of fungi from clinical specimens, p. 709–722. *In* Murray PR (ed.), *Manual of Clinical Microbiology*, 7th ed. American Society for Microbiology, Washington, DC.
3. **Sutton DA.** 2007. Specimen collection, transport, and processing: mycology, p 1728–1736. *In* Murray PR, Baron EJ, Jorgensen JH, Landry ML, Pfaller MA (ed), *Manual of Clinical Microbiology*, 9th ed. ASM Press, Washington, DC.
4. **Mawhorter SD, Curley GV, Kursh ED, Farver CE.** 2000. Prostatic and central nervous system histoplasmosis in an immunocompetent host: case report and review of the prostatic histoplasmosis literature. *Clin Infect Dis* **30:**595–598.
5. **Neal PM, Nikolai A.** 2008. Systemic blastomycosis diagnosed by prostate needle biopsy. *Clin Med Res* **6:**24–28.
6. **Sohail MR, Andrews PE, Blair JE.** 2005. Coccidioidomycosis of the male genital tract. *J Urol* **173:**1978–1982.
7. **Watts B, Argekar P, Saint S, Kauffman CA.** 2007. Building a diagnosis from the ground up. *N Engl J Med* **356:**1456–1462.
8. **Yurkanin JP, Ahmann F, Dalkin BL.** 2006. Coccidioidomycosis of the prostate: a determination of incidence, report of 4 cases, and treatment recommendations. *J Infect* **52:**e19–e25.
9. **Joint Commission on Accreditation of Healthcare Organizations.** 2009. IM.6.240. Clinical Laboratory Improvement Act Subpart K. Joint Commission on Accreditation of Healthcare Organizations, Oakbrook Terrace, IL.
10. **Larone DH.** 2011. *Medically Important Fungi: A Guide to Identification*, 5th ed. ASM Press, Washington, DC.
11. **Reimer LG, Wilson ML, Weinstein MP.** 1997. Update on detection of bacteremia and fungemia. *Clin Microbiol Rev* **10:**444–465.
12. **Richardson M, Lass-Flörl C.** 2008. Changing epidemiology of systemic fungal infections. *Clin Microbiol Infect* **14**(Suppl 4)**:** 5–24.
13. **Chiarini A, Palmeri A, Amato T, Immordino R, Distefano S, Giammanco A.** 2008. Detection of bacterial and yeast species with the Bactec 9120 automated system with routine use of aerobic, anaerobic, and fungal media. *J Clin Microbiol* **46:**4029–4033.
14. **Cockerill FR, III, Wilson JW, Vetter EA, Goodman KM, Torgerson CA, Harmsen WS, Schleck CD, Ilstrup DM, Washington JA, II, Wilson WR.** 2004. Optimal testing parameters for blood cultures. *Clin Infect Dis* **38:**1724–1730.
15. **Lee A, Mirrett S, Reller LB, Weinstein MP.** 2007. Detection of bloodstream infections in adults: how many blood cultures are needed? *J Clin Microbiol* **45:**3546–3548.
16. **Washington JA II, Ilstrup DM.** 1986. Blood cultures: issues and controversies. *Rev Infect Dis* **8:**792–802.
17. **Baron EJ, Weinstein MP, Dunne WM, Yagupsky P, Welch DF, Wilson DM.** 2005. *Cumitech 1C: Blood Cultures IV.* Coordinating ed, Baron EJ. ASM Press, Washington, DC.
18. **Kellogg JA, Manzella JP, Bankert DA.** 2000. Frequency of low-level bacteremia in children from birth to fifteen years of age. *J Clin Microbiol* **38:**2181–2185.
19. **Szymczak EG, Barr JT, Durbin WA, Goldmann DA.** 1979. Evaluation of blood culture procedures in a pediatric hospital. *J Clin Microbiol* **9:**88–92.
20. **Lamy B, Dargère S, Arendrup MC, Parienti JJ, Tattevin P.** 2016. How to optimize the use of blood cultures for the diagnosis of bloodstream infections? A state-of-the art. *Front Microbiol* **7:**697.
21. **Barenfanger J, Drake C, Lawhorn J, Verhulst SJ.** 2004. Comparison of chlorhexidine and tincture of iodine for skin antisepsis in preparation for blood sample collection. *J Clin Microbiol* **42:**2216–2217.
22. **Arendrup MC, Sulim S, Holm A, Nielsen L, Nielsen SD, Knudsen JD, Drenck NE, Christensen JJ, Johansen HK.** 2011. Diagnostic issues, clinical characteristics, and outcomes for patients with fungemia. *J Clin Microbiol* **49:**3300–3308.
23. **Gaitanis G, Magiatis P, Hantschke M, Bassukas ID, Velegraki A.** 2012. The *Malassezia* genus in skin and systemic diseases. *Clin Microbiol Rev* **25:**106–141.
24. **Gokbolat E, Oz Y, Metintas S.** 2017. Evaluation of three different bottles in BACTEC 9240 automated blood culture system and direct identification of *Candida* species to shorten the turnaround time of blood culture. *J Med Microbiol* **66:** 470–476.
25. **Kosmin AR, Fekete T.** 2008. Use of fungal blood cultures in an academic medical center. *J Clin Microbiol* **46:**3800–3801.
26. **Mess T, Daar ES.** 1997. Utility of fungal blood cultures for patients with AIDS. *Clin Infect Dis* **25:**1350–1353.
27. **Mirrett S, Reller LB, Petti CA, Woods CW, Vazirani B, Sivadas R, Weinstein MP.** 2003. Controlled clinical comparison of BacT/ALERT standard aerobic medium with BACTEC standard aerobic medium for culturing blood. *J Clin Microbiol* **41:**2391–2394.
28. **Mirrett S, Hanson KE, Reller LB.** 2007. Controlled clinical comparison of VersaTREK and BacT/ALERT blood culture systems. *J Clin Microbiol* **45:**299–302.

29. **Morello JA, Matushek SM, Dunne WM, Hinds DB.** 1991. Performance of a BACTEC nonradiometric medium for pediatric blood cultures. *J Clin Microbiol* **29:**359–362.
30. **Petti CA, Zaidi AK, Mirrett S, Reller LB.** 1996. Comparison of Isolator 1.5 and BACTEC NR660 aerobic 6A blood culture systems for detection of fungemia in children. *J Clin Microbiol* **34:**1877–1879.
31. **Witebsky FG, Gill VJ.** 1995. Fungal blood culture systems: which ones and when to use them. *Clin Microbiol Newsl* **17:**161–164.
32. **Hellinger WC, Cawley JJ, Alvarez S, Hogan SF, Harmsen WS, Ilstrup DM, Cockerill FR, III.** 1995. Clinical comparison of the Isolator and BacT/Alert aerobic blood culture systems. *J Clin Microbiol* **33:**1787–1790.
33. **Creger RJ, Weeman KE, Jacobs MR, Morrissey A, Parker P, Fox RM, Lazarus HM.** 1998. Lack of utility of the lysis-centrifugation blood culture method for detection of fungemia in immunocompromised cancer patients. *J Clin Microbiol* **36:** 290–293.
34. **Cockerill FR, III, Torgerson CA, Reed GS, Vetter EA, Weaver AL, Dale JC, Roberts GD, Henry NK, Ilstrup DM, Rosenblatt JE.** 1996. Clinical comparison of Difco ESP, Wampole Isolator, and Becton Dickinson Septi-Chek aerobic blood culturing systems. *J Clin Microbiol* **34:**20–24.
35. **Procop GW, Cockerill FR, III, Vetter EA, Harmsen WS, Hughes JG, Roberts GD.** 2000. Performance of five agar media for recovery of fungi from isolator blood cultures. *J Clin Microbiol* **38:**3827–3829.
36. **Fisher JF, Newman CL, Sobel JD.** 1995. Yeast in the urine: solutions for a budding problem. *Clin Infect Dis* **20:**183–189.
37. **Bain BJ, Clark DM, Lampert IA, Wilkins BS.** 2001. *Bone Marrow Pathology*, 3rd ed. Wiley-Blackwell, New York, NY.
38. **Duong S, Dezube BJ, Desai G, Eichelberger K, Qian Q, Kirby JE.** 2009. Limited utility of bone marrow culture: a ten-year retrospective analysis. *Lab Med* **40:**37–38.
39. **Mermel LA, Allon M, Bouza E, Craven DE, Flynn P, O'Grady NP, Raad II, Rijnders BJ, Sherertz RJ, Warren DK.** 2009. Clinical practice guidelines for the diagnosis and management of intravascular catheter-related infection: 2009 update by the Infectious Diseases Society of America. *Clin Infect Dis* **49:**1–45.
40. **Maki DG, Weise CE, Sarafin HW.** 1977. A semiquantitative culture method for identifying intravenous-catheter-related infection. *N Engl J Med* **296:**1305–1309.
41. **Hubbard TW, de Triquet JM.** 1992. Brush-culture method for diagnosing tinea capitis. *Pediatrics* **90:**416–418.
42. **Chern KC, Meisler DM, Wilhelmus KR, Jones DB, Stern GA, Lowder CY.** 1996. Corneal anesthetic abuse and *Candida* keratitis. *Ophthalmology* **103:**37–40.
43. **Tanure MA, Cohen EJ, Sudesh S, Rapuano CJ, Laibson PR.** 2000. Spectrum of fungal keratitis at Wills Eye Hospital, Philadelphia, Pennsylvania. *Cornea* **19:**307–312.
44. **Sonntag HG.** 2002. Sampling and transport of specimens for microbial diagnosis of ocular infections. *Dev Ophthalmol* **33:**362–367.
45. **Kwon-Chung KJ, Bennett J.** 1992. *Medical Mycology*. Lea & Febiger, Philadelphia, PA.
46. **Reimer LG, Carroll KC.** 1998. Role of the microbiology laboratory in the diagnosis of lower respiratory tract infections. *Clin Infect Dis* **26:**742–748.
47. **Wolf J, Daley AJ.** 2007. Microbiological aspects of bacterial lower respiratory tract illness in children: typical pathogens. *Paediatr Respir Rev* **8:**204–210.
48. **Müller FM, Seidler M.** 2010. Characteristics of pathogenic fungi and antifungal therapy in cystic fibrosis. *Expert Rev Anti Infect Ther* **8:**957–964.
49. **Blyth CC, Harun A, Middleton PG, Sleiman S, Lee O, Sorrell TC, Meyer W, Chen SC.** 2010. Detection of occult *Scedosporium* species in respiratory tract specimens from patients with cystic fibrosis by use of selective media. *J Clin Microbiol* **48:**314–316.
50. **Carroll K, Reimer L.** 1996. Microbiology and laboratory diagnosis of upper respiratory tract infections. *Clin Infect Dis* **23:**442–448.
51. **Chapin-Robertson K, Dahlberg SE, Edberg SC.** 1992. Clinical and laboratory analyses of Cytospin-prepared Gram stains for recovery and diagnosis of bacteria from sterile body fluids. *J Clin Microbiol* **30:**377–380.
52. **Shanholtzer CJ, Schaper PJ, Peterson LR.** 1982. Concentrated Gram stain smears prepared with a Cytospin centrifuge. *J Clin Microbiol* **16:**1052–1056.
53. **Cimbaluk D, Scudiere J, Butsch J, Jakate S.** 2005. Invasive candidal enterocolitis followed shortly by fatal cerebral hemorrhage in immunocompromised patients. *J Clin Gastroenterol* **39:**795–797.
54. **Kouklakis G, Dokas S, Molyvas E, Vakianis P, Efthymiou A.** 2001. *Candida* colitis in a middle-aged male receiving permanent haemodialysis. *Eur J Gastroenterol Hepatol* **13:** 735–736.
55. **Forbes BA, Sahm DF, Weissfeld AS.** 2007. *Bailey & Scott's Diagnostic Microbiology*, 12th ed. Mosby Elsevier, St. Louis, MO.

Reagents, Stains, and Media: Mycology*

MARK D. LINDSLEY

118

A variety of stains, media, and reagents are available to the mycology laboratory for the detection, isolation, characterization, and identification of yeasts and moulds. Familiarity with the composition and characteristics of these materials is critical to the diagnostic approach when processing specimens from patients with suspected mycotic diseases.

The direct microscopic examination of properly stained clinical material is rapid and cost-effective and may provide a presumptive identification of the etiologic agent, guiding the laboratory in the selection of media that best support fungal growth and sporulation *in vitro* (1–3). Stained preparations made from fungal cultures are essential for definitive identification. It is important to note that when processing patient specimens, universal precautions should be observed and work should be performed in a biosafety hood under biosafety level 2 (BSL2) conditions, particularly when working with blood and other body fluids that may also contain the blood-borne pathogens, human immunodeficiency virus, hepatitis B virus, and hepatitis C virus (4–6). Manipulation and identification of mould isolates under BSL2 conditions is desirable to reduce cross-contamination of cultures, to protect the laboratory environment, and to prevent exposure to potentially harmful agents. However, different biohazard requirements may apply in different countries.

Environmental samples, such as soil, suspected of containing the infectious mould forms of *Histoplasma* sp., *Blastomyces* sp., or *Coccidioides* sp. should be cultured and manipulated under BSL3 conditions (6). Likewise, BSL3 conditions should be used to handle mould isolates known to be *Histoplasma* sp., *Blastomyces* sp., or *Coccidioides* sp. from any source (patient or environmental).

Many media are available for the primary inoculation and cultivation of fungi from clinical specimens. No one specific medium or combination of media is adequate for all specimens. Media should be carefully selected on the basis of specimen type and suspected fungal agents (1, 3, 7–11). If the specimen is from a nonsterile site, it is important to include media that contain inhibitory substances such as chloramphenicol, gentamicin, and/or cycloheximide. Chloramphenicol or gentamicin inhibits most bacterial contaminants, while cycloheximide inhibits most saprobic moulds. Remember that cycloheximide may also inhibit some important opportunistic fungi such as *Fusarium*, *Scopulariopsis*, *Pseudallescheria*, *Trichosporon*, some *Aspergillus* spp., *Talaromyces* (formerly *Penicillium*) *marneffei*, mucoraceous fungi, some dematiaceous fungi, and yeasts such as *Cryptococcus* species and some *Candida* species. Therefore, it is necessary to select media both with and without inhibitory agents for the primary inoculation of the specimen. The Clinical and Laboratory Standards Institute (CLSI) Standard M54-A (12) is an excellent source for determining the selection and use of fungal medium.

Benomyl is a fungicide that selectively inhibits many genera of ascomycetes but not the growth of basidiomycetes, mucormycetes, and others (13). When it is added to fungal medium (10 μg/ml) such as Sabouraud dextrose agar or potato dextrose agar, resistance to benomyl is of particular use in differentiating moulds, particularly those that are not producing identifiable sporulating structures. Benomyl may also be added to media to inhibit the growth of unwanted moulds in environmental specimens. In particular, benomyl has been added to birdseed agar medium for the isolation of *Cryptococcus gattii* from environmental soil samples (14).

Media can be dispensed into containers such as 25- by 150-mm screw-cap tubes or 100-mm diameter petri dishes. Tubed media (slants and deeps) offer maximum safety and resistance to dehydration and contamination but have a small surface area for inoculation. Because of the enhanced safety aspects of tubed media, this is the required format for transporting fungal isolates to reference laboratories for further identification, when necessary. Petri plates, unlike tubed agar, offer the advantage of a large surface area for isolation and dilution of inhibitory substances in the specimens, but they must be poured thick, with at least 25 ml of medium, to resist dehydration during extended incubation periods. Because plates are vented, they are more likely to become contaminated during incubation. Plates may be placed in gas-permeable bags or sealed with gas-permeable tape (Shrink Seals; Scientific Device Laboratory, Des Plaines, IL) to offset this disadvantage. The gas-permeable tape also secures the lid of plated media, preventing the accidental removal of the lid outside the biosafety cabinet. Another format, in which medium is poured into a flat-bottom flask (Bactiflask, Remel, ThermoScientific,

*This chapter contains information presented in chapter 115 by Mark D. Lindsley, James W. Snyder, Ronald M. Atlas, and Mark T. LaRocco in the 11th edition of this *Manual*.

Waltham, MA; Mycoflask, BD Diagnostics BBL, Sparks, MD), provides the combination of an increase in surface area of the plated medium with the safety of tubed medium. Flasked media may be particularly useful when culturing dimorphic pathogens. Because of their propensity to crack and break, petri dishes or plastic flasks should never be used to transport fungal isolates to reference laboratories.

Once inoculated, cultures are incubated at 25 to 30°C. When specimens are derived from deep-site locations such as tissue biopsy, bronchoalveolar lavage (BAL), cerebrospinal fluid, etc., duplicate cultures may be prepared and incubated at 35 to 37°C to encourage faster growth of pathogenic fungi. Fungal cultures should be incubated for 4 to 6 weeks before being regarded as negative; however, many cultures can be read as early as 24 h after inoculation. For example, most yeasts are detected within 5 or fewer days, and dermatophytes are detected within 1 week. However, dematiaceous and dimorphic fungi may require 2 to 4 weeks. Therefore, to account for differences in growth rates, fungal cultures should be examined at regular intervals (e.g., daily during the first week, three times the second week, twice at 3 weeks, and once at 4 weeks) rather than being evaluated once at the end of 4 weeks. While growth may be observed within the first few weeks of incubation, incubation should be continued for the original plate, after subculture, to allow for the emergence of slower-growing pathogenic organisms. Manipulation of cultures must be performed inside a certified biological safety cabinet to prevent contamination of the plate and exposure of personnel to potentially hazardous fungi.

Each new lot of medium, whether purchased or prepared in-house, must be subjected to a quality control protocol that verifies appearance, pH, and performance (12, 15). Both positive and negative control strains need to be included in quality assurance testing protocols (12, 15). Media for primary isolation should be tested for optimal growth of several fungal pathogens. Selective media should be tested with strains known to be susceptible and resistant to the inhibitory agent in the media, while differential media should be evaluated with fungi that produce both positive and negative reactions. Many media are also commercially available as prepared plates or tubes. Although manufacturers perform quality control testing, clinical laboratories still need to ensure that media meet performance standards. Some widely used commercially prepared media may be exempt from routine quality assurance testing, when proof of quality assurance testing is provided by the media manufacturer. Nonexempt media still require specific quality assurance testing. A list of media in these categories can be found in CLSI documents M22-A3 and M54-A (12, 15). These requirements apply to those working in the United States; regulations may differ in other countries. Accrediting agencies in the United States, such as Centers for Medicare and Medicaid Services through the Clinical Laboratory Improvement Act or College of American Pathologists, no longer recognize the exempt status of certain media from quality assurance testing. Therefore, clinical laboratories that undergo inspection by accrediting agencies must perform quality assurance testing on all lots of media used in the laboratory.

Unless stated otherwise, the reagents and media listed in this chapter should be prepared by dissolving the components in the stated liquid with a magnetic stirring bar. The standard sterilization technique of autoclaving at 121°C at 15 lb/in^2 for 15 min should be used when needed. However, certain solutions, such as those containing antibiotics or carbohydrates, cannot be autoclaved because they will be denatured. These solutions are sterilized by filtration through a 0.22-μm-pore-size filter and added to the post-sterilized media after being cooled sufficiently; *Candida* chromogenic agars can be heated in a microwave.

Storage of prepared reagents in sterile, airtight, screw-cap containers is recommended. Some reagents require storage in dark containers, and some need to be stored refrigerated (2 to 8°C) instead of at room temperature. Special storage instructions are given when appropriate. Standard safety precautions should be taken when preparing the reagents. Follow the safety guidelines for the chemicals being used, in addition to the laboratory safety protocols.

The stains, media, and reagents listed in this chapter include those commonly used and a few specialized items. While outside the focus of this chapter, it is important to mention the usefulness of histopathology in the diagnosis of fungal infections (16). Several of the stains listed below—Fontana-Masson stain, methenamine silver stain, mucicarmine stain, and periodic acid-Schiff stain—are also used in the histopathological diagnosis of fungal infections (17). For more specific information not included here, refer to the literature cited in the chapter.

REAGENTS

■ *N*-Acetyl-L-cysteine (NALC) (0.5%)

NALC (Alpha Tec Systems, Inc.) is a mucolytic agent used for digestion of sputum specimens submitted for detection of *Pneumocystis jirovecii* cysts and/or trophozoites by microscopic examination. This compound can also be used for preparing samples for microscopic examination for a wide range of fungi. Sodium citrate (0.1 M) is included in the mixture to exert a stabilizing effect on the acetyl-L-cysteine. Formulations containing sodium hydroxide (NaOH) should be avoided because of adverse effects on fungal organisms.

■ Dithiothreitol (Sputolysin), 0.0065 M

Dithiothreitol is a mucolytic agent that can be purchased commercially and has been used to prepare sputum specimens for detection of *P. jirovecii*. Equal volumes of sputum and dithiothreitol are mixed and incubated at 35°C. The mixture is periodically mixed vigorously until nearly liquefied (complete liquefaction disperses the cells of *P. jirovecii*, making microscopic detection difficult). As with NALC, dithiothreitol can be useful for preparing samples for microscopic examination of a wide range of fungi. Formulations containing NaOH should be avoided because of adverse effects on fungal organisms.

■ Potassium hydroxide (KOH)

Wet mounts prepared in 10% KOH are used to distinguish fungi in thick mucoid specimens or in specimens that contain keratinous material such as skin, hair, and nails. Nails may require stronger alkaline treatment (up to 25%) to digest the nail prior to microscopic examination (see chapter 126 for more details). While the proteinaceous components of the host cells are partially digested, the fungal cell wall is left intact and more apparent. An aliquot of specimen is added to a drop of 10% or 20% KOH, which can be preserved with 0.1% thimerosal (Sigma Chemical Co.). The slide is held at room temperature for 5 to 30 min after the addition of KOH, depending on the specimen type, to allow digestion to occur. Digestive capabilities can be enhanced with gentle heating or the addition of 40% dimethyl sulfoxide (18). Solutions of NaOH (10% or 25% with added glycerin) may be used as alternatives to potassium hydroxide for the direct microscopic examination of hair, skin, and nails for dermatophyte-mediated infections. Visualization of fungal elements may be enhanced by the addition of lactophenol cotton blue or glucan-binding fluorescent brighteners such as calcofluor white, which bind to chitin, a major component of the fungal cell wall, as discussed below.

STAINS

■ Alcian blue stain

Alcian blue and the more commonly used mucicarmine stain (see below) are mucopolysaccharide stains. These are useful for visualizing the polysaccharide capsule produced by *Cryptococcus* species in histological sections of tissue.

Basic Procedure

Deparaffinized sections are stained in Alcian blue (1 g in 100 ml of acetic acid, 3% solution) for 30 min, washed in running tap water, and then rinsed in distilled water. The sections are counterstained in nuclear fast red (0.1 g in 100 ml of aluminum sulfate, 5% solution). After dehydration through 95% and absolute alcohol, the sections are cleared with xylene and mounted in Permount (Fisher Scientific). Capsular polysaccharides stain blue against a pink background.

■ Ascospore stain

Ascomycetous fungi may produce ascospores when grown on media that promote their formation. Visualization of ascospores can be accomplished with a differential staining procedure consisting of malachite green and safranin. Ascospores stain green, and the vegetative portion of the fungus stains red. The Kinyoun acid-fast stain (see chapter 31) may also be used for visualizing ascospores, as these structures tend to be acid fast.

Basic Procedure

A thin smear of growth is applied to a glass slide and heat fixed. The slide is flooded with malachite green (5 g in 100 ml of distilled water) for 3 min, washed with tap water, decolorized with 95% ethyl alcohol for 30 s, and counterstained with aqueous safranin (5%) for 30 s. The slide is washed with tap water, allowed to air dry, and examined at ×400 to ×1,000 magnification.

■ Calcofluor white

Calcofluor white and related compounds such as Uvitex 2B and Blankophor are nonspecific, nonimmunological fluorochromes that bind to β-1,3 and β-1,4 polysaccharides, specifically cellulose and chitin of fungal cell walls. Like the auramine-rhodamine stain, calcofluor white has become commonplace in microbiology laboratories because of the rapidity with which specimens can be observed. The fluorochrome can be mixed with KOH to clear specimens for easier observation of fungal elements. Fungal elements appear bluish white against a dark background when excited with UV or blue-violet radiation. Optimal fluorescence occurs with UV excitation. A barrier filter such as 510, 520, or 530 should be used for eye protection. Organisms impart a blue-white to green fluorescence (20) depending on the combination of excitation and barrier filters used. Typical *P. jirovecii* cysts are 5 to 8 μm in diameter, round, and uniform in size, and they exhibit a characteristic peripheral cyst wall staining with an intense "double parenthesis-like" structure (19, 20). Yeast cells are differentiated from *P. jirovecii* by budding and intense staining. Care must be used in interpreting the calcofluor white staining results because nonspecific reactions may be observed. Cotton fibers fluoresce strongly and must be differentiated from fungal hyphae. Additionally, tissues such as brain biopsy specimens from patients with tumors may fluoresce and resemble hyphae suggestive of *Aspergillus* or other moulds with branching hyphae.

Basic Procedure

Calcofluor white may be purchased from multiple mycological media and chemical suppliers either as premixed or in powdered form (see list of suppliers at the end of the chapter). KOH (10%) is mixed in equal proportion with calcofluor white solution (0.1 g of calcofluor white M2R and 0.05 g of Evans blue in 100 ml of water). The specimen is covered with this mixture and a coverslip is applied. Allow the slide to sit for 5 to 10 minutes prior to viewing the slide to permit the tissue to clear and the stain to interact with the fungal elements. Some nail and tissue preparations may require a longer incubation time (up to 30 minutes) for clearing to occur. Alternatively, the slides may be gently warmed on a slide warmer to speed up the clearing process. For optimal results the slide should be viewed as soon as the tissue has cleared. The preparation is examined with a fluorescent microscope containing appropriate excitation and barrier filters at ×100 to ×400 magnification. Darkly pigmented fungi may stain poorly with calcofluor white because of the pigmentation, which may mask the fluorescence.

■ Colloidal carbon wet mounts (India ink, nigrosin)

Colloidal carbon wet mounts are used for visualization of encapsulated microorganisms, especially *Cryptococcus* species. The polysaccharide capsule of organisms is refractory to the particles of ink, and capsules appear as clear halos around the organism. Artifacts such as erythrocytes, leukocytes, and talc particles from gloves or bubbles following a myelogram may displace the colloidal suspension and mimic yeast (false positive). These artifacts make it necessary to perform a careful examination of the wet mount for properties consistent with the organisms (e.g., rounded forms with buds of various sizes and double-contoured cell walls). Interpretation can also be hindered if the emulsion with the colloid suspension is too thick, blocking transmission of light.

Basic Procedure

Mix equal parts of the patient's cerebrospinal fluid with either commercial art India ink or nigrosin on a slide. Add a coverslip and examine at ×100 to ×1,000 magnification. Care must be taken not to contaminate India ink supplied in larger volumes. Limited-volume or individual-use dispensers can be purchased through many of the media and reagent distributers.

■ Fontana-Masson stain

The Fontana-Masson stain was originally developed for demonstrating melanin granules in mammalian tissue. It has a mycological application in detecting dematiaceous (melanin-containing) fungi, and to a lesser extent *Cryptococcus neoformans/gattii*, in histological sections. Fungal elements appear brown to brownish black against a reddish background.

Basic Procedure

A silver solution is prepared by adding concentrated ammonium hydroxide to 10% silver nitrate until the precipitated form disappears. Deparaffinized sections of tissue are hydrated and placed in heated silver solution for 30 to 60 min.

The slides are then rinsed in distilled water and toned in gold chloride (0.2 g in 100 ml of distilled water) for 10 min, followed by fixation in 5% sodium thiosulfate for 5 min. The sections are dehydrated through increasing concentrations of alcohol, cleared in xylene, and mounted with a coverslip.

■ Giemsa stain

The Giemsa stain is used for the detection of intracellular yeast forms of *Histoplasma capsulatum* in bone marrow and buffy coat specimens. The fungus is usually seen as small oval yeast cells, often contained within macrophages, and stains blue; a hyaline halo represents poorly staining cell wall. The stain can also be used to visualize the trophozoite of *P. jirovecii*.

Basic Procedure

A thin smear is prepared on a glass slide and placed in 100% methanol for 1 min. The slide is drained and then flooded with freshly prepared Giemsa stain (stock Giemsa stain diluted 1:10 with phosphate-buffered water). After 5 min, the slide is rinsed with distilled water and air dried. Examine at ×100 to ×400 magnification.

■ Lacto-fuchsin

Lacto-fuchsin is a mounting fluid that can be used as an alternative to the widely used lactophenol cotton blue (below). It stains fungal structures more quickly, and the refractive index of the lacto-fuchsin mounting medium is such that fungal structures may be more visible (21). Fungal structures stain pink to red. Lacto-fuchsin stain has a prolonged drying time; to prevent movement that could disrupt the microscopic structures of the mould, the coverslip should be ringed with nail polish.

Basic Procedure

Lacto-fuchsin is made by dissolving 0.1 g of acid fuchsin in 100 ml of lactic acid (85%). For a more permanent mount, polyvinyl alcohol may be added to the solution. Commercial preparations can be obtained from companies listed at the end of this chapter.

■ Lactophenol cotton blue

Lactophenol cotton blue (LPCB) is a basic mounting medium for fungi consisting of phenol, lactic acid, glycerol, and aniline (cotton) blue dye. The solution may be filtered to remove precipitated dye and stored at room temperature. It is commonly used for the microscopic examination of fungal cultures by tease or tape preparation. LPCB with 10% polyvinyl alcohol (LPCB-PVA) makes an excellent permanent stain or fixative for mounting slide culture preparations (3).

Basic Procedure

Concentrated phenol (20% [vol/vol]) is added to a mixture of glycerol (40%), lactic acid (20%), and water (20%), followed by the addition of aniline blue (0.05 g). The solution may be filter sterilized to remove precipitated dye. A drop is added to a glass slide, and a tease or tape mount is prepared. Add a coverslip and examine at ×100 to ×400 magnification.

■ Lactophenol cotton blue and potassium hydroxide (10%)

The addition of KOH to the wet mount with LPCB is used for the same purpose as the KOH preparation (see above). However, LPCB enhances the visibility of fungi in the KOH solution because aniline blue stains the outer cell wall of fungi and lactic acid serves as an additional clearing agent. The phenol component in LPCB acts as a fungicide.

■ Methenamine silver stain

Methenamine silver stains are perhaps the most useful stains for visualizing fungi in tissue. Fungal elements are sharply delineated in black against a pale green or yellow background. They are specialized stains that are more often performed in the histology laboratory than in the microbiology laboratory. Grocott's modification of the Gomori methenamine silver stain is commonly used for the histopathological examination of deparaffinized tissues for fungi. A variation that can be used by counterstaining with the hematoxylin and eosin stain displays the silver-stained fungal structures within a host tissue reaction.

Basic Procedure

Stock methenamine silver nitrate solution is prepared by adding 3% methenamine (3 g in 100 ml of distilled water) to 5% silver nitrate (5 g in 100 ml of distilled water) until a white precipitate forms that clears upon shaking. This solution is then diluted 1:2 with distilled water, to which 5 ml of 5% photographic-grade borax is added. Prepared slides are oxidized in a solution of chromic acid (5 g in 100 ml of distilled water), neutralized in sodium bisulfite (1 g in 100 ml of distilled water), placed in the diluted methenamine silver nitrate solution, and heated in an oven to 58 to 60°C until the material turns yellowish brown. After being rinsed vigorously in distilled water, the slides are toned in gold chloride (0.1 g in 100 ml of distilled water). Unreduced silver is removed by placing the slides in a sodium thiosulfate solution (2 g in 100 ml of distilled water) and counterstained in 0.03% light green. Rinse, blot dry, and examine at ×100 to ×400 magnification.

■ Mucicarmine stain

The mucicarmine stain is useful for differentiating *C. neoformans* and *C. gattii* from other fungi of similar size and shape when found in samples of tissue. The mucopolysaccharide in the capsular material of the fungus stains deep rose to red, whereas the other tissue elements stain yellow. *Blastomyces dermatitidis* and *Rhinosporidium seeberi* may also react positively with this stain but are differentiated by the size of the yeast and the intensity of the staining reaction of the mucopolysaccharide capsule of *Cryptococcus*.

Basic Procedure

Fixed tissue sections on glass slides are stained first with Weigert's iron hematoxylin and then placed in a solution of mucicarmine (1 g of carmine combined with 0.5 g of anhydrous aluminum chloride in 2 ml of distilled water and then diluted in 100 ml of 50% ethanol) for 30 to 60 min. The slides are rinsed in distilled water and then counterstained in metanil yellow (0.25 g in 100 ml of distilled water). Rinse, blot dry, and examine at ×100 to ×400 magnification.

■ Periodic acid-Schiff (PAS) stain

The PAS stain is used to detect fungi in clinical specimens, especially yeast cells and hyphae in tissues. Fungi stain a bright pink-magenta or purple against an orange background if picric acid is used as the counterstain, or against a green background if light green is used. The procedure is a multistep method combining hydrolysis and staining. The periodic acid step hydrolyzes the cell wall aldehydes, which are then able to combine with the modified Schiff reagent, coloring the cell wall carbohydrates a bright pink-magenta. The PAS stain is an excellent general stain because most fungi in clinical material take up the stain. However, the PAS staining procedure is rather involved, requiring several different reagents and time-consuming steps, and has been replaced in many laboratories by the calcofluor white staining procedure. The PAS stain cannot be used with undigested respiratory secretions as mucin also stains bright pink-magenta.

Basic Procedure

The prepared slide is fixed in formalin ethanol for 1 min and is then air dried. The slide is then immersed in 5% periodic acid for 5 min, followed by 2 min in basic fuchsin (0.1 g of dye in 5 ml of 95% alcohol and 95 ml of H_2O). The slide is rinsed in water and immersed in zinc or sodium hydrosulfite solution for 10 min (1 g of zinc or sodium hydrosulfite in 0.5 g of tartaric acid and 100 ml of H_2O). Rinse in water and counterstain with saturated aqueous picric acid for 2 min or with light green stain (1 g of dye in 0.25 ml of acetic acid and 100 ml of 80% alcohol) for 5 s. Rinse, blot dry, and examine at ×100 to ×400 magnification.

■ Toluidine blue O

Toluidine blue O is used primarily for the rapid detection of *P. jirovecii* from lung biopsy specimen imprints and BAL specimens (22). Toluidine blue O stains the cysts of *P. jirovecii* reddish blue or dark purple against a light blue background. The cysts are often clumped and may be punched in, appearing crescent shaped. Trophozoites are not discernible. Although the silver stain, monoclonal antibody, and calcofluor white stains are also used, the toluidine blue O stain is easy and rapid and yields reliable results with appropriate specimens (e.g., BAL specimens).

Basic Procedure

After the slide is air dried, place it in the sulfation reagent (45 ml of glacial acetic acid mixed with 15 ml of concentrated sulfuric acid) for 10 min. Rinse in cold water for 5 min, drain, and place in toluidine blue O (0.3 g of dye in 60 ml of H_2O) for 3 min. Rinse in 95% ethanol, followed by absolute ethanol and then xylene. Examine at ×100 to ×1,000 magnification.

MEDIA

■ Agar slide culture plate

Microscopic morphology of a fungal isolate is best observed with the slide culture method, in which an approximately 15-by-15-mm square block of media is placed on a sterile microscope slide. The desired fungal organism is inoculated on each of the block's edges, covered with a sterile 22 × 22 mm coverslip, and incubated in an individual humidified chamber. When sufficient sporulation is present, the coverslip is removed and placed growth side down on a microscope slide containing a drop of lactophenol cotton blue or other appropriate mounting fluid. Fungal morphology is visualized microscopically at ×200 and ×400 magnification. Commercial sources are available with preformed slide culture setups. Agar and incubation temperature used should be selected on the basis of the optimum conditions to induce sporulation for the fungal organism used. This agar can be found commercially through Remel (Slide Culture Plate) and Hardy Diagnostics (Mycovue) as listed at the end of this chapter.

■ Acetate ascospore agar

Acetate ascospore agar is used for the cultivation of ascosporogenous yeasts such as *Saccharomyces cerevisiae*. A potassium acetate formulation has been shown to be a better sporulation medium than the previously used formulation with sodium acetate. Ascospores produced on this medium are visible microscopically after staining with Kinyoun carbol-fuchsin acid-fast stain.

■ Antifungal susceptibility testing media

Recent advances in methods for antifungal susceptibility testing have resulted in several media that are now used for this type of testing. See chapter 134 of this volume for a comprehensive review of this topic.

■ Birdseed agar

Birdseed agar is a selective and differential medium used for the isolation of *Cryptococcus* species, especially *C. neoformans* and *C. gattii*, which are unique in that they produce the enzyme phenol oxidase. The breakdown of the substrate (*Guizotia abyssinica* seeds or niger seed) produces melanin, which is absorbed into the yeast wall and imparts a tan to brown pigmentation of the colonies. Colonies of other yeasts are beige or cream in color. Chloramphenicol is the selective agent that inhibits bacteria and some fungi. Creatinine enhances melanization of some strains of *C. neoformans*.

■ Bismuth sulfite-glucose-glycine yeast (BiGGY) agar

BiGGY agar is a selective and differential medium used for the isolation and differentiation of *Candida* spp. Peptone, glucose, and yeast extract are the nutritive bases. *Candida* species reduce the bismuth sulfite to bismuth sulfide, which results in pigmentation of the yeast colony and, with some species, the surrounding medium. *Candida albicans* appears as brown to black colonies with no pigment diffusion and no sheen, whereas *Candida tropicalis* appears as dark brown colonies with black centers, black pigment diffusion, and sheen. Specific colonial morphologies and growth patterns of the different *Candida* species are also detected. The bismuth sulfite also acts as an inhibitor of bacterial growth, making the medium selective.

■ Blood-glucose-cysteine agar

A fungal isolate believed to be a thermally dimorphic pathogen can be identified by converting the mould phase to the yeast phase at 37°C. Blood-glucose-cysteine agar medium is used to promote the mould-to-yeast conversion of *Histoplasma capsulatum*, *Blastomyces dermatitidis*, *Paracoccidioides brasiliensis*, and *Sporothrix schenckii*. The medium contains tryptose blood agar base, L-cysteine, and defibrinated sheep blood. Penicillin is added to inhibit bacterial contamination.

■ Brain heart infusion agar (fungal formulation)

Brain heart infusion (BHI) agar with sheep blood is a medium used for the cultivation and isolation of all fungi including fastidious dimorphic fungi. The nutritive base is BHI agar with 10% sheep blood for added enrichment. The antibiotics chloramphenicol and gentamicin are added to make the medium selective by inhibiting bacteria. This medium does not inhibit saprophytic fungi. When attempting to isolate more fastidious moulds, a medium containing cycloheximide should be included to inhibit overgrowth by the saprophytic fungi.

■ Bromcresol purple milk solids glucose medium

Bromcresol purple milk solids glucose (Dermatophyte Milk Agar; Hardy Diagnostics) is a differential medium used for the identification of *Trichophyton* species. The medium's differential capacity is based on the type of growth (profuse versus restricted as compared to growth on standard nutrient media) and change in the pH indicator due to the production of alkaline by-products.

■ Caffeic agar

Caffeic agar is an adaptation of the birdseed agar, as discussed previously. Caffeic acid is the biologically active chemical in niger seed that causes the yeast colony of *C. neoformans* to turn brown (23).

■ Canavanine-glycine-bromthymol blue agar

Canavanine-glycine-bromthymol blue agar is a differential medium for distinguishing *C. neoformans* from *C. gattii*. The medium contains glycine, thiamine, L-canavanine sulfate, and bromthymol blue. A colony of *Cryptococcus* is streaked onto the surface of the agar and incubated at 30°C for 1 to 5 days. *C. gattii* (serotypes B and C) turns the medium cobalt blue, whereas *C. neoformans* var. *grubii* (serotype A) and *C. neoformans* var. *neoformans* (serotype D) leave the medium greenish yellow.

■ *Candida* chromogenic media

The introduction of chromogenic media has facilitated the direct and rapid identification of yeasts and is particularly useful for detecting and separating mixed cultures. These media contain chromogenic substrates that are hydrolyzed by species-specific enzymes, e.g., β-*N*-acetylhexosaminidase and, depending on the medium, a second enzyme, β-glucosidase or phosphatase, resulting in identification of yeasts to the species level based on colonial features and color development (24–26). Commercially available chromogenic media are summarized in Table 1.

A brief description of selected chromogenic agar products that are approved by the U.S. FDA for use in United States laboratories is provided as an overview of how different yeasts react with chromogenic substrates and the resultant characteristic colony color.

■ CHROMagar (BD BBL; BD Diagnostics Systems)

CHROMagar is a differential and selective medium used for the isolation and differentiation of clinically important yeasts. The nutritive base is peptone and glucose. Chloramphenicol makes the medium selective by inhibiting bacteria. The medium is available with and without fluconazole, the former providing the additional selection of fluconazole-resistant yeasts such as *Candida krusei*. A proprietary chromogenic mixture allows the differentiation of many yeast species. For example, *C. albicans* forms yellow-green to blue-green colonies. Colonial morphology and distinctive color patterns have been shown to make the presumptive identification of yeast species very reliable (24, 26). The medium has been shown to be more selective than Sabouraud agar and helpful in identifying mixed cultures of yeasts, and it may enhance the rapid assimilation of trehalose by *Candida glabrata* (26). The colonies on the medium should be evaluated at 48 h. Although *C. neoformans* and *Geotrichum* species can grow on this medium, definitive identification requires subculture to a nonselective medium followed by use of the appropriate biochemical and morphological characterization tools.

■ chromID candida agar (CAN2) (bioMérieux)

Colonies of *C. albicans* produce a blue color following the hydrolysis of a hexosaminidase chromogenic substrate in the presence of an inducer of the enzyme (bioMérieux patent). The hydrolysis of a second substrate (pink color) differentiates mixed cultures and indicates the need for identification of other species of yeast (bioMérieux patent).

■ Christensen's urea agar

The ability to hydrolyze urea is an important phenotypic characteristic for the presumptive identification of *Cryptococcus*, *Trichosporon*, and *Rhodotorula* spp. Urea hydrolysis also facilitates separation of certain dermatophytes, in particular *Trichophyton mentagrophytes* and *Trichophyton rubrum*. The medium contains 2% urea, with phenol red serving as the indicator.

■ Cornmeal agar with 1% dextrose

Cornmeal agar with 1% dextrose is used for the cultivation of fungi and the differentiation of *T. mentagrophytes* from *T. rubrum* on the basis of pigment production. The replacement of Tween 80 (polysorbate 80) with dextrose promotes the growth and production of a red pigment by *T. rubrum*.

■ Cornmeal agar with Tween 80

Cornmeal agar with Tween (polysorbate) 80 is used for the cultivation and differentiation of *Candida* species on the basis of morphological characteristics. Tween 80, a surfactant, is specifically incorporated in lieu of dextrose for the demonstration of pseudohyphal, chlamydospore, and

TABLE 1 Commercial sources of yeast chromogenic agar media

Medium	Manufacturer	Candida species identified[a]
Candida Diagnostic Agar (CDA)	Helier Scientific, Ltd.	*C. albicans*, *C. kefyr*, and *C. tropicalis*
Candida Chromogenic Agar	Laboratorios CONDA	*C. albicans*, *C. tropicalis*, and *C. krusei*
Candi*Select* 4	Bio-Rad Laboratories	*C. albicans* Presumptive identification: *C. glabrata*, *C. tropicalis*, and *C. krusei*
CHROMagar Candida	CHROMagar Microbiology	*C. albicans*, *C. tropicalis*, and *C. krusei*
BBL CHROMagar	BD Diagnostic Systems	*C. albicans*, *C. tropicalis*, and *C. krusei*
chromID Candida Agar	bioMérieux, Inc.	*C. albicans* Presumptive identification: *C. tropicalis*, *C. lusitaniae*, and *C. kefyr*
HardyCHROM Candida	Hardy Diagnostics	*C. albicans*, *C. tropicalis*, and *C. krusei* Presumptive identification: *C. glabrata*
HiCrome Candida Differential Agar	HiMedia Laboratories	*C. albicans*, *C. krusei*, *C. tropicalis*, and *C. glabrata*
Oxoid Brilliance Candida Agar	Oxoid Microbiology Products	*C. albicans*/*C. dubliniensis*, *C. krusei*, and *C. tropicalis* Presumptive identification: *C. glabrata*, *C. kefyr*, *C. parapsilosis*, and *C. lusitaniae*

[a]*Candida* species identified as provided by the manufacturer. Species that are presumptively identified require further testing for final identification.

arthrospore formation. Chlamydospore production is best obtained by subsurface inoculation, or by placing a coverslip over the yeast inoculum, creating a microaerobic environment. The basic nutrients for yeast growth are provided by cornmeal infusion.

■ Czapek-Dox agar

Czapek-Dox agar is a medium used for the differentiation of *Aspergillus* spp. (1, 2, 27). Sucrose is the sole carbon source, with sodium nitrate serving as the sole nitrogen source. Any bacteria or fungi that can use sodium nitrate as a nitrogen source can grow on this medium.

■ Dermatophyte test medium (DTM)

Dermatophyte test medium is used as a screening medium for the recovery, selection, and differentiation of dermatophytes (*Microsporum*, *Trichophyton*, and *Epidermophyton*) from keratinous specimens (hair, skin, and nails). Nitrogenous and carbonaceous compounds are provided by soy peptone. Cycloheximide inhibits saprophytic moulds, chloramphenicol inhibits many Gram-positive bacteria, and gentamicin inhibits Gram-negative bacteria. The morphology and microscopic characteristics are easily identified with this medium. Pigmentation cannot be discerned because of the presence of phenol red indicator. The medium is yellow and turns red with growth of dermatophytes. Because *Aspergillus* species and other saprophytic fungi can grow and produce pigment on this medium, it is recommended as a screening medium only.

■ Inhibitory mould agar

Inhibitory mould agar is a selective and enriched medium that is used for the general cultivation of cycloheximide sensitive fungi (e.g., *Cryptococcus* species, mucoraceous fungi, and *H. capsulatum*) from contaminated specimens. Casein and animal tissue provide growth nutrients. Yeast extract serves as a source of vitamins. Chloramphenicol inhibits many Gram-positive and Gram-negative bacteria. Gentamicin is another additive that inhibits some Gram-negative bacteria. This is an excellent medium for use in the primary cultivation of fungi and has been demonstrated to be more sensitive than the standard Sabouraud dextrose agar (28).

■ Lactritmel agar (Borelli's medium)

Lactritmel agar (Borelli's medium) is composed of whole wheat flour, skim milk, and honey, which favors the sporulation of most dermatophytes and the pigment production of *Trichophyton* species. The medium may also be used for the morphological examination of dematiaceous fungi.

■ Leeming and Notman medium

Leeming and Notman medium is used for the isolation and growth of lipodependent *Malassezia* species. The key components of the medium include ox bile, glycerol monostearate, glycerol, Tween 80, and cow's milk (whole fat) (29). The medium may serve as an alternative to Sabouraud glucose agar because not all species can grow on this medium, e.g., *M. globosa*, *M. restricta*, and *M. obtusa*, which require more complex media for their isolation.

■ Littman oxgall agar

Littman oxgall agar is a selective general-purpose medium used for the isolation of fungi from contaminated specimens. Crystal violet and streptomycin are the selective agents and inhibit bacteria. Oxgall restricts the spreading of fungal colonies. The isolation characteristics of this medium are similar to those of Sabouraud dextrose agar with chloramphenicol and inhibitory mould agar in that it allows the growth of fungi that are sensitive to cycloheximide.

■ Malt extract (2%) agar

This medium is used for the cultivation of yeasts and moulds. A variety of formulations have been described but typically include malt extract with agar; they are supplemented with peptone, glucose, maltose, and dextrin and/or glycerol. Malt agar is particularly useful for stimulating the production of macroconidia in *Microsporum canis*.

■ Mycobiotic or Mycosel agar

Mycobiotic (Remel) and Mycosel (BD Diagnostic Systems) are trade names for a selective medium principally formulated for the isolation of dermatophytes but also used for the isolation of other pathogenic fungi from specimens contaminated with saprophytic fungi and bacteria. The medium consists primarily of peptones from a pancreatic digest of soybean meal and dextrose. The selective agents are cycloheximide and chloramphenicol. Cycloheximide inhibits the faster-growing saprophytic fungi but is also inhibitory to some clinically relevant species. These inhibited fungi include some *Candida* and *Aspergillus* species, mucoraceous fungi, and *C. neoformans*. Chloramphenicol inhibits Gram-negative and Gram-positive organisms.

■ Niger seed agar

See birdseed agar.

■ Potato dextrose agar

Potato dextrose agar is a medium used to stimulate conidium production by fungi. The medium also stimulates pigment production in some dermatophytes. This medium is most commonly used with the slide culture technique to view morphological characteristics. Infusions from potatoes and dextrose provide nutrient factors for excellent growth. The incorporation of tartaric acid in the medium lowers the pH, thereby inhibiting bacterial growth.

■ Potato flake agar

Potato flake agar is a medium useful in the stimulation of conidia by fungi. Its advantages over potato dextrose agar may be preparation and stability. Potato flakes and dextrose provide the nutrient factors that allow excellent growth. The pH is adjusted to 5.6 to enhance growth of fungi and to inhibit bacterial growth. The medium may be made selective by the addition of cycloheximide and chloramphenicol.

■ Sabouraud brain heart infusion (SABHI)

SABHI agar is a general-purpose medium used for the isolation and cultivation of all fungi. The medium is a combination of brain heart infusion agar and Sabouraud dextrose agar. The combined formulation allows for the recovery of most fungi, including the yeast phase of dimorphic fungi. The inclusion of sheep blood provides essential growth factors for the more fastidious fungi and enhances the growth of *H. capsulatum*. Selectivity is attained by the addition of chloramphenicol, cycloheximide, penicillin, and/or streptomycin.

■ Sabouraud dextrose agar

Sabouraud dextrose agar was formulated by Sabouraud for cultivating dermatophytes. The medium consists of pancreatic digest of casein, peptic digest of animal tissue, and dextrose at 4% concentration, buffered to a pH of 5.6. Emmons modified the original formulation by reducing the dextrose concentration to 2% and adjusting the pH nearer to neutrality at 6.9 to 7.0. Antibiotic additives in various combinations include cycloheximide, chloramphenicol, gentamicin, ciprofloxacin, penicillin, and/or streptomycin, which inhibit some fungi and Gram-positive and Gram-negative bacteria to achieve selectivity for this medium. This medium is also available as a broth.

■ Soil extract agar

Soil extract agar is a medium composed of garden soil, yeast extract, and glucose. The primary use of this medium is to promote sporulation of some saprobic fungi and for mating strains of *B. dermatitidis* (2).

■ Trichophyton agars 1 to 7

Trichophyton agars are a set of seven media that facilitate the identification of *Trichophyton* species on the basis of their growth factor requirements. The basic ingredients in the media are listed below. Growth in all seven media is then scored on a scale of 1 to 4, and an identification is assigned.

1. Casamino Acids; vitamin-free
2. Casamino Acids plus inositol
3. Casamino Acids plus inositol and thiamine
4. Casamino Acids plus thiamine
5. Casamino Acids plus niacin
6. Ammonium nitrate
7. Ammonium nitrate plus histidine

■ V8 agar

V8 agar is a medium consisting of dehydrated potato flakes and V-8 juice (Campbell Soup Co., Camden, NJ) that induces early sporulation of some environmental fungi. The naturally low pH makes the medium inhibitory to most bacteria.

■ Water (tap) agar

This medium is nutritionally deficient (1% water-agar: 1 g of agar, 100 ml of sterile tap water) and promotes the sporulation of dematiaceous fungi, *Apophysomyces elegans*, and *Saksenaea vasiformis* (30). The medium can be supplemented with sterilized carnation leaves for the identification of *Fusarium* species (8).

■ Yeast carbon agar

Yeast carbon agar is a solid medium recommended for use in qualitative procedures for the classification of yeasts according to their ability to assimilate nitrogenous compounds. The yeast's carbon base provides amino acids, vitamins, trace elements, and salts that are necessary to support growth. The ability to assimilate nitrogen is tested by the addition of various nitrogen sources such as potassium nitrate. While this traditional method of yeast identification may still be used, newer and simpler commercial methods or molecular methods are available for identification.

■ Yeast extract phosphate agar with ammonia (Smith's medium)

Yeast extract phosphate agar with ammonia (Smith's medium) is used for the isolation and sporulation of *H. capsulatum* and *B. dermatitidis* from contaminated specimens. This consists of phosphate buffer (Na_2HPO_4, KH_2PO_4, and distilled water). It should be mixed well with the pH adjusted to 6.0 with 1 N HCl or 1 N NaOH and yeast extract agar solution. Before inoculation of specimens, 1 drop of ammonium hydroxide is applied to the agar surface and allowed to diffuse into the medium. The combination of ammonium hydroxide and chloramphenicol suppresses bacteria and many moulds and yeasts, thus permitting detection of the slowly growing dimorphic fungi.

APPENDIX

Commercial Manufacturers and Supplies of Fungal Media, Stains, and Reagents

Alpha Tec Systems, Inc.
P.O. Box 5435
Vancouver, WA 98668
800-221-6058
http://www.alphatecsystems.com

BD Diagnostic Systems
7 Loveton Circle
Sparks, MD 21152
800-675-0908
http://www.bd.com

bioMérieux, Inc.
100 Rodolphe St.
Durham, NC 27712
800-682-2666
http://www.biomerieux-diagnostics.com/

Bio-Rad Laboratories
5500 East Second St.
Benicia, CA 94510
800-224-6723
http://www.bio-rad.com/

CHROMagar
4 Place du 18 Juin 1940
75006 Paris
France
Tel: +33 1 45 48 05 05
Fax: +33 1 45 48 05 06
chromagar@chromagar.com
http://chromagar.com/

Fisher Scientific
2000 Park Lane Dr.
Pittsburgh, PA 15275
800-766-7000
http://www.fishersci.com

Fluka Chemika/Biochemika
Industriestrasse 25
9471 Buchs
Switzerland
41 (0) 81 755 25 11
webmaster@sial.com
https://www.lab-honeywell.com

Hardy Diagnostics
1430 West McCoy Lane
Santa Maria, CA 93455
800-266-2222
http://www.hardydiagnostics.com

HiMedia Laboratories Pvt. Ltd.
23 Vadhani Est. LBS Marg
Mumbai 400 086
India
91 22 40951919
info@himedialabs.com
http://www.himedialabs.com

Laboratorios Conda
c/La Forja, 9
28850 Torrejon de Ardoz, Madrid
Spain
Phone: +34 91 761 02 00
Fax: +34 91 656 82 28
http://www.condalab.com

Newcomer Supply Inc.
2505 Parview Road
Middleton, WI 53562-2579
Phone: 800-383-7799
Fax: 608-831-0866
http://newcomersupply.com

Oxoid Limited
Wade Road
Basingstoke, Hampshire RG24 8PW
United Kingdom
44 (0) 1256 841144
Fax: 44 (0) 1256 814626
www.oxoid.com/uk/blue

Helier Scientific Limited
SWT Institute for Renal Research
Wrythe Lane
Carshalton
London
SM5 1AA
United Kingdom
Telephone: +44 (0)208 296 3111
http://www.helierscientific.com

Remel
12076 Santa Fe Dr.
Lenexa, KS 66215
800-255-6730
http://www.remel.com/

Scientific Device Laboratory
411 Jarvis Ave.
Des Plaines, IL 60018
847-803-9495
http://www.scientificdevice.com

Sigma-Aldrich Corp.
3050 Spruce St.
St. Louis, MO 63103
314-771-5765
http://www.sigmaaldrich.com

The findings and conclusions in this report are those of the author(s) and do not necessarily represent the official position of the Centers for Disease Control and Prevention. Use of trade names and commercial sources is for identification only and does not imply endorsement by the Centers for Disease Control and Prevention.

REFERENCES

1. **McGinnis M.** 1980. *Laboratory Handbook of Medical Mycology.* Academic Press, New York, NY.
2. **Dismukes WE, Pappas PG, Sobel JD.** 2003. *Clinical Mycology.* Oxford University Press, Inc, New York, NY.
3. **Larone DH.** 2011. *Medically Important Fungi*, 5th ed. ASM Press, Washington, DC.
4. **Best M, Graham ML, Leitner R, Ouellette M, Ugwu K.** 2004. *Laboratory Biosafety Guidelines*, 3rd ed. Minister of Population and Public Health Branch Centre for Emergency Preparedness and Response, Ottawa, Canada.
5. **World Health Organization.** 2004. *Laboratory Biosafety Manual*, 3rd ed. World Health Organization, Geneva, Switzerland.
6. **Chosewood LC, Wilson DE.** 2009. *Biosafety in Microbiological and Biomedical Laboratories*, 5th ed. U.S. Department of Health and Human Services, Washington, DC.
7. **Atlas RM, Snyder JW.** 2006. *Handbook of Media for Clinical Microbiology*, 2nd ed. Taylor & Francis, Boca Raton, FL.
8. **Leslie JF, Summerell BA (ed).** 2006. *The Fusarium Laboratory Manual.* Blackwell Publishing, Ames, IA.
9. **St-Germain G, Summerbell R.** 2011. *Identifying Fungi: A Clinical Laboratory Handbook*, 2nd ed. Star Publishing Company, Belmont, CA.
10. **Campbell CK, Johnson EM, Warnock DW.** 2013. *Identification of Pathogenic Fungi*, 2nd ed. Wiley-Blackwell, West Sussex, United Kingdom.
11. **Kidd SE, Halliday CL, Alexou H, Ellis DH.** 2017. *Descriptions of Medical Fungi*, 3rd ed. Adelaide Medical Centre for Women and Children, Adelaide, Australia.
12. **Clinical and Laboratory Standards Institute.** 2012. *Principles and Procedures for Detection of Fungi in Clinical Specimens—Direct Examination and Culture. Standard M54-A.* Clinical and Laboratory Standards Institute, Wayne, PA.
13. **Summerbell RC.** 1993. The benomyl test as a fundamental diagnostic method for medical mycology. *J Clin Microbiol* **31:**572–577.
14. **Pham CD, Ahn S, Turner LA, Wohrle R, Lockhart SR.** 2014. Development and validation of benomyl birdseed agar for the isolation of *Cryptococcus neoformans* and *Cryptococcus gattii* from environmental samples. *Med Mycol* **52:**417–421..
15. **National Committee for Clinical Laboratory Standards.** 2004. *Quality Control for Commercially Prepared Microbiological Culture Media. Standard M22-A3.* National Committee for Clinical Laboratory Standards, Wayne, PA.
16. **Guarner J, Brandt ME.** 2011. Histopathologic diagnosis of fungal infections in the 21st century. *Clin Microbiol Rev* **24:**247–280.
17. **Chandler FW, Kaplan W, Ajello L.** 1980. *Color atlas and text of the histopathology of mycotic diseases.* Year Book, Chicago, IL.
18. **Dasgupta T, Sahu J.** 2012. Origins of the KOH technique. *Clin Dermatol* **30:**238–241, discussion 241–242.
19. **Hageage GJ Jr, Harrington BJ.** 1984. Use of calcofluor white in clinical mycology. *Lab Med* **15:**109–112.
20. **Kim YK, Parulekar S, Yu PK, Pisani RJ, Smith TF, Anhalt JP.** 1990. Evaluation of calcofluor white stain for detection of *Pneumocystis carinii. Diagn Microbiol Infect Dis* **13:**307–310..
21. **Carmichael JW.** 1955. Lacto-fuchsin: a new medium for mounting fungi. *Mycologia* **47:**611–611.
22. **Paradis IL, Ross C, Dekker A, Dauber J.** 1990. A comparison of modified methenamine silver and toluidine blue stains for the detection of *Pneumocystis carinii* in bronchoalveolar lavage specimens from immunosuppressed patients. *Acta Cytol* **34:**511–516.
23. **Vidotto V, Aoki S, Pontón J, Quindós G, Koga-Ito CY, Pugliese A.** 2004. A new caffeic acid minimal synthetic medium for the rapid identification of *Cryptococcus neoformans* isolates. *Rev Iberoam Micol* **21:**87–89.
24. **Odds FC, Bernaerts R.** 1994. CHROMagar Candida, a new differential isolation medium for presumptive identification of clinically important *Candida* species. *J Clin Microbiol* **32:**1923–1929.

25. **Murray MP, Zinchuk R, Larone DH.** 2005. CHROMagar Candida as the sole primary medium for isolation of yeasts and as a source medium for the rapid-assimilation-of-trehalose test. *J Clin Microbiol* **43:**1210–1212.
26. **Pincus DH, Orenga S, Chatellier S.** 2007. Yeast identification—past, present, and future methods. *Med Mycol* **45:**97–121.
27. **Ellis D, Davis S, Alexiou H, Handke R, Bartley R.** 2007. *Descriptions of Medical Fungi*, 2nd ed. Mycology Unit Women's and Children's Hospital, Adelaide, Australia.
28. **Scognamiglio T, Zinchuk R, Gumpeni P, Larone DH.** 2010. Comparison of inhibitory mold agar to Sabouraud dextrose agar as a primary medium for isolation of fungi. *J Clin Microbiol* **48:**1924–1925.
29. **Leeming JP, Notman FH.** 1987. Improved methods for isolation and enumeration of *Malassezia furfur* from human skin. *J Clin Microbiol* **25:**2017–2019.
30. **Padhye AA, Ajello L.** 1988. Simple method of inducing sporulation by *Apophysomyces elegans* and *Saksenaea vasiformis*. *J Clin Microbiol* **26:**1861–1863.

General Approaches for Direct Detection and Identification of Fungi*

H. RUTH ASHBEE

119

The frequency with which invasive fungal disease occurs has increased markedly over the last decade, and the ability to detect and identify the causative fungi rapidly is essential to the successful management of these diseases (1). While culturing the fungus has always been important to determine the etiology of the infection, other non-culture-based methods may provide more timely results and offer advantages over culture techniques. Non-culture-based methods that will be reviewed in this chapter include direct microscopic examination, antibody and antigen detection, detection of 1,3-β-D-glucan and other fungal metabolites, the use of mass spectrometry, and nucleic acid detection. Although these methods are helpful in clinical use, as yet they have not entirely replaced culture methods and should still be used in conjunction with appropriate culture-based methods (which are reviewed in chapters 117 and 118 of this *Manual*). Although cultures from invasive infections are only infrequently positive, when a culture is obtained it allows susceptibility testing and epidemiological comparisons not widely available via non-culture-based methods.

DIRECT MICROSCOPIC EXAMINATION

The ability to detect fungi in clinical material depends on several factors, including the quality of the specimen that is received into the laboratory. If very small samples are received, few fungi may be present, making detection and identification less reliable. Also, if material is not taken from a representative part of the lesion, fungi may not be present in the part sampled. If very small samples are received, generally culture should take precedence over direct microscopy as culture is more sensitive. The exceptions to this would be dermatological samples in which microscopy is diagnostic or if mucoraceous moulds are suspected, in which case microscopy may be positive in the absence of a positive culture. If the sample is large enough, then both direct microscopy and culture should be performed, as microscopy is better able to differentiate colonization, tissue invasion, and contamination. Conversely, only nonviable organisms may be present in specimens obtained while the patient is receiving antifungal therapy, and microscopy and molecular methods may be the only method for detecting the etiologic agent. Specimen quantity and quality may be compromised when multiple clinical laboratories process portions of the specimens. Good communication between microbiology, other pathology services, and the clinician can greatly enhance diagnostic accuracy.

Consideration of the patient's travel history and residence is also important when attempting to detect and identify fungal causes of disease due to the endemicity of certain diseases. Lifelong travel history is important in patients who do not normally reside in areas of endemicity as certain infections, for example, paracoccidioidomycosis and histoplasmosis (2), may reactivate decades later. Although mycetoma is reported worldwide, most cases come from tropical and subtropical regions around the Tropic of Cancer (3), and hence specific travel or residence details may improve diagnostic accuracy.

Examination of clinical material before any processing takes place may be very informative and should always be performed. Areas of caseous necrosis, microabscesses, grains, granules, and nodules should all be noted. Grains and granules may indicate mycetoma; granulomas and caseous necrosis indicate histoplasmosis; and microabscesses are seen with chronic disseminated or renal candidiasis. Grains and granules should be examined for color, shape, size, and consistency as these may be indicative of the etiological agent. For example, *Scedosporium apiospermum*, a common cause of eumycetoma, produces yellowish-white soft grains 1 to 2 mm in diameter, and *Trematosphaeria grisea* produces globose or lobed black grains 0.5 to 1 mm in diameter (3).

Microscopic examination of specimens can either be carried out with unfixed specimens or fixed, stained specimens. The use of unfixed specimens has the advantages of being quick and relatively simple to carry out, while the use of fixed, stained specimens may highlight features specific to certain fungi and also the host response in tissue, but they take longer to process and hence may delay reporting. Generally, if fixed, stained specimens are being examined, a general stain such as hematoxylin and eosin (H&E) will be used for screening. If fungi are suspected after examination of H&E, then stains that are specific for fungal structures, such as Gomori methenamine silver (GMS), can be used, and finally more specialized stains such as mucicarmine or Fontana-Masson, which will demonstrate characteristic structures in fungi of interest. A range of stains and procedures can be used to detect fungi (see Table 1), and the role

*This chapter contains information presented in chapter 114 by Yvonne Shea in the 10th edition of this *Manual*.

TABLE 1 Methods and stains available for direct microscopic and histological detection of fungi in clinical specimens

Method	Use	Time required (min)	Color of fungus	Comments
Stains and methods used directly on unfixed tissue or samples				
Potassium hydroxide (KOH)	Clearing and softening of specimen to make fungi more readily visible	5–30	Hyaline moulds and yeasts appear transparent, while dematiaceous moulds may display golden brown hyphae.	Can be used in combination with calcofluor for fluorescence microscopy.
Calcofluor white	Detection of all fungi and cysts of *Pneumocystis jirovecii*	1–2	Depending on which barrier filter is used, fungal elements appear blue-white or bright green against a dark background (Fig. 10 and 12). Cysts have "double parenthesis-like" structure in center.	Requires fluorescence microscope; collagen and swab fibers also fluoresce; fat droplets may look similar to yeast cells. Counterstain minimizes background fluorescence. Melanized fungi may not stain as effectively.
Diff-Quik	Also applied to other specimens, such as BAL fluid or CSF	2–3	Yeast cells and trophozoites appear blue purple (Fig. 15).	Differentiate from *Leishmania*; *Leishmania* has a kinetoplast and *Histoplasma* does not.
India ink, nigrosin	Detection of *Cryptococcus neoformans* in CSF	1	Capsules around yeast cells show as clear halos against a black background (Fig. 16).	When positive in CSF, diagnostic of meningitis. Negative in many cases of meningitis; not reliable
Stains used on heat or alcohol-fixed samples or tissues				
Giemsa stain	Primarily used for the examination of bone marrow and peripheral blood smears	15	Detects trophozoite stage of *P. jirovecii*	Detects intracellular *H. capsulatum* and fission yeast cells of *T. marneffei* (Fig. 26)
Gram stain	Detection of bacteria and fungi	3	Generally, yeasts and pseudohyphae stain Gram positive, and hyphae (septate and aseptate) appear Gram negative (Fig. 1–7). Some yeasts, especially *Cryptococcus*, may decolorize and appear either Gram negative or stippled.	*Cryptococcus* spp. stain weakly in some instances and exhibit only stippling. Often have orange amorphous material around yeast (Fig. 7). Not all fungi are detected.
Toluidine blue	Detection of *P. jirovecii* in respiratory specimens	25	Cyst walls are purple (Fig. 18).	The background and other fungi stain the same color.
Papanicolaou	Cytologic stain used primarily to detect malignant cells	30	Depending on cell type detected, background stains in subtle range of green blue, orange to pink hues. *Candida* stains gold, while other fungi may not stain at all.	Further stains should be performed.
Alcian blue	Detection of *C. neoformans* in CSF	2	Capsule stains blue against a pink background.	Mucopolysaccharide stain, not commonly used; like India ink, does not detect all cases.
Stains used on fixed tissues				
Hematoxylin and eosin (H&E)	General-purpose histologic stain	30–60	Fungal cytoplasm is pink and the nuclei are blue. Demonstrates natural pigment of dematiaceous fungi (Fig. 14, 17, and 24). Background tissue is red.	Permits visualization of host tissue response to the fungus. *Aspergillus* spp. and mucoraceous moulds stain well. The Splendore-Hoeppli phenomenon may be seen with some fungi, including *Basidiobolus* and *Sporothrix*.
Periodic acid-Schiff (PAS)	Detection of fungi	20–25	Fungi stain pink to red purple, nuclei may be blue depending on the counterstain used.	PAS stains glycogen, so other tissue structures can have a similar appearance to yeast cells.
Gomori methenamine silver (GMS)	Detection of fungi including *Pneumocystis*	5–60	Fungal elements including *Pneumocystis* cysts stain gray to black. Background is green (Fig. 9, 11, 13, and 21).	Often stains fungi too densely to observe structural details. Yeast cells and cysts of *Pneumocystis* may appear similar in size and shape.
Mucicarmine	Stains mucin	60	Stains capsule of *Cryptococcus* pinkish red.	May also stain cell walls of *B. dermatitidis* and *Rhinosporidium seeberi*
Fontana-Masson (FM)	Detection of melanin of dematiaceous fungi and *C. neoformans*	60	Cell walls black. Background pale pink.	Many non-dematiaceous fungi (some *Aspergillus*, mucoraceous moulds, and *Trichosporon* species) can be FM positive. If hyaline in H&E, examine morphology carefully.

of histopathological diagnosis has recently been comprehensively reviewed (4). Staining methodology is reviewed in chapter 118 of this *Manual.*

The Gram stain may be useful in diagnosis, primarily because it is commonly used in most laboratories; hence, laboratory staff are familiar with it, and it may enable differentiation of yeasts from moulds in the initial sample. Although Gram reactions can vary, yeast cells and pseudohyphae generally stain Gram positive and hyphae (septate and aseptate) stain Gram negative. The size and shape of budding yeast-like cells can indicate a presumptive genus identification. *Cryptococcus* yeast cells are generally very round and display an amorphous orange-staining material, presumably the capsule.

Familiarity with the appearance of certain fungi in tissue may be helpful when performing direct examination (see Table 2). *Aspergillus* hyphae tend to be of a consistent diameter (4 to 6 μm) and commonly demonstrate 45° branching, with 90° branching less common. *Fusarium* and *Scedosporium* species look very similar to *Aspergillus* species in tissue (5). Sporulation in tissue is rare, but it can be distinctive with certain fungi. For example, aleurioconidia can be indicative of *Aspergillus terreus*. *Fusarium* may produce a combination of hyphae and yeast-like structures, and *Scedosporium* may produce ovoid pigmented annelloconidia (4). When fungal stains show both unicellular forms and filaments that appear to be hyphae or pseudohyphae, infection with *Fusarium*, *Paecilomyces*, or *Sarocladium* species should be considered, although filamentous yeast should also be included in the differential diagnosis (6). Mucoraceous moulds have aseptate or sparsely septate hyphae with wide-angle branching. The hyphae often appear twisted and flattened due to the lack of hyphal support because of the absence of septa (7). The Splendore-Hoeppli phenomenon on H&E sections may be seen with blastomycosis and sporotrichosis as well as with infections caused by *Basidiobolus* and *Conidiobolus* species. This phenomenon is the deposition of amorphous, eosinophilic material in tissue that occurs as a result of the antigen-antibody reaction. Dematiaceous moulds may display multiple forms, such as septate hyphae with parallel walls, rounded forms arranged in chains, or muriform (sclerotic) bodies. The diagnosis of phaeohyphomycosis can be made only if pigmented hyphae are observed. Sometimes pigmentation can be observed by use of a traditional KOH preparation; however, care should be taken if these are stained with calcofluor, as this is not taken up well by melanized hyphae. Some structures can provide definitive diagnosis of the etiologic agent (e.g., spherules of *Coccidioides* spp.). Specimens obtained from patients treated with antifungal drugs may demonstrate atypical structures, such as variations of hyphal size within the same hyphae, lack of septation within the hyphae, or bulb forms within the hyphae or at the hyphal tips.

There are many artifacts that can be mistaken for fungal structures when performing direct microscopy. Lymphocytes in cerebrospinal fluid (8) may be mistaken for *Cryptococcus* species; fibers and debris may be mistaken for hyphae, as they can fluoresce with calcofluor white; and fat droplets may be confused with budding yeast-like cells. Experience reading direct microscopy may overcome these problems, and discussions with colleagues may be necessary when doubt persists. Alternatively, use of another method may help to differentiate artifacts from genuine findings.

A positive result on direct microscopy should be reported promptly with as much information included as necessary to clarify the result. For example, "Yeast cells seen" is more helpfully reported as "Microscopic appearance may represent commensal species, e.g., *Malassezia*" in a skin sample, if the characteristic broad-based budding associated with this genus has been seen. Examples of various characteristic structures seen in direct microscopy of clinical specimens from fungal infections are shown in Fig. 1 through 26. As well as direct microscopy, various methods can be used for detecting fungi in clinical samples and blood cultures; these are listed in Table 3.

ANTIBODY DETECTION

Antibody detection may be useful in a range of diseases, particularly when they occur in immunocompetent patients, although it may have limited use in immunocompromised patients. Several immunological techniques have been used to detect antibodies during fungal infections, including immunodiffusion (ID), countercurrent immunoelectrophoresis (CIE), enzyme-linked immunosorbent assays (ELISA), complement-fixation tests (CFTs), and most recently fluorescent-enzyme immunoassay (FEIA).

Aspergillus Species

Antibodies to *Aspergillus* can be detected in most healthy individuals due to exposure to spores in the air (9), but their role in diagnosing aspergillosis in patients who are immunocompromised is minimal. Please also refer to chapter 122 of this *Manual.* In contrast, in patients who are nonneutropenic and develop aspergillosis, antibody detection may be helpful. Various techniques have been used, including countercurrent immunoelectrophoresis and FEIA (10); these tests mainly measure IgG, but often use poorly defined antigen preparations, although recombinant antigens are used by one manufacturer (Platelia Aspergillus IgG; Bio-Rad, Hercules, CA). Antibody detection is helpful in diagnosing allergic bronchopulmonary aspergillosis (9), aspergilloma (11), and chronic cavitary aspergillosis (12), and their utility has recently been extensively reviewed (9). Although background levels of antibody do occur, by careful examination of the performance of tests, for example, with receiver operator curve analysis, it is possible to define a lower, nonsignificant level and also a level at which antibodies become indicative of disease (13).

An enzyme immunoassay (EIA) is available commercially for the measurement of *Aspergillus* IgG (Platelia Bio-Rad; Bio-Rad, Hercules, CA), which is CE marked but not FDA approved. The kit defines levels of antibody <5 units/ml as negative, ≥ 10 units/ml as positive, with levels in between as intermediate. However, from the data presented by the manufacturer evaluating the performance of the kit in patients with cystic fibrosis, it is not clear how the diagnosis of allergic bronchopulmonary aspergillosis was made and hence how reliable the figures are for sensitivity and specificity.

Blastomyces Species

Blastomyces yeasts produce two antigens, A antigen and WI-1 antigen, of which only the former is used in commercially available kits. Detection of antibodies to *Blastomyces* can be carried out by immunodiffusion, CFT, or ELISA, and there are commercially available assays or reagents in all these formats (Gibson Biosciences, Lexington, KY; IMMY, Norman, OH; Meridian Diagnostics, Cincinnati, OH). Immunodiffusion may be positive in around 28 to 64% of patients, but the CFT is less helpful with positivity in less than 20% of patients (14). With an EIA, antibodies were detected in 83% of patients with blastomycosis, but 47% of specimens from patients with histoplasmosis were also positive (15). A more promising study detecting antibodies

TABLE 2 Characteristic fungal morphology seen by direct examination of clinical specimens

Fungal morphology observed	Organism(s)	Diam range (μm)	Characteristic features	Geographic distribution
Yeast forms	*Histoplasma capsulatum*	2–5	Small; oval to round budding cells; often found clustered within histiocytes; difficult to detect when present in small numbers; often intracellular (Fig. 23)	1. Worldwide, eastern half of the United States (localized in Ohio and Mississippi River valleys) and throughout Mexico, Central and South America 2. Tropical areas of Africa (Gabon, Uganda, Kenya)
	Sporothrix species	2–6	Small; oval to round to cigar shaped; single or multiple buds present; uncommonly seen in clinical specimens (Fig. 21)	Most often reported from Mexico, Central and South America (Brazil), Asia (Japan). More widespread in temperate and tropical zones.
	Cryptococcus spp.	4–10	Cells vary in size; usually spherical but may be football shaped; buds usually single and "pinched off"; capsule may or may not be evident; rarely, pseudohyphal forms with or without capsule may be seen (Fig. 7, 15, and 16)	*Cryptococcus neoformans*: worldwide, especially Europe, Africa, Australia *Cryptococcus gattii*: tropical and subtropical areas, including Australia, America, South Africa, Central America
	Blastomyces dermatitidis	8–15	Cells usually large and spherical, double refractile; buds usually single, but several may remain attached to parent cells; buds connected by broad base (Fig. 22). Small forms in tissue have occasionally been reported, similar in size to *Histoplasma*.	Southeast and south-central United States, Great Lakes region, near St. Lawrence River
	Paracoccidioides brasiliensis	5–60	Cell usually large and surrounded by smaller buds around periphery (mariner's wheel appearance); smaller cells (2–5 μm) that resemble *H. capsulatum* may be present; buds have "pinched off" appearance (Fig. 25).	South and Central America
Yeast forms (fission)	*Talaromyces* (formerly *Penicillium*) *marneffei*	3	Fission yeast, not budding, elongated, curved with septa visible (Fig. 26)	Southeast Asia and China
Cysts and trophozoites	*Pneumocystis jirovecii*	1–4 4–5	Trophozoites: small pleomorphic forms Cysts: round to cup-shaped with up to 8 intracystic bodies (Fig. 18)	Worldwide
Spherules	*Coccidioides immitis*, *Coccidioides posadasii*	10–200	Spherules vary in size; some contain endospores, others are empty and collapsed; hyphae may be seen in cavitary lesions (Fig. 24).	Southwestern United States, Mexico, Central and South America (*C. posadasii* organisms are non-Californian strains)
Yeast forms and pseudohyphae or true hyphae	*Candida* spp.	3–4 (yeast forms); 5–10 (pseudohyphae)	Cells usually exhibit single budding (Fig. 4, 6); pseudohyphae, when present, are constricted at ends and remain attached like links of sausage (Fig. 4, 5); true hyphae, when present, have parallel walls and are separated.	Worldwide
Yeast forms and pseudohyphae	*Malassezia* species	3–8 (yeast forms); 5–10 (pseudohyphae)	Short, curved hyphal elements may be present with round, oval, or elongated yeast cells that are round at one end and flattened at point of conidiation (Fig. 8)	Worldwide

Wide pauciseptate hyphae	Mucoraceous moulds	10–30	Hyphae are large, ribbonlike, often fractured or twisted. Occasional septa may be present, branching usually at right angles (Fig. 3, 11, and 12). The Splendore-Hoeppli phenomenon on H&E sections may be seen with *Basidiobolus* and *Conidiobolus* species.	Entomophthorales: worldwide *Basidiobolus ranarum*: tropical areas of Asia, Africa, South America (mostly Brazil), Mexico, Australia (155) *Conidiobolus coronatus* and *C. incongruus*: tropical and subtropical regions of Africa and Southeast Asia (adults)
Hyaline (colorless) septate hyphae	Dermatophytes (skin and nails)	3–15	Hyaline septate hyphae commonly seen; chains of arthroconidia may be present (Fig. 19).	Worldwide
	Dermatophytes (hair)	3–12	Arthroconidia on periphery of hair shaft that produce sheaths indicate ectothrix infection. Arthroconidia formed by fragmentation of hyphae within hair shaft indicate endothrix infection. Long hyphal filaments or channels within hair shaft indicate favus hair infection.	
Hyaline septate hyphae	*Aspergillus* spp.	4–6	*Aspergillus* spp. are generally septate with consistent diameter throughout; often show repeated dichotomous, 45° angle branching (Fig. 1, 9, 10, 13, and 14).	Worldwide
	Scedosporium spp. (not eumycetoma), *Fusarium* spp., *Paecilomyces* spp.	3–12	Hyphae are septate, difficult to distinguish from other hyaline moulds. May exhibit less 45° angle and more 90° angle branching.	
Dematiaceous (darkly pigmented) septate hyphae	Dematiaceous fungi	1.5–6	Dematiaceous polymorphous hyphae, budding cells with single septa and chains of swollen rounded cells may be present. Occasionally, aggregates may be present when infection is caused by *Phialophora* or *Exophiala* spp. (Fig. 2).	*Hortaea werneckii*: subtropical coastal locations *Piedraia hortae*: tropical climates of Central and South America, Southeast Asia, and the South Pacific Islands *Rhinocladiella mackenziei*: Middle East *Cladophialophora bantiana* found in Asia
Sclerotic bodies (muriform cells)	*Cladophialophora carrionii*, *Fonsecaea compacta*, *Fonsecaea pedrosoi*, *Phialophora verrucosa*, *Rhinocladiella aquaspersa*	5–20	Brown, round to pleomorphic, thick-walled cells with transverse septa. Commonly, cells contain two fission plates that form tetrads of cells. Occasionally, branched septate hyphae may be found in addition to sclerotic bodies (Fig. 20).	Occurs worldwide, although the majority of reported cases are from tropical and subtropical regions of the Americas and Africa
Granules (white grain eumycetomas)	*Acremonium* and related spp. (*Sarocladium kiliense*, *Acremonium recifei*)	200–300	White, soft granule; cement-like matrix absent	Asia, North, South and Central America, Oceania, Europe
	Aspergillus nidulans	65–160	White, soft granule; cement-like matrix absent	Africa
	Fusarium spp. (*F. moniliforme*, *F. oxysporum* species complex, *F. solani* species complex)	80–200	White-yellowish color of the grains, edges are entire or lobed; surrounded by an eosinophilic homogeneous material. Hyphae comprising the granules are not embedded in cement.	Europe, South America, Caribbean, Africa, Asia
	Neotestudina rosatii	500–1000	Round, oval, or lobed white grains; compact with cement in the center	West Africa

(*Continued on next page*)

TABLE 2 Characteristic fungal morphology seen by direct examination of clinical specimens *(Continued)*

Fungal morphology observed	Organism(s)	Diam range (μm)	Characteristic features	Geographic distribution
	Pseudallescheria boydii	1000–2000	White-yellow, soft granules composed of hyphae and swollen cells at periphery in cement-like matrix (Fig. 17)	Worldwide, most common in North America
Granules (black grain eumycetomas)	*Curvularia* spp. (*C. geniculata*, *C. lunata)*	500–1,000	Black, hard grains with cement-like matrix at periphery	Worldwide
	Exophiala jeanselmei	500–1000	Black, soft granules, vacuolated, cement-like matrix absent, made of dark hyphae and swollen cells	Worldwide
	Falciformispora senegalensis, *Falciformispora tompkinsii*	400–600	Black, soft granules; cement-like matrix; in tissue sections, the central part consists of hyphae, and a black cement-like substance is seen at the periphery.	West Africa (specifically Senegal and Mauritania)
	Trematosphaeria grisea	300–600	Black and soft with a brown cement-like material in the periphery of the granules	India, Africa, Central and South America
	Madurella mycetomatis	500–900	Black to brown hard granules of two types: (i) rust brown, compact, and filled with cement-like matrix and (ii) deep brown, filled with numerous vesicles, 6–14 μm in diameter, cement-like matrix in periphery and central area of light-colored hyphae	India, Africa, and South America
	Medicopsis romeroi, *Biatriospora mackinnonii*	40–100 × 50–160	Black, soft granules composed of polygonal swollen cells at periphery, cement-like matrix	Africa, India, and South America

TABLE 3 Platforms for detection of fungi in blood cultures and clinical specimens

Platform	Detection from clinical specimens	Detection from blood cultures
Direct microscopy	Yes	Yes
Histopathological staining	Yes	No
Antibody detection	Yes	No
Antigen detection	Yes	No
β-D-Glucan	Yes	No
Fungal-specific metabolites	Yes	No
Mass spectrometry	Yes	Yes
Nucleic acid detection	Yes	Yes

to the BAD1 antigen, a surface protein antigen, showed a sensitivity of 88% and a specificity of 99%, with only 3 of 50 patients with histoplasmosis being positive (16). However, the authors commented that combination with antigen testing provided the best diagnostic method. Please also refer to information in chapter 125.

Candida Species

Detection of antibodies specific to *Candida* is problematic as a diagnostic tool, as many people will carry *Candida* as a commensal and hence have low levels of antibodies in the absence of disease (17). The main antigen used is mannan, a cell wall component, and various immunoglobulin classes, including IgG, IgM, and IgA, may be detected. Many studies have examined the sensitivity and specificity of antibody detection for diagnosis of invasive candidiasis and found disappointingly low figures (18, 19). Figures as low as 62% for sensitivity and 53% for specificity have been reported when antibodies alone are used for diagnosis, and hence most authors now recommend they be used in conjunction with *Candida* mannan antigen detection (19, 20).

Coccidioides Species

Diagnosis of coccidioidomycosis can be achieved with a range of methods including antibody or antigen detection or by culture. Although culture remains the gold standard method, the risks inherent to laboratory personnel dealing with cultures mean that use of other methods is to be encouraged. Antibodies to *Coccidioides* can be detected by various methods, including immunodiffusion (ID), latex agglutination (LA), CFT, and EIA. Historically, the tube precipitin (21) was also used, but has now been replaced by the ID test using the same antigens. The ID test detects mainly IgM antibodies to a β-glucosidase antigen ("heated coccidioidin"), which is positive early in disease, while the CFT detects IgG antibodies to a heat-labile chitinase antigen ("unheated coccidioidin"), which is useful in diagnosing acute and chronic disease and can also be used prognostically (22). Early studies indicated that in primary infection, precipitating antibodies peak by week 3 of infection, with approximately 90% of sera positive, but then decline rapidly, with only 10% of sera positive at 5 months. Complement-fixing antibodies will be detected in about 50% of sera by 1 month and continue to increase for several months (23). LA assays are available commercially from IMMY (Coccidioides Antibody Latex Agglutination; IMMY, Norman, OH) and the Medical Chemical Company (Coccidioides Latex Agglutination; Torrance, CA), but IMMY warns that false positives can occur and results should be checked by another method.

An EIA is also now available that detects both IgG and IgM and can be used with serum or CSF (Premier Coccidioides EIA; Meridian, Cincinnati, OH). The EIA has higher sensitivity than ID and CFT, but there has been concern about whether the increased sensitivity is associated with decreased specificity (24). One study found no false-positive results (25), whereas others have found false IgM-positive results in patients (26). This has led to the suggestion that the EIA should be used as a screening tool, with any positive results confirmed by another method (22). Please also refer to information in chapter 125.

Cryptococcus Species

Antibodies, including IgG, IgM, and IgA, produced against glucuronoxylomannan antigen and also crude antigenic preparations can be used to detect *Cryptococcus* in patients with cryptococcosis (27). They have been suggested to have prognostic value (28) and be a marker for reactivation of disease in solid-organ transplant recipients (29). However, their utility in diagnosis is limited as the polysaccharide capsular antigen may inhibit the synthesis of antibodies (30).

Histoplasma capsulatum

Detection of antibodies is an important component in establishing a diagnosis of histoplasmosis. Antibodies appear approximately 4 to 6 weeks after the primary acute infection and will decline over a 2- to 5-year period (31). Two tests have been widely used and evaluated, namely, ID and CFT.

The antigens used in the tests are extracted from histoplasmin, which is obtained from the mycelial phase of the fungus. Two antigens detected by the tests are the M antigen, which is a catalase (32), and the H antigen, which is a β-glucosidase (33).

The ID test, which is about 80% sensitive, detects precipitating antibodies to the antigens, resulting in the H and M "bands." The M band appears first during infection and can indicate either active or prior infection; it persists for several years. In contrast, the H band occurs during active infection, but it is only found in a minority of patients, although it may persist for 1 to 2 years. If both bands are detected, this is considered to be diagnostic for active infection (34).

The CFT uses histoplasmin and an antigen produced by the yeast phase to detect complement-fixing antibodies, which appear 3 to 6 weeks after infection. Up to 95% of patients with histoplasmosis will have a positive reaction in the CFT, although titers may be relatively low (35). Low titers may represent past infection, but titers of 1:32 or greater, or a 4-fold rise in titer, indicate active disease (31). Antibodies generally appear to the yeast antigen first and to histoplasmin later; they decline over several years in the absence of further exposure (34). The CFT is more sensitive than ID, but it is also subject to more cross-reactivity. Patients with aspergillosis, blastomycosis, candidiasis, coccidioidomycosis, paracoccidioidomycosis, tuberculosis, and other bacterial or viral diseases have been found to have positive reactions in the CFT (36). False-negative results can occur due to the presence of rheumatoid factor or cold agglutinins (37). A commercial LA assay is available from IMMY (Norman, OH) that has good sensitivity when used for diagnosis of acute histoplasmosis, but due to potential cross-reactivity the manufacturer recommends confirming results by ID or CFT. Various other kits and reagents are available from IMMY, Focus Diagnostics (Cypress, CA), and Meridian Diagnostics (Cincinnati, OH).

ANTIGEN DETECTION

Aspergillus Species

The main antigen used as a diagnostic marker in commercially available kits for invasive aspergillosis (IA) is galactomannan (GM), a carbohydrate molecule with a mannose backbone. GM is released from the cell wall of *Aspergillus* hyphae during growth *in vivo*, but it is probably not detectable in patients until angioinvasion has occurred (38). GM can be detected in serum, bronchoalveolar lavage (BAL), cerebrospinal fluid (39), and urine in infected patients. The Platelia Aspergillus GM antigen ELISA kit produced by Bio-Rad uses a monoclonal rat antibody (EBA-2) to coat microtiter wells and also to act as the detector antibody conjugated to peroxidase. The amount of GM in each sample is expressed as a ratio of the sample OD compared to the cutoff control OD; GM indices of >0.5 are considered positive (Platelia Aspergillus Ag kit insert). Although the manufacturers currently recommend a cutoff of 0.5 for BAL, many laboratories use a cutoff of 1, due to the improved sensitivity of the kit with BAL. The kit (which is CE marked and FDA approved) is currently approved for the detection of GM in serum and BAL and has been extensively studied in a range of different patient groups; sensitivities and specificities vary widely depending on the setting in which it is used. Studies in patients with hematological malignancies and patients who have undergone hematopoietic stem cell transplantation have generally resulted in higher sensitivity and specificity than patients with solid-organ transplantation. For patients with hematological malignancies, sensitivity figures of up to 100% have been reported in patients with proven or probable IA (40), although other groups have only found sensitivity of 17% in proven IA (41). A recent review, which analyzed data from 54 studies, found the sensitivity and specificity were 82% and 81%, respectively (42). Unsurprisingly, studies that used a higher cutoff reported higher specificity and lower sensitivity, but this difference was not statistically significant. The frequency of testing will also impact the utility of the test, and twice-weekly testing may be optimal (43). The Infectious Disease Society of America (IDSA) guidelines on aspergillosis recommend that the assay should be used for diagnosis of IA in patients with hematological malignancy and hematopoietic stem cell transplants, but it should not be used for screening in patients receiving mould-active prophylaxis (44).

Although GM is a useful marker for IA, there are many causes of false positivity. Piperacillin/tazobactam or amoxicillin with clavulanic acid (45), Plasma-lyte (46), and certain foodstuffs, including pasta, vegetables, and milk, have all been reported to cause false positives, although the problem with piperacillin/tazobactam has now largely been overcome. In addition, several other fungal genera are known to be reactive in the kit, including *Penicillium*, *Alternaria*, *Rhodotorula*, *Paecilomyces*, *Cryptococcus*, *Blastomyces*, and *Histoplasma*. Detection of GM may be reduced in patients with chronic granulomatous disease (47) and patients who are treated with mould-active antifungals (48).

In addition to its use for diagnosis, GM has been assessed as a prognostic tool. Early studies demonstrated that an increase in the GM index was associated with progression of disease (49) and that patients in whom the GM index remained high had significantly poorer outcomes than those in whom it decreased (50). It has also been shown that the initial level of the GM index in serum and the rate of decay in GM over the first week were predictive of time to mortality. In the first week, if the GM index increased by 1 unit, the risk of time to mortality increased by 25%, whereas a fall of 1 unit decreased the risk by 22% (51).

Although the GM ELISA is the most widely used assay for the diagnosis of IA, a lateral flow device has been developed (Isca Diagnostics, Truro, United Kingdom) that uses a monoclonal antibody, JF5, which binds to a protein epitope from an extracellular glycoprotein antigen produced by *Aspergillus fumigatus* (52). It was hypothesized that, by targeting a non-galactomannan antigen, the problems with cross-reactivity would be reduced. The monoclonal antibody is used for both the capture and detection of the antigen in serum or BAL, visualized with colloidal gold, and seen as a line that appears within 10 to 15 min of the sample being added to the LFD. As the antigen is only produced by growing hyphae, contamination of samples (e.g., BAL) with *Aspergillus* spores should not produce positive results. This has been confirmed in a meta-analysis where sensitivity and specificity in BAL (72 to 86% and 84 to 93%, respectively) are better than in serum (53 to 68% and 81 to 87%, respectively) (53).

A recent comparison of the LFD and GM for BAL samples reported a sensitivity of 88% and a specificity of 84 to 95% (54). Perhaps, more importantly, the LFD had a high negative predictive value of 95 to 96%, which might allow more informed decisions to be made about cessation of treatment.

Although the LFD has been described as a point-of-care test (52), the requirement to boil serum samples in a pH-buffered EDTA solution and centrifuge them during processing still means that testing must be done in a laboratory, although BAL samples may be processed directly. The kit is CE marked and FDA approval is currently being sought. Please also refer to information in chapter 122.

FIGURE 1 (Row 1, left) Gram stain of BAL specimen showing Gram-negative branching septate hyphae of *Aspergillus fumigatus*. Magnification, approximately ×1,000.

FIGURE 2 (Row 1, right) Gram stain of skin biopsy with Gram-variable branching hyphae of *Exophiala jeanselmei*. Magnification, approximately ×1,000.

FIGURE 3 (Row 2, left) Gram stain of skin biopsy with Gram-negative aseptate hyphae of the *Rhizopus microsporus* group. Magnification, approximately ×1,000.

FIGURE 4 (Row 2, right) Gram stain of sputum with *Candida albicans* showing Gram-positive budding yeast cells with pseudohyphae.

FIGURE 5 (Row 3, left) Gram stain of spleen demonstrating ghost-like budding yeast-like cells with pseudohyphae. Magnification, approximately ×1,000.

FIGURE 6 (Row 3, right) Gram stain of vaginal secretions with Gram-positive budding yeast cells of *Candida glabrata*.

FIGURE 7 (Row 4, left) Gram stain of skin abscess with *Cryptococcus neoformans* showing Gram-positive and Gram-variable budding yeast cells of variable size surrounded by amorphous orange halos.

FIGURE 8 (Row 4, right) Parker ink stain of skin lesion showing typical yeast cells and short, stubby hyphae of *Malassezia* spp. Magnification, approximately ×400.

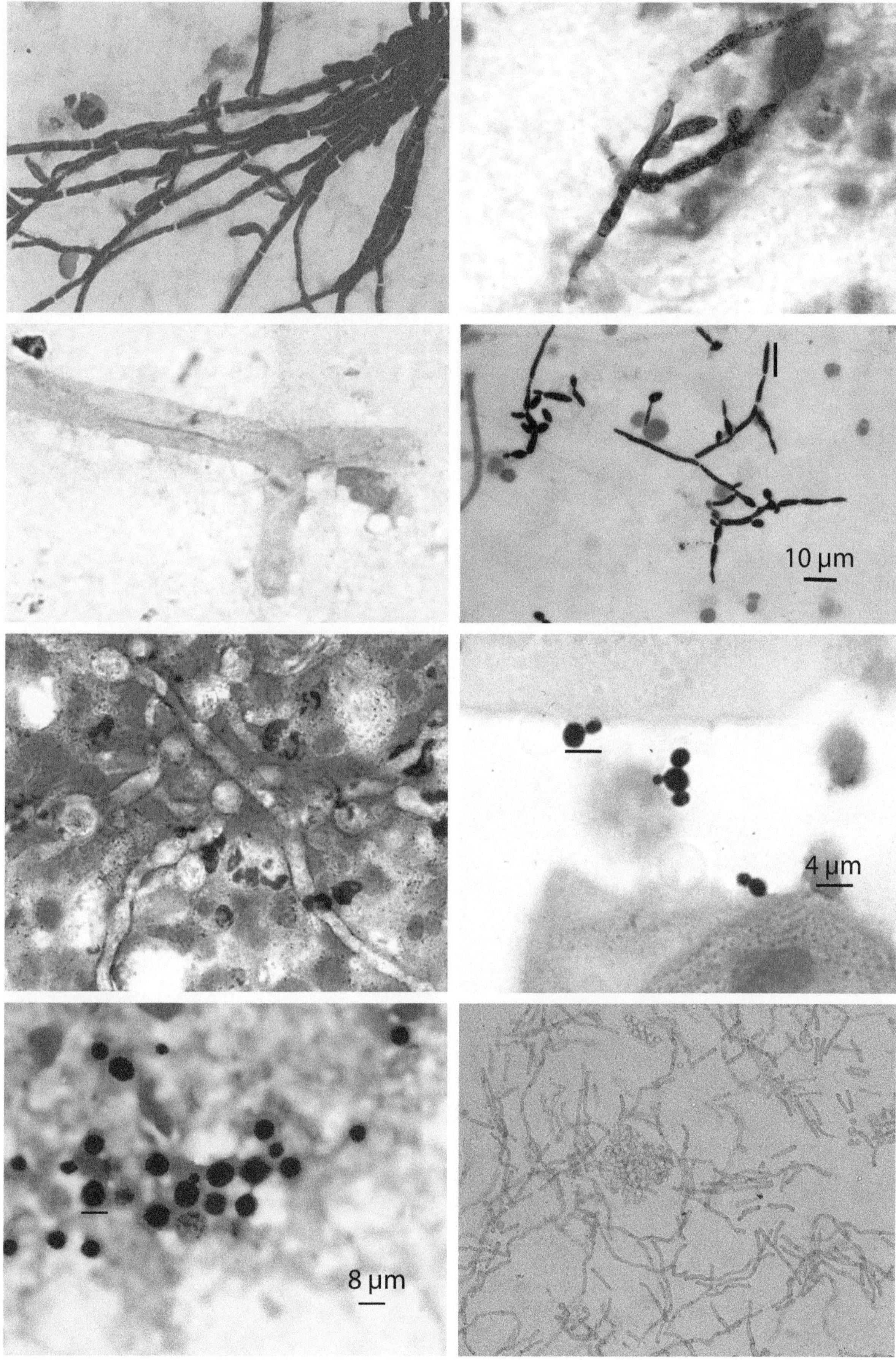
10 µm
4 µm
8 µm

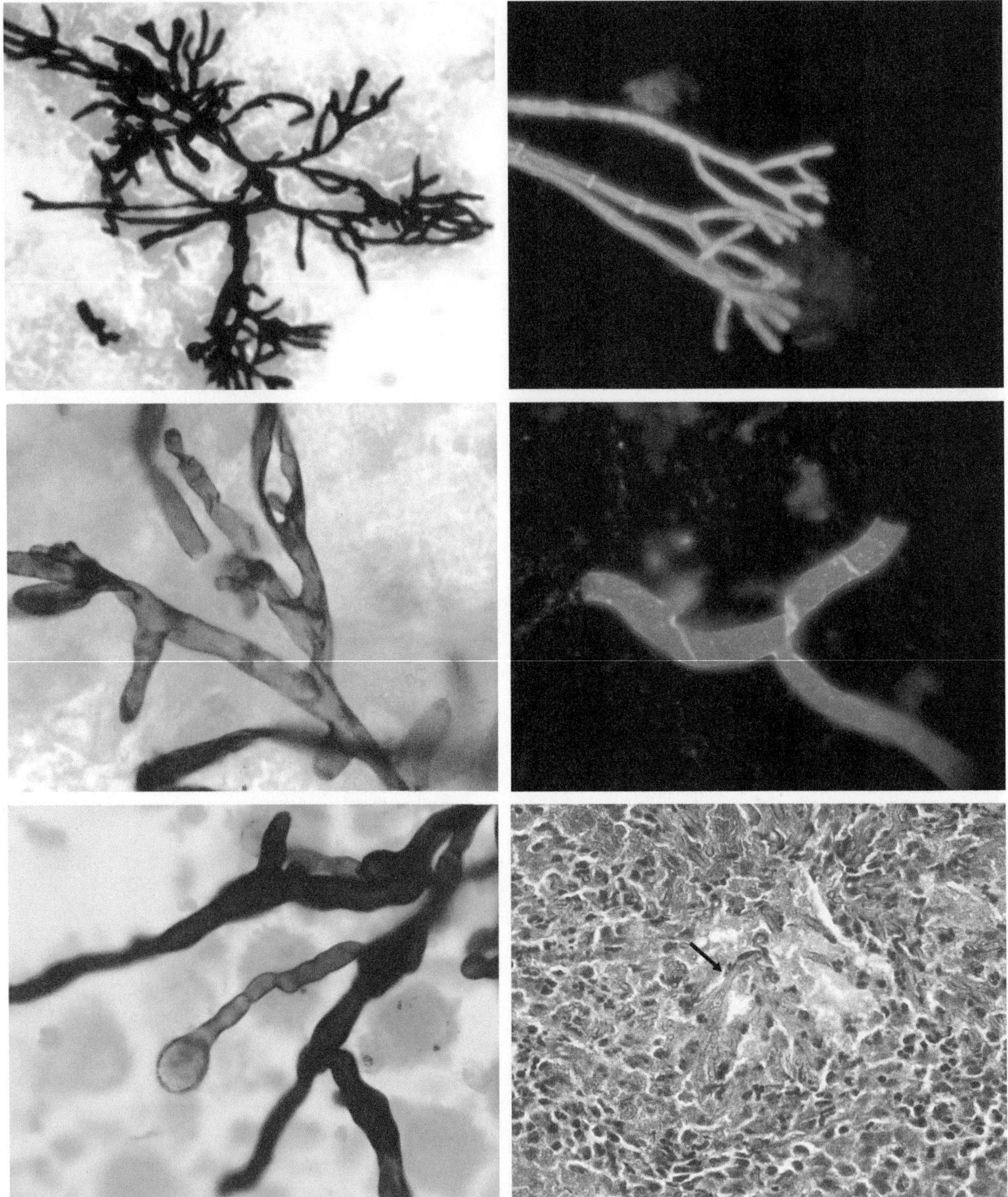

FIGURE 9 (Row 1, left) Gomori methenamine silver (GMS) stain of BAL specimen showing *Aspergillus fumigatus* dichotomously branching septate hyphae. Magnification, approximately ×400.
FIGURE 10 (Row 1, right) Calcofluor white stain of BAL specimen showing *Aspergillus fumigatus* dichotomously branching septate hyphae. Magnification, approximately ×500.
FIGURE 11 (Row 2, left) GMS stain of skin biopsy with *Rhizopus* spp. showing ribbonlike hyphae. Magnification, approximately ×400.
FIGURE 12 (Row 2, right) Calcofluor white stain of *Rhizopus* spp. showing ribbonlike hyphae. Magnification, approximately ×500.
FIGURE 13 (Row 3, left) GMS stain of lung biopsy specimen showing *Aspergillus fumigatus* with bulb formation at hyphal tip. Magnification, approximately ×1,000.
FIGURE 14 (Row 3, right) H&E stain of lung biopsy specimen showing *Aspergillus fumigatus* dichotomously branching septate hyphae (shown at arrow). Magnification, approximately ×400.

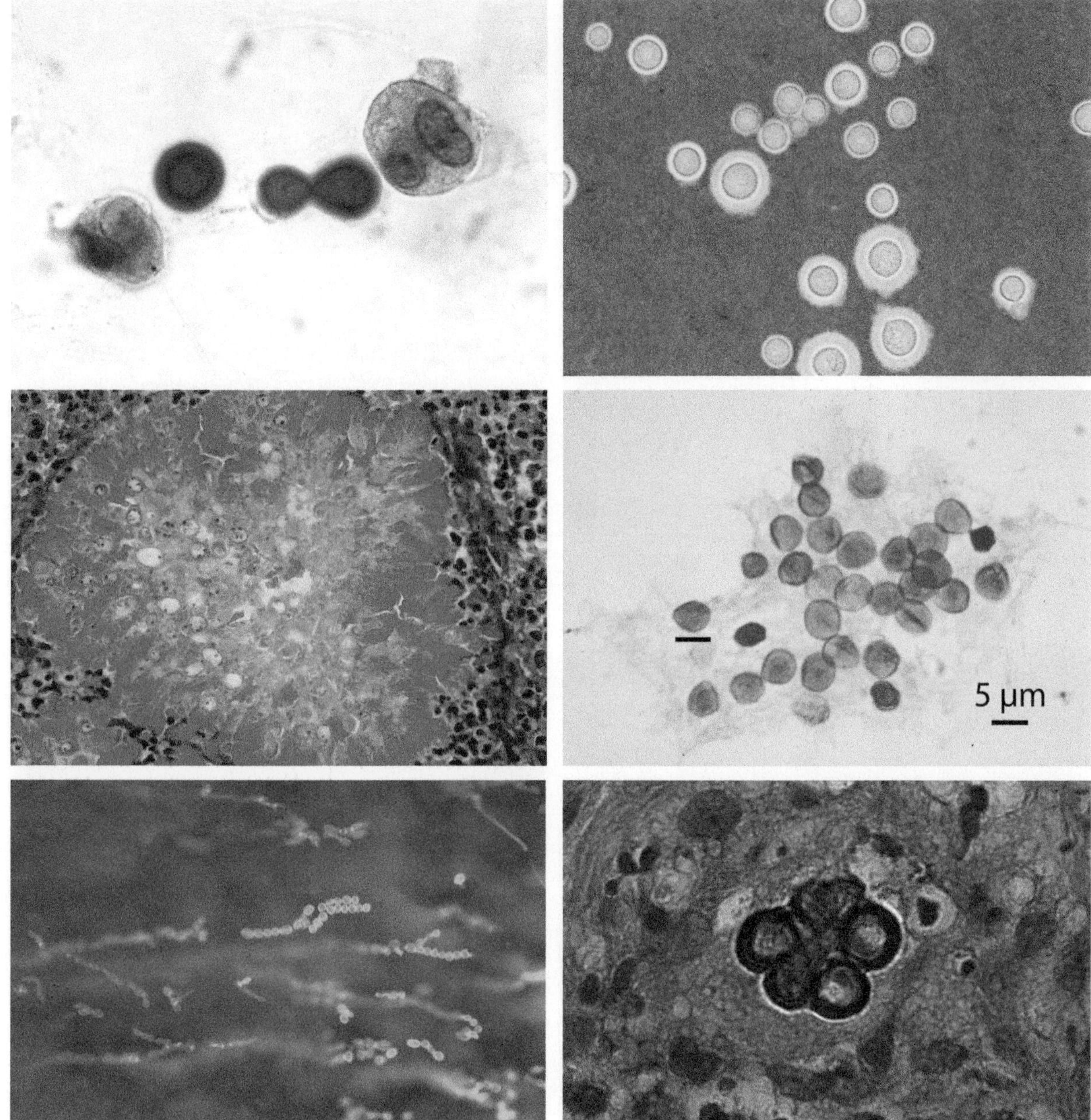

FIGURE 15 (Row 1, left) Diff-Quik stain of CSF with *Cryptococcus neoformans*. Magnification, approximately ×400.
FIGURE 16 (Row 1, right) India ink preparation of CSF showing encapsulated budding yeast cell of *Cryptococcus neoformans*. Magnification, approximately ×400.
FIGURE 17 (Row 2, left) H&E stain of eumycotic mycetoma granule of *Scedosporium apiospermum*. Magnification, approximately ×400.
FIGURE 18 (Row 2, right) Toluidine blue stain of BAL specimen showing cysts of *P. jirovecii*.
FIGURE 19 (Row 3, left) Calcofluor white stain of toenail specimen showing arthroconidia and hyphae of *Trichophyton rubrum*. Magnification, approximately ×200.
FIGURE 20 (Row 3, right) Muriform (sclerotic) cells (copper penny) in tissue of *Fonsecaea pedrosoi* chromoblastomycosis. Magnification, ×1,000.

Several studies have recently demonstrated that optimal sensitivity and specificity may be obtained when the GM test is combined with other tests such as PCR or β-D-glucan (55, 56).

Blastomyces Species

Diagnosis of blastomycosis is often made by culture, which is ultimately positive in over 80% of patients; however, due to the time taken for the culture to grow, other methods may also be used to give quicker results (57). Currently there is only one assay available to detect *Blastomyces* antigen, provided by MiraVista Diagnostics on a "fee for service" basis (MiraVista Diagnostics, Indianapolis, IN), which uses rabbit antibodies raised against whole cells of *B. dermatitidis* in the mould phase in a double-antibody sandwich assay (58). The assay

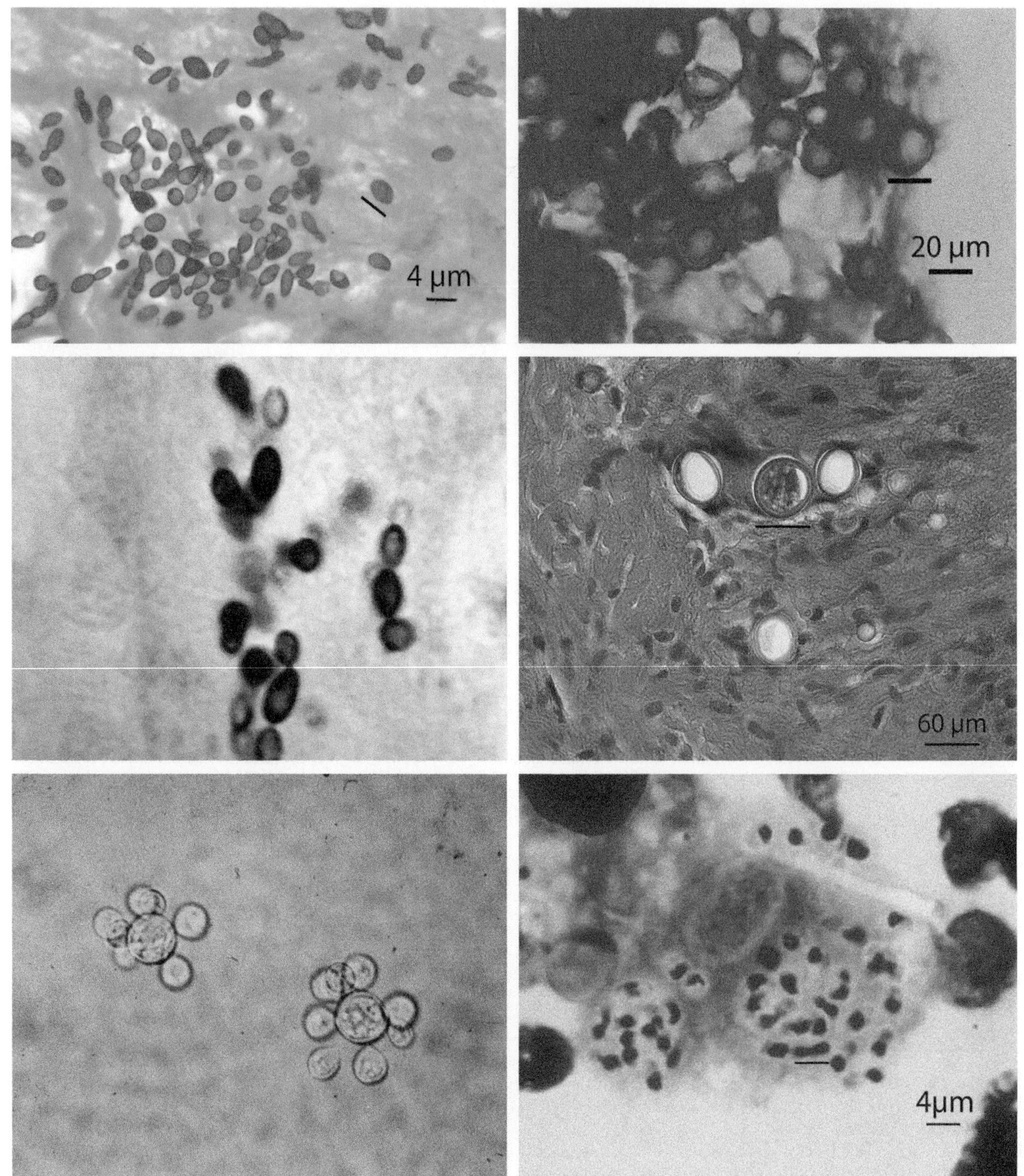

FIGURE 21 (Row 1, left) GMS stain of lymph node showing characteristic cigar-shaped yeast cells of *Sporothrix schenckii*.

FIGURE 22 (Row 1, right) Gram stain of abscess material showing large, broad-based, budding yeast cell with thick refractile wall characteristic of *Blastomyces dermatitidis*.

FIGURE 23 (Row 2, left) GMS stain of lymph node showing blastoconidia of *H. capsulatum*. Magnification, ×625.

FIGURE 24 (Row 2, right) H&E stain of *Coccidioides immitis*. Large, round, thick-walled spherules (10 to 80 μm in diameter) filled with endospores (2 to 5 μm in diameter). Young spherules have a clear center with peripheral cytoplasm and a prominent thick wall.

FIGURE 25 (Row 3, left) Bright-field photomicrograph of *Paracoccidioides brasiliensis* showing multiple budding yeast cells resembling mariner's wheels. Magnification, ×1,590.

FIGURE 26 (Row 3, right) Wright-Giemsa stain of BAL specimen showing characteristic fission yeast cells of *Talaromyces marneffei*.

can be used for most body fluids and has been evaluated mainly in urine, where sensitivity is higher than for serum (59). The drawback with the assay is the presence of cross-reactivity in a range of other mycoses, including histoplasmosis, paracoccidioidomycosis, infections with *Talaromyces marneffei*, cryptococcosis, and aspergillosis (http://www.miravistalabs.com/medical-testing/blastomycosis). A recent modification of the assay allowed quantification of antigen and increased its sensitivity when used with serum; however, it produced cross-reactivity in 96% of patients with histoplasmosis (60), which is problematic as the areas of endemicity for histoplasmosis and blastomycosis overlap in the United States. Due to the presence of such high rates of cross-reactivity, the utility of the *Blastomyces* antigen test is limited, although it may be useful to monitor therapeutic response or relapse (61). Please also refer to information in chapter 125.

Candida Species

Diagnosis of systemic candidiasis can be problematic as many people carry *Candida* as a commensal, and the presence of *Candida* colonization is often thought to affect the sensitivity and specificity of current diagnostic tests. The commercially available tests usually detect mannan or mannoproteins and include the Platelia Candida Ag EIA (Bio-Rad) and the CandTec LA test (Ramco Laboratories, Stafford, TX). Candida mannan is rapidly cleared from the circulation and hence frequent testing is important. A recent meta-analysis has examined the issues of sensitivity, specificity, and the effect of colonization on these parameters, mainly in studies that looked at both mannan antigen and antimannan antibody detection (20). One issue with the meta-analysis is the heterogeneity of the studies included, which is reflected in the wide ranges for the results reported. For mannan antigen detection alone, sensitivity ranged from 31 to 100%, with a median of 62% reported for the results. For antimannan antibodies, the figures were 44 to 100%, but when the two approaches were combined the median sensitivity was 86%. Sensitivity varied for different species of Candida, with the best results for *C. albicans*, followed by *C. glabrata* and *C. tropicalis*. Of note, they examined the effect of colonization of patients with *Candida* in four studies and found that neither colonization nor superficial candidiasis was associated with detection of mannan or antimannan antibodies. This led the authors to recommend that both mannan and anti-mannan antibodies should be used for the diagnosis of invasive candidiasis and that the combined approach was better than use of either technique alone.

Coccidioides Species

The most fully validated test available for detection of *Coccidioides* antigen is an EIA provided by MiraVista Laboratories on a "fee for service" basis (http://www.miravistalabs.com/wp-content/uploads/2012/09/315-TEST-PAGE-MVista-Coccidioides-Quantitative-Antigen-EIA.pdf). The MiraVista test uses antibodies against *Coccidioides* galactomannan and is suitable for use with urine, serum, plasma, BAL, CSF, and various other body fluids in patients with severe forms of disease (62). Treatment of serum and urine with EDTA to dissociate immune complexes improves the positivity in serum from 28 to 73%, but positivity in urine is only 50% (63). However, as with several other antigen detection assays for the endemic fungi, cross-reactions are common in patients with histoplasmosis or blastomycosis (63). Please also refer to information in chapter 125.

Cryptococcus Species

Detection of cryptococcal polysaccharide antigen in body fluids is an integral part of the diagnostic process for cryptococcal disease. The antigen detected is glucuronoxylomannan, which is the main component of the capsule and differs structurally between different serotypes. Classically, species of *Cryptococcus* were divided into five serotypes, A, B, C, D, and AD, but recently molecular studies have defined multiple species. It has been suggested that the names "*Cryptococcus neoformans* species complex" and "*C. gattii* species complex" should be adopted to reflect the genetic diversity already documented and prevent the need for multiple future name changes as further diversity is defined (64).

Commercially available kits for detection of cryptococcal antigen that have both FDA approval and CE marking for serum and CSF include enzyme immunoassays (Meridian and IMMY, Immuno-Mycologics, Norman, OK) and LA assays (Bio-Rad, IMMY, and Meridian). The sensitivity and specificity for the EIA and LA tests are high for both serum and CSF, where figures of >90% are commonly reported in studies (65, 66). Cryptococcal antigen may also be detected in BAL (67) and urine (68), although these samples are not currently routinely assayed. The presence of high initial CSF titers (≥1:1,024) in patients with HIV infection is known to carry a poor prognosis (69); although CSF titers decrease over time, they do so too slowly to be useful in monitoring therapy (70). Titers obtained from the same sample with different kits may vary, so laboratories should use kits from a single source.

Recently, the FDA approved a lateral flow device (52) for use with serum and CSF (IMMY, Immuno-Mycologics, Norman, OK). The LFD has been evaluated and shows enhanced sensitivity in serum when compared to both LA (71) and EIA (72). Several authors have noted that the titers obtained with the LFD are higher and hence are not comparable with results from other kits. Although not approved for use with urine or CSF, the LFD also has good activity in these sample types, ranging from sensitivities of 92 to 100% for urine (71, 72) and 99% in CSF (73). The advantage of the LFD is its lower cost compared to other kits (74) and its ease of use, particularly in resource-poor settings. A recent study demonstrated its superiority in diagnosing the disease in a multicenter evaluation in Africa (75); blood from finger pricks also has comparable accuracy to whole blood (76).

Multiple causes of false-positive and false-negative results have been documented in cryptococcal antigen kits. False-positive results have been attributed to disinfectants and soap (77), agar (78), bacterial infections (79), rheumatoid factor (80), systematic lupus erythematosus (81), and infection with *Geotrichum beigelii* (82), while false-negative results may be caused by low antigen titers (83) or high titers (84). Modifications of the tests have generally overcome these problems (84, 85). False-negative results due to high antigen titers are known as the prozone effect; for this reason, it is good practice to test specimens at neat and a 1:10 dilution. Recently, the occurrence of false-positive results at low titers with the lateral flow assay has been highlighted in several patients with no previous diagnosis of cryptococcal infection (86).

Histoplasma capsulatum

Histoplasmosis may be diagnosed with various methods, but as with other slow-growing fungi, diagnosis by culture may take several weeks to become positive (31). Other modalities for diagnosis include histopathology, antigen detection, antibody detection, and PCR. Please also refer to information in chapter 125. The first commercially available test for *Histoplasma* antigen (MiraVista Diagnostics) was originally developed in the mid-1980s as a radioimmunoassay, but it is now an EIA. The assay uses polyclonal rabbit antiserum against a polysaccharide antigen from *H. capsulatum* found in various body fluids during infection (87). The sensitivity of the assay varies with patient group, and most experience has been in patients with HIV infection and disseminated disease, in whom antigen is found in the urine and serum in 95% and 86% of patients, respectively. In other immunocompromised patients, the test is less sensitive, with 82% sensitivity in urine and 60% in serum (88). It is only useful in the early diagnosis of acute histoplasmosis, within 3 weeks of exposure. As well as disseminated histoplasmosis, the antigen test may also be useful in acute pulmonary disease, in which antigenemia and antigenuria were reported in 68% and 65% of patients, respectively (89). The utility of the test in other forms of histoplasmosis is much lower, with sensitivities of 15% or less for mediastinal or chronic pulmonary disease (88). In addition to serum and urine, the assay has also been evaluated in BAL and CSF. A recent study found that antigen could be detected in BAL from 94% of patients with histoplasmosis; in the same patients, urine and serum were positive in 79% and 65%, respectively (90). Although there have been no large studies assessing the sensitivity of antigen in CSF, it has been reported to have sensitivities ranging from 38 to 67% in small case series (91).

Antigen titers fall with successful treatment (92) and rise with relapses (93), so the test also has prognostic utility.

One of the major drawbacks with the antigen test is the frequency of false-positive results. Cross-reactivity in the urine test occurs in patients with blastomycosis, paracoccidioidomycosis, and in patients with *Talaromyces marneffei* infection; in serum, rheumatoid factor and treatment with rabbit antithymocyte globulin can cause false positives (31).

Although the antigen test from MiraVista is widely studied, other groups have also developed assays (94, 95). The latter group used commercially available polyclonal antibodies and found good correlations with both positive and negative samples when compared with the MiraVista test, but again the problem of cross-reactivity remained with *Blastomyces*, *Coccidioides*, and *Paracoccidioides*. Although monoclonal antibodies have been produced, overcoming the problem of specificity, they lack sensitivity and hence have not been further developed (96). An assay for urinary *Histoplasma* antigen has been developed by the Centers for Disease Control and Prevention and evaluated specifically for resource-limited settings; it demonstrated a sensitivity of 81% and specificity of 95% during evaluations (97).

There is now also a commercially available *Histoplasma* antigen test (ALPHA Histoplasma EIA) available from IMMY (Norman, OK), which is widely used by various diagnostic service providers. The assay had 97.6% agreement with the MiraVista test in urine; of the 24 discordant samples, 5 were considered false positive in the MiraVista test and a further 10 were below the limit of quantitation of the MiraVista assay (98).

The problems of cross-reactivity have led some workers to suggest that the detection of the urinary antigen should not be used as the sole method on which to base a diagnosis of histoplasmosis, but that it should be used in conjunction with other methods (31).

(1,3)-β-D-GLUCAN DETECTION

(1,3)-β-D-Glucan is a polysaccharide present in the cell wall of many fungi, including *Aspergillus*, *Candida*, and *Fusarium*; however, *Cryptococcus*, *Blastomyces*, and the mucoraceous moulds have very little or none. It is found in the blood of patients with invasive fungal infections, and its ability to activate factor G of the horseshoe crab coagulation pathway allows it to be measured and quantified. There are several commercially available assays (99), but the most widely available assay, and the only one with FDA approval and CE marking, is Fungitell, produced by Associates of Cape Cod (Associates of Cape Cod, Inc., Falmouth, MA) (100), which uses the coagulation cascade derived from the *Limulus* horseshoe crab as the detector method.

Early studies of the assay initially used a cutoff of 60 pg/ml (100). However, in a large multicenter study, the sensitivity and specificity were found to be 69.9% and 87.1%, respectively, at 60 pg/ml, and 64.4% and 92.4%, respectively, at 80pg/ml (101); the manufacturers now recommend interpreting <60 pg/ml as negative and ≥80 pg/ml as positive, with an indeterminate region in between (http://www.acciusa.com).

Clinical use of the assay has highlighted several important features. In one study, levels of β-D-glucan varied markedly between and within patients; optimal sensitivity, specificity, and accuracy occurred when two sequential samples had levels of ≥80 pg/ml, and successful clinical outcome did not always result in falls in β-D-glucan levels (102). A large retrospective study including 80 patients with proven and 36 patients with probable invasive fungal disease found that systemic antifungal therapy did not affect the sensitivity of the test. The test was more sensitive in IA than invasive candidiasis, but sensitivity was reduced in patients with either hematological malignancy or stem cell transplantation (103). Optimal sensitivity occurs when testing patients twice weekly (104). False-positive β-D-glucan results may be due to several factors, such as administration of intravenous immunoglobulins or albumin (103), hemodialysis using cellulose membranes (103), the use of glucan-containing gauzes or swabs, bacteremia, mucositis or graft-versus-host disease, and the use of various antibiotics (105).

One meta-analysis (106) included various β-D-glucan assays (including Fungitell, Glucatell [Associates of Cape Cod, Inc., Falmouth, MA], Fungitec [Seikagaku Corp., Tokyo, Japan], Wako BG [Wako Pure Chemicals Co., Osaka, Japan]) and documented a pooled sensitivity of 79.1% and a pooled specificity of 87.7% for the β-D-glucan assays for 365 patients with proven invasive fungal disease, but the ranges in the individual studies were very wide (sensitivity, 50 to 100%; specificity, 45 to 100%). Interestingly, they found no difference in sensitivity between patients with candidiasis or aspergillosis, in contrast to some single-center studies (103). A subsequent meta-analysis has largely confirmed these results (107). The IDSA guidelines for aspergillosis currently recommend the use of β-D-glucan for diagnosis, but point out that it is not specific to aspergillosis; the European Society for Clinical Microbiology and Infectious Diseases (ESCMID) guidelines support its use for the diagnosis of candidemia, invasive candidosis, and chronic disseminated candidosis (108).

Although not approved for use with BAL, several studies have found promising results when β-D-glucan testing is used in hematology-oncology patients (109), but disappointing results in solid-organ transplant recipients (110). It may also have use as a prognostic tool when used with a cutoff of 200 pg/ml, but this will require further evaluation (111).

β-D-Glucan testing of CSF proved useful in diagnosing and monitoring an outbreak of fungal meningitis caused by *Exserohilum rostratum* (112). With a cutoff value of 138 pg/ml, the sensitivity and specificity of the assay were 100% and 98%, respectively. Most patients in whom β-D-glucan levels declined remained asymptomatic after therapy; however, in those whose β-D-glucan levels remained high, outcomes were poorer, although there were relatively few patients in this group.

β-D-Glucan has also been used as a diagnostic marker for *Pneumocystis jirovecii*, both in HIV-positive and -negative patients (113, 114). Sensitivity and specificity in this setting were generally high, with sensitivities of 96.4 to 100% and specificities of 87.8 to 100%, although studies have used widely differing cutoff values to define positives (23.2 pg/ml [115]; 100 pg/ml [114]). The recent European Conference on Infections in Leukemia guidelines have given an AII recommendation for use of β-D-glucan as a diagnostic tool and stated that a negative β-D-glucan was sufficient to exclude *Pneumocystis* infection (116). Despite successful treatment in HIV patients, β-D-glucan levels do not decrease, so the assay cannot be used prognostically (115). The test performs better for diagnosis of *Pneumocystis* infections than for diagnosis of other invasive fungal infections, with a diagnostic odds ratio of 102.3 compared with 25.7 for other invasive fungal disease (117). A recent meta-analysis has found that while the sensitivity and specificity are high in both HIV-positive (92% and 78%, respectively) and HIV-negative (85% and 73%, respectively) groups, a negative result could only be used to exclude disease in the HIV-positive population (118).

Because of the risk of false positives in certain patient groups, it has been suggested that a negative β-D-glucan result might be more helpful in excluding these diagnoses and that a positive result should be treated cautiously (119).

FUNGAL-SPECIFIC METABOLITE DETECTION

Many fungal metabolites, as well as antigens, have been evaluated for their utility in detecting fungi in clinical specimens. Metabolites that have been assessed include D-arabinitol (120), D-mannitol (121), the ratio of D-arabinitol to L-arabinitol (122), gliotoxin (123), and 2-pentylfurane (124). The ratio of D-arabinitol to L-arabinitol in serum has recently been shown to be useful in detecting candidemia in the context of hematological neutropenic patients (19), while 2-pentylfurane has shown promise in diagnosing IA in a breath test (125). The ability to detect these metabolites by mass spectrometry may enable larger studies of their clinical utility (126), but to date none of these tests are available commercially.

MASS SPECTROMETRY

Matrix-assisted laser desorption ionization–time of flight (MALDI-TOF) mass spectrometry is increasingly used for the identification of both yeast and mould cultures after recovery on solid media (127, 128). However, the requirement to grow the organisms on solid media introduces a delay, and the ability to identify fungi directly in the original clinical sample is desirable. Identification of yeasts directly from blood cultures is desirable, but the presence of proteins and hemoglobin in blood cultures can interfere with the spectra produced and confuse the identification obtained (129). Despite this, several groups have developed methods for detection direct from blood cultures, but with varying success rates (130, 131), and several of the studies used simulated blood cultures (132, 133), which obviously differ significantly from those obtained in clinical practice.

One large two-center study with 346 positive yeast blood cultures found that direct MALDI-TOF identification yielded correct identifications for 95.9% of *C. albicans* and 86.5% of non-*C. albicans* species when compared with the conventional culture-based methods (134). This suggests that direct detection and identification of many *Candida* species following incubation of blood cultures is already feasible and may become the standard procedure relatively soon, although large-scale clinical evaluations in different patient groups are still required to confirm this.

Identification of moulds by MALDI-TOF has been more challenging than for yeasts, partly because mould colonies are composed of different structures, including hyphae, spores, and sporing structures, resulting in variability in the spectra produced. In addition, the sample preparation is more critical, and commercially available databases often contain limited numbers of species. The percentage of correct identifications for moulds ranges from 72 to 100%, depending on the system used (135). Many species of moulds, including the dermatophytes, *Aspergillus*, *Fusarium*, *Rhizopus*, *Paecilomyces*, various melanized fungi, and several other genera, can be identified by MALDI-TOF, but they usually require the construction of an in-house database (136, 137).

NUCLEIC ACID DETECTION

Nucleic acid detection for diagnosis of fungal infection and identification of the etiological agent has been actively pursued since the early 1990s. Theoretically, this method offers many advantages, including the ability to detect organisms present in small numbers or that cannot be cultured, the potential for automation, removal of the risks associated with culturing Category 3/Biosafety Level 3 fungi, decreased time for fungal identification, and detection of antifungal resistance in primary clinical samples (138). Moreover, it offers the potential to identify pathogens in biopsy samples that have been formalin fixed and even wax embedded. However, although there are many methods published (139–141), until recently there was little consensus about the optimal methods for specimen processing, extraction of DNA, target design, and quality control. Sensitivity and specificity varied considerably: for IA, sensitivity and specificity ranged from 58 to 80% and 78 to 95%, respectively (142); for invasive candidiasis, they were 95% and 92%, respectively (143). Partly because of this variability, the IDSA guidelines for aspergillosis only support the use of PCR when used in association with other diagnostic tests.

For IA, there are now recommendations from the European *Aspergillus* PCR Initiative (EAPCRI)/International Society for Human and Animal Mycology (ISHAM) working group, which have defined a set of standard recommendations for various parts of the assays for diagnostic PCR, rather than a standard PCR assay. They have reported standardized conditions when using whole blood, serum, and plasma as the diagnostic sample (144). For candidiasis, use of whole blood, rRNA, or P450 multicopy targets and an *in vitro* PCR detection limit of ≤10 CFU/ml were all associated with improved assay performance (143).

There are now many commercially available PCR assays for the diagnosis of IA on the market, including Septifast by Roche (Roche Diagnostics, Indianapolis, IN), which is able to detect several species of *Candida* and *A. fumigatus*, the MycAssay by Myconostica (Myconostica, Cambridge, United Kingdom), AsperGenius by Pathonostics (Maastricht, The Netherlands), and MycoGENIE by

Ademtech (Pessac, France). All four assays are CE marked. Septifast has been evaluated in both neutropenic (145) and non-neutropenic patients (146), but with disappointing results. There were false-positive and false-negative results for both *Candida* and *Aspergillus*; thus, the Septifast system has limited sensitivity and specificity and does not look promising for fungal infections.

The MycAssay *Aspergillus* has also been evaluated in several studies in intensive care unit (ICU) patients (146, 147) and high-risk hematology patients (148). The assay can be used with serum as a screening test or with BAL as a diagnostic test (http://www.myconostica.co.uk/aspergillus). In the setting of hematology patients, the sensitivity ranged from 50 to 80% and the specificity from 90.5 to 100%; the authors concluded that its performance was similar to the galactomannan assay (148). In the ICU setting, the sensitivity was higher (86.7 to 100%) and specificities of 87.6 to 92.9% (147) were reported, with increased sensitivity when multiple samples were examined (146). The MycAssay for *Pneumocystis* has also been reported to have a sensitivity and specificity of 100% in BAL in a comparative study (149).

The Pathonostics AsperGenius assay is validated for use with BAL and can be used to diagnose IA and detect azole resistance in the same sample. When compared with GM detection in BAL, it demonstrated sensitivity and specificity of 90% and 89%, respectively, in hematology patients and 80% and 93% in ICU patients (150). Although not validated in serum, sensitivity and specificity were found to be 79% and 100%, respectively, which suggests it may also be helpful when using a less invasive sample than BAL (151). A more recent study that examined its utility in plasma, using both spiked and clinical samples, found sensitivity and specificity of 80% and 78%, respectively, when a single positive result was taken as significant; if multiple samples were required to be significant, the study found 100% specificity but only 50% sensitivity (152).

Another *Aspergillus* PCR assay that has recently undergone evaluation is the MycoGENIE real-time PCR kit, which is used for diagnosis and concomitant detection of azole resistance, and uses either serum or BAL as a specimen (153). The assay was found to be relatively sensitive and specific both in BAL (93% and 90%, respectively) and in serum (100% and 85%, respectively), in addition to detecting all the resistant isolates that were tested.

One of the most promising assays for candidiasis is the T2Candida test (T2Biosystems, Lexington, KY), which is able to detect five *Candida* species directly from whole blood without the need for culture. Compared to various automated blood culture systems and against spiked blood samples, it had good sensitivity, good specificity, and reduced time to positivity (154). Other commercially available assays include Prove-it Sepsis (Mobidiag, Espoo, Finland) and Luminex (Chicago, IL), which provide detection/identification of fungi from blood cultures, and SeptiTest (Molzym, Bremen, Germany), Vyoo (Analytik Jena, Jena, Germany), Plex-ID (Omnica, Irvine, CA), Magicplex (Seegene, Seoul, Korea), and Iridica (Abbott, Maidenhead, United Kingdom), which can perform fungal detection/identification direct from blood samples.

The ESCMID guidelines on candidosis did not support the use of PCR for diagnosis of candidosis largely because of the lack of standardization of the assays and absence of large-scale clinical validations (108). With the development of newer assays and wider validation, this may change. Likewise, it remains to be seen if the forthcoming European Organization for Research and Treatment of Cancer (EORTC) definitions of invasive fungal disease will include positive PCR result(s) as a "mycological factor" for diagnosis.

The detection of other fungal infections with nucleic acid methods is still largely research based; they will need further development and validation before any are likely to be used clinically.

REFERENCES

1. **Garey KW, Rege M, Pai MP, Mingo DE, Suda KJ, Turpin RS, Bearden DT.** 2006. Time to initiation of fluconazole therapy impacts mortality in patients with candidemia: a multi-institutional study. *Clin Infect Dis* **43:**25–31.
2. **Ashbee HR, Evans EG, Viviani MA, Dupont B, Chryssanthou E, Surmont I, Tomsikova A, Vachkov P, Enero B, Zala J, Tintelnot KE; CMM Working Group on Histoplasmosis.** 2008. Histoplasmosis in Europe: report on an epidemiological survey from the European Confederation of Medical Mycology Working Group. *Med Mycol* **46:**57–65.
3. **Estrada R, Chávez-López G, Estrada-Chávez G, López-Martínez R, Welsh O.** 2012. Eumycetoma. *Clin Dermatol* **30:**389–396.
4. **Guarner J, Brandt ME.** 2011. Histopathologic diagnosis of fungal infections in the 21st century. *Clin Microbiol Rev* **24:**247–280.
5. **Lee S, Yun NR, Kim KH, Jeon JH, Kim EC, Chung DH, Park WB, Oh MD.** 2010. Discrepancy between histology and culture in filamentous fungal infections. *Med Mycol* **48:**886–888.
6. **Liu K, Howell DN, Perfect JR, Schell WA.** 1998. Morphologic criteria for the preliminary identification of *Fusarium*, *Paecilomyces*, and *Acremonium* species by histopathology. *Am J Clin Pathol* **109:**45–54.
7. **Christoff J, Galaydick J-L, Ramaprasad C, Pitrak D, Mullane KM.** 2010. Current diagnosis and management of mucormycoses. *Curr Fungal Infect Rep* **4:**8–16.
8. **McDonald R, Greenberg EN, Kramer R.** 1970. Cryptococcal meningitis. *Arch Dis Child* **45:**417–420.
9. **Page ID, Richardson M, Denning DW.** 2015. Antibody testing in aspergillosis—quo vadis? *Med Mycol* **53:**417–439.
10. **Agarwal R, Aggarwal AN, Sehgal IS, Dhooria S, Behera D, Chakrabarti A.** 2016. Utility of IgE (total and *Aspergillus fumigatus* specific) in monitoring for response and exacerbations in allergic bronchopulmonary aspergillosis. *Mycoses* **59:**1–6.
11. **Kawamura S, Maesaki S, Tomono K, Tashiro T, Kohno S.** 2000. Clinical evaluation of 61 patients with pulmonary aspergilloma. *Intern Med* **39:**209–212.
12. **Denning DW, Riniotis K, Dobrashian R, Sambatakou H.** 2003. Chronic cavitary and fibrosing pulmonary and pleural aspergillosis: case series, proposed nomenclature change, and review. *Clin Infect Dis* **37**(Suppl 3)**:**S265–S280.
13. **Barton RC, Hobson RP, Denton M, Peckham D, Brownlee K, Conway S, Kerr MA.** 2008. Serologic diagnosis of allergic bronchopulmonary aspergillosis in patients with cystic fibrosis through the detection of immunoglobulin G to *Aspergillus fumigatus*. *Diagn Microbiol Infect Dis* **62:**287–291.
14. **Klein BS, Vergeront JM, Kaufman L, Bradsher RW, Kumar UN, Mathai G, Varkey B, Davis JP.** 1987. Serological tests for blastomycosis: assessments during a large point-source outbreak in Wisconsin. *J Infect Dis* **155:**262–268.
15. **Bradsher RW, Pappas PG.** 1995. Detection of specific antibodies in human blastomycosis by enzyme immunoassay. *South Med J* **88:**1256–1259.
16. **Richer SM, Smedema ML, Durkin MM, Brandhorst TT, Hage CA, Connolly PA, Leland DS, Davis TE, Klein BS, Wheat LJ.** 2014. Development of a highly sensitive and specific blastomycosis antibody enzyme immunoassay using *Blastomyces dermatitidis* surface protein BAD-1. *Clin Vaccine Immunol* **21:**143–146.
17. **Mochon AB, Jin Y, Kayala MA, Wingard JR, Clancy CJ, Nguyen MH, Felgner P, Baldi P, Liu H.** 2010. Serological profiling of a *Candida albicans* protein microarray reveals permanent host-pathogen interplay and stage-specific responses during candidemia. *PLoS Pathog* **6:**e1000827.

18. **Ellis M, Al-Ramadi B, Bernsen R, Kristensen J, Alizadeh H, Hedstrom U.** 2009. Prospective evaluation of mannan and anti-mannan antibodies for diagnosis of invasive *Candida* infections in patients with neutropenic fever. *J Med Microbiol* **58:**606–615.
19. **Arendrup MC, Bergmann OJ, Larsson L, Nielsen HV, Jarløv JO, Christensson B.** 2010. Detection of candidaemia in patients with and without underlying haematological disease. *Clin Microbiol Infect* **16:**855–862.
20. **Mikulska M, Calandra T, Sanguinetti M, Poulain D, Viscoli C; Third European Conference on Infections in Leukemia Group.** 2010. The use of mannan antigen and anti-mannan antibodies in the diagnosis of invasive candidiasis: recommendations from the Third European Conference on Infections in Leukemia. *Crit Care* **14:**R222.
21. **Manitpisitkul W, McCann E, Lee S, Weir MR.** 2009. Drug interactions in transplant patients: what everyone should know. *Curr Opin Nephrol Hypertens* **18:**404–411.
22. **Ampel NM.** 2010. New perspectives on coccidioidomycosis. *Proc Am Thorac Soc* **7:**181–185.
23. **Pappagianis D, Zimmer BL.** 1990. Serology of coccidioidomycosis. *Clin Microbiol Rev* **3:**247–268.
24. **Nguyen C, Barker BM, Hoover S, Nix DE, Ampel NM, Frelinger JA, Orbach MJ, Galgiani JN.** 2013. Recent advances in our understanding of the environmental, epidemiological, immunological, and clinical dimensions of coccidioidomycosis. *Clin Microbiol Rev* **26:**505–525.
25. **Blair JE, Currier JT.** 2008. Significance of isolated positive IgM serologic results by enzyme immunoassay for coccidioidomycosis. *Mycopathologia* **166:**77–82.
26. **Blair JE, Mendoza N, Force S, Chang YH, Grys TE.** 2013. Clinical specificity of the enzyme immunoassay test for coccidioidomycosis varies according to the reason for its performance. *Clin Vaccine Immunol* **20:**95–98.
27. **Saha DC, Xess I, Zeng WY, Goldman DL.** 2008. Antibody responses to *Cryptococcus neoformans* in Indian patients with cryptococcosis. *Med Mycol* **46:**457–463.
28. **Diamond RD, Bennett JE.** 1974. Prognostic factors in cryptococcal meningitis: a study in 111 cases. *Ann Intern Med* **80:**176–181.
29. **Saha DC, Goldman DL, Shao X, Casadevall A, Husain S, Limaye AP, Lyon M, Somani J, Pursell K, Pruett TL, Singh N.** 2007. Serologic evidence for reactivation of cryptococcosis in solid-organ transplant recipients. *Clin Vaccine Immunol* **14:**1550–1554.
30. **Ma H, May RC.** 2009. Virulence in *Cryptococcus* species. *Adv Appl Microbiol* **67:**131–190.
31. **Kauffman CA.** 2007. Histoplasmosis: a clinical and laboratory update. *Clin Microbiol Rev* **20:**115–132.
32. **Zancopé-Oliveira RM, Reiss E, Lott TJ, Mayer LW, Deepe GS Jr.** 1999. Molecular cloning, characterization, and expression of the M antigen of *Histoplasma capsulatum*. *Infect Immun* **67:**1947–1953.
33. **Deepe GS Jr, Durose GG.** 1995. Immunobiological activity of recombinant H antigen from *Histoplasma capsulatum*. *Infect Immun* **63:**3151–3157.
34. **Guimarães AJ, Nosanchuk JD, Zancopé-Oliveira RM.** 2006. Diagnosis of histoplasmosis. *Braz J Microbiol* **37:**1–13.
35. **Wheat J, French MLV, Kohler RB, Zimmerman SE, Smith WR, Norton JA, Eitzen HE, Smith CD, Slama TG.** 1982. The diagnostic laboratory tests for histoplasmosis: analysis of experience in a large urban outbreak. *Ann Intern Med* **97:**680–685.
36. **Wheat J, French ML, Kamel S, Tewari RP.** 1986. Evaluation of cross-reactions in *Histoplasma capsulatum* serologic tests. *J Clin Microbiol* **23:**493–499.
37. **Johnson JE, Roberts GD.** 1976. Blocking effect of rheumatoid factor and cold agglutinins on complement fixation tests for histoplasmosis. *J Clin Microbiol* **3:**157–160.
38. **Hope WW, Kruhlak MJ, Lyman CA, Petraitiene R, Petraitis V, Francesconi A, Kasai M, Mickiene D, Sein T, Peter J, Kelaher AM, Hughes JE, Cotton MP, Cotten CJ, Bacher J, Tripathi S, Bermudez L, Maugel TK, Zerfas PM, Wingard JR, Drusano GL, Walsh TJ.** 2007. Pathogenesis of *Aspergillus fumigatus* and the kinetics of galactomannan in an in vitro model of early invasive pulmonary aspergillosis: implications for antifungal therapy. *J Infect Dis* **195:**455–466.
39. **Ikediobi ON, Shin J, Nussbaum RL, Phillips KA; UCSF Center for Translational and Policy Research on Personalized Medicine, Walsh JM, Ladabaum U, Marshall D.** 2009. Addressing the challenges of the clinical application of pharmacogenetic testing. *Clin Pharmacol Ther* **86:**28–31.
40. **Costa C, Costa JM, Desterke C, Botterel F, Cordonnier C, Bretagne S.** 2002. Real-time PCR coupled with automated DNA extraction and detection of galactomannan antigen in serum by enzyme-linked immunosorbent assay for diagnosis of invasive aspergillosis. *J Clin Microbiol* **40:**2224–2227.
41. **Buchheidt D, Hummel M, Schleiermacher D, Spiess B, Schwerdtfeger R, Cornely OA, Wilhelm S, Reuter S, Kern W, Südhoff T, Mörz H, Hehlmann R.** 2004. Prospective clinical evaluation of a LightCycler-mediated polymerase chain reaction assay, a nested-PCR assay and a galactomannan enzyme-linked immunosorbent assay for detection of invasive aspergillosis in neutropenic cancer patients and haematological stem cell transplant recipients. *Br J Haematol* **125:**196–202.
42. **Leeflang MM, Debets-Ossenkopp YJ, Wang J, Visser CE, Scholten RJ, Hooft L, Bijlmer HA, Reitsma JB, Zhang M, Bossuyt PM, Vandenbroucke-Grauls CM.** 2015. Galactomannan detection for invasive aspergillosis in immunocompromised patients. *Cochrane Database Syst Rev* **(12):**CD007394.
43. **Maertens J, Verhaegen J, Lagrou K, Van Eldere J, Boogaerts M.** 2001. Screening for circulating galactomannan as a noninvasive diagnostic tool for invasive aspergillosis in prolonged neutropenic patients and stem cell transplantation recipients: a prospective validation. *Blood* **97:**1604–1610.
44. **Patterson TF, Thompson GR III, Denning DW, Fishman JA, Hadley S, Herbrecht R, Kontoyiannis DP, Marr KA, Morrison VA, Nguyen MH, Segal BH, Steinbach WJ, Stevens DA, Walsh TJ, Wingard JR, Young JA, Bennett JE.** 2016. Practice guidelines for the diagnosis and management of aspergillosis: 2016 update by the Infectious Diseases Society of America. *Clin Infect Dis* **63:**e1–e60.
45. **Aubry A, Porcher R, Bottero J, Touratier S, Leblanc T, Brethon B, Rousselot P, Raffoux E, Menotti J, Derouin F, Ribaud P, Sulahian A.** 2006. Occurrence and kinetics of false-positive *Aspergillus* galactomannan test results following treatment with beta-lactam antibiotics in patients with hematological disorders. *J Clin Microbiol* **44:**389–394.
46. **Racil Z, Kocmanova I, Lengerova M, Winterova J, Mayer J.** 2007. Intravenous PLASMA-LYTE as a major cause of false-positive results of platelia *Aspergillus* test for galactomannan detection in serum. *J Clin Microbiol* **45:**3141–3142.
47. **Verweij PE, Weemaes CM, Curfs JH, Bretagne S, Meis JF.** 2000. Failure to detect circulating *Aspergillus* markers in a patient with chronic granulomatous disease and invasive aspergillosis. *J Clin Microbiol* **38:**3900–3901.
48. **Duarte RF, Sánchez-Ortega I, Cuesta I, Arnan M, Patiño B, Fernández de Sevilla A, Gudiol C, Ayats J, Cuenca-Estrella M.** 2014. Serum galactomannan-based early detection of invasive aspergillosis in hematology patients receiving effective antimold prophylaxis. *Clin Infect Dis* **59:**1696–1702.
49. **Boutboul F, Alberti C, Leblanc T, Sulahian A, Gluckman E, Derouin F, Ribaud P.** 2002. Invasive aspergillosis in allogeneic stem cell transplant recipients: increasing antigenemia is associated with progressive disease. *Clin Infect Dis* **34:**939–943.
50. **Han SB, Kim SK, Lee JW, Yoon JS, Chung NG, Cho B, Jeong DC, Kang JH, Kim HK, Lee DG, Lee HS, Im SA.** 2015. Serum galactomannan index for early prediction of mortality in immunocompromised children with invasive pulmonary aspergillosis. *BMC Infect Dis* **15:**271.
51. **Koo S, Bryar JM, Baden LR, Marty FM.** 2010. Prognostic features of galactomannan antigenemia in galactomannan-positive invasive aspergillosis. *J Clin Microbiol* **48:**1255–1260.
52. **Thornton CR.** 2010. Detection of invasive aspergillosis. *Adv Appl Microbiol* **70:**187–216.
53. **Pan Z, Fu M, Zhang J, Zhou H, Fu Y, Zhou J.** 2015. Diagnostic accuracy of a novel lateral-flow device in invasive aspergillosis: a meta-analysis. *J Med Microbiol* **64:**702–707.

54. **Hoenigl M, Prattes J, Spiess B, Wagner J, Prueller F, Raggam RB, Posch V, Duettmann W, Hoenigl K, Wölfler A, Koidl C, Buzina W, Reinwald M, Thornton CR, Krause R, Buchheidt D.** 2014. Performance of galactomannan, beta-d-glucan, *Aspergillus* lateral-flow device, conventional culture, and PCR tests with bronchoalveolar lavage fluid for diagnosis of invasive pulmonary aspergillosis. *J Clin Microbiol* **52:** 2039–2045.
55. **Arvanitis M, Anagnostou T, Mylonakis E.** 2015. Galactomannan and polymerase chain reaction-based screening for invasive aspergillosis among high-risk hematology patients: a diagnostic meta-analysis. *Clin Infect Dis* **61:**1263–1272.
56. **Boch T, Spiess B, Cornely OA, Vehreschild JJ, Rath PM, Steinmann J, Heinz WJ, Hahn J, Krause SW, Kiehl MG, Egerer G, Liebregts T, Koldehoff M, Klein M, Nolte F, Mueller MC, Merker N, Will S, Mossner M, Popp H, Hofmann WK, Reinwald M, Buchheidt D.** 2016. Diagnosis of invasive fungal infections in haematological patients by combined use of galactomannan, 1,3-β-D-glucan, *Aspergillus* PCR, multifungal DNA-microarray, and *Aspergillus* azole resistance PCRs in blood and bronchoalveolar lavage samples: results of a prospective multicentre study. *Clin Microbiol Infect* **22:**862–868.
57. **Smith JA, Kauffman CA.** 2010. Blastomycosis. *Proc Am Thorac Soc* **7:**173–180.
58. **Durkin M, Witt J, Lemonte A, Wheat B, Connolly P.** 2004. Antigen assay with the potential to aid in diagnosis of blastomycosis. *J Clin Microbiol* **42:**4873–4875.
59. **Bariola JR, Hage CA, Durkin M, Bensadoun E, Gubbins PO, Wheat LJ, Bradsher RW Jr.** 2011. Detection of *Blastomyces dermatitidis* antigen in patients with newly diagnosed blastomycosis. *Diagn Microbiol Infect Dis* **69:**187–191.
60. **Connolly P, Hage CA, Bariola JR, Bensadoun E, Rodgers M, Bradsher RW Jr, Wheat LJ.** 2012. *Blastomyces dermatitidis* antigen detection by quantitative enzyme immunoassay. *Clin Vaccine Immunol* **19:**53–56.
61. **Frost HM, Novicki TJ.** 2015. Blastomyces antigen detection for diagnosis and management of blastomycosis. *J Clin Microbiol* **53:**3660–3662.
62. **Durkin M, Connolly P, Kuberski T, Myers R, Kubak BM, Bruckner D, Pegues D, Wheat LJ.** 2008. Diagnosis of coccidioidomycosis with use of the *Coccidioides* antigen enzyme immunoassay. *Clin Infect Dis* **47:**e69–e73.
63. **Durkin M, Estok L, Hospenthal D, Crum-Cianflone N, Swartzentruber S, Hackett E, Wheat LJ.** 2009. Detection of *Coccidioides* antigenemia following dissociation of immune complexes. *Clin Vaccine Immunol* **16:**1453–1456.
64. **Kwon-Chung KJ, Bennett JE, Wickes BL, Meyer W, Cuomo CA, Wollenburg KR, Bicanic TA, Castañeda E, Chang YC, Chen J, Cogliati M, Dromer F, Ellis D, Filler SG, Fisher MC, Harrison TS, Holland SM, Kohno S, Kronstad JW, Lazera M, Levitz SM, Lionakis MS, May RC, Ngamskulrongroj P, Pappas PG, Perfect JR, Rickerts V, Sorrell TC, Walsh TJ, Williamson PR, Xu J, Zelazny AM, Casadevall A.** 2017. The case for adopting the "species complex" nomenclature for the etiologic agents of cryptococcosis. *MSphere* **2:**e00357-16.
65. **Gade W, Hinnefeld SW, Babcock LS, Gilligan P, Kelly W, Wait K, Greer D, Pinilla M, Kaplan RL.** 1991. Comparison of the PREMIER cryptococcal antigen enzyme immunoassay and the latex agglutination assay for detection of cryptococcal antigens. *J Clin Microbiol* **29:**1616–1619.
66. **Jaye DL, Waites KB, Parker B, Bragg SL, Moser SA.** 1998. Comparison of two rapid latex agglutination tests for detection of cryptococcal capsular polysaccharide. *Am J Clin Pathol* **109:**634–641.
67. **Baughman RP, Rhodes JC, Dohn MN, Henderson H, Frame PT.** 1992. Detection of cryptococcal antigen in bronchoalveolar lavage fluid: a prospective study of diagnostic utility. *Am Rev Respir Dis* **145:**1226–1229.
68. **Chapin-Robertson K, Bechtel C, Waycott S, Kontnick C, Edberg SC.** 1993. Cryptococcal antigen detection from the urine of AIDS patients. *Diagn Microbiol Infect Dis* **17:** 197–201.
69. **Brouwer AE, Teparrukkul P, Pinpraphaporn S, Larsen RA, Chierakul W, Peacock S, Day N, White NJ, Harrison TS.** 2005. Baseline correlation and comparative kinetics of cerebrospinal fluid colony-forming unit counts and antigen titers in cryptococcal meningitis. *J Infect Dis* **192:** 681–684.
70. **Powderly WG, Cloud GA, Dismukes WE, Saag MS.** 1994. Measurement of cryptococcal antigen in serum and cerebrospinal fluid: value in the management of AIDS-associated cryptococcal meningitis. *Clin Infect Dis* **18:**789–792.
71. **McMullan BJ, Halliday C, Sorrell TC, Judd D, Sleiman S, Marriott D, Olma T, Chen SC.** 2012. Clinical utility of the cryptococcal antigen lateral flow assay in a diagnostic mycology laboratory. *PLoS One* **7:**e49541.
72. **Lindsley MD, Mekha N, Baggett HC, Surinthong Y, Autthateinchai R, Sawatwong P, Harris JR, Park BJ, Chiller T, Balajee SA, Poonwan N.** 2011. Evaluation of a newly developed lateral flow immunoassay for the diagnosis of cryptococcosis. *Clin Infect Dis* **53:**321–325.
73. **Huang HR, Fan LC, Rajbanshi B, Xu JF.** 2015. Evaluation of a new cryptococcal antigen lateral flow immunoassay in serum, cerebrospinal fluid and urine for the diagnosis of cryptococcosis: a meta-analysis and systematic review. *PLoS One* **10:**e0127117.
74. **Nalintya E, Kiggundu R, Meya D.** 2016. Evolution of cryptococcal antigen testing: what is new? *Curr Fungal Infect Rep* **10:**62–67.
75. **Boulware DR, Rolfes MA, Rajasingham R, von Hohenberg M, Qin Z, Taseera K, Schutz C, Kwizera R, Butler EK, Meintjes G, Muzoora C, Bischof JC, Meya DB.** 2014. Multisite validation of cryptococcal antigen lateral flow assay and quantification by laser thermal contrast. *Emerg Infect Dis* **20:** 45–53.
76. **Williams DA, Kiiza T, Kwizera R, Kiggundu R, Velamakanni S, Meya DB, Rhein J, Boulware DR.** 2015. Evaluation of fingerstick cryptococcal antigen lateral flow assay in HIV-infected persons: a diagnostic accuracy study. *Clin Infect Dis* **61:**464–467.
77. **Blevins LB, Fenn J, Segal H, Newcomb-Gayman P, Carroll KC.** 1995. False-positive cryptococcal antigen latex agglutination caused by disinfectants and soaps. *J Clin Microbiol* **33:**1674–1675.
78. **Boom WH, Piper DJ, Ruoff KL, Ferraro MJ.** 1985. New cause for false-positive results with the cryptococcal antigen test by latex agglutination. *J Clin Microbiol* **22:**856–857.
79. **Chanock SJ, Toltzis P, Wilson C.** 1993. Cross-reactivity between *Stomatococcus mucilaginosus* and latex agglutination for cryptococcal antigen. *Lancet* **342:**1119–1120.
80. **Hay RJ, Mackenzie DW.** 1982. False positive latex tests for cryptococcal antigen in cerebrospinal fluid. *J Clin Pathol* **35:**244–245.
81. **Engler HD, Shea YR.** 1994. Effect of potential interference factors on performance of enzyme immunoassay and latex agglutination assay for cryptococcal antigen. *J Clin Microbiol* **32:**2307–2308.
82. **McManus EJ, Bozdech MJ, Jones JM.** 1985. Role of the latex agglutination test for cryptococcal antigen in diagnosing disseminated infections with *Trichosporon beigelii*. *J Infect Dis* **151:**1167–1169.
83. **Currie BP, Freundlich LF, Soto MA, Casadevall A.** 1993. False-negative cerebrospinal fluid cryptococcal latex agglutination tests for patients with culture-positive cryptococcal meningitis. *J Clin Microbiol* **31:**2519–2522.
84. **Gray LD, Roberts GD.** 1988. Experience with the use of pronase to eliminate interference factors in the latex agglutination test for cryptococcal antigen. *J Clin Microbiol* **26:** 2450–2451.
85. **Eng RH, Person A.** 1981. Serum cryptococcal antigen determination in the presence of rheumatoid factor. *J Clin Microbiol* **14:**700–702.
86. **Dubbels M, Granger D, Theel ES.** 2017. Low *Cryptococcus* antigen titers as determined by lateral flow assay should be interpreted cautiously in patients without prior diagnosis of cryptococcal infection. *J Clin Microbiol* **55:**2472–2479.

87. **Wheat LJ, Kohler RB, Tewari RP.** 1986. Diagnosis of disseminated histoplasmosis by detection of *Histoplasma capsulatum* antigen in serum and urine specimens. *N Engl J Med* **314:**83–88.
88. **Joseph Wheat L.** 2003. Current diagnosis of histoplasmosis. *Trends Microbiol* **11:**488–494.
89. **Swartzentruber S, Rhodes L, Kurkjian K, Zahn M, Brandt ME, Connolly P, Wheat LJ.** 2009. Diagnosis of acute pulmonary histoplasmosis by antigen detection. *Clin Infect Dis* **49:**1878–1882.
90. **Hage CA, Davis TE, Fuller D, Egan L, Witt JR III, Wheat LJ, Knox KS.** 2010. Diagnosis of histoplasmosis by antigen detection in BAL fluid. *Chest* **137:**623–628.
91. **Wheat LJ, Musial CE, Jenny-Avital E.** 2005. Diagnosis and management of central nervous system histoplasmosis. *Clin Infect Dis* **40:**844–852.
92. **Wheat LJ, Connolly-Stringfield P, Blair R, Connolly K, Garringer T, Katz BP, Gupta M.** 1992. Effect of successful treatment with amphotericin B on *Histoplasma capsulatum* variety capsulatum polysaccharide antigen levels in patients with AIDS and histoplasmosis. *Am J Med* **92:**153–160.
93. **Wheat LJ, Connolly-Stringfield P, Blair R, Connolly K, Garringer T, Katz BP.** 1991. Histoplasmosis relapse in patients with AIDS: detection using *Histoplasma capsulatum* variety capsulatum antigen levels. *Ann Intern Med* **115:**936–941.
94. **Gomez BL, Figueroa JI, Hamilton AJ, Ortiz BL, Robledo MA, Restrepo A, Hay RJ.** 1997. Development of a novel antigen detection test for histoplasmosis. *J Clin Microbiol* **35:**2618–2622.
95. **Cloud JL, Bauman SK, Neary BP, Ludwig KG, Ashwood ER.** 2007. Performance characteristics of a polyclonal enzyme immunoassay for the quantitation of *Histoplasma* antigen in human urine samples. *Am J Clin Pathol* **128:**18–22.
96. **Hamilton AJ, Bartholomew MA, Fenelon LE, Figueroa J, Hay RJ.** 1990. A murine monoclonal antibody exhibiting high species specificity for *Histoplasma capsulatum* var. *capsulatum*. *J Gen Microbiol* **136:**331–335.
97. **Scheel CM, Samayoa B, Herrera A, Lindsley MD, Benjamin L, Reed Y, Hart J, Lima S, Rivera BE, Raxcaco G, Chiller T, Arathoon E, Gómez BL.** 2009. Development and evaluation of an enzyme-linked immunosorbent assay to detect *Histoplasma capsulatum* antigenuria in immunocompromised patients. *Clin Vaccine Immunol* **16:**852–858.
98. **Theel ES, Jespersen DJ, Harring J, Mandrekar J, Binnicker MJ.** 2013. Evaluation of an enzyme immunoassay for detection of *Histoplasma capsulatum* antigen from urine specimens. *J Clin Microbiol* **51:**3555–3559.
99. **Hossain MA, Miyazaki T, Mitsutake K, Kakeya H, Yamamoto Y, Yanagihara K, Kawamura S, Otsubo T, Hirakata Y, Tashiro T, Kohno S.** 1997. Comparison between Wako-WB003 and Fungitec G tests for detection of (1→3)-beta-D-glucan in systemic mycosis. *J Clin Lab Anal* **11:**73–77.
100. **Odabasi Z, Mattiuzzi G, Estey E, Kantarjian H, Saeki F, Ridge RJ, Ketchum PA, Finkelman MA, Rex JH, Ostrosky-Zeichner L.** 2004. Beta-D-glucan as a diagnostic adjunct for invasive fungal infections: validation, cutoff development, and performance in patients with acute myelogenous leukemia and myelodysplastic syndrome. *Clin Infect Dis* **39:**199–205.
101. **Ostrosky-Zeichner L, Alexander BD, Kett DH, Vazquez J, Pappas PG, Saeki F, Ketchum PA, Wingard J, Schiff R, Tamura H, Finkelman MA, Rex JH.** 2005. Multicenter clinical evaluation of the (1→3) beta-D-glucan assay as an aid to diagnosis of fungal infections in humans. *Clin Infect Dis* **41:**654–659.
102. **Ellis M, Al-Ramadi B, Finkelman M, Hedstrom U, Kristensen J, Ali-Zadeh H, Klingspor L.** 2008. Assessment of the clinical utility of serial beta-D-glucan concentrations in patients with persistent neutropenic fever. *J Med Microbiol* **57:**287–295.
103. **Koo S, Bryar JM, Page JH, Baden LR, Marty FM.** 2009. Diagnostic performance of the (1→3)-beta-D-glucan assay for invasive fungal disease. *Clin Infect Dis* **49:**1650–1659.
104. **Wright WF, Overman SB, Ribes JA.** 2011. (1-3)-β-D-glucan assay: a review of its laboratory and clinical application. *Lab Med* **42:**679–685.
105. **Maertens JA, Blennow O, Duarte RF, Muñoz P.** 2016. The current management landscape: aspergillosis. *J Antimicrob Chemother 71*(suppl 2)**:**ii23–ii29.
106. **Karageorgopoulos DE, Vouloumanou EK, Ntziora F, Michalopoulos A, Rafailidis PI, Falagas ME.** 2011. β-D-glucan assay for the diagnosis of invasive fungal infections: a meta-analysis. *Clin Infect Dis* **52:**750–770.
107. **He S, Hang JP, Zhang L, Wang F, Zhang DC, Gong FH.** 2015. A systematic review and meta-analysis of diagnostic accuracy of serum 1,3-β-D-glucan for invasive fungal infection: focus on cutoff levels. *J Microbiol Immunol Infect* **48:**351–361.
108. **Cuenca-Estrella M, Verweij PE, Arendrup MC, Arikan-Akdagli S, Bille J, Donnelly JP, Jensen HE, Lass-Flörl C, Richardson MD, Akova M, Bassetti M, Calandra T, Castagnola E, Cornely OA, Garbino J, Groll AH, Herbrecht R, Hope WW, Kullberg BJ, Lortholary O, Meersseman W, Petrikkos G, Roilides E, Viscoli C, Ullmann AJ,** for the **ESCMID Fungal Infection Study Group (EFISG).** 2012. ESCMID* guideline for the diagnosis and management of *Candida* diseases 2012: diagnostic procedures. *Clin Microbiol Infect 18*(Suppl 7)**:**9–18.
109. **Rose SR, Vallabhajosyula S, Velez MG, Fedorko DP, VanRaden MJ, Gea-Banacloche JC, Lionakis MS.** 2014. The utility of bronchoalveolar lavage beta-D-glucan testing for the diagnosis of invasive fungal infections. *J Infect* **69:**278–283.
110. **Mutschlechner W, Risslegger B, Willinger B, Hoenigl M, Bucher B, Eschertzhuber S, Lass-Flörl C.** 2015. Bronchoalveolar lavage fluid (1,3)β-D-glucan for the diagnosis of invasive fungal infections in solid organ transplantation: A prospective multicenter study. *Transplantation* **99:**e140–e144.
111. **Reischies FM, Prattes J, Prüller F, Eigl S, List A, Wölfler A, Buzina W, Zollner-Schwetz I, Valentin T, Rabensteiner J, Flick H, Krause R, Raggam RB, Hoenigl M.** 2016. Prognostic potential of 1,3-beta-D-glucan levels in bronchoalveolar lavage fluid samples. *J Infect* **72:**29–35.
112. **Litvintseva AP, Lindsley MD, Gade L, Smith R, Chiller T, Lyons JL, Thakur KT, Zhang SX, Grgurich DE, Kerkering TM, Brandt ME, Park BJ.** 2014. Utility of (1-3)-β-D-glucan testing for diagnostics and monitoring response to treatment during the multistate outbreak of fungal meningitis and other infections. *Clin Infect Dis* **58:**622–630.
113. **Acosta J, Catalan M, del Palacio-Peréz-Medel A, Lora D, Montejo JC, Cuetara MS, Moragues MD, Ponton J, del Palacio A.** 2011. A prospective comparison of galactomannan in bronchoalveolar lavage fluid for the diagnosis of pulmonary invasive aspergillosis in medical patients under intensive care: comparison with the diagnostic performance of galactomannan and of (1→s3)-β-D-glucan chromogenic assay in serum samples. *Clin Microbiol Infect* **17:**1053–1060.
114. **Desmet S, Van Wijngaerden E, Maertens J, Verhaegen J, Verbeken E, De Munter P, Meersseman W, Van Meensel B, Van Eldere J, Lagrou K.** 2009. Serum (1-3)-beta-D-glucan as a tool for diagnosis of *Pneumocystis jirovecii* pneumonia in patients with human immunodeficiency virus infection or hematological malignancy. *J Clin Microbiol* **47:**3871–3874.
115. **Watanabe T, Yasuoka A, Tanuma J, Yazaki H, Honda H, Tsukada K, Honda M, Gatanaga H, Teruya K, Kikuchi Y, Oka S.** 2009. Serum (1→3) beta-D-glucan as a noninvasive adjunct marker for the diagnosis of Pneumocystis pneumonia in patients with AIDS. *Clin Infect Dis* **49:**1128–1131.
116. **Alanio A, Hauser PM, Lagrou K, Melchers WJ, Helweg-Larsen J, Matos O, Cesaro S, Maschmeyer G, Einsele H, Donnelly JP, Cordonnier C, Maertens J, Bretagne S; Fifth European Conference on Infections in Leukemia (ECIL-5), a joint venture of The European Group for Blood and Marrow Transplantation (EBMT), The European Organization for Research and Treatment of Cancer (EORTC), the Immunocompromised Host Society (ICHS), and the European LeukemiaNet (ELN).** 2016. ECIL guidelines for the diagnosis of *Pneumocystis jirovecii* pneumonia in patients with haematological malignancies and stem cell transplant recipients. *J Antimicrob Chemother* **71:**2386–2396.

117. **Onishi A, Sugiyama D, Kogata Y, Saegusa J, Sugimoto T, Kawano S, Morinobu A, Nishimura K, Kumagai S.** 2012. Diagnostic accuracy of serum 1,3-β-D-glucan for *Pneumocystis jiroveci* pneumonia, invasive candidiasis, and invasive aspergillosis: systematic review and meta-analysis. *J Clin Microbiol* **50:**7–15.
118. **Li WJ, Guo YL, Liu TJ, Wang K, Kong JL.** 2015. Diagnosis of pneumocystis pneumonia using serum (1-3)-β-D-Glucan: a bivariate meta-analysis and systematic review. *J Thorac Dis* **7:**2214–2225.
119. **Karageorgopoulos DE, Qu JM, Korbila IP, Zhu YG, Vasileiou VA, Falagas ME.** 2013. Accuracy of β-D-glucan for the diagnosis of *Pneumocystis jirovecii* pneumonia: a meta-analysis. *Clin Microbiol Infect* **19:**39–49.
120. **Christensson B, Sigmundsdottir G, Larsson L.** 1999. D-arabinitol—a marker for invasive candidiasis. *Med Mycol* **37:**391–396.
121. **Megson GM, Stevens DA, Hamilton JR, Denning DW.** 1996. D-mannitol in cerebrospinal fluid of patients with AIDS and cryptococcal meningitis. *J Clin Microbiol* **34:** 218–221.
122. **Larsson L, Pehrson C, Wiebe T, Christensson B.** 1994. Gas chromatographic determination of D-arabinitol/L-arabinitol ratios in urine: a potential method for diagnosis of disseminated candidiasis. *J Clin Microbiol* **32:**1855–1859.
123. **Kupfahl C, Michalka A, Lass-Flörl C, Fischer G, Haase G, Ruppert T, Geginat G, Hof H.** 2008. Gliotoxin production by clinical and environmental *Aspergillus fumigatus* strains. *Int J Med Microbiol* **298:**319–327.
124. **Chambers ST, Syhre M, Murdoch DR, McCartin F, Epton MJ.** 2009. Detection of 2-pentylfuran in the breath of patients with *Aspergillus fumigatus*. *Med Mycol* **47:**468–476.
125. **Chambers ST, Bhandari S, Scott-Thomas A, Syhre M.** 2011. Novel diagnostics: progress toward a breath test for invasive *Aspergillus fumigatus*. *Med Mycol* 49(Suppl 1): S54–S61.
126. **Havlicek V, Lemr K.** 2011. Fungal metabolites for microorganism classification by mass spectrometry, p 51–60. *In* Fenselau C (ed), *Rapid Characterization of Microorganisms by Mass Spectrometry*. American Chemical Society, Washington, DC.
127. **Marklein G, Josten M, Klanke U, Müller E, Horré R, Maier T, Wenzel T, Kostrzewa M, Bierbaum G, Hoerauf A, Sahl HG.** 2009. Matrix-assisted laser desorption ionization-time of flight mass spectrometry for fast and reliable identification of clinical yeast isolates. *J Clin Microbiol* **47:**2912–2917.
128. **Lau AF, Drake SK, Calhoun LB, Henderson CM, Zelazny AM.** 2013. Development of a clinically comprehensive database and a simple procedure for identification of molds from solid media by matrix-assisted laser desorption ionization-time of flight mass spectrometry. *J Clin Microbiol* **51:** 828–834.
129. **Giebel R, Worden C, Rust SM, Kleinheinz GT, Robbins M, Sandrin TR.** 2010. Microbial fingerprinting using matrix-assisted laser desorption ionization time-of-flight mass spectrometry (MALDI-TOF MS) applications and challenges. *Adv Appl Microbiol* **71:**149–184.
130. **Ferroni A, Suarez S, Beretti JL, Dauphin B, Bille E, Meyer J, Bougnoux ME, Alanio A, Berche P, Nassif X.** 2010. Real-time identification of bacteria and *Candida* species in positive blood culture broths by matrix-assisted laser desorption ionization-time of flight mass spectrometry. *J Clin Microbiol* **48:**1542–1548.
131. **Ferreira L, Sánchez-Juanes F, Porras-Guerra I, García-García MI, García-Sánchez JE, González-Buitrago JM, Muñoz-Bellido JL.** 2011. Microorganisms direct identification from blood culture by matrix-assisted laser desorption/ionization time-of-flight mass spectrometry. *Clin Microbiol Infect* **17:**546–551.
132. **Marinach-Patrice C, Fekkar A, Atanasova R, Gomes J, Djamdjian L, Brossas JY, Meyer I, Buffet P, Snounou G, Datry A, Hennequin C, Golmard JL, Mazier D.** 2010. Rapid species diagnosis for invasive candidiasis using mass spectrometry. *PLoS One* **5:**e8862.
133. **Yan Y, He Y, Maier T, Quinn C, Shi G, Li H, Stratton CW, Kostrzewa M, Tang YW.** 2011. Improved identification of yeast species directly from positive blood culture media by combining Sepsityper specimen processing and Microflex analysis with the matrix-assisted laser desorption ionization Biotyper system. *J Clin Microbiol* **49:**2528–2532.
134. **Spanu T, Posteraro B, Fiori B, D'Inzeo T, Campoli S, Ruggeri A, Tumbarello M, Canu G, Trecarichi EM, Parisi G, Tronci M, Sanguinetti M, Fadda G.** 2012. Direct MALDI-TOF mass spectrometry assay of blood culture broths for rapid identification of *Candida* species causing bloodstream infections: an observational study in two large microbiology laboratories. *J Clin Microbiol* **50:**176–179.
135. **Cassagne C, Normand AC, L'Ollivier C, Ranque S, Piarroux R.** 2016. Performance of MALDI-TOF MS platforms for fungal identification. *Mycoses* **59:**678–690.
136. **Sanguinetti M, Posteraro B.** 2017. Identification of molds by matrix-assisted laser desorption ionization-time of flight mass spectrometry. *J Clin Microbiol* **55:**369–379.
137. **Singh A, Singh PK, Kumar A, Chander J, Khanna G, Roy P, Meis JF, Chowdhary A.** 2017. Molecular and matrix-assisted laser desorption ionization-time of flight mass spectrometry-based characterization of clinically significant melanized fungi in India. *J Clin Microbiol* **55:**1090–1103.
138. **Spiess B, Seifarth W, Merker N, Howard SJ, Reinwald M, Dietz A, Hofmann WK, Buchheidt D.** 2012. Development of novel PCR assays to detect azole resistance-mediating mutations of the *Aspergillus fumigatus* cyp51A gene in primary clinical samples from neutropenic patients. *Antimicrob Agents Chemother* **56:**3905–3910.
139. **Melchers WJ, Verweij PE, van den Hurk P, van Belkum A, De Pauw BE, Hoogkamp-Korstanje JA, Meis JF.** 1994. General primer-mediated PCR for detection of *Aspergillus* species. *J Clin Microbiol* **32:**1710–1717.
140. **Yamakami Y, Hashimoto A, Yamagata E, Kamberi P, Karashima R, Nagai H, Nasu M.** 1998. Evaluation of PCR for detection of DNA specific for *Aspergillus* species in sera of patients with various forms of pulmonary aspergillosis. *J Clin Microbiol* **36:**3619–3623.
141. **Li Y, Gao L, Ding Y, Xu Y, Zhou M, Huang W, Jing Y, Li H, Wang L, Yu L.** 2013. Establishment and application of real-time quantitative PCR for diagnosing invasive aspergillosis via the blood in hematological patients: targeting a specific sequence of *Aspergillus* 28S-ITS2. *BMC Infect Dis* **13:**255.
142. **Cruciani M, Mengoli C, Loeffler J, Donnelly P, Barnes R, Jones BL, Klingspor L, Morton O, Maertens J.** 2015. Polymerase chain reaction blood tests for the diagnosis of invasive aspergillosis in immunocompromised people. *Cochrane Database Syst Rev* (9):CD009551.
143. **Avni T, Leibovici L, Paul M.** 2011. PCR diagnosis of invasive candidiasis: systematic review and meta-analysis. *J Clin Microbiol* **49:**665–670.
144. **White PL, Loeffler J, Barnes R, Donnelly JP.** 2012. Towards a standard for *Aspergillus* PCR - requirements, process and results. *Infectio* **16:**64–72.
145. **von Lilienfeld-Toal M, Lehmann LE, Raadts AD, Hahn-Ast C, Orlopp KS, Marklein G, Purr I, Cook G, Hoeft A, Glasmacher A, Stüber F.** 2009. Utility of a commercially available multiplex real-time PCR assay to detect bacterial and fungal pathogens in febrile neutropenia. *J Clin Microbiol* **47:**2405–2410.
146. **Guinea J, Padilla C, Escribano P, Muñoz P, Padilla B, Gijón P, Bouza E.** 2013. Evaluation of MycAssay™ Aspergillus for diagnosis of invasive pulmonary aspergillosis in patients without hematological cancer. *PLoS One* **8:**e61545.
147. **Torelli R, Sanguinetti M, Moody A, Pagano L, Caira M, De Carolis E, Fuso L, De Pascale G, Bello G, Antonelli M, Fadda G, Posteraro B.** 2011. Diagnosis of invasive aspergillosis by a commercial real-time PCR assay for *Aspergillus* DNA in bronchoalveolar lavage fluid samples from high-risk patients compared to a galactomannan enzyme immunoassay. *J Clin Microbiol* **49:**4273–4278.

148. **White PL, Perry MD, Moody A, Follett SA, Morgan G, Barnes RA.** 2011. Evaluation of analytical and preliminary clinical performance of Myconostica MycAssay Aspergillus when testing serum specimens for diagnosis of invasive Aspergillosis. *J Clin Microbiol* **49:**2169–2174.
149. **McTaggart LR, Wengenack NL, Richardson SE.** 2012. Validation of the MycAssay Pneumocystis kit for detection of *Pneumocystis jirovecii* in bronchoalveolar lavage specimens by comparison to a laboratory standard of direct immunofluorescence microscopy, real-time PCR, or conventional PCR. *J Clin Microbiol* **50:**1856–1859.
150. **Chong GL, van de Sande WW, Dingemans GJ, Gaajetaan GR, Vonk AG, Hayette MP, van Tegelen DW, Simons GF, Rijnders BJ.** 2015. Validation of a new *Aspergillus* real-time PCR assay for direct detection of *Aspergillus* and azole resistance of *Aspergillus fumigatus* on bronchoalveolar lavage fluid. *J Clin Microbiol* **53:**868–874.
151. **White PL, Posso RB, Barnes RA.** 2015. Analytical and clinical evaluation of the PathoNostics Aspergenius assay for detection of invasive aspergillosis and resistance to azole antifungal drugs during testing of serum samples. *J Clin Microbiol* **53:**2115–2121.
152. **White PL, Posso RB, Barnes RA.** 2017. Analytical and clinical evaluation of the PathoNostics Aspergenius assay for detection of invasive aspergillosis and resistance to azole antifungal drugs directly from plasma samples. *J Clin Microbiol* **55:**2356–2366.
153. **Dannaoui E, Gabriel F, Gaboyard M, Lagardere G, Audebert L, Quesne G, Godichaud S, Verweij PE, Accoceberry I, Bougnoux ME.** 2017. Molecular diagnosis of invasive aspergillosis and detection of azole resistance by a newly commercialized PCR kit. *J Clin Microbiol* **55:**3210–3218..
154. **Pfaller MA, Wolk DM, Lowery TJ.** 2016. T2MR and T2Candida: novel technology for the rapid diagnosis of candidemia and invasive candidiasis. *Future Microbiol* **11:**103–117.
155. **Ericson JE, Kaufman DA, Kicklighter SD, Bhatia J, Testoni D, Gao J, Smith PB, Prather KO, Benjamin DK Jr, Fluconazole Prophylaxis Study Team on behalf of the Best Pharmaceuticals for Children Act–Pediatric Trials Network Steering Committee.** 2016. Fluconazole prophylaxis for the prevention of candidiasis in premature infants: A meta-analysis using patient-level data. *Clin Infect Dis* **63:**604–610.

Candida, Cryptococcus, and Other Yeasts of Medical Importance*

ANDREW M. BORMAN AND ELIZABETH M. JOHNSON

120

Unicellular fungi which typically divide by budding have traditionally been referred to as yeasts. However, the term "yeast" is not a taxonomically valid unit, since a wide range of genetically unrelated organisms exhibit a yeast growth form, ranging from the black yeasts in the genus *Exophiala* to the yeast forms of several thermally dimorphic fungi in the genera *Histoplasma, Blastomyces, Paracoccidioides, Talaromyces,* and *Emergomyces* (1, 2). The genera discussed in this chapter are yeasts that have been classified in either the Ascomycota or the Basidiomycota, but with the exclusion of the thermally dimorphic fungi in the family Ajellomycetaceae and the genus *Talaromyces.*

TAXONOMY AND NOMENCLATURE

Yeast taxonomy is continually evolving. The rapidly expanding use of molecular identification strategies has permitted detailed phylogenetic analyses (see chapter 116), allowing more accurate delineation of taxonomic boundaries and the reclassification of many yeast species and genera. Molecular identification approaches have also further added to the taxonomic complexity via the delineation of a number of cryptic species and species complexes in many traditional *Candida* species that can be separated only based on DNA sequencing analysis. Additional taxonomic changes will also result from the Amsterdam Declaration (3), which proposed a major modification of Article 59 of the code of nomenclature that enforces the abandonment of the practice of assigning separate names to the anamorph (asexual) and teleomorph (sexual) states of an organism. From 2013, a fungus must retain a single name, with the decisions on which names should be retained being taken or ratified by the Nomenclature Committee for Fungi (4). The preexisting convention that the teleomorph name should always take precedence may lead to considerable confusion among medical mycologists who have previously ignored the convention, since it is usually the anamorph state that is isolated in the laboratory. However, additional changes to the code included, "Follow the principal [sic] of priority of publication when selecting the generic name to adopt," which seemingly ends the previous precedence of teleomorph over anamorph, with the caveat, "except where the younger generic name is far better known." Currently, working groups and committees established under the auspices of the International Commission on the Taxonomy of Fungi and the Nomenclature Committee for Fungi are working to propose lists of retained (protected) and rejected names for key genera, with only definitive changes being ratified. Input from the clinical community will certainly be required to determine the name to be retained (discussed in more detail in references 5 and 6).

Thus, although Kurtzman and Robnett (7) and Fell et al. (8) previously provided overviews on the phylogenetic relationships among ascomycetous and basidiomycetous yeasts, respectively, considerable taxonomic revisions are likely over the coming years, with taxonomic definitions based on sequence identities established over multiple loci. In this respect, it should be noted that a single rule for the degree of DNA sequence concordance necessary for two fungal isolates to be considered identical or different species is far from being established. With these uncertainties in mind, continued familiarity with both the teleomorph and anamorph names might be prudent.

Lists of currently valid anamorph and teleomorph names can be found at www.mycobank.org. A summary for the key pathogenic yeast species discussed in this chapter is presented in Table 1. Recent taxonomy changes among yeasts have also been reviewed (6).

Ascomycetous Yeasts

■ Genus *Candida*

The heterogeneous genus *Candida* belongs to the order Saccharomycetales within the ascomycetes. Currently, the genus contains more than 200 species, but it is clearly imperfect, since "*Candida*" species encompass at least 13 teleomorph genera. Due to the uncertainty surrounding final taxonomy, this chapter uses anamorph names for members of this genus, with teleomorph names displayed in parentheses, where known.

Candida albicans Species Complex

Candida albicans species complex comprises *C. albicans, Candida dubliniensis,* and *Candida africana. Candida albicans sensu stricto* is the most important pathogen in the complex and remains the major pathogen in this genus, in terms of

*This chapter incorporates material from chapter 117 by Susan A. Howell, Kevin C. Hazen, and Mary E. Brandt in the 11th edition of this *Manual.*

TABLE 1 Anamorph/teleomorph combinations and obsolete names for key pathogenic yeasts

Anamorphic species	Previous synonym or obsolete name	Teleomorph
Apiotrichum asahii	*Trichosporon asahii*	None
Apiotrichum loubieri	*Trichosporon loubieri*	None
Apiotrichum mycotoxinivorans	*Trichosporon mycotoxinivorans*	None
Candida albicans	*Oidium albicans, Monilia albicans*	None
Candida auris	None	None
Candida bracarensis	None	*Nakaseomyces bracarensis*
Candida catenulata	*Candida brumptii*	*Diutina catenulata*
Candida ciferrii	*Stephanoascus ciferrii*	*Trichomonascus ciferrii*
Candida famata	*Torulopsis candida*	*Debaryomyces hansenii*
Candida fermentati	*Torula fermentati*	*Meyerozyma caribbica*
Candida glabrata	*Cryptococcus glabratus*	*Nakaseomyces glabrata*
Candida guilliermondii	*Pichia guilliermondii*	*Meyerozyma guilliermondii*
Candida inconspicua	*Torulopsis inconspicua*	*Pichia cactophila*
Candida kefyr	*Candida pseudotropicalis, Candida macedoniensis*	*Kluyveromyces marxianus*
Candida krusei	*Issatchenkia orientalis*	*Pichia kudriavzevii*
Candida lipolytica	*Mycotorula lipolytica*	*Yarrowia lipolytica*
Candida lusitaniae	*Candida obtusa, Candida parapsilosis* var. *obtusa*	*Clavispora lusitaniae*
Candida nivariensis	None	*Nakaseomyces nivariensis*
Candida norvegensis	*Candida mycoderma var. annulata*	*Pichia norvegensis*
Candida pintolopesii	*Candida slooffiae, Torulopsis pintolopesii*	*Kazachstania telluris*
Candida pelliculosa	*Hansenula anomala, Pichia anomala*	*Wickerhamomyces anomalus*
Candida pulcherrima	*Torula pulcherrima*	*Metschnikowia pulcherrima*
Candida robusta	More than 100	*Saccharomyces cerevisiae*
Candida rugosa	*Mycoderma rugose, Torula rugosa*	*Diutina rugosa*
Candida utilis	*Torulopsis utilis, Pichia jadinii, Hansenual jadinii, Lindnera jadinii*	*Cyberlindnera jadinii*
Candida zeylanoides	*Monilia zelanoides*	None
Cutaneotrichosporon cutaneum	*Trichosporon cutaneum*	None
Cutaneotrichosporon dermatis	*Trichosporon dermatis*	None
Cutaneotrichosporon mucoides	*Trichosporon mucoides*	None
Saprochaete capitata	*Geotrichum capitatum, Trichosporon capitatum, Dipodascus capitatus, Blastoschizomyces capitatus*	*Magnusiomyces capitatus*
Rhodotorula minuta	*Torula minuta*	*Cystobasidium minuta*
Rhodotorula slooffiae	None	*Cystobasidium slooffiae*

both virulence and epidemiology (9–13). *Candida dubliniensis* has many phenotypic and genotypic similarities to *C. albicans* but exhibits reduced virulence in several *in vivo* models (14, 15). *Candida africana* is a germ tube-positive, chlamydospore-negative yeast which is closely related to *C. albicans* (16) but which seems almost exclusively restricted to the female genital tract in humans (15) and shows less virulence than both *C. albicans* and *C. dubliniensis in vivo* (15).

Non-*C. albicans* Species

According to most recent epidemiological surveys, some 8 to 10 non-*C. albicans* species are frequently encountered in the clinical setting (9–12), with several of these more common species being recognized as species complexes. *Candida parapsilosis* is a species complex currently comprising three species: *C. parapsilosis, Candida orthopsilosis,* and *Candida metapsilosis* (17). The recent teleomorph genus *Meyerozyma* includes *Candida guilliermondii* (teleomorph *Meyerozyma guilliermondii*) and *Candida fermentati* (teleomorph *Meyerozyma caribbica*) (18, 19). The *Candida glabrata* species complex (teleomorph *Nakaseomyces*) includes *C. glabrata* and the closely related but phenotypically distinguishable *Candida bracarensis* and *Candida nivariensis* (20). The *Candida rugosa* species complex (teleomorph *Diutina*) includes the species *C. rugosa, Candida pseudorugosa, Candida pararugosa, Candida mesorugosa,* and *Candida neorugosa* (21). *Candida catenulata* also has a *Diutina* teleomorph. For *Candida tropicalis,* neither a documented teleomorph nor cryptic species have so far been described (6).

A large number of other *Candida* species are infrequently encountered in the medical setting, many of which are increasingly commonly reported using their teleomorph names, after taxonomic reassignments driven by DNA sequencing studies. These include *Candida norvegensis* (*Pichia norvegensis*), *Candida inconspicua* (*Pichia cactophila*), *Candida ciferri* (*Trichomonoascus ciferrii*), *Candida famata* (*Debaryomyces hansenii*), *Candida guilliermondii* var. *membranifaciens* (*Kodamaea ohmeri*), *Candida kefyr* (*Kluyveromyces marxianus*), *Candida krusei* (*Pichia kudriavzevii*), *Candida lipolytica* (*Yarrowia lipolytica*), *Candida lusitaniae* (*Clavispora lusitaniae*), *Candida pelliculosa* (*Wickerhamomyces anomalus*), and *Candida utilis* (*Cyberlindnera jadinii*). *Candida zeylanoides* has no known teleomorph.

Rare species known mainly from single case reports include *Candida aaseri* and *C. pseudoaaseri,* which are close genetic relatives (22). *Candida subhashii* is genetically most closely related to the *C. parapsilosis* species complex, *C. tropicalis, C. albicans,* and *C. dubliniensis* (23). *Candida tunisiensis* and *Hanseniaspora opuntiae* were also recently identified among clinical isolates from hospitals in Tunisia (24). Of particular interest is the hitherto-rare *Candida haemulonii* species complex, comprising *C. haemulonii, Candida pseudohaemulonii, Candida duobushaemulonii,* and in particular *Candida auris.* Originally described in 2009 in association with otitis externa (25), the multidrug-resistant and highly pathogenic C. *auris* has simultaneously emerged on three continents as an important nosocomial pathogen, with evidence of high levels of inter- and intrahospital transmission (13, 26, 27) and distinct, geographically constrained clonal lineages (26–28).

■ Genus *Saccharomyces*

Although the wine-making industry has spent considerable effort investigating the taxonomy of the genus *Saccharomyces*, the principal medically relevant species is *Saccharomyces cerevisiae*.

■ Genus *Saprochaete*

Saprochaete capitata is the currently valid name for *Blastoschizomyces capitatus* (29), a taxon derived from the combination of the obsolete taxa *Blastoschizomyces pseudotrichosporon* and *Trichosporon capitatum* (30). The teleomorph is *Magnusiomyces capitatus* (29). Older names for this fungus are *Geotrichum capitatum*, *Trichosporon capitatum* (anamorph), and *Dipodascus capitatus* (teleomorph). Although the genus *Saprochaete* contains at least a dozen species, *S. capitata* is the principal species encountered in the clinical setting.

Basidiomycetous Yeasts

■ Genus *Cryptococcus*

Historically, five serotypes had been recognized within *Cryptococcus neoformans* and C. *gattii*. Serotype A was proposed as C. *neoformans* var. *grubii*, and serotype D as a distinct variety, *Cryptococcus neoformans* var. *neoformans*. The A/D serotype was recognized as an intervarietal C. *grubii*/C. *neoformans* hybrid. Serotypes B and C were recognized as the distinct species *Cryptococcus gattii*. Serotypes A and D were found to produce the teleomorphic state *Filobasidiella neoformans*, and serotypes B and C produce the teleomorph originally named *Filobasidiella bacillispora*. A number of recent phylogenetic studies have resulted in the proposal for a complete reorganization of the species complexes previously designated *Cryptococcus neoformans* and C. *gattii* (31). The name *Cryptococcus neoformans* was retained to describe species formerly referred to as *Cryptococcus neoformans* var. *grubii*; *Cryptococcus deneoformans* was erected to encompass serotype D isolates (formerly C. *neoformans* var. *neoformans*); and at least five cryptic species are recognized in C. *gattii* species complex, namely, C. *gattii*, *Cryptococcus deuterogattii*, *Cryptococcus tetragattii*, *Cryptococcus decagattii*, and *Cryptococcus bacillisporus*. While these newly erected species differ in prevalence, pathogenicity, and antifungal susceptibility and are represented as distinct lineages in most recent molecular analyses (31, 32), other workers have argued that such studies revealed more genetic variation than can be encompassed in only seven species and that the proposal for seven species is premature (33).

An increasing number of non-C. *neoformans* species have been described anecdotally as occasional agents of human infection, including *Cryptococcus adeliensis*, *Cryptococcus albidus*, *Cryptococcus curvatus*, *Cryptococcus diffluens*, *Cryptococcus flavescens*, *Cryptococcus luteolus*, *Cryptococcus laurentii*, *Cryptococcus liquefaciens*, *Cryptococcus terreus*, and *Cryptococcus uniguttulatus* (*Filobasidium uniguttulatum*). Many of these species have recently been reassigned to alternative Tremellomycete genera, including *Naganishia* (C. *adeliensis*, C. *albidus*, C. *diffluens*, and C. *liquefaciens*), *Hannaella* (C. *luteolus*), *Solicoccozyma* (C. *terreus*), and *Papiliotrema* (C. *laurentii* and C. *flavescens*) (34).

■ Genus *Malassezia*

Fifteen *Malassezia* species have been isolated from human and animal skin. The species most commonly seen in the clinical laboratory include *Malassezia furfur*, *Malassezia globosa*, *Malassezia slooffiae*, *Malassezia sympodialis*, *Malassezia obtusa*, and *Malassezia pachydermatis* (35, 36). *Malassezia* species are basidiomycetous yeasts of the subphylum Ustilaginomycotina (class Malasseziomycetes), most of which are lipophilic. Species identification is best achieved by DNA sequencing (35).

■ Genus "*Pseudozyma*"

Historically, at least 20 "*Pseudozyma*" species were recognized, most of which are environmental organisms, classified in the family Ustilaginaceae. However, the genus is now obsolete, following the demonstration that the type species of "*Pseudozyma*" (*Pseudozyma prolifica*) is synonymous with *Ustilago maydis* (36). The major human pathogens are *Pseudozyma aphidis*, *Pseudozyma antarctica*, and *Pseudozyma parantarctica*, which were recently transferred to the teleomorph genus *Moesziomyces*, and *Pseudozyma thailandica*, which is more closely related to *Macalpinomyces* spp. (36).

■ Genus "*Rhodotorula*"

Until recently, more than 60 species of *Rhodotorula* were listed in the Mycobank database. However, the historical genus *Rhodotorula* is clearly polyphyletic (37). The major clinically relevant species are *Rhodotorula mucilaginosa*, *Rhodotorula minuta*, *Rhodotorula glutinis*, *Rhodotorula slooffiae*, and *Rhodotorula dairenensis*. *R. mucilaginosa*, *R. dairenensis*, and *R. glutinis* are retained in *Rhodotorula*; *R. minuta* and *R. slooffiae* have been reclassified in *Cystobasidium* (37).

■ Genus "*Sporobolomyces*"

Sporobolomyces is another historical genus of environmental basidiomycetous yeasts that is now known to be polyphyletic (37). The three species that have been reported from human infection (*Sporobolomyces roseus*, *Sporobolomyces holsaticus*, and *Sporobolomyces salmonicolor*; the latter two species having the teleomorphs *Sporidiobolus johnsonii* [homothallic] and *Sporidiobolus salmonicolor* [heterothallic], respectively) are retained in *Sporobolomyces*. The other species previously classified in *Sporobolomyces* have been redistributed among more than 10 different basidiomycete genera (37).

■ Genus "*Trichosporon*"

Although 37 valid species were listed in the Mycobank database at the writing of the last edition of this *Manual*, the genus is now known to be polyphyletic (34). *Trichosporon asahii*, *Trichosporon asteroides*, *Trichosporon cutaneum*, *Trichosporon dermatis*, *Trichosporon inkin*, *Trichosporon jirovecii*, *Trichosporon loubieri*, *Trichosporon mucoides*, *Trichosporon mycotoxinivorans*, and *Trichosporon ovoides* have all been associated with human infections (38). *T. asahii*, *T. asteroides*, and *T. ovoides* are retained in *Trichosporon*, *T. loubieri* and *T. mycotoxinivorans* have been reclassified in *Apiotrichum*, and *T. cutaneum*, *T. mucoides*, *T. dermatis*, and *T. jirovecii* belong to the new genus *Cutaneotrichosporon* (34).

DESCRIPTION OF THE AGENTS

A key monograph on yeast taxonomy published in 1998 listed approximately 700 species (39). However, the startling discovery of over 200 novel species from a single study examining the flora of beetle guts indicated that the true number of yeast species was likely to be much greater (40), and the equivalent monograph in 2011 described over 1,500 species (41). Indeed, a simple PubMed search conducted in November 2017 with the search term "yeast sp. nov." returned over 220 additional novel species, of mainly environmental origin, described since 2015 (personal observation). Since morphology is a poor predictor of phylogenetic relationships and identity in yeasts (31, 34, 36–38), a detailed description of all of the etiological agents is beyond the scope of a single chapter. Here, the general features of the various genera of pathogenic yeasts are described, with specific reference only to features that are useful in distinguishing isolates at the genus level.

Growth on fungal media can be detected as early as 24 hours for many species of yeast; however, colonies usually are visible in 48 to 72 hours as white to cream colored or tan. Cultures of yeasts are moist, creamy, or glabrous to membranous in texture. Several produce a capsule that makes the colony mucoid. With rare exceptions, aerial hyphae are not produced. Colonies may be hyaline, brightly colored, or darkly pigmented due to the presence of melanins. The latter group, referred to as phaeoid fungi and belonging to the class Eurotiomycetes, is discussed in chapter 127; also, dimorphic fungal pathogens possessing a yeast phase in tissue are discussed in chapter 125.

In general, yeasts are unicellular, eukaryotic budding cells, generally round to oval or, less often, elongate or irregular in shape. They multiply principally by the production of blastoconidia (buds), such that a typical medically important yeast is composed of a progenitor cell with one or more attached progeny. When blastoconidia are produced one from the other in a linear fashion without separating, a structure termed a pseudohypha is formed. Under certain circumstances, such as growth under reduced oxygen tension, some yeasts may produce true septate hyphae, while a small number also produce large, refractile resting spores known as chlamydospores.

Ascomycetous Yeasts

■ Genus *Candida* and Its Teleomorphs

Blastoconidia of *Candida* spp. vary in shape, from round to oval to elongate. Occasional initial isolates, especially from patients receiving antimicrobial agents, may be highly pleomorphic. Asexual reproduction is by multilateral budding, and true mycelium may be present. Several species of *Candida*, most notably *C. albicans*, are diploid (42). The appearance of pseudohyphae and attachment of blastoconidia are important characteristics to observe in the identification of *Candida* spp. Figure 1 illustrates these morphologic features and other characteristics of the most common clinical species. Observation of germ tubes and chlamydospores is also helpful in identifying *C. albicans*. Most *Candida* spp. grow well aerobically at 25 to 30°C, and many grow at 37°C or above. Colonies are creamy in texture and may become more membranous and convoluted with age. In general, colonies are white to cream colored or tan, although a reddish colony variant of *C. glabrata*, which would otherwise have been confused with *Rhodotorula*, has been described (43). Many isolates of *C. albicans* produce "colonies with feet" (i.e., colonies with short marginal extensions; also known as "spiking") on blood agar, while most other yeasts do not, with the exception that this might be observed in 25% of isolates of *C. tropicalis* and *C. krusei* (44). The key physiologic properties of the most common pathogenic *Candida* spp. are listed in Table 2.

■ Genus *Saccharomyces*

Saccharomyces cerevisiae is the most common species of this genus recovered in the clinical laboratory. Multilateral budding yeast cells are round to oval, and short rudimentary (occasionally well-developed) pseudohyphae may be formed (Fig. 1). Other physiologic properties are listed in Table 2. Assimilation of raffinose by *S. cerevisiae* is noteworthy. Very few other yeast species encountered in the clinical laboratory utilize this carbon source.

■ Genus *Saprochaete*

Macroscopically, colonies are glabrous with radiating edges, white to cream colored, and shiny. Microscopically, isolates produce true hyphae, pseudohyphae, and annelloconidia resembling arthroconidia. Based on morphological features alone, *S. capitata* can be difficult to separate from *Trichosporon* and *Cutaneotrichosporon* spp., and physiological tests are needed. *S. capitata* is nonfermentative and can be differentiated from *Trichosporon* spp. by growth on Sabouraud glucose agar at 45°C, growth on cycloheximide-containing agar at room temperature, and failure to hydrolyze urea.

Basidiomycetous Yeasts

■ Genus *Cryptococcus*

Cryptococcus species are round to somewhat oval yeast-like fungi ranging greatly in size, from 3.5 to 8 μm or more in diameter, with a single bud and a narrow neck between the parent and daughter cell (Fig. 3). Unusually large yeast cells (up to 60 μm) have been observed, and this size appears to be associated with higher incubation temperatures (45). Occasionally, several buds are seen. The cell wall is quite fragile, and it is not unusual to find collapsed or crescent-shaped cells, especially in stained tissue sections. Cells are characterized by the presence of a polysaccharide (galactoxylomannan) capsule varying from a wide halo to a nearly undetectable, lighter zone around the cells, depending on the strain and the medium used. Colonies typically are mucoid due to the presence of capsular material, become dry and duller with age, and exhibit a wide range of color (cream, tan, pink, or yellow) that may darken with age. Strains possessing only a slight capsule may appear similar to colonies of *Candida* spp. Historically, canavanine-glycine-bromthymol blue agar was recommended for separating serotypes A and D from serotypes B and C (46, 47). However, standard biochemical laboratory tests are unable to fully differentiate *C. neoformans* and *C. deneoformans* or the five species in the *C. gattii* complex (31).

■ Genus *Malassezia*

Most *Malassezia* species require lipid for growth; only *M. pachydermatis* can grow independently of lipid supplementation of the media. Van Abbe (48) and Leeming and Notman (49) have designed media optimal for the growth and isolation of all of the *Malassezia* spp. (see chapter 118 for recipes). These media are not commercially available, and the alternative of overlaying Sabouraud glucose agar with a few drops of sterile olive oil has been used, but some of the more fastidious species do not survive on this medium (50). The inoculated media should be incubated aerobically at 32 to 35°C in a moist atmosphere for up to 2 weeks to permit development of the slower-growing species. Colonies are cream to beige, are smooth to deeply folded, and have a brittle texture that frequently makes it difficult to mix the colony into a suspension. *Malassezia* is distinguished microscopically from other yeasts by the formation of a prominent monopolar bud scar or collarette resulting from the continued formation of daughter cells at that site (Fig. 2b).

These structures are absent from *C. glabrata*, which could otherwise be confused with *Malassezia* species due to its small size and typical unipolar budding (Fig. 1g). Sympodial

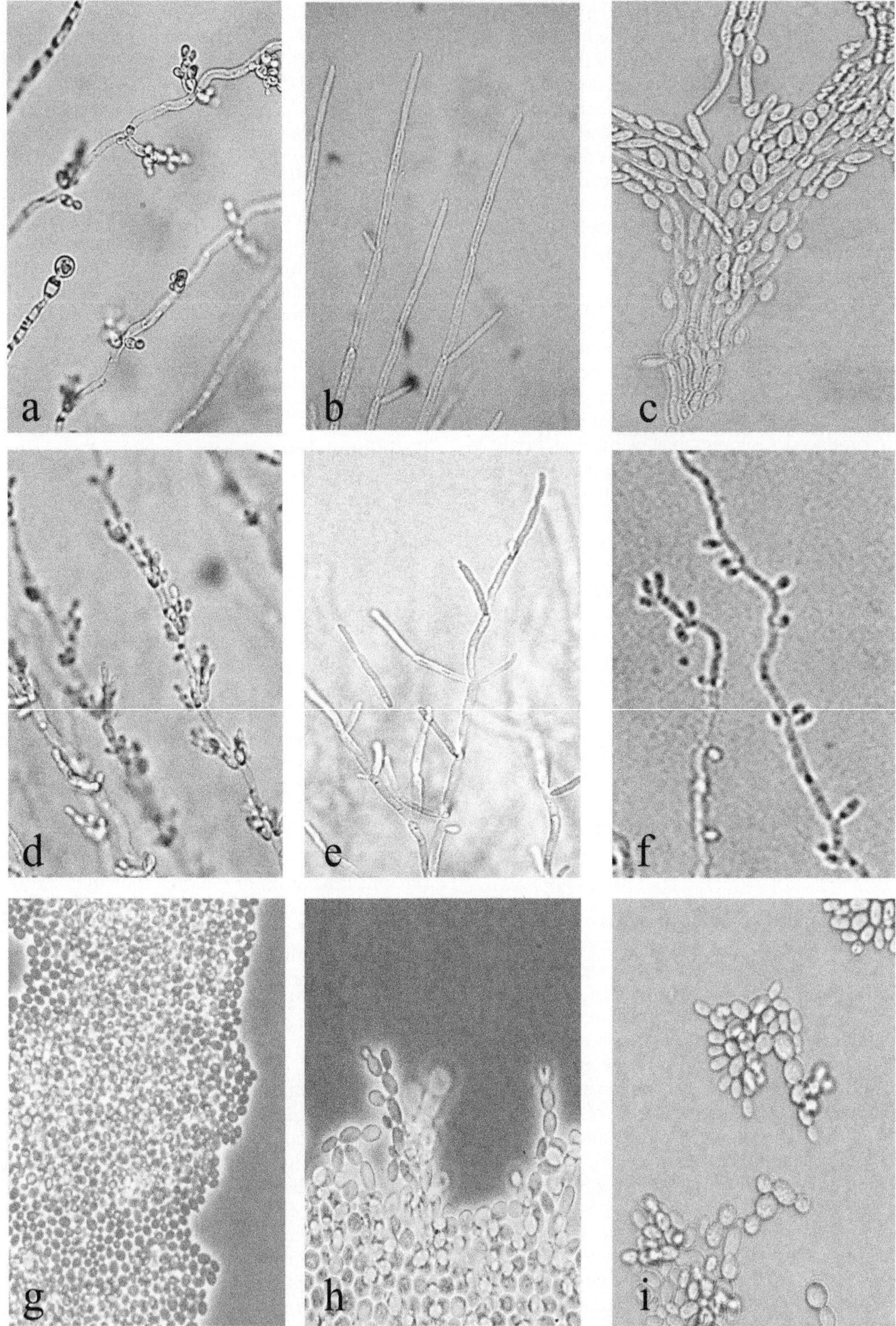

FIGURE 1 Morphological features of some common pathogenic yeast species on cornmeal agar at 24 to 48 hours and ambient temperature. (a) *Candida albicans*: blastoconidia, chlamydospores, true hyphae, and pseudohyphae. (b) *Candida krusei*: extremely elongated, rarely branched pseudohyphae arising at 45°, with few blastoconidia. (c) *Candida kefyr*: large numbers of elongate pseudohyphae and blastospores produced in a characteristic "logjam." (d) *Candida lusitaniae*: short, distinctly curved pseudohyphae with blastoconidia formed at, and occasionally between, septa. (e) *Candida parapsilosis*: elongated, delicately curved pseudohyphae with branches arising at nearly 90°, with blastoconidia at septa. (f) *Candida tropicalis*: blastoconidia formed at septa and between septa. (g) *Candida glabrata*: no true- or pseudomycelium; small oval budding cells only. (h) *Saccharomyces cerevisiae*: large oval to elongated blastospores, sometimes arranged as poorly formed pseudohyphae. (i) *Rhodotorula* spp.: large round to oval blastoconidia, occasionally in short chains. Magnification, ×400. (Photographs courtesy of Adrien Szekely.)

TABLE 2 Cultural and biochemical characteristics of yeasts frequently isolated from clinical specimens[a]

Species	Growth at 37°C	Pellicle in broth	Pseudohyphae or true hyphae	Chlamydospores	Germ tubes	Capsule, India ink	Assimilation of: Glucose	Maltose	Sucrose	Lactose	Galactose	Melibiose	Cellobiose	Inositol	Xylose	Raffinose	Trehalose	Dulcitol	Fermentation of: Glucose	Malose	Sucrose	Lactose	Galactose	Trehalose	Urease	KNO_3 utilization	Phenol oxidase	Ascospores
Candida and related genera																												
Candida albicans	+	–	+	+[b]	+	–	+	+	V	–	+	–	–	–	+	–	+	–	F	F	–	–	F	F	–	–	–	–
C. auris	+	–	V	–	–	–	+	+	+	–	–	+	–	–	–	+	+	ND	ND	ND	ND	ND	ND	ND	ND	ND	ND	–
C. catenulata	V	–	+	–	–	–	+	+	–	–	+	–	–	–	+	–	–	–	F*	–	–	–	–	–	–	–	–	–
C. dubliniensis	+	–	+	+[b]	+	–	+	+	+	–	+	–	–	–	V	–	+	–	F	F	–	–	F	F	–	–	–	–
C. famata	+	–	–	–	–	–	+	+	+	V	+	+	+	–	+	+	+	V	W	–	W	–	–	W	–	–	–	V
C. glabrata	+	–	–	–	–	–	+	+	–	–	–	–	–	–	–	–	+	–	F	–	–	–	–	F	–	–	–	–
C. guilliermondii	+	–	+	–	–	–	+	+	+	–	+	+	+	–	+	+	+	+	F	–	F	–	F*	F	–	–	–	V
C. kefyr	+	–	+	–	–	–	+	–	+	+	+	–	V	–	V	+	V	–	F	–	F	F*	F	–	–	–	–	–
C. krusei[c]	+	+	+	–	–	–	+	–	–	–	–	–	–	–	–	–	–	–	F	–	–	–	–	–	V	–	–	V
C. lambica	V	+	+	–	–	–	+	–	–	–	–	–	–	–	+	–	–	–	F	–	–	–	–	–	–	–	–	V
C. lipolytica[c]	+	+	+	–	–	–	+	–	–	–	–	–	–	–	–	–	–	–	–	–	–	–	–	–	+	–	–	V
C. lusitaniae[d]	+	–	+	–	–	–	+	+	+	–	+	–	+	–	+	–	+	–	F	–	F	–	F	F	–	–	–	V
C. parapsilosis[e]	+	–	+	–	–	–	+	+	+	–	+	–	–	–	+	–	+	–	F	–	–	–	–	–	–	–	–	–
C. pelliculosa	V	–	–	–	–	–	+	+	+	–	+	–	+	–	+	–	+	–	F	F*	F	–	F	–	–	+	–	+
C. pintolopesii[f]	+	–	–	–	–	–	+	–	–	–	–	–	–	–	–	–	–	–	–	–	F	–	–	–	–	–	–	–
C. rugosa	+	–	+	–	–	–	+	–	–	–	+	–	–	–	V	–	–	–	–	–	–	–	–	–	–	–	–	–
C. tropicalis[d,e]	+	+	+	–[g]	–	–	+	+	+	–	+	–	+	–	+	–	+	–	F	F	F	–	F*	F*	–	–	–	–
C. zeylanoides	–	V	+	–	–	–	+	–	–	–	V	–	V	–	–	–	+	–	–	–	–	–	–	–	–	–	–	–
Cryptococcus and related genera																												
Cryptococcus neoformans	+	–	R	–	–	+	+	+	+	–	+	–	+	+	+	V	+	+	–	–	–	–	–	–	+	–	+	–
Filobasidium uniguttulatum	–	–	–	–	–	+	+	+	+	–	V	–	V	+	+	V	V	–	–	–	–	–	–	–	+	–	–	–
Hannaella luteola	–	–	–	–	–	+	+	+	+	–	+	+	+	+	+	+	+	+	–	–	–	–	–	–	+	–	–	–
Naganishia albida	V	–	–	–	–	+	+	+	+	V	V	+	+	+	+	+	+	V	–	–	–	–	–	–	+	–	–	–
Papiliotrema laurentii	V	–	–	–	–	+	+	+	+	+	+	V	+	+	+	V	+	+	–	–	–	–	–	–	+	+	–	–
Solicoccozyma terrea	V	–	–	–	–	+	+	V	–	V	V	–		+	+	+	+	V	–	–	–	–	–	–	+	+	–	–

(*Continued on next page*)

TABLE 2 Cultural and biochemical characteristics of yeasts frequently isolated from clinical specimens[a] *(Continued)*

Species	Growth at 37°C	Pellicle in broth	Pseudohyphae or true hyphae	Chlamydospores	Germ tubes	Capsule, India ink	Assimilation of: Glucose	Maltose	Sucrose	Lactose	Galactose	Melibiose	Cellobiose	Inositol	Xylose	Raffinose	Trehalose	Dulcitol	Fermentation of: Glucose	Malose	Sucrose	Lactose	Galactose	Trehalose	Urease	KNO3 utilization	Phenol oxidase	Ascospores
Trichosporon and related genera																												
Cutaneotrichosporon mucoides	+		+	−	−	−	+	+	+	+	+	+	+	+	+	+	+	+	−	−	−	−	−	−	+	−	−	−
Trichosporon asahii	+		+	−	−	−	+	+	V	+	+	−	+	V	V	−	V	−	−	−	−	−	−	−	+	+	−	−
Trichosporon ovoides	V		+	−	−	−	+	+	+	+	+	+	+	+	+	+	+	−	−	−	−	−	−	−	+	−	−	−
Others																												
Geotrichum candidum[h]	V	+	+	−	−	−	+	−	−	−	+	−	−	−	+	−	−	−	−	−	−	−	−	−	−	−	−	−
Prototheca wickerhamii[h]	+	−	−	−	−	−	+	−	−	−	+	−	−	−	−	−	+	−	−	−	−	−	−	−	−	−	−	−
Rhodotorula glutinis	+	−	−	−	−	V	+	+	+	−	V	−	+	−	+	+	+	−	−	−	−	−	−	−	+	+	−	−
Rhodotorula rubra	+	−	−	−	−	V	+	+	+	−	+	−	V	−	+	+	+	−	−	−	−	−	−	−	+	−	−	−
Saccharomyces cerevisiae	+	−	V	−	−	−	+	+	+	−	+	−	−	−	−	+	V	−	F	F	F	−	F	F*	−	−	−	+
Saprochaete capitata	+	+	+	−	−	−	+	−	−	−	+	−	−	−	−	−	−	−	−	−	−	−	−	−	−	−	−	−
Sporobolomyces salmonicolor	V	+	V	−	−	−	+	+	+	−	V	−	+	−	W	−	+	−	−	−	−	−	−	−	+	+	−	−

[a]Modified from reference 168 and references therein. +, growth greater than that of the negative control; −, negative reaction; V, variation in reactions in an isolate-dependent manner; *, some isolates may give the opposite reaction; R, rare; F, the sugar is fermented (i.e., gas is produced); W, weak reaction.

[b]*C. albicans* typically produces single and no more than two terminal chlamydospores, while some isolates of *C. dubliniensis* will produce terminal chlamydospores in pairs, triplets, and clusters. See the text for additional methods to differentiate *C. dubliniensis* and *C. albicans*.

[c]*C. lipolytica* assimilates erythritol; *C. krusei* does not. Maximum growth temperatures are 43 to 45°C for *C. krusei* and 33 to 37°C for *C. lipolytica*.

[d]*C. lusitaniae* assimilates rhamnose; *C. tropicalis* usually does not.

[e]*C. parapsilosis* assimilates L-arabinose; *C. tropicalis* usually does not.

[f]C. pintolopesii is a thermophilic yeast capable of growth at 40 to 42°C.

[g]Rare strains of *C. tropicalis* produce teardrop-shaped chlamydospores.

[h]Not yeasts but may be confused with several yeast genera.

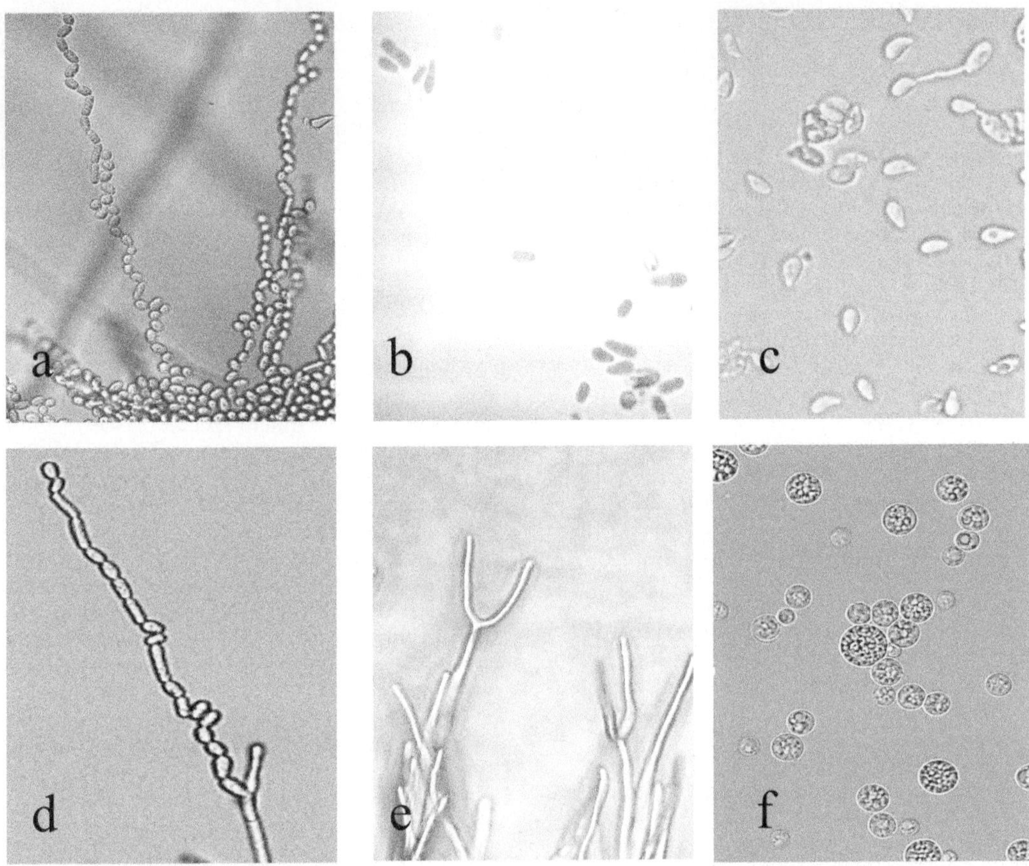

FIGURE 2 Morphological features of less common pathogenic yeast and yeast-like organisms on cornmeal agar at 24 to 48 hours and ambient temperature. (a) *Trichosporon* spp.: chains of arthroconidia with blastoconidia formed at the corners of arthroconidia. (b) *Malassezia furfur*: bottle-shaped, budding yeasts with annelloconidia and collarettes. (c) Ballistoconidia of *Sporobolomyces* spp. (d and e) Arthroconidia (d) and characteristic dichotomous branching (e) of *Geotrichum candidum* (*Galactomyces geotrichum*). (f) Sporangia of *Prototheca wickerhamii* containing sporangiospores. Magnification, ×400. (Photographs courtesy of Adrien Szekely.)

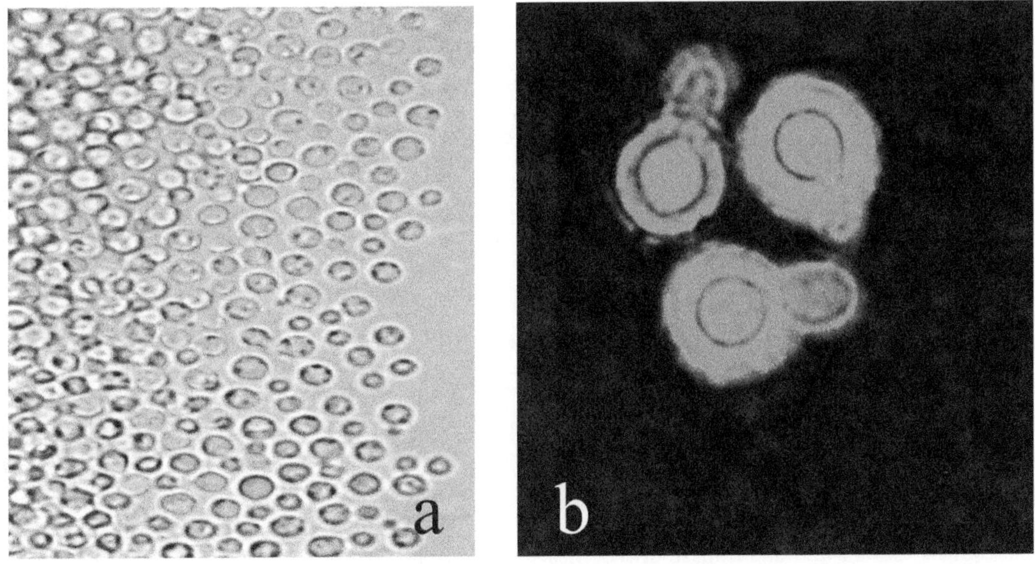

FIGURE 3 (a) Appearance of *Cryptococcus neoformans* on cornmeal agar at 48 hours and ambient temperature. Magnification, ×400. (b) India ink preparation of *Cryptococcus neoformans*. Magnification, ×1,000.

budding has been observed in cultures of M. *sympodialis* and M. *japonica*. The species vary in shape from spherical to oval or elongated, have thick cell walls, and range in length from 1.5 μm to 8 μm.

■ Genus "*Pseudozyma*"

Members of the former genus *Pseudozyma* are basidiomycetous plant pathogens and are usually found in the environment. They form moist, beige to tan, wrinkled colonies on routine media. *Moesziomyces aphidis* forms rough green colonies on CHROMagar *Candida* medium after 48 hours of incubation at 37°C. Growth is inhibited on cycloheximide-containing media. Microscopically, they demonstrate fusiform, spindle-shaped blastoconidia.

■ Genus "*Rhodotorula*"

Rhodotorula spp. and species in the allied genus *Cystobasidium* (37) share many similar physiologic and morphologic properties with *Cryptococcus* spp., as they are round to oval-shaped, multilateral budding yeasts (Fig. 1i) with capsules, although capsules, when present, are typically small. *Rhodotorula* spp. differ from cryptococci due to their obvious carotenoid pigment, producing colonies that are markedly orange-red to salmon pink. However, a large number of other nonpathogenic genera classified in Pucciniomycotina possess carotenoids and thus have similar colonial appearances (37).

■ Genus "*Sporobolomyces*"

Similar to *Rhodotorula* and *Cystobasidium* spp., colonies are soft and typically shades of salmon pink (37). Budding oval to ellipsoidal yeasts, pseudohyphae, and ballistoconidia on large sterigmata may be seen. When ballistoconidia are ejected, they can be found, often among droplets of condensation, on the inside of the lid of the petri dish (Fig. 2c).

■ Genus "*Trichosporon*" and Allied Genera *Apiotrichum* and *Cutaneotrichosporon*

Trichosporon, *Apiotrichum*, and *Cutaneotrichosporon* yeasts grow easily on standard mycological laboratory media; colonies usually appear within a week on solid media and are cream colored. There is considerable variation in colonial appearance, with mature colonies that may be dry, moist, shiny, folded, cerebriform, or elevated, with or without marginal zones with age.

They produce blastoconidia of various shapes, well-developed hyphae, pseudohyphae, and arthroconidia (Fig. 2a). *Apiotrichum loubieri* also produces one- and two-celled giant cells (51), while *Apiotrichum mycotoxinivorans* produces giant cells with as many as eight cells, depending on the growth medium (K. C. Hazen, D. G. Moore, and D. E. Padgett, unpublished observation). In cases where isolates produce only a few blastoconidia, differentiation from *Geotrichum* spp. and other arthrosporic moulds may be difficult (Fig. 2d and e).

EPIDEMIOLOGY AND TRANSMISSION

Most medically important yeasts are found as commensal organisms on humans and warm-blooded animals and in the environments they inhabit (reviewed in references 42 and 52). Environmental sampling of foods, plants, potable water, and juices (pasteurized and unpasteurized) has revealed an amazing array of yeast species known as opportunistic pathogens. In all cases, the presence of these yeasts could be attributed to direct and indirect contamination by warm-blooded animals. For example, Arias et al. (53) noted the presence of C. *parapsilosis*, C. *tropicalis*, C. *lusitaniae*, C. *zeylanoides*, and several other yeast species in single-strength orange juice that had been pasteurized but subsequently contaminated. These and many similar observations demonstrate that immunocompromised patients are repeatedly exposed to potential yeast pathogens other than those residing as part of their normal microbiota, and care should be exercised in preparing foods and in monitoring the level of contamination associated with devices or creams that may be applied to the patient (54, 55). Parenteral nutrition fluids and devices are particularly prone to contamination with yeasts, especially C. *parapsilosis* (56). It is also noteworthy that the hospital environment can contribute to the development of colonization with *Candida* species as well as facilitating the replacement of less virulent colonizing species with more virulent species (57–59).

With the possible exception of C. *auris* (58, 59), person-to-person transmission has a negligible impact on disease development, except in nosocomial outbreaks, in which hands or fomites are often the source. Invasive yeast infections are associated with opportunism; thus, the yeasts causing disease must be present when the conditions are such that disease can be initiated. Several studies have shown that transmission of yeasts through sexual contact (including oral) does occur, but establishment of the transferred organisms in the recipient is affected by a variety of factors, most notably the recipient's current normal microbiota and immunological and antifungal status (60, 61).

■ Genus *Candida*

Candida species are ubiquitous, being found on many plants and as normal flora of the alimentary tracts of mammals and mucocutaneous membranes of humans (42). Essentially, all areas of the gastrointestinal tract of humans can harbor *Candida*. The most commonly isolated species (50 to 70% of yeast isolates) from the gastrointestinal tract of humans is C. *albicans*, followed by C. *tropicalis*, C. *parapsilosis*, C. *krusei*, and C. *glabrata* (62).

Candidemia is the third or fourth most common hospital-acquired bloodstream infection in the United States and much of the rest of the developed world and accounts for more than half of all episodes of sepsis in nonneutropenic patients in intensive care units (ICUs) and surgical wards (10, 63). Most cases of candidemia are caused by one of five species—*Candida albicans*, C. *tropicalis*, C. *parapsilosis*, C. *glabrata*, or C. *krusei*—although the proportions of each species vary according to geographic location, precise patient population, patient age, and the existence of prior antifungal therapy (reviewed in reference 64). In the United States, the implementation of stringent protocols for central line catheter placement and maintenance has contributed enormously to decreases in the prevalence of candidemia in many institutions (65). However, the proportion of candidemia caused by non-C. *albicans* species, particularly C. *glabrata*, is rising in the United States. The PATH (Prospective Antifungal Therapy) Alliance registry reported results from more than 3,000 patients from 2004 to 2008, showing that the proportion of candidemia caused by non-C. *albicans Candida* species (58%) was higher than that caused by C. *albicans* (42%). C. *glabrata* was the predominant non-C. *albicans* cause of candidemia, accounting for 26.7% of all candidemias (66), and was associated with the poorest patient outcomes of all of the non-C. *albicans* species examined (67). Older adults were more likely to be infected with C. *glabrata* than children, and associated risk factors were patient age, severity of underlying disease, use of broad-spectrum antibiotics, central venous catheters, and length of stay in the ICU, with the link to the use of fluconazole being strong only in cancer centers (67). Several avian species have been reported as nonhuman hosts or vectors for *C. glabrata* carriage (reviewed in reference 20). *C. parapsilosis* has a greater incidence of bloodstream infections in children than in adults (67), but this organism is a known pathogen of the young (68).

Candida africana was reported as a new cause of vaginitis in 2009 (39), with isolates identified from Africa, Spain, Germany, and Italy, and its restriction to specimens from the female genital tract has also been confirmed in the United Kingdom (15). In fact, vulvovaginal candidiasis, which affects nearly 75% of women of reproductive age, is one of the most frequent presentations of *Candida* infection.

In the past 8 years, *Candida auris* has emerged simultaneously on three continents as an important novel cause of health care-related infections, with geographically restricted clonal lineages and high inter- and intrahospital transmission rates (25–28). A wide variety of deep-seated infections in addition to candidemia have been reported, and this multidrug-resistant organism has been shown to persist in hospital environments and also cause long-term colonization of patients in high-intensity care settings, leading to specific guidelines for the management of patients with this organism (27, 58, 59).

■ Genus *Cryptococcus*

Cryptococcus neoformans affects immunocompromised hosts worldwide, with *C. neoformans* var. *grubii* (serotype A; now *C. neoformans*) being the most commonly isolated type, although *C. deneoformans* (formerly *C. neoformans* serotype D) is more commonly isolated in Europe (31). The five species in the *C. gattii* complex predominantly infect immunocompetent hosts in areas where the organism is endemic, although approximately 10% of AIDS cases in Botswana and parts of sub-Saharan Africa are infected with members of this species complex, in particular *C. bacillisporus* and *C. tetragattii* (31, 69).

C. neoformans was first detected in the environment in the late 19th century, when Sanfelice recovered the yeast from peach juice. Since then, however, *C. neoformans* and *C. deneoformans* have been most frequently associated with pigeon (and other bird) droppings and soils contaminated with these droppings (31). The yeast usually is not found in fresh droppings but is most evident in bird excreta that have accumulated over long periods of time on window ledges, vacant buildings, and other roosting sites (69). The environmental habitat of members of the *C. gattii* species complex was originally identified as being the gum tree, *Eucalyptus camaldulensis*; however, a number of other plant families have been identified as sources (31). *C. gattii* species complex isolates have been reported from subtropical areas and from temperate areas of Europe, Asia, Oceana, Africa, North America, and Central and South America (31).

■ Genus *Malassezia*

Conflicting data exist concerning the epidemiological distribution of *Malassezia* spp. in humans and other animals, largely depending on whether culture-based or nucleic acid-based approaches were employed to assess the distribution of the 15 members of this genus (reviewed in reference 70). The most common species according to most studies are *M. furfur, M. pachydermatis, M. sympodialis, M. globosa, M. obtusa, M. restricta,* and *M. slooffiae,* although there appear to be geographical variations in species distribution. While many culture-based studies have attempted to prove associations between *Malassezia* spp. and various dermatological conditions, non-culture-based studies showed that *M. globosa* and *M. restricta* are virtually omnipresent on human skin (70). Colonization of pet dogs of health care workers with *M. pachydermatis*, a frequent colonizer of canine auditory canals, has been linked to outbreaks of systemic *Malassezia* infections in neonates (71).

CLINICAL SIGNIFICANCE

■ Genus *Candida*

Candida spp. present in clinical specimens can reflect environmental contamination, colonization, or actual disease processes. An accurate diagnosis requires proper handling of clinical material, thus ensuring that specimens reach the laboratory in a timely fashion and have been taken and stored in an appropriate manner. *Candida* spp. that are normal flora can invade tissue and produce life-threatening pathology in patients whose immune defenses have been altered by disease or iatrogenic intervention.

Candida albicans is the most common species isolated from nearly all forms of candidiasis (42, 64). Contributing to its high association with disease is its high prevalence in the normal population, as described above. In addition, *C. albicans* appears to possess a number of virulence properties that assist successful parasitism, which include the expression of proteases, adhesins, invasins, and surface integrins, the ability to form biofilms, metabolic adaptation, phenotypic switching, thigmotropism, and the secretion of a wide variety of hydrolytic enzymes (reviewed in references 72 and 73).

Only *C. tropicalis* (reviewed in reference 74) and *C. auris* (13, 75) appear to possess virulence similar to that of *C. albicans*, both in humans and in animal and invertebrate models of infection. Other medically important *Candida* spp. encountered with lower frequencies in clinical specimens include *C. blankii, C. (Diutina) catenulata, C. (Trichomonascus) ciferrii, C. dubliniensis, C. (Pichia) eremophila, C. (Cyberlindnera) fabianii, C. famata (Debaromyces hansenii), C. (Nakaseomyces) glabrata, C. glaebosa, C. (Meyerozyma) guilliermondii, C. haemulonii, C. inconspicua (Pichia cactophila), C. kefyr (Kluyveromyces marxianus), C. krusei (Pichia kudriavzevii), C. lambica, C. (Yarrowia) lipolytica, C. (Clavispora) lusitaniae, C. (Pichia) norvegensis, C. parapsilosis* species complex, *C. pelliculosa (Wickerhamomyces anomalus), C. (Metschnikowia) pulcherrima, C. (Diutina) rugosa* species complex, *C. utilis (Cyberlindnera jadinii),* and *C. zeylanoides* (11, 12, 55, 66, 67, 76). Fluconazole is one of the primary drugs used to treat candidiasis, but *C. krusei* is inherently resistant, isolates of *C. auris* are also frankly resistant, and isolates of *C. (Nakaseomyces) glabrata* may vary in susceptibility. Two other fluconazole-resistant species, *C. inconspicua (Pichia cactophila)* and *C. (Pichia) norvegensis*, are rarer agents of candidiasis. *C. (Nakaseomyces) glabrata* is emerging as a significant pathogen, with a relatively high proportion of strains exhibiting reduced susceptibility to fluconazole. Recently, strains resistant to echinocandin drugs have also been noted (reviewed in reference 20). *C. glabrata* is regarded as a symbiont of humans and can be isolated routinely from the oral cavity and genitourinary, alimentary, and respiratory tracts of most individuals. It has been associated with all possible presentations of deep-seated and systemic, disseminated disease (reviewed in reference 20). It is also recovered often from urine specimens and has been estimated to account for as much as 20% of *Candida* urinary tract infections (77). Because it may be slow growing, routine urine cultures should be incubated for at least 2 days. Two further cryptic yeast species, *C. nivariensis* and *C. bracarensis*, constitute a species complex with *C. glabrata* within the genus *Nakaseomyces* (20, 78). Both species have been reported from cases of oropharyngeal and vulvovaginal candidiasis (20), and *C. nivariensis* in particular appears to be an emerging cause of deep infections with isolates from certain countries reported to have elevated MICs of all of the triazole drugs (78).

Candida dubliniensis was originally isolated from the oropharynges of HIV-positive patients but may also be recovered from blood, urine, vaginal, or other specimen sites, especially if the patient is immunocompromised (reviewed in reference 79). Acute pseudomembranous oral candidiasis is the presentation seen in patients with compromised cell-mediated immunity; indeed, mucocutaneous forms of candidiasis are often related to defects in cell-mediated immunity, while systemic spread is generally associated with neutropenia (79). However, despite its genetic relatedness to *C. albicans*, a variety of studies have demonstrated that *C. dublinienesis* is significantly less prevalent in clinical samples than *C. albicans* and is less virulent in a variety of infection models (14, 15, 79). *C. parapsilosis* species complex (17), comprising *C. parapsilosis sensu stricto* and the cryptic species *C. metapsilosis* and *C. orthopsilosis*, is particularly associated with neonatal infections (reviewed in references 80–82), although a wide variety of clinical presentations have been described, including vulvovaginal candidiasis. In all settings, *C. orthopsilosis* and particularly *C. metapsilosis* are much less prevalent than *C. parapsilosis* (80, 82) and are less virulent in animal models of infection (80, 81, 83).

It is beyond the scope of this chapter to individually itemize the ranges of clinical presentations reported for the vast array of less common non-*C. albicans Candida* spp. reported in limited case studies or anecdotal case reports in the literature. For further information concerning the spectra of diseases caused by those organisms, the reader is referred to a variety of studies which have examined the epidemiology and clinical outcomes of infections caused by rare *Candida* spp. (10, 55, 66, 67, 84–86).

■ Genus *Cryptococcus*

Cryptococcus neoformans var. *grubii*, *C. neoformans* var. *neoformans*, *C. deneoformans* (formerly serotype D), and members of the *C. gattii* species complex are considered the principal human pathogens (34, 87–90). Infections are most common in patients with advanced HIV disease or who are receiving exogenous immunosuppression (87–90). The clinical presentation in AIDS patients appears to be similar regardless of the species (*C. neoformans* versus *C. gattii*) causing the infection. Initial cryptococcal infection begins by inhalation of the fungus into the lungs, usually followed by hematogenous spread to the brain and meninges. Involvement of the skin, bones, and joints is seen, and *C. neoformans* is often cultured from the urine of patients with disseminated infection. In nearly 45% of AIDS patients, cryptococcosis was reported as the first AIDS-defining illness. As none of the presenting signs or symptoms of cryptococcal meningitis (e.g., headache, fever, and malaise) are sufficiently characteristic to distinguish it from other infections that occur in patients with AIDS, determining cryptococcal antigen titers, performing direct microscopy, and culturing blood and cerebrospinal fluid (CSF) are useful in making a diagnosis (91). In patients without HIV infection, cryptococcosis may occur in association with underlying conditions such as lupus erythematosis, sarcoidosis, leukemia, lymphomas, Cushing's syndrome, end-stage liver disease, renal insufficiency, organ transplant, and receipt of tumor necrosis factor inhibitors (90). Such patients are generally more likely to develop pulmonary disease without multifocal dissemination. Species within the *C. gattii* complex are more likely to cause infections in nonimmunocompromised patients, and this complex has been associated with outbreaks in humans and other mammals (92, 93), although compromised immune status appears to be a significant risk factor for infections with certain *C. gattii* complex species (34, 92, 93). In North America, 38% (Canada) to 59% (United States) of individuals infected with *C. gattii* were immunocompromised (92, 93).

An increasing number of non-*C. neoformans*/*C. gattii* species, many of which have been assigned to alternative Tremellomycete genera, have been sporadically implicated in human disease. Approximately 80% of reported infections involved *Cryptococcus* (*Papiliotrema*) *laurentii* or *C.* (*Naganishia*) *albidus* (94, 95). Similar to infections with *C. neoformans*/*C. gattii*, most patients had a history of impaired immunity caused by neutropenia, malignancy, prior organ transplant, or recent corticosteroid use, and an additional risk factor for infection was the use of invasive vascular devices (94, 95). Clinical manifestations were also similar to infections with *C. neoformans*/*C. gattii* with fungemia (39% of cases) and central nervous system involvement (32%), although pulmonary, gastrointestinal, ocular, and cutaneous lesions were also reported (94, 95).

Additional anecdotal reports have identified *C.* (*Naganishia*) *liquefaciens* from a case of central venous catheter-associated fungemia (96), *C. uniguttulatus* (*Filobasidium uniguttulatum*) from a case of ventriculitis (97), subcutaneous cryptococcosis due to *C.* (*Naganishia*) *diffluens* (98), and *C. curvatus* associated with central nervous system infection (99).

■ Genus *Malassezia*

Yeasts belonging to the genus *Malassezia* are isolated from the skin of warm-blooded animals and humans as commensals but can be agents of dermatological diseases. *Malassezia sympodialis*, *M. slooffiae*, *M. globosa*, and *M. restricta* are the most frequent human colonizers (70, 100). The main causative agents of the skin infection pityriasis versicolor are *M. globosa*, *M. sympodialis*, *M. slooffiae*, *M. furfur*, and occasionally *M. restricta* (reviewed in reference 70). Other dermatological diseases, including seborrheic dermatitis, atopic eczema, psoriasis, and folliculitis, have been associated with a similar array of *Malassezia* species (70, 100, 101), often because there was a clinical response following antifungal therapy with a reduction in yeast numbers. However, because *Malassezia* may be present on the skin in high numbers and there are no other characteristic features to guide laboratory diagnosis, the exact role of the organisms in these diseases remains unclear. Similar concerns exist regarding reports of onychomycosis caused by *Malassezia* species (70). In addition, *Malassezia* spp. have, in rare cases, caused systemic infections, usually of neonates in ICUs, patients receiving total parenteral nutrition with lipid supplementation, or profoundly immunocompromised patients in the ICU (70, 100). In virtually all cases, the organism concerned was reported as either *M. furfur* or *M. pachydermatis* (reviewed in references 70 and 100).

■ Genus "*Pseudozyma*"

The first description of *Pseudozyma* as a human pathogen came in 2003, when the species *P. antarctica*, *P. parantarctica* (both now reclassified in *Moesziomyces* [36]), and *P.* (probably *Macalpinomyces*) *thailandica* were isolated from the blood of three Thai patients (reviewed in references 102 and 103). Two additional cases of fungemia due to *P.* (*Moesziomyces*) *aphidis* were reported from the United States and from India (102, 103). Three additional new species, which were originally named *Pseudozyma crassa* (now *Triodiomyces crassa* [36]) and *Pseudozyma siamensis* and *Pseudozyma alboarmeniaca* (now both *Ustilago* [36]), were also isolated from blood of Thai patients (104). Risk factors for infection mirror those of other less common yeast infections and include neutropenia, chemotherapy, thrombocytopenia, and the presence of indwelling catheters. Although the main manifestation of infection with these organisms is fungemia (102–104), they have also been isolated from brain abscess and pleural fluid associated with pulmonary infection (reviewed in references 102 and 103).

■ Genus "*Rhodotorula*"

Rhodotorula spp. are normal inhabitants of moist skin and can be recovered from wide-ranging environmental sources, including various foods and beverages, and aquatic environments, including shower curtains, bathtub grout, toothbrushes, salt and fresh water (105), and swimming pools (106). In 2008, a systemic review of clinical cases (107) listed 128 cases of infection with *Rhodotorula* spp.; the majority (79%) were fungemia, but other cases included ocular infections, peritonitis associated with peritoneal dialysis, and meningitis (107). The principal risk factors for infection were immunosuppression or malignancy and complications due to indwelling central venous catheters. The overall reported mortality of *Rhodotorula* infection, however, was less than 15%.

■ Genus *Saccharomyces*

Historically thought to be nonpathogenic, *Saccharomyces cerevisiae* is another emerging fungal pathogen, reported to cause thrush, vulvovaginitis, empyema, and fungemia (86, 108, 109). Person-to-person contact and exposure to commercial strains associated with health foods, probiotics, and baking may contribute to the ability of the organisms to colonize and infect human hosts (108, 110), with immunosuppression (109), ICU stay (108), total parenteral nutrition (108), and central venous catheters (110) being important risk factors for development of fungemia.

■ Genus *Saprochaete*

The environmental yeast *Saprochaete* is usually found in climates with hot, dry summers and mild, wet winters. Most infections have been reported from southern Europe, particularly in Italy, Spain, and France below a northern latitude of 44°. *S. capitata* is recognized as an emerging cause of invasive fungal disease in immunosuppressed patients but has also been reported in patients with continuous ambulatory dialysis, renal transplant, endocarditis, spondylodiscitis, and osteomyelitis (111). It is widely distributed in nature, has been recovered as normal skin flora and from the gastrointestinal tract, and has been associated with onychomycosis (112). A systematic review of the literature published in 2015 listed more than 100 cases of infection caused by *S. capitata* (111). The vast majority of patients were neutropenic at the time of infection, and in 75% of cases, the organism was isolated from blood cultures. Mortality from invasive disease is high in neutropenic patients (crude mortality of 60% [111]), and survival is associated with neutrophil count recovery and prompt appropriate antifungal therapy.

■ Genus "*Sporobolomyces*"

Three species of *Sporobolomyces* (*S. roseus*, *S. holsaticus*, and *S. salmonicolor*), which are normally encountered as environmental organisms, have been sporadically associated with cases of human disease (reviewed in reference 113). Disease manifestations reported to date include dermatitis, allergic alveolitis, deep-seated infections and fungemias in patients with AIDS or other immunocompromising conditions, endogenous endophthalmitis, and meningitis.

■ Genus "*Trichosporon*"

Yeasts of the polyphyletic "genus" *Trichosporon* (34) are distributed widely in nature and can cause both superficial and systemic infections and also allergic pneumonitis in humans. Superficial infections (white piedra) are characterized by nodules of approximately 0.5 mm attached to the hair shafts on the head, axilla, or genital area and are caused mainly by *T. inkin*, *T. ovoides*, *T.* (*Cutaneotrichosporon*) *cutaneum*, and *T.* (*Apiotrichum*) *loubieri*, with *T. inkin* predominating in genital infections (reviewed in reference 114). *T. asahii* and *T.* (*Cutaneotrichosporon*) *mucoides* are thought to be the major causes of summer-type hypersensitivity pneumonitis in Japan, a condition that results from inhalation of arthroconidia present in the homes of the patients (115).

Conversely, most systemic human infections are caused by *T. asahii*, *T. inkin*, *T.* (*Cutaneotrichosporon*) *dermatis*, and *T.* (*Cutaneotrichosporon*) *mucoides* (116). *T.* (*Apiotrichum*) *loubieri* is an apparently rare cause of disseminated trichosporonosis (51, 117), and *T.* (*Apiotrichum*) *mycotoxinivorans* has emerged as a novel pathogen capable of colonization and infection of the airways of patients with cystic fibrosis (118). In a systematic review of 203 confirmed cases of invasive *Trichosporon* infection (116), *T. asahii* was by far the most common species isolated from invasive trichosporonosis, and dissemination following fungemia occurred in nearly 80% of cases. The major risk factors for infection were hematological disease and especially neutropenia, solid organ transplantation, autoimmune disease, nonhematological malignancies, polytrauma, presence of central venous catheters, corticosteroid use, and surgery. Outbreaks in neonates, especially in preterm infants, have also been reported (116). Numerous breakthrough infections have been observed (116) in patients receiving echinocandin antifungals (to which all basidiomycete yeasts are resistant [Table 3]) or amphotericin B (to which individual *Trichosporon* species have different susceptibilities). Mortality rates of 40 to 90% have been reported, depending on the underlying condition of the patient, immune recovery, antifungal regimen, and primary versus breakthrough infection (reviewed in references 114 and 116).

COLLECTION, TRANSPORT, AND STORAGE OF SPECIMENS

No special practices for collection or transport of specimens from patients with suspected yeast infection need to be followed. Chapter 117 of this *Manual* describes standard practices for collection, transport, and storage. However, when specimens are collected and sent to the laboratory, consideration should be given to the possibility that a particular fungus is highly infectious (e.g., the mould form of *Histoplasma* spp.) or has unusual growth requirements (e.g., lipids for *Malassezia* species). Such information regarding the suspected etiologic agent should be provided to the laboratory.

Transportation of specimens should be undertaken as soon as possible. If a long delay is anticipated, specimens should be stored at 4°C. Yeasts can withstand normal refrigeration temperatures.

TABLE 3 Antifungal susceptibilities

Organism	MIC (μg/ml) of drug[a]								Reference(s)
	AmB	5FC	Flucon	Itra	Vori	Pos	Casp	Terb	
Candida albicans	0.06–1.0	1.0[b]	0.25–64	0.06–4	0.015–1	0.03–0.12[c]	0.015–0.125	0.03–128[b]	263,[c] 264
C. auris	0.125–8	ND	4–>64	0.03–2	0.03–16	0.015–8	0.015–8[d]	ND	265
C. dubliniensis	0.05–0.38	0.12	0.12–64	0.015–0.5	0.008–0.5	0.03[c]	ND	ND	2, 116, 263[c]
C. glabrata	0.125–4	ND	1–>64	0.125–4	0.03–1	0.03–4.0[c]	0.015–0.5	>128[b]	263,[c] 264
C. guilliermondii	0.06–32	0.06–4	0.5–>128	0.06–>8	0.06–>8	0.06–8	0.03–>8	0.625–100[b]	256, 266
C. haemulonii	0.5–32	ND	2–128	0.125–4	0.03–2	ND	0.125–0.25	ND	267
C. kefyr	0.5[b]	0.03–16[b]	0.5–1[b]	0.25–0.5[b]	0.03[b]	0.03[c]	ND	0.5–50[b]	263[c]
C. krusei	0.03–16	0.06–64	32–64[b]	0.5[b]	0.5–1.0[b]	0.03–0.25[c]	0.03–2.0	8–32[b]	263,[c] 268
C. lusitaniae	1.5–2.0	0.004–>32	0.064–6.0	0.004–0.5	0.003–0.09	0.03[c]	4–8	ND	255, 263,[c] 269
C. parapsilosis	0.125–1	1.0[b]	0.25–8	0.015–2	0.015–1	0.03–0.12[c]	0.06–2	0.125–2[b]	263,[c] 264
C. pelliculosa	0.12–1	ND	2–16	0.06–1	0.03–0.5	ND	0.03–0.25	ND	270
C. rugosa	0.5–1.0	0.12–1.0	1–8	0.03–0.12	0.03–0.06	0.03[c]	ND	ND	2, 116, 263[c]
C. tropicalis	0.06–1	1.0[b]	0.05–32	0.03–4	0.03–1	0.03–>16[c]	0.015–0.125	1.0[b]	263,[c] 264
Cryptococcus neoformans	0.5–1[b]	2–8[b]	2–8[b]	0.5[b]	0.25[b]	0.125–0.5	>8	2–8[b]	255
Kodamaea ohmeri	0.25–0.5	ND	2–32	0.125–0.5	0.3–0.5	ND	0.125–0.25	ND	271
Malassezia dermatis	0.03–0.12	ND	2	0.016-0.03	0.12	0.03–0.5[c]	ND	0.03–4	101, 263[c]
M. furfur	0.12–16	>64	2–32	0.03–25	0.03–16	0.03–32[c]	ND	0.03–50	101, 263[c]
M. globosa	0.10–4	ND	12.5–50	0.016–6.3	0.03–0.12	0.03–0.06[c]	ND	0.06–16	101, 263[c]
M. japonica	ND	ND	ND	0.016	ND	ND	ND	ND	101
M. nana	ND	ND	ND	0.016	ND	ND	ND	ND	101
M. obtusa	0.03–0.06	ND	2	0.016–1.6	0.03–0.06	0.03[c]	ND	0.03–64	101, 263[c]
M. pachydermatis	0.12	>64	4–16	0.016–6.3	0.03–0.25	0.12[c]	ND	0.03–50	101, 263[c]
M. restricta	4–8	ND	0.5–1	0.016–6.3	0.03	0.03[c]	ND	0.06–4	101, 263[c]
M. slooffiae	0.5–8	>64	1–4	0.016–0.8	0.03–0.25	0.03[c]	ND	0.03–25	101, 263[c]
M. sympodialis	0.06–0.5	>64	0.25–16	0.016–0.2	0.03–0.125	0.03–0.06[c]	ND	0.03–6.3	101, 263[c]
M. yamatoensis	ND	ND	ND	0.016	ND	ND	ND	ND	101
Rhodotorula glutinis	0.25–0.5	ND	64	2–16	2–16	0.06[c]	ND	ND	263,[c] 272
R. mucilaginosa	0.5–1	ND	0.5–>64	0.25–4	0.25–4	ND	ND	ND	2, 116
Saccharomyces cerevisiae	0.5[b]	0.125[b]	0.25–>64	0.015–>4	0.03[b]	0.015–>4	4–8	0.125[b]	255, 273
Saprochaete capitata	0.5–2.0	0.25–0.5	16–32	0.12–0.50	0.25–0.5	0.03-0.25[b]	ND	ND	274, 263[c]
Sporobolomyces salmonicolor	0.25–16	ND	8–64	0.25–0.5	0.12–0.25	ND	ND	ND	272
Trichosporon asahii	025–1.0	22.2[e]	1–16	0.12–1	0.12–1	0.03–0.25[c]	>8	ND	2, 116,[e] 263,[c] 275
T. asteroides	0.25–4.0	0.5–64	0.125–1	0.03–0.12	0.03–0.06	ND	2–>16	ND	273
T. ovoides	0.03	35.3	4.4	0.02	ND	ND	ND	ND	2, 116
Cutaneotrichosporon cutaneum	0.012	6.25	2.2	0.01	ND	ND	ND	ND	2, 116
C. mucoides	1	50[e]	2–64	0.25–2	0.12–0.16	ND	ND	ND	2, 116,[e] 272

[a]Abbreviations: AmB, amphotericin B; 5FC, 5-fluorocytosine; Flucon, fluoconazole; Itra, itraconazole; Vori, voriconazole; Pos, posaconazole; Casp, caspofungin; Terb, terbinafine; ND, not determined.
[b]MICs taken from https://mycology.adelaide.edu.au/descriptions/yeasts/.
[c]MICs taken from reference 269 for posaconazole.
[d]MIC ranges given for the alternative echinocandins micafungin and anidulafungin.
[e]MICs taken from reference 2 for 5-fluorocytosine.

DIRECT EXAMINATION

The appropriate examination of a clinical specimen is essential before proper processing of the material. In addition, it often aids the mycologist and the physician to obtain a preliminary identification and to either rule in or out certain pathogenic yeasts. Some methods are universal to the preliminary observation of fungi in a specimen (e.g., Gram stain, calcofluor stain, 20% potassium hydroxide [KOH]). If 20% KOH is used in a preparation, neither India ink nor Gram stain may be added. Chapter 118 describes in more detail the various stains and examination procedures used in the mycology laboratory.

Microscopy

During microscopic examination of a specimen for yeasts, structures may be observed that may aid in identification (Fig. 1 and 4): (i) size and shape of the organism, (ii) morphology of the bud attachment site and number of buds, (iii) presence or absence of a capsule, (iv) thickness of the cell wall, (v) presence of pseudohyphae, and (vi) presence of arthroconidia. A great deal of information can be gleaned from careful direct microscopic examination of an appropriately prepared and stained specimen.

KOH

Wet mounts prepared in a 10 to 30% KOH solution may be used to distinguish fungi in mucoid secretions, in normally sterile, deep tissues obtained after biopsies, or in skin, hair, or nail. The KOH digests the proteinaceous material, leaving the fungal elements intact. Gentle warming speeds the process, but care should be taken when strong concentrations of KOH are used, because the KOH rapidly crystallizes if overheated or left for prolonged periods before examination. The specimen is prepared by placing an aliquot on a slide, adding a drop of KOH, and placing a coverslip on top. Enough KOH should be present to completely cover the specimen. For tissues, skin, and nail, the specimen may be gently squashed while excess KOH is removed. In these thick materials, this makes visualization of the fungus easier. Hairs should always be viewed without squashing to obtain maximal information about the type of fungal invasion. Dimethyl sulfoxide (40% [vol/vol] in distilled water) may be added to the KOH reagent to facilitate clearing without the need for heating or incubation, but the specimen should be examined quickly. Bubbles can be confused with yeast cells. Budding cells with internal heterogeneous material should be seen in order to enhance

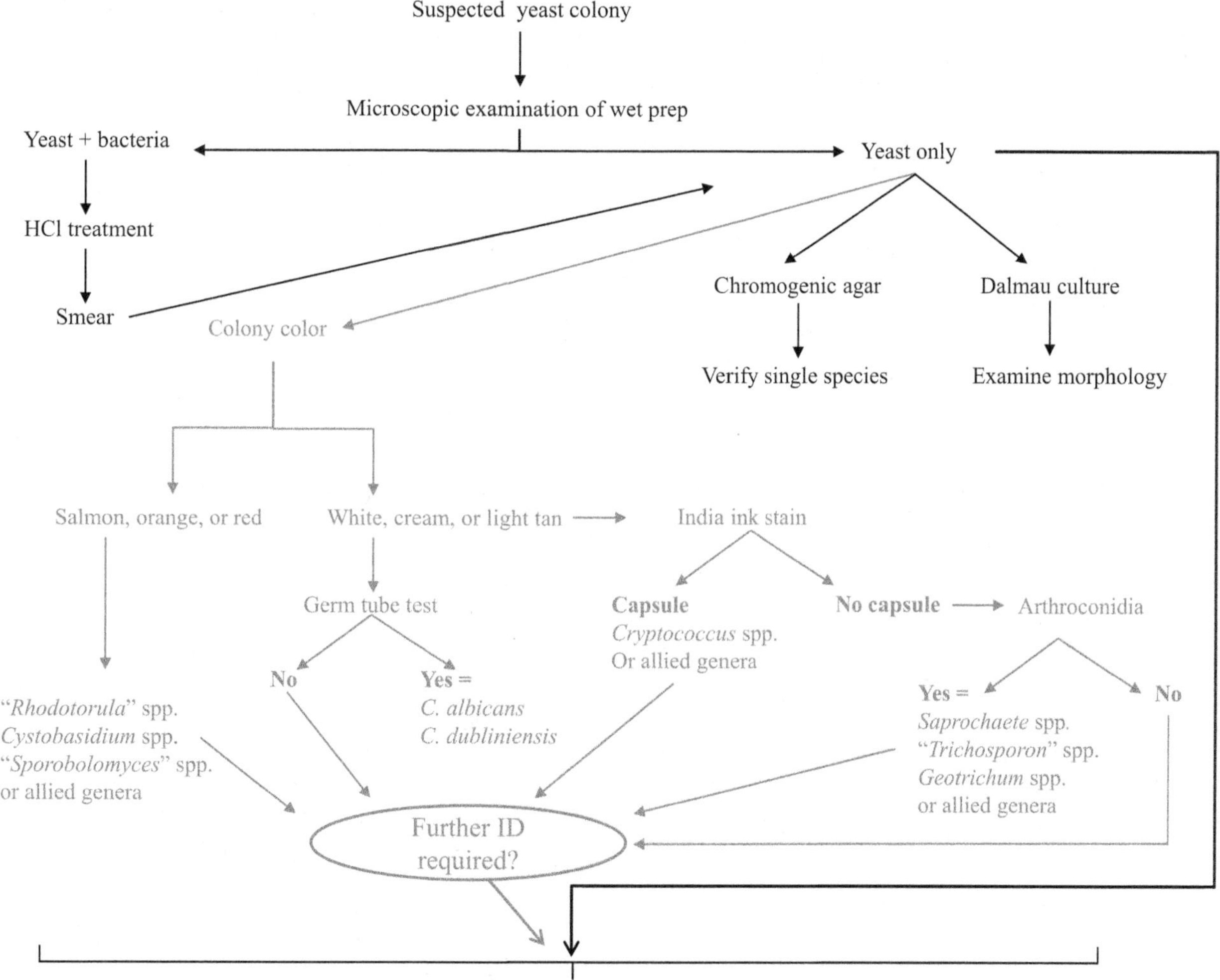

FIGURE 4 Scheme for identification of yeasts from clinical specimens. Traditional methods are shown in beige.

confidence that the object is a yeast cell. Round and oval objects lacking buds are common in tissue specimens and could be erroneously identified as yeasts.

The calcofluor stain (Blankophore; Uvitex 2B) fluoresces bright green under filtered UV light and facilitates detection of fungus as it binds to chitin in the cell wall (119). The specimen is prepared as described above except that a drop of calcofluor is added at the time of mounting in KOH (or after digestion in KOH for at least 1 h in the case of nail specimens). The diagnostic feature of pityriasis versicolor seen by direct microscopic examination of skin scrapings is the presence of short, nonbranching, blunt-ended *Malassezia* hyphae among *Malassezia* yeasts ("spaghetti and meatballs").

India Ink

India ink is used to examine specimens of CSF, urine, and other body fluids for the presence of *Cryptococcus* species (Fig. 3). Generally, it is not useful on primary specimens, such as sputum or other highly cellular material, that do not allow even distribution of the ink. India ink is used to visualize capsules that are transparent by bright-field illumination alone, as the ink is excluded from the capsule, showing a clear halo around the yeast. Artifacts such as erythrocytes, lymphocytes, or talc from gloves appear to cause a halo effect; therefore, careful examination for the presence of yeast cells and bud formation is essential. The specimen is prepared by placing a drop of the centrifuged sediment of a fluid specimen on a slide, adding a drop of Pelikan India ink or nigrosin solution, and placing a coverslip on top. While this method is relatively rapid and is generally satisfactory, a preferred method is to place a coverslip on the specimen and place a drop of ink on the side of the coverslip to allow the ink to diffuse underneath. This provides a gradient of ink which will contain an optimal region to detect a capsule. India ink solution should be replaced regularly as it becomes contaminated, or alternatively, a solution of 10% nigrosin in 10% formalin (using appropriate safety precautions) can be prepared.

Yeast in Tissue Sections

The appearance of fungus in histopathology sections has been reviewed (120). *C. neoformans* can be distinguished from other nondematiaceous yeasts in fixed tissue by the use of a Fontana-Masson stain, which detects melanin precursors in the cell wall. Mucicarmine stains the capsule, which helps to distinguish *Cryptococcus* spp. from yeasts with similar morphologies. *C. neoformans* yeast cells in tissue are typically rounder than yeasts of *Candida* species and tend to vary in size.

Yeasts can be visualized in tissue using Gomori's silver stain, although they stain blackish and some of the internal detail may be difficult to see. Periodic acid-Schiff stain is also useful; fungal material stains reddish.

A variety of methods have been described for the detection and identification of yeast in formalin-fixed tissue blocks using DNA-based technologies (121–123). Although these methods are largely in the experimental stage, they appear promising in offering potentially much higher sensitivity than conventional approaches. However, the quality and quantity of extracted fungal DNA are affected by formalin fixation methods, and care must be taken to limit the likelihood of amplifying fungi that may have contaminated the surface of paraffin-embedded blocks. Generally, discarding the first two wax curls cut from blocks is advisable to reduce the likelihood of contamination by commensal yeasts (personal observation).

Antigen Detection

Signs and symptoms of invasive yeast infections generally overlap those of bacterial infections, necessitating development of rapid non-culture-based methods for diagnosis. See chapter 119 for a comprehensive review of antigen testing. Non-culture-based tests for discriminating fungal versus bacterial infection and for detection of specific genera have been developed. Of all of these tests, the cryptococcal antigen test has proven the most successful.

The unique composition of the fungal cell wall makes it particularly well suited to being a focus for fungal serological tests. Many of the more common pathogenic yeasts contain β-1,3-glucan in the wall. Several commercial kits, the Fungitell (Associates of Cape Cod Inc., East Falmouth, MA; available in the United States and Europe), Fungitec G (Seikagaku Corp., Kogyo, Tokyo, Japan; Japan only), B-G-Star (Maruha Nichiro Foods, Inc., Tokyo, Japan; Japan only), and the Wako test (Wako Pure Chemical Industries Ltd., Tokyo, Japan; Japan only), are available for detection of β-1,3-glucan, although individual tests have different cutoffs (124). Repeat testing of patients with negative results is recommended, as single-test positive results provide generally good sensitivities and specificities (125) and repeatedly negative tests have a high negative predictive value. Repeat testing of patients who test positive also improves the specificity of the test (125–127) and may have value in assessing therapeutic success or failure (127). A positive test, however, does not provide information about the specific etiology, which is a weakness if tailored antifungal therapy is desired. Cryptococci do not contain β-1,3-glucan, so this test is not positive in patients with cryptococcal infection, and it also performs poorly in patients with the infective yeast form of *Blastomyces* spp.

■ Genus *Candida*

With the exception of cryptococcal antigen tests for serum and CSF, efforts to develop other genus- or species-specific antigen detection systems have focused primarily on candidemia and disseminated candidiasis. Aside from dipsticks for testing of vaginal secretions, no commercially available tests have been developed for body fluids and tissues other than blood and CSF. Carbohydrate antigens have provided useful targets for several commercial kits for the detection of disseminated candidiasis. Protein antigens have also been investigated. Another antigen, D-arabinitol, has been under investigation for over a decade and has been incorporated into the COBAS FARA II centrifugal autoanalyzer (Roche Diagnostic Systems, Montclair, NJ) (128). While only a limited number of laboratories have evaluated D-arabinitol as a marker for candidiasis, the antigen appears promising at least in certain patient groups (129). D-Arabinitol levels appear to correlate with therapeutic success (130).

The Platelia *Candida* Ag test (Bio-Rad Laboratories, Marnes-La-Coquette, France) utilizes a monoclonal antibody, EB-CA1, which targets an α-1,2-oligomannoside common among multiple species of *Candida*. The test has shown reasonable sensitivity and high specificities, although they vary from study to study and by *Candida* species. Several studies (129–131) have recommended that both the antigen and the antibody tests (Platelia *Candida* Ab) be performed to maximize early diagnosis of invasive candidiasis. The specificity of the antigen test can be further enhanced by including a test for a second antigen, β-1,2-oligomannan, which is found in only a limited number of *Candida* species: *C. albicans*, *C. glabrata*, and *C. tropicalis* (132). *C. dubliniensis* variably expresses the antigen (133). The Serion ELISA Antigen *Candida*

(Institut Virion/Serion GmbH, Wurzburg, Germany) is a qualitative and quantitative immunoassay for the detection of *Candida* antigen in serum or plasma. A corresponding assay, the Serion ELISA Classic *Candida albicans* IgG/IgM/IgA, measures serum antibody directed against *C. albicans*. These assays were evaluated and compared with the Platelia antigen/antibody assays and β-D-glucan (134). Although the Serion antigen test discriminated between patients with candidiasis and uninfected controls, in this study, its discriminatory power was lower than that of the Platelia test. These assays have been available in Europe for some time but are not approved for use in the United States.

The Pastorex *Candida* (Bio-Rad) and Cand-Tec (Ramco Inc., Stafford, TX) are agglutination tests that detect *Candida* antigen in human specimens, although their performance characteristics are likely to limit clinical utility. Their performance was reviewed recently (135).

■ Genus *Cryptococcus*

Methods for the detection of cryptococcal antigen (capsular galactoxylomannan) in serum and CSF have been available for over 2 decades; they can detect *C. neoformans* var. *grubii* and var. *neoformans*, *C. deneoformans*, and *C. gattii* species complex. During this time, commercial tests have evolved to overcome early problems with specificity and sensitivity. The chief problem was false positives due to rheumatoid factor. Once this factor is destroyed, the sensitivity and specificity of the current generation of cryptococcal antigen tests are high. Latex agglutination-based antigen detection kits include the Remel *Cryptococcus* antigen test (Remel, Lenexa, KS), CALAS (cryptococcal antigen latex agglutination system; Meridian Bioscience, Inc., Cincinnati, OH), the IMMY latex-*Cryptococcus* antigen test (Abacus ALS, Meadowbrook, Queensland, Australia), Pastorex Crypto Plus (Bio-Rad Laboratories, Marnes-La-Coquette, France), the Crypto-LA test (Wampole Laboratories, Cranbury, NJ), and the Eiken latex test (Eiken, Tokyo, Japan). The Premier cryptococcal antigen test (Meridian) is an enzyme immunoassay-based assay. The newest format is a lateral flow assay (LFA) (IMMY cryptococcal LFA; Abacus ALS, Meadowbrook, Queensland, Australia). These tests have been recommended as the primary evaluative tool in lieu of an India ink stain for screening CSF in suspected cases of cryptococcal meningitis, due to the low sensitivity of the India ink stain. Several studies have demonstrated superior sensitivity of the LFA device (136), coupled with shorter time to results, and the ability to test urine samples and to be used in finger prick testing (137, 138). Moreover, certain latex agglutination tests based on monoclonal antibodies appear to be insufficiently sensitive to detect a proportion of infections due to *C. gattii* or *C. neoformans*/*C. gattii* hybrids (139). However, a recent study highlighted possible issues with the clinical interpretation of positive but low-titer LFA results in patients with no prior evidence of infection (140). Finally, the utility of all of these tests in detecting infections with non-*C. neoformans* species previously assigned to this genus but now known to be accommodated in alternative Tremellomycete genera is unknown.

False-positive tests due to causes other than rheumatoid factor have also been observed. These have been associated with disseminated *Trichosporon* infections, *Capnocytophaga canimorsus* septicemia, malignancy, *Rothia* (formerly *Stomatococcus*) bacteremia, some soaps and disinfectants, and hydroxyethyl starch used in fluid resuscitation (141–147).

Monitoring a decrease in antigen titer as an indication of effective anticryptococcal therapy has been suggested. However, while the titer may decrease after initiation of therapy in non-HIV patients, it may remain greater than 200 despite microbiological clearance (148). The same authors (148) proposed that the return of CSF glucose, chloride, and leukocyte count to normal levels might be better indicators of successful treatment. Mycological sterility is also a useful indicator of successful therapy.

■ Specific Tests for Invasive Infections Caused by Other Yeasts

To date, little effort has been devoted to developing serologic tests for detection of invasive infections caused by yeasts other than *Candida* and *Cryptococcus* species. With the growing awareness of bloodstream infections caused by *Trichosporon* species, a possible strategy is to use the serum cryptococcal antigen test in combination with compatible signs and symptoms and underlying disease to suggest a diagnosis of trichosporonosis.

Nucleic Acid Detection

Detection in Positive Blood Cultures

The U.S. Food and Drug Administration has approved several commercially available peptide nucleic acid fluorescent *in situ* hybridization (PNA FISH) kits (AdvanDx, Woburn, MA) for identification of yeasts directly from positive blood cultures. The probes specifically detect *C. albicans*, *C. glabrata*, or *C. tropicalis* as individual species or detect a yeast species group (e.g., *C. albicans* and *C. parapsilosis* fluoresce green with the Yeast Traffic Light PNA FISH kit) in blood cultures by targeting species-specific rRNA sequences. Nucleic acid peptides that mimic 26S rRNA are used to hybridize to target rRNA. The probes are also coupled to a fluorophore that is detectable when the probe binds to its target. Several studies have shown that the *C. albicans* PNA FISH assay has a specificity approaching 100% (149–151). However, the manufacturer's package insert notes that the *C. albicans* probe can cross-react with *C. orthopsilosis*. In the most comprehensive study, the test was found to have excellent sensitivity (99%), specificity (100%), positive predictive value (100%), and negative predictive value (99.3%) (149). The test can rapidly (1.5 hours) indicate whether *C. albicans* is present and can thus indicate whether a non-*C. albicans* yeast is present (reviewed in reference 151). Other PNA FISH assays are similarly rapid, although recent modifications to the probes and reagents have resulted in a second-generation assay (QuickFISH) that shortens the assay to 30 minutes. The test does not replace subculture, because blood cultures may contain mixed species; therefore, PNA FISH-positive blood cultures should be subcultured to ensure that no other yeast species is present.

The FilmArray blood culture identification system (bioMérieux, Marcy l'Etoile, France) is an automated system which utilizes nested multiplex PCR to identify pathogens in positive blood cultures; it is FDA approved and CE marked. The test panel includes *C. albicans*, *C. glabrata*, *C. krusei*, *C. parapsilosis*, and *C. tropicalis* and can potentially identify polymicrobial infections in less than 2 h from positive blood culture bottles (152). Similarly, the Prove-it Sepsis assay (Mobidiag, Helsinki, Finland) combines broad-range PCR with microarray-based detection for the identification of *C. albicans*, *C. glabrata*, *C. parapsilosis*, *C. tropicalis*, *C. guilliermondii*, *C. lusitaniae*, and *C. krusei* in positive blood cultures. Additional species, including at least *C. dubliniensis*, *C. pelliculosa*, *C. kefyr*, *C. norvegensis*, *C. haemulonii*, and *Saccharomyces cerevisiae*, are covered in a "pan-yeast" assay. Studies using genuine clinical samples in conjunction with spiked blood cultures reported sensitivity and specificity of 99% and 98%, respectively (153).

The Luminex xTAG multiplex PCR assay (Luminex Molecular Diagnostics, Ontario, Canada) detects as many as 23 fungi in a single sample, using microsphere suspension technology with beads containing an individual probe designed to hybridize to a different amplified fungal DNA sequence. This assay was tested for the detection of *Candida* species in positive blood culture bottles (154, 155), showing 100% sensitivity and 99% specificity.

Detection Directly from Clinical Samples

Most assays for the direct detection of fungal DNA in human body fluids without prior culture have been directed at diagnosis of invasive candidiasis. White et al. (156) and Lau et al. (157) have reviewed methods for the rapid diagnosis of invasive candidiasis, including PCR-based methods. A meta-analysis of 54 published studies that used whole blood for PCR diagnosis of invasive candidiasis (158) found that the pooled sensitivity of these assays was 95% and the specificity was 92%. However, a lack of standardization and validation has previously hindered the acceptance of these tests as diagnostic criteria for fungal infections, although this may be somewhat circumvented by the availability of commercial assays (reviewed in references 135 and 159).

The time required to identify a pathogen could be shortened if more efficient methods of detecting fungal DNA in a specimen were developed. Real-time PCR can detect candidemia much earlier than conventional blood culture, but it does not always detect all cases of systemic infection with all species (160–163). Bennett (164) and Halliday et al. (159) provide a balanced discussion on the use of this technique, which is likely to be used alongside blood culture protocols while it is developed further.

In Europe, the LightCycler SeptiFast Test M (Roche Diagnostics GmbH, Mannheim, Germany) is available to detect five species of *Candida* and *Aspergillus fumigatus* DNA in whole blood using broad-range internal transcribed spacer (ITS) PCR and melting curves. Summaries of published studies with the LightCycler SeptiFast Test M and several other commercial tests available in Europe for experimental purposes are provided in references 135, 157, and 165. Additional recent molecular approaches for the rapid diagnosis of septicemia, including SeptiTest (Molzym GmbH, Bremen, Germany) and Vyoo (SIRS-Lab, Jena, Germany), are reviewed in detail in reference 166. The only FDA-approved DNA probe test is the Affirm VPIII microbial identification test (Becton Dickinson, Franklin Lakes, NJ), for use in the detection and identification of *Candida* species, *Gardnerella vaginalis*, and *Trichomonas vaginalis* nucleic acid in vaginal fluid specimens from patients with symptoms of vaginitis (167). The Affirm assay was significantly more likely to identify *Candida* than wet mounts of vaginal fluid (11 versus 7%). The T2 *Candida* panel (T2 Biosystems, Lexington, MA) was recently approved for direct detection of five *Candida* species in blood samples. T2MR is a magnetic resonance-based system for detection of sepsis agents (reviewed in reference 168) with reported detection limits of 1 to 3 CFU/ml and a clinical specificity of 99.4% (reviewed in reference 169) for the common *Candida* species included in the assay (*C. albicans*/*C. tropicalis*, *C. glabrata*/*C. krusei*, and *C. parapsilosis*).

ISOLATION PROCEDURES

Processing of specimens for fungal recovery is usually performed in conjunction with and as an extension of the processing procedure for recovery of bacteria. The principal difference is the selection of media for primary plating, which is discussed in chapter 118. Most media used for the recovery of fungi contain an antibacterial agent such as chloramphenicol or gentamicin; however, incorporation of cycloheximide (Acti-Dione) should be avoided, as only *C. albicans*, some species of *Trichosporon* and related genera, and *Malassezia* species are able to grow in the presence of this agent. One processing step that has unproven advantages for isolation of yeasts from sputum specimens is the use of mucolytic agents (*N*-acetyl-L-cysteine or Sputolysin).

There are, however, yeast infections for which specialized processing steps should be considered. For example, recovery of *C. neoformans* from blood or bone marrow is enhanced if lysis-centrifugation followed by inoculation onto solid media is used (170). For some yeasts, a medium supplement may be needed to either enhance or support growth during primary culture. For example, if *C. neoformans* is suspected from a respiratory specimen, setting up primary media that include a niger seed or related medium will enhance detection. Similarly, if *Malassezia* species are suspected, the primary culture plate should be supplemented with an olive oil overlay applied with a swab before inoculation. *Malassezia pachydermatis* will grow without the overlay, but the overlay is required to grow *M. furfur*. This may not be successful for other *Malassezia* species, as they are more fastidious. The detection of bile-dependent and bile-enhanced isolates of *C. glabrata* is enhanced by the addition of 8 μg/ml of fluconazole to the primary medium. This selects for bile-dependent isolates which have defects in the ergosterol synthesis pathway and are fluconazole resistant (171). This becomes a particularly powerful method when combined with a primary medium containing a chromogenic indicator used for presumptive identification of some yeasts (e.g., CHROMagar) (172).

The appropriate selection of isolation media is essential, even though detection of infectious agents using molecular methods is becoming more commonplace in the diagnostic setting. Successful culture is still necessary to perform antifungal susceptibility tests, for preservation in culture collections, for epidemiological studies, and for strain typing, if appropriate.

IDENTIFICATION

Historical Approaches to Yeast Identification

Historically, a systematic and laborious approach to yeast identification was employed in most microbiology laboratories. This consisted of initial macro- and microscopic examination of isolates of suspected pathogenic yeasts, followed by a rapid germ tube test (Fig. 5) to identify isolates of the most common *Candida* species, *C. albicans* (and *C. dubliniensis*). In parallel, the purity of isolates was verified, often using chromogenic agars (Fig. 4). Once pure

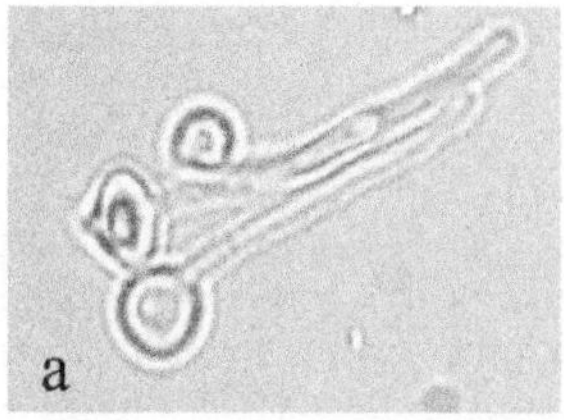

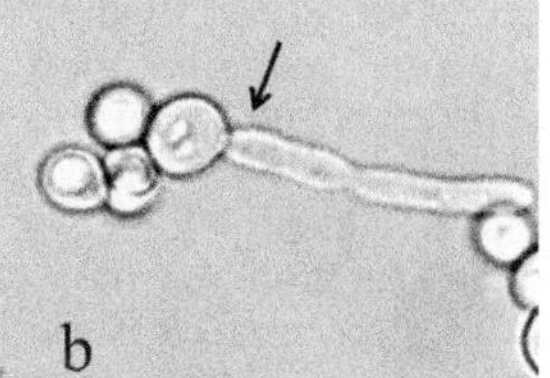

FIGURE 5 Germ tube test. (a) Germ tube formation of *Candida albicans*; (b) blastoconidial germination with constriction (arrow) of *Candida tropicalis* not seen with true germ tubes of *C. albicans*. Magnification, ×800. (Courtesy of B. A. Davis.)

isolates were obtained, morphological studies using specialized media were conducted to stimulate isolates to produce a range of morphological traits that could be used in conjunction with biochemical tests to produce an identification code that was central to most commercial yeast identification systems. The mainstay of yeast identification to the species level was the carbohydrate assimilation test (Table 2), for which several reliable commercial kits, such as API 20C AUX (bioMérieux SA, Marcy l'Etoile, France), API ID 32C (not available in the United States), Auxacolor 2 (Bio-Rad, Hercules, CA), and automated and semiautomated systems (e.g., ID 32C and Vitek 2 YST, produced by bioMérieux), are available (reviewed in references 173 and 174). The tests measure the ability of a yeast isolate to use a specific carbohydrate as the sole source of carbon in the presence of oxygen. In addition, numerous commercial rapid phenotypic tests designed to identify single or several *Candida* species have been described (173). Historically, a large range of adjunctive approaches have also been employed to aid yeast identification, including nitrate, urease, phenol oxidase, and rapid trehalose tests, carbohydrate fermentation tests, and induction of the formation of ascospores and their morphological characterization. These have been reviewed extensively in previous editions of this book (173 and references therein) and, for reasons described below, are not discussed in detail here. This chapter concentrates only on aspects that are still relevant to current approaches to yeast identification.

A large number of studies have compared the accuracy of phenotype and biochemical identifications with those obtained using molecular methods based upon PCR amplification and sequencing of various loci (11, 12, 174–180), pyrosequencing of ribosomal DNA (rDNA) genes (76, 77, 181–184), or, more recently, proteomic approaches using commercial matrix-assisted laser desorption ionization–time of flight mass spectrometry (MALDI-TOF MS) platforms (185–187). In a recent meta-analysis of such studies (188), conventional commercial methods were found to be reasonably accurate in identifying isolates of the more common *Candida* species, provided that they were producing typical biochemical profiles (11, 12, 174–178, 188), but were less useful for the rarer pathogenic yeast species (11, 12, 175, 176, 178, 188) and failed to identify cryptic species in many common species complexes or to delineate closely related species (11, 12, 15, 76, 78, 179, 180, 189). These failings result from a combination of issues, which include the fact that rare yeast pathogens are frequently not represented in databases that accompany the conventional commercial yeast identification platforms (reviewed in reference 181), the failure of restricted biochemical assimilation profiles to delineate closely related species or variants that behave unusually (11, 77, 188, 189), and, at least to some degree, laboratories failing to supplement biochemical profiles with appropriate morphological analyses (12).

The accurate identification of yeast isolates has always been important for epidemiological reasons (15, 26, 66, 67, 78, 190, 191), and also because *in vitro* patterns of antifungal susceptibility are known to vary substantially between different *Candida* species (9, 26, 78, 191, 192) (Table 3; see also chapter 134 of this *Manual*). Historically, the clinical impact of erroneous identifications could be mitigated by performing susceptibility testing on individual isolates. However, more recently, the importance of robust identification was compounded by surveys that examined the wild-type MIC distributions and epidemiological cutoff values for many key species and antifungal agents (192–198). Combined with analyses of the antifungal susceptibility profiles of yeast isolates from cases of therapeutic failure which harbor established antifungal drug resistance mutations, those studies demonstrated that it is inappropriate to apply generalized clinical breakpoints for a given antifungal agent to all yeast species (see for example reference 196). Subsequently, species-specific breakpoints for the interpretation of yeast antifungal drug susceptibility testing involving the echinocandins and the azoles fluconazole and voriconazole have been proposed for many common *Candida* spp. (194–200). Incorrect identification of these species will now have potentially profound effects on the interpretation of MIC data and subsequent therapeutic interventions. For these reasons, this chapter focuses principally on identification strategies based on genomic and proteomic methods, which have been proven to yield much more reliable identifications than the conventional biochemical methods employed previously.

Purity of Cultures

Before any additional tests are performed, it is essential to ensure that the culture is pure. A Gram stain of the culture can verify purity, but often, bacterial contamination can be detected by simple wet preparation examination. If the culture is mixed with bacteria, the isolate should be inoculated on a blood agar plate or Sabouraud dextrose agar containing antibiotics and individual colonies should be subcultured for purity or, alternatively, treated with hydrochloric acid (Fig. 4). The HCl procedure is performed by inoculating a colony into three tubes of Sabouraud glucose broth (each containing 5 ml). A capillary pipette is used to add 4 drops of 1 N HCl to the first tube, 2 drops to the second tube, and 1 drop to the third tube. After incubation at 25°C for 24 to 48 hours, 0.1 ml of each broth is subcultured onto fresh Sabouraud dextrose agar plates.

More than one yeast species may be recovered from a clinical specimen, especially if the specimen is from a normally nonsterile site (12, 201). In addition, multiple yeast species may be responsible for fungemia episodes. Careful attention to colonial morphology and microscopic characteristics can offer clues to a mixed population. Subculturing individual isolates to additional media can be helpful (201), and the use of a chromogenic medium may delineate the presence of more than one yeast species.

Chromogenic Agars

Presumptive identification of one or two yeast species based on colony characteristics can be obtained with chromogenic agar media (reviewed in references 135 and 174). CHROMagar *Candida* (CHROMagar France, Paris, France; distributed in the United States by Becton Dickinson/BBL, Sparks, MD) allows differentiation of more than 10 species and is marketed for the presumptive identification of *C. albicans*, *C. tropicalis*, *C. glabrata*, and *C. krusei*. Colony identification is based on the differential release of chromogenic breakdown products from various substrates following exoenzyme activity. It is important to recognize that identifications are presumptive, as many species exhibit considerable variations in colony appearance (202). The directions of the manufacturer must be strictly followed, as is the case for any rapid test based on exoenzyme activity. Incubation time and temperature significantly affect the colony appearance. The medium is useful for the detection of mixed yeast infections, which are particularly common with isolates from mucosal sites and are selective for fungi over bacteria. Other chromogenic media are now commercially available (see chapter 118). ChromID Candida (bioMérieux) and CandiSelect 4 (Bio-Rad, Marnes-La-Coquette, France) perform similarly to CHROMagar. Brilliance *Candida* agar (formerly Oxoid chromogenic *Candida* agar; Thermo Fisher Scientific, Basingstoke, United Kingdom) and HiChrome *Candida* differential agar (HiMedia Laboratories, Mumbai, India) were introduced recently. However, no one medium detects all instances of mixed yeast blood cultures (203, 204). CHROMagar and ChromID Candida are FDA approved.

Morphology Studies

Determining the morphology of isolates on cornmeal-Tween agar, rice agar, potato carrot bile agar (Bio-Rad, Marnes-La-Coquette, France), or other similar agars offers the opportunity to correlate morphologic characteristics with identifications obtained using genomic or proteomic approaches. These characteristics, which form part of the identification code for many commercially available biochemical testing kits, coupled with demonstration of purity on chromogenic agar, are useful adjuncts to genomic and proteomic approaches, as they can provide additional levels of reassurance that morphologies match the genomic and proteomic profiles (see for example references 12 and 205). Microscopic examination should reveal the thick-walled chlamydospores of *C. albicans*/*C. dubliniensis*; attention should be given to factors such as the size and shape of the pseudohyphae, the arrangement of blastoconidia along the pseudohyphae, and the presence of capsules (Fig. 1 and Table 2).

Germ Tube Test

One of the most valuable and simple tests for the rapid presumptive identification of *C. albicans* and *C. dubliniensis* is the germ tube test (Fig. 5a). The test is considered presumptive because not all isolates of *C. albicans* will be germ tube positive, and false positives may be obtained, especially with *C. tropicalis*, despite well-trained staff (206). Microscopic observation of the preparation reveals that the short hyphal initials produced by *C. albicans* are not constricted at the junction of the blastoconidium and germ tube. *Candida tropicalis* can produce hyphal initials, but the blastoconidia are larger than those of *C. albicans*, and there is a definite constriction where the hyphal initial joins the blastoconidium (Fig. 5b). Optimum conditions are obtained by using colonies grown on Sabouraud glucose agar or blood agar at 30°C for 24 to 48 hours (unpublished observations). The test is performed by first lightly touching a colony with a bacteriological loop so that a thin film of organism is obtained, transferring the inoculum into the test substrate (e.g., fetal bovine serum), and then incubating at 37°C for up to 3 hours. Germ tube tests should be read between 2 and 3 hours to prevent clumping of hyphal initials and to reduce the number of false positives. In addition, a heavy inoculum of yeasts and the presence of bacteria can each lead to false-negative results.

Molecular Methods

The obvious advantages of using molecular methods are the improved accuracy, as described above, and speed. If in-house Sanger sequencing is employed, results can be available within 12 hours of colony isolation, whereas traditional biochemical methods usually take several days. However, development of molecular databases and standardization remain issues that are starting to be addressed (see below).

Conventional (Sanger) DNA Sequencing

DNA sequencing is increasingly being used for definitive identification of unknown yeast isolates. In order to develop a universal genetic identification system for yeasts, the most reproducible, specific, and sensitive sequence for comparison must be employed, and most research has focused on the multicopy rDNA regions. The large subunit, specifically the D1/D2 region, was shown to be highly discriminatory for the ascomycetous yeasts (7) and, similarly, for the basidiomycetous yeasts (8, 207), although differentiation of some closely related species in the latter study (207) was achieved using the ITS and intergenic sequence regions. Other studies have also used the ITS1 and ITS2 regions (208, 209). Chen et al. demonstrated that the ITS2 sequence alone can be sufficient for discriminating *Candida* species (210). However, most existing data concern sequencing of 26S rDNA or ITS1, two regions for which the publicly available databases currently have the most comprehensive coverage (reviewed in reference 211). Linton et al. (11) conducted a study assessing the value of direct 26S rDNA sequencing using over 3,000 isolates submitted to the Mycology Reference Laboratory of the United Kingdom. All 153 isolates that could not be identified using the Auxacolor 2 kit were unambiguously identified using 26S DNA sequencing. Similarly, Ciardo et al. (212) demonstrated that ITS1 sequencing was superior to the ID 32C system in a prospective study employing 1,648 yeast isolates. Both loci allow the differentiation of cryptic species within key *Candida* species complexes (11, 12, 15, 78) and identify all currently described *Malassezia* spp. (35). These two DNA loci also have phylogenetic value and have been used extensively to help define novel species and taxonomic affiliations from both clinical and environmental samples (34, 36, 37, 211) and to identify geographically constrained, clonal lineages of *C. auris* (28). However, certain genera are fully resolved only by the inclusion of additional non-rDNA loci (34, 36, 37). Central to such approaches is the availability of comprehensive databases of accurately identified reference sequences against which a test sequence can be compared (157, 176). Two widely used databases are GenBank (http://www.ncbi.nlm.nih.gov/blast) and the Centraalbureau voor Schimmelcultures yeast database (http://www.westerdijkinstitute.nl/), with the latter containing databases for strains held in the culture collection. Lau et al. (157) highlighted the need to be aware of how the genetic database being used is maintained. GenBank contains unrefereed sequences, and errors are known to occur, whereas the Centraalbureau voor Schimmelcultures has a curated ITS sequence database, and a comprehensive ITS-based, curated database constructed using controlled reference isolates is under constant development under the auspices of an International Society of Human and Animal Mycology working group dedicated to the molecular identification of pathogenic fungi (213) (http://its.mycologylab.org). Reference texts such as the *Atlas of Clinical Fungi* (214) have useful restriction maps of ribosomal operons for described fungi. Molecular approaches and guidelines to fungal identification are described in CLSI documents MM03-02 and MM18-A (215, 216).

Two commercial systems for DNA sequencing and analysis are available. Hall et al. (217) demonstrated good concordance between the MicroSeq D2 large-subunit rDNA sequencing system (ABI) and the API 20C AUX system, with most of the discrepancies being attributable to a lack of available data in the relevant databases. The SmartGene Fungi system (SmartGene, Lausanne, Switzerland) is another commercial database used for identifying unknown isolates. In a recent evaluation with 2,938 specimens, 79% of 169 isolates that could not be identified using phenotypic tests were identified to species level using ITS sequencing and the SmartGene IDNS database (218). About half of the sequenced isolates were common pathogens with atypical biochemical profiles, and the remainder were rare yeast species. Neither system is FDA approved.

Pyrosequencing

Pyrosequencing is a novel method for rapid determination of a short stretch of DNA sequence that has been examined as a potentially fast identification method. This technique typically generates 20 to 40 nucleotide sequences in a 96-well microtiter plate format in as little as 90 minutes, after an initial PCR amplification stage that can be performed on relatively crude extracts of fungal genomic DNA (reviewed in reference 176). Thus, full identification from a starting colony can be achieved in less than 6 h. Montero et al. (184) identified 69.1% of 133 isolates representing 43 yeast species by sequencing of the hypervariable ITS region, as judged by comparison of identifications with those obtained using traditional methods, as it was not possible to identify the *Trichosporon* or *Cryptococcus* isolates to species level. In contrast, Boyanton et al. (181) obtained 100% agreement between pyrosequencing and traditional identification methods for 60 isolates of the species *C. albicans*, *C. dubliniensis*, *C. glabrata*, *C. guilliermondii*, *C. krusei*, *C. lusitaniae*, *C. parapsilosis*, and *C. tropicalis*. Similarly, Borman et al. demonstrated that pyrosequencing of 35 bp of the ITS2 region correctly identified most clinically important *Candida* species in a panel of nearly 500 test isolates encompassing over 40 distinct species (76) and was able to accurately resolve cryptic species in several key pathogenic *Candida* species complexes (15, 78, 189). More recent studies have also shown that the same approach can be successful with *Malassezia* spp. and other non-*Candida* yeasts (182, 183). Finally, pyrosequencing can be performed directly from positive blood cultures, without the need to first isolate and culture the yeast on mycological media (219), raising the possibility of even more rapid identification of the causative pathogens.

DNA-Based Methods That Do Not Involve Direct Sequencing

Restriction enzyme analysis (REA), karyotyping using pulsed-field gel electrophoresis, and the use of species-specific probes have all been used to identify yeast species and have been reviewed (174). However, the majority of these techniques were developed before discovery of many of the cryptic species complexes and thus may not be able to distinguish among them.

Microarrays for fungal identification have been produced using the ITS regions. Leinberger et al. (220) identified *C. albicans*, *C. dubliniensis*, *C. krusei*, *C. tropicalis*, *C. guilliermondii*, and *C. lusitaniae*. A method using a further modification of this principle was able to distinguish *C. parapsilosis*, *C. orthopsilosis*, and *C. metapsilosis* from among 24 other fungal pathogens, including 10 other *Candida* species (221), and coupling of microarray technology with flowthrough hybridization approaches was recently shown to improve sensitivity and reduce processing time (222). Other rapid identification systems developed include the DiversiLab system of automated repetitive sequence-based PCR (bioMérieux). This method uses primers against noncoding repetitive sequences; amplified products are separated on a microfluidic chip to generate a fingerprint of intensity of fluorescence versus migration time. This technique was used to screen 115 clinical isolates of *Candida* species by sequence analysis of the contiguous ITS region and yielded 99% concordant results with conventional molecular identification methods (223), although correct identification is dependent on a comprehensive library of species fingerprints for comparison. The Luminex multianalyte profiling platform enables the simultaneous screening for a range of fungal pathogens and has been used to identify *Candida* isolates from pure cultures (224) and directly from a number of types of clinical specimens (225), including positive blood cultures (155).

MALDI-TOF MS-Based Methods

An alternative method to DNA-based technologies is MALDI-TOF MS. Traditionally, this method required a pure colony of yeast and produced a mass spectrum fingerprint characteristic of the organism (see for example references 185–187 and 205; reviewed in reference 186). Several commercial platforms with accompanying mass-spectral databases are available; most data have been published concerning the Bruker Biotyper (Bruker Daltonics) and Vitek MS (bioMérieux) systems (see for example references 226 and 227), both of which have received FDA clearance. Although several studies have demonstrated that identification success is affected by the quality and/or age of the culture and also the extraction method used to prepare cultures for MS (205, 226, 228), extremely rapid methods that reliably identify most species of pathogenic yeasts directly from primary cultures and that allow robust identification in less than 15 minutes have been described (205). Indeed, Fraser et al. reported the accurate identification (compared to conventional rDNA sequencing in conjunction with pyrosequencing) of 99.8% of 6,343 isolates encompassing 71 different yeast species using the Bruker Biotyper platform and the accompanying commercial database supplemented with additional in-house reference spectra (205). MALDI-TOF MS can readily discriminate most species complexes within *Candida* (205, 226–228), with the exception of *C. albicans*/*C. africana*. Notably, with supplemented databases (https://biological-mass-spectrometry-identification.com/msi/), the technique also robustly identifies pathogenic non-*Candida* species, including *Trichosporon* and allied genera (229) and the various species within *Cryptococcus* (230, 231). Although the need for supplementation of commercial databases with additional in-house spectral profiles for the rarer, emerging species of pathogenic yeasts is potentially a limitation of MALDI-TOF MS (205, 226–231), the recent description of transferable databases (231) and online Web applications for identification of fungi by MALDI-TOF (232) (https://biological-mass-spectrometry-identification.com/msi/) are likely to mostly circumvent such issues.

In most cases of candidiasis, the organism burden in blood or other clinical samples is too low to allow direct MALDI-TOF MS approaches. Recently, however, the technique was used to assess the identification of 346 yeasts directly from positive blood culture bottles following centrifugation to concentrate the yeast cells and washing (233), with reported sensitivities for detection and identification of 96% for *C. albicans*, 94% for *C. parapsilosis*, 87% for *C. tropicalis*, 84% for *C. glabrata*, and 75% for *C. krusei* (234). Similar successes have been reported using positive blood cultures prepared by lysis-filtration or lysis-centrifugation (234, 235), in all cases with the reported time to result being significantly reduced compared with that of conventional approaches (233–235), and in most cases with results being available within 24 hours of the blood culture setup. MALDI-TOF MS is thus rapidly becoming the new gold standard method for the identification of pathogenic yeasts, as it offers the multiple advantages of simplicity, speed, robustness, and low cost per test (after machine acquisition costs) (205, 236).

Troubleshooting Difficult Identifications

Laboratories that employ traditional carbohydrate assimilation-based identification systems frequently encounter yeast isolates that do not fit easily into a specific species. These isolates will most likely be either relatively common species that produce atypical profiles or rarer species that are not included in the databases that accompany the commercial tests (11, 12, 17, 25, 76, 84, 174, 179, 188). For the common species, examination of morphology on cornmeal/Dalmau agar is often useful, and this is an essential adjunct to all identification approaches (including molecular and proteomic approaches), as it will aid the laboratory to identify inconsistencies between identification and morphology (see for example reference 12 and discussion therein). Clinically relevant isolates that consistently fail to be identified by conventional tests should be sent to a reference laboratory for DNA sequencing or MALDI-TOF MS analysis.

Laboratories that already employ molecular approaches will encounter isolates that fail to be identified much less frequently (see above). When rDNA sequencing-based approaches are used, identification failures typically result from lack of representation of that particular organism in the database that has been used for comparison. In such cases, successful identification can usually be achieved by sequencing of several different loci (for example, the 28S rDNA gene, ITS1, and ITS2) and interrogation of several databases, including both curated and public, synchronized ones. In rare instances, identification failure might be due to the yeast isolate in question being a novel, hitherto-undescribed taxon. In such cases, isolates should be sent to a reference laboratory for full phylogenetic analyses. For laboratories that currently employ MALDI-TOF MS approaches, identification failures usually result from the absence of reference spectra for that particular organism from the commercial databases supplied with the particular platform. The public sharing of extended, transferrable reference databases (231) and the availability of online MS identification tools (232) should hopefully extend the range of yeast species that can be identified. When an organism cannot be identified by MALDI-TOF MS even after interrogation of all of the current reference databases and despite producing good-quality spectra, then it should be formally identified by rDNA sequencing approaches, at a reference laboratory if necessary. Once a robust molecular identification has been achieved, reference spectra for this organism can be created and used to supplement the MALDI-TOF MS database in question. Our laboratory has adopted the practice of "validating" such in-house spectra only after a second, independent isolate has been encountered and shown to be the same species by both MALDI-TOF MS and rDNA sequencing.

ORGANISMS RESEMBLING YEASTS

Occasionally, organisms such as moulds and algae may grow on mycological media and produce colonies that resemble those produced by yeasts. However, careful attention to morphologic characteristics differentiates them. Examples of such organisms recovered from clinical specimens that can be superficially confused with yeasts include *Geotrichum* spp., black yeasts in the extended genus *Exophiala*, and *Prototheca* species. *Geotrichum candidum* (*Galactomyces geotrichum*; dry, white colonies) can be distinguished from members of *Trichosporon* and related genera by blastoconidium production and dichotomous branching (Fig. 2e). Black yeasts are discussed elsewhere in this *Manual*. *Prototheca* species (white to cream colored, dull or moist to mucoid colonies) are ubiquitous, achlorophyllous algae living on decaying organic material that rarely produce disease in humans and animals (237), causing principally cutaneous infections or deeper infections in immunocompromised hosts (238, 239). *P. wickerhamii* is recovered most often from human infections (Fig. 2f).

TYPING SYSTEMS

In order to understand the epidemiology of infection, to distinguish between endogenous and exogenous infection (and, in the latter case, to locate the source), to examine transmission, or to monitor the spread of drug resistance, it is necessary to be able to distinguish between isolates within a species. Successful strain typing depends on the choice of technique(s) and experimental conditions for maximum discrimination, which has to be established for each species tested.

DNA-based typing methods began in the 1980s with REA, which required careful selection of the enzyme used to maximize discrimination. Other methods quickly followed: Southern blotting using species-specific or generic probes, karyotyping, pulsed-field gel electrophoresis–REA, and random amplified polymorphic DNA analysis. These methods are all subject to discrepancies due to mutation or laboratory reproducibility and have been reviewed (240–243). Most of these techniques have been superseded by more accurate and reproducible methods, such as microsatellite typing and multilocus sequence typing (MLST). Gil-Lamaignere et al. (240) and Taylor et al. (241) have critically reviewed the limitations and applications of these techniques.

Microsatellite typing is the amplification of short tandem repeat sequences that are polymorphic. This is a fast typing method but cannot be used to estimate isolate relatedness unless the bands are sequenced and the content compared (for example, see reference 242). MLST, which uses the sequences of six to eight selected housekeeping genes and identifies polymorphic nucleotide sites, can be used to establish population structures by assessing variation in sequence for a set number of genes, and this has enabled the development of databases for interlaboratory comparisons. The method has been used to type a number of yeast species (244–246) and recently demonstrated the spread of *Cryptococcus gattii* from Vancouver Island in Canada to the northwest United States (247). MLST has been used to develop a consensus typing scheme for *C. gattii* and *C. neoformans* (248) and for *Candida albicans* (246). MLST has been used to demonstrate that most patients with *C. albicans* carried the same strain at multiple sites or over time and to confirm that microvariation could be detected over time when some isolates are stored (249). However, while MLST provided detail on the population structure of clinical isolates of *C. glabrata* from Taiwan, greater typing discrimination was achieved using pulsed-field gel electrophoresis–REA (250).

A commercial platform, DiversiLab (bioMérieux, France), has been developed for identification and strain typing of microbial pathogens, including fungi (223), based on PCR amplification of repetitive sequence elements (rep-PCR) that are duplicated throughout the fungal genome followed by fluidic chip separation of amplicons according to length. Although rep-PCR has the advantage of being applicable to any fungal species using universal PCR primers, it possesses less discriminatory power than microsatellite and MLST-based approaches (243, 251) and is not FDA approved.

Recently, the development of next-generation high-throughput sequencing approaches has facilitated low-cost, rapid whole-genome sequencing approaches in fungi, where all nucleotide polymorphisms detected throughout the whole genome can be used to infer relatedness and investigate potential fungal outbreaks. Whole-genome sequencing represents the pinnacle of fungal strain typing and has been successfully employed to investigate the global epidemiology of *Candida auris* (26) and *Cryptococcus gattii* (252) and outbreaks of *C. auris* (26) and *Saprochaete clavata* (253).

SEROLOGIC TESTS

Genus *Candida*

Invasive *Candida* infections are life threatening, but detection by relatively noninvasive methods such as blood culture is problematic. A test for detection of antibody to *Candida* mannan is available (e.g., using the Platelia *Candida* antibody enzyme immunoassay kit [Bio-Rad Laboratories]). Although such tests have poor sensitivity and specificity (157), at least in part due to the presence of *Candida* species as part of the commensal flora and antibodies against cell wall components that may be found in colonized individuals, they are recommended for the diagnosis of candidemia and chronic disseminated candidiasis (254). The utility of these tests is maximized when they are combined with detection of antigen levels, because the antibody and antigen levels may show an inverse correlation during disease progression. More detail on antigen testing is presented above.

ANTIMICROBIAL SUSCEPTIBILITIES

Details of susceptibility testing methods, antifungal resistance profiles, and mechanisms of resistance are described in other chapters of this *Manual*. Table 3 contains the MICs from a number of sources for 36 yeast species. The references in Table 3 have all used CLSI methods, with the following exceptions: the article by Lass-Flörl et al. (255), who followed EUCAST methodology; the *Atlas of Clinical Fungi* (2); and Ashbee's review (101), which contains data from published work. The data on *Malassezia* from Ashbee's review have been included because there is little information on the susceptibility of these organisms. Species-specific susceptibility breakpoints have been determined for several species of *Candida* and the major classes of antifungal drugs (194–200). Most species of *Candida* are susceptible to the echinocandins (190), although there is some variation within species in susceptibility to caspofungin (256), and echinocandin resistance has begun to emerge in *C. glabrata* (see for example reference 257). *C. krusei* is intrinsically resistant to fluconazole but is susceptible to posaconazole and voriconazole, while some strains of *C. glabrata* may have elevated MICs of fluconazole. *C. norvegensis* and *C. inconspicua* are also fluconazole resistant (9, 177, 190, 191, 194). Virtually all isolates of the emerging pathogen *C. auris* reported to date also have very elevated MICs of fluconazole, with distinct resistance mutations reported for the different geographically restricted clades (26). In addition, individual isolates with additional resistance to amphotericin B or the echinocandins have been described (reviewed in references 27 and 58). Few *Candida* species are resistant *in vitro* to amphotericin B, although *C. lusitaniae* may exhibit secondary resistance. Therefore, the clinical response to this drug may be poor despite *in vitro* susceptibility tests indicating that strains are susceptible (258, 259). Although clinically relevant breakpoints have not been established for susceptibility testing of yeasts against amphotericin B, epidemiological cutoff values have been reported (260).

Reference 113 reviews current information about diagnosis, antifungal susceptibility testing, and treatment of invasive fungal infections due to rare yeasts other than *Candida* species. The MICs of a variety of antifungal agents for common human *Trichosporon* species have been reviewed extensively (116). Echinocandin antifungals are ineffective against all species of basidiomycetous yeasts (*Cryptococcus, Trichosporon, Rhodotorula, Sporobolomyces,* and allied genera).

EVALUATION, INTERPRETATION, AND REPORTING OF RESULTS

As taxonomic relationships and rules are revised, the names of organisms change. To prevent confusion, it is recommended that clinical reports include the more familiar species names alongside any new classification being used. At this time, rather than change the name of *Candida* genus organisms from names that are deeply entrenched in the literature and in the minds of physicians and laboratorians, this *Manual* retains their *Candida* genus taxon as well as the teleomorph name. This is likely to change in the near future, and laboratory workers should familiarize themselves with newer names as they are introduced.

As in clinical bacteriology, the significance of isolating a species known to be a member of the normal microbiota or a common contaminant depends on numerous factors, including but not limited to the patient's underlying disease, geographic and hospital environment, specimen site, preceding antimicrobial and device management, specimen collection and quality, and specimen processing. In general, the isolation of yeasts from normally sterile body sites is suggestive of infection, but the influence of the method of collection (e.g., *C. albicans* in CSF collected by lumbar puncture) must be considered. The more challenging decision about significance is when the yeast is present in specimens obtained from nonsterile body sites.

Review of the literature reveals a surprising lack of evidence-based studies regarding development of criteria for establishing significance in nonsterile body sites, although some guidance in the interpretation of culture results is provided elsewhere (261). Clinical microbiology laboratories typically apply bacterial criteria to assess specimens for possible fungal infection. An example of this is to not report yeasts unless they are predominating over bacteria. However, there are several problems with this approach. First, yeasts are not as abundant as bacteria in the normal microbiota, so an increase in relative abundance may reflect yeast infection. Roughly 10 times more bacteria than yeast can occupy the same volume of tissue. Second, a specimen from a patient who is receiving antibacterial agents may contain more abundant yeasts, the reporting of which may mislead the patient's physician about the yeasts' significance. Third, when the abundance of a yeast is considered insufficient to warrant further investigation, the species may not be reported. This could lead to unfortunate consequences, because certain yeasts, such as *C. tropicalis,* are considered particularly aggressive in immunocompromised patients.

Two specimens that are particularly problematic are sputum and urine (clean catch, indwelling catheter, and "in-and-out" catheter). The significance of *Candida* species in sputum, regardless of quantity, has been questioned (262). The presence of these yeasts in sputum has little significance, as the respiratory tract is frequently colonized by *Candida* species in patients receiving ventilatory support. The latest Infectious Diseases Society of America guidelines recommend that antifungal therapy not be initiated on the basis of a positive respiratory tract culture, and in cases where *Candida* pneumonia is suspected, histopathological evidence should be sought (63). Similarly, the presence of a few *C. neoformans* CFU in sputum does not necessarily imply etiologic significance unless patient information strongly suggests cryptococcosis. To prevent unnecessary testing but still provide useful information to physicians, Barenfanger et al. (262) recommend reporting "yeast, not *Cryptococcus*" for all respiratory secretion specimens in which a rapidly growing yeast is obtained and reserving full identification for patients in whom candidal pneumonia is indicated by histopathology. Patients for whom the limited form of identification was used were found to experience a shorter hospital stay, received fewer antifungals, had a lower mortality rate, and incurred fewer expenses. This approach allows physicians the opportunity to request further identification if desired. A similar approach to reporting rapidly growing yeasts isolated from routine urine specimens (urinary tract infection is the only presentation) could also be used. The significance of yeasts in urine must be examined in the context of the clinical setting and whether therapy would be desirable (63). If the patient is asymptomatic and there is no predisposing condition, the situation should be monitored. If a predisposing condition is identified, treatment may be justified, but for patients with higher risk factors, such as neonates or immunocompromised patients with fever and risk of candidemia, treatment should be commenced. Fluconazole is the front-line therapy unless *C. krusei* or *C. glabrata* infection is suspected; in these cases, a short course of oral flucytosine, intravenous amphotericin B deoxycholate, or irrigation of the bladder with amphotericin B may be indicated (63).

Although yeast species express different antifungal profiles, especially for the expanding spectrum of new antifungal agents (113) (Table 3), the most commonly isolated *Candida* species are generally susceptible to the triazoles, the polyenes, and the echinocandins. The exceptions for the triazoles are *C. glabrata*, *C. auris*, and *C. krusei* (*C. parapsilosis* isolates are occasionally resistant to the echinocandins). *C. krusei* is relatively rarely isolated from infections. Thus, the need to identify rapidly growing yeasts present in clinically significant quantities from nonsterile sites can be limited to performing a rapid screen for *C. glabrata*. It is more important to obtain a yeast's antifungal susceptibility profile if there is failure to respond to antifungal therapy or if an azole-resistant isolate is suspected (63).

REFERENCES

1. **Dukik K, Muñoz JF, Jiang Y, Feng P, Sigler L, Stielow JB, Freeke J, Jamalian A, Gerrits van den Ende B, McEwen JG, Clay OK, Schwartz IS, Govender NP, Maphanga TG, Cuomo CA, Moreno LF, Kenyon C, Borman AM, de Hoog S.** 2017. Novel taxa of thermally dimorphic systemic pathogens in the Ajellomycetaceae (Onygenales). *Mycoses* **60:**296–309.
2. **De Hoog GS, Guarro J, Gene J, Figueras MJ (ed).** 2014. *Atlas of Clinical Fungi*, 4th ed. Centraalbureau voor Schimmelcultures, Baarn, The Netherlands.
3. **Hawksworth DL, et al.** 2011. The Amsterdam Declaration on Fungal Nomenclature. *IMA Fungus* **2:**105–112.
4. **Hawksworth DL.** 2011. A new dawn for the naming of fungi: impacts of decisions made in Melbourne in July 2011 on the future publication and regulation of fungal names. *IMA Fungus* **2:**155–162.
5. **de Hoog GS, Haase G, Chaturvedi V, Walsh TJ, Meyer W, Lackner M.** 2013. Taxonomy of medically important fungi in the molecular era. *Lancet Infect Dis* **13:**385–386.
6. **Brandt ME, Lockhart SR.** 2012. Recent taxonomic developments with *Candida* and other opportunistic yeasts. *Curr Fungal Infect Rep* **6:**170–177.
7. **Kurtzman CP, Robnett CJ.** 1997. Identification of clinically important ascomycetous yeasts based on nucleotide divergence in the 5′ end of the large-subunit (26S) ribosomal DNA gene. *J Clin Microbiol* **35:**1216–1223.
8. **Fell JW, Boekhout T, Fonseca A, Scorzetti G, Statzell-Tallman A.** 2000. Biodiversity and systematics of basidiomycetous yeasts as determined by large-subunit rDNA D1/D2 domain sequence analysis. *Int J Syst Evol Microbiol* **50:**1351–1371.
9. **Pfaller MA, Diekema DJ, Messer SA, Boyken L, Hollis RJ.** 2003. Activities of fluconazole and voriconazole against 1,586 recent clinical isolates of *Candida* species determined by broth microdilution, disk diffusion, and Etest methods: report from the ARTEMIS Global Antifungal Susceptibility Program, 2001. *J Clin Microbiol* **41:**1440–1446.
10. **Pfaller MA, Diekema DJ.** 2007. Epidemiology of invasive candidiasis: a persistent public health problem. *Clin Microbiol Rev* **20:**133–163.
11. **Linton CJ, Borman AM, Cheung G, Holmes AD, Szekely A, Palmer MD, Bridge PD, Campbell CK, Johnson EM.** 2007. Molecular identification of unusual pathogenic yeast isolates by large ribosomal subunit gene sequencing: 2 years of experience at the United Kingdom Mycology Reference Laboratory. *J Clin Microbiol* **45:**1152–1158.
12. **Borman AM, Szekely A, Palmer MD, Johnson EM.** 2012. Assessment of accuracy of identification of pathogenic yeasts in microbiology laboratories in the United Kingdom. *J Clin Microbiol* **50:**2639–2644.
13. **Borman AM, Szekely A, Johnson EM.** 2016. Comparative pathogenicity of United Kingdom isolates of the emerging pathogen *Candida auris* and other key pathogenic *Candida* species. *mSphere* **1:**e00189-16.
14. **Moran GP, Coleman DC, Sullivan DJ.** 2012. *Candida albicans* versus *Candida dubliniensis*: why is *C. albicans* more pathogenic? *Int J Microbiol* **2012:**205921.
15. **Borman AM, Szekely A, Linton CJ, Palmer MD, Brown P, Johnson EM.** 2013. Epidemiology, antifungal susceptibility, and pathogenicity of *Candida africana* isolates from the United Kingdom. *J Clin Microbiol* **51:**967–972.
16. **Romeo O, Criseo G.** 2011. *Candida africana* and its closest relatives. *Mycoses* **54:**475–486.
17. **Tavanti A, Davidson AD, Gow NA, Maiden MC, Odds FC.** 2005. *Candida orthopsilosis* and *Candida metapsilosis* spp. nov. to replace *Candida parapsilosis* groups II and III. *J Clin Microbiol* **43:**284–292.
18. **Vaughan-Martini A, Kurtzman CP, Meyer SA, O'Neill EB.** 2005. Two new species in the *Pichia guilliermondii* clade: *Pichia caribbica* sp. nov., the ascosporic state of *Candida fermentati*, and *Candida carpophila* comb. nov. *FEMS Yeast Res* **5:**463–469.
19. **Kurtzman CP, Suzuki M.** 2010. Phylogenetic analysis of ascomycete yeasts that form coenzymen Q-9 and the proposal of the new genera *Babjeviella*, *Meyerozyma*, *Millerozyma*, *Priceomyces*, and *Scheffersomyces*. *Mycoscience* **51:**2–14.
20. **Angoulvant A, Guitard J, Hennequin C.** 2016. Old and new pathogenic *Nakaseomyces* species: epidemiology, biology, identification, pathogenicity and antifungal resistance. *FEMS Yeast Res* **16:**fov114.
21. **Padovan AC, Melo AS, Colombo AL.** 2013. Systematic review and new insights into the molecular characterization of the *Candida rugosa* species complex. *Fungal Genet Biol* **61:**33–41.
22. **Pfüller R, Gräser Y, Erhard M, Groenewald M.** 2011. A novel flucytosine-resistant yeast species, *Candida pseudoaaseri*, causes disease in a cancer patient. *J Clin Microbiol* **49:** 4195–4202.
23. **Adam H, Groenewald M, Mohan S, Richardson S, Bunn U, Gibas CF, Poutanen S, Sigler L.** 2009. Identification of a new species, *Candida subhashii*, as a cause of peritonitis. *Med Mycol* **47:**305–311.

24. **Eddouzi J, Hofstetter V, Groenewald M, Manai M, Sanglard D.** 2013. Characterization of a new clinical yeast species, *Candida tunisiensis* sp. nov., isolated from a strain collection from Tunisian hospitals. *J Clin Microbiol* **51:**31–39.
25. **Satoh K, Makimura K, Hasumi Y, Nishiyama Y, Uchida K, Yamaguchi H.** 2009. *Candida auris* sp. nov., a novel ascomycetous yeast isolated from the external ear canal of an inpatient in a Japanese hospital. *Microbiol Immunol* **53:**41–44.
26. **Lockhart SR, Etienne KA, Vallabhaneni S, Farooqi J, Chowdhary A, Govender NP, Colombo AL, Calvo B, Cuomo CA, Desjardins CA, Berkow EL, Castanheira M, Magobo RE, Jabeen K, Asghar RJ, Meis JF, Jackson B, Chiller T, Litvintseva AP.** 2017. Simultaneous emergence of multidrug-resistant *Candida auris* on 3 continents confirmed by whole-genome sequencing and epidemiological analyses. *Clin Infect Dis* **64:**134–140.
27. **Chowdhary A, Sharma C, Meis JF.** 2017. *Candida auris*: a rapidly emerging cause of hospital-acquired multidrug-resistant fungal infections globally. *PLoS Pathog* **13:**e1006290.
28. **Borman AM, Szekely A, Johnson EM.** 2017. Isolates of the emerging pathogen *Candida auris* present in the UK have several geographic origins. *Med Mycol* **55:**563–567.
29. **De Hoog GS, Smith MT.** 2004. Ribosomal gene phylogeny and species delimitation in *Geotrichum* and its teleomorphs. *Stud Mycol* **50:**489–515.
30. **Salkin IF, Gordon MA, Samsonoff WM, Rieder CL.** 1985. *Blastoschizomyces capitatus*, a new combination. *Mycotaxon* **22:**365–380.
31. **Hagen F, Khayhan K, Theelen B, Kolecka A, Polacheck I, Sionov E, Falk R, Parnmen S, Lumbsch HT, Boekhout T.** 2015. Recognition of seven species in the *Cryptococcus gattii/Cryptococcus neoformans* species complex. *Fungal Genet Biol* **78:**16–48.
32. **Hagen F, et al.** 2017. Importance of resolving fungal nomenclature: the case of multiple pathogenic species in the *Cryptococcus* genus. *mSphere* **2:**e00238-17.
33. **Kwon-Chung KJ, Bennett JE, Wickes BL, Meyer W, Cuomo CA, Wollenburg KR, Bicanic TA, Castañeda E, Chang YC, Chen J, Cogliati M, Dromer F, Ellis D, Filler SG, Fisher MC, Harrison TS, Holland SM, Kohno S, Kronstad JW, Lazera M, Levitz SM, Lionakis MS, May RC, Ngamskulrongroj P, Pappas PG, Perfect JR, Rickerts V, Sorrell TC, Walsh TJ, Williamson PR, Xu J, Zelazny AM, Casadevall A.** 2017. The case for adopting the "species complex" nomenclature for the etiologic agents of cryptococcosis. *mSphere* **2:**00357-16.
34. **Liu XZ, Wang QM, Göker M, Groenewald M, Kachalkin AV, Lumbsch HT, Millanes AM, Wedin M, Yurkov AM, Boekhout T, Bai FY.** 2015. Towards an integrated phylogenetic classification of the Tremellomycetes. *Stud Mycol* **81:**85–147.
35. **Honnavar P, Prasad GS, Ghosh A, Dogra S, Handa S, Rudramurthy SM.** 2016. *Malassezia arunalokei* sp. nov., a novel yeast species isolated from seborrheic dermatitis patients and healthy individuals from India. *J Clin Microbiol* **54:**1826–1834.
36. **Wang QM, Begerow D, Groenewald M, Liu XZ, Theelen B, Bai FY, Boekhout T.** 2015. Multigene phylogeny and taxonomic revision of yeasts and related fungi in the Ustilaginomycotina. *Stud Mycol* **81:**55–83.
37. **Wang QM, Yurkov AM, Göker M, Lumbsch HT, Leavitt SD, Groenewald M, Theelen B, Liu XZ, Boekhout T, Bai FY.** 2015. Phylogenetic classification of yeasts and related taxa within Pucciniomycotina. *Stud Mycol* **81:**149–189.
38. **Colombo AL, Padovan AC, Chaves GM.** 2011. Current knowledge of *Trichosporon* spp. and trichosporonosis. *Clin Microbiol Rev* **24:**682–700.
39. **Kurtzman CP, Fell JW.** 1998. *The Yeasts: A Taxonomic Study*, 4th ed. Elsevier, Amsterdam, The Netherlands.
40. **Boekhout T.** 2005. Biodiversity: gut feeling for yeasts. *Nature* **434:**449–451.
41. **Kurtzman CP, Fell JW, Boekhout T.** 2011. *The Yeasts: A Taxonomic Study*, 5th ed. Elsevier, Amsterdam, The Netherlands.
42. **Calderone RA (ed).** 2002. *Candida and Candidiasis*. ASM Press, Washington, DC.
43. **Peltroche-Llacsahuanga H, von Oy S, Haase G.** 2002. First isolation of reddish-pigmented *Candida (Torulopsis) glabrata* from a clinical specimen. *J Clin Microbiol* **40:**1116–1118.
44. **Buschelman B, Jones RN, Pfaller MA, Koontz FP, Doern GV.** 1999. Colony morphology of *Candida* spp. as a guide to species identification. *Diagn Microbiol Infect Dis* **35:**89–91.
45. **Love GL, Boyd GD, Greer DL.** 1985. Large *Cryptococcus neoformans* isolated from brain abscess. *J Clin Microbiol* **22:**1068–1070.
46. **Kwon-Chung KJ, Polacheck I, Bennett JE.** 1982. Improved diagnostic medium for separation of *Cryptococcus neoformans* var. *neoformans* (serotypes A and D) and *Cryptococcus neoformans* var. *gattii* (serotypes B and C). *J Clin Microbiol* **15:**535–537.
47. **McTaggart L, Richardson SE, Seah C, Hoang L, Fothergill A, Zhang SX.** 2011. Rapid identification of *Cryptococcus neoformans var. grubii*, *C. neoformans var. neoformans*, and *C. gattii* by use of rapid biochemical tests, differential media, and DNA sequencing. *J Clin Microbiol* **49:**2522–2527.
48. **Van Abbe NJ.** 1964. The investigation of dandruff. *J Soc Cosmet Chem* **15:**609–630.
49. **Leeming JP, Notman FH.** 1987. Improved methods for isolation and enumeration of *Malassezia furfur* from human skin. *J Clin Microbiol* **25:**2017–2019.
50. **Midgley G.** 2000. The lipophilic yeasts: state of the art and prospects. *Med Mycol* **38**(Suppl 1)**:**9–16.
51. **Padhye AA, Verghese S, Ravichandran P, Balamurugan G, Hall L, Padmaja P, Fernandez MC.** 2003. *Trichosporon loubieri* infection in a patient with adult polycystic kidney disease. *J Clin Microbiol* **41:**479–482.
52. **Limon JJ, Skalski JH, Underhill DM.** 2017. Commensal fungi in health and disease. *Cell Host Microbe* **22:**156–165.
53. **Arias CR, Burns JK, Friedrich LM, Goodrich RM, Parish ME.** 2002. Yeast species associated with orange juice: evaluation of different identification methods. *Appl Environ Microbiol* **68:**1955–1961.
54. **Lupetti A, Tavanti A, Davini P, Ghelardi E, Corsini V, Merusi I, Boldrini A, Campa M, Senesi S.** 2002. Horizontal transmission of *Candida parapsilosis* candidemia in a neonatal intensive care unit. *J Clin Microbiol* **40:**2363–2369.
55. **Pfaller MA.** 1996. Nosocomial candidiasis: emerging species, reservoirs, and modes of transmission. *Clin Infect Dis* **22**(Suppl 2)**:**S89–S94.
56. **Trofa D, Gácser A, Nosanchuk JD.** 2008. *Candida parapsilosis*, an emerging fungal pathogen. *Clin Microbiol Rev* **21:**606–625.
57. **Bonassoli LA, Svidzinski TI.** 2002. Influence of the hospital environment on yeast colonization in nursing students. *Med Mycol* **40:**311–313.
58. **Chowdhary A, Voss A, Meis JF.** 2016. Multidrug-resistant *Candida auris*: 'new kid on the block' in hospital-associated infections? *J Hosp Infect* **94:**209–212.
59. **Tsay S, Kallen A, Jackson BR, Chiller TM, Vallabhaneni S.** 2017. Approach to the investigation and management of patients with *Candida auris*, an emerging multidrug-resistant yeast. *Clin Infect Dis* **66:**306–311.
60. **Dromer F, Improvisi L, Dupont B, Eliaszewicz M, Pialoux G, Fournier S, Feuillie V.** 1997. Oral transmission of *Candida albicans* between partners in HIV-infected couples could contribute to dissemination of fluconazole-resistant isolates. *AIDS* **11:**1095–1101.
61. **Reed BD, Zazove P, Pierson CL, Gorenflo DW, Horrocks J.** 2003. *Candida* transmission and sexual behaviors as risks for a repeat episode of *Candida* vulvovaginitis. *J Womens Health (Larchmt)* **12:**979–989.
62. **Suhr MJ, Hallen-Adams HE.** 2015. The human gut mycobiome: pitfalls and potentials—a mycologist's perspective. *Mycologia* **107:**1057–1073.
63. **Pappas PG, Kauffman CA, Andes DR, Clancy CJ, Marr KA, Ostrosky-Zeichner L, Reboli AC, Schuster MG, Vazquez JA, Walsh TJ, Zaoutis TE, Sobel JD.** 2016. Clinical practice guideline for the management of candidiasis: 2016 update by the Infectious Diseases Society of America. *Clin Infect Dis* **62:**409–417.
64. **Guinea J.** 2014. Global trends in the distribution of *Candida* species causing candidemia. *Clin Microbiol Infect* **20**(Suppl 6)**:**5–10.

65. **Srinavasan A, Wise M, Bell M, Cardo D, Edwards J, Fridkin S, Jernigan J, Kallen A, McDonald LC, Patel PR, Pollock D, Centers for Disease Control and Prevention (CDC).** 2011. Vital signs: central line-associated blood stream infections—United States, 2001, 2008, and 2009. *MMWR Morb Mortal Wkly Rep* **60:**243–248.
66. **Pfaller M, Neofytos D, Diekema D, Azie N, Meier-Kriesche HU, Quan SP, Horn D.** 2012. Epidemiology and outcomes of candidemia in 3648 patients: data from the Prospective Antifungal Therapy (PATH Alliance®) registry, 2004-2008. *Diagn Microbiol Infect Dis* **74:**323–331.
67. **Pfaller MA, Andes DR, Diekema DJ, Horn DL, Reboli AC, Rotstein C, Franks B, Azie NE.** 2014. Epidemiology and outcomes of invasive candidiasis due to non-*albicans* species of *Candida* in 2,496 patients: data from the Prospective Antifungal Therapy (PATH) Registry 2004–2008. *PLoS One* **9:**e101510.
68. **Pammi M, Holland L, Butler G, Gacser A, Bliss JM.** 2013. *Candida parapsilosis* is a significant neonatal pathogen: a systematic review and meta-analysis. *Pediatr Infect Dis J* **32:**e206–e216.
69. **Heitman J, Kozel TR, Kwon-Chung KJ, Perfect JR, Casadevall A (ed).** 2011. *Cryptococcus: From Human Pathogen to Model Yeast.* ASM Press, Washington, DC.
70. **Gaitanis G, Magiatis P, Hantschke M, Bassukas ID, Velegraki A.** 2012. The *Malassezia* genus in skin and systemic diseases. *Clin Microbiol Rev* **25:**106–141.
71. **Chang HJ, Miller HL, Watkins N, Arduino MJ, Ashford DA, Midgley G, Aguero SM, Pinto-Powell R, von Reyn CF, Edwards W, McNeil MM, Jarvis WR, Pruitt R.** 1998. An epidemic of *Malassezia* pachydermatis in an intensive care nursery associated with colonization of health care workers' pet dogs. *N Engl J Med* **338:**706–711.
72. **Höfs S, Mogavero S, Hube B.** 2016. Interaction of *Candida albicans* with host cells: virulence factors, host defense, escape strategies, and the microbiota. *J Microbiol* **54:**149–169.
73. **Brown AJ, Brown GD, Netea MG, Gow NA.** 2014. Metabolism impacts upon *Candida* immunogenicity and pathogenicity at multiple levels. *Trends Microbiol* **22:**614–622.
74. **Zuza-Alves DL, Silva-Rocha WP, Chaves GM.** 2017. An update on *Candida tropicalis* based on basic and clinical approaches. *Front Microbiol* **8:**1927.
75. **Ben-Ami R, Berman J, Novikov A, Bash E, Shachor-Meyouhas Y, Zakin S, Maor Y, Tarabia J, Schechner V, Adler A, Finn T.** Multidrug-resistant *Candida haemulonii* and *C. auris*, Tel Aviv, Israel. *Emerg Infect Dis.* **23:**195–203.
76. **Borman AM, Linton CJ, Oliver D, Palmer MD, Szekely A, Johnson EM.** 2010. Rapid molecular identification of pathogenic yeasts by pyrosequencing analysis of 35 nucleotides of internal transcribed spacer 2. *J Clin Microbiol* **48:**3648–3653.
77. **Fidel PL Jr, Vazquez JA, Sobel JD.** 1999. *Candida glabrata*: review of epidemiology, pathogenesis, and clinical disease with comparison to *C. albicans*. *Clin Microbiol Rev* **12:**80–96.
78. **Borman AM, Petch R, Linton CJ, Palmer MD, Bridge PD, Johnson EM.** 2008. *Candida nivariensis*, an emerging pathogenic fungus with multidrug resistance to antifungal agents. *J Clin Microbiol* **46:**933–938.
79. **Sullivan DJ, Moran GP, Coleman DC.** 2005. *Candida dubliniensis*: ten years on. *FEMS Microbiol Lett* **253:**9–17.
80. **da Silva BV, Silva LB, de Oliveira DB, da Silva PR, Ferreira-Paim K, Andrade-Silva LE, Silva-Vergara ML, Andrade AA.** 2015. Species distribution, virulence factors, and antifungal susceptibility among *Candida parapsilosis* complex isolates recovered from clinical specimens. *Mycopathologia* **180:**333–343.
81. **Turner SA, Butler G.** 2014. The *Candida* pathogenic species complex. *Cold Spring Harb Perspect Med* **4:**a019778.
82. **Constante CC, Monteiro AA, Alves SH, Carneiro LC, Machado MM, Severo LC, Park S, Perlin DS, Pasqualotto AC.** 2014. Different risk factors for candidemia occur for *Candida* species belonging to the *C. parapsilosis* complex. *Med Mycol* **52:**403–406.
83. **Németh T, Tóth A, Szenzenstein J, Horváth P, Nosanchuk JD, Grózer Z, Tóth R, Papp C, Hamari Z, Vágvölgyi C, Gácser A.** 2013. Characterization of virulence properties in the *C. parapsilosis sensu lato* species. *PLoS One* **8:**e68704.
84. **Walsh TJ, Groll A, Hiemenz J, Fleming R, Roilides E, Anaissie E.** 2004. Infections due to emerging and uncommon medically important fungal pathogens. *Clin Microbiol Infect* **10**(Suppl 1)**:**48–66.
85. **Colombo AL, Júnior JNA, Guinea J.** 2017. Emerging multidrug-resistant *Candida* species. *Curr Opin Infect Dis* **30:**528–538.
86. **Miceli MH, Díaz JA, Lee SA.** 2011. Emerging opportunistic yeast infections. *Lancet Infect Dis* **11:**142–151.
87. **McMullan BJ, Sorrell TC, Chen SC.** 2013. *Cryptococcus gattii* infections: contemporary aspects of epidemiology, clinical manifestations and management of infection. *Future Microbiol* **8:**1613–1631.
88. **La Hoz RM, Pappas PG.** 2013. Cryptococcal infections: changing epidemiology and implications for therapy. *Drugs* **73:**495–504.
89. **Byrnes EJ, III, Bartlett KH, Perfect JR, Heitman J.** 2011. *Cryptococcus gattii*: an emerging fungal pathogen infecting humans and animals. *Microbes Infect* **13:**895–907.
90. **Pappas PG.** 2013. Cryptococcal infections in non-HIV-infected patients. *Trans Am Clin Climatol Assoc* **124:**61–79.
91. **Chuck SL, Sande MA.** 1989. Infections with *Cryptococcus neoformans* in the acquired immunodeficiency syndrome. *N Engl J Med* **321:**794–799.
92. **Iverson SA, Chiller T, Beekmann S, Polgreen PM, Harris J.** 2012. Recognition and diagnosis of *Cryptococcus gattii* infections in the United States. *Emerg Infect Dis* **18:**1012–1015.
93. **Harris J, Lockhart S, Chiller T.** 2012. *Cryptococcus gattii*: where do we go from here? *Med Mycol* **50:**113–129.
94. **Khawcharoenporn T, Apisarnthanarak A, Mundy LM.** 2007. Non-neoformans cryptococcal infections: a systematic review. *Infection* **35:**51–58.
95. **Smith N, Sehring M, Chambers J, Patel P.** 2017. Perspectives on non-neoformans cryptococcal opportunistic infections. *J Community Hosp Intern Med Perspect* **7:**214–217.
96. **Takemura H, Ohno H, Miura I, Takagi T, Ohyanagi T, Kunishima H, Okawara A, Miyazaki Y, Nakashima H.** 2015. The first reported case of central venous catheter-related fungemia caused by *Cryptococcus liquefaciens*. *J Infect Chemother* **21:**392–394.
97. **McCurdy LH, Morrow JD.** 2001. Ventriculitis due to *Cryptococcus uniguttulatus*. *South Med J* **94:**65–66.
98. **Kantarcioğlu AS, Boekhout T, De Hoog GS, Theelen B, Yücel A, Ekmekci TR, Fries BC, Ikeda R, Koslu A, Altas K.** 2007. Subcutaneous cryptococcosis due to *Cryptococcus diffluens* in a patient with sporotrichoid lesions: case report, features of the case isolate and in vitro antifungal susceptibilities. *Med Mycol* **45:**173–181.
99. **Tarumoto N, Sakai J, Kodana M, Kawamura T, Ohno H, Maesaki S.** 2016. Identification of disseminated cryptococcosis using MALDI-TOF MS and clinical evaluation. *Med Mycol J* **57:**E41–E46.
100. **Velegraki A, Cafarchia C, Gaitanis G, Iatta R, Boekhout T.** 2015. *Malassezia* infections in humans and animals: pathophysiology, detection, and treatment. *PLoS Pathog* **11:**e1004523.
101. **Ashbee HR.** 2007. Update on the genus *Malassezia*. *Med Mycol* **45:**287–303.
102. **Prakash A, Wankhede S, Singh PK, Agarwal K, Kathuria S, Sengupta S, Barman P, Meis JF, Chowdhary A.** 2014. First neonatal case of fungaemia due to *Pseudozyma aphidis* and a global literature review. *Mycoses* **57:**64–68.
103. **Siddiqui W, Ahmed Y, Albrecht H, Weissman S.** 2014. Pseudozyma spp catheter-associated blood stream infection, an emerging pathogen and brief literature review. *BMJ Case Rep* bcr-2014-206369.
104. **Mekha N, Takashima M, Boon-long J, Cho O, Sugita T.** 2014. Three new basidiomycetous yeasts, *Pseudozyma alboarmeniaca* sp. nov., *Pseudozyma crassa* sp. nov., and *Pseudozyma siamensis* sp. nov., isolated from Thai patients. *Microbiol Immunol* **58:**9–14.
105. **Wirth F, Goldani LZ.** 2012. Epidemiology of *Rhodotorula*: an emerging pathogen. *Interdiscipl Perspect Infect Dis* **2012:**465717.

106. **Jankowski M, Charemska A, Czajkowski R.** 2017. Swimming pools and fungi: an epidemiology survey in Polish indoor swimming facilities. *Mycoses* **60:**736-738.
107. **Tuon FF, Costa SF.** 2008. *Rhodotorula* infection. a systematic review of 128 cases from literature. *Rev Iberoam Micol* **25:**135–140.
108. **Muñoz P, Bouza E, Cuenca-Estrella M, Eiros JM, Pérez MJ, Sánchez-Somolinos M, Rincón C, Hortal J, Peláez T.** 2005. *Saccharomyces cerevisiae* fungemia: an emerging infectious disease. *Clin Infect Dis* **40:**1625–1634.
109. **Popiel KY, Wong P, Lee MJ, Langelier M, Sheppard DC, Vinh DC.** 2015. Invasive *Saccharomyces cerevisiae* in a liver transplant patient: case report and review of infection in transplant recipients. *Transpl Infect Dis* **17:**435–441.
110. **Cassone M, Serra P, Mondello F, Girolamo A, Scafetti S, Pistella E, Venditti M.** 2003. Outbreak of *Saccharomyces cerevisiae* subtype boulardii fungemia in patients neighboring those treated with a probiotic preparation of the organism. *J Clin Microbiol* **41:**5340–5343.
111. **Mazzocato S, Marchionni E, Fothergill AW, Sutton DA, Staffolani S, Gesuita R, Skrami E, Fiorentini A, Manso E, Barchiesi F.** 2015. Epidemiology and outcome of systemic infections due to saprochaete capitata: case report and review of the literature. *Infection* **43:**211–215.
112. **D'Antonio D, Romano F, Iacone A, Violante B, Fazii P, Pontieri E, Staniscia T, Caracciolo C, Bianchini S, Sferra R, Vetuschi A, Gaudio E, Carruba G.** 1999. Onychomycosis caused by *Blastoschizomyces capitatus*. *J Clin Microbiol* **37:**2927–2930.
113. **Arendrup MC, Boekhout T, Akova M, Meis JF, Cornely OA, Lortholary O, European Society of Clinical Microbiology and Infectious Diseases Fungal Infection Study Group, European Confederation of Medical Mycology.** 2014. ESCMID and ECMM joint clinical guidelines for the diagnosis and management of rare invasive yeast infections. *Clin Microbiol Infect* **20**(Suppl 3)**:**76–98.
114. **Mariné M, Brown NA, Riaño-Pachón DM, Goldman GH.** 2015. On and under the skin: emerging basidiomycetous yeast infections caused by *Trichosporon* species. *PLoS Pathog* **11:**e1004982.
115. **Nishiura Y, Nakagawa-Yoshida K, Suga M, Shinoda T, Guého E, Ando M.** 1997. Assignment and serotyping of *Trichosporon* species: the causative agents of summer-type hypersensitivity pneumonitis. *J Med Vet Mycol* **35:**45–52.
116. **de Almeida Júnior JN, Hennequin C.** 2016. Invasive *Trichosporon* infection: a systematic review on a re-emerging fungal pathogen. *Front Microbiol* **7:**1629.
117. **Marty FM, Barouch DH, Coakley EP, Baden LR.** 2003. Disseminated trichosporonosis caused by *Trichosporon loubieri*. *J Clin Microbiol* **41:**5317–5320.
118. **Hickey PW, Sutton DA, Fothergill AW, Rinaldi MG, Wickes BL, Schmidt HJ, Walsh TJ.** 2009. *Trichosporon mycotoxinivorans*, a novel respiratory pathogen in patients with cystic fibrosis. *J Clin Microbiol* **47:**3091–3097.
119. **Monheit JE, Cowan DF, Moore DG.** 1984. Rapid detection of fungi in tissues using calcofluor white and fluorescence microscopy. *Arch Pathol Lab Med* **108:**616–618.
120. **Guarner J, Brandt ME.** 2011. Histopathologic diagnosis of fungal infections in the 21st century. *Clin Microbiol Rev* **24:**247–280.
121. **Muñoz-Cadavid C, Rudd S, Zaki SR, Patel M, Moser SA, Brandt ME, Gómez BL.** 2010. Improving molecular detection of fungal DNA in formalin-fixed paraffin-embedded tissues: comparison of five tissue DNA extraction methods using panfungal PCR. *J Clin Microbiol* **48:**2147–2153.
122. **Rickerts V, Khot PD, Myerson D, Ko DL, Lambrecht E, Fredricks DN.** 2011. Comparison of quantitative real time PCR with sequencing and ribosomal RNA-FISH for the identification of fungi in formalin fixed, paraffin-embedded tissue specimens. *BMC Infect Dis* **11:**202–214.
123. **Buitrago MJ, Aguado JM, Ballen A, Bernal-Martinez L, Prieto M, Garcia-Reyne A, Garcia-Rodriguez J, Rodriguez-Tudela JL, Cuenca-Estrella M.** 2013. Efficacy of DNA amplification in tissue biopsy samples to improve the detection of invasive fungal disease. *Clin Microbiol Infect* **19:**E271–E277.
124. **He S, Hang JP, Zhang L, Wang F, Zhang DC, Gong FH.** 2015. A systematic review and meta-analysis of diagnostic accuracy of serum 1,3-β-D-glucan for invasive fungal infection: focus on cutoff levels. *J Microbiol Immunol Infect* **48:**351–361.
125. **Odabasi Z, Mattiuzzi G, Estey E, Kantarjian H, Saeki F, Ridge RJ, Ketchum PA, Finkelman MA, Rex JH, Ostrosky-Zeichner L.** 2004. Beta-D-glucan as a diagnostic adjunct for invasive fungal infections: validation, cutoff development, and performance in patients with acute myelogenous leukemia and myelodysplastic syndrome. *Clin Infect Dis* **39:**199–205.
126. **Tran T, Beal SG.** 2016. Application of the 1,3-β-D-glucan (Fungitell) assay in the diagnosis of invasive fungal infections. *Arch Pathol Lab Med* **140:**181–185.
127. **McCarthy MW, Petraitiene R, Walsh TJ.** 2017. Translational development and application of (1→3)-β-D-glucan for diagnosis and therapeutic monitoring of invasive mycoses. *Int J Mol Sci* **18:**1124.
128. **Yeo SF, Zhang Y, Schafer D, Campbell S, Wong B.** 2000. A rapid, automated enzymatic fluorometric assay for determination of D-arabinitol in serum. *J Clin Microbiol* **38:**1439–1443.
129. **Arendrup MC, Bergmann OJ, Larsson L, Nielsen HV, Jarløv JO, Christensson B.** 2010. Detection of candidaemia in patients with and without underlying haematological disease. *Clin Microbiol Infect* **16:**855–862.
130. **Ellepola AN, Morrison CJ.** 2005. Laboratory diagnosis of invasive candidiasis. *J Microbiol* **43:**65–84.
131. **Sendid B, Caillot D, Baccouch-Humbert B, Klingspor L, Grandjean M, Bonnin A, Poulain D.** 2003. Contribution of the Platelia *Candida*-specific antibody and antigen tests to early diagnosis of systemic *Candida tropicalis* infection in neutropenic adults. *J Clin Microbiol* **41:**4551–4558.
132. **Sendid B, Jouault T, Coudriau R, Camus D, Odds F, Tabouret M, Poulain D.** 2004. Increased sensitivity of mannanemia detection tests by joint detection of α- and β-linked oligomannosides during experimental and human systemic candidiasis. *J Clin Microbiol* **42:**164–171.
133. **Hazen KC, Wu JG, Masuoka J.** 2001. Comparison of the hydrophobic properties of *Candida albicans* and *Candida dubliniensis*. *Infect Immun* **69:**779–786.
134. **Lunel FM, Mennink-Kersten MA, Ruegebrink D, van der Lee HA, Donnelly JP, Blijlevens NM, Verweij PE.** 2009. Value of *Candida* serum markers in patients with invasive candidiasis after myeloablative chemotherapy. *Diagn Microbiol Infect Dis* **64:**408–415.
135. **Marcos JY, Pincus DH.** 2013. Fungal diagnostics: review of commercially available methods, p 25–54. *In* O'Connor L, Glynn B (ed), *Fungal Diagnostics: Methods and Protocols. Methods in Molecular Biology*, vol 968. Springer Science and Business Media, New York, NY.
136. **Hansen J, Slechta ES, Gates-Hollingsworth MA, Neary B, Barker AP, Bauman S, Kozel TR, Hanson KE.** 2013. Large-scale evaluation of the immuno-mycologics lateral flow and enzyme-linked immunoassays for detection of cryptococcal antigen in serum and cerebrospinal fluid. *Clin Vaccine Immunol* **20:**52–55.
137. **Rivet-Dañon D, Guitard J, Grenouillet F, Gay F, Ait-Ammar N, Angoulvant A, Marinach C, Hennequin C.** 2015. Rapid diagnosis of cryptococcosis using an antigen detection immunochromatographic test. *J Infect* **70:**499–503.
138. **McMullan BJ, Halliday C, Sorrell TC, Judd D, Sleiman S, Marriott D, Olma T, Chen SC.** 2012. Clinical utility of the cryptococcal antigen lateral flow assay in a diagnostic mycology laboratory. *PLoS One*. **7:**e49541
139. **Tintelnot K, Hagen F, Han CO, Seibold M, Rickerts V, Boekhout T.** 2015. Pitfalls in serological diagnosis of *Cryptococcus gattii* infections. *Med Mycol* **53:**874–879.
140. **Dubbels M, Granger D, Theel ES.** 2017. Low *Cryptococcus* antigen titers as determined by lateral flow assay should be interpreted cautiously in patients without prior diagnosis of cryptococcal infection. *J Clin Microbiol* **55:**2472–2479.
141. **Campbell CK, Payne AL, Teall AJ, Brownell A, Mackenzie DW.** 1985. Cryptococcal latex antigen test positive in patient with *Trichosporon beigelii* infection. *Lancet* **ii:**43–44.

142. **Blevins LB, Fenn J, Segal H, Newcomb-Gayman P, Carroll KC.** 1995. False-positive cryptococcal antigen latex agglutination caused by disinfectants and soaps. *J Clin Microbiol* **33:**1674–1675.
143. **Chanock SJ, Toltzis P, Wilson C.** 1993. Cross-reactivity between *Stomatococcus mucilaginosus* and latex agglutination for cryptococcal antigen. *Lancet* **342:**1119–1120.
144. **Hopfer RL, Perry EV, Fainstein V.** 1982. Diagnostic value of cryptococcal antigen in the cerebrospinal fluid of patients with malignant disease. *J Infect Dis* **145:**915.
145. **Millon L, Barale T, Julliot M-C, Martinez J, Mantion G.** 1995. Interference by hydroxyethyl starch used for vascular filling in latex agglutination test for cryptococcal antigen. *J Clin Microbiol* **33:**1917–1919.
146. **Westerink MA, Amsterdam D, Petell RJ, Stram MN, Apicella MA.** 1987. Septicemia due to DF-2. Cause of a false-positive cryptococcal latex agglutination result. *Am J Med* **83:**155–158.
147. **Dalle F, Charles PE, Blanc K, Caillot D, Chavanet P, Dromer F, Bonnin A.** 2005. *Cryptococcus neoformans* galactoxylomannan contains an epitope(s) that is cross-reactive with *Aspergillus* galactomannan. *J Clin Microbiol* **43:**2929–2931.
148. **Lu H, Zhou Y, Yin Y, Pan X, Weng X.** 2005. Cryptococcal antigen test revisited: significance for cryptococcal meningitis therapy monitoring in a tertiary chinese hospital. *J Clin Microbiol* **43:**2989–2990.
149. **Wilson DA, Joyce MJ, Hall LS, Reller LB, Roberts GD, Hall GS, Alexander BD, Procop GW.** 2005. Multicenter evaluation of a *Candida albicans* peptide nucleic acid fluorescent in situ hybridization probe for characterization of yeast isolates from blood cultures. *J Clin Microbiol* **43:**2909–2912.
150. **Stone NR, Gorton RL, Barker K, Ramnarain P, Kibbler CC.** 2013. Evaluation of PNA-FISH yeast traffic light for rapid identification of yeast directly from positive blood cultures and assessment of clinical impact. *J Clin Microbiol* **51:**1301–1302.
151. **Klingspor L, Lindback E, Ullberg M, Özenci V.** 2017. Seven years of clinical experience with the Yeast Traffic Light PNA FISH: assay performance and possible implications on antifungal therapy. *Mycoses* **61:**179–185.
152. **Altun O, Almuhayawi M, Ullberg M, Ozenci V.** 2013. Clinical evaluation of the FilmArray blood culture identification panel in identification of bacteria and yeasts from positive blood culture bottles. *J Clin Microbiol* **51:**4130–4136.
153. **Aittakorpi A, Kuusela P, Koukila-Kähkölä P, Vaara M, Petrou M, Gant V, Mäki M.** 2012. Accurate and rapid identification of *Candida* spp. frequently associated with fungemia by using PCR and the microarray-based Prove-it Sepsis assay. *J Clin Microbiol* **50:**3635–3640.
154. **Babady NE, Miranda E, Gilhuley KA.** 2011. Evaluation of Luminex xTAG fungal analyte-specific reagents for rapid identification of clinically relevant fungi. *J Clin Microbiol* **49:**3777–3782.
155. **Balada-Llasat JM, LaRue H, Kamboj K, Rigali L, Smith D, Thomas K, Pancholi P.** 2012. Detection of yeasts in blood cultures by the Luminex xTAG fungal assay. *J Clin Microbiol* **50:**492–494.
156. **White PL, Perry MD, Barnes RA.** 2009. An update on the molecular diagnosis of invasive fungal disease. *FEMS Microbiol Lett* **296:**1–10.
157. **Lau A, Chen S, Sleiman S, Sorrell T.** 2009. Current status and future perspectives on molecular and serological methods in diagnostic mycology. *Future Microbiol* **4:**1185–1222.
158. **Avni T, Leibovici L, Paul M.** 2011. PCR diagnosis of invasive candidiasis: systematic review and meta-analysis. *J Clin Microbiol* **49:**665–670.
159. **Halliday CL, Kidd SE, Sorrell TC, Chen SC.** 2015. Molecular diagnostic methods for invasive fungal disease: the horizon draws nearer? *Pathology* **47:**257–269.
160. **Khlif M, Mary C, Sellami H, Sellami A, Dumon H, Ayadi A, Ranque S.** 2009. Evaluation of nested and real-time PCR assays in the diagnosis of candidaemia. *Clin Microbiol Infect* **15:**656–661.
161. **McMullan R, Metwally L, Coyle PV, Hedderwick S, McCloskey B, O'Neill HJ, Patterson CC, Thompson G, Webb CH, Hay RJ.** 2008. A prospective clinical trial of a real-time polymerase chain reaction assay for the diagnosis of candidemia in nonneutropenic, critically ill adults. *Clin Infect Dis* **46:**890–896.
162. **Wellinghausen N, Siegel D, Winter J, Gebert S.** 2009. Rapid diagnosis of candidaemia by real-time PCR detection of *Candida* DNA in blood samples. *J Med Microbiol* **58:**1106–1111.
163. **Lau A, Halliday C, Chen SC, Playford EG, Stanley K, Sorrell TC.** 2010. Comparison of whole blood, serum, and plasma for early detection of candidemia by multiplex-tandem PCR. *J Clin Microbiol* **48:**811–816.
164. **Bennett J.** 2008. Is real-time polymerase chain reaction ready for real use in detecting candidemia? *Clin Infect Dis* **46:**897–898.
165. **Elges S, Arnold R, Liesenfeld O, Kofla G, Mikolajewska A, Schwartz S, Uharek L, Ruhnke M.** 2017. Prospective evaluation of the SeptiFAST multiplex real-time PCR assay for surveillance and diagnosis of infections in haematological patients after allogeneic stem cell transplantation compared to routine microbiological assays and an in-house real-time PCR method. *Mycoses* **60:**781–788.
166. **Marco F.** 2017. Molecular methods for septicemia diagnosis. *Enferm Infecc Microbiol Clin* **35:**586–592.
167. **Brown HL, Fuller DD, Jasper LT, Davis TE, Wright JD.** 2004. Clinical evaluation of Affirm VPIII in the detection and identification of *Trichomonas vaginalis*, *Gardnerella vaginalis*, and *Candida* species in vaginitis/vaginosis. *Infect Dis Obstet Gynecol* **12:**17–21.
168. **Posch W, Heimdörfer D, Wilflingseder D, Lass-Flörl C.** 2017. Invasive candidiasis: future directions in non-culture based diagnosis. *Expert Rev Anti Infect Ther* **15:**829–838.
169. **Perlin DS, Wiederhold NP.** 2017. Culture-independent molecular methods for detection of antifungal resistance mechanisms and fungal identification. *J Infect Dis.* **216**(Suppl. 3)**:**S458–S465.
170. **Geha DJ, Roberts GD.** 1994. Laboratory detection of fungemia. *Clin Lab Med* **14:**83–97.
171. **Hazen KC, Stei J, Darracott C, Breathnach A, May J, Howell SA.** 2005. Isolation of cholesterol-dependent *Candida glabrata* from clinical specimens. *Diagn Microbiol Infect Dis* **52:**35–37.
172. **Patterson TF, Revankar SG, Kirkpatrick WR, Dib O, Fothergill AW, Redding SW, Sutton DA, Rinaldi MG.** 1996. Simple method for detecting fluconazole-resistant yeasts with chromogenic agar. *J Clin Microbiol* **34:**1794–1797.
173. **Howell SA, Hazen KC, Brandt ME.** 2015. *Candida, Cryptococcus* and other yeasts of medical importance, p 1984–2014. *In* Jorgensen JH, Pfaller MA, Carroll KC, Funke G, Landry ML, Richter SS, Warnock DW (ed), *Manual of Clinical Microbiology*, 11th ed. ASM Press, Washington, DC.
174. **Pincus DH, Orenga S, Chatellier S.** 2007. Yeast identification—past, present, and future methods. *Med Mycol* **45:**97–121.
175. **Latouche GN, Daniel HM, Lee OC, Mitchell TG, Sorrell TC, Meyer W.** 1997. Comparison of use of phenotypic and genotypic characteristics for identification of species of the anamorph genus *Candida* and related teleomorph yeast species. *J Clin Microbiol* **35:**3171–3180.
176. **Borman AM, Linton CJ, Miles SJ, Johnson EM.** 2008. Molecular identification of pathogenic fungi. *J Antimicrob Chemother* **61**(Suppl 1)**:**i7–i12.
177. **Pfaller MA, Woosley LN, Messer SA, Jones RN, Castanheira M.** 2012. Significance of molecular identification and antifungal susceptibility of clinically significant yeasts and moulds in a global antifungal surveillance programme. *Mycopathologia* **174:**259–271.
178. **Cendejas-Bueno E, Gomez-Lopez A, Mellado E, Rodriguez-Tudela JL, Cuenca-Estrella M.** 2010. Identification of pathogenic rare yeast species in clinical samples: comparison between phenotypical and molecular methods. *J Clin Microbiol* **48:**1895–1899.
179. **Criseo G, Scordino F, Romeo O.** 2015. Current methods for identifying clinically important cryptic *Candida* species. *J Microbiol Methods* **111:**50–56.

180. **Cafarchia C, Gasser RB, Figueredo LA, Latrofa MS, Otranto D.** 2011. Advances in the identification of *Malassezia*. *Mol Cell Probes* **25:**1–7.
181. **Boyanton BL, Jr, Luna RA, Fasciano LR, Menne KG, Versalovic J.** 2008. DNA pyrosequencing-based identification of pathogenic *Candida* species by using the internal transcribed spacer 2 region. *Arch Pathol Lab Med* **132:**667–674
182. **Kim JY, Hahn HJ, Choe YB, Lee YW, Ahn KJ, Moon KC.** 2013. Molecular biological identification of malassezia yeasts using pyrosequencing. *Ann Dermatol* **25:**73–79.
183. **Pannanusorn S, Elings MA, Römling U, Fernandez V.** 2012. Pyrosequencing of a hypervariable region in the internal transcribed spacer 2 to identify clinical yeast isolates. *Mycoses* **55:**172–180
184. **Montero CI, Shea YR, Jones PA, Harrington SM, Tooke NE, Witebsky FG, Murray PR.** 2008. Evaluation of pyrosequencing technology for the identification of clinically relevant non-dematiaceous yeasts and related species. *Eur J Clin Microbiol Infect Dis* **27:**821–830.
185. **Lima-Neto R, Santos C, Lima N, Sampaio P, Pais C, Neves RP.** 2014. Application of MALDI-TOF MS for requalification of a *Candida* clinical isolates culture collection. *Braz J Microbiol* **45:**515–522.
186. **Bader O, Weig M, Taverne-Ghadwal L, Lugert R, Gross U, Kuhns M.** 2011. Improved clinical laboratory identification of human pathogenic yeasts by matrix-assisted laser desorption ionization time-of-flight mass spectrometry. *Clin Microbiol Infect* **17:**1359–1365.
187. **Turhan O, Ozhak-Baysan B, Zaragoza O, Er H, Sarıtas ZE, Ongut G, Ogunc D, Colak D, Cuenca-Estrella M.** 2017. Evaluation of MALDI-TOF-MS for the identification of yeast isolates causing bloodstream infection. *Clin Lab* **63:**699–703.
188. **Posteraro B, Efremov L, Leoncini E, Amore R, Posteraro P, Ricciardi W, Sanguinetti M.** 2015. Are the conventional commercial yeast identification methods still helpful in the era of new clinical microbiology diagnostics? A meta-analysis of their accuracy. *J Clin Microbiol* **53:**2439–2450.
189. **Borman AM, Linton CJ, Oliver D, Palmer MD, Szekely A, Odds FC, Johnson EM.** 2009. Pyrosequencing analysis of 20 nucleotides of internal transcribed spacer 2 discriminates *Candida parapsilosis, Candida metapsilosis,* and *Candida orthopsilosis*. *J Clin Microbiol* **47:**2307–2310.
190. **Pfaller MA, Jones RN, Doern GV, Fluit AC, Verhoef J, Sader HS, Messer SA, Houston A, Coffman S, Hollis RJ, SENTRY Participant Group (Europe).** 1999. International surveillance of blood stream infections due to *Candida* species in the European SENTRY Program: species distribution and antifungal susceptibility including the investigational triazole and echinocandin agents. *Diagn Microbiol Infect Dis* **35:**19–25.
191. **Pfaller MA, Jones RN, Messer SA, Edmond MB, Wenzel RP, SCOPE Participant Group.** 1998. National surveillance of nosocomial blood stream infection due to species of *Candida* other than *Candida albicans*: frequency of occurrence and antifungal susceptibility in the SCOPE Program. *Diagn Microbiol Infect Dis* **30:**121–129.
192. **Arendrup MC, Denning DW, Pfaller MA, Diekema DJ, Rex JH.** 2007. Does one voriconazole breakpoint suit all *Candida* species? *J Clin Microbiol* **45:**2093–2094.
193. **Arendrup MC, Kahlmeter G, Rodriguez-Tudela JL, Donnelly JP.** 2009. Breakpoints for susceptibility testing should not divide wild-type distributions of important target species. *Antimicrob Agents Chemother* **53:**1628–1629.
194. **Pfaller MA, Diekema DJ.** 2010. Wild-type MIC distributions and epidemiological cutoff values for fluconazole and *Candida*: time for new clinical breakpoints? *Curr Fungal Infect Rep* **4:**168–174.
195. **Pfaller MA, Andes D, Arendrup MC, Diekema DJ, Espinel-Ingroff A, Alexander BD, Brown SD, Chaturvedi V, Fowler CL, Ghannoum MA, Johnson EM, Knapp CC, Motyl MR, Ostrosky-Zeichner L, Walsh TJ.** 2011. Clinical breakpoints for voriconazole and *Candida* spp. revisited: review of microbiologic, molecular, pharmacodynamic, and clinical data as they pertain to the development of species-specific interpretive criteria. *Diagn Microbiol Infect Dis* **70:**330–343.
196. **Pfaller MA, Boyken L, Hollis RJ, Kroeger J, Messer SA, Tendolkar S, Diekema DJ.** 2011. Wild-type MIC distributions and epidemiological cutoff values for posaconazole and voriconazole and *Candida* spp. as determined by 24-hour CLSI broth microdilution. *J Clin Microbiol* **49:**630–637.
197. **Clinical and Laboratory Standards Institute (CLSI).** 2012. Reference method for broth dilution antifungal susceptibility testing of yeasts; 4th informational supplement. Document M27-S4. Clinical and Laboratory Standards Institute, Wayne, PA.
198. **Diekema DJ, Pfaller MA.** 2012. Utility of antifungal susceptibility testing and clinical correlations, p. 131–158. *In* Hall GS (ed), *Interactions of Yeasts, Moulds, and Antifungal Agents: How to Detect Resistance*. Springer Science and Business Media, New York, NY.
199. **Arendrup MC, Cuenca-Estrella M, Lass-Flörl C, Hope WW.** 2013. Breakpoints for antifungal agents: an update from EUCAST focussing on echinocandins against *Candida* spp. and triazoles against *Aspergillus* spp. *Drug Resist Updat* **16:**81–95.
200. **Pfaller MA, Diekema DJ, Andes D, Arendrup MC, Brown SD, Lockhart SR, Motyl M, Perlin DS, CLSI Subcommittee for Antifungal Testing.** 2011. Clinical breakpoints for the echinocandins and *Candida* revisited: integration of molecular, clinical, and microbiological data to arrive at species-specific interpretive criteria. *Drug Resist Updat* **14:** 164–176.
201. **Yamane N, Saitoh Y.** 1985. Isolation and detection of multiple yeasts from a single clinical sample by use of Pagano-Levin agar medium. *J Clin Microbiol* **21:**276–277.
202. **Pfaller MA, Houston A, Coffmann S.** 1996. Application of CHROMagar Candida for rapid screening of clinical specimens for *Candida albicans, Candida tropicalis, Candida krusei,* and *Candida* (*Torulopsis*) *glabrata*. *J Clin Microbiol* **34:**58–61.
203. **Letscher-Bru V, Meyer M-H, Galoisy A-C, Waller J, Candolfi E.** 2002. Prospective evaluation of the new chromogenic medium Candida ID, in comparison with Candiselect, for isolation of molds and isolation and presumptive identification of yeast species. *J Clin Microbiol* **40:**1508–1510.
204. **Willinger B, Hillowoth C, Selitsch B, Manafi M.** 2001. Performance of candida ID, a new chromogenic medium for presumptive identification of *Candida* species, in comparison to CHROMagar Candida. *J Clin Microbiol* **39:**3793–3795.
205. **Fraser M, Brown Z, Houldsworth M, Borman AM, Johnson EM.** 2016. Rapid identification of 6328 isolates of pathogenic yeasts using MALDI-ToF MS and a simplified, rapid extraction procedure that is compatible with the Bruker Biotyper platform and database. *Med Mycol* **54:**80–88.
206. **Dealler SF.** 1991. *Candida albicans* colony identification in 5 minutes in a general microbiology laboratory. *J Clin Microbiol* **29:**1081–1082.
207. **Scorzetti G, Fell JW, Fonseca A, Statzell-Tallman A.** 2002. Systematics of basidiomycetous yeasts: a comparison of large subunit D1/D2 and internal transcribed spacer rDNA regions. *FEMS Yeast Res* **2:**495–517.
208. **Chen YC, Eisner JD, Kattar MM, Rassoulian-Barrett SL, Lafe K, Bui U, Limaye AP, Cookson BT.** 2001. Polymorphic internal transcribed spacer region 1 DNA sequences identify medically important yeasts. *J Clin Microbiol* **39:** 4042–4051.
209. **Turenne CY, Sanche SE, Hoban DJ, Karlowsky JA, Kabani AM.** 1999. Rapid identification of fungi by using the ITS2 genetic region and an automated fluorescent capillary electrophoresis system. *J Clin Microbiol* **37:**1846–1851.
210. **Chen YC, Eisner JD, Kattar MM, Rassoulian-Barrett SL, LaFe K, Yarfitz SL, Limaye AP, Cookson BT.** 2000. Identification of medically important yeasts using PCR-based detection of DNA sequence polymorphisms in the internal transcribed spacer 2 region of the rRNA genes. *J Clin Microbiol* **38:**2302–2310.
211. **Kurtzman CP, Mateo RQ, Kolecka A, Theelen B, Robert V, Boekhout T.** 2015. Advances in yeast systematics and phylogeny and their use as predictors of biotechnologically important metabolic pathways. *FEMS Yeast Res* **15:**fov050.

212. **Ciardo DE, Schär G, Böttger EC, Altwegg M, Bosshard PP.** 2006. Internal transcribed spacer sequencing versus biochemical profiling for identification of medically important yeasts. *J Clin Microbiol* **44:**77–84.
213. **Irinyi L, et al.** 2015. International Society of Human and Animal Mycology (ISHAM)-ITS reference DNA barcoding database—the quality controlled standard tool for routine identification of human and animal pathogenic fungi. *Med Mycol* **53:**313–337.
214. **de Hoog GS, Guarro J, Gene J, Figueras MJ.** 2011. *Atlas of Clinical Fungi*, ed 3.1. Centraalbureau voor Schimmelcultures, Utrecht, The Netherlands.
215. **Clinical and Laboratory Standards Institute.** 2006. Molecular diagnostic methods for infectious diseases; approved guideline—2nd ed. CLSI document MM03-02, 2nd ed. Clinical and Laboratory Standards Institute, Wayne, PA.
216. **Clinical and Laboratory Standards Institute.** 2008. Interpretive criteria for identification of bacteria and fungi by DNA target sequencing; approved guideline. CLSI Document MM18-A. Clinical and Laboratory Standards Institute, Wayne, PA.
217. **Hall L, Wohlfiel S, Roberts GD.** 2003. Experience with the MicroSeq D2 large-subunit ribosomal DNA sequencing kit for identification of commonly encountered, clinically important yeast species. *J Clin Microbiol* **41:**5099–5102.
218. **Slechta ES, Hohmann SL, Simmon K, Hanson KE.** 2012. Internal transcribed spacer region sequence analysis using SmartGene IDNS software for the identification of unusual clinical yeast isolates. *Med Mycol* **50:**458–466.
219. **Quiles-Melero I, García-Rodriguez J, Romero-Gómez MP, Gómez-Sánchez P, Mingorance J.** 2011. Rapid identification of yeasts from positive blood culture bottles by pyrosequencing. *Eur J Clin Microbiol Infect Dis* **30:**21–24.
220. **Leinberger DM, Schumacher U, Autenrieth IB, Bachmann TT.** 2005. Development of a DNA microarray for detection and identification of fungal pathogens involved in invasive mycoses. *J Clin Microbiol* **43:**4943–4953.
221. **Campa D, Tavanti A, Gemignani F, Mogavero CS, Bellini I, Bottari F, Barale R, Landi S, Senesi S.** 2008. DNA microarray based on arrayed-primer extension technique for identification of pathogenic fungi responsible for invasive and superficial mycoses. *J Clin Microbiol* **46:**909–915.
222. **Li C, Ding X, Liu Z, Zhu J.** 2017. Rapid identification of *Candida* spp. frequently involved in invasive mycoses by using flow-through hybridization and Gene Chip (FHGC) technology. *J Microbiol Methods* **132:**160–165.
223. **Wise MG, Healy M, Reece K, Smith R, Walton D, Dutch W, Renwick A, Huong J, Young S, Tarrand J, Kontoyiannis DP.** 2007. Species identification and strain differentiation of clinical *Candida* isolates using the DiversiLab system of automated repetitive sequence-based PCR. *J Med Microbiol* **56:**778–787.
224. **Deak E, Etienne KA, Lockhart SR, Gade L, Chiller T, Balajee SA.** 2010. Utility of a Luminex-based assay for multiplexed, rapid species identification of *Candida* isolates from an ongoing candidemia surveillance. *Can J Microbiol* **56:**348–351.
225. **Landlinger C, Preuner S, Willinger B, Haberpursch B, Racil Z, Mayer J, Lion T.** 2009. Species-specific identification of a wide range of clinically relevant fungal pathogens by use of Luminex xMAP technology. *J Clin Microbiol* **47:**1063–1073.
226. **Lee HS, Shin JH, Choi MJ, Won EJ, Kee SJ, Kim SH, Shin MG, Suh SP.** 2017. Comparison of the Bruker Biotyper and VITEK MS matrix-assisted laser desorption/ionization time-of-flight mass spectrometry systems using a formic acid extraction method to identify common and uncommon yeast isolates. *Ann Lab Med* **37:**223–230.
227. **Wang H, Fan YY, Kudinha T, Xu ZP, Xiao M, Zhang L, Fan X, Kong F, Xu YC.** 2016. A comprehensive evaluation of the Bruker Biotyper MS and Vitek MS matrix-assisted laser desorption ionization-time of flight mass spectrometry systems for identification of yeasts, Part of the National China Hospital Invasive Fungal Surveillance Net (CHIF-NET) study, 2012 to 2013. *J Clin Microbiol* **54:**1376–1380.
228. **Cassagne C, Cella AL, Suchon P, Normand AC, Ranque S, Piarroux R.** 2013. Evaluation of four pretreatment procedures for MALDI-TOF MS yeast identification in the routine clinical laboratory. *Med Mycol* **51:**371–377.
229. **de Almeida JN, Jr, Favero Gimenes VM, Francisco EC, Machado Siqueira LP, Gonçalves de Almeida RK, Guitard J, Hennequin C, Colombo AL, Benard G, Rossi F.** 2017. Evaluating and improving Vitek MS for identification of clinically relevant species of *Trichosporon* and the closely related genera *Cutaneotrichosporon* and *Apiotrichum*. *J Clin Microbiol* **55:**2439–2444.
230. **Firacative C, Trilles L, Meyer W.** 2012. MALDI-TOF MS enables the rapid identification of the major molecular types within the *Cryptococcus neoformans/C. gattii* species complex. *PLoS One* **7:**e37566.
231. **Danesi P, Drigo I, Iatta R, Firacative C, Capelli G, Cafarchia C, Meyer W.** 2014. MALDI-TOF MS for the identification of veterinary non-*C. neoformans-C. gattii Cryptococcus* spp. isolates from Italy. *Med Mycol* **52:** 659–666.
232. **Normand AC, Becker P, Gabriel F, Cassagne C, Accoceberry I, Gari-Toussaint M, Hasseine L, De Geyter D, Pierard D, Surmont I, Djenad F, Donnadieu JL, Piarroux M, Ranque S, Hendrickx M, Piarroux R.** 2017. Validation of a new web application for identification of fungi by use of matrix-assisted laser desorption ionization-time of flight mass spectrometry. *J Clin Microbiol* **55:** 2661–2670.
233. **Spanu T, Posteraro B, Fiori B, D'Inzeo T, Campoli S, Ruggeri A, Tumbarello M, Canu G, Trecarichi EM, Parisi G, Tronci M, Sanguinetti M, Fadda G.** 2012. Direct MALDI-TOF mass spectrometry assay of blood culture broths for rapid identification of *Candida* species causing bloodstream infections: an observational study in two large microbiology laboratories. *J Clin Microbiol* **50:**176–179.
234. **Fothergill A, Kasinathan V, Hyman J, Walsh J, Drake T, Wang YF.** 2013. Rapid identification of bacteria and yeasts from positive-blood-culture bottles by using a lysis-filtration method and matrix-assisted laser desorption ionization-time of flight mass spectrum analysis with the SARAMIS database. *J Clin Microbiol* **51:**805–809.
235. **Idelevich EA, Grünastel B, Becker K.** 2017. Rapid detection and identification of candidemia by direct blood culturing on solid medium by use of lysis-centrifugation method combined with matrix-assisted laser desorption ionization–time of flight mass spectrometry (MALDI-TOF MS). *J Clin Microbiol* **55:**97–100.
236. **van Belkum A, Welker M, Pincus D, Charrier JP, Girard V.** 2017. Matrix-assisted laser desorption ionization–time of flight mass spectrometry in clinical microbiology: what are the current issues? *Ann Lab Med* **37:**475–483.
237. **Pfaller MA, Diekema DJ.** 2005. Unusual fungal and pseudofungal infections of humans. *J Clin Microbiol* **43:**1495–1504.
238. **Sykora T, Horakova J, Buzzasyova D, Sladekova M, Poczova M, Sufliarska S.** 2014. Protothecal peritonitis in child after bone marrow transplantation: case report and literature review of paediatric cases. *New Microbes New Infect* **2:** 156–160.
239. **Ramírez I, Nieto-Ríos JF, Ocampo-Kohn C, Aristizábal-Alzate A, Zuluaga-Valencia G, Muñoz Maya O, Pérez JC.** 2016. Protothecal bursitis after simultaneous kidney/liver transplantation: a case report and review. *Transpl Infect Dis* **18:**266–274.
240. **Gil-Lamaignere C, Roilides E, Hacker J, Müller FM.** 2003. Molecular typing for fungi—a critical review of the possibilities and limitations of currently and future methods. *Clin Microbiol Infect* **9:**172–185.
241. **Taylor JW, Geiser DM, Burt A, Koufopanou V.** 1999. The evolutionary biology and population genetics underlying fungal strain typing. *Clin Microbiol Rev* **12:**126–146.
242. **Foulet F, Nicolas N, Eloy O, Botterel F, Gantier JC, Costa JM, Bretagne S.** 2005. Microsatellite marker analysis as a typing system for *Candida glabrata*. *J Clin Microbiol* **43:** 4574–4579.

243. **Saghrouni F, Ben Abdeljelil J, Boukadida J, Ben Said M.** 2013. Molecular methods for strain typing of *Candida albicans*: a review. *J Appl Microbiol* **114:**1559–1574.
244. **Chen KW, Chen YC, Lin YH, Chou HH, Li SY.** 2009. The molecular epidemiology of serial *Candida tropicalis* isolates from ICU patients as revealed by multilocus sequence typing and pulsed-field gel electrophoresis. *Infect Genet Evol* **9:**912–920.
245. **Cliff PR, Sandoe JA, Heritage J, Barton RC.** 2008. Use of multilocus sequence typing for the investigation of colonisation by *Candida albicans* in intensive care unit patients. *J Hosp Infect* **69:**24–32.
246. **Odds FC, Jacobsen MD.** 2008. Multilocus sequence typing of pathogenic *Candida* species. *Eukaryot Cell* **7:**1075–1084.
247. **Byrnes EJ III, Bildfell RJ, Frank SA, Mitchell TG, Marr KA, Heitman J.** 2009. Molecular evidence that the range of the Vancouver Island outbreak of *Cryptococcus gattii* infection has expanded into the Pacific Northwest in the United States. *J Infect Dis* **199:**1081–1086.
248. **Meyer W, Aanensen DM, Boekhout T, Cogliati M, Diaz MR, Esposto MC, Fisher M, Gilgado F, Hagen F, Kaocharoen S, Litvintseva AP, Mitchell TG, Simwami SP, Trilles L, Viviani MA, Kwon-Chung J.** 2009. Consensus multi-locus sequence typing scheme for *Cryptococcus neoformans* and *Cryptococcus gattii*. *Med Mycol* **47:** 561–570.
249. **Odds FC, Davidson AD, Jacobsen MD, Tavanti A, Whyte JA, Kibbler CC, Ellis DH, Maiden MCJ, Shaw DJ, Gow NAR.** 2006. *Candida albicans* strain maintenance, replacement, and microvariation demonstrated by multilocus sequence typing. *J Clin Microbiol* **44:**3647–3658.
250. **Lin CY, Chen YC, Lo HJ, Chen KW, Li SY.** 2007. Assessment of *Candida glabrata* strain relatedness by pulsed-field gel electrophoresis and multilocus sequence typing. *J Clin Microbiol* **45:**2452–2459.
251. **Diab-Elschahawi M, Forstner C, Hagen F, Meis JF, Lassnig AM, Presterl E, Klaassen CH.** 2012. Microsatellite genotyping clarified conspicuous accumulation of *Candida parapsilosis* at a cardiothoracic surgery intensive care unit. *J Clin Microbiol* **50:**3422–3426.
252. **Firacative C, Roe CC, Malik R, Ferreira-Paim K, Escandón P, Sykes JE, Castañón-Olivares LR, Contreras-Peres C, Samayoa B, Sorrell TC, Castañeda E, Lockhart SR, Engelthaler DM, Meyer W.** 2016. MLST and whole-genome-based population analysis of *Cryptococcus gattii* VGIII links clinical, veterinary and environmental strains, and reveals divergent serotype specific sub-populations and distant ancestors. *PLoS Negl Trop Dis* **10:**e0004861.
253. **Vaux S, Criscuolo A, Desnos-Ollivier M, Diancourt L, Tarnaud C, Vandenbogaert M, Brisse S, Coignard B, Dromer F, Geotrichum Investigation Group.** 2014. Multicenter outbreak of infections by *Saprochaete clavata*, an unrecognized opportunistic fungal pathogen. *mBio* **5:** e02309-14.
254. **Cuenca-Estrella M, Verweij PE, Arendrup MC, Arikan-Akdagli S, Bille J, Donnelly JP, Jensen HE, Lass-Flörl C, Richardson MD, Akova M, Bassetti M, Calandra T, Castagnola E, Cornely OA, Garbino J, Groll AH, Herbrecht R, Hope WW, Kullberg BJ, Lortholary O, Meersseman W, Petrikkos G, Roilides E, Viscoli C, Ullmann AJ, ESCMID** Fungal Infection Study Group. 2012. ESCMID guideline for the diagnosis and management of *Candida* diseases 2012: diagnostic procedures. Clin Microbiol Infect **18**(Suppl 7): 9–18.
255. **Lass-Flörl C, Mayr A, Perkhofer S, Hinterberger G, Hausdorfer J, Speth C, Fille M.** 2008. Activities of antifungal agents against yeasts and filamentous fungi: assessment according to the methodology of the European Committee on Antimicrobial Susceptibility Testing. *Antimicrob Agents Chemother* **52:**3637–3641.
256. **Pfaller MA, Boyken L, Hollis RJ, Messer SA, Tendolkar S, Diekema DJ.** 2006. *In vitro* susceptibilities of *Candida* spp. to caspofungin: four years of global surveillance. *J Clin Microbiol* **44:**760–763.
257. **Alexander BD, Johnson MD, Pfeiffer CD, Jiménez-Ortigosa C, Catania J, Booker R, Castanheira M, Messer SA, Perlin DS, Pfaller MA.** 2013. Increasing echinocandin resistance in *Candida glabrata*: clinical failure correlates with presence of *FKS* mutations and elevated minimum inhibitory concentrations. *Clin Infect Dis* **56:**1724–1732.
258. **Kollia K, Arabatzis M, Kostoula O, Kostourou A, Velegraki A, Belessiotou E, Lazou A, Kostourou A.** 2003. *Clavispora (Candida) lusitaniae* susceptibility profiles and genetic diversity in three tertiary hospitals (1998–2001). *Int J Antimicrob Agents* **22:**458–460.
259. **Atkinson BJ, Lewis RE, Kontoyiannis DP.** 2008. *Candida lusitaniae* fungemia in cancer patients: risk factors for amphotericin B failure and outcome. *Med Mycol* **46:**541–546.
260. **Pfaller MA, Espinel-Ingroff A, Canton E, Castanheira M, Cuenca-Estrella M, Diekema DJ, Fothergill A, Fuller J, Ghannoum M, Jones RN, Lockhart SR, Martin-Mazuelos E, Melhem MS, Ostrosky-Zeichner L, Pappas P, Pelaez T, Peman J, Rex J, Szeszs MW.** 2012. Wild-type MIC distributions and epidemiological cutoff values for amphotericin B, flucytosine, and itraconazole and *Candida* spp. as determined by CLSI broth microdilution. *J Clin Microbiol* **50:** 2040–2046.
261. **Borman AM, Johnson EM.** 2014. Interpretation of fungal culture results. *Curr Fungal Infect Rep* **8:**312–321.
262. **Barenfanger J, Arakere P, Cruz RD, Imran A, Drake C, Lawhorn J, Verhulst SJ, Khardori N.** 2003. Improved outcomes associated with limiting identification of *Candida* spp. in respiratory secretions. *J Clin Microbiol* **41:**5645–5649.
263. **Cantón E, Pemán J, Espinel-Ingroff A, Martín-Mazuelos E, Carrillo-Muñoz A, Martínez JP.** 2008. Comparison of disc diffusion assay with the CLSI reference method (M27-A2) for testing in vitro posaconazole activity against common and uncommon yeasts. *J Antimicrob Chemother* **61:** 135–138.
264. **González GM, Elizondo M, Ayala J.** 2008. Trends in species distribution and susceptibility of bloodstream isolates of *Candida* collected in Monterrey, Mexico, to seven antifungal agents: results of a 3-year (2004 to 2007) surveillance study. *J Clin Microbiol* **46:**2902–2905.
265. **Arendrup MC, Prakash A, Meletiadis J, Sharma C, Chowdhary A.** 2017. Comparison of EUCAST and CLSI reference microdilution MICs of eight antifungal compounds for *Candida auris* and associated tentative epidemiological cutoff values. *Antimicrob Agents Chemother* **61:**e00485-17.
266 **Pfaller MA, Diekema DJ, Messer SA, Boyken L, Hollis RJ, Jones RN, International Fungal Surveillance Participant Group.** 2003. In vitro activities of voriconazole, posaconazole, and four licensed systemic antifungal agents against *Candida* species infrequently isolated from blood. *J Clin Microbiol* **41:**78–83.
267. **Kim MN, Shin JH, Sung H, Lee K, Kim EC, Ryoo N, Lee JS, Jung SI, Park KH, Kee SJ, Kim SH, Shin MG, Suh SP, Ryang DW.** 2009. *Candida haemulonii* and closely related species at 5 university hospitals in Korea: identification, antifungal susceptibility, and clinical features. *Clin Infect Dis* **48:**e57–e61.
268. **Pfaller MA, Diekema DJ, Gibbs DL, Newell VA, Nagy E, Dobiasova S, Rinaldi M, Barton R, Veselov A, Global Antifungal Surveillance Group.** 2008. *Candida krusei*, a multidrug-resistant opportunistic fungal pathogen: geographic and temporal trends from the ARTEMIS DISK Antifungal Surveillance Program, 2001 to 2005. *J Clin Microbiol* **46:**515–521.
269. **Favel A, Michel-Nguyen A, Datry A, Challier S, Leclerc F, Chastin C, Fallague K, Regli P.** 2004. Susceptibility of clinical isolates of *Candida lusitaniae* to five systemic antifungal agents. *J Antimicrob Chemother* **53:**526–529.
270. **da Matta DA, de Almeida LP, Machado AM, Azevedo AC, Kusano EJ, Travassos NF, Salomão R, Colombo AL.** 2007. Antifungal susceptibility of 1000 *Candida* bloodstream isolates to 5 antifungal drugs: results of a multicenter study conducted in São Paulo, Brazil, 1995–2003. *Diagn Microbiol Infect Dis* **57:**399–404.

271. **Lee JS, Shin JH, Kim MN, Jung SI, Park KH, Cho D, Kee SJ, Shin MG, Suh SP, Ryang DW.** 2007. *Kodamaea ohmeri* isolates from patients in a university hospital: identification, antifungal susceptibility, and pulsed-field gel electrophoresis analysis. *J Clin Microbiol* **45:**1005–1010.
272. **Serena C, Mariné M, Pastor FJ, Nolard N, Guarro J.** 2005. In vitro interaction of micafungin with conventional and new antifungals against clinical isolates of *Trichosporon, Sporobolomyces* and *Rhodotorula*. *J Antimicrob Chemother* **55:**1020–1023.
273. **Barchiesi F, Arzeni D, Fothergill AW, Di Francesco LF, Caselli F, Rinaldi MG, Scalise G.** 2000. In vitro activities of the new antifungal triazole SCH 56592 against common and emerging yeast pathogens. *Antimicrob Agents Chemother* **44:**226–229.
274. **Gadea I, Cuenca-Estrella M, Prieto E, Diaz-Guerra TM, Garcia-Cia JI, Mellado E, Tomas JF, Rodriguez-Tudela JL.** 2004. Genotyping and antifungal susceptibility profile of *Dipodascus capitatus* isolates causing disseminated infection in seven hematological patients of a tertiary hospital. *J Clin Microbiol* **42:**1832–1836.
275. **Chagas-Neto TC, Chaves GM, Melo AS, Colombo AL.** 2009. Bloodstream infections due to *Trichosporon* spp.: species distribution, *Trichosporon asahii* genotypes determined on the basis of ribosomal DNA intergenic spacer 1 sequencing, and antifungal susceptibility testing. *J Clin Microbiol* **47:**1074–1081.

Pneumocystis

MELANIE T. CUSHION AND M. ALI RAI

121

The yeast-like fungi in the genus *Pneumocystis* are extracellular, host-obligate, host-specific, and typically restricted to the lung tissues of mammals, although extrapulmonary manifestations have been reported (1, 2). Once known collectively by the single genus and species "*Pneumocystis carinii*," it is now understood that distinct species of *Pneumocystis* infect different mammalian hosts. Current evidence suggests *Pneumocystis* can exist with little consequence in hosts with intact immune systems (3), but debilitation of the immune system, induced by various means including infectious or immunosuppressive agents, congenital defects, malnutrition, and more recently by treatment with new immunotherapeutics (4), can lead to organism proliferation within the lung alveoli, colonization, and potentially a lethal pneumonia if untreated. No species of *Pneumocystis* can be cultivated continuously outside the mammalian lung, which impedes diagnostic capabilities as well as basic scientific research. Limited therapy is available to treat the pneumonia, since these fungi are not susceptible to such antifungal drugs as amphotericin B, the azoles, or the echinocandins.

TAXONOMY

Taxonomic problems have plagued the organisms known as "*Pneumocystis carinii*" since their original description in 1909 by Carlos Chagas, who mistakenly identified the cyst forms as life cycle stages of the protozoan parasite *Trypanosoma cruzi*. In 1914, these organisms were provided an identity of their own and given the binomial epithet that reflected their predilection for the lung, *pneumo-*; the characteristic morphological form, *-cystis*; and, to honor the Italian investigator Antonio Carini, who provided the slides for study, *carinii*. The *P. carinii* organisms were presumed to be a protozoan parasite at the time of identification; the question of their potential fungal nature was first raised in the 1950s, and the controversy of their protozoan or fungal nature continued to the late 20th century. A more detailed early history of *Pneumocystis* identification and nomenclature can be found in reference 5.

The most recent phylogenetic classification based on gene comparisons with other fungi places *Pneumocystis carinii* in the phylum Ascomycota; subphylum Taphrinomycotina; class Pneumocystidomycetes; order Pneumocystidales; genus *Pneumocystis* (6). Within the Taphrinomycotina are the genera *Taphrina* (plant pathogens), *Neolecta* (associated with trees; may be parasitic), *Pneumocystis*, and *Schizosaccharomyces* (fission yeasts).

Pneumocystis species all appear to contain similar life cycle stages, although the clusters of organisms removed from the lungs of the different species can vary in presentation and size. For example, clusters of *P. jirovecii* can be much larger than those obtained from rodent lungs, stain more intensely with Wright-Giemsa-like stains, and form multilayered "mats" composed of several layers of organisms that hinder identification of individual life cycle stages (see Fig. 3B, D, and F for example). The term "*Pneumocystis carinii*" was thought to represent a single zoonotic species until 1976, at which time Frenkel described serological differences between human- and rat-derived organisms that he suggested were representative of distinct species (7). It is now clear that the organism first identified as *Pneumocystis carinii* is a collection of many species within the genus *Pneumocystis* that likely number in the hundreds to thousands. Almost every mammal examined to date appears to harbor at least one species of *Pneumocystis* that is not found in any other mammal. Five *Pneumocystis* species have been formally described per the International Code of Botanical Nomenclature: *Pneumocystis carinii* and *P. wakefieldiae* (8) are found in rats; *P. murina* is found in the lungs of mice (9); *P. jirovecii* is found in humans (5, 10); and *P. oryctolagi* resides in rabbits (11). The name *P. jirovecii*, though first resisted by some groups, has gained widespread acceptance within the scientific and clinical communities.

DESCRIPTION OF THE AGENTS

The terminology used to describe the various life cycle stages of *Pneumocystis* bears remnants of its earlier classification as a protozoan parasite. This discussion uses terms more suitable for its fungal identity, but identifies those commonly found in the literature for continuity. Three developmental forms are generally recognized: the trophic form (trophozoite), 1 to 4 μm (Fig. 1A); the sporocyte (precyst), 5 to 6 μm (Fig. 1B); and the ascus (cyst), 5 to 8 μm (Fig. 1C–E). *Pneumocystis* spp. reproduce extracellularly within the mammalian lung alveoli. The trophic forms appear ameboid in structure in electron micrographs, but in freshly prepared specimens they are ellipsoidal and often occur in clusters with other trophic forms and developmental stages. The nucleus and often the

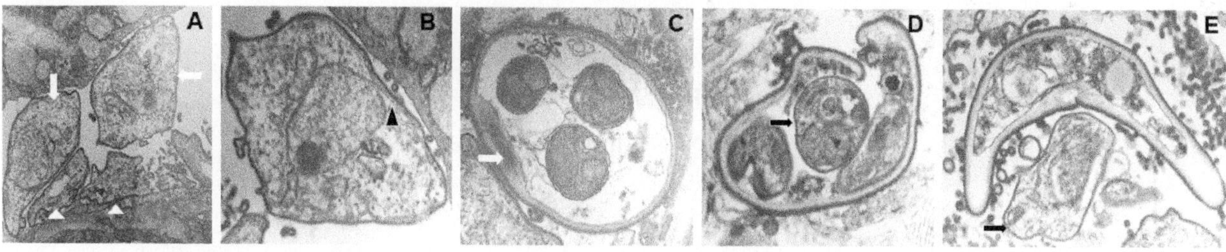

FIGURE 1 Electron micrographs of the major developmental forms of *Pneumocystis*. (A) Trophic form attached to type I pneumocytes (arrowheads) and two larger trophic forms in the alveolar lumen (arrows); (B) sporocyte (precyst), note thickening of the cell wall (arrowhead); (C) ascus (cyst) with three visible spores (intracystic bodies) and characteristic thickening of the cell wall (arrow); (D) ascus with a spore that is apparently excysting (arrow), with two remaining; (E) collapsed ascus with no remaining spores, but with a released trophic form in the immediate vicinity (arrow). (Magnification, ×10,000.)

mitochondrion are visible in rapid Wright-Giemsa-stained specimens by light microscopy. The trophic forms do not stain with fungal stains designed to complex with the cell wall, such as methenamine silver. The sporocyte is smaller than the mature cyst and frequently oval in shape. This stage contains a rigid cell wall that is lacking in the trophic forms and is stained with methenamine and other fungal wall stains. At the sporocyte stage, the nuclei are at varying levels of nuclear division (from two to eight nuclei) but have not yet been compartmentalized into separate spore structures. Aggregates of mitochondrion can also be seen in this stage. The mature cyst is spherical in shape; it contains eight spores (although these may not all be visible) and a thick cell wall that excludes certain stains such as the rapid Wright-Giemsa, and it can be visualized with cell wall-complexing stains such as methenamine silver. The cyst/ascus is considered the diagnostic morphological form. All developmental forms are often found in large, multilayered, tightly adherent aggregates or clusters in clinical specimens, making identification of each stage difficult (see Fig. 3B, D, and F).

EPIDEMIOLOGY AND TRANSMISSION

Early animal studies showed that *Pneumocystis* infection was likely transmitted by an airborne route. Immunosuppressed, *Pneumocystis*-free rats could acquire the infection from infected rats housed in the same room or from infected cage mates (12). Air sampling studies using quantitative PCR, conducted around patients admitted with *Pneumocystis* pneumonia (PCP), showed the highest levels of detection within 1 m of the patients' heads (13). Although levels decreased with increasing distance from the patient source, samples were still positive in corridors outside the patients' rooms. Importantly, the genotypes of the *P. jirovecii* infecting the patients were the same as the genotypes outside the immediate patient area, confirming that the potential sources of transmission were these patients. These data provide evidence that supports historical and more recent descriptions of outbreaks in renal transplant units (14–16) and other clinical settings where patient-to-patient transmission can occur, such as among heart transplant recipients (17).

The agent of transmission appears to be the cyst (ascus) form, as experiments using mice with infections composed almost exclusively of trophic forms could not transmit the infection (18).

Putative Life Cycle

Histochemical and ultrastructural studies form the basis of the current understanding of the life cycle of *Pneumocystis*, due to a historic lack of a long-term cultivation method outside the lung. Thus, any life cycle should be considered presumptive until it is possible to perform definitive kinetic analyses. There is no evidence for an intracellular phase, although the organisms can be frequently observed within macrophages as a result of the host response to the infection. Despite numerous attempts to find an environmental cycle or external reservoir for *Pneumocystis*, none has been identified. A growing body of evidence suggests that the reservoir for *Pneumocystis* is its mammalian host, a situation similar to other host-dependent pathogens like *Entamoeba histolytica* or *Mycobacterium tuberculosis*. Studies in humans and animal models support a role for neonates and immune-competent hosts as potential reservoirs that are colonized transiently or longer term (3).

A schematic of a proposed life cycle, based on several histological and ultrastructural studies, can be found in Fig. 2, with a detailed description provided in the legend. The various life cycle stages of *Pneumocystis* are most often found together in large adherent clusters that resemble biofilms *in vivo* (Fig. 2B). The *in vitro* formation of biofilms by *P. murina* and *P. carinii* provides support for the formation of these structures *in vivo*, which could be responsible for intransigent infections that are unresponsive to current therapies (19). Trophic forms are presumed to be the vegetative stages of the *Pneumocystis* life cycle; they reproduce asexually by binary fission, not budding as most yeast do. It is likely that they also participate in the sexual mode of reproduction using a process similar to yeast mating-type systems, although these processes are not fully defined. Several fungal meiosis-specific and mating-type gene homologs have been identified in genomic *Pneumocystis* databases (20).

The finding that *P. jirovecii*, *P. murina*, and *P. carinii* all contain a single genomic region with only three genes involved in differentiation lends credence to the existence of a homothallic sexual cycle, suggesting that these fungi do not need to seek a complementary mating type (heterothallism) (21).

After the mating process, which involves two mating types, *mam2* and *ste3*, nuclear fusion occurs and is followed by meiosis and sporogenesis, resulting in formation of the precyst, or sporocyte. Following meiosis, an additional mitotic replication occurs, with subsequent compartmentalization of the nuclei and organelles into eight ascospores. The end product of sporogenesis is the spherical cyst, or ascus, containing the eight spores. The process of spore release has not been described, but it may involve a localized thickening at one pole of the ascus. It should be noted that, unlike other fungi, all the developmental stages of *Pneumocystis* contain a double membrane.

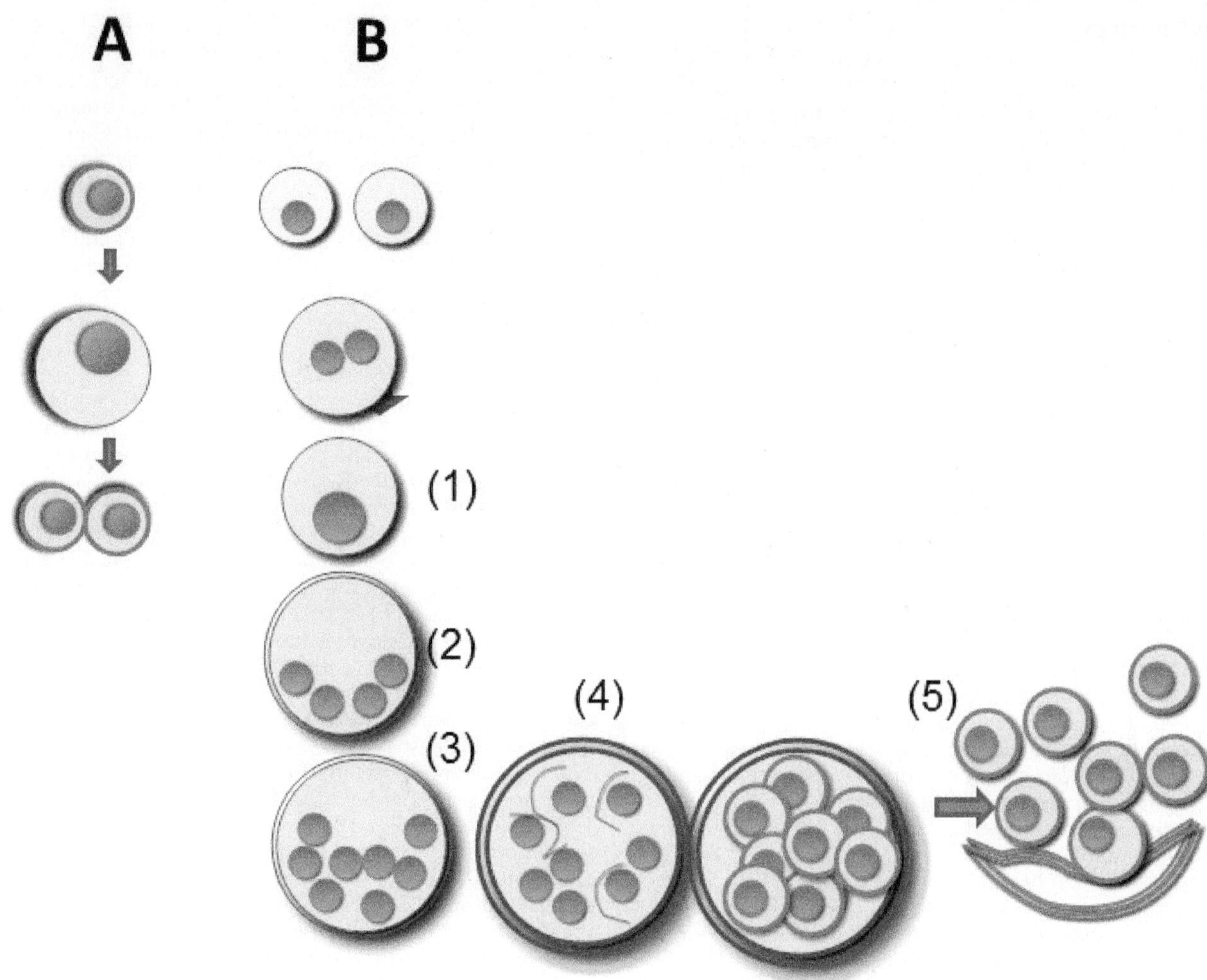

FIGURE 2 Proposed life cycle of *Pneumocystis*. (A) Asexual replication cycle of *Pneumocystis*. Trophic forms undergo binary fission after mitotic replication of the nucleus. (B) Putative sexual cycle of *Pneumocystis*: (1) Map3 and Mam2 (opposite mating types) fuse and undergo karyogamy resulting in a diploid zygote; (2) the zygote then undergoes meiosis, resulting in four nuclei; (3) additional postmeiotic mitosis increases the number of nuclei to eight; (4) the nuclei and mitochondria (not shown) are compartmentalized by invagination of the inner plasma membrane, resulting in eight spores; (5) spores are released from the ascus (cyst) and presumably enter into the vegetative phase of the cycle.

Transmission

Evidence from several different studies suggests that (i) *Pneumocystis* is transmitted by an airborne route; (ii) it is likely to be acquired early in life; (iii) it is transmitted among immunologically intact individuals; (iv) immunosuppressed and infected hosts can transmit the infection to immunologically intact hosts; and (v) transmission requires a short period of exposure and low numbers of organisms (22).

Experimental evidence indicates that very few organisms are required to initiate *Pneumocystis* infection and that these fungi are very efficient in their method of transmission. Studies have shown that fewer than 10 *P. carinii* organisms were sufficient to establish a fulminant infection in immunosuppressed rats (23), and a 1-day period of exposure was all that was needed to transmit the infection from an infected *scid/scid* mouse to an uninfected *scid/scid* mouse (24). The once widespread prevalence of *Pneumocystis* in commercial colonies housing healthy rats supports the very efficient dissemination of the infection throughout the members of a colony and also demonstrates that the organism thrives in the immune-competent host (25). Today, the animal husbandry practices of commercial vendors have all but eliminated *Pneumocystis* from their housing facilities. Transmission from infected patients to immune-competent health care workers has been reported (26). Evidence that healthy human populations may also serve as reservoirs or sources of infection is accumulating. A recent study conducted in humans without underlying lung disease or immunosuppression found that 20% of the oropharyngeal wash samples from 50 individuals were positive for *P. jirovecii* by nested PCR targeting the mitochondrial large subunit ribosomal gene (27). In a study of 851 non-HIV-infected patients with pneumonia in China, *P. jirovecii* was detected in 14.5% by methenamine silver staining and in 24% by PCR (28). Although direct proof of mother-to-child transmission was lacking, a recent study reported that three out of four children had transient colonization with *P. jirovecii* during the first 6 months after birth, while only half of the mothers were positive by nested PCR targeting the mitochondrial large subunit rRNA (mtLSU-rRNA) gene (29).

Epidemiology

Beard et al. reported that the expansion of *P. jirovecii* carrying a double mutation in the DHPS gene in selected HIV-infected human populations provided strong support for transmission of *P. jirovecii* via a person-to-person route, and that this was illustrative of a positive selective mechanism as well (30). Previous and recent epidemiological surveys showing the clustering of specific *P. jirovecii* genotypes with patients' place of residence or in clinical settings (many in renal transplant units) are consistent with the hypothesis of person-to-person transmission of *P. jirovecii* via the airborne route. A report from Japan documented a PCP outbreak in a renal transplantation unit, with 27 cases in a single year that could be traced by molecular methods back to the outpatient clinic (31). The median incubation time was estimated to be 53 days, with a range of 7 to 188 days. Several such outbreaks have been reported over the past 2 decades, providing a cautionary note for immunosuppressed patients gathering in a community setting, as well as for appropriate prophylaxis therapy for susceptible populations. In some cases, the mortality rate was as high as 50% (32). Surprisingly, investigators recently showed that most cases of *Pneumocystis* colonization in renal transplant patients were detected beyond 2 years after transplant rather than within the initial 2-year time period (32). However, a recent report on the epidemiology of *P. jirovecii* colonization in families showed only a 3.3% detection in children of HIV-infected adults, whose colonization rate was 11.4%, suggesting that merely close contact with potential reservoirs is not sufficient to induce this state (33).

Serological studies performed in the 1970s through the 1980s showed *P. jirovecii* was encountered early in life (34, 35). Most human beings become seropositive to *P. jirovecii* organisms or antigens by the age of 2 to 4 years. Vargas et al. detected *P. jirovecii* DNA in nasopharyngeal aspirates in 24 of 72 infants (32%) suffering from mild respiratory infections (36). Seroconversion developed in 67 of 79 (85%) of the same cohort of infants by 20 months of age. Thus, serological testing has not been useful for the diagnosis of PCP.

Colonization

Emerging reports of the detection of *P. jirovecii* in populations without underlying immunosuppression, as well as populations who have chronic underlying diseases that have not been historically associated with its presence, may suggest colonization or expansion of host range or the result of a new immunotherapeutic, such as ibrutinib, a small-molecule drug that is used to treat B cell cancers (37–40). Colonization, carriage, asymptomatic infection, and subclinical infection have all been used to describe the presence of *Pneumocystis* organisms or DNA in the absence of PCP. The effects of the presence of low numbers of *P. jirovecii* on the host have yet to be determined, and the role of carriage in mild respiratory infections, chronic lung disease, and progression to PCP is now being actively investigated. The most common underlying conditions associated with the presence of *P. jirovecii* in non-HIV-positive individuals include asthma and chronic lung diseases, chronic obstructive pulmonary disease, cystic fibrosis, Epstein-Barr virus infection, lupus erythematosus, high-dose corticosteroid therapy, anti-tumor necrosis factor-α therapies for rheumatoid arthritis, thyroiditis, ulcerative colitis, and pregnancy. Children appear to have a higher rate of colonization than adults do. Serological studies showed early exposure occurred during the first few years of life; 32% of colonized infants manifested mild respiratory symptoms in a large study in Chile (36). Studies from the same group suggested an association with sudden infant death syndrome, but this was not supported by subsequent investigations. Should the presence of *P. jirovecii* be confirmed as a causal agent in the underlying pathogenesis of any of these diseases, treatment of this cofactor could improve patient outcome. Currently, there is an ongoing discussion about the gene targets of PCR and the cutoff values for copy numbers for the correct diagnosis of colonization versus infection (41); the mtLSU-rRNA gene is favored for detection, with lower and upper cutoff values of 3.9×10^5 copies/ml and 3.2×10^6 copies/ml differentiating PCP and colonization (41).

CLINICAL SIGNIFICANCE

In the late 1980s, it was estimated that 75% of people living with AIDS developed PCP (42). Since the advent of antiretroviral therapy and prophylaxis, the proportion has decreased substantially. Recent incidence among patients with AIDS in Western Europe and the United States is <1 case per 100 person-years (43, 44). However, PCP remains the leading opportunistic infection associated with AIDS patients, even in the era of highly active antiretroviral therapy (HAART) (45). The mortality rate associated with PCP prior to and after the era of HAART (1996 forward) has not changed significantly in the United States, with an average of 10 to 13.5% (46, 47). In developing countries and within urban American cities, the mortality is much higher despite the availability of HAART (48, 49). The latter study reports that the mortality rate for a medically underserved population in Atlanta, Georgia, from 1996 to 2006 was 37%, while patients who required aggressive intervention such as mechanical ventilation experienced an 80% mortality rate from PCP. In patients with cancer and other non-HIV diseases, there has been little improvement in mortality rates, and often these patients fared more poorly than patients with HIV. In one such study, the mortality of non-HIV-infected patients with PCP was 48%, while HIV-infected patients experienced a 17% mortality (50). The mortality rate of *P. jirovecii* pneumonia in rheumatoid arthritis patients receiving eight immunosuppressive therapies in Japan averaged about 15.5%, with the highest mortality in patients who received tacrolimus; only one patient treated with golimumab, a human monoclonal antibody that targets tumor necrosis factor alpha, developed PCP and did not die (51). Although the incidence of PCP in pediatric populations has declined, PCP and its association with immune reconstitution inflammatory syndrome (IRIS) (52) cause significant clinical problems in these populations and in vulnerable adult populations worldwide.

Within the mammalian lung, the trophic forms of *Pneumocystis* adhere to the type I pneumocytes, presumably through macromolecular bridges (53, 54). Type I cells are responsible for the gas exchange between the alveolar capillaries and the alveolar lumen. Besides attachment to the type I cells, the various developmental stages of the parasite adhere to one another, producing large clusters that extend outwardly into the alveolar lumen. In severe, untreated infections, most of the alveoli are filled with organisms. Direct attachment to the cells responsible for gas exchange, combined with the accumulation of organisms within the alveoli, results in impaired gas exchange and altered lung compliance as well as other physiologic changes associated with the pneumonia, such as hypoxia (55).

Histopathologic findings can be characterized by two traits: (i) alveolar interstitial thickening and (ii) a frothy, eosinophilic, honeycombed exudate in the lumina of the lung. The interstitial thickening is a result of hyperplasia and hypertrophy of the type II pneumocyte, interstitial edema, mononuclear cell infiltration, and in some cases mild fibrosis. The exudate is apparent upon staining with hematoxylin and eosin, which does not stain the organisms but clearly permits visualization of the eosinic exudate. Methenamine silver or another yeast cell wall stain (e.g., toluidine blue) must be used to visualize the cyst/ascus form of the organism, considered the diagnostic stage.

Immune Reconstitution Inflammatory Syndrome

Treatment with antiretroviral therapy improves immune function, with a concomitant increase of CD4 cells within a few months after start of therapy. This improvement in immune responses can be accompanied by a paradoxical, exaggerated inflammatory response manifested against infectious or noninfectious agents that often results in clinical worsening, referred to as IRIS (52). IRIS occurs more frequently in adults, but has been reported in children. In adults, IRIS has been associated with patients harboring mycobacterial infections; PCP; cryptococcal infections; cytomegalovirus, varicella virus, or herpes simplex virus infections; or progressive multifocal leukoencephalopathy.

Presentation in Children

PCP is a less common manifestation among HIV-infected children than in previous years (52), but it is increasing in preterm infants (56). The highest incidence occurs during the first year of life, peaking at 3 to 6 months of age (52). Although a significant and dramatic decline in PCP infection rates in United States infants has been reported by the CDC and Perinatal AIDS Collaborative Transmission Study *Pneumocystis*, it remains a deadly neonatal disease in Africa, where postmortem analysis showed that 44% of children who died between 2000 and 2001 had PCP (57). Recent data indicate that *P. jirovecii* is a significant cause of pneumonia in HIV-infected children without appropriate antiretroviral therapy or prophylactic treatment, with high mortality rates ranging from 28 to 63% (58).

PCP was first described in children and was considered a pediatric infection in its early history (59). Prominent epidemics of "interstitial plasma cell pneumonia" in undernourished children housed in suboptimal conditions after World War II were manifestations of the disease that was later identified as *P. jirovecii* pneumonia. The infection in these children was characterized by a plasma cell infiltrate, in contrast to the type II cell hypertrophy and scanty mononuclear infiltrate described in adults with the pneumonia.

Clinical features of PCP in children include fever, tachypnea, dyspnea, and cough. Onset can be acute or subtle, associated with nonspecific conditions such as mild cough, loss of appetite, diarrhea, and weight loss. Fever may or may not be present, but most children will exhibit rapid breathing with short, shallow breaths at the time the pneumonia is visible by radiographic methods. Bilateral basilar rales, respiratory distress, and hypoxia are often evident on physical exam. In HIV-infected children, four clinical variables are independently associated with PCP: age younger than 6 months, a respiratory rate greater than 59 breaths per minute, arterial percentage hemoglobin saturation less than or equal to 92%, and the absence of vomiting (52, 60).

Most children manifest frank hypoxia, with low arterial oxygen pressure of less than 30 mmHg. The $CD4^+$ count is often less than 200 cells/mm^3 but can be higher. Children older than 5 years have a percent $CD4^+$ of less than 15%. Like adults, children will often have bilateral diffuse parenchymal infiltrates with a ground-glass appearance, but such manifestations may be altogether lacking or mild.

Presentation in Adults

Adults with PCP frequently present with dyspnea, nonproductive cough, inability to breathe deeply, chest tightness, and night sweats (55, 61). A low-grade fever (e.g., 38.5°C) and tachypnea are often present, while hemoptysis or sputum production is rare. On physical examination, few pronounced abnormalities are detected, but various degrees of respiratory distress, small respiratory volumes, and fine basilar rales can be observed. Patients with AIDS often have a more insidious progression to clinical disease than patients who are not infected with HIV but are immunosuppressed.

The chest radiograph may appear normal or reflect a disease state. Diffuse, symmetrical, interstitial infiltrates are most commonly present, while focal infiltrates, lobar consolidations, cavities, and nodules are less common. Infiltrates in early infection may be widely distributed, but consolidation increases as the disease progresses. Administration of aerosolized pentamidine as a prophylactic measure has been associated with increased frequency of apical infiltrates and pneumothoraces. The severity of abnormalities on the chest radiograph is considered prognostic and can be correlated with higher mortality.

If the radiograph is normal or unchanged from a prior radiograph, a test for the diffusing capacity of the lung for carbon monoxide (DL_{CO}) is recommended if the patient's symptoms consist of a nonproductive cough or shortness of breath, with or without fever. If the DL_{CO} (corrected for hemoglobin) is $\leq$75% of the predicted value or decreased $\geq$20% from baseline, the patient should undergo diagnostic evaluation or bronchoscopy or both (62).

The oxygenation impairment induced by pneumocystosis can be detected in most patients by a widening of the alveolar-arterial oxygen gradient [(A-a)DO_2] correlated with severity of disease and respiratory alkalosis (62). However, it should be noted that a significant number of patients can have a normal (A-a)DO_2 gradient at rest. Impaired diffusing capacity, alterations in lung compliance, total lung capacity, vital capacity, and hypoxemia are other physiologic changes that may be associated with *P. jirovecii* infection (55). Abnormalities in surfactant proteins also occur in infected individuals, with increases in surfactant protein A and D the most notable, since these proteins are considered components of innate immunity (63).

High-Resolution Computerized Tomography

Chest radiography (X ray) has been used to diagnose PCP, but the findings of ground-glass infiltrates and other characteristics are not definitive for the pneumonia, and about one-third of patients with PCP have normal radiographic findings. High-resolution computerized tomography of PCP patients reveals extensive ground-glass opacity with a central distribution in a background of interlobular septal thickening, a mosaic pattern, or diffuse distribution in some patients (64). In some rare cases, unusual multiple nodular changes are observed (65). Pulmonary cysts of varying shapes and sizes are increasingly detected in up to one-third of patients on chemoprophylaxis. In some cases, a reversed halo sign may be indicative of PCP. Such a finding is observed as a round area of ground-glass attenuation surrounded by a crescent or ring of consolidation. First described as being specific for cryptogenic organizing pneumonia, it can be observed in several other infectious and noninfectious diseases.

Extrapulmonary Pneumocystosis

The incidence of *Pneumocystis* organisms in sites other than the lung has been reported in 0.6 to 3% of postmortem examinations of patients with pulmonary *P. jirovecii* infections (1, 2). This is likely an underestimate due to the limited number of autopsies currently performed, the lack of suspicion of extrapulmonary pneumocystosis, and the efficacy of current antiviral therapies resulting in increased immune function. Methenamine silver staining or immunofluorescent kits served to identify the cyst/ascus stage of *Pneumocystis* in tissue samples and fine-needle aspirates in antemortem cases. The lymph nodes were the most frequent site of extrapulmonary involvement in a series of 52 patients (44%), followed by the spleen, bone marrow, and liver (33%). *P. jirovecii* has been detected in the adrenal glands, gastrointestinal tract, genitourinary tract, thyroid, ear, liver, pancreas, eyes, skin, and other sites. Infection of multiple extrapulmonary sites was associated with a rapidly fatal outcome. Pathological findings correlated with the organ where the infection was present. For example, retinal cotton wool spots were reported in infected eyes, and pancytopenia was observed in patients with bone marrow lesions.

COLLECTION, TRANSPORT, AND STORAGE OF SPECIMENS

P. jirovecii pneumonia should be considered in immunocompromised patients who present with fever, respiratory symptoms, or infiltrates on chest X ray. While mostly restricted to the lung, *P. jirovecii* has been found as extrapulmonary masses (e.g., pleura, intra-abdominal) in HIV-positive patients and should be included in a differential diagnosis in these patients. As no symptoms are specific for PCP, a definitive diagnosis is usually made by morphologic identification of the organism, though molecular methods are gaining importance for detection and diagnosis. Algorithms for clinical evaluation and treatment of PCP and differential diagnosis for HIV-associated pneumonias have been published, and the reader is referred to these reviews for further details (66).

Because *P. jirovecii* cannot be cultured, the diagnosis of PCP relies on efficient sampling as most diagnostic methods still rely on microscopic techniques. The fungus can be detected in a variety of respiratory specimens, including induced sputum, bronchoalveolar lavage fluid (BALF), tracheal aspirate fluid, tissue obtained by transbronchial biopsy, cellular material obtained by bronchial brush, pleural fluid, and tissue obtained by open thorax lung biopsy. The diagnostic yield is dependent on the underlying disease state of the patient and the expertise of the staff obtaining the sample. In some hospitals where the staff were trained to obtain sputum samples and there was a large population with AIDS, 80% of diagnoses of PCP were made from induced sputum (67). In contrast, the diagnostic yield from non-AIDS patients can be quite low, and bronchoalveolar lavage or other methods may be needed to ensure an appropriate diagnosis (59). Multiple slides from non-AIDS patients should be examined, especially when there is a high degree of suspicion. Hospitals serving a diverse population often rely on methods other than induced sputum. A notable drawback of using induced sputum as the primary procedure for the diagnosis of PCP is the lack of information concerning other infections or disease processes that may be present in the lung. The diagnosis of extrapulmonary pneumocystosis relies on accurate sampling of the infected organ and subsequent staining of the histological sections. For infants and young children who are unable to produce sputum or in whom this method is not warranted, tracheal aspirate fluid, open thorax lung biopsy, or respiratory specimens must be obtained by a special pediatric bronchoscopy service (68).

Bronchoalveolar Lavage

Fluid obtained by bronchoalveolar lavage is sufficiently liquid and does not require treatment with mucolytic agents. Twenty to 30 ml should be concentrated by centrifugation at 3,000 × *g* for 15 min. The resultant pellet is reconstituted in 0.5 to 1.0 ml of buffer or saline, and a sterile wooden applicator is used to smear the sediment on glass slides, which are then fixed in absolute methanol, acetone, or a commercial fixative in rapid staining kits. Samples in limited quantities can be concentrated by use of a Cytospin Centrifuge (ThermoScientific, Waltham, MA) or equivalent. Addition of 1 drop of 22% bovine serum albumin to 500 μl of sample will aid in adherence to the slide. Slides are air dried and then processed for staining. Morphological criteria for recognition of *P. jirovecii* stained by various procedures are discussed below and summarized in Table 1.

Induced Sputum Collection

Sputum collection is best done in a centralized facility by pulmonary function laboratory technicians, respiratory therapists, or specially trained assistants. Deep inhalation of nebulized 3% sodium chloride solution by the patient will result in osmotic accumulation of fluid in and irritation of the respiratory passages with subsequent coughing and expectoration of bronchoalveolar contents. The patient should vigorously brush the teeth, tongue, and gums with a toothbrush and normal saline for 5 to 10 minutes prior to sputum induction, followed by thorough rinsing, to remove as much cellular debris of oral origin as possible. Toothpaste should not be used, as it can interfere with subsequent processing and staining of the specimen. The induced sputum specimen is usually mucoid and translucent in appearance; only rarely is it purulent. When *P. jirovecii* clusters are present in the unstained sputum, they are typically 0.1 to 0.2 mm in diameter and cream to light tan in color. Sputum smeared directly on slides and subsequently stained was shown to be a less sensitive method than treatment with a mucolytic agent followed by concentration of the specimen (69).

Induced sputum is mucolyzed by the addition of an equal volume (at least 2 ml) of freshly prepared 0.0065 M dithiothreitol (Stat-Pak Sputolysin; Caldon-Biotech, Carlsbad, CA) or 0.5% *N*-acetyl-L-cysteine and incubation on a rotary shaker at 35°C with intermittent vigorous vortexing until the specimen is almost completely liquefied (complete liquefaction will lead to dispersal of the *P. jirovecii* clusters, making microscopic detection more difficult). Some protocols require the addition of a clearing reagent for optimal results (e.g., the LIGHT DIAGNOSTICS *Pneumocystis carinii* DFA Kit [Millipore Sigma, Billerica, MA]). The specimen is then concentrated by centrifugation at 3,000 × *g* for 5 min, and the sediment is smeared on glass slides, which are air dried and heat fixed by exposure to a heating block (50 to 60°C). Prolonged heat fixation (~30 min) is important in fixing the material to the slide, since most of the natural cellular adhesions are removed during mucolysis. Slides containing the fixed material are then stained and examined microscopically (see below). Samples can be concentrated with a Cytospin Centrifuge, as described for BALF (above).

Open Thorax Lung Biopsy

Open thorax lung biopsy is the most invasive of the sampling procedures and is not routinely performed.

TABLE 1 Comparison of stains used to detect *P. jirovecii*

Stain	Time to perform stain	Cyst wall	Trophic and other forms	Advantage(s)	Disadvantage(s)
Giemsa	30 to 60 min	Unstained; cyst wall appears as a clear ring around spores/intracystic bodies	Nuclei stain red-purple; cytoplasm stains light to dark blue, depending on thickness and depth of cluster	Inexpensive; stain simple to perform; stains all life cycle stages of *Pneumocystis*; stains most other pathogens (e.g., bacteria, parasites, fungi) and host cells	Experienced reader required to distinguish *Pneumocystis* clumps from stained host cells
Rapid Giemsa-like stains (e.g., Diff-Quik, Hema 3)	<5 min				
Fluorescein-conjugated monoclonal antibody kits (direct and indirect immunofluorescence)	15 to 30 min	Stains and fluoresces apple green; cyst contents usually unstained (appear black) or dull; fold in cyst wall sometimes apparent, giving a crinkled, raisin-like appearance	Stained; appear as small polygons or spheres outlined in apple green; nuclei may stain; clusters can stain with a diffuse green glow	Recommended for less experienced personnel; immunofluorescent staining is sensitive and specific for *Pneumocystis*	Requires fluorescence microscope; reagents are expensive
Methenamine silver (Gomori/Grocott)	30 min (microwave); 1 to 2 h (rapid); 6 to 24 h (conventional)	Stains brown to black; cyst wall thickenings (double comma) and fold in the cyst wall stain dark brown to black; does not differentiate empty cysts from cysts with spores	Unstained	Easy to detect cysts; host cells not stained	Prolonged staining time for conventional method; moderate costs; strong acids used; only the cyst form is stained; stains other fungi
Toluidine blue O/cresyl echt violet	1 to 6 h	Stains violet to purple; cyst wall thickenings and folds stain darker violet to purple; does not differentiate empty cysts from cysts with spores	Unstained	Easy to detect cysts; host cells not stained	Prolonged staining time; moderate costs; strong acids used; only the cyst is stained; stains other fungi
Calcofluor white	<5 min	Stains blue-white or green, depending on filter; cyst wall and thickenings intensely fluorescent	Unstained	Cyst fluoresces brilliantly; simple to perform; inexpensive	Requires fluorescence microscope; strong alkali used; only cyst is stained; stains other fungi; some expertise is required to distinguish *Pneumocystis* cysts from other fungi.
Gram-Weigert	<5 min	Unstained wall; intracystic bodies stain purple	Trophic forms faintly visible	Commonly available in cytopathology laboratories	Faint staining; can be overcome by experienced observer, but better stains are available.
Papanicolaou	1 to 6 h	Unstained wall; intracystic bodies stain purple	Trophic forms faintly visible	Commonly available in cytopathology laboratories	Faint staining; can be overcome by experienced observer, but better stains are available.

This technique also suffers from a lack of sensitivity (66). However, should the laboratory receive such a specimen, the tissue should be blotted onto sterile gauze to reduce excess fluid (which would interfere with a diagnostic imprint) and used to make touch imprints by pressing several cut surfaces onto sterile glass slides. The remainder of the tissue can be used for histological sections, for microbiological cultures, or for nucleic acid extractions and subsequent PCR techniques. Glass slides with touch imprints should be air dried and then treated with absolute methanol or fixatives included in commercial kits of rapid Wright-Giemsa-like stains, such as Protocol Hema 3 (Fisher Scientific Inc., Cincinnati, OH). Infected tissue stained in this manner will reveal the presence of clusters of trophic forms and cysts with reddish-purple nuclei and blue cytoplasm; cysts are surrounded by a halo of dye exclusion (see "Microscopic Identification" for a more detailed description). Slides should be fixed in acetone or a vendor-recommended fixative for immunofluorescent staining. Alternatively, a more concentrated sample can be achieved by a tissue homogenization with table-top instruments like the gentleMACS Dissociator (Miltenyi Biotec) or the Stomacher Lab Blender (Tekmar Inc., Cincinnati, OH) and with use of vendor recommendations for tissue type and weights. Slides are prepared with 10-µl drops of the homogenate, which are then air dried, fixed, and stained as desired.

Transbronchial Biopsy

Fiber-optic bronchoscopy with transbronchial biopsy is the most common invasive technique for collection of tissue; however, like open thorax lung biopsy, this procedure is rarely performed today. Tissue should be handled as described for open thorax lung biopsy above.

Nasopharyngeal Aspirates and Oropharyngeal Washes

A number of studies in humans reported the ability to detect *P. jirovecii*-specific DNA in nasopharyngeal aspirates (36, 70) and oropharyngeal washes (71) after amplification by PCR with *P. jirovecii*-specific primers. These minimally invasive techniques have been shown to have high sensitivity, specificity, positive predictive value, and negative predictive values for diagnosis of *P. jirovecii* pneumonia versus microscopic methods when used in conjunction with quantitative PCR techniques. Handling of oropharyngeal washes and nasopharyngeal aspirates is presented here because the use of PCR for the diagnosis of infectious diseases is becoming widespread. These methods will be extremely useful for sampling of pediatric populations, in which more invasive techniques of sampling are problematic or where the yield is low.

Oropharyngeal wash samples are obtained by gargling with 10 ml of sterile physiologic saline (0.9% NaCl) for 1 min (27, 72). Samples are then centrifuged at 2,900 × *g* for 5 min and kept frozen at −20°C until DNA is extracted. After digestion with proteinase K at 56°C for 2 h, DNA or RNA can be extracted with any number of commercial kits available.

Nasopharyngeal aspirates are collected with a suction catheter and sterile saline (36). If the amount of collected specimen is small or it is highly viscous, sterile saline should be washed through the catheter to dilute the specimen or added to the final collection tube. The sample can then be treated with a mucolytic agent and subsequently stained (as described above) or prepared for the PCR by DNA or RNA extraction (described below).

DIRECT EXAMINATION AND IDENTIFICATION

Microscopy

A variety of stains have been used for the identification of *P. jirovecii* organisms. One of the most common stains used by pathologists for tissue sections, hematoxylin and eosin, does not stain the organism but rather the foamy exudates within the lung alveoli, often described as honeycombed in appearance. Stains that illustrate the morphology of the organism by microscopic examination are those used for diagnosis in the clinical laboratory.

A common staining procedure used for the diagnosis of PCP is methenamine silver, which also stains other fungi (Table 1; Fig. 3C). Cell wall and membrane polysaccharides of fungi are oxidized to aldehydes by treatment with periodic acid, which in turn reduce the silver ion to metallic silver at alkaline pH. Addition of gold salts stabilizes the complex, and excess silver is removed by a sodium thiosulfate rinse. Variations of the methenamine silver stain (e.g., Grocott, Gomori) are used for both tissue sections and bodily fluids such as BALF or induced sputum (73–75). Disadvantages to the use of the silver staining process have been the instability of solutions, the capricious nature of the metal impregnation, and the length of time required for staining (1 to 2 h or 6 to 24 h; see Table 1). These disadvantages have been largely overcome with kits using standardized laboratory microwave ovens for controlled processing and supplied reagents (e.g., rapidmicrobiology, Gomori's Methenamine Silver Staining Kit for Fungi Detection; Merck Millipore, Darmstadt, Germany). Unlike other pathogenic fungi, *P. jirovecii* does not bud, and this feature can be used to discriminate between these organisms and other fungi found in the lung that do bud, e.g., *Histoplasma capsulatum*. Silver-stained cysts have a distinctive black, cup-shaped morphology against green-colored host cell architecture. In some staining reactions, cyst wall thickenings appear as a double-comma morphology. More often, the folds in the wall stain a dark brown to black to produce a crinkled, raisin-like appearance (Fig. 3C). Intracystic daughter forms cannot be seen with this stain, and cysts that are empty (nonviable) appear the same as those with the full contingent of eight spores.

Other stains that complex with components of the cyst wall include periodic acid-Schiff, toluidine blue, cresyl echt violet, and calcofluor. The reactions to some of the more commonly used stains are described in Table 1. Cresyl echt violet stain produces results similar to toluidine blue O (Fig. 3E) and has the same drawbacks, since a mixture of sulfuric acid and glacial acetic acid is necessary for the step prior to staining with the dye. Cysts/asci stained by toluidine blue are similar in appearance to those stained with methenamine silver, except for the light purple color. Staining with calcofluor, whether in commercial kits (e.g., Fungi-fluor; Polysciences, Inc., Warrington, PA) or prepared in-house, can produce variable effects. Designed to detect only the cysts, excitation at 420 to 490 nm with a suppression filter of 515 nm produces a yellow-green or apple-green fluorescence, often with a characteristic double-parentheses staining body within the cyst/asci (Fig. 3A). Excitation in the UV range (340 to 380 nm) with a suppression filter of 430 nm produces a fluorescent blue color that is not as intense and is sometimes difficult to visualize. Refer to the vendor instructions for optimal filter requirements.

In contrast to the cyst wall stains, Giemsa and rapid Giemsa-like stains do not stain the cyst/ascus wall, but instead stain the nuclei of all the various life cycle stages

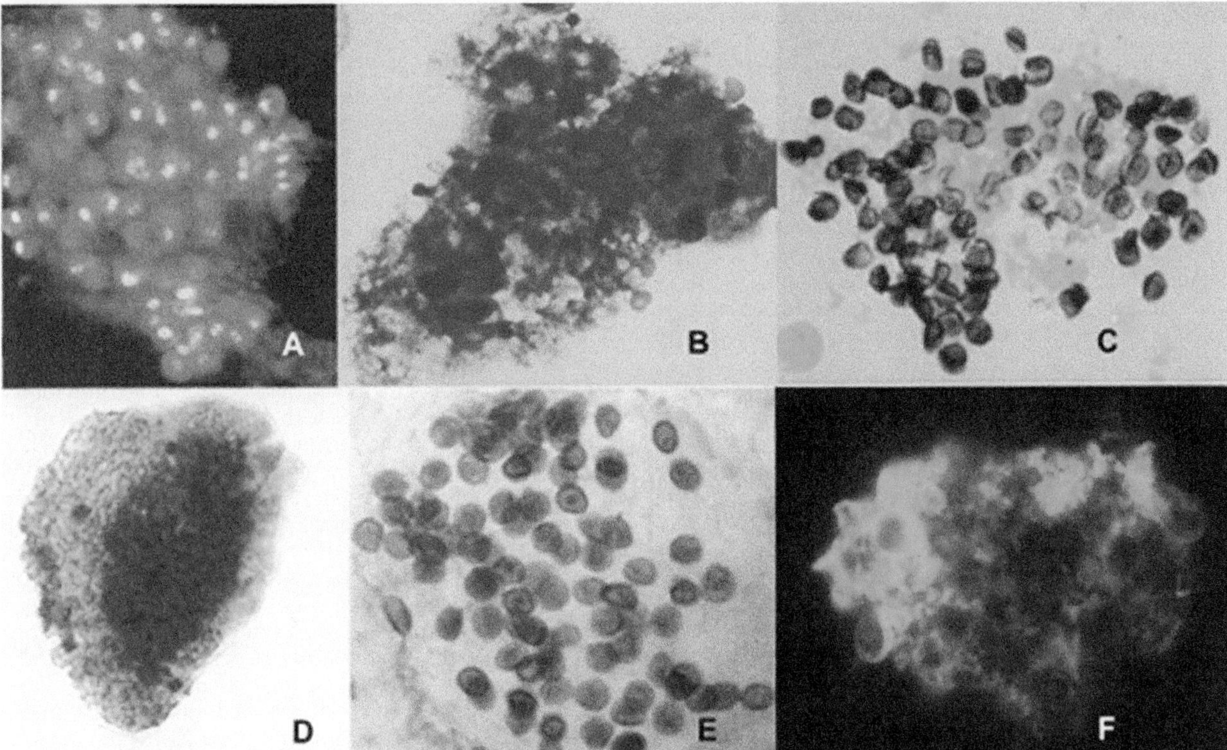

FIGURE 3 Morphology and tinctorial characteristics of *P. jirovecii* in clinical samples stained with various stains (magnification, ×960, unless stated otherwise). (A) Calcofluor stain of BALF. Cyst walls with internal thickenings (double comma) are highly fluorescent (color varies with barrier filter used). (B) Rapid Giemsa-like (Diff-Quick) stain of BALF. Thick cluster of mostly trophic forms (2 to 3 μm) with small reddish-purple nuclei and light blue to red-violet cytoplasm. Boundaries of trophic forms are rarely discernible with this stain. Trophic forms overlay each other to produce darker staining blue cytoplasm. Large dark purple host nuclei are admixed in the cluster. (C) Gomori methenamine silver stain (Grocott) of organisms from BALF. Cyst walls and thickenings (double comma) can be observed as well as collapsed cup shapes and crinkled raisin-like appearance. Note the lack of budding. Trophic forms are not stained with silver-based stains. (D) Papanicolaou stain of BALF. Note the distinctive alveolar cast morphology; magnification, ×400. (E) Toluidine blue O stain of *P. jirovecii* in BALF. Cyst walls are stained light purple. The crinkled appearance of the cysts is illustrated with this stain, as well as darker central staining body. Note the lack of budding with this and other cyst wall stains. Trophic forms are not stained. (F) Direct fluorescent antibody stain of organism cluster from BALF. Note apple-green fluorescence distributed unevenly over the cluster, with accumulation on a cyst wall (lower left of cluster). Structures within the cysts are unstained and appear black.

a reddish purple and the cytoplasm a light blue (Fig. 3B). The cyst wall excludes the dyes and appears with a circumscribed clear zone surrounding the reddish purple nuclei of the daughter forms within. Note the thick mat-type appearance, characteristic of the human infection. Lung cells are often present; their nuclei are much larger than those of *Pneumocystis* and stain a deep reddish purple (Fig. 3B). The rapid variants of the Giemsa stain are recommended for the diagnosis of PCP using BALF, induced sputum, or impression imprints because of the low cost, ease, and rapidity of the staining procedure. Commercial kits such as Protocol Hema 3 (Fisher Scientific Co., Cincinnati, OH) produce similar results. The staining procedure requires less than a minute to perform and all forms of the organism are detected. Since there are approximately 10-fold more trophic forms than cysts, the sensitivity of detection is likely to be increased. This stain also permits assessment of specimen quality of BALFs by demonstration of host alveolar macrophages, which should be present in a productive sample. In addition, the distinctive Giemsa-stained morphological appearance of other organisms likely to be encountered in the lung environment, such as *H. capsulatum*, permits rapid diagnosis of pulmonary infections caused by these pathogens, which may not be detected with other stains. Because background host cells will also stain, training and expertise in interpreting cellular elements in Giemsa-stained preparations are necessary. Laboratories with a lower volume of *P. jirovecii* specimens may prefer to use immunofluorescent staining or one of the other stains described in Table 1.

Direct and indirect fluorescein-conjugated monoclonal anti-*P. jirovecii* antibodies used for immunofluorescent assay (IFA) are targeted to a family of surface glycoproteins that contain both common and distinct epitopes, within and among *Pneumocystis* species (76). Depending on the monoclonal antibody supplied with the kit, staining may target only the cyst form or all forms of the organism. Since trophic forms are more numerous than cysts, kits using those antibodies directed to all forms of the organism, such as Millipore/Sigma's LIGHT DIAGNOSTICS *Pneumocystis carinii* DFA Kit or Bio-Rad's MONOFLUO

Pneumocystis jirovecii IFA Test Kit, direct immunofluorescence assays for the detection of all *P. jirovecii* life cycle forms, are more sensitive. The typical fluorophore conjugated to the antibody or used in an indirect assay is fluorescein isothiocyanate, which produces a brilliant apple-green color. The staining reaction shows a diffuse surface pattern distributed over the entire cluster of organisms (Fig. 3F) and often stains the matrix in which the organisms are embedded. Single cysts/asci will usually appear with a distinctive rim of fluorescence and duller interior fluorescence. It should be noted that kits using a direct staining procedure may not react with *P. jirovecii* on slides fixed in ethanol, and fixation in acetone or vendor recommendations for fixation should be followed.

Papanicolaou stain, frequently used for cytopathological specimens, stains the clusters of extracellular organisms a greenish color, although thick clusters of organisms can collect the stain and appear bicolored with pink to purple and green/turquoise staining as in Fig. 3D. A diagnostic criterion is the presence of distinctive alveolar casts, as shown in panel D. Organism architecture is better observed with the Giemsa-like stains. Gram's stain produces a negative (pink) reaction with poorly defined organism morphology.

However, it is worth noting that low fungal burden, which would limit the microscopic observations found especially in the non-HIV population, could lead to a false negative and a missed diagnosis. Therefore, it is critical to take the whole clinical scenario in perspective along with the histopathological picture.

Serum (1→3)-β-D-Glucan

An assay that measures the serum levels of (1→3)-β-D-glucan (BG) in patients suspected to have *P. jirovecii* is proving to be a successful diagnostic modality, especially for patients who cannot produce appropriate sputum samples or when bronchoscopy may not be safe (77). BG is a component of the ascus (cyst) cell wall and is secreted in significant amounts during infection with *Pneumocystis* spp. Except for *Cryptococcus* and Mucormycetes, most other fungi also secrete BG during infection, but the high amounts observed during infection with *P. jirovecii* have proven to be a useful diagnostic modality. A licensed detection kit uses a modification of the *Limulus* amebocyte lysate pathway. The Fungitell assay reagent (Associates of Cape Cod, Falmouth, MA) is processed to eliminate factor C and is therefore specific for BG (http://www.acciusa.com/clinical/fungitell/index.html). The reagent does not react with other polysaccharides, including beta-glucans with different glycosidic linkages. At present, the Fungitell assay is indicated for presumptive diagnosis of fungal infection and should be used in conjunction with other diagnostic procedures.

Other kits that measure BG include Endosafe-PTS (Charles River Laboratories, Charleston, SC), Fungitec-G (Seikagaku Biobusiness, Tokyo, Japan), beta-Glucan Test (Waco Pure Chemical Industries, Osaka, Japan), and BGSTAR β-Glucan Test (Maruha, Tokyo, Japan). The Endosafe-PTS and beta-Glucan Test kits are intended for research purposes only and not for clinical use. Only the Fungitell assay is FDA approved for use on serum in the United States.

Normal human serum contains low levels of BG, typically 10 to 40 pg/ml, presumably from commensal yeasts present in the alimentary canal and gastrointestinal tract. Values below 60 pg/ml are considered negative for fungal infection; those between 60 and 79 pg/ml are "indeterminate," while values of >80 pg/ml are positive for a fungal infection. The negative predictive value of the test (99.8%) greatly helps to exclude *Pneumocystis* infection in patients who cannot undergo bronchoscopy or in whom the clinical suspicion for *P. jirovecii* pneumonia is low (78).

Cutoff levels specifically for the diagnosis of *P. jirovecii* pneumonia vary slightly. Studies have reported that elevated plasma BG levels of >80 pg/ml have a high predictive value for diagnosis of *P. jirovecii* pneumonia in AIDS patients with respiratory symptoms (79), while another study suggested a threshold of 100 pg/ml (80). One meta-analysis that evaluated the use of BG for diagnosis of *P. jirovecii* pneumonia in a variety of patient settings found the sensitivity to be 94.7% with a range of cutoffs (77). The recommendation from this study was to use a slightly higher cutoff level than the >80 pg/ml that is recommended in general for fungal infections, e.g., 100 pg/ml. Other studies have proposed cutoffs ranging from 300 pg/ml for diagnosis in AIDS-positive patients (81) to a cutoff level for discrimination of 33.5 pg/ml (82).

It is very important to follow the vendor's instructions for handling of patient serum as there can be the potential for environmental contaminants. Serum is the only sample type that is currently approved for use with the Fungitell assay. Serum that is hemolyzed, lipemic, or visually icteric or turbid is not suitable for use with the Fungitell assay. Because a fungal infection is a dynamic process, repeat testing, typically two to three times per week, improves sensitivity. False-positive results have been attributed to infusion of human blood products (immunoglobulins or albumin) (83), use of antibiotics including amoxicillin-clavulanate or piperacillin-tazobactam (84, 85), hemodialysis with cellulose membranes (86), thrombocyte infusion with leukocyte-removing filters (87), serious bacterial infections (88), and severe mucositis (89). It has been argued that as BG is present in some supports, including cellulose filters used in manufacturing, which can possibly explain the false-positive results associated with it (87). Having said that, the full extent of cross-reactivity remains undeciphered, confounded even more when the test is ordered in populations having high risks for false positivity (90). Hence, it is critical that even though the BG assay has high sensitivity for patients with PCP, it should only be used as a rule-out test and positive results should be confirmed with a *Pneumocystis*-specific assay.

In another study, BG was found to be the most reliable serologic biomarker for PCP diagnosis, followed by KL-6, LDH, and SAM. The BG/KL-6 combination test was the most accurate serologic approach for PCP diagnosis, with 94.3% sensitivity and 89.6% specificity (91).

It should be cautioned that measurement of BG levels has not been shown to track with therapeutic efficacy and should not be employed for this purpose. Also, although a high BG level is likely to be diagnostic for PCP, another confirmatory test is recommended at this time.

Nucleic Acid Detection

Amplification of *P. jirovecii* DNA for the diagnosis of PCP in the clinical laboratory setting is a subject of keen interest, though no tests have been approved by the FDA as of this printing (92). Although not available in the United States for clinical use, many have been CE marked and are available outside the United States. With the advent of real-time PCR, detection of *P. jirovecii* is a more sensitive and specific method than microscopic detection methods and the standard PCR or nested PCR techniques (93). However, with this high degree of sensitivity, diagnosis should be in conjunction with clinical manifestations of PCP, as colonization with these organisms can be detected by these highly sensitive assays (3). PCR methods can also be used for identification of potentially resistant strains or species of the organism by targeting specific genes, such as that encoding dihydropteroate synthase, for mutations associated with resistance (94). Although the significance of infections with multiple genotypes of *P. jirovecii* is currently unclear, PCR-based detection systems would also be able to detect PCP caused by single or multiple genotypes. Quantitative PCR tests for PCP or TaqMan probes are available (e.g., *Pneumocystis jirovecii* Detection Kits, Norgen Biotek Corp.; RealStar *Pneumocystis jirovecii* PCR Kit, Altona Diagnostics, San Francisco, CA), as are multiplex real-time PCR assays that purport to have the ability for both diagnosis and DHPS mutations (PneumoGenius, PathoNostics, The Netherlands); none have been approved for clinical use in the United States, although several are available as CE marked outside the United States.

In-house detection of *P. jirovecii* by PCR typically targets the mtLSU-rRNA gene, intertranscribed spacer regions, or the major surface glycoprotein (MSG) family of genes (95, 96). The mtLSU-rRNA and MSG genes are present in multiple copies per organism and provide the most sensitive target for detection. DNA can be isolated from clinical samples by using commercial kits such as the PhaseLock System (Eppendorf Scientific, Westbury, NY) or a series of products designed for the clinical laboratory by vendors such as Qiagen (Valencia, CA). The primers targeting the mtLSU-rRNA and PCR conditions are listed in Table 2 for standard PCR.

A commercial real-time PCR assay, the MycAssay Pneumocystis kit (Myconostica Ltd., Cambridge, United Kingdom), was evaluated against direct immunofluorescence microscopy, real-time PCR (*cdc2* gene of *P. jirovecii*), and conventional PCR directed to the mtLSU-rRNA gene (93). Bronchoalveolar lavage samples were liquefied with BD BBL MycoPrep (BD Diagnostics, Sparks, MD) prior to DNA extraction with a MycXtra fungal DNA extraction kit (Myconostica). The kit contains proprietary reagents including primers and a molecular beacon targeting the mtLSU-rRNA. The test is considered positive if the cycle threshold (CT) value is <39.0 and negative if the CT is 39.0, or undetermined (failure to cross the threshold) without exponential amplification, while exponential amplification with CT values of <39.0 is considered positive. The MycAssay was superior to all other methods, including the *cdc2* real-time PCR assay (100% sensitivity, 86% specificity) and the mtLSU-rRNA conventional PCR and sequencing assay (100% sensitivity, 98.5% specificity), with 100% positive and negative predictive values. At present, the MycAssay is not for sale for diagnostic use in the United States, but it is available outside the United States.

Another highly sensitive and almost fully automated real-time PCR assay targets the multicopy MSG genes on a BD MAX platform (BD Diagnostics, Sparks, MD) (96). After treatment with dithiothreitol for liquefaction of respiratory specimens, the samples are loaded into extraction tubes and DNA or RNA is automatically extracted and added to the PCR master mix, where the MSG target gene, internal control (Texas Red), and a sample process control (Cy5) are amplified. The limit of detection is 10 copies/ml of a plasmid per PCR, which equated to 500 copies in BALF. Accurate quantitation was observed over a 7- to 8-log range. This fully automated method showed a good quantitative correlation with the reference PCR (R^2 = 0.82). This method permits pre-aliquotting of PCR reagents; allows the use of the entire system outside a specified PCR area, reducing cross-contamination; and requires little technician input, reducing potential human error. Like other nucleic acid-based detection methods, the BD Max platform has not yet received FDA approval. The use of such kits demands evaluation in the clinical setting and should be approached with caution. Thresholds of each assay to distinguish colonization versus infection remain a concern. In a recent study using

TABLE 2 PCR detection of *Pneumocystis*: suggested primers and conditions

Gene target	Primers	Sequence (5′ to 3′)	Expected product size (bp)	Conditions
mtLSU-rRNA				
Primary[a]	pAZ102-E pAZ102-H	GATGGCTGTTTCCAAGCCCA GTGTACGTTGCAAAGTACTC	346	94°C × 1 min; 55°C × 1 min; 72°C × 2 min; 40 cycles; termination: 72°C × 5 min
Nested[b]	pAZ102-X pAZ102-Y	GTGAAATACAAATCGGACTAGG TCACTTAATATTAATTGGGGAGC	267	94°C × 1 min; 55°C × 1 min; 72°C × 2 min; 35 cycles; termination: 72°C × 5 min
DHPS[c]				
Round 1	F1 B_{45}	CCTGGTATTAAACCAGTTTTGCC CAATTTAATAAATTTCTTTCCAAATAGCATC		94°C × 5 min; 92°C × 30 s; 52°C × 30 s; 72°C × 1 min; 35 cycles; termination: 72°C × 5 min
Round 2	A_{HUM} BN	GCGCCTACACATATTATGGCCATTTTAAATC GGAACTTTCAACTTGGCAACCAC	300	94°C × 5 min; 92°C × 30 s; 55°C × 30s; 72°C × 1 min; 35 cycles; termination: 72°C × 5 min

[a]Mitochondrial large subunit rRNA; from reference 111.
[b]From reference 112.
[c]Dihydropteroate synthase gene; from references 30 and 113.

real-time PCR with mtLSU-rRNA as the target gene, cutoff values of 1.6×10^3 copies/ml and an upper cutoff level of 2×10^4 copies/ml achieved 100% sensitivity and 100% specificity for determining colonization versus infection. Combined with a 100-pg/ml threshold for BG, these suggested copy numbers could discriminate PCP from colonization (95).

ISOLATION PROCEDURES

Detection of *Pneumocystis* by growth in artificial media or tissue culture is not a diagnostic option, since no species of this genus can be continuously cultivated outside the mammalian lung.

TYPING SYSTEMS

There is no consensus for a typing system for *P. jirovecii*.

SEROLOGIC TESTS

Serological assays to detect anti-*P. jirovecii* antibodies are useful for epidemiological studies but not for diagnosis of PCP. Most human beings become seropositive for *P. jirovecii* antibodies early in their childhood, between 2 and 4 years of age, and likely come in contact with the organism many times over during their lifetime. In some cases, a rise in antibody titer can be detected in some PCP patients over time; in others, antibody titers can just as frequently drop or remain the same.

A number of other laboratory tests have been used for the diagnosis of PCP, but none provides a definitive diagnosis. These include an increased arterial-alveolar gradient, an elevation of serum lactic dehydrogenase levels, and gallium and diethylenetriamine pentaacetic scans. The latter two tests are not routinely used due to higher costs. Reduced S-adenosylmethionine (AdoMet) levels have been reported to reflect infection with *P. jirovecii* (97–99); however, another study conducted to evaluate the diagnostic utility of AdoMet versus BG levels found that AdoMet levels did not discriminate between infected and noninfected patients, while BG levels correlated with a high level of sensitivity and specificity with a cutoff of 60 pg/ml (100).

ANTIMICROBIAL SUSCEPTIBILITIES

Two drugs comprise the mainstay of therapy for acute PCP, trimethoprim-sulfamethoxazole (TMP-SMX) and pentamidine isethionate (66). Secondary treatments, such as atovaquone and clindamycin-primaquine, have been used for milder forms of the disease, and treatment with corticosteroids has been used to improve clinical outcome in some patients. However, there have been significant rates of relapse and recurrence with such second-line therapies (101).

The initial approach to treatment is determined primarily by the level of oxygenation and/or A-a gradient. Mild disease is classified as patients who have an A-a gradient of <35 mmHg and/or a partial pressure of arterial oxygen of >70 mmHg. In these patients, oral therapy is recommended. Moderate-disease patients have an A-a gradient of >35 and <45 and/or a partial pressure of arterial oxygen >60 mmHg and <70 mmHg. In these patients, oral therapy is also recommended unless there are issues with oral absorption. Severe disease is when patients have an A-a gradient of >45 mmHg and/or the oxygen partial pressure is <60 mmHg. In this category, patients should receive intravenous therapy until they are clinically stable (e.g., oxygen partial pressure of >60 mmHg, respiratory rate <25) and can then be transitioned to an oral regimen.

TMP-SMX is a drug combination that targets the enzymes dihydrofolate reductase (trimethoprim) and dihydropteroate synthase (sulfamethoxazole), both integral steps in the folic acid pathway. The standard therapeutic dose of TMP-SMX is 15 to 20 mg/kg intravenously or orally daily in three or four divided doses. Steroids are an important adjunctive therapy for patients with moderate to severe infections associated with HIV infection. It is thought that deleterious inflammatory responses are reduced with their administration. Steroids are usually given in high doses for 5 to 7 days, with a reduction in dose and continued treatment for an additional 2 weeks. Steroid treatment may be started at the same time as therapy and withdrawn before antimicrobial treatment is complete. The drug of first choice for PCP prophylaxis is also TMP-SMX, with a daily or thrice-weekly administration of 960 mg (102). If patients are intolerant to TMP-SMX, oral dapsone (100 mg/day), aerosolized pentamidine (300 mg every 4 weeks), or oral atovaquone (at least 1,500 mg/day) is recommended.

Pentamidine is a cationic diamidine that was first used to treat African trypanosomiasis, or sleeping sickness, and later found to be efficacious as PCP therapy. The mode of action of this drug is not known but may involve suppression of mitochondrial activity, inhibition of topoisomerases, or binding of the minor groove of DNA (103). Pentamidine and TMP-SMX have significant side effects including nephrotoxicity and, in the case of TMP-SMX, severe rash, fever, and neutropenia, which often necessitate a change to alternative treatment. In a study of HIV-1-infected patients with first episode PCP, only 64% completed TMP-SMX treatment (104). Neither drug is considered pneumocysticidal. Administration of pentamidine via an aerosolized route delivers the drug efficiently to the areas of infection, but it has been shown to be less effective than other drugs in the treatment of PCP and is associated with dispersal of *P. jirovecii* and other respiratory pathogens.

PCP remains refractory to most common antifungal drugs such as the azoles or amphotericin B. Echinocandins, BG inhibitors, are a relatively new family of antifungal drugs that are fungicidal against candidal infections and fungistatic against *Aspergillus* infections (105). Reports of the efficacy of echinocandins for PCP have been contradictory, due in large part to the anecdotal nature of the reports (106, 107). Systematic studies of three clinically available echinocandins—caspofungin, anidulafungin, and micafungin—in rodent models of PCP revealed dramatic reductions in cysts/asci, but much less of an effect on trophic forms, suggesting that their use as monotherapies would not be efficacious, but they may provide benefit in combination with TMP-SMX (18).

Mutations in the DHPS gene of *P. jirovecii* associated with sulfa resistance in other pathogens have been identified in about 50% of the PCP isolates in certain geographic areas (108). The presence of the mutations in the DHPS gene of *P. jirovecii* was associated with previous TMP-SMX therapy, but the impact of the mutations in terms of outcome and response to therapy is not yet clear.

It may become desirable in the future to track the emergence of *P. jirovecii* strains that are resistant to TMP-SMX or to evaluate the potential for therapeutic response. In anticipation of this goal, the primers targeting the regions of the dihydropteroate gene (DHPS) associated with sulfa resistance in other pathogens are shown in Table 2. The nucleotide (nt) positions at which the mutations occur are nt 165 and nt 171. Changes at these nucleotide positions result in changes in amino acids. The following are the four genotypes for this target gene: genotype 1, nt 165 (A)/nt 171 (C) = Thr/Pro; genotype 2, nt 165 (G)/nt 171 (C) = Ala/Pro; genotype 3, nt 165 (A)/nt 171 (T) = Thr/Ser; and genotype 4, nt 165 (G)/nt 171 (T) = Ala/Ser. The last genotype, GT, represents a double mutation in the DHPS gene that has been associated with drug resistance and is emerging as the dominant genotype for *P. jirovecii* isolates in some areas. Although atovaquone resistance in PCP has been associated with mutations in the mitochondrial cytochrome b_1 gene (109), resistance to TMP-SMX is much more problematic, and identification of mutations in the DHPS gene will likely be the more critical factor in the clinical setting (110).

EVALUATION, INTERPRETATION, AND REPORTING OF RESULTS

The microscopic demonstration of *P. jirovecii* in tissue and fluids by staining with Gomori methenamine silver or a rapid variant of the Wright-Giemsa stain, by IFA, or by other stains such as Papanicolaou stain should be considered sufficient for diagnosis. In many cases, the fungi are present as large clusters of organisms, in which it may be difficult to differentiate the life cycle stages within the dense assemblage if using the Wright-Giemsa or Papanicolaou stains. Because of this, it is recommended that a stain that only visualizes the cyst form of *Pneumocystis* (e.g., Gomori methenamine silver) should be used for diagnosis because it is easier to interpret. The rapid stains can be used as a preliminary diagnostic technique, followed by the definitive cyst stain. IFA can be helpful in laboratories that are less familiar with *P. jirovecii* morphology, but this requires a fluorescence microscope, which may not always be available. The outcome of IFA staining depends on the monoclonal antibody target. Some kits use monoclonal antibodies targeting the surface glycoprotein present on all the life cycle stages, but these also stain the dense matrix in which *P. jirovecii* is embedded, resulting in a highly fluorescent mass with little detail. Since there are no other species of the genus that are known to cause pneumonia in humans, the presence of these fungi can be reported as *P. jirovecii* or *Pneumocystis* spp. The name "*Pneumocystis carinii*" should not be used, as this species infects rats. Treatment should be initiated upon demonstration of *P. jirovecii* by microscopic methods and based on clinical evaluation of the patient. Moderate to severe PCP is treated with a combination of corticosteroids and intravenous TMP-SMX, clindamycin/primaquine, or pentamidine. Mild to moderate PCP is treated with TMP-SMX, TMP-dapsone, pentamidine, atovaquone, or clindamycin/primaquine (62).

REFERENCES

1. **Ng VL, Yajko DM, Hadley WK.** 1997. Extrapulmonary pneumocystosis. *Clin Microbiol Rev* **10:**401–418.
2. **Telzak EE, Cote RJ, Gold JW, Campbell SW, Armstrong D.** 1990. Extrapulmonary *Pneumocystis carinii* infections. *Rev Infect Dis* **12:**380–386.
3. **Morris A, Norris KA.** 2012. Colonization by *Pneumocystis jirovecii* and its role in disease. *Clin Microbiol Rev* **25:**297–317.
4. **Mori S, Sugimoto M.** 2015. *Pneumocystis jirovecii* pneumonia in rheumatoid arthritis patients: risks and prophylaxis recommendations. *Clin Med Insights Circ Respir Pulm Med* **9**(Suppl 1)**:**29–40.
5. **Redhead SA, Cushion MT, Frenkel JK, Stringer JR.** 2006. Pneumocystis and *Trypanosoma cruzi*: nomenclature and typifications. *J Eukaryot Microbiol* **53:**2–11.
6. **Hibbett DS, et al.** 2007. A higher-level phylogenetic classification of the Fungi. *Mycol Res* **111:**509–547.
7. **Frenkel JK.** 1976. *Pneumocystis jiroveci* n. sp. from man: morphology, physiology, and immunology in relation to pathology. *Natl Cancer Inst Monogr* **43:**13–30.
8. **Cushion MT, Keely SP, Stringer JR.** 2004. Molecular and phenotypic description of *Pneumocystis wakefieldiae* sp. nov., a new species in rats. *Mycologia* **96:**429–438.
9. **Keely SP, Fischer JM, Cushion MT, Stringer JR.** 2004. Phylogenetic identification of *Pneumocystis murina* sp. nov., a new species in laboratory mice. *Microbiology* **150:**1153–1165.
10. **Frenkel JK.** 1999. Pneumocystis pneumonia, an immunodeficiency-dependent disease (IDD): a critical historical overview. *J Eukaryot Microbiol* **46:**89S–92S.
11. **Dei-Cas E, Chabé M, Moukhlis R, Durand-Joly I, Aliouat el M, Stringer JR, Cushion M, Noël C, de Hoog GS, Guillot J, Viscogliosi E.** 2006. *Pneumocystis oryctolagi* sp. nov., an uncultured fungus causing pneumonia in rabbits at weaning: review of current knowledge, and description of a new taxon on genotypic, phylogenetic and phenotypic bases. *FEMS Microbiol Rev* **30:**853–871.
12. **Hughes WT.** 1982. Natural mode of acquisition for de novo infection with *Pneumocystis carinii*. *J Infect Dis* **145:**842–848.
13. **Choukri F, Menotti J, Sarfati C, Lucet JC, Nevez G, Garin YJ, Derouin F, Totet A.** 2010. Quantification and spread of *Pneumocystis jirovecii* in the surrounding air of patients with Pneumocystis pneumonia. *Clin Infect Dis* **51:**259–265.
14. **Inkster T, Dodd S, Gunson R, Imrie L, Spalding E, Packer S, Deighan C, Daly C, Coia J, Imtiaz T, McGuffie C, Wilson R, Bal AM.** 2017. Investigation of outbreaks of *Pneumocystis jirovecii* pneumonia in two Scottish renal units. *J Hosp Infect* **96:**151–156.
15. **Chapman JR, Marriott DJ, Chen SC, MacDonald PS.** 2013. Post-transplant *Pneumocystis jirovecii* pneumonia—a re-emerged public health problem? *Kidney Int* **84:**240–243.
16. **Mulpuru S, Knoll G, Weir C, Desjardins M, Johnson D, Gorn I, Fairhead T, Bissonnette J, Bruce N, Toye B, Suh K, Roth V.** 2016. Pneumocystis pneumonia outbreak among renal transplant recipients at a North American transplant center: risk factors and implications for infection control. *Am J Infect Control* **44:**425–431.
17. **Vindrios W, Argy N, Le Gal S, Lescure FX, Massias L, Le MP, Wolff M, Yazdanpanah Y, Nevez G, Houze S, Dorent R, Lucet JC.** 2017. Outbreak of *Pneumocystis jirovecii* infection among heart transplant recipients: molecular investigation and management of an inter-human transmission. *Clin Infect Dis* **65:**1120–1126.
18. **Cushion MT, Linke MJ, Ashbaugh A, Sesterhenn T, Collins MS, Lynch K, Brubaker R, Walzer PD.** 2010. Echinocandin treatment of pneumocystis pneumonia in rodent models depletes cysts leaving trophic burdens that cannot transmit the infection. *PLoS One* **5:**e8524.
19. **Cushion MT, Collins MS.** 2011. Susceptibility of Pneumocystis to echinocandins in suspension and biofilm cultures. *Antimicrob Agents Chemother* **55:**4513–4518.
20. **Ma L, Chen Z, Huang da W, Kutty G, Ishihara M, Wang H, Abouelleil A, Bishop L, Davey E, Deng R, Deng X, Fan L, Fantoni G, Fitzgerald M, Gogineni E, Goldberg JM, Handley G, Hu X, Huber C, Jiao X, Jones K, Levin JZ, Liu Y, Macdonald P, Melnikov A, Raley C, Sassi M, Sherman BT, Song X, Sykes S, Tran B, Walsh L, Xia Y, Yang J, Young S, Zeng Q, Zheng X, Stephens R, Nusbaum C, Birren BW, Azadi P, Lempicki RA, Cuomo CA, Kovacs JA.** 2016. Genome analysis of three *Pneumocystis* species reveals adaptation mechanisms to life exclusively in mammalian hosts. *Nat Commun* **7:**10740.
21. **Almeida JM, Cissé OH, Fonseca Á, Pagni M, Hauser PM.** 2015. Comparative genomics suggests primary homothallism of Pneumocystis species. *MBio* **6:**e02250-14.
22. **Cushion MT.** 2004. Pneumocystis: unraveling the cloak of obscurity. *Trends Microbiol* **12:**243–249.
23. **Cushion MT, Linke MJ, Collins M, Keely SP, Stringer JR.** 1999. The minimum number of *Pneumocystis carinii* f. sp. *carinii* organisms required to establish infections is very low. *J Eukaryot Microbiol* **46:**111S.

24. **Gigliotti F, Harmsen AG, Wright TW.** 2003. Characterization of transmission of *Pneumocystis carinii* f. sp. *muris* through immunocompetent BALB/c mice. *Infect Immun* **71:** 3852–3856.
25. **Cushion MT, Kaselis M, Stringer SL, Stringer JR.** 1993. Genetic stability and diversity of *Pneumocystis carinii* infecting rat colonies. *Infect Immun* **61:**4801–4813.
26. **Nevez G, Le Gal S, Noel N, Wynckel A, Huguenin A, Le Govic Y, Pougnet L, Virmaux M, Toubas D, Bajolet O.** 2017. Investigation of nosocomial pneumocystis infections: usefulness of longitudinal screening of epidemic and post-epidemic pneumocystis genotypes. *J Hosp Infect* **99:**332–345.
27. **Medrano FJ, Montes-Cano M, Conde M, de la Horra C, Respaldiza N, Gasch A, Perez-Lozano MJ, Varela JM, Calderon EJ.** 2005. *Pneumocystis jirovecii* in general population. *Emerg Infect Dis* **11:**245–250.
28. **Sun L, Huang MJ, An YJ, Guo ZZ.** 2009. [An epidemiologic study on Pneumocystis pneumonia in non-HIV infected patients in China]. *Zhonghua Liu Xing Bing Xue Za Zhi* **30:**348–351.
29. **Vera C, Aguilar YA, Vélez LA, Rueda ZV.** 2017. High transient colonization by *Pneumocystis jirovecii* between mothers and newborn. *Eur J Pediatr* **176:**1619–1627.
30. **Beard CB, Carter JL, Keely SP, Huang L, Pieniazek NJ, Moura IN, Roberts JM, Hightower AW, Bens MS, Freeman AR, Lee S, Stringer JR, Duchin JS, del Rio C, Rimland D, Baughman RP, Levy DA, Dietz VJ, Simon P, Navin TR.** 2000. Genetic variation in *Pneumocystis carinii* isolates from different geographic regions: implications for transmission. *Emerg Infect Dis* **6:**265–272.
31. **Yazaki H, Goto N, Uchida K, Kobayashi T, Gatanaga H, Oka S.** 2009. Outbreak of *Pneumocystis jiroveci* pneumonia in renal transplant recipients: *P. jiroveci* is contagious to the susceptible host. *Transplantation* **88:**380–385.
32. **Fritzsche C, Riebold D, Fuehrer A, Mitzner A, Klammt S, Mueller-Hilke B, Reisinger EC.** 2013. *Pneumocystis jirovecii* colonization among renal transplant recipients. *Nephrology (Carlton)* **18:**382–387.
33. **Spencer L, Ukwu M, Alexander T, Valadez K, Liu L, Frederick T, Kovacs A, Morris A.** 2008. Epidemiology of Pneumocystis colonization in families. *Clin Infect Dis* **46:** 1237–1240.
34. **Peglow SL, Smulian AG, Linke MJ, Pogue CL, Nurre S, Crisler J, Phair J, Gold JW, Armstrong D, Walzer PD.** 1990. Serologic responses to *Pneumocystis carinii* antigens in health and disease. *J Infect Dis* **161:**296–306.
35. **Pifer LL, Hughes WT, Stagno S, Woods D.** 1978. *Pneumocystis carinii* infection: evidence for high prevalence in normal and immunosuppressed children. *Pediatrics* **61:**35–41.
36. **Vargas SL, Hughes WT, Santolaya ME, Ulloa AV, Ponce CA, Cabrera CE, Cumsille F, Gigliotti F.** 2001. Search for primary infection by *Pneumocystis carinii* in a cohort of normal, healthy infants. *Clin Infect Dis* **32:**855–861.
37. **Kaur N, Mahl TC.** 2007. *Pneumocystis jiroveci* (*carinii*) pneumonia after infliximab therapy: a review of 84 cases. *Dig Dis Sci* **52:**1481–1484.
38. **Tanaka M, Sakai R, Koike R, Komano Y, Nanki T, Sakai F, Sugiyama H, Matsushima H, Kojima T, Ohta S, Ishibe Y, Sawabe T, Ota Y, Ohishi K, Miyazato H, Nonomura Y, Saito K, Tanaka Y, Nagasawa H, Takeuchi T, Nakajima A, Ohtsubo H, Onishi M, Goto Y, Dobashi H, Miyasaka N, Harigai M.** 2012. *Pneumocystis jirovecii* pneumonia associated with etanercept treatment in patients with rheumatoid arthritis: a retrospective review of 15 cases and analysis of risk factors. *Mod Rheumatol* **22:**849–858.
39. **Ahn IE, Jerussi T, Farooqui M, Tian X, Wiestner A, Gea-Banacloche J.** 2016. Atypical *Pneumocystis jirovecii* pneumonia in previously untreated patients with CLL on single-agent ibrutinib. *Blood* **128:**1940–1943.
40. **Chamilos G, Lionakis MS, Kontoyiannis DP.** 2017. Call for action: invasive fungal infections associated with ibrutinib and other small molecule kinase inhibitors targeting immune signaling pathways. *Clin Infect Dis* **66:**140–148.
41. **Hoarau G, Le Gal S, Zunic P, Poubeau P, Antok E, Jaubert J, Nevez G, Picot S.** 2017. Evaluation of quantitative FTD-*Pneumocystis jirovecii* kit for Pneumocystis infection diagnosis. *Diagn Microbiol Infect Dis* **89:**212–217.
42. **Hay JW, Osmond DH, Jacobson MA.** 1988. Projecting the medical costs of AIDS and ARC in the United States. *J Acquir Immune Defic Syndr* **1:**466–485.
43. **Buchacz K, Baker RK, Palella FJ Jr, Chmiel JS, Lichtenstein KA, Novak RM, Wood KC, Brooks JT, HOPS Investigators.** 2010. AIDS-defining opportunistic illnesses in US patients, 1994–2007: a cohort study. *AIDS* **24:** 1549–1559.
44. **Buchacz K, Lau B, Jing Y, Bosch R, Abraham AG, Gill MJ, Silverberg MJ, Goedert JJ, Sterling TR, Althoff KN, Martin JN, Burkholder G, Gandhi N, Samji H, Patel P, Rachlis A, Thorne JE, Napravnik S, Henry K, Mayor A, Gebo K, Gange SJ, Moore RD, Brooks JT, North American AIDS Cohort Collaboration on Research and Design (NA-ACCORD) of IeDEA.** 2016. Incidence of AIDS-defining opportunistic infections in a multicohort analysis of HIV-infected persons in the United States and Canada, 2000–2010. *J Infect Dis* **214:**862–872.
45. **Maini R, Henderson KL, Sheridan EA, Lamagni T, Nichols G, Delpech V, Phin N.** 2013. Increasing Pneumocystis pneumonia, England, UK, 2000–2010. *Emerg Infect Dis* **19:** 386–392.
46. **Radhi S, Alexander T, Ukwu M, Saleh S, Morris A.** 2008. Outcome of HIV-associated Pneumocystis pneumonia in hospitalized patients from 2000 through 2003. *BMC Infect Dis* **8:**118.
47. **Walzer PD, Evans HE, Copas AJ, Edwards SG, Grant AD, Miller RF.** 2008. Early predictors of mortality from *Pneumocystis jirovecii* pneumonia in HIV-infected patients: 1985–2006. *Clin Infect Dis* **46:**625–633.
48. **Fisk DT, Meshnick S, Kazanjian PH.** 2003. *Pneumocystis carinii* pneumonia in patients in the developing world who have acquired immunodeficiency syndrome. *Clin Infect Dis* **36:**70–78.
49. **Tellez I, Barragán M, Franco-Paredes C, Petraro P, Nelson K, Del Rio C.** 2008. *Pneumocystis jiroveci* pneumonia in patients with AIDS in the inner city: a persistent and deadly opportunistic infection. *Am J Med Sci* **335:**192–197.
50. **Monnet X, Vidal-Petiot E, Osman D, Hamzaoui O, Durrbach A, Goujard C, Miceli C, Bourée P, Richard C.** 2008. Critical care management and outcome of severe Pneumocystis pneumonia in patients with and without HIV infection. *Crit Care* **12:**R28.
51. **Yoshida Y, Takahashi Y, Minemura N, Ueda Y, Yamashita H, Kaneko H, Mimori A.** 2012. Prognosis of pneumocystis pneumonia complicated in patients with rheumatoid arthritis (RA) and non-RA rheumatic diseases. *Mod Rheumatol* **22:**509–514.
52. **Mofenson LM, Brady MT, Danner SP, Dominguez KL, Hazra R, Handelsman E, Havens P, Nesheim S, Read JS, Serchuck L, Van Dyke R, Centers for Disease Control and Prevention, National Institutes of Health, HIV Medicine Association of the Infectious Diseases Society of America, Pediatric Infectious Diseases Society, American Academy of Pediatrics.** 2009. Guidelines for the prevention and treatment of opportunistic infections among HIV-exposed and HIV-infected children: recommendations from CDC, the National Institutes of Health, the HIV Medicine Association of the Infectious Diseases Society of America, the Pediatric Infectious Diseases Society, and the American Academy of Pediatrics. *MMWR Recomm Rep* **58**(RR-11):1–166.
53. **Kottom TJ, Burgess JW, Limper AH.** 2011. *Pneumocystis carinii* interactions with lung epithelial cells and matrix proteins induce expression and activity of the PcSte20 kinase with subsequent phosphorylation of the downstream cell wall biosynthesis kinase PcCbk1. *Infect Immun* **79:**4157–4164.
54. **Limper AH, Standing JE, Hoffman OA, Castro M, Neese LW.** 1993. Vitronectin binds to *Pneumocystis carinii* and mediates organism attachment to cultured lung epithelial cells. *Infect Immun* **61:**4302–4309.

55. **Huang L, Crothers K.** 2009. HIV-associated opportunistic pneumonias. *Respirology* **14:**474–485.
56. **Rojas P, Friaza V, García E, de la Horra C, Vargas SL, Calderón EJ, Pavón A.** 2017. Early acquisition of *Pneumocystis jirovecii* colonization and potential association with respiratory distress syndrome in preterm newborn infants. *Clin Infect Dis* **65:**976–981.
57. **Madhi SA, Cutland C, Ismail K, O'Reilly C, Mancha A, Klugman KP.** 2002. Ineffectiveness of trimethoprim-sulfamethoxazole prophylaxis and the importance of bacterial and viral coinfections in African children with *Pneumocystis carinii* pneumonia. *Clin Infect Dis* **35:**1120–1126.
58. **Punpanich W, Groome M, Muhe L, Qazi SA, Madhi SA.** 2011. Systematic review on the etiology and antibiotic treatment of pneumonia in human immunodeficiency virus-infected children. *Pediatr Infect Dis J* **30:**e192–e202.
59. **Gajdusek DC.** 1957. *Pneumocystis carinii*: etiologic agent of interstitial plasma cell pneumonia of premature and young infants. *Pediatrics* **19:**543–565.
60. **Fatti GL, Zar HJ, Swingler GH.** 2006. Clinical indicators of *Pneumocystis jiroveci* pneumonia (PCP) in South African children infected with the human immunodeficiency virus. *Int J Infect Dis* **10:**282–285.
61. **Huang YS, Yang JJ, Lee NY, Chen GJ, Ko WC, Sun HY, Hung CC.** 2017. Treatment of *Pneumocystis jirovecii* pneumonia in HIV-infected patients: a review. *Expert Rev Anti Infect Ther* **15:**873–892.
62. **Walzer PD, Smulian AG.**2010. *Pneumocystis* species, p 3377–3390. *In* G.L. Mandell JEB, Dolin R (ed), *Mandell, Douglas and Bennet's Principles and Practice of Infectious Diseases*. Churchill Livingstone Elsevier, Philadelphia, PA.
63. **Chou CW, Lin FC, Tsai HC, Chang SC.** 2014. The impact of concomitant pulmonary infection on immune dysregulation in *Pneumocystis jirovecii* pneumonia. *BMC Pulm Med* **14:**182.
64. **Kanne JP, Yandow DR, Meyer CA.** 2012. *Pneumocystis jiroveci* pneumonia: high-resolution CT findings in patients with and without HIV infection. *AJR Am J Roentgenol* **198:**W555-W561.
65. **Czarniak P, Załuska-Leśniewska I, Zagożdżon I, Zurowska A.** 2013. Difficulties in diagnosing severe *Pneumocystis jiroveci* pneumonia after rituximab therapy for steroid-dependent nephrotic syndrome. *Pediatr Nephrol* **28:**987–988.
66. **Kovacs JA, Gill VJ, Meshnick S, Masur H.** 2001. New insights into transmission, diagnosis, and drug treatment of *Pneumocystis carinii* pneumonia. *JAMA* **286:**2450–2460.
67. **Hadley WK, Ng VL.** 1999. *Pneumocystis*, p 1200–1211. *In* Murray PM, Baron EJ, Pfaller MA, Tenover FC, Yolken RH. (ed), *Manual of Clinical Microbiology*, 7th ed ASM Press, Washington, DC.
68. **Birriel JA Jr, Adams JA, Saldana MA, Mavunda K, Goldfinger S, Vernon D, Holzman B, McKey RM Jr.** 1991. Role of flexible bronchoscopy and bronchoalveolar lavage in the diagnosis of pediatric acquired immunodeficiency syndrome-related pulmonary disease. *Pediatrics* **87:**897–899.
69. **Ng VL, Gartner I, Weymouth LA, Goodman CD, Hopewell PC, Hadley WK.** 1989. The use of mucolysed induced sputum for the identification of pulmonary pathogens associated with human immunodeficiency virus infection. *Arch Pathol Lab Med* **113:**488–493.
70. **To KK, Wong SC, Xu T, Poon RW, Mok KY, Chan JF, Cheng VC, Chan KH, Hung IF, Yuen KY.** 2013. Use of nasopharyngeal aspirate for diagnosis of pneumocystis pneumonia. *J Clin Microbiol* **51:**1570–1574.
71. **Tsolaki AG, Miller RF, Wakefield AE.** 1999. Oropharyngeal samples for genotyping and monitoring response to treatment in AIDS patients with *Pneumocystis carinii* pneumonia. *J Med Microbiol* **48:**897–905.
72. **Respaldiza N, Montes-Cano MA, Friaza V, Muñoz-Lobato F, Medrano FJ, Varela JM, Calderon E, De la Horra C.** 2006. Usefulness of oropharyngeal washings for identifying *Pneumocystis jirovecii* carriers. *J Eukaryot Microbiol* **53**(Suppl 1): S100–S101.
73. **Chandra P, Delaney MD, Tuazon CU.** 1988. Role of special stains in the diagnosis of *Pneumocystis carinii* infection from bronchial washing specimens in patients with the acquired immune deficiency syndrome. *Acta Cytol* **32:**105–108.
74. **Mahan CT, Sale GE.** 1978. Rapid methenamine silver stain for Pneumocystis and fungi. *Arch Pathol Lab Med* **102:** 351–352.
75. **Schumann GB, Swensen JJ.** 1991. Comparison of Papanicolaou's stain with the Gomori methenamine silver (GMS) stain for the cytodiagnosis of *Pneumocystis carinii* in bronchoalveolar lavage (BAL) fluid. *Am J Clin Pathol* **95:** 583–586.
76. **Keely SP, Stringer JR.** 2009. Complexity of the MSG gene family of *Pneumocystis carinii*. *BMC Genomics* **10:**367.
77. **Karageorgopoulos DE, Qu JM, Korbila IP, Zhu YG, Vasileiou VA, Falagas ME.** 2011. Accuracy of beta-D-glucan for the diagnosis of *Pneumocystis jirovecii* pneumonia: a meta-analysis. *Clin Microbiol Infect* **19:**39–49.
78. **Held J, Koch MS, Reischl U, Danner T, Serr A.** 2011. Serum (1→3)-β-D-glucan measurement as an early indicator of *Pneumocystis jirovecii* pneumonia and evaluation of its prognostic value. *Clin Microbiol Infect* **17:**595–602.
79. **Wood BR, Komarow L, Zolopa AR, Finkelman MA, Powderly WG, Sax PE.** 2013. Test performance of blood beta-glucan for *Pneumocystis jirovecii* pneumonia in patients with AIDS and respiratory symptoms. *AIDS* **27:**967–972.
80. **Damiani C, Le Gal S, Lejeune D, Brahimi N, Virmaux M, Nevez G, Totet A.** 2011. Serum (1→3)-beta-D-glucan levels in primary infection and pulmonary colonization with *Pneumocystis jirovecii*. *J Clin Microbiol* **49:**2000–2002.
81. **Salerno D, Mushatt D, Myers L, Zhuang Y, de la Rua N, Calderon EJ, Welsh DA.** 2014. Serum and bal beta-D-glucan for the diagnosis of Pneumocystis pneumonia in HIV positive patients. *Respir Med* **108:**1688–1695.
82. **Tasaka S, Hasegawa N, Kobayashi S, Yamada W, Nishimura T, Takeuchi T, Ishizaka A.** 2007. Serum indicators for the diagnosis of pneumocystis pneumonia. *Chest* **131:** 1173–1180.
83. **Ikemura K, Ikegami K, Shimazu T, Yoshioka T, Sugimoto T.** 1989. False-positive result in Limulus test caused by Limulus amebocyte lysate-reactive material in immunoglobulin products. *J Clin Microbiol* **27:**1965–1968.
84. **Marty FM, Lowry CM, Lempitski SJ, Kubiak DW, Finkelman MA, Baden LR.** 2006. Reactivity of (1→3)-beta-d-glucan assay with commonly used intravenous antimicrobials. *Antimicrob Agents Chemother* **50:**3450–3453.
85. **Hachem RY, Kontoyiannis DP, Chemaly RF, Jiang Y, Reitzel R, Raad I.** 2009. Utility of galactomannan enzyme immunoassay and (1,3) beta-D-glucan in diagnosis of invasive fungal infections: low sensitivity for *Aspergillus fumigatus* infection in hematologic malignancy patients. *J Clin Microbiol* **47:**129–133.
86. **Kanda H, Kubo K, Hamasaki K, Kanda Y, Nakao A, Kitamura T, Fujita T, Yamamoto K, Mimura T.** 2001. Influence of various hemodialysis membranes on the plasma (1→3)-beta-D-glucan level. *Kidney Int* **60:**319–323.
87. **Nagasawa K, Yano T, Kitabayashi G, Morimoto H, Yamada Y, Ohata A, Usami M, Horiuchi T.** 2003. Experimental proof of contamination of blood components by (1→3)-beta-D-glucan caused by filtration with cellulose filters in the manufacturing process. *J Artif Organs* **6:**49–54.
88. **Pickering JW, Sant HW, Bowles CA, Roberts WL, Woods GL.** 2005. Evaluation of a (1→3)-beta-D-glucan assay for diagnosis of invasive fungal infections. *J Clin Microbiol* **43:**5957–5962.
89. **Ellis M, Al-Ramadi B, Finkelman M, Hedstrom U, Kristensen J, Ali-Zadeh H, Klingspor L.** 2008. Assessment of the clinical utility of serial beta-D-glucan concentrations in patients with persistent neutropenic fever. *J Med Microbiol* **57:**287–295.
90. **Koo S, Bryar JM, Page JH, Baden LR, Marty FM.** 2009. Diagnostic performance of the (1→3)-beta-D-glucan assay for invasive fungal disease. *Clin Infect Dis* **49:**1650–1659.

91. **Esteves F, Calé SS, Badura R, de Boer MG, Maltez F, Calderón EJ, van der Reijden TJ, Márquez-Martín E, Antunes F, Matos O.** 2015. Diagnosis of Pneumocystis pneumonia: evaluation of four serologic biomarkers. *Clin Microbiol Infect* **21:**379.e1–10.
92. **Doyle L, Vogel S, Procop GW.** 2017. Pneumocystis PCR: it is time to make PCR the test of choice. *Open Forum Infect Dis* **4:**ofx193.
93. **McTaggart LR, Wengenack NL, Richardson SE.** 2012. Validation of the MycAssay Pneumocystis kit for detection of *Pneumocystis jirovecii* in bronchoalveolar lavage specimens by comparison to a laboratory standard of direct immunofluorescence microscopy, real-time PCR, or conventional PCR. *J Clin Microbiol* **50:**1856–1859.
94. **Huang L, Welsh DA, Miller RF, Beard CB, Lawrence GG, Fox M, Swartzman A, Bensley MR, Carbonnet D, Davis JL, Chi A, Yoo BJ, Jones JL.** 2006. *Pneumocystis jirovecii* dihydropteroate synthase gene mutations and human immunodeficiency virus-associated Pneumocystis pneumonia. *J Eukaryot Microbiol* **53**(Suppl 1):S114–S116.
95. **Damiani C, Le Gal S, Da Costa C, Virmaux M, Nevez G, Totet A.** 2013. Combined quantification of pulmonary *Pneumocystis jirovecii* DNA and serum (1→3)-β-D-glucan for differential diagnosis of pneumocystis pneumonia and Pneumocystis colonization. *J Clin Microbiol* **51:**3380–3388.
96. **Dalpke AH, Hofko M, Zimmermann S.** 2013. Development and evaluation of a real-time PCR assay for detection of *Pneumocystis jirovecii* on the fully automated BD MAX platform. *J Clin Microbiol* **51:**2337–2343.
97. **Skelly M, Merali S, Clarkson AB.** 2011. Pneumocystis pneumonia and S-adenosylmethionine plasma levels. *J Infect* **62:**490–492, author reply 493–495.
98. **Skelly MJ, Holzman RS, Merali S.** 2008. S-adenosylmethionine levels in the diagnosis of *Pneumocystis carinii* pneumonia in patients with HIV infection. *Clin Infect Dis* **46:**467–471.
99. **Skelly M, Hoffman J, Fabbri M, Holzman RS, Clarkson AB Jr, Merali S.** 2003. S-adenosylmethionine concentrations in diagnosis of *Pneumocystis carinii* pneumonia. *Lancet* **361:**1267–1268.
100. **de Boer MG, Gelinck LB, van Zelst BD, van de Sande WW, Willems LN, van Dissel JT, de Jonge R, Kroon FP.** 2011. β-D-glucan and S-adenosylmethionine serum levels for the diagnosis of Pneumocystis pneumonia in HIV-negative patients: a prospective study. *J Infect* **62:**93–100.
101. **Patel N, Koziel H.** 2004. *Pneumocystis jiroveci* pneumonia in adult patients with AIDS: treatment strategies and emerging challenges to antimicrobial therapy. *Treat Respir Med* **3:** 381–397.
102. **Neumann S, Krause SW, Maschmeyer G, Schiel X, von Lilienfeld-Toal M, Infectious Diseases Working Party (AGIHO), German Society of Hematology and Oncology (DGHO).** 2013. Primary prophylaxis of bacterial infections and *Pneumocystis jirovecii* pneumonia in patients with hematological malignancies and solid tumors: guidelines of the Infectious Diseases Working Party (AGIHO) of the German Society of Hematology and Oncology (DGHO). *Ann Hematol* **92:**433–442.
103. **Barrett MP, Gemmell CG, Suckling CJ.** 2013. Minor groove binders as anti-infective agents. *Pharmacol Ther* **139:**12–23.
104. **Fisk M, Sage EK, Edwards SG, Cartledge JD, Miller RF.** 2009. Outcome from treatment of *Pneumocystis jirovecii* pneumonia with co-trimoxazole. *Int J STD AIDS* **20:**652–653.
105. **Kauffman CA, Carver PL.** 2008. Update on echinocandin antifungals. *Semin Respir Crit Care Med* **29:**211–219.
106. **Kamboj M, Weinstock D, Sepkowitz KA.** 2006. Progression of *Pneumocystis jiroveci* pneumonia in patients receiving echinocandin therapy. *Clin Infect Dis* **43:**e92–e94.
107. **Waters L, Nelson M.** 2007. The use of caspofungin in HIV-infected individuals. *Expert Opin Investig Drugs* **16:**899–908.
108. **Beard CB, Roux P, Nevez G, Hauser PM, Kovacs JA, Unnasch TR, Lundgren B.** 2004. Strain typing methods and molecular epidemiology of Pneumocystis pneumonia. *Emerg Infect Dis* **10:**1729–1735.
109. **Kazanjian P, Armstrong W, Hossler PA, Lee CH, Huang L, Beard CB, Carter J, Crane L, Duchin J, Burman W, Richardson J, Meshnick SR.** 2001. *Pneumocystis carinii* cytochrome b mutations are associated with atovaquone exposure in patients with AIDS. *J Infect Dis* **183:**819–822.
110. **Montesinos I, Delforge ML, Ajjaham F, Brancart F, Hites M, Jacobs F, Denis O.** 2017. Evaluation of a new commercial real-time PCR assay for diagnosis of *Pneumocystis jirovecii* pneumonia and identification of dihydropteroate synthase (DHPS) mutations. *Diagn Microbiol Infect Dis* **87:**32–36.
111. **Wakefield AE, Pixley FJ, Banerji S, Sinclair K, Miller RF, Moxon ER, Hopkin JM.** 1990. Amplification of mitochondrial ribosomal RNA sequences from *Pneumocystis carinii* DNA of rat and human origin. *Mol Biochem Parasitol* **43:** 69–76.
112. **Tia T, Putaporntip C, Kosuwin R, Kongpolprom N, Kawkitinarong K, Jongwutiwes S.** 2012. A highly sensitive novel PCR assay for detection of *Pneumocystis jirovecii* DNA in bronchoalveloar lavage specimens from immunocompromised patients. *Clin Microbiol Infect* **18:**598–603.
113. **Lane BR, Ast JC, Hossler PA, Mindell DP, Bartlett MS, Smith JW, Meshnick SR.** 1997. Dihydropteroate synthase polymorphisms in *Pneumocystis carinii*. *J Infect Dis* **175:** 482–485.

Aspergillus, Talaromyces, and *Penicillium*

SHARON C.-A. CHEN, WIELAND MEYER, TANIA C. SORRELL, AND CATRIONA L. HALLIDAY

122

ASPERGILLUS SPECIES

Taxonomy

The genus *Aspergillus* is classified in the family Trichocomaceae of the Ascomycota. Taxonomic assignment of members of this genus has evolved substantially, with over 350 species now described (1, 2) (http://www.aspergilluspenicillium.org). The majority (64%) of species show no sexual reproduction (3), with the anamorphic (asexual) genus *Aspergillus sensu stricto* being phylogenetically related to the anamorphic genera *Penicillium sensu stricto* and *Paecilomyces* (4).

Raper and Fennell in 1965 first classified 132 *Aspergillus* species into 18 subgroups (*Aspergillus candidus*, *A. clavatus*, *A. cervinus*, *A. cremeus*, *A. flavipes*, *A. flavus*, *A. fumigatus*, *A. glaucus*, *A. nidulans*, *A. niger*, *A. ochraceus*, *A. ornatus*, *A. restrictus*, *A. sparsus*, *A. terreus*, *A. ustus*, *A. versicolor*, and *A. wentii*) and 18 varieties based on their morphological characters (5). With advancements in molecular phylogeny, however, taxonomic changes in species classification have been made, resulting in new subdivisions, subgenera, and sections (1, 2). Using multigene phylogeny based on four genetic loci—(i) β-tubulin, (ii) calmodulin, (iii) the internal transcribed spacer (ITS) and large subunit of the ribosomal DNA (rDNA) gene cluster, and (iv) RNA polymerase II subunit RPB2—Peterson established five subgenera, *Aspergillus*, *Circumdati*, *Fumigati*, *Nidulantes*, and *Ornati*. These subgenera were further subdivided into 16 sections (*Aspergillus*, *Candidi*, *Cervini*, *Clavati*, *Circumdati*, *Cremei*, *Falvi*, *Flavipedes*, *Fumigati*, *Nidulantes*, *Nigri*, *Restricti*, *Sparsi*, *Terrei*, *Usti*, and *Versicolores*), either retaining formerly recognized sections or reclassifying them (6). This restructuring resulted in a number of important changes within the genus, including the fact that specific groups of aspergilli now contain uniseriate and biseriate species as well as species characterized by different colony colors. This was not the case previously, when phenotypic characteristics such as colony color were used as key features to separate different groups of aspergilli. The application of this polyphasic phylogenetic species concept has led to the discovery and description of new cryptic or sibling species within the most frequent pathogens, e.g., *A. lentulus* (7) and *A. alabamensis* (8). In the latest taxonomic revisions, Samson et al. (1), Chen et al. (2), and Kocsube et al. (9) extended the work of Peterson (6) and grouped more than 350 species into eight subgenera (*Aspergillus*, *Fumigati*, *Circumdati*, *Candidi*, *Terrei*, *Nidulantes*, *Warcupi*, and *Ornati*), which are subdivided into sections or species complexes.

Molecular work established sequence-based associations between the anamorph (asexual) and teleomorph (sexual) stages for aspergilli (where relevant) independent of whether mating occurs. At the time of writing, the anamorphic species of the genus *Aspergillus* are associated with 10 teleomorphic genera (*Cristaspora*, *Hemisartorya*, *Emericella*, *Eurotium*, *Fennellia*, *Neocarpenteles*, *Neopetromyces*, *Neosartorya*, *Petromyces*, and *Saitoa*) within the taxon Trichocomaceae (9). Peterson had suggested splitting the genus *Aspergillus* based on the teleomorph states associated with particular monophyletic lineages (6); however, this would have deemphasized the most common morphological features associated with the genus *Aspergillus*. With the establishment of the "one fungus = one name" principle in 2011 at the International Botanic Congress in Melbourne, Australia, a new International Code of Nomenclature for Algae, Fungi, and Plants (10), and the abolition of the priority of the teleomorph designation for fungi (11), the naming of *Aspergillus* species is still strongly debated. The *Aspergillus* Working Group of the International Society for Human and Animal Mycology (ISHAM) in 2012 agreed to retain the name *Aspergillus* and not adopt the teleomorph nomenclature (*sensu* Raper and Fennell [5]) by adopting a "wide *Aspergillus*" concept. This decision has significant consequences, as it results in the loss of the well-known teleomorph genera *Emericella*, *Eurotium*, and *Neosartorya*. The argument for maintaining *Aspergillus* for the whole genus is ensuring stability for nomenclature of most medically important *Aspergillus* species and their clinical interpretation. Pitt and Taylor (12), on the other hand, following Peterson's (6) original suggestion to adopt a teleomorph-based nomenclature (i.e., the "narrow *Aspergillus*" concept), which will preserve this genus for a small group or related species and takes into account that those species are morphologically discordant, provide a more consistent taxonomy. This approach results in the assignment of more taxonomically consistent genera that are monophyletic and convey precise morphological and physiological characteristics (13). Discussions are ongoing whether to use the anamorph name for the whole genus ("side *Aspergillus*" concept) or to split the genus according to teleomorph form ("narrow *Aspergillus*" concept). In this chapter, however, we follow the current official view on nomenclature advocated by the International Commission of *Penicillium* and *Aspergillus* by using the anamorphic name followed by its teleomorph stage in parentheses (http://www.aspergilluspenicillium.org).

The majority of human infections due to known *Aspergillus* species are caused by *A. fumigatus* (teleomorph synonym: *Neosartorya fumigata*), followed by *A. flavus* (teleomorph synonym: *Petromyces flavus*), *A. terreus*, and *A. niger*. In addition, at least another 48 *Aspergillus* species have been implicated in disease (14). These uncommon but important pathogens are shown in Table 1. The phylogenetic relationships, based on ITS1 and ITS2 rDNA sequence analysis, of most of these species are shown in Fig. 1.

TABLE 1 Known uncommon pathogenic *Aspergillus* species

Anamorph	Teleomorph (synonym)
Aspergillus acidus	
A. aculeatu	
A. alabamensis	
A. alliaceus	*Petromyces alliaceus*
A. avenaceus	
A. brasiliensis	
A. caesiellus	
A. calidoustus	
A. candidus	
A. carneus	
A. chevalieri	*Eurotium chevalieri*
A. clavato-nanicus	
A. clavatus	
A. conicus	
A. deflectus	
A. fischeri (formerly *A. fischerianus*)	*Neosartorya fischeri*
A. flavipes	*Fennellia flavipes*
A. fumigatiaffinis	
A. fumisynnematus	
A. glaucus	*Eurotium herbariorum*
A. granulosus	
A. montevidensis (formerly *A. hollandicus*)	*Eurotium amstelodami*
A. janus	
A. japonicus	
A. lentulus	
A. nidulans	*Emericella nidulans*
A. niveus	*Fennellia nivea*
A. nomius	*Petromyces nomius*
A. ochraceopetaliformis	
A. ochraceus	
A. oryzae	
A. persii	
A. pseudoglaucus (formerly *A. reptans*)	*Eurotium repens*
A. restrictus	
A. rugulosus (formerly *A. rubrobrunneus*)	*Emericella rugulosa*
A. sclerotiorum	
A. sydowii	
A. tamari	
A. quadrilineatus (formerly *A. tetrazonus*)	*Emericella quadrilineata*
A. spinosus	*Neosartorya spinosa*
A. thermomutatus	*Neosartorya pseudofischeri*
A. tritici	
A. tubingensis	
A. udagawae	*Neosartorya udagawae*
A. unguis	*Emericella unguis*
A. ustus	
A. versicolor	
A. viridinutans	

Description of the Agent

Aspergillus species are ubiquitous. They grow rapidly and form powdery colonies on mycological media. Colony color varies with species and is influenced by growth conditions and factors such as whether vegetative hyphae, conidial heads, and/or sexual structures are present. The color of the aerial part of the colony may also be different from that exhibited by the portion in the growth medium. The growth rates of *Aspergillus* species and their colony diameters in media at a certain age are important features to aid species identification, as well as the appearance of the colony at its margins. The margins can be sharply delineated or thin and diffuse, smooth over their entirety or irregularly lobed, and submerged or aerial. The texture of the colony surface, which ranges from velvety to floccose to granular and which may show a zonation, is also used to assist with species designation (14) (see "Identification").

Aspergillus spp. form nonseptate stipes or conidiophores (walls), which commonly terminate in a vesicle (distinct inflated part) from which phialides are produced synchronously. They reproduce via conidia, which are formed in dry chains on the end of the phialides. The phialides can be formed directly from the vesicle (uniseriate) or alternatively they can form metulae (intermediate series of cells) (biseriate) (14). Figure 2 provides a schematic of the important structural features of aspergilli. Morphological characteristics of clinically relevant sections and species are listed in Table 2.

Epidemiology and Transmission

Aspergillus species are environmental saprophytes that thrive in decaying vegetation and are readily cultured from soil, water, certain foods, and air. Although conidia are continually inhaled from the environment, they are eliminated from healthy hosts via mucociliary clearance or following phagocytosis by alveolar macrophages (15). In hosts with altered lung function, e.g., in those with cystic fibrosis, they may colonize the respiratory tract or cause allergic or invasive pulmonary disease. Severely immunocompromised individuals are at particular risk of invasive pulmonary aspergillosis, which may spread to contiguous sites or disseminate to other body sites via the bloodstream (16, 17).

In health care facilities, *Aspergillus* has been cultured from unfiltered air, ventilation systems, dust, food, hospital water supplies, and related wet environments, including shower outlets (18–20). Numerous outbreaks of hospital-acquired invasive infection have been described, mostly following inhalation of airborne spores originating from construction or demolition activities (21, 22). Aerosolization of water from contaminated sources or surfaces may also occur (19, 20, 23). Warris and Verweij have proposed control measures for the prevention of waterborne infection in hospitals, though the importance of water as a source of hospital outbreaks remains uncertain (23). Most outbreaks are associated with invasive pulmonary aspergillosis, but clusters of surgical wound and skin infections have also been described (24). In some studies, identification of a common source was supported by molecular genotyping (18, 21), though in addition to clonally related genotypes and microvariants, multiple genotypes have typically been found in clinical and environmental samples (25). Not all researchers have detected genetic relatedness between environmental and clinical isolates (23). Concentrations of airborne fungi in patient care areas during outbreak investigations have ranged from 0 to >100 spores/m^3. Though higher concentrations of airborne spores have been associated with outbreaks (25), a threshold below which patients

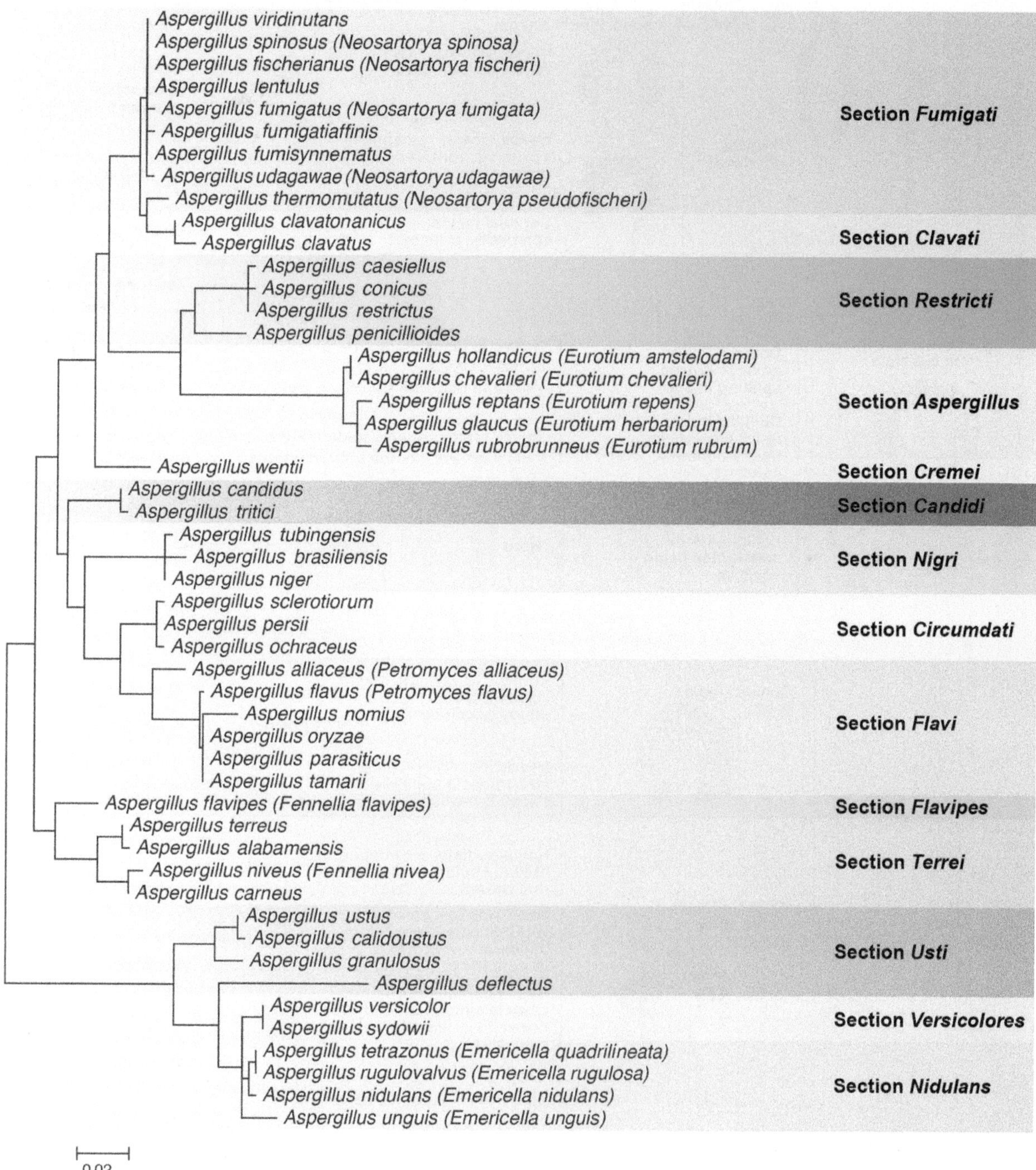

FIGURE 1 Maximum-likelihood tree of pathogenic *Aspergillus* species according to the *Atlas of Clinical Fungi*, version 4.1 (http://www.clinicalfungi.org), based on ITS1 and ITS2 sequences of the rDNA gene obtained from GenBank using the program MEGA, version 7.0. Teleomorph names are given in parentheses.

are considered safe has not been determined. Determining this threshold is problematic due to use of variable sampling methods, rapid temporal variation in spore counts, delayed sampling as a result of delays in clinical presentation after exposure, and differences in host susceptibility to infection (18). In a 10-year air sample analysis of *Aspergillus* prevalence, Falvey and Streifel concluded that routine air sampling was not an effective means of predicting hospital-acquired infections, although a transient spike may indicate a potential in-house source of contamination (26). The Centers for Disease Control and Prevention and the Healthcare Infection Control Practices Advisory Committee have published guidelines on prevention of aspergillosis in health care facilities (22).

A. fumigatus is the most common cause of invasive aspergillosis, accounting for at least 65% of cases, especially in the highest-risk group, patients with hematological malignancies (27–30). Other pathogenic species include members of the *A. flavus*, *A. terreus*, and *A. niger* species complexes and, infrequently, *A. nidulans* and *A. ustus* (31–33). *A. flavus* infections are more common in developing countries and in arid climates, where they comprise the

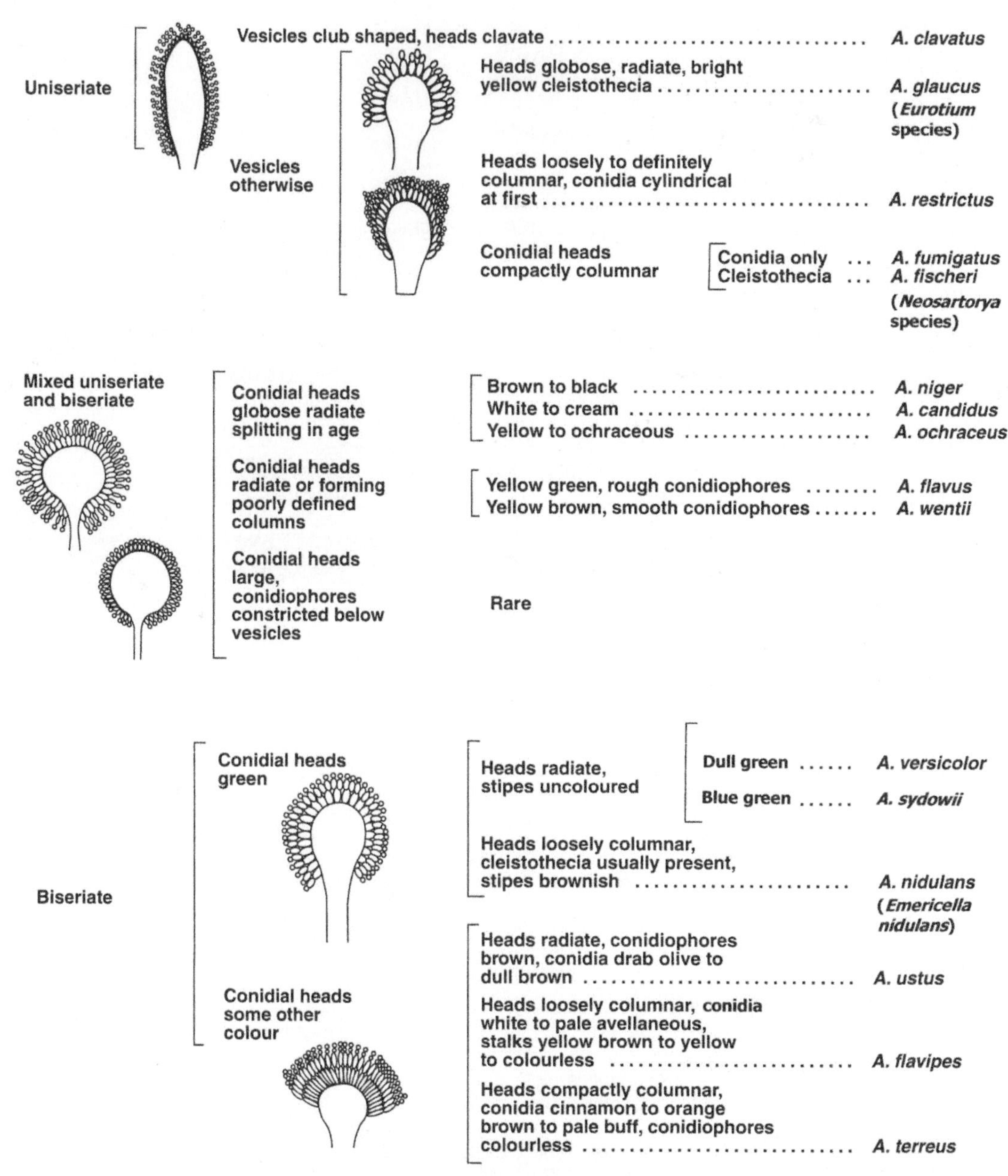

FIGURE 2 Key to representative species of *Aspergillus*.

majority of cases of allergic aspergillosis, trauma-associated endophthalmitis, and sino-orbital-cerebral disease (28, 34, 35), while in other regions, *A. terreus* may be the most frequent species (36). Nosocomial outbreaks of aspergillosis are most common in patients with hematological cancers and are almost always caused by *A. fumigatus* or *A. flavus* (19, 21). In the U.S.-based Transplant-Associated Infection Surveillance Network (TRANSNET) study conducted from 2001 to 2006, 67% of isolates were identified as *A. fumigatus*; cryptic species of *A. fumigatus* comprised 6% of this complex (30).

Clinical Significance

Aspergilli can cause disease as a result of ingestion of mycotoxins or other metabolites (see chapter 129); direct inoculation into traumatized skin, eyes, or other sites; and inhalation of spores causing hypersensitivity or invasive disease. Infection may also affect the ears, causing otomycosis. Aspergillosis most commonly involves the lungs, but almost every organ can be involved as a result of primary infection, contiguous spread, or dissemination (37). Lung infection presents as a spectrum of disease, depending on the extent of immunosuppression, genetic factors, and structural abnormalities within the respiratory system. Certain species are associated with specific forms of disease (Table 3).

Invasive aspergillosis, the second most common hospital-acquired fungal infection after invasive candidiasis (38), is associated with high morbidity and mortality especially in patients with hematological malignancies or allogeneic stem cell or lung transplants (39, 40). Other groups at increased risk and with poor outcomes include patients who have had heart, liver, and, less commonly, renal transplants; patients receiving immunomodulators such as infliximab or tumor necrosis factor alpha inhibitors; patients

TABLE 2 Characteristics of some medically important *Aspergillus* species grown on identification media

Section[a] and species	Seriation		Colony color	Microscopic features[b]	Comments[c]
	Uniseriate	Biseriate			
Fumigati					
Aspergillus fumigatus sensu stricto (teleomorph: *Neosartorya fumigata*)	+		Dark blue-green to gray-turquoise; slate gray with age; reverse variable (Fig. 3B)	Conidiophore: up to 300 μm long and 5–8 μm wide, smooth, noncolored or greenish Vesicle: dome-shaped, 20–30 μm diameter, phialides on upper half only Head: strongly columnar	Characteristic blue-green colonies, growth at 50°C (growth temperature range, 15–50°C) Columnar heads with single layer of phialides Sterile, white, fast-growing or glabrous cerebriform slow-growing variants confirmed by thermotolerance and DNA sequencing
A. felis	+/−		Floccose, usually white with poor sporulation	Conidia: subglobose to globose, smooth to echinulate, 2–3.5 μm diameter (Fig. 3C) Morphology similar to *A. fumigatus sensu stricto*	Cryptic relatively new species within *A. fumigatus* species complex. Distinguished from *A. fumigatus sensu stricto* by inability to grow at 50°C
A. lentulus	+		Suede-like to floccose, usually white, interspersed with gray-green colonies; reverse yellow, no diffusible pigment (Fig. 3D)	Stipes: 250–300 μm long, 2–7 μm wide, smooth, sometimes sinuous and often constricted at the neck, colorless Vesicle: diminutive, 8–10 μm wide, hyaline, subclavate or subglobose, fertile over only half of the area, few short flask-shaped phialides Head: short columnar Conidia: fewer than 6 or 7 per chain, globose to ellipsoidal, rough with ornamentation, 2.5–3 μm diameter, bluish to olive green (Fig. 3E)	Cryptic relatively new species within *A. fumigatus* species complex. Slow-sporulating, white Does not grow at 50°C (growth temperature range, 10–45°C)
A. thermomutatus (teleomorph: *N. pseudofischeri*)	+		Suede-like to floccose, usually white to pale yellow with slow to poor conidiation	Morphologically similar to *A. fumigatus sensu stricto*	Cryptic relatively new species within *A. fumigatus* species complex. Slow-sporulating, white
A. udagawae (teleomorph: *N. udagawae*)	+		Suede-like to floccose, usually white to pale yellow with slow to poor conidiation	Morphologically similar to *A. fumigatus sensu stricto*	Cryptic relatively new species within *A. fumigatus* species complex. Slow-sporulating, white
Flavi					
A. flavus (teleomorph: *Petromyces flavus*)	+	+	Yellow to dark yellowish green (Fig. 3F)	Conidiophore: 400–850 μm long, 20 μm wide, roughened, uncolored Vesicle: subglobose/globose, 25–45 μm diameter Head: loosely radiate or splitting into columns with age (Fig. 3G) Conidia: globose or ellipsoidal, roughened, 3–6 μm diameter	Heads vary in size and seriation, growth usually enhanced at 37°C, brown to black sclerotia may be present, colony color influenced by culture medium additions such as yeast extract Toxigenic
Flavipedes					
A. flavipes (teleomorph: *Fennellia flavipes*)		+	White with patches of yellow or pale grayish buff; reverse yellow to golden brown	Conidiophore: 150–400 μm long, 4–8 μm wide, smooth to rough, uncolored to pale brown Vesicle: subglobose, 10–290 μm diameter Head: radiate to loose columnar Conidia: globose, smooth, 2–3 μm diameter Cleistothecia and Hülle cells rare	Distinguished from *A. terreus* by slower-growing colonies, metulae usually formed over entire vesicle with radiate to loosely columnar heads

(Continued on next page)

TABLE 2 Characteristics of some medically important *Aspergillus* species grown on identification media *(Continued)*

Section[a] and species	Seriation: Uniseriate	Seriation: Biseriate	Colony color	Microscopic features[b]	Comments[c]
Nidulantes					
A. nidulans (teleomorph: *Emericella nidulans*)		+	Dark green if mainly conidial; buff to purple brown if cleistothecial; reverse: deep red to purple	Conidiophore: 70–150 μm long, 3–6 μm wide, smooth, brown Vesicle: hemispherical, 8–12 μm diameter Head: phialides on upper part, columnar Conidia: globose, rough, 3–4 μm diameter Cleistothecia: reddish brown, globose, 100–250 μm (Fig. 3H) Hülle cells: globose Ascospores: lenticular with 2 longitudinal crests ca. 5 μm long, red purple Conidial heads, ascocarps and Hülle cells similar to those of *E. nidulans*. Ascospores also similar but have 2 major and 2 minor equatorial crests	Distinguished by red-brown cleistothecia, abundant Hülle cells, red-purple ascospores with 2 crests, short conidia, and short metulae Toxigenic
A. quadrilineatus (teleomorph: *Emericella quadrilineata*)		+	Olive green to grayish purple; reverse purple		Distinguished from *E. nidulans* by 4 crests on ascospores
Nigri					
A. niger		+	Black with white margin, yellow surface mycelium; reverse uncolored or pale yellow	Conidiophore: 400–3,000 μm long, 15–20 μm wide, smooth, uncolored to brownish near tip Vesicle: globose, 30–75 μm diameter Head: radiate, then splitting into columns with age Conidia: globose with thick walls, brownish black, rough, 4–5 μm diameter	Frequent cause of otomycosis, sometimes associated with intracavitary colonization, especially in diabetes mellitus
A. tubingensis		+/–	Conidial heads in gray black-brown shades, borne on long conidiophores; reverse white	Conidiophore: 2–3 mm long, smooth and coarse, diameter 15–20 μm. Conidial heads: spherical to radiate, mostly 200–300 μm; Conidia: spherical, 3.0–3.5 μm in diam, becoming progressively darker and rougher Sclerotia produced in some strains, spherical to subspherical, cream coloured, becoming pinkish buff, sometimes darkening to almost black with age, usually 500–800 μm in diameter	Slow-sporulating, white Commonly involved in pulmonary disorders and otomycosis Distinguishable from other members of section *Nigri* by *benA* or *CaM gene* sequencing

(Continued on next page)

TABLE 2 Characteristics of some medically important *Aspergillus* species grown on identification media *(Continued)*

Section[a] and species	Seriation: Uniseriate	Seriation: Biseriate	Colony color	Microscopic features[b]	Comments[c]
Terrei					
A. terreus		+	Tan to cinnamon brown	Conidiophore: 100–150 μm long, 4.5–6 μm wide, smooth, uncolored Vesicle: dome shaped, 10–16 μm diameter, phialides on upper half Head: columnar Conidia: globose/subglobose, smooth, 2 μm diameter, solitary single-celled conidia, commonly sessile on submerged hyphae	Distinctive features: cinnamon-colored colonies, columnar heads and solitary accessory conidia Often resistant to amphotericin B
Usti					
A. ustus		+	Brown-gray or olive gray; reverse yellow, dull red or purplish	Conidiophore: 75–400 μm long, 4–7 μm wide, smooth, becoming brown Vesicle: globose/subglobose, 7–16 μm diameter, fertile over upper two-thirds Head: radiate to loosely columnar Conidia: globose, rough, 3–4.5 μm diameter Irregular Hülle cells often present (Fig. 31)	Hülle cells are distinguishing feature when present. Brown conidiophores
A. deflectus		+	Slow growing, mouse gray with pinkish margins or patches of yellow	Conidiophore: 40–125 μm long, 2.5–3.5 μm wide, smooth, red-brown Vesicle: hemispherical, 5–7 μm in diameter, bent at right angle to stipe Head: phialides on upper surface, columnar Conidia; globose, 3–3.5 μm diameter, smooth to rough Hülle cells sometimes present	Vesicle bent almost at right angle to stipe is distinguishing feature. Rare human pathogen
Versicolores					
A. versicolor		+	Green/gray-green or tan with patches of pink or yellow; reverse variable, often deep red	Vesicle: ovate to elliptical, 9–16 μm diameter Head: radiate to loosely columnar Conidia: globose, echinulate, 2.5–3 μm diameter Hülle cells globose	Distinguished by slow growing, green-tan or variably colored colonies and small biseriate vesicles
Less common pathogens					
Aspergillus					
A. glaucus (teleomorph: *Eurotium herbariorum* and other spp.)	+		Deep green mixed with bright yellow; reverse uncolored or pale yellow	Conidiophore: 200–300 μm long, 7–12 μm wide, smooth, uncolored to pale brown Vesicle: globose, 15–30 μm diameter Head: large radiate Conidia; subglobose, echinulate, 5 μm diameter Cleistothecia: thin walled, yellow, globose, 75–150 μm ascospores smooth or rough, with furrow and rounded or frilled crests	Formerly called glaucus group Osmophilic Reproduction enhanced on high-sugar media Growth poor at 37°C Readily identified by ascospore morphology rather than by conidial head features Members include *E. umbrosus*, *E. ruber*, *E. repens* *E. umbrosus* is reported as cause of farmer's lung (anamorph: *A. glaucus*)

(Continued on next page)

TABLE 2 Characteristics of some medically important *Aspergillus* species grown on identification media (*Continued*)

Section[a] and species	Seriation		Colony color	Microscopic features[b]	Comments[c]
	Uniseriate	Biseriate			
Restricti					
A. restrictus	+		Dull olive green to brownish green, very slow growing	Conidiophore: 80–200 μm long, 4–8 μm wide, smooth or rough, uncolored Vesicle: hemispherical, 8–20 μm diameter Head: phialides on upper third, columnar Conidia: cylindrical to ellipsoidal, rough, 4–7 μm long, 3–4 μm wide	Very slow growth on standard media distinguishes this from *A. fumigatus*, slightly enhanced growth on high-sugar media, no growth at 37°C, cylindrical conidia developing to long, adherent columns
Candidi					
A. candidus	+	+	White to cream	Conidiophore: mostly 200–500 μm long, 7–10 μm wide, smooth to rough, uncolored Vesicle: globose/subglobose, 17–35 μm diameter Head: fertile over entire surface, radiate Conidia: globose, smooth, 3–4 μm diameter Sclerotia: sometimes, present, reddish purple	Distinguished from all colored aspergilli by white, slow-growing colonies; however, be cautious about white, slow-growing forms of poor sporulators of *A. fumigatus* species complex.

[a]Modern concepts have replaced group names with subgenera and sections.
[b]Refer to "Taxonomy" above for descriptions of terms.
[c]Only species producing potent toxins are noted as toxigenic, but other species may produce toxins of lesser significance.

TABLE 3 Clinical categorization of *Aspergillus* infection and major causative species[a]

Clinical presentation	Syndromes	Associations
Allergic (hypersensitivity)	ABPA; SAFS[b]	*Aspergillus fumigatus* (*A. terreus*); *Aspergillus* spp.; asthma
Saprophytic	Aspergilloma	*A. fumigatus*; preexisting cavities, tuberculosis
	Otomycosis	*A. niger* is predominant cause
	Onychomycosis	*A. versicolor* complex and *A. sydowii* are common causes
Semi-invasive[c] (hyphal invasion of tissue)	Chronic necrotizing pulmonary aspergillosis	*A. fumigatus*; structural lung disease
	Keratitis	*A. fumigatus*, *A. flavus*, and other species
Invasive[d]	Rhinosinusitis (rhino-orbital/cerebral disease) (acute invasive, chronic invasive, chronic granulomatous forms; aspergilloma)	*A. fumigatus*, *A. flavus* *A. flavus* is the commonest cause in developing countries. Granulomatous sinusitis (Sudan, India, Pakistan, Saudi Arabia) *A. flavus* (90%), *A. fumigatus*, *A. niger* *A. fumigatus*, *A. flavus*, *A. nidulans*, *A. terreus*
	Invasive bronchial aspergillosis (superficial, pseudomembranous or ulcerative tracheobronchitis)	Lung transplantation, AIDS
	Invasive pulmonary aspergillosis	*A. fumigatus*, *A. terreus*, *A. flavus*
	Hyphal invasion (pyogranulomatous inflammation/necrosis)	Immunosuppression, no neutropenia: GVHD, SOT, CGD, HIV/AIDS, corticosteroids
	Angioinvasion (coagulative necrosis, hemorrhagic infarction)	Prolonged, severe neutropenia

[a]See reference 37. Abbreviations: CGD, chronic granulomatous disease; IPA, invasive pulmonary aspergillosis; GVHD, graft-versus-host disease; SAFS, severe asthma with fungal sensitization; SOT, solid organ transplant.
[b]SAFS can be caused by fungi other than *Aspergillus*; it does not meet serological criteria for ABPA (37).
[c]As defined by Chakrabarti et al. (28) and Thompson and Patterson (16).
[d]Classified by Hope et al. (37) on the basis of tissue invasion by hyphae (with or without angioinvasion).

with advanced AIDS, malnutrition, or other underlying qualitative and quantitative immune cell defects; and patients requiring hemodialysis. Critically ill patients in intensive care units and patients with chronic respiratory tract disease such as cystic fibrosis are also at risk of invasive pulmonary aspergillosis (17, 27–30, 41).

In diagnosing aspergillosis, positive cultures (or antigen- or nucleic acid-based tests) for *Aspergillus* from clinical specimens may not in themselves indicate a pathological process. The distinction between colonization of the respiratory tract and invasive disease is particularly difficult in highly immunosuppressed patients and those with chronic airway disease (42, 43), but the probability of requiring treatment increases with increasing immunosuppression. To enable standardization in assisting diagnosis, and for the purpose of clinical trials in patients with hematological malignancies, consensus definitions of proven and probable aspergillosis are published by the European Organization for Research and Treatment of Cancer and the Mycoses Study Group (EORTC/MSG). These incorporate host immune status, lung imaging (computerized tomography) findings, antigen-based biomarker tests, and histology and culture findings, but not, as yet, nucleic acid detection tests (44). Criteria have also been developed for diagnosis of invasive aspergillosis in patients with chronic obstructive lung disease and for the entity of chronic pulmonary aspergillosis (45–47). Demonstration of hyphae in tissue or other clinical samples and culture of a heavy growth of *Aspergillus* from a single specimen or the same species from multiple specimens point to invasive disease in the appropriate clinical context. Culture of at least three good-quality sputum specimens is recommended whenever fungal infection is suspected. Antigen- and nucleic acid-based diagnostics are discussed below.

Collection, Transport, and Storage of Specimens

Methods to collect appropriate clinical specimens (see chapter 117) are especially important for diagnosis of invasive pulmonary aspergillosis due to uncertainty in differentiation of *Aspergillus* colonization (or even contamination) from *Aspergillus* disease. Diagnosis can be difficult (38, 47) and appears to be most problematic in nonneutropenic hosts and in patients with compromised airways (e.g., lung transplant recipients). The most convincing evidence of aspergillosis is provided by recovery of the fungus from lung tissue and other sterile sites and/or by histopathologic demonstration of hyphae in tissue. However, nonsterile specimens such as sputum and bronchoalveolar lavage (BAL) fluid are frequent specimens submitted for culture where recovery of aspergilli may reflect colonization (48). Culture results should be interpreted in combination with an assessment of clinical, radiographic, and other diagnostic tests.

Other than the respiratory tract, *Aspergillus* can be recovered from culture of any body site, including sinus, cerebrospinal fluid (CSF), skin, other tissue, the eye, and heart valves. In *Aspergillus* endocarditis, as with other invasive infections, blood cultures are typically negative. Conversely, positive blood cultures for *Aspergillus* are often indicative of contamination even in populations at high risk for invasive aspergillosis (49), although they uncommonly are helpful in disseminated infection, and cases of fungemia, especially *A. terreus* fungemia, have been described (50). All specimens should be transported to the laboratory as soon as practicable for culture and other diagnostic testing. For detection of *Aspergillus* DNA in archived samples, such as paraffin-embedded (PE) tissue, tissue should be sent in thin (approximately 10- by 10-μm) sections in a sterile receptacle (51). It is advisable to discard the first section due to possible contamination with fungal spores.

Direct Examination

Microscopy

Microscopic examination of fresh and/or stained specimens of tissue, BAL fluid, sputum, tissue aspirates, and other specimens may reveal fungal structures, but this method is insensitive, and specimens are often positive only in advanced disease. Hyphal elements can be observed using routine potassium hydroxide preparations or with a fluorescent stain such as calcofluor white or Blankophor P. In tissue biopsy sections, hyphae may be seen if specific fungal stains are used, including Gomori methenamine silver or Grocott's stain and periodic acid-Schiff. In hematoxylin and eosin (H&E)-stained tissue, hyphae can also be visualized, although care must be taken not to traumatize tissue. Viable hyphae are typically basophilic to amphophilic, while damaged or necrotic hyphae are more often eosinophilic (52).

Although species identification of *Aspergillus* is not possible, microscopy provides relevant preliminary diagnostic information; some assessment of fungal morphology and demonstration of fungal hyphae in tissue are requirements of the EORTC/MSG classification for a "proven" fungal infection (44). *Aspergillus* hyphae are typically hyaline, septate, and 6 μm in diameter and branch dichotomously at acute (~45°C) angles, although not all the above features may be evident (see Fig. 3A for an H&E-stained section of lung). Hyphae have smooth parallel walls with no or slight constrictions at the septa (14, 52). Where invasion has occurred, hyphae may extend throughout the tissue and form parallel or radial arrays. Aspergilli in chronic lung cavities grow as tangled masses of hyphae and may exhibit atypical hyphal features, such as swellings measuring up to 12 μm in diameter or the absence of conspicuous septa. Unusual features, such as swelling of the terminal portion of the hyphae, may also be seen in patients who have received antifungal therapy, especially with the echinocandin class.

Adventitial forms (conidia, ascomata, and other asexual structures [Fig. 2]) of *Aspergillus* may be recognized in histopathologic sections to allow presumptive identification of the fungus. For example, in tissue, *A. terreus* displays distinctive aleurioconidia along the lateral hyphal walls (53). Calcium oxalate crystals have been associated with *A. niger* infection (54). However, culture, immunohistochemical staining, or nucleic acid amplification is required to identify the pathogen. The specificity of microscopic methods is low for distinguishing non-*Aspergillus* hyaline moulds from *Aspergillus* (55). *In situ* hybridization techniques using a specific fluorescent antibody that binds to fungal elements in tissue may aid diagnosis; in one study, *Fusarium* was distinguished from *Aspergillus* elements in tissue sections with a 100% positive predictive value (PPV) (56), although the use of immunohistochemistry has not been validated for this purpose.

Antigen Detection

Galactomannan (GM) is a major polysaccharide constituent of the cell walls of *Aspergillus*, most *Penicillium* (*Talaromyces*) species, and certain other moulds which is released *in vivo* from growing hyphae. Commercial assays for GM are standardized and are well validated. The Platelia *Aspergillus* enzyme-linked immunosorbent assay (ELISA) (Bio-Rad Laboratories, Hercules, CA) is a double sandwich enzyme immunoassay that has been cleared by the U.S. Food and Drug Administration (FDA) for diagnostic use and that utilizes the rat monoclonal antibody (MAb) EBA-2, directed against the galactofuranoside side chain of the GM antigen (reviewed in reference 57), and it is data on this test that resulted in inclusion of GM in the revised EORTC/MSG definitions of invasive aspergillosis in immunosuppressed patients and in both hematology and solid organ transplant patients (44, 57–63). These definitions were developed for use in clinical and epidemiological research; in clinical practice, they must be taken in context with clinical-pathologic descriptions and classifications (see "Clinical Significance"). Although the EORTC/MSG definitions include GM detection in plasma, serum, BAL fluid, or CSF, extensive clinical validations have only been performed for serum and, following release of a newer format of the above assay from Bio-Rad, BAL fluid (for reviews, meta-analyses, and systematic analyses, see references 58–62).

Based on a meta-analysis, the sensitivity and specificity of serum GM in adult patients, using a cutoff optical density index (ODI) of 0.5 for the diagnosis of invasive aspergillosis, are 71% and 89%, respectively, with a low PPV of 26 to 53% but high negative predictive value (NPV) of 95 to 98% (58), suggesting that GM is more suitable as a screening to exclude aspergillosis than as a diagnostic test. The sensitivity and specificity of serum GM testing vary substantially in different studies, mainly due to differences in study design and study populations. It is much more sensitive when used for samples from neutropenic and hematopoietic stem cell transplant recipients than for patients with solid organ transplants or critically ill patients with chronic obstructive pulmonary disease (64–67), As a diagnostic test in patients with hematological malignancies, the specificity and PPV increased to 98.6% when two separate and consecutive samples were positive at an ODI of at least 0.5 (68). This ODI is used because the goals are to minimize the risk of invasive aspergillosis by "screening" out patients unlikely to have disease. Maertens et al. have further recommended that a single positive GM index of ≥0.7 should prompt a diagnostic workup (68). The use of mould-active antifungal agents reduces the sensitivity of the serum GM test (69), and false positives have occurred in patients receiving piperacillin-tazobactam (although the frequency of false-positive results appears to be reduced with newer formulations of this antimicrobial agent), in those receiving amoxicillin-clavulanate in association with *Bifidobacteria* in the gut of neonates, and in those who have ingested foods containing GM (66). Some non-*Aspergillus* moulds may yield positive GM results (*Talaromyces marneffei*, *Histoplasma capsulatum*, *Fusarium oxysporum*, *Paecilomyces* species, and *Alternaria* species) (61). One systematic review of 19 studies that employed the use serum GM testing concluded that in children, the sensitivity, specificity, and PPV were highly variable when this test was used both as a screening tool and as a diagnostic test in patients with symptoms; the NPVs were 85 to 100% for screening and 70 to 100% in the diagnostic setting (70).

Recently, three systematic reviews and meta-analyses of the utility of GM in BAL fluid in patients with hematological malignancies or mixed comorbidities were published (60–62). All of them acknowledged limitations of the studies analyzed but concluded that the BAL GM assay was more sensitive than the serum GM assay, though the overall recommendations for a cutoff ODI for BAL fluid positive samples differed: 1.0 was recommended by Zou et al. (60), and 1.5 was recommended by Heng et al. (61), but Guo et al. arrived at no consensus (62). Data regarding the effect of mould-active agents on level of BAL GM are conflicting, and standardization across studies is needed to resolve these differences (61). Nonetheless, the positivity threshold is recommended to be at least 1.0 in BAL fluid for assessment of diagnosis (http://www.fda.gov/downloads/Drugs/GuidanceComplianceRegulatoryInformation/Guidances/UCM420248.pdf). There is also evidence that BAL GM is more sensitive and specific than serum GM in critically ill patients with chronic obstructive pulmonary disease, though the proposed cutoff of 0.8 for the ODI requires confirmation (71).

Aspergillus Antigen Detection Using Lateral Flow Technology

A simple test that is more specific than the GM assay and that does not require specific equipment has been developed as a rapid diagnostic test, although the current need for pretreatment (heating, centrifugation, and addition of a buffer solution) steps in testing serum (but not BAL fluid) samples reduces its utility as a point-of-care test. This *Aspergillus* lateral flow assay, the AspLFD test (OLM Diagnostics, Newcastle-upon-Tyne, United Kingdom), relies on binding of a mouse MAb (JF5) to an extracellular glycoprotein of *Aspergillus*, which is present in cell walls of growing germ tubes and secreted at growing hyphal tips but absent from ungerminated conidia (72, 73). The MAb JF5 does not cross-react with fungal antigens that cross-react with the MAb EB-A2 used in the GM assay, namely, those of *T. marneffei*, *H. capsulatum*, *F. oxysporum*, and *Alternaria* species, but does demonstrate cross-reactivity against *Paecilomyces* and non-*Talaromyces Penicillium* species (72). Testing of samples from patients with hematological malignancies suggests that the AspLFD assay (OLM Diagnostics) is as specific as, but may be more sensitive than, the GM assay (74–76) and that both sensitivity and specificity may be improved by using it in combination with PCR-based assays (76). A meta-analysis reported a pooled sensitivity of 68% (95% confidence interval [CI], 52 to 81%), specificity of 87% (95%, CI 80 to 92%), and diagnostic odds ratio (DOR) of 11.9 (95% CI, 3.54 to 39.96) for distinguishing proven or probable aspergillosis from absence of disease (74).

The use of the test on BAL fluid has also been evaluated in a number of studies and in different patient populations, including solid organ transplant recipients and patients with underlying respiratory disease. The results were summarized in the meta-analysis (74) described above with a pooled sensitivity of 85% (95% CI, 76 to 93%), specificity of 93% (95% CI, 89% to 96%), and DOR of 65.94 (95% CI, 27.21 to 159.81%) for invasive aspergillosis. Overall, the assay sensitivity was lower in patients with hematologic malignancies (67% sensitivity) than in other patient groups, most likely due to the use of antifungal prophylaxis in these patients. As for serum testing, combining the assay with other fungal biomarker tests has been shown to increase sensitivity substantially (76, 77).

It should be noted that, at the time of writing, commercial availability of the AspLFD assay (OLM Diagnostics) is still pending . The test is CE marked and is for investigational use but has not yet been approved by the FDA for diagnostic purposes.

(1,3)-β-D-Glucan

Besides tests to detect *Aspergillus* GM and, now, novel *Aspergillus*-specific antigens (68), colorimetric detection of (1,3)-β-D-glucan in the serum of patients represents another strategy for diagnosis of invasive aspergillosis. As with *Aspergillus* GM, detection of (1,3)-β-D-glucan has been added as a diagnostic criterion in the EORTC/MSG assessment for probability of invasive aspergillosis (44). This antigen is a major component of the fungal cell wall, and circulating (1,3)-β-D-glucan can be quantified in the serum of patients with invasive aspergillosis (78–81). Concentrations approaching 1 pg of antigen/ml can be detected, with a level of ≥80 ng/ml (Fungitell Assay; Associates of Cape Cod, Inc., Falmouth, MA) being considered indicative of fungal infection. Other assays (e.g., Fungitec-G; Seikagaku Corporation, Tokyo, Japan) have been commercialized in Asia, but only the Fungitell assay (Associates of Cape Cod, Inc.) is approved and cleared by the FDA for diagnostic use. (1,3)-β-D-Glucan assays are approved for use in serum only.

However, the inability of the test to discriminate between *Aspergillus*-related infections and those caused by other fungi—i.e., its low PPV (approximately 50% at best)—is a key limitation of the assay for diagnosing aspergillosis. The sensitivity, specificity, and NPV of the assay for any systemic fungal infection are described to be approximately 93, 77, and 98%, respectively (79). In four meta-analyses encompassing a variety of fungal infections in hematology and other patient populations, the pooled sensitivity was 60 to 80%, with a specificity of 80 to 90% (78–82); in one analysis, the positive likelihood ratio was 5.2, and the negative likelihood ratio was 0.29 (82). A recent meta-analysis of six cohort studies restricted to hematology-oncology patients reported that where two consecutive tests were required, the sensitivity and specificity were 49.6% (95% CI, 34.0 to 65.3%) and 98.9% (95% CI, 97.4 to 99.5%), respectively. The estimated positive and negative predictive values for any invasive fungal disease with a prevalence of 10% were 83.5% and 94.6%, respectively (78). Different (1,3)-β-D-glucan assays were noted to have similar accuracy for the diagnosis of fungal infection.

Data indicate that the sensitivity for invasive aspergillosis ranges widely, from 60 to 100%. Despite these limitations, the serum (1,3)-β-D-glucan test may be useful as a negative predictor of aspergillosis if combined with more specific tests; exposure to mould-active antifungal agents reduces the sensitivity of the test (80–82). Conversely, false-positive results are common under conditions of hemodialysis (cellulose membranes), treatment with immunoglobulin products, and exposure to glucan-containing material (57, 82). Cross-reactivity with amoxicillin-clavulanic acid and cell wall components of Gram-positive organisms has occurred. Test results should be interpreted within the clinical context, and further validation is required to determine its usefulness for monitoring therapeutic response. (1,3)-β-D-Glucan testing in BAL fluid has not been extensively investigated but appears to have poor specificity for aspergillosis (77).

Nucleic Acid Detection

Aspergillus DNA can be detected in clinical specimens either by nucleic acid amplification methods specifically targeting *Aspergillus* or by panfungal PCR assays followed by DNA sequencing for species identification. The former has the better sensitivity and faster turnaround time (no need for DNA sequencing), but panfungal assays have broader diagnostic potential. Both strategies may identify *Aspergillus* spp. directly in tissue, blood, CSF, and respiratory samples (51, 83–85) with good overall sensitivity and specificity, although with wide interstudy variability in performance (40 to 100% for sensitivity; 60 to 100% for specificity) (reviewed in references 57 and 86). Technical advances in amplicon detection methods have enabled real-time detection and quantification of *Aspergillus* DNA (quantitative PCR) using TaqMan, LightCycler, high-resolution melting curve analysis, or nucleic acid sequence-based amplification; these methods are detailed elsewhere (57, 87, 88). Multiple in-house PCR assays targeting various genetic sequences (18S rDNA, ITS region, and mitochondrial DNA) have been developed for detection of *Aspergillus* spp. in clinical specimens, but substantial variation in results were observed across studies due to lack of standardization of PCR methods, including the procedure of DNA extraction. These factors have, so far, prevented the inclusion of PCR within the current EORTC/MSG microbiological criterion for invasive aspergillosis.

Prior to initiatives by the European *Aspergillus* PCR Initiative (EAPCRI) working group of the ISHAM to address the above limitations of *Aspergillus* PCR assays (see below), Mengoli et al. undertook a systematic review to assess assays for their (i) diagnostic value (specifically, DORs) or (ii) role in screening for invasive aspergillosis (89). Sixteen studies that employed PCR on blood, serum, or plasma samples (>10,000 samples from 1,618 patients at high risk for invasive aspergillosis) were included. The meta-analysis showed that a single PCR-negative result was sufficient to exclude a diagnosis of proven or probable aspergillosis if PCR was used as a screening tool from the start of the at-risk period. Two positive PCR results are required to maximize specificity. The calculated pooled sensitivity was 75% (95% CI, 54 to 88%), the specificity was 87% (95% CI, 78 to 93%), the PPV was 15.2 to 81%, and the NPV was >97%. There was great heterogeneity in the patient population studied, PCR method, nature of samples (e.g., whole blood versus serum), and volume of sample tested (89); 1-ml serum volumes yielded superior sensitivity (100% versus 76.5%) compared with standard 100-μl volumes (90).

PCR performed on BAL fluid samples has good potential to assist diagnosis of invasive pulmonary aspergillosis (61, 91, 92). A recent evaluation of a real-time pan-*Aspergillus* PCR in lung transplant patients showed a sensitivity and specificity of 100% and 88%, respectively, with similar performance characteristics noted for an *A. fumigatus*-specific PCR (91). Despite assay differences, studies have demonstrated a high NPV and good sensitivity, with variable PPVs reflecting differences in diagnostic certainty.

The derivation of standardized protocols for each PCR step, especially for DNA extraction, by the EAPCRI with international collaboration (93, 94) has allowed multicenter clinical validation of PCR assays. Notably, the following factors are critical in influencing the quality and success of *Aspergillus* PCR assays: the type of specimen, the volume of specimen, the DNA fungal extraction method, and the potential for automation of the PCR process itself (to increase sensitivity). There was no significant difference in sensitivity between the use of whole blood and the use of serum for PCR-based diagnosis of aspergillosis, although in some studies there was a trend for whole blood to be more sensitive (85 to 91% versus 79%) and specific (96%) and to show earlier positive results (36 days versus 15 days) compared with serum (95, 96). Against this finding is the reduced false-positivity rate using serum, which is also easier to process. The optimum sample type should be determined by the local requirement. A later meta-analysis demonstrated higher diagnostic accuracy for studies that were compliant with the EAPCRI recommendations (97). Most cases included in these studies stemmed from hematology patients; the performance of PCR testing in serum from patients with other types of immunosuppression is uncertain.

A further advance is the availability of several commercial multiplex real-time PCR assays, such as AsperGenius (PathoNostics, Maastricht, the Netherlands), RenDx Fungiplex (Renshaw Diagnostics, Ltd., Glasgow, United Kingdom), PLEX-ID Broad Fungal Assay (Abbott, Abbott Park, IL), and MycoGENIE (Ademtech-Bioparc BioGalien, Pessac, France) (98–100). However, some of these kits are not cleared by the FDA for diagnostic use, although the MycoGENIE assay is CE *in vitro* diagnostic use compliant (100). Another, the MycAssay *Aspergillus* assay (Myconostica, Manchester, United Kingdom), is a platform that allows standardized detection using quality-controlled reagents. In high-risk hematology patients, the kit had a sensitivity of 65% and specificity of 95% with serum and BAL fluid (101). In nonhematology patients with invasive lung aspergillosis, the sensitivity, specificity, PPV, and NPV for lower respiratory tract samples were 86.7%, 87.6%, 34.1%, and 92.2%, respectively; sensitivity increased when multiple samples were analyzed (102). The median time to detection of *Aspergillus* was 4 hours. The AsperGenius (PathoNostics) kit allows the specific detection of *A. fumigatus* complex, *A. terreus*, and other *Aspergillus* species by targeting the 28S rRNA gene. It is able also to detect the most prevalent *CYP51* gene mutations in *A. fumigatus*—namely, the TR34, L98H, Y121F, and T289A mutations, which are known to confer resistance (99) (see "*In Vitro* Antifungal Susceptibility Testing" below).

Clinical Utility of Combined Antigen Detection and Nucleic Acid Amplification Test

The above descriptions of GM and (1,3)-β-D-glucan antigen and *Aspergillus* PCR testing for the diagnosis of invasive aspergillosis have highlighted a number of limitations of these tests. Test performance can vary considerably, and the (1,3)-β-D-glucan test is not specific for *Aspergillus* spp. However, substantive progress has been made in standardizing *Aspergillus* PCR procedures to enable its wider deployment.

It is clear from numerous publications that it is the use of these tests in combination that assists in the earlier diagnosis of invasive aspergillosis, including in children with hematologic cancers (70). In a recent randomized trial of the *Aspergillus* GM and *Aspergillus* PCR versus culture and histology methods in high-risk hematology patients, the use of GM and PCR to direct therapy reduced the use of empiric antifungals, enabled more diagnosis of probable aspergillosis a median of 4 days earlier, and was most effective in patients receiving fluconazole, itraconazole, or no antifungal prophylaxis (103). Rogers et al. demonstrated that addition of PCR to GM monitoring in the setting of hematological malignancy provided greater diagnostic accuracy for invasive aspergillosis (104). Others have reported that GM or PCR can diagnose invasive aspergillosis a median of 2 to 9 days earlier than culture and high-resolution computerized tomography scans in up to 88.8% of patients (95, 105) and that both serum GM and PCR testing led to greater sensitivity in diagnosing invasive aspergillosis in hematology patients (105, 106), with a meta-analysis showing the association of both GM and PCR to be highly suggestive of active infection (PPV, 88%). The combined use of the *Aspergillus* lateral flow test (OLM Diagnostics) with *Aspergillus* PCR yielded a 100% sensitivity and 100% specificity for proven or probable aspergillosis in an early retrospective clinical study (76).

Isolation Procedures

Aspergillus species are not fastidious in their growth requirements. They are typically easily recovered on standard mycological media and will also grow on bacteriological media such as blood agar. On occasions where respiratory tract specimens may be inoculated on media selective for certain non-*Aspergillus* moulds (e.g., dichloran rose bengal agar for selective isolation of *Scedosporium* species [107]), and where the presence of *Aspergillus* organisms may be clinically relevant, it should be noted that growth of aspergilli is inhibited on these media.

Most identification schemes utilize specific media and incubation conditions for the description of characteristics, such as colony color and size (diameter) (Fig. 3). *Aspergillus* species usually grow without difficulty at 25°C but also at higher temperatures. Although isolation procedures do not require specific biohazard precautions, it is good laboratory practice to handle all culture material in a class II biosafety cabinet to avoid dispersal of spores through the environment and cross-contamination. The culture process usually requires several days.

Identification

Culture-based identification of aspergilli remains important despite increasing use of molecular and proteomic tools. Diagnostic features of the more common pathogenic species and species complex are summarized in Table 2. For keys to taxa and additional information, see also the work of de Hoog et al. (14). Figure 2 presents a diagrammatic key to several species. Some species commonly produce sexual structures (i.e., cleistothecia and ascospores), which may aid identification. The respective teleomorph synonyms of common *Aspergillus* species are given in parentheses (e.g., *Emericella* and *Neosartorya* [Table 2]).

Phenotypic identification of *Aspergillus* requires the assessment of both macroscopic and microscopic morphological characteristics. Inoculation media and incubation conditions affect the morphological characteristics of *Aspergillus* species. Czapek yeast autolysate agar and/or 2% malt extract agar (Oxoid), with or without 20% sucrose, is recommended for identification and characterization (1). Isolates are usually inoculated at three points and incubated at 25°C (1, 14). Most species sporulate within 7 days, but

FIGURE 3 (A) H&E-stained section of lung showing *Aspergillus* hyphae with smooth hyaline which are septate and branch dichotomously at acute angles. (B) Colonies of *Aspergillus fumigatus* on potato dextrose agar showing typical blue-green surface pigmentation with a suede-like surface consisting of a dense felt of conidiophores. (C) Conidiophores of *Aspergillus fumigatus* are columnar (up to 400 by 50 μm long) but may be shorter and are uniseriate. The vesicle is conical and sports a singe row of phialides on the upper two-thirds. Conidia are produced in basipetal succession with long chains and are globose to subglobose. (D) Culture of *Aspergillus lentulus*. Colonies are suede-like to floccose, white, and interspersed with gray-green patches of conidia (conidiation is slow to poor). (E) Conidiophores of *Aspergillus lentulus* are short, columnar, and uniseriate. Stipes are narrower than those of *Aspergillus fumigatus*. Vesicles are subglobose and are smaller (6 to 25 μm in diameter) than those of *A. fumigatus* (10 to 26 μm). (F) Culture of *Aspergillus flavus*. Colonies are granular, flat, often with radial grooves, and yellow at first but quickly becoming bright to dark yellow-green with age. (G) Biseriate head of *Aspergillus flavus*. (H) *Aspergillus nidulans* (*Emericella nidulans*) showing cleistothecia. (I) *Aspergillus ustus* showing biseriate head, brown stipe, and Hülle cells.

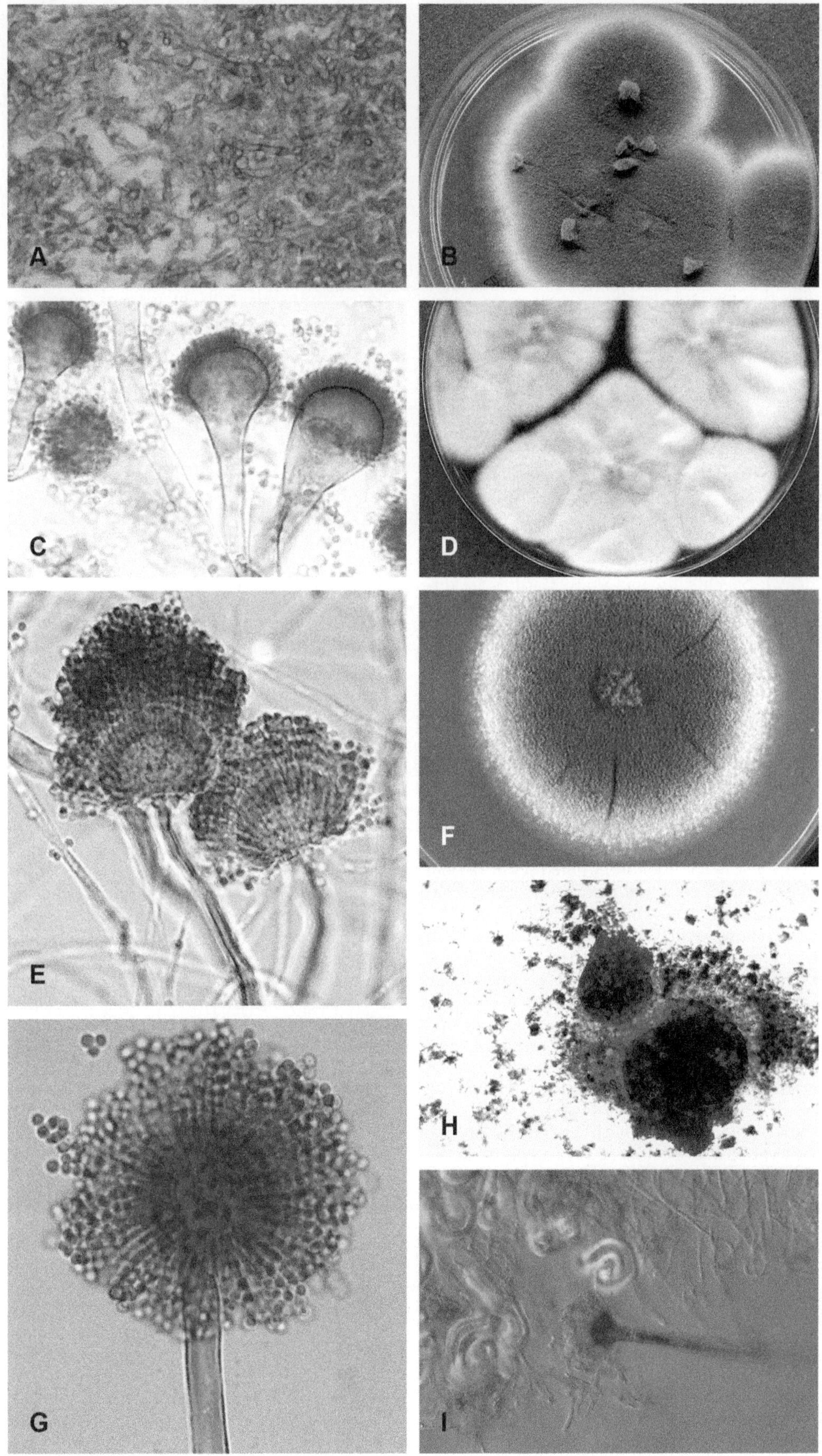
A
B
C
D
E
F
G
H
I

the teleomorph form takes longer to develop. Descriptions are primarily based on colony pigmentation and morphology of the conidial head with reference to those in expert monographs (4, 8).

Macroscopic Features

Important colony characteristics, recorded after 7 days, include growth rate, texture, degree of sporulation, surface and reverse colony color, the presence of exudate droplets and diffusible pigments, and the production of sclerotia, Hülle cells, and cleistothecia or ascospores (Fig. 3B to I) (1, 14, 108). Isolates that are not identifiable should be retained for longer for possible development of ascomata or other structures that may aid identification.

Microscopic Features

Microscopic mounts are best made from conidiophores produced on malt extract agar after 7 to 10 days, using sticky tape flag or slide culture preparations in lactic acid (1, 108). Lactophenol is no longer recommended for mounting because it is corrosive and the phenol is toxic, but lactofuchsin is still widely used (1). *Aspergillus* conidia are hydrophobic, and a drop of 70% alcohol is usually required to remove air bubbles and excess conidia. Key features are hyaline hyphae showing distinctive conidial heads with flask-shaped phialides arranged in whorls on a vesicle (Fig. 2). Specifically, important features are differences in size, shape, color, and wall ornamentation of various structures, including the stipe, shape and size of vesicles, and arrangement of phialides. A stipe or conidiophore arises either directly from the vegetative hyphae or from a specialized hyphal cell called a foot cell; it is typically nonseptate and varies in color, length, and wall ornamentation according to species. The stipe ends in a variably shaped (globose, subglobose, hemispherical, pear-shaped, or clavate [club-shaped]), swollen vesicle (Fig. 2); either the entire vesicle or its upper portion is covered with phialides, which give rise to the conidia. Conidial head morphology in *Aspergillus* is either uniseriate, where the phialides arise directly from the vesicle, or biseriate, where they arise from an intermediate series of cells, the metulae, or a combination of both, as occurs in *A. flavus* (Fig. 2; Table 2).

The conidia themselves may be borne in a single column (columnar), or columns may be split, with some arising at right angles to the stipe (radiate). A dissecting microscope is required to make this distinction. Conidia are usually ellipsoidal or globose, may be echinulate, and vary in size, color, and wall markings depending on the species. Differential interference contrast microscopy is recommended for best observation of conidiophore characteristics (1, 108).

Sclerotia are firm, fruiting-body-like structures comprising swollen hyphal cells but without internal spores. Hülle cells are variably globose with very thick refractile walls (Fig. 3I). They commonly occur within the growing mycelium near the colony center, where their presence is indicated by droplets of exudate. They are often associated with cleistothecial ascomata (Table 2). The interiors of cleistothecia are filled with asci and ascospores. Shape, color, size, and wall features of these structures are important in distinguishing the different teleomorph forms.

Poorly Sporulating Species or Variants

Where sporulation is poor, morphological identification may be problematic, although incubation at 25°C in light and allowing the cultures to experience the normal diurnal cycles of light and dark may help to induce sporulation (109, 110). Poorly sporulating isolates are not uncommonly recovered from clinical specimens (109), including those from patients with aspergillosis and with cystic fibrosis. When this occurs, *A. fumigatus* species complex could be considered if an atypical, sometimes waxy or cerebriform mould was grown at 45°C (all members of section *Fumigati* grow at this elevated temperature [Table 2]); it is now well established that various cryptic species such as *A. lentulus* and *A. thermomutatus* and other closely related sibling species of *A. fumigatus* demonstrate a poorly sporulating phenotype (7, 109). *A. lentulus* does exhibit smaller vesicles (Table 2; Fig. 3E) and, unlike *A. fumigatus*, cannot grow at 48 or 50°C, but in practice it cannot be distinguished by morphological methods alone from *A. fumigatus* without scanning electron microscopy or other sophisticated microscopy. As *A. lentulus* has low *in vitro* susceptibilities to the azoles, amphotericin B, and caspofungin (7), it is important to accurately identify all clinically significant isolates. Since the discovery of *A. lentulus* as a new species, subsequent screening studies of "*A. fumigatus*" isolates have uncovered pathogens misidentified as *A. fumigatus*, including *A. viridinutans*, *A. felis*, and *A. udagawae* (30, 109; summarized in reference 111); these isolates also demonstrate variable susceptibility to antifungal drugs *in vitro* and are associated with high mortality rates (see "Antimicrobial Susceptibilities" below) (111, 112). As for *A. lentulus*, phenotypic identification methods alone will not differentiate them from *A. fumigatus*.

Molecular Identification

Where conventional phenotypic methods cannot identify *Aspergillus* isolates or identification is uncertain (e.g., with nonsporulating isolates) due to overlapping morphological features, DNA sequencing is often helpful. Comparative multilocus sequence analysis is the gold standard for molecular identification, as no single gene can be relied on (1). The ITS region, including the 5.8S rRNA gene regions, is generally more discriminatory than the D1-D2 domain of the 28S subunit for the identification of aspergilli (110, 113, 114), with the ITS1-5.8S-ITS2 region being the universal DNA barcode marker for fungi (115). However, the ITS region does not contain enough variation for distinguishing species within some *Aspergillus* clades, and hence, the use of other gene targets for species identification, including the β-tubulin, rodlet A, and mitochondrial cytochrome *b* genes, may be necessary (1, 109, 111, 112, 116). The ISHAM *Aspergillus* Working Group recommends the use of a comparative sequencing-based identification method that uses the ITS regions for species complex-level identification and of a protein-coding locus (β-tubulin region) for identification of species within each *Aspergillus* species complex (1). This approach successfully identified 218 *Aspergillus* isolates collected for TRANSNET (30) and 278 (86.3%) isolates in the FILPOP study in Spain (33). However, the *benA* primers preferentially amplify the *tubC* paralogue for some species in the Nigri section (117), although this locus may be too variable to be used for phylogenetic reconstruction (14). The calmodulin gene, *CaM*, has recently been suggested as a candidate secondary identification marker in *Aspergillus*, as it is easy to amplify and distinguishes all species when used in combination with ITS sequencing (1). To improve species identification based on ITS sequencing, sequences may be searched against the RefSeq database (https://www.ncbi.nlm.nih.gov/refseq/), which contains only verified ITS sequences (118).

Non-sequence-based identification methods include real-time PCR and *Aspergillus* species-specific microsphere-based assays using Luminex xMAP technology

(Luminex Corp., Austin, TX). In addition, the three major species within section *Fumigati* (*A. fumigatus*, *A. lentulus*, and *A. udagawae*) can be accurately distinguished by PCR-restriction fragment length polymorphism (RFLP) analysis of the *benA* gene (119). Alonso et al. developed a real-time PCR followed by combined probe hybridization and high-resolution melting analysis to identify section *Fumigati* and non-*Fumigati Aspergillus* isolates; the detection limit was 10^2 conidia/ml (87). Microsphere-based Luminex (Luminex Corp.) assays have also enabled species complex-level identification as well as differentiation of species within the *A. fumigatus* complex (120).

The preciseness of reporting of an identification of *Aspergillus* depends on (i) the clinical need to accurately identify the fungus species (e.g., recovery from a tissue biopsy compared with recovery from sputum) and (ii) access to molecular identification methods. In smaller laboratories, the use of the term "species complex" aids correct identification, since isolates are relatively reliably identified to the section level by morphological methods. For example, a laboratory can identify a fungus as "*A. fumigatus* species complex" by phenotypic methods and indicate that molecular identification is required to identify the isolate as a species within the complex.

MALDI-TOF Methods

Identification of mould cultures using matrix-assisted laser desorption ionization–time-of-flight mass spectrometry (MALDI-TOF MS) is increasingly undergoing evaluation to reduce the turnaround time for identification of *Aspergillus* cultures in clinical laboratories. Despite initial technical difficulties in analyte preparation posed by the relatively complicated morphology and the *Aspergillus* cell wall, the technology has utility not only for identifying isolates to the species complex level but also for identifying species including "cryptic" *Aspergillus* species and, in some cases, delineating strain variation (121–127). There are now several well-described standardized preanalytical sample preparation methods described for filamentous fungi (122, 123). For *Aspergillus* species, mechanical disruption by bead beating of cells and conidia prior to on-target lysis is recommended to ensure highly discriminatory spectra (124, 125). Furthermore, a robust and extensive database of reference spectra is required for accurate species identification (126, 128). Many commercial databases have few species and intraspecies strain representations and need to be supplemented with an in-house library incorporating well-validated spectra from adequate numbers of species and from sufficient numbers of strains representing each species for accurate identification (121, 122, 126–128).

Bille et al. reported an overall identification rate for *Aspergillus* spp. of 98.4% (63/64 isolates) using the Andromas system (Andromas SA, Paris, France), and Alanio et al. reported an identification rate of 98.6% (138/140 isolates) (128, 129). Becker et al. correctly identified 99.6% of *Aspergillus* isolates ($n = 256$) to species level, compared with conventional methods, which correctly identified only 87.9% (126). The only isolate unable to be identified by MALDI-TOF MS was not available in the database. Hettick et al. used MALDI-TOF MS to derive spectra for 12 *Aspergillus* species and five different strains of *A. flavus*; classification of each species and strain of *Aspergillus* tested was achieved with 100% accuracy (130) when invasive *Aspergillus* isolates were analyzed.

All studies have stressed the need for adequate sample preparation for MALDI-TOF MS and the construction of libraries of robust spectra from known strains, independent of the MALDI-TOF MS system (reviewed in reference 121). Use of MALDI-TOF MS has not been approved for the identification of *Aspergillus* or other moulds by the FDA, and it is unlikely that industry will invest in strengthening filamentous fungi identification capacity. Plans are under way to develop a curated, publicly accessible MALDI-TOF MS database via the internet (126).

Typing Systems

Genotyping of *Aspergillus* is central to the understanding of epidemiological relationships between clinical and environmental isolates and to identifying the origin and tracking the spread of nosocomial infections (see "Epidemiology and Transmission" above), especially in responding to public health situations (131). Genotyping also assists in determining if a patient is colonized or infected with the same strain over long periods or becomes recolonized or reinfected by different strains. Many methods are described for the typing of *Aspergillus*; these include random amplified polymorphic DNA (RAPD) analysis, RFLP analysis, DNA fingerprinting, amplified fragment length polymorphism (AFLP) analysis, multilocus microsatellite typing (MLMT), multilocus sequence typing (MLST), and a simple single-locus sequence typing involving the gene encoding for cell surface protein (CSP). Most data are based on the typing of *A. fumigatus*, with the reference typing method being analysis of short tandem repeats (STR) based on microsatellite analysis (see below) (132).

RAPD analysis has been used to differentiate between isolates of *A. fumigatus* (133) and other species, including *A. flavus* (134) and *A. terreus* (135). RFLP analysis was likewise first applied to the genotyping of *A. fumigatus* using XhoI and SalI enzymes and then to species identification among a heterogeneous *Aspergillus* group, where it correctly identified *A. flavus* isolates (136). DNA fingerprinting has utility in genotyping using probes such as those containing retrotransposon-like elements, namely, Afut1, Afut2, and Afut4 (137–139), while clinical and environmental *A. flavus* isolates from a neonatal intensive care unit have been successfully typed with the species-specific probe pAF28 (140). AFLP analysis is another approach that has determined genetic diversity within *A. fumigatus* (141) and within the sections *Flavi* (142) and *Nigri* (143). Widespread application of these methods, in particular, RAPD and AFLP, has been hampered by a low degree of interlaboratory reproducibility due to their reliance on pattern-based typing techniques.

MLMT analysis using four, and later nine, different microsatellite markers was developed to form the STRAf scheme for genotyping *A. fumigatus* (132); this approach has been extended to include other species, including *A. flavus* (six or seven markers) (144, 145), *A. niger* (six markers), and *A. nidulans* (seven markers) (146, 147). More recent studies confirmed the high-resolution genotyping results for *A. flavus* (145, 148). Hadrich et al., using six STR markers, found that among 63 clinical isolates, the marker AFLA1 had the highest discriminatory power (14 distinct alleles; discriminatory or *D* value, 0.903) (145). STR typing has also been developed for *A. terreus*. By using a test set of 244 *A. terreus* isolates and a panel of eight STR markers, 79 genotypes of this species complex were identified with high discriminatory value; when the test was extended to analyze 63 Austrian clinical isolates, 68.2% comprised three genotypes (36). Kathuria et al. used nine STR markers to identify 75 genotypes among 101 Indian *A. terreus* complex strains (149).

MLST analysis with a panel of seven genetic loci has also been applied for strain typing of *A. fumigatus* (150). CSP typing (21) is a useful molecular tool but has lower discriminatory power than MLMT. Strain variation is a result of both repeat number variation and nucleotide sequence variation. In one study, CSP typing was compared with PCR fingerprinting using minisatellite (core sequence of the bacteriophage M13)-specific and microsatellite [$(GTG)_5$ and $(GACA)_4$]-specific single primers and MLMT analysis to differentiate between *A. fumigatus* strains; only MLMT separated all clinical and environmental isolates implicated in a case cluster (21).

MLMT, MLST, and CSP typing are all highly reproducible and yield unambiguous and portable data. Microsatellite-based approaches and MLST analysis are species specific. Recently, a new genotyping method based on hypervariable tandem repeats with exons of surface protein coding genes has been reported to offer high-level discrimination of *A. fumigatus*, where 96 genotypes were distinguished among 126 unrelated isolates with a *D* value of 0.994 (151). Finally, whole-genome sequencing technologies have very good potential to provide state-of-the-art means of comparative analysis of *Aspergillus* genomes, including tracking of azole-resistant isolates (152).

Serologic Tests

The detection of *Aspergillus* GM and *Aspergillus*-specific recombinant proteins in serum and other body fluids is discussed in "Antigen Detection" above. Methods to detect other *Aspergillus* antigens or anti-*Aspergillus* antibodies against these antigens, including determining reactivity in skin tests, have also been developed, but their clinical utility is less well defined (153). The main reasons for this are related to the nature and purity of the antigen. Although antigen preparations may be available commercially, their quality is variable, and they demonstrate cross-reactivity with non-*Aspergillus* antigens. However, hybridoma technology and monoclonal antibody-based detection systems have changed the state of immunodiagnosis of aspergillosis. In particular, measurement of *Aspergillus*-specific antibodies is important in the diagnostic pathway for the more chronic forms of aspergillosis, allergic bronchopulmonary aspergillosis (ABPA) and chronic pulmonary aspergillosis.

A number of reviews detail the candidate *Aspergillus* antigens for incorporation into immunoassays (72, 153, 154). Antigens tested include somatic preparations, either crude or purified whole-cell mycelial extracts, *Aspergillus* metabolites, mannoproteins, and expressed and purified recombinant antigens. One purified somatic antigen, a 19-kDa basic protein, was shown to be a major circulating antigen in the urine of patients with invasive aspergillosis (72). This protein was also present in the serum of patients with aspergillomas. Molecular characterization has subsequently shown it to be Aspf1, an IgE-binding protein (and potent allergen) related to the mitogillin family of cytotoxins. Other potential serodiagnostic antigens include an 18-kDa ribonuclease, 88-kDa dipeptidyl peptidase, 33-kDa alkaline protease, the recombinant mannoproteins antigens Afmp1 and Afmp2, and a recombinant 19-kDa Cu-Zn superoxide dismutase (153, 155, 156). Another *Aspergillus* protein, chitosanase CnsB, has also attracted attention as a potential antigen for antibody-based diagnostics (157). Various test formats have been exploited to detect antibodies to these antigens. Double immunodiffusion and counterimmunoelectrophoresis were initially used, but these have now been replaced by commercial ELISAs and immunofluorescence assays (153, 157).

However, rather than detecting antigen, most serological evaluations have focused on detecting antibody responses to these antigens. Although many assays proved sensitive, their routine use has been limited by substantial interlaboratory variability, cross-reactivity between different fungi, the type of antigen used in the assay, and, importantly, the inability to mount diagnostic antibody responses in immunocompromised hosts. Nonetheless, in one study, IgG anti-*A. fumigatus*-specific mitogillin was detected by ELISA in the serum of all (32 of 32) patients with aspergilloma and in 64% (31 of 42) of patients with invasive pulmonary aspergillosis (158); serum IgG and IgM antibodies were found in only 1.3% of healthy volunteers. However, the optimal cutoff value for the ELISA is not clearly established. Humoral antibody responses to Afmp1 detected by ELISA were demonstrated with high sensitivity (100%) for patients with aspergilloma, whereas in invasive aspergillosis, the sensitivity was only 33.3% (156). Combined immune responses to Afmp1 and Afmp2 may increase sensitivity (159). Recent work showed that total antibody specific to *Aspergillus*-specific thioredoxin reductase (GliT) was detected in nonneutropenic patients with invasive aspergillosis with a sensitivity of 81% and specificity of 96% (160). Whether the detection of *Aspergillus* IgG antibodies is of clinical value in the diagnosis of invasive aspergillosis in high-risk patients is uncertain; one study found that baseline IgG responses to a number of recombinant antigens were higher in patients with aspergillosis than in controls (161), while another concluded that measuring *Aspergillus* IgG levels is of little value (162). Further studies are required to determine their diagnostic potential.

Measurement of *Aspergillus*-specific antibody responses, however, has greater utility in chronic and allergic forms of aspergillosis and aspergilloma. For example, detection of circulating antibodies may aid diagnosis of ABPA in patients with cystic fibrosis and in those with severe asthma with fungal sensitization (Table 3). Anti-*A. fumigatus* IgE and IgG and *A. fumigatus* precipitins are established markers of ABPA and are criteria included in its diagnosis (reviewed in reference 153). Further, immunoglobulin subclass measurements may add valuable information. Recently, detection of specific IgE to recombinant *A. fumigatus* allergens, such as those of the rAspf family, and detection of the thymus activation-regulated chemokine TARC/CCL17 have been identified as new biomarkers of ABPA (163). Consensus opinion indicates that measurements of serum IgG subclasses, especially IgG4, against *A. fumigatus* are useful in screening for and classifying ABPA, at least in cystic fibrosis patients, whereas IgA measurement could be useful to determine prognosis of ABPA (163, 164). Quantitation of serum IgG4 may improve specificity of diagnosis. Further, the biomarker TARC has shown greater test accuracy for ABPA diagnosis than antibody responses. Anti-*A. fumigatus* IgE and IgG may be measured by commercial assays, such as the ImmunoCap assay (Phadia, Uppsala, Sweden) and the Platelia *Aspergillus* IgG assay (Bio-Rad, Marnes-la-Coquette, France); in a recent study, both these ELISAs were more sensitive than counterimmunoelectrophoresis (>93% versus 63%) in diagnosing ABPA (165).

Newer assays for measuring *Aspergillus* antibodies have become available. One study compared the efficacy of an indirect hemagglutination assay designed to detect *Aspergillus* agglutinating antibodies (ELI.H.A. *Aspergillus* indirect hemagglutination; EliTech Microbio, Signes, France) with an agar double-diffusion system to detect *Aspergillus* precipitins to diagnose chronic pulmonary aspergillosis. Concordance of a positive or negative test result was good, although titers varied with method. The EliTech assay (EliTech Microbio) was rapid and user friendly but was not easy to read (153). The *Aspergillus* Western blot IgG kit (LDBiodiagnostics, Lyon, France) has been shown to have a sensitivity of 88.6% and specificity of 84% for the diagnosis of chronic forms of aspergillosis in nonimmunocompromised hosts (166). Many of these assays have not yet been cleared by the FDA for diagnostic use.

Antimicrobial Susceptibilities

Drugs Used to Treat Invasive Aspergillosis

Amphotericin B, the triazoles (voriconazole, posaconazole, and isavuconazole), and echinocandins form the backbone for treatment of invasive aspergillosis, although itraconazole can be useful in the more chronic forms of disease. Consensus opinion informed by a landmark randomized, controlled trial recommends voriconazole as first-line therapy (167) for invasive pulmonary aspergillosis as well as extrapulmonary and disseminated infection (168). Oral voriconazole is preferred for step-down or maintenance therapy. Other antifungals approved for treating aspergillosis are lipid amphotericin B formulations (e.g., the liposomal compound, for primary therapy or salvage treatment) (168) and the echinocandins, although only caspofungin is licensed for this indication in many countries (169) (also for primary and salvage therapy). Posaconazole, amphotericin B, and caspofungin have been used in salvage therapy, all with response rates between 40 and 50%. Recently, isavuconazole was shown to be noninferior to voriconazole for the primary treatment of invasive aspergillosis (170) and is licensed by the FDA as an alternative to voriconazole for these infections. Though there are insufficient data to recommend antifungal combinations for primary and salvage treatment, a clinical trial of voriconazole versus voriconazole-anidulafungin for initial treatment of proven or probable aspergillosis showed a trend towards improved survival in hematology patients (171). For detailed treatment practices for aspergillosis, the reader is referred to the 2016 Infectious Diseases Society of America guidelines document (168).

In Vitro Antifungal Susceptibility Testing

In vitro susceptibility testing of *Aspergillus* isolates may help guide therapy. Resistance to azoles, the only orally active group of antifungals for aspergillosis, used to be uncommon and was limited to patients receiving long-term azole therapy or prophylaxis; in one study, there was a positive correlation between prolonged itraconazole use and high MICs of posaconazole (172). Given the increasing azole resistance among both clinical and environmental *A. fumigatus* isolates in some countries (173), routine testing of aspergilli for antifungal susceptibility in these regions is important for clinical decisions and to monitor trends. The prevalence of azole resistance is relatively high in Europe and variable in the rest of the world (0.55 to 11.2%) (174). Rates of azole resistance were 5.8% in the ARTEMIS global surveillance study (175, 176), up to 20% in the United Kingdom (173), and 20 to 30% in the Netherlands and Germany (174, 177). Knowledge of susceptibility patterns for new and cryptic species other than *A. fumigatus* is likewise important, as resistance rates can reach 40% (33).

The majority of azole-resistant *A. fumigatus* (and other *Aspergillus* species) isolates were found to contain an alteration in the target protein sterol 14a-demethylase (or Cyp51), inhibiting drug binding. These changes are a result of single nucleotide polymorphisms in the gene *CYP51A*, encoding the protein leading to amino acid substitutions. Mutational hot spots confirmed to cause resistance have been located at amino acid positions G54 and L98, among others, and the L98 alterations require a tandem repeat (TR) in the promoter region of *CYP51A* to cause resistance; this is referred to as the TR/L98 mutation (173). Mechanisms of azole and echinocandin resistance are detailed in chapter 133.

Methods and MIC Determinations

In the past few years, standardization of two reference methods for susceptibility testing of conidium-forming moulds has provided guidelines for antifungal susceptibility testing of *Aspergillus*. These methods are (i) the Clinical and Laboratory Standards Institute (CLSI) M38-A2 method and (ii) the European Committee on Antimicrobial Susceptibility Testing (EUCAST) standard (178, 179) (see chapter 134). With either approach, MIC determinations (and minimum fungicidal concentration determinations) are relatively straightforward for azoles and amphotericin B due to the growth-versus-no-growth pattern of inhibition, and MICs obtained by these reference methods are in close agreement.

Interpretative CLSI breakpoints to recognize susceptibility or resistance have not yet been established for any drugs for *Aspergillus*. Nonetheless, amphotericin B, itraconazole, voriconazole, posaconazole, and the echinocandins are active *in vitro* and demonstrate the lowest MICs (33, 180). Using the EUCAST method, clinical breakpoints (CBPs) for amphotericin B, voriconazole, posaconazole, itraconazole, and most recently isavuconazole have been published, primarily for *A. fumigatus* (181–184); epidemiological cutoff (ECOFF) MICs of wild-type *Aspergillus* strains have also been published (183–185). See chapter 134.

Importantly, MICs may vary with species and with geographic region. However, *A. terreus* is considered resistant to amphotericin B, as this species is a poor target for this drug; MICs are as high as 16 μg/ml, and routine susceptibility testing is not required for this species. Infections due to *A. terreus* are associated with poorer responses to amphotericin B than those caused by, e.g., *A. fumigatus*, although overall, there is no clear correlation of amphotericin B MICs with clinical response, since there is a narrow distribution of MICs with no clear resistance phenotype (186).

With regard to the correlation of azole MICs and clinical outcomes, earlier work observed good correlation between high MICs and treatment failure in animal models of invasive aspergillosis (187). Recently, voriconazole MICs were predictive of treatment results in *A. terreus* murine infections (188). However, in another study, there was no relationship between increasing MICs and response to voriconazole in mice with *A. fumigatus* infection (189). Baddley et al. observed that voriconazole MICs exceeding the ECOFF value (i.e., 1 μg/ml) were not associated with increased mortality in patients with *A. fumigatus* infection receiving voriconazole (190), and for other *Aspergillus* species, correlation of azole MICs and outcome is also uncertain (191). Nonetheless, in patients with very high MICs (e.g., a MIC of 16 μg/ml for itraconazole), case fatality rates may be as high as 88%.

Susceptibility endpoints for the echinocandins against *A. fumigatus* by the CLSI method may be uncertain due to significant trailing growth. Thus, a minimum effective concentration (MEC) is employed, where the MEC is the lowest concentration leading to macroscopically aberrant growth in the form of microcolonies or granular growth compared to the growth control wells. MEC determination is time-consuming and requires a microscope to determine morphological changes, and interlaboratory reproducibility is suboptimal. Correlation between MECs and *in vivo* outcomes is uncertain. One report found clinical failure and *in vivo* resistance in an animal model for an isolate with an MEC in the wild-type range (192). There are no CBPs for the echinocandins with EUCAST.

In practice, both reference methods, although easily performed by specialist mycology laboratories, are not suitable for use in most clinical laboratories, as they require extensive training. Commercial kits for susceptibility testing of *Aspergillus*, such as the Etest (AB Biodisk, Solna, Sweden) or other gradient strip methods, are useful. The Etest has excellent correlation with the CLSI reference method for voriconazole (193) and between 80 and 100% agreement for itraconazole and posaconazole (194, 195). The Sensititre Yeast YO10 system (incorporating prefilled trays of nine antifungal agents [Trek ThermoFisher Diagnostics, Cleveland, OH]) is based on the CLSI method. The visual endpoint allows easier reading, and it shows good correlation with the azoles and amphotericin and the echinocandins (195). Another approach is to use azole-containing agars, such as multiwell surveillance plates (VIPcheck, Nijmegen, the Netherlands) (see chapter 133), to screen for azole resistance; this technique has been evaluated for *A. fumigatus* (173). Cross-resistance between azoles occurs in up to 74% of cases (173, 176). Research methods include isothermal microcalorimetry for real-time susceptibility testing (196). Genotypic susceptibility testing of *A. fumigatus* is performed in many specialist laboratories (see chapter 134).

Evaluation, Interpretation, and Reporting of Results

The diagnostic mycology laboratory's aims are to provide timely, clinically meaningful information using accurate and up-to-date methods. The criteria proposed by the EORTC/MSG for the analysis of patient data in clinical trials will help to standardize result interpretation. Identification of *Aspergillus* fungi to species level should be undertaken when they are recovered from sterile specimens and from patients at high risk of invasive aspergillosis. Certain species may be more resistant to antifungal agents. The *A. terreus* complex is resistant to amphotericin B, while the *A. nidulans* complex and *A. ustus* are less susceptible to many agents than *A. fumigatus* (53, 197). *Aspergillus* recovered from nonsterile specimens, including BAL fluid and sputum, in immunocompetent patients may not be responsible for disease and may not require species identification. Workup of isolates should involve dialogue between the requesting clinician and the microbiologist.

Diagnosis of invasive aspergillosis remains difficult, as clinical and radiological features are nonspecific. Although diagnosis is more straightforward when *Aspergillus* is visualized in and cultured from clinical specimens, more often it relies collectively on non-culture-based tests in the setting of appropriate host risk factors, clinical presentation, and radiological findings. The conventional approach for patients at risk for aspergillosis is to administer antifungal agents empirically when a diagnosis has not yet been made. However, the increasing availability and use of biomarkers of infection, in particular *Aspergillus* GM and PCR, either alone or in combination, have led to the increasing adoption of a preemptive diagnostic-driven management approach incorporating the use of antifungal drugs. Using these biomarkers, prospective screening for infection in feasibility studies, including one randomized, controlled clinical trial, demonstrates the utility of further diagnostic workup (96, 103) and has led to earlier diagnosis of aspergillosis without decreasing mortality.

Despite progress made by the EUCAST movement in defining CBPs and ECOFF values for antifungal agents, correlation between MICs and clinical outcomes is not yet established. Interpretation of MIC testing of *Aspergillus* remains problematic. Nonetheless, given the rise in azole resistance among *A. fumigatus* in many countries, susceptibility testing of azoles against this species is warranted in these regions and in cases where there is therapeutic failure. The widespread use of EUCAST methods is limited by the expertise and training needed to perform these tests. Useful information regarding expected antifungal susceptibility may be obtained by identifying the fungus to species level (e.g., *A. lentulus*).

TALAROMYCES AND PENICILLIUM SPECIES

Taxonomy and Position of *Talaromyces marneffei* (formerly *Penicillium marneffei*)

Early work on the taxonomy of the genus *Penicillium* (otherwise referred to as *Penicillium sensu lato*) is based on the studies of Thom (198) and Raper and Thom (199). The genus contains over 250 species (http://www.aspergilluspenicillium.org). These species have traditionally been separated based on their morphology, specifically, conidiophore branching, into four anamorphic subgenera—*Aspergilloides*, *Furcatum*, *Penicillium*, and *Biverticillium*—within the family Trichocomaceae (4, 200). However, more recent multigene phylogenetic analyses have shown that three of these subgenera, *Aspergilloides*, *Furcatum*, and *Penicillium* (i.e., *Penicillium sensu stricto*), are polyphyletic, whereas the fourth, *Biverticillium*, forms a monophyletic group (201), which is characterized by the presence of symmetrical biverticillate conidiophores (202). The distinctive morphological and physiological features of *Biverticillium* have resulted in its evolving taxonomic status and suggestions to separate the subgenus *Biverticillium* from *Penicillium sensu stricto* (4, 200–202).

Rationale for Separation of Members of *Biverticillium* from *Penicillium sensu lato*

Penicillium sensu lato is associated with two teleomorphic genera: *Eupenicillium* (now synonymous with *Penicillium senso stricto*) and *Talaromyces* (now the teleomorph stage of *Biverticillium*). These two teleomorph genera are separated by distinctive ascomata. The sclerotium-like ascomata of *Penicillium sensu stricto* are thick-walled isodiametric cells maturing over several months and forming in most cases no ascospores, whereas *Talaromyces* cells are characterized by soft ascomatal walls comprising multiple layers of interwoven hyphae leading to mature ascomata within weeks. In comparison with *Penicillium senso stricto*, the members of *Talaromyces* often have darker green conidia, produce pigmented and encrusted aerial hyphae, and show yellow, orange, or red to purple colony color on reverse. Additionally, phylogenetic studies have increasingly provided evidence that *Penicillium sensu stricto* and *Talaromyces* should be considered subfamilies, as demonstrated by genetic relatedness analysis employing the fungal rRNA and calmodulin genes (203–206). The subdivision of these genera was finally confirmed using a multigene approach (201).

As mentioned above for "*Aspergillus*," the ability to correlate anamorphic and teleomorphic genera with modern taxonomic tools has led to the "one fungus = one name" concept (10). By removing the primacy of the teleomorph name over the anamorph-typified name (11), this has likewise had a major impact on what was known as the genus *Penicillium*. The name *Penicillium* is now used for *Penicillium sensu stricto* (i.e., comprising the subgenera *Aspergilloides*,

Furcatum, and *Penicillium*), while the term *Talaromyces* is now defined as a pleomorphic genus name, representative of the anamorphic species formerly within the *Penicillium* subgenus *Biverticillium* (207).

It is notable that the only species known to be a human and animal pathogen is *Talaromyces* (formerly *Penicillium*) *marneffei*, a member of the subgenus *Biverticillium*. This species is dimorphic, growing as a yeast at 37°C in the host and as a filamentous fungus at 25°C in the environment. As a result of the revised nomenclature, *P. marneffei* is now correctly classified as *T. marneffei* (Segretain, Capponi & Sureau) Samson, Yilmaz, Frisvad & Seifert, comb. nov. MycoBank MB560656 (207, 208), rendering *P. marneffei* [Segretain, Capponi & Sureau *apud* Segretain (1959)] the basonym of the new taxonomic assignment.

Epidemiology and Transmission

T. marneffei is a particular health problem in areas of endemicity for this organism in tropical Asia, especially Thailand, northeastern India, China, Hong Kong, Vietnam, and Taiwan (209–212). Although the disease is found predominantly in HIV/AIDS patients (209), its epidemiology is changing with better control of HIV infection globally, and non-HIV-infected individuals, including those with cell-mediated immunodeficiency, and patients receiving monoclonal antibody therapies (e.g., anti CD-20) and kinase inhibitors are also vulnerable (213). Its presence in HIV infection is an AIDS-defining illness.

The ecological reservoir of *T. marneffei* remains an enigma. A key question is whether human disease occurs as a result of zoonotic (animal) or sapronotic (environmental) transmission. Although *T. marneffei* was initially isolated from a bamboo rat, *Rhizomys sinensis*, in Vietnam in 1956 (214), exposure to soil and decaying material, especially under humid and rainy conditions, is likely the critical risk factor (209); agricultural occupations have been independently associated with increased risk (215). Yet, despite extensive efforts, attempts to recover the organism from soil have met with only limited success (209, 216), and proof of an environmental reservoir is still lacking. Conversely, it has been recovered from environments associated with bamboo rats of the genera *Rhizomys* and *Cannomys*, suggesting that these rodents are a key facet of the *T. marneffei* life cycle. When MLMT analysis was used to genotype this fungus, isolates from bamboo rats and humans shared identical genotypes (209, 217). This suggests that either rodents are vectors for human infections or both humans and rodents are infected from an as-yet-unidentified environmental source.

Patients are infected by inhalation of *T. marneffei* conidia; thus, pulmonary alveolar macrophages are the primary host defense. The fungus proliferates within phagocytic cells, resulting in granulomas in immunocompetent hosts. In HIV/AIDS, infection typically develops in advanced HIV infection, where the $CD4^+$ cell count is <50 cells/ml.

Clinical Significance

T. marneffei now ranks as the third most common opportunistic infection in HIV/AIDS in regions of endemicity (186). Its prevalence has increased in areas where HIV infection is on the rise (209, 218). Although uncommon, infections have been reported in other immunocompromised patients, including those with kidney transplants and systemic lupus erythematosus and those with primary or acquired immunodeficiency (213, 218–220). Immunosuppressed patients traveling to areas of endemicity should be vigilant with regard to risks of *T. marneffei* infection (221). Disseminated infection in HIV/AIDS, especially in those with CD4 counts below 100×10^9/liter, is typical, with involvement of the skin (60 to 85% of cases), lungs (pneumonia, including cavitation), liver, and joints. Most cases present with fever, weight loss, lymphadenopathy, and skin lesions—these are most often on the face, neck, and oral cavity, but they can affect any region, including the trunk and genitalia (209). The rash is typically an umbilicated papular rash with central necrosis but can be atypical, being flesh colored with no necrosis (222).

The fungus can be isolated from skin lesions or from blood, bone, or bone marrow. Presumptive diagnosis is made by visualization of yeast-like *T. marneffei* cells in Wright-stained smears of skin lesions or in biopsy specimens from these sites (223–225).

Collection, Transport, and Storage of Specimens

The methods of collection, transport, and storage of specimens are similar to those for other fungal pathogens (see chapter 117).

Direct Examination

Microscopy

Direct visualization of the organism in tissue or fine-needle aspiration samples of affected sites establishes presumptive diagnosis. Rapid diagnosis is enabled through cytological examination of lung biopsy imprint smears, lung aspirates, lymph node aspirates, skin smears, and even sputum. The yeast form is typically stained by methenamine silver or periodic acid-Schiff stain but can also be visualized by Giemsa and H&E stains (225, 226). Wright-stained bone marrow aspirates, often performed in the workup of HIV-positive patients with unexplained fever, are useful in these patients. Histiocytes are seen, with or without granuloma formation, and may contain few to many intracellular yeast-form cells (225); these are oval to elliptical (3 to 8 μm in diameter) with a distinctive clear central septum (226). This and the absence of budding help distinguish the condition from histoplasmosis and toxoplasmosis (14, 224). A specific indirect fluorescent-antibody reagent for rapid identification of *T. marneffei* in histologic sections using rabbit antiglobulin against yeast antigens of *T. marneffei* has also been developed (227).

Nucleic Acid Detection

A number of molecular techniques have been developed to directly detect and identify *T. marneffei* in clinical specimens. Many are in-house assays. Methods include single-step PCR and nested PCR assays to detect *T. marneffei* in PE tissue, skin, blood, BAL fluid, and other specimens. Most assays target the *T. marneffei* 18S rRNA and ITS gene region (228–230). The ability of one nested 18S rRNA PCR assay to directly identify the fungus in PE tissue was evaluated using inner primers (Pm1 and Pm2) specific to *T. marneffei*. Amplification of a species-specific fragment of ~400 bp was successful for tissue from all 14 patients studied as well as for tissue from 10 bamboo rats with *T. marneffei* infection, with an analytical sensitivity of 14 fg/μl (229). In a follow-up study, the same assay successfully detected *T. marneffei* DNA in BAL fluid and fresh lung tissue with good sensitivity and specificity in a mouse model of infection (230). In other studies, a multiplex ligation-dependent probe amplification assay detected *T. marneffei* DNA in PE tissue with high specificity (231), as has a loop-mediated isothermal amplification assay (232). Recently, Hien et al. evaluated a real-time PCR assay for the detection of the *T. marneffei* *MP1* gene in the plasma of AIDS patients with penicillosis;

the diagnostic sensitivity was 70.4% and the specificity was 100%, with a limit of detection of 100 *T. marneffei* cells per ml of plasma (233). The *MP1* gene encodes a *T. marneffei*-specific cell wall mannoprotein (234).

Isolation Procedures

Culture remains the gold standard method of diagnosis, even though it is slow and requires collection of clinical specimens with invasive procedures. *T. marneffei* is easily cultured from clinical specimens and grows well on Sabouraud dextrose agar without cycloheximide; culture of bone marrow is the most sensitive (100%), followed by skin culture (90%) and blood culture (76%) (212). Mould-to-yeast conversion is achieved by subculturing onto brain heart infusion agar and incubating at 37°C (226). Identification of *T. marneffei* is based on colony morphology (see below). In Europe, Australia, and New Zealand, *T. marneffei* is classed as a risk group 3 pathogen. Therefore, specimens and cultures should be handled in a containment level 3 (or above) facility to avoid inhalation of conidia or accidental inoculation into skin.

Identification

Members of the genus *Talaromyces* are ubiquitous laboratory moulds and are grown easily from most nonsterile specimens, especially respiratory specimens. Differentiation of *T. marneffei* from other penicillia is not usually problematic, since *T. marneffei* is thermally dimorphic. Diagnosis is made by observing the conversion of the mould to yeast form at 37°C or the reverse at 25°C.

Colonies on Sabouraud dextrose agar at 25°C are fast growing, downy, and white with yellowish-green conidial heads. Colonies become grayish pink to brown with age and produce a diffusible brown-red pigment that is particularly evident on the reverse (Fig. 4), which is an early indication that an isolate may be *T. marneffei*. However, red pigment may be produced by nonpathogenic *Penicillium* species, including *P. citrinum*, *P. janthellum*, *P. purpurogenum*, and *P. rubrum*. Colonies on brain heart infusion agar (37°C) are rough, glabrous, and tan colored. Microscopic yeast-like cells are spherical to elliptical and are 2 to 6 μm in diameter.

Morphology of *T. marneffei* is distinctive: hyaline smooth-walled conidiophores with terminal verticils comprising three to five metulae (secondary branches) with conidia, each bearing three to seven phialides. Conidia are globose to subglobose, 2 to 3 μm in diameter, smooth walled, and produced in basipetal succession from the phialides, producing a typical "penicillus," or brush-like fruiting structure (14, 226).

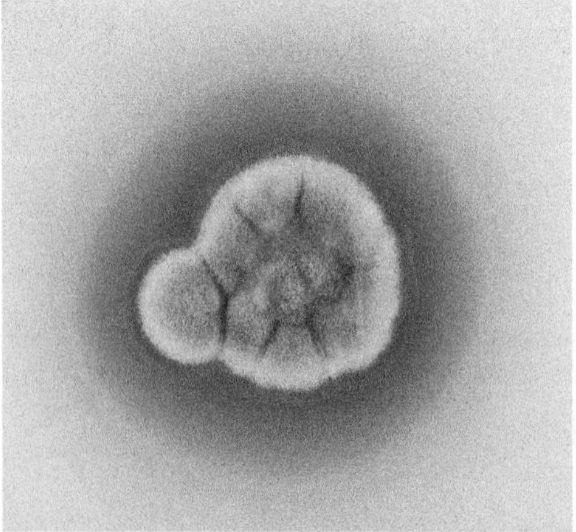

FIGURE 4 White colonies of *Talaromyces marneffei* on Sabouraud dextrose agar (25°C) with yellow-green conidial heads. With age, the diffusible brownish-red to wine-red pigment is evident.

Together with direct detection of the fungus in clinical specimens, molecular tools enable *T. marneffei* cultures to be identified by PCR in combination with DNA sequencing or probe hybridization and distinguished from other *Penicillium* species that may be incidentally present. Since species identification can be problematic within the genera *Penicillium* and *Talaromyces*, a polyphasic approach is recommended. Morphological approaches should be combined with molecular strategies. Assays typically amplify one or more of the 18S rRNA, ITS region, β-tubulin, calmodulin, actin, or RNA polymerase genes (209). Introduction of molecular methods of identification would depend on clinical need. MALDI-TOF MS has been investigated for its utility in identification of both the mould and yeast forms. However, correct identification is reliant on access to reference spectra, which are currently not available in commercial databases (235).

Typing Systems

Genotyping systems have been developed to (i) study the population structure and genetic diversity of *T. marneffei* and (ii) investigate clusters of infection should they arise. An MLMT system was developed using 23 genetic loci (236) and applied to clinical isolates from Southeast Asia; 21 of 23 tested loci were polymorphic, revealing a high degree of genetic diversity. A clear separation between the population of strains from the eastern region (China, Hong Kong, and Indonesia) and from the western region (Thailand and India) was evident, with the eastern clade being more polymorphic than the western clade (236). An independent study confirmed the clustering of isolates from these regions into two clades (237). The separation of these clades may be due to potential isolation of these populations or for reasons not yet known.

In addition to MLMT, MLST analysis incorporating eight genetic loci (transcription factor [*AbaA*], catalase [*CpeA*], homeodomain transcription factor [*StlA*], isocitrate lyase [*Icl1*], polyaromatic amino acid biosynthesis [*PAA*], NADH-dependent glutamate synthase [*NGS*], lovastatin nonaketide synthase [*LNS*], cell wall mannoprotein [*MP1*], and a gene fragment of the cytochrome oxidase subunit 1 gene [*COX1*] of the *T. marneffei* mitochondrial genome) has also been evaluated as a typing tool. In one study, no nucleotide polymorphisms were observed within the *COX1*, *AbaA*, and *NGS* loci. However, the remaining five loci showed a high degree of genetic diversity and again indicated geographic separation between isolates from China and Thailand, but also mixed clades. Identical MLST types between different patients have been shown, supporting an asexual mode of reproduction (238).

Serologic Tests

Serologic tests may help in diagnosis of infection, although no standardized commercial tests are available. Assays have been developed to detect antibodies to *T. marneffei*, *T. marneffei* antigen, or both in serum and other body fluids in various test formats, including immunodiffusion, indirect immunofluorescence, and ELISA (209, 223).

Immunodiffusion tests to detect precipitin antibodies using *T. marneffei* mycelial exoantigens had low sensitivities when they were used with serum in HIV-positive patients (239). When an indirect fluorescent approach for detecting

IgG antibodies against germinating conidia and yeast forms was used, patients with *T. marneffei* infection were shown to have higher titers (>160) than those without (≤40) (240). An ELISA-based antibody test using recombinant *T. marneffei* mannoprotein Mp1p diagnosed infection with 65 to 80% sensitivity and 100% specificity (234, 241); however, combining Mp1p-based antigen and antibody testing yielded a sensitivity of 88%, a PPV of 100%, and an NPV of 96% (241). In another study, a similar double-antibody sandwich ELISA for Mp1p antigen enabled diagnosis of disseminated penicilliosis in 9.3% of HIV-infected patients (242).

Other methods of serum antigen detection include a *T. marneffei*-specific latex agglutination test (sensitivity, 76%). When this test was used with the immunodiffusion test, the sensitivity increased to 82%. The specificity of both test formats is 100% (239). False-positive results have been rarely observed using the Platelia *Aspergillus* ELISA for GM, which uses a MAb to *A. fumigatus* (243). In-house ELISAs and latex agglutination formats have also been used to detect and quantitate *T. marneffei* antigen in urine with high sensitivity (94.6 to 97.3%) and specificity (>97%) at a cutoff titer of 1:40 for the ELISA (244). In one study, a capture ELISA was evaluated with 53 patients with culture-confirmed penicilliosis and 240 controls. When the ELISA was tested on serum, the diagnostic sensitivity, specificity, and accuracy were 92.45%, 97.5%, and 96.59%, respectively (245).

Antimicrobial Susceptibilities

Early treatment of *T. marneffei* infection is critical to reduce mortality of this infection. *In vitro* susceptibilities help guide therapy despite the absence of formal clinical breakpoints for antifungal drugs. *T. marneffei* appears to be susceptible *in vitro* to itraconazole, the older azole ketoconazole, flucytosine, voriconazole, and posaconazole. Amphotericin B is less active, and fluconazole is the least active. Some strains have high MICs of fluconazole (up to 16 mg/liter) and are considered resistant (246, 247). Testing of 39 *T. marneffei* strains from China revealed that voriconazole MICs were low (MIC range, 0.004 to 0.25 mg/liter; geometric mean, 0.04 mg/liter), with geometric mean MICs of itraconazole, terbinafine, amphotericin B, and fluconazole of 0.11, 0.15, <0.65, and 4.1 mg/liter, respectively (248). A more recent study evaluated the susceptibility of *T. marneffei* to posaconazole in comparison with other agents; posaconazole showed good activity against both yeast and mycelial forms (MIC ranges, 0.001 to 0.002 mg/liter and 0.004 to 0.063 mg/liter, respectively) (246). Clinical responses appear to correlate with susceptibility to azoles. A retrospective study in HIV patients has shown voriconazole to be effective and well tolerated for disseminated infection (249). The results for amphotericin B are difficult to assess, but amphotericin B, voriconazole, and itraconazole have all been used to treat penicillosis. The echinocandins are also active against *T. marneffei*; *in vitro*, the drugs are more active against the mycelial, rather than the yeast, form (246, 247). Micafungin has demonstrated synergy with itraconazole (65% of strains) and amphotericin B (50%) but not with fluconazole (250).

Other *Penicillium* (and *Talaromyces*) Species

As many *Penicillium* species are completely or strongly inhibited at 37°C, they rarely cause human infection. Even repeated isolation of *Penicillium* from patient specimens does not necessarily indicate an etiological role. This includes the isolation of the fungus from patients with chronic lung disorders, including bronchiectasis and cystic fibrosis, where *Penicillium* can colonize airways for prolonged periods. The role of penicillia in allergy and hypersensitivity pneumonitis is well established (251). Nonetheless, infections due to a range of *Penicillium* and *Talaromyces* species, resulting in keratitis, otomycosis, peritonitis, pneumonia, and endocarditis, are reported, typically after the fungus is repeatedly isolated. Species implicated in infection include *P. citrinum, P. commune, P. chrysogenum, P. aurantiogriseum, P. brevicompactum, T. verrucosum, T. piceus, T. pururogenus,* and *T. rugulosus* (14, 252).

Identification of *Penicillium* species requires expertise with growth of an isolate on several media and careful microscopic examination. No thermal dimorphism is displayed. Isolates are inoculated at three points on Czapek Dox agar, 2% malt extract agar, and/or 25% glycerol nitrate agar and incubated at 25°C. Colonies are fast growing, in shades of green (sometimes white), consisting of a dense felt of conidiophores. Most species sporulate within 7 days. Microscopic mounts are best made using a sticky tape flag or slide culture mounted in lactophenol cotton blue. A drop of alcohol is often needed to remove bubbles and excess conidia. Molecular techniques may be required for species identification. The phylogenetic relationships of penicillia based on sequence variation within the ITS1-ITS2 region are shown in Fig. 5.

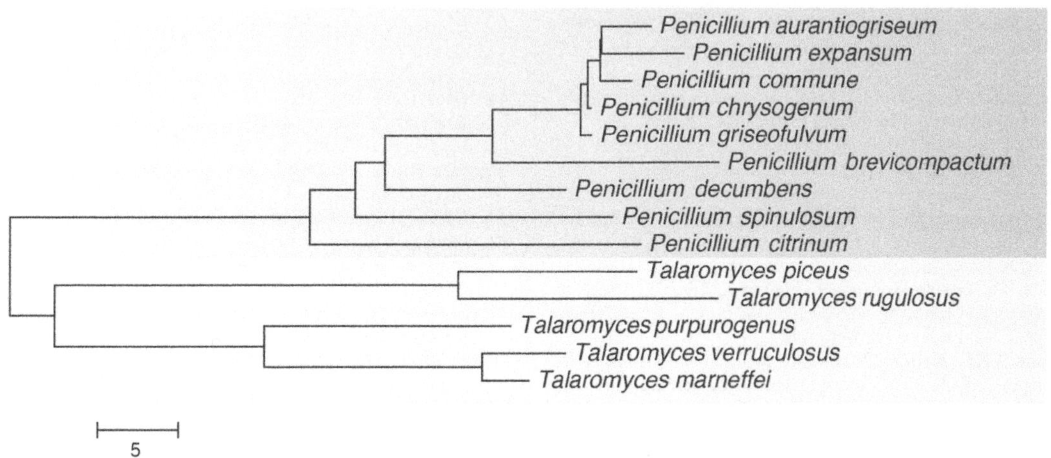

FIGURE 5 Neighbor-joining tree of pathogenic *Penicillium* and *Talaromyces* species according to the *Atlas of Clinical Fungi*, version 4.1 (http://www.clinicalfungi.org), based on ITS1 and ITS2 sequences of the rDNA gene cluster obtained from GenBank using MEGA, version 7.0 (253).

Evaluation, Interpretation, and Reporting of Results

T. marneffei is the only member of the genus *Talaromyces* that has been linked unequivocally to human infection. For the present, diagnosis of infection caused by this fungus should include a minimum of a positive culture, direct smear, and molecular detection and identification in a patient with a plausible clinical and exposure history. Most other *Penicillium/Talaromyces* species have low potential for causing human infection.

We thank David Ellis for his generous assistance with preparation of the photographs for Fig. 3B, C, D, E, F, and G and Fig. 4. We also thank Jos Houbraken, Sybren de Hoog, and John Taylor for their helpful comments on the current taxonomy and Carolina Firacative for her help in the preparation of Fig. 1 and 5.

REFERENCES

1. **Samson RA, Visagie CM, Houbraken J, Hong SB, Hubka V, Klaassen CHW, Perrone G, Seifert KA, Susca A, Tanney JB, Varga J, Kocsube S, Szigeti G, Yaguchi T, Frisvad JC.** 2014. Phylogeny, identification and nomenclature of the genus *Aspergillus*. *Stud Mycol* **78:**141–173.
2. **Chen AJ, Frisvad JC, Sun BD, Varga J, Kocsube S, Dijksterhuis J, Kim DH, Hong SB, Houbraken J, Samson RA.** 2016. *Aspergillus* section *Nidulantes* (formerly *Emericella*): polyphasic taxonomy, chemistry and biology. *Stud Mycol* **84:**1–118.
3. **Dyer P, O'Gorman CM.** 2011. A fungal sexual revolution: *Aspergillus* and *Penicillium* show the way. *Curr Opin Microbiol* **14:**649–654.
4. **Samson RA, Pitt JI.** 2000. *Integration of Modern Taxonomic Methods for Penicilium and Aspergillus Classification*. Harwood Scientific Publishers, Amsterdam, The Netherlands.
5. **Raper KB, Fennell DI.** 1965. *The Genus Aspergillus*. Williams & Wilkins Co, Baltimore, MD.
6. **Peterson SW.** 2008. Phylogenetic analysis of *Aspergillus* species using DNA sequences of four loci. *Mycologia* **100:**205–226.
7. **Balajee SA, Gribskov JL, Hanley E, Nickle D, Marr KA.** 2005. *Aspergillus lentulus* sp. nov., a new sibling species of *A. fumigatus*. *Eukaryot Cell* **4:**625–632.
8. **Balajee SA, Baddley JW, Peterson SW, Nickle D, Varga J, Boey A, Lass-Florl C, Frisvad JC, Samson RA, ISHAM Working Group on *A. terreus*.** 2009. *Aspergillus alabamensis*, a new clinically relevant species in the section *Terrei*. *Eukaryot Cell* **8:**713–722.
9. **Kocsube S, Perrone G, Magista D, Houbraken J, Varga J, Szigeti G, Hubka V, Hong SB, Frisvad JC, Samson RA.** 2016. *Aspergillus* is monophyletic: evidence from multiple gene phylogenies and extrolites profiles. *Stud Mycol* **85:**199–213.
10. **Hawksworth DL, Crous PW, Redhead SA, Reynolds DR, Samson RA, Seifert KA, Taylor JW, Wingfield MJ.** 2011. The Amsterdam Declaration on Fungal Nomenclature. *IMA Fungus* **2:**105–112.
11. **Norvell LL.** 2011. Fungal nomenclature. 1. Melbourne approves a new code. *Mycotaxon* **116:**481–490.
12. **Pitt JI, Taylor JW.** 2014. *Aspergillus*, its sexual states and the new International Code of Nomenclature. *Mycologia* **106:**1051–1062.
13. **Taylor JW, Göker M, Pitt JI.** 2016. Choosing one name for pleomorphic fungi: the example of *Aspergillus* versus *Eurotium*, *Neosartorya* and *Emericella*. *Taxon* **65:**593–601.
14. **de Hoog GS, Guarro J, Gene J, Figueras MJ.** 2011. *Atlas of Clinical Fungi*. version 4.1.4. Westerdijk Fungal Biodiversity Institute, Utrecht, The Netherlands.
15. **Dagenais TRT, Keller NP.** 2009. Pathogenesis of *Aspergillus fumigatus* in invasive aspergillosis. *Clin Microbiol Rev* **22:** 447–465.
16. **Thompson GR, III, Patterson TF.** 2011. Pulmonary aspergillosis: recent advances. *Semin Respir Crit Care Med* **32:** 673–681.
17. **Baddley JW.** 2011. Clinical risk factors for invasive aspergillosis. *Med Mycol* **49**(Suppl 1)**:**S7–S12.
18. **Vonberg RP, Gastmeier P.** 2006. Nosocomial aspergillosis in outbreak settings. *J Hosp Infect* **63:**246–254.
19. **Warris A, Gaustad P, Meis JF, Voss A, Verweij PE, Abrahamsen TG.** 2001. Recovery of filamentous fungi from water in a pediatric bone marrow transplantation unit. *J Hosp Infect* **47:**143–148.
20. **Anaissie EJ, Costa SF.** 2001. Nosocomial aspergillosis is waterborne. *Clin Infect Dis* **33:**1546–1548.
21. **Kidd SE, Ling LM, Meyer W, Morrissey CO, Chen SCA, Slavin MA.** 2009. Molecular epidemiology of invasive aspergillosis: lessons learned from an outbreak investigation in an Australian hematology unit. *Infect Control Hosp Epidemiol* **30:**1223–1226.
22. **Weber DJ, Peppercorn A, Miller MB, Sickbert-Benett E, Rutala WA.** 2009. Preventing healthcare-associated *Aspergillus* infections: review of recent CDC/HICPAPC recommendations. *Med Mycol* **47**(Suppl 1)**:**S199–S209.
23. **Warris A, Verweij PE.** 2005. Clinical implications of environmental sources for *Aspergillus*. *Med Mycol* **43**(Suppl 1)**:**S59–S65.
24. **Gastmeier P, Stamm-Balderjahn S, Hansen S, Nitzschke-Tiemann F, Zuschneid I, Groneberg K, Rüden H.** 2005. How outbreaks can contribute to prevention of nosocomial infection: analysis of 1,022 outbreaks. *Infect Control Hosp Epidemiol* **26:**357–361.
25. **Guinea J, García de Viedma D, Peláez T, Escribano P, Muñoz P, Meis JF, Klaassen CH, Bouza E.** 2011. Molecular epidemiology of *Aspergillus fumigatus*: an in-depth genotypic analysis of isolates involved in an outbreak of invasive aspergillosis. *J Clin Microbiol* **49:**3498–3503.
26. **Falvey DG, Streifel AJ.** 2007. Ten-year air sample analysis of *Aspergillus* prevalence in a university hospital. *J Hosp Infect* **67:**35–41.
27. **Burgos A, Zaoutis TE, Dvorak CC, Hoffman JA, Knapp KM, Nania JJ, Prasad P, Steinbach WJ.** 2008. Invasive aspergillosis: a multicenter retrospective analysis of 139 contemporary cases. *Pediatrics* **121:**e1286–e1294.
28. **Chakrabarti A, Chatterjee SS, Das A, Shivaprakash MR.** 2011. Invasive aspergillosis in developing countries. *Med Mycol* **49**(Suppl 1)**:**S35–S47.
29. **Steinbach WJ, Marr KA, Anaissie EJ, Azie N, Quan SP, Meier-Kriesche HU, Apewokin S, Horn DL.** 2012. Clinical epidemiology of 960 patients with invasive aspergillosis from the PATH Alliance registry. *J Infect* **65:**453–464.
30. **Balajee SA, Kano R, Baddley JW, Moser SA, Marr KA, Alexander BD, Andes D, Kontoyiannis DP, Perrone G, Peterson S, Brandt ME, Pappas PG, Chiller T.** 2009. Molecular identification of *Aspergillus* species collected for the Transplant-Associated Infection Surveillance Network. *J Clin Microbiol* **47:**3138–3141.
31. **Van Der Linden JW, Warris A, Verweij PE.** 2011. *Aspergillus* species intrinsically resistant to antifungal agents. *Med Mycol* **49**(Suppl 1)**:**S82–S89.
32. **Binder U, Lass-Florl C.** 2013. New insights into invasive aspergillosis—from pathogen to the disease. *Curr Pharm Des* **19:**3679–3688.
33. **Alastruey-Izquierdo A, Mellado E, Pelaez T, Peman J, Zapico S, Alvarez M, Rodriguez-Tudela JL, Cuenca-Estrella M, FILPOP Study Group.** 2013. Population-based survey of filamentous fungi and antifungal resistance in Spain (FILPOP Study). *Antimicrob Agents Chemother* **57:**3380–3387.
34. **Chakrabarti A, Shivaprakash MR, Singh R, Tarai B, George VK, Fomda BA, Gupta A.** 2008. Fungal endophthalmitis: fourteen years' experience from a center in India. *Retina* **28:**1400–1407.
35. **Slavin MA, Chakrabarti A.** 2012. Opportunistic fungal infections in the Asia Pacific region. *Med Mycol* **50:**18–25.
36. **Lackner M, Coassin S, Haun M, Binder U, Kronenberg F, Haas H, Jank M, Maurer E, Meis JF, Hagen F, Lass-Florl C.** 2016. Geographically predominant genotypes of *Aspergillus terreus* species complex in Austria: a microsatellite typing study. *Clin Microbiol Infect* **22:**270–276.
37. **Hope WW, Walsh TJ, Denning DW.** 2005. The invasive and saprophytic syndromes due to *Aspergillus* spp. *Med Mycol* **43**(Suppl 1)**:**S207–S238.

38. **Perfect JR, Cox GM, Lee JY, Kauffman CA, de Repentigny L, Chapman SW, Morrison VA, Pappas P, Hiemenz JW, Stevens DA.** 2001. The impact of culture isolation of *Aspergillus* species: a hospital-based survey of aspergillosis. *Clin Infect Dis* **33:**1824–1833.
39. **Kontoyiannis DP, Marr KA, Park BJ, Alexander BA, Anaissie EJ, Walsh TJ, Ito J, Andes DR, Baddley JW, Brown JM, Brumble LM, Freifeld AG, Hadley S, Herwaldt LA, Kauffman CA, Knapp K, Lyon GM, Morrison V, Papanicolaou G, Patterson TF, Perl TM, Schuster MG, Walker R, Wannemuehler KA, Wingard JR, Chiller TM, Pappas PG.** 2010. Prospective surveillance for invasive fungal infections in hematopoietic stem cell transplant recipients, 2001–2006: overview of the Transplant-Associated Infection Surveillance Network (TRANSNET) Database. *Clin Infect Dis* **50:**1091–1100.
40. **Pappas PG, Alexander BA, Andes DR, Hadley S, Kauffman CA, Freifeld A, Anaissie EJ, Brumble LM, Herwaldt L, Ito J, Kontoyiannis DP, Lyon GM, Marr KA, Morrison VA, Park BJ, Patterson TF, Perl TM, Oster RA, Schuster MG, Walker R, Walsh TJ, Wannemuehler KA, Chiller TM.** 2010. Invasive fungal infections among organ transplant recipients: results of the transplant-associated infection surveillance network (TRANSET). *Clin Infect Dis* **50:**1101–1111.
41. **Baddley JW, Stephens JM, Ji X, Gao X, Schlamm H, Tarallo M.** 2013. Aspergillosis in intensive care unit (ICU) patients: epidemiology and economic outcomes. *BMC Infect Dis* **13:**29.
42. **Guinea J, Torres-Narbona M, Gijón P, Muñoz P, Pozo F, Peláez T, de Miguel J, Bouza E.** 2010. Pulmonary aspergillosis in patients with chronic obstructive pulmonary disease: incidence, risk factors, and outcome. *Clin Microbiol Infect* **16:**870–877.
43. **Solé A, Morant P, Salavert M, Pemán J, Morales P, Valencia Lung Transplant Group.** 2005. *Aspergillus* infections in lung transplant recipients: risk factors and outcome. *Clin Microbiol Infect* **11:**359–365.
44. **De Pauw B, Walsh TJ, Donnelly JP, Stevens DA, Edwards JE, Calandra T, Pappas PG, Maertens J, Lortholary O, Kauffman CA, Denning DW, Patterson TF, Maschmeyer G, Bille J, Dismukes WE, Herbrecht R, Hope WW, Kibbler CC, Kullberg BJ, Marr KA, Muñoz P, Odds FC, Perfect JR, Restrepo A, Ruhnke M, Segal BH, Sobel JD, Sorrell TC, Viscoli C, Wingard JR, Zaoutis T, Bennett JE.** 2008. Revised definitions of invasive fungal disease from the European Organisation for Research and Treatment of Cancer/Invasive Fungal Infections Cooperative Group and the National Institute of Allergy and Infectious Diseases Mycoses Study Group (EORTC/MSG) Consensus Group. *Clin Infect Dis* **46:**1813–1821.
45. **Bulpa P, Dive A, Sibille Y.** 2007. Invasive pulmonary aspergillosis in patients with chronic obstructive pulmonary disease. *Eur Respir J* **30:**782–800.
46. **Felton TW, Baxter C, Moore CB, Roberts SA, Hope WW, Denning DW.** 2010. Efficacy and safety of posaconazole for chronic pulmonary aspergillosis. *Clin Infect Dis* **51:**1383–1391.
47. **Barton RC, Hobson RP, McLoughlin H, Morris A, Datta B.** 2013. Assessment of the significance of respiratory culture of *Aspergillus* in the non-neutropenic patient. A critique of published diagnostic criteria. *Eur J Clin Microbiol* **32:**923–928.
48. **Bouza E, Guinea J, Pelaez T, Perez-Molina J, Alcala L, Munoz P.** 2005. Workload due to *Aspergillus fumigatus* and significance of the organism in the microbiology laboratory of a general hospital. *J Clin Microbiol* **43:**2075–2079.
49. **Simoneau E, Kelly M, Labbe AC, Roy J, Laverdiere M.** 2005. What is the clinical significance of positive blood cultures with *Aspergillus* spp. in hematopoeitic stem cell transplant recipients? A 23-year experience. *Bone Marrow Transplant* **35:**303–306.
50. **Giannella M, Muñoz P, Guinea J, Escribano P, Rodríguez-Créixems M, Bouza E.** 2013. Growth of *Aspergillus* in blood cultures: proof of invasive aspergillosis in patients with chronic obstructive pulmonary disease? *Mycoses* **56:**488–490.
51. **Lau A, Chen S, Sorrell T, Carter D, Malik R, Martin P, Halliday C.** 2007. Development and clinical application of a panfungal PCR assay to detect and identify fungal DNA in tissue specimens. *J Clin Microbiol* **45:**380–385.
52. **Chandler FW, Watts JC.** 1987. *Pathologic Description of Fungal Infections*. American Society of Clinical Pathologists, Inc., Chicago, IL.
53. **Walsh TJ, Petraitis V, Petraitiene R, Field-Ridley A, Sutton D, Ghannoum M, Sein T, Schaufele R, Peter J, Bacher J, Casler H, Armstrong D, Espinel-Ingroff A, Rinaldi MG, Lyman CA.** 2003. Experimental pulmonary aspergillosis due to *Aspergillus terreus*: pathogenesis and treatment of an emerging fungal pathogen resistant to amphotericin B. *J Infect Dis* **188:**305–319.
54. **Severo LC, Geyer GR, de Silvo Porto N, Wagner MB, Londero AT.** 1997. Pulmonary *Aspergillus niger* intracavitary colonization. Report of 23 cases and a review of the literature. *Rev Iberoam Micol* **14:**104–110.
55. **Shah AA, Hazen KC.** 2013. Diagnostic accuracy of histopathologic and cytopathologic examination of *Aspergillus* species. *Am J Clin Pathol* **139:**55–61.
56. **Hayden RT, Isotalo PA, Parrett T, Wolk DM, Qian X, Roberts CD, Lloyd RV.** 2003. In situ hybridisation for the differentiation of *Aspergillus*, *Fusarium* and *Pseudallescheria* species in tissue section. *Diagn Mol Pathol* **12:**21–26.
57. **Lau A, Chen S, Sleiman S, Sorrell T.** 2009. Current status and future perspectives on molecular and serological methods in diagnostic mycology. *Future Microbiol* **4:**1185–1222.
58. **Pfeiffer CD, Fine JP, Safdar N.** 2006. Diagnosis of invasive aspergillosis using a galactomannan assay: a meta-analysis. *Clin Infect Dis* **42:**1417–1427.
59. **Leeflang MM, Debets-Ossenkopp YJ, Visser CE, Scholten RJ, Hooft L, Bijlmer HA, Reitsma JB, Bossuyt PMM, Vandenbroucke-Grauis CM.** 2008. Galactomannan detection for invasive aspergillosis in immunocompromised patients. *Cochrane Database Syst Rev*.
60. **Zou M, Tang L, Zhao S, Zhao Z, Chen L, Chen P, Huang Z, Li J, Chen L, Fan X.** 2012. Systematic review and meta-analysis of detecting galactomannan in bronchoalveolar lavage fluid for diagnosing invasive *aspergillosis*. *PLoS One* **7:**e43347.
61. **Heng SC, Morrissey O, Chen SC, Thursky K, Manser RL, Nation RL, Kong DC, Slavin M.** 2015. Utility of bronchoalveolar lavage fluid galactomannan alone or in combination with PCR for the diagnosis of invasive aspergillosis in adult haematology patients: a systematic review and meta-analysis. *Crit Rev Microbiol* **41:**124–134.
62. **Guo YL, Chen YQ, Wang K, Qin SM, Wu C, Kong JC.** 2010. Accuracy of BAL galactomannan in diagnosing invasive aspergillosis: a bivariate meta-analysis and systemic review. *Chest* **138:**817–824.
63. **López-Medrano F, Fernández-Ruiz M, Silva JT, Carver PL, van Delden C, Merino E, Pérez-Saez MJ, Montero M, Coussement J, de Abreu Mazzolin M, Cervera C, Santos L, Sabé N, Scemla A, Cordero E, Cruzado-Vega L, Martín-Moreno PL, Len Ó, Rudas E, de León AP, Arriola M, Lauzurica R, David M, González-Rico C, Henríquez-Palop F, Fortún J, Nucci M, Manuel O, Paño-Pardo JR, Montejo M, Muñoz P, Sánchez-Sobrino B, Mazuecos A, Pascual J, Horcajada JP, Lecompte T, Moreno A, Carratalà J, Blanes M, Hernández D, Fariñas MC, Andrés A, Aguado JM, Spanish Network for Research in Infectious Diseases (REIPI), the Group for the Study of Infection in Transplant Recipients (GESITRA) of the Spanish Society of Clinical Microbiology and Infectious Diseases (SEIMC), the Study Group for Infections in Compromised Hosts (ESGICH) of the European Society of Clinical Microbiology and Infectious Diseases (ESCMID), and the Swiss Transplant Cohort Study (STCS).** 2016. Clinical presentation and determinants of mortality of invasive pulmonary aspergillosis in kidney transplant recipients: a multinational cohort study. *Am J Transplant* **16:**3220–3234.
64. **Fortun J, Martin-Davila P, Alvarez ME, Norman F, Sanchez-Sousa A, Gajate L, Barcena R, Nuno SJ, Moreno S.** 2009. False-positive results of *aspergillus* galactomannan antigenemia in liver transplant recipients. *Transplantation* **87:**256–260.

65. **Husain S, Kwak EJ, Obman A, Wagener MM, Kusne S, Stout JE, McCurry KR, Singh N.** 2004. Prospective assessment of Platelia *Aspergillus* galactomannan antigen for the diagnosis of invasive aspergillosis in lung transplant recipients. *Am J Transplant* **4:**796–802.
66. **Marchetti O, Lamoth F, Mikulska M, Viscoli C, Verweij P, Bretagne S, European Conference on Infections in Leukaemia (ECIL) Laboratory Working Groups.** 2012. ECIL recommendations for the use of biological markers for the diagnosis of invasive fungal diseases in leukemic patients and hematopoietic SCT recipients. *Bone Marrow Transplant* **47:**846–854.
67. **Meersseman W, Vandecasteele SJ, Wilmer A, Verbeken E, Peetermans WE, Van Wijngaerden E.** 2004. Invasive aspergillosis in critically ill patients without malignancy. *Am J Respir Crit Care Med* **170:**621–625.
68. **Maertens JA, Klont R, Masson C, Theunissen K, Meersseman W, Lagrou K, Heinen C, Crepin B, Van Eldere J, Tabouret M, Donnelly JP, Verweij PE.** 2007. Optimisation of the cutoff value for the *Aspergillus* double-sandwich enzyme immunoassay. *Clin Infect Dis* **44:**1329–1336.
69. **Duarte RF, Sánchez-Ortega I, Cuesta I, Arnan M, Patiño B, Fernández de Sevilla A, Gudiol C, Ayats J, Cuenca-Estrella M.** 2014. Serum galactomannan-based early detection of invasive aspergillosis in hematology patients receiving effective antimold prophylaxis. *Clin Infect Dis* **59:**1696–1702.
70. **Lehrnbecher T, Robinson PD, Fisher BT, Castagnola E, Groll AH, Steinbach WJ, Zaoutis TE, Negeri ZF, Beyene J, Phillips B, Sung L.** 2016. Galactomannan, β-D-glucan, and polymerase chain reaction-based assays for the diagnosis of invasive fungal disease in pediatric cancer and hematopoietic stem cell transplantation: a systematic review and meta-analysis. *Clin Infect Dis* **63:**1340–1348.
71. **He H, Ding L, Sun B, Li F, Zhan Q.** 2012. Role of galactomannan determinations in bronchoalveolar lavage fluid samples from critically ill patients with chronic obstructive pulmonary diseases for the diagnosis of invasive pulmonary aspergillosis: a prospective study. *Crit Care* **16:**R138.
72. **Thornton CR.** 2010. Detection of invasive aspergillosis. *Adv Appl Microbiol* **70:**187–216.
73. **Thornton CR.** 2008. Development of an immunochromatographic lateral flow device for rapid serodiagnosis of invasive aspergillosis. *Clin Vaccine Immunol* **15:**1095–1105.
74. **Pan Z, Fu M, Zhang J, Zhou H, Fu Y, Zhou J.** 2015. Diagnostic accuracy of a novel lateral flow device in invasive aspergillosis: a meta-analysis. *J Med Microbiol* **64:**702–707.
75. **Held J, Schmidt T, Thornton CR, Kotter E, Bertz H.** 2013. Comparison of a novel *Aspergillus* lateral-flow device and the Platelia galactomannan assay for the diagnosis of invasive aspergillosis following haematopoietic stem cell transplantation. *Infection* **41:**1163–1169.
76. **White PL, Parr C, Thornton C, Barnes RA.** 2013. Evaluation of real-time PCR, galactomannan enzyme-linked immunosorbent assay (ELISA), and a novel lateral-flow device for diagnosis of invasive aspergillosis. *J Clin Microbiol* **51:** 1510–1516.
77. **Hoenigl M, Prattes J, Spiess B, Wagner J, Prueller F, Raggam RB, Posch V, Duettmann WK, Wölfler A, Koidl C, Buzina W, Reinwald M, Thornton CR, Krause R, Buchheidt D.** 2014. Performance of galactomannan, beta-D-glucan, *Aspergillus* lateral-flow device, conventional culture, and PCR tests with bronchoalveolar lavage fluid for diagnosis of invasive pulmonary aspergillosis. *J Clin Microbiol* **52:**2039–2045.
78. **Lamoth F, Cruciani M, Mengoli C, Castagnola E, Lortholary O, Richardson M, Marchetti O, Third European Conference on Infections in Leukemia (ECIL-3).** 2012. β-Glucan antigenemia assay for the diagnosis of invasive fungal infections in patients with hematological malignancies: a systematic review and meta-analysis of cohort studies from the Third European Conference on Infections in Leukemia (ECIL-3). *Clin Infect Dis* **54:**633–643.
79. **Persat F, Ranque S, Derouin F, Michel-Nguyen A, Picot S, Sulahian A.** 2008. Contribution of the (1→3)-β-D-glucan assay for diagnosis of invasive fungal infections. *J Clin Microbiol* **46:**1009–1013.
80. **Lu Y, Chen YQ, Guo YL, Qin SM, Wu C, Wang K.** 2011. Diagnosis of invasive fungal disease using serum (1,3)-β-D-glucan: a bivariate meta-analysis. *Intern Med* **50:**2783–2791.
81. **Onishi A, Sugiyama D, Kogata Y, Saegusa J, Sugimoto T, Kawano S, Morinobu A, Nishimura K, Kumagai S.** 2012. Diagnostic accuracy of serum 1,3-β-D-glucan for *Pneumocystis jirovecii* pnuemonia, invasive candidiasis, and invasive aspergillosis: systematic review and meta-analysis. *J Clin Microbiol* **50:**7–15.
82. **Karageorgopoulos DE, Vouloumanou EK, Ntziora F, Michalopoulos A, Rafailidis PI, Falagas ME.** 2011. β-D-Glucan assay for the diagnosis of invasive fungal infections: a meta-analysis. *Clin Infect Dis* **52:**750–770.
83. **Hendolin PH, Paulin L, Koukila-Kahkola P, Anttila VJ, Malmberg H, Richardson M, Ylikski J.** 2000. Panfungal PCR and multiplex liquid hybridization for detection of fungi in tissue specimens. *J Clin Microbiol* **38:**4186–4192.
84. **Hummel M, Spiess B, Kentouche K, Niggemann S, Bohm C, Reuter S, Kiehl M, Morz H, Hehlmann R, Buchheidt D.** 2006. Detection of *Aspergillus* DNA in cerebrospinal fluid from patients with cerebral aspergillosis by a nested PCR assay. *J Clin Microbiol* **44:**3989–3993.
85. **Badiee P, Kordbacheh P, Alborzi A, Ramzi M, Shakiba E.** 2008. Molecular detection of invasive aspergillosis in hematologic malignancies. *Infection* **36:**580–584.
86. **Halliday CL, Kidd SE, Sorrell TC, Chen SC-A.** 2015. Molecular diagnostic methods for invasive fungal disease: the horizon draws nearer. *Pathology* **47:**257–269.
87. **Alonso M, Escribano P, Guinea J, Recio S, Simon A, Pelaez T, Bouza E, Garcia de Viedma D.** 2012. Rapid detection and identification of *Aspergillus* from lower respiratory tract specimens by use of a combined probe-high resolution melting analysis. *J Clin Microbiol* **50:**3238–3243.
88. **Alanio A, Bretagne S.** 2014. Difficulties with molecular diagnostic tests for mould and yeast infections: where do we stand? *Clin Microbiol Infect* **20**(Suppl 6)**:**36–41.
89. **Mengoli C, Cruciani M, Barnes RA, Loeffler J, Donnelly JP.** 2009. Use of PCR for diagnosis of invasive aspergillosis: systematic review and meta-analysis. *Lancet Infect Dis* **9:**89–96.
90. **Suarez F, Lortholary O, Buland S, Rubio MT, Ghez D, Mahé V, Quesne G, Poirée S, Buzyn A, Varet B, Berche P, Bougnoux M.** 2008. Detection of circulating *Aspergillus fumigatus* DNA by real-time PCR assay of large serum volumes improves early diagnosis of invasive aspergillosis in high-risk adult patients under hematologic surveillance. *J Clin Microbiol* **46:**3772–3777.
91. **Luong MH, Clancy CJ, Vadnerkar A, Kwak EJ, Silveira F, Wissel MW, Grantham KJ, Shields JK, Crespo M, Pilewski J, Toyoda Y, Kleiboeker SB, Pakstis D, Reddy SK, Walsh TJ, Nguyen MH.** 2011. Comparison of an *Aspergillus* real-time polymerase chain reaction assay with galactomannan testing of bronchoalveolar lavage fluid for the diagnosis of invasive pulmonary aspergillosis in lung transplant recipients. *Clin Infect Dis* **52:**1218–1226.
92. **Kawazu M, Kanda Y, Goyama S, Takeshita M, Nannya Y, Niino M, Komeno Y, Nakamoto T, Kurokawa M, Tsujino S, Ogawa S, Aoki K, Chiba S, Motokura T, Ohishi N, Hirai H.** 2003. Rapid diagnosis of invasive pulmonary aspergillosis by quantitative polymerase chain reaction using bronchial lavage fluid. *Am J Hematol* **72:**27–30.
93. **White PL, Bretagne S, Klingspor L, Melchers WJG, McCulloch E, Schulz B, Finnstrom N, Mengoli C, Barnes RA, Donnelly JP, Loeffler J, European** Aspergillus **PCR Initiative.** 2010. *Aspergillus* PCR: one step closer to standardization. *J Clin Microbiol* **48:**1231–1240.
94. **White PL, Mengoli C, Bretagne S, Cuenca-Estrella M, Finnstrom N, Klingspor L, Melchers WJG, McCulloch E, Barnes RA, Donnelly JP, Loeffler J, European** Aspergillus **PCR Initiative (EAPCRI).** 2011. Evaluation of *Aspergillus* PCR protocols for testing serum specimens. *J Clin Microbiol* **49:**3842–3848.
95. **Springer J, Morton CO, Perry M, Heinz W, Paholcsek M, Alzheimer M, Rogers TR, Barnes RA, Einsele H, Loeffler J, White PL.** 2013. Multicentre comparison of serum and whole blood specimens for detection of *Aspergillus* DNA in high risk hematological patients. *J Clin Microbiol* **51:** 1445–1450.

96. **Springer J, White PL, Hamilton S, Michel D, Barnes RA, Einsele H, Loffler J.** 2016. Comparison of performance characteristics of *Aspergillus* PCR in a range of blood-based samples in accordance with international methodological recommendations. *J Clin Microbiol* **54:**705–711.
97. **Arvanitis M, Anagnostou T, Mylonakis E.** 2015. Galactomannan and polymerase chain reaction-based screening for invasive aspergillosis among high risk hematology patients: a diagnostic meta-analysis. *Clin Infect Dis* **61:**1263–1272.
98. **White PL, Hibbitts SJ, Perry MD, Green J, Stirling E, Woodford N, McNay G, Stevenson R, Barnes RA.** 2014. Evaluation of a commercially developed semiautomated PCR-surface-enhanced Raman scattering assay for diagnosis of invasive fungal disease. *J Clin Microbiol* **52:**3536–3543.
99. **Chong GL, van de Sande W, Dingemans G, Gaajetaan G, Vonk A, Hayette M-P, van Tegelen D, Simons G, Rijnders B.** 2015. Validation of a new *Aspergillus* real-time PCR assay for direct detection of *Aspergillus* and azole resistance of *Aspergillus fumigatus* on bronchoalveolar lavage fluid. *J Clin Microbiol* **53:**868–874.
100. **Dannaoui E, Gabriel F, Gaboyard M, Lagardere G, Audebert L, Quesne G, Godichaud S, Verweij P, Accoceberry I, Bougnoux M-E.** 2017. Molecular diagnosis of invasive aspergillosis and detection of azole resistance by a newly commercialized PCR kit. *J Clin Microbiol* **55:**3210–3218.
101. **White PL, Perry MD, Moody A, Follett SA, Morgan G, Barnes RA.** 2011. Evaluation of analytical and preliminary clinical performance of Myconostica MycAssay *Aspergillus* when testing serum specimens for diagnosis of invasive aspergillosis. *J Clin Microbiol* **49:**2169–2174.
102. **Guinea J, Padilla C, Escribano E, Munoz P, Padilla B, Gijon P, Bouza E.** 2013. Evaluation of MycAssay™ *Aspergillus* for diagnosis of invasive pulmonary aspergillosis in patients without hematological cancer. *PLoS One* **8:**e61545.
103. **Morrissey CO, Chen SC, Sorrell TC, Milliken S, Bardy PG, Bradstock KF, Szer J, Halliday CL, Gilroy NM, Moore J, Schwarer AP, Guy S, Bajel A, Tramontana AR, Spelman T, Slavin MA.** 2013. Galactomannan and PCR versus culture and histology for directing use of antifungal treatment for invasive aspergillosis in high-risk haematology patients: a randomized controlled trial. *Lancet Infect Dis* **13:** 519–528.
104. **Rogers TR, Morton CO, Springer J, Conneally E, Heinz W, Kenny C, Frost S, Einsele H, Loeffler J.** 2013. Combined real-time PCR and galactomannan surveillance improves diagnosis of invasive aspergillosis in high risk patients with hematological malignancies. *Br J Haematol* **161:**517–524.
105. **Aguado JM, et al.** 2014. Serum galactomannan versus a combination of galactomannan and polymerase chain reaction-based *Aspergillus* DNA detection for early therapy of invasive aspergillosis in high-risk hematological patients: a randomized controlled trial. *Clin Infect Dis* **60:**405–414.
106. **Wingard JR, Carter SL, Walsh TJ, Kurtzberg J, Small TN, Baden LR, Gersten ID, Mendizabal AM, Leather HL, Confer DL, Maziarz RT, Stadtmauer EA, Bolaños-Meade J, Brown J, Dipersio JF, Boeckh M, Marr KA, Blood and Marrow Transplant Clinical Trials Network.** 2010. Randomized, double-blind trial of fluconazole versus voriconazole for prevention of invasive fungal infection after allogeneic hematopoietic cell transplantation. *Blood* **116:**5111–5118.
107. **Rainer J, Kaltseis J, de Hoog SG, Summerbell RC.** 2008. Efficacy of a selective isolation procedure for members of the *Pseudallescheria boydii* complex. *Antonie van Leeuwenhoek* **93:**315–322.
108. **Kidd S, Halliday C, Alexiou H, Ellis D.** 2016. *Descriptions of Medical Fungi*, 3rd ed. Newstyle Printing, Mile End, Australia.
109. **Balajee SA, Gribskov J, Brandt M, Ito J, Fothergill A, Marr KA.** 2005. Mistaken identity: *Neosartorya pseudofischeri* and its anamorph masquerading as *Aspergillus fumigatus*. *J Clin Microbiol* **43:**5996–5999.
110. **Balajee SA, Lindsley MD, Iqbal N, Ito J, Pappas PG, Brandt ME.** 2007. Nonsporulating clinical isolates identified as *Petromyces alliaceus* (anamorph *Aspergillus alliaceus*) by morphological and sequence-based methods. *J Clin Microbiol* **45:**2701–2703.
111. **Talbot JJ, Barrs VR.** 2017. One-health pathogens in the *Aspergillus viridinutans* complex. *Med Mycol* **56:**1–12.
112. **Álvarez-Pérez S, Mellado E, Serrano D, Blanco JL, Garcia ME, Kwon M, Muñoz P, Cuenca-Estrella M, Bouza E, Peláez T.** 2013. Polyphasic characterization of fungal isolates from a published case of invasive aspergillosis reveals misidentification of *Aspergillus felis* as *Aspergillus viridinutans*. *J Med Microbiol* **62:**474–478.
113. **Ciardo DE, Lucke K, Imhof A, Bloemberg GV, Bottger EC.** 2010. Systematic internal transcribed spacer sequence analysis for identification of clinical mold isolates in diagnostic mycology: a 5-year study. *J Clin Microbiol* **48:**2809–2813.
114. **Hinrikson HP, Hurst SF, de Aguirre L, Morrison CJ.** 2005. Molecular methods for the identification of *Aspergillus* species. *Med Mycol* **43**(Suppl 1)**:**S129–S137.
115. **Schoch CL, Seifert KA, Huhndorf S, Robert V, Spouge JL, Levesque CA, Chen W, Fungal Barcoding Consortium.** 2012. Nuclear ribosomal internal transcribed spacer (ITS) region as a universal DNA barcode marker for Fungi. *Proc Natl Acad Sci USA* **109:**6241–6246.
116. **Balajee SA, Houbraken J, Verweij PE, Hong SB, Yaghuchi T, Varga J, Samson RA.** 2007. *Aspergillus* species identification in the clinical setting. *Stud Mycol* **59:**39–46.
117. **Hubka V, Kolarik M.** 2012. β-Tubulin paralogue *tub*C is frequently misidentified as the *ben*A gene in *Aspergillus* section *Nigri* taxonomy: primer specificity testing and taxanomic consequences. *Persoonia* **29:**1–10.
118. **Schoch CL, Robbertse B, Robert V, Vu D, Cardinali G, Irinyi L, Meyer W, Nilsson RH, Hughes K, Miller AN, Kirk PM, Abarenkov K, Aime MC, Ariyawansa HA, Bidartondo M, Boekhout T, Buyck B, Cai Q, Chen J, Crespo A, Crous PW, Damm U, De Beer ZW, Dentinger BT, Divakar PK, Dueñas M, Feau N, Fliegerova K, Garcia MA, Ge ZW, Groenewald JZ, Groenewald M, Grube M, Gryzenhout M, Gueidan C, Guo L, Hambleton S, Hamelin R, Hansen K, Hofstetter V, Hong SB, Houbraken J, Hyde KD, Inderbitzin P, Johnston PR, Karunarathna SC, Kõljalg U, Kovács GM, Kraichak E, Krizsan K, Kurtzman CP, Larsson KH, Leavitt S, Letcher PM, Liimatainen K, Liu JK, Lodge DJ, Luangsa-ard JJ, Lumbsch HT, Maharachchikumbura SS, Manamgoda D, Martin MP, Minnis AM, Moncalvo JM, Mulè G, Nakasone KK, Niskanen T, Olariaga I, Papp T, Petkovits T, Pino-Bodas R, Powell MJ, Raja HA, Redecker D, Sarmiento-Ramirez JM, Seifert KA, Shrestha B, Stenroos S, Stielow B, Suh SO, Tanaka K, Tedersoo L, Terreria MT, Udayanga D, Untereiner WA, Diéguez Uribeondo J, Subbarao KV, Vágvölgyi C, Visagie C, Voigt K, Walker DM, Weir BS, Weiß M, Wijayawardene NN, Wingfield MJ, Xu JP, Yang ZL, Zhang N, Zhuang WY, J, Subbarao KV, bbarao KV, Vroos S, Stielow B, Suh SO, Tanaka K, Tedersoo L, Terreria MT, Udayanga D, Untereiner WA, DieguezJM, Federhen S.** 2014. Finding needles in haystacks: linking scientific names, reference specimens and molecular data for Fungi. *Database* **2004:**bau061.
119. **Staab JF, Balajee SA, Marr KA.** 2009. *Aspergillus* section Fumigati typing by PCR-restriction fragment polymorphism. *J Clin Microbiol* **47:**2079–2083.
120. **Etienne KA, Gade L, Lockhart S, Diekema DJ, Messer SA, Pfaller MA, Balajee SA.** 2009. Screening of a large global *Aspergillus fumigatus* species complex collection by using a species-specific microsphere-based Luminex assay. *J Clin Microbiol* **47:**4171–4172.
121. **Clark AE, Kaleta EJ, Arora A, Wolk DM.** 2013. Matrix-assisted laser desorption ionization–time of flight mass spectrometry: a fundamental shift in the routine practice of clinical microbiology. *Clin Microbiol Rev* **26:**547–603.
122. **Lau AF, Drake SK, Calhoun LB, Henderson CM, Zelazny AM.** 2013. Development of a clinically comprehensive database and a simple procedure for identification of molds from solid media by matrix-assisted laser desorption ionization-time of flight mass spectrometry. *J Clin Microbiol* **51:**828–834 .
123. **Cassagne C, Ranque S, Normand A-C, Fourquet P, Thiebault S, Planard C, Hendrickx M, Piarroux R.** 2011. Mold routine identification in the clinical laboratory by matrix-assisted laser desorption ionization time-of-flight mass spectrometry. *PLoS One* **6:**e28425.

124. **Bader O.** 2013. MALDI-TOF-MS-based species identification and typing approaches in medical mycology. *Proteomics* **13:**788–799.
125. **Rizzato C, Lombardi L, Zoppo M, Lupetti A, Tavanti A.** 2015. Pushing the limits of MALDI-TOF mass spectrometry: beyond fungal species identification. *J Fungi* **1:**367–383.
126. **Becker PT, de Bel A, Martiny D, Ranque S, Piarroux R, Cassagne C, Detandt M, Hendrickx M.** 2014. Identification of filamentous fungi isolates by MALDI-TOF mass spectrometry: clinical evaluation of an extended reference spectra library. *Med Mycol* **52:**826–834.
127. **Sleiman S, Halliday CL, Chapman B, Brown M, Nitschke J, Lau AF, Chen SC-A.** 2016. Performance of matrix-assisted laser desorption ionization-time of flight mass spectrometry for identification of *Aspergillus*, *Scedosporium*, and *Fusarium* spp. in the Australian clinical setting. *J Clin Microbiol* **54:**2182–2186.
128. **Alanio A, Beretti JL, Dauphin B, Mellado E, Quesne G, Lacroix C, Amara A, Berche P, Nassif X, Bougnoux ME.** 2011. Matrix-assisted laser desorption ionization time-of-flight mass spectrometry for fast and accurate identification of clinically relevant *Aspergillus* species. *Clin Microbiol Infect* **17:**750–755.
129. **Bille E, Dauphin B, Leto J, Bougnoux ME, Beretti JL, Lotz A, Suarez S, Meyer J, Join-Lambert O, Descamps P, Grall N, Mory F, Dubreuil L, Berche P, Nassif X, Ferroni A.** 2012. MALDI-TOF MS Andromas strategy for the routine identification of bacteria, mycobacteria, yeasts, *Aspergillus* spp. and positive blood cultures. *Clin Microbiol Infect* **18:**1117–1125.
130. **Hettick JM, Green BJ, Buskirk AD, Kashon ML, Slaven JE, Janotka E, Blachere FM, Schmechel D, Beezhold DH.** 2008. Discrimination of *Aspergillus* isolates at the species and strain level by matrix-assisted laser desorption/ionization time-of-flight mass spectrometry fingerprinting. *Anal Biochem* **380:**276–281.
131. **Singh A, Goering RV, Simjee S, Foley SL, Zervos MJ.** 2006. Application of molecular techniques to the study of hospital infection. *Clin Microbiol Rev* **19:**512–530.
132. **de Valk HA, Meis JFGM, Curfs IM, Muehlethaler K, Mouton JW, Klaassen CHW.** 2005. Use of a novel panel of nine short tandem repeats for exact and high-resolution fingerprinting of *Aspergillus fumigatus* isolates. *J Clin Microbiol* **43:**4112–4120.
133. **Aufauvre-Brown A, Cohen J, Holden DW.** 1992. Use of randomly amplified polymorphic DNA markers to distinguish isolates of *Aspergillus fumigatus*. *J Clin Microbiol* **30:**2991–2993.
134. **Diaz-Guerra TM, Mellado E, Cuenca-Estrella M, Gaztelurrutia L, Navarro JI, Rodríguez Tudela JL.** 2000. Genetic similarity among one *Aspergillus flavus* strain isolated from a patient who underwent heart surgery and two environmental strains obtained from the operating room. *J Clin Microbiol* **38:**2419–2422.
135. **Lass-Flörl C, Grif K, Kontoyiannis DP.** 2007. Molecular typing of *Aspergillus terreus* isolates collected in Houston, Texas, and Innsbruck, Austria: evidence of great genetic diversity. *J Clin Microbiol* **45:**2686–2690.
136. **Moody SF, Tyler BM.** 1990. Restriction enzyme analysis of mitochondrial DNA of the *Aspergillus flavus* group: *A. flavus*, *A. parasiticus*, and *A. nomius*. *Appl Environ Microbiol* **56:**2441–2452.
137. **Neuveglise C, Sarfati J, Latge J, Paris S.** 1996. Afut1, a retrotransposon-like element from *Aspergillus fumigatus*. *Nucleic Acids Res* **24:**1428–1434.
138. **Paris S, Latge JP.** 2001. Afut2, a new family of degenerate gypsy-like retrotransposon from *Aspergillus fumigatus*. *Med Mycol* **39:**195–198.
139. **Semighini CP, Delmas G, Park S, Amstrong D, Perlin D, Goldman GH.** 2001. New restriction fragment length polymorphism (RFLP) markers for *Aspergillus fumigatus*. *FEMS Immunol Med Microbiol* **31:**15–19.
140. **James MJ, Lasker BA, McNeil MM, Shelton M, Warnock DW, Reiss E.** 2000. Use of a repetitive DNA probe to type clinical and environmental isolates of *Aspergillus flavus* from a cluster of cutaneous infections in a neonatal intensive care unit. *J Clin Microbiol* **38:**3612–3618.
141. **Warris A, Klaassen CHW, Meis JFGM, de Ruiter MT, de Valk HA, Abrahamsen TG, Gaustad P, Verweij PE.** 2003. Molecular epidemiology of *Aspergillus fumigatus* isolates recovered from water, air, and patients shows two clusters of genetically distinct strains. *J Clin Microbiol* **41:**4101–4106.
142. **Montiel D, Dickinson MJ, Lee HA, Dyer PS, Jeenes DJ, Roberts IN, James S, Fuller LJ, Matsuchima K, Archer DB.** 2003. Genetic differentiation of the *Aspergillus* section *flavi* complex using AFLP fingerprints. *Mycol Res* **107:**1427–1434.
143. **Perrone G, Mule G, Susca A, Battilani P, Pietri A, Logrieco A.** 2006. Ochratoxin A production and amplified fragment length polymorphism analysis of *Aspergillus carbonarius*, *Aspergillus tubingensis*, and *Aspergillus niger* strains isolated from grapes in Italy. *Appl Environ Microbiol* **72:**680–685.
144. **Tran-Dinh N, Carter D.** 2000. Characterization of microsatellite loci in the aflatoxigenic fungi *Aspergillus flavus* and *Aspergillus parasiticus*. *Mol Ecol* **9:**2170–2172.
145. **Hadrich I, Neji S, Drira I, Trabelsi H, Mahfoud N, Ranque S, Makni F, Ayadi A.** 2013. Microsatellite typing of *Aspergillus flavus* in patients with various clinical presentations of aspergillosis. *Med Mycol* **51:**586–591.
146. **Hosid E, Grishkan I, Frenkel Z, Wasser SP, Nevo E, Korol A.** 2005. Microsatellite markers for assessing DNA polymorphism of *Emericella nidulans* in nature. *Mol Ecol Notes* **5:**647–649.
147. **Esteban A, Leong SL, Tran-Dinh N.** 2005. Isolation and characterization of six polymorphic microsatellite loci in *Aspergillus niger*. *Mol Ecol Notes* **5:**375–377.
148. **Rudramurthy SM, de Valk HA, Chakrabarti A, Meis JF, Klaassen CH.** 2011. High resolution genotyping of clinical *Aspergillus flavus* isolates from India using microsatellites. *PLoS One* **6:**e16086.
149. **Kathuria S, Sharma C, Singh P, Agarwal P, Agarwal K, Hagen F, Meis J, Chowdhary A.** 2015. Molecular epidemiology and in vitro antifungal susceptibility of *Aspergillus terreus* species complex isolates in Delhi, India: evidence of genetic diversity by amplified fragment length polymorphism and microsatellite typing. *PLoS One* **10:**e0118997.
150. **Bain JM, Tavanti A, Davidson AD, Jacobsen MD, Shaw D, Gow NAR, Odds FC.** 2007. Multilocus sequence typing of the pathogenic fungus *Aspergillus fumigatus*. *J Clin Microbiol* **45:**1469–1477.
151. **Garcia-Rubio R, Gil H, Monteiro M, Pelaez T, Mellado E.** 2016. A new *Aspergillus fumigatus* typing method based on hypervariable tandem repeats located within exons of surface protein coding genes (TRESP). *PLoS One* **11:**e0163869 .
152. **Hagiwara D, Takahashi H, Watanabe A, Takahashi-Nakaguchi A, Kawamoto S, Kamei K, Gonoi T.** 2014. Whole genome comparison of *Aspergillus fumigatus* strains serially isolated from patients with aspergillosis. *J Clin Microbiol* **52:**4202–4209.
153. **Richardson MD, Page ID.** 2017. *Aspergillus* serology: have we arrived yet? *Med Mycol* **55:**48–55.
154. **Lindsley MD, Warnock DW, Morrison CJ.** 2006. Serological and molecular diagnosis of fungal infection, p 569–605. *In* Detrick B, Hamilton RG, Folds JD (ed), *Manual of Molecular and Clinical Laboratory Immunology*, 7th ed. ASM Press, Washington, DC.
155. **Holdom MD, Lechenne B, Hay RJ, Hamilton AJ, Monod M.** 2010. Production and characterization of recombinant *Aspergillus fumigatus* Cu, Zn superoxide dismutase and its recognition by immune human sera. *J Clin Microbiol* **38:**558–562.
156. **Chan CM, Woo PCY, Leung ASP, Lau SKP, Che XY, Cao L, Yuen KY.** 2002. Detection of antibodies specific to an antigenic cell wall galactomannanprotein for serodiagnosis of *Aspergillus fumigatus* aspergillosis. *J Clin Microbiol* **40:**2041–2045.
157. **Beck J, Broniszewska M, Schwienbacher M, Ebel F.** 2014. Characterization of the *Aspergillus fumigatus* chitosanase CsnB and evaluation of tis potential use in serological diagnostics. *Int J Med Microbiol* **304:**696–702.
158. **Weig M, Frosch M, Tintelnot K, Haas A, Groß U, Linsmeier B, Heesemann J.** 2001. Use of recombinant mitogillin for improved serodiagnosis of *Aspergillus fumigatus*-associated disease. *J Clin Microbiol* **39:**1721–1730.

159. **Chong KTK, Woo PCY, Lau SKP, Huang Y, Yuen KY.** 2004. *AFMP2* encodes a novel immunogenic protein of the antigenic mannoprotein superfamily in *Aspergillus fumigatus*. *J Clin Microbiol* **42:**2287–2291.
160. **Shi LN, Li F, Lu J, Kong X, Wang S, Huang M, Shao H, Shao S.** 2012. Antibody specific to thioredoxin reductase a new biomarker for serodiagnosis of invasive aspergillosis in non-neutropenic patients. *Clin Chim Acta* **413:**938–943 .
161. **Du C, Wingard JR, Cheng S, Nguyen MH, Clancy CJ.** 2012. Serum IgG responses against *Aspergillus* proteins before hematopoetic stem cell transplantation or chemotherapy identify patients who develop invasive aspergillosis. *Biol Blood Marrow Transplant* **18:**1927–1934.
162. **Erdmann JH, Graf B, Blau IW, Fischer F, Timm G, Hemmati P, Arnold R, Penack O.** 2016. Anti-*Aspergillus* immunoglobulin G testing in serum of hematopoetic stem cell transplant recipients. *Transpl Infect Dis* **18:**354–360.
163. **Delhaes L, Frealle E, Pinel C.** 2010. Serum markers for allergic bronchopulmonary aspergillosis in cystic fibrosis; state of the art and further challenge. *Med Mycol* **48**(Suppl 1)**:** S77–S87.
164. **Baxter CG, Dunn G, Jones AM, Webb K, Gore R, Richardson MD, Denning DW.** 2013. Novel immunologic classification of aspergillosis in adult cystic fibrosis. *J Allergy Clin Immunol* **132:**560–566.e10.
165. **Baxter CG, Denning DW, Jones AM, Todd A, Moore CB, Richardson MD.** 2013. Performance of two *Aspergillus* IgG EIA assays compared with the precipitin tests in chronic and allergic aspergillosis. *Clin Microbiol Infect* **19:** E197–E204 .
166. **Fukutomi Y, Tanimoto H, Yasueda H, Taniguchi M.** 2016. Serological diagnosis of allergic bronchopulmonary mycosis: progress and challenges. *Allergol Int* **65:**30–36.
167. **Herbrecht R, Denning DW, Patterson TF, Bennett JE, Greene RE, Oestmann J-W, Kern WV, Marr KA, Ribaud P, Lortholary O, Sylvester R, Rubin RH, Wingard JW, Stark P, Durand C, Caillot D, Thiel E, Chandrasekar PH, Hodges MR, Schlamm H, Troke PF, De Pauw B.** 2002. Voriconazole versus amphotericin B for primary therapy of invasive aspergillosis. *N Engl J Med* **347:**408–415.
168. **Patterson TF, Thompson GR, III, Denning DW, Fishamn J, Hadley S, Herbrecht R, Kontoyiannis DP, Marr KA, Morrison VA, Nguyen MH, Segal BH, Steinbach WJ, Stevens DA, Walsh TJ, Wingard JR, Young J-AH, Bennett JE.** 2016. Practice guidelines for the diagnosis and management of aspergillosis: 2016 update by the Infectious Diseases Society of America. *Clin Infect Dis* **63:**e1–e60.
169. **Herbrecht R, Maertens J, Baila L, Aoun M, Heinz W, Martino R, Schwartz S, Ullmann AJ, Meert L, Paesmans M, Marchetti O, Akan H, Ameye L, Shivaprakash M, Viscoli C.** 2010. Caspofungin first-line therapy for invasive aspergillosis in allogeneic hematopoeitic stem cell transplant recipients: an European Organisation for Research and Treatment of Cancer study. *Bone Marrow Transplant* **45:** 1227–1233 .
170. **Maertens JA, Raad II, Marr KA, Patterson TF, Kontoyiannis DP, Cornely OA, Bow EJ, Rahav G, Neofytos D, Aoun M, Baddley JW, Giladi M, Heinz W, Herbrecht R, Hope W, Karthaus M, Lee DG, Lortholary O, Morrison VA, Oren I, Selleslag D, Shoham S, Thompson GR, III, Lee M, Maher R, Schmitt-Hoffman AH, Zeiher B, Ullmann AJ.** 2016. Isavuconazole versus voriconazole for primary treatment of invasive mould disease caused by *Aspergillus* and other filamentous fungi (SECURE): a phase 3, randomised-controlled, non-inferiority trial. *Lancet* **387:**760–769.
171. **Marr KA, Schlamm H, Rottinghaus S, Jagannatha S, Bow EJ, Wingard JR, Pappas P, Herbrecht R, Walsh TJ, Maertens J, Mycoses Study Group.** 2012. A randomized double blind study of combination antifungal therapy with voriconazole and anidulafungin versus voriconazole monotherapy for primary treatment of invasive aspergillosis, abstr LB-2812. *Abstr 22nd Eur Congr Microbiol Infect Dis*. Congrex Switzerland Ltd., Basel, Switzerland.
172. **Tashiro M, Izumikawa K, Hirano K, Ide S, Mihara T, Hosogaya N, Takazono T, Morinaga Y, Nakamura S, Kurihara S, Imamura Y, Miyazaki T, Nishino T, Tsukamoto M, Kakeya H, Yamamoto Y, Yanagihara K, Yasuoka A, Tashiro T, Kohno S.** 2012. Correlation between triazole treatment history and susceptibility in clinically isolated *Aspergillus fumigatus*. *Antimicrob Agents Chemother* **56:**4870–4875.
173. **Howard SJ, Arendrup MC.** 2011. Acquired antifungal drug resistance in *Aspergillus fumigatus*: epidemiology and detection. *Med Mycol* **49**(Suppl 1)**:**S90–S95.
174. **Garcia-Rubio R, Cuenca-Estrella M, Mellado E.** 2017. Triazole resistance in *Aspergillus* species: an emerging problem. *Drugs* **77:**599–613.
175. **Van der Linden JW, Snelders E, Kampinga GA, Rijnders BJ, Mattsson E, Debets-Ossenkopp YJ, Kuijper EJ, Van Tiel FH, Melchers WJ, Verweij PE.** 2011. Clinical implications of azole resistance in *Aspergillus fumigatus*, The Netherlands, 2007–2009. *Emerg Infect Dis* **17:**1846–1854.
176. **Lockhart SP, Frade JP, Etienne KA, Pfaller MA, Diekema DJ, Balajee SA.** 2011. Azole resistance in *Aspergillus fumigatus* isolates from the ARTEMIS global surveillance study is primarily due to the TR/L98H mutation in the *cyp51A* gene. *Antimicrob Agents Chemother* **55:**4465–4468.
177. **Steinmann J, Hamprecht A, Vehreschild MJGT, Cornely OA, Buchheidt D, Spiess B, Koldehoff M, Buer J, Meis JF, Rath PM.** 2015. Emergence of azole-resistant invasive aspergillosis in HSCT recipients in Germany. *J Antimicrob Chemother* **70:**1522–1526.
178. **National Committee for Clinical Laboratory Standards.** 2002. Reference method for broth dilution antifungal susceptibility testing of filamentous fungi, 2nd ed. Approved standard M38–A2. National Committee for Clinical Laboratory Standards, Wayne, PA.
179. **Subcommittee on Antifungal Susceptibility Testing (AFST) of the ESMID European Committee on Antimicrobial Susceptibility Testing (EUCAST).** 2008. EUCAST technical note on method for the determination of broth dilution minimum inhibitory concentrations of antifungal agents for conidia-forming molds. *Clin Microbiol Infect* **14:**982–984.
180. **Goncalves S, Stchigel AM, Cano J, Guarro J, Colombo A.** 2013. *In vitro* antifungal susceptibility of clinically relevant species belonging to *Aspergillus* section Flavi. *Antimicrob Agents Chemother* **57:**1944–1947.
181. **Hope WW, Cuenca-Estrella M, Lass-Florl C, Arendrup MC.** 2013. EUCAST technical note on voriconazole and *Aspergillus* spp. *Clin Microbiol Infect* **19:**E278–E280.
182. **Arendrup MC, Cuenca-Estrella M, Lass-Florl C, Hope WW.** 2013. Breakpoints for antifungal agents: an update from EUCAST focussing on echinocandins against *Candida* spp. and triazoles against *Aspergillus* spp. *Drug Resist Updat* **16:**81–95.
183. **Verweij PE, Howard SJ, Melchers W, Denning DW.** 2009. Azole-resistance in *Aspergillus*: proposed nomenclature and breakpoints. *Drug Resist Updat* **12:**141–147.
184. **Rodriguez-Tudela JL, Alcazar-Fuoli L, Mellado E, Alastruey-Izquierdo A, Monzon A, Cuenca-Estrella M.** 2008. Epidemiological cutoffs and cross-resistance to azole drugs in *Aspergillus fumigatus*. *Antimicrob Agents Chemother* **52:**2468–2472.
185. **Espinel-Ingroff A, Chowdhary A, Gonzalez GM, Lass-Florl C, Martin-Mazuelos E, Meis J, Pelaez T, Pfaller MA, Turnidge JT.** 2013. Multicentre study of isavuconazole MIC distributions and epidemiological cutoff values for *Aspergillus* spp. for the CLSI M38-A2 broth microdilution method. *Antimicrob Agents Chemother* **57:**3823–3828.
186. **Johnson EM, Oakley KL, Radford SA, Moore CB, Warn P, Warnock D, Denning DW.** 2000. Lack of correlation of in vitro amphotericin B susceptibility testing with outcome in a murine model of *Aspergillus* infection. *J Antimicrob Chemother* **45:**85–93.
187. **Denning DW, Radford SA, Oakley KL, Hall L, Johnson EM, Warnock DW.** 1997. Correlation between in vitro susceptibility testing to itraconazole and in vivo outcome of *Aspergillus fumigatus* infection. *J Antimicrob Chemother* **40:**401–414.

188. **Salas V, Javier Pastor F, Sutton DA, Calvo E, Mayayo E, Fothergill AW, Rinaldi MG, Guarro J.** 2013. MIC values of voriconazole are predictive of treatment results in murine infections by *Aspergillus terreus* species complex. *Antimicrob Agents Chemother* **57:**1532–1534.
189. **Salas V, Javier Pastor F, Calvo E, Sutton DA, Fothergill AW, Guarro J.** 2013. Evaluation of in vivo activity of voriconazole as predictive of in vivo outcome in a murine *Aspergillus fumigatus* infection model. *Antimicrob Agents Chemother* **57:**1404–1408.
190. **Baddley JW, Marr KA, Andes DR, Walsh TJ, Kauffman CA, Kontoyiannis DP, Ito JI, Balajee SA, Pappas PG, Moser SA.** 2009. Patterns of susceptibility of *Aspergillus* isolates recovered from patients enrolled in the transplant associates infection surveillance network. *J Clin Microbiol* **47:**3271–3275.
191. **Calvo E, Pastor FJ, Sutton DA, Fothergill AW, Rinaldi MG, Salas V, Guarro J.** 2012. Are epidemiologic cutoff values predictors of the in vivo efficacy of azoles in experimental aspergillosis? *Diagn Microbiol Infect Dis* **74:**158–165.
192. **Arendrup MC, Perkhofer S, Howard SJ, Garcia-Effron G, Vishukumar A, Perlin D, Lass-Flörl C.** 2008. Establishing in vitro-in vivo correlations for *Aspergillus fumigatus*: the challenge of azoles versus echinocandins. *Antimicrob Agents Chemother* **52:**3504–3511.
193. **Pfaller JB, Messer SA, Hollis RJ, Diekema DJ, Pfaller MA.** 2003. In vitro susceptibility testing of *Aspergillus* spp.: comparison of Etest and reference broth microdilution methods for determining voriconazole and itraconazole MICs. *J Clin Microbiol* **41:**1126–1129.
194. **Meletiadis J, Mouton JW, Meis JF, Bouman BA, Verweij PE.** 2002. Comparison of the Etest and the sensititre colorimetric methods with the NCCLS proposed standard for antifungal susceptibility testing of *Aspergillus* species. *J Clin Microbiol* **40:**2876–2885.
195. **Espinel-Ingroff A.** 2006. Comparison of three commercial assays and a modified disk diffusion assay with two broth microdilution reference assays for testing zygomyctes, *Aspergillus* spp., *Candida* spp., and *Cryptococcus neoformans* with posaconazole and amphotericin B. *J Clin Microbiol* **44:**3616–3622.
196. **Tafin UF, Meis JF, Trampuz A.** 2012. Isothermal microcalorimetry for antifungal susceptibility testing of *Mucorales*, *Fusarium* spp., and *Scedosporium* spp. *Diagn Microbiol Infect Dis* **73:**330–337.
197. **Kontoyiannis DP, Lewis RE, May GS, Osherov N, Rinaldi MG.** 2002. *Aspergillus nidulans* is frequently resistant to amphotericin B. *Mycoses* **45:**406–407.
198. **Thom C.** 1930. *The Penicillia*. Williams & Wilkins, Baltimore, MD.
199. **Raper KB, Thom C.** 1949. *Manual of the Penicillia*. Williams & Wilkins, Baltimore, MD.
200. **Pitt JI.** 1980. *The Genus Penicillium and Its Teleomorphic States. Eupenicillium and Talaromyces*. Academic Press, London, United Kingdom.
201. **Houbraken J, Samson RA.** 2011. Phylogeny of *Penicillium* and the segregation of Trichocomaceae into three families. *Stud Mycol* **70:**1–51.
202. **Visagie CM, Houbraken J, Frisvad JC, Hong SB, Klaassen CHW, Perrone G, Seifert KA, Varga J, Yaguchi T, Samson RA.** 2014. Identification and nomenclature of the genus *Penicillium*. *Stud Mycol* **78:**343–371.
203. **Berbee ML, Yoshimura A, Sugiyama J, Taylor JW.** 1995. Is *Penicillium* monophyletic? An evaluation of phylogeny in the family Trichocomaceae from 18S, 5.8S and ITS ribosomal DNA sequence data. *Mycologia* **87:**210–222.
204. **Ogawa H, Sugiyama J.** 2000. Evolutionary relationships of the cleistothecial genera with *Penicillium*, *Geosmithia*, *Merimbla* and *Sarophorum* anamorphs as inferred from 18S rDNA sequence divergence, p 149–161. *In* Samson RA, Pitt JI (ed), *Integration of Modern Taxonomic Methods for Penicillium and Aspergillus Classification*. Plenum Press, New York, NY.
205. **Peterson SW.** 2000. Phylogenetic analysis of *Penicillium* species based on ITS and LSU-rDNA nucleotide sequences, p 163–178. *In* Samson RA, Pitt JI (ed), *Integration of Modern Taxonomic Methods for Penicillium and Aspergillus Classification*. Plenum Press, New York, NY.
206. **Wang L, Zhuang WY.** 2007. Phylogenetic analyses of penicillia based on partial calmodulin gene sequences. *Biosystems* **88:**113–126.
207. **Yilmaz N, Visagie CM, Houbraken J, Frisvad JC, Samson RA.** 2014. Polyphasic taxonomy of the genus *Talaromyces*. *Stud Mycol* **78:**175–341.
208. **Segretain G.** 1959. Description d'une nouvelle espèce de penicillium: *Penicillium marneffei* n. sp. *Bull Soc Mycol Fr* **75:**412–416.
209. **Vanittanakom N, Cooper CR, Jr, Fisher MC, Sirisanthana T.** 2006. *Penicillium marneffei* infection and recent advances in the epidemiology and molecular biology aspects. *Clin Microbiol Rev* **19:**95–110.
210. **Le T, Wolbers M, Chi NH, Quang VM, Chinh NT, Lan NP, Lam PS, Kozal MJ, Shikuma CM, Day JN, Farrar J.** 2011. Epidemiology, seasonality, and predictors of outcome of AIDS-associated *Penicillium marneffei* infection in Ho Chi Minh City, Viet Nam. *Clin Infect Dis* **52:**945–952.
211. **Ustianowski AP, Sieu TP, Day JN.** 2008. *Penicillium marneffei* infection in HIV. *Curr Opin Infect Dis* **21:**31–36.
212. **Chan JFW, Lau SKP, Yuen KY, Woo PCY.** 2016. *Talaromyces (Penicillium) marneffei* infection in non-HIV infected patients. *Emerg Microbes Infect* **5:**e19.
213. **Chan JFW, Chan TSY, Gill G, Lam F, Trendell-Smith NJ, Sridhar S, Tse H, Lau SSKP, Hung I, Yuen KY, Woo PCY.** 2015. Disseminated infections with *Talaromyces marneffei* in non-AIDS patients given monoclonal antibodies against CD20 and kinase inhibitors. *Emerg Infect Dis* **21:** 1101–1106.
214. **Capponi M, Sureau P, Segretain G.** 1956. Penicillose de *Rhizomys sinensis*. *Bull Soc Pathol Exot* **49:**418–421.
215. **Bulterys PL, Le T, Quang VM, Nelson KE, Lloyd-Smith JO.** 2013. Environmental predictors and incubation period of AIDS-associated *Penicillium marneffei* infection in Ho Chi Minh City, Vietnam. *Clin Infect Dis* **56:**1273–1279.
216. **Li X, Yang Y, Zhang X, Zhou X, Lu S, Ma L, Lu C, Xi L.** 2011. Isolation of *Penicillium marneffei* from soil and wild rodents in Guangdong, SE China. *Mycopathologia* **172:** 447–451.
217. **Cao C, Liang L, Wang W, Luo H, Huang S, Liu D, Xu J, Henk DA, Fisher MC.** 2011. Common reservoirs for *Penicillium marneffei* infection in humans and rodents, China. *Emerg Infect Dis* **17:**209–214.
218. **Huynh TX, Nguyen HC, Dinh Nguyen HM, Do MT, Odermatt-Biays O, Degremont A, Malvy D.** 2003. *Penicillium marneffei* infection and AIDS. A review of 12 cases reported in the Tropical Diseases Centre, Ho Chi Minh City (Vietnam). *Sante* **13:**149–153.
219. **Chong YB, Tan LP, Robinson S, Lim SK, Ng KP, Keng TC, Kamarulzaman A.** 2012. Penicilliosis in lupus patients presenting with unresolved fever: a report of 2 cases and literature review. *Trop Biomed* **29:**270–276.
220. **Tang BS, Chan JF-W, Chen M, Tsang OT-Y, Mok MY, Lai RW-M, Lee R, Que T-L, Tse H, Li IW-S, To KK-W, Cheng VC-C, Chan EY-T, Zheng B, Yuen K-Y.** 2010. Disseminated penicillosis, recurrent bacteremic nonytyphoidal salmonellosis and burkholderiosis associated with acquired immunodeficiency due to autoantibody against gamma interferon. *Clin Vaccine Immunol* **17:**1132–1138.
221. **Hart J, Dyer JR, Clark BM, McLellan DG, Perera S, Ferrari P.** 2012. Travel-related disseminated *Penicillium marneffei* infection in a renal transplant patient. *Transpl Infect Dis* **14:**434–439.
222. **Xiang Y, Guo W, Liang K.** 2015. An unusual appearing skin lesion from *Penicillium marneffei* infection in an AIDS patient in central China. *Am J Trop Med Hyg* **93:**3.
223. **Marques SA, Robles AM, Tortorano AM, Tuculet MA, Negroni R, Mendes RP.** 2000. Mycoses associated with AIDS in the third world. *Med Mycol* **38**(Suppl 1)**:**269–279.
224. **Lim D, Lee YS, Chang AR.** 2006. Rapid diagnosis of *Penicillium marneffei* infection by fine needle aspiration cytology. *J Clin Pathol* **59:**443–444.
225. **Wong KF.** 2010. Marrow penicillinosis: a readily missed diagnosis. *Am J Clin Pathol* **134:**214–218.

226. **Ellis D, Davis S, Alexiou H, Handke R, Bartley R.** 2007. *Descriptions of Medical Fungi,* 2nd ed, p 108–109. Mycology Unit, Women's and Children's Hospital, North Adelaide, Australia.
227. **Kaufman L, Standard PG, Anderson SA, Jalbert M, Swisher BL.** 1995. Development of specific fluorescent-antibody test for tissue form of *Penicillium marneffei. J Clin Microbiol* **33:**2136–2138.
228. **Tsunemi Y, Takahashi T, Tamaki T.** 2003. *Penicllium marneffei* infection diagnoses by polymerase chain reaction from the skin specimen. *J Am Acad Dermatol* **49:**344–346.
229. **Zeng H, Li X, Chen X, Zhang J, Sun J, Xie Z, Xi L.** 2009. Identification of *Penicillium marneffei* in paraffin-embedded tissue using nested PCR. *Mycopathologia* **168:**31–35.
230. **Liu Y, Huang X, Yi X, He Y, Mylonakis E, Xi L.** 2016. Detection of *Talaromyces marneffei* from fresh tissue of an inhalational murine pulmonary model using nested PCR. *PLoS One* **11:**e0149634.
231. **Zhang JM, Sun JF, Feng PY, Li XQ, Lu CM, Lu S, Cai WY, Xi LY, de Hoog GS.** 2011. Rapid identification and characterization of *Penicillium marneffei* using multiplex ligation-dependent probe amplification (MLPA) in paraffin-embedded tissue samples. *J Microbiol Methods* **85:**33–39.
232. **Sun J, Li X, Zeng H, Xie Z, Lu C, Xi L, de Hoog GS.** 2010. Development and evaluation of loop-mediated isothermal amplification (LAMP) for the rapid diagnosis of *Penicillium marneffei* in archived tissue samples. *FEMS Immunol Med Microbiol* **58:**381–388.
233. **Hien HT, Thanh TT, Thu N, Nguyen A, Thanh NT, Lan N, Simmons C, Shikuma C, Chau N, Thwaites G, Le T.** 2016. Development and evaluation of a real-time polymerase chain reaction assay for rapid detection of *Talaromyces marneffei MP1* gene in human plasma. *Mycoses* **59:**773–780.
234. **Cao L, Chen DL, Lee C, Chan CM, Chan KM, Vanittanakom N, Tsang DN, Yuen KY.** 1998. Detection of specific antibodies to an antigenic mannoprotein for diagnosis of *Penicillium marneffei* penicillosis. *J Clin Microbiol* **36:**3028–3031.
235. **Lau S, Lam C, Ngan A, Chow W, Wu A, Tsang D, Tse C, Que T, Tang B, Woo P.** 2016. Matrix-assisted laser desorption ionization time-of-flight mass spectrometry for rapid identification of mould and yeast cultures of *Penicillium marneffei. BMC Microbiol* **16:**36.
236. **Fisher MC, Aanensen D, de Hoog S, Vanittanakom N.** 2004. Multilocus microsatellite typing system for *Penicillium marneffei* reveals spatially structured populations. *J Clin Microbiol* **42:**5065–5069.
237. **Lasker BA, Ran Y.** 2004. Analysis of polymorphic microsatellite markers for typing *Penicillium marneffei* isolates. *J Clin Microbiol* **42:**1483–1490.
238. **Lasker BA.** 2006. Nucleotide sequence-based analysis for determining the molecular epidemiology of *Penicillium marneffei. J Clin Microbiol* **44:**3145–3153.
239. **Kaufman L, Standard PG, Jalbert M, Kantipong P, Limpakarnjanarat K, Mastro TD.** 1996. Diagnostic antigenemia tests for penicillosis marneffei. *J Clin Microbiol* **34:**2503–2505.
240. **Yuen KY, Wong SS, Chau P, Tsang DN.** 1994. Serodiagnosis of *Penicillium marneffei* infection. *Lancet* **344:**444–445.
241. **Cao L, Chan KM, Chen D, Vanittanakom N, Lee C, Chan CM, Sirisanthana T, Tsang DN, Yuen KY.** 1999. Detection of cell wall mannoprtein Mp1p in culture supernatants of *Penicillium marneffei* and in sera of penicillinosis patients. *J Clin Microbiol* **37:**981–986.
242. **Wang YF, Xu HF, Han ZG, Zeng L, Liang CY, Chen XJ, Chen YJ, Cai JP, Hao W, Chan JFW, Wang M, Fu N, Che XY.** 2015. Serological surveillance for *Penicillium marneffei* infection in HIV-infected patients during 2004-2011 in Guangzhou, China. *Clin Microbiol Infect* **21:**484–489.
243. **Rimek D, Zimmermann T, Hartmann M, Prariyachatigul C, Kappe R.** 1999. Disseminated *Penicillium marneffei* infection in an HIV-positive female from Thailand in Germany. *Mycoses* **42**(Suppl 2)**:**25–28.
244. **Desakorn V, Simpson AJH, Wuthiekanun V, Sahassananda D, Rajanuwong A, Pitisuttithum P, Howe P, Smith MD, White NJ.** 2002. Development and evaluation of rapid urinary antigen detection tests for diagnosis of penicillosis marneffei. *J Clin Microbiol* **40:**3179–3183.
245. **Chaiyaroj SC, Chawengkirttikul R, Sirisinha S, Watkins P, Srinoulprasert Y.** 2003. Antigen detection assay for identification of *Penicillium marneffei* infection. *J Clin Microbiol* **41:**432–434.
246. **Lau SK, Lo GC, Lam CS, Chow WN, Ngan AH, Wu AK, Tsang DN, Tse CW, Que TL, Tang BS, Woo PC.** 2017. In vitro activity of posaconazole against *Talaromyces marneffei* by broth microdilution and Etest methods and comparison to itraconazole, voriconazole and anidulafungin. *Antimicrob Agents Chemother* **61:**e01480-16.
247. **Odabasi Z, Paetznick VL, Rodriguez JR, Chen E, Ostrosky-Zeichner L.** 2004. In vitro activity of anidulafungin against seleted clinically important mold isolates. *Antimicrob Agents Chemother* **48:**1912–1915.
248. **Liu D, Liang L, Chen J.** 2013. In vitro antifungal drug susceptibilities of *Penicllium marneffei* from China. *J Infect Chemother* **19:**776–778.
249. **Ouyang Y, Cai S, Liang H, Cao C.** 2017. Administration of voriconazole in disseminated *Talaromyces* (*Penicillium*) *marneffei* infection: a retrospective study. *Mycopathologia* **182:**569–575.
250. **Cao C, Liu W, Li R, Wan Z, Qiao J.** 2008. In vitro interactions of micafungin with amphotericin B, itraconazole or fluconazole against the pathogenic phase of *Penicillium marneffei. J Antimicrob Chemother* **63:**340–342.
251. **Horner WE, Helbling A, Salvaggio JE, Lehrer SB.** 1995. Fungal allergens. *Clin Microbiol Rev* **8:**161–179.
252. **Santos PE, Piontelli E, Shea YR, Galluzzo ML, Holland SM, Zelazko ME, Rosenzweig SD.** 2006. *Penicillium piceum* infection: diagnosis and successful treatment in chronic granulomatous disease. *Med Mycol* **44:**749–753.
253. **Kumar S, Stecher G, Tamura K.** 2016. MEGA7: molecular evolutionary genetics analysis version 7.0 for bigger datasets. *Mol Biol Evol* **33:**1870–1874.

Fusarium and Other Opportunistic Hyaline Fungi

SEAN X. ZHANG, KERRY O'DONNELL, AND DEANNA A. SUTTON

123

The opportunistic hyaline or lightly colored molds (also referred to as moniliaceous molds) constitute a phylogenetically diverse group of common to rare asexual and sexual fungi that typically occur as saprobes in soil, in air, or on plant litter or as facultative plant pathogens. Some may be recovered from patients without having any clinical significance. Others are isolated infrequently enough to challenge the proficiency of a diagnostic laboratory, and critical assessment is required to evaluate the significance of their recovery. While several of the genera treated in this chapter include species that have either lightly colored or dark (melanized) conidia, the emphasis is on fungi that grow in tissue in the form of hyaline or lightly colored, septate hyphae.

The term "fusariosis" is used to define infections caused by species of *Fusarium* (1) (Table 1), but the practice of coining disease names based on the fungal genus is disadvantageous when infections are caused by uncommon or rare pathogens. The wide variety of fungi involved makes it difficult to place the organisms into accessible groups, and problems arise when fungal names are changed. To avoid unnecessary changes to disease names based on a genus, two major disease groups have been proposed: hyalohyphomycosis and phaeohyphomycosis (2). Although the groups were defined as encompassing similar clinical spectra, they were distinguished by the presence of septate hyphae in tissue without (hyalohyphomycosis) or with (phaeohyphomycosis) pigmentation or melanin in the fungal cell wall. However, some fungi, such as *Scedosporium* species and *Neoscytalidium dimidiatum* [formerly *Scytalidium dimidiatum* (*Nattrassia mangiferae*)] (3), which form darkly pigmented colonies and conidia *in vitro*, produce hyaline or lightly pigmented hyphae in tissue. Similarly, rare fusariosis cases have been reported to produce darkly pigmented colonies *in vitro* and *in vivo* (4). The Fontana-Masson stain helps to detect melanin pigmentation of fungal elements in tissue, but the results are not always conclusive (see also the discussion in chapter 118). Some fungi with variable pigmentation may stain faintly or inconsistently. In practice, the terms for the disease categories have been used to designate infections caused by fungi that are either hyaline or pigmented (melanized, phaeoid, or dematiaceous) *in vitro*. Although it may be useful to have terms for broad categories of mycotic diseases, there are problems in categorizing fungi by color. A subcommittee of the International Society for Human and Animal Mycology (ISHAM) has suggested that fungal diseases be named by providing a specific description of the pathology and naming the causative agent, e.g., subcutaneous cyst caused by fungus *x* (5, 6).

TAXONOMY AND IDENTIFICATION

The opportunistic hyaline molds include an ever-increasing number of genera. Most do not produce a teleomorph (meiotic or sexual stage) in culture and comprise taxa that are either anamorphs of the Ascomycota and Basidiomycota, or genera for which no sexual state has been described (see chapter 116). Today, the relationships between many anamorphs and their sexual relatives are known through discovery of teleomorphs or are inferred by phylogenetic analysis of DNA sequence data. This knowledge is extremely important in understanding fungal relationships and has allowed placement of fungi thought to reproduce only asexually next to their sexual relatives in fungal phylogenies. Rapid developments in this area have focused on circumscribing monophyletic genera and recognition of genealogically exclusive phylogenetically distinct species, particularly among the fusaria (7–17). Teleomorphs may develop in culture by homothallic, self-fertile species (see chapter 116), but they may be difficult to obtain without the use of specialized media and extended incubation. Recent modifications relative to the naming of pleomorphic fungi, however, have prohibited the use of dual nomenclature after 1 January 2013 (18, 19), and many changes are to be expected regarding accepted taxa. One such significant change is the proposed unitary use of the name *Fusarium* over various teleomorph names (20), in part because fewer than 20% of fusaria are known to reproduce sexually. The majority of fusaria studied to date are presumed to be self-sterile or heterothallic, because PCR screens for mating type indicate that they possess only one of the two idiomorphs (i.e., *MAT1-1* and *MAT1-2*) required for sexual reproduction (21).

Most of the pathogenic molds considered in this chapter are classified in the form class Hyphomycetes (genera which bear free conidia) (22–24). Phenotypic identification of Hyphomycetes is based on morphology of the conidia and the mechanisms by which conidia are formed (conidiogenesis; see chapter 116). Three basic tools are necessary for practical observation of these features.

TABLE 1 Classification of *Fusarium* infections[a]

- I. Normal host
  - A. Keratitis
    - a. Trauma and penetration of cornea
    - b. Contamination of soft contact lenses, solutions, cases
    - c. Local immunosuppression by corticosteroid drops
  - B. Onychomycosis[b]
    - a. Distal subungual lesion in toenails in females
    - b. Lateral subungual onychomycosis
    - c. Proximal subungual onychomycosis
    - d. Paronychia-like reaction in proximal nail fold
  - C. Intertrigo[b]
  - D. Tinea pedis[b]
    - a. Interdigital infection
  - E. Hyperkeratotic plantar lesions[b]
  - F. Skin infections[b]
  - G. Surgical wound infections
  - H. Burns
  - I. Ulcers
  - J. Otitis media
  - K. Peritonitis (continuous ambulatory peritoneal dialysis)
  - L. Catheter-associated fungemia
  - M. Fungemia with or without organ involvement
  - N. Pneumonia
  - O. Sinusitis
  - P. Septic arthritis
  - Q. Thrombophlebitis
  - R. Endophthalmitis
  - S. Osteomyelitis
- II. Immunocompromised host
  - A. Endophthalmitis
  - B. Sinusitis
  - C. Pneumonia
  - D. Skin involvement
  - E. Fungemia
  - F. Disseminated infection
  - G. Brain abscess
  - H. Peritonitis

[a]Adapted from references 60, 69, 76, and 105. Patients infected with other fungi discussed in this chapter may present with similar clinical syndromes, and fungal structures in tissue may resemble those of *Aspergillus* species.

[b]Patients from whom a dermatophyte has not been isolated.

(i) An ocular micrometer is essential for determining sizes of conidia or sexual spores, when present. Identification of molds often requires comparison with published taxonomic descriptions in which size is a key criterion for species distinction. (ii) A dissecting microscope with magnification of up to ×60 and basal illumination is useful for examining colonies in plates or tubes for the presence of conidia in chains or slimy heads, specialized structures such as Hülle cells, sclerotia, conidiomata, or sexual fruiting bodies formed under aerial mycelium or embedded in the agar. (iii) Microscopic mounts that allow observation of how a fungus forms its conidia also are necessary. Slide culture preparations are excellent for many fungi and are generally necessary for those with small, delicate conidia (25, 26); however, rapidly growing species, such as those in the genus *Trichoderma*, should be examined early by tease mounts. Morphologic features important for identification of conidial fungi include (i) conidium size, shape, and pattern of septation; (ii) the color of conidia and conidiophore, whether light (hyaline) or dark (melanized or phaeoid); (iii) developmental aspects of conidiogenesis, including the nature of the conidiogenous cell; (iv) the mechanism of conidium liberation or dehiscence; and (v) features of a multihyphal structure producing conidia (i.e., conidioma, if present). Differences in conidial shape and septation are useful characters for preliminary distinction and have been used traditionally for grouping conidial fungi. Conidia may be nonseptate or may have one or more septa. Some fungi produce septate and nonseptate conidia. In genera such as *Fusarium*, where large multiseptate and much smaller septate or nonseptate conidia are produced, they are referred to as macro- and microconidia, respectively.

Conidia also vary in shape. Some macroconidia are long and narrow, as in *Fusarium*. Development of a conidium may occur by conversion of an existing cell or several cells (thallicarthric or arthrosporic) or may involve construction of a new wall or blowing out of a portion of a preexisting wall (blastic). Conidiogenesis usually occurs at a particular location on a conidiogenous cell. If development occurs at a site that remains fixed and gives rise to more than one conidium, then the site is referred to as stable or determinate. If conidia develop at new points on the conidiogenous cell (or axis), then the site is described as unstable or indeterminate. New sites may occur on an axis which lengthens (progressive) or shortens (retrogressive). Depending on the species, conidiogenous cells may produce a single conidium or multiple conidia. Sympodial development involves the development of a single conidium at successive sites on a lengthening axis. Phialides and annellides are specialized conidiogenous cells that produce multiple conidia. Conidia may be produced successively (serially) and develop in slimy masses or in chains, with the youngest at the base of the chain (basipetal). Although it is sometimes difficult to differentiate between the two types of cells, the annellide elongates and sometimes narrows during formation of each new conidium, leaving an often imperceptible series of rings or scars on the conidiogenous cell. Scrutiny of the conidiogenous locus by use of an oil immersion objective may be necessary to make this distinction. Holoblastic conidiogenesis, in which the inner and outer cell walls are involved, usually results in the formation of acropetal chains, with the youngest conidium at the tip of the chain. The distinction between acropetal and basipetal chains may be revealed by comparison of the size and wall morphologies of the distal and proximal conidia in the chain. The youngest conidium is recognizable by its smaller size, lighter color if the conidia are pigmented, and differences in wall ornamentation if the conidia are roughened. Some conidiogenous cells form multiple conidia simultaneously over the surface of the swollen cell. When mature, conidia detach by fission of a double septum (schizolytic dehiscence) or by sacrifice of a supporting cell (rhexolytic dehiscence), either by fracture of a thin-walled region or by lysis of the supporting cell. Lytic dehiscence typically occurs in the dermatophytes and related fungi.

The presence of different spore states can make identification difficult. Careful examination and sometimes subculture via a single spore or hyphal tip are required to assess whether the spore types represent different states of the same fungus or whether the isolate is contaminated with more than one species. Molds that produce more than one conidial state (i.e., synanomorphs) or sexual and conidial states are called pleomorphic fungi. These may be represented by simple yeast or yeast-like stages or by the formation of complex conidiomatal structures such as sporodochia (conidiophores borne crowded on a compact mass of hyphae or a hyphal stroma), synnemata (conidiophores aggregated into a compound stalk), or pycnidia (conidiogenous cells formed inside a round or oval fruiting body). Production of synanamorphs may be influenced by the agar medium used and may be lost upon repeated subculture.

The number of hyaline fungal species that have been reported to cause opportunistic infections in humans and other animals is increasing, and it is beyond the scope of this chapter to describe them all. Some reports identify the fungus only to the genus level, while others provide the fungus name but without salient details of its colony and microscopic features. A continuing and vexing problem is that authenticity of published reports cannot be verified if the fungus is inadequately described and illustrated and if isolates are not deposited in publicly accessible culture collections. This chapter describes the salient colony and microscopic features of medically important species in the genus *Fusarium* (see Table 2) and other selected hyaline opportunists (see Table 3). Detailed descriptions of species listed are found in several reference manuals (15, 26–36) as well as the current literature. Due to the rapid discovery of novel phylogenetically distinct species via multilocus sequence typing over the past decade, most clinically important species within *Fusarium* appear to be undescribed (37). Two Internet-accessible websites have been developed for identifying *Fusarium*, FUSARIUM-ID (http://isolate.fusariumdb.org/guide.php) (38) and Fusarium MLST (http://www.westerdijkinstitute.nl/fusarium/) (37). Identifications are conducted via BLASTn searches of either database using a partial translation elongation factor (1α) sequence of the unknown as the query, or sequences from several other loci.

CLINICAL SIGNIFICANCE

The spectrum of disease caused by hyaline molds is diverse. The disease is largely determined by the local and general immunologic and physiologic state of the host and may be symptomatic or asymptomatic. In most instances, the portal of entry for fungal propagules is likely the lungs or a break in the epidermis due to trauma. Exceptions to this include introduction by means of contaminated surgical instruments, intraocular lenses, prosthetic devices, or other contaminated materials or solutions associated with surgery or routine health care. Individuals whose resistance is lowered as a result of a severe debilitating disease or immunosuppressive therapy typically suffer from invasive pulmonary or paranasal sinus infections, but in some instances, the infecting fungus may spread to surrounding tissues or disseminate hematogenously to virtually any organ. Fungemia is uncommon except in disseminated *Fusarium* infections. Noninvasive forms of infection also have been noted in debilitated individuals as well as in individuals with apparently normal defense mechanisms. In such cases, the fungus colonizes a preexisting cavity in the lungs such as an ectatic bronchus, a tuberculous cavity, or a lung cyst. Other clinical syndromes usually occurring in immunocompetent individuals include chronic sinusitis, onychomycosis, subcutaneous abscess, keratitis, otomycosis, and allergic manifestations including bronchopulmonary mycosis and sinusitis in atopic patients.

Although the majority of saprobic and plant-pathogenic molds are not considered pathogenic for humans and other animals and appear unlikely to be able to adapt to or take advantage of risk factors predisposing to opportunistic infection, those capable of growing at or near body temperature must be considered to have latent pathogenic capability. The diversity of fungi that have invaded human tissue has increased dramatically in recent years, as reflected by new reports of proven infection. Moreover, certain fungi are isolated often enough to be suspicious for pathogenic potential. Still, there is a need for definitive evidence of infection due to a normally saprobic mold. The laboratory procedure for confirming fungal etiology includes (i) detection of hyphae in the specimen that are compatible with the morphology of the isolated mold, (ii) isolation of several colonies of the fungus or isolation of the same fungus from two or more specimens over time, (iii) accurate identification of the isolated mold, and (iv) confirmation of the mold's ability to grow at or near body temperature. It should be noted here, however, that some species that fail to grow at 35°C are capable of inciting systemic disease in profoundly immunocompromised individuals (39) and are frequently agents of cutaneous or subcutaneous mycoses. Species of *Fusarium* or other hyaline molds isolated from all deep tissue or body fluids must be considered potential invasive opportunistic pathogens. No fungal isolate should be discarded as a contaminant without thorough examination of the clinical specimen. Quality control measures are essential to ensure that isolation media are not contaminated (i.e., the fungus is growing from the specimen and not elsewhere on the agar medium). Close communication between microbiologists and physicians also is essential, especially for rare or unusual opportunists seen in individuals maintained on long-term immunosuppressive therapy.

COLLECTION, TRANSPORT, AND STORAGE OF SPECIMENS

Clinical specimens from patients with suspected mycosis should be collected with prudence and transported to the laboratory and processed as soon as possible by using the standard procedures described in chapter 117. Because of the diverse clinical manifestations, various sites may need to be examined for fungal elements. Biopsy material, transtracheal aspirates, and sputum samples collected in the early morning all may be useful specimens for the isolation and detection of hyaline molds, as are infected nails. Swabs taken from mucous membranes and skin lesions are not recommended. Although the reliability of determining whether an isolate is a possible pathogen is increased if cultures of two different specimens yield the same organism, histological examination and culture of a tissue biopsy are more informative. While blood cultures are generally of limited use for detecting invasive hyaline molds that produce dry conidia (microconidia in chains), such as *Aspergillus* (40), *Fusarium* and other species that produce abundant yeast-like microconidia may be reliably detected (41). For optimum recovery, the specimen should be inoculated onto several types of media and incubated at 28 to 30°C. Opportunistic molds are variably sensitive to cycloheximide, so media containing this selective agent should be used cautiously. Suspicious isolates, especially of uncommon species, should be tested for their ability to grow at 35 to 37°C. Potentially neurotropic species may also grow at 40°C and beyond (42, 43).

FUSARIUM SPECIES

Taxonomy

Fusarium species are ubiquitous soil saprobes and facultative plant pathogens that can cause infection or toxicosis in humans and other animals (15, 27, 44, 45). They belong to the order Hypocreales, family Nectriaceae. Clinically significant species are mostly heterothallic, with only the anamorphic (asexual) state seen in culture. Prior to the abandonment of dual nomenclature on 1 January 2013, *Fusarium* teleomorphs were classified in *Gibberella*, *Neocosmospora*, and other genera; however, these taxa should be reported under the *Fusarium* anamorph name (20). Several molecular

TABLE 2 Key phenotypic features of clinically significant *Fusarium* species[a]

Complex and species	Colonial form	Characteristic(s) of: Sporodochia[b]	Conidia	Macroconidia[c]	Microconidia	Chlamydospores
FSSC						
F. solani (FSSC 5)	White to cream; reverse usually colorless; rapid growth	White to cream colored when sporodochia are present	Long monophialides arising laterally from aerial hyphae, mostly with a rather distinct collarette	Moderately curved, with short, blunt apical and indistinctly pedicellate basal cells, mostly 3–5 septate	Abundant, oval, ellipsoid, reniform and fusiform with 0 to 1 septate	Present, singly or in pairs, terminal or intercalary or rough walled
F. petroliphilum (FSSC 1), *F. keratoplasticum* (FSSC 2), and several other unnamed species (Fig. 1A)[d]	Mostly cream, occasionally slightly blue-green, reddish, or lavender; floccose; rapid growth	Cream in confluent pionnotes	Long monophialides	Multiseptate, abundant, stout, thick walled; dorsal and ventral surfaces only almost parallel	Abundant, mostly 0 or 1 septate; oval to kidney-shaped in false heads	Present, single and pairs
F. falciforme (FSSC 3+4, formerly *Acremonium falciforme*)	Cream to pale brown, glabrous to velvety; slow growth; lavender reverse on SDA[e]	Seldom seen on PDA	Long monophialides	Poor conidial production; mostly lack foot cells	One to three celled	Present, often pale brown
F. lichenicola (formerly *Cylindrocarpon lichenicola*)	Initially white, then pale yellow to light brown; floccose; rapid growth	Seldom seen	Long monophialides	Straight, multiseptate, rounded at apices, truncate basal cells	Absent	Short chains and clusters, brown, rough
F. neocosmosporiellum (formerly *Neocosmospora vasinfecta*)[f]	Flat, thin, almost transparent, becoming punctate with production of orange to pale brown perithecia	Absent	Long monophialides	Absent on PDA	Similar to those seen in *F. petroliphilum*	As in *F. petroliphilum*
FOSC						
F. oxysporum (Fig. 1B)[g]	White to lavender, salmon tinge, lavender reverse; floccose; rapid growth	Orange, erumpent	Short monophialides	Multiseptate, slightly sickle-shaped, thin walled, delicate	Mostly 0 septate, oval to kidney shaped, in false heads only	Present, abundant, single and pairs
FFSC						
F. verticillioides (formerly *F. moniliforme*) (Fig. 1C)	White to lavender with lavender reverse; floccose; rapid growth	Usually absent on PDA, tan to orange on CLA	Medium-length monophialides	Multiseptate, almost straight	0 or 1 septate, oval to clavate, truncate, occur in false heads and chains	Absent
F. thapsinum	Morphologically indistinguishable from *F. verticillioides* except for yellow diffusing pigment on PDA, although not produced by all strains	Same as for *F. verticillioides*	Same as for *F. verticillioides*	Same as for *F. verticillioides*	Same as for *F. verticillioides*	Same as for *F. verticillioides*
F. napiforme	White to lavender, lavender reverse	Usually absent on PDA; tan on CLA	Medium-length monophialides	Multiseptate, falcate to almost straight	0 or 1 septate, ovoid to pyriform (pear shaped) to napiform (beet shaped) in false heads and short chains	Sparse, short chains or clusters

(*Continued on next page*)

TABLE 2 Key phenotypic features of clinically significant *Fusarium* species[a] *(Continued)*

Complex and species	Colonial form	Characteristic(s) of: Sporodochia[b]	Conidia	Macroconidia[c]	Microconidia	Chlamydospores
F. proliferatum (Fig. 1D)	White to lavender, lavender reverse; floccose; rapid growth	May be absent on PDA; tan on CLA	Monophialides and polyphialides	Multiseptate, falcate to almost straight	Oval to pyriform, truncate; occur in false heads	Absent
F. nygamai	White to lavender, lavender reverse; floccose; rapid growth; orange to violet spore mass common centrally	Orange on CLA	Monophialides and polyphialides; however, polyphialide production variable	Multiseptate, falcate to almost straight, thin walled	Oval to clavate, mostly 0 septate, in false heads and short chains (to 20 conidia in length)	Few to abundant, single, chains, clusters; smooth or rough, hyaline to yellow
FCSC						
F. chlamydosporum	White to pink to carmine, brown centrally with production of chlamydospores; floccose; rapid growth	Uncommon on PDA; tan to orange on CLA	Short monophialides and short polyphialides, often with three openings	Rare except on sporodochia	0–2 septate, fusiform, apiculate; may be slow to form in some strains on PDA	Abundant, brown, rough, in chains and clusters
FDSC						
F. dimerum (Fig. 1E)	Slimy, yeast-like due to conidial masses; aerial mycelium sparse to absent; salmon to light orange, reverse same or pale yellow; slow growth	Orange, well developed on CLA	Monophialides; conidiation on agar surface from lateral phialidic pegs	Abundant; 0- or 1 septate with septum in middle; curved	Ellipsoidal to ovoidal to curved, mostly one-celled	Derived from macroconidia; hyphal chlamydospores rare or absent
F. delphinoides (Fig. 1F)	Similar to *F. dimerum* except for reverse, which may be speckled with red-brown clumps of pigment	Same as for *F. dimerum*	Same as for *F. dimerum*	Can be 2 septate; when 1 septate, septum is off-center	Same as for *F. dimerum*	Same as for *F. dimerum*
FIESC						
Fusarium sp.[h]	Buff to light brown, reverse salmon; floccose; rapid growth	Orange, produced by some strains on CLA	Monophialides and polyphialides	Those produced in aerial mycelium almost straight; those produced in pionnotes[i] or sporodochia curved	0 septate, sparse or absent	Sparse, intercalary, single or chains

[a]On PDA after 4 days of incubation at 25°C unless otherwise noted. See references cited in the text for a more detailed description of the features noted in this table; the list is not inclusive.

[b]Cushion-shaped mats of hyphae, conidiophores, and macroconidia. CLA, carnation leaf agar.

[c]Most characteristic macroconidia for all species are those formed in sporodochia on carnation leaf agar; macroconidia formed in aerial mycelium on PDA are often smaller.

[d]At least 20 species within the FSSC have been implicated in mycoses of humans and other animals. *Fusarium petroliphilum* (FSSC 1), *F. keratoplasticum* (FSSC 2) and *F. falciforme* (FSSC 3+4) account for most infections caused by members of the FSSC (12, 49).

[e]SDA, Sabouraud dextrose agar.

[f]This microconidial, self-fertile or homothallic *Fusarium* species frequently produces perithecial fruiting bodies in culture. Perithecial, walls of textura angularis type, asci cylindrical, eight-spored (30 to 100 by 11 to 15 μm); ascospores one-celled, thick-walled, roughened, yellow to brown, globose to ellipsoidal (10 to 15 by 7 to 12 μm).

[g]The FOSC is phylogenetically diverse and comprises at least 26 two-locus sequence types associated with mycoses (53), including the widespread clonal lineage ST 33, recovered from hospital and other plumbing systems (14, 47).

[h]Of the 20 species within the FIESC that have been implicated in mycotic infections of humans and other animals (13), Latin binomials can be applied with confidence only to *F. equiseti* (FIESC 14) and *F. lacertarum* (FIESC 4). Although the names *F. incarnatum*, *F. pallidoroseum*, and *F. semitectum* are commonly applied to members of the FIESC, these names should not be used until it is determined what species they represent.

[i]A flat mass of macroconidia having a greasy or fatty appearance.

TABLE 3 Key phenotypic features of selected hyaline molds

Group and genus	Key features[a]	Etiologic agent(s)	Comments
Homothallic ascomycetes			
Achaetomium[b]	Colonies fast growing, white to yellowish with pink diffusible pigment (Fig. 1G). Conidia formed from minute phialides. Pale brown perithecia bearing thin-walled setae. Ascospores brown, smooth, fusoidal.	*A. strumarium*[b]	Growth at 42°C, neurotropic; compare with *Chaetomium*. Extended incubation often enhances perithecial production.
Amesia[b]	Colonies black owing to perithecia and masses of ascospores maturing within 7 days. Setae flexuous. Ascospores fusiform. Growth to 47°C; neurotropic.	*A. atrobrunnea*[b]	Formerly *Chaetomium atrobrunneum*
Aphanoascus[b]	Colonies moderately fast growing, yellowish-white, granular; cycloheximide tolerant. Cleistothecia globose, containing roughened ascospores; associated with a *Chrysosporium* anamorph consisting of terminal 1-celled sessile conidia and alternate arthroconidia.	*A. fulvescens*[b]	Compare with *Chrysosporium* and dermatophytes. Extended incubation often enhances cleistothecium production.
Cephalotheca[b]	Colonies moderately fast growing, velvety to lanose, orange-gray with light brown reverse. Homothallic or self-fertile ascomycete forming black, superficial, ciliated cleistothecia and small, brown, kidney-shaped, foveolate (delicately pitted) ascospores (Fig. 2D); associated with a *Phialemonium*-like anamorph (Fig. 2E).	*C. foveolata*[b]	UV light and extended incubation enhance cleistothecium production.
Chaetomium[b]	Colonies fast growing, yellowish-green to gray. Anamorph absent or conidia formed from phialides. Perithecia bearing coiled, straight, branched brown, or indistinct setae. Ascospores lemon-shaped, brown, smooth.	*C. globosum*[b] *C. perlucidum*[b]	*Chaetomium perlucidum* grows at 42°C and is neurotropic. Extended incubation enhances perithecium production.
Gymnascella[b]	Colonies yellowish-white, becoming bright yellow or yellowish-green or orange (Fig. 1H and 2A). Ascospores borne in naked clusters, smooth, pale yellow. Anamorph absent. Ascospores of *G. hyalinospora* are oblate and yellowish (Fig. 2B); those of *G. dankaliensis* are reddish-orange and ornamented with a thickened polar band and minute thickenings on the sides.	*G. hyalinospora*[b] *G. dankaliensis*[b]	*Gymnascella hyalinospora*, also known as *Narasimhella hyalinospora*, may give false-positive results for *Blastomyces dermatitidis* with GenProbe DNA probe.
Microascus[b]	Colonies moderately fast growing, hyaline, or gray-brown to black. Perithecia with necks (Fig. 2C), containing yellowish to reddish orange (straw colored) ascospores extruded in cirri; associated with a hyaline or phaeoid *Scopulariopsis* anamorphs.	*M. cirrosus*[b] *M. cinereus*[b] *M. trigonosporus*[b] *M. gracilis*[b]	Ascospores in the first three species listed are heart-shaped, orange-section shaped, and triangular, respectively. Also see *Scopulariopsis*.
Scopulariopsis[b]	Colonies white, buff (gray-brown in *S. asperula*). Conidiogenous cells' annellides formed on branched conidiophores with 1 or 2 levels of branching. Conidia 1-celled, globose, or ellipsoidal, in chains. *Scopulariopsis brevicaulis* produces buff or tan granular colonies, thick-walled smooth to coarsely roughened conidia that are truncate at the base and rounded or pointed at the tip (Fig. 4F). *Scopulariopsis candida* produces white colonies and smooth conidia. *Scopulariopsis cordiae* produces heart-shaped ascospores.	*S. brevicaulis* *S. candida* *S. asperula* *S. cordiae*[b]	Also see *Microascus*.
Thermoascus[b]	Colonies yellow-orange to reddish-orange, woolly to granular. Thermophilic with growth to 50°C. Cleistothecia produced; ascospores pale yellow, elliptical, thick-walled, rough. Anamorphs are *Paecilomyces*-like. *Thermoascus taitungiacus* produces conidia that are initially rectangular, becoming elliptical to subglobose.	*T. crustaceus*[b] *T. taitungiacus*[b]	*T. taitungiacus* does not grow at 20°C and has irregularly verrucose ascospores. *T. crustaceus* produces finely echinulate ascospores.
Filamentous basidiomycetes			
Coprinellus, *Coprinopsis*	Colonies fast growing, white, amber to tan, woolly; cycloheximide sensitive, benomyl resistant. Conidiophores short, bearing short fertile branches. Arthroconidia schizolytic, thin-walled, 1-celled, often adherent around the conidiophores. Sclerotia sometimes present.	*Coprinellus domesticus* *Coprinopsis cinerea*	Differs from *Arthrographis kalrae* by cycloheximide sensitivity and rapid growth rate. Formerly reported under the names *Hormographiella verticillata* and *H. aspergillata*.
Oxyporus	Colonies moderately fast growing at 35°C but poor growth at 25°C; white and woolly. Conidia absent. Confirm with sequencing.	*O. corticola*	White-rot decay fungus of woody angiosperms and gymnosperms.

(Continued on next page)

TABLE 3 Key phenotypic features of selected hyaline molds *(Continued)*

Group and genus	Key features[a]	Etiologic agent(s)	Comments
Phanerochaete	Colonies fast growing, white to buff to beige, woolly. Conidiophores with profuse branching, each branch terminating with a conidium. Conidia ellipsoidal, truncate, thick walled, smooth. Large (20–60 μm) globose chlamydospores and arthroconidia also present.	*P. chrysosporium*	Large globose chlamydospores similar to those produced by *Emmonsia parva* can be seen in sputum. Former name: *Sporotrichum pruinosum*
Quambalaria	Colonies moderately fast growing, white to lavender, red diffusible pigment often present; cycloheximide sensitive. Conidiophores solitary, forming conidia sympodially on small denticles on sides or at tips. Primary conidia bear 1–3 secondary conidia.	*Q. cyanescens*	Synonyms include *Fugomyces cyanescens*, *Sporothrix cyanescens*, *Cerinosterus cyanescens*.
Schizophyllum	Colonies fast growing, growth enhanced at 37°C, white, woolly or cottony, cycloheximide sensitive. Usually sterile. Hyphae bearing clamp connections resemble aspergilli and short, thin pegs or spicules, but both may be absent (Fig. 2G). Clamped isolates usually develop fan-shaped, gilled basidiocarps (mushrooms) on sporulation media after 3–6 weeks (Fig. 2H).	*S. radiatum* *S. commune*	Clinical picture resembles aspergillosis and clampless isolates by histopathology (Fig. 2F).
Tropicoporus	Colonies fast growing, woolly, yellowish-orange; they are cycloheximide and benomyl resistant. Setal hyphae are thick walled, and hyphal swellings are present; conidia are absent (Fig. 3A). Identification should be confirmed with sequencing.	*T. tropicalis*	Synonyms include *Inonotus tropicalis* and *Phellinus tropicalis*; wood-destroying poroid basidiomycete.
Hyphomycetes			
Acremonium	Colonies slow growing (usually <3 cm in 10 days), often white, cottony, fasciculate (spiky), glabrous or moist and pink or salmon colored. Conidiogenous cells solitary, slender (ca. 2 μm wide), mostly unbranched, awl (needle-shaped) phialides. Conidia 1-celled, straight or curved, in slimy masses.	*A. sclerotigenum* *A. egyptiacum* *A. implicatum* *A. recifei* *A. persicinum* *A. fusidioides* *Acremonium* spp.	Differs from *Fusarium* by low growth rate, narrower hyphae (mostly <2 μm in width), and slenderer needle-like phialides. Compare with *Coniochaeta*, *Phialemonium*, *Brunneomyces*, and *Chordomyces*.
Acrophialophora	Colonies fast growing, white, darkening to grayish brown centrally. Conidiophores brown, long, seta-like, echinulate. Conidiogenous cells flask-shaped phialides borne near the tip of conidiophores or on vegetative hyphae. Conidia in long chains, 1-celled, lemon-shaped, smooth or rough; distinct spiral bands may be visible.	*A. fusispora* *A. levis*	Growth at 40°C. Potentially neurotropic. Compare with *Paecilomyces* spp. and *Lomentospora (Scedosporium) prolificans*.
Arthrographis	Colonies slow growing, growth enhanced at 37°C, initially white and yeast-like, becoming hyphal and buff with a yellow reverse. Cycloheximide tolerant. Conidiophores dendritic (tree-like), bearing lateral branches. Arthroconidia formed by fragmentation of branches or from undifferentiated hyphae.	*A. kalrae* *A. curvata* *A. longispora* *A. chlamydospora* *A. globosa*	Compare with *Onychocola*, *Scytalidium*, *Coprinellus*, *Coprinopsis*, and *Neoscytalidium*.
Brunneomyces	Colonies gray centrally, yellowish-white at periphery. Polyphialides commonly present. Conidia in long, dry chains. Hyphae become dark brown, verrucose, and thick-walled with age.	*B. hominis*	Morphologically similar to *Acremonium*. *Brunneomyces hominis* only species in the genus with growth at 35°C.
Beauveria	Colonies slow to moderately fast growing, yellowish-white. Conidiogenous cells solitary, in whorls, or in sporodochia, basally swollen, proliferating sympodially at the tip in a zigzag (geniculate) fashion. Conidia 1-celled, subglobose.	*B. bassiana*	Compare with *Parengyodontium album* and *Sporothrix*. *Beauveria bassiana* used for biological control of insects.
Chordomyces	Colonies white to cream, restricted, heaped growth on PDA. Prefers alkaline conditions. *C. albus* differs from *C. antarcticus* in that it does not produce synnemata in culture.	*C. albus* *C. antarcticus*	Morphologically similar to *Acremonium*; conidia in slimy heads.
Chrysosporium	Colonies slow to moderately fast growing, yellowish-white. Conidia 1-celled, smooth to roughened, aleurioconidia sessile or at the ends or on the sides of not swollen stalks (Fig. 3C). Arthroconidia sometimes present (see *Aphanoascus* and *Emmonsia*).	*C. zonatum*	Reports of infection by unnamed species are difficult to evaluate because isolates are not adequately described to confirm etiology.

(Continued on next page)

TABLE 3 Key phenotypic features of selected hyaline molds *(Continued)*

Group and genus	Key features[a]	Etiologic agent(s)	Comments
Coniochaeta	Colonies white to salmon, moist or fasciculate (spiky), or tan, darkening to black in patches. conidiogenous cells adelophialides (short, stumpy phialides without a basal septum), as well as awl-shaped phialides. *Coniochaeta mutabilis* forms brown chlamydospores, while *C. hoffmannii* does not.	*C. hoffmannii* *C. mutabilis*	Differs from *Acremonium* by predominance of adelo-phialides. Hyphal elements usually reported as hyaline. Also see chapter 127.
Cylindrocarpon	Colonies fast growing felty or cottony, yellowish-white, tan, orange or purple, sometimes with diffusing pigments. Conidiogenous cells awl-shaped phialides with a single opening, solitary, in branched structures or in sporodochia (conidiophores borne crowded in a compact mass of hyphae). Macroconidia straight or slightly curved with rounded ends, multicelled; microconidia not clearly distinguished from macroconidia. Chlamydospores sometimes present.	*C. destructans* *C. cyanescens*	Distinguished from *Fusarium* by production of macroconidia with rounded apical cells and absence of foot cells.
Metarhizium	Colonies moderately fast growing, becoming olivaceous green or buff. Conidiogenous cells cylindrical phialides borne on verticillately or irregularly branched conidiophores formed on sporodochia. Conidia cylindrical, smooth, yellowish-green, forming in adherent columns. Irregularly shaped appressoria may be present.	*M. anisopliae*	Biological control agent for insects
Myceliophthora	Mesophilic rather than thermophilic as for *Thermothelomyces thermophila*	*M. lutea*	Differs from *Chrysosporium* by swollen stalks; conidia smooth at maturity.
Myriodontium	Colonies moderately fast growing, yellowish-white, often zonate, powdery. Conidia formed at the ends of narrow stalks borne at right angles to the fertile hyphae.	*M. keratinophilum*	Differs from *Chrysosporium* by stalks borne at right angles.
Nannizziopsis	Colonies slow to moderately fast growing, yellowish-white. Conidia 1-celled, smooth to roughened, aleurioconidia sessile or at the ends or on the sides of unswollen stalks. Arthroconidia sometimes present.		Hosts as follows:
		N. arthrosporioides	Water dragon
		N. barbata	Coastal bearded dragon
		N. chlamydospora	Inland bearded dragon
		N. crocodili	Saltwater crocodile
		N. dermatitidis	Chameleons, geckos
		N. draconii	Inland bearded dragon,
		N. guarroi	Green iguana, inland bearded dragon, lizard, snake,
		N. hominis	Humans
		N. infrequens	Humans
		N. pluriseptata	Skink lizard
		N. vriesii	Lizard
Onychocola	Colonies restricted, raised, yellowish-white to grayish-white, cycloheximide tolerant (Fig. 3F). Conidia 1- or 2-celled cylindrical or swollen arthroconidia forming in adherent chains, detaching by schizolysis or lysis of thin-walled cells. Brown knobby setae often present (Fig. 3G).	*O. canadensis*	Differs from *Neoscytalidium dimidiatum* (see chapter 127), *Coprinellus*, and *Coprinopsis* by adherent chains, slow growth, and cycloheximide tolerance.
Ophidiomyces	Colonies slow to moderately fast growing, yellowish-white. Conidia 1-celled, smooth to roughened, aleurioconidia sessile or at the ends or on the sides of unswollen stalks. Arthroconidia sometimes present.	*O. ophiodiicola*	Emerging pathogen of captive and wild snakes
Paecilomyces	Section *Paecilomyces* includes the thermotolerant *P. variotii* and morphs of *Byssochlamys* and *Thermoascus* with fast-growing yellowish-brown, buff, or orange colonies (Fig. 3H). Phialides formed on verticillately branched condiophores. Conidia 1-celled, in chains.	*P. variotii* *P. formosus* *P. javanicus* *P. fumosoroseus*	*Thermoascus* species also produce a *Paecilomyces*-like anamorph
Parananannizziopsis	Colonies slow to moderately fast growing, yellowish-white. Conidia 1-celled, smooth to roughened, aleurioconidia sessile or at the ends or on the sides of unswollen stalks. Arthroconidia sometimes present.		Hosts as follows:
		P. australiensis	Northern tuatara, coastal bearded dragon, aquatic file snake
		P. californiensis	Tentacled snake
		P. crustacea	Tentacled snake
		P. longispora	Tentacled snake

(Continued on next page)

TABLE 3 Key phenotypic features of selected hyaline molds *(Continued)*

Group and genus	Key features[a]	Etiologic agent(s)	Comments
Parengyodontium	Colonies slow to moderately fast growing, yellowish-white. Conidiogenous cells solitary or borne in whorls, basally swollen, tapering at the tip and proliferating sympodially in a zigzag (geniculate) fashion. Conidia 1-celled, subglobose.	*P. album*	Compare with *Beauveria*. Formerly *Engyodontium album*.
Phialemonium	Colonies slow growing, white to grayish. Conidiogenous cells adelophialides, as well as awl-shaped phialides. *Phialemonium ovobatum* produces a green diffusible pigment.	*P. obovatum* *P. atrogriseum* *P. inflatum* *P. globosum*	Compare with *Acremonium* and *Coniochaeta*. Also see chapter 127.
Phialemoniopsis	Colonies slow growing, yellowish-white to grayish (Fig. 4C); conidiogenous cells adelophialides and awl-shaped phialides.	*P. curvata* *P. pluriloculosa* *P. cornearis* *P. ocularis*	Compare with *Phialemonium* and *Coniochaeta*.
Purpureocillium	Slower growth than for *Paecilomyces* spp., maximum growth temperature 25–33°C, conidia lilac-colored (Fig. 4A), chlamydospores absent (Fig. 4B).	*P. lilacinum*	Compare with *Paecilomyces* and *Rasamsonia*.
Rasamsonia	Colonies moderately fast growing with enhanced growth at 35°C. Cream to buff. Stipes and metulae rough. Cuneiform (wedge-shaped) to ellipsoidal conidia borne on rough-walled phialides lacking narrow necks as in *Penicillium* and *Paecilomyces* (Fig. 3D).	*R. argillacea*	Syn. *Penicillium argillaceum/Geosmithia argillacea*. Compare conidia with those of *Paecilomyces crustaceus*.
Sarocladium	Phylogenetically distinct from *Acremonium*. Several species form ochre-brown colors on SDA. Conidiogenous cells adelophialides or long slender phialides.	*S. kiliense* *S. strictum* *S. bacillisporum*	Compare with *Acremonium* and *Chordomyces*.
Thermothelomyces	Colonies fast growing, thermophilic (up to 50°C); cinnamon brown. One to three conidia formed on small denticles borne on the sides or at the ends of short, swollen stalks (Fig.3E). Conidia initially smooth and hyaline; brown and rough at maturity.	*T. thermophila*	Differs from *Chrysosporium* by swollen stalks. Formerly *Myceliophthora thermophila*.
Trichoderma	Colonies fast growing, cottony or woolly, white becoming yellowish-green to dark green, sometimes with a yellow diffusing pigment (Fig. 4G). Conidiogenous cells flask-shaped or cylindrical phialides, single or in whorls; conidia green, smooth, ellipsoidal to subglobose (Fig. 4H).	*T. longibrachiatum* *T. citrinoviride* *T. harzianum*	The *T. longibrachiatum* and *T. harzianum* clades both contain multiple species.
Coelomycetes			
Colletotrichum	Colonies fast growing, woolly, tan to gray-brown, occasionally greenish and sometimes with lavender shades, with honey-colored masses of conidia. Brown appressoria usually present; acervuli conidiomata, conidiogenous cells phialidic. Conidia hyaline, aseptate, straight to curved; also formed in aerial mycelium. Setae and sclerotia may be present.	C. gloeosporioides *C. coccodes* *C. dematium*	Colonies may be darker with better sporulation on potato carrot agar. Compare *C. dematium* with *Fusarium*. Resolution of crytic species in progress.
Phoma	Colonies pale to tan to gray-brown, woolly; pycnidial conidiomata, usually dark, separate or aggregated, ostioles single to several, immersed or semi-immersed, mostly thin walled. Conidiogenous cells phialidic, conidia 1-celled, small, hyaline, often guttulate.	Several species reported in the literature but most not well documented	Species-level identification difficult. Many taxonomic revisions have taken place and new genera added for closely related *Phoma*-like species. See references 212 and 214. See chapter 127 for additional coelomycetous genera.

[a]On PDA after 4 days of incubation at 25°C unless otherwise noted. See references cited in the text for a more detailed description of the features noted in this table; the list is not inclusive.

[b]Produces sexual reproductive structures in culture.

phylogenetic studies have shown that fusaria that were once considered individual species by morphologic features are now known to represent species complexes (SCs) (7, 8, 14–17, 38, 46, 47). Multilocus phylogenetic studies have revealed that the most frequently recovered clinically important fusaria are nested within the *Fusarium solani* SC (FSSC) (Fig. 1A). This SC comprises over 60 phylogenetically distinct species within three major clades, with the human and veterinary isolates being restricted to clade 3 (12, 48). Clade 3 was also shown to be associated with four major species-level lineages, designated groups 1 through 4, with many strains clustered in groups 1 and 2 (8, 17, 49). Subsequently, more robust typing studies identified 34 species within clade 3 of the FSSC (12). Because Latin binomials could not be applied to most of the species within this complex, species and multilocus haplotypes were distinguished by an *ad hoc* nomenclature using Arabic numbers and lowercase roman letters, respectively. The most important clinically relevant species within the FSSC are *F. petroliphilum* (FSSC 1), *F. keratoplasticum* (FSSC 2) (50), *F. falciforme* (FSSC 3+4), *F. solani sensu stricto* (FSSC 5) (51), *F. lichenicola* (FSSC 16), and *F. neocosmosporiellum* (FSSC 8, formerly *Neocosmospora vasinfecta*) (52). Although the *Fusarium oxysporum* SC (FOSC) is best known as an economically devastating group of vascular wilt pathogens on a wide range of agriculturally important plant hosts (53), it is also one of the more common *Fusarium* SCs responsible for human disease (Fig. 1B). The FOSC is also phylogenetically diverse (54). Multilocus sequence typing and amplified fragment length polymorphism analyses of over 100 isolates from the environment, hospital bronchoscopy, and water sources and clinical isolates revealed a geographically widespread clonal lineage comprising >70% of isolates genotyped (14). These studies have further supported hospital water distribution systems as a potential source of nosocomial infection (55, 56). Several medically important species are included within the species-rich *F. fujikuroi* SC (FFSC) as defined by multilocus genotyping (7, 9, 10). These include *F. verticillioides* (Fig. 1C), *F. proliferatum* (Fig. 1D), *F. napiforme*, and *F. nygamai*. Another morphologically and phylogenetically diverse group of fusaria includes those previously referred to as *F. semitectum* or *F. incarnatum*, which are nested within the *F. incarnatum-F. equiseti* SC (FIESC) (11). Multilocus phylogenetic studies have demonstrated that this complex encompasses at least 28 species (13), but Latin binomials could be applied to only three of them with confidence (*F. equiseti* = FIESC 14, *F. lacertarum* = FIESC 4, and *F. scirpi* = FIESC 9). For this reason, an *ad hoc* informal nomenclature was developed for all of the species within this complex. The *F. chlamydosporum* SC (FCSC) is also phylogenetically diverse and comprises at least four species based on multilocus genotyping (13). Similarly, the *Fusarium dimerum* SC (FDSC) (Fig. 1E and F) currently contains seven named and two unnamed species (57). Colonies produced by members of the FDSC are unlike those in the aforementioned SCs in that they frequently show slower growth, and aerial mycelium is either absent or only sparsely developed, so colonies appear mucoid to slimy (usually some shade of orange).

Description of the Agents

As can be seen from the taxonomic discussion, the *Fusarium* species cited as etiologic agents of human and animal disease mostly fall within six SCs. Based upon our current understanding of the genus, the most common species within these complexes are as follows: the FSSC includes *F. falciforme*, *F. petroliphilum*, *F. keratoplasticum*, *F. solani* (restricted to phylogenetic species FSSC 5); the FOSC includes *F. oxysporum* (phylogenetically diverse, but species limits are not currently resolved); and the FFSC includes *F. verticillioides*, *F. thapsinum*, and *F. proliferatum*. Fusaria within three other SCs are rarely encountered as mycotic agents. These include the FIESC, which includes mostly unnamed phylogenetic species usually reported incorrectly as *F. incarnatum*, *F. pallidoroseum*, or *F. semitectum*; the FDSC, which includes *F. dimerum* and *F. delphinoides*; and the FCSC, which includes *F.* cf. *chlamydosporum*. See also Table 2.

Epidemiology and Transmission

There are numerous toxic secondary metabolites produced by *Fusarium* species that have been implicated in human disease, especially associated with the consumption of contaminated grain (see chapter 129). Alimentary toxic aleukia was described in individuals who ate grain contaminated with trichothecene mycotoxins produced by *F. sporotrichioides* or *F. poae* (58). Besides orally ingested mycotoxins, systemic effects of exposure to inhaled mycotoxins have also been attributed to *Fusarium*, although these effects have been much less well characterized (59). The more common clinical presentation in human disease is associated with fusarial conidia gaining access to the host and germinating and subsequent tissue invasion by hyphae. The portal of entry, however, is unknown in most cases of invasive infection. Ingestion or access through mucosal membranes may occur in some (60, 61). Disseminated infection may also follow onychomycosis, often associated with cellulitis (62). Hospital water supply and distribution systems have also been implicated as a source of infection in immunocompromised patients by Anaissie et al. (55) and O'Donnell et al. (14). The most common mode of transmission, however, appears to be inhalation of airborne conidia (63).

Although invasive infection by *Fusarium* is uncommon, an increased incidence of disseminated infection has been reported in neutropenic patients with hematologic cancer, in recipients of solid-organ transplants, and in allogeneic hematopoietic stem cell transplant (HSCT) recipients (1, 41, 45, 61, 64–73). The incidence of fusariosis among allogeneic HSCT recipients varied between 4.21 and 5.0 cases per 1,000 in human leukocyte antigen-matched related transplant recipients and 20.19 cases per 1,000 in human leukocyte antigen-mismatched transplant recipients (72). Among allogeneic HSCT recipients, a trimodal distribution was observed: a first peak before engraftment, a second peak at a median of 62 days after transplantation, and a third peak >1 year after transplantation. The actuarial survival was 13% (median, 13 days), with persistent neutropenia (hazard ratio of 5.43) and use of corticosteroids (hazard ratio of 2.18) being the most important factors associated with poor outcome (69, 72).

Clinical Significance

Fusarium species can cause a spectrum of diseases in both healthy and immunocompromised hosts. A frequent infection in the healthy host is keratitis resulting from trauma and penetration of the cornea, contamination of soft contact lenses and/or solutions (11, 49, 70, 74–76), or local immunosuppression by corticosteroid drops (70). The keratitis outbreaks recognized in Hong Kong (76), Singapore (75), and the United States (49) in 2005 and 2006 in contact lens wearers using ReNu with MoistureLoc solution (Bausch & Lomb, Rochester, NY) resulted in the largest investigation and molecular characterization of fusarial keratitis isolates to date and clearly demonstrated that these strains occurred in nearly the full spectrum of clinically significant fusarial SCs. Other presentations in the immunocompetent host include those listed in Table 1. Cutaneous lesions in various stages of evolution (72, 77), fungemia (78), rhinocerebral involvement, pneumonia, endogenous endophthalmitis (79, 80), and combinations of these are common clinical findings in disseminated fusarial disease (41, 45, 61, 69–73, 81, 82). Unlike in invasive cases of aspergillosis, recovery of *Fusarium* species from the blood in disseminated disease approaches 60% (41, 71). Members of the FSSC are the most frequently cited agents of disease, and most cases involve keratitis (27, 83). Although multiple species within the FSSC have been reported as *F. solani*, this name should be applied only to the phylogenetic species FSSC 5 (51). Mayayo et al. (84) consider members of

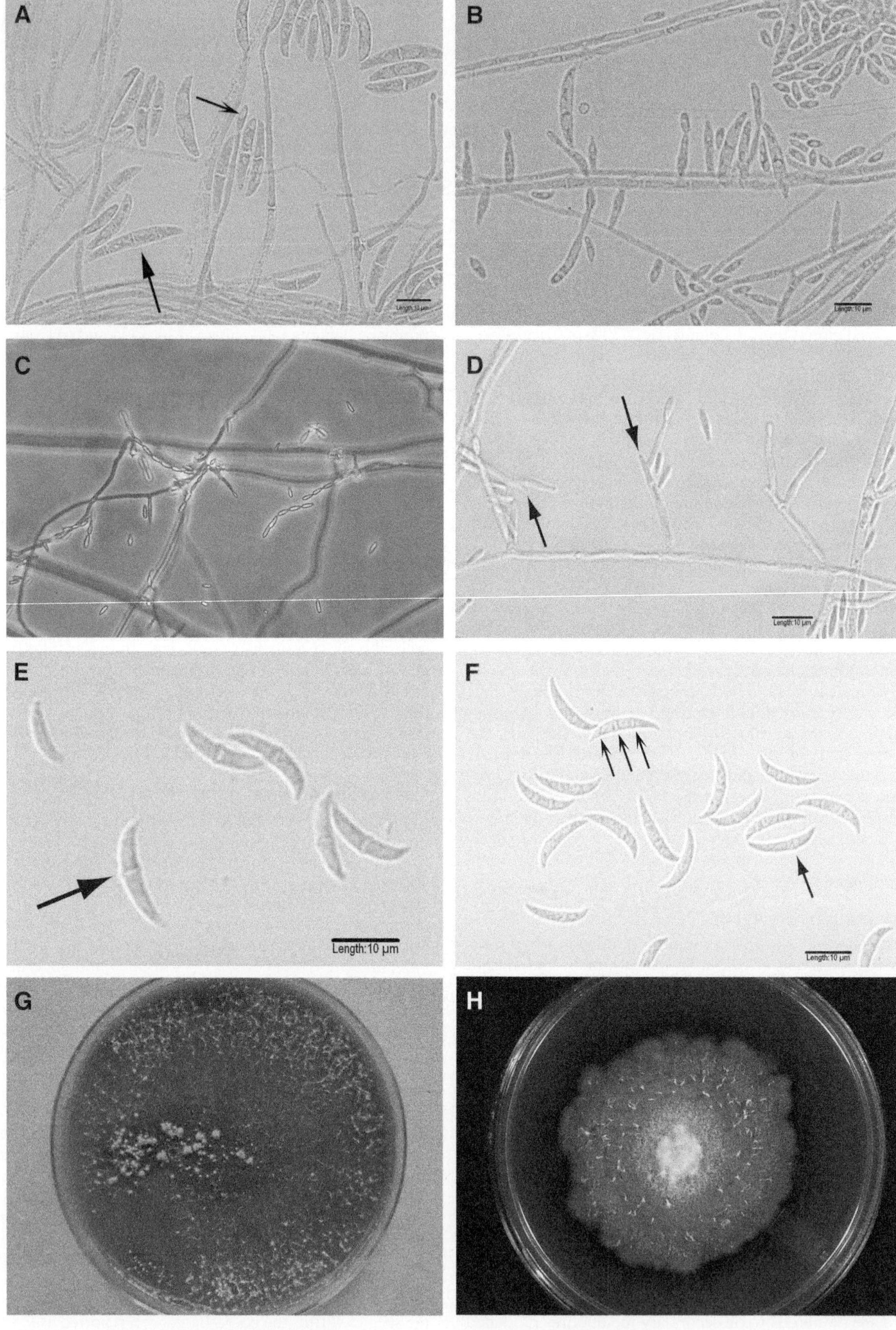
A
B
C
D
E
Length:10 µm
F
G
H

this SC to be the most virulent, and it has been suggested that their ability to produce cyclosporines may contribute to their pathogenicity (85). Members of the FOSC (14) and *F. verticillioides* (86) in the FFSC appear to be the next most common organisms recovered, with a similar spectrum of infection. *Fusarium verticillioides* was the most frequently isolated species in deep-seated infections in Italy (87). Because the name *F. moniliforme* was used for *F. verticillioides* and several other species within the FFSC, the identity of the etiological agent reported under the former name in the older clinical case reports can be verified only by DNA typing strains archived in culture collections. See references 27, 37, 57, and 87–89 for a more complete list of *Fusarium* species reported as etiologic agents in human and animal disease.

Collection, Transport, and Storage of Specimens

Methods of collection, transport, and storage of specimens are detailed in chapter 117. Like invasive aspergillosis, invasive *Fusarium* infections are difficult to diagnose and usually require a combination of clinical, cultural, and radiographic findings. However, unlike *Aspergillus*, *Fusarium* is more frequently recovered from blood, nails, and skin lesions of immunocompromised or immunosuppressed patients (60, 90). The recovery from a normally sterile site and microscopic evidence of invasive growth in tissue provide the most convincing evidence of invasive fusariosis.

Direct Examination

Microscopy

In direct examination of tissues, hyphae of *Fusarium* species resemble those of *Aspergillus*, *Paecilomyces*, or *Scedosporium* species in size (3 to 6 mm in width), septation, branching pattern, and predilection for vascular invasion. The hyphae are irregular in width and may show areas of collapse. Hyphae exhibit both dichotomous branching (i.e., branching at 45°), as is commonly seen in invasive aspergillosis, and branching at right angles (91, 92). Microconidia and, rarely, macroconidia and yeast-like polyblastic conidia, as well as phialides, may be found in blood vessel lumens or in aerated tissues (92). Immunohistological methods may help to distinguish between infections caused by some hyaline molds, but cross-reactivity is problematic, and serological tests are not in common use (93). Definitive diagnosis requires isolation and identification of the fungus, along with demonstration of fungal elements in tissue.

Antigen Detection

No commercial system is available for detection of genus-specific or species-specific antigens released by *Fusarium* species in human infection. The diagnostic utility of polyclonal fluorescent-antibody reagents to members of the FSSC in tissue sections from patients with invasive fusariosis was evaluated, but extensive cross-staining was observed with sections containing aspergilli, *Purpureocillium lilacinum*, and *Pseudallescheria boydii* (94).

In one study, 9 of 11 hematological patients with disseminated or deep-seated *Fusarium* infections had repeated serum-positive reactions with the Platelia *Aspergillus* galactomannan enzyme-linked immunosorbent assay (Bio-Rad, Marnes-La-Coquette, France) in the absence of *Aspergillus* spp. (95). Exoantigen extracted from *Fusarium* species including *F. oxysporum*, *F. proliferatum*, *F. falciforme*, and *F. verticillioides* produced positive reactions when tested undiluted by the galactomannan enzyme-linked immunosorbent assay *in vitro* (95), suggesting that *Fusarium* species may produce an exoantigen that is cross-reactive with the Platelia *Aspergillus* assay. Antigens prepared from *F. verticillioides* were also found to cause borderline cross-reactivity with the Platelia *Candida* antigen assay (Bio-Rad) (96). This reactivity appeared to be specific for *F. verticillioides*, since extracts prepared from members of the FSSC and FOSC showed no cross-reactivity *in vitro*.

Although (1→3)-β-D-glucan is not immunogenic, it is an important cell wall polysaccharide in most fungi that can be detected in serum via activation of a β-D-glucan-sensitive proteolytic coagulation cascade. Circulating (1→3)-β-D-glucan can be detected in the blood of patients with *Fusarium* fungemia and pneumonia (97, 98), although the presence of this marker is not specific for *Fusarium* (99). The sensitivity for detection of *Fusarium* infection was found to be 100% at a cutoff value of 60 pg/ml among three patients with invasive fusariosis (98). The clinical experience of (1→3)-β-D-glucan detection in patients with invasive fusariosis is limited, but the test is of value for patients with suspicion of invasive fungal infection as part of the diagnostic workup. In a mouse model, (1→3)-β-D-glucan remains high throughout the infection, suggesting that this marker may provide a specific and sensitive diagnostic tool for detecting invasive fusariosis (100). False-positive reactions of (1→3)-β-D-glucan are known to occur in some patients. These include subjects who had experienced renal failure and who were undergoing hemodialysis with cellulose membranes (101), subjects treated with certain immunoglobulin products (102), and specimens (or subjects) exposed to glucan-containing gauze or related materials (103). This underscores the need to combine (1→3)-β-D-glucan monitoring with clinical examination of the patient and other diagnostic procedures, such as high-resolution computed tomography scans, when making a diagnosis.

Nucleic Acid Detection

While most fusaria can be identified as members of this genus utilizing microscopic and macroscopic features, accurate identification of most isolates to the species level requires molecular data. However, with the exception of two Web-accessible databases dedicated to the identification of fusaria, only a very limited number of molecular

FIGURE 1 (A) A member of the FSSC. Microconidia are borne on long monophialides (thin arrow). Macroconidia borne in the aerial mycelium are also present (thick arrow). (B) A member of the FOSC bearing microconidia on short monophialides. A few macroconidia are also present. (C) Chains of microconidia produced by *Fusarium verticillioides* in the FFSC. (D) *Fusarium proliferatum* in the FFSC. Note polyphialides (arrows) with more than one conidiogenous locus per cell. Truncate conidia borne in chains and false heads are also present. (E) Two-celled macroconidia of *Fusarium dimerum* in the FDSC with a centrally located septum. (F) Macroconidia of *Fusarium delphinoides* in the FDSC. Note that the septum in two-celled conidia is off-center (thick arrow) and that a macroconidium with three septa (thin arrows) and four cells is also present. (G) Colony of *Achaetomium strumarium* showing yellowish surface mycelium and pink pigment on cornmeal agar after 5 weeks. (H) Glabrous and sterile colony of *Gymnascella hyalinospora* described in reference 142 when grown on PDA for 15 days at 30°C.

tools have been developed. In one study using PCR, *Fusarium* DNA was detected in tissues in a mouse model of disseminated fusariosis (104). In another study, a panfungal PCR was designed based on the 18S rRNA gene sequence and applied to ocular specimens from three patients with suspected bacterial or fungal endophthalmitis. Although *Fusarium* was detected in spiked specimens, no clinical samples from patients with *Fusarium* endophthalmitis were analyzed (105). PCR-based identification was also applied to *Fusarium* isolates obtained from patients with onychomycosis (106). Furthermore, *Fusarium* DNA was detected in patients' formalin-fixed paraffin-embedded tissue samples with histopathology results using real-time quantitative PCR assays (107). The *Fusarium* species identified were the same as those known to cause disseminated fusariosis in immunocompromised patients.

Panfungal PCR systems that detect a wide range of fungi, including *Fusarium*, have been developed. In one study, the PCR was positive with blood samples from a patient with invasive fusariosis, and blood cultures were positive for members of the FSSC (108). Luminex microbead hybridization technology using 75 genus-specific hybridization probes has recently been reported to detect a variety of fungal pathogens from blood and pulmonary samples, including *Fusarium* (109). As with other opportunistic fungi, molecular methods such as PCR appear to have promise for the detection and identification of fusaria causing infections; however, the value of these tools in the management of patients remains to be investigated.

Isolation Procedures

In general, *Fusarium* species can be recovered easily on routine mycological media without specific growth requirements. Given the aggressive nature of fusaria in neutropenic, immunocompromised individuals, however, the use of a medium for direct plating of specimens that can aid an early diagnosis by displaying consistent morphological features, such as potato dextrose agar (PDA), is highly recommended. Most *Fusarium* species grow rapidly on PDA in the absence of cycloheximide, which can be inhibitory. See chapter 117 for detailed information on specimen collection and processing.

Identification

For the limited number of *Fusarium* species that can be identified using phenotypic data, microscopic features of phialide shape, number conidiogenous loci on the conidiogenous cells (i.e., monophialides or polyphialides), formation of conidia in heads or chains, micro- and macroconidial shape and septation, presence and arrangement of chlamydospores, colony features (including growth rates and color of colony obverse and reverse [110]), and color of conidia en masse are important characters. However, considerable proficiency is required to identify *Fusarium* species with certainty, and a reference laboratory should be consulted. Although fusaria grow well on most mycological media, the medium can profoundly influence the colony topography, color, and conidium development. Synthetic nutrient agar, PDA, and tap water agar supplemented with either sterilized carnation leaves or potassium chloride are widely employed (45, 111). It is important to note that use of rich media such as PDA to maintain isolates can result in cultural degeneration. Alternatively, molecular tools are being developed to help identify clinical *Fusarium* isolates (37, 106, 112). With the wide application of matrix-assisted laser desorption ionization–time-of-flight mass spectrometry (MALDI-TOF MS) in clinical microbiology laboratories, this technique may allow the rapid and accurate genus- and species-level identification of *Fusarium* isolates (113, 114). A recently recommended biosafety level (BSL) classification for fusaria is either BSL1 or BSL2, depending upon the species (27). Clinical isolates should be handled in a biological safety cabinet.

Typing Systems

As for *Aspergillus* and *Candida*, multilocus DNA typing systems have been developed to differentiate clinically and veterinary important isolates of *Fusarium* (46, 47, 115, 116). Recently, the Clinical and Laboratory Standards Institute published a document for identification of bacteria and fungi by DNA target sequencing (117), and a consortium of international experts assembled as an ISHAM working group on fungal identification has provided clinical laboratories with initial recommendations for molecular typing of *Aspergillus*, *Fusarium*, and the Mucorales (118). These single-locus (internal transcribed spacer [ITS]) guidelines for placing fusaria within an SC are based upon knowledge gained from multilocus sequencing (ITS and large-subunit [LSU] ribosomal DNA, *TEF-1*, β-tubulin [β-*TUB*], calmodulin [CAM], and second largest subunit of RNA polymerase [*RPB2*]) analyzed by phylogenetic methods (8–14). These guidelines propose that if the ITS sequence yields >99% identity with a type or reference strain by comparative sequence analysis with GenBank/EMBL/DDBJ, then the isolate can be placed within one of the six SCs. DNA sequence data from some of the loci mentioned above are essential for identification of most clinically important fusaria to the species level (118). In addition to NCBI GenBank, which is a valuable resource but challenging to use, because many *Fusarium* sequences are misidentified (119), two dedicated websites are available for identifying fusaria via the Internet (37, 38).

Serologic Tests

Conventional serologic tests have been developed and used to measure exposure of specific patient populations to *Fusarium*, most commonly in the setting of occupational exposure or indoor dampness problems (120–122). In these populations, immunoglobulin G (IgG) directed against *Fusarium* can be detected. Elevated levels of IgE and IgG antibody directed against *F. oxysporum* were found in a patient with allergic bronchopulmonary mycosis due to this pathogen (123). Anti-*Fusarium* antibodies have not been evaluated as a diagnostic tool for patients with invasive fusariosis.

Antimicrobial Susceptibilities

The typical antifungal susceptibility profiles of *Fusarium* species indicate relative resistance to most antifungal agents (124). The MICs of amphotericin B and triazoles are elevated relative to those for *Aspergillus* species. *In vitro* studies show relatively high MICs of amphotericin B and itraconazole for members of the FSSC (MIC_{90}s, 4 and >8 μg/ml, respectively) and FOSC (MIC_{90}s, 1.0 and >8 μg/ml, respectively) (125). Universal *in vitro* resistance was found within clade 3 of the FSSC (126), and testing of this SC by the European Committee on Antimicrobial Susceptibility Testing method indicated a lack of activity by any agent tested (127). Voriconazole, posaconazole, itraconazole, and ravuconazole show variable to no *in vitro* activity against clinical isolates of *Fusarium* (128, 129). In one series, voriconazole was active against an unidentified member of the FSSC (reported as *F. solani*), *F. oxysporum*, *F. proliferatum*, and *F. verticillioides* (reported as *F. moniliforme*) (MIC_{90}, 2 μg/ml) but was not fungicidal against most isolates (130, 131). Although voriconazole and posaconazole exhibit only modest activity *in vitro* against isolates of *Fusarium*, both of these triazoles have been used successfully in some patients with amphotericin B-refractory fusariosis (132–134). The newest licensed triazole, isavuconazole, failed to show good *in vitro* activity against *Fusarium* species (135, 136). The echinocandins show no meaningful activity against *Fusarium in vitro* (137, 138); the *fks1* gene appears to confer intrinsic resistance to echinocandins in an unidentified member of the FSSC (139). *In vitro* testing of rarely encountered *Fusarium* species in the FFSC, FCSC, and FIESC showed that terbinafine was the most active agent except for a member of the FIESC (reported as *F. incarnatum*), against which amphotericin B was the most active agent (88, 140). In contrast, terbinafine showed high MIC_{90}s against members of the FSSC and FOSC (141). Synergy studies in a murine model with *F. oxysporum* showed prolonged survival and reduced fungal burden with a combination of amphotericin B and posaconazole (142); silver nitrate also exhibited *in vitro* activity against several fusaria from ocular infections (143).

Evaluation, Interpretation, and Reporting of Results

Early diagnosis of fusariosis is often key to appropriate management strategies, and the recovery of a *Fusarium* isolate should be reported to the clinician long before a final identification is made. With few exceptions, fusaria identified by phenotypic features and/or ITS ribosomal DNA sequence data should be reported as members of one of the SCs.

OTHER OPPORTUNISTIC HYALINE MOLDS

Taxonomy

Other opportunistic hyaline molds known to cause human or animal disease are distributed among numerous genera. A few are homothallic ascomycetes and filamentous basidiomycetes; however, the majority are conidial morphologies of the Ascomycota. Most are hyaline or only lightly pigmented; however, some, like *Acrophialophora*, become dark centrally. Others, such as *Phialemonium*, *Phialemoniopsis* (144), and *Coniochaeta* (formerly *Lecythophora*) (145), have been treated as agents of phaeohyphomycosis but are included here because they are frequently pale in culture. A few coelomycetous genera, such as *Colletotrichum* and *Phoma*, are also included. Unlike the hyphomycetes, which produce exposed conidiophores, coelomycetes produce conidia within semienclosed or enclosed structures known as acervuli or pycnidia, respectively. Infections caused by coelomycetes are typically acquired as a result of some type of implantation of the fungus following trauma rather than by inhalation (146, 147). While continued molecular characterization is placing many of these fungi within more appropriate phylogenetic classifications, Table 3 provides an overview of the fungi included in this chapter based on their phenotypic features. In keeping with the new International Code of Nomenclature for algae, fungi, and plants, in which dual nomenclature for pleomorphic fungi allowed under Article 59 was abandoned (148), only the most widely accepted anamorph or teleomorph name is used here (Table 3), even though making anamorph and teleomorph connections is still relevant (149).

Description of the Agents

Ascomycetes

Homothallic Ascomycetes

Homothallic, or self-fertile, ascomycetes that can reproduce sexually, in part because they possess both mating type idiomorphs (i.e., *MAT1-1* and *MAT1-2*), include genera that produce cleistothecia (ascomata without openings or ostioles), such as *Thermoascus*, *Aphanoascus*, and *Cephalotheca*, those that produce perithecia (ascomata with ostioles), such as *Achaetomium* (Fig. 1G), *Chaetomium*, *Microascus* (Fig. 2C), and *Scopulariopsis*, and species whose ascospores are borne in naked clusters, as in *Gymnascella*. *Thermoascus* species are nonostiolate, thermophilic ascomycetes with growth to 50°C. They produce pale yellow, elliptical, thick-walled ascospores and *Paecilomyces*-like morphologies. *Aphanoascus* is a keratinolytic ascomycete characterized by yellowish, lens-shaped reticulate ascospores and *Chrysosporium*- or *Malbranchea*-like morphologies. *Cephalotheca foveolata* is characterized by cleistothecial ascomata covered with yellow to brown hairs, foveolate ascospores that are delicately pitted or dimpled, as seen by scanning electron microscopy (Fig. 2D), and a *Phialemonium*-like morphology (Fig. 2E) (150). *Achaetomium* and *Chaetomium* produce brown lemon-shaped to fusiform ascospores within ascomata that are ornamented with hairs (or setae), especially around the upper part near the opening, with some species forming *Acremonium*- or *Humicola*-like morphologies. *Microascus*, *Scopulariopsis*, and related species produce yellowish to reddish orange, variously shaped ascospores extruded in long cirri (like toothpaste squeezed from a tube). Phenotypic identification of species in *Microascus* is based primarily on features of the perithecia, such as size and length of necks, and on ascospore shape. Recent molecular studies on *Scopulariopsis* and *Microascus* reveal that they are in separate lineages, with the former being mostly pale (with the exception of *S. asperula*) and the latter being dark. In addition, both genera contain perithecium-forming homothallic species (151–153). *Scopulariopsis brevicaulis* is the most common species in this annellidic genus (28, 152, 154) (see Fig. 4F). Members of the genus *Scopulariopsis* are common soil fungi that are noted for their deterioration of cellulosic substrates. Only a few species are reliably reported from human infections, and many have been moved to the genus *Microascus* based on molecular phylogenetic data (151–153).

Gymnascella species produce clusters of ascospores surrounded by yellow or orange filaments, but discrete ascomata are not formed (Fig. 1H and 2A and B). A case and reference isolate of this species both yielded false-positive results in the Gen-Probe test for *Blastomyces dermatitidis* (155).

Basidiomycetes

***Schizophyllum* and other genera**

Filamentous basidiomycetes are uncommon causes of human disease and are still poorly characterized. However, those that have been well documented are included in genera that may remain sterile in culture. A clinical isolate may be confirmed as a basidiomycete by the presence of clamp connections on the hyphae, but these diagnostic structures may be lacking. A nonsporulating hyaline mold may be suspected as a basidiomycete when the isolate is fast growing, displays growth on benomyl agar, grows at 37°C, and fails to grow on medium with cycloheximide (156). A positive urease test result may also suggest basidiomycetous affinities;

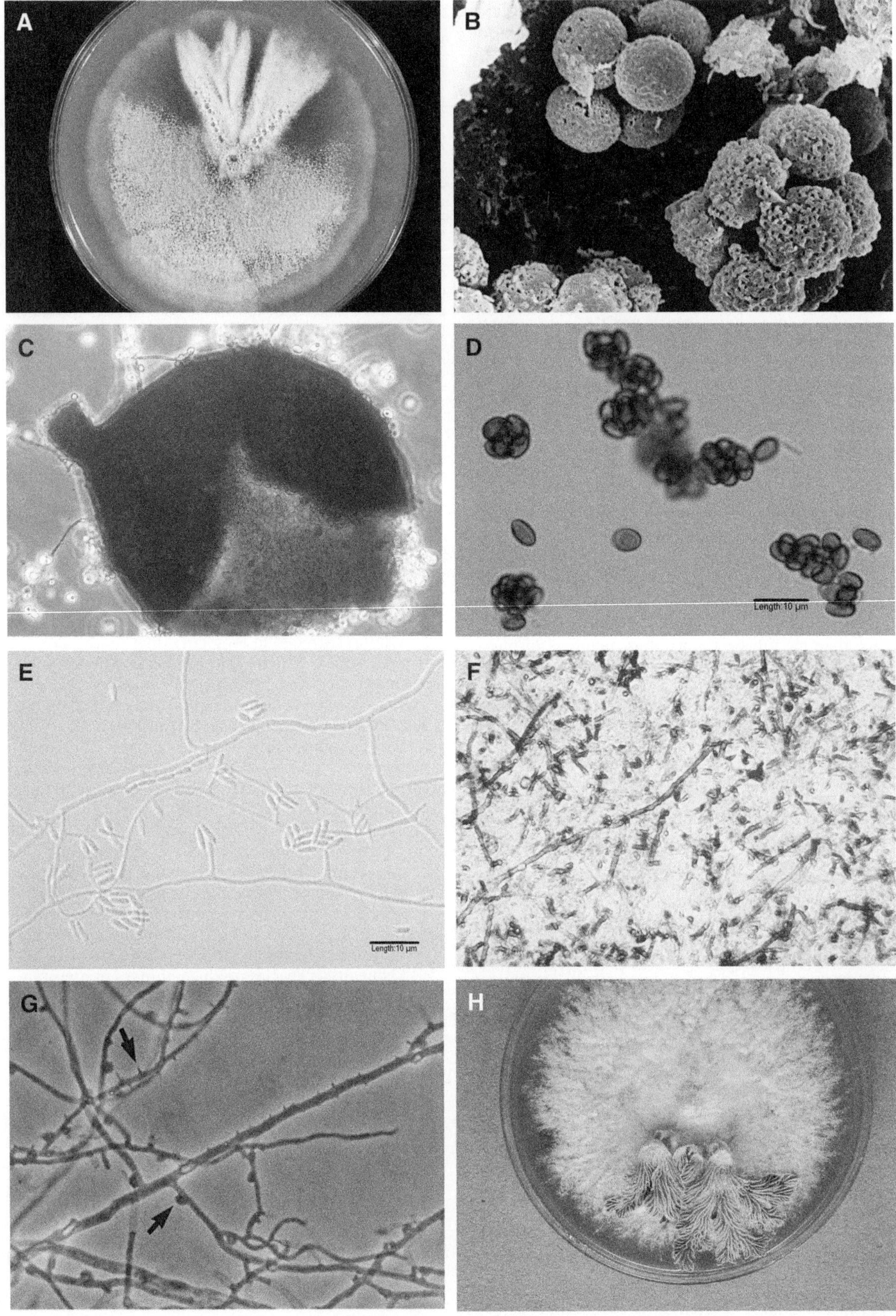
A
B
C
D
Length:10 µm
E
Length:10 µm
F
G
H

however, bacterial contamination should always be considered when positive results are being evaluated.

Schizophyllum commune has long been recognized as a significant cause of allergic sinusitis, allergic bronchopulmonary mycosis, and a related allergic disease and as an occasional cause of invasive infection in both immunocompetent and immunosuppressed patients (157). Recent molecular characterization of clinical isolates in the genus *Schizophyllum* has shown that the more common clinical species is *S. radiatum* rather than *S. commune* (158). In culture, isolates of either *S. radiatum* or *S. commune* may be dikaryotic, producing diagnostic spicules and clamp connections on the hyphae (Fig. 2G), as well as basidiocarps (mushrooms) when incubated under light (Fig. 2H). Other isolates are monokaryotic, remaining sterile, lacking clamps, and sometimes lacking spicules. When spicules are absent, hyphae of *Schizophyllum* spp. resemble those of *Aspergillus* species or other molds both in culture and in tissue (156, 159, 160) (Fig. 2F). Monokaryotic isolates are difficult to identify phenotypically, and molecular characterization is necessary for species confirmation (160, 161).

Other uncommon basidiomycetes causing disease in humans and other animals include *Tropicoporus tropicalis*, formerly *Inonotus tropicalis* (Fig. 3A) (162, 163), *Oxyporus corticola* (164), *Ceriporia lacerata* (165), *Irpex lacteus* (166), a *Perenniporia* sp. (167), *Volvariella volvacea* (168), *Coprinellus*/*Coprinopsis* (*Coprinus*) species with arthroconidium-forming *Hormographiella* morphs (169, 170), the *Sporothrix*-like *Quambalaria cyanescens* (171) (previously reported as *Sporothrix cyanescens* [161]), *Cerinosterus cyanescens* (172), and *Fugomyces cyanescens* (33). Another basidiomycete whose pathogenic potential remains to be determined is *Phanerochaete chrysosporium* (formerly *Sporotrichum pruinosum*) (173).

Hyphomycetes

Acremonium, Sarocladium, Coniochaeta, Phialemonium, and *Phialemoniopsis*

Fungi belonging to the genera *Acremonium*, *Sarocladium*, *Coniochaeta* (formerly *Lecythophora*), and *Phialemonium* form single-celled conidia in slimy masses or chains from long slender phialides or short, intercalary conidiogenous cells referred to as adelophialides; conidia are also formed from *Sporodochium*-like masses in *Phialemoniopsis*. The polyphyletic genus *Acremonium*, formerly called *Cephalosporium*, includes approximately 100 species associated with soil, insects, sewage, rhizospheres of plants, and other environmental substrates. Molecular data have provided evidence for restructuring of the genus along phylogenetic lines (27, 174, 175), and this is currently in progress. The most frequently encountered clinical species in the United States include *Acremonium kiliense* and the *A. sclerotigenum*-*A. egyptiacum* group (176). A more recent phylogenetic overview of *Acremonium* and related taxa has placed several clinical species in the genus *Sarocladium*, e.g., *Sarocladium kiliense*, *S. strictum*, and *S. bacillisporum* (177). The genera *Brunneomyces* and *Chordomyces* were also recently erected for several unnamed species formerly classified in the genus *Acremonium* (178). The genus *Lecythophora*, which contained two clinically significant species, *Lecythophora hoffmannii* and *L. mutabilis*, was transferred to the genus *Coniochaeta* based on the name's priority, and in keeping with the elimination of dual nomenclature after 1 January 2013. It now contains nine species, including *Coniochaeta hoffmannii* and *C. mutabilis* (145). Human etiologic agents in the genus *Phialemonium* previously included *Phialemonium obovatum* and *P. curvatum* (27). *P. obovatum* is retained in the genus, and new species added include *P. atrogriseum* (*Acremonium atrogriseum*), *P. inflatum* (*Paecilomyces inflatus*), *P. globosum*, and *P. limoniforme* (144, 179). However, species that produced *Sporodochium*-like morphs (species previously considered *P. curvatum*) were transferred to the genus *Phialemoniopsis*, which now includes *Phialemoniopsis curvata*, *P. pluriloculosa*, *P. cornearis*, *P. ocularis*, and *P. hongkongensis* (144). Three species of *Phialemonium* were formerly distinguished by conidial shape and colony color, including a green diffusing pigment in *P. obovatum* (180). However, based on PCR-restriction fragment length polymorphism banding patterns that indicated a close relationship between *P. curvatum* and *P. dimorphosporum*, the latter species was synonymized as *P. curvatum* (181). Subsequently, these species were transferred to *Phialemoniopsis* and are distinguished from other genera by the production of *Sporodochium*-like conidiomata. As many of the aforementioned genera are very similar morphologically, identification to the species level is very difficult without molecular data. Thus, many reports of infection are based on unidentified species (15, 175). The genus *Phaeoacremonium*, including *Phaeoacremonium parasiticum* and some other species associated with human infection, is distinguished from *Acremonium* by its brownish-pigmented hyphae and conidiophores (see chapter 127). The genera *Coniochaeta* and *Phialemonium* differ from *Acremonium* by their formation of short, stumpy phialides without basal septa (called adelophialides) in addition to the more spindle-shaped phialides (180), but these distinctions are not always readily observed. *Coniochaeta mutabilis* differs from *C. hoffmannii* in forming brown chlamydospores on sporulation media (145).

Arthrographis, Onychocola, Scytalidium and *Neoscytalidium*

The genera *Arthrographis*, *Onychocola*, *Scytalidium*, and *Neoscytalidium* are hyaline and/or dark arthroconidium-forming fungi. The thermotolerant *Arthrographis kalrae* is a rare opportunist recovered from skin, lung, corneal ulcer, and sinus (33, 182, 183). Because initial growth is often yeast-like, an isolate may not be recognized as a pleomorphic mold and thus may be incorrectly subjected to tests commonly used for yeast identification. Additional species include *A. curvata*, *A. longispora*, *A. chlamydospora*, and *A. globosa* (184). *Onychocola canadensis* (Fig. 3F and G) is a cycloheximide-tolerant hyphomycete. *Scytalidium cuboideum* (*Arthrographis cuboidea*), recently reported from respiratory specimens, including a lung mass and a nasal sinus,

FIGURE 2 (A) The isolate of *Gymnascella hyalinospora* shown in Fig. 1H turned yellow on oatmeal agar with clusters of ascospores after 15 days at 30°C. (B) Ascospores of *G. hyalinospora* observed by scanning electron microscopy. Magnification, ×6,000. (C) Perithecium of *Microascus*. (D) Brown ascospores of *Cephalotheca foveolata* formed after 8 weeks on carnation leaf agar at 25°C. (E) *C. foveolata* producing a *Phialemonium*-like morph consisting of adelophialides (reduced phialides without a septum) and ellipsoidal conidia. (F) Tissue section stained with Gomori methenamine silver stain showing monokaryotic (clampless) hyphae of *Schizophyllum commune*/*radiatum* in a pulmonary fungus ball. (G). *S. commune*/*radiatum* in a slide culture preparation showing clamp connections and narrow pegs or spicules (arrows). Magnification, ×580. (H) Dikaryotic culture of *S. commune*/*radiatum* showing development of gilled fruiting bodies on PDA after 7 weeks in the light.

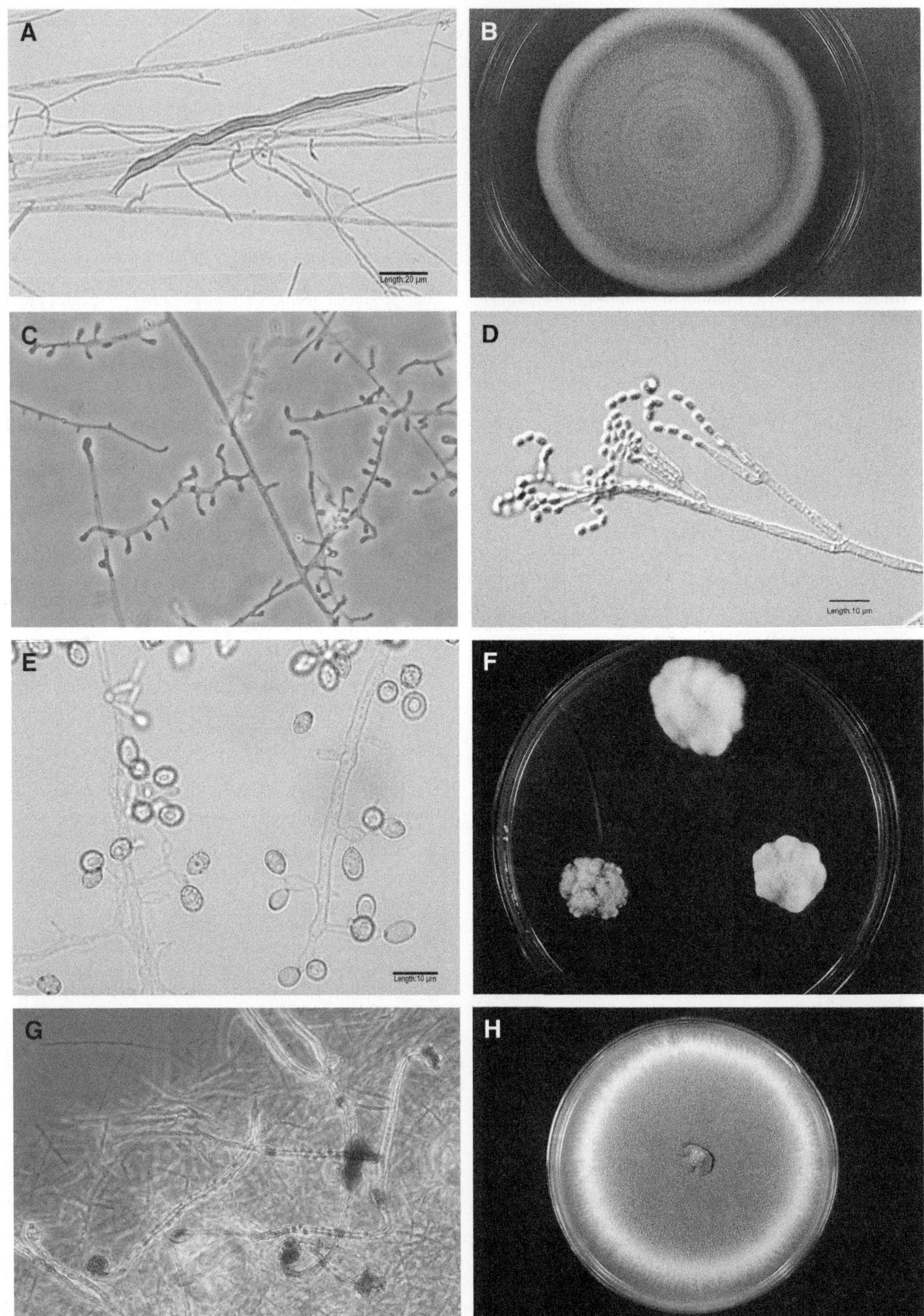

FIGURE 3 (A) Setal hyphae of *Tropicoporus tropicalis* produced on potato flakes agar after 10 days at 25°C. Bar, 20 μm. (B) Colony of *Chrysosporium zonatum* on PDA after 14 days at 37°C. (C) Conidia of *C. zonatum* formed on short curved stalks. (D) Rough-walled stipe, metulae, and phialides of *Rasamsonia argillacea*. Note that conidia are initially cuneiform (wedge-shaped). Bar, 10 μm. (E) Conidia of *Thermothelomyces thermophila* in varying stages of maturity. Mature conidia are dark and rough. Bar, 10 μm. (F) Culture of three different isolates of *Onychocola canadensis* after 5 weeks on Mycosel agar. (G). Setae (appendages) of *O. canadensis*. (H) Colony of *Paecilomyces variotii* on PDA after 7 days.

is differentiated from other species in the genus by orange colonies and its yellow cuboid arthroconidia. Although it is not known to cause disease, growth at 37°C suggests potential pathogenicity (185). *Neoscytalidium* (*Scytalidium*) *dimidiatum* includes the hyaline mold formerly known as *Scytalidium hyalinum* and so is also mentioned here (186).

Beauveria and *Parengyodontium*

Beauveria and *Parengyodontium* (formerly *Engyodontium*) species produce solitary conidia borne sympodially. The *Beauveria bassiana* SC comprises insect pathogens with limited virulence for humans (187). *Parengyodontium album* is closely related (27) and was segregated from the genus *Beauveria*. Recent molecular studies have shown that *Parengyodontium* (*Engyodontium*) *album* isolates form a monophyletic cluster and are separate from other *Engyodontium* species; thus the new genus designation (188).

Chrysosporium, *Myceliophthora*, *Thermothelomyces*, *Myriodontium*, *Nannizziopsis*, *Paranannizziopsis*, and *Ophidiomyces*

Members of the genera *Chrysosporium* (Fig. 3B and C), *Myceliophthora*, *Thermothelomyces*, *Myriodontium*, and *Nannizziopsis* (Fig. 3E) produce solitary, usually single-celled conidia that are called aleurioconidia because of the lytic method of conidium dehiscence (30). Members of these genera are related to the dermatophytes and the dimorphic pathogens, sharing with them a tolerance to cycloheximide and producing teleomorphs that are classified in the ascomycete order Onygenales (30, 32). *Myceliophthora* was separated into four genera, with the most common clinical species now being in *Thermothelomyces* as *Thermothelomyces thermophila* (formerly *M. thermophila*) (189). The recently described family within the Onygenales, Nannizziopsiaceae, contains the genera *Nannizziopsis*, *Paranannizziopsis*, and *Ophidiomyces* (formerly in *Chrysosporium*) (190, 191).

Metarhizium and *Trichoderma*

A multilocus phylogenetic analysis of the *Metarhizium anisopliae* complex, an insect pathogen of wide distribution, revealed that it comprises multiple species-level lineages (192). A taxonomic revision of the genus was made by Driver et al. in 2000 (193), and more recent generic and species boundaries were defined in keeping with "One Fungus/One Name" by Kepler et al. (194). Conidia are produced in chains that adhere together, in contrast to *Trichoderma* species, which form conidia in slimy heads. Morphological criteria for recognition of the *Trichoderma longibrachiatum* clade include (i) fast-growing yellowish green colonies on PDA; (ii) a strong yellow diffusing pigment present at 30°C but absent at 40°C; (iii) hyphae sparingly branched and forming phialides that are mostly solitary, longer, and more gradually tapered (cylindrical); and (iv) smooth oblong to ellipsoidal conidia (Fig. 4G and H). Intercalary phialides and chlamydospores are common. An oligonucleotide barcode program, *Trich*OKEY, was published in 2006 for sequence-based identification (195). Recent molecular studies have elucidated clinically relevant species (196), defined SCs (197), and provided a list of accepted *Trichoderma* names (198).

Paecilomyces, *Purpureocillium*, *Acrophialophora*, and *Rasamsonia*

The polyphyletic species of *Paecilomyces* occur worldwide as soil saprophytes, insect parasites, and agents of biodeterioration. Recent studies show that the medically significant species *Paecilomyces variotii* is actually a complex comprising five species, with *P. variotii* and *P. formosus* being the most important clinically (199). Their affinities are within the ascomycete family *Trichocomaceae*, which also includes *Penicillium*, *Talaromyces*, and *Aspergillus*. The genus *Thermoascus* (*Thermoascaceae*) also contains *Paecilomyces*-like morphologies. The colony (Fig. 3H) and morphological features of the *P. variotii* complex are described in Table 3. A similar species, *P. marquandii*, which produces a yellow diffusing pigment, cannot grow at 37°C and has not been documented as an agent of disease (200), was recently transferred to the genus *Metarhizium* (194). *Purpureocillium* is a new genus for the medically important *Paecilomyces lilacinus*, now placed within the family Ophiocordycipitaceae (201). Colonies are typically lilac, the growth rate is lower than that of *Paecilomyces* spp., the maximum growth temperature is 25 to 33°C, and chlamydospores are absent.

Acrophialophora is a thermotolerant and potentially neurotropic genus widespread in temperate to tropical regions. Colonies are initially pale but darken centrally at maturity. Also described under the name *Paecilomyces fusisporus*, *Acrophialophora* differs from *Paecilomyces* by producing unbranched, erect, brown, echinulate conidiophores that are fertile at the apex and anchored by a foot cell and basally swollen monophialidic or occasionally polyphialidic conidiogenous cells. Conidia are borne in chains, and distinct spiral bands may be present (202). The organism may superficially resemble *Lomentospora* (*Scedosporium*) *prolificans* (203, 204). Recent molecular studies have shown that the genus includes three species, *Acrophialophora fusispora*, *A. levis*, and *A. seudatica*, with *A. levis* being the most common clinically (205).

Rasamsonia is a new genus in the family *Trichocomaceae* that accommodates thermotolerant or thermophilic species segregated from *Geosmithia* (206). It is distinguished from *Penicillium* and *Talaromyces* species by roughened stipes, metulae, and phialides and by cuneiform to ellipsoidal conidia (Fig. 3D). *Rasamsonia argillacea*, under the name *Geosmithia argillacea*, caused a disseminated disease in a German shepherd dog (207) and is an emerging agent in cystic fibrosis patients (208) and those with chronic granulomatous disease (209). A recent phylogenetic study of the genus has differentiated this complex into six clinically important species (210).

Coelomycetous Fungi

Coelomycetous fungi are being documented as agents of disease more frequently, particularly in patients maintained on long-term immunosuppressive therapy. Infections are typically acquired through some type of direct implantation of the fungus, in contrast to inhalation as with the hyphomycetous genera. Two of the more common genera addressed here are *Colletotrichum* and *Phoma*; however, a review of the recent taxonomic revisions of many genera is beyond the scope of this chapter (211, 212). *Colletotrichum* species are acervular coelomycetes occasionally recovered as agents of disease. They produce fast-growing colonies of various shades that are most easily recognized in the laboratory by the production of brown, variably shaped appressoria. Honey-colored masses of conidia may be present in culture, as well as setae and sclerotia in some species. Cano et al. described the salient features seen in clinical strains (213). Studies are currently ongoing to resolve cryptic species (214). Species in the genus *Phoma* are pycnidial coelomycetes that may be pale or darker in culture. They are usually recognized by small dark pycnidia that form on the surface or are immersed in the agar. Boerema et al. published a *Phoma* identification manual (215); however, species differentiation is best handled in a reference laboratory.

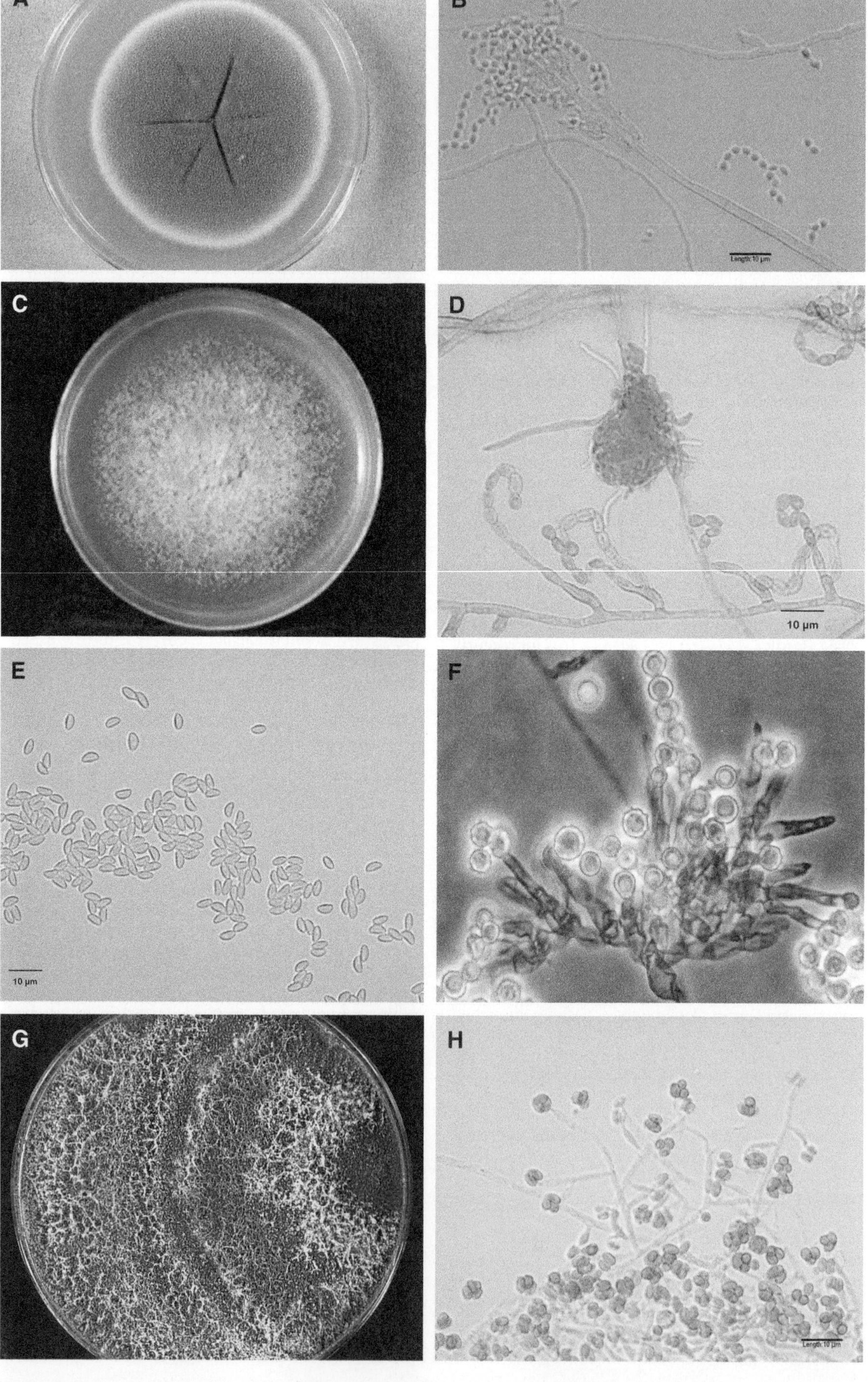
A
B
Length 10 µm
C
D
10 µm
E
10 µm
F
G
H
Length 10 µm

Two recent reviews of coelomycetous fungi seen in clinical laboratories cite several species documented to cause disease, give salient features for their phenotypic identification, and provide *in vitro* antifungal susceptibility data for selected genera and species (216, 217). Also, see chapter 127 for additional coelomycetous genera.

Epidemiology and Transmission

The methods of transmission and sources of infection for the other opportunistic hyaline molds are similar to those seen in aspergillosis and fusariosis, and acquisition is typically through inhalation or traumatic implantation. Coelomycetous fungi, although ubiquitous, are mostly reported from cases of keratitis and subcutaneous mycoses in immunocompromised individuals (218) and appear to be acquired primarily through external inoculation (146).

Clinical Significance

Ascomycetes

Homothallic Ascomycetes

Species of *Chaetomium*, *Amesia*, and *Achaetomium* (Fig. 1G) are neurotropic agents causing cerebral infections (42, 43, 219), while *Chaetomium globosum* occurs most commonly as a contaminant or as a rare agent of onychomycosis (6, 33). *Microascus* spp. are also agents of deep infections, including endocarditis (220) and a brain abscess (221) caused by *Microascus cinereus*, disseminated infections caused by *M. cirrosus*, and a fatal pneumonia caused by *M. trigonosporus* (222). *Scopulariopsis brevicaulis* (Fig. 4F) and other species are occasional agents of onychomycosis (30, 32, 154). They are also rarely invasive, causing otomycosis, keratitis, prosthetic valve endocarditis, sinusitis, pneumonia, brain abscess, and subcutaneous and bone invasion in immunocompetent and immunosuppressed individuals (27, 223–228). *Scopulariopsis candida* and *S. acremonium* have been reported from invasive sinusitis, but few details concerning the latter species were provided in the report (229, 230). Brain abscesses caused by *Fuscoannellis carbonaria*, *Microascus croci*, or *Microascus paisii*, all formerly known as *S. brumptii* (151), and invasive cutaneous infections caused by *Microascus cirrosus* have been reported to occur in liver transplant and bone marrow recipients (224, 231). A case of fatal *S. acremonium* was reported to occur in a lung transplant recipient (232). Numerous other species recovered from mostly respiratory specimens with growth at 37 to 40°C, though not substantiated as etiologic agents, are noted in recent publications (151–153). Additional rarely implicated genera include *Gymnascella* (Fig. 1H and 2A and B) and *Cephalotheca* (Fig. 2D and E). Please see references 27, 155, 220–222, 224, and 233.

Basidiomycetes

Schizophyllum and Other Genera

Filamentous basidiomycetes, as well as species of smuts that may appear yeast-like (Ustilaginaceae and Tilletiaceae), are commonly isolated from respiratory specimens and sometimes from blood; however, their significance can be difficult to evaluate (156, 234).

Schizophyllum radiatum is recognized as a significant cause of allergy-related sinusitis and pulmonary disease, including allergic bronchopulmonary mycosis and bronchial mucoid impaction (156, 159, 160, 235–238), as well as infections of the brain, lungs, and buccal mucosa in both immunocompetent and immunosuppressed patients (33, 156, 237, 239, 240). *Coprinus cinereus* has been reported under its anamorph name, *Hormographiella aspergillata*, from prosthetic valve endocarditis, fatal lung infections in leukemic patients, a lung abscess in a patient with non-Hodgkin's lymphoma, keratomycosis in a dog, and cutaneous lesions (33, 169, 170, 241, 242). *Tropicoporus tropicalis*, formerly *Inonotus tropicalis*, was reported as an agent of osteomyelitis in a patient with X-linked chronic granulomatous disease (162, 163) and has also been detected in an additional patient with this disease (D. Sutton, unpublished data). *Ceriporia lacerata* was reported in four cases from pulmonary sites (165), *Irpex lacteus* was recovered from a pulmonary abscess in an immunosuppressed child (166), a *Perennipora* sp. was the etiologic agent in a pulmonary fungal ball (167), and *Volvariella volvacea* incited invasive disease and death in a Hodgkin's lymphoma patient (168). The *Sporothrix*-like organism *Quambalaria cyanescens* was reported in an augmentation mammoplasty (243). See reference 157 for a recent review of basidiomycetous fungi and human disease.

Hyphomycetes

Acremonium, *Sarocladium*, *Coniochaeta*, *Phialemonium*, and *Phialemoniopsis*

Many reports concerning *Acremonium* involve infections of the nail, skin, eye, or mycetoma (see also chapter 128) (27, 30); however, many of these species are now classified in other genera. Localized and disseminated infections have been reported to occur in patients following valve replacement, dialysis, or transplantation or in patients with hematologic or solid organ malignancies (6, 15, 27, 175, 244, 245). Fungemia is common. Several cases of invasive disease caused by *Sarocladium* (*Acremonium*) *strictum* have been reported (246–248). *C. mutabilis* was reported to cause prosthetic valve endocarditis in a diabetic patient (249), and *C. hoffmannii* was reported to cause chronic sinusitis in an HIV-infected patient (250). *Phialemonium obovatum* was an agent of endocarditis (251), *P. hongkongensis* a subcutaneous nodule in a patient with underlying liver cirrhosis (252), while arthritis, fungemia, endovascular infections, and ophthalmitis have been reported for *Phialemoniopsis curvata* (*Phialemonium curvatum*) (181, 253–255).

Arthrographis, *Onychocola*, *Scytalidium*, and *Neoscytalidium*

The thermotolerant species *Arthrographis kalrae* is a rare opportunist recovered from skin, lung, corneal ulcer, and sinus (33, 182, 183). *Onychocola canadensis* (Fig. 3F and G) causes distal subungual onychomycosis or, less commonly,

FIGURE 4 (A) Colony of *Purpureocillium lilacinum* on PDA after 14 days. (B) Verticillate conidiophores of *P. lilacinum* bearing whorls of phialides. Bar, 10 μm. (C) Yellowish colony of *Phialemoniopsis curvata* on potato flakes agar after 14 days at 25°C. (D) *Microascus gracilis* showing asexual morph and an immature perithecium after 10 days on PDA at 25°C. (E) Ascospores of *M. gracilis* that developed on PDA after 18 days at 25°C. Bar, 10 μm. (F) Rough-walled conidia in chains formed on annellides of *Scopulariopsis brevicaulis*. Note branched conidiogenous cells. Magnification, ×580. (G) Colony of *Trichoderma longibrachiatum* on PDA after 4 days at 37°C. (H) Green, oval conidia of *T. longibrachiatum*. Bar, 10 μm.

white superficial onychomycosis and infection of the glabrous skin (30, 32, 256, 257). Although *O. canadensis* is a relatively uncommon agent of onychomycosis, more than 60 isolates from nails have been recorded from New Zealand, Australia, Europe, and the United States, with two additional cases from Spain (258). The growth of *Scytalidium cuboideum* at 37°C suggests its pathogenic potential (185).

Beauveria and *Parengyodontium*

Beauveria bassiana has caused several cases of fungal keratitis (259, 260). A recent molecular study comparing clinical keratitis isolates with Environmental Protection Agency-registered strains showed that these strains were unrelated (261, 262). An isolate that failed to grow at 35°C also caused disseminated disease in a patient with acute lymphoblastic leukemia (39). *Parengyodontium album* was the cause of two cases of endocarditis (263), one of which occurred in a bovine valve replacement (188).

Chrysosporium, *Myceliophthora*, *Thermothelomyces*, *Myriodontium*, *Nannizziopsis*, *Paranannizziopsis*, and *Ophidiomyces*

The thermotolerant species *Chrysosporium zonatum* is an etiologic agent of human pneumonia and osteomyelitis (264) (Fig. 3B and C). In a review of human infections caused by *Emmonsia* and *Chrysosporium*, it was reported that those caused by *Chrysosporium* typically occur in immunocompromised individuals (265). The thermophilic species *Thermothelomyces* (*Myceliophthora*) *thermophila* (Fig. 3E) (189) has been reported to cause fatal aortic vasculitis in two patients. It was isolated from the brain of a patient who developed a bacterial cerebral abscess after trauma and severe osteomyelitis following a pitchfork injury (266–269). The *Chrysosporium* anamorph of the *Nannizziopsis vriesii* complex, also known as CANV and *C. ophiodiicola* (240), has been transferred to *Nannizziopsis*, *Paranannizziopsis*, and *Ophidiomyces*. *Nannizziopsis hominis* appears to be the only human-associated species (270).

Metarhizium and *Trichoderma* species

The *Metarhizium anisopliae* complex contains multiple phylogenetically distinct species that are widely distributed insect pathogens. They are also documented to cause keratitis, sinusitis, invasive infections, and disseminated skin lesions (271–274). Species of *Trichoderma* in the section *Longibrachiatum*, which includes *Trichoderma longibrachiatum* (Fig. 4G and H) and *T. citrinoviride*, appear to be the most important pathogenic species (275–278). A recent review of 73 clinical isolates has advanced our understanding of species recovered in a clinical setting, including the new species *T. bissettii* (196).

Paecilomyces, *Purpureocillium*, *Acrophialophora*, and *Rasamsonia*

Mycoses caused by *Paecilomyces variotii* and *Purpureocillium lilacinum* include cutaneous and subcutaneous infections, pulmonary infection, pyelonephritis, sinusitis, cellulitis, endocarditis, and fungemia in both immunocompetent and immunocompromised patients (6, 15, 27, 279–281). The clinical manifestations, treatment options, and outcomes for *P. lilacinum* infections have been reviewed (282, 283). The species has also been noted to reside in water distribution systems, including those of a bone marrow transplant unit (201). The genus *Acrophialophora* has been responsible for cases of keratitis (255), pulmonary infections (255, 256), as a colonizer in patients with cystic fibrosis (257, 258), and a brain abscess in a child with leukemia (202). A recent molecular reevaluation confirms that the genus includes three species: *Acrophialophora fusispora* (conspecific with *A. naniana* and *Masoniella indica*), *A. levis*, and *A. seudatica* (*Ampullifera seudatica*), with *A. levis* being the most common clinically (205). *Rasamsonia argillacea* (formerly *Geosmithia argillacea*) has been described as an emerging cause of invasive fungal infection in human chronic granulomatous disease (209, 284) and has also been reported to cause a pulmonary and aortic graft infection in an immunocompetent patient (285). It is now considered an SC comprising *R. argillacea sensu stricto*, *R. piperina*, *R. aegroticola*, and *R. eburnea* (210), with *R. aegroticola* being the most common species to colonize airways of cystic fibrosis patients (286).

Coelomycetous Fungi

Colletotrichum species are primarily phytopathogens but occasionally are recovered as agents of keratitis (27). There are also rare reports of subcutaneous infection following trauma (218). A case of phaeohyphomycotic cysts caused by *Phoma* species was reported (287). Numerous other genera are being recovered from clinical specimens, and reviews of these from the United States (217) and France (216) have been reported.

Collection, Transport, and Storage of Specimens

Methods of collection, transport, and storage of specimens are detailed in chapter 117. As with other invasive mycoses, infections are difficult to diagnose and usually require a combination of clinical, culture, and radiographic findings. The recovery from a normally sterile site and microscopic evidence of invasive growth in tissue provide the most convincing evidence of disease.

Direct Examination

Microscopy

Histopathological findings for most opportunistic hyaline molds, including species of *Aspergillus*, *Fusarium*, and *Pseudallescheria*, are typically indistinguishable (93, 227). Ascospores may occasionally be observed, as was demonstrated with *Gymnascella* (155), and clamp connections may also be present in tissue sections with *Schizophyllum commune* (239). Budding forms are rarely observed (92, 244, 245).

Antigen Detection

Detection of (1→3)-β-D-glucan (97, 99) in patients with invasive hyalohyphomycosis may assist with an early diagnosis, but monitoring of this marker needs to be combined with clinical examination of the patient and other diagnostic procedures, such as high-resolution computed tomography scanning.

Nucleic Acid Detection

Nucleic acid detection has the potential to detect a variety of hyaline molds directly in clinical samples, but its application in clinical diagnosis is still limited. Luminex microbead hybridization technology has been reported to detect a variety of fungal pathogens from clinical blood and pulmonary samples (109). This method appears to have promise for the early detection and identification of various invasive fungal pathogens.

Isolation Procedures

Opportunistic hyaline molds are usually cultured easily on routine mycological media, and there are no specific growth requirements; however, media with and without cycloheximide should be employed. The fungicide benomyl at a final concentration of 10 mg/ml in the culture medium has shown utility in distinguishing filamentous basidiomycetes, which are tolerant to benomyl, from ascomycetes, which may be sensitive to this fungicide (288). Coelomycetous fungi grow well on most fungal media; however, they are notorious for remaining sterile without extended incubation (up to several weeks for some genera) (146). See chapters 117 and 118 for detailed information on appropriate media for initial plating and isolation.

Identification

More detailed descriptions of these hyaline fungi are found in several identification manuals and in the references cited therein (26–35). Many can be identified to the genus level with little difficulty; however, identification of most clinically relevant molds to the species level requires DNA sequence data. Furthermore, MALDI-TOF MS has the potential to speed up the genus- and species-level identification (113). See Table 3 for salient phenotypic features of the organisms reviewed. The use of DNA sequence data to identify isolates that remain sterile in culture is largely dependent on the accuracy of and interpretation of data in publicly accessible databases such as NCBI GenBank (https://www.ncbi.nlm.nih.gov/genbank/), Westerdijk Fungal Biodiversity Institute (formerly CBS; http://www.westerdijkinstitute.nl/), and ISHAM database (http://its.mycologylab.org/). The validity of this approach was demonstrated by DNA sequence-based identification of several nonsporulating molds (289); this approach will continue to be used more widely.

Typing Systems

Although comparative sequence analysis of clinical isolates is becoming more common in large tertiary-care and research centers, it is far from standardized. Various methods of DNA extraction are available (290), and several different genes or portions thereof may be sequenced (8–14, 17, 57, 117, 118, 291, 292). It should be highlighted, however, that numerous database entries in public databases are incorrect, making comparative sequence analysis without phenotypic correlation a challenge that requires that the top sequence matches be examined critically (118). On the other hand, molecular characterization has become the gold standard for classification of species for taxonomic categorization and will continue to provide a better understanding of the evolutionary relationships of clinically significant fungi (8–14, 57, 293). Furthermore, whole-genome sequencing technology could become a new standard for fungal genome typing as demonstrated in a recent study determining the source of a multinational outbreak of bloodstream infections caused by the fungus *Sarocladium kiliense* (294).

Serologic Tests

Serologic procedures currently have little clinical utility in the diagnosis of uncommon hyaline opportunistic fungi.

Antimicrobial Susceptibilities

Uncommon hyaline molds display various antifungal susceptibility patterns. Susceptibility testing of uncommon molds is useful for empirical antifungal therapy; however, isolates should be assessed individually for appropriate patient management. For published *in vitro* data, see references relating to the genera of interest. *Chaetomium* infections that failed to respond to treatment with amphotericin B alone or in combination with itraconazole have been reported (295). However, voriconazole and the experimental triazoles ravuconazole and albaconazole showed potent activity *in vitro* against *Chaetomium* spp., with MICs less than 0.5 μg/ml (295); however, the echinocandin micafungin was not active *in vitro*. Evaluation of antifungal activity against 44 clinical isolates of filamentous basidiomycetous fungi, including *Schizophyllum commune* ($n = 5$), *Coprinus* spp. ($n = 8$), *Bjerkandera adusta* ($n = 14$), and sterile, uncharacterized basidiomycetes ($n = 17$), demonstrated low MICs of amphotericin B, itraconazole, voriconazole, and posaconazole, in contrast to those of fluconazole and flucytosine (296). No statistically significant differences among the genera were noted.

Antifungals, including amphotericin B and itraconazole, have limited *in vitro* activity against *Scopulariopsis* spp., and conflicting results have been reported for voriconazole and terbinafine (141, 297). A promising interaction was observed between terbinafine and fluconazole, itraconazole, and voriconazole *in vitro* against isolates of *S. brevicaulis*, although clinical experience with combination therapy is very limited (298). When *Paecilomyces* species were evaluated by the European Committee on Antimicrobial Susceptibility Testing method (127, 299), amphotericin B, itraconazole, and the echinocandins showed poor activity against 27 strains of *P. lilacinum*; however, the newer triazoles voriconazole, ravuconazole, and posaconazole and the allylamine terbinafine showed low MIC_{90}s. In contrast, low MICs of all of the agents listed above, except for voriconazole and ravuconazole, were obtained for 31 strains of *P. variotii* (300). There are very limited data on *in vitro* activity of isavuconazole against uncommon hyaline molds. In one study, no activity and very limited activity were observed against *S. kiliense* and *P. lilacinum*, respectively (301).

Evaluation, Interpretation, and Reporting of Results

The early diagnosis of invasive hyalohyphomycosis caused by fusaria and other hyaline molds is often key to appropriate management strategies. Identification of uncommon hyaline molds should always be evaluated in light of the patient's immune status as well as the anatomic site of recovery and frequency of isolation.

We thank Lynne Sigler, University of Alberta Microfungus Collection & Herbarium, Devonian Botanic Garden, Edmonton, Alberta, Canada, for her helpful comments and review of this section.

The mention of firm names or trade products does not imply that they are endorsed or recommended by the U.S. Department of Agriculture over other firms or similar products not mentioned. The USDA is an equal opportunity provider and employer.

This chapter is dedicated to Deanna A. Sutton (deceased 4 July 2017) for her kindness and devotion and for her strong spirit of collegial collaboration; her numerous contributions to the field of diagnostic clinical mycology will always be remembered.

REFERENCES

1. **Nir-Paz R, Strahilevitz J, Shapiro M, Keller N, Goldschmied-Reouven A, Yarden O, Block C, Polacheck I.** 2004. Clinical and epidemiological aspects of infections caused by *Fusarium* species: a collaborative study from Israel. *J Clin Microbiol* **42:**3456–3461.
2. **Ajello L.** 1986. Hyalohyphomycosis and phaeohyphomycosis: two global disease entities of public health importance. *Eur J Epidemiol* **2:**243–251.

3. **Tan DH, Sigler L, Gibas CF, Fong IW.** 2008. Disseminated fungal infection in a renal transplant recipient involving *Macrophomina phaseolina* and *Scytalidium dimidiatum*: case report and review of taxonomic changes among medically important members of the Botryosphaeriaceae. *Med Mycol* **46:**285–292.
4. **Kantarcioglu AS, Summerbell RC, Sutton DA, Yücell A, Sarikaya E, Kaner G, Iscimen A, Altas K.** 2010. A dark strain in the *Fusarium solani* species complex isolated from primary subcutaneous sporotrichioid lesions associated with traumatic inoculation via a rose bush thorn. *Med Mycol* **48:**103–109.
5. **Odds FC, Arai T, Disalvo AF, Evans EG, Hay RJ, Randhawa HS, Rinaldi MG, Walsh TJ.** 1992. Nomenclature of fungal diseases: a report and recommendations from a subcommittee of the International Society for Human and Animal Mycology (ISHAM). *J Med Vet Mycol* **30:**1–10.
6. **Zhang SX, O'Donnell K, Sutton DA.** 2015. *Fusarium* and other opportunistic hyaline fungi, p 2057–2086. *In* Jorgensen JH, Pfaller MA, Carroll KC, Funke G, Landry ML, Richter SS, Warnock DW (ed), *Manual of Clinical Microbiology*, 11th ed. ASM Press, Washington, DC.
7. **Nirenberg HI, O'Donnell K.** 1998. New *Fusarium* species and combinations within the *Gibberella fujikuroi* species complex. *Mycologia* **90:**434–458.
8. **O'Donnell K.** 2000. Molecular phylogeny of the *Nectria haematococca-Fusarium solani* species complex. *Mycologia* **92:**919–938.
9. **O'Donnell K, Cigelnik E, Nirenberg HI.** 1998. Molecular systematics and phylogeography of the *Gibberella fujikuroi* species complex. *Mycologia* **90:**465–493.
10. **O'Donnell K, Nirenberg HI, Aoki T, Cigelnik E.** 2000. A multigene phylogeny of the *Gibberella fujikuroi* species complex: detection of additional phylogenetically distinct species. *Mycoscience* **41:**61–78.
11. **O'Donnell K, Sarver BA, Brandt M, Chang DC, Noble-Wang J, Park BJ, Sutton DA, Benjamin L, Lindsley M, Padhye A, Geiser DM, Ward TJ.** 2007. Phylogenetic diversity and microsphere array-based genotyping of human pathogenic fusaria, including isolates from the multistate contact lens-associated U.S. keratitis outbreaks of 2005 and 2006. *J Clin Microbiol* **45:**2235–2248.
12. **O'Donnell K, Sutton DA, Fothergill A, McCarthy D, Rinaldi MG, Brandt ME, Zhang N, Geiser DM.** 2008. Molecular phylogenetic diversity, multilocus haplotype nomenclature, and in vitro antifungal resistance within the *Fusarium solani* species complex. *J Clin Microbiol* **46:**2477–2490.
13. **O'Donnell K, Sutton DA, Rinaldi MG, Gueidan C, Crous PW, Geiser DM.** 2009. Novel multilocus sequence typing scheme reveals high genetic diversity of human pathogenic members of the *Fusarium incarnatum-F. equiseti* and *F. chlamydosporum* species complexes within the United States. *J Clin Microbiol* **47:**3851–3861.
14. **O'Donnell K, Sutton DA, Rinaldi MG, Magnon KC, Cox PA, Revankar SG, Sanche S, Geiser DM, Juba JH, van Burik JA, Padhye A, Anaissie EJ, Francesconi A, Walsh TJ, Robinson JS.** 2004. Genetic diversity of human pathogenic members of the *Fusarium oxysporum* complex inferred from multilocus DNA sequence data and amplified fragment length polymorphism analyses: evidence for the recent dispersion of a geographically widespread clonal lineage and nosocomial origin. *J Clin Microbiol* **42:**5109–5120.
15. **Summerbell RC.** 2003. *Aspergillus, Fusarium, Sporothrix, Piedraia*, and their relatives, p 237–498. *In* Howard DH (ed), *Fungi Pathogenic for Humans and Animals*, 2nd ed. Marcel Dekker, Inc, New York, NY.
16. **Summerbell RC, Schroers HJ.** 2002. Analysis of phylogenetic relationship of *Cylindrocarpon lichenicola* and *Acremonium falciforme* to the *Fusarium solani* species complex and a review of similarities in the spectrum of opportunistic infections caused by these fungi. *J Clin Microbiol* **40:**2866–2875.
17. **Zhang N, O'Donnell K, Sutton DA, Nalim FA, Summerbell RC, Padhye AA, Geiser DM.** 2006. Members of the *Fusarium solani* species complex that cause infections in both humans and plants are common in the environment. *J Clin Microbiol* **44:**2186–2190.
18. **Hawksworth DL.** 2011. A new dawn for the naming of fungi: impacts of decisions made in Melbourne in July 2011 on the future publication and regulation of fungal names. *IMA Fungus* **2:**155–162.
19. **Norvell LL.** 2011. Fungal nomenclature. 1. Melbourne approves a new code. *Mycotaxon* **116:**481–490.
20. **Geiser DM, et al.** 2013. One fungus, one name: defining the genus *Fusarium* in a scientifically robust way that preserves longstanding use. *Phytopathology* **103:**400–408.
21. **Kerényi Z, Moretti A, Waalwijk C, Oláh B, Hornok L.** 2004. Mating type sequences in asexually reproducing *Fusarium* species. *Appl Environ Microbiol* **70:**4419–4423.
22. **Guarro J, GenéJ, Stchigel AM.** 1999. Developments in fungal taxonomy. *Clin Microbiol Rev* **12:**454–500.
23. **Kirk PM, Cannon PG, David JC, Stalpers JA.** 2001. *Ainsworth & Bisby's Dictionary of the Fungi*, 9th ed. CABI Bioscience, Surrey, United Kingdom.
24. **Seifert K, Morgan-Jones G, Gams W, Kendrick B.** 2011. *The Genera of Hyphomycetes. CBS Biodiversity Series 9.* CBS-KNAW Fungal Biodiversity Centre, Utrecht, The Netherlands.
25. **Larone DH.** 2011. *Medically Important Fungi: A Guide to Identification*, 5th ed. ASM Press, Washington, DC.
26. **Sutton DA, Fothergill AW, Rinaldi MG.** 1998. *Guide to Clinically Significant Fungi*. Williams & Wilkins, Baltimore, MD.
27. **De Hoog GS, Guarro J, Gene J, Figueras MJ.** 2009. *Atlas of Clinical Fungi*, 3rd ed. Centraalbureau voor Schimmelcultures, Baarn, The Netherlands.
28. **Domsch KH, Gams W, Anderson TH.** 2007. *Compendium of Soil Fungi*, 2nd ed. IHW-Verlag, Eching, Germany.
29. **Ellis D, Davis S, Alexiou H, Handke R, Bartley R.** 2007. *Descriptions of Medical Fungi*, 2nd ed. Nexus Print Solutions, Adelaide, Australia.
30. **Kane J, Summerbell R, Sigler L, Krajden S, Land G.** 1997. *Laboratory Handbook of Dermatophytes*. Star Publishing Co., Belmont, CA.
31. **Samson RA, Hoekstra ES, Frisvad J, Filtenborg O.** 2000. *Introduction to Food and Airborne Fungi*, 6th ed. Centraalbureau voor Schimmelcultures, Utrecht, The Netherlands.
32. **Sigler L.** 2003. Ascomycetes: the *Onygenaceae* and other fungi from the order *Onygenales*, p 195–236 *In* Howard DH (ed), *Fungi Pathogenic for Humans and Animals*, 2nd ed. Marcel Dekker, Inc., New York, NY.
33. **Sigler L.** 2003. Miscellaneous opportunistic fungi: *Microascaceae* and other ascomycetes, hyphomycetes, coelomycetes and basidiomycetes, p 637–676. *In* Howard DH (ed), *Fungi Pathogenic for Humans and Animals*, 2nd ed. Marcel Dekker, Inc., New York, NY.
34. **St-Germain G, Summerbell R.** 2010. *Identifying fungi: a clinical laboratory handbook*, 2nd ed. Star Publishing Co, Belmont, CA.
35. **Ulloa M, Hanlin RT.** 2000. *Illustrated Dictionary of Mycology*. The American Phytopathological Society, St. Paul, MN.
36. **Campbell CK, Johnson EM, Warnock DW.** 2013. *Identification of Pathogenic Fungi*, 2nd ed. Wiley-Blackwell, West Sussex, United Kingdom.
37. **O'Donnell K, Sutton DA, Rinaldi MG, Sarver BA, Balajee SA, Schroers HJ, Summerbell RC, Robert VA, Crous PW, Zhang N, Aoki T, Jung K, Park J, Lee YH, Kang S, Park B, Geiser DM.** 2010. Internet-accessible DNA sequence database for identifying fusaria from human and animal infections. *J Clin Microbiol* **48:**3708–3718.
38. **Geiser D, del Mar Jimenez-Gasco M, Kang S, Makalowska I, Veeraraghavan N, Ward TJ, Zhang N, Kuldau GA, O'Donnell K.** 2004. FUSARIUM-ID v.1.0: a DNA sequence database for identifying *Fusarium*. *Eur J Plant Pathol* **110:**473–479.
39. **Tucker DL, Beresford CH, Sigler L, Rogers K.** 2004. Disseminated *Beauveria bassiana* infection in a patient with acute lymphoblastic leukemia. *J Clin Microbiol* **42:**5412–5414.
40. **Duthie R, Denning DW.** 1995. *Aspergillus* fungemia: report of two cases and review. *Clin Infect Dis* **20:**598–605.
41. **Rabodonirina M, Piens MA, Monier MF, Guého E, Fière D, Mojon M.** 1994. *Fusarium* infections in immunocompromised patients: case reports and literature review. *Eur J Clin Microbiol Infect Dis* **13:**152–161.

42. **Abbott SP, Sigler L, McAleer R, McGough DA, Rinaldi MG, Mizell G.** 1995. Fatal cerebral mycoses caused by the ascomycete *Chaetomium strumarium*. *J Clin Microbiol* **33:**2692–2698.
43. **Barron MA, Sutton DA, Veve R, Guarro J, Rinaldi M, Thompson E, Cagnoni PJ, Moultney K, Madinger NE.** 2003. Invasive mycotic infections caused by *Chaetomium perlucidum*, a new agent of cerebral phaeohyphomycosis. *J Clin Microbiol* **41:**5302–5307.
44. **Leslie JF, Summerell BF (ed).** 2006. *The Fusarium Laboratory Manual*. Blackwell Publishing, Ames, IA.
45. **Nelson PE, Dignani MC, Anaissie EJ.** 1994. Taxonomy, biology, and clinical aspects of *Fusarium* species. *Clin Microbiol Rev* **7:**479–504.
46. **Abd-Elsalam KA, Guo JR, Schnieder F, Asran-Amal AM, Verreet JA.** 2004. Comparative assessment of genotyping methods for study genetic diversity of *Fusarium oxysporum* isolates. *Pol J Microbiol* **53:**167–174.
47. **Godoy P, Cano J, Gené J, Guarro J, Höfling-Lima AL, Lopes Colombo A.** 2004. Genotyping of 44 isolates of *Fusarium solani*, the main agent of fungal keratitis in Brazil. *J Clin Microbiol* **42:**4494–4497.
48. **Short DP, O'Donnell K, Zhang N, Juba JH, Geiser DM.** 2011. Widespread occurrence of diverse human pathogenic types of the fungus *Fusarium* detected in plumbing drains. *J Clin Microbiol* **49:**4264–4272.
49. **Chang DC, Grant GB, O'Donnell K, Wannemuehler KA, Noble-Wang J, Rao CY, Jacobson LM, Crowell CS, Sneed RS, Lewis FM, Schaffzin JK, Kainer MA, Genese CA, Alfonso EC, Jones DB, Srinivasan A, Fridkin SK, Park BJ, Fusarium Keratitis Investigation Team, Fusarium Keratitis Investigation Team.** 2006. Multistate outbreak of *Fusarium keratitis* associated with use of a contact lens solution. *JAMA* **296:**953–963.
50. **Short DP, O'Donnell K, Thrane U, Nielsen KF, Zhang N, Juba JH, Geiser DM.** 2013. Phylogenetic relationships among members of the *Fusarium solani* species complex in human infections and the descriptions of *F. keratoplasticum* sp. nov. and *F. petroliphilum* stat. nov. *Fungal Genet Biol* **53:** 59–70.
51. **Schroers HJ, Samuels GJ, Zhang N, Short DP, Juba J, Geiser DM.** 2016. Epitypification of *Fusisporium* (*Fusarium*) *solani* and its assignment to a common phylogenetic species in the *Fusarium solani* species complex. *Mycologia* **108:** 806–819.
52. **O'Donnell K, Rooney AP, Proctor RH, Brown DW, McCormick SP, Ward TJ, Frandsen RJ, Lysøe E, Rehner SA, Aoki T, Robert VA, Crous PW, Groenewald JZ, Kang S, Geiser DM.** 2013. Phylogenetic analyses of RPB1 and RPB2 support a middle Cretaceous origin for a clade comprising all agriculturally and medically important fusaria. *Fungal Genet Biol* **52:**20–31.
53. **Pietro AD, Madrid MP, Caracuel Z, Delgado-Jarana J, Roncero MI.** 2003. *Fusarium oxysporum*: exploring the molecular arsenal of a vascular wilt fungus. *Mol Plant Pathol* **4:** 315–325.
54. **O'Donnell K, Gueidan C, Sink S, Johnston PR, Crous PW, Glenn A, Riley R, Zitomer NC, Colyer P, Waalwijk C, Lee T, Moretti A, Kang S, Kim HS, Geiser DM, Juba JH, Baayen RP, Cromey MG, Bithell S, Sutton DA, Skovgaard K, Ploetz R, Corby Kistler H, Elliott M, Davis M, Sarver BA.** 2009. A two-locus DNA sequence database for typing plant and human pathogens within the *Fusarium oxysporum* species complex. *Fungal Genet Biol* **46:**936–948.
55. **Anaissie EJ, Kuchar RT, Rex JH, Francesconi A, Kasai M, Müller FM, Lozano-Chiu M, Summerbell RC, Dignani MC, Chanock SJ, Walsh TJ.** 2001. Fusariosis associated with pathogenic fusarium species colonization of a hospital water system: a new paradigm for the epidemiology of opportunistic mold infections. *Clin Infect Dis* **33:**1871–1878.
56. **Warris A, Gaustad P, Meis JF, Voss A, Verweij PE, Abrahamsen TG.** 2001. Recovery of filamentous fungi from water in a paediatric bone marrow transplantation unit. *J Hosp Infect* **47:**143–148.
57. **Schroers HJ, O'Donnell K, Lamprecht SC, Kammeyer PL, Johnson S, Sutton DA, Rinaldi MG, Geiser DM, Summerbell RC.** 2009. Taxonomy and phylogeny of the *Fusarium dimerum* species group. *Mycologia* **101:**44–70.
58. **Munkvold GP.** 2017. *Fusarium* species and their associated mycotoxins, p 51–106. *In* Moretti A, Susca A (ed), *Mycotoxigenic Fungi: Methods and Protocols*. Humana Press, New York, NY.
59. **Kuhn DM, Ghannoum MA.** 2003. Indoor mold, toxigenic fungi, and *Stachybotrys chartarum*: infectious disease perspective. *Clin Microbiol Rev* **16:**144–172.
60. **Boutati EI, Anaissie EJ.** 1997. *Fusarium*, a significant emerging pathogen in patients with hematologic malignancy: ten years' experience at a cancer center and implications for management. *Blood* **90:**999–1008.
61. **Nucci M, Anaissie E.** 2006. Emerging fungi. *Infect Dis Clin North Am* **20:**563–579.
62. **Girmenia C, Arcese W, Micozzi A, Martino P, Bianco P, Morace G.** 1992. Onychomycosis as a possible origin of disseminated *Fusarium solani* infection in a patient with severe aplastic anemia. *Clin Infect Dis* **14:**1167.
63. **Raad I, Tarrand J, Hanna H, Albitar M, Janssen E, Boktour M, Bodey G, Mardani M, Hachem R, Kontoyiannis D, Whimbey E, Rolston K.** 2002. Epidemiology, molecular mycology, and environmental sources of *Fusarium* infection in patients with cancer. *Infect Control Hosp Epidemiol* **23:** 532–537.
64. **Ascioglu S, Rex JH, de Pauw B, Bennett JE, Bille J, Crokaert F, Denning DW, Donnelly JP, Edwards JE, Erjavec Z, Fiere D, Lortholary O, Maertens J, Meis JF, Patterson TF, Ritter J, Selleslag D, Shah PM, Stevens DA, Walsh TJ, Invasive Fungal Infections Cooperative Group of the European Organization for Research and Treatment of Cancer, Mycoses Study Group of the National Institute of Allergy and Infectious Diseases.** 2002. Defining opportunistic invasive fungal infections in immunocompromised patients with cancer and hematopoietic stem cell transplants: an international consensus. *Clin Infect Dis* **34:**7–14.
65. **Baddley JW, Stroud TP, Salzman D, Pappas PG.** 2001. Invasive mold infections in allogeneic bone marrow transplant recipients. *Clin Infect Dis* **32:**1319–1324.
66. **Girmenia C, Pagano L, Corvatta L, Mele L, del Favero A, Martino P, Gimema Infection Programme.** 2000. The epidemiology of fusariosis in patients with haematological diseases. *Br J Haematol* **111:**272–276.
67. **Grossi P, Farina C, Fiocchi R, Dalla Gasperina D, Italian Study Group of Fungal Infections in Thoracic Organ Transplant Recipients.** 2000. Prevalence and outcome of invasive fungal infections in 1,963 thoracic organ transplant recipients: a multicenter retrospective study. *Transplantation* **70:**112–116.
68. **Lionakis MS, Kontoyiannis DP.** 2004. The significance of isolation of saprophytic molds from the lower respiratory tract in patients with cancer. *Cancer* **100:**165–172.
69. **Nucci M.** 2003. Emerging moulds: *Fusarium*, *Scedosporium* and *Zygomycetes* in transplant recipients. *Curr Opin Infect Dis* **16:**607–612.
70. **Nucci M, Anaissie EJ.** 2009. Hyalohyphomycosis, p 309–327. *In* Anaissie EJ, McGinnis MR, Pfaller MA (ed), *Clinical Mycology*, 2nd ed. Elsevier, London, United Kingdom.
71. **Nucci M, Anaissie EJ, Queiroz-Telles F, Martins CA, Trabasso P, Solza C, Mangini C, Simões BP, Colombo AL, Vaz J, Levy CE, Costa S, Moreira VA, Oliveira JS, Paraguay N, Duboc G, Voltarelli JC, Maiolino A, Pasquini R, Souza CA.** 2003. Outcome predictors of 84 patients with hematologic malignancies and *Fusarium* infection. *Cancer* **98:**315–319.
72. **Nucci M, Marr KA, Queiroz-Telles F, Martins CA, Trabasso P, Costa S, Voltarelli JC, Colombo AL, Imhof A, Pasquini R, Maiolino A, Souza Cármino CA, Anaissie E.** 2004. *Fusarium* infection in hematopoietic stem cell transplant recipients. *Clin Infect Dis* **38:**1237–1242.
73. **Sampathkumar P, Paya CV.** 2001. *Fusarium* infection after solid-organ transplantation. *Clin Infect Dis* **32:**1237–1240.

74. **Imamura Y, Chandra J, Mukherjee PK, Lattif AA, Szczotka-Flynn LB, Pearlman E, Lass JH, O'Donnell K, Ghannoum MA.** 2008. *Fusarium* and *Candida albicans* biofilms on soft contact lenses: model development, influence of lens type, and susceptibility to lens care solutions. *Antimicrob Agents Chemother* **52:**171–182.
75. **Khor WB, Aung T, Saw SM, Wong TY, Tambyah PA, Tan AL, Beuerman R, Lim L, Chan WK, Heng WJ, Lim J, Loh RS, Lee SB, Tan DT.** 2006. An outbreak of *Fusarium* keratitis associated with contact lens wear in Singapore. *JAMA* **295:**2867–2873.
76. **Rao SK, Lam PT, Li EY, Yuen HK, Lam DS.** 2007. A case series of contact lens-associated *Fusarium* keratitis in Hong Kong. *Cornea* **26:**1205–1209.
77. **Hay RJ.** 2007. *Fusarium* infections of the skin. *Curr Opin Infect Dis* **20:**115–117.
78. **Yücesoy M, Ergon MC, Oren H, Gülay Z.** 2004. Case report: a *Fusarium* fungaemia. *Mikrobiyol Bul* **38:**265–271. [In Turkish.]
79. **Rezai KA, Eliott D, Plous O, Vazquez JA, Abrams GW.** 2005. Disseminated *Fusarium* infection presenting as bilateral endogenous endophthalmitis in a patient with acute myeloid leukemia. *Arch Ophthalmol* **123:**702–703.
80. **Tiribelli M, Zaja F, Filì C, Michelutti T, Prosdocimo S, Candoni A, Fanin R.** 2002. Endogenous endophthalmitis following disseminated fungemia due to *Fusarium solani* in a patient with acute myeloid leukemia. *Eur J Haematol* **68:** 314–317.
81. **Nucci M, Anaissie E.** 2007. *Fusarium* infections in immunocompromised patients. *Clin Microbiol Rev* **20:**695–704.
82. **Prins C, Chavaz P, Tamm K, Hauser C.** 1995. Ecthyma gangrenosum-like lesions: a sign of disseminated *Fusarium* infection in the neutropenic patient. *Clin Exp Dermatol* **20:**428–430.
83. **Sponsel WE, Graybill JR, Nevarez HL, Dang D.** 2002. Ocular and systemic posaconazole(SCH-56592) treatment of invasive *Fusarium solani* keratitis and endophthalmitis. *Br J Ophthalmol* **86:**829–830.
84. **Mayayo E, Pujol I, Guarro J.** 1999. Experimental pathogenicity of four opportunist *Fusarium* species in a murine model. *J Med Microbiol* **48:**363–366.
85. **Sugiura Y, Barr JR, Barr DB, Brock JW, Elie CM, Ueno Y, Patterson DG, Jr, Potter ME, Reiss E.** 1999. Physiological characteristics and mycotoxins of human clinical isolates of *Fusarium* species. *Mycol Res* **103:**1462–1468.
86. **Azor M, Gené J, Cano J, Sutton DA, Fothergill AW, Rinaldi MG, Guarro J.** 2008. In vitro antifungal susceptibility and molecular characterization of clinical isolates of *Fusarium verticillioides* (*F. moniliforme*) and *Fusarium thapsinum*. *Antimicrob Agents Chemother* **52:**2228–2231.
87. **Tortorano AM, Prigitano A, Dho G, Esposto MC, Gianni C, Grancini A, Ossi C, Viviani MA.** 2008. Species distribution and in vitro antifungal susceptibility patterns of 75 clinical isolates of *Fusarium* spp. from northern Italy. *Antimicrob Agents Chemother* **52:**2683–2685.
88. **Azor M, Gené J, Cano J, Manikandan P, Venkatapathy N, Guarro J.** 2009. Less-frequent *Fusarium* species of clinical interest: correlation between morphological and molecular identification and antifungal susceptibility. *J Clin Microbiol* **47:**1463–1468.
89. **O'Donnell K, Sutton DA, Wiederhold N, Robert VA, Crous PW, Geiser DM.** 2016. Veterinary fusarioses within the United States. *J Clin Microbiol* **54:**2813–2819.
90. **Musa MO, Al Eisa A, Halim M, Sahovic E, Gyger M, Chaudhri N, Al Mohareb F, Seth P, Aslam M, Aljurf M.** 2000. The spectrum of *Fusarium* infection in immunocompromised patients with haematological malignancies and in non-immunocompromised patients: a single institution experience over 10 years. *Br J Haematol* **108:**544–548.
91. **Chandler FW, Watts JC.** 1987. *Pathologic Diagnosis of Fungal Infections*. American Society of Clinical Pathologists, Inc., Chicago, IL..
92. **Liu K, Howell DN, Perfect JR, Schell WA.** 1998. Morphologic criteria for the preliminary identification of *Fusarium*, *Paecilomyces*, and *Acremonium* species by histopathology. *Am J Clin Pathol* **109:**45–54.
93. **Guarner J, Brandt ME.** 2011. Histopathologic diagnosis of fungal infections in the 21st century. *Clin Microbiol Rev* **24:**247–280.
94. **Kaufman L, Standard PG, Jalbert M, Kraft DE.** 1997. Immunohistologic identification of *Aspergillus* spp. and other hyaline fungi by using polyclonal fluorescent antibodies. *J Clin Microbiol* **35:**2206–2209.
95. **Tortorano AM, Esposto MC, Prigitano A, Grancini A, Ossi C, Cavanna C, Cascio GL.** 2012. Cross-reactivity of *Fusarium* spp. in the *Aspergillus* galactomannan enzyme-linked immunosorbent assay. *J Clin Microbiol* **50:**1051–1053.
96. **Rimek D, Singh J, Kappe R.** 2003. Cross-reactivity of the PLATELIA *CANDIDA* antigen detection enzyme immunoassay with fungal antigen extracts. *J Clin Microbiol* **41:** 3395–3398.
97. **Odabasi Z, Mattiuzzi G, Estey E, Kantarjian H, Saeki F, Ridge RJ, Ketchum PA, Finkelman MA, Rex JH, Ostrosky-Zeichner L.** 2004. β-D-glucan as a diagnostic adjunct for invasive fungal infections: validation, cut-off development, and performance in patients with acute myelogenous leukemia and myelodysplastic syndrome. *Clin Infect Dis* **39:**199–205.
98. **Ostrosky-Zeichner L, Alexander BD, Kett DH, Vazquez J, Pappas PG, Saeki F, Ketchum PA, Wingard J, Schiff R, Tamura H, Finkelman MA, Rex JH.** 2005. Multicenter clinical evaluation of the (1→3)beta-D-glucan assay as an aid to diagnosis of fungal infections in humans. *Clin Infect Dis* **41:**654–659.
99. **Obayashi T, Kawai T, Yoshida M, Mori T, Goto H, Yasuoka A, Shimada K, Iwasaki H, Teshima H, Kohno S, Horiuchi A, Ito A, Yamaguchi H.** 1995. Plasma (1→3)-beta-D-glucan measurement in diagnosis of invasive deep mycosis and fungal febrile episodes. *Lancet* **345:**17–20.
100. **Khan ZU, Ahmad S, Theyyathel AM.** 2008. Diagnostic value of DNA and (1→3)-beta-D-glucan detection in serum and bronchoalveolar lavage of mice experimentally infected with *Fusarium oxysporum*. *J Med Microbiol* **57:**36–42.
101. **Kato A, Takita T, Furuhashi M, Takahashi T, Maruyama Y, Hishida A.** 2001. Elevation of blood (1→3)-beta-D-glucan concentrations in hemodialysis patients. *Nephron* **89:**15–19.
102. **Ikemura K, Ikegami K, Shimazu T, Yoshioka T, Sugimoto T.** 1989. False-positive result in *Limulus* test caused by *Limulus* amebocyte lysate-reactive material in immunoglobulin products. *J Clin Microbiol* **27:**1965–1968.
103. **Nakao A, Yasui M, Kawagoe T, Tamura H, Tanaka S, Takagi H.** 1997. False-positive endotoxemia derives from gauze glucan after hepatectomy for hepatocellular carcinoma with cirrhosis. *Hepatogastroenterology* **44:**1413–1418.
104. **Hue FX, Huerre M, Rouffault MA, de Bievre C.** 1999. Specific detection of *Fusarium* species in blood and tissues by a PCR technique. *J Clin Microbiol* **37:**2434–2438.
105. **Jaeger EE, Carroll NM, Choudhury S, Dunlop AA, Towler HM, Matheson MM, Adamson P, Okhravi N, Lightman S.** 2000. Rapid detection and identification of *Candida*, *Aspergillus*, and *Fusarium* species in ocular samples using nested PCR. *J Clin Microbiol* **38:**2902–2908.
106. **Ninet B, Jan I, Bontems O, Léchenne B, Jousson O, Lew D, Schrenzel J, Panizzon RG, Monod M.** 2005. Molecular identification of *Fusarium* species in onychomycoses. *Dermatology* **210:**21–25.
107. **Salehi E, Hedayati MT, Zoll J, Rafati H, Ghasemi M, Doroudinia A, Abastabar M, Tolooe A, Snelders E, van der Lee HA, Rijs AJ, Verweij PE, Seyedmousavi S, Melchers WJ.** 2016. Discrimination of aspergillosis, mucormycosis, fusariosis, and scedosporiosis in formalin-fixed paraffin-embedded tissue specimens by use of multiple real-time quantitative PCR assays. *J Clin Microbiol* **54:**2798–2803.
108. **Van Burik JA, Myerson D, Schreckhise RW, Bowden RA.** 1998. Panfungal PCR assay for detection of fungal infection in human blood specimens. *J Clin Microbiol* **36:**1169–1175.
109. **Landlinger C, Preuner S, Willinger B, Haberpursch B, Racil Z, Mayer J, Lion T.** 2009. Species-specific identification of a wide range of clinically relevant fungal pathogens by use of Luminex xMAP technology. *J Clin Microbiol* **47:**1063–1073.

110. **Kornerup A, Wanscher JH.** 1983. *Methuen Handbook of Colour*. Eyre Methuen Ltd., London, United Kingdom.
111. **Nelson PE, Toussoun TA, Marasas WFO.** 1983. *Fusarium Species: an Illustrated Manual of Identification*. Pennsylvania State University Press, State College, PA.
112. **Wang H, Xiao M, Kong F, Chen S, Dou HT, Sorrell T, Li RY, Xu YC.** 2011. Accurate and practical identification of 20 *Fusarium* species by seven-locus sequence analysis and reverse line blot hybridization, and an *in vitro* antifungal susceptibility study. *J Clin Microbiol* **49:**1890–1898.
113. **Lau AF, Drake SK, Calhoun LB, Henderson CM, Zelazny AM.** 2013. Development of a clinically comprehensive database and a simple procedure for identification of molds from solid media by matrix-assisted laser desorption ionization-time of flight mass spectrometry. *J Clin Microbiol* **51:**828–834.
114. **De Carolis E, Posteraro B, Lass-Flörl C, Vella A, Florio AR, Torelli R, Girmenia C, Colozza C, Tortorano AM, Sanguinetti M, Fadda G.** 2012. Species identification of *Aspergillus, Fusarium* and *Mucorales* with direct surface analysis by matrix-assisted laser desorption ionization time-of-flight mass spectrometry. *Clin Microbiol Infect* **18:**475–484.
115. **Healy M, Reece K, Walton D, Huong J, Frye S, Raad II, Kontoyiannis DP.** 2005. Use of the DiversiLab System for species and strain differentiation of *Fusarium* species isolates. *J Clin Microbiol* **43:**5278–5280.
116. **Schmidt AL, Mitter V.** 2004. Microsatellite mutation directed by an external stimulus. *Mutat Res* **568:**233–243.
117. **Clinical and Laboratory Standards Institute.** 2008. Interpretive criteria for identification of bacteria and fungi by DNA target sequencing: approved guideline. CLSI document MM18-A. Clinical and Laboratory Standards Institute, Wayne, PA.
118. **Balajee SA, Borman AM, Brandt ME, Cano J, Cuenca-Estrella M, Dannaoui E, Guarro J, Haase G, Kibbler CC, Meyer W, O'Donnell K, Petti CA, Rodriguez-Tudela JL, Sutton D, Velegraki A, Wickes BL.** 2009. Sequence-based identification of *Aspergillus, Fusarium*, and *Mucorales* species in the clinical mycology laboratory: where are we and where should we go from here? *J Clin Microbiol* **47:**877–884.
119. **O'Donnell K, Ward TJ, Robert VA, Crous PW, Geiser DM, Kang S.** 2015. DNA sequence-based identification of *Fusarium*: current status and future directions. *Phytoparasitica* **43:**583–595.
120. **Jaakkola MS, Laitinen S, Piipari R, Uitti J, Nordman H, Haapala AM, Jaakkola JJ.** 2002. Immunoglobulin G antibodies against indoor dampness-related microbes and adult-onset asthma: a population-based incident case-control study. *Clin Exp Immunol* **129:**107–112.
121. **Lappalainen S, Pasanen AL, Reiman M, Kalliokoski P.** 1998. Serum IgG antibodies against *Wallemia sebi* and *Fusarium* species in Finnish farmers. *Ann Allergy Asthma Immunol* **81:**585–592.
122. **Rydjord B, Hetland G, Wiker HG.** 2005. Immunoglobulin G antibodies against environmental moulds in a Norwegian healthy population shows a bimodal distribution for *Aspergillus versicolor*. *Scand J Immunol* **62:**281–288.
123. **Saini SK, Boas SR, Jerath A, Roberts M, Greenberger PA.** 1998. Allergic bronchopulmonary mycosis to *Fusarium vasinfectum* in a child. *Ann Allergy Asthma Immunol* **80:**377–380.
124. **Alastruey-Izquierdo A, Cuenca-Estrella M, Monzón A, Mellado E, Rodríguez-Tudela JL.** 2008. Antifungal susceptibility profile of clinical *Fusarium* spp. isolates identified by molecular methods. *J Antimicrob Chemother* **61:**805–809.
125. **Espinel-Ingroff A.** 2001. Comparison of the E-test with the NCCLS M38-P method for antifungal susceptibility testing of common and emerging pathogenic filamentous fungi. *J Clin Microbiol* **39:**1360–1367.
126. **Azor M, Gené J, Cano J, Guarro J.** 2007. Universal in vitro antifungal resistance of genetic clades of the *Fusarium solani* species complex. *Antimicrob Agents Chemother* **51:**1500–1503.
127. **Lass-Flörl C, Mayr A, Perkhofer S, Hinterberger G, Hausdorfer J, Speth C, Fille M.** 2008. Activities of antifungal agents against yeasts and filamentous fungi: assessment according to the methodology of the European Committee on Antimicrobial Susceptibility Testing. *Antimicrob Agents Chemother* **52:**3637–3641.
128. **Pfaller MA, Messer SA, Hollis RJ, Jones RN, SENTRY Participants Group.** 2002. Antifungal activities of posaconazole, ravuconazole, and voriconazole compared to those of itraconazole and amphotericin B against 239 clinical isolates of *Aspergillus* spp. and other filamentous fungi: report from SENTRY Antimicrobial Surveillance Program, 2000. *Antimicrob Agents Chemother* **46:**1032–1037.
129. **Diekema DJ, Messer SA, Hollis RJ, Jones RN, Pfaller MA.** 2003. Activities of caspofungin, itraconazole, posaconazole, ravuconazole, voriconazole, and amphotericin B against 448 recent clinical isolates of filamentous fungi. *J Clin Microbiol* **41:**3623–3626.
130. **Arikan S, Lozano-Chiu M, Paetznick V, Nangia S, Rex JH.** 1999. Microdilution susceptibility testing of amphotericin B, itraconazole, and voriconazole against clinical isolates of *Aspergillus* and *Fusarium* species. *J Clin Microbiol* **37:** 3946–3951.
131. **Clancy CJ, Nguyen MH.** 1998. In vitro efficacy and fungicidal activity of voriconazole against *Aspergillus* and *Fusarium* species. *Eur J Clin Microbiol Infect Dis* **17:**573–575.
132. **Lozano-Chiu M, Arikan S, Paetznick VL, Anaissie EJ, Loebenberg D, Rex JH.** 1999. Treatment of murine fusariosis with SCH 56592. *Antimicrob Agents Chemother* **43:**589–591.
133. **Perfect JR, Marr KA, Walsh TJ, Greenberg RN, DuPont B, de la Torre-Cisneros J, Just-Nübling G, Schlamm HT, Lutsar I, Espinel-Ingroff A, Johnson E.** 2003. Voriconazole treatment for less-common, emerging, or refractory fungal infections. *Clin Infect Dis* **36:**1122–1131.
134. **Raad II, Hachem RY, Herbrecht R, Graybill JR, Hare R, Corcoran G, Kontoyiannis DP.** 2006. Posaconazole as salvage treatment for invasive fusariosis in patients with underlying hematologic malignancy and other conditions. *Clin Infect Dis* **42:**1398–1403.
135. **González GM.** 2009. In vitro activities of isavuconazole against opportunistic filamentous and dimorphic fungi. *Med Mycol* **47:**71–76.
136. **Guinea J, Peláez T, Recio S, Torres-Narbona M, Bouza E.** 2008. In vitro antifungal activities of isavuconazole (BAL4815), voriconazole, and fluconazole against 1,007 isolates of zygomycete, *Candida, Aspergillus, Fusarium*, and *Scedosporium* species. *Antimicrob Agents Chemother* **52:**1396–1400.
137. **Arikan S, Lozano-Chiu M, Paetznick V, Rex JH.** 2001. In vitro susceptibility testing methods for caspofungin against *Aspergillus* and *Fusarium* isolates. *Antimicrob Agents Chemother* **45:**327–330.
138. **Pfaller MA, Marco F, Messer SA, Jones RN.** 1998. In vitro activity of two echinocandin derivatives, LY303366 and MK-0991 (L-743,792), against clinical isolates of *Aspergillus, Fusarium, Rhizopus*, and other filamentous fungi. *Diagn Microbiol Infect Dis* **30:**251–255.
139. **Katiyar SK, Edlind TD.** 2009. Role for Fks1 in the intrinsic echinocandin resistance of *Fusarium solani* as evidenced by hybrid expression in *Saccharomyces cerevisiae*. *Antimicrob Agents Chemother* **53:**1772–1778.
140. **Clinical and Laboratory Standards Institute.** 2008. Reference method for broth dilution antifungal susceptibility testing of filamentous fungi; Approved standard, 2nd ed. Clinical and Laboratory Standards Institute, Wayne, PA.
141. **Garcia-Effron G, Gomez-Lopez A, Mellado E, Monzon A, Rodriguez-Tudela JL, Cuenca-Estrella M.** 2004. In vitro activity of terbinafine against medically important non-dermatophyte species of filamentous fungi. *J Antimicrob Chemother* **53:**1086–1089.
142. **Ruíz-Cendoya M, Mariné M, Rodríguez MM, Guarro J.** 2009. Interactions between triazoles and amphotericin B in treatment of disseminated murine infection by *Fusarium oxysporum*. *Antimicrob Agents Chemother* **53:**1705–1708.
143. **Xu Y, Pang G, Gao C, Zhao D, Zhou L, Sun S, Wang B.** 2009. In vitro comparison of the efficacies of natamycin and silver nitrate against ocular fungi. *Antimicrob Agents Chemother* **53:**1636–1638.
144. **Perdomo H, García D, Gené J, Cano J, Sutton DA, Summerbell R, Guarro J.** 2013. *Phialemoniopsis*, a new genus of Sordariomycetes, and new species of *Phialemonium* and *Lecythophora*. *Mycologia* **105:**398–421.

145. **Khan Z, Gené J, Ahmad S, Cano J, Al-Sweih N, Joseph L, Chandy R, Guarro J.** 2013. *Coniochaeta polymorpha*, a new species from endotracheal aspirate of a preterm neonate, and transfer of *Lecythophora* species to *Coniochaeta*. *Antonie van Leeuwenhoek* **104:**243–252.
146. **Sutton DA.** 1999. Coelomycetous fungi in human disease. A review: clinical entities, pathogenesis, identification and therapy. *Rev Iberoam Micol* **16:**171–179.
147. **Sutton DA.** 2008. Rare and emerging agents of hyalohyphomycosis. *Curr Fungal Infect Rep* **2:**134–142.
148. **McNeill J, Barrie FR, Buck WR, Demoulin V, Greuter W, Hawksworth DL, Herendeen PS, Knapp S, Markold K, Prado J, Prud'homme van Reine WF, Smith FG, Wiersema J, Turland NJ.** 2012. *International Code of Nomenclature for Algae, Fungi and Plants (Melbourne Code)*. International Association for Plant Taxonomy and Koeltz Scientific Books, Königstein, Germany.
149. **de Hoog GS, Chaturvedi V, Denning DW, Dyer PS, Frisvad JC, Geiser D, Gräser Y, Guarro J, Haase G, Kwon-Chung KJ, Meis JF, Meyer W, Pitt JI, Samson RA, Taylor JW, Tintelnot K, Vitale RG, Walsh TJ, Lackner M, ISHAM Working Group on Nomenclature of Medical Fungi.** 2015. Name changes in medically important fungi and their implications for clinical practice. *J Clin Microbiol* **53:**1056–1062.
150. **Yaguchi T, Sano A, Yarita K, Suh MK, Nishimura K, Udagawa S-I.** 2006. A new species of *Cephalotheca* isolated from a Korean patient. *Mycotaxon* **96:**309–322.
151. **Jagielski T, Sandoval-Denis M, Yu J, Yao L, Bakuła Z, Kalita J, Skóra M, Krzyściak P, de Hoog GS, Guarro J, Gené J.** 2016. Molecular taxonomy of scopulariopsis-like fungi with description of new clinical and environmental species. *Fungal Biol* **120:**586–602.
152. **Sandoval-Denis M, Gené J, Sutton DA, Cano-Lira JF, de Hoog GS, Decock CA, Wiederhold NP, Guarro J.** 2016. Redefining *Microascus, Scopulariopsis* and allied genera. *Persoonia* **36:**1–36.
153. **Sandoval-Denis M, Sutton DA, Fothergill AW, Cano-Lira J, Gené J, Decock CA, de Hoog GS, Guarro J.** 2013. *Scopulariopsis*, a poorly known opportunistic fungus: spectrum of species in clinical samples and *in vitro* responses to antifungal drugs. *J Clin Microbiol* **51:**3937–3943.
154. **Abbott SP, Sigler L.** 2001. Heterothallism in the Microascaceae demonstrated by three species in the *Scopulariopsis brevicaulis* series. *Mycologia* **93:**1211–1220.
155. **Iwen PC, Sigler L, Tarantolo S, Sutton DA, Rinaldi MG, Lackner RP, McCarthy DI, Hinrichs SH.** 2000. Pulmonary infection caused by *Gymnascella hyalinospora* in a patient with acute myelogenous leukemia. *J Clin Microbiol* **38:**375–381.
156. **Sigler L, Abbott SP.** 1997. Characterizing and conserving diversity of filamentous basidiomycetes from human sources. *Microbiol Cult Collect* **13:**21–27.
157. **Chowdhary A, Kathuria S, Agarwal K, Meis JF.** 2014. Recognizing filamentous basidiomycetes as agents of human disease: a review. *Med Mycol* **52:**782–797.
158. **Siqueira JP, Sutton D, Gené J, García D, Guevara-Suarez M, Decock C, Wiederhold N, Guarro J.** 2016. *Schizophyllum radiatum*, an emerging fungus from human respiratory tract. *J Clin Microbiol* **54:**2491–2497.
159. **Amitani R, Nishimura K, Niimi A, Kobayashi H, Nawada R, Murayama T, Taguchi H, Kuze F.** 1996. Bronchial mucoid impaction due to the monokaryotic mycelium of *Schizophyllum commune*. *Clin Infect Dis* **22:**146–148.
160. **Sigler L, de la Maza LM, Tan G, Egger KN, Sherburne RK.** 1995. Diagnostic difficulties caused by a nonclamped *Schizophyllum commune* isolate in a case of fungus ball of the lung. *J Clin Microbiol* **33:**1979–1983.
161. **Sigler L, Harris JL, Dixon DM, Flis AL, Salkin IF, Kemna M, Duncan RA.** 1990. Microbiology and potential virulence of *Sporothrix cyanescens*, a fungus rarely isolated from blood and skin. *J Clin Microbiol* **28:**1009–1015.
162. **Davis CM, Noroski LM, Dishop MK, Sutton DA, Braverman RM, Paul ME, Rosenblatt HM.** 2007. Basidiomycetous fungal *Inonotus tropicalis* sacral osteomyelitis in X-linked chronic granulomatous disease. *Pediatr Infect Dis J* **26:** 655–656.
163. **Sutton DA, Thompson EH, Rinaldi MG, Iwen PC, Nakasone KK, Jung HS, Rosenblatt HM, Paul ME.** 2005. Identification and first report of *Inonotus (Phellinus) tropicalis* as an etiologic agent in a patient with chronic granulomatous disease. *J Clin Microbiol* **43:**982–987.
164. **Brockus CW, Myers RK, Crandell JM, Sutton DA, Wickes BL, Nakasone KK.** 2009. Disseminated *Oxyporus corticola* infection in a German shepherd dog. *Med Mycol* **47:**862–868.
165. **Chowdhary A, Agarwal K, Kathuria S, Singh PK, Roy P, Gaur SN, de Hoog GS, Meis JF.** 2013. Clinical significance of filamentous basidiomycetes illustrated by isolates of the novel opportunist *Ceriporia lacerata* from the human respiratory tract. *J Clin Microbiol* **51:**585–590.
166. **Buzina W, Lass-Flörl C, Kropshofer G, Freund MC, Marth E.** 2005. The polypore mushroom *Irpex lacteus*, a new causative agent of fungal infections. *J Clin Microbiol* **43:** 2009–2011.
167. **Chowdhary A, Agarwal K, Kathuria S, Singh PK, Roy P, Gaur SN, Rodrigues AM, de Hoog GS, Meis JF.** 2012. First human case of pulmonary fungal ball due to a *Perenniporia* species (a basidiomycete). *J Clin Microbiol* **50:**3786–3791.
168. **Salit RB, Shea YR, Gea-Banacloche J, Fahle GA, Abu-Asab M, Sugui JA, Carpenter AE, Quezado MM, Bishop MR, Kwon-Chung KJ.** 2010. Death by edible mushroom: first report of *Volvariella volvacea* as an etiologic agent of invasive disease in a patient following double umbilical cord blood transplantation. *J Clin Microbiol* **48:**4329–4332.
169. **Lagrou K, Massonet C, Theunissen K, Meersseman W, Lontie M, Verbeken E, Van Eldere J, Maertens J.** 2005. Fatal pulmonary infection in a leukaemic patient caused by *Hormographiella aspergillata*. *J Med Microbiol* **54:**685–688.
170. **Verweij PE, van Kasteren M, van de Nes J, de Hoog GS, de Pauw BE, Meis JF.** 1997. Fatal pulmonary infection caused by the basidiomycete *Hormographiella aspergillata*. *J Clin Microbiol* **35:**2675–2678.
171. **de Beer ZW, Begerow D, Bauer R, Pegg GS, Crous PW, Wingfield MJ.** 2006. Phylogeny of the *Quambalariaceae* fam. nov., including important *Eucalyptus* pathogens in South Africa and Australia. *Stud Mycol* **55:**289–298.
172. **Middelhoven WJ, Guého E, de Hoog GS.** 2000. Phylogenetic position and physiology of *Cerinosterus cyanescens*. *Antonie van Leeuwenhoek* **77:**313–320.
173. **Khan ZU, Randhawa HS, Kowshik T, Gaur SN, de Vries GA.** 1988. The pathogenic potential of *Sporotrichum pruinosum* isolated from the human respiratory tract. *J Med Vet Mycol* **26:**145–151.
174. **Glenn AE, Bacon CW, Price R, Hanlin RT.** 1996. Molecular phylogeny of *Acremonium* and its taxonomic implications. *Mycologia* **88:**369–383.
175. **Guarro J, Gams W, Pujol I, Gené J.** 1997. *Acremonium* species: new emerging fungal opportunists—in vitro antifungal susceptibilities and review. *Clin Infect Dis* **25:**1222–1229.
176. **Perdomo H, Sutton DA, García D, Fothergill AW, Cano J, Gené J, Summerbell RC, Rinaldi MG, Guarro J.** 2011. Spectrum of clinically relevant *Acremonium* species in the United States. *J Clin Microbiol* **49:**243–256.
177. **Summerbell RC, Gueidan C, Schroers HJ, de Hoog GS, Starink M, Rosete YA, Guarro J, Scott JA.** 2011. *Acremonium* phylogenetic overview and revision of *Gliomastix, Sarocladium*, and *Trichothecium*. *Stud Mycol* **68:**139–162.
178. **Giraldo A, Gene J, Sutton DA, Wiederhold N, Guarro J.** 2017. New *Acremonium*-like species in the Bionectriaceae and Plectosphaerellaceae. *Mycol Prog* **16:**349–368.
179. **Crous PW, et al.** 2015. Fungal Planet description sheets: 320-370. *Persoonia* **34:**167–266.
180. **Gams W, McGinnis MR.** 1983. *Phialemonium*, a new anamorphic genus intermediate between *Phialophora* and *Acremonium*. *Mycologia* **75:**977–987.
181. **Guarro J, Nucci M, Akiti T, Gené J, Cano J, Barreiro MD, Aguilar C.** 1999. *Phialemonium* fungemia: two documented nosocomial cases. *J Clin Microbiol* **37:**2493–2497.
182. **Chin-Hong PV, Sutton DA, Roemer M, Jacobson MA, Aberg JA.** 2001. Invasive fungal sinusitis and meningitis due to *Arthrographis kalrae* in a patient with AIDS. *J Clin Microbiol* **39:**804–807.

183. **Perlman EM, Binns L.** 1997. Intense photophobia caused by *Arthrographis kalrae* in a contact lens-wearing patient. *Am J Ophthalmol* **123:**547–549.
184. **Giraldo A, Gené J, Sutton DA, Madrid H, Cano J, Crous PW, Guarro J.** 2014. Phylogenetic circumscription of Arthrographis (Eremomycetaceae, Dothideomycetes). *Persoonia* **32:**102–114.
185. **Giraldo A, Sutton DA, Gené J, Fothergill AW, Cano J, Guarro J.** 2013. Rare arthroconidial fungi in clinical samples: *Scytalidium cuboideum* and *Arthropsis hispanica*. *Mycopathologia* **175:**115–121.
186. **Crous PW, Slippers B, Wingfield MJ, Rheeder J, Marasas WF, Philips AJ, Alves A, Burgess T, Barber P, Groenewald JZ.** 2006. Phylogenetic lineages in the Botryosphaeriaceae. *Stud Mycol* **55:**235–253.
187. **Rehner SA, Buckley E.** 2005. A *Beauveria* phylogeny inferred from nuclear ITS and EF1-alpha sequences: evidence for cryptic diversification and links to *Cordyceps* teleomorphs. *Mycologia* **97:**84–98.
188. **Tsang CC, Chan JFW, Pong WM, Chen JHK, Ngan AHY, Cheung M, Lai CKC, Tsang DNC, Lau SKP, Woo PCY.** 2016. Cutaneous hyalohyphomycosis due to *Parengyodontium album* gen. et comb. nov. *Med Mycol* **54:**699–713.
189. **Marin-Felix Y, Stchigel AM, Miller AN, Guarro J, Cano-Lira JF.** 2015. A re-evaluation of the genus Myceliophthora (Sordariales, Ascomycota): its segregation into four genera and description of *Corynascus fumimontanus* sp. nov. *Mycologia* **107:**619–632.
190. **Rajeev S, Sutton DA, Wickes BL, Miller DL, Giri D, Van Meter M, Thompson EH, Rinaldi MG, Romanelli AM, Cano JF, Guarro J.** 2009. Isolation and characterization of a new fungal species, *Chrysosporium ophiodiicola*, from a mycotic granuloma of a black rat snake (*Elaphe obsoleta obsoleta*). *J Clin Microbiol* **47:**1264–1268.
191. **Stchigel AM, Sutton DA, Cano-Lira JF, Cabañes FJ, Abarca L, Tintelnot K, Wickes BL, García D, Guarro J.** 2013. Phylogeny of chrysosporia infecting reptiles: proposal of the new family Nannizziopsiaceae and five new species. *Persoonia* **31:**86–100.
192. **Bischoff JF, Rehner SA, Humber RA.** 2009. A multilocus phylogeny of the *Metarhizium anisopliae* lineage. *Mycologia* **101:**512–530.
193. **Driver F, Milner RJ, Trueman JWH.** 2000. A taxonomic revision of *Metarhizium* based on a phylogenetic analysis of rDNA sequence data. *Mycol Res* **104:**134–150.
194. **Kepler RM, Humber RA, Bischoff JF, Rehner SA.** 2014. Clarification of generic and species boundaries for Metarhizium and related fungi through multigene phylogenetics. *Mycologia* **106:**811–829.
195. **Druzhinina IS, Kopchinskiy AG, Kubicek CP.** 2006. The first 100 *Trichoderma* species characterized by molecular data. *Mycoscience* **47:**55–64.
196. **Sandoval-Denis M, Sutton DA, Cano-Lira JF, Gené J, Fothergill AW, Wiederhold NP, Guarro J.** 2014. Phylogeny of the clinically relevant species of the emerging fungus *Trichoderma* and their antifungal susceptibilities. *J Clin Microbiol* **52:**2112–2125.
197. **Bissett J, Gams W, Jaklitsch W, Samuels GJ.** 2015. Accepted *Trichoderma* names in the year 2015. *IMA Fungus* **6:** 263–295.
198. **Jaklitsch WM, Voglmayr H.** 2015. Biodiversity of *Trichoderma* (Hypocreaceae) in Southern Europe and Macaronesia. *Stud Mycol* **80:**1–87.
199. **Houbraken J, Verweij PE, Rijs AJ, Borman AM, Samson RA.** 2010. Identification of *Paecilomyces variotii* in clinical samples and settings. *J Clin Microbiol* **48:**2754–2761.
200. **Sigler L, Verweij PE.** 2003. *Aspergillus*, *Fusarium*, and other opportunistic moniliaceous fungi, p 1726–1760. *In* Murray PR, Baron EJ, Jorgensen JH, Pfaller MA, Yolken RH (ed), *Manual of Clinical Microbiology*, 8th ed. ASM Press, Washington, DC.
201. **Luangsa-ard J, Houbraken J, van Doorn T, Hong SB, Borman AM, Hywel-Jones NL, Samson RA.** 2011. *Purpureocillium*, a new genus for the medically important *Paecilomyces lilacinus*. *FEMS Microbiol Lett* **321:**141–149.
202. **Al-Mohsen IZ, Sutton DA, Sigler L, Almodovar E, Mahgoub N, Frayha H, Al-Hajjar S, Rinaldi MG, Walsh TJ.** 2000. *Acrophialophora fusispora* brain abscess in a child with acute lymphoblastic leukemia: review of cases and taxonomy. *J Clin Microbiol* **38:**4569–4576.
203. **Guarro J, Gené J, Sigler L, Sutton DA, Arthur S, Steed LL.** 2002. *Acrophialophora fusispora* misidentified as *Scedosporium prolificans*. *J Clin Microbiol* **40:**3544–3545; author reply, 3545.
204. **Sigler L, Sutton DA.** 2002. *Acrophialophora fusispora* misidentified as *Scedosporium prolificans*. *J Clin Microbiol* **40:**3544–3545; author reply, 3545.
205. **Sandoval-Denis M, Gené J, Sutton DA, Wiederhold NP, Guarro J.** 2015. *Acrophialophora*, a poorly known fungus with clinical significance. *J Clin Microbiol* **53:**1549–1555.
206. **Houbraken J, Spierenburg H, Frisvad JC.** 2012. *Rasamsonia*, a new genus comprising thermotolerant and thermophilic *Talaromyces* and *Geosmithia* species. *Antonie van Leeuwenhoek* **101:**403–421.
207. **Grant DC, Sutton DA, Sandberg CA, Tyler RD, Jr, Thompson EH, Romanelli AM, Wickes BL.** 2009. Disseminated *Geosmithia argillacea* infection in a German shepherd dog. *Med Mycol* **47:**221–226.
208. **Barton RC, Borman AM, Johnson EM, Houbraken J, Hobson RP, Denton M, Conway SP, Brownlee KG, Peckham D, Lee TW.** 2010. Isolation of the fungus *Geosmithia argillacea* in sputum of people with cystic fibrosis. *J Clin Microbiol* **48:**2615–2617.
209. **Machouart M, Garcia-Hermoso D, Rivier A, Hassouni N, Catherinot E, Salmon A, Debourgogne A, Coignard H, Lecuit M, Bougnoux ME, Blanche S, Lortholary O.** 2011. Emergence of disseminated infections due to *Geosmithia argillacea* in patients with chronic granulomatous disease receiving long-term azole antifungal prophylaxis. *J Clin Microbiol* **49:**1681–1683.
210. **Houbraken J, Giraud S, Meijer M, Bertout S, Frisvad JC, Meis JF, Bouchara JP, Samson RA.** 2013. Taxonomy and antifungal susceptibility of clinically important *Rasamsonia* species. *J Clin Microbiol* **51:**22–30.
211. **Chen Q, Jiang JR, Zhang GZ, Cai L, Crous PW.** 2015. Resolving the *Phoma* enigma. *Stud Mycol* **82:**137–217.
212. **de Gruyter J, Woudenberg JH, Aveskamp MM, Verkley GJ, Groenewald JZ, Crous PW.** 2013. Redisposition of phoma-like anamorphs in Pleosporales. *Stud Mycol* **75:**1–36.
213. **Cano J, Guarro J, Gené J.** 2004. Molecular and morphological identification of *Colletotrichum* species of clinical interest. *J Clin Microbiol* **42:**2450–2454.
214. **Cannon PF, Damm U, Johnston PR, Weir BS.** 2012. Colletotrichum— current status and future directions. *Stud Mycol* **73:**181–213.
215. **Boerema GH, de Gruyter J, Noordeloos ME, Hamers MEC (ed).** 2004. *Phoma Identification Manual. Differentiation of Specific and Infra-Specific Taxa in Culture*. CABI Publishing, Cambridge, MA.
216. **Guégan S, Garcia-Hermoso D, Sitbon K, Ahmed S, Moguelet P, Dromer F, Lortholary O, French Mycosis Study Group.** 2016. Ten-year experience of cutaneous and/or subcutaneous infections due to Coelomycetes in France. *Open Forum Infect Dis* **3:**ofw106.
217. **Valenzuela-Lopez N, Sutton DA, Cano-Lira JF, Paredes K, Wiederhold N, Guarro J, Stchigel AM.** 2017. Coelomycetous fungi in the clinical setting: morphological convergence and cryptic diversity. *J Clin Microbiol* **55:**552–567.
218. **Guarro J, Svidzinski TE, Zaror L, Forjaz MH, Gené J, Fischman O.** 1998. Subcutaneous hyalohyphomycosis caused by *Colletotrichum gloeosporioides*. *J Clin Microbiol* **36:**3060–3065.
219. **Aribandi M, Bazan C, III, Rinaldi MG.** 2005. Magnetic resonance imaging findings in fatal primary cerebral infection due to *Chaetomium strumarium*. *Australas Radiol* **49:**166–169.
220. **Célard M, Dannaoui E, Piens MA, Guého E, Kirkorian G, Greenland T, Vandenesch F, Picot S.** 1999. Early *Microascus cinereus* endocarditis of a prosthetic valve implanted after *Staphylococcus aureus* endocarditis of the native valve. *Clin Infect Dis* **29:**691–692.

221. **Baddley JW, Moser SA, Sutton DA, Pappas PG.** 2000. *Microascus cinereus* (anamorph *Scopulariopsis*) brain abscess in a bone marrow transplant recipient. *J Clin Microbiol* **38:**395–397.
222. **Mohammedi I, Piens MA, Audigier-Valette C, Gantier JC, Argaud L, Martin O, Robert D.** 2004. Fatal *Microascus trigonosporus* (anamorph *Scopulariopsis*) pneumonia in a bone marrow transplant recipient. *Eur J Clin Microbiol Infect Dis* **23:**215–217.
223. **Aznar C, de Bievre C, Guiguen C.** 1989. Maxillary sinusitis from *Microascus cinereus* and *Aspergillus repens*. *Mycopathologia* **105:**93–97.
224. **Krisher KK, Holdridge NB, Mustafa MM, Rinaldi MG, McGough DA.** 1995. Disseminated *Microascus cirrosus* infection in pediatric bone marrow transplant recipient. *J Clin Microbiol* **33:**735–737.
225. **Marques AR, Kwon-Chung KJ, Holland SM, Turner ML, Gallin JI.** 1995. Suppurative cutaneous granulomata caused by *Microascus cinereus* in a patient with chronic granulomatous disease. *Clin Infect Dis* **20:**110–114.
226. **Migrino RQ, Hall GS, Longworth DL.** 1995. Deep tissue infections caused by *Scopulariopsis brevicaulis*: report of a case of prosthetic valve endocarditis and review. *Clin Infect Dis* **21:**672–674.
227. **Phillips P, Wood WS, Phillips G, Rinaldi MG.** 1989. Invasive hyalohyphomycosis caused by *Scopulariopsis brevicaulis* in a patient undergoing allogeneic bone marrow transplant. *Diagn Microbiol Infect Dis* **12:**429–432.
228. **Schinabeck MK, Ghannoum MA.** 2003. Human hyalohyphomycoses: a review of human infections due to *Acremonium* spp., *Paecilomyces* spp., *Penicillium* spp., and *Scopulariopsis* spp. *J Chemother* **15**(Suppl 2)**:**5–15.
229. **Ellison MD, Hung RT, Harris K, Campbell BH.** 1998. Report of the first case of invasive fungal sinusitis caused by *Scopulariopsis acremonium*: review of *Scopulariopsis* infections. *Arch Otolaryngol Head Neck Surg* **124:**1014–1016.
230. **Kriesel JD, Adderson EE, Gooch WM, III, Pavia AT.** 1994. Invasive sinonasal disease due to *Scopulariopsis candida*: case report and review of scopulariopsosis. *Clin Infect Dis* **19:**317–319.
231. **Patel R, Gustaferro CA, Krom RA, Wiesner RH, Roberts GD, Paya CV.** 1994. Phaeohyphomycosis due to *Scopulariopsis brumptii* in a liver transplant recipient. *Clin Infect Dis* **19:**198–200.
232. **Wuyts WA, Molzahn H, Maertens J, Verbeken EK, Lagrou K, Dupont LJ, Verleden GM.** 2005. Fatal *Scopulariopsis* infection in a lung transplant recipient: a case report. *J Heart Lung Transplant* **24:**2301–2304.
233. **Ustun C, Huls G, Stewart M, Marr KA.** 2006. Resistant *Microascus cirrosus* pneumonia can be treated with a combination of surgery, multiple anti-fungal agents and a growth factor. *Mycopathologia* **162:**299–302.
234. **Romanelli AM, Sutton DA, Thompson EH, Rinaldi MG, Wickes BL.** 2010. Sequence-based identification of filamentous basidiomycetous fungi from clinical specimens: a cautionary note. *J Clin Microbiol* **48:**741–752.
235. **Buzina W, Lang-Loidolt D, Braun H, Freudenschuss K, Stammberger H.** 2001. Development of molecular methods for identification of *Schizophyllum commune* from clinical samples. *J Clin Microbiol* **39:**2391–2396.
236. **Clark S, Campbell CK, Sandison A, Choa DI.** 1996. *Schizophyllum commune*: an unusual isolate from a patient with allergic fungal sinusitis. *J Infect* **32:**147–150.
237. **Kamei K, Unno H, Ito J, Nishimura K, Miyaji M.** 1999. Analysis of the cases in which *Schizophyllum commune* was isolated. *Nippon Ishinkin Gakkai Zasshi* **40:**175–181. [In Japanese.].
238. **Sigler L, Bartley JR, Parr DH, Morris AJ.** 1999. Maxillary sinusitis caused by medusoid form of *Schizophyllum commune*. *J Clin Microbiol* **37:**3395–3398.
239. **Rihs JD, Padhye AA, Good CB.** 1996. Brain abscess caused by *Schizophyllum commune*: an emerging basidiomycete pathogen. *J Clin Microbiol* **34:**1628–1632.
240. **Roh ML, Tuazon CU, Mandler R, Kwon-Chung KJ, Geist CE.** 2005. Sphenocavernous syndrome associated with *Schizophyllum commune* infection of the sphenoid sinus. *Ophthal Plast Reconstr Surg* **21:**71–74.
241. **Rampazzo A, Kuhnert P, Howard J, Bornand V.** 2009. *Hormographiella aspergillata* keratomycosis in a dog. *Vet Ophthalmol* **12:**43–47.
242. **Surmont I, Van Aelst F, Verbanck J, De Hoog GS.** 2002. A pulmonary infection caused by *Coprinus cinereus* (*Hormographiella aspergillata*) diagnosed after a neutropenic episode. *Med Mycol* **40:**217–219.
243. **Fan X, Xiao M, Kong F, Kudinha T, Wang H, Xu YC.** 2014. A rare fungal species, *Quambalaria cyanescens*, isolated from a patient after augmentation mammoplasty—environmental contaminant or pathogen? *PLoS One* **9:**e106949.
244. **Schell WA, Perfect JR.** 1996. Fatal, disseminated *Acremonium strictum* infection in a neutropenic host. *J Clin Microbiol* **34:**1333–1336.
245. **Warris A, Wesenberg F, Gaustad P, Verweij PE, Abrahamsen TG.** 2000. *Acremonium strictum* fungaemia in a paediatric patient with acute leukaemia. *Scand J Infect Dis* **32:** 442–444.
246. **Foell JL, Fischer M, Seibold M, Borneff-Lipp M, Wawer A, Horneff G, Burdach S.** 2007. Lethal double infection with *Acremonium strictum* and *Aspergillus fumigatus* during induction chemotherapy in a child with ALL. *Pediatr Blood Cancer* **49:**858–861.
247. **Keynan Y, Sprecher H, Weber G.** 2007. *Acremonium* vertebral osteomyelitis: molecular diagnosis and response to voriconazole. *Clin Infect Dis* **45:**e5–e6.
248. **Miyakis S, Velegraki A, Delikou S, Parcharidou A, Papadakis V, Kitra V, Papadatos I, Polychronopoulou S.** 2006. Invasive *Acremonium strictum* infection in a bone marrow transplant recipient. *Pediatr Infect Dis J* **25:**273–275.
249. **Drees M, Wickes BL, Gupta M, Hadley S.** 2007. *Lecythophora mutabilis* prosthetic valve endocarditis in a diabetic patient. *Med Mycol* **45:**463–467.
250. **Marriott DJ, Wong KH, Aznar E, Harkness JL, Cooper DA, Muir D.** 1997. *Scytalidium dimidiatum* and *Lecythophora hoffmannii*: unusual causes of fungal infections in a patient with AIDS. *J Clin Microbiol* **35:**2949–2952.
251. **Gavin PJ, Sutton DA, Katz BZ.** 2002. Fatal endocarditis in a neonate caused by the dematiaceous fungus *Phialemonium obovatum*: case report and review of the literature. *J Clin Microbiol* **40:**2207–2212.
252. **Tsang CC, Chan JF, Ip PP, Ngan AH, Chen JH, Lau SK, Woo PC.** 2014. Subcutaneous phaeohyphomycotic nodule due to *Phialemoniopsis hongkongensis* sp. nov. *J Clin Microbiol* **52:**3280–3289.
253. **Dan M, Yossepowitch O, Hendel D, Shwartz O, Sutton DA.** 2006. *Phialemonium curvatum* arthritis of the knee following intra-articular injection of a corticosteroid. *Med Mycol* **44:**571–574.
254. **Proia LA, Hayden MK, Kammeyer PL, Ortiz J, Sutton DA, Clark T, Schroers HJ, Summerbell RC.** 2004. *Phialemonium*: an emerging mold pathogen that caused 4 cases of hemodialysis-associated endovascular infection. *Clin Infect Dis* **39:**373–379.
255. **Weinberger M, Mahrshak I, Keller N, Goldscmied-Reuven A, Amariglio N, Kramer M, Tobar A, Samra Z, Pitlik SD, Rinaldi MG, Thompson E, Sutton D.** 2006. Isolated endogenous endophthalmitis due to a sporodochial-forming *Phialemonium curvatum* acquired through intracavernous autoinjections. *Med Mycol* **44:**253–259.
256. **Gupta AK, Horgan-Bell CB, Summerbell RC.** 1998. Onychomycosis associated with *Onychocola canadensis*: ten case reports and a review of the literature. *J Am Acad Dermatol* **39:**410–417.
257. **Sigler L, Abbott SP, Woodgyer AJ.** 1994. New records of nail and skin infection due to *Onychocola canadensis* and description of its teleomorph *Arachnomyces nodosetosus* sp. nov. *J Med Vet Mycol* **32:**275–285.
258. **Llovo J, Prieto E, Vazquez H, Muñoz A.** 2002. Onychomycosis due to *Onychocola canadensis*: report of the first two Spanish cases. *Med Mycol* **40:**209–212.
259. **Kisla TA, Cu-Unjieng A, Sigler L, Sugar J.** 2000. Medical management of *Beauveria bassiana* keratitis. *Cornea* **19:** 405–406.

260. **McDonnell PJ, Werblin TP, Sigler L, Green WR.** 1984. Mycotic keratitis due to *Beauveria alba*. *Cornea* **3:**213–216.
261. **Pariseau B, Nehls S, Ogawa GS, Sutton DA, Wickes BL, Romanelli AM.** 2010. *Beauveria* keratitis and biopesticides: case histories and a random amplification of polymorphic DNA comparison. *Cornea* **29:**152–158.
262. **Tu EY, Park AJ.** 2007. Recalcitrant *Beauveria bassiana* keratitis: confocal microscopy findings and treatment with posaconazole (Noxafil). *Cornea* **26:**1008–1010.
263. **Augustinsky J, Kammeyer P, Husain A, deHoog GS, Libertin CR.** 1990. *Engyodontium album* endocarditis. *J Clin Microbiol* **28:**1479–1481.
264. **Roilides E, Sigler L, Bibashi E, Katsifa H, Flaris N, Panteliadis C.** 1999. Disseminated infection due to *Chrysosporium zonatum* in a patient with chronic granulomatous disease and review of non-*Aspergillus* fungal infections in patients with this disease. *J Clin Microbiol* **37:**18–25.
265. **Anstead GM, Sutton DA, Graybill JR.** 2012. Adiaspiromycosis causing respiratory failure and a review of human infections due to *Emmonsia* and *Chrysosporium* spp. *J Clin Microbiol* **50:**1346–1354.
266. **Bourbeau P, McGough DA, Fraser H, Shah N, Rinaldi MG.** 1992. Fatal disseminated infection caused by *Myceliophthora thermophila*, a new agent of mycosis: case history and laboratory characteristics. *J Clin Microbiol* **30:**3019–3023.
267. **Destino L, Sutton DA, Helon AL, Havens PL, Thometz JG, Willoughby RE, Jr, Chusid MJ.** 2006. Severe osteomyelitis caused by *Myceliophthora thermophila* after a pitchfork injury. *Ann Clin Microbiol Antimicrob* **5:**21.
268. **Farina C, Gamba A, Tambini R, Beguin H, Trouillet JL.** 1998. Fatal aortic *Myceliophthora thermophila* infection in a patient affected by cystic medial necrosis. *Med Mycol* **36:**113–118.
269. **Tekkök IH, Higgins MJ, Ventureyra EC.** 1996. Posttraumatic gas-containing brain abscess caused by *Clostridium perfringens* with unique simultaneous fungal suppuration by *Myceliophthora thermophila*: case report. *Neurosurgery* **39:**1247–1251.
270. **Sigler L, Hambleton S, Paré JA.** 2013. Molecular characterization of reptile pathogens currently known as members of the chrysosporium anamorph of *Nannizziopsis vriesii* complex and relationship with some human-associated isolates. *J Clin Microbiol* **51:**3338–3357.
271. **Burgner D, Eagles G, Burgess M, Procopis P, Rogers M, Muir D, Pritchard R, Hocking A, Priest M.** 1998. Disseminated invasive infection due to *Metarrhizium anisopliae* in an immunocompromised child. *J Clin Microbiol* **36:** 1146–1150.
272. **de García MC, Arboleda ML, Barraquer F, Grose E.** 1997. Fungal keratitis caused by *Metarhizium anisopliae* var. *anisopliae*. *J Med Vet Mycol* **35:**361–363.
273. **Osorio S, de la Cámara R, Monteserin MC, Granados R, Oña F, Rodriguez-Tudela JL, Cuenca-Estrella M.** 2007. Recurrent disseminated skin lesions due to *Metarrhizium anisopliae* in an adult patient with acute myelogenous leukemia. *J Clin Microbiol* **45:**651–655.
274. **Revankar SG, Sutton DA, Sanche SE, Rao J, Zervos M, Dashti F, Rinaldi MG.** 1999. *Metarrhizium anisopliae* as a cause of sinusitis in immunocompetent hosts. *J Clin Microbiol* **37:**195–198.
275. **Chouaki T, Lavarde V, Lachaud L, Raccurt CP, Hennequin C.** 2002. Invasive infections due to *Trichoderma* species: report of 2 cases, findings of in vitro susceptibility testing, and review of the literature. *Clin Infect Dis* **35:** 1360–1367.
276. **Munoz FM, Demmler GJ, Travis WR, Ogden AK, Rossmann SN, Rinaldi MG.** 1997. *Trichoderma longibrachiatum* infection in a pediatric patient with aplastic anemia. *J Clin Microbiol* **35:**499–503.
277. **Richter S, Cormican MG, Pfaller MA, Lee CK, Gingrich R, Rinaldi MG, Sutton DA.** 1999. Fatal disseminated *Trichoderma longibrachiatum* infection in an adult bone marrow transplant patient: species identification and review of the literature. *J Clin Microbiol* **37:**1154–1160.
278. **Seguin P, Degeilh B, Grulois I, Gacouin A, Maugendre S, Dufour T, Dupont B, Camus C.** 1995. Successful treatment of a brain abscess due to *Trichoderma longibrachiatum* after surgical resection. *Eur J Clin Microbiol Infect Dis* **14:**445–448.
279. **Castro LG, Salebian A, Sotto MN.** 1990. Hyalohyphomycosis by *Paecilomyces lilacinus* in a renal transplant patient and a review of human *Paecilomyces* species infections. *J Med Vet Mycol* **28:**15–26.
280. **Chan-Tack KM, Thio CL, Miller NS, Karp CL, Ho C, Merz WG.** 1999. *Paecilomyces lilacinus* fungemia in an adult bone marrow transplant recipient. *Med Mycol* **37:**57–60.
281. **Williamson PR, Kwon-Chung KJ, Gallin JI.** 1992. Successful treatment of *Paecilomyces varioti* infection in a patient with chronic granulomatous disease and a review of *Paecilomyces* species infections. *Clin Infect Dis* **14:**1023–1026.
282. **Okhravi N, Lightman S.** 2007. Clinical manifestations, treatment and outcome of *Paecilomyces lilacinus* infections. *Clin Microbiol Infect* **13:**554.
283. **Pastor FJ, Guarro J.** 2006. Clinical manifestations, treatment and outcome of *Paecilomyces lilacinus* infections. *Clin Microbiol Infect* **12:**948–960.
284. **De Ravin SS, Challipalli M, Anderson V, Shea YR, Marciano B, Hilligoss D, Marquesen M, Decastro R, Liu YC, Sutton DA, Wickes BL, Kammeyer PL, Sigler L, Sullivan K, Kang EM, Malech HL, Holland SM, Zelazny AM.** 2011. *Geosmithia argillacea*: an emerging cause of invasive mycosis in human chronic granulomatous disease. *Clin Infect Dis* **52:**e136–e143.
285. **Doyon JB, Sutton DA, Theodore P, Dhillon G, Jones KD, Thompson EH, Fu J, Wickes BL, Koehler JE, Schwartz BS.** 2013. *Rasamsonia argillacea* pulmonary and aortic graft infection in an immune-competent patient. *J Clin Microbiol* **51:**719–722.
286. **Mouhajir A, Matray O, Giraud S, Mély L, Marguet C, Sermet-Gaudelus I, Le Gal S, Labbé F, Person C, Troussier F, Ballet JJ, Gargala G, Zouhair R, Bougnoux ME, Bouchara JP, Favennec L.** 2016. Long-term *Rasamsonia argillacea* complex species colonization revealed by PCR amplification of repetitive DNA sequences in cystic fibrosis patients. *J Clin Microbiol* **54:**2804–2812.
287. **Vasoo S, Yong LK, Sultania-Dudani P, Scorza ML, Sekosan M, Beavis KG, Huhn GD.** 2011. Phaeomycotic cysts caused by *Phoma* species. *Diagn Microbiol Infect Dis* **70:**531–533.
288. **Summerbell RC.** 1993. The benomyl test as a fundamental diagnostic method for medical mycology. *J Clin Microbiol* **31:**572–577.
289. **Pounder JI, Simmon KE, Barton CA, Hohmann SL, Brandt ME, Petti CA.** 2007. Discovering potential pathogens among fungi identified as nonsporulating molds. *J Clin Microbiol* **45:**568–571.
290. **Fredricks DN, Smith C, Meier A.** 2005. Comparison of six DNA extraction methods for recovery of fungal DNA as assessed by quantitative PCR. *J Clin Microbiol* **43:** 5122–5128.
291. **Pryce TM, Palladino S, Kay ID, Coombs GW.** 2003. Rapid identification of fungi by sequencing the ITS1 and ITS2 regions using an automated capillary electrophoresis system. *Med Mycol* **41:**369–381.
292. **Kwiatkowski NP, Babiker WM, Merz WG, Carroll KC, Zhang SX.** 2012. Evaluation of nucleic acid sequencing of the D1/D2 region of the large subunit of the 28S rDNA and the internal transcribed spacer region using SmartGene IDNS software for identification of filamentous fungi in a clinical laboratory. *J Mol Diagn* **14:**393–401.
293. **Hibbett DS, et al.** 2007. A higher-level phylogenetic classification of the Fungi. *Mycol Res* **111:**509–547.
294. **Etienne KA, Roe CC, Smith RM, Vallabhaneni S, Duarte C, Escadon P, Castaneda E, Gomez BL, de Bedout C, López LF, Salas V, Hederra LM, Fernandez J, Pidal P, Hormazabel JC, Otaiza-O'Ryan F, Vannberg FO, Gillece J, Lemmer D, Driebe EM, Englethaler DM, Litvintseva AP.** 2016. Whole-genome sequencing to determine origin of multinational outbreak of *Sarocladium kiliense* bloodstream infections. *Emerg Infect Dis* **22:**476–481.

295. **Serena C, Ortoneda M, Capilla J, Pastor FJ, Sutton DA, Rinaldi MG, Guarro J.** 2003. In vitro activities of new antifungal agents against *Chaetomium* spp. and inoculum standardization. *Antimicrob Agents Chemother* **47:**3161–3164.
296. **González GM, Sutton DA, Thompson E, Tijerina R, Rinaldi MG.** 2001. In vitro activities of approved and investigational antifungal agents against 44 clinical isolates of basidiomycetous fungi. *Antimicrob Agents Chemother* **45:**633–635.
297. **Steinbach WJ, Schell WA, Miller JL, Perfect JR, Martin PL.** 2004. Fatal *Scopulariopsis brevicaulis* infection in a paediatric stem-cell transplant patient treated with voriconazole and caspofungin and a review of *Scopulariopsis* infections in immunocompromised patients. *J Infect* **48:**112–116.
298. **Ryder NS.** 1999. Activity of terbinafine against serious fungal pathogens. *Mycoses* **42**(Suppl 2)**:**115–119.
299. **Lass-Florl C, Cuenca-Estrella M, Denning DW, Rodriguez-Tudela JL.** 2006. Antifungal susceptibility testing in *Aspergillus* spp. according to EUCAST methodology. *Med Mycol* **44**(Suppl 1)**:**S319–S325.
300. **Castelli MV, Alastruey-Izquierdo A, Cuesta I, Monzon A, Mellado E, Rodriguez-Tudela JL, Cuenca-Estrella M.** 2008. Susceptibility testing and molecular classification of *Paecilomyces* spp. *Antimicrob Agents Chemother* **52:**2926–2928.
301. **Pfaller MA, Rhomberg PR, Messer SA, Jones RN, Castanheira M.** 2015. Isavuconazole, micafungin, and 8 comparator antifungal agents' susceptibility profiles for common and uncommon opportunistic fungi collected in 2013: temporal analysis of antifungal drug resistance using CLSI species-specific clinical breakpoints and proposed epidemiological cutoff values. *Diagn Microbiol Infect Dis* **82:**303–313.

Agents of Systemic and Subcutaneous Mucormycosis and Entomophthoromycosis

DEA GARCIA-HERMOSO, ALEXANDRE ALANIO, OLIVIER LORTHOLARY, AND FRANÇOISE DROMER

124

Mucormycosis and entomophthoromycosis are invasive fungal infections caused by environmental pauciseptate filamentous fungi. Mucormycosis is caused by the ubiquitous *Mucorales* and mostly occurs in immunocompromised patients or those with diabetes mellitus. These fungi are responsible for rhinocerebral, pulmonary, cutaneous, or disseminated infections characterized by angioinvasion, necrosis, and severe prognosis despite current antifungal and surgical therapies. Entomophthoromycosis, which occurs mostly in apparently immunocompetent hosts, is caused by members of *Entomophthorales* (responsible for conidiobolomycosis) and *Basidiobolales* (responsible for basidiobolomycosis), both mostly found in warm climates. Entomophthoromycosis presents as subcutaneous infections with favorable outcome after prolonged azole therapy without surgery, although it is potentially associated with disfiguring lesions.

TAXONOMY

The classification of the kingdom of *Fungi* has been constantly modified over the last decades. Recently, a comprehensive phylogenetic study based on multigene sequence analyses (1) proposed a classification that accepts one kingdom, one subkingdom, seven phyla, 10 subphyla, 35 classes, 12 subclasses, and 129 orders. The most important modifications were the creation of subphylum *Dikarya*, which includes members of *Ascomycota* and *Basidiomycota*, and the redistribution of taxa located in phyla *Zygomycota* and *Chytridiomycota*. The etiological agents responsible for mucormycosis (order *Mucorales*) and those responsible for entomophthoromycosis (orders *Entomophthorales* and *Basidiobolales*) were traditionally assigned to the lower fungus phylum *Zygomycota*. In the study by Hibbett et al., this phylum is no longer accepted because of its polyphyletic nature (1). Taxa are redistributed between *Glomeromycota* and four new subphyla of uncertain position (*incertae sedis*): *Mucoromycotina* (which includes three orders, the core group of *Mucorales*, *Endogonales*, and *Mortierellales*), the *Entomophthoromycotina* (with the order *Entomophthorales*), the *Zoopagomycotina* (with the order *Zoopagales*), and finally, the subphylum *Kickxellomycotina* (which includes the orders *Kickxellales*, *Dimargaritales*, *Harpellales*, and *Asellariales*).

Over the last years, phylogenetic interactions among members of the order *Mucorales* have been studied (2–4). These studies have mainly shown the polyphyletic nature of families (*Thamnidiaceae*, *Mucoraceae*, and *Chaetocladiaceae*) and genera such as *Absidia* and *Mucor*. The family structure of *Mucorales* was recently studied on the basis of the phylogenetic analysis of four markers (5). *Rhizopodaceae* is one of the newly erected families, which includes the genus *Rhizopus* and other pathogenic genera.

Revisions of other genera have been published in recent years and will be detailed below (3, 6–10). Of note, the first analysis of a genome sequence from a member of the *Mucorales* (*Rhizopus arrhizus*) was published in 2009 (11). The genome annotation for the species *Mucor circinelloides* var. *circinelloides* is now available (http://www.broadinstitute.org).

Table 1 displays the *Mucorales* species that have been described as human pathogens or potential human pathogens, considering the new family structure published by Hoffmann et al. (5).

Recently, the subphylum *Entomophthoromycotina* was elevated to the phylum *Entomophthoromycota*. The monophyly of these organisms was then confirmed by multigene phylogeny analysis (12, 13). This newly erected phylum comprises more than 250 species distributed among three classes (*Basidiobolomycetes*, *Neozygitomycetes*, and *Entomophthoromycetes*) and six families (*Basidiobolaceae*, *Neozygitaceae*, *Ancylistaceae*, *Completoriaceae*, *Entomophthoraceae*, and *Meristracraceae*). There are more than 25 species in the genus *Conidiobolus*, but only three (*C. coronatus*, *C. lamprauges*, and *C. incongruus*) have been recovered from clinical specimens; in the genus *Basidiobolus*, *Basidiobolus ranarum* is the only species of the genus to provoke human disease (14, 15).

MUCORMYCOSIS

Epidemiology and Transmission

Mucorales are ubiquitous fungi widely distributed in the environment (soil, plants, and decaying organic material) (16). They are frequent pathogens of plants and contaminants of grains and food such as fruit or bread. Airborne spores are considered the infectious particles responsible for disease, particularly in immunocompromised individuals, explaining the most frequent body localizations (skin, sinuses, and lungs). A comprehensive study of cases

TABLE 1 Species of *Mucorales* (subphylum *Mucoromycotina*) involved in human mucormycosis

Family	Genus	Species
Lichtheimiaceae	*Lichtheimia*	*L. corymbifera* (syn., *Mycocladus corymbifer*; *Absidia corymbifera*)
		L. ramosa (syn., *Absidia ramosa*)
		L. ornata (syn., *Absidia ornata*)
	Rhizomucor	*R. pusillus*
Mucoraceae	*Mucor*	*M. circinelloides*
		M. indicus
		M. velutinosus
		M. irregularis (formerly *Rhizomucor variabilis* var. *variabilis*)
		M. ramosissimus
	Actinomucor	*Ac. elegans*
	Cokeromyces	*C. recurvatus*
Saksenaeaceae	*Saksenaea*	*S. vasiformis*
		S. erythrospora
		S. oblongispora
	Apophysomyces	*A. elegans*
		A. trapeziformis
		A. ossiformis
		A. variabilis
Rhizopodaceae	*Rhizopus*	*R. microsporus*
		R. arrhizus (syn., *R. oryzae*)
		R. schipperae
Syncephalastraceae	*Syncephalastrum*	*S. racemosum*
Cunninghamellaceae	*Cunninghamella*	*C. bertholletiae*
		C. echinulata

diagnosed in France noted that immunocompetent patients may develop posttrauma skin infections, representing up to 18% of all mucormycosis cases (17). In addition, necrotizing cutaneous cases have been recently reported after a tornado in Joplin, Missouri (18), or as a cause of infections following combat-related injuries in Afghanistan (19). These species are easily found as laboratory contaminants and can be a source of nosocomial infections, including outbreaks (20–25). Specific geographical distribution and environmental niches will be described for relevant species in the corresponding section.

Some reports have suggested an increasing incidence of mucormycosis, based on single-center studies (26–30). In a retrospective analysis of hospital records in France, our group recently provided a population-based estimate of mucormycosis incidence and trends for the country over a 10-year period (31). Using two available sources of information, we then better estimated the real burden of mucormycosis infections through a capture-recapture method (32) and found different incidences according to the region, suggesting local ecological specificities at a country level (33). The incidence significantly increased over time, with an average $0.9/10^6$ annual incidence rate different from the incidence reported in a population-based study in California in 1992 to 1993 ($1.7/10^6$) (34) and in Spain in 2005 ($0.43/10^6$) (35). Such an increasing trend was further confirmed in France (36). The sex ratio (M/F) (1.8 versus 1.1) and mean age (38.8 versus 57.1 years) differ in the review of 929 cases published between 1940 and 1999 and in France (31, 37).

Diabetes is a major risk factor (23% in France and up to 36% of the cases elsewhere, 20% with type 1 diabetes) (17, 37, 38), with a significant increase in the incidence of diabetes-associated mucormycosis recently documented in France (31) and in a tertiary care center in North India (39). In the latter study, 131 out of 178 cases were observed in uncontrolled diabetic patients (73.6%), and more importantly, mucormycosis led to the diagnosis of diabetes in 56 cases (42.7% of diabetes cases). Diabetes mellitus was also found in 15% (type 1 = 13%) of 157 pediatric cases (40). Diabetes was an independent risk factor for mucormycosis in patients with leukemia and/or bone marrow transplantation (27) and significantly influenced the occurrence of mucormycosis during solid organ transplantation (SOT) (17, 41). Of note, the most frequent clinical presentation of diabetes-associated mucormycosis is sinusitis. Among patients with hematological malignancies, which represented 50% of the cases in France (17), those with acute leukemia (profound neutropenia or relapse) or allogeneic stem cell transplantation are more prone to develop mucormycosis, the lungs being the most frequent site involved. Mucormycosis most often occurs more than 3 months after transplant in the setting of graft versus host disease (27, 28, 30, 42–46). Mucormycosis now represents 7% to 8% of invasive fungal infections in bone marrow transplant patients (47, 48). An increased incidence of mucormycosis was observed in patients with hematological malignancies or stem cell transplant in France (31), as already noted in the 1990s in one U.S. center (30). In that population, the potential role of prior exposure to antifungals such as voriconazole and caspofungin that lack activity against *Mucorales* has been reported (27, 28, 41, 49–52).

Mucormycosis represents 2% of invasive fungal infections during SOT, mostly in kidney transplantation (53). In a recent international prospective study of SOT recipients, renal failure, diabetes mellitus, and prior voriconazole and/or caspofungin use were associated with a higher risk of mucormycoses, whereas tacrolimus was associated with a lower risk (41). Liver transplant recipients were more likely to have disseminated disease and developed infection significantly earlier after transplantation than other SOT recipients.

Mucormycosis can also develop in HIV-infected patients or intravenous drug users. It can affect otherwise healthy individuals after cutaneous injuries with contaminated soil, in almost 20% of the cases in some studies. Finally, it may present as community-acquired or as a health care-related disease. A careful review of cases published between 1970 and 2008 revealed 169 mucormycosis cases associated with health care (with 29% of them in children), of which 72% were published after 1990 (21). Outbreaks of mucormycosis are rare but have been related to building construction and use of contaminated adhesive tape, ostomy bags, or wooden tongue depressors and more recently to contaminated "linen" (24).

Clinical Manifestations

Localized and disseminated diseases need to be differentiated (44). The most frequent localized forms are sinusitis and pneumonia, representing 25% to 39% and 24% to 30% of clinical sites involved, respectively, in three recent series (17, 37, 54). Dissemination rates vary from 3% to more than 50% in patients with hematological malignancies (depending to some extent on the underlying diseases and the site of infection) (37, 44, 45).

Sinus involvement (isolated sinusitis, rhinocerebral, and sinoorbital forms) is the most common presentation in diabetes patients and intravenous drug users, and pulmonary infection is the second most common presentation; the reverse is true in hematology patients (27, 37). Infection causes necrosis and hemorrhage and may be localized or associated with dissemination. Clinicoradiological presentation is similar to that of invasive aspergillosis in patients with hematological malignancies, although the presence of a reversed halo sign may be suggestive of (55, 56) but not specific to (57, 58) mucormycosis. In a recent study of 58 SOT patients with mucormycosis, pulmonary localization was present in 31 (53%), including 23 with localized infection (59).

Localized cutaneous lesions are most often encountered in immunocompetent hosts (37) and follow injury and contamination with airborne spores or soil (60–62) and, less often, surgery or burns (23). Local extension and hematogenous dissemination may occur. In contrast, skin lesions resulting from dissemination from other sites are rare.

Cerebral infection can complicate sinusitis or can occur independently, especially in intravenous drug users. Cognitive disturbances and focal neurological deficits are often present. Gastrointestinal lesions are described in 7% of cases and occur in low-birth-weight, premature infants and malnourished individuals and after peritoneal dialysis (37). They are responsible for abdominal pain and digestive hemorrhage, and complications include digestive tract perforation, peritonitis, and dissemination to the liver.

Treatment

■ Prophylaxis

In immunocompromised patients, there is no benefit of the prophylactic use of azoles such as fluconazole or itraconazole because of the lack of (major) activity against *Mucorales* (30, 45, 46). The best preventive measure is the reduction of environmental exposure, notably with the use of high-efficiency particulate air-filtered rooms (45). The specific role of posaconazole as a prophylactic agent against mucormycosis has not been demonstrated (63, 64), and there is no decreased incidence of the disease in the hematology population over recent years, although posaconazole has been available since 2007 (33). In addition, no study has yet investigated isavuconazole as prophylaxis of mucormycosis.

■ Curative treatment

In the review by Roden et al., survival of untreated patients was 3%, but 64% of patients who received antifungal therapy survived (37). Combined medical and radical surgical treatments, especially for rhinocerebral and skin localizations, in association with correction of the underlying disease wherever possible (i.e., acidosis, hyperglycemia, neutrophil recovery, and modulation of immunosuppressive therapy), offer the best chance of survival (65, 66).

Lipid derivatives of amphotericin B (AMB) given early in the course of the disease are probably more effective and better tolerated than AMB deoxycholate (67). Clinical response has been obtained with a high dose of liposomal AMB in patients who failed with conventional dosages (68, 69); therefore, one of the two available options (lipid complex or liposomal formulation) is the cornerstone first-line therapy (70, 71). In the United States, isavuconazole has been approved for the treatment of mucormycosis; in Europe, isavuconazole has recently been made available as a first-line alternative to lipid formulations of amphotericin B when the latter are inappropriate.

In addition, isavuconazole efficacy has been documented in a limited number of patients as a first-line therapy, with a 10% response rate at week 12 in the Vital study (72) versus 48% with liposomal amphotericin B in the AmBizygo trial (73). Posaconazole in its oral tablet or intravenous formulation can only be considered a second-line therapy; iron chelators such as deferasirox should not be used, and echinocandins in combination with polyenes are considered a second-line therapy option. Global case fatality rates vary from 47% to 84% (37), with those of rhinocerebral forms ranging from 20% to 69% (29, 39). Survival is reduced in cases of hematological malignancies compared with diabetes mellitus (17).

Collection, Transport, and Storage of Specimens

Mucormycosis is one of the most rapidly progressing invasive fungal infections. The diagnosis of mucormycosis should be considered an emergency because delaying therapy will affect outcome (74). Although clinical features are not specific, some early radiological features make the diagnosis of mucormycosis more probable than other invasive fungal infections, particularly invasive aspergillosis (58). A combination of well-known predisposing factors and clinical and/or radiological signs must alert the physician and prompt the institution of immediate diagnostic procedures. Since currently available methods developed for the diagnosis of invasive fungal infections are based on antigens that are not produced by *Mucorales* (75), the diagnosis relies mainly on direct examination and/or recovery of the fungus and/or detection of their nucleic acids in pathological tissues, body fluids, or exudates. Blood cultures are not appropriate for the diagnosis. In high-risk patients, specimens, preferentially from deep lesions and sterile sites, must be rapidly and aseptically collected in sufficient quantities. Larger volumes will increase the likelihood of fungal recovery and will allow more diagnostic procedures (direct examination, culture, DNA extraction for PCR, histopathology) as well as storage of the sample for further analyses. For rhinocerebral localization, nasal discharge or scraping, sinus aspirate, or a tissue specimen from an abnormally vascularized area should be obtained. For pulmonary localization, sputum, bronchial aspirate, and bronchoalveolar lavage fluids can be examined, taking into account the low sensitivity of these specimens (76, 77). Negative, transbronchial, or percutaneous computerized tomography-guided biopsies of pulmonary lesions can be performed, but the potential of induced morbidity must be kept in mind (78).

Separate specimens must be sent for microbiological and histological analysis, because formalin used for histopathology inhibits fungal growth. Direct examination remains the most rapid diagnostic technique, and culture is still an essential step to test susceptibility to antifungal drugs. Reliable identification at the species level still relies on obtaining the isolate in culture. The transport container should be sterile and humidified with a few drops of sterile saline. The specimen should not be refrigerated and should ideally be transported to the laboratory within 2 h after collection and processed rapidly, because *Mucorales* are easily damaged and sensitive to environmental stresses (79). Biopsy specimen grinding is deleterious for the *Mucorales* because of the coenocytic nature of the hyphae. Biopsy specimens should be sliced into small pieces of tissue that are then dispatched for direct examination and culture.

Direct Examination and Histopathology

Demonstration of hyphae in clinical samples provides strong evidence of mucormycosis because *Mucorales* are environmental airborne moulds that could be present in conidial form in nonsterile specimens, with false-positive cultures as a result. Direct examination is a key test for two reasons: (i) culture from clinical samples is frequently negative (80) and (ii) histology requires multiple steps that necessarily delay diagnosis.

■ Microscopy

Direct examination can be performed with wet mounts of the sample or after addition of chlorazol black. However, optical brightener (calcofluor white, Blankophor, or Uvitex 2B) that specifically stains the chitin contained in the cell wall, coupled with a clearing and dissociating agent, such as KOH, provides better sensitivity (76). It is always a good idea to examine the slides again the following day, especially in the presence of thick samples, because of possible false negatives resulting from insufficient dissociation of tissues.

The morphological characteristics suggestive of *Mucorales* hyphae are specific and can be differentiated from those of *Aspergillus*, *Fusarium*, or *Scedosporium*. Hyphae are large (5 to 25 μm), irregular, hyaline, non- or pauciseptate, and thin walled with a ribbon-like morphology. A twisted or folded appearance of the hyphae is frequently observed. In contrast to the acute (45°) branching pattern observed in hyalohyphomycetes, wide branching angles (≥90°) are suggestive of *Mucorales*. If hyphae are fragmented, the typical features are missing, which makes it difficult to make a reliable diagnosis based solely on direct microscopy. However, the same characteristic features can be observed in tissue samples after histopathological preparation based on Gomori methenamine-silver or periodic acid-Schiff staining. Of note, the detection of *Mucorales* is difficult with use of hematoxylin-eosin stain. Sometimes, if only a few hyphae are present and the tissue section contains cross-sections through the hyphae, it can produce the appearance of yeast or vacuole-like structures, making the morphology difficult to interpret. Classically, *Mucorales* are angioinvasive, with invasion of venous and arterial walls frequently associated with infarction of the surrounding tissue. The inflammatory response is varied, ranging from none at all to a neutrophil infiltrate alone, granulomatous response alone, or both together. Perineural invasion can also be observed (81). Immunohistochemistry techniques based on commercially available kits can be used in difficult cases (82).

Antigen Detection

There are currently no specific antigen detection methods available for the diagnosis of mucormycosis. Moreover, testing for the presence of β-D-glucan is not helpful.

Isolation Procedures

Recovery of *Mucorales* from clinical specimens is difficult, with positive culture in only 15 to 25% of cases (80). However, culture is suitable for the definite diagnosis of mucormycosis, especially in cases of negative direct examination, keeping in mind that the lack of galactomannan antigen detection may indirectly suggest the diagnosis of mucormycosis. Indeed, clinical or radiological features are not specific for invasive fungal infection, nor can they distinguish between mucormycosis and other invasive fungal infections due to *Aspergillus*, *Fusarium*, or *Scedosporium*, especially in the hematological setting. However, the therapeutic management is different, and isolation of a fungus is sometimes the unique diagnostic element. Culture is also of prime importance for identification to the species level, especially since morphological structures are not species specific in tissues, and for antifungal susceptibility testing of the isolate (83). Primarily, culture is typically performed on rich medium such as Sabouraud dextrose agar, with additional antibiotic to inhibit bacterial growth. Cycloheximide-containing media should not be used, because inhibition of fungal growth can be observed for some species. After inoculation, plates must be incubated between 25–30°C and 37°C to allow growth of thermotolerant and thermointolerant isolates (84). However, Sabouraud dextrose agar is often not appropriate for morphological identification purposes, and growth on potato dextrose agar (PDA) is more suitable.

Detection of Nucleic Acids in Clinical Materials

In many cases, histopathology and/or direct examination are positive but culture fails. Species identification is, however, important for epidemiological purposes and for species-specific antifungal susceptibility profiles. PCR-based molecular identification can be performed with formalin-fixed, paraffin-embedded (85) frozen or fresh tissue specimens. In formalin-fixed, paraffin-embedded tissues, extracted DNA is often of poor quality because of fragmentation after fixation (86). Furthermore, extracted DNA usually contains small amounts of fungal DNA relative to the large quantity of human DNA. Consequently, PCR-based identification must rely on amplification of small fragments of DNA that should ideally allow sequence discrimination between species upon sequencing. PCR based on internal transcribed spacer 1 (ITS1) and ITS2 primers followed by sequencing has been proposed in formalin-fixed, paraffin-embedded organs recovered from mice with experimental mucormycosis (87). It has also been evaluated in formalin-fixed, paraffin-embedded human tissues, with identification of *Mucorales* in 7/18 samples harboring non-septate hyphae, based on histopathological reporting (85). A seminested PCR technique based on the 18S ribosomal DNA loci has also been used with *Mucorales* identification in 13/23 samples for which nonseptate hyphae were observed by histology (88). This molecular tool has also been prospectively evaluated with identification of *Mucorales* in six samples, of which five were culture positive (89, 90). An approach based on real-time PCR has been developed based on cytochrome *b* locus amplification. It allowed discrimination between different genera of *Mucorales* using analysis of melting curves (identification of 35/62 formalin-fixed, paraffin-embedded tissue samples) (91). Quantitative PCR using multiple target-specific assays has been developed to detect and identify *Mucorales* in formalin-fixed, paraffin-embedded human tissues (92). Multiplex PCR coupled with electrospray ionization in direct-positive/culture-negative unfixed clinical samples seems potentially interesting, allowing genus and species identification (93).

Fluorescent dye-labeled oligonucleotides with direct hybridization (fluorescent *in situ* hybridization) on the pathologic tissue is a promising tool because it does not require DNA extractions or PCR amplification and can be performed on formalin-fixed, paraffin-embedded tissue samples. It uses fluorescent DNA probes that are specific for 5.8S or 18S RNA of different groups of fungi. After hybridization, fluorescence of the microorganism can be observed directly on the slide (94, 95). Localization of the fluorescence can provide additional information that can reinforce the diagnosis. This tool seems particularly adapted for when the yield of DNA extraction or the quality of the extracted DNA is poor. Indeed, PCR-negative, fluorescent, *in situ* hybridization-positive results have been observed (95).

PCR-Based Diagnosis in Serum: Mucormycosis Screening

In addition to the molecular methods developed for fungal identification from tissues, another strategy, inspired by the screening strategy for patients at risk of aspergillosis, is emerging for the diagnosis of mucormycosis. In a population with a relatively high prevalence of mucormycosis, one recent study proposed to screen sequential serum samples by PCR targeting *Mucorales* genes of *Rhizopus* spp., *Mucor* spp., *Rhizomucor* spp., and *Lichtheimia* spp. Using this method, the authors were able to establish the diagnosis of mucormycosis between 3 and 68 days before a diagnosis based on histopathology or culture (96). A retrospective analysis of 44 patients in a multicentric French study validated these findings. In addition, it showed that a negativation of the qPCR test was associated with a better prognosis than persistently positive qPCR during treatment (97). Based on the same qPCR assays, a screening strategy has been tested on burn patients with high risk of invasive wound mucormycosis (IWM). After retrospective analysis of patients with and without IWM, PCR was done twice a week, and patients were treated once the PCR became positive. The treatment was stopped after two negative PCR results. This strategy decreased the burden of IWM in this high-risk population and improved outcome (23). Other PCR assays have been proposed recently with different designs, allowing detection of a broader spectrum of *Mucorales* with a combination of two assays in serum, tissue (98, 99), or BAL (100).

All qPCR assays must be standardized and then could be proposed, as a standard, to diagnose early invasive mucormycosis and potentially be used in a screening strategy in high-risk patients.

Identification

■ Phenotypic identification

General Description

Routine identification of *Mucorales* to the species level is mainly based on the examination of their macroscopic and asexual microscopic characteristics, although some other criteria such as physiological tests (101) or maximum growth temperature can be used. The formation of zygospores is not useful in routine identification unless the species is homozygous. The use of media with high carbohydrate content favors production of an abundant mycelium, which inhibits the production of asexual fruiting bodies by which the species can be identified. Therefore, media such as 2% malt, potato dextrose, and cherry decoction (acidic) agars are recommended for subculture of most of the *Mucorales* species, although some of these media are not commercially available. To trigger sporulation in genera such as *Apophysomyces* or *Saksenaea*, which are emerging pathogens (102–104), nutritionally deficient media containing a low percentage of yeast extract solution are advisable (105). Multiple factors such as light and temperature also influence the growth, the morphology, and the sporulation of these fungi. Several species are thermotolerant, capable of growing at a temperature well over 40°C. Mycelial development of the *Mucorales* tends to be rapid (24 to 48 h) and extensive. Colony appearance varies according to the species, the age of the culture, and the mycological media used. It is recommended for an accurate morphological study of *Mucorales* to use subculture at 27 to 30°C. Macroscopic examination involves the description of the colonies (height, color, texture) and the sporangiophore spatial branching configuration that can be observed under a 10× objective or a binocular loupe. For microscopic characteristics, a detailed study of adhesive tape mounts or teased mounts (a small piece of mycelium plus fruiting bodies placed in a water drop and gently needle teased) is essential for the description of the sporulating structures of the species. Fungi in the order *Mucorales* are characterized by branched, nonseptate, wide mycelia (10 to 20 μm) with chitinous walls. Sexual reproduction occurs by means of zygospore formation after fusion of hyphal branches from the same (homothallic) or from sexually differentiated mycelia (heterothallic) (106). The mature zygospore is often thick walled and undergoes an obligatory dormant period before germination. Asexual multiplication is by means of nonmotile sporangiospores (endospores) borne in closed sac-like structures named sporangia. They can exist as multispored sporangia or sporangiola (small sporangia) having few (to one) spores. Sporangia are supported by specialized hyphae named sporangiophores. In some species, they arise from a branched system of rhizoids, which anchor the sporangiophore to the substratum. These rhizoids are connected by a rooting branch called a stolon. Additional morphological structures are the columellae (central axis of the sporangium) and the apophysis (a swelling of the sporangiophore just below the columella). Some species can produce thick-walled and/or thin-walled swollen structures named chlamydospores and oidia, respectively. The liberation of sporangiospores occurs by breakage or deliquescence of the sporangial wall (Fig. 1). Structures of *Mucorales* used for routine identification include branching of sporangiophores, type of sporangia (merosporangia or sporangiola), shape, color, presence or absence of apophyses and columellae, and presence or absence of rhizoids or chlamydospores.

Several potentially useful websites are available: www.msgercdoctorfungus.com; www.mycology.adelaide.edu.au; www.cbs.knaw.nl; http://www.mycobank.org.

Description of Specific Genera and Species

Morphological (macroscopic and microscopic) characteristics of those species frequently implicated in human infections are described below. Only major features are mentioned, from our own experience and from descriptions in specialized books (14, 20, 107). All colony morphology descriptions are made from subcultures on MEA (2% malt agar) at 30°C (unless otherwise specified). The colonies of *Mucorales* have mostly floccose textures with colors varying from white (*Saksenaea*) to yellow (*Mucor*), brownish (*Apophysomyces*), or gray (*Lichtheimia, Rhizomucor*). The woolly brown-beige colonies of *Actinomucor elegans* are the exception. *Rhizopus* produces high aerial mycelium, whereas *Rhizomucor* produces a low aerial turf of 2- to 3-μm-high mycelium. The morphology of sporangiophores (height, branching) can vary depending on the genus. It can be branched as in *Lichtheimia* or *Mucor*, irregularly branched

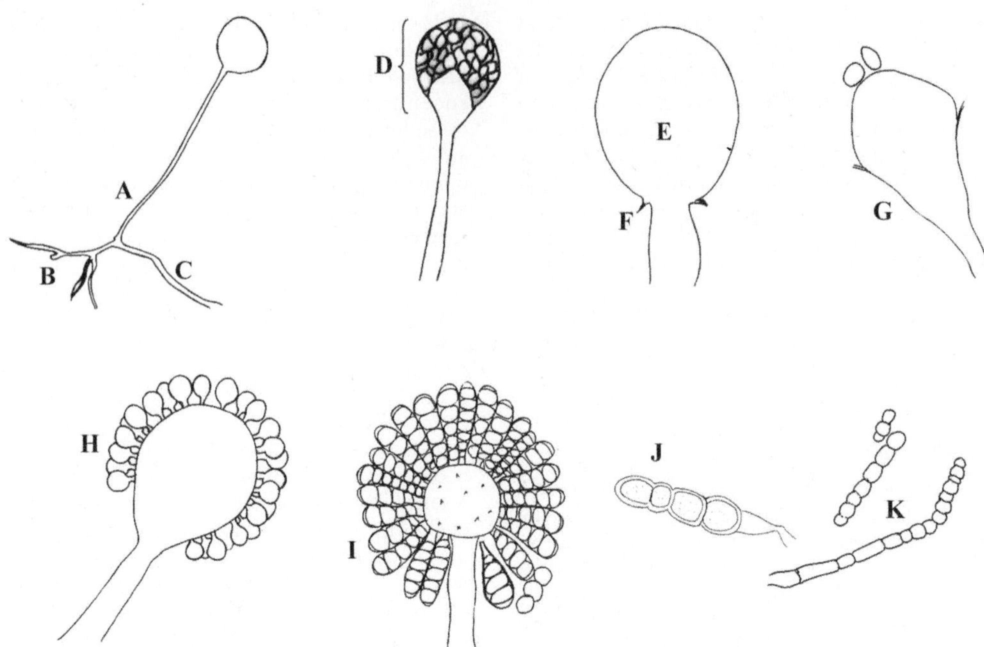

FIGURE 1 Schematic drawing of morphological structures observed in *Mucorales*. Sporangiophores (A) bear sporangia-containing sporangiospores (D), can be anchored to the substrate by rhizoids (B), and expand by means of stolons (C). The columella (E) is produced at the apex of the sporangiophore, and in some species, an apophysis (G) is present. For some species, after liberation of sporangiospores, a thin sporangium membrane may be visible (F). Sporangia with a single or few spores are called sporangiola (H), and sporangia with few spores aligned in rows are called merosporangia (I). Thick-walled chlamydospores (J) and oidia (thin-walled swollen vesicles) (K) can be observed. Drawings by Dea Garcia-Hermoso.

as in *Rhizomucor* and *Actinomucor*, or mostly unbranched as in *Rhizopus*. In addition, the site from which the sporangiophore arises (between rhizoids or directly from the stolon) is a supplementary clue for the identification of the different genera (Fig. 2). A morphological key to the principal genera of *Mucorales* is illustrated in Fig. 3. The combination of asexual fruiting bodies and criteria such as maximum growth temperature is useful for the differentiation of these fungi to the species level. The phenotypic differences described below refer to species defined by nucleotide sequence analysis.

Family *Lichtheimiaceae*

Genus *Lichtheimia* Vuill. 1903 (formerly *Absidia* or *Mycocladus*). The genus *Absidia* has been revised on the basis of phylogenetic, physiological, and morphological characteristics (7). The thermotolerant species of *Absidia corymbifera*, *A. blakesleeana*, and *A. hyalospora* were placed in the new family of *Mycocladiaceae* and the genus *Mycocladus*. The same group suggested revision of the nomenclature rectification to create the family *Lichtheimiaceae* (instead of *Mycocladiaceae*) and the reassignment of the genus *Lichtheimia* in place of *Mycocladus* (108). The multigene sequence analysis of 38 isolates morphologically identified as *Lichtheimia corymbifera* uncovered the presence of a different species (named *L. ramosa*), which differs in morphology and nucleotide sequences from *L. corymbifera* (6). Of the five recognized species of the genus *Lichtheimia*, only *L. corymbifera*, *L. ornata*, and *L. ramosa* are of clinical relevance (8). These species seem to have a worldwide distribution and have been isolated from diverse substrates, including seeds, soil, and decaying vegetable debris. They produce white, fast-growing, woolly colonies, which become grayish brown with age. Maximum growth temperature is between 46°C and 52°C. *L. ramosa* differs from *L. corymbifera* and *L. ornata* by faster growth at high temperatures (8). Microscopically, sporangiophores are usually erect and highly branched and arise singly or in small corymbs from stolons, but they are not opposite the rhizoids as in *Rhizopus*. Rhizoids are present but generally indistinguishable. Multispored sporangia are small and spherical to pyriform. Columellae are hemispherical or ellipsoidal with a marked conical apophysis, and sporangiospores are smooth, hyaline, and ellipsoidal, cylindrical, or subglobose (2.73 by 2.24 μm in diameter) (Fig. 4). Giant cells of irregular shape are frequently present. The morphologies of sporangiophores and sporangiospores are very similar for the three pathogenic species, even though significant differences in the lengths, widths, and length to width ratios of the sporangiospores were previously reported (45).

Genus *Rhizomucor* Lucet & Costantin 1900. *Rhizomucor pusillus* and *R. miehei* are the pathogenic species of the genus *Rhizomucor*. Species of the genus *Rhizomucor* are frequently isolated from composting or fermenting organic matter (109). Macroscopically, *Rhizomucor* produces rapidly growing gray (*R. miehei*) to brown (*R. pusillus*) woolly colonies. Sporangiophores are single or branched and arise from aerial mycelium or from stolons. Rhizoids are present but often difficult to recognize. Sporangia are multispored; apophyses are absent, and most species are thermophilic. Sporangiospores are round, hyaline, and smooth walled (Fig. 5). The species differ in the size of sporangia, sucrose assimilation, and the ability to grow in presence of thiamine. *R. miehei* has smaller sporangia than *R. pusillus* (60 μm versus 100 μm in diameter) and fails to assimilate sucrose, and its growth depends on the presence of thiamine.

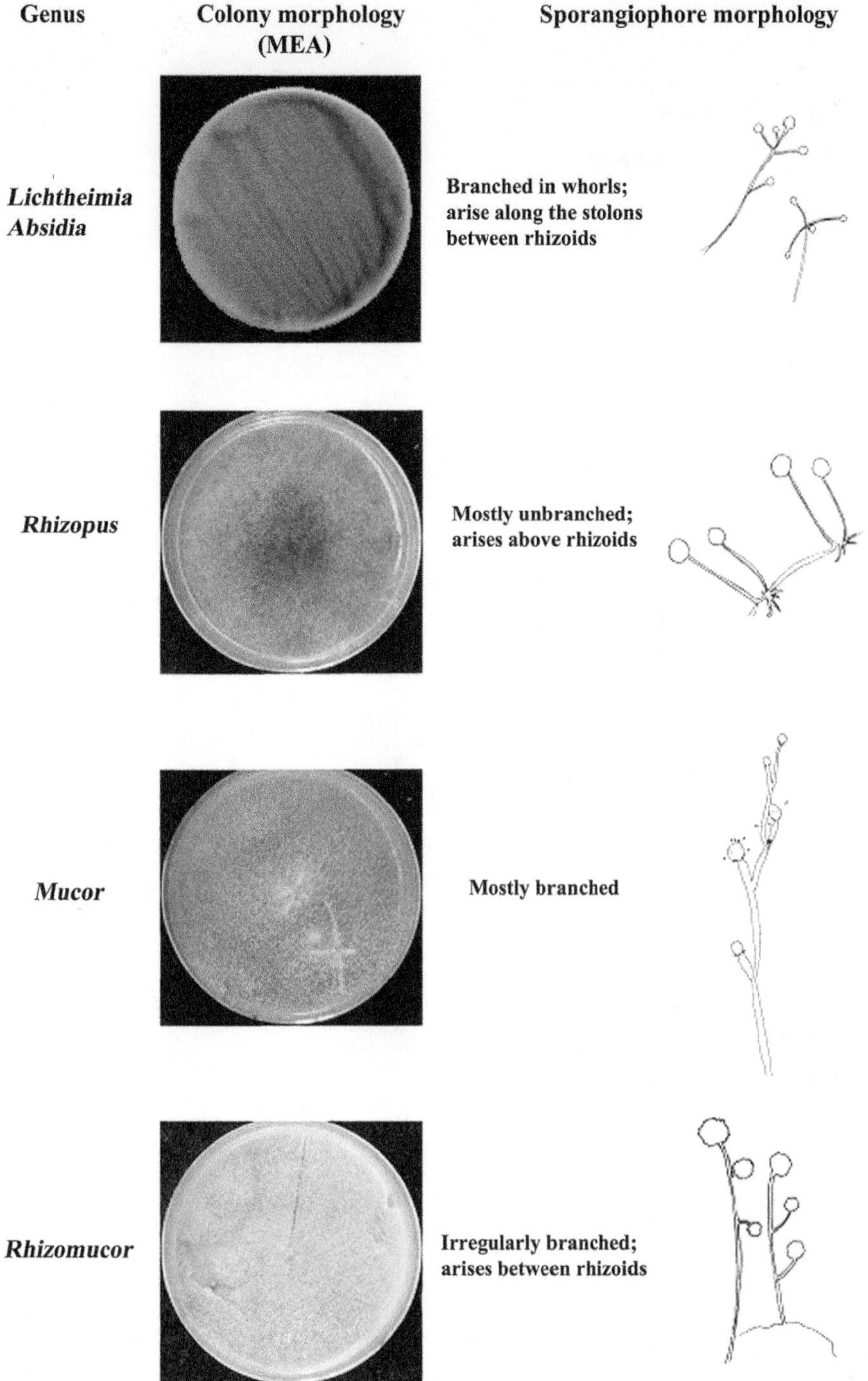

Genus
Colony morphology (MEA)
Sporangiophore morphology
Lichtheimia
Absidia
Branched in whorls; arise along the stolons between rhizoids
Rhizopus
Mostly unbranched; arises above rhizoids
Mucor
Mostly branched
Rhizomucor
Irregularly branched; arises between rhizoids

FIGURE 2 Culture variability of some of the genera of *Mucorales* and their branching development.

Family *Mucoraceae*

Genus *Mucor* Fresen. 1850. Four species are considered human pathogens: *Mucor circinelloides*, *M. irregularis* (formerly *R. variabilis* var. *variabilis*), *M. indicus*, and *M. ramosissimus* (10, 110).

Colonies of the genus *Mucor* are usually fast growing and white to yellow, becoming gray with time. Tall sporangiophores (they can reach several centimeters in height) are simple or branched, supporting multispored nonapophysate sporangia. Sporangiospores are hyaline and subspherical to ellipsoidal. In some species, residues of the sporangial wall (collarette) can be present, and some species can produce rhizoids and chlamydospores (Fig. 6).

Mucor circinelloides is a species complex comprising four varieties based mainly on differences in the shape of columellae and sporangiospores. Major phenotypic differences within the thermotolerant *Mucor* species involved in human infections are summarized in Table 2. Maximum growth temperatures for pathogenic *Mucor* species range from 35°C (*M. circinelloides*) to 42°C (*M. indicus*). The identification

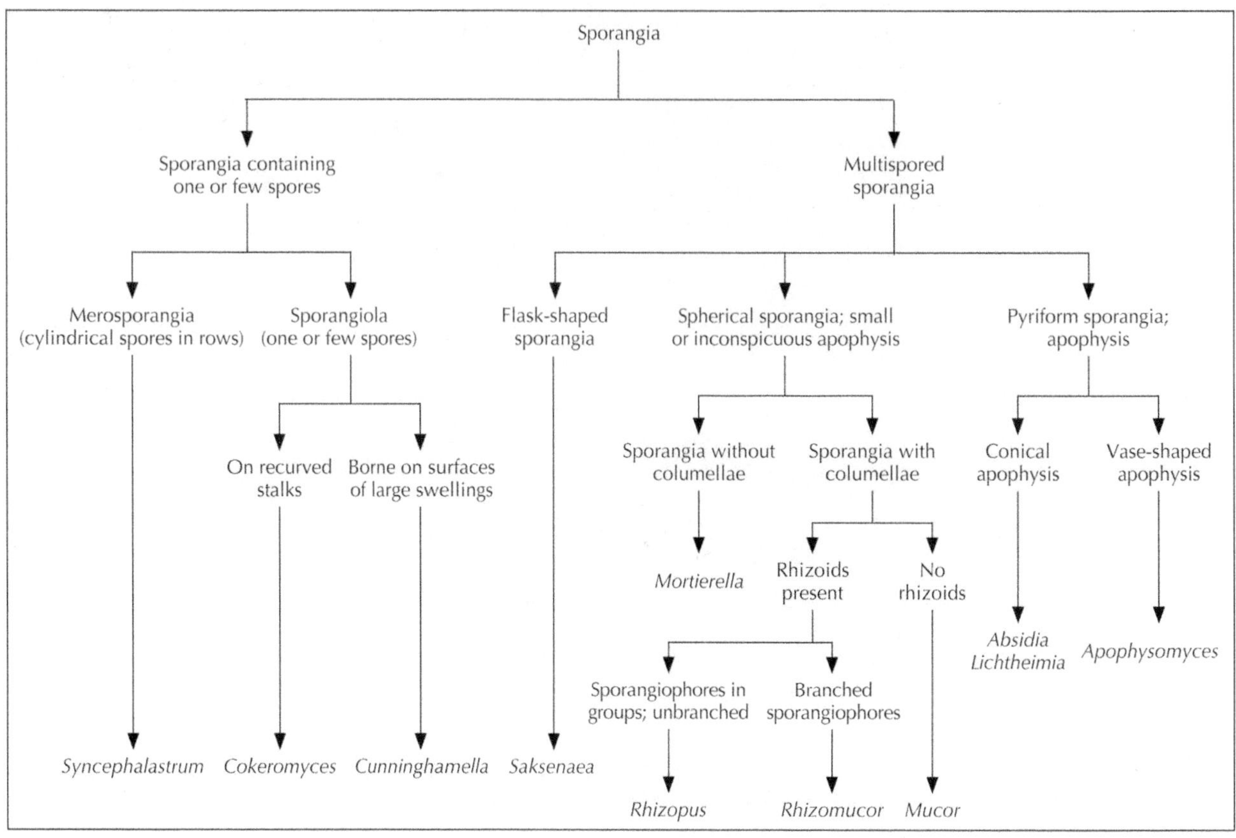

FIGURE 3 Flow diagram for the identification of the different genera of *Mucorales*.

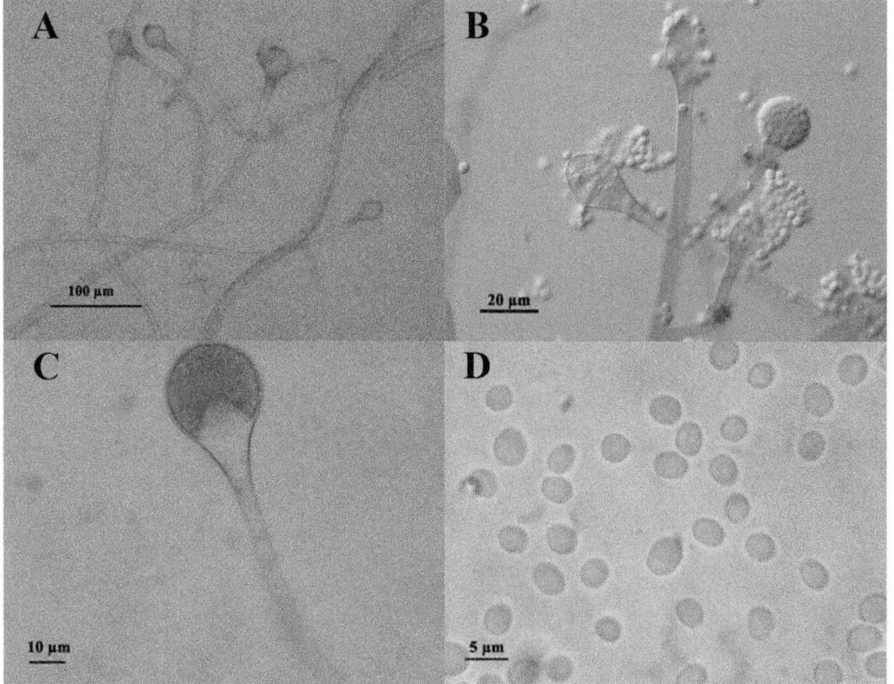

FIGURE 4 *Lichtheimia corymbifera*. (A) Branched sporangiophores; (B) hemispheric columellae and sporangiospores; (C) pyriform multispored sporangium and marked conical apophysis; (D) sporangiospores.

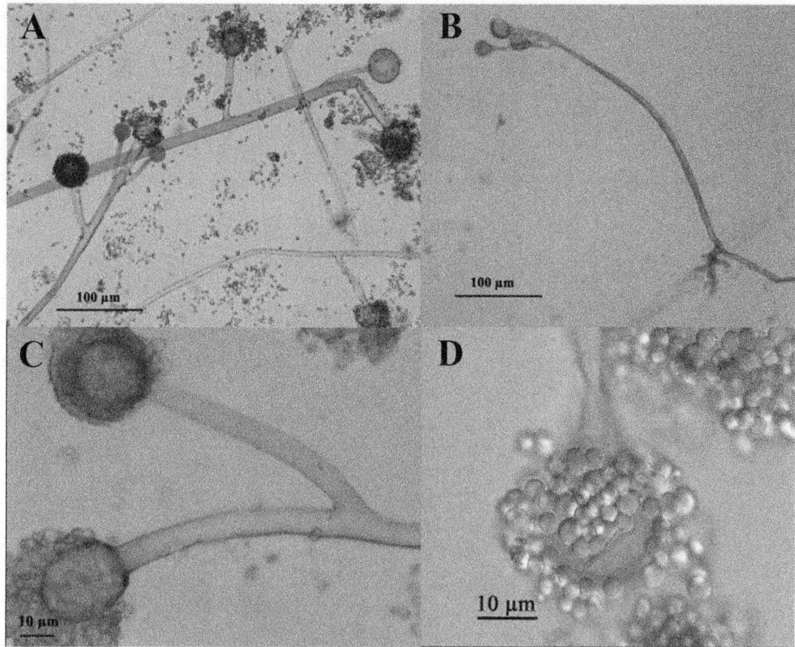

FIGURE 5 *Rhizomucor pusillus*. Sporangiophores with apical branching (A), simple rhizoids (B), and globose sporangia with round and smooth-walled sporangiospores (C and D) are shown.

of these species can be complicated under unsuitable growth conditions, which can induce morphological variations such as sterile sporangia, swelling in sporangiophores, and modifications in size and shape of sporangia, columellae, and sporangiospores (111).

Genus *Actinomucor* Schostak. 1898. The only species of the genus *Actinomucor* is *Actinomucor elegans*. This ubiquitous soil fungus has also been isolated from the rhizosphere of plants (oat, barley, wheat) and from mouse and rabbit dung (112). The three varieties of this

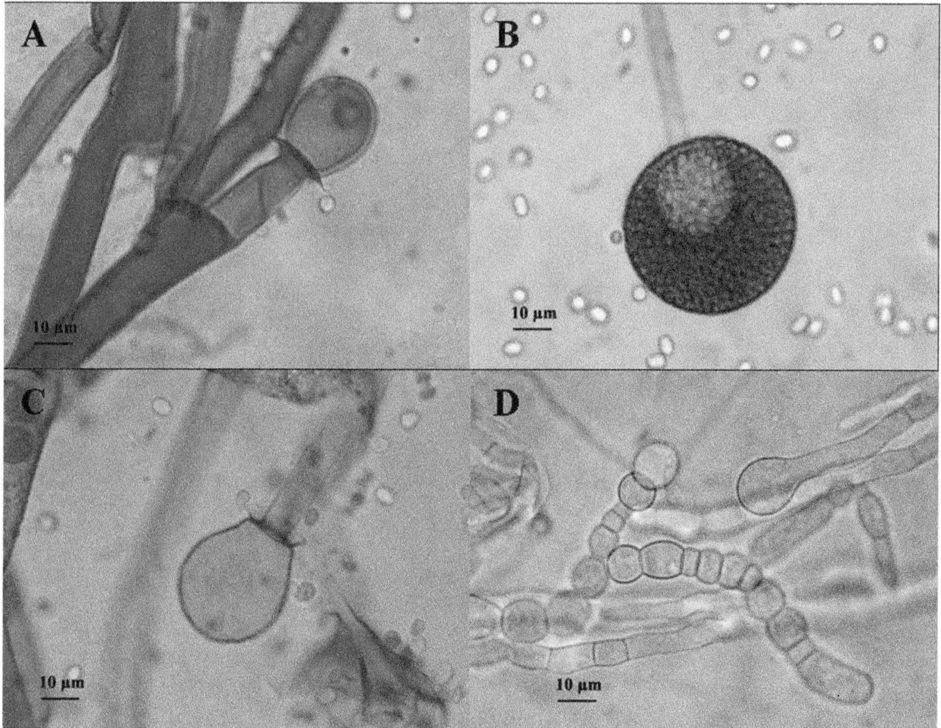

FIGURE 6 Micromorphology of *Mucor circinelloides*. (A) Sporangiophore; (B) sporangia; (B and C) ellipsoidal sporangiospores; (D) oidia.

TABLE 2 Macroscopic and microscopic features in *Mucor* species involved in human infection

Species	Colony morphology, height	Sporangiophore	Sporangia (diameter)	Columellae (shape)	Sporangiospores	Maximum growth temperature (°C)	Chlamydospores	Other characteristics
M. circinelloides	Light gray to brown, up to 6 mm	Repeatedly branched	Up to 80 μm	Obovoid to ellipsoidal	Ellipsoidal	36–40	Rare	Assimilation of ethanol
M. velutinosus	White-grayish, up to 2 mm	Sympodially branched	Up to 60 μm	Globose to conical	Verrucose, globose to subglobose	38	Abundant	Presence of rhizoids
M. irregularis (formerly *Rhizomucor variabilis* var. *variabilis*)	White to yellowish, up to 2 mm	Simple or once branched	Up to 100 μm	Irregular shape	Variable shape	38	Abundant	Presence of rhizoids
M. ramosissimus	Olive gray, up to 2 mm	Abundant swellings present	Up to 80 μm disposed on short lateral branches	Applanate	Smooth, subglobose to ellipsoidal	36	Absent	Presence of oidia in substrate mycelium
M. indicus	Deep yellow, up to 10 mm	Repeatedly branched	Up to 75 μm	Subglobose	Subglobose to cylindrical-ellipsoidal	42	Abundant	Light-dependent sporulation

species (var. elegans; var. kuwaitiensis; var. taiwanensis) are now considered synonyms (http://www.indexfungorum.org). *A. elegans* is an emerging pathogen responsible for few reported disseminated diseases (113–115) and superficial infections (116, 117). This species is involved in the fermentation of a cheese-like soybean product (*sufu*) popular in Vietnam and China (118, 119). Macroscopically, after 7 days of growth at 30°C colonies are floccose and white to cream colored. They become brown-beige with a woolly texture in older cultures. The distinctive microscopic features of the genus *Actinomucor* facilitate the morphological identification. Hyaline, verticillately branched sporangiophores with varied lengths terminate in sporangia. Whorls of branched sporangiophores may give rise to secondary sporangia or they can rebranch, terminating in subglobose columella. The deliquescent wall of sporangia may be smooth or spiny, enclosing spherical to ovoidal sporangiospores measuring 5 to 10 μm in diameter. Rhizoids and chlamydospores are present (Fig. 7).

Genus *Cokeromyces* Shanor 1950. *Cokeromyces recurvatus* remains a rare agent of mucormycosis. It has been mostly recovered from soil or from rabbit, rat, or lizard dung in North America (United States and Mexico). Colonies are slow growing (less than 1 mm high) and grayish to brown. Microscopic features include the presence of long, recurved, twisted stalks arising from terminal vesicles of unbranched sporangiophores, globose sporangiola (8 to 11 μm in diameter) borne on those stalks, and smooth-walled spherical sporangiospores 2 to 4 μm in size (Fig. 8). A yeast-like form can be obtained by subculturing on media such as brain heart infusion or yeast extract peptone agar. Yeast-like forms are thin to thick walled and spherical, measuring 10 to 100 μm in diameter. Some cells produce single buds across their entire surface, producing a ship's wheel appearance similar to that of *Paracoccidioides brasiliensis* (20). The species is homothallic and produces lemon-shaped zygospores.

Family *Saksenaeaceae*

Genus *Apophysomyces* P.C. Misra 1979. The members of the genus *Apophysomyces* are soil fungi with a tropical to subtropical distribution. They produce fast-growing white to gray colonies. General features are erect sporangiophores, unbranched and single, bearing multispored sporangia, usually pyriform, of 20 to 60 μm in diameter. Columellae are hemispherical, cylindrical, trapezoidal, or ellipsoidal; the sporangiophores are smooth walled. The production of prominent vase-shaped, bell-shaped, or funnel-shaped apophyses is a distinctive feature of this species (Fig. 9). Good growth is observed at 42°C (107). The use of poor-nutrient media (water-yeast extract medium) can improve sporulation, often lacking on primary isolation media (105). Until recently, *Apophysomyces* was considered a monotypic genus with *A. elegans* as the only species. The molecular diversity study performed by Alvarez and collaborators revealed three additional species (*A. variabilis*, *A. trapeziformis*, and *A. ossiformis*) of *Apophysomyces*, based on morphological, physiological, and phylogenetic differences (9).

Genus *Saksenaea* S. B. Saksena 1953. The genus *Saksenaea* is considered a complex of species. Alvarez et al. described two new species (*S. erythrospora* and *S. oblongispora*) different from *S. vasiformis*, long considered the only species in the genus (120). They are saprophytic fungi with a worldwide distribution first isolated from forest soil

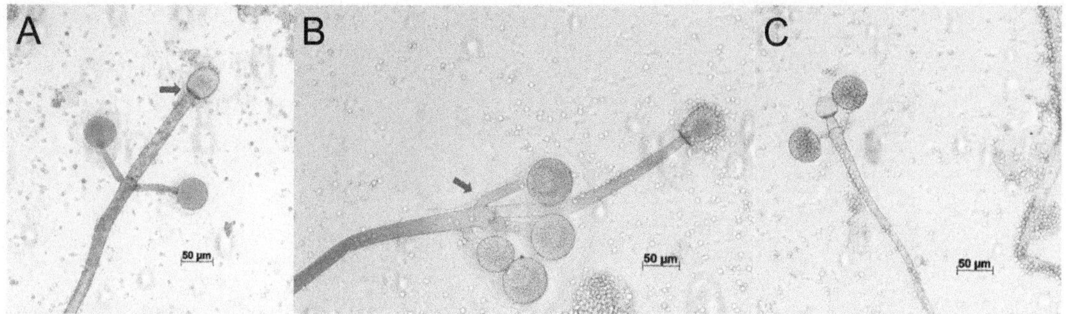

FIGURE 7 *Actinomucor elegans*. Branched sporangiophores. (A) Subglobose columella (arrow); (B) whorl of branched sporangiophores with secondary sporangia (arrow); (C) verticillately branched sporangiophore.

by Saksena (16). They produce white-grayish expanding colonies, with a maximum growth temperature of 44°C. The use of specific, poor-nutrient media (water-yeast extract medium) can induce sporulation, as suggested by Padhye and Ajello (105). Czapek medium at 30 or 37°C also induces sporulation. Microscopically, sporangiophores are unbranched with melanized rhizoids. The length of sporangiophore and sporangia, the shape and size of sporangiospores, and the maximum temperature for growth are useful parameters for the recognition of the different species. Figure 10 shows the distinctive flask-shaped multispored sporangia, which is a key feature for the identification of this genus.

Family *Rhizopodaceae*

Genus *Rhizopus* Ehrenb. 1821. *Rhizopus arrhizus* (syn., *R. oryzae*) and *Rhizopus microsporus* are the most common pathogenic species. This genus, commonly found in the air, soil, and compost, is characterized by the rapid production of white cottony colonies, which turn brownish to black with time because of the presence of pigmented sporangiophores and sporangia. Table 3 indicates useful features allowing the distinction between the pathogenic species of the genus *Rhizopus*. The sporangiophores are unbranched, arising singly or in groups, with well-developed rhizoids at the base, which distinguishes the genus *Rhizopus* from the genera *Lichtheimia* and *Rhizomucor*.

The microscopic features of *R. arrhizus* include single or clustered brown sporangiophores, of 1 to 2 mm in height, bearing multispored sporangia (150 to 170 µm in diameter). Columellae are ellipsoidal and brown to gray, and they generally have a truncate base. Rhizoids are well developed and easily observed under the stereomicroscope. Sporangiospores are angular and round to ellipsoidal, with longitudinal ridges 6 to 8 µm by 4.5 to 5.0 µm in size. Chlamydospores (10 to 35 µm in diameter) can be present (Fig. 11). This thermotolerant species can grow at 40°C but not at 45°C. *R. arrhizus* differs from the nonpathogenic *R. stolonifer*, which harbors longer sporangiophores (>2 mm) and larger columellae (up to 275 µm in diameter) and does not grow at 40°C (121).

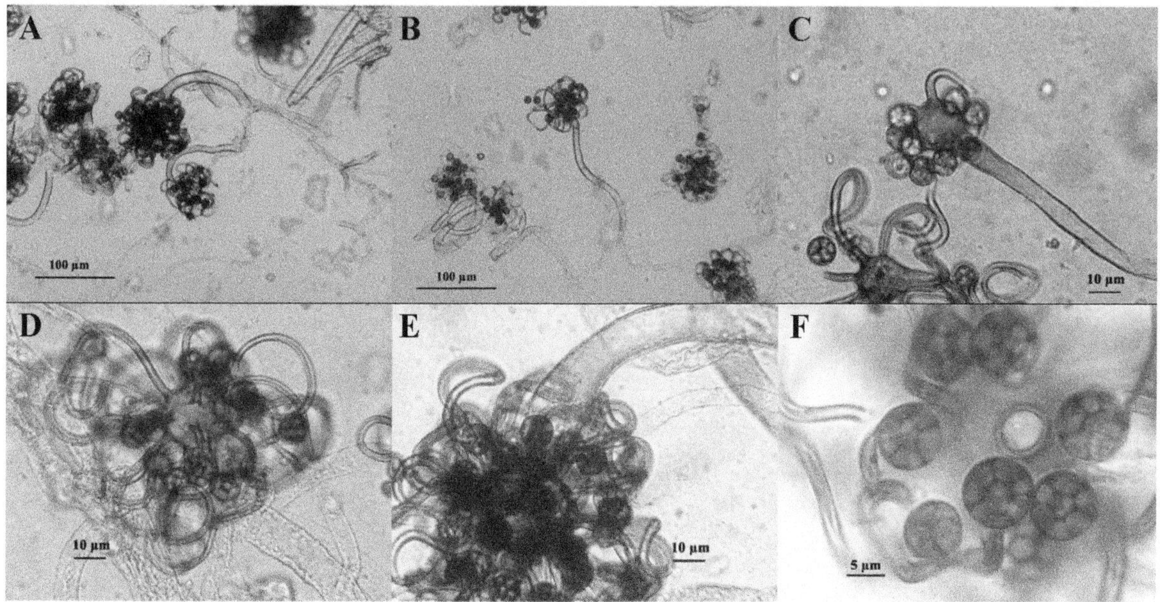

FIGURE 8 *Cokeromyces recurvatus*. (A and B) Mostly unbranched sporangiophores without rhizoids; (C) young sporangiolum; (D to F) recurved stalks arising from terminal vesicles and bearing few-spored sporangiola.

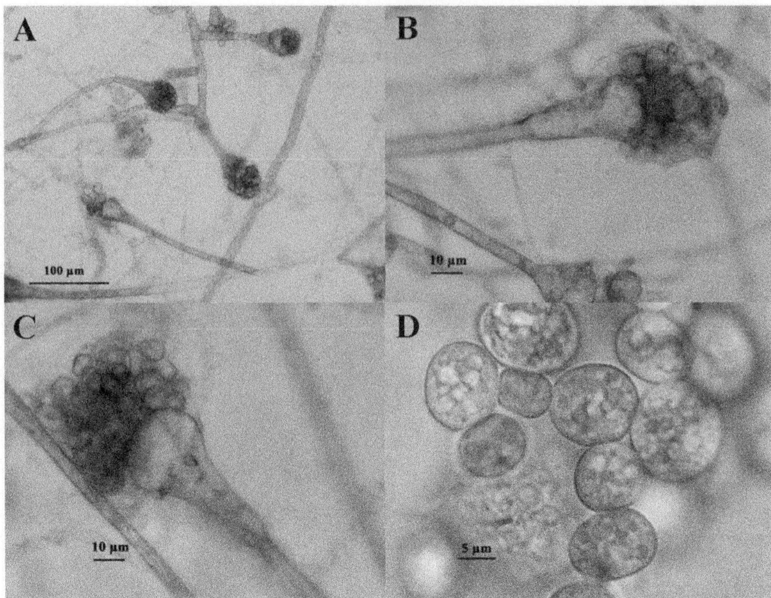

FIGURE 9 *Apophysomyces elegans.* (A) Unbranched sporangiophores bearing multispored sporangia with a vase-shaped apophysis (B and C); (D) cylindrical sporangiospores.

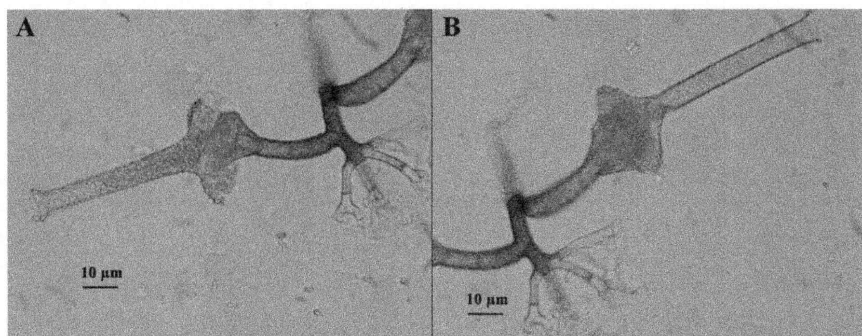

FIGURE 10 *Saksenaea vasiformis.* (A and B) Unbranched sporangiophores with dark rhizoids and typical multispored flask-shaped sporangia.

TABLE 3 Main characteristics allowing distinction among *Rhizopus* species

Species	Sporangiophores (height)	Sporangiospores (shape and ornamentation)	Growth temperature				
			30°C	37°C	40°C	45°C	50°C
R. arrhizus (syn., *R. oryzae*)	Often higher than 1 mm	Angular, round to ellipsoidal; striate	+	+	+	Neg	Neg
R. stolonifer			+	Neg	Neg	Neg	Neg
R. microsporus var. *microsporus*	Not exceeding 0.8 mm	Angular ellipsoidal; striate	+	+	+	+	Neg
R. microsporus var. *oligosporus*		Large, round; irregularly ornamented	+	+	+	Limited growth	Neg
R. microsporus var. *rhizopodiformis*		Small, round; spinulose	+	+	+	+	+
R. microsporus var. *chinensis*		Angular, homogeneous	+	+	+	+ (Sporangia immature)	Neg
R. microsporus var. *azygosporus*		Round; barely striate	+	+	+	+	+
R. schipperae		Round to ellipsoidal; striate	+	+	+	Very limited growth	Neg

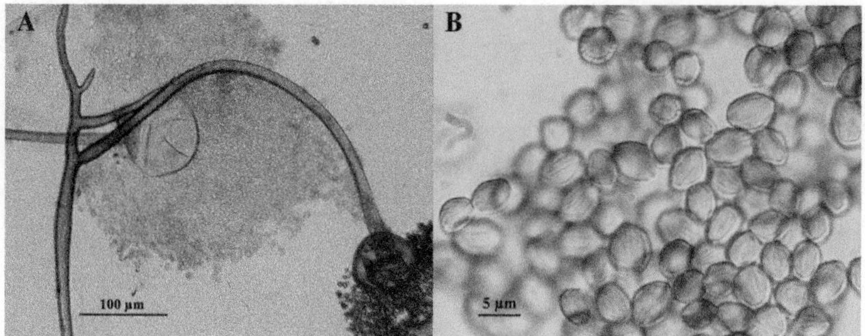

FIGURE 11 Typical microscopic features of *Rhizopus arrhizus*. (A) Melanized sporangiophore arising opposite rhizoids; (B) striate angular sporangiospores.

According to one recent U.S. epidemiological survey, *R. microsporus* is the second most frequent agent of mucormycosis (122). It can be isolated from soil or wood products. Colonies are pale brownish gray, with sporangiophores arising from stolons and measuring up to 400 µm in length (123). Sporangia are dark brown (up to 80 µm in diameter); columellae are conical, and sporangiospores are striate and angular to ellipsoidal (Fig. 12). In addition to the typical *R. microsporus* var. *microsporus*, there are three supplementary varieties: *R. microsporus* var. *chinensis*, *R. microsporus* var. *oligosporus*, and *R. microsporus* var. *rhizopodiformis*. They can be distinguished on the basis of the morphology of sporangiospores and temperature tolerance. These differences observed between varieties are not supported genetically (124). Table 3 indicates major differences among the species of the genus *Rhizopus*.

Family *Cunninghamellaceae*

Genus *Cunninghamella* Matr. 1903. Traditionally, *Cunninghamella bertholletiae* was considered the only clinically relevant species of the genus. Although rarely involved in human disease, *C. bertholletiae* has the capacity to infect immunocompetent individuals. Other species such as *C. elegans*, *C. echinulata* (125), and more recently *C. blakesleeana* (126) have also been implicated in cases of human mucormycoses. *C. bertholletiae* is a thermotolerant fungus isolated from soil. It produces white to dark gray expanding colonies. Sporangiophores are erect with lateral branching at the apical zone. Each branch produces a globose vesicle (up to 40 µm in diameter), which bears 1-spored sporangiola. At maturity, each sporangiola will become a finely echinulate spherical sporangiospore (7 to 11 µm in diameter) (Fig. 13). Key features for the identification of *C. bertholletiae* are essentially its growth at 45°C (with a maximum of 50°C) and the presence of monosporic sporangiola borne on terminal vesicles.

Family *Syncephalastraceae*

Genus *Syncephalastrum* J. Schröt. 1886. Species from the genus *Syncephalastrum* have a worldwide distribution

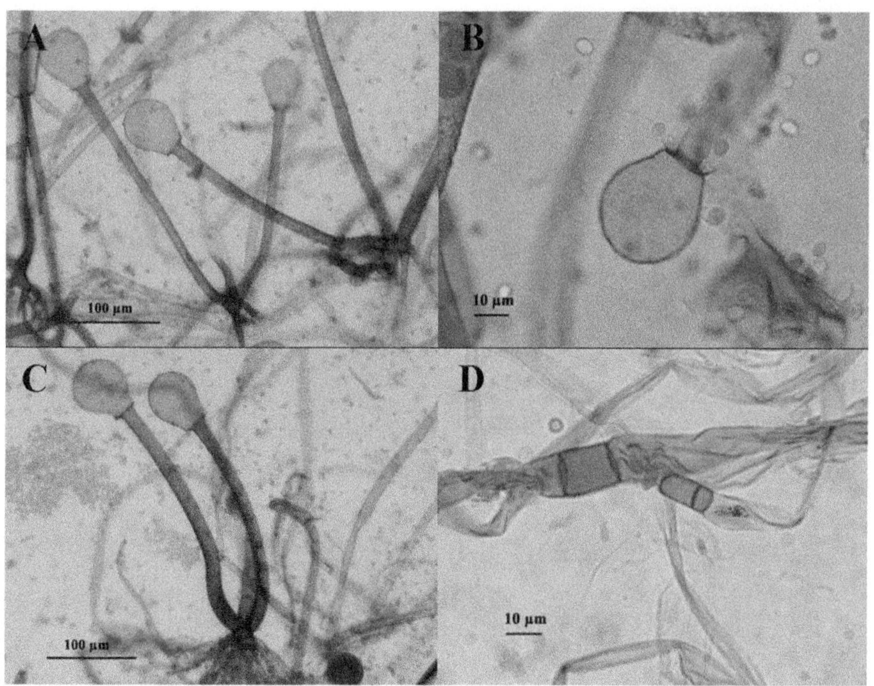

FIGURE 12 Short pigmented sporangiophores arising in pairs in *Rhizopus microsporus*. (A and C) Rhizoids; (B) conical columella; (D) chlamydospores.

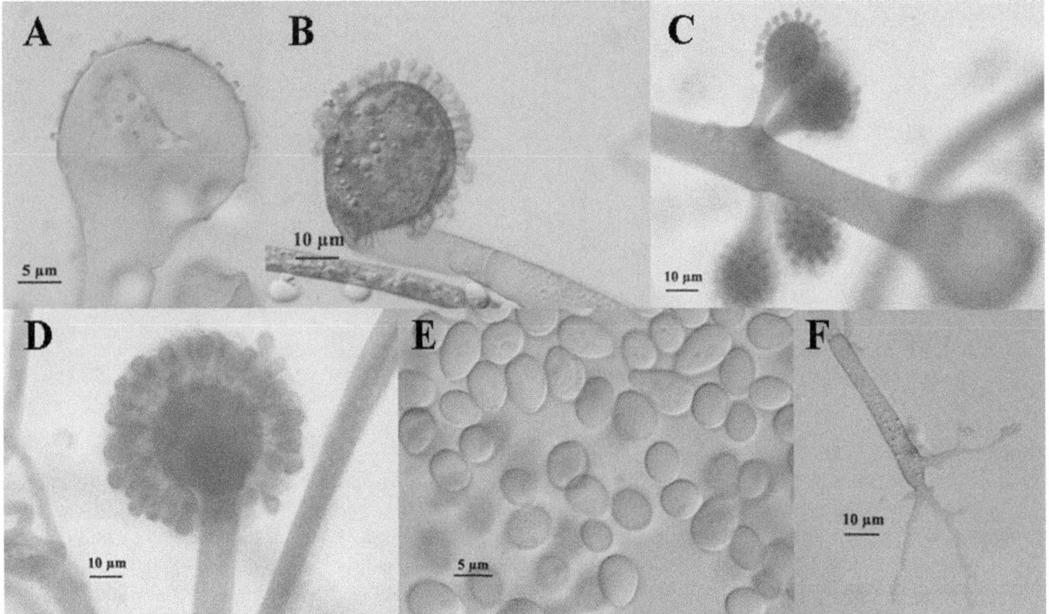

FIGURE 13 *Cunninghamella bertholletiae*. (A, B, and D) Development of single-spored sporangiola on the surface of globose vesicles, with frequent apical branching (C); (E) mature sporangiola grow to be single echinulate sporangiospores; (F) rhizoids.

and have been isolated from soil, plants, and diverse foodstuffs (16). The only species associated with cases of human infection is *S. racemosum*, which is described below.

In culture, *S. racemosum* grows rapidly and produces expanding white-grayish colonies, which turn darker due to the formation of sporangia and resemble the colonies formed by *Rhizopus* spp. The maximum temperature for growth is 40°C. Sporangiophores are short, erect, and mostly branched, arising from rhizoids and forming terminal globose vesicles. The whole surface of these vesicles is covered with cylindrical merosporangia containing (3 to 14) smooth-walled, spherical to ovoid merospores arranged in single rows (Fig. 14). This is a distinctive feature of the genus compared to other members of *Mucorales*.

■ Molecular identification

The species identification of *Mucorales* by phenotypic methods remains a difficult task because of the common

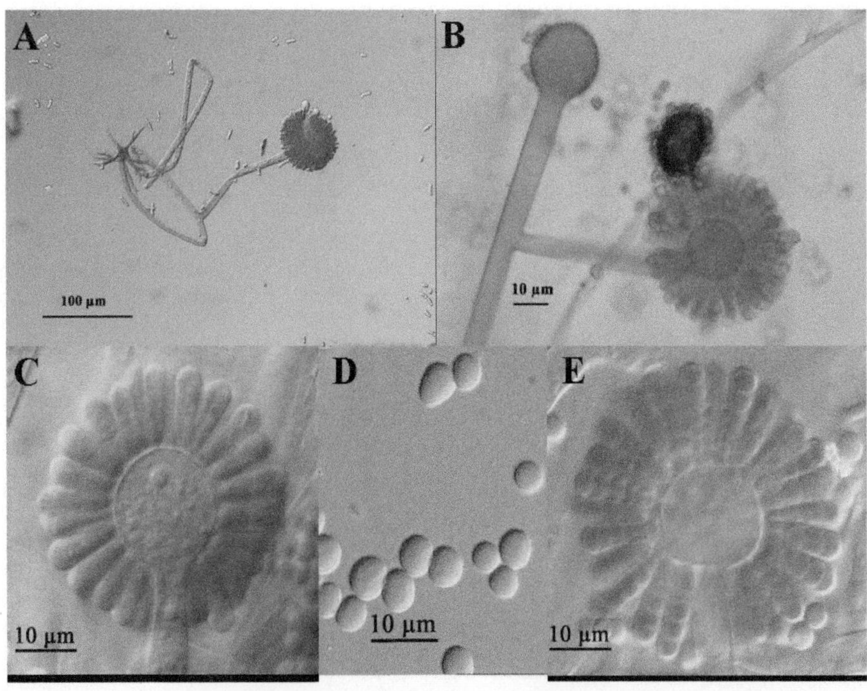

FIGURE 14 Short sporangiophores arising from rhizoids (A), terminal vesicles covered by merosporangia (B, C, and E), and merospores (D) characteristic of *Syncephalastrum racemosum*.

morphological features among the members of this group. In addition, some pathogenic species, such as members of *S. vasiformis* species complex and *A. elegans* species complex, regularly fail to sporulate on standard mycological media (127). Therefore, sequence-based identification is of interest because it provides fast and easily comparable data (128). In search of reliable DNA barcode markers for *Fungi*, Schoch and collaborators compared the performance of six markers: three nuclear ribosomal regions (ITS, ribosomal large subunit, ribosomal small subunit) and portions of three protein-coding genes on 17 fungal lineages. The ITS was finally proposed as the primary fungal barcode across all groups (129). Recently, a large phylogenetic study (more than 650 strains) validated the ITS marker as a useful barcode for the identification of *Mucorales*. Most of the accepted species that are currently taxonomically defined by morphology were well discriminated. However, the identity threshold of 99% defined by Balajee et al. in 2009 (130) did not cover the intraspecific variability of the clinically important species tested (124). Additional phylogenetic studies to delimit species boundaries and the analysis of intraspecies and interspecies variations are needed to define a new identity threshold to establish a reliable ITS-based identification for these organisms.

Typing Systems

By definition, typing methods are developed to study the diversity and relatedness of isolates (environmental or clinical isolates) within a given species. Few methods have been evaluated for the typing of clinical isolates of *Mucorales* (27, 131, 132). These methods proved to be inefficient because of their low discriminatory power. Whole-genome sequencing may provide the key to designing efficient typing methods in the future (102).

Serologic Tests

No commercial assays are available at this time. However, mucorales antigen can be used to detect mucorales-specific T cells (133). This test has been proposed as a diagnostic test for detection of mucorales-specific T cells in patients ($n = 3$) with invasive mucormycoses and not patients with other types of infection ($n = 17$) or without infection ($n = 8$). These T cells were detectable at the onset and during the course of the disease but not before diagnosis.

Antifungal Susceptibilities

In vitro antifungal susceptibility can be evaluated by the reference microdilution broth techniques from the CLSI (134) and the EUCAST (135) or, alternatively, by a commercially available test (Etest) (136). Although *Mucorales* share most antifungal susceptibility patterns, there is some specificity depending on genus and even species. AMB is the most active drug against the majority of *Mucorales*, as shown both *in vitro* (83, 137–141) and in animal models of infection (142–146). Among the new azoles, voriconazole has poor activity, which is highlighted by breakthrough mucormycosis in patients treated with voriconazole (147) and in experimental models (148). In contrast, posaconazole has relatively low MICs (83, 138, 139, 146, 149), and the *in vivo* efficacy of posaconazole has been demonstrated as curative and prophylactic treatment in animal models (150, 151). Isavuconazole has higher MICs than posaconazole (152) with values being in general one to three steps higher than those for posaconazole (153). However, animal models suggest that isavuconazole is effective as prophylaxis or curative treatment (154). Echinocandins have no significant *in vitro* activity (155, 156), even though *Rhizopus arrhizus* possesses the target enzyme for this class of compounds. *In vivo*, caspofungin alone exhibits modest efficacy (63), and it showed promising clinical efficacy in combination with AMB in some patients (111).

Evaluation, Interpretation, and Reporting of Results

Culture results should always be interpreted in light of the clinical presentation and along with the results of direct examination and/or histopathology. A positive culture of *Mucorales* can be due to contamination during collection of the sample or processing of the sample in the laboratory. A study in Spain showed that less than 8% of the *Mucorales* isolates recovered in the laboratory were from patients with invasive mucormycosis (35, 157). In the revised definitions of the EORTC/MSG study group for the diagnosis of invasive fungal infections, proven disease requires that "histopathologic, cytopathologic, or direct microscopic examination of a specimen obtained by needle aspiration or biopsy shows hyphae accompanied by evidence of associated tissue damage" or "the recovery of a mould by culture of a specimen obtained by a sterile procedure from a normally sterile and clinically or radiologically abnormal site consistent with an infectious disease process, excluding bronchoalveolar lavage fluid, a cranial sinus cavity specimen, and urine" (158). However, "the failure to meet the criteria for invasive fungal infection does not mean that there is none, only that there is insufficient evidence to support the diagnosis. This is the most compelling reason for not employing these definitions in daily clinical practice." One may thus have proof of an invasive fungal infection and a high suspicion of mucormycosis without evidence of the latter in the absence of positive culture. As mentioned before, attempts to establish the definite diagnosis are important to offer the best management for the patient.

ENTOMOPHTHOROMYCOSIS

Epidemiology and Transmission

Most members of the *Entomophthoromycota* are pathogens of arthropods and other animals. They are present in soil, decaying vegetables, and dung worldwide but more abundantly in the warm climates of Africa and Asia (20). Infections due to *Basidiobolus ranarum* are described in Asia (Indonesia, where the first cases were described, India, and Myanmar) and in several African countries (mostly Uganda and Nigeria but also Togo, Ghana, Cameroon, Benin, Saudi Arabia) but rarely in South America. *B. ranarum* has recently emerged with gastrointestinal presentations in the United States (159). Infections due to *Conidiobolus* spp. are described in Africa, Madagascar, Mayotte, India, China, Japan, and South America (160–162).

Clinical Manifestations

One of the major differences between mucormycosis and entomophthoromycosis is that the former occurs mainly in predisposed individuals, whereas the latter occurs mostly in apparently immunocompetent hosts.

B. ranarum is responsible for subcutaneous infections that mostly affect the limbs, buttocks, trunk, and perineum and less often the face and neck. The disease presents mostly in male children as a woody, hard, brawny, painless nodule that enlarges peripherally without affecting the overlying skin (163). Sporadic invasive infections with gastrointestinal involvement in adults (159, 164) and children (165) have been described worldwide. Of note, a small cluster has also been reported in Arizona (166) and such presentation may mimic malignancies (167–169). Disseminated infections are extremely rare (170).

In contrast to basidiobolomycosis, infections due to *Conidiobolus* spp. affect adults (mostly males) and outdoor workers and are usually limited to the nose and face. The onset of the infection is thought to take place in the nasal mucosa after inoculation of spores following a minor trauma. Swelling extends locally to the nose, the nasolabial folds, cheeks, eyebrows, the upper lip, and even the palate and pharynx, producing the characteristic facies in severe forms (171). A clinical staging system has now been proposed, split in atypical, early, intermediate, and late disease (172). Conjunctival inoculation of the fungus has been documented once in Brazil (173). Rare cases of dissemination have been reported in immunosuppressed individuals (174). Tissue lesions caused by *C. coronatus* and *C. incongruus* are similar (175).

Treatment and Outcome

Therapeutic strategies for basidiobolomycosis and conidiobolomycosis are not standardized because of the lack of clinical trials for these rare infections. Surgical excision, potassium iodide, and prolonged azole therapy have been used successfully for infection due to *Basidiobolus* (29, 160). For infections due to *Conidiobolus* spp., potassium iodide was historically used, with variable results. Prolonged oral azole therapy should now be used and is successful (161). More recently, a combination of itraconazole and potassium iodide has provided encouraging results, with 7 out of 10 patients who responded to the combination, including five patients with complete resolution (176).

Collection, Transport, and Storage of Specimens

As several differential diagnoses are possible, a confirmation of the fungal agent should be obtained; tissue biopsy specimens of the affected area are the best diagnostic specimens. The diagnosis relies on classical procedures combining direct examination and culture in unfixed samples and/or histology in fixed samples. In the gastrointestinal form of basidiobolomycosis, biopsy specimens obtained during endoscopy are the gold standard. Specimens should be processed immediately and should not be refrigerated (163).

Direct Examination

A direct examination of fresh specimens can be performed after dissolution of the tissue sample in KOH and staining with calcofluor white. For histology, classical stains, including hematoxylin and eosin, periodic acid-Schiff, and Gomori Grocott, could be performed. Typically, hyphae are broad, thin walled, and generally more septate than those of the *Mucorales*. Simultaneous acute and chronic inflammatory reactions are observed in the affected tissue. Hyphae can be observed with routine staining procedures. The presence of a Splendore-Hoeppli reaction associated with typical hyphae in tissue sections stained with hematoxylin-eosin is highly suggestive of entomophthoromycosis. The pink structure corresponds to a sheath of amorphous eosinophilic material around hyphal fragments. Even if the presence of a Splendore-Hoeppli phenomenon is strongly suggestive of entomophthoromycosis, it can be observed in various bacterial, fungal, and parasitic infections as well as in noninfectious diseases (177). In contrast to mucormycosis, there is typically no necrosis and no invasion of blood vessels.

Antigen Detection

No antigen tests are currently available for the detection of entomophthoromycosis.

Detection of Nucleic Acids in Clinical Materials

A PCR-based technique targeting *Basidiobolus* has been developed for the diagnosis of entomophthoromycosis in human samples (178).

Isolation Procedures

Biopsy samples should be sliced or minced (not ground) and placed on Sabouraud agar or PDA. Media containing cycloheximide should be avoided because of inhibition of *Basidiobolus* and *Conidiobolus* growth. Cultures must be incubated at both 37°C and 25 to 30°C because of the various optimum growth temperatures of these organisms. *Basidiobolus* grows well at 30°C but less rapidly at 37°C, whereas *Conidiobolus* spp. grow rapidly at 37°C (16).

Identification

■ Phenotypic identification

Members of *Entomophthoromycota* are characterized by the presence of coenocytic hyphae or short hyphal bodies and of primary and secondary conidia, which can be forcibly discharged at maturity. Primary conidia with papillate bases are produced straight from the thallus in repetitive cycles (14). They generate a germ tube or can produce smaller secondary conidia (similar in morphology to the primary conidia) in the presence of suitable substrate conditions. Villose conidia (old conidia with hair-like appendages) can also develop. Passive release of microconidia may also occur. In some species, thin sporangiophores bear capilliconidia at their apex. These spores are characterized by an adhesive tip. Zygospores (thick, bilayered, walled spores) are produced after conjugation of undifferentiated gametangia and can have beak-like appendages coming from gametangial remains (14, 20, 107). Sporulation occurs after 3 to 10 days of culture. Colonies are usually waxy or powdery with radial folds and with colors ranging from white to tan-brown (14, 20). A key feature of these fungi is their capacity to forcibly discharge conidia. Therefore, placing a cover slide inside the petri dish lid can be helpful to recover the papillate conidia. For a detailed description and additional information, see the taxonomic classification study by Ben-Ze'ev and Kenneth (179).

Class *Entomophthoromycetes*, Order *Entomophthorales*

Family *Ancylistaceae*

Genus *Conidiobolus* Bref. 1884. The genus *Conidiobolus* includes saprobes, facultative invertebrate, and vertebrate pathogens (13). The three species causing human conidiobolomycosis are *C. coronatus*, *C. incongruus*, and *C. lamprauges*.

Conidiobolus coronatus is a fast-growing fungus present in soil and on decaying leaves (107). It is most frequently isolated in the tropical forests of Africa (180). *C. coronatus* is an occasional pathogen of insects and has been recovered from diverse animals such as dolphins, chimpanzees, and horses (16).

Colonies are hyaline, radially folded, with an initially waxy appearance becoming powdery when mycelia become visible. The inside of the lid of the dish can be covered with conidia forcibly discharged by the conidiophores. These primary conidia are spherical (40 μm in diameter) and possess a prominent papilla. Villose conidia are present in older cultures (Fig. 15). Replicative, passively discharged microconidia are regularly produced (14). *C. coronatus* can

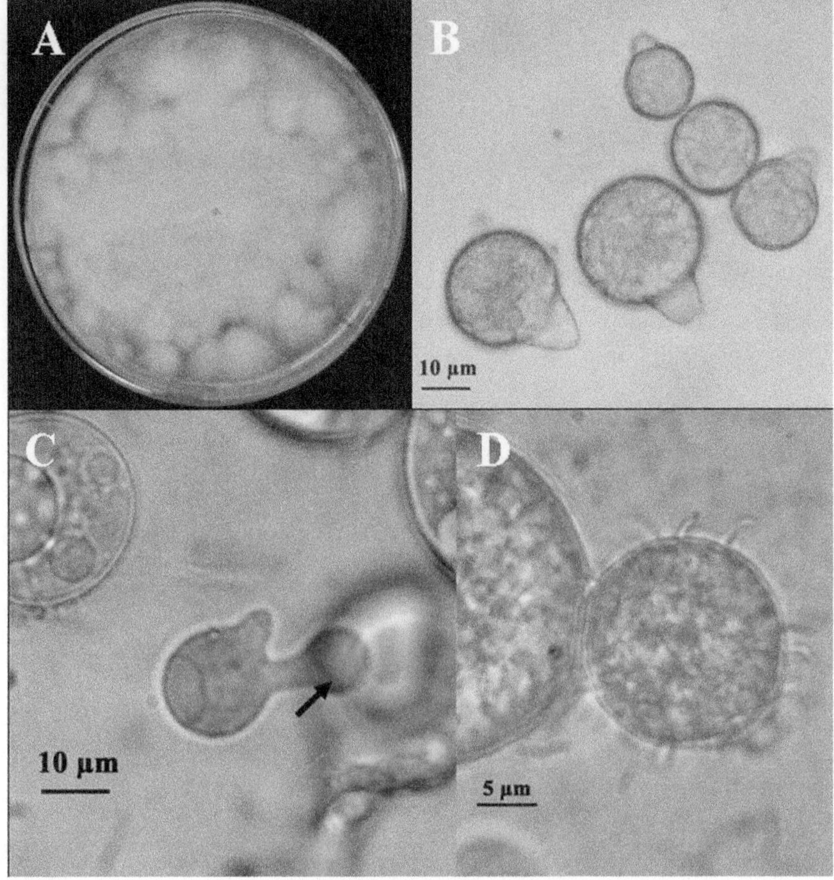

FIGURE 15 *Conidiobolus coronatus*. (A) Ten-day-old powdery colony on PDA medium; (B) primary conidia with papilla; (C) passively released secondary conidium (arrow); (D) villose conidium.

be differentiated from the two other pathogenic species by the absence of zygospores on PDA medium and the presence of villose conidia. Similarly, *C. incongruus* produces zygospores, which differ from those of *C. lamprauges* by the size and the formation of small globules inside the mature zygospores (181).

Order *Basidiobolales*

Family *Basidiobolaceae*

Genus *Basidiobolus*.

BASIDIOBOLUS RANARUM EIDEM. *Basidiobolus ranarum* is present in decaying fruit and vegetable matter (107). It can be present as a commensal in the intestinal tract of amphibians and reptiles (182). Colonies on PDA are yellowish and waxy, have radial folds, and do not form aerial mycelium when young. They grow well at 25 to 37°C. The microscopic examination after 7 to 10 days of culture reveals large aseptate mycelia, which can break up into free hyphal elements basically uninucleated. *B. ranarum* is homothallic. Sexual reproduction occurs by gametangial conjugation, producing thick-walled zygospores with lateral protuberances of gametangial remains (beaks) (Fig. 16). Primary conidiophores with swollen apices forcibly discharge spherical primary conidia. Secondary conidia are pyriform (clavate) and are passively released from the sporophore. These conidia possess a knob-like adhesive tip. Occasionally, elongated cells with a terminal adhesive tip (capilliconidia) are present (14, 180).

■ Molecular identification

There is no technique published for the molecular identification of *Entomophthoromycota*.

Typing Systems

To date, there is no typing method developed for *Entomophthoromycota*.

Serologic Tests

There are no commercially available diagnostic tests.

Antifungal Susceptibilities

In vitro susceptibility data are scarce, and some technical issues (such as inoculum preparation) remain to be addressed. Potassium iodide shows no *in vitro* activity despite *in vivo* efficacy (183). Both *Conidiobolus* and *Basidiobolus* species exhibit relatively high MICs when tested with AMB, azoles, and echinocandins (184–186). Recently, Tondolo and colleagues reported terbinafine as an active drug against *C. lamprauges* (186). Overall, *Basidiobolus* spp. are more susceptible than *Conidiobolus* spp. to the different antifungals tested.

Evaluation, Interpretation, and Reporting of Results

In areas of endemicity, final diagnosis is based on the combination of direct examination showing broad, thin-walled hyphae with a Splendore-Hoeppli phenomenon without necrosis or invasion of blood vessels. In case of positive cultures, results of antifungal susceptibility testing do not currently influence the therapeutic decision.

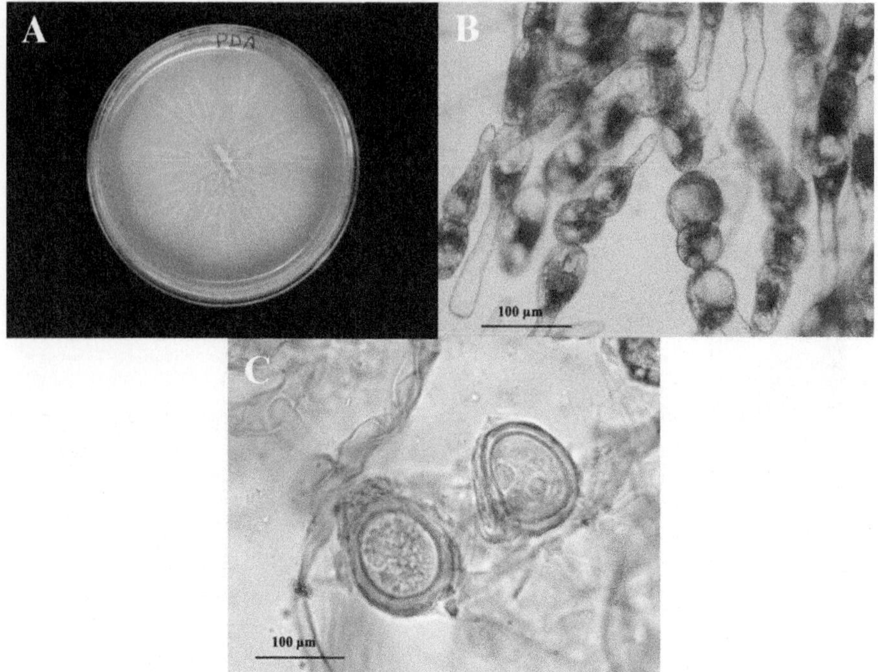

FIGURE 16 *Basidiobolus ranarum*. (A) Ten-day-old wrinkled colony on PDA medium; (B) uninucleated hyphal elements; (C) young zygospores.

REFERENCES

1. **Hibbett DS, et al.** 2007. A higher-level phylogenetic classification of the *Fungi*. *Mycol Res* **111:**509–547.
2. **O'Donnell K, Lutzoni F, Ward TJ, Benny GL.** 2001. Evolutionary relationships among mucoralean fungi (*Zygomycota*): evidence for family polyphyly on a large scale. *Mycologia* **93:**286–296.
3. **Voigt K, Cigelnik E, O'donnell K.** 1999. Phylogeny and PCR identification of clinically important Zygomycetes based on nuclear ribosomal-DNA sequence data. *J Clin Microbiol* **37:**3957–3964
4. **Voigt K, Wöstemeyer J.** 2001. Phylogeny and origin of 82 zygomycetes from all 54 genera of the *Mucorales* and *Mortierellales* based on combined analysis of actin and translation elongation factor EF-1alpha genes. *Gene* **270:**113–120.
5. **Hoffmann K, Pawłowska J, Walther G, Wrzosek M, de Hoog GS, Benny GL, Kirk PM, Voigt K.** 2013. The family structure of the *Mucorales*: a synoptic revision based on comprehensive multigene-genealogies. *Persoonia* **30:**57–76.
6. **Garcia-Hermoso D, Hoinard D, Gantier JC, Grenouillet F, Dromer F, Dannaoui E.** 2009. Molecular and phenotypic evaluation of *Lichtheimia corymbifera* (formerly *Absidia corymbifera*) complex isolates associated with human mucormycosis: rehabilitation of *L. ramosa*. *J Clin Microbiol* **47:**3862–3870.
7. **Hoffmann K, Discher S, Voigt K.** 2007. Revision of the genus *Absidia* (*Mucorales*, Zygomycetes) based on physiological, phylogenetic, and morphological characters; thermotolerant *Absidia* spp. form a coherent group, *Mycocladiaceae* fam. nov. *Mycol Res* **111:**1169–1183.
8. **Alastruey-Izquierdo A, Hoffmann K, de Hoog GS, Rodriguez-Tudela JL, Voigt K, Bibashi E, Walther G.** 2010. Species recognition and clinical relevance of the zygomycetous genus *Lichtheimia* (syn. *Absidia* pro parte, *Mycocladus*). *J Clin Microbiol* **48:**2154–2170.
9. **Alvarez E, Stchigel AM, Cano J, Sutton DA, Fothergill AW, Chander J, Salas V, Rinaldi MG, Guarro J.** 2010. Molecular phylogenetic diversity of the emerging mucoralean fungus *Apophysomyces*: proposal of three new species. *Rev Iberoam Micol* **27:**80–89.
10. **Alvarez E, Cano J, Stchigel AM, Sutton DA, Fothergill AW, Salas V, Rinaldi MG, Guarro J.** 2011. Two new species of *Mucor* from clinical samples. *Med Mycol* **49:**62–72.
11. **Ma LJ, Ibrahim AS, Skory C, Grabherr MG, Burger G, Butler M, Elias M, Idnurm A, Lang BF, Sone T, Abe A, Calvo SE, Corrochano LM, Engels R, Fu J, Hansberg W, Kim JM, Kodira CD, Koehrsen MJ, Liu B, Miranda-Saavedra D, O'Leary S, Ortiz-Castellanos L, Poulter R, Rodriguez-Romero J, Ruiz-Herrera J, Shen YQ, Zeng Q, Galagan J, Birren BW, Cuomo CA, Wickes BL.** 2009. Genomic analysis of the basal lineage fungus *Rhizopus oryzae* reveals a whole-genome duplication. *PLoS Genet* **5:**e1000549.
12. **Humber RA.** 2012. *Entomophthoromycota*: a new phylum and reclassification of entomophthoroid fungi. *Mycotaxon* **120:**477–492.
13. **Gryganskyi AP, Humber RA, Smith ME, Miadlikowska J, Wu S, Voigt K, Walther G, Anishchenko IM, Vilgalys R.** 2012. Molecular phylogeny of the *Entomophthoromycota*. *Mol Phylogenet Evol* **65:**682–694.
14. **de Hoog GS, Guarro J, Gené J, Figueras MJ.** 2011. *Atlas of Clinical Fungi CD-ROM, 3.1.* Centraalbureau voor Schimmelcultures, Utrecht, The Netherlands.
15. **Gryganskyi AP, Humber RA, Smith ME, Hodge K, Huang B, Voigt K, Vilgalys R.** 2013. Phylogenetic lineages in *Entomophthoromycota*. *Persoonia* **30:**94–105.
16. **Ribes JA, Vanover-Sams CL, Baker DJ.** 2000. Zygomycetes in human disease. *Clin Microbiol Rev* **13:**236–301.
17. **Lanternier F, Dannaoui E, Morizot G, Elie C, Garcia-Hermoso D, Huerre M, Bitar D, Dromer F, Lortholary O, French Mycosis Study Group.** 2012. A global analysis of mucormycosis in France: the RetroZygo Study (2005–2007). *Clin Infect Dis* **54**(Suppl 1)**:**S35–S43.
18. **Neblett Fanfair R, Benedict K, Bos J, Bennett SD, Lo YC, Adebanjo T, Etienne K, Deak E, Derado G, Shieh WJ, Drew C, Zaki S, Sugerman D, Gade L, Thompson EH, Sutton DA, Engelthaler DM, Schupp JM, Brandt ME, Harris JR, Lockhart SR, Turabelidze G, Park BJ.** 2012. Necrotizing cutaneous mucormycosis after a tornado in Joplin, Missouri, in 2011. *N Engl J Med* **367:**2214–2225.

19. **Warkentien T, Rodriguez C, Lloyd B, Wells J, Weintrob A, Dunne JR, Ganesan A, Li P, Bradley W, Gaskins LJ, Seillier-Moiseiwitsch F, Murray CK, Millar EV, Keenan B, Paolino K, Fleming M, Hospenthal DR, Wortmann GW, Landrum ML, Kortepeter MG, Tribble DR, Infectious Disease Clinical Research Program Trauma Infectious Disease Outcomes Study Group.** 2012. Invasive mold infections following combat-related injuries. *Clin Infect Dis* **55:**1441–1449.
20. **Kwon-Chung K, Bennett J.** 1982. *Medical Mycology*. Lea & Febiger, Philadelphia, PA.
21. **Rammaert B, Lanternier F, Zahar JR, Dannaoui E, Bougnoux ME, Lecuit M, Lortholary O.** 2012. Healthcare-associated mucormycosis. *Clin Infect Dis* **54**(Suppl 1)**:**S44–S54.
22. **Guarro J, Chander J, Alvarez E, Stchigel AM, Robin K, Dalal U, Rani H, Punia RS, Cano JF.** 2011. *Apophysomyces variabilis* infections in humans. *Emerg Infect Dis* **17:**134–135.
23. **Legrand M, Gits-Muselli M, Boutin L, Garcia-Hermoso D, Maurel V, Soussi S, Benyamina M, Ferry A, Chaussard M, Hamane S, Denis B, Touratier S, Guigue N, Fréalle E, Jeanne M, Shaal JV, Soler C, Mimoun M, Chaouat M, Lafaurie M, Mebazaa A, Bretagne S, Alanio A.** 2016. Detection of circulating *Mucorales* DNA in critically ill burn patients: preliminary report of a screening strategy for early diagnosis and treatment. *Clin Infect Dis* **63:**1312–1317.
24. **Duffy J, Harris J, Gade L, Sehulster L, Newhouse E, O'Connell H, Noble-Wang J, Rao C, Balajee SA, Chiller T.** 2014. Mucormycosis outbreak associated with hospital linens. *Pediatr Infect Dis J* **33:**472–476.
25. **Lee SC, Billmyre RB, Li A, Carson S, Sykes SM, Huh EY, Mieczkowski P, Ko DC, Cuomo CA, Heitman J.** 2014. Analysis of a food-borne fungal pathogen outbreak: virulence and genome of a *Mucor circinelloides* isolate from yogurt. *MBio* **5:**e01390–e14.
26. **Chayakulkeeree M, Ghannoum MA, Perfect JR.** 2006. Zygomycosis: the re-emerging fungal infection. *Eur J Clin Microbiol Infect Dis* **25:**215–229.
27. **Kontoyiannis DP, Lionakis MS, Lewis RE, Chamilos G, Healy M, Perego C, Safdar A, Kantarjian H, Champlin R, Walsh TJ, Raad II.** 2005. Zygomycosis in a tertiary-care cancer center in the era of Aspergillus-active antifungal therapy: a case-control observational study of 27 recent cases. *J Infect Dis* **191:**1350–1360.
28. **Marty FM, Cosimi LA, Baden LR.** 2004. Breakthrough zygomycosis after voriconazole treatment in recipients of hematopoietic stem-cell transplants. *N Engl J Med* **350:**950–952.
29. **Prabhu RM, Patel R.** 2004. Mucormycosis and entomophthoramycosis: a review of the clinical manifestations, diagnosis and treatment. *Clin Microbiol Infect* **10**(Suppl 1)**:**31–47.
30. **Marr KA, Carter RA, Crippa F, Wald A, Corey L.** 2002. Epidemiology and outcome of mould infections in hematopoietic stem cell transplant recipients. *Clin Infect Dis* **34:** 909–917.
31. **Bitar D, Van Cauteren D, Lanternier F, Dannaoui E, Che D, Dromer F, Desenclos JC, Lortholary O.** 2009. Increasing incidence of zygomycosis (mucormycosis), France, 1997–2006. *Emerg Infect Dis* **15:**1395–1401.
32. **Bitar D, Morizot G, Van Cauteren D, Dannaoui E, Lanternier F, Lortholary O, Dromer F.** 2012. Estimating the burden of mucormycosis infections in France (2005–2007) through a capture-recapture method on laboratory and administrative data. *Rev Epidemiol Sante Publique* **60:**383–387.
33. **Bitar D, Lortholary O, Dromer F, Coignard B, Che D.** 2013. Invasive fungal infections in hospital discharge data, metropolitan France, 2001–2010: incidence, lethality and trends. *Bull Epidemiol Hebd (Paris)* **2013:**109–114.
34. **Rees JR, Pinner RW, Hajjeh RA, Brandt ME, Reingold AL.** 1998. The epidemiological features of invasive mycotic infections in the San Francisco Bay area, 1992–1993: results of population-based laboratory active surveillance. *Clin Infect Dis* **27:**1138–1147.
35. **Torres-Narbona M, Guinea J, Martínez-Alarcón J, Muñoz P, Gadea I, Bouza E, MYCOMED Zygomycosis Study Group.** 2007. Impact of zygomycosis on microbiology workload: a survey study in Spain. *J Clin Microbiol* **45:**2051–2053.
36. **Bitar D, Lortholary O, Le Strat Y, Nicolau J, Coignard B, Tattevin P, Che D, Dromer F.** 2014. Population-based analysis of invasive fungal infections, France, 2001–2010. *Emerg Infect Dis* **20:**1149–1155.
37. **Roden MM, Zaoutis TE, Buchanan WL, Knudsen TA, Sarkisova TA, Schaufele RL, Sein M, Sein T, Chiou CC, Chu JH, Kontoyiannis DP, Walsh TJ.** 2005. Epidemiology and outcome of zygomycosis: a review of 929 reported cases. *Clin Infect Dis* **41:**634–653.
38. **Lanternier F, Lortholary O.** 2009. Zygomycosis and diabetes mellitus. *Clin Microbiol Infect* **15**(Suppl 5)**:**21–25.
39. **Chakrabarti A, Das A, Mandal J, Shivaprakash MR, George VK, Tarai B, Rao P, Panda N, Verma SC, Sakhuja V.** 2006. The rising trend of invasive zygomycosis in patients with uncontrolled diabetes mellitus. *Med Mycol* **44:**335–342.
40. **Zaoutis TE, Roilides E, Chiou CC, Buchanan WL, Knudsen TA, Sarkisova TA, Schaufele RL, Sein M, Sein T, Prasad PA, Chu JH, Walsh TJ.** 2007. Zygomycosis in children: a systematic review and analysis of reported cases. *Pediatr Infect Dis J* **26:**723–727.
41. **Singh N, Aguado JM, Bonatti H, Forrest G, Gupta KL, Safdar N, John GT, Pursell KJ, Muñoz P, Patel R, Fortun J, Martin-Davila P, Philippe B, Philit F, Tabah A, Terzi N, Chatelet V, Kusne S, Clark N, Blumberg E, Julia MB, Humar A, Houston S, Lass-Flörl C, Johnson L, Dubberke ER, Barron MA, Lortholary O.** 2009. Zygomycosis in solid organ transplant recipients: a prospective, matched case-control study to assess risks for disease and outcome. *J Infect Dis* **200:**1002–1011.
42. **Chamilos G, Marom EM, Lewis RE, Lionakis MS, Kontoyiannis DP.** 2005. Predictors of pulmonary zygomycosis versus invasive pulmonary aspergillosis in patients with cancer. *Clin Infect Dis* **41:**60–66.
43. **Pagano L, Caira M, Candoni A, Offidani M, Fianchi L, Martino B, Pastore D, Picardi M, Bonini A, Chierichini A, Fanci R, Caramatti C, Invernizzi R, Mattei D, Mitra ME, Melillo L, Aversa F, Van Lint MT, Falcucci P, Valentini CG, Girmenia C, Nosari A.** 2006. The epidemiology of fungal infections in patients with hematologic malignancies: the SEIFEM-2004 study. *Haematologica* **91:**1068–1075
44. **Nosari A, Oreste P, Montillo M, Carrafiello G, Draisci M, Muti G, Molteni A, Morra E.** 2000. Mucormycosis in hematologic malignancies: an emerging fungal infection. *Haematologica* **85:**1068–1071
45. **Pagano L, Offidani M, Fianchi L, Nosari A, Candoni A, Picardi M, Corvatta L, D'Antonio D, Girmenia C, Martino P, Del Favero A, GIMEMA (Gruppo Italiano Malattie EMatologiche dell'Adulto) Infection Program.** 2004. Mucormycosis in hematologic patients. *Haematologica* **89:**207–214
46. **Kontoyiannis DP, Wessel VC, Bodey GP, Rolston KV.** 2000. Zygomycosis in the 1990s in a tertiary-care cancer center. *Clin Infect Dis* **30:**851–856.
47. **Kontoyiannis DP, Marr KA, Park BJ, Alexander BD, Anaissie EJ, Walsh TJ, Ito J, Andes DR, Baddley JW, Brown JM, Brumble LM, Freifeld AG, Hadley S, Herwaldt LA, Kauffman CA, Knapp K, Lyon GM, Morrison VA, Papanicolaou G, Patterson TF, Perl TM, Schuster MG, Walker R, Wannemuehler KA, Wingard JR, Chiller TM, Pappas PG.** 2010. Prospective surveillance for invasive fungal infections in hematopoietic stem cell transplant recipients, 2001–2006: overview of the Transplant-Associated Infection Surveillance Network (TRANSNET) Database. *Clin Infect Dis* **50:**1091–1100.
48. **Neofytos D, Horn D, Anaissie E, Steinbach W, Olyaei A, Fishman J, Pfaller M, Chang C, Webster K, Marr K.** 2009. Epidemiology and outcome of invasive fungal infection in adult hematopoietic stem cell transplant recipients: analysis of Multicenter Prospective Antifungal Therapy (PATH) Alliance registry. *Clin Infect Dis* **48:**265–273.
49. **Blin N, Morineau N, Gaillard F, Morin O, Milpied N, Harousseau JL, Moreau P.** 2004. Disseminated mucormycosis associated with invasive pulmonary aspergillosis in a patient treated for post-transplant high-grade non-Hodgkin's lymphoma. *Leuk Lymphoma* **45:**2161–2163.

50. **Imhof A, Balajee SA, Fredricks DN, Englund JA, Marr KA.** 2004. Breakthrough fungal infections in stem cell transplant recipients receiving voriconazole. *Clin Infect Dis* **39:**743–746.
51. **Safdar A, O'Brien S, Kouri IF.** 2004. Efficacy and feasibility of aerosolized amphotericin B lipid complex therapy in caspofungin breakthrough pulmonary zygomycosis. *Bone Marrow Transplant* **34:**467–468.
52. **Girmenia C, Moleti ML, Micozzi A, Iori AP, Barberi W, Foà R, Martino P.** 2005. Breakthrough *Candida krusei* fungemia during fluconazole prophylaxis followed by breakthrough zygomycosis during caspofungin therapy in a patient with severe aplastic anemia who underwent stem cell transplantation. *J Clin Microbiol* **43:**5395–5396.
53. **Pappas PG, Alexander BD, Andes DR, Hadley S, Kauffman CA, Freifeld A, Anaissie EJ, Brumble LM, Herwaldt L, Ito J, Kontoyiannis DP, Lyon GM, Marr KA, Morrison VA, Park BJ, Patterson TF, Perl TM, Oster RA, Schuster MG, Walker R, Walsh TJ, Wannemuehler KA, Chiller TM.** 2010. Invasive fungal infections among organ transplant recipients: results of the Transplant-Associated Infection Surveillance Network (TRANSNET). *Clin Infect Dis* **50:** 1101–1111.
54. **Skiada A, Pagano L, Groll A, Zimmerli S, Dupont B, Lagrou K, Lass-Florl C, Bouza E, Klimko N, Gaustad P, Richardson M, Hamal P, Akova M, Meis JF, Rodriguez-Tudela JL, Roilides E, Mitrousia-Ziouva A, Petrikkos G, European Confederation of Medical Mycology Working Group on Zygomycosis.** 2011. Zygomycosis in Europe: analysis of 230 cases accrued by the registry of the European Confederation of Medical Mycology (ECMM) Working Group on Zygomycosis between 2005 and 2007. *Clin Microbiol Infect* **17:**1859–1867.
55. **Wahba H, Truong MT, Lei X, Kontoyiannis DP, Marom EM.** 2008. Reversed halo sign in invasive pulmonary fungal infections. *Clin Infect Dis* **46:**1733–1737.
56. **Legouge C, Caillot D, Chrétien ML, Lafon I, Ferrant E, Audia S, Pagès PB, Roques M, Estivalet L, Martin L, Maitre T, Bastie JN, Dalle F.** 2014. The reversed halo sign: pathognomonic pattern of pulmonary mucormycosis in leukemic patients with neutropenia? *Clin Infect Dis* **58:** 672–678.
57. **Georgiadou SP, Sipsas NV, Marom EM, Kontoyiannis DP.** 2011. The diagnostic value of halo and reversed halo signs for invasive mold infections in compromised hosts. *Clin Infect Dis* **52:**1144–1155.
58. **Marchiori E, Marom EM, Zanetti G, Hochhegger B, Irion KL, Godoy MCB.** 2012. Reversed halo sign in invasive fungal infections: criteria for differentiation from organizing pneumonia. *Chest* **142:**1469–1473.
59. **Sun HY, Aguado JM, Bonatti H, Forrest G, Gupta KL, Safdar N, John GT, Pursell KJ, Muñoz P, Patel R, Fortun J, Martin-Davila P, Philippe B, Philit F, Tabah A, Terzi N, Chatelet V, Kusne S, Clark N, Blumberg E, Julia MB, Humar A, Houston S, Lass-Florl C, Johnson L, Dubberke ER, Barron MA, Lortholary O, Singh N, Zygomycosis Transplant Study Group.** 2009. Pulmonary zygomycosis in solid organ transplant recipients in the current era. *Am J Transplant* **9:**2166–2171.
60. **Almaslamani M, Taj-Aldeen SJ, Garcia-Hermoso D, Dannaoui E, Alsoub H, Alkhal A.** 2009. An increasing trend of cutaneous zygomycosis caused by *Mycocladus corymbifer* (formerly *Absidia corymbifera*): report of two cases and review of primary cutaneous *Mycocladus* infections. *Med Mycol* **47:** 532–538.
61. **Vitrat-Hincky V, Lebeau B, Bozonnet E, Falcon D, Pradel P, Faure O, Aubert A, Piolat C, Grillot R, Pelloux H.** 2009. Severe filamentous fungal infections after widespread tissue damage due to traumatic injury: six cases and review of the literature. *Scand J Infect Dis* **41:**491–500.
62. **Lelievre L, Garcia-Hermoso D, Abdoul H, Hivelin M, Chouaki T, Toubas D, Mamez AC, Lantieri L, Lortholary O, Lanternier F, French Mycosis Study Group.** 2014. Post-traumatic mucormycosis: a nationwide study in France and review of the literature. *Medicine (Baltimore)* **93:**395–404.
63. **Cornely OA, Maertens J, Winston DJ, Perfect J, Ullmann AJ, Walsh TJ, Helfgott D, Holowiecki J, Stockelberg D, Goh YT, Petrini M, Hardalo C, Suresh R, Angulo-Gonzalez D.** 2007. Posaconazole vs. fluconazole or itraconazole prophylaxis in patients with neutropenia. *N Engl J Med* **356:**348–359.
64. **Ullmann AJ, Lipton JH, Vesole DH, Chandrasekar P, Langston A, Tarantolo SR, Greinix H, Morais de Azevedo W, Reddy V, Boparai N, Pedicone L, Patino H, Durrant S.** 2007. Posaconazole or fluconazole for prophylaxis in severe graft-versus-host disease. *N Engl J Med* **356:**335–347.
65. **Walsh TJ, Kontoyiannis DP.** 2008. Editorial commentary: what is the role of combination therapy in management of zygomycosis? *Clin Infect Dis* **47:**372–374.
66. **Tissot F, Agrawal S, Pagano L, Petrikkos G, Groll AH, Skiada A, Lass-Flörl C, Calandra T, Viscoli C, Herbrecht R.** 2017. ECIL-6 guidelines for the treatment of invasive candidiasis, aspergillosis and mucormycosis in leukemia and hematopoietic stem cell transplant patients. *Haematologica* **102:**433–444.
67. **Lanternier F, Lortholary O.** 2008. Liposomal amphotericin B: what is its role in 2008? *Clin Microbiol Infect* **14**(Suppl 4)**:**71–83.
68. **Björkholm M, Runarsson G, Celsing F, Kalin M, Petrini B, Engervall P, Magnus Björkholm, Gudmundur Runarss.** 2001. Liposomal amphotericin B and surgery in the successful treatment of invasive pulmonary mucormycosis in a patient with acute T-lymphoblastic leukemia. *Scand J Infect Dis* **33:** 316–319.
69. **Parkyn T, McNinch AW, Riordan T, Mott M.** 2000. Zygomycosis in relapsed acute leukaemia. *J Infect* **41:**265–268.
70. **Skiada A, Lanternier F, Groll AH, Pagano L, Zimmerli S, Herbrecht R, Lortholary O, Petrikkos GL, European Conference on Infections in Leukemia.** 2013. Diagnosis and treatment of mucormycosis in patients with hematological malignancies: guidelines from the 3rd European Conference on Infections in Leukemia (ECIL 3). *Haematologica* **98:**492–504.
71. **Cornely OA, Arikan-Akdagli S, Dannaoui E, Groll AH, Lagrou K, Chakrabarti A, Lanternier F, Pagano L, Skiada A, Akova M, Arendrup MC, Boekhout T, Chowdhary A, Cuenca-Estrella M, Freiberger T, Guinea J, Guarro J, de Hoog S, Hope W, Johnson E, Kathuria S, Lackner M, Lass-Flörl C, Lortholary O, Meis JF, Meletiadis J, Muñoz P, Richardson M, Roilides E, Tortorano AM, Ullmann AJ, van Diepeningen A, Verweij P, Petrikkos G, European Society of Clinical Microbiology and Infectious Diseases Fungal Infection Study Group, European Confederation of Medical Mycology.** 2014. ESCMID and ECMM joint clinical guidelines for the diagnosis and management of mucormycosis 2013. *Clin Microbiol Infect* **20**(Suppl 3)**:**5–26.
72. **Marty FM, Ostrosky-Zeichner L, Cornely OA, Mullane KM, Perfect JR, Thompson GR III, Alangaden GJ, Brown JM, Fredricks DN, Heinz WJ, Herbrecht R, Klimko N, Klyasova G, Maertens JA, Melinkeri SR, Oren I, Pappas PG, Ráčil Z, Rahav G, Santos R, Schwartz S, Vehreschild JJ, Young JH, Chetchotisakd P, Jaruratanasirikul S, Kanj SS, Engelhardt M, Kaufhold A, Ito M, Lee M, Sasse C, Maher RM, Zeiher B, Vehreschild MJGT, VITAL and FungiScope Mucormycosis Investigators.** 2016. Isavuconazole treatment for mucormycosis: a single-arm open-label trial and case-control analysis. *Lancet Infect Dis* **16:**828–837.
73. **Lanternier F, Poiree S, Elie C, Garcia-Hermoso D, Bakouboula P, Sitbon K, Herbrecht R, Wolff M, Ribaud P, Lortholary O, French Mycosis Study Group.** 2015. Prospective pilot study of high-dose (10 mg/kg/day) liposomal amphotericin B (L-AMB) for the initial treatment of mucormycosis. *J Antimicrob Chemother* **70:**3116–3123.
74. **Chamilos G, Lewis RE, Kontoyiannis DP.** 2008. Delaying amphotericin B-based frontline therapy significantly increases mortality among patients with hematologic malignancy who have zygomycosis. *Clin Infect Dis* **47:**503–509.
75. **Marchetti O, Lamoth F, Mikulska M, Viscoli C, Verweij P, Bretagne S, European Conference on Infections in Leukemia (ECIL) Laboratory Working Groups.** 2012. ECIL recommendations for the use of biological markers for the diagnosis of invasive fungal diseases in leukemic patients and hematopoietic SCT recipients. *Bone Marrow Transplant* **47:**846–854.

76. **Arendrup MC, Bille J, Dannaoui E, Ruhnke M, Heussel CP, Kibbler C.** 2012. ECIL-3 classical diagnostic procedures for the diagnosis of invasive fungal diseases in patients with leukaemia. *Bone Marrow Transplant* **47:**1030–1045.
77. **Glazer M, Nusair S, Breuer R, Lafair J, Sherman Y, Berkman N.** 2000. The role of BAL in the diagnosis of pulmonary mucormycosis. *Chest* **117:**279–282.
78. **Nosari A, Anghilieri M, Carrafiello G, Guffanti C, Marbello L, Montillo M, Muti G, Ribera S, Vanzulli A, Nichelatti M, Morra E.** 2003. Utility of percutaneous lung biopsy for diagnosing filamentous fungal infections in hematologic malignancies. *Haematologica* **88:**1405–1409
79. **Leber AL.** 2016. Mycology and Antifungal Susceptibility Testing. *In* Leber AL (ed.), *Clinical Microbiology Procedures Handbook*, vol. 2. sect. 8. ASM Press, Washington, DC.
80. **Lass-Flörl C.** 2009. Zygomycosis: conventional laboratory diagnosis. *Clin Microbiol Infect* **15**(Suppl 5)**:**60–65.
81. **Frater JL, Hall GS, Procop GW.** 2001. Histologic features of zygomycosis: emphasis on perineural invasion and fungal morphology. *Arch Pathol Lab Med* **125:**375–378
82. **Guarner J, Brandt ME.** 2011. Histopathologic diagnosis of fungal infections in the 21st century. *Clin Microbiol Rev* **24:**247–280.
83. **Almyroudis NG, Sutton DA, Fothergill AW, Rinaldi MG, Kusne S.** 2007. In vitro susceptibilities of 217 clinical isolates of zygomycetes to conventional and new antifungal agents. *Antimicrob Agents Chemother* **51:**2587–2590.
84. **Walsh TJ, Gamaletsou MN, McGinnis MR, Hayden RT, Kontoyiannis DP.** 2012. Early clinical and laboratory diagnosis of invasive pulmonary, extrapulmonary, and disseminated mucormycosis (zygomycosis). *Clin Infect Dis* **54**(Suppl 1)**:**S55–S60.
85. **Buitrago MJ, Aguado JM, Ballen A, Bernal-Martinez L, Prieto M, Garcia-Reyne A, Garcia-Rodriguez J, Rodriguez-Tudela JL, Cuenca-Estrella M.** 2013. Efficacy of DNA amplification in tissue biopsy samples to improve the detection of invasive fungal disease. *Clin Microbiol Infect* **19:**E271–E277.
86. **Cabaret O, Toussain G, Abermil N, Alsamad IA, Botterel F, Costa JM, Papon JF, Bretagne S.** 2011. Degradation of fungal DNA in formalin-fixed paraffin-embedded sinus fungal balls hampers reliable sequence-based identification of fungi. *Med Mycol* **49:**329–332.
87. **Schwarz P, Bretagne S, Gantier JC, Garcia-Hermoso D, Lortholary O, Dromer F, Dannaoui E.** 2006. Molecular identification of zygomycetes from culture and experimentally infected tissues. *J Clin Microbiol* **44:**340–349.
88. **Bialek R, Konrad F, Kern J, Aepinus C, Cecenas L, Gonzalez GM, Just-Nübling G, Willinger B, Presterl E, Lass-Flörl C, Rickerts V.** 2005. PCR based identification and discrimination of agents of mucormycosis and aspergillosis in paraffin wax embedded tissue. *J Clin Pathol* **58:**1180–1184.
89. **Rickerts V, Just-Nübling G, Konrad F, Kern J, Lambrecht E, Böhme A, Jacobi V, Bialek R.** 2006. Diagnosis of invasive aspergillosis and mucormycosis in immunocompromised patients by seminested PCR assay of tissue samples. *Eur J Clin Microbiol Infect Dis* **25:**8–13.
90. **Rickerts V, Mousset S, Lambrecht E, Tintelnot K, Schwerdtfeger R, Presterl E, Jacobi V, Just-Nübling G, Bialek R.** 2007. Comparison of histopathological analysis, culture, and polymerase chain reaction assays to detect invasive mold infections from biopsy specimens. *Clin Infect Dis* **44:**1078–1083.
91. **Hata DJ, Buckwalter SP, Pritt BS, Roberts GD, Wengenack NL.** 2008. Real-time PCR method for detection of zygomycetes. *J Clin Microbiol* **46:**2353–2358.
92. **Salehi E, Hedayati MT, Zoll J, Rafati H, Ghasemi M, Doroudinia A, Abastabar M, Tolooe A, Snelders E, van der Lee HA, Rijs AJ, Verweij PE, Seyedmousavi S, Melchers WJ.** 2016. Discrimination of aspergillosis, mucormycosis, fusariosis and scedosporiosis in formalin-fixed paraffin-embedded tissue specimens using multiple real-time quantitative PCR assays. *J Clin Microbiol* **54:**2798–2803.
93. **Alanio A, Garcia-Hermoso D, Mercier-Delarue S, Lanternier F, Gits-Muselli M, Menotti J, Denis B, Bergeron A, Legrand M, Lortholary O, Bretagne S, French Mycosis Study Group.** 2015. Molecular identification of *Mucorales* in human tissues: contribution of PCR electrospray-ionization mass spectrometry. *Clin Microbiol Infect* **21:**594.e1–594.e5.
94. **Hayden RT, Qian X, Procop GW, Roberts GD, Lloyd RV.** 2002. In situ hybridization for the identification of filamentous fungi in tissue section. *Diagn Mol Pathol* **11:**119–126.
95. **Rickerts V, Khot PD, Myerson D, Ko DL, Lambrecht E, Fredricks DN.** 2011. Comparison of quantitative real time PCR with sequencing and ribosomal RNA-FISH for the identification of fungi in formalin fixed, paraffin-embedded tissue specimens. *BMC Infect Dis* **11:**202.
96. **Millon L, Larosa F, Lepiller Q, Legrand F, Rocchi S, Daguindau E, Scherer E, Bellanger AP, Leroy J, Grenouillet F.** 2013. Quantitative polymerase chain reaction detection of circulating DNA in serum for early diagnosis of mucormycosis in immunocompromised patients. *Clin Infect Dis* **56:**e95–e101.
97. **Millon L, et al, French Mycosis Study Group.** 2016. Early diagnosis and monitoring of mucormycosis by detection of circulating DNA in serum: retrospective analysis of 44 cases collected through the French Surveillance Network of Invasive Fungal Infections (RESSIF). *Clin Microbiol Infect* **22:**810.e1–810.e8.
98. **Springer J, Goldenberger D, Schmidt F, Weisser M, Wehrle-Wieland E, Einsele H, Frei R, Löffler J.** 2016. Development and application of two independent real-time PCR assays to detect clinically relevant *Mucorales* species. *J Med Microbiol* **65:**227–234.
99. **Springer J, Lackner M, Ensinger C, Risslegger B, Morton CO, Nachbaur D, Lass-Flörl C, Einsele H, Heinz WJ, Loeffler J.** 2016. Clinical evaluation of a *Mucorales*-specific real-time PCR assay in tissue and serum samples. *J Med Microbiol* **65:**1414–1421.
100. **Springer J, White PL, Kessel J, Wieters I, Teschner D, Korczynski D, Liebregts T, Cornely OA, Schwartz S, Elgeti T, Meintker L, Krause SW, Posso RB, Heinz WJ, Fuhrmann S, Vehreschild JJ, Einsele H, Rickerts V, Loeffler J.** 2018. A Comparison of *Aspergillus* and *Mucorales* PCR testing of different bronchoalveolar lavage fluid fractions from patients with suspected invasive pulmonary fungal disease. *J Clin Microbiol* **56:**e01655–e17
101. **Schwarz P, Lortholary O, Dromer F, Dannaoui E.** 2007. Carbon assimilation profiles as a tool for identification of zygomycetes. *J Clin Microbiol* **45:**1433–1439.
102. **Etienne KA, Gillece J, Hilsabeck R, Schupp JM, Colman R, Lockhart SR, Gade L, Thompson EH, Sutton DA, Neblett-Fanfair R, Park BJ, Turabelidze G, Keim P, Brandt ME, Deak E, Engelthaler DM.** 2012. Whole genome sequence typing to investigate the Apophysomyces outbreak following a tornado in Joplin, Missouri, 2011. *PLoS One* **7:**e49989.
103. **Gomes MZ, Lewis RE, Kontoyiannis DP.** 2011. Mucormycosis caused by unusual mucormycetes, non-Rhizopus, -Mucor, and -Lichtheimia species. *Clin Microbiol Rev* **24:**411–445.
104. **Chakrabarti A, Singh R.** 2011. The emerging epidemiology of mould infections in developing countries. *Curr Opin Infect Dis* **24:**521–526.
105. **Padhye AA, Ajello L.** 1988. Simple method of inducing sporulation by *Apophysomyces elegans* and *Saksenaea vasiformis*. *J Clin Microbiol* **26:**1861–1863
106. **Gams W, Hoekstra E, Aptroot A.** 1998. *CBS Course of Mycology*. Centraalbureau voor Schimmelcultures, Baarn, The Netherlands.
107. **Ellis D, Davis S, Alexiou H, Handke R, Bartley R.** 2007. *Descriptions of Medical Fungi*, 2nd ed. Mycology Unit, Women's and Children's Hospital, Adelaide, Australia.
108. **Hoffmann K, Walther G, Voight K.** 2009. *Mycocladus* vs. *Lichtheimia*: a correction (*Lichtheimiaceae* fam. nov., *Mucorales*, *Mucoromycotina*). *Mycol Res* **113:**277–278.
109. **St-Germain G, Summerbell R.** 1996. *Identifying Filamentous Fungi. A Clinical Laboratory Handbook*. Star Publishing Company, Belmont, CA.
110. **Lu XL, Najafzadeh MJ, Dolatabadi S, Ran YP, Gerrits van den Ende AH, Shen YN, Li CY, Xi LY, Hao F, Zhang QQ, Li RY, Hu ZM, Lu GX, Wang JJ, Drogari-Apiranthitou M, Klaassen C, Meis JF, Hagen F, Liu WD, de Hoog GS.** 2013. Taxonomy and epidemiology of *Mucor irregularis*, agent of chronic cutaneous mucormycosis. *Persoonia* **30:**48–56.

111. **Schipper MAA.** 1976. On *Mucor circinelloides, Mucor racemosus* and related species. *Stud Mycol* **12:**1–40.
112. **Karimi K, Arzanlou M, Ahari AB, Ghazi M.** 2015. Phenotypic and molecular characterization of the causal agent of chafer beetle mortality in the wheat fields of the Kurdistan province, Iran. *J Plant Prot Res* **55:**227–234.
113. **Tully CC, Romanelli AM, Sutton DA, Wickes BL, Hospenthal DR.** 2009. Fatal *Actinomucor elegans* var. *kuwaitiensis* infection following combat trauma. *J Clin Microbiol* **47:**3394–3399.
114. **Mahmud A, Lee R, Munfus-McCray D, Kwiatkowski N, Subramanian A, Neofytos D, Carroll K, Zhang SX.** 2012. *Actinomucor elegans* as an emerging cause of Mucormycosis. *J Clin Microbiol* **50:**1092–1095.
115. **Dorin J, D'Aveni M, Debourgogne A, Cuenin M, Guillaso M, Rivier A, Gallet P, Lecoanet G, Machouart M.** 2017. Update on *Actinomucor elegans*, a mucormycete infrequently detected in human specimens: how combined microbiological tools contribute efficiently to a more accurate medical care. *Int J Med Microbiol* **307:**435–442.
116. **Davel G, Featherston P, Fernández A, Abrantes R, Canteros C, Rodero L, Sztern C, Perrotta D.** 2001. Maxillary sinusitis caused by *Actinomucor elegans*. *J Clin Microbiol* **39:**740–742.
117. **Khan ZU, Ahmad S, Mokaddas E, Chandy R, Cano J, Guarro J.** 2008. *Actinomucor elegans* var. *kuwaitiensis* isolated from the wound of a diabetic patient. *Antonie van Leeuwenhoek* **94:**343–352.
118. **Hesseltine CW.** 1991. Zygomycetes in food fermentations. *Mycologist* **5:**162–169.
119. **Han BZ, Kuijpers AFA, Thanh NV, Nout MJR.** 2004. Mucoraceous moulds involved in the commercial fermentation of Sufu Pehtze. *Antonie van Leeuwenhoek* **85:**253–257.
120. **Alvarez E, Garcia-Hermoso D, Sutton DA, Cano JF, Stchigel AM, Hoinard D, Fothergill AW, Rinaldi MG, Dromer F, Guarro J.** 2010. Molecular phylogeny and proposal of two new species of the emerging pathogenic fungus *Saksenaea*. *J Clin Microbiol* **48:**4410–4416.
121. **Schipper MAA.** 1984. A revision of the genus *Rhizopus* I. The *Rhizopus stolonifer*-group and *Rhizopus oryzae*. *Stud Mycol* **25:**1–19.
122. **Alvarez E, Sutton DA, Cano J, Fothergill AW, Stchigel A, Rinaldi MG, Guarro J.** 2009. Spectrum of zygomycete species identified in clinically significant specimens in the United States. *J Clin Microbiol* **47:**1650–1656.
123. **Schipper MAA, Stalpers JA.** 1984. A revision of the genus *Rhizopus* II. The *Rhizopus microsporus* group. *Stud Mycol* **25:**30–34.
124. **Walther G, Pawłowska J, Alastruey-Izquierdo A, Wrzosek M, Rodriguez-Tudela JL, Dolatabadi S, Chakrabarti A, de Hoog GS.** 2013. DNA barcoding in *Mucorales*: an inventory of biodiversity. *Persoonia* **30:**11–47.
125. **Lemmer K, Losert H, Rickerts V, Just-Nübling G, Sander A, Kerkmann ML, Tintelnot K.** 2002. [Molecular biological identification of *Cuninghamella* spec]. *Mycoses* **45**(Suppl 1)**:** 31–36.
126. **García-Rodríguez J, Quiles-Melero I, Humala-Barbier K, Monzon A, Cuenca-Estrella M.** 2012. Isolation of *Cunninghamella blakesleeana* in an immunodepressed patient. *Mycoses* **55:**463–465.
127. **Holland J.** 1997. Emerging zygomycoses of humans: *saksenaea vasiformis* and *Apophysomyces elegans*. *Curr Top Med Mycol* **8:**27–34
128. **Garcia-Hermoso D, Dannaoui E.** 2007. The *Zygomycetes*, p 159–183. *In* Kavanagh K (ed), *New Insights in Medical Mycology*. Springer Science, New York, NY.
129. **Schoch CL, et al, Fungal Barcoding Consortium, Fungal Barcoding Consortium Author List.** 2012. Nuclear ribosomal internal transcribed spacer (ITS) region as a universal DNA barcode marker for Fungi. *Proc Natl Acad Sci USA* **109:**6241–6246.
130. **Balajee SA, Borman AM, Brandt ME, Cano J, Cuenca-Estrella M, Dannaoui E, Guarro J, Haase G, Kibbler CC, Meyer W, O'Donnell K, Petti CA, Rodriguez-Tudela JL, Sutton D, Velegraki A, Wickes BL.** 2009. Sequence-based identification of *Aspergillus, fusarium*, and *mucorales* species in the clinical mycology laboratory: where are we and where should we go from here? *J Clin Microbiol* **47:**877–884.
131. **Abe A, Sone T, Sujaya IN, Saito K, Oda Y, Asano K, Tomita F.** 2003. rDNA ITS sequence of *Rhizopus oryzae*: its application to classification and identification of lactic acid producers. *Biosci Biotechnol Biochem* **67:**1725–1731.
132. **Chakrabarti A, Ghosh A, Prasad GS, David JK, Gupta S, Das A, Sakhuja V, Panda NK, Singh SK, Das S, Chakrabarti T.** 2003. *Apophysomyces elegans*: an emerging zygomycete in India. *J Clin Microbiol* **41:**783–788.
133. **Potenza L, Vallerini D, Barozzi P, Riva G, Forghieri F, Zanetti E, Quadrelli C, Candoni A, Maertens J, Rossi G, Morselli M, Codeluppi M, Paolini A, Maccaferri M, Del Giovane C, D'Amico R, Rumpianesi F, Pecorari M, Cavalleri F, Marasca R, Narni F, Luppi M.** 2011. Mucorales-specific T cells emerge in the course of invasive mucormycosis and may be used as a surrogate diagnostic marker in high-risk patients. *Blood* **118:**5416–5419.
134. **Clinical and Laboratory Standards Institute.** 2008. Reference Method for Broth Dilution Antifungal Susceptibility Testing of Filamentous Fungi: Approved Standard. Document M-38A2. Clinical and Laboratory Standards Institute, Wayne, PA.
135. **Subcommittee on Antifungal Susceptibility Testing of the ESCMID European Committee for Antimicrobial Susceptibility Testing.** 2008. EUCAST Technical Note on the method for the determination of broth dilution minimum inhibitory concentrations of antifungal agents for conidia-forming moulds. *Clin Microbiol Infect* **14:**982–984.
136. **Espinel-Ingroff A.** 2006. Comparison of three commercial assays and a modified disk diffusion assay with two broth microdilution reference assays for testing zygomycetes, *Aspergillus* spp., *Candida* spp., and *Cryptococcus neoformans* with posaconazole and amphotericin B. *J Clin Microbiol* **44:** 3616–3622.
137. **Dannaoui E, Meis JF, Mouton JW, Verweij PE, Eurofung Network.** 2002. In vitro susceptibilities of *Zygomycota* to polyenes. *J Antimicrob Chemother* **49:**741–744.
138. **Dannaoui E, Meletiadis J, Mouton JW, Meis JF, Verweij PE, Eurofung Network.** 2003. In vitro susceptibilities of zygomycetes to conventional and new antifungals. *J Antimicrob Chemother* **51:**45–52.
139. **Sun QN, Fothergill AW, McCarthy DI, Rinaldi MG, Graybill JR.** 2002. In vitro activities of posaconazole, itraconazole, voriconazole, amphotericin B, and fluconazole against 37 clinical isolates of zygomycetes. *Antimicrob Agents Chemother* **46:**1581–1582.
140. **Torres-Narbona M, Guinea J, Martínez-Alarcón J, Peláez T, Bouza E.** 2007. In vitro activities of amphotericin B, caspofungin, itraconazole, posaconazole, and voriconazole against 45 clinical isolates of zygomycetes: comparison of CLSI M38-A, Sensititre YeastOne, and the Etest. *Antimicrob Agents Chemother* **51:**1126–1129.
141. **Vitale RG, de Hoog GS, Schwarz P, Dannaoui E, Deng S, Machouart M, Voigt K, van de Sande WW, Dolatabadi S, Meis JF, Walther G.** 2012. Antifungal susceptibility and phylogeny of opportunistic members of the order *mucorales*. *J Clin Microbiol* **50:**66–75.
142. **Dannaoui E, Meis JF, Loebenberg D, Verweij PE.** 2003. Activity of posaconazole in treatment of experimental disseminated zygomycosis. *Antimicrob Agents Chemother* **47:**3647–3650.
143. **Ibrahim AS, Avanessian V, Spellberg B, Edwards JE Jr.** 2003. Liposomal amphotericin B, and not amphotericin B deoxycholate, improves survival of diabetic mice infected with *Rhizopus oryzae*. *Antimicrob Agents Chemother* **47:** 3343–3344.
144. **Sun QN, Najvar LK, Bocanegra R, Loebenberg D, Graybill JR.** 2002. In vivo activity of posaconazole against *Mucor* spp. in an immunosuppressed-mouse model. *Antimicrob Agents Chemother* **46:**2310–2312.

145. **Dannaoui E, Mouton JW, Meis JF, Verweij PE, Eurofung Network.** 2002. Efficacy of antifungal therapy in a nonneutropenic murine model of zygomycosis. *Antimicrob Agents Chemother* **46:**1953–1959.
146. **Salas V, Pastor FJ, Calvo E, Alvarez E, Sutton DA, Mayayo E, Fothergill AW, Rinaldi MG, Guarro J.** 2012. In vitro and in vivo activities of posaconazole and amphotericin B in a murine invasive infection by Mucor circinelloides: poor efficacy of posaconazole. *Antimicrob Agents Chemother* **56:**2246–2250.
147. **Spellberg B, Edwards J Jr, Ibrahim A.** 2005. Novel perspectives on mucormycosis: pathophysiology, presentation, and management. *Clin Microbiol Rev* **18:**556–569.
148. **Lewis RE, Liao G, Wang W, Prince RA, Kontoyiannis DP.** 2011. Voriconazole pre-exposure selects for breakthrough mucormycosis in a mixed model of *Aspergillus fumigatus-Rhizopus oryzae* pulmonary infection. *Virulence* **2:**348–355.
149. **Rodríguez MM, Pastor FJ, Sutton DA, Calvo E, Fothergill AW, Salas V, Rinaldi MG, Guarro J.** 2010. Correlation between in vitro activity of posaconazole and in vivo efficacy against *Rhizopus oryzae* infection in mice. *Antimicrob Agents Chemother* **54:**1665–1669.
150. **Salas V, Pastor FJ, Calvo E, Sutton DA, Chander J, Mayayo E, Alvarez E, Guarro J.** 2012. Efficacy of posaconazole in a murine model of disseminated infection caused by *Apophysomyces variabilis*. *J Antimicrob Chemother* **67:** 1712–1715.
151. **Salas V, Pastor FJ, Calvo E, Sutton D, García-Hermoso D, Mayayo E, Dromer F, Fothergill A, Alvarez E, Guarro J.** 2012. Experimental murine model of disseminated infection by *Saksenaea vasiformis*: successful treatment with posaconazole. *Med Mycol* **50:**710–715.
152. **Thompson GR III, Wiederhold NP.** 2010. Isavuconazole: a comprehensive review of spectrum of activity of a new triazole. *Mycopathologia* **170:**291–313.
153. **Arendrup MC, Jensen RH, Meletiadis J.** 2015. In vitro activity of isavuconazole and comparators against clinical isolates of the Mucorales order. *Antimicrob Agents Chemother* **59:**7735–7742.
154. **Luo G, Gebremariam T, Lee H, Edwards JE Jr, Kovanda L, Ibrahim AS.** 2014. Isavuconazole therapy protects immunosuppressed mice from mucormycosis. *Antimicrob Agents Chemother* **58:**2450–2453.
155. **Alastruey-Izquierdo A, Castelli MV, Cuesta I, Zaragoza O, Monzón A, Mellado E, Rodríguez-Tudela JL.** 2009. In vitro activity of antifungals against Zygomycetes. *Clin Microbiol Infect* **15**(Suppl 5)**:**71–76.
156. **Chakrabarti A, Shivaprakash MR, Curfs-Breuker I, Baghela A, Klaassen CH, Meis JF.** 2010. *Apophysomyces elegans*: epidemiology, amplified fragment length polymorphism typing, and in vitro antifungal susceptibility pattern. *J Clin Microbiol* **48:**4580–4585.
157. **Torres-Narbona M, Guinea J, Martínez-Alarcón J, Muñoz P, Peláez T, Bouza E.** 2008. Workload and clinical significance of the isolation of zygomycetes in a tertiary general hospital. *Med Mycol* **46:**225–230.
158. **De Pauw B, Walsh TJ, Donnelly JP, Stevens DA, Edwards JE, Calandra T, Pappas PG, Maertens J, Lortholary O, Kauffman CA, Denning DW, Patterson TF, Maschmeyer G, Bille J, Dismukes WE, Herbrecht R, Hope WW, Kibbler CC, Kullberg BJ, Marr KA, Muñoz P, Odds FC, Perfect JR, Restrepo A, Ruhnke M, Segal BH, Sobel JD, Sorrell TC, Viscoli C, Wingard JR, Zaoutis T, Bennett JE, European Organization for Research and Treatment of Cancer/Invasive Fungal Infections Cooperative Group, National Institute of Allergy and Infectious Diseases Mycoses Study Group (EORTC/MSG) Consensus Group.** 2008. Revised definitions of invasive fungal disease from the European Organization for Research and Treatment of Cancer/Invasive Fungal Infections Cooperative Group and the National Institute of Allergy and Infectious Diseases Mycoses Study Group (EORTC/MSG) Consensus Group. *Clin Infect Dis* **46:**1813–1821.
159. **Vikram HR, Smilack JD, Leighton JA, Crowell MD, De Petris G.** 2012. Emergence of gastrointestinal basidiobolomycosis in the United States, with a review of worldwide cases. *Clin Infect Dis* **54:**1685–1691.
160. **Cameron HM.** 1989. Entomophthoromycosis, p 186–198. *In* Mahgoub ES (ed), *Tropical Mycosis*. Janssen Research Council, Beerse, Belgium.
161. **Receveur MC, Roussin C, Mienniel B, Gasnier O, Rivière JP, Malvy D, Lortholary O.** 2005. [Rhinofacial entomophthoromycosis. About two new cases in Mayotte]. *Bull Soc Pathol Exot* **98:**350–353
162. **Kimura M, Yaguchi T, Sutton DA, Fothergill AW, Thompson EH, Wickes BL.** 2011. Disseminated human conidiobolomycosis due to *Conidiobolus lamprauges*. *J Clin Microbiol* **49:**752–756.
163. **Gugnani HC.** 1999. A review of zygomycosis due to *Basidiobolus ranarum*. *Eur J Epidemiol* **15:**923–929.
164. **Zavasky DM, Samowitz W, Loftus T, Segal H, Carroll K.** 1999. Gastrointestinal zygomycotic infection caused by *Basidiobolus ranarum*: case report and review. *Clin Infect Dis* **28:**1244–1248.
165. **Shreef K, Saleem M, Saeedd MA, Eissa M.** 2017. Gastrointestinal Basidiobolomycosis: an emerging, and a confusing, disease in children (a multicenter experience). *Eur J Pediatr Surg* **28:**194–199.
166. **Lyon GM, Smilack JD, Komatsu KK, Pasha TM, Leighton JA, Guarner J, Colby TV, Lindsley MD, Phelan M, Warnock DW, Hajjeh RA.** 2001. Gastrointestinal basidiobolomycosis in Arizona: clinical and epidemiological characteristics and review of the literature. *Clin Infect Dis* **32:**1448–1455.
167. **Sitterlé E, Rodriguez C, Mounier R, Calderaro J, Foulet F, Develoux M, Pawlotsky JM, Botterel F.** 2017. Contribution of ultra deep sequencing in the clinical diagnosis of a new fungal pathogen species: *basidiobolus meristosporus*. *Front Microbiol* **8:**334.
168. **Almoosa Z, Alsuhaibani M, AlDandan S, Alshahrani D.** 2017. Pediatric gastrointestinal basidiobolomycosis mimicking malignancy. *Med Mycol Case Rep* **18:**31–33.
169. **Abd El Maksoud WM, Bawahab MA, Ashraf TH, Al Shehri D, Mirza NI.** 2017. Surgical management of colonic basidiobolomycosis among adolescent and adult patients: presentation and outcome. *Colorectal Dis* **23:**296–303.
170. **Bigliazzi C, Poletti V, Dell'Amore D, Saragoni L, Colby TV.** 2004. Disseminated basidiobolomycosis in an immunocompetent woman. *J Clin Microbiol* **42:**1367–1369.
171. **Gugnani HC.** 1992. Entomophthoromycosis due to *Conidiobolus*. *Eur J Epidemiol* **8:**391–396.
172. **Blumentrath CG, Grobusch MP, Matsiégui PB, Pahlke F, Zoleko-Manego R, Nzenze-Afene S, Mabicka B, Sanguinetti M, Kremsner PG, Schaumburg F.** 2015. Classification of rhinoentomophthoromycosis into atypical, early, intermediate, and late disease: a proposal. *PLoS Negl Trop Dis* **9:**e0003984.
173. **Bittencourt AL, Marback R, Nossa LM.** 2006. Mucocutaneous entomophthoramycosis acquired by conjunctival inoculation of the fungus. *Am J Trop Med Hyg* **75:**936–938
174. **Walker SD, Clark RV, King CT, Humphries JE, Lytle LS, Butkus DE.** 1992. Fatal disseminated *Conidiobolus coronatus* infection in a renal transplant patient. *Am J Clin Pathol* **98:**559–564.
175. **Sharma NL, Mahajan VK, Singh P.** 2003. Orofacial conidiobolomycosis due to *Conidiobolus incongruus*. *Mycoses* **46:**137–140.
176. **Gupta M, Narang T, Kaur RJ, Manhas A, Saikia UN, Dogra S.** 2016. A prospective case series evaluating efficacy and safety of combination of itraconazole and potassium iodide in rhinofacial conidiobolomycosis. *Int J Dermatol* **55:**208–214.
177. **Hussein MR.** 2008. Mucocutaneous Splendore-Hoeppli phenomenon. *J Cutan Pathol* **35:**979–988.
178. **Gómez-Muñoz MT, Fernández-Barredo S, Martínez-Díaz RA, Pérez-Gracia MT, Ponce-Gordo F.** 2012. Development of a specific polymerase chain reaction assay for the detection of *Basidiobolus*. *Mycologia* **104:**585–591.

179. **Ben-Ze'ev I, Kenneth R.** 1982. Features-criteria of taxonomic value in the Entomophthorales. *Mycotaxon* **14:**393–455.
180. **Fromentin H, Ravisse P.** 1977. [Tropical entomophthoromycoses]. *Acta Trop* **34:**375–394
181. **Vilela R, Silva SM, Riet-Correa F, Dominguez E, Mendoza L.** 2010. Morphologic and phylogenetic characterization of *Conidiobolus lamprauges* recovered from infected sheep. *J Clin Microbiol* **48:**427–432.
182. **Okafor JI, Testrake D, Mushinsky HR, Yangco BG.** 1984. A *Basidiobolus* sp. and its association with reptiles and amphibians in southern Florida. *Sabouraudia* **22:**47–51.
183. **Yangco BG, Okafor JI, TeStrake D.** 1984. In vitro susceptibilities of human and wild-type isolates of *Basidiobolus* and *Conidiobolus* species. *Antimicrob Agents Chemother* **25:** 413–416.
184. **Guarro J, Aguilar C, Pujol I.** 1999. In-vitro antifungal susceptibilities of *Basidiobolus* and *Conidiobolus* spp. strains. *J Antimicrob Chemother* **44:**557–560.
185. **Taylor GD, Sekhon AS, Tyrrell DL, Goldsand G.** 1987. Rhinofacial zygomycosis caused by *Conidiobolus coronatus*: a case report including in vitro sensitivity to antimycotic agents. *Am J Trop Med Hyg* **36:**398–401.
186. **Tondolo JS, de Loreto ES, Dutra V, Nakazato L, de Paula DA, Zanette RA, Alves SH, Santurio JM.** 2013. In vitro susceptibility of *Conidiobolus lamprauges* recovered from sheep to antifungal agents. *Vet Microbiol* **166:**690–693.

Histoplasma, Blastomyces, Coccidioides, Paracoccidioides, and Other Dimorphic Fungi Causing Systemic Mycoses

GEORGE R. THOMPSON III AND BEATRIZ L. GÓMEZ

125

TAXONOMY

The dimorphic fungi causing systemic disease belong to the class *Eurotiomycetes*, order *Onygenales*. The *Onygenales* share several general characteristics: their sexual stages (teleomorphs) form rudimentary asci surrounded by a network of hyphae, which may have complex appendages, and their asexual (anamorph) species generally possess one of two forms, either unicellular aleurioconidia or arthroconidia in chains of alternately viable and nonviable cells.

The order *Onygenales* contains the families *Ajellomycetaceae* and *Onygenaceae*. The *Onygenaceae* and *Ajellomycetaceae* are well separated from the *Arthrodermataceae* (dermatophytes). This chapter covers the dimorphic members of the families *Onygenaceae* and *Ajellomycetaceae*. Nonpathogenic species of *Chrysosporium*, *Uncinocarpus*, and other related genera are not covered here. It should be noted that dual nomenclature for pleomorphic fungi has been discontinued (1), although it is likely that the widely recognized anamorph names for dimorphic fungi will be kept. The family *Ajellomycetaceae* contains the species *Ajellomyces dermatitidis*, *A. capsulatus*, and *A. duboisii*, the anamorphs of which have been placed in the genera *Blastomyces* (*Blastomyces dermatitidis*, *B. gilchristii*, *B. helicus*, *B. parvus*, *B. percursus*, and *B. silverae*), *Emmonsia* (*Emmonsia crescens* and *Ea. sola*), and *Histoplasma* (*Histoplasma capsulatum* and *H. duboisii*). The newer genera *Emergomyces* (*Emergomyces pasteurianus*, *Es. africanus*, *Es. orientalis*, *Es. canadensis*, and *Es. europaeus*) and *Emmonsiellopsis* (*Emmonsiellopsis terrestris* and *Emmonsiellopsis coralliformis*) contain some species that have no known teleomorphs (2, 3). *B. parvus* and *B. helicus* were previously assigned to the anamorph genus *Emmonsia*. DNA sequence data have placed *Paracoccidioides* (*Paracoccidioides brasiliensis* and *P. lutzii*) in the family *Ajellomycetaceae* as well (4). The family *Onygenaceae* contains the species *Coccidioides immitis* and *Coccidioides posadasii*. Molecular phylogenetic studies have indicated that species of the *Onygenales* are divided into several clades (descendants of a common ancestor). In all of these phylogenetic trees, pathogenic organisms are interspersed with nonpathogenic relatives, which suggests that the capacity to infect humans has arisen numerous times during the evolution of the *Onygenales*.

Histoplasma capsulatum

Historically, *H. capsulatum* was divided into three varieties: *H. capsulatum* var. *capsulatum*, a human pathogen found in North and South America; *H. capsulatum* var. *duboisii*, a human pathogen found in Africa (5); and *H. capsulatum* var. *farciminosum*, a pathogen of horses and mules found in parts of northern Africa and the Middle East. Phylogenetic studies defined at least eight clades within *H. capsulatum*: the North American class 1 (NAm 1), North American class 2 (NAm 2), Latin American group A (LAm A), Latin American group B (LAm B), Australian, Netherlands (Indonesian), Eurasian, and African clades (6). Seven of these eight clades comprise genetically and geographically distinct populations that can be regarded as phylogenetic species. The single exception, the Eurasian clade, originated from within the Latin American group A clade. *H. capsulatum* var. *farciminosum* was placed within the Eurasian clade. In addition to the seven phylogenetic species, another seven lineages represented by single isolates from Latin America were identified (6). These may represent additional phylogenetic species. Subsequent studies using also multilocus sequence typing of *H. capsulatum* in formalin-fixed paraffin-embedded tissues from cats living in regions where the fungus is not endemic revealed a new phylogenetic clade. The *H. capsulatum* sequences recovered from the cats were most closely related to the North American class 1 clade but clustered separately outside this clade, suggesting that the *H. capsulatum* strain infecting the animals may represent a separate clade or phylogenetic species (7). A later analysis of previous and new sequences of *Histoplasma*, using different phylogenetic and population genetics methods, led to a proposal of the new phylogenetic species LAm A1, LAm A2, LAm B1, LAm B2, RJ, and BAC-1, nested within the former Latin American group A clade (8). A recent analysis using additional sequence information led to partly different groupings and resulted in the proposal of the new species names *Histoplasma mississippiense* for NAm 1, *Histoplasma ohiense* sp. nov. for NAm 2, and *Histoplasma suramericanum* for LAm A and the restriction of *Histoplasma capsulatum sensu stricto* to the Panama (H81) lineage (9).

At this time, the disease African histoplasmosis is considered a distinct entity, but the taxonomic placement of *H. capsulatum* var. *duboisii* has been called into question by the finding of one *H. capsulatum* var. *capsulatum* isolate from South Africa that was placed in the African (*H. capsulatum* var. *duboisii*-containing) clade (6). The genome of *H. capsulatum* has an estimated size between 28 and 39 Mbp, and sequence assemblies are currently available for five strains (https://www.broadinstitute.org/fungal-genome-initiative/histoplasma-genome-project).

Blastomyces Species

Until recently, the genus *Blastomyces* consisted of *B. dermatitidis* and *B. gilchristii* (10). Since then, *B. percursus* (3, 11), *B. parvus* (formerly *Emmonsia parva*), *B. helicus* (formerly *Emmonsia helica*) (12), and *B. silverae* (13) have been proposed. Genotyping studies of *B. dermatitidis* have revealed an association between clinical phenotype and genetic groups—findings suggesting that genotyping of isolates may help to predict patient clinical associations (14), although this work had not been validated with newly identified species. Whole-genome sequence assemblies and annotations for *B. dermatitidis-B. gilchristii* strains, including the highly virulent clinical strain SLH14081 and the relatively avirulent strain ER-3 (15), are available via the Broad Institute page at https://www.broadinstitute.org/fungal-genome-initiative/blastomyces-genome-project.

Coccidioides Species

Phylogenetic studies have led to the recognition of two species within the genus *Coccidioides*. The species name *C. immitis* is now restricted to isolates from California and Washington State (16), while the name *C. posadasii* has been proposed for all other isolates belonging to this genus. These two taxa were initially thought not to interbreed; however, more recent evidence has shown that genetic exchange between these species has occurred, with evidence of hybridization and genetic introgression (17). Isolates from Venezuela, Mexico, and Brazil have undergone microsatellite typing, with two distinct clades being identified within these regions (18). More recent work using whole-genome sequencing has additionally identified genetically distinct subpopulations associated with specific geographic locales (19). Genome sequence assemblies and annotations of *C. immitis* and *C. posadasii* have been completed (20) and are now available at https://www.broadinstitute.org/scientific-community/science/projects/fungal-genome-initiative/coccidioides-genomes and http://fungidb.org/fungidb/.

Paracoccidioides Species

Phylogenetic analysis of *P. brasiliensis* showed that this fungus can be divided into at least three distinct species that appear to be confined to regions of endemicity: S1, PS2, and PS3 (21). The highly divergent Pb01-like group was named *Paracoccidioides lutzii* (22, 23), and very recently, names were also proposed for PS2 (*Paracoccidioides americana*), PS3 (*Paracoccidioides restrepiensis*), and a fifth phylogenetic species restricted to Venezuela, PS4 (24, 25) (*Paracoccidioides venezuelensis*) (26). Recent genomic and morphologic analyses strongly support the existence of a sexual cycle in species of the genus *Paracoccidioides* (27). Comparison of 18S and chitin synthetase sequences has indicated that *P. brasiliensis* is related to the uncultivable pathogen *Lacazia loboi*, the agent of lacaziosis (28) (see chapter 130). However, these sequences demonstrated sufficient differences for *Lacazia* to be kept as an independent genus (28).

The Broad Institute has completed the sequencing, assembly, and annotation (29) as well as a subsequent improved update (30) of the genomes of two reference strains of *P. brasiliensis* (Pb03 and Pb18) and one strain of *P. lutzii* (Pb01) (https://www.broadinstitute.org/fungal-genome-initiative/paracoccidioides-genome-project). Recently, the genome sequences of two additional strains of *P. brasiliensis* were released (strain PbCnh, this species' first assembled genome of mating type α/*MAT1-1*, and strain Pb300) (31).

Emergomyces Species

Significant taxonomic changes have occurred within *Ajellomycetaceae*, and a new genus has been recently proposed (*Emergomyces*).

Emergomyces contains *Es. pasteurianus* as the type species (formerly *Emmonsia pasteuriana*) and four recently identified species: *Es. africanus* (32), *Es. orientalis* (33), *Es. canadensis*, and *Es. europaeus* (3, 13). *Emergomyces* spp. have been found to cause disseminated disease in immunocompromised patients (34), and work to further characterize this newly described genus is ongoing. Whole-genome sequencing of *Es. africanus* (strain CBS136260) and its sister species *Es. pasteurianus* (strain CBS 101426) has been completed, and it shows that both contain the α mating-type locus (*MAT1-1*) (3).

Two former *Emmonsia* species have been moved to the genus *Blastomyces*. *Ea. parva* has been renamed *B. parvus*. *Ea. helica*, which was also recently described in an HIV-infected man in California (35), has been renamed *B. helicus*.

DESCRIPTION OF THE AGENTS

Histoplasma capsulatum

H. capsulatum is a thermally dimorphic fungus, displaying a filamentous mold form in the environment and in culture at temperatures below 35°C and a yeast phase in tissue and at temperatures above 35°C. The mold phase may contain two types of conidia (Fig. 1). Macroconidia are thick walled with a diameter of 8 to 15 µm and display characteristic tubercles or projections on their surfaces. Microconidia, smooth walled with a diameter of 2 to 4 µm, are the infectious particles (36, 37). The yeast phase develops as small oval budding cells with a diameter of 2 to 4 µm, often within macrophages (Fig. 2 and 3A). The yeast cell found in African histoplasmosis is thick walled and larger, 8 to 15 µm in diameter.

H. capsulatum is found in soils throughout the world. It grows best in soils with a high nitrogen content, particularly those enriched with bird or bat guano. Birds do not become colonized or infected with *H. capsulatum* (due to their high body temperatures), and their droppings are

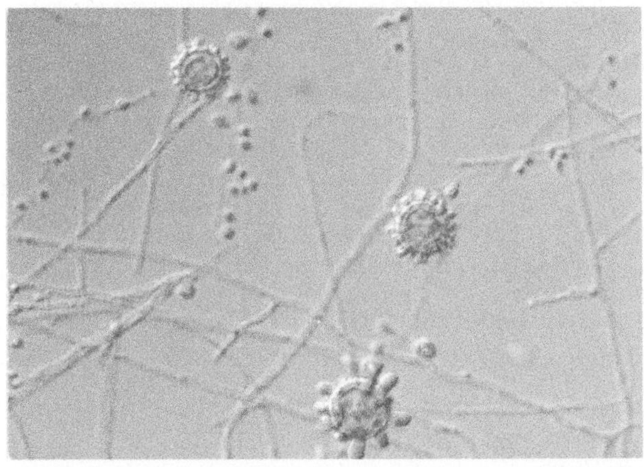

FIGURE 1 Mycelial phase of *H. capsulatum* showing tuberculate macroconidia and microconidia. Lactophenol cotton blue stain. Magnification, ~×245.

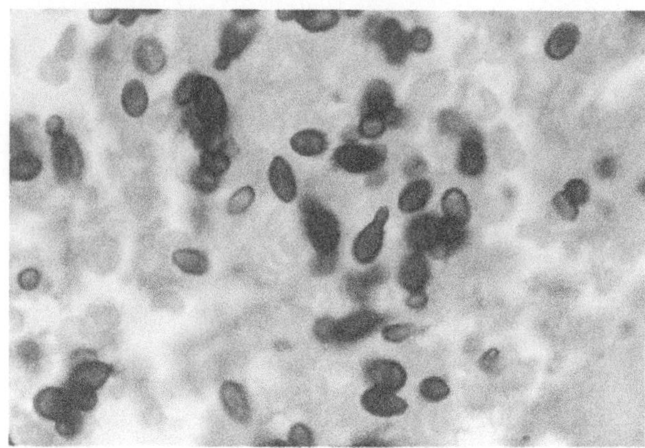

FIGURE 2 GMS stain showing blastoconidia of *H. capsulatum*. Magnification, ~×290.

primarily a nutrient source. Soil samples from sites where birds have roosted have remained contaminated for at least 10 years after the roost has been cleared (38).

Histoplasmosis is the most common endemic mycosis in North America, but it is also found throughout Central and South America (36, 39). In the United States, the disease is most prevalent in states surrounding the Mississippi and Ohio Rivers, but foci of endemicity exist throughout the eastern half of the continent. Other regions of endemicity include parts of Africa, Australia, and eastern Asia, in particular India and Malaysia.

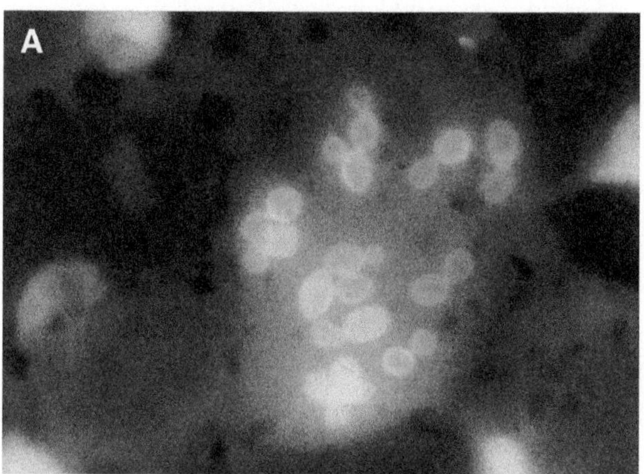

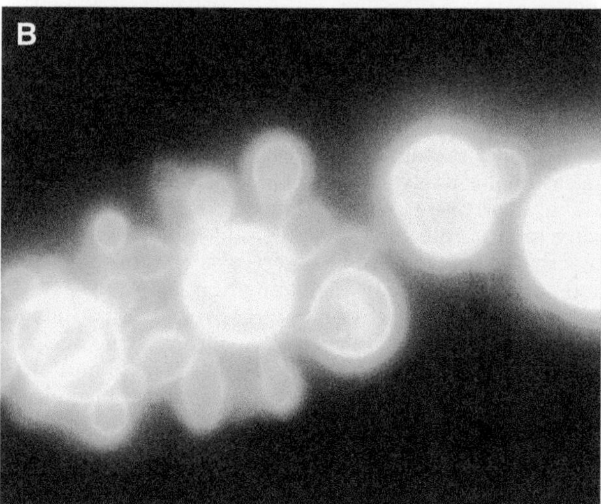

FIGURE 3 (A) Calcofluor white wet mount of sputum showing blastoconidia of *H. capsulatum*. Original magnification, ×475. Courtesy of the American Society of Clinical Pathology. (B) Calcofluor white wet mount of sputum showing blastoconidia of *P. brasiliensis*. Magnification, ~×255.

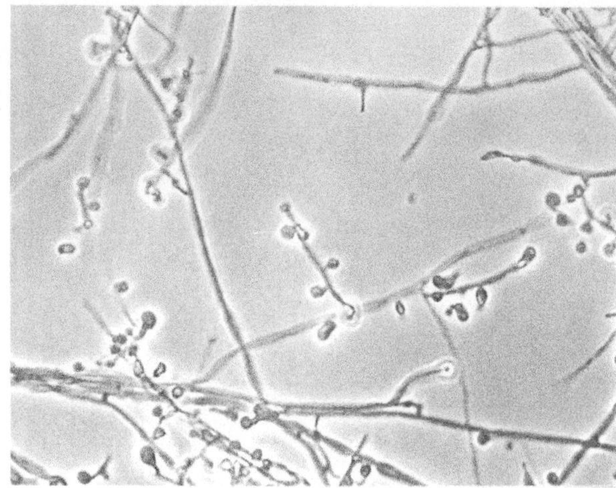

FIGURE 4 Mycelial phase of *B. dermatitidis*. Magnification, ~×240.

Blastomyces Species

B. dermatitidis, *B. gilchristii*, and *B. percursus* are thermally dimorphic, converting from the mold phase to the yeast phase under appropriate conditions of temperature and nutrition. At room temperature, a floccose white mold can be recovered (Fig. 4). The microconidia are oval or pyriform (pear shaped), with a diameter of 2 to 10 μm; no macroconidia are produced. Large, round, thick-walled yeast cells, 5 to 15 μm in size, with broad-based budding daughter cells are found in tissue and on appropriate media at 37°C (Fig. 5). Yeast cells may occur inside or outside macrophages. *B. helicus* and *B. silverae* have only recently been described and are phenotypically similar to *B. dermatitidis* (12).

B. parvus mold phase produces small single-celled conidia (about 4 μm in size) on the sides of the hyphae or on short side branches. Inside the host, the conidia transform into structures termed adiaspores, which resemble the spherules of

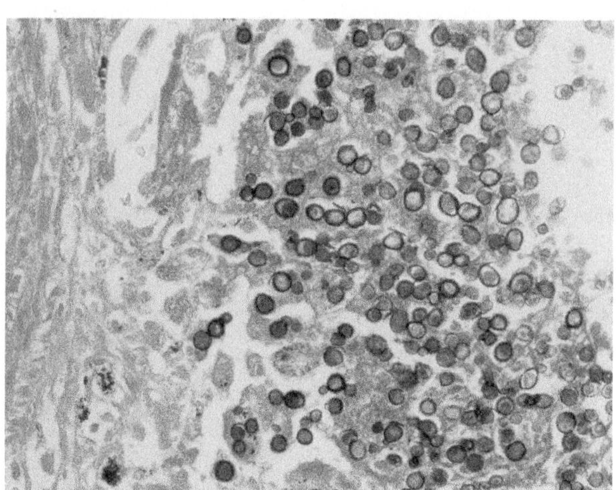

FIGURE 5 Blastoconidia of *B. dermatitidis*. GMS stain. Magnification, ~×290.

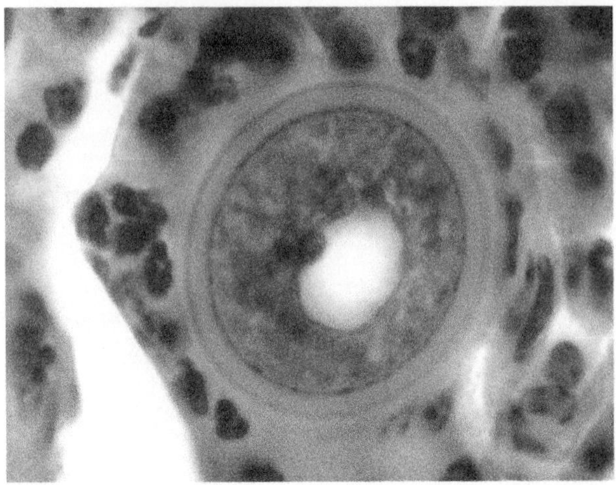

FIGURE 6 *B. parvus* adiaspore in mouse tissue. PAS stain. Magnification, ~×280.

Coccidioides species (Fig. 6). *B. parvus* adiaspores are smaller (10 to 25 μm) than those of *Adiaspiromyces crescens* and are produced at 40°C (40).

The natural habitat of *Blastomyces* spp. is the soil, particularly near waterways, although the ecology of *Blastomyces* has not been completely defined due to the difficulty in isolating the organism in nature (41). It appears to survive best in moist acidic soils with a high nitrogen and organic content. Higher soil temperatures and recent rainfall facilitate growth of the fungus.

The largest number of cases of blastomycosis has been reported from North America, but the disease is also endemic in Africa and parts of Central and South America. In the United States, the organism is most commonly found in states surrounding the Mississippi and Ohio Rivers; in Canada, the disease occurs in the provinces that border the Great Lakes (42).

Coccidioides Species

In the environment and in culture at room temperature, the *Coccidioides* fungus exists as a mold producing septate hyphae and arthroconidia that usually develop in alternate hyphal cells (Fig. 7). As the arthroconidia mature, the alternating disjunctor cells undergo lytic degradation, releasing the barrel-shaped arthroconidia, approximately 2 to 5 μm, which are the infectious particles. Inside the host and in special media, the arthroconidia transform into a structure called a spherule. A spherule is a large (up to 120 μm), thick-walled spherical structure containing hundreds to thousands of endospores, each approximately 2 to 4 μm, which can be released if the spherule ruptures (Fig. 8). Each endospore can develop into a spherule as well, continuing the process within the host.

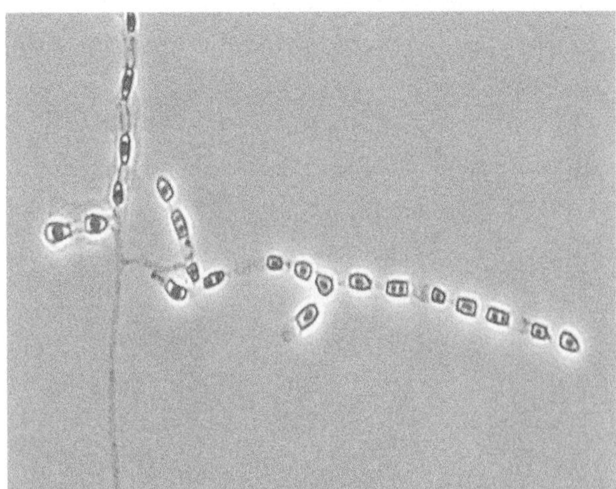

FIGURE 7 Mycelial phase of *C. immitis* showing alternating arthroconidia. Lactofuchsin stain. Magnification, ~×250.

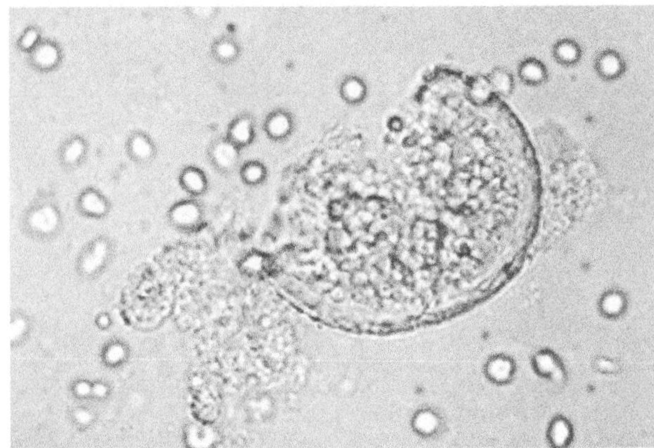

FIGURE 8 KOH preparation of pus from a lesion showing a *Coccidioides* spherule and endospores. Magnification, ~×290. Reprinted with permission from reference 154.

Coccidioides is a soil-inhabiting fungus with a restricted geographical distribution (43). It is confined to regions of the Western Hemisphere that correspond to the lower Sonoran desert life zone, and although an animal reservoir has been postulated, this has yet to be definitively demonstrated (44). In the United States, the region of endemicity includes central and southern California, southern Arizona, southern New Mexico, parts of Utah and Washington, and western Texas. The region of endemicity extends southwards into the desert regions of northern Mexico and parts of Central and South America (44).

Paracoccidioides Species

P. brasiliensis and *P. lutzii* are thermally dimorphic fungi. At room temperature, they grow as molds. Growth requires a lengthy incubation, of up to 30 days. Isolates incubated on rich media produce thin septate hyphae 1 to 3 μm in width with the appearance of interwoven threads and occasional chlamydospores. Under conditions of nutritional deprivation, some isolates produce conidia, which vary in structure from arthroconidia to microconidia of less than 5 μm and can be observed to be intercalary, septate, or pedunculated (originating from a narrower base). Conidia respond to temperature changes, germinating into hyphae at 20 to 24°C or converting into yeasts at 36°C on appropriate media. Yeast cells are mostly oval and characteristically display a mother cell surrounded by multiple buds, a structure thought to resemble a ship's pilot wheel (Fig. 3B and 9).

Although *Paracoccidioides* spp. have been isolated from soil, understanding of their precise environmental habitat remains limited. The region of endemicity extends from Mexico (23°N) to Argentina (34°S), sparing certain countries (Chile, Suriname, the Guianas, Nicaragua, Belize, and most of the Caribbean islands) within these latitudes. Within countries where the disease is endemic,

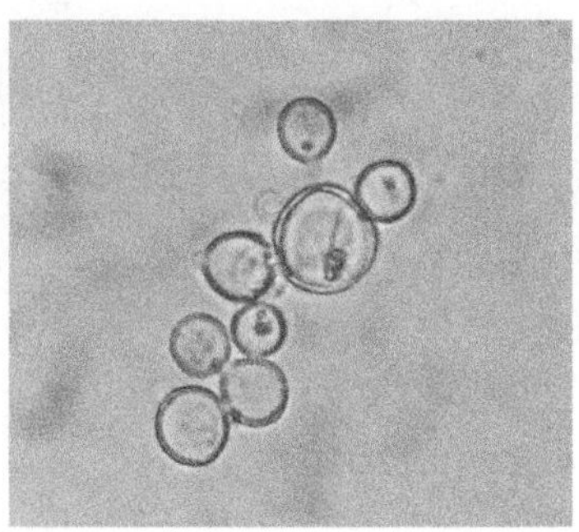

FIGURE 9 Wet mount showing blastoconidia of *P. brasiliensis*. Magnification, ~×290.

the mycosis is diagnosed only in areas with relatively well-defined ecologic characteristics (presence of tropical and subtropical forest, abundant watercourses, mild temperatures, high rainfall, and coffee and/or tobacco crops). The greatest numbers of reported cases have come from Brazil, Colombia, and Venezuela (45–47). *P. brasiliensis* has been repeatedly recovered from human clinical samples, from tissues of the nine-banded armadillo, *Dasypus novemcinctus*, and more rarely from the Northern naked-tailed armadillo (*Cabassous centralis*). Occasionally, *P. brasiliensis* has also been isolated from dogs and detected in other animal species (45).

Emmonsia Species

In the environment and in culture at room temperature, *Emmonsia* spp. exist as molds that produce small single-celled conidia (about 4 μm in size) on the sides of the hyphae or on short side branches. Inside the host, the conidia of *Ea. crescens* form adiaspores, as discussed above. Although adiaspores enlarge to become enormous, thick-walled structures, no endospores are produced, and the spores eventually die, failing to propagate *in vivo*, and thus probably do not disseminate from the lungs (48). Adiaspores can also be generated *in vitro* in rich media. Some of the *Ea. crescens* strains have been found to produce large (25- to 400-μm) multinucleate adiaspores at 37°C. The natural habitat of *Ea. crescens* is the soil, and infection has occurred in numerous rodents, fossorial mammals, and their predators. Human cases of infection or disease were initially rare but were reported from North, Central, and South America, as well as from several European and Asian countries and then more recently from South Africa. Previously, the majority of recent cases were reported from Brazil (40); however, in light of the reports from South Africa (49), the geographic extent of diseases caused by these fungi has become unclear.

Emergomyces Species

Es. pasteurianus (previously *Ea. pasteuriana*) does not produce adiaspores in tissue; rather, at 37°C on rich media, it produces structures that resemble budding yeast cells. The earliest cases of emergomycosis caused by the species now known as *Es. africanus* were diagnosed in the Western Cape province of South Africa, but molecular identification of dimorphic fungi in other regions has led to detection of cases in six of nine South African provinces and the Kingdom of Lesotho (50).

Emergomyces exists as a mold in the environment or when grown *in vitro* at a temperature less than 30°C (3, 51, 52). *In vivo*, in contrast, budding yeast cells are observed in infected tissue or when the organism is grown at 35°C in the laboratory (51). *Es. africanus*, *Es. pasteurianus*, and *Es. orientalis* grow at a minimum temperature of 6°C, with optimum growth at 24 to 27°C and a maximum temperature of 40°C. Morphologically, colonies appear beige and are slow growing and filamentous at room temperature. Conidiophores are short and unbranched, arising at right angles from thin-walled hyaline hyphae, and are slightly swollen at the top, sometimes with short, secondary conidiophores bearing a group of more than three conidia (3, 51). At human body temperature, colonies appear yeast-like: small, cream to smooth gray-brown, and heaped (3). Small oval yeast cells with narrow buds are formed; sometimes, larger cells with broader-based buds may also be present (3, 51).

EPIDEMIOLOGY AND TRANSMISSION

Histoplasmosis

Inhalation of microconidia is the usual mode of *H. capsulatum* infection in humans. The incubation period is 1 to 3 weeks. In cases of reinfection, the incubation period appears to be shorter (4 to 7 days after exposure). Histoplasmosis is not contagious, but there have been occasional reports of transmission from an organ donor to a recipient (53).

The major risk factor for infection is environmental exposure (37). The risk depends on several factors, including the nature of the environmental site, the activities performed, and the duration and degree of dust or soil exposure. Longer and more intense exposures usually result in more severe pulmonary disease. Most reported outbreaks have been associated with exposures to sites contaminated with *H. capsulatum* or have followed activities that disturbed accumulations of bird or bat guano (38).

Persons with underlying illnesses are at increased risk for some forms of histoplasmosis. Disseminated infection is more common among individuals with underlying cell-mediated immunological defects, including those with HIV infection, transplant recipients, and individuals receiving tumor necrosis factor alpha inhibitors for rheumatoid arthritis. Immunocompromised persons with histoplasmosis have a higher mortality rate than those who are not immunosuppressed (54).

Blastomycosis

Inhalation of conidia is the usual mode of infection leading to blastomycosis. The incubation period has been estimated to be 4 to 6 weeks, although in some cases, disease manifests only months following exposure (55). Blastomycosis is not contagious.

Outbreaks have been associated with occupational and recreational activities, often along streams or rivers, and have resulted from exposures to moist soil enriched with decaying vegetation. Apart from outbreaks, blastomycosis is more commonly seen in adults than in children. More men than women are affected, and most recently, a disproportionate number of Asians compared to non-Asians was found in a recent outbreak (56). The disease often occurs in individuals with an outdoor occupation or recreational interest.

B. dermatitidis is uncommon as an opportunistic pathogen, but it causes more-aggressive disease in persons with underlying cell-mediated immunological defects, such as those with HIV infection and transplant recipients.

Immunocompromised persons with blastomycosis have a higher mortality rate than those who are not immunosuppressed (57).

Coccidioidomycosis

Inhalation of arthroconidia is the usual mode of infection leading to coccidioidomycosis in humans. The incubation period is 1 to 3 weeks. In contrast to what is observed with histoplasmosis, once individuals have recovered from *Coccidioides* infection, they are usually immune to reinfection. The infection is not contagious, but occasional person-to-person spread has occurred via contaminated fomites (58) or by transmission from an organ donor to a recipient (59).

The major risk factor for infection is environmental exposure. The risk depends on a number of factors, including the nature of the environmental site, the activities performed, and the duration and degree of dust or soil exposure. Infection has been associated with ground-disturbing activities, such as building construction, landscaping, farming, archaeological excavation, and numerous recreational pursuits (60). Natural events that result in the generation of dust clouds, such as earthquakes and windstorms, have been associated with an increased risk of infection and have resulted in large outbreaks (61).

Disseminated infection is more common among those of black, Asian, or Filipino race and among pregnant women in the third trimester. Individuals with underlying cell-mediated immunological defects, such as those with AIDS and those receiving immunosuppressive medications, are also at increased risk of disease dissemination (62).

Paracoccidioidomycosis

Inhalation of conidia is the usual mode of infection leading to paracoccidioidomycosis in humans. The incubation period is unknown, but it is clear that the fungus can remain dormant for very long periods in the lymph nodes following asymptomatic primary infection. Paracoccidioidomycosis is not contagious (63).

Paracoccidioidomycosis predominates in adults, who account for 85 to 95% of cases, and in persons in agriculture-related occupations. The disease is more often diagnosed in males than in females (ratio of 15:1). Estrogen-mediated inhibition of the mold-to-yeast transformation could help to account for this (63). Sporadic cases have been reported in individuals with underlying immunosuppressive conditions, including HIV infection.

Adiaspiromycosis

Inhalation of conidia is the usual mode of infection leading to adiaspiromycosis in animals and humans, and even in cases with skin lesions, it is likely that such infection results from dissemination following inhalational exposure, given the systemic manifestations (including liver function abnormalities) (64). The incubation period is unknown, although circumstantial evidence has suggested that symptoms may develop 1 to 3 weeks following exposure. No risk factors have been identified.

Emergomycosis

Infection is presumed to follow inhalation of airborne propagules, and indeed, *Es. africanus* DNA has been frequently detected in air samples from an area of endemicity (Cape Town, South Africa) where cases of emergomycosis have been diagnosed (32). No similar epidemiological details are available for the other *Emergomyces* species. All cases of emergomycosis have occurred in immunocompromised patients, most commonly with defects in cell-mediated immunity caused by HIV infection.

CLINICAL SIGNIFICANCE

Histoplasmosis

There is a wide spectrum of clinical manifestations of histoplasmosis, ranging from a transient pulmonary infection that subsides without treatment to chronic pulmonary infection or to more widespread disseminated disease (36, 37). Many healthy individuals develop no symptoms when exposed to *H. capsulatum* in a setting of endemicity. Higher levels of exposure result in an acute symptomatic and often severe flu-like illness. The symptoms, which include fever, chills, headache, nonproductive cough, myalgia, pleuritic chest pain, loss of appetite, and fatigue, usually disappear within a few weeks. The most severe form of this disease is disseminated histoplasmosis. The clinical manifestations range from an acute illness that is fatal within a few weeks if left untreated (often seen in infants, persons with AIDS, and solid-organ transplant recipients) to an indolent, chronic illness that can affect a wide range of sites. Recent data also suggest that histoplasmosis is responsible for an increasing number of hospitalizations, likely from the growing immunosuppressed population (65).

Hepatic infection is common in nonimmunosuppressed individuals with disseminated histoplasmosis, and adrenal gland destruction is a frequent problem. Mucosal ulcers are found in over 60% of these patients. The mouth and throat are often affected, but lesions also occur on the lip, nose, and other sites. Central nervous system disease occurs in 5 to 20% of patients, presenting as chronic meningitis or focal brain lesions. In persons with AIDS, disseminated histoplasmosis is usually associated with low CD4 T-lymphocyte counts and presents with nonspecific symptoms, such as fever and weight loss. Mucosal lesions are uncommon, but multiple cutaneous lesions may be present. Central nervous system involvement occurs in 10 to 20% of cases (36, 37).

African Histoplasmosis

The clinical manifestations of African histoplasmosis differ from those of classical histoplasmosis. The illness is indolent at onset, and the predominant sites affected are the skin and bones, although more recent reports have shown disseminated infection in 77% of those affected (5). Individuals with more widespread infection involving the liver, spleen, and other organs have a febrile wasting illness that is fatal within weeks or months if left untreated. Multiple cutaneous lesions often develop on the face and trunk. These lesions often enlarge and ulcerate. Osteomyelitis occurs in about 30% of patients. The infection may spread into contiguous joints, causing arthritis, or into adjacent soft tissue, causing a purulent subcutaneous abscess.

Blastomycosis

Blastomycosis encompasses a wide clinical spectrum, ranging from a transient pulmonary infection that subsides without treatment to chronic pulmonary infection or to widespread disseminated disease (66). Acute pulmonary blastomycosis usually presents as a nonspecific flu-like illness, similar to that seen with community-acquired pneumonia or primary histoplasmosis or coccidioidomycosis. Otherwise healthy persons generally recover after 2 to

12 weeks of symptoms, but some infected individuals return months later with infection of other sites. Other patients with acute blastomycosis fail to recover and develop chronic pulmonary disease or disseminated infection.

The skin and bones are the most common sites of extrapulmonary disease. The skin is involved in more than 70% of cases, the lesions presenting either as raised verrucous lesions with irregular borders or as ulcers. The latter can also appear on the mucosa of the nose, mouth, and throat. Osteomyelitis occurs in about 30% of patients with disseminated infection, with the spine, ribs, and long bones being the most common sites of involvement. Arthritis occurs in about 10% of patients. Meningitis is rare, except in immunocompromised individuals. Other organs, such as the male genitourinary tract, adrenal glands, thyroid, liver, spleen, and gastrointestinal tract, are sometimes involved (55).

Coccidioidomycosis

Although a number of clinical manifestations may present after exposure, more than half of all infections are thought to be subclinical. Apparent illness is most commonly a subacute process known as valley fever (primary coccidioidal infection). Respiratory symptoms, such as cough, fever, chills, and fatigue, are common and may last weeks to months. In regions where the disease is endemic, primary coccidioidal pneumonia may account for 17 to 29% of all community-acquired pneumonia (67, 68). Up to 50% of patients develop a mild, diffuse erythematous or maculopapular rash covering the trunk and limbs within the first few days of the onset of symptoms, a clinical sign that may be useful for differentiating the patient's symptoms from those caused by bacterial pneumonia (69). More dramatic and persistent is the rash of erythema nodosum or erythema multiforme, which occurs in about 5% of infected persons. Otherwise healthy persons recover without treatment, their symptoms disappearing in a few weeks to months.

Fewer than 3% of infected individuals develop disseminated coccidioidomycosis. This progressive disease usually develops within 3 to 12 months of the initial infection, although it can occur much later following reactivation of a quiescent infection in an immunosuppressed individual. The clinical manifestations range from a fulminant illness that is fatal within a few weeks if left untreated to an indolent chronic disease that persists for months or years. One or more sites may be involved, but the skin, soft tissue, bones, joints, and meninges are most commonly affected. Cutaneous and subcutaneous lesions are common. Osteomyelitis occurs in about 40% of patients, with the spine, ribs, cranial bones, and ends of the long bones being the most common sites. The disease may spread into contiguous joints, causing arthritis, or into adjacent soft tissue, causing subcutaneous abscess formation. Meningitis is the most serious complication of coccidioidomycosis, occurring in 30 to 50% of patients with disseminated disease, and left untreated, it is almost universally fatal (70).

Paracoccidioidomycosis

Paracoccidioidomycosis encompasses a subclinical infection resulting from the initial contact with the fungus. The lungs are the usual initial site of *Paracoccidioides* infection, but the organism then spreads through the lymphatics to the regional lymph nodes. In most cases, the primary infection is asymptomatic. However, children and adolescents sometimes present with an acute disseminated form of infection in which superficial and/or visceral lymph node enlargement is the major manifestation. This presentation is also seen in immunocompromised patients. It has a poor prognosis.

The hallmarks of the chronic adult type of disease are significant lung involvement and extrapulmonary lesions. This is the predominant form occurring in approximately 90% of cases (63). In 80% of cases, the disease involves the lungs. The disease is slowly progressive and may take months or even years to become established. Ulcerative mucocutaneous lesions of the face, mouth, and nose are the most obvious presenting sign. Other sites of infection include the small or large intestine, liver and spleen, adrenal glands, bones and joints, central nervous system, and male genitourinary tract. In 60 to 80% of cases, active pulmonary involvement and residual fibrotic lesions are observed. A residual form is also recognized in 50 to 80% of cases and is represented by fibrotic scarring occurring at the sites of previously active lesions, which can alter respiratory function and incapacitate the patient. *Paracoccidioides* infection may become dormant and then be reactivated later under the influence of ill-defined conditions prevalent in rural settings, such as chronic alcoholism, malnutrition, and smoking (63).

Adiaspiromycosis

In most cases, adiaspiromycosis is a self-limited, localized pulmonary infection with few or no symptoms. Because the adiaspores enlarge but do not reproduce, symptoms and clinical signs depend upon the number of conidia inhaled. In some patients, the disease is discovered incidentally during the evaluation of other pulmonary conditions. However, nonproductive cough, dyspnea, and fever are not uncommon in those with adiaspiromycosis. Severe or even fatal cases are rare, although they have been reported (40), and they can occur in immunocompromised individuals, as recently reported (40, 71), with cutaneous manifestations and elevated liver function tests. A single outbreak of ocular adiaspiromycosis has also been reported (72).

Emergomycosis

The most common clinical manifestation of emergomycosis (previously described as disseminated emmonsiosis and best described for cases of *Es. africanus* infection) is the appearance of widespread cutaneous lesions, occurring in 95% of patients (50, 51).

COLLECTION, TRANSPORT, AND STORAGE OF SPECIMENS

Clinical Specimens

Methods of collection, transport, and storage of specimens are detailed in chapter 117. Tissue samples should be obtained when appropriate and should be divided and submitted for microbiological and histopathological examination. If possible, special tissue stains, such as the Grocott-Gomori methenamine silver (GMS) and periodic acid-Schiff (PAS) stains, should be requested. Since colonization with the dimorphic fungal pathogens does not occur, their microscopic detection and/or isolation in culture is consistent with proven infection. Blood, urine, and cerebrospinal fluid (CSF) can also be collected as appropriate for nucleic acid amplification, antigen, and/or antibody testing. The development of next-generation sequencing to detect cell-free pathogen DNA has received extensive attention and may be useful in the diagnosis of endemic fungal infections, although no data obtained via this method have yet been presented.

Histoplasma capsulatum

H. capsulatum organisms can be isolated from sputum or bronchoalveolar lavage fluid specimens in 60 to 85% of cases of chronic pulmonary histoplasmosis if multiple specimens are tested (73). In disseminated disease, useful specimens for culture include blood, urine, lymph node, and bone marrow samples. Bone marrow cultures are positive in over 75% of cases. Blood cultures collected with the Isolator lysis-centrifugation system (Wampole Laboratories, Princeton, NJ) or Bactec Mycolytic bottles (BD Diagnostic Systems, Franklin Lakes, NJ) show the greatest sensitivity. Biopsy specimens of oral, cutaneous, and gastrointestinal lesions, adrenal glands, or liver and spleen have also provided a diagnosis. *Histoplasma* meningitis is difficult to diagnose, with CSF cultures being positive in no more than two-thirds of cases. The best results are obtained when large volumes of CSF (10 to 20 ml) are cultured on multiple occasions.

Blastomyces Species

Sputum samples, bronchoalveolar lavage fluid, or lung biopsy specimens may be submitted. Skin biopsy specimens are useful in the diagnosis of cutaneous disease. Collection of urine after prostatic massage may be helpful in the diagnosis of genitourinary blastomycosis.

Coccidioides Species

In addition to lower respiratory tract samples, material for microscopy and culture can be collected from suppurative cutaneous and soft tissue lesions. Organisms can be recovered only infrequently from CSF (~30% or patients), and usually only after culture of large volumes (10 to 20 ml) (74).

Paracoccidioides Species

In addition to lower respiratory samples, material can be collected from oral or pharyngeal lesions, cutaneous lesions, lymph nodes, adrenal glands, and the gastrointestinal tract. With these specimens, a simple wet mount suffices to reveal *P. brasiliensis* in over 85% of the patients (63).

Emmonsia Species

The diagnosis of *Ea. crescens* is usually based on observing its unique histopathologic appearance, typically a single, large thick-walled adiaspore within a granuloma.

Emergomyces Species

Diagnosis of emergomycosis is currently made by detection of the yeast phase from affected tissue during histopathology examination or by isolation of the fungus from appropriate specimens, such as skin tissue, blood, bone marrow, respiratory tissue, liver tissue, and lymph nodes (75).

DIRECT EXAMINATION

Microscopy

Direct microscopic examination of clinical materials may provide a rapid presumptive diagnosis of a systemic fungal infection. However, it is important to appreciate that tissue-form cells of *Histoplasma* and *Blastomyces* can appear similar to each other as well as to yeast cells of various *Candida* species, *Cryptococcus neoformans*, *Cryptococcus gattii*, and *Talaromyces marneffei* (formerly *Penicillium marneffei*) and to endospores of *Coccidioides* species. It is often helpful to stain fresh, wet preparations of sputum, bronchoalveolar lavage fluid, CSF, urine, pus, or other material with calcofluor white, a fluorescent compound that binds to the fungal cell wall, to assist with preliminary evaluation.

Histoplasma capsulatum

Giemsa and Wright's stains can be used to detect yeast cells of *H. capsulatum* in blood or bone marrow smears. These cells can also be seen in tissue sections stained with GMS or PAS stain but usually not in those stained with hematoxylin and eosin (H&E). Detection of the small (2- to 4-μm) oval budding yeasts allows a presumptive diagnosis of histoplasmosis. Organisms can be found within macrophages or free in the tissues. It is unusual to find yeast cells on cytological examination of sputum or other respiratory tract fluids. The thick-walled, narrow-based budding yeast cells causing African histoplasmosis, approximately 10 to 15 μm in diameter, are about 4-fold larger than those of classical *H. capsulatum* in tissue sections and on occasion may be confused with *Blastomyces* spp.

Blastomyces Species

Direct calcofluor white or KOH mounts or Gram stains of sputum, tissues, and exudates often permit the detection of the large round yeast cells of *Blastomyces* spp. The broad-based buds often attain the same size as the parent cells before becoming detached. On occasion, larger "giant" yeast forms (>40 μm) or filamentous forms may be found in tissue. Histopathologic examination using PAS or GMS stain also can be of value. Adiaspores are observed in lung tissue in cases of *B. parvus* infection.

Coccidioides Species

Tissue sections should be stained with PAS stain, GMS stain, or H&E to permit the detection of the characteristic large, thick-walled spherules of *Coccidioides* species. Microscopic examination of wet preparations of sputum, bronchoalveolar lavage fluid, pus, or other samples treated with KOH is also helpful but is less sensitive. *Prototheca wickerhamii* may resemble small spherules, and *Rhinosporidium seeberi* may simulate larger ones.

Paracoccidioides Species

The characteristic translucent-walled yeast cells of *P. brasiliensis* with multiple buds can often be found on direct microscopic examination of sputum, bronchoalveolar lavage fluid, pus from draining lymph nodes, or tissue biopsy specimens. Staining of wet preparations with lactophenol cotton blue, methylene blue, Gram stain, or calcofluor white can be helpful. Tissue sections can be stained with PAS, GMS, or H&E stain.

Emmonsia Species

Tissue sections stained with PAS or GMS stain are most helpful in demonstrating the characteristic adiaspores in lung tissue for diagnosing adiaspore-producing fungi. It is important to appreciate that in the chronic stage the organism may collapse, forming various shapes that may resemble other fungi, helminths, or pollen grains. Adiaspores must also be distinguished from the spherules of *Coccidioides*. Adiaspores do not contain endospores, and adiaspores are typically much larger than empty *Coccidioides* spherules.

Emergomyces Species

A phenotypic difference between the species now placed in *Emergomyces* and the classic *Emmonsia* species (*Ea. crescens* and *B. parvus*) is that the former produce budding yeasts, while the latter produce adiaspores *in vitro* (51).

Antigen Detection

Histoplasma capsulatum

The *Histoplasma* polysaccharide antigen (HPA) test is a microtiter plate-based double-antibody sandwich enzyme immunoassay (EIA) to detect antigen in urine, serum, or CSF in cases of disseminated histoplasmosis with a sensitivity up to 95% (76). This test is also useful in the early diagnosis of acute pulmonary histoplasmosis and during treatment follow-up (77). Ten milliliters of urine, 5 ml of serum, or 1 ml of CSF is the preferred volume for the HPA test, although a minimum volume of 0.5 ml of any specimen is required for a single test. To obtain maximum test sensitivity, it is recommended that both serum and urine specimens be tested in parallel. Treatment success or failure may be assessed by collecting specimens at least 14 days after starting treatment and testing the newly acquired samples in parallel with the last specimen that was positive before initiation of treatment (78). This test is performed on a fee-for-service basis by several commercial laboratories. Since those assays were designed, a commercial *Histoplasma* antigen capture monoclonal antibody enzyme-linked immunosorbent assay (ELISA) (*Histoplasma* galactomannan monoclonal ELISA) has been developed by Immuno-Mycologics (IMMY; Norman, OK). The reagents have been evaluated in two laboratories in the United States and showed high performance in diagnosing histoplasmosis (79, 80), and they have now been tested in two Latin American countries (Colombia and Guatemala) with good sensitivity and specificity, 98% and 97%, respectively (81).

The detection of serum (1→3)-β-D-glucan, a component of the fungal cell wall, has undergone limited evaluation in histoplasmosis. Preliminary evidence suggests that it is useful in the detection of histoplasmosis (87% sensitivity and 65% specificity); however, a positive result must be confirmed with *Histoplasma*-specific testing (82).

Blastomyces Species

Blastomyces antigen testing is a microtiter plate-based double-antibody sandwich EIA to detect antigenuria and antigenemia in disseminated blastomycosis. The sensitivity is 89% in disseminated blastomycosis, with higher sensitivity in urine than in serum (83). However, specificity is modest and only 79% overall due to cross-reactivity with other endemic mycoses (84). Clinical reports have suggested a lower sensitivity, but serial urine testing is useful for monitoring disease (85). This test is provided on a fee-for-service basis by MiraVista Diagnostics.

The detection of serum (1→3)-β-D-glucan has been incompletely evaluated in blastomycosis; however, preliminary evidence suggests that it is not useful in the detection of *Blastomyces* (82).

Coccidioides Species

A coccidioidal urinary antigen test (MiraVista) has also been developed and exhibited a sensitivity of 71% in a largely immunosuppressed population (86). In a veterinary population, the sensitivity has been shown to be much lower (<20%) (87). Antigen testing may be useful in testing CSF (88). The sample requirements are the same as those for the HPA test.

Serum (1→3)-β-D-glucan has undergone limited evaluation in the detection of coccidioidomycosis and has a limited role (44% sensitivity) in patients with this mycosis (89).

Paracoccidioides Species

At present, paracoccidioidomycosis antigen testing is not available as a routine diagnostic test. A 43-kDa glycoprotein and an 87-kDa heat shock protein have been described as useful targets for serum antigen detection (90, 91). Several reports have described the detection of *P. brasiliensis* antigen in urine, CSF, and bronchoalveolar fluid samples (91). Others have noted that antigen levels in serum diminished or even disappeared during successful treatment (92).

Emmonsia Species

No antigen test exists at this time for the diagnosis of adiaspiromycosis.

Emergomyces Species

No antigen test exists at this time for the diagnosis of emergomycosis.

Nucleic Acid Detection in Clinical Materials

Only recently has a commercially available system become available for the detection of fungal nucleic acids in human clinical samples (GeneSTAT.MDx *Coccidioides* test) (see below). However, a number of in-house methods remain under investigation, several of which are highlighted in this section. Conserved regions of rRNA genes have been used as targets in a number of PCR-based detection assays. It is important to appreciate that amplification of conserved genes can result in products derived both from pathogenic fungi and from genetically related nonpathogenic fungal species. The nonspecific nucleic acids could arise from colonization of the original sample with saprophytic organisms, from contamination during sample collection, or from contamination of PCR reagents with fungal DNA. It is very important that the identity of amplicons detected using conserved genes be verified by direct sequencing. In more recent studies, genes specific for the fungus of interest have been chosen as PCR targets, thus eliminating this specificity problem.

Histoplasmosis

An increasing number of publications have described the use of PCR to detect *H. capsulatum* DNA in fixed paraffin-embedded tissue samples, blood, bronchial lavage fluids, bone marrow, and ophthalmic samples. Early studies targeted the internal transcribed spacer (ITS) rRNA gene region, but the use of targets unique to *H. capsulatum* has provided better assay specificity. Bialek et al. designed a nested PCR that targeted the gene coding for a unique 100-kDa protein of *H. capsulatum* (93), which has successfully been used to detect *H. capsulatum* DNA in clinical samples from patients with histoplasmosis in French Guiana and Colombia (sensitivity, 100%; specificity, 95%) (94, 95). The original format of nested or seminested PCR was recently adapted to real-time PCR with promising results (96). A consensus group recently started the evaluation of reproducibility of the most common in-house tests used (97). More recently, in a controlled histoplasmosis infection using an animal model, real-time PCR protocols targeting three protein-coding genes (100-kDa protein and H and M antigens) were evaluated, and it was concluded that the 100-kDa-protein and H-antigen molecular assays are promising tests for diagnosing this mycosis (98).

Blastomycosis

PCR assays of ribosomal genes, the ITS region, repetitive sequences, and species- or genus-specific genes have all been evaluated for the molecular detection of *B. dermatitidis* and *B. gilchristii*. The majority of these tests have been evaluated on paraffin-embedded tissue, although a real-time PCR assay to identify *B. dermatitidis-B. gilchristii* in culture specimens, bronchial washings, bronchoalveolar lavage fluid, pleural fluid, sputum, and blood has been published (99, 100).

Coccidioidomycosis

Various PCR assays have proven extremely sensitive and specific on isolate material (101). A PCR-based assay was recently granted approval by the Food and Drug Administration (FDA) for the detection of *Coccidioides* from clinical samples (GeneSTAT.MDx; available through DxNA LLC, St. George, UT). Few clinical studies have been published to date, although it appears that the sensitivity of PCR is similar to that of culture (~50%) (101, 102).

Paracoccidioidomycosis

The number of tests developed and evaluated so far for the detection of *P. brasiliensis* in clinical samples is very limited (103). The preferred target sequences have been gp43 and ribosomal RNA genes. A real-time PCR targeting the ITS-1 region was developed to detect *P. brasiliensis* DNA in both cultures and clinical specimens. Although this molecular test was evaluated with a small number of patients, the authors reported 100% sensitivity and specificity (104). A nested-PCR assay targeting the immunogenic gp43 gene was evaluated in the detection of *P. brasiliensis* DNA in lung homogenates from infected and uninfected mice, with 91% sensitivity (105). A test based on the 5′ nuclease assay using a fluorescent probe derived from the sequence of the gene coding for the *gp43* antigen was used and could detect at least 10 copies of this DNA sequence (106).

Adiaspiromycosis

A panfungal PCR targeting the ribosomal ITS-1 and -2 regions identified *Ea. crescens* from a bronchoalveolar lavage fluid sample of a patient with confirmed adiaspiromycosis (107); however, PCR testing for these organisms has thus far been limited.

Emergomycosis

Currently, no molecular tests for clinical samples are available, and culturing followed by sequencing is needed for molecular identification.

ISOLATION PROCEDURES

Biosafety

The mere lifting of a culture plate lid is often sufficient to cause the release of large numbers of conidia into the air, and screw-cap tubes or sealed plates should be used. Should a sporulating culture be dropped, millions of conidia may be dispersed. It is also important to note that local infections, including granuloma formation, have been reported following accidental percutaneous inoculation during injection of laboratory animals or during autopsies of humans with histoplasmosis, coccidioidomycosis, or blastomycosis.

All procedures involving the manipulation of sporulating cultures of *Coccidioides*, *Paracoccidioides*, *Blastomyces*, *Emergomyces*, *Emmonsia*, and *Histoplasma* species and the processing of soil or other environmental materials known or likely to contain these organisms should be performed inside a class II biological safety cabinet under conditions of biosafety level 3 containment. Biosafety level 2 practices and facilities are recommended for handling and processing clinical specimens and animal tissues (108). Hyaline molds of unknown identity should always be examined and manipulated inside a class II biosafety cabinet. Such molds should never be handled on an open laboratory bench.

Although *Emergomyces* and *Emmonsia* species have not been formally classified as risk group II or III pathogens, it is recommended that mycelial cultures of these fungi be handled carefully in a class II biosafety cabinet with additional use of personal protective equipment, e.g., N95 respirator masks (52).

Culture for Mold Phase

In general, the organisms discussed in this chapter can be readily cultivated in the mold phase on general fungal media such as Sabouraud dextrose agar or potato dextrose agar incubated at 25°C. Incubation at 37°C is also helpful to recover the yeast phase of most dimorphic organisms. Media containing antibiotics such as chloramphenicol or gentamicin should be used when clinical materials, such as sputum, that may be contaminated with bacteria are cultured. Media containing cycloheximide are useful for inhibiting saprophytic fungi and provide a differential tool in identification. Many unrelated saprophytic soil fungi fail to grow on media containing cycloheximide, fail to grow altogether at 37°C, or fail to convert to the yeast phase at 37°C. Screw-cap slants are preferable to plates for culturing dimorphic fungi. If plates are used, they should be sealed so that mold spores cannot escape into the ambient air. Seals that are permeable to air, such as Shrink Seals (Scientific Device Laboratory, Des Plaines, IL), are useful for this purpose. In general, colonies develop within 3 to 7 days, but some strains of *Histoplasma* and *Paracoccidioides* may require incubation for as long as 4 to 6 weeks.

Culture for Yeast Phase

Histoplasma, *Blastomyces*, and *Paracoccidioides* species can be recovered in the yeast phase by using appropriate media incubated at 37°C. At human body temperature, *Emergomyces* colonies appear yeast-like: small, cream to smooth grey-brown, and heaped (3).

Histoplasma capsulatum

The yeast phase of *H. capsulatum* can be recovered in rich media such as brain heart infusion agar (BHI) or BHI with blood (BHIB). Plates or slants should be incubated at 37°C under aerobic conditions for at least 4 weeks.

Blastomyces Species

The yeast phase of *B. dermatitidis-B. gilchristii* can be recovered in rich media such as BHI, BHIB, Pine's medium, or Kelley's agar by incubation at 37°C under aerobic conditions. Yeasts are usually visible within 1 week, but media should be held for at least 4 weeks before being discarded. *B. parvus* produces adiaspores *in vitro* when cultivated on Phytone yeast extract agar, BHI, or BHIB.

Paracoccidioides Species

The yeast phase of *Paracoccidioides* species can be recovered in media such as BHI, Pine's medium, or Kelley's agar by incubation at 37°C. The organism grows slowly, and plates or slants should be held for at least 4 weeks.

Emmonsia Species

Ea. crescens produces adiaspores *in vitro* when cultivated on Phytone yeast extract agar, BHI, or BHIB at 37 to 40°C.

Emergomyces Species

Es. pasteurianus produces yeast-like cells after culture on BHI at 37°C for approximately 10 days. The *Emergomyces* species recently recognized in South Africa do not produce adiaspores at 37°C or 40°C, although the mycelial cultures were converted to the yeast phase by incubating streaked or single-colony subcultures on BHI at 37°C after 10 to 14 days (51).

IDENTIFICATION

In general, these organisms are identified by their characteristic morphologic features, by conversion to the yeast phase, by DNA probe testing if available, and/or by direct DNA sequencing. Slide cultures should not be performed on suspected dimorphic isolates due to the possibility of laboratory infection from accidental inhalation of infectious conidia.

Histoplasma capsulatum

The mold phase can be recovered after incubation at 25°C. The colony is initially white or buff-brown. Both types may be isolated from the same patient, and eventually the brown type may convert to the white type. The brown type generally produces more of the characteristic tuberculate macroconidia than the white type. On subculture, only about 30% of macroconidia show tubercles. Microconidia are abundant in fresh isolates of *H. capsulatum*. After multiple subcultures, the production of both macroconidia and microconidia may be diminished. The presence of both macroconidia and microconidia is not required for identification of *H. capsulatum*, as authentic *H. capsulatum* isolates that fail to produce either macroconidia or microconidia have been recognized. Macroconidia but no microconidia can also be seen in the saprophytic fungus *Sepedonium* as well as in the related fungus *Renispora flavissima*. Authentic *H. capsulatum* isolates can be recognized by their thermal dimorphism as well as by their growth on inhibitory mold agar.

Once the characteristic morphology has been recognized, mold-phase *H. capsulatum* isolates can be confirmed by conversion to the yeast phase. The isolate is transferred to BHI or BHIB and incubated at 37°C for at least 7 to 10 days. Hyphal cells may form buds directly or develop enlarged, transitional cells that subsequently begin to bud. The microconidia may also convert to budding yeast cells. Complete conversion rarely is achieved, and multiple transfers to fresh BHI or BHIB medium may be required. The colony develops a white, smooth, yeast-like appearance, and microscopic examination reveals oval, budding yeasts approximately 1 to 3 by 3 to 5 μm. The cells have a narrower base of attachment between the bud and parent cell than do those of *B. dermatitidis*.

The AccuProbe test (Hologic, San Diego, CA) can also be used to confirm isolates as *H. capsulatum*. This test requires actively growing cultures: mold-phase cells not more than 4 weeks of age or yeast cells not older than 1 week. Isolates can be taken from solid media or broth cultures. In this assay, formation of specific DNA-RNA hybrids is quantitated in relative light units by use of a luminometer. Extracts that display values of >50,000 relative light units are considered positive. The AccuProbe test has largely replaced exoantigen testing for identification of *H. capsulatum*. Several studies have shown that this test is sensitive and specific for identification of *H. capsulatum* (109–111), although false-positive results can be obtained when isolates that are genetically related to the *Ajellomycetaceae* are tested (112). An exoantigen testing kit to identify the organism is commercially available from IMMY. African *Histoplasma* isolates display colonial morphology similar to that of non-African isolates and yield positive results in the AccuProbe test for *H. capsulatum* (111). Histopathologic examination of tissue forms is required to distinguish members of the African clade.

Blastomyces Species

At 25 to 30°C, isolates of *B. dermatitidis*-*B. gilchristii* produce a variety of forms, ranging from a fluffy white colony that is visible within 2 to 3 days to a glabrous, tan, nonconidiating colony that grows more slowly. Microscopic examination shows microconidia that are oval or pyriform, usually smooth walled, and formed on short lateral or terminal branches along the hyphae. *B. dermatitidis*-*B. gilchristii* also grow readily on inhibitory media containing cycloheximide. Conidia of the hyaline hyphomycete *Scedosporium apiospermum*, of some *Chrysosporium* species, and of the dermatophyte *Trichophyton rubrum* are morphologically similar and can be mistaken for *Blastomyces* species. These species either fail to grow at 37°C (some *Chrysosporium* species) or grow as molds when incubated at 37°C (*S. apiospermum* and *T. rubrum*).

The identification can be confirmed by conversion to the yeast phase. Generally, isolates of *B. dermatitidis*-*B. gilchristii* convert readily to the yeast phase on BHI, BHIB, or Pine's or Kelley's medium incubated at 37°C. Yeast cells are hyaline, smooth walled, and thick walled, generally 8 to 15 μm in diameter, with the bud connected to the parent cell by a broad base up to 4 to 5 μm in diameter. Conversion can be accomplished in 2 to 3 days, although occasional isolates may take several weeks. *B. parvus* produces hyphae at 37°C and produces smaller adiaspores (8 to 20 μm in diameter) at 40°C. *B. parvus* and *Ea. crescens* are indistinguishable in morphology and appearance at 25°C.

Identification can also be confirmed using the AccuProbe test for *Blastomyces*. False-positive *Blastomyces* Gen-Probe results were obtained with *P. brasiliensis* (113) and with *Gymnascella hyalinospora*, so care must be taken to distinguish these organisms. An exoantigen testing kit to identify the organism is commercially available from IMMY.

Coccidioides Species

At 25 to 30°C, isolates of *Coccidioides* species display considerable variation in colony morphology. Colonies can range from moist, glabrous, and grayish to abundant, floccose, and white. Colonies may become tan and even red with age (114). Microscopic examination shows hyphae that are thin and septate, with fertile (spore-producing) hyphae usually arising at right angles. Arthroconidia are hyaline, one-celled, short, cylindrical to barrel-shaped, moderately thick walled, smooth walled, and 2 to 8 by 3 to 5 μm. Arthroconidia alternate with thin-walled empty disjunctor cells. At maturity, the disjunctor cells undergo lytic degradation, releasing the arthroconidia. After this fragmentation, the arthroconidia may display frill-like remains of the disjunctor cells on each end. Isolates of *Coccidioides* grow well on inhibitory mold agar containing cycloheximide, which helps to distinguish this organism from similar soil saprophytes, such as *Malbranchea* species. It is also important to distinguish true alternate arthroconidia from aging mycelia that, due to cytoplasmic shrinkage, display an appearance that can be misinterpreted as arthroconidia. True arthroconidia eventually fragment and disperse; aging mycelia do not. The two species of *Coccidioides* cannot be readily distinguished morphologically.

When incubated at 37°C *in vitro*, the spherule/endospore form is produced. The organism can produce spherules *in vitro* when incubated at 37 to 40°C in appropriate media and increased CO_2 tension, but this procedure is rarely performed on routine clinical isolates.

The AccuProbe for *Coccidioides* may be used for confirmation of unknown isolates as *Coccidioides* species. This test is generally sensitive and specific, although pretreatment of isolates with formaldehyde leads to false-negative results (115). This test does not distinguish between the two species of *Coccidioides*.

Paracoccidioides Species

When incubated at 25 to 30°C, *Paracoccidioides* isolates display slow growth and produce a variety of forms, ranging from glabrous leathery, brownish, flat colonies with a few tufts of aerial mycelium to wrinkled, folded, floccose colonies to velvety, white-to-beige forms. The colonies are very similar in appearance to those of *B. dermatitidis*. Most strains grow for long periods of time without the production of conidia.

When cultures are transferred to 37°C on rich media such as BHI or Pine's or Kelley's agar, the resulting yeast colonies are generally folded (cerebriform) in appearance. Mycelial elements may be seen mixed with yeast cells. Conversion to the yeast phase also is quite slow. Yeasts are 2 to 30 μm in diameter and are oval or irregular in shape, displaying the characteristic "pilot's wheel" appearance of multiple thin-necked round buds developing around the parent cell. The walls are thinner than those of *B. dermatitidis* yeast cells, and the buds are not broad based.

Identification is usually confirmed by demonstrating thermal dimorphism. There is no commercial DNA probe test for *P. brasiliensis*. The AccuProbe test for *B. dermatitidis* cross-reacts with *P. brasiliensis* (111), so care must be taken when this test is used for isolates that may actually be *P. brasiliensis*. Slow-growing, nonsporulating isolates are more characteristic of *P. brasiliensis* than of *B. dermatitidis*.

Emmonsia Species

At 25°C, *Ea. crescens* grows as glabrous (waxy), colorless colonies, which produce yellowish white aerial mycelia in time. Some strains display pale orange to grayish orange aerial mycelia. The colonies often have areas that alternate between a tufted mycelium and a glabrous consistency. Reverse pigmentation is pale gray to grayish brown. On microscopic examination, the hyphae are septate and branching. Sporulation is enhanced on potato dextrose or Pablum cereal agar. Numerous conidia are produced either directly from the sides of the hyphae or on short stalks that branch at right angles from the hyphae. Each stalk bears a single terminal conidium. Sometimes the swollen end may bear one to three secondary spine-like pegs, which in turn form a secondary conidium in a flower-like arrangement (116). The conidia are round, oval, or pyriform and measure 2 to 4 μm by 3 to 5 μm. The conidial wall is smooth but may roughen with age. *B. parvus* and *A. crescens* are indistinguishable in morphology and appearance at 25°C.

A. crescens displays no hyphal growth at 37°C and forms larger adiaspores (20 to 140 μm in diameter) on BHI or Phytone yeast extract agar at this temperature.

Emergomyces Species

Es. pasteurianus displays some features at 25°C that are similar to those of *Ea. crescens* and *B. parvus*. At 37°C on BHIB, this species produces yeast-like cells that are oval or lemon shaped, budding on a narrow base, and 2 to 4 μm. The colonies are creamy and smooth. This species does not produce adiaspores *in vitro* or *in vivo* (117). Since the genus *Emergomyces* has only recently been proposed and described, it may be too early to give general guidelines for the recognition of each of its five species, *Es. pasteurianus*, *Es. africanus*, *Es. orientalis*, *Es. canadensis*, and *Es. europaeus*.

TYPING SYSTEMS

In general, typing systems have been used to show geographic differences among isolates and cryptic species. In some genera, diversity can be shown among isolates collected from a single geographic area.

Histoplasma capsulatum

Isolates can be divided into at least eight clades, as described earlier (6). This typing system can be used to place an unknown isolate into one of the major worldwide geographic groupings. For further delineation, restriction fragment length polymorphism (RFLP) typing with the yeast phase-specific nuclear gene *yps-3* and/or mitochondrial DNA probes and random amplified polymorphic DNA-based and ITS-based typing methods have been used in several studies (118). These studies have shown that considerable polymorphisms can be demonstrated among individual patient isolates from a particular geographic location (118), that animal and soil strains from Brazil display indistinguishable subtypes (119), and that strains from patients in Brazil, where mucocutaneous histoplasmosis is much more common than in the United States, display distinct ITS and *yps-3* subtypes not seen in strains from U.S. patients (120). Recently, a study compared multiple typing methods that have been developed to study *H. capsulatum* epidemiology in 51 environmental, animal, and human isolates from Brazil. The M13 PCR fingerprinting and PCR-RFLP analyses produced very similar results and separated the *H. capsulatum* isolates into three major groups (121). The use of genetic markers in the molecular epidemiology of histoplasmosis was recently published (122).

Blastomyces Species

In a study using RFLP analysis with several rRNA gene probes to study 59 isolates from the United States, India, and Africa, three major groups were defined. These groups were further divided using random amplified polymorphic DNA fingerprinting into 5, 15, and 12 types, respectively, that correlated with the geographic origin of the isolate (123). Interestingly, these studies showed that soil isolates collected from an outbreak of blastomycosis in Eagle River, WI, were not responsible for the majority of cases of disease in that outbreak. A study exploring polymorphisms in the promoter region upstream of the *BAD-1* virulence gene revealed further genetic diversity with large insertions in the promoter region (124). A modification in the taxonomy of this genus has recently been proposed, where some strains that might have previously been identified as *Emmonsia* species would now be classified as *Blastomyces* species (3). Isolates of *B. parvus* separate into two groups, one group isolated from the North American prairies and the second group from the desert southwest of the United States or from Italy.

Coccidioides Species

Two major clades, corresponding to the species *C. immitis* and *C. posadasii*, were defined when an extensive population sample, including isolates from Venezuela, Mexico, and Brazil, was studied by using a set of nine microsatellite markers (18). Typing of isolates to *C. immitis* (California) or *C. posadasii* (non-California) species can be accomplished by examining any of 17 sites fixed for alternate alleles (125). Microsatellite typing conducted with 121 clinical isolates from Arizona concluded that this disease in Arizona could not be linked to a dominant strain of *C. posadasii* (126). More recent work using whole-genome sequencing identified *C. posadasii* as the more ancient of the two species and demonstrated evidence of distinct geographic clades within Arizona (19).

Paracoccidioides Species

Multilocus sequence typing at eight loci demonstrated the existence of at least three distinct species within this organism (21). The *gp43* gene encoding a dominant glycoprotein antigen has been studied by several groups as a useful target for subtyping. In an earlier study, microsatellite sequences were compared as markers to discriminate among a set of *P. brasiliensis* human isolates causing either chronic or acute disease (127). These authors did not observe any clustering of isolates associated with either acute or chronic disease.

Emmonsia Species

Based on ITS sequences, isolates of *Ea. crescens* fall into two phylogenetic groups, North American and Eurasian, depending on the continents from which the isolates were obtained (1).

Emergomyces Species

Multilocus sequence typing (e.g., using sequences from ribosomal DNA large subunit, ITS, beta tubulin, and two other conserved genes) has been found useful for resolving groups within *Emergomyces* (3, 51).

SEROLOGIC TESTS

Histoplasmosis

Serologic tests have an important role in the rapid diagnosis of several forms of *H. capsulatum* infection but are most useful for persons with chronic pulmonary or disseminated histoplasmosis (128). Of the different methods that have been developed, the immunodiffusion (ID), complement fixation (CF), and latex agglutination (LA) tests are the most popular. The principal antigen used in these tests is histoplasmin, a soluble filtrate of mycelial-phase broth cultures. Histoplasmin contains *H. capsulatum* species-specific H and M antigens as well as C antigen. The H antigen is a β-glucosidase against which antibodies are formed during acute histoplasmosis. The M antigen is a catalase against which antibodies are produced during all phases of the disease. The H and M antigens were once thought to be specific proteins for the detection of anti-*H. capsulatum* antibodies. The M antigen, however, was found to be not specific unless used in a deglycosylated form.

The ID test is a qualitative method that detects precipitins to the H and M glycoprotein antigens of *H. capsulatum* present in histoplasmin. Both serum and CSF can be used. Patients with negative serum reactions during the acute phase of infection should have additional samples taken 3 to 4 weeks later. ID test kits and reagents are available from Gibson Laboratories (Lexington, KY), IMMY, and Meridian Bioscience (Cincinnati, OH). Commercial kits include mycelial-phase culture filtrates containing *H. capsulatum* H and M antigens, positive-control sera containing antibodies against both H and M antigens, and ID plates. Positive-control sera must be included each time the test is performed and must react with both the H and M antigens. The ID test is a useful screening procedure or can be used as an adjunct to the CF test. It is more specific but less sensitive than the CF test.

The CF test is a quantitative procedure in which two antigens are employed: histoplasmin and a suspension of intact Merthiolate-killed *H. capsulatum* yeast-phase cells. The latter is more sensitive (~80% versus ~20%) but less specific (~90% versus ~99%) than histoplasmin. Serum, peritoneal fluid, or CSF can be used in the CF test. Patients with negative serum reactions during the acute phase of infection should have additional samples taken 3 to 4 weeks later. No commercial kits are available, but antigens, antisera, and other reagents can be purchased from several commercial sources (e.g., IMMY and Meridian). Negative-control serum and positive-control serum from human histoplasmosis cases demonstrating a CF titer of 1:32 or greater with the homologous antigen should be tested each time the CF test is performed.

More recently, an ELISA for the detection of antibodies to *H. capsulatum* using metaperiodate-treated purified histoplasmin was reported to have sensitivities of 100% in acute disease, 90% in chronic disease, 89% in disseminated infection in individuals without HIV infection, 86% in disseminated disease in the setting of HIV infection, and 100% in mediastinal histoplasmosis (99). This test is, however, not commercially available.

An LA test using histoplasmin as antigen is commercially available (LA-Histo antibody system; IMMY). This semiquantitative test detects immunoglobulin M (IgM) antibodies and is used primarily for the presumptive diagnosis of acute histoplasmosis. It is less helpful for the detection of chronic infection. An EIA for IgM and IgG antibodies (MiraVista) has also been found useful to increase the sensitivity of diagnostic testing in *Histoplasma* meningitis (129).

Blastomycosis

Substantial improvement in the performance of serologic testing for blastomycosis has been achieved over the last 2 decades; however, current serologic testing is not useful for a definitive diagnosis of blastomycosis. Past work has focused on the use of two purified surface antigens of *B. dermatitidis*, one termed the A antigen and the other the WI-1 antigen. Both molecules are released from the yeast phase of *B. dermatitidis* by autolysis and can be recovered from culture filtrates. Immunological comparison of the two antigens has shown that they are very similar, but WI-1 is a 120-kDa protein that is not glycosylated, while the A antigen is a 135-kDa glycosylated protein (130).

However, serologic testing for blastomycosis lacks both the requisite sensitivity and specificity. Serologic testing by immunodiffusion measures the antibody to *B. dermatitidis* A antigen. This test is relatively specific, but sensitivity ranges from 28 to 64% (131). Patients with negative serum reactions during the acute phase of infection should have additional samples taken 3 to 4 weeks later.

CF testing has also been evaluated, although this test has shown even lower sensitivity and specificity (9 to 43%) (132). ID test kits and reagents are available from Gibson, MiraVista, and IMMY. Commercial kits include purified *B. dermatitidis* A antigen, positive-control serum containing antibodies against A antigen, and ID plates. The positive-control serum must be included each time the test is performed and must react with the homologous reference antigen to form the A precipitin line.

Coccidioidomycosis

Despite the fact that sensitive procedures such as EIA have been developed, the ID and CF tests remain the most reliable methods for the serologic diagnosis of coccidioidomycosis. The principal antigen used in these tests is a soluble filtrate of mycelial-phase broth cultures.

The simultaneous use of heated and unheated antigens permits the ID test to be employed to detect either IgM or IgG antibodies on a single plate. The immunodiffusion tube precipitin (IDTP) test utilizes heated coccidioidin as the antigen, detects IgM, and gives results comparable to those obtained with the classical tube precipitin test. It is most useful for diagnosing recent infection. The immunodiffusion complement fixation (IDCF) test utilizes unheated coccidioidin, detects IgG antibodies, and gives results comparable to those obtained by the CF method (see below). It is less sensitive but more specific than the CF test (133). Commercial kits are available (Gibson, IMMY, and Meridian) and include unheated and heat-treated coccidioidin antigens, positive-control sera containing IgM or IgG antibodies, and ID plates. The sensitivity of the IDTP and IDCF tests can be improved by 10-fold concentration of serum prior to testing. Positive-control sera must be included each time the test is performed and must react with the homologous reference antigen to form a precipitin line. The ID test is useful for initial screening of specimens and can be followed by other tests if positive.

The CF test is a sensitive quantitative method in which unheated coccidioidin is used to detect IgG antibodies. The major disadvantage of CF is that it is a laborious and time-consuming procedure that requires experienced personnel for optimum performance. No commercial kits are available, but reagents for in-house use can be obtained from several commercial sources (IMMY and Meridian). Negative-control serum and a positive-control serum from a human case of coccidioidomycosis (with a titer of ≥1:32) should be included each time the test is performed. Anticomplementary activity in serum samples can occur and may be resolved by subsequent ID testing. In addition to serum, the CF test can be performed with CSF, pleural, or joint fluid samples.

A qualitative LA test using heat-treated coccidioidin as antigen is available from several commercial sources (e.g., the LA-Cocci antibody system from IMMY and the *Coccidioides* latex agglutination system from Meridian). This test is simple and rapid to perform; however, the false-positive rate is higher than that observed with the IDTP and/or CF methods. It is not recommended for screening CSF specimens, because false-positive reactions can occur (134).

The Premier *Coccidioides* EIA (Meridian) is a qualitative test for detection of IgM and IgG antibodies in serum or CSF specimens. The antigen used in this test is a mixture of purified IDTP and CF antigens. False-positive reactions have been obtained with sera from some patients with blastomycosis and in patients with alternative diagnoses, and this test is now often used for "screening," with positive EIA results being evaluated by IDTP and IDCF tests for confirmation (135). Other EIAs have also been recently developed (MiraVista) with a favorable sensitivity; however, this test is less specific than ID (136).

Paracoccidioidomycosis

The most popular serologic methods for diagnosis of paracoccidioidomycosis are ID and CF, but other tests, such as ELISAs, counterimmunoelectrophoresis, dot blotting, and immunoblotting, have also been employed (137). The ID test demonstrates circulating antibodies in over 90% of cases. A reactive result allows a diagnosis to be made. The CF test allows a more precise evaluation of the patient's response to treatment, but cross-reactions with *H. capsulatum* antigens can occur. The principal antigens used in these tests are derived from culture filtrates of mycelial-phase or yeast-phase broth cultures of *P. brasiliensis*. The major diagnostic antigen in these preparations is a 43-kDa glycoprotein. Cell wall antigens have proved less useful than culture filtrate antigens, largely because wall antigens are dominated by cross-reactive galactomannan (137). Commercial mycelial-form culture filtrate antigen can be obtained for in-house use from IMMY. No commercial kits are available for this test. The CF test is performed with *P. brasiliensis* yeast-form culture filtrate antigen. No commercial kits or reagents are available.

Improvements in serodiagnosis include the detection of antibodies against chemically characterized and/or recombinant *P. brasiliensis* antigens, notably, gp43, pb27, and the 87-kDa heat shock protein. A combination of two recombinant products has resulted in increased sensitivity (92%) and specificity (88%) (138, 139). It has been found by double immunodiffusion that the serum from patients with paracoccidioidomycosis due to *P. brasiliensis* does not recognize antigen contained in the cell-free preparations of *P. lutzii*, unlike the serum from patients with paracoccidioidomycosis due to *P. lutzii*, which recognizes both antigens (*P. lutzii* and *P. brasiliensis*), suggesting that *P. lutzii* is antigenically more complex and has species-specific antigens but also shares common antigens with *P. brasiliensis* (140).

Adiaspiromycosis and Emergomycosis

No serologic tests are available for diagnosis of adiaspiromycosis or emergomycosis, although different methods are currently under active investigation.

ANTIMICROBIAL SUSCEPTIBILITIES

Established treatment options for *Histoplasma*, *Blastomyces*, *Emergomyces*, *Coccidioides*, and *Paracoccidioides* infections include amphotericin B and the triazoles voriconazole, posaconazole, itraconazole, and fluconazole. For isavuconazole, a new triazole, there are limited clinical data regarding the treatment of the endemic fungi, although it appears to be a useful alternative agent in selected cases (141). The echinocandins have a limited role in the treatment of endemic fungi and should not be used as monotherapy. *In vitro* antifungal susceptibility testing for dimorphic fungi remains unstandardized, and no susceptibility breakpoints have been determined for these organisms (142). Table 1 lists the *in vitro* susceptibilities of these organisms to established and investigational antifungal agents, as reported in studies that were performed in accordance with Clinical and Laboratory Standards Institute documents M38 (for filamentous fungi) (142) and M27 (for yeast) (143). Fluconazole treatment failures have been reported in some cases of histoplasmosis and coccidioidomycosis, partially attributed to organisms that demonstrated drug MICs of ≥64 μg/ml, although they remained responsive to itraconazole (144, 145).

EVALUATION, INTERPRETATION, AND REPORTING OF RESULTS

Histoplasmosis

The definitive diagnosis of histoplasmosis can be accomplished by direct microscopic detection of *H. capsulatum* in clinical specimens or its isolation in culture. However, isolation and identification may take 2 to 4 weeks.

Antigen detection complements other diagnostic methods for histoplasmosis and is particularly useful in immunocompromised patients with more extensive disease, often providing a rapid diagnosis before positive cultures can be identified. HPA has been detected in serum, urine, CSF, and bronchoalveolar lavage fluid specimens obtained from individuals with disseminated histoplasmosis. The sensitivity of antigen detection in disseminated histoplasmosis is higher in immunocompromised patients than in immunocompetent

TABLE 1 *In vitro* susceptibilities of dimorphic fungi to antifungal agents[a]

Fungus	Antifungal agent	MIC (μg/ml)	MIC_{90} (μg/ml)	Reference(s)
B. dermatitidis	Amphotericin B	≤0.03–1	0.5	155–157
	Fluconazole	1–64	NR	158
	Itraconazole	≤0.03–4	0.125	155–158
	Posaconazole	≤0.03–1	NR	158, 159
	Voriconazole	≤0.03–16	0.25	155–157
	Isavuconazole	0.5–4	NR	158
	Anidulafungin	2–8	NR	159
	Caspofungin	0.5–8	NR	159
Coccidioides spp.	Amphotericin B	0.125–4	0.5–1	156, 157, 160, 161
	Fluconazole	2–>64	64	157, 160, 161
	Itraconazole	0.125–16	1	156, 157, 161
	Posaconazole	0.06–16	1	158, 161, 162
	Voriconazole	≤0.03–8	0.25	156–158, 161
	Isavuconazole	0.125–1	0.5	158
	Caspofungin	8–64	32	160
H. capsulatum	Amphotericin B	≤0.03–2	0.25	155–157
	Fluconazole	≤0.125–64	NR	49
	Itraconazole	≤0.03–8	0.06	155–157
	Posaconazole	≤0.03–2	NR	158, 159
	Voriconazole	≤0.03–2	0.25	50, 155, 156
	Isavuconazole	0.125–2	2	158
	Anidulafungin	2–4	NR	159
	Caspofungin	0.5–4	NR	159
P. brasiliensis	Amphotericin B	0.125–4	NR	157
	Fluconazole	≤0.125–64	NR	157
	Itraconazole	≤0.03–1	NR	157
	Voriconazole	≤0.03–2	NR	157
	Isavuconazole	NR	NR	NR

[a]*Emergomyces* and *Emmonsia* susceptibility testing is limited, with few isolates tested thus far. NR, not reported.

patients and in patients with more severe illness. Antigen levels are higher in urine than in serum. For patients with AIDS and disseminated histoplasmosis, sensitivity is between 81% and 95% in urine and 86% in serum (146). Specificity is ~98%. Antigen has been detected in the CSF of patients with *Histoplasma* meningitis.

Antigen levels in the urine and serum decline with effective treatment, becoming undetectable in most patients (77). Failure of antigen concentrations to fall during treatment suggests therapeutic failure. In patients who have responded to treatment and in whom antigen levels have previously fallen, an increase in antigen levels in the urine or serum is suggestive of relapse.

The LA test for *Histoplasma* antibodies is most useful for the diagnosis of acute infection, positive results being obtained within 2 to 3 weeks after exposure. An LA titer of 1:16 is presumptive evidence of infection, and a titer of ≥1:32 is considered strong presumptive evidence of active or recent infection (110). Because false-positive reactions can occur, the results should be confirmed by the ID test. Low-titer results from single specimens should be interpreted with caution. In such cases, the test should be performed on another specimen collected 4 to 6 weeks later.

In the ID test, precipitins to the M antigen of *H. capsulatum* are the first to appear (4 to 8 weeks after exposure) and can be detected in up to 75% of persons with acute histoplasmosis. However, they can also be found in nearly all individuals with chronic pulmonary infection, as well as in those who have undergone a recent skin test with histoplasmin. Precipitins to the H antigen are specific for active disease but occur in fewer than 20% of cases. They usually disappear within the first 6 months of infection and are seldom, if ever, found in the absence of M precipitins. The presence of precipitins to both H and M antigens is highly suggestive of active histoplasmosis, regardless of other serologic test results.

The CF test is useful in the diagnosis of acute, chronic, disseminated, and meningeal forms of histoplasmosis. In acute infections, antibodies to the yeast antigen are the first to appear (about 4 weeks after exposure) and the last to disappear after resolution of the infection. Antibodies to histoplasmin appear later and reach lower titers than those observed for the yeast antigen. In contrast, histoplasmin titers are usually higher in persons with chronic histoplasmosis. CF test results can be difficult to interpret because cross-reactions can occur with sera from persons with blastomycosis, coccidioidomycosis, and other fungal infections. In such instances, titers usually range between 1:8 and 1:32 and reactions occur mainly against the yeast-form antigen. However, many serum samples from culture-confirmed cases of disseminated histoplasmosis yield titers in the same range. CF titers of 1:8 or greater with either antigen are considered presumptive evidence of histoplasmosis. Titers above 1:32 and rising titers in serial samples offer stronger evidence of infection.

Titers of CF antibodies to *H. capsulatum* decrease following resolution of the infection but increase in individuals with chronic progressive disease. However, clinical and microbiological findings should also be considered in assessing the patient's prognosis or making treatment decisions. In some patients, positive CF titers decline slowly and persist long after the disease has been cured. The significance of persistently elevated or fluctuating CF titers is unclear, as is the effect of antifungal treatment on antibody clearance (147).

Serologic tests are particularly useful in patients with *Histoplasma* meningitis. The detection of precipitins to H and M antigens in CSF specimens is sufficient to make a diagnosis in the appropriate clinical setting and often is the only positive diagnostic test.

Blastomycosis

Although microscopic examination and culture remain the most sensitive means of establishing the diagnosis of blastomycosis, serologic tests can also provide useful information. A positive reaction in an ID test using the A antigen of *B. dermatitidis* is suggestive of the blastomycosis (148). However, a negative ID test does not rule out the diagnosis, because the sensitivity of this method has been reported to range from ~30% for cases of localized infection to ~90% for cases of disseminated blastomycosis. In established cases of the disease, a decline in the number or the disappearance of precipitin lines is evidence of a favorable prognosis.

With urine specimens, the *Blastomyces* antigen test has been reported to have a sensitivity of 89% for disseminated infection and 100% for pulmonary disease, although recent experience has reported a lower sensitivity in clinical practice (85). However, cross-reactive antigens occurred in urine samples from all patients with paracoccidioidomycosis and from 96% of patients with histoplasmosis (83).

Coccidioidomycosis

Although the definitive laboratory diagnosis of coccidioidomycosis depends on microscopic examination and culture, serologic tests are of proven usefulness in diagnosis and management. A positive IDTP test result is indicative of acute coccidioidomycosis. IDTP-reactive IgM antibodies can be detected in up to 75% of cases within 1 week of symptom onset, and ~90% are positive within 3 weeks. Although infrequent, a positive IDTP test result within CSF is indicative of acute meningitis. In cases where the IDTP test is negative but the CF test is positive, patients should be investigated for microbiologic or histopathologic evidence of histoplasmosis or blastomycosis. In addition, sera should be obtained at 3-week intervals and examined by CF and ID tests for coccidioidomycosis, histoplasmosis, and blastomycosis if the patient has a history of travel to regions where the disease is endemic.

A positive IDCF test result is presumptive evidence of recent or chronic infection. IDCF-reactive IgG antibodies can usually be detected within 2 to 6 weeks after onset of symptoms. Although the IDCF test is generally not performed as a quantitative test, it can be used in this manner. Titers obtained using the quantitative IDCF are not identical to titers obtained from the CF test, but the observed trends are comparable.

The LA test is more sensitive than the IDTP test in detecting acute infection but is less specific. For this reason, a positive test result with undiluted serum should be confirmed by the ID and/or CF test.

The CF test does not become positive until about 4 to 12 weeks after infection, but CF antibodies persist for long periods in individuals with chronic pulmonary or disseminated coccidioidomycosis. Testing of serial specimens to detect rising or falling titers can reveal the progression or regression of illness and the response to antifungal treatment. A CF titer to coccidioidin at any dilution should be considered presumptive evidence of coccidioidomycosis. In most instances, the titer is proportional to the extent of the infection, and failure of the CF titer to fall during treatment of disseminated coccidioidomycosis is an ominous sign (149). Titers of 1:2 or 1:4 are usually indicative of early or residual disease. CF titers of >1:16 should lead to a careful assessment of the patient for possible spread of the disease beyond the respiratory tract (150). More than 60% of patients with disseminated coccidioidomycosis have CF titers of >1:32. However, false-negative results can occur in immunocompromised individuals, such as persons with AIDS. Patients with clinical presentations consistent with coccidioidomycosis but with negative or low serum CF titers should be retested at 3- to 4-week intervals.

The detection of CF antibodies in the CSF is usually diagnostic of coccidioidal meningitis and remains the single most useful test for diagnosis of that infection.

Antigen testing for coccidioidomycosis is insensitive and typically not used for diagnosis. When serology is negative in a severely immunocompromised patient suspected of underlying coccidioidomycosis, antigen testing may be useful (151).

Paracoccidioidomycosis

The definitive diagnosis of paracoccidioidomycosis depends on microscopic examination and culture. However, isolation and identification of *P. brasiliensis* from clinical specimens may take up to 4 weeks.

Serologic tests are useful for the rapid presumptive diagnosis of paracoccidioidomycosis, particularly in cases of disseminated infection (137). The ID test with yeast-form culture filtrate antigen is highly specific and is positive in 65 to 100% of cases of acute or chronic pulmonary infection or disseminated paracoccidioidomycosis. The CF test with yeast form culture filtrate antigen is less specific than the ID test, and cross-reactions can occur with cases of histoplasmosis. However, CF titers of ≥1:8 are considered presumptive evidence of paracoccidioidomycosis. Low CF titers are usually associated with localized infection, while higher titers are found in those with multifocal disease. Falling CF titers are often predictive of successful treatment, and high or fluctuating CF titers are suggestive of a poor prognosis. Some reports, however, have indicated that ID and CF results do not correlate well with the clinical status of the patient (152). Many efforts are under way to search for new serological markers for the diagnosis and monitoring of paracoccidioidomycosis, especially because of the recent advances in characterizing the taxonomy of the genus (153).

Adiaspiromycosis and Emergomycosis

The definitive diagnosis of adiaspiromycosis and emergomycosis can be accomplished by direct microscopic detection of *Emmonsia* or *Emergomyces* species in clinical specimens or their isolation in culture. No serological tests are currently available.

REFERENCES

1. **Hawksworth DL.** 2011. A new dawn for the naming of fungi: impacts of decisions made in Melbourne in July 2011 on the future publication and regulation of fungal names. *IMA Fungus* **2:**155–162.
2. **Peterson SW, Sigler L.** 1998. Molecular genetic variation in *Emmonsia crescens* and *Emmonsia parva*, etiologic agents of adiaspiromycosis, and their phylogenetic relationship to *Blastomyces dermatitidis* (*Ajellomyces dermatitidis*) and other systemic fungal pathogens. *J Clin Microbiol* **36:**2918–2925.
3. **Dukik K, Muñoz JF, Jiang Y, Feng P, Sigler L, Stielow JB, Freeke J, Jamalian A, Gerrits van den Ende B, McEwen JG, Clay OK, Schwartz IS, Govender NP, Maphanga TG, Cuomo CA, Moreno LF, Kenyon C, Borman AM, de Hoog S.** 2017. Novel taxa of thermally dimorphic systemic pathogens in the Ajellomycetaceae (Onygenales). *Mycoses* **60:**296–309.

4. **Untereiner WA, Scott JA, Naveau FA, Sigler L, Bachewich J, Angus A.** 2004. The Ajellomycetaceae, a new family of vertebrate-associated Onygenales. *Mycologia* **96:**812–821.
5. **Valero C, Gago S, Monteiro MC, Alastruey-Izquierdo A, Buitrago MJ.** 2018. African histoplasmosis: new clinical and microbiological insights. *Med Mycol* **56:**51–59.
6. **Kasuga T, White TJ, Koenig G, McEwen J, Restrepo A, Castañeda E, Da Silva Lacaz C, Heins-Vaccari EM, De Freitas RS, Zancopé-Oliveira RM, Qin Z, Negroni R, Carter DA, Mikami Y, Tamura M, Taylor ML, Miller GF, Poonwan N, Taylor JW.** 2003. Phylogeography of the fungal pathogen *Histoplasma capsulatum*. *Mol Ecol* **12:**3383–3401.
7. **Arunmozhi Balajee S, Hurst SF, Chang LS, et al.** 2013. Multilocus sequence typing of Histoplasma capsulatum in formalin-fixed paraffin-embedded tissues from cats living in non-endemic regions reveals a new phylogenetic clade. *Med Mycol* **51:**345–351.
8. **Teixeira MM, Patané JS, Taylor ML, Gómez BL, Theodoro RC, de Hoog S, Engelthaler DM, Zancopé-Oliveira RM, Felipe MS, Barker BM.** 2016. Worldwide phylogenetic distributions and population dynamics of the genus *Histoplasma*. *PLoS Negl Trop Dis* **10:**e0004732.
9. **Sepúlveda VE, Márquez R, Turissini DA, Goldman WE, Matute DR.** 2017. Genome sequences reveal cryptic speciation in the human pathogen *Histoplasma capsulatum*. *mBio* **8:**e013390-17.
10. **Meece JK, Anderson JL, Fisher MC, Henk DA, Sloss BL, Reed KD.** 2011. Population genetic structure of clinical and environmental isolates of *Blastomyces dermatitidis*, based on 27 polymorphic microsatellite markers. *Appl Environ Microbiol* **77:**5123–5131.
11. **Brown EM, McTaggart LR, Zhang SX, Low DE, Stevens DA, Richardson SE.** 2013. Phylogenetic analysis reveals a cryptic species *Blastomyces gilchristii*, sp. nov. within the human pathogenic fungus *Blastomyces dermatitidis*. *PLoS One* **8:**e59237. *CORRECTION PLoS One* **11:**e0168018.
12. **Schwartz IS, Wiederhold NP, Patterson TF, Sigler L.** 2017. *Blastomyces helicus*, an emerging dimorphic fungal pathogen causing fatal pulmonary and disseminated disease in humans and animals in western Canada and United States. *Open Forum Infect Dis* **4**(Suppl 1)**:**S83–S84.
13. **Jiang Y, Dukik K, Muñoz JF, Sigler L, Schwartz IS, Govender NP, Kenyon C, Feng P, van den Ende BG, Stielow JB, Stchigel AM, Lu H, de Hoog S.** 2018. Phylogeny, ecology and taxonomy of systemic pathogens and their relatives in *Ajellomycetaceae* (Onygenales): *Blastomyces*, *Emergomyces*, *Emmonsia*, *Emmonsiellopsis*. *Fungal Divers* **90:**245–291.
14. **Meece JK, Anderson JL, Gruszka S, Sloss BL, Sullivan B, Reed KD.** 2013. Variation in clinical phenotype of human infection among genetic groups of *Blastomyces dermatitidis*. *J Infect Dis* **207:**814–822.
15. **Muñoz JF, Gauthier GM, Desjardins CA, Gallo JE, Holder J, Sullivan TD, Marty AJ, Carmen JC, Chen Z, Ding L, Gujja S, Magrini V, Misas E, Mitreva M, Priest M, Saif S, Whiston EA, Young S, Zeng Q, Goldman WE, Mardis ER, Taylor JW, McEwen JG, Clay OK, Klein BS, Cuomo CA.** 2015. The dynamic genome and transcriptome of the human fungal pathogen *Blastomyces* and close relative *Emmonsia*. *PLoS Genet* **11:**e1005493.
16. **Litvintseva AP, Marsden-Haug N, Hurst S, Hill H, Gade L, Driebe EM, Ralston C, Roe C, Barker BM, Goldoft M, Keim P, Wohrle R, Thompson GR III, Engelthaler DM, Brandt ME, Chiller T.** 2015. Valley fever: finding new places for an old disease: *Coccidioides immitis* found in Washington State soil associated with recent human infection. *Clin Infect Dis* **60:**e1–e3.
17. **Neafsey DE, Barker BM, Sharpton TJ, Stajich JE, Park DJ, Whiston E, Hung CY, McMahan C, White J, Sykes S, Heiman D, Young S, Zeng Q, Abouelleil A, Aftuck L, Bessette D, Brown A, FitzGerald M, Lui A, Macdonald JP, Priest M, Orbach MJ, Galgiani JN, Kirkland TN, Cole GT, Birren BW, Henn MR, Taylor JW, Rounsley SD.** 2010. Population genomic sequencing of *Coccidioides fungi* reveals recent hybridization and transposon control. *Genome Res* **20:**938–946.
18. **Fisher MC, Koenig GL, White TJ, Taylor JW.** 2002. Molecular and phenotypic description of *Coccidioides posadasii* sp. nov., previously recognized as the non-California population of *Coccidioides immitis*. *Mycologia* **94:**73–84.
19. **Engelthaler DM, Roe CC, Hepp CM, Teixeira M, Driebe EM, Schupp JM, Gade L, Waddell V, Komatsu K, Arathoon E, Logemann H, Thompson GR III, Chiller T, Barker B, Keim P, Litvintseva AP.** 2016. Local population structure and patterns of Western Hemisphere dispersal for *Coccidioides* spp., the fungal cause of valley fever. *mBio* **7:**e00550-16.
20. **Sharpton TJ, Stajich JE, Rounsley SD, Gardner MJ, Wortman JR, Jordar VS, Maiti R, Kodira CD, Neafsey DE, Zeng Q, Hung CY, McMahan C, Muszewska A, Grynberg M, Mandel MA, Kellner EM, Barker BM, Galgiani JN, Orbach MJ, Kirkland TN, Cole GT, Henn MR, Birren BW, Taylor JW.** 2009. Comparative genomic analyses of the human fungal pathogens *Coccidioides* and their relatives. *Genome Res* **19:**1722–1731.
21. **Matute DR, McEwen JG, Puccia R, Montes BA, San-Blas G, Bagagli E, Rauscher JT, Restrepo A, Morais F, Niño-Vega G, Taylor JW.** 2006. Cryptic speciation and recombination in the fungus *Paracoccidioides brasiliensis* as revealed by gene genealogies. *Mol Biol Evol* **23:**65–73.
22. **Teixeira MM, Theodoro RC, de Carvalho MJ, Fernandes L, Paes HC, Hahn RC, Mendoza L, Bagagli E, San-Blas G, Felipe MS.** 2009. Phylogenetic analysis reveals a high level of speciation in the *Paracoccidioides* genus. *Mol Phylogenet Evol* **52:**273–283.
23. **Theodoro RC, Teixeira MM, Felipe MS, Paduan KS, Ribolla PM, San-Blas G, Bagagli E.** 2012. Genus *Paracoccidioides*: species recognition and biogeographic aspects. *PLoS One* **7:**e37694.
24. **Teixeira MM, Theodoro RC, Oliveira FF, et al.** 2014. *Paracoccidioides lutzii* sp. nov.: biological and clinical implications. *Med Mycol* **52:**19–28.
25. **Teixeira MM, Theodoro RC, Nino-Vega G, Bagagli E, Felipe MS.** 2014. *Paracoccidioides* species complex: ecology, phylogeny, sexual reproduction, and virulence. *PLoS Pathog* **10:**e1004397.
26. **Turissini DA, Gomez OM, Teixeira MM, McEwen JG, Matute DR.** 2017. Species boundaries in the human pathogen *Paracoccidioides*. *Fungal Genet Biol* **106:**9–25.
27. **Teixeira MM, Theodoro RC, Derengowski LS, Nicola AM, Bagagli E, Felipe MS.** 2013. Molecular and morphological data support the existence of a sexual cycle in species of the genus *Paracoccidioides*. *Eukaryot Cell* **12:**380–389.
28. **Herr RA, Tarcha EJ, Taborda PR, Taylor JW, Ajello L, Mendoza L.** 2001. Phylogenetic analysis of *Lacazia loboi* places this previously uncharacterized pathogen within the dimorphic Onygenales. *J Clin Microbiol* **39:**309–314.
29. **Muñoz JF, Gallo JE, Misas E, Priest M, Imamovic A, Young S, Zeng Q, Clay OK, McEwen JG, Cuomo CA.** 2014. Genome update of the dimorphic human pathogenic fungi causing paracoccidioidomycosis. *PLoS Negl Trop Dis* **8:**e3348.
30. **Desjardins CA, Champion MD, Holder JW, Muszewska A, Goldberg J, Bailão AM, Brigido MM, Ferreira ME, Garcia AM, Grynberg M, Gujja S, Heiman DI, Henn MR, Kodira CD, León-Narváez H, Longo LV, Ma LJ, Malavazi I, Matsuo AL, Morais FV, Pereira M, Rodríguez-Brito S, Sakthikumar S, Salem-Izacc SM, Sykes SM, Teixeira MM, Vallejo MC, Walter ME, Yandava C, Young S, Zeng Q, Zucker J, Felipe MS, Goldman GH, Haas BJ, McEwen JG, Nino-Vega G, Puccia R, San-Blas G, Soares CM, Birren BW, Cuomo CA.** 2011. Comparative genomic analysis of human fungal pathogens causing paracoccidioidomycosis. *PLoS Genet* **7:**e1002345.
31. **Muñoz JF, Farrer RA, Desjardins CA, Gallo JE, Sykes S, Sakthikumar S, Misas E, Whiston EA, Bagagli E, Soares CM, Teixeira MM, Taylor JW, Clay OK, McEwen JG, Cuomo CA.** 2016. Genome diversity, recombination, and virulence across the major lineages of *Paracoccidioides*. *mSphere* **1:**e00213-16.
32. **Schwartz IS, McLoud JD, Berman D, Botha A, Lerm B, Colebunders R, Levetin E, Kenyon C.** 2018. Molecular detection of airborne *Emergomyces africanus*, a thermally dimorphic fungal pathogen, in Cape Town, South Africa. *PLoS Negl Trop Dis* **12:**e0006174. *CORRECTION PLoS Negl Trop Dis* **12:**e0006468.

33. **Wang P, Kenyon C, de Hoog S, Guo L, Fan H, Liu H, Li Z, Sheng R, Yang Y, Jiang Y, Zhang L, Xu Y.** 2017. A novel dimorphic pathogen, *Emergomyces orientalis* (Onygenales), agent of disseminated infection. *Mycoses* **60:**310–319.
34. **Yang Y, Ye Q, Li K, Li Z, Bo X, Li Z, Xu Y, Wang S, Wang P, Chen H, Wang J.** 2017. Genomics and comparative genomic analyses provide insight into the taxonomy and pathogenic potential of novel *Emmonsia* pathogens. *Front Cell Infect Microbiol* **7:**105.
35. **Rofael M, Schwartz IS, Sigler L, Kong LK, Nelson N.** 2018. *Emmonsia helica* infection in HIV-infected man, California, USA. *Emerg Infect Dis* **24:**166–168.
36. **Kauffman CA.** 2011. Histoplasmosis, p 321–335. *In* Kauffman CA, Pappas PG, Sobel JD, Dismukes WE (ed), *Essentials of Clinical Mycology*, 2nd ed. Springer-Verlag, New York, NY.
37. **Deepe GS.** 2015. Histoplasma capsulatum, p 2948–2962. *In* Mandell GL, Bennett JE, Dollin R, Blaser MJ (ed), *Mandell, Douglas and Bennett's Principles and Practice of infectious Diseases*, 8th ed. Elsevier Churchill Livingstone, Philadelphia, PA.
38. **Lenhart SW, Schafer MP, Singal M, Hajjeh RA.** 2004. Histoplasmosis: protecting workers at risk. DHHS (NIOSH) publication no. 2005-109. National Institute for Occupational Safety and Health, Washington, DC. http://www.cdc.gov/niosh/docs/2005-109/pdfs/2005-109.pdf.
39. **Gómez BL.** 2011. Histoplasmosis: epidemiology in Latin America. *Curr Fungal Infect Rep* **5:**199.
40. **Anstead GM, Sutton DA, Graybill JR.** 2012. Adiaspiromycosis causing respiratory failure and a review of human infections due to *Emmonsia* and *Chrysosporium* spp. *J Clin Microbiol* **50:**1346–1354.
41. **Reed KD, Meece JK, Archer JR, Peterson AT.** 2008. Ecologic niche modeling of *Blastomyces dermatitidis* in Wisconsin. *PLoS One* **3:**e2034.
42. **Smith JA, Kauffman CA.** 2010. Blastomycosis. *Proc Am Thorac Soc* **7:**173–180.
43. **Thompson GR III.** 2011. Pulmonary coccidioidomycosis. *Semin Respir Crit Care Med* **32:**754–763.
44. **Brown J, Benedict K, Park BJ, Thompson GR III.** 2013. Coccidioidomycosis: epidemiology. *Clin Epidemiol* **5:**185–197.
45. **Restrepo A, González A, Agudelo CA.** 2011. Paracoccidioidomycosis, p 367–385. *In* Kauffman CA, Pappas PG, Sobel JD, Dismukes WE (ed), *Essentials of Clinical Mycology*, 2nd ed. Springer-Verlag, New York, NY.
46. **Restrepo A, Gómez BL, Tobón A.** 2012. Paracoccidioidomycosis: Latin America's own fungal disorder. *Curr Fungal Infect Rep* **6:**303–311.
47. **Martinez R.** 2017. New trends in paracoccidioidomycosis epidemiology. *J Fungi* **3:**1.
48. **Watts JC, Callaway CS, Chandler FW, Kaplan W.** 1975. Human pulmonary adiospiromycosis. *Arch Pathol* **99:**11–15.
49. **van Hougenhouck-Tulleken WG, Papavarnavas NS, Nel JS, Blackburn LY, Govender NP, Spencer DC, Lippincott CK.** 2014. HIV-associated disseminated emmonsiosis, Johannesburg, South Africa. *Emerg Infect Dis* **20:**2164–2166.
50. **Schwartz IS, Govender NP, Corcoran C, Dlamini S, Prozesky H, Burton R, Mendelson M, Taljaard J, Lehloenya R, Calligaro G, Colebunders R, Kenyon C.** 2015. Clinical characteristics, diagnosis, management, and outcomes of disseminated emmonsiosis: a retrospective case series. *Clin Infect Dis* **61:**1004–1012.
51. **Kenyon C, Bonorchis K, Corcoran C, Meintjes G, Locketz M, Lehloenya R, Vismer HF, Naicker P, Prozesky H, van Wyk M, Bamford C, du Plooy M, Imrie G, Dlamini S, Borman AM, Colebunders R, Yansouni CP, Mendelson M, Govender NP.** 2013. A dimorphic fungus causing disseminated infection in South Africa. *N Engl J Med* **369:**1416–1424.
52. **Maphanga TG, Britz E, Zulu TG, Mpembe RS, Naicker SD, Schwartz IS, Govender NP.** 2017. *In vitro* antifungal susceptibility of yeast and mold phases of isolates of dimorphic fungal pathogen *Emergomyces africanus* (formerly *Emmonsia* sp.) from HIV-infected South African patients. *J Clin Microbiol* **55:**1812–1820.
53. **Cuellar-Rodriguez J, Avery RK, Lard M, Budev M, Gordon SM, Shrestha NK, van Duin D, Oethinger M, Mawhorter SD.** 2009. Histoplasmosis in solid organ transplant recipients: 10 years of experience at a large transplant center in an endemic area. *Clin Infect Dis* **49:**710–716.
54. **Nacher M, Adenis A, Mc Donald S, Do Socorro Mendonca Gomes M, Singh S, Lopes Lima I, Malcher Leite R, Hermelijn S, Wongsokarijo M, Van Eer M, Marques Da Silva S, Mesquita Da Costa M, Silva M, Calvacante M, do Menino Jesus Silva Leitao T, Gómez BL, Restrepo A, Tobon A, Canteros CE, Aznar C, Blanchet D, Vantilcke V, Vautrin C, Boukhari R, Chiller T, Scheel C, Ahlquist A, Roy M, Lortholary O, Carme B, Couppié P, Vreden S.** 2013. Disseminated histoplasmosis in HIV-infected patients in South America: a neglected killer continues on its rampage. *PLoS Negl Trop Dis* **7:**e2319.
55. **Saccente M, Woods GL.** 2010. Clinical and laboratory update on blastomycosis. *Clin Microbiol Rev* **23:**367–381.
56. **Roy M, Benedict K, Deak E, Kirby MA, McNiel JT, Sickler CJ, Eckardt E, Marx RK, Heffernan RT, Meece JK, Klein BS, Archer JR, Theurer J, Davis JP, Park BJ.** 2013. A large community outbreak of blastomycosis in Wisconsin with geographic and ethnic clustering. *Clin Infect Dis* **57:**655–662.
57. **Pappas PG, Threlkeld MG, Bedsole GD, Cleveland KO, Gelfand MS, Dismukes WE.** 1993. Blastomycosis in immunocompromised patients. *Medicine (Baltimore)* **72:**311–325.
58. **Stagliano D, Epstein J, Hickey P.** 2007. Fomite-transmitted coccidioidomycosis in an immunocompromised child. *Pediatr Infect Dis J* **26:**454–456.
59. **Vucicevic D, Carey EJ, Blair JE.** 2011. Coccidioidomycosis in liver transplant recipients in an endemic area. *Am J Transplant* **11:**111–119.
60. **Nguyen C, Barker BM, Hoover S, Nix DE, Ampel NM, Frelinger JA, Orbach MJ, Galgiani JN.** 2013. Recent advances in our understanding of the environmental, epidemiological, immunological, and clinical dimensions of coccidioidomycosis. *Clin Microbiol Rev* **26:**505–525.
61. **Schneider E, Hajjeh RA, Spiegel RA, Jibson RW, Harp EL, Marshall GA, Gunn RA, McNeil MM, Pinner RW, Baron RC, Burger RC, Hutwagner LC, Crump C, Kaufman L, Reef SE, Feldman GM, Pappagianis D, Werner SB.** 1997. A coccidioidomycosis outbreak following the Northridge, Calif, earthquake. *JAMA* **277:**904–908.
62. **Ampel NM.** 2007. The complex immunology of human coccidioidomycosis. *Ann N Y Acad Sci* **1111:**245–258.
63. **Niño-Vega GA, et al.** 2017. Paracoccidioides spp. and Paracoccidioidomycosis, p 281–308. *In* Mora-Montes HM, Lopes-Becerra LM (ed), *Current Progress on Medical Mycology*. Springer International Publishing, Cham, Switzerland.
64. **Kenyon C, Corcoran C, Govender NP.** 2014. An *Emmonsia* species causing disseminated infection in South Africa. *N Engl J Med* **370:**284.
65. **Benedict K, Derado G, Mody RK.** 2016. Histoplasmosis-associated hospitalizations in the United States, 2001-2012. *Open Forum Infect Dis* **3:**ofv219.
66. **Chapman SW, Dismukes WE, Proia LA, Bradsher RW, Pappas PG, Threlkeld MG, Kauffman CA, Infectious Diseases Society of America.** 2008. Clinical practice guidelines for the management of blastomycosis: 2008 update by the Infectious Diseases Society of America. *Clin Infect Dis* **46:**1801–1812.
67. **Centers for Disease Control and Prevention.** 2009. Increase in coccidiodomycosis—California, 2000–2007. *MMWR Morb Mortal Wkly Rep* **58:**105–109.
68. **Sunenshine RH, Anderson S, Erhart L, Vossbrink A, Kelly PC, Engelthaler D, Komatsu K.** 2007. Public health surveillance for coccidioidomycosis in Arizona. *Ann N Y Acad Sci* **1111:**96–102.
69. **Kim MM, Blair JE, Carey EJ, Wu Q, Smilack JD.** 2009. Coccidioidal pneumonia, Phoenix, Arizona, USA, 2000-2004. *Emerg Infect Dis* **15:**397–401.
70. **Vincent T, Galgiani JN, Huppert M, Salkin D.** 1993. The natural history of coccidioidal meningitis: VA-Armed Forces cooperative studies, 1955-1958. *Clin Infect Dis* **16:**247–254.

71. **Pelegrin I, Ayats J, Xiol X, et al.** 2011. Disseminated adiaspiromycosis: case report of a liver transplant patient with human immunodeficiency infection, and literature review. *Transpl Infect Dis* **13:**507–514.
72. **Mendes MO, Moraes MA, Renoiner EI, Dantas MH, Lanzieri TM, Fonseca CF, Luna EJ, Hatch DL.** 2009. Acute conjunctivitis with episcleritis and anterior uveitis linked to adiaspiromycosis and freshwater sponges, Amazon region, Brazil, 2005. *Emerg Infect Dis* **15:**633–639.
73. **Kauffman CA.** 2009. Histoplasmosis. *Clin Chest Med* **30:**217–225.
74. **Mathisen G, Shelub A, Truong J, Wigen C.** 2010. Coccidioidal meningitis: clinical presentation and management in the fluconazole era. *Medicine (Baltimore)* **89:**251–284.
75. **Schwartz IS, Kenyon C, Feng P, Govender NP, Dukik K, Sigler L, Jiang Y, Stielow JB, Muñoz JF, Cuomo CA, Botha A, Stchigel AM, de Hoog GS.** 2015. Fifty years of *Emmonsia* disease in humans: the dramatic emergence of a cluster of novel fungal pathogens. *PLoS Pathog* **11:**e1005198.
76. **Connolly PA, Durkin MM, Lemonte AM, Hackett EJ, Wheat LJ.** 2007. Detection of histoplasma antigen by a quantitative enzyme immunoassay. *Clin Vaccine Immunol* **14:**1587–1591.
77. **Hage CA, Kirsch EJ, Stump TE, Kauffman CA, Goldman M, Connolly P, Johnson PC, Wheat LJ, Baddley JW.** 2011. Histoplasma antigen clearance during treatment of histoplasmosis in patients with AIDS determined by a quantitative antigen enzyme immunoassay. *Clin Vaccine Immunol* **18:**661–666.
78. **Azar MM, Hage CA.** 2017. Laboratory diagnostics for histoplasmosis. *J Clin Microbiol* **55:**1612–1620.
79. **Zhang X, Gibson B Jr, Daly TM.** 2013. Evaluation of commercially available reagents for diagnosis of histoplasmosis infection in immunocompromised patients. *J Clin Microbiol* **51:**4095–4101.
80. **Theel ES, Harring JA, Dababneh AS, Rollins LO, Bestrom JE, Jespersen DJ.** 2015. Reevaluation of commercial reagents for detection of Histoplasma capsulatum antigen in urine. *J Clin Microbiol* **53:**1198–1203.
81. **Cáceres DH, Samayoa BE, Medina NG, Tobón AM, Guzmán BJ, Mercado D, Restrepo A, Chiller T, Arathoon E, Gómez BL.** 2018. Multicenter validation of commercial antigenuria reagents to diagnose progressive disseminated histoplasmosis in people living with HIV/AIDS in two Latin American countries. *J Clin Microbiol* **56:**pii:e01959-17.
82. **Girouard G, Lachance C, Pelletier R.** 2007. Observations on (1-3)-beta-D-glucan detection as a diagnostic tool in endemic mycosis caused by *Histoplasma* or *Blastomyces*. *J Med Microbiol* **56:**1001–1002.
83. **Durkin M, Witt J, Lemonte A, Wheat B, Connolly P.** 2004. Antigen assay with the potential to aid in diagnosis of blastomycosis. *J Clin Microbiol* **42:**4873–4875.
84. **Wheat J, Wheat H, Connolly P, Kleiman M, Supparatpinyo K, Nelson K, Bradsher R, Restrepo A.** 1997. Cross-reactivity in *Histoplasma capsulatum* variety capsulatum antigen assays of urine samples from patients with endemic mycoses. *Clin Infect Dis* **24:**1169–1171.
85. **Frost HM, Novicki TJ.** 2015. Blastomyces antigen detection for diagnosis and management of blastomycosis. *J Clin Microbiol* **53:**3660–3662.
86. **Durkin M, Connolly P, Kuberski T, Myers R, Kubak BM, Bruckner D, Pegues D, Wheat LJ.** 2008. Diagnosis of coccidioidomycosis with use of the *Coccidioides* antigen enzyme immunoassay. *Clin Infect Dis* **47:**e69–e73.
87. **Kirsch EJ, Greene RT, Prahl A, Rubin SI, Sykes JE, Durkin MM, Wheat LJ.** 2012. Evaluation of *Coccidioides* antigen detection in dogs with coccidioidomycosis. *Clin Vaccine Immunol* **19:**343–345.
88. **Kassis C, Zaidi S, Kuberski T, Moran A, Gonzalez O, Hussain S, Hartmann-Manrique C, Al-Jashaami L, Chebbo A, Myers RA, Wheat LJ.** 2015. Role of coccidioides antigen testing in the cerebrospinal fluid for the diagnosis of coccidioidal meningitis. *Clin Infect Dis* **61:**1521–1526.
89. **Thompson GR III, Bays DJ, Johnson SM, Cohen SH, Pappagianis D, Finkelman MA.** 2012. Serum (1→3)-β-D-glucan measurement in coccidioidomycosis. *J Clin Microbiol* **50:**3060–3062.
90. **Marques da Silva SH, Queiroz-Telles F, Colombo AL, Blotta MH, Lopes JD, Pires De Camargo Z.** 2004. Monitoring gp43 antigenemia in paracoccidioidomycosis patients during therapy. *J Clin Microbiol* **42:**2419–2424.
91. **Marques da Silva SH, Colombo AL, Blotta MH, Lopes JD, Queiroz-Telles F, Pires de Camargo Z.** 2003. Detection of circulating gp43 antigen in serum, cerebrospinal fluid, and bronchoalveolar lavage fluid of patients with paracoccidioidomycosis. *J Clin Microbiol* **41:**3675–3680.
92. **Gómez BL, Figueroa JI, Hamilton AJ, Diez S, Rojas M, Tobón AM, Hay RJ, Restrepo A.** 1998. Antigenemia in patients with paracoccidioidomycosis: detection of the 87-kilodalton determinant during and after antifungal therapy. *J Clin Microbiol* **36:**3309–3316.
93. **Bialek R, Feucht A, Aepinus C, Just-Nübling G, Robertson VJ, Knobloch J, Hohle R.** 2002. Evaluation of two nested PCR assays for detection of *Histoplasma capsulatum* DNA in human tissue. *J Clin Microbiol* **40:**1644–1647.
94. **Muñoz C, Gómez BL, Tobón A, Arango K, Restrepo A, Correa MM, Muskus C, Cano LE, González A.** 2010. Validation and clinical application of a molecular method for identification of *Histoplasma capsulatum* in human specimens in Colombia, South America. *Clin Vaccine Immunol* **17:**62–67.
95. **Maubon D, Simon S, Aznar C.** 2007. Histoplasmosis diagnosis using a polymerase chain reaction method. Application on human samples in French Guiana, South America. *Diagn Microbiol Infect Dis* **58:**441–444.
96. **Imhof A, Schaer C, Schoedon G, et al.** 2003. Rapid detection of pathogenic fungi from clinical specimens using LightCycler real-time fluorescence PCR. *Eur J Clin Microbiol* **22:**558–560.
97. **Buitrago MJ, Canteros CE, Frías De León G, González Á, Marques-Evangelista De Oliveira M, Muñoz CO, Ramirez JA, Toranzo AI, Zancope-Oliveira R, Cuenca-Estrella M.** 2013. Comparison of PCR protocols for detecting *Histoplasma capsulatum* DNA through a multicenter study. *Rev Iberoam Micol* **30:**256–260.
98. **López LF, Muñoz CO, Cáceres DH, Tobón ÁM, Loparev V, Clay O, Chiller T, Litvintseva A, Gade L, González Á, Gómez BL.** 2017. Standardization and validation of real time PCR assays for the diagnosis of histoplasmosis using three molecular targets in an animal model. *PLoS One* **12:**e0190311.
99. **Sidamonidze K, Peck MK, Perez M, Baumgardner D, Smith G, Chaturvedi V, Chaturvedi S.** 2012. Real-time PCR assay for identification of *Blastomyces dermatitidis* in culture and in tissue. *J Clin Microbiol* **50:**1783–1786.
100. **Babady NE, Buckwalter SP, Hall L, Le Febre KM, Binnicker MJ, Wengenack NL.** 2011. Detection of *Blastomyces dermatitidis* and *Histoplasma capsulatum* from culture isolates and clinical specimens by use of real-time PCR. *J Clin Microbiol* **49:**3204–3208.
101. **Vucicevic D, Blair JE, Binnicker MJ, McCullough AE, Kusne S, Vikram HR, Parish JM, Wengenack NL.** 2010. The utility of *Coccidioides* polymerase chain reaction testing in the clinical setting. *Mycopathologia* **170:**345–351.
102. **Thompson GR III, Sharma S, Bays DJ, Pruitt R, Engelthaler DM, Bowers J, Driebe EM, Davis M, Libke R, Cohen SH, Pappagianis D.** 2013. Coccidioidomycosis: adenosine deaminase levels, serologic parameters, culture results, and polymerase chain reaction testing in pleural fluid. *Chest* **143:**776–781.
103. **Teles FR, Martins ML.** 2011. Laboratorial diagnosis of paracoccidioidomycosis and new insights for the future of fungal diagnosis. *Talanta* **85:**2254–2264.
104. **Buitrago MJ, Merino P, Puente S, Gomez-Lopez A, Arribi A, Zancopé-Oliveira RM, Gutierrez MC, Rodriguez-Tudela JL, Cuenca-Estrella M.** 2009. Utility of real-time PCR for the detection of *Paracoccidioides brasiliensis* DNA in the diagnosis of imported paracoccidioidomycosis. *Med Mycol* **47:**879–882.
105. **Bialek R, Ibricevic A, Aepinus C, Najvar LK, Fothergill AW, Knobloch J, Graybill JR.** 2000. Detection of *Paracoccidioides brasiliensis* in tissue samples by a nested PCR assay. *J Clin Microbiol* **38:**2940–2942.

106. **Semighini CP, de Camargo ZP, Puccia R, Goldman MH, Goldman GH.** 2002. Molecular identification of *Paracoccidioides brasiliensis* by 5′ nuclease assay. *Diagn Microbiol Infect Dis* **44:**383–386.
107. **Dot JM, Debourgogne A, Champigneulle J, Salles Y, Brizion M, Puyhardy JM, Collomb J, Plénat F, Machouart M.** 2009. Molecular diagnosis of disseminated adiaspiromycosis due to *Emmonsia crescens*. *J Clin Microbiol* **47:**1269–1273.
108. **CDC.** 2009. Biosafety in Microbiological and Biomedical Laboratories, 5th ed. U.S. Department of Health and Human Services, Washington, DC. http://www.cdc.gov/biosafety/publications/bmbl5/bmbl5_sect_viii_b.pdf.
109. **Hall GS, Pratt-Rippin K, Washington JA.** 1992. Evaluation of a chemiluminescent probe assay for identification of *Histoplasma capsulatum* isolates. *J Clin Microbiol* **30:**3003–3004.
110. **Stockman L, Clark KA, Hunt JM, Roberts GD.** 1993. Evaluation of commercially available acridinium ester-labeled chemiluminescent DNA probes for culture identification of *Blastomyces dermatitidis, Coccidioides immitis, Cryptococcus neoformans*, and *Histoplasma capsulatum*. *J Clin Microbiol* **31:**845–850.
111. **Padhye AA, Smith G, McLaughlin D, Standard PG, Kaufman L.** 1992. Comparative evaluation of a chemiluminescent DNA probe and an exoantigen test for rapid identification of *Histoplasma capsulatum*. *J Clin Microbiol* **30:**3108–3111.
112. **Brandt ME, Gaunt D, Iqbal N, McClinton S, Hambleton S, Sigler L.** 2005. False-positive *Histoplasma capsulatum* Gen-Probe chemiluminescent test result caused by a *Chrysosporium* species. *J Clin Microbiol* **43:**1456–1458.
113. **Padhye AA, Smith G, Standard PG, McLaughlin D, Kaufman L.** 1994. Comparative evaluation of chemiluminescent DNA probe assays and exoantigen tests for rapid identification of *Blastomyces dermatitidis* and *Coccidioides immitis*. *J Clin Microbiol* **32:**867–870.
114. **Sutton DA.** 2007. Diagnosis of coccidioidomycosis by culture: safety considerations, traditional methods, and susceptibility testing. *Ann N Y Acad Sci* **1111:**315–325.
115. **Sandhu GS, Kline BC, Stockman L, Roberts GD.** 1995. Molecular probes for diagnosis of fungal infections. *J Clin Microbiol* **33:**2913–2919.
116. **Sigler L.** 2005. Adiaspiromycosis and other infections caused by *Emmonsia* species, p 810–824. *In* Merz WG, Hay RJ (ed), *Topley and Wilson's Microbiology and Microbial Infections*, 10th ed. ASM Press, Washington, DC.
117. **Gori S, Drouhet E, Gueho E, Huerre M, Lofaro A, Parenti M, Dupont B.** 1998. Cutaneous disseminated mycosis in a patient with AIDS due to a new dimorphic fungus. *J Mycol Med* **8:**57–63.
118. **Taylor JW, Geiser DM, Burt A, Koufopanou V.** 1999. The evolutionary biology and population genetics underlying fungal strain typing. *Clin Microbiol Rev* **12:**126–146.
119. **Muniz MM, Pizzini CV, Peralta JM, Reiss E, Zancopé-Oliveira RM.** 2001. Genetic diversity of *Histoplasma capsulatum* strains isolated from soil, animals, and clinical specimens in Rio de Janeiro State, Brazil, by a PCR-based random amplified polymorphic DNA assay. *J Clin Microbiol* **39:**4487–4494.
120. **Karimi K, Wheat LJ, Connolly P, Cloud G, Hajjeh R, Wheat E, Alves K, Lacaz CDS, Keath E.** 2002. Differences in histoplasmosis in patients with acquired immunodeficiency syndrome in the United States and Brazil. *J Infect Dis* **186:**1655–1660.
121. **Muniz MM, Morais E Silva Tavares P, Meyer W, Nosanchuk JD, Zancope-Oliveira RM.** 2010. Comparison of different DNA-based methods for molecular typing of *Histoplasma capsulatum*. *Appl Environ Microbiol* **76:**4438–4447.
122. **Damasceno LS, Leitao TM, Taylor ML, Muniz MM, Zancope-Oliveira RM.** 2016. The use of genetic markers in the molecular epidemiology of histoplasmosis: a systematic review. *Eur J Clin Microbiol Infect Dis* **35:**19–27.
123. **McCullough MJ, DiSalvo AF, Clemons KV, Park P, Stevens DA.** 2000. Molecular epidemiology of *Blastomyces dermatitidis*. *Clin Infect Dis* **30:**328–335.
124. **Meece JK, Anderson JL, Klein BS, et al.** 2010. Genetic diversity in *Blastomyces dermatitidis*: implications for PCR detection in clinical and environmental samples. *Med Mycol* **48:**285–290.
125. **Koufopanou V, Burt A, Taylor JW.** 1997. Concordance of gene genealogies reveals reproductive isolation in the pathogenic fungus *Coccidioides immitis*. *Proc Natl Acad Sci USA* **94:**5478–5482.
126. **Jewell K, Cheshier R, Cage GD.** 2008. Genetic diversity among clinical *Coccidioides* spp. isolates in Arizona. *Med Mycol* **46:**449–455.
127. **Nascimento E, Martinez R, Lopes AR, de Souza Bernardes LA, Barco CP, Goldman MH, Taylor JW, McEwen JG, Nobrega MP, Nobrega FG, Goldman GH.** 2004. Detection and selection of microsatellites in the genome of *Paracoccidioides brasiliensis* as molecular markers for clinical and epidemiological studies. *J Clin Microbiol* **42:**5007–5014 .
128. **Lindsley MD, Warnock DW, Morrison CJ.** 2006. Serological and molecular diagnosis of fungal infection, p 569–605. *In* Rose NR, Hamilton RG, Detrick B (ed), *Manual of Molecular and Clinical Laboratory Immunology*, 7th ed. ASM Press, Washington, DC.
129. **Bloch KC, Myint T, Raymond-Guillen L, Hage CA, Davis TE, Wright PW, Chow FC, Woc-Colburn L, Khairy RN, Street AC, Yamamoto T, Albers A, Wheat LJ.** 2018. Improvement in diagnosis of histoplasma meningitis by combined testing for histoplasma antigen and immunoglobulin G and immunoglobulin M anti-histoplasma antibody in cerebrospinal fluid. *Clin Infect Dis* **66:**89–94.
130. **Soufleris AJ, Klein BS, Courtney BT, Proctor ME, Jones JM.** 1994. Utility of anti-WI-1 serological testing in the diagnosis of blastomycosis in Wisconsin residents. *Clin Infect Dis* **19:**87–92.
131. **Klein BS, Vergeront JM, Kaufman L, Bradsher RW, Kumar UN, Mathai G, Varkey B, Davis JP.** 1987. Serological tests for blastomycosis: assessments during a large point-source outbreak in Wisconsin. *J Infect Dis* **155:**262–268.
132. **Klein BS, Kuritsky JN, Chappell WA, Kaufman L, Green J, Davies SF, Williams JE, Sarosi GA.** 1986. Comparison of the enzyme immunoassay, immunodiffusion, and complement fixation tests in detecting antibody in human serum to the A antigen of *Blastomyces dermatitidis*. *Am Rev Respir Dis* **133:**144–148.
133. **Pappagianis D.** 2001. Serologic studies in coccidioidomycosis. *Semin Respir Infect* **16:**242–250.
134. **Pappagianis D, Krasnow RI, Beall S.** 1976. False-positive reactions of cerebrospinal fluid and diluted sera with the coccidioidal latex-agglutination test. *Am J Clin Pathol* **66:**916–921.
135. **Twarog M, Thompson GR III.** 2015. Coccidioidomycosis: recent updates. *Semin Respir Crit Care Med* **36:**746–755.
136. **Malo J, Holbrook E, Zangeneh T, Strawter C, Oren E, Robey I, Erickson H, Chahal R, Durkin M, Thompson C, Hoover SE, Ampel NM, Wheat LJ, Knox KS.** 2017. Enhanced antibody detection and diagnosis of coccidioidomycosis with the MiraVista IgG and IgM detection enzyme immunoassay. *J Clin Microbiol* **55:**893–901.
137. **Shikanai-Yasuda MA, Mendes RP, Colombo AL, Queiroz-Telles F, Kono ASG, Paniago AMM, Nathan A, Valle ACFD, Bagagli E, Benard G, Ferreira MS, Teixeira MM, Silva-Vergara ML, Pereira RM, Cavalcante RS, Hahn R, Durlacher RR, Khoury Z, Camargo ZP, Moretti ML, Martinez R.** 2017. Brazilian guidelines for the clinical management of paracoccidioidomycosis. *Rev Soc Bras Med Trop* **50:**715–740.
138. **Díez S, Gómez BL, McEwen JG, Restrepo A, Hay RJ, Hamilton AJ.** 2003. Combined use of *Paracoccidioides brasiliensis* recombinant 27-kilodalton and purified 87-kilodalton antigens in an enzyme-linked immunosorbent assay for serodiagnosis of paracoccidioidomycosis. *J Clin Microbiol* **41:**1536–1542.
139. **Fernandes VC, Coitinho JB, Veloso JM, Araújo SA, Pedroso EP, Goes AM.** 2011. Combined use of *Paracoccidioides brasiliensis* recombinant rPb27 and rPb40 antigens in an enzyme-linked immunosorbent assay for immunodiagnosis of paracoccidioidomycosis. *J Immunol Methods* **367:**78–84.
140. **Gegembauer G, Araujo LM, Pereira EF, Rodrigues AM, Paniago AM, Hahn RC, de Camargo ZP.** 2014. Serology of paracoccidioidomycosis due to *Paracoccidioides lutzii*. *PLoS Negl Trop Dis* **8:**e2986.

141. **Thompson GR III, Rendon A, Ribeiro Dos Santos R, Queiroz-Telles F, Ostrosky-Zeichner L, Azie N, Maher R, Lee M, Kovanda L, Engelhardt M, Vazquez JA, Cornely OA, Perfect JR.** 2016. isavuconazole treatment of cryptococcosis and dimorphic mycoses. *Clin Infect Dis* **63:**356–362.
142. **Clinical and Laboratory Standards Institute.** 2008. Reference method for broth dilution antifungal susceptibility testing of filamentous fungi; approved standard—2nd ed. CLSI document M38-A2. Clinical and Laboratory Standards Institute, Wayne, PA.
143. **Clinical and Laboratory Standards Institute.** 2008. Reference method for broth dilution antifungal susceptibility testing of yeasts; approved standard—3rd ed. CLSI document M27-A3. Clinical and Laboratory Standards Institute, Wayne, PA.
144. **Wheat LJ, Connolly P, Smedema M, Durkin M, Brizendine E, Mann P, Patel R, McNicholas PM, Goldman M.** 2006. Activity of newer triazoles against *Histoplasma capsulatum* from patients with AIDS who failed fluconazole. *J Antimicrob Chemother* **57:**1235–1239.
145. **Kriesel JD, Sutton DA, Schulman S, Fothergill AW, Rinaldi MG.** 2008. Persistent pulmonary infection with an azole-resistant *Coccidioides* species. *Med Mycol* **46:**607–610.
146. **Hage CA, Ribes JA, Wengenack NL, Baddour LM, Assi M, McKinsey DS, Hammoud K, Alapat D, Babady NE, Parker M, Fuller D, Noor A, Davis TE, Rodgers M, Connolly PA, El Haddad B, Wheat LJ.** 2011. A multicenter evaluation of tests for diagnosis of histoplasmosis. *Clin Infect Dis* **53:**448–454.
147. **Kauffman CA.** 2007. Histoplasmosis: a clinical and laboratory update. *Clin Microbiol Rev* **20:**115–132.
148. **Castillo CG, Kauffman CA, Miceli MH.** 2016. Blastomycosis. *Infect Dis Clin North Am* **30:**247–264.
149. **Stockamp NW, Thompson GR III.** 2016. Coccidioidomycosis. *Infect Dis Clin North Am* **30:**229–246.
150. **Thompson G III, Wang S, Bercovitch R, Bolaris M, Van Den Akker D, Taylor S, Lopez R, Catanzaro A, Cadena J, Chin-Hong P, Spellberg B.** 2013. Routine CSF analysis in coccidioidomycosis is not required. *PLoS One* **8:**e64249.
151. **Galgiani JN, Ampel NM, Blair JE, Catanzaro A, Geertsma F, Hoover SE, Johnson RH, Kusne S, Lisse J, MacDonald JD, Meyerson SL, Raksin PB, Siever J, Stevens DA, Sunenshine R, Theodore N.** 2016. 2016 Infectious Diseases Society of America (IDSA) clinical practice guideline for the treatment of coccidioidomycosis. *Clin Infect Dis* **63:**e112–e146.
152. **McKinsey DS, McKinsey JP, Northcutt N, Sarria JC.** 2009. Interlaboratory discrepancy of antigenuria results in 2 patients with AIDS and histoplasmosis. *Diagn Microbiol Infect Dis* **63:**111–114.
153. **da Silva JF, de Oliveira HC, Marcos CM, Assato PA, Fusco-Almeida AM, Mendes-Giannini MJS.** 2016. Advances and challenges in paracoccidioidomycosis serology caused by *Paracoccidioides* species complex: an update. *Diagn Microbiol Infect Dis* **84:**87–94.
154. **Verghese S, Arjundas D, Krishnakumar KC, et al.** 2002. Coccidioidomycosis in India: report of a second imported case. *Med Mycol* **40:**307–309.
155. **Espinel-Ingroff A.** 1998. In vitro activity of the new triazole voriconazole (UK-109,496) against opportunistic filamentous and dimorphic fungi and common and emerging yeast pathogens. *J Clin Microbiol* **36:**198–202.
156. **Li RK, Ciblak MA, Nordoff N, Pasarell L, Warnock DW, McGinnis MR.** 2000. In vitro activities of voriconazole, itraconazole, and amphotericin B against *Blastomyces dermatitidis*, *Coccidioides immitis*, and *Histoplasma capsulatum*. *Antimicrob Agents Chemother* **44:**1734–1736.
157. **McGinnis MR, Pasarell L, Sutton DA, Fothergill AW, Cooper CR Jr, Rinaldi MG.** 1997. In vitro evaluation of voriconazole against some clinically important fungi. *Antimicrob Agents Chemother* **41:**1832–1834.
158. **Thompson GR III, Wiederhold NP.** 2010. Isavuconazole: a comprehensive review of spectrum of activity of a new triazole. *Mycopathologia* **170:**291–313.
159. **Espinel-Ingroff A.** 1998. Comparison of In vitro activities of the new triazole SCH56592 and the echinocandins MK-0991 (L-743,872) and LY303366 against opportunistic filamentous and dimorphic fungi and yeasts. *J Clin Microbiol* **36:**2950–2956.
160. **González GM, Tijerina R, Najvar LK, Bocanegra R, Luther M, Rinaldi MG, Graybill JR.** 2001. Correlation between antifungal susceptibilities of *Coccidioides immitis* in vitro and antifungal treatment with caspofungin in a mouse model. *Antimicrob Agents Chemother* **45:**1854–1859.
161. **Thompson GR III, Barker BM, Wiederhold NP.** 2017. Large-scale evaluation of *in vitro* amphotericin B, triazole, and echinocandin activity against *Coccidioides* species from U.S. institutions. *Antimicrob Agents Chemother* **61:**e02634-16.
162. **González GM, Tijerina R, Najvar LK, Bocanegra R, Rinaldi M, Loebenberg D, Graybill JR.** 2002. In vitro and in vivo activities of posaconazole against *Coccidioides immitis*. *Antimicrob Agents Chemother* **46:**1352–1356.

Trichophyton, Microsporum, Epidermophyton, and Agents of Superficial Mycoses

ANDREW M. BORMAN AND RICHARD C. SUMMERBELL

126

TAXONOMY

For many years, the etiologic agents of dermatophytosis have been classified, along with some nonpathogenic relatives, in three genera: *Trichophyton*, *Microsporum*, and *Epidermophyton*, in the family *Arthrodermataceae* of the order Onygenales (1), phylum Ascomycota. These generic names were historically based on anamorphic (asexual state) names. Any dermatophytes capable of reproducing sexually, i.e., producing ascomata with asci and ascospores, also had historical teleomorph names in the genus *Arthroderma* or *Nannizzia* (2).

As part of the ongoing molecular revolution in biology, fungal taxonomy is ever more strongly influenced by our greatly increased understanding of population genetics (3). Dermatophytes show two population genetics patterns differing among species that have "population hosts" (4) in different zoological families, orders, or classes (5, 6). (A population host, which is the normal epidemiologic reservoir of the species, is distinguished from "occasional host" species that may acquire infection but that do not support ongoing populations; for example, *Microsporum canis* has mostly feline population hosts, and while humans are frequently infected by feline carriers, the species is seldom directly transmitted from human to human, making our species only an occasional host). Some dermatophyte species, including pathogens with population hosts in the rodent, rabbit, pig, dog, and cat families, are potentially sexual, with sexual reproduction occurring only off the host, i.e., on hair or other keratinous debris in contact with the ground. Other species, particularly those with human, ungulate, equine, or avian population hosts, have no access to a soil-based location suitable for sexual reproduction and host reinfection; not surprisingly, these species are found on investigation to be asexual and clonal. They consist, in all known cases, of genetically highly uniform isolates (7–9) sharing, where known, a single mating type factor (6, 10). Most appear to have evolved from a single strain of a sexual ancestral species that was able to make the rare successful switch to ongoing contagious infection of a new animal host. A few epidemiological and phenotypic characteristics in the clonal species appear to have undergone accelerated evolution due to strong selection for increased compatibility with the new host. This process has tended to produce differences allowing relatively easy laboratory identification of these species. At the same time, the basic cellular "housekeeping" genes investigated in phylogenetic taxonomic studies have evolved at a normal rate and thus strongly tend to resemble forms seen in ancestral species-complexes or in sibling species. This has led to considerable recent confusion about species concepts.

Fungal nomenclatural rules have evolved in parallel with novel taxonomic approaches, resulting in the "one fungus, one name" system (11) that came into force on 1 January 2013. Under that system, it appeared likely that the clinically familiar anamorph (*Trichophyton*, *Epidermophyton*, *Microsporum*) names would be chosen over *Arthroderma* for ongoing use in this group of fungi. However, recent multilocus phylogenetic studies of type and reference strains of members of *Arthrodermataceae*, while broadly supporting earlier phylogenies, demonstrated that *Trichophyton* is polyphyletic (12) and supported the recognition of seven genera of dermatophytes and dermatophyte relatives. Under this scheme, *Trichophyton* currently contains 16 species, *Epidermophyton* 1 species, *Nannizzia* 7 species, *Microsporum* 3 species, *Lophophyton* 1 species, *Paraphyton* 3 species, and *Arthroderma* 21 species. In this classification, almost all anthropophilic dermatophytes were retained in *Trichophyton* and *Epidermophyton*, together with several zoophilic species regularly associated with human infections. Conversely, most geophilic species and those zoophilic organisms that rarely cause human disease are divided among *Arthroderma*, *Lophophyton*, *Paraphyton*, and *Nannizzia*. Even with such multilocus approaches, certain recently diverged lineages are still narrowly delineated (for example, *Trichophyton tonsurans* and *Trichophyton equinum* [13]), suggesting that polyphasic approaches incorporating ecological, phenotypic, life cycle, and functional genomics features will be required to fully validate all species and definitively determine species borders. Moreover, it is likely that the geophilic dermatophytes have been insufficiently studied to date, raising the future possibility of numerous additional hitherto unsampled taxa. It is important to note that recent proteomic approaches support essentially the same phylogenies as those previously proposed based on phenotypic, clinical, and epidemiological characteristics (13). Since these recent taxonomic proposals have not been fully adopted in reporting practices by the medical mycology community, this chapter retains a relatively conservative approach to the ongoing taxonomic restructurings in this group of fungi. The list of heretofore recognized species is given in Table 1, with proposed new names given alongside

TABLE 1 Important characteristics of clinically isolated dermatophytes and dermatophytoids

Dermatophyte species and abundance (teleomorph name[s] if formation of sexual state is known)	Proposed new name (12)	Growth	Macromorphology	Micromorphology	BCP milk glucose (pH results for 7–10 days)	Urea test (7 days, broth)	Hair perforation	Other comments
Epidermophyton floccosum[a]	No change	Moderate to rapid	Flat, slightly granular at first, soon developing white puffs of degeneration; sandy to olive-brown (Fig. 18e); reverse pale to yellowish	Macroconidia abundant, club-shaped with broadly rounded apex, usually with fewer than 6 cells (Fig. 12); no microconidia formed; many chlamydospores in primary isolates	Alkaline	Pos	Neg	Invades skin and nails, rarely hair; no microconidia
Microsporum audouinii[b]	No change	Moderate to rapid	Flat to velvety, thin, pale salmon to pale brownish reverse	Rare, deformed macroconidia, often with beak, constricted mid-region, and at least trace granulation (Fig. 13); drop-shaped microconidia and aerial arthroconidia may be present; pectinate branching, apiculate terminal chlamydospores often seen	No pH change or alkaline	Neg	Neg	Poor growth and no or brownish pigment on polished rice medium; usually connected with patient or index patient in or recently from Africa; only children typically infected
Microsporum canis[a] (*Arthroderma otae*)	No change	Rapid	Flat to velvety, thin, pale to yellow (Fig. 18g), with yellow (rarely pale) reverse	Macroconidia thick-walled, roughened, and beaked (Fig. 14); microconidia drop-shaped	No pH change; macroconidia often abundant	Pos	Pos	Good growth and yellow pigment on polished rice medium; human infection usually from cat or dog. *M. canis* "distortum" phenotype has macroconidia distorted, bizarrely shaped. "*Microsporum equinum*" phenotype from horses has few, short macroconidia
Microsporum cookei complex[b] (includes *M. cookei* [*Arthroderma cajetani*], *M. mirabile* [*Arthroderma mirabile*])	All species moved to *Paraphyton*	Moderate to rapid	Granular to velvety; reverse wine-red	Macroconidia rough, thick-walled with cellular compartments rather than true cross walls (Fig. 15); microconidia drop-shaped	No pH change	Pos	Pos	Probably nonpathogenic; existing case reports poorly substantiated

(*Continued on next page*)

TABLE 1 Important characteristics of clinically isolated dermatophytes and dermatophytoids *(Continued)*

Dermatophyte species and abundance (teleomorph name[s] if formation of sexual state is known)	Proposed new name (12)	Growth	Macromorphology	Micromorphology	BCP milk glucose (pH results for 7–10 days)	Urea test (7 days, broth)	Hair perforation	Other comments
Microsporum ferrugineum[c]	No change	Slow	Flat or folded, waxy to slightly velvety; surface and reverse yellow, rusty or pale	No conidia; coarse, straight "bamboo" hyphae with prominent septa may be present	No pH change	Neg	Neg	Yellow colony on Lowenstein-Jensen medium (compare *Trichophyton soudanense*); geographically restricted to parts of Africa, Asia, and eastern Europe
Microsporum gallinae[c]	*Lophophyton gallinae*	Moderate to rapid	Flat to velvety; surface white tinged with pink; reverse red; red pigment diffuses into agar	Macroconidia smooth to slightly rough, often bent and with thickest cells near the apex, sometimes slightly rough; microconidia drop-shaped	No data	Neg	Neg	Rare; human infection usually from chicken Species may be an asexual phenotype within *A. grubyi* according to Gräser et al. (99)
Microsporum gypseum complex[a] (*Arthroderma gypseum*, *A. incurvatum*, *A. fulvum*, *Microsporum duboisii*)	All species moved to *Nannizzia*	Rapid	Granular, sandy in color, or occasionally light cinnamon or rosy buff; reverse usually pale to brownish	Macroconidia abundant, thin-walled, fusoid (tapered at both ends), roughened, with up to 6 septa (Fig. 16); microconidia drop-shaped, mostly formed along sparsely branched hyphae (a feature only noted if *M. racemosum* is queried)	No pH change	Pos	Pos	Human infection usually from soil contact
Microsporum nanum[b] (*Arthroderma obtusum*)	*Nannizzia nana*	Moderate to rapid	Powdery, sandy in color; reverse often reddish-brown	Macroconidia rough, usually only 1–3 cells long, egg-shaped to ellipsoidal	No data	Pos	Pos	Human infection usually from pig; now rare
Microsporum persicolor[b] (*Arthroderma persicolor*)	*Nannizzia persicolor*	Rapid	Powdery, sandy in color; reverse pale to yellowish, sometimes with rosy tones	Macroconidia fusoid (tapered on both ends), often absent or smooth-walled on Sabouraud agar but usually common and rough-walled on Sabouraud with added salt (3% or 5% NaCl) (Fig. 17); microconidia formed on pedicels (must be checked within 5 days)	No pH change	Pos	Pos	Usually poor growth at 37°C *in vitro*; rose to wine-red reverse on sugar-free media, e.g., glucose-free Sabouraud agar, human infection usually from soil (fomites from voles)
Microsporum praecox[b]	*Nannizzia praecox*	Rapid	Powdery, sandy in color, reverse yellow	See *M. gypseum*	No pH change	Pos	Neg	Uncommon

Microsporum racemosum[c] (*Arthroderma racemosum*)	Proposed as facultative synonym of *Paraphyton cookei*	Rapid	Powdery, sandy in color, reverse red	Macroconidia the same as *M. gypseum*; microconidia mostly formed in densely branched formations structured like grape clusters (racemes)	No pH change	Pos	Pos	Rare
Microsporum vanbreuseghemii[c] (*Arthroderma grubyi*)	*Lophophyton gallinae*	Rapid	Powdery, pinkish or buff; pale to yellow reverse	Macroconidia rough, thick-walled, cylindrical, often more than 8 cells long, with cellular compartments rather than true cross walls	No data	Pos	Pos	Rare Anamorph may be conspecific with phenotypically and epidemiologically different *M. gallinae* according to Gräser et al. (99)
Trichophyton ajelloi[b] (*Arthroderma uncinatum*)	*A. uncinatum*	Moderate to rapid	Powdery, rich tan to medium orange-brown in color; reverse pale, brownish or with purple-black pigment	Macroconidia smooth, thick-walled, cylindrical, often more than 7 cells long, with cellular compartments rather than true cross walls (Fig. 5)	No data	Pos	Pos	Nonpathogenic in humans
Trichophyton concentricum[c]	No change	Slow	Folded, honey-brown to reddish brown, glabrous or slightly velvety colony	No conidia	No data	Pos or neg	Neg	Only from indigenous Asian Austronesian/ Melanesian or indigenous Central and South American people with distinct tinea imbricata infection
Trichophyton equinum[b]	No change	Moderate to rapid	Flat to velvety colony with cream colored surface and yellow to red-brown reverse	Macroconidia uncommon, cylindrical to club-shaped, smooth; microconidia abundant, on small pedicels (examine before 5 days)	Alkaline	Pos	Usually neg, sometimes pos	Human infection usually from horse; has a nicotinic acid requirement except in autotrophic variant from Australia and New Zealand
Trichophyton erinacei Hedgehog form[b] (*Arthroderma benhamiae*)	No change	Rapid	Granular to powdery, yellow-cream to buff surface, yellow reverse	Macroconidia uncommon, club-shaped, smooth; microconidia nearly spherical, abundant, mostly produced in dense tufts; spiral appendages present	Alkaline	Neg (European/ New Zealand form) Pos (African form)	Pos	Human infection usually from hedgehog or its fomites; therefore, mostly restricted to regions with wild hedgehogs or to pet hedgehog owners
Trichophyton megninii[b]	No change	Moderate to rapid	Cottony, with white down sometimes suffused with rosy pigment; reverse red to red-brown	Macroconidia seldom seen, pencil-shaped; microconidia drop-shaped	Alkaline	Pos or weak pos	Neg	Region of endemicity in Portugal and nearby areas; requires histidine; considered a subtype of *T. rubrum* by Gräser et al. (99)

(*Continued on next page*)

TABLE 1 Important characteristics of clinically isolated dermatophytes and dermatophytoids *(Continued)*

Dermatophyte species and abundance (teleomorph name[s] if formation of sexual state is known)	Proposed new name (12)	Growth	Macromorphology	Micromorphology	BCP milk glucose (pH results for 7–10 days)	Urea test (7 days, broth)	Hair perforation	Other comments
T. mentagrophytes complex (zoophilic)[a] Inclusive of *T. mentagrophytes sensu stricto* (the former *T. mentagrophytes* var. *quinckeanum*) plus animal-adapted forms of *Trichophyton interdigitale* and the *Trichophyton* anamorph of *A. benhamiae* (*Arthroderma vanbreuseghemii*, *A. benhamiae*) Also includes rare species *Trichophyton eriotrephon* and probably *Trichophyton bullosum*	No change, but *Trichophyton* anamorph of *A. benhamiae* now proposed as *T. benhamiae*	Rapid	Granular to powdery, yellow-cream to buff surface (Fig. 18b), pale to red-brown reverse	Macroconidia uncommon, club-shaped, smooth; microconidia nearly spherical, abundant, mostly produced in dense tufts; spiral appendages present	Alkaline (rarely weak)	Pos	Pos	Human infection usually from rodent or rabbit Macroconidia induced on SGA + 3% or 5% sodium chloride (Fig. 6)
T. mentagrophytes complex (anthropophilic)[a] Inclusive of human-adapted forms of *T. interdigitale* and possibly of the *Trichophyton* anamorph of *A. benhamiae* (*A. vanbreuseghemii*, *A. benhamiae*)	No change, but *Trichophyton* anamorph of *A. benhamiae* now proposed as zoophilic *T. benhamiae*	Rapid	Powdery to cottony, yellow-cream to buff or white surface, pale to red-brown reverse	Macroconidia uncommon, club-shaped, smooth; microconidia nearly spherical or drop-shaped, abundant, produced mainly in dense tufts when round and on sparsely branched hyphae when drop-shaped; spiral appendages present but rare in very cottony isolates	Alkaline	Pos	Pos	Macroconidia often induced on SGA + 3% or 5% sodium chloride
T. mentagrophytes ("nodular" variant[b] formerly called *T. krajdenii*, now known to be a distinct morph of *T. interdigitale*)	No change	Moderate to slow	Cottony, cream to white surface often with yellow marginal zone (Fig. 18a), intense yellow reverse	Macroconidia rare, microconidia usually drop-shaped, sometimes also round; coiled, yellow "nodular bodies" and yellow pigment granules present in submerged mycelium; spiral appendages seldom seen	Alkaline	Pos	Pos	Although usually very different in morphology, this variant so far is not genetically distinguishable from other anthropophilic isolates of *T. interdigitale*

T. rubrum[a] (cosmopolitan variant)	No change	Moderate to slow	Cottony to velvety, white to reddish surface (Fig. 18c), typically wine red reverse (Fig. 18d) but yellow variants occasional Red color poorly formed in presence of common bacterial contamination	Macroconidia seldom seen, pencil-shaped (Fig. 8); microconidia drop-shaped, abundant, scanty or not formed; lateral hyphal projections often present	No pH change (alkalinity after 14 days)	Neg (rarely weak)	Neg	Melanoid variants secreting brown pigment rarely seen
T. rubrum (Afro-Asiatic variant[b] formerly called *T. raubitschekii*, *T. fluviomuniense*, or when microconidia absent, *T. kanei*)	No change	Moderate to slow	Powdery to low velvety, cream to deep red; reverse wine red	Macroconidia abundant (Fig. 7), club-shaped, sometimes with "rat-tail" extension; microconidia drop-shaped to round; many chlamydospores in primary isolates	No pH change (alkalinity after 14 days)	Pos	Neg	Although usually very different in morphology, this variant so far is genetically distinguished from typical *T. rubrum* only at microsatellite markers; often from upper body infection (tinea corporis, tinea cruris)
T. schoenleinii[c]	No change	Slow	Convoluted, slightly velvety whitish colony	No conidia seen; "favic chandeliers" or "nailhead hyphae" present	Alkaline	Variable	Neg	Very rare; associated with clinically recognizable "favus" lesions; now extirpated except in rural central Asia, rural Africa
Trichophyton simii[b] (*Arthroderma simii*)	No change	Rapid	Granular to powdery, yellow-cream to buff surface, pale to red-brown reverse	Macroconidia abundant, often with some cells swollen as chlamydospores; microconidia drop-shaped	Alkaline	Pos	Pos	Endemic to India and Africa; similar to zoophilic *T. mentagrophytes* but macroconidial number and shape are atypical; reference distinction is by mating or molecular study

(Continued on next page)

TABLE 1 Important characteristics of clinically isolated dermatophytes and dermatophytoids (*Continued*)

Dermatophyte species and abundance (teleomorph name[s] if formation of sexual state is known)	Proposed new name (12)	Growth	Macromorphology	Micromorphology	BCP milk glucose (pH results for 7–10 days)	Urea test (7 days, broth)	Hair perforation	Other comments
T. soudanense[b]	No change	Moderate to slow	Flat, bright yellow to (less commonly) wine-red colony with radial striations and star-like margin; uncommonly cottony; reverse yellow to wine red	Macroconidia not seen, microconidia drop-shaped, scarce, or absent; reflexive hyphal branches in radial striations	Alkaline, with small zone of clearing	Usually neg, occasionally pos	Neg	Endemic to sub-Saharan Africa but widely disseminated in cosmopolitan parts of Europe and Americas Dark colony on Lowenstein-Jensen medium (compare *M. ferrugineum*); may or may not grow on growth factor test media Considered a subtype of *T. rubrum* by Gräser and colleagues (104, 105)
Trichophyton terrestre complex[b] (*Arthroderma lenticulare*, *A. quadrifidum*, *A. insingulare*) Also similar, *Trichophyton eboreum* (*Arthroderma*), *Trichophyton thuringiense*	No change, although *Arthroderma* now proposed *T. eboreum* now *Arthroderma eboreum*	Moderate to rapid	Powdery white to cream or pinkish surface; pale or rarely yellow to red reverse	Macroconidia numerous, mostly small (5 or fewer cells) intergrading with large club-shaped microconidia in a continuous series (Fig. 9), so that 3-, 2-, and 1-celled conidia are present	Alkaline	Pos	Pos	No growth at 37°C *in vitro*; nonpathogenic
T. tonsurans[a]	No change	Moderate to slow	Powdery to velvety, white to yellowish or red-brown surface; reverse chestnut red-brown (Fig. 18f) and/or sulfur yellow, rarely pale	Macroconidia uncommon, small pencil- or club-shaped; microconidia abundant (Fig. 10), often on broad "match-stick" pedicels; "balloon forms" and "filiform branches" may be seen	Alkaline, sometimes weak	Pos	Usually neg, sometimes pos	Stimulated by thiamine; a form producing only macroconidia has been described

Trichophyton vanbreuseghemii[c] (*A. gertleri*)	*Arthroderma gertleri*	Moderate to slow	Buff colony, leathery, finely grainy; reverse whitish or pale yellow	Abundant macroconidia with cells of uneven length, tending to fragment into single cells; microconidia small, boxy	No data	Pos	Pos	Geophilic; very rare in clinical laboratory
Trichophyton verrucosum[a]	No change	Slow	Convoluted, slightly velvety whitish or less commonly tan to ochraceous colony	Macroconidia seldom seen, with "rat-tail extension"; microconidia round to drop-shaped; chains of symmetrical chlamydospores seen on milk solid media at 37° (Fig. 11)	Alkaline (may be weak) with broad zone of clearing	Neg	Neg	Human infection usually from cattle; growth stimulated at 37°C
Trichophyton violaceum[b]	No change	Slow	Glabrous (bald-looking), smooth or convoluted colony; purple-red, sometimes with white sectors; some East African isolates purely whitish	Macroconidia seldom seen; microconidia drop-shaped, formed mostly on thiamine medium or on sporulation media; chains of asymmetrical chlamydospores seen on milk solid media at 37°	No pH change or weak alkaline with small to broad zone of clearing (always broad after 14 days)	Pos or weak	Neg	Endemic to North Africa and Middle East but widely disseminated in cosmopolitan parts of Europe, Americas, and South Africa

[a]Common.
[b]Uncommon but likely to be seen by large labs in Americas and Europe.
[c]Unlikely to be seen except in region where endemic or proficiency test or soil isolation experiment.

the current names. Previous anamorph names and long-used *Arthroderma* names are included to facilitate comparison with earlier literature.

EPIDEMIOLOGY AND TRANSMISSION

Dermatophytes are keratinophilic fungi that are capable of invading the keratinous tissues of living animals. They are grouped into three categories based on host preference and natural habitat (Table 2) (14). Anthropophilic species almost exclusively infect humans; animals are rarely infected. Geophilic species are soil-associated organisms, and soil *per se* or soilborne keratinous debris (e.g., shed hairs, molted feathers) is a source of infection for humans as well as for other animals. Zoophilic species are essentially pathogens of nonhuman mammals or, rarely, birds; however, animal-to-human transmission is not uncommon. Understanding this ecological classification for case isolates may be helpful in determining the source of infection; e.g., human infections caused by *M. canis* are often the result of contact between susceptible children and newly acquired or stray kittens (15). Clinical species identification of dermatophytes assists in controlling infections that may have a family pet or other domesticated animal as an ongoing source of inoculum. Moreover, scalp infections with *M. canis* require a treatment regimen differing from that used for scalp infections caused by the more common agents of tinea capitis. This underscores the importance of correct identification of the etiological agent.

Some dermatophytes, e.g., *Trichophyton rubrum*, are cosmopolitan, whereas others, e.g., *Trichophyton concentricum*, are geographically limited (16). *T. concentricum* is found only in the Pacific Islands and regions in Southeast Asia and Central and South America. However, the ability of dermatophytes to spread to new geographical niches in conjunction with population movements should not be underestimated. In the United Kingdom, the large-scale introduction of *T. rubrum* and the historic emergence of *Microsporum audouinii* in rural areas could be correlated, respectively, with troop repatriation from the Far East and evacuation of children from major cities during the first and second world wars. Similarly, the reemergence of *T. tonsurans* as the preponderant agent of tinea capitis in British cities has been driven by large-scale immigration from the Caribbean (17). Thus, care should be taken against complacent assumptions based on historical epidemiological patterns.

Anthropophilic fungi are usually transmitted either directly through close human contact or indirectly through sharing of clothes, combs, brushes, towels, bedsheets, etc. Tinea capitis is highly contagious and may spread rapidly within a family, institution, or school. Transmission of tinea cruris is associated with shared clothing, towels, and sanitary facilities. The transmission of tinea pedis and tinea unguium often involves communal showers, baths, or other aquatic facilities but may depend on both environmental and host factors (18, 19). Acquisition of chronic *T. rubrum* tinea pedis has been suggested to require a dominant autosomal susceptibility gene (20).

Infections with geophilic dermatophytes involve transmission of soilborne inoculum to humans or other mammals. Outbreaks originating from infected soil with secondary human-to-human transmission have been reported (21). Infections by zoophilic species result from animal-to-human contact (cats, dogs, cattle, laboratory animals, etc.) or from indirect transmission involving fomites. The fungi may then be transmitted among humans to a limited extent, especially in institutions (22).

CLINICAL SIGNIFICANCE

The dermatophytoses (tinea or ringworm) generally manifest as infections of the keratinized tissues (hair, nails, skin, etc.) of humans, other mammals, and birds. Cutaneous infections resembling dermatophytoses may occasionally be caused by yeasts or by unrelated filamentous fungi that are normally saprobes or plant pathogens; these infections are referred to as opportunistic dermatomycoses (19).

Dermatophytes are among the very few fungal species that cause contagious, directly host-to-host-transmissible diseases of humans and animals. The transmission of these fungi is usually carried out by arthroconidia that have formed in or on infected host tissue. These conidia may be spread by direct skin-to-skin contact or via fomites containing free arthroconidia, shed skin scales, or hairs. Typical fomites include such divergent materials as hats, shoes, shower room floors, bedding, clothing of nursing staff in chronic care institutes, animal bedding/nesting material, and farm fenceposts used by animals for scratching. Tissue invasion is normally cutaneous; dermatophytes are usually unable to penetrate deeper tissues as a result of nonspecific inhibitory factors in serum (23), inhibition of fungal keratinases (24), a barrier formed of epidermal keratinocytes (25), and other immunological barriers (26, 27). In acute cases, there is a strong Th1 reaction mediated in part by CD4+ lymphocytes (28), while in chronic cases, there is an

TABLE 2 Grouping of dermatophytes on the basis of host preference and natural habitat[a]

Anthropophilic	Zoophilic	Geophilic
Epidermophyton floccosum	*Microsporum canis*	*Microsporum gypseum* (*Nannizzia gypsea*) complex
Microsporum audouinii	*M.* (*Lophophyton*) *gallinae*	*M.* (*Nannizzia*) *praecox*
M. ferrugineum	*M. nanum* (*Nannizzia nana*)	
Trichophyton concentricum	*M.* (*Nannizzia*) *persicolor*	*M. vanbreuseghemii* (*L. gallinae*)
T. megninii	*Trichophyton equinum*	*Trichophyton vanbreuseghemii* (*Arthroderma gertleri*)
T. mentagrophytes complex (velvety and cottony isolates)	*T. erinacei*	
T. rubrum	*T. mentagrophytes* complex (granular isolates)	
T. schoenleinii	*T. simii*	
T. soudanense	*T. verrucosum*	
T. tonsurans		
T. violaceum		

[a]Normally nonpathogenic, soil-associated dermatophytoids such as *T. terrestre* and *M. (Paraphyton) cookei* are not included in this table.

immediate hypersensitivity-type reaction characterized by high levels of IgE and IgG4 antibodies and production of Th2 cytokines by mononucleocytes (29).

Dermatophytes tend to grow in an annular fashion on most affected skin regions, producing a "ringworm" infection form with a more or less raised and erythematous active area at the periphery and a relatively scaly inactive zone at the center of established lesions. The organism can often only be isolated from the active, peripheral ring. Infection may range from mild to severe, partly as a consequence of the reaction of the host to the metabolic products of the fungus. Also important in determining the severity of infection are the virulence of the infecting strain, the anatomic location of the infection, the status of the host's immune system, and local environmental factors. Occasionally, especially in immunocompromised patients, subcutaneous tissue may be invaded, e.g., in Majocchi's granuloma, kerion, mycetoma-like processes (30, 31), or more rarely, a generalized systemic infection (32). A *T. rubrum* infection suggestive of cutaneous blastomycosis has been reported in an immunocompromised patient (33), and a fungal culture-negative, chronic ulcerated foot lesion was diagnosed by PCR and DNA sequencing as *T. rubrum* tinea pedis in a chronic granulomatous disease patient (34).

In brief, the principal current risk factors for common forms of dermatophytosis are age (youth for tinea capitis, advanced age for onychomycosis); family history of chronic dermatophytosis; participation in athletics featuring extensive body contact (e.g., wrestling, judo) or foot maceration (e.g., marathon running); barefoot use of communal aquatic facilities (showers, swimming areas); exchange of headgear, footwear, or inadequately cleaned bedding; contact with feral domestic animals (especially street kittens) or animals recently supplied by en masse breeding operations (especially cats, guinea pigs, rabbits, laboratory rats, and cattle); inhabitation of rodent-infested dwellings and, especially for children in developing countries, contact with livestock suffering from untreated dermatophytosis; and contact with barbering instruments that have not been effectively disinfected (20, 27, 35–42).

Anatomic Specificity

Infections caused by dermatophytes are named according to the anatomic location involved, e.g., tinea barbae (beard and moustache), tinea capitis (scalp, eyebrows, and eyelashes), tinea corporis (face, trunk, and major limbs), tinea cruris (groin, perineal, and perianal areas), tinea pedis (soles and toe webs), tinea manuum (palms), and tinea unguium (nails). Different dermatophyte species may produce clinically identical lesions; conversely, a single species may infect many anatomic sites.

Tinea barbae, usually caused by zoophilic fungi, e.g., *Trichophyton verrucosum* and granular, zoophilic forms of the *Trichophyton mentagrophytes* complex, is typically highly inflamed and may present as acute pustular folliculitis that can progress to suppurative boggy lesions (kerion). A less severe form that appears as dry, erythematous, scaly lesions also occurs. Tinea capitis may vary from highly erythematous, patchy, scaly areas with dull gray hair stumps to highly inflamed lesions with folliculitis, kerion formation, alopecia, and scarring. *T. tonsurans* and *M. canis* are the most common agents, depending on the precise geographic location (16, 17). Favus (tinea favosa), usually caused by *Trichophyton schoenleinii* but also potentially caused by *Trichophyton violaceum* or *Microsporum gypseum* (proposed *Nannizzia gypsea* [12]), is a now very rare chronic infection of the scalp and glabrous skin characterized by the formation of cup-shaped crusts (scutula) resembling honeycombs. Tinea corporis, which can be caused by any dermatophyte but is often associated with zoophiles, classically manifests as circular, erythematous lesions with scaly, raised, active, and often vesicular borders. Chronic lesions on the trunk and extremities usually are caused by *T. rubrum*, in particular by Afro-Asiatic forms of this fungus (formerly often called *Trichophyton raubitschekii*). Tinea cruris ("jock itch"), usually caused by *T. rubrum* or *Epidermophyton floccosum*, typically appears as scaly, erythematous to tawny brown, bilateral and asymmetric lesions extending down to the inner thigh and exhibiting a sharply marginated border frequently studded with small vesicles. Tinea pedis varies in appearance: the most common manifestation is maceration, peeling, itching, and painful fissuring between the fourth and fifth toes, but an acute inflammatory condition with vesicles and pustules can also occur, as can a hyperkeratotic chronic infection of the sole ("moccasin foot"). Members of the *T. mentagrophytes* complex frequently cause the more inflammatory type of infections, whereas *T. rubrum* usually causes the more chronic type. Infection of the sole by human-adapted forms of *Trichophyton interdigitale*, one of the members of the *T. mentagrophytes* complex, can be recognized by the formation of bullous vesicles in the thin skin of the plantar arch and along the sides of the feet and heel adjacent to the thick plantar stratum corneum (43). Tinea unguium, or nail infection by dermatophytes, is a subcategory of the more general phenomenon of onychomycosis, fungal nail infection. It is most often caused by *T. rubrum* and usually appears as thickened, deformed, friable, discolored nails with accumulated subungual debris. This type of presentation results from invasion of the underside of the distal nail and is therefore termed "distal-subungual onychomycosis." A less common infection type usually caused by *T. interdigitale* typically manifests, especially in its earlier stages, as "superficial white onychomycosis," i.e., white patches in the superficial portions of the nail. "Proximal-subungual tinea unguium" may also occur. This infection, in which the nail is subungually infected beginning near its point of origin in the area of the lunula, is usually caused by *T. rubrum* and often signals immunosuppression, e.g., AIDS (44).

COLLECTION, TRANSPORT, AND STORAGE OF SPECIMENS

Preliminary Patient Examination

In areas where tinea capitis caused by *M. canis* is common, patients may be examined with a Wood's lamp (filtered UV light with a wavelength of 365 nm) in a darkened room for the presence of bright green fluorescent hairs. These are ideal for collection as laboratory specimens, though in some cases diagnosis may be done by Wood's light alone. The fluorescent hairs, considered "Wood's light positive," typically show a small-arthroconidial, ectothrix type of hair invasion in direct microscopy. Apart from *M. canis*, *M. audouinii* and *Microsporum ferrugineum* also cause this type of fluorescent ectothrix infection. Hairs infected with *T. schoenleinii* may show a dull green color (42). The Wood's lamp can also be used to differentiate between dermatophytosis and nonfungal skin conditions that may be similar clinically, e.g., erythrasma. In erythrasma, the skin fluoresces orange to coral red, whereas in dermatophytosis, the skin is not fluorescent.

Sampling Preparations and Practice

Sufficient clinical material should be collected for both direct microscopic examination and culture. However, if clinical material is limiting in quantity, direct microscopic examination should always be preferred over fungal culture. It is the more sensitive technique (17), and the microscopic detection of fungal elements in dermatology specimens is diagnostic of fungal infection and should be sufficient to elicit antifungal therapy. Whenever feasible, aseptic technique is used to minimize contamination during the collection and transport of specimens, and the following equipment should be available: forceps for epilating hairs, sterile no. 15 scalpel blades or sharp curette, sterile nail clippers, scissors, sterile gauze squares, 70% alcohol for disinfection, sterile water for cleansing painful areas, and clean pill packets or clean paper envelopes to contain and transport the clinical specimens such as hairs, skin scrapings, or nail clippings. Black photographic paper or strong black paper may be used for collecting and better visualizing scrapings. After collection, the paper is folded, tightly taped in the corners, and placed in an envelope for transport. Several commercial transport package systems are available; MycoTrans (Biggar, Lanarkshire, United Kingdom) and Dermapak (Toddington, Bedfordshire, United Kingdom) are two of these. Closed tubes are not recommended for specimens, since they retain moisture, which may result in an overgrowth of bacterial as well as fungal contaminants. Disposable sterilized brushes have been recommended for collection of specimens from the scalp or from the fur of animals (45). Indeed, in the United States, disposable toothbrushes are often used to sample skin, with the bristle portion being pushed into the culture media in several locations after sampling. If histopathological processing is done, the nail plate may be placed in a 4% formaldehyde solution (46). Culture media (detailed below) may be inoculated directly on collection.

Hairs from the scalp should be epilated with sterile forceps. If the specimen is Wood's light positive, epilate only fluorescent hairs. Nonfluorescent hairs, especially those infected with endothrix fungi such as *T. tonsurans*, may need to be dug out with the tip of a sterile scalpel blade because the hairs often break off at scalp level and are thus difficult to grasp with a forceps. Rubbing with a sterile moistened swab has been successful with pediatric patients (47). In the rare event that favus is seen, the scutulum at the mouth of the hair follicle is suitable for culture and microscopic examination. In lower body dermatophytoses, lesions with defined borders should be preliminarily disinfected with alcohol or cleansed with sterile water, and then active border areas should be scraped with a scalpel (or toothbrush; see above) to collect epidermal scales. Where borders are not visible to indicate the area of maximal fungal activity, as in tinea manuum, the preliminarily cleansed infected area can be broadly scraped to obtain specimen from a variety of areas that may imperceptibly differ in current fungal activity. In vesicular tinea pedis, the tops of the vesicles can be removed with sterile scissors for direct examination and culture. Culture of the vesicle fluid is not recommended.

Nails should be disinfected with alcohol gauze squares. The most desirable material for culture in typical subungual onychomycosis is the waxy subungual debris, which contains the fungal elements. The highest proportion of viable elements for culturing is often found close to the juncture of the nail bed. To remove contaminating saprobic fungi and bacteria, the crumbly debris directly underneath the nail near the tips is removed with the scalpel before material is collected for culture. Some investigators will clip the nail short first and perform this scraping-away of contaminated material on the clipping. If the dorsal nail plate is diseased (superficial white onychomycosis), scrape and discard the outer surface before removing the underlying material for culture. In rare cases with a presentation consistent with *Trichophyton soudanense* endonyx nail infection (48), in which the internal strata of the nail plate are milky white but the upper and lower nail surfaces appear relatively unaffected, clippings may be taken or the milky area may be exposed and scraped.

Any specimen needing to be transported, or for any other reason not processed immediately, should be retained in the paper packets described above. Closed tubes are not recommended for specimens since they may retain moisture and may result in an overgrowth of contaminants. Dermatophytes in dry specimens of skin, hair, and nails may be stored for years in viable condition, provided the material is not subjected to temperature extremes.

LABORATORY TESTING OF SPECIMENS

Direct Microscopic Examination

Direct microscopic examination of skin, hair, and nails is the most rapid method of determining fungal etiology and is traditionally accomplished by examining the clinical material in 10% potassium hydroxide (KOH) (freely interchangeable with the cheaper sodium hydroxide [NaOH]) (49, 50). Another common procedure is to use 25% potassium or sodium hydroxide mixed with 5% glycerin to impede desiccation (49). Addition of fluorescent brighteners such as calcofluor white (Sigma-Aldrich, St. Louis, MO) or Blankophor (Blankophor GmbH, Ankum, Germany) significantly increases accuracy, especially where staff is not highly experienced in visual detection of fungal elements (51, 52). In nails, histopathology based on staining nail biopsy material with periodic acid-Schiff stain has been shown to have potential for generating results more accurate than those afforded by hydroxide-based direct microscopy (53). The suggestion, however, that biopsy/periodic acid-Schiff can also replace culturing (53) is unsound, in that this technique does not permit reliable distinction of dermatophytes from other nail-invading species (54).

Nail clippings should be aseptically cut into smaller fragments and, where possible, either pounded with a heavy object inside their collection packet or scraped with a sterile scalpel blade to release friable, flaky material containing the greatest amount of dermatophyte inoculum. Skin or nail scrapings, nail fragments, or hair roots are placed in 1 or 2 drops of one of the above-mentioned KOH or NaOH solutions on a clean glass slide. A coverslip is placed on top, and the preparation is heated gently (short of boiling) by being passed rapidly over a Bunsen burner or other heat source three or four times and then allowed to sit at room temperature for a few minutes for clearing. The exact time needed depends on the concentration of hydroxide used, the thickness of specimen fragments, and the exact amount of heat imparted by contact with the flame. A slide warmer set at 51 to 54°C may also be used to heat the slides for 1 h (49). Alternatively, samples may be incubated with alkali in closed sterile microtubes at room temperature for 1 to 2 h, prior to addition of fluorescent enhancer. Clearing is evident to the naked eye as a pronounced decrease in the opacity of the scraping. Laboratories using 10% KOH or NaOH solution for skin may find that nail scrapings require a stronger alkali solution (up to 25% KOH or NaOH). Demonstration of fungal elements may be facilitated by the use of glucan-binding fluorescent brighteners such as calcofluor white (50) or Congo red (49). These require a fluorescent microscope set up to visualize the specific fluorescence obtained. Calcofluor white is added directly to the

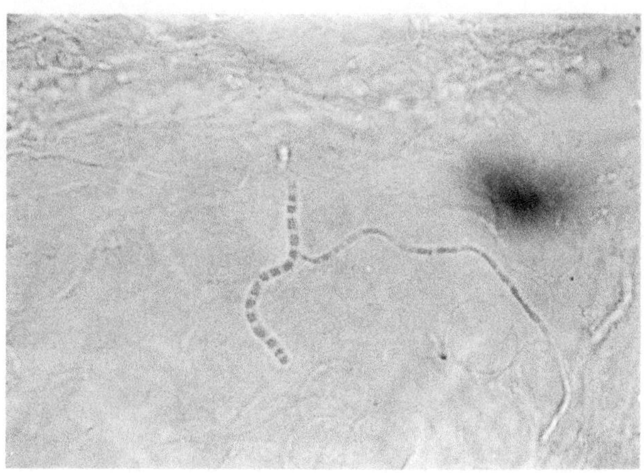

FIGURE 1 Dermatophyte hyphae in skin scraping. NaOH mount. Magnification, ×400.

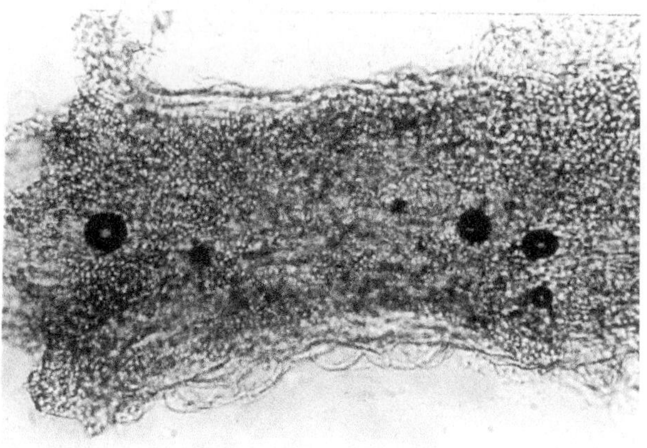

FIGURE 2 *Microsporum audouinii*, ectothrix type of hair invasion. Magnification, ×400.

KOH drop on the slide as an approximately equal drop of 0.1% solution (55). All preparations should be examined under low power and confirmed under high power.

Skin and nails infected by dermatophytes may reveal one or more of the following: hyaline hyphal fragments; septate, often branched hyphae; and chains of arthroconidia (Fig. 1). The appearance of infected hairs depends on the invading dermatophyte species. Hyphae invade the hairs, and arthroconidia are formed by fragmentation of these hyphae. The appearance and locations of the arthroconidia may suggest the infecting genera or species (Table 3), as may the sizes (42). Three main types of colonization (ectothrix, endothrix, and favic) are observed by direct microscopic examination. The terms "ectothrix" and "endothrix" refer to the location of the arthroconidia in relation to the hair shaft (ecto- and endo- meaning outside and inside, respectively), while "favic" refers to the distinctive infection caused by *T. schoenleinii*, a fungus that is now extremely rare except in some parts of central Asia and the African Sahel.

In ectothrix colonization, arthroconidia appear as a mosaic sheath around the hair or as chains on the surface of the hair shaft (Fig. 2). In *M. canis*, *M. audouinii*, and *M. ferrugineum* infections, colonized hairs fluoresce green under the Wood's lamp; other ectothrix infections (Table 3) are nonfluorescent. Endothrix hair invasion is observed as chains of arthroconidia filling the insides of shortened hair stubs (Fig. 3); hairs are Wood's lamp negative. In favic hairs, hyphae, air bubbles, or tunnels and fat droplets are observed within the hair (Fig. 4). These hairs are dull green under the Wood's lamp. In general, infected hairs from all infection types show hyphae within the hair shaft at some time during the course of infection, usually during the early stages.

TABLE 3 Hair invasion by dermatophytes on the human host

Ectothrix	Endothrix	Favic
Microsporum audouinii	*Trichophyton soudanense*	*Trichophyton schoenleinii*
M. canis	*T. tonsurans*	
M. ferrugineum	*T. violaceum*	
M. gypseum (*Nannizzia gypsea*) complex		
M. (*Nannizzia*) *praecox*		
T. megninii		
T. mentagrophytes complex		
T. verrucosum		

Isolation Procedures

Scrapings, hairs, and other materials collected as outlined above for direct examination are plated on selected isolation media and incubated at 32°C for optimal growth; temperatures between 24 and 32°C are also acceptable if the total incubation time is suitably adjusted to compensate for the slower outgrowth expected at lower temperatures. Generally from 5 to 15 skin or nail fragments are planted per plate or tube used for isolation, and these fragments are separated so that antibiotic-resistant mould or bacterial contaminants from one piece cannot overgrow the others. Hairs are also well separated. Cultures on primary isolation medium are routinely incubated at 25 to 30°C and examined weekly for up to 4 weeks.

The most common medium used for the isolation of dermatophytes is Sabouraud glucose agar (SGA) (original formulation with 4% glucose or Emmons' modification with 2% glucose), amended with chloramphenicol and cycloheximide to inhibit bacterial and saprobic fungal contamination. This type of medium is available commercially as, for example, Mycobiotic agar (Acumedia Manufacturers, Lansing, MI; Remel, Lenexa, KS; Delasco, Council Bluffs, IA), Mycosel (BD Diagnostic Systems, Sparks, MD), or

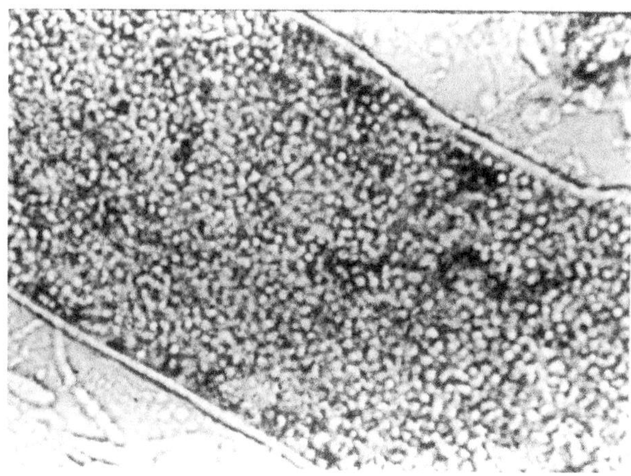

FIGURE 3 *Trichophyton tonsurans*, endothrix type of hair invasion. Magnification, ×1,000.

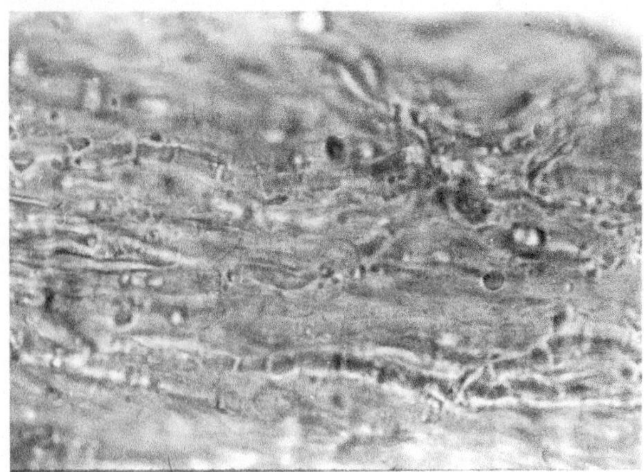

FIGURE 4 Hair infected by *Trichophyton schoenleinii* from a patient with favus. Magnification, ×1,000.

Dermasel Selective Supplement (Oxoid, Basingstoke, Hampshire, United Kingdom; note that Remel is currently the U.S. distributor for Oxoid). An alternative medium promoting more rapid conidiation and colony pigmentation development is potato flake agar amended with cycloheximide and chloramphenicol (Hardy Diagnostics, Santa Maria, CA). For the isolation of cycloheximide-susceptible fungi that cause clinical infections resembling dermatophytosis, any type of SGA with chloramphenicol (Remel, BD), inhibitory mould agar (BD, Remel, Hardy), or Littman oxgall agar (BD) is recommended (50). Inhibitory mould agar and Littman oxgall agar have the advantage of restricting contaminant colony diameters. For all media, the addition of gentamicin is recommended for specimens heavily contaminated by bacteria (56). SGA with cycloheximide, chloramphenicol, and gentamicin is routinely used as an isolation medium in some laboratories (49).

Additional and alternative media may be used in special circumstances. For example, vitamin-free casamino acids (BD)-erythritol-albumin agar medium plus cycloheximide, chloramphenicol, and gentamicin may be used for filament-positive skin and nail specimens, especially from body sites where *Candida* overgrowth may be a problem (e.g., groin, fingernails). This medium (currently not commercially available to our knowledge) prevents the common suppression of dermatophyte outgrowth by heavy inoculum of *Candida albicans*, *Candida parapsilosis*, and related biotin-requiring yeasts (57). Dermatophyte species with vitamin requirements (very uncommon in these types of cases) may grow poorly on it, and it is always used in combination with a cycloheximide-containing SGA.

Another primary isolation medium that may be used is dermatophyte test medium (DTM; available commercially from BD, Hardy, and Remel, among others [see chapter 118]). This selective medium screens for the presence of dermatophytes in heavily contaminated material (nails, etc.). The growth of dermatophytes causes a rise in pH, thus changing the phenol red indicator from yellow to red (58). The use of DTM should be combined with morphological study, since dermatophytoids (soilborne species that are usually nonpathogenic and thus are best not called dermatophytes) such as the *Trichophyton terrestre* complex (*Arthroderma insingulare*, *Arthroderma lenticulare*, *Arthroderma quadrifidum*), as well as various *Chrysosporium* species and other nondermatophytic fungi, can grow and turn the medium red (49, 59, 60). Rapid sporulation medium, mentioned above for potato flake agar, contains a pH indicator that works on a similar principle but turns from yellow to blue-green, leaving the red reverse pigment of typical *T. rubrum* visible (61). DTM may uncommonly give false-negative results with some *Microsporum* isolates (62).

Nucleic Acid-Based Direct Detection Techniques

Numerous techniques have been published for directly detecting dermatophyte DNA in tissue, but as yet none is established as a routine diagnostic procedure. This is mainly due to the relatively low cost of traditional procedures. However, in terms of accuracy, traditional procedures are by no means optimal; in onychomycosis, for example, they disclose at best ~85% of true-positive cases from the initial patient specimen, and this percentage is much lower in many laboratories (54). This has created a strong incentive for the development of molecular detection techniques. At present, a large number of primary studies related to rapid PCR of dermatological specimens for dermatophytosis and related mycoses (e.g., nondermatophyte filamentous fungal onychomycosis) have been published. Techniques employed include PCR-enzyme-linked immunosorbent assay (63), PCR-reverse line blot (64), PCR coupled with restriction fragment length polymorphism study (65), multiplex PCR (66), nested PCR (67), PCR based in part on a microsatellite locus permitting strain typing of *T. rubrum* (68), and direct PCR with sequencing (48). Also, related techniques such as real-time PCR (69–71) have been shown to work well in trial studies but need to prove themselves as consistently practical and cost-effective in interlaboratory studies related to routine diagnosis. Many of these techniques have been extensively discussed in the excellent review by Jensen and Arendrup (72). In unusual situations, molecular direct detection methods may be invaluable: for example, in a deep dermatophytosis case where all conventional tests had given negative results, *T. rubrum* was identified by means of a nested PCR study directed to amplifying a portion of the internal transcribed spacer (ITS) region from paraffin-embedded sections (73), and real-time PCR and sequencing unambiguously identified *T. rubrum* from biopsy samples in a culture-negative case of tinea pedis in a chronic granulomatous disease patient (34).

IDENTIFICATION

At present, the great majority of dermatophytes are identified phenotypically. Identification is often based on (i) colony characteristics in pure culture on SGA and (ii) microscopic morphology. These criteria alone, however, may be insufficient, since colonial appearance may vary or be similar for different species. Characteristic pigmentation may fail to appear, and isolates, especially *Trichophyton* species, may not sporulate. Special media may be required to stimulate pigment production; it may be necessary to use sporulation and physiologic tests in conjunction with morphology to identify the species correctly. The majority of isolates are easily identified when visual examination is combined with any needed testing for characteristic growth factor requirements; as a consequence, phenotypic studies remain the least expensive option for routine identification. However, although seldom practically applicable except in high-level reference laboratories, molecular identification strategies involving PCR amplification and sequencing of ITS regions (currently the "gold standard" for mould identification [75]) identify unusual isolates that are misbehaving phenotypically. Moreover, several recent studies have demonstrated that rapid and robust identification of most common dermatophytes is possible by matrix-assisted laser desorption ionization–time-of-flight mass spectrometry (MALDI-TOF). Indeed, MALDI-TOF identifications correlated much more closely with the results of ITS sequencing than with identifications based on conventional phenotypic approaches (13, 74).

Colony Characteristics

In observing gross colony morphology, note the color of the surface and the reverse of the colony, the texture of the surface (powdery, granular, woolly, cottony, velvety, or glabrous), the topography (elevation, folding, margins, etc.), and the rate of growth.

Microscopic Morphology

Microscopic morphology, especially the appearance and arrangement of the conidia (macroconidia or microconidia) and other structures, may be determined by teased mounts, sticky tape mounts, or slide culture preparations mounted in lactophenol cotton blue, in lactophenol aniline blue (phenol, an ingredient of lactophenol cotton blue and lactophenol aniline blue, is listed as a hazardous chemical; therefore, solutions containing phenol should be prepared, stored, and used in an approved chemical safety cabinet), in lacto-fuchsin (49), or in more permanent mounting fluids (75). Sometimes a special medium such as cornmeal or cornmeal-glucose agar, potato-glucose agar, SGA plus 3 to 5% NaCl (76, 77), pablum cereal agar (49), rapid sporulation medium (61), or lactrimel agar (78, 79) (see chapter 118) may be required to stimulate sporulation.

Physiological Tests

In Vitro Hair Perforation Test

The *in vitro* hair perforation test distinguishes between atypical isolates of the *T. mentagrophytes* complex and *T. rubrum* (80). It may also be used to assist in making other distinctions such as *M. canis* versus *M. audouinii* and *Microsporum (Nannizzia) praecox* versus *M. gypseum (N. gypsea)* (81). Hairs exposed to *T. mentagrophytes* complex members, *M. canis*, and *M. gypseum* show wedge-shaped perforations perpendicular to the hair shaft (a positive test result), whereas *T. rubrum*, *M. audouinii*, and *M. (N.) praecox* do not form these perforating structures.

Place short strands of human hair (ideally hair from a child under 18 months old) in petri dishes, and autoclave the dishes at 121°C for 10 min; add 25 ml of sterile distilled water and 2 or 3 drops of 10% sterilized yeast extract. Inoculate these plates with several fragments of the test fungus that has been grown on SGA; incubate the plates at 25°C, and examine them at regular intervals over a period of 21 days. Hairs may be examined microscopically for perforations by removing a few segments and placing them in a drop of lactophenol cotton blue mounting fluid. Gently heating the mounts aids in the detection of the fungus. A positive control test should always be run with a known perforating species; *M. canis* is recommended. Some hair samples may prove unsuitable for unknown reasons, e.g., possible prior contact with shampoos containing antifungal inhibitors.

Special Nutritional Requirements

Nutritional tests aid in the routine identification of *Trichophyton* species that seldom produce conidia or that resemble each other morphologically (82). Certain species have distinctive nutritional requirements, whereas others do not. The method employs a Casamino Acid basal medium that is vitamin free (*Trichophyton* agar 1 [T1]) and to which various vitamins are added, e.g., inositol (T2), thiamine plus inositol (T3), thiamine (T4), and nicotinic acid (T5). In addition, the series includes an ammonium nitrate basal medium (T6) to which histidine is added (T7). These media are available commercially in dehydrated form from BD Biosciences and in prepared form from Remel. A small fragment (about the size of the head of a pin) from the culture to be tested is placed on the surface of the basal medium (controls) and the media containing the vitamin and amino acid additives. Care must be taken to avoid transferring agar from the fungal inoculum to the nutritional media. Cultures are incubated at room temperature (or 37°C if *T. verrucosum* is suspected) and read after 7 and 14 days. The amount of growth is graded from 0 to 4+. Commonly observed reactions are summarized in Table 4.

TABLE 4 Dermatophyte nutritional response as elucidated by *Trichophyton* agars[a]

Species	Response by vitamin tests					Response by amino acid tests	
	1 Vitamin free	2 Inositol	3 Thiamine + inositol	4 Thiamine	5 Nicotinic acid	6 Aminoacid free	7 Histidine
Microsporum (Lophophyton) gallinae[b]						4	4
Trichophyton concentricum, 50%	4	4	4	4	4		
T. concentricum, 50%	2	2	4	4	2		
T. equinum var. *equinum*	0	0	0	0	4		
T. equinum var. *autotrophicum*	4	4	4	4	4		
T. megninii						0	4
T. soudanense	v	v	v	v	v	v	v
T. tonsurans	1	1	4	4	1		
T. verrucosum, 84%	1	2	4	2	1		
T. verrucosum, 16%	1	1	4	4	1		
T. violaceum (typical)	1	1	4	4	1		
T. violaceum (rare "*T. yaoundei*" form)	4	4	4	4	4		

[a]Only the growth responses for organisms with growth factor requirements and the selected organisms that must be most closely compared with them are included in this table. The numbers in the table body indicate the relative degree of growth according to traditional 1+ to 4+ visually approximated scale: 0, no growth; 1, slight growth, strongly nutrient-deprived colony morphology (very sparse, subsurface colonial growth only or colony diameter strongly reduced compared to Sabouraud agar control); 2, partially stimulated growth, but still significantly suppressed compared to that of the control; 4, growth comparable to that of the control (the table includes no 3+ reactions); v, variable.

[b]Blank spaces in the chart indicate growth responses that are not customarily examined but that are insignificantly different from control growth responses on Sabouraud agar.

Urea Hydrolysis

The ability to hydrolyze urea provides additional data to aid in distinguishing the typical, cosmopolitan form of *T. rubrum* (urease negative) from members of the *T. mentagrophytes* complex (typically urease positive) and from the urease-positive Afro-Asiatic or "granular" form of *T. rubrum*, formerly often called *T. raubitschekii* (83, 84). Christensen urea agar and broth may both be used; the broth appears to be the more sensitive of these alternatives (85). After the urea medium is inoculated, it is incubated at 25 to 30°C for up to 7 days. The tubes should be examined every 2 to 3 days for the color change from orange or pale pink to purple-red that indicates the presence of urease, a positive test result. Negative and positive controls should always be done on new batches of these media. See Table 1.

Growth on BCP-Milk Solids-Glucose Medium (BCPMSG)

This medium is available commercially as Dermatophyte Milk Agar (Hardy). Type of growth (profuse versus restricted) and a change in the pH indicator (BCP) indicating alkalinity are especially useful for distinguishing *T. rubrum* from the *T. mentagrophytes* complex, and *T. mentagrophytes* from *Microsporum* (*Nannizzia*) *persicolor* (49, 77, 86). *T. rubrum* shows restricted growth and produces no alkaline reaction on BCPMSG, whereas members of the *T. mentagrophytes* complex typically show profuse growth and an alkaline reaction. Although *M. persicolor* shows profuse growth, it does not result in an alkaline reaction. Other tests for distinguishing *T. mentagrophytes* and allies from *M.* (*N.*) *persicolor* are described elsewhere (87).

Cultures to be tested are inoculated onto slants of BCPMSG and examined for pH change and growth characteristics at the end of a 7-day incubation at 25°C. A color change from pale blue to violet purple indicates an alkaline reaction.

Growth on Polished Rice Grains

Unlike most dermatophytes, *M. audouinii* grows poorly on rice grains and produces a brownish discoloration of the rice (49, 87). This is a useful test for differentiating this species from *M. canis* and from other dermatophytes that typically grow and sporulate on rice grains. It may be especially useful in areas where *M. audouinii* is still endemic, e.g., sub-Saharan Africa, or where immigrants or travelers from such areas are reintroducing it.

The medium is prepared in 12-ml flasks by mixing 1 part raw unfortified rice grains and 3 parts water (88) or 8.0 g of rice grains and 125 ml of distilled water. Autoclave at 15 lb/in^2 for 15 min. Inoculate the surface of the rice, and incubate the sample for 2 weeks at 25 to 30°C.

Temperature Tolerance and Temperature Enhancement

Tests for temperature tolerance and enhancement are useful for distinguishing the *T. mentagrophytes* complex from *T. terrestre* complex (*A. insingulare*, *A. lenticulare*, *A. quadrifidum*) (89), *T. mentagrophytes* from *M.* (*N.*) *persicolor* (77), *T. verrucosum* from *T. schoenleinii* (42), and *T. soudanense* from *M. ferrugineum* (90). At 37°C, members of the *T. mentagrophytes* complex show good growth, whereas *T. terrestre* complex isolates do not grow, and *M.* (*N.*) *persicolor* generally grows poorly or not at all (a single atypical isolate with good growth has been observed); growth of *T. verrucosum* and *T. soudanense* is enhanced, but that of *T. schoenleinii* and *M. ferrugineum* is not.

Inoculate two slants of SGA with an equivalent fragment of the culture. Incubate one slant at room temperature (25 to 30°C) and one at 37°C. Compare the growth at the two temperatures when mature colonies appear at room temperature. Appropriate controls are recommended and should be compared first.

Molecular Identification Techniques

The recommendation of standard DNA barcodes (91) is in progress, with the ITS region 1 (ITS1) emerging as a key panfungal region for the molecular identification of moulds, including dermatophytes (92, 93). However, although PCR amplification and sequencing of ITS1 has proven efficacy for dermatophyte identification (93), several caveats remain. First, caution is required when comparing the sequences obtained with those in public synchronized databases, which are strewn with erroneously identified fungi. Second, relatively few conserved nucleotide positions separate the different *Trichophyton* species, principally due to the relatively slow evolution rate of the nuclear ribosomal repeat region. Many other nucleic-acid-based identification techniques for dermatophytes were published in previous years but have not been widely adopted to date. Some recent contenders for rapid, state-of-the-art species identification include PCR using a $(GACA)_4$ primer (94) and restriction fragment length polymorphism of the ITS 2 gene region (95).

DESCRIPTION OF ETIOLOGIC AGENTS

Characteristic features of dermatophyte species are presented in Table 1. The table also includes data on some similar but rarely or never pathogenic *Microsporum and Trichophyton* species that must be distinguished from pathogenic species.

Two types of conidia may be produced on the aerial mycelium of the dermatophytes: large multicellular, smooth or rough, thin- or thick-walled macroconidia and smaller unicellular, smooth-walled microconidia. The three genera are classically grouped according to the presence or absence of these two types of conidia and the appearance of the surface of the macroconidia, i.e., rough versus smooth. In reality, when atypical isolates and species are taken into account, the genera show considerable overlap in morphology (96). For this reason, it is often more convenient to identify isolates directly at the species level than it is to try to identify them at the genus level first. Identification of species is based on the microscopic appearance and arrangement of the conidia (Fig. 5 through 17), colonial morphology on SGA (Fig. 18), and physiological tests (Table 5).

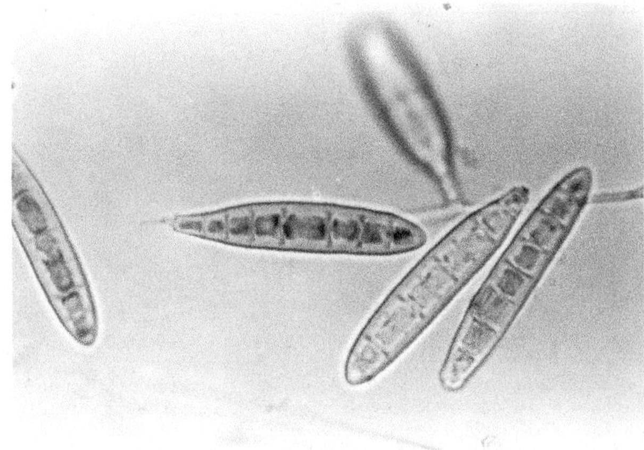

FIGURE 5 Smooth-walled macroconidia of *Trichophyton ajelloi* (*Arthroderma uncinatum*). Magnification, ×400.

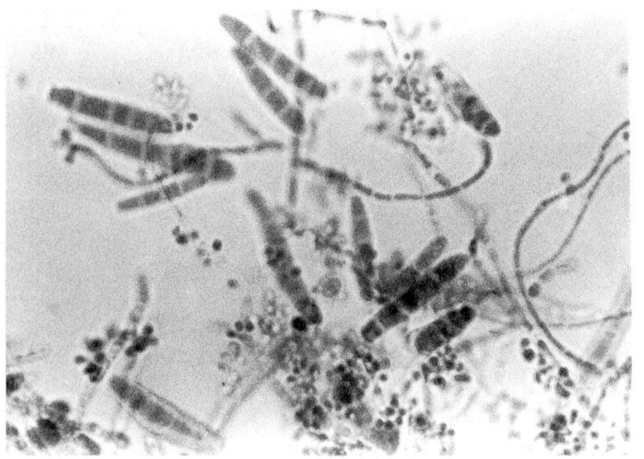

FIGURE 6 Macroconidia and microconidia of *Trichophyton mentagrophytes* complex on SGA with 5% NaCl. Magnification, ×400.

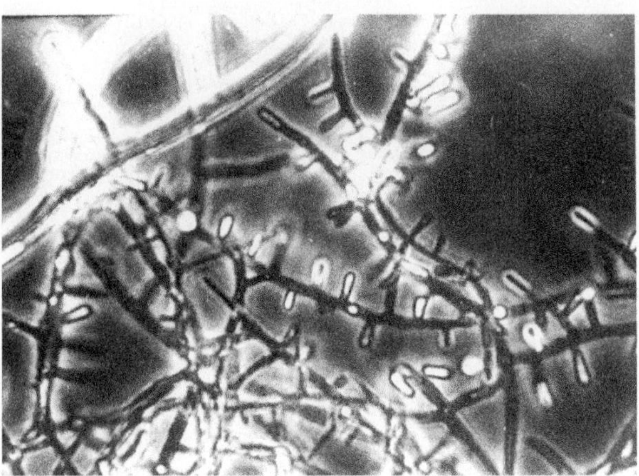

FIGURE 9 Clavate macroconidium, microconidia, and intermediate conidia of *Trichophyton terrestre*. Phase contrast; magnification, ×400.

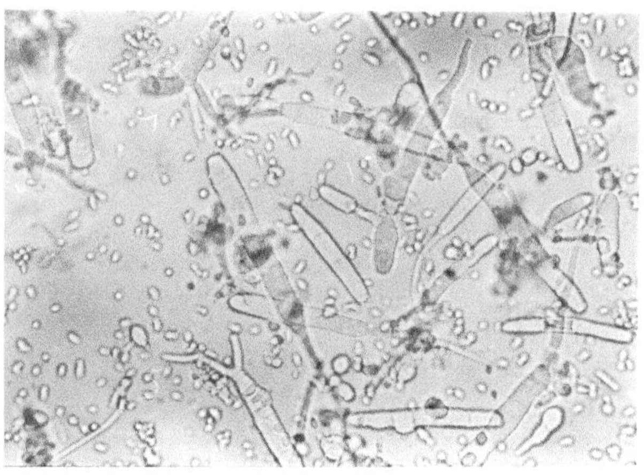

FIGURE 7 Smooth-walled macroconidia of Afro-Asiatic type *Trichophyton rubrum* (*Trichophyton raubitschekii*) from primary isolate on SGA. Magnification, ×1,000.

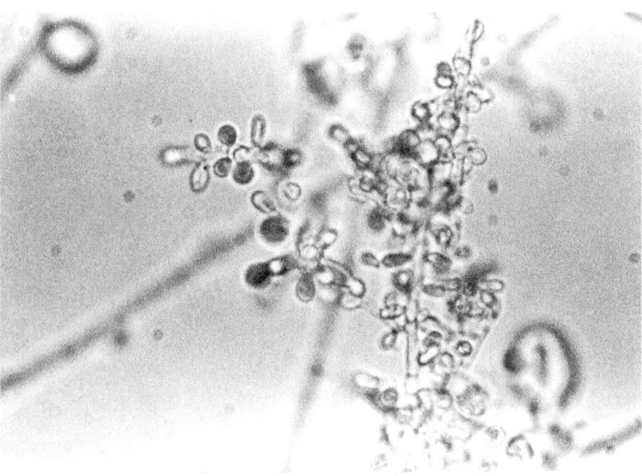

FIGURE 10 Microconidia with typical refractile cytoplasm of *Trichophyton tonsurans*. Magnification, ×400.

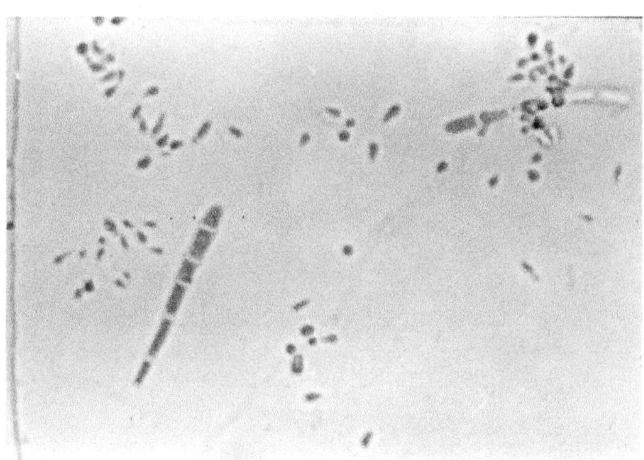

FIGURE 8 Long, narrow macroconidium and clavate to pyriform microconidia of *Trichophyton rubrum*. Magnification, ×400.

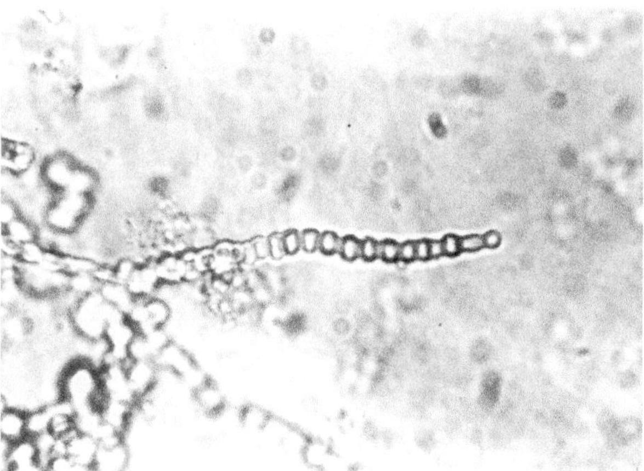

FIGURE 11 Characteristic chlamydospores produced by *Trichophyton verrucosum* or BCP-milk solids-yeast extract agar. Magnification, ×400.

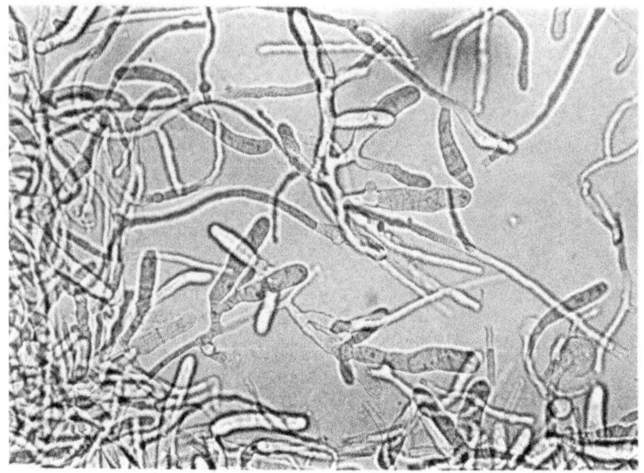

FIGURE 12 Macroconidia of *Epidermophyton floccosum* on SGA. Note the absence of microconidia. Magnification, ×400.

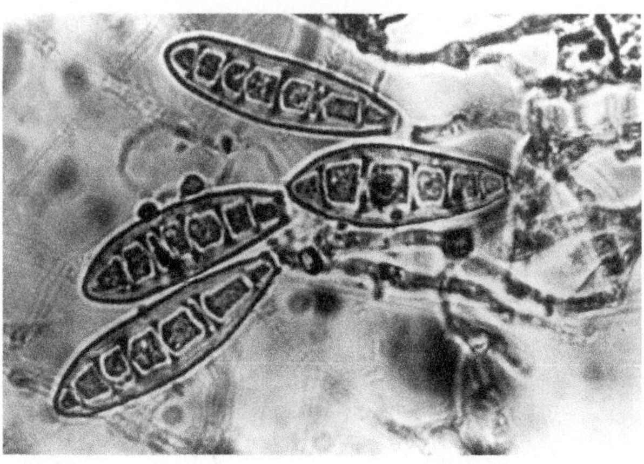

FIGURE 15 Macroconidia of *Microsporum* (*Paraphyton*) *cookei*, showing thick walls and pseudosepta. Magnification, ×400.

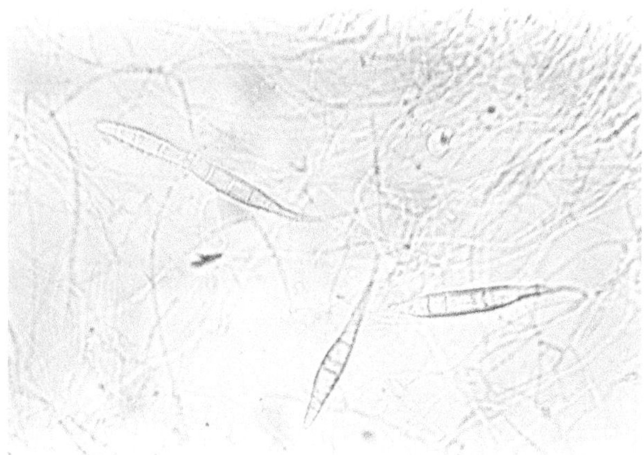

FIGURE 13 Macroconidia of *Microsporum audouinii* on SGA with 3% NaCl. Magnification, ×400.

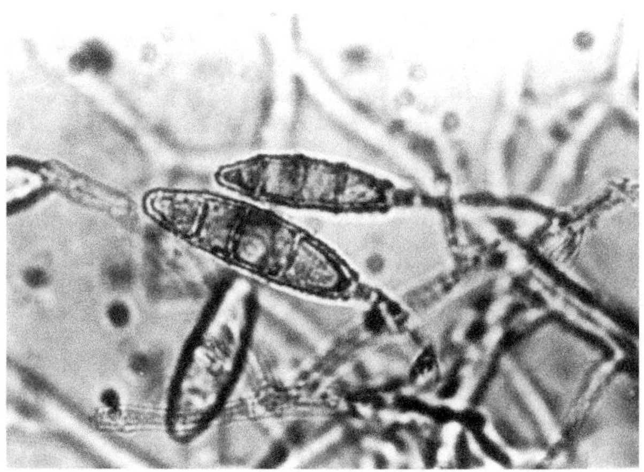

FIGURE 16 Macroconidia of *Microsporum gypseum* (*Nannizzia gypsea*). Magnification, ×400.

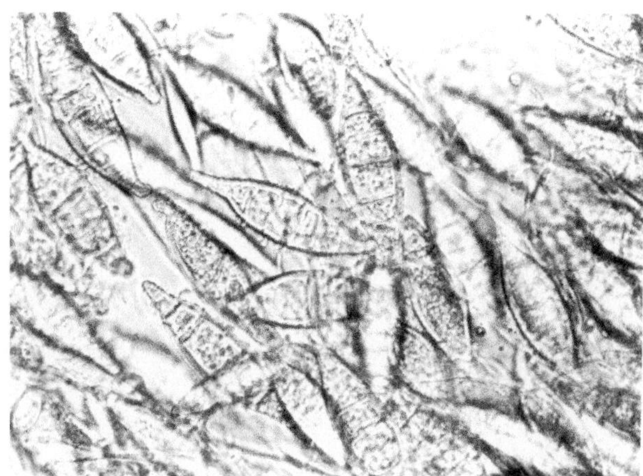

FIGURE 14 Macroconidia of *Microsporum canis* with rough thick walls. Magnification, ×400.

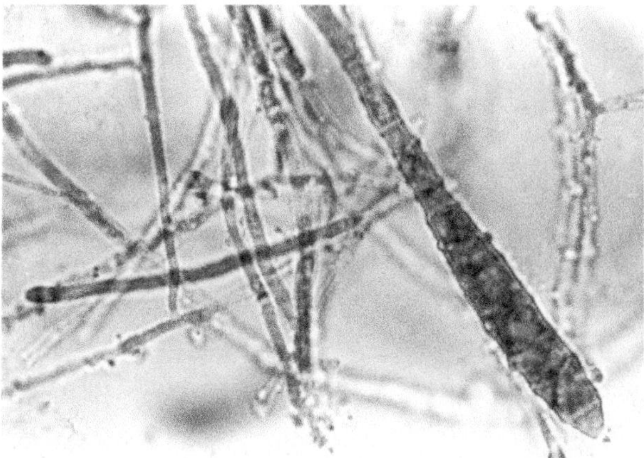

FIGURE 17 Rough-walled macroconidium of *Microsporum* (*Nannizzia*) *persicolor* on SGA with 3% NaCl. Magnification, ×1,000.

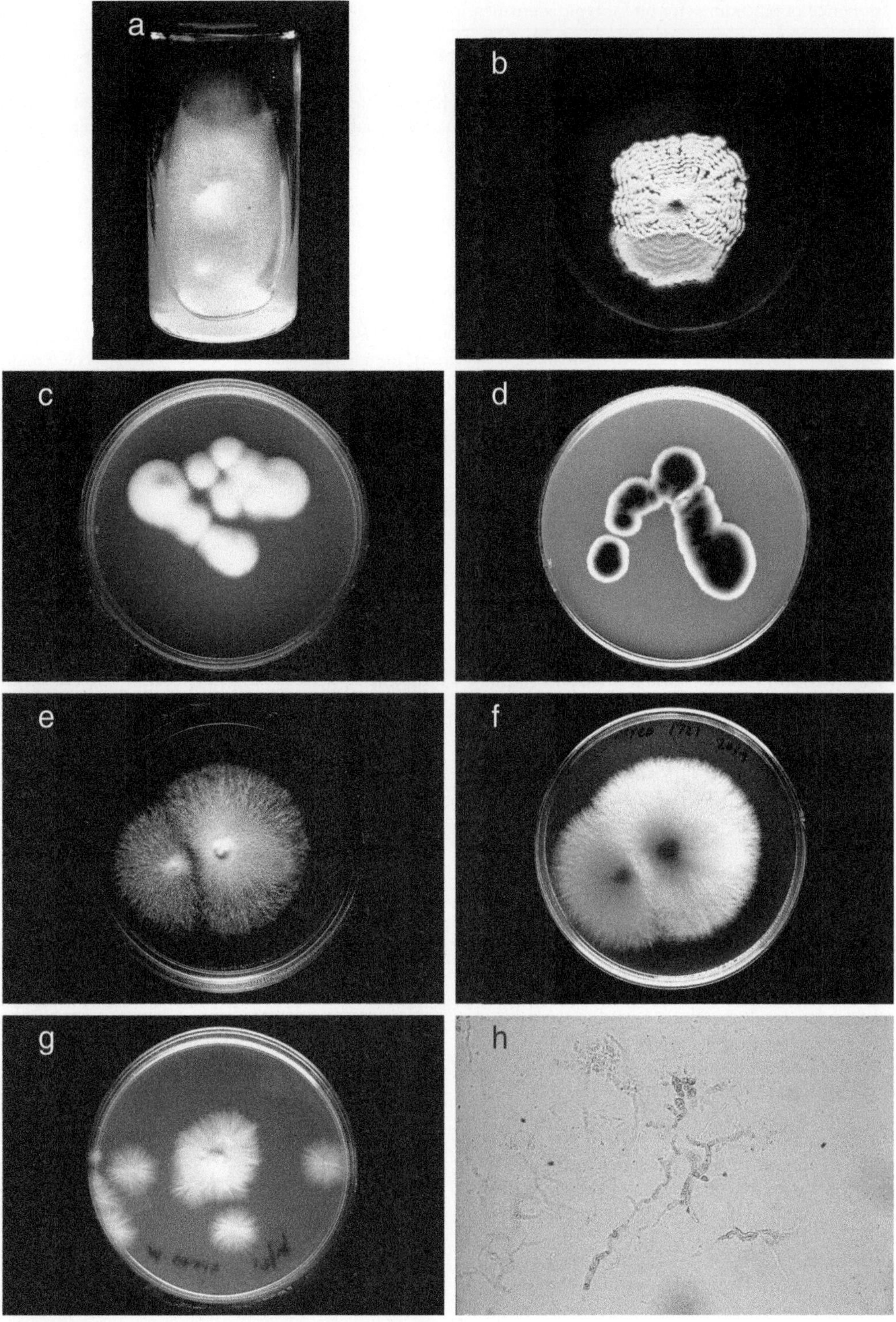

FIGURE 18 (a) *Trichophyton mentagrophytes* complex: "nodular" variant of *Trichophyton interdigitale* (formerly *Trichophyton krajdenii*), SGA, 12 days, showing typical bright yellow pigmentation. (b) *T. mentagrophytes* complex: granular, zoophilic type *T. interdigitale* (mating tester strain of *Arthroderma vanbreuseghemii*), 14 days. (c) *Trichophyton rubrum*, SGA, 10 days, surface showing cottony white mycelium. (d) *T. rubrum*, SGA, 10 days, reverse showing typical red pigment. (e) *T. tonsurans*, SGA, 14 days, surface showing low velvety texture, mixed white and brownish mycelium. (f) *T. tonsurans*, SGA, 14 days, reverse showing mixture of mahogany red-brown and sulfur yellow coloration. (g) *Microsporum canis*, SGA, 10 days, relatively flat colony showing pale striate margin and yellowish pigment near colony center. (h) Brown filaments of *Hortaea werneckii* in NaOH mount of scraping from tinea nigra. Magnification, ×400.

TABLE 5 Sequence of procedures for phenotypic identification of dermatophytes in pure culture[a]

1. Examine colony at day 7 and, if necessary, day 14 for colors of surface and reverse, topography, texture, and rate of growth. Proceed to step 2.
2. Prepare tease mounts and search for identifying microscopic morphology, especially presence, appearance, and arrangement of macroconidia and microconidia (consult Fig. 5 to 18 and Table 1). If the results are inconclusive, proceed to step 3.
3. Prepare slide cultures or transparent tape mounts and examine for characteristic morphology as indicated above if tease mounts do not provide sufficient information. Consider special media if sporulation is absent (potato glucose agar, lactrimel, BCPMSG, SGA with 3 to 5% NaCl). At the same time, proceed to step 4.
4. Perform as many of the following physiologic and other special tests as necessary for identification.
   a. Urease (ensure culture is bacteria-free!)
   b. Nutritional requirements if a *Trichophyton* sp. is suspected
   c. Growth on rice grains if an unusual *Microsporum* sp. is suspected
   d. Elevated temperature response (37° on SGA or, if *T. verrucosum* is suspected, BCPMSG)
   e. Special differentiation media: e.g., BCPMSG to distinguish *T. mentagrophytes* complex from *T. rubrum* and M. (*Nannizzia*) *persicolor*; Lowenstein-Jensen or BCPMSG to distinguish *T. soudanense* from *M. ferrugineum*; SGA + 3 to 5% NaCl to distinguish *T. mentagrophytes* complex from *M.* (*N.*) *persicolor* and atypical *T. rubrum*; DTM to distinguish nonsporulating dermatophytes from most other nonsporulating hyaline fungi
   f. *In vitro* hair perforation test
   g. Molecular or mating studies (to be performed in reference laboratories)

[a]It may be necessary to incubate cultures on brain heart infusion agar or BCPMSG to ensure the absence of antibiotic-resistant bacterial contamination before proceeding to step 4. Procedures are adapted from Weitzman and colleagues (19) and Kane et al. (49).

Existing Genera

Trichophyton Species

Macroconidia have smooth, thin to thick walls, are variable in shape (clavate, fusiform to cylindrical), vary in number of septa (1 to 12) and in size (8 to 86 by 4 to 14 μm), and are borne singly or in clusters. Microconidia, which are usually present and more numerous than macroconidia, may be globose, pyriform, or clavate and are borne singly along the sides of hyphae or in grapelike clusters. Though species in this genus generally produce microconidia more readily than macroconidia, two lineages producing macroconidia predominantly or exclusively have been described: (i) "*Trichophyton kanei*" (97), now known to be a variant of the Afro-Asiatic genotype of *T. rubrum*, and (ii) a variant all-macroconidial form of *T. tonsurans* (96). Fresh isolates of the dermatophytoid *T. ajelloi* may also produce many macroconidia and few or no microconidia. Some species such as *T. schoenleinii* rarely produce conidia of any kind in culture, and nonsporulating isolates of normally conidial species, especially *T. rubrum*, may also be frequently encountered, especially in primary cultures.

Microsporum Species

Microsporum species produce macroconidia and microconidia that may be rare or numerous, depending on the species and the substrate. The distinguishing characteristic is the macroconidium, which is typically rough walled (varying from minutely to conspicuously roughened). Macroconidia also vary in shape (obovate, fusiform to cylindrofusiform), number of septa (1 to 15), size (6 to 160 by 6 to 25 μm), and width of the cell wall. Microconidia are pyriform or clavate and usually are arranged singly along the sides of the hyphae. *Microsporum* species invade skin, hair, and rarely, nails. Under recent taxonomic proposals (12), only three species will be retained in *Microsporum*: *M. canis*, *M. audounii*, and *M. ferrugineaum*. Biological (teleomorphic) species within the *M. gypseum* complex, which are now encompassed in *Nannizzia* (12), can be provisionally recognized on the basis of colonial and microscopic features on Takashio's medium (98), but these species are best distinguished by mating or molecular testing.

E. floccosum

In *E. floccosum*, microconidia are lacking; only smooth-walled, broadly clavate macroconidia are produced, often with an abundance of intercalary and terminal chlamydospores in primary cultures. The macroconidia have one to six septa, are 20 to 40 μm long by 7 to 12 μm wide, and are borne singly or in clusters of two or three. *E. floccosum* is currently the only recognized *Epidermophyton* species; the former *Epidermophyton stockdaleae* is now considered a synonym of *Trichophyton ajelloi* (*Arthroderma uncinatum*) (12, 99).

Recently Proposed Additions

Nannizzia Species

Originally introduced with *Arthroderma* as the teleomorph state of several zoophilic and geophilic dermatophytes, *Nannizzia* has been reestablished as a distinct genus based on multilocus phylogenetic analyses (12 and references therein). *Nannizzia* species produce a range of micro- and macroconidia similar to those seen with *Microsporum* species, with macroconidia ranging from smooth and thin walled to thick walled and conspicuously roughened, and varying in shape from clavate to broadly cigar-shaped. The genus is now proposed to contain several of the rarer zoophilic and geophilic organisms previously accommodated in *Microsporum*, including *N. gypsea* (*M. gypseum*), *N. fulva* (*M. fulvum*), *N. persicolor* (*M. persicolor*), *N. incurvata* (*M. incurvatum*), and *N. nana* (*M. nanum*).

Paraphyton Species

The novel genus *Paraphyton* (12) was recently proposed to encompass the geophilic species previously classified in the *Microsporum cookei* complex (now *Paraphyton cookei*, *Paraphyton cookiellum*, *Paraphyton mirabile*); macroconidia are typically large, multicelled, roughened, and thick walled, whereas microconidia are smooth, thin walled and clavate.

Lophophyton gallinae

L. gallinae is the proposed new combination for *Microsporum gallinae* (12), the zoophilic species on poultry, which also has a morphologically distinct geophilic form; macroconidia of isolates from infections tend to be curved and proximally tapered, whereas those from soilborne isolates are large, thick walled, and rough walled.

Arthroderma Species

This genus, under recent proposals (12), contains zoophilic and geophilic species, most of which are completely nonpathogenic or extremely rare causes of human infection. Macroconidia, when produced, are multicelled and thick and rough walled; microconidia are smooth, thin walled, and clavate to subglobose.

STRAIN TYPING SYSTEMS

Dermatophyte strains within anthropophilic species tend to be very closely related, hindering the development of useful techniques for epidemiological analysis, but strains of *T. rubrum* were eventually distinguished by polymorphisms in the numbers of subrepeat elements in the ribosomal nontranscribed spacer region (100–103). In addition, the Afro-Asiatic lineage of *T. rubrum* was distinguished from the now-cosmopolitan epidemic *T. rubrum* form by means of a microsatellite marker designated T1 (104). More recently, an elegant system involving multiple microsatellite markers has been developed (105). Nontranscribed spacer polymorphisms can also be applied to distinguish *T. interdigitale* and *T. tonsurans* isolates (100, 106, 107). While it is beyond the scope of this chapter to review all current molecular differentiation techniques for dermatophytes or their applications in outbreaks, the multilocus genotyping system of Abdel-Rahman et al. (108) should be cited as an example of how such methods can foster the development of epidemiological insight.

ANTIMICROBIAL SUSCEPTIBILITIES

Dermatophytes can in principle be tested for susceptibility to antifungal drugs using the standard CLSI M38-A2 standard for moulds (109). A trial has shown that this type of methodology can be applied with good inter- and intralaboratory reproducibility to the commonly used drugs ciclopirox, fluconazole, griseofulvin, itraconazole, posaconazole, terbinafine, and voriconazole (110). However, drug resistance is very rarely encountered in dermatophytes, and treatment failures are almost always due to factors other than resistance (111). Thus, potentially burdensome requests for dermatophyte susceptibility testing should be closely screened for scientific and clinical appropriateness.

EVALUATION, INTERPRETATION, AND REPORTING OF LABORATORY RESULTS

For nonimmunocompromised patients, positive direct microscopy compatible with dermatophytosis is conventionally interpreted as presumptively indicating this condition in hair and in specimens other than those from nails, soles, and palms. The positive microscopic report itself conveys this information; it should be issued within 2 working days of specimen receipt. With soles and palms, people who have lived in tropical areas or who are of South Asian heritage may have dermatophytosis-like *Neoscytalidium* (112)—previously called *Scytalidium*, *Nattrassia*, and *Hendersonula* (see chapter 127)—infections, which are similar to dermatophytoses both clinically and in direct microscopy (49); no presumptive diagnosis can be inferred until the culture result is available. The direct microscopic result, however, is still reported immediately. For patients without risk factors for *Neoscytalidium*, qualified physicians may make presumptive diagnoses of dermatophytosis for sole and palm skin as for other skin sites. In onychomycosis, over 35 mould species may be involved in producing conditions clinically and microscopically resembling tinea unguium (49), particularly in geriatric patients. The presence of a nondermatophyte mould may be suspected upon direct microscopic examination, which often reveals intact distorted hyphae (as opposed to arthrospores) with pronounced terminal fronding or hyphal swellings. Microscopic results are still reported promptly, but culture results are of high interest. At the same time, outgrowth of known onychomycosis-causing nondermatophytes may or may not be significant, excepting the nail-infecting *Neoscytalidium* species, which are always considered significant when grown. The complexities of accurately reporting nondermatophytes from nail specimens are beyond the scope of this chapter but are discussed in light of rigorous validation studies on this topic by Summerbell et al. (54).

Isolation of a dermatophyte culture from lesional skin, hair, or nails is interpreted as diagnostic whether or not fungal elements are seen in the initial direct microscopy examination. Note that dermatophytoids such as *M. cookei* (*P. cookei*) and *T. terrestre* complex are presumed to be contaminants until proven otherwise; they are, however, reported along with the comment "normally nonpathogenic" when grown. These fungi have been the subjects of numerous false and questionable case reports in the literature, and there may be some confusion about their status. If such a fungus were to infect human epidermis, the gold standard for scientifically evidencing the case would be three successive, consistent repeat isolations of the fungus from the lesion in specimens collected on different days, plus demonstration of compatible fungal elements in direct microscopy of the affected tissue. No inferential diagnoses from lower-quality evidence should be accepted as conclusive, even if the patient is said to have been successfully treated. A common dermatophyte such as *T. rubrum* that failed to grow out in initial culture(s) is very likely to be the actual etiologic agent in such cases (54). In onychomycosis, in particular, true causal dermatophytes have only at best an ~75% chance of being grown from the initial specimen taken from any given patient; another ~15% will be recovered from a second specimen, while ~10% can only be detected by testing three or more serial specimens, something very seldom done in practice (54). Cycloheximide-tolerant dermatophytoids that grow (in any quantity whatsoever) from single, otherwise unproductive specimens should not be assumed to be causal simply because they share a genus name with dermatophyte species.

SUPERFICIAL MYCOSES

In the superficial mycoses, the causative fungi colonize the cornified layers of the epidermis or the suprafollicular portion of the hair. There is little tissue damage, and cellular response from the host generally is lacking. The diseases are largely cosmetic in impact, involving changes in the pigmentation of the skin (tinea versicolor or tinea nigra) or formation of nodules along the distal hair shaft (black piedra and white piedra).

In contrast to the agents of the dermatophytoses, the etiologic agents are diverse and unrelated.

Tinea versicolor (Pityriasis versicolor)

Tinea versicolor is an infection of the stratum corneum caused by a group of closely similar lipophilic yeast species of the *Malassezia furfur* complex. Members of this complex infecting human skin were often treated in former times as a single species but were then shown by molecular, physiological, and serotyping studies to be separate (113, 114). The complex includes *M. furfur* (synonyms: *Pityrosporum furfur* and *Pityrosporum ovale pro parte*), *M. sympodialis*, *M. globosa* (probable synonym *Pityrosporum orbiculare*), *M. restricta*,

M. slooffiae, *M. obtusa*, *M. dermatis*, *M. japonica*, and *M. yamatoensis* (6, 115). Some additional species have been reported from animals. In routine clinical reporting, referring to these organisms as members of the *M. furfur* complex is normally sufficient. *Malassezia pachydermatis*, which causes animal ear infections and occasional human iatrogenic fungemias, is not considered a member of the *M. furfur* complex and, if reported, is reported under its individual species name. It is easily distinguished from *M. furfur* complex members by its ability to grow on ordinary laboratory media such as Sabouraud agar (see comments on *Malassezia* culture, below). It is insignificant when grown from human skin except where investigations of catheter-related problems are involved.

Tinea versicolor lesions appear as scaly, discrete or concrescent, hypopigmented or hyperpigmented (fawn, yellow-brown, brown, or red) patches chiefly on the neck, torso, and limbs. The infection is largely cosmetic, becoming apparent when the skin fails to tan normally. The disease has a worldwide distribution: in tropical climates 30 to 35% of the population may be affected, while the incidence in areas of temperate climate is much lower, with only 1.0 to 4.0% of the population affected. *M. furfur* and related yeasts are found on the normal skin and elicit disease only under conditions, local or systemic, that favor the overgrowth of the organism.

The *M. furfur* complex has been associated with folliculitis (116), obstructive dacryocystitis (16), systemic infections in patients receiving intralipid therapy (117), and seborrheic dermatitis, especially in patients with AIDS (118). Excellent reviews are available on human infections caused by *Malassezia* species and on the characteristics of the genus (119–122). Additional information is also found in chapter 120 of this manual.

Direct Examination

The fungi are observed readily when scrapings are mounted in 10% KOH plus ink (123), 25% NaOH plus 5% glycerin, calcofluor white, or Kane's formulation (glycerol, 10 ml; Tween 80, 10 ml; phenol, 2.5 g; methylene blue, 1.0 g; distilled water, 480 ml). In cases where skin scrapings from unspecified body sites are examined, Kane's formulation has the advantage of vividly staining both fungi and the differential-diagnostic organisms causing erythrasma and pitted keratolysis. (These two bacterial infections, often confused with superficial mycosis, are mainly from intertriginous sites and foot soles, respectively.) Tinea versicolor is signaled in microscopy by the presence of "spaghetti and meatballs," i.e., short, septate, occasionally branching filaments 2.5 to 4 μm in diameter and of variable lengths intermingled with clusters of small, unicellular, oval or round budding yeast cells (Fig. 19). The yeasts show the presence of a collarette between mother and daughter cells (budding is phialidic and unipolar) and average 4 μm (up to 8 μm) in size.

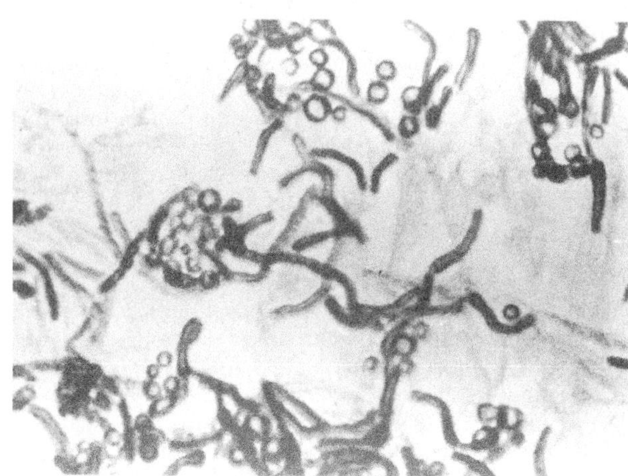

FIGURE 19 *Malassezia furfur* in skin scrapings from a lesion of tinea versicolor (Kane's stain). Magnification, ×1,000.

Isolation and Culture

Culture is not essential for identification unless the findings of direct microscopic examination are atypical or unless full species identification is desired for research purposes. Also, *M. furfur* complex members are part of the normal flora of the skin, and positive culture does not indicate infection. The species require exogenous lipid and do not grow on routine mycology media. If culture is desired, scrapings may be inoculated on Leeming-Notman medium, which uses whole milk as a major lipid source (124), on Dixon agar (125), or on modified Dixon agar, consisting of malt extract (3.6%), mycological peptone (Oxoid) (0.6%), desiccated ox bile (bile salts, Oxoid) (2%), Tween 40 (1%), glycerol (0.2%), oleic acid (0.2%), and agar (1.2%). Growth of the yeasts is slow; colonies are cream colored, glossy or rough, and raised (Fig. 20), later becoming dull, dry, and tan to brownish. Only budding yeast cells generally appear in culture (Fig. 21).

Tinea Nigra

Tinea nigra is characterized by the appearance, primarily on the palms of the hands and less commonly on the dorsa of the feet, of flat, sharply marginated, brownish black, nonscaly macules that may resemble melanoma (122).

The disease, almost always caused by *Hortaea werneckii* (*Phaeoannellomyces werneckii*, *Exophiala werneckii*, *Cladosporium werneckii*), is most common in tropical areas (126) but has been contracted occasionally in coastal areas in and near the southeastern United States (122, 127). Cases diagnosed outside the area of endemicity have mostly resulted from travel to the American tropics or the Caribbean islands (126). *H. werneckii* is related to the ascomycetous order Dothideales (128).

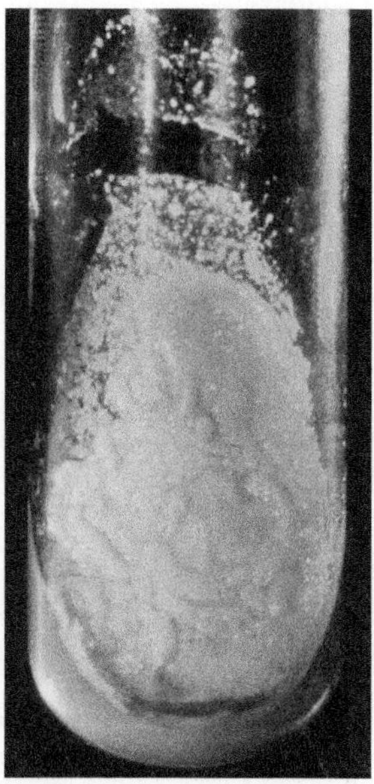

FIGURE 20 Culture of *Malassezia furfur* on Littman oxgall agar overlaid with oil.

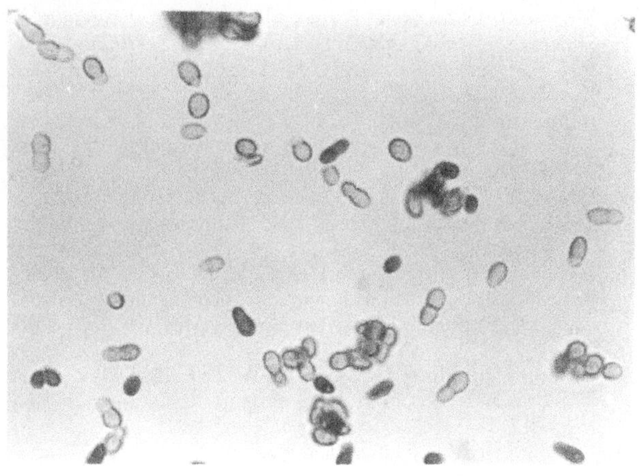
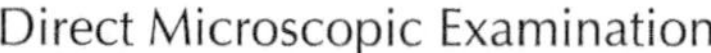

FIGURE 21 Microscopic appearance of *Malassezia furfur* yeast cells on Littman oxgall overlaid with olive oil. Magnification, ×400.

Direct Microscopic Examination

Microscopic examination of skin scrapings in KOH or NaOH reveals numerous light brown, frequently branching septate filaments of 1.5 to 5 μm in diameter (Fig. 18h); short, sinuous filaments; and budding cells, some septate.

Isolation

On SGA with or without antibiotics, *H. werneckii* grows slowly and usually appears within 2 to 3 weeks as moist, shiny olive to greenish black yeast-like colonies. The yeast-like cells are usually two-celled when reproductive and, instead of budding, produce new yeast cells from thick (up to 2 μm in diameter) distinctly annellated (multiply ringed as if wearing several bracelets) pegs. After 7 or more days, colonies may develop a fringe of thick, dark, conspicuously septate hyphae that also bear annellated fertile structures. These produce conidia that are indistinguishable from young yeast cells. The micromorphology of *H. werneckii* is described in more detail in chapter 127.

Black Piedra

Black piedra is a fungal infection of the scalp hair, less commonly of the beard or moustache, and rarely of axillary or pubic hairs. The disease is characterized by the presence of discrete, hard, gritty, dark brown to black nodules adhering firmly to the hair shaft (Fig. 22). It is found mostly in tropical regions in Africa, Asia, and Central and South America. Humans as well as other primates are infected (122, 126, 129).

The etiologic agent in humans is *Piedraia hortae*, an ascomycete (order Dothideales) forming nodules that serve as ascostromata containing locules that harbor the asci and ascospores.

Direct Microscopic Examination

Hair fragments containing one or more black nodules are placed in 25% KOH or NaOH with 5% glycerol. The preparation is heated gently and carefully squashed, trying not to break the coverslip because the nodules are very hard. A squashed preparation of a mature nodule should reveal compact masses of dark, septate hyphae and round to oval asci containing two to eight hyaline, aseptate banana-shaped (fusiform) ascospores that bear one or more appendages. The preparation should first be observed under low-power objective to reveal the dark mass of compacted hyphae around the surface of the hair, and then examined under the high-power objective to observe the asci and ascospores.

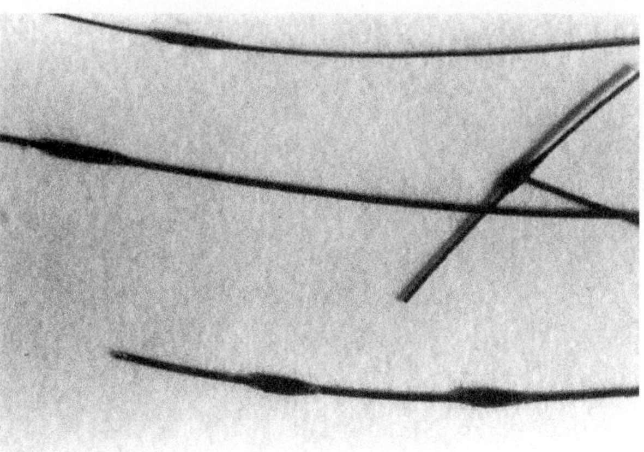

FIGURE 22 Black piedra nodules on scalp hair. NaOH mount. Magnification, ×100.

Isolation, Culture, and Identification

When ascospores are seen in direct specimen microscopy, culture is unnecessary. Otherwise, SGA with chloramphenicol or SGA with chloramphenicol and cycloheximide may be used for isolation. Some reports have indicated that cycloheximide may be inhibitory; however, others have used this antibiotic successfully. SGA amended with chloramphenicol alone may be used for successful isolation.

Colonies are very slow growing, appear dark brown to black, glabrous at first, and later covered with short dark brown to black aerial mycelium. They tend to be heaped in the center, with a flat periphery. Some colonies produce a reddish brown diffusible pigment on the agar. Microscopic examination reveals only highly septate dark hyphae and swollen intercalary cells. Conidia and ascospores are usually not found on routine mycological media.

White Piedra

White piedra is a fungal infection of the hair shaft characterized by the presence of soft white, yellowish, beige, or greenish nodules found chiefly on facial, axillary, or genital hairs (Fig. 23) and less commonly on the scalp, eyebrows, and eyelashes. Nodules may be discrete or more often coalescent, forming an irregular transparent sheath.

The infection occurs sporadically in North America and Europe and more commonly in South America, Africa, and Asia (126). Although white piedra is an uncommon

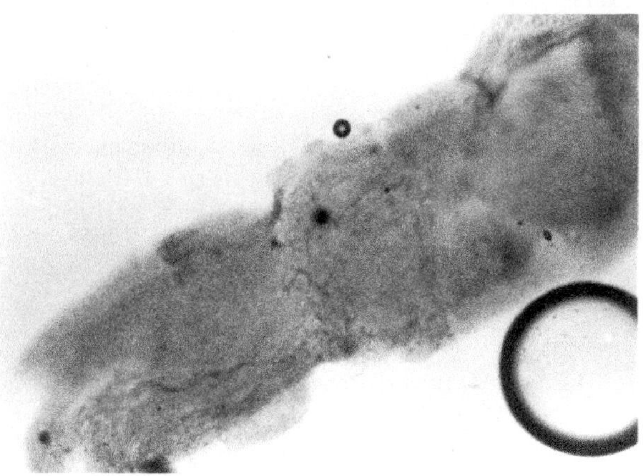

FIGURE 23 White piedra nodule on hair from the groin. Magnification, ×1,000.

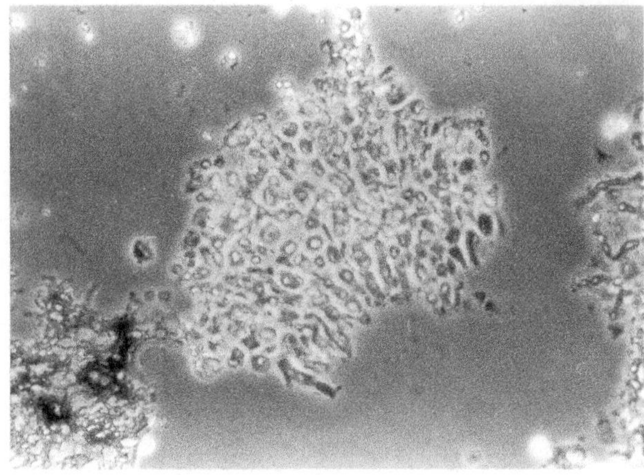

FIGURE 24 Arthroconidia from a crushed nodule of white piedra. Magnification, ×1,000.

infection, genital white piedra is occasionally but regularly seen in certain populations (122, 130).

Microscopic examination of hairs containing the adherent nodules mounted in 10% KOH or 25% NaOH-5% glycerin and squashed under a coverslip reveals intertwined hyaline septate hyphae, hyphae breaking up into oval or rectangular arthroconidia of 2 to 4 μm in diameter (Fig. 24), occasional blastoconidia, and bacteria that may surround the nodule as a zooglea (jelly-like mass).

The isolates were formerly described as *Trichosporon beigelii* or *Trichosporon cutaneum* (now *Cutaneotrichosporon cutaneum*) but are now correctly identified in most cases as *Trichosporon ovoides* (causes scalp hair white piedra), *Trichosporon inkin* (causes most cases of pubic white piedra), and *Trichosporon asahii* (131, 132). As with the *M. furfur* complex, these species form a complex of difficult to identify species whose distinction, except in demonstrated cases of piedra, is not known to have strong clinical implications in dermatologic mycology. They are also very common skin contaminants. Ordinarily, they may be reported from skin, hair, and nails of nonneutropenic patients simply as members of the genus *Trichosporon* and *Cutaneotrichosporon*, based on production of budding yeast cells, arthroconidia, and a positive urease test, unless a research-level identification of a proven etiologic agent is attempted. The causal agents of white piedra may be readily isolated on SGA with chloramphenicol or other isolation media containing antibacterial antibiotics. The isolation medium should not contain cycloheximide, since this drug is inhibitory to some of the species. Growth is rapid, yielding white to cream-colored colonies that exhibit a variety of colonial morphologies depending on the species. A description of the genus and characteristics of the species involved in white piedra are given in papers by Guého et al. (132, 133). More information about *Trichosporon* can be found in chapter 120 of this *Manual*.

REFERENCES

1. **Currah RS.** 1985. Taxonomy of the Onygenales: Arthrodermataceae, Gymnoascaceae, Myxotrichaceae and Onygenaceae. *Mycotaxon* **24:**1–216.
2. **Weitzman I, McGinnis MR, Padhye AA, Ajello L.** 1986. The genus *Arthroderma* and its later synonym *Nannizzia*. *Mycotaxon* **25:**505–518.
3. **Burnett J.** 2003. *Fungal Populations & Species*. Oxford University Press, Oxford, United Kingdom.
4. **Gupta AK, Kohli Y, Summerbell RC.** 2002. Exploratory study of single-copy genes and ribosomal intergenic spacers for distinction of dermatophytes. *Stud Mycol* **47:**87–96.
5. **Summerbell RC.** 2000. Form and function in the evolution of dermatophytes, p 30–43. *In* Kushwaha RKS, Guarro J (ed), *Biology of Dermatophytes and Other Keratinophilic Fungi*. Revista Iberoamericana de Micologia, Bilbao, Spain.
6. **Summerbell RC.** 2002. What is the evolutionary and taxonomic status of asexual lineages in the dermatophytes? *Stud Mycol* **47:**97–101.
7. **Gräser Y, Kuijpers AFA, Presber W, de Hoog GS.** 2000. Molecular taxonomy of the *Trichophyton rubrum* complex. *J Clin Microbiol* **38:**3329–3336.
8. **Mochizuki T, Watanabe S, Uehara M.** 1996. Genetic homogeneity of *Trichophyton mentagrophytes* var. *interdigitale* isolated from geographically distant regions. *J Med Vet Mycol* **34:** 139–143.
9. **Probst S, de Hoog GS, Gräser Y.** 2002. Development of DNA markers to explore host shifts in dermatophytes. *Stud Mycol* **47:**57–74.
10. **Summerbell RC, Weitzman I, Padhye A.** 2002. The *Trichophyton mentagrophytes* complex: biological species and mating type prevalences of North American isolates, and a review of the worldwide distribution and host associations of species and mating types. *Stud Mycol* **47:**75–86.
11. **Hawksworth DL.** 2011. A new dawn for the naming of fungi: impacts of decisions made in Melbourne in July 2011 on the future publication and regulation of fungal names. *IMA Fungus* **2:**155–162.
12. **de Hoog GS, Dukik K, Monod M, Packeu A, Stubbe D, Hendrickx M, Kupsch C, Stielow JB, Freeke J, Göker M, Rezaei-Matehkolaei A, Mirhendi H, Gräser Y.** 2017. Toward a novel multilocus phylogenetic taxonomy for the dermatophytes. *Mycopathologia* **182:**5–31.
13. **de Respinis S, Tonolla M, Pranghofer S, Petrini L, Petrini O, Bosshard PP.** 2013. Identification of dermatophytes by matrix-assisted laser desorption/ionization time-of-flight mass spectrometry. *Med Mycol* **51:**514–521.
14. **Ajello L.** 1960. Geographic distribution and prevalence of the dermatophytes. *Ann N Y Acad Sci* **89:**30–38.
15. **Hermoso de Mendoza M, Hermoso de Mendoza J, Alonso JM, Rey JM, Sanchez S, Martin R, Bermejo F, Cortes M, Benitez JM, Garcia WL, Garcia-Sanchez A.** 2010. A zoonotic ringworm outbreak caused by a dysgonic strain of *Microsporum canis* from stray cats. *Rev Iberoam Micol* **27:**62–65.
16. **Rippon JW.** 1985. The changing epidemiology and emerging patterns of dermatophyte species, p 208–234. *In* McGinnis MR (ed), *Current Topics in Medical Mycology*. Springer-Verlag, New York, NY.
17. **Borman AM, Campbell CK, Fraser M, Johnson EM.** 2007. Analysis of the dermatophyte species isolated in the British Isles between 1980 and 2005 and review of worldwide dermatophyte trends over the last three decades. *Med Mycol* **45:**131–141.
18. **Rosenthal SA.** 1974. The epidemiology of tinea pedis, p 515–526. *In* Robinson HM Jr (ed), *The Diagnosis and Treatment of Fungal Infections*. Charles C. Thomas, Springfield, IL.
19. **Weitzman I, Rosenthal SA, Silva-Hutner M.** 1988. Superficial and cutaneous infections caused by molds: dermatomycoses, p 33–97. *In* Wentworth BB (ed), *Diagnostic Procedures for Mycotic and Parasitic Infections*, 7th ed. American Public Health Association, Inc, Washington, DC.
20. **Zaias N, Tosti A, Rebell G, Morelli R, Bardazzi F, Bieley H, Zaiac M, Glick B, Paley B, Allevato M, Baran R.** 1996. Autosomal dominant pattern of distal subungual onychomycosis caused by *Trichophyton rubrum*. *J Am Acad Dermatol* **34:**302–304.
21. **Alsop J, Prior AP.** 1961. Ringworm infection in a cucumber greenhouse. *BMJ* **1:**1081–1083.
22. **Shah PC, Krajden S, Kane J, Summerbell RC.** 1988. Tinea corporis caused by *Microsporum canis*: report of a nosocomial outbreak. *Eur J Epidemiol* **4:**33–38.
23. **King RD, Khan HA, Foye JC, Greenberg JH, Jones HE.** 1975. Transferrin, iron, and dermatophytes. I. Serum dematophyte inhibitory component definitively identified as unsaturated transferrin. *J Lab Clin Med* **86:**204–212.
24. **Dei Cas E, Vernes A.** 1986. Parasitic adaptation of pathogenic fungi to mammalian hosts. *Crit Rev Microbiol* **13:** 173–218.

25. **Koga T.** 2003. Immune response in dermatophytosis. *Nippon Ishinkin Gakkai Zasshi* **44:**273–275. (In Japanese.)
26. **Ogawa H, Summerbell RC, Clemons KV, Koga T, Ran YP, Rashid A, Sohnle PG, Stevens DA, Tsuboi R.** 1998. Dermatophytes and host defence in cutaneous mycoses. *Med Mycol* **36**(Suppl 1)**:**166–173.
27. **Weitzman I, Summerbell RC.** 1995. The dermatophytes. *Clin Microbiol Rev* **8:**240–259.
28. **Koga T, Duan H, Urabe K, Furue M.** 2001. Immunohistochemical detection of interferon-gamma-producing cells in dermatophytosis. *Eur J Dermatol* **11:**105–107.
29. **Vermout S, Tabart J, Baldo A, Mathy A, Losson B, Mignon B.** 2008. Pathogenesis of dermatophytosis. *Mycopathologia* **166:**267–275.
30. **Barson WJ.** 1985. Granuloma and pseudogranuloma of the skin due to *Microsporum canis*. Successful management with local injections of miconazole. *Arch Dermatol* **121:**895–897.
31. **West BC, Kwon-Chung KJ.** 1980. Mycetoma caused by *Microsporum audouinii*. First reported case. *Am J Clin Pathol* **73:**447–454.
32. **Araviysky AN, Araviysky RA, Eschkov GA.** 1975. Deep generalized trichophytosis: Endothrix in tissues of different origin. *Mycopathologia* **56:**47–65.
33. **Squeo RF, Beer R, Silvers D, Weitzman I, Grossman M.** 1998. Invasive *Trichophyton rubrum* resembling blastomycosis infection in the immunocompromised host. *J Am Acad Dermatol* **39:**379–380.
34. **Durant J-F, Fonteyne P-A, Richez P, Marot L, Belkhir L, Tennstedt D, Gala JL.** 2009. Real-time PCR and DNA sequencing for detection and identification of *Trichophyton rubrum* as a cause of culture negative chronic granulomatous dermatophytosis. *Med Mycol* **47:**508–514.
35. **Adams BB.** 2002. Tinea corporis gladiatorum. *J Am Acad Dermatol* **47:**286–290.
36. **Aly R, Hay RJ, Del Palacio A, Galimberti R.** 2000. Epidemiology of tinea capitis. *Med Mycol* **38**(Suppl 1)**:**183–188.
37. **Connole MD, Yamaguchi H, Elad D, Hasegawa A, Segal E, Torres-Rodriguez JM.** 2000. Natural pathogens of laboratory animals and their effects on research. *Med Mycol* **38**(Suppl 1)**:** 59–65.
38. **Gupta AK, De Rosso JQ.** 1999. Management of onychomycosis in children. *Postgrad Med* (Spec No)**:**31–37.
39. **Hirose N, Shiraki Y, Hiruma M, Ogawa H.** 2005. An investigation of *Trichophyton tonsurans* infection in university students participating in sports clubs. *Nippon Ishinkin Gakkai Zasshi* **46:**119–123. (In Japanese.)
40. **Lacroix C, Baspeyras M, de La Salmonière P, Benderdouche M, Couprie B, Accoceberry I, Weill FX, Derouin F, Feuilhade de Chauvin M.** 2002. Tinea pedis in European marathon runners. *J Eur Acad Dermatol Venereol* **16:**139–142.
41. **Levy LA.** 1997. Epidemiology of onychomycosis in special-risk populations. *J Am Podiatr Med Assoc* **87:**546–550.
42. **Rippon JW.** 1988. *Medical Mycology: The Pathogenic Fungi and the Pathogenic Actinomycetes*, 3rd ed, p 169–275. The W B Saunders Co, Philadelphia, PA.
43. **Zaias N, Rebell G.** 2003. Clinical and mycological status of the *Trichophyton mentagrophytes* (*interdigitale*) syndrome of chronic dermatophytosis of the skin and nails. *Int J Dermatol* **42:**779–788.
44. **Daniel CR III, Norton LA, Scher RK.** 1992. The spectrum of nail disease in patients with human immunodeficiency virus infection. *J Am Acad Dermatol* **27:**93–97.
45. **Mackenzie DWR.** 1963. "Hairbrush diagnosis" in detection and eradication of non-fluorescent scalp ringworm. *BMJ* **2:**363–365.
46. **Suarez SM, Silvers DN, Scher RK, Pearlstein HH, Auerbach R.** 1991. Histologic evaluation of nail clippings for diagnosing onychomycosis. *Arch Dermatol* **127:**1517–1519.
47. **Head ES, Henry JC, Macdonald EM.** 1984. The cotton swab technic for the culture of dermatophyte infections: its efficacy and merit. *J Am Acad Dermatol* **11:**797–801.
48. **Tosti A, Baran R, Piraccini BM, Fanti PA.** 1999. "Endonyx" onychomycosis: a new modality of nail invasion by dermatophytes. *Acta Derm Venereol* **79:**52–53.
49. **Kane J, Summerbell RC, Sigler L, Krajden S, Land G.** 1997. *Laboratory Handbook of Dermatophytes and Other Filamentous Fungi from Skin, Hair and Nails*. Star Publishing Co., Belmont, CA.
50. **Robinson BE, Padhye AA.** 1988. Collection transport and processing of clinical specimens, p 11–32. *In* Wentworth BB (ed), *Diagnostic Procedures for Mycotic and Parasitic Infections*, 7th ed. American Public Health Association, Inc., Washington, DC.
51. **Haldane DJ, Robart E.** 1990. A comparison of calcofluor white, potassium hydroxide, and culture for the laboratory diagnosis of superficial fungal infection. *Diagn Microbiol Infect Dis* **13:**337–339.
52. **Hamer EC, Moore CB, Denning DW.** 2006. Comparison of two fluorescent whiteners, Calcofluor and Blankophor, for the detection of fungal elements in clinical specimens in the diagnostic laboratory. *Clin Microbiol Infect* **12:**181–184.
53. **Lawry MA, Haneke E, Strobeck K, Martin S, Zimmer B, Romano PS.** 2000. Methods for diagnosing onychomycosis: a comparative study and review of the literature. *Arch Dermatol* **136:**1112–1116.
54. **Summerbell RC, Cooper E, Bunn U, Jamieson F, Gupta AK.** 2005. Onychomycosis: a critical study of techniques and criteria for confirming the etiologic significance of nondermatophytes. *Med Mycol* **43:**39–59.
55. **McGinnis MR, Rex JH, Arikan S, Rodrigues L.** Examination of specimens page, Lab procedures section, Doctor Fungus website. https://drfungus.org/knowledge-base/laboratory-procedures/
56. **Taplin D.** 1965. The use of gentamicin in mycology media. *J Invest Dermatol* **45:**549–550.
57. **Fischer JB, Kane J.** 1974. The laboratory diagnosis of dermatophytosis complicated with *Candida albicans*. *Can J Microbiol* **20:**167–182.
58. **Taplin D, Zaias N, Rebell G, Blank H.** 1969. Isolation and recognition of dermatophytes on a new medium (DTM). *Arch Dermatol* **99:**203–209.
59. **Merz WG, Berger CL, Silva-Hutner M.** 1970. Media with pH indicators for the isolation of dermatophytes. *Arch Dermatol* **102:**545–547.
60. **Salkin IF.** 1973. Dermatrophye test medium: evaluation with nondermatophytic pathogens. *Appl Microbiol* **26:**134–137.
61. **Aly R.** 1994. Culture media for growing dermatophytes. *J Am Acad Dermatol* **31:**S107–S108.
62. **Moriello KA, Deboer DJ.** 1991. Fungal flora of the haircoat of cats with and without dermatophytosis. *J Med Vet Mycol* **29:**285–292.
63. **Beifuss B, Bezold G, Gottlöber P, Borelli C, Wagener J, Schaller M, Korting HC.** 2011. Direct detection of five common dermatophyte species in clinical samples using a rapid and sensitive 24-h PCR-ELISA technique open to protocol transfer. *Mycoses* **54:**137–145.
64. **Bergmans AM, Schouls LM, van der Ent M, Klaassen A, Böhm N, Wintermans RG.** 2008. Validation of PCR-reverse line blot, a method for rapid detection and identification of nine dermatophyte species in nail, skin and hair samples. *Clin Microbiol Infect* **14:**778–788.
65. **Bontems O, Hauser PM, Monod M.** 2009. Evaluation of a polymerase chain reaction-restriction fragment length polymorphism assay for dermatophyte and nondermatophyte identification in onychomycosis. *Br J Dermatol* **161:** 791–796.
66. **Brillowska-Dabrowska A, Saunte DM, Arendrup MC.** 2007. Five-hour diagnosis of dermatophyte nail infections with specific detection of *Trichophyton rubrum*. *J Clin Microbiol* **45:**1200–1204.
67. **Garg J, Tilak R, Singh S, Gulati AK, Garg A, Prakash P, Nath G.** 2007. Evaluation of pan-dermatophyte nested PCR in diagnosis of onychomycosis. *J Clin Microbiol* **45:** 3443–3445.
68. **Kardjeva V, Summerbell R, Kantardjiev T, Devliotou-Panagiotidou D, Sotiriou E, Gräser Y.** 2006. Forty-eight-hour diagnosis of onychomycosis with subtyping of *Trichophyton rubrum* strains. *J Clin Microbiol* **44:** 1419–1427.

69. **Arabatzis M, Bruijnesteijn van Coppenraet LE, Kuijper EJ, de Hoog GS, Lavrijsen AP, Templeton K, van der Raaij-Helmer EM, Velegraki A, Gräser Y, Summerbell RC.** 2007. Diagnosis of common dermatophyte infections by a novel multiplex real-time polymerase chain reaction detection/identification scheme. *Br J Dermatol* **157:**681–689.
70. **Bergmans AM, van der Ent M, Klaassen A, Böhm N, Andriesse GI, Wintermans RG.** 2010. Evaluation of a single-tube real-time PCR for detection and identification of 11 dermatophyte species in clinical material. *Clin Microbiol Infect* **16:**704–710.
71. **Gutzmer R, Mommert S, Küttler U, Werfel T, Kapp A.** 2004. Rapid identification and differentiation of fungal DNA in dermatological specimens by LightCycler PCR. *J Med Microbiol* **53:**1207–1214.
72. **Jensen RH, Arendrup MC.** 2012. Molecular diagnosis of dermatophyte infections. *Curr Opin Infect Dis* **25:**126–134.
73. **Nagao K, Sugita T, Ouchi T, Nishikawa T.** 2005. Identification of *Trichophyton rubrum* by nested PCR analysis from paraffin embedded specimen in trichophytia profunda acuta of the glabrous skin. *Nippon Ishinkin Gakkai Zasshi* **46:**129–132. (In Japanese.)
74. **Nenoff P, Erhard M, Simon JC, Muylowa GK, Herrmann J, Rataj W, Gräser Y.** 2013. MALDI-TOF mass spectrometry: a rapid method for the identification of dermatophyte species. *Med Mycol* **51:**17–24.
75. **Weeks RJ, Padhye AA.** 1982. A mounting medium for permanent preparations of microfungi. *Mykosen* **25:**702–704.
76. **Kane J, Fischer JB.** 1975. The effect of sodium chloride on the growth and morphology of dermatophytes and some other keratolytic fungi. *Can J Microbiol* **21:**742–749.
77. **Kane J, Sigler L, Summerbell RC.** 1987. Improved procedures for differentiating *Microsporum persicolor* from *Trichophyton mentagrophytes*. *J Clin Microbiol* **25:**2449–2452.
78. **Borelli D.** 1962. Medios caseros para micologia. *Arch Venez Med Trop Parasitol Med* **4:**301–310.
79. **Kaminski GW.** 1985. The routine use of modified Borelli's lactritmel agar (MBLA). *Mycopathologia* **91:**57–59.
80. **Ajello L, Georg LK.** 1957. *In vitro* hair cultures for differentiating between atypical isolates of *Trichophyton mentagrophytes* and *Trichophyton rubrum*. *Mycopathol Mycol Appl* **8:**3–17.
81. **Padhye AA, Young CN, Ajello L.** 1980. Hair perforation as a diagnostic criterion in the identification of *Epidermophyton*, *Microsporum* and *Trichophyton* species, p 115–120. *In Superficial Cutaneous and Subcutaneous Infections. Scientific publication no.* 396. Pan American Health Organization, Washington, DC.
82. **Georg LK, Camp LB.** 1957. Routine nutritional tests for the identification of dermatophytes. *J Bacteriol* **74:**113–121.
83. **Rosenthal SA, Sokolsky H.** 1965. Enzymatic studies with pathogenic fungi. *Dermatol Int* **4:**72–78.
84. **Sequeira H, Cabrita J, De Vroey C, Wuytack-Raes C.** 1991. Contribution to our knowledge of *Trichophyton megninii*. *J Med Vet Mycol* **29:**417–418.
85. **Kane J, Fischer JB.** 1971. The differentiation of *Trichophyton rubrum* and *T. mentagrophytes* by use of Christensen's urea broth. *Can J Microbiol* **17:**911–913.
86. **Summerbell RC, Rosenthal SA, Kane J.** 1988. Rapid method for differentiation of *Trichophyton rubrum*, *Trichophyton mentagrophytes*, and related dermatophyte species. *J Clin Microbiol* **26:**2279–2282.
87. **Padhye AA, Blank F, Koblenzer PJ, Spatz S, Ajello L.** 1973. *Microsporum persicolor* infection in the United States. *Arch Dermatol* **108:**561–562.
88. **Shadomy HJ, Philpot CM.** 1980. Utilization of standard laboratory methods in the laboratory diagnosis of problem dermatophytes. *Am J Clin Pathol* **74:**197–201.
89. **Padhye AA, Carmichael J.** 1971. The genus *Arthroderma* Berkeley. *Can J Bot* **49:**1525–1540.
90. **Weitzman I, Rosenthal S.** 1984. Studies in the differentiation between *Microsporum ferrugineum* Ota and *Trichophyton soudanense* Joyeux. *Mycopathologia* **84:**95–101.
91. **Summerbell RC, Moore MK, Starink-Willemse M, Van Iperen A.** 2007. ITS barcodes for *Trichophyton tonsurans* and *T. equinum*. *Med Mycol* **45:**193–200.
92. **Balajee SA, Borman AM, Brandt ME, Cano J, Cuenca-Estrella M, Dannaoui E, Guarro J, Haase G, Kibbler CC, Meyer W, O'Donnell K, Petti CA, Rodriguez-Tudela JL, Sutton D, Velegraki A, Wickes BL.** 2009. Sequence-based identification of *Aspergillus*, *Fusarium*, and *Mucorales* species in the clinical mycology laboratory: where are we and where should we go from here? *J Clin Microbiol* **47:**877–884.
93. **Li HC, Bouchara JP, Hsu MM, Barton R, Su S, Chang TC.** 2008. Identification of dermatophytes by sequence analysis of the rRNA gene internal transcribed spacer regions. *J Med Microbiol* **57:**592–600.
94. **Shehata AS, Mukherjee PK, Aboulatta HN, el-Akhras AI, Abbadi SH, Ghannoum MA.** 2008. Single-step PCR using (GACA)4 primer: utility for rapid identification of dermatophyte species and strains. *J Clin Microbiol* **46:**2641–2645.
95. **De Baere T, Summerbell R, Theelen B, Boekhout T, Vaneechoutte M.** 2010. Evaluation of internal transcribed spacer 2-RFLP analysis for the identification of dermatophytes. *J Med Microbiol* **59:**48–54.
96. **Padhye AA, Weitzman I, Domenech E.** 1994. An unusual variant of *Trichophyton tonsurans* var. *sulfureum*. *J Med Vet Mycol* **32:**147–150.
97. **Summerbell RC.** 1987. *Trichophyton kanei*, sp. nov. a new anthropophilic dermatophyte. *Mycotaxon* **28:**509–523.
98. **Demange C, Contet-Audonneau N, Kombila M, Miegeville M, Berthonneau M, De Vroey C, Percebois G.** 1992. *Microsporum gypseum* complex in man and animals. *J Med Vet Mycol* **30:**301–308.
99. **Gräser Y, de Hoog GS, Kuijpers AFA.** 2000. Recent advances in the molecular taxonomy of dermatophytes, p 17–21. *In* Kushwaha RKS, Guarro J (ed), *Biology of Dermatophytes and Other Keratinophilic Fungi.* Revista Iberoamericana de Micologia, Bilbao, Spain.
100. **Gupta AK, Kohli Y, Summerbell RC.** 2001. Variation in restriction fragment length polymorphisms among serial isolates from patients with *Trichophyton rubrum* infection. *J Clin Microbiol* **39:**3260–3266.
101. **Jackson CJ, Barton RC, Kelly SL, Evans EGV.** 2000. Strain identification of *Trichophyton rubrum* by specific amplification of subrepeat elements in the ribosomal DNA nontranscribed spacer. *J Clin Microbiol* **38:**4527–4534.
102. **Rad MM, Jackson C, Barton RC, Evans EG.** 2005. Single strains of *Trichophyton rubrum* in cases of tinea pedis. *J Med Microbiol* **54:**725–726.
103. **Yazdanparast A, Jackson CJ, Barton RC, Evans EG.** 2003. Molecular strain typing of *Trichophyton rubrum* indicates multiple strain involvement in onychomycosis. *Br J Dermatol* **148:**51–54.
104. **Ohst T, de Hoog S, Presber W, Stavrakieva V, Gräser Y.** 2004. Origins of microsatellite diversity in the *Trichophyton rubrum-T. violaceum* clade (Dermatophytes). *J Clin Microbiol* **42:**4444–4448.
105. **Gräser Y, Fröhlich J, Presber W, de Hoog S.** 2007. Microsatellite markers reveal geographic population differentiation in *Trichophyton rubrum*. *J Med Microbiol* **56:**1058–1065.
106. **Gaedigk A, Gaedigk R, Abdel-Rahman SM.** 2003. Genetic heterogeneity in the rRNA gene locus of *Trichophyton tonsurans*. *J Clin Microbiol* **41:**5478–5487.
107. **Mochizuki T, Ishizaki H, Barton RC, Moore MK, Jackson CJ, Kelly SL, Evans EG.** 2003. Restriction fragment length polymorphism analysis of ribosomal DNA intergenic regions is useful for differentiating strains of *Trichophyton mentagrophytes*. *J Clin Microbiol* **41:**4583–4588.
108. **Abdel-Rahman SM, Preuett B, Gaedigk A.** 2007. Multilocus genotyping identifies infections by multiple strains of *Trichophyton tonsurans*. *J Clin Microbiol* **45:**1949–1953.
109. **Clinical and Laboratory Standards Institute.** 2002. Reference method for broth dilution antifungal susceptibility testing of filamentous fungi; approved standard—2nd ed. Document M38-A2. CLSI, Wayne, PA.
110. **Ghannoum MA, Chaturvedi V, Espinel-Ingroff A, Pfaller MA, Rinaldi MG, Lee-Yang W, Warnock DW.** 2004. Intra- and interlaboratory study of a method for testing the antifungal susceptibilities of dermatophytes. *J Clin Microbiol* **42:**2977–2979.

111. **Gupta AK, Kohli Y.** 2003. Evaluation of *in vitro* resistance in patients with onychomycosis who fail antifungal therapy. *Dermatology* **207:**375–380.
112. **Crous PW, Slippers B, Wingfield MJ, Rheeder J, Marasas WF, Philips AJ, Alves A, Burgess T, Barber P, Groenewald JZ.** 2006. Phylogenetic lineages in the Botryosphaeriaceae. *Stud Mycol* **55:**235–253.
113. **Guého E, Midgley G, Guillot J.** 1996. The genus *Malassezia* with description of four new species. *Antonie van Leeuwenhoek* **69:**337–355.
114. **Guillot J, Hadina S, Guého E.** 2008. The genus *Malassezia*: old facts and new concepts. *Parassitologia* **50:**77–79.
115. **Sugita T, Tajima M, Takashima M, Amaya M, Saito M, Tsuboi R, Nishikawa A.** 2004. A new yeast, *Malassezia yamatoensis*, isolated from a patient with seborrheic dermatitis, and its distribution in patients and healthy subjects. *Microbiol Immunol* **48:**579–583.
116. **Bäck O, Faergemann J, Hörnqvist R.** 1985. *Pityrosporum* folliculitis: a common disease of the young and middle-aged. *J Am Acad Dermatol* **12:**56–61.
117. **Dankner WM, Spector SA, Fierer J, Davis CE.** 1987. *Malassezia* fungemia in neonates and adults: complication of hyperalimentation. *Rev Infect Dis* **9:**743–753.
118. **Groisser D, Bottone EJ, Lebwohl M.** 1989. Association of *Pityrosporum orbiculare* (*Malassezia furfur*) with seborrheic dermatitis in patients with acquired immunodeficiency syndrome (AIDS). *J Am Acad Dermatol* **20:**770–773.
119. **Batra R, Boekhout T, Guého E, Cabañes FJ, Dawson TL Jr, Gupta AK.** 2005. *Malassezia* Baillon, emerging clinical yeasts. *FEMS Yeast Res* **5:**1101–1113.
120. **Dawson TL Jr.** 2007. *Malassezia globosa* and *restricta*: breakthrough understanding of the etiology and treatment of dandruff and seborrheic dermatitis through whole-genome analysis. *J Investig Dermatol Symp Proc* **12:**15–19.
121. **Gupta AK, Batra R, Bluhm R, Boekhout T, Dawson TL Jr.** 2004. Skin diseases associated with *Malassezia* species. *J Am Acad Dermatol* **51:**785–798.
122. **Schwartz RA.** 2004. Superficial fungal infections. *Lancet* **364:**1173–1182.
123. **Cohen MM.** 1954. A simple procedure for staining tinea versicolor (*M. furfur*) with fountain pen ink. *J Invest Dermatol* **22:**9–10.
124. **Leeming JP, Notman FH.** 1987. Improved methods for isolation and enumeration of *Malassezia furfur* from human skin. *J Clin Microbiol* **25:**2017–2019.
125. **Crespo Erchiga V, Ojeda Martos A, Vera Casaño A, Crespo Erchiga A, Sanchez Fajardo F.** 2000. *Malassezia globosa* as the causative agent of pityriasis versicolor. *Br J Dermatol* **143:**799–803.
126. **Rippon JW.** 1988. *Medical Mycology: The Pathogenic Fungi and the Pathogenic Actinomycetes*, 3rd ed, p 154–168. The W B Saunders Co., Philadelphia, PA.
127. **Hughes JR, Moore MK, Pembroke AC.** 1993. Tinea nigra palmaris. *Clin Exp Dermatol* **18:**481–482.
128. **Hölker U, Bend J, Pracht R, Tetsch L, Müller T, Höfer M, de Hoog GS.** 2004. *Hortaea acidophila*, a new acid-tolerant black yeast from lignite. *Antonie van Leeuwenhoek* **86:**287–294.
129. **Gip L.** 1994. Black piedra: the first case treated with terbinafine (Lamisil). *Br J Dermatol* **130**(Suppl 43)**:**26–28.
130. **Kalter DC, Tschen JA, Cernoch PL, McBride ME, Sperber J, Bruce S, Wolf JE Jr.** 1986. Genital white piedra: epidemiology, microbiology, and therapy. *J Am Acad Dermatol* **14:**982–993.
131. **Douchet C, Thérizol-Ferly M, Kombila M, Duong TH, Gomez de Diaz M, Barrabes A, Richard-Lenoble D.** 1994. White piedra and *Trichosporon* species in equatorial Africa. III. Identification of *Trichosporon* species by slide agglutination test. *Mycoses* **37:**261–264.
132. **Guého E, Smith MT, de Hoog GS, Billon-Grand G, Christen R, Batenburg-van der Vegte WH.** 1992. Contributions to a revision of the genus *Trichosporon*. *Antonie van Leeuwenhoek* **61:**289–316.
133. **Guého E, de Hoog GS, Smith MT.** 1992. Neotypification of the genus *Trichosporon*. *Antonie van Leeuwenhoek* **61:**285–288.

Curvularia, Exophiala, Scedosporium, Sporothrix, and Other Melanized Fungi

JOSEP GUARRO, HUGO MADRID, AND SYBREN DE HOOG

127

This chapter covers most of the agents of phaeohyphomycosis, chromoblastomycosis, and sporotrichosis, as well as a number of agents of superficial and cutaneous disease. The genera discussed in this chapter belong to the ascomycetous orders Botryosphaeriales (*Lasiodiplodia*, *Macrophomina*, and *Neoscytalidium*), Calosphaeriales (*Pleurostoma*), Capnodiales (*Cladosporium* and *Hortaea*), Chaetothyriales (*Anthopsis*, *Arthrocladium*, *Cladophialophora*, *Cyphellophora*, *Exophiala*, *Fonsecaea*, *Knufia*, *Phialophora*, *Rhinocladiella*, and *Veronaea*), Diaporthales (*Diaporthe*), Dothideales (*Aureobasidium* and *Hormonema*), Microascales (*Knoxdaviesia*, *Microascus*, *Scedosporium*, *Scopulariopsis*, and *Triadelphia*), Ophiostomatales (*Ophiostoma* and *Sporothrix*), Pleosporales (*Alternaria*, *Bipolaris*, *Curvularia*, *Exserohilum*, and *Hongkongmyces*), Sordariales (*Phialemonium*, discussed in chapter 123, *Cladorrhinum*, "*Papulaspora*"), Togniniales (*Phaeoacremonium*), and Venturiales (*Ochroconis* and *Verruconis*). In this chapter, the genera are treated according to their ordinal relationships (Table 1). Definitions of mycological terms are provided in chapter 116.

The term dematiaceous applies to fungi with brown (containing melanin) hyphae and/or conidia in general (1), but it has been recommended in medical mycology to reserve this term for the rapidly growing members of Pleosporales only, as these are very different from Chaetothyriales in many respects. Also, the term phaeoid indicates brown hyphae; "phaeohyphomycosis" is an umbrella term for infections caused by moulds that display brownish yeast-like cells, pseudohyphae, or hyphae or a combination of these forms in host tissue (2). Conidia might be observed in infected tissue, but they are extremely uncommon (3). "Black yeasts and relatives" is preferably used to indicate members of Chaetothyriales and Dothideales only. The black yeasts are not a formal taxonomic group, but the term is applied to a wide range of unrelated melanized ascomycetous and basidiomycetous fungi that are able to produce budding yeast-like cells at some stage in their life cycle (2, 4).

Pleoanamorphism (multiple morphological forms) is particularly striking in members of the black yeasts and in the genera *Scedosporium* and *Triadelphia* (2, 5). These fungi are able to produce more than one asexual form of propagation ("synanamorphs" or "synasexual morphs"). These asexual states often were given separate names in the past, resulting in significant confusion. Further complication resulted from the fact that some fungi show either asexual or sexual morphs during different phases of their life cycle, which also used to be named separately (1, 2). Nowadays, fungal taxonomy is undergoing important changes because of the application of the "one fungus = one name" or "unitary nomenclature" concept, which should lead to a single name for a particular fungal species, giving priority to the oldest or most widely used name, depending on each particular case (6). Independently propagating asexual forms, then, are no longer assigned formal names, but the former generic names are used as descriptive nouns. Only a small percentage of clinically relevant fungal species are known to produce a sexual state ("teleomorph"), characterized by the formation of fruiting bodies with meiotic ascospores, under routine laboratory conditions. For each organism only a single sexual state can be produced (2).

TAXONOMY AND DESCRIPTION OF THE AGENTS

Botryosphaeriales

Lasiodiplodia

Lasiodiplodia is a phytopathogenic coelomycete genus characterized by spherical, thick-walled, often confluent fruiting bodies filled with asexual conidia. The conidia initially are ellipsoidal and hyaline but gradually become brown and develop a median septum at maturation. *Lasiodiplodia theobromae* (Fig. 1) (previously known as *Botryodiplodia theobromae*) is the only species well documented as an agent of human disease (7–9).

Macrophomina

Macrophomina phaseolina is a widespread plant pathogen affecting various economically important crops. It occasionally also infects immunocompromised humans. The fungus produces both dark sclerotia and pycnidia (globose to flask-shaped structures containing conidiogenous cells) on plant tissue, but clinical isolates only produce melanized mycelium and sclerotia in culture. Identification of this species is therefore mainly based on DNA sequence analyses (10, 11).

TABLE 1 Overview of the clinically relevant species of genera treated in this chapter and their attribution to the ordinal level

Order, genus, and species	Obsolete name(s), including sexual or asexual states recently synonymized by applying unitary nomenclature
Botryosphaeriales	
Lasiodiplodia theobromae	*Botryodiplodia theobromae, Diplodia theobromae*
Macrophomina phaseolina	*Macrophoma phaseolina, Tiarosporella phaseolina*
Neoscytalidium dimidiatum	*Scytalidium hyalinum, Hendersonula toruloidea, Scytalidium dimidiatum*
Calosphaeriales	
Pleurostoma	
repens	*Phialophora repens, Pleurostomophora repens*
richardsiae	*Phialophora richardsiae, Pleurostomophora richardsiae*
ochraceum	*Pleurostomophora ochracea*
Capnodiales	
Cladosporium	
cladosporioides	*Hormodendrum cladosporioides, Cladosporium herbarum f. hormodendroides*
oxysporum	*Cladosporium subtile, Cladosporium artocarpi, Cladosporium sorghi*
pseudocladosporioides	
sphaerospermum	
halotolerans	
tenuissimum	
subuliforme	
Hortaea werneckii	*Exophiala werneckii, Phaeoannellomyces werneckii*
Chaetothyriales	
Anthopsis deltoidea	
Arthrocladium fulminans	
Cladophialophora	
arxii	
bantiana	*Xylohypha bantiana, Cladosporium trichoides*
boppii	*Taeniolella boppii*
carrionii	*Cladosporium carrionii*
devriesii	*Cladosporium devriesii*
emmonsii	*Xylohypha emmonsii*
immunda	
modesta	
mycetomatis	
samoënsis	
saturnica	
Cyphellophora	
europaea	*Phialophora europaea*
fusarioides	*Pseudomicrodochium fusarioides*
laciniata	
ludoviensis	
pluriseptata	
suttonii	*Pseudomicrodochium suttonii*
Exophiala	
asiatica	
attenuata	
bergeri	
campbellii	
dermatitidis	*Wangiella dermatitidis*
equina	*Haplographium debellae-marengoi* var. *equinum*
hongkongensis	
jeanselmei	*Torula jeanselmei*
oligosperma	*Melanchlenus oligospermus*
phaeomuriformis	*Sarcinomyces phaeomuriformis*
polymorpha	
spinifera	*Phialophora spinifera*
xenobiotica	
Fonsecaea	
monophora	
nubica	
multimorphosa	
pedrosoi	*Hormodendrum pedrosoi, Fonsecaea compacta*
pugnacius	

(Continued on next page)

TABLE 1 Overview of the clinically relevant species of genera treated in this chapter and their attribution to the ordinal level *(Continued)*

Order, genus, and species	Obsolete name(s), including sexual or asexual states recently synonymized by applying unitary nomenclature
Knufia epidermidis	*Coniosporium epidermidis*
Phialophora	
americana	*Capronia semiimmersa*
chinensis	
ellipsoidea	
expanda	
macrospora	
tarda	
verrucosa	
Rhinocladiella	
mackenziei	*Ramichloridium mackenziei*
basitona	*Ramichloridium basitonum*
aquaspersa	*Acrotheca aquaspersa*
tropicalis	
similis	
Veronaea botryosa	
Diaporthales	
Diaporthe	
bougainvilleicola	*Phomopsis bougainvilleicola*
phaseolorum	*Phomopsis phaseoli*
phoenicicola	*Phomopsis phoenicicola*
longicolla	*Phomopsis longicolla*
Dothideales	
Aureobasidium	
pullulans	*Discosphaerina fulvida?*[a]
melanogenum	*Aureobasidium pullulans* var. *melanogenum*
Hormonema dematoides	*Sydowia polyspora?*
Microascales	
Knoxdaviesia dimorphospora	
Lomentospora prolificans	*Scedosporium prolificans*, *Scedosporium inflatum*
Microascus	
alveolaris	
brunneosporus	
campaniformis	
cinereus	*Scopulariopsis cinerea*
gracilis	
brunneosporus	
cirrosus	
croci	
gracilis	
intricatus	
paisi	
verrucosus	
Scedosporium	
apiospermum	*Monosporium apiospermum*
aurantiacum	
boydii	*Pseudallescheria boydii*
dehoogii	
Scopulariopsis	
asperula	
brevicaulis	*Microascus brevicaulis*
brumptii	
candida	
cordiae	
Triadelphia	
disseminata	
pulvinata	
Ophiostomatales	
Sporothrix	
brasiliensis	
chilensis	

(Continued on next page)

TABLE 1 Overview of the clinically relevant species of genera treated in this chapter and their attribution to the ordinal level *(Continued)*

Order, genus, and species	Obsolete name(s), including sexual or asexual states recently synonymized by applying unitary nomenclature
globosa	
luriei	*Sporothrix schenckii* var. *luriei*
pallida	
schenckii	
Ophiostoma piceae	
Pleosporales	
Alternaria	
alternata	*Alternaria tenuissima*
infectoria	*Lewia infectoria*
Bipolaris oryzae	
Curvularia	
americana	
australiensis	*Bipolaris australiensis, Cochliobolus australiensis, Drechslera australiensis,*
chlamydospora	
hawaiiensis	*Bipolaris hawaiiensis, Cochliobolus hawaiiensis, Drechslera hawaiiensis*
hominis	
muehlenbeckiae	
spicifera	*Bipolaris spicifera, Drechslera spicifera, Cochliobolus spicifer*
geniculata	*Cochliobolus geniculatus*
lunata	*Cochliobolus lunatus*
pseudolunata	
Exserohilum	
mcginnisii	
rostratum	*Setosphaeria rostrata*
longirostratum	
Hongkongmyces pedis	
Sordariales	
Achaetomium strumarium	*Chaetomium strumarium*
Chaetomium	
globosum	
perlucidum	
Cladorrhinum bulbillosum	*Papulaspora equi?*
Papulaspora equi	
Phialemonium obovatum	
Incertae sedis (Sordariomycetes class)	
Phialemoniopsis	*Phialemonium curvatum*
curvata	
Togniniales	
Phaeoacremonium	
alvesii	
amstelodamense	
griseorubrum	
inflatipes	
krajdenii	
minimum	
parasiticum	*Phialophora parasitica*
rubrigenum	
sphinctrophorum	
tardicrescens	
venezuelense	
Venturiales	
Ochroconis mirabilis	
Verruconis gallopava	*Ochroconis gallopava, Dactylaria gallopava, D. constricta* var. *gallopava*

[a]Names appearing with a question mark represent possible obsolete names that need to be corroborated by a thorough examination of type material and/or DNA sequence analyses.

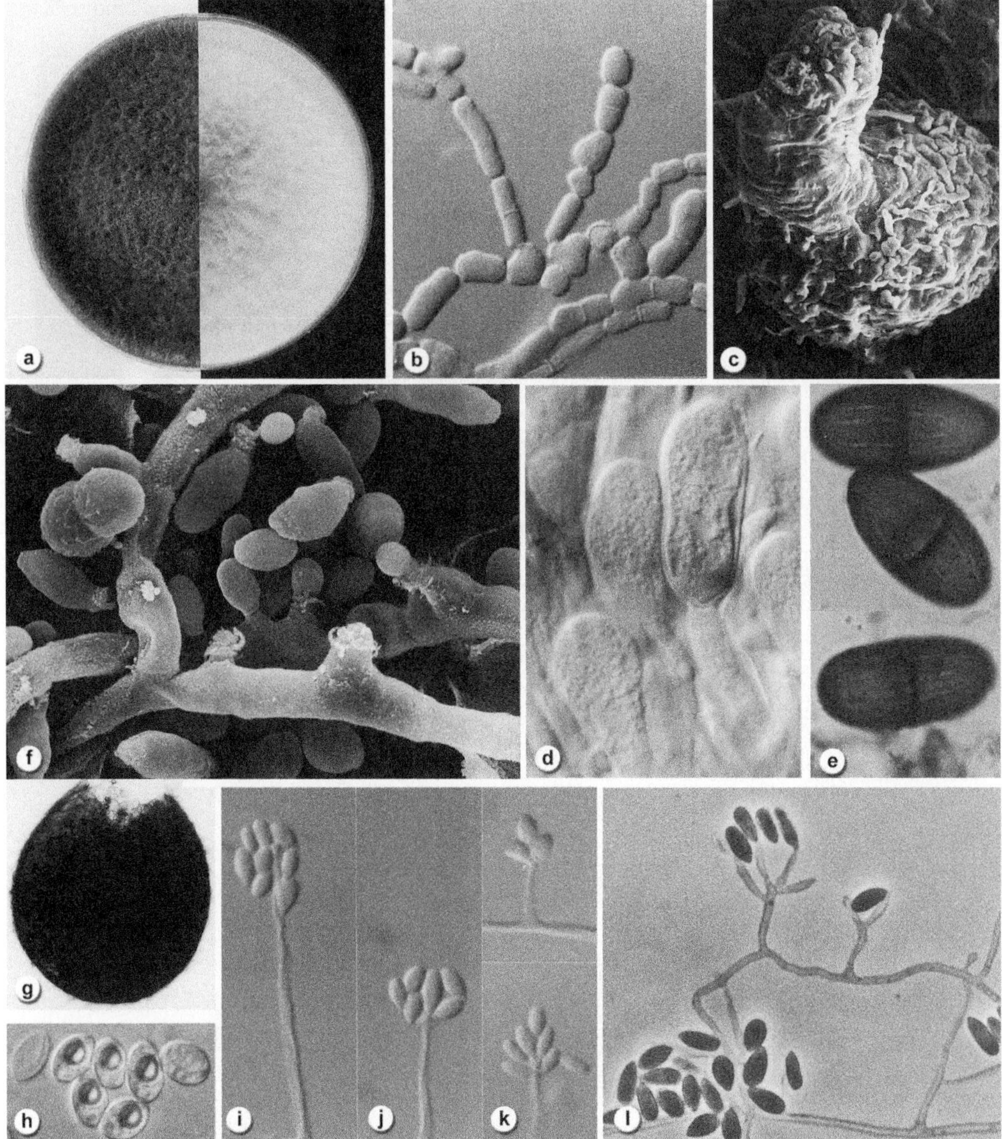

FIGURE 1 (a and b) *Neoscytalidium dimidiatum*; (c to e) *Lasiodiplodia theobromae*; (f) *Hortaea werneckii*; (g and h) *Scedosporium boydii* (sexual morph); (i to l) *Scedosporium boydii* (asexual morph). Reproduced from reference 2.

Neoscytalidium

Neoscytalidium dimidiatum (formerly known as *Scytalidium dimidiatum*) is a plant pathogen associated with a broad spectrum of infections in humans, especially affecting skin and nails (2). The fungus produces arthroconidia in culture, and some isolates also produce pycnidia under appropriate growth conditions. The coelomycetous synasexual morph has often been referred to as *Nattrassia mangiferae*, previously known as *Hendersonula toruloidea*. However, molecular studies have demonstrated that *N. dimidiatum* and *N. mangiferae* are two different species and that the latter actually belongs in the genus *Neofusicoccum* (10, 12).

Inside multilocular fruit bodies, hyaline, ellipsoidal conidia develop, which in part become brownish and have one or two septa. In culture, usually only a rapidly growing, jet black, floccose anamorph with dark arthroconidia is seen (Fig. 1); the pycnidia are only produced after 2 months of growth on a moistened plant leaf or on nutrient-poor culture media (2). Melaninless mutants, which also show reduced conidiation, were until recently referred to as *Neoscytalidium hyalinum* (= *Scytalidium hyalinum*) (13).

Calosphaeriales

Some melanized phialidic fungi were segregated from *Phialophora* on molecular grounds; these fungi now constitute small islands of clinical significance in the order Calosphaeriales, which otherwise contains plant-associated moulds. Infections are mostly of traumatic nature and are supposed to originate directly from the woody plant material of the fungal habitat (14).

Pleurostoma

Pleurostoma is a genus of mainly wood-inhabiting fungi. Hyphae are dark and bear pale, tapering phialides that may be single or aggregated in dense brushes; hyaline, slimy conidia are produced through small or large collaretes.

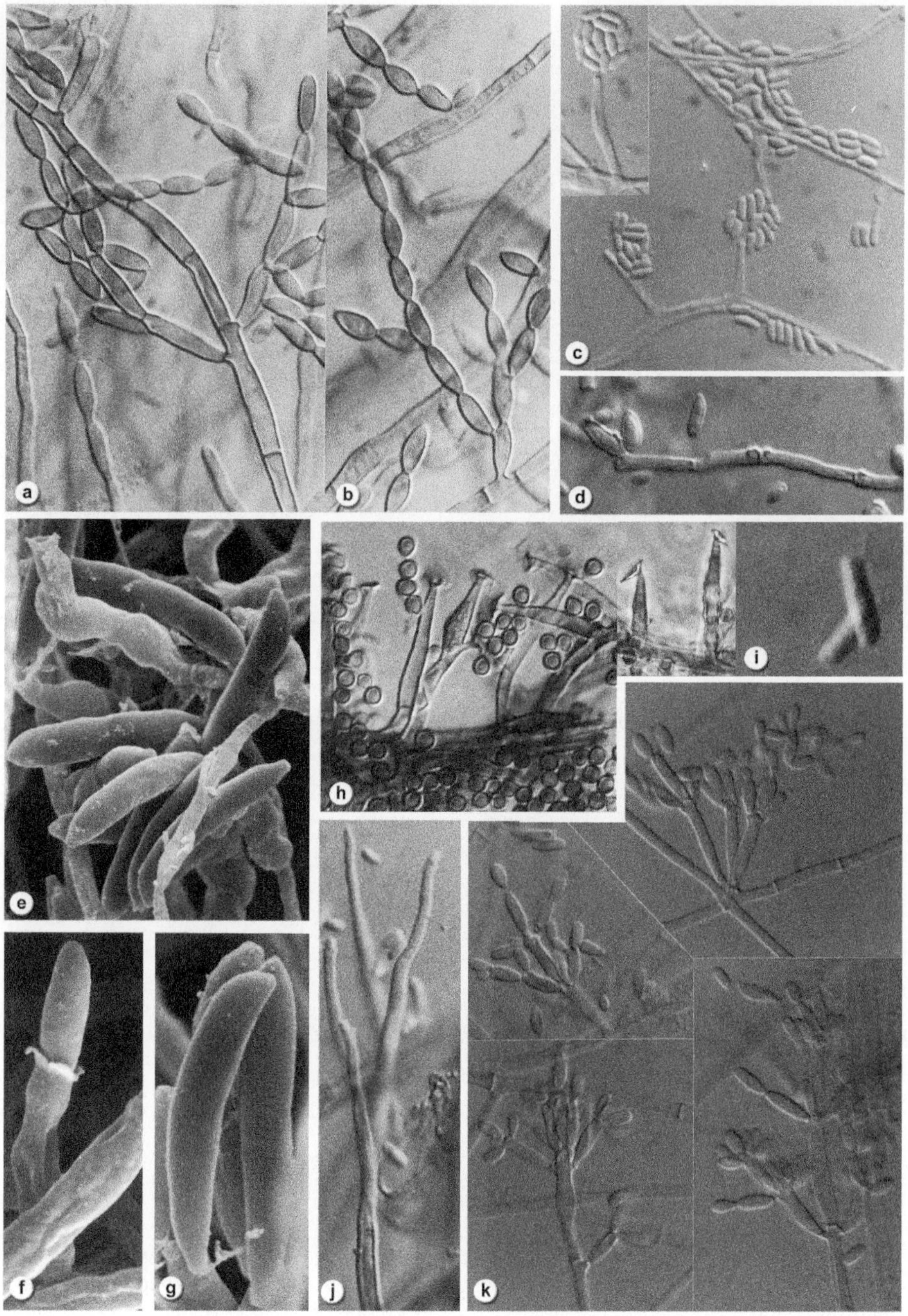

FIGURE 2 (a and b) *Cladophialophora bantiana*; (c) *Phialemoniopsis curvata*; (d) *Exophiala dermatitidis*; (e to g) *Cyphellophora pluriseptata*; (h and i) *Pleurostoma richardsiae*; (j) *Phaeoacremonium parasiticum*; (k) various pictures of *Fonsecaea pedrosoi*. Reproduced from reference 2.

Pleurostoma repens was occasionally reported from subcutaneous infections in humans. The second species of the genus also involved in human infections is *Pleurostoma richardsiae* (Fig. 2) (syn. *Phialophora richardsiae*), a soft-rot fungus on wood (14). The recently published species *Pleurostoma ochracea* is exceptional in producing yellow grains in mycetoma, which previously had been interpreted exclusively as being of bacterial nature (15). Clinically relevant *Pleurostoma* species were, until recently, named with the asexual morph name "*Pleurostomophora*" (14), but they were transferred to the sexually typified genus *Pleurostoma* in order to apply unitary nomenclature (16)

Capnodiales

Cladosporium

Species of *Cladosporium*, such as *Cladosporium cladosporioides* (Fig. 3), *C. oxysporum*, and *C. sphaerospermum*, are among the most common fungi in air and represent extremely common contaminants in the clinical laboratory, as well as allergens (2). The genus is characterized by branching acropetal chains of one-celled or septate conidia with dark scars; sexual states are rarely produced in culture. Several cladosporium-like genera have been described in recent years, but true *Cladosporium* spp. show distinctive

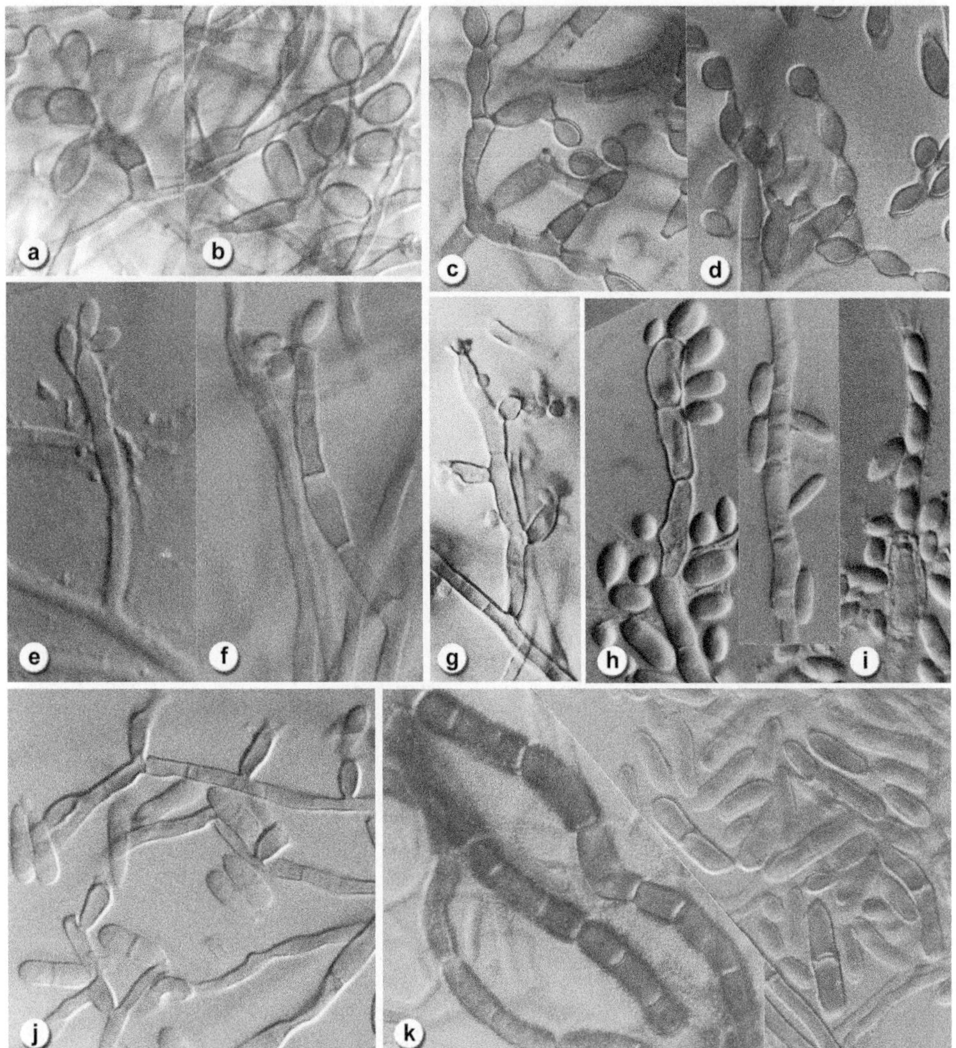

FIGURE 3 (a and b) *Rhinocladiella mackenziei;* (c and d) *Cladosporium cladosporioides;* (e and f) *Rhinocladiella aquaspersa;* (g) *Phialophora verrucosa;* (h and i) *Aureobasidium pullulans;* (j) *Verruconis gallopava;* (k) *Hormonema dematioides*. Reproduced from reference 2.

conidiogenous loci with a raised dome-shaped central zone surrounded by a rim. This has been referred to as "coronate" scar type in literature (17). *Cladosporium* spp. can be isolated from soil, plants, and water and have also been described as occasional human opportunists. Such cases need thorough evaluation, as infection by *Cladosporium* is highly unlikely. Several species probably associated with human disease are described in the reference book by de Hoog et al. (2). In a recent paper, 92 *Cladosporium* isolates obtained from diverse clinical specimens in United States were characterized by multilocus sequence analyses and morphology (18). The most frequently identified species were *C. halotolerans*, *C. tenuissimum*, and *C. pseudocladosporioides*.

Hortaea

Members of the genus *Hortaea* have rather wide hyphae that become profusely septate during growth of the fungus, and they have annellidic conidiogenesis from broad scars (2). The halophilic species *H. werneckii* (Fig. 1) lives in seawater, molluscs, evaporation ponds at the subtropical seashore, and other saline habitats and causes superficial infections. This fungus characteristically produces yeast-like, aseptate or septate elements (19). The clinical picture is known as tinea nigra (2) and is discussed in chapter 126. A second species, *H. thailandica*, has been described from leaves of *Syzygium* in Thailand (20).

Chaetothyriales

The rather small order Chaetothyriales is clinically highly relevant because many of its members are able to cause infections in humans (2). They are apparently widely distributed in nature, although difficult to isolate from environmental samples because of their slow growth rates (21).

Anthopsis

This is a small genus with peculiar ampulliform phialides that mostly appear inverted, with the collarettes near the base. The type species is *A. deltoidea*, a soilborne fungus with triangular conidia (22). A case of olecranon bursitis was attributed to this species (23), but molecular studies suggest that the clinical isolate represents a distinct, so far undescribed *Anthopsis* species (24).

Arthrocladium

The genus *Arthrocladium* currently includes four species mostly occurring on plant material and ant nests. One of them, *A. fulminans*, has been reported from infections in immunocompromised and otherwise healthy patients. Cultures of this fungus do not produce conidia, but moniliform hyphae and chlamydospore-like structures can be observed. Species identification relies on DNA sequence comparisons (25, 26).

Cladophialophora

This genus is characterized by the production of dry, rather coherent chains of conidia that usually lack dark scars. Conidiophores are mostly undifferentiated. This genus contains 11 pathogenic species (Table 1), many of which are almost exclusively known from humans and other warm-blooded animals (2, 27, 28). However, members of this genus also can be found in soil and on plant material (21, 27). The most significant species are *Cladophialophora bantiana* and *C. carrionii*. *C. bantiana*, a remarkable neurotropic mould, is recognizable by very long, poorly branched conidial chains and by an ability to grow at 40°C (Fig. 2; see also Fig. 5). This fungus can cause central nervous system phaeohyphomycosis and other infections in otherwise healthy individuals (2). It has a characteristic 558-bp intron at position 1768 of the small-subunit (SSU) ribosomal operon (29). *C. carrionii* is a common agent of chromoblastomycosis, with small conidia in profusely branched chains, and sometimes shows a phialidic synasexual state (2). Several clinically relevant *Cladophialophora* spp. were studied by de Hoog et al. (2) and Badali et al. (27, 28). They may be difficult to differentiate, and recent studies have revealed the existence of morphologically similar environmental siblings (21, 30). Accurate species identification in this group of fungi, therefore, should be supported by DNA sequence analyses.

Cyphellophora

Cyphellophora (including clinical species previously placed in *Pseudomicrodochium*) is a rather uncommon genus of phialidic hyphomycetes inhabiting soil, plant material, and river sediments (21, 31). Traditionally, they have been characterized by slender, curved, transversely septate conidia (2). Several phialophora-like species with one-celled conidia proved to cluster with *Cyphellophora* spp. and were therefore recently transferred to this genus (21, 32). All these fungi reside in Cyphellophoraceae, whereas the type species of *Phialophora* is a member of Herpotrichiellaceae (33). Cultures of *Cyphellophora* spp. are evenly melanized and show limited expansion growth. Conidia are generally produced from poorly developed collarettes alongside the hyphae, but discrete phialides also may be observed. Clinically relevant species, such as *Cyphellophora europaea*, *C. laciniata*, *C. pluriseptata*, and *C. reptans* (Fig. 2), are rare etiological agents of superficial mycoses (2). *Cyphellophora suttonii* was reported as the causative agent of a subcutaneous infection in a dog (34) and probably a respiratory tract infection in a human (35). *Cyphellophora ludoviensis* was recently reported from a case of chromoblastomycosis (36). The incidence of these fungi is probably low, but they are likely to be underdiagnosed.

Exophiala

Exophiala is the main genus of clinically relevant black yeasts. Strains usually show a high degree of morphological plasticity. Most isolates initially produce a yeast-like thallus but subsequently produce regular hyphae as well as filaments with frequent constrictions referred to as "moniliform hyphae." As a result, colonies are moist and slimy at first, becoming velvety to wooly with age. The process of conidium production is typically annellidic, from narrow, inconspicuous scars or extensions (4). Occasionally, a very slowly growing, meristematic morphology ("*Sarcinomyces*") can be observed (2, 37). Fresh isolates or strains cultivated on nutritionally deficient media frequently produce conidia in chains and may produce scattered or compacted phialides with huge collarettes (4, 38). The most frequently reported species are *Exophiala dermatitidis* (Fig. 2) and *E. jeanselmei sensu lato*. The latter has been subdivided into a number of taxa, such as *E. oligosperma*, *E. bergeri*, and *E. xenobiotica*, on molecular grounds; they are difficult to distinguish morphologically (39, 40). *E. dermatitidis* is recognizable morphologically by phialides without collarettes, which are wide and by conidiogenous cells with scar-like, very short, annellated zones. In addition, growth at 40°C and the inability to assimilate nitrate are characteristic (41). The related species *E. phaeomuriformis* differs by having a growth maximum at 38°C (37). The less frequent species *E. spinifera* can be recognized by the presence of large, stiff conidiophores (2). Recently, a similar species with reduced conidiogenous cells, *E. attenuata*, was described (39). DNA sequence analyses are strongly recommended for a reliable identification of *Exophiala* spp.

Fonsecaea

The genus *Fonsecaea* currently includes five pathogenic species, roughly characterized by dry, usually short, and more or less compact chains of conidia. In culture, *Fonsecaea* species mostly have one morphological form, but they may produce additional phialophora-like phialides with collarettes and rhinocladiella-like sympodial conidiophores (2). No budding cells are produced on routine media. *Fonsecaea pedrosoi* (Fig. 2, including the mutant *F. compacta*) is one of the main etiologic agents of human chromoblastomycosis. Two other agents of this disease, but also implicated in phaeohyphomycosis, *F. monophora* and *F. nubica* (42, 43), are morphologically indistinguishable but are recognized by DNA sequence analyses. A morphologically similar species, *F. pugnacius*, was recently reported from a case of chromoblastomycosis that disseminated to the central nervous system. Remarkably, the fungus produced meristematic cells in the skin but formed melanized hyphae in brain tissue (44). *Fonsecaea multimorphosa*, described from a cerebral infection in a cat, presents a cladophialophora-like synasexual state and chlamydospores in culture (45). In addition to these medically relevant species, *Fonsecaea* includes saprophytic, apparently nonpathogenic taxa, such as *F. erecta* and *F. minima*, which occur on plant material (46).

Knufia

Although most species of *Knufia* have been described as colonizers of rock and marble building walls, they are occasionally found as colonizers of human skin and nails. *Knufia epidermidis* (= *Coniosporium epidermidis*) has been reported from a superficial form of phaeohyphomycosis (47). Species of this genus show a high degree of morphological plasticity and may be able to produce phialides, arthroconidia, holoblastic conidia, endoconidia (conidia produced within an intercalary "mother cell"), and yeast-like budding elements in culture (48). *K. epidermidis* produces holoblastic conidia, arthroconidia, and meristematic cells in culture (47, 48).

Phialophora

In *Phialophora sensu stricto*, phialides appear as discrete conidiogenous cells in a poorly developed conidiogenous apparatus or as intercalary cells with lateral openings; they show conspicuous collarettes and produce unicellular, subglobose, tear-shaped, or (sub)cylindrical conidia in slimy masses. Moniliform hyphae and meristematic cells may also be observed. Yeast cells are typically absent in *Phialophora*, but budding conidia can be observed in certain species (49). The genus was phylogenetically heterogeneous because the type species, *P. verrucosa*, belongs in the family Herpotrichiellaceae, whereas many members of *Phialophora sensu lato* proved to be related to the genus *Cyphellophora*, which remained in an uncertain position within Chaeotothyriales. Réblová et al. (32) transferred many of those species to *Cyphellophora* and erected the family Cyphellophoraceae. In a recent phylogenetic study, five species were recognized in *Phialophora sensu stricto* by Li et al. (49). These fungi occur in association with diverse substrates, including plant debris, wood, straw, soil, and coal. In humans, these organisms are associated with different forms of phaeohyphomycosis, chromoblastomycosis, and occasionally mycetoma (2, 49). *Phialophora verrucosa*, with darkened, funnel-shaped collarettes (Fig. 3), is one of the best-known species of this genus. *Phialophora americana* differs mainly by having vase-shaped collarettes (33). Morphologically similar phialidic fungi belonging to other orders are now classified in genera such as *Cadophora*, *Gaeumannomyces*, *Phaeoacremonium*, and *Pleurostoma* (16, 21, 50).

Rhinocladiella

Rhinocladiella is characterized by melanized sympodial conidiophores bearing noncatenate one-celled conidia on denticles and occasionally shows exophiala-like budding cells in culture (51). It comprises five pathogenic species, *R. aquaspersa* (Fig. 3), *R. mackenziei* (Fig. 3), *R. basitona*, *R. similis*, and *R. tropicalis*, that are polyphyletic within the Chaetothyriales. *Rhinocladiella atrovirens* has been reported to cause cerebral phaeohyphomycosis in an AIDS patient (52), but as this species in a modern, molecular circumscription is limited to isolates growing on conifer wood in northern countries, that case probably concerned the sibling species *R. similis* (53). *Rhinocladiella aquaspersa* and *R. tropicalis* are rare agents of chromoblastomycosis, and the former species may also cause phaeohyphomycosis (36, 54). The neurotropic species *R. mackenziei* is endemic in the Middle East and is morphologically similar to *Pleurothecium obovoideum* (formerly *Ramichloridium obovoideum*). For a long time, these fungi were thought to be conspecific, but phylogenetically they belong in different orders of Ascomycota (*P. obovoideum* belongs to the Sordariales) (51). *R. basitona* has been reported from different forms of phaeohyphomycosis in humans (55).

Veronaea

The genus *Veronaea* includes one clinically relevant taxon, *V. botryosa*, as well as numerous saprophytes. *Veronaea botryosa* shows a conidiogenous apparatus similar to that of *Rhinocladiella* spp., consisting of a melanized, sympodial rachis with denticles. The conidia, however, are one-septate (2). Numerous cases of phaeohyphomycosis by this agent have been published, mostly involving the skin and subcutaneous tissue. Cases tend to be severe and many of them are associated with CARD9 immune disorder (56).

Diaporthales

Diaporthe

Diaporthe is a species-rich genus of plant pathogens, endophytes, and saprophytes with widespread geographical distribution (57). At least four members of this genus have been reported from human infections, *D. bougainvilleicola*, *D. phaseolorum*, *D. phoenicicola*, and *D. longicolla* (58–61), but some clinical isolates have been identified only to genus level (62, 63). Reports often used the asexual morph name *Phomopsis*, but the application of unitary nomenclature has given preference to *Diaporthe*, the name traditionally used for the sexual state (57). In culture, these fungi may produce pycnidia with two types of conidia, i.e., oval to fusoid "alpha conidia" and thin, curved or bent, elongated "beta conidia" (57). However, intraspecific morphological variability and the inability of some isolates to sporulate in culture often demand the use of DNA sequence data to achieve species-level identifications (61, 64).

Dothideales

The order Dothideales comprises numerous saprophytes that thrive well under conditions of decreased water activity, such as on sugary leaf surfaces, rocks, glass, and moist medical devices (65).

Aureobasidium

The genus *Aureobasidium* contains a number of saprophytic, black yeast-like species associated with diverse substrates, including soil, plant leaves, water, foodstuffs, and oligotrophic environments such as rocks and stone monument surfaces (4, 66). Two members of this genus, i.e., *A. pullulans* and *A. melanogenum*, are recognized as agents of phaeohyphomycosis in humans, ranging from mild cutaneous infections to invasive, life-threatening disease (67). *Aureobasidium* spp. are recognized by the production of budding yeast-like elements and both hyaline and thin-walled, as well as melanized and thick-walled hyphae, with segments becoming dark brown chlamydospores in age. Conidia are produced from both types of hyphae by blastic, synchronous conidiogenous cells. Endoconidia are sometimes also observed. *A. melanogenum* is easily distinguished from *A. pullulans* by the ability of the former to produce cultures that are characteristically black from the beginning owing to the abundant production of strongly melanized arthroconidia and dark synchronous conidia; in *A. pullulans*, evident melanization of the colonies usually takes about 2 weeks to develop, and colonies are typically pinkish but may develop radial dark brown areas (66).

Hormonema

One species of this genus, *H. dematioides*, has been reported as an occasional agent of phaeohyphomycosis. This fungus is morphologically similar to *Aureobasidium* but produces conidia in a basipetal succession with the youngest at the base, not synchronously as in *Aureobasidium* (2, 4). In addition, DNA sequence-based phylogenies proved that *Aureobasidium* and *Hormonema* are different genera (68).

Microascales

Among the clinically relevant genera of Microascales, *Knoxdaviesia*, *Lomentospora*, *Microascus*, *Scopulariopsis*, *Scedosporium*, and *Triadelphia* can be mentioned. Phylogenetic studies have recently determined great changes in the nomenclature of most of these genera.

Knoxdaviesia

This genus currently includes nine species, characterized by well-developed, brown, simple conidiophores bearing a whorl of phialides at the apex; conidia are (sub)hyaline, aseptate, and cylindrical to allantoid and are produced in slimy masses. One species of *Knoxdaviesia* has been reported from human infection, *K. dimorphospora*, which can easily be distinguished from other members of the genus by its production of a synasexual morph, with phialides appearing mostly laterally on undifferentiated hyphae, and ellipsoid, pale brown conidia. The typical robust brown conidiophores generate cylindrical conidia with an obtuse apex and a truncate base (69).

Lomentospora

A single medically relevant species in this genus is known, *L. prolificans*. This fungus was treated in earlier literature as "*Scedosporium prolificans*" (= *S. inflatum*) on account of its elongated annellidic conidiogenous cells and obovoid conidia produced in slimy masses (2). Molecular studies, however, proved that *L. prolificans* is phylogenetically distant from true *Scedosporium* species. Phenotypically, the production of more strongly melanized, rather flat colonies, the presence of a swollen basal zone in the conidiogenous cells and a high resistance to voriconazole separate *L. prolificans* from true *Scedosporium* spp. (70).

Microascus

The genus *Microascus* was previously considered to represent the sexual state of *Scopulariopsis*, but multilocus phylogenies proved the type species of these genera to belong in clearly separate clades, supporting their current status as different genera. Species of *Microascus* are characterized by dark brown to black, globose to ampulliform ascomata, with a papilla or a more or less developed neck; ascospores are one-celled, reniform to ellipsoid, triangular or quadrangular, straw-colored or light brown, with a conspicuous germ pore. The asexual states produce ampulliform to lageniform conidiogenous cells with a narrow cylindrical annellated zone, singly or on penicillate conidiophores; conidia are one celled, pale yellowish to dark brown, and smooth to finely roughened and appear in dry basipetal chains. Although a broad clinical spectrum has been associated with this genus in previous literature, most of the clinical isolates from a recent phylogenetic revision (71) originated from respiratory samples and synovial fluid. Species associated with human infections from that revision include *M. cinereus*, *M. gracilis*, *M. brunneosporus*, and other taxa listed in Table 1.

Scopulariopsis

Members of this genus are characterized by globose to pyriform, black ascomata with an ostiole, papillate or with a conspicuous neck; ascospores are one celled, asymmetrical, broadly reniform or lunate, with or without a conspicuous germ pore. The asexual states typically show annellides mostly arranged penicillately on conidiophores but sometimes appearing singly or in small groups on short stalks; conidia are one-celled, hyaline to brown, with a pointed or rounded apex and a truncate base, smooth to rough-walled, formed in basipetal dry chains (71). This genus includes several clinically relevant taxa, such as *S. asperula*, *S. brevicaulis*, and *S. candida*, implicated mostly in skin and nail infections, but occasionally also in deep, more severe disease (2). Species obtained from clinical samples, included in a recent revision (71), are listed in Table 1.

Scedosporium

Species of this genus are characterized by relatively fast growing, usually grayish colonies with abundant aerial mycelium and (sub)cylindrical, relatively long conidiophores with annellides; conidia are obovoid and subhyaline but tend to become brown with age. Conidia may also be produced laterally on undifferentiated hyphae or on short pedicels. In addition, a synnematous synasexual state is sometimes observed in culture. Sexual states of *Scedosporium* traditionally were placed in *Pseudallescheria* and typically consist of (sub)globose cleistothecia producing one-celled, fusiform to ellipsoid, melanized ascospores (2). When dual nomenclature was still in use, its application caused much confusion in this group of organisms (72, 73). One of the main clinically relevant species, *Scedosporium apiospermum*, used to be considered as the asexual state of *Pseudallescheria boydii* (2). However, it is currently accepted that *P. boydii* and *S. apiospermum* are two different species, the former homothallic and the latter heterothallic. The separation of these taxa is also supported by molecular data (72, 73). The application of unitary nomenclature led to the choice of *Scedosporium* as the correct name for this genus, and therefore certain names in *Pseudallescheria* needed to be transferred to *Scedosporium*. Currently, the main *Scedosporium* species of clinical importance are *S. apiospermum*, *S. aurantiacum*, *S. boydii*, and *S. dehoogii*, which are associated with various forms of phaeohyphomycosis and occasionally also mycetoma in humans (2, 70, 72, 73).

Triadelphia

This genus currently includes 17 species, most of which can produce multiple asexual morphs in culture. *Triadelphia* is polyphyletic, but many species have not been represented in molecular studies (74). Two species, *T. pulvinata* and *T. disseminata*, have been involved in phaeohyphomycoses in immunocompetent or immunocompromised individuals in Saudi Arabia. These species produce three synasexual morphs and can be distinguished by differences in the size and septation of conidia and by their internal transcribed spacer region (ITS) sequences (5, 75, 76).

Ophiostomatales

Ophiostomatales is a large order of plant-pathogenic and saprophytic fungi. Some of them are blue-stain fungi in wood and live in association with arthropods. Only a few species are human or animal pathogens. The main sexually typified genus is *Ophiostoma* (77).

Ophiostoma

This genus is characterized by the production of subglobose, dark perithecia with evanescent asci and long necks from which hyaline ascospores are extruded in slimy droplets. For decades a close phylogenetic relationship between *Ophiostoma* and *Sporothrix*, an important human pathogenic hyphomycete genus, has been recognized (78). Since multilocus phylogenetic studies revealed that clinically relevant *Sporothrix* species (including the type species, *S. schenckii*) belonged to a subclade within a broader *Ophiostoma sensu lato* clade, one of these genera had to be given priority under unitary nomenclature. *Sporothrix* is an older genus, but choosing it instead of *Ophiostoma* would require transferring over 100 species from the latter genus to the former one, including economically important plant pathogens. A choice was made to retain the name *Sporothrix* for the group containing *S. schenckii* and related species and to keep *Ophiostoma* as a species-rich, paraphyletic entity (77). Practically all clinically relevant Ophiostomatales belong to *Sporothrix sensu stricto*, except *Ophiostoma piceae*, which caused a fatal invasive infection in an immunocompromised patient. The fungus produced yeast-like cells and septate hyphae in tissue, and similar elements in cultures on routine mycological media. Morphological features were not remarkable, but chlamydospore-like cells and cycloheximide tolerance were reported. Species-level identification required DNA sequence analyses (79).

Sporothrix

In natural environments, or in cultures at 25°C, *Sporothrix schenckii* has colorless hyphae that produce poorly differentiated conidiophores bearing a cluster of thin denticles with hyaline, tear-shaped conidia at their tips. Additional subglobose to elongated, sessile conidia may or may not be present; conidia are the only melanized part of the fungus. The mould can be transformed *in vitro* to a stable yeast form at 37°C on enriched media such as chocolate agar or brain heart infusion agar. Occasional isolates are difficult to convert and may require multiple subcultures and extended incubation. Transition is observed in environmental as well as clinical isolates (2, 80, 81). The disease caused by this fungus is called "sporotrichosis" and ranges from localized fixed cutaneous lesions to lymphocutaneous or even disseminated disease, depending largely on the immunological status of the host (82).

Recent molecular studies have demonstrated that *S. schenckii sensu lato* is a complex of numerous phylogenetic species (83). The combination of phenotypic (morphology of the sessile pigmented conidia; growth at 30, 35, and 37°C; and assimilation of sucrose, raffinose, and ribitol) and genetic (analysis of the calmodulin gene sequences and other markers) approaches allows differentiation of some of these species. Apart from *S. schenckii sensu stricto*, the species *S. brasiliensis*, *S. globosa*, and *S. luriei* are also involved in human sporotrichosis (81, 84). *S. brasiliensis* is highly virulent and has caused large epidemics in Brazil; transmission occurs particularly through stray cats (85). *S. globosa* seems to be less aggressive and is mainly prevalent in Asia, where children in particular are infected (86), but some cases in the Americas also have been reported. *S. luriei* is a rare species that only has been reported from South Africa, India, and Italy (84). Recently, two additional *Sporothrix* spp., i.e., *S. pallida* and *S. chilensis*, have been reported from superficial infections involving human cornea and nails, respectively (87, 88).

Pleosporales

Most members of the order Pleosporales have rapidly expanding, floccose colonies, which show optimal conidium production on media poor in nutrients, such as oatmeal agar or potato carrot agar. Conidia are usually large and then easily visible with the aid of a stereomicroscope. Conidia are generally produced on septate, dark brown, erect, often geniculate (zig-zag–shaped) conidiophores with integrated conidiogenous cells showing minute pores ("tretic" conidiogenous cells). Conidia consist of several compartments. "True septa" are found in those conidia in which the outer wall and septum are continuous; such conidia are called "euseptate" (as in *Alternaria*). "False septa," in contrast, are observed in those conidia in which only the inner wall layers are involved in septation and the outer wall forms a sac-like structure around the individual cells; such conidia are called "distoseptate" (in *Bipolaris*, *Curvularia*, and *Exserohilum*) (89–91).

Alternaria

Since most clinical strains are very likely to belong to only two species complexes of *Alternaria*, *Alternaria infectoria* and *A. alternata*, isolates are easily identified down to the species complex level. Available criteria comprise characteristics of growth, sporulation, and morphology and very large differences in the ITS rDNA, which can be displayed by sequencing or by restriction fragment length polymorphisms (92). *A. infectoria* in tissue may present with hyaline yeast cells rather than melanized hyphae. Cultures of *A. infectoria*, in contrast to those of *A. alternata*, frequently exhibit creamish patches and show reduced sporulation. Conidia of *A. infectoria* bear long apical beaks that serve as secondary conidiophores. *A. alternata* displays conidia in chains (2, 90). The genus *Ulocladium*, associated with occasional cases of phaeohyphomycosis, was recently revealed by multilocus phylogenies to be synonymous with *Alternaria*. Species traditionally placed in *Ulocladium* usually show conidiophores more geniculate than those of *A. infectoria* and *A. alternata* and have more rounded conidia that are in contact with the conidiogenous cells from a narrow conidial base (2, 90, 92, 93).

Bipolaris

Relatively common opportunists traditionally treated in *Bipolaris* include *Bipolaris australiensis*, *B. hawaiiensis* (Fig. 4), and *B. spicifera*. They are characterized by large, ellipsoid to subcylindrical, rather straight conidia with conspicuous distosepta and a dark, flat basal scar (2, 89). These species, however, recently proved to belong to a phylogenetically and morphologically well-characterized group within the genus *Curvularia*, called the "*spicifera* clade" (91). These species are associated with a range of forms of phaeohyphomycosis, especially invasive and noninvasive sinusitis (2, 94). *Bipolaris oryzae*, a true member of *Bipolaris sensu stricto*, can cause corneal ulcers in humans (95). This fungus differs from *Curvularia sensu stricto* by producing long conidia that mostly appear gently curved but lack an asymmetrically swollen, darker intermediate cell (89, 96).

Curvularia

Members of this genus usually produce elongated conidia that are inconspicuously distoseptate (the outer and inner conidial wall layers can be seen in young conidia, but both layers usually appear too close together to be distinguished in mature ones with light microscopy) and often possess an intermediate, asymmetrically swollen cell that gives the conidia a typically curved appearance (89, 96). This typical conidial shape is observed in the type species, *C. lunata* (Fig. 4), and in several other species of clinical relevance, such as *C. aeria*, *C. americana*, *C. geniculata*, *C. hominis*, *C. muehlenbeckiae*, and *C. senegalensis* (89, 91, 96). Many species that produce conidia with conspicuous distosepta and lack an asymmetrically swollen intermediate cell, however, also cluster in *Curvularia*, as previously mentioned (96). The clinical spectrum of *Curvularia* spp. is quite broad, ranging from superficial skin infections and corneal ulcers to mycetoma and invasive phaeohyphomycoses (2, 94).

Exserohilum

Exserohilum is characterized by very long, distoseptate conidia with a distinct, protruding basal hilum (89). Three species have been recognized as opportunistic agents in humans and other vertebrates, i.e., *Exserohilum longirostratum*, *E. mcginnisii*, and *E. rostratum* (Fig. 4) (2, 94). These three species are phylogenetically closely related, and their

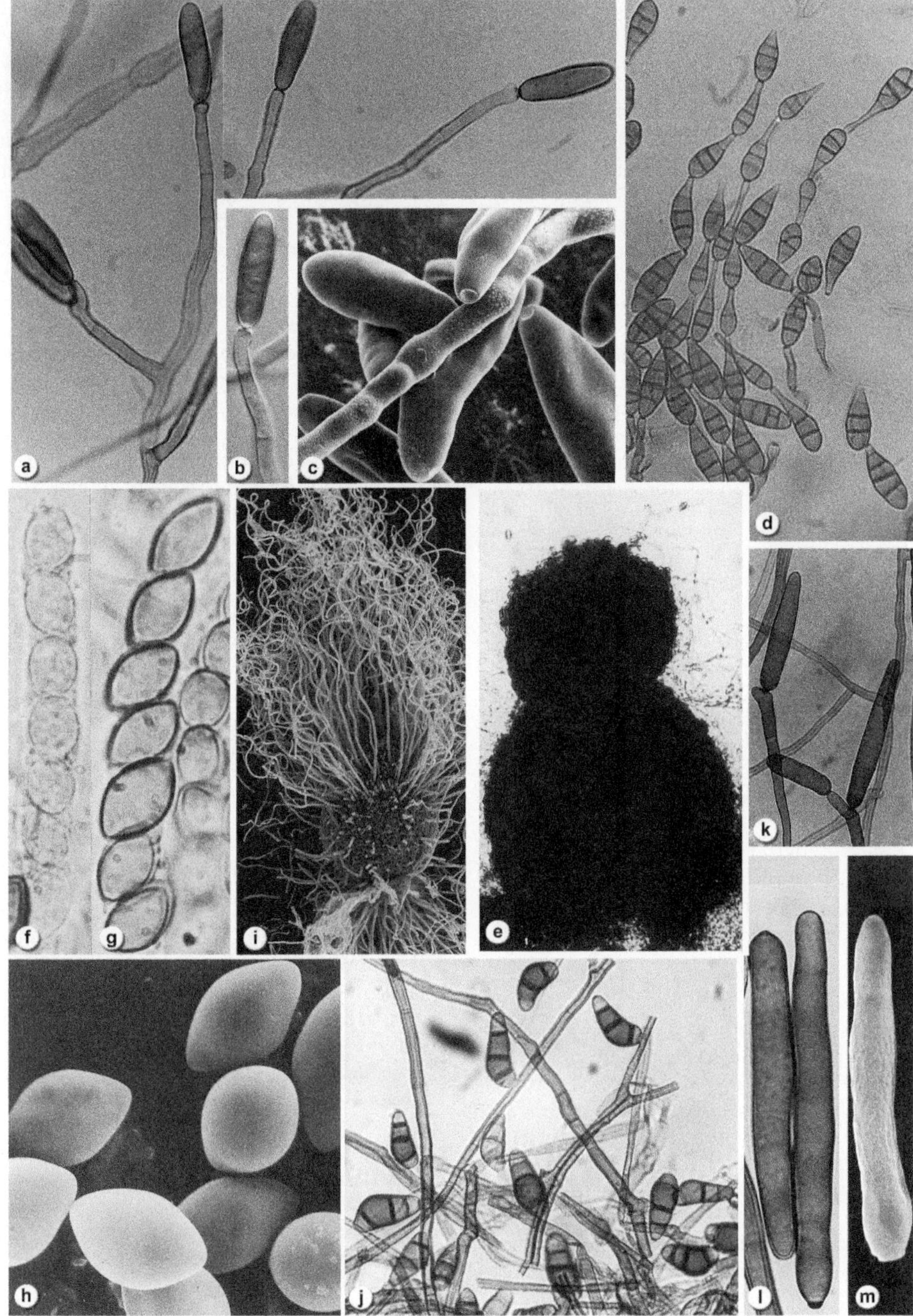

FIGURE 4 (a to c) *Curvularia hawaiiensis*; (d) *Alternaria alternata*; (e to h) *Achaetomium strumarium*; (i) *Chaetomium globosum*; (j) *Curvularia lunata*; (k to m) *Exserohilum rostratum*. Reproduced from reference 2.

boundaries deserve further study (97). The clinical spectrum of these fungi includes sinusitis, keratitis, endophthalmitis, peritonitis, endocarditis, and other deep-seated forms of phaeohyphomycosis (2, 94).

Hongkongmyces

The genus *Hongkongmyces* was recently erected to accommodate a sterile pleosporalean fungus isolated from a case of subcutaneous phaeohyphomycosis. The type species, *H. pedis*, was determined by DNA sequence data to be a member of Lindgomycetaceae, a family of Pleosporales that mostly encompasses aquatic fungi and does not include any other human pathogen (98).

Sordariales

Sordariales is a large and diverse order of ascomycetes. *Madurella mycetomatis* was proven to be a member of Sordariales, belonging in Chaetomiaceae (99); this species is treated in chapter 128. The genera *Phialemonium*, *Chaetomium*, and *Achaetomium* are treated in chapter 123. Currently, the genus *Phialemoniopsis* is *incertae sedis* in class Sordariomycetes (100).

Clinical strains producing bulbil-like clumps of strongly melanized cells often have been referred to as "*Papulaspora* spp." They may show a phialidic synasexual morph and do not produce sexual structures in culture. Molecular studies revealed that such "*Papulaspora*" strains often represent opportunistic members of Sordariales that are phylogenetically distant from the type species of *Papulaspora*, *P. sepedonioides* (Melanosporales) (101).

Cladorrhinum

Species of *Cladorrhinum* produce aseptate conidia in slimy masses mostly from intercalary conidiogenous cells with lateral phialidic openings ("pleurophialides"). Members of this genus are related to sexual morphs traditionally placed in the Lasiosphaeriaceae (102). The genus contains about eight species (103), and one of them, *C. bulbillosum*, has been reported from eye infections affecting humans and a horse (104–106). *C. bulbillosum* grows rapidly at 37°C and even at 40°C (107). This thermotolerance, the production of subglobose to tear-shaped conidia and abundant microsclerotia, and the absence of sterile setiform hyphae in culture characterize this species (104, 107). Some strains, however, remain sterile on mycological culture media and require DNA sequence analyses for identification (106, 107).

Togniniales

Phaeoacremonium

Phaeoacremonium is morphologically characterized by warted mycelium and slender, tubular, and often tapering or inflated brown phialides. Hyaline, slimy conidia are produced through inconspicuous collarettes. The sexual state was named *Togninia* and is characterized by perithecia with long necks and paraphyses, and 8-spored asci with hyaline, aseptate, ellipsoid to allantoid ascospores. Following unitary nomenclature, the name *Phaeoacremonium* was chosen for usage instead of the latter (108). Eleven species are associated with human disease (Table 1), *Phaeoacremonium parasiticum* (Fig. 2) being one of the most common.

Venturiales

Ochroconis (and *Verruconis*)

The genus *Ochroconis* is paraphyletic (a group of fungi that includes some, but not all, of the descendants from a common ancestor) in the family Sympoventuriaceae (109). All species have rust brown to olivaceous colonies and produce 1- to 3-septate conidia from small, open denticles inserted in low numbers on sympodial cells. Members of *Ochroconis sensu lato* are occasional agents of phaeohyphomycosis in various vertebrates, ranging from cutaneous lesions to deep-seated infections involving the lungs, brain, and other organs (110). Molecular distances within *Ochroconis sensu lato* are considerable; for this reason, the neurotropic species *O. gallopava* (Fig. 3), with hyaline, clavate, strongly ornamented conidia and growing well at 40°C, was reallocated to a separate genus, *Verruconis*, whereas mesophilic species were retained in *Ochroconis* (109).

EPIDEMIOLOGY AND TRANSMISSION

Phaeohyphomycosis

Phaeohyphomycoses are usually subcutaneous but can also be systemic or involve the central nervous system (111). Dematiaceous fungi are also able to cause superficial infections, such as those of the skin and nails (28, 67, 112). Infections of the central nervous system (CNS) are frequently manifested as brain abscesses or meningitis, which are usually fatal. In these infections, fungi can be present in the cerebrospinal fluid. Many cases are produced in immunocompetent patients. Typical symptoms include headache, neurologic deficits, and seizures. Common neurotropic species are *Cladophialophora bantiana*, *Ramichloridium mackenziei*, *Verruconis gallopava*, and *Exophiala dermatitidis*. The fungus probably disseminates from a primary pulmonary focus to the CNS, but other routes are possible, including dissemination from skin or subcutaneous lesions (43, 44, 113). The fungi most commonly involved in phaeohyphomycosis are *Exophiala xenobiotica*, *E. jeanselmei*, *E. dermatitidis*, *E. spinifera*, *C. bantiana*, and *Curvularia* spp. Superficial infections are mostly caused by *Alternaria* spp., *Neoscytalidium dimidiatum*, and black, yeast-like species such as *Exophiala oligosperma*, *Cyphellophora europaea*, and *Hortaea werneckii* (31, 112–114).

The route of (sub)cutaneous infection and keratitis is likely to be traumatic implantation, with the fungus causing an inflammatory reaction with pigmented hyphae and sometimes also yeast-like elements in tissue (111). In tinea nigra, by contrast, the etiological agent, *H. werneckii*, probably finds on the surface of human skin conditions of humidity, PH, salinity, etc., which are not too different from those of its natural habitats, favoring colonization of the stratum corneum (2, 19). Chromoblastomycosis leads to excessive proliferation of skin layers, with muriform cells being the invasive form. The development of either phaeohyphomycosis or chromoblastomycosis in black, yeast-like chaetothyrialean fungi is largely species specific, although certain etiological agents, e.g., *Phialophora verrucosa sensu lato*, may cause both types of infection (49, 115). The species that cause subcutaneous infections are often uncommon in the environment and occupy hitherto poorly known habitats. Some thermotolerant species seem to be associated with environmental xenobiotics or occur in animal feces (40, 116); others are found on slightly osmotic surfaces such as fruit (4). Psychrophilic species that cause infections in cold-blooded vertebrates are frequent in water of lakes and oceans, municipal drinking water, hospital water, and in river sediments (21, 117–119). In the indoor environment, *Exophiala* has been found in steam baths (120) and dishwashers (121). Members of the Pleosporales such as *Alternaria*, *Bipolaris*, *Curvularia*, and *Exserohilum* cause disease in numerous plant hosts but also occur as saprophytes on decaying plant material and in soil (89, 90). They may be encountered in allergic or invasive sinusitis of human and cattle, in lesions of the skin and subcutaneous tissue, in onychomycosis, keratomycosis, and other infections (2, 91, 92, 94, 95, 97, 114). Many members of the Dothideales are tolerant of extreme growth conditions and are found in Antarctic or Mediterranean rock (122) or in hypersaline ponds (65). These species can transition morphologically to a stress-tolerant, meristematic ecotype consisting of clumps of amorphous, thick-walled, highly melanized cells that may eventually fall apart into small cell clumps. Most clinically relevant Botryosphaeriales, Diaporthales, and Togniniales included in this chapter are plant pathogens (12, 57, 108), whereas the Microascales, Sordariales, and Venturiales treated here are mostly soilborne saprophytes, degraders of cellulose-rich substrates, and endophytes (70–73, 75, 101–107, 109, 110).

Chromoblastomycosis

Chromoblastomycosis is one of the most frequently found subcutaneous mycoses. It occurs usually in the tropical and subtropical regions, affecting mainly adult males working in agriculture or related activities. The fact that males are predominantly affected has been related to a possible role of human sex hormones, but probably occupational factors also favor exposure to the etiological agents (123, 124).

The fungus usually penetrates the cutaneous barrier through puncture wounds, usually by a thorn or a splinter. The fungal agents causing these infections are occasionally found on rotting plant material and in soil. Several reports have associated some of these fungi with palm trees and xerophyte plants, but recent sequencing data have proven that mostly other, strictly saprophytic relatives are concerned (30, 46). For example, in dry areas of Venezuela, cactus plant thorns carry *Cladophialophora yegresii*, while human cases are caused by *C. carrionii*. *C. yegresii* produces muriform cells in the spines morphologically similar to those known as the invasive form of *C. carrionii* in chromoblastomycosis. These cells may thus be regarded as an extremotolerant survival phase and are likely to play an essential role in the natural life cycle of these organisms (30). The ecology of the fungi causing chromoblastomycosis is still incompletely understood. *Fonsecaea* species are isolated in the evergreen forests of tropical areas, whereas *C. carrionii* is identified only in desert areas under arid climatic conditions (115, 124).

Sporotrichosis

Pathogenic *Sporothrix* species can be found in soil and thorny plants. Infection is mostly acquired through traumatic inoculation. Cases of primary pulmonary sporotrichosis are acquired by inhalation and commonly affect individuals with a history of alcohol abuse (125). *Sporothrix brasiliensis*, however, is particularly transmitted from bites or scratches from stray cats, which are considered a primary host of this fungus (85). Occasional outbreaks occur in different populations, such as gardeners, rural workers, armadillo hunters, and persons in contact with domestic cats. In Brazil, a large epidemic occurred because of expansion of *S. brasiliensis* (85). In the United States several outbreaks of sporotrichosis, associated with occupational or recreational exposure to sphagnum moss, have been reported; the largest occurred in 1988 and involved 84 patients (82). Most infections occur in otherwise healthy individuals, but *Sporothrix* infections have also been recognized as opportunistic in immunocompromised individuals (126).

CLINICAL SIGNIFICANCE

Disorders caused by the fungi described in this chapter are mainly localized and may occur in otherwise healthy hosts. The infections arise mostly after traumatic inoculation of contaminated material from the environment; less frequently, e.g., in the case of sinusitis, otitis, or growth in the mucus of lungs of patients with cystic fibrosis, asymptomatic or mostly mildly symptomatic colonization of cavities is observed. A number of the fungi treated in this chapter are typical opportunists, causing infections increasing in severity in individuals with impaired innate immunity and metabolic diseases such as diabetes. Such patients may have cutaneous infections by black yeasts that are otherwise found on cold-blooded animals (119), but the clinical course of such infections is usually mild (127–129). Infections also arise in patients with severe immunological disorders, neutropenic patients, solid-organ transplant recipients, or patients undergoing long-term corticosteroid therapy. This is particularly noted with *Scedosporium* species (70). Some species of Chaetothyriales (such as *Cladophialophora bantiana* and *Rhinocladiella mackenziei*) can cause deep or disseminated infections in hosts with no known immunosuppression. If untreated, such infections may take a chronic, fatal course after a destructive disease process (130). The frequency of these infections is low, but given the potentially severe course of the disease, as well as the sometimes very high degrees of resistance to antifungal drugs, attentiveness to these fungi is mandatory. Chromoblastomycosis is a relatively frequent infection with significant morbidity in rural subtropical regions (115). *Sporothrix* infections increase in severity with defects of acquired cellular immunity, such as AIDS (82, 126).

Among the specific disease entities caused by the melanized fungi are the following.

Phaeohyphomycosis

Superficial

Botryosphaeriales

Neoscytalidium dimidiatum is a common plant pathogen in the tropics and is regularly involved in syndromes very similar to dermatophytosis on skin and nails, usually leading to extensive hyperkeratosis (112).

Capnodiales

The halophilic species *Hortaea werneckii* can adhere to human skin, especially in the palms and soles, where superficial growth of the fungus leads to the formation of hyperpigmented maculae, causing a syndrome in the dead keratin layers known as tinea nigra (2, 19).

Chaetothyriales

Some species of the order Chaetothyriales cause occasional superficial infections in humans. *Cladophialophora boppii* has been reported from a case of onychomycosis (128). *Cyphellophora laciniata* and *C. pluriseptata* are occasionally isolated from human skin and nails (31), but their etiology has not unambiguously been proven. *Cyphellophora europaea* and various *Exophiala* spp. are involved in skin and nail infections, but because of their slow growth, they might be frequently overlooked (31, 127–129).

Dothideales

A rare tinea nigra-like infection of the facial skin caused by *Aureobasidium melanogenum* was recently reported in an otherwise healthy patient (67).

Microascales

Species of *Scopulariopsis* are frequently isolated from human skin and nails, often from asymptomatic individuals. However, several species, such as the common opportunist *S. brevicaulis*, can cause infection in keratinized tissues (2, 71). *Triadelphia pulvinata* was reported from eczematoid, scaly lesions in the eyelids of an otherwise healthy patient (75). Infections by this fungus have only been reported from Saudi Arabia.

Ophiostomatales

The recently described species *Sporothrix chilensis* is a soilborne fungus that may infect human nails (88).

Pleosporales

Alternaria alternata and *Curvularia* spp. are occasionally reported as agents of opportunistic onychomycosis, usually in patients with a history of ungueal trauma, exposure to soil, or immunosuppression (114, 131).

Cutaneous and Corneal

Botryosphaeriales

Lasiodiplodia theobromae is occasionally found to cause ocular infections following injury to the cornea (8). Cases of posttraumatic keratitis also have been attributed to

Macrophomina phaseolina and *Neoscytalidium dimidiatum* by Premamalini et al. (132) and Tendolkar et al. (133), respectively, but the identification of the etiological agents should be corroborated by further studies. A case of cutaneous infection caused by *M. phaseolina* in a child with acute myeloid leukemia was published by Srinivasan et al. (11).

Capnodiales

Species of *Cladosporium*, such as *C. cladosporioides* and *C. oxysporum*, are associated with allergic disease in the indoor environment, with numerous (sub)cutaneous and even deep infections, but there remains some doubt about their pathogenic role (2). Considering that *Cladosporium* spp. are extremely common laboratory contaminants, it would be convenient to corroborate the identity of any potential *Cladosporium* opportunist by *in situ* hybridization or immunohistochemistry.

Chaetothyriales

Cladophialophora emmonsii, *C. boppii*, and *C. saturnica* are rare agents of mild cutaneous infections (2, 27, 28); also, several *Exophiala* species, e.g., *E. xenobiotica*, *E. oligosperma*, and *E. bergeri*, may cause skin infections with various degrees of severity (40, 53, 113, 129). *Knufia epidermidis* so far has almost exclusively been found on human skin. The species may cause asymptomatic colonization, may be found in association with dermatophyte infections, or may cause mild cutaneous infections. The infection by this agent superficially resembles tinea nigra, but fungal elements of *K. epidermidis* may invade deeper layers of the skin, even reaching the basal membrane of the dermis (47), while in tinea nigra only the *stratum corneum* is involved. Certain *Exophiala* spp., such as *E. dermatitidis* and *E. jeanselmei*, are rare agents of keratitis, usually after traumatisms or surgery (134, 135).

Diaporthales

Diaporthe phoenicicola has been reported from a case of scleral keratitis after pterygium surgery (58). *Diaporthe longicolla* and *D. phaseolorum* have caused cutaneous lesions in transplant patients (59, 61).

Ophiostomatales

Sporothrix pallida, an environmental fungus mostly isolated from soil, has been reported as an etiological agent of keratitis in a corneal transplant recipient (87).

Pleosporales

One of the main recognized clinical entities associated with Pleosporales is cutaneous infection in immunosuppressed patients caused by *Alternaria* and mainly affecting patients on long-term steroid use, tacrolimus, or other immunosuppressive agents. Nearly all cases were caused by *Alternaria infectoria* and *A. alternata*, the two main saprophytic species of the genus (92), and certain infections attributed to *A. chlamydospora* probably concerned meristematic strains of *A. alternata* (114). Several cutaneous infections have been attributed to *A. tenuissima*, but this species is only doubtfully separate from *A. alternata* (92). *Exserohilum rostratum* and several *Curvularia* spp., such as *C. lunata*, *C. spicifera*, and *C. senegalensis*, can occasionally cause infections of the skin and cornea (91, 94, 136). *Bipolaris oryzae* also has been reported from keratitis (95).

Sordariales

Cladorrhinum bulbillosum is an agent of fungal keratitis. Three cases have been reported so far, and two of them followed local traumatisms. Human cases were reported by Zapater and Scattini (104) and Gajjar et al. (106); one case in a horse was reported by Chopin et al. (105). Several cases of corneal infections in a horse and humans have been attributed to *Papulaspora equi* (137, 138). BLAST searches, surprisingly, showed that the ITS sequence of the ex-type strain of *P. equi*, CBS 573.89 (GenBank accession JX280870), is 99% similar to that of the ex-type strain of *C. bulbillosum*, CBS 304.90 (GenBank FM955448). These results indicate that *P. equi* and *C. bulbillosum* probably are synonyms. We would like to corroborate this hypothesis by sequencing more loci and carrying out morphological studies of all available strains labeled with these names. If these names are synonyms, the correct name for the fungus is *C. bulbillosum* since *P. equi* is phylogenetically distant from the type species of *Papulaspora*, *P. sepedonioides* (101). *P. equi* probably represents strains of *C. bulbillosum* that are unable to produce phialides in culture but only show microsclerotia. Other strains of "*Papulaspora*" isolated from corneal infections in humans recently proved to be phylogenetically related to the ascomycete genus *Subramaniula* (101).

Subcutaneous

Botryosphaeriales

Rare cases of subcutaneous infection by *Lasiodiplodia theobromae* (7) and *Neoscytalidium dimidiatum* (139) have been reported. A subcutaneous granuloma in a cat was attributed to *Macrophomina* sp., but it is difficult to speculate about the identity of the etiological agent from the brief description and images in the clinical report (140).

Calosphaeriales

Human infections by *Pleurostoma richardsiae* mostly involve subcutaneous cysts, occasionally with bone involvement. Most patients have some underlying condition such as diabetes or transplantation (141). A case of yellow-grain mycetoma was caused by *P. ochracea* (15).

Chaetothyriales

Over 10 *Exophiala* spp. have been associated with subcutaneous lesions in humans (4, 38, 39, 113, 119). *Exophiala dermatitidis* is the most commonly encountered *Exophiala* species in clinical settings, causing infections of cutaneous and subcutaneous tissues mostly in immunocompromised patients (142). *Exophiala oligosperma* is a common etiologic agent of subcutaneous infections in immunosuppressed, elderly, diabetic, or otherwise debilitated individuals (143). *Exophiala jeanselmei* is considered mainly an agent of subcutaneous infections, including mycetoma, often in otherwise healthy individuals (40, 144). *Cladophialophora bantiana* and *C. mycetomatis* are also agents of mycetoma (27). Uncommon agents of subcutaneous phaeohyphomycosis in vertebrates include *Cladophialophora devriesii*, *C. immunda* (2, 27), *Cyphellophora suttonii* (34), and *Veronaea botryosa* (56). A case of olecranon bursitis attributed to *Anthopsis deltoidea* (23) was probably caused by an undescribed *Anthopsis* species (24).

Diaporthales

Diaporthe bougainvilleicola caused prepatellar bursitis in a renal transplant patient (60), and a *Diaporthe* sp. produced an abscess and osteomyelitis in a finger of a patient with diabetes and rheumatoid arthritis under prednisone treatment (62). A case of mycetoma with yellowish grains was caused by *Diaporthe phaseolorum* (64).

Microascales

Several species of *Scedosporium* are common causes of subcutaneous infections and mycetoma in temperate regions, especially in North America, having a predilection for the joints (145). *Lomentospora prolificans* and *Scopulariopsis* spp. are associated with diverse clinical manifestations, including subcutaneous infections (2, 70, 72, 73). *Knoxdaviesia dimorphospora* was recently reported from a case of olecranon bursitis (69).

Pleosporales

Members of the order Pleosporales (most commonly *Alternaria, Curvularia,* and *Exserohilum*) are able to cause subcutaneous infections, although more commonly they produce sinusitis with occasional cerebral involvement in otherwise healthy individuals (2, 94, 114). The recently described sterile fungus *Hongkongmyces pedis* caused a subcutaneous infection in the foot of a patient with an immunological disorder (98).

Togniniales

Members of the order Togniniales are typical agents of subcutaneous infections. Most of the 11 pathogenic species of *Phaeoacremonium* cause this type of infection, including cases of mycetoma and various forms of superficial and invasive phaeohyphomycosis. In addition, the genus includes numerous important plant pathogens (108).

Venturiales

Although the genus *Ochroconis* is mainly known for the neurotropic fungus *O. gallopavum* (currently named *Verruconis gallopava*), one species retained in *Ochroconis sensu stricto*, *O. mirabilis*, is an agent of cutaneous and subcutaneous infections in humans and other vertebrates (110, 146).

Systemic

Botryosphaeriales

Lasiodiplodia theobromae has been involved in a case of pneumonia (147). *Neoscytalidium dimidiatum* caused deep infections in immunocompromised patients (139, 148).

Chaetothyriales

A disease entity that is largely confined to Chaetothyriales is primary cerebral infection in immunocompromised or immunocompetent individuals, i.e., cerebritis in which the first symptoms of disease are of a neurologic nature. Hyphal elements that show melanization either directly or after Fontana-Masson staining are observed in abscesses in the brain parenchyma. The portal of entry may be the lung, but frequently symptoms are confined to the brain. Five species account for most nontraumatic brain infections. *Cladophialophora bantiana* has caused about one-third of the cases in otherwise healthy individuals (130). If untreated, the infections are fatal within 1 to 6 months. *Exophiala dermatitidis* is responsible for a striking number of fatal, neurotropic infections in young, healthy individuals, all in Asia (130, 142, 143). The other three species are *Cladophialophora modesta, Fonsecaea monophora,* and *Rhinocladiella mackenziei*. *R. mackenziei* is a remarkable fungus because it is exclusively known from fatal brain infections in the Middle East or from emigrants from that region (2, 130). Several patients had no known immune deficiency; the environmental niche of the species is unknown. Occasionally systemic dissemination is observed in patients with or without proven predisposing factors; these infections are fatal if they go untreated. Secondary cutaneous lesions often lead to marked eruptions with high morbidity. The disorder has been observed repeatedly in *Cladophialophora devriesii, C. modesta, C. arxii, Exophiala dermatitidis,* and *E. spinifera* (2, 130, 142, 149, 150). The last two species have capsule-like extracellular polysaccharides around yeast cells and have a high virulence in humans (151). The rare infections by *E. spinifera* can be localized, but in about one-half of the cases, fatal, disseminated mycoses are observed in adolescents (reviewed by de Hoog et al. [152]). *Exophiala dermatitidis* and, to a lesser extent, *E. phaeomuriformis* are regular pulmonary colonizers of patients with cystic fibrosis (153). *Exophiala asiatica* was reported from a case of disseminated infection in an immunocompetent patient (154).

The etiologic agents in cases of phaeohyphomycosis published under the name *Fonsecaea pedrosoi* should be reconsidered, since it has been observed that the second species of the genus, *F. monophora*, has a more diverse clinical spectrum that includes brain infection (42, 130). Occasionally, opportunistic infections including endocarditis and osteomyelitis caused by *Phialophora verrucosa* have been reported (155, 156). It is possible that some of these infections were attributable to a different *Phialophora* species. *Arthrocladium fulminans* was reported from a case of fatal disseminated disease in an immunocompromised patient (25) and from a case of arthritis and osteomyelitis in an otherwise healthy individual (26).

Dothideales

Aureobasidium pullulans has been implicated as an agent of catheter-related septicemia, peritonitis, and disseminated infection (2, 66, 157), and *Hormonema dematioides* has been implicated in a case of cutaneous lesions, fungemia, and peritonitis (2, 158).

Microascales

Relatively common deep and disseminated infections caused by *Scedosporium* are noted for immunosuppressed or otherwise healthy patients. The reported clinical spectrum of this genus has changed over time, from prevalently chronic mycetoma in otherwise healthy patients between 1911 and 1980 to systemic opportunistic infection after 1980 (145, 159). Systemic infections after solid-organ transplantation are relatively frequent. Osteomyelitis and arthritis are also relatively common (145, 159). Fisher et al. (160) were the first to describe an association of *S. apiospermum* with a near-drowning syndrome, which characteristically leads to delayed, potentially fatal brain infection after the patient has recovered from the primary effects of aspiration of polluted water. In severely compromised patients, cerebral dissemination may take place from local foci. *Scedosporium* species shows a high incidence in cystic fibrosis patients but occurs mostly as a colonizer in this population (145, 159).

Despite its rather frequent occurrence in clinical settings, the history of *Lomentospora prolificans*, one of the most virulent species of Microascales, is remarkably short (70). Malloch and Salkin described the first clinical cases in 1984 (161). Since then, numerous strains have been recovered, mostly from clinical cases with major immunosuppression, and since no older reports of cases in immunocompetent patients are known, the species is a truly emerging opportunist (162). The species has been reported from bone and soft tissue infections as well as from (secondary) cutaneous infection, fungemia, and endocarditis (2, 145, 159). The fungus may disseminate to visceral organs in immunocompromised individuals. A nosocomial outbreak has been described (163).

Triadelphia disseminata caused a fatal disseminated infection in a patient with acute myeloid leukemia. The fungus was recovered from blood cultures, and clinical and imagenological data suggested involvement of the lungs and brain (5, 76).

Ophiostomatales

Ophiostoma piceae caused a fatal invasive infection involving the lungs and brain in a patient with acute lymphoblastic leukemia. This fungus showed both elongated yeast-like elements and septate hyphae in tissue and in culture. Colonies were poorly pigmented at first but became dark with age. Microscopical examination did not show sporothrix-like sympodial conidiophores (79).

Pleosporales

A wide spectrum of invasive opportunistic infections has been attributed to *Curvularia*, including endocarditis, pulmonary infection, cerebral infection, and peritonitis (91, 96, 164, 165). *Exserohilum rostratum* caused a large iatrogenic outbreak because of injection with contaminated methylprednisolone preparations leading to numerous fatal cases of meningitis and CNS vasculitis (166).

Togniniales

Phaeoacremonium parasiticum is able to cause deep or disseminated infections in debilitated patients (108, 167).

Venturiales

Verruconis gallopava causes epizootic encephalitis in flocks of turkeys and chickens and can also cause pulmonary or invasive infections in immunocompetent and immunocompromised individuals (109–111).

Chromoblastomycosis

Chromoblastomycosis occurs in otherwise healthy patients; it is characterized by chronic, cutaneous to subcutaneous lesions and frequently with marked hyperplasia. A primary lesion is represented by a papula at the site of inoculation that slowly enlarges over time, becoming a plaque or a tumoral (cauliflower-like) lesion that can spread via the lymphatic system, although hematogenous dissemination has also been proposed. Lesions contain the typical and resistant subspherical and mostly cruciately septate muriform (sclerotic) bodies, indicative of chromoblastomycosis (115).

Three fungal species of Chaetothyriales account for virtually all cases of chromoblastomycosis: *Cladophialophora carrionii*, *Fonsecaea pedrosoi*, and *Phialophora verrucosa*. Infections by *C. carrionii* mainly occur in arid climates, probably acquired via traumatic inoculation of cactus spines (115). Occasionally *Cladophialophora boppii* (168) and, more recently, the new species *Cladophialophora samoënsis*, *Cyphellophora ludoviensis*, and *Rhinocladiella tropicalis* have also been reported as causes of chromoblastomycosis (27, 36). Infections by *P. verrucosa* mainly occur in tropical climatic zones (169). *Rhinocladiella aquaspersa* is a rare agent of chromoblastomycosis in Latin America (54). Systemic dissemination is very rare; a recent case caused by *Fonsecaea pugnacius* showed verrucous lesions in the right arm and face that developed during decades and contained typical muriform bodies. The infection disseminated later to the brain, where the fungus produced a phaeohyphomycotic mycelial phase (44).

Sporotrichosis

Sporotrichosis is a cutaneous to subcutaneous chronic infection that can undergo lymphatic spread. Musculoskeletal involvement and disseminated infection are relatively rare, as are the nasal and pulmonary infections that may arise from inhalation of conidia (82, 125). Most infections originate from traumatic implantation of the fungus. Some disseminated cases were observed in AIDS patients (126). In addition, infections have been described as being transmitted by animals (85, 170).

COLLECTION, TRANSPORT, AND STORAGE OF SPECIMENS

Collection, transport, and storage of specimens are described in chapter 117. Appropriate collection of specimens is essential for mycological study. There should be sufficient quantity for direct microscopic examination as well as for isolation.

DIRECT EXAMINATION

Microscopy

Melanization of vegetative cells or conidia, which results in colony coloration ranging from olive or gray to black, is caused by the deposition of dihydroxynaphthalene melanin in cell walls. This property occurs commonly among species classified in very different parts of the fungal kingdom. The amount of melanin expressed in host tissue may be very small and difficult to observe with traditional histologic stains. The use of the Fontana-Masson stain (see chapter 118) for demonstrating the presence of melanin is therefore recommended as a routine to distinguish fungi with melanized hyphae from those causing "hyalohyphomycosis," e.g., *Fusarium*. This does not apply for *Sporothrix* and *Scedosporium*, which are not melanized but are able to produce melanized conidia *in vitro*, *in vivo*, or both. *Sporothrix* has a characteristic "cigar-shaped" yeast form in tissue; the recognition of *Scedosporium* rests on methods other than histopathology.

There are numerous procedures for treating the specimen to enhance fungal detection, including treatment with potassium hydroxide or calcofluor white and Giemsa, Wright, or Gram stain (see chapter 118). Histopathology procedures using periodic acid-Schiff (PAS), hematoxylin and eosin, or methenamine silver enhance observation. Fontana-Masson staining is useful to detect melanization in cells that appear hyaline with light microscopy (171). To summarize, some characteristic features include the following.

Skin Infections

Pigmented hyphal fragments, occasionally melanized yeast-like cells, are visible in infected skin tissue (Fig. 5).

Sinusitis

In sinusitis, the sinuses are often occluded by amorphous fungus balls. Histologic examination reveals the presence of dense masses of pigmented, branched, and septate hyphae usually not invading the mucosa. Invasion of the mucosa mostly occurs in immunosuppressed individuals.

Cerebral Infection

In cases of cerebral infection, the hyphae are often poorly colored and scantily branched. In advanced cases, abscesses are formed (Fig. 5).

Disseminated Infection

Pigmented or poorly colored fungal elements such as hyphae or yeast-like cells can be observed in cases of disseminated infection (Fig. 6).

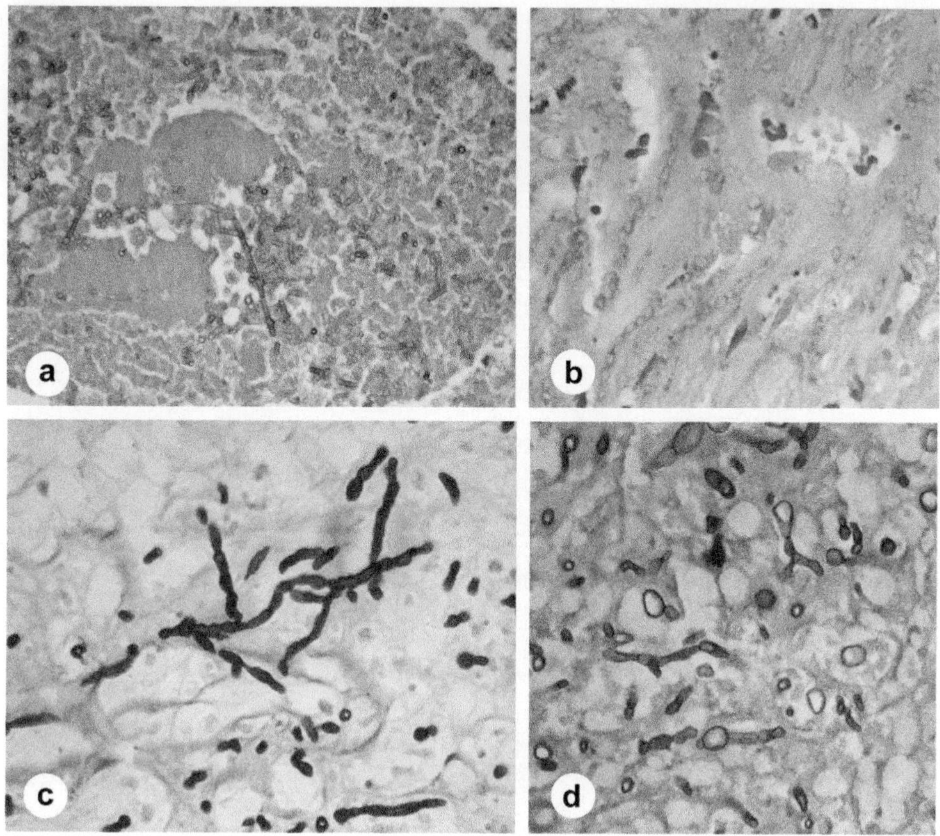

FIGURE 5 (a) Hematoxylin and eosin stain of subcutaneous nodule biopsy sample, showing branching hyphae of *Fonsecaea monophora*; (b to d) brain tissue showing irregular, branching, and septate hyphae of *Cladophialophora bantiana*, stained with hematoxylin and eosin stain (b), GMS stain (c), and PAS stain (d). Magnifications, ×250 (a) and ×400 (b to d). (Courtesy of E. Mayayo, Universitat Rovira i Virgili.)

Chromoblastomycosis

The hallmark of chromoblastomycosis is the presence of muriform or sclerotic cells in tissue sections or wet preparations of pus, scrapings, or biopsy samples. Muriform cells are swollen, spherical, dark brown, thick-walled cells that often develop a septum and may finally become divided by intersecting septa in more than one plane (Fig. 6).

Sporotrichosis

In sporotrichosis, hyaline, yeast-like cells are occasionally present, bearing slender daughter cells at very narrow bases. They are usually few in number and may easily be missed during microscopy, so Gomori methenamine silver (GMS) or PAS staining is therefore recommended; Fontana-Masson staining is negative (Fig. 6).

Antigen and Nucleic Acid Detection

There are few data for detection of antigens or nucleic acids in human clinical samples for diagnosis of the mycoses included in this chapter. The detection of (1→3)-β-D-glucan (BG), a fungal cell wall component, in serum and sterile body fluids is a useful marker of invasive fungal infections. The value of BD as a diagnostic adjunct has been proven in several studies about candidiasis and aspergillosis. However, patients with invasive infections by less common pathogens, such as species of *Alternaria*, *Cladosporium*, and *Scedosporium*, also have shown BG reactivity in serum (172). BG also showed high sensitivity and specificity for diagnosis of fungal meningitis caused by *Exserohilum rostratum* during an iatrogenic outbreak in the United States associated with contaminated steroid injections (173). In that study, BG levels correlated with clinical response, representing useful adjunctive data for the clinical management of patients.

A panfungal PCR assay has been developed that targets the ITS1 region of the rDNA gene cluster to detect fungal DNA in fresh and paraffin-embedded tissue specimens. This method was useful for identifying species of *Scedosporium*, *Exophiala*, and *Exserohilum*. PCR products were sequenced and compared with sequences in the GenBank database (174). Linked to the recent outbreak of *Exserohilum rostratum* infections due to injections of contaminated steroids in the United States, several molecular tests were developed for rapid identification of the fungus. Gade et al. (175) developed a test based on the detection of free-circulating fungal DNA from human fluids and subsequent PCR amplification, using panfungal and *Exserohilum*-specific primers that target the ITS2 region, and sequencing. This test proved to be more specific than cultures. A very sensitive *E. rostratum*-specific real-time PCR for rapid detection and quantification of the fungus in cerebrospinal fluid or brain tissues of patients with meningitis has also been developed (176).

ISOLATION PROCEDURES

Clinically relevant dematiaceous fungi grow well on standard mycological media, such as Sabouraud dextrose agar. This medium is adequate for isolation; however, it may be too rich in simple nutrients to stimulate sporulation properly; it generally favors growth of vegetative hyphae

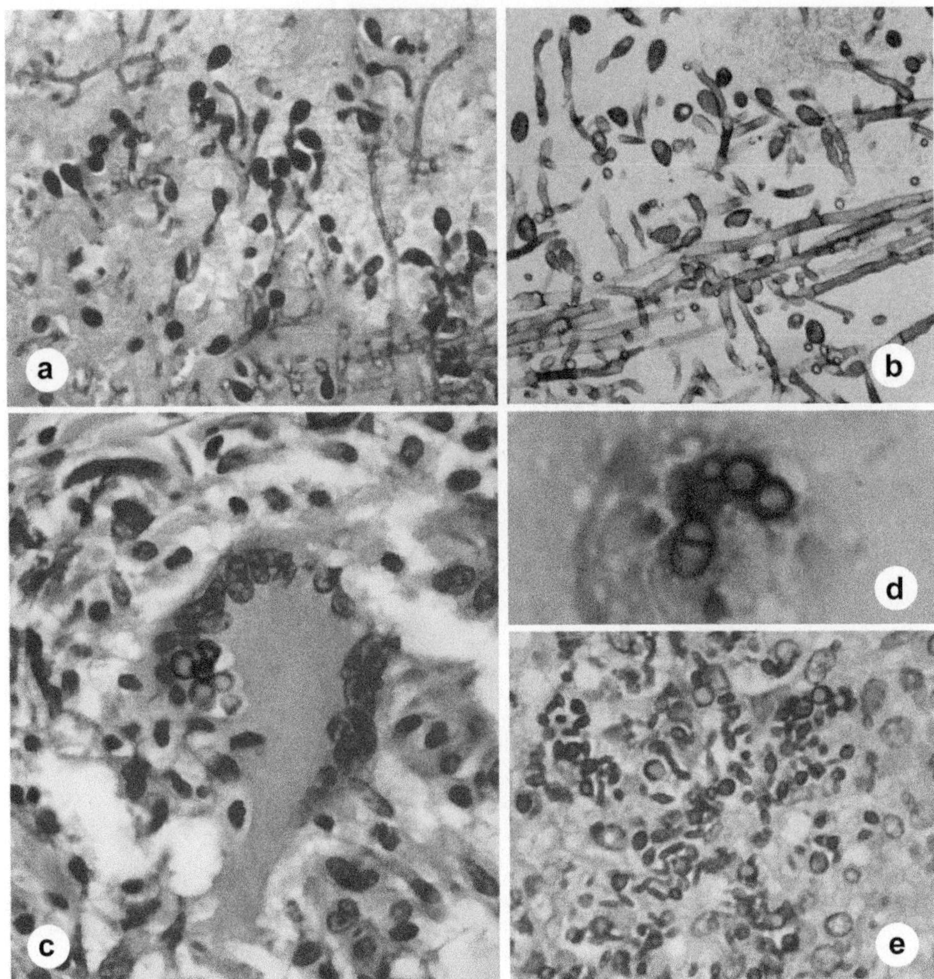

FIGURE 6 (a and b) Lung tissue with numerous conidia and hyphae of *Lomentospora prolificans* stained with PAS (a) and GMS (b); (c) PAS stain of a subcutaneous nodule biopsy sample, showing sclerotic cells of *Fonsecaea pedrosoi* within a giant cell; (d) PAS stain of a fine-needle aspirate of a subcutaneous nodule, showing sclerotic cells of *F. pedrosoi*; (e) PAS stain of a hepatic vessel, showing a massive embolization by *Sporothrix schenckii*, showing characteristic elongate cells. Magnifications, ×400. (Courtesy of E. Mayayo, Universitat Rovira i Virgili.)

instead of reproductive structures. The use of nutritionally poor media, such as cornmeal agar, potato carrot agar, oatmeal agar, or 2% water agar with moistened sterile wooden sticks, or moistened sterile filter paper stimulates the formation of reproductive structures. Once isolation has been achieved, if no sporulation is obtained, these nutrient-poor media are highly recommended. In the case of infection due to more than one agent, the strain that grows in a more limited manner may pass unnoticed for a long period. Therefore, a loopful of cells suspended in 0.1% Tween and streaked onto a fresh culture plate is useful to select an individual colony for identification.

For primary isolation, use of culture media with and without cycloheximide is recommended. This inhibitory substance is tolerated by many important dematiaceous pathogens, including members of the Chaetothyriales and Ophiostomatales, but numerous species in other taxonomic groups are sensitive (2, 21, 79).

IDENTIFICATION

For the identification of most of the species included in this chapter, the classical method is to grow the fungi in culture and to examine the relevant morphological characteristics described above. This method will mostly provide identification at the generic level. Further information on appropriate culture media is provided in chapter 118. Slide culture preparations using potato dextrose agar or cornmeal dextrose agar, to be handled only within a biological safety cabinet, are ideal for determining conidiogenesis. For morphological features of most of the fungi treated in this chapter, the reader is referred to the work of de Hoog et al. (2).

Molecular identification of most species is currently performed by sequencing of ribosomal genes and comparison with dedicated databases (177), such as those provided by the Westerdijk Fungal Biodiversity Institute (Utrecht, Netherlands; www.westerdijkinstitute.nl) and the International Society for Human and Animal Mycology (http://its.mycologylab.org/). Care should be taken when the GenBank database is used for identification in less known fungal groups because over 10% of the sequences may be incorrect (92). Sequences should be evaluated not only from a technical point of view but also nomenclaturally, i.e., by comparison with ex-type strains.

When ribosomal genes are used, the phylogenetic position of taxa can be established by sequencing the nuclear SSU (18S) or partial large subunit (28S) rRNA gene. These genes are mostly invariant between closely related species. In most fungal groups, species diagnostics are possible with ITS sequences. But application of this technique as a "gold standard" for melanized fungi is still in dispute. For some genera, such as *Alternaria*, numerous species described on the basis of morphology prove to be invariant in the ITS region. In this case the question remains as to whether ITS shows insufficient polymorphism or whether simply too many species have been introduced (93). In contrast, ITS-based species distinction with black yeasts provides satisfactory results (21, 129, 152). For some genera, such as *Sporothrix*, sequencing of the calmodulin gene is useful to gain resolution of species within the complex (81, 83, 84). In *Scedosporium* (72, 73) and *Phaeoacremonium* (167), β-tubulin gene sequencing is used for this purpose. A review about DNA sequence-based identification of fungi was published by Hibbet et al. (178).

In recent years, some studies have assessed the usefulness of matrix-assisted laser desorption ionization–time-of-flight mass spectrometry (MALDI-TOF MS) in the identification of filamentous fungi. These studies, recently reviewed by Sanguinetti and Posteraro (179), have considered mostly hyaline fungi and give overall rates of correct identification of 72 to 98.8%. MALDI-TOF MS identification has been studied in relatively few dematiaceous genera, such as *Exophiala* (180–182), *Lomentospora*, and *Scedosporium* (183), with promising results. However, this technique sometimes fails to discriminate phylogenetically closely related species, e.g., *Exophiala dermatitidis* from *E. phaeomuriformis* (181). Furthermore, commercial platforms have not provided reference mass spectrum databases covering the diversity of dematiaceous pathogens properly. A recent study by Singh et al. (184) evaluated MALDI-TOF MS in the identification of clinically relevant dematiaceous fungi isolated in 19 medical centers in India over a 4-year period. DNA sequence-based identifications revealed the presence of 29 dematiaceous pathogens, of which only six (20%) could be identified by MALDI-TOF MS with the commercial database of Bruker Daltonics (Bremen, Germany). An in-house database made the identification of 20 of the remaining isolates possible. As pointed out by Sanguinetti and Posteraro (179), comprehensive online-available databases are necessary for the widespread application of MALDI-TOF in the identification of filamentous fungal pathogens.

TYPING SYSTEMS

A diversity of high-resolution molecular typing systems has been developed in recent years. These have been applied mainly to epidemiological tracking of fungal pathogens in the hospital and the community but also to showing geographical differences among isolates and to detecting cryptic species.

Chaetothyriales

On the basis of a multigene phylogeny, it has been demonstrated that important phenotypic features have evolved independently several times in the order Chaetothyriales and that most of the clinically relevant species of *Cladophialophora* belong to a monophyletic group comprising two main clades (*carrionii* and *bantiana* clades) (27).

In a study that investigated the molecular diversity of oligotrophic and neurotropic members of the genus *Exophiala* with ITS sequences and M-13 fingerprint and SSU intron data, two main groups could be distinguished within *E. dermatitidis*. The environmental strains were mainly placed in one of these groups, while the clinical strains were in the second one. Interestingly, strains from East Asia that clustered in the clinical group caused severe brain and disseminated infections, and strains of the same group recovered from outside East Asia caused only a relatively mild fungemia (37).

The natural niche of *Fonsecaea*, one of the most common agents causing chromoblastomycosis, remains uncertain. To elucidate where and how patients acquire the infection, probably through traumatic inoculation, numerous isolates with *Fonsecaea*-like morphology from environmental sources were typed with randomly amplified polymorphic DNA methods. The results revealed a high degree of strain diversity and showed that most strains isolated from environments to which symptomatic human patients were exposed were found to be more closely related to species of *Cladophialophora* than to *Fonsecaea* (42).

Dothideales

Multilocus typing at four loci demonstrated the existence of at least five different sequence types in isolates of *Neoscytalidium dimidiatum*, of which two were detected exclusively in isolates from plants, two were found only in clinical isolates, and one was observed in isolates from humans and from a mango tree. This has been proposed as the possible source of infection in a case of mycetoma in an agricultural field worker and should be considered as a potential reservoir of pathogenic strains of the fungus (185).

Microascales

In numerous molecular studies, there has been a high genetic diversity among isolates of *Scedosporium* from different origins (reviewed in reference 159). However, recent multilocus sequence analyses have shown that such variability could be explained by the existence of numerous cryptic species in the *Pseudallescheria boydii* complex (72, 73). In contrast, in *L. prolificans* genetic variation seems to be low to absent.

Ophiostomatales

With *Sporothrix*, as with *Scedosporium*, numerous molecular studies (reviewed in reference 82) have proven the existence of a high level of intraspecific variability, with isolates mainly grouped according to their geographical origins. But recent multilocus studies have demonstrated that *S. schenckii sensu lato* comprises several phylogenetic species and morphospecies with a marked geographical distribution; i.e., *S. brasiliensis* isolates are mainly found in Brazil, and all the isolates from India tested molecularly belong to *S. globosa* (81, 83, 84). This likely correlates with the genetic and morphological diversity shown within *S. schenckii* by many authors.

Pleosporales

Whole genome sequencing (WGS) analyses have been used to assess the origin of a large outbreak of iatrogenic CNS infections caused by *Exserohilum rostratum* (186). The infections originated from contaminated vials of methylprednisolone produced by New England Compounding Center (NECC). WGS was used to detect single nucleotide polymorphisms (SNPs), and the sequences obtained were subjected to phylogenetic analyses, including 22 isolates from patients affected with meningitis and other infections, six isolates from contaminated NECC vials, and seven isolates unrelated to the outbreak. All isolates related to the outbreak showed almost identical genomes of 33.8 Mb, with a total of eight SNPs detected, but no more than two SNPs separating any two of the 28 genomes. These genomes were separated from the most closely related one, from an *E. rostratum* strain unrelated to the outbreak by about 136,000 SNPs (186).

SEROLOGIC TESTS

A latex agglutination test is commercially available (Immuno-Mycologics Inc., Norman, OK) for detecting antibodies against *S. schenckii*, particularly in disseminated cases; but despite a study (187) reporting a sensitivity of 90 to 94% and a specificity of 95 to 100%, the test has not been used widely. However, the detection of antibodies was demonstrated to be useful in the diagnosis of CNS sporotrichosis in several patients when culture-based diagnosis had failed (188).

ANTIFUNGAL SUSCEPTIBILITIES

In Vitro

The available *in vitro* data for dematiaceous fungi are increasing every day, and in general the antifungal susceptibilities of the most clinically relevant species are known. However, interpretive breakpoints have not been defined, and clinical correlation data are practically nonexistent.

Amphotericin B generally has good *in vitro* activity against most clinically important dematiaceous fungi, such as *Exophiala* (189) and *Alternaria* (190). However, some species have been consistently resistant *in vitro*, including *Scedosporium* spp. and *Scopulariopsis brumptii* (145, 191, 192). The azoles, in general, have demonstrated the most consistent *in vitro* activity against dematiaceous fungi (reviewed in reference 111) apart from *L. prolificans* (193).

The newer triazoles posaconazole and voriconazole have a broad spectrum of activity, being active against most of the fungi included in this chapter. The activities of these triazoles were similar against agents of chromoblastomycosis (194) and *Pseudallescheria boydii* complex (193). The activity of posaconazole is higher than that of voriconazole against *Alternaria* spp. (190), *Exophiala* spp. (189), and *Sporothrix* spp. (195), although against the last the activity of both drugs was very poor. Voriconazole was highly effective and considered the drug of choice during an outbreak of iatrogenic *Exserohilum rostratum* CNS infections in the United States (196). Isavuconazole has shown good *in vitro* activity against various dematiaceous pathogens, including species of *Alternaria*, *Bipolaris*, *Cladosporium*, *Curvularia*, *Exophiala*, *Fonsecaea*, and *Phialophora*, but not against *Scedosporium* spp. and *Lomentospora prolificans* (197). Terbinafine showed a clear fungicidal activity *in vitro* against filamentous fungi. Studies of *in vitro* activity against dematiaceous fungi are emerging and fairly broad-spectrum activity is seen, including against *Alternaria* and *Curvularia* (111). Echinocandins appear to have variable and species-dependent fungistatic activities for the dematiaceous fungi (198). Micafungin has demonstrated some moderate activity against *Scedosporium* spp. (192). The *in vitro* activities of the available antifungal drugs against selected dematiaceous fungi were reviewed by Revankar and Sutton (111).

In Vivo in Animal Models

Based on the small number of clinical cases produced by most of the fungi discussed in this chapter, the ideal treatment regimen against the infections that most of them produce is not yet known. Therefore, studies using different animal models have been designed to evaluate efficacy and/or corroborate the results obtained *in vitro*. Animal studies have demonstrated that posaconazole is generally the most effective against infections by less common moulds, including some of those included in this chapter (reviewed in reference by Guarro [199]).

Chromoblastomycosis

Recent studies using animal models of chromoblastomycosis that tested athymic mice demonstrated that posaconazole showed higher efficacy than the recommended drugs itraconazole and terbinafine against infections by *Fonsecaea pedrosoi* (200) and *Cladophialophora carrionii* (201); voriconazole did not work against the former species.

Scedosporiosis and *Lomentospora prolificans* infections

Voriconazole and posaconazole, but not amphotericin B, showed efficacy that correlated with *in vitro* MICs against *Scedosporium apiospermum*, *S. aurantiacum*, and *S. boydii*. No drug has shown efficacy against *L. prolificans* infections. The effects of double or triple antifungal drug combinations were tested against *L. prolificans* murine infections, and micafungin plus voriconazole or amphotericin B was the most effective, being able to prolong mouse survival and to reduce fungal load in the kidneys and brain. The combination of all three mentioned drugs was ineffective (202). In a few clinical cases, the combination of terbinafine and voriconazole demonstrated synergy and favorable results (162).

Phaeohyphomycosis

Different animal studies have evaluated the most useful antifungal drugs for treating disseminated infections produced by some clinically relevant fungi. Against *Fonsecaea monophora* (203) and *Exophiala dermatitidis* (204), posaconazole was better than amphotericin B and itraconazole. In an experimental treatment of *Neoscytalidium dimidiatum*, amphotericin B worked better than voriconazole and posaconazole (205). For the treatment of *Cladophialophora bantiana*, murine studies tested amphotericin B, micafungin, voriconazole, flucytosine, and posaconazole alone and in double and triple combinations. The only therapeutic regimen that was able to prolong animal survival for at least 10 months was the combination of three drugs (posaconazole, micafungin, and flucytosine) (206).

Sporotrichosis

Posaconazole showed excellent efficacy in experimental infections against the two most common species causing sporotrichosis, i.e., *S. schenckii* and *S. brasiliensis* (207).

EVALUATION, INTERPRETATION, AND REPORTING OF RESULTS

More than 100 species of melanized fungi have caused infection in humans and animals, and many of these are relatively rare as etiologic agents. As a result, few clinicians are familiar with these fungi and they are frequently overlooked. Infections caused by dematiaceous fungi are being diagnosed increasingly among healthy as well as immunocompromised patients. Concurrently, the expanding diversity of etiology within this group of fungi is becoming apparent.

Determining whether a particular dematiaceous fungus is involved in a disease process can be difficult because many of these fungi are occasionally recovered as contaminants from clinical specimens. Repeated recovery of a suspected etiologic agent is significant, while DNA sequence identity of clinical material and the isolate is highly supportive. Isolation of a dematiaceous fungus from a normally sterile body site should not be dismissed as contamination, particularly if colonies are numerous or more than one culture plate shows growth. If isolated from a nonsterile pulmonary specimen, such as sputum or bronchial lavage fluid, well-documented opportunists from genera such as *Cladophialophora, Fonsecaea, Scedosporium,* or *Verruconis,* which are not seen as contaminants, also are highly indicative. Correlation between culture and histopathology results should also be determined.

Failure to order fungus culture when tissues are collected during surgical procedures is an increasing problem in the management of these infections, and clinicians should order fungus culture whenever warranted. In the future, direct identification of fungal genera from tissue blocks by immunohistochemistry, *in situ* DNA hybridization, or DNA sequencing will be a promising approach to rapid detection and identification of these agents.

REFERENCES

1. **Ellis MB.** 1971. *Dematiaceous Hyphomycetes.* Commonwealth Mycological Institute, Kew, United Kingdom.
2. **de Hoog GS, Guarro J, Gené J, Figueras MJ.** 2000. *Atlas of Clinical Fungi,* 2nd ed. Centraalbureau voor Schimmelcultures, Utrecht, The Netherlands. (an online version of the latest edition is available at: www.clinicalfungi.org)
3. **Kimura M, Maenishi O, Ito H, Ohkusu K.** 2010. Unique histological characteristics of *Scedosporium* that could aid in its identification. *Pathol Int* **60:**131–136.
4. **de Hoog GS, Hermanides-Nijhof EJ.** 1977. The black yeasts and allied hyphomycetes. *Stud Mycol* **15:**1–222.
5. **Edathodu J, Al-Abdely HM, Althawadi S, Wickes BL, Thompson EH, Wiederhold NP, Madrid H, Guarro J, Sutton DA.** 2013. Invasive fungal infection due to *Triadelphia pulvinata* in a patient with acute myeloid leukemia. *J Clin Microbiol* **51:**3426–3429.
6. **Hawksworth DL, et al.** 2011. The Amsterdam declaration on fungal nomenclature. *IMA Fungus* **2:**105–112.
7. **Summerbell RC, Krajden S, Levine R, Fuksa M.** 2004. Subcutaneous phaeohyphomycosis caused by *Lasiodiplodia theobromae* and successfully treated surgically. *Med Mycol* **42:** 543–547.
8. **Saha S, Sengupta J, Banerjee D, Khetan A.** 2012. *Lasiodiplodia theobromae* keratitis: a case report and review of literature. *Mycopathologia* **174:**335–339.
9. **Gu HJ, Kim YJ, Lee HJ, Dong SH, Kim SW, Huh HJ, Ki CS.** 2016. Invasive fungal sinusitis by *Lasiodiplodia theobromae* in a patient with aplastic anemia: an extremely rare case report and literature review. *Mycopathologia* **181:**901–908.
10. **Tan DHS, Sigler L, Gibas CFC, Fong IW.** 2008. Disseminated fungal infection in a renal transplant recipient involving *Macrophomina phaseolina* and *Scytalidium dimidiatum*: case report and review of taxonomic changes among medically important members of the Botryosphaeriaceae. *Med Mycol* **46:**285–292.
11. **Srinivasan A, Wickes BL, Romanelli AM, Debelenko L, Rubnitz JE, Sutton DA, Thompson EH, Fothergill AW, Rinaldi MG, Hayden RT, Shenep JL.** 2009. Cutaneous infection caused by *Macrophomina phaseolina* in a child with acute myeloid leukemia. *J Clin Microbiol* **47:**1969–1972.
12. **Crous PW, Slippers B, Wingfield MJ, Rheeder J, Marasas WF, Philips AJ, Alves A, Burgess T, Barber P, Groenewald JZ.** 2006. Phylogenetic lineages in the Botryosphaeriaceae. *Stud Mycol* **55:**235–253.
13. **Huang S-K, Tangthirasunun N, Phillips AJL, Dai D-Q, Wanasinghe DN, Wen T-C, Bahkali AH, Hyde KD, Kang J-C.** 2016. Morphology and phylogeny of *Neoscytalidium orchidacearum* sp. nov. (Botryosphaeriaceae). *Mycobiology* **44:**79–84.
14. **Vijaykrishna D, Mostert L, Jeewon R, Gams W, Hyde KD, Crous PW.** 2004. *Pleurostomophora,* an anamorph of *Pleurostoma* (Calosphaeriales), a new anamorph genus morphologically similar to *Phialophora. Stud Mycol* **50:**387–396.
15. **Mhmoud NA, Ahmed SA, Fahal AH, de Hoog GS, Gerrits van den Ende AH, van de Sande WW.** 2012. *Pleurostomophora ochracea,* a novel agent of human eumycetoma with yellow grains. *J Clin Microbiol* **50:**2987–2994.
16. **Réblová M, Jaklitsch WM, Réblová K, Štěpánek V.** 2015. Phylogenetic reconstruction of the Calosphaeriales and Togniniales using five genes and predicted RNA secondary structures of ITS, and *Flabellascus tenuirostris* gen. et sp. nov. *PLoS One* **10:**e0144616.
17. **Bensch K, Braun U, Groenewald JZ, Crous PW.** 2012. The genus *Cladosporium. Stud Mycol* **72:**1–401.
18. **Sandoval-Denis M, Sutton DA, Martin-Vicente A, Cano-Lira JF, Wiederhold N, Guarro J, Gené J.** 2015. *Cladosporium* species recovered from clinical samples in the United States. *J Clin Microbiol* **53:**2990–3000.
19. **Piontelli E, Grixolli MA, Riquelme C, Jorquera M.** 1997. Notas micológicas: *Hortaea werneckii* en ambientes salinos del norte chileno. *Bol Micol* **12:**89–94.
20. **Crous PW, Schoch CL, Hyde KD, Wood AR, Gueidan C, de Hoog GS, Groenewald JZ.** 2009. Phylogenetic lineages in the Capnodiales. *Stud Mycol* **64:**17–47, S7.
21. **Madrid H, Hernández-Restrepo M, Gené J, Cano J, Guarro J, Silva V.** 2016. New and interesting chaetothyrialean fungi from Spain. *Mycol Prog* **15:**1179–1201.
22. **Marchisio VF, Fontana A, Mosca AML.** 1977. *Anthopsis deltoidea,* a new genus and species of Dematiaceae from soil. *Can J Bot* **55:**115–117.
23. **Kwon-Chung KJ, Droller DD.** 1984. Infection of the olecranon bursa by *Anthopsis deltoidea. J Clin Microbiol* **20:**271–273.
24. **Moussa TAA, Gerrits van den Ende BHG, Al Zahrani HS, Kadasa NMS, de Hoog SG, Dolatabadi S.** 2017. The genus *Anthopsis* and its phylogenetic position in Chaetothyriales. *Mycoses* **60:**254–259.
25. **Nascimento MM, Selbmann L, Sharifynia S, Al-Hatmi AM, Voglmayr H, Vicente VA, Deng S, Kargl A, Moussa TA, Al-Zahrani HS, Almaghrabi OA, de Hoog GS.** 2016. *Arthrocladium,* an unexpected human opportunist in Trichomeriaceae (Chaetothyriales). *Fungal Biol* **120:**207–218.
26. **Diallo A, Michaud C, Tabibou S, Raz M, Fernandez C, Lepidi H, Fournier PE, Stein A, Ranque S, Seng P.** 2017. *Arthrocladium fulminans* arthritis and osteomyelitis. *Am J Trop Med Hyg* **96:**698–700.
27. **Badali H, Gueidan C, Najafzadeh MJ, Bonifaz A, van den Ende AH, de Hoog GS.** 2008. Biodiversity of the genus *Cladophialophora. Stud Mycol* **61:**175–191.
28. **Badali H, Carvalho VO, Vicente V, Attili-Angelis D, Kwiatkowski IB, Gerrits Van Den Ende AH, De Hoog GS.** 2009. *Cladophialophora saturnica* sp. nov., a new opportunistic species of Chaetothyriales revealed using molecular data. *Med Mycol* **47:**51–62.
29. **Gerrits van den Ende AHG, de Hoog GS.** 1999. Variability and molecular diagnostics of the neurotropic species *Cladophialophora bantiana. Stud Mycol* **43:**151–162.
30. **de Hoog GS, Nishikaku AS, Fernandez-Zeppenfeldt G, Padín-González C, Burger E, Badali H, Richard-Yegres N, van den Ende AH.** 2007. Molecular analysis and pathogenicity of the *Cladophialophora carrionii* complex, with the description of a novel species. *Stud Mycol* **58:**219–234.
31. **Feng P, Lu Q, Najafzadeh MJ, Gerrits van den Ende AHG, Sun J, Li RY, Xi L, Vicente VA, Lai W, Lu C, de Hoog GS.** 2014. *Cyphellophora* and its relatives in *Phialophora*: biodiversity and possible role in human infection. *Fungal Divers* **65:**17–45.
32. **Réblová M, Untereiner WA, Réblová K.** 2013. Novel evolutionary lineages revealed in the Chaetothyriales (fungi) based on multigene phylogenetic analyses and comparison of its secondary structure. *PLoS One* **8:**e63547.
33. **de Hoog GS, Weenink XO, Gerrits van den Ende AHG.** 1999. Taxonomy of the *Phialophora verrucosa* complex with the description of four new species. *Stud Mycol* **43:**107–142.

34. **Ajello L, Padhye AA, Payne M.** 1980. Phaeohyphomycosis in a dog caused by *Pseudomicrodochium suttonii*. *Mycotaxon* **12:**131–136.
35. **Perfect JR, Schell WA.** 1996. The new fungal opportunists are coming. *Clin Infect Dis* **22**(Suppl 2)**:**S112–S118.
36. **Gomes RR, Vicente VA, Azevedo CM, Salgado CG, da Silva MB, Queiroz-Telles F, Marques SG, Santos DWCL, de Andrade TS, Takagi EH, Cruz KS, Fornari G, Hahn RC, Scroferneker ML, Caligine RB, Ramirez-Castrillon M, de Araújo DP, Heidrich D, Colombo AL, de Hoog GS.** 2016. Molecular epidemiology of agents of human chromoblastomycosis in Brazil with the description of two novel species. *PLoS Negl Trop Dis* **10:**e0005102.
37. **Matos T, Haase G, Gerrits van den Ende AHG, de Hoog GS.** 2003. Molecular diversity of oligotrophic and neurotropic members of the black yeast genus *Exophiala*, with accent on *E. dermatitidis*. *Antonie van Leeuwenhoek* **83:**293–303.
38. **Yong LK, Wiederhold NP, Sutton DA, Sandoval-Denis M, Lindner JR, Fan H, Sanders C, Guarro J.** 2015. Morphological and molecular characterization of *Exophiala polymorpha* sp. nov. isolated from sporotrichoid lymphocutaneous lesions in a patient with myasthenia gravis. *J Clin Microbiol* **53:**2816–2822.
39. **Vitale RG, de Hoog GS.** 2002. Molecular diversity, new species and antifungal susceptibilities in the *Exophiala spinifera* clade. *Med Mycol* **40:**545–556.
40. **De Hoog GS, Zeng JS, Harrak MJ, Sutton DA.** 2006. *Exophiala xenobiotica* sp. nov., an opportunistic black yeast inhabiting environments rich in hydrocarbons. *Antonie van Leeuwenhoek* **90:**257–268.
41. **Padhye AA, McGinnis MR, Ajello L.** 1978. Thermotolerance of *Wangiella dermatitidis*. *J Clin Microbiol* **8:**424–426.
42. **De Hoog GS, Attili-Angelis D, Vicente VA, Van Den Ende AH, Queiroz-Telles F.** 2004. Molecular ecology and pathogenic potential of *Fonsecaea* species. *Med Mycol* **42:**405–416.
43. **Najafzadeh MJ, Sun J, Vicente V, Xi L, van den Ende AH, de Hoog GS.** 2010. *Fonsecaea nubica* sp. nov, a new agent of human chromoblastomycosis revealed using molecular data. *Med Mycol* **48:**800–806.
44. **de Azevedo CMPS, Gomes RR, Vicente VA, Santos DWCL, Marques SG, do Nascimento MMF, Andrade CEW, Silva RR, Queiroz-Telles F, de Hoog GS.** 2015. *Fonsecaea pugnacius*, a novel agent of disseminated chromoblastomycosis. *J Clin Microbiol* **53:**2674–2685.
45. **Najafzadeh MJ, Vicente VA, Sun J, Meis JF, de Hoog GS.** 2011. *Fonsecaea multimorphosa* sp. nov, a new species of Chaetothyriales isolated from a feline cerebral abscess. *Fungal Biol* **115:**1066–1076.
46. **Nascimento MMF, Vicente VA, Bittencourt JVM, Gelinski JML, Prenafeta-Boldú FX, Romero-Güiza M, Fornari G, Gomes RR, Santos GD, Gerrits Van Den Ende AHG, de Azevedo CDMPS, De Hoog GS.** 2017. Diversity of opportunistic black fungi on babassu coconut shells, a rich source of esters and hydrocarbons. *Fungal Biol* **121:**488–500.
47. **Li DM, de Hoog GS, Saunte DM, van den Ende AH, Chen XR.** 2008. *Coniosporium epidermidis* sp. nov., a new species from human skin. *Stud Mycol* **61:**131–136.
48. **Tsuneda A, Hambleton S, Currah RS.** 2011. The anamorph genus *Knufia* and its phylogenetically allied species in *Coniosporium*, *Sarcinomyces* and *Phaeococcomyces*. *Botany* **89:**523–536.
49. **Li Y, Xiao J, de Hoog GS, Wang X, Wan Z, Yu J, Liu W, Li R.** 2017. Biodiversity and human-pathogenicity of *Phialophora verrucosa* and relatives in *Chaetothyriales*. *Persoonia* **38:**1–19.
50. **Gams W.** 2000. *Phialophora* and some similar morphologically little-differentiated anamorphs of divergent ascomycetes. *Stud Mycol* **45:**187–199.
51. **Arzanlou M, Groenewald JZ, Gams W, Braun U, Shin HD, Crous PW.** 2007. Phylogenetic and morphotaxonomic revision of *Ramichloridium* and allied genera. *Stud Mycol* **58:** 57–93.
52. **del Palacio-Hernanz A, Moore MK, Campbell CK, del Palacio-Perez-Medel A, del Castillo-Cantero R.** 1989. Infection of the central nervous system by *Rhinocladiella atrovirens* in a patient with acquired immunodeficiency syndrome. *J Med Vet Mycol* **27:**127–130.
53. **de Hoog GS, Vicente V, Caligiorne RB, Kantarcioglu S, Tintelnot K, Gerrits van den Ende AHG, Haase G.** 2003. Species diversity and polymorphism in the *Exophiala spinifera* clade containing opportunistic black yeast-like fungi. *J Clin Microbiol* **41:**4767–4778.
54. **Badali H, Bonifaz A, Barrón-Tapia T, Vázquez-González D, Estrada-Aguilar L, Oliveira NM, Sobral Filho JF, Guarro J, Meis JF, De Hoog GS.** 2010. *Rhinocladiella aquaspersa*, proven agent of verrucous skin infection and a novel type of chromoblastomycosis. *Med Mycol* **48:**696–703.
55. **Cai Q, Lv GX, Jiang Y-Q, Mei H, Hu S-Q, Xu H-B, Wu X-F, Shen Y-N, Liu W-D.** 2013. The first case of phaeohyphomycosis caused by *Rhinocladiella basitona* in an immunocompetent child in China. *Mycopathologia* **176:**101–105.
56. **Welfringer A, Vuong V, Argy N, Chochillon C, Deschamps L, Rollin G, Harent S, Joly V, Vindrios W, Descamps V.** 2017. A rare fungal infection: phaehyphomycosis due to *Veronaea botryosa* and review of literature. *Med Mycol Case Rep* **15:**21–24.
57. **Gomes RR, Glienke C, Videira SIR, Lombard L, Groenewald JZ, Crous PW.** 2013. *Diaporthe*: a genus of endophytic, saprobic and plant pathogenic fungi. *Persoonia* **31:** 1–41.
58. **Gajjar DU, Pal AK, Parmar TJ, Arora AI, Ganatra DA, Kayastha FB, Ghodadra BK, Vasavada AR.** 2011. Fungal scleral keratitis caused by *Phomopsis phoenicicola*. *J Clin Microbiol* **49:**2365–2368.
59. **García-Reyne A, López-Medrano F, Morales JM, García Esteban C, Martín I, Eraña I, Meije Y, Lalueza A, Alastruey-Izquierdo A, Rodríguez-Tudela JL, Aguado JM.** 2011. Cutaneous infection by *Phomopsis longicolla* in a renal transplant recipient from Guinea: first report of human infection by this fungus. *Transpl Infect Dis* **13:**204–207.
60. **Cariello PF, Wickes BL, Sutton DA, Castlebury LA, Levitz SM, Finberg RW, Thompson EH, Daly JS.** 2013. *Phomopsis bougainvilleicola* prepatellar bursitis in a renal transplant recipient. *J Clin Microbiol* **51:**692–695.
61. **Mattei AS, Severo CB, Guazzelli LS, Oliveira FM, Gené J, Guarro J, Cano J, Severo LC.** 2013. Cutaneous infection by *Diaporthe phaseolorum* in Brazil. *Med Mycol Case Rep* **2:** 85–87.
62. **Sutton DA, Timm WD, Morgan-Jones G, Rinaldi MG.** 1999. Human phaeohyphomycotic osteomyelitis caused by the coelomycete *Phomopsis* Saccardo 1905: criteria for identification, case history, and therapy. *J Clin Microbiol* **37:**807–811.
63. **Mandell KJ, Colby KA.** 2009. Penetrating keratoplasty for invasive fungal keratitis resulting from a thorn injury involving *Phomopsis* species. *Cornea* **28:**1167–1169.
64. **Iriart X, Binois R, Fior A, Blanchet D, Berry A, Cassaing S, Amazan E, Papot E, Carme B, Aznar C, Couppié P.** 2011. Eumycetoma caused by *Diaporthe phaseolorum* (*Phomopsis phaseoli*): a case report and a mini-review of *Diaporthe/Phomopsis* spp. invasive infections in humans. *Clin Microbiol Infect* **17:** 1492–1494.
65. **Zalar P, de Hoog GS, Gunde-Cimerman N.** 1999. Ecology of halotolerant dothideaceous black yeasts. *Stud Mycol* **43:** 38–48.
66. **Zalar P, Gostinčar C, de Hoog GS, Uršič V, Sudhadham M, Gunde-Cimerman N.** 2008. Redefinition of *Aureobasidium pullulans* and its varieties. *Stud Mycol* **61:**21–38.
67. **Chen W-T, Tu M-E, Sun PL.** 2016. Superficial phaeohyphomycosis caused by *Aureobasidium melanogenum* mimicking tinea nigra in an immunocompetent patient and review of published reports. *Mycopathologia* **181:**555–560.
68. **Humphries Z, Seifert KA, Hirooka Y, Visagie CM.** 2017. A new family and genus in *Dothideales* for *Aureobasidium*-like species isolated from house dust. *IMA Fungus* **8:**299–315.
69. **Guevara-Suarez M, Llaurado M, Pujol I, Mayayo E, Martin-Vicente A, Gené J.** 2018. Fungal olecranon bursitis in an immunocompetent patient by *Knoxdaviesia dimorphospora* sp. nov.: case report and review. *Mycopathologia* **183:**407–415.
70. **Lackner M, et al.** 2014. Proposed nomenclature for *Pseudallescheria*, *Scedosporium* and related genera. *Fungal Divers* **67:**1–10.

71. **Sandoval-Denis M, Gené J, Sutton DA, Cano-Lira JF, de Hoog GS, Decock CA, Wiederhold NP, Guarro J.** 2016. Redefining *Microascus, Scopulariopsis* and allied genera. *Persoonia* **36:**1–36.
72. **Gilgado F, Cano J, Gené J, Guarro J.** 2005. Molecular phylogeny of the *Pseudallescheria boydii* species complex: proposal of two new species. *J Clin Microbiol* **43:**4930–4942.
73. **Gilgado F, Cano J, Gené J, Sutton DA, Guarro J.** 2008. Molecular and phenotypic data supporting distinct species statuses for *Scedosporium apiospermum* and *Pseudallescheria boydii* and the proposed new species *Scedosporium dehoogii. J Clin Microbiol* **46:**766–771.
74. **Ma A-S, Soliman Z.** 2017. *Triadelphia moubasherii* sp. nov., from the gut of red palm weevils, *Rhynchophorus ferrugineus* Olivier. *Mycosphere* **8:**1228–1237.
75. **Al-Hedaithy SS.** 2001. First report of human infection due to the fungus *Triadelphia pulvinata. J Clin Microbiol* **39:** 3386–3389.
76. **Crous PW, et al.** 2015. Fungal Planet description sheets: 320–370. *Persoonia* **34:**167–266.
77. **de Beer ZW, Duong TA, Wingfield MJ.** 2016. The divorce of *Sporothrix* and *Ophiostoma*: solution to a problematic relationship. *Stud Mycol* **83:**165–191.
78. **de Beer ZW, Harrington TC, Vismer HF, Wingfield BD, Wingfield MJ.** 2003. Phylogeny of the *Ophiostoma stenoceras-Sporothrix schenckii* complex. *Mycologia* **95:**434–441.
79. **Bommer M, Hütter M-L, Stilgenbauer S, de Hoog GS, de Beer ZW, Wellinghausen N.** 2009. Fatal *Ophiostoma piceae* infection in a patient with acute lymphoblastic leukaemia. *J Med Microbiol* **58:**381–385.
80. **De Hoog GS.** 1974. The genera *Blastobotrys, Sporothrix, Calcarisporium* and *Calcarisporiella* gen. nov. *Stud Mycol* **7:**1–84.
81. **Marimon R, Cano J, Gené J, Sutton DA, Kawasaki M, Guarro J.** 2007. *Sporothrix brasiliensis, S. globosa,* and *S. mexicana,* three new *Sporothrix* species of clinical interest. *J Clin Microbiol* **45:**3198–3206.
82. **Barros MB, de Almeida Paes R, Schubach AO.** 2011. *Sporothrix schenckii* and sporotrichosis. *Clin Microbiol Rev* **24:** 633–654.
83. **Marimon R, Gené J, Cano J, Trilles L, Dos Santos Lazéra M, Guarro J.** 2006. Molecular phylogeny of *Sporothrix schenckii. J Clin Microbiol* **44:**3251–3256.
84. **Marimon R, Gené J, Cano J, Guarro J.** 2008. *Sporothrix luriei*: a rare fungus from clinical origin. *Med Mycol* **46:**621–625.
85. **Rodrigues AM, de Melo Teixeira M, de Hoog GS, Pacheco Schubach TM, Pereira SA, Ferreira Fernandes G, Lopes Bezerra LM, Felipe MS, Pires de Camargo Z.** 2013. Phylogenetic analysis reveals a high prevalence of *Sporothrix brasiliensis* in feline sporotrichosis. *PLoS Negl Trop Dis* **7:**e2281.
86. **Zhou X, Rodrigues AM, Feng P, de Hoog GS.** 2013. Global ITS diversity in the *Sporothrix schenckii* complex. *Fungal Divers* **66:**153–165.
87. **Morrison AS, Lockhart SR, Bromley JG, Kim JY, Burd EM.** 2013. An environmental *Sporothrix* as a cause of corneal ulcer. *Med Mycol Case Rep* **2:**88–90.
88. **Rodrigues AM, Cruz Choappa R, Fernandes GF, de Hoog GS, de Camargo ZP.** 2016. *Sporothrix chilensis* sp. nov. (Ascomycota: Ophiostomatales), a soil-borne agent of human sporotrichosis with mild-pathogenic potential to mammals. *Fungal Biol* **120:**246–264.
89. **Sivanesan A.** 1987. Graminicolous species of *Bipolaris, Curvularia, Drechslera, Exserohilum* and their teleomorphs. *Mycol Papers* **158:**1–261.
90. **Simmons EG.** 2007. *Alternaria*: an identification manual. *CBS Biodivers Ser* **6:**1–775. CBS Fungal Biodiversity Centre, Utrecht, The Netherlands.
91. **Madrid H, da Cunha KC, Gené J, Dijksterhuis J, Cano J, Sutton DA, Guarro J, Crous PW.** 2014. Novel *Curvularia* species from clinical specimens. *Persoonia* **33:**48–60.
92. **de Hoog GS, Horré R.** 2002. Molecular taxonomy of the *Alternaria* and *Ulocladium* species from humans and their identification in the routine laboratory. *Mycoses* **45:**259–276.
93. **Woudenberg JHC, Groenewald JZ, Binder M, Crous PW.** 2013. *Alternaria* redefined. *Stud Mycol* **75:**171–212.
94. **McGinnis MR, Rinaldi MG, Winn RE.** 1986. Emerging agents of phaeohyphomycosis: pathogenic species of *Bipolaris* and *Exserohilum. J Clin Microbiol* **24:**250–259.
95. **Wang L, Al-Hatmi AM, Lai X, Peng L, Yang C, Lai H, Li J, Meis JF, de Hoog GS, Zhuo C, Chen M.** 2016. *Bipolaris oryzae,* a novel fungal opportunist causing keratitis. *Diagn Microbiol Infect Dis* **85:**61–65.
96. **Manamgoda DS, Cai L, McKenzie HC, Crous PW, Madrid H, Chukeatirote E, Shivas RG, Tan YP, Hyde KD.** 2012. A phylogenetic and taxonomic re-evaluation of the *Bipolaris-Cochliobolus-Curvularia* complex. *Fungal Divers* **56:**131–144.
97. **Chowdhary A, Hagen F, Curfs-Breuker I, Madrid H, de Hoog GS, Meis JF.** 2015. In vitro activities of eight antifungal drugs against a global collection of genotyped *Exserohilum* isolates. *Antimicrob Agents Chemother* **59:**6642–6645.
98. **Tsang CC, Chan JFW, Trendell-Smith NJ, Ngan AHY, Ling IWH, Lau SKP, Woo PCY.** 2014. Subcutaneous phaeohyphomycosis in a patient with IgG4-related sclerosing disease caused by a novel ascomycete, *Hongkongmyces pedis* gen. et sp. nov.: first report of human infection associated with the family Lindgomycetaceae. *Med Mycol* **52:**736–747.
99. **de Hoog GS, Adelmann D, Ahmed AOA, van Belkum A.** 2004. Phylogeny and typification of *Madurella mycetomatis,* with a comparison of other agents of eumycetoma. *Mycoses* **47:**121–130.
100. **Perdomo H, García D, Gené J, Cano J, Sutton DA, Summerbell R, Guarro J.** 2013. *Phialemoniopsis,* a new genus of Sordariomycetes, and new species of *Phialemonium* and *Lecythophora. Mycologia* **105:**398–421.
101. **Ahmed SA, Khan Z, Wang XW, Moussa TAA, Al-Zahrani HS, Almaghrabi OA, Sutton DA, Ahmad S, Groenewald JZ, Alastruey-Izquierdo A, van Diepeningen A, Menken SBJ, Najafzadeh MJ, Crous PW, Cornely O, Hamprecht A, Vehreschild MJGT, Kindo AJ, de Hoog GS.** 2016. Chaetomium-like fungi causing opportunistic infections in humans: a possible role for extremotolerance. *Fungal Divers* **76:**11–26.
102. **Madrid H, Cano J, Gené J, Guarro J.** 2011. Two new species of *Cladorrhinum. Mycologia* **103:**795–805.
103. **Carmarán CC, Berretta M, Martínez S, Barrera V, Munaut F, Gasoni L.** 2015. Species diversity of *Cladorrhinum* in Argentina and description of a new species, *Cladorrhinum australe.* 2015. *Mycol Prog* **14:**94.
104. **Zapater RC, Scattini F.** 1979. Mycotic keratitis by *Cladorrhinum. Sabouraudia* **17:**65–69.
105. **Chopin JB, Sigler L, Connole MD, O'Boyle DA, Mackay B, Goldstein L.** 1997. Keratomycosis in a Percheron cross horse caused by *Cladorrhinum bulbillosum. J Med Vet Mycol* **35:** 53–55.
106. **Gajjar DU, Pal AK, Santos JM, Ghodadra BK, Vasavada AR.** 2011. Severe pigmented keratitis caused by *Cladorrhinum bulbillosum. Indian J Med Microbiol* **29:**434–437.
107. **Mouchacca J, Gams W.** 1993. The hyphomycete genus *Cladorrhinum* and its teleomorph connections. *Mycotaxon* **48:**415–440.
108. **Gramaje D, Mostert L, Groenewald JZ, Crous PW.** 2015. *Phaeoacremonium*: from esca disease to phaeohyphomycosis. *Fungal Biol* **119:**759–783.
109. **Samerpitak K, van der Linde E, Choi H-J, Gerrits van den Ende AHG, Machouart M, Gueidan C, de Hoog GS.** 2014. Taxonomy of *Ochroconis,* genus including opportunistic pathogens on humans and animals. *Fungal Divers* **65:**89–126.
110. **Giraldo A, Sutton DA, Samerpitak K, de Hoog GS, Wiederhold NP, Guarro J, Gené J.** 2014. Occurrence of *Ochroconis* and *Verruconis* species in clinical specimens from the United States. *J Clin Microbiol* **52:**4189–4201.
111. **Revankar SG, Sutton DA.** 2010. Melanized fungi in human disease. *Clin Microbiol Rev* **23:**884–928.
112. **Elewski BE.** 1996. Onychomycosis caused by *Scytalidium dimidiatum. J Am Acad Dermatol* **35:**336–338.
113. **Zeng JS, Sutton DA, Fothergill AW, Rinaldi MG, Harrak MJ, de Hoog GS.** 2007. Spectrum of clinically relevant *Exophiala* species in the United States. *J Clin Microbiol* **45:** 3713–3720.

114. **Pastor FJ, Guarro J.** 2008. *Alternaria* infections: laboratory diagnosis and relevant clinical features. *Clin Microbiol Infect* **14:**734–746.
115. **Queiroz-Telles F, de Hoog S, Santos DW, Salgado CG, Vicente VA, Bonifaz A, Roilides E, Xi L, Azevedo CM, da Silva MB, Pana ZD, Colombo AL, Walsh TJ.** 2017. Chromoblastomycosis. *Clin Microbiol Rev* **30:**233–276.
116. **de Hoog GS, Matos T, Sudhadham M, Luijsterburg KF, Haase G.** 2005. Intestinal prevalence of the neurotropic black yeast *Exophiala (Wangiella) dermatitidis* in healthy and impaired individuals. *Mycoses* **48:**142–145.
117. **Göttlich E, van der Lubbe W, Lange B, Fiedler S, Melchert I, Reifenrath M, Flemming H-C, de Hoog S.** 2002. Fungal flora in groundwater-derived public drinking water. *Int J Hyg Environ Health* **205:**269–279.
118. **Porteous NB, Grooters AM, Redding SW, Thompson EH, Rinaldi MG, de Hoog GS, Sutton DA.** 2003. Identification of *Exophiala mesophila* isolated from treated dental unit waterlines. *J Clin Microbiol* **41:**3885–3889.
119. **de Hoog GS, Vicente VA, Najafzadeh MJ, Harrak MJ, Badali H, Seyedmousavi S.** 2011. Waterborne *Exophiala* species causing disease in cold-blooded animals. *Persoonia* **27:** 46–72.
120. **Matos T, de Hoog GS, de Boer AG, de Crom I, Haase G.** 2002. High prevalence of the neurotrope *Exophiala dermatitidis* and related oligotrophic black yeasts in sauna facilities. *Mycoses* **45:**373–377.
121. **Zalar P, Novak M, de Hoog GS, Gunde-Cimerman N.** 2011. Dishwashers—a man-made ecological niche accommodating human opportunistic fungal pathogens. *Fungal Biol* **115:**997–1007.
122. **Selbmann L, de Hoog GS, Mazzaglia A, Friedmann EI, Onofri S.** 2005. Fungi at the edge of life: cryptoendolithic black fungi from Antarctic deserts. *Stud Mycol* **51:**1–26.
123. **Hernández-Hernández F, De Bievre C, Camacho-Arroyo I, Cerbon MA, Dupont B, Lopez-Martinez R.** 1995. Sex hormone effects on *Phialophora verrucosa* in vitro and characterization of progesterone receptors. *J Med Vet Mycol* **33:**235–239.
124. **Esterre P, Queiroz-Telles F.** 2006. Management of chromoblastomycosis: novel perspectives. *Curr Opin Infect Dis* **19:**148–152.
125. **Pluss JL, Opal SM.** 1986. Pulmonary sporotrichosis: review of treatment and outcome. *Medicine (Baltimore)* **65:**143–153.
126. **Donabedian H, O'Donnell E, Olszewski C, MacArthur RD, Budd N.** 1994. Disseminated cutaneous and meningeal sporotrichosis in an AIDS patient. *Diagn Microbiol Infect Dis* **18:**111–115.
127. **Saunte DM, Tarazooie B, Arendrup MC, de Hoog GS.** 2012. Black yeast-like fungi in skin and nail: it probably matters. *Mycoses* **55:**161–167.
128. **Brasch J, Dressel S, Müller-Wening K, Hügel R, von Bremen D, de Hoog GS.** 2011. Toenail infection by *Cladophialophora boppii*. *Med Mycol* **49:**190–193.
129. **Woo PCY, Ngan AHY, Tsang CCC, Ling IWH, Chan JFW, Leung SY, Yuen KY, Lau SKP.** 2013. Clinical spectrum of *Exophiala* infections and a novel *Exophiala* species, *Exophiala hongkongensis*. *J Clin Microbiol* **51:**260–267.
130. **Revankar SG, Sutton DA, Rinaldi MG.** 2004. Primary central nervous system phaeohyphomycosis: a review of 101 cases. *Clin Infect Dis* **38:**206–216.
131. **Vineetha M, Palakkal S, Sobhanakumari K, Celine MI, Letha V.** 2016. Verrucous onychomycosis caused by *Curvularia* in a patient with congenital pterygium. *Indian J Dermatol* **61:**701.
132. **Premamalini T, Ambujavalli BT, Vijayakumar R, Rajyoganandh SV, Kalpana S, Kindo AJ.** 2012. Fungal keratitis caused by *Macrophomina phaseolina*—A case report. *Med Mycol Case Rep* **1:**123–126.
133. **Tendolkar U, Tayal RA, Baveja SM, Shinde C.** 2015. Mycotic keratitis due to *Neoscytalidium dimidiatum*: a rare case. *Community Acquir Infect* **2:**142–144.
134. **Benaoudia F, Assouline M, Pouliquen Y, Bouvet A, Guého E.** 1999. *Exophiala (Wangiella) dermatitidis* keratitis after keratoplasty. *Med Mycol* **37:**53–56.
135. **Saeedi OJ, Iyer SA, Mohiuddin AZ, Hogan RN.** 2013. *Exophiala jeanselmei* keratitis: case report and review of literature. *Eye Contact Lens* **39:**410–412.
136. **Wilhelmus KR, Jones DB.** 2001. *Curvularia* keratitis. *Trans Am Ophthalmol Soc* **99:**111–130, discussion 130–132.
137. **Shadomy HJ, Dixon DM.** 1989. A new *Papulaspora* species from the infected eye of a horse: *Papulaspora equi* sp. nov. *Mycopathologia* **106:**35–39.
138. **Selvin SS, Korah SM, Michael JS, Raj PM, Jacob P.** 2014. Series of five cases of *Papulaspora equi* keratomycosis. *Cornea* **33:**640–643.
139. **Sigler L, Summerbell RC, Poole L, Wieden M, Sutton DA, Rinaldi MG, Aguirre M, Estes GW, Galgiani JN.** 1997. Invasive *Nattrassia mangiferae* infections: case report, literature review, and therapeutic and taxonomic appraisal. *J Clin Microbiol* **35:**433–440.
140. **Hasegawa T, Yoshida Y, Kosuge J, Haga T, Goto Y, Shinjo T, Uchida K, Yamaguchi R, Tateyama S, Takatori K.** 2005. Subcutaneous granuloma associated with *Macrophomina* species infection in a cat. *Vet Rec* **156:**23–24.
141. **Guého E, Bonnefoy A, Luboinski J, Petit J-C, de Hoog GS.** 1989. Subcutaneous granuloma caused by *Phialophora richardsiae*: case report and review of the literature. *Mycoses* **32:**219–223.
142. **Hohl PE, Holley HP Jr, Prevost E, Ajello L, Padbye AA.** 1983. Infections due to *Wangiella dermatitidis* in humans: report of the first documented case from the United States and a review of the literature. *Rev Infect Dis* **5:**854–864.
143. **Sudduth EJ, Crumbley AJ, Farrarn WE.** 1992. Phaeohyphomycosis due to *Exophiala* species: clinical spectrum of disease in humans. *Clin Infect Dis* **15:**639–644.
144. **Badali H, Najafzadeh MJ, van Esbroeck M, van den Enden E, Tarazooie B, Meis JF, de Hoog GS.** 2010. The clinical spectrum of *Exophiala jeanselmei*, with a case report and in vitro antifungal susceptibility of the species. *Med Mycol* **48:**318–327.
145. **Guarro J, Kantarcioglu AS, Horré R, Rodríguez-Tudela JL, Cuenca M, Berenguer J, de Hoog GS.** 2006. *Scedosporium apiospermum*: changing clinical spectrum of a therapy-refractory opportunist. *Med Mycol* **44:**295–327.
146. **Shi D, Lu G, Mei H, de Hoog GS, Samerpitak K, Deng S, Shen Y, Liu W.** 2016. Subcutaneous infection by *Ochroconis mirabilis* in an immunocompetent patient. *Med Mycol Case Rep* **11:**44–47.
147. **Woo PC, Lau SK, Ngan AH, Tse H, Tung ET, Yuen KY.** 2008. *Lasiodiplodia theobromae* pneumonia in a liver transplant recipient. *J Clin Microbiol* **46:**380–384.
148. **Willinger B, Kopetzky G, Harm F, Apfalter P, Makristathis A, Berer A, Bankier A, Winkler S.** 2004. Disseminated infection with *Nattrassia mangiferae* in an immunosuppressed patient. *J Clin Microbiol* **42:**478–480.
149. **González MS, Alfonso B, Seckinger D, Padhye AA, Ajello L.** 1984. Subcutaneous phaeohyphomycosis caused by *Cladosporium devriesii*, sp. nov. *Sabouraudia* **22:**427–432.
150. **Tintelnot K, von Hunnius P, de Hoog GS, Polak-Wyss A, Guého E, Masclaux F.** 1995. Systemic mycosis caused by a new *Cladophialophora* species. *J Med Vet Mycol* **33:** 349–354.
151. **Yurlova NA, de Hoog GS.** 2002. Exopolysaccharides and capsules in human pathogenic *Exophiala* species. *Mycoses* **45:**443–448.
152. **de Hoog GS, Poonwan N, Gerrits van den Ende AHG.** 1999. Taxonomy of *Exophiala spinifera* and its relationship to *E. jeanselmei*. *Stud Mycol* **43:**133–142.
153. **Kondori N, Gilljam M, Lindblad A, Jönsson B, Moore ER, Wennerås C.** 2011. High rate of *Exophiala dermatitidis* recovery in the airways of patients with cystic fibrosis is associated with pancreatic insufficiency. *J Clin Microbiol* **49:**1004–1009.
154. **Li DM, Li RY, De Hoog GS, Wang YX, Wang DL.** 2009. *Exophiala asiatica*, a new species from a fatal case in China. *Med Mycol* **47:**101–109.
155. **Duggan JM, Wolf MD, Kauffman CA.** 1995. *Phialophora verrucosa* infection in an AIDS patient. *Mycoses* **38:** 215–218.

156. **Turiansky GW, Benson PM, Sperling LC, Sau P, Salkin IF, McGinnis MR, James WD.** 1995. *Phialophora verrucosa*: a new cause of mycetoma. *J Am Acad Dermatol* **32:**311–315.
157. **Huang YT, Liaw SJ, Liao CH, Yang JL, Lai DM, Lee YC, Hsueh PR.** 2008. Catheter-related septicemia due to *Aureobasidium pullulans*. *Int J Infect Dis* **12:**e137–e139.
158. **Shin JH, Lee SK, Suh SP, Ryang DW, Kim NH, Rinaldi MG, Sutton DA.** 1998. Fatal *Hormonema dematioides* peritonitis in a patient on continuous ambulatory peritoneal dialysis: criteria for organism identification and review of other known fungal etiologic agents. *J Clin Microbiol* **36:** 2157–2163.
159. **Cortez KJ, Roilides E, Quiroz-Telles F, Meletiadis J, Antachopoulos C, Knudsen T, Buchanan W, Milanovich J, Sutton DA, Fothergill A, Rinaldi MG, Shea YR, Zaoutis T, Kottilil S, Walsh TJ.** 2008. Infections caused by *Scedosporium* spp. *Clin Microbiol Rev* **21:**157–197.
160. **Fisher JF, Shadomy S, Teabeaut JR, Woodward J, Michaels GE, Newman MA, White E, Cook P, Seagraves A, Yaghmai F, Rissing JP.** 1982. Near-drowning complicated by brain abscess due to *Petriellidium boydii*. *Arch Neurol* **39:**511–513.
161. **Malloch D, Salkin IF.** 1984. A new species of *Scedosporium* associated with osteomyelitis in humans. *Mycotaxon* **21:** 247–255.
162. **Rodriguez-Tudela JL, Berenguer J, Guarro J, Kantarcioglu AS, Horre R, de Hoog GS, Cuenca-Estrella M.** 2009. Epidemiology and outcome of *Scedosporium prolificans* infection, a review of 162 cases. *Med Mycol* **47:**359–370.
163. **Guerrero A, Torres P, Duran MT, Ruiz-Díez B, Rosales M, Rodríguez-Tudela JL.** 2001. Airborne outbreak of nosocomial *Scedosporium prolificans* infection. *Lancet* **357:** 1267–1268.
164. **Fernandez M, Noyola DE, Rossmann SN, Edwards MS.** 1999. Cutaneous phaeohyphomycosis caused by *Curvularia lunata* and a review of *Curvularia* infections in pediatrics. *Pediatr Infect Dis J* **18:**727–731.
165. **Pimentel JD, Mahadevan K, Woodgyer A, Sigler L, Gibas C, Harris OC, Lupino M, Athan E.** 2005. Peritonitis due to *Curvularia inaequalis* in an elderly patient undergoing peritoneal dialysis and a review of six cases of peritonitis associated with other *Curvularia* spp. *J Clin Microbiol* **43:**4288–4292.
166. **Kauffman CA, Pappas PG, Patterson TF.** 2013. Fungal infections associated with contaminated methylprednisolone injections. *N Engl J Med* **368:**2495–2500.
167. **Baddley JW, Mostert L, Summerbell RC, Moser SA.** 2006. *Phaeoacremonium parasiticum* infections confirmed by beta-tubulin sequence analysis of case isolates. *J Clin Microbiol* **44:**2207–2211.
168. **Borelli D.** 1983. "*Taeniolella boppii*", nova species, agente de cromomicosis. *Med Cutan Ibero Lat Am* **11:**227–232.
169. **Velazquez LF, Restrepo A, Calle G.** 1976. Cromomicosis: experiencia de doce años. *Acta Med Colomb* **1:**165–171.
170. **Saravanakumar PS, Eslami P, Zar FA.** 1996. Lymphocutaneous sporotrichosis associated with a squirrel bite: case report and review. *Clin Infect Dis* **23:**647–648.
171. **Guarner J, Brandt ME.** 2011. Histopathologic diagnosis of fungal infections in the 21st century. *Clin Microbiol Rev* **24:**247–280.
172. **Cuétara MS, Alhambra A, Moragues MD, González-Elorza E, Pontón J, del Palacio A.** 2009. Detection of (1→3)-β-D-glucan as an adjunct to diagnosis in a mixed population with uncommon proven invasive fungal diseases or with an unusual clinical presentation. *Clin Vaccine Immunol* **16:**423–426.
173. **Litvintseva AP, Lindsley MD, Gade L, Smith R, Chiller T, Lyons JL, Thakur KT, Zhang SX, Grgurich DE, Kerkering TM, Brandt ME, Park BJ.** 2014. Utility of (1-3)-β-D-glucan testing for diagnostics and monitoring response to treatment during the multistate outbreak of fungal meningitis and other infections. *Clin Infect Dis* **58:**622–630.
174. **Lau A, Chen S, Sorrell T, Carter D, Malik R, Martin P, Halliday C.** 2007. Development and clinical application of a panfungal PCR assay to detect and identify fungal DNA in tissue specimens. *J Clin Microbiol* **45:**380–385.
175. **Gade L, Scheel CM, Pham CD, Lindsley MD, Iqbal N, Cleveland AA, Whitney AM, Lockhart SR, Brandt ME, Litvintseva AP.** 2013. Detection of fungal DNA in human body fluids and tissues during a multistate outbreak of fungal meningitis and other infections. *Eukaryot Cell* **12:** 677–683.
176. **Zhao Y, Petraitiene R, Walsh TJ, Perlin DS.** 2013. A real-time PCR assay for rapid detection and quantification of *Exserohilum rostratum*, a causative pathogen of fungal meningitis associated with injection of contaminated methylprednisolone. *J Clin Microbiol* **51:**1034–1036.
177. **Clinical and Laboratory Standards Institute.** 2008. *Interpretive Criteria for Identification of Bacteria and Fungi by DNA Sequencing; Approved Guideline. CLSI document MM18-A.* Clinical and Laboratory Standards Institute, Wayne, PA.
178. **Hibbett D, Abarenkov K, Kõljalg U, Öpik M, Chai B, Cole J, Wang Q, Crous P, Robert V, Helgason T, Herr JR, Kirk P, Lueschow S, O'Donnell K, Nilsson RH, Oono R, Schoch C, Smyth C, Walker DM, Porras-Alfaro A, Taylor JW, Geiser DM.** 2016. Sequence-based classification and identification of Fungi. *Mycologia* **108:**1049–1068.
179. **Sanguinetti M, Posteraro B.** 2017. Identification of molds by matrix-assisted laser desorption ionization-time of flight mass spectrometry. *J Clin Microbiol* **55:**369–379.
180. **Kondori N, Erhard M, Welinder-Olsson C, Groenewald M, Verkley G, Moore ERB.** 2015. Analyses of black fungi by matrix-assisted laser desorption/ionization time-of-flight mass spectrometry (MALDI-TOF MS): species-level identification of clinical isolates of *Exophiala dermatitidis*. *FEMS Microbiol Lett* **362:**1–6.
181. **Özhak-Baysan B, Öğünç D, Döğen A, Ilkit M, de Hoog GS.** 2015. MALDI-TOF MS-based identification of black yeasts of the genus *Exophiala*. *Med Mycol* **53:**347–352.
182. **Borman AM, Fraser M, Szekely A, Larcombe DE, Johnson EM.** 2017. Rapid identification of clinically relevant members of the genus *Exophiala* by matrix-assisted laser desorption ionization-time of flight mass spectrometry and description of two novel species, *Exophiala campbelli* and *Exophiala lavatrina*. *J Clin Microbiol* **55:**1162–1176.
183. **Coulibaly O, Marinach-Patrice C, Cassagne C, Piarroux R, Mazier D, Ranque S.** 2011. *Pseudallescheria/Scedosporium* complex species identification by matrix-assisted laser desorption ionization time-of-flight mass spectrometry. *Med Mycol* **49:**621–626.
184. **Singh A, Singh PK, Kumar A, Chander J, Khanna G, Roy P, Meis JF, Chowdhary A.** 2017. Molecular and matrix-assisted laser desorption ionization-time of flight mass spectrometry characterization of clinically significant melanized fungi in India. *J Clin Microbiol* **55:**1090–1103.
185. **Madrid H, Ruíz-Cendoya M, Cano J, Stchigel A, Orofino R, Guarro J.** 2009. Genotyping and in vitro antifungal susceptibility of *Neoscytalidium dimidiatum* isolates from different origins. *Int J Antimicrob Agents* **34:**351–354.
186. **Litvintseva AP, Hurst S, Gade L, Frace MA, Hilsabeck R, Schupp JM, Gillece JD, Roe C, Smith D, Keim P, Lockhart SR, Changayil S, Weil MR, MacCannell DR, Brandt ME, Engelthaler DM.** 2014. Whole-genome analysis of *Exserohilum rostratum* from an outbreak of fungal meningitis and other infections. *J Clin Microbiol* **52:**3216–3222.
187. **Blumer SO, Kaufman L, Kaplan W, McLaughlin DW, Kraft DE.** 1973. Comparative evaluation of five serological methods for the diagnosis of sporotrichosis. *Appl Microbiol* **26:**4–8.
188. **Scott EN, Muchmore HG.** 1989. Immunoblot analysis of antibody responses to *Sporothrix schenckii*. *J Clin Microbiol* **27:**300–304.
189. **Fothergill AW, Rinaldi MG, Sutton DA.** 2009. Antifungal susceptibility testing of *Exophiala* spp.: a head-to-head comparison of amphotericin B, itraconazole, posaconazole and voriconazole. *Med Mycol* **47:**41–43.
190. **Badali H, De Hoog GS, Curfs-Breuker I, Andersen B, Meis JF.** 2009. *In vitro* activities of eight antifungal drugs against 70 clinical and environmental isolates of *Alternaria* species. *J Antimicrob Chemother* **63:**1295–1297.

191. **Gilgado F, Serena C, Cano J, Gené J, Guarro J.** 2006. Antifungal susceptibilities of the species of the *Pseudallescheria boydii* complex. *Antimicrob Agents Chemother* **50:**4211–4213.
192. **Lackner M, de Hoog GS, Verweij PE, Najafzadeh MJ, Curfs-Breuker I, Klaassen CH, Meis JF.** 2012. Species-specific antifungal susceptibility patterns of *Scedosporium* and *Pseudallescheria* species. *Antimicrob Agents Chemother* **56:**2635–2642.
193. **Carrillo AJ, Guarro J.** 2001. In vitro activities of four novel triazoles against *Scedosporium* spp. *Antimicrob Agents Chemother* **45:**2151–2153.
194. **González GM, Fothergill AW, Sutton DA, Rinaldi MG, Loebenberg D.** 2005. *In vitro* activities of new and established triazoles against opportunistic filamentous and dimorphic fungi. *Med Mycol* **43:**281–284.
195. **Marimon R, Serena C, Gené J, Cano J, Guarro J.** 2008. In vitro antifungal susceptibilities of five species of *Sporothrix*. *Antimicrob Agents Chemother* **52:**732–734.
196. **Pappas PG.** 2013. Lessons learned in the multistate fungal infection outbreak in the United States. *Curr Opin Infect Dis* **26:**545–550.
197. **Falci DR, Pasqualotto AC.** 2013. Profile of isavuconazole and its potential in the treatment of severe invasive fungal infections. *Infect Drug Resist* **6:**163–174.
198. **Espinel-Ingroff A.** 2003. In vitro antifungal activities of anidulafungin and micafungin, licensed agents and the investigational triazole posaconazole as determined by NCCLS methods for 12,052 fungal isolates: review of the literature. *Rev Iberoam Micol* **20:**121–136.
199. **Guarro J.** 2011. Lessons from animal studies for the treatment of invasive human infections due to uncommon fungi. *J Antimicrob Chemother* **66:**1447–1466.
200. **Calvo E, Pastor FJ, Mayayo E, Hernández P, Guarro J.** 2011. Antifungal therapy in an athymic murine model of chromoblastomycosis by *Fonsecaea pedrosoi*. *Antimicrob Agents Chemother* **55:**3709–3713.
201. **Calvo E, Pastor FJ, Salas V, Mayayo E, Capilla J, Guarro J.** 2012. Histopathology and antifungal treatment of experimental murine chromoblastomycosis caused by *Cladophialophora carrionii*. *J Antimicrob Chemother* **67:**666–670.
202. **Rodríguez MM, Calvo E, Serena C, Mariné M, Pastor FJ, Guarro J.** 2009. Effects of double and triple combinations of antifungal drugs in a murine model of disseminated infection by *Scedosporium prolificans*. *Antimicrob Agents Chemother* **53:**2153–2155.
203. **Calvo E, Pastor FJ, Rodríguez MM, Mayayo E, Salas V, Guarro J.** 2010. Murine model of a disseminated infection by the novel fungus *Fonsecaea monophora* and successful treatment with posaconazole. *Antimicrob Agents Chemother* **54:**919–923.
204. **Calvo E, Pastor FJ, Guarro J.** 2010. Antifungal therapies in murine disseminated phaeohyphomycoses caused by *Exophiala* species. *J Antimicrob Chemother* **65:**1455–1459.
205. **Ruíz-Cendoya M, Madrid H, Pastor J, Guarro J.** 2010. Evaluation of antifungal therapy in a neutropenic murine model of *Neoscytalidium dimidiatum* infection. *Int J Antimicrob Agents* **35:**152–155.
206. **Mariné M, Pastor FJ, Guarro J.** 2009. Combined antifungal therapy in a murine model of disseminated infection by *Cladophialophora bantiana*. *Med Mycol* **47:**45–49.
207. **Fernández-Silva F, Capilla J, Mayayo E, Guarro J.** 2012. Efficacy of posaconazole in murine experimental sporotrichosis. *Antimicrob Agents Chemother* **56:**2273–2277.

Fungi Causing Eumycotic Mycetoma*

SARAH ABDALLA AHMED, G. SYBREN DE HOOG,
AND WENDY W. J. VAN DE SANDE

128

Eumycetoma was recognized as a neglected tropical disease by the World Health Organization in 2016 (1). It is a chronic, granulomatous, progressive subcutaneous fungal disease characterized by the production of large masses of fungal material called grains, which are discharged through sinus tracts. Eumycetoma is seen more frequently in tropical and subtropical regions and is rare in temperate countries, where it usually occurs among immigrants from the tropics. Several hyaline and dematiaceous fungi can cause eumycetoma, and their distributions are greatly affected by climate, especially rainfall, and by socioeconomic conditions.

TAXONOMY AND DESCRIPTION OF THE AGENTS

All fungi known to cause eumycetoma belong to the phylum Ascomycota. Although for many species no ascus-producing state is known (2), their phylogenetic affiliation has been proven by DNA sequencing. Ordinal relationships are hypothesized on the basis of ribosomal small subunit (3) and internal transcribed spacer (ITS) DNA sequences (4) (Table 1; see also listing by order below). The etiologic agents described in this chapter are species that are isolated most commonly from human or lower-animal mycetoma. For species that are implicated as rare causative agents of mycetoma but more are common in other conditions, we refer to the corresponding chapters in this *Manual*.

Order Sordariales

Madurella Species

Madurella mycetomatis is the most common fungal causative agent of mycetoma (5) (Fig. 1A, B, and C). It is common in the arid climatic zone of Africa (Sudan, Mali, and Djibouti), and it is occasionally encountered in the Middle East and India. The taxonomy of *M. mycetomatis* was proved by a number of phylogenetic studies in which DNA sequences of the mitochondrial genome, the ribosomal DNA (rDNA) ITS, the beta-tubulin gene (*BT2*), and the RNA polymerase II subunit gene (*RPB2*) were determined (3, 6, 7). The complete genome has been sequenced for a Sudanese isolate (MM55) which has been deposited in the CBS-KNAW fungal collection of the Westerdijk Fungal Biodiversity Institute under the number CBS 131320 (8).

Based on the ITS, *BT2* and *RPB2* sequences, it appeared that several other species previously misidentified as *M. mycetomatis* belong to different *Madurella* species. These new *Madurella* species include *Madurella pseudomycetomatis*, *M. tropicana*, and *M. fahalii* (7, 9). Of these species, *M. fahalii* seemed to be more resistant to antifungal agents. Since these species could be differentiated only on the basis of molecular identification, it is not clear how many of the previous reported mycetoma cases attributed to *M. mycetomatis* might actually have been caused by a different *Madurella* species. *M. pseudomycetomatis* has been identified in Italy (7), Venezuela (10), and China (9).

Order Pleosporales

Falciformispora senegalensis (Previously Known as *Leptosphaeria senegalensis*) and *Falciformispora tompkinsii* (Previously Known as *L. tompkinsii*)

Based on the combined DNA sequence data set of the small ribosomal subunit (SSU), large ribosomal subunit (LSU), *RPB2*, and translation elongation factor 1-alpha (*TEF1*) genes, *Leptosphaeria senegalensis* and *L. tompkinsii* were found to cluster in the pleosporalean family Trematosphaeriaceae, with *Falciformispora lignatilis* as the closest relative. Therefore, *L. senegalensis* was renamed *Falciformispora senegalensis* and *L. tompkinsii* as *F. tompkinsii* (11). *F. senegalensis* is a dematiaceous filamentous fungus producing cleistothecia containing large asci with eight ascospores; each of the ascospores is ellipsoidal, has four septa, and is surrounded by a slime sheath (2) (Fig. 1D, E, and F). *F. senegalensis* and the related species *F. tompkinsii* cause mycetomata in the northern tropical portion of Africa, especially in Senegal and Mauritania, and in India (12–14).

Trematosphaeria grisea (Previously Known as *Madurella grisea*)

In 2004, it was demonstrated by molecular phylogeny and diagnostics that the members of the genus *Madurella* encompass a hidden diversity beyond the currently recognized species (3). Both an rRNA restriction fragment length polymorphism analysis and a species-specific ITS PCR were used for species distinction by Ahmed et al. (15, 16).

*Some of the material in this chapter was presented in chapter 125 by Abdalla O. A. Ahmed, G. Sybren de Hoog, and Wendy W. J. van de Sande in the 11th edition of this *Manual*.

TABLE 1 Overview of species causing eumycotic mycetoma

Order	Species	No. of isolates[a]	Prevalence[b]	Color of grains	Size of grains (mm)	Geographic distribution	Reference(s)
Sordariales	*Madurella mycetomatis*	2,032	C	Black	Up to 5.0 or more	East Africa, Middle East, India	5, 12, 47
Pleosporales	*Falciformispora senegalensis*	167	O	Black	0.5–2.0	West Africa, India	5, 12, 146
Pleosporales	*Trematosphaeria grisea*	116	O	Black	0.3–0.6	South America, India	5, 11, 14, 19, 20, 147–151
Microascales	*Scedosporium apiospermum* complex	83	O	White	0.2–2.0	North and South America, India	5, 36, 37, 152–157; chapter 127
Pleosporales	*Medicopsis romeroi*	22	O/R	Black			5, 11, 23–25, 126, 151
Pleosporales	*Nigrograna mackinnonii*	7	O/R	Black	0.3–1.0	Central and South America	5, 11, 151
Hypocreales	*Sarocladium kiliense* (Syn. *Acremonium kiliense*)		R	White			
Hypocreales	*Acremonium recifei*		R	White			158
Eurotiales	*Aspergillus flavus*	2	R	Green/ white			5, 159, 160 chapter 122
Eurotiales	*Aspergillus fumigatus*	2	R				5; chapter 122
Eurotiales	*Aspergillus nidulans*	1	R	White			5, 19; chapter 122
Chaetothyriales	*Cladiophialophora bantiana*		R				161; chapter 127
Chaetothyriales	*Cladiophialophora mycetomatis*		R	Black	0.5		162; chapter 127
Pleosporales	*Corynespora cassiicola*		R	Black			163
Pleosporales	*Curvularia geniculata*		R	Black	0.5–1.0	Worldwide	164, 165; chapter 127
Pleosporales	*Curvularia lunata*		R	Black	0.5–1.0	Worldwide	19, 166–168 chapter 127
Diaporthales	*Diaporthe phaseolorum*		R				169
Pleosporales	*Emmarelia grisea*		R	Black	0.3–0.6	India, Sri Lanka	151
Pleosporales	*Emmarelia paragrisea*		R	Black	0.3–0.6	India, Sri Lanka	151
Chaetothyriales	*Exophiala jeanselmei*	9	R	Black	0.5–1.0	Worldwide	5, 142, 170, 171; chapter 127
Pleosporales	*Falciformispora tompkinsii*		R	Black	0.5–1.0		11, 172
Hypocreales	*Fusarium falciforme*	3	R	White	0.2–0.5	Worldwide	5, 71, 173–176; chapter 123
Hypocreales	*Fusarium verticillioides* (Syn. *Fusarium monoliforme*)		R	White			143, 177 chapter 123
Hypocreales	*Fusarium oxysporum*		R	White			Chapter 123
Hypocreales	*Fusarium solani*		R	White			178; chapter 123
Saccharomycetales	*Geotrichum candidum*	1	R				5; chapter 120
Hypocreales	*Ilyonectria destructans*		R	White			179
Sordariales	*Madurella fahalii*		R	Black			7
Sordariales	*Madurella pseudomycetomatis*		R	Black			7, 9
Sordariales	*Madurella tropicana*		R	Black			7
Onygenales	*Microsporum audouini*	1	R	White			Chapter 126
Onygenales	*Microsporum canis*		R				66, 180–182; chapter 126
Pleosporales	*Neotestudina rosatii*	4	R	White			5
Diaporthales	*Phaeoacremonium krajdenii*		R	White			87; chapter 127
Diaporthales	*Phaeoacremonium parasiticum*		R				183; chapter 127
Diaporthales	*Phialophora cyanescens*		R	White			184; chapter 127
Diaporthales	*Phialophora verrucosa*		R	Black			Chapter 127
Calosphaeriales	*Pleurostomophora ochracea*		R	Yellow		Sudan	80; chapter 127
Pleosporales	*Pseudochaetosphaeronema larense*		R	Black			
Chaetothyriales	*Rhinocladiella atrovirens*	2	R				5
Hysteriales	*Rhytidhysteron rufulum*						14
Pleosporales	*Setosphaeria rostrata*		R				

[a]Numbers of isolates are from reference 5. In that study, a meta-analysis of 2,704 eumycetoma cases was performed. The species identification was unknown for 220 fungi. One should take into consideration that the species identification was based on histology and/or culturing. It is probable that molecular identification would be yield different numbers of isolates for each species.

[b]C, common (>5% of the reported cases worldwide were caused by this species); O, occasional (caused 1 to 5%); R, rare (caused <1%). Data according to reference 5.

Based on the rDNA sequence, the taxonomic position of *M. grisea* was changed to the order Pleosporales, and therefore, it should no longer be considered a sister species to *M. mycetomatis*, which is a member of the Sordariales. In 2013, the name was officially changed to *Trematosphaeria grisea* (11). Based on the combined molecular data set of the SSU gene, the LSU gene, *RPB2*, and *TEF1*, it was demonstrated that *M. grisea* formed a well-supported clade with *Trematosphaeria pertusa* (11); hence the renaming to *T. grisea*. *T. grisea* has been reported to occur as an etiologic agent of black-grain mycetoma in South America, India, Africa, and North and Central America (17–20), but older literature data need verification by sequencing (14). The fungus is a coelomycete, but conidial fruiting bodies may remain absent (Fig. 1G, H, and I). With strictly sterile cultures, molecular confirmation is required for identification, demonstrated by the finding that out of 31 fungal isolates deposited in either the National Collection of Pathogenic Fungi (NCPF, Bristol, United Kingdom) or the Institut Pasteur Culture Collection (UMIP, Paris, France) as *M. grisea*, 28 were in fact other pleosporalean agents of eumycetoma (*Nigrograna mackinnonii*, 8 isolates; *Medicopsis romeroi*, 10 isolates; *Rhytidhysteron rufulum*, 4 isolates; *E. grisea*, 5 isolates, *Emarellia paragrisea*, 1 isolate) (14).

Medicopsis romeroi (Previously Known as *Pyrenochaeta romeroi*)

Based on sequences of the 18S (small-subunit) rDNA and the 28S (large-subunit) rDNA, it has become clear that *Pyrenochaeta romeroi* is distantly related to the type species of *Pyrenochaeta* (*Pyrenochaeta nobilis*) (21). Therefore, *P. romeroi* was renamed as *Medicopsis romeroi* by de Gruyter et al. (22). *M. romeroi* is a coelomycetous anamorphic fungus. It might be misidentified as *T. grisea* when cultures lack pycnidia (2). Mycetomata caused by *M. romeroi* have been reported from Somalia, Saudi Arabia, India, Pakistan, and South America (14, 23–25). Colony appearance and microscopy of granules and fruiting bodies resemble those of *T. grisea*. This explains why at least 10 nonsporulating isolates of *M. romeroi* were misidentified as *T. grisea* in the past (14).

Nigrograna mackinnonii (Previously Known as *Pyrenochaeta mackinnonii*)

Molecular analysis of the rRNA genes also revealed that *Pyrenochaeta mackinnonii* is distant from the type species of *Pyrenochaeta* (*Pyrenochaeta nobilis*) (21, 22). Furthermore, *M. romeroi* (formerly *Pyrenochaeta romeroi*) and *P. mackinnonii* were found to be phylogenetically remote from each other, and therefore, *P. mackinnonii* was assigned to a different genus, *Nigrograna*, and renamed *N. mackinnonii* (27). Between 2014 and 2015, this species was named *Biatriospora mackinnonii* (11), but after a thorough taxonomic revision, it was changed back to *N. mackinnonii* in 2015 (26). The complete genome of *N. mackinnonii* has been sequenced from endophytic isolate E5202H, which was deposited in the American Type Culture Collection (ATCC) as SD-6893 (27). *N. mackinnonii* has been reported as the causative agent of mycetoma in patients from Costa Rica, Mexico, and Venezuela.

Emarellia grisea and *Emarellia paragrisea*

Based on the combined DNA sequence data of the LSU, ITS, *ACT*, *RPB2*, and *TEF1* genes, it was demonstrated that *Emarellia grisea* and *E. paragrisea* clustered among the pleosporalean causative agents of eumycetoma (14). In culture, these fungi produce only sterile, melanized hyphae. *E. grisea* causes mycetomata in India and Sri Lanka (14).

Neotestudina rosatii

Neotestudina rosatii has been isolated from soil from tropical countries; it is an ascomycete with spherical, deliquescent asci and rhomboid ascospores with one septum each (2) (Fig. 1J, K, and L). Mycetomata caused by *N. rosatii* have been described in Australia, Cameroon, Guinea, Senegal, and Somalia (25, 28).

Order Microascales

Scedosporium Species

The genus *Scedosporium* comprises a small group of rather variable species (29–31). The separation of the main species, *Scedosporium boydii* (previously known as *Pseudallescheria boydii*) and *S. apiospermum*, is still debated. Chen et al. (32) referred to both as a species complex. In addition, new species have been proposed, namely, *S. minutispora*, *S. aurantiacum*, and *S. dehoogii* (29, 30).

The *S. apiospermum* complex is associated with manure and polluted environments (33, 34) and has been known since the 1920s to be an agent of human mycetoma (35), mainly in temperate climates (36) and occurring mostly in the limbs (37). Subcutaneous infections frequently lack the formation of grains when the patients' immunity is impaired (38). In addition, arthritis is frequently observed, due to the predilection of this species for cartilaginous tissues (39–42).

Other Orders

Mycetoma can be caused by many different fungal species; most of these species are only rarely encountered in mycetoma (Table 1).

EPIDEMIOLOGY AND TRANSMISSION

The number of species involved in mycetoma is increasing, but little is known about the epidemiology and mode of transmission of these species. Case reports are indicative of the presence of certain species in particular geographical locations but do not provide a clear understanding of the environmental distribution of species and the possible ecological niches. In 2013, a meta-analysis was performed by van de Sande to estimate the prevalence of mycetoma, including 8,763 cases (5). Countries with a high prevalence were Mauritania (prevalence of 3.49 cases per 100,000 inhabitants) and Sudan (1.81 cases per 100,000 inhabitants) (5). Prevalence was relatively high in rural areas of countries where mycetoma is endemic (5).

The causal agents of eumycetoma are largely saprobes that live on hard plant materials, such as various types of thorns and spines, that are associated with soil (43–46). Segretain and Destombes (28, 47), using specific isolation media and techniques, showed that *F. senegalensis* and *F. tompkinsii* could be recovered from about 50% of the dry thorns of *Acacia* trees that they examined, particularly those that had been stained by mud during the rainy season. *N. rosatii* was isolated from sandy soil (25), and *M. mycetomatis* was isolated from soil and anthills (48, 49). It should be noted, however, that the identity of these fungi has not been verified with molecular methods; the possibility that environmental strains do not always belong to the same species as the clinical strains cannot be excluded. Using ITS sequencing, Badali et al. (50) reidentified a collection of *Exophiala jeanselmei* clinical and environmental strains. *E. jeanselmei* identification was confirmed in all mycetoma

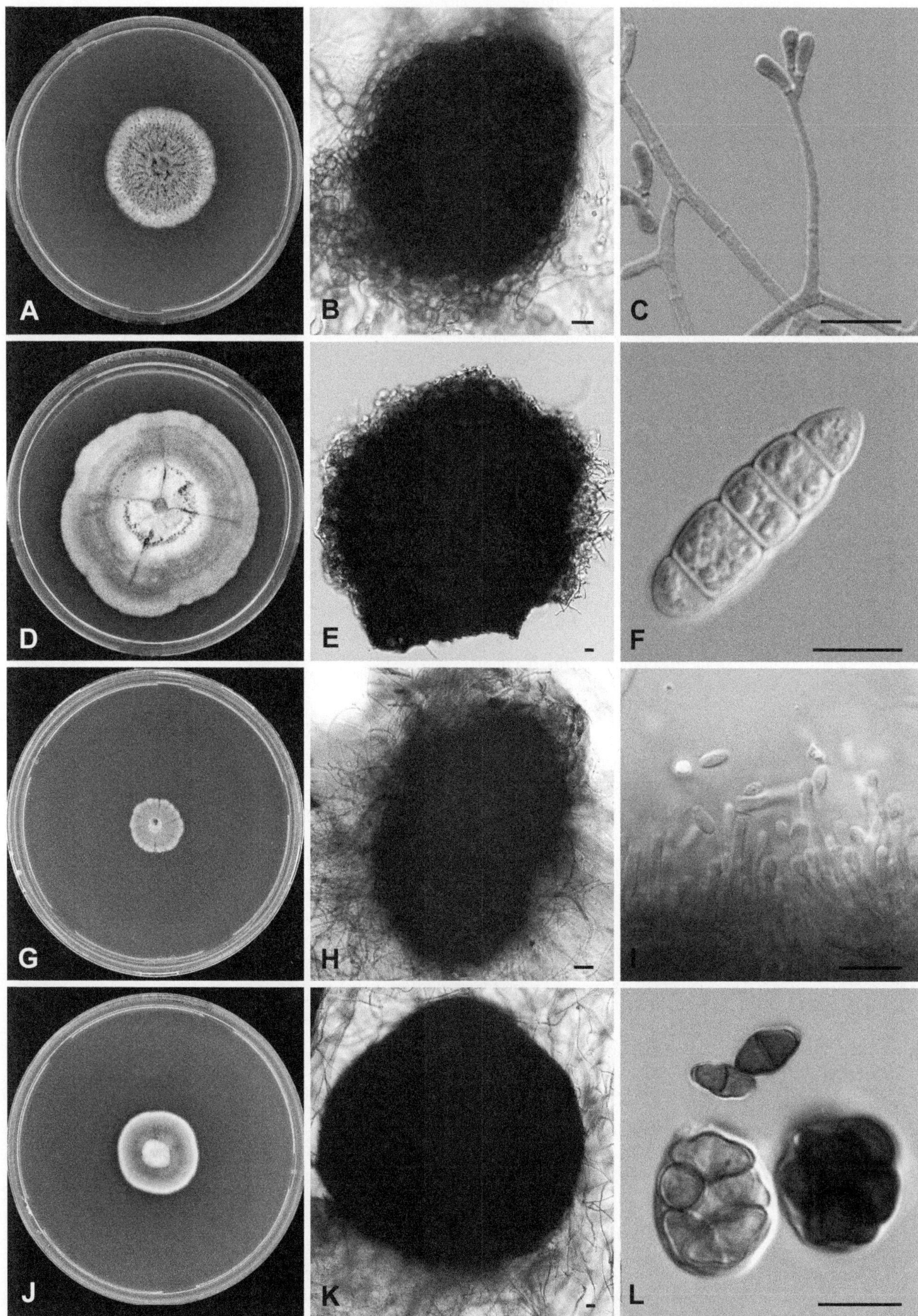
A
B
C
D
E
F
G
H
I
J
K
L

or mycetoma-like infections, while other environmental strains were found to belong to other *Exophiala* species, suggesting some predilection of particular species for human invasion. Another example of possible human predilection is *M. mycetomatis*, which is a common agent of black-grain mycetoma in the arid climate zones of East Africa. The direct isolation of this species from the environment is difficult (51), but its DNA could be present in both soil and thorns. Recently, phylogenetic findings even suggested dung as a possible new habitat for *M. mycetomatis* (52).

Borelli (53) isolated a sterile fungus, reported as *Madurella grisea* (now known as *T. grisea*), from soil in Venezuela; the ecological niche and clinical potential of this rare species have not yet been determined. Also, in relatively common fungi, such as *M. mycetomatis* and *Scedosporium* species, phenotypic identification alone is not enough to determine the exact epidemiology, since these apparently similar entities might hide significant diversity (see "Taxonomy and Description of the Agents" above).

Mycetoma may infect all people living in areas of endemicity but develops more commonly among persons who are in contact with contaminated materials, such as field workers, farmers, and fishermen. There is no obvious immune defect in mycetoma patients, although association with some rare immune defects does occur (54–58). This concerns single-nucleotide polymorphisms in genes involved in the functioning of the host's immune system, such as the chitinases AMCase and chitotriosidase, complement receptor 1 (CR1), the CC chemokine ligand 5 (CCR5), the chemokines interleukin 8 (CXCL8) and interleukin 10, the interleukin receptor CXCR2, metalloproteases 2 and 9, the nitric oxide synthase NOS2, and trombospondin 4, and in the sex hormone synthesis, such as cytochrome P450 subfamily 19 (CYP19) and catechol-O-methyltransferase (COMT) (54–58). The latter might explain why mycetoma is more common in males than females, as is also observed with many other opportunistic fungi.

Areas of endemicity are particularly located in tropical climate zones. *M. mycetomatis* is limited to semiarid to arid climates, while *Falciformispora* species are found in the rain forest. Locally acquired mycetomata in temperate climates invariably are caused by *S. apiospermum* complex. Cases observed in the United States and Europe caused by species other than *S. apiospermum* are imported by immigrants from tropical countries. For example, de Hoog et al. (59) reported cases in The Netherlands originating from Indonesia and Suriname, and Ahmed et al. (15) reported *M. mycetomatis* mycetoma cases seen in France but originating in Mali.

Climate has a definite influence on the prevalence and distribution of mycetoma. Rivers that flood each year during the wet season in many countries of Africa and Asia influence the distribution of the causal agents. Rainfall also aids the spread of the etiologic agents on organic matter (60).

CLINICAL SIGNIFICANCE

A mycetoma (61) is a localized, chronic, noncontiguous, granulomatous infection involving cutaneous and subcutaneous tissues and eventually, in some cases, bones. Mycetomata are generally confined to either the feet or the hands but occasionally affect sites such as the back, shoulders, and buttocks. Rarely, other body sites can be involved, such as the scalp, eye, jaw, and oral cavity (9, 62–64). The triad of a painless subcutaneous mass, sinuses, and discharge containing grains (masses of fungal organisms) (Fig. 2) is characteristic of mycetoma; however, a similar condition (actinomycetoma) may be caused by aerobic actinomycete bacteria.

The disease is more commonly seen in humans than in animals. Only a few cases of mycetoma involving animals, such as cats, dogs, horses, and goats, have been described in the literature (19, 65–69). Most cases occur in otherwise healthy patients. The development of mycetoma after an accidental implantation of the etiologic agent following surgery (70) and in a renal transplant recipient (71) has been reported.

A mycetoma develops after a traumatic injury by microbe-contaminated thorns, splinters, fish scales or fins, snake bites, insect bites, farm implements, and knives. The initial lesion is often characterized by a feeling of discomfort and pain at the point of inoculation. Weeks or months later, the subcutaneous tissue at the site of inoculation becomes indurated, abscesses develop, and fistulae may drain to the surface. As described above, mycetomata are characterized by swelling, granulomas, abscesses, and sinuses from which serosanguinous fluid containing fungal grains is discharged. Grains, which are not seen in other subcutaneous mycoses, can vary from approximately 0.2 to over 5 mm in diameter. The size, color, shape, and internal architecture of the grains vary depending on the etiologic agent. Some of the host material, especially at the periphery of the grain, provides a protective barrier for the fungus against antifungal agents and against components of humoral immune responses, such as antibodies.

A mycetoma develops slowly beneath thick fibrosclerous tissue. The subsequent phase of proliferation involves the invasion of muscles and intramuscular layers by portions of the sclerotium that break free from their parent structure. The granulomatous lesions can extend as deep as bone, where severe bone destruction, formation of small cavities, and complete remodeling may occur. Early osteolytic damage includes loss of the cortical margin and external erosion of the bone. As the infection progresses, blood, lymphatic vessels, and nerves may be damaged. Frequently, secondary bacterial infections and osteomyelitis producing total bone destruction occur. Pain in mycetoma is often associated with bone involvement and secondary bacterial infection.

Fungus balls in preexisting lung cavities are sometimes inappropriately called mycetomata (72, 73). In the absence of well-organized grains, they should be referred to as aspergillomas, or simply as fungus balls, depending on the etiologic agent (74). Similarly, mycelial aggregates formed by dermatophytes in cutaneous or subcutaneous tissues differ from grains of mycetomata by lacking granule ontogeny, a distinct Splendore-Hoeppli reaction (see "Microscopy" below) surrounding the mycelial aggregates, and the entry of the fungus from the hair follicles into deeper tissue following the rupture of the follicular epithelium. Such infections caused by dermatophytes have been referred to as pseudomycetomata (75).

FIGURE 1 Cultures of mycetoma-causative agents. (A) *M. mycetomatis* colony on Sabouraud dextrose agar. (B) *M. mycetomatis* sterile sclerotia. (C) *M. mycetomatis* phialides and minute conidia. (D) *F. senegalensis* colony on malt extract agar. (E) *F. senegalensis* ascomata. (F) *F. senegalensis* ascospore. (G) *T. grisea* colony on malt extract agar. (H) *T. grisea* pycnidia containing conidia. (I) *T. grisea* conidiophores and conidia. (J) *N. rosatii* colony on malt extract agar. (K) *N. rosatii* ascomata. (I) *N. rosatii* asci and ascospores.

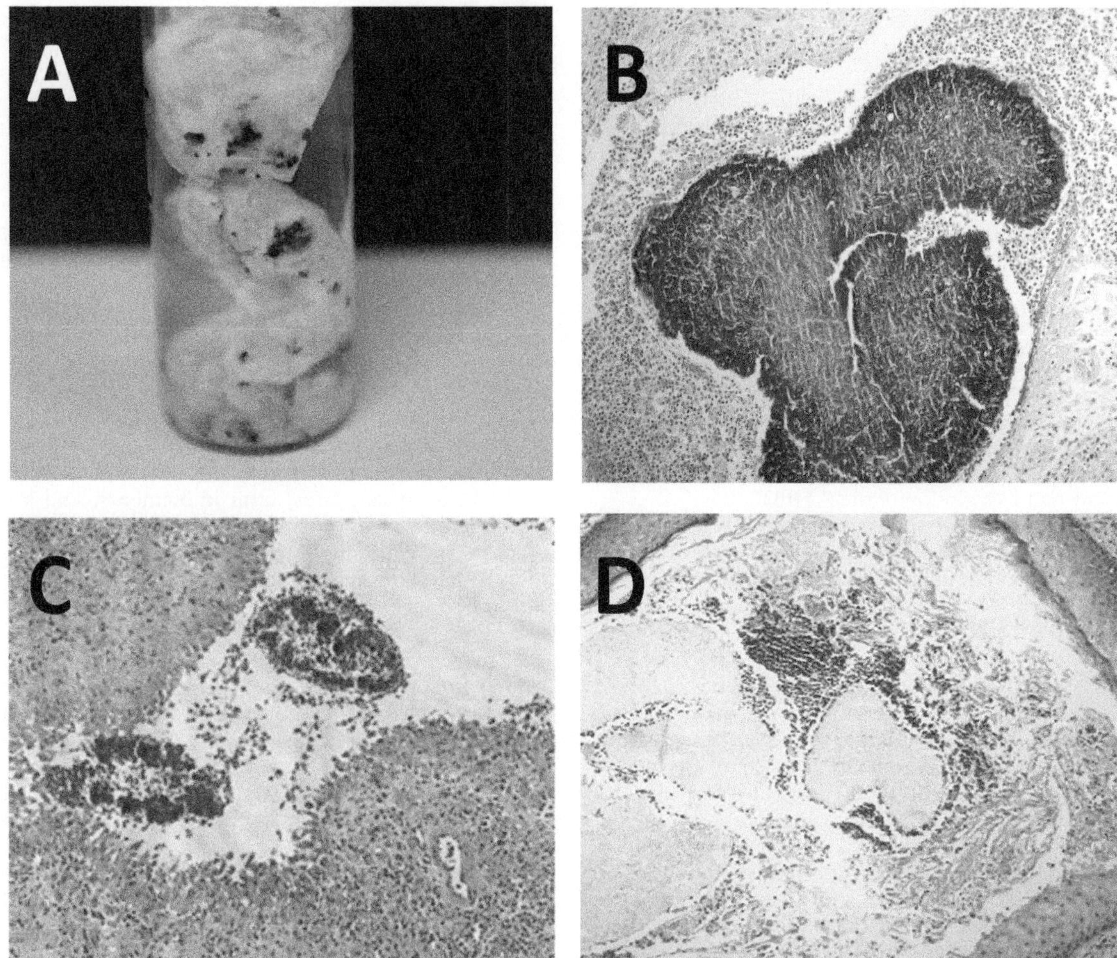

FIGURE 2 Grains of *M. mycetomatis* within subcutaneous tissue. (A) Black *M. mycetomatis* grains in formalin-fixed subcutaneous tissue. Magnification, ×1. Grains are clearly visible to the naked eye. (B) Black *M. mycetomatis* grain in subcutaneous tissue. Hematoxylin-eosin stained. Magnification, ×100. (C) Black *E. jeanselmei* grain in subcutaneous tissue. Hematoxylin-eosin stained. Magnification, ×100 (142). (D) White *Fusarium verticilloides* grain. Hematoxylin-eosin stained. Magnification, ×100 (143).

COLLECTION, TRANSPORT, AND STORAGE OF SPECIMENS

Different specimens can be obtained from patients with eumycetoma, but direct examination and culture of fungi causing mycetoma always require surgical tissue biopsies and/or bone curettage. Tissue materials should be divided and submitted for both microbiology and histopathology examination. It should be noted that tissue biopsy specimens without visible grains usually result in negative cultures. The best specimen for fungal culture is usually collected during surgery as an excisional or incisional biopsy specimen. Grains are not always present in tissue specimens obtained by a cutaneous biopsy procedure with local anesthesia. However, incisional biopsy specimens obtained under local anesthesia, when they contain grains, can also result in positive cultures. Grains collected with cotton swabs from the sinus tracts are not recommended, because such grains can be contaminated or dead.

Several grains are usually needed for direct examination and culture, and therefore, as much tissue as possible should be obtained. Tissue should be collected in sterile dry leakproof containers and transported to the laboratory as soon as possible at room temperature. If transport is delayed for more than 2 h, specimens can be refrigerated, but care should be taken, since long storage can result in no growth. Small biopsy samples can be covered with 2 to 3 ml of sterile saline to prevent drying during transportation to the laboratory.

DIRECT EXAMINATION

Microscopy (Grain Appearance)

The grains of eumycetomata are composed of septate mycelial filaments at least 2 to 5 μm in diameter. The mycelium may be distorted and unusual in form and size, and the cell walls of the fungi, especially toward the periphery of the grains, are thickened. Vesicles are frequently present, especially at the periphery of the grain. The mycelium of the grains may be embedded in a cement-like substance, depending on the species involved. The cement material is most likely composed of both fungal and host material. Wethered et al. (76) described the cement surrounding grains of *M. mycetomatis* as being an amorphous, electron-dense material with areas containing different-sized membrane-bound vesicular inclusions. Recently, Ibrahim et al. studied the composition of *M. mycetomatis* grains, which were found to contain melanin, heavy metals, proteins and lipids (77). It was suggested that the elements composing the grains in mycetoma may play a role in pathogenicity and resistance to antifungal agents (77, 78). Often, the grains elicit an immune response, known as the Splendore-Hoeppli reaction (61, 75), seen histologically in the form of an eosinophilic deposit of amorphous material around the grain. A similar tissue reaction in experimental eumycetoma in mice has been described (79).

As is shown in Table 1, grains are white or yellow-brown (white-grain mycetoma) when the agent produces mostly hyaline mycelia and black (black-grain mycetoma) in the case of melanized fungi. A single proven yellow-grain fungal mycetoma has been reported thus far, but earlier cases may have been incorrectly diagnosed as bacterial mycetomata (80). Reports of hyaline fungi such as *Acremonium kiliense* and *Fusarium solani* var. *coeruleum* forming black grains (81) are probably erroneous. Etiologic agents with melanized hyphae or conidia, such as *Phaeoacremonium inflatipes* and *S. apiospermum*, produce whitish grains in tissue (46, 82–84). Melanin production in *Phaeoacremonium* species is facultative, while in *Scedosporium*, dark pigmentation is limited to the conidia.

Black Grains

The color of black grains is probably caused by melanin, a high-molecular-weight compound that is anchored to extracellular proteins. A precursor for production of melanin in ascomycetous fungi is 1,8-dihydroxynaphthalene (DHN-melanin) (61, 85).

M. mycetomatis

In *M. mycetomatis*, melanin has been shown to be produced through the DHN pathway, and it offers the fungus protection against strong oxidants and antifungal drugs (78).

Although black grains might resemble each other, species-specific features can be noted. The grains produced by *M. mycetomatis* are reddish brown to black (Fig. 2A and B). They may reach 5 mm or more in diameter and are firm to hard. In tissue sections, the grains are compact, variable in size and shape, and frequently multilobulated. They are composed of hyphae 1.2 to 5 μm in diameter that terminate in enlarged hyphal cells at the periphery of the grains, which measure 12 to 15 μm in diameter. The cell wall pigment is minimal, but hyphal cells contain brown particles. The hyphae are embedded in a conspicuous brown matrix that is characteristic of *M. mycetomatis*. Some grains are vesicular and more regular in size and shape. The vesicles are predominantly visible in the peripheral zone in a dense, brown, cement-like matrix.

Falciformispora Species

The grains of the two *Falciformispora* species that cause mycetoma are indistinguishable from each other. They are black, 0.5 to 2 mm in size, and firm to hard. In tissue sections, the grains are round to polylobulated, with large vesicles. At the periphery, the mycelium is embedded in a black, cement-like substance. The central portion of each grain consists of a loose network of hyphae.

T. grisea

Grains of *T. grisea* are black, 0.3 to 0.6 mm in diameter, and soft to firm. In tissue sections, the grains are oval, lobulated, or reniform (kidney shaped), and sometimes vermiform (worm shaped). They are composed of a dense network of hyphae that are weakly pigmented in the center and brown to blackish brown in the peripheral region as the result of the presence of a brown, cement-like interstitial material.

M. romeroi

M. romeroi produces soft to firm black sclerotia that are oval, lobulated, sometimes vermiform, and about 1.0 mm in diameter. They resemble those of *T. grisea* (86).

Curvularia geniculata

Curvularia geniculata grains are black to dark brown, firm, and 0.5 to 1.0 mm or more in size. In tissue sections, grains are spherical, ovoid, or irregularly shaped and are often surrounded by a zone of epithelioid cells. The periphery of the grain is a dense, interwoven mass of dematiaceous mycelium and thick-walled, chlamydospore-like cells embedded in a cement-like substance. The interior of the grains is vacuolar and consists of a loose network of septate, hyphal filaments. The grains of *C. lunata* resemble those of *C. geniculata* in their morphologic characteristics.

E. jeanselmei

In host tissue, *E. jeanselmei* produces dark brown to black grains that are irregular in shape and fragile (Fig. 2C). Detached portions or fragments of the grains often are found within giant cells. When extruded through fistulae, the grains often look like worms (vermiform) because of their elongated shapes and irregular surfaces. In tissue sections, grains appear as hollow structures or as sinuous bands that are vermiform. The external surface is composed of brown, thick-walled hyphae and thick-walled chlamydospore-like cells. The grains are cement free. Within the hollow grains, smaller, degenerated hyphal fragments with leukocytes and giant cells may be seen.

White Grains

Scedosporium Species

Grains of *Scedosporium* species in tissue are white to yellowish white and soft to firm; they vary from globose to subglobose or lobulated and are 0.2 to 2.0 mm in diameter. They are composed of hyaline hyphae 1.5 to 5.0 μm in diameter that radiate from the center into terminal thick-walled cells 15 to 20 μm in diameter at the peripheries. The central portion of each grain consists of loosely interwoven hyaline mycelium.

Fusarium Species

The grains of *Fusarium* spp (Fig. 2D) are white to pale yellow, soft, and 0.2 to 0.5 mm in diameter. They are composed of slender, polymorphic, septate hyphae 1.5 to 2.0 μm in diameter with irregular bulbous swellings and peripheral cementing material.

N. rosatii

The sclerotia of *N. rosatii* are white to brownish white, 0.5 to 1.0 mm in diameter, and soft. In tissue sections, the sclerotia appear to be polyhedral to subregular and consist of hyphae, which are embedded in the peripheral cementing material. The grains demonstrate an eosinophilic border. The central portion of each grain consists of more or less disintegrated mycelium and chlamydospores.

Phaeoacremonium Species

Although *Phaeoacremonium* is a dematiaceous fungus and a well-known agent of phaeohyphomycosis, it seems that melanin production is facultative in eumycetoma. White-grain mycetoma caused by *P. krajdenii* has been reported by Hemashettar et al. (87).

Antigen Detection

There are currently no specific commercially available antigen tests for detecting any of the mycetoma-causative agents, but the panfungal (1→3)-β-D-glucan detection assay could be of use to monitor disease progression (see chapter 119). (1→3)-β-D-Glucan has been detected in serum of eumycetoma patients (88). Unfortunately, since (1→3)-β-D-glucan is panfungal, it cannot discriminate between the different causative agents (88). Furthermore, it also cannot discriminate between actinomycetoma and eumycetoma, as (1→3)-β-D-glucan has been detected in serum from both types (88).

Nucleic Acid Detection

Molecular diagnostics have been developed for selected agents. However, most of these molecular assays have been used for culture identification. Only recently have methods been developed to isolate DNA directly from fungal grains of M. *mycetomatis*. To isolate DNA directly from fungal grains, 2-mm metal beads are added to isolated grains and treated in a Bead-Beater for 2 minutes. DNA is isolated from the lysate with either the DNeasy plant mini-kit (Qiagen) or the ZR fungal/bacterial DNA miniprep kit (Zymo Research) (89). To identify M. *mycetomatis*, a classic PCR assay (16) and also isothermal amplification techniques, including rolling circle amplification (90), loop-mediated amplification (89), and recombinase polymerase amplification (89), have been developed.

PCR-based assays for rapid diagnosis of S. *apiospermum* infections from infected tissue are useful (91, 92). Willinger et al. (93) used molecular techniques for detection of S. *apiospermum* and similar organisms from fungus balls in the maxillary sinus. A multiplex PCR for direct detection of *Scedosporium* species in respiratory specimens has also been developed (94) (see chapter 127).

ISOLATION PROCEDURES

To maximize the chances of obtaining pure cultures of the etiologic agents, grains from the eumycotic mycetomata should be washed several times with saline containing antibacterial antibiotics, such as penicillin and streptomycin. The grains are then cultured on Sabouraud's glucose agar (SGA) containing chloramphenicol (50 mg/liter) and SGA containing chloramphenicol and cycloheximide (500 mg/liter) in petri dishes. Plates should be incubated at 25 and 37°C. Because many of the fungi that cause mycetoma grow slowly, culture plates should be incubated for 4 weeks before being discarded as negative. Identification of the isolated fungus is based on gross morphology of fruiting bodies and conidia, if present.

IDENTIFICATION

Morphological Identification

The mycological identification of most of fungi causing mycetoma can be achieved by studying the morphological characteristics described below and in chapters 122, 123, 126, and 127. For additional morphological features and simplified identification keys, readers are referred to specialized references such as the *Atlas of Clinical Fungi* (2). One should be careful when relying solely on morphological features. Many misidentifications have occurred in the past. Currently, molecular identification tools have been proven to be the most reliable in species identification (14).

M. mycetomatis

In culture, M. *mycetomatis* shows wide variation. Colonies are slow growing and white at first, becoming olivaceous, yellow, or brown; flat or dome-shaped; and velvety to glabrous, often with a rust-brown diffusible pigment (Fig. 1A). On nutritionally deficient media, sclerotial bodies 750 μm in diameter develop. These are black and consist of undifferentiated polygonal cells (Fig. 1B). On SGA, the mycelium is sterile. On nutritionally poor media, such as soil extract or hay infusion agar, about 50% of the isolates produce round to pyriform conidia 3 to 4 μm in diameter at the tips of phialides. The phialides are tapering, ranging from 3 to 15 μm in length, often with an inconspicuous collarette (Fig. 1C).

Falciformispora Species

F. senegalensis and *F. tompkinsii* grow rapidly and produce gray-brown colonies (Fig. 1D). The optimal growth temperature for *F. senegalensis* is 33°C, and that for *F. tompkinsii* is 36°C (11). On cornmeal agar, both species produce ascostromata that are nonostiolate (without natural opening), scattered, immersed or superficial, globose to subglobose, black, and covered with brown, smoothly bent hyphae (Fig. 1E). The asci, produced after prolonged incubation on plant stems, are eight-spored, clavate to cylindrical, and double walled . The major difference between the two species is found in the ascospores, which differ in size, shape, septation, and the nature of the gelatinous sheath that surrounds them (13, 95) (Fig. 1F).

T. grisea

T. grisea forms slow-growing, velvety colonies that are cerebriform, radially furrowed or smooth, and dark gray to olive brown to black (Fig. 1G). The reverses of the colonies are black. The optimal growth temperature is 30°C, and no growth is observed at 37°C (11). Microscopically, the hyphae are septate, light to dark brown, 1 to 3 μm in diameter, and nonsporulating. Chlamydospores are rare. Large moniliform hyphae, 3 to 5 μm in diameter, are often present. Some isolates of *T. grisea* have been described as producing abortive or fertile pycnidia (86, 96). Such isolates are morphologically indistinguishable from *N. mackinnonii* (97, 98), but rRNA ITS sequence data (3) show large differences between these species. Furthermore, the optimal growth temperature of *N. mackinnonii* is 24°C, which is lower than that of *T. grisea* (11). Environmental isolates of *T. grisea* are rapidly growing and produce conidiomata (pycnidia) after 8 weeks of incubation (Fig. 1I).

M. romeroi

Colonies of M. *romeroi* are fast growing and floccose to velvety, with a gray surface and whitish margin. The reverse of the colony is black, with no diffusible pigment. The optimal growth temperature is 33°C. On nutritionally deficient media such as oatmeal agar under near-UV light, pycnidia develop after 3 to 4 weeks. The pycnidia are subglobose, 80 to 160 μm in diameter, and dark brick to fawn, later becoming dark brown with short necks. They are ostiolate (with a natural opening), and setae around ostioles are septate and roughened and measure 80 to 100 by 3 μm. The conidiophores inside the conidiomata are sparse and have lateral branches. Conidiogenous cells are hyaline and are borne on branches or arise directly from cells lining the conidiomatal cavity, which produce hyaline to yellowish, shortly cylindrical conidia measuring 1 to 2 by 1.0 μm.

Scedosporium colonies grow rapidly and are floccose and white at first, becoming gray as conidia are produced.

With age, the colonies become dark grayish brown. Submerged ascocarps (cleistothecia) may be produced when isolates are grown on cornmeal agar and are visible macroscopically as small black dots. They are globose, nonostiolate, 140 to 200 μm in diameter, and often covered with brown, thick-walled, septate hyphae 2 to 3 μm wide. They have a wall 4 to 6 μm thick that is composed of two or three layers of interwoven, flattened, dark brown cells, each 2 to 6 μm wide. The cleistothecia open at maturity by an irregular rupture of the wall. The eight-spored asci are ellipsoidal to nearly spherical and 12 to 18 by 9 to 13 μm. The ascospores are ellipsoidal to oblate, are symmetrical or slightly flattened, measure 6 to 7 by 3.5 to 4.0 μm, are straw-colored, and have two germ pores. The anamorph produces conidia that are oval to clavate, truncate, and subhyaline, becoming pale gray to pale brown in masses. Conidia are produced singly. They remain attached at the tips of annellides. Annellations can be detected at the tips of conidiogenous cells as swollen rings. Some isolates also produce a graphium-like anamorph, which is characterized by rope-like bundles of hyphae with annellidic conidiogenesis. The hyphae are fused into long stalks known as synnemata. The conidia produced are hyaline, cylindric to clavate, and truncate at the base. A fungus consisting of elongate, multicellular conidia and described as *Polycytella hominis* (99) was recently proven to be a degenerate anamorph of *S. boydii* (100).

Colonies of *N. rosatii* are slow growing, attaining diameters of 25 to 28 mm in 2 weeks, and have an aerial mycelium that is grayish black to brownish black (Fig. 1J). On potato-carrot or cornmeal agar incubated at 30°C, most of the ascomata are submerged (Fig. 1K). The ascostromal walls are smooth and are surrounded by interwoven brown to hyaline hyphae. The eight-spored asci, 12 to 35 by 10 to 25 μm, are scattered in the central part of the ascostroma (Fig. 1L) and are globose to subglobose, thick walled, and bitunicate, becoming evanescent as the ascospores mature. The ascospores vary in size (9 to 12.5 by 4.5 to 8.0 μm) and shape, ranging from ellipsoidal to rhomboidal, asymmetrical, or slightly curved; they are constricted at the median transverse septum and have brown smooth walls.

Assimilation Patterns

To discriminate fungi causing mycetoma only on the basis of morpholical features is difficult. Therefore, some biochemical analyses can be performed to aid in the identification (Table 2). It is known that *M. mycetomatis* grows better

TABLE 2 Assimilation patterns of species causing eumycotic mycetoma

Test[a]	*M. mycetomatis*	*F. senegalensis*	*F. tompkinsii*	*T. grisea*	*M. romeroi*	*N. mackinnonii*
Growth at 37°C	+	+	+	−	+	−
Assimilation of:						
D-Galactose	+	+	+	+	+	+
Actidione	ND	+	+	+	+	−
D-Saccharose (sucrose)	+/−	+	+	+	+	+
N-Acetyl-glucosamine	+	+	+	+	+	+
DL-Lactate	ND	−	−	−	−	−
L-Arabinose	+	+	−	−	−	+/−
D-Cellobiose	+	+	+	+	+	+
D-Raffinose	W	+	+	+	+	+
D-Maltose	+	+	+	+	+	+
D-Trehalose	+	+	+	+	+	+
Potassium 2-keto-gluconate	+	−	+	+	+	+
methyl-D-Glucopyranoside	+/−	+	+	+	−	+
D-Mannitol	+	+/−	+	+	+	+
D-Lactose	+	+	−	−	−	−
Inositol	+/−	+/−	−	+	+	+
D-Sorbitol	+	+/−	−	+	+	+
D-Xylose	+	+	+	+	+	+
D-Ribose	+	−	−	−	−	+/−
Glycerol	+/−	−	−	−	−	−
L-Rhamnose	+	+	+	+	+	+
Palatinose	ND	+	+	+	+	+
Erythritol	+/−	−	+	+/−	+	+
D-Melibiose	−	−	+/−	+	+/−	+
Sodium glucuronate	ND	−	−	−	−	+/−
D-Melezitose	W	+	+	+	+	+
Potassium gluconate	+	−	−	−	−	−
Levulinate	ND	−	−	+/−	−	+
D-Glucose	+	+	+	+	+	+
L-Sorbose	W	+	W	+	+	−
Glucosamine	+	−	−	−	−	−
Esculin	−	+	+	+	W	+
Salt tolerance test (NaCl)	ND	20%	20%	20%	20%	20%
Laccase test	ND	+	−/W	+	+	+
Urease test	ND	+	+	+	+	+

[a]Data from reference 11. Results were positive (+), negative (−), weak (W), positive or negative (+/−), negative or positive (−/+), or not done (ND).

at 37 than at 30°C, with a maximum of 40°C, whereas *T. grisea* grows better at 30 than at 37°C. *M. mycetomatis* is slowly proteolytic and utilizes glucose, maltose, and galactose but not sucrose. It utilizes potassium nitrate, ammonium sulfate, asparagine, and urea, and it hydrolyzes starch. *T. grisea*, on the other hand, is weakly proteolytic and assimilates glucose, maltose, and sucrose but not lactose (Table 2).

The pleosporalean eumycetoma-causative agents *F. senegalensis*, *F. tompkinsii*, *T. grisea*, *M. romeroi*, *N. mackinnonii* and *P. larense* all are able to assimilate D-galactose, D-saccharose, *N*-acetylglucosamine, D-cellobiose, D-raffinose, D-maltose, D-trehalose, D-mannitol, L-rhamnose, D-melezitose, palatinose and D-glucose but not DL-lactate, potassium gluconate, sodium glucoronate, and glucosamine (11). *F. senegalensis* does not assimilate potassium-2-keto-gluconate, erythritol, or D-melibiose, whereas *F. tompkinsii*, *T. grisea*, *M. romeroi*, *N. mackinnonii*, and *P. larense* do (11). Furthermore, *F. senegalensis* is able to assimilate D-lactose, whereas the majority of the pleosporalean eumycetoma-causative agents do not. *F. tompkinsii* is the only species which does not assimilate inositol and sorbitol (11). *M. romeroi* is the only species that does not assimilate methyl-D-glucopyranoside, and *N. mackinnonii* is sensitive to cycloheximide and able to assimilate D-xylose (11).

Molecular Identification

Certain species (*T. grisea*, *M. mycetomatis*, *N. mackinnonii*, and *M. romeroi*) do not sporulate readily but can be recognized by molecular techniques (16, 101). Borman and coworkers developed a rapid protocol for identifying agents of black-grain mycetoma by sequence data of the rRNA ITS (102). The black yeast *E. jeanselmei* (50), *M. mycetomatis* (15), *Curvularia lunata*, *M. romeroi*, *N. mackinnonii* (103), and members of the genus *Phaeoacremonium* can be identified by using the same marker (104, 105). Wedde et al. (101) also developed specific primers based on rRNA ITS sequences for the identification of *Scedosporium* species. Given the large intraspecific variability of the species, a less variable region, such as the 26S rRNA operon (106), might also provide successful detection of *S. apiospermum*-like genotypes. Recently, Lu et al. developed and evaluated three molecular methods targeting the partial beta-tubulin gene for the identification of six closely related species of the *S. apiospermum* complex using quantitative real-time PCR, PCR-based reverse line blot, and loop-mediated isothermal amplification (107). Restriction fragment length polymorphism analysis of the beta-tubulin gene and ITS-based rolling circle amplification, loop-mediated isothermal amplification, and recombinase polymerase amplification were also used for identification of *M. mycetomatis* (89, 90), *M. fahalii* (90), *M. pseudomycetomatis* (90), *M. tropicana* (90), *F. senegalensis* (90), *F. tompkinsii* (90), *M. romeroi* (90), *T. grisea* (90), and *S. apiospermum* complex (108, 109).

TYPING SYSTEMS

Over the years, many molecular typing techniques have been established for a number of fungal species, including those causing mycetoma. Such techniques are useful not only in genotyping but also in accurate species identification (16). Genotyping enables differentiation of environmental and clinical isolates, and therefore, it is an important tool in understanding the environmental distribution of species and source of infection. Harun et al. (110) provided a comprehensive review of the methods used in the genotyping of *Scedosporium* species. van de Sande et al. (111) used an amplified fragment length polymorphism study to reveal clones of *Madurella* species differing in virulence and geographic distribution. Subspecific typing of *S. apiospermum* at the population level is not problematic, because of the large degree of heterogeneity. Rainer et al. (112) found with M-13 fingerprinting that nearly all strains analyzed belonged to different genotypes; several genotypes were recovered from a single sampling site. The high degree of polymorphism enabled Zouhair et al. (113) to monitor the dissemination of a strain colonizing the lungs of a patient with cystic fibrosis to cutaneous locations by using multilocus enzyme electrophoresis and randomly amplified polymorphic DNA. In a longitudinal study, Defontaine et al. (114) analyzed nine patients with cystic fibrosis, none of which were found to harbor strains that shared the same genotype.

SEROLOGIC TESTS

There are no commercially available assays for antigen or antibody detection of any of the individual mycetoma-causative agents, but some in-house-made antibody detection tests have been used in some locations where mycetoma is endemic (115–118). The clinical value of these tests is hampered by lack of standardized antigen preparations, sensitivity, and specificity. The most widely used assays for antibody detection in areas of endemicity are immunodiffusion and counterimmunoelectrophoresis (CIE) using crude antigens prepared from fungal hyphae (119). Using immunodiffusion, it was possible to differentiate patients with eumycetoma due to *M. mycetomatis* from patients with actinomycetoma (116). None of the sera from healthy controls from outside the area of endemicity reacted with the *M. mycetomatis* antigens, but when these antigens were used routinely as a diagnostic tool for mycetoma patients, they appeared not to be sensitive enough, since negative results in confirmed cases were frequent (116, 119). Using the same antigens, CIE seemed to be more sensitive, as demonstrated by the detection of antibodies present in patients infected with *M. mycetomatis* at concentrations at which the immunodiffusion test was negative (120).

Besides immunodiffusion and CIE, several enzyme-inked immunosorbent assays (ELISAs) have been developed. For these ELISAs, either whole-fungus cytoplasmatic extracts or recombinant proteins, such as the *M. mycetomatis* translationally controlled tumor protein, fructose bisphosphate aldolase, and pyruvate kinase (98, 121–123), are used. For most of the ELISAs, no clear distinction between patients and healthy controls could be demonstrated (121–123). Furthermore, sera from patients infected with *M. mycetomatis* also cross-reacted with antigens prepared from *S. boydii* (123). Only the ELISA developed by Wethered et al. (118) for *M. mycetomatis* cytoplasmic antigens could clearly differentiate between patients and healthy controls based on IgM antibody responses, but when this ELISA was repeated by Zaini et al. (123), again, no differentiation between patients and healthy controls was obtained. Also, the use of three recombinant *M. mycetomatis* antigens did not result in a reliable ELISA, as cross-reactivity was noted (121, 122). Recently, three immunodominant proteins of 45 kDa, 60 kDa, and 95 kDa with high specificity for *M. mycetomatis* were identified in a cytoplasmatic extract of *M. mycetomatis* (115). This preparation was tested with 100 patients in Sudan, but clinical use of this assay still needs to be evaluated (115). Of all the assays described, the CIE was deemed most reliable and was used for many years by the Mycetoma Research Centre in Khartoum, Sudan, as a routine diagnostic tool until problems with the reproducibility of the antigen preparation ended use of this assay.

ANTIMICROBIAL SUSCEPTIBILITIES

Limited antifungal susceptibility data are available for most fungi causing eumycotic mycetoma. However, for some species, such as M. *mycetomatis*, S. *apiospermum*, and E. *jeanselmei*, reasonable numbers of strains have been tested.

With the exception of S. *apiospermum* and *Fusarium* species, most fungi causing eumycotic mycetoma are susceptible *in vitro* to ketoconazole, itraconazole, voriconazole, and posaconazole. However, it should be noted that *in vitro* activities and clinical responses to these agents are variable (50, 124–129). Ketoconazole and itraconazole are the common agents used for the treatment of mycetoma, but the clinical response to them is poor (124, 125, 130, 131). The newer triazoles, such as voriconazole and posaconazole, have the highest *in vitro* and *in vivo* efficacy (125); however, treatment failure has also been reported, especially with voriconazole (129). As shown in Table 3, most mycetoma-causative agents have relatively high MICs for amphotericin B, fluconazole, terbinafine, 5-flucytosine, caspofungin, anidulafungin, and micafungin. In contrast, most species have relatively lower MICs for the azoles, with the lowest MICs for all species being those of posaconazole. However, it should be noted that antifungal susceptibilities of different azoles vary among different causative agents (Table 3), which make species identification essential for appropriate selection of antifungal therapy.

There is currently a large gap between the *in vitro* susceptibility data and clinical outcome. Only three studies have tested the efficacy of antifungal agents against eumycetoma in animals: two in the invertebrate *Galleria mellonella* (132), and one in mice. In both models, M. *mycetomatis* was the causative agent studied (132). In these three studies, it was demonstrated that although M. *mycetomatis* was highly susceptible *in vitro* to azole antifungal agents, no therapeutic efficacy was demonstrated for ketoconazole (132), itraconazole (132–134), voriconazole (132), or posaconazole (132). Higher MICs have been obtained for amphotericin B and terbinafine, but these antifungal agents showed some therapeutic efficacy in larvae of G. *mellonella* (132, 133) and mice (134). Combining amphotericin B, terbinafine, or itraconazole was antagonistic in G. *mellonella* larvae (133).

The management and prognosis of actinomycetoma differ from those of eumycetoma. Actinomycetoma is treated with antimicrobial therapy only, with a high success rate. Eumycetoma is treated with a combination of antifungal therapy and surgery, with limited success. Only limited patient-based studies have been performed to determine the outcome of antifungal treatment, and studies comparing different antifungal agents with clinical outcome are lacking. The first large clinical study to determine the therapeutic efficacy of itraconazole and fosravuconazole only started in 2017, and currently, no data are available from this study (135). Nevertheless, in summarizing the few published studies, we can draw some conclusions. In case of M. *mycetomatis* mycetoma, ketoconazole resulted in cure of only 5 out of 13 patients (130), while itraconazole resulted in cure of only one patient out of 13 (131). Since ketoconazole is now no longer approved for the treatment of fungal diseases, itraconazole has become the recommended antifungal agent (136, 137). Although the cure rates with itraconazole were not promising, all patients receiving regular treatments partially improved or had stable lesions. However, with newer azoles, such as posaconazole, better outcomes have been achieved (138). Negroni and his group treated six mycetoma patients with posaconazole; they were able to cure four patients, and the other two either were clinically improved or had stable mycetoma lesion (138). The only nonazole drug, which was evaluated clinically for treatment of mycetoma, is terbinafine. In the study by N'diaye et al., 20 patients were treated with terbinafine; 4 were cured, 12 showed clinical improvement, and 4 showed no effect (139). Based on these limited observations and the *in vitro* data summarized in Table 1, posaconazole seems to be a promising choice for the treatment of mycetoma, but properly designed clinical trials are needed to confirm this assumption.

In terms of drug discovery and drug development for eumycetoma, fosravuconazole is currently being explored in a large clinical trial (135). Fosravuconazole is a prodrug of ravuconazole, and M. *mycetomatis* appeared to be highly susceptible to this drug *in vitro* (140).

EVALUATION, INTERPRETATION, AND REPORTING OF RESULTS

Because agents of eumycotic mycetoma are soil or plant saprobes, their etiologic role in mycetoma must be carefully established. A definitive diagnosis is based on the demonstration of grains in tissue, which are expelled through draining sinuses. Grains may become entangled in gauze bandages placed over fistulae. Pus, exudate, or biopsy material should be examined for the presence of grains that are detectable with the naked eye. Their color, internal architecture, size, and shape give a fair indication of the identity of the possible etiologic agents.

Actinomycotic mycetomata are differentiated from eumycotic mycetomata by the examination of crushed, Gram-stained grains. Actinomycotic grains, as well as coccoid and bacillary forms, are composed of Gram-positive, interwoven, thin filaments, 0.5 to 1.0 μm in diameter. Grains of the eumycotic agents, on the other hand, are composed of broader, interwoven, septate hyphae, 2 to 5 μm in diameter, with many unusually shaped, swollen cells up to 15 μm in diameter, especially at the periphery of the grains. In many species, the grains are embedded in cement-like material.

Although the gross and microscopic characteristics of the grains provide insight into the identity of the etiologic agent or a particular group to which it belongs (141), definitive identification of the etiologic agent should be based on isolation of the same fungus from several grains. Clinical microbiology laboratories should avoid reporting patients' specimens as "black-grain mycetoma" or "pale-grain mycetoma," and isolation and identification of species involved should be attempted. Careful evaluation of culture results is important, especially when new or uncommon fast-growing species are reported, since some of these species might represent contamination during collection of specimens or isolation. On the other hand, physicians should avoid planning a patient's therapy based on grain morphology in clinical materials alone; rather, results of laboratory diagnosis with species identification should be awaited.

TABLE 3 *In vitro* susceptibilities of mycetoma-causative fungi[a]

Antifungal agent	*Madurella mycetomatis*[b]		*Trematosphaeria grisea*[c]		*Scedosporium boydii*[d]		*Falciforma senegalensis*[e]		*Medicopsis romeroi*[f]		*Exophiala jeanselmei*[g]	
	MIC_{50} (range)	No. of strains	MIC_{50} (range)	No. of strains	MIC_{50} (range)	No. of strains	MIC_{50} (range)	No. of strains	MIC_{50} (range)	No. of strains	MIC_{50} (range)	No. of strains
Amphotericin B	0.5 (<0.016–4)	34	8 (2– >16)	3	1 (0.25–2)	21	2 (2)	4	0.125 (0.125)	5	1 (0.25–2)	9
Ketoconazole	0.06 (<0.03–4)	38	1 (0.125–8)	11			0.5 (0.5–1)	4	8 (0.125–8)	7	1 (1–8)	2
Itraconazole	0.03 (<0.03–0.5)	38	0.5 (0.03–4)	11	0.25 (<0.03–4)	21	0.125 (0.125–0.25)	4	16 (0.125– >16)	7	0.125 (0.03–0.25)	11
Posaconazole	<0.03 (<0.03–0.125)	34	0.03 (0.03–0.25)	3	0.5 (ND[b])	30	0.06 (0.06–0.25)	4	0.5 (0.25–1)	5	0.03 (0.016–0.063)	9
Fluconazole	4 (0.25– >128)	34	64 (16–64)	3	16 (8–32)	21	64 (64–128)	4	>256 (>256)	5	16 (8–32)	9
Voriconazole	0.06 (<0.016–1)	34	0.25 (0.25–0.5)	3			0.25 (0.25–0.5)	4	0.125 (0.125–0.25)	5	1 (0.25–2)	9
Isavuconazole	0.03 (<0.016–0.25)	22									ND	
Ravuconazole	0.004 (<0.002–0.03)	23										
Terbinafine	8 (1– >16)	34									ND	
5-flucytosin	>64 (>64)	34	64 (16– >64)	3			32 (8–32)	4	8 (8–32)	5	ND	
Caspofungin	64 (16– >128)	17	>16 (8– >16)	3			16 (16– >16)	4	>16 (16– >16)	5	4 (2–8)	9
Anidulafungin	>128 (0.5 – >128)	17									0.5 (0.063–4)	9
Micafungin	> 128 (8– >128)	17									ND	

[a]MICs are in micrograms per milliliter. ND, data not available.
[b]Data from references 127, 140, and 185–190.
[c]Data from references 191 and 192.
[d]Data from references 193 and 194.
[e]Data from reference 192.
[f]Data from references 191 and 192.
[g]Data from references 190 and 195.

REFERENCES

1. **WHO.** 2013. The 17 neglected tropical diseases. http://www.who.int/neglected_diseases/diseases/en/. Accessed 21 March 2013.
2. **De Hoog GS, Guarro J, Gené J, Figueras MJ.** 2016. Atlas of clinical fungi, vol 4.1. Westerdijk FungalBio Diversity Institute, Utrecht, The Netherlands.
3. **de Hoog GS, Adelmann D, Ahmed AO, van Belkum A.** 2004. Phylogeny and typification of *Madurella mycetomatis*, with a comparison of other agents of eumycetoma. *Mycoses* **47:**121–130.
4. **Desnos-Ollivier M, Bretagne S, Dromer F, Lortholary O, Dannaoui E.** 2006. Molecular identification of black-grain mycetoma agents. *J Clin Microbiol* **44:**3517–3523.
5. **van de Sande WWJ.** 2013. Global burden of human mycetoma: a systematic review and meta-analysis. *PLoS Negl Trop Dis* **7:**e2550.
6. **van de Sande WW.** 2012. Phylogenetic analysis of the complete mitochondrial genome of *Madurella mycetomatis* confirms its taxonomic position within the order Sordariales. *PLoS One* **7:**e38654.
7. **de Hoog GS, van Diepeningen AD, Mahgoub S, van de Sande WW.** 2012. New species of *Madurella*, causative agents of black-grain mycetoma. *J Clin Microbiol* **50:**988–994.
8. **Smit S, Derks MF, Bervoets S, Fahal A, van Leeuwen W, van Belkum A, van de Sande WW.** 2016. Genome sequence of *Madurella mycetomatis* mm55, isolated from a human mycetoma case in Sudan. *Genome Announc* **4:**e00418-16.
9. **Yan J, Deng J, Zhou CJ, Zhong BY, Hao F.** 2010. Phenotypic and molecular characterization of *Madurella pseudomycetomatis* sp. nov., a novel opportunistic fungus possibly causing black-grain mycetoma. *J Clin Microbiol* **48:**251–257.
10. **Rojas OC, León-Cachón RB, Moreno-Treviño M, González GM.** 2017. Molecular identification of unusual mycetoma agents isolated from patients in Venezuela. *Mycoses* **60:**129–135.
11. **Ahmed SA, van de Sande WWJ, Stevens DA, Fahal A, van Diepeningen AD, Menken SB, de Hoog GS.** 2014. Revision of agents of black-grain eumycetoma in the order *Pleosporales*. *Persoonia* **33:**141–154.
12. **Destombes P, Mariat F, Rosati L, Segretain G.** 1977. Mycetoma in Somalia—results of a survey done from 1959 to 1964. *Acta Trop* **34:**355–373. [In French.]
13. **el-Ani AS.** 1966. A new species of *Leptosphaeria*, an etiologic agent of mycetoma. *Mycologia* **58:**406–411.
14. **Borman AM, Desnos-Ollivier M, Campbell CK, Bridge PD, Dannaoui E, Johnson EM.** 2016. Novel taxa associated with human fungal black-grain mycetomas: *Emarellia grisea* gen. nov., sp. nov., and *Emarellia paragrisea* sp. nov. *J Clin Microbiol* **54:**1738–1745.
15. **Ahmed AO, Desplaces N, Leonard P, Goldstein F, De Hoog S, Verbrugh H, van Belkum A.** 2003. Molecular detection and identification of agents of eumycetoma: detailed report of two cases. *J Clin Microbiol* **41:**5813–5816.
16. **Ahmed AO, Mukhtar MM, Kools-Sijmons M, Fahal AH, de Hoog S, van den Ende BG, Zijlstra EE, Verbrugh H, Abugroun ES, Elhassan AM, van Belkum A.** 1999. Development of a species-specific PCR-restriction fragment length polymorphism analysis procedure for identification of *Madurella mycetomatis*. *J Clin Microbiol* **37:**3175–3178.
17. **Butz WC, Ajello L.** 1971. Black grain mycetoma. A case due to *Madurella grisea*. *Arch Dermatol* **104:**197–201.
18. **Mackinnon JE, Ferrada LV, Montemayor L.** 1949. *Madurella grisea* n. sp., a new species of fungus producing black variety of maduromycosis in South America. *Mycopathol Mycol Appl* **4:**385–392.
19. **Mahgoub ES.** 1973. Mycetomas caused by *Curvularia lunata*, *Madurella grisea*, *Aspergillus nidulans*, and *Nocardia brasiliensis* in Sudan. *Sabouraudia* **11:**179–182.
20. **Montes LF, Freeman RG, McClarin W.** 1969. Maduromycosis due to *Madurella grisea*. Report of the fifth North American case. *Arch Dermatol* **99:**74–79.
21. **de Gruyter J, Woudenberg JH, Aveskamp MM, Verkley GJ, Groenewald JZ, Crous PW.** 2010. Systematic reappraisal of species in *Phoma* section *Paraphoma*, *Pyrenochaeta* and *Pleurophoma*. *Mycologia* **102:**1066–1081.
22. **de Gruyter J, Woudenberg JHC, Aveskamp MM, Verkley GJM, Groenewald JZ, Crous PW.** 2013. Redisposition of *Phoma*-like anamorphs in Pleosporales. *Stud Mycol* **75:**1–36.
23. **Borelli D.** 1959. *Pyrenochaeta romeroi* n. sp. *Rev Dermatol Venez* **1:**325–327.
24. **Klokke AH, Swamidasan G, Anguli R, Verghese A.** 1968. The causal agents of mycetoma in South India. *Trans R Soc Trop Med Hyg* **62:**509–516.
25. **Mariat F, Destombes P, Segretain G.** 1977. The mycetomas: clinical features, pathology, etiology and epidemiology. *Contrib Microbiol Immunol* **4:**1–39.
26. **Jaklitsch WM, Voglmayr H.** 2016. Hidden diversity in *Thyridaria* and a new circumscription of the Thyridariaceae. *Stud Mycol* **85:**35–64.
27. **Shaw JJ, Spakowicz DJ, Dalal RS, Davis JH, Lehr NA, Dunican BF, Orellana EA, Narváez-Trujillo A, Strobel SA.** 2015. Biosynthesis and genomic analysis of medium-chain hydrocarbon production by the endophytic fungal isolate *Nigrograna mackinnonii* E5202H. *Appl Microbiol Biotechnol* **99:**3715–3728.
28. **Segretain G, Destombes P.** 1961. Description of a new agent for maduromycosis, *Neotestudina rosatii*, n. gen., n. sp., isolated in Africa. *C R Hebd Seances Acad Sci* **253:**2577–2579. [In French.]
29. **Gilgado F, Cano J, Gené J, Guarro J.** 2005. Molecular phylogeny of the *Pseudallescheria boydii* species complex: proposal of two new species. *J Clin Microbiol* **43:**4930–4942.
30. **Gilgado F, Cano J, Gené J, Sutton DA, Guarro J.** 2008. Molecular and phenotypic data supporting distinct species statuses for *Scedosporium apiospermum* and *Pseudallescheria boydii* and the proposed new species *Scedosporium dehoogii*. *J Clin Microbiol* **46:**766–771.
31. **Rainer J, De Hoog GS.** 2006. Molecular taxonomy and ecology of *Pseudallescheria*, *Petriella* and *Scedosporium prolificans* (Microascaceae) containing opportunistic agents on humans. *Mycol Res* **110:**151–160.
32. **Chen M, Zeng J, De Hoog GS, Stielow B, Gerrits Van Den Ende AH, Liao W, Lackner M.** 2016. The 'species complex' issue in clinically relevant fungi: a case study in *Scedosporium apiospermum*. *Fungal Biol* **120:**137–146.
33. **de Hoog GS, Marvin-Sikkema FD, Lahpoor GA, Gottschall JC, Prins RA, Guého E.** 1994. Ecology and physiology of the emerging opportunistic fungi *Pseudallescheria boydii* and *Scedosporium prolificans*. *Mycoses* **37:**71–78.
34. **Fisher JF, Shadomy S, Teabeaut JR, Woodward J, Michaels GE, Newman MA, White E, Cook P, Seagraves A, Yaghmai F, Rissing JP.** 1982. Near-drowning complicated by brain abscess due to *Petriellidium boydii*. *Arch Neurol* **39:**511–513.
35. **Shear CL.** 1922. Life history of an undescribed ascomycete isolated from a granular mycetoma of man. *Mycologia* **14:**239–243.
36. **Castro LG, Belda W, Jr, Salebian A, Cucé LC.** 1993. Mycetoma: a retrospective study of 41 cases seen in São Paulo, Brazil, from 1978 to 1989. *Mycoses* **36:**89–95.
37. **Venugopal PV, Venugopal TV.** 1995. Pale grain eumycetomas in Madras. *Australas J Dermatol* **36:**149–151.
38. **Posteraro P, Frances C, Didona B, Dorent R, Posteraro B, Fadda G.** 2003. Persistent subcutaneous *Scedosporium apiospermum* infection. *Eur J Dermatol* **13:**603–605.
39. **Ginter G, de Hoog GS, Pschaid A, Fellinger M, Bogiatzis A, Berghold C, Reich EM, Odds FC.** 1995. Arthritis without grains caused by *Pseudallescheria boydii*. *Mycoses* **38:**369–371.
40. **Hayden G, Lapp C, Loda F.** 1977. Arthritis caused by *Monosporium apiospermum* treated with intraarticular amphotericin B. *Am J Dis Child* **131:**927.
41. **Lutwick LI, Rytel MW, Yañez JP, Galgiani JN, Stevens DA.** 1979. Deep infections from *Petriellidium boydii* treated with miconazole. *JAMA* **241:**272–273.
42. **Ochiai N, Shimazaki C, Uchida R, Fuchida S, Okano A, Ashihara E, Inaba T, Fujita N, Nakagawa M.** 2003. Disseminated infection due to *Scedosporium apiospermum* in a patient with acute myelogenous leukemia. *Leuk Lymphoma* **44:**369–372.
43. **Ajello L.** 1962. Epidemiology of human fungus infections, p 69–83. *In* Dalldorf G (ed), *Fungi and Fungous Diseases*. Charles C Thomas, Springfield, IL.

44. **Baylet R, Camain R, Rey M.** 1961. Champignons de mycétomes isolés des épineux au Sénégal. *Bull Soc Med Afr Noire Lang Fr* **6:**317–319.
45. **Emmons CW.** 1962. Soil reservoirs of pathogenic fungi. *J Wash Acad Sci* **52:**3–9.
46. **Mackinnon JE, Conti-Diaz IA, Gezuele E, Civila E.** 1971. Datos sobre ecologia de *Allescheria boydii*, Shear. *Rev Urug Pathol Clin Microbiol* **9:**37–43.
47. **Segretain G, Mariat F.** 1968. Recherches sur la presence d'agents de mycetomes dans le sol et sur les épineux du Senegal et de la Mauritanie. *Bull Soc Pathol Exot Filiales* **61:**194–202.
48. **Segretain G.** 1972. Recherches sur l'écologie de *Madurella mycetomi* au Senegal. *Bull Soc Fr Mycol Med* **14:**121–124.
49. **Thirumalachar MJ, Padhye AA.** 1968. Isolation of *Madurella mycetomi* from soil in India. *Hindustan Antibiot Bull* **10:** 314–318.
50. **Badali H, Najafzadeh MJ, Van Esbroeck M, van den Enden E, Tarazooie B, Meis JF, de Hoog GS.** 2009. The clinical spectrum of *Exophiala jeanselmei*, with a case report and in vitro antifungal susceptibility of the species. *Med Mycol* **48:**38–327.
51. **Ahmed A, Adelmann D, Fahal A, Verbrugh H, van Belkum A, de Hoog S.** 2002. Environmental occurrence of *Madurella mycetomatis*, the major agent of human eumycetoma in Sudan. *J Clin Microbiol* **40:**1031–1036.
52. **de Hoog GS, Ahmed SA, Najafzadeh MJ, Sutton DA, Keisari MS, Fahal AH, Eberhardt U, Verkleij GJ, Xin L, Stielow B, van de Sande WWJ.** 2013. Phylogenetic findings suggest possible new habitat and routes of infection of human eumyctoma. *PLoS Negl Trop Dis* **7:**e2229.
53. **Borelli D.** 1962. *Madurella mycetomi* y *Madurella grisea*. *Arch Venez Med Trop Parasitol Med* **4:**195–211.
54. **van de Sande WW, Fahal A, Tavakol M, van Belkum A.** 2010. Polymorphisms in catechol-O-methyltransferase and cytochrome p450 subfamily 19 genes predispose towards *Madurella mycetomatis*-induced mycetoma susceptibility. *Med Mycol* **48:**959–968.
55. **van de Sande WW, Fahal A, Verbrugh H, van Belkum A.** 2007. Polymorphisms in genes involved in innate immunity predispose toward mycetoma susceptibility. *J Immunol* **179:**3065–3074.
56. **Mhmoud NA, Fahal AH, van de Sande WW.** 2013. The association between the interleukin-10 cytokine and CC chemokine ligand 5 polymorphisms and mycetoma granuloma formation. *Med Mycol* **51:**527–533.
57. **Geneugelijk K, Kloezen W, Fahal AH, van de Sande WW.** 2014. Active matrix metalloprotease-9 is associated with the collagen capsule surrounding the *Madurella mycetomatis* grain in mycetoma. *PLoS Negl Trop Dis* **8:**e2754.
58. **Verwer PE, Notenboom CC, Eadie K, Fahal AH, Verbrugh HA, van de Sande WW.** 2015. A polymorphism in the chitotriosidase gene associated with risk of mycetoma due to *Madurella mycetomatis* mycetoma—a retrospective study. *PLoS Negl Trop Dis* **9:**e0004061.
59. **de Hoog GS, Buiting A, Tan CS, Stroebel AB, Ketterings C, Boer EJ, Naafs B, Brimicombe R, Nohlmans-Paulssen MKE, Fabius GTJ, Klokke AH, Visser LG** 1993. Diagnostic problems with imported cases of mycetoma in The Netherlands. *Mycoses* **36:**81–87.
60. **Destombes P, Ravisse P, Nazimoff O.** 1970. Summary of deep mycoses established in 20 years of histopathology in the Institut Pasteur de Brazzaville. *Bull Soc Pathol Exot* **63:** 315–324. [In French.]
61. **McGinnis MR.** 1996. Mycetoma. *Dermatol Clin* **14:**97–104.
62. **Suleiman AM, Fahal AH.** 2013. Oral cavity eumycetoma: a rare and unusual condition. *Oral Surg Oral Med Oral Pathol Oral Radiol* **115:**e23–e25.
63. **Joshi A, Acharya S, Anehosur VS, Tayaar AS, Gopalkrishnan K.** 2013. Oral eumycetoma of infancy: a rare presentation and a brief review. *J Craniomaxillofac Surg* **42:** 35–40.
64. **Gueye NN, Seck SM, Diop Y, Ndiaye Sow MN, Agboton G, Diakhate M, Dieng M, Dieng MT.** 2013. Orbital mycetoma: a case report. *J Fr Ophtalmol* **36:**435–441. [In French.]
65. **Brodey RS, Schryver HF, Deubler MJ, Kaplan W, Ajello L.** 1967. Mycetoma in a dog. *J Am Vet Med Assoc* **151:**442–451.
66. **Kano R, Edamura K, Yumikura H, Maruyama H, Asano K, Tanaka S, Hasegawa A.** 2009. Confirmed case of feline mycetoma due to *Microsporum canis*. *Mycoses* **52:**80–83.
67. **Lambrechts N, Collett MG, Henton M.** 1991. Black grain eumycetoma (*Madurella mycetomatis*) in the abdominal cavity of a dog. *J Med Vet Mycol* **29:**211–214.
68. **Lopez MJ, Robinson SO, Cooley AJ, Prichard MA, McGinnis MR.** 2007. Molecular identification of *Phialophora oxyspora* as the cause of mycetoma in a horse. *J Am Vet Med Assoc* **230:**84–88.
69. **Sun PL, Peng PC, Wu PH, Chiang YL, Ju YM, Chang CC, Wang PC.** 2013. Canine eumycetoma caused by *Cladophialophora bantiana* in a Maltese: case report and literature review. *Mycoses* **56:**376–381.
70. **Pankovich AM, Auerbach BJ, Metzger WI, Barreta T.** 1981. Development of maduromycosis (*Madurella mycetomi*) after nailing of a closed tibial fracture: a case report. *Clin Orthop Relat Res* (154)**:**220–222.
71. **Van Etta LL, Peterson LR, Gerding DN.** 1983. *Acremonium falciforme* (*Cephalosporium falciforme*) mycetoma in a renal transplant patient. *Arch Dermatol* **119:**707–708.
72. **Fahey PJ, Utell MJ, Hyde RW.** 1981. Spontaneous lysis of mycetomas after acute cavitating lung disease. *Am Rev Respir Dis* **123:**336–339.
73. **Hadjiliadis D, Sporn TA, Perfect JR, Tapson VF, Davis RD, Palmer SM.** 2002. Outcome of lung transplantation in patients with mycetomas. *Chest* **121:**128–134.
74. **Matsumoto T, Ajello L.** 1986. No granules, no mycetomas. *Chest* **90:**151–152.
75. **Ajello L, Kaplan W, Chandler FW.** 1980. *In Superficial, Cutaneous and Subcutaneous Infections*, p 135–140. Pan American Health Organization, Washington, D.C..
76. **Wethered DB, Markey MA, Hay RJ, Mahgoub ES, Gumaa SA.** 1987. Ultrastructural and immunogenic changes in the formation of mycetoma grains. *J Med Vet Mycol* **25:**39–46.
77. **Ibrahim AI, El Hassan AM, Fahal A, van de Sande WW.** 2013. A histopathological exploration of the Madurella mycetomatis grain. *PLoS One* **8:**e57774.
78. **van de Sande WW, de Kat J, Coppens J, Ahmed AO, Fahal A, Verbrugh H, van Belkum A.** 2007. Melanin biosynthesis in *Madurella mycetomatis* and its effect on susceptibility to itraconazole and ketoconazole. *Microbes Infect* **9:**1114–1123.
79. **Ahmed AO, van Vianen W, ten Kate MT, van de Sande WW, van Belkum A, Fahal AH, Verbrugh HA, Bakker-Woudenberg IA.** 2003. A murine model of *Madurella mycetomatis* eumycetoma. *FEMS Immunol Med Microbiol* **37:**29–36.
80. **Mhmoud NA, Ahmed SA, Fahal AH, de Hoog GS, Gerrits van den Ende AH, van de Sande WW.** 2012. *Pleurostomophora ochracea*, a novel agent of human eumycetoma with yellow grains. *J Clin Microbiol* **50:**2987–2994.
81. **Thianprasit M, Sivayathorn A.** 1984. Black dot mycetoma. *Mykosen* **27:**219–226.
82. **Crous PW, Gams W, Wingfield MJ, van Wyk PS.** 1996. *Phaeoacremonium* gen. nov. associated with wilt and decline diseases of woody hosts and human infections. *Mycologia* **88:**786–796.
83. **de Albornoz MB.** 1974. *Cephalosporium serrae*, an etiologic agent of mycetoma. *Mycopathol Mycol Appl* **54:**485–498. [In Spanish.]
84. **McGinnis MR, Padhye AA, Ajello L.** 1982. *Pseudallescheria boydii* Negroni et Fischer, 1943, and its later synonym *Petriellidium malloch*, 1970. *Mycotaxon* **14:**94–102.
85. **McGinnis M.** 1992. Black fungi: a model for understanding tropical mycosis, p 129–149. *In* Walker DH (ed), *Global Infectious Diseases: Prevention, Control, and Eradication*. Springer Verlag, New York, N.Y..
86. **Segretain G, Destombes P.** 1969. Recherche sur les mycetomes a Madurella grisea et Pyrenochaeta romeroi. *Sabouraudia* **7:**51–61.
87. **Hemashettar BM, Siddaramappa B, Munjunathaswamy BS, Pangi AS, Pattan J, Andrade AT, Padhye AA, Mostert L, Summerbell RC.** 2006. *Phaeoacremonium krajdenii*, a cause of white grain eumycetoma. *J Clin Microbiol* **44:**4619–4622.

88. **Fahal AH, Finkelman MA, Zhang Y, van de Sande WW.** 2016. Detection of (1→3)-β-D-glucan in eumycetoma patients. *J Clin Microbiol* **54:**2614–2617.
89. **Ahmed SA, van de Sande WW, Desnos-Ollivier M, Fahal AH, Mhmoud NA, de Hoog GS.** 2015. Application of isothermal amplification techniques for the identification of *Madurella mycetomatis*, the prevalent agent of human mycetoma. J Clin Microbiol **53:**3280–3285.
90. **Ahmed SA, van den Ende BH, Fahal AH, van de Sande WW, de Hoog GS.** 2014. Rapid identification of black grain eumycetoma causative agents using rolling circle amplification. *PLoS Negl Trop Dis* **8:**e3368.
91. **Hagari Y, Ishioka S, Ohyama F, Mihara M.** 2002. Cutaneous infection showing sporotrichoid spread caused by *Pseudallescheria boydii* (*Scedosporium apiospermum*): successful detection of fungal DNA in formalin-fixed, paraffin-embedded sections by seminested PCR. *Arch Dermatol* **138:**271–272.
92. **Mancini N, Ossi CM, Perotti M, Carletti S, Gianni C, Paganoni G, Matusuka S, Guglielminetti M, Cavallero A, Burioni R, Rama P, Clementi M.** 2005. Direct sequencing of *Scedosporium apiospermum* DNA in the diagnosis of a case of keratitis. *J Med Microbiol* **54:**897–900.
93. **Willinger B, Obradovic A, Selitsch B, Beck-Mannagetta J, Buzina W, Braun H, Apfalter P, Hirschl AM, Makristathis A, Rotter M.** 2003. Detection and identification of fungi from fungus balls of the maxillary sinus by molecular techniques. *J Clin Microbiol* **41:**581–585.
94. **Harun A, Blyth CC, Gilgado F, Middleton P, Chen SC, Meyer W.** 2011. Development and validation of a multiplex PCR for detection of *Scedosporium* spp. in respiratory tract specimens from patients with cystic fibrosis. *J Clin Microbiol* **49:**1508–1512.
95. **El-Ani AS, Gordon MA.** 1965. The ascospore sheath and taxonomy of *Leptosphaeria senegalensis*. *Mycologia* **57:**275–278.
96. **Mayorga R, Close de León JE.** 1966. On a limb from which spore bearing *Madurella grisea* was isolated from a black grained mycetoma in a Guatemalan. *Sabouraudia* **4:**210–214. [In French.]
97. **Borelli D.** 1976. *Pyrenochaeta mackinnonii* nova species agente de micetoma. *Castellania* **4:**227–234.
98. **Romero H, Mackenzie DW.** 1989. Studies on antigens from agents causing black grain eumycetoma. *J Med Vet Mycol* **27:**303–311.
99. **Campbell CK.** 1987. *Polycytella hominis* gen. et sp. nov., a cause of human pale grain mycetoma. *J Med Vet Mycol* **25:**301–305.
100. **Borman AM, Campbell CK, Linton CJ, Bridge PD, Johnson EM.** 2006. *Polycytella hominis* is a mutated form of *Scedosporium apiospermum*. *Med Mycol* **44:**33–39.
101. **Wedde M, Müller D, Tintelnot K, De Hoog GS, Stahl U.** 1998. PCR-based identification of clinically relevant *Pseudall escheria/Scedosporium* strains. *Med Mycol* **36:**61–67.
102. **Borman AM, Linton CJ, Miles SJ, Johnson EM.** 2008. Molecular identification of pathogenic fungi. *J Antimicrob Chemother* **61**(Suppl 1)**:**i7–i12.
103. **Santos DW, Padovan AC, Melo AS, Gonçalves SS, Azevedo VR, Ogawa MM, Freitas TV, Colombo AL.** 2013. Molecular identification of melanised non-sporulating moulds: a useful tool for studying the epidemiology of phaeohyphomycosis. *Mycopathologia* **175:**445–454.
104. **Mostert L, Groenewald JZ, Summerbell RC, Gams W, Crous PW.** 2006. Taxonomy and pathology of *Togninia* (*Diaporthales*) and its *Phaeoacremonium* anamorphs. *Stud Mycol* **54:**1–113.
105. **Mostert L, Groenewald JZ, Summerbell RC, Robert V, Sutton DA, Padhye AA, Crous PW.** 2005. Species of *Phaeoacremonium* associated with infections in humans and environmental reservoirs in infected woody plants. *J Clin Microbiol* **43:**1752–1767.
106. **Sandhu GS, Kline BC, Stockman L, Roberts GD.** 1995. Molecular probes for diagnosis of fungal infections. *J Clin Microbiol* **33:**2913–2919.
107. **Lu Q, Gerrits van den Ende AH, Bakkers JM, Sun J, Lackner M, Najafzadeh MJ, Melchers WJ, Li R, de Hoog GS.** 2011. Identification of *Pseudallescheria* and *Scedosporium* species by three molecular methods. *J Clin Microbiol* **49:**960–967.
108. **Lackner M, Najafzadeh MJ, Sun J, Lu Q, de Hoog GS.** 2012. Rapid identification of *Pseudallescheria* and *Scedosporium* strains by using rolling circle amplification. *Appl Environ Microbiol* **78:**126–133.
109. **Lackner M, Klaassen CH, Meis JF, van den Ende AH, de Hoog GS.** 2012. Molecular identification tools for sibling species of *Scedosporium* and *Pseudallescheria*. *Med Mycol* **50:**497–508.
110. **Harun A, Perdomo H, Gilgado F, Chen SC, Cano J, Guarro J, Meyer W.** 2009. Genotyping of *Scedosporium* species: a review of molecular approaches. *Med Mycol* **47:** 406–414.
111. **van de Sande WW, Gorkink R, Simons G, Ott A, Ahmed AO, Verbrugh H, van Belkum A.** 2005. Genotyping of *Madurella mycetomatis* by selective amplification of restriction fragments (amplified fragment length polymorphism) and subtype correlation with geographical origin and lesion size. *J Clin Microbiol* **43:**4349–4356.
112. **Rainer J, de Hoog GS, Wedde M, Gräser Y, Gilges S.** 2000. Molecular variability of *Pseudallescheria boydii*, a neurotropic opportunist. *J Clin Microbiol* **38:**3267–3273.
113. **Zouhair R, Defontaine A, Ollivier C, Cimon B, Symoens F, Hallet JN, Deunff J, Bouchara JP.** 2001. Typing of *Scedosporium apiospermum* by multilocus enzyme electrophoresis and random amplification of polymorphic DNA. *J Med Microbiol* **50:**925–932.
114. **Defontaine A, Zouhair R, Cimon B, Carrère J, Bailly E, Symoens F, Diouri M, Hallet JN, Bouchara JP.** 2002. Genotyping study of *Scedosporium apiospermum* isolates from patients with cystic fibrosis. *J Clin Microbiol* **40:**2108–2114.
115. **ELbadawi HS, Mahgoub E, Mahmoud N, Fahal AH.** 2016. Use of immunoblotting in testing *Madurella mycetomatis* specific antigen. *Trans R Soc Trop Med Hyg* **110:**312–316.
116. **Mahgoub ES.** 1964. The value of gel diffusions in the diagnosis of mycetoma. *Trans R Soc Trop Med Hyg* **58:**560–563.
117. **Murray IG, Mahgoub ES.** 1968. Further studies on the diagnosis of mycetoma by double diffusion in agar. *Sabouraudia* **6:**106–110.
118. **Wethered DB, Markey MA, Hay RJ, Mahgoub ES, Gumaa SA.** 1988. Humoral immune responses to mycetoma organisms: characterization of specific antibodies by the use of enzyme-linked immunosorbent assay and immunoblotting. *Trans R Soc Trop Med Hyg* **82:**918–923.
119. **Fahal A.** 2006. *Mycetoma—clinicopathological monograph*. Khartoum University Press, Khartoum, Sudan.
120. **Gumaa SA, Mahgoub ES.** 1975. Counterimmunoelectrophoresis in the diagnosis of mycetoma and its sensitivity as compared to immunodiffusion. *Sabouraudia* **13:**309–315.
121. **de Klerk N, de Vogel C, Fahal A, van Belkum A, van de Sande WW.** 2012. Fructose-bisphosphate aldolase and pyruvate kinase, two novel immunogens in *Madurella mycetomatis*. *Med Mycol* **50:**143–151.
122. **van de Sande WW, Janse DJ, Hira V, Goedhart H, van der Zee R, Ahmed AO, Ott A, Verbrugh H, van Belkum A.** 2006. Translationally controlled tumor protein from *Madurella mycetomatis*, a marker for tumorous mycetoma progression. *J Immunol* **177:**1997–2005.
123. **Zaini F, Moore MK, Hathi D, Hay RJ, Noble WC.** 1991. The antigenic composition and protein profiles of eumycetoma agents. *Mycoses* **34:**19–28.
124. **Ahmed AA, van de Sande WW, Fahal A, Bakker-Woudenberg I, Verbrugh H, van Belkum A.** 2007. Management of mycetoma: major challenge in tropical mycoses with limited international recognition. *Curr Opin Infect Dis* **20:**146–151.
125. **Ameen M, Arenas R.** 2009. Developments in the management of mycetomas. *Clin Exp Dermatol* **34:**1–7.
126. **Cerar D, Malallah YM, Howard SJ, Bowyer P, Denning DW.** 2009. Isolation, identification and susceptibility of *Pyrenochaeta romeroi* in a case of eumycetoma of the foot in the UK. *Int J Antimicrob Agents* **34:**613–614.
127. **van de Sande WW, Luijendijk A, Ahmed AO, Bakker-Woudenberg IA, van Belkum A.** 2005. Testing of the in vitro susceptibilities of *Madurella mycetomatis* to six antifungal agents by using the Sensititre system in comparison with a

viability-based 2,3-bis(2-methoxy-4-nitro-5-sulfophenyl)-5-[(phenylamino)carbonyl]-2H-tetrazolium hydroxide (XTT) assay and a modified NCCLS method. *Antimicrob Agents Chemother* **49:**1364–1368.

128. **Oliveira FM, Unis G, Hochhegger B, Severo LC.** 2013. *Scedosporium apiospermum* eumycetoma successfully treated with oral voriconazole: report of a case and review of the Brazilian reports on scedosporiosis. *Rev Inst Med Trop São Paulo* **55:**121–123.
129. **Cartwright KE, Clark TW, Hussain AM, Wiselka M, Borman A, Johnson EM.** 2011. Eumycetoma of the hand caused by *Leptosphaeria tompkinsii* and refractory to medical therapy with voriconazole. *Mycopathologia* **172:**311–315.
130. **Mahgoub ES, Gumaa SA.** 1984. Ketoconazole in the treatment of eumycetoma due to *Madurella mycetomii. Trans R Soc Trop Med Hyg* **78:**376–379.
131. **Fahal AH, Rahman IA, El-Hassan AM, Rahman ME, Zijlstra EE.** 2011. The safety and efficacy of itraconazole for the treatment of patients with eumycetoma due to *Madurella mycetomatis. Trans R Soc Trop Med Hyg* **105:**127–132.
132. **Kloezen W, Parel F, Brüggemann R, Asouit K, Helvert-van Poppel M, Fahal A, Mouton J, van de Sande W.** Amphotericin B and terbinafine but not the azoles prolong survival in *Galleria mellonella* larvae infected with *Madurella mycetomatis*. Med Mycol, in press.
133. **Eadie K, Parel F, Helvert-van Poppel M, Fahal A, van de Sande W.** 2017. Combining two antifungal agents does not enhance survival of *Galleria mellonella* larvae infected with *Madurella mycetomatis. Trop Med Int Health* **22:**696–702.
134. **van de Sande WW, van Vianen W, ten Kate M, Fahal A, Bakker-Woudenberg I.** 2015. Amphotericin B but not itraconazole is able to prevent grain formation in experimental *Madurella mycetomatis* mycetoma in mice. *Br J Dermatol* **173:**1561–1562.
135. **Drugs for Neglected Diseases Initiative.** 2016. Fosravuconazole. http://www.dndi.org/diseases-projects/portfolio/fosravuconazole/. Accessed 20-09-2016.
136. **European Medicines Agency.** 2013. Suspension of marketing authorisations for oral ketoconazole. http://www.ema.europa.eu/docs/en_GB/document_library/Referrals_document/Ketoconazole-containing_medicines/WC500168458.pdf.
137. **FDA.** 2013. FDA Drug Safety Communication: FDA limits usage of Nizoral (ketoconazole) oral tablets due to potentially fatal liver injury and risk of drug interactions and adrenal gland problems. Drug Safety Communications. 7-26-2013. FDA Washington, DC.
138. **Negroni R, Tobón A, Bustamante B, Shikanai-Yasuda MA, Patino H, Restrepo A.** 2005. Posaconazole treatment of refractory eumycetoma and chromoblastomycosis. *Rev Inst Med Trop São Paulo* **47:**339–346.
139. **N'Diaye B, Dieng MT, Perez A, Stockmeyer M, Bakshi R.** 2006. Clinical efficacy and safety of oral terbinafine in fungal mycetoma. *Int J Dermatol* **45:**154–157.
140. **Ahmed SA, Kloezen W, Duncanson F, Zijlstra EE, de Hoog GS, Fahal AH, van de Sande WW.** 2014. *Madurella mycetomatis* is highly susceptible to ravuconazole. *PLoS Negl Trop Dis* **8:**e2942.
141. **Rippon JW.** 1988. *Medical mycology: The Pathogenic Fungi and the Pathogenic Actinomycetes*, 3rd ed. W.B. Saunders Company, Philadelphia, Pa.
142. **Desoubeaux G, Millon A, Freychet B, de Muret A, Garcia-Hermoso D, Bailly E, Rosset P, Chandenier J, Bernard L.** 2013. Eumycetoma of the foot caused by *Exophiala jeanselmei* in a Guinean woman. *J Mycol Med* **23:**168–175.
143. **Bonifaz A, Saldaña M, Araiza J, Mercadillo P, Tirado-Sánchez A.** 2017. Two simultaneous mycetomas caused by *Fusarium verticillioides* and *Madurella mycetomatis. Rev Inst Med Trop São Paulo* **59:**e55.
144. **Ahmed A, Desplaces N, Leonard P, Goldstein F, de Hoog S, Verbrugh H, van Belkum A.** 2003. Eumycetoma caused by *Madurella mycetomatis* identified by PCR and sequencing: a report of two cases. *J Clin Microbiol* **41:**5813–5816.
145. **Lacroix C, de Kerviler E, Morel P, Derouin F, Feuilhade de Chavin M.** 2005. *Madurella mycetomatis* mycetoma treated successfully with oral voriconazole. *Br J Dermatol* **152:**1067–1068.
146. **Develoux M, Ndiaye B, Dieng MT.** 1995. Mycetomas in Africa. *Sante* **5:**211–217. [In French.]
147. **Vandepitte J, Beeckmans G, Ninane J.** 1956. First case of Madura foot caused by *Madurella grisea* in the Belgian Congo. *Ann Soc Belg Med Trop* **36:**493–497. [In French.]
148. **Machado LA, Rivitti MC, Cucé LC, Salebian A, Lacaz CS, Heins-Vaccari EM, Belda Júnior W, de Melo NT.** 1992. Black-grain eumycetoma due to *Madurella grisea*. A report of 2 cases. *Rev Inst Med Trop São Paulo* **34:**569–580. [In Portuguese.]
149. **Mackinnon JE, Ferrada-Urzúa LV, Montemayor L.** 1943. *Madurella grisea* n. sp. A new species of fungus producing the black variety of maduromycosis in South America. *Mycopathologia* **4:**384–393.
150. **Vanbreuseghem R.** 1956. A culture of *Madurella grisea* Mackinnon 1949 isolated in the Belgian Congo. *Ann Soc Belg Med Trop* **36:**467–477. [In French.]
151. **Borman AM, Desnos-Ollivier M, Miles S-J, Linton CJ, Campbell CK, Bridge PD, Dannaoui E, Johnson EM.** 2009. Molecular characterisation of the *Madurella grisea* complex reveals at least three new taxa associated with human mycetomas, abstr MO-01-3, p 241. The 17th Congress of the International Society for Human and Animal Mycology, 2009, Tokyo, Japan.
152. **Courtois G, De Loof C, Thys A, Vanbreuseghem R.** 1954. Nine cases of maduromycosis in the Belgian Congo caused by *Allescheria boydii, Monosporium apiospermum* and *Nocardia madurae. Ann Soc Belg Med Trop* **34:**371–395. [In French.]
153. **Horré R, Schumacher G, Marklein G, Stratmann H, Wardelmann E, Gilges S, De Hoog GS, Schaal KP.** 2002. Mycetoma due to *Pseudallescheria boydii* and co-isolation of *Nocardia abscessus* in a patient injured in road accident. *Med Mycol* **40:**525–527.
154. **Mohr JA, Muchmore HG.** 1968. Maduromycosis due to *Allescheria boydii. JAMA* **204:**335–336.
155. **Béraud G, Desbois N, Coyo C, Quist D, Rozé B, Savorit L, Cabié A.** 2015. Paradoxical response preceding control of *Scedosporium apiospermum* mycetoma with posaconazole treatment. *Infect Dis (Lond)* **47:**830–833.
156. **Porte L, Khatibi S, Hajj LE, Cassaing S, Berry A, Massip P, Linas MD, Magnaval JF, Sans N, Marchou B.** 2006. *Scedosporium apiospermum* mycetoma with bone involvement successfully treated with voriconazole. *Trans R Soc Trop Med Hyg* **100:**891–894.
157. **Shear CL.** 1922. Life history of an undescribed ascomycete from a granular mycetoma of man. *Mycologia* **14:**239–243.
158. **Koshi G, Padhye AA, Ajello L, Chandler FW.** 1979. *Acremonium recifei* as an agent of mycetoma in India. *Am J Trop Med Hyg* **28:**692–696.
159. **Ahmed SA, Abbas MA, Jouvion G, Al-Hatmi AM, de Hoog GS, Kolecka A, Mahgoub S.** 2015. Seventeen years of subcutaneous infection by *Aspergillus flavus*; eumycetoma confirmed by immunohistochemistry. *Mycoses* **58:**728–734.
160. **Mahgoub ES.** 1973. Can *Aspergillus flavus* cause maduromycetoma? *Bull Soc Pathol Exot* **66:**390–395.
161. **Bonifaz A, De Hoog S, McGinnis MR, Saúl A, Rodríguez-Cortés O, Araiza J, Cruz M, Mercadillo P.** 2009. Eumycetoma caused by *Cladophialophora bantiana* successfully treated with itraconazole. *Med Mycol* **47:**111–114.
162. **Badali H, Gueidan C, Najafzadeh MJ, Bonifaz A, van den Ende AH, de Hoog GS.** 2008. Biodiversity of the genus *Cladophialophora. Stud Mycol* **61:**175–191.
163. **Mahgoub E.** 1969. *Corynespora cassiicola*, a new agent of maduromycetoma. *J Trop Med Hyg* **72:**218–221.
164. **Bridges CH.** 1957. Maduromycotic mycetomas in animals; *Curvularia geniculata* as an etiologic agent. *Am J Pathol* **33:**411–427.
165. **Shinde RS, Hanumantha S, Mantur BG, Parande MV.** 2015. A rare case of mycetoma due to curvularia. *J Lab Physicians* **7:**55–57.
166. **Elad D, Orgad U, Yakobson B, Perl S, Golomb P, Trainin R, Tsur I, Shenkler S, Bor A.** 1991. Eumycetoma caused by *Curvularia lunata* in a dog. *Mycopathologia* **116:**113–118.

167. **Garg A, Sujatha S, Garg J, Parija SC, Thappa DM.** 2008. Eumycetoma due to *Curvularia lunata*. *Indian J Dermatol Venereol Leprol* **74:**515–516.
168. **Gunathilake R, Perera P, Sirimanna G.** 2014. *Curvularia lunata*: a rare cause of black-grain eumycetoma. *J Mycol Med* **24:**158–160.
169. **Iriart X, Binois R, Fior A, Blanchet D, Berry A, Cassaing S, Amazan E, Papot E, Carme B, Aznar C, Couppié P.** 2011. Eumycetoma caused by *Diaporthe phaseolorum* (*Phomopsis phaseoli*): a case report and a mini-review of *Diaporthe/Phomopsis* spp invasive infections in humans. *Clin Microbiol Infect* **17:**1492–1494.
170. **Pattanaprichakul P, Bunyaratavej S, Leeyaphan C, Sitthinamsuwan P, Sudhadham M, Muanprasart C, Feng P, Badali H, de Hoog GS.** 2013. An unusual case of eumycetoma caused by *Exophiala jeanselmei* after a sea urchin injury. *Mycoses* **56:**491–494.
171. **Neumeister B, Zollner TM, Krieger D, Sterry W, Marre R.** 1995. Mycetoma due to *Exophiala jeanselmei* and *Mycobacterium chelonae* in a 73-year-old man with idiopathic CD4+ T lymphocytopenia. *Mycoses* **38:**271–276.
172. **Venugopal PV, Venugopal TV.** 1990. *Leptosphaeria tompkinsii* mycetoma. *Int J Dermatol* **29:**432–433.
173. **Lee MW, Kim JC, Choi JS, Kim KH, Greer DL.** 1995. Mycetoma caused by *Acremonium falciforme*: successful treatment with itraconazole. *J Am Acad Dermatol* **32:**897–900.
174. **Halde C, Padhye AA, Haley LD, Rinaldi MG, Kay D, Leeper R.** 1976. *Acremonium falciforme* as a cause of mycetoma in California. *Sabouraudia* **14:**319–326.
175. **Milburn PB, Papayanopulos DM, Pomerantz BM.** 1988. Mycetoma due to *Acremonium falciforme*. *Int J Dermatol* **27:**408–410.
176. **Negroni R, López Daneri G, Arechavala A, Bianchi MH, Robles AM.** 2006. Clinical and microbiological study of mycetomas at the Muñiz hospital of Buenos Aires between 1989 and 2004. *Rev Argent Microbiol* **38:**13–18. [In Spanish.]
177. **Ajello L, Padhye AA, Chandler FW, McGinnis MR, Morganti L, Alberici F.** 1985. *Fusarium moniliforme*, a new mycetoma agent. Restudy of a European case. *Eur J Epidemiol* **1:** 5–10.
178. **Katkar VJ, Tankhiwale SS, Kurhade A.** 2011. *Fusarium soloni* mycetoma. *Indian J Dermatol* **56:**315–317.
179. **Zoutman DE, Sigler L.** 1991. Mycetoma of the foot caused by *Cylindrocarpon destructans*. *J Clin Microbiol* **29:**1855–1859.
180. **Chiapello LS, Dib MD, Nuncira CT, Nardelli L, Vullo C, Collino C, Abiega C, Cortes PR, Spesso MF, Masih DT.** 2011. Mycetoma of the scalp due to *Microsporum canis*: hystopathologic, mycologic, and immunogenetic features in a 6-year-old girl. *Diagn Microbiol Infect Dis* **70:**145–149.
181. **Kramer SC, Ryan M, Bourbeau P, Tyler WB, Elston DM.** 2006. Fontana-positive grains in mycetoma caused by *Microsporum canis*. *Pediatr Dermatol* **23:**473–475.
182. **Yager JA, Wilcock BP, Lynch JA, Thompson AR.** 1986. Mycetoma-like granuloma in a cat caused by *Microsporum canis*. *J Comp Pathol* **96:**171–176.
183. **Aguilar-Donis A, Torres-Guerrero E, Arenas-Guzmán R, Hernández-Hernández F, López-García L, Criales-Vera S, Teliz-Meneses MA.** 2011. Mycetoma caused by *Phaeoacremonium parasiticum*—a case confirmed with B-tubulin sequence analysis. *Mycoses* **54:**e615–e618.
184. **de Vries GA, de Hoog GS, de Bruyn HP.** 1984. *Phialophora cyanescens* sp. nov. with *Phaeosclera*-like synanamorph, causing white-grain mycetoma in man. *Antonie van Leeuwenhoek* **50:**149–153.
185. **Ahmed AO, van de Sande WW, van Vianen W, van Belkum A, Fahal AH, Verbrugh HA, Bakker-Woudenberg IA.** 2004. In vitro susceptibilities of *Madurella mycetomatis* to itraconazole and amphotericin B assessed by a modified NCCLS method and a viability-based 2,3-bis(2-methoxy-4-nitro-5- sulfophenyl)-5-[(phenylamino)carbonyl]-2H-tetrazolium hydroxide (XTT) assay. *Antimicrob Agents Chemother* **48:**2742–2746.
186. **Kloezen W, Meis JF, Curfs-Breuker I, Fahal AH, van de Sande WW.** 2012. In vitro antifungal activity of isavuconazole against *Madurella mycetomatis*. *Antimicrob Agents Chemother* **56:**6054–6056.
187. **van Belkum A, Fahal AH, van de Sande WW.** 2011. In vitro susceptibility of *Madurella mycetomatis* to posaconazole and terbinafine. *Antimicrob Agents Chemother* **55:**1771–1773.
188. **van de Sande WW, Fahal AH, Bakker-Woudenberg IA, van Belkum A.** 2010. *Madurella mycetomatis* is not susceptible to the echinocandin class of antifungal agents. *Antimicrob Agents Chemother* **54:**2738–2740.
189. **van de Sande WW, Fahal AH, Riley TV, Verbrugh H, van Belkum A.** 2007. In vitro susceptibility of *Madurella mycetomatis*, prime agent of Madura foot, to tea tree oil and artemisinin. *J Antimicrob Chemother* **59:**553–555.
190. **Venugopal PV, Venugopal TV, Ramakrishna ES, Ilavarasi S.** 1993. Antimycotic susceptibility testing of agents of black grain eumycetoma. *J Med Vet Mycol* **31:**161–164.
191. **Venugopal PV, Venugopal TV.** 1993. Treatment of eumycetoma with ketoconazole. *Australas J Dermatol* **34:**27–29.
192. **Ahmed SA, de Hoog GS, Stevens DA, Fahal AH, van de Sande WW.** 2015. In vitro antifungal susceptibility of coelomycete agents of black grain eumycetoma to eight antifungals. *Med Mycol* **53:**295–301.
193. **González GM, Tijerina R, Najvar LK, Bocanegra R, Rinaldi MG, Loebenberg D, Graybill JR.** 2003. Activity of posaconazole against *Pseudallescheria boydii*: in vitro and in vivo assays. *Antimicrob Agents Chemother* **47:**1436–1438.
194. **Walsh TJ, Peter J, McGough DA, Fothergill AW, Rinaldi MG, Pizzo PA.** 1995. Activities of amphotericin B and antifungal azoles alone and in combination against *Pseudallescheria boydii*. *Antimicrob Agents Chemother* **39:** 1361–1364.
195. **Badali H, Najafzadeh MJ, van Esbroeck M, van den Enden E, Tarazooie B, Meis JF, de Hoog GS.** 2010. The clinical spectrum of *Exophiala jeanselmei*, with a case report and in vitro antifungal susceptibility of the species. *Med Mycol* **48:**318–327.

Mycotoxins

JOANNA TANNOUS AND NANCY P. KELLER

129

Mycotoxins are secondary metabolites produced by many different species of ubiquitous fungi that have adverse effects on humans and animals. Secondary metabolites (SMs), also referred to as natural products, are not required for growth in laboratory conditions but afford protective roles for the producing fungi. These roles range from protection from predators to exclusion of other microbes for niche securement (1, 2). Current available data suggest that SMs assume a crucial role in microbial communication. Recent studies have led to the discovery that fungal interactions with other microbial species induce the production of new SMs by activating silent gene clusters (3–5). In the past few years, some SMs have also been reported as virulence factors in plant-fungal interactions and animal infections (6–8). Accordingly, many SMs are bioactive and cause damage when ingested by humans and animals. Not all toxic compounds produced by fungi are referred to as mycotoxins; for example, yeast and mushroom poisons are excluded by convention, compounds mainly inhibitory to bacteria are termed antibiotics, and those toxic to plants are called phytotoxins, although there can be overlap in toxicity to several kingdoms (9). Currently, more than 500 different mycotoxins have been discovered (10), and this number is increasing continuously with the application of modern mass spectrometry-based profiling and metabolomics workflows (11, 12). In this chapter, we review the most common mycotoxins and their relevance to sick building syndrome (SBS), bioterrorism, and food safety. We do not describe the impacts of mycotoxins on health, health costs, or the economy, as these topics have been reviewed extensively elsewhere (13–16). The reader is also referred to other recent reviews on mycotoxins (9, 17–19).

CHEMICAL CLASSIFICATION AND BIOSYNTHESIS OF MYCOTOXINS

The vast majority of mycotoxins, and indeed all fungal SMs, arise from a few well-known chemical precursors. Polyketides, like fatty acids, are synthesized from acyl-CoA, nonribosomal peptides from amino acids, alkaloids from prenylated aromatic amino acids utilizing a dimethylallyltryptophan synthase, and terpenes from isoprene. Figure 1 provides a listing of some of the most commonly encountered mycotoxins, their chemical class, and structure, and Table 1 presents the producing fungi. Among the biosynthetic categories cited above, the polyketide chemical class derived from acetate metabolism appears to dominate (20). It is important to mention that among the nine classes of mycotoxins shown in Fig. 1, only trichothecenes (terpene) and ergot alkaloids (nonribosomal peptide and prenylated tryptophan) do not belong to the polyketide family. However, some of the more uncommon mycotoxins are derived solely from terpene or nonribosomal peptide/alkaloid origins.

The structure, and in some cases biochemistry, of the most common mycotoxins was elucidated earlier than the genetics. However, within the last decade, the genes encoding the enzymes required to synthesize many common mycotoxins have been found (17). Very recently, a scalable platform has been developed to identify novel fungal SMs and assigned them to their corresponding biosynthetic gene clusters (21). The first mycotoxin gene clusters to be characterized were the aflatoxin cluster in both *Aspergillus flavus* and *A. parasiticus* (22, 23) and sterigmatocystin cluster in *A. nidulans* (24). The finding that the genes were clustered in a single genetic locus has turned out to be a hallmark of fungal SMs (20). The physical clustering of metabolic genes has a significant impact on their regulation (25). Therein, it is important to mention that gene clusters coding for mycotoxins' biosynthesis often, but not necessarily, include a gene encoding a transcription factor that specifically modulates the expression of the rest of the genes within the cluster. The molecular genetics of fungal secondary metabolite clusters has been the subject of many recent reviews (25–27). Figure 2 summarizes our current understanding of the gene clusters for the mycotoxins described in this chapter.

Aflatoxins

The aflatoxin class of mycotoxins was the first to be discovered and studied. Some of the most common aflatoxins (Fig. 1) are aflatoxins B_1, B_2, G_1, and G_2, named for their blue or green fluorescence under UV light (28), with aflatoxin B_1 being the most potent natural carcinogen known (29). There have been several recent reviews of aflatoxins and the producing fungi (30).

Aflatoxins are produced by several species of *Aspergillus*, in particular *A. flavus* and *A. parasiticus*. *A. flavus* is the most common contaminant of agricultural products, including cereals, rice, figs, nuts, and tobacco (31, 32).

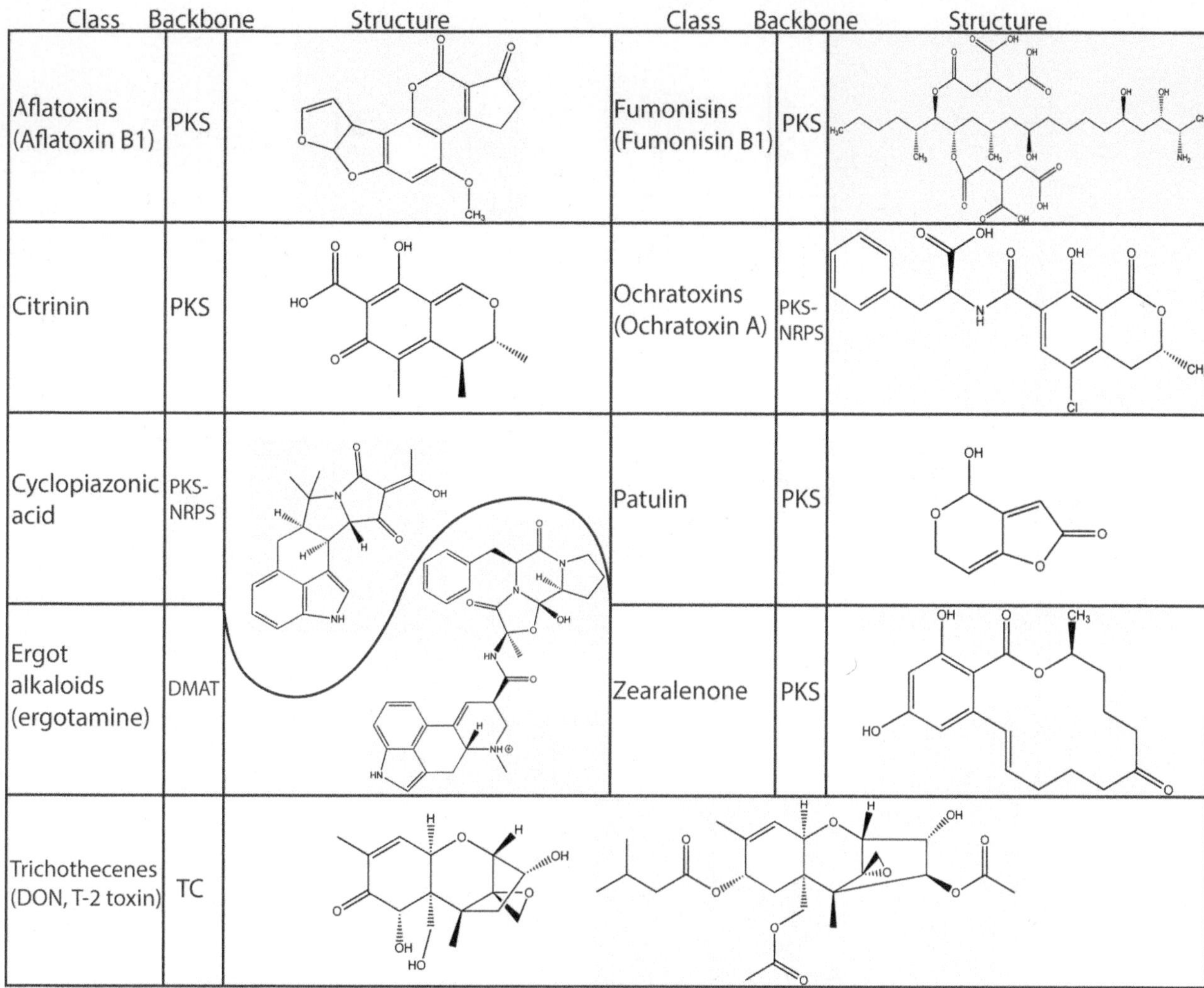

FIGURE 1 Classes of mycotoxins, the central enzyme in their biosyntheses, and the structures of examples of each. PKS, polyketide synthase; NRPS, nonribosomal peptide synthetase; DMAT, dimethylallyltryptophan synthase; TC, terpene cyclase; DON, deoxynivalenol (9).

TABLE 1 Simplified taxonomy of mycotoxin-producing fungi (180)

Mycotoxin class	Genera	Representative species
Aflatoxin	*Aspergillus, Penicillium*	*A. fumigatus, A. flavus, A. parasiticus, P. aurantiogriseum*
Citrinin	*Penicillium*	*P. citrinin, P. expansum*
Cyclopiazonic acid	*Aspergillus, Penicillium*	*P. griseofulvum, A. flavus*
Ergot alkaloid	*Aspergillus, Balansia, Claviceps, Epichloë, Neotyphodium*	*A. fumigatus, C. purpurea*
Fumonisin	*Gibberella, Fusarium*	*G. fujikuroi, F. proliferatum*
Ochratoxin	*Aspergillus, Penicillium*	*A. ochraceus, P. verrucosum*
Patulin	*Aspergillus, Paecilomyces, Penicillium*	*A. clavatus, Paecilomyces fulvus, Paecilomyces niveus, P. griseofulvum, P. expansum*
Trichothecene	*Stachybotrys*	*S. chartarum*
Zearalenone	*Gibberella, Fusarium*	*F. crookwellense, F. culmorum, G. zeae, F. incarnatum*

Contamination of crops can occur in the fields before harvest, especially in times of drought (32, 33), or during storage, depending upon the moisture content of the substrate and the humidity of the storage conditions (31, 34). Aflatoxin is mainly problematic in countries with tropical and subtropical climates where temperature and humidity conditions are optimal to fungus growth and toxin production (35). However, its danger has spread beyond its predicted geographical boundaries and has reached countries previously considered as relatively safe from this toxin (36). Aflatoxin contamination can be the cause of a variety of economic and health problems and is particularly problematic in developing countries (37). For instance, the presence of aflatoxin in grain significantly lowers the grain's value, as feed or an export commodity, because of the toxin's link to increased mortality in farm animals (38). Further, ingestion of aflatoxin by dairy cows can lead to the presence of aflatoxin M_1, a hydroxylated form of B_1, in their milk (39).

There are substantial differences in the susceptibilities of vertebrate species to aflatoxin exposure. One of the first indications of the effects of aflatoxins was observed in 1960, when more than 100,000 turkey poults died from aflatoxin-contaminated feed, an outbreak named "turkey X disease" (40). Other outbreaks have occurred in

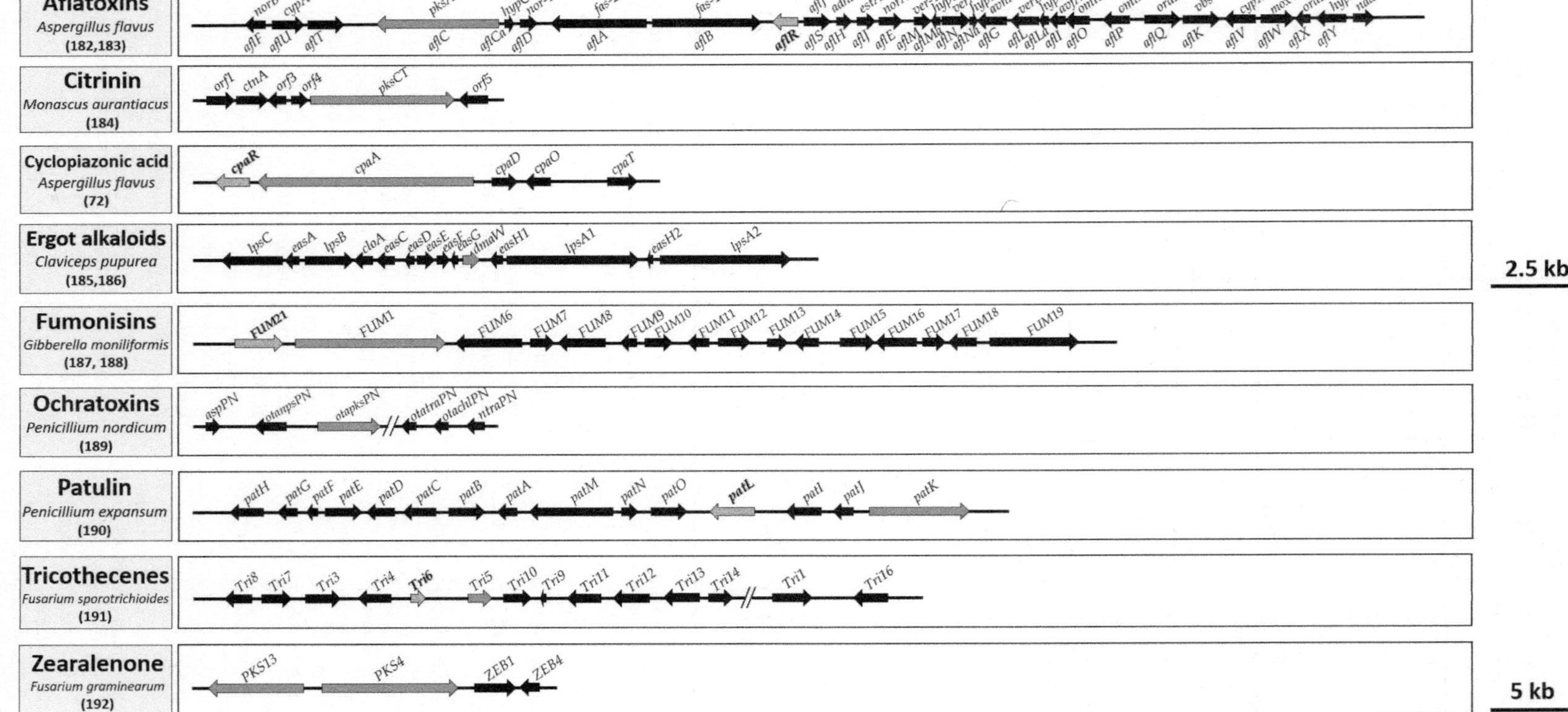
Aflatoxins
Aspergillus flavus
(182,183)
Citrinin
Monascus aurantiacus
(184)
Cyclopiazonic acid
Aspergillus flavus
(72)
Ergot alkaloids
Claviceps pupurea
(185,186)
Fumonisins
Gibberella moniliformis
(187, 188)
Ochratoxins
Penicillium nordicum
(189)
Patulin
Penicillium expansum
(190)
Tricothecenes
Fusarium sporotrichioides
(191)
Zearalenone
Fusarium graminearum
(192)
2.5 kb
5 kb

FIGURE 2 The genetic structure of the biosynthetic gene clusters for each of the major groups of mycotoxins in the particular species. The backbone genes are represented in blue and the specific transcription factors in gray. Each gene is represented as an arrow in the direction of transcription with the name of the gene above it. In the aflatoxin pathway gene cluster, the old gene names are labeled on top of the line and the new gene names are labeled below the line. Diagonal bisection of a cluster signifies that it is not contiguous. The 5-kb scale bar applies to all of the clusters except the ergot alkaloids cluster, to which the 2.5-kb scale bar applies.

ducklings and chickens (41), swine (42), and calves (43), due mostly to contaminated Brazilian peanut meal used as feed. The most recent notable outbreak of acute aflatoxicosis in humans was in Kenya in 2004 (44), followed by lesser yet significant outbreaks in 2005 and 2006 (45). These outbreaks illustrate the need for monitoring and regulation of the amount of mycotoxins in foods meant for human consumption, a luxury not normally available to developing countries. Aflatoxin contamination of pet food, particularly dog food, is a recurring problem in the United States and other countries (46). Many papers review the worldwide aflatoxin contamination of food and feed (47–49) and the recent advances in aflatoxin management technologies (50).

Citrinin

Citrinin (Fig. 1) is a simple, low-molecular-weight compound that crystallizes as lemon-colored needles. It was tested as an antibiotic and a treatment for ulcers (51) before the discovery of its mycotoxic effects. The most common organisms producing citrinin are *Penicillium citrinum*, *P. expansum*, *P. aurantiogriseum*, *P. camemberti* (used to produce cheese), *A. neoniveus*, *A. oryzae* (used to produce sake and soy sauce), *A. terreus*, and *Monascus* spp. (used to produce red food dyes) (52).

Citrinin, first isolated from *P. citrinum*, has been associated with Japanese yellow rice disease (53). It has also been found in various grains, peanuts, and fruits, and there is limited evidence of its surviving unchanged in cereal products (9). Citrinin-producing fungi are major producers of other classes of mycotoxins, including ochratoxin, aflatoxin, and patulin. Therefore, co-occurrence of citrinin with these fungal metabolites was reported in rice (54) and apples (55). Citrinin has demonstrated nephrotoxic effects on all animal species tested (56) and was shown to inhibit dehydrogenase activity in rats' kidneys, liver, and brain (57). The toxic effects of citrinin on the mammal reproductive system, especially on oocyte maturation, have also been reported (58–60). However, there have been no reported outbreaks of human citrinin poisoning, and its relevance to human health is unknown.

Cyclopiazonic acid

Cyclopiazonic acid (CPA) (Fig. 1) is an indole-tetramic acid mycotoxin produced by several species of *Penicillium* and *Aspergillus* (61, 62). It has demonstrated severe toxicity on all species tested, including rats (63), chickens (64), dogs (65), and pigs (66). By virtue of it cytotoxicity, CPA is considered a potential pathogenicity factor in the invasion of plant cells by *A. flavus* (67). Contamination of various food products, including grains, meats, and cheese, with CPA is sometimes coincident with aflatoxin contamination (68). As such, it is suspected that some of the symptoms of "turkey X disease" may have been due to the toxicity of co-contaminant CPA (69).

Interestingly, the CPA gene cluster is present in *A. flavus* but truncated in its close relative *A. oryzae* (70); this is reminiscent of repeated findings of truncated or mutated aflatoxin clusters in this species (71). *Aspergillus oryzae*, a species used in the manufacture of fermented rice products, does not produce CPA due to a deletion in the backbone gene of the cluster, or in some strains where the backbone gene is present, CPA is converted to a less toxic compound, 2-oxoCPA, by an enzyme not present in *A. flavus* (72). Little is known about its toxicity to humans, but it may affect the heart (73) and liver and is thought to cause "kodo poisoning" (74).

Ergot Alkaloids

Ergot alkaloids, produced by the ergot fungus *Claviceps purpurea*, are the causative agent of ergotism, or St. Anthony's fire, which can manifest either as a gangrenous or convulsive condition following ingestion of contaminated grains, especially rye (75). Two main classes of ergot alkaloids exist: lysergic acid derivatives and clavines. Both are indole alkaloids derived from tetracyclic ergoline. Lysergic acid, common to all ergot alkaloids, often forms amide, amino acid, or peptide derivatives, e.g., ergine, ergonovine, lysergic acid diethylamide, and ergovaline. The clavines contain the ergoline structure but do not have amino acid or peptide components, e.g., pergolide and lisuride (75). Semisynthetic ergot alkaloids have been developed through decades of research, which began with the series of lysergic acid derivatives that included the infamous hallucinogen LSD (76). Most recently, ergot alkaloids have been investigated for their anticancer potential (77) and their effect on serotonin and serotonin receptors (78, 79). A representative compound, ergotamine, is shown in Fig. 1.

Aspergillus, *Balansia*, *Claviceps*, *Epichloë*, and *Neotyphodium* spp. have been found to produce ergot alkaloids. *Aspergillus fumigatus* has been shown to produce fumigaclavines A, B, and C and festuclavine, first described for *C. purpurea* and later for *Neotyphodium* (80). Modern methods of cleaning grains have all but eliminated the threat to the human food chain. However, ergotism remains an important veterinary concern, as symptoms of gangrene, convulsions, and abortion in cattle, sheep, pigs, and chickens mimic those in humans (81).

Fumonisins

Fumonisins (Fig. 1) are among the most recently discovered mycotoxins. In the late 1970s and early 1980s it was determined that fumonisins produced by *Gibberella fujikuroi* were the cause of leukoencephalomalacia in horses (82) and hepatocarcinoma in rats (83). By 2002, there were 28 known fumonisin analogs, separated into groups A, B, C, and P (84). *Fusarium proliferatum*, *G. nygamai*, *A. niger*, and *Alternaria alternata* also produce these mycotoxins (85, 86).

Besides the syndromes mentioned above, fumonisins have been shown to cause pulmonary edema and hydrothorax in swine (87). In addition, numerous acute exposure studies bring information on the impact of fumonisins on pig intestine and have been recently reviewed (88). *G. fujikuroi*, the major producer of fumonisins, can have an important effect on the supply of corn, as it causes a variety of blights and rots depending on environmental conditions (89). Moreover, there is considerable concern and evidence that fumonisins cause several human diseases, particularly esophageal cancer (90). Likely due to these concerns, international monitoring systems are now in place for this metabolite (91), which, unfortunately, is often found in food and feed products, co-contaminated with aflatoxin (92). The recent review by Wang et al. (93) represents a must-read for anyone interested in fumonisin toxicity.

Ochratoxins

Ochratoxins A and B (Fig. 1) are produced by *Penicillium verrucosum* and *Aspergillus* spp., especially *A. ochraceus*. These toxins can be carcinogenic, immunosuppressive, and nephrotoxic (38, 94). Ochratoxin A, first discovered to be toxic to animals in 1965 (95), is more common than ochratoxin B and can be metabolized by cytochrome P450 in the liver (96). Ochratoxins are most often found contaminating barley, but they may be present in oats, rye, wheat, and coffee beans (9, 95, 97). They are of particular concern because they can be carried through the food chain, especially in milk and pork (98). Scandinavian countries, particularly Denmark, have had high incidence of porcine nephropathy and high levels of ochratoxin A contamination (99). After cereals, wine is the largest source of human exposure to ochratoxin A due contamination of grapes in the vineyards with fungal species belonging to the genus *Aspergillus* (100). Some studies speculate that ochratoxin A may contribute to Parkinson disease (101).

Patulin

Patulin (Fig. 1) was first isolated in the 1940s from *Penicillium griseofulvum*, and efforts were made to mass-produce it for its antibiotic effects (102). However, patulin was reclassified as a mycotoxin in the 1960s following discovery of its toxicity to plants and animals (9). Effects of acute poisoning, such as hematemesis, diarrhea, lethargy, tachypnea, massive atelectasis, and alveolar hemorrhages, were described in different animal species (103–105). At present, there are no documented cases of acute toxicity reported in humans. Chronic exposure to patulin was likewise associated with diverse toxic effects, mainly cytotoxicity and genotoxicity (106–108). Patulin occurs commonly in unfermented juice made from *P. expansum*-contaminated fruit (109), whereas ascladiol, its direct biosynthetic precursor, has been reported in alcoholic beverages, mainly apple cider (110). Though toxic at high concentrations *in vitro*, natural patulin poisoning in humans has yet to be proven (9). Nevertheless, due to concern of its prevalence in apple juice and other items preferentially consumed by children, several countries limit patulin levels in certain foods and beverages (111). A number of papers in recent years (112, 113) have reported the potential role of patulin as a virulence factor in apple infections. The reader is referred to recent reviews on the biosynthesis, pathogenicity, and toxicity of patulin (114, 115).

Trichothecenes

Trichothecene mycotoxins are SMs of a variety of *Fusarium*, *Myrothecium*, *Phomopsis*, *Stachybotrys*, *Trichoderma*, and *Trichothecium* spp., among others. Some of the most common and well-studied *Fusarium* trichothecenes (Fig. 1) are T-2 toxin, HT-2 toxin, diacetoxyscirpenol, nivalenol, and deoxynivalenol, also called DON or vomitoxin. DON is one of the most common mycotoxins found in grain, including barley, oats, rye, and wheat. When ingested in large quantities by livestock, it can cause nausea, vomiting, and diarrhea. Ingestion of smaller quantities results in weight loss and feed refusal (116). DON can also suppress bovine and porcine neutrophil function *in vitro* (117). *Stachybotrys chartarum* produces several trichothecenes, including verrucarins B and J, roridin E, satratoxins F, G, and H, and isosatratoxins F, G, and H (118, 119). *Stachybotrys*-contaminated straw was first described as causing a highly fatal equine disease (120) and has since become better known as a factor in SBS, discussed below. The exhaustive review of Pinton and Oswald (121) summarizes the available data concerning the toxicity of DON and other trichothecenes.

Zearalenone

Zearalenone (Fig. 1) is a nonsteroidal estrogen or phytoestrogen produced by various species of *Gibberella*, including *G. pulicaris* and *G. tricincta* (122). Zearalenone is a common contaminant of cereal crops worldwide and has been implicated in hyperestrogenism of farm animals as a result of digestion of moldy corn and grains (123). Some of the symptoms of hyperestrogenism are enlargement of the uterus and nipples, vaginal prolapse, and infertility (124). Recently zearalenone was proved to be immunotoxic, causing thymic atrophy with histological and thymocyte phenotype changes as well as a decrease in the B cell percentage in the spleen (125). In addition, several outbreaks of zearalenone poisoning of swine have been reported (126). Many recent studies have demonstrated that zearalenone induces reactive oxygen species generation, lipid peroxidation, oxidative DNA damage, and cell apoptosis (127, 128) and suggest that oxidative stress appears to be a key determinant of its *in vivo* and *in vitro* toxicity. Recently, resveratrol, an antioxidant phenolic compound, has been shown to exhibit significant protective effects on zearalenone-induced cell damage (129).

FOOD SAFETY

Consumption of moldy food products is the leading cause of mycotoxicoses in agricultural animals and humans alike. Contamination can occur at any point, ranging from the crop field through storage and shipping. The economic consequences of mycotoxin contamination are immense, and mycotoxins pose a higher chronic dietary risk than synthetic contaminants, plant toxins, food additives, or pesticide residues (130). Tables 1 and 2 list the mycotoxins discussed in this chapter and their common substrates. The reader should note that neither table is exhaustive, and other fungi and substrates can be involved in mycotoxin poisonings.

Regulation

Considering the difficulty of preventing mycotoxin contamination and the harmful effects of these deleterious molecules on human and animal health, many countries have

TABLE 2 Mycotoxins and their common food substrates (181)

Mycotoxin class	Barley	Cheese	Coffee beans	Corn	Fruits	Oats	Peanuts	Rice	Rye	Wheat
Aflatoxin				X			X	X		X
Citrinin	X			X		X		X	X	X
Cyclopiazonic acid		X		X			X			
Ergot alkaloid	X					X			X	X
Fumonisin				X						
Ochratoxin	X		X			X			X	X
Patulin					X					
Trichothecene				X						
Zearalenone				X						

TABLE 3 Major mycotoxins: pathological effects and toxicological reference values (131, 132, 182, 183)[a]

Mycotoxin class	Proven or suspected pathological effects	Established regulatory levels in food and feed (ppb)		Maximum tolerable daily intake per kg of body weight (JECFA)
		European Union	United States (FDA)	
Aflatoxin	Hepatotoxicity Carcinogenesis Hematopoietic effects Genotoxicity Immunotoxicity Teratogenesis	B1: 0.10–12 B1 + B2 + G1 + G2: 4–15 M1: 0.025–0.050	B1 + B2 + G1 + G2: 20 M1: 0.5 (action levels)	Consumption should be as low as reasonably achievable[b]
Citrinin	Nephrotoxicity Cytotoxicity Immunotoxicity Reprotoxicity Genotoxicity	NR	NR	–
Cyclopiazonic acid	Necrotic effects Carcinogenicity Neurotoxicity	NR	NR	–
Ergot alkaloid	Digestive disorders Convulsion Abortion	NR	NR	–
Fumonisin	Cancerogenicity Genotoxicity Hepatotoxicity Immunotoxicity Nephrotoxicity Reprotoxicity	200–4,000	2,000–4,000 (guidance level)	2 μg/kg/day
Ochratoxin	Nephrotoxicity Hepatotoxicity Immunotoxicity Neurotoxicity Teratogenesis Carcinogenesis	0.2–80	NR	0.005/0.0143 μg/kg/day
Patulin	Cytotoxicity Genotoxicity Immunotoxicity Reprotoxicity Teratogenicity	25–50	50 (action level)	0.4 μg/kg/day
Trichothecene (DON)	Hematopoietic effects Genotoxicity Immunotoxicity Neurotoxicity Nephrotoxicity Estrogenic effects	200–1,750	1,000–10,000 (guidance level)	1 μg/kg/day
Zearalenone	Immunotoxicity Reprotoxicity Teratogenicity	20–400	NR	0.2/0.5 μg/kg/day

[a]NR, not regulated.
[b]Aflatoxins exhibit carcinogenic and genotoxic effects without threshold; the only realistic approach is to reduce exposure to as low a level as possible without destroying the food matrix, following the ALARA (as low as reasonably achievable) principle.

enacted regulations for levels of mycotoxins in food and animal feed. Regulations for mycotoxins were first established in the late 1960s in the United States. Subsequently, new limits and regulations were set by the Federal Food, Drug, and Cosmetic Act, which is enforced by the Food and Drug Administration (FDA). The latter has established specific "action" levels for aflatoxin and "advisory" levels for other classes of mycotoxins (131). European countries were also among the first to set EU-harmonized regulations and limits for mycotoxins in food and feed (132). The regulatory guidelines for limiting mycotoxins differ between countries but have been summarized in compendia published by the Food and Agriculture Organization of the United Nations and more recently reviewed (111, 133). Table 3 summarizes the main mycotoxins, their major toxic effects, and toxicological reference values.

Detection

Because of the wide-ranging structural diversity of mycotoxins, serious health risks caused by these compounds, and their high chemical stability, it has been very crucial to develop vigorous and effective detection techniques. Mycotoxins are often present in smaller amounts than other interfering substances, requiring that each be separated from its substrate and studied by a unique assay. Generally, sample preparation consists of an extraction step and a purification step. Though this method is the most definitive, it is very expensive and time-consuming. Thus, newer screening methods for the presence of mycotoxins have been developed over the past decade. However, many of these screening methods are still plagued by cross-reactivity and require confirmation with more selective validated methods.

Several reviews exist on current detection methodologies (134, 135). Confirmatory tests and novel screening techniques include immunoassays such as enzyme-linked immunosorbent assay (ELISA), fluorescence polarization immunoassay, surface-plasmon resonance, and other conductometric measurements (136). High-performance liquid chromatography (HPLC) and gas chromatography are widely used, and since the introduction of atmospheric pressure ionization, liquid chromatography-mass spectrometry has become a routine technique for detecting the presence of mycotoxins, including trichothecenes, ochratoxins, zearalenone, fumonisins, and aflatoxins (137). The latest official methods, validated by the Association of Official Analytical Chemists International, are based on immunoaffinity column cleanup of conventional extracts, followed by fluorescently labeled HPLC (38). Over the past few years, novel approaches such as sensors and biosensors for mycotoxin detection have emerged as promising alternatives to classical analysis methods due to their high sensitivity and selectivity, usability, and low cost (138). Even though the performance and applicability of such techniques need some improvements, they were already proven to be potent tools for analysis of aflatoxins (139), ochratoxins (140), and zearalenone (141). The reader is referred to comprehensive reviews of recent developments in analytical protocols (142–144).

Effects of Climate Change

It is estimated that one-quarter to almost three-quarters of the world's crops are contaminated to some extent with mycotoxins, depending on country sampled (145, 146); this proportion varies from year to year, based on environmental factors. There is much evidence of the influence of environmental factors, mainly temperature, humidity, CO_2, drought, insect attack, and other plant stressors, on mycotoxin production by molds. Further, the pathogenicity of different molds may be additive, and competition between mold species may be temperature dependent (124). Each species and its ability to produce mycotoxins must be evaluated independently in its optimum growth conditions. For wheat species, infection of the cereal ears by *Gibberella* spp., particularly *G. zeae*, a predominant producer of DON, is enhanced by warm, humid weather (147). However, contamination with this same mycotoxin in maize is greater under abundant precipitation and lower air temperature, which are favorable for *Fusarium graminearum* and *F. culmorum* growth (148). At the other extreme, production of fumonisins and aflatoxins is greater under drought conditions. Warmer temperatures and fewer frost days result in more insect and plant pathogens surviving the winter and causing plants to be more susceptible to mold infestation. Considerable recent research has examined the impact of interactions of three main environmental factors: temperature, water availability, and CO_2 on the ecophysiology of mycotoxigenic fungi and mycotoxin production. The current literature is summarized in a recent review by Medina et al. (149). To conclude, climate and environmental changes in any particular region may result in radical changes in the amount and type of crop damage and mycotoxin contamination.

Current Practices and the Future of Prevention and Amelioration of Mycotoxin Contamination

Several different approaches are currently being developed to protect the food supply from mycotoxin contamination, including measures taken before, during, and after cultivation of crops, yet the most reliable preventive treatments are still cultural practices and humidity control in postharvest facilities. Though most breeding successes have been reported for wheat and barley, it is also essential to breed for resistance in other crops, such as corn and oats (150). Several laboratories have attempted to create transgenic lines resistant to various mycotoxigenic fungi, but none are in production. However, several reports suggest that Bt crops, i.e., those transgenically expressing insecticidal *Bacillus thuringiensis* toxins, are less susceptible to mycotoxin contamination due to decreased insect infestation (151). Indeed, insecticides have been shown to reduce the growth of *Aspergillus* and resultant accumulation of ochratoxin A (152).

One biological control discussed but not implemented to any degree is the application of mycoviruses, which are typically easily spread through asexual fungal spores. Though many mycoviruses have minimal effects on their host fungi, they have the potential to be used as vectors for resistance genes. This approach may expand with the increasing availability of virus-specific molecular detection methods (14). Additionally, a recent study shows that the application of nontoxigenic strains of *A. flavus* to corn plant whorls prior to tasseling significantly reduced aflatoxin accumulation, presumably through competition with toxigenic strains (153). This latter method appears promising and is being assessed in many different climates worldwide (154).

Natural extracts have proven to be a safe alternative for toxic chemical insecticides and for biological blocking agents whose efficiency is yet to be established (155). Several natural extracts, such as essential oils, organic and aqueous extracts from herbs and spices, have been described as having fungicidal and antimycotoxigenic activities (156–159). Their application in the food industry is being evoked through diverse methods such as edible films (160), active packaging (161), or by vapor contact (162).

Finally, recent studies have concentrated on degradation of mycotoxins following crop harvest. Many microorganisms, such as soil and water bacteria, fungi, protozoa, and specific enzymes isolated from microbial systems, degrade mycotoxins, specifically aflatoxins (163). The addition of sodium carbonate and other feed additives has demonstrated success, lowering mortality and reducing adverse effects of mycotoxin-contaminated feed in livestock (84, 164).

BIOTERRORISM

In response to concern about possible use of mycotoxins in bioterrorism, the Committee on Protection from Mycotoxins was formed by the U.S. National Research Council in 1982 (165). Following years of research, Ciegler proposed the use of mycotoxins as chemical weapons in 1986 (166). However, the choice of aflatoxin as a weapon of mass destruction is odd at best; the effects of aflatoxicosis, such as liver cancer, are too slow-acting to be effective during war.

Trichothecenes are much more suited for warfare than aflatoxins; they act immediately upon contact, and several milligrams can be lethal. Of historical note is the "yellow rain" incident of 1981 (167). The United States accused the Soviet Union of using nivalenol, DON, and T-2 toxin against Hmong tribesmen in Cambodia and Laos. However, it was later concluded that this "yellow rain" was not a weapon but the excreta of swarms of wild Asian honeybees (168).

The use of mycotoxins in bioterrorism has been assessed by several investigators in recent years (9, 169, 170). Aflatoxins and trichothecenes have been tested for combined toxicity and were found to have additive effects in most cases. The combination of these mycotoxins resulted in a synergistic effect in human bronchial epithelial cells (171). Interestingly, chlorine dioxide may be effective in the detoxification of trichothecenes, roridin A, and verrucarin A (172) in the case of widespread exposure. T-2 toxin, along with aflatoxin, received some notoriety as possible biological weapons used in the Gulf War (173). However, there is no clear data to support a role for either mycotoxin in ensuing illnesses from veterans of this war (174). Much of the data addressing mycotoxins in biological warfare remains classified and thus unresolved. In general, it is accepted that, while the presence of mycotoxin weapons may cause terror, the actual use of such weapons would not be effective or reliable in a time of war.

SICK BUILDING SYNDROME

SBS is a loosely defined term that applies to indoor environments suspected of causing a variety of health problems for occupants. The buildings usually have many issues, including water damage; improper heating, ventilation, and air conditioning systems; poor construction; and bacterial, fungal, and/or insect infestation. Symptoms may include eye, nose, and throat irritation, fatigue, headache, lack of concentration, frequent respiratory tract infections, shortness of breath, dizziness, and nausea (175). Mycotoxins are just one of many factors considered possible contributors to SBS. Several mycotoxin-producing fungi have been implicated, including *Alternaria*, *Aspergillus*, *Cladosporium*, *Chaetomium*, and *Penicillium* spp. One of the most widely investigated species is *S. chartarum*. For comprehensive reviews, see references 13 and 176.

For some decades, many reviews of SBS conclude that there is no evidence that molds inside buildings present a threat to life for healthy members of the general population in typical exposures (13, 175). A further argument against mycotoxins as the cause of SBS symptoms is that most mycotoxins are not volatile, and, therefore, widespread exposure is unlikely. Moreover, the conditions conducive for mold growth are not necessarily optimal for mycotoxin production, and fungi differ in their abilities to produce mycotoxins.

However, during the past 5 years, more studies have been conducted to evaluate the association between SBS symptoms and relevant toxins from indoor airborne fungi. The new findings contradict earlier reports and suggest a significant contribution of airborne mycotoxins to signs of illness and discomfort in healthy people (177, 178). Furthermore, newer studies using more sensitive detection technologies indicate that, in contrast to what was previously thought, many mycotoxins are volatile and at substantial concentrations (179). Thus, the contribution of mycotoxins to SBS still remains a somewhat open question.

CONCLUSIONS

There are several classes of mycotoxins, produced by a wide range of fungal species, which have been linked to various environmental issues such as SBS, veterinary problems, bioterrorism, and food safety. Over the past decade, there have been many developments in the processes for identifying mycotoxin contamination and advances in methods to control its production. Much research is yet needed to reduce the threat of mycotoxin-producing fungal species to the health of human, livestock, and plant populations and its resultant effects on the international economy.

REFERENCES

1. **Rohlfs M, Churchill AC.** 2011. Fungal secondary metabolites as modulators of interactions with insects and other arthropods. *Fungal Genet Biol* **48:**23–34.
2. **Combès A, Ndoye I, Bance C, Bruzaud J, Djediat C, Dupont J, Nay B, Prado S.** 2012. Chemical communication between the endophytic fungus *Paraconiothyrium variabile* and the phytopathogen *Fusarium oxysporum*. *PLoS One* **7:**e47313.
3. **Schroeckh V, Scherlach K, Nützmann HW, Shelest E, Schmidt-Heck W, Schuemann J, Martin K, Hertweck C, Brakhage AA.** 2009. Intimate bacterial-fungal interaction triggers biosynthesis of archetypal polyketides in *Aspergillus nidulans*. *Proc Natl Acad Sci USA* **106:**14558–14563.
4. **Nützmann HW, Reyes-Dominguez Y, Scherlach K, Schroeckh V, Horn F, Gacek A, Schümann J, Hertweck C, Strauss J, Brakhage AA.** 2011. Bacteria-induced natural product formation in the fungus *Aspergillus nidulans* requires Saga/Ada-mediated histone acetylation. *Proc Natl Acad Sci USA* **108:**14282–14287.
5. **Netzker T, Fischer J, Weber J, Mattern DJ, König CC, Valiante V, Schroeckh V, Brakhage AA.** 2015. Microbial communication leading to the activation of silent fungal secondary metabolite gene clusters. *Front Microbiol* **6:**299.
6. **Sugui JA, Pardo J, Chang YC, Zarember KA, Nardone G, Galvez EM, Müllbacher A, Gallin JI, Simon MM, Kwon-Chung KJ.** 2007. Gliotoxin is a virulence factor of *Aspergillus fumigatus*: gliP deletion attenuates virulence in mice immunosuppressed with hydrocortisone. *Eukaryot Cell* **6:**1562–1569.
7. **Kazan K, Gardiner DM, Manners JM.** 2012. On the trail of a cereal killer: recent advances in *Fusarium graminearum* pathogenomics and host resistance. *Mol Plant Pathol* **13:**399–413.
8. **De Bruyne L, Van Poucke C, Di Mavungu DJ, Zainudin NAIM, Vanhaecke L, De Vleesschauwer D, Turgeon BG, De Saeger S, Höfte M.** 2016. Comparative chemical screening and genetic analysis reveal tentoxin as a new virulence factor in *Cochliobolus miyabeanus*, the causal agent of brown spot disease on rice. *Mol Plant Pathol* **17:**805–817.
9. **Bennett JW, Klich M.** 2003. Mycotoxins. *Clin Microbiol Rev* **16:**497–516.
10. **Medeiros FH, Martins SJ, Zucchi TD, Melo IS, Batista LR, Machado JD.** 2012. Biological control of mycotoxin-producing molds. *Cienc Agrotec* **36:**483–497.
11. **Cano PM, Jamin EL, Tadrist S, Bourdaud'hui P, Péan M, Debrauwer L, Oswald IP, Delaforge M, Puel O.** 2013. New untargeted metabolic profiling combining mass spectrometry and isotopic labeling: application on *Aspergillus fumigatus* grown on wheat. *Anal Chem* **85:**8412–8420.
12. **Kildgaard S, Mansson M, Dosen I, Klitgaard A, Frisvad JC, Larsen TO, Nielsen KF.** 2014. Accurate dereplication of bioactive secondary metabolites from marine-derived fungi by UHPLC-DAD-QTOFMS and a MS/HRMS library. *Mar Drugs* **12:**3681–3705.
13. **Kuhn DM, Ghannoum MA.** 2003. Indoor mold, toxigenic fungi, and *Stachybotrys chartarum*: infectious disease perspective. *Clin Microbiol Rev* **16:**144–172.
14. **Pitt JI.** 2000. Toxigenic fungi: which are important? *Med Mycol* 38(Suppl 1)**:**17–22.
15. **Khlangwiset P, Wu F.** 2010. Costs and efficacy of public health interventions to reduce aflatoxin-induced human disease. *Food Addit Contam Part A Chem Anal Control Expo Risk Assess* **27:**998–1014.
16. **Wu F, Munkvold GP.** 2008. Mycotoxins in ethanol co-products: modeling economic impacts on the livestock industry and management strategies. *J Agric Food Chem* **56:**3900–3911.
17. **Woloshuk CP, Shim WB.** 2013. Aflatoxins, fumonisins, and trichothecenes: a convergence of knowledge. *FEMS Microbiol Rev* **37:**94–109.

18. **Ismaiel AA, Papenbrock J.** 2015. Mycotoxins: producing fungi and mechanisms of phytotoxicity. *Agriculture* **5:** 492–537.
19. **Adeyeye SAO.** 2016. Fungal mycotoxins in foods: a review. *Cogent Food Agric* **2:**1213127.
20. **Keller NP, Turner G, Bennett JW.** 2005. Fungal secondary metabolism—from biochemistry to genomics. *Nat Rev Microbiol* **3:**937–947.
21. **Clevenger KD, Bok JW, Ye R, Miley GP, Verdan MH, Velk T, Chen C, Yang K, Robey MT, Gao P, Lamprecht M, Thomas PM, Islam MN, Palmer JM, Wu CC, Keller NP, Kelleher NL.** 2017. A scalable platform to identify fungal secondary metabolites and their gene clusters. *Nat Chem Biol* **13:**895–901.
22. **Trail F, Mahanti N, Rarick M, Mehigh R, Liang SH, Zhou R, Linz JE.** 1995. Physical and transcriptional map of an aflatoxin gene cluster in *Aspergillus parasiticus* and functional disruption of a gene involved early in the aflatoxin pathway. *Appl Environ Microbiol* **61:**2665–2673.
23. **Yu J, Chang PK, Cary JW, Wright M, Bhatnagar D, Cleveland TE, Payne GA, Linz JE.** 1995. Comparative mapping of aflatoxin pathway gene clusters in *Aspergillus parasiticus* and *Aspergillus flavus*. *Appl Environ Microbiol* **61:**2365–2371.
24. **Brown DW, Yu JH, Kelkar HS, Fernandes M, Nesbitt TC, Keller NP, Adams TH, Leonard TJ.** 1996. Twenty-five coregulated transcripts define a sterigmatocystin gene cluster in *Aspergillus nidulans*. *Proc Natl Acad Sci USA* **93:**1418–1422.
25. **Yin W, Keller NP.** 2011. Transcriptional regulatory elements in fungal secondary metabolism. *J Microbiol* **49:**329–339.
26. **Palmer JM, Keller NP.** 2010. Secondary metabolism in fungi: does chromosomal location matter? *Curr Opin Microbiol* **13:**431–436.
27. **Brakhage AA.** 2013. Regulation of fungal secondary metabolism. *Nat Rev Microbiol* **11:**21–32.
28. **Wogan GN.** 1966. Chemical nature and biological effects of the aflatoxins. *Bacteriol Rev* **30:**460–470.
29. **Squire RA.** 1981. Ranking animal carcinogens: a proposed regulatory approach. *Science* **214:**877–880.
30. **Yu J.** 2012. Current understanding on aflatoxin biosynthesis and future perspective in reducing aflatoxin contamination. *Toxins (Basel)* **4:**1024–1057.
31. **Detroy RW, Lillehoj EB, Ciegler A.** 1971. Aflatoxin and related compounds, p. 3–178. *In* Ciegler A, Kadis S, Ajl SJ (ed), *Microbial Toxins*, vol VI, *Fungal Toxins*. Academic Press, New York, NY.
32. **Diener UL, Cole RJ, Sanders TH, Payne GA, Lee LS, Klich MA.** 1987. Epidemiology of aflatoxin formation by *Aspergillus flavus*. *Annu Rev Phytopathol* **25:**249–270.
33. **Klich MA.** 1987. Relation of plant water potential at flowering to subsequent cottonseed infection by *Aspergillus flavus*. *Phytopathology* **77:**739–741.
34. **Wilson DM, Payne GA.** 1994. Factors affecting *Aspergillus flavus* group infection and aflatoxin contamination of crops, p 309–325. *In* Eaton DL, Groopman JD (ed), *The Toxicology of Aflatoxins: Human Health, Veterinary and Agricultural Significance*. Academic Press, San Diego, CA.
35. **Groopman JD, Kensler TW, Wild CP.** 2008. Protective interventions to prevent aflatoxin-induced carcinogenesis in developing countries. *Annu Rev Public Health* **29:**187–203.
36. **Rodrigues I, Naehrer K.** 2012. A three-year survey on the worldwide occurrence of mycotoxins in feedstuffs and feed. *Toxins (Basel)* **4:**663–675.
37. **Gnonlonfin GJ, Hell K, Adjovi Y, Fandohan P, Koudande DO, Mensah GA, Sanni A, Brimer L.** 2013. A review on aflatoxin contamination and its implications in the developing world: a sub-Saharan African perspective. *Crit Rev Food Sci Nutr* **53:**349–365.
38. **Smith JE, Moss MO.** 1985. *Mycotoxins: Formation, Analyses and Significance*. John Wiley and Sons, Chichester, United Kingdom.
39. **Van Egmond HP.** 1989. Aflatoxin M1: occurrence, toxicity, regulation, p 11–55. *In* Van Egmond HP (ed), *Mycotoxins in Dairy Products*. Elsevier Applied Science, London, United Kingdom.
40. **Blount WP.** 1961. Turkey "X" disease. *Turkeys* **9:**52, 55–58, 61, 77.
41. **Asplin FD, Carnaghan RBA.** 1961. The toxicity of certain groundnut meals for poultry with special reference to their effect on ducklings and chickens. *Vet Rec* **73:**1215–1219.
42. **Harding JDJ, Done JT, Lewis G, Allcroft R.** 1963. Experimental groundnut poisoning in pigs. *Res Vet Sci* **4:**217–229.
43. **Loosemore RM, Markson LM.** 1961. Poisoning of cattle by Brazilian groundnut meal. *Vet Rec* **73:**813–814.
44. **Centers for Disease Control and Prevention (CDC).** 2004. Outbreak of aflatoxin poisoning—eastern and central provinces, Kenya, January–July 2004. *MMWR Morb Mortal Wkly Rep* **53:**790–793.
45. **Daniel JH, Lewis LW, Redwood YA, Kieszak S, Breiman RF, Flanders WD, Bell C, Mwihia J, Ogana G, Likimani S, Straetemans M, McGeehin MA.** 2011. Comprehensive assessment of maize aflatoxin levels in Eastern Kenya, 2005–2007. *Environ Health Perspect* **119:**1794–1799.
46. **Leung MC, Díaz-Llano G, Smith TK.** 2006. Mycotoxins in pet food: a review on worldwide prevalence and preventative strategies. *J Agric Food Chem* **54:**9623–9635.
47. **Elzupir AO, Alamer AS, Dutton MF.** 2015. The occurrence of aflatoxin in rice worldwide: a review. *Toxin Rev* **34:**37–42.
48. **Jalili M, Scotter M.** 2015. A review of aflatoxin M1 in liquid milk. *Iran J Health Saf Environ* **2:**283–295.
49. **Hove M, Van Poucke C, Njumbe-Ediage E, Nyanga LK, De Saeger S.** 2016. Review on the natural co-occurrence of AFB1 and FB1 in maize and the combined toxicity of AFB1 and FB1. *Food Control* **59:**675–682.
50. **Udomkun P, Wiredu AN, Nagle M, Müller J, Vanlauwe B, Bandyopadhyay R.** 2017. Innovative technologies to manage aflatoxins in foods and feeds and the profitability of application—a review. *Food Control* **76:**127–138.
51. **Lejeune P.** 1957. [Use of a new antibiotic, citrinin, in treatment of tropical ulcer]. *Ann Soc Belg Med Trop 1920* **37:**139–146.
52. **Chu FS.** 1991. Current immunochemical methods for mycotoxin analysis, p 140–157. *In* Vanderlaan M, Stanker LH, Watkins BE, Roberts DW (ed), *Immunoassays for Trace Chemical Analysis: Monitoring Toxic Chemicals in Humans, Food, and the Environment*. American Chemical Society, Washington, DC.
53. **Saito M, Enomoto M, Tatsuno T.** 1971. Yellowed rice toxins: luteroskyrin and related compounds, chlorine-containing compounds and citrinin, p 299–380. *In* Ciegler A, Kadis S, Ajl SJ (ed), *Microbial Toxins*, vol VI, *Fungal Toxins*. Academic Press, New York, NY.
54. **Nguyen MT, Tozlovanu M, Tran TL, Pfohl-Leszkowicz A.** 2007. Occurrence of aflatoxin B1, citrinin and ochratoxin A in rice in five provinces of the central region of Vietnam. *Food Chem* **105:**42–47.
55. **Martins ML, Gimeno A, Martins HM, Bernardo F.** 2002. Co-occurrence of patulin and citrinin in Portuguese apples with rotten spots. *Food Addit Contam* **19:**568–574.
56. **Carlton WW, Tuite J.** 1977. Metabolites of *P. viridicatum* toxicology, p 525–555. *In* Rodricks JV, Hesseltine CW, Mehlman MA (ed), *Mycotoxins in Human and Animal Health*. Pathotox Publications, Inc, Park Forest South, IL.
57. **Hashimoto K, Morita Y.** 1957. Inhibitory effect of citrinin (C13H1405) on the dehydrogenase system of rat's kidney, liver and brain tissue, specially concerning the mechanism of polyuria observed in the poisoned animal. *Jpn J Pharmacol* **7:**48–54.
58. **Chan WH, Shiao NH.** 2007. Effect of citrinin on mouse embryonic development *in vitro* and *in vivo*. *Reprod Toxicol* **24:**120–125.
59. **Chan WH.** 2008. Effects of citrinin on maturation of mouse oocytes, fertilization, and fetal development *in vitro* and *in vivo*. *Toxicol Lett* **180:**28–32.
60. **Wu Y, Zhang N, Li YH, Zhao L, Yang M, Jin Y, Xu YN, Guo H.** 2017. Citrinin exposure affects oocyte maturation and embryo development by inducing oxidative stress-mediated apoptosis. *Oncotarget* **8:**34525–34533.
61. **Holzapfel CW.** 1968. The isolation and structure of cyclopiazonic acid, a toxic metabolite of *Penicillium cyclopium* Westling. *Tetrahedron* **24:**2101–2119.

62. **Chang PK, Ehrlich KC, Fujii I.** 2009. Cyclopiazonic acid biosynthesis of *Aspergillus flavus* and *Aspergillus oryzae*. *Toxins (Basel)* **1:**74–99.
63. **Purchase IF.** 1971. The acute toxicity of the mycotoxin cyclopiazonic acid to rats. *Toxicol Appl Pharmacol* **18:**114–123.
64. **Dorner JW, Cole RJ, Lomax LG, Gosser HS, Diener UL.** 1983. Cyclopiazonic acid production by *Aspergillus flavus* and its effects on broiler chickens. *Appl Environ Microbiol* **46:**698–703.
65. **Nuehring LP, Rowland GN, Harrison LR, Cole RJ, Dorner JW.** 1985. Cyclopiazonic acid mycotoxicosis in the dog. *Am J Vet Res* **46:**1670–1676.
66. **Lomax LG, Cole RJ, Dorner JW.** 1984. The toxicity of cyclopiazonic acid in weaned pigs. *Vet Pathol* **21:**418–424.
67. **Chalivendra SC, DeRobertis C, Chang PK, Damann KE.** 2017. Cyclopiazonic acid is a pathogenicity factor for *Aspergillus flavus* and a promising target for screening germplasm for ear rot resistance. *Mol Plant Microbe Interact* **30:**361–373.
68. **Martins ML, Martins HM.** 1999. Natural and in vitro coproduction of cyclopiazonic acid and aflatoxins. *J Food Prot* **62:**292–294.
69. **Bradburn N, Coker RD, Blunden G.** 1994. The aetiology of turkey 'X' disease. *Phytochemistry* **35:**817.
70. **Shinohara Y, Tokuoka M, Koyama Y.** 2011. Functional analysis of the cyclopiazonic acid biosynthesis gene cluster in *Aspergillus oryzae* RIB 40. *Biosci Biotechnol Biochem* **75:**2249–2252.
71. **Lee YH, Tominaga M, Hayashi R, Sakamoto K, Yamada O, Akita O.** 2006. *Aspergillus oryzae* strains with a large deletion of the aflatoxin biosynthetic homologous gene cluster differentiated by chromosomal breakage. *Appl Microbiol Biotechnol* **72:**339–345.
72. **Kato N, Tokuoka M, Shinohara Y, Kawatani M, Uramoto M, Seshime Y, Fujii I, Kitamoto K, Takahashi T, Takahashi S, Koyama Y, Osada H.** 2011. Genetic safeguard against mycotoxin cyclopiazonic acid production in *Aspergillus oryzae*. *ChemBioChem* **12:**1376–1382.
73. **Schwinger RH, Brixius K, Bavendiek U, Hoischen S, Müller-Ehmsen J, Bölck B, Erdmann E.** 1997. Effect of cyclopiazonic acid on the force-frequency relationship in human nonfailing myocardium. *J Pharmacol Exp Ther* **283:**286–292.
74. **Antony M, Shukla Y, Janardhanan KK.** 2003. Potential risk of acute hepatotoxicity of kodo poisoning due to exposure to cyclopiazonic acid. *J Ethnopharmacol* **87:**211–214.
75. **Bennett JW, Bentley R.** 1999. Pride and prejudice: the story of ergot. *Perspect Biol Med* **42:**333–355.
76. **Floss HG.** 1976. [Recent advances in the chemistry and biosynthesis of ergot alkaloids]. *Cesk Farm* **25:**409–419.
77. **Floss HG.** 2006. From ergot to ansamycins-45 years in biosynthesis. *J Nat Prod* **69:**158–169.
78. **Reissig JE, Rybarczyk AM.** 2005. Pharmacologic treatment of opioid-induced sedation in chronic pain. *Ann Pharmacother* **39:**727–731.
79. **Winter JC, Kieres AK, Zimmerman MD, Reissig CJ, Eckler JR, Ullrich T, Rice KC, Rabin RA, Richards JB.** 2005. The stimulus properties of LSD in C57BL/6 mice. *Pharmacol Biochem Behav* **81:**830–837.
80. **Panaccione DG, Coyle CM.** 2005. Abundant respirable ergot alkaloids from the common airborne fungus *Aspergillus fumigatus*. *Appl Environ Microbiol* **71:**3106–3111.
81. **Lorenz K, Hoseney RC.** 1979. Ergot on cereal grains. *CRC Crit Rev Food Sci Nutr* **11:**311–354.
82. **Marasas WFO, Kellerman TS, Pienaar JG, Naudé TW.** 1976. Leukoencephalomalacia: a mycotoxicosis of *Equidae* caused by *Fusarium moniliforme* Sheldon. *Onderstepoort J Vet Res* **43:**113–122.
83. **Marasas WFO, Kriek NPJ, Fincham JE, van Rensburg SJ.** 1984. Primary liver cancer and oesophageal basal cell hyperplasia in rats caused by Fusarium moniliforme. *Int J Cancer* **34:**383–387.
84. **Rheeder JP, Marasas WFO, Vismer HF.** 2002. Production of fumonisin analogs by *Fusarium* species. *Appl Environ Microbiol* **68:**2101–2105.
85. **Desjardins AE, Plattner RD, Nelsen TC, Leslie JF.** 1995. Genetic analysis of fumonisin production and virulence of *Gibberella fujikuroi* mating population A (*Fusarium moniliforme*) on maize (*Zea mays*) seedlings. *Appl Environ Microbiol* **61:**79–86.
86. **Frisvad JC, Larsen TO, Thrane U, Meijer M, Varga J, Samson RA, Nielsen KF.** 2011. Fumonisin and ochratoxin production in industrial *Aspergillus niger* strains. *PLoS One* **6:**e23496.
87. **Harrison LR, Colvin BM, Greene JT, Newman LE, Cole JR Jr.** 1990. Pulmonary edema and hydrothorax in swine produced by fumonisin B1, a toxic metabolite of *Fusarium moniliforme*. *J Vet Diagn Invest* **2:**217–221.
88. **Pierron A, Alassane-Kpembi I, Oswald IP.** 2016. Impact of two mycotoxins deoxynivalenol and fumonisin on pig intestinal health. *Porcine Health Manag* **2:**21.
89. **Nelson PE, Desjardins AE, Plattner RD.** 1993. Fumonisins, mycotoxins produced by fusarium species: biology, chemistry, and significance. *Annu Rev Phytopathol* **31:**233–252.
90. **Sun G, Wang S, Hu X, Su J, Huang T, Yu J, Tang L, Gao W, Wang JS.** 2007. Fumonisin B1 contamination of home-grown corn in high-risk areas for esophageal and liver cancer in China. *Food Addit Contam* **24:**181–185.
91. **Xu L, Cai Q, Tang L, Wang S, Hu X, Su J, Sun G, Wang JS.** 2010. Evaluation of fumonisin biomarkers in a cross-sectional study with two high-risk populations in China. *Food Addit Contam Part A Chem Anal Control Expo Risk Assess* **27:**1161–1169.
92. **Sun G, Wang S, Hu X, Su J, Zhang Y, Xie Y, Zhang H, Tang L, Wang JS.** 2011. Co-contamination of aflatoxin B1 and fumonisin B1 in food and human dietary exposure in three areas of China. *Food Addit Contam Part A Chem Anal Control Expo Risk Assess* **28:**461–470.
93. **Wang X, Wu Q, Wan D, Liu Q, Chen D, Liu Z, Martínez-Larrañaga MR, Martínez MA, Anadón A, Yuan Z.** 2016. Fumonisins: oxidative stress-mediated toxicity and metabolism in vivo and in vitro. *Arch Toxicol* **90:**81–101.
94. **Kuiper-Goodman T.** 1990. Uncertainties in the risk assessment of three mycotoxins: aflatoxin, ochratoxin, and zearalenone. *Can J Physiol Pharmacol* **68:**1017–1024.
95. **Van Egmond HP, Speijers GJA.** 1994. Survey of data on the incidence and levels of ochratoxin A in food and animal feed worldwide. *Nat Toxins* **3:**125–144.
96. **Zepnik H, Pähler A, Schauer U, Dekant W.** 2001. Ochratoxin A-induced tumor formation: is there a role of reactive ochratoxin A metabolites? *Toxicol Sci* **59:**59–67.
97. **Wongworapat K, Ho MHT, Soontornjanagit M, Kawamura O.** 2016. Occurrence of ochratoxin A and ochratoxin B in commercial coffee in Vietnam and Thailand. *JSM Mycotoxins* **66:**1–6.
98. **Marquardt RR, Frohlich AA.** 1992. A review of recent advances in understanding ochratoxicosis. *J Anim Sci* **70:**3968–3988.
99. **Krogh P.** 1987. Ochratoxins in food, p 97–121. *In* Krogh P (ed), *Mycotoxins in Food*. Academic Press, London, United Kingdom.
100. **Dachery B, Manfroi V, Berleze KJ, Welke JE.** 2016. Occurrence of ochratoxin A in grapes, juices and wines and risk assessment related to this mycotoxin exposure. *Cienc Rural* **46:**176–183.
101. **Sava V, Reunova O, Velasquez A, Sanchez-Ramos J.** 2006. Can low level exposure to ochratoxin-A cause parkinsonism? *J Neurol Sci* **249:**68–75.
102. **Norstadt FA, McCalla TM.** 1969. Patulin production by *Penicillium urticae* Bainier in batch culture. *Appl Microbiol* **17:**193–196.
103. **Reddy CS, Chan PK, Hayes AW, Williams WL, Ciegler A.** 1979. Acute toxicity of patulin and its interaction with penicillic acid in dogs. *Food Cosmet Toxicol* **17:**605–609.
104. **Hayes AW, Phillips TD, Williams WL, Ciegler A.** 1979. Acute toxicity of patulin in mice and rats. *Toxicology* **13:**91–100.
105. **Tapia MO, Giordano AF, Soraci AL, Gonzalez CA, Denzoin LA, Ortega IO, Olson W, Murphy MJ.** 2006. Toxic effects of patulin on sheep. *J Anim Vet Adv* **5:**271–276.

106. **Mahfoud R, Maresca M, Garmy N, Fantini J.** 2002. The mycotoxin patulin alters the barrier function of the intestinal epithelium: mechanism of action of the toxin and protective effects of glutathione. *Toxicol Appl Pharmacol* **181:**209–218.
107. **Schumacher DM, Metzler M, Lehmann L.** 2005. Mutagenicity of the mycotoxin patulin in cultured Chinese hamster V79 cells, and its modulation by intracellular glutathione. *Arch Toxicol* **79:**110–121.
108. **de Melo FT, de Oliveira IM, Greggio S, Dacosta JC, Guecheva TN, Saffi J, Henriques JAP, Rosa RM.** 2012. DNA damage in organs of mice treated acutely with patulin, a known mycotoxin. *Food Chem Toxicol* **50:**3548–3555.
109. **Trucksess MW, Tang Y.** 2001. Solid phase extraction method for patulin in apple juice and unfiltered apple juice, p 205–213. *In* Trucksess MW, Pohland AF (ed), *Mycotoxin Protocols*. Humana Press, Totowa, NJ.
110. **Moss MO, Long MT.** 2002. Fate of patulin in the presence of the yeast *Saccharomyces cerevisiae*. *Food Addit Contam* **19:**387–399.
111. **van Egmond HP, Schothorst RC, Jonker MA.** 2007. Regulations relating to mycotoxins in food: perspectives in a global and European context. *Anal Bioanal Chem* **389:** 147–157.
112. **Barad S, Horowitz SB, Kobiler I, Sherman A, Prusky D.** 2014. Accumulation of the mycotoxin patulin in the presence of gluconic acid contributes to pathogenicity of *Penicillium expansum*. *Mol Plant Microbe Interact* **27:**66–77.
113. **Snini SP, Tannous J, Heuillard P, Bailly S, Lippi Y, Zehraoui E, Barreau C, Oswald IP, Puel O.** 2016. Patulin is a cultivar-dependent aggressiveness factor favouring the colonization of apples by *Penicillium expansum*. *Mol Plant Pathol* **17:**920–930.
114. **Puel O, Galtier P, Oswald IP.** 2010. Biosynthesis and toxicological effects of patulin. *Toxins (Basel)* **2:**613–631.
115. **Tannous J, Keller NP, Atoui A, El Khoury A, Lteif R, Oswald IP, Puel O.** 2017. Secondary metabolism in *Penicillium expansum*: emphasis on recent advances in patulin research. *Crit Rev Food Sci Nut* **2017 Mar 31:**1–17.
116. **Rotter BA, Prelusky DB, Pestka JJ.** 1996. Toxicology of deoxynivalenol (vomitoxin). *J Toxicol Environ Health* **48:**1–34.
117. **Takayama H, Shimada N, Mikami O, Murata H.** 2005. Suppressive effect of deoxynivalenol, a *Fusarium* mycotoxin, on bovine and porcine neutrophil chemiluminescence: an *in vitro* study. *J Vet Med Sci* **67:**531–533.
118. **Hinkley SF, Mazzola EP, Fettinger JC, Lam YF, Jarvis BB.** 2000. Atranones A–G, from the toxigenic mold *Stachybotrys chartarum*. *Phytochemistry* **55:**663–673.
119. **Jarvis BB, Sorenson WG, Hintikka EL, Nikulin M, Zhou Y, Jiang J, Wang S, Hinkley S, Etzel RA, Dearborn D.** 1998. Study of toxin production by isolates of *Stachybotrys chartarum* and *Memnoniella echinata* isolated during a study of pulmonary hemosiderosis in infants. *Appl Environ Microbiol* **64:**3620–3625.
120. **Forgacs J.**1972. Stachybotryotoxicosis, p 95–128. *In* Kadis S, Ciegler A, Ajl SJ (ed), *Microbial Toxins*, vol VI, *Fungal Toxins*. Academic Press, New York, NY.
121. **Pinton P, Oswald IP.** 2014. Effect of deoxynivalenol and other Type B trichothecenes on the intestine: a review. *Toxins (Basel)* **6:**1615–1643.
122. **El-Nezami H, Polychronaki N, Salminen S, Mykkänen H.** 2002. Binding rather than metabolism may explain the interaction of two food-grade *Lactobacillus* strains with zearalenone and its derivative (')alpha-earalenol. *Appl Environ Microbiol* **68:**3545–3549.
123. **Mirocha CJ, Pathre SV, Christensen CM.** 1977. Zearalenone, p 345–364. *In* Rodricks JV, Hesseltine CW, Mehlman MA (ed), *Mycotoxins in Human and Animal Health*. Pathotox Publishers Inc, Park Forest South, IL.
124. **Mirocha CJ, Schauerhamer B, Pathre SV.** 1974. Isolation, detection, and quantitation of zearalenone in maize and barley. *J Assoc Off Anal Chem* **57:**1104–1110.
125. **Hueza IM, Raspantini PCF, Raspantini LER, Latorre AO, Górniak SL.** 2014. Zearalenone, an estrogenic mycotoxin, is an immunotoxic compound. *Toxins (Basel)* **6:**1080–1095.
126. **Dacasto M, Rolando P, Nachtmann C, Ceppa L, Nebbia C.** 1995. Zearalenone mycotoxicosis in piglets suckling sows fed contaminated grain. *Vet Hum Toxicol* **37:**359–361.
127. **Venkataramana M, Chandra Nayaka S, Anand T, Rajesh R, Aiyaz M, Divakara ST, Murali HS, Prakash HS, Lakshmana Rao PV.** 2014. Zearalenone induced toxicity in SHSY-5Y cells: the role of oxidative stress evidenced by N-acetyl cysteine. *Food Chem Toxicol* **65:**335–342.
128. **Qin X, Cao M, Lai F, Yang F, Ge W, Zhang X, Cheng S, Sun X, Qin G, Shen W, Li L.** 2015. Oxidative stress induced by zearalenone in porcine granulosa cells and its rescue by curcumin in vitro. *PLoS One* **10:**e0127551.
129. **Sang Y, Li W, Zhang G.** 2016. The protective effect of resveratrol against cytotoxicity induced by mycotoxin, zearalenone. *Food Funct* **7:**3703–3715.
130. **Kuiper-Goodman T.** 1998. Food safety: mycotoxins and phycotoxins in perspective, p 25–48. *In* Miraglia M, van Edmond H, Brera C, Gilbert J (ed), *Mycotoxins and Phycotoxins—Developments in Chemistry, Toxicology and Food Safety*. Alaken Inc, Fort Collins, CO.
131. **Dohlman E.** 2003. Mycotoxin hazards and regulations, p 97–108. *In* Buzby J (ed), *International Trade and Food Safety: Economic Theory and Case Studies, Agricultural Economic Report 828*. USDA.
132. **European Commission.** 2006. Commission Regulation (EC) No. 401/2006 of 23 February 2006 laying down the methods of sampling and analysis for the official control of the levels of mycotoxins in foodstuffs. *Off J Eur Union* **70:**12–34.
133. **Food and Agriculture Organization (FAO).** 2004. Worldwide regulations for mycotoxins 2003: a compendium. *Food and Nutrition Paper 81*. FAO of the United Nations, Rome, Italy.
134. **Leslie JF, Bandyopadhyay R, Visconti A (ed).** 2008. *Mycotoxins: Detection Methods, Management, Public Health and Agricultural Trade*. CABI Publishing, Wallingford, UK.
135. **Turner NW, Bramhmbhatt H, Szabo-Vezse M, Poma A, Coker R, Piletsky SA.** 2015. Analytical methods for determination of mycotoxins: an update (2009–2014). *Anal Chim Acta* **901:**12–33.
136. **Cigić IK, Prosen H.** 2009. An overview of conventional and emerging analytical methods for the determination of mycotoxins. *Int J Mol Sci* **10:**62–115.
137. **Zöllner P, Mayer-Helm B.** 2006. Trace mycotoxin analysis in complex biological and food matrices by liquid chromatography-atmospheric pressure ionisation mass spectrometry. *J Chromatogr A* **1136:**123–169.
138. **Campàs M, Garibo D, Prieto-Simón B.** 2012. Novel nanobiotechnological concepts in electrochemical biosensors for the analysis of toxins. *Analyst (Lond)* **137:**1055–1067.
139. **Pohanka M, Malir F, Roubal T, Kuca K.** 2008. Detection of aflatoxins in capsicum spice using an electrochemical immunosensor. *Anal Lett* **41:**2344–2353.
140. **Alonso-Lomillo MA, Domínguez-Renedo O, Román LT, Arcos-Martínez MJ.** 2011. Horseradish peroxidase-screen printed biosensors for determination of Ochratoxin A. *Anal Chim Acta* **688:**49–53.
141. **Duca RC, Badea IA, David IG, Delaforge M, Vladescu L.** 2010. Redox behavior of zearalenone in various solvents. *Anal Lett* **43:**1287–1300.
142. **Chauhan R, Singh J, Sachdev T, Basu T, Malhotra BD.** 2016. Recent advances in mycotoxins detection. *Biosens Bioelectron* **81:**532–545.
143. **Anfossi L, Giovannoli C, Baggiani C.** 2016. Mycotoxin detection. *Curr Opin Biotechnol* **37:**120–126.
144. **Reverté L, Prieto-Simón B, Campàs M.** 2016. New advances in electrochemical biosensors for the detection of toxins: nanomaterials, magnetic beads and microfluidics systems. A review. *Anal Chim Acta* **908:**8–21.
145. **Mannon J, Johnson E.** 1985. Fungi down on the farm. *New Sci* **105:**12–16.
146. **Streit E, Naehrer K, Rodrigues I, Schatzmayr G.** 2013. Mycotoxin occurrence in feed and feed raw materials worldwide: long-term analysis with special focus on Europe and Asia. *J Sci Food Agric* **93:**2892–2899.

147. **Mirocha CJ, Christensen CM, Nelson GH.** 1971. F-2 (zearalenone) estrogenic mycotoxin from *Fusarium*, p 107–138. *In* Kadis S, Ciegler A, Ajl SJ (ed), *Microbial Toxins*, vol VII, *Algal and Fungal Toxins*. Academic Press, New York, NY.
148. **Kos J, Hajnal EJ, Šarić B, Jovanov P, Nedeljković N, Milovanović I, Krulj J.** 2017. The influence of climate conditions on the occurrence of deoxynivalenol in maize harvested in Serbia during 2013–2015. *Food Control* **73:** 734–740.
149. **Medina A, Akbar A, Baazeem A, Rodriguez A, Magan N.** 2017. Climate change, food security and mycotoxins: do we know enough? *Fungal Biol Rev* **31:**143–154.
150. **Cary JW, Rajasekaran K, Brown RL, Luo M, Chen ZY, Bhatnagar D.** 2011. Developing resistance to aflatoxin in maize and cottonseed. *Toxins (Basel)* **3:**678–696.
151. **Wu F.** 2006. Mycotoxin reduction in Bt corn: potential economic, health, and regulatory impacts. *Transgenic Res* **15:**277–289.
152. **Cozzi G, Haidukowski M, Perrone G, Visconti A, Logrieco A.** 2009. Influence of *Lobesia botrana* field control on black aspergilli rot and ochratoxin A contamination in grapes. *J Food Prot* **72:**894–897.
153. **Dorner JW.** 2009. Biological control of aflatoxin contamination in corn using a nontoxigenic strain of *Aspergillus flavus*. *J Food Prot* **72:**801–804.
154. **Degola F, Berni E, Restivo FM.** 2011. Laboratory tests for assessing efficacy of atoxigenic *Aspergillus flavus* strains as biocontrol agents. *Int J Food Microbiol* **146:**235–243.
155. **Ehrlich KC.** 2014. Non-aflatoxigenic *Aspergillus flavus* to prevent aflatoxin contamination in crops: advantages and limitations. *Front Microbiol* **5:**50.
156. **Kohiyama CY, Yamamoto Ribeiro MM, Mossini SAG, Bando E, Bomfim NS, Nerilo SB, Rocha GHO, Grespan R, Mikcha JMG, Machinski M Jr.** 2015. Antifungal properties and inhibitory effects upon aflatoxin production of *Thymus vulgaris L.* by *Aspergillus flavus* Link. *Food Chem* **173:**1006–1010.
157. **Kumar A, Shukla R, Singh P, Dubey NK.** 2010. Chemical composition, antifungal and antiaflatoxigenic activities of *Ocimum sanctum L.* essential oil and its safety assessment as plant based antimicrobial. *Food Chem Toxicol* **48:**539–543.
158. **Prakash B, Kedia A, Mishra PK, Dubey NK.** 2015. Plant essential oils as food preservatives to control moulds, mycotoxin contamination and oxidative deterioration of agri-food commodities: potentials and challenges. *Food Control* **47:**381–391.
159. **Kedia A, Dwivedy AK, Jha DK, Dubey NK.** 2016. Efficacy of *Mentha spicata* essential oil in suppression of *Aspergillus flavus* and aflatoxin contamination in chickpea with particular emphasis to mode of antifungal action. *Protoplasma* **253:**647–653.
160. **Mehyar GF, El Assi NM, Alsmairat NG, Holley RA.** 2014. Effect of edible coatings on fruit maturity and fungal growth on Berhi dates. *Int J Food Sci Technol* **49:**2409–2417.
161. **Manso S, Pezo D, Gómez-Lus R, Nerín C.** 2014. Diminution of aflatoxin B1 production caused by an active packaging containing cinnamon essential oil. *Food Control* **45:**101–108.
162. **Avila-Sosa R, Palou E, Jiménez Munguía MT, Nevárez-Moorillón GV, Navarro Cruz AR, López-Malo A.** 2012. Antifungal activity by vapor contact of essential oils added to amaranth, chitosan, or starch edible films. *Int J Food Microbiol* **153:**66–72.
163. **Wu Q, Jezkova A, Yuan Z, Pavlikova L, Dohnal V, Kuca K.** 2009. Biological degradation of aflatoxins. *Drug Metab Rev* **41:**1–7.
164. **Diaz GJ, Cortés A, Botero L.** 2009. Evaluation of the ability of a feed additive to ameliorate the adverse effects of aflatoxins in turkey poults. *Br Poult Sci* **50:**240–250.
165. **Desjardins AE.** 2009. From yellow rain to green wheat: 25 years of trichothecene biosynthesis research. *J Agric Food Chem* **57:**4478–4484.
166. **Ciegler A.** 1986. Mycotoxins: a new class of chemical weapons. *NBC Def Technol Int.* **1:**52–57.
167. **Rosen RT, Rosen JD.** 1982. Presence of four *Fusarium* mycotoxins and synthetic material in 'yellow rain': evidence for the use of chemical weapons in Laos. *Biomed Mass Spectrom* **9:**443–450.
168. **Nowicke JW, Meselson M.** 1984. Yellow rain—a palynological analysis. *Nature* **309:**205–206.
169. **Henghold WB II.** 2004. Other biologic toxin bioweapons: ricin, staphylococcal enterotoxin B, and trichothecene mycotoxins. *Dermatol Clin* **22:**257–262, v.
170. **Stark AA.** 2005. Threat assessment of mycotoxins as weapons: molecular mechanisms of acute toxicity. *J Food Prot* **68:**1285–1293.
171. **McKean C, Tang L, Billam M, Tang M, Theodorakis CW, Kendall RJ, Wang JS.** 2006. Comparative acute and combinative toxicity of aflatoxin B1 and T-2 toxin in animals and immortalized human cell lines. *J Appl Toxicol* **26:**139–147.
172. **Wilson SC, Brasel TL, Martin JM, Wu C, Andriychuk L, Douglas DR, Cobos L, Straus DC.** 2005. Efficacy of chlorine dioxide as a gas and in solution in the inactivation of two trichothecene mycotoxins. *Int J Toxicol* **24:**181–186.
173. **Zilinskas RA.** 1997. Iraq's biological weapons: the past as future? *JAMA* **278:**418–424.
174. **Ferguson E, Cassaday HJ.** 2002. Theoretical accounts of Gulf War Syndrome: from environmental toxins to psychoneuroimmunology and neurodegeneration. *Behav Neurol* **13:**133–147.
175. **Anonymous.** 2002. Adverse human health effects associated with molds in the indoor environment. American College of Occupational and Environmental Medicine, Arlington Heights, IL. http://www.acoem.org/guidelines/pdf/Mold-10-27-02.pdf.
176. **Straus DC.** 2011. The possible role of fungal contamination in sick building syndrome. *Front Biosci (Elite Ed)* **3:**562–580.
177. **Norbäck D, Markowicz P, Cai GH, Hashim Z, Ali F, Zheng YW, Lai XX, Spangfort MD, Larsson L, Hashim JH.** 2014. Endotoxin, ergosterol, fungal DNA and allergens in dust from schools in Johor Bahru, Malaysia: associations with asthma and respiratory infections in pupils. *PLoS One* **9:**e88303.
178. **Norbäck D, Hashim JH, Cai GH, Hashim Z, Ali F, Bloom E, Larsson L.** 2016. Rhinitis, ocular, throat and dermal symptoms, headache and tiredness among students in schools from Johor Bahru, Malaysia: associations with fungal DNA and mycotoxins in classroom dust. *PLoS One* **11:**e0147996.
179. **Aleksic B, Draghi M, Ritoux S, Bailly S, Lacroix M, Oswald IP, Bailly JD, Robine E.** 2017. Aerosolization of mycotoxins after growth of toxinogenic fungi on wallpaper. *Appl Environ Microbiol* **83:**AEM.01001-17.
180. **Dorner JW.** 2002. Recent advances in analytical methodology for cyclopiazonic acid. *Adv Exp Med Biol* **504:**107–116.
181. **Council for Agricultural Science and Technology.** 2003. Mycotoxins: risks in plant, animal, and human systems. Task Force Report. Council for Agricultural Science and Technology, Ames, Iowa.
182. **Ehrlich KC, Yu J, Cotty PJ.** 2005. Aflatoxin biosynthesis gene clusters and flanking regions. *J Appl Microbiol* **99:**518–527.
183. **Amaike S, Keller NP.** 2011. *Aspergillus flavus*. *Annu Rev Phytopathol* **49:**107–133.
184. **Wang C, Yang H, Chen M, Wang Y, Li F, Luo C, Zhao S, He D.** 2012. Real-time quantitative analysis of the influence of blue light on citrinin biosynthetic gene cluster expression in *Monascus*. *Biotechnol Lett* **34:**1745–1748.
185. **Lorenz N, Haarmann T, Pazoutová S, Jung M, Tudzynski P.** 2009. The ergot alkaloid gene cluster: functional analyses and evolutionary aspects. *Phytochemistry* **70:**1822–1832.
186. **Haarmann T, Machado C, Lübbe Y, Correia T, Schardl CL, Panaccione DG, Tudzynski P.** 2005. The ergot alkaloid gene cluster in *Claviceps purpurea*: extension of the cluster sequence and intra species evolution. *Phytochemistry* **66:**1312–1320.
187. **Proctor RH, Brown DW, Plattner RD, Desjardins AE.** 2003. Co-expression of 15 contiguous genes delineates a fumonisin biosynthetic gene cluster in *Gibberella moniliformis*. *Fungal Genet Biol* **38:**237–249.

188. **Brown DW, Butchko RAE, Busman M, Proctor RH.** 2007. The *Fusarium verticillioides* FUM gene cluster encodes a Zn(II)2Cys6 protein that affects FUM gene expression and fumonisin production. *Eukaryot Cell* **6:**1210–1218.
189. **Karolewiez A, Geisen R.** 2005. Cloning a part of the ochratoxin A biosynthetic gene cluster of *Penicillium nordicum* and characterization of the ochratoxin polyketide synthase gene. *Syst Appl Microbiol* **28:**588–595.
190. **Tannous J, El Khoury R, Snini SP, Lippi Y, El Khoury A, Atoui A, Lteif R, Oswald IP, Puel O.** 2014. Sequencing, physical organization and kinetic expression of the patulin biosynthetic gene cluster from *Penicillium expansum*. *Int J Food Microbiol* **189:**51–60.
191. **Kimura M, Tokai T, Takahashi-Ando N, Ohsato S, Fujimura M.** 2007. Molecular and genetic studies of *fusarium* trichothecene biosynthesis: pathways, genes, and evolution. *Biosci Biotechnol Biochem* **71:**2105–2123.
192. **Lysøe E, Bone KR, Klemsdal SS.** 2009. Real-time quantitative expression studies of the zearalenone biosynthetic gene cluster in *Fusarium graminearum*. *Phytopathology* **99:**176–184.

Lacazia, Lagenidium, Pythium, and *Rhinosporidium*

RAQUEL VILELA AND LEONEL MENDOZA

130

In the past 100 years, the microbial pathogens described in this chapter have been classified as fungal and/or parafungal protistan microbes (1–4). Based on their apparent epidemiological connection with water, they were at one point also placed in a new category of hydrophilic infectious agents (1). However, based on taxonomic and other morphological characteristics, these four anomalous species, *Lacazia, Lagenidium, Pythium,* and *Rhinosporidium,* were not well understood (1, 4). This frustrating situation fueled a strong controversy that has only recently been solved with the advent of molecular methodologies (5, 6). Despite the recent finding that both *Pithium insidiosum* and *Rhinosporidium seeberi* are protistan pathogens, they are still studied by medical mycologists, continuing a historical tradition. The finding of two members of the Oomycota affecting mammalian hosts, *Lagenidium* and *Paralagenidium,* alerted the medical community to the presence of a novel group of pathogens phenotypically similar to the fungi and indistinguishable from the clinical and pathological features displayed by *P. insidiosum* during infection. In addition, Vilela et al. (7) recently reported that the organism developing yeast-like cells in dolphin skin granulomas, long believed to be *Lacazia loboi,* was identified as a new *Paracoccidioides brasiliensis* variety. Based on ribosomal DNA phylogenetic analysis, the evolutionary location of the microbial pathogens discussed in this chapter is illustrated in Fig. 1. Table 1 summarizes the most prominent features of the pathogens covered in this section.

LACAZIA LOBOI

Taxonomy

Jorge de Oliveira Lobo first described lacaziosis (lobomycosis) in a patient from the state of Pernambuco, Brazil (8). He stated that the new pathogen was phenotypically similar to the parasitic stages of the genera *Blastomyces* and *Paracoccidioides.* The earliest attempts to isolate this pathogen in culture met with failure, and soon it became clear that this pathogen cannot be cultured (4, 9). This fact led to great controversy regarding its epidemiological and taxonomic affinities, reflected by the numerous names under which this pathogen has been known. In 1999, Taborda et al. (10) suggested the binomial *Lacazia loboi* to end more than 70 years of taxonomic ambiguity. Because the epithet "lobomycosis" was derived from the obsolete genus *Lobomyces* (4), Vilela et al. (11) suggested the name "lacaziosis" as a more suitable term. Their suggestion was based on the proposal by Taborda et al. (10) and the placement of *L. loboi* as a separate taxon from the genus *Paracoccidioides* (11–13). Initial phylogenetic studies placed *L. loboi* as the sister taxon to *P. brasiliensis* (5, 12), but besides the long branches described in phylogenetic analysis between these pathogens, there were not sufficient DNA sequences to support this claim. Vilela et al. (14), using at least five different loci and 20 *L. loboi* human strains, presented a strong argument for the phylogenetic placement of this pathogen as an independent taxon. Currently, human *L. loboi* is classified within the Ascomycota in the order Onygenales, family Ajellomycetaceae.

The first case of lacaziosis-like disease in dolphins was reported in 1971 (15). Based on clinical, histopathological, and serological analyses and the uncultivated nature of the pathogen, it was long believed to be the same as *L. loboi* in humans (4, 7). However, recent molecular analyses in different dolphins and geographical locations (16–18) clustered the DNA sequences of the yeast-like cells in dolphins with DNA sequences of cultivated *P. brasiliensis* isolates causing systemic infection in humans. A recent phylogenetic study using DNA sequences of six dolphins in the United States with granulomas and yeast-like cells confirmed previous reports (7). This study revealed that the interrogated dolphin DNA sequences, including those used in early analyses, clustered among the cultivated human *P. brasiliensis* isolates. Interestingly, the inclusion of these DNA sequences lowers the bootstrap support of human *L. loboi* DNA sequences as an independent species from the genus *Paracoccidioides.* Vilela et al. (7) argued that, as was previously suspected (4), perhaps the genus *Lacazia* is actually another *Paracoccidioides* species. Using phylogenetic analysis, the separation of the dolphin DNA from the cultivated *P. brasiliensis* was not possible; thus, Vilela and Mendoza (19) recently proposed the variety *P. brasiliensis* var. *ceti* and the disease name paracoccidioidomycosis ceti (7) to differentiate the uncultivated dolphin DNA sequences from the human cultivated *P. brasiliensis* strains (Table 1). The analysis of more DNA sequences and perhaps the complete genomes of both pathogens of humans and dolphins would reveal more insights into the evolutionary paths of these two neglected uncultivated fungal pathogens.

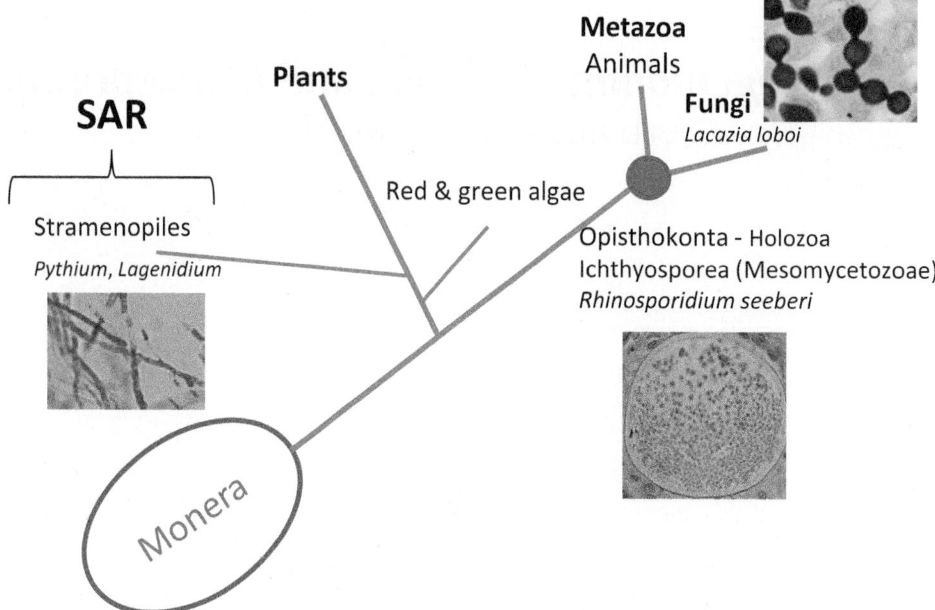

FIGURE 1 Phylogenetic location of the four groups of microbial pathogens studied in this chapter (based on small-subunit ribosomal DNA sequences). Forming a sister group, the Algae (Archaeplastida) and Stramenopiles (SAR) are placed basal to the plants (28). The latter includes the mammalian pathogenic Oomycota *Pythium* spp. and *Lagenidium* spp. They develop hypha-like elements, vesicles with biflagellate zoospores, and oogonia. *R. seeberi* is placed within the Opisthokonta, at the point where the Metazoa (animals) and Fungi diverged (red circle) (28). This uncultivated protist is characterized by the development of spherical phenotypes with endoconidia. *L. loboi* is an anomalous, uncultivated, ascomycetous fungus developing yeast-like cells in chains.

TABLE 1 Taxonomic, epidemiological, clinical, and mycological features of the neglected microbes *Lacazia loboi*, *Lagenidium*, *Paralagenidium*, *Paracoccidioides brasiliensis* var. *ceti*, *Pythium insidiosum*, and *Rhinosporidium seeberi*

Pathogen (host)	Taxonomy and phylogeny	Epidemiology	Clinical feature(s)	*In vivo* form	*In vitro* form
Lacazia loboi (humans only)	Ascomycete fungus located with the dimorphic Onygenales	Restricted to humans in South America. Hydrophilic	Parakeloidal skin lesions in head, arms, chest, low limbs	Lemon-shaped, yeast-like cells in chains, connected small tubes	Uncultivated
Paracoccidioides brasiliensis var. *ceti* (dolphins only)	Ascomycete fungus in the Onygenales, phylogenetically different from *L. loboi*	Restricted to dolphins in many oceans	Parakeloidal skin lesions on dolphins	Lemon-shaped, yeast-like cells in chains, connected small tubes	Uncultivated
Lagenidium and *Paralagenidium* species (humans and animals)	SAR supergroup. Stramenopiles, known as the water molds	Tropical, subtropical and temperate areas. Acquired in aquatic or terrestrial environments by trauma. Hydrophilic	Keratitis and ulcerate skin lesions; dissemination to large vessels and lungs has been mentioned.	Sparsely septate hyphae, ~8 to 20 μm; Splendore-Hoeppli phenomenon; prominent eosinophilia	Submerged colonies; sparsely septate hyphae, ~10 to 25 μm; some spherical structures; large biflagellate zoospores in water; sucrose negative
Pythium insidiosum (humans and animals)	SAR supergroup. Stramenopiles, known as the water molds	Tropical, subtropical and temperate areas. Acquired in aquatic or terrestrial environments by trauma. Hydrophilic	Keratitis, cutaneous, intestinal, and vascular; dissemination to other organs including lungs	Sparsely septate hyphae, ~4 to 10 μm; Hoeppli-Splendore phenomenon; prominent eosinophilia	Submerged colonies; sparsely septate hyphae, ~5 to 12 μm without fruiting bodies; biflagellate zoospores in water; sucrose positive
Rhinosporidium seeberi (humans and animals)	Opisthokonta, Ichthyosporea (Mesomycetozoea). Located at the Metazoa-Fungi divergence	All continents except Australia. Endemic in India and Sri Lanka. Acquired by trauma. Hydrophilic	Polypoidal mucosal and skin lesions; common in mouth, nares, and eyes	Spherical sporangia, with or without endospores, at different stages of development	Uncultivated

Description of the Agent

Because human *L. loboi* cannot be cultured, our knowledge of this pathogen is based on the morphological features observed in its parasitic stage. Its *in vivo* phenotype is characterized by the development of unicellular, thick-walled, lemon-shaped yeast-like cells that can be found forming chains of one, two, or more cells with occasional branching and characteristically connected by short tubules (Fig. 2). The yeast-like cells of *L. loboi* measure ~5 to 12 μm in diameter and can be easily observed with most stains. Interestingly, *L. loboi*'s *in vivo* phenotype is very similar to the parasitic stage of *P. brasiliensis*, a finding consistent with current phylogenetic analysis (7). The morphological features of *L. loboi* and the cross-reaction observed in serological tests of patient sera with lacaziosis and the antigens of *P. brasiliensis* led Lacaz et al. (4) to classify this pathogen in the genus *Paracoccidioides*. Electron-microscopic analysis of *L. loboi* showed thick chitinous yeast-like cell walls and an amorphous cytoplasmic content. Approximately 60% of the yeast-like cells observed lacked a defined cytoplasmic region, a finding in agreement with the result of viability studies.

Epidemiology and Transmission

Lacaziosis in humans (Jorge Lobo's disease) is known to occur only in patients inhabiting the tropical areas of the Americas (8). Although the majority of human patients with lacaziosis have been from Brazil, cases from Mexico, Central America, Colombia, Suriname, Venezuela, and other nearby countries have also been reported (4). Two European human patients apparently acquired the infection after contact with an infected bottle-nosed dolphin in an aquarium. In addition, American and Canadian patients were reported with the infection after visiting or working in the areas of endemicity (20, 21). Interestingly, an apparent lacaziosis case in a Greek woman with no history of traveling to the Americas was recently reported (22). The diagnosis was based on histological morphology. However, the yeast-like cells depicted in this particular patient lacked some of the morphological features observed in Fig. 2B and C. Moreover, no molecular testing was conducted to further authenticate the case.

It is believed that the infection is acquired through small traumatic skin lesions after contact with the pathogen near aquatic ecological niches. However, the real ecological niche of this pathogen is unknown. The disease seems to occur in apparently healthy hosts. It is quite possible that in nature, *L. loboi* cells could develop hyphae with propagules (perhaps conidia) similar to those in *P. brasiliensis* that may make contact with hosts through trauma, thus causing lacaziosis. Transmission of the disease from one patient to another is rare, but some cases of autoinoculation and accidental infection by physicians in contact with infected hosts have been reported (4, 23, 24). In addition, the disease can be experimentally reproduced in mice (25).

Clinical Significance

Infections caused by *L. loboi* are rarely observed in the tropical areas of endemicity in the Americas. Recent reports indicate that human cases of the disease are sporadic in the areas of endemicity and occur mainly in males. The number of cases so far reported is around 600, but its real occurrence could be higher. The disease is diagnosed in apparently healthy hosts inhabiting such areas. A genetic predisposition theory was abandoned after the finding that the number of cases in a Brazilian tribe with a high occurrence of the disease dramatically decreased when the tribe was moved to a new location. One common problem in the areas of endemicity is that patients with the disease do not seek medical attention until years after the initial infection, when the lesions have increased in size and spread to other skin areas. One explanation may be that the affected population is usually poor, with no access to health care, and that the lesions are rarely painful (4).

Frequently affected anatomical areas are the arms, ears, back, chest, face, and lower limbs. Some investigators believe that the distribution of lesions on cooler areas of skin in humans may indicate that the pathogen does not tolerate well a temperature of 37°C. Initially, a single small (0.5 to 1.0 cm in diameter), smooth, parakeloidal skin lesion develops. Some patients complain of slight pruritus at this stage. The infection is not life-threatening and evolves very slowly, sometimes over 20 or more years. Usually, when patients seek medical attention, they have

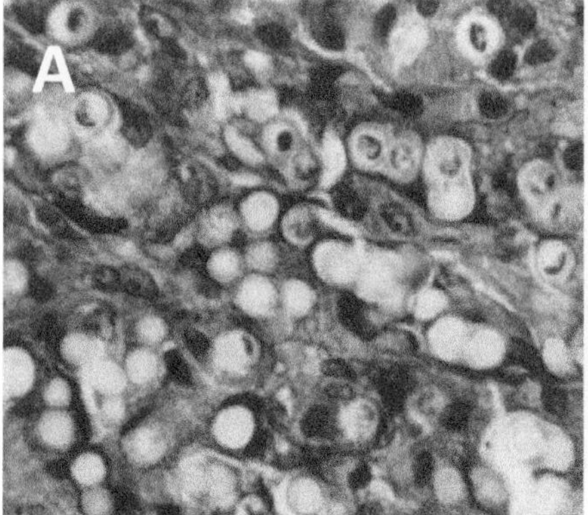

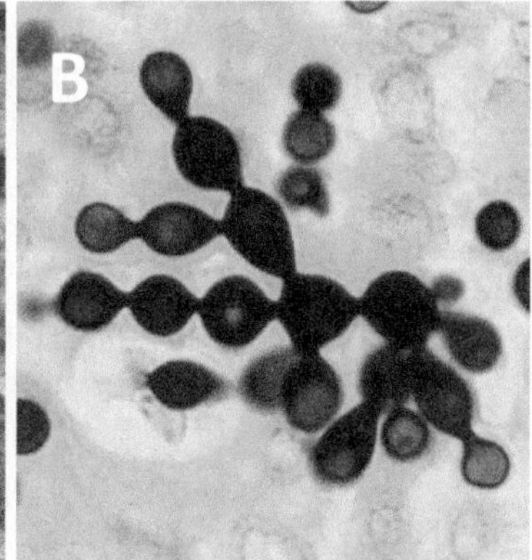

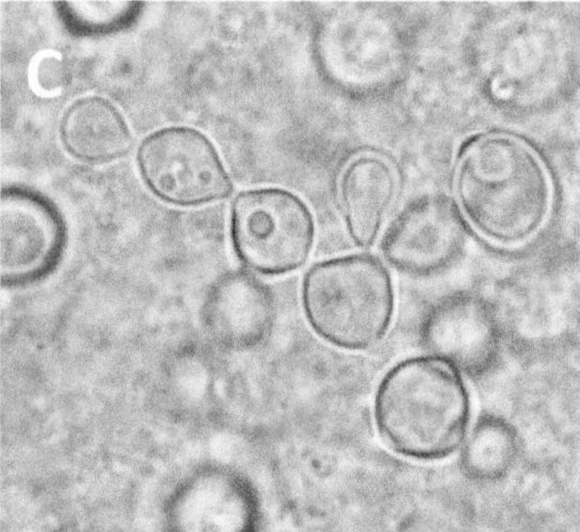

FIGURE 2 *L. loboi*. Histological sections stained with H&E (A) and silver stain (B) show the typical morphological features found in patients with cutaneous lacaziosis. (A) *L. loboi* yeast-like cells are poorly stained with H&E and are observed as empty round structures surrounded by an area of granulomatous reaction. Magnification, ×40. (B) The presence of abundant lemon-shaped yeast-like branching cells in chains connected with slender tubules is the main feature of *L. loboi* in silver-stained sections. Magnification, ×50. (C) A wet-mount preparation in 10% KOH shows numerous *L. loboi* yeast-like cells in chains, some of them containing small dancing bodies in their cytoplasm. Magnification, ×100.

already developed more than one lesion. In the chronic phase, the lesions are polymorphic. At least five clinical manifestations are recognized, including the typical parakeloidal type and the infiltrative, gummatous, ulcerated, and verrucous forms. However, Lacaz et al. (4) pointed out that two or more forms, including a macular type, could be found in a single patient. The differential diagnosis includes chromoblastomycosis, leishmaniasis, leprosy, neoplasia, paracoccidioidomycosis, and similar skin conditions.

Collection, Transport, and Storage of Specimens

The guidelines for the collection, processing, storage, and examination of specimens are provided in chapter 117. Clinical specimens collected in cases of lacaziosis are mostly biopsied tissues from the infected sites. *L. loboi* cannot be cultured; thus, clinical specimens from the infected areas are usually fixed in formaldehyde for histopathologic evaluation.

Direct Examination

Microscopy

In contrast to the systemic spread of *P. brasiliensis* infections, *L. loboi* is typically confined to cutaneous and subcutaneous tissues. The lesions are characterized by fibrosis and granulomatous reactions, with numerous histiocytes and giant cells containing numerous yeast-like cells of *L. loboi*. Areas of necrosis and the presence of other inflammatory cells have been reported. When tissue is stained with hematoxylin and eosin (H&E), the typical yeast-like cell arrangement in chains is not observed. Instead, *L. loboi* appears as oval to spherical, poorly stained cells or as round empty spaces with thick cell walls (Fig. 2A). Special fungal stains such as Gomori methenamine silver (GMS) and periodic acid-Schiff (PAS) should be used for the histopathological diagnosis of lacaziosis. With GMS, *L. loboi* yeast-like cells are dark or have the appearance of empty cells (Fig. 2B). The yeast-like cells are in chains of two or more cells and form branches, similar to the yeast cells observed in the infected tissue of patients with paracoccidioidomycosis. The cells are typically connected with small tubules, a feature also observed with other fungal stains, such as PAS (Fig. 2B and C). Similar microscopic features have been reported in paracoccidioidomycosis ceti in dolphins.

To visualize the etiologic agent of the disease in humans and dolphins using direct microscopy, biopsy specimens should be cut into pieces 2 to 5 mm in diameter. One or more pieces are then placed with 1 or 2 drops of 10 to 20% potassium hydroxide (KOH) on a glass slide with a coverslip. The slide should be heated without boiling and then held for about 15 min at room temperature before microscopic evaluation. In 10% KOH, *L. loboi* yeast-like cells appear in great quantities (Fig. 2C). Cells ~2 to 12 μm in diameter and uniform in size can be found as single yeast cells or as chains of three or more cells connected by tubules. In wet mounts, moving protoplasmic granules can also be detected within some of the yeast-like cells (Fig. 2C).

Nucleic Acid Detection

So far, there are no commercially available nucleic acid probes for the detection of this pathogen in clinical samples.

Isolation Procedures, Identification, and Typing Systems

Claims that *L. loboi* has been isolated in pure culture have not yet been validated. Most of the recovered organisms were fungal contaminants or *P. brasiliensis* (4, 9). The identification of the etiologic agent is based on the clinical features and the phenotypic characteristics on wet-mount preparations and/or histopathological analyses of the infected tissues. No typing systems for this organism exist at this time. However, in-house molecular procedures from suspected tissue, using primers previously used by others, could be of help to authenticate histopathological findings (9).

Serologic Tests

One major obstacle to developing serologic assays has been the lack of cultures. Thus, most of the serologic approaches in humans and dolphins have been carried out using parasitic forms in infected tissues as antigen or using cultures of closely related pathogens (4). These tests showed that *L. loboi* and *P. brasiliensis* var. *ceti* possess cross-reactive antigens in common with fungal pathogens such as *Blastomyces dermatitidis*, *Histoplasma capsulatum*, and cultivated *P. brasiliensis* (4). Mendoza et al. (26), using antigenic proteins derived from the yeast-like cells of *L. loboi* from experimentally infected mice, found that the antibodies in the sera of humans, dolphins, and mice with the disease detected a 193-kDa immunodominant protein. Although antibodies in these sera did react with a *P. brasiliensis* purified gp43 antigen (26), they did not detect the corresponding gp43 homologous antigen of the *L. loboi* parasitic stage. This finding suggests that the 193-kDa protein of *L. loboi* may have epitopes in common with gp43 of *P. brasiliensis*. It also implies that, although the 193-kDa antigen expressed during lacaziosis infection cross-reacts with the antibodies against gp43 of *P. brasiliensis*, it might be an entirely different antigenic protein. The role of this *L. loboi* antigenic protein in the pathogenesis of lacaziosis is under investigation. The use of *L. loboi* antigens in serological surveys to study the epidemiology of lacaziosis has been suggested (26). Although serology is not commercially available, the Biomedical Laboratory Diagnostics Program at Michigan State University has developed a Western blot assay that can be requested at https://bld.natsci.msu.edu/research/pythium-insidiosum/.

Antimicrobial Susceptibilities

Although antifungal therapy has cured some cases of lacaziosis, *L. loboi* is well known for its resistance to antimicrobial drugs, including most antifungals (4). This fact has left clinicians with only one choice: surgery. Due to the intractability of this organism to culture, susceptibility testing is not possible.

Evaluation, Interpretation, and Reporting of Results

Clinical samples from patients suspected of lacaziosis submitted to the laboratory comprise deep skin scrapings and tissue biopsies. The samples have to be processed as described above ("Direct Examination" and "Microscopy") and evaluated for the presence of uniform yeast-like cells connected by small tubules forming short chains. Because *P. brasiliensis* in the parasitic phase can also form yeast cells connected by tubules, the significant variation in size could be used to separate *L. loboi* from *P. brasiliensis*. The latter pathogen tends to develop large and small yeast cells in the infected tissues, whereas *L. loboi* yeast-like cells have a uniform size. In addition, the lack of fungal growth in culture could also be used as an aid in the diagnosis of this uncultivated pathogen. After laboratory evaluation of the clinical material, the presence of uniform yeast-like cells that yield no fungal growth in culture is used to confirm lacaziosis. This is particularly important for patients who have visited areas where the disease is endemic. The report of the results should include the finding of uniform yeast-like cells connected by tubules, the lack of fungal growth in culture, and the histopathological results of the evaluated tissue samples.

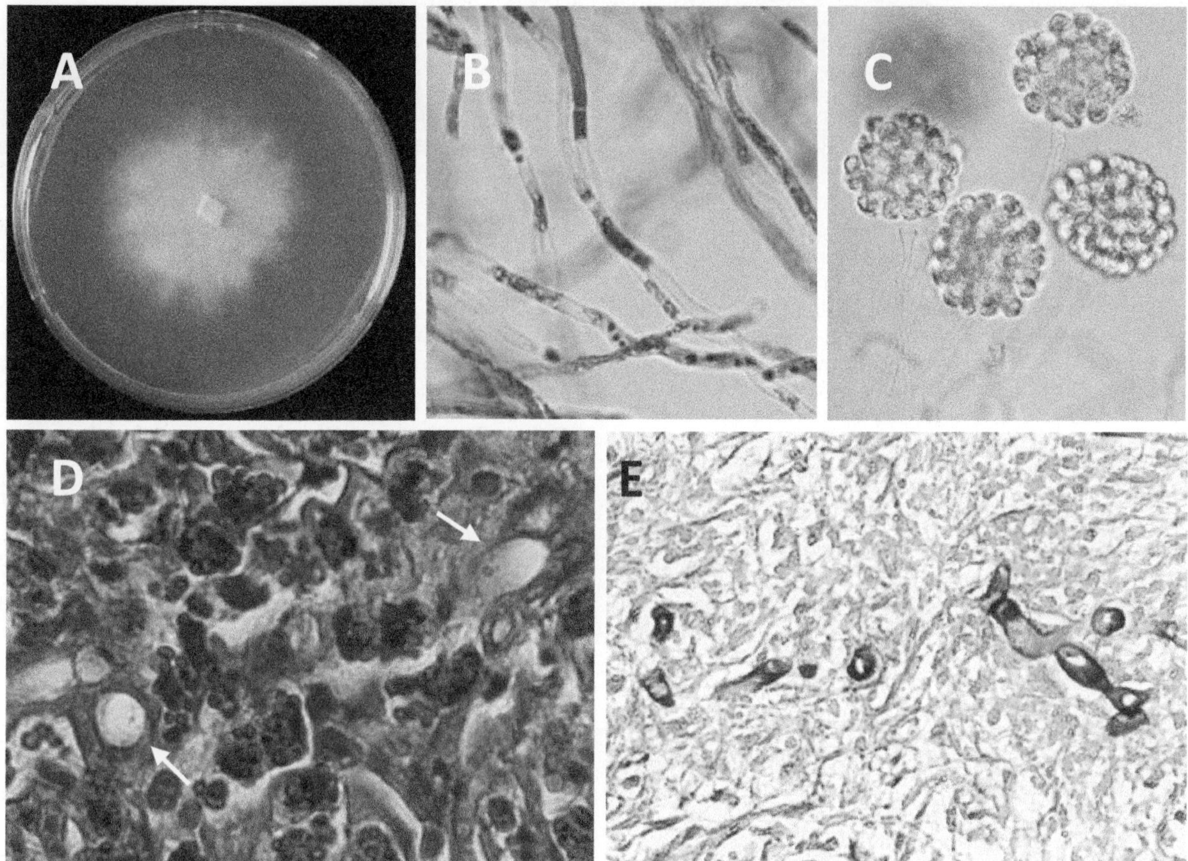

FIGURE 3 *P. insidiosum*. (A) Colony of *Pythium insidiosum* on SDA showing a submerged colony with few aerial mycelia. (B) Slender, sparsely septate hyphae without fruiting bodies from culture. Magnification, ×40. (C) Four vesicles of *P. insidiosum* containing numerous unhatched zoospores. Magnification, ×40. (D) Several eosinophils are observed around *P. insidiosum* hyphae from a case of horse subcutaneous pythiosis (arrows). Magnification, ×100. (E) Silver-stained hyphae showing the typical features of *P. insidiosum* in infected hosts. Magnification, ×50.

PYTHIUM INSIDIOSUM

Taxonomy

P. insidiosum was first reported more than 150 years ago in Indonesian equines (3), but successful isolation of this organism in pure culture was not possible until the beginning of the 20th century. Later, a similar organism was isolated again from horses, and the name *Hyphomyces destruens* was introduced. The finding that a strain from New Guinea (27) developed zoospores suggested that this pathogen was an organism in the genus *Pythium*. De Cock et al. (3) introduced the binomial *P. insidiosum*, and according to the current classification of eukaryotes, this pathogen was placed within the SAR (for "stramenopiles, alveolates, and rhizaria") supergroup (Fig. 1) (28). Phylogenetic studies (29, 30) showed that *P. insidiosum* isolates from around the world cluster according to their geographic origin. Thus, it is likely that *P. insidiosum* could be a phylogenetic complex of closely related species, or perhaps a complex of different strains belonging to a single species, *P. insidiosum* (31).

Description of the Agent

P. insidiosum can be readily isolated on most mycological media (3). This pathogen develops white submerged colonies with a characteristic radiate pattern and few or no aerial hyphae, very similar to the mammalian pathogenic *Lagenidium* spp. (Fig. 3A). The hyphae have perpendicular lateral branches measuring 4 to 10 μm in diameter and possess few cross-septa (Fig. 3B). Zoosporogenesis (development of zoospores) is possible only in water cultures containing various ions, including $Ca2^+$ (3, 32, 33). The structures in which the zoospores develop are termed vesicles (Fig. 3C).

Zoospores form by progressive cleavage and mature inside large vesicles (20 to 60 μm in diameter) (Fig. 3C). Once fully formed, the biflagellate zoospores mechanically break the sporangial wall, swim, and then encyst. It has been proposed that the zoospores may be the infectious units due to their motility. Zoospores are kidney-like in shape, and two unequal flagella arise from inside a lateral groove. Upon encystment, the zoospores lose their flagella and become spherical. Under the right conditions, the encysted zoospores develop a germ tube and form long filaments (32). *P. insidiosum* oogonia (sexual stage) have rarely been observed and are believed to represent a resistant stage in nature.

Epidemiology and Transmission

Infections caused by this hydrophilic pathogen have been recorded in tropical, subtropical, and some temperate areas of the world. In the Americas, pythiosis is common in tropical Central, North, and South America, with most cases reported in Brazil, Colombia, Costa Rica, the United States, and Venezuela (3, 32). In the United States, infections are more prevalent in animals and humans inhabiting southern states, such as Alabama, Georgia, Florida, Louisiana, Mississippi, North Carolina, South Carolina, and Texas. However, cases of the disease have also been reported in states farther north, including California, Illinois, Indiana, Kansas, New Jersey, Missouri, Tennessee, and Virginia, and as far north as Wisconsin and New York. In Asia, pythiosis has been reported in Japan, India, Indonesia, Pacific islands, South Korea, and Thailand and also in nearby areas such as Australia, New Guinea, and New Zealand. Tropical Africa is ideal for pythiosis; however, only one case, in a dog with the cutaneous form, was reported, in the northwest African country of Mali. This might suggest that the disease has been misdiagnosed in this geographic region (29).

Until recently, infections caused by *P. insidiosum* were considered exotic. The disease was believed to be restricted to animals in tropical regions with few or no occurrences in other geographical areas. Interestingly, in the last 10 years, the number of pythiosis cases has increased on all continents (3, 31). The finding that humans (32–37), dogs (38, 39), and other animals can be infected indicates that previously pythiosis was erroneously diagnosed as a fungal infection. Most cases of pythiosis occur in apparently healthy humans and animals. In Thailand, however, the disease in humans is associated with thalassemia or similar blood disorders (35).

The infection is acquired after *P. insidiosum* propagules enter the skin or the intestinal tract through traumatic lesions (32, 39). The infection is believed to be acquired from wet environments. Supabandhu et al. (40), Presser and Goss (41), and Rujirawat et al. (42) cultured and identified *P. insidiosum* from environmental samples, confirming the presence of this oomycete in wet agricultural environments in Thailand and the United States. In addition, cases of pythiosis in the absence of water suggest that *P. insidiosum* can cause infection after contact with resting spores from terrestrial environments. The transmission of *P. insidiosum* from one individual to another (human or animal or *vice versa*) has not been recorded. Only rabbits seem to be susceptible to experimental inoculation (43).

Clinical Significance

The clinical manifestations of pythiosis vary according to the infection site. Most patients with the disease state that they had a skin injury prior to the infection. The lesions caused by *P. insidiosum* in humans can be classified into superficial infections (keratitis); cutaneous and subcutaneous forms, including orbital pythiosis; and vascular forms that usually lead to systemic infection and death. Keratitis caused by *P. insidiosum* is similar to that caused by fungi and other etiologic agents (44–46). It begins with trauma to the superficial layers of the eye, followed by the development of conjunctivitis, photophobia, corneal ulcers, and hypopyon (pus in the interior chamber of the eye). Cutaneous and subcutaneous infection is characterized by the formation of granulomatous plaques and/or ulcerated swellings that remain localized. Once the pathogen has reached the subcutaneous tissues, itchy papules may develop. The orbital form of subcutaneous pythiosis is rare and has been observed mainly in children in Australia and the United States (47). Vascular pythiosis starts with a traumatic lesion, usually on the lower limbs, followed by dissemination of the pathogen to the nearby arteries (38, 47). Initially, the infected skin shows signs of dry gangrene, and the formation of painful necrotic ulcers in some patients has also been reported (34). Clinical symptoms are claudication (limping) of the affected limb, local ischemia, swelling, pain, and the absence of the dorsalis pedis pulse. As the infection progresses, an ascending arteritis, with the formation of thrombi and aneurysms of the large arteries, is the main feature. If not treated, *P. insidiosum* may spread through the arteries and reach the iliac and renal arteries and abdominal aorta, causing disseminated pythiosis. This form of pythiosis is more common in Thailand among patients with thalassemia, and it is usually life threatening (34, 36, 37). Human pythiosis should be differentiated from arteriosclerosis, diabetes mellitus, *Lagenidium* spp. cutaneous leishmaniasis, mycotic keratitis, subcutaneous tuberculosis, subcutaneous mucormycosis, and other mycoses associated with filamentous fungi.

Collection, Transport, and Storage of Specimens

The clinical specimens required for diagnosis of pythiosis vary according to the infected host and the clinical form (31, 34). The collection, transport, and storage of clinical samples from patients with infections caused by *P. insidiosum* are identical to those for samples from patients with *Lagenidium* spp. A portion of the small tissue samples used for microscopy can also be used to inoculate Sabouraud dextrose agar (SDA) plates. The pieces should be submerged into the agar and incubated at 37°C for 24 to 48 hours. *Lagenidium* spp. that are pathogenic for dogs, cats, and humans develop white-yellowish, flat, glabrous colonies (Fig. 4A), similar to those recovered in cases of pythiosis. The presence of broad, 9- to 18-µm, coenocytic hyphae displaying large spherical structures connected by short strands of hyphae is the main feature of strains recovered from dogs (Fig. 4B). A *Lagenidium* strain recovered recently in a case of human keratitis showed only broad, sparsely septate hyphae (48). Strains of *Lagenidium* displaying spherical structures connected by short strands of hyphae can be used to differentiate *P. insidiosum* from *Lagenidium* sp. (Fig. 4B); however, some mammalian pathogenic *Lagenidium* spp. develop only hyphae. Those cases have to be investigated using molecular methods (see below). So far, there is no typing system available for *Lagenidium* spp.

For patients with keratitis, scrapings of the affected eyes should be collected. Dryness of clinical specimens from keratitis patients could prevent the microscopic detection of the hyphal elements and subsequent culture of *Lagenidium* spp. Although swabs are not recommended, if collected they must be immediately transported at room temperature in tubes with high humidity (or containing small quantities of sterile distilled water) to the laboratory and should be processed upon arrival. The collected eye scrapings should be placed in small aseptic petri dishes and immediately transported at room temperature to be processed promptly upon arrival. Biopsy or necropsy samples are usually collected in sterile distilled water and transported at room temperature to the laboratory. Specimens collected from patients with cutaneous, subcutaneous, vascular, and disseminated lagenidiosis can also be placed in tubes containing sterile distilled water plus 100 U of penicillin/ml and 0.25 mg of streptomycin or 0.4 mg of chloramphenicol per ml. If these antibiotics are not available, the use of sterile distilled water is encouraged. Although some studies indicate that transportation or storage at 4°C of specimens from patients suspected of lagenidiosis did not interfere with the isolation of the pathogen in the laboratory, others report a considerable reduction in the number of positive cultures from samples stored at 4°C (31, 32). Consult chapter 117 for more information on collection.

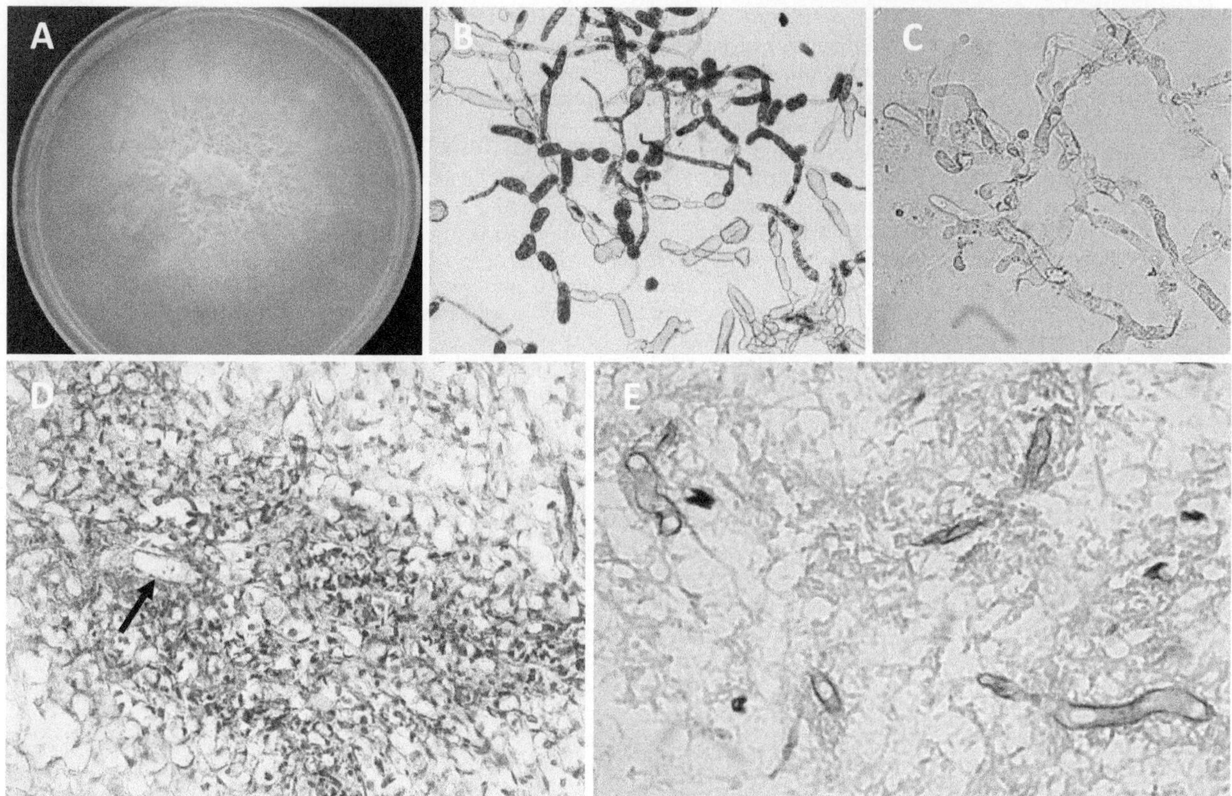

FIGURE 4 (A) Colony of *Lagenidium giganteum* recovered from a dog with cutaneous lagenidiosis on SDA. *L. giganteum* develops cream to white submerged colonies at 25 and 37°C. (B) Microscopically, ribbon-type hyphae highly constricted at septa are found in samples from SDA plates. In lactophenol blue stain, the presence of large spherical and oval structures is common in some isolates. Magnification, ×20. However, some strains may develop only hyphae. (C) A 10% KOH preparation from biopsied tissue depicting several broader hyphal elements without septa (magnification, ×40). (D) Histopathological H&E-stained tissue sample from cat infected with *L. deciduum* (*L. vilelae*). Magnification, ×40. Note the eosinophilic material (Splendore-Hoeppli phenomenon) around hyphae 12 to 18 μm in diameter (arrow). (E) Tissue sample from panel D stained with GMS showing *L. deciduum* broader ribbon-like hyphae. Magnification, ×40.

Direct Examination

Microscopy

Clinical specimens of *P. insidiosum* in 10% KOH characteristically show the presence of long (4.0 to 9.0 μm in diameter), hyaline, sparsely septate hyphal structures (Fig. 3B). Some hyphal elements may reach more than 15-μm lateral branches at a 90° angle, a typical feature of this oomycete. In histopathological preparations stained with H&E, *P. insidiosum* appears as short or long, hyaline, coenocytic (without septa) hyphae 6 to 10 μm in diameter (Fig. 3D). The fact that *in vivo* structures of *P. insidiosum* are detectable by H&E staining has been used to differentiate this oomycete from the hyphal elements developed by members of the order Enthomophthorales (genera *Basidiobolus* and *Conidiobolus*). In infected tissues, *P. insidiosum* triggers eosinophilic granulomas with giant cells, mast cells, and other inflammatory cells (Fig. 3D). The hyphal elements of *P. insidiosum* are found in the center of microabscesses with numerous eosinophils that usually degranulate over the organism's hyphae (Splendore-Hoeppli phenomenon) (Fig. 3D, arrows). The activation of an eosinophilic inflammatory response with the Splendore-Hoeppli phenomenon is a feature in common with the order Entomophthorales, from which it must be differentiated. Although most experts in the diagnosis of pythiosis agree that it is difficult to distinguish between the hyphal structures of *P. insidiosum* and those of the Entomophthorales, the poor staining capabilities in H&E, the ribbon-type morphology, and the bigger size of the zygomycetes hyphal filaments sometimes help to distinguish these fungi from *P. insidiosum*. *P. insidiosum*'s hyphal elements are well stained by GMS and appear as short or long, sparsely septate, tubular dark structures (Fig. 3E). Transversely sectioned, poorly stained (with GMS or PAS) hyphae can be also found as ring-shaped bodies.

The most important immunohistological tests for the specific identification of the hyphal elements of *P. insidiosum* in infected tissues have been the peroxidase and the immunofluorescence tests (49). Because the hyphal structures of *P. insidiosum* are difficult to differentiate from those in the fungi, especially the mucormycota and entomophthoromycota, these assays have been of paramount importance for the accurate identification of this oomycete in the absence of culture. Most of these assays are available through reference laboratories for pythiosis in the United States at Michigan State University (https://bld.natsci.msu.edu/research/pythium-insidiosum) and Pan American Veterinary Laboratories (http://www.pavlab.com/) and in other countries, such as Brazil and Thailand.

Nucleic Acid Detection

The first molecular approach for the diagnosis of *P. insidiosum* from clinical specimens was carried out on a patient with keratitis (44). The hyphal elements present in the specimen were identified by sequencing part of the 18S ribosomal DNA region using the NS1 and NS2 and internal transcriber spacer (ITS) universal primers. This approach has been successful on clinical specimens (36, 44). Grooters and Gee (50) introduced a PCR technique for the identification of *P. insidiosum* from cultures and from clinical specimens. A set of primers (PI-1 and PI-2) that amplified 105 bp of the ITS-1 region of *P. insidiosum* were tested. These primers have been used by several laboratories (36) and were entirely specific when tested against several filamentous fungi. Schurko et al. (51) introduced a dot-blot hybridization technique by constructing a 530-bp species-specific DNA probe for the detection of *P. insidiosum*. This DNA probe specifically binds to the intergenetic spacer 1 (IGS1) of this pathogen, and it did not hybridize with the genomic DNA from 23 other *Pythium* species, *Lagenidium gigantum*, or several pathogenic fungi, including the entomophthoromycete fungi *Conidiobolus coronatus* and *Basidiobolus ranarum*. This probe may be ideal for the detection of *P. insidiosum* from environmental samples and for the specific diagnosis of pythiosis from clinical specimens from susceptible hosts. Other similar in-house molecular assays targeting different DNA genes have been suggested, but they have limited availability (52).

Isolation Procedures, Identification, and Typing Systems

In contrast with the other hydrophilic pathogens covered in this chapter, *Lagenidium* spp. (see below) and *P. insidiosum* can be cultured on various media. The most common media used for the isolation of *P. insidiosum* are 2% SDA and broth with or without antibiotics (see "Collection, Transport, and Storage of Specimens"), blood agar, cornmeal agar (Difco), potato dextrose agar, and nutritive agar (Difco). Biopsy or necropsy tissues and kunkers (stony hard masses found only in horses with pythiosis) from patients suspected of having pythiosis are usually cut into small fragments 2 to 5 mm in diameter, placed into tubes containing sterile distilled water, and vigorously washed two or three times before plating. The small fragments are then physically pushed into the agar, and the plates are incubated at 25 and 37°C for 2 or more days. The relative humidity of the incubator should be enhanced by placing a beaker of water inside the chamber. Specimens that have been transported for more than 24 h can also be inoculated into tubes containing broth and then incubated at 37°C. Usually, cottony colonies surrounding the clinical specimens are detectable after 24 to 48 h of incubation (31). On solid medium, *P. insidiosum* develops only sparsely septate hyphae (Fig. 3B). The appearance of *P. insidiosum* on solid medium was previously described.

P. insidiosum can be identified definitively only if the isolate develops the characteristic oogonia (sexual stage) on culture plates. The formation of oogonia, however, is extremely rare, which further complicates the final identification of this pathogen in the clinical setting. Given that *Lagenidium* spp. and *P. insidiosum* display identical lesions in infected mammals, the development of zoospores in water as a definitive characteristic for the identification of *P. insidiosum* needs to be revisited. The identification of *P. insidiosum* using molecular methods with isolates and clinical specimens as described above is recommended (see "Nucleic Acid Detection Techniques" above). A drawback to this approach is that only a few laboratories possess these capabilities. Although the use of sugars has been evaluated to identify this pathogen in the clinical laboratory (53), there are currently no typing systems available for *P. insidiosum*.

Serologic Tests

Early serological tests showed that anti-*P. insidiosum* antibodies could be detected in the sera of infected hosts and, thus, could be used for the diagnosis of pythiosis. The most common assays for pythiosis are agglutination, enzyme-linked immunosorbent assay (ELISA), immunodiffusion, and Western blotting. Immunodiffusion has proven to be a very specific test, with several precipitin bands, but it is too insensitive and yields many false negatives, especially when performed with sera from humans and dogs with pythiosis (54). To overcome this drawback, an ELISA and a Western blot assay were later introduced (36, 38, 54–56). These assays are extremely sensitive in detecting anti-*P. insidiosum* IgG. However, it may cross-react with anti-*Lagenidium* spp. antibodies (57). Recently, an agglutination test was used for the rapid diagnosis of pythiosis. Although it proved to be a good screening test, it had a high rate of false positives and false negatives (58). The finding that antibodies in the sera of different hosts recognize different antigenic proteins when evaluated with several geographically divergent strains of *P. insidiosum* suggests frequent subclinical infections with multiple *P. insidiosum* strains (59). Recently, a rapid dry immunochromatographic test was evaluated (60). The test was able to detect anti-*P. insidiosum* antibodies in the sera of humans and animals with pythiosis, but its sensitive was lower (false negatives) than that of the traditional ELISA.

Antimicrobial Susceptibilities

P. insidiosum, like the other oomycetes (including *Lagenidium* spp.), does not possess ergosterol in its cytoplasmic membrane. Despite this obvious contraindication, amphotericin B and other antifungal drugs that target ergosterol have been used with mixed results. For instance, two children with orbital pythiosis were successfully treated with amphotericin B in Australia (47). However, this antifungal did not have an effect in humans from Thailand with the disease (35, 37). Recently, susceptibility testing on a strain isolated from a child in Tennessee with orbital pythiosis showed the strain to have low MICs of terbinafine and itraconazole (61). Although this combination of drugs was successfully used in this case, the same combination was less effective when tested in other humans and animals. One explanation for this contradiction is the possibility that these antifungal drugs may affect pathways other than sterols. The inconsistent results with most antifungal drugs for the treatment of pythiosis have led to the use of unconventional treatments such as immunotherapy (37). Immunotherapy has been found to be effective in 55% of humans and dogs and in 70% of equines with the disease (58). In addition, some investigators have evaluated *in vitro* combinations of several antifungals against *P. insidiosum*, with promising results (49, 62–64). These studies indicate that terbinafine plus fluconazole or ketoconazole (63) or terbinafine plus amphotericin B (64) substantially reduces the *in vitro* growth of *P. insidiosum*. However, these combinations of antifungal drugs have yet to be tested in clinical cases.

Evaluation, Interpretation, and Reporting of Results

Culture is the gold standard test for pythiosis. Because *P. insidiosum* morphological features in infected tissues are identical to those displayed by the fungal entomophthoromycetes *Conidiobolus* and *Basidiobolus*, wet mounts, histopathological examination of tissue sections, serological assays, and culture have to be evaluated as a whole for a proper interpretation and identification of this pathogen in the laboratory. For instance, the finding of sparsely septate hyaline hyphae in a wet-mount preparation must be confirmed by culture. Moreover, serological assays such as ELISA and Western blotting could detect anti-*P. insidiosum* antibodies in hosts with putative clinical diagnosis of pythiosis, but they should be interpreted with caution. *P. insidiosum* can cause subclinical infections in humans and animals inhabiting areas of endemicity. Thus, false positives have been found in apparently healthy individuals (58). When culture is not possible, the use of molecular approaches and/or immunohistochemical (peroxidase and immunofluorescence) tests could be of help. The presence of hyaline hyphae in wet-mount preparations and in histopathology should be reported as suggestive of pythiosis, whereas positive results in culture (development of zoospores in water cultures) or positive reactions in molecular assays and/or in immunohistochemical staining tests are reported as confirmatory tests of disease. In such cases the report of results should include the following: "Pythiosis caused by *P. insidiosum* confirmed by culture and supported by serological and/or molecular assays."

LAGENIDIUM AND *PARALAGENIDIUM SPECIES*

Taxonomy

Until recently, *P. insidiosum* was considered the only member of the Oomycota causing disease in mammalian hosts (3, 31). However, in 1999, several cases of novel *Lagenidium* mammalian-pathogenic species causing skin infection with dissemination to blood vessels were reported (57). The genus *Lagenidium* comprises oomycetous species affecting lower animals, such as crabs, mosquito larvae, nematodes, and others (57, 65, 66). Because members of the oomycetes develop hypha-like elements, they were known for a long time as the "aquatic fungi" (water molds). However, they are not true fungi. Currently, *Lagenidium* spp. are placed within the SAR supergroup (Fig. 1) (28). Although Dick (67), using phenotypic characteristics, recently questioned the validity of this genus, current phylogenetic studies have found that an *L. giganteum* isolate infecting dogs clustered with *L. giganteum* from mosquito larvae (68). This finding suggests that the classification of *Lagenidium* species based on morphology alone is problematic. At least three species were recently reported: *L. giganteum*, affecting dogs in the United States; *L. deciduum* (*L. vilelae*), affecting a cat in the United States; and *L. albertoi*, causing keratitis in a Thai man (69, 70). In addition, based on phylogenetic analysis, the genus *Paralagenidium* was also suggested for some strains recovered from dogs with lagenidiosis (70).

Description of the Agent

Lagenidium species can be readily isolated in media used to recover fungi in the clinical laboratory (57, 66). This is in contrast with some of the other pathogens covered in this chapter. On SDA, *Lagenidium* species develop well at 37°C and more slowly at 25°C. At 37°C, they develop white-yellow submerged colonies without aerial mycelia in less than 24 hours (Fig. 4A). Based on cases studied at Michigan State University, *Lagenidium* spp. developed 8- to 15-μm ribbon-type hyphae and spherical structures 20 to 45 μm in diameter (68, 69) (Fig. 4B). In liquid media, undifferentiated hyphae can develop vesicles at the tips of these structures. The vesicle increases in size as more protoplasmic material enters the vesicle, and zoospores are formed within the following 20 minutes. The species *Paralagenidium karlingii*, infecting dogs, thermotolerant *L. giganteum* isolates from dogs (different from thermosensitive *L. giganteum* from mosquitoes), *L. deciduum*, isolated from a cat, and *L. albertoi*, isolated from a Thai human patient, have been reported so far as pathogens of mammals (68–70). The presence of sexual structures in culture (oogonia) has not yet been reported.

Epidemiology and Transmission

So far, most cases of lagenidiosis in mammalian hosts have been reported in the United States (65, 66). A case of keratitis caused by a *Lagenidium* sp. in a Thai human patient was recently reported (48). In addition, an Australian dog case of lagenidiosis was also studied by us (unpublished data). In the United States, lagenidiosis occurs in the same areas reporting *P. insidiosum* infection (see below) (62, 65, 66). This includes the states bordering the Gulf of Mexico, as well as Arkansas, Georgia, Illinois, Indiana, Maryland, North Carolina, South Carolina, Tennessee, and Virginia, among others. *Lagenidium* completes its life cycle in wet environments, possibly using lower animal hosts or plants. Mammals with open skin injuries entering contaminated environments can be exposed to the zoospores developed by these species and could develop lagenidiosis. Transmission from one infected host to another has not been observed. Experimental infection in mice has been unsuccessful (58).

Clinical Significance

The organisms *Paralagenidium*, *Lagenidium*, and *P. insidiosum* have been recognized as emerging Oomycota pathogens causing invasive superficial, cutaneous, subcutaneous, and arterial infections (31). These pathogens have also been observed to cause systemic infection. The common sites of infection in humans and animals are the cornea, gastrointestinal tract, limbs, and other anatomical areas (48, 66). Mammal-pathogenic *Lagenidium* species have been reported in only three geographical areas (see above), but other tropical and subtropical regions may contain these pathogenic species as well.

Collection, Transport, and Storage of Specimens

See the corresponding text in the section on *P. insidiosum*.

Direct Examination

Microscopy

Small pieces of biopsy tissue cut into 5-mm blocks, scrapings of lesions in wet mounts, and cytological samples stained with Giemsa reveal the hyphal structures of *Paralagenidium* and *Lagenidium* spp. in infected tissues. In wet mounts, broad 9- to 18-μm, branched, sparsely septate hyphae (broader than those in *P. insidiosum*) are observed in cases of lagenidiosis (Fig. 4C). Differentiation in histopathological sections between *Paralagenidium*, *Lagenidium*, and *P. insidiosum* hyphae is difficult. Both trigger an eosinophilic granuloma (Fig. 4D and E), and although *Paralagenidium* and *Lagenidium* hyphae are broader than *P. insidiosum* hyphae, a definitive diagnosis can be made only by culture (Fig. 4A) (see the text above for *P. insidiosum*) or by the use of molecular tools. Hyphal elements from coenocytic fungi (Mucormycota and Entomophthoromycota) are readily observed in H&E staining; however, the Oomycota are more difficult to detect with this stain (31, 34). The use of

GMS stain is recommended in cases of lagenidiosis or paralagenidiosis (Fig. 4D). In culture, the microscopic features of some *Lagenidium* spp. causing lagenidiosis in dogs include oval and spherical structures, a morphological feature that could be used to separate these mammal-pathogenic oomycetes in the laboratory (Fig. 4B). However, there are some other *Lagenidium* strains that are pathogenic for mammals but lack these features, and thus, morphology alone would not provide an unequivocal distinction between these two organisms.

Isolation Procedures, Identification, and Typing Systems

Vilela et al. (53) found that pathogenic *Lagenidium* and *Paralagenidium* species, including the fungal pathogens *Basidiobolus*, *Conidiobolus*, and *Mucor*, did not utilize sucrose in culture, whereas *P. insidiosum* was sucrose positive on a medium containing sucrose. These authors propose the use of this simple test to putatively separate fungal and fungus-like pathogens in the clinical laboratory (53).

Serologic and DNA Tests

ELISA and Western blot assays have been tested in cases of lagenidiosis in both humans and lower animals (57). Although both assays detected the presence of antibodies in cases of lagenidiosis, the antigenic banding patterns observed in Western blots were very difficult to interpret, and ELISA had a strong cross-reaction with *P. insidiosum* antigens. Despite this limitation, the ELISA has been suggested to monitor the response to treatment because a decline in anti-*Lagenidium* antibodies has been demonstrated in cured cases (57). Specific primers for the identification of isolates and *Lagenidium* hyphae in biopsied tissue section have been described (57, 58). However, their specificity is not known.

Antimicrobial Susceptibilities

As previously mentioned, the oomycetes differ from the true fungi in several respects, one of which is that oomycetes lack sterols in their cytoplasmic membranes. Thus, *Pythium* spp. and *Lagenidium* spp. are intrinsically resistant to most antifungal drugs targeting this pathway. Thus, an early and accurate diagnosis is essential for a good response in infected hosts. Several antifungals have been tested *in vitro* using *Lagenidium* isolated from humans and lower animals (62). Unfortunately, the *in vivo* response has shown contradictory results.

Evaluation, Interpretation, and Reporting of Results

Cases of lagenidiosis with positive culture (Fig. 4A) have to be evaluated by microscopy, looking for the typical structures encountered in some strains (Fig. 4B). If the strain does not display fruiting bodies, the induction of zoospores must be performed (31, 33). The development of sporangia and biflagellate zoospores could be interpreted as proof that the isolate is an oomycete. So far, there are no reports of oomycetes as normal laboratory contaminants or normal microbiota of humans or lower animals. In addition, genomic DNA from the strain under investigation should be tested using molecular methods (see above) to further confirm the findings. The report of the case should include the following: (i) the presence of broad coenocytic hyphae in wet mounts and stained preparations from clinical samples, (ii) the development of zoospores from positive cultures, and (iii) the identification of the strain by morphology and DNA tools.

RHINOSPORIDIUM SEEBERI

Taxonomy

The first two cases of rhinosporidiosis were reported in 1900 by Guillermo Rodolfo Seeber in his M.D. thesis in Argentina (1, 2). He stated that in 1896, he had found two patients with nasal polyps containing an organism similar to that reported by Posadas in 1892 (coccidioidomycosis). He also mentioned that, in 1892, Malbran had studied a case of a nasal polyp showing a spherical microbe with identical morphological features. A nasal case of rhinosporidiosis observed by O'Kinealy in 1903 in India was studied in detail by Minchin and Fanthan in 1905 (2). These investigators suggested the binomial *Rhinosporidium kinealyi* to identify this pathogen. In 1912, Seeber introduced the name *Rhinosporidium seeberi* and called attention to its priority over *R. kinealyi*. In 1924, Ashworth (2) stated that the genus *Rhinosporidium*, proposed by Minchin and Fanthan, should be adopted and that, based on the description of Seeber (2) and the name *Coccidioides seeberia* reintroduced by Belou, the binomial *R. seeberi* has priority.

The fact that this pathogen has not been cultured led some investigators to extreme hypotheses recently reviewed by Vilela and Mendoza (71). The suggestion that *R. seeberi* is a cyanobacterium in the genus *Microcystis* is the most recent in a long list of similar views. This and other views have been challenged by several groups showing that morphological, cell cycle, and phylogenetic analyses all link this pathogen with the protistan eukaryotes (71). The placement of *R. seeberi* within the Mezomycetozoea came as a surprise. This group comprises orphan aquatic fish and amphibian parasites with spherical forms and endospores strikingly similar to those of *R. seeberi* (1, 5). Currently, this pathogen is part of the supergroup Opisthokonta (Ichthyosporea [Mesomycetozoea]) (28). By using the ribosomal DNA ITS, it was found that *R. seeberi* might include several species-specific strains that could represent new species (72).

Description of the Agent

This anomalous pathogen has resisted culture; thus, its morphological features are known only through *in vivo* microscopic and ultramicroscopic studies (1, 2, 5). In infected tissues, *R. seeberi* has a complex parasitic cell cycle. It appears as multiple spherical structures known as sporangia (cysts in most mesomycetozoans) in different stages of development (Fig. 5A and B). The *in vivo* life cycle starts with the release of hundreds of oval or spherical endospores, 7 to 15 μm in diameter, from a pore developed only in mature sporangia (MS) (Fig 5B). The endospores increase in size and progressively develop from juvenile sporangia (JS) (10 to 100 μm), to intermediate sporangia (IS) (100 to 150 μm), and then to MS (150 to more than 450 μm). The endospores are released from MS, and then the *in vivo* cycle is somehow reinitiated. Although the diameter of the sporangium has been used to identify the *in vivo* stages, the MS differs from other stages by the presence of well-developed endospores (Fig. 5B). The finding of mitotic figures within some sporangia in histological preparations has been mentioned (73). These authors found that the nuclei within IS synchronously divide without cytokinesis. A cell wall is developed around each endospore in large sporangia with thousands of nuclei, becoming an MS. Recently, Delfino et al. (74), using confocal microscopy and DAPI (4′,6-diamidino-2-phenylindole) staining, confirmed previous beliefs (73) about the synchronized nature of the nuclear division of *R. seeberi* (Fig. 5C).

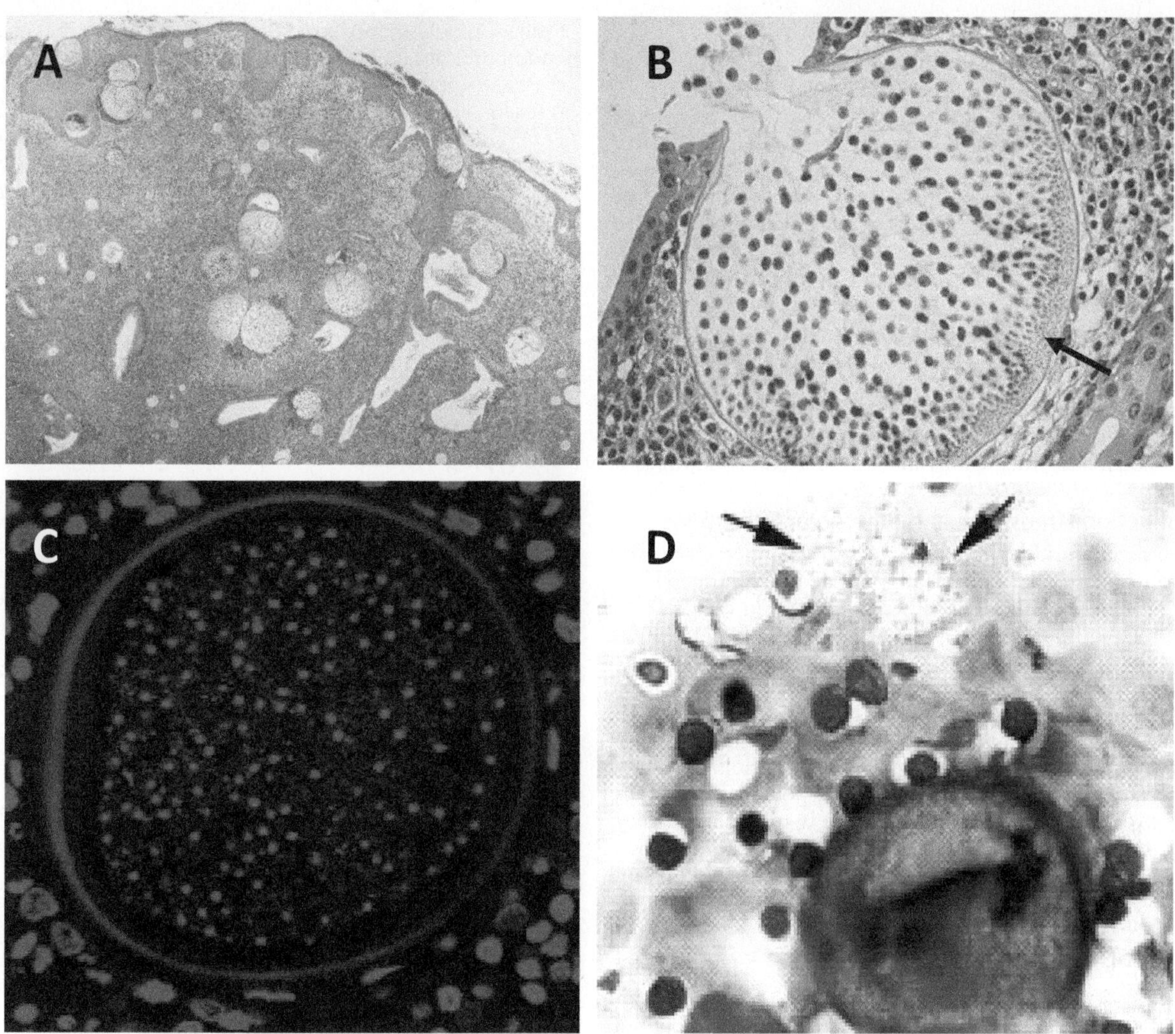

FIGURE 5 *R. seeberi.* (A) H&E-stained tissue sample from a nose polyp showing MS with endospores and JS of different sizes. Magnification, ×10. (B) Release of endospores from an MS. Note the presence of small endospores arising from the opposite site of the exit pore (arrow). Magnification, ×40. (C) Confocal microscopy of a tissue sample containing the *R. seeberi* parasitic stage stained with DAPI and actin dyes, showing an immature sporangium (74). Note the presence of multiple nuclei and the binding of the actin probe to the layer below the cell wall. Magnification, ×40. Courtesy of Delfino et al. (74). (D) Wright-Giemsa impression smear from a dog with nasal rhinosporidiosis. An immature collapsed sporangium may be observed in the lower section. Numerous endospores surrounded by a clear halo are shown near the top (arrows). Magnification, ×70. Courtesy of W. A. Meier.

Epidemiology and Transmission

Rhinosporidiosis usually occurs in most tropical and subtropical areas of the world except Australia (1). Although the infection was first recognized in Argentina, India and Sri Lanka show the highest occurrence of the disease (1, 74). Rhinosporidiosis occurs sporadically in other geographical areas, such as the Americas, Africa, Europe, and Asian countries, including the Middle East. Because some cases of rhinosporidiosis occur in dry areas, especially after sand storms, the hydrophilic nature of this pathogen has long been questioned (1, 2, 74). Based on accounts from patients with the disease, it is believed that rhinosporidiosis is acquired through contact with aquatic environments contaminated with *R. seeberi*, but the precise mechanism of infection from natural sources is unknown.

The finding linking *R. seeberi* to aquatic pathogens of fish and amphibians (5–7, 76) tends to confirm its hydrophilic nature. Most probably, this pathogen evolved from an aquatic niche, in which it still can be found, to terrestrial environments by the development of resistant spores. This is a very likely scenario, since the formation of zoospores, as in the other members of the Dermocystida, among which *R. seeberi* is phylogenetically located, has not been found (1, 2, 6, 75). The disease tends to occur as single cases, but two outbreaks of rhinosporidiosis in humans in Serbia (77) and in swans from Florida (78) have also been recorded. The resistant spores present in water and soil may gain entry through small cutaneous or mucocutaneous wounds and establish infection. Although the disease occurs in apparently normal hosts, some investigators have suggested associations with particular occupational and social conditions (1, 75). Little is known about the predisposing factors leading to the disease. The disease has not been induced in experimental animals, and transmission from one host to another has yet to be reported.

Clinical Significance

In addition to humans, rhinosporidiosis around the facial areas has been also reported in several animal species, including cattle, cats, dogs, goats, horses, river dolphins, and birds (1, 6). In humans, the most common clinical manifestation is the formation of painless polyps usually located on mucosal areas of the nose, eye, larynx, genitalia, and rectum. Multicentric skin lesions have been also recorded (1, 75). The disease is not life threatening, but it can cause breathing difficulties when the polyps obstruct the nose or laryngeal passages. Rhinorrhea and bleeding are common with polyps located in the nose. The slow-growing polypoidal masses are usually found as single or multiple, pedunculate (attached to the skin), sessile, red lesions that bleed easily. Pruritus of the affected areas is also common. The differential diagnosis includes bacterial and fungal infection, neoplasia, and other similar mucosal and skin conditions.

Collection, Transport, and Storage of Specimens

The guidelines for the collection, processing, storage, and examination of specimens are provided in chapter 117 of this *Manual*. Clinical specimens collected in cases of rhinosporidiosis are usually biopsy tissues from infected sites. Since *R. seeberi* cannot be cultured, clinical specimens are usually fixed in formaldehyde upon collection to be histopathologically evaluated later. Nonetheless, fresh samples should also be examined in the laboratory to rule out other etiologic agents and to confirm the histopathological findings. In these cases, biopsy specimens should be aseptically collected and transported immediately to the laboratory. For samples collected far from the laboratory, cooling (−80 to 4°C) of collected specimens for shipping or storage purposes may be necessary.

Direct Examination

Microscopy

Wet-mount preparations from clinical specimens from cases of rhinosporidiosis usually show the presence of mature and immature spherical sporangia and numerous endospores. Mature sporangia with endospores have thin cell walls and measure more than 400 μm in diameter. JS and IS are smaller and may have thicker cell walls. In fresh specimens treated only with water, the release of endospores from MS has been reported (6). A purification system to study *R. seeberi* phenotypes was recently proposed (1). The presence of *R. seeberi* sporangia and endospores can also be detected on smears stained with Giemsa or Gram stain (Fig. 5D). The spherical unstained elements of *R. seeberi* develop autofluorescence when viewed with a fluorescence microscope.

The parasitic spherical structures of this mesomycetozoan pathogen stain very well with H&E, but they also stain with GMS and PAS, a feature used by many in the past to suggest a link with the members of the kingdom Fungi. Biopsy tissue from polypoidal lesions stained with H&E is characterized by the presence of numerous sporangia at different stages of development (Fig. 5A and B). Hyperplasia of the mucous membranes and/or skin with fibrovascular and fibromyxomatous connective tissue containing numerous sporangia is the main feature of the infection. Inflammatory infiltrates of lymphocytes, neutrophils, plasma cells, and, more rarely, giant cells and eosinophils are usually observed in cases of nasal, ocular, and skin infections. JS and IS possess a central nucleus with a prominent nucleolus (73, 74). The collapse of defective sporangia may cause the formation of U-shaped structures. Some MS with numerous endospores are found near the mucosal epithelium, where they are transported from the internal infected areas by a transepidermal elimination phenomenon (Fig. 5A and B) (75). The cell wall of the MS is usually thin, and the enclosed endospores may contain clusters of 1- to 3-μm reddish spherical vesicles. Endospores have a mucoid capsule that does not stain in H&E preparations. The presence of a pore on the sporangial wall is also observed, depending on the plane of the sectioned tissue (Fig. 5B).

Nucleic Acid Detection

Currently, there are no available DNA-based techniques for the diagnosis of *R. seeberi*.

Isolation Procedures, Identification, and Typing Systems

Despite numerous reports claiming that *R. seeberi* has been isolated in pure culture, such claims have not yet been validated. Most of the organisms recovered from cases of rhinosporidiosis have proven to be fungal or bacterial contaminants (1, 75). Because *R. seeberi* has not yet been cultured, the identification of this pathogen is based on its phenotypic characteristics on wet-mount preparations and/or histopathological analyses. The morphological characteristics of *R. seeberi* in infected tissues are almost pathognomonic. Nonetheless, the organism's epidemiological features and the clinical signs of disease should be taken into consideration for a final diagnosis. Morphologically, the parasitic (spherule) stages of *Coccidioides immitis* and *C. posadasii* mimic the *R. seeberi* sporangia with endospores. However, the sporangium size range of *R. seeberi* (<400 to 4 μm), the epidemiological, clinical, and phylogenetic features of coccidioidomycosis, and the fact that *Coccidioides* species can be readily cultured categorically separate this pathogen from *R. seeberi*.

Serologic Tests

Although early investigators did not detect *R. seeberi* antibodies in the sera of infected hosts using endospores or sporangia as antigens, others suggested that the reason for the failure was the use of insensitive assays such as immunodiffusion. Using an immuno-electron-microscopic approach, it was shown for the first time that anti-*R. seeberi* antibodies react against a specific antigen in MS in the sera of patients with rhinosporidiosis (1, 75). Despite these efforts, there are no available serological diagnostic assays for rhinosporidiosis in the clinical setting.

Antimicrobial Susceptibilities

R. seeberi is resistant to most antifungal drugs (1, 75); however, the use of dapsone was found to be helpful in controlling some cases (1). Because this pathogen cannot be isolated in culture, susceptibility testing is not possible. Treatment is carried out by surgical removal of the infected tissues, but recurrences are common (1, 75, 79).

Evaluation, Interpretation, and Reporting of Results

The finding of spherical structures at different stages of development, some of them containing numerous endospores on histopathology, in cytological samples stained with Giemsa and Gram stains, and in wet-mount preparations, is suggestive of rhinosporidiosis. Since the *R. seeberi* spherical structures with endospores mimic the parasitic stage of *Coccidioides* species, a differential diagnosis is required, especially in the areas where coccidioidomycosis is endemic.

The finding of >300-μm spherical sporangia with endospores and negative cultures could be confirmatory of rhinosporidiosis. The report of the results should contain the finding of typical spherical structures that resisted culture.

REFERENCES

1. **Arseculeratne SN, Mendoza L.** 2005. *Rhinosporidium seeberi,* p 435–475. *In* Merz WG, Hay RJ (ed), *Topley and Wilson's Microbiology and Microbial Infections,* 10th ed, vol 3. *Medical Mycology.* Hodder Arnold, London, United Kingdom.
2. **Ashworth JH.** 1924. On *Rhinosporidium seeberi* (Wernicke, 1903) with special reference to its sporulation and affinities. *Trans R Soc Edinb* **53:**301–342.
3. **De Cock AW, Mendoza L, Padhye AA, Ajello L, Kaufman L.** 1987. *Pythium insidiosum* sp. nov., the etiologic agent of pythiosis. *J Clin Microbiol* **25:**344–349.
4. **Lacaz CDS, Baruzzi RG, De Rosa M.** 1986. *Doenca de Jorge Lôbo.* Editora da Universidade de São Paulo, Brazil. IPIS Gráfica e Editora, São Paulo, Brazil.
5. **Mendoza L, Silva V.** 2004. The use of phylogenetic analysis to investigate uncultivated microbes in medical mycology, p 275–298. *In* San-Blas G, Calderone RA (ed), *Pathogenic Fungi: Structural, Biology, and Taxonomy.* Caister Academic Press, Norfolk, United Kingdom.
6. **Mendoza L, Taylor JW, Ajello L.** 2002. The class Mesomycetozoea: a heterogeneous group of microorganisms at the animal-fungal boundary. *Annu Rev Microbiol* **56:**315–344.
7. **Vilela R, Bossart GD, St Leger JA, Dalton LM, Reif JS, Schaefer AM, McCarthy PJ, Fair PA, Mendoza L.** 2016. Cutaneous granulomas in dolphins caused by novel uncultivated *Paracoccidioides brasiliensis. Emerg Infect Dis* **22:**2063–2069.
8. **Lobo JO.** 1930. Nova especie de blastomycose. *Bras Med* **44:**1227.
9. **Vilela R, Martins JE, Pereira CN, Melo N, Mendoza L.** 2007. Molecular study of archival fungal strains isolated from cases of lacaziosis (Jorge Lobo's disease). *Mycoses* **50:**470–474.
10. **Taborda PR, Taborda VA, McGinnis MR.** 1999. *Lacazia loboi* gen. nov., comb. nov., the etiologic agent of lobomycosis. *J Clin Microbiol* **37:**2031–2033.
11. **Vilela R, Mendoza L, Rosa PS, Belone AF, Madeira S, Opromolla DV, de Resende MA.** 2005. Molecular model for studying the uncultivated fungal pathogen *Lacazia loboi. J Clin Microbiol* **43:**3657–3661.
12. **Herr RA, Tarcha EJ, Taborda PR, Taylor JW, Ajello L, Mendoza L.** 2001. Phylogenetic analysis of *Lacazia loboi* places this previously uncharacterized pathogen within the dimorphic Onygenales. *J Clin Microbiol* **39:**309–314.
13. **Teixeira MM, Theodoro RC, de Carvalho MJ, Fernandes L, Paes HC, Hahn RC, Mendoza L, Bagagli E, San-Blas G, Felipe MS.** 2009. Phylogenetic analysis reveals a high level of speciation in the *Paracoccidioides* genus. *Mol Phylogenet Evol* **52:**273–283.
14. **Vilela R, Rosa PS, Belone AF, Taylor JW, Diório SM, Mendoza L.** 2009. Molecular phylogeny of animal pathogen *Lacazia loboi* inferred from rDNA and DNA coding sequences. *Mycol Res* **113:**851–857.
15. **Migaki G, Valerio MG, Irvine B, Garner FM.** 1971. Lobo's disease in an atlantic bottle-nosed dolphin. *J Am Vet Med Assoc* **159:**578–582.
16. **Esperón F, García-Párraga D, Bellière EN, Sánchez-Vizcaíno JM.** 2012. Molecular diagnosis of lobomycosis-like disease in a bottlenose dolphin in captivity. *Med Mycol* **50:**106–109.
17. **Ueda K, et al.** 2013. Two cases of lacaziosis in bottlenose dolphins (*Tursiops truncates*) in Japan. *Case Rep Vet Med* **2013:**318438 https://www.hindawi.com/journals/crivem/2013/318548/
18. **Minakawa T, Ueda K, Tanaka M, Tanaka N, Kuwamura M, Izawa T, Konno T, Yamate J, Itano EN, Sano A, Wada S.** 2016. Detection of multiple budding yeast cells and a partial sequence of 43-kDa glycoprotein coding gene of *Paracoccidioides brasiliensis* from a case of lacaziosis in a female Pacific white-sided dolphin (*Lagenorhynchus obliquidens*). *Mycopathologia* **181:**523–529.
19. **Vilela R, Mendoza L.** 2018. Paracoccidioidomycosis ceti (*lacaziosis/lobomycosis*) in dolphins, p 177–196. *In* Seyedmousavi S, de Hoog GS, Guillot J, Verweij PE (ed), *Emerging and Epizootic Fungal Infections in Animals.* Springer, New York, NY.
20. **Burns RA, Roy JS, Woods C, Padhye AA, Warnock DW.** 2000. Report of the first human case of lobomycosis in the United States. *J Clin Microbiol* **38:**1283–1285.
21. **Elsayed S, Kuhn SM, Barber D, Church DL, Adams S, Kasper R.** 2004. Human case of lobomycosis. *Emerg Infect Dis* **10:**715–718.
22. **Papadavid E, Dalamaga M, Kapniari I, Pantelidaki E, Papageorgiou S, Pappa V, Tsirigotis P, Dervenoulas I, Stavrianeas N, Rigopoulos D.** 2012. Lobomycosis: a case from southeastern Europe and review of the literature. *J Dermatol Case Rep* **6:**65–69.
23. **Rosa PS, Soares CT, Belone AF, Vilela R, Ura S, Filho MC, Mendoza L.** 2009. Accidental Jorge Lobo's disease in a worker dealing with *Lacazia loboi* infected mice: a case report. *J Med Case Reports* **3:**67–71.
24. **Symmers WS.** 1983. A possible case of Lôbo's disease acquired in Europe from a bottle-nosed dolphin (*Tursiops truncatus*). *Bull Soc Pathol Exot* **76:**777–784.
25. **Belone AF, Madeira S, Rosa PS, Opromolla DV.** 2002. Experimental reproduction of the Jorge Lobo's disease in BALB/c mice inoculated with *Lacazia loboi* obtained from a previously infected mouse. *Mycopathologia* **155:**191–194.
26. **Mendoza L, Belone AF, Vilela R, Rehtanz M, Bossart GD, Reif JS, Fair PA, Durden WN, St Leger J, Travassos LR, Rosa PS.** 2008. Use of sera from humans and dolphins with lacaziosis and sera from experimentally infected mice for Western blot analyses of *Lacazia loboi* antigens. *Clin Vaccine Immunol* **15:**164–167.
27. **Austwick PK, Copland JW.** 1974. Swamp cancer. *Nature* **250:**84.
28. **Adl SM, Simpson AG, Lane CE, Lukeš J, Bass D, Bowser SS, Brown MW, Burki F, Dunthorn M, Hampl V, Heiss A, Hoppenrath M, Lara E, Le Gall L, Lynn DH, McManus H, Mitchell EA, Mozley-Stanridge SE, Parfrey LW, Pawlowski J, Rueckert S, Shadwick L, Schoch CL, Smirnov A, Spiegel FW.** 2012. The revised classification of eukaryotes. *J Eukaryot Microbiol* **59:**429–514.
29. **Rivierre C, Laprie C, Guiard-Marigny O, Bergeaud P, Berthelemy M, Guillot J.** 2005. Pythiosis in Africa. *Emerg Infect Dis* **11:**479–481.
30. **Schurko AM, Mendoza L, Lévesque CA, Désaulniers NL, de Cock AWAM, Klassen GR.** 2003. A molecular phylogeny of *Pythium insidiosum. Mycol Res* **107:**537–544.
31. **Gaastra W, Lipman LJ, De Cock AW, Exel TK, Pegge RB, Scheurwater J, Vilela R, Mendoza L.** 2010. *Pythium insidiosum*: an overview. *Vet Microbiol* **146:**1–16.
32. **Mendoza L, Hernandez F, Ajello L.** 1993. Life cycle of the human and animal oomycete pathogen *Pythium insidiosum. J Clin Microbiol* **31:**2967–2973.
33. **Chaiprasert A, Samerpitak K, Wanachiwanawin W, Thasnakorn P.** 1990. Induction of zoospore formation in Thai isolates of *Pythium insidiosum. Mycoses* **33:**317–323.
34. **Thianprasit M, Chaiprasert A, Imwidthaya P.** 1996. Human pythiosis. *Curr Top Med Mycol* **7:**43–54.
35. **Sathapatayavongs B, Leelachaikul P, Prachaktam R, Atichartakarn V, Sriphojanart S, Trairatvorakul P, Jirasiritham S, Nontasut S, Eurvilaichit C, Flegel T.** 1989. Human pythiosis associated with thalassemia hemoglobinopathy syndrome. *J Infect Dis* **159:**274–280.
36. **Vanittanakom N, Supabandhu J, Khamwan C, Praparattanapan J, Thirach S, Prasertwitayakij N, Louthrenoo W, Chiewchanvit S, Tananuvat N.** 2004. Identification of emerging human-pathogenic *Pythium insidiosum* by serological and molecular assay-based methods. *J Clin Microbiol* **42:**3970–3974.
37. **Wanachiwanawin W, Mendoza L, Visuthisakchai S, Mutsikapan P, Sathapatayavongs B, Chaiprasert A, Suwanagool P, Manuskiatti W, Ruangsetakit C, Ajello L.** 2004. Efficacy of immunotherapy using antigens of *Pythium insidiosum* in the treatment of vascular pythiosis in humans. *Vaccine* **22:**3613–3621.

38. **Grooters AM, Leise BS, Lopez MK, Gee MK, O'Reilly KL.** 2002. Development and evaluation of an enzyme-linked immunosorbent assay for the serodiagnosis of pythiosis in dogs. *J Vet Intern Med* **16:**142–146.
39. **Thomas RC, Lewis DT.** 1998. Pythiosis in dogs and cats. *Compend Contin Educ Pract Vet* **20:**63–74.
40. **Supabandhu J, Fisher MC, Mendoza L, Vanittanakom N.** 2008. Isolation and identification of the human pathogen *Pythium insidiosum* from environmental samples collected in Thai agricultural areas. *Med Mycol* **46:**41–52.
41. **Presser JW, Goss EM.** 2015. Environmental sampling reveals that *Pythium insidiosum* is ubiquitous and genetically diverse in North Central Florida. *Med Mycol* **53:**674–683.
42. **Rujirawat T, Sridapan T, Lohnoo T, Yingyong W, Kumsang Y, Sae-Chew P, Tonpitak W, Krajaejun T.** 2017. Single nucleotide polymorphism-based multiplex PCR for identification and genotyping of the oomycete *Pythium insidiosum* from humans, animals and the environment. *Infect Genet Evol* **54:**429–436.
43. **Miller RI, Campbell RS.** 1983. Experimental pythiosis in rabbits. *Sabouraudia* **21:**331–341.
44. **Badenoch PR, Coster DJ, Wetherall BL, Brettig HT, Rozenbilds MA, Drenth A, Wagels G.** 2001. *Pythium insidiosum* keratitis confirmed by DNA sequence analysis. *Br J Ophthalmol* **85:**496.
45. **Murdoch D, Parr D.** 1997. *Pythium insidiosum* keratitis. *Aust N Z J Ophthalmol* **25:**177–179.
46. **Virgile R, Perry HD, Pardanani B, Szabo K, Rahn EK, Stone J, Salkin I, Dixon DM.** 1993. Human infectious corneal ulcer caused by *Pythium insidiosum*. *Cornea* **12:**81–83.
47. **Triscott JA, Weedon D, Cabana E.** 1993. Human subcutaneous pythiosis. *J Cutan Pathol* **20:**267–271.
48. **Reinprayoon U, Permpalung N, Kasetsuwan N, Plongla R, Mendoza L, Chindamporn A.** 2013. *Lagenidium* sp. ocular infection mimicking ocular pythiosis. *J Clin Microbiol* **51:** 2778–2780.
49. **Brown CC, McClure JJ, Triche P, Crowder C.** 1988. Use of immunohistochemical methods for diagnosis of equine pythiosis. *Am J Vet Res* **49:**1866–1868.
50. **Grooters AM, Gee MK.** 2002. Development of a nested polymerase chain reaction assay for the detection and identification of *Pythium insidiosum*. *J Vet Intern Med* **16:**147–152.
51. **Schurko AM, Mendoza L, de Cock AW, Bedard JE, Klassen GR.** 2004. Development of a species-specific probe for *Pythium insidiosum* and the diagnosis of pythiosis. *J Clin Microbiol* **42:**2411–2418.
52. **Keeratijarut A, Lohnoo T, Yingyong W, Rujirawat T, Srichunrusami C, Onpeaw P, Chongtrakool P, Brandhorst TT, Krajaejun T.** 2015. Detection of the oomycete *Pythium insidiosum* by real-time PCR targeting the gene coding for exo-1,3-β-glucanase. *J Med Microbiol* **64:**971–977.
53. **Vilela R, Viswanathan P, Mendoza LA.** 2015. A biochemical screening approach to putatively differentiate mammalian pathogenic Oomycota species in the clinical laboratory. *J Med Microbiol* **64:**862–868.
54. **Krajaejun T, Kunakorn M, Niemhom S, Chongtrakool P, Pracharktam R.** 2002. Development and evaluation of an in-house enzyme-linked immunosorbent assay for early diagnosis and monitoring of human pythiosis. *Clin Diagn Lab Immunol* **9:**378–382.
55. **Mendoza L, Kaufman L, Mandy W, Glass R.** 1997. Serodiagnosis of human and animal pythiosis using an enzyme-linked immunosorbent assay. *Clin Diagn Lab Immunol* **4:**715–718.
56. **Mendoza L, Nicholson V, Prescott JF.** 1992. Immunoblot analysis of the humoral immune response to *Pythium insidiosum* in horses with pythiosis. *J Clin Microbiol* **30:**2980–2983.
57. **Grooters AM.** 2003. Pythiosis, lagenidiosis, and zygomycosis in small animals. *Vet Clin North Am Small Anim Pract* **33:**695–720, v.
58. **Mendoza L, Newton JC.** 2005. Immunology and immunotherapy of the infections caused by *Pythium insidiosum*. *Med Mycol* **43:**477–486.
59. **Chindamporn A, Vilela R, Hoag KA, Mendoza L.** 2009. Antibodies in the sera of host species with pythiosis recognize a variety of unique immunogens in geographically divergent *Pythium insidiosum* strains. *Clin Vaccine Immunol* **16:**330–336.
60. **Intaramat A, Sornprachum T, Chantrathonkul B, Chaisuriya P, Lohnoo T, Yingyong W, Jongruja N, Kumsang Y, Sandee A, Chaiprasert A, Banyong R, Santurio JM, Grooters AM, Ratanabanangkoon K, Krajaejun T.** 2016. Protein A/G-based immunochromatographic test for serodiagnosis of pythiosis in human and animal subjects from Asia and Americas. *Med Mycol* **54:**641–647.
61. **Shenep JL, English BK, Kaufman L, Pearson TA, Thompson JW, Kaufman RA, Frisch G, Rinaldi MG.** 1998. Successful medical therapy for deeply invasive facial infection due to *Pythium insidiosum* in a child. *Clin Infect Dis* **27:**1388–1393.
62. **Brown TA, Grooters AM, Hosgood GL.** 2008. In vitro susceptibility of *Pythium insidiosum* and a *Lagenidium* sp to itraconazole, posaconazole, voriconazole, terbinafine, caspofungin, and mefenoxam. *Am J Vet Res* **69:**1463–1468.
63. **Cavalheiro AS, Maboni G, de Azevedo MI, Argenta JS, Pereira DI, Spader TB, Alves SH, Santurio JM.** 2009. In vitro activity of terbinafine combined with caspofungin and azoles against *Pythium insidiosum*. *Antimicrob Agents Chemother* **53:**2136–2138.
64. **Cavalheiro AS, Zanette RA, Spader TB, Lovato L, Azevedo MI, Botton S, Alves SH, Santurio JM.** 2009. In vitro activity of terbinafine associated to amphotericin B, fluvastatin, rifampicin, metronidazole and ibuprofen against *Pythium insidiosum*. *Vet Microbiol* **137:**408–411.
65. **Grooters AM, Proia LA, Sutton DA, Hodgin EC.** 2004. Characterization of a previously undescribed *Lagenidium* pathogen associated with soft tissue infection: initial description of a new human oomycosis, abstr P-174. Focus on Fungal Infections 14, New Orleans, LA.
66. **Mendoza L, Vilela R.** 2013. The mammalian pathogenic oomycetes. *Curr Fungal Infect Rep* **7:**198–208.
67. **Dick MW.** 2001. *Straminipilous Fungi: Systematics of the Peronosporomycetes, Including Accounts of the Marine Straminipilous Protists, the Plasmodiophorids, and Similar Organisms.* Springer, New York, NY.
68. **Vilela R, Taylor JW, Walker ED, Mendoza L.** 2015. *Lagenidium giganteum* pathogenicity in mammals. *Emerg Infect Dis* **21:**290–297.
69. **Mendoza L, Taylor JW, Walker ED, Vilela R.** 2016. Description of three novel *Lagenidium* (Oomycota) species causing infection in mammals. *Rev Iberoam Micol* **33:**83–91.
70. **Spies CFJ, Grooters AM, Lévesque CA, Rintoul TL, Redhead SA, Glockling SL, Chen CY, de Cock AWAM.** 2016. Molecular phylogeny and taxonomy of *Lagenidium*-like oomycetes pathogenic to mammals. *Fungal Biol* **120:**931–947.
71. **Vilela R, Mendoza L.** 2012. The taxonomy and phylogenetics of the human and animal pathogen *Rhinosporidium seeberi*: a critical review. *Rev Iberoam Micol* **29:**185–199.
72. **Silva V, Pereira CN, Ajello L, Mendoza L.** 2005. Molecular evidence for multiple host-specific strains in the genus *Rhinosporidium*. *J Clin Microbiol* **43:**1865–1868.
73. **Mendoza L, Vilela R.** 2013. Presumptive synchronized nuclear divisions without cytokinesis in the *Rhinosporidium seeberi* parasitic life cycle. *Microbiology* **159:**1545–1551.
74. **Delfino D, Mendoza L, Vilela R.** 2016. *Rhinosporidium seeberi* nuclear cycle activities using confocal microscopy. *J Parasitol* **102:**60–68.
75. **Thianprasit M, Thagerngpol K.** 1989. Rhinosporidiosis. *Curr Top Med Mycol* **3:**64–85.
76. **Herr RA, Ajello L, Taylor JW, Arseculeratne SN, Mendoza L.** 1999. Phylogenetic analysis of *Rhinosporidium seeberi*'s 18S small-subunit ribosomal DNA groups this pathogen among members of the protoctistan Mesomycetozoa clade. *J Clin Microbiol* **37:**2750–2754.
77. **Radovanovic Z, Vukovic Z, Jankovic S.** 1997. Attitude of involved epidemiologists toward the first European outbreak of rhinosporidiosis. *Eur J Epidemiol* **13:**157–160.
78. **Kennedy FA, Buggage RR, Ajello L.** 1995. Rhinosporidiosis: a description of an unprecedented outbreak in captive swans (*Cygnus* spp.) and a proposal for revision of the ontogenic nomenclature of *Rhinosporidium seeberi*. *J Med Vet Mycol* **33:**157–165.
79. **Janardhanan J, Patole S, Varghese L, Rupa V, Tirkey AJ, Varghese GM.** 2016. Elusive treatment for human rhinosporidiosis. *Int J Infect Dis* **48:**3–4.

Microsporidia

RAINER WEBER, PETER DEPLAZES, AND ALEXANDER MATHIS

131

TAXONOMY

Microsporidia are obligate intracellular, unicellular, spore-forming eukaryotes. More than 200 microsporidial genera and approximately 1,500 species that are pathogenic in every major animal group have been identified (1–7). To date, nine genera (*Anncaliia*, *Encephalitozoon*, *Endoreticulatus*, *Enterocytozoon*, *Nosema*, *Pleistophora*, *Trachipleistophora*, *Tubulinosema*, and *Vittaforma*), as well as unclassified microsporidia, assigned to the collective group *Microsporidium* have been implicated in human infections (Table 1).

Microsporidia develop intracellularly exclusively and have no metabolically active stages outside the host cell. A life cycle (Fig. 1) involving a proliferative merogonic sequence followed by a sporogonic sequence results in environmentally resistant spores of unique structure. Mature spores contain a tubular extrusion apparatus (polar tube) for injecting infective spore contents (sporoplasm) into the host cell (8).

Microsporidia are true eukaryotes because they have a membrane-bound nucleus, an intracytoplasmic membrane system, and chromosome separation on mitotic spindles, but they are unusual eukaryotes in that they have bacterium-like ribosomes, no recognizable mitochondria, no peroxisomes, and simple vesicular Golgi membranes. Compared with those of other eukaryotes, the genomes of microsporidia are reduced in size and complexity (9, 10). The genome sizes of different microsporidia vary between 2.3 and 19.5 Mbp, and the number of chromosomes ranges from 7 to 16 (11). The compactness of the microsporidial genomes results from the loss of genes, from the reduction of coding and noncoding elements, from reorganization of genome structure, and from evolution of new gene functions (12–15).

Due to the absence of mitochondria in microscopical studies, it had been postulated that microsporidia are "ancient" protists that diverged before the mitochondrial endosymbiosis (16). However, genes related to mitochondrial functions were identified in *Encephalitozoon cuniculi* (9), and immunolocalization of the mitochondrial heat shock protein 70 in the microsporidian *Trachipleistophora hominis* revealed tiny organelles with double membranes, named mitosomes (17, 18). Genome-wide sequence and synteny analyses indicate that the organisms of the phylum Microsporidia belong to the kingdom of the Fungi (19), being derived from an endoparasitic chytrid ancestor on the earliest diverging branch of the fungal phylogenetic tree (20, 21). Recently, Microsporidia were proposed to be linked to (22) or placed within (23) the novel phylum Cryptomycota (24, 25), which phylogenetically represents intermediate fungal forms. Also, structural features of the organisms such as the presence of chitin in the spore wall, diplokaryotic nuclei, and electron-dense spindle plaques associated with the nuclear envelope suggest a possible relationship between fungi and microsporidia, whereas the life cycle of microsporidia is unique and dissimilar to that of other fungal species.

DESCRIPTION OF THE GENERA AND SPECIES

The species are illustrated in Fig. 1 and listed in Table 1.

Anncaliia spp. have diplokaryotic nuclei and develop in direct contact with host cell cytoplasm. Additionally, the organisms produce electron-dense extracellular secretions and vesiculotubular appendages. Three former members of the microsporidial genus *Brachiola* that are pathogenic in humans were transferred to the genus *Anncaliia* on the basis of novel ultrastructural and molecular data (26). Disporoblastic sporogony of *Anncaliia vesicularum* (formerly *Brachiola vesicularum*) produces 2.5- by 2-μm diplokaryotic spores containing 7 to 10 anisofilar coils of the polar filament arranged in one to three rows, usually two (27). On the basis of diplokaryotic nuclei, disporoblastic sporogony, and the formation of vesiculotubular secretions, *Nosema connori* and *Nosema algerae*, also discovered in human infections, have been reclassified as species of *Anncaliia*. Spores of *Anncaliia connori* measure 2.0 to 2.5 by 4.0 to 4.5 μm and contain polar tubes with 10 to 12 coils (28). Spores of *Anncaliia algerae* measure 3.7 to 5.4 by 2.3 to 3.9 μm and have 8 to 11 coils of the polar tube (29).

Encephalitozoon spp. develop intracellularly in parasitophorous vacuoles bounded by a membrane of presumed host cell origin. Nuclei of all stages are unpaired. Meronts divide repeatedly by binary fission and lie close to the vacuolar membrane. Sporonts appear free in the center of the vacuole and divide into two or four sporoblasts, which mature into spores. The spores measure 1.0 to 1.5 by 2.0 to 3.0 μm, and the polar tube has four to eight isofilar coils.

TABLE 1 Microsporidial species pathogenic in humans, and clinical manifestations

Microsporidial species	Clinical manifestations	
	Immunocompromised patients	Immunocompetent persons
Anncaliia algerae[a]	Myositis, nodular cutaneous lesions	Keratitis, vocal cord infection, myositis
Anncaliia connori[b]	Disseminated infection	Not described
Anncaliia vesicularum[c]	Myositis	Not described
Encephalitozoon cuniculi	Disseminated infection, keratoconjunctivitis, sinusitis, bronchitis, pneumonia, nephritis, hepatitis, peritonitis, intestinal infection, encephalitis, endocarditis	Encephalitis
Encephalitozoon hellem	Disseminated infection, keratoconjunctivitis, sinusitis, bronchitis, pneumonia, urogenital infection	Possibly diarrhea
Encephalitozoon intestinalis[d]	Chronic diarrhea, cholangiopathy, sinusitis, bronchitis, pneumonitis, nephritis, bone infection, nodular cutaneous lesions	Self-limiting diarrhea, asymptomatic carriers
Endoreticulatus spp.	Not described	Myositis, disseminated infection
Enterocytozoon bieneusi	Chronic diarrhea, wasting syndrome, "AIDS-cholangiopathy," cholangitis, acalculous cholecystitis, chronic sinusitis, pneumonia	Self-limiting diarrhea in adults and children, traveler's diarrhea, asymptomatic carriers
Microsporidium africanum, *M. ceylonensis*[e]	Not described	Corneal ulcer, keratitis
Nosema ocularum	Not described	Keratitis
Pleistophora sp.	Myositis	Not described
Pleistophora ronneafiei	Myositis	Not described
Trachipleistophora anthropophthera	Disseminated infection (including brain, heart, kidney), keratitis	Not described
Trachipleistophora hominis	Myositis, myocarditis, keratoconjunctivitis, sinusitis	Keratitis
Tubulinosema acridophagus	Disseminated infection, myositis, hepatitis; pulmonary, peritoneal, and skin infection	Not described
Vittaforma corneae[f]	Disseminated infection, urinary tract infection	Keratoconjunctivitis
Unidentified *Microsporidia* sp.	Ocular infection; keratitis after collagen cross-linking	Reactive arthritis

[a] Formerly *Brachiola algerae*, *Nosema algerae*.
[b] Formerly *Brachiola connori*, *Nosema connori*.
[c] Formerly *Brachiola vesicularum*.
[d] Formerly *Septata intestinalis*.
[e] *Microsporidium* is a collective generic name for microsporidia that cannot be classified because available information is not sufficient.
[f] Formerly *Nosema corneum*.

Encephalitozoon cuniculi was isolated from a range of animals before human infections were identified. Human isolates of three *Encephalitozoon* spp. and animal isolates of *E. cuniculi* are morphologically identical. In 1991, *Encephalitozoon hellem* was distinguished from *E. cuniculi* on the basis of different protein patterns (30). In 1993, *Septata intestinalis* was described and named on the basis of the unique morphological findings that the organisms are contained in intracellular vacuoles and that a pathogen-secreted fibrillar network surrounds the developing organisms, giving the vacuoles a septate appearance (31). Subsequently, on the basis of phylogenetic analyses, *S. intestinalis* was reclassified as *Encephalitozoon intestinalis*. Finally, on the basis of genetic analyses, four strains of *E. cuniculi* have been identified so far that partially differ in animal-host preferences and geographic distributions (32, 33).

Endoreticulatus spp. was proposed in two cases on the basis of genetic findings; ultrastructural results are not available (34, 35).

Enterocytozoon bieneusi develops in direct contact with host cell cytoplasm (Fig. 2). The proliferative and sporogonial forms are rounded multinucleate plasmodia with unpaired nuclei measuring up to 6 μm in diameter. The oval spores measure 0.7 to 1.0 by 1.1 to 1.6 μm. The polar tube, derived from electron-dense disks in sporonts, has five to seven isofilar coils that appear in two rows when seen in transverse section by transmission electron microscopy (36). Numerous genotypes have been identified, with differences in host specificity and zoonotic potential (37).

Nosema spp. develop in direct contact with host cell cytoplasm; nuclei are paired (diplokaryotic); divisions are by binary fission, and sporonts are disporoblastic. Only one species of human origin, *Nosema ocularum*, has been retained in this genus. It will probably require reclassification, but insufficient information is currently available for a new generic assignment. Spores measure 3 by 5 μm and have polar tubes with 9 to 12 coils.

Pleistophora spp., including *Pleistophora ronneafiei*, which is pathogenic in humans, have unpaired nuclei, and all stages are multinucleate plasmodia, which divide into smaller multinucleate segments. Meronts have a thick, amorphous coat, which separates from the surface in sporogony to form a sporophorous vesicle. Sporogonic divisions give rise to a large and variable number of spores, packaged in the persistent sporophorous vesicle. The spores contain polar tubes with 9 to 12 coils and measure 2 to 2.8 by 3.3 to 4.0 μm (38).

Trachipleistophora hominis forms spores in sporophorous vesicles; these arise from repeated binary fissions and not from multinucleate plasmodia. The vesicles, which contain 2 to more than 32 spores, enlarge as the number of spores increases. The nuclei are unpaired in all stages of development. The pear-shaped spores measure 2.4 by 4.0 μm and have about 11 anisofilar coils (39). *Trachipleistophora anthropophthera* is similar to *T. hominis* but appears to be dimorphic, as two different forms of sporophorous vesicles and spores have been observed (40).

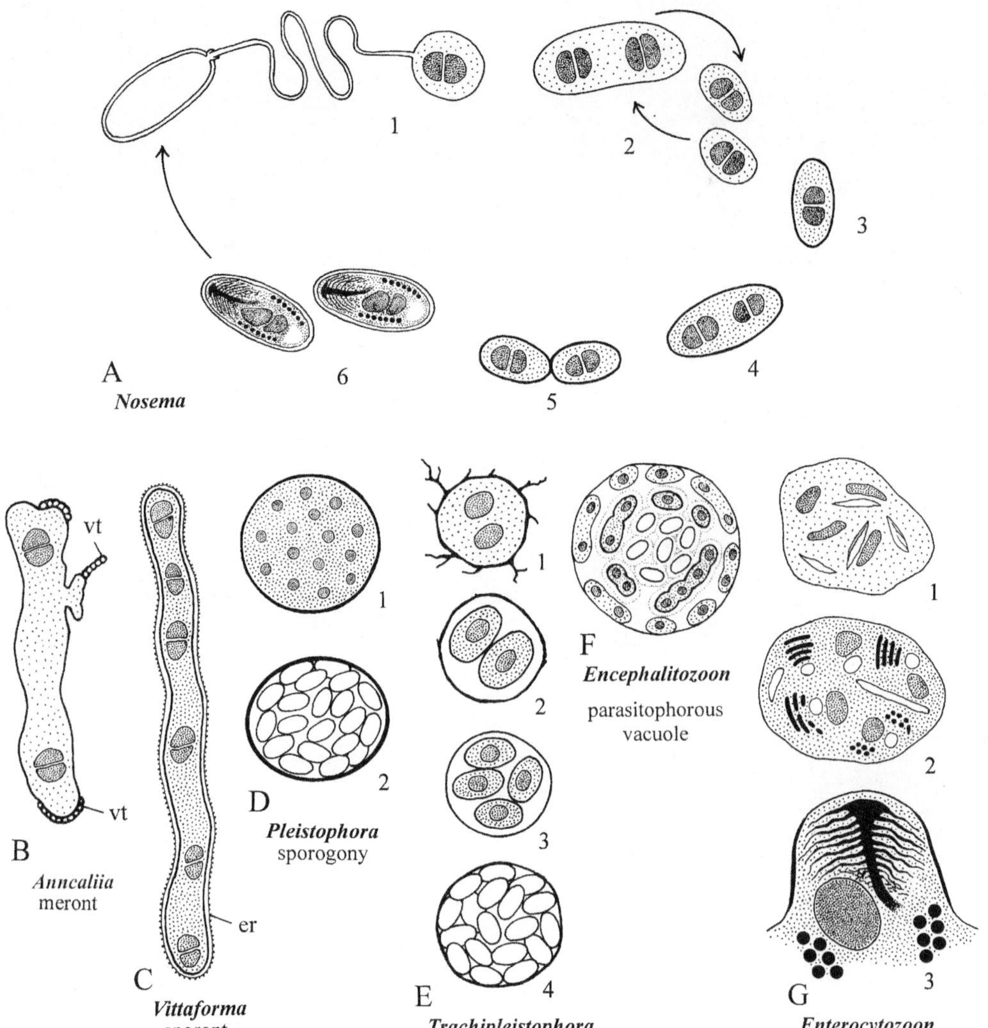

FIGURE 1 Generalized life cycle of microsporidia and identifying characteristics of the genera known to infect humans. Light stippling indicates merogonic stages; heavy stippling indicates sporogonic stages; no stippling indicates spores and sporoplasm. (A) Basic life cycle, illustrated by *Nosema*. Development may occur in direct contact with host cell cytoplasm (*Nosema*, *Anncaliia*, and *Enterocytozoon*) or in isolation by host cell membranes (*Vittaforma* and *Encephalitozoon*) or a cyst-like sporophorous vesicle of pathogen origin (*Pleistophora* and *Trachipleistophora*). (1) Sporoplasm: the infective stage emergent from the spore. It may have unpaired nuclei (monokaryotic) or two nuclei in close apposition (diplokaryotic), depending on the genus. (2) Merogony: proliferative stage. It may have a simple plasma membrane, but a surface coat is present in *Anncaliia*, *Pleistophora*, and *Trachipleistophora*. Division can be by binary or multiple fission into two or more individuals. (3) Sporont: the first stage of sporogony. If not already present, a surface coat is added (this step is delayed in *Enterocytozoon*). (4) Sporogony: divisions culminating in spore production. Binary or multiple fissions give rise to sporoblasts. (5) Sporoblasts: end products of sporogony, which mature into spores. (6) Spores: resistant stages for transmission. Spores are characterized by an extrusion apparatus (polar tube), which serves to conduct the sporoplasm into a host cell. The polar tube may be of uniform diameter (isofilar) or show a sharp decrease in diameter in the most posterior coils (anisofilar). (B to G) Identifying characteristics of genera. (B) *Anncaliia*. Members of this genus are diplokaryotic and disporoblastic; the life cycle is like that of *Nosema*, but meronts are bizarrely shaped and possess a surface coat with vesiculotubular structures (vt) embedded in it and extended from it. (C) *Vittaforma*. Members of this genus are diplokaryotic and polysporoblastic; all stages, including spores, are isolated in a close-fitting, ribosome-studded cisterna of host endoplasmic reticulum (er). (D) *Pleistophora*. Members of this genus are monokaryotic and polysporoblastic; meronts and sporonts are multinucleate stages called plasmodia; a thick surface coat is already present on meronts and sporonts (1); this coat separates from the sporogonial plasmodium to form a cyst-like vesicle, the sporophorous vesicle; the plasmodium divides within it to produce numerous spores (2). (E) *Trachipleistophora*. Members of this genus are monokaryotic and polysporoblastic. The meront surface coat has branched extensions (1); these are withdrawn when the coat separates to form the sporophorous vesicle around a uninucleate sporont; the sporont undergoes a series of binary fissions (2, 3) and finally encloses numerous spores (4). (F) *Encephalitozoon*. Members of this genus are monokaryotic and di- or tetrasporoblastic; all stages of the life cycle, developing from the sporoplasm, occur concurrently within a host cell vacuole (parasitophorous vacuole); merogonic stages are appressed against the vacuole wall; sporogonic stages are free; the vacuole is finally packed with spores, so that it superficially resembles a sporophorous vesicle. (G) *Enterocytozoon*. Members of this genus are monokaryotic and polysporoblastic; meronts (1) have irregular nuclei and lucent clefts; sporonts (2) are multinucleate with rounded nuclei and have highly characteristic electron-dense disks, which are polar tube precursors; all spore organelles are formed prematurely, so that constriction around the sets of organelles and a nucleus (3) gives rise directly to almost mature spores. The surface coat is deposited only during constriction.

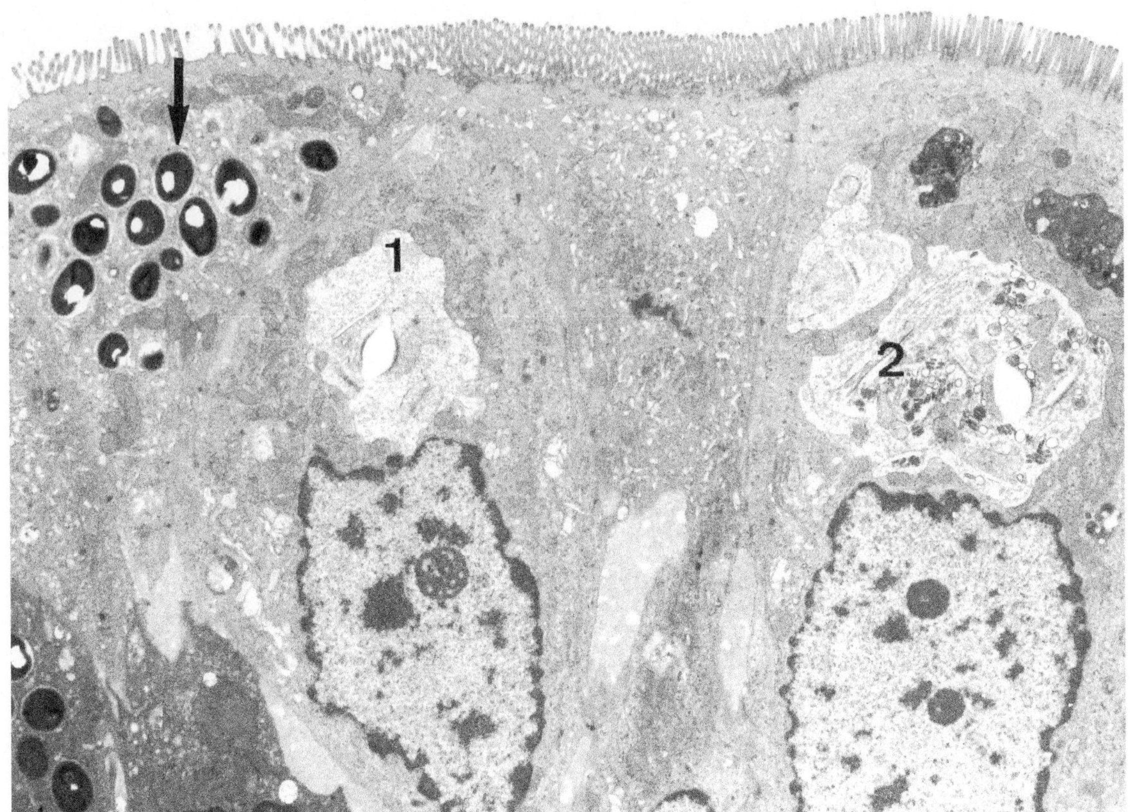

FIGURE 2 Transmission electron micrograph showing the duodenal epithelium of an HIV-infected patient infected with *Enterocytozoon bieneusi*. The different developmental stages between the enterocyte nuclei and the microvillus border include a proliferative plasmodium (1), late sporogonial plasmodia (2), and mature spores (arrow). Magnification, ×5,370. (Courtesy of M. A. Spycher, University Hospital, Zurich, Switzerland.)

Tubulinosema acridophagus was proposed on the basis of genetic analyses in two cases (41, 42) and additionally documented by electron microscopy in a recent case (43). Ultrastructurally, all developing stages are in direct contact with the host cell cytoplasm. Spore size ranges from 1.4 to 2.4 μm in length; nuclei are diplokaryotic, and polar filaments are anisofilar and contain 11 coils arranged mostly in single rows, although in some spores double rows are present.

Vittaforma corneae, originally classified as *Nosema corneum*, was transferred to a new genus on the basis of ultrastructural features (44). Nuclei are diplokaryotic; sporogony is polysporoblastic; sporonts are ribbon-shaped, and all stages, including spores, are individually enveloped by a cisterna of host endoplasmic reticulum studded with ribosomes. The spores contain polar tubes with five to seven coils and measure 1.2 by 3.8 μm (45).

Microsporidium is a collective generic name for microsporidia that cannot be classified because available information is not sufficient. *Microsporidium ceylonensis* and *Microsporidium africanum* have been assigned to the group name (46).

EPIDEMIOLOGY AND TRANSMISSION

Human microsporidial infections have been documented globally and have even been detected in ancient samples from Neanderthals (47). The sources of microsporidia infecting humans and their modes of transmission are uncertain, but ingestion of the environmentally highly resistant spores is probably the most important mode of transmission. Transmission by dust or aerosol has also been considered on the basis of respiratory or ocular infections (48, 49). Direct contact with water during bathing in hot spring spas was associated with microsporidial keratitis (50). Water contact was found to be a risk factor for microsporidiosis. DNA homologous to *E. bieneusi*, *E. intestinalis*, *V. corneae*, and other microsporidia have been detected in sewage effluent, groundwater, and surface water (51, 52), suggesting the potential for zoonotic and anthroponotic transmission. Furthermore, foodborne outbreaks associated with microsporidia have been reported (52, 53), and microsporidia pathogenic to humans have been detected in fresh food produce (spores and DNA) (54) and in milk specimens from dairy cows (DNA) (55). Studies with mammals suggest that *Encephalitozoon* spp. can be transmitted transplacentally from mother to offspring, but no congenitally acquired human infections have been reported.

Direct zoonotic transmission of microsporidia has not been verified but appears likely, because many microsporidial species can infect both humans and animals (3). *E. cuniculi* is considered to be a zoonotic pathogen: All four strains were detected in natural infections in rabbits, rodents, tamarins, cats, dogs, or a variety of wild animals (33); strains I ("rabbit strain"), II ("mouse strain"), and III ("dog strain") have been isolated from human immunodeficiency virus (HIV)-infected patients (3, 32, 33, 56).

Furthermore, strain IV ("human strain") was documented in a renal transplant recipient (57) but later also in cats and dogs (33). In addition to documentation in humans, *Encephalitozoon* spp. have been detected in psittacines kept in aviaries, in a variety of wild birds, including in feces of urban feral pigeons (58), in domestic animals in Mexico (59), and in gorillas in Uganda. *E. bieneusi*, discovered in humans, is increasingly being recognized in animals (wildlife, livestock, and companion animals). Genetic analyses of this pathogen revealed two major groups, one comprising anthroponotic genotypes and the other containing multiple genotypes with zoonotic potential (60, 61). Also, an insect-pathogenic microsporidian, *A. algerae*, was isolated from three patients (62, 63).

Organ transplants have been identified as a donor-derived source of microsporidial infection: *E. cuniculi* infections were diagnosed in three patients with a neurological symptom (64); *E. cuniculi* and *E. bieneusi* infections, in renal transplant recipients who presented with fever of unknown origin, diarrhea, or asymptomatic proteinuria and microhematuria (65–69).

CLINICAL SIGNIFICANCE

Although microsporidiosis appears to occur most frequently in persons infected with HIV, it is emerging in otherwise immunocompromised and in immunocompetent persons, causing intestinal, extraintestinal, and systemic infections (Table 1) (1, 2, 4, 6, 70). In the non-HIV-infected immunocompromised host, microsporidial infections were described in solid-organ transplant recipients (64, 65, 67), in allogeneic hematopoietic stem cell transplant recipients (71, 72), in patients with hematologic malignancies receiving monoclonal antibody therapy (73), in patients with rheumatic disease undergoing anti-tumor necrosis factor therapy (74), in the elderly (75), and in malnourished children (76). In immunocompetent persons, microsporidia have been associated with keratoconjunctivitis (77–79), keratoconjunctivitis in contact lens wearers (80) and after corneal collagen cross-linking (a noninvasive technique to treat keratoconus) (81), self-limiting diarrhea (82), and rarely cerebral infection (1, 64, 83–89). Microsporidia can also cause latent asymptomatic infections (90).

Microsporidiosis has been associated with abnormalities in structures and functions of infected organs, but the mechanisms of pathogenicity of the different microsporidial species are not sufficiently understood. Patients with severe cellular immunodeficiency appear to be at the highest risk for developing microsporidial disease. Unfortunately, little is known about immunity to this infection, although the importance of T cells has been demonstrated in experiments with athymic mice (91–93). It is not understood whether microsporidiosis in immunocompromised patients is primarily a reactivation of latent infection acquired prior to the state of suppressed immunity or whether microsporidial disease is caused by recently acquired infection.

Enterocytozoon bieneusi

E. bieneusi infects the enterocytes of the small intestine and epithelial cells of the biliary tree and respiratory tract. Clinical disease is probably caused by the continuous excess loss of epithelial cells. *Enterocytozoon* infection may be accompanied by alterations in small-bowel physiology such as decreased brush border sucrase, lactase, and maltase activities as well as malabsorption.

E. bieneusi is estimated to be one of the most important HIV-associated intestinal pathogens, present in 5 to 30% of patients with chronic diarrhea, weight loss, or cholangiopathy, particularly when CD4 lymphocyte counts are below 100/μl (94). Upper or lower respiratory tract infections have been detected in a few patients (95), but systemic infection due to *E. bieneusi* has not been documented. Case reports have documented that the organisms are also a cause of diarrhea in organ transplant recipients (96).

In immunocompetent adults and in children, *E. bieneusi* is associated with self-limited watery diarrhea (lasting up to 2 to 3 weeks), particularly among persons who reside or have traveled in tropical countries (97). Furthermore, the organisms have been identified among malnourished children in tropical areas (76) and elderly persons (residing in resource-rich countries) with acute or chronic diarrhea (75).

Encephalitozoon spp.

Encephalitozoon spp. infect epithelial and endothelial cells, fibroblasts, macrophages, and possibly other cell types, as reported for humans and mammals. Human encephalitozoonosis was first described in two children with a seizure disorder (83, 84). Cerebral infections have subsequently been substantiated (1, 64, 85–89). Unexpectedly, *E. cuniculi* endocarditis was diagnosed in a non-immunocompromised patient with a dual-chamber pacemaker (98).

The spectrum of recognized *E. cuniculi-* and *E. hellem-*associated disease in patients with AIDS, organ transplant recipients, and otherwise immunocompromised patients includes keratoconjunctivitis, intraocular infection, sinusitis, bronchiolitis, pneumonitis, nephritis, ureteritis, cystitis, prostatitis, urethritis, hepatitis, sclerosing cholangitis, peritonitis, diarrhea, and encephalitis (1, 30, 56, 85). Clinical manifestations may vary substantially, ranging from an asymptomatic carrier state to organ failure.

Encephalitozoon intestinalis infects primarily enterocytes, but the organism is also found in intestinal lamina propria, and dissemination to the kidneys, airways, and biliary tract appears to occur via infected macrophages (31). Chronic diarrhea and disseminated disease due to *E. intestinalis* have been diagnosed mainly in immunodeficient patients. A case of nodular cutaneous *E. intestinalis* infection was observed in a patient with AIDS (99). Furthermore, *E. intestinalis* has been detected in stool specimens from healthy children and adults, with or without diarrhea, living in Mexico (100), and among travelers with diarrhea returning from tropical countries (101).

Other Microsporidia

Different microsporidial species have been isolated from immunocompetent persons (1, 44) and from immunodeficient persons (45) with keratoconjunctivitis, keratitis, corneal ulcers (79), and reactive arthritis (102) (Table 1).

In immunocompromised patients, disseminated infections and myositis have been linked to infections with different microsporidia (Table 1), including *Pleistophora* spp. (103), *P. ronneafiei* (38), *T. hominis* (104), *A. vesicularum* (27), *A. algerae* (62, 105), and *T. acridophagus* (41, 42). *A. algerae* has also been isolated from erythematous skin nodules from a boy with acute lymphocytic leukemia (106). Myositis due to *Endoreticulatus* spp. was diagnosed in an otherwise healthy man in Thailand (34).

T. anthropophthera has been identified at autopsy in cerebral, cardiac, renal, pancreatic, thyroid, hepatic, splenic, lymphoid, and bone marrow tissue of patients with AIDS who initially presented with seizures (107). Disseminated infection due to *A. connori* was found at autopsy in a 4-month-old athymic male infant (28).

COLLECTION, TRANSPORT, AND STORAGE OF SPECIMENS

Spores of enteropathogenic microsporidia can be detected in stool specimens or duodenal aspirates that have been fixed in 10% formalin or in sodium acetate-acetic acid-formalin, fresh stool samples, or biopsy specimens. The spores of microsporidia causing disseminated infection can usually be detected in fresh or fixed urine sediments, other body fluids (including sputum, bronchoalveolar lavage fluid, nasal secretions, cerebrospinal fluid, and conjunctival smears), corneal scrapings, or tissue. For histologic examination, tissue specimens are fixed in formalin. For electron microscopy, fixation of tissue with glutaraldehyde is preferred. Collection of fresh material (without fixative) may be useful for cell culture and for molecular identification. Microsporidial spores are environmentally resistant and, if prevented from drying, can remain infectious for periods of up to several years (108).

DETECTION PROCEDURES

The most robust technique for the diagnosis of microsporidial infection is light-microscopic detection of the organisms themselves. Spores, the stages of microsporidia pathogenic in humans that are usually identified, are small, ranging in size from 1 to 4 μm. Evaluation of patients with suspected intestinal microsporidiosis should begin with light-microscopic examination of stool specimens, and microsporidia that cause systemic infection are best detected in urine sediments or other body fluids. Definitive species identification of microsporidia is made by electron microscopy and, preferably, genetic analysis (4, 6, 108).

Examination of Stool Specimens

Preparation of Smears, Staining, and Microscopic Examination

Smears are prepared with 10 to 20 μl of unconcentrated stool that is very thinly spread onto slides. Most of the coprological procedures that have been adapted for the concentration of ova and parasites (i.e., helminth eggs and protozoa) fail to concentrate microsporidial spores. The formalin-ethyl acetate concentration and different flotation methods remove significant amounts of fecal debris; smears prepared from these concentrates appear to be easier to read by light microscopy, but they are less sensitive (109).

The most commonly used stains are chromotrope-based stains (109) and chemofluorescent optical brightening agents (110, 111), including calcofluor white and other chemofluorescent stains. Regardless of which staining technique is utilized, the use of positive-control material is essential. The detection of microsporidial spores requires adequate illumination and magnification, i.e., magnification of ×630 or ×1,000 (oil immersion). The differences in the sizes of *Enterocytozoon* spores (1 to 1.5 μm) and *Encephalitozoon* spores (2 to 3 μm) often permit a tentative identification of the genus from light-microscopic examination of stool specimens.

Chromotrope-Based Staining Procedures

Microsporidial spores are ovoid and have a specific appearance when stained with chromotrope stains (Fig. 3 and 4, right panel) (109). The spore wall stains bright pinkish red; some spores appear transparent, and other spores show a distinct pinkish red-stained belt-like stripe that girds the spores diagonally or equatorially. Most background debris in stool specimens counterstains a faint green (or blue, depending on the staining technique). Some other fecal elements, such as parasite cysts (e.g., *Cyclospora*), yeasts, and some bacteria, may also stain reddish, but they are distinguished from microsporidial spores by their sizes, shapes, and staining patterns.

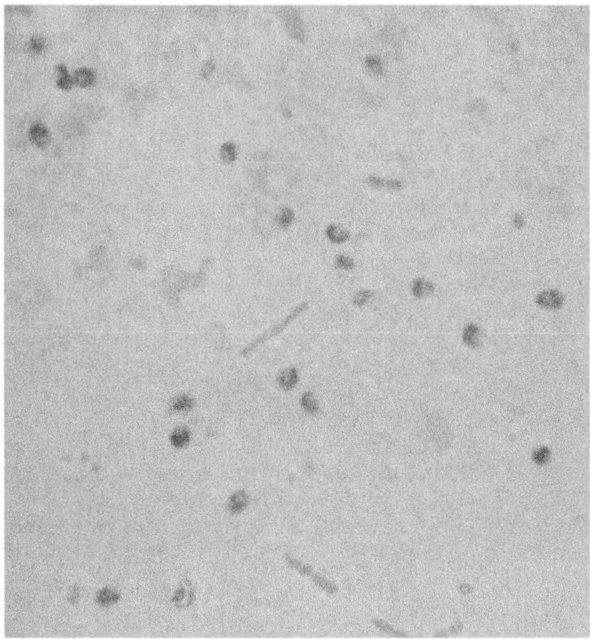

FIGURE 3 Smear of a stool specimen from a patient with AIDS and chronic diarrhea, showing pinkish red-stained spores of *Enterocytozoon bieneusi* that measure 0.7 to 1.0 by 1.1 to 1.6 μm. Chromotrope staining was used. Magnification, ×1,000 (oil immersion).

Several modifications of the original chromotrope-staining solution (109) have been proposed, including modifications of the counterstain and changes in the temperature of the standard chromotrope-staining solution and in the staining time (112). An acid-fast trichrome stain (113), which permits visualization of acid-fast cryptosporidial oocysts and microsporidial spores on the same slide, and a "quick-hot" Gram-chromotrope-staining technique (114) have also been developed.

Chemofluorescent Agents

Chemofluorescent optical brightening agents are chitin stains (see chapter 118 of this *Manual*), which require examination with a fluorescent microscope. With the correct wavelength illumination, the chitinous wall of the microsporidial spores fluoresces brightly, facilitating the detection of spores. However, staining is not specific, because small yeast cells, which may be present in fecal material, and other fecal elements may also be brightened. Some experience is necessary to distinguish the microsporidia.

Epidemiological comparisons of the chromotrope-staining technique with methods that use chemofluorescent optical brighteners indicate that these tests are robust for routine use and that the sensitivities of both methods are similarly high. Some laboratories use both staining techniques because the chromotrope stains result in a highly specific visualization of spores, whereas the chemofluorescent agents may be more sensitive but may produce false-positive results.

Immunofluorescent-Antibody Tests

Monoclonal antibodies against *Encephalitozoon* spp. (115) and *E. bieneusi* (116) have been generated, some of which have been evaluated for diagnostic purposes with stool specimens.

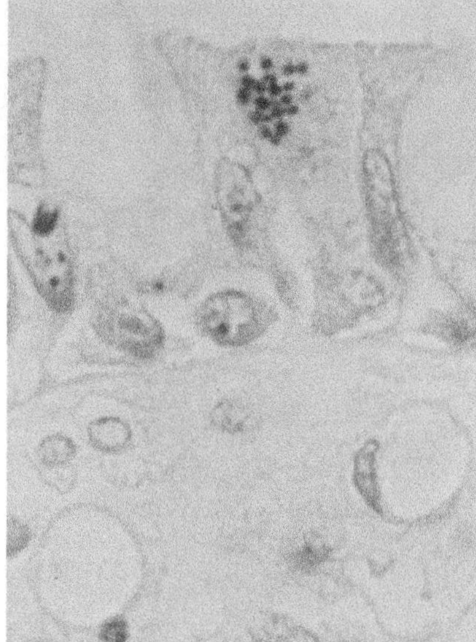
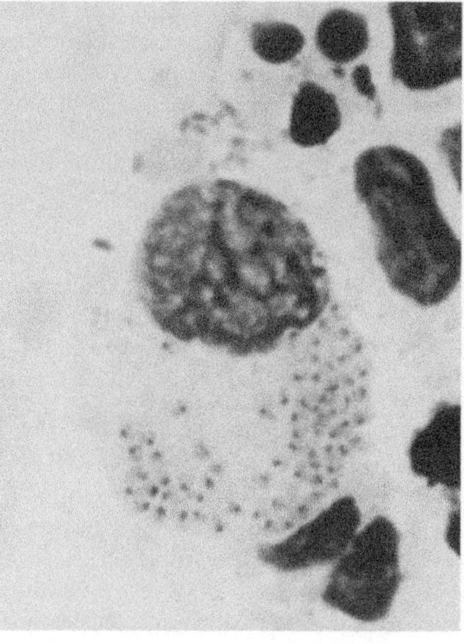
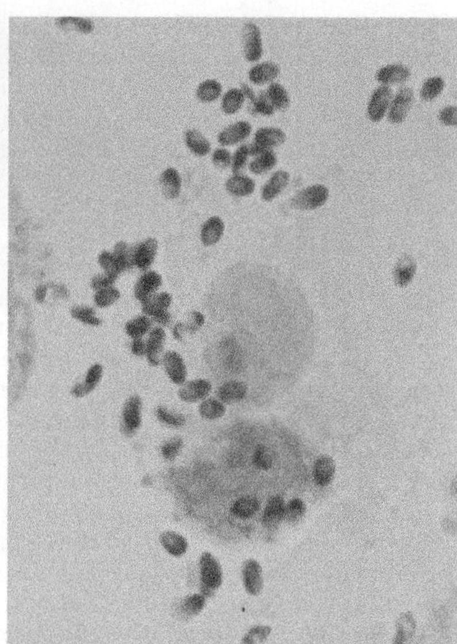

FIGURE 4 (Left) Terminal ileal tissue obtained by ileocolonoscopy from a patient with AIDS and chronic diarrhea due to *Enterocytozoon bieneusi* infection. Gram-labile microsporidial spores, measuring 0.7 to 1.0 by 1.1 to 1.6 μm, are found at a supranuclear location within small intestinal enterocytes. Brown-Brenn stain was used. Magnification, ×1,000. (Middle) Cytospin preparation of bronchoalveolar lavage fluid from a patient with AIDS and intestinal *E. bieneusi* infection, showing intracellular microsporidia. Giemsa stain was used. Magnification, ×1,000 (oil immersion). (Right) Urine sediment from a patient with AIDS and disseminated *Encephalitozoon cuniculi* infection, showing pinkish red-stained microsporidial spores measuring 1.0 to 1.5 by 2.0 to 3.0 μm. Chromotrope stain was used. Magnification, ×1,000 (oil immersion).

Recently, a commercial indirect fluorescent-antibody assay became available (Bordier Affinity Products, Switzerland; CE marked but not FDA approved). With PCR as gold standard, sensitivity and specificity of this indirect fluorescent-antibody assay for *E. bieneusi* were 95.2% and 100%, respectively; with the modified trichrome stain as gold standard, sensitivity and specificity were 100% and 99.4%, respectively (117).

Cytological Diagnosis

Microsporidial spores have been detected in sediments obtained by centrifugation of body fluids for 10 min at 500 × g, including duodenal aspirates, bile, biliary aspirates, urine (Fig. 4, right panel), bronchoalveolar lavage fluid (Fig. 4, middle panel), and cerebrospinal fluid, and in smears of conjunctival swabs, sputum, and nasal discharge. Microscopic examination of stained smears of centrifuged duodenal aspirate obtained during endoscopy is a highly sensitive technique for the diagnosis of intestinal microsporidiosis. Because microsporidial infection often involves multiple organs, the detection of microsporidia in virtually any tissue or body fluid should prompt a thorough search of other sites. Particularly for patients with suspected disseminated microsporidiosis, urine specimens should be examined (1, 108).

Examination of Biopsy Specimens and Corneal Scrapings

Examination of duodenal and terminal ileal tissue has resulted in the detection of intestinal microsporidia, but the pathogens are rarely found in colonic tissue sections. Microsporidial species causing disseminated infection have been found in almost every organ system (1, 6).

Only highly experienced pathologists have reliably and consistently identified microsporidia in tissue sections by using routine techniques such as hematoxylin and eosin staining. Ultrathin plastic sections stained with methylene blue-azure II-basic fuchsin or with toluidine blue may facilitate detection. In our experience, tissue Gram stains (Brown-Brenn or Brown-Hopps) have proved to be the most useful for the rapid and reliable identification of HIV-associated microsporidia in routine paraffin-embedded tissue sections (Fig. 4, left panel) and corneal scrapings (1, 48). The microsporidial spores are Gram variable, and they are readily identified because of the contrasting dark blue or reddish staining against a faint brown-yellow background. Others prefer a silver stain (Warthin-Starry stain) (118), the chromotrope-based staining technique, or chemofluorescent agents.

Molecular Techniques

Universal panmicrosporidian and genus- or species-specific PCR primer pairs that target the rRNA genes and their application in the diagnosis of intestinal microsporidial infection have been described (6, 119). The detection and identification of *E. bieneusi* and the different *Encephalitozoon* spp. have been successfully performed with fresh stool specimens, formalin-fixed stool specimens, intestinal tissue obtained by endoscopic biopsy, urine specimens, and other body fluids. A real-time PCR method was developed for quantitation of *E. bieneusi* DNA (120) and *E. intestinalis* DNA (121) in stool specimens. An assay based on the loop-mediated isothermal amplification technique (LAMP) was established for *E. bieneusi* (122). Furthermore, *in situ* hybridization to visualize *E. bieneusi* in tissue sections has been developed (123).

ISOLATION OF MICROSPORIDIA

Microsporidia cannot be grown axenically. *Encephalitozoon* spp., *T. hominis*, *V. corneae*, and *A. algerae* have been isolated with different cell culture systems, including RK-13 (rabbit kidney), MDCK (Madin-Darby canine kidney), MRC-5 (human embryonic lung fibroblast) cells, and other cells (46, 124, 125). Only short-term *in vitro* propagation has been accomplished with *E. bieneusi*. The isolation of microsporidia has no relevance for diagnostic purposes but is an important research tool.

IDENTIFICATION

The identification of microsporidia and their taxonomy have been based primarily upon ultrastructural characteristics. Microsporidial ultrastructure is unique and pathognomonic for the phylum; ultrastructural features can distinguish all microsporidial genera (Fig. 1) (46). Nevertheless, morphologic features alone do not sufficiently characterize all microsporidial species pathogenic for humans. The characterization of the three *Encephalitozoon* spp., which share most of their morphologic features, requires genetic analyses, which may also reveal subtype-specific variation (30, 32). Identification of novel microsporidial species can be achieved by phylogenetic analyses of gene sequences derived from PCRs with panmicrosporidian primers (3, 6, 23, 45, 119, 124, 126).

SEROLOGIC TESTS

Serologic assays (including the carbon immunoassay, indirect immunofluorescence test, enzyme-linked immunosorbent assay, and Western blot immunodetection) have been useful in detecting specific antibodies to *E. cuniculi* in several species of animals. However, the value of such tests for humans has been discussed controversially because of possible cross-reactivity of the spore wall antigens of the *Encephalitozoon* species. Furthermore, results of serologic studies with humans were not substantiated by the detection of organisms in individuals with antibody responses. By employing recombinant antigens of the polar tube of *E. cuniculi*, improved specificity was demonstrated, and the development of serodiagnostic tools seems feasible (127).

ANTIMICROBIAL SUSCEPTIBILITIES

Albendazole has been found to cause growth deformities of *Encephalitozoon* and *Vittaforma* and to reduce or eradicate the organisms propagated in cell cultures but does not destroy mature microsporidial spores; thus, these may sustain infection (128). Fumagillin, its analog TNP-470, nikkomycin Z, and fluoroquinolones have been shown *in vitro* to inhibit completely or partially the replication or spore germination of *Encephalitozoon* and *Vittaforma* (128, 129). *In vitro* systems to investigate *E. bieneusi* are not available.

Treatment studies with humans are limited, and only two randomized controlled trials have been conducted (130, 131). Albendazole can result in clinical cure of HIV-associated encephalitozoonosis in parallel with the cessation of spore excretion (130). A case report suggested treatment response of a disseminated *T. acridophagus* infection to albendazole (43). In contrast, albendazole is not effective against *Enterocytozoon* infection and does not reduce pathogen load, although previous observations had suggested that clinical improvement may occur in some patients. Orally applied fumagillin appeared to eliminate *E. bieneusi* in severely immunodeficient HIV-infected patients (131), in renal transplant recipients (132), and in stem cell transplant recipients (72), but serious adverse events have also been reported (131, 133).

Enterocytozoon bieneusi-associated diarrhea as well as systemic infection due to *Encephalitozoon* spp. is mainly observed in severely immunodeficient patients. Improvement of immune functions by antiretroviral therapy results in complete clinical response and normalization of intestinal architecture, which parallel the clearance of intestinal microsporidia (134).

Microsporidial keratoconjunctivitis may be a self-limiting disease (135, 136), may be cleared by repeated corneal swabbing or debridement (137–139), and may respond to systemic albendazole treatment (140) or to topical voriconazole application (141).

EVALUATION, INTERPRETATION, AND REPORTING OF RESULTS

Microsporidia are predominantly opportunistic pathogens capable of causing disease in severely immunodeficient HIV-infected persons (with CD4 cell counts below 200/μl) and otherwise immunocompromised patients, including organ transplant recipients. Therefore, stool examination or examination of other specimens is particularly indicated for these patient groups, and it is prudent to consider microsporidia as the etiologic agents when they are detected in clinical specimens from such patients. Furthermore, various microsporidial species may cause self-limited diarrhea or keratoconjunctivitis in immunocompetent and otherwise healthy persons.

Routine diagnosis of microsporidiosis is based upon microscopic detection of microsporidial spores. Although sensitive and specific, light-microscopic examination does not allow the identification of the organisms to the genus and species level. This can be achieved in most cases by electron microscopy, which is relatively insensitive for the detection of microsporidia because only small samples are examined and sampling errors may occur, or by PCR assays and further sequence analyses. Immunocompetent patients may excrete lower numbers of microsporidial spores in feces or urine; therefore, the threshold of the current light-microscopic detection procedures may not be sufficient for the reliable detection of microsporidia in this group.

REFERENCES

1. **Weber R, Bryan RT, Schwartz DA, Owen RL.** 1994. Human microsporidial infections. *Clin Microbiol Rev* **7:**426–461.
2. **Wittner M, Weiss LM.** 1999. *The Microsporidia and Microsporidiosis*. ASM Press, Washington, DC.
3. **Mathis A, Weber R, Deplazes P.** 2005. Zoonotic potential of the microsporidia. *Clin Microbiol Rev* **18:**423–445.
4. **Didier ES, Weiss LM.** 2011. Microsporidiosis: not just in AIDS patients. *Curr Opin Infect Dis* **24:**490–495.
5. **Vávra J, Lukeš J.** 2013. Microsporidia and 'the art of living together'. *Adv Parasitol* **82:**253–319.
6. **Weiss LM, Becnel JJ.** 2014. *Microsporidia: Pathogens of Opportunity*. John Wiley & Sons, Chichester, United Kingdom.
7. **Weber R, Deplazes P, Mathis A.** 2015. Microsporidia, p 2209–2219. *In* Jorgensen JH, Pfaller MA, Carroll KC, Funke G, Landry ML, Richter SS, Warnock DW (ed), *Manual of Clinical Microbiology*, 11th ed, vol 2. ASM Press, Washington, DC.
8. **Han B, Polonais V, Sugi T, Yakubu R, Takvorian PM, Cali A, Maier K, Long M, Levy M, Tanowitz HB, Pan G, Delbac F, Zhou Z, Weiss LM.** 2017. The role of microsporidian polar tube protein 4 (PTP4) in host cell infection. *PLoS Pathog* **13:**e1006341.
9. **Katinka MD, Duprat S, Cornillot E, Méténier G, Thomarat F, Prensier G, Barbe V, Peyretaillade E, Brottier P, Wincker P, Delbac F, El Alaoui H, Peyret P, Saurin W, Gouy M, Weissenbach J, Vivarès CP.** 2001. Genome sequence and gene compaction of the eukaryote parasite *Encephalitozoon cuniculi*. *Nature* **414:**450–453.

10. **Akiyoshi DE, Morrison HG, Lei S, Feng X, Zhang Q, Corradi N, Mayanja H, Tumwine JK, Keeling PJ, Weiss LM, Tzipori S.** 2009. Genomic survey of the non-cultivatable opportunistic human pathogen, *Enterocytozoon bieneusi*. *PLoS Pathog* **5:**e1000261.
11. **Williams BA, Lee RC, Becnel JJ, Weiss LM, Fast NM, Keeling PJ.** 2008. Genome sequence surveys of *Brachiola algerae* and *Edhazardia aedis* reveal microsporidia with low gene densities. *BMC Genomics* **9:**200.
12. **Heinz E, Williams TA, Nakjang S, Noël CJ, Swan DC, Goldberg AV, Harris SR, Weinmaier T, Markert S, Becher D, Bernhardt J, Dagan T, Hacker C, Lucocq JM, Schweder T, Rattei T, Hall N, Hirt RP, Embley TM.** 2012. The genome of the obligate intracellular parasite *Trachipleistophora hominis*: new insights into microsporidian genome dynamics and reductive evolution. *PLoS Pathog* **8:**e1002979.
13. **Corradi N.** 2015. Microsporidia: eukaryotic intracellular parasites shaped by gene loss and horizontal gene transfers. *Annu Rev Microbiol* **69:**167–183.
14. **Dean P, Hirt RP, Embley TM.** 2016. Microsporidia: why make nucleotides if you can steal them? *PLoS Pathog* **12:**e1005870.
15. **Williams TA, Nakjang S, Campbell SE, Freeman MA, Eydal M, Moore K, Hirt RP, Embley TM, Williams BA.** 2016. A recent whole-genome duplication divides populations of a globally distributed microsporidian. *Mol Biol Evol* **33:**2002–2015.
16. **Vossbrinck CR, Maddox JV, Friedman S, Debrunner-Vossbrinck BA, Woese CR.** 1987. Ribosomal RNA sequence suggests microsporidia are extremely ancient eukaryotes. *Nature* **326:**411–414.
17. **Williams BA, Hirt RP, Lucocq JM, Embley TM.** 2002. A mitochondrial remnant in the microsporidian *Trachipleistophora hominis*. *Nature* **418:**865–869.
18. **Vávra J.** 2005. "Polar vesicles" of microsporidia are mitochondrial remnants ("mitosomes")? *Folia Parasitol (Praha)* **52:** 193–195.
19. **Hibbett DS, et al.** 2007. A higher-level phylogenetic classification of the Fungi. *Mycol Res* **111:**509–547.
20. **James TY, et al.** 2006. Reconstructing the early evolution of Fungi using a six-gene phylogeny. *Nature* **443:**818–822.
21. **Lee SC, Corradi N, Byrnes EJ III, Torres-Martinez S, Dietrich FS, Keeling PJ, Heitman J.** 2008. Microsporidia evolved from ancestral sexual fungi. *Curr Biol* **18:**1675–1679.
22. **James TY, Pelin A, Bonen L, Ahrendt S, Sain D, Corradi N, Stajich JE.** 2013. Shared signatures of parasitism and phylogenomics unite Cryptomycota and microsporidia. *Curr Biol* **23:**1548–1553.
23. **Keeling PJ.** 2014. Phylogenetic place of Microsporidia in the tree of eukaryotes, p 195–202. *In* Weiss L, Becnel JJ (ed), *Microsporidia: Pathogens of Opportunity*. John Wiley & Sons, Chichester, United Kingdom.
24. **Jones MD, Forn I, Gadelha C, Egan MJ, Bass D, Massana R, Richards TA.** 2011. Discovery of novel intermediate forms redefines the fungal tree of life. *Nature* **474:**200–203.
25. **Jones MD, Richards TA, Hawksworth DL, Bass D.** 2011. Validation and justification of the phylum name *Cryptomycota* phyl. nov. *IMA Fungus* **2:**173–175.
26. **Franzen C, Nassonova ES, Schölmerich J, Issi IV.** 2006. Transfer of the members of the genus *Brachiola* (microsporidia) to the genus *Anncaliia* based on ultrastructural and molecular data. *J Eukaryot Microbiol* **53:**26–35.
27. **Cali A, Takvorian PM, Lewin S, Rendel M, Sian CS, Wittner M, Tanowitz HB, Keohane E, Weiss LM.** 1998. *Brachiola vesicularum*, n. g., n. sp., a new microsporidium associated with AIDS and myositis. *J Eukaryot Microbiol* **45:**240–251.
28. **Margileth AM, Strano AJ, Chandra R, Neafie R, Blum M, McCully RM.** 1973. Disseminated nosematosis in an immunologically compromised infant. *Arch Pathol* **95:**145–150.
29. **Cali A, Weiss LM, Takvorian PM.** 2004. An analysis of the microsporidian genus *Brachiola*, with comparisons of human and insect isolates of *Brachiola algerae*. *J Eukaryot Microbiol* **51:**678–685.
30. **Didier ES, Didier PJ, Friedberg DN, Stenson SM, Orenstein JM, Vee RW, Tio FO, Davis RM, Vossbrinck C, Millichamp N, Shadduck JA.** 1991. Isolation and characterization of a new human microsporidian, *Encephalitozoon hellem* (n. sp.), from three AIDS patients with keratoconjunctivitis. *J Infect Dis* **163:**617–621.
31. **Cali A, Kotler DP, Orenstein JM.** 1993. *Septata intestinalis* N. G., N. Sp., an intestinal microsporidian associated with chronic diarrhea and dissemination in AIDS patients. *J Eukaryot Microbiol* **40:**101–112.
32. **Didier ES, Vossbrinck CR, Baker MD, Rogers LB, Bertucci DC, Shadduck JA.** 1995. Identification and characterization of three *Encephalitozoon cuniculi* strains. *Parasitology* **111:**411–421.
33. **Hinney B, Sak B, Joachim A, Kváč M.** 2016. More than a rabbit's tale—*Encephalitozoon* spp. in wild mammals and birds. *Int J Parasitol Parasites Wildl* **5:**76–87.
34. **Suankratay C, Thiansukhon E, Nilaratanakul V, Putaporntip C, Jongwutiwes S.** 2012. Disseminated infection caused by novel species of Microsporidium, Thailand. *Emerg Infect Dis* **18:**302–304.
35. **Pariyakanok L, Satitpitakul V, Putaporntip C, Jongwutiwes S.** 2015. Femtosecond laser-assisted anterior lamellar keratoplasty in stromal keratitis caused by an Endoreticulatus-like microsporidia. *Cornea* **34:**588–591.
36. **Desportes I, Le Charpentier Y, Galian A, Bernard F, Cochand-Priollet B, Lavergne A, Ravisse P, Modigliani R.** 1985. Occurrence of a new Microsporidan: *Enterocytozoon bieneusi* n.g., n. sp., in the enterocytes of a human patient with AIDS. *J Protozool* **32:**250–254.
37. **Santín-Durán M.** 2015. *Enterocytozoon bieneusi*, p149–174. *In* Xiao L, Ryan U, Feng Y (ed), *Biology of Foodborne Parasites*. CRC Press.
38. **Cali A, Takvorian PM.** 2003. Ultrastructure and development of *Pleistophora ronneafiei* n. sp., a microsporidium (Protista) in the skeletal muscle of an immune-compromised individual. *J Eukaryot Microbiol* **50:**77–85.
39. **Hollister WS, Canning EU, Weidner E, Field AS, Kench J, Marriott DJ.** 1996. Development and ultrastructure of *Trachipleistophora hominis* n.g., n.sp. after in vitro isolation from an AIDS patient and inoculation into athymic mice. *Parasitology* **112:**143–154.
40. **Vávra J, Yachnis AT, Shadduck JA, Orenstein JM.** 1998. Microsporidia of the genus Trachipleistophora—causative agents of human microsporidiosis: description of *Trachipleistophora anthropophthera* n. sp. (Protozoa: Microsporidia). *J Eukaryot Microbiol* **45:**273–283.
41. **Choudhary MM, Metcalfe MG, Arrambide K, Bern C, Visvesvara GS, Pieniazek NJ, Bandea RD, Deleon-Carnes M, Adem P, Choudhary MM, Zaki SR, Saeed MU.** 2011. *Tubulinosema* sp. microsporidian myositis in immunosuppressed patient. *Emerg Infect Dis* **17:**1727–1730.
42. **Meissner EG, Bennett JE, Qvarnstrom Y, da Silva A, Chu EY, Tsokos M, Gea-Banacloche J.** 2012. Disseminated microsporidiosis in an immunosuppressed patient. *Emerg Infect Dis* **18:**1155–1158.
43. **Connors WJ, Carson JA, Chan WW, Parkins MD.** 2017. Albendazole-responsive disseminated *Tubulinosema acridophagus* in a patient with chronic lymphocytic leukaemia. *Clin Microbiol Infect* **23:**684–685.
44. **Silveira H, Canning EU.** 1995. *Vittaforma corneae* n. comb. for the human microsporidium *Nosema corneum* Shadduck, Meccoli, Davis & Font, 1990, based on its ultrastructure in the liver of experimentally infected athymic mice. *J Eukaryot Microbiol* **42:**158–165.
45. **Deplazes P, Mathis A, van Saanen M, Iten A, Keller R, Tanner I, Glauser MP, Weber R, Canning EU.** 1998. Dual microsporidial infection due to *Vittaforma corneae* and *Encephalitozoon hellem* in a patient with AIDS. *Clin Infect Dis* **27:**1521–1524.
46. **Canning EU.** 1993. Microsporidia, p 299–370. *In* Kreier JP (ed), *Parasitic Protozoa*, vol 6. Academic Press, London, United Kingdom.
47. **Weyrich LS, Duchene S, Soubrier J, Arriola L, Llamas B, Breen J, Morris AG, Alt KW, Caramelli D, Dresely V, Farrell M, Farrer AG, Francken M, Gully N, Haak W, Hardy K,**

Harvati K, Held P, Holmes EC, Kaidonis J, Lalueza-Fox C, de la Rasilla M, Rosas A, Semal P, Soltysiak A, Townsend G, Usai D, Wahl J, Huson DH, Dobney K, Cooper A. 2017. Neanderthal behaviour, diet, and disease inferred from ancient DNA in dental calculus. *Nature* **544:**357–361.

48. **Weber R, Kuster H, Visvesvara GS, Bryan RT, Schwartz DA, Lüthy R.** 1993. Disseminated microsporidiosis due to *Encephalitozoon hellem*: pulmonary colonization, microhematuria, and mild conjunctivitis in a patient with AIDS. *Clin Infect Dis* **17:**415–419.
49. **Lam TS, Wong MH, Chuang SK.** 2013. Microsporidial keratoconjunctivitis outbreak among athletes from Hong Kong who visited Singapore, 2012. *Emerg Infect Dis* **19:**516–517.
50. **Fan NW, Wu CC, Chen TL, Yu WK, Chen CP, Lee SM, Lin PY.** 2012. Microsporidial keratitis in patients with hot springs exposure. *J Clin Microbiol* **50:**414–418.
51. **Stentiford GD, Feist SW, Stone DM, Bateman KS, Dunn AM.** 2013. Microsporidia: diverse, dynamic, and emergent pathogens in aquatic systems. *Trends Parasitol* **29:**567–578.
52. **Stentiford GD, Becnel JJ, Weiss LM, Keeling PJ, Didier ES, Williams BA, Bjornson S, Kent ML, Freeman MA, Brown MJ, Troemel ER, Roesel K, Sokolova Y, Snowden KF, Solter L.** 2016. Microsporidia—emergent pathogens in the global food chain. *Trends Parasitol* **32:**336–348.
53. **Decraene V, Lebbad M, Botero-Kleiven S, Gustavsson AM, Löfdahl M.** 2012. First reported foodborne outbreak associated with microsporidia, Sweden, October 2009. *Epidemiol Infect* **140:**519–527.
54. **Jedrzejewski S, Graczyk TK, Slodkowicz-Kowalska A, Tamang L, Majewska AC.** 2007. Quantitative assessment of contamination of fresh food produce of various retail types by human-virulent microsporidian spores. *Appl Environ Microbiol* **73:**4071–4073.
55. **Kváč M, Tomanová V, Samková E, Koubová J, Kotková M, Hlásková L, McEvoy J, Sak B.** 2016. *Encephalitozoon cuniculi* in raw cow's milk remains infectious after pasteurization. *Foodborne Pathog Dis* **13:**77–79.
56. **Deplazes P, Mathis A, Müller C, Weber R.** 1996. Molecular epidemiology of *Encephalitozoon cuniculi* and first detection of *Enterocytozoon bieneusi* in faecal samples of pigs. *J Eukaryot Microbiol* **43:**93S.
57. **Talabani H, Sarfati C, Pillebout E, van Gool T, Derouin F, Menotti J.** 2010. Disseminated infection with a new genovar of *Encephalitozoon cuniculi* in a renal transplant recipient. *J Clin Microbiol* **48:**2651–2653.
58. **Bart A, Wentink-Bonnema EM, Heddema ER, Buijs J, van Gool T.** 2008. Frequent occurrence of human-associated microsporidia in fecal droppings of urban pigeons in Amsterdam, the Netherlands. *Appl Environ Microbiol* **74:**7056–7058.
59. **Bornay-Llinares FJ, da Silva AJ, Moura H, Schwartz DA, Visvesvara GS, Pieniazek NJ, Cruz-López A, Hernández-Jaúregui P, Guerrero J, Enriquez FJ.** 1998. Immunologic, microscopic, and molecular evidence of *Encephalitozoon intestinalis* (*Septata intestinalis*) infection in mammals other than humans. *J Infect Dis* **178:**820–826.
60. **Li W, Cama V, Akinbo FO, Ganguly S, Kiulia NM, Zhang X, Xiao L.** 2013. Multilocus sequence typing of *Enterocytozoon bieneusi:* lack of geographic segregation and existence of genetically isolated sub-populations. *Infect Genet Evol* **14:**111–119.
61. **Yang J, Song M, Wan Q, Li Y, Lu Y, Jiang Y, Tao W, Li W.** 2014. *Enterocytozoon bieneusi* genotypes in children in Northeast China and assessment of risk of zoonotic transmission. *J Clin Microbiol* **52:**4363–4367.
62. **Coyle CM, Weiss LM, Rhodes LV III, Cali A, Takvorian PM, Brown DF, Visvesvara GS, Xiao L, Naktin J, Young E, Gareca M, Colasante G, Wittner M.** 2004. Fatal myositis due to the microsporidian *Brachiola algerae*, a mosquito pathogen. *N Engl J Med* **351:**42–47.
63. **Visvesvara GS, Belloso M, Moura H, Da Silva AJ, Moura IN, Leitch GJ, Schwartz DA, Chevez-Barrios P, Wallace S, Pieniazek NJ, Goosey JD.** 1999. Isolation of *Nosema algerae* from the cornea of an immunocompetent patient. *J Eukaryot Microbiol* **46:**10S.
64. **Smith RM, Muehlenbachs A, Schaenmann J, Baxi S, Koo S, Blau D, Chin-Hong P, Thorner AR, Kuehnert MJ, Wheeler K, Liakos A, Jackson JW, Benedict T, da Silva AJ, Ritter JM, Rollin D, Metcalfe M, Goldsmith CS, Visvesvara GS, Basavaraju SV, Zaki S.** 2017. Three cases of neurologic syndrome caused by donor-derived microsporidiosis. *Emerg Infect Dis* **23:**387–395.
65. **Kicia M, Wesolowska M, Kopacz Z, Jakuszko K, Sak B, Kvetonova D, Krajewska M, Kvac M.** 2016. Prevalence and molecular characteristics of urinary and intestinal microsporidia infections in renal transplant recipients. *Clin Microbiol Infect* **22:**462.e5–9.
66. **Ladapo TA, Nourse P, Pillay K, Frean J, Birkhead M, Poonsamy B, Gajjar P.** 2014. Microsporidiosis in pediatric renal transplant patients in Cape Town, South Africa: two case reports. *Pediatr Transplant* **18:**E220–E226.
67. **Hocevar SN, Paddock CD, Spak CW, Rosenblatt R, Diaz-Luna H, Castillo I, Luna S, Friedman GC, Antony S, Stoddard RA, Tiller RV, Peterson T, Blau DM, Sriram RR, da Silva A, de Almeida M, Benedict T, Goldsmith CS, Zaki SR, Visvesvara GS, Kuehnert MJ, Microsporidia Transplant Transmission Investigation Team.** 2014. Microsporidiosis acquired through solid organ transplantation: a public health investigation. *Ann Intern Med* **160:**213–220.
68. **Nagpal A, Pritt BS, Lorenz EC, Amer H, Nasr SH, Cornell LD, Iqbal S, Wilhelm MP.** 2013. Disseminated microsporidiosis in a renal transplant recipient: case report and review of the literature. *Transpl Infect Dis* **15:**526–532.
69. **George B, Coates T, McDonald S, Russ G, Cherian S, Nolan J, Brealey J.** 2012. Disseminated microsporidiosis with *Encephalitozoon* species in a renal transplant recipient. *Nephrology (Carlton)* **17**(Suppl 1)**:**5–8.
70. **Ramanan P, Pritt BS.** 2014. Extraintestinal microsporidiosis. *J Clin Microbiol* **52:**3839–3844.
71. **Ambrosioni J, van Delden C, Krause KH, Bouchuiguir-Wafa C, Nagy M, Passweg J, Chalandon Y.** 2010. Invasive microsporidiosis in allogeneic haematopoietic SCT recipients. *Bone Marrow Transplant* **45:**1249–1251.
72. **Bukreyeva I, Angoulvant A, Bendib I, Gagnard JC, Bourhis JH, Dargère S, Bonhomme J, Thellier M, Gachot B, Wyplosz B.** 2017. *Enterocytozoon bieneusi* microsporidiosis in stem cell transplant recipients treated with Fumagillin 1. *Emerg Infect Dis* **23:**1039–1041.
73. **Desoubeaux G, Caumont C, Passot C, Dartigeas C, Bailly E, Chandenier J, Duong TH.** 2012. Two cases of opportunistic parasite infections in patients receiving alemtuzumab. *J Clin Pathol* **65:**92–95.
74. **Aikawa NE, Twardowsky AO, Carvalho JF, Silva CA, Silva IL, Ribeiro AC, Saad CG, Moraes JC, Toledo RA, Bonfá E.** 2011. Intestinal microsporidiosis: a hidden risk in rheumatic disease patients undergoing anti-tumor necrosis factor therapy combined with disease-modifying anti-rheumatic drugs? *Clinics (Sao Paulo)* **66:**1171–1175.
75. **Lores B, López-Miragaya I, Arias C, Fenoy S, Torres J, del Aguila C.** 2002. Intestinal microsporidiosis due to *Enterocytozoon bieneusi* in elderly human immunodeficiency virus—negative patients from Vigo, Spain. *Clin Infect Dis* **34:**918–921.
76. **Mor SM, Tumwine JK, Naumova EN, Ndeezi G, Tzipori S.** 2009. Microsporidiosis and malnutrition in children with persistent diarrhea, Uganda. *Emerg Infect Dis* **15:**49–52.
77. **Tan J, Lee P, Lai Y, Hishamuddin P, Tay J, Tan AL, Chan KS, Lin R, Tan D, Cutter J, Goh KT.** 2013. Microsporidial keratoconjunctivitis after rugby tournament, Singapore. *Emerg Infect Dis* **19:**1484–1486.
78. **Garg P.** 2013. Microsporidia infection of the cornea—a unique and challenging disease. *Cornea* **32**(Suppl 1)**:**S33–S38.
79. **Agashe R, Radhakrishnan N, Pradhan S, Srinivasan M, Prajna VN, Lalitha P.** 2017. Clinical and demographic study of microsporidial keratoconjunctivitis in South India: a 3-year study (2013–2015). *Br J Ophthalmol* **101:**1436–1439.
80. **Theng J, Chan C, Ling ML, Tan D.** 2001. Microsporidial keratoconjunctivitis in a healthy contact lens wearer without human immunodeficiency virus infection. *Ophthalmology* **108:**976–978.

81. **Gautam, Jhanji V, Satpathy G, Khokhar S, Agarwal T.** 2013. Microsporidial keratitis after collagen cross-linking. *Ocul Immunol Inflamm* **21:**495–497.
82. **Wright SG.** 2012. Protozoan infections of the gastrointestinal tract. *Infect Dis Clin North Am* **26:**323–339.
83. **Matsubayashi H, Koike T, Mikata I, Takei H, Hagiwara S.** 1959. A case of *Encephalitozoon*-like body infection in man. *AMA Arch Pathol* **67:**181–187.
84. **Bergquist NR, Stintzing G, Smedman L, Waller T, Andersson T.** 1984. Diagnosis of encephalitozoonosis in man by serological tests. *Br Med J (Clin Res Ed)* **288:**902.
85. **Weber R, Deplazes P, Flepp M, Mathis A, Baumann R, Sauer B, Kuster H, Lüthy R.** 1997. Cerebral microsporidiosis due to *Encephalitozoon cuniculi* in a patient with human immunodeficiency virus infection. *N Engl J Med* **336:**474–478.
86. **Mertens RB, Didier ES, Fishbein MC, Bertucci DC, Rogers LB, Orenstein JM.** 1997. *Encephalitozoon cuniculi* microsporidiosis: infection of the brain, heart, kidneys, trachea, adrenal glands, and urinary bladder in a patient with AIDS. *Mod Pathol* **10:**68–77.
87. **Okuyama H, Kanamori M, Watanabe M, Kumabe T, Tominaga T.** 2008. [Multiple intracerebral enhanced lesions strongly suspected to be microsporidiosis. A case report]. *No Shinkei Geka* **36:**645–650.
88. **Ditrich O, Chrdle A, Sak B, Chmelík V, Kubále J, Dyková I, Kváс M.** 2011. *Encephalitozoon cuniculi* genotype I as a causative agent of brain abscess in an immunocompetent patient. *J Clin Microbiol* **49:**2769–2771.
89. **Loignon M, Labrecque LG, Bard C, Robitaille Y, Toma E.** 2014. Cerebral microsporidiosis manifesting as progressive multifocal leukoencephalopathy in an HIV-infected individual—a case report. *AIDS Res Ther* **11:**20.
90. **Sak B, Kváč M, Kučerová Z, Květoňová D, Saková K.** 2011. Latent microsporidial infection in immunocompetent individuals—a longitudinal study. *PLoS Negl Trop Dis* **5:**e1162.
91. **Moretto MM, Khan IA, Weiss LM.** 2012. Gastrointestinal cell mediated immunity and the microsporidia. *PLoS Pathog* **8:**e1002775.
92. **Ghosh K, Weiss LM.** 2012. T cell response and persistence of the microsporidia. *FEMS Microbiol Rev* **36:**748–760.
93. **Szumowski SC, Troemel ER.** 2015. Microsporidia-host interactions. *Curr Opin Microbiol* **26:**10–16.
94. **Weber R, Ledergerber B, Zbinden R, Altwegg M, Pfyffer GE, Spycher MA, Briner J, Kaiser L, Opravil M, Meyenberger C, Flepp M.** 1999. Enteric infections and diarrhea in human immunodeficiency virus-infected persons: prospective community-based cohort study. Swiss HIV Cohort Study. *Arch Intern Med* **159:**1473–1480.
95. **Weber R, Kuster H, Keller R, Bächi T, Spycher MA, Briner J, Russi E, Lüthy R.** 1992. Pulmonary and intestinal microsporidiosis in a patient with the acquired immunodeficiency syndrome. *Am Rev Respir Dis* **146:**1603–1605.
96. **Agholi M, Hatam GR, Motazedian MH.** 2013. Microsporidia and coccidia as causes of persistence diarrhea among liver transplant children: incidence rate and species/genotypes. *Pediatr Infect Dis J* **32:**185–187.
97. **Breton J, Bart-Delabesse E, Biligui S, Carbone A, Seiller X, Okome-Nkoumou M, Nzamba C, Kombila M, Accoceberry I, Thellier M.** 2007. New highly divergent rRNA sequence among biodiverse genotypes of *Enterocytozoon bieneusi* strains isolated from humans in Gabon and Cameroon. *J Clin Microbiol* **45:**2580–2589.
98. **Filho MM, Ribeiro HB, Paula LJ, Nishioka SA, Tamaki WT, Costa R, Siqueira SF, Kawakami JT, Higuchi ML.** 2009. Images in cardiovascular medicine. Endocarditis secondary to microsporidia: giant vegetation in a pacemaker user. *Circulation* **119:**e386–e388.
99. **Kester KE, Turiansky GW, McEvoy PL.** 1998. Nodular cutaneous microsporidiosis in a patient with AIDS and successful treatment with long-term oral clindamycin therapy. *Ann Intern Med* **128:**911–914.
100. **Enriquez FJ, Taren D, Cruz-López A, Muramoto M, Palting JD, Cruz P.** 1998. Prevalence of intestinal encephalitozoonosis in Mexico. *Clin Infect Dis* **26:**1227–1229.
101. **Raynaud L, Delbac F, Broussolle V, Rabodonirina M, Girault V, Wallon M, Cozon G, Vivares CP, Peyron F.** 1998. Identification of *Encephalitozoon intestinalis* in travelers with chronic diarrhea by specific PCR amplification. *J Clin Microbiol* **36:**37–40.
102. **Mason E, Foster R, Wray L, McNulty A, Donovan B.** 2016. Reactive arthritis following a Microsporidia infection. *Int J STD AIDS* **27:**1239–1241.
103. **Ledford DK, Overman MD, Gonzalvo A, Cali A, Mester SW, Lockey RF.** 1985. Microsporidiosis myositis in a patient with the acquired immunodeficiency syndrome. *Ann Intern Med* **102:**628–630.
104. **Field AS, Marriott DJ, Milliken ST, Brew BJ, Canning EU, Kench JG, Darveniza P, Harkness JL.** 1996. Myositis associated with a newly described microsporidian, *Trachipleistophora hominis*, in a patient with AIDS. *J Clin Microbiol* **34:**2803–2811.
105. **Watts MR, Chan RC, Cheong EY, Brammah S, Clezy KR, Tong C, Marriott D, Webb CE, Chacko B, Tobias V, Outhred AC, Field AS, Prowse MV, Bertouch JV, Stark D, Reddel SW.** 2014. *Anncaliia algerae* microsporidial myositis. *Emerg Infect Dis* **20:**185–191.
106. **Visvesvara GS, Moura H, Leitch GJ, Schwartz DA, Xiao LX.** 2005. Public health importance of *Brachiola algerae* (Microsporidia)—an emerging pathogen of humans. *Folia Parasitol (Praha)* **52:**83–94.
107. **Yachnis AT, Berg J, Martinez-Salazar A, Bender BS, Diaz L, Rojiani AM, Eskin TA, Orenstein JM.** 1996. Disseminated microsporidiosis especially infecting the brain, heart, and kidneys. Report of a newly recognized pansporoblastic species in two symptomatic AIDS patients. *Am J Clin Pathol* **106:**535–543.
108. **Weber R, Schwartz DA, Deplazes P.** 1999. Laboratory diagnosis of microsporidiosis, p 315–362. *In* Wittner M (ed), *The Microsporidia and Microsporidiosis*. ASM Press, Washington, DC.
109. **Weber R, Bryan RT, Owen RL, Wilcox CM, Gorelkin L, Visvesvara GS, The Enteric Opportunistic Infections Working Group.** 1992. Improved light-microscopical detection of microsporidia spores in stool and duodenal aspirates. *N Engl J Med* **326:**161–166.
110. **Vávra J, Dahbiová R, Hollister WS, Canning EU.** 1993. Staining of microsporidian spores by optical brighteners with remarks on the use of brighteners for the diagnosis of AIDS associated human microsporidioses. *Folia Parasitol (Praha)* **40:**267–272.
111. **van Gool T, Snijders F, Reiss P, Eeftinck Schattenkerk JK, van den Bergh Weerman MA, Bartelsman JF, Bruins JJ, Canning EU, Dankert J.** 1993. Diagnosis of intestinal and disseminated microsporidial infections in patients with HIV by a new rapid fluorescence technique. *J Clin Pathol* **46:**694–699.
112. **Didier ES, Orenstein JM, Aldras A, Bertucci D, Rogers LB, Janney FA.** 1995. Comparison of three staining methods for detecting microsporidia in fluids. *J Clin Microbiol* **33:**3138–3145.
113. **Ignatius R, Lehmann M, Miksits K, Regnath T, Arvand M, Engelmann E, Futh U, Hahn H, Wagner J.** 1997. A new acid-fast trichrome stain for simultaneous detection of *Cryptosporidium parvum* and microsporidial species in stool specimens. *J Clin Microbiol* **35:**446–449.
114. **Moura H, Schwartz DA, Bornay-Llinares F, Sodré FC, Wallace S, Visvesvara GS.** 1997. A new and improved "quick-hot Gram-chromotrope" technique that differentially stains microsporidian spores in clinical samples, including paraffin-embedded tissue sections. *Arch Pathol Lab Med* **121:**888–893.
115. **Enriquez FJ, Ditrich O, Palting JD, Smith K.** 1997. Simple diagnosis of *Encephalitozoon* sp. microsporidial infections by using a panspecific antiexospore monoclonal antibody. *J Clin Microbiol* **35:**724–729.
116. **Accoceberry I, Thellier M, Desportes-Livage I, Achbarou A, Biligui S, Danis M, Datry A.** 1999. Production of monoclonal antibodies directed against the microsporidium *Enterocytozoon bieneusi*. *J Clin Microbiol* **37:**4107–4112.

117. **Ghoshal U, Khanduja S, Pant P, Ghoshal UC.** 2016. Evaluation of immunoflourescence antibody assay for the detection of *Enterocytozoon bieneusi* and *Encephalitozoon intestinalis*. *Parasitol Res* **115:**3709–3713.
118. **Field AS, Hing MC, Milliken ST, Marriott DJ.** 1993. Microsporidia in the small intestine of HIV-infected patients. A new diagnostic technique and a new species. *Med J Aust* **158:**390–394.
119. **Weiss LM.**2011. Microsporidiosis, p 598–614. *In* Palmer SR, Soulsby L, Torgerson PR, Brown DWG (ed), *Oxford Textbook of Zoonoses Biology, Clinical Practice, and Public Health Control.* Oxford University Press, New York, NY.
120. **Menotti J, Cassinat B, Porcher R, Sarfati C, Derouin F, Molina JM.** 2003. Development of a real-time polymerase-chain-reaction assay for quantitative detection of *Enterocytozoon bieneusi* DNA in stool specimens from immunocompromised patients with intestinal microsporidiosis. *J Infect Dis* **187:** 1469–1474.
121. **Menotti J, Cassinat B, Sarfati C, Liguory O, Derouin F, Molina JM.** 2003. Development of a real-time PCR assay for quantitative detection of *Encephalitozoon intestinalis* DNA. *J Clin Microbiol* **41:**1410–1413.
122. **Nasarudin SN, Zainudin NS, Bernadus M, Nawi AM, Hanafiah A, Osman E.** 2015. Loop-mediated isothermal amplification for rapid molecular detection of *Enterocytozoon bieneusi* in faecal specimens. *J Med Microbiol* **64:**1329–1334.
123. **Carville A, Mansfield K, Widmer G, Lackner A, Kotler D, Wiest P, Gumbo T, Sarbah S, Tzipori S.** 1997. Development and application of genetic probes for detection of *Enterocytozoon bieneusi* in formalin-fixed stools and in intestinal biopsy specimens from infected patients. *Clin Diagn Lab Immunol* **4:**405–408.
124. **Deplazes P, Mathis A, Baumgartner R, Tanner I, Weber R.** 1996. Immunologic and molecular characteristics of *Encephalitozoon*-like microsporidia isolated from humans and rabbits indicate that *Encephalitozoon cuniculi* is a zoonotic parasite. *Clin Infect Dis* **22:**557–559.
125. **Visvesvara GS.** 2002. In vitro cultivation of microsporidia of clinical importance. *Clin Microbiol Rev* **15:**401–413.
126. **Mathis A, Tanner I, Weber R, Deplazes P.** 1999. Genetic and phenotypic intraspecific variation in the microsporidian *Encephalitozoon hellem*. *Int J Parasitol* **29:**767–770.
127. **van Gool T, Biderre C, Delbac F, Wentink-Bonnema E, Peek R, Vivarès CP.** 2004. Serodiagnostic studies in an immunocompetent individual infected with *Encephalitozoon cuniculi*. *J Infect Dis* **189:**2243–2249.
128. **Didier ES.** 1997. Effects of albendazole, fumagillin, and TNP-470 on microsporidial replication in vitro. *Antimicrob Agents Chemother* **41:**1541–1546.
129. **Didier PJ, Phillips JN, Kuebler DJ, Nasr M, Brindley PJ, Stovall ME, Bowers LC, Didier ES.** 2006. Antimicrosporidial activities of fumagillin, TNP-470, ovalicin, and ovalicin derivatives in vitro and in vivo. *Antimicrob Agents Chemother* **50:**2146–2155.
130. **Molina JM, Chastang C, Goguel J, Michiels JF, Sarfati C, Desportes-Livage I, Horton J, Derouin F, Modaï J.** 1998. Albendazole for treatment and prophylaxis of microsporidiosis due to *Encephalitozoon intestinalis* in patients with AIDS: a randomized double-blind controlled trial. *J Infect Dis* **177:**1373–1377.
131. **Molina JM, Tourneur M, Sarfati C, Chevret S, de Gouvello A, Gobert JG, Balkan S, Derouin F, Agence Nationale de Recherches sur le SIDA 090 Study Group.** 2002. Fumagillin treatment of intestinal microsporidiosis. *N Engl J Med* **346:**1963–1969.
132. **Champion L, Durrbach A, Lang P, Delahousse M, Chauvet C, Sarfati C, Glotz D, Molina JM.** 2010. Fumagillin for treatment of intestinal microsporidiosis in renal transplant recipients. *Am J Transplant* **10:**1925–1930.
133. **Audemard A, Le Bellec ML, Carluer L, Dargère S, Verdon R, Castrale C, Lobbedez T, Hurault de Ligny B.** 2012. Fumagillin-induced aseptic meningoencephalitis in a kidney transplant recipient with microsporidiosis. *Transpl Infect Dis* **14:**E147–E149.
134. **Carr A, Marriott D, Field A, Vasak E, Cooper DA.** 1998. Treatment of HIV-1-associated microsporidiosis and cryptosporidiosis with combination antiretroviral therapy. *Lancet* **351:**256–261.
135. **Das S, Sahu SK, Sharma S, Nayak SS, Kar S.** 2010. Clinical trial of 0.02% polyhexamethylene biguanide versus placebo in the treatment of microsporidial keratoconjunctivitis. *Am J Ophthalmol* **150:**110–115.e2.
136. **Das S, Sharma S, Sahu SK, Nayak SS, Kar S.** 2012. Diagnosis, clinical features and treatment outcome of microsporidial keratoconjunctivitis. *Br J Ophthalmol* **96:**793–795.
137. **Fan NW, Lin PY, Chen TL, Chen CP, Lee SM.** 2012. Treatment of microsporidial keratoconjunctivitis with repeated corneal swabbing. *Am J Ophthalmol* **154:**927–933.e1.
138. **Das S, Wallang BS, Sharma S, Bhadange YV, Balne PK, Sahu SK.** 2014. The efficacy of corneal debridement in the treatment of microsporidial keratoconjunctivitis: a prospective randomized clinical trial. *Am J Ophthalmol* **157:**1151–1155.
139. **Thanathanee O, Athikulwongse R, Anutarapongpan O, Laummaunwai P, Maleewong W, Intapan PM, Suwan-Apichon O.** 2016. Clinical features, risk factors, and treatments of microsporidial epithelial keratitis. *Semin Ophthalmol* **31:**266–270.
140. **Sangit VA, Murthy SI, Garg P.** 2011. Microsporidial stromal keratitis successfully treated with medical therapy: a case report. *Cornea* **30:**1264–1266.
141. **Khandelwal SS, Woodward MA, Hall T, Grossniklaus HE, Stulting RD.** 2011. Treatment of microsporidia keratitis with topical voriconazole monotherapy. *Arch Ophthalmol* **129:**509–510.

ANTIFUNGAL AGENTS AND SUSCEPTIBILITY TEST METHODS

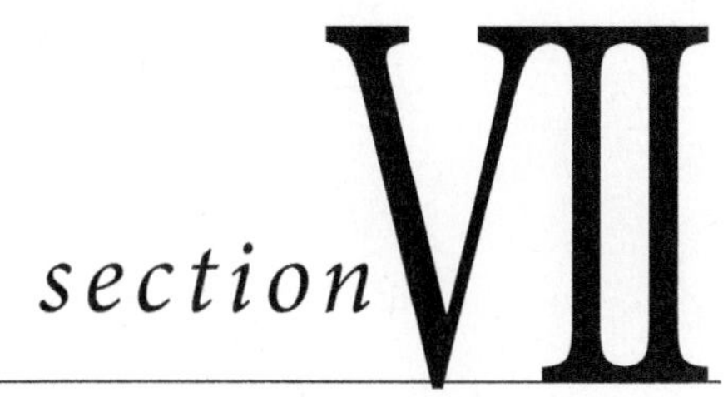

VOLUME EDITOR: DAVID W. WARNOCK

SECTION EDITORS: MARY E. BRANDT AND ELIZABETH M. JOHNSON

Antifungal Agents*

SHAWN R. LOCKHART AND ELIZABETH L. BERKOW

132

After a long period of slow development, we have recently seen the introduction of an important new class of antifungal agents (the echinocandins), expansion of the spectrum of an established class of agents through chemical modification (the triazoles), and the development of novel methods for delivering established agents (lipid-based formulations of amphotericin B). These developments have changed the standards of care for the treatment of many invasive fungal infections, particularly aspergillosis and candidiasis. This chapter reviews the four major families of antifungal drugs that are currently available for systemic administration: the allylamines, the azoles, the echinocandins, and the polyenes. The comparative activities of the major systemic antifungal agents against important groups of fungi are summarized in Table 1. This chapter also discusses the characteristics of the several other agents that can be used for the oral or parenteral treatment of superficial, subcutaneous, or systemic fungal infections. Novel agents that are currently in clinical trials are briefly reviewed.

ALLYLAMINES

The allylamines are a group of synthetic antifungal compounds effective in the topical and oral treatment of dermatophytoses. Two drugs, terbinafine and naftifine, are licensed for clinical use. Naftifine is available only as a topical preparation.

Mechanism of Action

The allylamines inhibit squalene epoxidase, a critical enzyme in the formation of ergosterol, the principal sterol in the membrane of susceptible fungal cells. The consequent accumulation of squalene leads to membrane disruption and cell death (1).

Terbinafine

Terbinafine (Lamisil; Novartis Pharmaceuticals) is a lipophilic drug that is available for oral or topical administration. It is widely used for the treatment of superficial fungal infections caused by dermatophytes.

Spectrum of Activity

Terbinafine is effective against several groups of pathogenic fungi, including dermatophytes (*Epidermophyton*, *Microsporum*, and *Trichophyton* spp.) (2–4) and dematiaceous fungi (5). It also has some activity against *Aspergillus* spp. (6), *Candida* spp. (7), *Blastomyces dermatitidis* and *Histoplasma capsulatum* (8), *Paracoccidioides brasiliensis* (9), *Talaromyces marneffei* (10), and *Sporothrix schenckii* (8).

Acquired Resistance

The development of resistance to terbinafine among dermatophytes even after prolonged exposure is rare.

Pharmacokinetics

Terbinafine is well absorbed after oral administration and is then rapidly and extensively distributed to body tissues (11). It reaches the stratum corneum as a result of diffusion through the dermis and epidermis and secretion in sebum. Diffusion from the nail bed is the major factor in its rapid penetration of nails. Terbinafine has been found to persist in nail for long periods after cessation of treatment. It is extensively metabolized by the human hepatic cytochrome P-450 (CYP) enzyme system, and the inactive metabolites are mostly excreted in the urine (12).

Clinical Use

Terbinafine is the drug of choice for dermatophyte infections of the skin and nails where topical treatment is considered inappropriate or has failed (13, 14). It is not as effective as itraconazole for treatment of fungal nail infections (onychomycosis) involving nondermatophytes, and it may not be as effective in scalp infections with *Microsporum canis*. Terbinafine has also proven effective in some patients with aspergillosis, chromoblastomycosis, and sporotrichosis (15), but it is not licensed for these indications. Anecdotal evidence suggests that the use of terbinafine in combination with voriconazole may be beneficial in the treatment of infections with *Lomentospora prolificans* (16, 17).

Drug Interactions

Although terbinafine is metabolized by the human hepatic CYP enzyme system, it does not inhibit most CYP enzymes at clinically relevant concentrations (12). Blood concentrations of terbinafine are reduced when it is given

*This chapter contains information presented by Shawn R. Lockhart and David W. Warnock in chapter 129 of the 11th edition of this *Manual*.

TABLE 1 Spectrum and extent of activity of commonly used systemic antifungal agents[a]

Organism	Activity[b] of:								
	Amphotericin	Fluconazole	Isavuconazole	Itraconazole	Posaconazole	Voriconazole	Anidulafungin	Caspofungin	Micafungin
Aspergillus spp.	+++	–	+++	++	+++	+++	++	++	++
B. dermatitidis	+++	+	+++	+++	+++	+++	–	–	–
Candida spp.									
C. albicans	+++	+++	+++	+++	+++	+++	+++	+++	+++
C. glabrata	+++	++	++	++	++	++	+++	+++	+++
C. krusei	++	–	+++	+++	+++	+++	+++	+++	+++
C. lusitaniae	++	+++	+++	+++	+++	+++	++	++	++
C. parapsilosis	+++	+++	+++	+++	+++	+++	++	++	++
C. tropicalis	+++	+++	+++	+++	+++	+++	+++	+++	+++
Coccidioides spp.	+++	+++	+++	+++	+++	+++	–	–	–
Cryptococcus spp.	+++	+++	+++	++	+++	+++	–	–	–
Fusarium spp.	++	–	+	+	++	++	–	–	–
H. capsulatum	+++	–	+++	+	++	++	–	–	–
Mucorales	++	–	++	–	++	–	–	–	–
P. brasiliensis	+++	++	+++	+++	+++	+++	–	–	–

[a]This table is a general overview for comparison of the activities of some systemic drugs against various fungi. Readers are referred to the text for more detailed information.

[b]–, no meaningful activity; +, occasional activity; ++, moderate activity but resistance is noted; +++, reliable activity with occasional resistance.

together with drugs, such as rifampin, that induce the hepatic CYP system.

Toxicity and Adverse Effects

Terbinafine produces few adverse reactions. These include abdominal discomfort, nausea, diarrhea, impairment of taste, and transient skin rashes (18). Rare, but serious, side effects include Stevens-Johnson syndrome and hepatotoxic reactions, including cholestasis and hepatitis.

AZOLES

The azoles are a large group of synthetic agents that contains many compounds that are effective in the topical treatment of dermatophyte infections and superficial forms of candidiasis; a number are suitable for systemic administration. Members of this group have in common an imidazole or triazole ring with *N*-carbon substitution. The systemic-use antifungals are the triazoles.

Mechanism of Action

Azole compounds inhibit a fungal CYP-dependent enzyme, lanosterol 14 α-demethylase, which is responsible for the conversion of lanosterol to ergosterol, the principal sterol in the membranes of susceptible fungal cells. This results in the accumulation of various toxic methylated sterols and the depletion of ergosterol, with subsequent disruption of membrane structure and function. The activity is essentially fungistatic, although voriconazole and itraconazole can exert fungicidal effects against *Aspergillus* and some other mold species at concentrations achieved with recommended dosages (19).

Several mechanisms of resistance have been described (see chapter 133). These include upregulation of multidrug efflux transporter genes, upregulation of the *ERG11* gene (which encodes the target enzyme, lanosterol 14 α-demethylase), and decreased affinity of this enzyme for azole agents due to either intrinsic or acquired amino acid substitutions (20, 21). Changes in other enzymes involved in the ergosterol biosynthesis pathway, such as loss of $\Delta^{5,6}$ sterol desaturase activity, may also contribute to azole resistance (20). When azole resistance is efflux mediated, there is often cross-resistance between all of the azoles.

Pharmacokinetics

With the exception of fluconazole and isavuconazole, food has a significant effect on the absorption of azole antifungals. Administration with lipid-rich food improves the absorption of ketoconazole, posaconazole, and the capsule formulation of itraconazole (22, 23). In contrast, absorption of voriconazole and the oral solution formulation of itraconazole is reduced when these agents are given with a high-fat meal (24).

Peak blood concentrations of azoles are typically reached within 2 to 3 h after oral administration. With fluconazole and posaconazole, blood levels increase in proportion to dosage (25). In contrast, increases in itraconazole dosage produce disproportionate changes in peak blood concentrations due to saturable first-pass metabolism in the liver (26). In adults, there is a disproportionate increase in blood levels of voriconazole with increasing oral and parenteral dosage (27). In children, however, increases in dosage produce proportional changes in drug levels, and clearance of the drug is more rapid (28).

Due to its low protein binding (about 12%), fluconazole attains high concentrations in most tissues and body fluids. Levels of the drug in cerebrospinal fluid (CSF) usually exceed 50% of the simultaneous blood concentration (27).

Likewise, voriconazole is extensively distributed into tissues, with CSF levels that are around 30 to 60% of the simultaneous blood concentration (29). Voriconazole and fluconazole concentrations in vitreous and aqueous fluids are around 40 to 50% of the simultaneous blood level, which make them useful for treating endophthalmitis (30). Levels of itraconazole in the CSF are minimal (22).

Levels of itraconazole in tissues, such as lung, liver, brain, and bone, are two to three times higher than in serum. High concentrations are also found in the stratum corneum as a result of drug secretion in sebum (31). Itraconazole has been found to persist in the skin and nails for weeks to months after the end of a course of treatment, thereby allowing intermittent pulse regimens for dermatophyte infections and onychomycosis (22, 31).

With the exception of fluconazole and posaconazole, the azoles are extensively metabolized by the human hepatic CYP enzyme system and are eliminated as inactive metabolites in the bile or urine. More than 90% of a dose of fluconazole is eliminated in the urine, predominantly as unchanged drug, which makes it useful for treating urinary tract infections caused by susceptible species (32). More than 75% of a dose of posaconazole is eliminated in the feces, predominantly as unchanged drug, with the remainder being excreted as glucuronidated derivatives in the urine (33). Itraconazole is unusual because its major metabolite, hydroxyitraconazole, is bioactive and has a spectrum of activity similar to that of the parent compound (34). This metabolite is found at serum concentrations about 2-fold higher than those of the parent drug (22).

Voriconazole is metabolized by several different hepatic CYP enzymes, primarily CYP-2C19, with more than 80% of a dose being eliminated as inactive metabolites in the urine (27). However, as a result of a point mutation in the gene encoding this enzyme, some persons are poor metabolizers while others are extensive metabolizers. About 3 to 5% of Caucasians and 15 to 20% of non-Indian Asians are poor metabolizers (35). Voriconazole blood concentrations are as much as 4-fold lower in individuals who metabolize the drug more extensively and can reach toxic levels in poor metabolizers.

Isavuconazole is metabolized by CYP-3A4 and CYP-3A5 and is eliminated in the feces (36). It exhibits linear pharmacokinetics and does not appear to require therapeutic drug monitoring.

Drug Interactions

Most azole antifungal agents are extensively metabolized by the human hepatic CYP enzyme system and are potent inhibitors of CYP-3A4; some also inhibit CYP-2C9 and CYP-2C19. Their coadministration with other drugs that are metabolized by these enzymes can result in increased blood concentrations of the azole, the interacting drug, or both (37). When an azole agent is discontinued, the change in metabolism that occurs may necessitate upward or downward adjustment of the dosage of the other drugs. Administration of azoles with drugs that are potent inducers of the human CYP enzyme system, such as rifampin, results in a marked reduction in blood concentrations of the azoles, especially itraconazole (37).

Fluconazole

Fluconazole (Diflucan; Pfizer) is a water-soluble bis-triazole available in both oral and parenteral formulations. It is used extensively as prophylaxis and in treating yeast infections, particularly in the treatment of candidiasis and cryptococcosis.

Spectrum of Activity

Fluconazole possesses the narrowest spectrum of all the azole antifungals currently available for systemic use. It is active against most *Candida* spp. and *Cryptococcus* spp. (38, 39). However, isolates of *Candida krusei* are intrinsically resistant, and *Candida glabrata* and *Candida auris* have decreased susceptibility (40). Fluconazole may have some limited *in vitro* activity against several dimorphic fungi in the mold phase (*B. dermatitidis*, *Coccidioides* spp., and *H. capsulatum*) (41). Fluconazole has no activity against *Aspergillus* spp., *Fusarium* spp., or Mucorales.

Acquired Resistance

There have been few reports of resistance developing in *Candida albicans* during short-term fluconazole treatment in patients with mucosal or deep-seated forms of candidiasis (42). In contrast, many strains of *C. glabrata* rapidly become resistant to fluconazole during treatment (42), and so do isolates of *C. auris* (43). In persons with AIDS, resistant strains of *C. albicans* have appeared following repeated courses of low-dose fluconazole treatment for oral or esophageal infection. However, with the widespread use of highly active antiretroviral treatment for HIV infection, resistant strains are now rarely encountered. There are a few reports of resistant strains of *Cryptococcus neoformans* from AIDS patients with relapsed infection following long-term maintenance treatment with fluconazole, but those cases are thought to be rare (44).

Clinical Use

Fluconazole is widely used in the treatment of mucosal and systemic candidiasis (45), coccidioidomycosis (46), and cryptococcosis (47). It is also recommended for the prevention of candidiasis in high-risk adult patients in intensive care units (45), as well as for the prevention of relapse of cryptococcal meningitis in persons with AIDS (47). Fluconazole is an alternative for the treatment of histoplasmosis and sporotrichosis but is less effective than itraconazole (48, 49).

Therapeutic Drug Monitoring

Serum concentrations of fluconazole are predictable from dosing and organ function, and routine monitoring of drug levels is not required (50).

Toxicity and Adverse Effects

Fluconazole is one of the least toxic and best-tolerated azole drugs, and side effects during treatment are rare. The most common patient complaints include headache, hair loss, and loss of appetite. Transient abnormalities of liver enzymes and rare serious skin reactions, including Stevens-Johnson syndrome, have been reported.

Isavuconazole

Isavuconazole (Cresemba; Astellas Pharma) is a second-generation broad-spectrum triazole compound available as an oral capsule or for intravenous administration. It is prescribed as a water-soluble prodrug, isavuconazonium sulfate, which is hydrolyzed by plasma esterases in the blood or gastrointestinal (GI) tract into the active compound isavuconazole. The intravenous formulation does not require cyclodextrin, making it an option for patients with renal impairment. Its chemical structure is similar to that of fluconazole and voriconazole. Isavuconazole has good oral availability, and food uptake has no effect on the plasma concentration. The drug exhibits linear pharmacokinetics and is highly protein bound and eliminated through the

GI tract, with less than 1% excreted in the urine. The half-life is approximately 80 to 100 hours, which allows once-daily dosing following loading (51). Tissue penetration was assessed in a rat model. The highest concentrations were reached in liver and bile, with good concentrations in brain, kidney, and intestinal mucosa and the lowest concentrations in bone and the lenses of the eyes (52).

Spectrum of Activity

Isavuconazole is active against *Candida* (53), *Cryptococcus* spp. (54), and non-*Candida* yeasts such as *Trichosporon*, *Rhodotorula*, and *Saccharomyces* (55). Isavuconazole has good activity against *Aspergillus* species (53, 56) and the endemic fungi (57, 58). Activity against dematiaceous molds is species dependent (57, 59, 60), as is the activity against the Mucorales (61, 62). It does not have good activity against *Scedosporium* spp. (57, 63), *L. prolificans* (63), or *Fusarium* spp. (57, 64).

Acquired Resistance

Clinical use of isavuconazole is just beginning, and therefore, not much acquired resistance has been noted. In a study of azole-resistant isolates of *Candida* species, isavuconazole MICs were increased, similar to what was seen with voriconazole (65). There is also evidence that the pan-azole-resistant isolates of *Aspergillus fumigatus* are resistant to isavuconazole as well (66).

Clinical Use

In the United States, isavuconazole has been approved for the treatment of aspergillosis and mucormycosis. In the phase III clinical trial, isavuconazole was found to be noninferior to voriconazole for the treatment of invasive aspergillosis (56). In the European Union, it is approved for use against invasive aspergillosis and for mucormycosis in patients for whom amphotericin B is inappropriate. In a phase III trial for the treatment of candidemia, isavuconazole failed to exhibit noninferiority to caspofungin. However, it was noninferior to fluconazole in a phase II trial of esophageal candidiasis (67). In another phase III trial, intravenous isavuconazole followed by oral isavuconazole was compared to caspofungin followed by oral voriconazole for the treatment of candidemia or invasive candidiasis. The results did not meet the noninferiority margin. In an open-label phase III trial against endemic mycoses and *Cryptococcus*, isavuconazole showed good clinical efficacy (58).

Therapeutic Drug Monitoring

The average trough level in patient groups during the phase III clinical trials exceeded the MIC_{90} for the majority of target organisms, and routine monitoring of drug levels is not currently thought to be required (68).

Toxicity and Adverse Effects

Isavuconazole is well tolerated. The most frequent side effects are abdominal pain, conjunctivitis, diarrhea, rhinitis, and nasopharyngitis (51). In a phase III head-to-head trial with voriconazole, fewer drug-related adverse events were reported with isavuconazole than with voriconazole (56).

Itraconazole

Itraconazole (Sporanox; Ortho-McNeil-Janssen Pharmaceuticals) is a lipophilic triazole drug available for oral or parenteral administration. It is extensively used, particularly in the treatment of superficial fungal infections, as well as in a range of subcutaneous and systemic infections.

Spectrum of Activity

Itraconazole has good activity against a broad spectrum of pathogenic fungi, including *Aspergillus* spp. (69–71), *Candida* spp. (69, 72, 73), many dematiaceous molds (5), dermatophytes (2–4), and dimorphic fungi (*B. dermatitidis*, *Coccidioides* spp., *H. capsulatum*, *P. brasiliensis*, *T. marneffei*, and *S. schenckii*) (9, 10, 41, 74). Itraconazole has modest activity against *C. neoformans* (69) but is ineffective against *Scedosporium* species (63) and most Mucorales (75).

Acquired Resistance

Itraconazole-resistant strains of *A. fumigatus* have been reported following treatment (76, 77). Of more concern are increasing reports of itraconazole resistance due to the environmentally acquired mutations in *cyp51A*, TR_{34}/L94H, and TR46/Y121F/T289A (78). This mutation has now been identified in isolates from Asia, Africa, North America, South America, and Australia and has become a serious problem in parts of Europe (79).

Clinical Use

Itraconazole has been widely used to treat various superficial fungal infections, including the dermatophytoses, onychomycosis, pityriasis versicolor, and mucosal and cutaneous forms of candidiasis. It is also effective in patients with paracoccidioidomycosis, chromoblastomycosis, sporotrichosis, and certain forms of phaeohyphomycosis. Despite its limitations, itraconazole continues to be a drug of choice in the management of mild to moderate forms of blastomycosis and histoplasmosis (49, 80). It was the first orally active drug for aspergillosis, but its use in seriously ill patients with life-threatening forms of this disease is not recommended (81). Itraconazole is the drug of choice for long-term maintenance treatment to prevent relapse in AIDS patients with histoplasmosis (49), but it is less effective than fluconazole as maintenance treatment in AIDS patients with cryptococcosis (47).

Therapeutic Drug Monitoring

Absorption of the capsule formulation of itraconazole after oral administration shows marked variation between individuals. Because low serum concentrations are often predictive of treatment failure, measurement of blood levels is advisable in situations where the drug is used to treat or prevent serious invasive fungal infections (50). For prophylaxis, a target trough concentration of >0.5 μg/ml has been proposed; for treatment, a trough of >1 to 2 μg/ml has been recommended (50).

Toxicity and Adverse Effects

Most side effects associated with itraconazole are mild and reversible. The most frequently reported adverse events are headache, loss of appetite, nausea, abdominal discomfort, diarrhea, skin rashes, and transient elevations of liver enzymes. Gastrointestinal intolerance is more common with itraconazole oral solution and is sometimes severe enough to necessitate discontinuation of treatment (26). Rare, but serious, side effects include Stevens-Johnson syndrome, hepatitis, and congestive heart failure.

Ketoconazole

Ketoconazole (Nizoral; Ortho-McNeil-Janssen Pharmaceuticals) is a lipophilic drug formulated for oral or topical use.

It is the only antifungal imidazole still available for systemic administration, but its main use is now as a topical agent.

Spectrum of Activity

Ketoconazole has useful activity against dermatophytes (82) and dimorphic fungi (*B. dermatitidis*, *Coccidioides* spp., *H. capsulatum*, *P. brasiliensis*, and *S. schenckii*) (83). It is also active against *Candida* spp. and *C. neoformans*, although it is less effective than the newer triazoles.

Acquired Resistance

Acquired resistance is rare, but several instances were documented in the 1980s among patients given long-term treatment for chronic mucocutaneous candidiasis due to *C. albicans*.

Clinical Use

Due to the availability of less toxic, more efficacious alternatives, ketoconazole is now little used, except in resource-limited environments. Ketoconazole remains a useful topical agent for dermatophytosis, cutaneous candidiasis, pityriasis versicolor, and seborrheic dermatitis (82).

Toxicity and Adverse Effects

Unwanted effects include loss of appetite, abdominal pain, nausea, and vomiting. Transient elevations of liver enzymes are common with oral ketoconazole, and fatal hepatitis is a rare but well-recognized adverse event. High doses of ketoconazole inhibit human adrenal and testicular steroid synthesis, with clinical consequences such as alopecia, gynecomastia, and impotence.

Posaconazole

Posaconazole (Noxafil; Merck) is a second-generation broad-spectrum triazole compound which is available as an oral suspension, an intravenous formulation, and a tablet. The new intravenous formulation allows the treatment in seriously ill patients for which there used to be a formulary advantage to voriconazole. Posaconazole is highly lipophilic and has a chemical structure similar to that of itraconazole.

Spectrum of Activity

Posaconazole is highly active against most *Aspergillus* spp. (70, 84), as well as *Candida* spp., *C. neoformans*, and *Trichosporon* spp. (39, 72, 85–87). It has potent activity against a number of dimorphic fungi, including *B. dermatitidis*, *Coccidioides* spp., *H. capsulatum*, *T. marneffei*, and *S. schenckii* (41, 57). It is less active against *Fusarium* spp. and *Scedosporium* spp. but appears to be effective against dematiaceous fungi (57, 63, 88). Unlike most other azole antifungals, posaconazole has significant activity against some Mucorales (75, 89–91).

Acquired Resistance

Posaconazole sometimes has activity against strains of *Aspergillus* and *Candida* spp. that show resistance to itraconazole, fluconazole, and/or voriconazole (92). Posaconazole resistance in *A. fumigatus* isolates harboring the TR_{34}/L98H mutation has been demonstrated (93).

Clinical Use

In the United States, the drug has been approved for the treatment of oropharyngeal candidiasis (including infections refractory to itraconazole and/or fluconazole), as well as for prophylaxis of invasive aspergillosis and candidiasis in high-risk patients, such as hematopoietic stem cell transplant (HSCT) recipients with graft-versus-host disease and neutropenic cancer patients. In the European Union, posaconazole has been licensed for similar indications, as well as for salvage treatment of invasive aspergillosis, coccidioidomycosis, chromoblastomycosis, *Fusarium* infections, and mycetoma. Other indications for which posaconazole has proved effective but is not currently licensed include histoplasmosis (94), coccidioidomycosis (95), and infections caused by Mucorales (91, 96).

Therapeutic Drug Monitoring

Similar to itraconazole and voriconazole, there appears to be a relationship between posaconazole trough serum concentrations and clinical response, and measurement of drug levels may therefore be useful (27, 50). For prophylaxis, a target trough concentration of >0.5 μg/ml has been proposed; for treatment, a trough of >0.5 to 1.5 μg/ml has been suggested (50). Oral uptake of posaconazole differs depending on the formulation used. It may not be necessary to monitor blood levels after either capsule administration or intravenous administration.

Toxicity and Adverse Effects

Posaconazole is well tolerated, even among patients receiving the drug for longer than 6 months (97). The most frequently reported side effects are gastrointestinal symptoms and headache. Transient transaminase abnormalities have also been reported. Rare cases of cholestasis or hepatic failure have occurred during treatment with posaconazole.

Voriconazole

Voriconazole (Vfend; Pfizer) is a second-generation broad-spectrum triazole compound available for oral or intravenous administration. Its chemical structure is similar to that of fluconazole.

Spectrum of Activity

Voriconazole is highly active against most *Aspergillus* spp., *Fusarium* spp., and *Scedosporium* spp. (57, 63, 70, 88), as well as *Candida* spp., *C. neoformans*, and *Trichosporon* spp. (39, 44, 72, 85, 86). Voriconazole has potent activity against a number of dimorphic fungi, including *B. dermatitidis*, *Coccidioides* spp., *H. capsulatum*, and *T. marneffei* (57, 74), as well as dematiaceous molds (57). Voriconazole is ineffective against Mucorales (75, 90).

Acquired Resistance

Some fluconazole-resistant strains of *Candida* spp. have shown reduced susceptibility to voriconazole, and essentially all *C. glabrata* isolates that are resistant to fluconazole should be considered nonsusceptible to voriconazole. *Aspergillus* isolates may acquire voriconazole resistance during long-term azole therapy, and environmentally acquired resistance in *A. fumigatus* is due to a TR_{34}/L98H mutation in the CYP-51A gene (76, 92, 98). The newly emerging mutation in *A. fumigatus*, TR_{46}/Y121/T289A, seems to be specific for voriconazole resistance (76, 92, 98).

Clinical Use

The availability of both an intravenous formulation and a well-absorbed oral formulation of voriconazole is a distinct advantage when seriously ill patients are being treated. In the United States, the drug has been approved for the treatment of invasive aspergillosis and has become the drug of choice for these infections (81). It is also licensed for the treatment of candidemia in nonneutropenic patients, for disseminated infections caused by *Candida* spp., and for esophageal candidiasis, as well as for salvage treatment of *Fusarium* and *Scedosporium* infections. In the European Union, voriconazole has been approved for similar indications. Because voriconazole has no activity against Mucorales, its use in immunocompromised patients has sometimes been associated with breakthrough infections caused by these organisms.

Therapeutic Drug Monitoring

Voriconazole serum concentrations are highly variable, largely due to differences in the rate of metabolism between individuals, and it may be beneficial to monitor drug levels (27, 50, 99). For prophylaxis, a target trough concentration of >0.5 μg/ml has been proposed; for treatment, a trough of >1 to 2 μg/ml has been recommended (50). To avoid toxicity, trough concentrations should not exceed 6 μg/ml.

Toxicity and Adverse Effects

Voriconazole is generally well tolerated. About 30% of patients experience transient visual disturbances and hallucinations, usually during the first week of treatment (99). Other side effects include skin rashes and transient abnormalities of liver enzymes. Rare, but serious, adverse effects include Stevens-Johnson syndrome, hepatic failure, and cardiovascular events.

ECHINOCANDINS

The echinocandins are semisynthetic lipopeptide antifungal agents that target the fungal cell wall. Three echinocandins have been approved for the treatment of serious fungal infections: anidulafungin, caspofungin, and micafungin. Due to their high molecular weight and low oral bioavailability, these drugs are available only as intravenous preparations. They are now widely used, particularly in the treatment of candidiasis.

Mechanism of Action

The echinocandins disrupt fungal cell wall synthesis by inhibiting the enzyme 1,3-β-D-glucan synthase. This results in inhibition of the formation of 1,3-β-D-glucan, an essential polysaccharide component of the cell wall of susceptible fungi. Inhibition leads to osmotic lysis of the cell and eventual cell death. Echinocandin drugs bind to Fksp, the major subunit of 1,3-β-D-glucan synthase, which is encoded by three *FKS* genes in *Candida* spp. (100). The echinocandins are fungicidal for *Candida* spp. but fungistatic for *Aspergillus* spp., where they block the growth of the apical tips of the hyphae (101).

Spectrum of Activity

The echinocandins have a limited spectrum of activity. They are highly active against a broad range of *Candida* spp., including fluconazole-resistant strains (72, 102, 103). *Candida parapsilosis*, *Candida lusitaniae*, and *Candida guilliermondii* have higher MICs of the echinocandins, but the clinical implications of these values are not yet clear (102, 104). The echinocandins are also active against *Aspergillus* spp., including those that are intrinsically resistant to amphotericin B (105, 106).

The echinocandins are ineffective against fungi that lack a significant amount of 1,3-β-D-glucan in their cell walls, including *C. neoformans* and *Trichosporon* spp., as well as *Fusarium* spp. and the Mucorales (107). Micafungin has been reported to be active against the mycelial forms of several dimorphic fungi, including *B. dermatitidis* and *H. capsulatum*, but is ineffective against the tissue forms of these pathogens (108).

Acquired Resistance

Acquired resistance is rare at present, but resistant strains of several *Candida* spp. have been recovered from patients for whom echinocandin treatment failed (43, 109, 110). Resistance has been associated with acquisition of mutations in the *FKS1* and/or *FKS2* genes that led to amino acid substitutions within the FKS1p and FKS2p subunits of 1,3-β-D-glucan synthase (103, 109, 111). These changes result in altered drug binding and confer cross-resistance to all echinocandin drugs. Mutations in the *FKS1* and *FKS2* genes are responsible for reduced susceptibility to caspofungin, micafungin, and anidulafungin in most *Candida* species (111). The highest rates of resistance have been detected in *C. glabrata*, especially in strains already resistant to fluconazole (103, 109, 112).

Pharmacokinetics

Blood concentrations of all three echinocandins increase in proportion to dosage (27, 113). These drugs are extensively distributed to body tissues, but levels in CSF and ocular tissue are negligible. The predominant differences among these agents lie in their metabolism and half-lives. Caspofungin and micafungin are largely metabolized by the liver and eliminated as inactive metabolites in the feces and urine (27, 114). Anidulafungin is not eliminated by hepatic metabolism but undergoes slow nonenzymatic degradation in the blood to an inactive open-ring peptide (115). Less than 1 to 3% of an echinocandin dose is excreted unchanged in the urine (27, 114, 116, 117). In adults, the half-life of caspofungin is about 9 to 10 h (117), while that of micafungin is 13 h (118), and that of anidulafungin is 18 to 27 h (115). The three echinocandins have a shorter half-life in children (119). The ratio of the 24-h area under the concentration-time curve to the MIC is a good indicator of the exposure-response relationship and should exceed 10 to 20 (120).

Drug Interactions

The echinocandins do not interact with the human hepatic CYP system, and their use has been associated with very few significant drug interactions.

Therapeutic Drug Monitoring

At this time, there is no established relationship between efficacy or toxicity of the echinocandins and serum concentrations (27, 50, 121). Routine monitoring of serum levels during treatment with these drugs is not required.

Toxicity and Adverse Effects

As a class, the echinocandins are well tolerated, and their use is associated with very few significant adverse effects (113, 116–118). The most common side effects are gastrointestinal, but they occur in only around 5% of patients. Occasional cases of infusion-related pain and phlebitis have been noted with anidulafungin and micafungin, but these are less common with caspofungin. Transient elevations of liver enzymes have been reported in a few patients.

Anidulafungin

Anidulafungin (Ecalta, Eraxis; Pfizer) was the first echinocandin to go into development and the most recent to be licensed for clinical use. It differs from caspofungin and micafungin in that it is insoluble in water. Anidulafungin is derived from a fermentation product of *Aspergillus nidulans* and is formulated for intravenous infusion.

Clinical Use

In the United States, anidulafungin is currently approved for the treatment of esophageal candidiasis, candidemia, and two invasive forms of candidiasis (abdominal abscesses and peritonitis). In the European Union, anidulafungin is approved for the treatment of invasive candidiasis in nonneutropenic patients. Anidulafungin has not been evaluated in sufficient numbers of neutropenic patients to determine its effectiveness in that group.

Caspofungin

Caspofungin (Cancidas; Merck) is a water-soluble lipopeptide, derived from a fermentation product of *Glarea lozoyensis*. It is formulated for intravenous infusion.

Clinical Use

In the United States, caspofungin is currently approved for the treatment of esophageal candidiasis, candidemia, and certain invasive forms of candidiasis, including abdominal abscesses, peritonitis, and pleural space infections. Caspofungin is also licensed for the salvage treatment of invasive aspergillosis in patients who have failed to respond to or are intolerant of other antifungal agents. Caspofungin is approved for the empiric treatment of presumed fungal infections in febrile neutropenic patients. It has similar indications in the European Union, with a license for the treatment of invasive candidiasis in adult and pediatric patients, salvage treatment of aspergillosis, and empiric treatment of febrile neutropenia in adult or pediatric patients.

Micafungin

Micafungin (Mycamine; Astellas Pharma, Fujisawa Healthcare) is a water-soluble antifungal agent, derived from a fermentation product of *Coleophoma empetri*. It is formulated for intravenous administration.

Clinical Use

In the United States, micafungin is currently approved for use in adults for the treatment of esophageal candidiasis, candidemia, and several invasive forms of candidiasis, including abdominal abscesses and peritonitis, and for prophylaxis of *Candida* infections in HSCT patients. In the European Union, the drug is approved for the treatment of esophageal candidiasis in adults and for invasive candidiasis in adults and children, including neonates. In addition, micafungin is licensed as prophylactic treatment to prevent *Candida* infections in HSCT recipients in the United States and the European Union. In Japan, the license includes respiratory and GI mycosis due to *Aspergillus* spp. Micafungin does have a black box warning in the European Union due to the development of hepatic tumors in rats following prolonged use, but this has not been seen in patients postmarketing.

POLYENES

Around 100 polyene antibiotics have been described, but few have been developed for clinical use. Amphotericin B and its lipid formulations are used for the treatment of systemic fungal infections. Nystatin, natamycin, and mepartricin are topical polyene agents used in the treatment of oral, vaginal, and ocular fungal infections. A liposomal formulation of nystatin entered clinical trials, but its development has ceased. The polyenes are large molecules that consist of a closed macrolide lactone ring. One side of the ring is composed of a rigid lipophilic chain with a variable number of conjugated double bonds, and on the opposite side there are a similar number of hydroxyl groups. Thus, the molecule is amphipathic, and this feature of its structure is believed to be important in its mechanism of action.

Mechanism of Action

The polyenes bind to sterols, principally ergosterol, in the membranes of susceptible fungal cells, causing impairment of membrane barrier function, leakage of cell constituents, metabolic disruption, and cell death (122). In addition to its membrane-permeabilizing effects, amphotericin B can cause oxidative damage to fungal cells through a cascade of oxidative reactions linked to lipoperoxidation of the cell membrane.

Amphotericin B

Amphotericin B (Fungizone; Apothecon) is a fermentation product of *Streptomyces nodosus* available for intravenous infusion. The conventional micellar suspension formulation of this drug (amphotericin B deoxycholate) is often associated with serious toxic side effects, particularly renal damage. During the 1990s, three new lipid-associated formulations of amphotericin B were developed in an effort to alleviate the infusion-related toxicity of the agent. These include the following: liposomal amphotericin B (Ambisome; Astellas Pharma, Gilead Sciences), in which the drug is encapsulated in phospholipid-containing liposomes; amphotericin B lipid complex (ABLC) (Abelcet; Enzon Pharmaceuticals), in which the drug is complexed with phospholipids to produce ribbon-like structures; and amphotericin B colloidal dispersion (ABCD) (Amphotec; Three Rivers Pharmaceuticals), in which the drug is packaged into small lipid disks containing cholesterol sulfate. These formulations possess the same broad spectrum of activity as the micellar suspension but are less nephrotoxic (123). There is also an encochleated amphotericin B in development (MAT2203; Matinas Biopharma). This lipid-based delivery mechanism allows oral administration and leads to good tissue penetration (124, 125). A phase II clinical trial against refractory mucocutaneous candidiasis is under way.

Spectrum of Activity

Amphotericin B is active against a broad spectrum of pathogenic fungi, including most *Aspergillus* spp. (81, 126), *Candida* spp. (72, 73), *Cryptococcus* spp. (39, 44, 54), and the Mucorales (75, 90). However, most isolates of *Aspergillus terreus* are resistant to amphotericin B (127, 128), as are isolates of *Aspergillus lentulus*, a new sibling species of *A. fumigatus* (129). *C. krusei* and *C. lusitaniae* also demonstrate reduced susceptibility to amphotericin B. Amphotericin B is effective against the dimorphic fungi (*B. dermatitidis*, *Coccidioides* spp., *H. capsulatum*, and *P. brasiliensis*) and many dematiaceous fungi (74, 130). Strains of *Scedosporium* spp., *L. prolificans*, *Fusarium* spp., and *Trichosporon* spp. are often intrinsically resistant to amphotericin B (63, 86, 131).

Acquired Resistance

Acquired resistance is rare, but amphotericin B-resistant strains of *C. albicans*, *C. glabrata*, *C. guilliermondii*, *Candida tropicalis*, *C. neoformans*, and especially *C. lusitaniae* with alterations in the cell membrane, including reduced amounts of ergosterol, have been reported following prolonged treatment (132). Resistance is also seen in the emerging species *Candida haemulonii*, *Candida duobushaemulonii*, and *C. auris* (133).

Pharmacokinetics

Amphotericin B is poorly absorbed after oral administration and must be administered as a slow intravenous infusion. The drug is widely distributed to many tissues, with the highest concentrations being found in the liver, spleen, and kidneys. Levels in CSF are less than 5% of the simultaneous blood concentration. Amphotericin B is mostly excreted as unchanged drug in the urine (21%) and feces (42%) (134). No metabolites have been identified. The drug is cleared very slowly, with the conventional deoxycholate formulation having a terminal half-life of around 127 h.

The pharmacokinetics of lipid-based formulations of amphotericin B are quite diverse. Maximal serum concentrations of the liposomal formulation are much higher than those of the deoxycholate formulation, while levels of ABCD and ABLC are lower due to more rapid distribution of the drug to tissue (123, 134). Administration of lipid-associated formulations of amphotericin B results in higher drug concentrations in the liver and spleen than are achieved with the conventional formulation (135). Renal concentrations of the drug are lower, and the nephrotoxic side effects are greatly reduced (136).

Clinical Use

Although other agents have subsequently been introduced, amphotericin B remains the treatment of choice for many serious fungal infections, including blastomycosis, coccidioidomycosis, histoplasmosis, sporotrichosis, cryptococcosis, and mucormycosis (46–49, 80). However, with the advent of voriconazole and the echinocandins, amphotericin B is no longer regarded as the drug of first choice for many cases of aspergillosis or candidiasis. The three lipid-based formulations of amphotericin B are currently licensed for treatment of invasive fungal infections in patients who are refractory to or intolerant of conventional amphotericin B. In addition, liposomal amphotericin B is licensed for the treatment of cryptococcal meningitis in persons with AIDS, as well as for the empirical treatment of presumed fungal infection in febrile neutropenic patients. Clinical experience with these preparations has demonstrated that they are safer and no less active than the conventional formulation, and for some infections, they are more effective, especially since the reduced toxicity allows them to be used at a higher dose.

Drug Interactions

Amphotericin B can augment the nephrotoxicity of many other agents, including aminoglycoside antibiotics and cyclosporine.

Therapeutic Drug Monitoring

Serum and tissue concentrations of amphotericin B show marked variation with formulation, especially among the lipid-based products, and there are few data relating either efficacy or toxicity to blood levels. Therefore, there is no need to monitor serum concentrations of amphotericin B during therapy (27, 50). However, due to the risk of toxicity, kidney function should be monitored.

Toxicity and Adverse Effects

Amphotericin B deoxycholate causes infusion-related reactions, including hypotension, fever, rigors, and chills, in approximately 70% of patients (123). The major adverse effect of the drug is nephrotoxicity. This is dose related and may occur in more than 80% of patients receiving treatment. The lipid-associated formulations all lower the risk of amphotericin B-induced renal failure (134, 136). However, infusion-related side effects, such as hypoxia and chills, are more common in patients treated with ABCD than with other formulations of amphotericin B. In contrast, infusion-related reactions are uncommon in patients receiving liposomal amphotericin B or ABLC (123, 134, 136).

OTHER MISCELLANEOUS AGENTS

Flucytosine

Flucytosine (5-fluorocytosine; Ancobon; Valeant Pharmaceuticals) is a synthetic fluorinated analogue of cytosine and the only available antifungal agent acting as an antimetabolite. In the United States, flucytosine is available as oral tablets; elsewhere, it is also available as an infusion for parenteral administration.

Mechanism of Action

Flucytosine disrupts pyrimidine metabolism and thus the synthesis of DNA, RNA, and proteins within susceptible fungal cells. Flucytosine is transported into these cells by the enzyme cytosine permease and there converted by cytosine deaminase to 5-fluorouracil (5-FU). Two mechanisms then account for the antifungal activity. The first involves the conversion of 5-FU into 5-fluoro-UTP, which is incorporated into fungal RNA in place of uridylic acid, with resulting inhibition of protein synthesis. The second mechanism involves the conversion of 5-FU to 5-fluoro-dUMP, which blocks the enzyme thymidylate synthetase, causing inhibition of fungal DNA synthesis. Fungi lacking cytosine deaminase are intrinsically resistant to flucytosine.

Spectrum of Activity

Flucytosine has a narrow spectrum of activity. It includes *Candida* spp., *C. neoformans*, and some dematiaceous fungi causing chromoblastomycosis (39, 44, 72, 73, 130). Primary resistance to flucytosine is very uncommon among *Candida* spp., occurring in around 2 to 3% of isolates (72, 73, 137).

Acquired Resistance

Monotherapy with flucytosine often leads to the induction of resistance among *Candida* spp. and *C. neoformans* (138).

Pharmacokinetics

Flucytosine is rapidly and almost completely absorbed after oral administration. The drug is widely distributed, with levels in most body tissues and fluids usually exceeding 50% of the simultaneous blood concentration (138). Flucytosine is primarily eliminated by renal excretion of unchanged drug. The serum half-life is between 3 and 6 h but may be greatly extended in renal failure, necessitating modification of the dosage regimen.

Clinical Use

Due to the risk of resistance, flucytosine is rarely administered as a single agent. It is most commonly used in combination with amphotericin B in the treatment of candidiasis and cryptococcosis (45, 47). Combination treatment with fluconazole has also been shown to be effective in AIDS-associated cryptococcal meningitis (47).

Drug Interactions

The antifungal activity of flucytosine is competitively inhibited by cytarabine (cytosine arabinoside), and the two drugs should not be administered together (138). Nephrotoxic drugs, such as amphotericin B, decrease the elimination of flucytosine, and serum concentrations of the latter should be monitored when these agents are administered together. Flucytosine is myelosuppressive (see below) and should be used with caution in patients receiving other drugs, such as zidovudine, that could enhance its immunosuppressive side effects.

Therapeutic Drug Monitoring

Regular monitoring of serum drug concentrations of flucytosine is advisable to reduce the risk of hepatotoxicity and hematological toxicity; this is essential when there is renal impairment. To avoid toxicity, a peak concentration of 100 μg/ml of flucytosine should not be exceeded (121). In contrast to toxicity, there are few data relating efficacy to blood levels for flucytosine. A reasonable goal is to maintain a postdose concentration of >25 μg/ml but <100 μg/ml (50, 121).

Toxicity and Adverse Effects

The most common, and least harmful, side effects of flucytosine are gastrointestinal and include nausea, diarrhea, vomiting, and abdominal pain. The most severe adverse effects include bone marrow depression and hepatotoxicity (138). These complications are more likely to occur if excessively high blood concentrations are maintained.

Griseofulvin

Griseofulvin (Gris-PEG; Pedinol Pharmacal Inc.) is an antifungal antibiotic derived from a number of *Penicillium* species, including *Penicillium griseofulvum*. Introduced in 1958, oral griseofulvin transformed the treatment of dermatophytosis.

Mechanism of Action

Griseofulvin is a fungistatic drug which binds to microtubular proteins and inhibits fungal cell mitosis (139).

Spectrum of Activity

The spectrum of useful activity is restricted to dermatophytes causing skin, nail, and hair infections (*Epidermophyton*, *Microsporum*, and *Trichophyton* spp.) (2, 3). Resistance has rarely been reported.

Pharmacokinetics

Absorption of griseofulvin from the gastrointestinal tract differs between individuals but is improved if the drug is given with a high-fat meal. Griseofulvin appears in the stratum corneum within a few hours of ingestion, as a result of secretion in perspiration. However, levels begin to fall soon after the drug is discontinued, and within 48 to 72 h, it can no longer be detected. Griseofulvin is metabolized by the liver to 6-desmethyl griseofulvin, which is excreted in the urine.

Clinical Use

Newer oral agents, such as terbinafine and itraconazole, are often preferred for nail infections, but griseofulvin remains a useful second-line agent for moderate to severe dermatophytoses of the skin and scalp hair, where topical treatment is considered inappropriate or has failed.

Drug Interactions

Absorption of griseofulvin is reduced in persons receiving concomitant treatment with barbiturates. Griseofulvin may decrease the effectiveness of oral anticoagulants, oral contraceptives, and cyclosporine.

Toxicity and Adverse Effects

In most cases, prolonged courses and high doses are well tolerated. Adverse effects occur in around 15% of patients and include headache, nausea, vomiting and abdominal discomfort, and rashes.

NOVEL ANTIFUNGAL AGENTS IN DEVELOPMENT

We are currently in an era of growth for new antifungal agents. New antifungal compounds including compounds with novel targets as well as promising improvements on existing antifungal drugs are currently in development. Discussed below are compounds that have reached at least phase II clinical trials.

APX001

APX001 (E1210; Amplyx) is a small-molecule inhibitor of glycophosphatidylinositol biosynthesis that exhibits potent broad-spectrum antifungal activity against *Candida* spp. and *Aspergillus* spp., as well as other molds that are difficult to treat, such as Mucorales, *Fusarium solani*, and *L. prolificans*. APX001 is also active against fungal isolates which are azole and/or echinocandin resistant, including the emerging pathogen *C. auris* (131, 140–142).

SCY-078

SCY-078 (MK-3118; Scynexis) is a structurally distinct class of β-1,3-D-glucan synthase inhibitor—a triterpene glucan synthase inhibitor—that has been developed to treat invasive fungal infections. Unlike current echinocandins, it is orally bioavailable, and its activity is not compromised by the most common mutations within the protein target Fks (143, 144). SCY-078 shows both *in vitro* and *in vivo* activity against the most common *Candida* species as well as against *C. auris*, *Aspergillus* spp., *Paecilomyces variotii*, and *L. prolificans* (145–147). Phase II studies targeting vaginal and invasive candidiasis have been completed. SCY-078 has recently been given a Qualified Infectious Disease Product designation by the Food And Drug Administration for invasive candidiasis and aspergillosis.

F901318

F901318 (F2G Ltd.) is a member of a new class of orotomide antifungal agents that inhibit an enzyme involved in pyrimidine biosynthesis, dihydroorotate dehydrogenase. It has been developed in both oral and intravenous formulations for the treatment of systemic mold infections. It shows potent activity against a broad range of filamentous and dimorphic fungi, including *Aspergillus* spp., *H. capsulatum*, *B. dermatitidis*, *Coccidioides immitis*, *Fusarium* spp., *T. marneffei*, and *L. prolificans* (148, 149). Of note, this agent is effective against azole-resistant *A. fumigatus* strains harboring the TR_{34}/L98H mutation both *in vitro* and *in vivo* (150, 151). Little or no activity is seen against *Candida* spp. or the Mucorales (148).

CD101

CD101 (rezafungin; Cidara Therapeutics) was developed to overcome the disadvantages of daily intravenous administration of an echinocandin while preserving the benefits of low toxicity and fungus-specific activity associated with this drug class. Adjustments to the echinocandin backbone chemical structure lowered the clearance of CD101 and afforded a longer compound half-life, about 3-fold longer than that of anidulafungin (152). Therefore, once-weekly intravenous administration provides appropriate systemic levels of CD101 for treatment of invasive fungal infections (153). This compound exhibits activity against echinocandin-resistant *Candida* spp., including *C. auris*, as well as *Aspergillus* spp. (154, 155). A phase II trial against invasive candidiasis has been completed.

VT-1598 and VT-1161

VT-1598 and VT-1161 (Viamet Pharmaceuticals) were developed as fungus-specific 14α-lanosterol demethylase inhibitors that selectively target fungal enzyme over human enzyme and result in fewer drug-drug interactions (156). VT-1161 shows potent *in vitro* and *in vivo* activity against *Candida* spp., *C. immitis*, *Coccidioides posadasii*, and *Trichophyton* spp. but is not active against *Aspergillus* spp. as monotherapy (157–160). VT-1598 displays an even broader antifungal range; it shows *in vitro* activity against *Candida* spp. including *C. auris*, *Cryptococcus* spp., *Aspergillus* spp., *Rhizopus oryzae*, *B. dermatitidis*, *Coccidioides* spp., and *H. capsulatum* (161–163).

Albaconazole

Albaconazole (Stiefel) is an oral agent that has demonstrated high levels of bioavailability and antifungal activity. It was evaluated in a phase I trial for tinea pedis and has completed a phase II trial for the treatment of toenail onychomycosis (164–166).

CONCLUSION

The recent surge in development of new antifungal agents has greatly increased the number of drugs available to combat the growing number of serious fungal infections. There are now few life-threatening conditions for which there is no effective treatment, and there are many for which there are several therapeutic options. However, we are seeing the emergence of multidrug-resistant yeasts, including *C. glabrata* and *C. auris*, so effective antifungal stewardship will be a challenge. With judicious use of the available agents, antifungal drug resistance can be mitigated. It remains to be seen which if any of the new antifungal agents in development will reach the marketplace.

REFERENCES

1. **Ryder NS.** 1991. Squalene epoxidase as a target for the allylamines. *Biochem Soc Trans* **19:**774–777.
2. **Favre B, Hofbauer B, Hildering KS, Ryder NS.** 2003. Comparison of in vitro activities of 17 antifungal drugs against a panel of 20 dermatophytes by using a microdilution assay. *J Clin Microbiol* **41:**4817–4819.
3. **Fernández-Torres B, Carrillo AJ, Martín E, Del Palacio A, Moore MK, Valverde A, Serrano M, Guarro J.** 2001. In vitro activities of 10 antifungal drugs against 508 dermatophyte strains. *Antimicrob Agents Chemother* **45:**2524–2528.
4. **Perea S, Fothergill AW, Sutton DA, Rinaldi MG.** 2001. Comparison of in vitro activities of voriconazole and five established antifungal agents against different species of dermatophytes using a broth macrodilution method. *J Clin Microbiol* **39:**385–388.
5. **McGinnis MR, Pasarell L.** 1998. In vitro evaluation of terbinafine and itraconazole against dematiaceous fungi. *Med Mycol* **36:**243–246.
6. **Schmitt HJ, Bernard EM, Andrade J, Edwards F, Schmitt B, Armstrong D.** 1988. MIC and fungicidal activity of terbinafine against clinical isolates of *Aspergillus* spp. *Antimicrob Agents Chemother* **32:**780–781.
7. **Ryder NS, Wagner S, Leitner I.** 1998. In vitro activities of terbinafine against cutaneous isolates of *Candida albicans* and other pathogenic yeasts. *Antimicrob Agents Chemother* **42:**1057–1061.
8. **Shadomy S, Espinel-Ingroff A, Gebhart RJ.** 1985. In-vitro studies with SF 86-327, a new orally active allylamine derivative. *Sabouraudia* **23:**125–132.
9. **Hahn RC, Fontes CJ, Batista RD, Hamdan JS.** 2002. In vitro comparison of activities of terbinafine and itraconazole against *Paracoccidioides brasiliensis*. *J Clin Microbiol* **40:**2828–2831.
10. **McGinnis MR, Nordoff NG, Ryder NS, Nunn GB.** 2000. In vitro comparison of terbinafine and itraconazole against *Penicillium marneffei*. *Antimicrob Agents Chemother* **44:**1407–1408.
11. **Kovarik JM, Mueller EA, Zehender H, Denouël J, Caplain H, Millerioux L.** 1995. Multiple-dose pharmacokinetics and distribution in tissue of terbinafine and metabolites. *Antimicrob Agents Chemother* **39:**2738–2741.
12. **Vickers AE, Sinclair JR, Zollinger M, Heitz F, Glänzel U, Johanson L, Fischer V.** 1999. Multiple cytochrome P-450s involved in the metabolism of terbinafine suggest a limited potential for drug-drug interactions. *Drug Metab Dispos* **27:**1029–1038.
13. **Darkes MJ, Scott LJ, Goa KL.** 2003. Terbinafine: a review of its use in onychomycosis in adults. *Am J Clin Dermatol* **4:**39–65.
14. **Krishnan-Natesan S.** 2009. Terbinafine: a pharmacological and clinical review. *Expert Opin Pharmacother* **10:**2723–2733.
15. **Revankar SG, Nailor MD, Sobel JD.** 2008. Use of terbinafine in rare and refractory mycoses. *Future Microbiol* **3:**9–17.
16. **Howden BP, Slavin MA, Schwarer AP, Mijch AM.** 2003. Successful control of disseminated *Scedosporium prolificans* infection with a combination of voriconazole and terbinafine. *Eur J Clin Microbiol Infect Dis* **22:**111–113.
17. **Bhat SV, Paterson DL, Rinaldi MG, Veldkamp PJ.** 2007. *Scedosporium prolificans* brain abscess in a patient with chronic granulomatous disease: successful combination therapy with voriconazole and terbinafine. *Scand J Infect Dis* **39:**87–90.
18. **Hall M, Monka C, Krupp P, O'Sullivan D.** 1997. Safety of oral terbinafine: results of a postmarketing surveillance study in 25,884 patients. *Arch Dermatol* **133:**1213–1219.
19. **Manavathu EK, Cutright JL, Chandrasekar PH.** 1998. Organism-dependent fungicidal activities of azoles. *Antimicrob Agents Chemother* **42:**3018–3021.
20. **Berkow EL, Lockhart SR.** 2017. Fluconazole resistance in *Candida* species: a current perspective. *Infect Drug Resist* **10:**237–245.
21. **Chowdhary A, Sharma C, Hagen F, Meis JF.** 2014. Exploring azole antifungal drug resistance in *Aspergillus fumigatus* with special reference to resistance mechanisms. *Future Microbiol* **9:**697–711.
22. **Heykants J, Van Peer A, Van de Velde V, Van Rooy P, Meuldermans W, Lavrijsen K, Woestenborghs R, Van Cutsem J, Cauwenbergh G.** 1989. The clinical pharmacokinetics of itraconazole: an overview. *Mycoses* **32**(Suppl 1)**:**67–87.
23. **Ezzet F, Wexler D, Courtney R, Krishna G, Lim J, Laughlin M.** 2005. Oral bioavailability of posaconazole in fasted healthy subjects: comparison between three regimens and basis for clinical dosage recommendations. *Clin Pharmacokinet* **44:**211–220.
24. **Purkins L, Wood N, Kleinermans D, Greenhalgh K, Nichols D.** 2003. Effect of food on the pharmacokinetics of multiple-dose oral voriconazole. *Br J Clin Pharmacol* **56**(Suppl 1)**:**17–23.
25. **Lipp HP.** 2011. Posaconazole: clinical pharmacokinetics and drug interactions. *Mycoses* **54**(Suppl 1)**:**32–38.
26. **Lestner J, Hope WW.** 2013. Itraconazole: an update on pharmacology and clinical use for treatment of invasive and allergic fungal infections. *Expert Opin Drug Metab Toxicol* **9:**911–926.
27. **Bellmann R, Smuszkiewicz P.** 2017. Pharmacokinetics of antifungal drugs: practical implications for optimized treatment of patients. *Infection* **45:**737–779.

28. **Walsh TJ, Karlsson MO, Driscoll T, Arguedas AG, Adamson P, Saez-Llorens X, Vora AJ, Arrieta AC, Blumer J, Lutsar I, Milligan P, Wood N.** 2004. Pharmacokinetics and safety of intravenous voriconazole in children after single- or multiple-dose administration. *Antimicrob Agents Chemother* **48:**2166–2172.
29. **Theuretzbacher U, Ihle F, Derendorf H.** 2006. Pharmacokinetic/pharmacodynamic profile of voriconazole. *Clin Pharmacokinet* **45:**649–663.
30. **Riddell J IV, Comer GM, Kauffman CA.** 2011. Treatment of endogenous fungal endophthalmitis: focus on new antifungal agents. *Clin Infect Dis* **52:**648–653.
31. **Cauwenbergh G, Degreef H, Heykants J, Woestenborghs R, Van Rooy P, Haeverans K.** 1988. Pharmacokinetic profile of orally administered itraconazole in human skin. *J Am Acad Dermatol* **18:**263–268.
32. **Thomas L, Tracy CR.** 2015. Treatment of fungal urinary tract infection. *Urol Clin North Am* **42:**473–483.
33. **Krieter P, Flannery B, Musick T, Gohdes M, Martinho M, Courtney R.** 2004. Disposition of posaconazole following single-dose oral administration in healthy subjects. *Antimicrob Agents Chemother* **48:**3543–3551.
34. **Odds FC, Bossche HV.** 2000. Antifungal activity of itraconazole compared with hydroxy-itraconazole in vitro. *J Antimicrob Chemother* **45:**371–373.
35. **Li X, Yu C, Wang T, Chen K, Zhai S, Tang H.** 2016. Effect of cytochrome P450 2C19 polymorphisms on the clinical outcomes of voriconazole: a systematic review and meta-analysis. *Eur J Clin Pharmacol* **72:**1185–1193.
36. **Kovanda LL, Maher R, Hope WW.** 2016. Isavuconazonium sulfate: a new agent for the treatment of invasive aspergillosis and invasive mucormycosis. *Expert Rev Clin Pharmacol* **9:** 887–897.
37. **Gubbins PO.** 2011. Triazole antifungal agents drug-drug interactions involving hepatic cytochrome P450. *Expert Opin Drug Metab Toxicol* **7:**1411–1429.
38. **Pfaller MA, Diekema DJ, Gibbs DL, Newell VA, Ellis D, Tullio V, Rodloff A, Fu W, Ling TA, Global Antifungal Surveillance Group.** 2010. Results from the ARTEMIS DISK Global Antifungal Surveillance Study, 1997 to 2007: a 10.5-year analysis of susceptibilities of *Candida* species to fluconazole and voriconazole as determined by CLSI standardized disk diffusion. *J Clin Microbiol* **48:**1366–1377.
39. **Espinel-Ingroff A, Chowdhary A, Cuenca-Estrella M, Fothergill A, Fuller J, Hagen F, Govender N, Guarro J, Johnson E, Lass-Flörl C, Lockhart SR, Martins MA, Meis JF, Melhem MS, Ostrosky-Zeichner L, Pelaez T, Pfaller MA, Schell WA, Trilles L, Kidd S, Turnidge J.** 2012. *Cryptococcus neoformans-Cryptococcus gattii* species complex: an international study of wild-type susceptibility endpoint distributions and epidemiological cutoff values for amphotericin B and flucytosine. *Antimicrob Agents Chemother* **56:**3107–3113.
40. **Pfaller MA, Messer SA, Hollis RJ, Boyken L, Tendolkar S, Kroeger J, Diekema DJ.** 2009. Variation in susceptibility of bloodstream isolates of *Candida glabrata* to fluconazole according to patient age and geographic location in the United States in 2001 to 2007. *J Clin Microbiol* **47:**3185–3190.
41. **González GM, Fothergill AW, Sutton DA, Rinaldi MG, Loebenberg D.** 2005. In vitro activities of new and established triazoles against opportunistic filamentous and dimorphic fungi. *Med Mycol* **43:**281–284.
42. **Sanglard D, Odds FC.** 2002. Resistance of *Candida* species to antifungal agents: molecular mechanisms and clinical consequences. *Lancet Infect Dis* **2:**73–85.
43. **Lockhart SR, Etienne KA, Vallabhaneni S, Farooqi J, Chowdhary A, Govender NP, Colombo AL, Calvo B, Cuomo CA, Desjardins CA, Berkow EL, Castanheira M, Magobo RE, Jabeen K, Asghar RJ, Meis JF, Jackson B, Chiller T, Litvintseva AP.** 2017. Simultaneous emergence of multidrug-resistant *Candida auris* on 3 continents confirmed by whole-genome sequencing and epidemiological analyses. *Clin Infect Dis* **64:**134–140.
44. **Govender NP, Patel J, van Wyk M, Chiller TM, Lockhart SR, Group for Enteric, Respiratory and Meningeal Disease Surveillance in South Africa (GERMS-SA).** 2011. Trends in antifungal drug susceptibility of *Cryptococcus neoformans* isolates obtained through population-based surveillance in South Africa in 2002-2003 and 2007-2008. *Antimicrob Agents Chemother* **55:**2606–2611.
45. **Pappas PG, Kauffman CA, Andes DR, Clancy CJ, Marr KA, Ostrosky-Zeichner L, Reboli AC, Schuster MG, Vazquez JA, Walsh TJ, Zaoutis TE, Sobel JD.** 2016. Clinical practice guideline for the management of candidiasis: 2016 update by the Infectious Diseases Society of America. *Clin Infect Dis* **62:**409–417.
46. **Hartmann CA, Aye WT, Blair JE.** 2016. Treatment considerations in pulmonary coccidioidomycosis. *Expert Rev Respir Med* **10:**1079–1091.
47. **Perfect JR, Dismukes WE, Dromer F, Goldman DL, Graybill JR, Hamill RJ, Harrison TS, Larsen RA, Lortholary O, Nguyen MH, Pappas PG, Powderly WG, Singh N, Sobel JD, Sorrell TC.** 2010. Clinical practice guidelines for the management of cryptococcal disease: 2010 update by the Infectious Diseases Society of America. *Clin Infect Dis* **50:**291–322.
48. **Kauffman CA, Bustamante B, Chapman SW, Pappas PG, Infectious Diseases Society of America.** 2007. Clinical practice guidelines for the management of sporotrichosis: 2007 update by the Infectious Diseases Society of America. *Clin Infect Dis* **45:**1255–1265.
49. **Wheat LJ, Freifeld AG, Kleiman MB, Baddley JW, McKinsey DS, Loyd JE, Kauffman CA, Infectious Diseases Society of America.** 2007. Clinical practice guidelines for the management of patients with histoplasmosis: 2007 update by the Infectious Diseases Society of America. *Clin Infect Dis* **45:**807–825.
50. **Andes D, Pascual A, Marchetti O.** 2009. Antifungal therapeutic drug monitoring: established and emerging indications. *Antimicrob Agents Chemother* **53:**24–34.
51. **Schmitt-Hoffmann A, Roos B, Maares J, Heep M, Spickerman J, Weidekamm E, Brown T, Roehrle M.** 2006. Multiple-dose pharmacokinetics and safety of the new antifungal triazole BAL4815 after intravenous infusion and oral administration of its prodrug, BAL8557, in healthy volunteers. *Antimicrob Agents Chemother* **50:**286–293.
52. **Schmitt-Hoffmann AH, Kato K, Townsend R, Potchoiba MJ, Hope WW, Andes D, Spickermann J, Schneidkraut MJ.** 2017. Tissue distribution and elimination of isavuconazole following single and repeat oral-dose administration of isavuconazonium sulfate to rats. *Antimicrob Agents Chemother* **61:**e01292-17.
53. **Astvad KMT, Hare RK, Arendrup MC.** 2017. Evaluation of the in vitro activity of isavuconazole and comparator voriconazole against 2635 contemporary clinical *Candida* and *Aspergillus* isolates. *Clin Microbiol Infect* **23:**882–887.
54. **Hagen F, Illnait-Zaragozi MT, Bartlett KH, Swinne D, Geertsen E, Klaassen CH, Boekhout T, Meis JF.** 2010. In vitro antifungal susceptibilities and amplified fragment length polymorphism genotyping of a worldwide collection of 350 clinical, veterinary, and environmental *Cryptococcus gattii* isolates. *Antimicrob Agents Chemother* **54:**5139–5145.
55. **Thompson GR III, Wiederhold NP, Sutton DA, Fothergill A, Patterson TF.** 2009. In vitro activity of isavuconazole against *Trichosporon, Rhodotorula, Geotrichum, Saccharomyces* and *Pichia* species. *J Antimicrob Chemother* **64:**79–83.
56. **Maertens JA, Raad II, Marr KA, Patterson TF, Kontoyiannis DP, Cornely OA, Bow EJ, Rahav G, Neofytos D, Aoun M, Baddley JW, Giladi M, Heinz WJ, Herbrecht R, Hope W, Karthaus M, Lee DG, Lortholary O, Morrison VA, Oren I, Selleslag D, Shoham S, Thompson GR III, Lee M, Maher RM, Schmitt-Hoffmann AH, Zeiher B, Ullmann AJ.** 2016. Isavuconazole versus voriconazole for primary treatment of invasive mould disease caused by *Aspergillus* and other filamentous fungi (SECURE): a phase 3, randomised-controlled, non-inferiority trial. *Lancet* **387:**760–769.
57. **González GM.** 2009. In vitro activities of isavuconazole against opportunistic filamentous and dimorphic fungi. *Med Mycol* **47:**71–76.

58. **Thompson GR III, Rendon A, Ribeiro Dos Santos R, Queiroz-Telles F, Ostrosky-Zeichner L, Azie N, Maher R, Lee M, Kovanda L, Engelhardt M, Vazquez JA, Cornely OA, Perfect JR.** 2016. Isavuconazole treatment of *Cryptococcosis* and dimorphic mycoses. *Clin Infect Dis* **63:**356–362.
59. **Najafzadeh MJ, Badali H, Illnait-Zaragozi MT, De Hoog GS, Meis JF.** 2010. In vitro activities of eight antifungal drugs against 55 clinical isolates of *Fonsecaea* spp. *Antimicrob Agents Chemother* **54:**1636–1638.
60. **Feng P, Najafzadeh MJ, Sun J, Ahmed S, Xi L, de Hoog GS, Lai W, Lu C, Klaassen CH, Meis JF.** 2012. In vitro activities of nine antifungal drugs against 81 *Phialophora* and *Cyphellophora* isolates. *Antimicrob Agents Chemother* **56:**6044–6047.
61. **Arendrup MC, Jensen RH, Meletiadis J.** 2015. In vitro activity of isavuconazole and comparators against clinical isolates of the *Mucorales* order. *Antimicrob Agents Chemother* **59:**7735–7742.
62. **Verweij PE, González GM, Wiederhold NP, Lass-Flörl C, Warn P, Heep M, Ghannoum MA, Guinea J.** 2009. In vitro antifungal activity of isavuconazole against 345 mucorales isolates collected at study centers in eight countries. *J Chemother* **21:**272–281.
63. **Lackner M, de Hoog GS, Verweij PE, Najafzadeh MJ, Curfs-Breuker I, Klaassen CH, Meis JF.** 2012. Species-specific antifungal susceptibility patterns of *Scedosporium* and *Pseudallescheria* species. *Antimicrob Agents Chemother* **56:**2635–2642.
64. **Guinea J, Peláez T, Recio S, Torres-Narbona M, Bouza E.** 2008. In vitro antifungal activities of isavuconazole (BAL4815), voriconazole, and fluconazole against 1,007 isolates of zygomycete, *Candida*, *Aspergillus*, *Fusarium*, and *Scedosporium* species. *Antimicrob Agents Chemother* **52:**1396–1400.
65. **Sanglard D, Coste AT.** 2016. Activity of isavuconazole and other azoles against *Candida* clinical isolates and yeast model systems with known azole resistance mechanisms. *Antimicrob Agents Chemother* **60:**229–238.
66. **Chowdhary A, Kathuria S, Randhawa HS, Gaur SN, Klaassen CH, Meis JF.** 2012. Isolation of multiple-triazole-resistant *Aspergillus fumigatus* strains carrying the TR/L98H mutations in the cyp51A gene in India. *J Antimicrob Chemother* **67:**362–366.
67. **Viljoen J, Azie N, Schmitt-Hoffmann AH, Ghannoum M.** 2015. A phase 2, randomized, double-blind, multicenter trial to evaluate the safety and efficacy of three dosing regimens of isavuconazole compared with fluconazole in patients with uncomplicated esophageal candidiasis. *Antimicrob Agents Chemother* **59:**1671–1679.
68. **Desai AV, Kovanda LL, Hope WW, Andes D, Mouton JW, Kowalski DL, Townsend RW, Mujais S, Bonate PL.** 2017. Exposure-response relationships for isavuconazole in patients with invasive aspergillosis and other filamentous fungi. *Antimicrob Agents Chemother* **61:**e01034-17.
69. **Pfaller MA, Boyken L, Hollis RJ, Messer SA, Tendolkar S, Diekema DJ.** 2005. In vitro susceptibilities of clinical isolates of *Candida* species, *Cryptococcus neoformans*, and *Aspergillus* species to itraconazole: global survey of 9,359 isolates tested by clinical and laboratory standards institute broth microdilution methods. *J Clin Microbiol* **43:**3807–3810.
70. **Espinel-Ingroff A, Diekema DJ, Fothergill A, Johnson E, Pelaez T, Pfaller MA, Rinaldi MG, Canton E, Turnidge J.** 2010. Wild-type MIC distributions and epidemiological cutoff values for the triazoles and six *Aspergillus* spp. for the CLSI broth microdilution method (M38-A2 document). *J Clin Microbiol* **48:**3251–3257.
71. **Masih A, Singh PK, Kathuria S, Agarwal K, Meis JF, Chowdhary A.** 2016. Identification by molecular methods and matrix-assisted laser desorption ionization–time of flight mass spectrometry and antifungal susceptibility profiles of clinically significant rare *Aspergillus* species in a referral chest hospital in Delhi, India. *J Clin Microbiol* **54:**2354–2364.
72. **Lockhart SR, Iqbal N, Cleveland AA, Farley MM, Harrison LH, Bolden CB, Baughman W, Stein B, Hollick R, Park BJ, Chiller T.** 2012. Species identification and antifungal susceptibility testing of *Candida* bloodstream isolates from population-based surveillance studies in two U.S. cities from 2008 to 2011. *J Clin Microbiol* **50:**3435–3442.
73. **Pfaller MA, Espinel-Ingroff A, Canton E, Castanheira M, Cuenca-Estrella M, Diekema DJ, Fothergill A, Fuller J, Ghannoum M, Jones RN, Lockhart SR, Martin-Mazuelos E, Melhem MS, Ostrosky-Zeichner L, Pappas P, Pelaez T, Peman J, Rex J, Szeszs MW.** 2012. Wild-type MIC distributions and epidemiological cutoff values for amphotericin B, flucytosine, and itraconazole and *Candida* spp. as determined by CLSI broth microdilution. *J Clin Microbiol* **50:**2040–2046.
74. **Li RK, Ciblak MA, Nordoff N, Pasarell L, Warnock DW, McGinnis MR.** 2000. In vitro activities of voriconazole, itraconazole, and amphotericin B against *Blastomyces dermatitidis*, *Coccidioides immitis*, and *Histoplasma capsulatum*. *Antimicrob Agents Chemother* **44:**1734–1736.
75. **Almyroudis NG, Sutton DA, Fothergill AW, Rinaldi MG, Kusne S.** 2007. In vitro susceptibilities of 217 clinical isolates of zygomycetes to conventional and new antifungal agents. *Antimicrob Agents Chemother* **51:**2587–2590.
76. **Howard SJ, Cerar D, Anderson MJ, Albarrag A, Fisher MC, Pasqualotto AC, Laverdiere M, Arendrup MC, Perlin DS, Denning DW.** 2009. Frequency and evolution of azole resistance in *Aspergillus fumigatus* associated with treatment failure. *Emerg Infect Dis* **15:**1068–1076.
77. **Burgel PR, Baixench MT, Amsellem M, Audureau E, Chapron J, Kanaan R, Honoré I, Dupouy-Camet J, Dusser D, Klaassen CH, Meis JF, Hubert D, Paugam A.** 2012. High prevalence of azole-resistant *Aspergillus fumigatus* in adults with cystic fibrosis exposed to itraconazole. *Antimicrob Agents Chemother* **56:**869–874.
78. **Mellado E, Garcia-Effron G, Alcázar-Fuoli L, Melchers WJ, Verweij PE, Cuenca-Estrella M, Rodríguez-Tudela JL.** 2007. A new *Aspergillus fumigatus* resistance mechanism conferring in vitro cross-resistance to azole antifungals involves a combination of *cyp51A* alterations. *Antimicrob Agents Chemother* **51:**1897–1904.
79. **Meis JF, Chowdhary A, Rhodes JL, Fisher MC, Verweij PE.** 2016. Clinical implications of globally emerging azole resistance in *Aspergillus fumigatus*. *Philos Trans R Soc Lond B Biol Sci* **371:**20150460.
80. **Chapman SW, Dismukes WE, Proia LA, Bradsher RW, Pappas PG, Threlkeld MG, Kauffman CA, Infectious Diseases Society of America.** 2008. Clinical practice guidelines for the management of blastomycosis: 2008 update by the Infectious Diseases Society of America. *Clin Infect Dis* **46:**1801–1812.
81. **Walsh TJ, Anaissie EJ, Denning DW, Herbrecht R, Kontoyiannis DP, Marr KA, Morrison VA, Segal BH, Steinbach WJ, Stevens DA, van Burik JA, Wingard JR, Patterson TF, Infectious Diseases Society of America.** 2008. Treatment of aspergillosis: clinical practice guidelines of the Infectious Diseases Society of America. *Clin Infect Dis* **46:**327–360.
82. **Gupta AK, Lyons DC.** 2015. The rise and fall of oral ketoconazole. *J Cutan Med Surg* **19:**352–357.
83. **Shadomy S, White SC, Yu HP, Dismukes WE.** 1985. Treatment of systemic mycoses with ketoconazole: in vitro susceptibilities of clinical isolates of systemic and pathogenic fungi to ketoconazole. *J Infect Dis* **152:**1249–1256.
84. **Baddley JW, Marr KA, Andes DR, Walsh TJ, Kauffman CA, Kontoyiannis DP, Ito JI, Balajee SA, Pappas PG, Moser SA.** 2009. Patterns of susceptibility of *Aspergillus* isolates recovered from patients enrolled in the Transplant-Associated Infection Surveillance Network. *J Clin Microbiol* **47:**3271–3275.
85. **Espinel-Ingroff A, Pfaller MA, Bustamante B, Canton E, Fothergill A, Fuller J, Gonzalez GM, Lass-Flörl C, Lockhart SR, Martin-Mazuelos E, Meis JF, Melhem MS, Ostrosky-Zeichner L, Pelaez T, Szeszs MW, St-Germain G, Bonfietti LX, Guarro J, Turnidge J.** 2014. Multilaboratory study of epidemiological cutoff values for detection of resistance in eight *Candida* species to fluconazole, posaconazole, and voriconazole. *Antimicrob Agents Chemother* **58:**2006–2012.

86. **Paphitou NI, Ostrosky-Zeichner L, Paetznick VL, Rodriguez JR, Chen E, Rex JH.** 2002. In vitro antifungal susceptibilities of *Trichosporon* species. *Antimicrob Agents Chemother* **46:**1144–1146.
87. **Pfaller MA, Castanheira M, Diekema DJ, Messer SA, Jones RN.** 2011. Wild-type MIC distributions and epidemiologic cutoff values for fluconazole, posaconazole, and voriconazole when testing *Cryptococcus neoformans* as determined by the CLSI broth microdilution method. *Diagn Microbiol Infect Dis* **71:**252–259.
88. **Espinel-Ingroff A, Colombo AL, Cordoba S, Dufresne PJ, Fuller J, Ghannoum M, Gonzalez GM, Guarro J, Kidd SE, Meis JF, Melhem TM, Pelaez T, Pfaller MA, Szeszs MW, Takahaschi JP, Tortorano AM, Wiederhold NP, Turnidge J.** 2016. International evaluation of MIC distributions and epidemiological cutoff value (ECV) definitions for *Fusarium* species identified by molecular methods for the CLSI broth microdilution method. *Antimicrob Agents Chemother* **60:**1079–1084.
89. **Greenberg RN, Mullane K, van Burik JA, Raad I, Abzug MJ, Anstead G, Herbrecht R, Langston A, Marr KA, Schiller G, Schuster M, Wingard JR, Gonzalez CE, Revankar SG, Corcoran G, Kryscio RJ, Hare R.** 2006. Posaconazole as salvage therapy for zygomycosis. *Antimicrob Agents Chemother* **50:**126–133.
90. **Espinel-Ingroff A, Chakrabarti A, Chowdhary A, Cordoba S, Dannaoui E, Dufresne P, Fothergill A, Ghannoum M, Gonzalez GM, Guarro J, Kidd S, Lass-Flörl C, Meis JF, Pelaez T, Tortorano AM, Turnidge J.** 2015. Multicenter evaluation of MIC distributions for epidemiologic cutoff value definition to detect amphotericin B, posaconazole, and itraconazole resistance among the most clinically relevant species of *Mucorales*. *Antimicrob Agents Chemother* **59:**1745–1750.
91. **Vehreschild JJ, Birtel A, Vehreschild MJ, Liss B, Farowski F, Kochanek M, Sieniawski M, Steinbach A, Wahlers K, Fätkenheuer G, Cornely OA.** 2013. Mucormycosis treated with posaconazole: review of 96 case reports. *Crit Rev Microbiol* **39:**310–324.
92. **van der Linden JW, Camps SM, Kampinga GA, Arends JP, Debets-Ossenkopp YJ, Haas PJ, Rijnders BJ, Kuijper EJ, van Tiel FH, Varga J, Karawajczyk A, Zoll J, Melchers WJ, Verweij PE.** 2013. Aspergillosis due to voriconazole highly resistant *Aspergillus fumigatus* and recovery of genetically related resistant isolates from domiciles. *Clin Infect Dis* **57:**513–520.
93. **Bueid A, Howard SJ, Moore CB, Richardson MD, Harrison E, Bowyer P, Denning DW.** 2010. Azole antifungal resistance in *Aspergillus fumigatus*: 2008 and 2009. *J Antimicrob Chemother* **65:**2116–2118.
94. **Restrepo A, Tobón A, Clark B, Graham DR, Corcoran G, Bradsher RW, Goldman M, Pankey G, Moore T, Negroni R, Graybill JR.** 2007. Salvage treatment of histoplasmosis with posaconazole. *J Infect* **54:**319–327.
95. **Kim MM, Vikram HR, Kusne S, Seville MT, Blair JE.** 2011. Treatment of refractory coccidioidomycosis with voriconazole or posaconazole. *Clin Infect Dis* **53:**1060–1066.
96. **van Burik JA, Hare RS, Solomon HF, Corrado ML, Kontoyiannis DP.** 2006. Posaconazole is effective as salvage therapy in zygomycosis: a retrospective summary of 91 cases. *Clin Infect Dis* **42:**e61–e65.
97. **Raad II, Graybill JR, Bustamante AB, Cornely OA, Gaona-Flores V, Afif C, Graham DR, Greenberg RN, Hadley S, Langston A, Negroni R, Perfect JR, Pitisuttithum P, Restrepo A, Schiller G, Pedicone L, Ullmann AJ.** 2006. Safety of long-term oral posaconazole use in the treatment of refractory invasive fungal infections. *Clin Infect Dis* **42:**1726–1734.
98. **Verweij PE, Chowdhary A, Melchers WJ, Meis JF.** 2016. Azole resistance in *Aspergillus fumigatus*: can we retain the clinical use of mold-active antifungal azoles? *Clin Infect Dis* **62:**362–368.
99. **Malani AN, Kerr LE, Kauffman CA.** 2015. Voriconazole: how to use this antifungal agent and what to expect. *Semin Respir Crit Care Med* **36:**786–795.
100. **Park S, Kelly R, Kahn JN, Robles J, Hsu MJ, Register E, Li W, Vyas V, Fan H, Abruzzo G, Flattery A, Gill C, Chrebet G, Parent SA, Kurtz M, Teppler H, Douglas CM, Perlin DS.** 2005. Specific substitutions in the echinocandin target Fks1p account for reduced susceptibility of rare laboratory and clinical *Candida* sp. isolates. *Antimicrob Agents Chemother* **49:**3264–3273.
101. **Sucher AJ, Chahine EB, Balcer HE.** 2009. Echinocandins: the newest class of antifungals. *Ann Pharmacother* **43:**1647–1657.
102. **Pfaller MA, Espinel-Ingroff A, Bustamante B, Canton E, Diekema DJ, Fothergill A, Fuller J, Gonzalez GM, Guarro J, Lass-Flörl C, Lockhart SR, Martin-Mazuelos E, Meis JF, Ostrosky-Zeichner L, Pelaez T, St-Germain G, Turnidge J.** 2014. Multicenter study of anidulafungin and micafungin MIC distributions and epidemiological cutoff values for eight *Candida* species and the CLSI M27-A3 broth microdilution method. *Antimicrob Agents Chemother* **58:**916–922.
103. **Pfaller MA, Castanheira M, Lockhart SR, Ahlquist AM, Messer SA, Jones RN.** 2012. Frequency of decreased susceptibility and resistance to echinocandins among fluconazole-resistant bloodstream isolates of *Candida glabrata*. *J Clin Microbiol* **50:**1199–1203.
104. **Lockhart SR, Pham CD, Kuykendall RJ, Bolden CB, Cleveland AA.** 2016. Candida lusitaniae MICs to the echinocandins are elevated but FKS-mediated resistance is rare. *Diagn Microbiol Infect Dis* **84:**52–54.
105. **Lockhart SR, Zimbeck AJ, Baddley JW, Marr KA, Andes DR, Walsh TJ, Kauffman CA, Kontoyiannis DP, Ito JI, Pappas PG, Chiller T.** 2011. In vitro echinocandin susceptibility of *Aspergillus* isolates from patients enrolled in the Transplant-Associated Infection Surveillance Network. *Antimicrob Agents Chemother* **55:**3944–3946.
106. **Pfaller MA, Boyken L, Hollis RJ, Kroeger J, Messer SA, Tendolkar S, Diekema DJ.** 2010. Wild-type minimum effective concentration distributions and epidemiologic cutoff values for caspofungin and *Aspergillus* spp. as determined by Clinical and Laboratory Standards Institute broth microdilution methods. *Diagn Microbiol Infect Dis* **67:**56–60.
107. **Espinel-Ingroff A.** 2003. In vitro antifungal activities of anidulafungin and micafungin, licensed agents and the investigational triazole posaconazole as determined by NCCLS methods for 12,052 fungal isolates: review of the literature. *Rev Iberoam Micol* **20:**121–136.
108. **Nakai T, Uno J, Ikeda F, Tawara S, Nishimura K, Miyaji M.** 2003. In vitro antifungal activity of micafungin (FK463) against dimorphic fungi: comparison of yeast-like and mycelial forms. *Antimicrob Agents Chemother* **47:**1376–1381.
109. **Alexander BD, Johnson MD, Pfeiffer CD, Jiménez-Ortigosa C, Catania J, Booker R, Castanheira M, Messer SA, Perlin DS, Pfaller MA.** 2013. Increasing echinocandin resistance in *Candida glabrata*: clinical failure correlates with presence of FKS mutations and elevated minimum inhibitory concentrations. *Clin Infect Dis* **56:**1724–1732.
110. **Shields RK, Nguyen MH, Press EG, Clancy CJ.** 2014. Abdominal candidiasis is a hidden reservoir of echinocandin resistance. *Antimicrob Agents Chemother* **58:**7601–7605.
111. **Perlin DS.** 2007. Resistance to echinocandin-class antifungal drugs. *Drug Resist Updat* **10:**121–130.
112. **Pham CD, Iqbal N, Bolden CB, Kuykendall RJ, Harrison LH, Farley MM, Schaffner W, Beldavs ZG, Chiller TM, Park BJ, Cleveland AA, Lockhart SR.** 2014. Role of FKS mutations in *Candida glabrata*: MIC values, echinocandin resistance, and multidrug resistance. *Antimicrob Agents Chemother* **58:**4690–4696.
113. **Song JC, Stevens DA.** 2016. Caspofungin: pharmacodynamics, pharmacokinetics, clinical uses and treatment outcomes. *Crit Rev Microbiol* **42:**813–846.
114. **Muilwijk EW, Lempers VJ, Burger DM, Warris A, Pickkers P, Aarnoutse RE, Brüggemann RJ.** 2015. Impact of special patient populations on the pharmacokinetics of echinocandins. *Expert Rev Anti Infect Ther* **13:**799–815.
115. **Damle BD, Dowell JA, Walsky RL, Weber GL, Stogniew M, Inskeep PB.** 2009. In vitro and in vivo studies to

characterize the clearance mechanism and potential cytochrome P450 interactions of anidulafungin. *Antimicrob Agents Chemother* **53:**1149–1156.

116. **Wagner C, Graninger W, Presterl E, Joukhadar C.** 2006. The echinocandins: comparison of their pharmacokinetics, pharmacodynamics and clinical applications. *Pharmacology* **78:**161–177.
117. **Stone JA, Holland SD, Wickersham PJ, Sterrett A, Schwartz M, Bonfiglio C, Hesney M, Winchell GA, Deutsch PJ, Greenberg H, Hunt TL, Waldman SA.** 2002. Single- and multiple-dose pharmacokinetics of caspofungin in healthy men. *Antimicrob Agents Chemother* **46:**739–745.
118. **Hebert MF, Smith HE, Marbury TC, Swan SK, Smith WB, Townsend RW, Buell D, Keirns J, Bekersky I.** 2005. Pharmacokinetics of micafungin in healthy volunteers, volunteers with moderate liver disease, and volunteers with renal dysfunction. *J Clin Pharmacol* **45:**1145–1152.
119. **Autmizguine J, Guptill JT, Cohen-Wolkowiez M, Benjamin DK Jr, Capparelli EV.** 2014. Pharmacokinetics and pharmacodynamics of antifungals in children: clinical implications. *Drugs* **74:**891–909.
120. **Andes D, Diekema DJ, Pfaller MA, Bohrmuller J, Marchillo K, Lepak A.** 2010. In vivo comparison of the pharmacodynamic targets for echinocandin drugs against *Candida* species. *Antimicrob Agents Chemother* **54:**2497–2506.
121. **Goodwin ML, Drew RH.** 2008. Antifungal serum concentration monitoring: an update. *J Antimicrob Chemother* **61:**17–25.
122. **Baginski M, Czub J.** 2009. Amphotericin B and its new derivatives—mode of action. *Curr Drug Metab* **10:**459–469.
123. **Hamill RJ.** 2013. Amphotericin B formulations: a comparative review of efficacy and toxicity. *Drugs* **73:** 919–934.
124. **Zarif L, Graybill JR, Perlin D, Najvar L, Bocanegra R, Mannino RJ.** 2000. Antifungal activity of amphotericin B cochleates against *Candida albicans* infection in a mouse model. *Antimicrob Agents Chemother* **44:**1463–1469.
125. **Delmas G, Park S, Chen ZW, Tan F, Kashiwazaki R, Zarif L, Perlin DS.** 2002. Efficacy of orally delivered cochleates containing amphotericin B in a murine model of aspergillosis. *Antimicrob Agents Chemother* **46:**2704–2707.
126. **Espinel-Ingroff A, Cuenca-Estrella M, Fothergill A, Fuller J, Ghannoum M, Johnson E, Pelaez T, Pfaller MA, Turnidge J.** 2011. Wild-type MIC distributions and epidemiological cutoff values for amphotericin B and *Aspergillus* spp. for the CLSI broth microdilution method (M38-A2 document). *Antimicrob Agents Chemother* **55:**5150–5154.
127. **Kathuria S, Sharma C, Singh PK, Agarwal P, Agarwal K, Hagen F, Meis JF, Chowdhary A.** 2015. Molecular epidemiology and in-vitro antifungal susceptibility of *Aspergillus terreus* species complex isolates in Delhi, India: evidence of genetic diversity by amplified fragment length polymorphism and microsatellite typing. *PLoS One* **10:**e0118997.
128. **Risslegger B, et al.** 2017. A prospective international *Aspergillus terreus* survey: an EFISG, ISHAM and ECMM joint study. *Clin Microbiol Infect* **23:**776.e1–776.e5.
129. **Alcazar-Fuoli L, Mellado E, Alastruey-Izquierdo A, Cuenca-Estrella M, Rodriguez-Tudela JL.** 2008. *Aspergillus* section *Fumigati*: antifungal susceptibility patterns and sequence-based identification. *Antimicrob Agents Chemother* **52:**1244–1251.
130. **Cuenca-Estrella M, Gomez-Lopez A, Mellado E, Buitrago MJ, Monzon A, Rodriguez-Tudela JL.** 2006. Head-to-head comparison of the activities of currently available antifungal agents against 3,378 Spanish clinical isolates of yeasts and filamentous fungi. *Antimicrob Agents Chemother* **50:**917–921.
131. **Castanheira M, Duncanson FP, Diekema DJ, Guarro J, Jones RN, Pfaller MA.** 2012. Activities of E1210 and comparator agents tested by CLSI and EUCAST broth microdilution methods against *Fusarium* and *Scedosporium* species identified using molecular methods. *Antimicrob Agents Chemother* **56:**352–357.
132. **Ellis D.** 2002. Amphotericin B: spectrum and resistance. *J Antimicrob Chemother* **49**(Suppl 1)**:**7–10.
133. **Kathuria S, Singh PK, Sharma C, Prakash A, Masih A, Kumar A, Meis JF, Chowdhary A.** 2015. Multidrug-resistant *Candida auris* misidentified as *Candida haemulonii*: characterization by matrix-assisted laser desorption ionization–time of flight mass spectrometry and DNA sequencing and its antifungal susceptibility profile variability by Vitek 2, CLSI broth microdilution, and Etest method. *J Clin Microbiol* **53:** 1823–1830.
134. **Stone NR, Bicanic T, Salim R, Hope W.** 2016. Liposomal amphotericin B (AmBisome®): a review of the pharmacokinetics, pharmacodynamics, clinical experience and future directions. *Drugs* **76:**485–500.
135. **Vogelsinger H, Weiler S, Djanani A, Kountchev J, Bellmann-Weiler R, Wiedermann CJ, Bellmann R.** 2006. Amphotericin B tissue distribution in autopsy material after treatment with liposomal amphotericin B and amphotericin B colloidal dispersion. *J Antimicrob Chemother* **57:** 1153–1160.
136. **Steimbach LM, Tonin FS, Virtuoso S, Borba HH, Sanches AC, Wiens A, Fernandez-Llimós F, Pontarolo R.** 2017. Efficacy and safety of amphotericin B lipid-based formulations—a systematic review and meta-analysis. *Mycoses* **60:**146–154.
137. **Pfaller MA, Messer SA, Boyken L, Huynh H, Hollis RJ, Diekema DJ.** 2002. In vitro activities of 5-fluorocytosine against 8,803 clinical isolates of *Candida* spp.: global assessment of primary resistance using National Committee for Clinical Laboratory Standards susceptibility testing methods. *Antimicrob Agents Chemother* **46:**3518–3521.
138. **Vermes A, Guchelaar HJ, Dankert J.** 2000. Flucytosine: a review of its pharmacology, clinical indications, pharmacokinetics, toxicity and drug interactions. *J Antimicrob Chemother* **46:**171–179.
139. **Gupta AK, Tu LQ.** 2006. Therapies for onychomycosis: a review. *Dermatol Clin* **24:**375–379.
140. **Hata K, Horii T, Miyazaki M, Watanabe NA, Okubo M, Sonoda J, Nakamoto K, Tanaka K, Shirotori S, Murai N, Inoue S, Matsukura M, Abe S, Yoshimatsu K, Asada M.** 2011. Efficacy of oral E1210, a new broad-spectrum antifungal with a novel mechanism of action, in murine models of candidiasis, aspergillosis, and fusariosis. *Antimicrob Agents Chemother* **55:**4543–4551.
141. **Pfaller MA, Duncanson F, Messer SA, Moet GJ, Jones RN, Castanheira M.** 2011. In vitro activity of a novel broad-spectrum antifungal, E1210, tested against *Aspergillus* spp. determined by CLSI and EUCAST broth microdilution methods. *Antimicrob Agents Chemother* **55:**5155–5158.
142. **Pfaller MA, Hata K, Jones RN, Messer SA, Moet GJ, Castanheira M.** 2011. In vitro activity of a novel broad-spectrum antifungal, E1210, tested against *Candida* spp. as determined by CLSI broth microdilution method. *Diagn Microbiol Infect Dis* **71:**167–170.
143. **Walker SS, Xu Y, Triantafyllou I, Waldman MF, Mendrick C, Brown N, Mann P, Chau A, Patel R, Bauman N, Norris C, Antonacci B, Gurnani M, Cacciapuoti A, McNicholas PM, Wainhaus S, Herr RJ, Kuang R, Aslanian RG, Ting PC, Black TA.** 2011. Discovery of a novel class of orally active antifungal beta-1,3-D-glucan synthase inhibitors. *Antimicrob Agents Chemother* **55:**5099–5106.
144. **Jiménez-Ortigosa C, Paderu P, Motyl MR, Perlin DS.** 2014. Enfumafungin derivative MK-3118 shows increased in vitro potency against clinical echinocandin-resistant *Candida* species and *Aspergillus* species isolates. *Antimicrob Agents Chemother* **58:**1248–1251.
145. **Berkow EL, Angulo D, Lockhart SR.** 2017. In vitro activity of a novel glucan synthase inhibitor, SCY-078, against clinical isolates of *Candida auris*. *Antimicrob Agents Chemother* **61:**e00435.
146. **Pfaller MA, Messer SA, Motyl MR, Jones RN, Castanheira M.** 2013. Activity of MK-3118, a new oral glucan synthase inhibitor, tested against *Candida* spp. by two international methods (CLSI and EUCAST). *J Antimicrob Chemother* **68:**858–863.
147. **Lamoth F, Alexander BD.** 2015. Antifungal activities of SCY-078 (MK-3118) and standard antifungal agents against

clinical non-*Aspergillus* mold isolates. *Antimicrob Agents Chemother* **59:**4308–4311.

148. **Oliver JD, Sibley GE, Beckmann N, Dobb KS, Slater MJ, McEntee L, du Pré S, Livermore J, Bromley MJ, Wiederhold NP, Hope WW, Kennedy AJ, Law D, Birch M.** 2016. F901318 represents a novel class of antifungal drug that inhibits dihydroorotate dehydrogenase. *Proc Natl Acad Sci USA* **113:**12809–12814.
149. **Hope WW, McEntee L, Livermore J, Whalley S, Johnson A, Farrington N, Kolamunnage-Dona R, Schwartz J, Kennedy A, Law D, Birch M, Rex JH.** 2017. Pharmacodynamics of the orotomides against *Aspergillus fumigatus*: new opportunities for treatment of multidrug-resistant fungal disease. *mBio* **8:**e01157-17.
150. **Wiederhold NP.** 2018. The antifungal arsenal: alternative drugs and future targets. *Int J Antimicrob Agents* **51:**333–339.
151. **Buil JB, et al.** 2016. Activity of F901318 against azole-resistant and difficult-to-treat Aspergillus species, poster P1605. 26th European Congress of Clinical Microbiology and Infectious Disease, Amsterdam, the Netherlands.
152. **Ong V, Hough G, Schlosser M, Bartizal K, Balkovec JM, James KD, Krishnan BR.** 2016. Preclinical evaluation of the stability, safety, and efficacy of CD101, a novel echinocandin. *Antimicrob Agents Chemother* **60:**6872–6879.
153. **Ong V, James KD, Smith S, Krishnan BR.** 2017. Pharmacokinetics of the novel echinocandin CD101 in multiple animal species. *Antimicrob Agents Chemother* **61:**e01626-16.
154. **Pfaller MA, Messer SA, Rhomberg PR, Castanheira M.** 2017. Activity of a long-acting echinocandin (CD101) and seven comparator antifungal agents tested against a global collection of contemporary invasive fungal isolates in the SENTRY 2014 Antifungal Surveillance Program. *Antimicrob Agents Chemother* **61:**e02045-16.
155. **Zhao Y, Perez WB, Jiménez-Ortigosa C, Hough G, Locke JB, Ong V, Bartizal K, Perlin DS.** 2016. CD101: a novel long-acting echinocandin. *Cell Microbiol* **18:**1308–1316.
156. **Hoekstra WJ, Garvey EP, Moore WR, Rafferty SW, Yates CM, Schotzinger RJ.** 2014. Design and optimization of highly-selective fungal CYP51 inhibitors. *Bioorg Med Chem Lett* **24:**3455–3458.
157. **Break TJ, Desai JV, Natarajan M, Ferre EMN, Henderson C, Zelazny AM, Siebenlist U, Hoekstra WJ, Schotzinger RJ, Garvey EP, Lionakis MS.** 2018. VT-1161 protects mice against oropharyngeal candidiasis caused by fluconazole-susceptible and -resistant *Candida albicans*. *J Antimicrob Chemother* **73:**151–155.
158. **Shubitz LF, Trinh HT, Galgiani JN, Lewis ML, Fothergill AW, Wiederhold NP, Barker BM, Lewis ER, Doyle AL, Hoekstra WJ, Schotzinger RJ, Garvey EP.** 2015. Evaluation of VT-1161 for treatment of coccidioidomycosis in murine infection models. *Antimicrob Agents Chemother* **59:**7249–7254.
159. **Warrilow AG, Hull CM, Parker JE, Garvey EP, Hoekstra WJ, Moore WR, Schotzinger RJ, Kelly DE, Kelly SL.** 2014. The clinical candidate VT-1161 is a highly potent inhibitor of *Candida albicans* CYP51 but fails to bind the human enzyme. *Antimicrob Agents Chemother* **58:**7121–7127.
160. **Garvey EP, Hoekstra WJ, Moore WR, Schotzinger RJ, Long L, Ghannoum MA.** 2015. VT-1161 dosed once daily or once weekly exhibits potent efficacy in treatment of dermatophytosis in a guinea pig model. *Antimicrob Agents Chemother* **59:**1992–1997.
161. **Wiederhold NP, et al.** 2017. The novel fungal Cyp51 inhibitor VT-1598 demonstrates potent in vitro activity against endemic fungi, *Aspergillus*, and *Rhizopus*, abstr 232. ASM Microbe, New Orleans, LA.
162. **Wiederhold NPTB, Patterson H, Yates CM, Schotzinger RJ, Garvey EP.** 2017. The novel fungal Cyp51 inhibitor VT-1598 demonstrates potent in vitro activity against *Candida* and *Cryptococcus* species, abstr 237. ASM Microbe, New Orleans, LA.
163. **Berkow ELLN, Peterson J, Garvey EP, Yates CM, Schotzinger RJ, Lockhart SR.** 2017. In vitro activity of a novel Cyp51 inhibitor VT-1598 against clinical isolates of *Candida auris*, abstr 304. ASM Microbe, New Orleans, LA.
164. **Dietz AJ, Barnard JC, van Rossem K.** 2014. A randomized, double-blind, multiple-dose, placebo-controlled, dose escalation study with a 3-cohort parallel group design to investigate the tolerability and pharmacokinetics of albaconazole in healthy subjects. *Clin Pharmacol Drug Dev* **3:**25–33.
165. **Sigurgeirsson B, van Rossem K, Malahias S, Raterink K.** 2013. A phase II, randomized, double-blind, placebo-controlled, parallel group, dose-ranging study to investigate the efficacy and safety of 4 dose regimens of oral albaconazole in patients with distal subungual onychomycosis. *J Am Acad Dermatol* **69:**416–425.e1.
166. **van Rossem K, Lowe JA.** 2013. A phase 1, randomized, open-label crossover study to evaluate the safety and pharmacokinetics of 400 mg albaconazole administered to healthy participants as a tablet formulation versus a capsule formulation. *Clin Pharmacol* **5:**23–31.

Mechanisms of Resistance to Antifungal Agents

DAVID S. PERLIN

133

Serious fungal infections result in over 1,350,000 deaths per year (1). Some fungal diseases are acute and severe, such as cryptococcal meningitis and invasive aspergillosis, while others are recurrent, such as *Candida* vaginitis and oral candidiasis in AIDS. The most serious fungal infections occur as a consequence of other serious health problems, such as asthma, AIDS, cancer, organ transplantation, and corticosteroid therapies (1). All require specialized testing for diagnosis and antifungal therapy. More than 90% of all reported fungal infection-related deaths result from species that belong to one of three genera: *Cryptococcus*, *Candida*, and *Aspergillus* (1). Failure to treat effectively often leads to death, serious chronic illness, or blindness. The global importance of fungal infections has led to a rise in the use of antifungal agents for the treatment and prevention of such infections. Unfortunately, treatment options for invasive fungal infections are limited, as there are few chemical classes represented by existing antifungal drugs.

Classes of antifungal drugs include polyenes, azoles, flucytosine (5FC), and echinocandins. The azoles (e.g., fluconazole, voriconazole, posaconazole, and isavuconazole) target ergosterol biosynthesis. Like cholesterol in mammalian cells, ergosterol is the major sterol in fungal plasma membrane. Polyenes, like amphotericin B, bind to ergosterol in the plasma membrane, where they form large pores that disrupt cell function. 5FC inhibits pyrimidine metabolism and DNA synthesis. Finally, the echinocandins (caspofungin, anidulafungin, and micafungin) are cell wall-active agents that inhibit the biosynthesis of β1,3-D-glucan, a major component of the fungal cell wall.

The expanding use of antifungal agents has led to rising drug resistance. The emergence of acquired drug resistance among susceptible fungal species negatively impacts patient management. A greater understanding of biological factors that contribute to mechanism-specific resistance is critical to the field of medical mycology. The biological and molecular nature of antifungal drug resistance mechanisms among major systemic drugs is the topic of this chapter.

DEFINING CLINICAL AND MICROBIOLOGICAL RESISTANCE

The development of antifungal resistance is complex and relies on multiple host and microbial factors. A discussion of drug resistance must distinguish between multifaceted clinical resistance and microbial resistance to antifungal agents.

"Clinical resistance" refers to therapeutic failure whereby a patient inadequately responds to an antifungal drug following administration at a standard dose. A variety of host, drug, pharmacological, and microbial factors contribute to therapeutic failure. A major factor is the immune status of the host. Antifungal drug action and the host immune system often must work synergistically to control and clear an infection. Patients with severe immune dysfunction are more refractory to treatment, as the antifungal drug must combat the infection without the positive benefit of the immune response. The presence of indwelling catheters, artificial heart valves, and other surgical devices contributes to refractory infections, as the infecting fungus attaches to these objects, creating resilient biofilms that resist drug therapy. The site of the infection also contributes to clinical resistance, as appropriate therapy requires that a drug reach its microbial target at a suitable concentration to inhibit growth or kill the organism. However, we still do not have a good understanding of drug penetration at the site of infection or within host reservoirs, with the result that some microorganisms are exposed to drug at inadequate levels. Finally, patient compliance with prescribed drug regimens is critical for effective treatment, as poor adherence reduces the effectiveness of the drug and contributes to development of persistent drug-tolerant cell populations.

"Microbiological resistance" refers to decreased susceptibility of a fungal strain to an antifungal agent, which is reflected in standardized *in vitro* susceptibility testing relative to susceptible standard reference strains. (The details of antifungal susceptibility testing according to guidelines established by the Clinical and Laboratory Standards Institute and the European Committee on Antimicrobial Susceptibility Testing are addressed in chapter 134.) Susceptibility testing provides a measure of the MIC, and resistance breakpoints refer to the drug concentrations that separate strains for which there is a high likelihood of treatment success from those organisms for which treatment is more likely to fail (2). However, interpreting the results of *in vitro* antifungal susceptibility testing can be problematic, as MICs above the breakpoint do not always directly correlate with response to antifungal therapy. This apparent discordance between *in vivo* and *in vitro* data is partially captured by the "90-60 rule," which maintains that infections due to susceptible strains respond to appropriate therapy in ~90% of cases, whereas infections due to resistant strains respond in ~60% of cases (3). Microbiologic resistance can be primary (intrinsic) or secondary (acquired). Primary resistance is found naturally among certain fungi without prior drug exposure. It may involve the mechanism responsible for acquired resistance or unknown mechanisms.

Primary Resistance

Antimicrobial agents are generally developed for efficacy against the most prominent pathogens causing disease (e.g., *Candida albicans*). Universal broad-spectrum activity (e.g., panfungal), while desirable, is rarely achieved, and there will always be a subset of species or naturally occurring variants of mostly susceptible species that are inherently resistant. Presently, there are more than 200 species of *Candida*, and while fewer than 40 are known to cause human infections (4), there is great genetic diversity that can impact drug action. The extended application of antifungal agents against a wide spectrum of mycoses can result in the selection of naturally occurring species with inherent resistance (5). Nevertheless, the overall selection of resistant species, subspecies, or less susceptible variants from the environment or from patient reservoirs occurs uncommonly (6). The unifying feature of intrinsic resistance is that the underlying resistance mechanism is inherent and not acquired during therapy.

Azoles

The azole antifungal agents are the most prominent example of drug selection for less susceptible species (7). Numerous global epidemiological studies have documented the impact of widespread triazole use on the distribution and shift of *Candida* species toward less susceptible organisms, like *C. glabrata* and *C. krusei*. In many regions where use of azoles (e.g., fluconazole) is prevalent, there has been a shift away from *C. albicans* as the predominant cause of invasive infections toward less susceptible non-*C. albicans* species (8). *C. glabrata*, which can rapidly acquire resistance to fluconazole and other azoles, is the species whose incidence has increased the most to account for a decrease in the prevalence of *C. albicans* (8). Similarly, fluconazole use is linked to emergence of the highly resistant species *C. krusei* (9) and *C. guilliermondii* (10). Most recently, *C. auris* has emerged as an important nosocomial multidrug-resistant species (11). In many cases, inherent resistance to fluconazole confers cross-resistance to more highly active triazoles, like voriconazole. This is not true for *Aspergillus* and other moulds that are resistant to fluconazole but susceptible to more highly active triazoles. However, breakthrough infections against triazole drugs have been reported for *A. ustus* (12) and *A. lentulus*, which show pleiotropic resistance to multiple antifungals (13). Sometimes a susceptible species develops a prevalent variant that is the source of resistant infections. In the bacterial world, the spread of drug-resistant strains from a common progenitor is commonly observed. Such transmission is not typically observed for fungal drug resistance. Notable exceptions include *C. auris* (11) and environmentally derived strains of azole-resistant *Aspergillus fumigatus* (14), which are spreading globally (15).

Echinocandins

Echinocandins are highly active against most *Candida* spp., but they have inherent reduced *in vitro* activity against the *C. parapsilosis* group (*C. parapsilosis sensu stricto*, *C. orthopsilosis*, and *C. metapsilosis*) and *C. guilliermondii* (16). Some breakthrough infections have been reported during therapy and have been attributed to the inherent reduced *in vitro* activity against these strains (17). Resistance to echinocandin drugs has also been described for *A. lentulus* (13) and *C. auris* (18). In some filamentous fungi, like *A. lentulus*, *A. ustus*, and *Fusarium* spp., there is resistance to azoles and echinocandin drugs, and occasionally resistance to polyenes.

Polyenes

The polyene drug amphotericin is fungicidal, and resistance rarely occurs. When it does, it is mostly due to selection of strains with intrinsic reduced susceptibility (MIC, >1 μg/ml), which correlates with the epidemiological cutoff values for most *Candida* species (19). The organisms *Scedosporium apiospermum*, *Fusarium* spp., *Trichosporon* spp., and *Sporothrix schenckii* are frequently resistant to amphotericin (7). Breakthrough infections have been reported for *C. rugosa* (20), *C. lusitaniae* (21), and *C. tropicalis* (22) and frequently for *C. auris* (23). Among the *Aspergillus* spp., primary resistance to amphotericin B has been reported for strains of *A. terreus* (24), *A. flavus* (25), and *A. ustus* (26).

In summary, drug pressure imparts powerful selection that results in infections by uncommon fungi with inherent reduced susceptibility to antifungal drugs. For many fungi, drug insensitivity reflects underlying resistance mechanisms that emerge in susceptible strains in response to drug action.

RESISTANCE TO AZOLES

Mechanism of Action of Azoles

Azoles inhibit the biosynthesis of ergosterol, the principal sterol in fungal cell membranes, by interfering with the action of lanosterol 14α-demethylase, which is encoded by *ERG11* (*Cyp51A* in *Aspergillus*). There are many licensed azole antifungal drugs (imidazoles and triazoles), yet the triazole drugs fluconazole, voriconazole, itraconazole, posaconazole, and isavuconazole are the most commonly prescribed drugs for prophylaxis or treatment of invasive fungal infections. Triazoles differ in their target affinities, which influences their spectrum of activity. Hence, fluconazole has the weakest interaction with its target and shows the narrowest spectrum of activity. It is active against many yeasts but has poor activity against moulds. The more highly active triazoles, like voriconazole, posaconazole, and isavuconazole, interact more strongly with the demethylase target and show broad-spectrum activity against yeasts and moulds, as well as activity against some fluconazole-resistant strains. Fluconazole and voriconazole are very similar in chemical structure, while posaconazole and itraconazole are more closely related. It is this moderate chemical diversity around a core unit that promotes cross-reactivity and, at times, differential susceptibility, which ultimately depends upon the nature of the resistance mechanism.

Epidemiology of Azole Resistance

Candida Species

The widespread use of fluconazole as a safe and effective antimycotic agent to treat HIV-infected patients in the preantiretroviral therapy era with oropharyngeal or esophageal candidiasis led to the emergence of resistance. A multitude of sentinel and population-based surveillance programs from more than 40 countries have contributed to our understanding of azole resistance (27, 28). Overall, the studies confirm that acquired resistance among susceptible species is low (1 to 3%), while resistance is more significant in non-*albicans Candida* species. Over a 10-year period ending in 2007, the ARTEMIS DISK Global Antifungal Surveillance Study examined clinical isolates of *Candida* spp. from 142 sites in 41 countries. For all *Candida* spp. isolates, 90.2% were susceptible to fluconazole, while 95.0% were susceptible to voriconazole. Among 128,625 isolates of *C. albicans*, 1.4% and 1.2% were resistant to fluconazole and voriconazole, respectively. In 23,305 clinical isolates of *C. glabrata*, there was a higher population of resistant isolates, 15.7% and 10% for fluconazole and voriconazole, respectively. There was a yearly trend upward for increased azole resistance among *C. glabrata* (29), and resistance to fluconazole varied by region (27, 28).

More recent global studies have affirmed the low level of acquired resistance. In the 2014 Taiwan Surveillance of Antimicrobial Resistance of Yeasts, involving 1,106 *Candida* isolates, 2.8% and 2.2% were resistant to fluconazole and voriconazole, respectively (30). In an Italian study involving 394 episodes of candidemia from 1998 to 2013, only 5% and 2.9% of isolates were resistant to fluconazole and voriconazole, respectively (31). The SENTRY Antifungal Surveillance Program reported for the Asia-Western Pacific region during 2012 to 2014 fluconazole resistance rates of 6.8%, 5.7%, and 3.6% for *C. glabrata*, *C. parapsilosis*, and *C. tropicalis*, respectively (32). In China from 2009 to 2013, rates of resistance to fluconazole, voriconazole, and itraconazole were 7.6%, 3.2%, and 1.8%, respectively (33). In a study of 3,181 yeasts causing vulvovaginal candidiasis in southern China from 2003 to 2012, the rate of resistance of *C. albicans* to fluconazole was 1.1%, while the rates of resistance of non-*C. albicans* strains to fluconazole and itraconazole were 11.8% and 2.5%, respectively (34). Azole resistance is notable with *C. guilliermondii* and *C. krusei*, and an overall increase in fluconazole resistance has been observed among *C. parapsilosis*, *C. guilliermondii*, *C. lusitaniae*, and *C. pelliculosa* (35). In South African hospitals during 2009 and 2010, 531 *C. parapsilosis* isolates were found, with a staggering 63% resistance to fluconazole and voriconazole (36). This contrasts with low fluconazole resistance among *C. parapsilosis* isolates in most U.S. institutions (37). For the emerging pathogen *C. auris*, among clinical isolates from 54 patients from Pakistan, India, South Africa, and Venezuela during 2012 to 2015, 93% were found to be resistant to fluconazole (23). Azole resistance among *Cryptococcus neoformans* is generally very low in developed countries (38), while in developing countries, fluconazole resistance is also low but more significant (39).

Aspergillus Species

Triazole-resistant strains of *A. fumigatus* were first reported in 1997 from patients in California treated with itraconazole (40). Azole-resistant *A. fumigatus* has now been reported in China, Canada, the United States, and several European countries. High rates in the United Kingdom (15 to 20%) (41) and in the Netherlands (5 to 7%) have been observed (42). Approximately 5% of *Aspergillus* isolates were found to be azole resistant in studies involving respiratory colonization of cystic fibrosis patients (43). The ARTEMIS global surveillance program reported a 5.8% resistance rate in 2008 and 2009 (44). The most recent global surveillance study revealed that 3.2% of *A. fumigatus* isolates were resistant to one or more azoles (45). Azole resistance among *A. fumigatus* is due to both acquired resistance during therapy and acquisition of resistant environmental variants (46, 47). Azole resistance linked to the environment has now been observed globally in at least 19 countries (45), including the United States (48). However, the rates may underestimate the global prevalence of *Aspergillus* drug resistance, especially among patients with chronic diseases. The true frequency of triazole resistance is unknown, because *A. fumigatus* is cultured from less than 30% of infected patients. PCR can more efficiently identify the presence of *Aspergillus* in respiratory specimens that are otherwise culture negative, and the simultaneous detection of characteristic drug resistance markers in these assays indicates that resistant strains are more prevalent than is reported as a result of culture (49).

MECHANISMS OF AZOLE RESISTANCE

The underlying molecular mechanisms responsible for acquired azole resistance have been extensively studied over the past several decades. Early studies elucidating the biological machinery central to resistance have evolved into eloquent descriptions of cellular regulatory mechanisms and circuitry that help modulate azole resistance mechanisms following exposure of a susceptible strain to drug. Many excellent reviews have covered this topic (50, 51). The general mechanisms and cellular mediators of drug resistance are summarized in Table 1 and include the following.

1. Reduced drug-target interaction
2. Increase in target copy number
3. Reduction of intracellular drug concentration mediated via drug efflux transporters and reduced uptake
4. Modification of other ergosterol biosynthesis pathway elements
5. Biofilms
6. Cell stress responses and drug tolerance

The biological responses revealing these resistance mechanisms involve adaptive cellular responses resulting in drug tolerance followed by modification of genetic regulatory elements. The relative contributions of individual mechanisms to development of resistance vary by genus and species. In some strains, a single dominant mechanism may prevail, while in others, stepwise development of high-level resistance involves a combination of resistance mechanisms. The contributions of specific resistance mechanisms include both multicomponent mechanisms and single dominant mechanisms among the major pathogens.

Drug Target Modification

Modification of the target Erg11p resulting in reduced affinity for drug is one of the most direct mechanisms of resistance. At least 60 amino acid substitutions in Erg11p from azole-resistant clinical isolates have been described (52, 53). The impact of individual substitutions determines the relative degree of resistance and cross-reactivity within the class. For example, Y132H, K143R, F145L, G450E, G464S, R467K, S405F, G448E, F449V, G450E, and G464S show reduced susceptibility to fluconazole and voriconazole (52) but not necessarily to the longer-chain drugs itraconazole and posaconazole. The contribution of many *ERG11* mutations to fluconazole resistance is weak, as some have a modest impact on azole resistance phenotypes (52). Furthermore, in diploid *C. albicans*, nucleotide mutations may occur as homozygous (both alleles) or heterozygous (single allele) substitutions, which can impact the resistance phenotype. In *C. neoformans*, strains resistant to fluconazole may contain characteristic mutations in the *ERG11* gene (54). In *A. fumigatus*, modification of the azole target lanosterol 14α-demethylase is the predominant mechanism underlying clinical resistance. A limited number of acquired

TABLE 1 Antifungal targets, drug resistance mechanisms, and effectors

Antifungal agent	Drug target	Mode of action	Resistance mechanism	Effectors of resistance
Triazoles • Fluconazole • Voriconazole • Itraconazole • Posaconazole • Isavuconazole	Lanosterol 14α-demethylase (Erg11, Cyp51A)	Blocks ergosterol biosynthesis	Altered drug affinity by Erg11 (Cyp51A) target	
			Upregulation of *ERG11* (*CYP51A*)	Upc2, LOH, aneuploidy
			Upregulation of CDR and MDR multidrug transporters	Tac1, Mrr1, SrbA, biofilms, Crz1, LOH, aneuploidy
			Other ergosterol biosynthesis genes (*ERG3*)	
			Biofilms; drug uptake	Hsp90, Sm11, Adh5, Csh1, Gca1, Bcr1, Gca2, Rlmp, Fks1
			Tolerance; heteroresistance	*HSP90*, post-translational modification
Polyenes • Amphotericin B • Nystatin	Binds ergosterol and forms aqueous pores	Forms large aqueous pores	Sterol depletion; biofilms	
Echinocandins • Caspofungin • Micafungin • Anidulafungin	β1,3-D-Glucan synthase (Fks1, Fks2)	Alters cell wall integrity by blocking β1,3-D-glucan biosynthesis	Modification of Fks1 and/or Fks2 subunits of glucan synthase	*MSH2*
			Biofilms	*FKS*
			Tolerance	*HSP90*, *CRZ1*, CHS, sphingolipids
5-Fluorocytosine (5FC)	Nucleic acids	Inhibits DNA/RNA synthesis	Uracil pyrophosphorylase (Fur1) Cytosine deaminase (Fcy1) Cytosine permease (Fcy2)	

[a]LOH, loss of heterozygosity.

amino acid substitutions have been described in Cyp51A, which confer a variety of triazole resistance phenotypes (46, 55). All modifications confer resistance to itraconazole, while others also confer some cross-resistance to voriconazole and posaconazole (Table 2). The most prominent modifications occur at the amino acids Gly54, Leu98, Gly138, F219, M220, and Gly448.

Environmentally Acquired Resistance Is a Major Factor

Resistance in *A. fumigatus* is largely due to mutation in Cyp51A at the codon for Leu98 and a tandem repeat (TR) of 34 bp in the promoter region (14), which confers pan-azole resistance (Table 2). The TR/L98H resistant isolates arose as a consequence of azole use in the agricultural

TABLE 2 Amino acid substitutions in *A. fumigatus* Cyp51A conferring triazole resistance and associated MICs[a]

Cyp51A locus	Amino acid substitution(s)	MIC (mg/liter) of:		
		Itraconazole	Voriconazole	Posaconazole
TR34/L98	H	>8	8	1–2
TR46/Y121/T289	F/A	>16	>16	1–2
F46	Y	>8	2–4	0.125–0.5
G54	E, R, V	>8	0.125–1	1–>8
H147	Y	>8	>8	0.5
M172	V	>8	2–4	0.125–0.5
P216	L	>8	1	1
F219	C	>8	1	1
M220	I, K, T	>8	0.5–4	0.5–>8
N248	T	>8	2	0.25
D255	E	>8	2	0.25
E427	G, K	>8	2–4	0.125–0.5
Y431	C	>8	4	1
G434	C	>8	4	1
G448	S	>8	>8	0.5–1

[a]Adapted from reference 46. Tandem repeat (TR) promoter designations include the number of bases.

world (56). This singular mechanism (14) has been identified in parts of Europe, India, Asia (57), and most recently in the United States (58), but it is only sporadically observed in patients that evolve resistance during therapy. In Denmark from 2010 to 2014, there was an increasing prevalence of azole resistance, with TR34/L98H being responsible for >50% of the azole resistance mechanisms (59). A second mechanism, TR46/Y121F/T289A, has been observed, which further suggests an environmental route of resistance selection (60).

Structural Modeling of Resistance

Nonsynonymous mutations in *CYP51A* (and *ERG11*) result in structural alterations to lanosterol 14-demethylase that reduce drug binding. Homology overlay modeling of Cyp51A and Erg11 using related high-resolution structural models has been used to describe the impact of specific amino acid substitutions on the interaction of triazole drugs with the target enzyme (61). Such models predict interactions based on different chemical structural properties of the various triazole drugs (e.g., voriconazole versus posaconazole). Most mutations are clustered in three hot spot mutation regions (62). The most prominent resistance-conferring substitutions alter the apparent interaction of drug with the heme cofactor. In *C. tropicalis*, a K143R substitution in Erg11 is strong and confers pan-azole resistance (63). However, many Erg11 amino acid replacements from fluconazole-resistant *C. albicans* strains are peripheral and are predicted to exert a relatively weak action and resulting phenotype. In *A. fumigatus* Cyp51A, the amino acids Gly54, Gly138, Pro216, Phe219, Met220, and Gly448, conferring triazole resistance, are predicted to lie in close proximity to the opening of one of two ligand access channels, which would allow azole compounds to enter the enzyme active site (64, 65) (Fig. 1). Modification of the channel openings is presumed to disturb the docking of azole molecules. The model helps predict why modification of Gly54 yields itraconazole and posaconazole resistance, yet the organism retains voriconazole susceptibility. Leu98 is located on a loop that partly forms an arch-like structure highly conserved among the members of the Cyp51 family of proteins (56, 64). Amino acid substitutions at this position are proposed to result in ligand-induced instability, which may account for strong resistance. Among azoles, the fluconazole was the weakest inhibitor, while posaconazole was the strongest (66).

Increasing the Target Abundance

Lanosterol 14α-demethylase is a key enzyme in the ergosterol biosynthesis pathway. In response to azole antifungals and/or sterol depletion, *Candida* strains may overexpress *ERG11* (67) and other genes involved in ergosterol

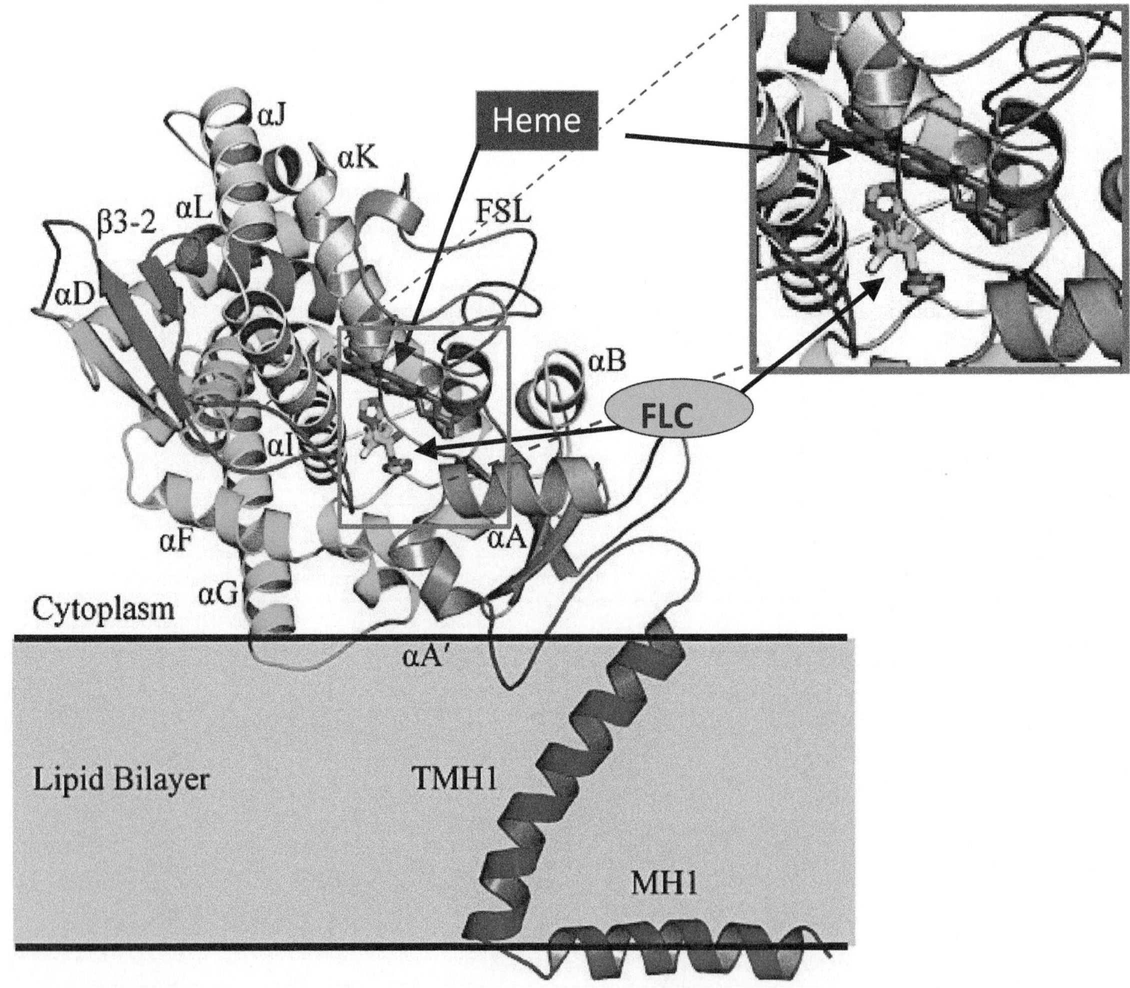

FIGURE 1 High-resolution structures of Erg11p complexed with fluconazole (FLC). (Adapted from reference 194.)

biosynthesis (68). An elevated abundance of target proteins decreases the effectiveness of azole drugs. Increased *ERG11* expression arises from *cis*-acting gain-of-function (GOF) mutations within the promoter region or from alterations in a *trans*-acting factor Upc2p (69). The *C. albicans* Upc2p is a Zn_2-Cys_6 cluster transcription factor homologous to *Saccharomyces cerevisiae* paralogues *UPC2* and *ECM22* (70, 71). Upc2p is required for upregulation of *ERG11* (72) and other sterol biosynthesis genes in response to sterol depletion (70, 71). Mutations in *UPC2* result in increased expression of *ERG11* and decreased fluconazole susceptibility (69, 71). Upc2p activates transcription of target genes by binding to a conserved sequence known as the sterol response element (SRE) (70). An 11-bp SRE was identified in the promoters of *ERG2* and *ERG3*; Upc2 and Ecm22 bind to this element. Induced overexpression of *ERG11* or *UPC2* increases resistance to azoles, while mutants lacking *UPC2* show no induction of *ERG* genes, and they are hypersusceptible to these drugs (71). In *C. albicans*, *UPC2* activity can increase up to 100-fold with prolonged azole exposure. The *UPC2* promoter also contains a putative SRE (70), and transcriptional regulation of *UPC2* expression occurs through Upc2p-dependent and -independent mechanisms (73). *UPC2* mutations may also potentiate resistance by influencing expression of other genes, including *MDR1*, which encodes an efflux transporter (69, 74). Stepwise enhancement of fluconazole resistance can involve constitutive high-level expression of *ERG11* and overexpression of drug transporters (75). Less is known about the regulation of Cyp51A in *A. fumigatus*, although overexpression of Cyp51A confers reduced azole susceptibility (76), as does overexpression of Cyp51B (77). The expression of Cyp51A appears to be regulated by the global Zn_2-Cys_6 transcription factor AtrR (78).

Reducing Cellular Drug Levels: Drug Efflux Transporters

Fungi encode numerous putative drug efflux transporters that have the potential to influence susceptibility to azole antifungal agents by reducing the effective cellular concentrations of drugs below their inhibitory thresholds. Overexpression of multidrug efflux transporters confers resistance to azole antifungal drugs (79). The two main classes of efflux pumps that contribute to azole resistance in fungi include ATP-binding cassette (ABC) transporters (e.g., *C. albicans* Cdr1 [CaCdr1] and CaCdr2), which use energy derived from ATP hydrolysis to transport drugs, and the major facilitator superfamily (MFS) transporters (e.g., CaMdr1), which utilize the plasma membrane electrochemical proton gradient to translocate substrates.

The ABC superfamily is one of the largest protein families known. Proteins in this family transport a wide variety of substrates across extracellular and intracellular membranes, including metabolic products, lipids and sterols, and drugs. A common feature of all ABC transporters is that they contain a transmembrane domain and the nucleotide-binding domain. The *C. albicans* genome contains at least 27 genes with ABC domains (80). Cdr1 was first identified as a transporter of unrelated cytotoxic drugs, and it was shown to be a major determinant of fluconazole resistance in *C. albicans* (81). The closely related transporter Cdr2 exhibits 84% amino acid homology with Cdr1 and confers resistance to azole antifungal agents. *CDR2* overexpression has been observed in resistant mutants that revert spontaneously to wild-type levels of susceptibility (82), suggesting that its impact on resistance is less pronounced than that of *CDR1*. In *C. glabrata*, azole resistance is almost exclusively due to enhanced drug efflux, which is a consequence of overexpression of transporter genes, including *C. glabrata CDR1* (*CgCDR1*) (83), *CgCDR2* (*PDH1*) (84), and *CgSNQ2* (85). In *C. glabrata*, petite mutants displaying a loss of mature mitochondria can become azole resistant through increased expression of *CgCDR1* and possibly *CgCDR2* (86). Similarly, in *C. neoformans*, the ABC transporter-encoding gene *CnAFR1* confers resistance to fluconazole (87). In *C. krusei*, *ABC1* is strongly upregulated in response to azole exposure, where it plays a role in intrinsic resistance (88). In *A. fumigatus*, overexpression of the ABC transporter AbcG1 (formerly Cdr1B) has been linked to wild-type azole resistance in *A. fumigatus* and appears to be important for resistance linked to certain Cyp51A mutations (89).

MFS transporters account for nearly half of the solute transporters encoded within the genomes of microorganisms. The *C. albicans* genome contains at least 95 open reading frames that may encode an MFS transporter (90). MFS transporters are single-polypeptide secondary carriers capable only of transporting small solutes in response to electrochemical ion gradients. In *C. albicans*, Mdr1 (91) was identified because it was overexpressed in azole-resistant isolates (79). Mdr1 confers lower-level resistance to fluconazole, in contrast to Cdr1, which is associated with efflux of a wider range of substrates at higher capacity. In *C. albicans*, *MDR1* is not significantly expressed, but it is induced by chemicals like benomyl, H_2O_2, and azoles (92). Another MFS transporter, Flu1, confers resistance to fluconazole, but its expression varies among azole-susceptible clinical isolates, and it does not appear to be an important factor in clinical resistance (93).

In summary, the relative contribution of different drug efflux transporters to azole resistance varies with expression level and the type of transporter. Overall, in *Candida*, high-level azole resistance most often correlates with overexpression of *CDR1*. However, it has been demonstrated in serial isolates from patients exposed to azoles that multifactorial resistance develops stepwise with drug exposure and involves CDR and/or MDR gene expression (94, 95) and other mechanisms, such as *ERG11* overexpression and specific ERG1 mutations. Similarly, the contribution of AbcG1 in *A. fumigatus* to resistance is unclear, and alternative mechanisms of non-Cyp51a-mediated triazole resistance may involve other transporters or novel mechanisms (41, 89).

Regulation of Azole Resistance

The underlying mechanism regulating drug pump overexpression is an important component for development of azole resistance phenotypes. A major emphasis in recent years has been placed on understanding regulatory circuits controlling the expression of these genes. It is well established for *C. albicans* and other *Candida* spp. that GOF mutations in the zinc cluster transcription factors Tac1 and Mrr1 regulate the expression of *CDR* and *MDR* genes, respectively (96, 97). Specific mutations in *TAC1* mediate the overexpression of the genes encoding the ABC transporters CDR1 and CDR2 (96, 98), while Mrr1 regulates the MFS transporter Mdr1 in azole-resistant isolates (99). In *C. glabrata*, CgPdr1p is a Zn_2-Cys_6 transcription factor involved in the regulation of the ABC transporter genes *CgCDR1*, *CgCDR2*, and *CgSNQ2* (100). GOF mutations in *CgPDR1* are responsible for intrinsic high expression of ABC transporters (101, 102). GOF mutations show high diversity among *CgPDR1* alleles from azole-resistant clinical isolates, with more than 65 nonsynonymous substitutions identified (102). Finally, mRNA stability is an important factor that contributes to message stability and sustained overexpression of *CDR1* in *C. albicans* isolates (103). In *A. fumigatus*, a related Zn_2-Cys_6 transcription factor, AtrR, mediates resistance via Cyp51A and AbcG1 (78).

Loss of Heterozygosity and Other Chromosomal Abnormalities

Azole resistance may occur when *C. albicans* upregulates and/or carries mutations in *ERG11* and *TAC1*. An increase in copy number can occur for these genes due to loss of heterozygosity. Chromosome 5 (Chr 5) rearrangements lead to homozygosity in *TAC1* but also in other regions, including *ERG11* (104). Azole resistance can result from segmental aneuploidy on Chr 5, which increases copy numbers of *TAC1*, *MTL*, and *ERG11* via formation of isochromosome 5L (98, 105). This genetic plasticity provides *C. albicans* with a dynamic response to azole drugs that is prevalent in resistant clinical isolates (106). The emergence of drug resistance is generally expected to be reflected within a resistant clonal population of cells. However, some strains display heteroresistance, which refers to variability in the response to a drug within a clonal cell population. Such strains are not detected by routine susceptibility testing and may be associated with therapeutic failure (107). In *C. neoformans* and *C. glabrata*, heteroresistance to fluconazole is an adaptive mode of azole resistance (107, 108). Heteroresistant cell populations respond differentially to drug and adapt in a stepwise manner to higher drug concentrations. *Cryptococcus* strains adapting to fluconazole may contain disomies of Chr 1. The duplication of Chr 1 causes overexpression of *ERG11* and the major transporter Afr1 (109). In the absence of drug, the strains return to their basal level of susceptibility by losing the extra copy of Chr 1, followed by loss of the extra copies of the remaining disomic chromosomes.

Azole Resistance and Virulence

The acquisition of drug resistance is often associated with a loss of fitness or virulence. In *C. albicans*, GOF mutations in Mrr1, Tac1, and Upc2 carry a fitness cost, suggesting that regulation of drug pumps is tightly controlled by the cell (110). In *A. fumigatus*, azole resistance also alters virulence (76, 111). Such virulence defects suggest that resistant strains should be self-limiting in a vast reservoir of highly fit wild-type strains. However, this does not appear to be the case for environmentally derived strains carrying the Cyp51A defects L98H/TR and TR46/Y121F/T289A. These strains maintain virulence and are spreading globally as infectious strains. In *C. glabrata*, in contrast to other mechanisms, GOF mutations in the transcription factor gene *PDR1* modulate host-pathogen interactions that increase virulence (102). Such GOF CgPDR1 mutations decrease adherence and uptake by macrophages, which allows evasion of the host's innate cellular immune response (112). Similarly, enhanced virulence is observed for azole-resistant strains of *C. glabrata* with mitochondrial DNA deficiency (petite mutants), which upregulate the ABC transporter genes *CgCDR1*, *CgCDR2*, and *CgSNQ2* (113).

Other ERG Genes and Mechanisms

ERG3 encodes a sterol $\Delta^{5,6}$-desaturase involved in sterol biosynthesis. Azole exposure results in the accumulation of 14α-methylated sterols and 14α-methylergosta-8,24(28)-dien-3,6-diol, and formation of the latter sterol metabolite is catalyzed by sterol $\Delta^{5,6}$-desaturase. Inactivation of *ERG3* suppresses toxicity, facilitating azole resistance (114). Clinical isolates of *C. albicans* resistant to both azoles and amphotericin B have been shown to have sterol depletion and defects in *ERG3* (115). However, inactivation of *ERG3* does not always result in azole resistance, as a null *ERG3* mutant of *C. glabrata* was not azole resistant (116), and in *A. fumigatus*, disruption of ERG3(A/B) had no effect on azole susceptibility (117). Finally, azole uptake may be mediated by specific transporters. Impairment of such transporters may be able to impart drug resistance, although this has not been observed clinically (118).

Biofilms

Biofilms are one of the most prevalent forms of microbial growth in nature, and they are often refractory to antifungal agents. *Candida* species are among the most common sources of fungal biofilm infections (119), and *C. albicans* is the most prominent biofilm producer (120), although other yeasts and filamentous fungi are important biofilm producers, including other *Candida* spp., *Cryptococcus*, *Blastoschizomyces*, *Trichosporon*, *Pneumocystis*, *Saccharomyces*, *Aspergillus*, and *Coccidioides* (120). The mature biofilm comprises a dense network of yeast and filamentous cells embedded in an exopolymeric matrix consisting of carbohydrates, proteins, and nucleic acids. The complex organization of the extracellular biofilm matrix is a major feature that distinguishes biofilm from planktonic cells (Fig. 2).

Candida biofilms are intrinsically resistant to azoles like fluconazole. The mechanisms for this resistance are multifactorial, involving both induction of drug efflux transporters and drug sequestration within the extensive matrix structure (120, 121) (Fig. 2). The drug efflux transporter genes *CDR* and *MDR* are upregulated during biofilm development (122, 123). However, a larger component of the multidrug resistance phenotype is imparted by drug sequestration within the extracellular matrix (124). A key constituent of the matrix is β1,3-D-glucan produced by glucan synthase, and key genes responsible for its delivery and arrangement in the matrix have been defined (124, 125). Extracellular glucan sequesters drug, thereby reducing the effective drug concentration at the cell membrane (126) (Fig. 2). Other cellular proteins, such as the alcohol dehydrogenases Adh5, Csh1, and Ifd6 and the glucoamylases CaGCA1 and CaGCA2, contribute to matrix production and resistance phenotypes (127). Heat shock protein 90 (Hsp90), a chaperone that regulates cellular signaling by stabilizing numerous client proteins involved in signal transduction (128), is important for biofilm health. Its depletion in *C. albicans* reduces biofilm growth and maturation, resulting in diminished resistance to azole antifungals (129). Impairment of Hsp90 function allows fluconazole to be effective in eradicating azole-insensitive biofilms (129). Collectively, matrix production is highly regulated and comprises a key resistance factor for *Candida* spp. (130), as well as *Aspergillus* biofilms (131).

MECHANISMS OF ECHINOCANDIN RESISTANCE

Echinocandin Antifungal Drugs

The cell wall-active echinocandin drugs anidulafungin, caspofungin, and micafungin are lipopeptides that inhibit glucan synthase, which catalyzes the biosynthesis of β1,3-D-glucan. Echinocandins are the recommended first-line treatment for invasive candidiasis (132). The β1,3-D-glucan synthase consists of a catalytic unit, Fks, and a regulatory component, Rho. Fks is encoded by three related genes, *FKS1*, *FKS2*, and *FKS3*. *FKS1* is essential in *C. albicans* (133) and other *Candida* spp., but in *C. glabrata*, *FKS1* and *FKS2*

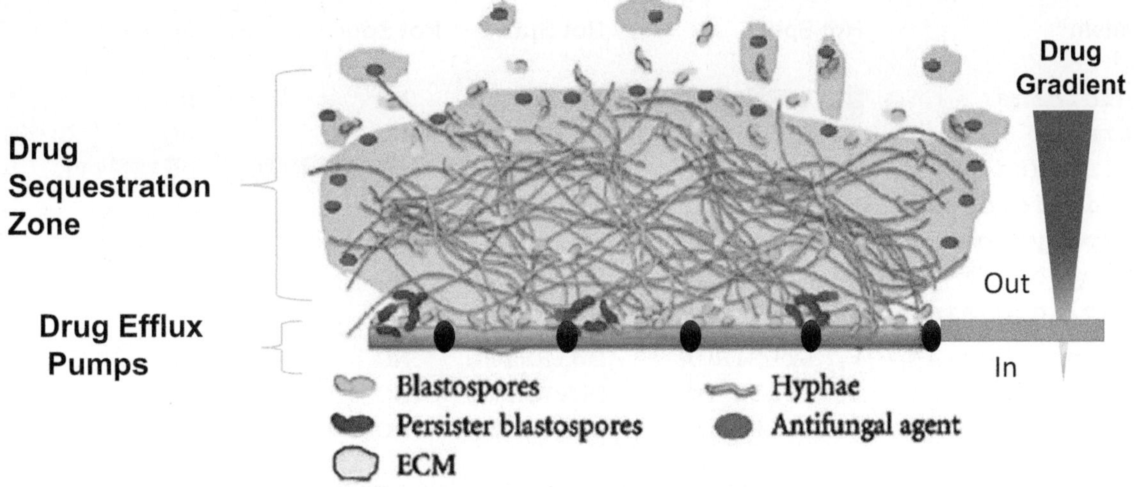

FIGURE 2 Schematic of biofilm composition and mechanisms of resistance showing effects on drug levels. (Adapted from reference 177.)

are functionally redundant (134). Echinocandin drugs are fungicidal against susceptible *Candida* spp. (135) but fungistatic against moulds, where they lyse the tips of growing hyphae but do not fully block growth (136). Echinocandin drugs are inactive against mucormycetes, *Cryptococcus* spp., and *Fusarium* spp. They are not affected by cross-resistance to other antifungal agents, which enables them to be effective against azole-resistant yeasts.

Epidemiology of Echinocandin Resistance

Clinical failures due to *Candida* spp. isolates resistant to echinocandin drugs are increasingly encountered, although their frequency remains relatively low (1 to 3%) with *C. albicans* and most other *Candida* spp. (137–139). Resistance of 7% has been reported for *C. auris* isolates (23), while the most significant resistance problem involves *C. glabrata*, where resistance is growing more severe, often as multidrug resistance (140). The widespread use of echinocandins and azoles has resulted in an epidemiologic shift, with *C. glabrata* emerging as the most dominant fungal bloodstream pathogen in some health care centers (141). Drug resistance generally occurs after prolonged therapy, but it can also occur early in therapy (142). The SENTRY Antimicrobial Surveillance Program reported echinocandin resistance of 8.0 to 9.3% among 1,669 bloodstream isolates of *C. glabrata* from 2006 to 2010 (29). Furthermore, in a 10-year study of *C. glabrata* bloodstream isolates, echinocandin resistance rose from 2 to 3% during 2001 to 2006 to >13% in the years 2009 and 2010 (143). Most recently, in an analysis of 1,385 *C. glabrata* cases in four metropolitan areas and 80 hospitals for the period 2008 to 2014, 6.0% were resistant, and the proportion of nonsusceptible isolates rose from 4.2% in 2008 to 7.8% in 2014. Alarmingly, 59% of nonsusceptible cases had no known prior echinocandin exposure, suggesting possible transmission (144). There appears to be regional variability, as large-scale surveillance programs in Europe (145) and the Asia-Western Pacific region (32) reported very low-level echinocandin resistance.

FKS Mechanism of Resistance

Clinical resistance resulting in breakthrough infections involves modification of Fks subunits of glucan synthase, and clinical breakpoints reflect this underlying mechanism (146). Unlike azoles, echinocandins are not substrates for multidrug transporters (147). Resistance-conferring amino acid substitutions in Fks subunits induce elevated MICs (148) and reduce the sensitivity of glucan synthase (i.e., the 50% inhibitory concentration) to drug 50- to 3,000-fold (149). In *C. albicans* and most other *Candida* spp., mutations occur in two highly conserved hot spot regions of *FKS1*. In *C. glabrata*, equivalent amino acid substitution in Fks1 and Fks2 confers resistance (Fig. 3). These limited regions encompass residues (*C. albicans*) Phe641 to Pro649 and Arg1361 (150). For *C. albicans*, amino acid changes at Ser641 and Ser645 are the most abundant (~90%) and cause the most pronounced resistance phenotype (151, 152). In *C. glabrata*, comparable mutations conferring resistance occur in both *FKS1* and *FKS2*, with S629P, F625S, D632E (FKS1), and S663P, F, or Y and F659S or V (FKS2) being the most prominent amino acid substitutions (151, 153). Echinocandin resistance may depend on the relative expression of *FKS* genes, which can vary more than 20-fold (154). Resistance conferred by *FKS2* can be reversed following treatment with the calcineurin inhibitor FK506 (134), which downregulates *FKS2* expression (155). A third potential hot spot region is exemplified by W695 of *S. cerevisiae* Fks1 and the equivalent residues, F695 and W760, from *Scedosporium* species and *Schizosaccharomyces pombe*, respectively (156). Its clinical significance for acquired resistance is unclear. Finally, amino acid substitutions in Fks1 of *C. albicans* may confer reduced fitness (134, 154), as they decrease glucan biosynthesis (154), resulting in altered cell wall morphology (157). A consequence of reduced fitness is that resistant strains compete poorly with wild-type counterparts (157), which may explain why resistance is generally associated with acquired *de novo* resistance and not transmission.

Hot Spot Polymorphisms and Inherent Reduced susceptibility

Candida parapsilosis complex (*C. parapsilosis sensu stricto*, *Candida orthopsilosis*, and *Candida metapsilosis*) and *C. guilliermondii* display higher echinocandin antifungal MICs (0.5 to 8 μg/ml) than other susceptible *Candida* species, which is reflected in resistance breakpoints (146). The clinical significance of intrinsic reduced susceptibility is

Organism	Fks1 Hot Spot1	Fks1 Hot Spot 2	Fks2 Hot Spot 1	Fks2 Hot Spot 2	Fks3 Hot Spot 1
C. albicans	F_{641}LTLSLRDP	DWIRRYTL	NO	NO	NO
C. krusei	F_{655}LILSIRDP	DWIRRYTL	NO	NO	NO
C. glabrata	F_{625}LILSIRDP	DWIRRYTL	F_{659}LILSLRDP	DWIRRYTL	NO
C. guilliermondii	F_{632}MALSIRDP	DWIRRYTL	NO	NO	NO
C. lipolytica	F_{662}LILSIRDP	DWIRRCVL	NO	NO	NO
C. tropicalis	F---LTLSIRDP	DWIRRYTL	NO	NO	NO
C. dubliniensis	F_{641}LTLSIRDP	DWIRRYTL	NO	NO	NO
*C. parapsilosis**	F_{652}LTLSIRDA	DWIRRYTL	NO	NO	NO
C. orthopsilosis	F---LTLSIRDA	DWVRRYTL	NO	NO	NO
C. metapsilosis	F---LTLSIRDA	DWIRRYTL	NO	NO	NO

NO: Not Observed **C. parapsilosis sensu stricto* ---: Incomplete sequence designation

Acquired Mutation Strong Resistance   Acquired Mutation Weak Resistance   Naturally occurring polymorphism

FIGURE 3 Fks amino acid substitutions and polymorphisms in hot spot regions conferring reduced susceptibility to echinocandin drugs among clinical isolates of *Candida* spp.

unclear, since patients with these infecting strains can be successfully treated at standard dosages (158), although clinical efficacy varies with patient population (17, 159). The mechanism underlying reduced echinocandin susceptibility involves naturally occurring polymorphisms in FKS hot spot regions, which confer moderately reduced sensitivity of glucan synthase to drug (160). In *C. parapsilosis* complex, the highly conserved proline at the distal edge of hot spot 1 (Pro660) is present as alanine (Fig. 3). Overall, it appears that naturally occurring Fks1 polymorphisms of non-*albicans Candida* spp. and other fungi account for reduced susceptibility to echinocandin drugs.

Biofilms

As with azole resistance, the glucan matrix acts to sequester echinocandin drugs, preventing them from reaching the cell membrane. Disruption of this process by genetic or chemical modification of β1,3-D-glucan synthase decreases drug sequestration in the matrix, rendering biofilms susceptible to antifungal agents (125). This mechanism accounts for a large fraction of the drug resistance phenotype during biofilm growth (161), and it is a factor in the observation of persister cells that may be encountered in the presence of drug. Transcription factors like Bcr1 govern biofilm formation (162) and *SMI1* biofilm matrix glucan production, as well as subsequent development of the drug resistance phenotype (125).

MECHANISMS OF POLYENE RESISTANCE

The polyene amphotericin B was the first antifungal agent approved in the United States (1957) to treat life-threatening invasive fungal infections (163). Polyene drugs bind the fungal-specific sterol ergosterol in the plasma membrane, resulting in the formation of high-conductance channels that allow ions and other cellular components to flow from the cell, causing cell death. For decades, it was a mainstay therapy for invasive fungal infections, including invasive aspergillosis, cryptococcosis, blastomycosis, candidemia, coccidioidomycosis, histoplasmosis, and mucormycosis. However, its avidity for sterols like cholesterol in animal cell membranes contributes to renal toxicity, and hence its relegation as a second-line antifungal option. Lipid formulations of amphotericin B overcome the most serious limitations but still suffer from issues of cost and potential toxicity.

Epidemiology of Polyene Resistance

Refractive therapeutic response to polyenes generally involves inherently insensitive moulds, such as *A. terreus*, *Pseudallescheria boydii*, *Scedosporium* spp., *Purpureocillium lilacinum*, and *Fusarium* spp. (164–166). Resistance among susceptible species is typically <1%. However, 35% of *C. auris* isolates were found to be resistant to amphotericin B (23). The prevalence of polyene resistance in *Aspergillus* species is low, with >98% of isolates being inhibited at 1 μg/ml (167). Less common *Aspergillus* species, such as *A. ustus* and *A. lentulus* (13, 166), show resistance to amphotericin B and other antifungal agents. Acquired resistance to polyenes among *Cryptococcus* and *Candida* strains is rare, although high MICs of amphotericin B and/or poor outcome have been reported for *C. albicans*, *C. krusei*, *C. rugosa* (20), *C. lusitaniae* (21), and *C. glabrata* (168, 169). In recent years, acquired resistance to amphotericin among *C. glabrata* has been identified as part of a multidrug resistance phenotype (170).

Mechanisms of Polyene Resistance

The mechanism of resistance to amphotericin B typically involves a reduced content of ergosterol in the cell membrane. Prior exposure to an azole, which lowers cellular sterol levels, can confer stable polyene resistance (171). Acquired resistance to amphotericin B has been most extensively evaluated in yeasts. Mutant yeast strains with defects in the sterol pathway genes *ERG1*, *ERG2*, *ERG3*, *ERG4*, *ERG6*, and *ERG11* are largely depleted of ergosterol, which confers varying levels of resistance (115, 168, 172). In *C. neoformans*, strains with defective sterol C8-isomerase activity and diminished sterol content exhibit reduced susceptibility to polyenes (173). In *C. albicans*, strains resistant to both azole antifungals and amphotericin B were found to be defective in *ERG3* (116, 174) and *ERG6* (175). However, in *A. fumigatus*, deletion of *ERG3* did not alter amphotericin B susceptibility (117). Resistance to amphotericin B appears to be more complex in *Aspergillus* spp. and likely involves other mechanisms (176). Biofilm formation is again an important factor that restricts drug entry, as highly hydrophobic drugs get trapped in the extensive glucan matrix (177).

MECHANISMS OF 5FC RESISTANCE

5FC is a prodrug that when taken up by cells is metabolized by organisms expressing cytosine deaminase to a toxic form of 5FC, which disrupts DNA and protein synthesis. 5FC is generally administered in combination with other antifungal agents (e.g., amphotericin or fluconazole) because of a high propensity for fungal cells to develop resistance, since it targets a nonessential salvage pathway. In yeasts, decreased activity of either cytosine deaminase or uracil phosphoribosyltransferase uracil plays a major role. In *C. albicans*, nucleotide polymorphism in the *FUR1* gene (uracil pyrophosphorylase) is responsible for resistance to 5FC and plays a major role in clinical resistance (178). In *C. lusitaniae*, inactivation of *FCY2* (cytosine permease), *FCY1* (cytosine deaminase), and *FUR1* genes yielded differential resistance to 5FC (179). In *C. glabrata*, high-level 5FC resistance is conferred by a wide array of mutations conferring null phenotypes for *FCY1* or *FUR1*, while low-level resistance was conferred by mutations in one or more *FCY2* permeases (180). In *C. glabrata*, the aquaglyceroporin-encoding genes *CgFPS1* and *CgFPS2* mediate 5FC resistance by decreasing drug accumulation within cells (181).

MICROBIAL DRIVERS OF RESISTANCE: DRUG ADAPTATION AND ESCAPE

The conversion of a drug-sensitive cell to a drug-resistant mutant requires acquisition of one or more resistance mechanisms. The pathway leading to genetically stable escape mutants is a multiphase process (Fig. 4). Initially, cells exposed to drug undergo a stress response, leading to induction of adaptive cellular pathways that protect a subset of cells (182). Such cells are tolerant of drug, which allows them to develop genetically stable resistance mechanisms that increase the *in vitro* MIC and promote escape (183). The mechanisms promoting drug tolerance are diverse (Fig. 5). Hsp90 is a cellular stress modulator that plays a role in promoting cell adaptation in *Candida* species, especially to azoles (184). Compromising Hsp90 can block the emergence of azole resistance (185). Inhibition of glucan biosynthesis by the echinocandins induces stress tolerance pathways, including cell wall integrity, *PKC*, Ca^{2+}-calcineurin-Crz1, and *HOG* (186) (Fig. 5). Modulation of sphingolipid biosynthesis can lead to a mixed susceptibility phenotype in which strains are resistant to caspofungin and hypersensitive to micafungin (187). Hsp90 also helps orchestrate tolerance to echinocandin drugs through calcineurin and Crz1 (188). Echinocandin action strongly results in compensatory increases in chitin synthesis.

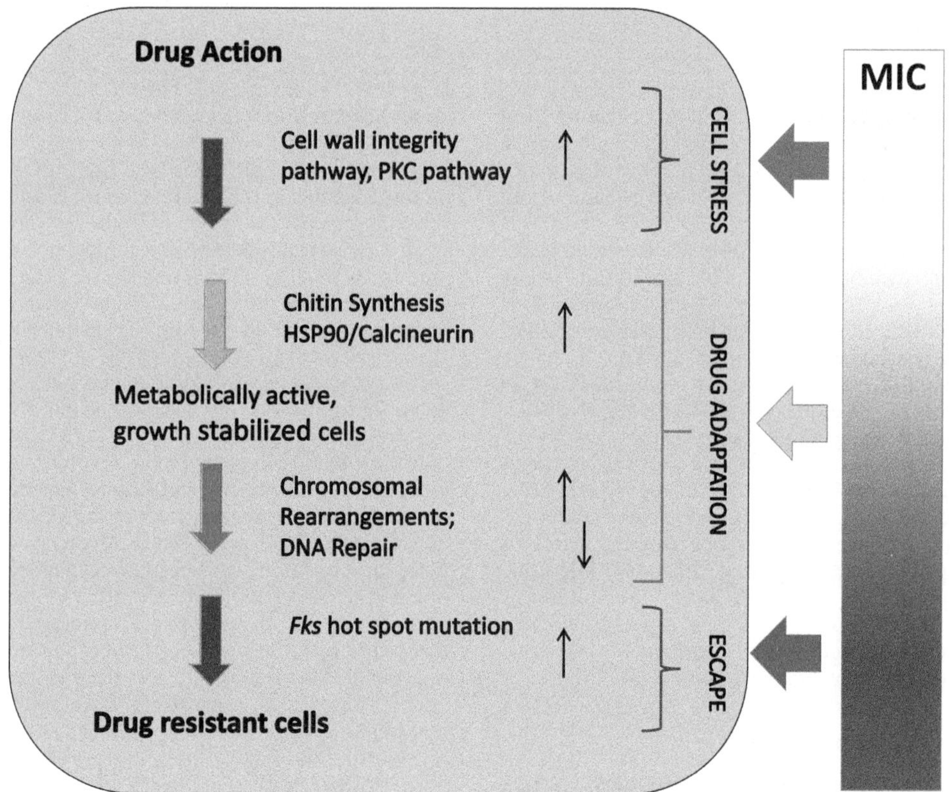

FIGURE 4 Evolution of drug resistance. Drug action results in cell stress, which through cell membrane and/or cell wall receptors activates downstream mechanisms that stabilize a subset of cells, resulting in drug adaptation and elevated *in vitro* MICs. In time, the cells develop well-characterized mechanisms leading to drug escape and clinical drug resistance.

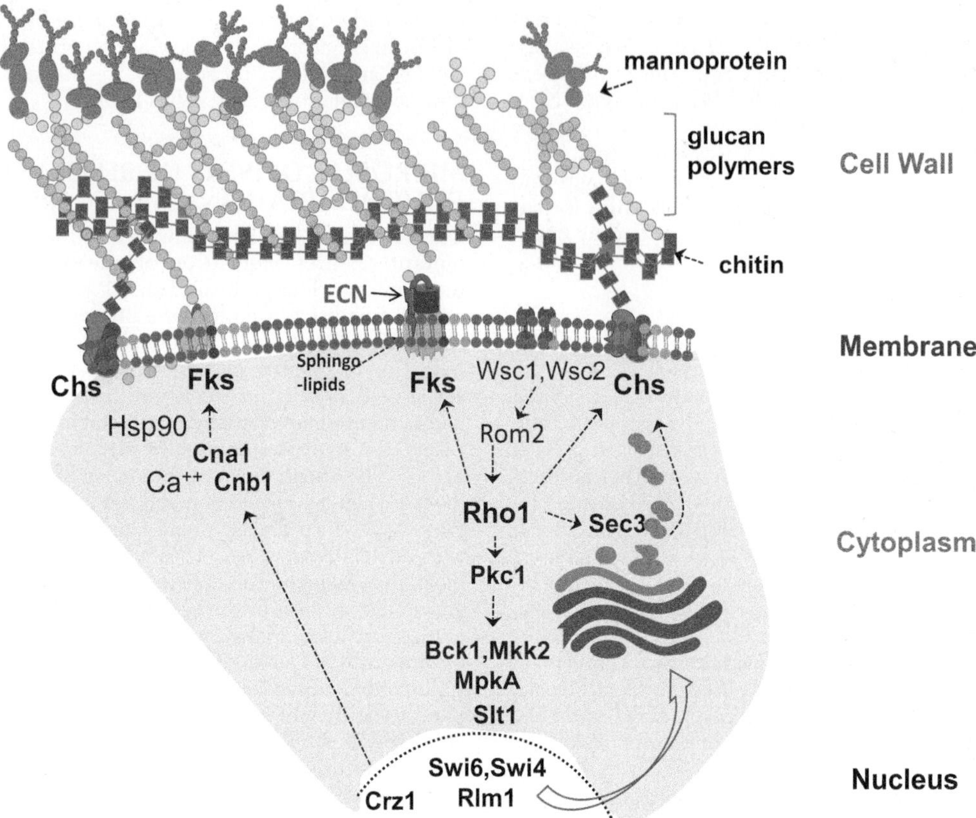

FIGURE 5 Schematic overview of major cellular processes induced in response to inhibition of glucan synthase (Fks) by echinocandin drugs, resulting in cell wall stress and drug tolerance.

Cell wall mutants with higher basal chitin contents are less susceptible to caspofungin (189). Paradoxical growth at very high drug levels (190) is also linked to compensatory responses in chitin biosynthesis (191). Heteroresistance may result from nonheritable epigenetic events, which contributes to variable MICs in a clonal population.

Collectively, adaptive responses stabilize cells in the presence of drug, leading to a drug-tolerant cell population. A consequence of drug tolerance is a physiological state that allows cells to ultimately break through drug action by forming stable resistance mutations (e.g., *FKS*). Recently, it was established for *C. glabrata* that more than 50% of clinical isolates carry a mutator phenotype due to defects in DNA mismatch repair, which increases the spontaneous mutation rate, leading to rapid induction of drug resistance (175). This mechanism is not specific to any drug class, as it can promote azole, echinocandin, and polyene resistance. In some settings, it appears to be a contributing factor for development of multidrug resistance (192). It is important to note that acquisition of drug resistance does not always carry a fitness cost. For example, in *C. glabrata*, GOF mutations in transcription factor PDR1 that confer azole resistance are associated with enhanced virulence (193).

SUMMARY AND PERSPECTIVE

As the global burden of fungal infections rises, antifungal therapy remains a critical element of patient management. However, treatment choices are restricted due to the limited classes of antifungal agents and by antifungal resistance. The mechanisms contributing to resistance are largely well characterized. They include reducing the drug-target interaction by modifying the target (drug affinity changes or target abundance) or reducing the effective cellular content of drug (via ABC or MFS drug pumps or a biofilm glucan trap). *C. albicans* shows a full complement of resistance mechanisms, yet not all mechanisms are present in all fungal strains despite the genetic potential. For example, the expression of drug transporter genes is more important for azole resistance in *C. glabrata* than development of target site mutations. In contrast, echinocandin resistance in all *Candida* strains is dependent on development of target site mutations, while drug pumps play no effective role. Azole resistance in *Aspergillus* is mostly influenced by target site mutations, while in some strains, drug pumps and unknown mechanisms may play a significant role. Much is known about the genetic regulatory elements that influence expression of the drug target genes *ERG11 and FKS*, as well as prominent ABC and MFS transporters. In some strains, point mutations in transcription factors are sufficient to upregulate expression, while in others, large-scale changes in chromosomes, including isochromosome formation, alter the transcriptional profiles. Heteroresistance has emerged as an important transient mechanism to modulate cell susceptibility to drugs, especially with azoles.

Fungal cells are highly dynamic and adapt to environmental challenges, including antifungal agents. Biofilms convert normally susceptible planktonic cells into highly resistant cell communities and create persister cells that seed resistance. Compensatory mechanisms, such as enhanced chitin biosynthesis, following echinocandin action help ensure cell wall integrity. Furthermore, a wide range of cellular stress response pathways contribute to cell stability and the development of drug-adapted persister cells that have the potential to escape therapy by induction of permanent resistance mechanisms.

A detailed understanding of the principal resistance mechanisms and the factors that contribute to their evolution is important for developing new diagnostic approaches to more easily identify drug resistance and create new strategies for therapeutic intervention that prevent and overcome resistance. Advances in molecular diagnostic tools now make it highly feasible to rapidly determine genus and species while simultaneously assessing mutations conferring drug resistance. Furthermore, by interfering with adaptive responses, it may be possible to develop combination drug regimens that both overcome and prevent resistance.

REFERENCES

1. **Brown GD, Denning DW, Gow NA, Levitz SM, Netea MG, White TC.** 2012. Hidden killers: human fungal infections. *Sci Transl Med* **4:**165rv13.
2. **Turnidge J, Paterson DL.** 2007. Setting and revising antibacterial susceptibility breakpoints. *Clin Microbiol Rev* **20:** 391–408.
3. **Rex JH, Pfaller MA.** 2002. Has antifungal susceptibility testing come of age? *Clin Infect Dis* **35:**982–989.
4. **Johnson EM.** 2009. Rare and emerging *Candida* species. *Curr Fungal Infect Rep* **3:**152–159.
5. **Lewis RE.** 2009. Overview of the changing epidemiology of candidemia. *Curr Med Res Opin* **25:**1732–1740.
6. **Tortorano AM, Kibbler C, Peman J, Bernhardt H, Klingspor L, Grillot R.** 2006. Candidaemia in Europe: epidemiology and resistance. *Int J Antimicrob Agents* **27:**359–366.
7. **Pfaller MA, Diekema DJ.** 2004. Rare and emerging opportunistic fungal pathogens: concern for resistance beyond *Candida albicans* and *Aspergillus fumigatus*. *J Clin Microbiol* **42:** 4419–4431.
8. **Diekema D, Arbefeville S, Boyken L, Kroeger J, Pfaller M.** 2012. The changing epidemiology of healthcare-associated candidemia over three decades. *Diagn Microbiol Infect Dis* **73:**45–48.
9. **Hope W, Morton A, Eisen DP.** 2002. Increase in prevalence of nosocomial non-*Candida albicans* candidaemia and the association of *Candida krusei* with fluconazole use. *J Hosp Infect* **50:**56–65.
10. **Pfaller MA, Diekema DJ, Mendez M, Kibbler C, Erzsebet P, Chang SC, Gibbs DL, Newell VA.** 2006. *Candida guilliermondii*, an opportunistic fungal pathogen with decreased susceptibility to fluconazole: geographic and temporal trends from the ARTEMIS DISK antifungal surveillance program. *J Clin Microbiol* **44:**3551–3556.
11. **Chowdhary A, Sharma C, Meis JF.** 2017. *Candida auris*: a rapidly emerging cause of hospital-acquired multidrug-resistant fungal infections globally. *PLoS Pathog* **13:**e1006290.
12. **Pavie J, Lacroix C, Hermoso DG, Robin M, Ferry C, Bergeron A, Feuilhade M, Dromer F, Gluckman E, Molina JM, Ribaud P.** 2005. Breakthrough disseminated *Aspergillus ustus* infection in allogeneic hematopoietic stem cell transplant recipients receiving voriconazole or caspofungin prophylaxis. *J Clin Microbiol* **43:**4902–4904.
13. **Balajee SA, Gribskov JL, Hanley E, Nickle D, Marr KA.** 2005. *Aspergillus lentulus* sp. nov., a new sibling species of *A. fumigatus*. *Eukaryot Cell* **4:**625–632.
14. **Snelders E, van der Lee HA, Kuijpers J, Rijs AJ, Varga J, Samson RA, Mellado E, Donders AR, Melchers WJ, Verweij PE.** 2008. Emergence of azole resistance in *Aspergillus fumigatus* and spread of a single resistance mechanism. *PLoS Med* **5:**e219.
15. **Meis JF, Chowdhary A, Rhodes JL, Fisher MC, Verweij PE.** 2016. Clinical implications of globally emerging azole resistance in *Aspergillus fumigatus*. *Philos Trans R Soc Lond B Biol Sci* **371:**20150460.
16. **Pfaller MA, Castanheira M, Messer SA, Moet GJ, Jones RN.** 2011. Echinocandin and triazole antifungal susceptibility profiles for *Candida* spp., *Cryptococcus neoformans*, and *Aspergillus fumigatus*: application of new CLSI clinical breakpoints and epidemiologic cutoff values to characterize resistance in the SENTRY Antimicrobial Surveillance Program (2009). *Diagn Microbiol Infect Dis* **69:**45–50.
17. **Kabbara N, Lacroix C, Peffault de Latour R, Socié G, Ghannoum M, Ribaud P.** 2008. Breakthrough *C. parapsilosis* and *C. guilliermondii* blood stream infections in allogeneic hematopoietic stem cell transplant recipients receiving long-term caspofungin therapy. *Haematologica* **93:** 639–640.
18. **Arendrup MC, Prakash A, Meletiadis J, Sharma C, Chowdhary A.** 2017. Comparison of EUCAST and CLSI reference microdilution MICs of eight antifungal compounds for *Candida auris* and associated tentative epidemiological cutoff values. *Antimicrob Agents Chemother* **61:**e00485-17.
19. **Pfaller MA, Espinel-Ingroff A, Canton E, Castanheira M, Cuenca-Estrella M, Diekema DJ, Fothergill A, Fuller J, Ghannoum M, Jones RN, Lockhart SR, Martin-Mazuelos E, Melhem MS, Ostrosky-Zeichner L, Pappas P, Pelaez T, Peman J, Rex J, Szeszs MW.** 2012. Wild-type MIC distributions and epidemiological cutoff values for amphotericin B, flucytosine, and itraconazole and *Candida* spp. as determined by CLSI broth microdilution. *J Clin Microbiol* **50:** 2040–2046.
20. **Lopes Colombo A, Azevedo Melo A, Crespo Rosas RF, Salomão R, Briones M, Hollis RJ, Messer SA, Pfaller MA.** 2003. Outbreak of *Candida rugosa* candidemia: an emerging pathogen that may be refractory to amphotericin B therapy. *Diagn Microbiol Infect Dis* **46:**253–257.
21. **Atkinson BJ, Lewis RE, Kontoyiannis DP.** 2008. *Candida lusitaniae* fungemia in cancer patients: risk factors for amphotericin B failure and outcome. *Med Mycol* **46:**541–546.
22. **Woods RA, Bard M, Jackson IE, Drutz DJ.** 1974. Resistance to polyene antibiotics and correlated sterol changes in two isolates of *Candida tropicalis* from a patient with an amphotericin B-resistant funguria. *J Infect Dis* **129:**53–58.
23. **Lockhart SR, Etienne KA, Vallabhaneni S, Farooqi J, Chowdhary A, Govender NP, Colombo AL, Calvo B, Cuomo CA, Desjardins CA, Berkow EL, Castanheira M, Magobo RE, Jabeen K, Asghar RJ, Meis JF, Jackson B, Chiller T, Litvintseva AP.** 2017. Simultaneous emergence of multidrug-resistant *Candida auris* on 3 continents confirmed by whole-genome sequencing and epidemiological analyses. *Clin Infect Dis* **64:**134–140.
24. **Steinbach WJ, Benjamin DK, Jr, Kontoyiannis DP, Perfect JR, Lutsar I, Marr KA, Lionakis MS, Torres HA, Jafri H, Walsh TJ.** 2004. Infections due to *Aspergillus terreus*: a multicenter retrospective analysis of 83 cases. *Clin Infect Dis* **39:**192–198.
25. **Koss T, Bagheri B, Zeana C, Romagnoli MF, Grossman ME.** 2002. Amphotericin B-resistant *Aspergillus flavus* infection successfully treated with caspofungin, a novel antifungal agent. *J Am Acad Dermatol* **46:**945–947.
26. **Azzola A, Passweg JR, Habicht JM, Bubendorf L, Tamm M, Gratwohl A, Eich G.** 2004. Use of lung resection and voriconazole for successful treatment of invasive pulmonary *Aspergillus ustus* infection. *J Clin Microbiol* **42:**4805–4808.
27. **Pfaller MA, Diekema DJ, Gibbs DL, Newell VA, Bijie H, Dzierzanowska D, Klimko NN, Letscher-Bru V, Lisalova M, Muehlethaler K, Rennison C, Zaidi M, Global Antifungal Surveillance Group.** 2009. Results from the ARTEMIS DISK Global Antifungal Surveillance Study, 1997 to 2007: 10.5-year analysis of susceptibilities of noncandidal yeast species to fluconazole and voriconazole determined by CLSI standardized disk diffusion testing. *J Clin Microbiol* **47:** 117–123.
28. **Pfaller MA, Messer SA, Hollis RJ, Boyken L, Tendolkar S, Kroeger J, Diekema DJ.** 2009. Variation in susceptibility of bloodstream isolates of *Candida glabrata* to fluconazole according to patient age and geographic location in the United States in 2001 to 2007. *J Clin Microbiol* **47:**3185–3190.

29. **Pfaller MA, Castanheira M, Lockhart SR, Ahlquist AM, Messer SA, Jones RN.** 2012. Frequency of decreased susceptibility and resistance to echinocandins among fluconazole-resistant bloodstream isolates of *Candida glabrata*: results from the SENTRY Antimicrobial Surveillance Program (2006–2010) and the Centers for Disease Control and Prevention Population-Based Surveillance (2008–2010). *J Clin Microbiol* **50:**1199–1203.
30. **Zhou ZL, Lin CC, Chu WL, Yang YL, Lo HJ, Hospitals T, TSARY Hospitals.** 2016. The distribution and drug susceptibilities of clinical *Candida* species in TSARY 2014. *Diagn Microbiol Infect Dis* **86:**399–404.
31. **Caggiano G, Coretti C, Bartolomeo N, Lovero G, De Giglio O, Montagna MT.** 2015. *Candida* bloodstream infections in Italy: changing epidemiology during 16 years of surveillance. *BioMed Res Int* **2015:**256580.
32. **Pfaller MA, Messer SA, Jones RN, Castanheira M.** 2015. Antifungal susceptibilities of *Candida, Cryptococcus neoformans* and *Aspergillus fumigatus* from the Asia and Western Pacific region: data from the SENTRY antifungal surveillance program (2010-2012). *J Antibiot (Tokyo)* **68:**556–561.
33. **Zhang L, Zhou S, Pan A, Li J, Liu B.** 2015. Surveillance of antifungal susceptibilities in clinical isolates of *Candida* species at 36 hospitals in China from 2009 to 2013. *Int J Infect Dis* **33:**1–4.
34. **Liu XP, Fan SR, Peng YT, Zhang HP.** 2014. Species distribution and susceptibility of *Candida* isolates from patient with vulvovaginal candidiasis in Southern China from 2003 to 2012. *J Mycol Med* **24:**106–111.
35. **Pfaller MA, Diekema DJ, Gibbs DL, Newell VA, Ellis D, Tullio V, Rodloff A, Fu W, Ling TA, Global Antifungal Surveillance Group.** 2010. Results from the ARTEMIS DISK Global Antifungal Surveillance Study, 1997 to 2007: a 10.5-year analysis of susceptibilities of *Candida* species to fluconazole and voriconazole as determined by CLSI standardized disk diffusion. *J Clin Microbiol* **48:**1366–1377.
36. **Govender NP, Patel J, Magobo RE, Naicker S, Wadula J, Whitelaw A, Coovadia Y, Kularatne R, Govind C, Lockhart SR, Zietsman IL, TRAC-South Africa Group.** 2016. Emergence of azole-resistant *Candida parapsilosis* causing bloodstream infection: results from laboratory-based sentinel surveillance in South Africa. *J Antimicrob Chemother* **71:**1994–2004.
37. **Grossman NT, Pham CD, Cleveland AA, Lockhart SR.** 2015. Molecular mechanisms of fluconazole resistance in *Candida parapsilosis* isolates from a U.S. surveillance system. *Antimicrob Agents Chemother* **59:**1030–1037.
38. **Pfaller MA, Castanheira M, Diekema DJ, Messer SA, Jones RN.** 2011. Wild-type MIC distributions and epidemiologic cutoff values for fluconazole, posaconazole, and voriconazole when testing *Cryptococcus neoformans* as determined by the CLSI broth microdilution method. *Diagn Microbiol Infect Dis* **71:**252–259.
39. **Govender NP, Patel J, van Wyk M, Chiller TM, Lockhart SR, Group for Enteric, Respiratory and Meningeal Disease Surveillance in South Africa (GERMS-SA).** 2011. Trends in antifungal drug susceptibility of *Cryptococcus neoformans* isolates obtained through population-based surveillance in South Africa in 2002–2003 and 2007–2008. *Antimicrob Agents Chemother* **55:**2606–2611.
40. **Denning DW, Radford SA, Oakley KL, Hall L, Johnson EM, Warnock DW.** 1997. Correlation between in-vitro susceptibility testing to itraconazole and in-vivo outcome of *Aspergillus fumigatus* infection. *J Antimicrob Chemother* **40:**401–414.
41. **Bueid A, Howard SJ, Moore CB, Richardson MD, Harrison E, Bowyer P, Denning DW.** 2010. Azole antifungal resistance in *Aspergillus fumigatus*: 2008 and 2009. *J Antimicrob Chemother* **65:**2116–2118.
42. **van der Linden JW, Snelders E, Kampinga GA, Rijnders BJ, Mattsson E, Debets-Ossenkopp YJ, Kuijper EJ, Van Tiel FH, Melchers WJ, Verweij PE.** 2011. Clinical implications of azole resistance in *Aspergillus fumigatus*, The Netherlands, 2007-2009. *Emerg Infect Dis* **17:**1846–1854.
43. **Mortensen KL, Jensen RH, Johansen HK, Skov M, Pressler T, Howard SJ, Leatherbarrow H, Mellado E, Arendrup MC.** 2011. *Aspergillus* species and other molds in respiratory samples from patients with cystic fibrosis: a laboratory-based study with focus on *Aspergillus fumigatus* azole resistance. *J Clin Microbiol* **49:**2243–2251.
44. **Lockhart SR, Frade JP, Etienne KA, Pfaller MA, Diekema DJ, Balajee SA.** 2011. Azole resistance in *Aspergillus fumigatus* isolates from the ARTEMIS global surveillance study is primarily due to the TR/L98H mutation in the *cyp51A* gene. *Antimicrob Agents Chemother* **55:**4465–4468.
45. **van der Linden JW, Arendrup MC, Warris A, Lagrou K, Pelloux H, Hauser PM, Chryssanthou E, Mellado E, Kidd SE, Tortorano AM, Dannaoui E, Gaustad P, Baddley JW, Uekötter A, Lass-Flörl C, Klimko N, Moore CB, Denning DW, Pasqualotto AC, Kibbler C, Arikan-Akdagli S, Andes D, Meletiadis J, Naumiuk L, Nucci M, Melchers WJ, Verweij PE.** 2015. Prospective multicenter international surveillance of azole resistance in *Aspergillus fumigatus*. *Emerg Infect Dis* **21:**1041–1044.
46. **Howard SJ, Arendrup MC.** 2011. Acquired antifungal drug resistance in *Aspergillus fumigatus*: epidemiology and detection. *Med Mycol* **49(**Suppl 1**):**S90–S95.
47. **Denning DW, Perlin DS.** 2011. Azole resistance in *Aspergillus*: a growing public health menace. *Future Microbiol* **6:**1229–1232.
48. **Pham CD, Reiss E, Hagen F, Meis JF, Lockhart SR.** 2014. Passive surveillance for azole-resistant *Aspergillus fumigatus*, United States, 2011-2013. *Emerg Infect Dis* **20:**1498–1503.
49. **Denning DW, Park S, Lass-Florl C, Fraczek MG, Kirwan M, Gore R, Smith J, Bueid A, Moore CB, Bowyer P, Perlin DS.** 2011. High-frequency triazole resistance found In nonculturable *Aspergillus fumigatus* from lungs of patients with chronic fungal disease. *Clin Infect Dis* **52:**1123–1129.
50. **Cowen LE, Sanglard D, Howard SJ, Rogers PD, Perlin DS.** 2015. Mechanisms of antifungal drug resistance. *Cold Spring Harb Perspect Med* **5:**a019752.
51. **Whaley SG, Berkow EL, Rybak JM, Nishimoto AT, Barker KS, Rogers PD.** 2017. Azole antifungal resistance in *Candida albicans* and emerging non-albicans *Candida* species. *Front Microbiol* **7:**2173.
52. **Flowers SA, Colón B, Whaley SG, Schuler MA, Rogers PD.** 2015. Contribution of clinically derived mutations in ERG11 to azole resistance in *Candida albicans*. *Antimicrob Agents Chemother* **59:**450–460.
53. **Zhang L, Yang HF, Liu YY, Xu XH, Ye Y, Li JB.** 2013. Reduced susceptibility of *Candida albicans* clinical isolates to azoles and detection of mutations in the ERG11 gene. *Diagn Microbiol Infect Dis* **77:**327–329.
54. **Sionov E, Chang YC, Garraffo HM, Dolan MA, Ghannoum MA, Kwon-Chung KJ.** 2012. Identification of a *Cryptococcus neoformans* cytochrome P450 lanosterol 14α-demethylase (Erg11) residue critical for differential susceptibility between fluconazole/voriconazole and itraconazole/posaconazole. *Antimicrob Agents Chemother* **56:**1162–1169.
55. **Verweij PE, Howard SJ, Melchers WJ, Denning DW.** 2009. Azole-resistance in *Aspergillus*: proposed nomenclature and breakpoints. *Drug Resist Updat* **12:**141–147.
56. **Verweij PE, Snelders E, Kema GH, Mellado E, Melchers WJ.** 2009. Azole resistance in *Aspergillus fumigatus*: a side-effect of environmental fungicide use? *Lancet Infect Dis* **9:**789–795.
57. **Verweij PE, Chowdhary A, Melchers WJ, Meis JF.** 2016. Azole resistance in *Aspergillus fumigatus*: can we retain the clinical use of mold-active antifungal azoles? *Clin Infect Dis* **62:**362–368.
58. **Hurst SF, Berkow EL, Stevenson KL, Litvintseva AP, Lockhart SR.** 2017. Isolation of azole-resistant *Aspergillus fumigatus* from the environment in the south-eastern USA. *J Antimicrob Chemother* **72:**2443–2446.
59. **Jensen RH, Hagen F, Astvad KM, Tyron A, Meis JF, Arendrup MC.** 2016. Azole-resistant *Aspergillus fumigatus* in Denmark: a laboratory-based study on resistance mechanisms and genotypes. *Clin Microbiol Infect* **22:**570.e1–9.

60. **van der Linden JW, Camps SM, Kampinga GA, Arends JP, Debets-Ossenkopp YJ, Haas PJ, Rijnders BJ, Kuijper EJ, van Tiel FH, Varga J, Karawajczyk A, Zoll J, Melchers WJ, Verweij PE.** 2013. Aspergillosis due to voriconazole highly resistant *Aspergillus fumigatus* and recovery of genetically related resistant isolates from domiciles. *Clin Infect Dis* **57:**513–520.
61. **Xiao L, Madison V, Chau AS, Loebenberg D, Palermo RE, McNicholas PM.** 2004. Three-dimensional models of wild-type and mutated forms of cytochrome P450 14α-sterol demethylases from *Aspergillus fumigatus* and *Candida albicans* provide insights into posaconazole binding. *Antimicrob Agents Chemother* **48:**568–574.
62. **Favre B, Didmon M, Ryder NS.** 1999. Multiple amino acid substitutions in lanosterol 14alpha-demethylase contribute to azole resistance in *Candida albicans*. *Microbiology* **145:** 2715–2725.
63. **Xisto MI, Caramalho RD, Rocha DA, Ferreira-Pereira A, Sartori B, Barreto-Bergter E, Junqueira ML, Lass-Flörl C, Lackner M.** 2017. Pan-azole-resistant *Candida tropicalis* carrying homozygous erg11 mutations at position K143R: a new emerging superbug? *J Antimicrob Chemother* **72:**988–992.
64. **Snelders E, Karawajczyk A, Schaftenaar G, Verweij PE, Melchers WJ.** 2010. Azole resistance profile of amino acid changes in *Aspergillus fumigatus* CYP51A based on protein homology modeling. *Antimicrob Agents Chemother* **54:**2425–2430.
65. **Fraczek MG, Bromley M, Bowyer P.** 2011. An improved model of the *Aspergillus fumigatus* CYP51A protein. *Antimicrob Agents Chemother* **55:**2483–2486.
66. **Hargrove TY, Friggeri L, Wawrzak Z, Qi A, Hoekstra WJ, Schotzinger RJ, York JD, Guengerich FP, Lepesheva GI.** 2017. Structural analyses of *Candida albicans* sterol 14α-demethylase complexed with azole drugs address the molecular basis of azole-mediated inhibition of fungal sterol biosynthesis. *J Biol Chem* **292:**6728–6743.
67. **Song JL, Harry JB, Eastman RT, Oliver BG, White TC.** 2004. The *Candida albicans* lanosterol 14-alpha-demethylase (ERG11) gene promoter is maximally induced after prolonged growth with antifungal drugs. *Antimicrob Agents Chemother* **48:**1136–1144.
68. **Henry KW, Nickels JT, Edlind TD.** 2000. Upregulation of ERG genes in *Candida species* by azoles and other sterol biosynthesis inhibitors. *Antimicrob Agents Chemother* **44:** 2693–2700.
69. **Flowers SA, Barker KS, Berkow EL, Toner G, Chadwick SG, Gygax SE, Morschhäuser J, Rogers PD.** 2012. Gain-of-function mutations in UPC2 are a frequent cause of ERG11 upregulation in azole-resistant clinical isolates of *Candida albicans*. *Eukaryot Cell* **11:**1289–1299.
70. **MacPherson S, Akache B, Weber S, De Deken X, Raymond M, Turcotte B.** 2005. *Candida albicans* zinc cluster protein Upc2p confers resistance to antifungal drugs and is an activator of ergosterol biosynthetic genes. *Antimicrob Agents Chemother* **49:**1745–1752.
71. **Silver PM, Oliver BG, White TC.** 2004. Role of *Candida albicans* transcription factor Upc2p in drug resistance and sterol metabolism. *Eukaryot Cell* **3:**1391–1397.
72. **Oliver BG, Song JL, Choiniere JH, White TC.** 2007. *cis*-acting elements within the *Candida albicans* ERG11 promoter mediate the azole response through transcription factor Upc2p. *Eukaryot Cell* **6:**2231–2239.
73. **Hoot SJ, Oliver BG, White TC.** 2008. *Candida albicans* UPC2 is transcriptionally induced in response to antifungal drugs and anaerobicity through Upc2p-dependent and -independent mechanisms. *Microbiology* **154:**2748–2756.
74. **Znaidi S, Weber S, Zin Al-Abdin O, Bomme P, Saidane S, Drouin S, Lemieux S, De Deken X, Robert F, Raymond M.** 2008. Genomewide location analysis of *Candida albicans* Upc2p, a regulator of sterol metabolism and azole drug resistance. *Eukaryot Cell* **7:**836–847.
75. **Marr KA, Lyons CN, Rustad TR, Bowden RA, White TC.** 1998. Rapid, transient fluconazole resistance in *Candida albicans* is associated with increased mRNA levels of CDR. *Antimicrob Agents Chemother* **42:**2584–2589.
76. **Arendrup MC, Mavridou E, Mortensen KL, Snelders E, Frimodt-Møller N, Khan H, Melchers WJ, Verweij PE.** 2010. Development of azole resistance in *Aspergillus fumigatus* during azole therapy associated with change in virulence. *PLoS One* **5:**e10080.
77. **Buied A, Moore CB, Denning DW, Bowyer P.** 2013. High-level expression of cyp51B in azole-resistant clinical *Aspergillus fumigatus* isolates. *J Antimicrob Chemother* **68:**512–514.
78. **Hagiwara D, Miura D, Shimizu K, Paul S, Ohba A, Gonoi T, Watanabe A, Kamei K, Shintani T, Moye-Rowley WS, Kawamoto S, Gomi K.** 2017. A novel Zn2-Cys6 transcription factor AtrR plays a key role in an azole resistance mechanism of *Aspergillus fumigatus* by co-regulating cyp51A and cdr1B expressions. *PLoS Pathog* **13:**e1006096.
79. **Sanglard D, Kuchler K, Ischer F, Pagani JL, Monod M, Bille J.** 1995. Mechanisms of resistance to azole antifungal agents in *Candida albicans* isolates from AIDS patients involve specific multidrug transporters. *Antimicrob Agents Chemother* **39:**2378–2386.
80. **Braun BR, van Het Hoog M, d'Enfert C, Martchenko M, Dungan J, Kuo A, Inglis DO, Uhl MA, Hogues H, Berriman M, Lorenz M, Levitin A, Oberholzer U, Bachewich C, Harcus D, Marcil A, Dignard D, Iouk T, Zito R, Frangeul L, Tekaia F, Rutherford K, Wang E, Munro CA, Bates S, Gow NA, Hoyer LL, Köhler G, Morschhäuser J, Newport G, Znaidi S, Raymond M, Turcotte B, Sherlock G, Costanzo M, Ihmels J, Berman J, Sanglard D, Agabian N, Mitchell AP, Johnson AD, Whiteway M, Nantel A.** 2005. A human-curated annotation of the *Candida albicans* genome. *PLoS Genet* **1:**e1.
81. **Shukla S, Saini P, Smriti, Jha S, Ambudkar SV, Prasad R.** 2003. Functional characterization of *Candida albicans* ABC transporter Cdr1p. *Eukaryot Cell* **2:**1361–1375.
82. **Sanglard D, Ischer F, Monod M, Bille J.** 1997. Cloning of *Candida albicans* genes conferring resistance to azole antifungal agents: characterization of CDR2, a new multidrug ABC transporter gene. *Microbiology* **143:**405–416.
83. **Sanglard D, Ischer F, Calabrese D, Majcherczyk PA, Bille J.** 1999. The ATP binding cassette transporter gene CgCDR1 from *Candida glabrata* is involved in the resistance of clinical isolates to azole antifungal agents. *Antimicrob Agents Chemother* **43:**2753–2765.
84. **Izumikawa K, Kakeya H, Tsai HF, Grimberg B, Bennett JE.** 2003. Function of *Candida glabrata* ABC transporter gene, PDH1. *Yeast* **20:**249–261.
85. **Torelli R, Posteraro B, Ferrari S, La Sorda M, Fadda G, Sanglard D, Sanguinetti M.** 2008. The ATP-binding cassette transporter-encoding gene CgSNQ2 is contributing to the CgPDR1-dependent azole resistance of *Candida glabrata*. *Mol Microbiol* **68:**186–201.
86. **Brun S, Bergès T, Poupard P, Vauzelle-Moreau C, Renier G, Chabasse D, Bouchara JP.** 2004. Mechanisms of azole resistance in petite mutants of *Candida glabrata*. *Antimicrob Agents Chemother* **48:**1788–1796.
87. **Sanguinetti M, Posteraro B, La Sorda M, Torelli R, Fiori B, Santangelo R, Delogu G, Fadda G.** 2006. Role of AFR1, an ABC transporter-encoding gene, in the in vivo response to fluconazole and virulence of *Cryptococcus neoformans*. *Infect Immun* **74:**1352–1359.
88. **Katiyar SK, Edlind TD.** 2001. Identification and expression of multidrug resistance-related ABC transporter genes in *Candida krusei*. *Med Mycol* **39:**109–116.
89. **Paul S, Diekema D, Moye-Rowley WS.** 2017. Contributions of both ATP-binding cassette transporter and Cyp51A proteins are essential for azole resistance in *Aspergillus fumigatus*. *Antimicrob Agents Chemother* **61:**e02748-16.
90. **Gaur M, Puri N, Manoharlal R, Rai V, Mukhopadhayay G, Choudhury D, Prasad R.** 2008. MFS transportome of the human pathogenic yeast *Candida albicans*. *BMC Genomics* **9:**579.
91. **Goldway M, Teff D, Schmidt R, Oppenheim AB, Koltin Y.** 1995. Multidrug resistance in *Candida albicans*: disruption of the BENr gene. *Antimicrob Agents Chemother* **39:**422–426.
92. **Sasse C, Schillig R, Reimund A, Merk J, Morschhäuser J.** 2012. Inducible and constitutive activation of two polymorphic promoter alleles of the *Candida albicans* multidrug efflux pump MDR1. *Antimicrob Agents Chemother* **56:**4490–4494.

93. **Calabrese D, Bille J, Sanglard D.** 2000. A novel multidrug efflux transporter gene of the major facilitator superfamily from *Candida albicans* (FLU1) conferring resistance to fluconazole. *Microbiology* **146:**2743–2754.
94. **Lopez-Ribot JL, McAtee RK, Lee LN, Kirkpatrick WR, White TC, Sanglard D, Patterson TF.** 1998. Distinct patterns of gene expression associated with development of fluconazole resistance in serial *Candida albicans* isolates from human immunodeficiency virus-infected patients with oropharyngeal candidiasis. *Antimicrob Agents Chemother* **42:**2932–2937.
95. **Franz R, Kelly SL, Lamb DC, Kelly DE, Ruhnke M, Morschhäuser J.** 1998. Multiple molecular mechanisms contribute to a stepwise development of fluconazole resistance in clinical *Candida albicans* strains. *Antimicrob Agents Chemother* **42:**3065–3072.
96. **Coste AT, Karababa M, Ischer F, Bille J, Sanglard D.** 2004. TAC1, transcriptional activator of CDR genes, is a new transcription factor involved in the regulation of *Candida albicans* ABC transporters CDR1 and CDR2. *Eukaryot Cell* **3:**1639–1652.
97. **Schubert S, Barker KS, Znaidi S, Schneider S, Dierolf F, Dunkel N, Aïd M, Boucher G, Rogers PD, Raymond M, Morschhäuser J.** 2011. Regulation of efflux pump expression and drug resistance by the transcription factors Mrr1, Upc2, and Cap1 in *Candida albicans*. *Antimicrob Agents Chemother* **55:**2212–2223.
98. **Coste A, Turner V, Ischer F, Morschhäuser J, Forche A, Selmecki A, Berman J, Bille J, Sanglard D.** 2006. A mutation in Tac1p, a transcription factor regulating CDR1 and CDR2, is coupled with loss of heterozygosity at chromosome 5 to mediate antifungal resistance in *Candida albicans*. *Genetics* **172:**2139–2156.
99. **Riggle PJ, Kumamoto CA.** 2006. Transcriptional regulation of MDR1, encoding a drug efflux determinant, in fluconazole-resistant *Candida albicans* strains through an Mcm1p binding site. *Eukaryot Cell* **5:**1957–1968.
100. **Vermitsky JP, Edlind TD.** 2004. Azole resistance in *Candida glabrata*: coordinate upregulation of multidrug transporters and evidence for a Pdr1-like transcription factor. *Antimicrob Agents Chemother* **48:**3773–3781.
101. **Ferrari S, Sanguinetti M, Torelli R, Posteraro B, Sanglard D.** 2011. Contribution of CgPDR1-regulated genes in enhanced virulence of azole-resistant *Candida glabrata*. *PLoS One* **6:**e17589.
102. **Ferrari S, Ischer F, Calabrese D, Posteraro B, Sanguinetti M, Fadda G, Rohde B, Bauser C, Bader O, Sanglard D.** 2009. Gain of function mutations in CgPDR1 of *Candida glabrata* not only mediate antifungal resistance but also enhance virulence. *PLoS Pathog* **5:**e1000268.
103. **Manoharlal R, Gaur NA, Panwar SL, Morschhäuser J, Prasad R.** 2008. Transcriptional activation and increased mRNA stability contribute to overexpression of CDR1 in azole-resistant *Candida albicans*. *Antimicrob Agents Chemother* **52:**1481–1492.
104. **Selmecki AM, Dulmage K, Cowen LE, Anderson JB, Berman J.** 2009. Acquisition of aneuploidy provides increased fitness during the evolution of antifungal drug resistance. *PLoS Genet* **5:**e1000705.
105. **Coste A, Selmecki A, Forche A, Diogo D, Bougnoux ME, d'Enfert C, Berman J, Sanglard D.** 2007. Genotypic evolution of azole resistance mechanisms in sequential *Candida albicans* isolates. *Eukaryot Cell* **6:**1889–1904.
106. **Coste AT, Crittin J, Bauser C, Rohde B, Sanglard D.** 2009. Functional analysis of *cis-* and *trans*-acting elements of the *Candida albicans* CDR2 promoter with a novel promoter reporter system. *Eukaryot Cell* **8:**1250–1267.
107. **Ben-Ami R, Zimmerman O, Finn T, Amit S, Novikov A, Wertheimer N, Lurie-Weinberger M, Berman J.** 2016. Heteroresistance to fluconazole is a continuously distributed phenotype among *Candida glabrata* clinical strains associated with *in vivo* persistence. *mBio* **7:**e00655-16.
108. **Sionov E, Lee H, Chang YC, Kwon-Chung KJ.** 2010. *Cryptococcus neoformans* overcomes stress of azole drugs by formation of disomy in specific multiple chromosomes. *PLoS Pathog* **6:**e1000848.
109. **Sionov E, Chang YC, Garraffo HM, Kwon-Chung KJ.** 2009. Heteroresistance to fluconazole in *Cryptococcus neoformans* is intrinsic and associated with virulence. *Antimicrob Agents Chemother* **53:**2804–2815.
110. **Sasse C, Dunkel N, Schäfer T, Schneider S, Dierolf F, Ohlsen K, Morschhäuser J.** 2012. The stepwise acquisition of fluconazole resistance mutations causes a gradual loss of fitness in *Candida albicans*. *Mol Microbiol* **86:**539–556.
111. **Mavridou E, Meletiadis J, Arendrup M, Melchers W, Mouton J, Verweij P.** 2010. Impact of CYP51A mutations associated with azole-resistance on in vitro growth rates and in vivo virulence of clinical Aspergillus fumigatus isolates, abstr O345. *In* 20th European Congress of Clinical Microbiology and Infectious Diseases, Vienna, Austria.
112. **Vale-Silva L, Ischer F, Leibundgut-Landmann S, Sanglard D.** 2013. Gain-of-function mutations in PDR1, a regulator of antifungal drug resistance in *Candida glabrata*, control adherence to host cells. *Infect Immun* **81:**1709–1720.
113. **Ferrari S, Sanguinetti M, De Bernardis F, Torelli R, Posteraro B, Vandeputte P, Sanglard D.** 2011. Loss of mitochondrial functions associated with azole resistance in *Candida glabrata* results in enhanced virulence in mice. *Antimicrob Agents Chemother* **55:**1852–1860.
114. **Kelly SL, Lamb DC, Kelly DE, Manning NJ, Loeffler J, Hebart H, Schumacher U, Einsele H.** 1997. Resistance to fluconazole and cross-resistance to amphotericin B in *Candida albicans* from AIDS patients caused by defective sterol delta5,6-desaturation. *FEBS Lett* **400:**80–82.
115. **Sanglard D, Ischer F, Parkinson T, Falconer D, Bille J.** 2003. *Candida albicans* mutations in the ergosterol biosynthetic pathway and resistance to several antifungal agents. *Antimicrob Agents Chemother* **47:**2404–2412.
116. **Geber A, Hitchcock CA, Swartz JE, Pullen FS, Marsden KE, Kwon-Chung KJ, Bennett JE.** 1995. Deletion of the *Candida glabrata* ERG3 and ERG11 genes: effect on cell viability, cell growth, sterol composition, and antifungal susceptibility. *Antimicrob Agents Chemother* **39:**2708–2717.
117. **Alcazar-Fuoli L, Mellado E, Garcia-Effron G, Buitrago MJ, Lopez JF, Grimalt JO, Cuenca-Estrella JM, Rodriguez-Tudela JL.** 2006. Aspergillus fumigatus C-5 sterol desaturases Erg3A and Erg3B: role in sterol biosynthesis and antifungal drug susceptibility. *Antimicrob Agents Chemother* **50:**453–460.
118. **Esquivel BD, Smith AR, Zavrel M, White TC.** 2015. Azole drug import into the pathogenic fungus *Aspergillus fumigatus*. *Antimicrob Agents Chemother* **59:**3390–3398.
119. **Kumamoto CA.** 2002. *Candida* biofilms. *Curr Opin Microbiol* **5:**608–611.
120. **Ramage G, Mowat E, Jones B, Williams C, Lopez-Ribot J.** 2009. Our current understanding of fungal biofilms. *Crit Rev Microbiol* **35:**340–355.
121. **Fanning S, Mitchell AP.** 2012. Fungal biofilms. *PLoS Pathog* **8:**e1002585.
122. **Ramage G, Bachmann S, Patterson TF, Wickes BL, López-Ribot JL.** 2002. Investigation of multidrug efflux pumps in relation to fluconazole resistance in *Candida albicans* biofilms. *J Antimicrob Chemother* **49:**973–980.
123. **Mukherjee PK, Chandra J, Kuhn DM, Ghannoum MA.** 2003. Mechanism of fluconazole resistance in *Candida albicans* biofilms: phase-specific role of efflux pumps and membrane sterols. *Infect Immun* **71:**4333–4340.
124. **Nett JE, Sanchez H, Cain MT, Andes DR.** 2010. Genetic basis of *Candida* biofilm resistance due to drug-sequestering matrix glucan. *J Infect Dis* **202:**171–175.
125. **Desai JV, Bruno VM, Ganguly S, Stamper RJ, Mitchell KF, Solis N, Hill EM, Xu W, Filler SG, Andes DR, Fanning S, Lanni F, Mitchell AP.** 2013. Regulatory role of glycerol in *Candida albicans* biofilm formation. *mBio* **4:**e00637-12.
126. **Nett JE, Crawford K, Marchillo K, Andes DR.** 2010. Role of Fks1p and matrix glucan in *Candida albicans* biofilm resistance to an echinocandin, pyrimidine, and polyene. *Antimicrob Agents Chemother* **54:**3505–3508.
127. **Nobile CJ, Nett JE, Hernday AD, Homann OR, Deneault JS, Nantel A, Andes DR, Johnson AD, Mitchell AP.** 2009. Biofilm matrix regulation by *Candida albicans* Zap1. *PLoS Biol* **7:**e1000133.

128. **Shapiro RS, Zaas AK, Betancourt-Quiroz M, Perfect JR, Cowen LE.** 2012. The Hsp90 co-chaperone Sgt1 governs *Candida albicans* morphogenesis and drug resistance. *PLoS One* **7:**e44734.
129. **Robbins N, Uppuluri P, Nett J, Rajendran R, Ramage G, Lopez-Ribot JL, Andes D, Cowen LE.** 2011. Hsp90 governs dispersion and drug resistance of fungal biofilms. *PLoS Pathog* **7:**e1002257.
130. **Silva S, Henriques M, Martins A, Oliveira R, Williams D, Azeredo J.** 2009. Biofilms of non-*Candida albicans Candida* species: quantification, structure and matrix composition. *Med Mycol* **47:**681–689.
131. **Beauvais A, Fontaine T, Aimanianda V, Latgé JP.** 2014. *Aspergillus* cell wall and biofilm. *Mycopathologia* **178:**371–377.
132. **Pappas PG, Kauffman CA, Andes DR, Clancy CJ, Marr KA, Ostrosky-Zeichner L, Reboli AC, Schuster MG, Vazquez JA, Walsh TJ, Zaoutis TE, Sobel JD.** 2016. Executive summary: clinical practice guideline for the management of candidiasis: 2016 update by the Infectious Diseases Society of America. *Clin Infect Dis* **62:**409–417.
133. **Mio T, Adachi-Shimizu M, Tachibana Y, Tabuchi H, Inoue SB, Yabe T, Yamada-Okabe T, Arisawa M, Watanabe T, Yamada-Okabe H.** 1997. Cloning of the *Candida albicans* homolog of *Saccharomyces cerevisiae* GSC1/FKS1 and its involvement in beta-1,3-glucan synthesis. *J Bacteriol* **179:**4096–4105.
134. **Katiyar SK, Alastruey-Izquierdo A, Healey KR, Johnson ME, Perlin DS, Edlind TD.** 2012. Fks1 and Fks2 are functionally redundant but differentially regulated in *Candida glabrata*: implications for echinocandin resistance. *Antimicrob Agents Chemother* **56:**6304–6309.
135. **Ernst EJ, Klepser ME, Ernst ME, Messer SA, Pfaller MA.** 1999. In vitro pharmacodynamic properties of MK-0991 determined by time-kill methods. *Diagn Microbiol Infect Dis* **33:**75–80.
136. **Bowman JC, Hicks PS, Kurtz MB, Rosen H, Schmatz DM, Liberator PA, Douglas CM.** 2002. The antifungal echinocandin caspofungin acetate kills growing cells of *Aspergillus fumigatus* in vitro. *Antimicrob Agents Chemother* **46:**3001–3012.
137. **Pfaller MA, Rhomberg PR, Messer SA, Jones RN, Castanheira M.** 2015. Isavuconazole, micafungin, and 8 comparator antifungal agents' susceptibility profiles for common and uncommon opportunistic fungi collected in 2013: temporal analysis of antifungal drug resistance using CLSI species-specific clinical breakpoints and proposed epidemiological cutoff values. *Diagn Microbiol Infect Dis* **82:**303–313.
138. **Dannaoui E, Desnos-Ollivier M, Garcia-Hermoso D, Grenouillet F, Cassaing S, Baixench MT, Bretagne S, Dromer F, Lortholary O, French Mycoses Study Group.** 2012. *Candida* spp. with acquired echinocandin resistance, France, 2004-2010. *Emerg Infect Dis* **18:**86–90.
139. **Castanheira M, Woosley LN, Diekema DJ, Messer SA, Jones RN, Pfaller MA.** 2010. Low prevalence of *fks1* hot spot 1 mutations in a worldwide collection of *Candida* strains. *Antimicrob Agents Chemother* **54:**2655–2659.
140. **Ostrosky-Zeichner L.** 2013. *Candida glabrata* and FKS mutations: witnessing the emergence of the true multidrug-resistant *Candida*. *Clin Infect Dis* **56:**1733–1734.
141. **Lortholary O, Desnos-Ollivier M, Sitbon K, Fontanet A, Bretagne S, Dromer F, French Mycosis Study Group.** 2011. Recent exposure to caspofungin or fluconazole influences the epidemiology of candidemia: a prospective multicenter study involving 2,441 patients. *Antimicrob Agents Chemother* **55:**532–538.
142. **Fekkar A, Meyer I, Brossas JY, Dannaoui E, Palous M, Uzunov M, Nguyen S, Leblond V, Mazier D, Datry A.** 2013. Rapid emergence of echinocandin resistance during *Candida kefyr* fungemia treatment with caspofungin. *Antimicrob Agents Chemother* **57:**2380–2382.
143. **Alexander BD, Johnson MD, Pfeiffer CD, Jiménez-Ortigosa C, Catania J, Booker R, Castanheira M, Messer SA, Perlin DS, Pfaller MA.** 2013. Increasing echinocandin resistance in *Candida glabrata*: clinical failure correlates with presence of FKS mutations and elevated minimum inhibitory concentrations. *Clin Infect Dis* **56:**1724–1732.
144. **Vallabhaneni S, Cleveland AA, Farley MM, Harrison LH, Schaffner W, Beldavs ZG, Derado G, Pham CD, Lockhart SR, Smith RM.** 2015. Epidemiology and risk factors for echinocandin nonsusceptible *Candida glabrata* bloodstream infections: data from a large multisite population-based candidemia surveillance program, 2008-2014. *Open Forum Infect Dis* **2:**ofv163.
145. **Dellière S, Healey K, Gits-Muselli M, Carrara B, Barbaro A, Guigue N, Lecefel C, Touratier S, Desnos-Ollivier M, Perlin DS, Bretagne S, Alanio A.** 2016. Fluconazole and echinocandin resistance of *Candida glabrata* correlates better with antifungal drug exposure rather than with MSH2 mutator genotype in a French cohort of patients harboring low rates of resistance. *Front Microbiol* **7:**2038.
146. **Pfaller MA, Diekema DJ, Andes D, Arendrup MC, Brown SD, Lockhart SR, Motyl M, Perlin DS, CLSI Subcommittee for Antifungal Testing.** 2011. Clinical breakpoints for the echinocandins and *Candida* revisited: integration of molecular, clinical, and microbiological data to arrive at species-specific interpretive criteria. *Drug Resist Updat* **14:**164–176.
147. **Niimi K, Maki K, Ikeda F, Holmes AR, Lamping E, Niimi M, Monk BC, Cannon RD.** 2006. Overexpression of *Candida albicans* CDR1, CDR2, or MDR1 does not produce significant changes in echinocandin susceptibility. *Antimicrob Agents Chemother* **50:**1148–1155.
148. **Arendrup MC, Perlin DS.** 2014. Echinocandin resistance: an emerging clinical problem? *Curr Opin Infect Dis* **27:**484–492.
149. **Garcia-Effron G, Park S, Perlin DS.** 2009. Correlating echinocandin MIC and kinetic inhibition of *fks1* mutant glucan synthases for *Candida albicans*: implications for interpretive breakpoints. *Antimicrob Agents Chemother* **53:**112–122.
150. **Park S, Kelly R, Kahn JN, Robles J, Hsu MJ, Register E, Li W, Vyas V, Fan H, Abruzzo G, Flattery A, Gill C, Chrebet G, Parent SA, Kurtz M, Teppler H, Douglas CM, Perlin DS.** 2005. Specific substitutions in the echinocandin target Fks1p account for reduced susceptibility of rare laboratory and clinical *Candida* sp. isolates. *Antimicrob Agents Chemother* **49:**3264–3273.
151. **Perlin DS.** 2011. Current perspectives on echinocandin class drugs. *Future Microbiol* **6:**441–457.
152. **Arendrup MC, Perlin DS, Jensen RH, Howard SJ, Goodwin J, Hope W.** 2012. Differential in vivo activities of anidulafungin, caspofungin, and micafungin against *Candida glabrata* isolates with and without FKS resistance mutations. *Antimicrob Agents Chemother* **56:**2435–2442.
153. **Pham CD, Iqbal N, Bolden CB, Kuykendall RJ, Harrison LH, Farley MM, Schaffner W, Beldavs ZG, Chiller TM, Park BJ, Cleveland AA, Lockhart SR.** 2014. Role of FKS mutations in *Candida glabrata*: MIC values, echinocandin resistance, and multidrug resistance. *Antimicrob Agents Chemother* **58:**4690–4696.
154. **Garcia-Effron G, Lee S, Park S, Cleary JD, Perlin DS.** 2009. Effect of *Candida glabrata* FKS1 and FKS2 mutations on echinocandin sensitivity and kinetics of 1,3-beta-D-glucan synthase: implication for the existing susceptibility breakpoint. *Antimicrob Agents Chemother* **53:**3690–3699.
155. **Eng WK, Faucette L, McLaughlin MM, Cafferkey R, Koltin Y, Morris RA, Young PR, Johnson RK, Livi GP.** 1994. The yeast FKS1 gene encodes a novel membrane protein, mutations in which confer FK506 and cyclosporin A hypersensitivity and calcineurin-dependent growth. *Gene* **151:**61–71.
156. **Johnson ME, Katiyar SK, Edlind TD.** 2011. New Fks hot spot for acquired echinocandin resistance in *Saccharomyces cerevisiae* and its contribution to intrinsic resistance of *Scedosporium* species. *Antimicrob Agents Chemother* **55:**3774–3781.
157. **Ben-Ami R, Garcia-Effron G, Lewis RE, Gamarra S, Leventakos K, Perlin DS, Kontoyiannis DP.** 2011. Fitness and virulence costs of *Candida albicans* FKS1 hot spot mutations associated with echinocandin resistance. *J Infect Dis* **204:**626–635.

158. **Kale-Pradhan PB, Morgan G, Wilhelm SM, Johnson LB.** 2010. Comparative efficacy of echinocandins and non-echinocandins for the treatment of *Candida parapsilosis* Infections: a meta-analysis. *Pharmacotherapy* **30:**1207–1213.
159. **Forrest GN, Weekes E, Johnson JK.** 2008. Increasing incidence of *Candida parapsilosis* candidemia with caspofungin usage. *J Infect* **56:**126–129.
160. **Garcia-Effron G, Katiyar SK, Park S, Edlind TD, Perlin DS.** 2008. A naturally occurring proline-to-alanine amino acid change in Fks1p in *Candida parapsilosis*, *Candida orthopsilosis*, and *Candida metapsilosis* accounts for reduced echinocandin susceptibility. *Antimicrob Agents Chemother* **52:** 2305–2312.
161. **Nett JE, Sanchez H, Cain MT, Ross KM, Andes DR.** 2011. Interface of *Candida albicans* biofilm matrix-associated drug resistance and cell wall integrity regulation. *Eukaryot Cell* **10:**1660–1669 doi:EC.05126-11 [pii] 10.1128/EC.05126-11.
162. **Nobile CJ, Nett JE, Andes DR, Mitchell AP.** 2006. Function of *Candida albicans* adhesin Hwp1 in biofilm formation. *Eukaryot Cell* **5:**1604–1610.
163. **Zotchev SB.** 2003. Polyene macrolide antibiotics and their applications in human therapy. *Curr Med Chem* **10:**211–223.
164. **Kanafani ZA, Perfect JR.** 2008. Antimicrobial resistance: resistance to antifungal agents: mechanisms and clinical impact. *Clin Infect Dis* **46:**120–128.
165. **Walsh TJ, Petraitis V, Petraitiene R, Field-Ridley A, Sutton D, Ghannoum M, Sein T, Schaufele R, Peter J, Bacher J, Casler H, Armstrong D, Espinel-Ingroff A, Rinaldi MG, Lyman CA.** 2003. Experimental pulmonary aspergillosis due to *Aspergillus terreus*: pathogenesis and treatment of an emerging fungal pathogen resistant to amphotericin B. *J Infect Dis* **188:**305–319.
166. **Balajee SA, Weaver M, Imhof A, Gribskov J, Marr KA.** 2004. *Aspergillus fumigatus* variant with decreased susceptibility to multiple antifungals. *Antimicrob Agents Chemother* **48:**1197–1203.
167. **Espinel-Ingroff A, Cuenca-Estrella M, Fothergill A, Fuller J, Ghannoum M, Johnson E, Pelaez T, Pfaller MA, Turnidge J.** 2011. Wild-type MIC distributions and epidemiological cutoff values for amphotericin B and *Aspergillus* spp. for the CLSI broth microdilution method (M38-A2 document). *Antimicrob Agents Chemother* **55:**5150–5154.
168. **Hull CM, Bader O, Parker JE, Weig M, Gross U, Warrilow AG, Kelly DE, Kelly SL.** 2012. Two clinical isolates of *Candida glabrata* exhibiting reduced sensitivity to amphotericin B both harbor mutations in ERG2. *Antimicrob Agents Chemother* **56:**6417–6421.
169. **Hull CM, Parker JE, Bader O, Weig M, Gross U, Warrilow AG, Kelly DE, Kelly SL.** 2012. Facultative sterol uptake in an ergosterol-deficient clinical isolate of *Candida glabrata* harboring a missense mutation in ERG11 and exhibiting cross-resistance to azoles and amphotericin B. *Antimicrob Agents Chemother* **56:**4223–4232.
170. **Farmakiotis D, Tarrand JJ, Kontoyiannis DP.** 2014. Drug-resistant *Candida glabrata* infection in cancer patients. *Emerg Infect Dis* **20:**1833–1840.
171. **Vazquez JA, Arganoza MT, Boikov D, Yoon S, Sobel JD, Akins RA.** 1998. Stable phenotypic resistance of *Candida* species to amphotericin B conferred by preexposure to subinhibitory levels of azoles. *J Clin Microbiol* **36:**2690–2695.
172. **Vandeputte P, Tronchin G, Larcher G, Ernoult E, Bergès T, Chabasse D, Bouchara JP.** 2008. A nonsense mutation in the ERG6 gene leads to reduced susceptibility to polyenes in a clinical isolate of *Candida glabrata*. *Antimicrob Agents Chemother* **52:**3701–3709.
173. **Kelly SL, Lamb DC, Taylor M, Corran AJ, Baldwin BC, Powderly WG.** 1994. Resistance to amphotericin B associated with defective sterol $\Delta^{8\to7}$ isomerase in a *Cryptococcus neoformans* strain from an AIDS patient. *FEMS Microbiol Lett* **122:**39–42.
174. **Miyazaki Y, Geber A, Miyazaki H, Falconer D, Parkinson T, Hitchcock C, Grimberg B, Nyswaner K, Bennett JE.** 1999. Cloning, sequencing, expression and allelic sequence diversity of ERG3 (C-5 sterol desaturase gene) in *Candida albicans*. *Gene* **236:**43–51.
175. **Healey KR, Zhao Y, Perez WB, Lockhart SR, Sobel JD, Farmakiotis D, Kontoyiannis DP, Sanglard D, Taj-Aldeen SJ, Alexander BD, Jimenez-Ortigosa C, Shor E, Perlin DS.** 2016. Prevalent mutator genotype identified in fungal pathogen *Candida glabrata* promotes multi-drug resistance. *Nat Commun* **7:**11128.
176. **Blum G, Perkhofer S, Haas H, Schrettl M, Würzner R, Dierich MP, Lass-Flörl C.** 2008. Potential basis for amphotericin B resistance in *Aspergillus terreus*. *Antimicrob Agents Chemother* **52:**1553–1555.
177. **Ramage G, Rajendran R, Sherry L, Williams C.** 2012. Fungal biofilm resistance. *Int J Microbiol* **2012:**528521.
178. **Hope WW, Tabernero L, Denning DW, Anderson MJ.** 2004. Molecular mechanisms of primary resistance to flucytosine in *Candida albicans*. *Antimicrob Agents Chemother* **48:**4377–4386.
179. **Papon N, Noël T, Florent M, Gibot-Leclerc S, Jean D, Chastin C, Villard J, Chapeland-Leclerc F.** 2007. Molecular mechanism of flucytosine resistance in *Candida lusitaniae*: contribution of the FCY2, FCY1, and FUR1 genes to 5-fluorouracil and fluconazole cross-resistance. *Antimicrob Agents Chemother* **51:**369–371.
180. **Edlind TD, Katiyar SK.** 2010. Mutational analysis of flucytosine resistance in *Candida glabrata*. *Antimicrob Agents Chemother* **54:**4733–4738.
181. **Costa C, Ponte A, Pais P, Santos R, Cavalheiro M, Yaguchi T, Chibana H, Teixeira MC.** 2015. New mechanisms of flucytosine resistance in *C. glabrata* unveiled by a chemogenomics analysis in *S. cerevisiae*. *PLoS One* **10:**e0135110.
182. **Shor E, Perlin DS.** 2015. Coping with stress and the emergence of multidrug resistance in fungi. *PLoS Pathog* **11:**e1004668.
183. **Perlin DS, Shor E, Zhao Y.** 2015. Update on antifungal drug resistance. *Curr Clin Microbiol Rep* **2:**84–95.
184. **Cowen LE.** 2009. Hsp90 orchestrates stress response signaling governing fungal drug resistance. *PLoS Pathog* **5:**e1000471.
185. **Cowen LE, Carpenter AE, Matangkasombut O, Fink GR, Lindquist S.** 2006. Genetic architecture of Hsp90-dependent drug resistance. *Eukaryot Cell* **5:**2184–2188.
186. **Munro CA, Selvaggini S, de Bruijn I, Walker L, Lenardon MD, Gerssen B, Milne S, Brown AJ, Gow NA.** 2007. The PKC, HOG and Ca2+ signalling pathways co-ordinately regulate chitin synthesis in *Candida albicans*. *Mol Microbiol* **63:**1399–1413.
187. **Healey KR, Katiyar SK, Raj S, Edlind TD.** 2012. CRS-MIS in *Candida glabrata*: sphingolipids modulate echinocandin-Fks interaction. *Mol Microbiol* **86:**303–313.
188. **Singh SD, Robbins N, Zaas AK, Schell WA, Perfect JR, Cowen LE.** 2009. Hsp90 governs echinocandin resistance in the pathogenic yeast *Candida albicans* via calcineurin. *PLoS Pathog* **5:**e1000532.
189. **Walker LA, Munro CA, de Bruijn I, Lenardon MD, McKinnon A, Gow NA.** 2008. Stimulation of chitin synthesis rescues *Candida albicans* from echinocandins. *PLoS Pathog* **4:**e1000040.
190. **Stevens DA, Espiritu M, Parmar R.** 2004. Paradoxical effect of caspofungin: reduced activity against *Candida albicans* at high drug concentrations. *Antimicrob Agents Chemother* **48:**3407–3411.
191. **Stevens DA, Ichinomiya M, Koshi Y, Horiuchi H.** 2006. Escape of *Candida* from caspofungin inhibition at concentrations above the MIC (paradoxical effect) accomplished by increased cell wall chitin; evidence for beta-1,6-glucan synthesis inhibition by caspofungin. *Antimicrob Agents Chemother* **50:**3160–3161.
192. **Healey KR, Jimenez Ortigosa C, Shor E, Perlin DS.** 2016. Genetic drivers of multidrug resistance in *Candida glabrata*. *Front Microbiol* **7:**1995.
193. **Vale-Silva LA, Moeckli B, Torelli R, Posteraro B, Sanguinetti M, Sanglard D.** 2016. Upregulation of the adhesin gene EPA1 mediated by PDR1 in *Candida glabrata* leads to enhanced host colonization. *mSphere* **1:**e00065-15.
194. **Sagatova AA, Keniya MV, Wilson RK, Monk BC, Tyndall JD.** 2015. Structural insights into binding of the antifungal drug fluconazole to *Saccharomyces cerevisiae* lanosterol 14α-demethylase. *Antimicrob Agents Chemother* **59:**4982–4989.

Susceptibility Test Methods: Yeasts and Filamentous Fungi*

ELIZABETH M. JOHNSON AND MAIKEN CAVLING-ARENDRUP

134

ANTIFUNGAL SUSCEPTIBILITY TESTING

Rationale

The groups of antifungal agents licensed for the systemic treatment of invasive fungal infection currently include the polyene amphotericin B and its three lipid formulations; the azoles fluconazole, isavuconazole, itraconazole, ketoconazole, posaconazole, and voriconazole; the echinocandins anidulafungin, caspofungin, and micafungin; the pyrimidine flucytosine; and the allylamine terbinafine (see chapter 132). With their increasing use has come the recognition of innate resistance to one or more agents in some isolates of yeast and mold and the emergence of resistance during therapy (1–9). Moreover, a recent worrying development has been the emergence of strains of *Aspergillus fumigatus* with cross-resistance to therapeutic triazole drugs due to environmental exposure to agricultural azoles, the emergence of *Candida glabrata* with acquired resistance to echinocandins following increased use of these agents, and the global emergence of *Candida auris*, a yeast that is often fluconazole resistant and can readily develop resistance to other agents and that has caused large health care-related outbreaks in high-dependency units on five continents (10, 11). As a result, clinical laboratories are now asked to assume a larger role in the selection and monitoring of antifungal chemotherapy. Thus, accurate and predictive antifungal susceptibility testing has become imperative and is now so widely accepted as a useful tool for informing decision making during the management of patients with invasive fungal infections that recommendations for testing appear in management guidelines (12, 13).

To be clinically useful, the requirements of *in vitro* susceptibility tests are that they should (i) provide a reproducible and reliable indication of the activities of antifungal agents, (ii) provide results that correlate with *in vivo* activity and therefore help to predict the likely outcome of therapy, (iii) provide a means with which to detect the development of resistance during therapy by applying clinical breakpoints, (iv) act as a surveillance tool for monitoring the development of resistance mechanisms among a normally susceptible wild-type population of organisms by adopting species-specific epidemiological cutoff values (ECOFFs/ECVs), and (v) have value as a screening tool to predict the therapeutic potential of newly discovered investigational agents. To provide this information, there has to be a careful analysis of the pharmacokinetic and pharmacodynamic interactions of the drug, as well as host-organism interactions.

The basic methodology of reference antifungal susceptibility testing has remained stable since the introduction in the early 1990s of the first standardized broth dilution method (National Committee for Clinical Laboratory Standards [NCCLS] M27-P) (14), which has since been modified to include a microdilution method conducted in a microtiter plate (CLSI M27-A3) (15). The accepted reference methods published by the Committee for Clinical and Laboratory Standards (CLSI) Subcommittee on Antifungal Susceptibility Testing and the Subcommittee on Antifungal Susceptibility Testing of the European Society of Clinical Microbiology and Infectious Diseases European Committee for Antimicrobial Susceptibility Testing (EUCAST) are now well established (14–20). The CLSI subcommittee has developed reference methods for broth macro- and microdilution susceptibility testing of yeasts (CLSI M27-A3 document) and molds (CLSI M38-A2 document), as well as disk diffusion methods for yeasts (CLSI M44-A2 document) and molds (CLSI M51-A document) (15, 16, 19, 20), while EUCAST has developed broth microdilution methods for fermentative yeast (E.Def 7.3 document) and for conidia-forming molds (E.Def 9.3 document) (17, 18). The main differences between the EUCAST and CLSI reference methods were the EUCAST recommendation of a higher glucose and inoculum concentration and for yeast, a shorter incubation time and a spectrophotometer reading rather than 2 days of incubation and visual reading as recommended by CLSI. However, as experience with these methods has become more widespread and their impact better understood, there have been changes. Thus, evaluation of the CLSI M27 method (15) for yeast susceptibility testing suggested that, in agreement with the EUCAST reference method (17) for most yeast species, results with fluconazole, amphotericin B, and the echinocandins could be evaluated after 24 h of incubation, thus reducing the total time to result from 72 to 48 h (15, 21–23). Studies also suggested that, in line with EUCAST methodology, posaconazole and voriconazole MICs for *Candida* spp. could also be read at 24 h (24).

*This chapter contains information presented in chapter 131 by E. M. Johnson, A. Espinel-Ingroff, and M. A. Pfaller in the 10th edition of this *Manual*.

TABLE 1 Clinical breakpoints for *Candida* spp. according to CLSI (previous and revised breakpoints) and EUCAST[a]

Drug	CLSI			EUCAST species-specific breakpoints (mg/liter)	
	M27-S3 non-species-specific breakpoints (mg/liter)	M27-S4 species-specific breakpoints (mg/liter)			
Amphotericin				≤1	
Anidulafungin	≤2	≤0.25; >0.5	*C. albicans*, *C. krusei*, *C. tropicalis*	≤0.03; >0.03	*C. albicans*
		≤0.125; >0.25	*C. glabrata*	≤0.06; >0.06	*C. glabrata*, *C. krusei*, *C. tropicalis*
		≤2; >4	*C. parapsilosis*	≤0.002; 4	*C. parapsilosis*[b]
Caspofungin	≤2			—[c]	
Micafungin	≤2	≤0.25; >0.5	*C. albicans*, *C. krusei*, *C. tropicalis*	≤0.016; >0.03	*C. albicans*
		≤0.06; >0.125	*C. glabrata*	≤0.03; >0.03	*C. glabrata*
		≤2; >4	*C. parapsilosis*	≤0.002; 2	*C. parapsilosis*[b]
Fluconazole	≤8; >32	≤2; >4	*C. albicans*, *C. parapsilosis*, *C. tropicalis*	≤2; >4	*C. albicans*, *C. parapsilosis*, *C. tropicalis*
		SDD: ≤32; >32	*C. glabrata*[d]	≤0.02; 32	*C. glabrata*[b]
Itraconazole	≤0.125; >0.5			—	
Posaconazole	—	—		≤0.06; >0.06	*C. albicans*, *C. parapsilosis*, *C. tropicalis*
Voriconazole	≤1; >2	≤0.125; >0.5	*C. albicans*, *C. parapsilosis*, *C. tropicalis*	≤0.125; >0.125	*C. albicans*, *C. parapsilosis*, *C. tropicalis*
			≤0.5; >1	*C. krusei*	

[a]Breakpoints are presented as S ≤ X, R > Y (except for the revised fluconazole breakpoint for *C. glabrata*). The I category (if present) is readily interpreted as the values between the S and the R breakpoints. Data from references 25–28, 80, 82.

[b]The entire wild-type population of *C. parapsilosis* is classified by EUCAST as intermediate (I) to anidulafungin and micafungin, and the wild-type population of *C. glabrata* is likewise classified as I to fluconazole. This is to accommodate use of these compounds in some clinical situations.

[c]EUCAST breakpoints for caspofungin have not been established due to an unacceptable variation of MIC ranges obtained using different lots of pure substance and across laboratories and time. However, because there is substantial evidence suggesting cross-resistance between anidulafungin and caspofungin, EUCAST recommends that isolates categorized as anidulafungin-susceptible can be regarded as susceptible to caspofungin until drug-specific EUCAST breakpoints are available for caspofungin.

[d]The wild-type population of *C. glabrata* is classified by CLSI as susceptible dose dependent (SDD) to fluconazole to accommodate use of fluconazole at elevated doses in some clinical situations.

The most significant development has been the introduction of species-specific breakpoints for the systemically active antifungal agents, together with the revision of the CLSI breakpoints based on the 24-h reading that has brought them in line with those proposed by EUCAST and has been published in document CLSI M27-S4 and now revised and extended in document M60 (23, 25–28, 173) and Table 1.

Basic Test Principles

MIC

In its simplest form, susceptibility testing is a measure of the potency of an agent to inhibit the growth *in vitro* of an organism, and the MIC is the lowest concentration of the agent able to inhibit growth to a predetermined degree. Growth inhibition may be determined in a broth format, usually in microtiter plates, or on solid agar by either incorporation of the agent into the agar base or impregnation into a disk or strip applied to the surface of a previously inoculated plate. Solid agar incorporation is particularly useful in the high-throughput testing required for surveillance screening of environmental isolates, and commercial plates with four wells containing breakpoint concentrations of three different antifungal agents and a control well have been validated (VIPCheck, Nijmegen, the Netherlands) (29) (Fig. 1). However, *in vitro* susceptibility testing is heavily influenced by a number of technical variables, including inoculum size and preparation, medium formulation and pH, duration and temperature of incubation, and the criterion used for MIC endpoint determination, all of which have to be considered when developing and interpreting test methods (30–34). In addition, antifungal susceptibility testing is complicated by problems unique to fungi, such as slow growth rates (relative to bacteria) and the ability of certain fungi (dimorphic) to grow either as a unicellular yeast form that produces blastoconidia or as a hyphal or filamentous fungal form that may have the ability to produce conidia or sporangiospores. Finally, the basic properties of the antifungal agents themselves, such as solubility, chemical stability, modes of action, and the tendency to produce partial inhibition of growth over a wide range of concentrations above the MIC, must be taken into account.

Minimum Fungicidal/Lethal Concentration

Many of the patients contracting invasive fungal infections are immunocompromised and thus unable to mount a significant immune response. Therefore, it has been postulated that antifungal agents that demonstrate fungicidal activity at concentrations that can be achieved *in vivo* may provide better outcomes than those agents that are fungistatic and thus rely on some host phagocytic cell activity to remove the remaining viable pathogens. It has thus been reported that the clinical outcome is significantly better for patients with invasive candidiasis due to *Candida albicans* and treated with an echinocandin (fungicidal) compared to those receiving fluconazole (fungistatic), despite the fact that *C. albicans* is susceptible to both (35, 36). Standard testing parameters are not yet available for evaluation of the

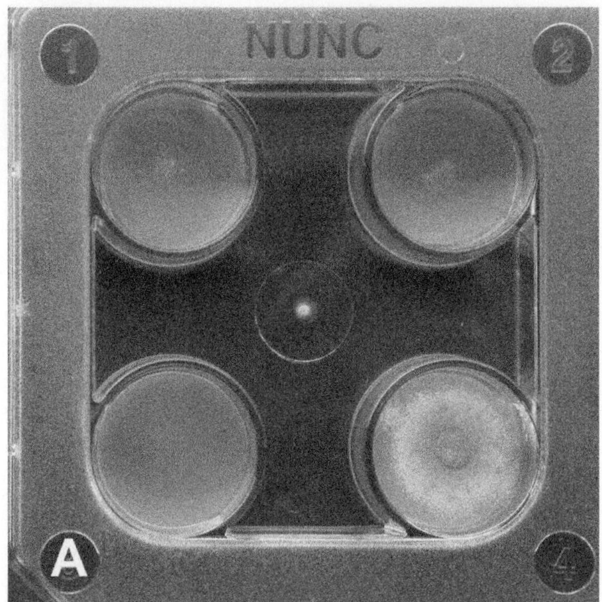

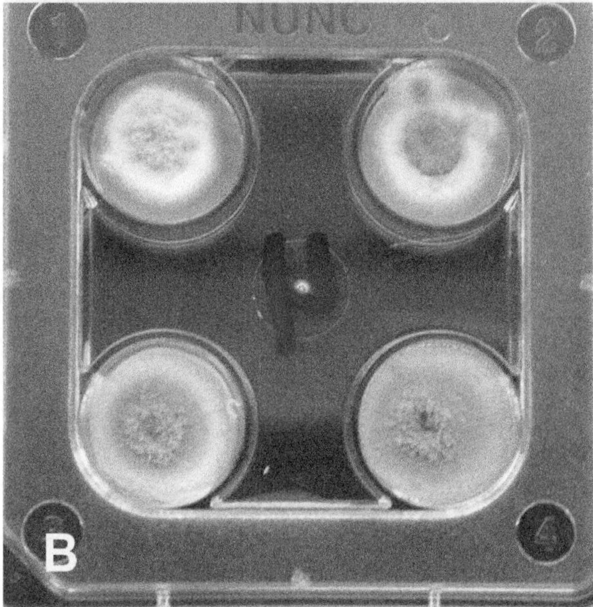

FIGURE 1 Azole agar screening plate. The four wells contain itraconazole, 4 mg/liter (ITR) (top-left well); voriconazole, 1 mg/liter (VRC) (top-right well); posaconazole, 0.5 mg/liter (PSC) (bottom-left well); or no antifungal compound (control) (bottom-right well). The upper agar multidish (A) is inoculated with a wild-type azole-susceptible *A. fumigatus* isolate, whereas the lower agar multidish (B) is inoculated with a multiazole-resistant *A. fumigatus* isolate. (Plates have been incubated 2 days.)

fungicidal activity of antifungal agents. The determination of minimum fungicidal concentrations (MFCs) requires the subculturing onto an agar medium of fixed volumes from each MIC tube or well that shows complete inhibition of growth. The criteria for MFC determination vary in different publications, and the MFC has been described as the lowest drug concentration resulting in either no growth or three to five colonies. The clinical relevance and the development of standard guidelines for MFC determination still need to be addressed (37, 38).

Clinical Resistance and Clinical Breakpoint Setting

Wild-Type Distribution

Within any group of organisms tested by a defined method with any given drug there is usually a distribution of MIC results that may be modal, bimodal, or occasionally appear to be quite random. Often, further taxonomic studies of those species complexes that appear to have a random MIC distribution further delineate taxonomic groupings within the complex that each display separate susceptibility profiles, such as *Scedosporium aurantiacum* within the *Scedosporium apiospermum* complex (39) and *Aspergillus lentulus* within the *A. fumigatus* complex (40). In most fungal species, the MICs of the majority of organisms are concentrated in a small number of doubling dilutions, and rules have been defined to predict less susceptible outliers. Susceptibility characteristics of a population can be described by defining the range of MIC values encountered and calculating the value at which 50% (MIC_{50}) and 90% (MIC_{90}) of the population is inhibited. However, when constructing wild-type distribution curves, one must always be aware of the inherent variability of even well-standardized and controlled testing. Arendrup and colleagues (41) tested a single isolate of *C. glabrata* with a fluconazole MIC of 2.0 mg/liter, as assessed by the EUCAST susceptibility testing method, a total of 45 times. They found MIC results spanning three 2-fold dilutions ranging from 2.0 to 8.0 mg/liter, almost directly mirroring those results produced when 35 *C. glabrata* isolates were tested. It was postulated that variation within the wild-type population could be explained solely by test variation allowing for a doubling dilution on each occasion. Therefore, in a normal distribution the MIC_{50} reflects the susceptibility of the entire wild-type population and is a useful predictor of species susceptibility.

Microbiological Resistance and Epidemiological Cutoff Values

In the absence of interpretable clinical outcome data to predict clinical breakpoints, the wild-type distributions can be used to define ECOFF/ECV. This provides an indication of the normal susceptibility patterns encountered with a given drug-organism combination and thus confirms whether a given isolate conforms to the predicted wild-type susceptibility profile or is displaying a less susceptible or non-wild-type phenotype. An MIC above the ECOFF/ECV cannot be explained by inherent test variation. Such outlier organisms can most often be found to harbor resistance mechanisms (42). Clinical breakpoints should therefore not be set higher than ECOFF/ECV unless there is supporting clinical evidence to demonstrate that such isolates do respond to standard therapy (43). In some cases clinical breakpoints can reflect the need to achieve higher than normal blood concentrations for a given drug to achieve good outcomes. CLSI has used the term "susceptible dose dependent" (SDD) for such isolates. Such categorization has been used with itraconazole and fluconazole where there is clear clinical evidence that higher doses, and therefore higher blood concentrations, can influence the outcome in isolates with MICs above the usual susceptible range (44). When this supporting clinical evidence is lacking, isolates with MIC results only just in excess of the normal wild-type MIC_{50} may be described as having intermediate susceptibility, which means that the currently available data do not allow the organism to be categorized as either fully susceptible or resistant. EUCAST has a slightly different terminology and has not adopted the SDD category. In line with the antibacterial classification of susceptibility (S), I and R are used. The I category is assigned for isolates/species that may respond to treatment under certain conditions (e.g., high drug concentration at the target site) to accommodate use of the antifungal compound in some clinical situations. Another important point to consider when setting breakpoints is that they should not divide wild-type distributions of important target species because this would lead to random classification of isolates with identical susceptibility (41). Species-specific breakpoints have been introduced to prevent this occurrence while not incorrectly classifying other groups and to acknowledge that virulence differs across various species. Table 1 shows a comparison of the species-specific breakpoints for yeast isolates accepted by the CLSI and EUCAST.

Clinical Breakpoints and Determinants Associated with Outcome

The following parameters are considered when setting breakpoints: (i) standard dosing, (ii) species-specific MIC distributions, (iii) ECOFFs/ECVs, (iv) pharmacokinetic-pharmacodynamic analyses, and (v) clinical experience and MIC-outcome relationships. In the ideal situation, all of these data would be available; however, more often, breakpoints are selected based on less than perfect datasets usually comprising MIC distributions, some pharmacokinetic and pharmacodynamic information, and clinical experience from infections involving wild-type isolates. Breakpoint setting therefore is not an exact science, and classification of isolates into S, I, and R based on clinical breakpoints does not *per se* predict outcome because other factors, including severity of the infection and underlying disease, timing of therapy, and virulence of the organisms, all influence the outcome. Susceptibility classification, however, predicts the likelihood of a successful outcome. It has been suggested that for antifungal therapy of yeast infections the "90-60 rule" should be applied, which suggests that infections due to susceptible organisms respond 90% of the time, while those due to resistant organisms respond in 60% of cases (45). The same may not be true of chronic or invasive mold infections. The lack of adjunctive host response in the neutropenic patient may have an additional adverse impact on the likely outcome, and it is well recognized that removal of intravenous catheters can positively influence outcome irrespective of the choice of antifungal therapy (35, 46, 47). For systemic therapy, dose, dosing interval, route of administration, and effect of coadministration of other drugs have a direct impact on achievable blood levels, and it is usually considered that blood levels should be several times in excess of the MIC for successful outcome. For example, a dose/MIC ratio of 25 (using the higher MICs obtained with 48-h CLSI reading) or 100 (using the lower MICs obtained with EUCAST and CLSI with 24-h reading) was found to correlate well with successful outcome of treatment with fluconazole and was supportive of the suggested breakpoint (26, 38, 48). It is becoming increasingly recognized that monitoring of blood levels for some drugs is therefore an important part of the management of patients, particularly those treated with the triazole agents itraconazole, posaconazole, and voriconazole (49).

When agents are used topically, such as in the treatment of cutaneous and mucosal forms of candidiasis, otomycosis, and mycotic keratitis, different, higher breakpoints may be more applicable because local concentrations of the agent may be many-fold in excess of the MIC of the infecting organism. An example of this is the topical treatment of mycotic keratitis, where topical agents such as 0.15% (1,500 mg/liter) amphotericin B, 1% (10,000 mg/liter) natamycin, 1% (10,000 mg/liter) voriconazole, and 2% (20,000 mg/liter) econazole would greatly exceed the *in vitro* susceptibility cutoffs for most organisms. However, although local concentrations may be high, there are other complexities, and consideration has to be given to issues such as tissue penetration and duration of contact, so to date, breakpoint setting for topical therapy has not been formally addressed.

STANDARDIZED BROTH DILUTION METHODS FOR YEASTS

Currently, there are two internationally recognized broth dilution methods for testing yeasts such as *Candida* spp. Broth microdilution testing (Table 2) has become the most widely used reference technique for antifungal susceptibility testing; this approach is described in the CLSI M27-A3 document (15) and the EUCAST E.Def 7.3 document (17) and is also outlined below.

Standard Medium

The test medium recommended for both established reference methods is the Roswell Park Memorial Institute (RPMI) 1640 broth medium with L-glutamine and a pH indicator and without sodium bicarbonate (04-525Y from BioWhittaker, Walkersville, MD, and American Biorganics, Inc., Niagara Falls, NY; and R-6504 from Sigma Chemical Co., St. Louis, MO). The medium should be buffered to a pH of 7.0 at 25°C with morpholinepropanesulfonic acid (MOPS; final molarity at pH 7.0, 0.165). This medium is suitable for testing most fungi (15, 16), but it may not be optimal to support the growth of some strains of *Cryptococcus neoformans* or to determine amphotericin B MICs (50). RPMI medium containing a higher concentration of 2% dextrose is the basal medium used in EUCAST testing because it allows faster growth of the yeast, thus facilitating the determination of MICs at 24 h (17). This modification to include glucose at a final concentration of 20 g/liter is also included in CLSI M27-S4 as a suggestion to simplify endpoint determination (25).

Drug Stock Solutions

Antifungal powders can be obtained directly from the drug manufacturers or from reputable commercial sources. Clinical intravenous or oral preparations should not be used. Antifungal stock solutions should be prepared at concentrations at least 10 times the highest concentration to be tested (e.g., 1,280 mg/liter for fluconazole and flucytosine). Solutions of standard powders of hydrophilic substances are prepared in distilled water. For testing non-water-soluble agents, sufficient drug standard should be weighed to prepare a solution 100 times the desired final concentration. EUCAST and CLSI methodology specifies the use of dimethyl sulfoxide for all non-water-soluble agents, which allows storage of prepared plates for up to 6 months without loss of potency (51). The actual amount to be weighed must be adjusted according to the specific biological activity of each standard. Amphotericin B solutions must be protected from light, and drug stock solutions prepared with solvents should be allowed to stand for 30 min before use.

The sterile stock solutions may be stored in small volumes in sealed, sterile polypropylene or polyethylene vials, ideally at −70°C or below and no higher than −20°C; caspofungin can be stored at −80°C for 3 to 6 months without significant loss of activity. Vials should be removed as needed and used on the same day. The use of quality control (QC) strains such as those listed in Table 3 is mandatory in evaluating drug activity (15, 17).

TABLE 2 CLSI M27-A3 document and EUCAST E.Def 7.2 broth microdilution guidelines for antifungal susceptibility testing of yeasts[a]

Parameter	CLSI M27-A3 microdilution modification	EUCAST EDef 7.2
Test organism	Yeast	Yeast
Broth medium	RPMI 1640 broth buffered with MOPS buffer (0.165 M) and 0.2% dextrose to pH 7.0 at 25°C	RPMI 1640 broth buffered with MOPS buffer (0.165 M) and 2.0% dextrose to pH 7.0 at 25°C
Microdilution plates	Sterile plastic, disposable 96-well plates with 300-μl-capacity round-bottomed wells	Sterile plastic, disposable 96-well plates with 300-μl-capacity flat-bottomed wells
Medium modifications	Yeast nitrogen base broth (pH 7.0) with MOPS provides better growth for *C. neoformans* RPMI 1640 with 2% dextrose	*Cryptococcus* spp. tested as for other yeast and read if optical density value is above 0.2. If not, repeat test but incubate at 30°C.
Drug dilutions	Additive 2× 2-fold drug dilutions with medium (fluconazole and flucytosine [5FC]), or 100× with solvent (amphotericin B, other azoles, anidulafungin, caspofungin, and micafungin)	Prepared according to ISO recommendations
Drug dilution ranges:		
5FC and fluconazole	0.12–64 mg/liter	0.12–64 mg/liter
Other azoles	0.03–16 mg/liter	0.015–8 mg/liter
Amphotericin B and echinocandins	0.03–16 mg/liter	0.03–16 mg/liter
Storage of prepared plates	Sealed in plastic bags and stored at −70°C or below for up to 6 mo	Sealed in plastic bags or aluminum foil and stored at −70°C or below for up to 6 mo or −20°C for not more than 1 mo
Inoculum preparation	Five colonies from 24-h (*Candida* spp.) or 48-h (*C. neoformans*) cultures on Sabouraud dextrose agar or potato dextrose agar	Five colonies (>1 mm) from 18- to 24-h cultures suspended in 5 ml sterile distilled water
Stock inoculum suspension	Adjusted by spectrophotometer at 530 nm by addition of sterile distilled water to match the turbidity of a 0.5 McFarland standard (1 to 5 × 10^6 CFU/ml)	Adjusted by spectrophotometer at 530 nm by addition of sterile distilled water to match the turbidity of a 0.5 McFarland standard (1 to 5 × 10^6 CFU/ml)
Test inoculum	Mix stock inoculum on a vortex for 15 s, then 1:1,000 dilution (1:20 followed by 1:50 dilution) with medium of the stock inoculum suspension	1:10 dilution in sterile distilled water of the stock inoculum suspension
Plate inoculation	100 μl of diluted test inoculum plus 100 μl of 2× drug concn; final concn, 0.5 × 10^3 to 2.5 × 10^3 CFU/ml	100 μl of diluted test inoculum plus 100 μl of 2× drug concn; final concn, 0.5–2.5 × 10^5 CFU/ml
Growth control(s)	100 μl of diluted inoculum plus 100 μl of drug-free medium (or plus 2% of solvent)	100 μl of diluted inoculum plus 100 μl of drug-free medium (or plus 2% of solvent)
Sterility control	Column 12 of the plate can be used to perform the sterility control (drug-free medium only, no inoculum).	Column 12 of the plate can be used to perform the sterility control (drug-free medium only, no inoculum + 100 μl of sterile distilled water used to make inocula).
QC strains	Select QC strains that have MICs that fall near the midrange for all drugs tested. Rules have been established for QC testing based on frequency of testing.	At least two QC strains with results close to the middle range
Incubation	Incubate at 35°C	Without agitation in ambient air at 35 ± 2°C
Time of reading	Amphotericin B, 24 or 48 h; fluconazole, 24 or 48 h; echinocandins, 24 h only; 5FC and other azoles, 48 h	24 ± 2 h all drugs, 48 h for *Cryptococcus* spp. If plates show absorbance ≤0.2 indicating poor growth, reincubate for further 12–24 h. Failure to reach absorbance of 0.2 after this time is a failed test. For *Cryptococcus*, repeat test at 30°C.
MIC determination	Visual assessment with the aid of a reading mirror	Spectrophotometric assessment at 530 nm (or, alternatively, 405 or 450 nm). The value of the inoculum-free control should be subtracted from the readings of the other wells.
Amphotericin B	Lowest drug concn that prevents any discernible growth (100% inhibition)	≥90% inhibition as compared to drug-free control
5FC, azoles, caspofungin, and other echinocandins	Lowest drug concn that shows prominent (~50%) decrease in turbidity	≥50% inhibition as compared to drug-free control
Reading modification[b]	*C. neoformans* MICs determined spectrophotometrically at 492 nm after 48 h of incubation	

[a]Data from references 15, 17.
[b]CLSI M27-A3 document includes this reading modification when using the broth microdilution method with yeast nitrogen base broth and a 10^4 CFU/ml inoculum.

TABLE 3 MIC ranges for commonly used QC and reference isolates for CLSI and EUCAST broth microdilution methods[a]

QC or reference isolates	Antifungal agent	MIC range (mg/liter)		
		EUCAST E.Def 7.2 and 9.1	CLSI M27-A3 and M38-A2 24 h, microdilution	CLSI M27-A3 and M38-A2 48 h, microdilution
QC isolates				
Candida parapsilosis ATCC 22019	Amphotericin B	0.12–1.0	0.25–2.0	0.5–4.0
	Anidulafungin	0.25–1.0	0.25–2.0	0.5–2.0
	Caspofungin	NA	0.25–1.0	0.5–4.0
	Flucytosine (5FC)	0.12–0.5	0.06–0.25	0.12–0.5
	Fluconazole	0.5–2.0	0.5–4.0	1.0–4.0
	Itraconazole	0.03–0.12	0.06–0.5	0.06–0.5
	Ketoconazole	NA	0.03–0.25	0.06–0.5
	Micafungin	NA	0.5–2.0	0.5–4.0
	Posaconazole	0.015–0.06	0.03–0.25	0.03–0.25
	Voriconazole	0.015–0.06	0.016–0.12	0.03–0.25
Candida krusei ATCC 6258	Amphotericin B	0.12–1.0	0.5–2.0	1.0–4.0
	Anidulafungin	≤0.06	0.03–0.12	0.03–0.12
	Caspofungin	NA	0.12–1.0[b]	0.25–1.0[b]
	Flucytosine (5FC)	1.0–4.0	4.0–16	8.0–32
	Fluconazole	16–64	8.0–64	16–128
	Itraconazole	0.03–0.12	0.12–1.0	0.25–1.0
	Micafungin	NA	0.5–2.0	0.12–0.5
	Ketoconazole	NA	0.12–1.0	0.25–1.0
	Posaconazole	0.015–0.06	0.06–0.5	0.12–1.0
	Voriconazole	0.03–0.25	0.06–0.5	0.12–1.0
Paecilomyces variotti ATCC MYA-3630	Amphotericin B	NA	NA	1.0–4.0
	Anidulafungin (MEC)	NA	≥0.015	NA
	Itraconazole	NA	NA	0.06–0.5
	Posaconazole	NA	NA	0.03–0.25
	Voriconazole	NA	NA	0.015–0.12
Reference isolates				
Aspergillus flavus ATCC 204304	Amphotericin B	0.5–2.0	NA	0.5–4.0
	Itraconazole	0.12–0.5	NA	0.25–0.5
	Posaconazole	0.12–0.5	NA	0.06–0.5
	Ravuconazole	NA	NA	0.5–4.0
	Voriconazole	0.5–2.0	NA	0.5–4
Aspergillus flavus ATCC MYA-3631	Amphotericin B	NA	NA	1.0–8.0
	Posaconazole	NA	NA	0.12–1.0
	Voriconazole	NA	NA	0.5–2.0
Aspergillus fumigatus ATCC MYA-3626	Amphotericin B	NA	NA	0.5–4.0
	Anidulafungin (MEC)	NA	≤0.015	NA
	Posaconazole	NA	NA	0.25–2.0
	Voriconazole	NA	NA	0.25–1.0
Aspergillus fumigatus ATCC MYA-3627	Amphotericin B	NA	NA	0.5–4.0
	Itraconazole	NA	NA	>16
	Voriconazole	NA	NA	0.25–1.0
Aspergillus terreus ATCC MYA-3633	Amphotericin B	NA	NA	2.0–8.0
	Anidulafungin (MEC)	NA	≤0.015	NA
	Voriconazole	NA	NA	0.25–1.0
Fusarium moniliforme ATCC MYA-3629	Amphotericin B	NA	NA	2.0–8.0
	Anidulafungin (MEC)	NA	≥8.0	NA
	Itraconazole	NA	NA	>16
	Posaconazole	NA	NA	0.5–2.0
	Voriconazole	NA	NA	1.0–4.0
Fusarium solani ATCC 3636	Anidulafungin (MEC)	NA	≥8.0	NA
Scedosporium apiospermum ATCC MYA-3635	Amphotericin B	NA	NA	4.0–16
	Posaconazole	NA	NA	1.0–4.0
	Voriconazole	NA	NA	0.5–2.0
S. apiospermum ATCC MYA-3634	Anidulafungin (MEC)	NA	NA	1.0–4.0

(Continued on next page)

TABLE 3 MIC ranges for commonly used QC and reference isolates for CLSI and EUCAST broth microdilution methods[a] *(Continued)*

QC or reference isolates	Antifungal agent	MIC range (mg/liter) EUCAST E.Def 7.2 and 9.1	CLSI M27-A3 and M38-A2 24 h, microdilution	CLSI M27-A3 and M38-A2 48 h, microdilution
Trichophyton mentagrophytes MRL 1957 ATCC MYA-4439	Ciclopirox	NA	NA	0.5–2.0 (4 days)
	Griseofulvin	NA	NA	0.12–0.5 (4 days)
	Itraconazole	NA	NA	0.03–0.25 (4 days)
	Posaconazole	NA	NA	0.03–0.25 (4 days)
	Terbinafine	NA	NA	0.002–0.008 (4 days)
	Voriconazole	NA	NA	0.03–0.25 (4 days)
Trichophyton rubrum MRL 666 ATCC MYA-4438	Ciclopirox	NA	NA	0.5–2.0 (4 days)
	Fluconazole	NA	NA	0.5–4.0 (4 days)
	Voriconazole	NA	NA	0.008–0.06 (4 days)

[a]Data from EUCAST E.Def 7.2 and 9.1 and CLSI M27-S3, M38-A2, and M27-S4 (15–18, 80, 82). NA, not available. Data for additional strains are available in these publications.

[b]The QC range for caspofungin and *C. krusei* ATCC 6258 was established using data generated in 2010 from 15 reference laboratories. Since then, caspofungin susceptibility testing has been associated with significant variation, the reason for which has not yet been fully elucidated. The clinical breakpoints approved in the CLSI M27-S4 document are based on the use of high-potency caspofungin powder for which the 24-h MIC range (mode) for the *C. krusei* ATCC 6258 was 0.06–0.25 mg/liter (0.125 mg/liter). Misclassification of susceptible isolates may therefore occur despite acceptable performance of the QC strain according to the range above (80).

Preparation of Inocula

Inocula should be prepared by the spectrophotometric method (52) as outlined in Table 2. The inoculum suspension is prepared by picking five colonies, each at least 1 mm in diameter, ideally from 24-h-old cultures of *Candida* spp. or 48-h-old cultures of *C. neoformans*. These are then suspended in 5 ml of sterile 0.85% NaCl or sterile distilled water for the EUCAST method and vigorously shaken on a vortex mixer. The turbidity of the cell suspension measured at 530 nm is adjusted with the appropriate suspension medium to match the transmittance produced by a 0.5 McFarland barium sulfate standard. This procedure produces a cell suspension containing 1×10^6 to 5×10^6 CFU/ml. For the CLSI method, this is then diluted 1:1,000 with RPMI medium to provide the 2× test inoculum (1×10^3 to 5×10^3 CFU/ml). The 2× inoculum is diluted 1:1 when the wells are inoculated to achieve the desired final inoculum size (0.5×10^3 to 2.5×10^3 CFU/ml). For the EUCAST method, which utilizes a higher final inoculum, a working suspension is prepared from a 1:10 dilution of the standardized suspension in sterile distilled water to produce 1×10^5 to 5×10^5 CFU/ml.

Drug Dilutions and Performance of Microdilution Test for Yeasts

For hydrophobic drugs dissolved in solvents other than water (e.g., the polyenes, the echinocandins, and the azoles except some formulations of fluconazole), intermediate test drug dilutions are prepared from stock solutions to be 100 times the strength of the final drug concentration, with 100% dimethyl sulfoxide used as a diluent (e.g., 1,600 to 3 mg/liter). Dilutions should be prepared according to ISO recommendations (53). This procedure prevents precipitation of agents with low solubility in aqueous media. Alternative dilution schemes may be used if they are shown to perform as well as the reference method (54). Despite careful procedures, itraconazole and some other agents do not remain completely solubilized upon dilution into aqueous media, which makes the use of QC procedures vital to minimize inaccuracies. For water-soluble drugs, such as flucytosine and some formulations of fluconazole, dilutions are prepared from the stock to be 10 times the final test drug concentrations directly in RPMI medium according to the additive, 2-fold drug dilution schema (15) (e.g., 640 to 1.2 mg/liter for fluconazole and flucytosine). The 10× and 100× drug concentrations should be diluted 1:5 and 1:50, respectively, with RPMI to achieve the 2× drug concentrations needed for the microdilution test; after the inoculation step the drug concentrations are 16 to 0.03 mg/liter for amphotericin B and triazoles and 64 to 0.12 mg/liter for fluconazole and flucytosine. Because the echinocandins are potent at lower concentrations and to encompass the EUCAST breakpoints, drug dilution series from 4.0 to 0.08 mg/liter are recommended for these compounds.

The broth microdilution test is performed by using sterile, disposable, multiwell microdilution polystyrene plates (96 U-shaped wells for CLSI or flat-bottom plates for EUCAST). Differential binding capacity has been observed for untreated or tissue/cell culture plates, and most EUCAST data for breakpoint setting have been generated with treated plates. A multichannel pipette (or a large dispensing instrument for 96-well trays) is used to dispense the 2× drug concentrations in 100-μl volumes into the wells of columns 1 to 10 of the microdilution plates. Column 1 contains the highest drug concentration, and column 10 contains the lowest drug concentration. Microdilution trays can be sealed in plastic bags and stored frozen at −70°C (or −80°C) for up to 6 months or at −20°C for not more than 1 month (15, 17, 51). Each well is inoculated on the day of the test with 100 μl of the corresponding 2× inoculum, which brings the drug dilutions and inoculum densities to the final test concentrations (final volume in each well, 200 μl). The growth control wells (column 11) contain 100 μl of sterile drug-free medium (for water-soluble agents) or 100 μl of sterile drug-free medium with 2% solvent (for non-water-soluble agents) and are inoculated with 100 μl of the corresponding 2× inoculum. The QC yeasts are tested in the same manner as the other isolates and are included each time an isolate is tested. Row 12 of the microdilution plate can be used for the sterility control (drug-free medium only).

Incubation and Determination of Microdilution MICs for Yeasts

The microdilution plates are incubated at 35°C in ambient air. For the EUCAST method, 24 h of incubation is recommended, provided the optical density increase compared to the background level is ≥0.2. For the CLSI method and in most instances when testing *Candida* spp., results with fluconazole, posaconazole, voriconazole, amphotericin B, and the echinocandins can also be evaluated after 24 h (15, 21–24). The breakpoints suggested for fluconazole, voriconazole, and the echinocandins are based on a 24-h reading (25).

The determination of MIC endpoints is a critical step in antifungal susceptibility testing, especially with the azoles (for yeasts) and echinocandins (for yeasts and molds). For the CLSI methodology, the endpoint reading is undertaken by eye, whereas the flat-bottom plates used for EUCAST testing allow a nonsubjective spectrophotometric reading and cutoff defined by a fixed percentage of the optical density achieved in the corresponding control well. The recommended absorbance for reading the plates is 530 nm, although others can be used (e.g., 405 or 450 nm), and the value of the blank background should be deducted from the readings for the other wells. For the CLSI methodology, the growth in each well is compared with that in the growth control (drug-free) well with the aid of a reading mirror (e.g., Cooke Engineering Co., Alexandria, VA). The MIC for amphotericin B is defined as the lowest concentration at which a complete absence of growth (optically clear) is observed, i.e., 100% inhibition or ≥90% inhibition if read with a spectrophotometer for the EUCAST method.

The partial inhibition or trailing that is observed with fungistatic compounds such as the azoles prevents adoption of a complete absence-of-growth endpoint. Moreover, the highest degree of reproducibility is obtained if the steepest part of the growth inhibition curve is taken as the endpoint. Therefore, the MIC of the azoles, echinocandins, and flucytosine is defined as the lowest concentration at which prominent growth inhibition is observed (≥50% inhibition as compared to the growth control well) for both standards. For visual interpretation, agitation of the microdilution trays is highly recommended prior to MIC determination; this step facilitates the visual estimate of prominent growth inhibition (55).

Heavily trailing endpoints are seen with about 5% of isolates when reading fluconazole MICs at 48 h, but studies of the *in vivo* response of such isolates in animal models of infection and in patients with oropharyngeal candidiasis suggest that they respond in the same way to low-dose fluconazole therapy as fully susceptible strains (44, 56).

Macrodilution

Broth macrodilution tests are adequate for the testing of all antifungal agents and are suitable for small laboratories in which the volume of these tests is low. Only the steps and testing conditions that are relevant to the macrodilution test are discussed in detail here (Table 2). Each intermediate drug concentration solution is further diluted (1:10) in RPMI medium to obtain 10 times the final strength. This step reduces the final solvent concentration to 10%. The 10× drug dilutions are dispensed in 0.1-ml volumes into round-bottom, snap-cap, sterile polystyrene tubes (12 by 75 mm; e.g., Falcon 2054; Becton Dickinson Labware, Lincoln Park, NJ); these tubes can be stored at −60°C or lower for 3 to 6 months. On the day of the test, each tube is inoculated with a 0.9-ml volume of the corresponding diluted yeast inoculum suspension. This step brings the drug dilutions to the final test drug concentrations mentioned above and the corresponding solvent to 1% in each MIC tube. The stock inoculum suspensions are prepared and adjusted as described above for the microdilution test and are then diluted 1:2,000 with RPMI to provide an inoculum of 0.5×10^3 to 2.5×10^3 CFU/ml. The growth control tube(s) is inoculated with a 0.9-ml volume of the inoculum suspension(s) and a 0.1-ml volume(s) of drug-free medium with 1% of the corresponding solvent. The QC yeasts are tested in the same manner as the other isolates and are included each time an isolate is tested. In addition, 1 ml of uninoculated drug-free medium (for water-soluble agents) or drug-free medium with 1% of the corresponding solvent is included as a sterility control.

Incubation and Determination of Macrodilution MICs for Yeasts

The MIC tubes are incubated at 35°C without agitation for 24 to 48 h (*Candida*) or 70 to 74 h (*C. neoformans*) in ambient air; the turbidity or growth in each tube is visually graded. For amphotericin B, the MIC is read as the lowest concentration that prevents any discernible growth. For azoles and flucytosine, the MIC is defined as the lowest drug concentration that causes a prominent decrease in turbidity to about 50% relative to that of the growth control (Table 2) (15).

Quality Control for Yeast Testing

QC of MIC tests is essential to good laboratory practice. *Candida parapsilosis* ATCC 22019 and *Candida krusei* ATCC 6258 are frequently selected as the QC strains according to the CLSI and EUCAST guidelines for such selection. However, the EUCAST guidelines caution against use of these as QC strains when testing caspofungin because they are not sufficiently sensitive in detecting variation in caspofungin potency, so for this drug *C. albicans* ATCC 64548 or ATCC 64550 is preferred (17, 51). Table 3 summarizes the expected MIC ranges of 10 antifungal agents for these QC isolates (15, 25). Each new batch of medium and lot of macrodilution tubes and microdilution trays should be checked with one of the two QC strains to determine if the MICs are within these ranges. In addition, the overall performance of the test system should be monitored by testing either or both QC isolates each day on which a test is performed for each drug. Details regarding corrective measures when the MICs for the QC isolates are not within the expected ranges are found in the CLSI M27-A3 document (15) and the EUCAST 7.3 document (17). A selection of potentially useful reference strains has been deposited with the American Type Culture Collection (ATCC) (Table 3).

YEAST GENERA OTHER THAN *CANDIDA*

Although the CLSI and EUCAST methods only provide suggested breakpoints for the most common human-pathogenic *Candida* spp. (see Table 1), with certain caveats these methods are broadly suitable for most fermentative yeasts. However, there are certain issues with nonfermentative yeast species such as *Cryptococcus* spp., *Cutaneotrichosporon* spp., *Dipodascus* (previously *Geotrichum*) spp., *Malassezia* spp., *Pichia* spp., *Yarrowia lipolytica*, *Rhodotorula* spp., *Saprochaete* spp., *Sporobolomyces* spp., and *Trichosporon* spp. Moreover, they have not been validated for the yeast forms of endemic dimorphic molds. The CLSI method (15) and EUCAST method (17) do encompass the testing of *Cryptococcus* spp. Because they are slower growing than *Candida* spp., a 72-h incubation period is advised (15), or with EUCAST methodology the plates can be read when the optical density exceeds 0.2. It is suggested that if this value is not reached, then tests should be repeated with incubation of the trays at 30°C. Moreover, there is a suggestion in CLSI M27-S4 (25) for the use of yeast nitrogen base glucose (YNBG) broth, which may enhance the growth of *C. neoformans*, thus facilitating the determination of MICs. A recent study examined a number of parameters for testing a range of nonfermentative yeast species. These included growth medium (RPMI versus YNBG), glucose at 0.2 or 2%, shaken or static, a different nitrogen source, incubation temperature (30 versus 35°C), and inoculum size (10^3, 10^4, or 10^5 CFU/ml). It concluded that the use of YNBG medium, shaking, and a lower incubation temperature enhanced the growth rate of *Cryptococcus* spp. and most of the other nonfermentative yeast species tested. This allowed reading after 24 h and more consistent endpoint determination; however, there were no significant differences in MICs obtained by the different methods (50). Two large global studies utilized the CLSI M27-A3 method in RPMI medium read at 72 h to define ECVs for fluconazole, itraconazole, posaconazole, and voriconazole (57, 58). The largest of these (58) reported susceptibility patterns for more than 3,000 isolates of *C. neoformans* and more than 700 isolates of *Cryptococcus gattii*. A much smaller subset of isolates was tested in YNBG medium, and the modal MIC was higher for fluconazole, as has been noted previously (59), which suggests some variability of susceptibility test results using different methodologies.

Most *Malassezia* spp. do not grow in RPMI medium, because they require a lipid-rich environment, and to date, there is not a standard method validated through a consensus procedure. *Malassezia pachydermatis* grows in RPMI medium but is slower growing than most fermentative yeast species, although microdilution testing and a number of other procedures have been reported in the literature. However, this has resulted in conflicting results in terms of both absolute MIC values and interpretive results, and there are no established breakpoints for this genus. To date, susceptibility testing of *Malassezia* is still investigational and is not recommended for clinical practice (60, 61).

SPECIAL CONSIDERATIONS

Amphotericin B

Amphotericin B MICs determined by the microdilution methods are clustered between 0.25 and 1.0 mg/liter for 94% of clinical yeast isolates, and ≥1.0 mg/liter is often used as a breakpoint for this drug. The difference in amphotericin B MICs for susceptible and potentially resistant isolates is often no more than a doubling dilution, so caution should be exercised in the interpretation of results. Although it has been suggested that antibiotic medium 3 provides reliable detection of resistant isolates, lot-to-lot variability has been documented (62). In addition, this medium did not improve the detection of potentially amphotericin B-resistant isolates recovered from patients with candidemia who had failed amphotericin B therapy (microbiological failure) (63). Etest methodology may more readily detect amphotericin B resistance *in vitro* (64). Further optimization is needed but is difficult due to the lack of isolates with confirmed resistance mechanisms.

Caspofungin

There are ongoing issues with the validity of performing microdilution testing with caspofungin by either the CLSI or EUCAST methodology (65, 66). In a multicenter study of data from 17 laboratories analyzing up to 11,550 *Candida* isolates, wide discrepancies were found for most species in modal values, as well as truncated and bimodal distributions. Despite examination of many testing parameters, including caspofungin powder source, storage time and temperature, solvent, and MIC determination, no single source of this variability could be established (66). In general, the efficacy of the three echinocandins against *Candida* isolates is uniform in the sense that resistance mutations confer resistance across all three compounds. Therefore, both anidulafungin and micafungin have been evaluated as markers for caspofungin resistance (28, 67, 68). However, differential activity has been demonstrated for some *C. glabrata* strains where *FKS* mutations have conferred resistance to anidulafungin and caspofungin but not to micafungin *in vitro* and in animal models (42). Therefore, the recommendation at this time is to use anidulafungin as a marker of echinocandin susceptibility or resistance and to retest *C. glabrata* isolates for susceptibility to micafungin if they are found to be anidulafungin resistant (66). EUCAST has only proposed interpretative breakpoints for anidulafungin and micafungin (43, 69).

CLSI AND EUCAST BREAKPOINTS FOR *CANDIDA* SPP.

There is now a considerable body of data indicating that standardized antifungal susceptibility testing (15, 17) for *Candida* spp. and some triazoles, amphotericin B, and the echinocandins provides results that have predictive utility consistent with the 90-60 rule. Interpretive MIC breakpoints (Table 1) have been established for isolates tested by the CLSI M27-A3 method for fluconazole, voriconazole, anidulafungin, caspofungin, and micafungin following some correlation with clinical data predominantly from patients with oropharyngeal candidiasis, candidemia in nonneutropenic patients, and some more invasive infections but also taking into account ECVs (25, 70, 71). Breakpoints for yeast isolates tested by the EUCAST E.Def 7.3 method are available for amphotericin B, fluconazole, itraconazole, posaconazole, voriconazole, anidulafungin, and micafungin (19, 43, 69, 72–77). Considerable effort has been expended on rationalization of the discrepant CLSI and EUCAST breakpoints for yeast isolates, because there was concern that the results of two very similar methods should be interpreted with different breakpoint criteria (23, 24, 26, 27, 78–80). This is especially true since the publication of CLSI M27-A3, which like EUCAST E.Def 7.3, allows the reading of results at 24 h, which has led to lower CLSI MICs for most drug-organism combinations (as illustrated also by the lower QC ranges for the 24-h reading) (15). Changes to the CLSI breakpoints were published in a supplement to the reference method, CLSI document M27-S4 (25), and have now been slightly revised in document M80 (174); these, together with the EUCAST breakpoints, are presented in Table 1. Breakpoints are species-specific, which makes accurate species identification a vital part of breakpoint interpretation. Harmonization has been achieved for many drug-organism combinations; where differences remain is mainly dependent on differences in the endpoints achieved by the two methods (e.g., for anidulafungin).

Fluconazole inhibits the majority (~90%) of *Candida* spp. at concentrations of ≤2 mg/liter, so this is the breakpoint for susceptibility for the majority of species; 4.0 mg/liter is considered SDD (CLSI terminology)/I (EUCAST terminology), and ≥8 mg/liter is considered resistant. The SDD/I designation for fluconazole encompasses isolates in which susceptibility is dependent on achievable peak levels in serum of 40 to 60 mg/liter at fluconazole dosages of 800 mg/day versus the expected peak levels of ≤30 mg/liter at lower dosages. The pharmacodynamic parameter that predicts efficacy for fluconazole is ~100 (area under the concentration-time curve [AUC]/MIC ratio). Fluconazole MICs for *C. glabrata*, *C. krusei*, and *C. auris* are generally higher than for other species, at 4 to 16, 16 to ≥64, and 8 to ≥64 mg/liter, respectively (11, 81). The recommendation is that these species are not good targets for standard dosing of fluconazole, but because *C. glabrata* is not fully resistant, the *C. glabrata* wild-type population is classified as SDD/I to accommodate use of fluconazole at higher doses in some clinical situations (17, 25, 44). In contrast, *C. krusei* and *C. auris* should be considered innately resistant and should not be treated with fluconazole (11, 25).

Species-specific breakpoints for itraconazole have been set by EUCAST for *C. albicans*, *C. parapsilosis*, and *Candida tropicalis* (72) but are not addressed in CLSI M27-S4 or M60; however, non-species-specific breakpoints for this agent were included in CLSI M27-S3 (82). Itraconazole is generally quite active *in vitro*, with CLSI MICs of 0.01 to 1.0 mg/liter or less for most yeast isolates, except for *C. glabrata* (0.06 to 8 mg/liter) and *C. krusei* (0.5 to 2 mg/liter). Overall, ≥99% of isolates of *Candida* spp. are inhibited by ≤1 mg/liter, so this was the suggested CLSI resistance breakpoint (83). Isolates with an MIC of ≤0.125 mg/liter were considered susceptible, while those with an MIC of 0.5 mg/liter were classified as SDD. For itraconazole, an MIC within the SDD range indicates the need for higher serum concentrations for an optimal response. The need for species-specific breakpoints has been recognized by CLSI, and species-specific CLSI ECVs have been published that may assist in detecting and monitoring any acquired resistance development (70).

For voriconazole, a consensus susceptible breakpoint of ≤0.12 mg/liter has been agreed upon by CLSI and EUCAST groups for most *Candida* spp. documented, but whereas the CLSI document specifies an SDD of 0.5 mg/liter and a resistant breakpoint of ≥1.0 mg/liter (Table 1), EUCAST classifies isolates with MICs of >0.12 mg/liter as resistant. Isolates for which the voriconazole MIC is ≥1.0 mg/liter (CLSI resistant endpoint) are mostly *C. glabrata*, for which there are no accepted breakpoints, but also include non-*Candida* genera such as *Sporobolomyces salmonicolor* and *Rhodotorula rubra*, as well as some *C. albicans* isolates (81). Pharmacokinetics and pharmacodynamic parameters indicate that 24-h free-drug AUC/MIC ratios of 24 and 75 to 100 are predictive of the 50% effective dose and a 2-log CFU reduction, respectively. Recommended doses would produce free-drug AUCs of ~20 μg h/ml (84). However, voriconazole has nonlinear and variable pharmacokinetics, and the coefficient of variation of the AUC has been estimated to be 74 to 100%. Monte Carlo simulations showed that a target free-drug AUC/MIC of 24 would inhibit 99% of isolates with an MIC of ≤0.5 mg/liter if standard treatment were given intravenously and 99% of isolates with MICs of ≤0.25 mg/liter if treatment were given orally (75).

The EUCAST group has also addressed breakpoints for posaconazole for *Candida* spp. and suggests a susceptible breakpoint of ≤0.06 mg/liter and a resistant breakpoint of >0.12 mg/liter, again based on careful evaluation of known wild-type distributions and the pharmacokinetic parameters of the drug (74). A multilaboratory analysis of ECVs of eight *Candida* spp. to fluconazole, posaconazole, and voriconazole suggests that breakpoints should be higher if assessed by the CLSI methodology (85).

Reevaluation of the clinical CLSI breakpoints for the echinocandins following the analysis of accumulated data suggested that the previous CLSI breakpoint threshold of ≤2.0 mg/liter as susceptible and ≥2.0 mg/liter as nonsusceptible were too high for most *Candida* spp. This led to the misclassification as susceptible of a significant number of isolates from infections that were refractory to echinocandin therapy and had known *FKS* mutations, which are recognized as a marker for echinocandin resistance (79). Thus, with the exception of *C. parapsilosis* and *Candida guilliermondii*, lower drug- and species-specific CLSI breakpoints have been suggested for the echinocandins (see Table 1). The CLSI breakpoints differ between the three echinocandins and are lower for *C. glabrata* than for most other *Candida* spp. Applying these new lower breakpoints to 15,269 isolates of *Candida* spp. from 100 centers worldwide collected over an 8-year period from 2001 to 2009, Pfaller and colleagues detected a significant number of isolates with non-wild-type resistance patterns that would have been missed by applying the higher clinical breakpoints (28). At present, EUCAST has refrained from setting breakpoints for caspofungin due to significant variation associated with *in vitro* testing of this compound (66). The EUCAST breakpoints for anidulafungin and micafungin are lower than those proposed by the CLSI because the EUCAST method provides lower MICs than are obtained by CLSI. Hence, for both methods, the breakpoints basically mirror the ECOFFs/ECVs, and the differences are method driven. Anidulafungin is considered a good marker for caspofungin susceptibility until the reproducibility issue has been solved and breakpoints can be established for this agent (68). Differential activity has, however, been demonstrated for micafungin and *C. glabrata*, because some weaker mutations elevate the anidulafungin and caspofungin MIC but not the micafungin MIC and are not associated with efficacy loss in an animal model (42). Hence, anidulafungin is the preferred testing agent for caspofungin and anidulafungin susceptibility. In contrast to CLSI, EUCAST has classified the wild-type population of *C. parapsilosis* as intermediate, acknowledging the higher MIC values related to the intrinsic alteration in the target gene and the fact that unlike for the other species, echinocandins were not superior to fluconazole for *C. parapsilosis*. However, *C. parapsilosis* and other members of the species complex demonstrate low virulence, which in clinical practice abrogates the consequences of elevated MICs, and therefore it is considered safe to use echinocandins as first-line agents for this species.

The breakpoints suggested for amphotericin B are ≤1.0 mg/liter (susceptible) and >1.0 mg/liter (resistant) (73). These have been applied historically, and numerous publications support their application, although very little clinical experience exists for *Candida* isolates with MICs above 1 mg/liter. Additional ECOFF values for drug-organism combinations not addressed here are available in tabulated form on the EUCAST website by accessing MIC distributions and ECOFFs (http://www.eucast.org/antifungal_susceptibility_testing_afst) or in CLSI document M59 (174).

ALTERNATIVE APPROACHES FOR YEASTS

Although the CLSI and EUCAST methods for *in vitro* susceptibility testing were essential for standardization and for improving interlaboratory reproducibility, they may not be the best methods for testing all organisms or all drugs or for routine use in clinical laboratories. Once reference methods become established, this allows the introduction of commercially available methods that produce comparative results. The methods that have been most frequently applied to antifungal susceptibility testing are listed in Table 4.

TABLE 4 Methods used for antifungal susceptibility testing[a]

Test method	Means of endpoint determination
Broth macrodilution (yeasts)	Visual comparison of turbidity (≥50% inhibition) with that of growth control (CLSI M27-A3 document)
Broth microdilution (yeasts)	Visual comparison of turbidity (≥50% inhibition) with that of growth control (CLSI M27-A3 document)
Colorimetric microdilution (yeasts [YeastOne] and molds)	Visual observation of color change
Spectrophotometric microdilution (yeasts)	Turbidimetric MIC determination by spectrophotometer (EUCAST E.Def 7.2)
Macro- and microdilution (filamentous fungi)	Visual comparison of growth (50% inhibition or more [nondermatophytes] or 80% or more [dermatophytes] or MEC) with that of growth control (M38-A2 document, EUCAST E.Def 9.1)
Agar macrodilution (yeasts and molds, standard dishes)	Visual
Agar diffusion (yeasts and molds)	Zone diameter (visual)
Disk (yeasts and molds)	Zone diameter (visual) (CLSI M44-A2, M51-A1)
Antifungal gradient strip (e.g., Etest) (yeast and molds)	Ellipse of inhibition (visual)

[a]Data from references 15–20.

Colorimetric Methods

Colorimetric indicators or fluorescent dyes can facilitate determination of MIC endpoints. Commercial (Sensititre YeastOne, ASTY, and Fungitest) and noncommercial (tetrazolium salt methods and substrate uptake indicators) procedures have been adapted for antifungal susceptibility testing (86–89). The Sensititre YeastOne YO2IVD plate (TREK Diagnostic Systems, Inc., Cleveland, OH) follows the same microdilution format as the CLSI reference method; it has been approved by the U.S. Food and Drug Administration (FDA) and is CE-marked for the testing of nonfastidious yeast species with fluconazole, itraconazole, voriconazole, flucytosine, and caspofungin, with the ability to include a QC organism on the same plate. Other systemic antifungal agents included on the Sensititre YeastOne YO9 plate, such as amphotericin B, posaconazole, anidulafungin, and micafungin, are available for nondiagnostic use in the United States, but the same range of antifungals on Sensititre YeastOne Y10 has been CE marked for use in Europe. Reading of endpoints is enhanced by the inclusion of alamarBlue as the oxidation-reduction colorimetric indicator. If wells remain blue, there is no growth; pink wells indicate growth, and purple wells indicate partial inhibition. Agreement to within 2 doubling dilutions with reference broth microdilution MICs has been excellent with posaconazole and voriconazole (95.4%) and with anidulafungin, caspofungin, and micafungin (100%), all read after 24-h incubation (87, 89). Evaluation against the CLSI microdilution method using the most recent clinical breakpoints and epidemiological cutoff values for the echinocandins with 404 isolates of *Candida* spp. showed excellent (100%) essential agreement and close agreement with categorical values. For *C. albicans*, categorical agreement ranged from 93.6% (caspofungin) to 99.6% (micafungin) with less than 1% very major or major errors (90). For *C. glabrata* and *C. krusei* and caspofungin, it was somewhat less optimal (87.9 and 69.1%, respectively). More recent studies have included large numbers of echinocandin-resistant isolates with known *FKS* mutations and applying species-specific ECVs for anidulafungin, caspofungin, and micafungin, 88.9%, 91.4%, and 93.8% of isolates, respectively, were correctly classified (91).

Vitek 2 Yeast Susceptibility Testing

In an effort to automate yeast susceptibility testing, bioMérieux (Hazelwood, MO) developed the Vitek 2 yeast susceptibility test, a commercial test system based on spectrophotometric analysis and incorporating a card-based miniaturized version of the doubling-dilution reference method. This was shown to produce reproducible, rapid, and accurate results consistent with those produced by the CLSI broth microdilution method for amphotericin B, flucytosine, fluconazole, and voriconazole with several hundred isolates of *Candida* spp. (92, 93). One study investigated the potential of the Vitek 2 system to specifically detect resistance to fluconazole and voriconazole in 36 isolates of *C. albicans* and 86 isolates of *C. glabrata* with well-characterized resistance mechanisms (94). The Vitek 2 system exhibited excellent agreement with the reference broth microdilution method for detecting resistance, with overall categorical agreement of 97.5% for both fluconazole and voriconazole. In a study of 154 isolates, including some resistant to the azoles and amphotericin B, Cuenca-Estrella and colleagues (95) compared the Vitek 2 antifungal susceptibility testing system with the CLSI and EUCAST broth dilution reference methods and with the Sensititre YeastOne and Etest techniques. With essential agreement to within 2 doubling dilutions of >95% for *Candida* spp. and 92% for *C. neoformans*, they concluded that the Vitek 2 system was a reliable technique to determine antifungal susceptibility of yeast species and, moreover, was a more rapid and easier alternative to the reference procedures. The average time to reading was 15.5 h for *Candida* spp. and 34 h for *Cryptococcus*. Recently, caspofungin has been included in the panel. A drawback is that the MIC range that can be reported is ≤0.25 to ≥4 mg/liter and thus does not include the revised breakpoint for *C. glabrata* (S: ≤0.125 mg/liter), and hence susceptible and intermediate isolates cannot be discriminated. A recent study evaluated the performance of the Vitek 2 system for caspofungin testing using a well-defined panel of wild-type and resistant mutants of the five most common *Candida* spp. If *C. glabrata* isolates with an MIC of ≤0.25 were considered susceptible, there were no misclassifications of susceptible wild-type isolates. However, 19.4% (6/31) of isolates harboring *FKS* hot-spot resistance mutations were misclassified as susceptible (76). The AST-YS05 card for use with the Vitek 2 system, which contains fluconazole, voriconazole, and caspofungin, is available in the United States and Europe.

Flow Cytometry

Flow cytometric methods also have been adapted for antifungal susceptibility testing by introducing DNA-binding vital dyes into the culture to detect fungal cell damage after exposure to an antifungal agent. MICs determined by this approach have been comparable to those obtained by the CLSI M27-A3 methods (77). Although these methods produce faster results (4 to 6 h), the need for a flow cytometer for MIC determination precludes their use in small laboratories; moreover, they are not FDA approved or CE marked.

Standardized Disk Diffusion Method for Yeasts

Worldwide, the most commonly used technique for antibacterial susceptibility testing is the disk diffusion test, which yields a quantitative result (zones of inhibition) and a qualitative interpretive category (e.g., susceptible or resistant) based on correlation of zone sizes obtained with organisms with known MICs. Agar disk diffusion testing is a simple, flexible, and cost-effective alternative to broth dilution testing. The CLSI Subcommittee on Antifungal Susceptibility Testing has developed a disk diffusion method (Table 5) for testing *Candida* spp. with caspofungin, fluconazole, posaconazole, and voriconazole, although interpretive criteria are only available for caspofungin, fluconazole, and voriconazole, and as yet there are no commercially available FDA-approved disks (CLSI M44-A2 document) (19). Extensive worldwide testing with fluconazole and voriconazole as part of a global survey suggests that this method performs very well (96). It has also demonstrated good performance with caspofungin (97). The M44 disk test method has also been shown to be a useful approach for determining the susceptibility of *C. neoformans* and other genera of yeast (96, 98). Zone interpretive criteria have been approved for fluconazole, voriconazole, caspofungin, and micafungin (CLSI M44-S3, now replaced by M60) (99, 173).

Standard Medium

The CLSI M44-A2 document includes instructions for preparing Mueller-Hinton agar supplemented with 2% glucose to improve growth and 0.5 mg/liter of methylene blue to produce sharper zone definition (19). The pH of the medium should be 7.2 to 7.4 at room temperature after gelling, and the surface of the agar should be moist but without moisture droplets. The medium can be prepared and poured with the two supplements, or the supplements can be added to commercially prepared Mueller-Hinton agar plates; the latter enables the use of routine agar plates from the bacteriology laboratory.

Preparation of Inocula

The CLSI M44-A2 method employs an inoculum suspension adjusted to the turbidity of a 0.5 McFarland standard by the spectrophotometer, as described above for broth dilution standard methods (Table 2) (15).

Performance of Disk Diffusion Method for Yeasts

The agar plates are inoculated within 15 min of adjusting the inoculum suspension, as follows (Table 5). Briefly, a sterile cotton swab is dipped into the undiluted inoculum suspension, rotated several times, and pressed firmly against the inside wall of the tube above the fluid level to remove excess fluid. The entire dried agar surface is evenly streaked in three directions, swabbing the rim of the plate as the final step. The lid of the plate should be left ajar to allow the agar surface to dry for no more than 15 min. Fluconazole (25 μg), posaconazole (5 μg), voriconazole (1 μg), caspofungin (5 μg), and micafungin (10 μg) disks are dispensed onto the inoculated agar surface. Disks must be pressed down to ensure complete contact with the agar and distributed evenly so they are not closer than 24 mm from center to center. After the disks are placed, they cannot be moved, because drug diffusion is almost instantaneous. Plates should be incubated within 15 min after disks have been placed (19).

Incubation and Determination of Disk Diffusion Zone Diameters for Yeasts

After 20 to 24 h of incubation at 35°C, the resulting inhibition zones should be uniformly circular, and a confluent lawn of growth should be present. The plates are read above a black, nonreflecting background illuminated with reflected light (19). The zone diameters surrounding the disks are measured to the nearest whole millimeter at the point at which there is prominent reduction in growth. Pinpoint microcolonies at the zone edge or large colonies within a zone are encountered frequently and should be ignored. If growth is insufficient, the plates should be read at 48 h (Table 5) (19). QC zone diameter limits have been defined for fluconazole, posaconazole, voriconazole, and caspofungin when testing *Candida* spp. (99).

Agar-Based Alternative Approaches for Yeasts

Gradient Strip Testing

The Etest (bioMérieux; Marcy l'Etoile, France, and Durham, NC) was the first antifungal gradient strip test to be produced, but Liofilchem strips are now also commercially available in some European countries and North Africa (Launch Diagnostics, Kent, United Kingdom). Such tests are based on the diffusion of a stable concentration gradient of an antimicrobial agent from a plastic strip onto an agar medium. There are commercially available gradient strips for amphotericin B, fluconazole, flucytosine, ketoconazole, itraconazole, isavuconazole, posaconazole, voriconazole,

TABLE 5 CLSI M44-A2 document guidelines for antifungal disk diffusion susceptibility testing of *Candida* spp.[a]

Parameter	Description
Agar medium	Mueller-Hinton agar + 2% dextrose and 0.5 μg of methylene blue dye/ml
Inoculum preparation	From 24-h cultures on Sabouraud dextrose agar as described in Table 2 for broth micro- and macrodilution methods
Test medium	Stock inoculum suspension, adjusted by spectrophotometer at 530 nm to match the turbidity of a 0.5 McFarland standard: 1×10^6 to 5×10^6 CFU/ml
Disk contents	Caspofungin, 5 μg; fluconazole, 25 μg; posaconazole, 5 μg; voriconazole, 1 μg
Incubation conditions	20–24 h at 35°C
Reading zone diameter	To the nearest whole millimeter at the point at which there is prominent reduction in growth. Pinpoint microcolonies at the zone edge or large colonies within the zone should be ignored.

[a]Data from CLSI M44-A2 (19).

anidulafungin, caspofungin, and micafungin. For clinical use, the FDA has approved fluconazole, itraconazole, voriconazole, and flucytosine Etest strips; all gradient strips are CE marked. Agreement of Etest and reference MICs has been species, drug (68, 100), and medium dependent. The medium that provides the best performance for Etest MICs is solidified RPMI medium supplemented with 2% glucose, and reading requires expertise and close adherence to the manufacturer's instructions with the proviso on reading *C. glabrata* and *C. krusei* outlined below. If a clear zone is seen, the MIC can easily be read where the zone of inhibition intersects the strip. Problems can arise when inexperienced readers incorrectly interpret faint background growth of small colonies within the zone as resistance. This is most often seen with fluconazole, and if an isolate is unexpectedly found to be fluconazole resistant by Etest, it should be retested by a reference method. In this regard, it is crucial to ensure that a pure culture is used; for example, with a mixture of *C. albicans* and *C. glabrata*, the susceptibility of the more susceptible *C. albicans* would be read, and the smaller *C. glabrata* colonies in the *C. albicans* inhibition zone could be mistaken for trailing that should be ignored. The Etest may be useful in testing yeasts suspected of being potentially resistant to amphotericin B (64, 101). This method has also been evaluated and found to correlate well with CLSI methodology for testing the susceptibilities of *Candida* spp. to triazoles and echinocandins (102–104). It is clear that the breakpoints developed for the reference tests cannot necessarily be applied to results obtained with the commercial methods. A recent study suggests that if the modified CLSI breakpoints for caspofungin are applied to Etest results for some isolates of *C. glabrata* and *C. krusei*, a significant number will be misclassified as intermediate (105). This finding has been confirmed for *C. glabrata* when evaluating the clinical response for patients with infections involving isolates with MICs just above the CLSI breakpoint (106).

Direct Susceptibility Testing

Although most published susceptibility data have been derived following subculture of organisms, there have been attempts to perform tests directly on blood samples from patients with fungemia, thus further reducing the incubation time required to complete the test (107, 108). In a study of 195 prospectively collected and 133 laboratory-simulated specimens of a wide range of clinically relevant yeast species, Guinea and colleagues were able to show high rates of agreement between direct Etest results obtained within 24 h and the reference CLSI M27-A3 method obtained in 48 to 72 h for fluconazole, voriconazole, isavuconazole, and caspofungin (108).

Proteomics and Antifungal Susceptibility Testing

Early work suggests that proteomic methodology can be used to detect the presence of resistance to several classes of antifungal drugs (109, 110). The protein composition of yeast cells varies in relation to the inhibition of cell growth in varying drug concentrations, and analysis of such changes could be exploited to herald a new generation of antifungal susceptibility testing. Marinach and colleagues (109) studied the effect of different fluconazole concentrations on the spectral profiles produced by one reference and 16 other strains of *C. albicans* with different susceptibilities to fluconazole and different resistance mechanisms. They analyzed deviations from the control spectra that were quantifiable to produce minimal profile change concentration endpoints representing the lowest drug concentration at which mass spectrum profile changes can be detected. There was a high degree of correlation (100% ± 2 doubling dilutions, 94% ± 1 doubling dilution) between minimal profile change concentration results and MIC results obtained with the standard CLSI methodology, and only one isolate would have been in a different susceptibility category (minor error). This methodology has also been applied to an analysis of caspofungin susceptibility testing of 34 yeast and 10 mold isolates with and without known resistance-associated *FKS* mutations (110). As in earlier tests, minimal profile change concentration results were compared with MIC (or minimum effective concentration [MEC] for the molds) results obtained by the appropriate CLSI methodology. There was 100% essential agreement (± 2 dilutions) for both yeast and mold isolates and 94.1% categorical agreement.

Matrix-assisted laser desorption ionization–time of flight mass spectrometry-based methods appear to be a reliable and reproducible tool for antifungal susceptibility testing with results analyzed after 15 h of incubation as compared to 24 h for CLSI and EUCAST methods; moreover, objective analyses are produced for both yeast and mold isolates. Although currently as labor-intensive and time-consuming as a full susceptibility testing method, such a process has the potential to be adapted to breakpoint testing to provide an early surveillance test for antifungal drug resistance in a given isolate or as a screening tool for emerging resistance within a population, but the method still awaits multicenter validation and inclusion of all relevant antifungal compounds (110, 111).

Molecular Methods

Multiple mechanisms lead to reduced susceptibility or overt resistance to azole antifungal drugs in *Candida* species; these include changes in cell wall composition leading to reduced uptake, increased efflux, upregulation of target gene production, and mutation in the target enzymes (see chapter 133). One or more of these may be present in a cell, and stepwise acquisition appears to be common (112, 113). Thus, any method for molecular determination of resistance must be a multiplex system and must also be capable of determining not just the presence but the upregulation of housekeeping genes. Recent application of whole-genome sequencing techniques has facilitated detection of known resistance mutations, but such methods are currently the province of research laboratories (11). Resistance to echinocandins usually centers on mutations of two hot-spot regions of the FKS1 gene, although other mutations have been induced in the laboratory setting (43). These are easier to detect by simple sequencing, including pyrosequencing (114). A recent study attests to the utility of a Luminex-based multiplex assay that can be used for high-throughput screening and proved to be 100% concordant with DNA sequencing results on 102 isolates of *C. glabrata* with mutations in the FKS1 and FKS2 hot-spot domains (115). However, molecular techniques are unable to detect previously uncharacterized mechanisms of resistance and thus should always be confirmed by phenotypic testing.

STANDARDIZED BROTH DILUTION METHODS FOR MOLDS

Antifungal susceptibility testing of molds is becoming increasingly important due to the range of emerging opportunistic pathogens and the reporting of both innate and emergent resistance among the most common mold pathogens (1). Both CLSI (M38-A2) (16) and EUCAST (E.Def 9.1) (18) have developed broth microdilution methods for filamentous fungi that are similar to those for yeast and are summarized in Table 6.

TABLE 6 CLSI M38-A2 document for filamentous fungi and EUCAST broth microdilution guidelines for antifungal susceptibility testing of conidia-forming molds[a]

Parameter	CLSI M38-A2	EUCAST E.Def.9.1N
Test organism	Filamentous fungi	Conidia-forming molds
Broth medium	RPMI-1640 broth buffered with MOPS buffer (0.165 M) and 0.2% dextrose to pH 7.0 at 25°C	RPMI-1640 broth buffered with MOPS buffer (0.165 M) and 2.0% glucose to pH 7.0 at 25°C
Microdilution plates	Sterile plastic, disposable 96-well plates with 300-μl-capacity, round-bottomed wells	Sterile plastic, disposable 96-well plates with 300-μl-capacity, flat-bottomed wells
Drug dilutions	Additive 2× 2-fold drug dilutions with solvent	Additive 2× 2-fold drug dilutions with solvent in double-strength RPMI to allow for dilution factor when inoculum is added
Drug dilution ranges		
Azoles	0.03–16 mg/liter	0.015–8 mg/liter
Amphotericin B	0.03–16 mg/liter	0.03–16 mg/liter
Echinocandins	0.015–8.0 mg/liter	0.03–16 mg/liter
Dermatophyte testing		
Ciclopirox	0.06–32 mg/liter	
Griseofulvin, fluconazole	0.125–64 mg/liter	
Itraconazole, voriconazole, terbinafine	0.001–0.5 mg/liter	
Posaconazole	0.004–8.0 mg/liter	
Storage of prepared plates	Sealed in plastic bags and stored at −70°C or below for up to 6 mo	Sealed in plastic bags or aluminum foil and stored at −70°C or below for up to 6 mo (echinocandins no more than 2 mo) or at −20°C for not more than 1 mo (not echinocandins)
Inoculum preparation	Incubate test isolates on potato dextrose agar (oatmeal agar for *Trichophyton rubrum*) for 7 days at 35°C or until good sporulation is obtained, which may be 48 h for some genera. Flood with 1 ml of sterile 0.85% saline (addition of 0.01 ml Tween 20 will help for *Aspergillus* spp.); gently probe the colony with the tip of the pipette. Allow to settle for 3–5 min, then withdraw upper homogeneous suspension to sterile tube. Vortex mix for 15 s.	Incubate test organisms on potato dextrose agar slants (or other sporulation-enhancing medium) at 35°C for 2 to 5 days or longer if required. Cover colonies with 5 ml of sterile water + 0.1% Tween 20, rub with sterile cotton swab, then transfer suspension to sterile tube. Homogenize on a vortex mixer for 15 s, then dilute as appropriate for hemocytometer counting. If suspension contains hyphae, filter through 11-μm filter, or if clumps remain, revortex for further 15 s.
Stock inoculum suspension	Optical density adjusted by spectrophotometer at 530 nm by addition of sterile saline to 0.09–0.13 for *Aspergillus* spp., *Paecilomyces* spp., *Exophiala dermatitidis*, and *Sporothrix schenckii*; 0.15–0.17 for *Fusarium* spp., *Scedosporium apiospermum*, *Verruconis* (previously *Ochroconis*) *gallopava*, *Cladophialophora bantiana*, and mucoraceous molds; and 0.25–0.3 for *Curvularia* (previously *Bipolaris*) spp. and *Alternaria* spp.	Count conidia on a hemocytometer and adjust with sterile distilled water to give 2×10^6 to 5×10^6 CFU/ml.
Test inoculum	Dilute suspension 1:50 in medium to produce 2× final inoculum 0.4×10^4 to 5×10^4 CFU/ml (Note: *Scedosporium*, *Curvularia* [previously *Bipolaris*], and *Alternaria* may require a lower [50%] dilution factor).	Dilute suspension 1:10 with sterile distilled water to obtain a final working inoculum of 2×10^5 to 5×10^5 CFU/ml; use within 30 min
Plate inoculation	100 μl of diluted test inoculum plus 100 μl of 2× drug concn; final concn	100 μl of diluted test inoculum plus 100 μl of 2× drug concn; final concn
Inoculum verification	Plate 0.01 ml of a 1:10 dilution, or neat for dermatophytes, onto Sabouraud dextrose agar and incubate at 28–30°C; observe daily and count when colonies become visible up to 5 days.	Remove 20 μl from the growth control well immediately after inoculating, dilute in 2 ml of sterile distilled water with 0.1% Tween, homogenize with vortex mixer, spread 100 μl on suitable agar plate, and incubate for 24–48 h, after which there should be 50–250 colonies.
Growth control(s)	100 μl of diluted inoculum plus 100 μl of drug-free medium (or plus 2% of solvent)	100 μl of diluted inoculum plus 100 μl of drug-free medium (or plus solvent)
Sterility control	Column 12 of the plate can be used to perform the sterility control (drug-free medium only, no inoculum).	Column 12 of the plate can be used to perform the sterility control (drug-free medium only, no inoculum).
QC strains	Select QC strains that have MICs that fall near the midrange for all drugs tested. Rules have been established for QC testing based on frequency of testing.	At least two QC strains with results close to the middle range

(Continued on next page)

TABLE 6 CLSI M38-A2 document for filamentous fungi and EUCAST broth microdilution guidelines for antifungal susceptibility testing of conidia-forming molds[a] *(Continued)*

Parameter	CLSI M38-A2	EUCAST E.Def.9.1N
Incubation	Incubate at 35°C without agitation or 30°C if more suitable for the species tested.	Without agitation in ambient air at 35 ± 2°C
Time of reading	21–74 h depending on species; echinocandins, 24 h or as soon as there is confluent growth in the control well	24–48 h; Mucorales should be read at 24 h; other molds at 48 h, occasionally 72 h to allow sufficient growth in control well
MIC or MEC determination	Visual assessment with the aid of a reading mirror	Visual assessment with the aid of a reading mirror
Amphotericin B, itraconazole, posaconazole, ravuconazole, voriconazole	Lowest drug concn that prevents any discernible growth (100% inhibition)	Lowest drug concn that prevents any discernible growth (100% inhibition). Ignore single colonies on the surface and "skipped wells."
Echinocandins	MEC, which is the lowest concn of drug that leads to the growth of small, round, compact hyphal forms, compared to confluent growth in the control	MEC, which is the lowest concn in which abnormal, short, and branched hyphal clusters are observed in contrast to the long, unbranched hyphal elements seen in the growth control
Ciclopirox, griseofulvin, terbinafine	80% growth reduction compared to control	
Colorimetric modification	Addition of 2× concn of colorimetric indicator, modified resazurin, to 2× concn RPMI medium when preparing the plates may help endpoint interpretation with itraconazole.	

[a]Data from references 16, 18.

Microdilution

Standard Medium and Drug Stock Solutions

The test medium employed by the CLSI method is the same MOPS-buffered standard RPMI recommended for yeast testing and for the EUCAST method supplemented with 2% glucose. Drug stock solutions are prepared as described above for yeast testing (15, 17) and in the CLSI M38-A3 and EUCAST E.Def 9.1 documents (16, 18).

Preparation of Inocula

Since nongerminated conidia are easier to prepare and standardize, this is the method of inoculum preparation described, and it is broadly similar in both documents. For the CLSI method, the inoculum for each isolate is prepared by first growing the mold on potato dextrose agar slants (oatmeal agar for *Trichophyton rubrum*) for 7 days at 35°C or until good sporulation is obtained, which may be 48 h for some genera. Each slant is then flooded with 1 ml of sterile 0.85% saline (addition of 0.01 ml of Tween 20 will help for *Aspergillus* spp.), and the surface of the colony is gently probed with the tip of the pipette. The resulting mixture is withdrawn, and the heavy particles are allowed to settle for 3 to 5 min. The upper homogeneous suspension, containing the mixture of nongerminated conidia or sporangiospores and hyphal fragments, is aliquoted and mixed for 15 s with a vortex. The turbidity is measured with a spectrophotometer at 530 nm, and the optical density adjusted by addition of sterile saline to 0.09 to 0.13 for *Aspergillus* spp., *Paecilomyces* spp., *Exophiala dermatitidis*, and *Sporothrix schenckii*; to 0.15 to 0.17 for *Fusarium* spp., *S. apiospermum*, *Scolecobasidium gallopavum* (formerly *Ochroconis gallopava*), *Cladophialophora bantiana*, and mucoraceous molds; and to 0.25 to 0.3 for *Curvularia* (previously *Bipolaris*) spp. and *Alternaria* spp. Stock inoculum suspensions are then diluted 1:50 in medium to obtain 2× the final inoculum of 0.4×10^4 to 5×10^4 CFU/ml. Certain genera (e.g., *Scedosporium*, *Lomentospora*, *Curvularia*, and *Alternaria*) may require a lower (50%) dilution factor (16).

The EUCAST method differs by utilizing a higher inoculum, which is prepared by counting in a hemocytometer, except for *Aspergillus*, for which spectrophotometric determination is a valid alternative (72). Conidia are harvested in 5 ml of sterile water plus 0.1% Tween 20 by rubbing 2- to 5-day growth at 35°C on potato dextrose agar slants (or other suitable selective agar) with a sterile cotton swab and then transferring the suspension to a sterile tube and homogenizing it on a vortex mixer for 15 s. The resulting suspension is diluted as appropriate for hemocytometer counting. Suspensions containing clumps should be vortexed for a further 15 s and if hyphae are present should be filtered through an 11-μm pore size filter. The inoculum is adjusted with sterile distilled water to give a 2×10^6 to 5×10^6 CFU/ml suspension, which is diluted 1:10 with sterile distilled water to obtain a final working inoculum of 2×10^5 to 5×10^5 CFU/ml, which must be used within 30 min.

Drug Dilutions and Performance of Microdilution Test for Molds

Drug dilutions are prepared and dispensed in sterile, disposable, multiwell microdilution trays, as described above for yeast testing. On the day of the test, each well is inoculated with 100-μl volumes of the diluted conidial or sporangiospore suspensions.

Incubation and Determination of Broth Microdilution MICs for Molds

All microdilution trays are incubated at 35°C without agitation, and MICs are determined visually after 21 to 74 h. Most mucoraceous molds should be read at 24 h and most other opportunistic fungi at 48 h; occasionally, 72 to 74 h may be required to allow sufficient growth in the control wells. Testing of the dimorphic fungi should only be undertaken at the designated hazard containment level for the organism and may require 5 to 7 days of incubation. The MIC endpoint criterion for molds is the lowest drug concentration that shows complete growth inhibition when testing amphotericin B, itraconazole, voriconazole, and posaconazole. Endpoint determination with the echinocandin agents is difficult to assess and requires microscopic evaluation (see below) of the MEC, which for most molds is read at 21 to 26 h and at 46 to 72 h for *Scedosporium* and *Lomentospora* spp.

Echinocandins: MEC

When the echinocandins are tested, most *Aspergillus* isolates show trailing growth, and conventional MIC determination could categorize these trailing isolates as resistant to caspofungin. A more careful examination of the microdilution wells reveals the presence of compact, round microcolonies. Under microscopic examination, these microcolonies correspond to significant morphologic alterations. The hyphae grow abnormally as short, highly branched filaments with swollen germ tubes. Kurtz and colleagues (116) defined the concentration of drug producing these morphologic changes as the MEC to distinguish it from conventional MICs. A multicenter study demonstrated that caspofungin MECs were reliable endpoints in 14 of 17 laboratories (117), and in another study in 8 of these laboratories, evaluating anidulafungin MECs against a variety of mold species provided reliable endpoints (118). More recently, an international study involving five laboratories was able to determine wild-type distributions and epidemiological cutoff points for caspofungin against *Aspergillus* spp. (119). However, it is notable that broth microdilution testing failed to identify an animal-model-confirmed resistant isolate from a patient failing therapy as non-wild type, even though this isolate failed to produce an inhibition ellipse with a caspofungin Etest strip (120). Consequently, because conflicting results have been reported from some laboratories, caution and further refinement of this testing approach are needed (117).

Macrodilution

There is good agreement between results obtained by both micro- and macrodilution methods for molds (121). This test format may be more suitable for testing organisms that require longer incubation periods due to problems with evaporation from the microtiter plates on prolonged incubation. Macrodilution testing conditions are described in the CLSI M38-A2 document (17). Briefly, inoculum stock suspensions and drug dilutions are prepared as for the microdilution test. The 100-fold drug dilutions should be diluted 1:10 with RPMI to achieve 10 times the strength needed for the macrodilution test. The stock inoculum suspensions are diluted 1:100 with medium to obtain 0.4×10^4 to 5×10^4 CFU/ml. The 10× drug concentrations are dispensed into 12- by 75-mm sterile tubes in 0.1-ml volumes. Each tube is inoculated on the day of the test with 0.9 ml of the corresponding suspension. Tubes are incubated at 35°C without agitation and observed for the presence or absence of visible growth. The MICs are determined as described above for the microdilution method for molds.

Quality Control for Mold Testing

Either one of the QC yeast organisms or the QC *Paecilomyces variotii* ATCC MYA-3630 isolate may be tested in the same manner as the other mold isolates or as described above for yeasts and should be included each time an isolate is evaluated with any antifungal agent. In addition, other molds have been selected as reference isolates by CLSI and EUCAST (Table 3) (17, 19).

Expected Results and Interpretation of Breakpoints for Molds

EUCAST has published clinical breakpoints for selected *Aspergillus* spp. with amphotericin B and the mold-active azoles (Table 7). Some CLSI ECVs for molds are available in document M59 (174). Clinical failures in the treatment of aspergillosis have been convincingly documented for the azoles, whereas few correlations have been reported for both aspergillosis and hyalohyphomycosis and amphotericin B MICs of >2 mg/liter (2, 122–124). There were also failures and breakthrough infections with molds reported in patients on caspofungin therapy (120, 125). Moreover, there were experiences with treating infections with other groups of fungi, such as *Scedosporium*, where the finding of greater *in vitro* susceptibility to voriconazole than to amphotericin B translates into better clinical outcomes in patients treated with this drug (126).

Amphotericin B MICs determined by either reference method are ≤1.0 mg/liter for most mold species, including most mucoraceous molds (7, 127, 128). High amphotericin B MICs (>2 mg/liter) have been reported for *Purpureocillium lilacinum*, most *Scedosporium* and *Pseudallescheria* spp., *Lomentospora prolificans*, and some isolates of *Alternaria* spp., *Aspergillus* spp. (especially *A. terreus* and *A. flavus*), *Fusarium* spp., *Talaromyces* (formerly *Penicillium*) *marneffei*, *Phialophora* spp., and *S. schenckii* (7, 39, 128, 129), and infections with these species are often refractory to treatment (130).

The EUCAST breakpoints for amphotericin B with *A. fumigatus* and *Aspergillus niger* are ≤1.0 mg/liter (susceptible) and >2.0 mg/liter (resistant) (Table 7). *A. terreus* has not been assigned breakpoints because it is not considered a good target for amphotericin B, and caution should be exercised for *A. flavus* because MICs are similar to those for *A. terreus* and variable efficacy has been reported in an

TABLE 7 EUCAST breakpoints for *Aspergillus* species

Antifungal compound	Breakpoint[a] (mg/liter)				
	A. flavus	*A. fumigatus*	*A. nidulans*	*A. niger*	*A. terreus*
Amphotericin	IE[b]	1/2	Note	1/2	Poor target
Itraconazole	1/2	1/2	1/2	IE[b]	1/2
Posaconazole	IE[b]	0.125/0.25[c]	IE[b]	IE[b]	Note[d]
Voriconazole	Note[d]	1/2	Note[d]	Note[d]	Note[d]

[a]Breakpoints are presented as S ≤ X, R >Y (except for the revised fluconazole breakpoint for *C. glabrata*). The I category (if present) is readily interpreted as the values between the S and the R breakpoints.

[b]IE (insufficient evidence): MICs are higher than for *A. fumigatus*. There is insufficient evidence that this species is a good target for treatment.

[c]Provided sufficient drug levels can be achieved.

[d]Note that the MICs exhibited by this species are similar to those exhibited by *A. fumigatus*, but clinical data are insufficient to establish a breakpoint.

animal model (131). Finally, for *Aspergillus nidulans*, insufficient clinical data are available for breakpoint selection.

MICs of itraconazole are also usually ≤1.0 for *A. fumigatus* and ≤2.0 mg/liter for most other molds; the exceptions are its high MICs for *Aspergillus ustus/calidoustus* (some isolates), *Fusarium solani*, *Fusarium oxysporum*, *P. lilacinum*, *S. schenckii*, *L. prolificans*, *Trichoderma longibrachiatum*, and many mucoraceous molds (7, 129, 132). EUCAST has established itraconazole breakpoints for *A. flavus*, *A. fumigatus*, *A. nidulans*, and *A. terreus* (S, ≤1 mg/liter; R, >2 mg/liter) (Table 7). Azole resistance in *A. fumigatus* isolates has been associated with target gene mutations (*cyp51A* gene), efflux pumps, and upregulation of the target gene and with HapE mutations (see chapter 133). CYP51A alterations may confer resistance to itraconazole only or to itraconazole and posaconazole or may induce pan-azole resistance. Recently, a novel resistant genotype was found in the environment (TR_{46}/Y121F/T289A) which displays high-level voriconazole and isavuconazole resistance but variable itraconazole and posaconazole susceptibility (133). Therefore, combined itraconazole and voriconazole susceptibility testing may serve as an initial azole-resistance screening panel in *Aspergillus*.

Voriconazole, isavuconazole, and posaconazole display an extended spectrum of antimold activity, and particularly for isavuconazole and posaconazole, good *in vitro* activity against the mucoraceous molds has been reported (127, 128, 134–136). Publications have agreed on epidemiological breakpoints for *A. fumigatus* tested by the CLSI and EUCAST methods (137–139). The consensus epidemiological cutoff results were ≤1.0 mg/liter for itraconazole and voriconazole and ≤0.25 mg/liter for posaconazole. For isavuconazole the EUCAST ECOFF was 2 mg/liter, whereas the CLSI/ECV was 1 mg/liter (140). The EUCAST breakpoints reflect these accepted ECOFFs: voriconazole breakpoints are ≤1.0 mg/liter (susceptible) and >2.0 mg/liter (resistant) for *A. fumigatus*, *A. flavus*, *A. nidulans*, and *A. terreus*, while posaconazole breakpoints are ≤0.125 mg/liter (susceptible) and >0.25 mg/liter (resistant) for *A. fumigatus* and *A. terreus* (Table 7). The breakpoints for posaconazole and isavuconazole are conservative and one step below the ECOFF due to the pharmcokinetic/pharmacodynamic data suggesting that the wild-type MIC is only just covered and suggesting for posaconazole specifically, the variable bioavailability of the current oral solution. Publications have cited resistance to itraconazole and some cross-resistance to voriconazole in *A. fumigatus* from certain chronic clinical conditions necessitating long-term use of these agents (2, 141). More recently, there have been reports from the Netherlands and subsequently from many other countries of primary azole resistance in clinical *A. fumigatus* isolates, and the Netherlands was the first country to revise the national treatment guidelines recommending combination therapy as the first-line therapy due to high levels of resistance. This has been linked to the significant environmental use of azoles for plant protection, and a correlation of frequency of such resistant isolates in the environment (most of which harbor the unique TR_{34}/L98H/L98H or TR_{46}/Y121F/T289A alterations) with the proportional global use of antifungal pesticides has been established.

Resistance frequencies therefore vary. (For recent reviews, see reference 9 and chapter 133 of this *Manual*.) MICs/MECs of the echinocandins are usually <1.0 mg/liter for most *Aspergillus* spp. (121, 142). However, a study that tested 81 isolates of *A. flavus* by the EUCAST methodology found them to be uniformly resistant to caspofungin, anidulafungin, and micafungin, with MIC_{50} results at >16.0 mg/liter (142). In contrast, a study employing the CLSI methodology reported that 95% of 432 isolates of *A. flavus* yielded a caspofungin MIC of ≤0.25 mg/liter (120). Higher MICs/MECs are often reported for other mold species for which the echinocandins usually demonstrate low to moderate activity (39, 142). However, MICs of <1.0 mg/liter have been reported for some isolates of dimorphic fungi, *Acremonium* spp., *Phialophora* spp., and *S. apiospermum* (142, 143).

For the echinocandins, *Aspergillus* spp. have been characterized as susceptible or nonsusceptible based on their wild-type distributions and ECVs, and based on large numbers of isolates in a multicenter collaboration, species-specific caspofungin ECVs were proposed, ranging from 0.25 to 1.0 mg/liter (121). However, unacceptable variation in the MIC range for caspofungin against *Aspergillus* is found if various publications are compared across laboratories and time, as has been reported for caspofungin testing of *Candida*. Until this variability has been reduced to an acceptable level, it will not be meaningful to adopt ECOFFs/ECVs or to attempt to establish breakpoints (144–147). Because there are clinical data to suggest that *A. fumigatus* isolates may acquire echinocandin resistance and that infections due to such isolates may fail therapy, it is of the utmost importance to optimize and validate echinocandin testing of *Aspergillus* (120).

Broth Microdilution Method for Dermatophytes

Susceptibility testing of dermatophytes has lagged behind that of other molds, but the M38-A2 broth microdilution method has been successfully adapted, with minor modifications, to the testing of dermatophytes (148). This is an important step forward because terbinafine-resistant *T. rubrum* has been reported (149). The method modifications include the use of oatmeal agar for inoculum preparation when testing *T. rubrum* to induce conidium formation, and 4 to 5 days of incubation at 35°C for MIC determination (80% growth inhibition endpoints). Two isolates of *Trichophyton* spp. have been validated as reference strains (Table 3).

Colorimetric Methods

The YeastOne method has also been evaluated for molds, and it appears to be a suitable method producing results that are comparable to reference methods (150–152). The measurement of metabolic activity by reading the alamarBlue color change (optical density) produced when tetrazolium salts (yellow) are cleaved to their formazan derivative (purple), using a microtiter plate spectrophotometer, has also been evaluated for molds (153, 154). Again, further evaluations, including interlaboratory studies, are needed with more isolates and species, and particularly important, such studies should whenever possible include wild-type as well as resistant isolates for as many species as possible.

Agar-Based Alternative Approaches for Filamentous Fungi

As for yeasts, agar-based methods have been applied to susceptibility testing of molds, including agar dilution, disk diffusion, and Etest methods and semisolid agar (155–157).

Agar Dilution Methods

Agar dilution methods involve the preparation of 10× double dilutions of the agent, which are incorporated into molten agar. Drug-containing plates are inoculated with suspensions of the organism being tested. In one study, results with an itraconazole-resistant isolate tested by agar incorporation and broth microdilution correlated well with the outcome in a mouse model of infection (156). Since standard methods are not available, the size of the inoculum varies among the different studies. Such methods are particularly useful for the high throughput required for environmental surveillance and for initial and early screening for azole resistance of clinical cultures, because testing can be done directly from the primary plate before a pure culture is available. Plates with four wells containing different concentrations of three antifungal agents in RPMI-1640 with 2% glucose agar (itraconazole 4 mg/liter, posaconazole 0.5 mg/liter, and voriconazole 1 mg/liter) and a control well have been developed and validated in a multicenter study (VIPcheck, Neijmegen, the Netherlands) (29). Surveillance plates are inoculated with 25 μl of a standardized test suspension and examined after 24 and 48 h of incubation at 37°C. Provided that sufficient growth is observed on the drug-free control agar after 48 h and that there is no growth on the azole-containing agars, the isolate can be reported as itraconazole, posaconazole, isavuconazole, and voriconazole susceptible. The use of such screening plates may reduce the number of isolates that need further reference testing by 90% and at the same time provide an early indication of azole susceptibility patterns (Fig. 1).

Disk Diffusion Method

The disk diffusion methodology has been evaluated for amphotericin B, anidulafungin, caspofungin, micafungin, itraconazole, posaconazole, and voriconazole against a wide range of opportunistic pathogenic molds (157–160). The CLSI subcommittee published an approved method for testing caspofungin, amphotericin B, and the triazoles against nondermatophyte filamentous fungi (document M51-A1) (20). It is similar to that for yeasts (document M44-A2) (19) but employs Mueller-Hinton agar not supplemented with methylene blue or increased dextrose, because in a collaborative multicenter study these conditions were found to be unsuitable for many molds (158). The inoculum concentration is prepared as for CLSI M38-A3, and plates are inoculated in the same way as for the yeast disk diffusion methodology. After incubation at 35°C for 16 to 24 h for mucoraceous molds, 24 h for *Aspergillus* spp., and 48 h for other molds, there should be a confluent lawn of growth surrounding a circular inhibition zone, which is measured to the nearest whole millimeter (158). Good levels of overall categorical agreement were found as compared to CLSI M38 results when testing large numbers of isolates from many mold species. However, there were reservations about using amphotericin B disks except with mucoraceous molds, and the itraconazole disks should not be used to test mucoraceous molds but are suitable for other genera (158). Three strains have been selected as QC isolates (*A. fumigatus* ATCC MYA-3626, *P. variotii* ATCC MYA-3630, and *C. krusei* ATCC 6258) for which zone diameter ranges have been established for amphotericin B, itraconazole, posaconazole, and voriconazole (161).

Etest and Other Gradient Strips

Numerous studies have assessed the utility of Etest for testing mold pathogens (159, 162–166). Since the trailing effect is not a major problem for azole testing against most molds, Etest inhibition ellipses are usually sharp and MICs are easily interpreted. In contrast, with the echinocandins there may be quite heavy background growth within the inhibition zone, but much heavier growth within the inhibition ellipse may indicate resistance (120). Overall, comparisons of the Etest and CLSI M38-A methods have demonstrated better agreement when testing the triazoles (>90%) than amphotericin B (>80%). Amphotericin B Etest MICs for *A. flavus*, *S. apiospermum*, and *L. prolificans* are usually higher than reference values, especially after 48 h of incubation (164). In a case study, an isolate of *A. fumigatus* was found to be multiresistant to azoles with corresponding genetic mutation and also appeared resistant to caspofungin by Etest, with an MIC of >32 mg/liter, although this resistance had not been detected by broth microdilution testing (120). On molecular testing, the isolate was shown to have upregulation in the expression of the *FKS* gene and displayed reduced susceptibility to caspofungin in an animal model of infection. The reliability of the Etest method and the clinical relevance of its MICs for molds should be addressed. Although Etest strips for amphotericin B, anidulafungin, ketoconazole, posaconazole, voriconazole, and caspofungin are commercially available, the U.S. FDA has not to date approved any antifungal strip for clinical use in susceptibility testing of molds.

Molecular Tests

The application of molecular methods to the detection of resistance in isolates of filamentous fungi has proved to be easier in mold isolates than in yeast because resistance mechanisms appear to be fewer. A multiplex PCR assay to detect the three most frequent *A. fumigatus cyp51A* gene mutations leading to triazole resistance and cross-resistance has been developed (167). A commercially available multiplex assay, AsperGenius (PathoNostics B.V. Maastricht, The Netherlands), has been developed and is CE marked for use on clinical bronchoalveolar lavage samples for the detection and differentiation of *Aspergillus* spp. and the detection of four azole resistance markers in *A. fumigatus* samples. Such a test could be beneficial particularly in the azole-naive setting, because it includes the most common environmental resistance mechanism also seen in isolates from invasive infections (TR_{34}/L98H and TR_{46}/Y121F/T289A), and publications attest to its clinical utility (168, 169). However, in the setting of chronic aspergillosis, a huge variety of CYP51A mutations have been associated with mono-, multi-, or pan-azole resistance, and up to 40% of the resistant isolates were found to have other underlying mechanisms apart from target gene mutations, thereby rendering the negative predictive value of absence of mutations unacceptably low (2, 170). The molecular mechanisms behind echinocandin resistance in *Aspergillus* are less well understood. *FKS1* gene mutations have been induced in laboratory strains and shown to confer resistance but have so far not been detected in clinical isolates. Moreover, additional mechanisms not involving the *FKS* target gene have been found in isolates exposed to cell wall digestion and subsequently cultured in the presence of caspofungin (171). Gene expression profiling by Northern blotting and real-time PCR has revealed overexpression of the *FKS1* gene leading to reduced susceptibility in an isolate of *A. fumigatus* from a patient who had failed caspofungin therapy (120).

Fungicidal Activity

A CLSI study demonstrated that laboratories can reliably perform MFC testing (37) and time-kill curves. In contrast to what is observed with yeasts, the azoles appear to have a certain degree of fungicidal activity, as mentioned above, for a variety of common and rare opportunistic mold pathogens. MFCs of <0.03 to >16 mg/liter have been reported with the triazoles for various mold species (7, 37).

However, standardization of this procedure is needed to reliably assess the potential value of the MFC endpoint in patient management. These standardization efforts should include the correlation of *in vitro* results with the clearing of target organs of the infecting organism in animal models and the further clinical relevance of MFC data. Studies incorporating an indicator of metabolic activity [2,3-bis(2-methoxy-4-nitro-5-sulfophenyl)-2H-tetrazolium-5-carboxanilide] in microdilution broth-based formats examined fungicidal activity of amphotericin B and voriconazole and revealed a concentration-dependent sigmoid pattern of fungicidal effects (172). Such developments will need careful evaluation and standardization.

SUMMARY AND CONCLUSIONS

A great deal of progress has been achieved in the field of antifungal susceptibility testing with both yeast and filamentous fungi since testing began in earnest in the early 1980s. Standardized broth macrodilution and microdilution methods are available for testing molds and yeasts, as are standardized disk diffusion methods for systemically active antifungal drugs. Progress is also being made in establishing the relationship between test results and patient responses to therapy in varied clinical settings and with many of the currently available antifungal agents. Breakpoints are available for common yeast species with most systemically active drugs, and there are some breakpoints for *A. fumigatus*. Moreover, some commercial methods have been approved for the antifungal susceptibility testing of *Candida* spp., but care should be taken in selecting appropriate breakpoints based on the ECOFF/ECV for these methods, which may vary from those produced by the standardized reference tests. Often, identifying the yeast or mold pathogen to the species level is sufficient to direct initial therapy (see chapter 132), but given the increasing problem of resistance to azole antifungals in *A. fumigatus* in many countries, the use of drug-containing screening agars is to be encouraged for primary isolates to provide an early indication of resistance while isolates are being purified for reference testing. The strong move toward consensus in the standardized methodology employed and the principles by which breakpoints are selected in the United States and Europe has meant that internationally agreed upon breakpoints can be applied for some drug-fungus combinations. This has helped to improve surveillance of resistance patterns worldwide and will help in the further development of clinically relevant breakpoints.

REFERENCES

1. **Pfaller MA, Diekema DJ.** 2004. Rare and emerging opportunistic fungal pathogens: concern for resistance beyond *Candida albicans* and *Aspergillus fumigatus*. *J Clin Microbiol* **42:**4419–4431.
2. **Howard SJ, Cerar D, Anderson MJ, Albarrag A, Fisher MC, Pasqualotto AC, Laverdiere M, Arendrup MC, Perlin DS, Denning DW.** 2009. Frequency and evolution of azole resistance in *Aspergillus fumigatus* associated with treatment failure. *Emerg Infect Dis* **15:**1068–1076.
3. **Pfaller MA, Castanheira M, Lockhart SR, Ahlquist AM, Messer SA, Jones RN.** 2012. Frequency of decreased susceptibility and resistance to echinocandins among fluconazole-resistant bloodstream isolates of *Candida glabrata*. *J Clin Microbiol* **50:**1199–1203.
4. **Van Der Linden JWM, Warris A, Verweij PE.** 2011. *Aspergillus* species intrinsically resistant to antifungal agents. *Med Mycol* **49**(Suppl 1)**:**S82–S89.
5. **Arendrup MC, Perlin DS.** 2014. Echinocandin resistance: an emerging clinical problem? *Curr Opin Infect Dis* **27:**484–492.
6. **Arendrup MC, Patterson TF.** 2017. Multidrug-resistant *Candida*: epidemiology, molecular mechanisms, and treatment. *J Infect Dis* **216**(suppl_3)**:**S445–S451.
7. **Borman AM, Fraser M, Palmer MD, Szekely A, Houldsworth M, Patterson Z, Johnson EM.** 2017. MIC distributions and evaluation of fungicidal activity for amphotericin B, itraconazole, voriconazole, posaconazole and caspofungin and 20 species of pathogenic filamentous fungi determined using CLSI broth dilution method. *J Fungi (Basel)* **3:**E27.
8. **Wang E, Farmakiotis D, Yang D, McCue DA, Kantarjian HM, Kontoyiannis DP, Mathisen MS.** 2015. The ever-evolving landscape of candidaemia in patients with acute leukaemia: non-susceptibility to caspofungin and multidrug resistance are associated with increased mortality. *J Antimicrob Chemother* **70:**2362–2368.
9. **Verweij PE, Chowdhary A, Melchers WJ, Meis JF.** 2016. Azole resistance in *Aspergillus fumigatus*: can we retain the clinical use of mould-active antifungal azoles? *Clin Infect Dis* **62:**362–368.
10. **Chowdhary A, Sharma C, Meis JF.** 2017. *Candida auris*: a rapidly emerging cause of hospital-acquired multidrug-resistant fungal infections globally. *PLoS Pathog* **13:**e1006290.
11. **Lockhart SR, Etienne KA, Vallabhaneni S, Farooqi J, Chowdhary A, Govender NP, Colombo AL, Calvo B, Cuomo CA, Desjardins CA, Berkow EL, Castanheira M, Magobo RE, Jabeen K, Asghar RJ, Meis JF, Jackson B, Chiller T, Litvintseva AP.** 2017. Simultaneous emergence of multidrug-resistant *Candida auris* on 3 continents confirmed by whole-genome sequencing and epidemiological analyses. *Clin Infect Dis* **64:**134–140.
12. **Cuenca-Estrella M, Verweij PE, Arendrup MC, Arikan-Akdagli S, Bille J, Donnelly JP, Jensen HE, Lass-Flörl C, Richardson MD, Akova M, Bassetti M, Calandra T, Castagnola E, Cornely OA, Garbino J, Groll AH, Herbrecht R, Hope WW, Kullberg BJ, Lortholary O, Meersseman W, Petrikkos G, Roilides E, Viscoli C, Ullman J, ESCMID Fungal Infection Study Group (EFISG).** 2012. ESCMID guidelines for the diagnosis and management of Candida diseases 2012: diagnostic procedures. *Clin Microbiol Infect* **Supp 7:**9–18.
13. **Arendrup MC, Bille J, Dannaoui E, Ruhnke M, Heussel CP, Kibbler C.** 2012. ECIL-3 classical diagnostic procedures for the diagnosis of invasive fungal diseases in patients with leukaemia. *Bone Marrow Transplant* **47:**1030–1045.
14. **National Committee for Clinical Laboratory Standards.** 1992. Reference method for broth dilution antifungal susceptibility testing of yeasts. Proposed standard. NCCLS document M27-P. National Committee for Clinical Laboratory Standards, Wayne, PA.
15. **Clinical and Laboratory Standards Institute.** 2008. Reference method for broth dilution antifungal susceptibility testing of yeasts, 3rd ed. Approved standard. CLSI document M27-A3. Clinical and Laboratory Standards Institute, Wayne, PA.
16. **Clinical and Laboratory Standards Institute.** 2008. Reference method for broth dilution antifungal susceptibility testing of filamentous fungi, 2nd ed. Approved standard. NCCLS document M38-A2. Clinical and Laboratory Standards Institute, Wayne, PA.
17. **Arendrup MC, Meletiadis J, Mouton JW, Guinea J, Lagrou K, Hamal P, Subcommittee on Antifungal Susceptibility Testing (AFST) of the ESCMID European Committee for Antimicrobial Susceptibility Testing (EUCAST).** 2017. EUCAST definitive document E.DEF 7.3.1: method for the determination of broth dilution minimum inhibitory concentrations of antifungal agents for yeasts. http://www.eucast.org.
18. **Arendrup MC, Meletiadis J, Mouton JW, Lagrou K, Hamal P, Guinea J, Subcommittee on Antifungal Susceptibility Testing (AFST) of the ESCMID European Committee for Antimicrobial Susceptibility Testing (EUCAST).** 2017. EUCAST definitive document E.DEF 9.3.1: method for the determination of broth dilution minimum inhibitory concentrations of antifungal agents for conidia forming moulds. http://www.eucast.org.

19. **Clinical and Laboratory Standards Institute.** 2009. Method for antifungal disk diffusion susceptibility testing of yeasts, 2nd ed. Approved guideline. Document M44-A2. Clinical and Laboratory Standards Institute, Wayne, PA.
20. **Clinical and Laboratory Standards Institute.** 2010. Method for antifungal disk diffusion susceptibility testing of non-dermatophyte filamentous fungi. Approved standard. CLSI document M51-A1. Clinical and Laboratory Standards Institute, Wayne, PA.
21. **Ostrosky-Zeichner L, Rex JH, Pfaller MA, Diekema DJ, Alexander BD, Andes D, Brown SD, Chaturvedi V, Ghannoum MA, Knapp CC, Sheehan DJ, Walsh TJ.** 2008. Rationale for reading fluconazole MICs at 24 hours rather than 48 hours when testing *Candida* spp. by the CLSI M27-A2 standard method. *Antimicrob Agents Chemother* **52:**4175–4177.
22. **Espinel-Ingroff A, Canton E, Peman J, Rinaldi MG, Fothergill AW.** 2009. Comparison of 24-hour and 48-hour voriconazole MICs as determined by the Clinical and Laboratory Standards Institute broth microdilution method (M27-A3 document) in three laboratories: results obtained with 2,162 clinical isolates of *Candida* spp. and other yeasts. *J Clin Microbiol* **47:**2766–2771.
23. **Pfaller MA, Andes D, Diekema DJ, Espinel-Ingroff A, Sheehan D, CLSI Subcommittee for Antifungal Susceptibility Testing.** 2010. Wild-type MIC distributions, epidemiological cutoff values and species-specific clinical breakpoints for fluconazole and *Candida*: time for harmonization of CLSI and EUCAST broth microdilution methods. *Drug Resist Updat* **13:**180–195.
24. **Pfaller MA, Boyken LB, Hollis RJ, Kroeger J, Messer SA, Tendolkar S, Diekema DJ.** 2011. Validation of 24-hour posaconazole and voriconazole MIC readings versus the CLSI 48-hour broth microdilution reference method: application of epidemiological cutoff values to results from a global *Candida* antifungal surveillance program. *J Clin Microbiol* **49:**1274–1279.
25. **Clinical and Laboratory Standards Institute.** 2012 Reference method for broth dilution antifungal susceptibility testing of yeast, 4th informational supplement. CLSI document M27-S4. Clinical and Laboratory Standards Institute, Wayne, PA.
26. **Pfaller MA, Diekema DJ, Sheehan DJ.** 2006. Interpretive breakpoints for fluconazole and *Candida* revisited: a blueprint for the future of antifungal susceptibility testing. *Clin Microbiol Rev* **19:**435–447.
27. **Pfaller MA, Andes D, Arendrup MC, Diekema DJ, Espinel-Ingroff A, Alexander BD, Brown SD, Chaturvedi V, Fowler CL, Ghannoum MA, Johnson EM, Knapp CC, Motyl MR, Ostrosky-Zeichner L, Walsh TJ.** 2011. Clinical breakpoints for voriconazole and *Candida* spp. revisited: review of microbiologic, molecular, pharmacodynamic, and clinical data as they pertain to the development of species-specific interpretive criteria. *Diagn Microbiol Infect Dis* **70:**330–343.
28. **Pfaller M, Boyken L, Hollis R, Kroeger J, Messer S, Tendolkar S, Diekema D.** 2011. Use of epidemiological cutoff values to examine 9-year trends in susceptibility of *Candida* species to anidulafungin, caspofungin, and micafungin. *J Clin Microbiol* **49:**624–629.
29. **Arendrup MC, Verweij PE, Mouton JW, Lagrou K, Meletiadis J.** 2017. Multicentre validation of 4-well azole agar plates as a screening method for detection of clinically relevant azole-resistant *Aspergillus fumigatus*. *J Antimicrob Chemother* **72:**3325–3333.
30. **Nguyen MH, Yu CY.** 1999. Influence of incubation time, inoculum size, and glucose concentrations on spectrophotometric endpoint determinations for amphotericin B, fluconazole, and itraconazole. *J Clin Microbiol* **37:**141–145.
31. **Rambali B, Fernandez JA, Van Nuffel L, Woestenborghs F, Baert L, Massart DL, Odds FC.** 2001. Susceptibility testing of pathogenic fungi with itraconazole: a process analysis of test variables. *J Antimicrob Chemother* **48:**163–177.
32. **Gomez-Lopez A, Aberkane A, Petrikkou E, Mellado E, Rodriguez-Tudela JL, Cuenca-Estrella M.** 2005. Analysis of the influence of Tween concentration, inoculum size, assay medium, and reading time on susceptibility testing of *Aspergillus* spp. *J Clin Microbiol* **43:**1251–1255.
33. **Johnson EM.** 2008. Issues in antifungal susceptibility testing. *J Antimicrob Chemother* **61**(Suppl 1)**:**i13–i18.
34. **Arendrup MC.** 2013. *Candida* and candidaemia. Susceptibility and epidemiology. *Dan Med J* **60:**B4698.
35. **Andes DR, Safdar N, Baddley JW, Playford G, Reboli AC, Rex JH, Sobel JD, Pappas PG, Kullberg BJ, Mycoses Study Group.** 2012. Impact of treatment strategy on outcomes in patients with candidemia and other forms of invasive candidiasis: a patient-level quantitative review of randomized trials. *Clin Infect Dis* **54:**1110–1122.
36. **Reboli AC, Rotstein C, Pappas PG, Chapman SW, Kett DH, Kumar D, Betts R, Wible M, Goldstein BP, Schranz J, Krause DS, Walsh TJ, Anidulafungin Study Group.** 2007. Anidulafungin versus fluconazole for invasive candidiasis. *N Engl J Med* **356:**2472–2482.
37. **Espinel-Ingroff A, Chaturvedi V, Fothergill A, Rinaldi MG.** 2002. Optimal testing conditions for determining MICs and minimum fungicidal concentrations of new and established antifungal agents for uncommon molds: NCCLS collaborative study. *J Clin Microbiol* **40:**3776–3781.
38. **Pfaller MA, Sheehan DJ, Rex JH.** 2004. Determination of fungicidal activities against yeasts and molds: lessons learned from bactericidal testing and the need for standardization. *Clin Microbiol Rev* **17:**268–280.
39. **Lackner M, de Hoog GS, Verweij PE, Najafzadeh MJ, Curfs-Breuker I, Klaassen CH, Meis JF.** 2012. Species-specific antifungal susceptibility patterns of *Scedosporium* and *Pseudallescheria* species. *Antimicrob Agents Chemother* **56:** 2635–2642.
40. **Balajee SA, Nickle D, Varga J, Marr KA.** 2006. Molecular studies reveal frequent misidentification of *Aspergillus fumigatus* by morphotyping. *Eukaryot Cell* **5:**1705–1712.
41. **Arendrup MC, Kahlmeter G, Rodriguez-Tudela JL, Donnelly JP.** 2009. Breakpoints for susceptibility testing should not divide wild-type distributions of important target species. *Antimicrob Agents Chemother* **53:**1628–1629.
42. **Arendrup MC, Perlin DS, Jensen RH, Howard SJ, Goodwin J, Hope W.** 2012. Differential *in vivo* activities of anidulafungin, caspofungin, and micafungin against *Candida glabrata* isolates with and without FKS resistance mutations. *Antimicrob Agents Chemother* **56:**2435–2442.
43. **Arendrup MC, Cuenca-Estrella M, Lass-Flörl C, Hope WW.** 2013. Breakpoints for antifungal agents: an update from EUCAST focussing on echinocandins against *Candida* spp. and triazoles against *Aspergillus* spp. *Drug Resist Updat* **16:**81–95.
44. **Rex JH, Pfaller MA, Galgiani JN, Bartlett MS, Espinel-Ingroff A, Ghannoum MA, Lancaster M, Odds FC, Rinaldi MG, Walsh TJ, Barry AL, Subcommittee on Antifungal Susceptibility Testing of the National Committee for Clinical Laboratory Standards.** 1997. Development of interpretive breakpoints for antifungal susceptibility testing: conceptual framework and analysis of *in vitro-in vivo* correlation data for fluconazole, itraconazole, and *Candida* infections. *Clin Infect Dis* **24:**235–247.
45. **Rex JH, Pfaller MA.** 2002. Has antifungal susceptibility testing come of age? *Clin Infect Dis* **35:**982–989.
46. **Pappas PG, Kauffman CA, Andes DR, Clancy CJ, Marr KA, Ostrosky-Zeichner L, Reboli AC, Schuster MG, Vazquez JA, Walsh TJ, Zaoutis TE, Sobel JD.** 2016. Clinical practice guideline for the management of candidiasis: 2016 update by the Infectious Disease Society of America. *Clin Infect Dis* **62:**e1–e50.
47. **Cornely OA, Bassetti M, Calandra T, Garbino J, Kullberg BJ, Lortholary O, Meersseman W, Akova M, Arendrup MC, Arikan-Akdagli S, Bille J, Castagnola E, Cuenca-Estrella M, Donnelly JP, Groll AH, Herbrecht R, Hope WW, Jensen HE, Lass-Flörl C, Petrikkos G, Richardson MD, Roilides E, Verweij PE, Viscoli C, Ullmann AJ, ESCMID Fungal Infection Study Group.** 2012. ESCMID* guideline for the diagnosis and management of *Candida* diseases 2012: non-neutropenic adult patients. *Clin Microbiol Infect* **18**(Suppl 7)**:**19–37.
48. **Rodríguez-Tudela JL, Almirante B, Rodríguez-Pardo D, Laguna F, Donnelly JP, Mouton JW, Pahissa A, Cuenca-Estrella M.** 2007. Correlation of the MIC and dose/MIC ratio of fluconazole to the therapeutic response of patients with mucosal candidiasis and candidemia. *Antimicrob Agents Chemother* **51:**3599–3604.

49. **Ashbee HR, Barnes RA, Johnson EM, Richardson MD, Gorton R, Hope WW.** 2014. Therapeutic drug monitoring (TDM) of antifungal agents: guidelines from the British Society for Medical Mycology. *J Antimicrob Chemother* **69:**1162–1176.
50. **Zaragoza O, Mesa-Arango AC, Gómez-López A, Bernal-Martínez L, Rodríguez-Tudela JL, Cuenca-Estrella M.** 2011. Process analysis of variables for standardization of antifungal susceptibility testing of nonfermentative yeasts. *Antimicrob Agents Chemother* **55:**1563–1570.
51. **Arendrup MC, Rodriguez-Tudela JL, Park S, Garcia-Effron G, Delmas G, Cuenca-Estrella M, Gomez-Lopez A, Perlin DS.** 2011. Echinocandin susceptibility testing of *Candida* spp. Using EUCAST EDef 7.1 and CLSI M27-A3 standard procedures: analysis of the influence of bovine serum albumin supplementation, storage time, and drug lots. *Antimicrob Agents Chemother* **55:**1580–1587.
52. **Pfaller MA, Burmeister L, Bartlett MS, Rinaldi MG.** 1988. Multicenter evaluation of four methods of yeast inoculum preparation. *J Clin Microbiol* **26:**1437–1441.
53. **International Organization for Standards (ISO).** 2006. Clinical laboratory testing and in vitro diagnostic test systems. Susceptibility testing of infectious agents and evaluation of performance of antimicrobial susceptibility test devices. Part 1. Reference method for testing the *in vitro* activity of antimicrobial agents against rapidly growing aerobic bacteria involved in infectious diseases. ISO 20776–1. ISO, Geneva, Switzerland.
54. **Gomez-Lopez A, Arendrup MC, Lass-Floerl C, Rodriguez-Tudela JL, Cuenca-Estrella M.** 2010. Multicenter comparison of the ISO standard 20776-1 and the serial 2-fold dilution procedures to dilute hydrophilic and hydrophobic antifungal agents for susceptibility testing. *J Clin Microbiol* **48:**1918–1920.
55. **Anaissie EJ, Paetznick VL, Ensign LG, Espinel-Ingroff A, Galgiani JN, Hitchcock CA, LaRocco M, Patterson T, Pfaller MA, Rex JH, Rinaldi MG.** 1996. Microdilution antifungal susceptibility testing of *Candida albicans* and *Cryptococcus neoformans* with and without agitation: an eight-center collaborative study. *Antimicrob Agents Chemother* **40:**2387–2391.
56. **Arthington-Skaggs BA, Jradi H, Desai T, Morrison CJ.** 1999. Quantitation of ergosterol content: novel method for determination of fluconazole susceptibility of *Candida albicans*. *J Clin Microbiol* **37:**3332–3337.
57. **Pfaller MA, Castanheira M, Diekema DJ, Messer SA, Jones RN.** 2011. Wild-type MIC distributions and epidemiologic cutoff values for fluconazole, posaconazole, and voriconazole when testing *Cryptococcus neoformans* as determined by the CLSI broth microdilution method. *Diagn Microbiol Infect Dis* **71:**252–259.
58. **Espinel-Ingroff A, Aller AI, Canton E, Castañón-Olivares LR, Chowdhary A, Cordoba S, Cuenca-Estrella M, Fothergill A, Fuller J, Govender N, Hagen F, Illnait-Zaragozi MT, Johnson E, Kidd S, Lass-Flörl C, Lockhart SR, Martins MA, Meis JF, Melhem MS, Ostrosky-Zeichner L, Pelaez T, Pfaller MA, Schell WA, St-Germain G, Trilles L, Turnidge J.** 2012. *Cryptococcus neoformans-Cryptococcus gattii* species complex: an international study of wild-type susceptibility endpoint distributions and epidemiological cutoff values for fluconazole, itraconazole, posaconazole, and voriconazole. *Antimicrob Agents Chemother* **56:**5898–5906.
59. **Chong HS, Dagg R, Malik R, Chen S, Carter D.** 2010. *In vitro* susceptibility of the yeast pathogen cryptococcus to fluconazole and other azoles varies with molecular genotype. *J Clin Microbiol* **48:**4115–4120.
60. **Peano A, Pasquetti, M, Tizzani P, Chiavassa E, Guillot J, Johnson E.** 2017. Methodological issues in antifungal susceptibility testing of *Malassezia pachydermatis*. *J. Fungi* **3:**1–15.
61. **Arendrup MC, Boekhout T, Akova M, Meis JF, Cornely OA, Lortholary O, European Society of Clinical Microbiology and Infectious Diseases Fungal Infection Study Group, European Confederation of Medical Mycology.** 2014. ESCMID and ECMM joint clinical guidelines for the diagnosis and management of rare invasive yeast infections. *Clin Microbiol Infect* **20**(Suppl 3)**:**76–98.
62. **Lozano-Chiu M, Nelson PW, Lancaster M, Pfaller MA, Rex JH.** 1997. Lot-to-lot variability of antibiotic medium 3 used for testing susceptibility of *Candida* isolates to amphotericin B. *J Clin Microbiol* **35:**270–272.
63. **Nguyen MH, Clancy CJ, Yu VL, Yu YC, Morris AJ, Snydman DR, Sutton DA, Rinaldi MG.** 1998. Do *in vitro* susceptibility data predict the microbiologic response to amphotericin B? Results of a prospective study of patients with *Candida* fungemia. *J Infect Dis* **177:**425–430.
64. **Wanger A, Mills K, Nelson PW, Rex JH.** 1995. Comparison of Etest and National Committee for Clinical Laboratory Standards broth macrodilution method for antifungal susceptibility testing: enhanced ability to detect amphotericin B-resistant *Candida* isolates. *Antimicrob Agents Chemother* **39:**2520–2522.
65. **Arendrup MC, Garcia-Effron G, Buzina W, Mortensen KL, Reiter N, Lundin C, Jensen HE, Lass-Flörl C, Perlin DS, Bruun B.** 2009. Breakthrough *Aspergillus fumigatus* and *Candida albicans* double infection during caspofungin treatment: laboratory characteristics and implication for susceptibility testing. *Antimicrob Agents Chemother* **53:**1185–1193.
66. **Espinel-Ingroff A, Arendrup MC, Pfaller MA, Bonfietti LX, Bustamante B, Canton E, Chryssanthou E, Cuenca-Estrella M, Dannaoui E, Fothergill A, Fuller J, Gaustad P, Gonzalez GM, Guarro J, Lass-Flörl C, Lockhart SR, Meis JF, Moore CB, Ostrosky-Zeichner L, Pelaez T, Pukinskas SR, St-Germain G, Szeszs MW, Turnidge J.** 2013. Interlaboratory variability of caspofungin MICs for *Candida* spp. using CLSI and EUCAST methods: should the clinical laboratory be testing this agent? *Antimicrob Agents Chemother* **57:**5836–5842.
67. **Pfaller MA, Messer SA, Diekema DJ, Jones RN, Castanheira M.** 2014. Use of micafungin as a surrogate marker to predict susceptibility and resistance to caspofungin among 3,764 clinical isolates of *Candida* by use of CLSI methods and interpretive criteria. *J Clin Microbiol* **52:**108–114.
68. **Shields RK, Nguyen MH, Press EG, Updike CL, Clancy CJ.** 2013. Anidulafungin and micafungin MIC breakpoints are superior to that of caspofungin for identifying FKS mutant *Candida glabrata* strains and echinocandin resistance. *Antimicrob Agents Chemother* **57:**6361–6365.
69. **Arendrup MC, Rodriguez-Tudela JL, Lass-Flörl C, Cuenca-Estrella M, Donnelly JP, Hope W, European Committee on Antimicrobial Susceptibility Testing - Subcommittee on Antifungal Susceptibility Testing (EUCAST-AFST).** 2011. EUCAST technical note on anidulafungin. *Clin Microbiol Infect* **17:**E18–E20.
70. **Pfaller MA, Espinel-Ingroff A, Canton E, Castanheira M, Cuenca-Estrella M, Diekema DJ, Fothergill A, Fuller J, Ghannoum M, Jones RN, Lockhart SR, Martin-Mazuelos E, Melhem MS, Ostrosky-Zeichner L, Pappas P, Pelaez T, Peman J, Rex J, Szeszs MW.** 2012. Wild-type MIC distributions and epidemiological cutoff values for amphotericin B, flucytosine, and itraconazole and *Candida* spp. as determined by CLSI broth microdilution. *J Clin Microbiol* **50:**2040–2046.
71. **Pfaller MA, Boyken L, Hollis RJ, Kroeger J, Messer SA, Tendolkar S, Jones RN, Turnidge J, Diekema DJ.** 2010. Wild-type MIC distributions and epidemiological cutoff values for the echinocandins and *Candida* spp. *J Clin Microbiol* **48:**52–56.
72. **Arendrup MC, Meletiadis J, Mouton JW, Guinea J, Cuenca-Estrella M, Lagrou K, Howard SJ, Arendrup MC, Meletiadis J, Howard SJ, Mouton J, Guinea J, Lagrou K, Arikan-Akdagli S, Barchiesi F, Hamal P, Järv H, Lass-Flörl C, Mares M, Matos T, Muehlethaler K, Rogers TR, Torp Andersen C, Verweij P, Subcommittee on Antifungal Susceptibility Testing (AFST) of the ESCMID European Committee for Antimicrobial Susceptibility Testing (EUCAST).** 2016. EUCAST technical note on isavuconazole breakpoints for *Aspergillus*, itraconazole breakpoints for *Candida* and updates for the antifungal susceptibility testing method documents. *Clin Microbiol Infect* **22:**571.e1–571.e4.
73. **Lass-Flörl C, Arendrup MC, Rodriguez-Tudela JL, Cuenca-Estrella M, Donnelly P, Hope W, European Committee on Antimicrobial Susceptibility Testing-Subcommittee on Antifungal Susceptibility Testing.** 2011. EUCAST technical note on amphotericin B. *Clin Microbiol Infect* **17:**E27–E29.

74. **Arendrup MC, Cuenca-Estrella M, Donnelly JP, Hope W, Lass-Flörl C, Rodriguez-Tudela JL, European Committee on Antimicrobial Susceptibility Testing - Subcommittee on Antifungal Susceptibility Testing (EUCAST-AFST).** 2011. EUCAST technical note on posaconazole. *Clin Microbiol Infect* **17:**E16–E17.
75. **Subcommittee on Antifungal Susceptibility Testing of the ESCMID European Committee for Antimicrobial Susceptibility Testing.** 2008. EUCAST technical note on voriconazole. *Clin Microbiol Infect* **14:**985–987.
76. **Astvad KM, Perlin DS, Johansen HK, Jensen RH, Arendrup MC.** 2013. Evaluation of caspofungin susceptibility testing by the new Vitek 2 AST-YS06 yeast card using a unique collection of FKS wild-type and hot spot mutant isolates, including the five most common *Candida* species. *Antimicrob Agents Chemother* **57:**177–182.
77. **Chaturvedi V, Ramani R, Pfaller MA.** 2004. Collaborative study of the NCCLS and flow cytometry methods for antifungal susceptibility testing of *Candida albicans*. *J Clin Microbiol* **42:**2249–2251.
78. **Cuesta I, Bielza C, Cuenca-Estrella M, Larrañaga P, Rodríguez-Tudela JL.** 2010. Evaluation by data mining techniques of fluconazole breakpoints established by the Clinical and Laboratory Standards Institute (CLSI) and comparison with those of the European Committee on Antimicrobial Susceptibility Testing (EUCAST). *Antimicrob Agents Chemother* **54:**1541–1546.
79. **Pfaller MA, Diekema DJ, Andes D, Arendrup MC, Brown SD, Lockhart SR, Motyl M, Perlin DS, CLSI Subcommittee for Antifungal Testing.** 2011. Clinical breakpoints for the echinocandins and *Candida* revisited: integration of molecular, clinical, and microbiological data to arrive at species-specific interpretive criteria. *Drug Resist Updat* **14:**164–176 .
80. **Pfaller MA, Espinel-Ingroff A, Boyken L, Hollis RJ, Kroeger J, Messer SA, Tendolkar S, Diekema DJ.** 2011. Comparison of the broth microdilution (BMD) method of the European Committee on Antimicrobial Susceptibility Testing with the 24-hour CLSI BMD method for testing susceptibility of *Candida* species to fluconazole, posaconazole, and voriconazole by use of epidemiological cutoff values. *J Clin Microbiol* **49:**845–850.
81. **Pfaller MA, Messer SA, Boyken L, Hollis RJ, Rice C, Tendolkar S, Diekema DJ.** 2004. *In vitro* activities of voriconazole, posaconazole, and fluconazole against 4,169 clinical isolates of *Candida* spp. and *Cryptococcus neoformans* collected during 2001 and 2002 in the ARTEMIS global antifungal surveillance program. *Diagn Microbiol Infect Dis* **48:**201–205.
82. **Clinical and Laboratory Standards Institute.** 2008. Reference method for broth dilution antifungal susceptibility testing of yeasts, 3rd informational supplement. Supplement M27-S3. Clinical and Laboratory Standards Institute, Wayne, PA.
83. **Pfaller MA, Boyken L, Hollis RJ, Messer SA, Tendolkar S, Diekema DJ.** 2005. *In vitro* susceptibilities of clinical isolates of *Candida* species, *Cryptococcus neoformans*, and *Aspergillus* species to itraconazole: global survey of 9,359 isolates tested by Clinical and Laboratory Standards Institute broth microdilution methods. *J Clin Microbiol* **43:**3807–3810.
84. **Andes D, Marchillo K, Stamstad T, Conklin R.** 2003. *In vivo* pharmacokinetics and pharmacodynamics of a new triazole, voriconazole, in a murine candidiasis model. *Antimicrob Agents Chemother* **47:**3165–3169.
85. **Espinel-Ingroff A, Pfaller MA, Bustamante B, Canton E, Fothergill A, Fuller J, Gonzalez GM, Lass-Flörl C, Lockhart SR, Martin-Mazuelos E, Meis JF, Melhem MS, Ostosky-Zeichner L, Pelaez T, Szeszs MW, St-Germain G, Bonfietti LX, Guarro J, Turnidge J.** 2014. A multilaboratory study of epidemiological cutoff values for detection of resistance in eight *Candida* spp. to fluconazole, posaconazole, and voriconazole. *Antimicrob Agents Chemother* **58:**2006–2012.
86. **Davey KG, Holmes AD, Johnson EM, Szekely A, Warnock DW.** 1998. Comparative evaluation of FUNGITEST and broth microdilution methods for antifungal drug susceptibility testing of *Candida* species and *Cryptococcus neoformans*. *J Clin Microbiol* **36:**926–930.
87. **Espinel-Ingroff A, Pfaller M, Messer SA, Knapp CC, Holliday N, Killian SB.** 2004. Multicenter comparison of the Sensititre YeastOne colorimetric antifungal panel with the NCCLS M27-A2 reference method for testing new antifungal agents against clinical isolates of *Candida* spp. *J Clin Microbiol* **42:**718–721.
88. **Pfaller MA, Arikan S, Lozano-Chiu M, Chen Y, Coffman S, Messer SA, Rennie R, Sand C, Heffner T, Rex JH, Wang J, Yamane N.** 1998. Clinical evaluation of the ASTY colorimetric microdilution panel for antifungal susceptibility testing. *J Clin Microbiol* **36:**2609–2612.
89. **Pfaller MA, Chaturvedi V, Diekema DJ, Ghannoum MA, Holliday NM, Killian SB, Knapp CC, Messer SA, Miskov A, Ramani R.** 2008. Clinical evaluation of the Sensititre YeastOne colorimetric antifungal panel for antifungal susceptibility testing of the echinocandins anidulafungin, caspofungin, and micafungin. *J Clin Microbiol* **46:**2155–2159.
90. **Pfaller MA, Chaturvedi V, Diekema DJ, Ghannoum MA, Holliday NM, Killian SB, Knapp CC, Messer SA, Miskou A, Ramani R.** 2012. Comparison of the Sensititre YeastOne colorimetric antifungal panel with CLSI microdilution for antifungal susceptibility testing of the echinocandins against *Candida* spp., using new clinical breakpoints and epidemiological cutoff values. *Diagn Microbiol Infect Dis* **73:** 365–368.
91. **Espinel-Ingroff A, Alvarez-Fernandez M, Cantón E, Carver PL, Chen SC, Eschenauer G, Getsinger DL, Gonzalez GM, Govender NP, Grancini A, Hanson KE, Kidd SE, Klinker K, Kubin CJ, Kus JV, Lockhart SR, Meletiadis J, Morris AJ, Pelaez T, Quindós G, Rodriguez-Iglesias M, Sánchez-Reus F, Shoham S, Wengenack NL, Borrell Solé N, Echeverria J, Esperalba J, Gómez-G de la Pedrosa E, García García I, Linares MJ, Marco F, Merino P, Pemán J, Pérez Del Molino L, Roselló Mayans E, Rubio Calvo C, Ruiz Pérez de Pipaon M, Yagüe G, Garcia-Effron G, Guinea J, Perlin DS, Sanguinetti M, Shields R, Turnidge J.** 2015. Multicenter study of epidemiological cutoff values and detection of resistance in *Candida* spp. to anidulafungin, caspofungin, and micafungin using the Sensititre YeastOne colorimetric method. *Antimicrob Agents Chemother* **59:** 6725–6732 .
92. **Pfaller MA, Diekema DJ, Procop GW, Rinaldi MG.** 2007. Multicenter comparison of the VITEK 2 yeast susceptibility test with the CLSI broth microdilution reference method for testing fluconazole against *Candida* spp. *J Clin Microbiol* **45:**796–802.
93. **Pfaller MA, Diekema DJ, Procop GW, Rinaldi MG.** 2007. Multicenter comparison of the VITEK 2 antifungal susceptibility test with the CLSI broth microdilution reference method for testing amphotericin B, flucytosine, and voriconazole against *Candida* spp. *J Clin Microbiol* **45:**3522–3528.
94. **Posteraro B, Martucci R, La Sorda M, Fiori B, Sanglard D, De Carolis E, Florio AR, Fadda G, Sanguinetti M.** 2009. Reliability of the Vitek 2 yeast susceptibility test for detection of *in vitro* resistance to fluconazole and voriconazole in clinical isolates of *Candida albicans* and *Candida glabrata*. *J Clin Microbiol* **47:**1927–1930.
95. **Cuenca-Estrella M, Gomez-Lopez A, Alastruey-Izquierdo A, Bernal-Martinez L, Cuesta I, Buitrago MJ, Rodriguez-Tudela JL.** 2010. Comparison of the Vitek 2 antifungal susceptibility system with the Clinical and Laboratory Standards Institute (CLSI) and European Committee on Antimicrobial Susceptibility Testing (EUCAST) broth microdilution reference methods and with the Sensititre YeastOne and Etest techniques for *in vitro* detection of antifungal resistance in yeast isolates. *J Clin Microbiol* **48:**1782–1786.
96. **Pfaller MA, Diekema DJ, Gibbs DL, Newell VA, Meis JF, Gould IM, Fu W, Colombo AL, Rodriguez-Noriega E, Global Antifungal Surveillance Study.** 2007. Results from the ARTEMIS DISK Global Antifungal Surveillance Study, 1997 to 2005: an 8.5-year analysis of susceptibilities of *Candida* species and other yeast species to fluconazole and voriconazole determined by CLSI standardized disk diffusion testing. *J Clin Microbiol* **45:**1735–1745.

97. **Lozano-Chiu M, Nelson PW, Paetznick VL, Rex JH.** 1999. Disk diffusion method for determining susceptibilities of *Candida* spp. to MK-0991. *J Clin Microbiol* **37:**1625–1627.
98. **Pfaller MA, Messer SA, Boyken L, Rice C, Tendolkar S, Hollis RJ, Diekema DJ.** 2004. Evaluation of the NCCLS M44-P disk diffusion method for determining susceptibilities of 276 clinical isolates of *Cryptococcus neoformans* to fluconazole. *J Clin Microbiol* **42:**380–383.
99. **Clinical and Laboratory Standards Institute.** 2009. Zone diameter interpretive standards and corresponding minimal inhibitory concentration (MIC) interpretive breakpoints. Informational supplement M44S3. Clinical and Laboratory Standards Institute, Wayne, PA.
100. **Axner-Elings M, Botero-Kleiven S, Jensen RH, Arendrup MC.** 2011. Echinocandin susceptibility testing of *Candida* isolates collected during a 1-year period in Sweden. *J Clin Microbiol* **49:**2516–2521.
101. **Peyron F, Favel A, Michel-Nguyen A, Gilly M, Regli P, Bolmström A.** 2001. Improved detection of amphotericin B-resistant isolates of *Candida lusitaniae* by Etest. *J Clin Microbiol* **39:**339–342.
102. **Pfaller MA, Messer SA, Mills K, Bolmström A, Jones RN.** 2001. Evaluation of Etest method for determining caspofungin (MK-0991) susceptibilities of 726 clinical isolates of *Candida* species. *J Clin Microbiol* **39:**4387–4389.
103. **Pfaller MA, Messer SA, Mills K, Bolmström A, Jones RN.** 2001. Evaluation of Etest method for determining posaconazole MICs for 314 clinical isolates of *Candida* species. *J Clin Microbiol* **39:**3952–3954.
104. **Ranque S, Lachaud L, Gari-Toussaint M, Michel-Nguyen A, Mallié M, Gaudart J, Bertout S.** 2012. Interlaboratory reproducibility of Etest amphotericin B and caspofungin yeast susceptibility testing and comparison with the CLSI method. *J Clin Microbiol* **50:**2305–2309.
105. **Arendrup MC, Pfaller MA, Danish Fungaemia Study Group.** 2012. Caspofungin Etest susceptibility testing of *Candida* species: risk of misclassification of susceptible isolates of *C. glabrata* and *C. krusei* when adopting the revised CLSI caspofungin breakpoints. *Antimicrob Agents Chemother* **56:**3965–3968.
106. **Shields RK, Nguyen MH, Press EG, Updike CL, Clancy CJ.** 2013. Caspofungin MICs correlate with treatment outcomes among patients with *Candida glabrata* invasive candidiasis and prior echinocandin exposure. *Antimicrob Agents Chemother* **57:**3528–3535.
107. **Chang HC, Chang JJ, Chan SH, Huang AH, Wu TL, Lin MC, Chang TC.** 2001. Evaluation of Etest for direct antifungal susceptibility testing of yeasts in positive blood cultures. *J Clin Microbiol* **39:**1328–1333.
108. **Guinea J, Recio S, Escribano P, Torres-Narbona M, Peláez T, Sánchez-Carrillo C, Rodríguez-Créixems M, Bouza E.** 2010. Rapid antifungal susceptibility determination for yeast isolates by use of Etest performed directly on blood samples from patients with fungemia. *J Clin Microbiol* **48:**2205–2212 .
109. **Marinach C, Alanio A, Palous M, Kwasek S, Fekkar A, Brossas J-Y, Brun S, Snounou G, Hennequin C, Sanglard D, Datry A, Golmard J-L, Mazier D.** 2009. MALDI-TOF MS-based drug susceptibility testing of pathogens: the example of *Candida albicans* and fluconazole. *Proteomics* **9:** 4627–4631.
110. **De Carolis E, Vella A, Florio AR, Posteraro P, Perlin DS, Sanguinetti M, Posteraro B.** 2012. Use of matrix-assisted laser desorption ionization-time of flight mass spectrometry for caspofungin susceptibility testing of *Candida* and *Aspergillus* species. *J Clin Microbiol* **50:**2479–2483.
111. **Vella A, De Carolis E, Vaccaro L, Posteraro P, Perlin DS, Kostrzewa M, Posteraro B, Sanguinetti M.** 2013. Rapid antifungal susceptibility testing by matrix-assisted laser desorption ionization-time of flight mass spectrometry analysis. *J Clin Microbiol* **51:**2964–2969.
112. **Sanglard D, Coste A, Ferrari S.** 2009. Antifungal drug resistance mechanisms in fungal pathogens from the perspective of transcriptional gene regulation. *FEMS Yeast Res* **9:** 1029–1050.
113. **Jensen RH, Astvad KM, Silva LV, Sanglard D, Jørgensen R, Nielsen KF, Mathiasen EG, Doroudian G, Perlin DS, Arendrup MC.** 2015. Stepwise emergence of azole, echinocandin and amphotericin B multidrug resistance *in vivo* in *Candida albicans* orchestrated by multiple genetic alterations. *J Antimicrob Chemother* **70:**2551–2555.
114. **Wiederhold NP, Grabinski JL, Garcia-Effron G, Perlin DS, Lee SA.** 2008. Pyrosequencing to detect mutations in *FKS1* that confer reduced echinocandin susceptibility in *Candida albicans*. *Antimicrob Agents Chemother* **52:** 4145–4148.
115. **Pham CD, Bolden CB, Kuykendall RJ, Lockhart SR.** 2014. Development of a Luminex-based multiplex assay for detection of mutations conferring resistance to echinocandins in *Candida glabrata*. *J Clin Microbiol* **52:**790–795.
116. **Kurtz MB, Heath IB, Marrinan J, Dreikorn S, Onishi J, Douglas C.** 1994. Morphological effects of lipopeptides against *Aspergillus fumigatus* correlate with activities against (1,3)-β-D-glucan synthase. *Antimicrob Agents Chemother* **38:**1480–1489.
117. **Odds FC, Motyl M, Andrade R, Bille J, Cantón E, Cuenca-Estrella M, Davidson A, Durussel C, Ellis D, Foraker E, Fothergill AW, Ghannoum MA, Giacobbe RA, Gobernado M, Handke R, Laverdière M, Lee-Yang W, Merz WG, Ostrosky-Zeichner L, Pemán J, Perea S, Perfect JR, Pfaller MA, Proia L, Rex JH, Rinaldi MG, Rodriguez-Tudela JL, Schell WA, Shields C, Sutton DA, Verweij PE, Warnock DW.** 2004. Interlaboratory comparison of results of susceptibility testing with caspofungin against *Candida* and *Aspergillus* species. *J Clin Microbiol* **42:**3475–3482.
118. **Espinel-Ingroff A, Fothergill A, Ghannoum M, Manavathu E, Ostrosky-Zeichner L, Pfaller MA, Rinaldi MG, Schell W, Walsh TJ.** 2007. Quality control and reference guidelines for CLSI broth microdilution method (M38-A document) for susceptibility testing of anidulafungin against molds. *J Clin Microbiol* **45:**2180–2182.
119. **Espinel-Ingroff A, Fothergill A, Fuller J, Johnson E, Pelaez T, Turnidge J.** 2011. Wild-type MIC distributions and epidemiological cutoff values for caspofungin and *Aspergillus* spp. for the CLSI broth microdilution method (M38-A2 document). *Antimicrob Agents Chemother* **55:** 2855–2859.
120. **Arendrup MC, Perkhofer S, Howard SJ, Garcia-Effron G, Vishukumar A, Perlin D, Lass-Flörl C.** 2008. Establishing *in vitro-in vivo* correlations for *Aspergillus fumigatus*: the challenge of azoles versus echinocandins. *Antimicrob Agents Chemother* **52:**3504–3511.
121. **Espinel-Ingroff A, Dawson K, Pfaller M, Anaissie E, Breslin B, Dixon D, Fothergill A, Paetznick V, Peter J, Rinaldi M.** 1995. Comparative and collaborative evaluation of standardization of antifungal susceptibility testing for filamentous fungi. *Antimicrob Agents Chemother* **39:** 314–319.
122. **Astvad KMT, Jensen RH, Hassan TM, Mathiasen EG, Thomsen GM, Pedersen UG, Christensen M, Hilberg O, Arendrup MC.** 2014. First detection of TR46/Y121F/T289A and TR34/L98H alterations in *Aspergillus fumigatus* isolates from azole-naive patients in Denmark despite negative findings in the environment. *Antimicrob Agents Chemother* **58:**5096–5101.
123. **Espinel-Ingroff A, Canton E, Peman J.** 2009. Updates in antifungal susceptibility testing of filamentous fungi. *Curr Fungal Infect Rep* **3:**133–141.
124. **Lass-Flörl C, Kofler G, Kropshofer G, Hermans J, Kreczy A, Dierich MP, Niederwieser D.** 1998. *In-vitro* testing of susceptibility to amphotericin B is a reliable predictor of clinical outcome in invasive aspergillosis. *J Antimicrob Chemother* **42:**497–502.
125. **Madureira A, Bergeron A, Lacroix C, Robin M, Rocha V, de Latour RP, Ferry C, Devergie A, Lapalu J, Gluckman E, Socié G, Ghannoum M, Ribaud P.** 2007. Breakthrough invasive aspergillosis in allogeneic haematopoietic stem cell transplant recipients treated with caspofungin. *Int J Antimicrob Agents* **30:**551–554.

126. **Troke P, Aguirrebengoa K, Arteaga C, Ellis D, Heath CH, Lutsar I, Rovira M, Nguyen Q, Slavin M, Chen SCA, Global Scedosporium Study Group.** 2008. Treatment of scedosporiosis with voriconazole: clinical experience with 107 patients. *Antimicrob Agents Chemother* **52:**1743–1750.
127. **Alastruey-Izquierdo A, Castelli MV, Cuesta I, Monzon A, Cuenca-Estrella M, Rodriguez-Tudela JL.** 2009. Activity of posaconazole and other antifungal agents against *Mucorales* strains identified by sequencing of internal transcribed spacers. *Antimicrob Agents Chemother* **53:**1686–1689.
128. **Drogari-Apiranthitou M, Mantopoulou F-D, Skiada A, Kanioura L, Grammatikou M, Vrioni G, Mitroussia-Ziouva A, Tsakris A, Petrikkos G.** 2012. *In vitro* antifungal susceptibility of filamentous fungi causing rare infections: synergy testing of amphotericin B, posaconazole and anidulafungin in pairs. *J Antimicrob Chemother* **67:**1937–1940.
129. **Espinel-Ingroff A, Johnson E, Hockey H, Troke P.** 2008. Activities of voriconazole, itraconazole and amphotericin B *in vitro* against 590 moulds from 323 patients in the voriconazole phase III clinical studies. *J Antimicrob Chemother* **61:**616–620.
130. **Sahi H, Avery RK, Minai OA, Hall G, Mehta AC, Raina P, Budev M.** 2007. *Scedosporium apiospermum* (*Pseudoallescheria boydii*) infection in lung transplant recipients. *J Heart Lung Transplant* **26:**350–356.
131. **Barchiesi F, Spreghini E, Sanguinetti M, Giannini D, Manso E, Castelli P, Girmenia C.** 2013. Effects of amphotericin B on *Aspergillus flavus* clinical isolates with variable susceptibilities to the polyene in an experimental model of systemic aspergillosis. *J Antimicrob Chemother* **68:** 2587–2591.
132. **Espinel-Ingroff A.** 2001. *In vitro* fungicidal activities of voriconazole, itraconazole, and amphotericin B against opportunistic moniliaceous and dematiaceous fungi. *J Clin Microbiol* **39:**954–958.
133. **Vermeulen E, Maertens J, Schoemans H, Lagrou K.** 2012. Azole-resistant *Aspergillus fumigatus* due to TR46/Y121F/T289A mutation emerging in Belgium, July 2012. *Euro Surveill* **17:**20326. https://www.eurosurveillance.org/content/10.2807/ese.17.48.20326-en.
134. **Dannaoui E, Meletiadis J, Mouton JW, Meis JF, Verweij PE, Eurofung Network.** 2003. *In vitro* susceptibilities of zygomycetes to conventional and new antifungals. *J Antimicrob Chemother* **51:**45–52.
135. **Arendrup MC, Jensen RH, Meletiadis J.** 2015. *In vitro* activity of isavuconazole and comparators against clinical isolates of the Mucorales order. *Antimicrob Agents Chemother* **59:**7735–7742.
136. **Marty FM, Ostrosky-Zeichner L, Cornely OA, Mullane KM, Perfect JR, Thompson GR III, Alangaden GJ, Brown JM, Fredricks DN, Heinz WJ, Herbrecht R, Klimko N, Klyasova G, Maertens JA, Melinkeri SR, Oren I, Pappas PG, Ráčil Z, Rahav G, Santos R, Schwartz S, Vehreschild JJ, Young JH, Chetchotisakd P, Jaruratanasirikul S, Kanj SS, Engelhardt M, Kaufhold A, Ito M, Lee M, Sasse C, Maher RM, Zeiher B, Vehreschild MJGT, VITAL and FungiScope Mucormycosis Investigators.** 2016. Isavuconazole treatment for mucormycosis: a single-arm open-label trial and case-control analysis. *Lancet Infect Dis* **16:**828–837.
137. **Rodriguez-Tudela JL, Alcazar-Fuoli L, Mellado E, Alastruey-Izquierdo A, Monzon A, Cuenca-Estrella M.** 2008. Epidemiological cutoffs and cross-resistance to azole drugs in *Aspergillus fumigatus*. *Antimicrob Agents Chemother* **52:**2468–2472.
138. **Pfaller MA, Diekema DJ, Ghannoum MA, Rex JH, Alexander BD, Andes D, Brown SD, Chaturvedi V, Espinel-Ingroff A, Fowler CL, Johnson EM, Knapp CC, Motyl MR, Ostrosky-Zeichner L, Sheehan DJ, Walsh TJ, Clinical and Laboratory Standards Institute Antifungal Testing Subcommittee.** 2009. Wild-type MIC distribution and epidemiological cutoff values for *Aspergillus fumigatus* and three triazoles as determined by the Clinical and Laboratory Standards Institute broth microdilution methods. *J Clin Microbiol* **47:**3142–3146.
139. **Espinel-Ingroff A, Diekema DJ, Fothergill A, Johnson E, Pelaez T, Pfaller MA, Rinaldi MG, Canton E, Turnidge J.** 2010. Wild-type MIC distributions and epidemiological cutoff values for the triazoles and six *Aspergillus* spp. for the CLSI broth microdilution method (M38-A2 document). *J Clin Microbiol* **48:**3251–3257.
140. **Espinel-Ingroff A, Chowdhary A, Gonzalez GM, Lass-Flörl C, Martin-Mazuelos E, Meis J, Peláez T, Pfaller MA, Turnidge J.** 2013. Multicenter study of isavuconazole MIC distributions and epidemiological cutoff values for *Aspergillus* spp. for the CLSI M38-A2 broth microdilution method. *Antimicrob Agents Chemother* **57:**3823–3828.
141. **Verweij PE, Howard SJ, Melchers WJ, Denning DW.** 2009. Azole-resistance in *Aspergillus*: proposed nomenclature and breakpoints. *Drug Resist Updat* **12:**141–147.
142. **Cuenca-Estrella M, Gomez-Lopez A, Mellado E, Monzon A, Buitrago MJ, Rodriguez-Tudela JL.** 2009. Activity profile *in vitro* of micafungin against Spanish clinical isolates of common and emerging species of yeasts and molds. *Antimicrob Agents Chemother* **53:**2192–2195.
143. **Espinel-Ingroff A.** 2003. *In vitro* antifungal activities of anidulafungin and micafungin, licensed agents and the investigational triazole posaconazole as determined by NCCLS methods for 12,052 fungal isolates: review of the literature. *Rev Iberoam Micol* **20:**121–136.
144. **Pfaller MA, Boyken L, Hollis RJ, Kroeger J, Messer SA, Tendolkar S, Diekema DJ.** 2010. Wild-type minimum effective concentration distributions and epidemiologic cutoff values for caspofungin and *Aspergillus* spp. as determined by Clinical and Laboratory Standards Institute broth microdilution methods. *Diagn Microbiol Infect Dis* **67:**56–60.
145. **Arabatzis M, Kambouris M, Kyprianou M, Chrysaki A, Foustoukou M, Kanellopoulou M, Kondyli L, Kouppari G, Koutsia-Karouzou C, Lebessi E, Pangalis A, Petinaki E, Stathi A, Trikka-Graphakos E, Vartzioti E, Vogiatzi A, Vyzantiadis T-A, Zerva L, Velegraki A.** 2011. Polyphasic identification and susceptibility to seven antifungals of 102 *Aspergillus* isolates recovered from immunocompromised hosts in Greece. *Antimicrob Agents Chemother* **55:**3025–3030.
146. **Fuller J, Schofield A, Jiwa S, Sand C, Jansen B, Rennie R.** 2010. Caspofungin Etest endpoint for *Aspergillus* isolates shows poor agreement with the reference minimum effective concentration. *J Clin Microbiol* **48:**479–482.
147. **Pfaller MA, Castanheira M, Messer SA, Moet GJ, Jones RN.** 2011. Echinocandin and triazole antifungal susceptibility profiles for *Candida* spp., *Cryptococcus neoformans*, and *Aspergillus fumigatus*: application of new CLSI clinical breakpoints and epidemiologic cutoff values to characterize resistance in the SENTRY Antimicrobial Surveillance Program (2009). *Diagn Microbiol Infect Dis* **69:**45–50.
148. **Ghannoum MA, Isham NC, Chand DV.** 2009. Susceptibility testing of dermatophytes. *Curr Fungal Infect Rep* **32:**142–146.
149. **Yamada T, Maeda M, Alshahni MM, Tanaka R, Yaguchi T, Bontems O, Salamin K, Fratti M, Monod M.** 2017. Terbinafine resistance of *Trichophyton* clinical isolates caused by specific point mutations in the squalene epoxidase gene. *Antimicrob Agents Chemother* **61:**e00115-17.
150. **Castro C, Serrano MC, Flores B, Espinel-Ingroff A, Martín-Mazuelos E.** 2004. Comparison of the Sensititre YeastOne colorimetric antifungal panel with a modified NCCLS M38-A method to determine the activity of voriconazole against clinical isolates of *Aspergillus* spp. *J Clin Microbiol* **42:**4358–4360.
151. **Linares MJ, Charriel G, Solís F, Rodriguez F, Ibarra A, Casal M.** 2005. Susceptibility of filamentous fungi to voriconazole tested by two microdilution methods. *J Clin Microbiol* **43:**250–253.
152. **Martín-Mazuelos E, Pemán J, Valverde A, Chaves M, Serrano MC, Cantón E.** 2003. Comparison of the Sensititre YeastOne colorimetric antifungal panel and Etest with the NCCLS M38-A method to determine the activity of amphotericin B and itraconazole against clinical isolates of *Aspergillus* spp. *J Antimicrob Chemother* **52:**365–370.

153. **Hawser SP, Jessup C, Vitullo J, Ghannoum MA.** 2001. Utility of 2,3-bis(2-methoxy-4-nitro-5-sulfophenyl)-5-[(phenylamino)carbonyl]-2H-tetrazolium hydroxide (XTT) and minimum effective concentration assays in the determination of antifungal susceptibility of *Aspergillus fumigatus* to the lipopeptide class compounds. *J Clin Microbiol* **39:**2738–2741.
154. **Meletiadis J, Meis JFGM, Mouton JW, Donnelly JP, Verweij PE.** 2000. Comparison of NCCLS and 3-(4,5-dimethyl-2-Thiazyl)-2, 5-diphenyl-2H-tetrazolium bromide (MTT) methods of *in vitro* susceptibility testing of filamentous fungi and development of a new simplified method. *J Clin Microbiol* **38:**2949–2954.
155. **Kuzucu C, Rapino B, McDermott L, Hadley S.** 2004. Comparison of the semisolid agar antifungal susceptibility test with the NCCLS M38-P broth microdilution test for screening of filamentous fungi. *J Clin Microbiol* **42:**1224–1227.
156. **Denning DW, Radford SA, Oakley KL, Hall L, Johnson EM, Warnock DW.** 1997. Correlation between *in-vitro* susceptibility testing to itraconazole and *in-vivo* outcome of *Aspergillus fumigatus* infection. *J Antimicrob Chemother* **40:**401–414.
157. **Arikan S, Paetznick V, Rex JH.** 2002. Comparative evaluation of disk diffusion with microdilution assay in susceptibility testing of caspofungin against *Aspergillus* and *Fusarium* isolates. *Antimicrob Agents Chemother* **46:**3084–3087.
158. **Espinel-Ingroff A, Arthington-Skaggs B, Iqbal N, Ellis D, Pfaller MA, Messer S, Rinaldi M, Fothergill A, Gibbs DL, Wang A.** 2007. Multicenter evaluation of a new disk agar diffusion method for susceptibility testing of filamentous fungi with voriconazole, posaconazole, itraconazole, amphotericin B, and caspofungin. *J Clin Microbiol* **45:**1811–1820.
159. **Serrano MC, Ramírez M, Morilla D, Valverde A, Chávez M, Espinel-Ingroff A, Claro R, Fernández A, Almeida C, Martín-Mazuelos E.** 2004. A comparative study of the disc diffusion method with the broth microdilution and Etest methods for voriconazole susceptibility testing of *Aspergillus* spp. *J Antimicrob Chemother* **53:**739–742.
160. **Martos AI, Martín-Mazuelos E, Romero A, Serrano C, González T, Almeida C, Puche B, Cantón E, Pemán J, Espinel-Ingroff A.** 2012. Evaluation of disk diffusion method compared to broth microdilution for antifungal susceptibility testing of 3 echinocandins against *Aspergillus* spp. *Diagn Microbiol Infect Dis* **73:**53–56.
161. **Espinel-Ingroff A, Canton E, Fothergill A, Ghannoum M, Johnson E, Jones RN, Ostrosky-Zeichner L, Schell W, Gibbs DL, Wang A, Turnidge J.** 2011. Quality control guidelines for amphotericin B, itraconazole, posaconazole, and voriconazole disk diffusion susceptibility tests with nonsupplemented Mueller-Hinton agar (CLSI M51-A document) for nondermatophyte filamentous fungi. *J Clin Microbiol* **49:**2568–2571.
162. **Colosi IA, Faure O, Dessaigne B, Bourdon C, Lebeau B, Colosi HA, Pelloux H.** 2012. Susceptibility of 100 filamentous fungi: comparison of two diffusion methods, Neo-Sensitabs and E-test, for amphotericin B, caspofungin, itraconazole, voriconazole and posaconazole. *Med Mycol* **50:**378–385.
163. **Szekely A, Johnson EM, Warnock DW.** 1999. Comparison of E-test and broth microdilution methods for antifungal drug susceptibility testing of molds. *J Clin Microbiol* **37:** 1480–1483.
164. **Espinel-Ingroff A.** 2001. Comparison of the E-test with the NCCLS M38-P method for antifungal susceptibility testing of common and emerging pathogenic filamentous fungi. *J Clin Microbiol* **39:**1360–1367.
165. **Espinel-Ingroff A, Rezusta A.** 2002. E-test method for testing susceptibilities of *Aspergillus* spp. to the new triazoles voriconazole and posaconazole and to established antifungal agents: comparison with NCCLS broth microdilution method. *J Clin Microbiol* **40:**2101–2107.
166. **Pfaller JB, Messer SA, Hollis RJ, Diekema DJ, Pfaller MA.** 2003. *In vitro* susceptibility testing of *Aspergillus* spp.: comparison of Etest and reference microdilution methods for determining voriconazole and itraconazole MICs. *J Clin Microbiol* **41:**1126–1129.
167. **Garcia-Effron G, Dilger A, Alcazar-Fuoli L, Park S, Mellado E, Perlin DS.** 2008. Rapid detection of triazole antifungal resistance in *Aspergillus fumigatus*. *J Clin Microbiol* **46:**1200–1206.
168. **Chong G-L, van de Sande WWJ, Dingemans GJ, Gaajetaan GR, Vonk AG, Hayette M-P, van Tegelen DWE, Simons GFM, Rijnders BJ.** 2015. Validation of a new *Aspergillus* real-time PCR assay for direct detection of *Aspergillus* and azole resistance of *Aspergillus fumigatus* on bronchoalveolar lavage fluid. *J Clin Microbiol* **53:**868–874.
169. **White PL, Posso RB, Barnes RA.** 2015. An analytical and clinical evaluation of the PathoNostics AsperGenius assay for the detection of invasive aspergillosis and resistance to azole antifungal drugs during testing of serum samples. *J Clin Microbiol* **53:**2115–2121.
170. **Bueid A, Howard SJ, Moore CB, Richardson MD, Harrison E, Bowyer P, Denning DW.** 2010. Azole antifungal resistance in *Aspergillus fumigatus*: 2008 and 2009. *J Antimicrob Chemother* **65:**2116–2118.
171. **Gardiner RE, Souteropoulos P, Park S, Perlin DS.** 2005. Characterization of *Aspergillus fumigatus* mutants with reduced susceptibility to caspofungin. *Med Mycol* **43**(Suppl 1):S299–S305.
172. **Meletiadis J, Antachopoulos C, Stergiopoulou T, Pournaras S, Roilides E, Walsh TJ.** 2007. Differential fungicidal activities of amphotericin B and voriconazole against *Aspergillus* species determined by microbroth methodology. *Antimicrob Agents Chemother* **51:**3329–3337.
173. **Clinical and Laboratory Standards Institute.** 2017. *Performance Standards for Antifungal Susceptibility Testing of Yeast.* CLSI Suppl. M60. Clinical and Laboratory Standards Institute, Wayne, PA.
174. **Clinical and Laboratory Standards Institute.** 2018. *Epidemiological Cutoff Values for Antifungal Susceptibility Testing*, 2nd ed. CLSI Suppl. M59. Clinical and Laboratory Standards Institute, Wayne, PA.

PARASITOLOGY

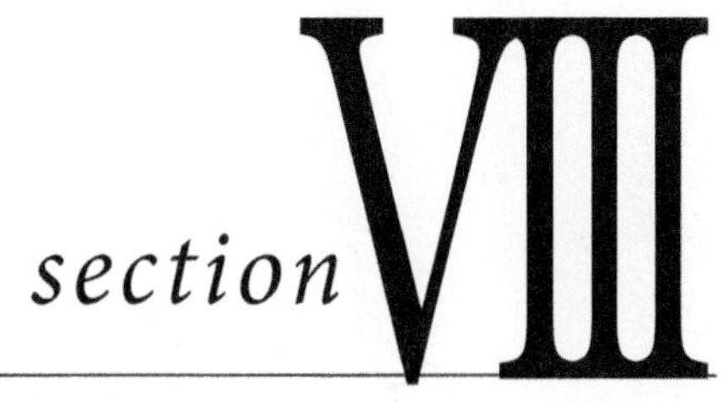

VOLUME EDITOR: DAVID W. WARNOCK

SECTION EDITORS: BOBBI S. PRITT AND GARY W. PROCOP

GENERAL

PARASITES

Taxonomy and Classification of Human Eukaryotic Parasites

SINA M. ADL AND BLAINE A. MATHISON

135

The eukaryotic parasites of medical importance are classically known as protozoan, arthropod, and helminthic parasites; the last includes nematodes, cestodes, trematodes, and acanthocephalans. Historically, fungi such as Microsporidia and *Pneumocystis* were included among the parasites, but they are placed among the fungi herein. The previous edition of this *Manual* carried the classical taxonomy as far as was possible despite the modern transformation of eukaryote classification. In this edition, we have adopted the system already used in research and by biologists for over a decade. To facilitate the transition for clinical microbiologists who are unfamiliar with these changes, we provide the names from the previous edition alongside the modern ones.

The modern classification of biological species intends to reflect an evolutionary history of living organisms. The Linnaean hierarchical classification system continues to be used in botany and zoology, governed by the rules of the International Code of Zoological Nomenclature and the International Code of Nomenclature for Algae, Fungi, and Plants (no longer botany), each with its overseeing body. That was fine when the biology of eukaryotes was divided into plants (and fungi) and animals, but since this is no longer the case, a new approach was necessary to accommodate the diversity of protists from which all other groups diverge. Rules and established practice of both systems of nomenclature are irreconcilably in conflict, so they can be applied to all eukaryotes only if one ignores rules, or if one develops two parallel classifications. In contrast, the modern system allows parasitologists, as well as botanists and zoologists, to keep classical traditions and incorporates them into the classification of protist diversity. For those who are interested in further in-depth reading, works by Adl et al. (1, 2) provide an adequate summary of the background for the system currently used. Additional discussion has also been provided by Adl et al. (3). The biggest change with the modern system is that most of the artificially rigidly named higher-ranked levels of complexity (e.g., kingdom, phylum, class, and order) are no longer formally assigned among the protists, and only genus and species designations are formally retained. However, the higher levels are often retained among animal taxonomists. In the zoological code, the higher ranks are not required, and there is little agreement about which level these ranks apply to. The hierarchy in the classification described herein reflects our current understanding of how monophyletic lineages (i.e., clades) are related, as indicated by phylogenetic trees (1). Clades are defined simply as a group of organisms believed to have evolved from a common ancestor. Many of the familiar clade names, like Apicomplexa, Endamoebidae, and Trypanosomatidae, retain the ending for ease of communication, but they are no longer linked to named hierarchy descriptors like order, class, or phylum.

One might ask why all the fuss about classification is necessary if it is just a way of organizing species. The reason is that there are patterns inherited through species lineages. When the sequence of lineages derived from other lineages (phylogenetics) is correctly deduced, it will reflect the genetic information carried with modification into successive taxonomic groups. When species are correctly placed in the classification, one can deduce a great amount of information from their position in the classification. It is not dissimilar from the classification of elements in the periodic table. That is how the periods (or patterns) are identified, and it helps with learning and remembering. The patterns discernible in the biological classification include those related to organisms' ecological function, the biochemistry of metabolic pathways, cell biology and cell membrane chemistry, host cell penetration, and ability to evade host immune response. For example, if a species is incorrectly placed in the classification, then group-specific pharmacology will be ineffective until research is directed at its metabolism according to its correct placement in the classification. So how should a clinical microbiologist use this new system, especially when teaching future generations of technologists, residents, and fellows? One recommendation that is commonly adopted is to provide a brief discussion of the highest level of organization, the supergroups, and then reference the familiar names of the other clades (e.g., Apicomplexa). The names for the lowest clades—genus and species—are retained, thus simplifying communication with clinicians and other microbiologists. This approach can be illustrated using the well-known parasites causing malaria. For most purposes, one could state that these are parasites in the clade Apicomplexa (i.e., apicomplexan parasites), genus *Plasmodium*. This is essentially the wording used today, with the exception that the clade Apicomplexa is no longer referred to as a phylum. When it is desirable to provide the full lineage as it is currently understood based on genetic analyses, one lists the clades in order of highest (supergroup) to lowest (species) separated by a colon (e.g., SAR: Apicomplexa: Aconoidasida: Haemosporida: *Plasmodium*).

MODERN CLASSIFICATION OF EUKARYOTES

Eukaryotes are now divided into five monophyletic lineages called supergroups, of which four include human parasites: SAR, Excavata, Amoebozoa, and Opisthokonta (Fig. 1). As discussed above, these supergroups replace the previous kingdoms that encompassed the eukaryotes (the plants, animals, and fungi). Protists are clades within the eukaryotes and are defined as species with a unicellular organization without cell differentiation into tissues (i.e., all eukaryotes without an embryology) (1). Using this definition, protists include what were known as protozoan parasites, free-living protozoa, fungi, and most algae. Thus, clades that encompass the multicellular organisms are the animals, plants, and the brown macro-algae. Where cell differentiation occurs in protists, it is limited to sexual cells with complementary mating types, an alternate vegetative morphology (such as a trophozoite), and quiescent or resistant stages such as cysts or spores. Dispersal occurs by cysts (from mitosis and vegetative reproduction) or by spores (from meiosis and sexual reproduction); the classical literature did not use these terms consistently. The morphology of protists is varied, including cells with a cell wall or without, with motility or without. Motile cells can move by gliding on surfaces, by amoeboid crawling locomotion, or by swimming in liquid with a motility organelle called a cilium (commonly but incorrectly referred to as a flagellum). Unfortunately, the term "flagellum" continues to be applied indiscriminately to the motility organelle in both prokaryotes and eukaryotes. However, the molecular structures and mechanisms of motion generation of the bacterial flagellum and the eukaryotic cilium are unrelated and dissimilar. Thus, they are sensitive to different pharmaceuticals. For the purposes of this chapter, we use the correct terminology. Unlike bacterial flagella (with assembled flagellin monomers and an anchoring molecular motor), the eukaryotic cilium consists of tubulin monomers in a complex assembly, with additional cytoskeletal and regulatory molecules, and a very complex anchor that includes basal bodies and fibrous roots made of diverse families of

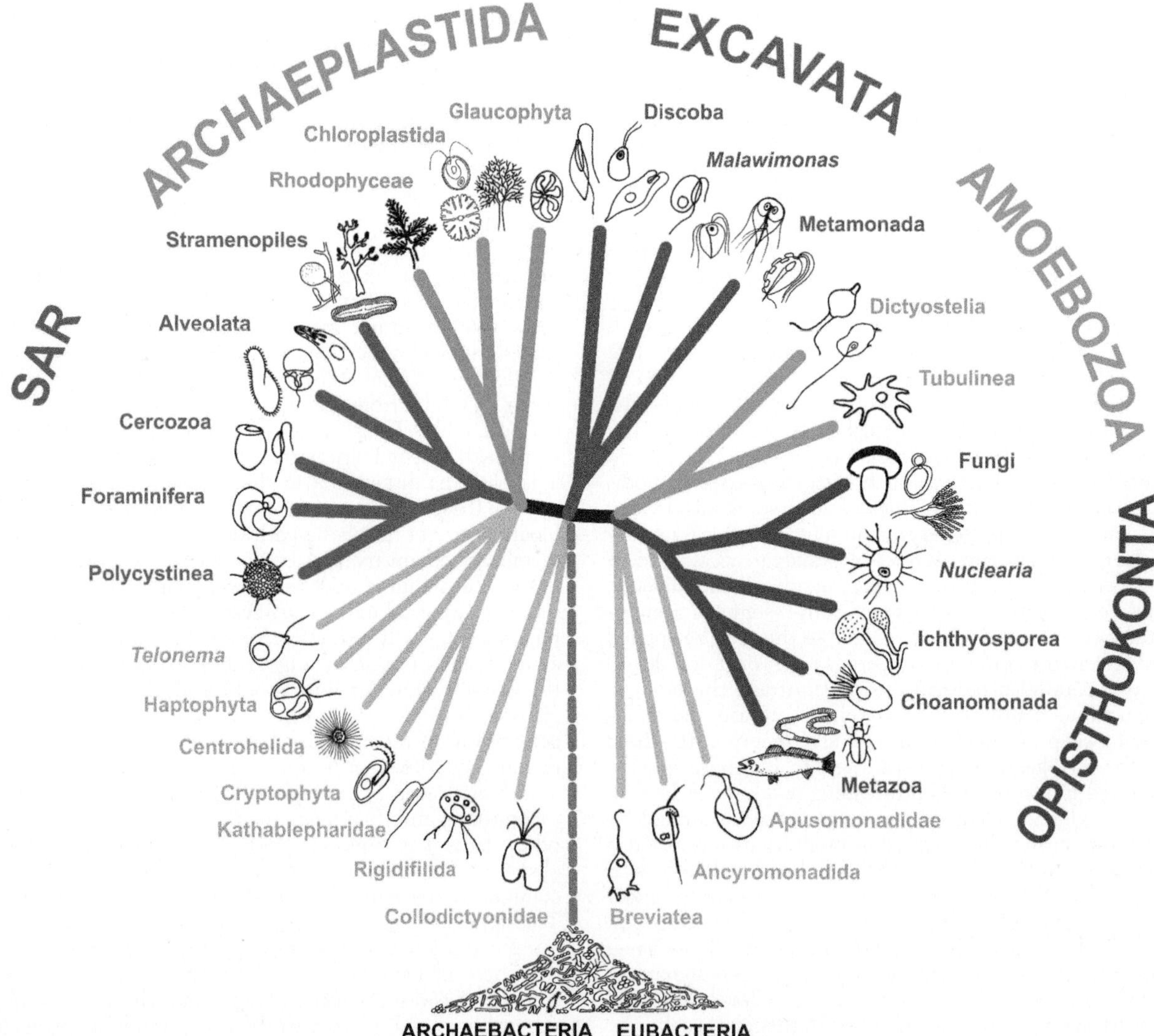

FIGURE 1 The modern classification of eukaryotes. The five monophyletic lineages known as supergroups are labeled.

cytoskeletal molecules that are phylogenetically relevant and diverse in their morphology. Most protists have one or more cilium in at least part of their life cycle; the cilia are absent (secondarily lost) in many Amoebozoa and in families scattered across the supergroups. Ameboid locomotion occurs in diverse phyla, not only in the Amoebozoa. Gliding locomotion occurs in species with or without cilia, and it is observed in many taxa.

Here, we outline the composition of the five supergroups of protists with examples that might be familiar. The multicellular worms that are parasitic to humans are also described. The Opisthokonta include the fungi, the animals, and several protist clades that are key to understanding the origin of animal and fungal metabolism and the origin of multicellularity in animals. The Amoebozoa include primarily genera with amoeboid locomotion, but some include ciliated stages in their life cycle. Important examples in this supergroup are the genera *Entamoeba*, *Endolimax*, *Iodamoeba*, *Acanthamoeba*, *Balamuthia*, and *Sappinia* (Table 1). The Amoebozoa and the Opisthokonta have a common origin and are called the Amorphea (Greek, "without form") due to their ancestrally unconstrained cell shape. The Excavata include many parasitic lineages. Many are well known to clinical microbiologists, such as *Giardia*, *Trichomonas*,

TABLE 1 Protistan parasites detected in humans[a]

Representative organism(s)[b]	Name in previous edition[c]	Modern classification	Supergroup
Giardia duodenalis (syn. *G. intestinalis*, *G. lamblia*)[d]	Metamonada (P): Trepomonadea (C): Diplomonadida (O)	Metamonada: Fornicata: Diplomonadida: Giardiinae	Excavata
Enteromonas hominis	Metamonada (P): Diplomonadida (O)	Metamonada: Fornicata: Diplomonadida: Hexamitinae	Excavata
Chilomastix[e] *mesnili*, *Retortamonas*[e] *intestinalis*	Metamonada (P): Retortamonadida (O)	Metamonada: Fornicata: Retortamonadida	Excavata
Dientamoeba fragilis	Metamonada (P): Trichomonadida (O)	Metamonada: Parabasalia: Tritrichomonadea	Excavata
Trichomonas vaginalis, *T. tenax*, *Tetratrichomonas empyemagena*, *Pentatrichimonas hominis*	Metamonada (P): Trichomonadida (O)	Metamonada: Parabasalia: Trichomonadea	Excavata
Naegleria fowleri, other *Naegleria* spp.	Heterolobosea (C): Schizopyrenida (O)	Discicristata: Heterolobosea: Tetramitia	Excavata
Leishmania donovani, *L. infantum*, *L. major*, *L. tropica*, *L. braziliensis*, *L. mexicana*, *L. aethiopica*, *L. archibaldi*, *L. amazonensis*, *L. colombiensis*, *L. garnhami*, *L. guyanensis*, *L. killicki*, *L. lainsoni*, *L. naiffi*, *L. panamensis*, *L. peruviana*, *L. pifanoi*, *L. shawi*	Trypanosomatida (O)	Discicristata: Euglenozoa: Kinetoplastea: Trypanosomatida	Excavata
Trypanosoma cruzi, ***T. brucei gambiense***,[f] ***T. brucei rhodesiense***,[f] *T. rangeli*	Trypanosomatida (O)	Discicristata: Euglenozoa: Kinetoplastea: Trypanosomatida	Excavata
Acanthamoeba castellanii, *A. astronyxis*, *A. culbertsoni*, *A. hatchetti*, *A. healyi*, *A. polyphaga*, *A. rhysodes*, other *Acanthamoeba* spp., ***Balamuthia mandrillaris***, *Sappinia diploidea*	Amoebaea (C): Acanthopodida (O) (free-living and opportunistic amoebae)	Discosea: Longamoebia: Centramoebida	Amoebozoa
Entamoeba histolytica, ***E. coli***, ***E. dispar***, ***E. hartmanni***, *E. bangladeshi*, *E. nuttalli*, *E. gingivalis*, *E. moshkovskii*, *E. chattoni*,[g] *E. polecki*,[g] *Endolimax nana*, *Iodamoeba bütschlii*	Archamoebae (C): Euamoebida (O)	Archamoebae: Entamoebida	Amoebozoa
Cryptosporidium parvum, *C. bailey*, *C. canis*, *C. felis*, ***C. hominis***, *C. meleagridis*, other species	Apicomplexa (P): Coccidea (C): Eimeriida (O)	Apicomplexa: Conoidasida: Cryptosporidium	SAR
Toxoplasma gondii, ***Cyclospora cayetanensis***, *Cystoisopora* (formerly *Isospora*) *belli*, *Sarcocystis hominis*, *S. suihominis*	Apicomplexa (P): Coccidea (C): Eimeriida (O)	Apicomplexa: Conoidasida: Coccidia: Eimeriorina	SAR
Babesia microti, *B. duncani*, *B. divergens*, *B. gibsoni*, other *Babesia* spp., ***Theileria* spp.**	Apicomplexa (P): Coccidea (C): Piroplasmida (O)	Apicomplexa: Aconoidasida: Piroplasmorida	SAR
Plasmodium knowlesi, *P. cynomolgi*, ***P. falciparum***, ***P. malariae***, ***P. ovale***, ***P. vivax***	Apicomplexa (P): Coccidea (C): Haemosporida (O)	Apicomplexa: Aconoidasida: Haemospororida	SAR
Neobalantidium* (formerly *Balantidium*) *coli	Ciliophora (P): Trichostomatia (O)	Ciliophora: Litostomatea: Trichostomatia	SAR
***Blastocystis* spp.** (designation *hominis* no longer recommended for clinical reporting)	Blastocystea (C)	Stramenopiles: *Blastocystis*	SAR

[a]An update to the classification of protists can be found in Adl et al. (25).
[b]The most common pathogens are in boldface.
[c]The formerly used ranks phylum, class, and order are abbreviated P, C, and O, respectively. These ranks are not used in the modern classification system and were arbitrarily assigned in the previous edition.
[d]The *Giardia* morphotype is most probably two cryptic species.
[e]The genera *Chilomastix* and *Retortamonas* are often confused or misidentified based on morphology, as revealed by phylogenetic studies.
[f]The two subspecies of *T. brucei* are *T. brucei gambiense* and *T. brucei rhodesiense*, but sometimes the literature lists them as *T. gambiense* and *T. rhodesiense*.
[g]*E. chattoni* is a variant of *E. polecki*.

trypanosomes, and *Leishmania*. The Archaeplastida include the green algae and the red algae and do not contain any human parasites; they are not discussed further here.

Finally, the SAR supergroup includes three very diverse monophyletic clades, the Stramenopiles, the Alveolata, and the Rhizaria (the last of which is divided into the Cercozoa, Foraminifera, and Polycystinea). The SAR and the Archaeplastida, together with a few other taxa not discussed in this chapter, form a monophyletic cluster of supergroups and clades called the Diaphoretickes (Greek, "diverse"). The Stramenopiles include *Blastocystis*, along with the brown algae and a variety of plant parasites. The Alveolata include the Ciliophora (e.g., *Balantidium*), the Dinoflagellata, and the Apicomplexa (parasitic genera historically called the Sporozoa). The Apicomplexa have the remnant of a chloroplast that has retained a small number of coding genes in most species. This plastid was of green algal origin; therefore, the enzymes differ from those of the mitochondrion and of the nuclear eukaryotic genes. This organelle has become a potential candidate for new pharmaceuticals targeted at these gene products. Important apicomplexan parasites include *Cryptosporidium*, *Toxoplasma*, *Cyclospora*, *Sarcocystis*, *Babesia*, and *Plasmodium*. The last lineage in the SAR supergroup is the Rhizaria, which does not include any human parasites.

CLASSIFICATION OF PARASITIC PROTISTS

Specific information about parasitic protists can be found in later chapters in this *Manual*. In this section, we outline basic characters of the parasitic protists by clade (Table 1) and the state of their classification at the level of family and genus. Species are identified by sequencing of the 18S small rRNA gene regions and phylogenetic analysis, and the species identification is verified against reference sequences.

Giardia, *Enteromonas*, *Chilomastix*, *Retortamonas*, *Dientamoeba*, *Trichomonas*, and *Pentatrichomonas*

The genera *Giardia*, *Enteromonas*, *Chilomastix*, *Retortamonas*, *Dientamoeba*, *Trichomonas*, and *Pentatrichomonas* belong to the supergroup Excavata (2) and are anaerobic or microaerophilic. The mitochondria are reduced, without a chromosome, and incapable of respiration. These reduced mitochondria are called hydrogenosomes and mitosomes, depending on the functions retained. All feed by pinocytosis unless stated otherwise. All are responsible for intestinal infections, except *Trichomonas vaginalis* (a genitourinary parasite) and *Trichomonas tenax* (an oral parasite). *Giardia* (Metamonada: Fornicata: Diplomonadida: Giardiinae) has a pair of nuclei and four cilia, and the organisms appear as two mirror-image halves. Giardiinae are obligate intestinal parasites in many mammals and birds. *Enteromonas* (Diplomonadida: Hexamitinae) has lost the mirror-image arrangement and retains one nucleus and two cilia. It uses a different codon for glutamine (TAR). It has a feeding groove (cytostome). *Chilomastix* and *Retortamonas* are intestinal parasites, as are all species in the Retortamonadida except one known free-living species. The two genera are morphologically distinguished by having four cilia (*Chilomastix*) or two cilia (*Retortamonas*). However, phylogenetic studies do not support the monophyly of this group, and they are thus considered separate lineages.

Dientamoeba, *Trichomonas*, and *Pentatrichomonas* are Excavata genera that belong to the Parabasalia. They have hydrogenosomes and cytoskeletal elements (parabasal body) that link the cilia basal bodies to the Golgi apparatus. There are additional complex cytoskeletal structures to facilitate gliding in viscous fluids. The trophozoite *Dientamoeba* (Parabasalia: Tritrichomonadea) is without cilia, has two nuclei, and does not form cysts. *Trichomonas* and *Pentatrichomonas* (Parabasalia: Trichomonadea) also do not form cysts. *Pentatrichomonas* has six cilia and feeds by pinocytosis of the intestinal fluids and phagocytosis of bacteria. *Trichomonas* is one of the most common sexually transmitted protist pathogens in humans. More recently, a number of Parabasalia species were described from human respiratory tract infections.

Naegleria, *Leishmania*, and *Trypanosoma*

Naegleria, *Leishmania*, and *Trypanosoma* belong to the Excavata in a clade called the Discicristata (2). In addition to many shared traits (apomorphies) in the arrangement of the cytoskeleton, they have mitochondria with flat or disc-shaped cristae.

Naegleria (Heterolobosea: Tetramitia) has two locomotive forms; one is the amoeboid trophozoite, and the other is the dispersal ciliated form. Although both forms are capable of pinocytosis, only the amoeboid form is capable of phagocytosis of bacteria. It is a free-living bacterium-feeding amoeba typically found in soil or encysted in freshwater sediments and disturbed resuspended sediment. Some strains of *Naegleria fowleri* are opportunistic parasites that cause primary amebic meningoencephalitis.

Both *Leishmania* and *Trypanosoma* (Euglenozoa: Kinetoplastea) have one cilium emerging from a tubular feeding structure (cytostome) capable of pinocytosis. Their taxonomy has been revised recently (4). The mitochondrion has a characteristic mass of DNA that consists of multiple copies of the circular chromosome entangled like chain mail (catenated). There are two types, maxicircles and minicircles. Maxicircles are catenated replicated copies of the mitochondrial circular chromosome, numbering in the dozens, each 20 to 40 kb in size. The minicircles are 0.5 to 1 kb in size, numbering in the thousands, and code for guide RNA. The mitochondrial pre-mRNA from the maxicircles requires substantial editing of the genetic code before the mRNA can be usefully translated into a protein. The editing occurs by insertion or deletion of uridine by the guide RNA from the minicircles. The complexity of RNA editing in the mitochondria of Euglenozoa is perplexing.

Trypanosoma organisms infect vertebrate hosts and are transmitted by sanguivorous (hematophagous) insect vector species (with very few exceptions). The *Trypanosoma* species are subdivided into nine clades (no longer subgenera). The clade *Trypanozoon* has three species: *Trypanosoma brucei*, *T. evansi*, and *T. equiperdum*. However, new results show that the latter two are strains or subspecies of *T. brucei* (this eliminates the need for the subgenus). In humans, *T. brucei* species complex members are responsible for sleeping sickness and are transmitted by the tsetse fly (*Glossina* spp.) through the salivary glands. The causative agents are *Trypanosoma brucei rhodesiense* and *T. brucei gambiense*. *Trypanosoma cruzi* causes Chagas disease and is transmitted by insects from the subfamily Triatominae (kissing bugs); the insect feces on the host skin contain infective cells that can penetrate host tissues. *T. cruzi* can be further subdivided into clusters based on phylogenetic analysis of mitochondrial or nuclear genes. Recent studies tend to accept three *T. cruzi* species clusters instead of seven.

Leishmania organisms infect vertebrate hosts, most commonly Canidae, Procaviidae (four known species), Rodentia, and humans. They are transmitted by at least 93 species of sand flies (*Phlebotomus*) in the Old World and by at least 33 species of sand flies (*Lutzomyia*) in the Americas. Both genera of sand flies are sanguivorous and belong to the Diptera (Psychodidae: Phlebotominae). Only females bite a host for a blood meal. Some species of the sand flies are more specific about choice of prey to bite, whereas others are less selective. There are about 53 species of *Leishmania*, with about 20 being infective to humans. The infective promastigote form has a cilium and occurs in the intestinal tract of the sand fly. The amastigote form (without cilium) is found as an intracellular parasite of blood mononuclear phagocytes and in the circulatory system.

Acanthamoeba, Balamuthia, Entamoeba, Endolimax, and *Iodamoeba*

The amoeboid protist genera *Acanthamoeba*, *Balamuthia*, *Entamoeba*, *Endolimax*, and *Iodamoeba* belong to the supergroup Amoebozoa (2). *Acanthamoeba* and *Balamuthia* (Discosea: Longamoebia: Centramoebida) are flat and elongated, with pseudopodia and characteristic subpseudopodia. They feed on bacteria by phagocytosis in the soil, forming resistant cysts for quiescence and dispersal. Both genera have species that can be opportunistic parasites in humans causing granulomatous amoebic encephalitis. The genus *Entamoeba* (Archamoebae: Entamoebidae) can probably be subdivided into several clades by molecular phylogenetic studies. There are very few free-living isolates, with species being found in animal oral cavity and intestinal samples. There are few organelles (the organisms are without cilia, centrioles, or peroxisomes), and notably, the mitochondria are reduced to noncoding mitosomes that do not contribute to respiration or energy generation. The endomembrane and secretory membranes are greatly reduced. These species feed on gut bacteria by phagocytosis. Dispersal is by cysts that form in stools. *Endolimax* and *Iodamoeba* are related to the Entamoebidae and similarly have reduced nonaerobic mitochondria, with cyst dispersal. The genus *Endolimax* has been found in the intestines of various animals, where it feeds on bacteria by phagocytosis, with one species, *Endolimax nana*, being found in human samples. *Iodamoeba bütschlii* occurs in human intestines and feeds by phagocytosis on bacteria and yeasts.

Babesia, Plasmodium, Cryptosporidium, Cyclospora, Cystoisospora, Sarcocystis, and *Toxoplasma*

The genera *Babesia*, *Plasmodium*, *Cryptosporidium*, *Cyclospora*, *Cystoisospora*, *Sarcocystis*, and *Toxoplasma* belong to the Apicomplexa (Alveolata: Apicomplexa) clade in the supergroup SAR (2). The Apicomplexa are a lineage of genera that are parasites of vertebrate and invertebrate animals and of a few protists, such as ciliates and foraminifera (5). Key characteristics are flattened vesicles against the cell membrane at least in one life cycle stage, and an apical complex for host cell penetration. Locomotion is typically by gliding and body flexion. Nutrition is by pinocytosis.

The Aconoidasida (*Babesia* and *Plasmodium*) lack the conoid of the apical complex in the asexual motile form. In Haemosporida, the motile diploid zygotes (ookinetes) retain the conoid. Macrogametes and microgametes form independently, with a heteroxenous life cycle. *Plasmodium* (Aconoidasida: Haemosporida) is responsible for malaria and requires a vertebrate host and an insect vector. Asexual reproduction is by schizogony. The motile zygote retains the conoid. Microgametes move with a cilium, and oocyst nuclear divisions form sporozoites. *Babesia* (Aconoidasida: Piroplasmorida) are hemolytic blood parasites of vertebrates, and some species infect humans. The conoid and cilium are always absent, but the polar ring of the apical complex is present. Piroplasmorida are without an oocyst stage, and sexuality is probably associated with large pseudopodium-like extensions (known as Strahlen).

The Conoidasida (*Cryptosporidium*, *Cyclospora*, *Cystoisospora*, *Sarcocystis*, and *Toxoplasma*) have an apical complex, including the conoid, in all or most asexual stages. Cells move by gliding, with flexion or undulation of pellicular ridges, and microgametes may have a cilium for motility. Classification within the Conoidasida is still in flux, but at least three clades are recognized: (i) the Coccidia, (ii) the Gregarinasina, and (iii) *Cryptosporidium*. Species of *Cryptosporidium* are responsible for respiratory and intestinal tract infections in many mammals. Oocysts have a feeder attachment organelle. The oocysts are without sporocysts and form four naked sporozoites; the microgametes are without cilia. The life cycle is completed in one host, and cysts are excreted through feces. Typically, ingested oocysts excyst in the duodenum. A second form of transmission occurs via inhaling contaminated fomites. The remaining genera (*Cyclospora*, *Cystoisospora*, *Sarcocystis*, and *Toxoplasma*) belong to the Coccidia in the Eimeriorina (Conoidasida: Coccidia: Eimeriorina). They are characterized by having a zygote that is rarely motile, with gamete maturation occurring intracellularly, a microgamont that releases many microgametes with a cilium, and oocysts that form a sporocyst for dispersal of sporozoites; syzygy is absent. *Cyclospora cayetanensis* infects humans, and other species are known to infect primates. *Cystoisospora* has been found in mammals. *Sarcocystis* infects reptiles and birds too, but mostly mammals. All three genera cause intestinal infections in their hosts. *Toxoplasma* is an obligate intracellular parasite of all warm-blooded animals, wherein it infects host tissues; Felidae (cats) are the definitive host, where sexual reproduction occurs.

Neobalantidium

The genus *Neobalantidium*, previously known as *Balantidium*, belongs to the clade Ciliophora of the Alveolata in the supergroup SAR (6). *Neobalantidium* occurs in several mammals, where it is an intestinal endosymbiont that is often nonpathogenic and asymptomatic. It forms cysts in excreted feces, and it is normally transmitted through the oral-fecal route. Excystment occurs in the intestines where the trophozoite ingests bacteria by phagocytosis. *Neobalantidium coli* (Ciliophora: Litostomatea: Trichostomatia) is the only ciliate (i.e., Ciliophora) known to be a human parasite. All genera of the Trichostomatia are typically vertebrate endosymbionts. They have the characteristic ciliature of the Litostomatea.

Blastocystis

The genus *Blastocystis* belongs to the Stramenopiles in the SAR supergroup. *Blastocystis* stands alone without further classification in the Stramenopiles as a genus of anaerobic commensals or parasites of the intestinal tract of many (maybe even all) vertebrates and some invertebrates (7). Cells lack morphology and appear yeast-like, although slightly amoeboid forms have been observed. The remnant of the mitochondrion retains a small number of genes, and its metabolism has received considerable attention. Trophozoites feed on intestinal fluids, and a cyst form also exists. Species are nonspecific to hosts, and infections can include several genetic varieties. The convention of naming species of *Blastocystis* by the host species is therefore not supported by phylogenetic studies. For this reason, the species epithet "*hominis*" is no longer considered valid; instead, the clade to which it belongs is identified by the DNA sequence of the

18S small rRNA gene. While researchers tend to refer to *Blastocystis* genotypes or subtypes based on sequence data, these genetic types are morphologically indistinguishable by light microscopy, and therefore it is most practical for the clinical microbiologist to simply report "*Blastocystis* sp." on stool parasite examination reports.

CLASSIFICATION OF PARASITIC WORMS AND ARTHROPODS

Within the supergroup Opisthokonta, the animals fall within the Holozoa (Holozoa: Metazoa: Animalia). The Holozoa include several protist clades, as well as the Metazoa. The Metazoa include the sponges and the Animalia. Within the Animalia, species parasitic to humans occur in the Bilateria (animals with bilateral body symmetry and three basic germ layers). Within the Bilateria, they belong to the Protostomia (at gastrulation of the embryo, the blastopore becomes the mouth opening). The Protostomia are divided basically into three clades (Table 2). One includes the arrow worms (Chaetognatha); they are not discussed here. Another includes the Arthropoda, Nematoda, Priapulida, and other lineages and is named the Ecdysozoa (with growth through molting and a tubular digestive tract). The last includes Mollusca, Annelida, Platyhelminthes (including cestodes and trematodes), and other lineages in a clade named the Spiralia (with spiral cleavage of cells in early embryogenesis). Within the Spiralia, the human parasites we are concerned with occur in the Lophotrochozoa (with a larval stage that possesses a lophophore, at least ancestrally, that has a tuft of tentacles bearing cilia around the mouth opening). The term Lophotrochozoa is used by some incorrectly to refer to all the Spiralia. The five groups of parasites discussed below belong to the Protostomia. The Acanthocephala, Trematoda, and Cestoda belong to the Lophotrochozoa, and the Nematoda and Arthropoda belong to the Ecdysozoa.

Acanthocephala

Commonly called thorny-headed worms, the Acanthocephala are endoparasitic worms evolutionarily derived from the free-living rotifers and placed together in the clade Syndermata (Platyhelminthes: Syndermata: Acanthocephala) (8). The Acanthocephala are further subdivided into three clades: the Archiacanthocephala, the Eoacanthocephala, and the Palaeacanthocephala (9). The spined proboscis in the adult is used to attach to the intestine wall of the definitive host, and transmission is through eggs in feces. The intermediate host is typically an arthropod, and definitive hosts are Gnathostomata (jawed vertebrates), Actinopterygii (ray-finned fish), amphibians, and mammals, including livestock and humans. There about 1,100 described species, but many others exist in hosts that have not been studied. Human infections are uncommon, and *Moniliformis moniliformis* (Archiacanthocephala: Moniliformidae) is the most common species encountered in clinical labs. However, six others have been implicated in human infections (10, 11), including *Macracanthorhynchus hirudinaceus*, *M. ingens*, *Acanthocephalus bufonis*, *Corynosoma strumosum*, *Plagiorhynchus* sp., and *Bolbosoma* species.

TABLE 2 Classification of Protostomia (Animalia: Bilateria) animals relevant to human parasites

Classification	Members
Chaetognatha	Arrow worms (no known human parasites)
Ecdysozoa	Arthropoda, Nematoda, Priapulida, and others
Spiralia: Lophotrochozoa	Acanthocephala, Cestoda, Trematoda

Trematoda

There are two subclasses of Trematoda (Platyhelminthes: Neodermata: Trematoda), all obligate parasites (12). The Aspidogastrea infect molluscs, and the Digenea (commonly called flukes) are parasites of molluscs and vertebrates. They are characterized by a syncytial tegument and two suckers, one ventral and one oral. About 80 families are recognized, and about 6,000 species have been described so far, but about 13 species occur in humans with any frequency (Table 3), affecting more than 250 million people. There are several genera, called tissue flukes, that cause foodborne infections, while the *Schistosoma* species infect from a snail host through contact with infected freshwater bearing the parasites and pass through the blood; thus, they are called blood flukes. Unlike other flukes, which are monoecious (hermaphroditic), the *Schistosoma* are dioecious, with separate male and female sexes.

Cestoda

Commonly called tapeworms, all Cestoda (Platyhelminthes: Neodermata: Cestoda) are obligate enteric parasites. There are at least 19 orders that can be distinguished by molecular phylogenies (13–15), but the arrangement of genera into monophyletic families remains in flux as research continues. There are more than 7,000 known species, but many others exist in various animals. Two orders contain species that infect humans (Table 4). Pseudophyllidea adults have multiple segments (proglottids) and two sucking grooves (bothria). The segments have characteristic midventral genital and uterine pores, with a bilobed ovary, and characteristic egg morphology. The family Diphyllobothriidae includes species parasitic to humans, which can be definitive (*Dibothriocephalus*, *Diphyllobothrium*, *Adenocephalus*) or incidental (*Spirometra*) hosts, but its classification is in flux, as it is paraphyletic. Mammals are the definitive hosts, with copepods or copepods and fish as intermediate hosts. The second order, the Cyclophyllidea, holds 15 families, and there are at least 3,100 known species. The order contains the Taeniidae, which include genera of medical importance, such as *Taenia* and *Echinococcus*. There are five other families of significance in the Cyclophyllidea (Table 4). They are characterized by multiple proglottid segments, four suckers on the scolex for attachment to the host, a genital opening on one side (except for the Dilepididae, where there are openings on both sides), and a compact yolk gland posterior to the ovary.

Nematoda

Commonly called roundworms, the Nematoda belong to the Ecdysozoa, the sister clade to the Lophotrochozoa. At least 20,000 species are described, but most estimates expect about 1 million species to exist. Their large diversity is due to the fact that they inhabit all habitats, from the deep sea to the mountain peaks, across all latitudes. They are classified into five clades (labelled I to V), each with a name (16–19). Clades III to V and related lineages are grouped together in a parent clade called the Chromadoria. The phylogeny of the orders and families of nematodes is still in flux, particularly for the Chromadoria and clade III, as the research has not been completed. Vertebrate parasites must have originated independently at least four times. They occur in the Trichinellida and Dioctophymatida

TABLE 3 Trematoda (Animalia: Spiralia: Lophotrochozoa: Platyhelminthes: Neodermata: Trematoda: Digenea)

Species[a]	Classification in previous edition	Modern classification (order and family)
Schistosoma mansoni*, *S. guineensis*, *S. haematobium*, *S. japonicum*, *S. intercalatum, *S. mekongi*, *S. bovis*, *S. malayensis*, *S. mattheei*, *Schistosoma* spp., *Austrobilharzia terrigalensis*, *Bilharziella polonica*, *Gigantobilharzia sturniae*, *G. huttoni*, *Heterobilharzia americana*, *Microbilharzia variglandis*, *Orientobilharzia turkestanicum*, *Trichobilharzia* spp.	Diplostomida: Schistosomatidae	Strigeatida: Schistosomatidae
Clinostomum complanatum	Diplostomida: Clinostomidae	Diplostomida: Clinostomidae
Alaria alata, *A. americana*, *Diplostomum spathaceum*, *Neodiplostomum seoulensis*	Diplostomida: Diplostomatidae	Strigeatida: Diplostomatidae
Philophthalmus spp.		Echinostomida: Philophthalmidae
Gastrodiscoides hominis, *Watsonius watsoni*	Plagiorchiida: Zygocotylidae	Echinostomida: Paramphistomidae
Echinostoma hortense, *E. echinatum*, *E. macrorchis*, *E. revolutum*, *E. ilocanum*, *E. perfoliatum*, *Acanthoparyphium kurogamo*, *A. tyosenense*, *Artyfechinostomum malayanum*, *Echinoparyphium recurvatum*, *Echinochasmus* spp., *Hypoderaeum conoideum*	Plagiorchiida: Echinostomatidae	Echinostomida: Echinostomatidae
Fasciola hepatica, *F. gigantica*, ***Fasciolopsis buski***	Plagiorchiida: Fasciolidae	Echinostomida: Fasciolidae
Apophallus donicus, *Centrocestus cuspidatus*, *C. formosanus*, *Cryptocotyle lingua*, *Haplorchis* spp., *Heterophyes heterophyes*, *Heterophyes* spp., *Metagonimus yokogawai*, *M. takahashii*, *M. miyatai*, *Pygidiopsis summa*, *Stellantchasmus falcatus*, *Stichodora* spp.	Plagiorchiida: Heterophyidae	Opisthorchiida: Heterophyidae
Clonorchis sinensis*, *Opisthorchis felineus*, *O. viverrini	Plagiorchiida: Opisthorchidae	Opisthorchiida: Opisthorchiidae
Phaneropsolus bonnie, *P. spinicirrus*, *P. molenkampi*	Plagiorchiida: Lecithodendriidae	Plagiorchiida: Lecithodendriidae
Paragonimus westermani*, *P. heterotremus*, *P. kellicotti, *P. uterobilateralis*, *P. africanus*, *P. mexicanus* complex, *P. miyazakii*, *P. ohirai*, *P. pulmonalis*, *P. skrjabini*	Plagiorchiida: Paragonimidae	Plagiorchiida: Troglotrematidae
Dicrocoelium dendriticum, *Eurytrema pancreaticum*	Plagiorchiida: Dicrocoeliidae	Plagiorchiida: Dicrocoeliidae
Plagiorchis spp.	Plagiorchiida: Plagiorchiidae	Plagiorchiida: Plagiorchiidae
Nanophyetus salmincola	Plagiorchiida: Troglotrematiidae	Plagiorchiida: Troglotrematiidae
Achillurbainia spp.	Plagiorchiida: Achillurbainiidae	Plagiorchiida: Achillurbainiidae

[a]More important species are in boldface; less common species are in lightface.

TABLE 4 Cestoda (Animalia: Spiralia: Lophotrochozoa: Platyhelminthes: Neodermata: Cestoda)

Species[a]	Classification (order and family)
Dibothriocephalus latus*, *D. nihonkaiensis, *D. dendriticus*, *D. dalliae*, ***Adenocephalus pacificus***, *Diphyllobothrium stemmacephalum*, *D. balaennopterae*	Pseudophyllidea: Diphyllobothriidae (26)
Bertiella mucronata, *B. studeri*, *Inermicapsifer cubensis*, *I. madagascariensis*, *Mathevotaenia symmetrica*	Cyclophyllidea: Anoplocephalidae
Buginetta alouattae, *Raillietina celebensis*, *R. demerariensis*	Cyclophyllidea: Davaineidae
Dipylidium caninum	Cyclophyllidea: Dipylidiidae
Hymenolepis nana, *Hymenolepis diminuta*	Cyclophyllidea: Hymenolepididae
Mesocestoides variabilis, *M. lineatus*	Cyclophyllidea: Mesocestoidae
Taenia saginata*, *T. solium, *T. asiatica*, *T. serialis*, *T. multiceps*, ***Echinococcus granulosus*, *E. multilocularis***, *E. vogeli*, *E. oligarthrus*, *E. canadensis*, *E. ortleppi*	Cyclophyllidea: Taeniidae

[a]More important species are in boldface; less common species are in lightface.

(Dorylaimia, clade I); in all six groups of clade III (Spirurina, clade III), namely, the Ascaridomorpha, the Spiruromorpha, the Rhigonematomorpha, the Oxyuridomorpha, the Gnathostomatomorpha, and the Dracunculoidea; in the Panagrolaimomorpha (Tylenchina, clade IV); and in the Rhabditomorpha (Rhabditina, clade V). None are known in the Enoplia (clade II) or other lineages within the Chromadoria. Only about 16 species infect humans with any frequency (Table 5).

Arthropoda

The arthropods also belong to the Ecdysozoa, and they are divided into the subphyla Trilobitomorpha (trilobites; all extinct), Chelicerata (scorpions, spiders, mites, ticks, and relatives), Crustacea (crabs, shrimp, crayfish, and pentatomids), Myriapoda (centipedes and millipedes), and Hexapoda (including the insects), plus a few extinct taxa of uncertain affinities (20). Medically important taxa occur in all four extant subphyla, with obligate parasites in Crustacea, Chelicerata, and Hexapoda.

Myriapoda contains four extant classes, and several groupings of these classes have been proposed (21). Only two classes have medically important species: Chilopoda (centipedes) and Diplopoda (millipedes). Some centipedes (especially members of the order Scolopendromorpha) can have venomous bites. Millipedes produce poisonous defensive secretions or serve as intermediate hosts for parasites, such as *M. ingens* (Acanthocephala).

TABLE 5 Nematoda (Animalia: Ecdysozoa: Nematoda)

Species[a]	Classification [order (suborder)[b]: family]
Clade I: Dorylaimia	
Capillaria philippinensis, ***C. hepatica***, *C. aerophila*	Trichocephalida: Capillariidae
Trichinella spiralis, ***T. pseudospiralis***, ***T. nativa***, *T. nelsoni*, *T. britovi*, *T. papuae*, *Trichinella* spp.	Trichocephalida: Trichinellidae
Anatrichosoma spp.	Trichocephalida: Trichosomoididae
Trichuris trichiura	Trichocephalida: Trichuridae
Dioctophyme renale, *Eustrongylides* spp.	Dioctophymatida: Dioctophymatidae
Haycocknema perplexum	Muspiceida: Robertdollfusidae
Clade III: Chromadoria: Spururina	
Ascaris lumbricoides (syn. *A. suum*), *Baylisascaris procyonis*, *Lagochilascaris minor*	Ascaridida: Ascarididae
Anisakis simplex, ***Anisakis* spp.**, ***Pseudoterranova decepiens***, ***Pseudoterranova* spp.**, *Contracaecum* spp.	Ascaridida: Anisakidae
Toxocara cati, ***T. canis***, *Toxascaris leonina*	Ascaridida: Toxocaridae
Enterobius vermicularis	Oxyurida: Oxyuridae
Dracunculus medinensis	Camallanida: Dracunculidae
Brugia malayi, *B. timori*, *Brugia* spp., *Dirofilaria immitis*, *D. repens*, *D. tenuis*, *D. ursi*, ***Mansonella perstans***, ***M. ozzardi***, *M. streptocerca*, ***Onchocerca volvulus***, *O. lupi*, ***Wuchereria bancrofti***	Spirurida: Onchocercidae
Gnathostoma hispidum, *G. spinigerum*	Spirurida: Gnathostomatidae
Thelazia callipaeda, *T. californiensis*, *T. gulosa*	Spirurida: Thelaziidae
Physaloptera spp.	Spirurida: Physalopteridae
Gongylonema pulchrum	Spirurida: Gongylonematidae
Clade V: Chromadoria: Rhabditina	
Halicephalobus gingivalis, *Pelodera* spp.	Rhabditida (Rhabditida): Rhabditidae
Strongyloides stercoralis, *S. fuelleborni*, *Oesophagostomum* spp.	Rhabditida (Strongylida): Strongylidae
Mammomonogamus laryngeus	Rhabditida (Strongylida): Syngamidae
Ancylostoma duodenale, ***A. ceylanicum***, *A. braziliense*, *A. caninum*, ***Necator americanus***	Rhabditida (Strongylida): Ancylostomatidae
Angiostrongylus cantonensis, *A. costaricensis*	Rhabditida (Strongylida): Metastrongylidae
Trichostrongylus spp.	Rhabditida (Strongylida): Trichostrongylidae

[a]More important species are in boldface; less common species are in lightface.
[b]Suborders are given for Rhabditida, as these groups have been traditionally been placed in separate orders.

The Crustacea species of medical importance occur within the classes Maxillopoda and Malacostraca. Examples include copepods (Maxillopoda: Copepoda) as intermediate hosts of *Dracunculus medinensis* (Nematoda Guinea worm) and diphyllobothriid cestodes (tapeworms) and various crabs and crayfish (Malacostraca: Eumalacostraca: Decapoda) as intermediate hosts of *Paragonimus* spp. (a trematode fluke). Pentastomes, which are commonly referred to as tongue worms (Maxillopoda: Pentastomida: Porocephalida), are the causal agents of visceral pentastomiasis (Table 6).

The Chelicerata are divided into two classes: Merostomata contain the horseshoe crabs (Xiphosura) and the extinct sea scorpions (Eurypterida), and Arachnida includes spiders, scorpions, mites, and ticks. Only the class Arachnida contains medically important species. The phylogeny of Arachnida and of Acari in particular remains in flux and requires further research (22). Arachnids can be medically important in a variety of ways. A few spiders (Araneae) and many scorpions (Scorpionida) can inflict potentially life-threatening bites and stings, respectively. Some spiders (e.g., tarantulas in the family Theraphosidae) possess urticating hairs. Dust mites (Acari: Pyroglyphidae) and their feces can cause severe allergic reactions. The most medically important arachnids are the obligate ectoparasitic ticks and mites in the subclass Acari (Table 6), including *Sarcoptes scabiei* (the causal agent of scabies), hard ticks (Ixodidae), and soft ticks (Argasidae). Ticks are vectors of many serious disease-causing agents, including *Borrelia burgdorferi* (Lyme disease), *Babesia* spp. (babesiosis), *Rickettsia rickettsiae* (Rocky Mountain spotted fever), relapsing fever spirochetes, and Crimean-Congo hemorrhagic fever virus, among many others (23).

Hexapoda contains two classes: Entognatha (which contains microscopic soil-dwelling animals of no medical importance) and Insecta (insects), the most diverse class of extant animals. There are approximately 28 extant orders of insects, depending on the classification scheme used (24), roughly eight of which contain medically important species. There is a vast multitude of ways in which insects can be of medical importance, most notably as vectors of many agents of debilitating diseases, including the agents of malaria and plague and numerous arboviruses, or as intermediate hosts for helminthic infections (see chapter 151 for a comprehensive review of insects and other arthropods of medical importance). The focus of Table 6 is the ectoparasites most commonly encountered by clinical, diagnostic, and reference laboratories. Insect ectoparasites of humans are found in the orders Hemiptera (true bugs), Psocodea (Psocoptera + Phthiraptera [Anoplura + Mallophaga], the lice), Diptera (flies), and Siphonaptera (fleas, all of which are obligate parasites of mammals or birds as adults) (Table 6) (23).

It is remarkable that despite the millions of eukaryotic species estimated, so few of the pathogenic genera have species that infect humans. Modern specimen analysis is

TABLE 6 Arthropoda (Animalia: Ecdysozoa)

Representative genus and species	Order and family	Medical importance
Crustacea: Class Maxillopoda, subclass Pentastomida		
Armillifer armillatus, *A. grandis*, *Porocephalus crotali*	Porocephalida: Porocephalidae	Agents of pentastomiasis
Linguatula serrata	Porocephalida: Linguatulidae	Agents of pentastomiasis
Class Arachnida, subclass Acari (mites and ticks)		
Sarcoptes scabiei	Sarcoptiformes: Sarcoptidae (itch mites)	Agent of scabies
Ornithonyssus bacoti, *O. bursa*, *O. sylviarum*, *Dermanyssus gallinae*, *Liponyssoides sanguineus*, *Laelaps echidnina*	Mesostigmata: Macronyssidae, Dermanyssidae, Laelapidae (avian, rodent mites)	Zoonotic biting mites
Pyemotes tritici	Trombidiformes: Pyemotidae (itch mites)	Zoonotic biting mites
Demodex folliculorum, *D. brevis*	Trombidiformes: Demodicidae (follicle mites)	Agents of demodicosis
Leptotrombidium spp.	Trombidiformes: Trombiculidae (chiggers)	Vectors of agent of scrub typhus
Cheyletiella spp.	Trombidiformes: Cheyletidae (cheyletiellid mites)	Zoonotic biting mites
Ixodes scapularis, *I. pacificus*, *I. ricinus*, *I. holocyclus*, *Dermacentor variabilis*, *D. andersoni*, *Rhipicephalus sanguineus*, *Amblyomma americanum*, *A. maculatum*, *Hyalomma marginatum*, *H. truncatum*, *Haemaphysalis spinigera*, *H, hystricis*, *H. bispinosa*	Ixodida: Ixodidae (hard ticks)	Vectors of agents of babesiosis, Lyme borreliosis, ehrlichiosis, anaplasmosis, boutonneuse fever, Tidewater spotted fever, tularemia, Colorado tick fever, Crimean-Congo hemorrhagic fever, tick-borne encephalitis, Kyasanur Forest disease, Powassan virus fever, many others; agents of tick paralysis
Ornithodoros turicata, *O. hermsi*, *O. moubata*, *O. savignyi*, *Otobius megnini*	Ixodida: Argasidae (soft ticks)	Vectors of tick-borne relapsing fever spirochetes
Class Hexapoda, subclass Insecta		
Cimex lectularius, *C. hemipterus*, *C. pilosellus*, *C. adjunctus*	Hemiptera: Cimicidae (bed and bat bugs)	Nuisance pests
Triatoma infestans, *Rhodnius prolixus*, *Panstrongylus megistus*	Hemiptera: Reduviidae (assassin bugs)	Vectors of agent of Chagas disease
Pediculus humanus humanus, *P. h. capitis*	Psocodea: Pediculidae (primate sucking lice)	Vectors of agents of epidemic typhus, trench fever, louse-borne relapsing fever; nuisance pests
Pthirus pubis	Psocodea: Pthiridae (pubic lice)	Nuisance pests
Musca domestica, *M. autumnalis*, *Fannia* spp.	Diptera: Muscidae and Fanniidae (house flies)	Facultative myiasis; vectors of agents of thelaziasis
Phormia spp., *Cochliomyia hominovorax*, *C. macellaria*, *Calliphora* spp., *Chrysomya bezziana*, *Auchmeromyia senegalensis*	Diptera: Calliphoridae (blow flies)	Facultative myiasis
Sarcophaga spp., *Wohlfahrtia vigil*, *W. opaca*	Diptera: Sarcophagidae (flesh flies)	Facultative myiasis
Cuterebra spp., *Dermatobia hominis*, *Oestrus ovis*, *Gasterophilus* spp., *Hypoderma* spp.	Diptera: Oestridae (bot flies)	Obligatory myiasis
Xenopsylla cheopis, *Pulex irritans*, *Ctenocephalides felis*, *C. canis*	Siphonaptera: Pulicidae (human, cat, dog, and rodent fleas)	Vectors of agents of plague, feline rickettsiae, and murine typhus; intermediate hosts of *Dipylidium*, *Hymenolepis*
Tunga penetrans, *T. trimamillata*	Siphonaptera: Tungidae (chigoe fleas)	Agents of tungiasis

discovering new opportunistic pathogens related to known pathogenic groups, but others unrelated to known pathogenic genera will continue to be encountered. We are now able to identify environmental strains of concern within species, so that markers can be developed.

REFERENCES

1. **Adl SM, Simpson AGB, Farmer MA, Andersen RA, Anderson OR, Barta JR, Bowser SS, Brugerolle G, Fensome RA, Fredericq S, James TY, Karpov S, Kugrens P, Krug J, Lane CE, Lewis LA, Lodge J, Lynn DH, Mann DG, McCourt RM, Mendoza L, Moestrup O, Mozley-Standridge SE, Nerad TA, Shearer CA, Smirnov AV, Spiegel FW, Taylor MF.** 2005. The new higher level classification of eukaryotes with emphasis on the taxonomy of protists. *J Eukaryot Microbiol* **52:**399–451.
2. **Adl SM, Leander BS, Simpson AGB, Archibald JM, Anderson OR, Bass D, Bowser SS, Brugerolle G, Farmer MA, Karpov S, Kolisko M, Lane CE, Lodge DJ, Mann DG, Meisterfeld R, Mendoza L, Moestrup Ø, Mozley-Standridge SE, Smirnov AV, Spiegel F.** 2007. Diversity, nomenclature, and taxonomy of protists. *Syst Biol* **56:**684–689.
3. **Adl SM, Simpson AG, Lane CE, Lukeš J, Bass D, Bowser SS, Brown MW, Burki F, Dunthorn M, Hampl V, Heiss A, Hoppenrath M, Lara E, Le Gall L, Lynn DH, McManus H, Mitchell EA, Mozley-Stanridge SE, Parfrey LW, Pawlowski J, Rueckert S, Shadwick L, Schoch CL, Smirnov A, Spiegel FW.** 2012. The revised classification of eukaryotes. *J Eukaryot Microbiol* **59:**429–514.
4. **Votýpka J, d'Avila-Levy CM, Grellier P, Maslov DA, Lukeš J, Yurchenko V.** 2015. New approaches to systematics of Trypanosomatidae: criteria for taxonomic (re)description. *Trends Parasitol* **31:**460–469.

5. **Seeber F, Steinfelder S.** 2016. Recent advances in understanding apicomplexan parasites. *F1000 Res* **5:**1369.
6. **Pomajbíková K, Oborník M, Horák A, Petrželková KJ, Grim JN, Levecke B, Todd A, Mulama M, Kiyang J, Modrý D.** 2013. Novel insights into the genetic diversity of Balantidium and Balantidium-like cyst-forming ciliates. *PLoS Negl Trop Dis* **7:**e2140.
7. **Casero RD, Mongi F, Sánchez A, Ramírez JD.** 2015. Blastocystis and urticaria: examination of subtypes and morphotypes in an unusual clinical manifestation. *Acta Trop* **148:**156–161.
8. **Sielaff M, Schmidt H, Struck TH, Rosenkranz D, Mark Welch DB, Hankeln T, Herlyn H.** 2016. Phylogeny of Syndermata (syn. Rotifera): mitochondrial gene order verifies epizoic Seisonidea as sister to endoparasitic Acanthocephala within monophyletic Hemirotifera. *Mol Phylogenet Evol* **96:**79–92.
9. **Weber M, Wey-Fabrizius AR, Podsiadlowski L, Witek A, Schill RO, Sugár L, Herlyn H, Hankeln T.** 2013. Phylogenetic analyses of endoparasitic Acanthocephala based on mitochondrial genomes suggest secondary loss of sensory organs. *Mol Phylogenet Evol* **66:**182–189.
10. **Ashford RW, Crewe W.** 2003. *The Parasites of Homo sapiens—an Annotated Checklist of the Protozoa, Helminths and Arthropods for Which We Are a Home*, 2nd ed. Taylor & Francis, London, United Kingdom..
11. **Mathison BA, Bishop HS, Sanborn CR, Dos Santos Souza S, Bradbury R.** 2016. *Macracanthorhynchus ingens* infection in an 18-month-old child in Florida: a case report and review of acanthocephaliasis in humans. *Clin Infect Dis* **63:**1357–1359.
12. **Kostadinova A, Pérez-del-Olmo A.** 2014. The systematics of the trematoda. *Adv Exp Med Biol* **766:**21–44.
13. **Waeschenbach A, Webster BL, Littlewood DT.** 2012. Adding resolution to ordinal level relationships of tapeworms (Platyhelminthes: Cestoda) with large fragments of mtDNA. *Mol Phylogenet Evol* **63:**834–847.
14. **Caira JN, Jensen K, Waeschenbach A, Olson PD, Littlewood DTJ.** 2014. Orders out of chaos—molecular phylogenetics reveals the complexity of shark and stingray tapeworm relationships. *Int J Parasitol* **44:**55–73.
15. **Sharma S, Lyngdoh D, Roy B, Tandon V.** 2016. Molecular phylogeny of Cyclophyllidea (Cestoda: Eucestoda): an in-silico analysis based on mtCOI gene. *Parasitol Res* **115:** 3329–3335.
16. **Smythe AB, Sanderson MJ, Nadler SA.** 2006. Nematode small subunit phylogeny correlates with alignment parameters. *Syst Biol* **55:**972–992.
17. **Hodda M.** 2007. Phylum Nematoda. *Zootaxa* **1668:**265–293.
18. **Petrov NB, Pegova AN, Manylov OG, Vladychenskaya NS, Mugue NS, Aleshin VV.** 2007. Molecular phylogeny of Gastrotricha on the basis of a comparison of the 18S rRNA genes: rejection of the hypothesis of a relationship between Gastrotricha and Nematoda. *Mol Biol* **41:**445–452.
19. **Blaxter M.** 2011. Nematodes: the worm and its relatives. *PLoS Biol* **9:**e1001050 CORRECTION *PLoS Biol* **9**.
20. **Regier JC, Shultz JW, Zwick A, Hussey A, Ball B, Wetzer R, Martin JW, Cunningham CW.** 2010. Arthropod relationships revealed by phylogenomic analysis of nuclear protein-coding sequences. *Nature* **463:**1079–1083.
21. **Miyazawa H, Ueda C, Yahata K, Su ZH.** 2014. Molecular phylogeny of Myriapoda provides insights into evolutionary patterns of the mode in post-embryonic development. *Sci Rep* **4:**4127.
22. **Pepato AR, Klimov PB.** 2015. Origin and higher-level diversification of acariform mites—evidence from nuclear ribosomal genes, extensive taxon sampling, and secondary structure alignment. *BMC Evol Biol* **15:**178.
23. **Goddard J.** 2012. *Physician's Guide to Arthropods of Medical Importance*, 6th ed. CRC Press, Boca Raton, FL.
24. **BugGuide.** Identification, images, and information for insects, spiders, and their kin for the United States and Canada. Iowa State University, Ames, IA. http://bugguide.net/node/view/52 Accessed 30 August 2017.
25. **Adl SM, et al.** 2019. Revisions to the classification, nomenclature, and diversity of eukaryotes. *J Eukaryot Microbiol* **66,** in press.
26. **Waeschenbach A, Brabec J, Scholz T, Littlewood DTJ, Kuchta R.** 2017. The catholic taste of broad tapeworms—multiple routes to human infection. *Int J Parasitol* **47:**831–843.

Specimen Collection, Transport, and Processing: Parasitology

ROBYN Y. SHIMIZU AND LYNNE S. GARCIA

136

Routine diagnostic parasitology generally includes laboratory procedures designed to detect organisms within clinical specimens by using morphological criteria rather than culture, biochemical tools, and/or physical growth characteristics (Table 1). Parasite identification is frequently based on bright-field microscopic analysis of concentrated and/or stained preparations. Small organisms often require high magnification, such as with oil immersion (×1,000). Furthermore, new commercial test kits designed especially for detection of DNA or antigens in feces (e.g., coproantigens of *Giardia intestinalis*, *G. lamblia*, *G. duodenalis*, *Cryptosporidium* spp., and *Entamoeba histolytica* [Table 2] or circulating *Plasmodium* antigens in blood) have expanded the methodological repertoire. In addition to methods for direct parasite detection (morphology, antigens, and nucleic acid amplification tests [NAAT]), methods for indirect detection of parasite infections demonstrating specific antibodies directed to a variety of native or recombinant parasite antigens have been developed and made commercially available (Table 3). Diagnostic techniques are available to detect a large range of protozoan and helminth species in different clinical specimens. An important precondition for reliable diagnostic results is the proper collection, processing, and examination of clinical specimens. Based on the biology of the parasites and the procedural features of the tests, multiple specimens must often be submitted and examined before the suspected organism(s) is found and its identity is confirmed or a suspected infection can be excluded.

SPECIMEN COLLECTION AND TRANSPORT

Various collection methods are available for specimens suspected of containing parasites or parasitic elements (Tables 4, 5, 6, and 7) (1–7). When collection methods are selected, the decision should be based on a thorough understanding of the value and limitations of each. The final laboratory results are based on parasite recovery and identification and depend on the initial handling of the specimen. Unless the appropriate specimens are properly collected and processed, these infections may not be detected. Therefore, specimen rejection criteria have become much more important for all diagnostic microbiology procedures. Diagnostic laboratory results based on improperly collected specimens may require inappropriate expenditures of time and supplies and mislead the physician. As a part of any continuous quality improvement program for the laboratory, the generation of test results must begin with stringent criteria for specimen acceptance or rejection. In addition, diagnostic laboratories should provide clear information on preanalytical requirements to the physician.

All fresh specimens should be handled carefully, since each specimen represents a potential source of infectious material. Proper training of laboratory personnel is mandatory. Safety precautions should include personal protective equipment; proper labeling of reagents; specific areas designated for specimen handling (fume hoods to reduce chemical exposure or biological safety cabinets may be necessary under certain circumstances, such as parasite cultures); proper containers for centrifugation; acceptable discard policies; appropriate policies of no eating, drinking, or smoking in work areas; and, if applicable, correct techniques for organism culture and/or animal inoculation. Appropriate biosafety precautions should be followed; this is particularly important when blood and other body fluids are being handled (8, 9). The U.S. Centers for Disease Control and Prevention (CDC) has provided additional guidelines for processing specimens when hemorrhagic fever viruses, such as Ebola virus, are suspected (https://www.cdc.gov/vhf/ebola/laboratory-personnel/safe-specimen-management.html).

Collection of Fresh Stool

Collection of stool for parasite detection should always be performed before barium is used for radiological examination. Stool specimens containing the opaque, chalky sulfate suspension of barium are unacceptable for examination, and intestinal protozoa may be undetectable for 5 to 10 days after barium is given to the patient. Certain substances and medications also interfere with the detection of intestinal protozoa, including mineral oil, bismuth, antibiotics (metronidazole and tetracyclines), antimalarial agents, and nonabsorbable antidiarrheal preparations. After administration of any of these compounds, parasites may not be recovered for a week to several weeks. Therefore, specimen collection should be delayed for 5 to 10 days or at least 2 weeks after barium or antibiotics, respectively, are administered (1, 2, 10, 11). Some laboratories add the following comment to their negative reports: "Certain antibiotics such as metronidazole or tetracycline may interfere with the recovery of intestinal parasites, particularly the protozoa."

Fecal specimens should be collected in clean, wide-mouthed containers; often, a waxed cardboard or plastic

TABLE 1 Body sites and possible parasites recovered[a]

Site	Parasites
Blood	
RBC	*Plasmodium* spp., *Babesia* spp.
Leukocytes	*Leishmania* spp., *Toxoplasma gondii*
Whole blood/plasma	*Trypanosoma* spp., microfilariae
Bone marrow	*Leishmania* spp., *Trypanosoma cruzi*, *Plasmodium* spp., *Toxoplasma gondii*
Central nervous system	*Taenia solium* (cysticerci), *Echinococcus* spp., *Naegleria fowleri*, *Acanthamoeba* spp., *Balamuthia mandrillaris*, *Toxoplasma gondii*, microsporidia,[b] *Trypanosoma* spp.
Intestinal tract	*Entamoeba histolytica*, *Entamoeba dispar*, *Entamoeba coli*, *Entamoeba hartmanni*, *Endolimax nana*, *Iodamoeba bütschlii*, *Blastocystis* spp., *Giardia duodenalis* (*G. lamblia*, *G. intestinalis*), *Chilomastix mesnili*, *Dientamoeba fragilis*, *Pentatrichomonas hominis*, *Balantidium coli*, *Cryptosporidium* spp., *Cyclospora cayetanensis*, *Cystoisospora belli*, *Enterocytozoon bieneusi*,[b] *Encephalitozoon* spp.,[b,c] *Sarcocystis* spp., *Ascaris lumbricoides*, *Enterobius vermicularis*, hookworm, *Strongyloides stercoralis*, *Trichuris trichiura*, *Hymenolepis nana*, *Hymenolepis diminuta*, *Taenia saginata*, *Taenia solium*, *Diphyllobothrium* spp., *Clonorchis sinensis*, *Opisthorchis* spp., *Paragonimus* spp., *Schistosoma* spp., *Fasciolopsis buski*, *Fasciola hepatica*, *Metagonimus yokogawai*, *Heterophyes heterophyes*
Liver, spleen	*Echinococcus* spp., *Entamoeba histolytica*, *Leishmania* spp., microsporidia,[b] *Capillaria hepatica*, *Clonorchis sinensis*/*Opisthorchis* spp., *Fasciola hepatica*
Lungs	*Cryptosporidium* spp.,[c] *Echinococcus* spp., *Paragonimus* spp., *Toxoplasma gondii*, helminth larvae of *Ascaris lumbricoides*, *Strongyloides stercoralis*, hookworm, *Toxocara* spp.
Muscle	*Trichinella*, *Taenia solium* (cysticerci), *Trypanosoma cruzi*, microsporidia,[b] *Sarcocystis* spp.
Skin and cutaneous ulcers	*Leishmania* spp., *Acanthamoeba* spp., *Balamuthia mandrillaris*, *Onchocerca volvulus*, microfilariae, *Sarcoptes scabiei*, *Dermatobia hominis*, *Tunga penetrans*
Urogenital system	*Trichomonas vaginalis*, *Schistosoma* spp., microsporidia,[b] microfilariae
Eyes	*Acanthamoeba* spp., *Toxoplasma gondii*, *Loa loa*, microsporidia,[b] *Thelazia* spp., *Taenia solium* (cysticercosis), *Dirofilaria* spp.

[a]Parasites include trophozoites, cysts, oocysts, spores, adults, larvae, eggs, and amastigote and trypomastigote stages. This table does not include every possible parasite that could be found in a particular body site. However, the most likely organisms are listed.
[b]Traditionally classified with the protozoa, microsporidia are reclassified with the fungi.
[c]Disseminated in severely immunosuppressed individuals.

container with a tight-fitting lid is selected for this purpose. The specimens should not be contaminated with water or urine because water may contain free-living organisms that can be mistaken for human parasites, and urine may destroy motile organisms. Stool specimen containers should be placed in plastic bags when transported to the laboratory for testing. If postal delivery services are used, any diagnostic specimens must be packed according to national or international rules (e.g., labeling with UN code 3373; three-container approach). Specimens should be identified with the patient's name and identification number, physician's name, and the date and time the specimen was collected. The specimen must also be accompanied by a request form indicating which laboratory procedures should be performed. In addition to the presumptive diagnosis and travel history, state of U.S. residence may be helpful information (e.g., if *Babesia* is being considered in the differential diagnosis) and should accompany the test request. In some situations, it may be necessary to contact the physician for additional patient history.

In the past, it has been recommended that a normal examination for stool parasites before therapy include three specimens. The use of three specimens, collected as outlined above, has also been recommended for posttherapy examinations. However, a patient who has received treatment for a protozoan infection should be checked 3 to 4 weeks after therapy, and those treated for *Taenia* infections should be checked 5 to 6 weeks after therapy. In many cases, the posttherapy specimens are not collected, often as a cost containment measure; if the patient becomes symptomatic again, additional specimens can be submitted (3, 4).

Although some recommend collection of only one or two specimens, there are differences of opinion regarding this approach. It has also been suggested that three specimens be pooled and examined as a single specimen; again, this approach is somewhat controversial. However, physicians should be aware that the probability of detecting clinically relevant parasites in a single stool specimen may be as low as 50 to 60%, but the probability of detection is >95% if three samples are examined (4).

If a series of three specimens is collected, they should be submitted on separate days. If possible, the specimens should be submitted every other day; otherwise, the series of three specimens should be submitted within no more than 10 days. If a series of six specimens is requested, the specimens should also be collected on separate days or within no more than 14 days (1). Many organisms, particularly the intestinal protozoa, do not appear in the stool in consistent numbers on a daily basis, and the series of three specimens is considered the minimum for an adequate examination. Multiple specimens from the same patient should not be submitted on the same day. One possible exception would be a patient who has severe, watery diarrhea, in whom any organisms present might be missed because of a tremendous dilution factor related to fluid loss. These specimens should be accepted only after consultation with the physician. It is also not recommended that the three specimens be submitted one each day for 3 consecutive days; however, use of this collection time frame would not be cause to reject the specimens.

To evaluate patients who are at risk for giardiasis, the negative predictive value of some of the immunoassays on a single stool specimen is not sufficiently high to exclude the possibility of a *Giardia* infection. In cases in which the clinical suspicion for *Giardia* infection is moderate or high and the first assay yields a negative result, testing of a second specimen is recommended (12).

TABLE 2 Commercially available kits for immunodetection of parasitic organisms or antigens in stool samples[a]

Organism and kit name	Manufacturer and/or distributor	Type of test[b]	Comment(s)[c]
Cryptosporidium spp.			Detects *C. hominis*, different *C. parvum* genotypes, and other species, depending on intensity of the infection
ProSpecT *Cryptosporidium* microplate assay	Remel/Thermo Scientific	EIA	Can be used with unpreserved, frozen, or formalin-preserved stool. Stool in Cary-Blair transport medium is also acceptable. http://www.thermofisher.com
Xpect *Cryptosporidium* kit	Remel/Thermo Scientific	IC(Rapid)	Can be used with unpreserved, frozen, or preserved stool
PARA-TECT *Cryptosporidium*	Medical Chemical Corp.	EIA	Can be used with unpreserved, frozen, SAF-preserved, formalin-preserved, or selected single-vial-preserved stool; http://www.med-chem.com
Crypto-CELISA	Cellabs	EIA	Can be used with unpreserved, frozen, SAF-preserved, or formalin-preserved stool; http://www.cellabs.com.au
Crypto Cel	Cellabs	DFA	Can be used with unpreserved, frozen, or formalin-preserved stool
Cryptosporidium II test	TechLab/Alere	EIA	Can be used with unpreserved, frozen, SAF-preserved, or formalin-preserved stool. Transport media such as Cary-Blair or C&S are also acceptable. https://alere.com/en/home.html
Entamoeba histolytica			Differentiates between *E. histolytica* and *E. dispar*
Entamoeba histolytica II Test	TechLab/ Alere	EIA	Requires unpreserved or frozen stool
Entamoeba histolytica Quik Chek	TechLab/Alere	IC(Rapid)	Requires unpreserved or frozen stool; differentiates between *E. histolytica* and *E. dispar*
Entamoeba CELISA Path	Cellabs	EIA	Requires unpreserved or frozen stool. Transport media such as Cary-Blair and C&S are acceptable
Entamoeba histolytica/E. dispar group			Does not differentiate *E. histolytica* from *E. dispar*
ProSpecT *Entamoeba histolytica*	Remel/Thermo Scientific	EIA	Requires unpreserved or frozen stool. Cary-Blair transport medium is acceptable.
Giardia spp.			
ProSpecT *Giardia*, ProSpecT *Giardia* EZ	Remel/Thermo Scientific	EIA	Can be used with unpreserved, frozen, SAF-preserved, or formalin-preserved stool
PARA-TECT *Giardia*	Medical Chemical	EIA	Can be used with unpreserved, frozen, SAF-preserved, formalin-preserved, or selected single-vial-preserved stool
Giardia-CELISA	Cellabs	EIA	Can be used with unpreserved, frozen, SAF-preserved, or formalin-preserved stool
Giardia-Cel	Cellabs	DFA	Can be used with unpreserved, frozen, SAF-preserved, or formalin-preserved stool
Xpect *Giardia*	Remel/Thermo Scientific	IC	Can be used with unpreserved, frozen, or formalin-preserved stool
Giardia II	TechLab/Alere	EIA	Can be used with unpreserved, frozen, or formalin-preserved stool
Cryptosporidium and *Giardia* (combination tests)			
ProSpecT *Giardia/Cryptosporidium*	Remel/Thermo Scientific	EIA	Can be used with unpreserved, frozen, or formalin-preserved stool
Merifluor *Cryptosporidium/Giardia*	Meridian Bioscience	DFA	Can be used with unpreserved, frozen, SAF-preserved, or formalin-preserved stool; http://www.meridianbioscience.com
PARA-TECT *Cryptosporidium/Giardia* DFA	Medical Chemical	DFA	Can be used with unpreserved, frozen, SAF-preserved, formalin-preserved, and selected single-vial-preserved stool
Crypto/Giardia-Cel	Cellabs	DFA	Can be used with fresh, frozen, or formalin-preserved stool
ImmunoCard STAT! *Cryptosporidium/Giardia*	Meridian Bioscience	IC(Rapid)	Can be used with fresh, frozen, or formalin-preserved stool
Xpect Giardia/Cryptosporidium	Remel/Thermo Scientific	IC(Rapid)	Can be used with fresh, frozen, or formalin-preserved stool
Giardia/Cryptosporidium Chek	TechLab/Alere	EIA	Can be used with fresh, frozen, or formalin-preserved stool
Giardia/Cryptosporidium Quick Chek	TechLab/Alere	IC(Rapid)	Can be used with fresh, frozen, or formalin-preserved stool
Giardia/Cryptosporidium/Entamoeba histolytica	TechLab/Alere	EIA	Can be used with fresh or frozen stool. Differentiates between *E. histolytica* and *E. dispar*
Triage Parasite Panel	Biosite Diagnostics, Inc.	IC (Rapid)	Requires unpreserved or frozen stool; combination test with *Giardia* and *E. histolytica/E. dispar* group; does not differentiate between *E. histolytica* and *E. dispar*

[a]This is not a complete listing of all available products but reflects readily available information. It is important to review package inserts; the use of other fecal fixatives not mentioned in the package insert must be validated prior to use.
[b]EIA, enzyme immunoassay; DFA, direct fluorescent antibody; IC(Rapid), immunochromatography (membrane flow cartridge).
[c]URLs are given only the first time the company name appears in the table.

TABLE 3 Commercially available kits or antigens for immunodetection of specific serum antibodies[a]

Disease (organism)	Manufacturer and/or distributor[b]	Type of test[c]	Comment(s)
Protozoa			
Toxoplasmosis (*Toxoplasma gondii*)			See chapter 141 for serologic tests.
Amebiasis (*Entamoeba histolytica*)	Biotrin Int.	EIA	Serology is considered the best diagnostic tool for extraintestinal amebiasis. Early extraintestinal infections may be missed (follow-ups recommended); infections with *E. dispar* do not induce detectable antibodies.
	Bordier Affinity	EIA	
	Chemicon Int.	EIA	
	NovaTec	EIA	
	Scimedx Corp.	EIA	
Chagas' disease (*Trypanosoma cruzi*)	Hemagen Diagnostics	EIA	
	InBios	EIA, IC	
	NovaTec	EIA	
	Operon	EIA	
	Oxford Biosystems	EIA	
	Scimedx Corp.		
Leishmaniasis	Bordier Affinity Products	EIA	Most useful for visceral leishmaniasis
	NovaTec	EIA	
	Scimedx Corp.	EIA	
Helminths[d]			
Ascariasis	NovaTec	EIA	Cross-reactions in cases of other helminthic infections
	Oxford Biosystems	EIA	
	Scimedx Corp.	EIA	
Cysticercosis (*Taenia solium*)	NovaTec	EIA	Cross-reactions in cases of other helminthic infections (especially echinococcosis) may occur.
	Scimedx Corp.	EIA	
Schistosomiasis (*Schistosoma* spp.)	Bordier Affinity Products	EIA	
	NovaTec	EIA	
	Oxford Biosystems	EIA	
	Scimedx Corp.	EIA	
Cystic echinococcosis (*Echinococcus granulosus*)	Bordier Affinity Products	EIA	Not species-specific. Cases of alveolar echinococcosis cross-react. False-positive reactions may occur for patients with other helminth infections (especially cysticercosis).
	Launch Diagnostics	EIA	
	Oxford Biosystems	EIA	
Alveolar echinococcosis (*E. multilocularis*)	Bordier Affinity Products	EIA	Screening test for alveolar echinococcosis; cases of cystic echinococcosis may cross-react.
Strongyloidiasis (*Strongyloides stercoralis*)	Bordier Affinity Products	EIA	Cross-reactions in patients with other helminth infections may occur.
	InBios	EIA	
	Scimedx Corp.	EIA	
Toxocariasis (*Toxocara canis*)	Bordier Affinity Products	EIA	
	NovaTec	EIA	
	Scimedx Corp.	EIA	
Trichinellosis (*Trichinella spiralis*)	Oxford Biosystems	EIA	Numerous cross-reactions with other helminth infections may occur.
	Scimedx Corp.	EIA	
Filariasis	Bordier Affinity Products	EIA	
	NovaTec	EIA	

[a]This is not a complete listing of all available products but reflects readily available information.

[b]Biotrin Int., http://www.biotrin.com; Bordier Affinity Products, http://www.bordier.ch; Chemicon Int., http://www.fishersci.com; Hemagen, http://www.hemagen.com; InBios, http://www.inbios.com; Launch Diagnostics Limited, http://launchdiagnostics.com; NovaTec, http://www.novatec-id.com; Operon, http://operon.es; Oxford Biosystems and Cadama, http://oxfordbiosystems.com; Scimedx Corp., http://scimedx.com.

[c]Abbreviations: EIA, enzyme immunoassay; IC, rapid immunochromatography (dipstick, cartridge, or other rapid test formats).

[d]Due to broad cross-reactivity, especially with the nematodes, use of serologic testing is not recommended.

TABLE 4 Specimen preparation and procedures, recommended stain(s) and relevant parasites, and additional information[a]

Body site	Procedure and specimens	Recommended methods and relevant parasites	Additional information
Blood	Microscopy[b]: thin and thick blood films. Fresh blood (preferred) or EDTA-blood (fill EDTA tube completely with blood and then mix)	Giemsa stain for all blood parasites; hematoxylin-based stain (sheathed microfilariae) Malaria: thick and thin blood films are definitely recommended and should be prepared within 30 to 60 min of blood collection via venipuncture (other tests may be used complementarily)	Most drawings and descriptions of blood parasites are based on Giemsa-stained blood films. Although Wright's stain (or Wright-Giemsa combination stain) works, intracytoplasmic inclusions (stippling) in malaria may not be visible, and the organisms' colors may not match the descriptions. However, with other stains (those listed previously, in addition to some "quick" blood stains), the organisms should be detectable on the blood films.
	Concentration methods: EDTA-blood Antigen detection: EDTA-blood for malaria, serum or plasma for circulating antigens (hemolyzed blood can interact in some tests)	Buffy coat, membrane filtration (microfilariae), fresh blood films for detection of moving microfilariae or trypanosomes Commercial immunoassay test kits for malaria and some microfilariae. Sensitivity is not higher than for thick films for *Plasmodium* spp., much more sensitive for *Leishmania* spp. (peripheral blood is used from immunodeficient patients only).	The use of blood collected with anticoagulant (rather than fresh) has direct relevance to the morphology of malaria organisms seen in peripheral blood films. If the blood smears are prepared after more than 1 h, intracytoplasmic inclusions may not be visible, even if the correct pH buffers are used. Also, if blood is kept at room temperature (with the stopper removed), the male microgametocyte may exflagellate and fertilize the female macrogametocyte, and development continues within the tube of blood (as it would in the mosquito host). The ookinete may actually resemble *Plasmodium falciparum* gametocytes, while the microgametocyte fragments resemble spirochetes.
	Nucleic acid amplification[c]: EDTA-blood, ethanol-fixed or unfixed thin and thick blood films, coagulated blood, possibly with hemolyzed or frozen blood samples	Sequencing of product is often used for species or genotype identification.	So far, no commercial tests approved by the FDA are available; high laboratory standards are needed (may work with frozen, coagulated, or hemolyzed blood samples).
	Specific antibody detection: serum or plasma, anticoagulated or coagulated blood (hemolyzed blood can cause problems in some tests)	Most commonly used are EIA (many test kits commercially available), EITB (commercially available for some parasites), and IFA.	Many laboratories use in-house tests; only a few fully defined antigens are available; sensitivities and specificities of the tests should be documented by the laboratory.
Bone marrow	Biopsy samples or aspirates Microscopy: thin and thick films with aspirate collected in EDTA	Giemsa stain for all blood parasites	*Leishmania* sp. amastigotes are recovered in cells of the reticuloendothelial system; if films are not prepared directly after sample collection, infected cells may disintegrate. Sensitivity of microscopy is low; use only in combination with other methods. Culture for *Leishmania* spp., *Trypanosoma cruzi*, or *Toxoplasma*
	Cultures: sterile material in EDTA or culture medium Nucleic acid amplification: aspirate in EDTA	Media or tissue culture lines must be used for specific organisms	If available, molecular amplification tests for blood parasites including *Leishmania* and *Toxoplasma* and other possible parasites can be performed
Central nervous system	Microscopy: spinal fluid and CSF (wet examination, stained smears), brain biopsy (touch or squash preparations, stained)	Stains: Giemsa (trypanosomes, *Toxoplasma*); Giemsa, trichrome, or calcofluor (amebae [for *Naegleria*, PAM; for *Acanthamoeba* spp. or *Balamuthia mandrillaris*, GAE]); Giemsa, acid-fast, PAS, modified trichrome, silver methenamine (microsporidia) (tissue Gram stains also recommended for microsporidia in routine histologic preparations); H&E, routine histology (larval cestodes, *Taenia solium* [cysticerci], *Echinococcus* spp.)	If CSF is received (with no suspect organism suggested), Giemsa is the best choice; however, trichrome, modified trichrome or calcofluor is also recommended as a second stain (amebic cysts, microsporidia). If brain biopsy material is received (particularly from an immunocompromised patient), NAAT is recommended for diagnosis and identification to the species or genotype level.

(Continued on next page)

TABLE 4 Specimen preparation and procedures, recommended stain(s) and relevant parasites, and additional information[a] *(Continued)*

Body site	Procedure and specimens	Recommended methods and relevant parasites	Additional information
	Culture: sterile aspirate or biopsy material (in physiological saline) Nucleic acid amplification: aspirate or biopsy material, native, frozen, or fixed in ethanol	Free-living amebae (exception: *Balamuthia mandrillaris* does not grow in the routine agar/bacterial overlay method). *Toxoplasma* can be cultured in tissue culture media. Protozoa and helminths; species and genotype characterization	A small amount of the sample should always be stored frozen for molecular analyses in case the results of the other methods are inconclusive.
Cutaneous ulcers	Microscopy: aspirate, biopsy material (smears, touch or squash preparations, histologic sections)	Giemsa (*Leishmania* spp.); H&E, routine histology (*Acanthamoeba* spp., *Balamuthia mandrillaris*, *Entamoeba histolytica*)	Most likely causative parasites would be *Leishmania* spp., which stain with Giemsa. PAS or methenamine silver stain (GMS) could be used to differentiate *Histoplasma capsulatum* (PAS+, GMS+) from *Leishmania* spp. (PAS−, GMS−) in tissue. Sensitivity of microscopy may be low.
	Cultures (less common)	*Leishmania* spp., free-living amebae (often bacterial contamination)	In immunocompromised patients, skin ulcers have been documented with amebae as causative agents.
	Nucleic acid amplification: aspirate, biopsy material, native, frozen, or fixed in ethanol	*Leishmania* spp. (species identification), free-living amebae	Cultures of material from cutaneous ulcers may be contaminated with bacteria; nucleic acid amplification would be the method of choice.
Eye	Microscopy: biopsy material (smears, touch or squash preparations), scrapings, contact lens, sediment of lens solution Culture: native material (see above) in PBS supplemented with antibiotics if possible to avoid bacterial growth Nucleic acid amplification: native material in physiological saline or PBS, ethanol, or frozen	Calcofluor (*Acanthamoeba* sp. cyst only, microsporidia); Giemsa (amebic trophozoites, cysts); modified trichrome (preferred) or silver methenamine stain, PAS, modified acid-fast (microsporidial spores); H&E, routine histology (cysticerci, *Loa loa*, *Toxoplasma*, *Dirofilaria* spp.) Cultures: free-living amebae (except *Balamuthia*) and *Toxoplasma* Free-living amebae, *Toxoplasma*, microsporidial species and genotype identification	Macroscopic examination of adult helminth worms may be useful for identification prior to routine histology. *Acanthamoeba* has been implicated as a cause of keratitis. Although calcofluor stains the cyst walls, it does not stain the trophozoites. Therefore, in suspected cases of amebic keratitis, both stains should be used. H&E (routine histology) can be used to detect and confirm cysticercosis. The adult worm of *Loa loa*, when removed from the eye, can be macroscopically examined or can be stained and examined by routine histology. Microsporidium identification to the species or genotype level is done by nucleic acid amplification and sequence analyses; however, the spores can be found by routine light microscopy with modified trichrome and/or calcofluor stain. Sensitivity of microscopic methods may be low.
Intestinal tract	Stool and other intestinal material Microscopy: stool, sigmoidoscopy material, duodenal contents (all fresh or preserved (see Table 4), direct wet smear, concentration methods Adult worms or tapeworm segments (proglottids)	Concentration methods: formalin-ethyl acetate sedimentation of formalin-, SAF-, or single-vial fixative-preserved stool samples (most protozoa); flotation or combined sedimentation flotation methods (helminth ova); agar or Baermann concentration (larvae of *Strongyloides*; unpreserved stool required) Direct wet smear (direct examination of unpreserved fresh material is also used); (motile protozoan trophozoites; helminth eggs and protozoan cysts may also be detected) Stains: trichrome or iron hematoxylin (intestinal protozoa); modified trichrome (microsporidia); modified acid fast (*Cryptosporidium* spp., *Cyclospora*, *Cystoisospora* spp.) Adhesive cellulose tape, no stain (*Enterobius vermicularis*)	Stool fixation with formalin or single-vial fixative preserves protozoan morphology, allows prolonged storage (room temperature) and long transportation, and prevents hatching of *Schistosoma* sp. eggs but makes *Strongyloides* larval concentration impossible and impedes further NAAT analyses. Taeniid eggs cannot be identified to the species level. Stool fixation is necessary if there is a delay in examination of stool. Microsporidia: confirmation to the species or genotype level requires molecular testing; however, modified trichrome and/or calcofluor stain can be used to confirm the presence of spores. Four to six consecutive negative tapes are required to rule out infection with pinworm (*Enterobius vermicularis*). Pediatricians often treat based on symptoms alone.

(Continued on next page)

TABLE 4 Specimen preparation and procedures, recommended stain(s) and relevant parasites, and additional information[a] *(Continued)*

Body site	Procedure and specimens	Recommended methods and relevant parasites	Additional information
		Carmine stains (rarely used for adult worms or cestode segments). Proglottids can usually be identified to the genus level (*Taenia* spp., *Diphyllobothrium* spp., *Hymenolepis* spp.) without using tissue stains	Worm segments can be stained with special stains. India ink injection of *Taenia* proglottids may be necessary for visualization of uterine branches. However, after dehydration through alcohols and xylenes (or xylene substitutes), the sexual organs and the branched uterine structure are visible, allowing identification of the proglottid to the species level. Lactophenol clearing may be useful.
	Antigen detection: fresh native or frozen material; suitability of fixation is test dependent Nucleic acid detection: native material, fresh, frozen or ethanol fixed Biopsy material Microscopy: fixed for histology or touch or squash preparations for staining Nucleic acid detection: see above	Commercial immunoassays (Table 2), e.g., EIA, FA, cartridge formats (*Entamoeba histolytica*, the *Entamoeba histolytica/E. dispar* group, *Giardia* spp., and *Cryptosporidium* spp.). In-house tests for *Taenia solium* and *Taenia saginata*. Availability of commercial kits will become more readily available. Primers for genus or species identification of most helminths and protozoa are published. H&E, routine histology (*Entamoeba histolytica*, *Cryptosporidium* spp., *Cyclospora*, *Cystoisospora* spp., *Giardia*, microsporidia); less common findings include *Schistosoma* spp., hookworm, and *Trichuris*.	Coproantigens can be detected in the prepatent period and independently from egg excretion. Due to potential inhibition after DNA extraction from stool samples, concentration or isolation methods may be required before DNA extraction. However, some DNA isolation kits facilitate isolation of high-quality DNA from stool. Sequence analyses may be required for species or genotype identification. Special stains may be helpful for the identification of microsporidia (tissue Gram stains, silver stains, PAS, and Giemsa) or coccidia (modified acid-fast stain).
Liver and spleen	Biopsy samples or aspirates Microscopy: unfixed material in physiological saline; fixed for histology Culture or animal inoculation: sterile preparation of native material Nucleic acid detection: native material, frozen or ethanol fixed	Examination of wet smears for *Entamoeba histolytica* (trophozoites), protoscolices of *Echinococcus* spp. or eggs of *Capillaria hepatica*. Giemsa stain (*Leishmania* spp., other protozoa and microsporidia); H&E (routine histology) For *Leishmania* spp. (not common) Intraperitoneal inoculation of *E. multilocularis* cyst material for viability test after long-term chemotherapy Species or genotype identification (e.g., *Echinococcus* spp.)	Definite risks are associated with punctures (aspirates and/or biopsy) of spleen or liver lesions (*Echinococcus* spp.). Always keep a small amount of material frozen for nucleic acid analysis. Most laboratories do not perform culture or testing using animal inoculation.
Respiratory tract	Sputum, induced sputum, nasal and sinus discharge, bronchoalveolar lavage fluid, transbronchial aspirate, tracheobronchial aspirate, brush biopsy sample, open-lung biopsy sample Microscopy: unfixed material, treated for smear preparation Nucleic acid detection: unfixed native material, frozen or fixed in ethanol	Helminth larvae (*Ascaris*, *Strongyloides*), eggs (*Paragonimus* spp., *Capillaria* spp.), or hooklets (*Echinococcus* spp.) can be recovered in unstained respiratory specimens. Stains: Giemsa for many protozoa, including *Toxoplasma*, modified acid-fast stains (*Cryptosporidium* spp.); modified trichrome (microsporidia) Routine histology (H&E; silver methenamine stain, PAS, modified acid-fast, tissue Gram stains for helminths, protozoa, and microsporidia)	Immunoassay reagents (FA) are available for diagnosis of pulmonary cryptosporidiosis. Routine histologic procedures allow identification of any of the helminths or helminth eggs in the lung. Disseminated toxoplasmosis and microsporidiosis are well documented, with organisms being found in many different respiratory specimens.
Muscle	Biopsy material Microscopy: unfixed, touch, and squash preparations or fixed for histology and EM PCR: unfixed or native, frozen, or ethanol fixed	Larvae of *Trichinella* can be identified unstained (species identification with single larvae by molecular analysis). H&E, routine histology (*Trichinella*, cysticerci); PAS, modified acid-fast, tissue Gram stains, EM (rare microsporidia). Microsporidial identification to the species level requires subsequent sequencing.	If *Trypanosoma cruzi* organisms are present in the striated muscle, they could be identified in routine histology preparations. Modified trichrome and/or calcofluor stain can be used to confirm the presence of microsporidial spores. Larvae of *Trichinella* may be detected in heavy infections only. Biopsies are not recommended as standard procedures.

(Continued on next page)

TABLE 4 Specimen preparation and procedures, recommended stain(s) and relevant parasites, and additional information[a] *(Continued)*

Body site	Procedure and specimens	Recommended methods and relevant parasites	Additional information
Skin	Aspirates, skin snips, scrapings, biopsy samples	See "Cutaneous ulcer" (above)	Any of the parasites can be identified by routine histology procedures, but the sensitivities of these methods may be low.
	Microscopy: direct exam, wet examination, stained smear (or fixed for histology or EM) Nucleic acid detection: unfixed native, frozen or fixed in ethanol	Wet preparations (microfilariae), Giemsa-stained smears or H&E, routine histology (*Onchocerca volvulus*, *Dipetalonema streptocerca*, *Dirofilaria repens*, other larvae causing cutaneous larva migrans [zoonotic *Strongyloides*, hookworms], *Leishmania* spp., *Acanthamoeba* spp., *Entamoeba histolytica*, microsporidia, *Balamuthia mandrillaris* and arthropods [*Sarcoptes scabiei* and other mites]) Primers for most parasite species are available	
Amniotic fluid	Microscopy: stained smear	Giemsa-stained smear	Only applicable to confirm suspected prenatal *Toxoplasma* infections
	Nucleic acid detection: native material		Nucleic acid amplification is the method of choice
	Culture	Various tissue culture media can be used	
Urogenital system	Vaginal discharge, saline swab, transport swab (no charcoal), air-dried smear for FA, urethral discharge, prostatic secretions, urine (single unpreserved, 24-h unpreserved, or early-morning specimen). Microscopy: wet smears, smears of urine sediment, stained smears Cultivation: vaginal or urethral discharge or swab preparations Nucleic acid detection: native material, frozen or fixed in ethanol	Giemsa, lateral flow immunoassay, NAAT (*Trichomonas vaginalis*); Delafield's hematoxylin (microfilariae); modified trichrome (microsporidia); H&E, routine histology, PAS, acid-fast, tissue Gram stains (microsporidia). Direct examination of urine sediment for *Schistosoma haematobium* eggs or microfilariae Identification and propagation of *T. vaginalis* (commercial plastic envelope culture systems available); moving trophozoites can be detected microscopically (or in Giemsa-stained smears)	Although *T. vaginalis* is probably the most common parasite identified, there are others to consider, the most recently implicated organisms being in the microsporidial group. Microfilariae could also be recovered and stained. Fixation of urine with formalin prevents hatching of *Schistosoma* eggs. Material must be put into culture medium immediately after collection; do not cool or freeze.

[a]CSF, cerebrospinal fluid; EIA, enzyme immunoassay; EITB, enzyme-linked immunoelectrotransfer blotting (Western blotting); EM, electron microscopy; FA, fluorescent antibody; GAE, granulomatous amebic encephalitis; GI, gastrointestinal; H&E, hematoxylin and eosin; IFA, indirect immunofluorescence assay; PAM, primary amebic encephalitis; PAS, periodic acid-Schiff stain; PBS, phosphate-buffered saline.

[b]Many parasites or parasite stages may be detected in standard histologic sections of tissue material. However, species identification is difficult, and additional examinations may be required. Usually, these techniques are not considered first-line methods. Additional methods like EM are carried out only by specialized laboratories and are not available for standard diagnostic purposes. EM examination for species identification has largely been replaced by NAAT.

[c]Material/specimens suitable for nucleic acid detection: native (unfixed), in saline, PBS, or ethanol, or frozen; formalin should be avoided. Whenever possible, a portion of the sample should be reserved in case additional testing is necessary.

Fresh specimens are mandatory for the recovery of motile trophozoites (amebae, flagellates, or ciliates). The protozoan trophozoite stage is normally found in cases of diarrhea; the intestinal tract contents move through the system too rapidly for cyst formation to occur. Once the stool specimen is passed from the body, trophozoites do not encyst but may disintegrate if not examined or preserved within a short time after passage. However, most helminth eggs and larvae, coccidian oocysts, and microsporidial spores survive for extended periods. Liquid specimens should be examined within 30 min of passage, not 30 min from the time they reach the laboratory. If meeting this general recommendation is not possible, the specimen should be placed in one of the available fixatives (2). Soft (semiformed) specimens may have a mixture of protozoan trophozoites and cysts and should be examined within 1 h of passage; again, if this time frame is not possible, fixatives should be used. Immediate examination of formed specimens is not as critical; in fact, if the specimen is examined any time within 24 h after passage, the protozoan cysts should still be intact.

Preservation of Stool

If there are delays from the time of specimen passage until examination in the laboratory, the use of stool fixative should be considered. To preserve protozoan morphology and prevent the continued development of some helminth eggs and larvae, the stool specimens can be placed in fixative either immediately after passage (by the patient or hospital staff, using a collection kit). Several fixatives are

TABLE 5 Fecal specimens for parasites: options for collection and processing

Option	Pros	Cons
Although physicians can order stools for parasitology when deemed appropriate, many laboratories include in their protocols the rejection of stools from inpatients who have been in-house for >3 days.	Patients may become symptomatic with diarrhea after they have been inpatients for a few days; symptoms are usually not attributed to parasitic infections but are generally due to other causes.	There is always a chance that the problem is related to a nosocomial parasitic infection (rare), but *Cryptosporidium* spp., *Giardia*, and microsporidia may be possible.
Examination of a single stool (O&P examination)	If parasites are detected in the first sample or if the patient becomes asymptomatic after collection of the first stool, subsequent specimens may not be necessary. However, with some intestinal parasitic infections, patients may alternate with constipation and diarrhea.	Diagnosis from examination of a single stool specimen depends on the parasite load in the specimen. Of organisms present, 40–60% are found with only a single stool exam; two O&P examinations are acceptable, but three specimens are more sensitive; any patient remaining symptomatic would require additional testing. In a series of three stool specimens, frequently not all three specimens are positive and/or may be positive for different organisms (may be a cost-effective approach).
Examination of a second stool specimen only after the first one is negative and the patient is still symptomatic (O&P examination)	With additional examinations, yield of protozoa increases (*Entamoeba histolytica*, 22.7%; *Giardia*, 11.3%; and *Dientamoeba fragilis*, 31.1%).	Assumes that the second (or third) stool specimen is collected within the recommended 10-day time frame for a series of stools; protozoa are shed periodically. May be inconvenient for the patient, and the correct diagnosis might be delayed.
Examination of a single stool and a *Giardia* immunoassay	If the examinations are negative and the patient's symptoms subside, further testing is likely not required.	Patients may exhibit symptoms sporadically, so it may be difficult to rule out parasitic infections with only a single stool and immunoassay. If the patient remains symptomatic, even if the *Giardia* immunoassay is negative, other protozoa may be missed (*Cryptosporidium* spp., *E. histolytica*/*E. dispar*, and *D. fragilis*).
Pooling of three specimens for examination; one concentration and one permanent stain are performed. The laboratory pools the specimens.	Three specimens are collected over 7–10 days, which may save time and expense.	Procedure not recommended. Decreases strongly the sensitivity of the procedure; organisms present in low numbers may be missed due to the dilution factor.
Permanent stained smears are performed, one from each of the three specimens; subsequently, three specimens are pooled for a single concentration on the pooled specimen.	Three specimens are collected over 7–10 days; would maximize recovery of protozoa in areas of the U.S. where these organisms are most common.	Might miss light helminth infection (eggs and larvae) due to the pooling procedure.
Three stool specimens are collected, but samples of stool from all three are put into a single vial (patient is given a single vial only).	Pooling of the specimens would require only a single vial.	Absolutely not recommended. Lack of sensitivity; proper mixing of specimen and fixative complicates patient collection and depends on patient compliance.
Immunoassays are performed only for selected patients[a] (children <5 yr old, children attending day care centers, patients with immunodeficiencies, and patients involved in diarrheal outbreaks) for intestinal protozoa.	Would be more cost-effective than performing immunoassay procedures on all specimens.	The competence and the information needed to group patients are often not available in the laboratory. Ordering guidelines for clients are highly recommended.
Automated molecular panels performed on majority of patients other than those for which the O&P is recommended (travelers, those who live in countries where the organism is endemic, those who live in large cities within U.S.)	As parasitic panels expand, this option may become more commonly used. If the patient remains symptomatic with negative results, then additional testing could be performed.	Specific automated panels may be seen in Table 7 in chapter 138. The organisms included in various panels include *Giardia*, *Cryptosporidium*, *Cyclospora*, *Entamoeba histolytica* complex, and *Entamoeba histolytica*. Panels under development will include *Blastocystis* spp., *Dientamoeba fragilis*, microsporidia, and *Strongyloides*.

[a]It is difficult to recognize an early outbreak situation in which screening of all specimens for *Giardia*, *Cryptosporidium* spp., or both may be relevant. If it appears that an outbreak is in the early stages, performing the immunoassays or NAAT on request can be changed to screening all stools.

TABLE 6 Approaches to stool parasitology: test ordering[a]

Patient and/or situation	Test ordered	Follow-up test ordered
Patients with diarrhea and HIV or other cause of immune deficiency	*Cryptosporidium* or *Giardia/Cryptosporidium* immunoassay[b,c] (see Table 2) or NAAT	If immunoassays or NAAT are negative and symptoms continue, special tests for microsporidia (modified trichrome stain) and coccidia (modified acid-fast stain) and O&P examination should be performed.
Potential waterborne outbreak from (municipal) water supply Patient with diarrhea (nursery school, day care center, camper or backpacker) Patient from area in the United States where *Giardia* is the most common organism found	*Giardia* or *Giardia/Cryptosporidium* immunoassay[b,c] or NAAT	If immunoassays or NAAT are negative and symptoms continue, special tests for microsporidia and coccidia and O&P examination should be performed.
Patient with diarrhea and relevant travel history Patient with diarrhea who is a past or present resident of a developing country Patient in area of the U.S. where parasites other than *Giardia* are found	O&P examination, *Entamoeba histolytica* immunoassay, *Cryptosporidium* or *Giardia/Cryptosporidium* immunoassay,[b,c] test or NAAT, and *Strongyloides stercoralis* (even in the absence of eosinophilia)	If O&P examinations are negative and symptoms continue, perform stains for coccidia and microsporidia.
Patient with unexplained eosinophilia (may be low or high); may or may not have diarrhea; may be immunocompromised, often due to receipt of steroids; patient may present with hyperinfection and severe diarrhea (symptoms may also include pneumonia and/or episodes of sepsis and/or meningitis).	O&P examination with emphasis on helminths (stool in fixative for sedimentation/flotation techniques); it is very important to make sure that an infection with *Strongyloides* has been ruled out—particularly if the patient is immunosuppressed or may become immunosuppressed from therapy, etc. (unfixed stool, Baermann concentration, or agar plate culture).	If the O&P examinations are negative, agar plate cultures for *Strongyloides* are recommended, particularly if the history is suggestive for this infection. The serological detection of specific antibody is an additional diagnostic option.
Patient with diarrhea (suspected foodborne outbreak)	Test for *Cyclospora cayetanensis* (modified acid-fast stain, autofluorescence)	If test is negative and symptoms continue, special procedures for microsporidia and other coccidia and O&P examination should be performed.

[a]Modified from reference 1.
[b]Depending on the particular immunoassay kit or panel used, various single or multiple organisms may be included. Selection of a particular kit depends on many variables such as clinical relevance, cost, ease of performance, training, personnel availability, number of test orders, training of physician clients, sensitivity, specificity, equipment, and time to result. Very few laboratories handle this type of testing in exactly the same way. Many options are clinically relevant and acceptable for patient care.
[c]Two stool specimens should be tested using an immunoassay in order to rule out an infection with *Giardia*; fecal immunoassays may also be negative in cases with a low parasite load.

available; however, regardless of the fixative selected, adequate mixing of the specimen and preservative is mandatory. Specimens preserved in stool fixatives should be stored at room temperature. It is also important to use the correct ratio of stool and fixative to ensure proper fixation. Commercial vials are marked with a "fill-to" line for the addition of stool to the container.

Historically, a formalin vial and a fixative vial containing polyvinyl alcohol (PVA) were used for collection; however, there are currently many fixative options, including one-vial and two-vial combinations. When selecting an appropriate fixative, one should keep in mind that a permanent stained smear is mandatory for a complete examination for parasites (1, 2, 9, 10, 13) (see chapter 137). The fixative must be compatible with the kit or the method selected. It is also important to remember that disposal regulations for compounds containing mercury are becoming stricter; each laboratory must check applicable regulations to help determine fixative options.

Formalin

Formalin is an all-purpose fixative appropriate for helminth eggs and larvae and for protozoan cysts. Two concentrations are commonly used: 5%, which is recommended for preservation of protozoan cysts, and 10%, which is recommended for helminth eggs and larvae. Although 5% is often recommended for all-purpose use, most commercial manufacturers provide 10%, which is more likely to kill all helminth eggs. To help maintain organism morphology, the formalin can be buffered with sodium phosphate buffers (i.e., neutral formalin). Selection of specific formalin formulations is at the user's discretion. Aqueous formalin permits the examination of the specimen as a wet mount only, a technique much less accurate than a stained smear for the identification of intestinal protozoa.

Protozoan cysts (not trophozoites), coccidian oocysts, helminth eggs, and larvae are well preserved for long periods in 10% aqueous formalin. Formalin heated to 60°C can be used for specimens containing helminth eggs, since

TABLE 7 Fecal fixatives: pros and cons

Stool preservative	Pros	Cons
Formalin	Good overall fixative for stool concentration. Easy to prepare; long shelf life. Concentrated sediment can be used with different stains[a] but not with all immunoassays (see Table 2).	Does not preserve trophozoites well. Does not adequately preserve organism morphology for a good permanent stained smear; not optimal for all immunoassays; not appropriate for molecular diagnosis (PCR).
SAF	Can be used for concentration and permanent stained smears. Contains no mercury compounds. Easy to prepare; long shelf life. Concentrated sediment can be used with most of the new immunoassay methods and special stains.	Poor adhesive properties; albumin-coated slides recommended. Protozoan morphology is better if iron hematoxylin stain is used for permanent stained smears (trichrome is not quite as good). May be a bit more difficult to use; however, this is really not a limiting factor. Not appropriate for molecular detection tests.
Schaudinn's fixative (mercury base)	Fixation of slides prepared from fresh fecal specimens or samples from the intestinal mucosal surfaces. Provides excellent fixation of protozoan trophozoites and cysts.	Not generally recommended for concentration procedures. Contains mercuric chloride; creates disposal problems. Poor adhesive qualities with liquid or mucoid specimens.
PVA (mercury base)	Can prepare permanent stained smears and perform concentration techniques (less common). Provides excellent fixation of protozoan trophozoites and cysts. Specimens can be shipped to the laboratory for subsequent examination; organism morphology excellent after processing. Suitable for NAAT. This formulation is considered the gold standard against which all other fixatives are evaluated (organism morphology after permanent staining).	*Trichuris trichiura* eggs and *Giardia* cysts are not concentrated as easily as from formalin-based fixative. *Strongyloides stercoralis* larval morphology is poor (better from formalin-based preservation). *Cystoisospora* sp. oocysts may not be visible from PVA-fixed material (better from formalin-based preservation). Contains mercury compounds and may pose a disposal problem (chemical waste). May turn white and gelatinous when it begins to dehydrate or when refrigerated. Difficult to prepare in the laboratory. Specimens containing PVA cannot be used with the immunoassay methods.
Modified PVA (copper or zinc base)	Can prepare permanent stained smears and perform concentration techniques (less common). Many workers prefer the zinc substitutes over those prepared with copper sulfate. Does not contain mercury compounds.	Overall protozoan morphology of trophozoites and cysts is not as good when they are fixed in modified PVA, compared with organisms fixed in mercuric chloride-based fixatives. Zinc-based fixatives appear to be some of the better alternatives. Staining characteristics of protozoa are not consistent; some are good, and some are poor. Organism identification may be difficult, particularly with small protozoan cysts (*Endolimax nana*).
Single-vial systems (with or without PVA)	Can prepare permanent stained smears and perform concentration techniques. Can perform immunoassays. May not contain formalin or mercury compounds. Unless organism numbers are rare, acceptable organism recovery and identification are possible.	Overall protozoan morphology of trophozoites and cysts is not as good as that of organisms fixed with mercuric chloride-based fixative; similar to modified PVA options. Staining characteristics of protozoa are not consistent; some are good, and some are poor. Identification of *Endolimax nana* cysts may be difficult. Additional training may be required to recognize the organisms because the overall morphology is not comparable to that seen with mercury-based fixatives. Not all immunoassays can be performed from stool specimens in these fixatives. However, in spite of the cons, single-vial systems are becoming more widely used for concentrations, permanent stained smears, and fecal immunoassays.
	Concentration, permanent stains, some immunoassays, and some molecular testing can be performed.	

[a]Modified acid-fast and modified trichrome stains.

in cold formalin, some thick-shelled eggs may continue to develop, become infective, and remain viable for long periods. Several grams of fecal material should be thoroughly mixed in 5% or 10% formalin (ratio, 1:10).

Formaldehyde vapor concentrations must be monitored and maintained at concentrations below the 8-hour time-weighted average. In the United States, these limits are 0.75 ppm and the 15-minute short-term exposure limit (i.e., 2.0 ppm) (1). However, these limits may vary from country to country. Generally, the amount of formaldehyde used in microbiology is quite small; laboratory monitoring values are usually well below the required maximum concentrations. Initial monitoring must be repeated any time there is a change in production, equipment, process, personnel, or control measures that may result in new or additional exposure to formaldehyde. Stool fixatives that contain formaldehyde indicate that fact on the label. A number of single-vial fixative collection systems are now available; although they may not contain formaldehyde, the actual formulas are proprietary.

SAF

Both the concentration and the permanent stained smear can be performed with specimens in sodium acetate-acetic acid-formalin (SAF). It is a liquid fixative, much like the 10% formalin described above. The sediment is used to prepare the permanent smear, and it is frequently recommended that the stool material be placed on an albumin-coated slide to improve adherence to the glass (14, 15).

SAF is considered a "softer" fixative than mercuric chloride. The organism morphology is not quite as sharp after staining as that of organisms originally fixed in solutions containing mercuric chloride. The pairing of SAF-fixed material with iron hematoxylin staining provides better organism morphology than does staining of SAF-fixed material with trichrome (personal observation). Although SAF has a long shelf life and is easy to prepare, the smear preparation technique may be a bit more difficult for less experienced personnel who are not familiar with fecal specimen techniques. Laboratories that have considered using only a single preservative have selected this option. Helminth eggs and larvae, protozoan trophozoites and cysts, coccidian oocysts, and microsporidian spores can be recovered using this method.

Schaudinn's Fluid

Schaudinn's fluid containing mercuric chloride can be used with fresh stool specimens or samples from the intestinal mucosal surface. Many laboratories that receive specimens from in-house patients (with no delay in delivery times) often select this approach. Permanent stained smears are then prepared from fixed material. A concentration technique using Schaudinn's fluid-preserved material is also available but is not widely used (1, 10, 11).

PVA

PVA is a plastic resin that is normally incorporated into Schaudinn's fixative. The PVA powder serves as an adhesive for the stool material (i.e., when the stool-PVA mixture is spread onto the glass slide, it adheres because of the PVA component). Fixation is still accomplished by Schaudinn's fluid itself. Perhaps the greatest advantage in the use of PVA is that a permanent stained smear can be prepared. Like SAF, PVA fixative solution is recommended as a means of preserving cysts and trophozoites for later examination and permits specimens to be shipped (by regular mail service) from any location in the world to a laboratory for subsequent examination. PVA is particularly useful for liquid specimens and should be used at a ratio of 3 parts PVA to 1 part fecal specimen (16).

Modified PVA

Although fixatives that do not contain mercury compounds have been developed, some of the substitute compounds have not provided the quality of fixation necessary for good protozoan morphology on the permanent stained smear. Copper sulfate has been tried but does not provide results equal to those seen with mercuric chloride (17). Zinc sulfate has proven to be an acceptable mercury substitute and is used with trichrome stain. Substitutes containing zinc have become widely available; each manufacturer has a proprietary formula for the fixative (18, 19).

Single-Vial Collection Systems

Several manufacturers now have available single-vial stool collection systems, similar to SAF or modified PVA methods. From the single vial, both the concentration and permanent stained smear can be prepared. It is also possible to perform immunoassays from some of these vials. Ask the manufacturer about all diagnostic capabilities (concentration, permanent stained smear, immunoassay procedures, and molecular analyses) and for specific information indicating that there are no formula components that would interfere with any of the methods. Like the zinc substitutes, these formulas are proprietary (19). New formulations continue to be developed, and some of them appear to adhere to the slide without the use of albumin or PVA. These formulations may be used to perform concentrations and some of the immunoassays and to prepare permanent stained smears. There are several commercially available single-vial fixatives for stool specimens that are mercury and formalin free, preserve morphology, and alleviate many disposal and monitoring problems encountered by laboratories. A single-vial fixative that is mercury, formalin, and PVA free is also commercially available.

Collection of Blood

Depending on the life cycle, a number of parasites may be recovered in a blood specimen, either whole blood, buffy coat preparations, or various types of concentrations (2, 10, 11). These parasites include *Plasmodium* spp., *Babesia* spp., *Trypanosoma* spp., *Leishmania* spp., *Toxoplasma gondii*, and microfilariae. Although some organisms may be motile in fresh whole blood, species identification is normally accomplished from the examination of permanent stained thin and/or thick blood films. Blood films can be prepared from fresh whole blood collected with no anticoagulants, anticoagulated blood, or sediment from the various concentration procedures.

Unless it is certain that well-prepared slides will be available, it is necessary to request a tube of fresh blood (EDTA anticoagulant is preferred) and prepare the smears. The tube should be filled with blood to provide the proper blood/anticoagulant ratio. For detection of intracytoplasmic inclusions (e.g., stippling), the smears should be prepared within 1 h after the specimen is drawn. After that time, stippling may not be visible on stained films; however, the overall organism morphology will still be excellent. Most laboratories routinely use commercially available blood collection tubes; preparation of EDTA collection tubes in-house is neither necessary nor cost-effective.

The time the specimen was drawn should be clearly indicated on the tube of blood and also on the result report. The physician will then be able to correlate the results with any fever pattern (most likely seen in a semi-immune patient with past exposure to malaria with antibodies) or other symptoms that the patient may have. In immunologically naive patients or travelers with no previous exposure to malaria, there may be no periodicity at all; symptoms will mimic many other infections or medical problems. There should also be comments on the test result report sent back to the physician stating that one negative specimen does not rule out the possibility of a parasitic infection (1, 20).

Collection of Specimens from Other Body Sites

Although clinical specimens for examination can be obtained from many other body sites, these specimens, and the appropriate diagnostic methods, are not as common as routine stool specimens and blood specimens (21, 22). Most specimens from other body sites (Table 1) are submitted as fresh specimens for further testing.

DIRECT DETECTION BY ROUTINE METHODS

Intestinal Tract Specimens

The most common specimen submitted to the diagnostic laboratory is the stool specimen, and the most commonly performed procedure in parasitology is the ova and parasite (O&P) examination, which is composed of three separate protocols: the direct wet mount, the concentration, and the permanent stained smear. The direct wet mount requires fresh stool, is designed to allow the detection of motile protozoan trophozoites, and is examined microscopically at low and high dry magnifications (×100, entire 22- by 22-mm coverslip [larvae, larger helminth eggs]; ×400, one-third to one-half of a 22- by 22-mm coverslip [protozoan cysts and/or trophozoites, smaller helminth eggs]). If the specimens are received in the laboratory in stool collection fixatives, the direct wet preparation may be eliminated from the routine O&P examination.

The second part of the O&P examination is the concentration, which is designed to facilitate the recovery of protozoan cysts, coccidian oocysts, microsporidial spores, and helminth eggs and larvae. Both flotation (zinc sulfate, zinc chloride, and others) and sedimentation methods are available, the most common procedure being the formalin-ethyl acetate sedimentation method (formerly called the formalin-ether method). The concentrated specimen is examined as a wet preparation, with or without iodine (personal preference), using low and high dry magnifications (×100 and ×400) as indicated for the direct wet smear examination. It is important to remember that large, heavy helminth eggs (unfertilized *Ascaris* eggs) or eggs that are operculated (trematode and some cestode eggs) do not float optimally when flotation fluids with densities of <1.35 are used; both the surface film and sediment must be examined by this method. It is also important to note that the flotation media with high densities may change the morphological characteristics of some parasites.

The third part of the O&P examination is the permanent stained smear, which is designed to facilitate the identification of intestinal protozoa. Several staining methods are available, the two most common being the Wheatley modification of Gomori's tissue trichrome and the iron hematoxylin stains. This part of the O&P examination is critical for the confirmation of suspicious objects seen in the wet examination and identification of protozoa that might not have been seen in the wet preparation. The permanent stained smears are examined using oil immersion objectives (×600 for screening and ×1,000 for final review of ≥300 oil immersion fields).

Other specimens from the intestinal tract, such as duodenal aspirates or drainage, mucus from the Entero-Test capsule technique, and sigmoidoscopy material, can also be examined as wet preparations and as permanent stained smears after processing with either trichrome or iron hematoxylin staining. Adult and pediatric Entero-Test capsules are currently available from Nutri-Link Ltd., Newton Abbot, United Kingdom (www.nutri-linkltd.co.uk). Although not all laboratories examine these types of specimens, they are included to give some idea of the possibilities for diagnostic testing.

Amniotic Fluid

Methods for the diagnosis of congenital *T. gondii* infection are summarized in chapter 141. Amniotic fluid collected under sterile conditions allows both mouse or tissue culture inoculation and molecular diagnosis. NAAT is the recommended test of choice for the detection of *Toxoplasma* in amniotic fluid.

Urogenital Tract Specimens

The identification of *Trichomonas vaginalis* is historically based on the microscopic examination of wet preparations of vaginal and urethral discharges and prostatic secretions or urine sediment. Multiple specimens may have to be examined before the organisms are detected. These specimens are diluted with a drop of saline and examined under low power (×100) and reduced illumination for the presence of motile organisms; as the jerky motility begins to diminish, it may be possible to observe the undulating membrane, particularly under high dry power (×400). Culture systems (InPouch TV; BioMed Diagnostics, White City, OR) that allow direct inoculation, transport, culture, and microscopic examination are available commercially (1, 23). Rapid tests that allow detection of *T. vaginalis* antigens and molecular testing kits (e.g., DNA probes and nucleic acid amplification methods) are also commercially available.

Stained smears such as Papanicolaou- or Giemsa-stained smears can be used, but they are usually not necessary for the identification of this organism and can be difficult to interpret. If a dry smear is received by the laboratory, it can be fixed with absolute methanol and stained with Giemsa stain; this approach is not optimal, but the smear can be examined and may confirm a positive infection. The number of false-positive and false-negative results reported on the basis of stained smears strongly suggests the value of confirmation by observation of motile organisms from the direct mount, from appropriate culture media, or via direct detection by more sensitive antigen detection or molecular methods (Table 3) (5).

Examination of urinary sediment may be indicated in certain filarial infections. Administration of the drug diethylcarbamazine (Hetrazan) has been reported to enhance the recovery of microfilariae from urine. The triple-concentration technique is recommended for the recovery of microfilariae (1). The membrane filtration technique can also be used with urine for the recovery of microfilariae (1). *Schistosoma haematobium* eggs can be concentrated by centrifugation of urine specimens; a membrane filter technique for the egg recovery has also been useful (1). Fresh samples or fixed samples in formalin should be used to prevent hatching of eggs.

Microsporidial spores of *Encephalitozoon* spp. can also be recovered from urine sediment. This organism primarily infects the intestinal tract but can also disseminate to the kidneys in immunocompromised individuals.

Respiratory Tract Specimens

Sputum (expectorated or induced), bronchoalveolar lavage or washings, and transtracheal secretions may be submitted for examination for parasites (1, 24). Organisms that may be detected and may cause pneumonia, pneumonitis, or Loeffler's syndrome include the migrating larval stages of *Ascaris lumbricoides*, *Strongyloides stercoralis*, and hookworm; the eggs of *Paragonimus* spp.; *Echinococcus granulosus* hooklets; *E. histolytica*, *Entamoeba gingivalis*, and *Trichomonas tenax* trophozoites; *Cryptosporidium* sp. oocysts; and possibly the microsporidia. In a *Paragonimus* infection, the sputum may be viscous and tinged with brownish flecks, which are clusters of eggs ("iron filings"), and may be streaked with blood. Sputum is usually examined as a wet mount (saline or iodine), using low and high dry power (×100 and ×400). The specimen can be concentrated before preparation of the wet mount. If the sputum is thick, mucolytic agents or an equal amount of 3% sodium hydroxide (NaOH) (or undiluted chlorine bleach) can be added; the specimen is thoroughly mixed and then centrifuged at 500 × *g* for 5 min. NaOH should not be used if one is looking for *Entamoeba* spp. or *T. tenax*. After centrifugation, the supernatant fluid is discarded, and the sediment can be examined as a wet mount with saline or iodine. If examination has to be delayed for any reason, the sputum should be fixed in 5 or 10% formalin to preserve helminth eggs or larvae or in PVA fixative to be stained later for protozoa.

Aspirates

The examination of aspirated material for the diagnosis of parasitic infections may be extremely valuable, particularly when routine testing methods have failed to demonstrate the organisms. These specimens should be transported to the laboratory immediately after collection. Aspirates include liquid specimens collected from a variety of sites where organisms might be found. The aspirates most commonly processed in the parasitology laboratory include fine-needle and duodenal aspirates.

Fine-needle aspirates may be submitted for slide preparation, culture, and/or molecular analyses. Aspirates of cysts and abscesses for amebae may require concentration by centrifugation, digestion, microscopic examination for motile organisms in direct preparations, and cultures and microscopic evaluation of stained preparations. Antigen detection and PCR are other possibilities, depending on individual laboratory testing options.

Bone marrow aspirates for *Leishmania* sp. amastigotes, *Trypanosoma cruzi* amastigotes, or *Plasmodium* spp. require Giemsa staining or the use of other stains for blood and tissues. Examination of these specimens may confirm an infection that has been missed by examination of routine blood films. In certain situations, culture, immunoassays for antigen detection, and PCR also provide more sensitive results (24).

Biopsy Specimens

Biopsy specimens are recommended for the microscopic detection of tissue parasites (Table 5). The following may be used for this purpose in addition to standard histologic preparations: impression smears and teased and squash preparations of biopsy tissue from skin, muscle, cornea, intestine, liver, lung, and brain. Tissue to be examined by permanent sections or electron microscopy should be fixed as specified by the laboratories that will process the tissue. In certain cases, a biopsy may be the only means of confirming a suspected parasitic infection. Specimens that are going to be examined as fresh material rather than as tissue sections should be kept moist in saline and submitted to the laboratory immediately.

Detection of parasites in tissue depends in part on specimen collection and on having sufficient material to perform the recommended diagnostic procedures. Biopsy specimens are usually quite small and may not be representative of the diseased tissue. Using multiple tissue samples often improves diagnostic results. To optimize the yield from any tissue specimen, all areas should be examined by as many procedures as possible. Tissues are obtained by invasive procedures, many of which are very expensive and lengthy; consequently, these specimens deserve the most comprehensive procedures possible.

Tissue submitted in a sterile container in sterile saline or on a sterile sponge dampened with saline may be used for cultures or molecular analyses of protozoa after mounts for direct examination or impression smears for staining have been prepared. Bacteriological transport media should be avoided. If cultures for parasites are to be made, sterile slides should be used for smear and mount preparation.

Blood

Depending on the life cycle, a number of parasites may be recovered in a blood specimen, either whole blood, buffy coat preparations, or various types of concentrations (1). Although some organisms may be motile in fresh whole blood, species identification is normally accomplished from the examination of permanent stained blood films, both thick and thin films. Blood films can be prepared from fresh whole blood collected with no anticoagulants, anticoagulated blood, or sediment from the various concentration procedures. The recommended stain of choice is Giemsa stain; however, the parasites can also be seen on blood films stained with Wright's stain or Wright-Giemsa stain. Delafield's hematoxylin stain is used to stain the microfilarial sheath; in some cases, Giemsa stain may not provide sufficient staining to allow visualization of the sheath; however, other characteristics (e.g., size, nuclear arrangement) can be used for identification.

Thin Blood Films

In any examination of thin blood films for parasitic organisms, the initial screen should be carried out with the low-power objective (×100) of a microscope. Microfilariae may be missed if the entire thin film is not examined. Microfilariae are rarely present in large numbers, and frequently, only a few organisms are present in each thin film preparation. Microfilariae are commonly found at the edges of the thin film or at the feathered end of the film because they are carried to these sites during spreading of the blood. The feathered end of the film, where the erythrocytes (RBCs) are drawn out into one single, distinctive layer of cells, should be examined for the presence of malaria parasites and trypanosomes. In these areas, the morphology and size of the infected RBCs are most clearly seen.

Depending on the training and experience of the microscopist, examination of the thin film usually takes 15 to 20 min (≥300 oil immersion fields) for the thin film at a magnification of ×1,000. Although some people use a 50× or 60× oil immersion objective to screen stained blood films, there is some concern that small parasites, such as *Plasmodium* spp., *Babesia* spp., and *Leishmania* spp., may be missed at this lower total magnification (×500 or ×600) compared with the ×1,000 total magnification obtained using the more traditional 100× oil immersion objective. Because people tend to scan blood films at different rates, it is important to examine a minimum of 300 oil immersion fields. If something suspicious has been seen in the thick film, the number of fields examined on the thin film is often considerably greater than 300. The request for blood film examination should always be considered a stat procedure, with all reports (negative as well as positive) being relayed by telephone to the physician as soon as possible. If the result is positive, appropriate governmental public health agencies (local, state, and federal) should be notified within a reasonable time frame in accordance with guidelines and laws.

Both malaria and *Babesia* infections have been missed with automated differential instruments, and in those cases, therapy was delayed. Although these instruments are not designed to detect intracellular blood parasites, the inability of the automated systems to discriminate between uninfected RBCs and those infected with parasites may pose serious diagnostic problems (25). Some modern hematology analyzers based on flow-cytometric principles can combine multiple parameters into an algorithm that can suggest the presence of intracellular parasites. A positive flag would then alert the staff to closely review the blood slide for organisms (26).

Thick Blood Films

In the preparation of a thick blood film, the highest concentration of blood cells is in the center of the film. The examination should be performed at low magnification to detect microfilariae more readily. Examination of a thick film usually requires 5 to 10 min (approximately 300 oil immersion fields). The search for malarial organisms and trypanosomes is best done under oil immersion (magnification, ×1,000). Intact RBCs are frequently seen at the very periphery of the thick film; such cells, if infected, may prove useful in malaria diagnosis, since they may demonstrate the characteristic morphology necessary to identify the organisms to the species level.

Blood Stains

For accurate identification of blood parasites, a laboratory should develop proficiency in the use of at least one good staining method. It is better to select one method that will provide reproducible results than to use several on a hit-or-miss basis. Blood films should be stained as soon as possible, since prolonged storage may result in stain retention. Delay in staining positive malarial smears may result in failure to demonstrate typical staining characteristics for individual species.

The most common stains are of two types. Wright's stain (or Wright-Giemsa) has the fixative in combination with the staining solution, so that both fixation and staining occur at the same time; therefore, the thick film must be laked before staining. In Giemsa stain, the fixative and stain are separate; therefore, the thin film must be fixed with absolute methanol before staining.

Buffy Coat Films

Trypanosomes, occasionally *H. capsulatum* (a fungus that manifests as small oval yeast cells resembling those of *Leishmania* amastigote stages), and, in immunocompromised patients, potentially *T. gondii* and *Leishmania* spp. (*Leishmania infantum*, *L. chagasi*, and *L. donovani*) are detected within the large mononuclear cells in the buffy coat (a layer of leukocytes resulting from centrifugation of whole anticoagulated blood). The amastigote form of *Leishmania* spp. possesses a kinetoplast, a nucleus that stains dark red-purple, and the cytoplasm stains light blue. *H. capsulatum* appears as a large dot of nuclear material (dark red-purple) surrounded by a clear halo area. Trypanosomes in the peripheral blood also concentrate with the buffy coat cells (1).

Screening Methods

Microhematocrit centrifugation with use of the QBC malaria test, a glass capillary tube, and closely fitting plastic insert (QBC malaria blood tubes; Becton Dickinson, Tropical Disease Diagnostics, Sparks, MD) has been used for the detection of blood parasites. Tubes precoated with acridine orange provide a stain that induces fluorescence in the parasites. At the end of centrifugation of 50 to 60 μl of capillary or venous blood (5 min in a QBC centrifuge, 14,387 × *g*), parasites or RBCs containing parasites are concentrated in a 1- to 2-mm region near the top of the RBC column and are held close to the wall of the tube by the plastic float, making them readily visible by fluorescence microscopy. This method automatically prepares a concentrated smear, which represents the distance between the float and the walls of the tube. Once the tube is placed in the plastic holder (Para-viewer) and immersion oil is applied to the top of the hematocrit tube (no coverslip is necessary), the tube is examined with a 40× to 60× oil immersion objective (which must have a working distance of 0.3 mm or greater) (1). The cost of the equipment and the level of technical expertise required may limit use of this test method.

Antigen Detection and Molecular Detection for Blood Parasites

Several antigen detection tests are available. Many among them are designed for rapid and individual diagnoses. Most of the kits are not available in the United States but have proven to be very useful in other countries (27). Rapid tests are available to diagnose specifically *Plasmodium falciparum* or, on a genus level, *Plasmodium* sp. infections. These tests are simple to perform and can be applied during the more time-consuming microscopic identification of the thin and thick blood smears. However, one has to be aware that false-positive and false-negative reactions do occur (28–30). The general recommendation is to use these tests only in addition to the microscopic examination of thick and thin blood smears. Various molecular methods (e.g., PCR, DNA/RNA hybridization, and sequencing) have been described in the scientific literature. Although the methods are more sensitive than standard microscopic examinations of blood films, they are not routinely used for malaria diagnosis.

Knott Concentration

The Knott concentration procedure is used primarily to detect the presence of microfilariae in the blood, especially when a light infection is suspected. Aqueous formalin is added to anticoagulated blood and centrifuged at 300 × *g* to concentrate microfilaria. The sediment is examined microscopically (magnifications of ×100 and ×400). A thick prep can be made with the remainder of the sediment. Microfilariae will be nonmotile in the wet smear; however, they will exhibit diagnostic morphologic characteristics when stained. The disadvantage of the procedure is that the microfilariae are killed by the formalin and are therefore not seen as motile organisms.

Membrane Filtration Technique

The membrane filtration technique (25-mm Nuclepore filter [5-μm porosity]) has proved highly efficient in demonstrating filarial infections when microfilariae are of low density. It has also been successfully used in field surveys (1).

Culture Methods

Very few clinical laboratories offer specific culture techniques for parasites. The methods for *in vitro* culture are often complex, while quality control is difficult and not really feasible for the routine diagnostic laboratory. In certain institutions, some techniques may be available, particularly where consultative services are provided and for research purposes.

Few parasites can be routinely cultured, and the only procedures that are in general use are for *E. histolytica*, *Naegleria fowleri*, *Acanthamoeba* spp., *Trichomonas vaginalis*, *T. gondii*, *T. cruzi*, *Encephalitozoon* spp., and the leishmanias. These procedures are usually available only after consultation with the laboratory and on special request. Commercial tests are available only for *T. vaginalis* (InPouch TV; BioMed Diagnostics, White City, OR).

Animal Inoculation and Xenodiagnosis

Most routine clinical laboratories do not have the animal care facilities necessary to provide animal inoculation capabilities for the diagnosis of parasitic infections. Host specificity for many animal parasite species is well known and limits the types of animals available for these procedures. For certain suspected infections, animal inoculation may be requested and can be very helpful in making the diagnosis, although animal inoculation certainly does not take the place of other, more routine procedures. Mouse inoculation with amniotic fluid was used in the past for diagnosis of congenital toxoplasmosis; this method, however, has mostly been replaced by NAAT.

Xenodiagnosis is a technique that uses the arthropod host as an indicator of infection. Uninfected reduviid bugs are allowed to feed on the blood of a patient who is suspected of having Chagas' disease (*T. cruzi* infection). After 30 to 60 days, feces from the bugs are examined over a 3-month time frame for the presence of developmental stages of the parasite, which are found in the hindgut of the vector. This type of procedure is used primarily in South America for fieldwork, and the appropriate bugs are raised in various laboratories specifically for this purpose.

Antigen Detection

The detection of parasite-specific antigen is indicative of current infection. Immunoassays are generally simple to perform. Some formats allow the processing of large numbers of tests at one time, thereby reducing overall costs; others are specially designed for rapid individual diagnoses. A major disadvantage of antigen detection is that in most cases the method can detect only a single pathogen at one time. Therefore, additional parasitological examinations must be performed to detect other parasitic pathogens. The current commercially available immunoassays for the detection of intestinal protozoa have excellent sensitivity and specificity compared with routine microscopy (31–34). Specific ordering approaches using both immunoassays and routine O&P examinations are listed in Table 6. Rapid tests for the diagnosis of malaria should be used only in parallel with the examination of thick and thin blood smears.

Parasite Nucleic Acid Detection

Molecular testing is becoming more readily available for most diagnostic laboratories. Assays for *T. vaginalis*, *E. histolytica*, *E. histolytica* complex, *Giardia*, *Cyclospora*, and *Cryptosporidium* spp. are commercially available and approved by the Food and Drug Administration (FDA). Intestinal gastrointestinal panels are available that can test simultaneously for multiple gastrointestinal pathogens, including bacterial, viral, and parasitic pathogens. As with antigen detection, only select pathogens can be detected, and other pathogens may be missed. Specific automated panels are listed in chapter 138. Additional panels for *Blastocystis* spp., *Dientamoeba fragilis*, microsporidia and *S. stercoralis* are under development.

Nucleic acid-based diagnostic tests (with their inherent potential for highly efficient and specific amplification of DNA) have been developed for almost all species of parasites. However, only a few are routinely used in diagnostic settings. The main reason for this minor role in diagnostic parasitology is the fact that many parasite stages can be adequately diagnosed using established, more traditional techniques (microscopy, detection of antigens and antibodies, and *in vitro* cultivation) that are generally less expensive and technically less demanding than NAAT. Therefore, diagnosis by NAAT is of great value in cases in which these techniques are insufficient, that is, in cases in which (i) the immune response is not informative (e.g., acute infections, short-term follow-up after therapy, and congenital infections), (ii) high sensitivity is needed because of low parasite levels (e.g., cutaneous leishmaniasis), or (iii) morphologically indistinguishable organisms need to be identified (e.g., *E. histolytica/Entamoeba dispar* and eggs of taeniid tapeworms).

Diagnostic NAAT may become more widespread when simple, fully standardized (commercial) test kits are available and costs are reduced through the implementation of pre- and post-NAAT automated techniques. Furthermore, it is possible not only to detect and identify but also to quantify organisms and determine their genotypes by analyzing the diagnostic NAAT product. Indeed, NAAT coupled with genetic characterization is already widely used in parasitology to address questions such as those concerning parasite host range and host specificity, means of transmission, and molecular epidemiology. Such genotyping applications should increase in the future with increasing knowledge of the relationship between genetic variation in parasites and features such as virulence or drug resistance. An important limitation of NAAT-based diagnosis is the fact that sensitivity dramatically decreases with material stored for more than 1 day in formalin due to the fragmentation (fragment length of a few hundred base pairs) of the DNA. However, by selecting primers that yield products as short as possible, sensitivity might be reasonably high. Therefore, it seems to be the best choice to avoid formalin fixation if NAAT analyses have to be considered. Such tests, however, are not yet widely available in parasitology.

APPENDIX

Parasite Images

Parasite image library and parasitological resources (accessed 5 October 2017)

University of Delaware
http://www.udel.edu/mls/dlehman/medt372/index.html

Centers for Disease Control and Prevention
http://www.cdc.gov/dpdx/

Oregon Public Health Laboratories Parasite Image Library
http://public.health.oregon.gov/LaboratoryServices/ImageLibrary/Pages/parlib.aspx

American Society of Parasitologists
https://www.amsocparasit.org/parasite-images

Parasitology Information (accessed 5 October 2017)

Centers for Disease Control and Prevention
http://www.cdc.gov/dpdx/az.html

World Health Organization
http://www.who.int

Medical Chemical Corporation
http://www.med-chem.com

NCBI National Library of Medicine (PubMed)
http://www.ncbi.nlm.nih.gov/entrez/query.fcgi

U.S. Air Force Public Health Information and Resources
http://www.phsource.us

Atlas of Human Intestinal Protozoa
http://www.atlas-protozoa.com

Swiss Tropical and Public Health Institute
http://www.parasite-diagnosis.ch/home

REFERENCES

1. **Garcia LS.** 2016. *Diagnostic Medical Parasitology*, 6th ed. ASM Press, Washington, DC.
2. **Garcia LS.** 2009. *Practical Guide to Diagnostic Parasitology*, 2nd ed. ASM Press, Washington, DC.
3. **Hiatt RA, Markell EK, Ng E.** 1995. How many stool examinations are necessary to detect pathogenic intestinal protozoa? *Am J Trop Med Hyg* **53:**36–39.

4. **Marti H, Koella JC.** 1993. Multiple stool examinations for ova and parasites and rate of false-negative results. *J Clin Microbiol* **31:**3044–3045.
5. **Chernesky M, Morse S, Schachter J.** 1999. Newly available and future laboratory tests for sexually transmitted diseases (STDs) other than HIV. *Sex Transm Dis* **26**(Suppl)**:**S8–S11.
6. **Weber R, Schwartz DA, Deplazes P.** 1999. Laboratory diagnosis of microsporidiosis, p 315–362. *In* Wittner ML, Weiss LM (ed), *The Microsporidia and Microsporidiosis.* ASM Press, Washington, DC.
7. **Leber AL (ed).** 2016. *Clinical Microbiology Procedures Handbook*, 4th ed. ASM Press, Washington, D.C.
8. **Occupational Safety and Health Administration.** 1991. Occupational exposure to bloodborne pathogens. 29 CFR 1910.1030. *Fed Regist* **56:**64004–64182.
9. **U.S. Department of Health and Human Services.** 2009. *Biosafety in Microbiological and Biomedical Laboratories*, 5th ed. U.S. Government Printing Office, Washington, DC.
10. **Markell EK, John DT, Krotoski WA.** 1999. *Medical Parasitology*, 8th ed. WB Saunders Co, Philadelphia, PA.
11. **Melvin DM, Brooke MM.** 1982. Laboratory procedures for the diagnosis of intestinal parasites, 3rd ed. U.S. Department of Health, Education, and Welfare publication (CDC) 82-8282. U.S. Government Printing Office, Washington, DC.
12. **Hanson KL, Cartwright CP.** 2001. Use of an enzyme immunoassay does not eliminate the need to analyze multiple stool specimens for sensitive detection of *Giardia lamblia*. *J Clin Microbiol* **39:**474–477.
13. **National Committee for Clinical Laboratory Standards/ Clinical and Laboratory Standards Institute.** 2005. Procedures for the recovery and identification of parasites from the intestinal tract. Approved standard M28-A2. Clinical and Laboratory Standards Institute, Wayne, PA.
14. **Scholten TH, Yang J.** 1974. Evaluation of unpreserved and preserved stools for the detection and identification of intestinal parasites. *Am J Clin Pathol* **62:**563–567.
15. **Yang J, Scholten T.** 1977. A fixative for intestinal parasites permitting the use of concentration and permanent staining procedures. *Am J Clin Pathol* **67:**300–304.
16. **Brooke MM, Goldman M.** 1949. Polyvinyl alcohol-fixative as a preservative and adhesive for protozoa in dysenteric stools and other liquid material. *J Lab Clin Med* **34:**1554–1560.
17. **Horen WP.** 1981. Modification of Schaudinn fixative. *J Clin Microbiol* **13:**204–205.
18. **Garcia LS, Shimizu RY, Brewer TC, Bruckner DA.** 1983. Evaluation of intestinal parasite morphology in polyvinyl alcohol preservative: comparison of copper sulfate and mercuric chloride bases for use in Schaudinn fixative. *J Clin Microbiol* **17:**1092–1095.
19. **Garcia LS, Shimizu RY, Shum A, Bruckner DA.** 1993. Evaluation of intestinal protozoan morphology in polyvinyl alcohol preservative: comparison of zinc sulfate- and mercuric chloride-based compounds for use in Schaudinn's fixative. *J Clin Microbiol* **31:**307–310.
20. **National Committee for Clinical Laboratory Standards.** 2000. Use of blood film examination for parasites. Approved standard M15-A. National Committee for Clinical Laboratory Standards, Wayne, PA.
21. **Winn WC, Allen SD, Janda WM, Koneman EW, Procop GW, Schreckenberger PC, Woods G.** 2006. *Color Atlas and Textbook of Diagnostic Microbiology*, 6th ed. J. B. Lippincott Co., Philadelphia, PA.
22. **John DT, Petri WA.** 2006. *Medical Parasitology*, 9th ed. The W.B. Saunders Co., Philadelphia, PA.
23. **Beal C, Goldsmith R, Kotby M, Sherif M, el-Tagi A, Farid A, Zakaria S, Eapen J.** 1992. The plastic envelope method, a simplified technique for culture diagnosis of trichomoniasis. *J Clin Microbiol* **30:**2265–2268.
24. **Mathis A, Deplazes P.** 1995. PCR and in vitro cultivation for detection of *Leishmania* spp. in diagnostic samples from humans and dogs. *J Clin Microbiol* **33:**1145–1149.
25. **Garcia LS, Shimizu RY, Bruckner DA.** 1986. Blood parasites: problems in diagnosis using automated differential instrumentation. *Diagn Microbiol Infect Dis* **4:**173–176.
26. **Hanscheid T, Grobusch MP.** 2017. Modern hematology analyzers are very useful for diagnosis of malaria and, crucially, may help avoid misdiagnosis. *J Clin Microbiol* **55:**3303–3304.
27. **World Health Organization.** 2017. WHO-FIND malaria RDT evaluation programme. http:www.who.int/malaria/areas/diagnosis/rapid-diagnostic-tests/rdt-evaluation-programme/en/. Accessed 20 November 2017.
28. **Bell D, Go R, Miguel C, Walker J, Cacal L, Saul A.** 2001. Diagnosis of malaria in a remote area of the Philippines: comparison of techniques and their acceptance by health workers and the community. *Bull World Health Organ* **79:**933–941.
29. **Craig MH, Bredenkamp BL, Williams CH, Rossouw EJ, Kelly VJ, Kleinschmidt I, Martineau A, Henry GF.** 2002. Field and laboratory comparative evaluation of ten rapid malaria diagnostic tests. *Trans R Soc Trop Med Hyg* **96:**258–265.
30. **Mathison BA, Pritt BS.** 2017. Update on malaria diagnostics and test utilization. *J Clin Microbiol* **55:**2009–2017.
31. **Aldeen WE, Carroll K, Robison A, Morrison M, Hale D.** 1998. Comparison of nine commercially available enzyme-linked immunosorbent assays for detection of *Giardia lamblia* in fecal specimens. *J Clin Microbiol* **36:**1338–1340.
32. **Garcia LS, Shimizu RY.** 1997. Evaluation of nine immunoassay kits (enzyme immunoassay and direct fluorescence) for detection of *Giardia lamblia* and *Cryptosporidium parvum* in human fecal specimens. *J Clin Microbiol* **35:**1526–1529.
33. **Garcia LS, Shimizu RY.** 2000. Detection of *Giardia lamblia* and *Cryptosporidium parvum* antigens in human fecal specimens using the ColorPAC combination rapid solid-phase qualitative immunochromatographic assay. *J Clin Microbiol* **38:**1267–1268.
34. **Garcia LS, Shimizu RY, Bernard CN.** 2000. Detection of *Giardia lamblia, Entamoeba histolytica/Entamoeba dispar*, and *Cryptosporidium parvum* antigens in human fecal specimens using the triage parasite panel enzyme immunoassay. *J Clin Microbiol* **38:**3337–3340.

Reagents, Stains, and Media: Parasitology

ANDREA J. LINSCOTT AND SUSAN E. SHARP

137

The evaluation of clinical specimens for ova and parasites in the clinical laboratory can involve the use of direct macroscopic examination of the specimen and microscopic examination of fresh and preserved specimens, as well as culture for some parasitic organisms. These examinations necessitate the use of a variety of stains, reagents, and media, the most common of which are discussed in this chapter.

Because many parasitic organisms cannot be cultured, microscopic examination is the mainstay of diagnostic parasitology. Examination after proficient staining of fresh and unconcentrated specimens, as well as preserved and/or concentrated specimens with permanent stained preparations, most often provides a rapid and accurate diagnosis. A variety of reagents and stains are available for these purposes, and each laboratory must decide which ones to use to best serve its patient population. In addition, because most specimens are submitted in fixatives and preservatives, the reader should note the specific interference of polyvinyl alcohol (PVA) and mercury reagents with immunoassays that are commonly used for parasitic diagnosis. As immunoassays and nucleic acid amplification assays become more commonly used for the detection of parasites, reagents needed to perform these tests must be considered.

Caution should be taken when reagents are used in the parasitology laboratory. Many routinely used compounds can be dangerous if not handled appropriately. For example, formalin and formaldehyde solutions can cause severe skin irritation and, if swallowed, can cause violent vomiting and diarrhea; mercury compounds are local irritants and systemic poisons that can be absorbed through the skin; phenol is a skin irritant, and exposure to large amounts can affect the central nervous system; and xylene can cause serious skin irritation, with extended exposure causing gastrointestinal, neurologic, and tissue damage (1). It is also important to remember that reagents that contain formalin and/or mercury require special disposal. Proper disposal should be carried out using state and federal regulatory guidelines.

REAGENTS

All of the following reagents are preservatives and/or fixatives. Table 1 lists several types of preservatives along with their content, specific permanent stained smears that can be performed, and immunoassays for which they can be used, and additional comments concerning the fixative. Today, most clinical laboratories purchase premixed, packaged vials of preservatives and fixatives/adhesives that can be either inoculated with fecal sample sent to the laboratory or sent home with the patient for home collection. A list of commercially available transport vials can be found in Table 2.

Formalin Preparations

Formalin

Formalin has been used in parasitology as an all-purpose preservative for concentration procedures. However, formalin should not be used to prepare smears for permanent stains, because the reagent does not adequately preserve organism morphology (2). Formalin is easy to prepare and has a long shelf life. It is most routinely used as a preservative for stool and duodenal aspirate specimens. Formalin works well to preserve the morphologies of helminth ova and larvae and those of protozoan cysts, oocysts, and spores, although it does not preserve protozoan trophozoites well. Although both 5% and 10% solutions of formalin are currently used (5% for the best preservation of protozoan stages and 10% for ova and larvae), the 10% formulation is most widely used in clinical parasitology today. A formalin vial is often paired with a vial containing a fixative such as PVA or Schaudinn's to ensure that a permanent stained smear can be prepared and read. Formalin (10%) is prepared as indicated below.

Formaldehyde (37% to 40% HCHO solution) .... 100 ml
Saline (0.85% NaCl) OR distilled water .... 900 ml

Buffered formalin

Formalin buffered with sodium and potassium phosphates can be used to help maintain the morphology of parasites for long-term storage and is used for concentration procedures. To make buffered formalin, mix the following dry ingredients and store in a tightly closed container. Add 0.8 g of this mixture to 1 liter of 10% (or 5%) formalin.

Sodium phosphate, dibasic (Na_2HPO_4) .... 6.1 g
Potassium phosphate, monobasic (KH_2PO_4)........ 0.15 g

Merthiolate-iodine-formalin

Protozoa and helminth ova and larvae can be distinguished on direct wet mounts after stool and duodenal aspirate

TABLE 1 Preservatives used in diagnostic parasitology (intestinal tract specimens)

Preservative	Use		
	Concentrated examination	Permanent stained smear	Immunoassays[a]
5% or 10% formalin	Yes	No	Yes (EIA, FA, rapid)
5% or 10% buffered formalin	Yes	No	Yes (EIA, FA, rapid)
MIF	Yes	Polychrome IV stain[b]	No (no published data for immunoassay systems)
SAF	Yes	Iron hematoxylin, trichrome (not as good)	Yes (EIA, FA, rapid)
Hg-PVA[c]	Yes	Trichrome or iron hematoxylin	No (PVA plastic powder interferes with immunoassays)
Cu-PVA[d]	Yes	Trichrome or iron hematoxylin	No (PVA plastic powder interferes with immunoassays)
Zn-PVA[e]	Yes	Trichrome or iron hematoxylin	Some, but not all; PVA plastic powder interferes with immunoassays
Single-vial systems[f]	Yes	Trichrome or iron hematoxylin	Some, but not all. If no PVA or mercury, may be compatible with fecal immunoassays
Schaudinn's (without PVA)[c]	No	Trichrome or iron hematoxylin	No (mercury interferes with immunoassays)

[a]EIA, enzyme immunoassay; FA, fluorescence assay.

[b]This stain can be used in place of trichrome for staining fecal smears preserved with MIF, PVA, or SAF. It is available commercially.

[c]PVA (plastic powder used as "glue" to attach stool onto the glass slide; no fixation properties per se) and Schaudinn's fixative (mercuric chloride base) are still considered the gold standard against which all other fixatives are evaluated for organism morphology after permanent staining. Additional fixatives prepared with non-mercuric chloride-based compounds are being developed and tested.

[d]This modification uses a copper sulfate base rather than mercuric chloride.

[e]This modification uses a zinc base rather than mercuric chloride and apparently works well with both trichrome and iron hematoxylin stains.

[f]These modifications use a combination of ingredients (including zinc) but are prepared from proprietary formulas. The aim is to provide a fixative that can be used for the fecal concentration and permanent stained smear. Acceptability for use with immunoassays for *Giardia duodenalis* and *Cryptosporidium* species varies, so proper use should be verified with the manufacturer's package insert. Testing for *E. histolytica* and/or the *E. histolytica/E. dispar* group still requires fresh or frozen specimens.

specimens are fixed in merthiolate-iodine-formalin (MIF). MIF allows not only fixation but also staining of the organisms. MIF can be used to perform concentration procedures. This method requires that the two stock solutions listed below be combined into a fresh working solution immediately before use. In addition, after specimens have been mixed with MIF, the mixture must be left undisturbed for 24 h before preparation of smears from the bottom two layers of the three layers that will form. Parasitological examination of specimens placed in MIF can be performed for several weeks after preservation, making it very useful for field surveys. MIF is also readily available commercially.

Solution I (store in brown bottle)

Distilled water .... 50 ml
Formaldehyde .... 5 ml
Thimerosal (tincture of merthiolate, 1:1,000) ..... 40 ml
Glycerol .... 1 ml

Solution II (Lugol's solution) (good for several weeks in a tightly stoppered brown bottle)

Distilled water .... 100 ml
Potassium iodide crystals (KI) .... 10 g
Iodine crystals (add after KI dissolves) .... 5 g

TABLE 2 Commercially available collection/transport vials for the recovery of parasites[a]

Company	Preservative	Fixative	Single-vial system
Alpha-Tec Systems (http://www.alphatecsystems.com; accessed 8/5/17)	10% formalin	SAF Zn-PVA	Proto-fix CLR
Medical Chemical Corporation (http://www.med-chem.com/; accessed 8/5/17)	10% formalin MIF	Cu-PVA LV-PVA Zn-PVA SAF	Total-Fix universal fixative (no mercury, formalin, or PVA)
Meridian Bioscience (http://www.meridianbioscience.com/; accessed 8/5/17)	10% formalin	LV-PVA SAF Zn-PVA	EcoFix universal fixative (no mercury or formalin; contains PVA)
Remel (http://www.remel.com; accessed 8/5/17)	5% formalin 10% formalin	PVA SAF Zn-PVA	
Scientific Device Laboratory (http://www.scientificdevice.com; accessed 8/5/17)		PVA SAF	Parasafe
VWR (http://VWR.com; accessed 8/5/17)			Alcorfix

[a]LV-PVA, low-velocity PVA. Website access dates are in month/day/year format.

Combine 9.4 ml of solution I with 0.6 ml of solution II just before use.

PVA-Containing Preservatives and Fixatives

PVA acts as an adhesive for stool material, allowing the stool to adhere to glass slides. Several modifications are commercially available. The compound accompanying the PVA, specifically, mercuric chloride, zinc sulfate, or cupric sulfate, acts as the preservative and allows fixation of protozoan cysts and trophozoites for use with trichrome or iron hematoxylin stains for permanent smears. All PVA-containing preservatives interfere with immunoassays. PVA is not an appropriate reagent to use for stool specimen concentration and should be paired with a reagent vial (formalin, MIF, or sodium acetate-acetic acid-formalin [SAF]) that can be used for that purpose.

■ Hg-PVA

The Hg-PVA fixative uses mercuric chloride as the preservative. Protozoan morphology is best preserved with PVA-incorporating mercury compounds. However, due to the toxic nature of mercury compounds and the difficulty in preparation, most laboratories no longer prepare Hg-PVA.

■ Zn-PVA

The Zn-PVA fixative uses zinc sulfate in place of mercury as a preservative and fixative for protozoans. Specimens treated with Zn-PVA may also be stained with trichrome or iron hematoxylin stains for permanent smears.

■ Cu-PVA

The Cu-PVA fixative uses cupric sulfate in place of mercury as a preservative and fixative for protozoans. Specimens treated with Cu-PVA may also be stained with trichrome or iron hematoxylin stains for permanent smears.

Studies have shown that zinc sulfate provides a satisfactory, but not equal, substitute for mercury in the permanent staining procedures and that copper sulfate does not preserve morphology equal to that seen with mercuric chloride (3, 4).

■ Schaudinn's fixative/solution

Schaudinn's solution is a fixative made of mercuric chloride, distilled water, and 95% ethyl alcohol that gives excellent morphological preservation of protozoan organisms. It is used primarily in the preparation of permanent stained smears for parasitological examination from fresh, nonpreserved specimens. Specimens fixed in Schaudinn's solution can be used with either trichrome or iron hematoxylin stains. As with Hg-PVA, due to the toxic nature of mercuric compounds and the difficulty of preparing this fixative, Schaudinn's solution is not routinely made in the clinical microbiology laboratory. In addition, Schaudinn's fixative is becoming increasingly more difficult to purchase commercially. Many laboratories are opting to use a mercury-free or low-level-mercury single vial that can be used to prepare both a concentration and a preparation for permanent stained smears. See "Nonmercury or low-level-mercury, nonformalin fixatives: single-vial systems" below.

■ Sodium acetate-acetic acid-formalin

SAF is very similar to formalin in that it is a liquid fixative and contains no mercury. However, unlike formalin, SAF can be used for both concentration techniques and permanent stained smears. The sediment from the concentration procedure is used for both the wet preparation and the permanent stain. Albumin-coated slides allow better adhesion of the concentrated material to the slide and are recommended for use with SAF. SAF is an acceptable substitute for PVA or Schaudinn's solution for permanent smears stained with either trichrome or iron hematoxylin. SAF is available commercially and has a long shelf life, but it can also readily be made in the laboratory by mixing the reagents listed below.

Sodium acetate .... 1.5 g
Glacial acetic acid.. 2.0 ml
Formaldehyde (37% to 40% HCHO solution)..... 4.0 ml
Distilled water.. 92.0 ml

■ Nonmercury or low-level-mercury, nonformalin fixatives: single-vial systems

Several nonmercury, nonformalin proprietary fixatives are commercially available for both concentration of stool specimens and the preparation of permanently stained smears (Medical Chemical Corporation, Torrance, CA; Meridian Bioscience, Cincinnati, OH). There is also a low-level-mercury, nonformalin proprietary fixative available that can be used as described above (Alpha-Tec, Vancouver, WA). Another formalin-free single-collection device is Alcorfix, which is used in conjunction with a Mini Parasep solvent-free collection tube for concentration. Alcorfix has been evaluated and is used by several large reference laboratories (5). This product in manufactured by Apacor (Berkshire, United Kingdom) and is distributed in the United States by VWR. The beauty of these systems is that only one vial is needed to prepare both a concentration and a permanent stained smear and that the vials can be discarded along with other biohazardous waste in the laboratory. Acceptability for use in fecal immunoassays varies (check with manufacturers for specific uses). Special stains are also available for use with some of these fixatives.

STAINS

Table 3 lists the stains that are most commonly used to detect and aid in the identification of parasitic organisms. Figures 1 through 5 illustrate staining properties of parasites

TABLE 3 Stains used for parasitic identification

Organism	Stain(s) used for detection
Cryptosporidium spp., *Cystoisospora belli*, *Cyclospora cayetanensis*	Modified acid-fast stain (Fig. 1)
Cystoisospora and *Cyclospora* oocysts, *Sarcocystis* sporocysts	Autofluorescence with no stain using fluorescent microscopy (Fig. 2)
Cyclospora	Modified safranin stain
Naegleria spp., *Acanthamoeba* spp., *Balamuthia* spp.	Calcofluor white stain using fluorescent microscopy, trichrome stain
Acanthamoeba	Modified Field's stain, trichrome stain
Blood parasites (agents of malaria, microfilariae, and *Leishmania*, *Babesia*, and *Trypanosoma* spp.)	Giemsa or Wright's stain (rapid blood stains are also acceptable) (Fig. 3)
Microfilariae (specifically for sheaths and nuclei)	Delafield's hematoxylin stain; Giemsa stain also acceptable except for *Wuchereria bancrofti*
Parasitic helminth eggs/larvae and protozoan cysts	Iodine (Fig. 4)
Intestinal protozoan parasites	Iron hematoxylin stain, trichrome stain (Fig. 5)

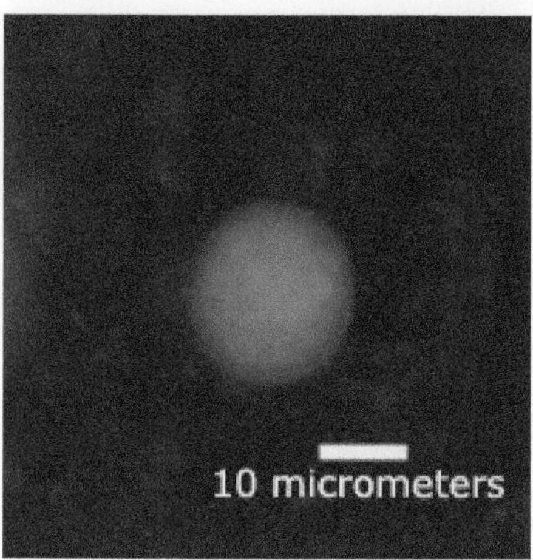

FIGURE 1 Autofluorescence of an oocyst of *Cyclospora* seen using UV microscopy.

using various stains mentioned below. The descriptions of and procedures for stains used in parasitology are listed below. A list of commercially available parasitology stains can be found in Table 4.

■ Iodine (Lugol's or D'Antoni's)

A solution of iodine can be used for preparing direct or concentrated wet mounts for parasitological examination.

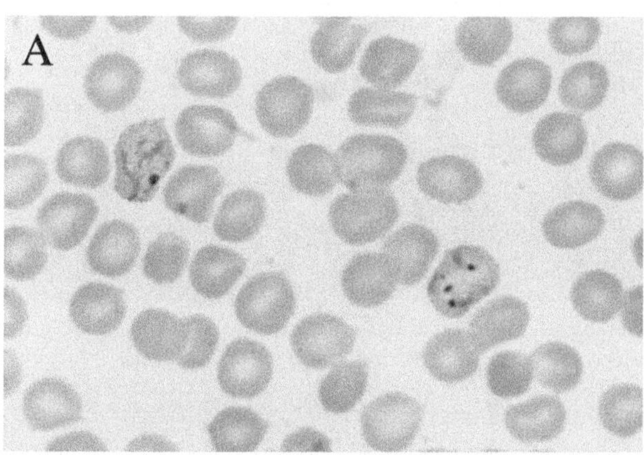

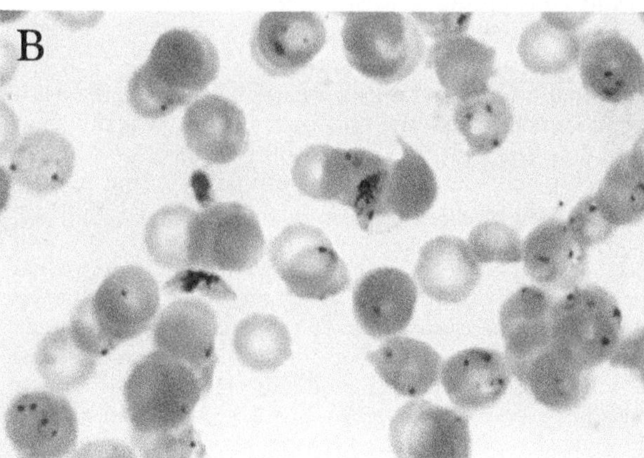

FIGURE 2 (A) Giemsa-stained peripheral blood smear showing dark pink Schüffner's dots and ring trophozoites. (B) Giemsa-stained gametocytes in a peripheral blood smear.

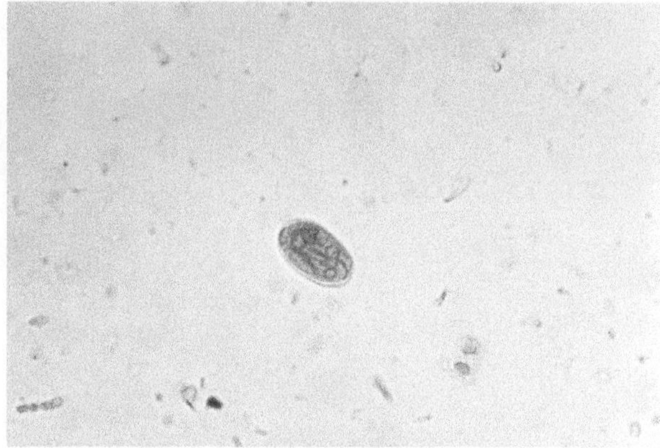

FIGURE 3 *Giardia* cyst stained golden brown with iodine stain.

These nonspecific dyes allow the differentiation of parasitic cysts from leukocytes, the former of which retain the iodine and appear light brown. Iodine can easily overstain eggs; thus, a wet prep without iodine should be used to detect eggs. Iodine stains can be purchased commercially for use in routine parasitology. These solutions should be stored in dark containers in a dark environment. D'Antoni's iodine preparation has the advantage of use without further dilution, whereas Lugol's iodine must be diluted into a working solution (1:5 dilution in distilled water) before use. Working solutions of both iodine preparations fade with time and should be discarded and replaced when their dark tea color lightens.

Basic procedure

Place 1 drop of iodine on a slide; add to this a small amount of fecal specimen and mix until homogeneous. The iodine stains fecal material immediately, and the timing of this step is not important. Place a coverslip on top of the suspension and view under a magnification of ×100. Examine any suspicious material under a ×400 magnification.

Acid-Fast Stains (Modified)

Cryptosporidium, *Cystoisospora belli*, and *Cyclospora cayetanensis* are coccidian parasites that can cause diarrheal disease in humans. These organisms are more easily detected

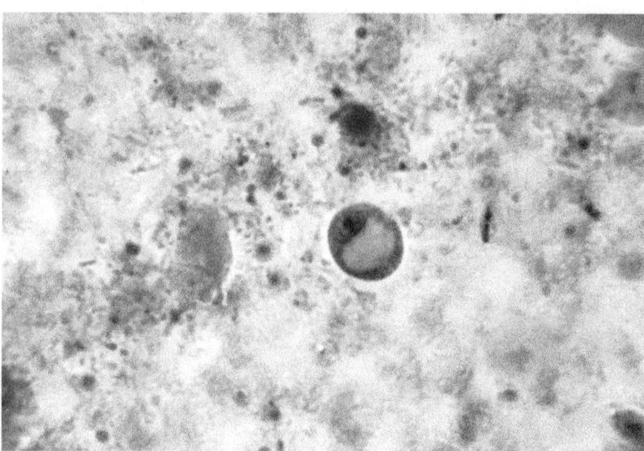

FIGURE 4 *Iodamoeba* cyst stained blue with trichrome stain. Note that the karyosome stains darker blue and the vacuole stains light blue.

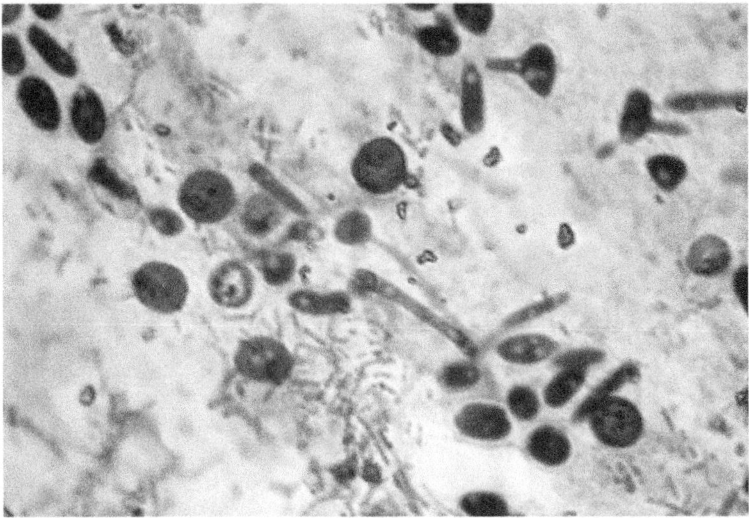

FIGURE 5 *Cryptosporidium* oocyst stained bright red with acid-fast stain. Bacteria and yeasts stain blue.

when a modified acid-fast stain is used. The modification to the acid-fast stains is the use of decolorizing agents that are less harsh than those used for staining mycobacteria. The carbol fuchsin and counterstain (methylene blue) reagents used for mycobacteria can be used for staining coccidian parasites; however, the decoloring agents are not interchangeable. In the modified acid-fast staining procedures, a 1% solution of sulfuric acid (1 ml of sulfuric acid in 99 ml of water) is used, as opposed to the 3% solution used in the acid-fast bacillus Kinyoun staining procedure, and a 5% sulfuric acid solution (5 ml of concentrated sulfuric acid in 95 ml of distilled water) is used, as opposed to the 3% HCl solution in 95% ethanol that is used in the acid-fast bacillus Ziehl-Neelsen staining procedure.

TABLE 4 Commercially available stains for the detection of parasites

Company[a]	Stains
Alpha-Tec Systems (http://www.alphatecsystems.com, accessed 8/5/17)	Cryptosporidium stain set Giemsa stain and buffer Proto-fix stain set Wheatley's trichrome stain
Hardy Diagnostics (http://hardydiagnostic.com, accessed 8/5/17)	Giemsa stain and buffer Iodine alcohol Wheatley's trichrome stain
Medical Chemical Corporation (http://www.med-chem.com, accessed 8/5/17)	D'Antoni iodine Iron hematoxylin stain Giemsa stain and buffer Wheatley's modified Gomori trichrome
Meridian Bioscience (http://www.meridianbioscience.com, accessed 8/5/17)	EcoStain Trichrome stain
Remel (http://www.remel.com, accessed 8/5/17)	Trichrome stain Trichrome quick stain
Scientific Device Laboratory (http://www.scientificdevic.com, accessed 8/5/17)	StainQuick trichrome Cryptosporidium Kinyoun stain Trichrome stain

[a]Access dates are in the format month/day/year.

■ Modified Kinyoun stain (cold method)

Basic procedure (modified Kinyoun stain)
Apply specimen (1 or 2 drops) to a slide, allow it to air dry, and fix with absolute methanol for 1 min. Apply carbol fuchsin to the slide for 5 min, and then rinse the slide with 50% ethanol, followed by a water rinse. Add sulfuric acid (1%) decolorizer for 2 min, and rinse the slide again with water. Add methylene blue for 1 min, and then rinse the slide again with water. Air dry the slide and examine at ×100 to ×1,000 magnification.

■ Modified Ziehl-Neelsen stain (hot method)

Apply specimen (1 or 2 drops) to a slide, allow it to air dry, and then dry it on a heating block (70°C) for 5 min. Place the slide on a rack and flood it with carbol fuchsin. With an alcohol lamp or Bunsen burner, gently heat the slide until steam appears. Allow the specimen to stain for 5 min and then rinse. Decolorize with 5% sulfuric acid for 30 seconds and rinse. Counterstain with methylene blue for 1 minute and rinse. The slide is then air dried and examined at ×100 to ×1,000 magnification.

Blood Film Stains

■ Giemsa and Wright's stains

Examination of blood films for parasites includes the use of two common stains, the Giemsa stain and Wright's stain, both derivatives of the original Romanowsky stain. These stains are very similar, differing primarily in that no fixative is included in the Giemsa stain and the blood film must be fixed with absolute methanol before staining. Erythrocytic stippling, seen in some malaria infections, can be seen using only the Giemsa stain (6). Although stock solutions of these stains can be prepared in the laboratory, the procedure is very cumbersome and involves grinding of powdered stain with methanol and/or glycerol with a mortar and pestle, days to weeks of storage with shaking, and removal of supernatant or filtering before use. In addition, it is recommended that the Giemsa stain be prepared fresh each day of use by diluting the stain stock solution with phosphate-buffered water, pH 7 to 7.2 (7). Alternatively, Giemsa, Wright's, and Wright-Giemsa stains are readily available from commercial suppliers in liquid form and may need only dilution in a buffer solution. Blood films may be stained manually, but many laboratories rely on automated hematologic instruments for staining of thin (not thick) blood films, with acceptable results. These stains allow the detection of blood parasites, including the agent of malaria, microfilariae, and *Leishmania*, *Babesia*, and *Trypanosoma* species. Although for many years, Giemsa stain has been the stain of choice, the parasites can also be seen on blood films stained with Wright's stain, a Wright-Giemsa combination stain, or one of the more rapid stains, such as Diff-Quik (American Scientific Products, McGaw Park, IL), Wright's Dip Stat stain (Medical Chemical Corp.), or Field's stain. It is more appropriate to use a stain with which you are familiar than Giemsa stain, which is somewhat complicated to use. Polymorphonuclear leukocytes can serve as the quality control organism for any of the blood stains. Any parasites present will stain like the polymorphonuclear leukocytes, regardless of the stain used.

Basic procedure

Cover the surface of a thin blood film with stain for 1 to 3 min. Add an equal volume of buffered water to the slide and mix by gently blowing on the surface of the slide. Wait 4 to 8 min and flood the slide with buffered water. Coplin jars with stain can also be used. Allow the slide to dry and examine it under ×1,000 magnification. Thick films must be laked in distilled water or treated with saponin before performance of the staining procedure (8, 9). Satisfactorily stained smears show the following characteristics for Giemsa and Wright's stains: erythrocytes, pale red and light tan, reddish, or buff, respectively; nuclei of leukocytes, purple with pale purple cytoplasm and bright blue with contrasting light cytoplasm, respectively; eosinophilic granules, bright purple-red and bright red, respectively; and neutrophilic granules, deep pink-purple and pink or light purple, respectively.

Hematoxylin Stains

■ Delafield's hematoxylin stain

Delafield's hematoxylin stain is used for thin and concentrated blood films for the detection of microfilariae and may show greater detail of the nuclei and sheaths than Giemsa and Wright's stains. Although the stain is not procedurally difficult to prepare, it does involve an aging process of 1 week followed by 1 month before it can be used. Delafield's hematoxylin stain is not readily available commercially and is used only in special circumstances. Preparation of the stain involves dissolving 180 g of aluminum ammonium sulfate in 1 liter of distilled water, heating until dissolved, and cooling (ammonium alum). Hematoxylin crystals (4 g) are dissolved in 25 ml of 95% ethyl alcohol, and the solution is then added to 400 ml of the ammonium alum. The solution is then covered with a cotton plug and exposed to sunlight and air for 1 week, after which it is filtered. To this solution, 100 ml each of glycerol and 95% ethyl alcohol is added. This solution is placed in sunlight for at least 1 month (10).

Basic procedure

Allow the specimen on a slide to air dry. Lake blood films with distilled water for 15 min and fix in absolute methanol for 5 min, followed by air drying. Stain for 10 to 15 min and rinse in water. Air dry, add a coverslip with mounting fluid, and examine the slide under ×1,000 magnification.

■ Iron hematoxylin stain

Iron hematoxylin stains are used for the detection, identification, and enumeration of intestinal protozoan parasites. There are many derivations of the iron hematoxylin stain, all of which can be used with fresh fecal specimens, fixed specimens containing PVA, or specimens preserved in Schaudinn's solution or SAF to make permanent stained smears. Solutions of hematoxylin-ethanol and ferrous ammonium sulfate-hydrochloric acid are combined in equal parts to make a working iron hematoxylin stain, and both solutions are available commercially.

Basic procedure

Place prepared slides in 70% ethanol for 5 min. If mercury-based fixatives are being used, place the slide in 70% ethanol with iodine for 5 min and then again in 70% ethanol for 5 min more (the last two steps are not necessary for non-mercury-based fixatives). Wash the slide in running tap water for 10 min and place it in iron hematoxylin working solution for 5 min. After this staining step, wash again in running tap water for 10 min and then place the slide in the following reagents for 5 min each: 70% ethanol, 95% ethanol, 100% ethanol (twice), and xylene (or a substitute) (twice). Add Permount, and add a coverslip. Examine the slide under ×1,000 magnification.

■ Trichrome stain (Wheatley trichrome stain)

The Wheatley trichrome stain, a modification of the Gomori tissue stain, is used for the detection, identification, and enumeration of intestinal protozoan parasites (11). This stain uses chromotrope 2R and light green SF stains to visually distinguish internal elements of protozoan parasitic cysts and trophozoites. Trichrome staining is usually performed on fixed fecal specimens containing PVA or Schaudinn's solution-preserved specimens. MIF- or SAF-preserved specimens may also be stained with the trichrome stain, as well as specimens preserved with single-vial systems. In addition, some proprietary stains are also available that may work better with these and other fixatives to make permanent stained preparations. Trichrome stain can be easily prepared in the laboratory or purchased from a commercial supplier.

Basic procedure

Place a prepared slide in 70% ethanol for 5 min. For mercury-based fixatives only, place the slide in 70% ethanol with iodine for 1 minute (fresh specimens) or for as long as 10 min (PVA-fixed air-dried specimens). Then place the slide again in 70% ethanol for 5 min (twice). Place in trichrome stain for 10 min, followed by a 1- to 3-s rinse in 90% ethanol with acetic acid. Dip the slide several times in 100% ethanol, and then place it in 100% ethanol for 3 min (twice), followed by xylene for 5 to 10 min (twice). Add Permount, and add a coverslip. Dry overnight or for 1 h at 37°C. Examine under ×1,000 magnification. If 95% alcohol is substituted for 100% ethanol and xylene substitutes are used, it is important to increase the dehydration times for both the alcohol and xylene substitutes by at least 5 to 10 min.

■ Acid-fast trichrome stain

The acid-fast trichrome staining technique allows the detection of acid-fast coccidia (*Cryptosporidium* spp., *C. belli*, and *C. cayetanensis*) (12). Smears prepared from fresh or preserved fecal material can be used in this staining procedure.

TABLE 5 Media used for cultivation of parasites

Medium	Organism(s)	Comment(s)
Acanthamoeba monoxenic culture	*Acanthamoeba* and *Naegleria* species	Acanthamoeba medium plus nonnutrient agar overlaid with *Escherichia coli* or *Enterobacter aerogenes* Used for cerebrospinal fluid, tissue, or soil samples
Balamuth's aqueous egg yolk infusion medium	Intestinal amebae	Cannot grow *Balamuthia*; *Balamuthia* grows only in cell culture lines
Boeck and Drbohlav's Locke-egg-serum (LES) medium	Intestinal amebae	Inspissated egg base slant with serum and rice powder
Buffered charcoal-yeast extract agar	*Acanthamoeba* species	Some manufacturers' media support growth better than others. Some of these media support growth of trophozoites and/or cysts.
Cysteine-peptone-liver-maltose medium	*Trichomonas vaginalis*	Methylene blue dye is added to aid visualization of the organisms.
Defined medium (16, 17) for pathogenic *Naegleria* species	*Naegleria fowleri*	Defined medium
DGM-21A medium	*Acanthamoeba* species	Defined medium
Diamond's Trypticase-yeast extract-maltose (TYM) complete medium, Diamond's complete medium modified by Klass	*Trichomonas vaginalis*	TYM contains no antibiotics; a nonselective medium Klass modification contains penicillin G, streptomycin sulfate, and amphotericin B to inhibit bacterial overgrowth.
Evans' modified Tobie's medium	*Leishmania* species and *Trypanosoma cruzi*	Uses beef extract, defibrinated horse blood, and phenol red as a pH indicator
InPouch TV (Biomed Diagnostics, Inc.)	*Trichomonas vaginalis*	Commercially available
Lash's casein hydrolysate-serum medium	*Trichomonas vaginalis*	Contains beef blood serum, which is absent from other media for *T. vaginalis*
LYI-S-2 medium	*Entamoeba histolytica*	Similar to TYI-S-33
M-11 medium	*Acanthamoeba culbertsoni*	Defined medium containing 11 amino acids
Modified Columbia agar	*Trichomonas vaginalis*	Solid agar medium; *T. vaginalis* colonies change pH and appearance of the agar plates.
Nelson's medium	*Naegleria fowleri*	Contains fetal calf serum, which is necessary for growth of *N. fowleri*
NIH medium	*Leishmania* and *Trypanosoma* species	Similar to Evans' modified Tobie's medium
Novy-MacNeal-Nicolle (NNN) medium	*Leishmania* and *Trypanosoma* species	NaCl base agar medium
NNN medium with Offutt's modifications	*Leishmania* species	Contains blood in base medium, differentiating it from NNN medium
4 N medium	*Leishmania* and *Trypanosoma* species	Uses a sugar base Uses NIH medium overlay
Nonnutrient agar with live or dead bacteria	*Acanthamoeba* species	Some manufacturers' media support growth better than others.
Proteose peptone-yeast extract-glucose (PPYG) medium	*Acanthamoeba* species	Basic medium to support growth of *Acanthamoeba* species
Peptone-yeast extract-glucose medium	*Acanthamoeba* species	Similar to PPYG medium
SCGYEM medium (16)	*Naegleria fowleri*	Undefined medium
Schneider's *Drosophila* medium with 30% fetal calf serum	*Leishmania* and *Trypanosoma* species	Liquid medium; less costly than blood-based agars
Trichomonas culture system	*Trichomonas vaginalis*	Commercially available
Trypticase soy agar with 5% sheep, rabbit, or horse blood	*Acanthamoeba* species	Some manufacturers' media support growth better than others.
TYI-S-33 medium	*Entamoeba histolytica*	Contains no antibiotics; a nonselective medium
TYSGM-9 medium	*Entamoeba histolytica*	Contains penicillin G and streptomycin sulfate to inhibit bacterial overgrowth
U.S. Army Medical Research Unit	*Leishmania* species	Particularly useful in isolation of *Leishmania brasiliensis* complex
Yeager's LIT (liver infusion tryptose) medium	*Trypanosoma cruzi*	Hemin and antibiotics are added to isolate *T. cruzi* from triatoma gut specimens.
YI-S medium	*Entamoeba histolytica*	Similar to TYI-S-33 medium

Basic procedure

Place a prepared, air-dried slide in absolute methanol for 5 to 10 min and then again allow it to air dry. Place the slide in carbol fuchsin solution for 10 min before rinsing in tap water. Decolorize with 0.5% acid-alcohol and rinse in tap water. Place the slide in trichrome stain for 30 min at 37°C. Rinse the slide in acid-alcohol for 10 s, and then dip it several times in 95% alcohol for 10 s. Place the slide in 95% alcohol for 30 s and then allow it to air dry. Examine at ×1,000 magnification.

Other Stains

■ Modified Field's stain

Modified Field's stain facilitates the identification of *Acanthamoeba* species. This stain was evaluated and shown to give very good contrast compared with other stains, such as Wright's, Giemsa, Ziehl-Neelsen, and trichrome stains. For information on preparation and use of modified Field's stain, refer to the article by Pirehma and colleagues (13).

■ Modified safranin stain

Modified safranin stain allows the detection of *Cyclospora* oocysts in formalin-fixed specimens and fecal concentrates. The stain most commonly used in the past for these organisms was the modified acid-fast stain; however, tremendous variations in staining properties can be seen with this stain. The modified safranin stain reportedly uniformly stains oocysts of *Cyclospora*. It has also been shown to be fast, reliable, and easy to perform (14).

Basic procedure

Place a prepared, thin smear of stool on a 60°C slide warmer until dried. Cover smear with a 1% safranin solution and heat in a microwave oven at full power (650 W) for 30 to 60 s. Rinse the smear with tap water for 30 s, counterstain with 1% aqueous methylene blue for 1 min, rinse with tap water, and air dry. Examine at ×1,000 magnification.

■ Calcofluor white stain

Calcofluor white, one of a number of optical brighteners, binds to cellulose and chitin and fluoresces best when exposed to long-wavelength UV light. These properties allow its use in detecting fungi, including *Pneumocystis jirovecii*, and free-living amebae like *Naegleria*, *Acanthamoeba*, and *Balamuthia* species, as well as the larvae of *Dirofilaria* species (its cuticle contains chitin). Calcofluor white is available through several commercial suppliers and is also easily made in the laboratory by following the manufacturer's recommendations.

Basic procedure

Place the specimen on a slide and allow it to air dry. Fix the slide in methanol for 1 to 2 min, rinse with distilled water, and allow it to air dry. Add 1 or 2 drops of 10% KOH, place 1 or 2 drops of calcofluor white solution on the specimen for 3 min, and view the slide with a fluorescent microscope and barrier filter (300 to 412 nm) at ×100 to ×400 magnification.

MEDIA

Cultures can be performed for only a few parasitic organisms, including *Acanthamoeba* species, *Naegleria fowleri*, *Plasmodium* species, intestinal amebae (like *Entamoeba histolytica*), *Trichomonas vaginalis*, *Leishmania* species, and *Trypanosoma* species (7). However, most clinical diagnostic microbiology laboratories do not provide parasite cultures. Cultures of these organisms are done only at large reference laboratories or research facilities. The exception is *T. vaginalis*, for which commercial products have been adapted for the routine laboratory. Many of the media listed in Table 5 are not commercially available but are listed for reference. Additional information regarding these media is available in the literature (1, 2, 13, 15).

REFERENCES

1. **Garcia LS.** 2016. *Diagnostic Medical Parasitology*, 6th ed, p 219–228. ASM Press, Washington, DC.
2. **Garcia LS.** 2016. *Diagnostic Medical Parasitology*, 6th ed, p 183–194. ASM Press, Washington, DC.
3. **Garcia LS, Shimizu RY, Shum A, Bruckner DA.** 1993. Evaluation of intestinal protozoan morphology in polyvinyl alcohol preservative: comparison of zinc sulfate- and mercuric chloride-based compounds for use in Schaudinn's fixative. *J Clin Microbiol* **31:**307–310.
4. **Garcia LS, Shimizu RY, Brewer TC, Bruckner DA.** 1983. Evaluation of intestinal parasite morphology in polyvinyl alcohol preservative: comparison of copper sulfate and mercuric chloride bases for use in Schaudinn fixative. *J Clin Microbiol* **17:**1092–1095.
5. **Couturier BA, Jensen R, Arias N, Heffron M, Gubler E, Case K, Gowans J, Couturier MR.** 2015. Clinical and analytical evaluation of a single-vial stool collection device with formalin-free fixative for improved processing and comprehensive detection of gastrointestinal parasites. J Clin Microbiol 53:2539–2548.
6. **Fritsche TR, Pritt BS.** 2016. Medical parasitology, p 1231–1283. *In* Henry JB (ed), *Clinical Diagnosis and Management by Laboratory Methods*, 23rd ed. The W. B. Saunders Company, Philadelphia, PA.
7. **Garcia LS, Johnston SP, Linscott AJ, Shimizu RY.** 2008. *Cumitech 46: Laboratory Procedures for Diagnosis of Blood-Borne Parasitic Diseases*. Coordinating ed, Garcia LS. ASM Press, Washington, DC.
8. **Gleeson RM.** 1997. An improved method for thick film preparation using saponin as a lysing agent. *Clin Lab Haematol* **19:**249–251.
9. **Hira PR.** 1977. Wuchereria bancrofti: the staining of the microfilarial sheath in Giemsa and haematoxylin for diagnosis. *Med J Zambia* **11:**93–96.
10. **Garcia LS.** 2012. *Diagnostic Medical Parasitology*, 6th ed, p 152–153. ASM Press, Washington, DC.
11. **Wheatley WB.** 1951. A rapid staining procedure for intestinal amoebae and flagellates. *Am J Clin Pathol* **21:**990–991.
12. **Ignatius R, Lehmann M, Miksits K, Regnath T, Arvand M, Engelmann E, Futh U, Hahn H, Wagner J.** 1997. A new acid-fast trichrome stain for simultaneous detection of *Cryptosporidium parvum* and microsporidial species in stool specimens. *J Clin Microbiol* **35:**446–449.
13. **Pirehma M, Suresh K, Sivanandam S, Khairul Anuar AK, Ramakrishnan K, Suresh Kumar GS.** 1999. Field's stain—a rapid staining method for *Acanthamoeba* spp. *Parasitol Res* **85:**791–793.
14. **Visvesvara GS, Moura H, Kovacs-Nace E, Wallace S, Eberhard ML.** 1997. Uniform staining of *Cyclospora* oocysts in fecal smears by a modified safranin technique with microwave heating. *J Clin Microbiol* **35:**730–733.
15. **Clark CG, Diamond LS.** 2002. Methods for cultivation of luminal parasitic protists of clinical importance. *Clin Microbiol Rev* **15:**329–341.
16. **Schuster FL.** 2002. Cultivation of pathogenic and opportunistic free-living amebas. *Clin Microbiol Rev* **15:**342–354.
17. **Visvesvara GS, Garcia LS.** 2002. Culture of protozoan parasites. *Clin Microbiol Rev* **15:**327–328.

General Approaches for Detection and Identification of Parasites

LYNNE S. GARCIA, GRAEME P. PALTRIDGE, AND ROBYN Y. SHIMIZU

138

This chapter discusses various approaches and diagnostic methods currently used for the diagnosis of parasitic infections. Assuming that clinical specimens have been properly collected and processed according to specific specimen rejection and acceptance criteria, the examination of prepared wet mounts, concentrated specimens, permanent stained smears, thick and thin blood films, and various culture materials can provide critical information leading to organism identification and confirmation of the suspected cause of clinical disease (1–6). Nucleic acid amplification and molecular assays are also becoming more widely used. With the exception of a few fecal immunoassay and molecular diagnostic kits, the majority of this diagnostic work depends on the knowledge and microscopy skills of the microbiologist. The field of diagnostic parasitology has taken on greater importance during the past few years for a number of reasons. Expanded world travel has increased the potential levels of exposure to a number of infectious agents, as well as expanding epidemiologic boundaries and organism changes in pathogenicity. It is important to be aware of organisms commonly found within certain areas of the world and the makeup of the patient population being serviced at your institution, particularly if immunocompromised patients are frequently seen as a part of your routine patient population. It is also important for the physician and microbiologist to recognize and understand the efficacy of any diagnostic method for parasite recovery and identification. Specific information on specimen collection and processing can be found in chapter 136. In order to become proficient in diagnostic medical parasitology, there is no substitute for performing extensive bench work and the required microscopy associated with this type of testing.

STOOL SPECIMENS

For review, see the lists of options for the collection of fecal specimens in chapter 136, Table 3 and Table 6. Algorithms for the processing of stool specimens are presented in Fig. 1, 2, and 3. The procedures that normally make up the ova and parasite (O&P) examination are provided below and include the direct wet mount in saline, the concentration, and the permanent stained smear (1–4, 6–16).

Direct Wet Mount in Saline

The purpose of a direct wet mount is to confirm the possibility of infection with certain protozoa and helminths, to assess the worm burden of the patient, and to look for organism motility (Table 1) (1, 6, 7, 10, 11, 14). Any fresh stool specimens that have not been refrigerated and that have been delivered to the laboratory within specified time frames are acceptable for testing; however, it is much more important to examine liquid or soft stools than formed stools. Liquid and soft stools are much more likely to contain motile protozoan trophozoites than cysts, which do not demonstrate motility. Low-power examination (magnification, ×100) of the entire coverslip preparation (22 mm by 22 mm) and high dry power examination (magnification, ×400) of at least one-third to one-half of the coverslip area are recommended before the preparation is considered negative. Often, results from the direct smear examination should be considered presumptive; however, some organisms (*Giardia duodenalis* [*G. lamblia*, *G. intestinalis*] cysts and trophozoites, *Entamoeba coli* cysts, *Iodamoeba bütschlii* cysts, helminth eggs and larvae, and *Cystoisospora belli* oocysts) can be definitively identified. Reports of results obtained by this method should be considered preliminary, with the final report being made available after the results of the concentration wet mount and permanent stained smear, both of which are more sensitive methods than the direct wet smear, have been obtained. It is important to remember that direct wet smears are not relevant for concentration sediments, since the specimen has been subjected to various solutions that kill the organisms. Although liquid or very soft fresh stools should be examined by the laboratory within 30 minutes of passage, this is often not practical, and stools are collected in fecal preservatives for submission.

If iodine is added to the preparation for increased contrast, the organisms will be killed and motility will be lost. Specimens that arrive in the laboratory in stool preservatives do not require a direct smear examination; proceed to the concentration and permanent stained smear. Examination of the wet mount using iodine is not required but is the decision of each user performing this type of microscopy.

Concentration Wet Mount

The purpose of the concentration method is to separate parasites from fecal debris and to concentrate any parasites present through either sedimentation or flotation (1, 6–8, 10, 11, 14). The sedimentation concentration is the most common method used; all organisms will be found in the concentrated sediment. Use of the flotation is more limited,

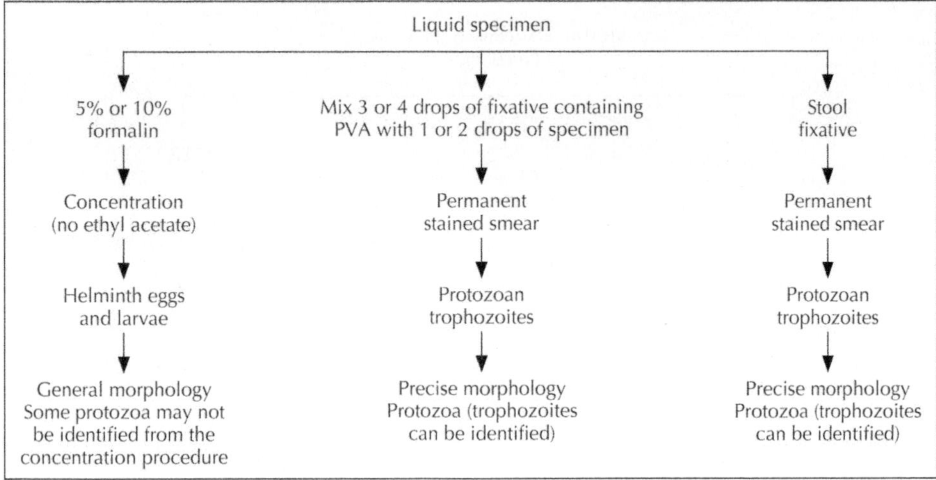

FIGURE 1 Processing liquid stool for O&P examination. Either PVA or Schaudinn's fixative can be used for the preparation of the permanent stained smear. Organism motility is seen when saline is used; iodine kills the organisms, so motility will no longer be visible. The use of ethyl acetate may remove the entire specimen and pull it into the layer of debris that will be discarded (liquid specimen normally contains mucus); the liquid should be centrifuged at 500 × *g* for 10 min (normal centrifugation time), but ethyl acetate should not be used in the procedure. In general, laboratories have switched to nonmercury substitutes; the original Schaudinn's fixative contains mercuric chloride. However, in some instances the term "Schaudinn's fixative" is still used to describe not the original fixative but a formulation that is prepared with a copper or zinc base or other proprietary compounds. When fixatives are selected, it is important to know the contents in order to comply with disposal regulations. (Reprinted from reference 10.)

since not all parasites will float, and centrifugation speeds and time are critical for success. The concentration is specifically designed to allow recovery of protozoan cysts, coccidian oocysts, microsporidian spores (now classified with the fungi), and helminth eggs and larvae (Table 2). Any stool specimen that is fresh or preserved is acceptable for testing. Wet mounts prepared from concentrated stool are examined in the same manner as that used for the direct wet mount method (Fig. 4). The addition of too much iodine may obscure helminth eggs (the eggs may resemble debris);

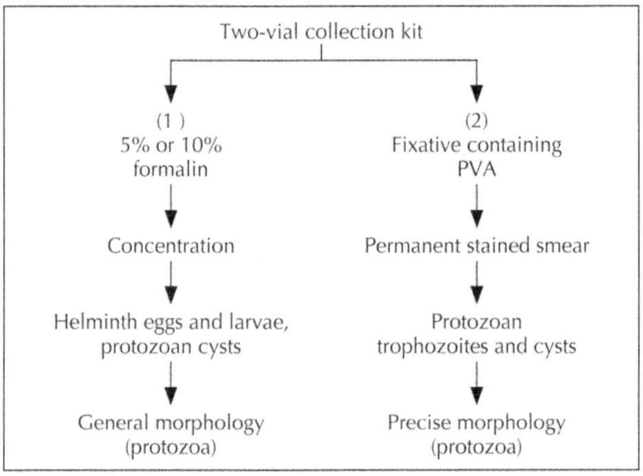

Two-vial collection kit

(1) 5% or 10% formalin	(2) Fixative containing PVA
Concentration	Permanent stained smear
Helminth eggs and larvae, protozoan cysts	Protozoan trophozoites and cysts
General morphology (protozoa)	Precise morphology (protozoa)

FIGURE 2 Processing preserved stool for O&P examination (two-vial collection kit). The formalin can be buffered or nonbuffered, depending on the laboratory protocol in use. Fixative prepared with mercuric chloride provides the best organism preservation. Alternatives are available, including zinc-based PVA, copper sulfate-based PVA, SAF, and the one of the single-vial fixatives that requires no adhesive (PVA or albumin). (Reprinted from reference 10.)

the use of iodine is an individual decision. Often, results from the concentration examination should be considered presumptive; however, some organisms (*G. duodenalis* [*G. lamblia*, *G. intestinalis*] cysts, *E. coli* cysts, *I. bütschlii* cysts, helminth eggs and larvae, and *C. belli* oocysts) can be definitively identified. As with the direct wet mount, results obtained by the concentration wet mount should be considered preliminary, with the definitive report being made available after the results of the permanent stained smear are obtained.

The formalin-ethyl acetate sedimentation concentration procedure is the most commonly used procedure, and the recommended centrifugation speed and time are 500 × *g* and 10 min, respectively. In this procedure, the use of ether has been replaced with ethyl acetate. However, it is important to remember that ethyl acetate should not be used for liquid specimens or those containing a great deal of mucus. The ethyl acetate may pull the liquid or mucus specimen contents into the debris layer, which will be discarded. Although the recovery of parasites from a liquid specimen or one containing a great deal of mucus may not be successful, this simple centrifugation approach is still recommended. The standard zinc sulfate flotation procedure does not detect operculated or heavy eggs; when this method is used, both the surface film and sediment should be examined before a negative result is reported.

Permanent Stained Smears

Trichrome, Iron-Hematoxylin, or Iron-Hematoxylin/Carbol Fuchsin

The permanent stained smear provides contrasting colors for both the background debris and the parasites present (Fig. 4, Table 3, Table 4, and Table 5) (1, 6, 7, 10, 11, 14). Permanent stained stool smears are designed to allow examination and recognition of detailed organism morphology under oil immersion magnification (magnification, ×1,000).

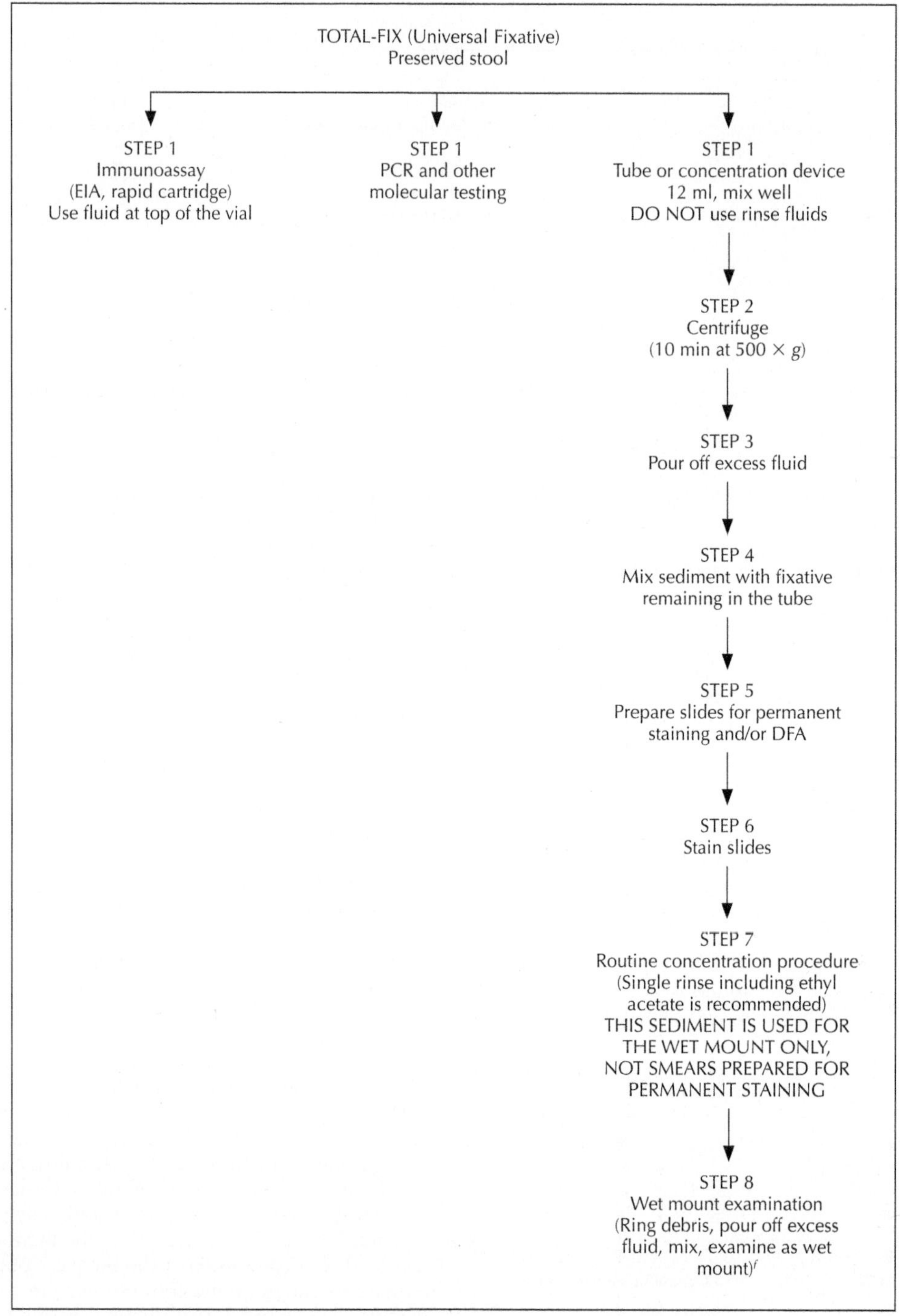

FIGURE 3 Processing preserved stool for O&P examination (one-vial collection kit). There are single-vial collection systems for which the formulas are proprietary; however, many contain zinc sulfate as one of the key ingredients. With the exception of SAF, compatibility of these fixatives with immunoassay reagents is not always possible, particularly if the fixative contains PVA. Other options include TOTAL-FIX (single-vial fixative with no mercury, formalin, or PVA) (Medical Chemical Corp.) and Ecofix (Meridian Biosciences, Cincinnati, OH). This figure provides three options for testing. In some cases, in-house validation procedures need to be performed prior to use. Commercial validation procedures are under way and should be available in the near future for some of these products. It is always important to read the package brochure carefully regarding the need for additional validation procedures.

TABLE 1 Diagnostic characteristics of organisms in wet mounts

Specimen	Characteristics to observe in: Protozoa	Helminths
Stool Other specimens from gastrointestinal tract Specimens from urogenital system	Size Shape Stage (trophozoite, precyst, cyst, oocyst) Motility (fresh specimens only) Refractility Cytoplasm inclusions (chromatoidal bars, glycogen vacuoles, axonemes, axostyles, median bodies, sporozoites)	Egg, larva, or adult: size, internal structure Egg: embryonated, opercular shoulders, abopercular thickenings or projections, hooklets, polar filaments, spines Larva: head and tail morphology, digestive tract Adult: nematode, cestode, or trematode

TABLE 2 Identification of helminth eggs[a]

Description	Identification
1. Eggs small (~25–40 μm)	
A. Operculate, generally oval, shoulders (egg, <35 μm); *Clonorchis*, operculated shoulders, bile stained, may be an abopercular knob, miracidium present but difficult to see	*Clonorchis* (*Opisthorchis*) spp. (Chinese liver fluke) or intestinal flukes (*Heterophyes* or *Metagonimus yokogawai*)
B. Thick, radially striated shell (six-hooked oncosphere, individual eggs resemble those of *Taenia* spp.; eggs passed in egg packets containing 6–10 eggs; each egg is 25–40 μm)	*Dipylidium caninum* (dog, cat tapeworm); egg packets could measure >150 μm
C. Thick, radially striated shell (six-hooked oncosphere may not be visible in every egg from formalinized fecal specimens) (eggs cannot be identified to species level without special stains) (each egg is 30–47 μm)	*Taenia* spp. (*T. saginata*, beef tapeworm; *T. solium*, pork tapeworm)
D. Thin eggshell, clear space between developing shell and embryo, spherical or subspherical, containing a six-hooked oncosphere; polar filaments (filamentous strands) present between thin egg shell and embryo (each egg is 31–43 μm)	*Hymenolepis nana* (dwarf tapeworm)
2. Eggs medium (~40–100 μm)	
A. Egg barrel-shaped, with clear polar plugs (each egg is 50–54 by 20–23 μm)	*Trichuris trichiura* (whipworm)
B. Egg flattened on one side, may contain larva (each egg is 70–85 by 60–80 μm)	*Enterobius vermicularis* (pinworm)
C. Egg with thick, tuberculated (bumpy) capsule (in decorticate eggs, capsule may be missing) (each egg is 45–75 by 35–50 μm)	*Ascaris lumbricoides* (large roundworm), fertilized eggs
D. Egg bluntly rounded at ends, thin shell (contains developing embryo at the 8–16 ball stage of development) (each egg is 56–75 by 36–40 μm)	Hookworm
E. Operculate, operculum break in shell sometimes hard to see, smooth transition from shell to operculum; small "bump" may be seen at abopercular end (each egg is 58–75 by 40–50 μm)	*Diphyllobothrium* spp. (broad fish tapeworm)
F. Thin eggshell, clear space between developing shell and embryo, spherical or subspherical, containing a six-hooked oncosphere; no polar filaments (filamentous strands) present between thin eggshell and embryo (each egg is 70–85 by 60–80 μm)	*Hymenolepis diminuta* (rat tapeworm)
3. Eggs large (~100–180 μm)	
A. Egg with opercular shoulders into which the operculum fits (looks like teapot lid and flange into which lid fits), abopercular end somewhat thickened—not always visible (each egg is 80–120 by 48–60 μm); egg has been described as "urn-shaped."	*Paragonimus* spp. (lung fluke)
B. Egg tapered at one or both ends; long thin shell containing developing embryo (each egg is 73–95 by 40–50 μm)	*Trichostrongylus* spp.
C. Egg with thick, tuberculated (bumpy) capsule (in decorticate eggs, capsule may be missing) (each egg is 85–95 by 43–47 μm)	*Ascaris lumbricoides* (large roundworm); unfertilized eggs
D. Egg spined, ciliated miracidium larva may be seen, lateral spine very short (each egg is 70–100 by 55–65 μm)	*Schistosoma japonicum* (blood fluke, stool) *Schistosoma mekongi* (rounder and smaller than *S. japonicum*); measure 50–65 by 30–55 μm
E. Egg spined, ciliated miracidium larva may be seen, spine terminal (each egg is 112–170 by 40–70 μm)	*Schistosoma haematobium* (blood fluke, urine)
F. Egg spined, ciliated miracidium larva may be seen, spine terminal (each egg is 140–240 by 50–85 μm)	*Schistosoma intercalatum* (blood fluke, stool)
G. Egg spined, ciliated miracidium larva may be seen, large lateral spine (each egg is 114–180 by 45–70 μm)	*Schistosoma mansoni* (blood fluke, stool)
H. Egg >85 μm, operculum break in shell sometimes hard to see; smooth transition from shell to operculum; egg passed in undeveloped stage (each egg is 130–140 by 80–85 μm)	*Fasciolopsis buski* (giant intestinal fluke) or *Fasciola hepatica* (sheep liver fluke) or *Echinostoma* spp.

[a]This table does not include every possible helminth that could be found as a human parasite; however, the most likely helminth infections are included.

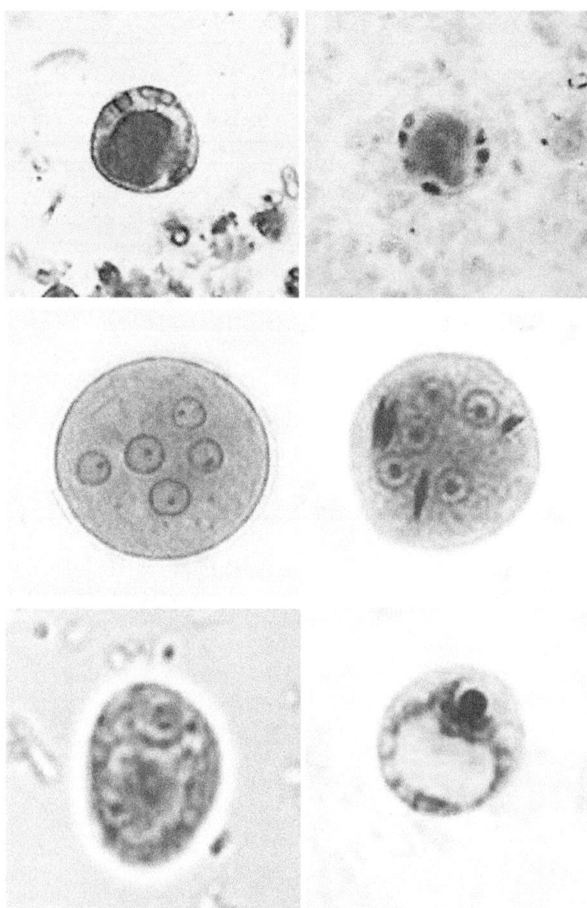

FIGURE 4 Examples of iodine staining wet mounts (left) and permanent staining with Wheatley's trichrome stain (right). (Top row) *Blastocystis* spp. central body forms. (Middle row) *E. coli* cysts. (Bottom row) *I. bütschlii* cysts. Note that in the *Blastocystis* spp. and *I. bütschlii* preparations, the central body area and large glycogen vacuole clearly stain with iodine.

This method is primarily designed to allow the recovery and identification of the more common intestinal protozoan trophozoites and cysts, excluding the coccidia (unless the iron-hematoxylin/carbol fuchsin method is used) and microsporidia. Oil immersion examination of a minimum of 300 oil immersion fields is recommended; additional fields may be required if suspect organisms have been seen in the wet mounts. The use of a specific time for slide examination is not recommended, since each microbiologist screens the slides at a different rate. Although review of 300 fields seems like a time-consuming procedure, it takes less time than one would assume. This is particularly true for a trained microscopist in microbiology. Based on their expertise, the patient population, and the percentage of positive specimens, different laboratories may approach the examination of permanent stained smears by using different guidelines. Some laboratories may use a 60× oil immersion objective for screening purposes (magnification, ×600); however, it is important to examine a sufficient number of fields at a total magnification of ×1,000 before reporting the specimen as negative (no parasites seen).

Modified Acid-Fast Staining

The modified acid-fast staining method is used to provide contrasting colors for the background debris and the parasites present and to allow examination and recognition of the acid-fast characteristic of the organisms under high dry magnification (magnification, ×400) (1, 6, 7, 10, 11, 14). Organisms that can be identified with this stain are *Cryptosporidium* spp., *Cyclospora cayetanensis*, and *C. belli*. It is important to remember that *C. cayetanensis* stains much more acid-fast variable than *Cryptosporidium* spp. (Fig. 5). However, occasionally one can see acid-fast variability with *Cryptosporidium*, particularly if the decolorizer is too strong (17). A 1% acid destain is sufficient to provide excellent results for all of the Apicomplexa. Although some microsporidian spores are acid-fast positive, their small size makes recognition very difficult; modified trichrome stains are recommended for the detection of microsporidian spores. Oil immersion examination of a minimum of 300 oil immersion fields is recommended.

Both modified Ziehl-Neelsen and Kinyoun acid-fast staining methods are excellent for staining oocysts. Limitations of the procedure are generally related to specimen handling, including proper collection, centrifugation speed and time, and the percent acid used for the destain step. Another excellent option is the modified safranin method (1).

Modified Trichrome

Modified trichrome stains were primarily designed to allow recovery and identification of microsporidial spores from centrifuged stool specimens; internal morphology (horizontal and diagonal stripes of the polar tubule) may be seen in some spores under oil immersion (magnification, ×1,000) (Fig. 6). Any stool specimen that is submitted fresh or preserved in formalin, sodium acetate-acetic acid-formalin (SAF), or the single-vial fixative is acceptable. Polyvinyl alcohol (PVA)-fixed specimens are unacceptable. Oil immersion examination of a minimum of 300 oil immersion

TABLE 3 Diagnostic characteristics of organisms in permanent stained smears

Specimen	Characteristics to observe in: Protozoa	Helminths
Stool, other specimens from gastrointestinal tract, urogenital system	Size, shape, stage (trophozoite, precyst, cyst, oocyst, spore) Nuclear arrangement, cytoplasm inclusions (chromatoidal bars, vacuoles, axonemes, axostyles, median bodies, sporozoites, polar tubules) *Balantidium coli* trophozoites and cysts may not be visible due to excess stain retention.	Eggs, larvae, and/or adults may not be identified because of excess stain retention or distortion

TABLE 4 Key to identification of intestinal amebae (permanent stained smear)

1. Trophozoites present	2
Cysts present	7
2. Trophozoites measure >12 μm	3
Trophozoites measure <12 μm	4
3. Karyosome central, compact; peripheral nuclear chromatin evenly arranged; "clean" cytoplasm	*Entamoeba histolytica*[a]
Karyosome eccentric, spread out; peripheral nuclear chromatin unevenly arranged; "dirty" cytoplasm	*Entamoeba coli*
4. Peripheral nuclear chromatin	5
Other than above	6
5. Karyosome central, compact (nucleus looks like a target); peripheral nuclear chromatin evenly arranged; "clean" cytoplasm	*Entamoeba hartmanni*
Karyosome large, blot-like; extensive nuclear variation (nuclear variants may include those with peripheral chromatin)	*Endolimax nana*
6. No peripheral chromatin, karyosome large, junky cytoplasm	*Iodamoeba bütschlii*
No peripheral chromatin, karyosome variable, clean cytoplasm	*Endolimax nana*
7. Cysts measure >10 μm (including any shrinkage "halo")	8
Cysts measure <10 μm (including any shrinkage "halo")	10
8. Single *Entamoeba*-like nucleus with large inclusion mass	*Entamoeba polecki*[b]
Multiple nuclei	9
9. Four *Entamoeba*-like nuclei; chromatoidal bars have smooth, rounded ends	*Entamoeba histolytica*[a]
Five or more *Entamoeba*-like nuclei, chromatoidal bars have sharp, pointed ends (chromatoidal bars often not present)	*Entamoeba coli*
10. Single nucleus (may be "basket" nucleus), large glycogen vacuole	*Iodamoeba bütschlii*[c]
Multiple nuclei	11
11. Four *Entamoeba*-like nuclei, chromatoidal bars have smooth, rounded ends (nuclei may also number only two)	*Entamoeba hartmanni*
Four karyosomes, no peripheral chromatin, round to oval shape	*Endolimax nana*[d]

[a]*Entamoeba histolytica* refers to the *E. histolytica-E. dispar* group or complex. *E. histolytica* (pathogenic) can be determined by finding RBCs in the cytoplasm of the trophozoites. Otherwise, on the basis of morphological grounds, *E. histolytica* (pathogen) and *E. dispar* (nonpathogen) cannot be differentiated. A report should read: *Entamoeba histolytica-E. dispar* group (or complex).

[b]It is very difficult to differentiate *Entamoeba polecki* trophozoites from those of the *E. histolytica-E. dispar* group, *E. coli*, or *E moshkovskii*.

[c]Although some *I. bütschlii* cysts are larger than 10 μm, the majority of cysts measure 9 to 10 μm, and the typical glycogen vacuole ensures the proper identification.

[d]*E. nana* and *Dientamoeba fragilis* (flagellate; see Table 5) often mimic one another, especially the trophozoite forms. However, since *D. fragilis* is classified as a flagellate, it appears in Table 5.

TABLE 5 Key to identification of intestinal flagellates

1. Trophozoites present	2
Cysts present[a]	7
2. Pear shaped	3
Shape other	6
3. Two nuclei, sucking disk present	*Giardia duodenalis* (*G. lamblia*, *G. intestinalis*)
One nucleus present	4
4. Costa length of body	*Pentatrichomonas hominis*
No costa	5
5. Cytostome present, >10 μm	*Chilomastix mesnili*
Cytostome present, <10 μm	*Retortamonas intestinalis* or *Enteromonas hominis*
6. Ameba shaped, one or two fragmented nuclei	*Dientamoeba fragilis*
Oval, one nucleus	*Enteromonas hominis*
7. Oval or round cyst	8
Lemon-shaped cyst	9
8. Four nuclei, median bodies, axoneme, >10 μm	*Giardia duodenalis* (*G. lamblia*, *G. intestinalis*)
Two nuclei, no fibrils, <10 μm	*Enteromonas hominis*
9. One nucleus, (shepherd's) crook fibril	*Chilomastix mesnili*
One nucleus, bird's beak fibril	*Retortamonas intestinalis*

[a]Although *Dientamoeba fragilis* now has a confirmed stage in the life cycle, the number of cysts in any one fecal smear is very low (~1%), so it is not included in this key. The trophozoite resembles more closely an ameba; however, it is placed in this table per classification as a flagellate.

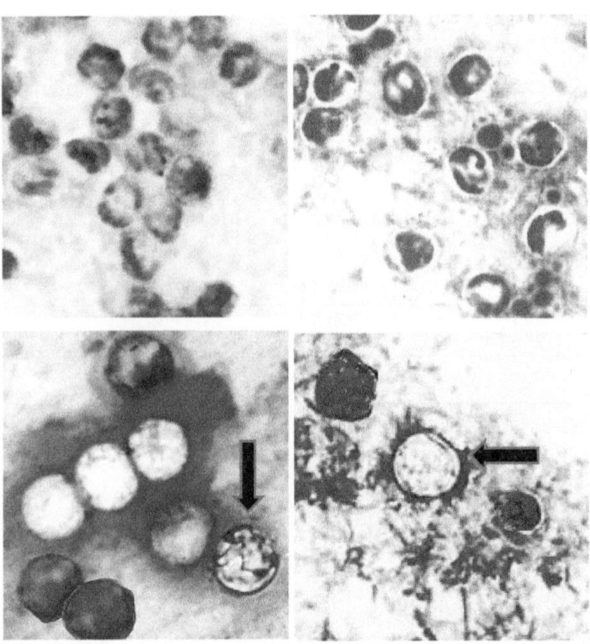

FIGURE 5 Modified acid-fast stains. (Top row) *Cryptosporidium* spp. oocysts, 4 to 6 μm. (Note that the curved sporozoites can be seen in a few of the oocysts. These oocysts are immediately infectious when passed.) (Bottom row) *C. cayetanensis* oocysts, 8 to 10 μm. These oocysts are not immediately infectious when passed. Note that some of the *Cyclospora* oocysts do not stain (modified acid-fast stain variable); also, some oocysts look like wrinkled cellophane (arrows).

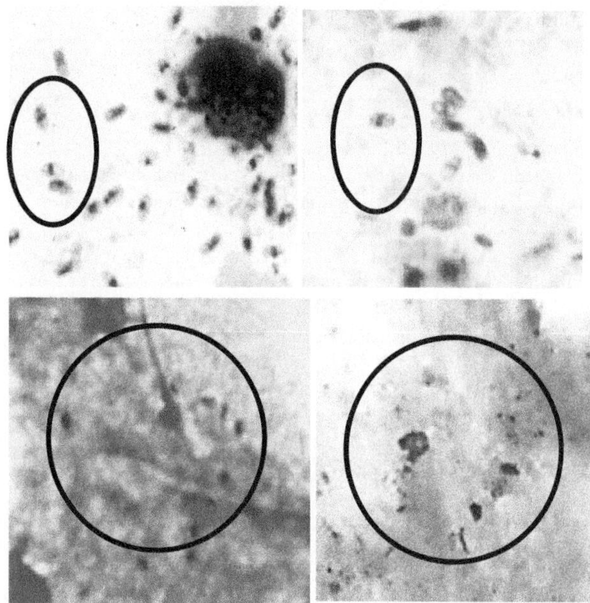

FIGURE 6 Modified trichrome stains. (Top row) Microsporidian spores, 1.5 to 2.5 μm; note the horizontal or diagonal lines within the spores (oval), evidence of the polar tubules. The left panel shows the Weber blue counterstain, while the right shows the Weber green counterstain. (Bottom row) Microsporidian spores from eye specimens. (Left) Gram stain (note the resemblance to bacteria). (Right) Corneal scraping stained with a Gram stain (again, note the resemblance to bacteria). Misidentifications can result in inappropriate therapy and serious sequelae for the patient.

fields is recommended. The identification of microsporidial spores may be possible; however, their small size makes recognition difficult, particularly in infections with few organisms in the clinical specimen. Identification to the species level requires electron microscopy or molecular methods such as PCR (see chapter 131).

Immunoassay Methods

Immunoassay reagents are available commercially for several of the protozoan parasites, including *G. duodenalis* (*G. lamblia*, *G. intestinalis*), *Cryptosporidium* spp., the *Entamoeba histolytica*-*E. dispar* group, and *E. histolytica* (Table 6). These methods (enzyme immunoassay [EIA], fluorescent-antibody assay, and immunochromatographic assay [cartridge]) are designed to detect the antigens of selected organisms; a negative result does not rule out the possibility that these organisms or antigens are present in low numbers or that other intestinal parasites are agents causing disease, including *Dientamoeba fragilis*, the microsporidia, and helminth parasites (1, 18–20) (Fig. 7). Immunoassay reagents are currently under development, as are trials for *D. fragilis* and *Blastocystis* spp. Fecal immunoassays for the microsporidia are available; however, none are currently approved by the Food and Drug Administration (FDA) for use within the United States.

There are other products available with a valid CE marking; a valid CE marking affixed to a product indicates that it complies with the relevant European New Approach product safety directives. The directives contain the essential requirements that a product must meet to be sold in the European Union.

Molecular Methods

In January 2013, the FDA approved the first test that can simultaneously detect 11 common viral, bacterial, and parasitic (*Cryptosporidium* and *Giardia*) causes of infectious gastroenteritis from a single patient sample (xTAG gastrointestinal pathogen panel; Luminex, Inc., Austin, TX). A number of molecular systems are now available (Table 7) (21).

There are also several molecular tests that are in clinical trials for the detection of selected gastrointestinal parasites. These tests are molecular gastrointestinal panels and target the most commonly occurring bacterial, viral, and parasitic stool pathogens. Although there are laboratory-developed tests for most parasites, these are not commercially available or are available only in specialized testing centers. When such tests are used, attention should be given to the use of internal amplification controls to detect inhibition, since common specimens, such as blood and stool, contain PCR inhibitors. Thorough validation is required before these are implemented for clinical testing.

TABLE 6 Commercially available immunoassays for detection of intestinal parasites[a]

Fresh stool		Preserved in 5–10% formalin, SAF, or other single-vial system	
No concentration	Concentration	No concentration	Concentration
EIA	DFA[c]	EIA	DFA
Cryptosporidium spp.	*Cryptosporidium* spp.	*Cryptosporidium* spp.	*Cryptosporidium* spp.
G. lamblia[b]	*G. lamblia*[b]	*G. lamblia*[b]	*G. lamblia*[b]
E. histolytica		Immunochromatographic assay (cartridge format)	
E. histolytica-*E. dispar* group		*Cryptosporidium* spp.	
Immunochromatographic assay (cartridge format)		*G. lamblia*[b]	
Cryptosporidium spp.			
G. lamblia[b]			
E. histolytica-*E. dispar* group			
E. histolytica			

[a]There are other products available with a valid CE marking; a valid CE marking affixed to a product indicates that it complies with the relevant European New Approach product safety directives. The directives contain the essential requirements that a product must meet to be sold in the European Union.

[b]Diagnostic kits retain the *Giardia lamblia* designation.

[c]DFA, direct fluorescent-antibody assay.

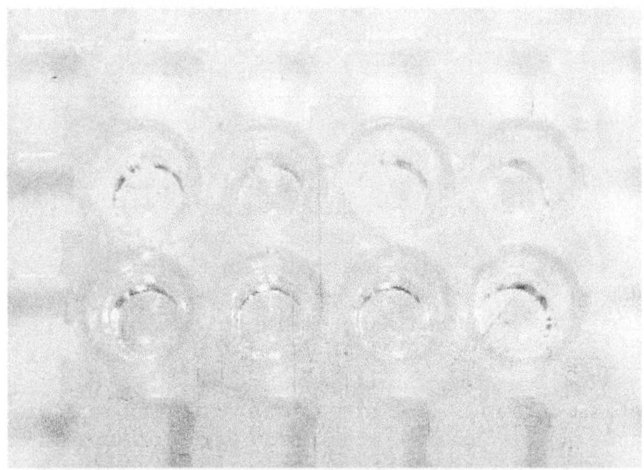

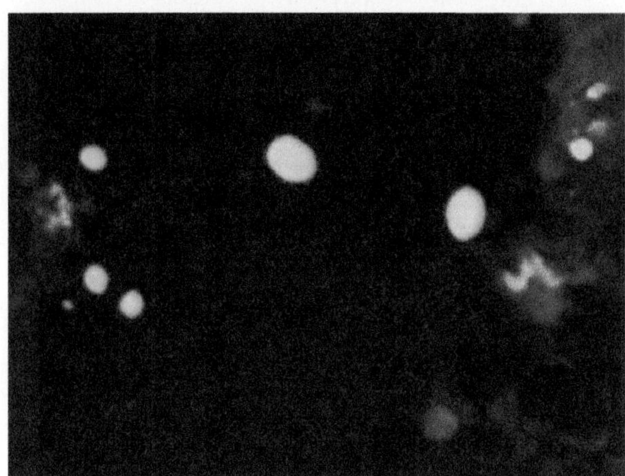

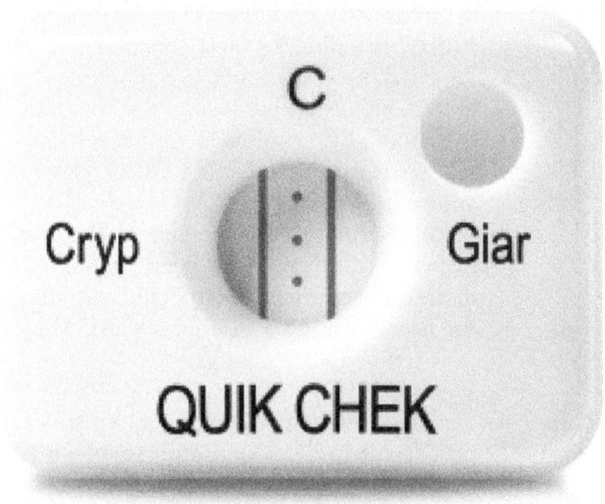

FIGURE 7 Examples of fecal immunoassays. (Top) Example of an enzyme immunoassay plate; these often come as 96-well trays or individual cup rows that can be inserted into a holder (courtesy of TECHLAB, Inc., Blacksburg, VA, and Alere North America, Orlando, FL). (Middle) Example of a combination *Giardia-Cryptosporidium* fluorescent assay (large organisms are *Giardia* cysts, smaller organisms are *Cryptosporidium* oocysts) (courtesy of Medical Chemical Corporation, Torrance, CA). (Bottom) Example of a rapid cartridge for the detection of *Giardia* and/or *Cryptosporidium* (courtesy of TECHLAB, Inc., Blacksburg, VA, and Alere North America, Orlando, FL). Note that in this cartridge, both the *Cryptosporidium* and *Giardia* lines are positive, as is the dot control line.

ADDITIONAL TECHNIQUES FOR STOOL EXAMINATION

Although the routine O&P examination consisting of the direct wet mount, the concentration, and the permanent stained smear is an excellent procedure recommended for the detection of most intestinal parasites, several other diagnostic techniques are available for the recovery and identification of specific parasitic organisms (1, 6, 7, 10, 11, 14). Most laboratories do not routinely offer all of these techniques, but many can be performed relatively simply and inexpensively. Occasionally, it is necessary to examine stool specimens visually for the presence of scolices and proglottids of cestodes and adult nematodes and trematodes to confirm the diagnosis and/or for species identification (Table 8). A method for the recovery of these stages is described in this chapter.

Culture of Larval-Stage Nematodes

Nematode infections giving rise to larval stages that hatch in soil or in tissues may be diagnosed by using fecal culture methods to concentrate the larvae (1, 6, 7, 10, 11, 14). *Strongyloides stercoralis* larvae are the most common larvae found in stool specimens. Depending on the fecal transit time through the intestine and the patient's condition, rhabditiform and filariform larvae may be present. Caution must be exercised when larval cultures are handled, because infective filariform larvae may be present. If there is a delay in the preservation of the stool specimen, embryonated ova as well as larvae of hookworm may be present. Culture of feces for larvae is useful for (i) revealing their presence when they are too scant to be detected by concentration methods; (ii) distinguishing whether the infection is due to *S. stercoralis* or hookworm on the basis of rhabditiform larval morphology by allowing hookworm egg hatching to occur, releasing first-stage larvae; and (iii) allowing the development of larvae into the filariform stage for further differentiation.

Fecal culture methods are especially helpful for the detection of light infections with hookworm, *S. stercoralis*, and *Trichostrongylus* spp. and for the specific identification of parasites. Also, such techniques are useful for obtaining a large number of infective-stage larvae for research purposes. One enhanced recovery method, the agar plate culture for *Strongyloides*, and several culture techniques are described in this chapter. Since these procedures are less common, brief descriptions are included.

Agar Plate Culture for *S. stercoralis*

The agar plate culture is recommended for the recovery of *S. stercoralis* larvae; it tends to be more sensitive than some of the other diagnostic methods and, with the exception of molecular methods, is currently the method of choice (1, 6, 7, 10, 11). Approximately 2 g of fresh stool (about 1 in. [25 mm] in diameter) is placed in the center of the agar plate, and the plate is sealed to prevent accidental infections and held for 2 days at room temperature. As the larvae crawl over the agar, they carry bacteria with them, thus creating visible tracks over the agar. The plates are examined under the microscope for confirmation of the presence of larvae, the surface of the agar is then washed with 10% formalin, and final confirmation of larval identification is made via wet examination of the sediment from the formalin washings. Although specific agar formulations are often provided, any agar plate where the bacterial colonies are easily seen can be used for this purpose. However, it is recommended that the plates be drier rather than very moist, to avoid bacterial swarming, which could obscure the tracking on the agar surface.

TABLE 7. FDA-approved and cleared molecular diagnostic tests for parasites[a]

Test (company)	Description	Comments
APTIMA (Gen-Probe, San Diego, CA) *Trichomonas vaginalis*	Nucleic acid test that uses target capture, transcription-mediated amplification, and hybridization protection assay technologies	High sensitivity and specificity; does not require organism viability or motility; therapeutic failure or success cannot be determined since nucleic acid may persist following therapy; qualitative results
Affirm VPIII microbial identification test (Becton Dickinson Co., Franklin Lakes, NJ) *Trichomonas vaginalis*	Two single-stranded nucleic acid probes for each organism, capture probe, and a color development probe for each target	Vaginitis: *Candida* spp., *Gardnerella vaginalis*, *Trichomonas vaginalis*. Positive = visible blue color reaction on the organism-specific bead embedded in the Probe Analysis Card; organism presence or absence cannot be used as a test for therapeutic success or failure.
BD MAX CT/GC/TV vaginal panel (Becton Dickinson Co., Franklin Lakes, NJ) *Chlamydia trachomatis* *Neisseria gonorrhoeae* *Trichomonas vaginalis*	Multiplex TaqMan-based PCR technology; moderate complexity	Allows simultaneous detection of organisms from a single test; male/female urine samples, vaginal swabs, endocervical swabs. Results in <3 h; reagents stored at room temperature. Panel cannot be used as a test for therapeutic success or failure.
BD MAX enteric parasite panel (Becton Dickinson Co., Sparks, MD) *Giardia lamblia* *Cryptosporidium* (*C. hominis*, *C. parvum*) *Entamoeba histolytica*	Multiplex qualitative *in vitro* diagnostic test. Automates sample lysis, nucleic acid extraction and concentration, reagent rehydration, nucleic acid amplification, and detection of the target nucleic acid sequence using real-time PCR. Amplified targets are detected with hydrolysis probes labeled with quenched fluorophores.	Simultaneously and differentially detects DNA from *Giardia lamblia*, *Cryptosporidium* (*C. hominis*, *C parvum*), *Entamoeba histolytica*. As with all PCR-based *in vitro* diagnostic tests, extremely low levels of target below the analytical sensitivity of the assay may be detected, but results may not be reproducible. False negatives may also occur if the level of organism nucleic acid is below the threshold of detection. Qualitative test; not used for monitoring therapy.
BioFire Film Array gastrointestinal panel (bioMérieux, Marcy l'Étoile, France) *Cryptosporidium* spp. *Cyclospora cayetanensis* *Entamoeba histolytica* *Giardia lamblia*	Consists of automated nucleic acid extraction, reverse transcription, amplification, and analysis. The panel contains two assays (Crypt 1 and Crypt 2) for detection of *Cryptosporidium* spp.	Results available in 1 h per run (i.e., per specimen). Each FilmArray pouch contains an internal nucleic acid extraction control and a PCR control. *E. histolytica* may cross-react with *E. dispar* when present at higher levels. Detection of approximately 23 different *Cryptosporidium* spp. occurs, including the most common species of human clinical relevance (i.e., *C. hominis* and *C. parvum*), as well as several less common species (e.g., *C. meleagridis*, *C. felis*, *C. canis*, *C. cuniculus*, *C. muris*, and *C. suis*). Nested PCR and melting curve.
Luminex xTAG gastrointestinal pathogen panel (Luminex, Inc., Austin, TX) *Cryptosporidium* spp. (*C. hominis*, *C. parvum* only) *Entamoeba histolytica* *Giardia lamblia*	Multiplexed nucleic acid test for the simultaneous qualitative detection and identification of multiple viral, parasitic, and bacterial nucleic acids in human stool specimens	Organisms do not have to be viable. The performance of this test has not been established for monitoring treatment of infection with any of the panel organisms. PCR plus xTAG (fluorescent-bead-based detection).
Nanosphere Verigene Enteric Pathogen Panel (recently acquired by Luminex); Verigene EP Flex (Nanosphere [now Luminex], Northbrook, IL) (estimated release, 2018) *Blastocystis* spp. *Cryptosporidium* spp. *Cyclospora cayetanensis* *Dientamoeba fragilis* *Entamoeba histolytica* *Giardia lamblia* Microsporidia *Strongyloides stercoralis*	PCR + gold nanoparticle hybridization; qualitative, hybridization-based assay	Closed, fully automated system; one cartridge, multiple reporting configurations; removes preanalytic step of physician test selection; increased sensitivity of pathogen detection
SMART Leish PCR assay (Walter Reed Army Institute of Research, U.S. Army Medical Materiel Development Activity, Cepheid USA, Inc., Cepheid, Sunnyvale, CA)	Qualitative test using real-time PCR for amplification of DNA sequences unique to the organism that causes cutaneous leishmaniasis	Can provide consistent results when microscopy and culture results are negative at day 30

[a]There are other products available with a valid CE marking; a valid CE marking affixed to a product indicates that it complies with the relevant European New Approach product safety directives. The directives contain the essential requirements that a product must meet to be sold in the European Union.

TABLE 8 Additional helminth recovery and identification techniques (other than O&P examination)

Organism	Specimen	Procedure
Nematodes		
S. stercoralis Hookworm *Trichostrongylus* spp.	Fresh stool, not refrigerated (all organisms can be recovered by any of the procedures in the column to the right)	Harada-Mori filter paper strip Filter paper/slant culture Charcoal culture Baermann test Agar plate culture (primarily for *S. stercoralis*)
Hookworm *Ascaris lumbricoides* *Trichuris trichiura*	Fresh stool, refrigeration acceptable	Direct smear (Beaver)[a] Dilution egg count (Stoll)[a] Either method acceptable for estimation of worm burden[a]
Enterobius vermicularis	Scotch tape preparations, paddles, anal swab, other collection devices	Direct microscopic examination
Trematodes		
Schistosoma spp.	Fresh stool, not refrigerated Fresh urine (24-h and single collection)	Egg hatching test Egg viability test
Cestodes		
Tapeworms	Proglottids (gravid in alcohol) Stool in 5 to 10% formalin	India ink injection Scolex search

[a]Although these two methods have been used in the past, currently the World Health Organization recommendation is the Kato-Katz thick fecal smear method, with the McMaster egg count method being an excellent alternative for monitoring large-scale eradication programs. In the majority of diagnostic laboratories, none of these procedures are routinely performed; generally their use is limited to relevant geographic areas and/or studies (27).

Baermann Technique

Another method of examining a stool specimen suspected of having small numbers of *Strongyloides* larvae is the use of a modified Baermann apparatus. The Baermann technique uses a funnel apparatus and relies on the principle that active larvae migrate from a fresh fecal specimen that has been placed on a wire mesh with several layers of gauze, which are in contact with tap water (1). Larvae migrate through the gauze into the water and settle to the bottom of the funnel, where they can be collected and examined. The main difference between this method and the Harada-Mori and petri dish methods is the greater amount of fresh stool used, possibly providing a better chance of larval recovery in a light infection. Besides being used for patient fecal specimens, this technique can be used to examine soil specimens for the presence of larvae. However, the agar plate method is considered a more sensitive method for the recovery of *S. stercoralis* larvae.

Harada-Mori Filter Paper Strip Culture

To detect light infections with hookworm, *S. stercoralis*, and *Trichostrongylus* spp., as well as to facilitate specific identification, the Harada-Mori filter paper strip culture technique is very useful (1, 6, 7, 10, 11). The technique requires filter paper (a strip cut to fit into a 15-ml test tube); fresh fecal material (about the size of a raisin to a small grape) is added to the middle of the filter paper, and the filter paper is inserted into a test tube. Moisture is provided by adding water to the tube (within a half-inch of the stool, but not covering the stool), which continuously soaks the filter paper by capillary action. Incubation under suitable conditions favors hatching of ova and/or development of larvae. Fecal specimens to be cultured should not be refrigerated, since some parasites are susceptible to cold and may fail to develop after refrigeration. Also, caution must be exercised in handling the filter paper strip itself, since infective *Strongyloides* larvae may migrate upward as well as downward on the paper strip.

Filter Paper/Slant Culture Technique (Petri Dish)

An alternative technique for culturing *Strongyloides* larvae is a filter paper/slant culture on a microscope slide placed in a glass or plastic petri dish (1, 6, 7, 10, 11). As with the techniques described above, sufficient moisture is provided by continuous soaking of filter paper in water. Fresh stool material is placed on filter paper, which is cut to fit the dimensions of a standard (1 by 3 in.) (2.5 cm by 7.6 cm) microscope slide. The filter paper is then placed on a slanted glass slide in a glass or plastic petri dish containing water. This technique allows direct examination of the culture system with a dissecting microscope to look for nematode larvae and free-living stages of *S. stercoralis* in the fecal mass or the surrounding water without having to sample the preparation.

Egg Studies and Scolex Search

Estimation of Worm Burdens

The only human parasites for which it is reasonably possible to correlate egg production with adult worm burdens are *Ascaris lumbricoides*, *Trichuris trichiura*, and the hookworms (*Necator americanus* and *Ancylostoma duodenale*). The specific instances in which information on approximate worm burdens is useful are when one is determining the intensity of infection, deciding on possible chemotherapy, and evaluating the efficacies of the drugs administered. With current therapy, the need for the monitoring of therapy through egg counts is no longer as relevant. A number of methods have been described (1, 6, 7, 10).

Hatching of Schistosome Eggs

When schistosome eggs are recovered from either urine or stool, they should be carefully examined to determine viability. The presence of living miracidia within the eggs indicates an active infection that may require therapy. The viability of the miracidia can be determined in two ways: (i) the cilia of the flame cells (primitive excretory cells) may be seen on a wet smear by using high dry power and are usually actively moving, and (ii) the miracidia may be released from the eggs by the use of a hatching procedure (1). The eggs usually hatch within several hours when placed in 10 vol of dechlorinated or spring water (hatching may begin soon after contact with the water). The eggs that are recovered in the urine (24-h specimen collected with no preservatives) are easily obtained from the sediment and can be examined under the microscope to determine viability. A sidearm flask is recommended, but an Erlenmeyer flask is an acceptable substitute.

Because adult worms occasionally reside in veins other than their normal site, both urine and stool specimens must be collected. Specimens should be collected without preservatives and should not be refrigerated prior to processing. Hatching does not occur until the saline is removed and nonchlorinated water is added. If a stool concentration is performed, saline should be used throughout the procedure to prevent premature hatching. The light must not be too close to the side arm or top layer of water in the Erlenmeyer flask. Excess heat kills the miracidia. The lamp light mimics the sun shining on a water source, and the hatched larvae tend to swim toward the light (*S. mansoni* more so than *S. haematobium* and *S. japonicum*). The absence of live miracidia does not rule out the presence of schistosome eggs. Nonviable eggs or eggs that failed to hatch are not detected by this method. Microscopic examination of direct or concentrated specimens should be used to detect the presence or absence of eggs. Egg viability can be determined by placing some stool or urine sediment (the same material used for the hatching flask) on a microscope slide. Low-power magnification (×100) can be used to locate the eggs. Individual eggs can be examined with high dry magnification (×400); moving cilia on the flame cells (primitive excretory system) confirm egg viability.

Search for Tapeworm Scolices

Since therapy for the elimination of tapeworms is usually very effective, a search for the tapeworm scolex is rarely requested and is no longer clinically relevant. However, stool specimens may have to be examined for the presence of scolices and gravid proglottids of cestodes for proper species identification. Specific methods can be found in various publications (1, 6, 7, 11).

EXAMINATION OF OTHER SPECIMENS FROM THE INTESTINAL TRACT

Examination for Pinworm

A roundworm parasite that has a worldwide distribution and that is commonly found in children is *Enterobius vermicularis*, known as pinworm or seatworm. The adult female worm migrates out of the anus, usually at night, and deposits her eggs on the perianal area. The adult female (8 to 13 mm long) may occasionally be found on the surface of a stool specimen or on the perianal skin. Since the eggs are usually deposited around the anus, they are not commonly found in feces and must be detected by other diagnostic techniques. Diagnosis of pinworm infection is usually based on the recovery of typical eggs, which are described as thick-shelled, football-shaped eggs with one slightly flattened side. Often each egg contains a fully developed embryo and becomes infective within a few hours after being deposited. Commercial collection devices are available and can be used for specimen collection, similar to the approach with cellulose tape indicated below (1). Many clinicians may treat patients on the basis of clinical symptoms without confirmation of the suspected diagnosis of pinworm infection.

Cellulose Tape and Anal Swab Preparations

The most widely used procedure for the diagnosis of pinworm infection is the cellulose tape (adhesive cellophane tape) method (1, 9, 12, 13). Specimens should be obtained in the morning, before the patient bathes or goes to the bathroom. The tape is applied to the anal folds and is then placed sticky side down on a microscope slide for examination. At least six consecutive negative slides should be observed before the patient is considered free of infection. The use of up to six tapes is no longer considered practical; if children are symptomatic, pediatricians will usually treat without actual egg confirmation. The anal swab technique (1) is also available for the detection of pinworm infections; however, most laboratories prefer the cellulose tape method if one of the options is selected.

Sigmoidoscopy Material

Material obtained from sigmoidoscopy can be helpful in the diagnosis of amebiasis that has not been detected by routine fecal examinations, and the procedure is recommended for this purpose. However, usually a series of at least three routine stool examinations for parasites should be performed for each patient before a sigmoidoscopy examination is done (1).

Material from the mucosal surface should be aspirated or scraped and must not be obtained with cotton-tipped swabs. At least six representative areas of the mucosa should be sampled and examined (six samples, six slides). Usually, the amount of material is limited and should be processed immediately to ensure the best examination possible (Table 9). If the amount of material limits the examination to one procedure, the use of one of the fecal fixatives is highly recommended for the subsequent preparation of permanent stains.

Although the fecal immunoassays are generally not validated for or performed on sigmoidoscopy specimens, they can be used on fecal specimens for the detection of the *E. histolytica-E. dispar* group or confirmation of the pathogen *E. histolytica*. However, this testing requires fresh or frozen stool; preserved stool is not acceptable.

It is recommended that a parasitology specimen tray (containing Schaudinn's fixative, a liquid fixative containing PVA, 5 or 10% formalin, or one of the single-vial fixatives) be provided or that a trained technologist be available at the time of sigmoidoscopy to prepare the slides.

Direct Saline Mount

If there is no lag time after collection and a microscope is available in the immediate vicinity, some of the material should be examined as a direct saline mount for the presence of motile trophozoites (1). A drop of material is mixed with a drop of 0.85% sodium chloride and is examined under low-intensity light for the characteristic movement of amebae. It may take time for the organisms to become acclimated to this type of preparation; thus, motility may not be obvious for several minutes. There will be epithelial cells, macrophages, and possibly polymorphonuclear leukocytes (PMNs) and erythrocytes, which require a careful examination to reveal amebae.

Since specific identification of protozoan organisms can be difficult when only the direct saline mount is used, this technique should be used only when there is sufficient material left to prepare permanent stained smears.

Permanent Stained Smear

Most of the material obtained at sigmoidoscopy can be smeared (gently) onto a slide and immediately immersed in SAF or one of the single-vial fixatives (1). These slides can then be stained with trichrome or iron hematoxylin stain and examined for specific cell morphology, either protozoan or otherwise. The procedure and staining times are identical to those for routine fecal smears.

TABLE 9 Recovery of parasites from other intestinal tract specimens

Source	Organisms	Procedure[a]
Sigmoidoscopy specimens		
Unpreserved	Ameba trophozoites (motility)	Direct wet mount, immunoassay tests[b]
Air-dried smears	Coccidia	Modified acid-fast stain
	Microsporidia	Modified trichrome, optical brighteners, immunoassay tests[c]
Preserved 5–10% formalin or SAF or a single-vial fixative	Helminth eggs and larvae (rare), ameba and flagellate cysts[d] and trophozoites (SAF and a single-vial fixative)	Concentration wet mount, immunoassay tests
	Coccidia	Modified acid-fast smear, immunoassay tests
	Microsporidia	Modified trichrome, optical brighteners, immunoassay tests[c]
Fixative with polyvinyl alcohol	Helminth eggs and larvae (rare), ameba and flagellate cysts[d]	Wet mount
	Ameba and flagellate cysts[d] and trophozoites	Permanent stained smear
Schaudinn's fixative	Ameba and flagellate cysts[d] and trophozoites	Permanent stained smear
Duodenal specimens[e]		
Unpreserved	Helminth eggs and larvae, trophozoites (motility) of *Giardia*	Direct wet mount
Entero-Test capsule[f]		
Preserved 5–10% formalin or SAF or a single-vial fixative	Helminth eggs and larvae, *Giardia* trophozoites	Concentration wet mount, immunoassay tests (depending on validation documentation)
		Permanent stained smear
Entero-Test capsule[f]	Coccidia	Modified acid-fast smear, immunoassay tests
	Microsporidia	Modified trichrome, optical brighteners, immunoassay tests[c]
Fecal fixatives containing polyvinyl alcohol (adhesive)	Flagellate trophozoites	Permanent stained smear
Anal impression smear	Pinworm adult and eggs	No stain, cellulose tape preparation and other collection devices
Adult worm or segments	Helminth adult worms or proglottids	Carmine stain (rarely used), India ink
Tissue biopsy specimen	Helminth eggs, larvae, and adults; protozoan cysts; trophozoites; oocysts; sporozoites; and spores	Touch preparations, squash preparations, permanent stains, histology

[a]Molecular tests are available for certain organisms; collection options will vary (fresh, Cary-Blair, some single-vial fecal preservatives). Some of these collection vial options may require in-house validation prior to clinical use.

[b]Immunoassay tests for the *Entamoeba histolytica-E. dispar* group or *Entamoeba histolytica* require fresh or frozen stool; preserved stool specimens are not acceptable for testing. Immunoassays for *Cryptosporidium* spp. and *Giardia lamblia* (name designation on commercial kits) are approved for use on stool; immunoassay use for other intestinal tract specimens (sigmoidoscopy) may or may not be appropriate, depending on specimen source, consistency, volume, and appropriate validation documentation.

[c]Some genus-specific immunoassay reagents for the microsporidia are available commercially but are not FDA approved.

[d]Although cysts may be present in stool, sigmoidoscopy specimens are often obtained from patients with severe diarrhea or dysentery. In these cases, the cyst forms are usually absent; trophozoites are the most likely stage seen, particularly in the case of *E. histolytica*.

[e]Duodenal specimens are often submitted as aspirates; in such cases, the volume may be sufficient to perform concentrations. However, if small amounts of duodenal mucus and/or biopsy material are obtained, squash preparations preserved with Schaudinn's fixative are preferred. This approach may require the use of slides precoated with albumin to facilitate adhesion. Mucus obtained from the Entero-Test capsule string may be treated as a fresh specimen; the string can also be immediately placed in preservative after retrieval, and the mucus can be processed as a permanent stained smear from a number of fixative options (with and without polyvinyl alcohol).

[f]The Entero-Test capsule commercial availability varies over time; currently it is not in production.

Duodenal Contents

Duodenal Drainage

In infections with *G. duodenalis* (*G. lamblia*, *G. intestinalis*) or *S. stercoralis*, routine stool examinations may not reveal the organisms. Duodenal drainage material can be submitted for examination (Table 8) (1).

A fresh, unpreserved specimen should be submitted to the laboratory; the amount may vary from <0.5 ml to several milliliters of fluid. The specimen may be centrifuged (at 500 × *g* for 10 min) and should be examined immediately as a wet mount for motile organisms (iodine may be added later to facilitate identification of any organisms present). If the specimen cannot be completely examined within 2 h after it is taken, any remaining material should be preserved in one of the fecal fixatives for permanent staining.

If the duodenal fluid contains mucus, this is where the organisms tend to be found. Therefore, centrifugation of the specimen is important, and the sedimented mucus should be examined. *Giardia* trophozoites may be caught in mucus strands, and the movement of the flagella on the trophozoites may be the only subtle motility seen for these flagellates. *Strongyloides* larvae are usually very motile. Immunoassay methods for *Cryptosporidium* spp. and *G. duodenalis* (*G. lamblia*, *G. intestinalis*) can also be used with fresh or formalinized material; however, duodenal fluid is not included in many of the package inserts as an acceptable specimen.

If the amount of duodenal material submitted is very small, rather than using any of the specimen for a wet smear examination, permanent stains can be prepared. This approach provides a more permanent record, and the potential problems with unstained organisms, very minimal motility, and a lower-power examination can be avoided by using oil immersion examination of the stained specimen at a magnification of ×1,000.

Duodenal Capsule Technique (Entero-Test)

A method of sampling duodenal contents that eliminates the need for intestinal intubation consists of the use of a length of nylon yarn coiled inside a gelatin capsule with a weight on the end that is swallowed (1, 6, 7, 11). The capsule is swallowed and allowed to progress into the duodenum while retaining one end of the yarn, usually taped to the patient's cheek. After approximately 60 minutes, the yarn is retrieved. The bile-stained mucus from the string should be examined immediately as a wet mount for motile organisms. If the specimen cannot be completely examined within an hour after the yarn has been removed, the material should be preserved in SAF, in one of the single-vial fixatives, or in fixative containing PVA. Mucus smears should be prepared. However, it appears that both the pediatric and adult capsules are no longer being manufactured; however, this could change in the future.

UROGENITAL SPECIMENS

Several parasites may be recovered and identified from urogenital specimens. Although the most common pathogens are probably *Trichomonas vaginalis* and *Schistosoma haematobium*, other organisms, such as the microsporidia, are becoming much more important (Table 10). Also, the membrane filtration for the recovery of microfilariae can be performed from urine.

TABLE 10 Detection of urogenital parasites

Organism(s)	Procedure
Trichomonas vaginalis	Wet mount (motility)
	Culture
	Giemsa stain (if dry smear submitted—prefix in absolute methanol and allow smear to dry prior to staining)
	Direct fluorescent antibody
	DNA probe
	Latex agglutination
	Enzyme-linked immunoassay
	Rapid immunochromatographic assay (dipstick)
Schistosoma haematobium	Wet mount (urine sediment)
	Membrane filtration
	Tissue section (squash prep and/or histology section)
Microfilariae	Knott concentration
	Membrane filtration (Nuclepore filter)
	Giemsa stain
	Delafield's hematoxylin stain
Microsporidia	Modified trichrome stain[a]
	Optical brighteners (calcofluor white)[a]
	Immunoassay tests[a,b]
	Routine histology
	Electron microscopy or molecular methods for identification to the genus and species levels

[a]Staining procedures and fluorescent-antibody tests for organism detection performed on centrifuged sediment (500 × *g* for 10 min).

[b]Immunoassays are available commercially but are not yet FDA approved for use within the United States.

Direct Wet Mount

The identification of *T. vaginalis* is usually based on the examination of a wet preparation of vaginal and urethral discharges and prostatic secretions or urine sediment and may require the testing of multiple specimens to confirm the diagnosis. These specimens are diluted with a drop of saline and are examined under low power and reduced illumination for the presence of actively motile organisms. As the jerky motility begins to diminish, it may be possible to observe the undulating membrane, particularly under high dry power (magnification, ×400). However, wet mounts are considered very insensitive for the confirmation of trichomoniasis (1). Molecular test options are becoming more common and are considerably more sensitive.

While the membrane filtration technique can be used for the recovery of microfilariae, the examination of urinary sediment may be indicated in certain filarial infections. The occurrence of microfilariae in urine has been reported with increasing frequency in *Onchocerca volvulus* infections in Africa. Detailed directions for the membrane filtration procedure can be found in several publications (1, 6, 7, 10, 11).

The membrane filtration technique can also be used with urine for the recovery of *Schistosoma haematobium* eggs (1). This approach uses a 25-mm Nuclepore filter (5-μm porosity) (1, 6, 10, 11).

The use of stained smears is usually not necessary for the identification of *T. vaginalis*. The high number of false-positive and false-negative results reported on the basis of stained smears strongly suggests the value of confirmation by observation of motile organisms from the direct mount, from appropriate culture media (1, 6, 7, 10), or from direct detection with immunoassay reagents (1).

Stained smears may be prepared from material obtained from the membrane filtration techniques used for the recovery of microfilariae; Delafield's hematoxylin or Giemsa stain may be used. It is important to remember that Giemsa stain may not adequately stain the sheath, and correct identification of the organisms may require staining with a hematoxylin-based stain.

Some microsporidial infections can also be diagnosed from the examination of urine sediment that has been stained by one of the modified trichrome methods or by using optical brightening agents such as calcofluor white (1). Multiple methods are recommended for confirmation of the diagnosis. It is recommended that any patient suspected of microsporidiosis submit both stool and urine for examination.

Culture

Specimens from women for culture (for *T. vaginalis*) may consist of vaginal exudate collected from the posterior fornix on cotton-tipped applicator sticks or genital secretions collected on polyester sponges. Specimens from men can include semen, urethral samples collected with a polyester sponge, or urine. Urine samples collected from the patient should be the specimen first voided in the morning. It is critical that clinical specimens be inoculated into culture medium as soon as possible after collection (1, 13). Another approach is use of the plastic envelope methods (*Trichomonas* culture system [Empyrean Diagnostics, Mountain View, CA] or InPouch TV [BioMed Diagnostics, San Jose, CA]), which are simplified techniques for transport and culture (4). The control strain *T. vaginalis* ATCC 30001 should be available when these cultures are used for clinical specimens. Many media for the isolation of *T. vaginalis* are available, and some of these can be purchased commercially and have relatively long shelf lives, particularly those used for the plastic envelope methods.

If no trophozoites are seen after 4 days of incubation, then the tubes should be discarded and the culture should be reported as negative. Results for patient specimens should not be reported as positive unless control cultures are positive. Since culture may take as long as 3 to 4 days and the clinical specimens may contain nonviable organisms, it is recommended that microscopic examination of wet smears be performed as well (dead organisms may be present, although they will be difficult to see).

Antigen Detection (*T. vaginalis*)

The culture method is considered very sensitive for the diagnosis of trichomoniasis; however, due to the time and effort involved, some laboratories have decided to use some of the new immunoassay detection kits (1). The Osom Trichomonas Rapid Test (Genzyme Diagnostics, Cambridge, MA) is an immunochromatographic method for antigen detection using the dipstick format. Results are available within 10 min, and according to the manufacturer, there is 95% agreement with the reference standard (culture and wet mount). The Affirm VPIII DNA probe technology (Becton Dickinson Co., Franklin Lakes, NJ) offers a dependable, rapid means for the early identification of three organisms causing vaginitis: *Candida* species, *Gardnerella vaginalis*, and *T. vaginalis*. Also, the APTIMA *T. vaginalis* assay (GenProbe, San Diego, CA) is available. Other molecular options can be seen in Table 7.

SPECIMENS FROM OTHER BODY SITES

Molecular methods may or may not be available for the individual organisms mentioned; certainly molecular tests will generally be more sensitive, especially when the organisms present in the clinical specimen are rare. When routine testing methods have failed to demonstrate the organisms, the examination of aspirated material for the diagnosis of parasitic infections may be extremely valuable (Table 11). Specimens should be transported to the laboratory immediately after collection. Aspirates include liquid specimens collected from a variety of sites as well as fine-needle aspirates and duodenal aspirates. Fine-needle aspirates are often collected by the cytopathology staff who process the specimens, or they may be collected and sent to the laboratory directly for slide preparation and/or culture. Fluid specimens collected by bronchoscopy include bronchoalveolar lavage and bronchial washing fluids.

Procedural details for processing sigmoidoscopic aspirates and scrapings for the recovery of *E. histolytica* and techniques for preparation of duodenal aspirate material are presented above.

Biopsy specimens are recommended for use in the diagnosis of parasitic infections in tissues (Table 11). In addition to standard histologic preparations, impression smears and teased and squash preparations of biopsy tissue from the following can be used: skin, muscle, cornea, intestine, liver, lung, and brain. Tissue to be examined as permanent sections or by electron microscopy should be fixed as specified by the laboratories that will process the tissue, and in certain cases, testing of a biopsy specimen may be the only means of confirming a suspected parasitic problem. Specimens that are going to be examined as fresh material rather than as tissue sections should be kept moist in saline and submitted to the laboratory immediately.

Detection of parasites in tissue depends on specimen collection and the retrieval of sufficient material for examination. Biopsy specimens are usually quite small and may not be representative of the diseased tissue. Multiple tissue samples often improve diagnostic results. To optimize the yield from any tissue specimen, examine all areas and use as many procedures as possible. Tissues are obtained from invasive procedures, many of which are very expensive and lengthy: consequently, these specimens deserve the most comprehensive procedures possible.

Tissue submitted in a sterile container on a sterile sponge dampened with saline may be used for cultures of protozoa after mounts for direct examination or touch or impression smears for staining have been prepared. If cultures for parasites will be made, sterile slides should be used for smear and mount preparation, or cultures should be inoculated prior to smear preparation.

Detached ciliary tufts (ciliocytophthoria) have been seen in a variety of body fluids (especially peritoneal and amniotic fluids; also respiratory specimens). These tufts are the remnants of ciliated epithelium that are found as a part of normal cellular turnover in a number of sites: respiratory tract and sinuses, ventricles of the brain, central canal of the spinal cord, and epithelia of the male and female reproductive tracts. The tufts are motile, measure 10 to 15 μm in diameter, and can be confused with ciliated or flagellated protozoa. However, when they are carefully examined on a stained smear, there is no internal structure like that seen in protozoa (1).

Bone Marrow

Bone marrow aspirates to be evaluated for *Leishmania* amastigotes, *Trypanosoma cruzi* amastigotes (African trypanosomiasis organisms are not relevant), *Plasmodium* spp., or *Toxoplasma gondii* (bone marrow is a less common site for this organism) require Giemsa staining. However, if stained with a hematoxylin-Giemsa combination or other blood stains, the organisms will be visible as well. If specimens are to be processed for culture, it is important to maintain sterility of the specimen prior to inoculation of media for parasitology cultures. After inoculation of appropriate media, the remaining specimen can be processed for smear preparation and staining.

Brain and Cerebrospinal Fluid

Generally, when cerebrospinal fluid or brain aspirates or biopsy specimens are received, the most likely parasites include the free-living amebae *Acanthamoeba* spp., *Balamuthia mandrillaris*, *Naegleria fowleri*, and *Sappinia* spp. The use of nonnutrient agar (with bacterial overlays) cultures is recommended for *Acanthamoeba* spp. and *N. fowleri*; quality control cultures with known positive organisms are recommended as a basis for acceptable interpretation of patient culture results. *Sappinia* spp. also grow in the culture system consisting of nonnutrient agar with a bacterial overlay. If free-living ameba cultures are ordered for central nervous system specimens, the agar plates should be incubated at 37°C (room air, no CO_2) (1, 6, 7, 10). Unfortunately, cultures for *B. mandrillaris* are difficult to perform; consultation with the U.S. Centers for Disease Control and Prevention (CDC) is recommended if this infection is suspected. The remaining specimen can then be processed for smear preparation and staining. Although *T. gondii* would also be seen in stained smears, one could also use immunospecific reagents, cell line culture, or PCR. Spinal fluid should not be diluted before examination. Impression smears or touch preparations from tissues should be prepared and stained with a blood stain. The material is

TABLE 11 Specimen, possible parasite recovered, and appropriate tests (other than intestinal tract)[a]

Body site	Specimen	Possible parasite(s)	Tests
Bone marrow	Aspirate	*Leishmania* spp., *Trypanosoma cruzi*, *Plasmodium* spp., *Toxoplasma gondii*	Giemsa, culture (if relevant), PCR for sensitivity in early, late infections
Brain	Tissue biopsy specimen, cerebrospinal fluid	*Naegleria* spp., *Acanthamoeba* spp., *Sappinia* spp.	Giemsa, trichrome, culture, PCR genus ID
		Balamuthia mandrillaris, *Entamoeba histolytica*	Giemsa, trichrome
		Toxoplasma gondii	Giemsa, immunospecific reagent, culture, PCR
		Microsporidia (*Encephalitozoon* spp., *Trachipleistophora anthropophthera*)	Modified trichrome, acid-fast stain, Giemsa, optical brightening agent (calcofluor white), histology[b] (methenamine silver, PAS, tissue Gram stains), PCR, electron microscopy
		Taenia solium (cysticerci), *Echinococcus* spp.	Routine histology[b]
Eye	Cornea, conjunctiva, contact lens, lens solutions[c]	Microsporidia (*Encephalitozoon* spp., *Trachipleistophora* spp., *Anncaliia* sp., *Nosema* spp., *Microsporidium* spp.)	Acid-fast stain, Giemsa, modified trichrome, methenamine silver, optical brightening agent (calcofluor white), histology[b] (methenamine silver, PAS, tissue Gram stains), electron microscopy
		Acanthamoeba spp.	Giemsa, trichrome, culture, calcofluor white (cysts only), PCR for genus ID
		Toxoplasma gondii	Giemsa, immunospecific reagent, culture
	Larval or adult worms	*Loa loa*, *Dipetalonema*, *Thelazia*, *Dirofilaria immitis*, *Gnathostoma* spp., *Toxocara canis*, *Taenia solium* (cysticerci), *Echinococcus* spp.	Direct examination, routine histology[b]
	Fly larvae, adult lice	Myiasis, louse infestation	Direct examination
Kidney, bladder	Biopsy specimens	Microsporidia (*Encephalitozoon* spp., *Enterocytozoon bieneusi*)	Modified trichrome, acid-fast stain, Giemsa, optical brightening agent (calcofluor white), histology[b] (methenamine silver, PAS, tissue Gram stains), electron microscopy
		Schistosoma haematobium	Direct examination
	Adult worm, eggs	*Dioctophyma renale*	Direct examination
Liver, spleen	Aspirates, biopsy specimens	*Echinococcus* spp.	Wet mount, routine histology[b]
		Clonorchis sp., *Opisthorchis* spp., *Capillaria hepatica*, *Toxocara canis*, *T. cati*	Routine histology[b]
		Toxoplasma gondii, *Leishmania donovani*	Giemsa, culture
		Cryptosporidium spp.	Modified acid-fast stain, immunospecific reagents
		Microsporidia (*Encephalitozoon* spp., *Enterocytozoon bieneusi*)	Modified trichrome, acid-fast stain, Giemsa, optical brightening agent (calcofluor white), histology[b] (methenamine silver, PAS, tissue Gram stains), electron microscopy
		Entamoeba histolytica[d]	Wet mount, trichrome
Lymph node, lymphatics	Aspirates, biopsy specimens	*Toxoplasma gondii*, *Trypanosoma cruzi*, *Trypanosoma brucei rhodesiense*, *T. brucei gambiense*	Direct examination, routine histology,[b] Giemsa, culture
		Microsporidia	Modified trichrome, acid-fast stain, Giemsa, optical brightening agent (calcofluor white), histology[b] (methenamine silver, PAS, tissue Gram stains), electron microscopy
		Wuchereria bancrofti, *Brugia malayi*, *Brugia* spp.	Thick blood films, concentration, membrane filtration

(Continued on next page)

TABLE 11 Specimen, possible parasite recovered, and appropriate tests (other than intestinal tract)[a] *(Continued)*

Body site	Specimen	Possible parasite(s)	Tests
Lung	Sputum (expectorated or induced), bronchoalveolar lavage fluid, transbronchial aspirates, brush biopsy specimens, open lung biopsy specimens	*Ascaris lumbricoides*, *Strongyloides stercoralis*, hookworm, *Paragonimus* spp., *Echinococcus granulosus*	Wet mount, routine histology[b]
		Microsporidia (*Encephalitozoon* spp., *Enterocytozoon bieneusi*)	Modified trichrome, acid-fast stain, Giemsa, optical brightening agent (calcofluor white), histology[b] (methenamine silver, PAS, tissue Gram stains), electron microscopy
		Toxoplasma gondii	Giemsa, immunospecific reagent, culture
		Cryptosporidium spp.	Modified acid-fast stain, immunospecific reagent
	Saliva	*Entamoeba gingivalis*, *Trichomonas tenax*	Trichrome
Muscle	Biopsy specimen	*Trichinella* spp.	Wet examination, squash preparation, routine histology[b]
		Microsporidia (*Pleistophora* spp., *Nosema* spp., *Trachipleistophora hominis*)	Modified trichrome, acid-fast stain, Giemsa, optical brightening agent (calcofluor white), histology[b] (methenamine silver, PAS, tissue Gram stains), electron microscopy
		Sarcocystis spp., *Baylisascaris procyonis*, *Ancylostoma* spp., *Taenia solium* (cysticerci), *Taenia* (*Multiceps*) (coenurus), *Echinococcus* spp., *Spirometra* (spargana), *Onchocerca volvulus* (nodules), *Gnathostoma* spp., *Trypanosoma cruzi*	Routine histology[b]
Nasopharynx, sinus cavities	Scraping, biopsy specimens, aspirates	Microsporidia (*Encephalitozoon* spp., *Enterocytozoon bieneusi*, *Trachipleistophora hominis*)	Modified trichrome, acid-fast stain, Giemsa, optical brightening agent (calcofluor white), histology[b] (methenamine silver, PAS, tissue Gram stains), electron microscopy
		Acanthamoeba spp.	Giemsa, trichrome, culture, calcofluor white (cysts only)
		Naegleria spp.	Giemsa, trichrome, culture
		Leishmania spp.	Giemsa, culture
Rectal tissue	Scraping, aspirate, biopsy specimens	*Schistosoma mansoni*, *S. japonicum*	Direct examination
Skin	Skin snips	*Onchocerca volvulus*, *Mansonella streptocerca*	Giemsa, routine histology[b]
	Scraping, aspirates, biopsy specimen	*Leishmania* spp.	Giemsa, culture, routine histology[b]
		Acanthamoeba spp.	Giemsa, trichrome, culture, calcofluor (cysts only)
		Entamoeba histolytica, *Schistosoma* spp.	Routine histology[b]

[a]This table does not include every possible parasite that could be found in a particular body site. Parasite stages include trophozoites, cysts, oocysts, spores, adults, larvae, eggs, hooklets, amastigotes, and trypomastigotes. Although PCR methods have been used in the research setting for most of the organisms listed in the table, reagents are generally not commercially available. When available, molecular methods are recommended for enhanced sensitivity and specificity. In other cases, serologies may be recommended rather than routine testing on various tissues (*Toxoplasma*).

[b]Routine histology can be used for the detection and identification of many parasites. In some cases, it may be the only means of diagnosis.

[c]Although eye specimens are much preferred, free-living amebae have been cultured from patient contact lenses and lens solutions; we would not reject these specimens. An exception is unopened commercial lens care solutions; these solutions should be rejected.

[d]The examination of abscess aspirates for the presence of *E. histolytica* trophozoites is an uncommon procedure and not always reliable in diagnosing extraintestinal amebiasis; serologic tests are preferred.

pressed between two slides, with the smear resulting when the slides are pulled apart (one across the other). The smears are allowed to air dry and are then processed like a thin blood film (fixed in absolute methanol and stained with one of the blood stains).

Patients with primary amebic meningoencephalitis are rare, but the examination of spinal fluid may reveal the amebae, usually *N. fowleri*. Unspun sedimented spinal fluid should be placed on a slide, under a coverslip, and observed for motile amebae; smears can also be stained with trichrome, Wright's, or one of the blood stains. Spinal fluid, exudate, or tissue fragments can be examined by light microscopy or phase-contrast microscopy. Care must be taken not to confuse leukocytes with actual organisms and vice versa. The spinal fluid may be clear early in the infection or appear cloudy or purulent (with or without erythrocytes), with a cell count ranging from a few hundred to more than 20,000 leukocytes (primarily neutrophils) per ml. Failure to find bacteria in this type of spinal fluid should alert one to the possibility of primary amebic meningoencephalitis; however, false-positive bacterial Gram stains have been reported due to the excess debris. Isolation of these organisms from tissues can be done by using special media. When spinal fluid is placed in a counting chamber, organisms that settle to the bottom of the chamber tend to round up and look very much like leukocytes. For this reason, it is better to examine the spinal fluid on a slide directly under a coverslip, not in a counting chamber.

Possible infection with microsporidia (the most likely organism is *Encephalitozoon* spp.; less common is *Trachipleistophora anthropophthera*) should also be considered. Specific methods include modified trichrome, acid-fast, and blood stains; a nonspecific optical brightening agent (calcofluor white); routine histology (methenamine silver, periodic acid-Schiff [PAS], and tissue Gram stains); and electron microscopy. Electron microscopy or immunospecific reagents are required to identify the microsporidia to the genus and species levels.

Helminth parasite stages such as *Taenia solium* cysticerci and hydatid cysts of *Echinococcus* spp. are generally identified through examination of routine histologic slides; however, confirmation of hydatid disease could also be made from the hooklets seen in the hydatid cyst fluid contents.

Eyes

Eye specimens could include those from the cornea, conjunctiva, contact lens, or contact lens solutions. Although eye specimens are preferred, *Acanthamoeba* spp. have been cultured from patient contact lenses and opened lens solution. These specimens are acceptable; however, due to risk management issues, the laboratory should not accept unopened commercial lens care solutions. These solutions could be referred to laboratories or agencies, such as the FDA, that handle testing and approval of commercial products. Also, the presence of *Acanthamoeba* in a lens solution does not automatically equate to *Acanthamoeba* keratitis; it is only suggestive at best. A corneal scraping is recommended. After appropriate media have been inoculated, smears from acceptable specimens should be prepared and stained using a blood stain or trichrome stains. Although *T. gondii* could be seen in stained smears, one could also use an immunospecific reagent or PCR for confirmation. Most individuals who are infected with *T. gondii* do not develop ocular disease; however, two populations are at risk, immunocompromised patients with HIV and neonates who have been exposed transplacentally to the mother's acute infection.

Also, microsporidia are highly suspect from this body site, and specific methods include modified trichrome, acid-fast, and blood stains; a nonspecific optical brightening agent (calcofluor white); routine histology (methenamine silver, PAS, and tissue Gram stains); and electron microscopy. Electron microscopy or immunospecific reagents are required to identify the microsporidia to the genus and species levels, which could include *Encephalitozoon* spp., *Trachipleistophora* spp., *Nosema* spp., *Vittaforma* spp., *Anncaliia* spp., and *Microsporidium* spp. These eye infections are frequently seen in immunocompetent individuals with no underlying disease. It is also important to recognize the possible confusion between microsporidial spores and bacteria on a Gram-stained smear or cytology preparation, particularly when the culture plates are negative.

Ocular diseases caused by nematodes include onchocerciasis, loiasis, dirofilariasis, gnathostomiasis, theileriasis, and toxocariasis. Diagnosis of onchocerciasis can be accomplished by confirming the presence of microfilariae in a corneal biopsy or from the microscopic examination of multiple skin snips. The diagnosis of loiasis can be confirmed from the detection of circulating microfilariae of *Loa loa* in the blood or direct eye examination for the presence of the adult worm. Ocular disease can occur with the migration of *Dirofilaria immitis* larvae through periorbital or palpebral tissue; however, laboratory diagnosis of this infection is uncommon. Diagnosis of infections with *Gnathostoma* spp. and *Toxocara canis* is difficult but should be considered in patients with marked eosinophilia and elevated IgE. In the case of visceral and ocular larva migrans, serology for toxocariasis is essential; molecular methods, if available, are highly sensitive.

Eye disease can also be caused by cestodes, including *T. solium* (cysticercosis) and *Echinococcus* spp. (hydatid disease). These infections are generally identified through direct ophthalmoscopic demonstration of the larval *T. solium*, computed tomography scans for hydatid cysts, or examination of routine histologic slides.

Ocular myiasis and infestations of the eyelashes with lice are also possible; laboratory personnel may be asked to identify various fly larvae (*Dermatobia*, *Gasterophilus*, *Oestrus*, *Cordylobia*, *Chrysomyia*, *Wohlfahrtia*, *Cochliomyia*, and *Hypoderma*) and/or lice (*Pediculus humanus corporis* or *P. humanus capitis* [documented, but rare], *Phthirus* [*Pthirus*] *pubis* [more common], or *Demodex* spp. [blepharitis]).

Kidneys and Bladder

The kidneys serve as the primary site for the adult worm *Dioctophyma renale*. These worms generally live in the pelvis of the right kidney or in body cavities. Although these organisms have been isolated from dogs in many areas of the world, they tend to be uncommon in humans. Infections can be confirmed at autopsy, by the migration of worms from the urethra, by discharge of worms from the skin over an abscessed kidney, or by recovery of eggs in the urine. Possible infection with microsporidia (the most likely organism is *Encephalitozoon* spp.; less common is *Enterocytozoon bieneusi*) should also be considered. Specific methods include modified trichrome, acid-fast, and blood stains; a nonspecific optical brightening agent (calcofluor white); routine histology (methenamine silver, PAS, and tissue Gram stains); and electron microscopy. Electron microscopy or immunospecific reagents are required to identify the microsporidia to the genus and species levels.

Mucosa from the bladder wall may reveal eggs of *Schistosoma haematobium* (tissue squash preparation) when they are not recovered in the urine. The eggs in the bladder wall should be checked for viability by either a hatching technique or microscopic observation of the functioning flame cells within the miracidium larva; the hatching test is most appropriate for a urine specimen (1).

Liver and Spleen

Although the liver and spleen can serve as sites for a number of organisms as the secondary site, specific organisms that need to be considered for these organs as primary sites include *Leishmania donovani*, *T. gondii*, *Echinococcus* spp., *T. canis*, *Toxocara cati*, *Capillaria hepatica*, *Clonorchis* spp.,

Opisthorchis spp., *Cryptosporidium* spp., *E. histolytica*, *Encephalitozoon* spp., and *Encephalitozoon intestinalis* (liver). Typical methods for diagnosis include wet mounts, routine histology, blood stains, culture, modified acid-fast stains, immunospecific reagents, and trichrome stains (routine and modified).

Examination of aspirates from liver abscesses may reveal trophozoites of *E. histolytica*; however, demonstration of the organisms may be difficult (1). Liver aspirate material should be taken from the margin of the abscess rather than the necrotic center. The organisms are often trapped in the viscous pus or debris and do not exhibit typical motility. A minimum of two separate portions of exudate should be removed (more than two are recommended). The first portion of the aspirate, usually yellowish white, rarely contains organisms. The last portion of the aspirated abscess material is reddish and is more likely to contain amebae. The best material to be examined is that obtained from the actual wall of the abscess. The Amebiasis Research Unit, Durban, South Africa, has recommended the use of proteolytic enzymes to free the organisms from the aspirate material.

After the addition of the enzyme streptodornase to the thick pus (10 U/ml of pus), the mixture is incubated at 37°C for 30 min and shaken repeatedly. After centrifugation (500 × *g* for 5 min), the sediment may be examined microscopically as wet mounts or may be used to inoculate culture media. Some of the aspirate can be mixed directly with fixative on a slide and examined as a permanent stained smear; damaged red blood cells (RBCs) may or may not be seen in trophozoites from these sites (1, 22). In a suspected case of extraintestinal amebiasis, many laboratories prefer to use a serologic diagnostic approach.

Aspiration of cyst material for the diagnosis of hydatid disease is generally performed by using the recommended percutaneous aspiration, injection, and reaspiration method. Cyst aspiration has proven to be safe when performed carefully, particularly with radiologic guidance. Aspirated fluid usually contains hydatid sand (intact and degenerating scolices, hooklets, and calcareous corpuscles). Some older cysts contain material that resembles curded cottage cheese, and the hooklets may be very difficult to see. Some of this material can be diluted with saline or 10% KOH or concentrated HCl; usually, scolices or daughter cysts will have disintegrated. However, the diagnosis can be made from seeing the hooklets under high dry power (magnification, ×400) or with special stains. The absence of scolices or hooklets does not rule out the possibility of hydatid disease, since some cysts are sterile and contain no scolices and/or daughter cysts. Histologic examination of the cyst wall should be able to confirm the diagnosis.

Confirmation of leishmaniasis in liver or spleen can be accomplished using routine histology, culture, and molecular methods; culture and molecular identification are available through the CDC.

Lungs

Expectorated Sputum and Induced Sputum

Although it is not one of the more common specimens, expectorated sputum may be submitted for examination for parasites (Table 11). Organisms in sputum that may be detected and that may cause pneumonia, pneumonitis, or Loeffler's syndrome include the migrating larval stages of *Ascaris lumbricoides*, *S. stercoralis*, and hookworm; the eggs of *Paragonimus* spp.; *Echinococcus granulosus* hooklets; the protozoa *E. histolytica* and *Cryptosporidium* spp.; and possibly the microsporidia (1). In a *Paragonimus* infection, the sputum may be viscous and tinged with brownish flecks ("iron filings"), which are clusters of eggs, and may be streaked with blood. Although *Entamoeba gingivalis* and *Trichomonas tenax* may be found in sputum, they are generally indicators of poor oral hygiene and/or periodontal disease, not pulmonary disease.

A sputum specimen should be collected properly so that the laboratory receives a "deep sputum" sample from the lower respiratory tract for examination rather than a specimen that is primarily saliva from the mouth. If the sputum is not induced, then the patient should receive specific instructions regarding collection.

Care should be taken not to confuse *E. gingivalis*, which may be found in the mouth and saliva, with *E. histolytica*, which could result in an incorrect suspicion of pulmonary abscess. *E. gingivalis* usually contains ingested PMNs, while *E. histolytica* may contain ingested erythrocytes but not PMNs. More commonly, *E. histolytica* with ingested RBCs can be seen from intestinal specimens. *T. tenax* is also found in saliva from the mouth and thus would be an incidental finding and normally not an indication of pulmonary problems.

Direct Wet Mount

Sputum is usually examined as a wet mount (saline or iodine), using low and high dry power (magnifications, ×100 and ×400, respectively). The specimen is not concentrated before preparation of the wet mount. If the sputum is thick, an equal amount of 3% sodium hydroxide (or undiluted chlorine bleach) can be added; the specimen is thoroughly mixed and then centrifuged. However, NaOH destroys any protozoan trophozoites that might be present. After centrifugation, the supernatant fluid is discarded, and the sediment can be examined as a wet mount with saline or iodine. If examination must be delayed for any reason, the sputum should be fixed in 5 or 10% formalin to preserve helminth eggs or larvae or in one of the fecal fixatives to be stained later for protozoa. Another option is the use of a dithiothreitol-based product such as Sputasol (Oxoid code SR0233A; Remel, Lenexa, KS). Sputasol is formulated to break down mucus and liberate organisms without killing them.

Permanent Stained Smears

If *Cryptosporidium* spp. are suspected (which is rare), then modified acid-fast or immunoassay techniques normally used for stool specimens can be used (1). Trichrome or iron hematoxylin stains of material may aid in differentiating *E. histolytica* from *E. gingivalis*, and Giemsa stain may better define larvae and juvenile worms.

Bronchoscopy Aspirates

Fluid specimens collected by bronchoscopy may be lavage or washing fluids, with bronchoalveolar lavage fluids being preferred. Specimens are usually concentrated by centrifugation prior to microscopic examination of stained preparations. Organisms that may be detected in such specimens are *Paragonimus* spp., *S. stercoralis*, *T. gondii*, *Cryptosporidium* spp., and the microsporidia.

If *T. gondii* is suspected, one of the blood stains, immunospecific reagents, and/or culture (tissue culture) can be used to confirm the diagnosis. A number of cell lines have been used (human foreskin fibroblast is one example), and most routine cell lines work well for the growth and isolation of this organism.

Lymph Nodes and Lymphatics

Material from lymph nodes and lymphatics may confirm parasitic infections (toxoplasmosis, Chagas' disease, trypanosomiasis, microsporidiosis, or filariasis) and should be processed as follows. Fluid material can be examined under low power (magnification, ×100) and high dry power (magnification, ×400) as a wet mount (diluted with saline) for the presence of motile organisms.

Material obtained from lymph nodes should be processed for tissue sectioning and as touch preparations that should be processed as thin blood films and stained with one of the blood stains. Appropriate culture media can also be inoculated; again, it is important to be sure that the specimen has been collected under sterile conditions.

If microsporidia are suspected, modified trichrome stains can be used; calcofluor white and immunoassay methods (currently under development) are also excellent options (1). If *T. gondii* is suspected, Giemsa stain, immunospecific reagents, and/or culture (tissue culture) can be used to confirm the diagnosis.

Specific filarial infections generally are caused by *Wuchereria bancrofti*, *Brugia malayi*, and *Brugia* spp. In most cases, the microfilariae can be recovered and identified through examination of thick blood films, specific concentration sediment, and/or membrane filtration methods (1).

Muscle

Muscle is considered the primary site for the following organisms: *Sarcocystis* spp., microsporidia (*Pleistophora* spp., *Trachipleistophora hominis*, or *Nosema* spp.), *Gnathostoma* spp., *Trichinella* sp. larvae, and cestode larval forms (coenurus [*Taenia* spp.], cysticercosis [*T. solium*], and sparganum). *T. cruzi* amastigotes can also be found primarily in cardiac and/or skeletal muscle. *Baylisascaris procyonis* and *Ancylostoma* spp. are also possibilities, as are hydatid cysts (*Echinococcus* spp.). In most cases, biopsy specimens processed by routine histologic methods are the most appropriate specimens for examination and confirmation of the causative agent.

The presumptive diagnosis of trichinosis is often based on patient history: ingestion of raw or rare pork, walrus meat, bear meat, or horse meat; diarrhea followed by edema and muscle pain; and the presence of eosinophilia. Generally, the suspected food is not available for examination. The diagnosis may be confirmed by finding larval *Trichinella* spp. in a muscle biopsy specimen. The encapsulated larvae can be seen in fresh muscle if small pieces are pressed between two slides and examined under the microscope (1). Larvae are usually most abundant in the diaphragm, masseter muscle, or tongue and may be recovered from these muscles at necropsy. Routine histologic sections can also be prepared.

Human infection with any of the larval cestodes may present diagnostic problems, and frequently, the larvae are referred for identification after surgical removal (1). In addition to *E. granulosus* (hydatid disease) and the larval stage of *Taenia solium* (cysticercosis), other larval cestodes occasionally cause human disease. The larval stage of tapeworms of the genus *Taenia* (*Multiceps*), a parasite of dogs and wild canids, is called a coenurus and may cause human coenurosis. The coenurus resembles a cysticercus but is larger and has multiple scolices developing from the germinal membrane surrounding the fluid-filled bladder. These larvae occur in extraintestinal locations, including the eye, central nervous system, and muscle.

Human sparganosis is caused by the larval stages of tapeworms of the genus *Spirometra*, which are parasites of various canine and feline hosts; these tapeworms are closely related to the genus *Diphyllobothrium*. Sparganum larvae are elongated, ribbon-like larvae without a bladder and with a slightly expanded anterior end lacking suckers. These larvae are usually found in superficial tissues or nodules, although they may cause ocular sparganosis, a more serious disease.

Finding prominent calcareous corpuscles in the tapeworm tissue frequently supports the diagnosis of larval cestodes; specific identification usually depends on referral to specialists.

Nasopharynx and Sinus Cavities

Organisms that might be found in these body sites include the microsporidia, *Acanthamoeba* spp., and *Naegleria*. Specimens submitted for examination could include scrapings, aspirates, and/or biopsy specimens. A number of the special stains include modified trichrome, acid-fast, and tissue Gram stains. Giemsa, calcofluor white, and regular trichrome stains are also appropriate. If *Naegleria* or *Acanthamoeba* spp. are suspected, culture is highly recommended. In certain cases of mucocutaneous leishmaniasis, *Leishmania* spp. could also be found from these body sites. One of the blood stains is recommended for confirmation in both aspirates and biopsy specimens; cultures are also an option (1).

Rectal Tissue

Often when a patient has an old, chronic infection or a light infection with *Schistosoma mansoni* or *Schistosoma japonicum*, the eggs may not be found in the stool and an examination of the rectal mucosa may reveal the presence of eggs. The fresh tissue should be compressed between two microscope slides and examined under the low power of the microscope (low-intensity light) (1). Critical examination of these eggs should be made to determine whether living miracidia are still within them. Treatment may depend on the viability of the eggs; for this reason, the condition of the eggs should be reported to the physician.

Skin

The use of skin snips is the method of choice for the diagnosis of human filarial infections with *O. volvulus* and *Mansonella streptocerca* (1, 7). Microfilariae of both species occur chiefly in the skin, although *O. volvulus* microfilariae may be found rarely in the blood and occasionally in the urine. Skin snip specimens should be thick enough to include the outer part of the dermal papillae. With a surgical blade, a small slice may be cut from a skin fold held between the thumb and forefinger, or a slice may be taken from a small "cone" of skin pulled up with a needle. Significant bleeding should not occur, and there should be just a slight oozing of fluid. Corneal-scleral punches (either Holth or Walser type) have been found to be successful in taking skin snips of uniform size and depth and an average weight of 0.8 mg (range, 0.4 mg to 1.2 mg); this procedure is easy to perform and is painless. In African onchocerciasis, it is preferable to take skin snips from the buttock region (above the iliac crest); in Central American onchocerciasis, the preferred skin snip sites are from the shoulders (over the scapula).

Skin snips are placed immediately in a drop of normal saline or distilled water and are covered so that they will not dry; teasing of the specimen with dissecting needles is not necessary but may facilitate release of the microfilariae. Microfilariae tend to emerge more rapidly in saline; however, in either solution, the microfilariae usually emerge within 30 min to 1 h and can be examined with low-intensity light and the 10× objective of the microscope. To see definitive morphological details of the microfilariae, the snip preparation should be allowed to dry, fixed in absolute methyl alcohol, and stained with Giemsa or one of the other blood stains.

Skin biopsy specimens used for the diagnosis of cutaneous amebiasis (*Entamoeba histolytica* or *Acanthamoeba* spp.) and cutaneous leishmaniasis should be processed for tissue sectioning and subsequently stained by the hematoxylin-and-eosin technique (21).

Although cutaneous disease is an unusual presentation for schistosomiasis, it does occur with skin lesions as the only manifestation. Based on routine histologic examination of skin biopsies, eggs can be found in the cellular infiltrate from within the lesion. When patients with unusual skin lesions are being evaluated, a complete history may reveal travel to an area where schistosomiasis is endemic.

Material containing intracellular *Leishmania* organisms can be aspirated from below the ulcer bed through the uninvolved skin, not from the surface of the ulcer. The surface of the ulcer must be thoroughly cleaned before specimens are taken; any contamination of the material with bacteria or fungi may prevent recovery of the organism from culture. Aspirated material is placed on a slide and stained with Giemsa or one of the blood stains.

Some prefer to perform a punch biopsy through the active margin of the lesion (after cleaning the lesion); good results have also been seen with the use of dermal scrapings from the bottoms of the ulcers. When microscopic examinations of dermal scrapings of both the ulcer bottom and active margins are combined, the sensitivity of diagnosis may increase to 94% (23). Aspirate culture has been shown to be the most sensitive method for the diagnosis of patients with chronic ulcers. However, any successful culture depends on the prevention of contamination with bacteria and/or fungi; sampling of the ulcer must be done correctly in order to prevent false-negative culture results.

BLOOD

Depending on the life cycle, a number of parasites may be recovered in a blood specimen, either whole blood or buffy coat preparations, or following concentration by various types of procedures. These parasites include *Plasmodium*, *Babesia*, and *Trypanosoma* species, *L. donovani*, and microfilariae. Although some organisms may be motile in fresh, whole blood, species identification is usually accomplished from the examination of permanent stained thick and thin blood films. Blood films can be prepared from fresh, whole blood collected with no anticoagulants, anticoagulated blood (EDTA is recommended; heparin is acceptable, but organism morphology is not as good; other anticoagulants are not recommended), or sediment from the various concentration procedures. Although for many years Giemsa stain has been the stain of choice, the parasites can also be seen on blood films stained with Wright's stain, a Wright-Giemsa combination stain, or one of the more rapid stains, such as Diff-Quik (American Scientific Products, McGaw Park, IL), Wright's Dip Stat stain (Medical Chemical Corp., Torrance, CA), or Field's stain. It is more appropriate for personnel to use a stain with which they are familiar rather than having to use Giemsa stain, which is somewhat more complicated to use. PMNs serve as the quality control cell for any of the blood stains. Any parasites present stain like the PMN nuclear and cytoplasmic material, regardless of the stain used. Delafield's hematoxylin stain is often used to stain the microfilarial sheath; in some cases, Giemsa stain does not provide sufficient stain quality to allow differentiation of the microfilariae (Table 11). As with other clinical specimens, when blood is being handled, standard precautions should be observed (1, 4, 5, 15, 24).

Preparation of Thick and Thin Blood Films

Microfilariae and trypanosomes can be detected in fresh blood by their characteristic shape and motility; however, specific identification of the organisms requires a permanent stain. Two types of blood films are recommended. Thick films allow a larger amount of blood to be examined, which increases the possibility of detecting light infections (1, 5, 13). However, only experienced workers can usually make species identification with a thick film, particularly in the case of malaria, and the morphological characteristics of blood parasites are best seen in thin films.

The accurate examination of thick and thin blood films and identification of parasites depend on the use of absolutely clean, grease-free slides for preparation of all blood films. Old (unscratched) slides should be cleaned first in detergent and then with 70% ethyl alcohol; new slides should additionally be cleaned with alcohol (use gauze, not cotton) and allowed to dry before use.

Thick and thin blood films should be handled on a STAT basis (ordering, collection, processing, examination, reporting). Blood films should be prepared when the patient is admitted or seen in the emergency room or clinic; typical fever patterns are frequently absent, and the patient may not be suspected of having malaria. If malaria remains a possible diagnosis, after the first set of negative smears, samples should be taken at intervals of 6 to 8 h for at least 3 successive days. Often, after a day or two, other etiologic agents may be suspected and no additional blood specimens will be received. Another option is to collect blood immediately on admission; if the initial blood films are negative, daily specimens should be collected for 2 additional days (ideally between paroxysms if present; however, there is often no periodicity seen). Using either collection option, quality patient care depends on the fact that both the physician and laboratory staff know that one negative set of blood films does not eliminate *Plasmodium* spp. as possible etiologic agents.

After a fingerstick, the blood should flow freely; blood that has to be "milked" from the finger is diluted with tissue fluids, which decrease the number of parasites per field. An alternative approach to the fingerstick is collection of fresh blood containing anticoagulant (preferably EDTA) for the preparation of blood films. Ideally, the smears should be prepared within 1 h after the specimen is drawn. After that time, stippling may not be visible on stained films and other morphologic changes will occur the longer the blood stands; however, the overall organism morphology may still be acceptable within 1 to 2 h. After 4 to 6 h, parasites may be lost.

The time at which the specimen was drawn should be clearly indicated on the tube of blood and on the result report. The physician will then be able to correlate the results with any symptoms that the patient may have. There should also be some indication on the slip that is sent back to the physician that one negative specimen does not rule out the possibility of a parasitic infection.

Thick Blood Films

The thick film should be prepared as follows. Place 2 or 3 small drops of capillary blood directly from the fingerstick (no anticoagulant) on an alcohol-cleaned slide. With the corner of another slide and using a circular motion, mix the drops and spread them over an area 2 cm in diameter. Continue stirring for 30 s to prevent the formation of fibrin strands that may obscure the parasites after staining. If blood containing an anticoagulant is used, 1 or 2 drops may be spread over an area about 2 cm in diameter; it is not necessary to continue stirring for 30 s, since there will be no formation of fibrin strands. If too much blood is used or any grease remains on the slide, the blood may flake off during staining. Allow the film to air dry (room temperature) in a dust-free area. Never apply heat to a thick film, since heat fixes the blood, causing the erythrocytes to remain intact during staining; the result is stain retention and an inability to identify the parasites. However, the thick films can be placed in a 37°C incubator for 10 to 15 min to dry; this seems to work quite well. Do not make the films too thick; one should be able to see newsprint through the wet film prior to drying. After the thick films are thoroughly dry, they can be laked to remove the hemoglobin. To lake the films, place them in buffer solution before staining for 10 min or directly into a dilute, buffered aqueous Giemsa stain. If thick films are to be stained at a later time, they should be laked before storage (1). Although not as commonly used, other methods for the preparation of combination thick-thin blood films are available (1, 6, 7).

Thin Blood Films

The thin blood film is routinely used for specific parasite identification, although the number of organisms per field is much lower than the number in the thick film. The thin film is prepared exactly as one used for a differential count, and a well-prepared film is thick at one end and thin at the other (one layer of evenly distributed erythrocytes with no cell overlap). The thin, feathered end should be at least 2 cm long, and the film should occupy the central area of the slide, with free margins on both sides. Holes in the film indicate the presence of grease on the slide. After the film has air dried (do not apply heat), it may be stained. The necessity for fixation before staining depends on the stain selected.

Staining Blood Films

For accurate identification of blood parasites, a laboratory should develop proficiency in the use of at least one good staining method (1, 6–12). Since prolonged storage may result in stain retention, blood films should be stained on the same day as or within a few days of collection. If thick blood films are not prepared or received, it is possible to stain one of the thin blood films as a thick film and examine the thick portion of the thin film. During staining, the RBCs are laked, thus leaving the white blood cells, platelets, and any parasites present.

Wright's stain has the fixative in combination with the staining solution, so that both fixation and staining occur at the same time; therefore, the thick film must be laked before staining. In aqueous Giemsa stain, the fixative and stain are separate; thus, the thin film must be fixed with absolute methanol before staining.

When slides are removed from either type of staining solution, they should be dried in a vertical position. After being air dried, they may be examined under oil immersion by placing the oil directly on the uncovered blood film. If slides are going to be stored for a considerable length of time for teaching or legal purposes, they should be protected with a cover glass by being mounted in a medium such as Permount. Blood films that have been stained with any of the Romanowsky stains and that have been mounted with Permount or other resinous mounting media are susceptible to fading of the basophilic elements and generalized loss of stain intensity. An antioxidant, such as 1% (by volume) 2,6-di-*t*-butyl-*p*-cresol (butylated hydroxytoluene; Sigma-Aldrich), can be added to the mounting medium. Without the addition of this antioxidant, mounted stained blood films eventually become pink; stained films protected with this compound generally remain unchanged in color for many years.

Giemsa Stain

Each new lot number of Giemsa stain should be tested for optimal staining times before being used on patient specimens. If the blood cells appear to be adequately stained, the timing and stain dilution should be appropriate to demonstrate the presence of malaria and other parasites. The use of prepared liquid stain or stain prepared from the powder depends on personal preference; there is apparently little difference between the two preparations.

The commercial liquid stain or the stock solution prepared from powder should be diluted approximately the same amount to prepare the working stain solution (1, 5). Stock Giemsa liquid stain is diluted 1:10 with buffer for both thick and thin blood films, with dilutions ranging from 1:10 to 1:50. Staining times usually match the dilution factor (e.g., 1:20 for 20 min or 1:50 for 50 min). Some people prefer to use the longer method with more dilute stain for both thick and thin films. The phosphate buffer used to dilute the stock stain should be neutral or slightly alkaline (pH 7.0 to 7.2). Phosphate buffer solution may be used to obtain the right pH. In some laboratories, the pH of tap water may be satisfactory and may be used for the entire staining procedure and the final rinse.

Giemsa stain colors the blood components as follows: erythrocytes, pale red; nuclei of leukocytes, purple with pale purple cytoplasm; eosinophilic granules, bright purple-red; and neutrophilic granules, deep pink-purple. In malaria parasites, the cytoplasm stains blue and the nuclear material stains red or purple-red. Schüffner's dots and other inclusions in the erythrocytes stain red but can vary. The nuclear and cytoplasmic staining characteristics of the other blood parasites, such as *Babesia* spp., trypanosomes, and leishmaniae, are like those of the malaria parasites and white blood cells. While the sheath of microfilariae may not always stain with Giemsa, the nuclei within the microfilaria itself stain blue to purple.

Wright's Stain

Wright's stain is available in liquid form and powder form, which must be dissolved in anhydrous, acetone-free methyl alcohol before use. Since Wright's stain contains alcohol, the thin blood films do not require fixation before staining. Thick films stained with Wright's stain are usually inferior to those stained with Giemsa solution. Great care should also be taken to avoid excess stain precipitate on the slide during the final rinse. Before staining, thick films must be laked in distilled water (to rupture and remove erythrocytes) and air dried. The staining procedure is the same as that for thin films, but the staining time is usually somewhat longer and must be determined for each batch of stain. Wright's stain colors blood components as follows: erythrocytes, light tan, reddish, or buff; nuclei of leukocytes, bright blue with contrasting light cytoplasm; eosinophilic granules, bright red; and neutrophilic granules, pink or light purple.

In malaria parasites, the cytoplasm stains pale blue and the nuclear material stains red. Schüffner's dots and other inclusions in the erythrocytes usually do not stain or stain very pale with Wright's stain. Nuclear and cytoplasmic staining characteristics of the other blood parasites, such as *Babesia* spp., trypanosomes, and leishmaniae, are like those seen in the malaria parasites. While the sheath of microfilariae may not always stain with Wright's stain, the nuclei within the microfilaria itself stain pale to dark blue.

Other Stains for Blood

Although Giemsa and Wright's stains are excellent options, the parasites can also be seen on blood films stained with a Wright-Giemsa combination stain or one of the more rapid stains, such as Diff-Quik (American Scientific Products),

Wright's Dip Stat stain (Medical Chemical Corp.), or Field's stain. PMNs serve as the quality control for any of the blood stains. Any parasites present stain like the PMNs, regardless of the stain used. With any of the blood stains, color variations are common.

Inactivation of Ebola Virus

The CDC has recommended the addition of Triton X-100 and heat inactivation at 56°C prior to testing specimens from patients suspected to have a potential Ebola infection, in addition to performing enhanced safety procedures, such as using personal protective equipment and a certified class II biosafety cabinet. Using the CDC-recommended inactivation procedure for Ebola virus with a combination of heat and Triton X-100 on the detection of *Plasmodium falciparum* by BinaxNOW rapid diagnostic test and real-time PCR resulted in no loss of performance for either test following inactivation. This inactivation procedure enhances safety for laboratory staff handling specimens suspected to contain Ebola virus without compromising the validity of diagnostic tests for malaria (http://www.cdc.gov/vhf/ebola/hcp/interim-guidance-specimen-collection-submission-patients-suspected-infection-ebola.html; accessed 3 August 2017). For thin blood films, a 15-min absolute methanol fixation was found to inactivate Ebola virus; thus, prior inactivation treatment of the blood is not required.

Proper Examination of Thin and Thick Blood Films

In cases where malaria parasites have not been indicated as the suspect organism, the initial screen of the thin blood film should be carried out with the low-power objective of a microscope, because microfilariae may be missed if the entire thin film is not examined. Microfilariae are rarely present in large numbers, and frequently, only a few organisms occur in each thin film preparation. Microfilariae are commonly found at the edges of the thin film or at the feathered end of the film, because they are carried to these sites during the process of spreading the blood. This approach to thin film examination is particularly important in cases where a suspect organism has not been indicated. The feathered end of the film where the erythrocytes are drawn out into one single, distinctive layer of cells should be examined for the presence of malaria parasites and trypanosomes. In these areas, the morphology and size of the infected erythrocytes are most clearly seen.

In the case of a suspected malaria diagnosis, the request for blood film examination should always be considered a STAT procedure, with all reports (negative as well as positive) being sent to the physician as soon as possible (1, 5). Examination of the thin film should include viewing of 200 to 300 oil immersion fields at a magnification of ×1,000. Although some people use a 50× or 60× oil immersion objective to screen stained blood films, there is some concern that small parasites such as *Plasmodium* spp., *Babesia* spp., or *L. donovani* may be missed at this lower total magnification (×500 or ×600), although they are usually detected at the total magnification of ×1,000 obtained with the more traditional 100× oil immersion objective. Because people tend to scan blood films at different rates, it is important to examine a minimum number of fields, regardless of the time that it takes to perform this procedure. If something suspicious has been seen in the thick film, often the number of fields examined on the thin film may be considerably greater than 300.

Diagnostic problems with the use of automated differential instruments have been reported (1). Both malaria and *Babesia* infections can be missed with these instruments, and therapy is therefore delayed. Because these instruments are not designed to detect intracellular blood parasites, any reliance on the automated systems for discrimination between uninfected erythrocytes and those infected with parasites may pose serious diagnostic problems.

In the preparation of a thick blood film, the greatest concentration of blood cells is in the center of the film. A search for parasitic organisms on the entire thick film should be carried out initially at low magnification (10× objective) to detect microfilariae more readily. Examination of a thick film usually requires 3 to 5 min (approximately 100 oil immersion fields). The search for malarial organisms and trypanosomes is best done under oil immersion (total magnification, ×1,000). Close examination of the very periphery of the thick film may reveal intact erythrocytes; such cells, if infected, may prove useful in malaria diagnosis, since the characteristic morphology necessary to identify the organisms to the species level is more easily seen.

Immunochromatographic Tests for Malaria

Immunochromatography relies on the migration of liquid across the surface of a nitrocellulose membrane. Using monoclonal antibodies prepared against a malaria antigen target that has been incorporated onto the strip of nitrocellulose, these tests are based on the capture of parasite antigen from peripheral blood. Currently, the malaria antigens used for these rapid diagnostic tests are histidine-rich protein 2 (HRP-2), parasite lactate dehydrogenase (pLDH), and *Plasmodium* aldolase (Table 12). These dipsticks offer the possibility of more rapid, nonmicroscopic methods for malaria diagnosis. The tests are easy to perform and interpret; however, there are a number of questions that remain concerning the relevant uses for this type of testing, especially considering the fact that the Binax Now malaria test (Alere, Inc., Waltham, MA) is now FDA approved. A positive-control specimen is also available.

Sensitivity remains a problem, particularly for nonimmune populations. Parasite densities of >100 parasites/μl (0.002% parasitemia) should be detected and are reasonable targets to expect from dipsticks for *P. falciparum* diagnosis. However, this level of sensitivity is at the lower end of the capability of most devices using capture methods for HRP-2 or pLDH. This level of sensitivity is probably as good as that which clinical laboratory staff in nonspecialized laboratories with limited exposure to malaria cases could expect to provide using microscopy diagnosis. One of the potential benefits is for inexperienced evening staff, for whom the dipstick identification of a life-threatening parasitemia with *P. falciparum* could prevent a missed infection. However, a negative test cannot be accepted and requires confirmation by microscopic examination of both thick and thin blood films for the detection of parasitemia below the present threshold of detection by these rapid tests. Also, there are rare false positives for patients with certain rheumatologic disorders; this is noted in the package insert and has been confirmed by users in this patient population. The U.S. military has conducted FDA-approved trials because of possible use of the devices in the field.

Concentration Procedures

Buffy Coat Films

L. donovani, trypanosomes, and *Histoplasma capsulatum* (a fungus with intracellular elements resembling those of *L. donovani*) may occasionally be detected in the peripheral blood. The

TABLE 12 Techniques for the recovery and identification of blood parasites (EDTA or heparin)[a] (28, 29)

Organism	Procedure	Stain
Malaria parasites	Thick and thin films	Giemsa, Wright's, Field's, rapid stains
	QBC[b]	Stain not relevant (centrifugation, acridine orange, microscopy)
	SD BIOLINE[c]	Stain not relevant (HRP-2 immunochromatographic assay)
	Binax Now Malaria[d]	Stain not relevant (HRP-2 and aldolase immunochromatographic assay)
	PATH IC Falciparum malaria IC[e]	Stain not relevant (HRP-2 immunochromatographic assay)
	Malaria Ag-CELISA[f]	Stain not relevant (HRP-2 immunochromatographic assay)
	Rapimal dipstick[f]	Stain not relevant (HRP-2 immunochromatographic assay)
	Rapimal cassette[f]	Stain not relevant (HRP-2 immunochromatographic assay)
	OptiMAL[g]	Stain not relevant (pLDH immunochromatographic assay)
Babesia spp.	Thick and thin films	Giemsa, Wright's, Field's, rapid stains
Microfilariae	Thick and thin films, Knott concentration, membrane filtration, gradient centrifugation	Giemsa, Wright's, or Delafield's hematoxylin
	QBC[b]	Stain not relevant
	Binax Now ICT Filariasis[d]	Rapid dipstick format
	Filariasis Ag-CELISA[f]	EIA
	TropBio[h]	Rapid dipstick format
Trypanosomes	Thick and thin films, buffy coat smears, triple centrifugation, culture	Giemsa, Wright's, Field's, rapid stains
	QBC[b]	Stain not relevant
Leishmaniae	Thick and thin films, buffy coat smears, culture	Giemsa, Wright's, Field's, rapid stains

[a]Molecular techniques are still experimental and are not always available; it is always important to verify FDA approval within the United States (contact the manufacturer). For those working outside the United States, there are many other commercially available immunoassays for malaria detection; however, numerous publications are available for those specifically listed in the table. A valid CE marking affixed to a product indicates that it complies with the relevant European New Approach product safety directives. The directives contain the essential requirements that a product must meet to be sold in the European Union. WHO Prequalification will become the determinant of procurement eligibility of malaria rapid diagnostic tests as of 31 December 2017 (http://www.who.int/malaria/news/2016/rdt-procurement-criteria/en/) (accessed 14 September 2017).

[b]QBC blood parasite detection method (Becton Dickinson Tropical Disease Diagnostics, Sparks, MD).

[c]SD BIOLINE rapid test for *P. falciparum* malaria (Standard Diagnostics, Inc./BIOLINE/Alere, Waltham, MA) (CE marked). This test is not licensed for diagnostic use in the United States. This test is a dipstick format.

[d]Binax Now Malaria (all four *Plasmodium* species) (Alere, Inc., Waltham, MA) (FDA), Binax Now ICT Filariasis (*Wuchereria bancrofti*) (Binax, Inc., Portland, ME) (not available for U.S. and European Union use). These tests are in a dipstick format, and positive controls are available for both tests.

[e]PATH IC Falciparum malaria IC test (PATH, Seattle, WA). This test is in a dipstick format.

[f]Filariasis Ag-CELISA (*Wuchereria bancrofti*), Malaria Ag-CELISA (*P. falciparum*). Rapimal dipstick (*P. falciparum*), Rapimal cassette (*P. falciparum*) (CE marked) (Cellabs, Sydney, New South Wales, Australia).

[g]OptiMAL (differentiates between *P. falciparum* and *P. vivax*) (Flow, Inc., Portland, OR). This test is in a dipstick format.

[h]TropBio (James Cook University, Townsville, Queensland, Australia).

parasite or fungus is found in the large mononuclear cells that are found in the buffy coat (a layer of leukocytes resulting from centrifugation of whole citrated blood). The nuclear material stains dark red-purple, and the cytoplasm is light blue (*L. donovani*). *H. capsulatum* appears as a dot of nuclear material (dark red-purple) surrounded by a clear halo area, while *L. donovani* organisms contain a kinetoplast. Trypanosomes in the peripheral blood also concentrate with the buffy coat cells.

Alcohol-cleaned slides should be used for preparation of the blood films. A microhematocrit tube can also be used; the tube is carefully scored and snapped at the buffy coat interface, and the leukocytes are prepared as a thin film. The tube can also be examined prior to removal of the buffy coat under low and high dry powers of the microscope. If trypanosomes are present, the motility may be observed in the buffy coat. Microfilaria motility is also visible.

QBC Microhematocrit Centrifugation Method

Microhematocrit centrifugation with use of the QBC malaria tube, a glass capillary tube and closely fitting plastic insert (QBC malaria blood tubes; Becton Dickinson Tropical Disease Diagnostics, Sparks, MD), has been used for the detection of blood parasites (1). At the end of centrifugation of 50 to 60 μl of capillary or venous blood (5 min in a QBC centrifuge, 14,387 × g), parasites or erythrocytes containing parasites are concentrated into a 1- to 2-mm region near the top of the erythrocyte column and are held close to the wall of the tube by the plastic float, thereby making them readily visible by microscopy. Tubes precoated with acridine orange provide a stain that induces fluorescence in the parasites. This method automatically prepares a concentrated smear that represents the distance between the float and the walls of the tube. Once the tube is placed into the plastic holder (Paraviewer) and immersion oil is applied onto the top of the hematocrit tube (no coverslip is necessary), the tube is examined with a 40× to 60× oil immersion objective (it must have a working distance of 0.3 mm or greater).

Although a malaria infection could be detected by this method (which is much more sensitive than the thick or the thin blood smear), appropriate thick and thin blood films need to be examined to accurately identify the species of the organism causing the infection.

Knott Concentration

The Knott concentration procedure is used primarily to detect the presence of microfilariae in the blood, especially when a light infection is suspected (1, 6–11). The disadvantage of the procedure is that the microfilariae are killed by the formalin and are therefore not seen as motile organisms. An alternative blood concentration is the citrate-saponin method, where microfilaria can be seen as actively motile organisms—until killed for staining with dilute acetic acid—and where they remain straightened out, which aids in detecting identification landmarks (25).

Membrane Filtration Technique

The membrane filtration technique is highly efficient in demonstrating filarial infections when microfilaremias are of low density. This method is unsatisfactory for the isolation of *Mansonella perstans* microfilariae because of their small size. A 3-μm-pore-size filter could be used for recovery of this organism. Other filters with similar pore sizes are not as satisfactory as the Nuclepore filter (1).

Delafield's Hematoxylin

Some of the material that is obtained from the concentration procedures can be allowed to dry as thick and thin films and then stained with Delafield's hematoxylin, which demonstrates greater nuclear detail as well as the microfilarial sheath, if present. In addition, fresh thick films of blood containing microfilariae can be stained by this hematoxylin technique (1).

Triple-Centrifugation Method for Trypanosomes

The triple-centrifugation procedure may be valuable in demonstrating the presence of trypanosomes in the peripheral blood when the parasitemia is light (1). After repeated centrifugation of the supernatant, the sediment is examined as a wet preparation or is stained as a thin blood film.

SUMMARY

This chapter covers various approaches and diagnostic methods currently in use for the diagnosis of parasitic infections. If clinical specimens have been properly collected and processed according to specific specimen rejection and acceptance criteria, the examination of prepared wet mounts, concentrated specimens, permanent stained smears, blood films, and various culture materials provides detailed information leading to parasite identification and confirmation of the suspected etiologic agent (1, 2, 4, 6–14, 21, 26). Although other tests, such as immunoassay diagnostic kits, continue to become available commercially, the majority of medical parasitology diagnostic work depends on the knowledge and microscopy skills of the microbiologist. Continued development of molecular methods will provide added sensitivity and specificity for the detection of human parasitic infections.

REFERENCES

1. **Garcia LS.** 2016. *Diagnostic Medical Parasitology*, 6th ed. ASM Press, Washington, DC.
2. **Hiatt RA, Markell EK, Ng E.** 1995. How many stool examinations are necessary to detect pathogenic intestinal protozoa? *Am J Trop Med Hyg* **53:**36–39.
3. **Morris AJ, Wilson ML, Reller LB.** 1992. Application of rejection criteria for stool ovum and parasite examinations. *J Clin Microbiol* **30:**3213–3216.
4. **Jorgensen JH, Pfaller MA, Carroll KC, Funke G, Landry ML, Richter SS, Warnock DW (ed).** 2011. *Manual of Clinical Microbiology*, 11th ed. ASM Press, Washington, DC.
5. **National Committee for Clinical Laboratory Standards.** 2000. Laboratory diagnosis of blood-borne parasitic diseases. Approved guideline M15-A. National Committee for Clinical Laboratory Standards, Wayne, PA.
6. **Garcia LS (ed).** 2010. *Clinical Microbiology Procedures Handbook*, 3rd ed. ASM Press, Washington, DC.
7. **Leber AL (ed).** 2016. *Clinical Microbiology Procedures Handbook*, 4th ed. ASM Press, Washington, DC.
8. **Ash LR, Orihel TC.** 1991. *Parasites: A Guide to Laboratory Procedures and Identification*. ASCP Press, Chicago, IL.
9. **Beaver PC, Jung RC, Cupp EW.** 1984. *Clinical Parasitology*, 9th ed. Lea & Febiger, Philadelphia, PA.
10. **Garcia LS.** 2009. *Practical Guide to Diagnostic Parasitology*, 2nd ed. ASM Press, Washington, DC.
11. **Isenberg HD (ed).** 2004. *Clinical Microbiology Procedures Handbook*, 2nd ed. ASM Press, Washington, DC.
12. **Winn WC, Allen SD, Janda WM, Koneman EW, Procop GW, Schreckenberger PC, Woods G.** 2006. *Color Atlas and Textbook of Diagnostic Microbiology*, 6th ed. JB Lippincott Co., Philadelphia, PA.
13. **John DT, Petri WA.** 2006. *Medical Parasitology*, 9th ed. The WB Saunders Co., Philadelphia, PA.
14. **Melvin DM, Brooke MM.** 1982. *Laboratory Procedures for the Diagnosis of Intestinal Parasites*, 3rd ed. U.S. Department of Health, Education, and Welfare publication no. (CDC) 82-8282. Government Printing Office, Washington, DC.
15. **National Committee for Clinical Laboratory Standards.** 1997. Protection of laboratory workers from instrument biohazards and infectious disease transmitted by blood, body fluids, and tissue. Approved guideline M29-A. National Committee for Clinical Laboratory Standards, Wayne, PA.
16. **National Committee for Clinical Laboratory Standards.** 1997. Procedures for the recovery and identification of parasites from the intestinal tract. Approved guideline M28-A. National Committee for Clinical Laboratory Standards, Wayne, PA.
17. **Nielsen CK, Ward LA.** 1999. Enhanced detection of *Cryptosporidium parvum* in the acid-fast stain. *J Vet Diagn Invest* **11:**567–569.
18. **Katanik MT, Schneider SK, Rosenblatt JE, Hall GS, Procop GW.** 2001. Evaluation of ColorPAC *Giardia/Cryptosporidium* rapid assay and ProSpecT *Giardia/Cryptosporidium* microplate assay for detection of *Giardia* and *Cryptosporidium* in fecal specimens. *J Clin Microbiol* **39:**4523–4525.
19. **Kehl KSC.** 1996. Screening stools for *Giardia* and *Cryptosporidium*: are antigen tests enough? *Clin Microbiol Newsl* **18:**133–135.
20. **Sharp SE, Suarez CA, Duran Y, Poppiti RJ.** 2001. Evaluation of the Triage Micro Parasite Panel for detection of *Giardia lamblia*, *Entamoeba histolytica/Entamoeba dispar*, and *Cryptosporidium parvum* in patient stool specimens. *J Clin Microbiol* **39:**332–334.
21. **Binnicker MJ.** 2015. Multiplex molecular panels for diagnosis of gastrointestinal infection: performance, result interpretation, and cost-effectiveness. *J Clin Microbiol* **53:**3723–3728.
22. **Orozco E, Guarneros G, Martinez-Palomo A, Sánchez T.** 1983. *Entamoeba histolytica*. Phagocytosis as a virulence factor. *J Exp Med* **158:**1511–1521.
23. **Ramírez JR, Agudelo S, Muskus C, Alzate JF, Berberich C, Barker D, Velez ID.** 2000. Diagnosis of cutaneous leishmaniasis in Colombia: the sampling site within lesions influences the sensitivity of parasitologic diagnosis. *J Clin Microbiol* **38:**3768–3773.
24. **Code of Federal Regulations.** 2016. Title 29. Labor. Subtitle B. Regulations Relating to Labor. Chapter XVII. Occupational Safety and Health Administration, Department of Labor. Part 1910. Occupational safety and health standards. 29 CFR 1910.1030. https://www.gpo.gov/fdsys/pkg/CFR-2018-title29-vol6/xml/CFR-2018-title29-vol6-sec1910-1030.xml.
25. **McQuay RM.** 1970. Citrate-saponin-acid method for the recovery of microfilariae from blood. *Am J Clin Pathol* **54:**743–746.
26. **Freeman, K, Hema M, Tsertsvadze A, Royle P, McCarthy N, Taylor-Philips S, Manuel R, Mason J.** 2017. Multiplex tests to identify gastrointestinal bacteria, viruses and parasites in people with suspected gastroenteritis: a systematic review and economic analysis. *Health Technol Assess* **21:**1–188.
27. **Levecke B, Behnke JM, Ajjampur SS, Albonico M, Ame SM, Charlier J, Geiger SM, Hoa NT, Kamwa Ngassam RI, Kotze AC, McCarthy JS, Montresor A, Periago MV, Roy S, Tchuem Tchuenté LA, Thach DT, Vercruysse J.** 2011. A comparison of the sensitivity and fecal egg counts of the McMaster egg counting and Kato-Katz thick smear methods for soil-transmitted helminths. *PLoS Negl Trop Dis* **5:**e1201.
28. **World Health Organization.** 2017. Malaria rapid diagnostic test performance. Results of WHO product testing of malaria RDTs: round 7 (2017). http://www.who.int/malaria/publications/atoz/978924151268/en/ (accessed 8 October 2018).
29. **Mathison BA, Pritt BS.** 2017. Update on malaria diagnostics and test utilization. *J Clin Microbiol* **55:**2009–2017.

Plasmodium and *Babesia*

BOBBI S. PRITT

139

Plasmodium and *Babesia* are intraerythrocytic protozoan parasites that cause malaria and babesiosis, respectively. Both are transmitted through the bite of an infected arthropod and cause significant human morbidity and mortality worldwide. Although they differ in their epidemiology and life cycle, there is overlap between both the clinical and diagnostic features of these two parasites, and for these reasons, they are discussed together in this chapter.

TAXONOMY

Plasmodium and *Babesia* are apicomplexan parasites within the supergroup SAR, Alveolata clade (1). Within the Alveolata, these two genera belong to the Apicomplexa clade (formerly Sporozoa), a large complex group of eukaryotic single-celled parasites characterized by a specialized apical complex used for host cell penetration and an apicoplast (2). The apicoplast is a plastid organelle thought to have been acquired by an ancient secondary endosymbiosis of a red alga and its chloroplast. Unlike its chloroplast precursor, the apicoplast is not involved in photosynthesis and instead is thought to be involved in the synthesis of heme, lipids, and isoprenoids (2). Within the Apicomplexa, *Plasmodium* falls within the Haemosporida (SAR: Alveolata: Apicomplexa: Aconoidasida: Haemosporida: *Plasmodium*) and *Babesia* falls within the Piroplasmorida (SAR: Alveolata: Apicomplexa: Aconoidasida: Piroplasmorida: *Babesia*). See chapter 135 for further information about these taxonomic placements.

PLASMODIUM

Description of the Agent

Members of the *Plasmodium* genus infect a wide range of birds, mammals, reptiles, and amphibians worldwide using blood-feeding dipteran vectors (3). Despite there being at least 200 named *Plasmodium* species, only 4 are considered major causes of human malaria: *P. falciparum*, *P. vivax*, *P. malariae*, and *P. ovale* (4). These species designations were originally based on morphologic characteristics, with *P. ovale* being one of the last to be described due to its morphologic similarities to *P. vivax* (5). Recently, multilocus genetic analysis identified the presence of polymorphisms in *P. ovale*, leading to the description of classic and variant strains (6). It is now widely accepted that *P. ovale* comprises two closely related subspecies that coexist in the same geographic regions without interbreeding: *Plasmodium ovale curtisi* (classic strain) and *P. ovale wallikeri* (variant strain) (7). These two subspecies are morphologically indistinguishable but have been reported to differ in duration of latency (8).

In addition to the human malaria species, humans may occasionally become infected with simian malaria species (9). *Plasmodium knowlesi* was recognized as a significant cause of human infections in 2004 (10), being responsible for 27.7% of cases in Malaysian Borneo hospitals in one report (11). While this species predominantly infects macaque monkeys (genus *Macaca*), is it now known to cause human cases throughout parts of Southeast Asia (12). Individual cases have also been reported from western travelers to Southeast Asia, including individuals from Finland, Sweden, Austria, Spain, Great Britain, and the United States (13). Another simian parasite, *Plasmodium cynomolgi*, has been reported as a rare cause of human malaria in Southeast Asia (9).

Epidemiology and Transmission

Malaria is arguably one of the most important infectious diseases in the world, with nearly half of the world's population at risk of acquiring this disease (4). According to the World Health Organization (WHO), extensive global control efforts have produced a 21% reduction in malaria incidence and a 29% reduction in mortality rates between 2010 and 2015, leading to significant life expectancy gains in endemic regions (4). Unfortunately, there were still an estimated 212 million new cases and 429,000 deaths in 2015 (4). Approximately 92% of deaths occur in sub-Saharan Africa, where a close link between malaria mortality and poverty is observed. Seventy percent of deaths occur in children less than 5 years of age (4).

Malaria is found primarily in the tropics and subtropics today (Table 1). However, it was once widespread throughout many temperate regions, including Europe and North America (14). The *Plasmodium* parasite is transmitted primarily through the bite of an infected *Anopheles* mosquito (Fig. 1), and competent mosquito vectors are found throughout the world. A list of countries with endemic malaria is available through the U.S. Centers for Disease Control and Prevention (CDC) Yellow Book (15).

TABLE 1 Characteristics of *Plasmodium* spp. infections[a]

Diagnostic criteria	*P. falciparum*	*P. malariae*	*P. vivax*	*P. ovale*	*P. knowlesi*
Incubation period (days)	8–11	18–40	10–17	10–17	9–12[b]
Fever cycle	36–48 h, "malignant tertian or subtertian"	72 h, "benign quartan"	44–48 h, "benign tertian"	48 h, "tertian"	24 h, "quotidian"
Stage of erythrocyte infected	All stages	Old cells	Young cells	Young cells	All stages
Degree of possible parasitemia	High	Low, <2%	Low, <2%	Low, <2%	High
Sequestration of infected erythrocytes	Yes	No	No	No	Possibly[b]
Usual degree of disease severity	Moderate to severe, life-threatening	Mild to moderate	Moderate to severe, occasionally life-threatening	Mild	Moderate to severe, life-threatening
Degree of anemia	Severe	Mild to moderate	Moderate to severe	Mild	Severe
Involvement of the central nervous system	Common	Rare	Occasional	Rare	Common
Nephrotic syndrome	Rare	Common	Occasional	Rare	Rare
Degree of host inflammatory response	High	Low	Very high	Low	High
Relapses	No	No, but recrudescences ≤50 years later	Yes	Yes	Not likely[b]
Area of endemicity	Large range; tropics and subtropics, especially Africa and Asia	Narrow range; tropics	Large range; tropics, subtropics, and temperate regions; relatively absent from West Africa	Tropics; sub-Saharan Africa and Southeast Asia	Narrow range; Southeast Asia
Proportion in endemic area	80–90%	0.5–3%	50–80%	5–8%	1–60%

[a]Adapted from references 13, 23, and 36.
[b]Information is lacking due to the limited number of reported human cases.

Today, cases of malaria in the United States and Europe are almost exclusively imported from individuals traveling from countries with ongoing malaria transmission, although occasional autochthonous cases have been reported (16–19). In the United States, the majority of imported malaria is detected in individuals who travel to regions of endemicity to visit friends and relatives (20). These individuals often do not consider themselves to be at risk for malaria and do not commonly seek travel advice from their physician or take malaria prophylaxis (21). They also demonstrate behavioral and travel patterns which place them at heightened risk for infection, including travel to remote regions and extended stays (21). The CDC reported 1,724 cases of malaria with symptom onset in 2014, with 5 fatalities (20). This is similar to the number of cases observed in 2013 (n = 1,741) (20). When the purpose of travel was known, people visiting friends and relatives were the largest group of infected individuals (44.9%), followed by refugees/immigrants (8.5%), business travelers (6.6%), missionaries and their dependents (6.0%), students/teachers (3.9%), and tourists (3.7%) (20). Of the cases in which the infecting species was known, *P. falciparum* was responsible for the majority of cases (66.1%), followed by *P. vivax* (13.3%), *P. ovale* (5.2%), and *P. malariae* (2.7%). Less than 1% had infections due to two species (20).

Less common means of malaria transmission are through blood transfusion and transplacental transmission. In 2014, the CDC detected no transfusion-related cases of malaria and one congenitally acquired case, making these extremely rare means of transmission in the United States (20). In most nonendemic countries, the blood supply is partially protected through use of screening questionnaires that defer individuals from donating blood if they have recently traveled to malaria-endemic countries or have had malaria recently. In the United States, the American Association of Blood Banks recommends that individuals traveling to areas of endemicity be deferred from donating blood products for 1 year after their return and that previously infected patients and those living in malaria-endemic regions for 5 years or more be deferred for 3 years after successful treatment (22). In some European countries and Australia, antigen detection methods are used to screen individuals with possible exposure to malaria, thus shortening the potential deferral time; in comparison, there are no assays that are approved or cleared by the U.S. Food and Drug Administration (FDA) for malaria donor blood screening (22).

Clinical Significance

Patients are asymptomatic for the initial 7- to 30-day incubation period during which parasites replicate in the liver (23). It is only with subsequent infection and destruction of host erythrocytes that parasite antigens such as glucose phosphate isomerase are released into the blood and stimulate cytokine production and resultant fever. The classic malarial fever paroxysm begins with rigors and chills, followed by an abrupt onset of fever which lasts for 1 to 2 hours. The paroxysm resolves with profuse sweating and a return to normal temperature. With time, infected

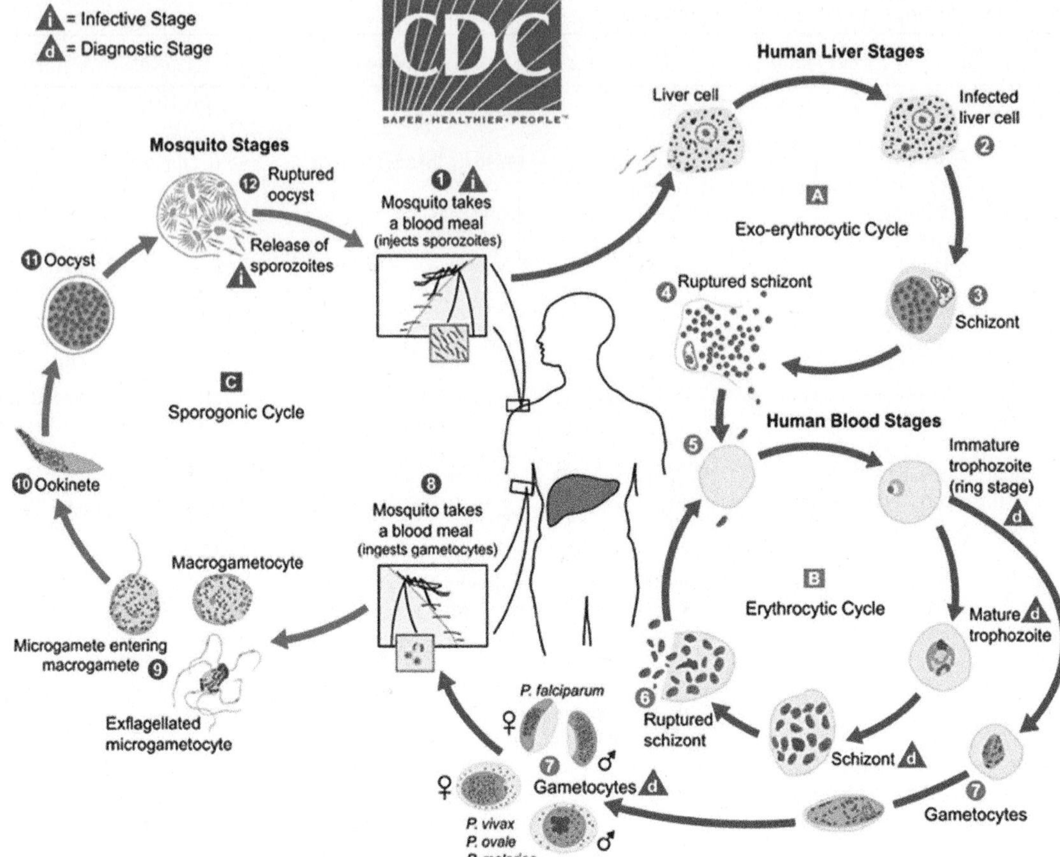

FIGURE 1 The *Plasmodium* parasite is transmitted to humans when an infected female *Anopheles* mosquito takes a blood meal and inoculates sporozoites into the bloodstream (1). Sporozoites infect hepatocytes (2) and undergo asexual reproduction to form schizonts (3) in a process called exoerythrocytic schizogony (A). After 5 to 15 days, liver schizonts rupture to release hundreds of thousands of merozoites into the blood (4), which then infect erythrocytes (5). *P. vivax* and *P. ovale* have a dormant hypnozoite stage which may remain in the liver and cause relapsing disease weeks to months later, while other human *Plasmodium* species do not have this stage. In erythrocytes, merozoites undergo asexual reproduction to form trophozoites and then schizonts in a process called erythrocytic schizogony (B). Schizonts rupture to release merozoites, which then infect other erythrocytes (6). This process is repeated every 1 to 3 days, resulting in the production of thousands to millions of infected erythrocytes in several days. Some merozoite-infected erythrocytes do not undergo asexual reproduction but instead develop into male microgametocytes and female macrogametocytes (7). When ingested by a female *Anopheles* mosquito during a blood meal (8), microgametocytes exflagellate to release microgametes, which penetrate macrogametes and form zygotes (9) via sexual reproduction in the sporogonic cycle (C). Zygotes become motile and elongated to form ookinetes (10), which invade the mosquito's midgut wall and develop into oocysts (11). Over a period of 8 to 15 days, oocysts grow, rupture, and release thousands of sporozoites (12), which travel to the mosquito's salivary glands to be inoculated into a new human host during the mosquito's next blood meal (1). Life cycle courtesy of the CDC DPDx (http://cdc.gov/dpdx/).

cells may begin to rupture in synchrony, producing the classic (but infrequently observed) "tertian" or "quartan" fever cycles (Table 1). Fever is commonly preceded or accompanied by severe headache, malaise, and myalgias (23).

Infection can range from mild or asymptomatic disease, usually in individuals with preexisting immunity, to severe, life-threatening disease. Severe malaria is associated with high mortality and is defined by the presence of one or more features including impaired consciousness, multiple convulsions, respiratory distress, shock, abnormal bleeding, jaundice, hypoglycemia, acidosis, severe anemia, renal impairment, hyperlactatemia, and hyperparasitemia (more than 100,000 parasites/μl of blood) (24, 25). Young children, nonimmune individuals, and pregnant women and their fetuses are at greatest risk of severe disease (25).

P. falciparum infection has the highest morbidity and mortality of the four human *Plasmodium* species, being responsible for nearly all cases of severe malaria and malaria deaths worldwide (23). *P. knowlesi* and, less commonly, *P. vivax* can also cause fatal infections (24). The high morbidity and mortality of *P. falciparum* infection are attributed in part to the parasite's ability to infect and destroy all stages of erythrocytes, leading to high levels of parasitemia and resultant severe anemia, splenomegaly, and jaundice. In contrast, the other *Plasmodium* species preferentially infect older erythrocytes (*P. malariae*) or young erythrocytes (*P. vivax* and *P. ovale*) and cause a lesser degree of total erythrocyte destruction (23).

P. falciparum virulence is also attributed to a phenomenon called cytoadherence, which is accomplished through insertion of parasite-derived adhesion molecules from the *P. falciparum* erythrocyte membrane protein 1 (PfEMP1) family onto the surface of infected erythrocytes during later stages of parasite development. The PfEMP1 molecules allow for clumping of uninfected erythrocytes around infected erythrocytes (rosetting) and receptor-mediated cytoadherence of infected erythrocytes to endothelial cells (sequestration) (26). Accumulation of infected erythrocytes within the microvasculature is associated with metabolic acidosis, hypoxia, and release of detrimental inflammatory cytokines, particularly in the lung, kidney, and brain. During pregnancy, a special form of cytoadhesion occurs between infected erythrocytes and syncytiotrophoblasts in the placenta (26). Symptoms resulting from the high *P. falciparum* parasitemia and sequestration in the microvasculature include acute renal failure, respiratory distress, abortion, intrauterine growth retardation, mental status changes, coma, and death. Other *Plasmodium* species do not sequester and generally cause less severe disease (23). Prior to the advent of highly effective artemisinin combination treatments (ACT), even uncomplicated *falciparum* malaria was associated with a case-specific mortality rate of 0.1%, and delays in treatment or drug resistance increased the mortality rate to approximately 1% (24). Today, the mortality rate associated with uncomplicated *falciparum* malaria is less than 1% when ACT is used (24).

Additional species-associated manifestations include splenic rupture (*P. vivax*), nephrotic syndrome (*P. malariae* in children), hypoglycemia (*P. falciparum* in children), extensive erythrocyte destruction with hemoglobinuria and kidney failure ("blackwater fever," *P. falciparum*), recrudescent disease (*P. malariae*), and relapses due to reactivation of hypnozoites in the liver (*P. ovale* and *P. vivax*) (23). Fatal cases have also been reported in infections with *P. knowlesi*. Given that *Plasmodium* infection can cause a diverse spectrum of symptoms including gastrointestinal and respiratory manifestations, it is essential that malaria be considered in the differential diagnosis for anyone with fever and recent exposure to malaria-endemic areas (27, 28).

Collection, Transport, and Storage of Specimens

Since *P. falciparum* infection can cause rapidly progressive, fatal disease, blood collection and testing for malaria should always be performed on a STAT basis (29–31). Preparation of thick and thin blood films is considered the "gold standard" for diagnosis of malaria. If a laboratory does not have the expertise to perform examination of thin and thick blood films, then consideration should be given to the use of rapid antigen tests for preliminary screening (see "Clinical and Laboratory Diagnosis" section below) or to rapid transport to a neighboring laboratory that can receive and test the blood shortly after it is drawn. Testing options for malaria should be available 7 days a week on a 24-hour basis (30, 31).

Blood is ideally collected via finger prick with immediate (bedside) preparation of thick and thin smears. However, it is more common in nonendemic settings to collect blood by venipuncture for rapid transport to the laboratory (30). EDTA is the preferred anticoagulant because the use of other anticoagulants such as heparin may cause significant parasite distortion (30). Prolonged storage in EDTA may also cause parasite distortion, parasite maturation into sexual life cycle stages, and loss of diagnostic features such as stippling; therefore, blood films should be prepared within 1 hour of collection (30, 32). A single set of blood films may be insufficient to detect *Plasmodium* parasites. The Clinical and Laboratory Standards Institute (CLSI) recommends preparation of two thin and two thick blood films upon initial evaluation of the patient, with preparation and examination of repeat films every 6 to 8 hours if necessary for up to 3 days before excluding malaria from the clinical differential diagnosis (30). Similarly, the CDC recommends that repeat blood films be examined for nonimmune individuals every 12 to 24 hours for a total of three evaluations before ruling out malaria (27).

Additional EDTA whole blood may be refrigerated for supplemental testing such as PCR if necessary. Unfortunately, parasite morphology rapidly degrades in stored blood and is not usually adequate for later identification or species determination by morphologic methods. Chapters 136 and 138 of this *Manual* and the CLSI guidelines for diagnosis of blood-borne parasites (30) provide detailed directions for collecting and preparing blood films. Requests for blood films should be accompanied by important patient information such as clinical signs and symptoms, travel history, and receipt of malaria chemoprophylaxis or therapeutic antimalarial agents which might suppress parasitemia or alter parasite morphology.

Clinical and Laboratory Diagnosis

Clinical features alone are not diagnostic for malaria, and thus parasite-specific testing is recommended for definitive diagnosis (33). A number of different modalities may be used for laboratory diagnosis of malaria, of which microscopic examination of thick and thin blood films remains the gold standard (27, 33). Rapid antigen detection tests are also widely available and form an integral part of the WHO's strategy for combating malaria worldwide (34). When available, molecular amplification techniques may also be used for sensitive and specific detection of infection (35). Serology plays little role in the diagnosis of acute infection but is used for blood donor screening and epidemiologic studies (36).

Direct Examination

Microscopy: Giemsa-Stained Blood Films

Microscopic examination of Giemsa-stained thick and thin blood films is the gold standard method for malaria diagnosis. Accurate interpretation of this time-honored method relies on the availability of trained and experienced microscopists, high-quality reagents, and well-maintained light microscopes. The thick film contains 1 to 2 drops of blood that have been lysed (laked) on the slide by placement into a hypotonic solution (30). This releases intracellular parasites and allows for examination of 20 to 30 layers of blood. The thick blood film is approximately 10 to 20 times more sensitive than the thin film, with a reported detection threshold of 10 to 50 parasites/μl of blood, or approximately 0.0002 to 0.001% parasitemia, assuming a total erythrocyte count of 5×10^6/μl of blood (37). Given this high sensitivity, the thick film is ideal for screening and parasite detection. Under field conditions, the estimated sensitivity may be somewhat lower (100 to 500 parasites/μl of blood) (37, 38).

Given the greater sensitivity of the thick film compared to the thin film, efforts should be made to quickly prepare and examine the thick film so that it can be used as the primary screening method. A common mistake is to use too much blood on the slide, thus requiring longer times for the film to dry. A well-made thick film should be approximately 1.5 to 2.0 cm in diameter and of a thickness through which newsprint can barely be read (30). Drying of the thick film can be enhanced by placing the slides in a laminar flow hood or under the gentle breeze from a fan.

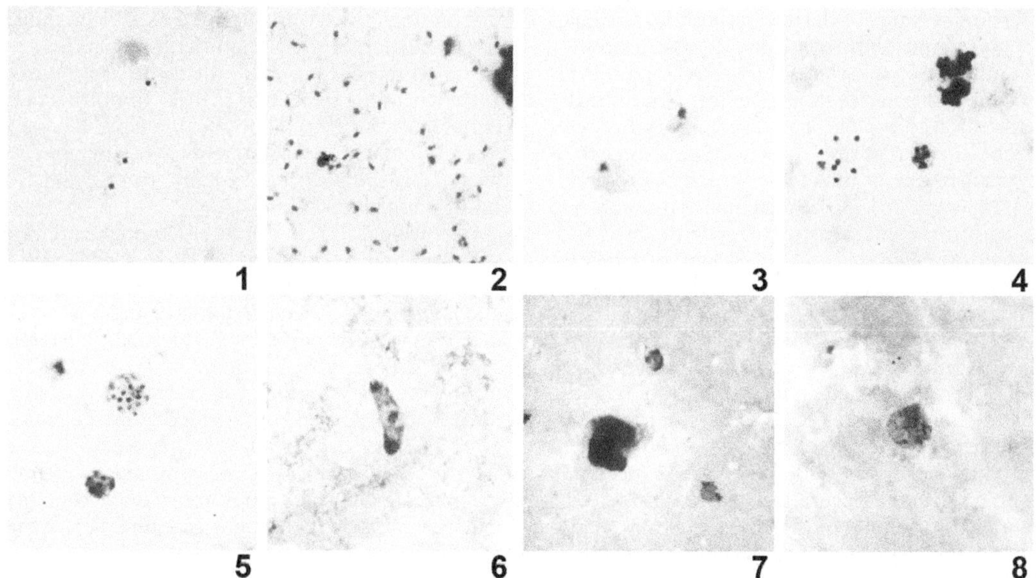

FIGURE 2 *Plasmodium* morphology on thick blood films encompasses the entire spectrum of forms, including trophozoites, schizonts, and gametocytes. Shown are *P. falciparum* early trophozoites in a moderate (1) and heavy (2) infection, *P. vivax* early trophozoites (3), *P. malariae* (4) and *P. vivax* (5) schizonts, and *P. falciparum* (6), *P. malariae* (7), and *P. vivax* (8) gametocytes. Neutrophils are shown for size comparison in panels 4 and 7. (Giemsa, 1,000×).

Exposure to heat is not recommended since it may cause fixation of the blood and interfere with the laking process (30). Gently scratching grooves into the carrier slide with the edge of another glass slide while spreading the blood to the appropriate diameter facilitates adhesion to the slide and obviates the need for extended drying times without negatively impacting the microscopic morphology (39); films may be safely stained as soon as the film is visibly dry (generally within 30 minutes).

Thin films are made in the same manner as hematology blood films. A single drop of blood is spread on the slide in such a manner as to produce a feathered edge. The films are then fixed in methanol prior to staining (30).

Staining of thick and thin films is best performed with Giemsa at a pH of 7.0 to 7.2 to highlight potential stippling and other features of the parasites (30) (see chapter 137 for further information on malaria stains). Wright-Giemsa may also be used but is typically performed at a pH of 6.8, which does not adequately highlight Schüffner's stippling and Maurer's clefts. The Field stain is useful for rapid diagnosis but is not recommended for routine use in nonendemic settings (36). The CDC provides additional guidance for processing specimens when hemorrhagic fever viruses such as Ebola virus are suspected (https:cdc.gov/vhf/ebola/healthcare-us/laboratories/safe-specimen-management.html). After staining, a well-prepared thick film should have a relatively clean background of lysed erythrocytes, leukocyte nuclei, and platelets, while thin films demonstrate pale blue-gray to light pink erythrocytes and a well-formed feathered edge. Parasites have pale to deep blue cytoplasm and pink-red chromatin (30).

Both thick and thin slides should first be screened at low power using the 10× objective for identification of microfilariae, followed by examination under oil immersion with the 100× objective (30). Examination of 200 to 300 microscopic fields on thick and thin films using the 100× objective should be performed before reporting a specimen as negative (30). Considerable practice is required to accurately differentiate parasites from platelets, stain debris, and leukocyte granules on the thick film (Fig. 2), but the additional training effort is rewarded by the increased sensitivity that this method provides. The species of the infecting organism can be determined using the thick film but is best accomplished using the thin film. Thin films provide ideal erythrocyte and parasite morphology for species determination since they are fixed in methanol prior to staining, thus maintaining the structure of the erythrocytes and intraerythrocytic parasites (30). The area of the thin film that provides optimal parasite morphology is where the erythrocytes have minimal overlap and maintain their central pallor (Fig. 3); parasites outside of this region may be considerably distorted. Species determination is made using a number of morphologic features including the size and shape of the infected erythrocyte, the presence of intracytoplasmic inclusions (e.g., stippling), the stages of the parasite present in peripheral blood, and the specific characteristics of each parasite stage (Table 2, Fig. 4 to 8). Atlases and other resources are widely available for differentiating the various *Plasmodium* species (29, 36, 40–42).

The size of the infected erythrocytes is a particularly important feature for determining the infecting *Plasmodium* species, since enlarged infected erythrocytes are characteristic of *P. ovale* and *P. vivax* infection, particularly in the later parasite stages, while small to normal-sized infected erythrocytes are characteristic of *P. malariae* and *P. falciparum* infection. Thus, the size of the infected cell can quickly allow the microscopist to halve the number of species in their differential. The presence of Schüffner's stippling supports the diagnosis of *P. ovale* and *P. vivax* infection. Care must be taken, however, not to confuse the finer Schüffner's dots with the larger, coarser Maurer's clefts that may occur in *P. falciparum* infections. Stippling and Maurer's clefts are most commonly seen when smears are made shortly after blood collection and the pH of the Giemsa stain is 7.0 to 7.2 (30).

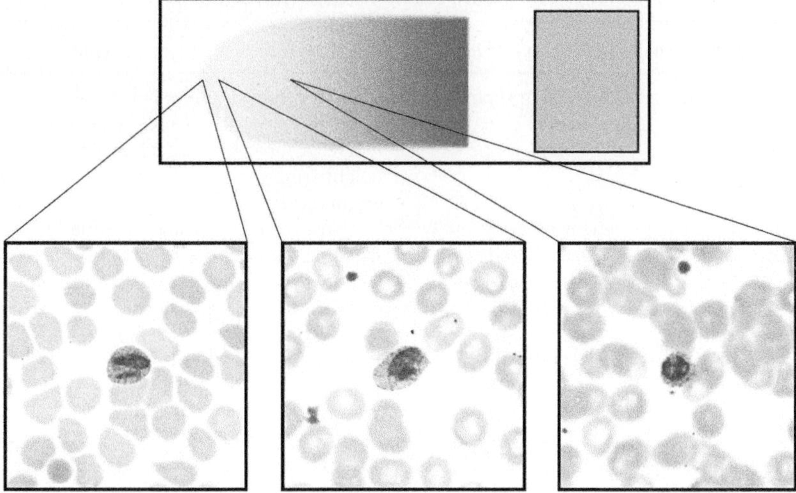

FIGURE 3 The ideal location for microscopic examination of a thin film is the region of the feathered edge where the erythrocytes have minimal overlap and maintain their central pallor (middle). In this location, the erythrocyte infected with *P. ovale* is clearly enlarged and ovoid. When similar cells are examined in regions of the film that are too thin (left) or thick (right), the morphology is distorted and may be misleading.

The life cycle stages present are also very useful for species identification. Infection with *P. falciparum* usually consists solely of early trophozoites ("rings") and, less commonly, gametocytes; intermediate stages (maturing trophozoites and schizonts) are only rarely seen since they are sequestered in the microvascular beds. When intermediate stages of *P. falciparum* are present, they may indicate severe, overwhelming infection. In contrast to *P. falciparum*, a spectrum of forms including late-stage trophozoites and schizonts are commonly seen with other species (36).

When examining peripheral blood films, it is important to remember that mixed malaria infections are not uncommon and that *P. falciparum* may be found in conjunction with less virulent species in the same patient. It is also important to remember that other microorganisms may be seen on peripheral blood films such as *Babesia* intraerythrocytic parasites (see the section on *Babesia* below) and extracellular microfilariae (chapter 147), trypanosomes (chapter 140), and *Borrelia* spirochetes (chapter 61). Intraleukocytic *Ehrlichia*/*Anaplasma* morulae may also be seen on the peripheral blood film, although this is not the preferred method for detection of these bacteria (see chapter 67).

When *Plasmodium* species are identified, it is important to quantify the degree of parasitemia to help guide initial therapy, predict patient prognosis, and monitor response to treatment. This may be done using either the thin or thick film, and formulas for this purpose are widely available (29, 30, 36, 41, 43). When using the thick film for quantitation, it is common practice to express the number of parasites in relation to a standard number of leukocytes per microliter of blood (8,000/μl), although it is preferable to substitute the patient's actual leukocyte count when known. Results are reported as the number of parasites per microliter of blood. When using the thin film, results are reported as the percentage of infected erythrocytes in the fields examined (number of infected cells counted/total number of erythrocytes counted × 100). When calculating the degree of parasitemia with either the thick or thin film, it is important to not include parasite sexual stages (gametocytes) in the total count since they are not infectious to humans and are not killed by most antimalarial drugs. With the thin film, it is also important to count consecutive fields, even if they do not include parasites, and to not count extracellular parasites. Multiply infected erythrocytes are only counted as a single infected cell. Regardless of the method used for calculating the degree of parasitemia, it is important to use the same method for initial and posttreatment specimens (38). Given the possibility of interobserver variability, it may be prudent to limit the number of individuals performing the assessment on sequential specimens from the same patient.

Microscopy: Other Methods

Other microscopic methods are less commonly used for the identification of malaria parasites in whole blood, including stains for nucleic acid and hemozoin (Table 3). Of these, the most commonly used is acridine orange (AO), a DNA-binding fluorescent dye that is excited at 490 nm, producing a yellow or apple-green fluorescence (38). Use of this method requires a fluorescence microscope or light microscope with the appropriate adaptor. Identification of infected cells is relatively straightforward since mature erythrocytes lack DNA and do not produce a fluorescent signal, while parasites contain DNA and fluoresce brightly. However, leukocyte nuclei and Howell-Jolly bodies within erythrocytes also fluoresce, occasionally making identification of low parasite levels challenging. A number of studies found AO staining to have a similar sensitivity and specificity to traditional Giemsa-stained thick films, with the ability to reliably detect <100 parasites/μl (0.002% parasitemia) (38). This method may also allow for more rapid screening than with traditional Giemsa-stained films (37, 38, 44). Another technique that uses AO staining is the centrifugal quantitative buffy coat (QBC Diagnostics, Becton Dickinson, Franklin Lakes, NJ). In this method, whole blood is stained with AO and spun in a microhematocrit tube that contains an internal float. The buffy coat and adjacent red blood cell layer in the microcentrifuge tube are then directly examined using a fluorescence

TABLE 2 Comparative morphology of *Plasmodium* spp. in Giemsa-stained thin films[a]

Diagnostic criteria	*P. falciparum*	*P. malariae*[b]	*P. vivax*	*P. ovale*	*P. knowlesi*
Size and shape of infected erythrocytes	Normal size and shape	Normal or slightly smaller size, normal shape	Normal or enlarged size, may appear molded against neighboring erythrocytes	Normal or enlarged size, frequently oval, may be fimbriated	Normal size and shape
Cytoplasmic inclusions	Occasional Maurer's clefts; larger "comma-shaped," and less numerous than Schüffner's	Ziemann's dots rarely seen; requires deliberate over-staining	Schüffner's dots/ stippling; may not be present in early trophozoites	Dark Schüffner's/ James' dots/ stippling; may not be present in early trophozoites	Irregular stippling in late trophozoites and schizonts
Parasite stages in peripheral blood	Early trophozoites and gametocytes	All stages	All stages	All stages	All stages
Multiply infected erythrocytes	Common	Rare	Occasional	Occasional	Common
Early trophozoite characteristics	Delicate rings, <1/3 diameter of the erythrocyte, frequently with double chromatin dots ("head phone" form); often at edge of erythrocyte ("appliqué/accolé form")	Rings ≤1/3 diameter of the erythrocyte; chromatin dot may appear unattached in center of ring ("bird's eye" form)	Rings ≥1/3 diameter of the erythrocyte; larger chromatin dot than *P. falciparum*	Rings ≥1/3 diameter of the erythrocyte; similar to *P. vivax*	Rings ≤1/3 diameter of the erythrocyte; double chromatin dots, rare appliqué forms; resembles *P. falciparum* early trophozoites
Mature trophozoites	Not typically seen in peripheral blood, compact thick rings	Compact cytoplasm; round, oval, basket, or band-shaped; dark brown pigment	Ameboid trophozoites, fine golden-brown pigment	More compact and less ameboid than *P. vivax*, dark brown pigment	Slightly ameboid; band forms common; scattered clumps of golden-brown pigment; resembles *P. malariae* mature trophozoites
Schizont characteristics	Not typically seen in peripheral blood, 8–24 merozoites	6–12 merozoites, often radially arranged around central pigment ("rosette" or "daisy head" schizont)	12–24 merozoites	6–14 merozoites	10–16 merozoites
Gametocyte characteristics	Crescent- or banana-shaped; distorting the shape of the erythrocyte	Round to oval; filling most of the erythrocyte	Round to oval; filling most of the erythrocyte	Round to oval; filling most of the erythrocyte	Round to oval; filling most of the erythrocyte

[a]Adapted from references 13, 23, and 36.
[b]Identification of *P. malariae* in patients with recent travel to Southeast Asia should raise the possibility of *P. knowlesi* infection, given the morphologic similarities of these two parasites. In this situation, severe clinical disease and a high parasite burden are consistent with *P. knowlesi* infection.

microscope with a specialized long-focal-length objective (38). Clinical studies using the quantitative buffy coat show the best sensitivity and specificity for detecting *P. falciparum*, since the early trophozoites are easily identified within the red cell layer (38). Lower sensitivities have been reported for other species since mature trophozoites, schizonts, and gametocytes of these parasites may be hidden in the granulocyte layer. Also, the early trophozoites of all species may be indistinguishable, and thus definitive species identification is not always possible. When using any of the DNA-binding fluorescent dyes, it is important not to mistake positively staining nuclear debris and Howell-Jolly bodies for parasites (38).

Rarely, malaria pigment (hemozoin) is detected via dark-field microscopy or in histologic tissue sections. In tissue sections, the pigment is concentrated within infected sequestered erythrocytes and macrophages in the capillaries of infected organs, such as the lung, kidney, liver, brain, and placenta (Fig. 9).

Antigen Detection

During the past decade, there has been a marked expansion of commercially available immunochromatographic tests for rapid detection of *Plasmodium* antigens (38, 45, 46). These tests, commonly referred to as rapid diagnostic tests (RDTs), are rapid and relatively easy to use, and many are stable in field conditions (46).

The antigens most commonly detected by the commercially available RDTs are parasite lactate dehydrogenase (pLDH), *P. falciparum* histidine-rich protein 2 (Pf-HRP2), and *Plasmodium* aldolase (36). Some tests specifically detect *P. falciparum* and/or *P. vivax*, while others offer only pan-*Plasmodium* results. There are no specific tests for *P. ovale*, *P. malariae*, or *P. knowlesi* (45). At this time, the

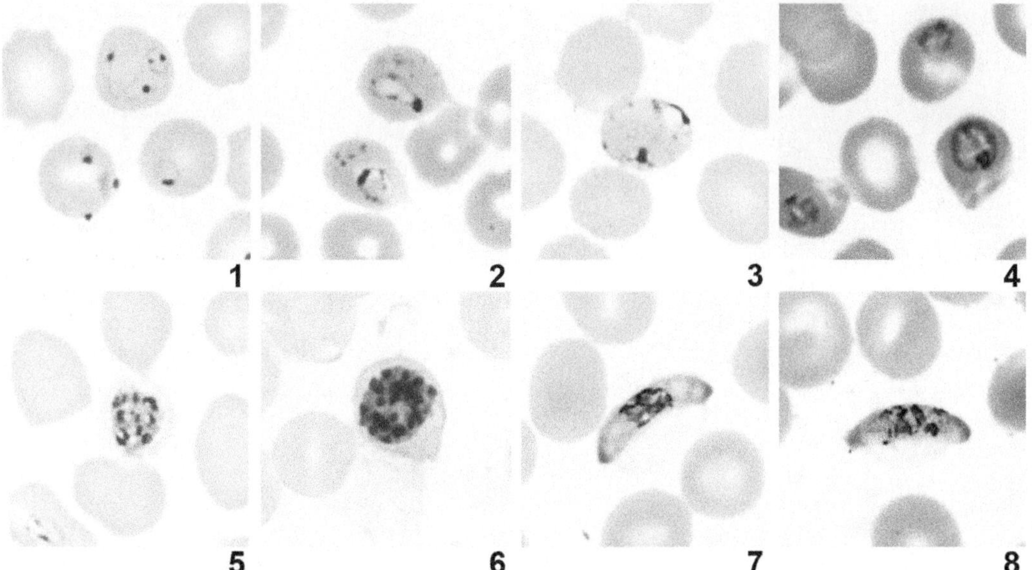

FIGURE 4 *P. falciparum*, successive developmental stages in Giemsa-stained thin blood films: early stage trophozoites/rings with a "headphone" form (1), rings with Maurer's clefts (2), rings with appliqué forms and Maurer's clefts (3), maturing trophozoites (4), early stage schizont (5), mature schizont (6) (courtesy of the CDC DPDx), macrogametocyte (7), and microgametocyte (8). Rings (1, 2, 3) and, less commonly, gametocytes (7, 8) are found in peripheral blood, while other stages (4 to 6) are typically sequestered in the microvasculature.

only FDA-approved RDT is the BinaxNow malaria test (Alere, Inc., Waltham, MA) which targets Pf-HRP2 antigen and a pan-malarial antigen. However, numerous tests are commercially available outside the United States, including several CE-marked tests (46, 47).

In general, malaria RDTs perform almost as well as microscopy for detection of *P. falciparum* at moderate or high parasite levels but suffer from lower sensitivity for detection of non-*P. falciparum* infections and low levels of parasitemia for all species (38, 45, 46). While parasite levels of 100 parasites/μl (0.002% parasitemia) are commonly seen in the clinical setting, many RDTs cannot reliably detect parasites at this level, even when the infecting species is *P. falciparum* (38, 45). The WHO, the Foundation for Innovative New Diagnostics, and the Special Programme for Research and Training in Tropical Diseases launched a massive study in 2006, comparing commercial RDTs for their ability to detect *P. falciparum* and *P. vivax* at high

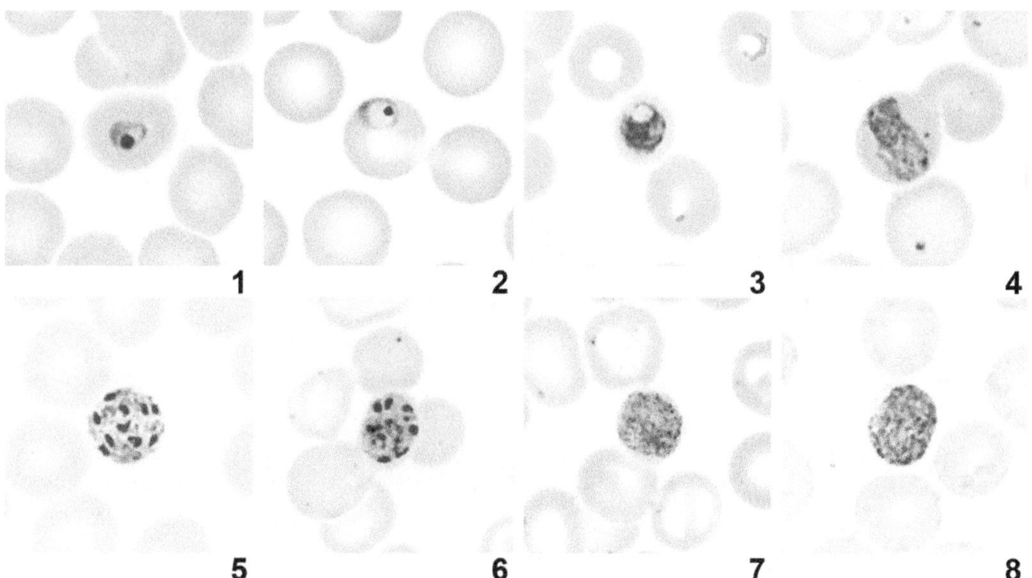

FIGURE 5 *P. malariae*, successive developmental stages in Giemsa-stained thin blood films: early stage trophozoite/ring (1), "bird's eye" ring form (2), mature trophozoites with "basket" form (3), mature trophozoite with "band" form (4), mature schizont (5), mature schizont showing rosette form with central pigment (6), macrogametocyte (7), and microgametocyte (8).

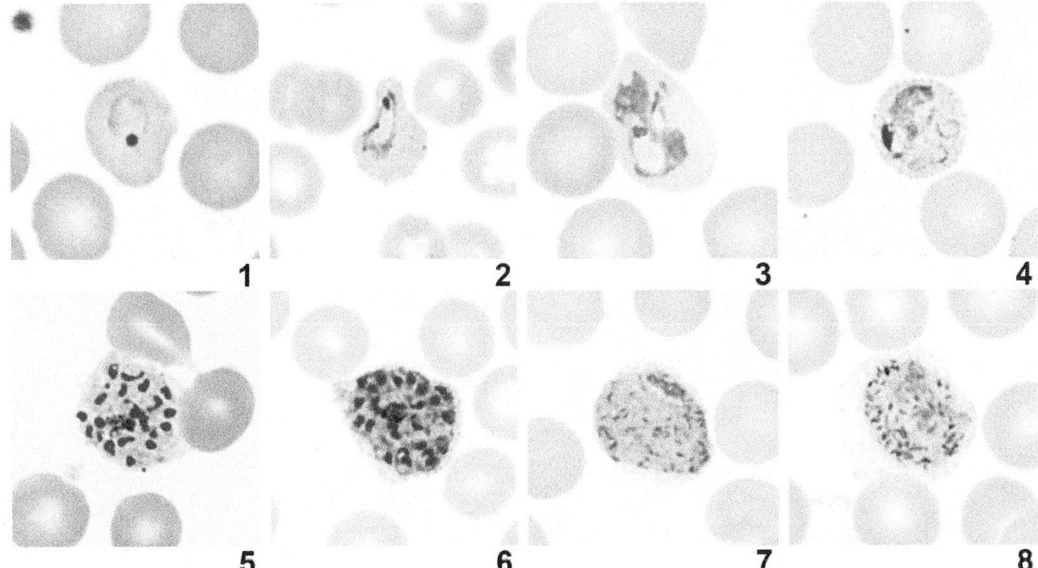

FIGURE 6 *P. vivax*, successive developmental stages in Giemsa-stained thin blood films: early stage trophozoite/ring, (1), maturing ring (2), mature ameboid trophozoites (3, 4), mature schizonts (5, 6), macrogametocyte (7), and microgametocyte (8). Note the Schüffner's dots (2, 4, 6, 8) and frequent molding of infected cells to neighboring erythrocytes. The infected erythrocytes are slightly larger than noninfected cells.

(2,000 to 5,000 parasites/μl) and low (200 parasites/μl) concentrations (46). Their 6 published rounds of product testing, including analyses of over 120 RDTs, clearly demonstrated that RDT performance varies widely by kit, manufacturer, and even lot number (34). In these studies, the FDA-approved BinaxNow malaria test had 100% sensitivity for detection of *P. falciparum* at high levels but sensitivities of 91.1%, 85%, and 10% for detection of *P. falciparum* at low levels, *P. vivax* at high levels, and *P. vivax* at low levels, respectively (34). Some RDTs demonstrated superior sensitivity and specificity to the BinaxNow test but are not approved for *in vitro* diagnostic use in the United States (34).

Despite their advantages, some caveats concerning RDT use should be noted. As with many immunochromatographic assays, false-positive results may be observed in the presence of autoantibodies such as rheumatoid factor. Also, antigen may be detected for days after

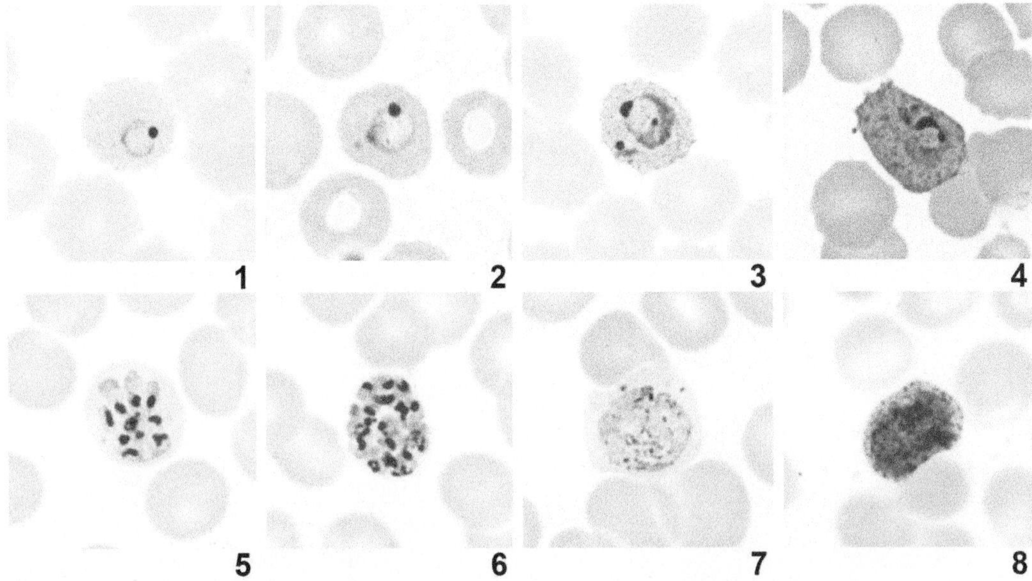

FIGURE 7 *P. ovale*, successive developmental stages in Giemsa-stained thin blood films: early stage trophozoite/ring (1, 2), developing trophozoite (3), mature trophozoite with "comet cell" morphology (4), early stage schizont (5), mature schizont (6), macrogametocyte (7), and microgametocyte (8). Note the Schüffner's dots (3, 4, 8) and oval/elongated shape of the infected cells (4, 6, 8). The infected erythrocytes are slightly larger than noninfected cells.

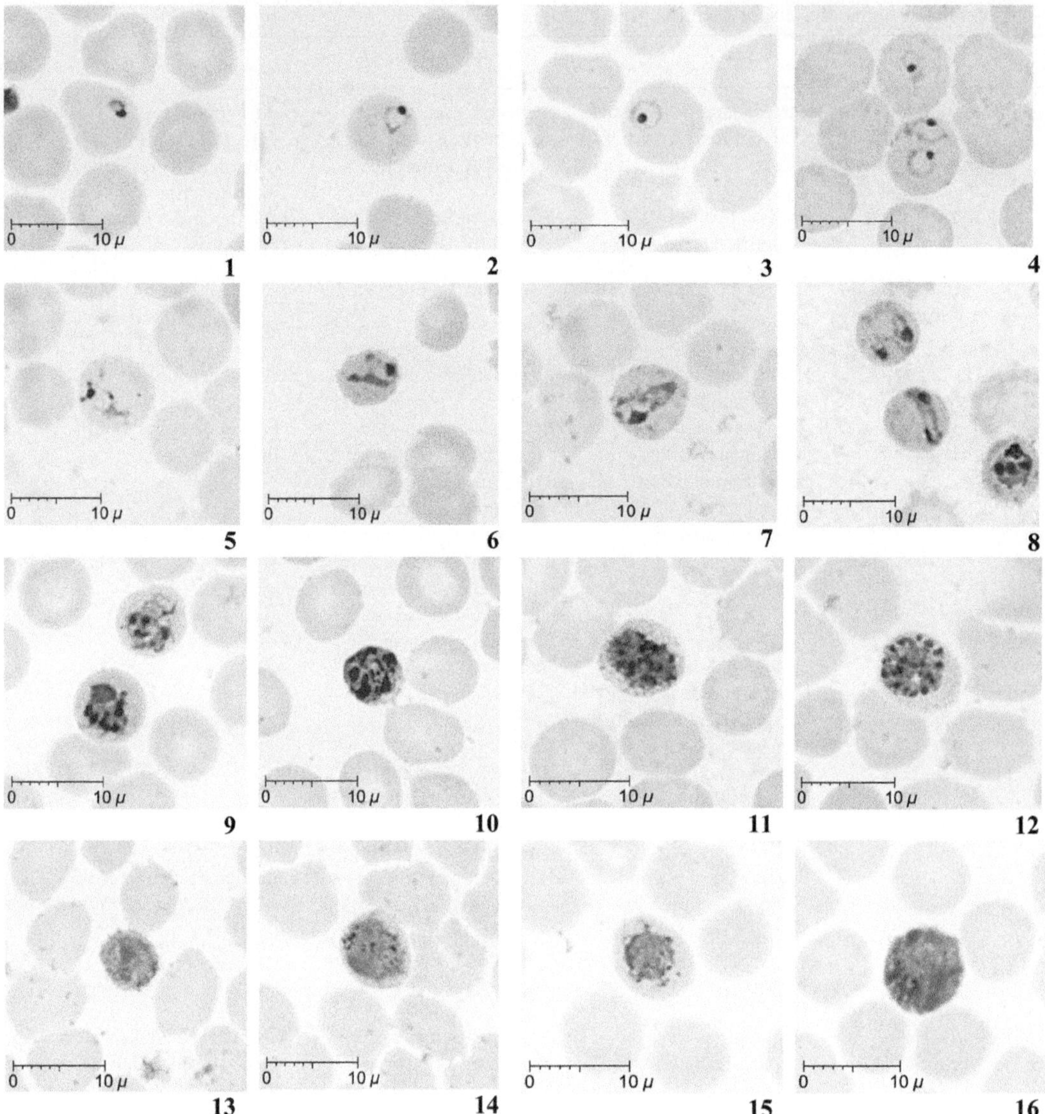

FIGURE 8 *P. knowlesi*, successive developmental stages in Giemsa-stained thin blood films: early stage trophozoites/rings (1, 2), developing trophozoite (3), developing trophozoites with "band" form (4), early stage schizont (5), mature schizont (6), mature macrogametocyte (7), mature microgametocyte (8). Images reproduced from figures in reference 42 with permission.

successful treatment, and therefore RDTs should not be used to monitor outcomes of treatment (45). In contrast, false-negative results have been reported with parasite deletions of *pfhrp2* or closely related *pfhrp3* when RDTs detecting Pf-HRP2 are used (48). Decreased sensitivity for *P. falciparum* has been reported for pregnant women, presumably due to sequestration of parasite antigens in the placenta (49).

Given the limitations of RDTs, it is widely recommended that all results be confirmed with standard thick and thin blood films (36, 38). In nonendemic settings such as the United States and Europe, laboratories that may benefit from RDT use include those that lack the expertise to interpret traditional blood films or desire a more rapid diagnostic method for general or point-of-care testing (50–52). RDTs may be particularly beneficial in STAT laboratories and during the evening shift, when expertise for sensitive detection of blood parasites using thick films is lacking; in these settings, the ability to immediately detect cases with high *P. falciparum* parasitemia may be life-saving.

Nucleic Acid Detection

A variety of nucleic acid detection methods have been described, including DNA/RNA hybridization, PCR, nucleic acid sequence-based amplification, and loop-mediated isothermal amplification (LAMP) (35). Of these, the most commonly used method is PCR, with the 18S small subunit ribosomal RNA gene being the most common target (35). Numerous conventional (53–55) and real-time PCR formats (56–60) have been described for *Plasmodium* detection, species/subspecies differentiation (including *P. ovale curtisi* and *P. ovale wallikeri*), and identification of parasite resistance markers to antimalarial drugs (see "Treatment and Prevention" below). Most PCR assays are laboratory developed, although some CE-marked commercial test kits exist, including the Artus Malaria RG PCR

TABLE 3 Comparison of malaria diagnostic direct methods[a]

Method	Test	Advantages	Disadvantages	Comments	References
Giemsa stain	Thick film	Screens large volume of blood; high sensitivity	Subjective; species differentiation is not easily accomplished	Gold standard for detection; requires experienced and skilled microscopists	23, 30, 36, 39, 41, 43
	Thin film	Preserves parasite morphology; good for species determination	Subjective; less sensitive than the thick film for screening	Gold standard for species determination; requires experienced and skilled microscopists	
Fluorescent DNA/RNA stains	AO- or BCP-stained films	May decrease screening time	Nonspecific stain; may be hard to interpret	Requires fluorescence microscope	44, 128
	QBC Malaria (AO-stained blood in microhematocrit tube)	Rapid, screens large volume of blood; best sensitivity and specificity for *P. falciparum* Separation of blood components and parasites by centrifugation facilitates screening.	Nonspecific stain; may be hard to interpret Species determination and calculation of percent parasitemia is difficult; less sensitive for non-*P. falciparum* species since stages other than early trophozoites may be obscured in the granulocyte layer	Requires centrifuge, fluorescence microscope, or fluorescent adaptor for light microscope	38, 129–131
	Flow cytometry	Automated	Variable sensitivity		132
Hemozoin detection	Dark-field microscopy	No stain used; abundant pigment in macrophages suggests poor prognosis	Poor sensitivity		38, 133, 134
	Histology/FFPE tissues	Allows for correlation with morphologic features	Requires tissue biopsy; hemozoin may be confused with formalin or anthracotic pigment		135
Antigen detection	Kits for detection of HRP-2, aldolase, and parasite LDH	Rapid, ease of use and interpretation; some kits appropriate for field use	Relatively expensive compared to blood films, variable sensitivity for low percent parasitemia and non-*P. falciparum* infections	Performance characteristics vary widely by kit	46
Nucleic acid detection	DNA/RNA hybridization	Nonamplification technique; does not require the same degree of contamination controls as PCR	Poor sensitivity, expensive, requires sophisticated equipment and facilities for high-complexity testing	First nucleic acid detection method; not widely used clinically	136, 137
	PCR	High sensitivity and specificity, equal to or exceeding thick film; some assay designs give excellent detection of mixed infections	Expensive, requires sophisticated equipment and facilities for high complexity testing; potential for amplicon contamination; not usually performed rapidly	Multiple laboratory-developed methods; no FDA-cleared/approved tests; clinical availability limited to reference and public health laboratories	35, 53, 57–59, 138
	LAMP	Sensitivity and specificity comparable to PCR, some tests suitable for field use	Expensive (but less than PCR); no commercial options at this time	Not widely used clinically; no FDA-cleared/approved tests	35, 139

[a]AO, acridine orange; BCP, benzothiocarboxypurine; FFPE, formalin-fixed, paraffin-embedded; HRP-2, histidine-rich protein 2; LDH, lactate dehydrogenase; QBC, quantitative buffy coat

kit (Qiagen, Helsinki, Finland), RealStar Malaria PCR kit (Altona Diagnostics, Hamburg, Germany), Geno-Sen's Malaria Real Time PCR kit for *P. vivax* (Genome Diagnostics, New Delhi, India), and the Malaria RealAMP kit (Osang HealthCare, Anyang, Republic of Korea). The Loopamp Malaria Pan/Pf detection kit (Eiken Chemical, Tokyo, Japan) and Illumigene Malaria (Meridian Bioscience, London, United Kingdom) are also CE-marked and use LAMP for detection of *Plasmodium* species to the genus level. The Loopamp also has primers for specific detection of *P. falciparum*. Unfortunately, no nucleic acid amplification tests have been approved or cleared by the FDA for *in vitro* diagnostic use.

Although there is tremendous variability between published assays, PCR-based tests are generally recognized as having improved sensitivity over the traditional thick film, with detection limits below 10 parasites/μl of blood. Scientists at the National Institute for Medical Research in London, United Kingdom, have described a nested conventional PCR test capable of detecting at least 6 parasites/μl (61),

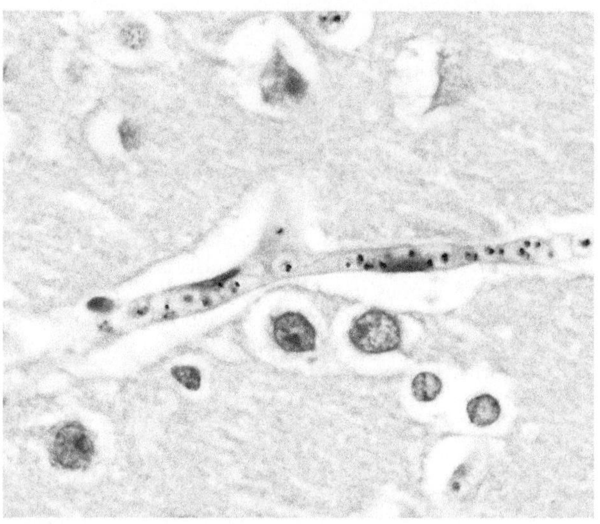

FIGURE 9 Cerebral malaria due to *P. falciparum* on tissue section (hematoxylin and eosin, ×400). The capillary in the center of the image contains multiple infected erythrocytes, seen primarily by their brown-black hemozoin pigment.

while a reverse transcriptase quantitative real-time PCR test has a reported detection limit of 0.002 parasites/μl (35, 62). A quantitated *P. falciparum* standard is available through the WHO (63) which can be used to determine the analytical sensitivity of new and existing molecular assays.

PCR-based tests for detection of *Plasmodium* nucleic acid are primarily limited to specialized reference or public health laboratories and are not generally suited for rapid diagnosis in the clinical setting. However, they may be useful for detection of low parasitemia, confirmation of suspected infection, differentiation of *Plasmodium* from *Babesia* parasites, *Plasmodium* species determination, and sensitive detection of mixed infections (36).

Despite the potential advantages of PCR assays, implementation in endemic resource-limited settings poses many challenges due to the associated expense and need for highly specialized equipment and facilities. Fortunately, isothermal amplification techniques such as nucleic acid sequence-based amplification and LAMP offer simpler and less-expensive tests for detection of *Plasmodium* DNA and RNA, respectively (64, 65). One recently described innovative electricity-free system utilizes a calcium oxide-based heat-generating reaction within an improvised thermos for malaria LAMP testing (66). Other methods of *Plasmodium* nucleic acid amplification that may be suitable for resource-limited settings include the nucleic acid lateral flow immunoassay (67) and the PCR-based enzyme-linked immunosorbent assay (68). Further studies are needed to determine the performance characteristics of these alternative assay designs in a variety of clinical settings.

When positive results are obtained with malaria nucleic acid tests, thick or thin blood films should be examined so that the percent parasitemia can be determined. Quantitative PCR may one day replace the subjective manual parasite counts that suffer from a lack of interobserver reproducibility. Unfortunately, quantitative PCR results do not correlate well with the conventionally obtained percent parasitemia. This is because conventional counts do not include gametocytes and extracellular forms, and multiply infected cells are only counted once; in contrast, PCR detects nucleic acid from each parasite in the specimen.

Serologic Tests

Serologic testing plays little role in the diagnosis of acute malaria given that antibodies are frequently absent at the time of patient presentation. Also, a positive test indicates previous exposure but does not differentiate between acute and past infection. For these reasons, serology has its greatest utility in epidemiologic studies, blood donor screening (69), and occasionally for evaluating relapsing, recrudescent, or untreated malaria in nonimmune patients. Indirect fluorescent antibody (IFA) tests using antigens prepared from the four human *Plasmodium* species have been previously described (70, 71) and are available at specialized testing facilities. These tests are time-consuming and subjective but are highly sensitive and specific.

Other Diagnostic Laboratory Methods

Other nonconventional techniques for laboratory diagnosis include laser-desorption mass spectrometry (72) for detection of hemozoin in whole blood and, recently, detection of hemozoin-generated vapor nanobubbles across intact skin (73). These techniques hold promise for rapid and affordable malaria testing in the future.

Treatment and Prevention

A number of drugs are used to treat malaria, including chloroquine, mefloquine, quinine, quinidine, atovaquone-proguanil (Malarone), and artemether-lumefantrine (Coartem) (27, 74). Treatment decisions are based on the clinical severity of disease, region where infection was acquired, drug resistance (when known), and species of infecting parasite (27, 74). When infection is with either *P. ovale* or *P. vivax*, primaquine must be administered in addition to a standard antimalarial agent to eradicate the dormant liver hypnozoite forms formed by these parasites, thus underscoring the need for accurate species identification by the laboratory (27). Partial or complete red cell exchange transfusion may also be used for patients with parasitemia of ≥10%. This approach is supported by the American Society for Apheresis but is no longer recommended by the CDC (28).

Unfortunately, parasite resistance to antimalarial medications is a serious problem worldwide (75–77). Chloroquine was a mainstay of treatment and prophylaxis for many years, but due to widespread *P. falciparum* resistance, it has been supplanted with other drugs such as atovaquone-proguanil, doxycycline, sulfadoxine-pyrimethamine, and Malarone for *P. falciparum* therapy (76). Chloroquine-susceptible *P. falciparum* is now only found in Mexico, the Caribbean, and parts of the Middle East and Central America (75, 76). *P. falciparum* resistance to mefloquine and sulfadoxine-pyrimethamine, as well as *P. vivax* tolerance to chloroquine and primaquine, has also been detected in some regions of endemicity (75, 76, 78, 79). Only rare instances of quinine resistance have been reported, allowing this drug to remain a therapy for severe malaria (80, 81). Artemisinin compounds (e.g., artesunate, artemether) have been recognized as superior drugs for malaria treatment and are now recommended by the WHO as first-line therapy for both uncomplicated and complicated disease in combination with other antimalarial agents (ACT) (74, 77). Recently, decreased *in vivo* susceptibility to artemisinin compounds has been detected in *P. falciparum* strains along the Thai-Cambodian border (greater Mekong subregion), a historic site for emerging resistance to antimalarial agents (77, 82). Outside the greater Mekong subregion, significant levels of ACT failure are primarily due to resistance to the partner drug rather than to the artemisinin component. Full (high-level) artemisinin resistance has not yet been documented (77). Containment interventions are urgently needed to prevent global spread of these partially resistant *P. falciparum* artemisinin-resistant strains.

Antimalaria resistance may be detected by using *in vitro* susceptibility testing (83), although this method is not available clinically. A more practical approach is through molecular detection of single-nucleotide polymorphisms that have been associated with antimalarial resistance, such as *dhps/dhft* (sulfadoxine/pyrimethamine), *Pfcrt* (chloroquine), *Pfmdr* (chloroquine, mefloquine, and quinine), and *PfATPase6/pfmdr* and *PfKelch13* (artemisinin) (78), using PCR (60) and DNA microarray formats (76, 77, 81, 84). A number of government laboratories perform molecular amplification and sequencing for detection of known mutations associated with antimalarial resistance for treatment and/or epidemiologic purposes including those in the United States (CDC), Canada, the United Kingdom, the European Union, and China (27). See chapter 154 for further discussion of susceptibility test methods of parasites.

Evaluation, Interpretation, and Reporting of Results

Detection of malaria parasites by any diagnostic method is considered a critical result and must be reported to the clinical team immediately. The final report for blood smear evaluation should include the *Plasmodium* species and calculated degree of parasitemia. It is important to convey when a mixed infection or late-stage forms of *P. falciparum* are suspected since these findings may have treatment implications. Similarly, parasite loads above 100,000 parasites/μl (approximately 2% parasitemia) in nonimmune individuals is indicative of severe disease requiring urgent therapy (24). Parasite levels above 10% may suggest a role for exchange transfusion, although this is no longer recommended by the CDC (27, 28). It may be useful to relay to the clinical team that a single set of negative blood films does not exclude the diagnosis of malaria and that serial smears should be performed if clinically indicated (30).

Examination of serial blood films is recommended in patients with malaria to monitor the response to treatment. The frequency of repeat blood film examinations is typically based on the clinical severity of the patient's illness, with at least daily monitoring recommended for patients with severe malaria (27). It is important to note that asexual forms of the parasites may be seen in repeat blood films for 2 to 3 days following appropriate treatment and that the degree of parasitemia may rise during the first 12 to 24 hours of treatment. However, if the level of parasitemia does not fall by 75% in the first 36 to 48 hours of treatment or parasites are still present after day 3, then parasite resistance or lack of patient compliance with treatment should be considered (25, 27). Gametocytes may circulate for 2 weeks or more since they are not killed by most antimalarial drugs and therefore should be excluded from the parasite count or reported separately (27).

If expertise for *Plasmodium* species determination or differentiation between *Plasmodium* and *Babesia* parasites is not available in the primary laboratory, it is important to inform the clinician that *Plasmodium* or *Babesia* parasites are identified and that blood and/or films are being sent to a reference or public health laboratory for further analysis. It is important to mention that the potentially deadly *P. falciparum* cannot be excluded in the preliminary report. The CDC's Division of Parasitic Diseases and Malaria provides a rapid telediagnostic service (http://cdc.gov/dpdx/contact.html) at no cost for both national and international patients (27).

BABESIA

Description of the Agent

Members of the genus *Babesia* infect a wide range of wild and domestic animals worldwide using primarily ixodid tick vectors (85). Despite there being over 100 named *Babesia* species, only a few are known to regularly infect humans (85). *Babesia microti* is responsible for the vast majority of human cases in the United States. Infection with *Babesia duncani* and *B. duncani*-like organisms has also been reported in Washington, Oregon, and California (86–88), and rare cases of *B. divergens*-like organisms (e.g., strain MO-1) have been detected in Kentucky, Missouri, and Washington (85, 89). *B. divergens*-like organisms have also been detected in cottontail rabbits on Nantucket Island (90). In Europe, *B. divergens* causes the majority of cases, with fewer cases attributable to *B. venatorum* and *B. microti* (91–94). Elsewhere, a number of *Babesia* species have been detected in humans, including *B. microti*-like organisms in Taiwan (95) and Japan (96), *B. venatorum* in China (97), a new *Babesia* sp., the KO-1 strain, in South Korea (98), and incompletely characterized species in Mexico, Brazil, Colombia, Egypt, Mozambique, South Africa, and India (85). Rare unverified human cases have also been attributed to *B. canis* and *B. bovis* (99).

Traditionally, *Babesia* species were classified into small and large forms based on size, with *B. microti* and *B. divergens* grouped together as "small form" species (trophozoites of <2.5 μm) (91). Later, genetic analysis of the 18S rRNA gene was used to clarify *Babesia* phylogeny and divide the piroplasms into four to five clades (91, 100). Most recently, the genome of *B. microti* has been sequenced, showing it to be the smallest genome of any Apicomplexan parasite sequenced to date (comprising approximately 3,500 genes) (101, 102). These studies also revealed that *B. microti* is genetically distant from other *Babesia* species and may constitute a separate genus (85).

Epidemiology and Transmission

In contrast to malaria, babesiosis is a disease of the temperate regions, including parts of North America and Europe. In the United States, classic "hot spots" for babesiosis due to *B. microti* include the Northeast coast (e.g., Martha's Vineyard, Nantucket, and Long Island), upper Midwest states, and areas of the Atlantic and South-Central states, while a small number of cases due to other *Babesia* species have been described in Missouri, Kentucky, Washington, Oregon, and California (85). National U.S. surveillance was begun in 18 endemic states and New York City on 1 January 2011 (103), with 1,124 probable and confirmed cases reported in the first year. The majority of cases were reported by just seven states; in ascending order, these were Minnesota, Rhode Island, Connecticut, Wisconsin, New Jersey, Massachusetts, and New York. The majority of patients were ≥60 years of age (range 1 to 98 years), and most did not recall a tick bite (103). The most recent CDC surveillance report for babesiosis in the United States described 1,744 cases, with 94% being residents of the seven states listed above (104). Given that most infections with *Babesia* are asymptomatic, the actual number of infections is probably much greater than reported.

Significantly fewer cases of babesiosis have been reported in Europe. To date, 30 or more cases of babesiosis due to *B. divergens* have been reported, primarily from patients in France, Great Britain, and Ireland, while only sporadic cases of babesiosis due to *B. venatorum* and *B. microti* infection have been documented (85, 105). *B. divergens* is primarily a bovine babesiosis that has a significant economic impact on the livestock industry (106).

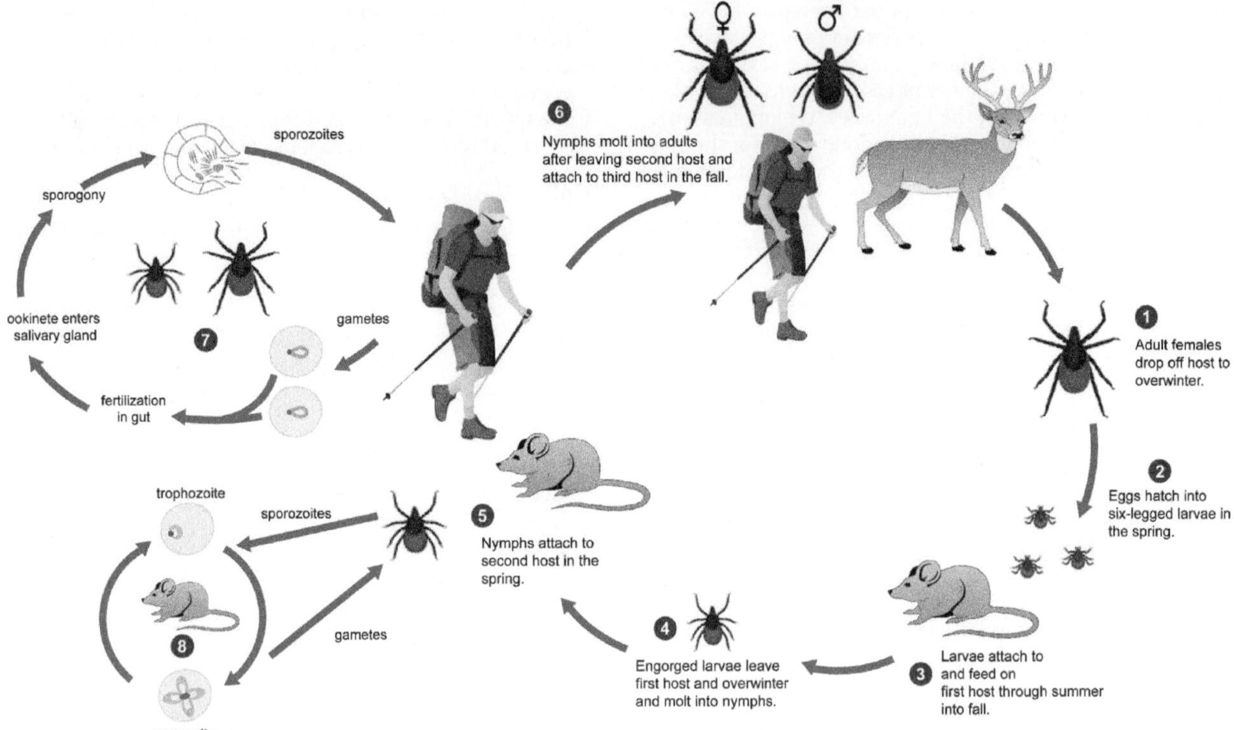

FIGURE 10 Life cycle of *I. scapularis* and *B. microti*. *I. scapularis* has a four-stage life cycle that generally lasts 2 years and includes vertebrate hosts (including rodents, deer, or humans), where each mobile tick stage has a blood meal on a different individual host. During the first year, mated adult female ticks detach from the vertebrate host to overwinter (1) and lay eggs in the spring. Eggs hatch in spring (2), and larvae attach to their first vertebrate host, usually small rodents or birds (3). The six-legged larvae feed on the first host, generally in late summer, and may become infected with *B. microti* while taking a blood meal. Engorged larvae leave the host and overwinter and molt into nymphs (4). In the spring of the second year, nymphs attach to a second vertebrate host (e.g., rodents, deer, or humans) (5) and in the fall leave the second host to molt into adults and attach to a third vertebrate host, such as deer and humans (6). *B. microti* has a two-host life cycle including *I. scapularis* as the definitive host and a vertebrate intermediate host. In the tick (7), gametes ingested while taking a blood meal undergo sexual reproduction, leading to the eventual formation of infectious sporozoites. In the mammalian host (e.g., rodents or humans) (8), sporozoites initiate the erythrocytic cycle, resulting in the formation of trophozoites that divide asexually by budding. Subsequently, trophozoites transform into merozoites and perpetuate the erythrocytic cycle, or gametes which are ingested by ticks during a blood meal initiate the sexual cycle. All mobile stages of *I. scapularis* may acquire *B. microti* parasites from infected first or second vertebrate hosts, but only nymphs and adults transmit parasites. Figure and credit used by permission (127).

Most cases of babesiosis are acquired through the bite of an infected ixodid tick (Fig. 10). In nature, disease is maintained between invertebrate and vertebrate hosts. Humans readily become infected but are considered dead-end hosts. *Ixodes scapularis* (the blacklegged or deer tick) and *I. ricinus* (the castor bean or sheep tick) are the most common vectors in the United States and Europe, respectively (85). The primary vertebrate host in the life cycle of *B. microti* in the United States is the white-footed mouse, *Peromyscus leucopus*, and other rodents and shrews may serve as the host for *B. microti* cases in Europe (85). The primary hosts for *B. divergens* and *B. venatorum* in Europe are cattle and deer, respectively. Following a tick bite, *Babesia* sporozoites enter the blood and directly infect circulating erythrocytes to form trophozoites resembling malarial parasites. There is no liver stage as seen in malaria and thus no latent exoerythrocytic forms. Trophozoites divide asexually via budding rather than schizogony as in malaria to form similar-appearing merozoites and gametocytes (99). Lysis of infected erythrocytes releases merozoites into the blood, where they infect new erythrocytes. As with malaria, sexual reproduction with fertilization of the gametes occurs in the gut of the arthropod host. Fertilized gametes migrate across the intestinal wall and travel to the salivary glands to develop into sporoblasts. The final step in maturation occurs when the tick takes a blood meal; sporozoites develop from the sporoblasts and are injected into the host during the final hours of feeding. The seasonality of babesiosis corresponds with the activity of the tick vectors, with most cases occurring in the spring, summer, and fall (85).

Less commonly, human babesiosis is acquired through receipt of infected blood products (107) or by vertical transmission across the placenta (108). Blood transfusion is recognized as an increasingly important source of infection (85, 107, 109), with six cases of transfusion-related *B. microti* infection identified in the United States in 2014 (104). The largest review of transfusion-related babesiosis in the United States identified 159 cases from 1979 to 2009, with 156 cases due to *B. microti* and 3 due to *B. duncani* (109). Recently, a case of probable transfusion transmission of *B. divergens*-like organisms has also been reported (110). Significantly fewer cases of transfusion-transmitted babesiosis have been reported in Europe (107). As expected, most implicated blood donations were collected during times of the year that ticks are active; however, a number of cases occurred from blood donated in the winter. In the latter cases, the original infections were presumably acquired by donors during the tick-biting season and remained dormant in the blood for months without causing symptoms. Most transfusion-transmitted cases have been associated with the receipt of whole blood, but cases associated with whole blood-derived platelets have also been reported (107, 109). The American Red Cross estimates that the risk of transfusion-transmitted babesiosis is approximately 1 in 100,000 donations in endemic states, and 1 in 18,000 donations in highly endemic areas (107, 111, 112).

Clinical Significance

Babesiosis due to *B. microti* and *B. duncani*/*B. duncani*-like parasites can manifest as asymptomatic or mild infection to life-threatening illness (85). In patients with a functioning spleen, *B. microti* infection is generally mild; when present, symptoms may include fever and a nonspecific influenza-like illness. Severe disease is most commonly seen in asplenic patients and may be associated with high fever, chills, night sweats, myalgia, hemolytic anemia, hematuria, hepatosplenomegaly, and jaundice. Life-threatening complications include disseminated intravascular coagulation, acute renal or respiratory failure, congestive heart failure, and coma. In addition to asplenia, immunosuppression and advanced age are risk factors for severe disease (91).

Patients infected with *B. divergens* in Europe are generally asplenic or immunocompromised and present with severe disease. Most infections with *B. divergens*-like agents in the United States have similar characteristics. At this time, only a small number of infections with *B. venatorum* have been reported, but preliminary evidence suggests that disease is relatively mild (91).

Treatment and Prevention

Treatment is only recommended for cases of symptomatic babesiosis (113). Oral azithromycin and atovaquone are recommended for mild to moderate disease, while intravenous clindamycin and oral quinine are used for severe babesiosis (113). Red cell exchange transfusion may also be used for patients with severe disease and/or parasitemia of ≥10% (113, 114).

Disease is prevented primarily through measures to avoid tick bites in areas of endemicity, such as applying tick repellents containing *N*,*N*-diethyl-meta-toluamide to exposed skin and permethrin to clothing, avoiding tick habitats such as deciduous forests and tall grasses, and performing frequent "tick checks" to locate and remove attached ticks (105). This is especially important for patients at risk for severe disease such as immunocompromised and asplenic individuals (105). Measures can also be taken to minimize tick habitat around dwellings, such as keeping grass mowed short, removing leaf litter, and spraying vegetation with acaricides. Community education can be an important component of disease prevention strategies in areas of high endemicity (105).

Prevention of transfusion-related cases is mostly through blood donor questionnaire screening; those with a history of babesiosis are deferred indefinitely from donating blood (105). The number of transfusion-related cases appears to be on the rise in the United States, and there is a need for a viable and cost-effective screening method for blood products (112). At this time, there is no FDA-approved test for this purpose (107, 112). However, the American Red Cross has been screening blood donations obtained in regions of high endemicity in the United States under an investigational protocol since 2012. Under this protocol, specimens are tested using PCR and serologic-based tests. Reactive specimens are tested using a second, more sensitive PCR and Western blotting. The American Red Cross reports detecting infected donors in approximately 1 out of every 300 donations in regions of endemicity (111).

Collection, Transport, and Storage of Specimens

Collection and transport of whole blood specimens for babesiosis testing are performed in the same manner as for malaria. It is important to remember that *I. scapularis*, the main vector of *B. microti*, is also a vector for other tick-borne pathogens such as *Anaplasma phagocytophilum* and *Borrelia burgdorferi*, the agents of anaplasmosis and Lyme disease, respectively, and consideration should be given to concurrent testing for these agents (115). Importantly, recent studies indicate that coinfection with *B. microti* and *B. burgdorferi* promotes transmission of *B. microti* from ticks to humans and results in greater disease severity (115).

Requests for blood films should be accompanied by important patient information such as clinical signs and symptoms, state of residence, travel history, immune status, and presence or absence of a functioning spleen.

Direct Examination

Microscopy

As with malaria, the traditional method for diagnosis of babesiosis is microscopic examination of Giemsa-stained thick and thin blood films (85, 114). Further details regarding the preparation and use of blood films are provided in the previous section on malaria.

Babesia spp. parasites may present a diagnostic challenge on blood films due to the many morphologic similarities they share with *Plasmodium* species (specifically *P. falciparum*) on thick and thin films (Fig. 11, 12). However, a number of diagnostic features can be used to differentiate between *Babesia* and *Plasmodium* in most instances (Table 4). In general, *Babesia* parasites demonstrate greater pleomorphism in size and shape than *P. falciparum* parasites, with ovoid, elliptical, pear, racket, and spindle shapes commonly seen. Extracellular forms are also common. Rarely, classic tetrads ("Maltese crosses") are seen. It is important to note that

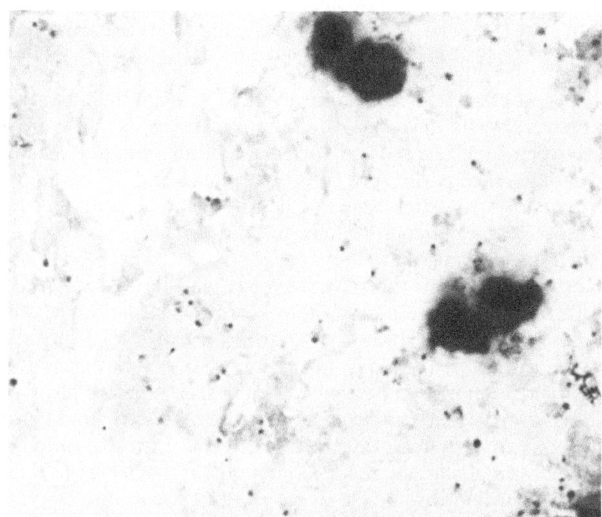

FIGURE 11 *Babesia* morphology on thick blood film consists of ring forms resembling trophozoites of *P. falciparum*. Some pleomorphism is apparent.

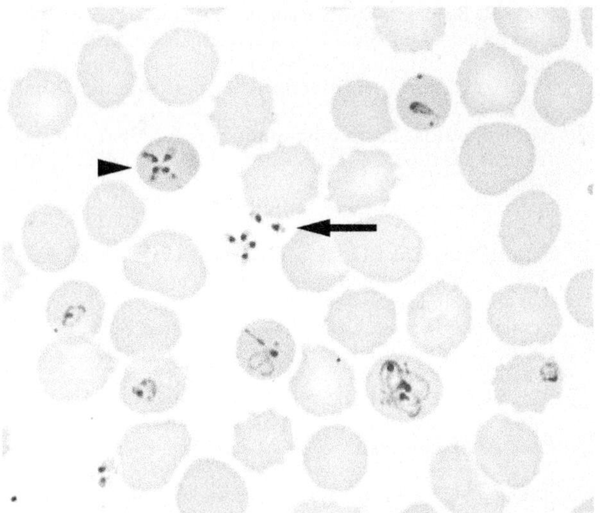

FIGURE 12 *Babesia* morphology on thin blood film. Note the presence of small intraerythrocytic ring forms resembling early trophozoites of *P. falciparum*, as well as thicker and markedly pleomorphic ring forms. Characteristic extracellular forms (arrow) and a tetrad form (arrowhead) are also seen.

only ring-type forms are seen in babesiosis. The presence of stippling, hemozoin pigment, schizonts, or plasmodial-type gametocytes excludes the diagnosis of babesiosis. It is not possible to differentiate the various human *Babesia* species by morphology; this requires molecular methods.

When the morphology is insufficient for differentiation of *Babesia* and *Plasmodium* parasites, it is helpful to obtain a complete travel history, examine multiple blood samples for parasites, or perform an alternative detection method (e.g., PCR).

Determining the degree of parasitemia may be useful for patient management. Parasitemia levels usually vary between 1 and 10% but may reach up to 80% (85, 91). Monitoring the parasite load in conjunction with treatment may be especially important in immunocompromised and asplenic patients who are at risk for prolonged or relapsing disease (116).

Nucleic Acid Detection

Nucleic acid amplification assays such as PCR offer increased sensitivity over blood film examination and may be useful in instances of low parasitemia and when parasite morphology is inconclusive. Assays have been described for *B. microti* (35, 117–120) and *B. divergens* (120). A real-time PCR assay for detection of *B. microti* reports a detection limit of approximately 0.0001% parasitemia, which is superior to the detection limit of thick films (0.0002 to 0.001% parasitemia) (35). Sequencing of 18s ribosomal DNA has also been used for molecular characterization of *Babesia* species (92, 120). There are no FDA-cleared/approved or CE-marked *Babesia* PCR assays at this time.

Isolation Procedures

In rare instances, it may be necessary to inoculate the blood from a patient with suspected babesiosis into a laboratory animal such as a golden hamster (*B. microti*) (119, 121) or gerbil (*B. divergens*) (92, 106) to confirm the presence of a low-level infection or to determine the viability of an organism detected only by DNA testing. This is rarely performed in the clinical laboratory but may be available following consultation at the CDC or at other specialized centers.

Serologic Tests

Serologic testing plays little role in the diagnosis of acute babesiosis but may be useful for epidemiologic studies, blood donor screening, and in cases of chronic disease. Antibodies to *B. microti* typically appear 2 weeks after the onset of illness and may be detectable for several years after infection (85). The IFA (122, 123) is the recommended method for detection of serum antibodies against *B. microti* and has a relatively high sensitivity (88 to 96%) and specificity (90 to 100%) (122). Premade slides for *B. microti* IFA testing are commercially available in the United States and Europe through various manufacturers including Bio Nuclear Diagnostics Inc. (Toronto, ON), Focus Diagnostics (Cypress, CA), Fuller Laboratories (Fullerton, CA), Genoprice Gentaur (Kampenhout, Belgium), and Invitech (Cambridgeshire, England). Interpretation of IFA results is subjective, and the cutoff titer for defining a positive result varies by laboratory; titers of 1:128 to 1:256 may be associated with a higher specificity (124). Low antibody titers or negative results may be seen when serum is obtained early in disease or when patients are immunosuppressed or asplenic, while false positives may occur in patients with connective tissue disorders (e.g., rheumatoid arthritis). *B. microti* IFA serology does not demonstrate significant cross-reactivity with antibodies to *B. duncani*, *B. divergens*, or *B. venatorum* (122), so specific assays must be used for these organisms (125, 126).

TABLE 4 Comparative morphology of *Babesia* spp. and *P. falciparum*

Diagnostic features	*P. falciparum*	*Babesia* spp.
Size of infected RBC[a]	Normal	Normal
Parasite stages in peripheral blood	Ring forms, less commonly crescent-shaped gametocytes; may see high parasitemia; other stages only rarely seen	Ring forms only; heavy infections common
Parasite characteristics	Delicate rings, <1/3 diameter of the RBC; may have headphone and applique forms; multiply infected RBCs common	Delicate rings, 1/3–1/6 diameter of the RBC; pleomorphic with ovoid, spindled, and ameboid forms; multiply infected RBCs common; single or multiple chromatin dots; rarely tetrad forms
RBC inclusions	Occasionally Maurer's clefts	None
Extracellular forms	Rare	Common
Pigment	Brown-black hemozoin	None
Fever cycle	36–48 hours	No periodicity
Area of endemicity	Tropical and subtropical regions	Temperate regions

[a]RBC, red blood cell (erythrocyte).

Evaluation, Interpretation, and Reporting of Results

Detection of *Babesia* parasites by any diagnostic method should be considered a clinically significant result and be promptly reported to the clinical team. The final blood film report should ideally include the calculated degree of parasitemia. When the blood film examination is negative, the report may include a statement that a single set of negative blood films does not exclude the diagnosis of babesiosis and that serial smears should be performed if clinically indicated.

If expertise for differentiation of *Babesia* and *Plasmodium* parasites is not available in the primary laboratory, it is important to inform the clinician that *Plasmodium* or *Babesia* parasites are identified and blood and/or films are being sent to a reference or public health laboratory for further analysis.

REFERENCES

1. **Adl SM, Simpson AG, Lane CE, Lukeš J, Bass D, Bowser SS, Brown MW, Burki F, Dunthorn M, Hampl V, Heiss A, Hoppenrath M, Lara E, Le Gall L, Lynn DH, McManus H, Mitchell EA, Mozley-Stanridge SE, Parfrey LW, Pawlowski J, Rueckert S, Shadwick L, Schoch CL, Smirnov A, Spiegel FW.** 2012. The revised classification of eukaryotes. *J Eukaryot Microbiol* **59:**429–493.
2. **Waller RF, McFadden GI.** 2005. The apicoplast: a review of the derived plastid of apicomplexan parasites. *Curr Issues Mol Biol* **7:**57–79.
3. **Perkins SL.** 2014. Malaria's many mates: past, present, and future of the systematics of the order *Haemosporida*. *J Parasitol* **100:**11–25.
4. **World Health Organization.** 2016. *World Malaria Report 2016*. http://apps.who.int/iris/bitstream/10665/252038/1/9789241511711-eng.pdf?ua=1. Accessed 21 May 2017.
5. **Collins WE, Jeffery GM.** 2005. *Plasmodium ovale*: parasite and disease. *Clin Microbiol Rev* **18:**570–581.
6. **Sutherland CJ, Tanomsing N, Nolder D, Oguike M, Jennison C, Pukrittayakamee S, Dolecek C, Hien TT, do Rosário VE, Arez AP, Pinto J, Michon P, Escalante AA, Nosten F, Burke M, Lee R, Blaze M, Otto TD, Barnwell JW, Pain A, Williams J, White NJ, Day NP, Snounou G, Lockhart PJ, Chiodini PL, Imwong M, Polley SD.** 2010. Two nonrecombining sympatric forms of the human malaria parasite *Plasmodium ovale* occur globally. *J Infect Dis* **201:**1544–1550.
7. **Simner PJ.** 2017. Medical parasitology taxonomy update: January 2012 to December 2015. *J Clin Microbiol* **55:**43–47.
8. **Nolder D, Oguike MC, Maxwell-Scott H, Niyazi HA, Smith V, Chiodini PL, Sutherland CJ.** 2013. An observational study of malaria in British travellers: *plasmodium ovale wallikeri* and *Plasmodium ovale curtisi* differ significantly in the duration of latency. *BMJ Open* **3:**e002711.
9. **Coatney GR, Collins WE, Warren MW, Contacos PG.** 1971. *The Primate Malarias*. National Institute of Allergy and Infectious Diseases, Bethesda, MD.
10. **Singh B, Kim Sung L, Matusop A, Radhakrishnan A, Shamsul SS, Cox-Singh J, Thomas A, Conway DJ.** 2004. A large focus of naturally acquired *Plasmodium knowlesi* infections in human beings. *Lancet* **363:**1017–1024.
11. **Cox-Singh J, Davis TM, Lee KS, Shamsul SS, Matusop A, Ratnam S, Rahman HA, Conway DJ, Singh B.** 2008. *Plasmodium knowlesi* malaria in humans is widely distributed and potentially life threatening. *Clin Infect Dis* **46:**165–171.
12. **Singh B, Daneshvar C.** 2013. Human infections and detection of *Plasmodium knowlesi*. *Clin Microbiol Rev* **26:**165–184.
13. **Kantele A, Jokiranta TS.** 2011. Review of cases with the emerging fifth human malaria parasite, *Plasmodium knowlesi*. *Clin Infect Dis* **52:**1356–1362.
14. **Linscott AJ.** 2011. Malaria in the United States: past and present. *Clin Microbiol Newsl* **33:**49–52.
15. **Centers for Disease Control and Prevention.** 2017. *CDC Yellow Book 2018*. https://wwwnc.cdc.gov/travel/page/yellowbook-home. Accessed 21May 2017.
16. **Romi R, Boccolini D, Menegon M, Rezza G.** 2012. Probable autochthonous introduced malaria cases in Italy in 2009-2011 and the risk of local vector-borne transmission. *Euro Surveill* **17:**20325. https://eurosurveillance.org/content/10.2807/ese.17.48.20325-en.
17. **Andriopoulos P, Economopoulou A, Spanakos G, Assimakopoulos G.** 2013. A local outbreak of autochthonous *Plasmodium vivax* malaria in Laconia, Greece: a re-emerging infection in the southern borders of Europe? *Int J Infect Dis* **17:**e125–e128.
18. **Shkurti K, Vyshka G, Velo E, Boçari A, Kokici M, Kraja D.** 2013. Imported malaria in Albania and the risk factors that could allow its reappearance. *Malar J* **12:**197.
19. **Centers for Disease Control and Prevention (CDC).** 2004. Multifocal autochthonous transmission of malaria: Florida, 2003. *MMWR Morb Mortal Wkly Rep* **53:**412–413.
20. **Mace KE, Arguin PM.** 2017. Malaria surveillance: United States, 2014. *MMWR Surveill Summ* **66:**1–24.
21. **Pavli A, Maltezou HC.** 2010. Malaria and travellers visiting friends and relatives. *Travel Med Infect Dis* **8:**161–168.
22. **Stramer SL, Hollinger FB, Katz LM, Kleinman S, Metzel PS, Gregory KR, Dodd RY.** 2009. Emerging infectious disease agents and their potential threat to transfusion safety. *Transfusion* **49**(Suppl 2)**:**1S–29S.
23. **John DT, Petri WA.** 2006. *Markell and Voge's Medical Parasitology*, 9th ed, p 79–106. Saunders Elsevier, St. Louis, MO.
24. **World Health Organization.** 2014. Severe malaria. *Trop Med Int Health* **19**(Suppl 1)**:**7–131.
25. **Trampuz A, Jereb M, Muzlovic I, Prabhu RM.** 2003. Clinical review: severe malaria. *Crit Care* **7:**315–323.
26. **Rowe JA, Claessens A, Corrigan RA, Arman M.** 2009. Adhesion of *Plasmodium falciparum*-infected erythrocytes to human cells: molecular mechanisms and therapeutic implications. *Expert Rev Mol Med* **11:**e16.
27. **Centers for Disease Control and Prevention.** 2017. Malaria. https://www.cdc.gov/malaria/. Accessed 21 May 2017.
28. **Tan KR, Wiegand RE, Arguin PM.** 2013. Exchange transfusion for severe malaria: evidence base and literature review. *Clin Infect Dis* **57:**923–928.
29. **Garcia LS.** 2009. *Practical Guide to Diagnostic Parasitology*, 2nd ed. ASM Press, Washington, DC.
30. **Clinical and Laboratory Standards Institute.** 2000. M15-A laboratory diagnosis of blood-borne parasitic diseases. Approved guideline, vol 12. CLSI/NCCLS, Wayne, PA.
31. **Mathison BA, Pritt BS.** 2017. Update on malaria diagnostics and test utilization. *J Clin Microbiol* **55:**2009–2017.
32. **Garcia LS, Bruckner DA.** 1997. *Diagnostic Medical Parasitology*, 3rd ed. ASM Press, Washington, DC.
33. **World Health Organization.** 2015. *Guidelines for the Treatment of Malaria*, 3rd ed. World Health Organization Press, Geneva, Switzerland.
34. **Foundation for Innovative New Diagnostics (FIND).** 2012. Malaria rapid diagnostic test performance. Results of WHO product testing of malaria RDTs: Round 4 (2012). TDR/World Health Organization Press, Geneva, Switzerland.
35. **Vasoo S, Pritt BS.** 2013. Molecular diagnostics and parasitic disease. *Clin Lab Med* **33:**461–503.
36. **Garcia LS.** 2007. *Diagnostic Medical Parasitology*, 5th ed. ASM Press, Washington, DC.
37. **Ochola LB, Vounatsou P, Smith T, Mabaso ML, Newton CR.** 2006. The reliability of diagnostic techniques in the diagnosis and management of malaria in the absence of a gold standard. *Lancet Infect Dis* **6:**582–588.
38. **Moody A.** 2002. Rapid diagnostic tests for malaria parasites. *Clin Microbiol Rev* **15:**66–78.
39. **Norgan AP, Arguello HE, Sloan LM, Fernholz EC, Pritt BS.** 2013. A method for reducing the sloughing of thick blood films for malaria diagnosis. *Malar J* **12:**231.
40. **Ash LR, Orihel TC.** 2007. *Ash & Orihel's Atlas of Human Parasitology*, 5th ed. ASCP Press, Chicago, IL.
41. **World Health Organization.** 2000. *Bench Aids for the Diagnosis of Malaria Infections*. World Health Organization Press, Geneva, Switzerland.

42. **Lee KS, Cox-Singh J, Singh B.** 2009. Morphological features and differential counts of *Plasmodium knowlesi* parasites in naturally acquired human infections. *Malar J* **8:**73.
43. **Garcia LS, Isenberg HD.** 2007. *Clinical Microbiology Procedures Handbook*, 2nd ed. ASM Press, Washington, DC.
44. **Keiser J, Utzinger J, Premji Z, Yamagata Y, Singer BH.** 2002. Acridine Orange for malaria diagnosis: its diagnostic performance, its promotion and implementation in Tanzania, and the implications for malaria control. *Ann Trop Med Parasitol* **96:**643–654.
45. **Wilson ML.** 2012. Malaria rapid diagnostic tests. *Clin Infect Dis* **54:**1637–1641.
46. **World Health Organization.** 2017. WHO-FIND malaria RDT evaluation programme. http://www.who.int/malaria/areas/diagnosis/rapid-diagnostic-tests/rdt-evaluation-programme/en/. Accessed 21 May 2017.
47. **World Health Organization.** 2016. WHO list of prequalified *in vitro* diagnostic products. http://www.who.int/diagnostics_laboratory/evaluations/160324_prequalified_product_list.pdf. Accessed 21 May 2017.
48. **World Health Organization.** 2016. False-negative RDT results and implications of new reports of *P. falciparum* histidine-rich protein 2/3 gene deletions. http://www.who.int/malaria/publications/atoz/information-note-hrp2-based-rdt/en/. Accessed 21 May 2017.
49. **Fried M, Muehlenbachs A, Duffy PE.** 2012. Diagnosing malaria in pregnancy: an update. *Expert Rev Anti Infect Ther* **10:**1177–1187.
50. **DiMaio MA, Pereira IT, George TI, Banaei N.** 2012. Performance of BinaxNOW for diagnosis of malaria in a U.S. hospital. *J Clin Microbiol* **50:**2877–2880.
51. **Ota-Sullivan K, Blecker-Shelly DL.** 2013. Use of the rapid BinaxNOW malaria test in a 24-hour laboratory associated with accurate detection and decreased malaria testing turnaround times in a pediatric setting where malaria is not endemic. *J Clin Microbiol* **51:**1567–1569.
52. **Bobenchik A, Shimizu-Cohen R, Humphries RM.** 2013. Use of rapid diagnostic tests for diagnosis of malaria in the United States. *J Clin Microbiol* **51:**379.
53. **Mixson-Hayden T, Lucchi NW, Udhayakumar V.** 2010. Evaluation of three PCR-based diagnostic assays for detecting mixed *Plasmodium* infection. *BMC Res Notes* **3:**88.
54. **Luchavez J, Espino F, Curameng P, Espina R, Bell D, Chiodini P, Nolder D, Sutherland C, Lee KS, Singh B.** 2008. Human infections with *Plasmodium knowlesi*, the Philippines. *Emerg Infect Dis* **14:**811–813.
55. **Tanomsing N, Imwong M, Sutherland CJ, Dolecek C, Hien TT, Nosten F, Day NP, White NJ, Snounou G.** 2013. Genetic marker suitable for identification and genotyping of *Plasmodium ovale curtisi* and *Plasmodium ovale wallikeri*. *J Clin Microbiol* **51:**4213–4216.
56. **Swan H, Sloan L, Muyombwe A, Chavalitshewinkoon-Petmitr P, Krudsood S, Leowattana W, Wilairatana P, Looareesuwan S, Rosenblatt J.** 2005. Evaluation of a real-time polymerase chain reaction assay for the diagnosis of malaria in patients from Thailand. *Am J Trop Med Hyg* **73:**850–854.
57. **Shokoples SE, Ndao M, Kowalewska-Grochowska K, Yanow SK.** 2009. Multiplexed real-time PCR assay for discrimination of *Plasmodium* species with improved sensitivity for mixed infections. *J Clin Microbiol* **47:** 975–980 .
58. **Cnops L, Jacobs J, Van Esbroeck M.** 2011. Validation of a four-primer real-time PCR as a diagnostic tool for single and mixed *Plasmodium* infections. *Clin Microbiol Infect* **17:**1101–1107.
59. **Johnston SP, Pieniazek NJ, Xayavong MV, Slemenda SB, Wilkins PP, da Silva AJ.** 2006. PCR as a confirmatory technique for laboratory diagnosis of malaria. *J Clin Microbiol* **44:**1087–1089.
60. **Farcas GA, Soeller R, Zhong K, Zahirieh A, Kain KC.** 2006. Real-time polymerase chain reaction assay for the rapid detection and characterization of chloroquine-resistant *Plasmodium falciparum* malaria in returned travelers. *Clin Infect Dis* **42:**622–627.
61. **Snounou G, Viriyakosol S, Zhu XP, Jarra W, Pinheiro L, do Rosario VE, Thaithong S, Brown KN.** 1993. High sensitivity of detection of human malaria parasites by the use of nested polymerase chain reaction. *Mol Biochem Parasitol* **61:**315–320.
62. **Kamau E, Tolbert LS, Kortepeter L, Pratt M, Nyakoe N, Muringo L, Ogutu B, Waitumbi JN, Ockenhouse CF.** 2011. Development of a highly sensitive genus-specific quantitative reverse transcriptase real-time PCR assay for detection and quantitation of plasmodium by amplifying RNA and DNA of the 18S rRNA genes. *J Clin Microbiol* **49:**2946–2953.
63. **Padley DJ, Heath AB, Sutherland C, Chiodini PL, Baylis SA, Collaborative Study Group.** 2008. Establishment of the 1st World Health Organization International Standard for *Plasmodium falciparum* DNA for nucleic acid amplification technique (NAT)-based assays. *Malar J* **7:**139.
64. **Mens PF, Schoone GJ, Kager PA, Schallig HD.** 2006. Detection and identification of human *Plasmodium* species with real-time quantitative nucleic acid sequence-based amplification. *Malar J* **5:**80.
65. **Sirichaisinthop J, Buates S, Watanabe R, Han ET, Suktawonjaroenpon W, Krasaesub S, Takeo S, Tsuboi T, Sattabongkot J.** 2011. Evaluation of loop-mediated isothermal amplification (LAMP) for malaria diagnosis in a field setting. *Am J Trop Med Hyg* **85:**594–596.
66. **LaBarre P, Hawkins KR, Gerlach J, Wilmoth J, Beddoe A, Singleton J, Boyle D, Weigl B.** 2011. A simple, inexpensive device for nucleic acid amplification without electricity: toward instrument-free molecular diagnostics in low-resource settings. *PLoS One* **6:**e19738.
67. **Mens PF, van Amerongen A, Sawa P, Kager PA, Schallig HD.** 2008. Molecular diagnosis of malaria in the field: development of a novel 1-step nucleic acid lateral flow immunoassay for the detection of all 4 human *Plasmodium* spp. and its evaluation in Mbita, Kenya. *Diagn Microbiol Infect Dis* **61:**421–427.
68. **Laoboonchai A, Kawamoto F, Thanoosingha N, Kojima S, Scott Miller RR, Kain KC, Wongsrichanalai C.** 2001. PCR-based ELISA technique for malaria diagnosis of specimens from Thailand. *Trop Med Int Health* **6:**458–462.
69. **Reesink HW.** 2005. European strategies against the parasite transfusion risk. *Transfus Clin Biol* **12:**1–4.
70. **Sulzer AJ, Wilson M.** 1971. The indirect fluorescent antibody test for the detection of occult malaria in blood donors. *Bull World Health Organ* **45:**375–379.
71. **She RC, Rawlins ML, Mohl R, Perkins SL, Hill HR, Litwin CM.** 2007. Comparison of immunofluorescence antibody testing and two enzyme immunoassays in the serologic diagnosis of malaria. *J Travel Med* **14:**105–111.
72. **Demirev PA, Feldman AB, Kongkasuriyachai D, Scholl P, Sullivan D Jr, Kumar N.** 2002. Detection of malaria parasites in blood by laser desorption mass spectrometry. *Anal Chem* **74:**3262–3266.
73. **Lukianova-Hleb EY, Campbell KM, Constantinou PE, Braam J, Olson JS, Ware RE, Sullivan DJ Jr, Lapotko DO.** 2014. Hemozoin-generated vapor nanobubbles for transdermal reagent- and needle-free detection of malaria. *Proc Natl Acad Sci USA* **111:**900–905.
74. **World Health Organization.** 2015. *Guidelines for the Treatment of Malaria*, 3rd ed.. http://www.who.int/malaria/publications/atoz/9789241549127/en/. Accessed 21 May 2017.
75. **Freedman DO.** 2008. Clinical practice. Malaria prevention in short-term travelers. *N Engl J Med* **359:**603–612.
76. **Worldwide Antimalarial Resistance Network (WWARN).** 2017. Malaria drug resistance. http://www.wwarn.org/about-us/malaria-drug-resistance. Accessed 15 October 2017.
77. **World Health Organization.** 2017. Artemisinin and artemisinin-based combination therapy resistance status report, April 2017. http://apps.who.int/iris/bitstream/10665/255213/1/WHO-HTM-GMP-2017.9-eng.pdf?ua=1. Accessed 15 October 2017.
78. **Sá JM, Chong JL, Wellems TE.** 2011. Malaria drug resistance: new observations and developments. *Essays Biochem* **51:**137–160.

79. **Price RN, von Seidlein L, Valecha N, Nosten F, Baird JK, White NJ.** 2014. Global extent of chloroquine-resistant *Plasmodium vivax*: a systematic review and meta-analysis. *Lancet Infect Dis* **14:**982–991.
80. **Pradines B, Pistone T, Ezzedine K, Briolant S, Bertaux L, Receveur MC, Parzy D, Millet P, Rogier C, Malvy D.** 2010. Quinine-resistant malaria in traveler returning from Senegal, 2007. *Emerg Infect Dis* **16:**546–548.
81. **Björkman A, Phillips-Howard PA.** 1990. The epidemiology of drug-resistant malaria. *Trans R Soc Trop Med Hyg* **84:**177–180.
82. **Dondorp AM, Nosten F, Yi P, Das D, Phyo AP, Tarning J, Lwin KM, Ariey F, Hanpithakpong W, Lee SJ, Ringwald P, Silamut K, Imwong M, Chotivanich K, Lim P, Herdman T, An SS, Yeung S, Singhasivanon P, Day NP, Lindegardh N, Socheat D, White NJ.** 2009. Artemisinin resistance in *Plasmodium falciparum* malaria. *N Engl J Med* **361:**455–467.
83. **Rieckmann KH, Campbell GH, Sax LJ, Ema JE.** 1978. Drug sensitivity of *plasmodium falciparum*. An *in-vitro* microtechnique. *Lancet* **1:**22–23.
84. **Steenkeste N, Dillies MA, Khim N, Sismeiro O, Chy S, Lim P, Crameri A, Bouchier C, Mercereau-Puijalon O, Beck HP, Imwong M, Dondorp AM, Socheat D, Rogier C, Coppée JY, Ariey F.** 2009. FlexiChip package: an universal microarray with a dedicated analysis software for high-thoughput SNPs detection linked to anti-malarial drug resistance. *Malar J* **8:**229.
85. **Vannier EG, Diuk-Wasser MA, Ben Mamoun C, Krause PJ.** 2015. Babesiosis. *Infect Dis Clin North Am* **29:**357–370.
86. **Herwaldt BL, de Bruyn G, Pieniazek NJ, Homer M, Lofy KH, Slemenda SB, Fritsche TR, Persing DH, Limaye AP.** 2004. *Babesia divergens*-like infection, Washington State. *Emerg Infect Dis* **10:**622–629.
87. **Persing DH, Herwaldt BL, Glaser C, Lane RS, Thomford JW, Mathiesen D, Krause PJ, Phillip DF, Conrad PA.** 1995. Infection with a babesia-like organism in northern California. *N Engl J Med* **332:**298–303.
88. **Conrad PA, Kjemtrup AM, Carreno RA, Thomford J, Wainwright K, Eberhard M, Quick R, Telford SR III, Herwaldt BL.** 2006. Description of *Babesia duncani* n.sp. (Apicomplexa: Babesiidae) from humans and its differentiation from other piroplasms. *Int J Parasitol* **36:**779–789.
89. **Herwaldt B, Persing DH, Précigout EA, Goff WL, Mathiesen DA, Taylor PW, Eberhard ML, Gorenflot AF.** 1996. A fatal case of babesiosis in Missouri: identification of another piroplasm that infects humans. *Ann Intern Med* **124:**643–650.
90. **Goethert HK, Telford SR III.** 2003. Enzootic transmission of *Babesia divergens* among cottontail rabbits on Nantucket Island, Massachusetts. *Am J Trop Med Hyg* **69:**455–460.
91. **Gray J, Zintl A, Hildebrandt A, Hunfeld KP, Weiss L.** 2010. Zoonotic babesiosis: overview of the disease and novel aspects of pathogen identity. *Ticks Tick Borne Dis* **1:**3–10.
92. **Herwaldt BL, Cacciò S, Gherlinzoni F, Aspöck H, Slemenda SB, Piccaluga P, Martinelli G, Edelhofer R, Hollenstein U, Poletti G, Pampiglione S, Löschenberger K, Tura S, Pieniazek NJ.** 2003. Molecular characterization of a non-*Babesia divergens* organism causing zoonotic babesiosis in Europe. *Emerg Infect Dis* **9:**942–948.
93. **Häselbarth K, Tenter AM, Brade V, Krieger G, Hunfeld KP.** 2007. First case of human babesiosis in Germany: clinical presentation and molecular characterisation of the pathogen. *Int J Med Microbiol* **297:**197–204.
94. **Hildebrandt A, Hunfeld KP, Baier M, Krumbholz A, Sachse S, Lorenzen T, Kiehntopf M, Fricke HJ, Straube E.** 2007. First confirmed autochthonous case of human *Babesia microti* infection in Europe. *Eur J Clin Microbiol Infect Dis* **26:**595–601.
95. **Shih CM, Liu LP, Chung WC, Ong SJ, Wang CC.** 1997. Human babesiosis in Taiwan: asymptomatic infection with a *Babesia microti*-like organism in a Taiwanese woman. *J Clin Microbiol* **35:**450–454.
96. **Wei Q, Tsuji M, Zamoto A, Kohsaki M, Matsui T, Shiota T, Telford SR III, Ishihara C.** 2001. Human babesiosis in Japan: isolation of *Babesia microti*-like parasites from an asymptomatic transfusion donor and from a rodent from an area where babesiosis is endemic. *J Clin Microbiol* **39:**2178–2183.
97. **Jiang JF, Zheng YC, Jiang RR, Li H, Huo QB, Jiang BG, Sun Y, Jia N, Wang YW, Ma L, Liu HB, Chu YL, Ni XB, Liu K, Song YD, Yao NN, Wang H, Sun T, Cao WC.** 2015. Epidemiological, clinical, and laboratory characteristics of 48 cases of "*Babesia venatorum*" infection in China: a descriptive study. *Lancet Infect Dis* **15:**196–203.
98. **Kim JY, Cho SH, Joo HN, Tsuji M, Cho SR, Park IJ, Chung GT, Ju JW, Cheun HI, Lee HW, Lee YH, Kim TS.** 2007. First case of human babesiosis in Korea: detection and characterization of a novel type of *Babesia* sp. (KO1) similar to ovine babesia. *J Clin Microbiol* **45:**2084–2087.
99. **Hunfeld KP, Hildebrandt A, Gray JS.** 2008. Babesiosis: recent insights into an ancient disease. *Int J Parasitol* **38:**1219–1237.
100. **Criado-Fornelio A, Martinez-Marcos A, Buling-Saraña A, Barba-Carretero JC.** 2003. Molecular studies on *Babesia, Theileria* and *Hepatozoon* in southern Europe. Part II. Phylogenetic analysis and evolutionary history. *Vet Parasitol* **114:**173–194.
101. **Cornillot E, Hadj-Kaddour K, Dassouli A, Noel B, Ranwez V, Vacherie B, Augagneur Y, Brès V, Duclos A, Randazzo S, Carcy B, Debierre-Grockiego F, Delbecq S, Moubri-Ménage K, Shams-Eldin H, Usmani-Brown S, Bringaud F, Wincker P, Vivarès CP, Schwarz RT, Schetters TP, Krause PJ, Gorenflot A, Berry V, Barbe V, Ben Mamoun C.** 2012. Sequencing of the smallest Apicomplexan genome from the human pathogen *Babesia microti*. *Nucleic Acids Res* **40:**9102–9114.
102. **Cornillot E, Dassouli A, Garg A, Pachikara N, Randazzo S, Depoix D, Carcy B, Delbecq S, Frutos R, Silva JC, Sutton R, Krause PJ, Mamoun CB.** 2013. Whole genome mapping and re-organization of the nuclear and mitochondrial genomes of *Babesia microti* isolates. *PLoS One* **8:**e72657.
103. **Centers for Disease Control and Prevention (CDC).** 2012. Babesiosis surveillance: 18 states, 2011. *MMWR Morb Mortal Wkly Rep* **61:**505–509.
104. **Centers for Disease Control and Prevention.** 2016. Surveillance for babesiosis: United States, 2014 annual summary. https://www.cdc.gov/parasites/babesiosis/resources/babesiosis_surveillance_summary_2016.pdf. Accessed 21 May 2017.
105. **Vannier E, Krause PJ.** 2012. Human babesiosis. *N Engl J Med* **366:**2397–2407.
106. **Zintl A, Mulcahy G, Skerrett HE, Taylor SM, Gray JS.** 2003. *Babesia divergens*, a bovine blood parasite of veterinary and zoonotic importance. *Clin Microbiol Rev* **16:**622–636.
107. **Leiby DA.** 2011. Transfusion-transmitted *Babesia* spp.: bull's-eye on *Babesia microti*. *Clin Microbiol Rev* **24:**14–28.
108. **Joseph JT, Purtill K, Wong SJ, Munoz J, Teal A, Madison-Antenucci S, Horowitz HW, Aguero-Rosenfeld ME, Moore JM, Abramowsky C, Wormser GP.** 2012. Vertical transmission of *Babesia microti*, United States. *Emerg Infect Dis* **18:**1318–1321.
109. **Herwaldt BL, Linden JV, Bosserman E, Young C, Olkowska D, Wilson M.** 2011. Transfusion-associated babesiosis in the United States: a description of cases. *Ann Intern Med* **155:**509–519.
110. **Burgess MJ, Rosenbaum ER, Pritt BS, Haselow DT, Ferren KM, Alzghoul BN, Rico JC, Sloan LM, Ramanan P, Purushothaman R, Bradsher RW.** 2017. Possible transfusion-transmitted *Babesia divergens*-like/MO-1 infection in an Arkansas patient. *Clin Infect Dis* **64:**1622–1625.
111. **American Red Cross.** 2017. Infectious disease testing: babesiosis (*Babesia microti*) antibody and NAT (2012). http://www.redcrossblood.org/learn-about-blood/blood-testing#babesia_test. Accessed 15 October 2017.
112. **Moritz ED, Winton CS, Tonnetti L, Townsend RL, Berardi VP, Hewins ME, Weeks KE, Dodd RY, Stramer SL.** 2016. Screening for *Babesia microti* in the U.S. blood supply. *N Engl J Med* **375:**2236–2245.
113. **Wormser GP, Dattwyler RJ, Shapiro ED, Halperin JJ, Steere AC, Klempner MS, Krause PJ, Bakken JS, Strle F, Stanek G, Bockenstedt L, Fish D, Dumler JS, Nadelman RB.** 2006. The clinical assessment, treatment, and prevention of Lyme disease, human granulocytic anaplasmosis, and babesiosis: clinical practice guidelines by the Infectious Diseases Society of America. *Clin Infect Dis* **43:**1089–1134.

114. **Sanchez E, Vannier E, Wormser GP, Hu LT.** 2016. Diagnosis, treatment, and prevention of Lyme disease, human granulocytic anaplasmosis, and babesiosis: a review. *JAMA* **315:**1767–1777.
115. **Diuk-Wasser MA, Vannier E, Krause PJ.** 2016. Coinfection by *Ixodes* tick-borne pathogens: ecological, epidemiological, and clinical consequences. *Trends Parasitol* **32:**30–42.
116. **Krause PJ, Gewurz BE, Hill D, Marty FM, Vannier E, Foppa IM, Furman RR, Neuhaus E, Skowron G, Gupta S, McCalla C, Pesanti EL, Young M, Heiman D, Hsue G, Gelfand JA, Wormser GP, Dickason J, Bia FJ, Hartman B, Telford SR III, Christianson D, Dardick K, Coleman M, Girotto JE, Spielman A.** 2008. Persistent and relapsing babesiosis in immunocompromised patients. *Clin Infect Dis* **46:**370–376.
117. **Persing DH, Mathiesen D, Marshall WF, Telford SR, Spielman A, Thomford JW, Conrad PA.** 1992. Detection of *Babesia microti* by polymerase chain reaction. *J Clin Microbiol* **30:**2097–2103.
118. **Krause PJ, Telford S III, Spielman A, Ryan R, Magera J, Rajan TV, Christianson D, Alberghini TV, Bow L, Persing D.** 1996. Comparison of PCR with blood smear and inoculation of small animals for diagnosis of *Babesia microti* parasitemia. *J Clin Microbiol* **34:**2791–2794.
119. **Teal AE, Habura A, Ennis J, Keithly JS, Madison-Antenucci S.** 2012. A new real-time PCR assay for improved detection of the parasite *Babesia microti*. *J Clin Microbiol* **50:**903–908.
120. **Liu D.** 2013. *Molecular Detection of Human Parasitic Pathogens*. CRC Press, Boca Raton, FL.
121. **Brandt F, Healy GR, Welch M.** 1977. Human babesiosis: the isolation of *Babesia microti* in golden hamsters. *J Parasitol* **63:**934–937.
122. **Krause PJ, Telford SR III, Ryan R, Conrad PA, Wilson M, Thomford JW, Spielman A.** 1994. Diagnosis of babesiosis: evaluation of a serologic test for the detection of *Babesia microti* antibody. *J Infect Dis* **169:**923–926.d
123. **Chisholm ES, Ruebush TK II, Sulzer AJ, Healy GR.** 1978. *Babesia microti* infection in man: evaluation of an indirect immunofluorescent antibody test. *Am J Trop Med Hyg* **27:**14–19.
124. **Homer MJ, Aguilar-Delfin I, Telford SR III, Krause PJ, Persing DH.** 2000. Babesiosis. *Clin Microbiol Rev* **13:**451–469.
125. **Duh D, Jelovsek M, Avsic-Zupanc T.** 2007. Evaluation of an indirect fluorescence immunoassay for the detection of serum antibodies against *Babesia divergens* in humans. *Parasitology* **134:**179–185.
126. **Quick RE, Herwaldt BL, Thomford JW, Garnett ME, Eberhard ML, Wilson M, Spach DH, Dickerson JW, Telford SR III, Steingart KR, Pollock R, Persing DH, Kobayashi JM, Juranek DD, Conrad PA.** 1993. Babesiosis in Washington State: a new species of *Babesia? Ann Intern Med* **119:**284–290.
127. **Westblade LF, Simon MS, Mathison BA, Kirkman LA.** 2017. *Babesia microti*: from mice to ticks to an increasing number of highly susceptible humans. *J Clin Microbiol* **55:**2903–2912.
128. **Gay F, Traoré B, Zanoni J, Danis M, Fribourg-Blanc A.** 1996. Direct acridine orange fluorescence examination of blood slides compared to current techniques for malaria diagnosis. *Trans R Soc Trop Med Hyg* **90:**516–518.
129. **Long GW, Jones TR, Rickman LS, Trimmer R, Hoffman SL.** 1991. Acridine orange detection of *Plasmodium falciparum* malaria: relationship between sensitivity and optical configuration. *Am J Trop Med Hyg* **44:**402–405.
130. **Rickman LS, Long GW, Oberst R, Cabanban A, Sangalang R, Smith JI, Chulay JD, Hoffman SL.** 1989. Rapid diagnosis of malaria by acridine orange staining of centrifuged parasites. *Lancet* **1:**68–71.
131. **Spielman A, Perrone JB, Teklehaimanot A, Balcha F, Wardlaw SC, Levine RA.** 1988. Malaria diagnosis by direct observation of centrifuged samples of blood. *Am J Trop Med Hyg* **39:**337–342.
132. **van Vianen PH, van Engen A, Thaithong S, van der Keur M, Tanke HJ, van der Kaay HJ, Mons B, Janse CJ.** 1993. Flow cytometric screening of blood samples for malaria parasites. *Cytometry* **14:**276–280.
133. **Jamjoom GA.** 1983. Dark-field microscopy for detection of malaria in unstained blood films. *J Clin Microbiol* **17:**717–721.
134. **Jamjoom GA.** 1991. Improvement in dark-field microscopy for the rapid detection of malaria parasites and its adaptation to field conditions. *Trans R Soc Trop Med Hyg* **85:**38–39.
135. **Connor DH.** 1997. *Pathology of Infectious Diseases*. Appleton & Lange, Stamford, CT.
136. **Franzén L, Westin G, Shabo R, Aslund L, Perlmann H, Persson T, Wigzell H, Pettersson U.** 1984. Analysis of clinical specimens by hybridisation with probe containing repetitive DNA from *Plasmodium falciparum*. A novel approach to malaria diagnosis. *Lancet* **1:**525–528.
137. **Barker RH Jr, Suebsaeng L, Rooney W, Alecrim GC, Dourado HV, Wirth DF.** 1986. Specific DNA probe for the diagnosis of *Plasmodium falciparum* malaria. *Science* **231:**1434–1436.
138. **Singh B, Bobogare A, Cox-Singh J, Snounou G, Abdullah MS, Rahman HA.** 1999. A genus- and species-specific nested polymerase chain reaction malaria detection assay for epidemiologic studies. *Am J Trop Med Hyg* **60:**687–692.
139. **Han ET, Watanabe R, Sattabongkot J, Khuntirat B, Sirichaisinthop J, Iriko H, Jin L, Takeo S, Tsuboi T.** 2007. Detection of four *Plasmodium* species by genus- and species-specific loop-mediated isothermal amplification for clinical diagnosis. *J Clin Microbiol* **45:**2521–2528.

Leishmania and *Trypanosoma*

DAVID A. BRUCKNER AND JAIME A. LABARCA

140

Leishmania spp. and *Trypanosoma* spp. have a common ancestry and belong to the Trypanosomatida, found in the supergroup Excavata of the eukaryotes (Excavata: Discicristata: Euglenozoa: Kinetoplastea: Trypanosomatida) (1, 2). This is a group of unicellular organisms that have modified mitochondrial organelles and a single flagellum.

Leishmaniasis is principally a zoonosis, and the organisms are obligate intracellular parasites transmitted to humans by bites from an infected female sand fly. For *Leishmania* in the Old World, there is only one subgenus, *Leishmania*; however, in the New World, the genus has been split into subgenera (*Leishmania* and *Viannia*) according to the development of the organism in the digestive tract (peripyloric or suprapyloric) of the sand fly. Depending on the geographic area, many different species can infect humans, producing a variety of diseases (cutaneous, diffuse cutaneous, mucocutaneous, and visceral diseases) (Table 1).

Human *Trypanosoma* spp. are hemoflagellate protozoa that live in the blood and tissue of the human host. American trypanosomiasis (Chagas' disease) is produced by *Trypanosoma cruzi* and is confined to the Americas. *Trypanosoma rangeli* produces an asymptomatic infection and is also present only in the Americas. African trypanosomiasis (sleeping sickness, or human African trypanosomiasis) is caused by *Trypanosoma brucei gambiense* and *Trypanosoma brucei rhodesiense* and is confined to the central belt of Africa. African trypanosomes and *T. rangeli* are transmitted directly into the bite wound by salivary secretions from the insect vector, whereas *T. cruzi* is transmitted primarily through contamination of the bite wound with the feces and by fecal contamination of the food supply by the reduviid bug (Table 2). The first documented case of human trypanosomiasis caused by *Trypanosoma evansi* was detected in India (3).

LEISHMANIA SPP.

Recent estimates suggest that there are approximately 350 million people at risk of acquiring leishmaniasis, with 700,000 to 1 million new cases per year (4). New species of *Leishmania* are detected frequently. The taxonomy of leishmaniasis continues to be controversial and in a state of dynamic flux. Species differentiation is currently based on molecular techniques rather than geographical distribution and clinical presentation (5–7). The molecular techniques used for identification to species level include PCR amplification of chromosomal and kinetoplastic DNA, including specific protein-coding genes (6, 8). Diagnostically, many laboratories still rely on geographical distribution and clinical identification of specimens (Table 1).

Life Cycle and Morphology

The parasite has two distinct phases in its life cycle (amastigote and promastigote) (Fig. 1; see www.cdc.gov/dpdx/index.html for the complete life cycle). The amastigote stage (Leishman-Donovan body) is found in reticuloendothelial cells of the mammalian host. The amastigote form is small, is round or oval, measures 3 to 5 μm, and contains a large nucleus and small kinetoplast (Fig. 1 and 2). Under ideal microscopic conditions, the parabasal body may also be detected. This stage undergoes multiplication within the reticuloendothelial cells of the host.

Upon ingestion during a blood meal by the insect vector (sand fly), the amastigote transforms into the promastigote stage (Fig. 3). Promastigotes multiply in the gut of the sand fly, transform to metacyclic promastigotes, and migrate to the hypostome, where they are released when the next blood meal is taken. The complete life cycle in the sand fly is 4 to 18 days. Upon inoculation into the bite site, the promastigote changes to the amastigote form after being engulfed by tissue macrophages. This form change helps to defeat the host's immune response. Changes in the parasite's surface molecules play an important role in macrophage attachment and evasion of the host's immune response, including manipulating the macrophage's signaling pathways.

The life cycles of *Leishmania* organisms are similar for cutaneous, mucocutaneous, and visceral leishmaniasis, except that infected reticuloendothelial cells can be found throughout the body in visceral leishmaniasis.

Epidemiology and Transmission

All adult female sand flies transmitting leishmaniasis belong to the genus *Phlebotomus* in the Old World and *Lutzomyia* in the New World. There are >30 species of sand flies that can transmit leishmaniasis. The disease is considered primarily a zoonosis, with natural reservoirs including rodents, opossums, anteaters, sloths, and dogs. In certain areas of the world where the disease is endemic, the infection can be transmitted by a human-vector-human cycle. The infection

TABLE 1 Features of *Leishmania* organisms infecting humans

Proposed subgenus	Current subgenus and complex	Species	Disease type[a]	Recommended specimen	Geographic distribution
Euleishmania	*Leishmania*				
	L. major complex	*L. major*	CL	Skin biopsy	Afghanistan, Africa, Middle East, former USSR
	L. tropica complex	*L. tropica*	CL	Skin biopsy	Afghanistan, India, Turkey, former USSR
		L. killicki	CL	Skin biopsy	Algeria, Tunisia
		L. aethiopica	CL, DCL, MCL	Skin or mucosal biopsy	Ethiopia, Kenya, former USSR, Yemen
	L. mexicana complex	*L. amazonensis*	CL, DCL	Skin or mucosal biopsy	Brazil, Venezuela
		L. garnhami	CL	Skin biopsy	Venezuela
		L. mexicana	CL, DCL, MCL	Skin or mucosal biopsy	Belize, Guatemala, Mexico, Texas
		L. venezuelensis	CL	Skin biopsy	Venezuela
		L. pifanoi	CL, DCL	Skin or mucosal biopsy	Brazil, Venezuela
		L. waltoni	CL, DCL	Skin biopsy	Central and South America
	L. donovani complex	*L. archibaldi*	VL	Tissue[b]	Old World
		L. chagasi	VL	Tissue	New World
		L. donovani	VL, CL, MCL, DL	Tissue Skin or mucosal biopsy	Africa, Asia. South America
		L. infantum	VL	Tissue	Old World
	Viannia				
	L. braziliensis complex	*L. braziliensis*	CL, MCL	Skin or mucosal biopsy	Central and South America
		L. peruviana	CL	Skin biopsy	Colombia, Costa Rica, Panama
	L. guyanensis complex	*L. guyanensis*	CL, MCL	Skin or mucosal biopsy	Brazil, Colombia, French Guiana, Peru
		L. panamensis	CL	Skin biopsy	Colombia, Costa Rica, Peru
		L. shawii	CL	Skin biopsy	Brazil
		L. lainsoni	CL	Skin biopsy	Brazil
		L. naiffi	CL	Skin biopsy	Brazil, Caribbean Islands
		L. lindenbergi	CL	Skin biopsy	Brazil
	L. enriettii complex	*L. martiniquensis*	CL, DL, VL	Skin biopsy Tissue	Caribbean Islands, Thailand
		L. siamensis	CL	Skin biopsy	Thailand
Paraleishmania		*L. colombiensis*	CL, VL	Skin biopsy Tissue	Colombia, Panama, Venezuela

[a]CL, cutaneous leishmaniasis; DCL, diffuse cutaneous leishmaniasis; DL, diffuse leishmaniasis; MCL, mucocutaneous leishmaniasis; VL, visceral leishmaniasis.
[b]Bone marrow, liver, lymph node, spleen.

may also be transmitted by direct contact with an infected lesion or mechanically through bites by stable or dog flies (*Stomoxys calcitrans*). If the blood meal of the fly is interrupted and it restarts its meal on another host, it can regurgitate part of the last meal with salivary juices into the bite site, thereby infecting that host. More than 66% of the new human cases of cutaneous leishmaniasis occur in Afghanistan, Algeria, Brazil, Colombia, Iran, and Syria (4). Autochthonous human infections have been described in Texas and Oklahoma (8). Most of the diagnosed cases of mucocutaneous leishmaniasis are from Bolivia, Brazil, Ethiopia, and Peru (4).

Visceral leishmaniasis may exist as an endemic, epidemic, and sporadic disease. The disease is a zoonosis

TABLE 2 Characteristics of agents of trypanosomiasis

Characteristic	*T. brucei rhodesiense*	*T. brucei gambiense*	*T. cruzi*	*T. rangeli*
Vector	Tsetse fly (*Glossina*)	Tsetse fly (*Glossina*)	Reduviid bug (*Panstrongylus, Rhodnius, Triatoma*)	Reduviid bug (*Rhodnius*)
Primary reservoir	Animals	Humans	Animals	Animals
Illness	Acute, <9 mo	Chronic, months to years	Acute, chronic	Asymptomatic
Epidemiology[a]	Anthropozoonosis	Anthroponosis	Anthropozoonosis	Anthropozoonosis
Diagnostic stage	Trypomastigote	Trypomastigote	Trypomastigote, amastigote	Trypomastigote
Recommended specimen(s)	Blood, CSF, chancre, and lymph node aspirate	Blood, CSF, chancre, and lymph node aspirate	Blood, chagoma, and lymph node aspirate	Blood

[a]Anthropozoonosis, transmission involving a human-animal-human cycle; anthroponosis, transmission involving a human-human cycle.

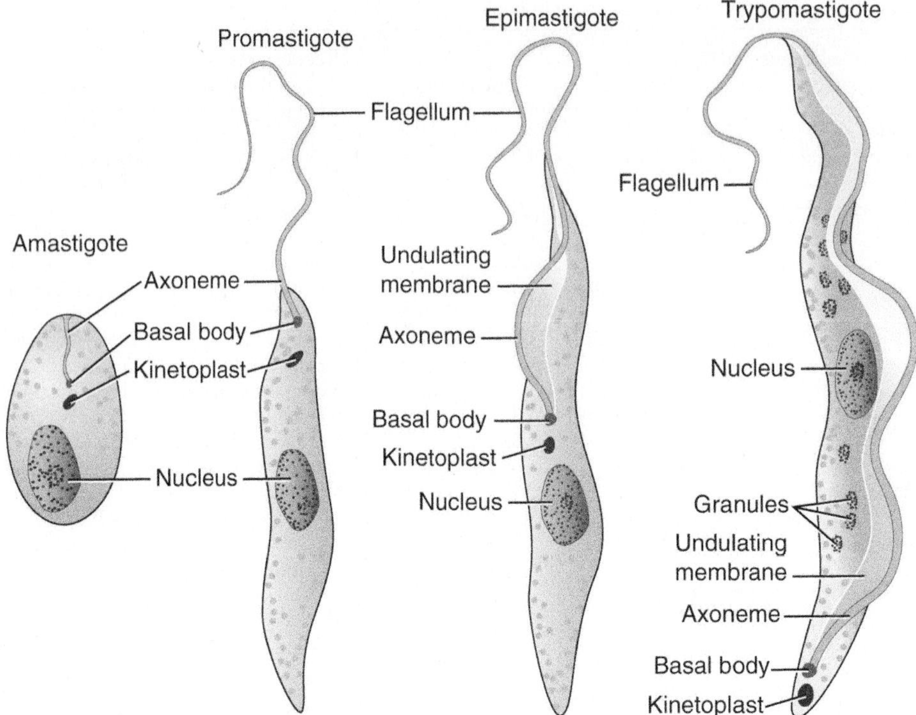

FIGURE 1 Life cycle stages of *Leishmania* and *Trypanosoma* found in human and insect hosts.

except in India and Brazil, where kala-azar is an anthroponosis (9, 10). Natural reservoirs are wild members of the *Canidae* and various rodents for *Leishmania donovani*; dogs, other members of the *Canidae*, and rats for *Leishmania infantum*; and members of the *Canidae* and cats for *Leishmania chagasi* in the Americas. Individuals with post-kala-azar dermal leishmaniasis (PKDL) may be very important reservoirs for maintaining the infection during interendemic cycles. More than 90% of the cases of visceral leishmaniasis are found in Brazil, Ethiopia, India, Kenya, Somalia, and Sudan (4). Bangladesh, India, and Nepal have established kala-azar elimination programs with a target date of 2020 (9, 10).

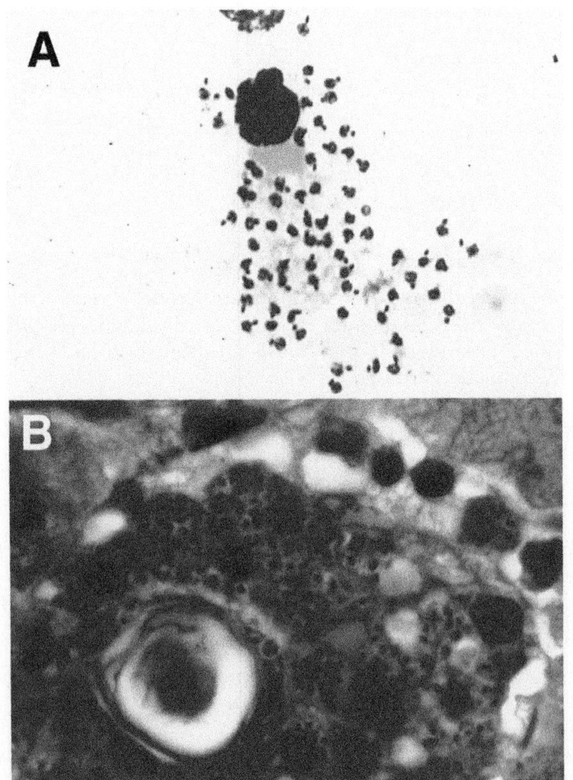

FIGURE 2 (A) *L. donovani* amastigotes from a spleen press preparation (Giemsa stain); (B) *L. donovani* in liver (hematoxylin and eosin stain).

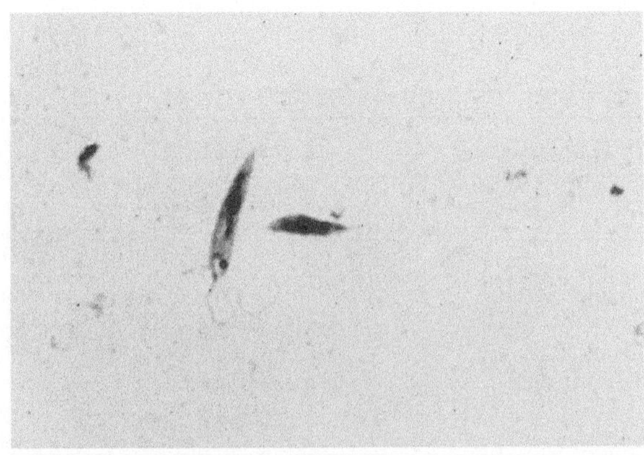

FIGURE 3 *L. donovani* promastigotes (Giemsa stain).

Clinical Significance

Depending on the species involved, infection with *Leishmania* spp. can result in cutaneous, diffuse cutaneous, mucocutaneous, or visceral disease (Table 1). A large number of disease variations have been described, which makes classical disease categories confusing (6, 11). In areas of endemicity, *Leishmania* coinfection of human immunodeficiency virus (HIV)-positive patients is common. Of coinfected patients who remain severely immunocompromised, approximately one-quarter die within the first month of being diagnosed with leishmaniasis. The leishmanial infection manifests itself like an opportunistic infection, and parasites are detected in atypical sites. The use of highly active antiretroviral therapy has significantly improved the prognosis of patients infected with HIV and visceral leishmaniasis (11, 12). Antiretroviral therapy and treatment for leishmaniasis can be given concomitantly; however, patients must be closely monitored for immune reconstitution inflammatory syndrome and the potential for increased drug toxicity (11).

The first sign of cutaneous disease is the appearance of a firm, painless papule at or near the insect bite site (13). The incubation period may be as short as 2 weeks (*Leishmania major*) or as long as several months to 3 years (*Leishmania tropica* and *Leishmania aethiopica*). Papules may be intensely pruritic and will grow to 2 cm or more in diameter. Lesions may progress from a simple papule or erythematous macule to a nodule and ulcerate within days to weeks. In simple cutaneous leishmaniasis, the infection remains localized at the insect bite site, where a definite self-limiting granulomatous response develops. Lesions have been mistaken for basal cell carcinoma, tropical pyoderma, sporotrichosis, and cutaneous mycobacterial infections. Lesions may spontaneously heal over time (months to years) with possible residual scarring. The patient should be watched for development of satellite lesions and lymphatic spread and should also be evaluated for the potential risk of developing mucocutaneous leishmaniasis, at which time drug therapy may be recommended (11). The propensity of developing lymphatic spread or mucocutaneous leishmaniasis is dependent on the immunocompetence of the patient and the geographic area of acquisition of the infection (Table 1).

Mucocutaneous leishmaniasis is produced most often by the *Leishmania braziliensis* complex. At the beginning, the primary lesions may be similar to those found in infections of cutaneous leishmaniasis. Chronic nasal congestion and secretions are a prominent manifestation of mucocutaneous leishmaniasis. Mouth, palatal, pharyngeal, and laryngeal involvement may also occur as the infection develops. Untreated primary lesions may develop into the mucocutaneous form in up to 80% of the cases. Metastatic spread to the nasal or oral mucosa may occur in the presence of the active primary lesion or many years later, after the primary lesion has healed. Mucosal lesions do not heal spontaneously, and secondary bacterial infections are frequent and may be fatal. A small number of mucocutaneous leishmaniasis cases with *L. donovani* and *L. aethiopica* have been reported. Differential diagnosis has included lymphoma, midline granuloma, Wegener's granulomatosis, paracoccidioidomycosis, histoplasmosis, cutaneous mycobacterial infection, syphilis, and leprosy.

Clinical features of the visceral disease vary from asymptomatic, self-resolving infections to frank visceral leishmaniasis. The incubation period may be as short as 10 days and as long as 2 years; usually it is 2 to 4 months. Common symptoms include fever, anorexia, malaise, weight loss, and frequently diarrhea. Visceral leishmaniasis is an important opportunistic infection in individuals infected with HIV. Concomitant HIV infection dramatically increases the risk of developing active visceral leishmaniasis in asymptomatic individuals (12). Individuals coinfected with HIV may not exhibit common symptoms seen in immunocompetent individuals. Common clinical signs include nontender hepatomegaly and splenomegaly, lymphadenopathy, and occasional acute abdominal pain; darkening of facial, hand, foot, and abdominal skin (kala-azar) is often seen in light-skinned persons in India. Anemia, cachexia, and marked enlargement of liver and spleen are noted as the disease progresses. Death may ensue after a few weeks or after 2 to 3 years in chronic cases. The majority of infected individuals are asymptomatic or have very few or minor symptoms that resolve without therapy. There has been a significant increase in leishmaniasis in organ transplant recipients since 1990. Most of the reported cases in organ transplant recipients have been visceral leishmaniasis, with a much smaller number of mucocutaneous leishmaniasis cases and, rarely, cutaneous leishmaniasis cases (14). Differential diagnosis in the acute stage includes amebic liver abscess, Chagas' disease, malaria, typhoid, typhus, and schistosomiasis. Subacute or chronic disease has been confused with malnutrition, bacteremia, brucellosis, histoplasmosis, leukemia, lymphoma, malaria, mononucleosis, and schistosomiasis.

Postdermal leishmaniasis, or PKDL, is a condition seen in India and Sudan in some patients unsuccessfully treated for visceral leishmaniasis. PKDL usually occurs 6 months or later after completion of therapy. This syndrome is rarely seen in Latin America but has been reported to occur in patients coinfected with HIV. The macular or hypopigmented dermal lesions are associated with few parasites, whereas erythematous and nodular lesions are associated with abundant parasites. This condition must be differentiated from leprosy, syphilis, and yaws.

Diagnosis

In areas where the disease is endemic, the diagnosis may be made on clinical grounds. Prolonged fever, progressive weight loss, anemia, leukopenia, hypergammaglobulinemia, and pronounced hepatomegaly and splenomegaly are highly suggestive of visceral leishmaniasis. The development of one or more chronic skin lesions with a history of exposure in an area of endemicity is suggestive of cutaneous leishmaniasis. In many areas of the world where the disease is endemic, laboratory testing (microscopy, culture, PCR, antigen tests, and serology) is almost impossible to obtain. Definitive diagnosis has depended on detecting either the amastigotes in clinical specimens or the promastigotes in culture; however, the ability to detect infections by molecular methods and sequence the gene product to identify the infecting organism to species level has changed this picture (8). Whenever leishmaniasis is suspected, multiple specimens should be taken and all of the diagnostic techniques should be employed if possible. When infected cells are present in low numbers in specimens (*L. braziliensis* complex infections), one method maybe successful in detecting the infection while others may be negative.

Collection of Specimens

All cutaneous lesions should be thoroughly cleaned with 70% alcohol, and extraneous debris, the eschar, and exudates should be removed. After debridement, with precautions being taken to prevent bleeding, the base of the ulcer can be scraped with a scalpel blade to obtain an exudate for slide preparation, culture, or nucleic acid amplification tests (NAAT). Specimens can be collected from the margin of the lesion by aspiration, scraping, or punch biopsy or by making a slit with a scalpel blade. Material scraped from the wall of the slit should be smeared onto a number of slides. NAAT methods for the diagnosis of leishmaniasis have used a variety of specimens (15–17). NAAT has been shown to be more sensitive than direct microscopy, histology, and culture, but availability is limited mainly to large hospitals or clinics. The NAAT methods have not been standardized, and multicenter studies to validate these tests have not been done (6, 15–17). Laboratorians may want to contact their local, state, or national public health laboratories or the U.S. Centers for Disease Control and Prevention (CDC) for diagnostic information and assistance with specimen selection and available tests. The CDC website https://www.cdc.gov/parasites/leishmaniasis/resources/pdf/cdc_diagnosis_guide_leishmaniasis_2016.pdf contains a practical guide for laboratory diagnosis of leishmaniasis. It is highly recommended that laboratories not rely on one diagnostic method but use multiple methods for diagnosis (culture, direct microscopy, histology, NAAT, and serology if available).

The core of tissue from a punch biopsy can be used to make imprints or touch preparations on a slide. A tissue core should also be submitted for histological examination. Recognition of amastigotes in tissues is more difficult than in smears or imprints because the organisms tend to be crowded within the cells, appear smaller, and are cut at various angles. Fine-needle aspiration can also be performed by using a sterile syringe containing sterile preservative-free buffered saline (0.1 ml) and a 26-gauge needle. The needle is inserted under the outer border of the lesion, the needle is rotated several times, and tissue fluid is aspirated into the needle. Tissue obtained by splenic puncture yields the highest rate of positive specimens for visceral leishmaniasis; however, this procedure carries significant risk to the patient, particularly those with coagulation disorders. Other specimens for the detection of visceral leishmaniasis include lymph node aspirates, liver biopsy specimens, sternal aspirates, iliac crest bone marrow specimens, and buffy coat preparations of venous blood. Amastigotes with reticuloendothelial cells have been detected in bronchoalveolar lavage fluid, pleural effusions, and biopsy specimens collected from the gastrointestinal tracts and oropharynges of HIV-positive patients. Individuals with PKDL have large numbers of parasites in the skin, particularly those with erythematous and nodular lesions.

Direct Examination

Microscopic Detection

Amastigote stages are found within macrophages or close to disrupted cells (Fig. 2). This stage can be recognized by its shape, size, staining characteristics, and especially the presence of an intracytoplasmic kinetoplast. The cytoplasm stains light blue and the nucleus and kinetoplast stain red or purple with Giemsa stain. Amastigotes detected in tissue sections stained with hematoxylin and eosin can be differentiated from intracellular fungal organisms because they do not stain positive with periodic acid-Schiff, mucicarmine, or Gomori methenamine silver stain. Intracellular fungal organisms do not have a kinetoplast that can be seen in amastigote stages. Amastigotes are more difficult to recognize in tissue sections than they are in properly prepared tissue imprints or smears, where the whole organism can be observed. Sensitivity varies from 15 to 70% (18).

Nucleic Acid Detection

Molecular techniques for the detection of leishmanial DNA or RNA have been used for diagnosis, prognosis, and species identification (18). Most of the molecular diagnostic tests are laboratory-developed tests. The FDA has approved SMART Leish PCR for the detection of cutaneous leishmaniasis (Cepheid, Sunnyvale, CA). These methods are considered more sensitive than slide examination or culture, particularly for the detection of the agents of mucocutaneous leishmaniasis, which are difficult to culture (6, 15–17, 19, 20). Generally, organisms in mucocutaneous lesions are scant and difficult to detect microscopically. Because infections caused by the *Leishmania* subgenus *Viannia* are considered more aggressive and are more likely to result in treatment failure, molecular techniques to identify the organism to the species and strain levels can be very important for therapy. Multilocus enzyme electrophoresis and multilocus sequence typing have been used to identify *Leishmania* species and strains, but this depended on having culturable isolates, and in some cases these methods were not discriminative enough. To improve isolate identification, various rRNA and DNA targets, such as mini-exon or spliced leader sequences, the rRNA internal transcribed spacer, the 7SL-RNA gene, the heat shock protein 70 gene, and the cytochrome *b* gene, have been used. A great target is kinetoplastic DNA, because there are more than 10,000 copies per organism, thereby increasing the likelihood of detection; however, minicircle heterogeneity is an issue (8). Use of multiple targets may be necessary due to gene polymorphism within the target sequences (6, 8, 18). Sensitivity varies from 80 to 100% depending on the method used (18). The CDC should be consulted before specimen collection, as they can provide molecular diagnostic testing (https://www.cdc.gov/parasites/leishmaniasis/index.html).

Culture

If material is to be cultured, it must be collected aseptically. Tissues should be minced prior to culture. Culture media successfully employed to recover organisms include Novy-MacNeal-Nicolle medium (NNN) and Schneider's *Drosophila* medium supplemented with 30% fetal bovine serum (21). Cultures, incubated at 25°C, should be examined twice weekly for the first 2 weeks and once a week thereafter for up to 4 weeks before the culture is declared negative. Promastigote stages can be detected microscopically in wet mounts and then stained with Giemsa stain to observe their morphology. Most laboratories do not offer culture; however, it is important to recover the isolate for species identification and drug susceptibility information. Sensitivity varies from 44 to 58%, with recovery being the poorest in cases of mucocutaneous leishmaniasis (18). The CDC should be consulted before specimen collection, as they can provide transport for specimen cultures (https://www.cdc.gov/parasites/leishmaniasis/index.html).

Animal Inoculation

Animals such as the golden hamster can be inoculated with patient material. Animals are inoculated intranasally for cutaneous and mucocutaneous leishmaniasis and intraperitoneally for visceral leishmaniasis. It may take 2 to 3 months before an animal becomes positive. A combination of tissue smears, PCR (if available), culture, and animal inoculation may be needed to optimize the laboratory diagnosis of the infection. Regulations and financial costs make this diagnostic method impractical nowadays. Sensitivity varies from 44 to 52% (18).

Skin Testing

The leishmanin (Montenegro) test (not available in Canada or the United States), a delayed-type hypersensitivity reaction, is useful for epidemiological surveys of a population to identify groups at risk of infection. This test may be available from clinics and institutions in areas of endemicity. The heavier the parasite burden and the longer the patient has been infected, the more likely a positive skin test is. Although skin test antigens are commercially available outside the United States, there is a lack of product standardization and stability. Positive reactions are usually seen in cutaneous and mucocutaneous leishmaniasis; however, patients with active visceral and diffuse cutaneous leishmaniasis exhibit negative reactions. Post-kala-azar patients may also exhibit a negative reaction. This test is of no value for the diagnosis of visceral leishmaniasis. Sensitivity varied from 82 to 89% for cutaneous leishmaniasis to 100% for patients with mucocutaneous and diffuse cutaneous leishmaniasis (18).

Serologic and Antigen Tests

Serologic tests are available; however, they are not very useful for the diagnosis of mucocutaneous and visceral leishmaniasis. In kala-azar, there is a large increase in gamma globulins, both immunoglobulin G (IgG) and IgM. This is the basis for the aldehyde or Formol-gel test, which has been used as a screening test in areas of endemicity (22). The addition of 1 drop of formalin to 1 ml of serum promotes the precipitation of immunoglobulins. A number of serologic tests, including indirect fluorescent-antibody (IFA) testing, enzyme-linked immunoassays (ELISAs), and immunoblot tests have been developed for diagnostic purposes; however, they are not widely available except in areas of endemicity (8, 18, 23, 24). Sensitivity varied from 28 to 93% depending on the method, the antigen used, and the *Leishmania* species being detected (18, 24).

An ELISA, dipstick test, and rapid immunochromatographic strip using *L. infantum/L. chagasi* recombinant k39 antigen had a sensitivity of 37 to 100% in diagnosing visceral leishmaniasis in immunocompetent people (18). Visceral leishmaniasis patients coinfected with HIV may have no detectable antileishmania antibodies (12). Serologic testing is available at some referral laboratories and the CDC.

The detection of urinary antigens has been used for the diagnosis of visceral leishmaniasis, with a sensitivity of 41 to 86% (8, 18, 24, 25).

Treatment and Prevention

Lesions in simple cutaneous leishmaniasis generally heal spontaneously. Treatment options have included cryotherapy, heat, photodynamic therapy, surgical excision of lesions, and chemotherapy (11). Chemotherapeutics include azoles (fluconazole, ketoconazole, and posaconazole), amphotericin B, miltefosine, paromomycin, pentavalent antimonials, and pentamidine (11). The FDA has approved miltefosine for the treatment of cutaneous leishmaniasis. Treatment is advocated to reduce scarring in areas of cosmetic importance and to prevent dissemination and/or relapse of the infection. Although the optimal treatment for cutaneous leishmaniasis is unknown, therapy in the area of endemicity may consist of injections of antimonial compounds. Intralesional antimonial therapy may be given to patients with a limited number of cutaneous lesions (three or fewer), whereas intramuscular or intravenous therapy should be given for more disseminated infections. Topical therapy should not be advocated for mucocutaneous infections. Response to therapy varies depending on the species of *Leishmania* and the type of disease (11, 26). Patients with *L. (V.) braziliensis* infection, which is noted for its chronicity, latency, and metastasis with mucosal membrane involvement, have been found to be PCR positive up to 11 years posttherapy (27). Therapy may be individualized and may include pentavalent antimonial compound, liposomal amphotericin B, and miltefosine, which may be used in combination.

Visceral leishmaniasis can be fatal if not treated, and individuals coinfected with HIV must be treated aggressively (11). In addition, the individual may have to be treated for life to prevent relapse of visceral leishmaniasis. Drugs most commonly used to treat visceral leishmaniasis include amphotericin B, miltefosine, paromomycin, and pentavalent antimonials (sodium stibogluconate and meglumine antimonite). Liposomal amphotericin B (approved by the FDA for visceral leishmaniasis) has the highest therapeutic efficacy, whereas resistance to antimonial drugs is common in India and Nepal. Miltefosine is an effective oral agent, although failure rates as high as 30% have been reported (26).

If the patient is not clinically improving, follow-up smears and cultures should be done 1 to 2 weeks posttherapy. PCR testing can also be used to monitor the progress of therapy, but there are no standards for monitoring, and this is not used as routine follow-up (11, 26, 28).

In areas where leishmaniasis is endemic, vaccination is still a major goal for eliminating leishmaniasis. Inoculating the serous exudate from naturally acquired lesions of cutaneous leishmaniasis into an inconspicuous area of the body of a nonimmune person has been effective; however, vaccines against other forms of leishmaniasis have not worked. Vaccination with exudates from individuals with mucocutaneous leishmaniasis should never be tried due to the extensive pathology associated with this infection. Other possible prevention methods include spraying dwellings with insecticides, applying insect repellents to the skin, wearing protective clothing, and the use of fine-mesh bed netting. Reservoir control has been unsuccessful in most areas, although in areas where canines may be a reservoir host, pyrethroid-impregnated collars are being used to prevent infections. Individuals with lesions should be warned to protect the lesion from insect bites, and patients should be educated about the possibility of autoinoculation or infection.

AMERICAN TRYPANOSOMIASIS

■ *Trypanosoma cruzi*

American trypanosomiasis (Chagas' disease) is a zoonosis caused by *T. cruzi* primarily in Latin America. There are 65 million persons at risk of infection in 21 American countries and 28,000 new cases per year (29, 30). Over 60% of Chagas' disease cases can be found in Argentina, Brazil, and Mexico. Patients can present with either acute or chronic disease. Chagas' disease was considered a disease of rural areas; however, it is now ubiquitous due to social pattern changes, including rural to urban migration and migration of infected persons to areas where Chagas' disease would not usually be suspected. Transmission was thought to be primarily through vector bites, but fecal contamination of the food supply by the vector is a significant source of infection also. Transmission can occur *in utero*, which is a diagnostic problem when the infected mother migrates to an area where the disease is not endemic. A very serious problem is disease acquisition through blood transfusion and organ transplantation (31, 32). A large number of infected patients with positive serology can remain asymptomatic (30, 33).

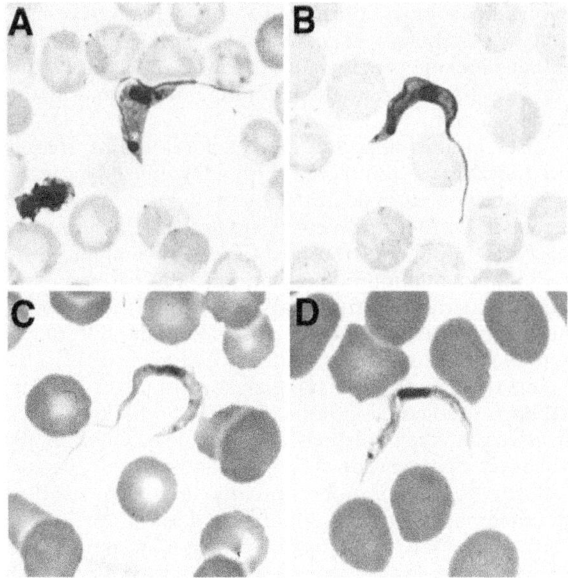

FIGURE 4 (A and B) *T. cruzi* trypomastigotes; (C and D) *T. brucei gambiense* trypomastigotes.

Life Cycle and Morphology

Trypomastigotes (Fig. 4 and 5) are ingested by the reduviid bug (triatomids, kissing bugs, or conenose bugs) as it obtains a blood meal. The trypomastigotes transform into epimastigotes (Fig. 1, 4, and 5) that multiply in the posterior portion of the midgut. After 8 to 10 days, metacyclic trypomastigotes develop from the epimastigotes. These metacyclic trypomastigotes passed in the feces of the reduviid bug are the infectious stage for humans (see www.cdc.gov/dpdx/index.html for the complete life cycle). Transmission by blood or blood product transfusion is a serious concern in areas of endemicity, and serologic screening of blood donors can be used, whereas in areas where the disease is not endemic, questionnaires have been used to defer prospective donors from areas of endemicity. Blood donor units are routinely screened for Chagas' disease antibodies using FDA-approved tests (Abbott Prism Chagas and Ortho T. cruzi ELISA). Transmission from solid organ donors and vertical transmission from pregnant mothers to the fetus can occur. Foodborne outbreaks have also occurred when food was contaminated with vector feces (30).

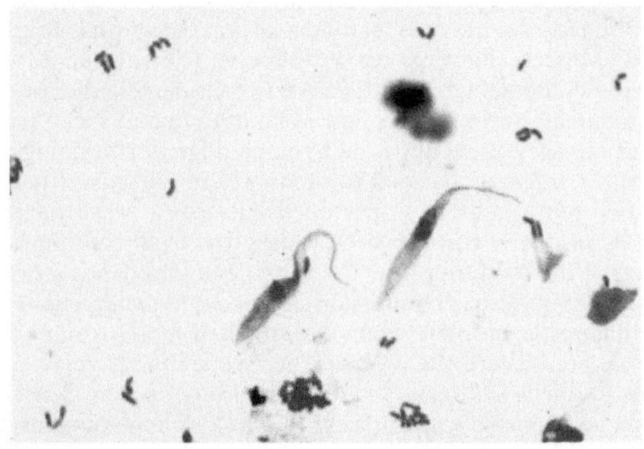

FIGURE 5 *T. cruzi* epimastigotes (Giemsa stain).

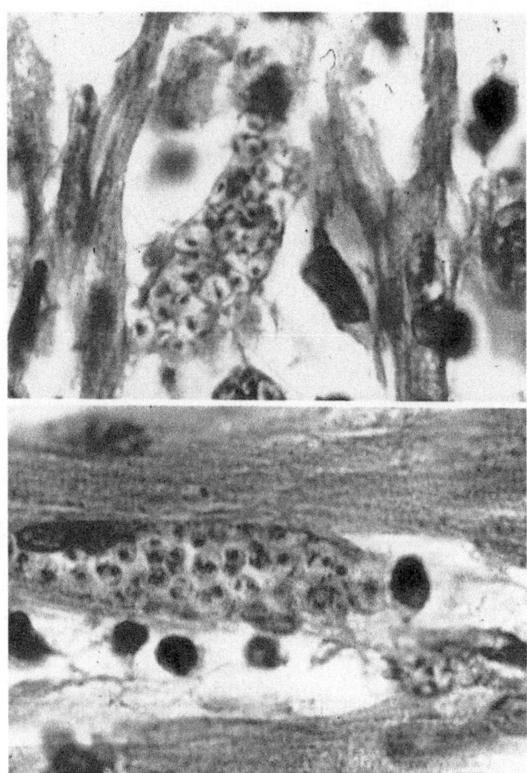

FIGURE 6 *T. cruzi* amastigotes in heart muscle (hematoxylin and eosin stain).

Humans contract Chagas' disease when the reduviid bug defecates while taking a blood meal and metacyclic trypomastigotes in the feces are rubbed or scratched into the bite wound or onto mucosal surfaces. In humans, *T. cruzi* can be found in two forms, as amastigotes and trypomastigotes (Fig. 1, 4, and 6). The trypomastigote form is present in the blood and infects any nucleated host cell but preferentially transforms to the amastigote stage in skeletal and cardiac muscle. The amastigote form multiplies within the cell, eventually destroying the cell, and both amastigotes and trypomastigotes are released into the blood.

The trypomastigote is spindle shaped and approximately 20 μm long, and it characteristically assumes a C or U shape in stained blood films (Fig. 4). Trypomastigotes occur in the blood in two forms, a long, slender form and a short, stubby one. The short, stubby form is thought to be the infectious form for the vector. The nucleus is situated in the center of the body, with a large, oval kinetoplast located at the posterior end. A flagellum arises from the basal body and extends along the outer edge of an undulating membrane until it reaches the anterior end of the body, where it projects as a free flagellum. When the trypomastigotes are stained with Giemsa stain, the cytoplasm stains blue and the nucleus, kinetoplast, and flagellum stain red or violet.

The amastigote (2 to 6 μm in diameter) is indistinguishable from those found in leishmanial infections. It contains a large nucleus and a rod-shaped kinetoplast that stains red or violet with Giemsa stain, and the cytoplasm stains blue.

Epidemiology and Transmission

Chagas' disease is a zoonosis occurring throughout the Americas, including Central and South America and California, Louisiana, and Texas in the United States

(30, 34). It involves reduviid bugs living in close association with reservoirs (dogs, cats, armadillos, opossums, raccoons, and rodents). Human infections occur mainly in rural areas where poor sanitary and socioeconomic conditions and poor housing provide excellent breeding places for reduviid bugs. Chagas' disease is found in 21 countries in the Americas. A number of autochthonous cases have been identified in the United States (34–36). Infections in the United States may be limited by the habit of the reduviid bug of not immediately defecating on the host after acquiring the blood meal. Due to population mobility (infected patients migrating from areas of endemicity), the infection can be found in many regions where the disease is not endemic, such as Spain and Japan, where physicians may not consider this infection in their diagnostic differential.

The disease distribution has been broken into two ecological zones: the southern cone (South America), where the reduviid vector lives inside the human home, and the northern cone (Central America and Mexico), where the reduviid bug lives inside and outside the home. Strains of *T. cruzi* have large differences in infectivity, potential vectors, antigenicity, histotropism, pathogenicity, and response to therapy (32). Based on molecular epidemiology, *T. cruzi* has been broken into six genotypes or discrete typing units (TcI to TcVI) (37). Most human infections are due to type TcII in the southern cone, whereas in the northern cone, type TcI predominates.

Clinical Significance

In addition to contracting *T. cruzi* infections through the insect bite wound or exposed mucous membranes, one can be infected by blood transfusion, placental transfer, organ transplant, and accidental ingestion of parasitized reduviid bugs or their feces in food or drink (31). Most congenital infections are asymptomatic. A localized inflammatory reaction may ensue at the infection site with development of a chagoma (erythematous subcutaneous nodule) or Romaña's sign (edema of the eyelids and conjunctivitis).

The incubation period following exposure is usually 1 to 2 weeks. Most patients have nonspecific symptoms or no symptoms at all. Acute systemic signs occur around the second to third week of infection and are characterized by high fevers, hepatosplenomegaly, myalgia, erythematous rash, acute myocarditis, lymphadenopathy, and subcutaneous edema of face, legs, and feet. The acute phase of Chagas' disease in immunosuppressed patients is manifested as acute myocarditis or acute encephalitis with a high mortality rate. Most acute cases are never detected and resolve over a period of 2 to 3 months into an asymptomatic chronic stage (indeterminate phase or clinical latency period). These patients remain infected for life unless treated. Approximately 70% of individuals with chronic Chagas' infection remain asymptomatic (indeterminate phase); however, they are still capable of transmitting the infection. The remaining 30% of individuals with chronic Chagas' infection develop myocarditis or symptoms associated with denervation of the digestive tract (30). Chronic Chagas' disease signs may develop years or decades after undetected infection or after the diagnosis of acute disease. The most frequent clinical sign of chronic Chagas' disease is cardiomyopathy manifested by cardiomegaly and conduction changes. Patients who acquire the infection orally (foodborne infection) have a higher incidence of myocarditis and mortality. Some patients are more likely to develop megaesophagus or megacolon. Gastrointestinal Chagas' disease is rare outside Argentina, Bolivia, Brazil, Chile, and Paraguay (southern cone countries). The "mega" condition has been associated with the destruction of ganglion cells, resulting in dysmotility and causing dysphagia, aspiration, and regurgitation in patients with megaesophagus and severe constipation in patients with megacolon. In chronic Chagas' disease, autoimmunity may also be responsible for tissue destruction in addition to the tissue destruction caused by the parasite. Reactivation of Chagas' disease in HIV-positive patients usually leads to very high parasitemia and can occur in other immunosuppressed patients (30). Central nervous system (CNS) involvement is seldom observed, but in HIV-coinfected individuals, CNS involvement is frequently noted, and acute fatal meningoencephalitis and granulomatous encephalitis have been described for these patients.

Congenital transmission from mother to fetus can occur in both acute and chronic phases of the disease. Congenital infections can cause abortion, prematurity, neurological sequelae, and mental deficiency (38, 39). Infants of seropositive mothers should be monitored for up to a year after birth to rule out infection. Transmission of the infection during transplantation of solid organs and other tissues from seropositive donors has become a significant problem (30). Although transplantation of any organ or tissue from a seropositive donor should be regarded as infectious, the risk of transmission of the infection is dependent on other factors. Some recipients do not develop infections; however, all should be serially monitored for signs of infection.

Diagnosis

Health care personnel working with specimens from patients suspected of having Chagas' disease should follow the guidelines for blood-borne pathogens using universal precautions. Trypomastigotes are highly infectious.

Patients with chronic Chagas' disease who become immunosuppressed (i.e., those with HIV infection and those receiving organ transplants) should be monitored weekly for the first few months and monthly thereafter for a year or more for reactivation of infection.

Collection of Specimens

The definitive diagnosis depends on demonstration of trypomastigotes in the blood, amastigote stages in tissues, or positive PCR and serologic tests (Table 3). Aspirates from chagomas and enlarged lymph nodes can be examined for amastigotes and trypomastigotes. Histological examination of biopsy specimens may also be done. Trypomastigotes may be easily detected in the blood in acute disease; however, in chronic disease, this stage is rare or absent, except during febrile episodes. Trypomastigotes are at their highest concentration in the blood during the febrile crises. Trypomastigotes appear in the blood about 10 days after infection and persist through the acute phase. Laboratorians may want to contact their local, state, or national public health laboratory or the CDC for diagnostic information and help with specimen selection and available tests (www.cdc.gov/parasites/chagas/health_professionals/index.html).

Direct Examination

Microscopic Detection

Trypomastigotes may be detected in wet mounts of blood or by using thin and thick blood films or the buffy coat concentration technique (21, 40). The thick blood film concentrates diagnostic stages using approximately the same amount of blood used for the thin film into a much smaller viewing area. The microhematocrit method uses two to

TABLE 3 Diagnostic methods to detect Chagas' infections

Method[a]	Use during infection stage		
	Acute	Indeterminate	Chronic
Direct			
Direct microscopy	+	−	−
Thick and thin blood films	+	−	−
PCR	+	+	+
Blood culture	+	−	−
Xenodiagnosis	+	+	+
Indirect			
IFA (IgM and IgG)	+	+	+
EIA	−	+	+
IHA	−	+	+
RIPA/WB	−	+	+

[a]IFA, indirect fluorescent-antibody assay; EIA, enzyme immunoassay; IHA, indirect hemagglutinin assay; RIPA, radioimmunoprecipitation assay; WB, Western blotting.

three times the amount of blood and concentrates trypomastigotes into the buffy coat region. The stain of choice is Giemsa for both amastigote and trypomastigote stages. Amastigotes which can be readily seen in hematoxylin-and-eosin-stained tissue can be differentiated from fungal organisms (*Histoplasma*) because they do not stain positive with periodic acid-Schiff, mucicarmine, or Gomori methenamine silver stain. Amastigotes are detected primarily in skeletal and cardiac muscle cells. In areas where kala-azar occurs, amastigote stages look similar, and infections with *L. donovani* and *T. cruzi* must be differentiated by PCR, immunoassay, culture (epimastigote in *T. cruzi* versus promastigote in *L. donovani*), serologic tests, animal inoculation, or xenodiagnosis techniques (30, 32). Patient history, including geographic and/or travel history, and confirmation of organisms in striated muscle rather than reticuloendothelial tissues are very strong evidence for *T. cruzi* rather than *L. donovani* as the causative agent.

Nucleic Acid Detection

Although not routinely available except in specialized centers, NAAT (not FDA approved) has been used to detect as few as one trypomastigote in 20 ml of blood and has been useful in treatment follow-up (34–37, 39, 41, 42). It is not diagnostically useful for identifying patients in the indeterminate or chronic phase of infection (43). To improve identification of positive patients, real-time PCR using multiple gene targets has been advocated. Multiple targets are needed due to polymorphism within the gene targets. PCR-based methods have not been standardized, and multicenter studies to validate these tests have not been done. The primary target for many NAAT has been kinetoplastic DNA due to the large number of copies per organism, thereby increasing the chance of detection of the infection. There have been few studies where various PCR methods used for diagnostic purposes have been compared, as most are laboratory-developed tests.

Culture and Animal Inoculation

Aspirates, blood, and tissues can also be cultured. The medium of choice is NNN (21). Cultures, incubated at 25°C, should be examined for epimastigote stages twice weekly during the first 2 weeks and once per week thereafter for up to 4 weeks before they are considered negative. If available, laboratory animals (rats or mice) can be inoculated and the blood can be observed for trypomastigotes or tested by PCR.

Xenodiagnosis

Xenodiagnosis is used less frequently than in the past for clinical diagnosis of Chagas' disease in areas of endemicity. Other diagnostic methods, such as molecular testing, have proved to be more useful. Trypanosome-free reduviid bugs are allowed to feed on individuals suspected of having Chagas' disease. The feces, hemolymph, hindgut, and salivary glands can be examined microscopically for flagellated forms over a period of 3 months, or PCR methods can be used to detect infected bugs and provide a rapid diagnosis. Xenodiagnosis is positive in less than 50% of seropositive patients. Some patients may develop a severe anaphylactic reaction to the reduviid bug's salivary secretion.

Serologic Tests

Serologic testing is used primarily to detect indeterminate and chronic infections (43). To detect congenital infections due to vertical transmission of the parasite when direct microscopy and PCR tests are negative, serology tests should be used at 9 to 12 months after birth (38). This reduces the effect of passively transferred maternal antibody. Many congenital *T. cruzi* infections are asymptomatic until later in life, when chronic sequelae are manifested.

Serologic tests using blood and saliva for the diagnosis of Chagas' disease include complement fixation (Guerreiro-Machado test), chemiluminescence, IFA testing, indirect hemagglutination, and ELISA (30, 32, 38, 44). Many of these tests use an epimastigote antigen, and cross-reactions have been noted for patients infected with *T. rangeli*, *Leishmania* spp., *Toxoplasma gondii*, and hepatitis. The use of synthetic peptides and recombinant proteins has improved the sensitivity and specificity of the serodiagnostic techniques. Several diagnostic enzyme immunoassay and immunochromatographic methods using parasite lysate and recombinant antigens have been approved by the FDA for screening blood donors and patients. The FDA and American Association of Blood Banks require that donated blood be screened for Chagas' antibodies, and it is recommended that the United Network for Organ Sharing test tissue donors for the presence of Chagas' antibodies. Due to lack of sensitivity, specificity, and cross-reactivity with antibody from other infections, it is recommended that any positive serologic test be confirmed using a second test that employs different antigens (31, 43). This will help to reduce the number of false-positive tests.

Follow-up blood specimens should be reexamined 1 to 2 months after therapy by the techniques described above. A difficult problem associated with serology is that of determining whether a patient has been reinfected or whether treatment has been unsuccessful, because the IgG response remains elevated for a prolonged period of time. Therapeutic monitoring by serologic methods has largely been replaced by molecular methods. Serologic testing is available at referral laboratories and the CDC.

Treatment and Prevention

Benznidazole (Radamil, Ragonil, Rochagan) and nifurtimox (Lampit) can reduce the severity or eliminate Chagas' disease (33, 39, 45, 46). Benznidazole has been approved by the FDA for use in the United States. Other drugs, including allopurinol, fluconazole, itraconazole, ketoconazole, and posaconazole, have been used to treat a limited number of patients (46). Treatment is more beneficial for patients with acute infection than those with chronic disease. The progression of pathologic sequelae can be slowed and mortality decreased but not eliminated in chronic Chagas' disease. This may be due to failure to eliminate the infection or to immune processes already set in motion.

Response to therapy can be monitored by measuring the reduction in parasite load by PCR (33, 39, 41, 45, 47). Surgery has been successfully used to treat cases of chagasic heart disease, megaesophagus, and megacolon (30).

Heart transplantation has been used to treat end-stage Chagas' cardiomyopathy since 1985 (48). It is a leading indicator for organ transplants in Central and South America.

Until recently, control of Chagas' disease has been achieved mainly through the use of insecticides to eliminate the reduviid vector. Construction of reduviid-proof dwellings and health education are essential for effective control programs. Vector control, education, and improved housing conditions have reduced the infected population from over 20 million to 6 to 8 million in areas of endemicity. Bed nets are also effective in preventing infections. Serologic screening of blood products for transfusion from areas in which the disease is endemic is highly recommended. An alternative approach to serologic testing for blood donors is the use of questionnaires to defer prospective donors from areas of endemicity. Vaccines are unavailable.

■ *Trypanosoma rangeli*

T. rangeli infects humans and other vertebrates in both Central and South America and is often found in areas where *T. cruzi* is also present (49). Human infections are asymptomatic, and trypomastigotes have been noted to persist in the blood for longer than a year. *T. rangeli* and *T. cruzi* can use the same triatomid vector to transmit infections. *T. rangeli* infections can be transmitted by inoculation of triatomid saliva during feeding or by the vector's feces (50). In some areas, *T. rangeli* infections are five to six times more frequent than infections with *T. cruzi*. Trypomastigotes can be detected from the blood of infected patients by using thin and thick blood smears and buffy coat concentration techniques. The parasites can be stained with Giemsa or Wright stain. Microscopically, the trypomastigote cannot be differentiated from African trypanosomes, which do not occur in the Americas. *T. rangeli* trypomastigotes can be differentiated from *T. cruzi* trypomastigotes based on the smaller size of the kinetoplast. PCR methods have been used to detect infections in humans and vectors (51). Infections can also be detected by xenodiagnosis. In addition, blood can be cultured (Tobies medium or NNN) (21) or injected into laboratory animals (mice) and examined for epimastigotes and trypomastigotes, respectively. Although there are no serologic tests to detect *T. rangeli* infections, serologic cross-reactions have been noted to occur with tests for *T. cruzi*.

To differentiate between the two infections, clinical history, serologic testing using acute- and convalescent-phase sera or different test methods, PCR, or microscopic analysis of blood may have to be used. There are no treatment recommendations for *T. rangeli* infections.

AFRICAN TRYPANOSOMIASIS

African trypanosomiasis is limited to the tsetse fly belt of Central Africa, where there are over 60 million people at risk for African trypanosomiasis (52). Fewer than 10,000 cases are reported per annum (2,800 cases in 2015). The WHO has targeted human African trypanosomiasis for elimination in 2020 (52, 53). The West African (Gambian) form of sleeping sickness, noted for its chronicity and responsible for 99% of the sleeping sickness cases, is caused by *T. brucei gambiense*, whereas the East African (Rhodesian) form, noted for its acute morbidity and mortality within months of infection, is caused by *T. brucei rhodesiense*. *T. brucei gambiense* infections can last for months to years, with slow CNS involvement. In some areas of endemicity, civil strife has disrupted both the health care infrastructure and vector control, which has led to a resurgence of this disease.

Life Cycle and Morphology

T. brucei rhodesiense and *T. brucei gambiense* are closely related and morphologically indistinguishable. In the past, differentiation was based on clinical signs and geographic area; however, differentiation can now be accomplished using molecular methods. *T. brucei rhodesiense* is associated with enhanced morbidity and mortality and treatment options are also different.

The trypomastigote forms (Fig. 1 and 4) in the blood range from long, slender-bodied organisms with a long flagellum to short, fat, stumpy forms without a free flagellum (14 to 33 μm long and 1.5 to 3.5 μm wide). The short, stumpy forms are the infective stage for the tsetse fly (see www.cdc.gov/dpdx/index.html for the complete life cycle).

Using Giemsa or Wright stain, the granular cytoplasm stains pale blue and contains dark blue granules and possibly vacuoles. The centrally located nucleus stains reddish. The kinetoplast is located at the organism's posterior end and stains reddish; the remaining intracytoplasmic flagellum (axoneme) may not be visible. The flagellum arises from the kinetoplast, as does the undulating membrane. The flagellum runs along the edge of the undulating membrane until the undulating membrane merges with the trypanosome body at the organism's anterior end. At this point, the flagellum becomes free to extend beyond the body. Trypanosomal forms are ingested by the tsetse fly when a blood meal is taken and transform to epimastigotes (Fig. 1). The organisms multiply in the gut of the fly, and after approximately 2 weeks, the organisms migrate back to the salivary glands. Humans are infected when metacyclic forms from the salivary glands are introduced into the bite site as the blood meal is taken by the tsetse fly. The trypomastigote has the ability to change the surface coat of the outer membrane, helping the organism evade the host's humoral immune response (54).

Epidemiology and Transmission

The development cycle in the tsetse fly varies from 12 to 30 days and averages 20 days. Fewer than 10% of tsetse flies become infective after obtaining blood from infected patients. Both female and male tsetse flies can transmit the infection. Infections can also occur through organ transplants, via placental transfer from mother to fetus, and by needlesticks.

Although there is no evidence of animal-to-human transmission of *T. brucei gambiense*, trypanosomal strains isolated from hartebeest, kob, chickens, dogs, cows, and domestic pigs in West Africa are identical to those isolated from humans in the same area. Evidence suggests that transmission may be entirely interhuman. The tsetse fly vectors of Rhodesian trypanosomiasis are game feeders (including cattle) that may transmit the disease from human to human or from animal to human.

There is molecular evidence of multistrain introduction of the infection with parasites of the *T. brucei* complex that can have epidemiological implications as to virulence, pathogenicity, and response to therapy (55). It is also suggested that human leukocyte antigen plays a critical role in the progression of the infection and disease (56).

Clinical Significance

After a bite by an infected tsetse fly, a local inflammatory reaction that resolves spontaneously within 1 to 2 weeks can be detected at the bite site. The bite site chancre can be painful, presenting as an erythematous indurated nodule that may ulcerate. The trypomastigotes gain entrance to the bloodstream, causing a symptom-free, low-grade parasitemia that may continue for many months. The infection may self-cure during this period without development of symptoms or lymph node invasion. Chancres may be confused with insect bites and bacterial skin infections, with resolution occurring within a few weeks.

The clinical course and disease progression are more acute with *T. brucei rhodesiense* than with *T. brucei gambiense* infections (57). Diagnostic symptoms include irregular fever, lymph node enlargement (particularly those of the posterior triangle of the neck, known as Winterbottom's sign, which is prominent in *T. brucei gambiense* infections), delayed sensation to pain (Kerandel's sign), and transient erythematous skin rashes 6 to 8 weeks postinfection. In addition to lymph node involvement, the spleen and liver become enlarged. Stage I of African trypanosomiasis is when the trypomastigotes multiply in the subcutaneous tissues, blood, and lymph (hemolymphatic phase). Stage II occurs when the trypomastigotes cross the blood-brain barrier to initiate infection of the central nervous system (neurologic phase). With Gambian trypanosomiasis, the blood lymphatic stage (stage I) may last for years before the sleeping sickness syndrome occurs (CNS involvement, meningoencephalitis stage, stage II). When symptoms occur in a patient infected with Gambian trypanosomiasis, the patient is already in the advanced stages of disease with CNS involvement.

Laboratory findings include anemia, granulocytopenia, increased sedimentation rate, and marked increases in serum IgM. The sustained high IgM levels are a result of the parasite producing variable antigen types to evade the patient's defense system (57). In an immunocompetent host, the lack of elevated serum IgM rules out African trypanosomiasis. Diagnostic differential may include brucellosis, CNS lymphoma, HIV infection, leishmaniasis, malaria, meningitis, relapsing fever, toxoplasmosis, tuberculosis, and typhoid fever.

Upon trypomastigote invasion of the CNS, the sleeping sickness stage of the infection is initiated (stage II). Gambian trypanosomiasis is characterized by steady, progressive meningoencephalitis, behavioral changes, apathy, confusion, coordination loss, and somnolence. *T. brucei rhodesiense* produces a more rapid, fulminating disease, and death may occur before there is extensive CNS involvement. In the terminal phase of the disease, the patient becomes emaciated, leading to profound coma and death, usually from secondary infections. Cerebrospinal fluid (CSF) findings include increased protein and IgM levels, lymphocytosis, and morular cells of Mott. Morular (mulberry) cells are altered plasma cells whose cytoplasm is filled with proteinaceous droplets. Morular cells are not seen in all patients; however, they are highly suggestive of CNS stage II disease. Besides finding trypomastigotes in the CSF, World Health Organization criteria for CNS involvement include a white blood cell count greater than 5 cells and increased protein levels in the CNS fluid. The diagnostic differential may include cryptococcosis, HIV, meningitis, Parkinson's disease, psychiatric disorders, viral encephalitis, and space-occupying lesions.

Diagnosis

Because most infections occur in rural areas, sophisticated diagnostic techniques are not readily available and diagnosis is dependent on simple direct detection methods. Definitive diagnosis depends upon demonstration of trypomastigotes in blood, lymph node aspirates, sternum bone marrow, chancre fluid, and CSF. Trypomastigotes can be more readily detected in body fluids in infections due to *T. brucei rhodesiense* than in those due to *T. brucei gambiense* because of substantially higher parasitemias. Due to periodic fevers, parasite numbers in the blood vary, and a number of techniques must be used to detect the trypomastigotes. Laboratorians may want to contact their local, state, or national public health laboratory or the CDC for diagnostic information and help with specimen selection and available tests (https://www.cdc.gov/parasites/sleepingsickness/health_professionals/index.html#dx).

Collection of Specimens

Trypomastigotes are highly infectious, and health care personnel must be cautious and adhere to guidelines for blood-borne pathogens using universal precautions when handling blood, CSF, or aspirates. Microscopic specimens should be examined as rapidly as possible due to potential lysis of trypomastigotes. Serial exams of fluids may be necessary to detect trypomastigotes, especially with Gambian trypanosomiasis. Blood can be collected from either fingersticks or venipuncture. Venous blood should be collected in a tube containing EDTA. Multiple blood exams should be performed before trypanosomiasis is ruled out. Parasites are found in high numbers in the blood during the febrile period and in low numbers in the afebrile periods. CSF should always be collected to rule out CNS involvement. If CSF is examined, a volume greater than 1 ml, preferably 5 ml or more, should be collected. In cases in which trypomastigotes are present in undetectable numbers in the blood, they may be seen in aspirates of inflamed lymph nodes; however, attempts to demonstrate them in tissue are not practical. Blood and CSF specimens should be examined every 6 months during therapy to evaluate the clinical response and for up to 2 years after therapy.

Direct Examination

Microscopic Detection

In addition to thin and thick blood films, a buffy coat concentration method is recommended to detect the parasites. Parasites can be detected on thick blood smears when numbers are greater than 2,000/ml, with the hematocrit capillary tube concentration or quantitative buffy coat method when numbers are greater than 100/ml, and on an anion-exchange column when numbers are greater than 4/ml. Unfortunately, anion exchange is not easily adapted to clinical laboratories or field studies (58). In suspected and confirmed cases of trypanosomiasis, a lumbar puncture is mandatory to rule out CNS involvement (stage II). CSF examination must be conducted by using centrifuged sediments. The CSF should be examined immediately, because the trypomastigotes begin to autolyze within 10 minutes. Detection of trypomastigotes in the CSF allows immediate classification of stage II illness (CNS involvement).

Nucleic Acid Detection

Referral laboratories use molecular methods (PCR, not FDA approved) to detect infections and differentiate species, but these methods are not routinely used in the field (57, 59). The PCR-based methods have not been standardized, and multicenter institutional studies to validate these tests have not been done. There have been few studies in which the various PCR methods used for diagnostic purposes have been compared.

Culture and Animal Inoculation

Small laboratory animals (rats and guinea pigs) have been used to detect infections. *T. brucei rhodesiense* is more adaptable to cultivation (Tobies medium) (21) and animal infection than *T. brucei gambiense*; however, cultivation is not practical for most diagnostic laboratories.

Serologic Tests

Serologic techniques (not FDA approved) that have been used for epidemiologic screening include IFA, ELISA, indirect hemagglutination assay, the card agglutination trypanosomiasis test (CATT), LATEX/T. b. gambiense, and immunochromatographic assays (Hat Sero-K-SeT and SD Boline HAT 1.0) (57, 60). Serologic tests are normally used for screening, with the definitive diagnosis of infection being dependent on microscopic observation of trypomastigotes. CATT is effective in screening the population for suspected cases of *T. brucei gambiense* infection but not *T. brucei rhodesiense* infection. CATT requires refrigeration, making it difficult to use in rural areas, whereas the immunochromatographic method does not require electricity, making it easier to use in field settings. Major serodiagnostic problems with CATT include false-positive results due to malarial infections and the fact that many in the population have elevated antibody levels due to exposure to animal trypanosomes that are noninfectious to humans. CATT does not differentiate between current and past infections (53). Markedly elevated serum and CSF IgM concentrations are of diagnostic value. CSF antibody titers should be interpreted with caution because of the lack of reference values and the possibility of CSF containing serum due to a traumatic tap. Intrathecal production of immunoglobulins can be found in a number of neuroinflammatory diseases. LATEX/IgM has been developed for field use to measure CSF concentrations of IgM (58).

ELISA has been used to detect antigen in serum and CSF. Biomarker tests (antigen detection) are not widely used due to the limited sensitivity of the test when there are limited numbers of trypomastigotes in the blood or CSF (61, 62). This method could also be used for clinical staging of the disease to determine whether there was CNS infection and as a follow-up to therapy.

Treatment and Prevention

All patients determined to have active infections should be treated. The drugs used and the course of treatment are dependent on the trypanosomal species and the clinical stage of the disease (63). Suramin (Bayer 205; Naphuride or Antrypol) is the drug of choice for treating the early blood or lymphatic stage of *T. brucei rhodesiense* infections, whereas pentamidine isethionate (Lomidine) or suramin is the drug of choice for treating the early stages of *T. brucei gambiense* infections (57). Melarsoprol (Mel B or Arsobal) is the drug of choice when CNS involvement is suspected with *T. brucei rhodesiense* infections. This drug may be given with a corticosteroid to reduce possible encephalopathy.

Difluoromethylornithine (eflornithine; Ornidyl) is a cytostatic drug effective against the acute and late stages of *T. brucei gambiense* infections. It can be used alone or with oral nifurtimox. Difluoromethylornithine is not effective against late-stage *T. brucei rhodesiense* infections. The effectiveness of therapy can be judged microscopically by the absence of trypomastigotes in the blood, lymph fluid, or CSF and by a decrease in CSF white blood cells (56). CSF antibodies (IgM) decrease, as do levels of interleukin-10, after successful therapy (64). Any individual treated for African trypanosomiasis should be monitored every 6 months for 2 years after completion of therapy. *T. brucei gambiense* relapses may be treated with difluoromethylornithine or melarsoprol.

Population screening programs have been used to control *T. brucei gambiense* infections. The use of vector control measures has met with limited success. The most effective control measures include an integrated approach to reduce the human reservoir of infection and the use of insecticide and fly traps (57). The use of DEET (*N*,*N*-diethyl-*m*-toluamide) and permethrin-impregnated clothing or other insect repellents has not proved to be particularly effective against tsetse flies, but it does prevent other insect bites. Tsetse flies are attracted to clothing with bright and dark colors (blue and black). Persons visiting areas in which the infection is endemic should wear protective clothing (long-sleeved shirts and long trousers). Vaccines are not available.

OTHER TRYPANOSOMES INFECTING HUMANS

Trypanosoma congolense

Only one case of human infection with *Trypanosoma congolense* has been reported and confirmed by DNA identification (65). The patient had a mixed infection with *T. brucei* and was successfully treated with pentamidine.

Trypanosoma evansi

The first human case of *T. evansi* infection was diagnosed in India (3, 66). This organism is normally considered a parasite of animals (buffalo, camels, cattle, horses, and rats) and has a very wide geographic distribution (Africa, Asia, and Central and South America). The infection is transmitted mechanically by blood-sucking insects such as stable flies or horseflies. In animals, the incubation period is 5 to 60 days and the severity of the disease varies from no symptoms to weakness, weight loss, anemia, abortions, and death. In the abovementioned human case, the patient complained of transient fevers and sensory disorders. Fever peaks were noted every 7 to 10 days, and large numbers of parasites were detected in the blood at the time of fevers. No parasites were observed in the CSF. The patient was successfully treated with suramin. Normally, human serum has natural trypanolytic activity, but this patient was determined to have a mutation in apolipoprotein L1 (APOL1), which has trypanolytic activity (67). Laboratory diagnosis is usually done by examination of blood and lymph node aspirates or biopsy specimens. *T. evansi* can be cultured in mice and rats (68).

T. evansi cannot be differentiated from *T. brucei gambiense*, *T. brucei rhodesiense*, or *T. rangeli* microscopically.

Trypanosoma lewisi

Human cases of *Trypanosoma lewisi* infection have been described in India and Thailand in pediatric patients (69–72). Trypomastigotes were detected in the blood of these patients. In these cases, the patients fully recovered from the infection with no therapy. Symptoms included prolonged fever, thrombocytopenia hepatosplenomegaly, and elevated liver enzymes. The prevalence of this infection in humans is unknown.

The kinetoplast is subterminal to the posterior end of the trypomastigote, and the nucleus is found at the anterior end, terminating where the flagellum is free of the trypomastigote body. *T. lewisi* infection is a natural infection of wild rats and is considered nonpathogenic. The intermediate host is the flea, where the parasite multiplies in the gut and gives rise to epimastigotes that are found in the rectum and feces. The infection is passed to susceptible rats by ingestion of fleas or their feces. Human infections are thought to be transmitted in a similar fashion.

REFERENCES

1. **Adl SM, Simpson AG, Lane CE, Lukeš J, Bass D, Bowser SS, Brown MW, Burki F, Dunthorn M, Hampl V, Heiss A, Hoppenrath M, Lara E, Le Gall L, Lynn DH, McManus H, Mitchell EAD, Mozley-Stanridge SE, Parfrey LW, Pawlowski J, Rueckert S, Shadwick L, Schoch CL, Smirnov A, Spiegel FW.** 2012. The revised classification of eukaryotes. *J Eukaryot Microbiol* **59:**429–514. *ERRATUM J Eukaryot Microbiol* **60:**321.
2. **Votýpka J, d'Avila-Levy CM, Grellier P, Maslov DA, Lukeš J, Yurchenko V.** 2015. New approaches to systematics of Trypanosomatidae: criteria for taxonomic (re)description. *Trends Parasitol* **31:**460–469.
3. **World Health Organization.** 2005. A new form of human trypanosomiasis in India. Description of the first human case in the world caused by *Trypanosoma evansi*. *Wkly Epidemiol Rec* **80:**62–63.
4. **World Health Organization.** 2018. Leishmaniasis. World Health Organization, Geneva, Switzerland. http://www.who.int/mediacentre/factsheets/fs375/en/ (Accessed 14 March 2018.)
5. **Leelayoova S, Siripattanapipong S, Manomat J, Piyaraj P, Tan-Ariya P, Bualert L, Mungthin M.** 2017. Leishmaniasis in Thailand: a review of causative agents and situations. *Am J Trop Med Hyg* **96:**534–542.
6. **Akhoundi A, Downing T, Votypka J, Kuhls K. Lukes J, Cannet A, Ravel C, Marty P, Delaunay P, Kasbari M, Granouillac B, Gradoni L, Sereno D.** 2017. *Leishmania* infections: molecular targets and diagnosis. *Mol Aspects Med* **57:**1–29.
7. **Schönian G, Mauricio I, Cupolillo E.** 2010. Is it time to revise the nomenclature of *Leishmania*? *Trends Parasitol* **26:**466–469.
8. **Clarke CF, Bradley KK, Wright JH, Glowicz J.** 2013. Case report: emergence of autochthonous cutaneous leishmaniasis in northeastern Texas and southeastern Oklahoma. *Am J Trop Med Hyg* **88:**157–161.
9. **Bhattacharya SK, Dash AP.** 2017. Elimination of kala-azar from the southeast Asia region. *Am J Trop Med Hyg* **96:**802–804.
10. **Harhay MO, Olliaro PL, Costa DL, Costa CHN.** 2011. Urban parasitology: visceral leishmaniasis in Brazil. *Trends Parasitol* **27:**403–409.
11. **Aronson N, Herwaldt BL, Libman M, Pearson R, Lopez-Velez R, Weina P, Carvalho EM, Ephros M, Jeronimo S, Magill A.** 2016. Diagnosis and treatment of leishmaniasis: clinical practice guidelines by the Infectious Disease Society of America (IDSA) and the American Society of Tropical Medicine and Hygiene (ASTMH). *Clin Infect Dis* **63:**e202–e264.
12. **Pagliano P, Esposito S.** 2017. Visceral leishmaniosis in immunocompromised host: an update and literature review. *J Chemother* **29:**261–266.
13. **Saldanha MG, Queiroz A, Machado PRL, de Carvalho LP, Scott P, de Carvalho Filho EM, Arruda S.** 2017. Characterization of the histopathologic features in patients in the early and late phases of cutaneous leishmaniasis. *Am J Trop Med Hyg* **96:**645–652.
14. **Gajurel K, Dhakal R, Deresinski S.** 2017. Leishmaniasis in solid organ and hematopoietic stem cell transplant recipients. *Clin Transplant* **31:**e12867.
15. **de Almeida ME, Koru O, Steurer F, Herwaldt BL, da Silva AJ.** 2017. Detection and differentiation of *Leishmania* spp. in clinical specimens by use of a SYBR green-based real-time PCR assay. *J Clin Microbiol* **55:**281–290.
16. **Gomes CM, Cesetti MV, de Paula NA, Vernal S, Gupta G, Sampaio RN, Roselino AM.** 2017. Field validation of SYBR green- and TaqMan-based real-time PCR using biopsy and swab samples to diagnose American tegumentary leishmaniasis in an area where *Leishmania (Viannia) braziliensis* is endemic. *J Clin Microbiol* **55:**526–534.
17. **Siriyasatien P, Chusri S, Kraivichian K, Jariyapan N, Hortiwakul T, Silpapojakul K, Pym AM, Phumee A.** 2016. Early detection of novel *Leishmania* species DNA in the saliva of two HIV-infected patients. *BMC Infect Dis* **16:**89.
18. **Torpiano P, Pace D.** 2015. Leishmaniasis: diagnostic issues in Europe. *Expert Rev Anti Infect Ther* **13:**1123–1138.
19. **Neitzke-Abreu HC, Venazzi MS, Bernal MVZ, Reinhold-Castro KR, Vagetti F, Mota CA, Silva NR, Aristides SMA, Silveira TGV, Lonardoni MVC.** 2013. Detection of DNA from *Leishmania (Viannia)*: accuracy of polymerase chain reaction for the diagnosis of cutaneous leishmaniasis. *PLoS One* **8:**e62473.
20. **Paiva-Cavalcanti M, Morais RC, Pessoa-e-Sivla R, Trajano-Silva LA, Albuquerque SC, Tavares DH, Castro MC, Silva RF, Pereira VR.** 2015. Leishmaniasis diagnosis: an update on the use of immunological and molecular tools. *Cell Biosci* **5:**31.
21. **Leber A (ed).** 2015. *Clinical Microbiology Procedures Handbook*, 4th ed. ASM Press, Washington, DC.
22. **Napier LE.** 2012. A new serum test for kala-azar. 1922. *Indian J Med Res* **136:**830–846.
23. **Sato CM, Sanchez MC, Celeste BJ, Duthie MS, Guderian J, Reed SG, de Brito ME, Campos MB, de Souza Encarnação HV, Guerra J, de Mesquita TG, Pinheiro SK, Ramasawmy R, Silveira FT, de Assis Souza M, Goto H.** 2017. Use of recombinant antigens for sensitive serodiagnosis of American tegumentary leishmaniasis caused by different *Leishmania* species. *J Clin Microbiol* **55:**495–503.
24. **Bhattacharyya T, Marlais T, Miles MA.** 2017. Diagnostic antigens for visceral leishmaniasis: clarification of nomenclatures. *Parasit Vectors* **10:**178–180.
25. **Ghosh P, Bhaskar KRH, Hossain F, Khan MA, Vallur AC, Duthie MS, Hamano S, Salam MA, Huda MM, Khan MG, Coler RN, Reed SG, Mondal D.** 2016. Evaluation of diagnostic performance of rK28 ELISA using urine for diagnosis of visceral leishmaniasis. *Parasit Vectors* **9:**383–390.
26. **Srivastava S, Mishra J, Gupta AK, Singh A, Shankar P, Singh S.** 2017. Laboratory confirmed miltefosine resistant cases of visceral leishmaniasis from India. *Parasit Vectors* **10:**49–59.
27. **Mendonça MG, de Brito MEF, Rodrigues EHG, Bandeira V, Jardim ML, Abath FGC.** 2004. Persistence of *Leishmania* parasites in scars after clinical cure of American cutaneous leishmaniasis: is there a sterile cure? *J Infect Dis* **189:**1018–1023.
28. **Trajano-Silva LAM, Pessoa-E-Silva R, Gonçalves-de-Albuquerque SDC, Morais RCS, Costa-Oliveira CND, Goes TC, Paiva-Cavalcanti M.** 2017. Standardization and evaluation of a duplex real-time quantitative PCR for the detection of *Leishmania infantum* DNA: a sample quality control approach. *Rev Soc Bras Med Trop* **50:**350–357.
29. **Pan American Health Organization.** 2018. Chagas disease. Pan American Health Organization, Washington, DC. https://www.paho.org/hq/index.php?option=com_topics&view=article&id=10&Itemid=40473&lang=en.
30. **Bern C.** 2015. Chagas' Disease. *N Engl J Med* **373:**456–466.
31. **World Health Organization.** 2018. Chagas disease (American trypanosomiasis). World Health Organization, Geneva, Switzerland. http://www.who.int/mediacentre/factsheets/fs340/en/
32. **Balouz V, Agüero F, Buscaglia CA.** 2017. Chagas disease diagnostic applications: present knowledge and future steps. *Adv Parasitol* **97:**1–45.

33. **Forsyth CJ, Hernandez S, Olmedo W, Abuhamidah A, Traina MI, Sanchez DR, Soverow J, Meymandi SK.** 2016. Safety profile of nifurtimox for treatment of Chagas disease in the United States. *Clin Infect Dis* **63:**1056–1062.
34. **Garcia MN, Burroughs H, Gorchakov R, Gunter SM, Dumonteil E, Murray KO, Herrera CP.** 2017. Molecular identification and genotyping of *Trypanosoma cruzi* DNA in autochthonous Chagas disease patients from Texas, USA. *Infect Genet Evol* **49:**151–156.
35. **Gunter SM, Murray KO, Gorchakov R, Beddard R, Rossmann SN, Montgomery SP, Rivera H, Brown EL, Aguilar D, Widman LE, Garcia MN.** 2017. Likely autochthonous transmission of *Trypanosoma cruzi* to humans in south central Texas, USA. *Emerg Infect Dis* **23:**500–503.
36. **Montgomery SP, Parise ME, Dotson EM, Bialek SR.** 2016. What do we know about Chagas disease in the United States? *Am J Trop Med Hyg* **95:**1225–1227.
37. **Muñoz-San Martín C, Apt W, Zulantay I.** 2017. Real-time PCR strategy for the identification of *Trypanosoma cruzi* discrete typing units directly in chronically infected human blood. *Infect Genet Evol* **49:**300–308.
38. **Abras A, Muñoz C, Ballart C, Berenguer P, Llovet T, Herrero M, Tebar S, Pinazo MJ, Posada E, Martí C, Fumadó V, Bosch J, Coll O, Juncosa T, Ginovart G, Armengol J, Gascón J, Portús M, Gállego M.** 2017. Towards a new strategy for diagnosis of congenital *Trypanosoma cruzi* infection. *J Clin Microbiol* **55:**1396–1407.
39. **Murcia L, Simón M, Carrilero B, Roig M, Segovia M.** 2017. Treatment of infected women of childbearing age prevents congenital *Trypanosoma cruzi* infection by eliminating the parasitemia detected by PCR. *J Infect Dis* **215:**1452–1458.
40. **Strout RG.** 1962. A method for concentrating hemoflagellates. *J Parasitol* **48:**100.
41. **Wei B, Chen L, Kibukawa M, Kang J, Waskin H, Marton M.** 2016. Development of a PCR assay to detect low level Trypanosoma cruzi in blood specimens collected with PAXgene blood DNA tubes for clinical trials treating Chagas disease. *PLoS Neg Trop Dis* **10:**e0005146.
42. **Seiringer P, Pritsch M, Flores-Chavez M, Marchisio E, Helfrich K, Mengele C, Hohnerlein S, Bretzel G, Löscher T, Hoelscher M, Berens-Riha N.** 2017. Comparison of four PCR methods for efficient detection of *Trypanosoma cruzi* in routine diagnostics. *Diagn Microbiol Infect Dis* **88:**225–232.
43. **do Brasil PEAA, Castro R, de Castro L.** 2016. Commercial enzyme-linked immunosorbent assay versus polymerase chain reaction for the diagnosis of chronic Chagas disease: a systematic review and meta-analysis. *Mem Inst Oswaldo Cruz Rio de Janeiro* **111:**1–19.
44. **Abras A, Gállego M, Llovet T, Tebar S, Herrero M, Berenguer P, Ballart C, Martí C, Muñoz C.** 2016. Serological diagnosis of chonic Chagas disease: is it time for a change? *J Clin Microbiol* **54:**1566–1572.
45. **Morillo CA, Waskin H, Sosa-Estani S, Del Carmen Bangher M, Cuneo C, Milesi R, Mallagray M, Apt W, Beloscar J, Gascon J, Molina I, Echeverria LE, Colombo H, Perez-Molina JA, Wyss F, Meeks B, Bonilla LR, Gao P, Wei B, McCarthy M, Yusuf S, STOP-CHAGAS Investigators.** 2017. Benznidole and posaconazole in eliminating parasites in asymptomatic *T. cruzi* carriers: the STOP-CHAGAS Trial. *J Am Coll Cardiol* **69:**939–947.
46. **Rodriguez JB, Falcone BN, Szajnman SH.** 2016. Detection and treatment of *Trypanosoma cruzi*: a patent review (2011-2015). *Expert Opin Ther Pat* **26:**993–1015.
47. **Alvarez MG, Bertocchi GL, Cooley G, Albareda MC, Viotti R, Perez-Mazliah DE, Lococo B, Eiro MC, Laucella SA, Tarleton RL.** 2016. Treatment success in Trypanosoma cruzi infection is predicted by early changes in serially monitored parasite-specific T and B cell responses. *PLoS Neg Trop Dis* **10:**e0004657.
48. **Benatti RD, Oliveira GH, Bacal F.** 2017. Heart transplantation for Chagas cardiomyopathy. *J Heart Lung Transplant* **36:**597–603.
49. **Guhl F, Vallejo GA.** 2003. *Trypanosoma* (*Herpetosoma*) *rangeli* Tejera, 1920: an updated review. *Mem Inst Oswaldo Cruz* **98:**435–442.
50. **Chiurillo MA, Crisante G, Rojas A, Peralta A, Dias M, Guevara P, Añez N, Ramírez JL.** 2003. Detection of *Trypanosoma cruzi* and *Trypanosoma rangeli* infection by duplex PCR assay based on telomeric sequences. *Clin Diagn Lab Immunol* **10:**775–779.
51. **Da Silva FM, Noyes H, Campaner M, Junqueira ACV, Coura JR, Añez N, Shaw JJ, Stevens JR, Teixeira MMG.** 2004. Phylogeny, taxonomy and grouping of *Trypanosoma rangeli* isolates from man, triatomines and sylvatic mammals from widespread geographical origin based on SSU and ITS ribosomal sequences. *Parasitology* **129:**549–561.
52. **World Health Organization.** Human African trypanosomiasis. World Health Organization, Geneva, Switzerland. http://www.who.int/trypanosomiasis_african/en/ (Accessed 18 July 2018.)
53. **Bisser S, Lumbala C, Nguertoum E, Kande V, Flevaud L, Vatunga G, Boelaert M, Buscher P, Josenando T, Bessell PR, Bieler S, Ndung'u JM.** 2016. Sensitivity and specificity of a prototype rapid diagnostic test for the detection of Trypanosoma brucei gambiense infection: a multi-centric prospective study. *PLOS Neg Trop Dis* **10:**e0004608.
54. **Dubois ME, Demick KP, Mansfield JM.** 2005. Trypanosomes expressing a mosaic variant surface glycoprotein coat escape early detection by the immune system. *Infect Immun* **73:**2690–2697.
55. **Balmer O, Caccone A.** 2008. Multiple-strain infections of *Trypanosoma brucei* across Africa. *Acta Trop* **107:**275–279.
56. **Gineau L, Courtin D, Camara M, Ilboudo H, Jamonneau V, Dias FC, Tokplonou L, Milet J, Mendonça PB, Castelli EC, Camara O, Camara M, Favier B, Rouas-Freiss N, Moreau P, Donadi EA, Bucheton B, Sabbagh A, Garcia A.** 2016. Human leukocyte antigen-G: a promising prognostic marker of disease progression to improve the control of human African trypanosomiasis. *Clin Infect Dis* **63:**1189–1197.
57. **Buscher P, Cecchi G, Jamonneau V, Priotto G.** 2017. Human African trypanosomiasis. *Lancet* **390:**2397–2409.
58. **Chappuis F, Loutan L, Simarro P, Lejon V, Büscher P.** 2005. Options for field diagnosis of human African trypanosomiasis. *Clin Microbiol Rev* **18:**133–146.
59. **Ngotho M, Kagira JM, Gachie BM, Karanja SM, Waema MW, Maranga DN, Maina NW.** 2015. Loop mediated isothermal amplification for detection of *Trypanosoma brucei gambiense* in urine and saliva samples in nonhuman primate model. *BioMed Res Int* **2015:**867846.
60. **Büscher P, Gilleman Q, Lejon V.** 2013. Rapid diagnostic test for sleeping sickness. *N Engl J Med* **368:**1069–1070.
61. **Lejon V, Roger I, Mumba Ngoyi D, Menten J, Robays J, N'siesi FX, Bisser S, Boelaert M, Büscher P.** 2008. Novel markers for treatment outcome in late-stage *Trypanosoma brucei gambiense* trypanosomiasis. *Clin Infect Dis* **47:**15–22.
62. **Sullivan L, Wall SJ, Carrington M, Ferguson MAJ.** 2013. Proteomic selection of immunodiagnostic antigens for human African trypanosomiasis and generation of a prototype lateral flow immunodiagnostic device. *PLoS Negl Trop Dis* **7:**e2087.
63. **Eyford BA, Ahmad R, Enyaru JC, Carr SA, Pearson TW.** 2013. Identification of trypanosome proteins in plasma from African sleeping sickness patients infected with *T. b. rhodesiense*. *PLoS One* **8:**e71463.
64. **Lejon V, Büscher P.** 2005. Review article: cerebrospinal fluid in human African trypanosomiasis: a key to diagnosis, therapeutic decision and post-treatment follow-up. *Trop Med Int Health* **10:**395–403.
65. **Truc P, Jamonneau V, N'Guessan P, N'Dri L, Diallo PB, Cuny G.** 1998. *Trypanosoma brucei* ssp. and *T congolense*: mixed human infection in Côte d'Ivoire. *Trans R Soc Trop Med Hyg* **92:**537–538.
66. **Van Vinh Chau N, Buu Chau L, Desquesnes M, Herder S, Phu Huong Lan N, Campbell JI, Van Cuong N, Yimming B, Chalermwong P, Jittapalapong S, Ramon Franco J, Tri Tue N, Rabaa MA, Carrique-Mas J, Pham Thi Thanh T, Tran Vu Thieu N, Berto A, Thi Hoa N, Van Minh Hoang N, Canh Tu N, Khac Chuyen N, Wills B, Tinh Hien T, Thwaites GE, Yacoub S, Baker S.** 2016. A clinical and epidemiological investigation of the first reported human

infection with the zoonotic parasite *Trypanosoma evansi* in Southeast Asia. *Clin Infect Dis* **62:**1002–1008.

67. **Vanhollebeke B, Truc P, Poelvoorde P, Pays A, Joshi PP, Katti R, Jannin JG, Pays E.** 2006. Human *Trypanosoma evansi* infection linked to a lack of apolipoprotein L-I. *N Engl J Med* **355:**2752–2756.
68. **Kaur R, Gupta VK, Dhariwal AC, Jain DC, Shiv L.** 2007. A rare case of trypanosomiasis in a two month old infant in Mumbai, India. *J Commun Dis* **39:**71–74.
69. **Sarataphan N, Vongpakorn M, Nuansrichay B, Autarkool N, Keowkarnkah T, Rodtian P, Stich RW, Jittapalapong S.** 2007. Diagnosis of a *Trypanosoma lewisi*-like (*Herpetosoma*) infection in a sick infant from Thailand. *J Med Microbiol* **56:**1118–1121.
70. **Verma A, Manchanda S, Kumar N, Sharma A, Goel M, Banerjee PS, Garg R, Singh BP, Balharbi F, Lejon V, Deborggraeve S, Singh Rana UV, Puliyel J.** 2011. *Trypanosoma lewisi* or *T. lewisi*-like infection in a 37-day-old Indian infant. *Am J Trop Med Hyg* **85:**221–224.
71. **de Sousa MA.** 2014. On opportunist infections by *Trypanosoma lewisi* in humans and its differential diagnosis from *T. cruzi* and *T. rangeli*. *Parasitol Res* **113:**4471–4475.
72. **Lun ZR, Wen YZ, Uzureau P, Lecordier L, Lai DH, Lan YG, Desquesnes M, Geng GQ, Yang TB, Zhou WL, Jannin JG, Simarro PP, Truc P, Vincendeau P, Pays E.** 2015. Resistance to normal human serum reveals *Trypanosoma lewisi* as an underestimated human pathogen. *Mol Biochem Parasitol* **199:**58–61.

Toxoplasma

JAMES B. McAULEY AND KAMALJIT SINGH

141

Toxoplasmosis is caused by infection with the parasite *Toxoplasma gondii*. It is one of the most common parasitic infections in humans and is most typically asymptomatic. However, in certain clinical situations, it can cause severe and disabling disease, making accurate and timely diagnosis vital.

TAXONOMY

T. gondii is classified in the Apicomplexa: Conoidasida: Coccidia: Eimeriorina, genus *Toxoplasma*. See chapter 135.

LIFE CYCLE

T. gondii is a protozoan parasite that infects most species of warm-blooded animals, including humans, through ingestion of tissue cysts or plants contaminated by oocysts. Members of the cat family Felidae are the only known definitive hosts for the sexual stages of *T. gondii* and thus are the main reservoirs of infection. The three stages of this obligate intracellular parasite are (i) tachyzoites (trophozoites), which rapidly proliferate and destroy infected cells during acute infection; (ii) bradyzoites, which slowly multiply in tissue cysts; and (iii) sporozoites in oocysts (Fig. 1). Tachyzoites and bradyzoites occur in body tissues; oocysts are excreted in cat feces (Fig. 2). Cats become infected with *T. gondii* by consuming infected animals or animal products or by ingestion of oocysts. Cats that are allowed to roam outside are much more likely to become infected than domestic cats that are confined indoors. After tissue cysts or oocysts are ingested by the cat, viable organisms are released and invade epithelial cells of the small intestine, where they undergo an asexual cycle followed by a sexual cycle and then form oocysts, which are then excreted. The unsporulated (i.e., noninfective) oocyst takes 1 to 5 days after excretion to become sporulated (infective). Although cats shed oocysts for only 1 to 2 weeks, large numbers may be shed, often exceeding 100,000 per g of feces. Oocysts can survive in the environment for several months to more than a year and are remarkably resistant to disinfectants, freezing, and drying but are killed by heating to 70°C for 10 min (1).

EPIDEMIOLOGY AND TRANSMISSION

Serologic prevalence data indicate that toxoplasmosis is one of the most common infections of humans throughout the world (2). Because *T. gondii* organisms are rarely detected in humans with toxoplasmosis, serologic examination is used to indicate the presence of the infection by detecting *Toxoplasma*-specific antibodies. The prevalence of positive serologic titers increases with age. In many areas of the world, infection is more common in warm climates and at lower altitudes than in cold climates and mountainous regions. This distribution is probably related to conditions favoring the sporulation and survival of oocysts. Variations in the prevalence of infection between geographic areas and between population groups within the same locale are also probably due to differences in exposure. A high prevalence of infection in France (50 to 85%) has been related to a preference for eating raw or undercooked meat. However, a high prevalence in Central America has been related to the frequency of stray cats in a climate favoring the survival of oocysts. In U.S. military recruits in 1962, seroprevalence rates of up to 30% were found in people living along the sea coast, with rates of less than 1% in people from the Rocky Mountains and the desert Southwest. More recent data comparing antibody prevalence in U.S. military recruits in 1962 and 1989 indicated a one-third decrease in seropositivity (3). The overall seroprevalence in the United States as determined with specimens collected by the Third National Health and Nutritional Assessment Survey (NHANES III) between 1988 and 1994 among persons 12 or more years of age was found to be 22.5%, with seroprevalence among women of childbearing age (15 to 44 years) being 15% (4). More recently, in an analysis of NHANES data, *T. gondii* seroprevalence was shown to have declined in U.S.-born persons 12 to 49 years old from 14.1% in 1988 to 1994 to 9.0% in 1999 to 2004 (5).

Human infection may be acquired in several ways: (i) ingestion of undercooked contaminated meat containing *T. gondii* cysts; (ii) ingestion of oocysts from hands, food, soil, or water contaminated with cat feces; (iii) organ transplantation or blood transfusion; (iv) transplacental transmission; and (v) accidental inoculation of tachyzoites. The two major routes of transmission of *Toxoplasma* to humans are oral and congenital. In humans, ingesting either the tissue cyst or the oocyst results in the rupture of the cyst wall (6), which releases organisms that invade the intestinal epithelium, disseminate throughout the body, and multiply intracellularly. The host cell dies and releases

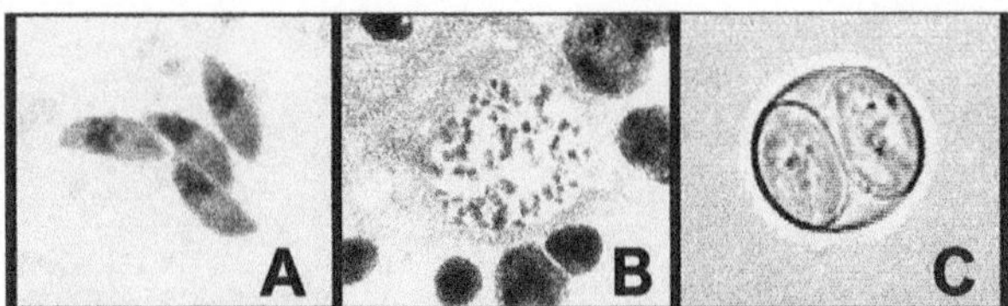

FIGURE 1 Three life stages of *T. gondii*. (A) Tachyzoites stained with Giemsa stain. (B) Cyst with bradyzoites in brain tissue stained with Giemsa stain. (C) Sporulated oocysts, unstained. Photographs courtesy of J. P. Dubey, U.S. Department of Agriculture, Beltsville, MD.

tachyzoites, which invade adjacent cells and continue the process. The tachyzoites are pressured by the host's immune response to transform into bradyzoites and form tissue cysts, most commonly in skeletal muscle, myocardium, and brain; these cysts may remain throughout the life of the host. Recrudescence of clinical disease may occur if the host becomes immunosuppressed and the cysts rupture, releasing the parasites.

Recently, researchers have begun to appreciate that differences in transmission, reactivation, and disease severity may also be explained by different genotypes of *T. gondii* which occur in different parts of the world (7).

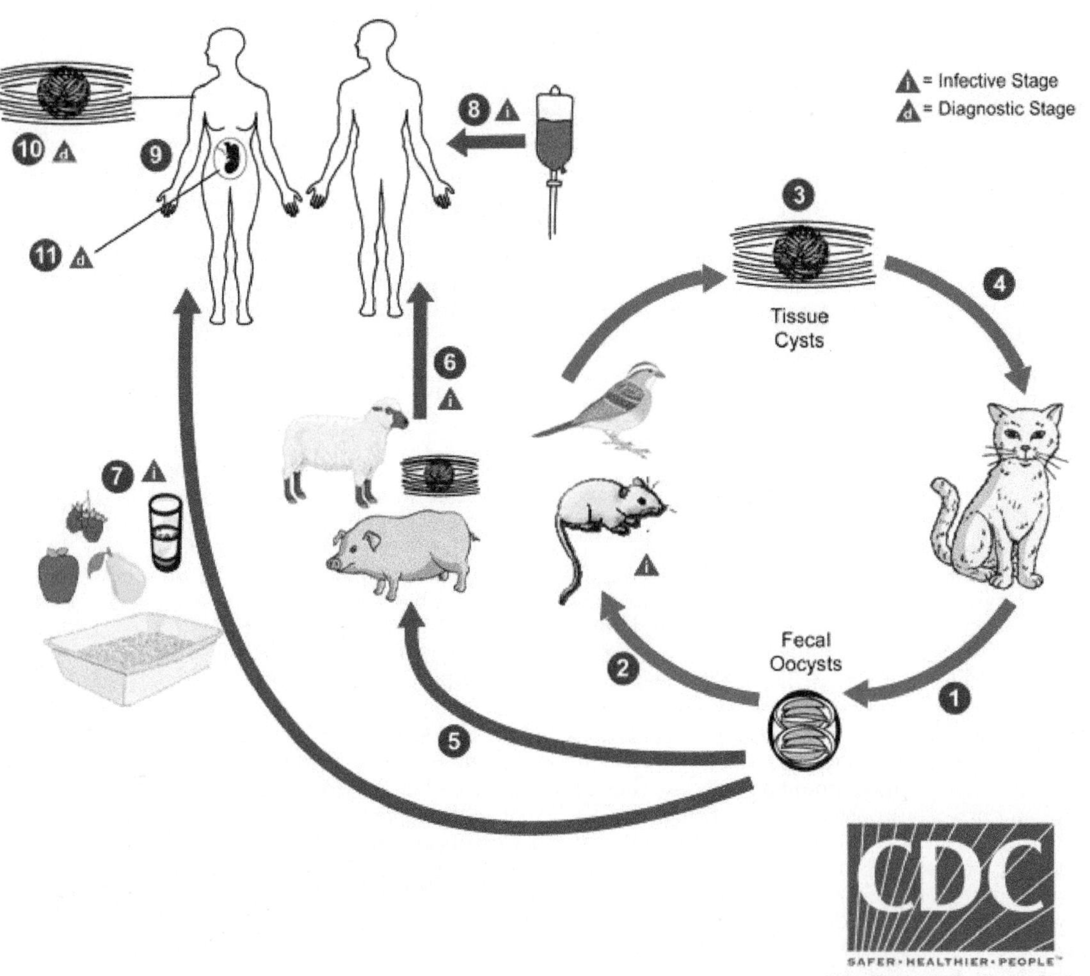

FIGURE 2 Life cycle of *T. gondii*. (1) Unsporulated oocysts are shed in the cat's feces; although oocysts are usually shed for only 1 to 2 weeks, large numbers may be shed. (2) Intermediate hosts in nature (including birds and rodents) become infected after ingesting soil, water, or plant material contaminated with oocysts. (3) Oocysts transform into tachyzoites, which localize in neural and muscle tissue and develop into tissue cyst bradyzoites. (4) Cats become infected after consuming intermediate hosts harboring tissue cysts or by ingestion of sporulated oocysts. (5) Animals bred for human consumption and wild game may also become infected with tissue cysts after ingestion of sporulated oocysts in the environment. Humans can become infected by any of several routes: (6) eating undercooked meat of animals harboring tissue cysts; (7) consuming food or water contaminated with cat feces or coming into contact with contaminated substances (such as feces-contaminated soil or the litter box of a pet cat); (8) blood transfusion or organ transplantation; (9) transplacentally from mother to fetus. (10) Diagnosis is usually achieved by serology, although tissue cysts may be observed in stained biopsy specimens. (11) Diagnosis of congenital infections can be achieved by detecting *T. gondii* DNA in amniotic fluid using molecular methods, such as PCR.

Prevention

Risk factors for *T. gondii* infection identified in epidemiologic studies include eating raw or undercooked pork, mutton, lamb, beef, ground meat products, oysters, clams, mussels, or wild game meat; kitten ownership; cleaning the cat litter box; contact with soil (gardening and yard work); and eating raw or unwashed vegetables or fruits (1, 4, 8–10). Recommendations for prevention of toxoplasmosis for all persons, including pregnant women, were originally discussed at a conference at the U.S. Centers for Disease Control and Prevention (CDC) and published (1), and these now have been updated (see the Division of Parasitic Diseases and Malaria web page: http://www.cdc.gov/parasites/toxoplasmosis/prevent.html). These recommendations included the following: (i) food should be cooked to safe temperatures (beef, lamb, and veal roasts and steaks to at least 145°F with a 3-minute rest; pork, ground meat, and wild game to 160°F; poultry to at least 165°F with a 3-minute rest); (ii) fruits and vegetables should be peeled or washed thoroughly before eating; (iii) cutting boards, dishes, counters, utensils, and hands should always be washed with hot soapy water after they have contacted raw meat, poultry, or seafood or unwashed fruits or vegetables; (iv) individuals should wear gloves when gardening and during any contact with soil or sand, because cat waste might be in soil or sand, and should wash hands afterwards. Pregnant women should avoid changing cat litter; pregnant women who must change cat litter should use gloves and then wash their hands thoroughly. The litter box should be changed daily, because *T. gondii* oocysts require more than one day to become infectious. Pregnant women should be encouraged to keep their cats inside and not adopt or handle stray cats. Cats should be fed only canned or dried commercial food or well-cooked table food, not raw or undercooked meats. Several outbreaks have been reported in association with drinking untreated water contaminated by oocysts. Freezing meats for several days at subzero (0°F) temperatures greatly reduces the risk of infection (1).

CLINICAL SIGNIFICANCE

Toxoplasmosis can be categorized into four groups: (i) infection acquired in the immunocompetent patient; (ii) infection acquired or reactivated in the immunodeficient patient; (iii) congenital infection; and (iv) ocular infection. Methods of diagnosis and their interpretations may differ for each clinical category.

Acquired infection with *Toxoplasma* in immunocompetent individuals is generally an asymptomatic infection. However, 10 to 20% of patients with acute infection may develop cervical lymphadenopathy and/or a flu-like illness. The clinical course is benign and self-limited; symptoms usually resolve within weeks or months.

Immunodeficient patients often have central nervous system (CNS) disease but may have myocarditis or pneumonitis. In patients with AIDS, toxoplasmic encephalitis is the most common cause of intracerebral mass lesions and is thought to be due most often to reactivation of chronic infection. Toxoplasmosis in patients being treated with immunosuppressive drugs may be due to either newly acquired or reactivated latent infection (11, 12).

Congenital toxoplasmosis results from an acute primary infection acquired by the mother during pregnancy. The incidence and severity of congenital toxoplasmosis vary with the trimester during which infection was acquired (13). Because treatment of the mother may reduce the severity of manifestations in the infant due to congenital infection, prompt and accurate diagnosis is extremely important. Many infants with subclinical infection at birth will subsequently develop signs or symptoms of congenital toxoplasmosis; however, prompt treatment may help prevent subsequent symptoms.

Ocular toxoplasmosis, an important cause of chorioretinitis in the United States, may be the result of congenital or acquired infection (14). Acquired infection is now thought to be more common than congenital infection and can be seen in immunocompetent and immunocompromised hosts. Congenitally infected patients can be asymptomatic until the second or third decade of life, when lesions develop in the eye, presumably due to cyst rupture and subsequent release of tachyzoites and bradyzoites. Chorioretinitis is characteristically bilateral in patients with congenital infection but is often unilateral in individuals with acute acquired *T. gondii* infection.

Recent data have suggested an association between *T. gondii* infection and various neurologic or psychiatric syndromes, including schizophrenia, Alzheimer's disease, and even suicide (15–17). These findings are intriguing but require further study to validate.

COLLECTION, TRANSPORT, AND STORAGE OF SPECIMENS

Serum, plasma, cerebrospinal fluid (CSF), ocular fluid, and amniotic fluid may be tested for antibodies and/or parasite DNA (2).

Collection for Determination of Parasite DNA

Blood samples should be collected with an anticoagulant; CSF, ocular fluid, and amniotic fluids do not need an anticoagulant. All samples should be shipped and stored at 4°C prior to testing.

Collection for Antibody Determination

Blood specimens to be tested for the presence of antibodies should be allowed to clot and centrifuged, and the serum should be removed and shipped to a reference laboratory. Hemolysis does not seem to interfere with the antibody reaction in most tests. At least 3 ml of serum and 1 ml of CSF should be submitted. Specimens may be stored up to 1 week at 4°C or frozen for longer storage. Specimens may be shipped at ambient temperature for overnight delivery or using a cold pack or frozen if there will be delays in transit. To avoid evaporation of small volumes, ocular fluids should be stored and shipped frozen. CSF and ocular fluid should be tested in parallel with a serum sample drawn on the same date. Long-term storage should take place at −20°C or below.

If the determination of immune status is the reason for testing, a single serum specimen is satisfactory; acute- and convalescent-phase specimens are not necessary. In situations in which determining the time of infection is important, specimens drawn at least 3 weeks apart may or may not be useful. In most cases, detection of an increasing immunoglobulin G (IgG) or IgM titer is not possible because the titers have already reached a plateau by the time the initial sample is drawn. If two specimens are to be compared, they should be tested in parallel. Results from tests done at different times, in different laboratories, or with different procedures should not be compared quantitatively, only qualitatively as positive or negative.

For tests other than serology, a reference laboratory should be contacted for instructions before specimens are collected, to ensure proper collection and handling.

DIRECT EXAMINATION

Microscopy

Only very rarely can the diagnosis of toxoplasmosis be documented by the observation of parasites in patient specimens (18, 19). Secretions, excretions, body fluids, and tissues are potential specimens for direct observation of parasites but are generally unrewarding. Fluid specimens such as heparinized blood or CSF should be centrifuged, and the sediment should be smeared on a microscope slide. The slides should be air dried, fixed in methanol, and stained with Giemsa for microscopic examination. Tachyzoites may be observed as free organisms or within host cells, such as leukocytes. Well-preserved tachyzoites are crescent shaped and stain well, but degenerating organisms may be oval and stain poorly. Tissue imprints stained with Giemsa may reveal *T. gondii* cysts.

Antigen Detection

Immunologic techniques have been used to identify parasites in tissue sections or tissue cultures; fluorescein isothiocyanate- or peroxidase-labeled antisera may be useful in detecting tachyzoites in tissue sections. EIA antigen detection techniques lack sensitivity for human samples and are not recommended.

Nucleic Acid Detection

Nucleic acid amplification testing (NAAT) for *Toxoplasma* DNA detection is an increasingly important technology for detection of congenital infections, ocular disease in immunocompetent patients, and toxoplasmic encephalitis in AIDS patients (20–28). The most important use of NAAT is for prenatal diagnosis of congenital toxoplasmosis using amniotic fluid. When maternal serological results indicate potential infection during pregnancy, NAAT of amniotic fluid has been particularly important for the confirmation of fetal infection, performing better than traditional methods of inoculation of mice and tissue culture cells and fetal blood testing for IgM (29, 30). NAAT technology for *Toxoplasma* is offered at the Toxoplasma Serology Laboratory, Palo Alto, CA (http://www.pamf.org/serology/), and by a few commercial laboratories. Commercial systems are now available (ELITe MGB) and compare favorably to reference laboratory systems (31). The repeated-sequence AF146257 gene target (also known as *Rep529*) has largely replaced other NAAT targets, such as the B1 gene. The requestor should be aware that the reliability of NAAT tests may vary widely (20, 32–35). NAAT testing by low-density microarrays has been used successfully in the evaluation of granulomatous lymphadenitis (36). Recently, loop-mediated isothermal amplification has been used to detect *Toxoplasma* DNA in blood (37).

Cell-Mediated Immune Responses

T-cell response has been studied in newborns with congenital toxoplasmosis, and a recent study suggested that measurement of interferon gamma production by T cells in response to stimulation by specific *Toxoplasma* antigens may add to the diagnosis of congenital infection (38). The interferon gamma release assay has been used successfully to detect cell-mediated responses in congenitally infected infants (39).

ISOLATION PROCEDURES

Parasites can be isolated with limited success by inoculating patient tissue or body fluids into either mice or tissue culture cells (40). Fresh tissue samples are ground in saline with a mortar and pestle and inoculated intraperitoneally into mice or directly into tissue culture flasks. The mice should be monitored for 4 to 6 weeks; if the organism is virulent for mice, the parasites can often be demonstrated in the peritoneal fluid after 5 to 10 days. However, if the organism is relatively avirulent for mice, as is usually the case, the mice may not be killed by the infection. If they survive for 6 weeks, serum samples should be obtained for serologic testing. If antibodies are present, the mouse brain should be examined for the presence of *T. gondii* cysts. If cysts are not observed, the murine host may not have been the ideal host. Inoculate additional mice with brain homogenate from the initially inoculated mice and observe and recheck after 6 weeks. *T. gondii* grows in a variety of tissue culture cells. A cytopathic effect may be detected on direct examination after 24 to 96 h in culture. Giemsa staining may reveal parasite structure, but parasitized cells may be difficult to detect. Immunofluorescence allows more sensitive detection of the organisms. The following procedure has been used with some success for parasite isolation from amniotic fluids (2, 41). Centrifuge a 10-ml sample of amniotic fluid at 1,000 × *g*. Resuspend the sediment in 8 ml of minimum essential medium. Inoculate 1 ml into coverslip cultures of human embryonic fibroblast cell line MRC5 in 24-well plates. Incubate the cultures for 96 h with one change of medium at 24 h; fix the cultures with cold acetone. Examine the coverslips by indirect immunofluorescence for the presence of *T. gondii*. The use of tissue culture cells for isolation permits a more rapid diagnosis than mouse inoculation; both methods can be useful for diagnosing congenital toxoplasmosis.

SEROLOGIC TESTS

Serologic testing for *T. gondii*-specific antibodies is the most commonly used method for diagnosis of toxoplasmosis. Many tests for the detection of antibodies to *Toxoplasma* have been used since Sabin and Feldman developed the methylene blue dye test (DT) (2, 35, 42). Commercial kits for agglutination tests, indirect fluorescent antibody (IFA) tests, and enzyme immunoassays (EIA) are available worldwide. Multiple platforms, including multiplex microarrays, semiautomated immunoassays, etc., allow testing of large numbers of specimens and of multiple pathogens in high-volume laboratories (43, 44). Because of difficulties in obtaining specimens from patients with clinically documented toxoplasmosis, commercial kit sensitivity and specificity may be based not on documented case specimens but rather on a comparison of results obtained with another kit. Consequently, the true sensitivity and specificity of a kit are generally not known or determined. The rates stated by the manufacturer or published in articles may vary depending upon the samples chosen for testing. Sensitivity and specificity rates determined in prospective studies, when random samples are tested as received for *Toxoplasma* testing, will usually differ from those determined in retrospective studies, when the samples have been chosen as either clear positive or negative specimens, which decreases the probability of detecting false-positive or false-negative reactions.

When laboratory personnel decide to initiate *Toxoplasma*-specific antibody testing or when they decide to switch to a different antibody detection kit, the user must carefully review the manufacturer's package insert and published literature for information on the sensitivity and specificity rates. The user should perform an in-laboratory comparison of kits by using positive and negative samples confirmed by a toxoplasmosis reference laboratory. Tables 1 and 2 list

TABLE 1 *Toxoplasma* IgG kits available commercially in the United States

Type of test and company[a]	Kit	Reference(s)
IFA		
GenBio	ImmunoFA Toxoplasma IgG	
Hemagen	Virgo Toxo IgG	
Inverness	Toxoplasma IgG	
Meridian	Toxoplasma IgG	
EIA		
Abbott Labs	IMx Toxo IgG	18, 38, 50, 52, 67, 93
	AxSYM Toxo IgG	24, 42, 84, 89, 105
Bayer Diagnostics	Immuno1	93
	Advia Centaur	86
Beckman Coulter	Access Toxo G	19
bioMérieux Vitek	Vidas Toxo IgG	38, 42, 52, 89, 100, 105, 106
Bio-Rad	Platelia Toxo G	52, 89
Biotecx	OptiCoat Toxo IgG ELISA	
Biotest Diagnostics	Toxo IgG	
Diagnostic Products Corp.	Immulite Toxoplasma IgG	24, 32, 106
Diamedix	Toxoplasma IgG	
DiaSorin	Toxoplasma IgG	
	Liaison	107
GenBio	Immunodot Torch	
Hemagen	Toxoplasma IgG	
Inverness	Toxo IgG II	
Roche Diagnostics	Elecsys Toxo IgG	
Trinity Biotech	Captia Toxoplasma gondii IgG	
Teco Diagnostics	Toxoplasma IgG	
Latex		
Biokit	Toxogen	

[a]Abbott Labs, Diagnostics Division, North Chicago, IL 60064; Ani Labsystems Lyd., Tiilitie 3, 01720 Vantaa, Finland; Bayer Diagnostics, 511 Benedict Ave., Tarrytown, NY 10591; Beckman Coulter, 4300 N. Harbor Blvd., Fullerton, CA 92834; Biokit USA, 113 Hartwell Ave., Lexington, MA 02173; bioMérieux, 595 Anglum Dr., Hazelwood, MO 63042; BioRad, 4000 Alfred Nobel Dr., Hercules, CA 94547; Biotecx Laboratories, 6023 S. Loop East, Houston, TX 77033; Biotest Diagnostics Corp., 66 Ford Rd., Suite 131, Denville, NJ 07834; Diagnostic Products Corp., 5700 W. 96th St., Los Angeles, CA 90045; Diamedix Corp., 2140 N. Miami Ave., Miami, FL 33127; DiaSorin, P.O. Box 285, Stillwater, MN 55082; GenBio, 15222A Avenue of Science, San Diego, CA 92128; Hemagen Diagnostics, 34-40 Bear Hill Rd., Waltham, MA 02154; Inverness Medical Professional Diagnostics, 2 Research Way, Princeton, NJ 08540; Meridian Bioscience, 3471 River Hills Dr., Cincinnati, OH 45244; Roche Diagnostics Corp., 9115 Hague Rd., Indianapolis, IN 46250; Teco Diagnostics, 1268 N. Lakeview Ave., Anaheim, CA 92807.

commercial kits available in the United States and references to published evaluations. However, the test kit industry is in a great deal of flux; company and kit names may change.

In the United States, initial testing for the presence of IgG antibodies in most laboratories is usually performed with an EIA or IFA commercial kit. Results may be stated in international units (based on the WHO international standard reference serum for *Toxoplasma* [36, 45] distributed by the Public Health Wales, Singleton Hospital [Swansea SA2 8QA, Wales, United Kingdom; http://www.wales.nhs.uk/]), as an index (specific to each kit), as an optical density value (specific to each kit), or as a geometric mean titer. Numerical results are not comparable from kit to kit; comparison may be made only qualitatively as negative (nonreactive or not infected) or positive (reactive or infected). Although elevated *Toxoplasma*-specific IgG levels have been suggested as an indicator of recent infection, high levels may last for many years after primary infection and should not be relied upon for this purpose.

To more definitely distinguish acute and chronic infections, detection of *Toxoplasma*-specific IgM antibodies has been used. The most important use of IgM test results is that a negative reaction essentially excludes recent infection. A guide to the general interpretation of *Toxoplasma* IgG and IgM serology results is presented in Table 3. IFA IgM titers generally increase within 1 week of the onset of symptoms and revert to negative within 6 to 9 months of infection. False-positive reactions caused by rheumatoid factor and false-negative reactions caused by blockage by *Toxoplasma*-specific IgG may occur in IFA for IgM and indirect EIA for IgM when whole serum samples are tested. To decrease the effects of these interfering factors, specimens should be treated to obtain only the IgM fraction for testing.

The IgM capture EIA eliminates potential interference by IgG and other isotypes by binding only IgM antibodies; unbound antibodies are removed by washing, thus eliminating the need for serum fractionation. The most important advantage of the IgM capture EIA compared to IFA is the increased detection of congenital infections: the IgM ELISA was positive for 73% of serum samples from newborn infants with proven congenital toxoplasmosis, whereas only 25% of the same serum samples were positive by an IFA IgM test (46). Although the capture EIA system is more efficient at detecting acute infections, some persons may have undetectable or low-level IgM antibodies, and some persons may have detectable IgM antibodies beyond 2 years postinfection (2, 47). Therefore, determining the relative time of infection is not possible with this system alone. Many commercial companies market an EIA kit for IgM; some use the indirect EIA format with a serum pretreatment step, while others use the IgM capture format. False-positive IgM reactions due to unknown factors may be a problem with commercially available kits (48).

TABLE 2 *Toxoplasma* IgM kits available commercially in the United States

Type of test and company[a]	Kit	Reference(s)
IFA		
GenBio	ImmunoFA Toxoplasma IgM	
Hemagen	Virgo Toxo IgM	
Inverness	Toxoplasma gondii IgM	
Meridian	Toxoplasma IgM	
EIA		
Abbott Labs	IMx Toxo IgM	20, 52, 67, 71, 108
	AxSYM Toxo IgM	19, 42, 89, 109
Bayer Diagnostics	Immuno1	
	Advia Centaur	86
Beckman Coulter	Access Toxo M	19, 20, 29, 69
bioMérieux Vitek	Vidas Toxo IgM	5, 19, 42, 52, 89, 108, 109
Bio-Rad	Platelia Toxo IgM	20, 52, 68, 89, 108
Biotecx	OptiCoat Toxo IgM	
Biotest Diagnostics	Toxo IgM	
Biokit	Toxoplasma IgM	
Diagnostic Products Corp.	Immulite	32, 106
Diamedix	Toxoplasma IgM	107
DiaSorin	Toxoplasma IgM	
	Liaison	89
Hemagan	Toxoplasma IgM	
Trinity Biotech	Captia Toxoplasma gondii IgM	
Inverness	Toxo IgM	
Teco Diagnostics	Toxoplasma IgG	

[a]Abbott Labs, Diagnostics Division, North Chicago, IL 60064; Bayer Diagnostics, 511 Benedict Ave., Tarrytown, NY 10591; Beckman Coulter, 4300 N. Harbor Blvd., Fullerton, CA 92834; Biokit USA, 113 Hartwell Ave., Lexington, MA 02173; bioMérieux, 595 Anglum Dr., Hazelwood, MO 63042; BioRad, 4000 Alfred Nobel Dr., Hercules, CA 94547; Biotecx Laboratories, 6023 S. Loop East, Houston, TX 77033; Biotest Diagnostics Corp., 66 Ford Rd., Suite 131, Denville, NJ 07834; Diagnostic Products Corp., 5700 W. 96th St., Los Angeles, CA 90045; Diamedix Corp., 2140 N. Miami Ave., Miami, FL 33127; DiaSorin, P.O. Box 285, Stillwater, MN 55082; GenBio, 15222A Avenue of Science, San Diego, CA 92128; Hemagen Diagnostics, 34-40 Bear Hill Rd., Waltham, MA 02154; Inverness Medical Professional Diagnostics, 2 Research Way, Princeton, NJ 08540; Meridian Bioscience, 3471 River Hills Dr., Cincinnati, OH 45244; Teco Diagnostics, 1268 N. Lakeview Ave., Anaheim, CA 92807.

The *Toxoplasma* IgG avidity test is an additional tool to help discriminate between past and recently acquired infection (2, 25, 34, 38, 49–52). The test is based on the observation that during acute infection, IgG antibodies bind antigen weakly or have low avidity, while patients with chronic infection have more strongly binding (high-avidity) antibodies. Depending on the method used, a high-avidity result indicates an infection that is more than 5 months old. However, a low-avidity result does not indicate a recently acquired infection, because low-avidity antibodies may be detectable for a year postinfection. The Vidas Toxo avidity assay by bioMérieux is the only kit approved by the Food and Drug Administration (FDA). Multiple commercial kits are available outside the United States, including those from Ani Labsystems (53), bioMérieux (24, 54), and DiaSorin (55).

TABLE 3 Guide to general interpretation of *Toxoplasma* serology results obtained with IgG and IgM commercial assays

IgG result	IgM result	Report/interpretation for humans except infants
Negative	Negative	No serological evidence of infection with *Toxoplasma*
Negative	Equivocal	Possible early acute infection or false-positive IgM reaction. Obtain a new specimen for IgG and IgM testing. If results for the second specimen remain the same, the patient is probably not infected with *Toxoplasma*.
Negative	Positive	Possible acute infection or false-positive IgM result. Obtain a new specimen for IgG and IgM testing. If results for the second specimen remain the same, the IgM reaction is probably a false positive.
Equivocal	Negative	Indeterminate: obtain a new specimen for testing or retest this specimen for IgG in a different assay.
Equivocal	Equivocal	Indeterminate: obtain a new specimen for both IgG and IgM testing.
Equivocal	Positive	Possible acute infection with *Toxoplasma*. Obtain a new specimen for IgG and IgM testing. If results for the second specimen are the same or if the IgG becomes positive, both specimens should be sent to a reference laboratory with experience in the diagnosis of toxoplasmosis for further testing.
Positive	Negative	Infected with *Toxoplasma* for more than 1 year
Positive	Equivocal	Infected with *Toxoplasma* for probably more than 1 year, or false-positive IgM reaction. Obtain a new specimen for IgM testing. If results for the second specimen are the same, both specimens should be sent to a reference laboratory with experience in the diagnosis of toxoplasmosis for further testing.
Positive	Positive	Possible recent infection within the last 12 months, or false-positive IgM reaction. Send the specimen to a reference laboratory with experience in the diagnosis of toxoplasmosis for further testing.

Other tests may be of assistance in determining current infection. Assays for *Toxoplasma*-specific IgA antibodies should always be performed in addition to IgM assays for newborns suspected of having congenital infection (56–58). Results of IgA testing in adults have been less consistent (59). The presence of *Toxoplasma*-specific IgE antibodies may also contribute to the determination of acute infections, although reports concerning the utility of IgE antibody detection have been mixed (60, 61). Immunoblot assays may be useful in determining congenital infections (62, 63) and ocular infections (64). These and other assays (33, 35, 65) are available in the United States at the Toxoplasma Serology Laboratory, Palo Alto Medical Foundation [Palo Alto, CA; http://www.pamf.org/serology/; phone, (650) 853-4828], and at many of the *Toxoplasma* reference laboratories in Europe (for example, National Reference Centre for Toxoplasmosis, Maison Blanche Hospital, University Reims Champagne-Ardenne, France; http://cnrtoxoplasmose.chu-reims.fr/?lang=en).

A guideline for the clinical use and interpretation of serologic tests for *T. gondii* was published (66) by the Clinical and Laboratory Standards Institute (formerly called the National Committee for Clinical Laboratory Standards) and is available for purchase at www.clsi.org.

CLINICAL USE OF DIAGNOSTIC TESTS

There are four groups of patients for whom diagnosis of toxoplasmosis is critical: pregnant women with infection during gestation, congenitally infected newborns, patients with chorioretinitis, and immunocompromised individuals. The selection of diagnostic tests depends on the patient's immune status and clinical presentation.

Determination of Immune Status

An algorithm for serological testing for immune status and acute acquired infection is shown in Fig. 3. Three situations in which baseline information about an individual's immune status would be useful include the following: (i) before conceiving a child; (ii) before receiving immunosuppressive therapy; and (iii) after the initial determination of HIV-1-positive status. Screening one serum specimen with a sensitive test for IgG antibodies, such as a DT, IFA test, or EIA, is sufficient. A negative test result indicates that the patient has not been infected. A positive result of any degree indicates infection with *T. gondii* at some undetermined time.

Diagnosis of Acute Acquired Infections

For immunocompetent patients with suspected acute infection, the patient's serum specimen should be tested for the presence of *Toxoplasma*-specific antibodies (Fig. 3). A negative result in a DT, IgG IFA test, or IgG EIA essentially excludes the diagnosis of acute *Toxoplasma* infection. The presence of typical lymphadenopathy suggestive of acute toxoplasmosis, together with a positive IgG EIA (or DT or IgG IFA test) and IgM EIA antibodies, is indicative of acute infection (54, 67, 68). Very rarely, early after infection, a person may present with a positive IgM and a negative IgG, which will soon turn positive. Demonstration of seroconversion from a negative titer to a positive titer or of a more-than-4-fold increase in titer confirms the diagnosis

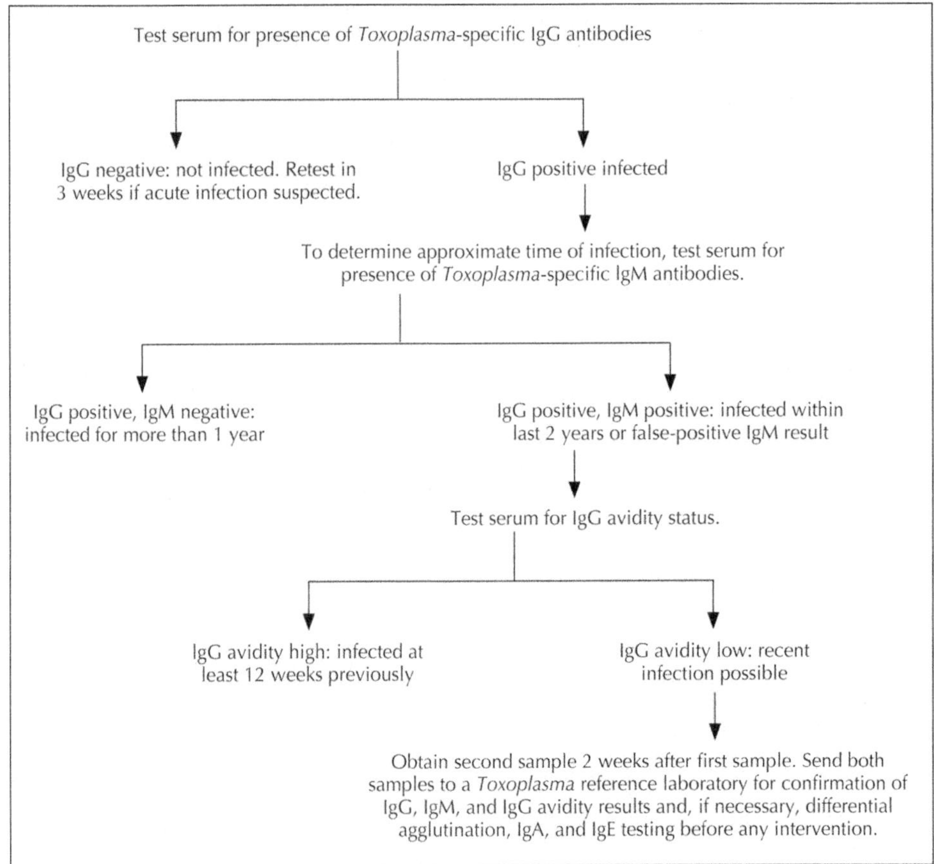

FIGURE 3 Algorithm for the serodiagnosis of toxoplasmosis in people more than 1 year of age.

of recent infection when specimens drawn several (≥3) weeks apart are tested in parallel with the same test. However, such situations are rare, because specimens are usually drawn after titers have peaked, too late to observe titer changes after initial infection.

Confirmatory IgM testing to confirm acute infection can be performed with an IgM capture EIA or IgM immunosorbent agglutination assay and an IgG avidity assay to provide additional evidence for or against acute infection when IgG antibodies are present (2, 35, 69). A negative IgM test essentially rules out infection in the previous 6 months. A positive IgM titer combined with a positive IgG titer may be suggestive of acute infection, due to persistent IgM antibodies, or may be a false-positive reaction.

Diagnosis during Pregnancy

Congenital toxoplasmosis occurs when a woman passes the infection to her fetus after acquiring a primary infection during pregnancy or, more rarely, when a pregnant woman is immunocompromised and a previously acquired infection is reactivated. Congenital toxoplasmosis can also occur, as more recently described, when second infection occurs with a different genotype (7, 42, 70). The rate of transmission of infection to the fetus ranges from 11% in the first trimester to 90% in the late third trimester, with an overall transmission rate of approximately 30 to 50% (13). In France and Austria, the prevention, diagnosis, and treatment of congenital toxoplasmosis begin with mandatory serologic testing of all women before or soon after conception. The cost-effectiveness of adopting this approach for all pregnant women in the United States is controversial, although modeling suggests that it may be cost-effective; this approach does serve as a model for managing individual pregnant patients (32, 71, 72).

Immunocompetent women who have IgG antibody before conception are generally considered immune and so at very little risk for transmission of infection to the fetus (28). As noted above, newer research suggests that infection with a second genotype may occasionally lead to congenital transmission. Women who are seronegative are considered at risk for infection and in France are tested monthly during pregnancy for IgG antibody. If a woman is first tested after conception and has *Toxoplasma*-specific IgG antibodies, IgG avidity testing, and possibly the differential agglutination (of acetone [AC]-fixed versus formalin [HS]-fixed tachyzoites [AC/HS]) test, should be done to determine if acute infection has occurred during pregnancy (2, 42) (Fig. 3). A high-avidity result in the first 12 weeks of pregnancy essentially rules out an infection acquired during gestation. A low-avidity result cannot be used as an indicator of recent infection, because some individuals have persistent low IgG avidity for many months after infection. Immunodiagnosis of acute infection in a pregnant woman should be confirmed by a toxoplasmosis reference laboratory prior to intervention (13, 28, 32, 34, 38, 42).

When the diagnosis of acute toxoplasmosis has been made in a pregnant woman, she can be treated and the fetus can be tested for evidence of infection. The strategy used by Daffos et al. (73) involved initiating treatment with spiramycin once acute maternal infection was indicated and then obtaining amniotic fluid and fetal blood samples between 20 and 26 weeks of gestation for testing (Fig. 4). Amniotic fluid PCR (at 18 weeks gestation or later) is the recommended test of choice to establish the intrauterine diagnosis of congenital toxoplasmosis (13, 28, 49, 74–77), as fetal blood sampling does not improve the diagnostic yield and increases the risk of fetal loss. In addition, fetal ultrasound examinations were performed every 2 to 4 weeks until delivery to search for several nonspecific signs of infection: cerebral or hepatic calcifications, hydrocephalus, hepatomegaly, or ascites.

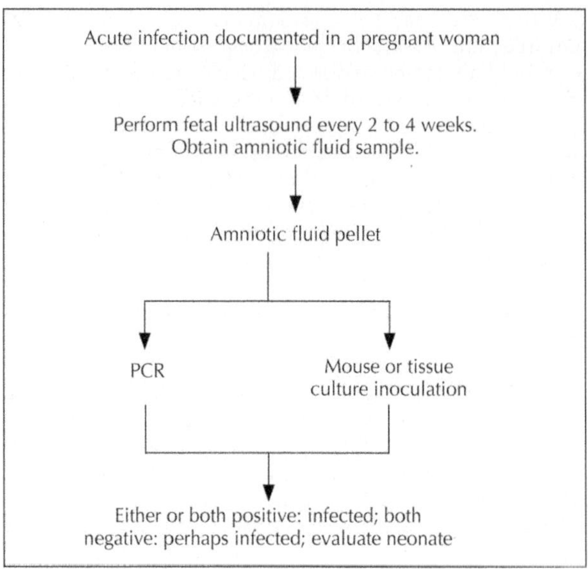

FIGURE 4 Algorithm for the diagnosis of antenatal congenital toxoplasmosis.

If collected, fetal blood should be tested for *Toxoplasma*-specific IgG, IgM, and IgA antibodies. Clotted blood should be inoculated into mice or tissue culture cells to demonstrate parasitemia. Nonspecific markers of infection should be evaluated; these include leukocytes, eosinophils, platelets, total IgM, gamma-glutamyltransferase, and lactate dehydrogenase (74). Most infected fetuses have one or more abnormal nonspecific tests, most commonly an elevated total IgM level or an elevated gamma-glutamyltransferase level (63, 72, 74, 78). Demonstrating *Toxoplasma*-specific IgM or IgA antibodies in fetal serum or isolating the parasite from fetal leukocytes is a definitive diagnosis of fetal infection.

Diagnosis in Newborns

Diagnosis of *Toxoplasma* infection in the newborn is made through a combination of serologic testing, amniotic fluid PCR, and radiologic tests (13, 28, 63, 74, 79–81). PCR should be performed on amniotic fluid for the detection of *T. gondii* DNA when serologic or fetal ultrasound tests are suggestive of acute infection during pregnancy (Fig. 5).

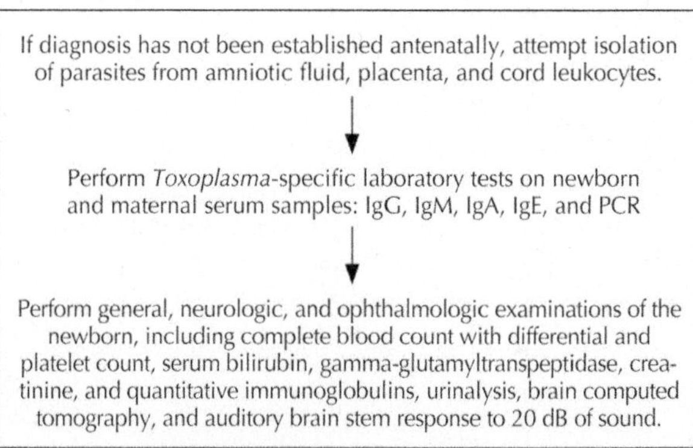

FIGURE 5 Algorithm for the diagnosis of neonatal toxoplasmosis.

The preferred time for amniocentesis is at 18 weeks gestation or later if acute infection was diagnosed after 18 weeks. The child's serum should be tested for *Toxoplasma*-specific IgG, IgM, and IgA antibodies. CSF should be analyzed for cells, glucose, protein, total IgG antibody, and *Toxoplasma*-specific IgG and IgM antibodies and directly examined for *T. gondii* tachyzoites. A child suspected of having congenital toxoplasmosis should have a thorough general, neurologic, and ophthalmologic examination and a computed tomographic scan of the head (magnetic resonance imaging does not demonstrate calcifications). Because the diagnosis can take several months to confirm, clinicians may have to treat patients based upon early signs, symptoms, and serology while awaiting definitive confirmation. Although the complexity of diagnosing congenital infection necessitates the use of multiple costly laboratory tests, the benefit of early diagnosis and treatment and the cost of unnecessary treatment justify establishing the correct diagnosis.

Persistent or increasing IgG antibody levels in the infant compared with the mother as measured by the DT or IFA test and/or positive results for *Toxoplasma*-specific IgM or IgA are diagnostic of congenital infection. Demonstration by IgG and IgM Western blots of serum antibodies in the newborn that are directed against unique *Toxoplasma* epitopes not found in the mother's serum is also evidence of congenital infection (34, 35, 42, 51, 82).

Placental leak can occasionally lead to false-positive IgM or IgA measurements in the newborn. Positive tests for these antibodies usually must be confirmed by repeat testing for IgM at 2 to 4 days of life and repeat testing for IgA at 10 days of life. Passively transferred maternal IgG has a half life of approximately 1 month. Maternal antibodies can be detected for several months and have been reported up to 1 year of age. The untreated congenitally infected newborn will begin to produce *Toxoplasma*-specific IgG antibody within approximately 3 months. Treatment of the infected child may delay antibody production until 9 months of age and on rare occasion may prevent production altogether. Persistence of a positive IgG result at 12 months of life in the child confirms infection. Demonstration of a decrease in antibody load (*Toxoplasma*-specific IgG antibody divided by total IgG) can be helpful in differentiating maternal antibody from fetal antibody.

PCR for *Toxoplasma* DNA in CSF or demonstration of IgM antibody or local *Toxoplasma*-specific IgG antibody production in CSF not contaminated with peripheral blood can help confirm the diagnosis of congenital toxoplasmosis. The calculation is made by dividing the *Toxoplasma*-specific antibody titer in the body fluid by the *Toxoplasma*-specific antibody titer in the serum and multiplying the result by the concentration of gamma globulin in serum divided by the concentration of gamma globulin in the body fluid. A result of 4 or greater corresponds to significant antibody production.

A long-term prospective study is under way in the United States to define optimal therapeutic regimens for the treatment of congenital toxoplasmosis (8, 83). Clinicians should contact Rima McLeod at University of Chicago Hospitals, Chicago, IL [phone, (773) 834-4152], regarding the treatment of infected children.

Diagnosis of Ocular Infection

Toxoplasma chorioretinitis results from both acute infection and congenital infection (84, 85). Patients with chorioretinitis caused by reactivation of congenital toxoplasmosis tend to have low levels of IgG antibody and negative IgM antibodies. In contrast, patients with active chorioretinitis as a result of acute infection have both detectable IgM and IgG antibodies. In addition to demonstrating IgG antibody to *Toxoplasma* in the serum of a person with compatible eye lesions, demonstration of the local production of antibody and detection of parasite DNA in aqueous humor have been used to document active ocular toxoplasmosis (2, 21, 24, 86). When the formula described above is used to calculate results obtained in eye fluids and with results obtained in serum, a value of 8 or greater suggests acute ocular toxoplasmosis. If the serum DT titer is greater than 1:1,000, it is usually not possible to calculate local antibody production.

Diagnosis in Immunocompromised Hosts

A wide variety of immunosuppressed hosts, including hematologic and solid organ transplant recipients, patients with AIDS, and those with autoimmune disorders, have been described as having severe, often fatal, toxoplasmosis. The disease is most often related to reactivation of latent infection and commonly involves the CNS, although a wide spectrum of clinical manifestations have been reported. Diagnosis can be very difficult for these patients, as IgM antibody is usually not detectable and the presence of IgG antibody only confirms chronic infection. In the absence of serologic evidence of acute infection, diagnosis can be confirmed by tissue biopsy and demonstration of the organism histologically or cytologically as replicating within tissue, by detection of *T. gondii* DNA by PCR in a site such as peripheral blood, amniotic fluid, CSF, bronchoalveolar fluid, or aqueous humor, or by myocardial biopsy, in which the encysted organism would not be present as part of a latent infection.

Persons undergoing organ or bone marrow transplantation can benefit from pretransplant testing for *Toxoplasma*-specific IgG antibodies to determine immune status, because they are at risk for acute acquired infection if they are seronegative before transplantation or for reactivation if they are seropositive before transplantation (2, 87). Those with acute acquired infection will usually develop detectable *Toxoplasma*-specific IgG and IgM antibodies, while those with reactivation will not have a detectable *Toxoplasma*-specific IgM response. Serial measurement of *Toxoplasma* DNA in peripheral blood by PCR has been advocated by some as a supplement to serology for monitoring for development of toxoplasmosis in bone marrow transplant patients (22, 23). Seronegative recipients of heart transplants from seropositive donors can develop toxoplasmic myocarditis that mimics organ rejection.

Toxoplasmic encephalitis is the most frequent opportunistic CNS infection in AIDS patients and is uniformly fatal if untreated. Among people who died with AIDS from 1992 through 1997 in the United States, 7.2% developed toxoplasmic encephalitis during the course of AIDS (11, 88). It is recommended that all HIV-infected persons be tested for *Toxoplasma*-specific IgG antibodies soon after the diagnosis of HIV infection to detect latent infection (11, 88). If *Toxoplasma* seropositive, symptomatic patients who have a $CD4^+$ T-lymphocyte count of $<100/\mu l$ should be administered treatment as described in "Treatment" below. Most AIDS patients with toxoplasmic encephalitis have demonstrable IgG antibodies to *T. gondii*. However, approximately 3% of AIDS patients with toxoplasmic encephalitis do not have *Toxoplasma*-specific antibody in their serum. A lumbar puncture should be performed, if it can be done safely, and PCR examination for *T. gondii* DNA should be done. CSF can also be used for detection of Epstein-Barr virus, cytomegalovirus, and JC virus if primary CNS lymphoma, cytomegalovirus ventriculitis, and progressive multifocal leukoencephalopathy, respectively, are considered part of the differential diagnosis. Local production of *Toxoplasma*-specific IgG antibody in CSF has been demonstrated for persons with AIDS and for those with toxoplasmic encephalitis (34, 35). When the formula described above for toxoplasmosis in the newborn is used, a result greater than 1 corresponds to significant antibody production.

TREATMENT

In general, physicians treat *T. gondii* infection in four groups of patients: (i) pregnant women with acute infection to prevent fetal infection (13, 32, 72, 73, 81, 89, 90); (ii) congenitally infected infants (13, 79, 83, 91–93); (iii) immunosuppressed persons, usually with reactivated disease (11, 22, 23, 34, 88, 94–96); and (iv) patients with acute and recurrent ocular disease (84, 85, 97–100). Drugs are also prescribed for preventive or suppressive treatment in HIV-infected persons (11, 88). The currently recommended drugs work primarily against the actively dividing tachyzoite form of *T. gondii* and do not eradicate encysted organisms (bradyzoites).

The most common drug combination used to treat congenital toxoplasmosis consists of pyrimethamine and a sulfonamide (sulfadiazine is recommended in the United States), plus folinic acid in the form of leucovorin calcium to protect the bone marrow from the toxic effects of pyrimethamine. Pyrimethamine inhibits dihydrofolate reductase, which is important in the synthesis of folic acid and produces a reversible depression of the bone marrow. Sulfonamides inhibit synthesis of dihydrofolic acid, also important in the synthesis of folic acid. The two drugs work synergistically against *T. gondii*. Due to toxicity in early pregnancy, pyrimethamine and sulfadiazine therapy is generally recommended for use in pregnant women at ≥18 weeks of gestation (42, 65). After the 18th week, pyrimethamine and sulfadiazine may be given if fetal infection is confirmed by amniocentesis or cordocentesis. Spiramycin [available through the FDA; phone, (301) 796-0563 or (301) 796-1400; if no response, use (301) 796-3763] is recommended for pregnant women with acute toxoplasmosis when fetal infection has not been confirmed in an attempt to prevent transmission of *T. gondii* from the mother to the fetus (42, 65). Randomized prospective studies of treatment during acute infection in pregnant women have not been performed. Some researchers have questioned, or been unable to demonstrate, the effectiveness of treatment during pregnancy in preventing congenital infection (81, 101) or sequelae in infants (101). One hypothesis for the lack of effectiveness is that *T. gondii* tachyzoites transform into bradyzoites within days of infection, probably coinciding with the serological and cell-mediated responses (101). Therefore, by the time an infection is detected in a pregnant woman, tachyzoites may have already been transmitted to the fetus, inflicted damage, and converted to encysted bradyzoites, which do not respond to therapy. Nevertheless, a multicenter observational study found that the treatment of acute *T. gondii* infection in pregnancy was associated with a reduction of sequelae in infants but not a reduction in maternal-fetal transmission (68). Pyrimethamine and sulfadiazine (plus leucovorin) are the drugs generally used to treat infants with congenital toxoplasmosis and have led to improved outcomes compared with historic controls (42, 83).

In immunosuppressed persons with toxoplasmosis, a regimen of pyrimethamine and sulfadiazine plus leucovorin is the preferred treatment (11, 34, 65, 88). Clindamycin is a second alternative for use in combination with pyrimethamine and leucovorin in those who cannot tolerate sulfonamides (11, 65, 88, 96, 102). Leucovorin prevents the hematologic toxicities associated with pyrimethamine therapy. Atovaquone in combination with either pyrimethamine or sulfadiazine has sufficient activity to be considered for treatment in some less severely affected adult patients (65, 103). The role of other drugs in the treatment of systemic toxoplasmosis has not been defined by controlled trials. In general, alternative drugs such as azithromycin, clarithromycin, and dapsone should be used in combination with another drug, preferably pyrimethamine (33).

Because relapse often occurs after toxoplasmosis in HIV-infected patients, maintenance therapy (secondary prophylaxis) with pyrimethamine plus sulfadiazine (first choice) or pyrimethamine plus clindamycin (alternative) is recommended (10, 87). Secondary prophylaxis for toxoplasmosis may be discontinued in patients with a sustained increase in $CD4^+$ T-cell counts (e.g., 6 months) to >200 cells/μl in response to highly active antiretroviral therapy if the patient has completed the initial therapy and has no symptoms or signs attributable to toxoplasmosis. For prophylaxis to prevent an initial episode of *T. gondii* in *Toxoplasma*-seropositive persons with $CD4^+$ T-lymphocyte counts less than 100 cells/μl, trimethoprim-sulfamethoxazole is recommended as the first choice, with alternatives consisting of dapsone plus pyrimethamine, or atovaquone with or without pyrimethamine. Leucovorin is given with all regimens, including pyrimethamine (11, 88).

Pyrimethamine and sulfadiazine are often used for persons with ocular disease (85). Clindamycin in combination with other antiparasitic medications is also frequently prescribed for ocular disease (98). A variety of newer agents have been tried in the treatment of ocular toxoplasmosis, including atovaquone (104), rifabutin, azithromycin, and clarithromycin (100). In addition to antiparasitic drugs, physicians may add corticosteroids to reduce ocular inflammation. However, the optimal treatment for ocular toxoplasmosis remains to be defined by controlled trials.

REFERENCES

1. **Lopez A, Dietz VJ, Wilson M, Navin TR, Jones JL, Centers for Disease Control and Prevention.** 2000. Preventing congenital toxoplasmosis. *MMWR Recomm Rep* **49**(RR-2):59–68.
2. **Robert-Gangneux F, Dardé ML.** 2012. Epidemiology of and diagnostic strategies for toxoplasmosis. *Clin Microbiol Rev* **25**:264–296.
3. **Smith KL, Wilson M, Hightower AW, Kelley PW, Struewing JP, Juranek DD, McAuley JB.** 1996. Prevalence of *Toxoplasma gondii* antibodies in US military recruits in 1989: comparison with data published in 1965. *Clin Infect Dis* **23**: 1182–1183.
4. **Jones JL, Kruszon-Moran D, Wilson M, McQuillan G, Navin T, McAuley JB.** 2001. *Toxoplasma gondii* infection in the United States: seroprevalence and risk factors. *Am J Epidemiol* **154**:357–365.
5. **Jones JL, Kruszon-Moran D, Sanders-Lewis K, Wilson M.** 2007. *Toxoplasma gondii* infection in the United States, 1999–2004, decline from the prior decade. *Am J Trop Med Hyg* **77**:405–410.
6. **Muñoz-Zanzi CA, Fry P, Lesina B, Hill D.** 2010. *Toxoplasma gondii* oocyst-specific antibodies and source of infection. *Emerg Infect Dis* **16**:1591–1593.
7. **Lindsay DS, Dubey JP.** 2011. *Toxoplasma gondii*: the changing paradigm of congenital toxoplasmosis. *Parasitology* **138**:1829–1831.

8. **Boyer KM, Holfels E, Roizen N, Swisher C, Mack D, Remington J, Withers S, Meier P, McLeod R, the Toxoplasmosis Study Group.** 2005. Risk factors for *Toxoplasma gondii* infection in mothers of infants with congenital toxoplasmosis: implications for prenatal management and screening. *Am J Obstet Gynecol* **192:**564–571.
9. **Jones JL, Dargelas V, Roberts J, Press C, Remington JS, Montoya JG.** 2009. Risk factors for *Toxoplasma gondii* infection in the United States. *Clin Infect Dis* **49:**878–884.
10. **Jones JL, Lopez A, Wilson M, Schulkin J, Gibbs R.** 2001. Congenital toxoplasmosis: a review. *Obstet Gynecol Surv* **56:**296–305.
11. **Panel on Opportunistic Infections in HIV-Infected Adults and Adolescents.** Last updated 25 July 2018. Guidelines for the prevention and treatment of opportunistic infections in HIV-infected adults and adolescents. http://aidsinfo.nih.gov/contentfiles/lvguidelines/adult_oi.pdf. Accessed 12 October 2018.
12. **Schmidt-Hieber M, Zweigner J, Uharek L, Blau IW, Thiel E.** 2009. Central nervous system infections in immunocompromised patients: update on diagnostics and therapy. *Leuk Lymphoma* **50:**24–36.
13. **Maldonado YA, Read JS, Committee on Infectious Diseases.** 2017. Diagnosis, treatment, and prevention of congenital toxoplasmosis in the United States. *Pediatrics* **139:**e1–e50.
14. **Jones J, Holland GN.** 2010. Annual burden of ocular toxoplasmosis in the United States. *Am J Trop Med Hyg* **82:**464–465.
15. **Kusbeci OY, Miman O, Yaman M, Aktepe OC, Yazar S.** 2011. Could *Toxoplasma gondii* have any role in Alzheimer disease? *Alzheimer Dis Assoc Disord* **25:**1–3.
16. **Ling VJ, Lester D, Mortensen PB, Langenberg PW, Postolache TT.** 2011. *Toxoplasma gondii* seropositivity and suicide rates in women. *J Nerv Ment Dis* **199:**440–444.
17. **Arias I, Sorlozano A, Villegas E, de Dios Luna J, McKenney K, Cervilla J, Gutierrez B, Gutierrez J.** 2012. Infectious agents associated with schizophrenia: a meta-analysis. *Schizophr Res* **136:**128–136.
18. **Fricker-Hidalgo H, Brenier-Pinchart MP, Schaal JP, Equy V, Bost-Bru C, Pelloux H. 2007.** Value of *Toxoplasma gondii* detection in one hundred thirty-three placentas for the diagnosis of congenital toxoplasmosis. *Pediatr Infect Dis J* **26:**845–846.
19. **Palm C, Tumani H, Pietzcker T, Bengel D.** 2008. Diagnosis of cerebral toxoplasmosis by detection of *Toxoplasma gondii* tachyzoites in cerebrospinal fluid. *J Neurol* **255:**939–941.
20. **Bastien P, Jumas-Bilak E, Varlet-Marie E, Marty P, ANOFEL Toxoplasma-PCR Quality Control Group.** 2007. Three years of multi-laboratory external quality control for the molecular detection of *Toxoplasma gondii* in amniotic fluid in France. *Clin Microbiol Infect* **13:**430–433.
21. **Garweg JG.** 2005. Determinants of immunodiagnostic success in human ocular toxoplasmosis. *Parasite Immunol* **27:**61–68.
22. **Derouin F, Pelloux H, ESCMID Study Group on Clinical Parasitology.** 2008. Prevention of toxoplasmosis in transplant patients. *Clin Microbiol Infect* **14:**1089–1101.
23. **Edvinsson B, Lundquist J, Ljungman P, Ringden O, Evengard B.** 2008. A prospective study of diagnosis of *Toxoplasma gondii* infection after bone marrow transplantation. *APMIS* **116:**345–351.
24. **Fekkar A, Bodaghi B, Touafek F, Le Hoang P, Mazier D, Paris L.** 2008. Comparison of immunoblotting, calculation of the Goldmann-Witmer coefficient, and real-time PCR using aqueous humor samples for diagnosis of ocular toxoplasmosis. *J Clin Microbiol* **46:**1965–1967.
25. **Iqbal J, Khalid N.** 2007. Detection of acute *Toxoplasma gondii* infection in early pregnancy by IgG avidity and PCR analysis. *J Med Microbiol* **56:**1495–1499.
26. **Wallon M, Franck J, Thulliez P, Huissoud C, Peyron F, Garcia-Meric P, Kieffer F.** 2010. Accuracy of real-time polymerase chain reaction for *Toxoplasma gondii* in amniotic fluid. *Obstet Gynecol* **115:**727–733.
27. **Sterkers Y, Varlet-Marie E, Cassaing S, Brenier-Pinchart MP, Brun S, Dalle F, Delhaes L, Filisetti D, Pelloux H, Yera H, Bastien P.** 2010. Multicentric comparative analytical performance study for molecular detection of low amounts of *Toxoplasma gondii* from simulated specimens. *J Clin Microbiol* **48:**3216–3222.
28. **Pomares C, Montoya JG.** 2016. Laboratory diagnosis of congenital toxoplasmosis. *J Clin Microbiol* **54:**2448–2454.
29. **Foulon W, Pinon JM, Stray-Pedersen B, Pollak A, Lappalainen M, Decoster A, Villena I, Jenum PA, Hayde M, Naessens A.** 1999. Prenatal diagnosis of congenital toxoplasmosis: a multicenter evaluation of different diagnostic parameters. *Am J Obstet Gynecol* **181:**843–847.
30. **Hohlfeld P, Daffos F, Costa JM, Thulliez P, Forestier F, Vidaud M.** 1994. Prenatal diagnosis of congenital toxoplasmosis with a polymerase-chain-reaction test on amniotic fluid. *N Engl J Med* **331:**695–699.
31. **Robert-Gangneux F, Brenier-Pinchart MP, Yera H, Belaz S, Varlet-Marie E, Bastien P, Molecular Biology Study Group of the French National Reference Center for Toxoplasmosis.** 2017. Evaluation of *Toxoplasma* ELITe MGB Real-Time PCR assay for diagnosis of toxoplasmosis. *J Clin Microbiol* **55:**1369–1376.
32. **Guy EC, Pelloux H, Lappalainen M, Aspöck H, Hassl A, Melby KK, Holberg-Pettersen M, Petersen E, Simon J, Ambroise-Thomas P.** 1996. Interlaboratory comparison of polymerase chain reaction for the detection of *Toxoplasma gondii* DNA added to samples of amniotic fluid. *Eur J Clin Microbiol Infect Dis* **15:**836–839.
33. **Montoya JG, Remington JS.** 2008. Management of *Toxoplasma gondii* infection during pregnancy. *Clin Infect Dis* **47:**554–566.
34. **Montoya JF, Remington JS.** 2009. *Toxoplasma gondii*, p 3495–3526. *In* Mandell GL, Bennett JE, Dolin R (ed), *Principles and Practice of Infectious Diseases*, 7th ed. Churchill Livingstone, Inc, New York, NY.
35. **Montoya JG.** 2002. Laboratory diagnosis of *Toxoplasma gondii* infection and toxoplasmosis. *J Infect Dis* **185**(Suppl 1)**:**S73–S82.
36. **Odenthal M, Koenig S, Farbrother P, Drebber U, Bury Y, Dienes HP, Eichinger L.** 2007. Detection of opportunistic infections by low-density microarrays: a diagnostic approach for granulomatous lymphadenitis. *Diagn Mol Pathol* **16:**18–26.
37. **Lau YL, Meganathan P, Sonaimuthu P, Thiruvengadam G, Nissapatorn V, Chen Y.** 2010. Specific, sensitive, and rapid diagnosis of active toxoplasmosis by a loop-mediated isothermal amplification method using blood samples from patients. *J Clin Microbiol* **48:**3698–3702.
38. **Ciardelli L, Meroni V, Avanzini MA, Bollani L, Tinelli C, Garofoli F, Gasparoni A, Stronati M.** 2008. Early and accurate diagnosis of congenital toxoplasmosis. *Pediatr Infect Dis J* **27:**125–129.
39. **Chapey E, Wallon M, Debize G, Rabilloud M, Peyron F.** 2010. Diagnosis of congenital toxoplasmosis by using a whole-blood gamma interferon release assay. *J Clin Microbiol* **48:**41–45.
40. **Filisetti D, Cocquerelle V, Pfaff A, Villard O, Candolfi E.** 2010. Placental testing for *Toxoplasma gondii* is not useful to diagnose congenital toxoplasmosis. *Pediatr Infect Dis J* **29:**665–667.
41. **Derouin F, Thulliez P, Candolfi E, Daffos F, Forestier F.** 1988. Early prenatal diagnosis of congenital toxoplasmosis using amniotic fluid samples and tissue culture. *Eur J Clin Microbiol Infect Dis* **7:**423–425.
42. **Remington JS, McLeod R, Thulliez P, Desmonts G.** 2006. Toxoplasmosis, p 947–1091. *In* Remington JS, Klein JO (ed), *Infectious Diseases of the Fetus and Newborn Infant*, 6th ed. The W. B. Saunders Co., Philadelphia, PA.
43. **Villard O, Cimon B, L'Ollivier C, Fricker-Hidalgo H, Godineau N, Houze S, Paris L, Pelloux H, Villena I, Candolfi E, Network of the French National Reference Center for Toxoplasmosis.** 2016. Help in the choice of automated or semiautomated immunoassays for serological diagnosis of toxoplasmosis: evaluation of nine immunoassays by the French National Reference Center for Toxoplasmosis. *J Clin Microbiol* **54:**3034–3042.
44. **Baschirotto PT, Krieger MA, Foti L.** 2017. Preliminary multiplex microarray IgG immunoassay for the diagnosis of toxoplasmosis and rubella. *Mem Inst Oswaldo Cruz* **112:**428–436.
45. **Rigsby P, Rijpkema S, Guy EC, Francis J, Das RG.** 2004. Evaluation of a candidate international standard preparation for human anti-*Toxoplasma* immunoglobulin G. *J Clin Microbiol* **42:**5133–5138.

46. **Naot Y, Desmonts G, Remington JS.** 1981. IgM enzyme-linked immunosorbent assay test for the diagnosis of congenital *Toxoplasma* infection. *J Pediatr* **98:**32–36.
47. **Gras L, Gilbert RE, Wallon M, Peyron F, Cortina-Borja M.** 2004. Duration of the IgM response in women acquiring *Toxoplasma gondii* during pregnancy: implications for clinical practice and cross-sectional incidence studies. *Epidemiol Infect* **132:**541–548.
48. **Wilson M, Remington JS, Clavet C, Varney G, Press C, Ware D, The FDA Toxoplasmosis Ad Hoc Working Group.** 1997. Evaluation of six commercial kits for detection of human immunoglobulin M antibodies to *Toxoplasma gondii*. *J Clin Microbiol* **35:**3112–3115.
49. **Calderaro A, Peruzzi S, Piccolo G, Gorrini C, Montecchini S, Rossi S, Chezzi C, Dettori G.** 2009. Laboratory diagnosis of *Toxoplasma gondii* infection. *Int J Med Sci* **6:**135–136.d
50. **Pietkiewicz H, Hiszczyńska-Sawicka E, Kur J, Petersen E, Nielsen HV, Paul M, Stankiewicz M, Myjak P.** 2007. Usefulness of *Toxoplasma gondii* recombinant antigens (GRA1, GRA7 and SAG1) in an immunoglobulin G avidity test for the serodiagnosis of toxoplasmosis. *Parasitol Res* **100:**333–337.
51. **Remington JS, Thulliez P, Montoya JG.** 2004. Recent developments for diagnosis of toxoplasmosis. *J Clin Microbiol* **42:**941–945.
52. **Yamada H, Nishikawa A, Yamamoto T, Mizue Y, Yamada T, Morizane M, Tairaku S, Nishihira J.** 2011. Prospective study of congenital toxoplasmosis screening with use of IgG avidity and multiplex nested PCR methods. *J Clin Microbiol* **49:**2552–2556.
53. **Buffolano W, Lappalainen M, Hedman L, Ciccimarra F, Del Pezzo M, Rescaldani R, Gargano N, Hedman K.** 2004. Delayed maturation of IgG avidity in congenital toxoplasmosis. *Eur J Clin Microbiol Infect Dis* **23:**825–830.
54. **Montoya JG, Huffman HB, Remington JS.** 2004. Evaluation of the immunoglobulin G avidity test for diagnosis of toxoplasmic lymphadenopathy. *J Clin Microbiol* **42:**4627–4631.
55. **Petersen E, Borobio MV, Guy E, Liesenfeld O, Meroni V, Naessens A, Spranzi E, Thulliez P.** 2005. European multicenter study of the LIAISON automated diagnostic system for determination of *Toxoplasma gondii*-specific immunoglobulin G (IgG) and IgM and the IgG avidity index. *J Clin Microbiol* **43:**1570–1574.
56. **Carvalho FR, Silva DAO, Cunha-Júnior JP, Souza MA, Oliveira TC, Béla SR, Faria GG, Lopes CS, Mineo JR.** 2008. Reverse enzyme-linked immunosorbent assay using monoclonal antibodies against SAG1-related sequence, SAG2A, and p97 antigens from *Toxoplasma gondii* to detect specific immunoglobulin G (IgG), IgM, and IgA antibodies in human sera. *Clin Vaccine Immunol* **15:**1265–1271.
57. **Decoster A, Darcy F, Caron A, Vinatier D, Houze de L'Aulnoit D, Vittu G, Niel G, Heyer F, Lecolier B, Delcroix M, Monnier JC, Duhamel M, Capron A.** 1992. Anti-P30 IgA antibodies as prenatal markers of congenital toxoplasma infection. *Clin Exp Immunol* **87:**310–315.
58. **Wallon M, Dunn D, Slimani D, Girault V, Gay-Andrieu F, Peyron F.** 1999. Diagnosis of congenital toxoplasmosis at birth: what is the value of testing for IgM and IgA? *Eur J Pediatr* **158:**645–649.
59. **Nascimento FS, Suzuki LA, Rossi CL.** 2008. Assessment of the value of detecting specific IgA antibodies for the diagnosis of a recently acquired primary *Toxoplasma* infection. *Prenat Diagn* **28:**749–752.
60. **Foudrinier F, Villena I, Jaussaud R, Aubert D, Chemla C, Martinot F, Pinon JM.** 2003. Clinical value of specific immunoglobulin E detection by enzyme-linked immunosorbent assay in cases of acquired and congenital toxoplasmosis. *J Clin Microbiol* **41:**1681–1686.
61. **Kodym P, Machala L, Roháceová H, Sirocká B, Malý M.** 2007. Evaluation of a commercial IgE ELISA in comparison with IgA and IgM ELISAs, IgG avidity assay and complement fixation for the diagnosis of acute toxoplasmosis. *Clin Microbiol Infect* **13:**40–47.
62. **Jost C, Touafek F, Fekkar A, Courtin R, Ribeiro M, Mazier D, Paris L.** 2011. Utility of immunoblotting for early diagnosis of toxoplasmosis seroconversion in pregnant women. *Clin Vaccine Immunol* **18:**1908–1912.
63. **Pinon JM, Dumon H, Chemla C, Franck J, Petersen E, Lebech M, Zufferey J, Bessieres MH, Marty P, Holliman R, Johnson J, Luyasu V, Lecolier B, Guy E, Joynson DH, Decoster A, Enders G, Pelloux H, Candolfi E.** 2001. Strategy for diagnosis of congenital toxoplasmosis: evaluation of methods comparing mothers and newborns and standard methods for postnatal detection of immunoglobulin G, M, and A antibodies. *J Clin Microbiol* **39:**2267–2271.
64. **Robert-Gangneux F, Binisti P, Antonetti D, Brezin A, Yera H, Dupouy-Camet J.** 2004. Usefulness of immunoblotting and Goldmann-Witmer coefficient for biological diagnosis of toxoplasmic retinochoroiditis. *Eur J Clin Microbiol Infect Dis* **23:**34–38.
65. **Montoya JG, Liesenfeld O.** 2004. Toxoplasmosis. *Lancet* **363:**1965–1976.
66. **Clinical and Laboratory Standards Institute.** 2004. Clinical use and interpretation of serologic tests for *Toxoplasma gondii*. Approved guideline. Clinical and Laboratory Standards Institute, Wayne, PA.
67. **Montoya JG, Berry A, Rosso F, Remington JS.** 2007. The differential agglutination test as a diagnostic aid in cases of toxoplasmic lymphadenitis. *J Clin Microbiol* **45:**1463–1468.
68. **Montoya JG, Remington JS.** 1995. Studies on the serodiagnosis of toxoplasmic lymphadenitis. *Clin Infect Dis* **20:**781–789.
69. **Roberts A, Hedman K, Luyasu V, Zufferey J, Bessières MH, Blatz RM, Candolfi E, Decoster A, Enders G, Gross U, Guy E, Hayde M, Ho-Yen D, Johnson J, Lécolier B, Naessens A, Pelloux H, Thulliez P, Petersen E.** 2001. Multicenter evaluation of strategies for serodiagnosis of primary infection with *Toxoplasma gondii*. *Eur J Clin Microbiol Infect Dis* **20:**467–474.
70. **Boyer K, Hill D, Mui E, Wroblewski K, Karrison T, Dubey JP, Sautter M, Noble AG, Withers S, Swisher C, Heydemann P, Hosten T, Babiarz J, Lee D, Meier P, McLeod R, Toxoplasmosis Study Group.** 2011. Unrecognized ingestion of *Toxoplasma gondii* oocysts leads to congenital toxoplasmosis and causes epidemics in North America. *Clin Infect Dis* **53:**1081–1089.
71. **Stillwaggon E, Carrier CS, Sautter M, McLeod R.** 2011. Maternal serologic screening to prevent congenital toxoplasmosis: a decision-analytic economic model. *PLoS Negl Trop Dis* **5:**e1333.
72. **Hezard N, Marx-Chemla C, Foudrinier F, Villena I, Quereux C, Leroux B, Dupouy D, Talmud M, Pinon JM.** 1997. Prenatal diagnosis of congenital toxoplasmosis in 261 pregnancies. *Prenat Diagn* **17:**1047–1054.
73. **Daffos F, Forestier F, Capella-Pavlovsky M, Thulliez P, Aufrant C, Valenti D, Cox WL.** 1988. Prenatal management of 746 pregnancies at risk for congenital toxoplasmosis. *N Engl J Med* **318:**271–275.
74. **Pratlong F, Boulot P, Villena I, Issert E, Tamby I, Cazenave J, Dedet JP.** 1996. Antenatal diagnosis of congenital toxoplasmosis: evaluation of the biological parameters in a cohort of 286 patients. *Br J Obstet Gynaecol* **103:**552–557.
75. **Romand S, Chosson M, Franck J, Wallon M, Kieffer F, Kaiser K, Dumon H, Peyron F, Thulliez P, Picot S.** 2004. Usefulness of quantitative polymerase chain reaction in amniotic fluid as early prognostic marker of fetal infection with *Toxoplasma gondii*. *Am J Obstet Gynecol* **190:**797–802.
76. **Romand S, Wallon M, Franck J, Thulliez P, Peyron F, Dumon H.** 2001. Prenatal diagnosis using polymerase chain reaction on amniotic fluid for congenital toxoplasmosis. *Obstet Gynecol* **97:**296–300.
77. **Thalib L, Gras L, Romand S, Prusa A, Bessieres MH, Petersen E, Gilbert RE.** 2005. Prediction of congenital toxoplasmosis by polymerase chain reaction analysis of amniotic fluid. *BJOG* **112:**567–574.
78. **Desmonts G, Naot Y, Remington JS.** 1981. Immunoglobulin M-immunosorbent agglutination assay for diagnosis of infectious diseases: diagnosis of acute congenital and acquired *Toxoplasma* infections. *J Clin Microbiol* **14:**486–491.
79. **Guerina NG, Hsu H-W, Meissner HC, Maguire JH, Lynfield R, Stechenberg B, Abroms I, Pasternack MS, Hoff R, Eaton RB, Grady GF, The New England Regional Toxoplasma Working Group.** 1994. Neonatal serologic screening and early treatment for congenital *Toxoplasma gondii* infection. *N Engl J Med* **330:**1858–1863.

80. **Naessens A, Jenum PA, Pollak A, Decoster A, Lappalainen M, Villena I, Lebech M, Stray-Pedersen B, Hayde M, Pinon JM, Petersen E, Foulon W.** 1999. Diagnosis of congenital toxoplasmosis in the neonatal period: a multicenter evaluation. *J Pediatr* **135:**714–719.
81. **Robert-Gangneux F, Gavinet MF, Ancelle T, Raymond J, Tourte-Schaefer C, Dupouy-Camet J.** 1999. Value of prenatal diagnosis and early postnatal diagnosis of congenital toxoplasmosis: retrospective study of 110 cases. *J Clin Microbiol* **37:**2893–2898.
82. **Robert-Gangneux F, Commerce V, Tourte-Schaefer C, Dupouy-Camet J.** 1999. Performance of a Western blot assay to compare mother and newborn anti-*Toxoplasma* antibodies for the early neonatal diagnosis of congenital toxoplasmosis. *Eur J Clin Microbiol Infect Dis* **18:**648–654.
83. **McAuley J, Boyer KM, Patel D, Mets M, Swisher C, Roizen N, Wolters C, Stein L, Stein M, Schey W, Remington J, Meier P, Johnson D, Heydeman P, Holfels E, Withers S, Mack D, Brown C, Patton D, McLeod R.** 1994. Early and longitudinal evaluations of treated infants and children and untreated historical patients with congenital toxoplasmosis: the Chicago Collaborative Treatment Trial. *Clin Infect Dis* **18:**38–72.
84. **Holland GN.** 2003. Ocular toxoplasmosis: a global reassessment. Part I: epidemiology and course of disease. *Am J Ophthalmol* **136:**973–988.
85. **Holland GN.** 2004. Ocular toxoplasmosis: a global reassessment. Part II: disease manifestations and management. *Am J Ophthalmol* **137:**1–17.
86. **Talabani H, Asseraf M, Yera H, Delair E, Ancelle T, Thulliez P, Brézin AP, Dupouy-Camet J.** 2009. Contributions of immunoblotting, real-time PCR, and the Goldmann-Witmer coefficient to diagnosis of atypical toxoplasmic retinochoroiditis. *J Clin Microbiol* **47:**2131–2135.
87. **Schaffner A.** 2001. Pretransplant evaluation for infections in donors and recipients of solid organs. *Clin Infect Dis* **33**(Suppl 1)**:**S9–S14.
88. **Siberry GK, Abzug MJ, Nachman S, Brady MT, Dominguez KL, Handelsman E, Mofenson LM, Nesheim S, the Panel on Opportunistic Infections in HIV-Exposed and HIV-Infected Children.** 2013. Guidelines for the prevention and treatment of opportunistic infections in HIV-exposed and HIV-infected children. *Pediatr Infect Dis J* **32**(Suppl 2)**:**i-KK4.
89. **Cortina-Borja M, Tan HK, Wallon M, Paul M, Prusa A, Buffolano W, Malm G, Salt A, Freeman K, Petersen E, Gilbert RE, European Multicentre Study on Congenital Toxoplasmosis (EMSCOT).** 2010. Prenatal treatment for serious neurological sequelae of congenital toxoplasmosis: an observational prospective cohort study. *PLoS Med* **7:**e1000351.
90. **Foulon W, Villena I, Stray-Pedersen B, Decoster A, Lappalainen M, Pinon JM, Jenum PA, Hedman K, Naessens A.** 1999. Treatment of toxoplasmosis during pregnancy: a multicenter study of impact on fetal transmission and children's sequelae at age 1 year. *Am J Obstet Gynecol* **180:**410–415.
91. **Berrébi A, Assouline C, Bessières MH, Lathière M, Cassaing S, Minville V, Ayoubi JM.** 2010. Long-term outcome of children with congenital toxoplasmosis. *Am J Obstet Gynecol* **203:**552.e1–552.e6.
92. **Peyron F, Garweg JG, Wallon M, Descloux E, Rolland M, Barth J.** 2011. Long-term impact of treated congenital toxoplasmosis on quality of life and visual performance. *Pediatr Infect Dis J* **30:**597–600.
93. **European Multicentre Study on Congenital Toxoplasmosis.** 2003. Effect of timing and type of treatment on the risk of mother to child transmission of *Toxoplasma gondii*. *BJOG* **110:**112–120.
94. **Soave R.** 2001. Prophylaxis strategies for solid-organ transplantation. *Clin Infect Dis* **33**(Suppl 1)**:**S26–S31.
95. **Israelski DM, Remington JS.** 1993. Toxoplasmosis in the non-AIDS immunocompromised host. *Curr Clin Top Infect Dis* **13:**322–356.
96. **Luft BJ, Hafner R, Korzun AH, Leport C, Antoniskis D, Bosler EM, Bourland DD, Uttamchandani R, Fuhrer J, Jacobson J, Morlat P, Vilde J-L, Remington JS, ACTG 077p/ANRS 009 Study Team.** 1993. Toxoplasmic encephalitis in patients with the acquired immunodeficiency syndrome. *N Engl J Med* **329:**995–1000.
97. **Sauer A, de la Torre A, Gomez-Marin J, Bourcier T, Garweg J, Speeg-Schatz C, Candolfi E.** 2011. Prevention of retinochoroiditis in congenital toxoplasmosis: Europe versus South America. *Pediatr Infect Dis J* **30:**601–603.
98. **Engstrom RE Jr, Holland GN, Nussenblatt RB, Jabs DA.** 1991. Current practices in the management of ocular toxoplasmosis. *Am J Ophthalmol* **111:**601–610.
99. **Rothova A.** 1993. Ocular involvement in toxoplasmosis. *Br J Ophthalmol* **77:**371–377.
100. **Rothova A, Meenken C, Buitenhuis HJ, Brinkman CJ, Baarsma GS, Boen-Tan TN, de Jong PT, Klaassen-Broekema N, Schweitzer CM, Timmerman Z, de Vries J, Zaal MJ, Kijlstra A.** 1993. Therapy for ocular toxoplasmosis. *Am J Ophthalmol* **115:**517–523.
101. **Gilbert R, Dunn D, Wallon M, Hayde M, Prusa A, Lebech M, Kortbeek T, Peyron F, Pollak A, Petersen E.** 2001. Ecological comparison of the risks of mother-to-child transmission and clinical manifestations of congenital toxoplasmosis according to prenatal treatment protocol. *Epidemiol Infect* **127:**113–120.
102. **Dannemann B, McCutchan JA, Israelski D, Antoniskis D, Leport C, Luft B, Nussbaum J, Clumeck N, Morlat P, Chiu J, Vilde J-L, Orellana M, Feigal D, Bartok A, Heseltine P, Leedom J, Remington J, The California Collaborative Treatment Group.** 1992. Treatment of toxoplasmic encephalitis in patients with AIDS. A randomized trial comparing pyrimethamine plus clindamycin to pyrimethamine plus sulfadiazine. *Ann Intern Med* **116:**33–43.
103. **Chirgwin K, Hafner R, Leport C, Remington J, Andersen J, Bosler EM, Roque C, Rajicic N, McAuliffe V, Morlat P, Jayaweera DT, Vilde JL, Luft BJ, AIDS Clinical Trials Group 237/Agence Nationale de Recherche sur le SIDA Essai 039 Study Team.** 2002. Randomized phase II trial of atovaquone with pyrimethamine or sulfadiazine for treatment of toxoplasmic encephalitis in patients with acquired immunodeficiency syndrome: ACTG 237/ANRS 039 Study. *Clin Infect Dis* **34:**1243–1250.
104. **Pearson PA, Piracha AR, Sen HA, Jaffe GJ.** 1999. Atovaquone for the treatment of toxoplasma retinochoroiditis in immunocompetent patients. *Ophthalmology* **106:**148–153.
105. **Holland GN.** 2000. Ocular toxoplasmosis: new directions for clinical investigation. *Ocul Immunol Inflamm* **8:**1–7.
106. **Roux-Buisson N, Fricker-Hidalgo H, Foussadier A, Rolland D, Suchel-Jambon AS, Brenier-Pinchart MP, Pelloux H.** 2005. Comparative analysis of the VIDAS Toxo IgG IV assay in the detection of antibodies to *Toxoplasma gondii*. *Diagn Microbiol Infect Dis* **53:**79–81.
107. **Hofgärtner WT, Swanzy SR, Bacina RM, Condon J, Gupta M, Matlock PE, Bergeron DL, Plorde JJ, Fritsche TR.** 1997. Detection of immunoglobulin G (IgG) and IgM antibodies to *Toxoplasma gondii*: evaluation of four commercial immunoassay systems. *J Clin Microbiol* **35:**3313–3315.
108. **Vlaspolder F, Singer P, Smit A, Diepersloot RJ.** 2001. Comparison of Immulite with Vidas for detection of infection in a low-prevalence population of pregnant women in The Netherlands. *Clin Diagn Lab Immunol* **8:**552–555.
109. **Decoster A, Lambert N, Germaneau C, Masson C.** 2000. Sérodiagnostic de le toxoplasmose: comparaison de la trousse Access Toxo IgM II aux trousses Axsym Toxo IgM et Vidas Toxo IgM. *Ann Biol Clin (Paris)* **58:**721–727.

Pathogenic and Opportunistic Free-Living Amebae

JENNIFER R. COPE, IBNE KARIM M. ALI, AND GOVINDA S. VISVESVARA

142

Free-living amebae belonging to the genera *Naegleria*, *Acanthamoeba*, and *Balamuthia* can infect humans and other animals and cause potentially severe, life-threatening disease. Only one species of *Naegleria* (*Naegleria fowleri*), several species of *Acanthamoeba* (e.g., *Acanthamoeba castellanii*, *A. culbertsoni*, *A. hatchetti*, *A. healyi*, *A. polyphaga*, *A. rhysodes*, *A. astronyxis*, *A. lenticulata*, and *A. divionensis*), and the only known species of *Balamuthia*, *Balamuthia mandrillaris*, are known to cause central nervous system (CNS) disease (1, 2). *Acanthamoeba* spp. also cause infection of the human cornea, *Acanthamoeba* keratitis (3). Further, both *Acanthamoeba* spp. and *B. mandrillaris* have been identified as agents of cutaneous infections in humans (4). There have also been single case reports of human disease caused by *Sappinia pedata* and *Paravahlkampfia francinae* (5–7).

The concept that these free-living amebae may occur as human pathogens was proposed by Culbertson and colleagues, who isolated *Acanthamoeba* sp. strain A-1 (now designated *A. culbertsoni*) from tissue culture medium thought to contain an unknown virus (8). They also demonstrated the presence of amebae in brain lesions of mice and monkeys that died within a week after intracerebral inoculation with *A. culbertsoni*. Culbertson et al. hypothesized that similar infections might exist in nature in humans. In 1965, Fowler and Carter were the first to describe a fatal infection due to free-living amebae (*N. fowleri*) in the brain of an Australian patient (9).

TAXONOMY

Previously, classical taxonomic classification was based largely on morphologic, ecologic, and physiologic criteria. According to this system, *Acanthamoeba* and *Balamuthia*, along with a heterogeneous group of amebae that include both free-living (e.g., *Hartmannella*, *Vahlkampfia*, and *Vannella*) and parasitic (e.g., *Entamoeba*) amebae, were classified in the phylum Protozoa, subphylum Sarcodina, superclass Rhizopodea, class Lobosea, and order Amoebida. *Naegleria* was classified in the class Heterolobosea, order Schizopyrenida, and family Vahlkampfiidae. *Sappinia* was classified in the class Amoebozoa: Lobosea, order Euamoebida, and family Thecamoebidae. Recent information based on modern morphological approaches, biochemical pathways, and molecular phylogenetics has led to the abandonment of the older hierarchical systems consisting of the traditional taxa "kingdom," "phylum," "class," "subclass," "superorder," and "order" and replacement with a new classification system. According to this new schema, these eukaryotes have been classified into six clusters or "supergroups," namely, Amoebozoa, Opisthokonta, Rhizaria, Archaeplastida, Chromalveolata, and Excavata. *Acanthamoeba* and *Balamuthia* are included in the supergroup Amoebozoa: Acanthamoebidae; *Sappinia* is included in the supergroup Amoebozoa: Flabellinea: Thecamoebidae; and *N. fowleri* is included in the supergroup Excavata: Heterolobosea: Vahlkampfiidae (10). The classification of amebae presented here is supported by the International Society of Protistologists. However, other classification schemes may also be used. See chapter 135 for further information on parasitology taxonomy.

DESCRIPTION OF THE AGENTS

Acanthamoeba spp.

Acanthamoeba has two stages in its life cycle, a feeding and multiplying stage, known as the trophozoite, and the cyst (a dormant, resistant stage). The trophozoite measures 15 to 45 µm in length and produces from the surface of its body fine, tapering, hyaline projections called acanthopodia (see Fig. 5). The trophozoite is uninucleate, although binucleate forms are occasionally seen. The nucleus is characterized by a centrally located, large, dense nucleolus. It feeds on *Escherichia coli* or other Gram-negative bacteria and divides by binary fission. During cell division, the nucleus divides by conventional mitosis, in which the nucleolus and the nuclear membrane disappear. It has no flagellate stage but produces a double-walled cyst (10 to 25 µm) (see Fig. 6) with a wrinkled outer wall (the ectocyst) and a stellate, polygonal, or even round inner wall (the endocyst) (11). Cysts are resistant to many physical and chemical environmental pressures, including desiccation (12).

Historically, the genus *Acanthamoeba* was divided into three groups based on size and morphology. Because such morphological characteristics can change with environmental pressures and culture conditions, sequence analysis of the 18S rRNA gene is now used for the classification and diagnosis of *Acanthamoeba* infection, since it is present in multiple copies and is evolutionarily stable. In the case of *Acanthamoeba*, a substantial sequence variation was seen

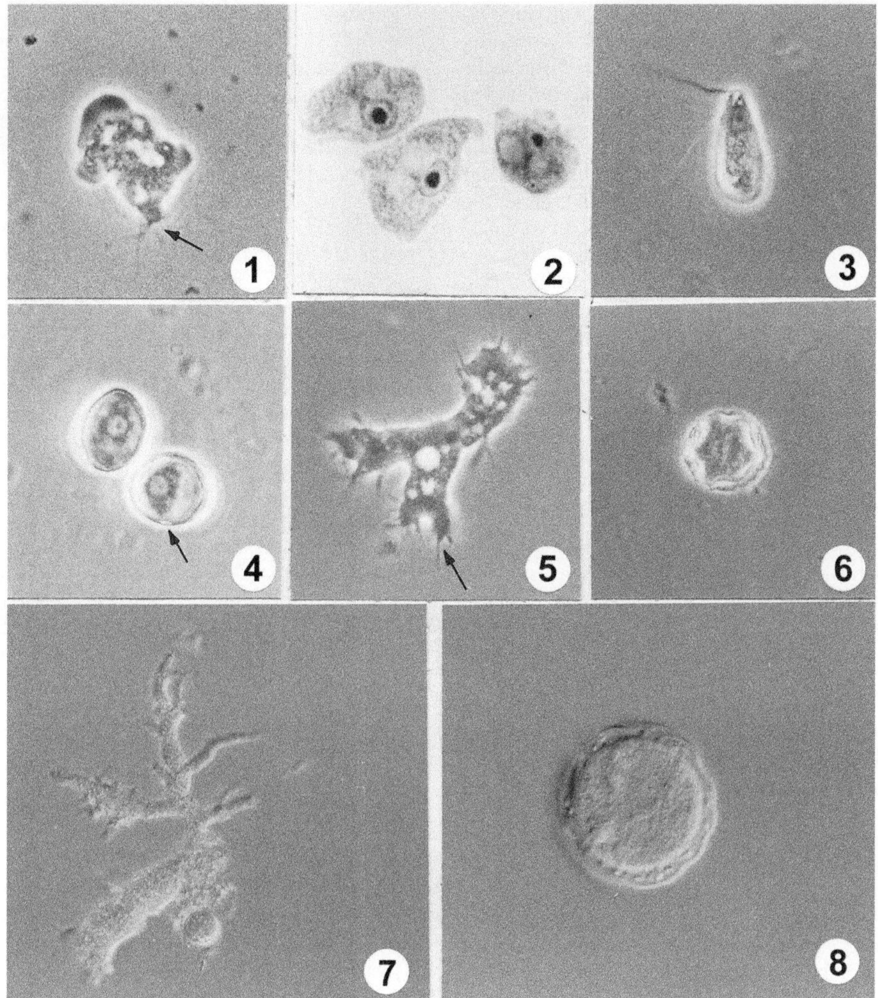

FIGURES 1 THROUGH 4 *N. fowleri*. (1) Trophozoite, phase contrast (note the uroid and filaments [arrow]); (2) trophozoite, trichrome stain; (3) biflagellate, phase contrast; (4) smooth-walled cyst, phase contrast (note the pore [arrow]). All magnifications, approximately ×835.
FIGURES 5 AND 6 *A. castellanii*. (5) Trophozoite, phase contrast (note the acanthopodia [arrow]); (6) double-walled cyst, phase contrast. Both magnifications, approximately ×835.
FIGURES 7 AND 8 *B. mandrillaris*. (7) Trophozoite, phase contrast; (8) cyst, phase contrast. Both magnifications, approximately ×1,140.

not only between the species but also within the same species, identified based on morphological features. *Acanthamoeba* is therefore classified into up to 20 genotypes known as T1 to T20 (13–16).

Naegleria

N. fowleri has three stages in its life cycle: a trophozoite, a flagellate, and a cyst. The trophozoite is a small, slug-like ameba measuring 10 to 25 μm long that exhibits an eruptive locomotion by producing smooth hemispherical bulges. The posterior end, termed the uroid, appears to be sticky and often has several trailing filaments. It is uninucleate and is characterized by a centrally located, large, dense nucleolus. It feeds on *E. coli* or other Gram-negative bacteria and divides by binary fission. During cell division, the nucleus divides by promitosis, in which the nucleolus elongates and divides into two polar bodies, and the nuclear membrane persists. During its life cycle, this ameba produces a transient pear-shaped biflagellate stage, resulting from altered environmental conditions, and smooth-walled cysts (Fig. 1 to 4). Cysts are usually spherical and measure 7 to 15 μm, and the cyst wall may have one or more pores plugged with a mucoid material (1).

Balamuthia

Balamuthia trophozoites are in general irregular in shape; a few, however, may be slug-like. They are uninucleate, but binucleate forms may occasionally be seen. The nucleus has a large, centrally located nucleolus. The pattern of nuclear division in *Balamuthia* is termed metamitosis, in which the nuclear membrane breaks down and the nucleolus eventually disappears. Occasionally, the nucleus of *Balamuthia*, especially in tissue sections, may have more than one nucleolus. Unlike *Acanthamoeba* and *N. fowleri*, *Balamuthia* is not known to feed on bacteria. In the laboratory, it feeds on mammalian tissue culture cells, such as monkey kidney cells, human lung fibroblasts, and human brain microvascular endothelial cells. Actively feeding amebae may be

12 to 60 μm long, with a mean length of 30 μm (Fig. 7). The trophic forms, either in axenic media or while feeding on tissue culture cells, produce broad pseudopodia without any clearly discernible movement. However, when tissue culture cells are destroyed, the trophozoites resort to a spider-like walking movement by producing finger-like determinate pseudopodia (17). Like *Acanthamoeba*, *Balamuthia* does not have a flagellate stage. Cysts are generally uninucleate and spherical and measure 6 to 30 μm in diameter (Fig. 8). Under a light microscope, each cyst appears to have an irregular and slightly wavy outer wall and a round inner wall. A layer of refractile granules immediately below the inner cyst wall is often seen in mature cysts. Under an electron microscope, the cyst wall can be seen to consist of three walls: a thin, irregular outer ectocyst; a thick, electron-dense inner endocyst; and a middle amorphous layer, the mesocyst (17, 18).

EPIDEMIOLOGY

Infection with *N. fowleri* was first described in 1965 in Australia and has now been identified in most parts of the world. In the United States, primary amebic meningoencephalitis (PAM) cases have been retrospectively identified as far back as 1931. From 1962 to 2015, 138 cases of PAM were reported in the United States, with a range of 0 to 8 cases annually (19). Generally, PAM mainly affects young males who dive and jump into warm freshwater (e.g., lakes and rivers) in the summer, when the water temperature is elevated, especially in the southern tier of the United States. The risk for infection might be reduced if appropriate measures to reduce the amount of water going up the nose are taken, such as holding the nose shut or using nose clips, not stirring up sediments while swimming, or avoiding water sports in freshwater lakes and other bodies of water (20). Recent occurrences of PAM in more northern states, such as Minnesota (21), Kansas, Indiana, and Maryland, indicate that the geographic range of *N. fowleri* is changing. It has been postulated that higher ambient water temperatures due to climate change might be responsible for the increasing geographic range of *N. fowleri* (21). PAM cases have also been associated with the use of tap water for nasal and sinus irrigation and recreation (22–24). *N. fowleri* prevention measures for nasal rinsing include using boiled, sterile, or filtered water.

Both *Acanthamoeba* and *Balamuthia* infections have been identified in many parts of the world. However, they are not associated with a particular time of the year. *Acanthamoeba* infections are found mostly in people with immunocompromising conditions, such as HIV infection, cancer, or organ transplantation (25–27), whereas infections with *Balamuthia* are found in both immunocompromised and immunocompetent individuals (28, 29). Recently, *B. mandrillaris* was identified as an agent of encephalitis in solid organ transplant recipients (30, 31). According to one report, Hispanic Americans have a high incidence of *B. mandrillaris* infection. It is not clearly known whether this is due to environmental factors, genetic predisposition, limited access to medical care, or other socioeconomic factors and pressures (32).

N. fowleri and *Acanthamoeba* spp. are commonly found in soil, freshwater, sewage, and sludge and even on dust in the air. Several species of *Acanthamoeba* have also been isolated from brackish water and seawater and from ear discharges, pulmonary secretions, nasopharyngeal mucosa samples, maxillary sinus samples, mandibular autografts, and stool samples. These amebae normally feed on bacteria and multiply in their environmental niche as free-living organisms. *Acanthamoeba* spp. have also been known to harbor *Legionella* spp., *Mycobacterium avium*, and other bacterial pathogens, such as *Listeria monocytogenes*, *Burkholderia pseudomallei*, *Vibrio cholerae*, and *E. coli* serotype O157, which signifies a potential expansion of the public health importance of these organisms (33, 34). Additionally, pure cultures of *A. polyphaga* have been used to isolate *Legionella pneumophila* (35), *Legionella anisa* (36), and *Mycobacterium massiliense* (37) from human clinical specimens, such as sputum, liver, and lung abscess specimens, and even from human feces. Obligate intracellular pathogens, such as *Chlamydia*, *Chlamydophila*, and *Chlamydia*-like bacteria, have been found in ~5% of *Acanthamoeba* isolates, and *Chlamydophila pneumophila*, a respiratory pathogen, can survive and grow within *Acanthamoeba* (33). Whether endosymbiont-bearing *Acanthamoeba* strains serve as reservoirs for these bacteria, some of which are potential pathogens for humans, is unknown.

Although *B. mandrillaris* has been isolated from soil, dust, and water (38–41) and its DNA found in the environment (42), not much is known about the environmental niche of *B. mandrillaris* and its feeding habits. It is, however, believed that its habitat is similar to those of *Acanthamoeba* and *Naegleria* and that it feeds on small amebae and possibly flagellates (43).

CLINICAL SIGNIFICANCE

Table 1 presents a list of clinical syndromes caused by free-living amebae infections.

Naegleria Meningoencephalitis

In 1966, Butt (44) described the first case of CNS infection caused by *N. fowleri* in the United States and coined the term "primary amebic meningoencephalitis." PAM is an acute fulminating disease with an abrupt onset that occurs generally in previously healthy children and young adults who had nasal exposure to freshwater an average of 5 days (range, 1 to 9 days) before the onset of symptoms (45). It is characterized by headache, fever, stiff neck, photophobia, and coma, leading to death within an average of 5.3 days (range, 1 to 18 days) after the onset of symptoms (45). The portal of entry of *N. fowleri* amebae is the nasal passages. When water containing *N. fowleri* enters the nose, the amebae make their way into the olfactory lobes via the cribriform plate and cause acute hemorrhagic necrosis,

TABLE 1 Clinical syndromes caused by free-living amebae infections

Organism	Neurologic clinical syndrome	Other clinical syndromes
Acanthamoeba spp.	GAE	Disseminated, cutaneous, sinusitis, osteomyelitis, pneumonia, keratitis
Balamuthia mandrillaris	GAE	Cutaneous
Naegleria fowleri	PAM	None described
Sappinia pedata	Encephalitis (1 case)	None described
Paravahlkampfia francinae	Meningoencephalitis (1 case)	None described

leading to destruction of the olfactory bulbs and the cerebral cortex. Only a few patients have survived. To date, there have been four well-documented survivors in the United States (46). On autopsy, large numbers of amebic trophozoites, many with ingested erythrocytes and brain tissue, are usually seen interspersed with brain tissue (Fig. 9). It is believed that *N. fowleri* directly ingests brain tissue by producing food cups, or amebostomes, as well as by exerting contact-dependent cytolysis, possibly mediated by a multicomponent system consisting of a heat-stable hemolytic protein, a heat-labile cytolysin, and/or phospholipase enzymes (47). Cysts of *N. fowleri* are not usually seen in brain tissue. It was thought that *N. fowleri* infects only humans until 1997, when a report of the first case of PAM causing death in a South American tapir was published, indicating that PAM can occur in animals other than humans (48). Additionally, a report of PAM deaths in Holstein cattle, associated with drinking of surface waters, indicates that PAM in animals is probably more common than is currently appreciated (49).

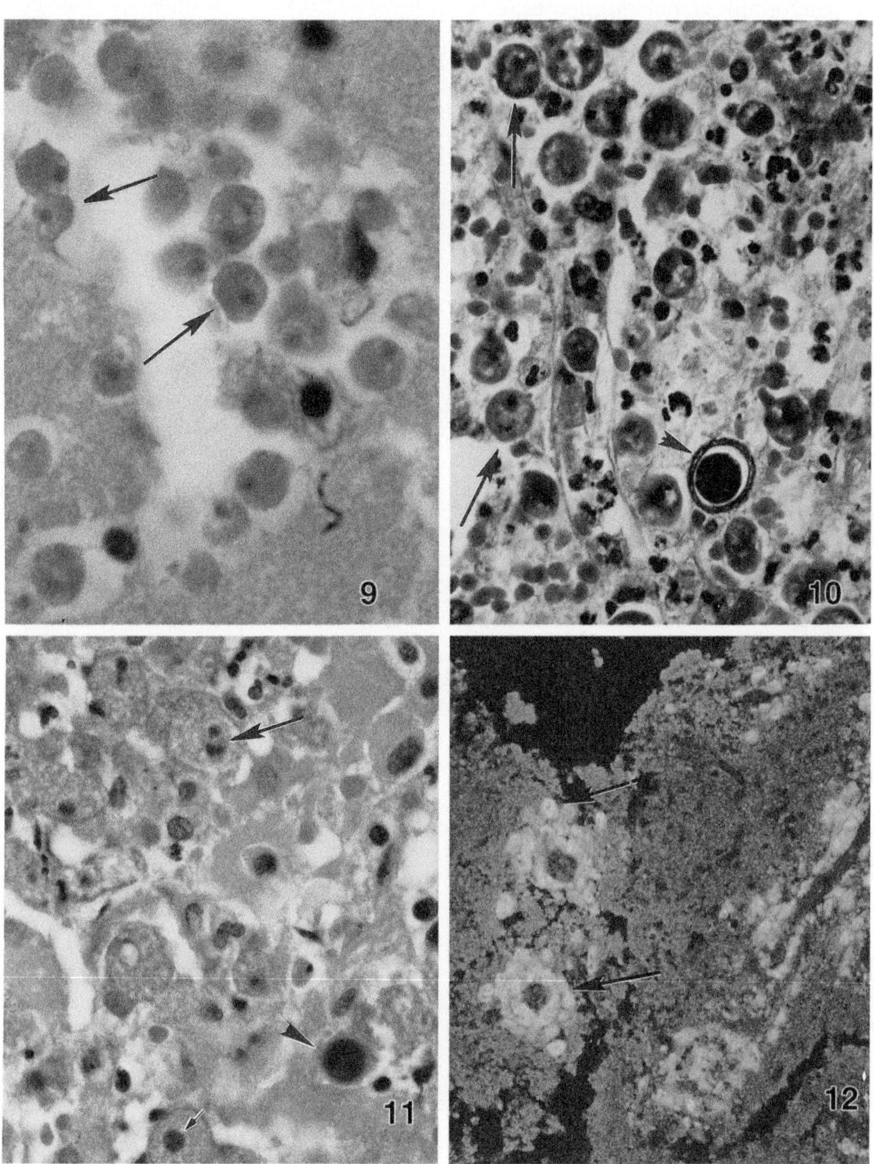

FIGURE 9 Large numbers of *N. fowleri* trophozoites (arrows) in a section of CNS tissue, showing extensive necrosis and destruction of brain tissue. Magnification, approximately ×564.

FIGURE 10 *A. culbertsoni* trophozoites (arrows) and a cyst (arrowhead) around a blood vessel in a section of CNS tissue from a GAE patient. Magnification, approximately ×489.

FIGURE 11 *B. mandrillaris* trophozoites and a cyst (arrowhead) in a brain section from a GAE patient. Note the double (small arrow) and triple (large arrow) nucleolar elements within the nuclei of the trophozoites. Magnification, approximately ×413.

FIGURE 12 Immunofluorescence localization of *B. mandrillaris* in a brain section from a GAE patient. Note the fluorescent amebae (arrows) around blood vessels. Magnification, approximately ×188.

Acanthamoeba Encephalitis and Other Manifestations

Several species of *Acanthamoeba* have been known to cause chronic granulomatous amebic encephalitis (GAE). It is characterized by headache, confusion, dizziness, drowsiness, seizures, and sometimes hemiparesis. Cerebral hemispheres are usually the most heavily affected CNS tissue. They are often edematous, with extensive hemorrhagic necrosis involving the temporal, parietal, and occipital lobes. Amebic trophozoites and cysts are usually scattered throughout the tissue. Many blood vessels are thrombotic and exhibit fibrinoid necrosis; they are also surrounded by polymorphonuclear leukocytes, amebic trophozoites, and cysts (Fig. 10). Multinucleated giant cells forming granulomas may be seen in immunocompetent patients. Some patients develop chronic ulcerative skin lesions, abscesses, or erythematous nodules (50). Other manifestations of *Acanthamoeba* infection include sinusitis, osteomyelitis, and pneumonia (26, 50, 51). It is believed that the route of invasion of and penetration into the CNS is hematogenous, probably from a primary focus in the lower respiratory tract or the skin (1). *Acanthamoeba* spp. also cause infections of the CNS of animals other than humans. Such infections have been recorded in gorillas, monkeys, dogs, ovines, bovines, horses, and kangaroos (1).

Balamuthia (Leptomyxid Ameba) Encephalitis

The pathology and pathogenesis of *B. mandrillaris* GAE are similar to those of *Acanthamoeba* GAE. Both trophozoites and cysts are found in CNS tissue (Fig. 11), and their sizes overlap those of *Acanthamoeba* trophozoites and cysts. Hence, it is difficult to differentiate *Balamuthia* from *Acanthamoeba* spp. in tissue sections under a light microscope. In some cases, *Balamuthia* trophozoites in tissue sections appear to have more than one nucleolus in the nucleus (Fig. 11). In such cases, it may be possible to distinguish *Balamuthia* amebae from *Acanthamoeba* organisms on the basis of nuclear morphology, since *Acanthamoeba* trophozoites have only one nucleolus. In most cases, immunohistochemical techniques, molecular testing, or both are necessary to identify *Balamuthia* organisms. *Balamuthia* amebae are antigenically distinct from *Acanthamoeba* organisms; they can easily be distinguished by immunofluorescence or other immunochemical assays (Fig. 12) (17, 18, 52). It is now known that a number of primates, including gorillas, gibbons, baboons, orangutans, and monkeys, as well as dogs, sheep, and horses, have died of CNS infections caused by *B. mandrillaris* (1, 53).

Acanthamoeba Keratitis

Acanthamoeba spp. also cause a painful vision-threatening disease of the human cornea, *Acanthamoeba* keratitis. If the infection is not treated promptly, it may lead to ulceration of the cornea, loss of visual acuity, and eventually blindness and enucleation (3, 50). *Acanthamoeba* keratitis is characterized by severe ocular pain, a 360° or partial paracentral stromal ring infiltrate, recurrent corneal epithelial breakdown, and a corneal lesion refractory to the commonly used ophthalmic antibacterial medications. *Acanthamoeba* keratitis in the early stages is frequently misdiagnosed as herpes simplex virus keratitis because of the irregular epithelial lesions, stromal infiltrative keratitis, and edema that are commonly seen in herpes simplex virus keratitis (3, 54). A nonhealing corneal ulcer is often the first clue that *Acanthamoeba* keratitis may be the problem.

The first case of *Acanthamoeba* keratitis in the United States was reported in 1973 in a south Texas rancher with a history of trauma to his right eye (55). Both the trophozoite and cyst stages of *A. polyphaga* were demonstrated to be present in corneal sections and were repeatedly cultured from corneal scrapings and biopsy specimens. Between 1973 and July 1986, 208 cases were diagnosed and reported to the U.S. Centers for Disease Control and Prevention (CDC) (56). The number of cases increased gradually between 1973 and 1984, and a dramatic increase began in 1985. A case-control study conducted in 1985–1986 (56) revealed that a major risk factor was the use of contact lenses, predominantly daily-wear or extended-wear soft lenses, and that patients with *Acanthamoeba* keratitis were significantly more likely than controls to use homemade saline solution instead of commercially prepared saline (78 and 30%, respectively), to disinfect their lenses less frequently than recommended by the lens manufacturers (72 and 32%), and to wear their lenses while swimming (63 and 30%). Based on a case-control study conducted by the CDC to investigate a recent increase in *Acanthamoeba* keratitis cases during 2004 to 2007, it was revealed that a national increase in the number of such cases was associated with the use of a specific multipurpose contact lens solution (57). Further, another study revealed that most contact lens solutions marketed in the United States do not have sufficient disinfection activity against *Acanthamoeba* spp. (58). More recent case-control studies of *Acanthamoeba* keratitis have shown that poor contact lens hygiene habits, such as "topping off" disinfecting solution in the case, sleeping in contact lenses, and storing lenses in water, are associated with infection (59, 60).

COLLECTION, HANDLING, AND STORAGE OF SPECIMENS

For isolation of *N. fowleri*, cerebrospinal fluid (CSF) and brain tissue (especially surrounding the nasal olfactory bulbs) should be obtained aseptically. For *Acanthamoeba* and *Balamuthia*, brain, lungs, and ulcerated skin tissues should be obtained aseptically. CSF is not ideal for *Acanthamoeba* and *Balamuthia* detection, since the amebae are not readily found in CSF. For *Acanthamoeba* in the case of *Acanthamoeba* keratitis, corneal scrapings or corneal biopsy tissue should be obtained aseptically. Specimens should be kept at room temperature (24 to 28°C) and should never be frozen if amebae are to be isolated and grown in culture. Tissues should be preserved in 10% neutral buffered formalin so that they can be examined histologically for amebae (52). CSF or tissue specimens kept frozen are appropriate for molecular detection. Personnel handling the specimens must take appropriate precautions, such as wearing laboratory coats, gloves, and eye protection glasses and working in a biological safety cabinet.

CLINICAL AND LABORATORY DIAGNOSIS

Methods of Examination

Direct Examination

Since no distinctive clinical features differentiate PAM from pyogenic or bacterial meningitis, direct examination of the sample as a wet mount preparation is of paramount importance in the diagnosis of PAM and other diseases caused by these amebae. In PAM, the CSF is usually pleocytotic, with a preponderance of polymorphonuclear leukocytes and no bacteria. The CSF pressure may be elevated. The CSF glucose level may be normal or slightly reduced, but the CSF protein level is increased. Microscopic detection of amebic organisms in the CSF is the quickest means of diagnosing PAM. CSF should be examined microscopically by an expert pathologist or microbiologist for the presence of *N. fowleri* amebae with directional movement. Since the amebae tend to attach to the surface of the container, the container should be shaken gently; then, a small drop of fluid should be placed on a clean microscope slide and covered with a number 1 coverslip. The CSF may have to be centrifuged at 500 × *g* for 5 min to concentrate the amebae. After the specimen has been centrifuged, most of the supernatant is carefully aspirated and the sediment is gently suspended in the remaining fluid. A drop of this suspension is prepared as described above for microscopic observation. Giemsa or trichrome staining should be performed on CSF smears to visualize the nuclear morphology of the amebae in order to eliminate false-positive results due to any sluggish movement seen with host macrophages. The slide preparation should be examined under a compound microscope with 10× and 40× lens objectives. Phase-contrast optics is preferable. If regular bright-field illumination is used, the slide should be examined under diminished light. The slide may be warmed to 35°C (to promote amebic movement), and amebae, especially *N. fowleri*, if present, can be detected by their active directional movements. Rarely, flagellates with two flagella may be seen.

Permanently Stained Preparations

A small drop of the sedimented CSF or other sample is placed in the middle of a slide, which is allowed to stand in a moist chamber for 5 to 10 min at 37°C. This will allow any amebae to attach to the surface of the slide. Several drops of warm (37°C) Schaudinn's fixative are dropped directly onto the sample, which is allowed to stand for 1 min. The slide is then transferred for 1 h to a Coplin jar containing the fixative. It may be stained with Wheatley's trichrome or Heidenhain's iron hematoxylin stain. Corneal scrapings smeared onto microscope slides may be fixed with methanol and stained with Hemacolor stain (Harleco, EM Industries, Inc.) (1, 61). CSF can also be processed via cytospinning whenever possible and stained with Wright-Giemsa stain. Amebae, if present, can be distinguished based on their nuclear morphology, and the result should be reported to the clinician immediately so that the patient can be treated appropriately. This is especially important in the case of PAM caused by *N. fowleri*. Gram staining is not useful in the detection of amebae, as it will also stain host cells. For example, a false-positive Gram stain may lead to inaccurate diagnosis and hence to inappropriate therapy. A recent report suggests the possibility of extra-CNS dissemination of *N. fowleri*, and therefore, the organism might pose a risk of transmission of PAM via organ transplantation (62). A few reports describing the transplantation of solid organs from donors infected with *B. mandrillaris* (30, 31) underscore the importance of a correct and timely diagnosis.

Antigen Detection

Pathogenic *N. fowleri* is morphologically indistinguishable from nonpathogenic *Naegleria* at the trophic stage. Differences between these amebae, however, have been demonstrated antigenically by the gel diffusion, immunoelectrophoretic, and immunofluorescence techniques, as well as by their isoenzyme patterns, and these techniques have been utilized to identify the amebae isolated in culture (1, 61). Similarly, antigenic differences have also been shown among various species of *Acanthamoeba* (50, 63). Additionally, *N. fowleri*, *Acanthamoeba* spp., and *B. mandrillaris* have been identified in tissue sections by histochemical methods (1, 21, 29, 30, 52, 62, 64, 65). There are currently no commercially available antigen detection test kits.

Nucleic Acid Detection in Clinical Materials

Acanthamoeba genotypes have been identified in corneal tissue, tear fluid, and brain and lung tissue, as well as in the environment. A number of studies have analyzed the mitochondrial DNA and 18S rRNA gene by conventional PCR and Sanger sequencing to understand the inter- and intraspecies diversity and phylogeny of *Acanthamoeba* spp. (1, 50, 61). However, only a few studies have used this technique to identify *Acanthamoeba* keratitis or *Acanthamoeba* GAE by using patient specimens (13, 14, 61, 64, 66, 67). This is probably because of the lack of reagents from commercial sources.

For the detection of *Acanthamoeba*, Booton et al. (13) used nuclear small subunit ribosomal DNA (rDNA) sequences and the genus-specific primers JDP1 (5′-GGCCCAGATCGTTTACCGTGAA-3′) and JDP2 (5′-TCTCACAAGCTGCTAGGGGAGTCA-3′), which amplify a region of the small subunit rDNA that permits genotypic identification of an *Acanthamoeba* isolate following sequence analysis.

In the case of *Balamuthia*, all isolates analyzed so far seem to be identical on the basis of their 18S rRNA gene sequences (68). A PCR assay for the detection of *B. mandrillaris* has been described (69). A PCR assay to detect *B. mandrillaris* in formalin-fixed archival tissue specimens has also been described (70).

In the case of *N. fowleri*, however, different isolates show similar nuclear 18S rRNA gene sequences, but variation in the internal transcribed spacer (ITS) sequences has been used to identify six different genotypes (I, II, III, IV, V, and VI) (71), although only three genotypes (I, II, and III) circulate in North America (72). Sequencing of the 5.8S rRNA gene and ITS1 and ITS2 of *N. fowleri* not only can differentiate *N. fowleri* from other *Naegleria* spp. and *Paravahlkampfia* spp. but also can be used in the genotypic analysis of *N. fowleri* strains (7, 22, 68, 71, 72). Recently, six microsatellite markers have been used in *N. fowleri* that show better resolution in strain typing than the 5.8S rRNA gene and ITS1 and ITS2 (73). The recently unraveled genome of *N. fowleri* (74, 75) offers great promise not only in elucidating the pathogenic mechanisms but also in the development of better drug targeting and thus increased survival of patients infected with this deadly pathogen.

A real-time multiplex PCR test that simultaneously identifies *Acanthamoeba*, *Balamuthia*, and *N. fowleri* in CSF and biopsy tissue specimens has been developed at the CDC (68). In this assay, PCR primers and TaqMan probes targeting three regions of the 18S rRNA gene are used. The real-time multiplex PCR assay is a fast, sensitive, and robust assay that detects all three pathogenic free-living amebae, *Acanthamoeba* spp., *B. mandrillaris*, and *N. fowleri*, simultaneously in a single specimen and has many advantages over conventional PCR. This test is being used at the CDC to identify *Acanthamoeba*, *Balamuthia*, and *N. fowleri* in patient specimens with great success. Because of its high sensitivity and specificity, this assay can specifically identify a single ameba in a specimen. Unfortunately, these molecular tests are not routinely available in clinical laboratories because of the lack of commercially available reagents.

ISOLATION

The recommended procedure for isolating free-living pathogenic amebae from biological specimens is as follows.

Note that the nonnutrient agar plate method is suitable only for *Acanthamoeba* and *Naegleria* cultures.

Materials

1. Page's ameba saline (11). Physiological saline and phosphate-buffered saline solutions that are normally available in clinical laboratories are not suitable, as the sodium chloride concentrations in these solutions will prevent the growth of amebae, especially *N. fowleri*.

2. Petri dishes containing 1.5% Difco agar made with Page's ameba saline (nonnutrient agar plate) (11). These plates can be stored at 4°C for up to 3 months. Chocolate agar with blood, Trypticase soy agar, and Lowenstein-Jensen agar have been used sometimes. These are not suitable because bacteria that coat the plates or bacteria from the clinical sample may overgrow and either prevent the growth of amebae, especially when they are present in small numbers, or obscure their presence.

3. Eighteen- to 24-h-old cultures of *E. coli* or *Enterobacter aerogenes*.

Preparation of Agar Plates

1. Remove the plates from the refrigerator and place them in a 37°C incubator for 30 min.

2. Add 0.5 ml of ameba saline to a slant culture of *E. coli* or *Enterobacter aerogenes*. Gently scrape the surface of the slant with a sterile bacteriologic loop (do not break the agar surface). Using a sterile Pasteur pipette, gently and uniformly suspend the bacteria. Add 2 or 3 drops of this suspension to the middle of a warmed (37°C) agar plate and spread the bacteria over the surface of the agar with a bacteriologic loop. The plate is then ready for inoculation.

Inoculation of Plates with Specimens

1. For CSF samples, centrifuge the CSF at 500 × *g* for 5 to 8 min. With a sterile serologic pipette, carefully transfer all but 0.5 ml of the supernatant to a sterile tube, and store the tube at 4°C for possible future use. Mix the sediment with the remaining fluid. With a sterile Pasteur pipette, place 2 or 3 drops in the center of the agar plate precoated with bacteria and incubate in room air at 37°C.

2. For tissue samples, finely mince a small piece of the tissue in a small amount of ameba saline. With a sterile Pasteur pipette, place 2 or 3 drops of the mixture in the center of the agar plate. Incubate the plate in room air at 37°C for CNS and lung tissues and at 30°C for tissues from other sites (e.g., skin and cornea).

3. Handle water and soil samples in the same manner as CSF and tissue specimens, respectively.

4. Control cultures are recommended for comparative purposes, although care should be exercised to prevent cross-contamination of patient cultures.

Examination of Plates

1. Using the low-power (10×) lens objective of a microscope, observe the plates daily for 7 days for amebae. Amebae can be seen as early as day 1.

2. If you see amebae anywhere, circle that area with a wax pencil. If there is interest in propagating the culture, using a fine spatula, cut a small piece of agar from the circled area and place it face down on the surface of a fresh agar plate precoated with bacteria; incubate as described above. Both *N. fowleri* and *Acanthamoeba* spp. can easily be cultivated in this way and, with periodic passages, maintained indefinitely. When the plate is examined under a microscope, the amebae will look like small blotches, and if they are observed carefully, their movement can be discerned. After 2 to 3 days of incubation, the amebae will start to encyst. If a plate is examined after 4 to 5 days of incubation, trophozoites as well as cysts will be visible. *B. mandrillaris*, however, will not grow on agar plates seeded with bacteria. While *B. mandrillaris* can be grown on monkey kidney or lung fibroblast cell lines, on human brain microvascular endothelial cells, and axenically in a complex medium (17, 18, 76–78), such techniques are not routinely available.

Identification and Culture

Identification of free-living amebae to the genus level is best achieved by conventional or real-time PCRs that are based on the rDNA sequences. However, PCRs may not be available in every diagnostic setting. In these situations, living organisms can be identified based on characteristic patterns of locomotion, morphologic features of the trophozoite and cyst forms, and results of enflagellation experiments. Immunofluorescence or immunoperoxidase tests using monoclonal or polyclonal antibodies (available at the CDC) are helpful in differentiating *Acanthamoeba* spp. from *B. mandrillaris* in fixed tissue (1, 27, 30, 52, 65, 79). Positive amebic cultures from ocular specimens may be considered presumptively positive for *Acanthamoeba*, since this is the only free-living ameba known to cause ocular infections.

Enflagellation Experiment

1. Mix 1 drop of the sedimented CSF containing amebae with about 1 ml of sterile distilled water in a sterile tube, or with a bacteriologic loop scrape the surface of a plate that is positive for amebae, transferring a loopful of scraping to a sterile tube that contains approximately 1 ml of distilled water.

2. Gently shake the tube and transfer a drop of this suspension to the center of a coverslip whose edges have been coated thinly with petroleum jelly. Place a microscope slide over the coverslip and invert the slide. Seal the edges of the coverslip with Vaspar. Place the slide in a moist chamber and incubate as before for 2 to 3 h. In addition, incubate the tube as described above.

3. Periodically examine the tube and the slide preparation microscopically for free-swimming flagellates. *N. fowleri* has a flagellate stage; *Acanthamoeba* spp. and *B. mandrillaris* do not. If the sample contains *N. fowleri*, about 30 to 50% of the amebae will have undergone transformation into pear-shaped biflagellate organisms (Fig. 3).

Other Culture Methods

Axenic Culture

Acanthamoeba spp. can easily be cultivated axenically, without the addition of serum or host tissue, in many different types of nutrient media, e.g., proteose peptone-yeast extract-glucose medium, Trypticase soy broth medium, and chemically defined medium (77). *N. fowleri*, however, requires media containing fetal calf serum or brain extract, e.g., Nelson's medium. A chemically defined medium has only recently been developed for *N. fowleri* (76). *B. mandrillaris* cannot be cultivated on agar plates with bacteria. It can, however, be cultivated on mammalian cell lines or a complex axenic medium (77).

Axenic cultures of *Acanthamoeba* spp. and *N. fowleri* can be established as follows. An actively growing 24- to 36-h-old ameba culture is scraped from the surface of the plate, suspended in 50 ml of ameba saline, and centrifuged at 500 × *g* for 5 min. The supernatant is aspirated, and the sediment is inoculated into proteose peptone-yeast extract-glucose medium or Nelson's medium, depending on the ameba isolate, and incubated at 37°C. Gentamicin, to a final concentration of 50 μg/ml, is added aseptically to the medium before the amebae are inoculated. Three subcultures into the antibiotic-containing medium at weekly intervals are usually sufficient to eliminate the associated bacteria (*E. coli* or *Enterobacter aerogenes*). Similarly, actively growing *B. mandrillaris* organisms on a mammalian cell culture may be used as a starting material to adapt them to grow in axenic medium containing Biosate peptone, yeast extract, *Torula* yeast RNA, Hanks' basal salt with calcium and magnesium, and vitamin mixture (78).

Cell Culture

Acanthamoeba spp., *B. mandrillaris*, and *N. fowleri* can also be inoculated onto many types of mammalian cell cultures. Shell vial cultures normally used in the isolation of viruses are suitable for the isolation of the amebae provided that antifungal agents (amphotericin B) are not included in the antibiotic mix. The amebae grow vigorously in these cell cultures and produce cytopathic effects somewhat similar to those caused by viruses (77, 78, 80). Because of such cytopathic effects, *Acanthamoeba* organisms were mistaken for transformed cell types presumed to contain viruses and were erroneously termed lipovirus and Ryan virus (1).

Animal Inoculation

Two-week-old Swiss Webster mice weighing 12 to 15 g each can be infected with these amebae. The mice are anesthetized with ether, and a drop of ameba suspension is instilled into their nostrils. Mice infected with *N. fowleri* die within 5 to 7 days after developing characteristic signs, such as ruffled fur, aimless wandering, partial paralysis, and finally coma and death. Mice infected with *Acanthamoeba* spp. and *B. mandrillaris* may die of acute disease within 5 to 7 days or may die of chronic disease after several weeks. In all cases, the presence of amebae in the mouse brain can be demonstrated either by culture or by histologic examination.

Serology

The serologic techniques discussed here have been developed as research tools and are not routinely available to clinical laboratories. Antibodies (detected by complement fixation, indirect fluorescent-antibody assay [IFA], precipitin, etc.) to *Acanthamoeba* spp. have been shown to be present in the sera of patients with GAE, upper respiratory tract distress, optic neuritis, macular disease, and keratitis (50, 61).

An antibody response to *N. fowleri*, however, has not yet been defined. Most patients with *N. fowleri* PAM die very shortly after infection, before they have time to produce detectable levels of antibody. In one case, however, in which the patient survived PAM, an antibody response was detected by 10 days after hospitalization, ultimately reaching a titer of 1:4,096 (81).

Since the recognition of *Balamuthia* GAE is relatively new, not much information is available on the serologic responses of patients infected with *Balamuthia*. According to a recent report, four patients with confirmed *Balamuthia* GAE infection had high titers of antibody to *Balamuthia*, whereas six serum specimens from patients with encephalitis of unknown causes (10% of the sera) had titers of 64 and above and none of the control sera had titers of 64 or above (29). According to Schuster et al. (82), IFA can be successfully used to screen GAE due to *Acanthamoeba* and *Balamuthia* in patients whose clinical presentation, laboratory results, and neuroimaging findings are suggestive of amoebic encephalitis, thus enabling an earlier diagnosis and earlier start of antimicrobial therapy. Recently, Kucerova et al. showed by SDS-PAGE and Western blot assay that several isolates, irrespective of their isolation from humans or animals or from different geographic locales, are basically similar, underscoring the similarity of the isolates (83).

TREATMENT

There is no single drug that is effective against systemic acanthamebiasis. A number of antimicrobials have shown efficacy against amebae *in vitro*, but there is no assurance that these drugs will be effective clinically. An important consideration in corneal infections is that drugs should be not only amebicidal but also cysticidal. As long as cysts remain viable, the infection can recur. *In vitro* studies indicate that chlorhexidine gluconate and polyhexamethyl biguanide have excellent amebicidal and cysticidal properties, and they have been used topically in the treatment of *Acanthamoeba* keratitis with success. Several patients with *Acanthamoeba* keratitis have been successfully treated with different drug combinations administered over a long period (61). Although a few patients with *Acanthamoeba* GAE have survived, most have died in spite of treatment with several drug combinations. The prognoses of patients without CNS infection but with disseminated cutaneous ulcers due to *Acanthamoeba* spp. are good. Some patients with *Acanthamoeba* CNS infections have also been cured with a combination of pharmaceuticals that included amikacin, voriconazole, sulfa drugs, and miltefosine (1, 66, 84).

Pathogenic *N. fowleri* is exquisitely susceptible to amphotericin B *in vitro*, and the minimum amebicidal concentrations were determined to be 0.02 to 0.078 μg/ml for three different clinical isolates of *N. fowleri* (1, 9, 61, 81). Although many patients with PAM have been treated with amphotericin B, only a few patients have survived after receiving intrathecal and intravenous injections of amphotericin B alone or in combination with other drugs (81, 85, 86).

In vitro studies indicate that *B. mandrillaris* is susceptible *in vitro* to pentamidine isothiocyanate and that patients with *B. mandrillaris* infection may benefit from treatment with this drug (4, 30, 31). Although most patients with *B. mandrillaris* GAE have died of this disease, several patients have survived after treatment initially with pentamidine isethionate and subsequently with a combination of sulfadiazine, clarithromycin, and fluconazole.

The anticancer and antiparasitic drug miltefosine and the antifungal drug voriconazole were tested *in vitro* against *B. mandrillaris*, *Acanthamoeba* spp., and *N. fowleri*. The ability of miltefosine and voriconazole to penetrate brain tissue and CSF and their low toxicity make them attractive possibilities in the treatment of the amebic encephalitides. In combination with other antimicrobials, these two drugs may form the basis of an optimal therapy for treatment of *Acanthamoeba*, *Balamuthia*, and *Naegleria* infections (80). For example, miltefosine in conjunction with other pharmaceuticals has been used in the successful treatment of *Acanthamoeba* (66), *Balamuthia* (87), and *N. fowleri* (85, 86).

EVALUATION, INTERPRETATION, AND REPORTING OF RESULTS

Most clinical laboratories rely on the agar plate technique for the isolation and identification of *N. fowleri* and

Acanthamoeba spp. An agar plate inoculated with patient CSF should be microscopically examined every day for the presence of amebae. If amebae are seen, an area with amebae should be scraped and inoculated into ~1 ml of distilled water and incubated at 37°C and examined every 10 min for 1 h. If flagellates are seen, the clinician should be informed that the CSF is positive for *Naegleria* (possibly *N. fowleri*) amebae. If no flagellates are seen, even after 2 h, then the amebae should be examined under high magnification (×400) for the presence of fine thorn-like processes (acanthopodia). The clinician should then be informed of the presence of amebae, probably *Acanthamoeba*. Wet-mount preparations should always be confirmed with permanently stained smears (trichrome, hematoxylin, or Giemsa-Wright). If other techniques, like real-time PCR, are available, then the identity of the amebae should be confirmed. Since many clinical laboratories do not have the necessary expertise and/or equipment, they usually send the specimens to an outside laboratory like the CDC for identification and interpretation. The CDC also offers Web-based rapid evaluation of digital images of specimens for expedited review and consultation through a telediagnostic service known as Laboratory Identification of Parasitic Diseases of Public Health Concern (DPDx). DPDx is a rapid means of obtaining a probable diagnosis from tissue sections or wet mounts of CSF and tissue. A molecular diagnosis is often needed with CSF or tissue specimens when the species-specific morphological features cannot be extracted from the digital images. Also, antimicrobial testing is currently not available in clinical laboratories and is only occasionally performed at CDC for research purposes. Antimicrobial testing is not routinely recommended for clinical isolates. Further, it is well known, at least for these free-living amebae, that what works *in vitro* may not always work *in vivo*. For example, fluconazole has no activity *in vitro* against *Balamuthia* but is one of the drugs of choice for treatment. Several patients have survived after receiving fluconazole given along with other drugs; this approach may represent synergistic activities.

Use of trade names is for identification only and does not imply endorsement by the Public Health Service or by the U.S. Department of Health and Human Services.

REFERENCES

1. **Visvesvara GS, Moura H, Schuster FL.** 2007. Pathogenic and opportunistic free-living amoebae: *Acanthamoeba* spp., *Balamuthia mandrillaris*, *Naegleria fowleri*, and *Sappinia diploidea*. *FEMS Immunol Med Microbiol* **50:**1–26.
2. **Visvesvara GS.** 2010. Amebic meningoencephalitides and keratitis: challenges in diagnosis and treatment. *Curr Opin Infect Dis* **23:**590–594.
3. **Clarke DW, Niederkorn JY.** 2006. The pathophysiology of *Acanthamoeba* keratitis. *Trends Parasitol* **22:**175–180.
4. **Bravo FGCJ, Gottuzo E, Visvesvara GS.** 2005. Cutaneous manifestations of infection by free-living amebas, p 49–55. *In* Tyring SKLO, Hengge UR (ed), *Tropical Dermatology*. Elsevier Churchill Livingstone, Philadelphia, PA.
5. **Gelman BB, Rauf SJ, Nader R, Popov V, Borkowski J, Chaljub G, Nauta HW, Visvesvara GS.** 2001. Amoebic encephalitis due to *Sappinia diploidea*. *JAMA* **285:**2450–2451.
6. **Qvarnstrom Y, da Silva AJ, Schuster FL, Gelman BB, Visvesvara GS.** 2009. Molecular confirmation of *Sappinia pedata* as a causative agent of amoebic encephalitis. *J Infect Dis* **199:**1139–1142.
7. **Visvesvara GS, Sriram R, Qvarnstrom Y, Bandyopadhyay K, Da Silva AJ, Pieniazek NJ, Cabral GA.** 2009. *Paravahlkampfia francinae* n. sp. masquerading as an agent of primary amoebic meningoencephalitis. *J Eukaryot Microbiol* **56:**357–366.
8. **Culbertson CG, Smith JW, Minner JR.** 1958. *Acanthamoeba*: observations on animal pathogenicity. *Science* **127:**1506.
9. **Carter RF.** 1972. Primary amoebic meningo-encephalitis. *Trans R Soc Trop Med Hyg* **66:**193–208.
10. **Adl SM, Simpson AG, Lane CE, Lukeš J, Bass D, Bowser SS, Brown MW, Burki F, Dunthorn M, Hampl V, Heiss A, Hoppenrath M, Lara E, Le Gall L, Lynn DH, McManus H, Mitchell EA, Mozley-Stanridge SE, Parfrey LW, Pawlowski J, Rueckert S, Shadwick L, Schoch CL, Smirnov A, Spiegel FW.** 2012. The revised classification of eukaryotes. *J Eukaryot Microbiol* **59:**429–514.
11. **Page FC.** 1988. *A New Key to Freshwater and Soil Gymnamoebae*. Freshwater Biological Association, Ambleside, Cumbria, England.
12. **Sriram R, Shoff M, Booton G, Fuerst P, Visvesvara GS.** 2008. Survival of *Acanthamoeba* cysts after desiccation for more than 20 years. *J Clin Microbiol* **46:**4045–4048.
13. **Booton GC, Visvesvara GS, Byers TJ, Kelly DJ, Fuerst PA.** 2005. Identification and distribution of *Acanthamoeba* species genotypes associated with nonkeratitis infections. *J Clin Microbiol* **43:**1689–1693.
14. **Qvarnstrom Y, Nerad TA, Visvesvara GS.** 2013. Characterization of a new pathogenic *Acanthamoeba* species, *A. byersi* n. sp., isolated from a human with fatal amoebic encephalitis. *J Eukaryot Microbiol* **60:**626–633.
15. **Stothard DR, Schroeder-Diedrich JM, Awwad MH, Gast RJ, Ledee DR, Rodriguez-Zaragoza S, Dean CL, Fuerst PA, Byers TJ.** 1998. The evolutionary history of the genus *Acanthamoeba* and the identification of eight new 18S rRNA gene sequence types. *J Eukaryot Microbiol* **45:**45–54.
16. **Corsaro D, Köhsler M, Montalbano Di Filippo M, Venditti D, Monno R, Di Cave D, Berrilli F, Walochnik J.** 2017. Update on *Acanthamoeba jacobsi* genotype T15, including full-length 18S rDNA molecular phylogeny. *Parasitol Res* **116:**1273–1284.
17. **Visvesvara GS, Schuster FL, Martinez AJ.** 1993. *Balamuthia mandrillaris*, N. G., N. Sp., agent of amebic meningoencephalitis in humans and other animals. *J Eukaryot Microbiol* **40:**504–514.
18. **Visvesvara GS, Martinez AJ, Schuster FL, Leitch GJ, Wallace SV, Sawyer TK, Anderson M.** 1990. Leptomyxid ameba, a new agent of amebic meningoencephalitis in humans and animals. *J Clin Microbiol* **28:**2750–2756.
19. **Cope JR, Ali IK.** 2016. Primary amebic meningoencephalitis: what have we learned in the last 5 years? *Curr Infect Dis Rep* **18:**31.
20. **Yoder JS, Eddy BA, Visvesvara GS, Capewell L, Beach MJ.** 2010. The epidemiology of primary amoebic meningoencephalitis in the USA, 1962-2008. *Epidemiol Infect* **138:**968–975.
21. **Kemble SK, Lynfield R, DeVries AS, Drehner DM, Pomputius WF, III, Beach MJ, Visvesvara GS, da Silva AJ, Hill VR, Yoder JS, Xiao L, Smith KE, Danila R.** 2012. Fatal *Naegleria fowleri* infection acquired in Minnesota: possible expanded range of a deadly thermophilic organism. *Clin Infect Dis* **54:**805–809.
22. **Yoder JS, Straif-Bourgeois S, Roy SL, Moore TA, Visvesvara GS, Ratard RC, Hill VR, Wilson JD, Linscott AJ, Crager R, Kozak NA, Sriram R, Narayanan J, Mull B, Kahler AM, Schneeberger C, da Silva AJ, Poudel M, Baumgarten KL, Xiao L, Beach MJ.** 2012. Primary amebic meningoencephalitis deaths associated with sinus irrigation using contaminated tap water. *Clin Infect Dis* **55:**e79–e85.
23. **Cope JR, Ratard RC, Hill VR, Sokol T, Causey JJ, Yoder JS, Mirani G, Mull B, Mukerjee KA, Narayanan J, Doucet M, Qvarnstrom Y, Poole CN, Akingbola OA, Ritter JM, Xiong Z, da Silva AJ, Roellig D, Van Dyke RB, Stern H, Xiao L, Beach MJ.** 2015. The first association of a primary amebic meningoencephalitis death with culturable *Naegleria fowleri* in tap water from a US treated public drinking water system. *Clin Infect Dis* **60:**e36–e42.
24. **Centers for Disease Control and Prevention (CDC).** 2013. Notes from the field: primary amebic meningoencephalitis associated with ritual nasal rinsing—St. Thomas, U.S. Virgin islands, 2012. *MMWR Morb Mortal Wkly Rep* **62:**903.

25. **Seijo Martinez M, Gonzalez-Mediero G, Santiago P, Rodriguez De Lope A, Diz J, Conde C, Visvesvara GS.** 2000. Granulomatous amebic encephalitis in a patient with AIDS: isolation of acanthamoeba sp. group II from brain tissue and successful treatment with sulfadiazine and fluconazole. *J Clin Microbiol* **38:**3892–3895.
26. **Brondfield MN, Reid MJ, Rutishauser RL, Cope JR, Tang J, Ritter JM, Matanock A, Ali I, Doernberg SB, Hilts-Horeczko A, DeMarco T, Klein L, Babik JM.** 2017. Disseminated *Acanthamoeba* infection in a heart transplant recipient treated successfully with a miltefosine-containing regimen: case report and review of the literature. *Transpl Infect Dis* **19:**e12661.
27. **Kaul DR, Lowe L, Visvesvara GS, Farmen S, Khaled YA, Yanik GA.** 2008. *Acanthamoeba* infection in a patient with chronic graft-versus-host disease occurring during treatment with voriconazole. *Transpl Infect Dis* **10:**437–441.
28. **Deetz TR, Sawyer MH, Billman G, Schuster FL, Visvesvara GS.** 2003. Successful treatment of *Balamuthia* amoebic encephalitis: presentation of 2 cases. *Clin Infect Dis* **37:**1304–1312.
29. **Schuster FL, Yagi S, Gavali S, Michelson D, Raghavan R, Blomquist I, Glastonbury C, Bollen AW, Scharnhorst D, Reed SL, Kuriyama S, Visvesvara GS, Glaser CA.** 2009. Under the radar: *Balamuthia* amebic encephalitis. *Clin Infect Dis* **48:**879–887.
30. **Gupte AA, Hocevar SN, Lea AS, Kulkarni RD, Schain DC, Casey MJ, Zendejas-Ruiz IR, Chung WK, Mbaeyi C, Roy SL, Visvesvara GS, da Silva AJ, Tallaj J, Eckhoff D, Baddley JW.** 2014. Transmission of *Balamuthia mandrillaris* through solid organ transplantation: utility of organ recipient serology to guide clinical management. *Am J Transplant* **14:**1417–1424.
31. **Farnon EC, Kokko KE, Budge PJ, Mbaeyi C, Lutterloh EC, Qvarnstrom Y, da Silva AJ, Shieh WJ, Roy SL, Paddock CD, Sriram R, Zaki SR, Visvesvara GS, Kuehnert MJ, Weiss J, Komatsu K, Manch R, Ramos A, Echeverria L, Moore A, Zakowski P, Kittleson M, Kobashigawa J, Yoder J, Beach M, Mahle W, Kanter K, Geraghty PJ, Navarro E, Hahn C, Fujita S, Stinson J, Trachtenberg J, Byers P, Cheung M, Jie T, Kaplan B, Gruessner R, Bracamonte E, Viscusi C, Gonzalez-Peralta R, Lawrence R, Fratkin J, Butt F, Balamuthia Transplant Investigation Teams.** 2016. Transmission of *Balamuthia mandrillaris* by organ transplantation. *Clin Infect Dis* **63:**878–888.
32. **Schuster FL, Glaser C, Honarmand S, Maguire JH, Visvesvara GS.** 2004. *Balamuthia* amebic encephalitis risk, Hispanic Americans. *Emerg Infect Dis* **10:**1510–1512.
33. **Fritsche TR, Horn M, Wagner M, Herwig RP, Schleifer KH, Gautom RK.** 2000. Phylogenetic diversity among geographically dispersed *Chlamydiales* endosymbionts recovered from clinical and environmental isolates of *Acanthamoeba* spp. *Appl Environ Microbiol* **66:**2613–2619.
34. **Greub G, Raoult D.** 2004. Microorganisms resistant to free-living amoebae. *Clin Microbiol Rev* **17:**413–433.
35. **Rowbotham TJ.** 1998. Isolation of *Legionella pneumophila* serogroup 1 from human feces with use of amebic cocultures. *Clin Infect Dis* **26:**502–503.
36. **La Scola B, Mezi L, Weiller PJ, Raoult D.** 2001. Isolation of *Legionella anisa* using an amoebic coculture procedure. *J Clin Microbiol* **39:**365–366.
37. **Adékambi T, Reynaud-Gaubert M, Greub G, Gevaudan MJ, La Scola B, Raoult D, Drancourt M.** 2004. Amoebal coculture of "*Mycobacterium massiliense*" sp. nov. from the sputum of a patient with hemoptoic pneumonia. *J Clin Microbiol* **42:**5493–5501.
38. **Dunnebacke TH, Schuster FL, Yagi S, Booton GC.** 2004. *Balamuthia mandrillaris* from soil samples. *Microbiology* **150:**2837–2842.
39. **Niyyati M, Lorenzo-Morales J, Rezaeian M, Martin-Navarro CM, Haghi AM, Maciver SK, Valladares B.** 2009. Isolation of *Balamuthia mandrillaris* from urban dust, free of known infectious involvement. *Parasitol Res* **106:**279–281.
40. **Schuster FL, Dunnebacke TH, Booton GC, Yagi S, Kohlmeier CK, Glaser C, Vugia D, Bakardjiev A, Azimi P, Maddux-Gonzalez M, Martinez AJ, Visvesvara GS.** 2003. Environmental isolation of *Balamuthia mandrillaris* associated with a case of amebic encephalitis. *J Clin Microbiol* **41:**3175–3180.
41. **Magnet A, Fenoy S, Galván AL, Izquierdo F, Rueda C, Fernandez Vadillo C, Del Aguila C.** 2013. A year long study of the presence of free living amoeba in Spain. *Water Res* **47:**6966–6972.
42. **Ahmad AF, Andrew PW, Kilvington S.** 2011. Development of a nested PCR for environmental detection of the pathogenic free-living amoeba *Balamuthia mandrillaris*. *J Eukaryot Microbiol* **58:**269–271.
43. **Tapia JL, Torres BN, Visvesvara GS.** 2013. *Balamuthia mandrillaris*: in vitro interactions with selected protozoa and algae. *J Eukaryot Microbiol* **60:**448–454.
44. **Butt CG.** 1966. Primary amebic meningoencephalitis. *N Engl J Med* **274:**1473–1476.
45. **Capewell LG, Harris AM, Yoder JS, Cope JR, Eddy BA, Roy SL, Visvesvara GS, Fox LM, Beach MJ.** 2015. Diagnosis, clinical course, and treatment of primary amoebic meningoencephalitis in the United States, 1937-2013. *J Pediatric Infect Dis Soc* **4:**e68–e75.
46. **Centers for Disease Control and Prevention (CDC).** 2017. Parasites—*Naegleria fowleri*—primary amebic meningoencephalitis (PAM)—amebic encephalitis. https://www.cdc.gov/parasites/naegleria/treatment.html. Accessed 9 August 2017.
47. **Marciano-Cabral F, Cabral GA.** 2007. The immune response to *Naegleria fowleri* amebae and pathogenesis of infection. *FEMS Immunol Med Microbiol* **51:**243–259.
48. **Lozano-Alarcón F, Bradley GA, Houser BS, Visvesvara GS.** 1997. Primary amebic meningoencephalitis due to *Naegleria fowleri* in a South American tapir. *Vet Pathol* **34:**239–243.
49. **Visvesvara GS, De Jonckheere JF, Sriram R, Daft B.** 2005. Isolation and molecular typing of *Naegleria fowleri* from the brain of a cow that died of primary amebic meningoencephalitis. *J Clin Microbiol* **43:**4203–4204.
50. **Marciano-Cabral F, Cabral G.** 2003. *Acanthamoeba* spp. as agents of disease in humans. *Clin Microbiol Rev* **16:**273–307.
51. **Im K, Kim DS.** 1998. Acanthamoebiasis in Korea: two new cases with clinical cases review. *Yonsei Med J* **39:**478–484.
52. **Guarner J, Bartlett J, Shieh WJ, Paddock CD, Visvesvara GS, Zaki SR.** 2007. Histopathologic spectrum and immunohistochemical diagnosis of amebic meningoencephalitis. *Mod Pathol* **20:**1230–1237.
53. **Rideout BA, Gardiner CH, Stalis IH, Zuba JR, Hadfield T, Visvesvara GS.** 1997. Fatal infections with *Balamuthia mandrillaris* (a free-living amoeba) in gorillas and other Old World primates. *Vet Pathol* **34:**15–22.
54. **Pfister DR, Cameron JD, Krachmer JH, Holland EJ.** 1996. Confocal microscopy findings of *Acanthamoeba keratitis*. *Am J Ophthalmol* **121:**119–128.
55. **Jones DB, Visvesvara GS, Robinson NM.** 1975. *Acanthamoeba polyphaga* keratitis and *Acanthamoeba* uveitis associated with fatal meningoencephalitis. *Trans Ophthalmol Soc UK* **95:**221–232.
56. **Stehr-Green JKBT, Bailey TM, Visvesvara GS.** 1989. The epidemiology of *Acanthamoeba* keratitis in the United States. *Am J Ophthalmol* **107:**331–336.
57. **Verani JR, Lorick SA, Yoder JS, Beach MJ, Braden CR, Roberts JM, Conover CS, Chen S, McConnell KA, Chang DC, Park BJ, Jones DB, Visvesvara GS, Roy SL, AcanthamoebaKeratitis Investigation Team.** 2009. National outbreak of *Acanthamoeba* keratitis associated with use of a contact lens solution, United States. *Emerg Infect Dis* **15:**1236–1242.
58. **Johnston SP, Sriram R, Qvarnstrom Y, Roy S, Verani J, Yoder J, Lorick S, Roberts J, Beach MJ, Visvesvara G.** 2009. Resistance of *Acanthamoeba* cysts to disinfection in multiple contact lens solutions. *J Clin Microbiol* **47:**2040–2045.
59. **Cope JR, Collier SA, Schein OD, Brown AC, Verani JR, Gallen R, Beach MJ, Yoder JS.** 2016. *Acanthamoeba* keratitis among rigid gas permeable contact lens wearers in the United States, 2005 through 2011. *Ophthalmology* **123:**1435–1441.

60. **Brown AC, Ross J, Jones DB, Collier SA, Ayers TL, Hoekstra RM, Backensen B, Roy SL, Beach MJ, Yoder JS.** 2018. Risk factors for *Acanthamoeba* keratitis—a multistate case-control study, 2008–2011. *Eye Contact Lens* **44**(Suppl 1): S173-S178.
61. **Schuster FL, Visvesvara GS.** 2004. Free-living amoebae as opportunistic and non-opportunistic pathogens of humans and animals. *Int J Parasitol* **34:**1001–1027.
62. **Roy SL, Metzger R, Chen JG, Laham FR, Martin M, Kipper SW, Smith LE, Lyon GM III, Haffner J, Ross JE, Rye AK, Johnson W, Bodager D, Friedman M, Walsh DJ, Collins C, Inman B, Davis BJ, Robinson T, Paddock C, Zaki SR, Kuehnert M, DaSilva A, Qvarnstrom Y, Sriram R, Visvesvara GS.** 2014. Risk for transmission of *Naegleria fowleri* from solid organ transplantation. *Am J Transplant* **14:**163–171.
63. **Martinez AJ, Visvesvara GS.** 1997. Free-living, amphizoic and opportunistic amebas. *Brain Pathol* **7:**583–598.
64. **Barete S, Combes A, de Jonckheere JF, Datry A, Varnous S, Martinez V, Ptacek SG, Caumes E, Capron F, Francès C, Gibert C, Chosidow O.** 2007. Fatal disseminated *Acanthamoeba lenticulata* infection in a heart transplant patient. *Emerg Infect Dis* **13:**736–738.
65. **Satlin MJ, Graham JK, Visvesvara GS, Mena H, Marks KM, Saal SD, Soave R.** 2013. Fulminant and fatal encephalitis caused by *Acanthamoeba* in a kidney transplant recipient: case report and literature review. *Transpl Infect Dis* **15:** 619–626.
66. **Aichelburg AC, Walochnik J, Assadian O, Prosch H, Steuer A, Perneczky G, Visvesvara GS, Aspöck H, Vetter N.** 2008. Successful treatment of disseminated *Acanthamoeba* sp. infection with miltefosine. *Emerg Infect Dis* **14:** 1743–1746.
67. **Taher EE, Méabed EMH, Abdallah I, Abdel Wahed WY.** 2018. *Acanthamoeba* keratitis in noncompliant soft contact lenses users: genotyping and risk factors, a study from Cairo, Egypt. *J Infect Public Health* **11:**377-383.
68. **Qvarnstrom Y, Visvesvara GS, Sriram R, da Silva AJ.** 2006. Multiplex real-time PCR assay for simultaneous detection of *Acanthamoeba* spp., *Balamuthia mandrillaris*, and *Naegleria fowleri*. *J Clin Microbiol* **44:**3589–3595.
69. **Booton GC, Carmichael JR, Visvesvara GS, Byers TJ, Fuerst PA.** 2003. Identification of *Balamuthia mandrillaris* by PCR assay using the mitochondrial 16S rRNA gene as a target. *J Clin Microbiol* **41:**453–455.
70. **Yagi S, Booton GC, Visvesvara GS, Schuster FL.** 2005. Detection of *Balamuthia* mitochondrial 16S rRNA gene DNA in clinical specimens by PCR. *J Clin Microbiol* **43:**3192–3197.
71. **De Jonckheere JF.** 2011. Origin and evolution of the worldwide distributed pathogenic amoeboflagellate *Naegleria fowleri*. *Infect Genet Evol* **11:**1520–1528.
72. **Zhou L, Sriram R, Visvesvara GS, Xiao L.** 2003. Genetic variations in the internal transcribed spacer and mitochondrial small subunit rRNA gene of *Naegleria* spp. *J Eukaryot Microbiol* **50**(Suppl)**:**522–526.
73. **Coupat-Goutaland B, Régoudis E, Besseyrias M, Mularoni A, Binet M, Herbelin P, Pélandakis M.** 2016. Population structure in *Naegleria fowleri* as revealed by microsatellite markers. *PLoS One* **11:**e0152434.
74. **Herman EK, Greninger AL, Visvesvara GS, Marciano-Cabral F, Dacks JB, Chiu CY.** 2013. The mitochondrial genome and a 60-kb nuclear DNA segment from *Naegleria fowleri*, the causative agent of primary amoebic meningoencephalitis. *J Eukaryot Microbiol* **60:**179–191.
75. **Zysset-Burri DC, Müller N, Beuret C, Heller M, Schürch N, Gottstein B, Wittwer M.** 2014. Genome-wide identification of pathogenicity factors of the free-living amoeba *Naegleria fowleri*. *BMC Genomics* **15:**496.
76. **Jayasekera S, Sissons J, Tucker J, Rogers C, Nolder D, Warhurst D, Alsam S, White JM, Higgins EM, Khan NA.** 2004. Post-mortem culture of *Balamuthia mandrillaris* from the brain and cerebrospinal fluid of a case of granulomatous amoebic meningoencephalitis, using human brain microvascular endothelial cells. *J Med Microbiol* **53:**1007–1012.
77. **Schuster FL.** 2002. Cultivation of pathogenic and opportunistic free-living amebas. *Clin Microbiol Rev* **15:**342–354.
78. **Schuster FL, Visvesvara GS.** 1996. Axenic growth and drug sensitivity studies of *Balamuthia mandrillaris*, an agent of amebic meningoencephalitis in humans and other animals. *J Clin Microbiol* **34:**385–388.
79. **Tavares M, Correia da Costa JM, Carpenter SS, Santos LA, Afonso C, Aguiar A, Pereira J, Cardoso AI, Schuster FL, Yagi S, Sriram R, Visvesvara GS.** 2006. Diagnosis of first case of *Balamuthia amoebic* encephalitis in Portugal by immunofluorescence and PCR. *J Clin Microbiol* **44:**2660–2663.
80. **Schuster FL, Guglielmo BJ, Visvesvara GS.** 2006. In-vitro activity of miltefosine and voriconazole on clinical isolates of free-living amebas: *Balamuthia mandrillaris*, *Acanthamoeba* spp., and *Naegleria fowleri*. *J Eukaryot Microbiol* **53:**121–126.
81. **Seidel JS, Harmatz P, Visvesvara GS, Cohen A, Edwards J, Turner J.** 1982. Successful treatment of primary amebic meningoencephalitis. *N Engl J Med* **306:**346–348.
82. **Schuster FL, Honarmand S, Visvesvara GS, Glaser CA.** 2006. Detection of antibodies against free-living amoebae *Balamuthia mandrillaris* and *Acanthamoeba* species in a population of patients with encephalitis. *Clin Infect Dis* **42:**1260–1265.
83. **Kucerova Z, Sriram R, Wilkins PP, Visvesvara GS.** 2011. Identification of antigenic targets for immunodetection of *Balamuthia mandrillaris* infection. *Clin Vaccine Immunol* **18:**1297–1301.
84. **Webster D, Umar I, Kolyvas G, Bilbao J, Guiot MC, Duplisea K, Qvarnstrom Y, Visvesvara GS.** 2012. Treatment of granulomatous amoebic encephalitis with voriconazole and miltefosine in an immunocompetent soldier. *Am J Trop Med Hyg* **87:**715–718.
85. **Linam WM, Ahmed M, Cope JR, Chu C, Visvesvara GS, da Silva AJ, Qvarnstrom Y, Green J.** 2015. Successful treatment of an adolescent with *Naegleria fowleri* primary amebic meningoencephalitis. *Pediatrics* **135:**e744–e748.
86. **Cope JR, Conrad DA, Cohen N, Cotilla M, DaSilva A, Jackson J, Visvesvara GS.** 2016. Use of the novel therapeutic agent miltefosine for the treatment of primary amebic meningoencephalitis: report of 1 fatal and 1 surviving case. *Clin Infect Dis* **62:**774–776.
87. **Martínez DY, Seas C, Bravo F, Legua P, Ramos C, Cabello AM, Gotuzzo E.** 2010. Successful treatment of *Balamuthia mandrillaris* amoebic infection with extensive neurological and cutaneous involvement. *Clin Infect Dis* **51:**e7–e11.

Intestinal and Urogenital Amebae, Flagellates, and Ciliates

SUSAN NOVAK-WEEKLEY AND AMY L. LEBER

143

Entamoeba histolytica and *Giardia duodenalis* infections are two of the most common protozoal infections seen worldwide and are of serious concern on a global scale due to their prevalence and the pathogenicity of their causative agents. *Trichomonas vaginalis* is also recognized as a very common sexually transmitted infection affecting millions of people around the world. Most of the other protozoa described in this chapter are nonpathogenic organisms. Nevertheless, detection and differentiation of nonpathogens from true pathogens in clinical specimens is useful in that their presence indicates exposure to fecal contamination, and further examination of additional specimens may reveal pathogenic protozoa. The pathogenic and nonpathogenic organisms are categorized as indicated in Table 1; however, reports of disease in patients infected with organisms considered nonpathogenic are found in the literature.

Microscopic examination of stool specimens continues to be one of the main tools used in the laboratory diagnosis of intestinal amebic, flagellate, and ciliate infections. The goal of microscopy is to identify pathogenic protozoa, differentiate between these and nonpathogenic species, and properly discriminate among various artifacts that may be present. Antigen detection methods such as enzyme immunoassays (EIAs), immunochromatographic assays, and direct fluorescent-antibody (DFA) assays are available for the detection of pathogens such as the *E. histolytica/Entamoeba dispar* group, *E. histolytica*, and *G. duodenalis*. Culture for the intestinal amebae is generally not feasible, readily available, or clinically relevant except in certain limited situations but is useful still in the diagnosis of *T. vaginalis*. Nucleic acid-based techniques have been developed, and reports in the literature for select pathogens are ever increasing. One of the most important developments related to the molecular detection of parasites is the advent of panels for detection of multiple agents of gastrointestinal disease, including combinations of bacterial, viral, and parasitic agents (1–3). More data are needed, particularly related to detection of intestinal parasites, to assess the performance of these systems and the potential impact they might have on outcomes; however, on the whole they appear more sensitive than conventional methods. With multiple multiplex molecular testing assays now widely available for organisms such as *E. histolytica*, *G. duodenalis*, and *Cryptosporidium* spp., their use is a viable alternative to other more conventional methods. These assays will be particularly useful to diagnose diseases such as amebiasis, where microscopy does not allow differentiation of pathogenic versus nonpathogenic *Entamoeba* spp. See the sections below and refer to chapters 7, 8, and 138 of this *Manual* for additional information.

AMEBAE

Taxonomy

The amebae that parasitize the intestinal tracts of humans belong to three genera: *Entamoeba*, *Endolimax*, and *Iodamoeba*. They all belong to the supergroup Amoebozoa (Archamoebae: Entamoebida). These organisms move by means of cytoplasmic protrusions called pseudopodia (see chapter 135 of this *Manual*). While *Dientamoeba fragilis* was once classified as an ameba, it is now grouped with the flagellates, but it is still identified microscopically on the basis of morphologic comparison to amebae.

Description of the Agents

Of the 11 species of intestinal amebae, *E. dispar*, *Entamoeba hartmanni*, *Entamoeba coli*, *Entamoeba polecki*, *Entamoeba gingivalis*, *Endolimax nana*, and *Iodamoeba bütschlii* are nonpathogenic for humans. To date, little is known about *Entamoeba moshkovskii* and *Entamoeba bangladeshi* in regard to their pathogenicity. *E. histolytica* is pathogenic for humans, causing invasive intestinal and extraintestinal amebiasis.

Epidemiology, Transmission, and Prevention

All amebae have a common and relatively simple life cycle. The cyst is the infectious form and is acquired by ingestion of contaminated material such as water and food or by direct fecal-oral transmission. Once the cyst reaches the intestinal tract, excystation occurs, releasing trophozoites. Encystment occurs in the colon, presumably when conditions become unfavorable for the trophozoites. Cysts are passed in the feces and remain viable in the environment for days to weeks in water and soil if protected from desiccation. Improvements in sanitary conditions are necessary to prevent infections in areas where the organisms are endemic. Research to develop a vaccine against *E. histolytica* is ongoing, but none is currently available.

TABLE 1 Intestinal and urogenital amebae, flagellates, and ciliates of humans[a]

Parasite	Pathogenic	Nonpathogenic
Amebae	*Entamoeba histolytica*[b]	*Entamoeba dispar*, *Entamoeba moshkovskii*[c], *Entamoeba bangladeshi*[d]
	Blastocystis sp.	*Entamoeba hartmanni*
		Entamoeba coli
		Entamoeba polecki
		Entamoeba gingivalis[e]
		Endolimax nana
		Iodamoeba bütschlii
Flagellates	*Giardia duodenalis*	*Chilomastix mesnili*
	Trichomonas vaginalis	*Pentatrichomonas (Trichomonas) hominis*
	Dientamoeba fragilis	*Trichomonas tenax*[e]
		Enteromonas hominis
		Retortamonas intestinalis
Ciliates	*Neobalantidium coli*	

[a]All organisms are intestinal with the exception of *T. vaginalis*.
[b]A distinction between *E. histolytica*, *E. dispar*, *E. moshkovskii*, and *E. bangladeshi* cannot be made on the basis of morphology unless ingested RBCs are seen in the cytoplasm of the trophozoite, indicative of *E. histolytica*.
[c]*E. moshkovskii* may be found in human stool specimens more predominantly in certain areas of endemicity. A free-living ameba, it is morphologically identical to *E. histolytica/E. dispar*, and its pathogenicity is still not fully understood (10, 36).
[d]*E. bangladeshi* has been recently identified from human stool specimens of both symptomatic and asymptomatic individuals. It is morphologically identical to *E. histolytica/E. dispar* (16).
[e]*E. gingivalis* and *T. tenax* are found in the oral cavity and related specimens.

Collection, Transport, and Storage of Specimens

For detection of amebae, laboratories predominantly receive stool specimens for examination. Both fresh and preserved specimens are useful for the diagnosis of infection, depending on the methodology employed and the circumstances of the laboratory. If fresh specimens are received for the detection of organism motility, they must be examined quickly; wet mounts for the detection of motility cannot be performed on preserved specimens. It is important to be aware that in most clinical and laboratory settings it is not feasible to examine fresh stool within the recommended time frame. The optimal solution is preservation of the specimen in a suitable fixative for stool parasites. Other sample types, such as aspirates and tissue samples, may be received and are appropriate for testing, depending on the organism suspected. For a more detailed description of collection, refer to chapter 136 of this *Manual*.

Direct Examination

Microscopy

All diagnostic stages of the amebae (trophozoite and cyst) can be detected in fecal specimens. The key morphologic features of amebae must be used to differentiate among the various species and to distinguish between somatic cells and other material. Trophozoites must be distinguished from epithelial cells and macrophages. Cysts must be distinguished from polymorphonuclear cells. Yeast, pollen, mold spores, food particles, and other debris present in feces may cause confusion (Table 2; Fig. 1 and 2).

Morphologic examination of fecal specimens can be accomplished with fresh wet mount preparations, wet mounts of concentrated material, and permanent-stained smears. Each of these three types of preparations may be useful for visualizing certain key characteristics. Stained and unstained wet mounts of concentrated material can also be useful for identification, particularly for certain cysts such as those of *E. coli* and *I. bütschlii*. Iodine provides color and contrast, both of which may aid in the identification of organisms in wet preparations. However, morphologic examination with permanent-stained smears by oil immersion microscopy (magnification, ×1,000) is the most useful procedure (4, 5).

Trophozoite motility is visible only in saline wet mounts of fresh feces and is often difficult to detect. The arrangement, size, and pattern of nuclear chromatin help differentiate species within the genus *Entamoeba* from other intestinal amebae. The size and position of the nuclear karyosome are also important morphologic features. A ring of nuclear chromatin surrounding the karyosome, resembling a bull's-eye, is characteristic of *Entamoeba*. *Endolimax*, *Iodamoeba*, and the flagellate *Dientamoeba* lack peripheral chromatin. The cytoplasm of the trophozoites may contain granules and ingested material such as red blood cells (RBCs), bacteria, yeasts, and molds. It is important to note that it is very difficult to differentiate *I. bütschlii* trophozoites from *E. nana* trophozoites. This is true even on the permanent-stained smear (6). The characteristics of cysts are less variable than those of trophozoites. To aid in differentiation among the genera, the cytoplasm should be examined for the presence of chromatoidal bodies and vacuoles, particularly the large glycogen vacuole seen in *I. bütschlii*.

Evaluation, Interpretation, and Reporting of Results

It is important to remember that identification may not be possible on the basis of one morphologic feature or the characteristics of a single organism in the preparation. Nuclear and cytoplasmic features can vary within species and may overlap between species, making identification a challenge. Mixed infections are not uncommon and can be missed in a cursory examination. A complete, overall assessment of the slide is necessary for correct identification. It is important to use an accurate micrometer to measure life cycle stages. Size is reliable only for the differentiation of *E. histolytica/E. dispar* from *E. hartmanni*. Also, on permanent-stained smears, shrinkage may occur, affecting the apparent size of the organism. Results of microscopy should clearly indicate the full taxonomic name of the organisms detected along with the forms of the organisms seen (trophozoites versus cysts). Quantitation of the amebae on the final report is not appropriate. The only exception to the lack of quantitation on direct examination is for *Blastocystis* spp. (see below).

E. histolytica

Description of the Agent

The development of axenic culture methods was a key step in confirming the existence of two species among organisms that had been identified as *E. histolytica* based solely on microscopic findings. Using organisms obtained by such cultures, Sargeaunt and Williams (7) performed isoenzyme analysis of several glycolytic enzymes and identified electrophoretic banding patterns, or zymodemes. Two groups were identified on the basis of these patterns: pathogenic zymodemes (invasive isolates) and nonpathogenic zymodemes (noninvasive isolates). The zymodeme patterns represent stable genetic differences and do not interconvert (8). Additional genetic, biochemical, and immunologic evidence has supported the existence of two distinct species. Diamond and Clark (9) redescribed the two species as

TABLE 2 Key features of trophozoites and cysts of common intestinal amebae and *Blastocystis*[a]

Organism	Trophozoites	Cysts
E. histolytica/E. dispar[e]	Size[b]: 12–60 μm (usually 15–20 μm); invasive forms, >20 μm Motility: Progressive, directional, rapid Nucleus[c]: 1; peripheral chromatin evenly distributed; karyosome small, compact, centrally located; may resemble *E. coli* Cytoplasm: Finely granular, like "ground glass"; may contain bacteria Note: RBCs in cytoplasm diagnostic for *E. histolytica* infection	Size: 10–20 μm; spherical, centrally located Cytoplasm: Chromatoidal bodies may be present; elongate with blunt rounded edges; may be round or oval Nucleus: Mature cyst, 4; immature, 1 or 2 nuclei; characteristics of the nuclei are more visible on permanent stained smears
E. hartmanni	Size: 5–12 μm Motility: Nonprogressive Nucleus: 1; peripheral chromatin like *E. histolytica/E. dispar*, may appear as solid ring; karyosome small, compact, centrally located or eccentric Cytoplasm: Finely granular, bacteria, no RBCs Note: Accurate measurement essential for differentiation from *E. histolytica/E. dispar*	Size: 5–10 μm; spherical Nucleus: Mature cyst, 4; immature cyst, 1 or 2 (very common); peripheral chromatin fine, evenly distributed, may be difficult to see; karyosome small, compact, centrally located Cytoplasm: Chromatoidal bodies usually present, like in *E. histolytica/E. dispar*
E. coli	Size: 15–50 μm (usually 2–25 μm) Motility: Sluggish, nondirectional Nucleus: 1; peripheral chromatin clumped and uneven, may be solid ring; karyosome large, not compact, diffuse, eccentric Cytoplasm: Granular, usually vacuolated; contains bacteria, yeast, no RBCs Note: Can resemble *E. histolytica/E. dispar*; coinfection seen; stained smear essential	Size: 10–35 μm; spherical, rarely oval or triangular Nucleus: Mature cyst, 8; occasionally ≥16; immature cyst, ≥2; peripheral chromatin coarsely granular, unevenly arranged; may resemble *E. histolytica/E. dispar*; karyosome small, usually eccentric but may be central Cytoplasm: Chromatoidal bodies less frequent than in *E. histolytica/E. dispar*; splintered, with rough, pointed ends Note: May be distorted on permanent-stained smear due to poor penetration of fixative
E. nana	Size: 6–12 μm Motility: Sluggish, nonprogressive Nucleus: 1; no peripheral chromatin; karyosome large, "blot like" Cytoplasm: Granular, vacuolated; may contain bacteria Note: May be tremendous nuclear variation; can mimic *E. hartmanni* and *D. fragilis*	Size: 5–10 μm; oval, may be round Nucleus: Mature cyst, 4; immature cyst, 2; no peripheral chromatin; karyosome smaller than those in trophozoites but larger than those in *Entamoeba* spp. Cytoplasm: Chromatoidal bodies rare; small granules occasionally seen
I. bütschlii	Size: 8–20 μm Motility: Sluggish, nonprogressive Nucleus: 1; no peripheral chromatin; karyosome large, may have "basket nucleus" Cytoplasm: Coarsely granular, may be highly vacuolated; bacteria, yeast, and debris may be seen Note: Stained smear essential; nucleus may appear to have a halo with chromatin granules fanning around karyosome	Size: 5–20 μm; oval to round Nucleus: Mature cyst, 1; no peripheral chromatin; karyosome large, usually eccentric Cytoplasm: No chromatoidal bodies; small granules occasionally present Note: Glycogen present, large, compact, well-defined mass; cysts may collapse owing to large glycogen vacuole space
Blastocystis spp.[d]	Very difficult to identify; rarely seen	Size: 2–200 μm; generally round Description: Usually characterized by a large, central body (looks like a large vacuole) surrounded by small, multiple nuclei; central body area can stain various colors (trichrome) or remain clear

[a]Adapted from reference 6.
[b]Size ranges are based on wet preparations (with permanent stains, organisms usually measure 1 to 2 μm less).
[c]Nuclear and cytoplasmic descriptions are based on permanent-stained smears.
[d]Description of central body form.
[e]Morphologic features listed for *E. histolytica/E. dispar* also apply to *E. moshkovskii* and *E. bangladeshi*.

E. histolytica Schaudinn 1903, which is the invasive human pathogen, and *E. dispar* Brumpt 1925, which is noninvasive and does not cause disease.

A third species of *Entamoeba*, *E. moshkovskii*, has been recognized and is generally considered a free-living amoeba that may be detected in human stool specimens. It is morphologically indistinguishable from *E. histolytica/E. dispar*. The epidemiology of *E. moshkovskii* is not well understood. Its prevalence varies depending on the population studied, from relatively rare up to nearly 50% of the identified *Entamoeba* spp. found in stool (10), and coinfections with *E. histolytica* and *E. dispar* are not

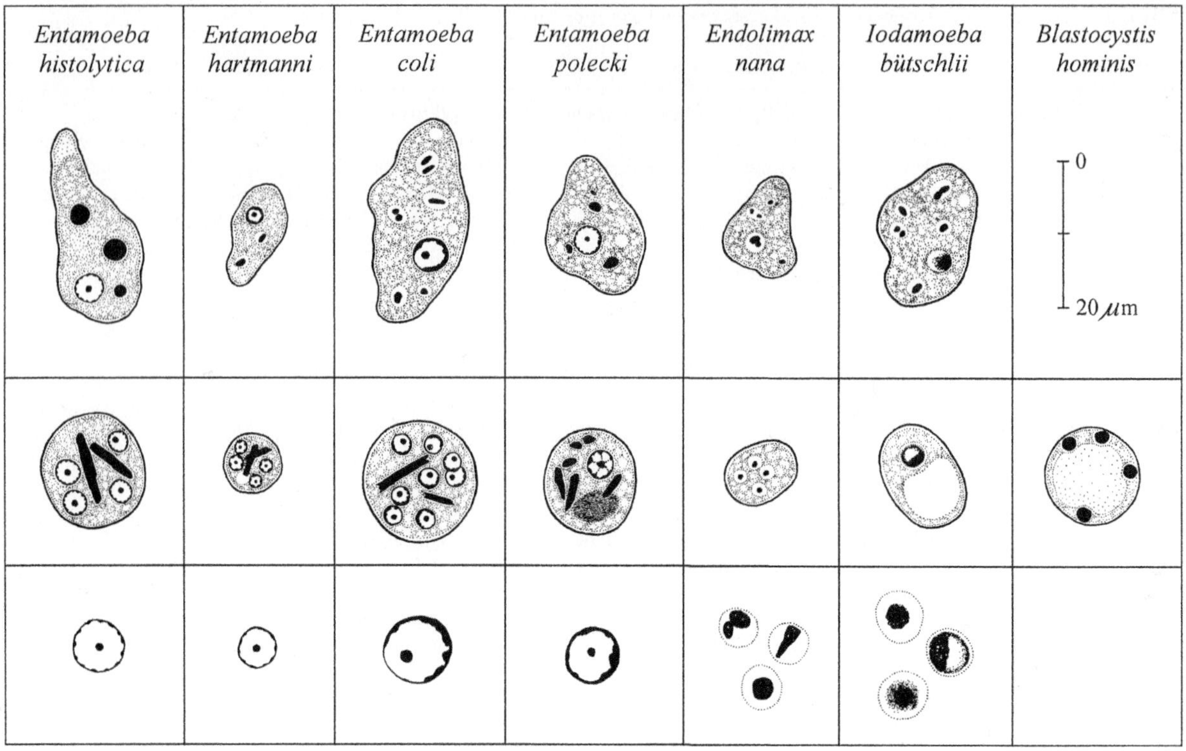

Entamoeba histolytica	*Entamoeba hartmanni*	*Entamoeba coli*	*Entamoeba polecki*	*Endolimax nana*	*Iodamoeba bütschlii*	*Blastocystis hominis*
						0 – 20 μm

FIGURE 1 Intestinal amebae of humans. (Top row) Trophozoites. *E. histolytica* is shown with ingested RBCs. This is the only microscopic finding that allows differentiation of the pathogenic species *E. histolytica* from the species *E. dispar*, *E. moshkovskii*, and *E. bangladeshi*. An ameboid form of *Blastocystis* spp. is rarely seen and is difficult to identify. (Middle row) Cysts. For *Blastocystis* spp. the central body form is depicted. (Bottom row) Trophozoite nuclei, shown in relative proportion.

uncommon (11). It has been reported as an agent associated with gastrointestinal disease in the absence of other known causes (11–14), and newly documented acquisition of *E. moshkovskii* in children has been associated with diarrhea (15). Most recently, Royer et al. (16) reported a fourth species, *E. bangladeshi* nov. sp., Bangladesh, which is also morphologically indistinguishable from *E. histolytica*/*E. dispar*. It was identified in stool specimens from symptomatic and asymptomatic children in Mirpur, Bangladesh; specimens were positive for *E. histolytica*/*E. dispar* by microscopy but negative by PCR targeting *E. histolytica*, *E. dispar*, and *E. moshkovskii*. More research is needed to understand the role of both *E. moshkovskii* and *E. bangladeshi* in human disease and the importance of laboratory diagnosis (10, 13, 16).

Epidemiology, Transmission, and Prevention

Among the estimated 500 million people infected each year with *E. histolytica*, there are approximately 50 million cases of colitis and liver abscess and 100,000 deaths (17). The discrepancy between the number of people infected with *E. histolytica* and the morbidity and mortality rates is explained by the existence of two morphologically similar yet distinct species: one capable of producing disease (*E. histolytica*) and the other not (*E. dispar*). *E. dispar* appears to be at least 10 times more common than *E. histolytica* (18). More precise determination of prevalence is possible using newer molecular methods to detect and differentiate among the species of *Entamoeba* and may change our understanding of the epidemiology of these infections (19).

E. histolytica can be found worldwide but is more prevalent in tropical and subtropical regions. In areas where the organism is endemic, up to 50% of people may be infected. In temperate climates with poor sanitation, infection rates can approach those seen in tropical regions. Humans are the primary reservoir; infection occurs by ingestion of cysts from material contaminated with feces, such as water and food. Sexual transmission also occurs.

Asymptomatic *E. histolytica* infection is equally distributed between the genders, while invasive amebiasis affects men predominantly. Groups with a higher incidence of amebiasis include immigrants from South and Central America and Southeast Asia (6). In the United States, the prevalence of amebiasis is estimated to be approximately 4 to 5%, with residents of the southern United States and institutionalized individuals being more likely than others to be infected (6). In one study, short-term travelers to areas where *E. histolytica* and *E. dispar* are endemic were found to be at higher risk of infection with the pathogenic species, *E. histolytica*, than were residents, who were more likely to harbor the nonpathogenic species, *E. dispar* (20). In homosexual males, the infection is often transmitted by sexual behavior, with up to 30% found to be infected with *E. histolytica*/*E. dispar* in some studies (21, 22). These infections are usually asymptomatic. Among human immunodeficiency virus (HIV)-infected patients in the United States, the incidence of diagnosed *E. histolytica* disease is low (13.5 cases per 10,000 person-years) (22). HIV-infected individuals in non-Western countries, such as Taiwan and Korea, have a higher risk of invasive amebiasis, in contrast to findings from the United States (23, 24). These differing rates of invasive disease may be attributed to the higher endemicity of *E. histolytica* in the Asia-Pacific regions (25).

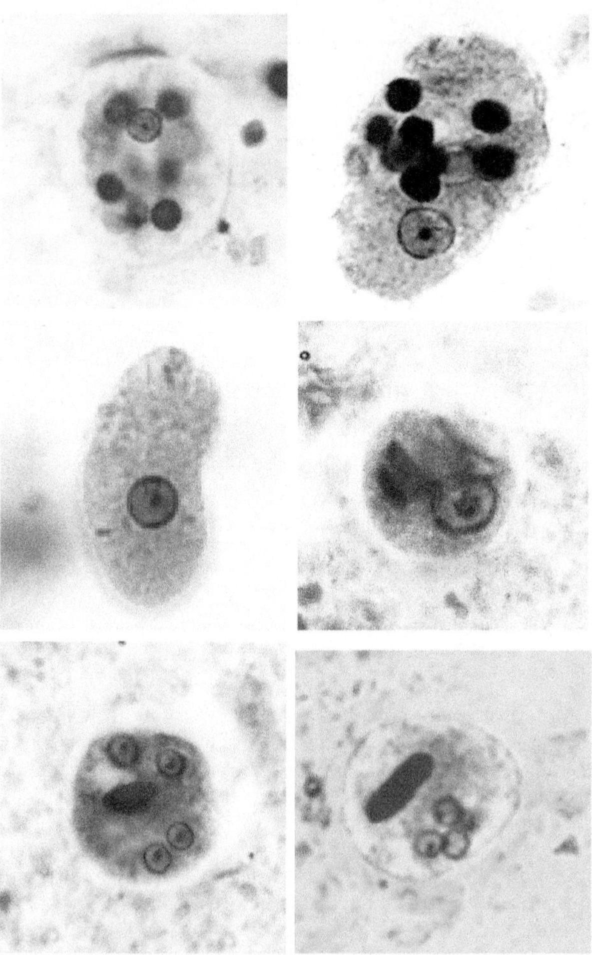

FIGURE 2 (Top row) *E. histolytica* trophozoites (organism on the right stained with iron-hematoxylin). Note the ingested RBCs in the cytoplasm. (Middle row) Left, *E. histolytica/E. dispar* trophozoite; right, *E. histolytica/E. dispar* precyst. (Bottom row) *E. histolytica/E. dispar* cysts. Trophozoites without ingested RBCs, precysts, and cysts cannot be identified to the species level on the basis of morphology. Organisms are stained with Wheatley's trichrome stain. (Courtesy of L. Garcia.)

Clinical Significance

Infection with *E. histolytica/E. dispar* can result in different clinical presentations: asymptomatic infection, symptomatic infection without extraintestinal tissue invasion, and symptomatic infection with extraintestinal tissue invasion. The majority of infections with *E. histolytica/E. dispar* are asymptomatic and are actually due to *E. dispar*. Individuals with such infections have a negative or weak serologic response and primarily pass cysts in their stools. Zymodeme analysis corroborates this and shows that most asymptomatic individuals are infected with the noninvasive species *E. dispar* (17, 26). However, it appears that infection with both *E. histolytica* and *E. dispar* can be asymptomatic, with cyst stages being passed in the stool (27). Asymptomatic *E. histolytica* infection may be due to the existence of genetically distinct invasive and noninvasive strains of *E. histolytica* (28).

Intestinal disease results from the penetration of the amebic trophozoites into the intestinal tissues. Approximately 10% of infected individuals have clinical symptoms, presenting as dysentery, colitis, or rarely, ameboma. The incubation period varies from a few days to several months. Various molecules such as adhesins, amebapores, and proteases have been associated with lysis of the colonic mucosa in intestinal amebiasis (29), and evidence supports the role of caspase-3-dependent apoptotic death as a major mechanism of host cell destruction (30). The 260-kDa galactose- or *N*-acetylgalactosamine-specific lectin of *E. histolytica* is an important virulence factor, mediating the attachment of the ameba to the intestinal epithelium and contact-dependent cytolysis (31). Symptoms of amebic dysentery include diarrhea with cramping, lower abdominal pain, low-grade fever, and the presence of blood and mucus in stool. The ulcers produced by intestinal invasion by trophozoites start as superficial localized lesions that deepen into the classic flask-shaped ulcers of amebic colitis. The ulcers are separated by segments of normal tissue but can coalesce. Amebae can be found at the advancing edges of the ulcer but usually not in the necrotic areas. Abdominal perforation and peritonitis are rare but serious complications. Rarely, a more chronic presentation-associated *E. histolytica* infection can occur that is characterized by intermittent diarrhea over a long period, weight loss, and abdominal pain which can be misdiagnosed as ulcerative colitis or irritable bowel syndrome. Ameboma is a mass of granulation tissue with peripheral fibrosis and a core of inflammation related to amebic chronic infection and is a relatively rare complication with amebic colitis. It resembles a tumor-like lesion and may be mistaken for malignancy.

Extraintestinal disease occurs with the hematogenous spread of *E. histolytica*. It can occur with or without previous symptomatic intestinal infection. The liver is the most common site of extraintestinal disease, followed by the lungs, pericardium, brain, and other organs. Symptoms can be acute or gradual and may include low-grade fever, right-upper-quadrant pain, and weight loss. Up to 5% of individuals with intestinal symptoms develop liver abscess. However, up to 50% of individuals with liver abscess have no history of gastrointestinal disease. Cutaneous amebiasis, involving the skin and soft tissues, occurs usually in association with dysenteric diarrhea and liver abscess. It can arise by direct extension of *E. histolytica* trophozoites from the colon and rectum to the perianal or genital regions. Other mechanisms of transmission include sexual transmission, direct inoculation by scratching, and following drainage from ruptured abscesses (32, 33).

Direct Examination

The laboratory diagnosis of amebiasis can be made by the examination of feces, material obtained from sigmoidoscopy, tissue biopsy specimens, and abscess aspirates. Serologic testing is also useful for the diagnosis of extraintestinal amebiasis. The choice of methods used by each laboratory is dependent on the available resources, funding, and clinical need. A summary of the laboratory techniques and their performance characteristics is presented in Table 3.

Microscopy

As discussed above, the most important part of the standard microscopic examination of stool and other specimens is the permanent-stained smear. Direct wet preparations and concentration procedures may also be useful (Fig. 1 and Table 2; see also chapter 138 of this *Manual*). Detection of trophozoites and cysts does not, however, allow differentiation of the pathogenic species, *E. histolytica*, from the nonpathogenic species, *E. dispar* (Fig. 1 and 2). The presence of ingested RBCs in the cytoplasm of the trophozoites is commonly regarded as diagnostic of *E. histolytica* infection.

TABLE 3 Sensitivity and specificity of diagnostic tests for amebiasis[a]

Test Specimen type	Clinical presentation		
	Colitis		Liver abscess
	Sensitivity (%)	Specificity (%)	Sensitivity (%)
Microscopy			
Stool	>60	10–50	<10
Abscess fluid	NA[b]	NA	<25
Culture with isoenzyme analysis	Lower than antigen or PCR tests	Gold standard	<25
Antigen detection (ELISA)[c]			
Stool	>95	>95	Usually negative
Serum	65 (early)	>90	~75 (late); ~100 (first 3 days)
Abscess fluid	NA	NA	~100 (before treatment)
Saliva	Not done	Not done	70
PCR			
Stool	70–>95[d]	>90	Rarely done
Antibody detection (ELISA)			
Serum	>90	>85	70–80 (acute stage); >90 (convalescent stage)

[a]Adapted from reference 36 with permission.
[b]NA, not available.
[c]ELISA, enzyme-linked immunosorbent assay.
[d]Sensitivities of PCR assays are dependent on comparator methods and PCR techniques with real-time demonstrating increased sensitivity over conventional PCR.

However, the majority of patient samples do not contain trophozoites with ingested RBCs (18). In addition to concerns about sensitivity, Haque et al. (34) found that 16% of *E. dispar* isolates had ingested RBCs; thus, this distinction between the two species is not absolute and may affect specificity (35, 36). In tissue specimens, only the trophozoite is found, and its presence is considered diagnostic of invasive *E. histolytica* disease.

Antigen Detection

For a more definitive differentiation of *E. histolytica* and *E. dispar*, methods other than microscopy are necessary. Zymodeme analysis can accomplish this differentiation, but it requires culture of the organisms from the specimen and is too expensive and complex for routine laboratory use. Antigen-based methods for the detection of *E. histolytica*/*E. dispar* are commercially available in the United States, including one that detects *E. histolytica*/*E. dispar*, *G. duodenalis*, and *Cryptosporidium parvum* in an immunochromatographic cartridge format (37). The antigen assays offer a more sensitive method for detection than microscopy and, depending on the kit used, allow specific detection of *E. histolytica* (18). A listing of commercially available parasite antigen detection kits is given in chapter 138 of this *Manual* and has been recently reviewed (6, 18, 38).

The antigen detection assays are designed for use with fresh, fresh-frozen, or unfixed human fecal specimens. As mentioned previously, depending on the kit used, the group *E. histolytica*/*E. dispar* or the individual species can be detected in the feces. Of the available kits, Abbott (formerly Alere/TechLab, Blacksburg, VA; FDA cleared) offers an *E. histolytica*-specific EIA kit, *E. histolytica* II, which detects the Gal- or GalNAc-binding lectin specific to the pathogenic species (34, 39). A rapid point-of-care test which is specific for *E. histolytica* adherence lectin (*E. Histolytica* Quik Chek; TechLab, Inc., Blacksburg, VA; FDA cleared) has been reported and would be particularly useful in the developing world (40, 41). All the antigen detection methods are relatively simple and are more sensitive and specific than microscopy (Table 3) (34, 37, 42). In comparison to amplified methods such as PCR, antigen detection using stool specimens may be less sensitive and specific for detection of *E. histolytica*/*E. dispar*, depending on the population studied (43, 44). To date, none of the available products can be used with preserved stool (i.e., formalin), because the fixative appears to denature the antigens. Although some reports of the use of preserved stool have appeared (45), more work is needed to identify additional antigens that withstand fixation before it would be practical to offer antigen tests in laboratories that receive only preserved stool specimens. Antigen assays have been used to test a number of other sample types such as serum, pus, and saliva (46, 47); the detection of antigen in serum may prove to be a sensitive means of diagnosing amebic liver abscess and intestinal disease (36, 47). Because fewer than 10% of patients with amebic liver abscesses have concurrent intestinal disease with amebae detectable in the stool, methods such as routine ova and parasite examination are not useful. Microscopic examination or culture of pus from liver abscesses likewise lacks sensitivity. In a study by Haque et al. (47), serum antigen detection by using the TechLab *E. histolytica* II kit was a sensitive method for diagnosis with samples collected prior to treatment with metronidazole. Serum antigenemia appears to clear after treatment, suggesting possible utility to monitor therapy; however, this use is still experimental (36, 47).

Nucleic Acid Detection Techniques

Nucleic acid amplification techniques, such as PCR, have been developed for the detection and differentiation of *E. histolytica* and *E. dispar*. The most common genomic targets include the rRNA- or species-specific episomal repeats. Conventional PCR has been applied to specimens such as stool, liver, and brain aspirates and cerebrospinal fluid and can detect both trophozoite and cyst DNA (48–52). More recently, real-time PCR has been used for the detection of *E. histolytica* and *E. dispar* (43, 53). Haque et al. reported on the use of *E. histolytica* real-time PCR on blood, saliva, and urine samples for detection of amebic liver abscess and amebic colitis, finding that a combination of testing both urine and saliva increased diagnostic sensitivity, with 97% and 89% for amebic liver abscess and colitis cases detected, respectively; blood was less sensitive, being positive in 49% of amebic liver abscess cases and 36% of colitis cases examined (54). Several researchers have reported methods for multiplex molecular detection and differentiation among the *Entamoeba* spp., including *E. histolytica*, *E. dispar*, and *E. moshkovskii* (18, 48, 55, 56). Use of such a multiplex assay would permit a more accurate diagnosis than microscopy and allow targeted therapy for only true *E. histolytica* infections. As mentioned previously, simultaneous detection from stool of multiple intestinal parasites or multiple organisms, including bacteria and viruses, is of interest because there is significant overlap in the clinical presentations. Reports include detection of various combinations including *E. histolytica*, *G. duodenalis*, and *C. parvum* using real-time PCR (57) and *E. histolytica*, *G. duodenalis*, *Cryptosporidium* spp., and *D. fragilis* using tandem multiplex real-time PCR (58). At the time of writing there are three FDA-cleared multiplex molecular tests and others that are CE marked (Table 4). The xTAG gastrointestinal panel (Luminex Molecular Diagnostics, Austin, TX) is designed for testing unpreserved stool or stool samples in Cary Blair transport medium, detecting 11 agents of gastroenteritis including the parasites *G. duodenalis*, *Cryptosporidium* spp., and *E. histolytica*. It is a bead-based assay utilizing nucleic acid extraction followed by endpoint PCR amplification and bead-based detection. The BioFire FilmArray GI panel (bioMérieux, Salt Lake City, UT) is designed for testing on stool in Cary Blair medium and detects 22 targets including the parasites *G. duodenalis*, *Cryptosporidium* spp., *E. histolytica*, and *Cyclospora cayetanensis*. The platform is a sample-to-answer technology utilizing a nested real-time PCR (1). The BD Max enteric parasite panel (Becton Dickinson, Sparks, MD) uses unpreserved or preserved stool samples in Cary Blair medium. The assay uses automated extraction and multiplex real-time PCR for detection of *G. duodenalis*, *Cryptosporidium* spp., and *E. histolytica* (2, 59). The initial reports for all of these tests demonstrate their utility, but the numbers of parasite detections, particularly for *E. histolytica*, are low (Table 4). A recent publication including the FilmArray GI panel demonstrated the utility of panels to detect parasitic pathogens (*C. cayetanensis*) that are not initially suspected by the care provider (60), demonstrating the power of the syndromic testing approach. As more data are generated and other FDA-cleared multiplex molecular tests are made available, the multiplex molecular approach will have a significant impact on many aspects of laboratory diagnosis of amebiasis and other gastrointestinal parasites.

PCR on stool specimens using laboratory-developed assays has proven to be more sensitive and specific than microscopy and at least as sensitive as antigen detection, depending on the study (Table 3) (36, 43, 61). For routine use in clinical laboratories, a PCR method would ideally involve a relatively simple sample preparation procedure and allow the use of preserved material. Different extraction techniques, some of which are relatively simple, and the use of fresh and preserved material have been reported (62–64). Stool can present challenges due to the presence of PCR inhibitors (65), so the inclusion of an amplification control is useful (57).

Serologic Tests

Serologic testing is a valuable aid, in conjunction with antigen detection or PCR, for the diagnosis of symptomatic, invasive disease. Multiple serologic methods have been used, including indirect hemagglutination, complement fixation, latex agglutination, and EIA (18, 36). These methods are most useful in populations where *E. histolytica* is not endemic. Of patients with biopsy-proven intestinal amebiasis, 85% have serum antibodies. For patients with extraintestinal disease, serologic tests have a sensitivity approaching 99%. For asymptomatic intestinal diseases, serology is generally not useful unless the patient has invasive infection. People infected with *E. dispar* do not produce detectable antibodies. After cure of invasive amebiasis, serum antibodies may persist for up to 10 years; this can complicate diagnosis in areas where infection is endemic (66).

EIAs for the detection of immunoglobulin M (IgM) and IgG are widely used, and most are based on the detection

TABLE 4 Commercially available molecular amplification panels with stool parasite targets[a]

Assay	Manufacturer	Parasite targets	Other targets	References
xTAG gastrointestinal panel PCR[b,c]	Luminex; Austin, TX	*Giardia*, *Cryptosporidium*, *E. histolytica*	8 bacteria 3 viruses	3, 134, 268
BioFire FilmArray gastroenteritis panel[b,c]	bioMérieux, Salt Lake City, UT	*Giardia*, *Cryptosporidium*, *E. histolytica*, *Cyclospora*	11 bacteria 5 viruses	1, 268
BD Max enteric parasite panel[b,c]	Becton Dickinson and Co.; Sparks, MD	*Giardia*, *Cryptosporidium*, *E. histolytica*	Separate bacterial and viral panels	2, 139, 140
Ridagene stool panel PCR[c]	R-Biopharm AG, Darmstadt, Germany	*Giardia*, *Cryptosporidium*, *E. histolytica*, *Dientamoeba*		250
Gastrofinder Smart 17 Fast[c]	PathoFinder B.V., The Netherlands	*Giardia*, *Cryptosporidium*, *E. histolytica*, *Dientamoeba*	9 bacteria 4 viruses	269
Gastrointestinal parasite panel[c]	AusDiagnostics, Beaconsfield, Australia	*Giardia*, *Cryptosporidium*, *E. histolytica*, *Dientamoeba*, *Cyclospora*, *Blastocystis* spp.		58, 269
Allplex gastrointestinal panel 4-parasite[c]	SeeGene, Seoul, Korea	*Giardia*, *Cryptosporidium*, *E. histolytica*, *Dientamoeba*, *Cyclospora*, *Blastocystis* spp.	Available in various combinations with bacterial and viral	269
NaniCHIP GIP[c]	Savyon Diagnostics, Ashdod, IL	*Giardia*, *Cryptosporidium*, *E. histolytica*, *Dientamoeba*, *Blastocystis* spp.	Microarray with other enteric bacteria	270

[a]List may not be all-inclusive.
[b]FDA cleared *in vitro* diagnostic test.
[c]CE certified *in vitro* diagnostic test.

of antilectin antibodies, which appear over 1 week after symptoms of *E. histolytica* infection (36). Indirect hemagglutination is useful and highly specific but may lack sensitivity compared to EIAs (36). Several investigators have reported the utility of IgA antibody testing and a link to partial immunity in individuals with detectable antilectin IgA (47, 67, 68). There are several commercially available serologic kits for diagnosis of amebiasis, some of which are available in the United States. For a review of serologic testing, see the article by Fotedar et al. (18) and also refer to chapter 8 in this *Manual*.

Treatment

On the basis of the 1997 World Health Organization conference, treatment is not recommended for *E. dispar* infections; if *E. histolytica/E. dispar* is detected (no differentiation of species) in symptomatic patients, the physician must evaluate the total clinical presentation to decide whether treatment is indicated. The detection of *E. histolytica* requires treatment of the patient regardless of the symptoms. The use of diagnostics that are species specific (i.e., antigen detection or PCR) allows for targeted chemotherapy.

The drugs used for the treatment of amebiasis are of two classes: luminal amebicides for cysts (paromomycin, iodoquinol, and diloxanide furoate) and tissue amebicides for trophozoites (metronidazole, tinidazole, and dehydroemetine) (69). Invasive disease should be treated with a tissue amebicide followed by a luminal amebicide. Tissue amebicides are not appropriate for treatment of asymptomatic infections (cysts). No high-level resistance to amebicides has been detected to date. Follow-up stool examination is always necessary because of potential treatment failures. Chemoprophylaxis is never appropriate because it may lead to drug resistance and limit the utility of drugs such as metronidazole (17, 70).

Evaluation, Interpretation, and Reporting of Results

Laboratory reporting of *Entamoeba* infection must account for the ability of a particular methodology to detect and differentiate pathogenic and nonpathogenic species. This is based on the report of a World Health Organization panel of experts which made recommendations concerning the reporting and treatment of amebiasis (17). If a microscopic diagnosis is made on the basis of the detection of trophozoites and/or cysts and no method is used to differentiate the two species, the report should indicate "*E. histolytica/E. dispar* detected." Laboratory reports must indicate whether trophozoites and/or cysts are present, due to differences in therapy (6).

With the increasing awareness of other *Entamoeba* spp., reporting as *E. histolytica/E. dispar* complex (*E. histolytica*, *E. dispar*, *E. moshkovskii*, and *E. bangladeshi*) might be considered, but care must be taken to convey the proper interpretation of these results, reflecting the lack of differentiation of the pathogenic and nonpathogenic species. Laboratories may also choose to further test stools with *E. histolytica/E. dispar* detected with an *E. histolytica*-specific test such as antigen or PCR. This reflexive testing could allow more specific and appropriate treatment and be a cost-effective testing algorithm.

Antigen detection methods may or may not allow species differentiation, and the laboratory report should accurately reflect these facts. Reporting of PCR results which are specific for *E. histolytica* or other *Entamoeba* spp. such as *E. dispar* should state that nucleic acid was detected or not detected. Due to the ability of amplified methods to detect nonviable organisms, the use of PCR for determination of treatment failure should be interpreted cautiously. PCR does not allow for the determination of the parasite forms present, in contrast to the TechLab *E. histolytica* II.

NONPATHOGENIC AMEBAE

The other species of intestinal amebae are considered nonpathogenic; except for *E. polecki*, they have a worldwide distribution and are more prevalent in warmer climates. They must, however, be differentiated from the pathogenic species *E. histolytica*. A permanently stained smear is often essential to accomplish this goal (Table 2; Fig. 1).

E. hartmanni is a separate species that is morphologically similar to *E. histolytica/E. dispar* (Fig. 3). Size is the key differentiating characteristic. *E. coli* trophozoites may be difficult to differentiate from *E. histolytica/E. dispar* trophozoites on wet preparations. The mature cyst of *E. coli* may be refractory to fixation, making it less visible in permanent-stained smears but still detectable by the wet mount method (Fig. 4). It has been reported as the most common ameba isolated from human stool specimens. *E. polecki* is associated with pigs, and in certain areas of the world, such as Papua New Guinea, it is the most common human intestinal parasite. The trophozoite shares characteristics with both *E. histolytica/E. dispar* and *E. coli*; the cyst normally has one nucleus. *E. gingivalis* was the first parasitic ameba of humans to be described. It is found in the soft tartar between teeth and can be recovered from sputum. In the trophozoite, the cytoplasm often contains ingested leukocytes. A cyst form has not been observed.

E. nana, like *E. hartmanni*, is one of the smaller intestinal amebae. It is seen in most populations as frequently as *E. coli*. There is a great deal of nuclear variation, and it can mimic *D. fragilis* and *E. hartmanni* (Fig. 5). The cysts of

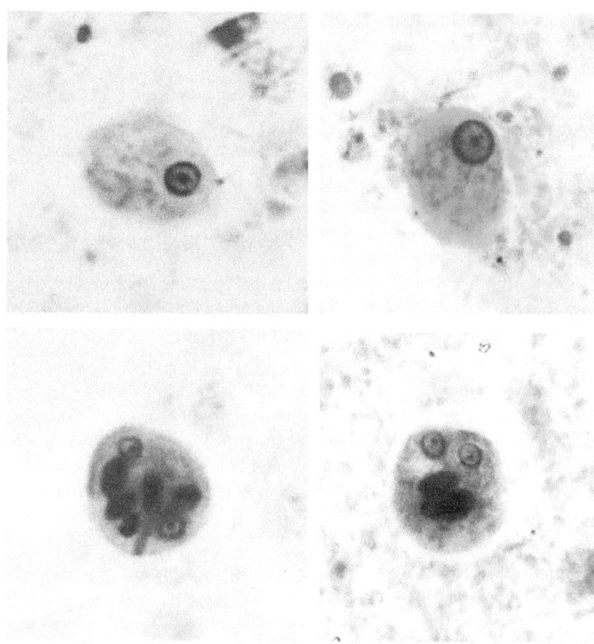

FIGURE 3 (Top row) *Entamoeba hartmanni* trophozoites (note the "bull's-eye" nucleus, very clear with compact karyosome). (Bottom row) *E. hartmanni* cysts (note that they often stop at two nuclei and contain many chromatoidal bars). All organisms are stained with Wheatley's trichrome stain. (Courtesy of L. Garcia).

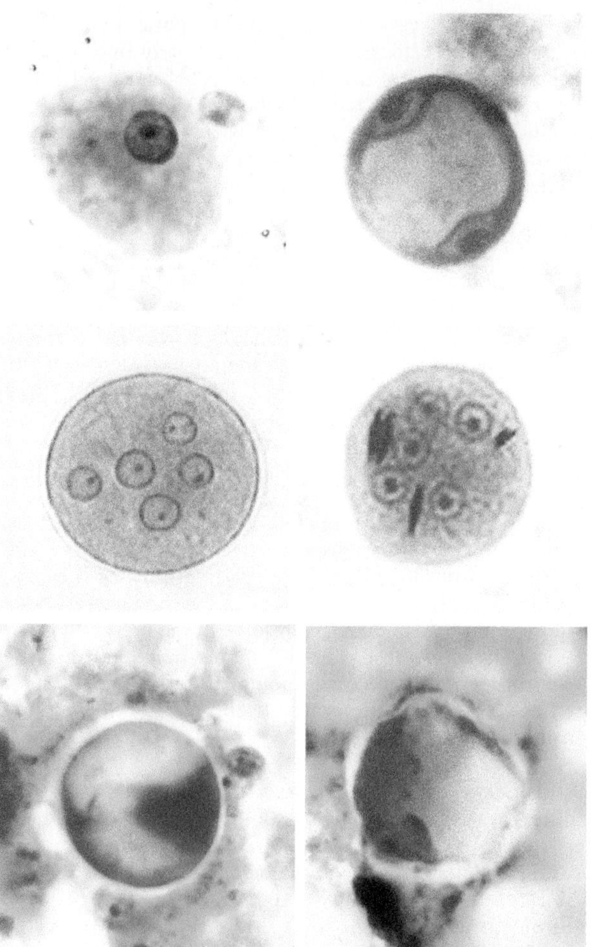

FIGURE 4 (Top row) Left, *Entamoeba coli* trophozoite (note the uneven nuclear chromatin and large, blot-like karyosome); right, *E. coli* precyst (note the two enlarged nuclei, one at each side of the cyst). (Middle row) Left, *E. coli* cyst, iodine wet mount preparation (note the clarity of five of the eight nuclei and typical color using iodine); right, *E. coli* cyst (note that this morphology is exceptionally good and not always seen). (Bottom row) *E. coli* cysts. Cysts do not preserve well with most fixatives; they often appear shrunken and distorted and display varying colors from red to purple to blue. Consequently, these cysts are often seen in a concentration wet mount but are not clearly seen on the permanent-stained smear. Organisms are stained with Wheatley's trichrome stain unless indicated otherwise. (Courtesy of L. Garcia.)

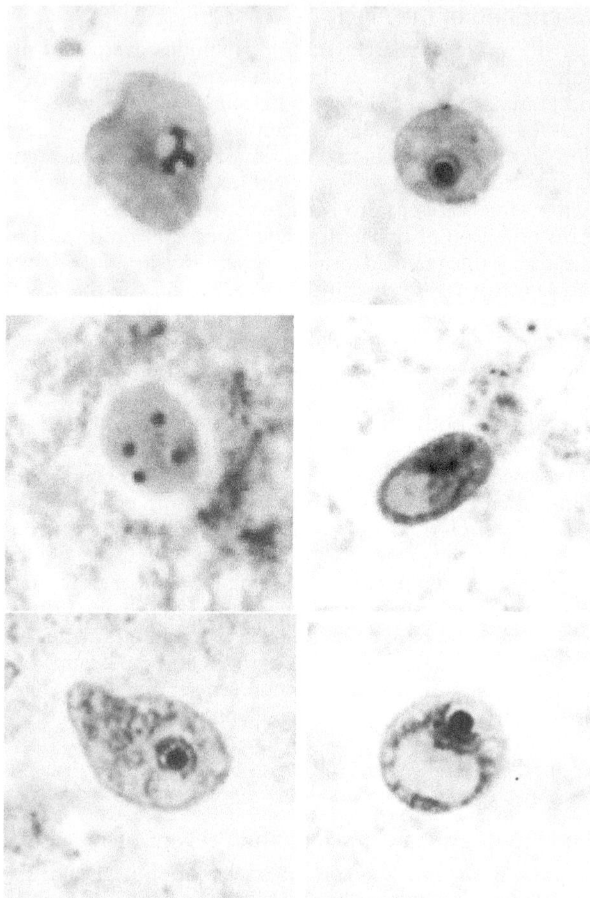

FIGURE 5 (Top row) Left, *Endolimax nana* trophozoite (note the nuclear karyosome variation, which is typical in *E. nana*); right, *E. nana* trophozoite (note the more normal karyosome; occasionally, there may also appear to be some peripheral nuclear chromatin. (Middle row) Left, *E. nana* cyst (note the typical four karyosomes); right, *E. nana* cyst (note the four karyosomes, but also vacuole; cysts containing a single vacuole are not that rare). (Bottom row) Left, *Iodamoeba bütschlii* trophozoite; right, *I. bütschliii* cyst (note the single karyosome and large glycogen cyst). Organisms are stained with Wheatley's trichrome stain. (Courtesy of L. Garcia.)

E. nana are usually oval, and both the trophozoites and the cysts are commonly present in fecal material. *I. bütschlii* has the same distribution as other nonpathogenic amebae but is less common than *E. coli* and *E. nana*. The trophozoite of *I. bütschlii* may be similar to that of *E. nana*, and differentiation between them is difficult. The cyst is very characteristic; it is round to oval and may contain a large glycogen vacuole (Fig. 5).

Treatment is not recommended for infections with any of the nonpathogenic amebae; however, it is important to report nonpathogenic amebae to the health care provider. The presence of these organisms indicates exposure to contaminated food or water, and therefore pathogenic parasites may still be present and additional studies may be warranted. Methods of prevention of infection with all these amebae include improved personal hygiene and improved sanitary conditions.

BLASTOCYSTIS SPECIES

Taxonomy

The taxonomic classification of *Blastocystis* spp. (formerly *Blastocystis hominis*) was first described in 1912 but has changed multiple times and is still somewhat unclear (71, 72). *Blastocystis* spp. are in supergroup SAR (Stramenopiles: *Blastocystis*) (see chapter 135 in this *Manual*). Molecular studies indicate that *Blastocystis* spp. are closely related to *Proteromonas lacertae* (73–75). Though *P. lacertae* is a flagellate, interestingly, *Blastocystis* spp. do not possess a flagellum and are nonmotile. Genetic, biochemical, and immunologic analyses have revealed that great diversity exists within the genus (76–78). Studies have shown that *Blastocystis* spp. in humans and animals can be divided into 12 or more species (78).

Description of the Agent

The life cycle of *Blastocystis* spp. includes cyst, central body (also referred to as the vacuolar form), amoeboid, and granular forms. All but the granular form have been observed in human stool specimens, with the central body form being the most commonly seen. Humans are infected by ingestion of the cyst form, with excystation occurring in the large intestine to release the central body form. Transformation of the central body form can produce the granular or the ameboid form and vice versa (6). The exact nature of the life cycle of this organism and the infective form have yet to be confirmed experimentally. *Blastocystis* spp. are capable of pseudopod extension and retraction. They reproduce by binary fission or sporulation, are strictly anaerobic, and are capable of ingesting bacteria and other debris. Both thin- and thick-walled cysts have been observed. The thick-walled cysts are thought to be responsible for external transmission via the fecal-oral route; the thin-walled cysts are thought to cause autoinfection (79). The cyst form is the most recently described form of the life cycle stages; they can vary in shape but are mostly ovoid or spherical and can vary depending on whether the cyst is observed in fresh stool or in culture (75). The central body form is the most common form found in clinical stool samples. The membrane-bound central body can occupy up to 90% of the cell and may function in reproduction. The amebic form is more difficult to see but has been observed in diarrheal stool specimens (6). The ameboid form is rarely reported, and the granular form can be seen when culturing the parasite.

Epidemiology, Transmission, and Prevention

Blastocystis spp. are common intestinal parasites of humans and animals, with a worldwide distribution (75). It is estimated that over 1 billion humans are infected, with the majority being asymptomatic (80). Depending on the geographic location, *Blastocystis* may be detected in 1 to 40% of fecal specimens. Human-to-human, animal-to-human, and waterborne modes of transmission have been proposed (75, 78, 81, 82).

Clinical Significance

The role of *Blastocystis* spp. in human disease is an area of continuing study, with data supporting and refuting their pathogenicity being published (83–85). Since many genotypes appear to exist, with 9 of 17 subtypes found in humans, there is evidence of possibly pathogenic and nonpathogenic species (75, 86). More recently, metagenomic analysis of the human gut microbiome has been used to study the prevalence, genetic diversity, and associations with disease states (87, 88). These types of analyses do not rely on growth of the organism and are able to more fully assess the true numbers of infected individuals and have shown the incredible level of genetic diversity within the genus. More such studies are needed, but initial data show that the associations with disease states such as irritable bowel disease, irritable bowel syndrome, and obesity may not hold up when analyzed using large-scale comparative metagenomics (88, 89). While this scientific debate continues, clinicians may decide to treat patients with *Blastocystis* spp. infection, particularly when it is present in large numbers in the absence of other pathogens. The most common symptoms associated in this setting include recurrent diarrhea without fever, vomiting, and abdominal pain. The symptoms may be more pronounced and prolonged in patients with underlying conditions such as HIV infection, neoplasia, and abnormal intestinal tract function (90, 91). Other studies suggest that symptomatic patients receiving treatment for *Blastocystis* spp. infection may improve due to the elimination of another, undetected pathogen (83). In a study of HIV-infected individuals, Albrecht et al. (92) concluded that even in patients with severe underlying immunodeficiencies, *Blastocystis* spp. are not pathogenic and detection does not justify treatment.

Direct Examination

Microscopy

Diagnosis of infection is made by detection of the organism, typically the central body form, by routine microscopic stool examination (Table 2; Fig. 1 and 6).While this is the most commonly used method, it lacks sensitivity when compared to other methods, such as PCR (93). The size of the central body form can vary tremendously, from 2 to 200 μm. Extensive size variation exists within and between isolates. The vacuolar form contains a large central vacuole that occupies approximately 90% of the cell (75, 94). Examination of permanent-stained smears is the procedure of choice. Exposure to water before fixation (for the concentration method) lyses the trophozoites and central body forms, yielding false-negative results. Some type of quantitation (few, moderate, or many) should be included in the laboratory report. Direct wet mounts using iodine as a stain are not recommended, because trichrome staining is more sensitive (75).

Other Diagnostic Methods

Culture of the organism from stool is possible and has been reported to be more sensitive than microscopy but is not routinely available (81). A serologic response to *Blastocystis* spp. has been detected using techniques such as EIA and fluorescent-antibody testing (75, 95, 96). It is suggested that this antibody response supports the role of *Blastocystis* spp. as human pathogens but is not useful for diagnosis and

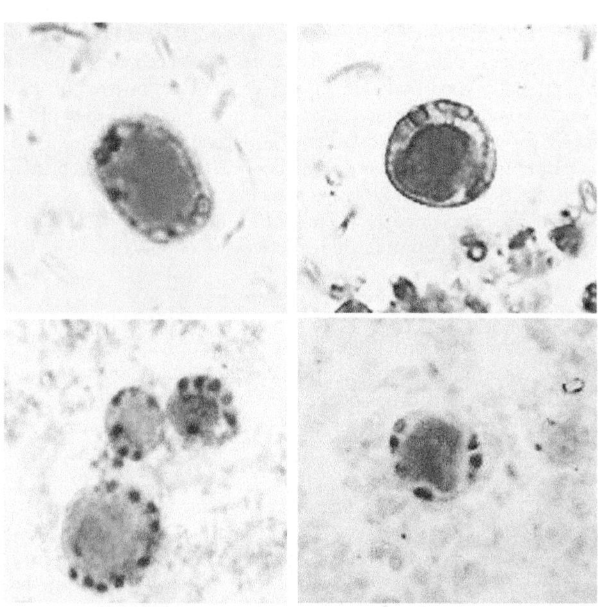

FIGURE 6 (Top row) *Blastocystis* spp. central body forms (note the central body area stained with iodine; also note peripheral nuclei). (Bottom row) *Blastocystis* spp. central body forms stained with Wheatley's trichrome stain. (Courtesy of L. Garcia).

should be limited to epidemiological and serologic studies. In asymptomatic individuals, a serologic response may require exposure of up to 2 years before it is detectable (97). A review by Tan describes in detail molecular approaches to the diagnosis and characterization of *Blastocystis* spp. (75). Molecular approaches to organism detection are more sensitive but are still not routinely available in the clinical laboratory setting (89). As pointed out by Stensvold et al., due to the commonality of asymptomatic infections along with prolonged carriage, the routine use of molecular methods for detection of *Blastocystis* spp. either by themselves or in a multiplex molecular panel along with known pathogens such as *E. histolytica* probably does not make sense at present (89).

Treatment

Until the role of *Blastocystis* spp. as intestinal pathogens is clearly established, treatment decisions must be based on the overall clinical presentation. Current recommendations for treatment include the use of metronidazole and trimethoprim-sulfamethoxazole, but nitazoxanide, tinidazole, paromomycin, iodoquinol, and ketoconazole have also been used therapeutically (98). Metronidazole appears to be the most appropriate choice at present. *In vitro* data on the susceptibility of *Blastocystis* spp. to various drugs are limited (85), but resistance to metronidazole has been reported (99, 100). A failure to clear organisms from the stool has been demonstrated in patients treated with metronidazole and trimethoprim-sulfamethoxazole.

Evaluation, Interpretation, and Reporting of Results

For most laboratories, testing and reporting for *Blastocystis* spp. are limited to detection of the organism by microscopic means. There can be confusion in identifying *Blastocystis* spp. correctly, since the organism can be confused with yeast, fat globules, and even *Cyclospora*. It is not necessary to state the form of the organism present (i.e., central body form). This is the sole intestinal parasite that should be routinely reported with quantitation to aid clinicians in determining its clinical significance. Additional commentary may be added to the laboratory report explaining the role of *Blastocystis* spp. in disease and the need to exclude other causes of the clinical condition.

FLAGELLATES

Taxonomy

Controversy exits regarding the proper nomenclature of eukaryotic flagella. The recommendation from some in the scientific community is to refer to them as cilia, but this has not been widely adopted within the clinical microbiology arena. For discussion purposes here, they will continue to be referred to as flagella.

Several flagellates are pathogenic to humans, and others are harmless intestinal tract commensals. Classification of the flagellates is as follows: *G. duodenalis* is in the supergroup Excavata (Metamonada: Fornicata: Diplomonadida: Giardiinae); *Enteromonas hominis* is in the supergroup Excavata (Metamonada: Fornicata: Diplomonadida: Hexamitinae); *Chilomastix mesnili* and *Retortamonas intestinalis* are in the supergroup Excavata (Metamonada: Fornicata: Retortamonadida); *T. vaginalis* is in the supergroup Excavata (Metamonada: Parabasalia: Trichomonadida) (Fig. 7; see chapter 135 in this *Manual*).

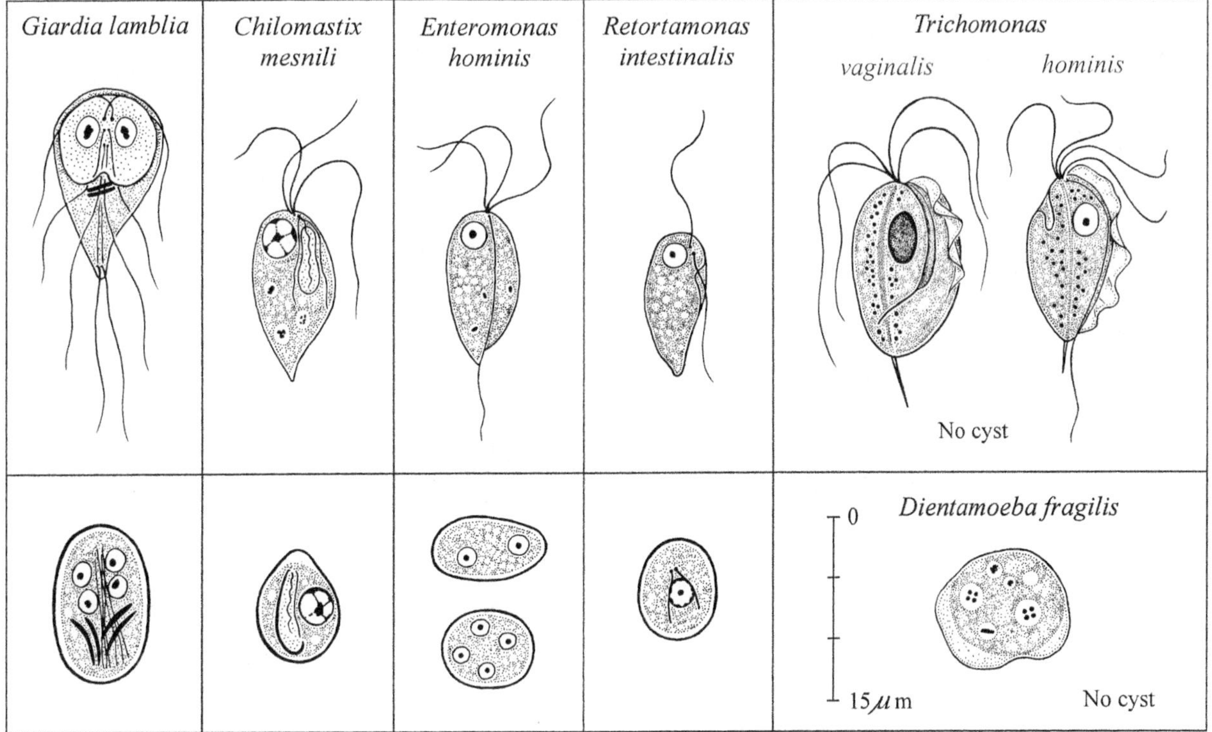

FIGURE 7 Intestinal and urogenital flagellates of humans. (Top row) Trophozoites. *T. vaginalis* is found in urogenital sites; all other flagellates are intestinal. (Bottom row) Cysts. *D. fragilis* trophozoite is shown; cyst stage is not shown.

Description of the Agents

Some flagellates are commensals that reside in the intestinal tract and are harmless to the individual. The flagellates that are pathogenic to humans include *G. duodenalis*, *D. fragilis*, and *T. vaginalis*. The nonpathogenic organisms are *C. mesnili*, *E. hominis*, *R. intestinalis*, and *Pentatrichomonas* (*Trichomonas*) *hominis*. As mentioned above, *D. fragilis* has been reclassified as a flagellate and appears to be closely related to the trichomonads.

Epidemiology, Transmission, and Prevention

Transmission of flagellates, with the exception of *T. vaginalis*, is initiated via the ingestion of contaminated food or water. Of the members of the six genera, all except for *Trichomonas* spp. are transmitted in a cyst form; however, the role of the cyst form in the transmission of *D. fragilis* infections is unclear. To date, only a trophozoite form has been observed for *Trichomonas* spp. Once in the intestine, the organism excysts, releasing trophozoites that attach to the intestinal epithelium. Completion of the life cycle in humans culminates in the release of viable cysts into the environment via the feces. Infection with any of the flagellates indicates exposure to feces regardless of the pathogenicity of the organism; preventing this exposure is the key. Measures to improve sanitary conditions are necessary to prevent the spread of infection. As yet, no human flagellate vaccines are available.

Collection, Transport, and Storage of Specimens

For the detection of flagellates and ciliates, laboratories predominantly receive stool specimens for microscopic examination. String test samples (Entero-Test; Nutri-Link Ltd., United Kingdom) can be submitted for *Giardia* as well, which is described in detail below. Fresh or preserved specimens can be submitted, but preserved stool is the specimen of choice for most routine clinical laboratories. If fresh specimens are submitted and observed for motility, they must be examined within a specific time period depending on the consistency of the stool. Stool specimens for immunoassay or DFA assay can be fixed in formalin, which can also be used for an ova and parasite exam if immunoassays are negative for *G. duodenalis*. Additional information on specimen collection and transport can be found in chapter 136 of this *Manual*.

Direct Examination

Microscopy

In the clinical laboratory, wet preparations and permanent-stained smears of fecal material are still the predominant specimens used to diagnose infections with flagellates. The flagellates have greater morphologic diversity relative to one another than do the amebae (described above), making determination of the genus easier (Table 5; Fig. 7). To aid in the identification of the trophozoite, key features to be noted are the shape, size, number, and position of flagella; the number of nuclei; and the presence of a spiral groove, cytostome, and characteristic features such as a sucking disk or undulating membrane. Typically, the size, shape, and number of nuclei are diagnostic characteristics used to identify cysts. Examination of permanent-stained smears is always recommended for diagnosis of infection because the wet mount may not be reflective of all organisms and stages present in the specimen.

Other Diagnostic Methods

Antigen-based tests for organisms such as *G. duodenalis* have increased in popularity over the years due to their ease of use and increased throughput compared to microscopy. In addition, nucleic acid amplification methods have been developed to detect *T. vaginalis* in clinical samples and *G. duodenalis* in water and clinical samples but are not yet routinely available in the clinical laboratory. Both antigen and amplification tests for the flagellates will be discussed in more detail below. Serologic assays are available for the diagnosis of *G. duodenalis* infection but are not routinely used in the clinical setting.

Evaluation, Interpretation, and Reporting of Results

It is important that a representative portion of the slide, either a wet mount or a permanent smear, be scanned before a final opinion on a specimen is given. It is also important to use an accurate micrometer to measure life cycle stages. Reports of microscopy results should clearly indicate the full taxonomic names of the organisms detected, along with the forms of the organisms seen (trophozoites versus cysts) (4). Quantitation of the number of organisms seen is not appropriate for the flagellates.

G. duodenalis

Taxonomy

G. duodenalis is in the supergroup Excavata (Metamonada: Fornicata: Diplomonadida: Giardiinae) (see chapter 135 of this *Manual*).

Description of the Agent

G. duodenalis is an intestinal flagellate that infects both humans and animals and is the most common cause of intestinal parasitosis in humans worldwide. Because the literature refers to this organism as *Giardia lamblia*, *Giardia intestinalis*, and *G. duodenalis*, there has been debate about the classification and nomenclature of this flagellate. There is an extensive review of taxonomy related to *Giardia* which explores in depth the taxonomy of this genus (101). Currently, *G. duodenalis* is the accepted species name in regard to human infections. According to Feng and Xiao, there are six species: *G. agilis*, *G. ardeae*, *G. muris*, *G. microti*, *G. psittaci*, and *G. duodenalis* (101).

It is now accepted that there is considerable genetic diversity within *G. duodenalis*. Based on molecular biology, the genus *Giardia* is subdivided into major genotypes containing subgenotypes. The major genotypes of *G. duodenalis* that are associated with human infections are assemblages A and B. Assemblage A is associated with a mixture of both human and animal isolates, whereas assemblage B is typically associated with human isolates only. Most zoonotic animal-to-human infections occur with assemblage A (102).

Epidemiology, Transmission, and Prevention

Infection with *G. duodenalis* occurs through fecal-oral transmission or the ingestion of cysts in contaminated food or water, and an inoculum of only 10 to 100 cysts is sufficient for human infection (103). Individuals more commonly infected in developed countries are children in day care centers, hikers, and immunocompromised individuals. Among immunocompromised individuals, infections have been documented in people with AIDS and hypogammaglobulinemia and those affected by malnutrition. Prevalence rates for this pathogen range from 1 to 7% in industrialized countries and from 5 to 50% in developing countries. Of the intestinal flagellates, *G. duodenalis* is the flagellate most frequently isolated in the United States. In high-risk domestic settings, such as day care centers, prevalence rates can reach 90% (104). A *Giardia* vaccine is

TABLE 5 Key features of trophozoites and cysts of common intestinal and urogenital flagellates[a]

Organism	Trophozoites	Cysts
D. fragilis	Size[b]: 5–15 µm; shaped like amebae Motility: Nonprogressive; pseudopodia are angular Flagella: Internalized (only visible by electron microscopy) Nucleus[c]: 1 (40%) or 2 (60%); no peripheral chromatin; karyosome clusters of 4–8 granules Note: Trophozoites not visible in unstained preparation; variation in size between trophozoites can exist on the same smear; cytoplasm is finely granular, and vacuoles may be present	Size[d]: ~5–8 µm; shape is oval to round; inner organism about 5 µm; cyst has an inner and outer wall; rare in human specimens Nucleus: 1 or 2 Note[d]: Cyst has a distinct wall with an irregular inner (cyst) wall located directly adjacent to encysted parasite; peritrophic space present between outer cyst wall and encysted parasite
G. duodenalis	Size: 10–20 µm long, 5–15 µm wide; pear shaped Motility: Falling leaf Flagella: 4 lateral, 2 ventral, 2 caudal Nucleus: 2; not easily visualized in wet preparations; small central karyosomes present Note: Sucking disk is prominent on ventral side of trophozoite; organism is spoon shaped from side view; two axonemes are present	Size: 8–19 µm long, 7–10 µm wide; oval, ellipsoidal, or round Nucleus: 4 nuclei usually located on one end; not distinct in unstained preparation; no peripheral chromatin; karyosomes smaller than those in trophozoite Cytoplasm: Staining can cause shrinkage where cytoplasm pulls away from the cyst wall; 4 median bodies present Note: Axoneme may be present
C. mesnili	Size: 6–24 µm long, 4–8 µm wide; pear shaped Motility: Stiff, rotary Flagella: 3 anterior, 1 in cytostome Nucleus: 1; not visible in unstained preparation Cytoplasm: Prominent cytostome extends over 1/3 to 1/2 of body; spiral groove across ventral surface can be hard to see; vacuoles present	Size: 6–10 µm long, 4–6 µm wide; lemon shaped with anterior hyaline knob Nucleus: Same as trophozoite; difficult to see in unstained preparation; indistinct central karyosome present Cytoplasm: Curved fibril alongside cytostome known as "shepherd's crook"
P. hominis	Size: 5–15 µm long, 7–10 µm wide; pear shaped Motility: Jerky, rapid Flagella: 3–5 anterior, 1 posterior (extends beyond end of body) Nucleus: 1; not visible in unstained preparation Cytoplasm: Central longitudinal axostyle; undulating membrane runs the entire length of body Note: May have tremendous nuclear variation; can mimic *E. hartmanni* and *D. fragilis*	No cyst stage
T. vaginalis	Size: 7–23 µm long, 5–15 µm wide Motility: Jerky, rapid Flagella: 3–5 anterior, 1 posterior Nucleus: 1; not visible in unstained preparation Note: Undulating membrane extends 1/2 the length of body; no free posterior flagella	No cyst stage
E. hominis	Size: 4–10 µm long, 5–6 µm wide; oval Motility: Jerky Flagella: 3 anterior, 1 posterior Nucleus: 1; not visible in unstained preparation Note: One side of the body is flat; posterior flagellum extends free posteriorly or laterally	Size: 4–10 µm long, 4–6 µm wide; elongate or oval in shape Nucleus: 1–4; not visible in stained preparation; nuclei are polar Note: Resemble *E. nana* cysts; fibrils or flagella usually not seen
R. intestinalis	Size: 4–9 µm long, 3–4 µm wide; pear shaped or oval Motility: Jerky Flagella: 1 anterior, 1 posterior Nucleus: 1; not visible in unstained preparation Note: Very difficult to identify; rarely seen; prominent cytostome which extends half the length of body	Size: 4-9 µm long, 5 µm wide; pear or lemon shaped Nucleus: 1; not visible in unstained preparation Note: Resemble *Chilomastix* cysts; bird beak fibril arrangement; shadow outline of cytostome with supporting fibrils extends above nucleus

[a]Adapted from reference 6.
[b]Size ranges are based on wet preparations (with permanent stains, organisms usually measure 1 to 2 µm less).
[c]Nuclear and cytoplasmic descriptions are based on permanent-stained smears.
[d]Though the cyst form has been described in the literature, it must still be independently verified.

available for dogs and cats; this may affect the prevalence of infections in humans (105).

Infection occurs when viable cysts are ingested, excyst, and transform into trophozoites. After excystation, the trophozoite, which appears to have a propensity for the duodenum, attaches to the mucosal epithelium. Trophozoites attach to the epithelium via a sucking disk located on the ventral side of the parasite. During the course of infection, the parasites remain attached to the epithelium and do not invade the mucosa. In the intestine, trophozoites divide by binary fission to produce two identical daughter trophozoites. As they move down toward the large intestine, the trophozoites encyst, and infective cysts are excreted into the environment (6).

Clinical Significance

The majority of individuals infected with G. *duodenalis* are asymptomatic. Asymptomatic versus symptomatic infection may be due to the existence of two strains of *Giardia* with different levels of virulence. Preliminary studies have grouped G. *duodenalis* into two groups, group A and group B. Group A appears to be more pathogenic and is associated with symptomatic infection. Isoenzyme and molecular studies show that group A and group B differ from one another and appear to be no more related than *E. histolytica* and *E. dispar*. The genes homologous between group A and group B *Giardia* isolates show an identity of approximately 81 to 89% (106–108). In symptomatic individuals, acute G. *duodenalis* infections can mimic infections with other protozoal, viral, and bacterial pathogens. After an incubation period of approximately 12 to 20 days, patients can experience nausea, chills, low-grade fever, epigastric pain, and a sudden onset of watery diarrhea. Diarrhea is often explosive and presents as foul smelling without the presence of blood, cellular exudate, or mucus. Individuals can develop subacute or chronic infections with symptoms such as recurrent diarrhea, abdominal discomfort and distention, belching, and heartburn. In patients with chronic cases of giardiasis, diarrhea can lead to dehydration, malabsorption, and impairment of pancreatic function (109). Prevalence varies depending on geographical region (110).

Studies have shown that *Giardia* infections in nonendemic settings can be associated with chronic fatigue and irritable bowel syndrome years later. Though the prevalence of *Giardia* decreases over time, the organism can elicit longer-term complications in some patients (111). Large multicenter studies in countries where *Giardia* is endemic found that the organism is not associated with diarrheal disease (112–114). The increase in this evidence has caused some confusion in the *Giardia* research community. One plausible explanation of the lack of diarrheal disease in these endemic settings is that immunological responses are established early on, during the first 2 years of life. *Giardia* is seemingly regarded as a commensal in many countries, in older children and adults, where there is endemicity of the parasite (115).

Direct Examination

Microscopy

Diagnosis of G. *duodenalis* infection is often established by the microscopic examination of stool for the presence of cysts and/or trophozoites, though many laboratories have migrated to antigen-based assays. Stained smears are more helpful in identifying the trophozoite stage of the infection, although this stage can be identified in wet mount preparations (Table 5; Fig. 7 and 8). Examination of stool specimens may not be diagnostic because cyst forms can be trapped in mucus, making them difficult to detect on smears. Also, the excretion pattern of cysts can be cyclical. In these instances, other methods, such as the string test (Entero-Test; Nutri-Link, Ltd., United Kingdom), should be used to obtain clinical samples. The string test procedure consists of a patient swallowing a weighted capsule containing gelatin and a tightly wound string. After approximately 5 h, the string is removed from the patient and the adherent material is examined as a wet mount or permanent smear (6). Endoscopy can also be used to collect clinical specimens. Because this procedure is invasive, it is used only for diagnosis of disease in patients with perplexing clinical presentations (104).

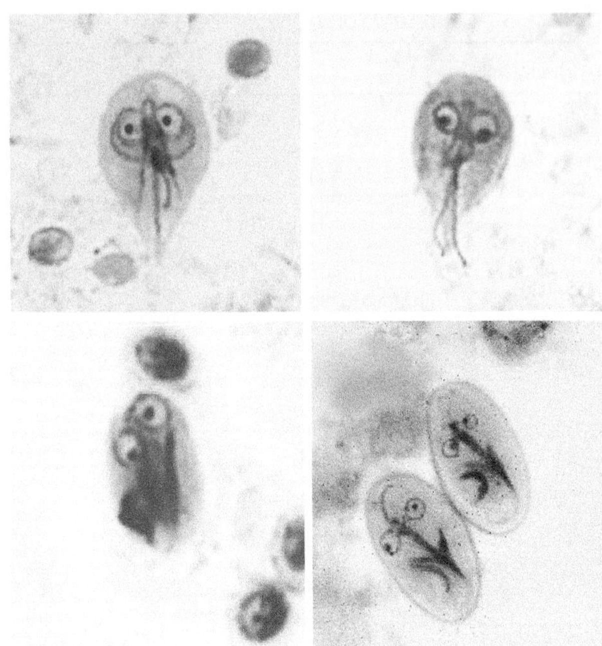

FIGURE 8 (Top row) *Giardia duodenalis* (*G. lamblia*, *G. intestinalis*) trophozoites (note the teardrop shape, two nuclei, linear axonemes, and curved median bodies). (Bottom row) *G. duodenalis* (*G. lamblia*, *G. intestinalis*) cysts (note that although there are multiple nuclei, they are not in the frame of focus in these images). All organisms (except the cyst on the right, iron hematoxylin) stained with Wheatley's trichrome stain. (Courtesy of L. Garcia.)

Antigen Detection

Several assays exist for the detection of G. *duodenalis* in stool specimens, such as EIAs, DFA, and immunochromatographic assays (6, 116). These methods, on average, have fairly high specificities (90 to 100%) and sensitivities that range from 63 to 100% (117–122). Although these methods have proven to be fairly sensitive and specific compared to the routine staining of fecal smears (trichrome staining), other important pathogens may be missed if a wet mount and permanent-stained smear are not examined. The DFA assay widely used is the Merifluor reagent assay (Meridian Bioscience, Inc., Cincinnati, OH), but it requires the availability of a fluorescent microscope. DFA assays on average have a sensitivity and specificity of >95%.

Immunoassays are available and can be useful for testing large numbers of patient specimens. Various studies have shown the performance of EIAs to be excellent compared to that of the ova and parasite exam (118, 123, 124).

Several commercially available immunoassays are on the market (6, 121, 125, 126).

It is very important to note that if a patient is immunocompromised, has traveled, or is suspected of coming into contact with an unusual pathogen, the ova and parasite examination should be performed. Some studies suggest that the use of an immunoassay does not necessarily eliminate the need for more than one stool specimen. Positive specimens from asymptomatic patients may be missed if only one stool specimen is tested using an immunoassay (127). Some immunoassays are affected by specimens contaminated with blood. It was documented in one study that blood can interfere with the performance of the ProSpecT assay and potentially cause false-positive results (119). Immunochromatographic detection methods have also been developed for use in the clinical laboratory (37, 123, 127–129). The ImmunoCard STAT (Meridian Bioscience, Inc.) has been developed to detect *G. duodenalis* and *C. parvum* antigens in stool specimens by using rapid solid-phase qualitative immunochromatography. It is recommended that patients who are negative by the ImmunoCard STAT and remain symptomatic be tested using a routine ova and parasite exam (128). The Triage Micro parasite panel (Biosite Diagnostics, Inc. [Alere]) is a rapid immunoassay that can detect not only *G. duodenalis* antigens but also those of *E. histolytica*/*E. dispar* and *C. parvum* in stool specimens (130). Antigens in stool specimens are immobilized on a membrane containing specific antibodies to the respective intestinal parasites. The formation of color bars occurs on a specific area of the membrane depending on the parasite present in the stool. Laboratories should check with the manufacturer's package insert to determine what specimens, formal fixed or fresh, are compatible with each assay. The Quik Check (TechLab) is also available for rapid diagnosis of *Giardia* and *Cryptosporidium*. Although several methods are now available for the detection of *G. duodenalis*, parameters such as workload, skill levels of technologists, and the availability of necessary equipment should be considered in choosing a specific method, along with performance characteristics of the assay (131). Refer to chapter 138 of this *Manual* for a complete list of currently available assays for *Giardia* detection in the clinical laboratory. Soares et al. have written a fairly recent review of various methods and respective performance characteristics for several assays for the detection of *Giardia* in clinical samples (116).

Nucleic Acid Detection Techniques

Several molecular assays currently exist for the detection of *G. duodenalis* infection in clinical samples (1, 2, 57, 58, 102, 132–141) (see Table 4). Table 4 also lists which assays are FDA approved. One group has developed an oligonucleotide microarray with excellent sensitivity and specificity for the detection of *G. duodenalis* and other intestinal parasites in stool specimens. The assay was also able to discriminate between *Giardia* assemblages A and B (142). A multiplex PCR assay to detect specific genotypes of *G. duodenalis* has also been developed which may potentially aid in epidemiologic investigations of outbreaks (25). In one study the BD Max had a sensitivity of 98.2% and a specificity of 99.5% compared to in-house PCR and bidirectional sequencing in addition to DFA (2). The BioFire FilmArray GI panel in one study had a sensitivity of 100% and specificity of 99.5% compared to alternate PCR and sequencing (1). It is important to note that one study showed a decrease in sensitivity using the BD Max assay, but frozen specimens were used, which may confound the results (139).

Because of the potential for contamination of municipal water supplies, routine monitoring of water for parasitic protozoa is recommended as a public health control measure. *G. duodenalis* cysts can remain viable for 2 to 3 months in cold water and are fairly resistant to killing by routine chlorine treatments. DFA assays are commonly used to detect *G. duodenalis* cysts in water samples, but PCR is also being used for this purpose (143). The advantage of PCR is the increased sensitivity compared to those of fluorescence assays or assays that use special stains. Research continues to enhance the ability of investigators to detect viable organisms, which is a better indication of poor water quality (144).

Treatment

For individuals diagnosed with giardiasis, the treatment of choice is metronidazole, tinidazole, or nitazoxanide (69). Alternatives include paromomycin, furazolidone, and quinacrine or other nitroimidazoles such as ornidazole and secnidazole (145). In most immunocompetent hosts, infection is self-limiting; however, treatment lessens the duration of symptoms and prevents transmission. Other drugs that have been used to treat giardiasis are albendazole, mebendazole, and bacitracin (146), and there are other therapeutics on the horizon. Albendazole, mebendazole, and paromomycin have lower activity against *Giardia* than do the nitroimidazoles (145). Resistance to metronidazole and other agents has been observed clinically and *in vitro* (70). *In vitro* resistance-testing assays are available but lack the standardization required for the clinical laboratory (147).

Evaluation, Interpretation, and Reporting of Results

As with any of the organisms mentioned in this chapter, it is important to evaluate more than one stool specimen for the presence of *G. duodenalis*. For *Giardia*, this could include up to five or six stool specimens to increase the chance of recovery. This is especially important for diagnosing *G. duodenalis* infection, since organisms can be passed in the stool intermittently on a cyclical basis. During the staining procedure, the cysts can be shrunken or distorted, which may impact the ability of the clinical laboratory scientists to read the smear. Several techniques are available for the diagnosis of giardiasis in the clinical laboratory. Some methods might offer somewhat better sensitivity but need to fit into the overall workflow of the laboratory. EIAs offer somewhat enhanced sensitivity but cannot always replace the ova and parasite exam due to the prevalence of other pathogens in the patient population being tested. Adding assays, such as the EIA or amplified molecular testing, might increase detection of *Giardia* but add to the bottom-line cost per test if the physicians continue to order a routine ova and parasite exam as well.

D. fragilis

Taxonomy

D. fragilis is currently in the supergroup Excavata (Metamonada: Parabasalia: Trichomonadida) (148) (see chapter 135 in this *Manual*).

Description of the Agent

Despite the lack of external flagella, this parasite is currently classified as a flagellate but has historically been grouped with the amebae. Electron microscopy and antigenic analysis have aided in the classification of this organism and have demonstrated that it is closely related to

Trichomonas and *Histomonas* species. Phylogenetic analysis of small-subunit rRNA sequences has also confirmed the relationship between *D. fragilis* and *Histomonas* (149, 150). *D. fragilis* possesses a trophozoite, precyst, and cyst stage (148, 151). Historically, degenerative forms of *D. fragilis* have often been confused with the existence of a precyst form or stage (148). For years it was accepted that there was no cyst form for *D. fragilis*. It was confirmed with the help of a rodent model that a cyst stage is present. Cyst forms were detected after oral inoculation of mice in 2013 (152), and in 2014 cyst forms of *D. fragilis* were found in human specimens and documented in the published literature (151). The authors comment that the cyst form in human specimens appearing to be rare could perhaps indicate that this may not be the predominant transmissible stage for *D. fragilis* (148, 151).

Epidemiology, Transmission, and Prevention

D. fragilis is found worldwide and is known to cause a noninvasive diarrheal illness in humans. Based on the current literature, two major genotypes of *D. fragilis* exist: genotype 1 and genotype 2. Genotype 1 appears to be the most common of the two genotypes (148). Colonization in humans is similar to that seen with other intestinal parasites; typically, the cecum and the proximal part of the colon are affected. The mode of transmission of *D. fragilis* is still uncertain; one hypothesis concerning the spread of *D. fragilis* is that transmission occurs within the eggs of *Enterobius vermicularis* or *Ascaris lumbricoides* (153). Several historical studies provided circumstantial evidence to support *E. vermicularis* as a vector, documenting a greater-than-expected coinfection rate with the two organisms (154).

More recent studies support the role of *E. vermicularis* in transmission (155, 156). Though DNA is present in *E. vermicularis* ova, some researchers believe that this does not prove the viability of *D. fragilis* DNA and that additional animal studies should be performed to prove that the ova can result in *D. fragilis* infection (157). Munasinghe et al. have shown via animal experiments that *E. vermicularis* is not an absolute requirement for *D. fragilis* infection (152).

Though *D. fragilis* has a worldwide distribution, prevalence rates for this organism vary substantially from 0% in Prague, Czech Republic, to 42% in Germany (154). There appears to be a higher prevalence in certain groups of individuals such as missionaries, Native Americans living in Arizona, and institutionalized individuals (158). In the United States, the prevalence is reported to be quite low. This may be due to underreporting attributable to difficulties associated with identifying the organism in clinical samples. In addition, Johnson and Clark (159) identified two genetically distinct types of *D. fragilis* with a resulting sequence divergence of approximately 2% (159, 160). The degree of divergence appears to be similar to that seen with *E. histolytica* and *E. dispar*. Since asymptomatic infections occur, this finding may lend support to the possibility that two distinct species exist, though there is no consensus on this matter (154, 159).

Clinical Significance

The frequency of symptomatic disease ranges from 15 to 25% in adults, and symptomatic disease is more common in children, in whom up to 90% of those infected have clinical signs (104, 161, 162). Symptoms include fatigue, insufficient weight gain, diarrhea (often intermittent), abdominal pain, anorexia, and nausea. Studies have linked *D. fragilis* infection to biliary infection (163), irritable bowel syndrome (29), allergic colitis (164), and diarrhea in HIV-infected patients (165). One case report describes a patient who presented in the emergency room with acute appendicitis which was attributed to *D. fragilis* infection (166). Some individuals, mainly children, also experience unexplained peripheral blood eosinophilia (6, 167). Diarrhea is seen predominantly during the first 1 to 2 weeks after the onset of disease. The number of *D. fragilis* organisms can vary greatly from day to day, which is similar to other intestinal protozoa. Abdominal pain can persist for 1 to 2 months (161). Although *D. fragilis* has been implicated in the above-mentioned clinical situations, the organism is also isolated from patients with no apparent clinical symptoms. In addition, the lack of an animal model affects researchers' ability to detect specific pathological manifestations (154).

Direct Detection

Microscopy

Diagnosis of *D. fragilis* infection is similar to that of infections with other intestinal protozoa, and detection of the trophozoite in fresh or preserved stool is warranted to establish infection. Laboratories using direct microscopy may be at a disadvantage, since the trophozoite can degenerate rapidly if not placed in fixative as soon as possible. Nonfixed trophozoites can appear rounded and refractile and are more difficult to identify microscopically. Morphologically, the trophozoite of *D. fragilis* contains one or two nuclei (binucleate), with two nuclei being more common (Table 5; Fig. 7 and 9). A number of fixatives and stains can be used, but safranin and modified iron hematoxylin appear to be the best combination. Stark et al. provide a thorough discussion of appropriate fixatives and stains for *D. fragilis* (148).

Other Diagnostic Methods

Culture has been shown to be more sensitive than microscopy; however, it is not recommended for the routine clinical laboratory (154). Culture of *D. fragilis* is accomplished with the use of xenic culture systems where the organism is grown in the presence of bacterial flora derived from the patients' stool specimen. Axenic cultures do not support the growth of *D. fragilis* (148). Antigen and antibody techniques have been used as diagnostic tools for the detection of *D. fragilis* but are not commercially available (58, 168, 169). *D. fragilis* DNA has been detected using PCR with fresh, unpreserved stool. Molecular techniques have the promise of being more sensitive than microscopy (58, 170–172). As mentioned previously, multiplex PCR assays are being developed for the detection of other parasites including *D. fragilis* (58). Several PCR assays are available for the detection of *D. fragilis* (148, 173), though none to date are FDA approved in the United States. One assay exhibited a sensitivity of 92 to 100% and specificity of 100%, showing great promise for use of molecular assays for the detection of this pathogen (173).

Treatment

Stark et al. provide a complete summary of therapeutic regimens for the treatment of *D. fragilis* (148). Iodoquinol is commonly used to treat patients with *D. fragilis* in the United States; however, the exact mode of action is unknown (148, 174). The CDC recommends tetracycline, though the recommendation is based on limited case reports in the literature (175). Alternative choices include paromomycin and metronidazole (174). Additional therapeutic options include diphetarsone, carbarsone, erythromycin,

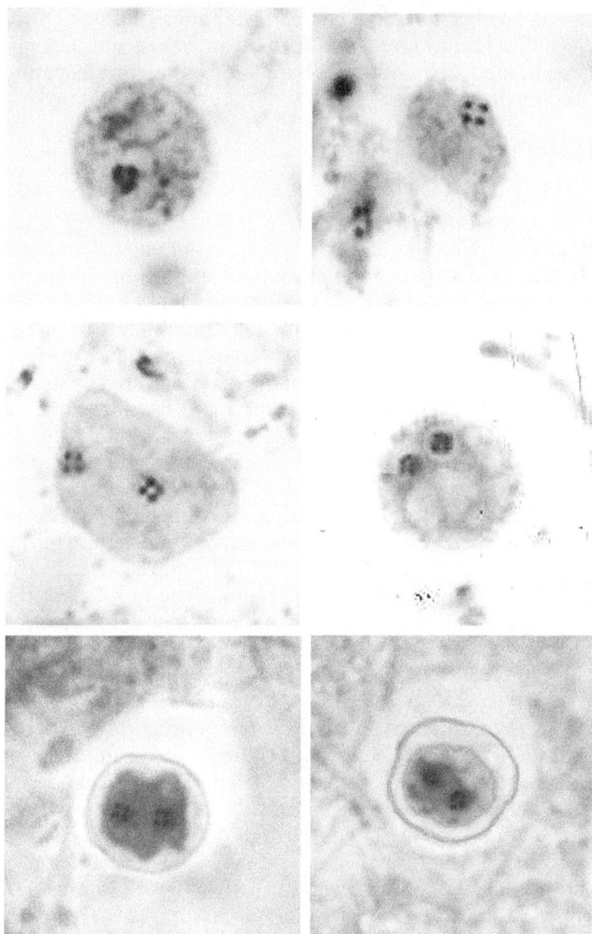

FIGURE 9 (Top row) *Dientamoeba fragilis* trophozoites (note the single, fragmented nucleus; if the nucleus has not yet fragmented, it will resemble *Endolimax nana*). (Middle row) *D. fragilis* trophozoites (note the two fragmented nuclei). (Bottom row) *D. fragilis* cysts (note that they appear to be shrunken with a cyst wall; there are only about 1% cysts on a human fecal smear, so diagnosis still relies on the trophozoite morphology on the stained smear). All organisms (with the exception of the trophozoite with two nuclei on the right, which was stained with iron hematoxylin) stained with Wheatley's trichrome stain. (Courtesy of L. Garcia.)

hydroxyquinoline, and secnidazole (154, 176). It is important to note that though several therapeutic agents are currently used to treat dientamoebiasis, there have been very few randomized, double-blinded, controlled trials using most of the aforementioned agents (148). One randomized, double-blinded, placebo-controlled clinical trial found that metronidazole treatment of children is not associated with improved clinical outcomes (177). If *E. vermicularis* is detected concomitantly, the patient should be treated for that organism as well (161).

Evaluation, Interpretation, and Reporting of Results

The recovery of *D. fragilis* is greatly enhanced by the collection of at least three stool specimens (4, 104). Trophozoites have been recovered from soft and formed stools, indicating the need to evaluate all types of samples (161). Low incidence of *D. fragilis* in a community setting may be due to the inability of the laboratory to accurately identify the organism.

T. vaginalis

Taxonomy

T. vaginalis is a flagellate in supergroup Excavata (Metamonada: Parabasalia: Trichomonadida) (see chapter 135 of this *Manual*). Unlike the other flagellates, which inhabit the intestinal tract, *T. vaginalis* infects the urogenital tract.

Description of the Agent

The life cycle of *T. vaginalis* includes only the trophozoite stage; there is no cyst stage. The organism is similar in morphology to the other trichomonads and is characterized as a pear shape with a prominent axostyle and an undulating membrane that stops halfway down the side of the trophozoite (Table 5; Fig. 7 and 10). It is a facultative anaerobe that divides by binary fission, and it cannot survive long outside the host.

Epidemiology, Transmission, and Prevention

T. vaginalis is a pathogenic flagellate that infects the urogenital tracts of males and females. The infection is primarily a sexually transmitted infection. According to the CDC, *T. vaginalis* is the most prevalent nonviral sexually transmitted infection in the United States, with estimated infections reaching 3.7 million a year (175), and is thought to be the most common curable sexually transmitted infection among sexually active young women. Worldwide, there are an estimated 250 million cases of *Trichmonas* infection each year, with an overall estimated prevalence of 4.5% (178). Prevalence is estimated to be higher in women (8%) than in men (1%) (178, 179). It is hypothesized that hormones in women may play a large role in terms of infection and persistence of *Trichomonas* infections. The incidence of trichomoniasis differs depending on the population examined, varying from 5 to 60% in various studies. Factors such as lower socioeconomic status, multiple sex partners, and poor personal hygiene are linked to a higher incidence of infection. The prevalence of trichomoniasis appears to be higher in older women as shown by several studies (180–182). This is in contrast to the prevalence of other common sexually transmitted diseases (STDs) such as chlamydia where prevalence is typically higher in younger women. One study screened male patients to assess the prevalence in that population. The percentage prevalence was approximately 6.6%, though the prevalence was higher

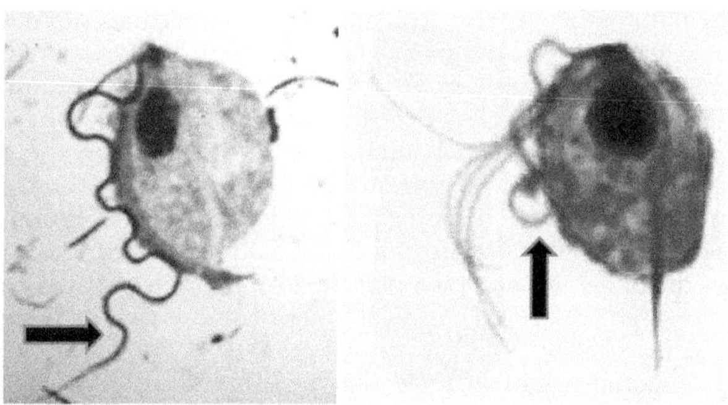

FIGURE 10 (Left) *Pentatrichomonas hominis* (note that the undulating membrane/arrow goes to the bottom of the organism, nonpathogen). (Right) *Trichomonas vaginalis* (note that the undulating membrane/arrow only goes halfway down the organism, pathogen). Both organisms stained with Giemsa stain. (Courtesy of L. Garcia.)

in males that were an average age of 39.9 years old (180). This parallels what is seen in women, as described above. Several studies have described the relationship between *T. vaginalis* and the possibility of lethal prostate cancer (183–185). Some researchers are exploring the use of a serodiagnostic test that would identify those at risk for prostate cancer related to seropositivity for *T. vaginalis* (186).

The estimated infection rates cited in the literature may be too low because (i) trichomoniasis is not a reportable disease in the United States and other countries, (ii) the infection, particularly in men, can be asymptomatic, and (iii) laboratory tests used for diagnosis vary in their sensitivities. Despite these rates of infection and their serious medical consequences, trichomoniasis has not received adequate attention from public health and STD prevention programs (187). In the United States the CDC has categorized *T. vaginalis* as a neglected parasitic infection.

Clinical Significance

Infection with *T. vaginalis* in females can result in vaginitis, cervicitis, and urethritis (187). The vaginal discharge is classically described as copious, liquid, greenish, frothy, and foul smelling. The onset of symptoms, such as intense vaginal and vulvar pruritus and discharge, is often sudden and occurs during or after menstruation. The vaginal pH is usually elevated above the normal pH of 4.5, and dysuria occurs in 20% of women with *T. vaginalis* infection. Infection has also been associated with premature rupture of membranes, premature birth, other adverse pregnancy outcomes, and posthysterectomy cuff infections (188–190). Up to 50% of infected women are asymptomatic carriers. In men, the most common symptomatic presentation is urethritis, though it is estimated that the majority of infections are asymptomatic. Due to the asymptomatic nature of this disease, these carriers can serve as an important reservoir for transmission and also remain at risk for developing the disease. Untreated *Trichomonas* infections can last for months or even years (191). Trichomoniasis has been implicated as a cofactor in the transmission of HIV (192, 193). In one study, men with symptomatic *Trichomonas* urethritis were found to have increased HIV concentrations in seminal plasma compared to HIV-infected men without urethritis (194). The CDC recommends routine screening of HIV-infected women for *T. vaginalis* because of the adverse events associated with HIV and *T. vaginalis* infection (195). However, routine screening of asymptomatic infection for *T. vaginalis* is currently not recommended. Screening asymptomatic patients in high-prevalence settings such as correctional facilities or STD clinics might be considered. There are no data currently to support routine screening in these high-prevalence settings or to show whether there would be an impact on the burden of infection in these communities (195). Some studies suggest that prevalence might dictate which testing method for *Trichomonas* is chosen. In one study the use of the rapid OSOM test (discussed in detail below) had poor performance in a low-prevalence setting, therefore suggesting a molecular approach in these settings (196).

Neonates can acquire the organism during passage through the infected birth canal (187). Reports have also documented *T. vaginalis* as a cause of neonatal pneumonia (197). Bilateral conjunctivitis in a male without genital infection was recently reported (198). One case of cerebral trichomoniasis was documented in a neonate with seizures and multiorgan failure. *T. vaginalis* was isolated from the cerebrospinal fluid (199). Multilocus sequence typing has been used to characterize different strains of *T. vaginalis*. Techniques such as this can be useful for population-based studies and perhaps strain selection for future vaccine development (200).

Direct Detection

Microscopy

The diagnosis of *T. vaginalis* infection is commonly based on the examination of wet preparations of vaginal and urethral discharges, prostatic secretions, and urine sediments. Permanent stains such as Papanicolaou and Giemsa stains can be used, but the organisms may be difficult to recognize (201). For wet preparations, vaginal specimens are routinely collected during a speculum examination, but studies suggest that self-collected or tampon-collected specimens may be used successfully (202, 203). Specimens should be mixed with a drop of physiologic saline and examined microscopically within 1 h under low power (magnification, ×100) with reduced illumination. Specimens should never be refrigerated. The presence of actively motile organisms with jerky motility is diagnostic. The movement of the undulating membrane may be seen as the motility of the trophozoite diminishes. Polymorphonuclear cells are often present. The sensitivity of the wet preparation test with vaginal specimens is between 50 and 70%, depending on the skill of the microscopist and other factors. The sensitivity of microscopy in males is low, and additional testing, such as culture of urethral swab, urine, and semen, is required for optimal sensitivity. Perhaps the most important factor affecting the sensitivity of wet mount testing is the time between collection and examination of the specimen. Viability of the organism is essential for the detection of motility on the wet mount and drops off precipitously with time. Amies transport medium can maintain the viability for culture of *T. vaginalis* on swabs held at room temperature for 24 ± 6 h before inoculation of the specimen into a culture pouch (204). Because the morphology of *P. hominis*, a nonpathogenic intestinal flagellate, is very similar to that of *T. vaginalis*, care must be taken to ensure that specimens are not contaminated with fecal material.

Culture

Culture has greater sensitivity (>80%) than the wet mount method and is considered the gold standard method for the detection of *T. vaginalis*. Specimens must be collected properly and inoculated immediately into the appropriate medium, such as modified Diamond's, Trichosel, or Hollander's medium. Due to cost and convenience, this approach is not routinely used. Culture systems (InPouch TV; BioMed Diagnostics, San Jose, CA, and the system of Empyrean Diagnostics, Inc., Mountain View, CA) that allow direct inoculation, transport, culture, and microscopic examination are commercially available (205, 206). In situations where immediate transport of specimens is not feasible, the use of these transport/culture devices should be encouraged. Studies have also shown that a delayed inoculation protocol is as sensitive as immediate inoculation, allowing the results of microscopy to be used to determine whether further culture is necessary (207). Serologic testing is not useful for the diagnosis of trichomoniasis.

Antigen Detection

Several antigen detection methods have been developed for *T. vaginalis* and offer the advantage of being rapid and easy to perform. A latex agglutination test (TV Latex; Kalon Biological, Guildford, Surrey, United Kingdom) has been shown to have excellent sensitivity (208) but is not available in the United States. An immunofluorescence assay (Light Diagnostics *T. vaginalis* DFA; Chemicon International, Temecula, CA) is available in the United States for testing directly from patient samples. An immunochromatographic capillary flow assay is available commercially for the qualitative detection of *T. vaginalis* antigens from vaginal swabs. The OSOM *Trichomonas* rapid test kit (Genzyme Corporation, Cambridge, MA) is a dipstick assay that provides results in 10 min. In published studies, the OSOM test has demonstrated good sensitivity (67 to 94.7%) and specificity (98.8 to 100%) compared to various comparator assays, including wet mount, culture, and amplified testing (209–215). This assay would perhaps be more suitable for a clinic setting where more rapid results are desirable (216). A rapid point-of-care test is being developed for *T. vaginalis*. This assay features novel electrochemical endpoint detection and in initial studies appears to have high sensitivity and specificity (217).

Nucleic Acid Detection Techniques

Various nucleic acid detection techniques are available for the detection of *T. vaginalis* in clinical specimens. The choice of methodology depends on many factors, whether a point-of-care test is necessary for instances when the patient might not come back to the physician's office (STD clinic) or other clinical settings where follow-up is not an issue and where a molecular test may be more suitable. The Affirm VPIII assay (Becton Dickinson and Company, Sparks, MD) is a direct DNA probe test (nonamplified) for the detection of organisms from vaginal swabs associated with vaginosis/vaginitis (218–220). It tests for the three most common syndromes associated with increased vaginal discharge: bacterial vaginosis (*Gardnerella vaginalis*), candidiasis (*Candida albicans*), and trichomoniasis (*T. vaginalis*). According to the manufacturer's package insert, the assay has a sensitivity and specificity of 90% and 98%, respectively, compared with wet mount and culture for *T. vaginalis* (package insert, Affirm VPIII, version no. 670160JAAG; Becton Dickinson). In a clinical evaluation of vaginal swab specimens from both symptomatic and asymptomatic females, the Affirm assay detected more *T. vaginalis*-positive samples than wet mount testing, although the difference was not statistically significant (221). It is important to note that the Affirm VPIII assay (Becton Dickinson) is less sensitive than molecular testing (181, 220, 222, 223). Andrea and Chapin compared the Gen-Probe (Hologic) Aptima *T. vaginalis* (ATV) (Hologic) assay to the Affirm VPIII (Becton Dickinson) assay and showed the sensitivity of the ATV assay to be 100% and the Affirm VPIII assay to be 63.4% (181).

Nucleic acid amplification tests have been available for the diagnosis of *T. vaginalis* for the past several years, and data show many of these assays to be superior to other methods for the clinical diagnosis of *Trichomonas* infections (182, 187, 211, 224–235). In the United States there are currently five FDA-cleared amplified molecular assays available for the detection of *T. vaginalis*: (i) Xpert TV (approved for male urine and female endocervical and self-collected vaginal swabs) (Cepheid, Sunnyvale, CA), (ii) Quidel Solana *Trichomonas* assay (San Diego, CA) (approved for female vaginal and urine specimens), (iii) ATV assay (Hologic, San Diego, CA) (approved for male urine and female vaginal swab and urine specimens), (iv) BD ProbeTec TV assay (Becton Dickinson, Sparks, MD) (approved for female endocervical swab, patient-collected vaginal swab in a physician setting, and female urine specimens), and (v) the BD Max vaginal panel (approved for vaginal swab) and the BD Max CT/GC/TV assay (Becton Dickinson, Sparks, MD) (approved for female endocervical swab, vaginal swab, and urine and male urine specimens) (236–238). Most of these assays are CE marked as well. The Cepheid Xpert TV assay is a PCR-based assay that detects *T. vaginalis* using PCR on the GeneXpert system and according to the manufacturer is the only FDA-approved assay for both male and female specimens (both asymptomatic and symptomatic patients) (216, 236, 239). The total assay time is approximately 40 min. The Quidel Solana *Trichomonas* assay (performed on the Solana instrument) is a rapid point-of-care test approved for vaginal and urine specimens (symptomatic and asymptomatic patients), with results in less than 40 min. The assay uses helicase-dependent amplification and fluorescent-based probe detection (240). The Hologic ATV assay (Hologic, San Diego, CA) can be performed on both the automated Panther and Tigris instruments, and studies have shown the performance of the assay to be superior to other standard methodologies (181, 182, 235). The ATV assay detects rRNA by transcription-mediated amplification and is approved for testing of a wide variety of specimens such as clinician-collected vaginal specimens, endocervical swabs, ThinPrep liquid-based cytology samples, and urine samples (235). In addition to testing on adults, molecular testing is being used for the detection of *Trichomonas* in specimens collected from children (241). Some researchers have also evaluated the ATV assay for the diagnosis of anorectal *T. vaginalis* using rectal swabs (180, 242). One study compared the Affirm VPIII assay to the Hologic ATV assay and found the sensitivity of the ATV to be 98.1% and that of the Affirm VPIII to be 46.3% (220). Becton Dickinson has an assay called the BD *T. vaginalis* Qx, which can be performed on their automated BD Viper system (238). According to one study, the assay has a sensitivity and specificity of 98.3% and 99.0%, respectively, compared to patient infected status (238). The BD Max has a multiplex assay for the detection of *Neisseria gonorrhoeae*, *Chlamydia trachomatis*, and *T. vaginalis* (237). Another assay available outside the United States is the Seeplex Anyplex II STI-5 detection kit (Seegene, Seoul, Korea), which detects *T. vaginalis* and other pathogens (243). Detection employs six pairs of dual priming oligonucleotide primers targeted to unique genes of the specific pathogen. It is not clear if this assay will be FDA approved in the United States. Similar to the Affirm VPIII, Becton Dickinson manufactures another vaginal panel on the BD Max. The BD Max vaginal panel is a qualitative PCR assay using fluorogenic target-specific hybridization probes that amplify specific DNA targets such as organisms associated with bacterial vaginosis and other organisms such as certain *Candida* spp. and *T. vaginalis*. Specimen collection is achieved via the BD Max UVE, which is part of the assay system. Gaydos et al. reported that the BD Max vaginal panel had a sensitivity of ~93.1% and specificity of 99.3% for *Trichomonas*. Sensitivity and specificity were similar whether the specimen was collected by the physician or self-collected by the patient. Patient self-collection is a consideration in some settings where a pelvic exam might be challenging (244, 245).

While the wet mount method provides a rapid result at a low cost, tests with increased sensitivities, such as nucleic acid probes and amplification tests, may be indicated because of the impact of *T. vaginalis* infections on pregnancy and the link with HIV transmission (204, 233). The use of alternative specimen types such as urine makes amplified testing an important advancement for diagnosis of trichomoniasis. An algorithm to reflex specimens with negative wet mounts to culture or a more sensitive methodology may be a useful diagnostic approach (212). Because the true prevalence of *T. vaginalis* is unknown and the prevalence appears to be higher in older women, it is important for laboratories and clinicians to be aligned in regard to which patients should be tested (182).

Treatment

The recommended treatment for *T. vaginalis* infections is metronidazole or tinidazole (69, 246). For metronidazole, oral therapy is recommended over topical treatment. Tinidazole may be used as a first-line agent or for refractory cases previously treated with metronidazole (247). For treatment during pregnancy, metronidazole is the recommended therapy; however, it should be used cautiously, as data do not suggest that metronidazole treatment results in a reduction in perinatal morbidity (246, 248). All sexual partners of infected individuals should also receive treatment. Treatment failure with metronidazole is usually due to noncompliance or reinfection. True resistance to metronidazole has been documented and appears to be increasing (247, 249). While not routinely available, methods have been published for the *in vitro* determination of susceptibility. These methods have not been standardized, and the results can vary based on assay conditions (250, 251).

Evaluation, Interpretation, and Reporting of Results

A laboratory finding that is positive for *T. vaginalis* is considered diagnostic of trichomoniasis. As discussed above, both microscopy and culture are prone to lower sensitivities due to issues related to sampling and transport. Laboratories should have strict rejection criteria for *Trichomonas* culture and wet mount specimens that do not arrive within the specified time or transport conditions; such policies improve sensitivity, ensuring more accurate results. Microscopy, culture, and antigen tests have a lower sensitivity than molecular assays; therefore, a negative result by any of these methods should be viewed cautiously and evaluated in conjunction with clinical symptoms.

With testing for *Trichomonas*, such as antigen detection and direct molecular probes or amplified tests, reported results should reflect the analyte that is detected. For example, a positive result for *T. vaginalis* by a direct DNA probe assay should state "*T. vaginalis* DNA detected." If testing is expanded to differing sample types, such as urine testing by amplified methods, the report should clearly state the specimen tested.

In the United States if home brew assays are used for the diagnosis of *T. vaginalis*, it is required that the result be labeled to indicate its status as an in-house test in accordance with CLIA regulations as follows: "This test was developed and its performance characteristics determined by [Laboratory Name]. It has not been cleared or approved by the U. S. Food and Drug Administration." This would also apply to off-label usage of FDA-approved tests where certain sample times are not validated by the manufacturer. Any off-label use of an assay with a sample type not validated by the manufacturer needs to be validated in-house by the laboratory before any patient reporting.

NONPATHOGENIC FLAGELLATES

C. mesnili is found worldwide and is generally considered nonpathogenic. *C. mesnili* has both a trophozoite and a cyst stage. The organism is acquired through the ingestion of contaminated food or water and resides in the cecum and/or colon of the infected human or animal. The trophozoite is 6 to 24 μm long and contains a characteristic spiral groove that runs longitudinally along the body (Table 4; Fig. 7 and 11). Motility of the organism can sometimes be seen in fresh preparations, and the spiral groove may be exposed as the organism turns. Flagella are difficult to see in stained preparations. The trophozoite contains one nucleus, with a cytostome or oral groove in close proximity. The pear-shaped cyst retains the cytoplasmic organelles of the trophozoite, with a single nucleus and curved cytostomal fibril. Observing the organism in permanent-stained preparations makes identification more definitive.

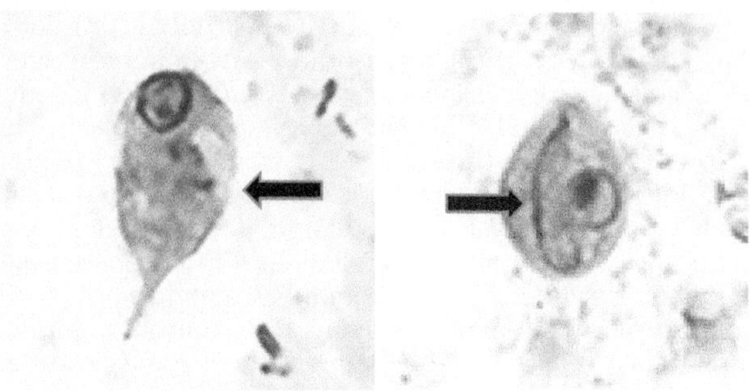

FIGURE 11 (Left) *Chilomastix mesnili* trophozoite (note the clear feeding groove or cytostome/arrow). (Right) *C. mesnili* cyst. Note the curved fibril called the shepherd's crook/arrow. Also note the typical pear or lemon shape of the cyst. Both organisms stained with Wheatley's trichrome stain. (Courtesy of L. Garcia.)

P. hominis, formerly referred to as *Trichomonas hominis*, is a nonpathogenic flagellate, and only the trophozoite stage has been observed. Although the organism is cosmopolitan in nature and is recovered from individuals with diarrhea, it is still considered nonpathogenic. The trophozoites typically inhabit the cecum. They are pyriform and contain an undulating membrane that runs the length of the parasite. The use of permanent smears is recommended for observation of these organisms in clinical specimens. The trophozoites may stain weakly, making them difficult to detect on stained smears (6).

Two additional nonpathogenic intestinal flagellates are *E. hominis* and *R. intestinalis*. They are both found in warm or temperate climates, and infection is acquired through the ingestion of cysts. When clinical specimens are examined, it is important to note that cysts of *E. hominis* can resemble those of *E. nana*, although *E. nana* cysts containing two nuclei are rare. Because of the small sizes of *E. hominis* and *R. intestinalis*, it is difficult to detect these organisms even when permanent-stained smears are examined. This may lead to the underreporting of both organisms. *R. intestinalis* has been recovered from the pancreatic juice of a patient with small lesions of the pancreatic duct (252).

In general, treatment is not recommended for infections with the nonpathogenic flagellates. Improved personal hygiene and sanitary conditions are key methods for the prevention of infection. As with intestinal nonpathogenic amebae, it is important to report the presence of nonpathogenic flagellates if they are present in clinical specimens. The presence of these organisms can indicate exposure to a contaminated food or water source, and additional testing may be indicated.

CILIATES

Neobalantidium coli

Taxonomy

N. coli is a ciliate which belongs to the supergroup SAR (Ciliophora: Litostomatea) (see chapter 135 of this *Manual*).

Members of the phylum Ciliophora are protozoa that possess cilia in at least one stage of their life cycles. They also have two types of nuclei, one macronucleus and one or more micronuclei. Over the past several years, molecular analysis has aided in the characterization of the genus *Neobalantidium* (253–255). Sequences of the genus are on file at GenBank based on the small subunit rRNA. There is a question as to whether the species isolated from humans, *N. coli*, and pigs, *Neobalantidium suis*, are the same species (253).

Description of the Agent

This organism has both the trophozoite and cyst forms as part of its life cycle (Table 6; Fig. 12). The cyst form is the infective stage. After ingestion of the cysts and excystation, trophozoites secrete hyaluronidase, which aids in the invasion of the tissue. The trophozoite, which is oval and covered with cilia, is easily seen in wet mount preparations under low-power magnification. The cytoplasm contains both a macronucleus and a micronucleus, in addition to two contractile vacuoles. Motile trophozoites can be observed in fresh wet preparations, but the specimen must be observed soon after collection. The trophozoite is somewhat pear shaped and also contains vacuoles that may harbor debris such as cell fragments and ingested bacteria. Cyst formation takes place as the trophozoite moves down the large intestine.

Epidemiology, Transmission, and Prevention

N. coli exists in animal reservoirs such as pigs and chimpanzees, with pigs being the primary reservoir (253). The organism is the only pathogenic ciliate and the largest pathogenic protozoan known to infect humans. Transmission occurs by the fecal-oral route following ingestion of the cysts in contaminated food or water. Infection is more common in warmer climates and in areas where humans are in close contact with pigs. As with other intestinal protozoa, poor sanitary conditions lead to a higher incidence of infection. Prevalence of *Neobalantidium* varies by geographic location but overall is estimated to be between 0.02 and 1% (256). High-prevalence areas include parts of the Middle East, Papua New Guinea and West Irian, Latin America, and the Philippines (257, 258).

TABLE 6 Key features of the ciliate *N. coli*

Stage	Characteristics
Trophozoite	Shape and size: Ovoid with tapering anterior end; 50–100 μm long, 40–70 μm wide Motility: Rotary, boring; may be rapid Nuclei: 1 large kidney-bean-shaped macronucleus may not be distinct in unstained preparation; 1 small round micronucleus adjacent to macronucleus, difficult to see Cytoplasm: May be vacuolated; may contain ingested bacteria and debris; anterior cytostome Cilia: Body surface covered with longitudinal rows of cilia; longer near cytostome Note: May be confused with helminth eggs or debris on a permanent-stained smear; concentration or sedimentation examination recommended
Cyst	Shape and size: Spherical or oval; 50–70 μm in diam Nuclei: 1 large macronucleus, 1 micronucleus, difficult to see Cytoplasm: Vacuoles are visible in young cysts; in older cysts, internal structure appears granular Cilia: Difficult to see within the thick cyst wall

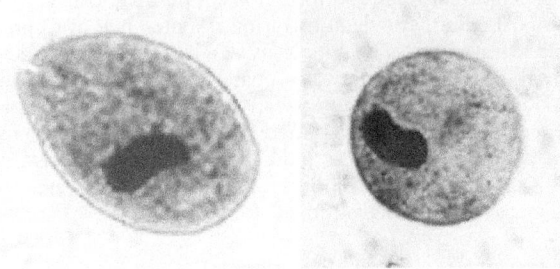

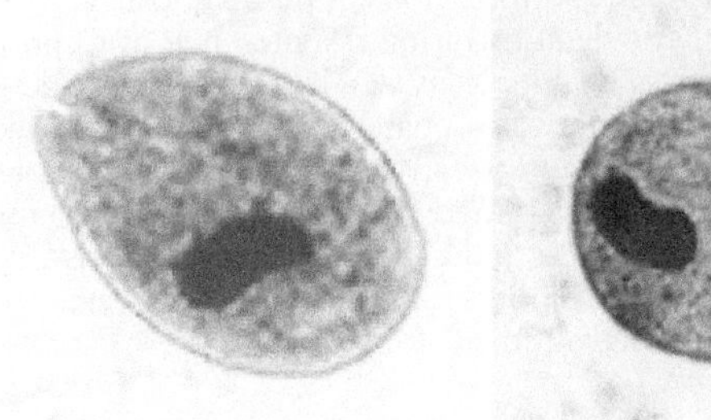

FIGURE 12 (Left) *Neobalantidium coli* trophozoite (note the large macronucleus; the micronucleus is not visible). (Right) *N. coli* cyst (note the large macronucleus; the micronucleus is not visible). All organisms stained with Wheatley's trichrome stain. (Courtesy of L. Garcia.)

Clinical Significance

Infection with *N. coli* is usually asymptomatic; however, symptomatic infection can occur, resulting in bouts of dysentery similar to amebiasis (6, 259). Infection with *Neobalantidium* can be described in three ways: (i) asymptomatic host carrying the disease; (ii) chronic infection, nonbloody diarrhea, including other symptoms such as cramping and abdominal pain; and (iii) fulminating disease consisting of mucoid and bloody stools (253). In addition, colitis caused by *N. coli* is often indistinguishable from that caused by *E. histolytica*. Symptoms typically include diarrhea, nausea, vomiting, headache, and anorexia. Fluid loss can be dramatic, as seen in some patients with cryptosporidiosis. The organism can invade the submucosa of the large bowel, and ulcerative abscesses and hemorrhagic lesions can occur. The shallow ulcers and submucosal lesions that result from invasion are prone to secondary infection by bacteria and can be problematic for the patient (260, 261). Death due to invasive *N. coli* infection has been reported (260). Infections associated with extraintestinal sites have been described (260–262). There have been several reports of *Neobalantidium* spreading from the intestine to the lung. Most of these cases have occurred in patients that are either elderly or immunocompromised. The disease presents as a pneumonia-like illness. In these documented cases, *Neobalantidium* has been recovered from specimens such as bronchial secretions and bronchial lavage specimens. It is hypothesized that extraintestinal colonization can occur between the lymphatic or circulatory system, perforation through the colon, or through aspiration of fluid from the oral cavity (253). One case describes an individual with vertebral osteomyelitis and myelopathy, which is the first documented case of infection in the bone (263). *Neobalantidium* is very rare in the urinary tract but was documented in an elderly man with chronic kidney disease and in a patient with chronic obstructive pulmonary disease (264, 265). The first liver abscess was reported in a patient in India (266). Albeit rare, there have been documented cases of polymicrobial keratitis with *N. coli* (267).

Direct Examination

Microscopy

Either ova and parasite examination of feces or histological examination of intestinal biopsy specimens establishes the diagnosis of *N. coli* infections. The diagnosis can be established only by demonstrating the presence of trophozoites in stool or tissue samples (262). It is very easy to identify these organisms in wet preparations and concentrated stool samples. Conversely, it can be challenging to identify *N. coli* from trichrome-stained permanent smears because the organisms are so large and have a tendency to overstain. This makes the organism less discernible and increases the chance of misidentification.

Treatment

The treatment of choice for *N. coli* infection is tetracycline, although it is considered an investigational drug when used in this context (69). Metronidazole and iodoquinol are therapeutic alternatives used in some cases (6). Nitazoxanide, which is a broad-spectrum antiparasitic drug, may be another alternative for treatment (253).

Evaluation, Interpretation, and Reporting of Results

The recovery of *N. coli* in humans is fairly uncommon despite its worldwide distribution. Pulmonary infections can occur, but the clinical laboratory scientist needs to make sure that this organism is not confused with motile ciliated epithelial cells that can be present in respiratory specimens. *Neobalantidium* spp. in wet mounts are very active parasites with uniform ciliation.

SUMMARY

Clinical laboratories are now given more choices for testing in diagnostic parasitology, with assays ranging from microscopy, culture, antigen detection, and nucleic acid amplification techniques for detection of the intestinal and urogenital amebae, flagellates, and ciliates. Molecular biology has the promise to deliver more sensitive and specific methods, with the availability of an FDA-cleared assay for detection of *T. vaginalis* from genital specimens and multiplex assays for *E. histolytica*, *G. duodenalis*, *Cryptosporidium* spp., and *Blastocystis* spp. detection from stool. As more multiplex assays become available for diagnosis of syndromes such as infectious gastroenteritis, their utility and impact on patient outcomes will become clearer. In addition to these amplification tests, rapid point-of-care tests are available for organisms such as *T. vaginalis*. Results can now be available in real time for the clinician to manage patients directly in the exam setting. While these new test modalities are exciting, clinical laboratories are still faced with using microscopy for routine work-up for stool specimens due to the lack of commercially available testing for all the relevant organisms. Some laboratories have switched to antigen-based methods, but many still rely on microscopy because antigen-based methods cannot detect all potential pathogens in a given stool specimen. Microscopy, as we know, cannot differentiate between pathogenic and nonpathogenic amebae and the different genotypes of *Giardia*. The diagnostic landscape continues to change with an increase in options that the clinical parasitology laboratory has for the diagnosis of intestinal and urogenital parasitic infections.

REFERENCES

1. **Buss SN, Leber A, Chapin K, Fey PD, Bankowski MJ, Jones MK, Rogatcheva M, Kanack KJ, Bourzac KM.** 2015. Multicenter evaluation of the BioFire FilmArray gastrointestinal panel for etiologic diagnosis of infectious gastroenteritis. *J Clin Microbiol* **53:**915–925.
2. **Madison-Antenucci S, Relich RF, Doyle L, Espina N, Fuller D, Karchmer T, Lainesse A, Mortensen JE, Pancholi P, Veros W, Harrington SM.** 2016. Multicenter evaluation of BD Max enteric parasite real-time PCR assay for detection of *Giardia duodenalis*, *Cryptosporidium hominis*, *Cryptosporidium parvum*, and *Entamoeba histolytica*. *J Clin Microbiol* **54:**2681–2688.
3. **Mengelle C, Mansuy JM, Prere MF, Grouteau E, Claudet I, Kamar N, Huynh A, Plat G, Benard M, Marty N, Valentin A, Berry A, Izopet J.** 2013. Simultaneous detection of gastrointestinal pathogens with a multiplex Luminex-based molecular assay in stool samples from diarrhoeic patients. *Clin Microbiol Infect* **19:**E458–E465.
4. **Clinical and Laboratory Standards Institute.** 2005. Recovery and identification of parasites from the intestinal tract. Approved guidelines M28-A2, 2nd ed, vol 25. Clinical and Laboratory Standards Institute, Wayne, PA.
5. **Leber A (ed).** 2016. *Clinical Microbiology Procedures Handbook*. ASM Press, Washington, DC.
6. **Garcia LS.** 2016. *Diagnostic Medical Parasitology*, 6th ed. ASM Press, Washington, DC.
7. **Sargeaunt PG, Williams JE.** 1978. Electrophoretic isoenzyme patterns of *Entamoeba histolytica* and *Entamoeba coli*. *Trans R Soc Trop Med Hyg* **72:**164–166.
8. **Ortner S, Clark CG, Binder M, Scheiner O, Wiedermann G, Duchêne M.** 1997. Molecular biology of the hexokinase isoenzyme pattern that distinguishes pathogenic *Entamoeba histolytica* from nonpathogenic *Entamoeba dispar*. *Mol Biochem Parasitol* **86:**85–94.
9. **Diamond LS, Clark CG.** 1993. A redescription of *Entamoeba histolytica* Schaudinn, 1903 (Emended Walker, 1911) separating it from *Entamoeba dispar* Brumpt, 1925. *J Eukaryot Microbiol* **40:**340–344.
10. **Heredia RD, Fonseca JA, López MC.** 2012. *Entamoeba moshkovskii* perspectives of a new agent to be considered in the diagnosis of amebiasis. *Acta Trop* **123:**139–145.
11. **Ali IK, Hossain MB, Roy S, Ayeh-Kumi PF, Petri WA Jr, Haque R, Clark CG.** 2003. *Entamoeba moshkovskii* infections in children, Bangladesh. *Emerg Infect Dis* **9:**580–584.
12. **Clark CG, Diamond LS.** 1991. The Laredo strain and other '*Entamoeba histolytica*-like' amoebae are *Entamoeba moshkovskii*. *Mol Biochem Parasitol* **46:**11–18.
13. **Fotedar R, Stark D, Marriott D, Ellis J, Harkness J.** 2008. *Entamoeba moshkovskii* infections in Sydney, Australia. *Eur J Clin Microbiol Infect Dis* **27:**133–137.
14. **Herbinger KH, Fleischmann E, Weber C, Perona P, Löscher T, Bretzel G.** 2011. Epidemiological, clinical, and diagnostic data on intestinal infections with *Entamoeba histolytica* and *Entamoeba dispar* among returning travelers. *Infection* **39:**527–535.
15. **Shimokawa C, Kabir M, Taniuchi M, Mondal D, Kobayashi S, Ali IK, Sobuz SU, Senba M, Houpt E, Haque R, Petri WA Jr, Hamano S.** 2012. *Entamoeba moshkovskii* is associated with diarrhea in infants and causes diarrhea and colitis in mice. *J Infect Dis* **206:**744–751.
16. **Royer TL, Gilchrist C, Kabir M, Arju T, Ralston KS, Haque R, Clark CG, Petri WA Jr.** 2012. *Entamoeba bangladeshi* nov. sp., Bangladesh. *Emerg Infect Dis* **18:**1543–1544.
17. **World Health Organization.** 1997. Amoebiasis. *Wkly Epidemiol Rec* **72:**97–99.
18. **Fotedar R, Stark D, Beebe N, Marriott D, Ellis J, Harkness J.** 2007. Laboratory diagnostic techniques for *Entamoeba* species. *Clin Microbiol Rev* **20:**511–532.
19. **Ximénez C, Morán P, Rojas L, Valadez A, Gómez A.** 2009. Reassessment of the epidemiology of amebiasis: state of the art. *Infect Genet Evol* **9:**1023–1032.
20. **Walderich B, Weber A, Knobloch J.** 1997. Differentiation of *Entamoeba histolytica* and *Entamoeba dispar* from German travelers and residents of endemic areas. *Am J Trop Med Hyg* **57:**70–74.
21. **Ortega HB, Borchardt KA, Hamilton R, Ortega P, Mahood J.** 1984. Enteric pathogenic protozoa in homosexual men from San Francisco. *Sex Transm Dis* **11:**59–63.
22. **Lowther SA, Dworkin MS, Hanson DL.** 2000. *Entamoeba histolytica/Entamoeba dispar* infections in human

immunodeficiency virus-infected patients in the United States. *Clin Infect Dis* **30:**955–959.

23. **Hung CC, Chen PJ, Hsieh SM, Wong JM, Fang CT, Chang SC, Chen MY.** 1999. Invasive amoebiasis: an emerging parasitic disease in patients infected with HIV in an area endemic for amoebic infection. *AIDS* **13:**2421–2428.
24. **Oh MD, Lee K, Kim E, Lee S, Kim N, Choi H, Choi MH, Chai JY, Choe K.** 2000. Amoebic liver abscess in HIV-infected patients. *AIDS* **14:**1872–1873.
25. **Hung CC, Deng HY, Hsiao WH, Hsieh SM, Hsiao CF, Chen MY, Chang SC, Su KE.** 2005. Invasive amebiasis as an emerging parasitic disease in patients with human immunodeficiency virus type 1 infection in Taiwan. *Arch Intern Med* **165:**409–415.
26. **Wilson M, Schantz P, Pieniazek N.** 1995. Diagnosis of parasitic infections: immunologic and molecular methods, p 1159–1170. *In* Murray PR, Baron EJ, Pfaller MA (ed), *Manual of Clinical Microbiology*, 6th ed. ASM Press, Washington, DC.
27. **Bruckner DA.** 1992. Amebiasis. *Clin Microbiol Rev* **5:**356–369.
28. **Zaki M, Clark CG.** 2001. Isolation and characterization of polymorphic DNA from *Entamoeba histolytica*. *J Clin Microbiol* **39:**897–905.
29. **Espinosa-Cantellano M, Martínez-Palomo A.** 2000. Pathogenesis of intestinal amebiasis: from molecules to disease. *Clin Microbiol Rev* **13:**318–331.
30. **Ralston KS, Petri WA Jr.** 2011. Tissue destruction and invasion by *Entamoeba histolytica*. *Trends Parasitol* **27:**254–263.
31. **Petri WA Jr, Smith RD, Schlesinger PH, Murphy CF, Ravdin JI.** 1987. Isolation of the galactose-binding lectin that mediates the *in vitro* adherence of *Entamoeba histolytica*. *J Clin Invest* **80:**1238–1244.
32. **Kenner BM, Rosen T.** 2006. Cutaneous amebiasis in a child and review of the literature. *Pediatr Dermatol* **23:**231–234.
33. **Magaña ML, Fernández-Díez J, Magaña M.** 2008. Cutaneous amebiasis in pediatrics. *Arch Dermatol* **144:**1369–1372.
34. **Haque R, Neville LM, Hahn P, Petri WA Jr.** 1995. Rapid diagnosis of *Entamoeba* infection by using *Entamoeba* and *Entamoeba histolytica* stool antigen detection kits. *J Clin Microbiol* **33:**2558–2561.
35. **Tanyuksel M, Tachibana H, Petri WA.** 2001. Amebiasis, an emerging disease, p 197–202. *In* Scheld WM, Craig WA, Hughes JM (ed), *Emerging Infections 5*. ASM Press, Washington, DC.
36. **Tanyuksel M, Petri WA Jr.** 2003. Laboratory diagnosis of amebiasis. *Clin Microbiol Rev* **16:**713–729.
37. **Garcia LS, Shimizu RY, Bernard CN.** 2000. Detection of *Giardia lamblia*, *Entamoeba histolytica/Entamoeba dispar*, and *Cryptosporidium parvum* antigens in human fecal specimens using the triage parasite panel enzyme immunoassay. *J Clin Microbiol* **38:**3337–3340.
38. **McHardy IH, Wu M, Shimizu-Cohen R, Couturier MR, Humphries RM.** 2014. Detection of intestinal protozoa in the clinical laboratory. *J Clin Microbiol* **52:**712–720.
39. **Petri WA Jr, Jackson TF, Gathiram V, Kress K, Saffer LD, Snodgrass TL, Chapman MD, Keren Z, Mirelman D.** 1990. Pathogenic and nonpathogenic strains of *Entamoeba histolytica* can be differentiated by monoclonal antibodies to the galactose-specific adherence lectin. *Infect Immun* **58:**1802–1806.
40. **Korpe PS, Stott BR, Nazib F, Kabir M, Haque R, Herbein JF, Petri WA Jr.** 2012. Evaluation of a rapid point-of-care fecal antigen detection test for *Entamoeba histolytica*. *Am J Trop Med Hyg* **86:**980–981.
41. **Verkerke HP, Hanbury B, Siddique A, Samie A, Haque R, Herbein J, Petri WA Jr.** 2015. Multisite clinical evaluation of a rapid test for *Entamoeba histolytica* in stool. *J Clin Microbiol* **53:**493–497.
42. **Ong SJ, Cheng MY, Liu KH, Horng CB.** 1996. Use of the ProSpecT microplate enzyme immunoassay for the detection of pathogenic and non-pathogenic *Entamoeba histolytica* in faecal specimens. *Trans R Soc Trop Med Hyg* **90:**248–249 .
43. **Roy S, Kabir M, Mondal D, Ali IK, Petri WA Jr, Haque R.** 2005. Real-time-PCR assay for diagnosis of *Entamoeba histolytica* infection. *J Clin Microbiol* **43:**2168–2172.
44. **Stark D, van Hal S, Fotedar R, Butcher A, Marriott D, Ellis J, Harkness J.** 2008. Comparison of stool antigen detection kits to PCR for diagnosis of amebiasis. *J Clin Microbiol* **46:**1678–1681.
45. **Yau YC, Crandall I, Kain KC.** 2001. Development of monoclonal antibodies which specifically recognize *Entamoeba histolytica* in preserved stool samples. *J Clin Microbiol* **39:**716–719.
46. **Abd-Alla MD, Jackson TF, Reddy S, Ravdin JI.** 2000. Diagnosis of invasive amebiasis by enzyme-linked immunosorbent assay of saliva to detect amebic lectin antigen and anti-lectin immunoglobulin G antibodies. *J Clin Microbiol* **38:**2344–2347.
47. **Haque R, Mollah NU, Ali IK, Alam K, Eubanks A, Lyerly D, Petri WA Jr.** 2000. Diagnosis of amebic liver abscess and intestinal infection with the TechLab *Entamoeba histolytica* II antigen detection and antibody tests. *J Clin Microbiol* **38:**3235–3239.
48. **Evangelopoulos A, Spanakos G, Patsoula E, Vakalis N, Legakis N.** 2000. A nested, multiplex, PCR assay for the simultaneous detection and differentiation of *Entamoeba histolytica* and *Entamoeba dispar* in faeces. *Ann Trop Med Parasitol* **94:**233–240.
49. **Qvarnstrom Y, James C, Xayavong M, Holloway BP, Visvesvara GS, Sriram R, da Silva AJ.** 2005. Comparison of real-time PCR protocols for differential laboratory diagnosis of amebiasis. *J Clin Microbiol* **43:**5491–5497 .
50. **Rivera WL, Tachibana H, Silva-Tahat MR, Uemura H, Kanbara H.** 1996. Differentiation of *Entamoeba histolytica* and *E. dispar* DNA from cysts present in stool specimens by polymerase chain reaction: its field application in the Philippines. *Parasitol Res* **82:**585–589.
51. **Solaymani-Mohammadi S, Lam MM, Zunt JR, Petri WA Jr.** 2007. *Entamoeba histolytica* encephalitis diagnosed by PCR of cerebrospinal fluid. *Trans R Soc Trop Med Hyg* **101:**311–313.
52. **Zengzhu G, Bracha R, Nuchamowitz Y, Cheng-I W, Mirelman D.** 1999. Analysis by enzyme-linked immunosorbent assay and PCR of human liver abscess aspirates from patients in China for *Entamoeba histolytica*. *J Clin Microbiol* **37:**3034–3036.
53. **Blessmann J, Buss H, Nu PA, Dinh BT, Ngo QT, Van AL, Alla MD, Jackson TF, Ravdin JI, Tannich E.** 2002. Real-time PCR for detection and differentiation of *Entamoeba histolytica* and *Entamoeba dispar* in fecal samples. *J Clin Microbiol* **40:**4413–4417.
54. **Haque R, Kabir M, Noor Z, Rahman SM, Mondal D, Alam F, Rahman I, Al Mahmood A, Ahmed N, Petri WA Jr.** 2010. Diagnosis of amebic liver abscess and amebic colitis by detection of *Entamoeba histolytica* DNA in blood, urine, and saliva by a real-time PCR assay. *J Clin Microbiol* **48:**2798–2801.
55. **Khairnar K, Parija SC.** 2007. A novel nested multiplex polymerase chain reaction (PCR) assay for differential detection of *Entamoeba histolytica*, *E. moshkovskii* and *E. dispar* DNA in stool samples. *BMC Microbiol* **7:**47.
56. **Santos HL, Bandyopadhyay K, Bandea R, Peralta RH, Peralta JM, Da Silva AJ.** 2013. LUMINEX®: a new technology for the simultaneous identification of five *Entamoeba* spp. commonly found in human stools. *Parasit Vectors* **6:**69.
57. **Verweij JJ, Blangé RA, Templeton K, Schinkel J, Brienen EA, van Rooyen MA, van Lieshout L, Polderman AM.** 2004. Simultaneous detection of *Entamoeba histolytica*, *Giardia lamblia*, and *Cryptosporidium parvum* in fecal samples by using multiplex real-time PCR. *J Clin Microbiol* **42:**1220–1223.
58. **Stark D, Al-Qassab SE, Barratt JL, Stanley K, Roberts T, Marriott D, Harkness J, Ellis JT.** 2011. Evaluation of multiplex tandem real-time PCR for detection of *Cryptosporidium* spp., *Dientamoeba fragilis*, *Entamoeba histolytica*, and *Giardia intestinalis* in clinical stool samples. *J Clin Microbiol* **49:**257–262.
59. **Johnson LR, Starkey CR, Palmer J, Taylor J, Stout S, Holt S, Hendren R, Bock B, Waibel E, Tyree G, Miller GC.** 2008. A comparison of two methods to determine the presence of high-risk HPV cervical infections. *Am J Clin Pathol* **130:**401–408.
60. **Buss SN, Alter R, Iwen PC, Fey PD.** 2013. Implications of culture-independent panel-based detection of *Cyclospora cayetanensis*. *J Clin Microbiol* **51:**3909.
61. **Haque R, Ali IK, Akther S, Petri WA Jr.** 1998. Comparison of PCR, isoenzyme analysis, and antigen detection for diagnosis of *Entamoeba histolytica* infection. *J Clin Microbiol* **36:**449–452.

62. **Paglia MG, Visca P.** 2004. An improved PCR-based method for detection and differentiation of *Entamoeba histolytica* and *Entamoeba dispar* in formalin-fixed stools. *Acta Trop* **92:**273–277.
63. **Troll H, Marti H, Weiss N.** 1997. Simple differential detection of *Entamoeba histolytica* and *Entamoeba dispar* in fresh stool specimens by sodium acetate-acetic acid-formalin concentration and PCR. *J Clin Microbiol* **35:**1701–1705.
64. **Verweij JJ, Blotkamp J, Brienen EA, Aguirre A, Polderman AM.** 2000. Differentiation of *Entamoeba histolytica* and *Entamoeba dispar* cysts using polymerase chain reaction on DNA isolated from faeces with spin columns. *Eur J Clin Microbiol Infect Dis* **19:**358–361.
65. **Monteiro L, Bonnemaison D, Vekris A, Petry KG, Bonnet J, Vidal R, Cabrita J, Mégraud F.** 1997. Complex polysaccharides as PCR inhibitors in feces: *Helicobacter pylori* model. *J Clin Microbiol* **35:**995–998.
66. **Joyce MP, Ravdin JI.** 1988. Antigens of *Entamoeba histolytica* recognized by immune sera from liver abscess patients. *Am J Trop Med Hyg* **38:**74–80.
67. **Haque R, Ikm A, Petri WA Jr.** 2000. Salivary antilectin IgA antibodies in a cohort of children residing in an endemic area of Bangladesh. *Arch Med Res* **31**(Suppl)**:**S41–S43.
68. **Stanley SL Jr.** 2001. Protective immunity to amebiasis: new insights and new challenges. *J Infect Dis* **184:**504–506.
69. **The Medical Letter.** 2013. *Drugs for Parasitic Infections*, 3rd ed. The Medical Letter, New Rochelle, NY.
70. **Upcroft P, Upcroft JA.** 2001. Drug targets and mechanisms of resistance in the anaerobic protozoa. *Clin Microbiol Rev* **14:**150–164.
71. **Cavalier-Smith T.** 1998. A revised six-kingdom system of life. *Biol Rev Camb Philos Soc* **73:**203–266.
72. **Silberman JD, Sogin ML, Leipe DD, Clark CG.** 1996. Human parasite finds taxonomic home. *Nature* **380:**398.
73. **Arisue N, Hashimoto T, Yoshikawa H, Nakamura Y, Nakamura G, Nakamura F, Yano TA, Hasegawa M.** 2002. Phylogenetic position of *Blastocystis hominis* and of stramenopiles inferred from multiple molecular sequence data. *J Eukaryot Microbiol* **49:**42–53.
74. **Hoevers JD, Snowden KF.** 2005. Analysis of the ITS region and partial *ssu* and *lsu* rRNA genes of *Blastocystis* and *Proteromonas lacertae*. *Parasitology* **131:**187–196.
75. **Tan KS.** 2008. New insights on classification, identification, and clinical relevance of *Blastocystis* spp. *Clin Microbiol Rev* **21:**639–665.
76. **Clark CG.** 1997. Extensive genetic diversity in *Blastocystis hominis*. *Mol Biochem Parasitol* **87:**79–83.
77. **Mansour NS, Mikhail EM, el Masry NA, Sabry AG, Mohareb EW.** 1995. Biochemical characterisation of human isolates of *Blastocystis hominis*. *J Med Microbiol* **42:**304–307.
78. **Noël C, Dufernez F, Gerbod D, Edgcomb VP, Delgado-Viscogliosi P, Ho LC, Singh M, Wintjens R, Sogin ML, Capron M, Pierce R, Zenner L, Viscogliosi E.** 2005. Molecular phylogenies of *Blastocystis* isolates from different hosts: implications for genetic diversity, identification of species, and zoonosis. *J Clin Microbiol* **43:**348–355.
79. **Moe KT, Singh M, Howe J, Ho LC, Tan SW, Ng GC, Chen XQ, Yap EH.** 1996. Observations on the ultrastructure and viability of the cystic stage of *Blastocystis hominis* from human feces. *Parasitol Res* **82:**439–444.
80. **Scanlan PD, Knight R, Song SJ, Ackermann G, Cotter PD.** 2016. Prevalence and genetic diversity of *Blastocystis* in family units living in the United States. *Infect Genet Evol* **45:**95–97.
81. **Leelayoova S, Rangsin R, Taamasri P, Naaglor T, Thathaisong U, Mungthin M.** 2004. Evidence of waterborne transmission of *Blastocystis hominis*. *Am J Trop Med Hyg* **70:**658–662.
82. **Yoshikawa H, Abe N, Iwasawa M, Kitano S, Nagano I, Wu Z, Takahashi Y.** 2000. Genomic analysis of *Blastocystis hominis* strains isolated from two long-term health care facilities. *J Clin Microbiol* **38:**1324–1330.
83. **Markell EK, Udkow MP.** 1986. Blastocystis hominis: pathogen or fellow traveler? *Am J Trop Med Hyg* **35:**1023–1026.
84. **Sheehan DJ, Raucher BG, McKitrick JC.** 1986. Association of *Blastocystis hominis* with signs and symptoms of human disease. *J Clin Microbiol* **24:**548–550.
85. **Zierdt CH.** 1991. *Blastocystis hominis*: past and future. *Clin Microbiol Rev* **4:**61–79.
86. **Yan Y, Su S, Lai R, Liao H, Ye J, Li X, Luo X, Chen G.** 2006. Genetic variability of *Blastocystis hominis* isolates in China. *Parasitol Res* **99:**597–601.
87. **Gentekaki E, Curtis BA, Stairs CW, Klimeš V, Eliáš M, Salas-Leiva DE, Herman EK, Eme L, Arias MC, Henrissat B, Hilliou F, Klute MJ, Suga H, Malik SB, Pightling AW, Kolisko M, Rachubinski RA, Schlacht A, Soanes DM, Tsaousis AD, Archibald JM, Ball SG, Dacks JB, Clark CG, van der Giezen M, Roger AJ.** 2017. Extreme genome diversity in the hyper-prevalent parasitic eukaryote *Blastocystis*. *PLoS Biol* **15:**e2003769.
88. **Beghini F, Pasolli E, Truong TD, Putignani L, Cacciò SM, Segata N.** 2017. Large-scale comparative metagenomics of *Blastocystis*, a common member of the human gut microbiome. *ISME J* **11:**2848–2863.
89. **Stensvold CR, Clark CG.** 2016. Current status of *Blastocystis*: a personal view. *Parasitol Int* **65**(6 Pt B)**:**763–771.
90. **Horiki N, Kaneda Y, Maruyama M, Fujita Y, Tachibana H.** 1999. Intestinal blockage by carcinoma and *Blastocystis hominis* infection. *Am J Trop Med Hyg* **60:**400–402.
91. **Udkow MP, Markell EK.** 1993. *Blastocystis hominis*: prevalence in asymptomatic versus symptomatic hosts. *J Infect Dis* **168:**242–244.
92. **Albrecht H, Stellbrink HJ, Koperskl K, Greten H.** 1995. *Blastocystis hominis* in human immunodeficiency virus-related diarrhea. *Scand J Gastroenterol* **30:**909–914.
93. **Poirier P, Wawrzyniak I, Albert A, El Alaoui H, Delbac F, Livrelli V.** 2011. Development and evaluation of a real-time PCR assay for detection and quantification of *Blastocystis* parasites in human stool samples: prospective study of patients with hematological malignancies. *J Clin Microbiol* **49:**975–983.
94. **Yaicharoen R, Ngrenngarmlert W, Wongjindanon N, Sripochang S, Kiatfuengfoo R.** 2006. Infection of *Blastocystis hominis* in primary schoolchildren from Nakhon Pathom province, Thailand. *Trop Biomed* **23:**117–122.
95. **Garavelli PL, Zierdt CH, Fleisher TA, Liss H, Nagy B.** 1995. Serum antibody detected by fluorescent antibody test in patients with symptomatic *Blastocystis hominis* infection. *Recenti Prog Med* **86:**398–400.
96. **Zierdt CH, Zierdt WS, Nagy B.** 1995. Enzyme-linked immunosorbent assay for detection of serum antibody to *Blastocystis hominis* in symptomatic infections. *J Parasitol* **81:**127–129.
97. **Kaneda Y, Horiki N, Cheng X, Tachibana H, Tsutsumi Y.** 2000. Serologic response to *Blastocystis hominis* infection in asymptomatic individuals. *Tokai J Exp Clin Med* **25:**51–56.
98. **Centers for Disease Control and Prevention.** 2017. DPDx - laboratory identification of parasitic disease of public health concern: *Blastocystis hominis*. https://www.cdc.gov/dpdx/blastocystis/index.html. Accessed 28 October 2017.
99. **Haresh K, Suresh K, Khairul Anuar A, Saminathan S.** 1999. Isolate resistance of *Blastocystis hominis* to metronidazole. *Trop Med Int Health* **4:**274–277.
100. **Yakoob J, Jafri W, Jafri N, Islam M, Asim Beg M.** 2004. *In vitro* susceptibility of *Blastocystis hominis* isolated from patients with irritable bowel syndrome. *Br J Biomed Sci* **61:** 75–77.
101. **Feng Y, Xiao L.** 2011. Zoonotic potential and molecular epidemiology of *Giardia* species and giardiasis. *Clin Microbiol Rev* **24:**110–140.
102. **Guy RA, Xiao C, Horgen PA.** 2004. Real-time PCR assay for detection and genotype differentiation of *Giardia lamblia* in stool specimens. *J Clin Microbiol* **42:**3317–3320.
103. **Rendtorff RC.** 1978. The experimental transmission of *Giardia lamblia* among volunteer subjects, p 64–81. *In* Jacubowski W, Hoff W (ed), *Waterborne Transmission of Giardiasis 1978*. EPA 600/9-79-001. U.S. Environmental Protection Agency, Washington, DC.
104. **Panosian CB.** 1988. Parasitic diarrhea. *Infect Dis Clin North Am* **2:**685–703.
105. **Olson ME, Ceri H, Morck DW.** 2000. Giardia vaccination. *Parasitol Today* **16:**213–217.

106. **Monis PT, Andrews RH, Mayrhofer G, Ey PL.** 1999. Molecular systematics of the parasitic protozoan *Giardia intestinalis*. *Mol Biol Evol* **16:**1135–1144.
107. **Paintlia AS, Descoteaux S, Spencer B, Chakraborti A, Ganguly NK, Mahajan RC, Samuelson J.** 1998. *Giardia lamblia* groups A and B among young adults in India. *Clin Infect Dis* **26:**190–191.
108. **Paintlia AS, Paintlia MK, Mahajan RC, Chakraborti A, Ganguly NK.** 1999. A DNA-based probe for differentiation of *Giardia lamblia* group A and B isolates from northern India. *Clin Infect Dis* **28:**1178–1180.
109. **Carroccio A, Montalto G, Iacono G, Ippolito S, Soresi M, Notarbartolo A.** 1997. Secondary impairment of pancreatic function as a cause of severe malabsorption in intestinal giardiasis: a case report. *Am J Trop Med Hyg* **56:**599–602.
110. **Zylberberg HM, Green PH, Turner KO, Genta RM, Lebwohl B.** 2017. Prevalence and predictors of giardia in the United States. *Dig Dis Sci* **62:**432–440.
111. **Hanevik K, Wensaas KA, Rortveit G, Eide GE, Mørch K, Langeland N.** 2014. Irritable bowel syndrome and chronic fatigue 6 years after *Giardia* infection: a controlled prospective cohort study. *Clin Infect Dis* **59:**1394–1400.
112. **Platts-Mills JA, Babji S, Bodhidatta L, Gratz J, Haque R, Havt A, McCormick BJ, McGrath M, Olortegui MP, Samie A, Shakoor S, Mondal D, Lima IF, Hariraju D, Rayamajhi BB, Qureshi S, Kabir F, Yori PP, Mufamadi B, Amour C, Carreon JD, Richard SA, Lang D, Bessong P, Mduma E, Ahmed T, Lima AA, Mason CJ, Zaidi AK, Bhutta ZA, Kosek M, Guerrant RL, Gottlieb M, Miller M, Kang G, Houpt ER, MAL-ED Network Investigators.** 2015. Pathogen-specific burdens of community diarrhoea in developing countries: a multisite birth cohort study (MAL-ED). *Lancet Glob Health* **3:**e564–e575.
113. **Donowitz JR, Alam M, Kabir M, Ma JZ, Nazib F, Platts-Mills JA, Bartelt LA, Haque R, Petri WA Jr.** 2016. A prospective longitudinal cohort to investigate the effects of early life giardiasis on growth and all cause diarrhea. *Clin Infect Dis* **63:**792–797.
114. **Kotloff KL, Nataro JP, Blackwelder WC, Nasrin D, Farag TH, Panchalingam S, Wu Y, Sow SO, Sur D, Breiman RF, Faruque AS, Zaidi AK, Saha D, Alonso PL, Tamboura B, Sanogo D, Onwuchekwa U, Manna B, Ramamurthy T, Kanungo S, Ochieng JB, Omore R, Oundo JO, Hossain A, Das SK, Ahmed S, Qureshi S, Quadri F, Adegbola RA, Antonio M, Hossain MJ, Akinsola A, Mandomando I, Nhampossa T, Acácio S, Biswas K, O'Reilly CE, Mintz ED, Berkeley LY, Muhsen K, Sommerfelt H, Robins-Browne RM, Levine MM.** 2013. Burden and aetiology of diarrhoeal disease in infants and young children in developing countries (the Global Enteric Multicenter Study, GEMS): a prospective, case-control study. *Lancet* **382:**209–222.
115. **Hanevik K.** 2016. Editorial commentary: *Giardia lamblia*: pathogen or commensal? *Clin Infect Dis* **63:**798–799.
116. **Soares R, Tasca T.** 2016. Giardiasis: an update review on sensitivity and specificity of methods for laboratorial diagnosis. *J Microbiol Methods* **129:**98–102.
117. **Garcia LS, Shimizu RY.** 1997. Evaluation of nine immunoassay kits (enzyme immunoassay and direct fluorescence) for detection of *Giardia lamblia* and *Cryptosporidium parvum* in human fecal specimens. *J Clin Microbiol* **35:**1526–1529.
118. **Johnston SP, Ballard MM, Beach MJ, Causer L, Wilkins PP.** 2003. Evaluation of three commercial assays for detection of *Giardia* and *Cryptosporidium* organisms in fecal specimens. *J Clin Microbiol* **41:**623–626.
119. **Katanik MT, Schneider SK, Rosenblatt JE, Hall GS, Procop GW.** 2001. Evaluation of ColorPAC *Giardia/Cryptosporidium* rapid assay and ProSpecT *Giardia/Cryptosporidium* microplate assay for detection of *Giardia* and *Cryptosporidium* in fecal specimens. *J Clin Microbiol* **39:**4523–4525.
120. **Maraha B, Bonten M, Fiolet H, Stobberingh E.** 2000. The impact of microbiological cultures on antibiotic prescribing in general internal medicine wards: microbiological evaluation and antibiotic use. *Clin Microbiol Infect* **6:**99–102.
121. **Youn S, Kabir M, Haque R, Petri WA Jr.** 2009. Evaluation of a screening test for detection of *Giardia* and *Cryptosporidium* parasites. *J Clin Microbiol* **47:**451–452.
122. **Goñi P, Martín B, Villacampa M, García A, Seral C, Castillo FJ, Clavel A.** 2012. Evaluation of an immunochromatographic dip strip test for simultaneous detection of *Cryptosporidium* spp, *Giardia duodenalis*, and *Entamoeba histolytica* antigens in human faecal samples. *Eur J Clin Microbiol Infect Dis* **31:**2077–2082.
123. **Garcia LS, Shimizu RY.** 2000. Detection of *Giardia lamblia* and *Cryptosporidium parvum* antigens in human fecal specimens using the ColorPAC combination rapid solid-phase qualitative immunochromatographic assay. *J Clin Microbiol* **38:**1267–1268.
124. **Maraha B, Buiting AG.** 2000. Evaluation of four enzyme immunoassays for the detection of *Giardia lamblia* antigen in stool specimens. *Eur J Clin Microbiol Infect Dis* **19:**485–487 .
125. **Garcia LS, Garcia JP.** 2006. Detection of *Giardia lamblia* antigens in human fecal specimens by a solid-phase qualitative immunochromatographic assay. *J Clin Microbiol* **44:**4587–4588.
126. **Christy NC, Hencke JD, Escueta-De CA, Nazib F, von Thien H, Yagita K, Ligaba S, Haque R, Nozaki T, Tannich E, Herbein JF, Petri WA, Jr.** 2012. Multisite performance evaluation of an enzyme-linked immunosorbent assay for detection of *Giardia*, *Cryptosporidium*, and *Entamoeba histolytica* antigens in human stool. *J Clin Microbiol* **50:**1762–1763.
127. **Hanson KL, Cartwright CP.** 2001. Use of an enzyme immunoassay does not eliminate the need to analyze multiple stool specimens for sensitive detection of *Giardia lamblia*. *J Clin Microbiol* **39:**474–477.
128. **Garcia LS, Shimizu RY, Novak S, Carroll M, Chan F.** 2003. Commercial assay for detection of *Giardia lamblia* and *Cryptosporidium parvum* antigens in human fecal specimens by rapid solid-phase qualitative immunochromatography. *J Clin Microbiol* **41:**209–212.
129. **Pillai DR, Kain KC.** 1999. Immunochromatographic strip-based detection of *Entamoeba histolytica-E. dispar* and *Giardia lamblia* coproantigen. *J Clin Microbiol* **37:**3017–3019.
130. **Sharp SE, Suarez CA, Duran Y, Poppiti RJ.** 2001. Evaluation of the Triage Micro Parasite Panel for detection of *Giardia lamblia*, *Entamoeba histolytica/Entamoeba dispar*, and *Cryptosporidium parvum* in patient stool specimens. *J Clin Microbiol* **39:**332–334.
131. **Minak J, Kabir M, Mahmud I, Liu Y, Liu L, Haque R, Petri WA Jr.** 2012. Evaluation of rapid antigen point-of-care tests for detection of *Giardia* and *Cryptosporidium* species in human fecal specimens. *J Clin Microbiol* **50:**154–156.
132. **Amar CF, Dear PH, Pedraza-Díaz S, Looker N, Linnane E, McLauchlin J.** 2002. Sensitive PCR-restriction fragment length polymorphism assay for detection and genotyping of *Giardia duodenalis* in human feces. *J Clin Microbiol* **40:**446–452.
133. **Nantavisai K, Mungthin M, Tan-ariya P, Rangsin R, Naaglor T, Leelayoova S.** 2007. Evaluation of the sensitivities of DNA extraction and PCR methods for detection of *Giardia duodenalis* in stool specimens. *J Clin Microbiol* **45:**581–583.
134. **Claas EC, Burnham CA, Mazzulli T, Templeton K, Topin F.** 2013. Performance of the xTAG® gastrointestinal pathogen panel, a multiplex molecular assay for simultaneous detection of bacterial, viral, and parasitic causes of infectious gastroenteritis. *J Microbiol Biotechnol* **23:**1041–1045.
135. **Zebardast N, Yeganeh F, Gharavi MJ, Abadi A, Seyyed Tabaei SJ, Haghighi A.** 2016. Simultaneous detection and differentiation of *Entamoeba histolytica*, *E. dispar*, *E. moshkovskii*, *Giardia lamblia* and *Cryptosporidium* spp. in human fecal samples using multiplex PCR and qPCR-MCA. *Acta Trop* **162:**233–238.
136. **Batra R, Judd E, Eling J, Newsholme W, Goldenberg SD.** 2016. Molecular detection of common intestinal parasites: a performance evaluation of the BD Max™ enteric parasite panel. *Eur J Clin Microbiol Infect Dis* **35:**1753–1757.
137. **Albert MJ, Rotimi VO, Iqbal J, Chehadeh W.** 2016. Evaluation of the xTAG gastrointestinal pathogen panel assay for the detection of enteric pathogens in Kuwait. *Med Princ Pract* **25:**472–476.

138. **Wessels E, Rusman LG, van Bussel MJ, Claas EC.** 2014. Added value of multiplex Luminex gastrointestinal pathogen panel (xTAG® GPP) testing in the diagnosis of infectious gastroenteritis. *Clin Microbiol Infect* **20:**O182–O187.
139. **Mölling P, Nilsson P, Ennefors T, Ögren J, Florén K, Thulin Hedberg S, Sundqvist M.** 2016. Evaluation of the BD Max enteric parasite panel for clinical diagnostics. *J Clin Microbiol* **54:**443–444.
140. **Perry MD, Corden SA, Lewis White P.** 2017. Evaluation of the BD MAX enteric parasite panel for the detection of *Cryptosporidium parvum/hominis, Giardia duodenalis* and *Entamoeba histolytica. J Med Microbiol* **66:**1118–1123.
141. **Perry MD, Corden SA, Howe RA.** 2014. Evaluation of the Luminex xTAG gastrointestinal pathogen panel and the Savyon diagnostics gastrointestinal infection panel for the detection of enteric pathogens in clinical samples. *J Med Microbiol* **63:**1419–1426.
142. **Wang Z, Vora GJ, Stenger DA.** 2004. Detection and genotyping of *Entamoeba histolytica, Entamoeba dispar, Giardia lamblia,* and *Cryptosporidium parvum* by oligonucleotide microarray. *J Clin Microbiol* **42:**3262–3271.
143. **Rochelle PA, De Leon R, Stewart MH, Wolfe RL.** 1997. Comparison of primers and optimization of PCR conditions for detection of *Cryptosporidium parvum* and *Giardia lamblia* in water. *Appl Environ Microbiol* **63:**106–114.
144. **Weiss JB.** 1995. DNA probes and PCR for diagnosis of parasitic infections. *Clin Microbiol Rev* **8:**113–130.
145. **Gardner TB, Hill DR.** 2001. Treatment of giardiasis. *Clin Microbiol Rev* **14:**114–128.
146. **Marshall MM, Naumovitz D, Ortega Y, Sterling CR.** 1997. Waterborne protozoan pathogens. *Clin Microbiol Rev* **10:**67–85.
147. **Sousa MC, Poiares-Da-Silva J.** 1999. A new method for assessing metronidazole susceptibility of *Giardia lamblia* trophozoites. *Antimicrob Agents Chemother* **43:**2939–2942.
148. **Stark D, Barratt J, Chan D, Ellis JT.** 2016. *Dientamoeba fragilis,* the neglected trichomonad of the human bowel. *Clin Microbiol Rev* **29:**553–580.
149. **Gerbod D, Edgcomb VP, Noël C, Zenner L, Wintjens R, Delgado-Viscogliosi P, Holder ME, Sogin ML, Viscogliosi E.** 2001. Phylogenetic position of the trichomonad parasite of turkeys, *Histomonas meleagridis* (Smith) Tyzzer, inferred from small subunit rRNA sequence. *J Eukaryot Microbiol* **48:**498–504.
150. **Silberman JD, Clark CG, Sogin ML.** 1996. *Dientamoeba fragilis* shares a recent common evolutionary history with the trichomonads. *Mol Biochem Parasitol* **76:**311–314.
151. **Stark D, Garcia LS, Barratt JL, Phillips O, Roberts T, Marriott D, Harkness J, Ellis JT.** 2014. Description of *Dientamoeba fragilis* cyst and precystic forms from human samples. *J Clin Microbiol* **52:**2680–2683.
152. **Munasinghe VS, Vella NG, Ellis JT, Windsor PA, Stark D.** 2013. Cyst formation and faecal-oral transmission of *Dientamoeba fragilis*: the missing link in the life cycle of an emerging pathogen. *Int J Parasitol* **43:**879–883.
153. **Burrows RB, Swerdlow MA.** 1956. *Enterobius vermicularis* as a probable vector of *Dientamoeba fragilis. Am J Trop Med Hyg* **5:**258–265.
154. **Johnson EH, Windsor JJ, Clark CG.** 2004. Emerging from obscurity: biological, clinical, and diagnostic aspects of *Dientamoeba fragilis. Clin Microbiol Rev* **17:**553–570.
155. **Ögren J, Dienus O, Löfgren S, Iveroth P, Matussek A.** 2013. *Dientamoeba fragilis* DNA detection in *Enterobius vermicularis* eggs. *Pathog Dis* **69:**157–158.
156. **Röser D, Nejsum P, Carlsgart AJ, Nielsen HV, Stensvold CR.** 2013. DNA of *Dientamoeba fragilis* detected within surface-sterilized eggs of *Enterobius vermicularis. Exp Parasitol* **133:**57–61.
157. **Clark CG, Röser D, Stensvold CR.** 2014. Transmission of *Dientamoeba fragilis*: pinworm or cysts? *Trends Parasitol* **30:**136–140.
158. **Yang J, Scholten T.** 1977. *Dientamoeba fragilis*: a review with notes on its epidemiology, pathogenicity, mode of transmission, and diagnosis. *Am J Trop Med Hyg* **26:**16–22.
159. **Johnson JA, Clark CG.** 2000. Cryptic genetic diversity in *Dientamoeba fragilis. J Clin Microbiol* **38:**4653–4654.
160. **Peek R, Reedeker FR, van Gool T.** 2004. Direct amplification and genotyping of *Dientamoeba fragilis* from human stool specimens. *J Clin Microbiol* **42:**631–635.
161. **Butler WP.** 1996. *Dientamoeba fragilis.* An unusual intestinal pathogen. *Dig Dis Sci* **41:**1811–1813.
162. **Schure JM, de Vries M, Weel JF, van Roon EN, Faber TE.** 2013. Symptoms and treatment of *Dientamoeba fragilis* infection in children, a retrospective study. *Pediatr Infect Dis J* **32:**e148–e150.
163. **Talis B, Stein B, Lengy J.** 1971. *Dientamoeba fragilis* in human feces and bile. *Isr J Med Sci* **7:**1063–1069.
164. **Cuffari C, Oligny L, Seidman EG.** 1998. *Dientamoeba fragilis* masquerading as allergic colitis. *J Pediatr Gastroenterol Nutr* **26:**16–20.
165. **Lainson R, da Silva BA.** 1999. Intestinal parasites of some diarrhoeic HIV-seropositive individuals in North Brazil, with particular reference to *Isospora belli* Wenyon, 1923 and *Dientamoeba fragilis* Jepps & Dobell, 1918. *Mem Inst Oswaldo Cruz* **94:**611–613.
166. **Schwartz MD, Nelson ME.** 2003. *Dientamoeba fragilis* infection presenting to the emergency department as acute appendicitis. *J Emerg Med* **25:**17–21.
167. **Gray TJ, Kwan YL, Phan T, Robertson G, Cheong EY, Gottlieb T.** 2013. *Dientamoeba fragilis*: a family cluster of disease associated with marked peripheral eosinophilia. *Clin Infect Dis* **57:**845–848.
168. **Chan F, Stewart N, Guan M, Robb I, Fuite L, Chan I, Diaz-Mitoma F, King J, MacDonald N, Mackenzie A.** 1996. Prevalence of *Dientamoeba fragilis* antibodies in children and recognition of a 39 kDa immunodominant protein antigen of the organism. *Eur J Clin Microbiol Infect Dis* **15:**950–954 .
169. **Chan FT, Guan MX, Mackenzie AM.** 1993. Application of indirect immunofluorescence to detection of *Dientamoeba fragilis* trophozoites in fecal specimens. *J Clin Microbiol* **31:**1710–1714.
170. **Stark D, Beebe N, Marriott D, Ellis J, Harkness J.** 2005. Detection of *Dientamoeba fragilis* in fresh stool specimens using PCR. *Int J Parasitol* **35:**57–62.
171. **Stark D, Beebe N, Marriott D, Ellis J, Harkness J.** 2006. Evaluation of three diagnostic methods, including real-time PCR, for detection of *Dientamoeba fragilis* in stool specimens. *J Clin Microbiol* **44:**232–235.
172. **Calderaro A, Gorrini C, Montecchini S, Peruzzi S, Piccolo G, Rossi S, Gargiulo F, Manca N, Dettori G, Chezzi C.** 2010. Evaluation of a real-time polymerase chain reaction assay for the laboratory diagnosis of giardiasis. *Diagn Microbiol Infect Dis* **66:**261–267.
173. **Stark D, Roberts T, Ellis JT, Marriott D, Harkness J.** 2014. Evaluation of the EasyScreen™ enteric parasite detection kit for the detection of *Blastocystis* spp., *Cryptosporidium* spp., *Dientamoeba fragilis, Entamoeba* complex, and *Giardia intestinalis* from clinical stool samples. *Diagn Microbiol Infect Dis* **78:**149–152.
174. **Anonymous.** 2010. Treatment Guidelines from Medical Letter: Drugs for Parasitic Infections, vol 8 (Suppl).
175. **Centers for Disease Control and Prevention.** 2017. Trichomoniasis treatment and care. https://www.cdc.gov/std/trichomonas/treatment.htm. Accessed 28 October 2017.
176. **Girginkardeşler N, Coşkun S, Cüneyt Balcioğlu I, Ertan P, Ok UZ.** 2003. *Dientamoeba fragilis,* a neglected cause of diarrhea, successfully treated with secnidazole. *Clin Microbiol Infect* **9:**110–113.
177. **Röser D, Simonsen J, Stensvold CR, Olsen KE, Bytzer P, Nielsen HV, Mølbak K.** 2014. Metronidazole therapy for treating dientamoebiasis in children is not associated with better clinical outcomes: a randomized, double-blinded and placebo-controlled clinical trial. *Clin Infect Dis* **58:** 1692–1699.
178. **Poole DN, McClelland RS.** 2013. Global epidemiology of *Trichomonas vaginalis. Sex Transm Infect* **89:**418–422 (Erratum, **90:**75.)
179. **Schwebke JR, Hook EW III.** 2003. High rates of *Trichomonas vaginalis* among men attending a sexually transmitted diseases clinic: implications for screening and urethritis management. *J Infect Dis* **188:**465–468.

180. **Munson KL, Napierala M, Munson E, Schell RF, Kramme T, Miller C, Hryciuk JE.** 2013. Screening of male patients for *Trichomonas vaginalis* with transcription-mediated amplification in a community with a high prevalence of sexually transmitted infection. *J Clin Microbiol* **51:**101–104 .
181. **Andrea SB, Chapin KC.** 2011. Comparison of Aptima *Trichomonas vaginalis* transcription-mediated amplification assay and BD affirm VPIII for detection of *T. vaginalis* in symptomatic women: performance parameters and epidemiological implications. *J Clin Microbiol* **49:**866–869.
182. **Ginocchio CC, Chapin K, Smith JS, Aslanzadeh J, Snook J, Hill CS, Gaydos CA.** 2012. Prevalence of *Trichomonas vaginalis* and coinfection with *Chlamydia trachomatis* and *Neisseria gonorrhoeae* in the United States as determined by the Aptima *Trichomonas vaginalis* nucleic acid amplification assay. *J Clin Microbiol* **50:**2601–2608.
183. **Stark JR, Judson G, Alderete JF, Mundodi V, Kucknoor AS, Giovannucci EL, Platz EA, Sutcliffe S, Fall K, Kurth T, Ma J, Stampfer MJ, Mucci LA.** 2009. Prospective study of *Trichomonas vaginalis* infection and prostate cancer incidence and mortality: Physicians' Health Study. *J Natl Cancer Inst* **101:**1406–1411.
184. **Sutcliffe S, Giovannucci E, Alderete JF, Chang TH, Gaydos CA, Zenilman JM, De Marzo AM, Willett WC, Platz EA.** 2006. Plasma antibodies against *Trichomonas vaginalis* and subsequent risk of prostate cancer. *Cancer Epidemiol Biomarkers Prev* **15:**939–945.
185. **Mitteregger D, Aberle SW, Makristathis A, Walochnik J, Brozek W, Marberger M, Kramer G.** 2012. High detection rate of *Trichomonas vaginalis* in benign hyperplastic prostatic tissue. *Med Microbiol Immunol (Berl)* **201:**113–116.
186. **Neace CJ, Alderete JF.** 2013. Epitopes of the highly immunogenic *Trichomonas vaginalis* α-actinin are serodiagnostic targets for both women and men. *J Clin Microbiol* **51:** 2483–2490.
187. **Schwebke JR, Burgess D.** 2004. Trichomoniasis. *Clin Microbiol Rev* **17:**794–803.
188. **Cotch MF, Pastorek JG II, Nugent RP, Yerg DE, Martin DH, Eschenbach DA, The Vaginal Infections and Prematurity Study Group.** 1991. Demographic and behavioral predictors of *Trichomonas vaginalis* infection among pregnant women. *Obstet Gynecol* **78:**1087–1092.
189. **Minkoff H, Grunebaum AN, Schwarz RH, Feldman J, Cummings M, Crombleholme W, Clark L, Pringle G, McCormack WM.** 1984. Risk factors for prematurity and premature rupture of membranes: a prospective study of the vaginal flora in pregnancy. *Am J Obstet Gynecol* **150:** 965–972.
190. **Soper DE, Bump RC, Hurt WG.** 1990. Bacterial vaginosis and Trichomoniasis vaginitis are risk factors for cuff cellulitis after abdominal hysterectomy. *Am J Obstet Gynecol* **163:**1016–1021; discussion 1021–1013.
191. **Peterman TA, Tian LH, Metcalf CA, Malotte CK, Paul SM, Douglas JM Jr, RESPECT-2 Study Group.** 2009. Persistent, undetected *Trichomonas vaginalis* infections? *Clin Infect Dis* **48:**259–260.
192. **Jackson DJ, Rakwar JP, Bwayo JJ, Kreiss JK, Moses S.** 1997. Urethral *Trichomonas vaginalis* infection and HIV-1 transmission. *Lancet* **350:**1076.
193. **Laga M, Manoka A, Kivuvu M, Malele B, Tuliza M, Nzila N, Goeman J, Behets F, Batter V, Alary M, Heyward WL, Ryder RW, Piot P.** 1993. Non-ulcerative sexually transmitted diseases as risk factors for HIV-1 transmission in women: results from a cohort study. *AIDS* **7:**95–102.
194. **Hobbs MM, Kazembe P, Reed AW, Miller WC, Nakata E, Zimba D, Daly CC, Chakraborty H, Cohen MS, Hoffman I.** 1999. *Trichomonas vaginalis* as a cause of urethritis in Malawian men. *Sex Transm Dis* **26:**381–387.
195. **Mississippi State Medical Association.** 2015. Sexually transmitted diseases: summary of 2015 CDC treatment guidelines. *J Miss State Med Assoc* **56:**372–375.
196. **Munson KL, Napierala M, Munson E.** 2016. Suboptimal *Trichomonas vaginalis* antigen test performance in a low-prevalence sexually transmitted infection community. *J Clin Microbiol* **54:**500–501.
197. **McLaren LC, Davis LE, Healy GR, James CG.** 1983. Isolation of *Trichomonas vaginalis* from the respiratory tract of infants with respiratory disease. *Pediatrics* **71:**888–890.
198. **Abdolrasouli A, Croucher A, Roushan A, Gaydos CA.** 2013. Bilateral conjunctivitis due to *Trichomonas vaginalis* without genital infection: an unusual presentation in an adult man. *J Clin Microbiol* **51:**3157–3159.
199. **Hamilton H, Pontiff KL, Bolton M, Bradbury RS, Mathison BA, Bishop H, de Almeida M, Ogden BW, Barnett E, Rastanis D, Klar AL, Uzodi A.** 2018. *Trichomonas vaginalis* brain abscess in a neonate. *Clin Infect Dis* **66:**604–607.
200. **Cornelius DC, Robinson DA, Muzny CA, Mena LA, Aanensen DM, Lushbaugh WB, Meade JC.** 2012. Genetic characterization of *Trichomonas vaginalis* isolates by use of multilocus sequence typing. *J Clin Microbiol* **50:**3293–3300.
201. **Krieger JN, Tam MR, Stevens CE, Nielsen IO, Hale J, Kiviat NB, Holmes KK.** 1988. Diagnosis of trichomoniasis. Comparison of conventional wet-mount examination with cytologic studies, cultures, and monoclonal antibody staining of direct specimens. *JAMA* **259:**1223–1227.
202. **Heine RP, Wiesenfeld HC, Sweet RL, Witkin SS.** 1997. Polymerase chain reaction analysis of distal vaginal specimens: a less invasive strategy for detection of *Trichomonas vaginalis*. *Clin Infect Dis* **24:**985–987.
203. **Schwebke JR, Morgan SC, Pinson GB.** 1997. Validity of self-obtained vaginal specimens for diagnosis of trichomoniasis. *J Clin Microbiol* **35:**1618–1619.
204. **Hook EW III.** 1999. *Trichomonas vaginalis*: no longer a minor STD. *Sex Transm Dis* **26:**388–389.
205. **Borchardt KA, Smith RF.** 1991. An evaluation of an InPouch TV culture method for diagnosing *Trichomonas vaginalis* infection. *Genitourin Med* **67:**149–152.
206. **Draper D, Parker R, Patterson E, Jones W, Beutz M, French J, Borchardt K, McGregor J.** 1993. Detection of *Trichomonas vaginalis* in pregnant women with the InPouch TV culture system. *J Clin Microbiol* **31:**1016–1018.
207. **Schwebke JR, Venglarik MF, Morgan SC.** 1999. Delayed versus immediate bedside inoculation of culture media for diagnosis of vaginal trichomonosis. *J Clin Microbiol* **37:**2369–2370.
208. **Adu-Sarkodie Y, Opoku BK, Danso KA, Weiss HA, Mabey D.** 2004. Comparison of latex agglutination, wet preparation, and culture for the detection of *Trichomonas vaginalis*. *Sex Transm Infect* **80:**201–203.
209. **Campbell L, Woods V, Lloyd T, Elsayed S, Church DL.** 2008. Evaluation of the OSOM *Trichomonas* rapid test versus wet preparation examination for detection of *Trichomonas vaginalis* vaginitis in specimens from women with a low prevalence of infection. *J Clin Microbiol* **46:**3467–3469.
210. **Huppert JS, Batteiger BE, Braslins P, Feldman JA, Hobbs MM, Sankey HZ, Sena AC, Wendel KA.** 2005. Use of an immunochromatographic assay for rapid detection of *Trichomonas vaginalis* in vaginal specimens. *J Clin Microbiol* **43:**684–687.
211. **Huppert JS, Mortensen JE, Reed JL, Kahn JA, Rich KD, Miller WC, Hobbs MM.** 2007. Rapid antigen testing compares favorably with transcription-mediated amplification assay for the detection of *Trichomonas vaginalis* in young women. *Clin Infect Dis* **45:**194–198.
212. **Pattullo L, Griffeth S, Ding L, Mortensen J, Reed J, Kahn J, Huppert J.** 2009. Stepwise diagnosis of *Trichomonas vaginalis* infection in adolescent women. *J Clin Microbiol* **47:**59–63.
213. **Kurth A, Whittington WL, Golden MR, Thomas KK, Holmes KK, Schwebke JR.** 2004. Performance of a new, rapid assay for detection of *Trichomonas vaginalis*. *J Clin Microbiol* **42:**2940–2943.
214. **Pillay A, Lewis J, Ballard RC.** 2004. Evaluation of Xenostrip-Tv, a rapid diagnostic test for *Trichomonas vaginalis* infection. *J Clin Microbiol* **42:**3853–3856.
215. **Jones HE, Lippman SA, Caiaffa-Filho HH, Young T, van de Wijgert JH.** 2013. Performance of a rapid self-test for detection of *Trichomonas vaginalis* in South Africa and Brazil. *J Clin Microbiol* **51:**1037–1039.
216. **Harding-Esch EM, Nori AV, Hegazi A, Pond MJ, Okolo O, Nardone A, Lowndes CM, Hay P, Sadiq ST.** 2017. Impact of deploying multiple point-of-care tests with a 'sample first'

approach on a sexual health clinical care pathway. A service evaluation. *Sex Transm Infect* **93:**424–429.

217. **Pearce DM, Styles DN, Hardick JP, Gaydos CA.** 2013. A new rapid molecular point-of-care assay for *Trichomonas vaginalis*: preliminary performance data. *Sex Transm Infect* **89:**495–497.
218. **Byun SW, Park YJ, Hur SY.** 2016. Affirm VPIII microbial identification test can be used to detect *Gardnerella vaginalis*, *Candida albicans* and *Trichomonas vaginalis* microbial infections in Korean women. *J Obstet Gynaecol Res* **42:**422–426 .
219. **Mulhem E, Boyanton BL Jr, Robinson-Dunn B, Ebert C, Dzebo R.** 2014. Performance of the Affirm VP-III using residual vaginal discharge collected from the speculum to characterize vaginitis in symptomatic women. *J Low Genit Tract Dis* **18:**344–346.
220. **Cartwright CP, Lembke BD, Ramachandran K, Body BA, Nye MB, Rivers CA, Schwebke JR.** 2013. Comparison of nucleic acid amplification assays with BD affirm VPIII for diagnosis of vaginitis in symptomatic women. *J Clin Microbiol* **51:**3694–3699.
221. **Brown HL, Fuller DD, Jasper LT, Davis TE, Wright JD.** 2004. Clinical evaluation of affirm VPIII in the detection and identification of *Trichomonas vaginalis*, *Gardnerella vaginalis*, and *Candida* species in vaginitis/vaginosis. *Infect Dis Obstet Gynecol* **12:**17–21.
222. **Chapin K, Andrea S.** 2011. APTIMA® *Trichomonas vaginalis*, a transcription-mediated amplification assay for detection of *Trichomonas vaginalis* in urogenital specimens. *Expert Rev Mol Diagn* **11:**679–688.
223. **Gaydos CA, Klausner JD, Pai NP, Kelly H, Coltart C, Peeling RW.** 2017. Rapid and point-of-care tests for the diagnosis of *Trichomonas vaginalis* in women and men. *Sex Transm Infect* **93**(S4)**:**S31–S35.
224. **Van Der Pol B.** 2016. Clinical and laboratory testing for *Trichomonas vaginalis* infection. *J Clin Microbiol* **54:**7–12.
225. **Hardick J, Yang S, Lin S, Duncan D, Gaydos C.** 2003. Use of the Roche LightCycler instrument in a real-time PCR for *Trichomonas vaginalis* in urine samples from females and males. *J Clin Microbiol* **41:**5619–5622.
226. **Lin PR, Shaio MF, Liu JY.** 1997. One-tube, nested-PCR assay for the detection of *Trichomonas vaginalis* in vaginal discharges. *Ann Trop Med Parasitol* **91:**61–65.
227. **Munson E, Napierala M, Olson R, Endes T, Block T, Hryciuk JE, Schell RF.** 2008. Impact of *Trichomonas vaginalis* transcription-mediated amplification-based analyte-specific-reagent testing in a metropolitan setting of high sexually transmitted disease prevalence. *J Clin Microbiol* **46:**3368–3374.
228. **Nye MB, Schwebke JR, Body BA.** 2009. Comparison of APTIMA *Trichomonas vaginalis* transcription-mediated amplification to wet mount microscopy, culture, and polymerase chain reaction for diagnosis of trichomoniasis in men and women. *Am J Obstet Gynecol* **200:**188.e1—188.e7.
229. **Riley DE, Roberts MC, Takayama T, Krieger JN.** 1992. Development of a polymerase chain reaction-based diagnosis of *Trichomonas vaginalis*. *J Clin Microbiol* **30:**465–472.
230. **Kaydos SC, Swygard H, Wise SL, Sena AC, Leone PA, Miller WC, Cohen MS, Hobbs MM.** 2002. Development and validation of a PCR-based enzyme-linked immunosorbent assay with urine for use in clinical research settings to detect *Trichomonas vaginalis* in women. *J Clin Microbiol* **40:**89–95.
231. **Lawing LF, Hedges SR, Schwebke JR.** 2000. Detection of trichomonosis in vaginal and urine specimens from women by culture and PCR. *J Clin Microbiol* **38:**3585–3588.
232. **Kaydos-Daniels SC, Miller WC, Hoffman I, Banda T, Dzinyemba W, Martinson F, Cohen MS, Hobbs MM.** 2003. Validation of a urine-based PCR-enzyme-linked immunosorbent assay for use in clinical research settings to detect *Trichomonas vaginalis* in men. *J Clin Microbiol* **41:**318–323.
233. **Schwebke JR, Lawing LF.** 2002. Improved detection by DNA amplification of *Trichomonas vaginalis* in males. *J Clin Microbiol* **40:**3681–3683.
234. **Hardick A, Hardick J, Wood BJ, Gaydos C.** 2006. Comparison between the Gen-Probe transcription-mediated amplification *Trichomonas vaginalis* research assay and real-time PCR for *Trichomonas vaginalis* detection using a Roche LightCycler instrument with female self-obtained vaginal swab samples and male urine samples. *J Clin Microbiol* **44:**4197–4199.
235. **Schwebke JR, Hobbs MM, Taylor SN, Sena AC, Catania MG, Weinbaum BS, Johnson AD, Getman DK, Gaydos CA.** 2011. Molecular testing for *Trichomonas vaginalis* in women: results from a prospective U.S. clinical trial. *J Clin Microbiol* **49:**4106–4111.
236. **Mudau M, Peters RP, De Vos L, Olivier DH, Davey DD, Mkwanazi ES, McIntyre JA, Klausner JD, Medina-Marino A.** 2017. High prevalence of asymptomatic sexually transmitted infections among human immunodeficiency virus-infected pregnant women in a low-income South African community. *Int J STD AIDS* **29:**324–333.
237. **Van Der Pol B, Williams JA, Fuller D, Taylor SN, Hook EW III.** 2017. Combined testing for chlamydia, gonorrhea, and trichomonas by use of the BD Max CT/GC/TV assay with genitourinary specimen types. *J Clin Microbiol* **55:**155–164.
238. **Van Der Pol B, Williams JA, Taylor SN, Cammarata CL, Rivers CA, Body BA, Nye M, Fuller D, Schwebke JR, Barnes M, Gaydos CA.** 2014. Detection of *Trichomonas vaginalis* DNA by use of self-obtained vaginal swabs with the BD ProbeTec Qx assay on the BD Viper system. *J Clin Microbiol* **52:**885–889.
239. **Badman SG, Vallely LM, Toliman P, Kariwiga G, Lote B, Pomat W, Holmer C, Guy R, Luchters S, Morgan C, Garland SM, Tabrizi S, Whiley D, Rogerson SJ, Mola G, Wand H, Donovan B, Causer L, Kaldor J, Vallely A.** 2016. A novel point-of-care testing strategy for sexually transmitted infections among pregnant women in high-burden settings: results of a feasibility study in Papua New Guinea. *BMC Infect Dis* **16:**250.
240. **Gaydos CA, Schwebke J, Dombrowski J, Marrazzo J, Coleman J, Silver B, Barnes M, Crane L, Fine P.** 2017. Clinical performance of the Solana® point-of-care *Trichomonas* assay from clinician-collected vaginal swabs and urine specimens from symptomatic and asymptomatic women. *Expert Rev Mol Diagn* **17:**303–306.
241. **Bandea CI, Joseph K, Secor EW, Jones LA, Igietseme JU, Sautter RL, Hammerschlag MR, Fajman NN, Girardet RG, Black CM.** 2013. Development of PCR assays for detection of *Trichomonas vaginalis* in urine specimens. *J Clin Microbiol* **51:**1298–1300.
242. **Cosentino LA, Campbell T, Jett A, Macio I, Zamborsky T, Cranston RD, Hillier SL.** 2012. Use of nucleic acid amplification testing for diagnosis of anorectal sexually transmitted infections. *J Clin Microbiol* **50:**2005–2008.
243. **Lee SJ, Park DC, Lee DS, Choe HS, Cho YH.** 2012. Evaluation of Seeplex® STD6 ACE detection kit for the diagnosis of six bacterial sexually transmitted infections. *J Infect Chemother* **18:**494–500.
244. **Gaydos CA, Beqaj S, Schwebke JR, Lebed J, Smith B, Davis TE, Fife KH, Nyirjesy P, Spurrell T, Furgerson D, Coleman J, Paradis S, Cooper CK.** 2017. Clinical validation of a test for the diagnosis of vaginitis. *Obstet Gynecol* **130:**181–189.
245. **Gaydos CA, Jett-Goheen M, Barnes M, Dize L, Hsieh YH.** 2016. Self-testing for *Trichomonas vaginalis* at home using a point-of-care test by women who request kits via the Internet. *Sex Health* .
246. **Workowski KA, Berman S, Centers for Disease Control and Prevention (CDC).** 2010. Sexually transmitted diseases treatment guidelines, 2010. *MMWR Recomm Rep* **59**(RR-12)**:**1–110. (Erratum, **60:**18.)
247. **Cudmore SL, Delgaty KL, Hayward-McClelland SF, Petrin DP, Garber GE.** 2004. Treatment of infections caused by metronidazole-resistant *Trichomonas vaginalis*. *Clin Microbiol Rev* **17:**783–793.
248. **Klebanoff MA, Carey JC, Hauth JC, Hillier SL, Nugent RP, Thom EA, Ernest JM, Heine RP, Wapner RJ, Trout W, Moawad A, Leveno KJ, Miodovnik M, Sibai BM, Van Dorsten JP, Dombrowski MP, O'Sullivan MJ, Varner M, Langer O, McNellis D, Roberts JM, National Institute of Child Health and Human Development Network of Maternal-Fetal Medicine Units.** 2001. Failure of metronidazole to prevent

preterm delivery among pregnant women with asymptomatic *Trichomonas vaginalis* infection. *N Engl J Med* **345:**487–493.

249. **Sobel JD, Nagappan V, Nyirjesy P.** 1999. Metronidazole-resistant vaginal trichomoniasis: an emerging problem. *N Engl J Med* **341:**292–293.
250. **Borchardt KA, Li Z, Zhang MZ, Shing H.** 1996. An *in vitro* metronidazole susceptibility test for trichomoniasis using the InPouch TV test. *Genitourin Med* **72:**132–135.
251. **Meri T, Jokiranta TS, Suhonen L, Meri S.** 2000. Resistance of *Trichomonas vaginalis* to metronidazole: report of the first three cases from Finland and optimization of *in vitro* susceptibility testing under various oxygen concentrations. *J Clin Microbiol* **38:**763–767.
252. **Kawamura O, Kon Y, Naganuma A, Iwami T, Maruyama H, Yamada T, Sonobe K, Horikoshi T, Kusano M, Mori M.** 2001. *Retortamonas intestinalis* in the pancreatic juice of a patient with small nodular lesions of the main pancreatic duct. *Gastrointest Endosc* **53:**508–510.
253. **Schuster FL, Ramirez-Avila L.** 2008. Current world status of *Balantidium coli*. *Clin Microbiol Rev* **21:**626–638.
254. **Strüder-Kypke MC, Kornilova OA, Lynn DH.** 2007. Phylogeny of trichostome ciliates (*Ciliophora, Litostomatea*) endosymbiotic in the Yakut horse (*Equus caballus*). *Eur J Protistol* **43:**319–328.
255. **Strüder-Kypke MC, Wright AD, Foissner W, Chatzinotas A, Lynn DH.** 2006. Molecular phylogeny of litostome ciliates (*Ciliophora, Litostomatea*) with emphasis on free-living haptorian genera. *Protist* **157:**261–278.
256. **Esteban JG, Aguirre C, Angles R, Ash LR, Mas-Coma S.** 1998. Balantidiasis in Aymara children from the northern Bolivian Altiplano. *Am J Trop Med Hyg* **59:**922–927.
257. **Solaymani-Mohammadi S, Rezaian M, Hooshyar H, Mowlavi GR, Babaei Z, Anwar MA.** 2004. Intestinal protozoa in wild boars (*Sus scrofa*) in western Iran. *J Wildl Dis* **40:**801–803.
258. **Yazar S, Altuntas F, Sahin I, Atambay M.** 2004. Dysentery caused by *Balantidium coli* in a patient with non-Hodgkin's lymphoma from Turkey. *World J Gastroenterol* **10:**458–459.
259. **Castro J, Vazquez-Iglesias JL, Arnal-Monreal F.** 1983. Dysentery caused by *Balantidium coli*: report of two cases. *Endoscopy* **15:**272–274.
260. **Currie AR.** 1990. Human balantidiasis. A case report. *S Afr J Surg* **28:**23–25.
261. **Knight R.** 1978. Giardiasis, isosporiasis and balantidiasis. *Clin Gastroenterol* **7:**31–47.
262. **Ladas SD, Savva S, Frydas A, Kaloviduris A, Hatzioannou J, Raptis S.** 1989. Invasive balantidiasis presented as chronic colitis and lung involvement. *Dig Dis Sci* **34:**1621–1623.
263. **Dhawan S, Jain D, Mehta VS.** 2013. *Balantidium coli*: an unrecognized cause of vertebral osteomyelitis and myelopathy. *J Neurosurg Spine* **18:**310–313.
264. **Karuna T, Khadanga S.** 2014. A rare case of urinary balantidiasis in an elderly renal failure patient. *Trop Parasitol* **4:** 47–49.
265. **Kaur S, Gupta A.** 2016. Urinary balantidiasis: a rare incidental finding in a patient with chronic obstructive pulmonary disease. *J Cytol* **33:**169–171.
266. **Kapur P, Das AK, Kapur PR, Dudeja M.** 2016. *Balantidium coli* liver abscess: first case report from India. *J Parasit Dis* **40:**138–140.
267. **Hazarika M, Pai H V, Khanna V, Reddy H, Tilak K, Chawla K.** 2016. Rare case of polymicrobial keratitis with *Balantidium coli*. *Cornea* **35:**1665–1667.
268. **Khare R, Espy MJ, Cebelinski E, Boxrud D, Sloan LM, Cunningham SA, Pritt BS, Patel R, Binnicker MJ.** 2014. Comparative evaluation of two commercial multiplex panels for detection of gastrointestinal pathogens by use of clinical stool specimens. *J Clin Microbiol* **52:**3667–3673.
269. **Zhang H, Morrison S, Tang YW.** 2015. Multiplex polymerase chain reaction tests for detection of pathogens associated with gastroenteritis. *Clin Lab Med* **35:**461–486.
270. **Ken Dror S, Pavlotzky E, Barak M.** 2016. Evaluation of the NanoCHIP® gastrointestinal panel (GIP) test for simultaneous detection of parasitic and bacterial enteric pathogens in fecal specimens. *PLoS One* **11:**e0159440.

Cystoisospora, Cyclospora, and *Sarcocystis*

DAVID S. LINDSAY AND LOUIS M. WEISS

144

The parasites traditionally referred to as coccidia that develop in the intestines of humans—*Cystoisospora belli*, *Cyclospora cayetanensis*, and *Sarcocystis* spp.—are in the SAR supergroup (Apicomplexa: Conoidasida: Coccidia: Eimeriorina) in the current taxonomic scheme used by protozoologists (1, 2). They have varied life cycles (Fig. 1 to 5), epidemiology, treatment requirements, and diagnostic methods. Oocysts of these coccidia are found in the feces of humans (Table 1), and diagnosis is based ultimately on demonstrating oocysts (*Cystoisospora belli* or *Cyclospora cayetanensis*) or sporocysts (*Sarcocystis* spp.) in human stool samples. Sarcocysts can be demonstrated in tissue sections of muscle biopsies or muscle samples collected at autopsy.

TAXONOMY

The use of molecular methods to evaluate the phylogenetics and genetic diversity of parasites has resulted in a revision of the coccidial parasites. The intestinal parasites covered in this chapter are in the SAR supergroup (Apicomplexa: Conoidasida: Coccidia: Eimeriorina) (1, 2). The names of individual parasites have remained unchanged from those used in the last version of this text.

DESCRIPTION OF THE PATHOGENS

Life Cycles

Cystoisospora belli

The life cycle is direct (monoxenous), but evidence exists that it can be facultatively heteroxenous (use two hosts). *C. belli* oocysts are passed in the feces unsporulated or partially sporulated (Fig. 1C and D and 2A and B). Oocysts generally complete sporulation within 72 h, although sporulation time varies between 24 h and more than 5 days, depending on temperature and humidity. Sporulated oocysts contain two sporocysts, each with four sporozoites, although *Caryospora*-like oocysts of *C. belli* (containing one sporocyst with eight sporozoites) have been reported and can comprise up to 5% of the sporulated oocysts in a sample (3). The prepatent period, the time it takes for unsporulated oocysts to appear in the feces after sporulated oocysts are ingested, is 9 to 17 days (4). The patent period, the time from when oocysts are first excreted in the feces until they can no longer be observed in the feces, is quite variable and depends on the immune status of the infected individual. Oocysts can usually be found for 30 to 50 days in immunocompetent patients, while immunosuppressed patients may continue to shed oocysts for 6 months or more (5). Recurrence of oocyst shedding is common. This prolonged oocyst shedding in immunosuppressed patients is presumably due to recycling of one or more schizogenous stages or activation of dormant extraintestinal monozoic tissue cysts (Fig. 4).

Developmental stages of *C. belli* have been reported for intestinal biopsy specimens of the duodenum, jejunum, and occasionally ileum, and oocysts can be aspirated directly from the duodenal contents. Intestinal development occurs predominantly in epithelial cells, although schizonts (meronts) are occasionally reported from the lamina propria or submucosa (6). At least two generations of schizonts, as well as macrogametocytes (female sexual stage), microgametocytes (male sexual stage), and unsporulated oocysts, have been observed.

C. belli sporozoites/merozoites can travel extraintestinally, becoming dormant as single-organism-containing tissue cysts (Fig. 4) in a variety of tissues, including lamina propria, mesenteric lymph nodes, liver, and spleen (7–9). These cysts are commonly termed monozoic tissue cysts (7). Monozoic tissue cysts in histological sections are thick walled and measure 12 to 22 by 8 to 10 μm, and each contains a single dormant sporozoite or merozoite of about 8 to 10 by 5 μm (7, 8). Presumably, the monozoic tissue cysts are capable of reactivating patent infections once immunity wanes. Monozoic tissue cysts can be present in the lamina propria in the absence of oocysts in stool samples (9). *C. belli* zoites were observed in blood smears from an HIV-infected patient that had chronic diarrhea and disseminated monozoic tissue cysts (9).

The existence of these monozoic tissue cysts has led to speculation that a paratenic (transport) host may be involved in the life cycle of *C. belli* (7). Paratenic hosts are known to occur in the *Cystoisospora* species that infect cats and dogs (7), and it is probable that they occur in the life cycle of *C. belli*.

This chapter contains information presented by David S. Lindsay and Louis M. Weiss in chapter 141 of the 11th edition of this *Manual*.

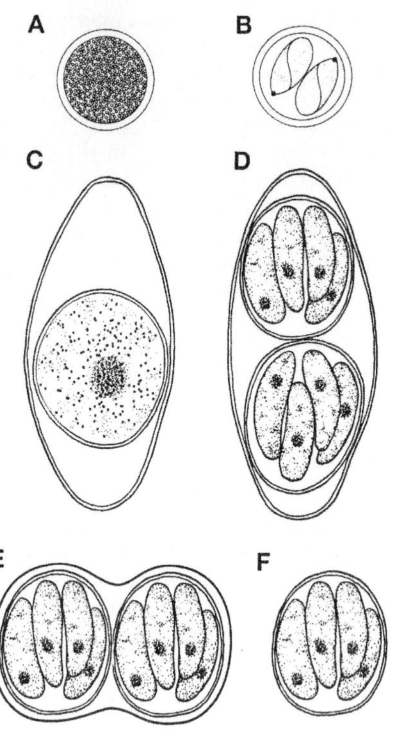

FIGURE 1 Line drawings of unsporulated and sporulated oocysts of *Cyclospora cayetanensis* (A and B) and *Cystoisospora belli* (C and D) and a sporulated oocyst (E) and sporocyst (F) of a *Sarcocystis* species from humans. Bar, 10 µm.

Cystoisospora natalensis

The life cycle is unknown but presumably monoxenous (direct). The oocysts are smaller and more spherical than those of *C. belli* (Table 1). Oocysts are passed in the stool unsporulated. At ambient temperature, oocysts can complete sporulation within 24 h (10). The prepatent and patent periods of *C. natalensis* are unknown. One individual passed unsporulated oocysts for at least 4 days (11).

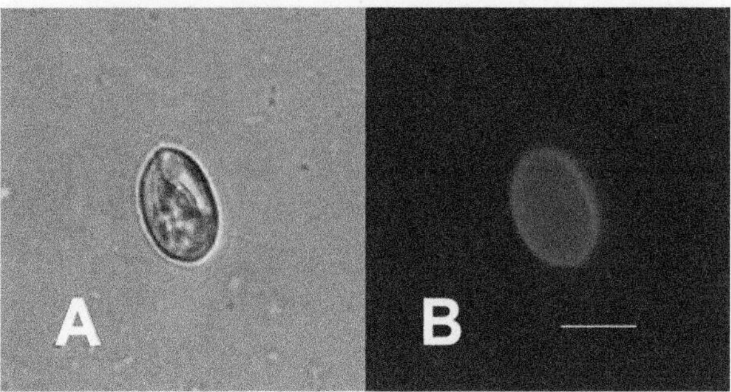

FIGURE 3 Sporocyst of a *Sarcocystis* species in a stool sample viewed with differential interference contrast microscopy (A) and autofluorescence using UV light (B). Bar, 10 µm. Courtesy of Alice E. Houk, Department of Biomedical Sciences and Pathobiology, Virginia Tech, Blacksburg, VA.

The validity of this species is questionable because oocysts of *C. natalensis* have been reported only for patients from South Africa and no reports of *C. natalensis* appear in the literature after 1955 (10, 11).

Cyclospora cayetanensis

The life cycle is monoxenous and involves only humans as hosts. Oocysts are passed in the stool unsporulated (Fig. 1A and 2C). At room temperature (23 to 25°C), small numbers of oocysts may sporulate within 10 to 12 days (12) (Fig. 1B). However, many oocysts require 3 to 4 weeks for sporozoites to fully develop. Sporulated *C. cayetanensis* oocysts contain two sporocysts, each with two sporozoites. A structure termed a Stieda body is present in the end of each sporocyst. There are no Stieda bodies in the sporocysts of *C. belli* or *Sarcocystis* species (Fig. 1). The precise prepatent period is not yet known. However, the onset of clinical signs following infection generally averages 7 to 8 days postinfection and lasts 2 to 3 weeks, but this may range from 1 to more than 100 days. The length of time that oocysts are shed in the feces is highly variable. Oocysts may be shed in the feces for anywhere from 7 days to several months. Relapse of diarrhea can occur in up to

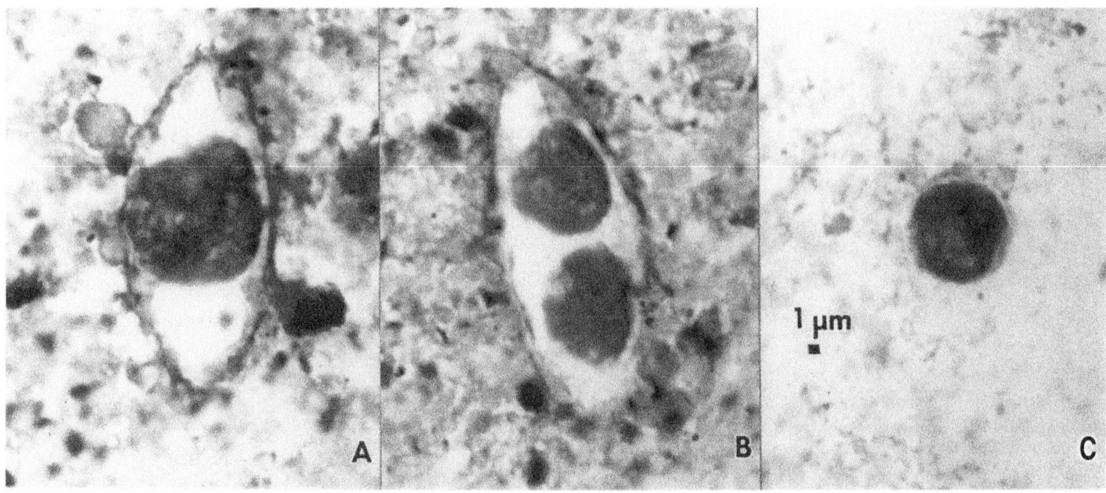

FIGURE 2 Modified Kinyoun's acid-fast-stained smears demonstrating a *Cystoisospora belli* oocyst with a sporont (A), a *C. belli* oocyst with two sporoblasts (B), and a *Cyclospora cayetanensis* oocyst with a sporont (C). Bar, 10 µm.

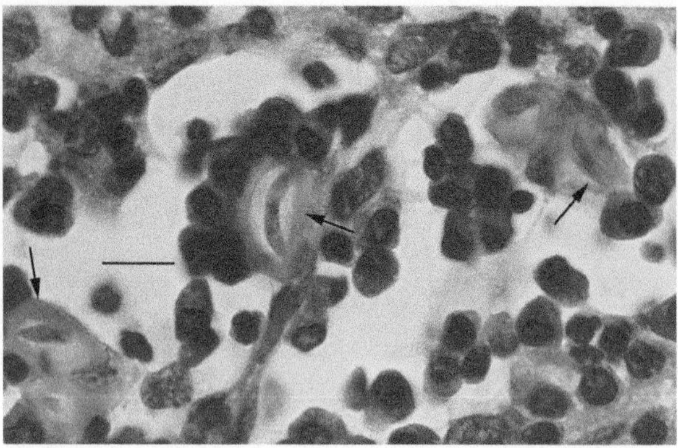

FIGURE 4 Hematoxylin and eosin-stained tissue section demonstrating several monozoic tissue cysts (arrows) of *Cystoisospora belli*. Note the thick wall that surrounds each single zoite. Bar, 10 μm.

25% of infected individuals (13). Indigenous infections are confined primarily to tropical, subtropical, or warm temperate regions of the world. Outbreaks occur in other areas of the world because of contaminated foodstuffs obtained from regions of endemicity.

Developmental stages of *C. cayetanensis* generally occur within epithelial cells of the lower duodenum and jejunum (14–16). There are two asexual generations followed by sexual stages and oocysts. Stages develop in a supranuclear location within enterocytes (16). An experimental attempt to infect seven healthy human volunteers by oral administration of microscopically confirmed sporulated oocysts of *C. cayetanensis* was not successful, as none of the patients developed clinical signs or shed oocysts in their stools (17).

Sarcocystis hominis

The life cycle is heteroxenous. Humans are definitive hosts for *S. hominis*, and bovids are the intermediate hosts. Infection occurs when raw or undercooked meat containing sarcocysts is ingested. Known intermediate hosts include cattle (*Bos taurus*), American bison (*Bison bison*), water buffaloes (*Bubalus bubalis*), and wisents (European bison; *Bison bonasus*). These intermediate hosts harbor sarcocysts (muscle cysts) that are infective when ingested by humans. Infective bradyzoites (dormant merozoite-like stages) are present in the sarcocysts. The bradyzoites penetrate the human intestinal epithelium and develop as sexual stages (macrogametocytes and microgametocytes) in cells in the lamina propria of the intestine. Fertilization occurs, and the oocysts sporulate in the lamina propria. The oocysts are *Cystoisospora*-like and contain two sporocysts, each with four sporozoites. The oocyst wall often ruptures as the oocyst makes its way to the intestinal lumen. This results in the shedding of individual sporocysts in the feces (Fig. 3). Individual sporocysts contain four sporozoites. Both oocysts with two sporocysts and individual sporocysts can be seen in the feces of humans with intestinal *Sarcocystis* infection (Fig. 1E and F).

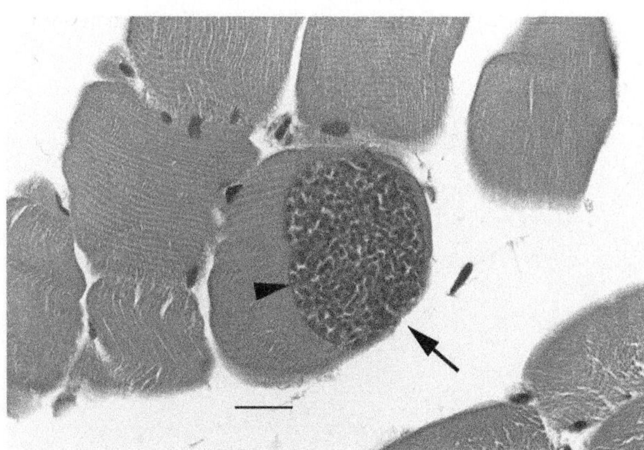

FIGURE 5 Sarcocyst (arrow) of a *Sarcocystis* species in a skeletal muscle biopsy specimen from a male Dutch patient obtained during an outbreak of muscular sarcocystosis (49) among visitors to Tioman Island off the east coast of Malaysia. A sarcocyst wall (arrowhead) surrounds hundreds of bradyzoites. Note the lack of inflammatory response. The patient's traveling partner was also confirmed to be positive by muscle biopsy. Bar, 10 μm. Courtesy of Douglas H. Esposito and Clifton Drew, National Center for Emerging and Zoonotic Infectious Diseases, CDC, Atlanta, GA.

Oocysts and sporocysts are fully sporulated when passed in the feces. For human volunteers, the prepatent period has been reported to be 8 to 39 days, and patent infections can last as long as 18 months. *S. hominis* occurs on all continents, anywhere cattle or buffaloes have access to human feces and humans ingest raw or undercooked beef or buffalo meat.

Sarcocystis suihominis

The life cycle is similar to that described above for *S. hominis*, except that pigs are the intermediate hosts. The prepatent period is 9 to 10 days, and patency is in excess of 36 days. *S. suihominis* presumably occurs on all continents, anywhere swine have access to human feces and humans ingest raw or undercooked pork.

Muscle Infection due to *Sarcocystis* spp.

Sarcocysts have now been reported as incidental findings from tissue sections of both skeletal and cardiac muscle of approximately 100 humans worldwide. Humans become infected after ingesting *Sarcocystis* species sporocysts in contaminated food or water. One to two generations of precystic schizogony presumably occur in endothelial cells in capillaries throughout the body. The final generation of merozoites penetrates striated muscle cells and transforms into metrocytes. Metrocytes divide by endodyogeny to produce bradyzoites within the sarcocyst. Clinical signs probably arise from schizogony occurring in endothelial cells of capillaries and the host reaction to developing sarcocysts in muscles (i.e., eosinophilic myositis). There are several distinct structural types of sarcocysts present in human muscles (18), suggesting that as many definitive hosts may be able to produce sporocysts infective for humans. Many of these sarcocysts appear similar to sarcocysts found in nonhuman primates (19). *Sarcocystis nesbitti* DNA has been demonstrated in muscle biopsies from individuals that have traveled to Malaysia and developed muscular sarcocystosis (20). It is believed that snakes are the definitive host for *S. nesbitti* and that monkeys are the true intermediate hosts.

EPIDEMIOLOGY, TRANSMISSION, AND PREVENTION

Cystoisospora belli

C. belli is found primarily in tropical, subtropical, and warm temperate regions, but reports of indigenous infections have been published from temperate areas as well. Most cases of infection in temperate areas involve foreign travel or anal

TABLE 1 Structural data for *Cystoisospora, Cyclospora,* and *Sarcocystis* oocysts and sporocysts found in stool samples from humans

Species	Mean size (range) (μm)[a]	
	Oocysts	Sporocysts
Cystoisospora belli	32 × 14 (20–36 × 10–19)	14 × 10 (12–17 × 7–11)
Cystoisospora natalensis	Not given (25–30 × 21–24)	17 × 12 (not given)
Cyclospora cayetanensis	9 × 9 (8–10 × 8–10)	6 × 4 (6–7 × 3–4)
Sarcocystis hominis	19 × 15 (not given)	15 × 9 (13–17 × 8–11)
Sarcocystis suihominis	19 × 13 (19–20 × 12–15)	14 × 11 (12–14 × 10–11)

[a]Data have been rounded to the nearest micrometer.

sexual contact. Transmission is via ingestion of sporulated oocysts and possibly the ingestion of raw or undercooked tissues from unknown paratenic hosts. An outbreak of *C. belli* infections involving approximately 90 patients was reported in the city of Antofagasta, Chile, in 1977 (21). It was associated with ingestion of vegetables contaminated with irrigation water from a sewage treatment plant (21). Improving sanitation and water quality in areas of endemicity will decrease transmission of *C. belli.*

Cyclospora cayetanensis

C. cayetanensis is endemic in Central and South America, the Caribbean, Mexico, Indonesia, Asia, Nepal, Africa, India, southern Europe, and the Middle East. In areas of endemicity, there is an increased risk of *C. cayetanensis* infection with contact with soil (22) and water (23, 24). In the United States, cyclosporiasis is a nationally notifiable disease, and health care providers should report suspected and confirmed cases of infection to public health authorities. Health care providers must specifically order testing for *C. cayetanensis* because testing for *C. cayetanensis* is not routinely done in most U.S. laboratories, even when stool is tested for parasites. Infections in most temperate areas are correlated with the consumption of imported, contaminated fruits and vegetables, such as basil, raspberries, lettuce, mesclun, and snow peas. Two large outbreaks of cyclosporiasis occurred in the United States during the summer of 2013 (25). One was concentrated in Iowa (153 cases) and Nebraska (86 cases) and linked to a restaurant-associated salad mix that contained iceberg lettuce, romaine lettuce, red cabbage, and carrots (25). The other was associated with fresh cilantro (25) and was associated with a restaurant (22 of 30 patrons) in a large outbreak in Texas (278 cases). The CDC reported an increase in the numbers of *C. cayetanensis* cases in the United States in 2017. They reported that 1,065 cases had been reported as of October 2017, compared to 88 in the year 2016 (26). The patients came from 40 states, and 56% of patients reported no history of foreign travel (26). The reasons for this increase in number of total *C. cayetanensis* cases over previous years have not been identified and are under investigation.

Individuals in areas of endemicity should wear gloves when gardening to prevent exposure to oocysts of *C. cayetanensis*. Better washing of produce may help to remove *C. cayetanensis* oocysts, but many fruits are delicate. Most of the produce items implicated as transmitting *C. cayetanensis* are consumed raw, which does not lend itself to prevention by thermal means. Nonthermal treatments such as high hydrostatic pressure have been shown to inactivate *Toxoplasma gondii* oocysts, and these methods may be effective in inactivating *C. cayetanensis* on produce.

Sarcocystis Species

Human intestinal *Sarcocystis* species are potentially present in any region in the world where cattle, buffaloes, and swine have access to human feces and the life cycle can be maintained. The cycle has not been detected in the United States. Cultural habits that include ingestion of raw meat or undercooked meat products help to maintain this life cycle in areas where *Sarcocystis* species are endemic. Cooking meat to an internal temperature of more than 67°C kills *T. gondii* tissue cysts in the meat (27), and this temperature should also kill tissue cysts of human-infective *Sarcocystis* species in meat products. Preventing cattle, buffaloes, and swine from consuming human feces will also break the cycle in areas of endemicity.

Most cases of human muscular *Sarcocystis* species infection (Fig. 5) have been reported from the Far East, particularly Malaysia (28–30). One study of 100 consecutive autopsy cases from Malaysia found that 21% of tongue sections were positive for sarcocysts (30). This is probably an underrepresentation of the true prevalence because only a small amount of muscle can be examined histologically. Humans become infected by ingesting sporocysts in contaminated water (28) or food.

Consumption of raw horse meat containing sarcocysts identified as *Sarcocystis fayeri* was reported in a study of six outbreaks of food poisoning in Japan during 2009 and 2010 (21). Diarrhea occurs around an hour after meat containing *S. fayeri* sarcocysts is ingested (31). A 15-kDa protein toxin was identified in horse meat samples obtained from outbreaks, and studies demonstrated that it was homologous to the actin-depolymerizing factor of *T. gondii* and *Eimeria tenella* and that the toxin caused food poisoning in the laboratory assays (32).

CLINICAL SIGNIFICANCE

Cystoisospora belli

C. belli can cause serious and sometimes fatal disease in immunocompetent individuals. Symptoms of *C. belli* infection include diarrhea, steatorrhea, headache, fever, malaise, abdominal pain, vomiting, dehydration, and weight loss (6, 12, 33). Blood is not usually present in the feces. Eosinophilia is observed in many patients. The disease is often chronic, with parasites present in the feces or biopsy specimens for several months to years. Recurrences are common and can occur as long as 10 years after apparently successful treatment and resolution of clinical symptoms (34). Disease is more severe in infants and young children.

Clinical disease from *C. belli* infection is usually more severe in immunocompromised patients than in immunocompetent patients. *C. belli* infection produces diarrhea in AIDS patients that is often very fluid and secretory-like and leads to dehydration requiring hospitalization. Fever and weight loss are also common findings. Other opportunistic pathogens are also common copathogens in these patients. *C. belli* superinfection of the small bowel was seen in a patient who was immunosuppressed with systemic corticosteroids to aid in treatment of eosinophilic gastroenteritis (35). *C. belli* has been observed in both renal transplant (36) and liver transplant (37) patients. *C. belli*-induced intestinal lesions and responses to chemotherapy are usually similar to those observed in immunocompetent patients. *C. belli* has been observed in patients with concurrent Hodgkin's disease (6), non-Hodgkin's lymphoproliferative disease (38), human T-cell leukemia virus type 1-associated adult T-cell leukemia (39), and acute lymphoblastic leukemia and human T-cell leukemia virus type 1-associated T-cell lymphoma (40). These patients respond to specific anti-*C. belli* treatment. Extraintestinal cyst-like stages have been documented for AIDS patients and may play a role in relapse of infection (7). These usually contain a single merozoite-like stage (Fig. 4) and are called monozoic tissue cysts. Many thousands of these stages can be present (7). A case of parasitemia with zoites present in blood smears has been reported in an HIV patient with chronic diarrhea (9).

Infections with *C. belli* in the gallbladder epithelium (41–43) and endometrial epithelium (44) have been reported, and oocysts have been observed in bile samples (45). Clinical signs in patients with parasites in these locations are not specific for coccidiosis, and parasites are located after tissue biopsy as part of a diagnostic workup. Infection of the biliary tract with *C. belli* was the first HIV-related opportunistic infection in one patient, and it may have represented an AIDS-defining infection in that case (43). The parasites probably reach these extraintestinal sites as merozoites from the gut or zoites from extraintestinal locations, and the epithelial cells of these tissues are permissive to parasite entrance and multiplication.

Cyclospora cayetanensis

Nonbloody, watery diarrhea is the main clinical symptom of *C. cayetanensis* infection. Symptoms of nausea, fatigue, abdominal cramps, and fever were reported in more than 50% of clinical cases in one foodborne outbreak (13). Headache and vomiting also occurred in 30% to 45% of these patients (13). Some individuals can be infected and show no clinical signs. In most immunocompetent patients, typical symptoms of cyclosporiasis include cycles of diarrhea with anorexia, malaise, nausea, and cramping and periods of apparent remission. A diagnosis of cyclosporiasis should be considered in patients who have prolonged or remitting-relapsing diarrheal illness, and health care providers should specifically order testing for *C. cayetanensis*, whether testing is requested by ova and parasite examination or by gastrointestinal pathogen multiplex panel test that detects *C. cayetanensis*. Several stool specimens may be required because the presence of an oocyst wall and sporocyst wall hinders extraction of DNA from *C. cayetanensis* parasites and oocysts may be shed intermittently and at low levels. Positive cases should be reported to local health departments.

C. cayetanensis infection can be associated with biliary disease in both immunosuppressed patients and immunologically normal patients (46). Developmental stages of *C. cayetanensis* have been seen in the gallbladder epithelium of AIDS patients with acalculous cholecystitis (47). Oocysts can be observed in the bile of patients with active biliary disease.

Intestinal *Sarcocystis* Infections

Clinical *Sarcocystis* spp. infections in humans can manifest either as intestinal disease if infected meat is ingested or as muscular disease if sporocysts are ingested (48). Intestinal disease occurs soon after consumption of infected meat (3 to 6 h) and is characterized by nausea, abdominal pain, and diarrhea. Intestinal disease can be more severe in individuals who have additional enteropathogens present in the gut. Experimental studies with human volunteers have produced more-severe disease in those who have ingested pork containing *S. suihominis* than in those who have ingested beef containing *S. hominis* (48). Some individuals can be infected and show no clinical signs.

Muscular *Sarcocystis* Infections

Muscular *Sarcocystis* spp. infections (Fig. 5) in humans are usually subclinical or associated with only mild clinical signs and are usually considered incidental findings (49, 50). Clinical case reports are from Southeast Asia. Three outbreaks of acute muscular sarcocystosis have been reported from Malaysia (28, 29, 51). In the first reported outbreak, clinical signs associated with muscular *Sarcocystis* spp. infection occurred in 7 of 15 members of a U.S. combat unit (28). The signs developed about 3 weeks after the troops returned from the jungle and were fever, myalgias, bronchospasm, fleeting pruritic rashes, transient lymphadenopathy, and subcutaneous nodules. Eosinophilia, elevated erythrocyte sedimentation rate, and elevated levels of muscle creatine kinase were present in these troops (28). The second (29) and third (51) outbreaks occurred in travelers returning from Tioman Island off the east coast of Malaysia. The second outbreak, during the summer of 2011, was in 32 patients, most of whom were from Germany (approximately 50%), other European countries, North America, and Asia. Within days or weeks of returning home, most patients experienced fever and muscle pain (29). All had peripheral eosinophilia, and most had elevated serum creatinine phosphokinase levels (29). The third outbreak was reported in 100 patients returning from Tioman Island and occurred during July and August of 2011 and 2012. Most patients experienced fever and myalgia, while fewer had arthralgia, asthenia, headache, cough, and diarrhea (51).

COLLECTION, TRANSPORT, AND STORAGE OF SPECIMENS

The results obtained in the diagnostic laboratory are only as good as the material presented for testing. Choosing the appropriate sample and sample fixative is extremely important (52). Universal precautions should be followed when fresh stool samples are handled. If samples are to be sent to another laboratory for diagnosis, they should be fixed in an appropriate fixative. A 5% or 10% formalin solution is an appropriate fixative for stools suspected of containing intestinal coccidia. Formalin fixation does not interfere with some of the immunodetection methods currently employed to detect *Cryptosporidium* spp. and *Giardia duodenalis*; interference is a drawback of polyvinyl alcohol fixative. Oocyst structure lasts for several months when stools are stored at 4°C in formalin fixatives.

DIRECT EXAMINATION

Microscopy

Oocysts of *C. belli* and *C. cayetanensis* and sporocysts of *Sarcocystis* species are readily identified in fresh unstained wet mounts on the basis of their characteristic sizes and morphologies (Table 1; Fig. 1). This is especially true if oocysts and sporocysts are present in large numbers. Autofluorescence of oocysts of *C. belli* and *C. cayetanensis* and oocysts and sporocysts of *Sarcocystis* spp. (Fig. 3) is an especially useful tool (53, 54) and has replaced many of the staining techniques previously used for these parasites in laboratories equipped with appropriate fluorescent microscopes.

Concentration techniques, such as formalin-ethyl acetate (rarely formalin-ether) sedimentation or sucrose centrifugal flotation, are helpful when few oocysts are present. Sucrose centrifugal flotation has been found to be superior to formalin-ether sedimentation for demonstrating oocysts of *C. cayetanensis* (55), and this is likely the case for oocysts of *C. belli* and sporocysts of *Sarcocystis* spp. as well. Few laboratories employ sucrose concentration, and fortunately, direct wet smears can be very useful: their utility approaches that of sucrose centrifugal flotation when coupled with autofluorescence examination (55). Staining procedures may adversely affect the autofluorescence of oocysts and sporocysts.

Stained fecal smears have been widely used to demonstrate *C. cayetanensis* oocysts and, to a lesser extent, *C. belli* oocysts (53, 56). *C. belli* and *C. cayetanensis* oocysts stain red with the modified Kinyoun acid-fast stain, and this method is widely used (Fig. 2). The main drawbacks are that staining can be variable and some oocysts do not stain (57). Oocysts usually do not stain with trichrome, chromotrope, or Gram-chromotrope stain (57). Some *C. cayetanensis* oocysts stain light blue with Giemsa stain (57). Variations on the safranin staining technique stain *C. cayetanensis* oocysts orange or pinkish orange, and heating and other treatments have been used to increase the staining frequency of oocysts. Flow cytometry has been used to detect *C. cayetanensis* oocysts in human stool samples (58). The results of flow cytometry examination were similar to those of microscopy, and preparation times for the two methods were similar (58).

A single negative stool specimen is not conclusive in the examination of stools for coccidial parasites; a total of three or more stool specimens collected on subsequent days need to be examined before coccidial infection can be ruled out. Liquid stool samples can be concentrated by centrifugation, and the pellet may be used for examination by use of wet mounts, concentration techniques, or stained smears. Large numbers of oocysts may make diagnosis less challenging but do not always translate directly to the severity of clinical signs. Some individuals may excrete oocysts and be asymptomatic.

Cases of muscular *Sarcocystis* spp. infection are diagnosed on the detection of sarcocysts in muscle samples taken from biopsy specimens or postmortem samples. Muscle samples that have been frozen can be thawed and fixed in 10% formalin solution and processed routinely for hematoxylin and eosin staining with minimal or no loss of sarcocyst structure.

Culture

In vitro culture of intestinal coccidial parasites is most often used as a tool to study developmental biology or to identify active chemotherapeutic agents. It presently has limited use in diagnosis of active human infection.

Only minimal development of *C. belli* occurs in human (ileocecal adenocarcinoma [HCT-8 cells] or epithelial carcinoma of the lung [A549]) or mammalian (African green monkey kidney [Vero] or Madin-Darby bovine kidney) cell cultures (59). No reports on development of *C. cayetanensis* in cell culture have been published. Bradyzoites of *S. suihominis* undergo sexual development and produce oocysts in cell culture (60). Vascular schizont stages of human *Sarcocystis* species have not been reported for *in vitro* systems, but continuous cultures of the asexual stages of several mammalian and avian species have been reported. Cultures of asexual stages of human *Sarcocystis* species are needed to produce DNA and antigens for diagnosis.

Antigen Detection

The inability to produce life cycle stages of these organisms in cell culture has blocked the development of a reliable source of diagnostic antigens and has limited the usefulness of antigen detection for these coccidial parasites of humans.

Nucleic Acid Detection

Several research laboratories have developed nucleic acid-based detection tests for target gene regions (*18S rRNA*, *28S rRNA*, *ITS1*, *ITS2*, and *cox1*) to demonstrate infection with *C. belli*, *C. cayetanensis*, or *Sarcocystis* species in stool and tissue samples. Commercially available multiplex gastrointestinal panels that detect DNA of important bacterial and viral pathogens and four protozoan pathogens including *C. cayetanensis* (but not *C. belli* or *Sarcocystis* species) are now used by many diagnostic laboratories.

Gene sequencing can be used to identify the parasites detected and, in some cases, to determine parasite genotype.

Detection of *C. belli* by PCR with primers based on *ITS* and *18S rRNA* sequences has been reported (61, 62). Three different genotypes of *C. belli* can be identified with PCR and restriction fragment length polymorphism by MboII digestion (62). Coinfection of a single patient with two different genotypes has been observed (62). Molecular diagnosis of cystoisosporiasis employing extended-range PCR screening has been proven to detect *C. belli* in biopsy material from a patient who was fecal examination and histological examination negative on initial testing (63). Developmental stages were eventually observed in biopsy material and confirmed the findings (63). A real-time PCR using *ITS2* sequences has been developed to detect *C. belli* in stool samples (61).

Much attention has been placed on molecular methods to detect *C. cayetanensis* oocysts in stools, in water samples, and on produce because of the numerous outbreaks of *C. cayetanensis* infections (64). The *18S rRNA* gene is presently the most frequently used target. Because *C. cayetanensis* is closely related to *Eimeria* species (65) from vertebrates, it is important that tests designed to detect *C. cayetanensis* in water or on produce be examined for cross-reactivity to *Eimeria* spp. (66). *Cyclospora* species infecting mammals other than humans may also be present in water samples or on produce, and proofs of specificity are needed for these tests designed to look at environmental sources of *C. cayetanensis* and to detect *C. cayetanensis* oocysts on produce.

Quantitative PCR assays have been developed for *C. cayetanensis* oocysts in stool samples (67). This method detected DNA of the *18S rRNA* gene from as little as one oocyst of *C. cayetanensis*.

Sarcocystis DNA from sporocysts in human stool and in muscle obtained by biopsy can be detected with PCR and identified by sequencing of PCR products. Quantitative PCR assays have not been reported for *Sarcocystis* species in the stools of humans or in muscle samples.

SEROLOGIC TESTS

Serologic tests are of minimal value for diagnosis of intestinal infections with *C. belli*, *C. cayetanensis*, *S. hominis*, or *S. suihominis* because few serum antibodies are produced for stages that develop in the intestine. The inability to obtain usable quantities of antigens from these parasites hinders development of antibody-based stool diagnostic tests. Antibody tests have more promise for detecting muscular *Sarcocystis* infections in patients because of the development of presarcocyst schizont stages in the host's vascular system, stimulating an antibody response (68). Antibody-based diagnostic tests are commonly used to detect *Sarcocystis* species infection in the central nervous system of horses and to study the prevalence of *Sarcocystis* infection in several intermediate host species.

TREATMENT

Cystoisospora belli

The drug of choice for the treatment of *C. belli* is trimethoprim-sulfamethoxazole. A dose of trimethoprim (160 mg)-sulfamethoxazole (800 mg) two to four times a day for 10 to 14 days results in clearance of parasites, a decrease in diarrhea, and a decrease in abdominal pain within a mean of 2.5 days after treatment (69). Before the advent of combination antiretroviral therapy (cART), it was recommended that patients with HIV-1 infection and CD4$^+$ cell counts of less than 200 should receive secondary prophylaxis with trimethoprim (320 mg)-sulfamethoxazole (1,600 mg) once daily or three times a week to prevent relapse. In most cases, secondary prophylaxis is not needed once the CD4$^+$ count exceeds 200. However, a recent study described eight cases of chronic *C. belli* infection that persisted despite standard trimethoprim-sulfamethoxazole therapy, secondary prophylaxis, and good immunological and virological response to cART (70). Four patients died, two remained clinically ill, and two recovered (71).

For patients unable to tolerate sulfonamides because of allergy or intolerance, there is no standard treatment. Pyrimethamine at a dose of 50 to 75 mg/day is an effective alternative treatment for patients with sulfonamide allergies (72). Secondary prophylaxis using pyrimethamine at 25 mg/day can be used for patients not on cART (72). Pyrimethamine should be given with folinic acid (5 to 10 mg/day) to minimize bone marrow suppression. Another alternative agent is ciprofloxacin, a fluoroquinolone that inhibits topoisomerase. In a randomized study of 22 patients with cystoisosporiasis and HIV infection, all the 10 patients who received trimethoprim-sulfamethoxazole had a cessation of diarrhea within 2 days, and 10 of 12 patients who received ciprofloxacin (500 mg twice daily) had a cessation of diarrhea within 4.5 days (73). All three patients (two with diarrhea and one without) who had persistent *C. belli* oocysts in their stools responded to trimethoprim-sulfamethoxazole treatment (73). In patients who responded to ciprofloxacin, continued prophylaxis with ciprofloxacin prevented recurrence of disease (73). Nitazoxanide has been used to treat *C. belli* infections (74, 75). Two patients who were given 500 mg of nitazoxanide twice daily for 3 days were oocyst negative after treatment (75). A patient treated with 500 mg of nitazoxanide twice daily for 7 days became oocyst negative by day 14 after treatment (74). Treatment failure was observed in a patient with biliary cystoisosporiasis and malabsorption when 2 g of nitazoxanide was given orally twice daily (76). Treatment failure was likely due to the lack of absorption of nitazoxanide and poor levels of the drug in the serum (76). Elevations in liver function tests and nausea are potential side effects of orally administered nitazoxanide.

In a study of eight AIDS patients with *C. belli* enteritis treated with diclazuril, 200 mg/day for 7 days, treatment resulted in resolution of diarrhea in four of eight patients (70). Diclazuril, 300 mg twice a day, was reported to successfully treat *C. belli* in an AIDS patient who was hypersensitive to trimethoprim-sulfamethoxazole and pyrimethamine, and in this case, when the dose was decreased to 300 mg/day, the diarrhea recurred (77). Treatment with other antiprotozoal agents, such as metronidazole, tinidazole, quinacrine, and furazolidone, appears to be of little value for this infection.

Cyclospora cayetanensis

The drug of choice for the treatment of *C. cayetanensis* infection is trimethoprim (160 mg)-sulfamethoxazole (800 mg) given twice daily for 7 days (78, 79). Clearance of parasites, a decrease in diarrhea, and a decrease in abdominal pain occurred within a mean of 2.5 days after treatment. Patients on cART likely do not need secondary prophylaxis.

For patients unable to tolerate sulfonamides because of allergy or intolerance, there is no standard treatment. Nitazoxanide has been evaluated for activity against *C. cayetanensis*, and in these studies, its efficacy for the treatment of cyclosporiasis has been approximately 70% (80, 81). It should be appreciated, however, that only a few patients with cyclosporiasis were treated in any of these studies (80, 81). Another alternative agent is ciprofloxacin, a fluoroquinolone that inhibits topoisomerase. In a randomized study of 20 patients with cyclosporiasis, all of the 9 patients who received trimethoprim-sulfamethoxazole had a cessation of diarrhea within 3 days, and 10 of 11 who received ciprofloxacin (500 mg twice daily) had a cessation of diarrhea within 4 days; however, only 7 of 11 patients treated with ciprofloxacin cleared the organism from the stool (73). Anecdotal data suggest that the following drugs are ineffective: albendazole, azithromycin, pyrimethamine, nalidixic acid, norfloxacin, tinidazole, metronidazole, quinacrine, tetracycline, doxycycline, and diloxanide furoate (L. M. Weiss et al., unpublished data).

Sarcocystis hominis, *Sarcocystis suihominis*, and Muscular *Sarcocystis* spp.

There is no known treatment or prophylaxis for intestinal infection, myositis, vasculitis, or related lesions due to sarcocystosis in humans. It is clear that individuals who travel to Malaysia (28, 29) should take precautions and not drink water or consume food that has not been boiled or cooked to kill potentially contaminating *Sarcocystis* spp. sporocysts. Supportive therapy is indicated for patients with intestinal *Sarcocystis* spp. infection and severe diarrhea.

There is a case report of albendazole having efficacy in an outbreak of eosinophilic myositis due to *Sarcocystis* spp. (28). It is likely that steroids have a role in decreasing the inflammatory response in cases of myositis and vasculitis due to *Sarcocystis* spp. infection, but this has never been evaluated in a controlled trial.

Treatment Failure

There are no documented reports of drug-resistant strains of *C. belli*, *C. cayetanensis*, or *Sarcocystis* species. Development of resistance to trimethoprim-sulfamethoxazole has been suggested in one study of eight AIDS patients with *C. belli*, but other factors such as antigen-specific immune deficiency or generalized reduction in gut immunity could not be excluded (71). It appears that treatment failures are most likely to be related to poor drug absorption or distribution than to true drug resistance.

EVALUATION, INTERPRETATION, AND REPORTING OF RESULTS

Both *C. belli* and *C. cayetanensis* are usually identified by stool examination and are rarely misidentified in human feces. Quantitation of the number of organisms found per high-power field is not required. Stool examinations that are reported as negative should indicate that at least three stool examinations are needed to detect organisms in 95% of infected individuals and that a single specimen may miss as many as 30% of infected patients. If acid-fast or similar stains are done on the stool examination and are positive, then this should be indicated in the report. Computer report notes can indicate that trimethoprim-sulfamethoxazole is the drug of choice for treatment of these parasites. PCR can be used for the identification of these organisms but is not commercially available for *C. belli* or *Sarcocystis* spp. and should be indicated as an experimental test. Serology is not currently used for diagnosis of these diseases in humans. Of the coccidia discussed here, only *C. cayetanensis* is reportable to state health departments and the CDC, as it has been associated with outbreaks and the contamination of human food sources.

S. hominis and *S. suihominis* can be identified by their characteristic morphology in stool specimens or in tissue biopsy specimens. They cannot be identified to the species level on the basis of sporocyst structure and can only be identified as *Sarcocystis* spp. Because of the rarity of these infections, confirmation of the observed organisms should be obtained from experts in parasitology. Laboratory reports should indicate whether expert confirmation of the identity of these organisms has been obtained.

REFERENCES

1. **Adl SM, Simpson AG, Lane CE, Lukeš J, Bass D, Bowser SS, Brown MW, Burki F, Dunthorn M, Hampl V, Heiss A, Hoppenrath M, Lara E, Le Gall L, Lynn DH, McManus H, Mitchell EA, Mozley-Stanridge SE, Parfrey LW, Pawlowski J, Rueckert S, Shadwick L, Schoch CL, Smirnov A, Spiegel FW.** 2012. The revised classification of eukaryotes. *J Eukaryot Microbiol* **59:**429–493.
2. **Simner PJ.** 2016. Medical parasitology taxonomy update: January 2012 to December 2015. *J Clin Microbiol* **55:**43–47.
3. **Jongwutiwes S, Putaporntip C, Charoenkorn M, Iwasaki T, Endo T.** 2007. Morphologic and molecular characterization of *Isospora belli* oocysts from patients in Thailand. *Am J Trop Med Hyg* **77:**107–112.
4. **Ferreira LF, Coutinho SG, Argento CA, da SILVA J.** 1962. Experimental human coccidial enteritis by *Isospora belli* Wenyon, 1923. A study based on the infection of 5 volunteers. *Hospital (Rio J)* **62:**795–804.
5. **Mughal TI, Khan MY.** 1991. *Isospora belli* diarrhea as a presenting feature of AIDS. *Saudi Med J* **12:**433–434.
6. **Brandborg LL, Goldberg SB, Breidenbach WC.** 1970. Human coccidiosis—a possible cause of malabsorption. *N Engl J Med* **283:**1306–1313.
7. **Lindsay DS, Houk AE, Mitchell SM, Dubey JP.** 2014. Developmental biology of *Cystoisospora* (Apicomplexa: Sarcocystidae) monozoic tissue cysts. *J Parasitol* **100:**392–398.
8. **Michiels JF, Hofman P, Bernard E, Saint Paul MC, Boissy C, Mondain V, LeFichoux Y, Loubiere R.** 1994. Intestinal and extraintestinal *Isospora belli* infection in an AIDS patient. A second case report. *Pathol Res Pract* **190:**1089–1093, discussion 1094.
9. **Velásquez JN, di Risio CA, Etchart CB, Chertcoff AV, Nigro MG, Pantano ML, Ledesma BA, Vittar N, Carnevale S.** 2016. First report of *Cystoisospora belli* parasitemia in a patient with acquired immunodeficiency syndrome. *Acta Parasitol* **61:**172–177.
10. **Elsdon-Dew R.** 1953. *Isospora natalensis* (sp. nov.) in man. *J Trop Med Hyg* **56:**149–150.
11. **Dodds SE, Elsdon-Dew R.** 1955. Further observations on human coccidiosis in Natal. *S Afr J Lab Clin Med* **1:**104–109.
12. **Smith HV, Paton CA, Mitambo MM, Girdwood RW.** 1997. Sporulation of *Cyclospora* sp. oocysts. *Appl Environ Microbiol* **63:**1631–1632.
13. **Milord F, Lampron-Goulet E, St-Amour M, Levac E, Ramsay D.** 2012. *Cyclospora cayetanensis*: a description of clinical aspects of an outbreak in Quebec, Canada. *Epidemiol Infect* **140:**626–632.
14. **Bendall RP, Lucas S, Moody A, Tovey G, Chiodini PL.** 1993. Diarrhoea associated with cyanobacterium-like bodies: a new coccidian enteritis of man. *Lancet* **341:**590–592.
15. **Ortega YR, Nagle R, Gilman RH, Watanabe J, Miyagui J, Quispe H, Kanagusuku P, Roxas C, Sterling CR.** 1997. Pathologic and clinical findings in patients with cyclosporiasis and a description of intracellular parasite life-cycle stages. *J Infect Dis* **176:**1584–1589.
16. **Sun T, Ilardi CF, Asnis D, Bresciani AR, Goldenberg S, Roberts B, Teichberg S.** 1996. Light and electron microscopic identification of *Cyclospora* species in the small intestine. Evidence of the presence of asexual life cycle in human host. *Am J Clin Pathol* **105:**216–220.
17. **Alfano-Sobsey EM, Eberhard ML, Seed JR, Weber DJ, Won KY, Nace EK, Moe CL.** 2004. Human challenge pilot study with *Cyclospora cayetanensis*. *Emerg Infect Dis* **10:**726–728.
18. **Beaver PC, Gadgil K, Morera P.** 1979. *Sarcocystis* in man: a review and report of five cases. *Am J Trop Med Hyg* **28:**819–844.
19. **Tappe D, Abdullah S, Heo CC, Kannan Kutty M, Latif B.** 2013. Human and animal invasive muscular sarcocystosis in Malaysia—recent cases, review and hypotheses. *Trop Biomed* **30:**355–366.
20. **Lau YL, Chang PY, Tan CT, Fong MY, Mahmud R, Wong KT.** 2014. *Sarcocystis nesbitti* infection in human skeletal muscle: possible transmission from snakes. *Am J Trop Med Hyg* **90:**361–364.
21. **Karanis P, Kourenti C, Smith H.** 2007. Waterborne transmission of protozoan parasites: a worldwide review of outbreaks and lessons learnt. *J Water Health* **5:**1–38.
22. **Chacín-Bonilla L.** 2008. Transmission of *Cyclospora cayetanensis* infection: a review focusing on soil-borne cyclosporiasis. *Trans R Soc Trop Med Hyg* **102:**215–216.
23. **Dowd SE, John D, Eliopolus J, Gerba CP, Naranjo J, Klein R, López B, de Mejía M, Mendoza CE, Pepper IL.** 2003. Confirmed detection of *Cyclospora cayetanesis, Encephalitozoon intestinalis* and *Cryptosporidium parvum* in water used for drinking. *J Water Health* **1:**117–123.
24. **Baldursson S, Karanis P.** 2011. Waterborne transmission of protozoan parasites: review of worldwide outbreaks—an update 2004–2010. *Water Res* **45:**6603–6614.
25. **DeVignes-Kendrick M, Reynolds K, Gaul L, Klein K, Irvin K, Wellman A, Hardin A, Williams I, Wiegand R, Harris J, Parise M, Abanyie F, Harvey RR, Centers for Disease Control and Prevention (CDC).** 2013. Outbreaks of cyclosporiasis—United States, June–August 2013. *MMWR Morb Mortal Wkly Rep* **62:**862.
26. **CDC.** Cyclosporiasis outbreak investigations—United States, 2017. https://www.cdc.gov/parasites/cyclosporiasis/outbreaks/2017/index.html
27. **Dubey JP, Kotula AW, Sharar A, Andrews CD, Lindsay DS.** 1990. Effect of high temperature on infectivity of *Toxoplasma gondii* tissue cysts in pork. *J Parasitol* **76:**201–204.
28. **Arness MK, Brown JD, Dubey JP, Neafie RC, Granstrom DE.** 1999. An outbreak of acute eosinophilic myositis attributed to human *Sarcocystis* parasitism. *Am J Trop Med Hyg* **61:**548–553.
29. **Centers for Disease Control and Prevention (CDC).** 2012. Notes from the field: acute muscular sarcocystosis among returning travelers—Tioman Island, Malaysia, 2011. *MMWR Morb Mortal Wkly Rep* **61:**37–38.
30. **Wong KT, Pathmanathan R.** 1992. High prevalence of human skeletal muscle sarcocystosis in south-east Asia. *Trans R Soc Trop Med Hyg* **86:**631–632.

31. **Furukawa M, Minegishi Y, Izumiyama S, Yagita K, Mori H, Uemura T, Etoh Y, Maeda E, Sasaki M, Ichinose K, Harada S, Kamata Y, Otagiri M, Sugita-Konishi Y, Ohnishi T.** 2016. The development of a novel, validated, rapid and simple method for the detection of *Sarcocystis fayeri* in horse meat in the sanitary control setting. *Biocontrol Sci* **21:**131–134.
32. **Irikura D, Saito M, Sugita-Konishi Y, Ohnishi T, Sugiyama KI, Watanabe M, Yamazaki A, Izumiyama S, Sato H, Kimura Y, Doi R, Kamata Y.** 2017. Characterization of *Sarcocystis fayeri*'s actin-depolymerizing factor as a toxin that causes diarrhea. *Genes Cells* **22:**825–835.
33. **Trier JS, Moxey PC, Schimmel EM, Robles E.** 1974. Chronic intestinal coccidiosis in man: intestinal morphology and response to treatment. *Gastroenterology* **66:**923–935.
34. **Jongwutiwes S, Sampatanukul P, Putaporntip C.** 2002. Recurrent isosporiasis over a decade in an immunocompetent host successfully treated with pyrimethamine. *Scand J Infect Dis* **34:**859–862.
35. **Navaneethan U, Venkatesh PG, Downs-Kelly E, Shen B.** 2012. *Isospora belli* superinfection in a patient with eosinophilic gastroenteritis—a diagnostic challenge. *J Crohn's Colitis* **6:**236–239.
36. **Koru O, Araz RE, Yilmaz YA, Ergüven S, Yenicesu M, Pektaş B, Tanyüksel M.** 2007. Case report: *Isospora belli* infection in a renal transplant recipent. *Turkiye Parazitol Derg* **31:**98–100.
37. **Atambay M, Bayraktar MR, Kayabas U, Yilmaz S, Bayindir Y.** 2007. A rare diarrheic parasite in a liver transplant patient: *Isospora belli*. *Transplant Proc* **39:**1693–1695.
38. **Hallak A, Yust I, Ratan Y, Adar U.** 1982. Malabsorption syndrome, coccidiosis, combined immune deficiency, and fulminant lymphoproliferative disease. *Arch Intern Med* **142:**196–197.
39. **Greenberg SJ, Davey MP, Zierdt WS, Waldmann TA.** 1988. *Isospora belli* enteric infection in patients with human T-cell leukemia virus type I-associated adult T-cell leukemia. *Am J Med* **85:**435–438.
40. **Ud Din N, Torka P, Hutchison RE, Riddell SW, Wright J, Gajra A.** 2012. Severe *Isospora (Cystoisospora) belli* diarrhea preceding the diagnosis of human T-cell-leukemia-virus-1-associated T-cell lymphoma. *Case Rep Infect Dis* **2012:**640104.
41. **Lai KK, Goyne HE, Hernandez-Gonzalo D, Miller KA, Tuohy M, Procop GW, Lamps LW, Patil DT.** 2016. *Cystoisospora belli* infection of the gallbladder in immunocompetent patients: a clinicopathologic review of 18 cases. *Am J Surg Pathol* **40:**1070–1074.
42. **French AL, Beaudet LM, Benator DA, Levy CS, Kass M, Orenstein JM.** 1995. Cholecystectomy in patients with AIDS: clinicopathologic correlations in 107 cases. *Clin Infect Dis* **21:**852–858.
43. **Walther Z, Topazian MD.** 2009. *Isospora* cholangiopathy: case study with histologic characterization and molecular confirmation. *Hum Pathol* **40:**1342–1346.
44. **de Otazu RD, García-Nieto L, Izaguirre-Gondra E, Mayayo E, Ciani S, Nogales FF.** 2004. Endometrial coccidiosis. *J Clin Pathol* **57:**1104–1105.
45. **Bialek R, Binder N, Dietz K, Knobloch J, Zelck UE.** 2002. Comparison of autofluorescence and iodine staining for detection of *Isospora belli* in feces. *Am J Trop Med Hyg* **67:**304–305.
46. **Sifuentes-Osornio J, Porras-Cortés G, Bendall RP, Morales-Villarreal F, Reyes-Terán G, Ruiz-Palacios GM.** 1995. *Cyclospora cayetanensis* infection in patients with and without AIDS: biliary disease as another clinical manifestation. *Clin Infect Dis* **21:**1092–1097.
47. **Zar FA, El-Bayoumi E, Yungbluth MM.** 2001. Histologic proof of acalculous cholecystitis due to *Cyclospora cayetanensis*. *Clin Infect Dis* **33:**e140–e141.
48. **Fayer R.** 2004. *Sarcocystis* spp. in human infections. *Clin Microbiol Rev* **17:**894–902.
49. **Mehrotra R, Bisht D, Singh PA, Gupta SC, Gupta RK.** 1996. Diagnosis of human *sarcocystis* infection from biopsies of the skeletal muscle. *Pathology* **28:**281–282.
50. **Van den Enden E, Praet M, Joos R, Van Gompel A, Gigasse P.** 1995. Eosinophilic myositis resulting from sarcocystosis. *J Trop Med Hyg* **98:**273–276.
51. **Esposito DH, Freedman DO, Neumayr A, Parola P.** 2012. Ongoing outbreak of an acute muscular *Sarcocystis*-like illness among travellers returning from Tioman Island, Malaysia, 2011–2012. *Euro Surveill* **17:**20310.
52. **Garcia LS, Bruckner DA.** 1997. *Diagnostic Medical Parasitology*, 3rd ed, p 593–607. ASM Press, Washington, DC.
53. **Eberhard ML, Pieniazek NJ, Arrowood MJ.** 1997. Laboratory diagnosis of *Cyclospora* infections. *Arch Pathol Lab Med* **121:**792–797.
54. **Lindquist HD, Bennett JW, Hester JD, Ware MW, Dubey JP, Everson WV.** 2003. Autofluorescence of *Toxoplasma gondii* and related coccidian oocysts. *J Parasitol* **89:**865–867.
55. **Kimura K, Kumar Rai S, Takemasa K, Ishibashi Y, Kawabata M, Belosevic M, Uga S.** 2004. Comparison of three microscopic techniques for diagnosis of *Cyclospora cayetanensis*. *FEMS Microbiol Lett* **238:**263–266.
56. **Parija SC, Shivaprakash MR, Jayakeerthi SR.** 2003. Evaluation of lacto-phenol cotton blue (LPCB) for detection of *Cryptosporidium*, *Cyclospora* and *Isospora* in the wet mount preparation of stool. *Acta Trop* **85:**349–354.
57. **Visvesvara GS, Moura H, Kovacs-Nace E, Wallace S, Eberhard ML.** 1997. Uniform staining of *Cyclospora* oocysts in fecal smears by a modified safranin technique with microwave heating. *J Clin Microbiol* **35:**730–733.
58. **Dixon BR, Bussey JM, Parrington LJ, Parenteau M.** 2005. Detection of *Cyclospora cayetanensis* oocysts in human fecal specimens by flow cytometry. *J Clin Microbiol* **43:**2375–2379.
59. **Oliveira-Silva MB, Lages-Silva E, Resende DV, Prata A, Ramirez LE, Frenkel JK.** 2006. *Cystoisospora belli*: in vitro multiplication in mammalian cells. *Exp Parasitol* **114:**189–192.
60. **Mehlhorn H, Heydorn AO.** 1979. Electron microscopical study on gamogony of *Sarcocystis suihominis* in human tissue cultures. *Z Parasitenkd* **58:**97–113.
61. **ten Hove RJ, van Lieshout L, Brienen EA, Perez MA, Verweij JJ.** 2008. Real-time polymerase chain reaction for detection of *Isospora belli* in stool samples. *Diagn Microbiol Infect Dis* **61:**280–283.
62. **Resende DV, Pedrosa AL, Correia D, Cabrine-Santos M, Lages-Silva E, Meira WSF, Oliveira-Silva MB.** 2011. Polymorphisms in the 18S rDNA gene of *Cystoisospora belli* and clinical features of cystoisosporosis in HIV-infected patients. *Parasitol Res* **108:**679–685.
63. **Murphy SC, Hoogestraat DR, Sengupta DJ, Prentice J, Chakrapani A, Cookson BT.** 2011. Molecular diagnosis of cystoisosporiasis using extended-range PCR screening. *J Mol Diagn* **13:**359–362.
64. **Lalonde LF, Gajadhar AA.** 2008. Highly sensitive and specific PCR assay for reliable detection of *Cyclospora cayetanensis* oocysts. *Appl Environ Microbiol* **74:**4354–4358.
65. **Relman DA, Schmidt TM, Gajadhar A, Sogin M, Cross J, Yoder K, Sethabutr O, Echeverria P.** 1996. Molecular phylogenetic analysis of *Cyclospora*, the human intestinal pathogen, suggests that it is closely related to *Eimeria* species. *J Infect Dis* **173:**440–445.
66. **Jinneman KC, Wetherington JH, Hill WE, Adams AM, Johnson JM, Tenge BJ, Dang NL, Manger RL, Wekell MM.** 1998. Template preparation for PCR and RFLP of amplification products for the detection and identification of *Cyclospora* sp. and *Eimeria* spp. oocysts directly from raspberries. *J Food Prot* **61:**1497–1503.
67. **Varma M, Hester JD, Schaefer FW III, Ware MW, Lindquist HD.** 2003. Detection of *Cyclospora cayetanensis* using a quantitative real-time PCR assay. *J Microbiol Methods* **53:**27–36.
68. **Dubey JP, Calero-Bernal R, Rosenthal BM, Speer CA, Fayer R.** 2015. *Sarcocystosis of Animals and Humans*, 2nd ed. CRC Press, Boca Raton, FL.
69. **Pape JW, Verdier RI, Johnson WD Jr.** 1989. Treatment and prophylaxis of *Isospora belli* infection in patients with the acquired immunodeficiency syndrome. *N Engl J Med* **320:**1044–1047.

70. **Kayembe K, Desmet P, Henry MC, Stoffels P.** 1989. Diclazuril for *Isospora belli* infection in AIDS. *Lancet* **333:**1397–1398.
71. **Boyles TH, Black J, Meintjes G, Mendelson M.** 2012. Failure to eradicate *Isospora belli* diarrhoea despite immune reconstitution in adults with HIV—a case series. *PLoS One* **7:**e42844.
72. **Weiss LM, Perlman DC, Sherman J, Tanowitz H, Wittner M.** 1988. *Isospora belli* infection: treatment with pyrimethamine. *Ann Intern Med* **109:**474–475.
73. **Verdier RI, Fitzgerald DW, Johnson WD Jr, Pape JW.** 2000. Trimethoprim-sulfamethoxazole compared with ciprofloxacin for treatment and prophylaxis of *Isospora belli* and *Cyclospora cayetanensis* infection in HIV-infected patients. A randomized, controlled trial. *Ann Intern Med* **132:**885–888.
74. **Doumbo O, Rossignol JF, Pichard E, Traore HA, Dembele TM, Diakite M, Traore F, Diallo DA.** 1997. Nitazoxanide in the treatment of cryptosporidial diarrhea and other intestinal parasitic infections associated with acquired immunodeficiency syndrome in tropical Africa. *Am J Trop Med Hyg* **56:**637–639.
75. **Romero Cabello R, Guerrero LR, Muñóz García MR, Geyne Cruz A.** 1997. Nitazoxanide for the treatment of intestinal protozoan and helminthic infections in Mexico. *Trans R Soc Trop Med Hyg* **91:**701–703.
76. **Bialek R, Overkamp D, Rettig I, Knobloch J.** 2001. Case report: nitazoxanide treatment failure in chronic isosporiasis. *Am J Trop Med Hyg* **65:**94–95.
77. **Limson-Pobre RN, Merrick S, Gruen D, Soave R.** 1995. Use of diclazuril for the treatment of isosporiasis in patients with AIDS. *Clin Infect Dis* **20:**201–202.
78. **Madico G, McDonald J, Gilman RH, Cabrera L, Sterling CR.** 1997. Epidemiology and treatment of *Cyclospora cayetanensis* infection in Peruvian children. *Clin Infect Dis* **24:**977–981.
79. **Pape JW, Verdier RI, Boncy M, Boncy J, Johnson WD Jr.** 1994. *Cyclospora* infection in adults infected with HIV. Clinical manifestations, treatment, and prophylaxis. *Ann Intern Med* **121:**654–657.
80. **Diaz E, Mondragon J, Ramirez E, Bernal R.** 2003. Epidemiology and control of intestinal parasites with nitazoxanide in children in Mexico. *Am J Trop Med Hyg* **68:**384–385.
81. **Fox LM, Saravolatz LD.** 2005. Nitazoxanide: a new thiazolide antiparasitic agent. *Clin Infect Dis* **40:**1173–1180.

Cryptosporidium

LIHUA XIAO AND VITALIANO CAMA

145

Cryptosporidium spp. are protozoan parasites that inhabit the brush borders of the gastrointestinal and respiratory epithelium of various vertebrates, causing enterocolitis, diarrhea, and cholangiopathy in humans (1). In immunocompetent children and adults, cryptosporidiosis is usually a short-term illness accompanied by watery diarrhea, nausea, vomiting, and weight loss. In immunocompromised persons, however, the infection can be protracted and life-threatening. In developing countries, cryptosporidiosis is one of the most important causes of moderate to severe diarrhea and diarrhea-associated death (2–4). *Cryptosporidium* spp. are well-recognized water- and foodborne pathogens in industrialized nations, having caused many outbreaks of human illness (5, 6).

TAXONOMY

Cryptosporidium spp. are members of the Conoidasida group of the Apicomplexa (Alveolata: Apicomplexa). Phylogenetically, they are more related to the Gregarinasina group than to the Coccidia, which includes *Cyclospora*, *Cystoisospora*, *Sarcocystis*, and *Toxoplasma* (7).

The taxonomy of *Cryptosporidium* has gone through revisions as the result of extensive molecular genetic studies and biologic characterizations of parasites from various animals (8). There are over 30 established *Cryptosporidium* species. Some of the species commonly found in vertebrates include *Cryptosporidium hominis* and *C. viatorum* in humans; *C. parvum* in humans and preweaned ruminants; *C. andersoni*, *C. bovis*, and *C. ryanae* in weaned calves and adult cattle; *C. ubiquitum* and *C. xiaoi* in sheep and goats; *C. suis* and *C. scrofarum* in pigs; *C. canis* in dogs; *C. felis* in cats; *C. cuniculus* in rabbits; *C. wrairi* and *C. homai* in guinea pigs; *C. muris*, *C. tyzzeri*, and *C. proliferans* in rodents; *C. fayeri* and *C. macropodum* in marsupials; *C. meleagridis*, *C. baileyi*, *C. galli*, and *C. avium* in birds; *C. varanii* and *C. serpentis* in reptiles; *C. fragile* in amphibians; and *C. molnari* and *C. scophthalmi* in fish. There are also many host-adapted *Cryptosporidium* genotypes that do not yet have species names, such as *Cryptosporidium* horse, skunk, and chipmunk genotypes I and II and deer mouse genotypes I to III (8). These species and genotypes biologically, morphologically, and phylogenetically belong to three groups: intestinal, gastric, and piscine species and genotypes (9). Only some of these *Cryptosporidium* species and genotypes, almost all of them from mammals, have been found in humans (10).

DESCRIPTION OF THE AGENT

Cryptosporidium spp. are intracellular protozoan parasites that primarily infect epithelial cells of the intestine and biliary ducts, especially the ileum and colon. In severely immunosuppressed persons, the entire gastrointestinal tract and sometimes the respiratory tract are involved. The involvement of the respiratory system in immunocompetent persons may be more common than previously believed, although its role in cryptosporidiosis transmission is not yet clear (11). The infection site varies according to species, but almost the entire development of *Cryptosporidium* spp. occurs between the two lipoprotein layers of the membrane of the epithelial cells.

Cryptosporidium infections in humans or other susceptible hosts start with the ingestion of oocysts, which, unlike those from *Cyclospora* spp. and *Cystoisospora* spp., are fully sporulated upon excretion (Fig. 1). Upon contact with gastric and duodenal fluid, four sporozoites are liberated from each excysted oocyst, invade the epithelial cells, develop into trophozoites surrounded by a parasitophorous vacuole, and undergo two or three generations of asexual multiplication and one generation of sexual reproduction, leading to the formation of new oocysts. The latter sporulate *in situ*, are excreted into the environment with feces, and can initiate infection in a new host upon ingestion without further development (Fig. 1). The time from ingestion of infective oocysts to the completion of endogenous development and excretion of new oocysts varies with species, hosts, and infection doses; it is usually 4 to 10 days. In addition to the classic coccidian developmental stages, a gregarine-like extracellular stage was described, which supposedly can go through multiplication via syzygy, a sexual reproduction process involving the end-to-end fusion of two or more parasites (7).

Currently, over 20 *Cryptosporidium* species and genotypes have been found in humans, including *C. hominis*, *C. parvum*, *C. meleagridis*, *C. felis*, *C. canis*, *C. cuniculus*, *C. ubiquitum*, *C. viatorum*, *C. muris*, *C. suis*, *C. scrofarum*, *C. fayeri*, *C. andersoni*, *C. bovis*, *C. xiaoi*, *C. tyzzeri*, *C. erinacei*, and *Cryptosporidium* horse, skunk, mink, and chipmunk I genotypes (12). Humans are most frequently infected with *C. hominis* and *C. parvum*. The former almost exclusively infects humans and non-human primates and thus is considered an anthroponotic parasite, whereas the

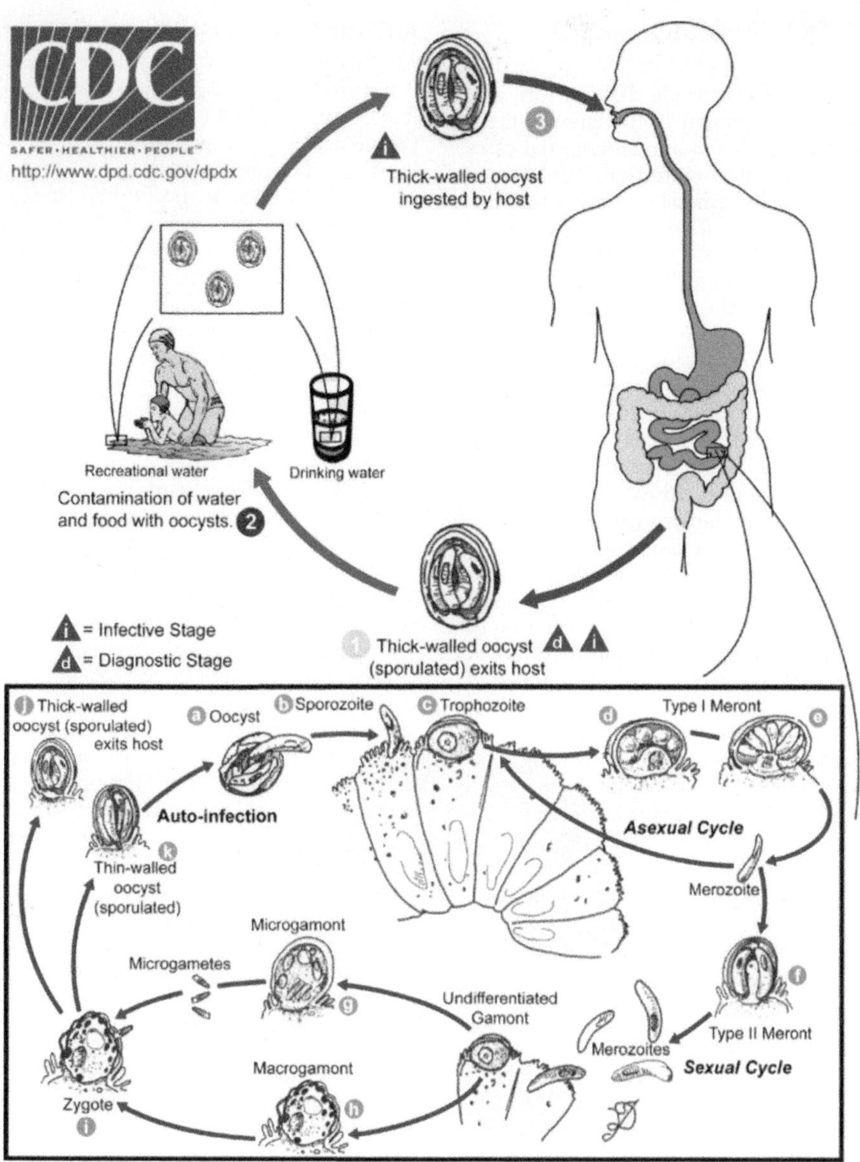

FIGURE 1 Life cycle of *Cryptosporidium* spp. Sporulated oocysts, containing four sporozoites, are excreted by the infected host through feces and possibly other routes, such as respiratory secretions (1). Transmission of *Cryptosporidium* spp. in humans occurs mainly through contact with infected persons (for *C. hominis* and *C. parvum*) or animals (mostly for *C. parvum*) and consumption of contaminated water and food (2). Following ingestion (and possibly inhalation) by a suitable host (3), excystation (a) occurs. The sporozoites are released and parasitize epithelial cells (b, c) of the gastrointestinal tract or other tissues, such as the respiratory tract. In these cells, the parasites undergo asexual multiplication (schizogony or merogony) (d, e, f) and then sexual multiplication (gametogony), producing microgamonts (male) (9) and macrogamonts (female) (h). Upon fertilization of the macrogamonts by the microgametes (i), oocysts (j, k) develop and then sporulate in the infected host. Two different types of oocysts are produced, the thick-walled type, which is commonly excreted from the host (j), and the thin-walled oocyst (k), which is primarily involved in autoinfection. Oocysts are infective upon excretion, thus permitting direct and immediate fecal-oral transmission (courtesy of DPDx: http://www.cdc.gov/dpdx/).

latter mostly infects humans and ruminants and thus is considered a zoonotic pathogen. Other species, such as *C. meleagridis*, *C. felis*, *C. canis*, *C. cuniculus*, *C. ubiquitum*, *C. viatorum*, *C. muris*, and chipmunk genotype I, are less common. The remaining *Cryptosporidium* species and genotypes have been found in only a few human cases (10, 13). These *Cryptosporidium* spp. infect both immunocompetent and immunocompromised persons. The distribution of these species in humans is different among geographic areas and socioeconomic conditions, with *C. meleagridis*, *C. canis*, *C. felis*, and *C. viatorum* being seen mostly in humans in developing countries, *C. ubiquitum* and chipmunk genotype I being seen mostly in industrialized nations, and *C. cuniculus* being seen mostly in the United Kingdom (10, 12, 14, 15). This is probably the result of differences in infection sources and transmission routes.

EPIDEMIOLOGY, TRANSMISSION, AND PREVENTION

Cryptosporidium spp. have a worldwide distribution, and their oocysts are ubiquitously present in the environment. In the United States, the number of annual reported cases of cryptosporidiosis has increased more than 2-fold since 2004; there were 2,769 to 3,787 annual reported cases during 1999 to 2002, 3,505 to 8,269 during 2003 to 2005, 6,479 to 11,657 during 2006 to 2008, 7,656 to 8,951 during 2009 to 2010, and 8,008 to 9,313 during 2011 to 2012 (16–20). Currently, it is estimated that there are about ~750,000 cases of cryptosporidiosis in the United States each year, as 98.6% of cases remain undiagnosed or unreported (6). The estimated annual cost of hospitalization alone due to cryptosporidiosis in the United States is $45 million, with a per-case cost of $16,797 (21). In developing countries, cryptosporidiosis is one of the most important causes of moderate to severe diarrhea and diarrhea-associated mortality in young children (2–4). Humans can acquire cryptosporidiosis through several transmission routes, such as direct contact with infected persons or animals and consumption of contaminated water (drinking or recreational) or food (10, 15, 22). However, the relative contribution of each in the transmission of *Cryptosporidium* infection in humans is unclear. In response to this and the increased national reporting of cryptosporidiosis in recent years, the U.S. Centers for Disease Control and Prevention (CDC) in 2010 launched CryptoNet, the first molecular tracking system for a parasitic infection (https://www.cdc.gov/parasites/crypto/cryptonet.html) (23). CryptoNet is aimed at the efficient use of existing infrastructure to facilitate the systematic collection and real-time sharing of epidemiologic data and molecular characterization of *Cryptosporidium* isolates. This allows improved understanding of *Cryptosporidium* transmission and investigations of cryptosporidiosis outbreaks.

Susceptible Populations

In developing countries, human *Cryptosporidium* infection occurs mostly in children younger than 2 years and is one of the top five causes of diarrhea in this age group (2, 3, 14). Immunity against cryptosporidiosis occurrence develops over increased age and repeated exposures, and there is no apparent species-specific protection against clinical cryptosporidiosis (24). In industrialized nations, pediatric cryptosporidiosis in children occurs later than it does in developing countries, probably due to delayed exposures to contaminated environments as a result of better hygiene (15, 25). Cryptosporidiosis is also common in elderly people attending nursing homes, where person-to-person transmission probably plays a major role in the spread of *Cryptosporidium* infections (25, 26). In the general population, a substantial number of adults are susceptible to *Cryptosporidium* infection, as sporadic infections occur in all age groups in the United States and United Kingdom, and traveling to developing countries and consumption of contaminated food or water can frequently lead to infection (23, 27–30). Cryptosporidiosis is common in immunocompromised persons, including AIDS patients, persons with primary immunodeficiency, and cancer and transplant patients undergoing immunosuppressive therapy (31–38). Hemodialysis patients with chronic renal failure and renal transplant patients commonly develop cryptosporidiosis (32, 38–43). In HIV-positive persons, the occurrence of cryptosporidiosis increases as the $CD4^+$ lymphocyte cell counts fall, especially below 200 cells/μl (44–46).

Anthroponotic versus Zoonotic Transmission

Contact with persons with diarrhea has been identified as a major risk factor for sporadic cryptosporidiosis in industrialized countries (28, 30, 47–49). This is supported by the high prevalence of cryptosporidiosis in day care facilities and nursing homes and among mothers with young children in these countries. Studies in the United States and Europe have further shown that cryptosporidiosis is more common in homosexual men than in persons in other HIV transmission categories (50), indicating that direct person-to-person or anthroponotic transmission of cryptosporidiosis is common.

Only a few case-control studies have assessed the role of zoonotic transmission in the acquisition of cryptosporidiosis in humans. In industrialized countries, contact with farm animals (especially cattle) is a major risk factor for sporadic cases of human cryptosporidiosis (23, 28, 47, 48, 51, 52). Similarly, contact with farm animals has been identified as a risk factor for *Cryptosporidium* infection in AIDS patients and immunocompetent persons in China, Ethiopia, and Nigeria (45, 53–55). The role of companion animals in the transmission of human *Cryptosporidium* infection in humans is probably less important (56, 57). However, direct transmission of *C. canis* or *C. felis* between dogs or cats and humans has been reported (58, 59).

The distribution of *C. parvum* and *C. hominis* in humans is a reflection of the role of different transmission routes in cryptosporidiosis epidemiology. Thus far, studies conducted in developing countries have shown a predominance of *C. hominis* in children or HIV-positive adults. This is also true for most areas in the United States, Canada, Australia, and Japan. In Europe and New Zealand, however, several studies have shown almost equal prevalence of *C. parvum* and *C. hominis* in both immunocompetent and immunocompromised persons (10, 14, 15). In contrast, children in the Mideast are mostly infected with *C. parvum* (60–62). The differences in the distribution of *Cryptosporidium* species in humans are considered an indication of differences in infection sources (8, 10, 12, 63); the occurrence of *C. hominis* in humans is most likely due to anthroponotic transmission, whereas *C. parvum* in a population can be the result of both anthroponotic and zoonotic transmission. Thus, in most developing countries, it is possible that anthroponotic transmission of *Cryptosporidium* plays a major role in human cryptosporidiosis, whereas in Europe, Australia, New Zealand, and rural areas of the United States, both anthroponotic and zoonotic transmissions could be important.

Recent subtyping studies based on sequence analyses of the gene encoding the 60-kDa glycoprotein (gp60) have shown that many *C. parvum* infections in humans are not results of zoonotic transmission (10). Among several *C. parvum* subtype families identified, IIa and IIc are the two most common families. The former has been identified in both humans and ruminants and thus can be a zoonotic pathogen, whereas the latter has been seen mainly in humans (9, 10) and thus is an anthroponotic pathogen. In developing countries, most *C. parvum* infections in children and HIV-positive persons are caused by the subtype family IIc, with IIa being largely absent, indicating that anthroponotic transmission of *C. parvum* is common in these areas (9, 10, 14). In contrast, both IIa and IIc subtype families are seen in humans in developed countries, with the former being far more common than the latter. Even in the United Kingdom, where zoonotic transmission is known to play a significant role in the transmission of human cryptosporidiosis, anthroponotic transmission of *C. parvum* also occurs (64). Another *C. parvum* subtype family commonly found in sheep and goats, IId, is the dominant *C. parvum* subtype family in humans in Mideast countries (60). Results of multilocus subtyping support the conclusions of gp60 subtyping studies (65, 66).

Waterborne Transmission

Epidemiologic studies have frequently identified water as a major route of *Cryptosporidium* transmission in industrialized nations (67). Seasonal variations in the incidence of human *Cryptosporidium* infection in the United States and Europe have been partially attributed to waterborne transmission (23, 25, 27, 28, 68). In the United States, there is a late summer peak in sporadic cases of cryptosporidiosis (19, 20, 23, 25, 28), which is largely due to recreational activities such as swimming and water sports (69). The role of water in *Cryptosporidium* infection in developing countries is less clear. In most tropical countries, *Cryptosporidium* infections in children peak during the rainy season, indicating that waterborne transmission could play a potential role in the transmission of cryptosporidiosis in these areas (14). In a study conducted in a slum in southern India, however, drinking bottled water was not associated with reduced occurrence of cryptosporidiosis in children (70).

Numerous waterborne outbreaks of cryptosporidiosis have occurred in the United States, Canada, the United Kingdom, France, Australia, Japan, and other industrialized nations (5, 71–75). These include outbreaks associated with both drinking water and recreational water (swimming pools and water parks). After the massive cryptosporidiosis outbreak in Milwaukee, WI, in 1993, the water industry has adopted more stringent treatments of source water. Currently, the number of drinking water-associated outbreaks is in decline in the United States and United Kingdom, and most outbreaks in the United States are associated with recreational water (23, 25, 69, 74). Even though five *Cryptosporidium* species are commonly found in humans, *C. parvum* and *C. hominis* are responsible for most cryptosporidiosis outbreaks, with *C. hominis* being responsible for more outbreaks than *C. parvum* (10). This is also the case for the United Kingdom, where *C. parvum* and *C. hominis* are both common in the general population. Recently, there was one drinking water-associated cryptosporidiosis outbreak caused by *C. cuniculus* (76). An outbreak of *C. meleagridis* also occurred in a high school dormitory in Japan, although the role of waterborne transmission in the occurrence of the outbreak was not clear (77).

Foodborne Transmission

Foodborne transmission is also important in cryptosporidiosis epidemiology. *Cryptosporidium* oocysts have been isolated often from fruits, vegetables, and shellfish (78–82). Direct contamination of food by fecal materials from animals or food handlers has been implicated in several foodborne outbreaks of cryptosporidiosis in industrialized nations. In most instances, human infections were usually due to consumption of contaminated fresh produce and unpasteurized apple cider or milk (83–88).

Very few case-control studies have examined the role of contaminated food as a risk factor in the acquisition of *Cryptosporidium* infection in areas where the organism is endemic. A pediatric study in Brazil failed to show any association between *Cryptosporidium* infection and diet or type of food hygiene (89), although a participatory risk assessment of zoonotic *Cryptosporidium* infection on dairy farms in urban Dagoretti in Nairobi, Kenya, suggested that consumption of vegetables contaminated by dairy cattle is a potential risk factor (90). Case-control studies conducted in the United States, the United Kingdom, and Australia have shown lower prevalence of *Cryptosporidium* infection in immunocompetent persons with frequent consumptions of raw vegetables, probably because of acquired immunity as a result of repeated historical exposures to the pathogen in *Cryptosporidium*-contaminated fresh produce (28, 47, 49, 91). It is estimated that about 8% of *Cryptosporidium* infections in the United States are foodborne (6).

Prevention

As for any pathogens that are transmitted by the fecal-oral route, good hygiene is the key in preventing the acquisition of *Cryptosporidium* infection (22, 92, 93). In particular, immunosuppressed persons should take necessary precautions in preventing the occurrence of cryptosporidiosis (94). This includes washing hands before preparing food and after going to the bathroom, changing diapers, and coming into contact with calves, lambs, goat kids, pets, or soil (including gardening); refraining from drinking water from lakes and rivers, swallowing water in recreational activities, and consuming unpasteurized milk, milk products, and juices; and following safe-sex practices (avoiding oral-anal contact). During cryptosporidiosis outbreaks or when a community advisory to boil water is issued, individuals should boil water for 1 minute to kill the parasite or use a tap water filter capable of removing particles less than 1 μm in diameter. Immunosuppressed persons also should avoid eating raw shellfish and should not eat uncooked vegetable salads and unpeeled fruits when traveling to developing countries (94).

CLINICAL SIGNIFICANCE

In developing countries, frequent symptoms of cryptosporidiosis in children include diarrhea, abdominal cramps, nausea, vomiting, headache, fatigue, and low-grade fever (14). The diarrhea can be voluminous and watery but usually resolves within 1 to 2 weeks without treatment. Not all infected children have diarrhea or other gastrointestinal symptoms, and the occurrence of diarrhea in children with cryptosporidiosis is as low as 30% in community-based studies (24, 95). Even subclinical cryptosporidiosis exerts a significant adverse effect on child growth, as infected children with no clinical symptoms experience growth faltering, both in weight and in height (14, 31). Children can have multiple episodes of cryptosporidiosis, implying that anti-*Cryptosporidium* immunity in children is short-lived or incomplete (24, 96). Cryptosporidiosis has been associated with increased mortality in developing countries (2, 97), and globally, cryptosporidiosis was the second most important cause of diarrhea-associated mortality in children under 5 years old in 2015 (4).

Unlike in developing countries, immunocompetent persons with sporadic cryptosporidiosis in industrialized nations, including children and adults, are more likely to have diarrhea (15, 31). The median number of stools per day during the worst period of the infection is 7 to 9.5 (91). Other common symptoms include abdominal pain, nausea, vomiting, and low-grade fever. The duration of illness has a mean or median of 9 to 21 days, with a median loss of 5 work or study days and hospitalization of 7 to 22% of patients (27, 29, 91). Patients infected with *C. hominis* are more likely to have joint pain, eye pain, recurrent headache, dizziness, and fatigue than those infected with *C. parvum* (98). There are significant differences among different *Cryptosporidium* species and *C. hominis* subtype families in clinical manifestations of pediatric cryptosporidiosis (96).

Cryptosporidiosis in immunocompromised persons, including AIDS patients, is frequently associated with chronic, life-threatening diarrhea (44). Sclerosing cholangitis and other biliary involvements are also common in AIDS and other immunocompromised patients with cryptosporidiosis (35, 99, 100). In severely immunocompromised persons, respiratory system involvement is common (101). Cryptosporidiosis in AIDS patients is associated with increased mortality and shortened survival (102). Different *Cryptosporidium* species and *C. hominis* subtype families are associated with different clinical manifestations in HIV-positive persons in developing countries (103).

COLLECTION, TRANSPORT, AND STORAGE OF SPECIMENS

Currently, most active *Cryptosporidium* infections are diagnosed by analysis of stool specimens. Stool specimens are usually collected fresh or in fixative solutions, such as 10% buffered formalin and polyvinyl alcohol (PVA) (104). However, stool specimens fixed in formalin and mercury-based preservatives (such as low-viscosity PVA) cannot be used for molecular diagnosis (105). For outbreak investigations, *Cryptosporidium* spp. present are frequently genotyped and subtyped by PCR methods, which require the use of fresh or frozen stool specimens or stools stored in Cary-Blair transport medium or preserved in PCR-friendly preservatives such as ethanol-based fixatives, zinc PVA, and 2.5% potassium dichromate. It is recommended that multiple specimens (three specimens passed at intervals of 2 to 3 days) from each patient be examined whenever possible if *Cryptosporidium* infection is suspected and the examination of initial stool specimen is negative by microscopy, immunoassays, or PCR (104). Examinations of intestinal or biliary biopsy specimens and sputum or bronchoalveolar lavage fluid are sometimes used in the diagnosis of cryptosporidiosis in AIDS patients (104, 106).

DIRECT EXAMINATION

In clinical laboratories, *Cryptosporidium* spp. in stool specimens are commonly detected by microscopic examinations of oocysts, immunologic detection of antigens, and PCR detection of nucleic acids (107).

Microscopy

Stool specimens can be examined directly for *Cryptosporidium* oocysts by microscopy of direct wet mounts or stained fecal materials if the number of oocysts in specimens is high. *Cryptosporidium* oocysts in humans are generally 4 to 6 μm. Occasionally, *C. muris* oocysts are also found, which are more elongated and 6 to 8 μm and require the accurate measurement of a substantial number of oocysts in diagnosis. Oocysts present can be concentrated by using ethyl acetate sedimentation or sodium chloride or sucrose flotation methods (104). Direct wet mounts or wet mounts from concentrated stools can be examined by microscopy in several ways. *Cryptosporidium* oocysts can be detected by bright-field microscopy. This allows the observation of oocyst morphology and more accurate measurement of oocysts, which is frequently needed in biologic studies. Differential interference contrast can be used in microscopy, which produces better images and visualization of internal structures of oocysts. Due to the small size of *Cryptosporidium* oocysts, microscopic examination of wet mounts is not a very sensitive technique.

More often, *Cryptosporidium* oocysts in concentrated stool specimens are detected by microscopy after staining of the fecal smears. Many special stains have been used in the detection of *Cryptosporidium* oocysts, but modified acid-fast and auramine phenol stains are the most commonly used ones (107), especially in developing countries, because of their low cost, ease of use, lack of need for special microscopes, and simultaneous detection of several other pathogens, such as *Cystoisospora* (formerly *Isospora*) and *Cyclospora* (Fig. 2). Two widely used stains are the modified Ziehl-Neelsen acid-fast stain and the modified Kinyoun's acid-fast stain. Oocysts stain bright red to purple against a blue or green background (Fig. 2).

Direct fluorescent-antibody assays (DFA) have been used increasingly in *Cryptosporidium* oocyst detection by microscopy, especially in industrialized nations. Compared to acid-fast staining, DFA has higher sensitivity and specificity (104). Many commercial DFA kits are marketed for the diagnosis of *Cryptosporidium*, most of which include reagents allowing simultaneous detection of *Giardia* cysts (Table 1). Oocysts appear apple green against a dark background in immunofluorescence microscopy (Fig. 3). It has been shown that most antibodies in commercial DFA kits react with oocysts of almost all *Cryptosporidium* species, ensuring a broad *Cryptosporidium* species detection range of the assays (108).

Compared to that of DFA, the sensitivity of most microscopic methods is probably low. The detection limit for the combination of ethyl acetate concentration and DFA was shown to be 10,000 oocysts per gram of liquid stool and 50,000 oocysts per gram of formed stool (109, 110). A similar sensitivity was achieved with fecal specimens from dogs (111). The sensitivity of modified acid-fast staining was 10-fold lower than that of DFA (110), probably because acid-fast stains do not consistently stain all oocysts (112). The sensitivity of the DFA can be significantly improved by the incorporation of an oocyst isolation step using an immunomagnetic separation technique (104).

Antigen Detection

Cryptosporidium infection can also be diagnosed by the detection of *Cryptosporidium* antigens in stool specimens by immunoassays (107). Antigen capture-based enzyme immunoassays (EIAs) have been used in the diagnosis of cryptosporidiosis since 1990. In recent years, EIAs have gained popularity because they do not require experienced microscopists and can be used to screen a large number of samples (107). In clinical laboratories, several commercial EIA kits are commonly used (Table 2). High specificity (99 to 100%) has generally been reported for these EIA kits (113). Sensitivities, however, have been reported to range from 70% (114) to 94 to 100% (113, 115). Most EIA kits have been evaluated only with human stool specimens, presumably from patients infected with *C. hominis* or *C. parvum* (113). Studies should be conducted to evaluate their performance in the detection of human-pathogenic *Cryptosporidium* species that are significantly divergent from *C. hominis* and *C. parvum*, such as *C. canis* and *C. felis* (113). The usefulness of commercial EIA kits in the detection of *Cryptosporidium* spp. in animals may also be compromised by the specificity of the antibodies.

In recent years, several lateral-flow immunochromatographic assays have been marketed for rapid detection of *Cryptosporidium* in stool specimens (Table 3). In evaluation studies, these assays have been shown to have high specificities (>90%) and sensitivities (98 to 100%) (116–119). However, sensitivities of 68 to 75% were shown in some studies for some assays (114, 120–122).

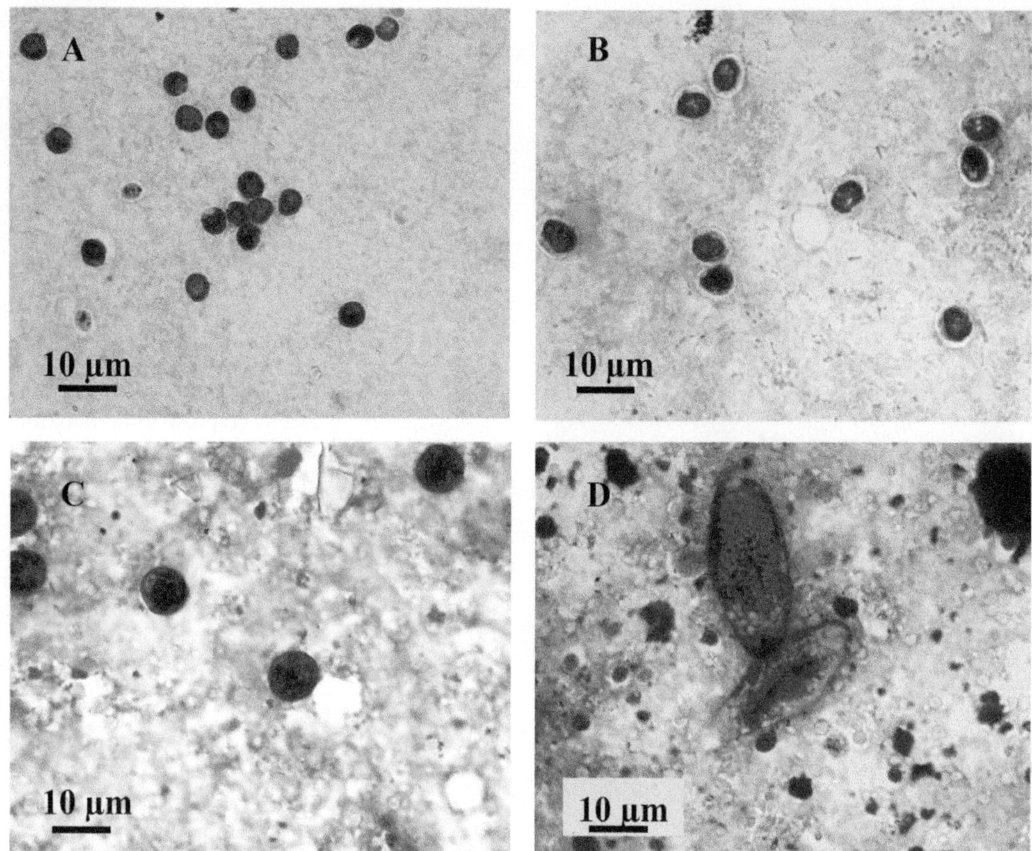

FIGURE 2 Oocysts of *Cryptosporidium hominis* (4 to 6 µm) (A), *Cryptosporidium muris* (6 to 8 µm) (B), *Cyclospora cayetanensis* (8 to 10 µm) (C), and *Cystoisospora belli* (20 to 30 by 10 to 20 µm) (D) stained with modified Ziehl-Neelsen acid-fast stain.

High false-positive rates of several rapid assays in clinical diagnosis of cryptosporidiosis in the United States have been reported (123, 124). This has prompted the Council of State and Territorial Epidemiologists to change the case definition of rapid-assay-positive cases from confirmed cases to probable cases. It has also been shown recently that some rapid assay kits have low sensitivity (<35%) in detecting some *Cryptosporidium* species other than *C. hominis* and *C. parvum* (122).

PCR Detection

Molecular techniques, especially PCR and PCR-related methods, have been developed and used in the detection and differentiation of *Cryptosporidium* spp. for many years (104). Some of the PCR assays for *Cryptosporidium* spp. are commercially available, most as part of the gastrointestinal or multiplex enteric panel assays targeting major diarrheal pathogens (Table 4). They offer high sensitivity and specificity and the ability to detect coinfections (125–132), and they may lead to more frequent detection of *Cryptosporidium*, which is not commonly ordered in tests of diarrheal pathogens (133, 134). While the BD Max enteric parasite panel, Fast-Track Diagnostics stool parasite kit, and G-DiaParaTrio PCR kit target only three major diarrheal protozoa, they could be useful in targeted investigations of parasite-associated diarrhea cases in developing countries (135–139). With reductions in prices, the use of these gastrointestinal panel assays in outbreak investigations and studies of disease burdens is expected to increase in the near future. The utility of in-house multiplex quantitative PCRs in the assessment of causes of diarrhea has been demonstrated in the analysis of stool specimens from European soldiers deployed in Mali and reanalysis of stool specimens from the Global Enteric Multicenter Study (140, 141).

TYPING SYSTEMS

Genotyping and subtyping have been used in characterizations of *Cryptosporidium* infections, especially in cryptosporidiosis surveillance and outbreak investigations.

TABLE 1 Commercial immunofluorescence assays for microscopy detection of *Cryptosporidium* oocysts in stool specimens

Product	Manufacturer or distributor	Regulatory status[a]
Merifluor *Cryptosporidium*/*Giardia*	Meridian Biosciences, U.S., http://www.meridianbioscience.com	FDA/CE
Crypto Cel	Cellabs, Australia, http://www.cellabs.com.au	CE
Cryptosporidium/*Giardia* DFA	IVD Research Inc., U.S., http://www.ivdresearch.com	FDA

[a]FDA, assay cleared by the U.S. Food and Drug Administration and commercially available in the United States; CE, assay cleared by Conformité Européenne.

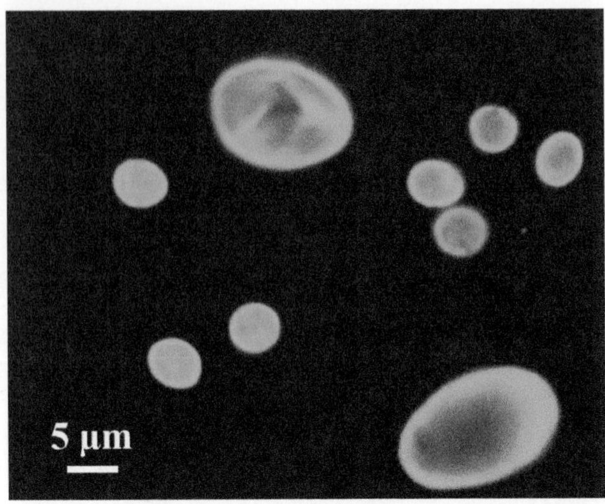

FIGURE 3 *C. hominis* oocysts (4 to 6 µm) and *Giardia duodenalis* cysts (11 to 14 µm by 7 to 10 µm) under immunofluorescence microscopy.

Although species-level identification is not needed for patient management, given that individual *Cryptosporidium* species have unique host ranges, identifying the *Cryptosporidium* species can provide insight into possible exposures and infection sources (8, 10, 12). Several small-subunit (SSU) rRNA gene-based genus-specific PCR-restriction fragment length polymorphism-based genotyping or sequencing tools are available for the differentiation of various *Cryptosporidium* species (142, 143). Other genotyping techniques are designed mostly for the differentiation of *C. parvum* and *C. hominis* and thus cannot detect and differentiate other *Cryptosporidium* spp. or genotypes (10, 12). In recent years, SSU rRNA-based qPCR assays have been increasingly used in genotyping *C. hominis*, *C. parvum*, and *C. cuniculus* (144–150). One SSU rRNA-based qPCR assay has a melting curve analysis developed for rapid genotyping of five common *Cryptosporidium* species in human specimens (151).

Several gp60 (also known as gp40/15) gene-based subtyping tools have also been developed to characterize the diversity within *C. parvum* or *C. hominis* (8, 10, 12). The genetic heterogeneity in this gene is represented by sequence differences among subtype families and variations in the number of trinucleotide repeats (TCA, TCG, or TCT) in the beginning of the gene among subtypes within each subtype family. A nomenclature system is used in naming *Cryptosporidium* subtypes (8, 10). The name of *Cryptosporidium* subtypes starts with the subtype family designation (Ia, Ib, Id, Ie, If, etc., for *C. hominis*; IIa, IIb, IIc, IId, etc., for *C. parvum*). This is followed by the number of TCA (represented by the letter A), TCG (represented by the letter G), or TCT (represented by the letter T) repeats. Thus, the name IbA10G2 indicates that the subtype belongs to the *C. hominis* Ib subtype family and has 10 copies of the TCA repeat and 2 copies of the TCG repeat in the trinucleotide repeat region of the gene. Subtyping tools are now routinely used in the investigation of cryptosporidiosis outbreaks (72, 73, 75, 84, 152–160). Subtyping *C. parvum* and *C. hominis* based on gp60 sequence analysis is a key component of the current molecular surveillance system CryptoNet, which has facilitated the investigations of recent cryptosporidiosis outbreaks in the United States (74, 159, 161).

High-resolution multilocus subtyping tools have been developed for *C. parvum* and *C. hominis* (162–164). With the recent development of next-generation sequence techniques and procedures for isolation and enrichment of pure *Cryptosporidium* DNA (165–168), whole-genome sequencing has been increasingly used in advanced characterizations of *Cryptosporidium* specimens (169–173). These new tools are needed in advanced typing of some dominant gp60 subtypes, such as IbA10G2 of *C. hominis* and IIaA15G2R1 of *C. parvum* (163, 171, 173, 174). Whole-genome sequencing of human-pathogenic *Cryptosporidium* spp. will be incorporated in the next-generation CryptoNet.

ISOLATION PROCEDURES

The *in vitro* cultivation of *Cryptosporidium* spp. remains inefficient despite recent advances (175). The low parasite yields and oocyst production have limited the usefulness of parasite culture in the isolation and diagnosis of *Cryptosporidium* spp. As a result, isolation and cultivation of *Cryptosporidium* spp. are not practiced in clinical laboratories. *In vitro* cultivation of early *Cryptosporidium* developmental stages in several epithelial cell lines (HCT-8, MDBK, Caco-2, etc.) has been used widely in research studies to assess potential drugs and oocyst disinfection methods and to characterize parasite development, differentiation, and biochemistry (176, 177). The recent development of procedures for long-term maintenance of *C. parvum* using cryopreservation for long-term storage of sporozoites and hollow-fiber technology or bioengineered three-dimensional human intestinal tissue for *in vitro* cultivation could promote the isolation of *Cryptosporidium* spp. for diagnosis and typing (178–180).

TABLE 2 Commercial enzymatic immunoassays for the detection of *Cryptosporidium* antigens in stool specimens[a]

Product	Manufacturer(s) or distributor(s)	Regulatory status[b]
Cryptosporidium II, *Giardia/Cryptosporidium* Quik Chek, *Giardia/Cryptosporidium* Chek ELISA	TechLab, U.S., http://www.techlab.com; Alere, U.S., http://www.alere.com	FDA/CE
ProSpecT *Cryptosporidium*, ProSpecT *Giardia/Cryptosporidium*	Thermo Fisher Scientific, U.S., https://www.thermofisher.com	FDA/CE
Ridascreen *Cryptosporidium*	R-Biopharm, Germany, http://www.r-biopharm.com/products/clinical-diagnostics	CE
Tri Combo Parasite Screen (*Cryptosporidium*, *Giardia*, *Entamoeba histolytica*)	TechLab, U.S., http://www.techlab.com; Alere, U.S., http://www.alere.com	FDA

[a]Almost all of the assays have been evaluated using only clinical stool specimens from *C. hominis* and *C. parvum*. Their sensitivity and specificity for other *Cryptosporidium* species are unknown.

[b]FDA, assay cleared by the U.S. Food and Drug Administration and commercially available in the United States; CE, assay cleared by Conformité Européenne.

TABLE 3 Commercial immunochromatography assays for the detection of *Cryptosporidium* antigens in stool specimens[a]

Product	Manufacturer or distributor	Regulatory status[b]
ImmunoCard STAT! *Cryptosporidium/Giardia* Rapid Assay	Meridian Bioscience, U.S., http://www.meridianbioscience.com	FDA/CE
Xpect *Cryptosporidium* Xpect *Giardia/Cryptosporidium*	Thermo Fisher Scientific, U.S., https://www.thermofisher.com	FDA/CE
Crypto-Strip Crypto/*Giardia* Duo-Strip	Coris BioConcept, Belgium, http://www.corisbio.com	CE
Crypto Kit	Cypress Diagnostics, Belgium, http://www.diagnostics.be	CE
Cryptosporidium parvum (Crypto) Crypto + *Giardia* Crypto + *Giardia* + *Entamoeba*	CerTest Biotec, Spain, http://www.certest.es	CE
Stick Crypto Stick Crypto-*Giardia* Stick Crypto-*Giardia*-*Entamoeba*	Operon, Spain, http://www.operon.es	CE
RIDA Quick *Cryptosporidium* RIDA Quick *Cryptosporidium/Giardia* Combi RIDA Quick *Cryptosporidium/Giardia/Entamoeba* Combi (dipstick or cassette)	R-Biopharm, Germany, http://www.r-biopharm.com/products/clinical-diagnostics	CE
IVD *Cryptosporidium* antigen detection assay	IVD Research Inc., U.S., http://www.ivdresearch.com	FDA

[a]Almost all of the assays have been evaluated using only clinical stool specimens from *C. hominis* and *C. parvum*. Their sensitivity and specificity for other *Cryptosporidium* species are unknown.
[b]FDA, assay cleared by the U.S. Food and Drug Administration and commercially available in the United States; CE, assay cleared by Conformité Européenne.

TREATMENT

Nitazoxanide is the only U.S. Food and Drug Administration-approved drug for the specific treatment of cryptosporidiosis in immunocompetent persons (181). Supportive oral or intravenous rehydration and antimotility agents are widely used whenever severe diarrhea is associated with cryptosporidiosis. Clinical trials have demonstrated that nitazoxanide can shorten clinical disease and reduce parasite loads (182, 183). It has been used effectively in the treatment of clinical cryptosporidiosis in both industrialized nations and developing countries (184, 185). This drug, however, is not effective in the treatment of *Cryptosporidium* infections in immunodeficient patients (182, 186). For this population, paromomycin and spiramycin have been used in the treatment of some patients, but their efficacy remains unproven (183, 186, 187).

In industrialized nations, the most effective treatment and prophylaxis for cryptosporidiosis in AIDS patients is the use of highly active antiretroviral therapy (HAART) (183, 187, 188). It is also an effective prevention for cryptosporidiosis in HIV-positive persons in developing countries (189, 190). It is believed that the eradication and prevention of the infection are related to the replenishment of $CD4^+$ cells in treated persons and the antiparasitic activities of the protease inhibitors (such as indinavir, nelfinavir, and ritonavir) used in HAART (187, 191). Relapse of cryptosporidiosis is common in AIDS patients who have

TABLE 4 Commercial enteric panel assays for the detection of *Cryptosporidium* DNA in stool specimens

Product	Manufacturer or distributor	Regulatory status[a]
BD Max enteric parasite panel[b]	Becton Dickinson, U.S., http://www.bd.com/en-us	FDA/CE
BioFire FilmArray gastrointestinal panel[c]	BioFire, U.S., http://www.biofiredx.com	FDA/CE
xTag gastrointestinal pathogen panel[c]	Luminex Molecular Diagnostics, Inc., U.S., https://www.luminexcorp.com	FDA/CE
Faecal Pathogens M[d] Faecal Bacteria and Parasites[d] Faecal Pathogens A[d] Faecal Pathogens B[d] Faecal Pathogens C[d] Parasites (assays for HighPlex 384 platform)[d]	AusDiagnostics Pty Ltd, Australia, http://www.ausdiagnostics.com	CE
G-DiaPara[e]	Diagenode Diagnostics, Belgium, https://www.diagenodediagnostics.com	CE
FTD Stool Parasites[c]	Fast Track Diagnostics Ltd., Malta, http://www.fast-trackdiagnostics.com	CE
NanoCHIP gastrointestinal panel[c]	Savyon Diagnostics, Israel, http://savyondiagnostics.com	CE
EntericBio DX[f] EntericBio Parasite Panel 1[f] EntericBio Gastro Panel 2[f]	Serosep, Ireland, http://www.serosep.com	CE
Viasure, *Cryptosporidium*[f]	CerTest Biotec, Spain, http://certest.es	CE
Cryptosporidium Tyzzer kit[f]	Liferiver, U.S., http://www.liferiverbiotech.com	CE

[a]FDA, assay cleared by the U.S. Food and Drug Administration and commercially available in the United States; CE, assay cleared by Conformité Européenne.
[b]Reported to detect *C. hominis* and *C. parvum*.
[c]Reported to detect *Cryptosporidium* spp.
[d]Reported to detect *C. hominis*, *C. parvum*, *C. wrairi*, and *C. meleagridis* but not *C. felis*, *C. muris*, and *C. baileyi*.
[e]Reported to detect *C. parvum*.
[f]Reported to detect *Cryptosporidium*.

stopped taking HAART (192). Recent reports have shown that cryptosporidiosis is still common in HIV-positive patients receiving HAART in developing countries, although at lower frequencies than those generally reported in untreated HIV patients (53, 54, 193–195).

The development of effective therapy against cryptosporidiosis has received increased attention after the recent identification of cryptosporidiosis as a primary cause of moderate to severe diarrhea and diarrhea-associated mortality in young children in developing countries (196–198). With improved understanding of *Cryptosporidium* metabolism and increased research in this area, several *Cryptosporidium* targets have shown promises in drug development, including calcium-dependent protein kinases, phosphatidylinositol-4-OH and other kinases, and lactate dehydrogenase. Several selective inhibitors of these *Cryptosporidium* enzymes have been identified in a series of recent studies (177, 199–204). Several groups of existing drugs for other pathogens have been identified as potential repurposed drugs for the treatment of cryptosporidiosis (197).

EVALUATION, INTERPRETATION, AND REPORTING OF RESULTS

Cryptosporidiosis is a notifiable disease in most states in the United States and in some other industrialized countries, although only about 1.4% of actual cases are diagnosed in the United States (6, 15). Thus, the detection of the pathogen in stools or tissues should be reported to the local health department in addition to the physicians. Because most routine diagnostic tests cannot differentiate *Cryptosporidium* species, the detection of *Cryptosporidium* oocysts or antigens in stools or other specimens should be reported as *Cryptosporidium* positive without referring to the nature of species involved. From a public health point of view, the reporting of significant numbers of cases above background levels in industrialized nations indicates the likely occurrence of outbreaks of cryptosporidiosis or false positivity of diagnostic kits (205–209). In situations like this, it is crucial to have the test results verified with a confirmatory test such as DFA or PCR and to report them to the state or local public health department. The inclusion of both positive and negative controls in each test run and stringently following the recommended procedures will reduce the occurrence of test errors. In the United States, patients positive for *Cryptosporidium* by immunochromatographic assay-based rapid tests are considered by the Council of State and Territorial Epidemiologists as probable cryptosporidiosis cases. The diagnostic result requires the confirmation by a second assay, such as DFA, EIA, or PCR. In Minnesota and Tennessee, state regulations require that all *Cryptosporidium*-positive specimens be submitted to state public health laboratories for confirmatory testing and molecular characterizations.

The findings and conclusions in this report are those of the authors and do not necessarily represent the views of the Centers for Disease Control and Prevention.

REFERENCES

1. **Checkley W, White AC Jr, Jaganath D, Arrowood MJ, Chalmers RM, Chen XM, Fayer R, Griffiths JK, Guerrant RL, Hedstrom L, Huston CD, Kotloff KL, Kang G, Mead JR, Miller M, Petri WA Jr, Priest JW, Roos DS, Striepen B, Thompson RC, Ward HD, Van Voorhis WA, Xiao L, Zhu G, Houpt ER.** 2015. A review of the global burden, novel diagnostics, therapeutics, and vaccine targets for *Cryptosporidium*. *Lancet Infect Dis* **15:**85–94.
2. **Kotloff KL, Nataro JP, Blackwelder WC, Nasrin D, Farag TH, Panchalingam S, Wu Y, Sow SO, Sur D, Breiman RF, Faruque AS, Zaidi AK, Saha D, Alonso PL, Tamboura B, Sanogo D, Onwuchekwa U, Manna B, Ramamurthy T, Kanungo S, Ochieng JB, Omore R, Oundo JO, Hossain A, Das SK, Ahmed S, Qureshi S, Quadri F, Adegbola RA, Antonio M, Hossain MJ, Akinsola A, Mandomando I, Nhampossa T, Acácio S, Biswas K, O'Reilly CE, Mintz ED, Berkeley LY, Muhsen K, Sommerfelt H, Robins-Browne RM, Levine MM.** 2013. Burden and aetiology of diarrhoeal disease in infants and young children in developing countries (the Global Enteric Multicenter Study, GEMS): a prospective, case-control study. *Lancet* **382:** 209–222.
3. **Platts-Mills JA, Babji S, Bodhidatta L, Gratz J, Haque R, Havt A, McCormick BJ, McGrath M, Olortegui MP, Samie A, Shakoor S, Mondal D, Lima IF, Hariraju D, Rayamajhi BB, Qureshi S, Kabir F, Yori PP, Mufamadi B, Amour C, Carreon JD, Richard SA, Lang D, Bessong P, Mduma E, Ahmed T, Lima AA, Mason CJ, Zaidi AK, Bhutta ZA, Kosek M, Guerrant RL, Gottlieb M, Miller M, Kang G, Houpt ER, MAL-ED Network Investigators.** 2015. Pathogen-specific burdens of community diarrhoea in developing countries: a multisite birth cohort study (MAL-ED). *Lancet Glob Health* **3:**e564–e575.
4. **GBD Diarrhoeal Diseases Collaborators.** 2017. Estimates of global, regional, and national morbidity, mortality, and aetiologies of diarrhoeal diseases: a systematic analysis for the Global Burden of Disease Study 2015. *Lancet Infect Dis* **17:**909–948.
5. **Efstratiou A, Ongerth JE, Karanis P.** 2017. Waterborne transmission of protozoan parasites: review of worldwide outbreaks. An update 2011–2016. *Water Res* **114:**14–22.
6. **Scallan E, Hoekstra RM, Angulo FJ, Tauxe RV, Widdowson MA, Roy SL, Jones JL, Griffin PM.** 2011. Foodborne illness acquired in the United States—major pathogens. *Emerg Infect Dis* **17:**7–15.
7. **Ryan U, Paparini A, Monis P, Hijjawi N.** 2016. It's official—*Cryptosporidium* is a gregarine: what are the implications for the water industry? *Water Res* **105:**305–313.
8. **Ryan U, Fayer R, Xiao L.** 2014. *Cryptosporidium* species in humans and animals: current understanding and research needs. *Parasitology* **141:**1667–1685.
9. **Xiao L, Feng Y.** 2008. Zoonotic cryptosporidiosis. *FEMS Immunol Med Microbiol* **52:**309–323.
10. **Xiao L.** 2010. Molecular epidemiology of cryptosporidiosis: an update. *Exp Parasitol* **124:**80–89.
11. **Sponseller JK, Griffiths JK, Tzipori S.** 2014. The evolution of respiratory cryptosporidiosis: evidence for transmission by inhalation. *Clin Microbiol Rev* **27:**575–586.
12. **Xiao L, Feng Y.** 2017. Molecular epidemiologic tools for waterborne pathogens Cryptosporidium spp. and Giardia duodenalis. *Food Waterborne Parasitol* **8–9:**14–32.
13. **Elwin K, Hadfield SJ, Robinson G, Chalmers RM.** 2012. The epidemiology of sporadic human infections with unusual cryptosporidia detected during routine typing in England and Wales, 2000–2008. *Epidemiol Infect* **140:**673–683.
14. **Squire SA, Ryan U.** 2017. *Cryptosporidium* and *Giardia* in Africa: current and future challenges. *Parasit Vectors* **10:**195.
15. **Cacciò SM, Chalmers RM.** 2016. Human cryptosporidiosis in Europe. *Clin Microbiol Infect* **22:**471–480.
16. **Yoder JS, Beach MJ, Centers for Disease Control and Prevention.** 2007. Cryptosporidiosis surveillance—United States, 2003–2005. *MMWR Surveill Summ* **56:**1–10.
17. **Hlavsa MC, Watson JC, Beach MJ.** 2005. Cryptosporidiosis surveillance—United States 1999–2002. *MMWR Surveill Summ* **54:**1–8.
18. **Yoder JS, Harral C, Beach MJ, Centers for Disease Control and Prevention.** 2010. Cryptosporidiosis surveillance—United States, 2006–2008. *MMWR Surveill Summ* **59:**1–14.
19. **Yoder JS, Wallace RM, Collier SA, Beach MJ, Hlavsa MC, Centers for Disease Control and Prevention.** 2012. Cryptosporidiosis surveillance—United States, 2009–2010. *MMWR Surveill Summ* **61:**1–12.

20. **Painter JE, Hlavsa MC, Collier SA, Xiao L, Yoder JS, Centers for Disease Control and Prevention.** 2015. Cryptosporidiosis surveillance—United States, 2011–2012. *MMWR Suppl* **64**(3):1–14.
21. **Collier SA, Stockman LJ, Hicks LA, Garrison LE, Zhou FJ, Beach MJ.** 2012. Direct healthcare costs of selected diseases primarily or partially transmitted by water. *Epidemiol Infect* **140:**2003–2013.
22. **Ryan U, Zahedi A, Paparini A.** 2016. *Cryptosporidium* in humans and animals—a one health approach to prophylaxis. *Parasite Immunol* **38:**535–547.
23. **Yoder JS, Beach MJ.** 2010. *Cryptosporidium* surveillance and risk factors in the United States. *Exp Parasitol* **124:**31–39.
24. **Kattula D, Jeyavelu N, Prabhakaran AD, Premkumar PS, Velusamy V, Venugopal S, Geetha JC, Lazarus RP, Das P, Nithyanandhan K, Gunasekaran C, Muliyil J, Sarkar R, Wanke C, Ajjampur SS, Babji S, Naumova EN, Ward HD, Kang G.** 2017. Natural history of cryptosporidiosis in a birth cohort in Southern India. *Clin Infect Dis* **64:**347–354.
25. **Painter JE, Gargano JW, Yoder JS, Collier SA, Hlavsa MC.** 2016. Evolving epidemiology of reported cryptosporidiosis cases in the United States, 1995–2012. *Epidemiol Infect* **144:**1792–1802.
26. **Mor SM, DeMaria A Jr, Griffiths JK, Naumova EN.** 2009. Cryptosporidiosis in the elderly population of the United States. *Clin Infect Dis* **48:**698–705.
27. **Dietz V, Vugia D, Nelson R, Wicklund J, Nadle J, McCombs KG, Reddy S.** 2000. Active, multisite, laboratory-based surveillance for *Cryptosporidium parvum*. *Am J Trop Med Hyg* **62:**368–372.
28. **Roy SL, DeLong SM, Stenzel SA, Shiferaw B, Roberts JM, Khalakdina A, Marcus R, Segler SD, Shah DD, Thomas S, Vugia DJ, Zansky SM, Dietz V, Beach MJ, Emerging Infections Program FoodNet Working Group.** 2004. Risk factors for sporadic cryptosporidiosis among immunocompetent persons in the United States from 1999 to 2001. *J Clin Microbiol* **42:**2944–2951.
29. **Goh S, Reacher M, Casemore DP, Verlander NQ, Chalmers R, Knowles M, Williams J, Osborn K, Richards S.** 2004. Sporadic cryptosporidiosis, North Cumbria, England, 1996–2000. *Emerg Infect Dis* **10:**1007–1015.
30. **Pintar KD, Pollari F, Waltner-Toews D, Charron DF, McEwen SA, Fazil A, Nesbitt A.** 2009. A modified case-control study of cryptosporidiosis (using non-*Cryptosporidium*-infected enteric cases as controls) in a community setting. *Epidemiol Infect* **137:**1789–1799.
31. **Chalmers RM, Davies AP.** 2010. Minireview: clinical cryptosporidiosis. *Exp Parasitol* **124:**138–146.
32. **Krause I, Amir J, Cleper R, Dagan A, Behor J, Samra Z, Davidovits M.** 2012. Cryptosporidiosis in children following solid organ transplantation. *Pediatr Infect Dis J* **31:**1135–1138.
33. **Al-Qobati SA, Al-Maktari MT, Bin Al-Zoa AM, Derhim M.** 2012. Intestinal parasitosis among Yemeni patients with cancer, Sana'a, Yemen. *J Egypt Soc Parasitol* **42:**727–734.
34. **Hassanein SM, Abd-El-Latif MM, Hassanin OM, Abd-El-Latif LM, Ramadan NI.** 2012. *Cryptosporidium* gastroenteritis in Egyptian children with acute lymphoblastic leukemia: magnitude of the problem. *Infection* **40:**279–284.
35. **Domenech C, Rabodonirina M, Bleyzac N, Pagès MP, Bertrand Y.** 2011. Cryptosporidiosis in children with acute lymphoblastic leukemia on maintenance chemotherapy. *J Pediatr Hematol Oncol* **33:**570–572.
36. **Sulżyc-Bielicka V, Kołodziejczyk L, Jaczewska S, Bielicki D, Kładny J, Safranow K.** 2012. Prevalence of *Cryptosporidium* sp. in patients with colorectal cancer. *Pol Przegl Chir* **84:**348–351.
37. **Lanternier F, Amazzough K, Favennec L, Mamzer-Bruneel MF, Abdoul H, Tourret J, Decramer S, Zuber J, Scemla A, Legendre C, Lortholary O, Bougnoux ME, ANOFEL Cryptosporidium National Network and Transplant Cryptosporidium Study Group.** 2017. *Cryptosporidium* spp. infection in solid organ transplantation: the nationwide "TRANSCRYPTO" study. *Transplantation* **101:**826–830.
38. **Bonatti H, Barroso LF II, Sawyer RG, Kotton CN, Sifri CD.** 2012. *Cryptosporidium* enteritis in solid organ transplant recipients: multicenter retrospective evaluation of 10 cases reveals an association with elevated tacrolimus concentrations. *Transpl Infect Dis* **14:**635–648.
39. **Raja K, Abbas Z, Hassan SM, Luck NH, Aziz T, Mubarak M.** 2014. Prevalence of cryptosporidiosis in renal transplant recipients presenting with acute diarrhea at a single center in Pakistan. *J Nephropathol* **3:**127–131.
40. **Dey A, Ghoshal U, Agarwal V, Ghoshal UC.** 2016. Genotyping of *Cryptosporidium* species and their clinical manifestations in patients with renal transplantation and human immunodeficiency virus infection. *J Pathogens* **2016:**2623602
41. **Hawash YA, Dorgham LS, Amir AM, Sharaf OF.** 2015. Prevalence of intestinal protozoa among Saudi patients with chronic renal failure: a case-control study. *J Trop Med* **2015:**563478.
42. **Mohaghegh MA, Hejazi SH, Ghomashlooyan M, Kalani H, Mirzaei F, Azami M.** 2017. Prevalence and clinical features of *Cryptosporidium* infection in hemodialysis patients. *Gastroenterol Hepatol Bed Bench* **10:**137–142.
43. **Bhadauria D, Goel A, Kaul A, Sharma RK, Gupta A, Ruhela V, Gupta A, Vardhan H, Prasad N.** 2015. *Cryptosporidium* infection after renal transplantation in an endemic area. *Transpl Infect Dis* **17:**48–55.
44. **Hunter PR, Nichols G.** 2002. Epidemiology and clinical features of *Cryptosporidium* infection in immunocompromised patients. *Clin Microbiol Rev* **15:**145–154.
45. **Akinbo FO, Okaka CE, Omoregie R, Dearen T, Leon ET, Xiao L.** 2012. Molecular epidemiologic characterization of *Enterocytozoon bieneusi* in HIV-infected persons in Benin City, Nigeria. *Am J Trop Med Hyg* **86:**441–445.
46. **Shimelis T, Tassachew Y, Lambiyo T.** 2016. *Cryptosporidium* and other intestinal parasitic infections among HIV patients in southern Ethiopia: significance of improved HIV-related care. *Parasit Vectors* **9:**270.
47. **Hunter PR, Hughes S, Woodhouse S, Syed Q, Verlander NQ, Chalmers RM, Morgan K, Nichols G, Beeching N, Osborn K.** 2004. Sporadic cryptosporidiosis case-control study with genotyping. *Emerg Infect Dis* **10:**1241–1249.
48. **Pollock KG, Ternent HE, Mellor DJ, Chalmers RM, Smith HV, Ramsay CN, Innocent GT.** 2010. Spatial and temporal epidemiology of sporadic human cryptosporidiosis in Scotland. *Zoonoses Public Health* **57:**487–492.
49. **Valderrama AL, Hlavsa MC, Cronquist A, Cosgrove S, Johnston SP, Roberts JM, Stock ML, Xiao L, Xavier K, Beach MJ.** 2009. Multiple risk factors associated with a large statewide increase in cryptosporidiosis. *Epidemiol Infect* **137:**1781–1788.
50. **Hellard M, Hocking J, Willis J, Dore G, Fairley C.** 2003. Risk factors leading to *Cryptosporidium* infection in men who have sex with men. *Sex Transm Infect* **79:**412–414.
51. **Lake IR, Harrison FC, Chalmers RM, Bentham G, Nichols G, Hunter PR, Kovats RS, Grundy C.** 2007. Case-control study of environmental and social factors influencing cryptosporidiosis. *Eur J Epidemiol* **22:**805–811.
52. **Snel SJ, Baker MG, Venugopal K.** 2009. The epidemiology of cryptosporidiosis in New Zealand, 1997–2006. *N Z Med J* **122:**47–61.
53. **Adamu H, Petros B, Zhang G, Kassa H, Amer S, Ye J, Feng Y, Xiao L.** 2014. Distribution and clinical manifestations of *Cryptosporidium* species and subtypes in HIV/AIDS patients in Ethiopia. *PLoS Negl Trop Dis* **8:**e2831.
54. **Wang L, Zhang H, Zhao X, Zhang L, Zhang G, Guo M, Liu L, Feng Y, Xiao L.** 2013. Zoonotic *Cryptosporidium* species and *Enterocytozoon bieneusi* genotypes in HIV-positive patients on antiretroviral therapy. *J Clin Microbiol* **51:**557–563.
55. **Yang Y, Zhou YB, Xiao PL, Shi Y, Chen Y, Liang S, Yihuo WL, Song XX, Jiang QW.** 2017. Prevalence of and risk factors associated with *Cryptosporidium* infection in an underdeveloped rural community of southwest China. *Infect Dis Poverty* **6:**2.
56. **Lucio-Forster A, Griffiths JK, Cama VA, Xiao L, Bowman DD.** 2010. Minimal zoonotic risk of cryptosporidiosis from pet dogs and cats. *Trends Parasitol* **26:**174–179.

57. **de Lucio A, Bailo B, Aguilera M, Cardona GA, Fernández-Crespo JC, Carmena D.** 2017. No molecular epidemiological evidence supporting household transmission of zoonotic *Giardia duodenalis* and *Cryptosporidium* spp. from pet dogs and cats in the province of Álava, Northern Spain. *Acta Trop* **170:**48–56.
58. **Beser J, Toresson L, Eitrem R, Troell K, Winiecka-Krusnell J, Lebbad M.** 2015. Possible zoonotic transmission of *Cryptosporidium* felis in a household. *Infect Ecol Epidemiol* **5:**28463.
59. **Xiao L, Cama VA, Cabrera L, Ortega Y, Pearson J, Gilman RH.** 2007. Possible transmission of *Cryptosporidium* canis among children and a dog in a household. *J Clin Microbiol* **45:**2014–2016.
60. **Nazemalhosseini-Mojarad E, Feng Y, Xiao L.** 2012. The importance of subtype analysis of *Cryptosporidium* spp. in epidemiological investigations of human cryptosporidiosis in Iran and other Mideast countries. *Gastroenterol Hepatol Bed Bench* **5:**67–70.
61. **Iqbal J, Khalid N, Hira PR.** 2011. Cryptosporidiosis in Kuwaiti children: association of clinical characteristics with *Cryptosporidium* species and subtypes. *J Med Microbiol* **60:**647–652.
62. **Alyousefi NA, Mahdy MA, Lim YA, Xiao L, Mahmud R.** 2013. First molecular characterization of *Cryptosporidium* in Yemen. *Parasitology* **140:**729–734.
63. **Chalmers RM, Smith RP, Hadfield SJ, Elwin K, Giles M.** 2011. Zoonotic linkage and variation in *Cryptosporidium parvum* from patients in the United Kingdom. *Parasitol Res* **108:**1321–1325.
64. **Hunter PR, Hadfield SJ, Wilkinson D, Lake IR, Harrison FC, Chalmers RM.** 2007. Correlation between subtypes of *Cryptosporidium parvum* in humans and risk. *Emerg Infect Dis* **13:**82–88.
65. **Drumo R, Widmer G, Morrison LJ, Tait A, Grelloni V, D'Avino N, Pozio E, Cacciò SM.** 2012. Evidence of host-associated populations of *Cryptosporidium parvum* in Italy. *Appl Environ Microbiol* **78:**3523–3529.
66. **Quílez J, Vergara-Castiblanco C, Monteagudo L, del Cacho E, Sánchez-Acedo C.** 2013. Host association of *Cryptosporidium parvum* populations infecting domestic ruminants in Spain. *Appl Environ Microbiol* **79:**5363–5371.
67. **Chalmers RM.** 2012. Waterborne outbreaks of cryptosporidiosis. *Ann Ist Super Sanita* **48:**429–446.
68. **McLauchlin J, Amar C, Pedraza-Díaz S, Nichols GL.** 2000. Molecular epidemiological analysis of *Cryptosporidium* spp. in the United Kingdom: results of genotyping *Cryptosporidium* spp. in 1,705 fecal samples from humans and 105 fecal samples from livestock animals. *J Clin Microbiol* **38:**3984–3990.
69. **Hlavsa MC, Roberts VA, Anderson AR, Hill VR, Kahler AM, Orr M, Garrison LE, Hicks LA, Newton A, Hilborn ED, Wade TJ, Beach MJ, Yoder JS, CDC.** 2011. Surveillance for waterborne disease outbreaks and other health events associated with recreational water—United States, 2007–2008. *MMWR Surveill Summ* **60:**1–32.
70. **Sarkar R, Ajjampur SS, Prabakaran AD, Geetha JC, Sowmyanarayanan TV, Kane A, Duara J, Muliyil J, Balraj V, Naumova EN, Ward H, Kang G.** 2013. Cryptosporidiosis among children in an endemic semiurban community in southern India: does a protected drinking water source decrease infection? *Clin Infect Dis* **57:**398–406.
71. **Baldursson S, Karanis P.** 2011. Waterborne transmission of protozoan parasites: review of worldwide outbreaks. An update 2004–2010. *Water Res* **45:**6603–6614 .
72. **DeSilva MB, Schafer S, Kendall Scott M, Robinson B, Hills A, Buser GL, Salis K, Gargano J, Yoder J, Hill V, Xiao L, Roellig D, Hedberg K.** 2016. Communitywide cryptosporidiosis outbreak associated with a surface water-supplied municipal water system—Baker City, Oregon, 2013. *Epidemiol Infect* **144:**274–284.
73. **Widerström M, Schönning C, Lilja M, Lebbad M, Ljung T, Allestam G, Ferm M, Björkholm B, Hansen A, Hiltula J, Långmark J, Löfdahl M, Omberg M, Reuterwall C, Samuelsson E, Widgren K, Wallensten A, Lindh J.** 2014. Large outbreak of *Cryptosporidium hominis* infection transmitted through the public water supply, Sweden. *Emerg Infect Dis* **20:**581–589.
74. **Hlavsa MC, Roberts VA, Kahler AM, Hilborn ED, Mecher TR, Beach MJ, Wade TJ, Yoder JS, Centers for Disease Control and Prevention.** 2015. Outbreaks of illness associated with recreational water—United States, 2011–2012. *MMWR Morb Mortal Wkly Rep* **64:**668–672.
75. **Mahon M, Doyle S.** 2017. Waterborne outbreak of cryptosporidiosis in the South East of Ireland: weighing up the evidence. *Ir J Med Sci* **186:**989–994.
76. **Puleston RL, Mallaghan CM, Modha DE, Hunter PR, Nguyen-Van-Tam JS, Regan CM, Nichols GL, Chalmers RM.** 2014. The first recorded outbreak of cryptosporidiosis due to *Cryptosporidium cuniculus* (formerly rabbit genotype), following a water quality incident. *J Water Health* **12:**41–50.
77. **Asano Y, Karasudani T, Okuyama M, Takami S, Oseto M, Inouye H, Yamamoto K, Aokage J, Saiki N, Fujiwara M, Shiraishi M, Uchida K, Saiki H, Suzuki M, Yamamoto T, Udaka M, Kan K, Matsuura S, Kimura M.** 2006. An outbreak of gastroenteritis associated with *Cryptosporidium meleagridis* among high school students of dormitory in Ehime, Japan. *Annu Rep Ehime Prefect Inst Public Health Environ Sci* **9:**21–25.
78. **Budu-Amoako E, Greenwood SJ, Dixon BR, Barkema HW, McClure JT.** 2011. Foodborne illness associated with *Cryptosporidium* and *Giardia* from livestock. *J Food Prot* **74:** 1944–1955.
79. **Robertson LJ, Gjerde B.** 2001. Occurrence of parasites on fruits and vegetables in Norway. *J Food Prot* **64:**1793–1798.
80. **Fayer R, Dubey JP, Lindsay DS.** 2004. Zoonotic protozoa: from land to sea. *Trends Parasitol* **20:**531–536.
81. **Dixon B, Parrington L, Cook A, Pollari F, Farber J.** 2013. Detection of *Cyclospora*, *Cryptosporidium*, and *Giardia* in ready-to-eat packaged leafy greens in Ontario, Canada. *J Food Prot* **76:**307–313.
82. **Hong S, Kim K, Yoon S, Park WY, Sim S, Yu JR.** 2014. Detection of *Cryptosporidium parvum* in environmental soil and vegetables. *J Korean Med Sci* **29:**1367–1371.
83. **Gherasim A, Lebbad M, Insulander M, Decraene V, Kling A, Hjertqvist M, Wallensten A.** 2012. Two geographically separated food-borne outbreaks in Sweden linked by an unusual *Cryptosporidium parvum* subtype, October 2010. *Euro Surveill* **17:**20318.
84. **McKerr C, Adak GK, Nichols G, Gorton R, Chalmers RM, Kafatos G, Cosford P, Charlett A, Reacher M, Pollock KG, Alexander CL, Morton S.** 2015. An outbreak of *Cryptosporidium parvum* across England & Scotland associated with consumption of fresh pre-cut salad leaves, May 2012. *PLoS One* **10:**e0125955.
85. **Rosenthal M, Pedersen R, Leibsle S, Hill V, Carter K, Roellig DM, Centers for Disease Control and Prevention.** 2015. Notes from the field: cryptosporidiosis associated with consumption of unpasteurized goat milk—Idaho, 2014. *MMWR Morb Mortal Wkly Rep* **64:**194–195.
86. **Robinson TJ, Scheftel JM, Smith KE.** 2014. Raw milk consumption among patients with non-outbreak-related enteric infections, Minnesota, USA, 2001–2010. *Emerg Infect Dis* **20:**38–44.
87. **Åberg R, Sjöman M, Hemminki K, Pirnes A, Räsänen S, Kalanti A, Pohjanvirta T, Caccio SM, Pihlajasaari A, Toikkanen S, Huusko S, Rimhanen-Finne R.** 2015. *Cryptosporidium parvum* caused a large outbreak linked to Frisee salad in Finland, 2012. *Zoonoses Public Health* **62:**618–624.
88. **Centers for Disease Control and Prevention.** 2011. Cryptosporidiosis outbreak at a summer camp—North Carolina, 2009. *MMWR Morb Mortal Wkly Rep* **60:**918–922.
89. **Pereira MD, Atwill ER, Barbosa AP, Silva SA, García-Zapata MT.** 2002. Intra-familial and extra-familial risk factors associated with *Cryptosporidium parvum* infection among children hospitalized for diarrhea in Goiânia, Goiás, Brazil. *Am J Trop Med Hyg* **66:**787–793.
90. **Grace D, Monda J, Karanja N, Randolph TF, Kang'ethe EK.** 2012. Participatory probabilistic assessment of the risk to human health associated with cryptosporidiosis from urban dairying in Dagoretti, Nairobi, Kenya. *Trop Anim Health Prod* **44**(Suppl 1)**:**33–40.

91. **Robertson B, Sinclair MI, Forbes AB, Veitch M, Kirk M, Cunliffe D, Willis J, Fairley CK.** 2002. Case-control studies of sporadic cryptosporidiosis in Melbourne and Adelaide, Australia. *Epidemiol Infect* **128:**419–431.
92. **Julian TR.** 2016. Environmental transmission of diarrheal pathogens in low and middle income countries. *Environ Sci Process Impacts* **18:**944–955.
93. **Shrivastava AK, Kumar S, Smith WA, Sahu PS.** 2017. Revisiting the global problem of cryptosporidiosis and recommendations. *Trop Parasitol* **7:**8–17.
94. **Kaplan JE, Benson C, Holmes KK, Brooks JT, Pau A, Masur H, Centers for Disease Control and Prevention, National Institutes of Health, HIV Medicine Association of the Infectious Diseases Society of America.** 2009. Guidelines for prevention and treatment of opportunistic infections in HIV-infected adults and adolescents: recommendations from CDC, the National Institutes of Health, and the HIV Medicine Association of the Infectious Diseases Society of America. *MMWR Recomm Rep* **58**(RR-4)**:**1–207.
95. **Certad G, Viscogliosi E, Chabé M, Cacciò SM.** 2017. Pathogenic mechanisms of *Cryptosporidium* and *Giardia*. *Trends Parasitol* **33:**561–576.
96. **Cama VA, Bern C, Roberts J, Cabrera L, Sterling CR, Ortega Y, Gilman RH, Xiao L.** 2008. *Cryptosporidium* species and subtypes and clinical manifestations in children, Peru. *Emerg Infect Dis* **14:**1567–1574.
97. **Sarkar R, Tate JE, Ajjampur SS, Kattula D, John J, Ward HD, Kang G.** 2014. Burden of diarrhea, hospitalization and mortality due to cryptosporidial infections in Indian children. *PLoS Negl Trop Dis* **8:**e3042.
98. **Hunter PR, Hughes S, Woodhouse S, Nicholas R, Syed Q, Chalmers RM, Verlander NQ, Goodacre J.** 2004. Health sequelae of human cryptosporidiosis in immunocompetent patients. *Clin Infect Dis* **39:**504–510.
99. **De Angelis C, Mangone M, Bianchi M, Saracco G, Repici A, Rizzetto M, Pellicano R.** 2009. An update on AIDS-related cholangiopathy. *Minerva Gastroenterol Dietol* **55:**79–82.
100. **Rahman M, Chapel H, Chapman RW, Collier JD.** 2012. Cholangiocarcinoma complicating secondary sclerosing cholangitis from cryptosporidiosis in an adult patient with CD40 ligand deficiency: case report and review of the literature. *Int Arch Allergy Immunol* **159:**204–208.
101. **Tali A, Addebbous A, Asmama S, Chabaa L, Zougaghi L.** 2011. Respiratory cryptosporidiosis in two patients with HIV infection in a tertiary care hospital in Morocco. *Ann Biol Clin (Paris)* **69:**605–608.
102. **Bern C, Kawai V, Vargas D, Rabke-Verani J, Williamson J, Chavez-Valdez R, Xiao L, Sulaiman I, Vivar A, Ticona E, Navincopa M, Cama V, Moura H, Secor WE, Visvesvara G, Gilman RH.** 2005. The epidemiology of intestinal microsporidiosis in patients with HIV/AIDS in Lima, Peru. *J Infect Dis* **191:**1658–1664.
103. **Cama VA, Ross JM, Crawford S, Kawai V, Chavez-Valdez R, Vargas D, Vivar A, Ticona E, Navincopa M, Williamson J, Ortega Y, Gilman RH, Bern C, Xiao L.** 2007. Differences in clinical manifestations among *Cryptosporidium* species and subtypes in HIV-infected persons. *J Infect Dis* **196:**684–691.
104. **Chalmers RM, Katzer F.** 2013. Looking for *Cryptosporidium*: the application of advances in detection and diagnosis. *Trends Parasitol* **29:**237–251.
105. **Abdelsalam IM, Sarhan RM, Hanafy MA.** 2017. The impact of different copro-preservation conditions on molecular detection of *Cryptosporidium* species. *Iran J Parasitol* **12:**274–283.
106. **Nétor Velásquez J, Marta E, Alicia di Risio C, Etchart C, Gancedo E, Victor Chertcoff A, Bruno Malandrini J, Germán Astudillo O, Carnevale S.** 2012. Molecular identification of protozoa causing AIDS-associated cholangiopathy in Buenos Aires, Argentina. *Acta Gastroenterol Latinoam* **42:**301–308.
107. **Chalmers RM, Atchison C, Barlow K, Young Y, Roche A, Manuel R.** 2015. An audit of the laboratory diagnosis of cryptosporidiosis in England and Wales. *J Med Microbiol* **64:**688–693.
108. **Yu JR, O'Hara SP, Lin JL, Dailey ME, Cain G, Lin JL.** 2002. A common oocyst surface antigen of *Cryptosporidium* recognized by monoclonal antibodies. *Parasitol Res* **88:** 412–420.
109. **Webster KA, Smith HV, Giles M, Dawson L, Robertson LJ.** 1996. Detection of *Cryptosporidium parvum* oocysts in faeces: comparison of conventional coproscopical methods and the polymerase chain reaction. *Vet Parasitol* **61:**5–13.
110. **Weber R, Bryan RT, Bishop HS, Wahlquist SP, Sullivan JJ, Juranek DD.** 1991. Threshold of detection of *Cryptosporidium* oocysts in human stool specimens: evidence for low sensitivity of current diagnostic methods. *J Clin Microbiol* **29:**1323–1327.
111. **Rimhanen-Finne R, Enemark HL, Kolehmainen J, Toropainen P, Hänninen ML.** 2007. Evaluation of immunofluorescence microscopy and enzyme-linked immunosorbent assay in detection of *Cryptosporidium* and *Giardia* infections in asymptomatic dogs. *Vet Parasitol* **145:**345–348.
112. **Garcia LS, Brewer TC, Bruckner DA.** 1987. Fluorescence detection of *Cryptosporidium* oocysts in human fecal specimens by using monoclonal antibodies. *J Clin Microbiol* **25:**119–121.
113. **Chalmers RM, Campbell BM, Crouch N, Charlett A, Davies AP.** 2011. Comparison of diagnostic sensitivity and specificity of seven *Cryptosporidium* assays used in the UK. *J Med Microbiol* **60:**1598–1604.
114. **Johnston SP, Ballard MM, Beach MJ, Causer L, Wilkins PP.** 2003. Evaluation of three commercial assays for detection of *Giardia* and *Cryptosporidium* organisms in fecal specimens. *J Clin Microbiol* **41:**623–626.
115. **Bialek R, Binder N, Dietz K, Joachim A, Knobloch J, Zelck UE.** 2002. Comparison of fluorescence, antigen and PCR assays to detect *Cryptosporidium parvum* in fecal specimens. *Diagn Microbiol Infect Dis* **43:**283–288.
116. **El-Moamly AA, El-Sweify MA.** 2012. ImmunoCard STAT! cartridge antigen detection assay compared to microplate enzyme immunoassay and modified Kinyoun's acid-fast staining technique for detection of *Cryptosporidium* in fecal specimens. *Parasitol Res* **110:**1037–1041.
117. **Karadam SY, Ertug S, Ertabaklar H.** 2016. Comparative evaluation of three methods (microscopic examination, direct fluorescent antibody assay, and immunochromatographic method) for the diagnosis of Giardia intestinalis from stool specimens. *Turkiye Parazitol Derg* 40:22–25.
118. **Banisch DM, El-Badry A, Klinnert JV, Ignatius R, El-Dib N.** 2015. Simultaneous detection of *Entamoeba histolytica/dispar*, *Giardia duodenalis* and cryptosporidia by immunochromatographic assay in stool samples from patients living in the Greater Cairo Region, Egypt. *World J Microbiol Biotechnol* **31:**1251–1258.
119. **Fleece ME, Heptinstall J, Khan SS, Kabir M, Herbein J, Haque R, Petri WA Jr.** 2016. Evaluation of a rapid lateral flow point-of-care test for detection of *Cryptosporidium*. *Am J Trop Med Hyg* **95:**840–841.
120. **Weitzel T, Dittrich S, Möhl I, Adusu E, Jelinek T.** 2006. Evaluation of seven commercial antigen detection tests for *Giardia* and *Cryptosporidium* in stool samples. *Clin Microbiol Infect* **12:**656–659.
121. **Goñi P, Martín B, Villacampa M, García A, Seral C, Castillo FJ, Clavel A.** 2012. Evaluation of an immunochromatographic dip strip test for simultaneous detection of *Cryptosporidium* spp, *Giardia duodenalis*, and *Entamoeba histolytica* antigens in human faecal samples. *Eur J Clin Microbiol Infect Dis* **31:**2077–2082.
122. **Agnamey P, Sarfati C, Pinel C, Rabodoniriina M, Kapel N, Dutoit E, Garnaud C, Diouf M, Garin JF, Totet A, Derouin F, ANOFEL Cryptosporidium National Network.** 2011. Evaluation of four commercial rapid immunochromatographic assays for detection of *Cryptosporidium* antigens in stool samples: a blind multicenter trial. *J Clin Microbiol* **49:**1605–1607.
123. **Robinson TJ, Cebelinski EA, Taylor C, Smith KE.** 2010. Evaluation of the positive predictive value of rapid assays used by clinical laboratories in Minnesota for the diagnosis of cryptosporidiosis. *Clin Infect Dis* **50:**e53–e55.

124. **Roellig DM, Yoder JS, Madison-Antenucci S, Robinson TJ, Van TT, Collier SA, Boxrud D, Monson T, Bates LA, Blackstock AJ, Shea S, Larson K, Xiao L, Beach M.** 2017. Community laboratory testing for *Cryptosporidium*: multicenter study retesting public health surveillance stool samples positive for *Cryptosporidium* by rapid cartridge assay with direct fluorescent antibody testing. *PLoS One* **12:**e0169915.
125. **Buss SN, Leber A, Chapin K, Fey PD, Bankowski MJ, Jones MK, Rogatcheva M, Kanack KJ, Bourzac KM.** 2015. Multicenter evaluation of the BioFire FilmArray gastrointestinal panel for etiologic diagnosis of infectious gastroenteritis. *J Clin Microbiol* **53:**915–925.
126. **Ken Dror S, Pavlotzky E, Barak M.** 2016. Evaluation of the NanoCHIP® Gastrointestinal Panel (GIP) test for simultaneous detection of parasitic and bacterial enteric pathogens in fecal specimens. *PLoS One* **11:**e0159440.
127. **Mengelle C, Mansuy JM, Prere MF, Grouteau E, Claudet I, Kamar N, Huynh A, Plat G, Benard M, Marty N, Valentin A, Berry A, Izopet J.** 2013. Simultaneous detection of gastrointestinal pathogens with a multiplex Luminex-based molecular assay in stool samples from diarrhoeic patients. *Clin Microbiol Infect* **19:**E458–E465.
128. **Albert MJ, Rotimi VO, Iqbal J, Chehadeh W.** 2016. Evaluation of the xTAG gastrointestinal pathogen panel assay for the detection of enteric pathogens in Kuwait. *Med Princ Pract* **25:**472–476.
129. **Wessels E, Rusman LG, van Bussel MJ, Claas EC.** 2014. Added value of multiplex Luminex Gastrointestinal Pathogen Panel (xTAG® GPP) testing in the diagnosis of infectious gastroenteritis. *Clin Microbiol Infect* **20:**O182–O187.
130. **Navidad JF, Griswold DJ, Gradus MS, Bhattacharyya S.** 2013. Evaluation of Luminex xTAG gastrointestinal pathogen analyte-specific reagents for high-throughput, simultaneous detection of bacteria, viruses, and parasites of clinical and public health importance. *J Clin Microbiol* **51:**3018–3024.
131. **McAuliffe G, Bissessor L, Williamson D, Moore S, Wilson J, Dufour M, Taylor S, Upton A.** 2017. Use of the EntericBio Gastro Panel II in a diagnostic microbiology laboratory: challenges and opportunities. *Pathology* **49:**419–422.
132. **Goldfarb DM, Dixon B, Moldovan I, Barrowman N, Mattison K, Zentner C, Baikie M, Bidawid S, Chan F, Slinger R.** 2013. Nanolitre real-time PCR detection of bacterial, parasitic, and viral agents from patients with diarrhoea in Nunavut, Canada. *Int J Circumpolar Health* **72:**19903.
133. **Ryan U, Paparini A, Oskam C.** 2017. New technologies for detection of enteric parasites. *Trends Parasitol* **33:**532–546.
134. **Duong VT, Phat VV, Tuyen HT, Dung TT, Trung PD, Minh PV, Tu TP, Campbell JI, Le Phuc H, Ha TT, Ngoc NM, Huong NT, Tam PT, Huong DT, Xang NV, Dong N, Phuong T, Hung NV, Phu BD, Phuc TM, Thwaites GE, Vi LL, Rabaa MA, Thompson CN, Baker S.** 2016. Evaluation of Luminex xTAG gastrointestinal pathogen panel assay for detection of multiple diarrheal pathogens in fecal samples in Vietnam. *J Clin Microbiol* **54:**1094–1100.
135. **Batra R, Judd E, Eling J, Newsholme W, Goldenberg SD.** 2016. Molecular detection of common intestinal parasites: a performance evaluation of the BD Max™ enteric parasite panel. *Eur J Clin Microbiol Infect Dis* **35:**1753–1757.
136. **Madison-Antenucci S, Relich RF, Doyle L, Espina N, Fuller D, Karchmer T, Lainesse A, Mortensen JE, Pancholi P, Veros W, Harrington SM.** 2016. Multicenter evaluation of BD Max enteric parasite real-time PCR assay for detection of *Giardia duodenalis*, *Cryptosporidium hominis*, *Cryptosporidium parvum*, and *Entamoeba histolytica*. *J Clin Microbiol* **54:**2681–2688.
137. **Mölling P, Nilsson P, Ennefors T, Ögren J, Florén K, Thulin Hedberg S, Sundqvist M.** 2016. Evaluation of the BD Max enteric parasite panel for clinical diagnostics. *J Clin Microbiol* **54:**443–444.
138. **McAuliffe GN, Anderson TP, Stevens M, Adams J, Coleman R, Mahagamasekera P, Young S, Henderson T, Hofmann M, Jennings LC, Murdoch DR.** 2013. Systematic application of multiplex PCR enhances the detection of bacteria, parasites, and viruses in stool samples. *J Infect* **67:**122–129.
139. **Laude A, Valot S, Desoubeaux G, Argy N, Nourrisson C, Pomares C, Machouart M, Le Govic Y, Dalle F, Botterel F, Bourgeois N, Cateau E, Leterrier M, Le Pape P, Morio F.** 2016. Is real-time PCR-based diagnosis similar in performance to routine parasitological examination for the identification of *Giardia intestinalis*, *Cryptosporidium parvum/Cryptosporidium hominis* and *Entamoeba histolytica* from stool samples? Evaluation of a new commercial multiplex PCR assay and literature review. *Clin Microbiol Infect* **22:**190.e1–190.e8.
140. **Liu J, Platts-Mills JA, Juma J, Kabir F, Nkeze J, Okoi C, Operario DJ, Uddin J, Ahmed S, Alonso PL, Antonio M, Becker SM, Blackwelder WC, Breiman RF, Faruque AS, Fields B, Gratz J, Haque R, Hossain A, Hossain MJ, Jarju S, Qamar F, Iqbal NT, Kwambana B, Mandomando I, McMurry TL, Ochieng C, Ochieng JB, Ochieng M, Onyango C, Panchalingam S, Kalam A, Aziz F, Qureshi S, Ramamurthy T, Roberts JH, Saha D, Sow SO, Stroup SE, Sur D, Tamboura B, Taniuchi M, Tennant SM, Toema D, Wu Y, Zaidi A, Nataro JP, Kotloff KL, Levine MM, Houpt ER.** 2016. Use of quantitative molecular diagnostic methods to identify causes of diarrhoea in children: a reanalysis of the GEMS case-control study. *Lancet* **388:**1291–1301.
141. **Frickmann H, Warnke P, Frey C, Schmidt S, Janke C, Erkens K, Schotte U, Köller T, Maaßen W, Podbielski A, Binder A, Hinz R, Queyriaux B, Wiemer D, Schwarz NG, Hagen RM.** 2015. Surveillance of food- and smear-transmitted pathogens in European soldiers with diarrhea on deployment in the tropics: experience from the European Union Training Mission (EUTM) Mali. *BioMed Res Int* **2015:**573904.
142. **Xiao L, Escalante L, Yang C, Sulaiman I, Escalante AA, Montali RJ, Fayer R, Lal AA.** 1999. Phylogenetic analysis of *Cryptosporidium* parasites based on the small-subunit rRNA gene locus. *Appl Environ Microbiol* **65:**1578–1583.
143. **Ryan U, Xiao L, Read C, Zhou L, Lal AA, Pavlasek I.** 2003. Identification of novel *Cryptosporidium* genotypes from the Czech Republic. *Appl Environ Microbiol* **69:**4302–4307.
144. **Hadfield SJ, Chalmers RM.** 2012. Detection and characterization of *Cryptosporidium cuniculus* by real-time PCR. *Parasitol Res* **111:**1385–1390.
145. **Hadfield SJ, Robinson G, Elwin K, Chalmers RM.** 2011. Detection and differentiation of *Cryptosporidium* spp. in human clinical samples by use of real-time PCR. *J Clin Microbiol* **49:**918–924.
146. **Staggs SE, Beckman EM, Keely SP, Mackwan R, Ware MW, Moyer AP, Ferretti JA, Sayed A, Xiao L, Villegas EN.** 2013. The applicability of TaqMan-based quantitative real-time PCR assays for detecting and enumerating *Cryptosporidium* spp. oocysts in the environment. *PLoS One* **8:**e66562.
147. **Mary C, Chapey E, Dutoit E, Guyot K, Hasseine L, Jeddi F, Menotti J, Paraud C, Pomares C, Rabodonirina M, Rieux A, Derouin F, ANOFEL Cryptosporidium National Network.** 2013. Multicentric evaluation of a new real-time PCR assay for quantification of *Cryptosporidium* spp. and identification of *Cryptosporidium parvum* and *Cryptosporidium hominis*. *J Clin Microbiol* **51:**2556–2563.
148. **Burnet JB, Ogorzaly L, Tissier A, Penny C, Cauchie HM.** 2012. Novel quantitative TaqMan real-time PCR assays for detection of *Cryptosporidium* at the genus level and genotyping of major human and cattle-infecting species. *J Appl Microbiol* **114:**1211–1222.
149. **Yang R, Murphy C, Song Y, Ng-Hublin J, Estcourt A, Hijjawi N, Chalmers R, Hadfield S, Bath A, Gordon C, Ryan U.** 2013. Specific and quantitative detection and identification of *Cryptosporidium hominis* and *C. parvum* in clinical and environmental samples. *Exp Parasitol* **135:**142–147.
150. **Bouzid M, Elwin K, Nader JL, Chalmers RM, Hunter PR, Tyler KM.** 2016. Novel real-time PCR assays for the specific detection of human infective *Cryptosporidium* species. *Virulence* **7:**395–399.
151. **Li N, Neumann NF, Ruecker N, Alderisio KA, Sturbaum GD, Villegas EN, Chalmers R, Monis P, Feng Y, Xiao L.** 2015. Development and evaluation of three real-time PCR assays for genotyping and source tracking *Cryptosporidium* spp. in water. *Appl Environ Microbiol* **81:**5845–5854.

152. **Utsi L, Smith SJ, Chalmers RM, Padfield S.** 2016. Cryptosporidiosis outbreak in visitors of a UK industry-compliant petting farm caused by a rare *Cryptosporidium parvum* subtype: a case-control study. *Epidemiol Infect* **144:**1000–1009.
153. **Roelfsema JH, Sprong H, Cacciò SM, Takumi K, Kroes M, van Pelt W, Kortbeek LM, van der Giessen JW.** 2016. Molecular characterization of human *Cryptosporidium* spp. isolates after an unusual increase in late summer 2012. *Parasit Vectors* **9:**138.
154. **Galuppi R, Piva S, Castagnetti C, Sarli G, Iacono E, Fioravanti ML, Caffara M.** 2016. *Cryptosporidium parvum*: from foal to veterinary students. *Vet Parasitol* **219:**53–56. *CORRIGENDUM Vet Parasitol* **221:**59.
155. **Ng-Hublin JS, Hargrave D, Combs B, Ryan U.** 2015. Investigation of a swimming pool-associated cryptosporidiosis outbreak in the Kimberley region of Western Australia. *Epidemiol Infect* **143:**1037–1041.
156. **Kinross P, Beser J, Troell K, Silverlås C, Björkman C, Lebbad M, Winiecka-Krusnell J, Lindh J, Löfdahl M.** 2015. *Cryptosporidium parvum* infections in a cohort of veterinary students in Sweden. *Epidemiol Infect* **143:**2748–2756. *CORRIGENDUM Epidemiol Infect* **143:**2757.
157. **Goñi P, Almagro-Nievas D, Cieloszyk J, Lóbez S, Navarro-Marí JM, Gutiérrez-Fernández J.** 2015. Cryptosporidiosis outbreak in a child day-care center caused by an unusual *Cryptosporidium hominis* subtype. *Enferm Infecc Microbiol Clin* **33:**651–655.
158. **Deshpande AP, Jones BL, Connelly L, Pollock KG, Brownlie S, Alexander CL.** 2015. Molecular characterization of *Cryptosporidium parvum* isolates from human cryptosporidiosis cases in Scotland. *Parasitology* **142:**318–325.
159. **Hlavsa MC, Roellig DM, Seabolt MH, Kahler AM, Murphy JL, McKitt TK, Geeter EF, Dawsey R, Davidson SL, Kim TN, Tucker TH, Iverson SA, Garrett B, Fowle N, Collins J, Epperson G, Zusy S, Weiss JR, Komatsu K, Rodriguez E, Patterson JG, Sunenshine R, Taylor B, Cibulskas K, Denny L, Omura K, Tsorin B, Fullerton KE, Xiao L.** 2017. Using molecular characterization to support investigations of aquatic facility-associated outbreaks of cryptosporidiosis—Alabama, Arizona, and Ohio, 2016. *MMWR Morb Mortal Wkly Rep* **66:**493–497.
160. **Cope JR, Prosser A, Nowicki S, Roberts MW, Roberts JM, Scheer D, Anderson C, Longsworth A, Parsons C, Goldschmidt D, Johnston S, Bishop H, Xiao L, Hill V, Beach M, Hlavsa MC.** 2015. Preventing community-wide transmission of *Cryptosporidium*: a proactive public health response to a swimming pool-associated outbreak—Auglaize County, Ohio, USA. *Epidemiol Infect* **143:**3459–3467.
161. **Hlavsa MC, Roberts VA, Kahler AM, Hilborn ED, Wade TJ, Backer LC, Yoder JS, Centers for Disease Control and Prevention.** 2014. Recreational water-associated disease outbreaks—United States, 2009–2010. *MMWR Morb Mortal Wkly Rep* **63:**6–10.
162. **Feng Y, Tiao N, Li N, Hlavsa M, Xiao L, Doern GV.** 2014. Multilocus sequence typing of an emerging *Cryptosporidium hominis* subtype in the United States. *J Clin Microbiol* **52:**524–530.
163. **Li N, Xiao L, Cama VA, Ortega Y, Gilman RH, Guo M, Feng Y.** 2013. Genetic recombination and *Cryptosporidium hominis* virulent subtype IbA10G2. *Emerg Infect Dis* **19:**1573–1582.
164. **Chalmers RM, Robinson G, Hotchkiss E, Alexander C, May S, Gilray J, Connelly L, Hadfield SJ.** 2017. Suitability of loci for multiple-locus variable-number of tandem-repeats analysis of *Cryptosporidium parvum* for inter-laboratory surveillance and outbreak investigations. *Parasitology* **144:**37–47.
165. **Hadfield SJ, Pachebat JA, Swain MT, Robinson G, Cameron SJ, Alexander J, Hegarty MJ, Elwin K, Chalmers RM.** 2015. Generation of whole genome sequences of new *Cryptosporidium hominis* and *Cryptosporidium parvum* isolates directly from stool samples. *BMC Genomics* **16:**650.
166. **Guo Y, Li N, Lysén C, Frace M, Tang K, Sammons S, Roellig DM, Feng Y, Xiao L.** 2015. Isolation and enrichment of *Cryptosporidium* DNA and verification of DNA purity for whole-genome sequencing. *J Clin Microbiol* **53:**641–647.
167. **Andersson S, Sikora P, Karlberg ML, Winiecka-Krusnell J, Alm E, Beser J, Arrighi RB.** 2015. It's a dirty job—a robust method for the purification and de novo genome assembly of *Cryptosporidium* from clinical material. *J Microbiol Methods* **113:**10–12.
168. **Troell K, Hallström B, Divne AM, Alsmark C, Arrighi R, Huss M, Beser J, Bertilsson S.** 2016. *Cryptosporidium* as a testbed for single cell genome characterization of unicellular eukaryotes. *BMC Genomics* **17:**471.
169. **Feng Y, Li N, Roellig DM, Kelley A, Liu G, Amer S, Tang K, Zhang L, Xiao L.** 2017. Comparative genomic analysis of the IId subtype family of *Cryptosporidium parvum*. *Int J Parasitol* **47:**281–290.
170. **Ifeonu OO, Chibucos MC, Orvis J, Su Q, Elwin K, Guo F, Zhang H, Xiao L, Sun M, Chalmers RM, Fraser CM, Zhu G, Kissinger JC, Widmer G, Silva JC.** 2016. Annotated draft genome sequences of three species of *Cryptosporidium*: *Cryptosporidium meleagridis* isolate UKMEL1, *C. baileyi* isolate TAMU-09Q1 and *C. hominis* isolates TU502_2012 and UKH1. *Pathog Dis* **74:**ftw080.
171. **Guo Y, Tang K, Rowe LA, Li N, Roellig DM, Knipe K, Frace M, Yang C, Feng Y, Xiao L.** 2015. Comparative genomic analysis reveals occurrence of genetic recombination in virulent *Cryptosporidium hominis* subtypes and telomeric gene duplications in *Cryptosporidium parvum*. *BMC Genomics* **16:**320.
172. **Liu S, Roellig DM, Guo Y, Li N, Frace MA, Tang K, Zhang L, Feng Y, Xiao L.** 2016. Evolution of mitosome metabolism and invasion-related proteins in *Cryptosporidium*. *BMC Genomics* **17:**1006.
173. **Sikora P, Andersson S, Winiecka-Krusnell J, Hallström B, Alsmark C, Troell K, Beser J, Arrighi RB.** 2017. Genomic variation in IbA10G2 and other patient-derived *Cryptosporidium hominis* subtypes. *J Clin Microbiol* **55:**844–858.
174. **Feng Y, Torres E, Li N, Wang L, Bowman D, Xiao L.** 2013. Population genetic characterisation of dominant *Cryptosporidium parvum* subtype IIaA15G2R1. *Int J Parasitol* **43:** 1141–1147.
175. **Hijjawi N.** 2010. *Cryptosporidium*: new developments in cell culture. *Exp Parasitol* **124:**54–60.
176. **Teichmann K, Kuliberda M, Schatzmayr G, Pacher T, Zitterl-Eglseer K, Joachim A, Hadacek F.** 2016. In vitro inhibitory effects of plant-derived by-products against *Cryptosporidium parvum*. *Parasite* **23:**41.
177. **Castellanos-Gonzalez A, Sparks H, Nava S, Huang W, Zhang Z, Rivas K, Hulverson MA, Barrett LK, Ojo KK, Fan E, Van Voorhis WC, White AC Jr.** 2016. A novel calcium-dependent kinase inhibitor, bumped kinase inhibitor 1517, cures cryptosporidiosis in immunosuppressed mice. *J Infect Dis* **214:**1850–1855.
178. **Morada M, Lee S, Gunther-Cummins L, Weiss LM, Widmer G, Tzipori S, Yarlett N.** 2016. Continuous culture of *Cryptosporidium parvum* using hollow fiber technology. *Int J Parasitol* **46:**21–29.
179. **DeCicco RePass MA, Chen Y, Lin Y, Zhou W, Kaplan DL, Ward HD.** 2017. Novel bioengineered three-dimensional human intestinal model for long-term infection of *Cryptosporidium parvum*. *Infect Immun* **85:**e00731-16.
180. **Paziewska-Harris A, Schoone G, Schallig H.** 2017. Long-term storage of *Cryptosporidium parvum* for in vitro culture. *J Parasitol* **104:**96–100.
181. **Sparks H, Nair G, Castellanos-Gonzalez A, White AC Jr.** 2015. Treatment of *Cryptosporidium*: what we know, gaps, and the way forward. *Curr Trop Med Rep* **2:**181–187.
182. **Bailey JM, Erramouspe J.** 2004. Nitazoxanide treatment for giardiasis and cryptosporidiosis in children. *Ann Pharmacother* **38:**634–640.
183. **Rossignol JF.** 2010. *Cryptosporidium* and *Giardia*: treatment options and prospects for new drugs. *Exp Parasitol* **124:** 45–53.
184. **McLeod C, Morris PS, Snelling TL, Carapetis JR, Bowen AC.** 2014. Nitazoxanide for the treatment of infectious diarrhoea in the Northern Territory, Australia 2007–2012. *Rural Remote Health* **14:**2759.

185. **Ali S, Mumar S, Kalam K, Raja K, Baqi S.** 2014. Prevalence, clinical presentation and treatment outcome of cryptosporidiosis in immunocompetent adult patients presenting with acute diarrhoea. *J Pak Med Assoc* **64:**613–618.
186. **Abubakar I, Aliyu SH, Arumugam C, Usman NK, Hunter PR.** 2007. Treatment of cryptosporidiosis in immunocompromised individuals: systematic review and meta-analysis. *Br J Clin Pharmacol* **63:**387–393.
187. **Pantenburg B, Cabada MM, White AC Jr.** 2009. Treatment of cryptosporidiosis. *Expert Rev Anti Infect Ther* **7:**385–391.
188. **Zardi EM, Picardi A, Afeltra A.** 2005. Treatment of cryptosporidiosis in immunocompromised hosts. *Chemotherapy* **51:**193–196.
189. **Werneck-Silva AL, Prado IB.** 2009. Gastroduodenal opportunistic infections and dyspepsia in HIV-infected patients in the era of highly active antiretroviral therapy. *J Gastroenterol Hepatol* **24:**135–139.
190. **Mengist HM, Taye B, Tsegaye A.** 2015. Intestinal parasitosis in relation to $CD4^+$ T cells levels and anemia among HAART initiated and HAART naive pediatric HIV patients in a model ART center in Addis Ababa, Ethiopia. *PLoS One* **10:**e0117715.
191. **Kaniyarakkal V, Mundangalam N, Moorkoth AP, Mathew S.** 2016. Intestinal parasite profile in the stool of HIV positive patients in relation to immune status and comparison of various diagnostic techniques with special reference to *Cryptosporidium* at a tertiary care hospital in South India. *Adv Med* **2016:**3564359.
192. **Maggi P, Larocca AM, Quarto M, Serio G, Brandonisio O, Angarano G, Pastore G.** 2000. Effect of antiretroviral therapy on cryptosporidiosis and microsporidiosis in patients infected with human immunodeficiency virus type 1. *Eur J Clin Microbiol Infect Dis* **19:**213–217.
193. **Akinbo FO, Okaka CE, Omoregie R, Adamu H, Xiao L.** 2013. Unusual *Enterocytozoon bieneusi* genotypes and *Cryptosporidium hominis* subtypes in HIV-infected patients on highly active antiretroviral therapy. *Am J Trop Med Hyg* **89:**157–161.
194. **Ukwah BN, Ezeonu IM, Ezeonu CT, Roellig D, Xiao L.** 2017. *Cryptosporidium* species and subtypes in diarrheal children and HIV-infected persons in Ebonyi and Nsukka, Nigeria. *J Infect Dev Ctries* **11:**173–179.
195. **Nsagha DS, Njunda AL, Assob NJC, Ayima CW, Tanue EA, Kibu OD, Kwenti TE.** 2016. Intestinal parasitic infections in relation to $CD4^+$ T cell counts and diarrhea in HIV/AIDS patients with or without antiretroviral therapy in Cameroon. *BMC Infect Dis* **16:**9.
196. **Chellan P, Sadler PJ, Land KM.** 2017. Recent developments in drug discovery against the protozoal parasites *Cryptosporidium* and *Toxoplasma*. *Bioorg Med Chem Lett* **27:**1491–1501.
197. **Shoultz DA, de Hostos EL, Choy RK.** 2016. Addressing *Cryptosporidium* infection among young children in low-income settings: the crucial role of new and existing drugs for reducing morbidity and mortality. *PLoS Negl Trop Dis* **10:**e0004242.
198. **Debnath A, McKerrow JH.** 2017. Editorial: drug development for parasite-induced diarrheal diseases. *Front Microbiol* **8:**577.
199. **Manjunatha UH, Vinayak S, Zambriski JA, Chao AT, Sy T, Noble CG, Bonamy GMC, Kondreddi RR, Zou B, Gedeck P, Brooks CF, Herbert GT, Sateriale A, Tandel J, Noh S, Lakshminarayana SB, Lim SH, Goodman LB, Bodenreider C, Feng G, Zhang L, Blasco F, Wagner J, Leong FJ, Striepen B, Diagana TT.** 2017. A *Cryptosporidium* PI(4)K inhibitor is a drug candidate for cryptosporidiosis. *Nature* **546:**376–380.
200. **Zhang H, Guo F, Zhu G.** 2015. *Cryptosporidium* lactate dehydrogenase is associated with the parasitophorous vacuole membrane and is a potential target for developing therapeutics. *PLoS Pathog* **11:**e1005250.
201. **Hulverson MA, Vinayak S, Choi R, Schaefer DA, Castellanos-Gonzalez A, Vidadala RSR, Brooks CF, Herbert GT, Betzer DP, Whitman GR, Sparks HN, Arnold SLM, Rivas KL, Barrett LK, White AC Jr, Maly DJ, Riggs MW, Striepen B, Van Voorhis WC, Ojo KK.** 2017. Bumped-kinase inhibitors for cryptosporidiosis therapy. *J Infect Dis* **215:**1275–1284.
202. **Arnold SLM, Choi R, Hulverson MA, Schaefer DA, Vinayak S, Vidadala RSR, McCloskey MC, Whitman GR, Huang W, Barrett LK, Ojo KK, Fan E, Maly DJ, Riggs MW, Striepen B, Van Voorhis WC.** 2017. Necessity of bumped kinase inhibitor gastrointestinal exposure in treating *Cryptosporidium* infection. *J Infect Dis* **216:**55–63.
203. **Huang W, Choi R, Hulverson MA, Zhang Z, McCloskey MC, Schaefer DA, Whitman GR, Barrett LK, Vidadala RSR, Riggs MW, Maly DJ, Van Voorhis WC, Ojo KK, Fan E.** 2017. 5-Aminopyrazole-4-carboxamide based compounds prevent the growth of *Cryptosporidium parvum*. *Antimicrob Agents Chemother* **61:**e00020-17.
204. **Osman KT, Ye J, Shi Z, Toker C, Lovato D, Jumani RS, Zuercher W, Huston CD, Edwards AM, Lautens M, Santhakumar V, Hui R.** 2017. Discovery and structure activity relationship of the first potent *cryptosporidium* FIKK kinase inhibitor. *Bioorg Med Chem* **25:**1672–1680.
205. **Centers for Disease Control and Prevention.** 1999. False-positive laboratory tests for *Cryptosporidium* involving an enzyme-linked immunosorbent assay—United States, November 1997–March 1998. *MMWR Morb Mortal Wkly Rep* **48:**4–8.
206. **Centers for Disease Control and Prevention.** 2002. Manufacturer's recall of rapid assay kits based on false positive *Cryptosporidium* antigen tests—Wisconsin, 2001–2002. *MMWR Morb Mortal Wkly Rep* **51:**189.
207. **Centers for Disease Control and Prevention.** 2004. Manufacturer's recall of rapid cartridge assay kits on the basis of false-positive *Cryptosporidium* antigen tests—Colorado, 2004. *MMWR Morb Mortal Wkly Rep* **53:**198.
208. **Doing KM, Hamm JL, Jellison JA, Marquis JA, Kingsbury C.** 1999. False-positive results obtained with the Alexon ProSpecT *Cryptosporidium* enzyme immunoassay. *J Clin Microbiol* **37:**1582–1583.
209. **Fournet N, Deege MP, Urbanus AT, Nichols G, Rosner BM, Chalmers RM, Gorton R, Pollock KG, van der Giessen JW, Wever PC, Dorigo-Zetsma JW, Mulder B, Mank TG, Overdevest I, Kusters JG, van Pelt W, Kortbeek LM.** 2013. Simultaneous increase of *Cryptosporidium* infections in the Netherlands, the United Kingdom and Germany in late summer season, 2012. *Euro Surveill* **18:**20348.

Nematodes

HARSHA SHEOREY, BEVERLEY-ANN BIGGS, AND NORBERT RYAN

146

Nematodes are unsegmented cylindrical worms with a body cavity containing an alimentary canal and genital system; the sexes are separate. They lack circular muscles and move by flexing their bodies. There are four larval stages and the adult worm. In most instances, the third-stage larva is the infective stage.

Infections caused by intestinal nematodes, including the soil-transmitted helminths (STH), are the most common infections globally, with more than 1.5 billion people infected, especially in resource-poor settings where sanitation is inadequate and in tropical and subtropical regions. These parasites are a major cause of poor health, with the greatest morbidity in women and children, and are included in the list of neglected tropical diseases by the World Health Organization (WHO) (1). By definition, the STH infections are ascariasis, trichuriasis, and hookworm infection. Although *Strongyloides* also has a soil-transmitted cycle, it differs from other helminths in its capacity to reproduce within a human host. However, there is a compelling argument that strongyloidiasis should also be considered in conjunction with the STH (2) and that control measures be included in STH treatment programs in areas where the disease is endemic (3). In developed countries, groups such as immigrants and refugees, travelers, and war veterans often unknowingly harbor helminths for years after leaving an area of endemicity. This has implications for provision of health services and necessitates action to formulate guidelines for managing infections that are not commonly seen in these countries (e.g., guidelines formulated within Australia [4]). Global efforts to target STH infections in children with school-based chemotherapy have reduced their prevalence in many lower- and middle-income countries (3) (http://www.who.int/intestinal_worms/en/). Chronic morbidity in humans from STH infections can be reduced by periodic treatment with anthelmintics in high-risk populations. However, monitoring and evaluation of treatment programs are labor-intensive, and newer technologies are needed for assessing program effectiveness. Because deworming programs need to distinguish between populations where parasitic infection is controlled and those where further treatment is required, multiparallel quantitative PCR or similar high-throughput molecular diagnostics may provide new and important diagnostic information in future (5).

Conventional laboratory diagnosis is based primarily on microscopic examination of feces and differentiation of species based on morphology of eggs or larvae detected (Fig. 1 to 3). The sensitivity of microscopy is influenced by the method of processing, e.g., direct microscopy, formalin-ethyl acetate concentration, or Kato-Katz smear, and is affected by factors such as variability of the number of eggs or larvae excreted. Occasionally, adult worms may be processed by histology, and features of both the adult worm and the eggs may be used in identifying the parasite (Fig. 4). Molecular diagnosis for intestinal nematodes (including real-time multiplexed PCR) (6) is gradually being introduced but is not routinely available in diagnostic laboratories at the time of writing. There are issues with sensitivity of assays for *Strongyloides* in particular; in chronic infection, numbers of larvae may be low, and they are intermittently excreted in feces. In particular, the number of eggs produced by *Strongyloides* is estimated at only 30 to 50 per day. This exceptionally low yield compared to the output of the STH accounts for some of the diagnostic difficulties encountered in screening for this species. Furthermore, due to small sample size for PCR assays, sensitivity is likely to remain low unless multiple stool samples are tested (7).

The subject of preventive chemotherapy was recently updated by the WHO (1). Global trends and management options for *Strongyloides* infection (including prophylaxis of at-risk groups prior to immune suppression) have been updated (8–10). For details about susceptibility testing for parasites, consult chapter 154.

TAXONOMY OF NEMATODES

There are a variety of morphological features which form the basis for taxonomy of nematodes. At the anterior end, mouth parts may possess structures for attachment or penetration. These may include spines, hooks, or cutting plates. The pharyngeal cavity may be short, hollowed out, or long and capillary. Esophageal shape also varies, but the esophagus usually ends in a muscular bulb. In the male, features of the tail may include caudal papillae and copulatory spicules (sclerotized copulatory aids). In the majority of cases, males carry more taxonomically useful information than females; the latter may often be unidentifiable to species level in the absence of males. Studies strongly suggest that nematodes are actually related to the arthropods and priapulids in a newly recognized group, the Ecdysozoa. All these nematodes belong to the kingdom Animalia, phylum

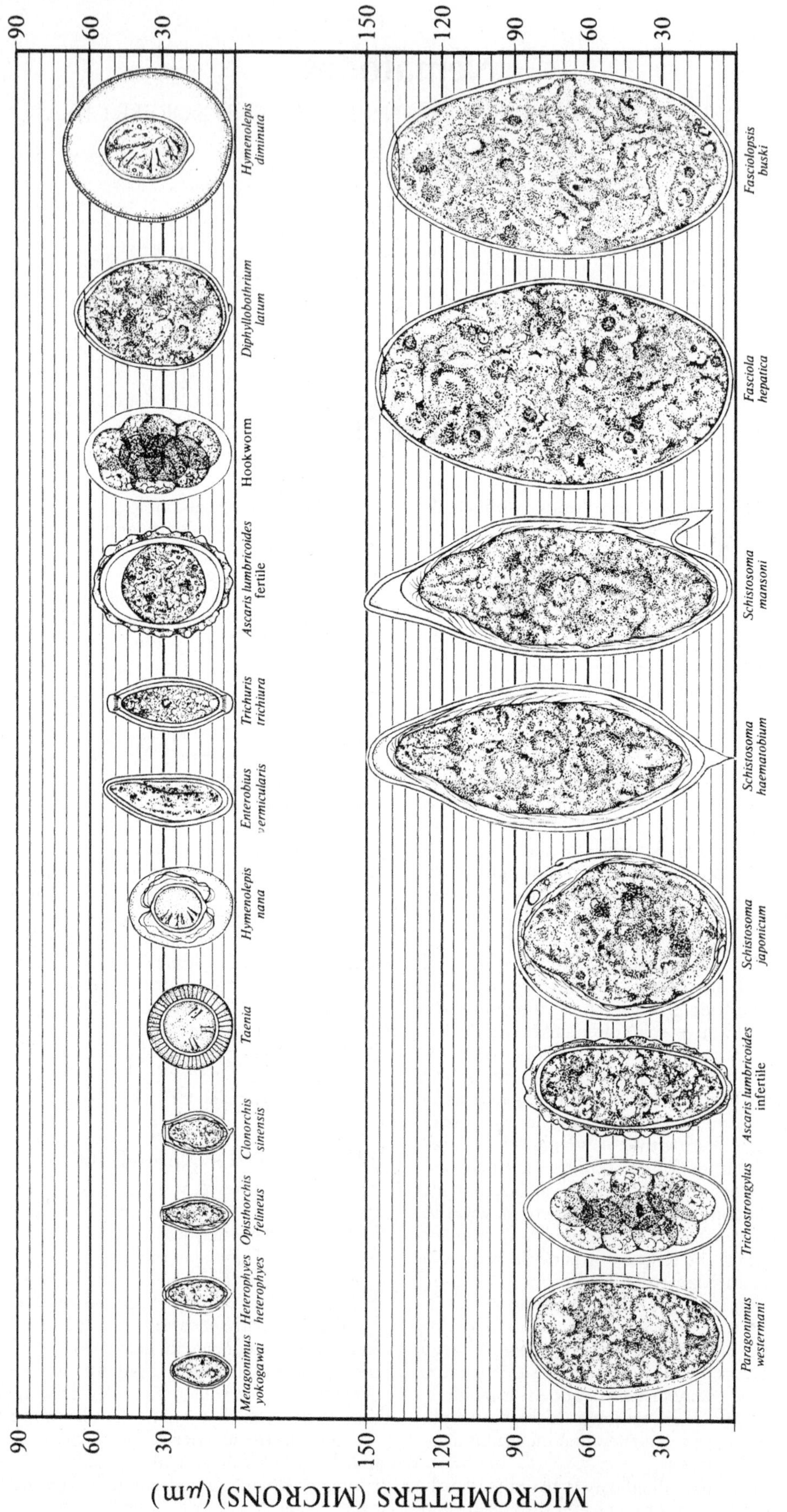

FIGURE 1 Relative sizes of helminth eggs.

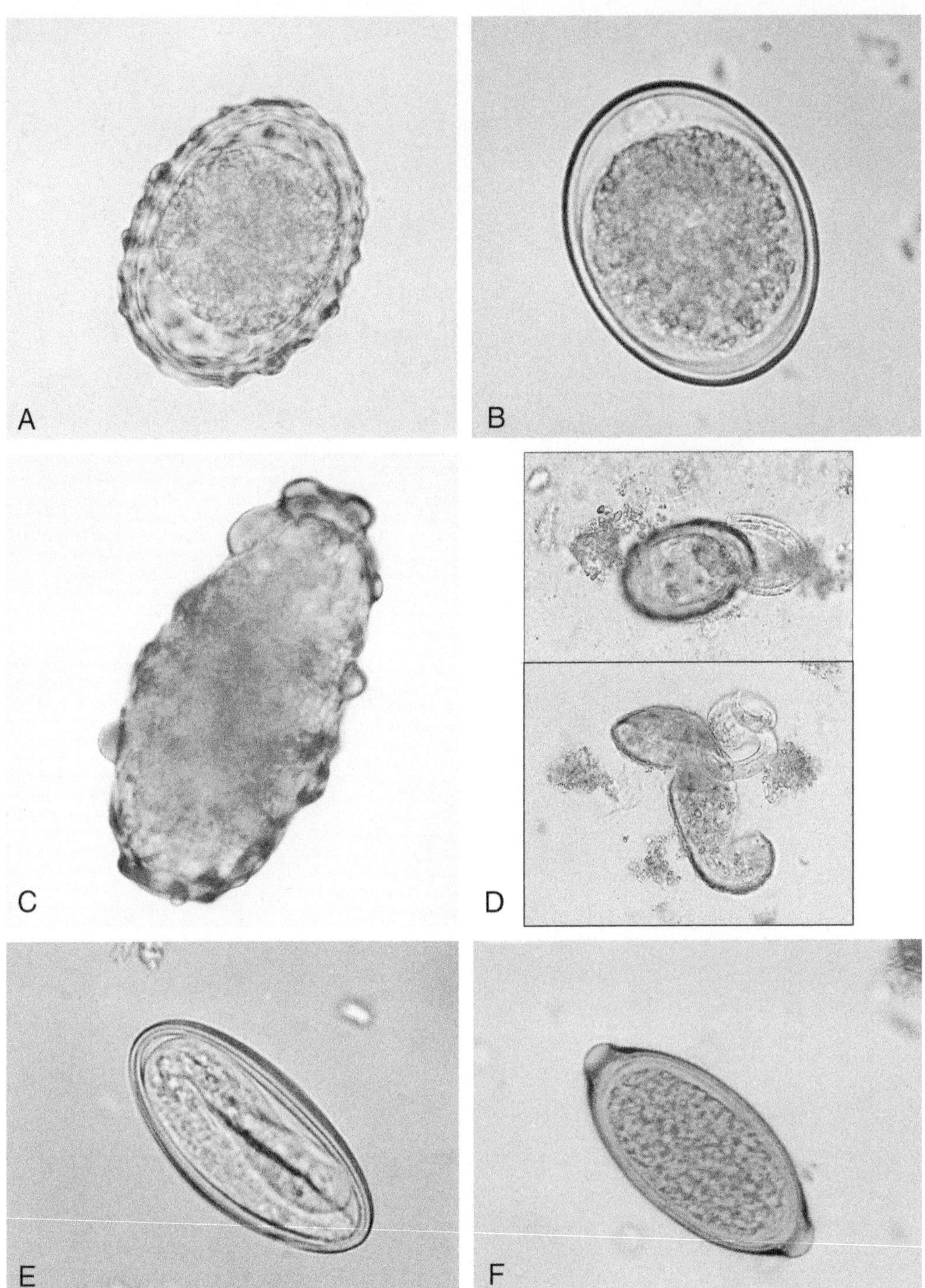

FIGURE 2 Eggs of various intestinal nematodes (magnification, ×850). (A) Fertile egg of *A. lumbricoides*. (B) Decorticated fertile egg of *A. lumbricoides*. (C) Infertile egg of *A. lumbricoides*. (D) Fertile eggs of *A. lumbricoides* with hatching larvae. Courtesy of Pam Smith, Royal Darwin Hospital. (E) Embryonated infective egg of *E. vermicularis*. (F) Egg of *T. trichiura* with polar plugs.

Nemathelminthes (Nematoda). As new molecular techniques are applied, the taxonomy of nematodes is changing and constantly being updated (see chapter 135 and reference 11 for details).

The list of nematode infections described in detail below is by no means exhaustive but includes those commonly affecting humans on a worldwide scale. This chapter mainly focuses on the STH along with *Strongyloides stercoralis* and *Enterobius vermicularis*. From time to time, other less common species may be encountered, and the assistance of reference laboratories covering both human and veterinary diagnostic services may be required.

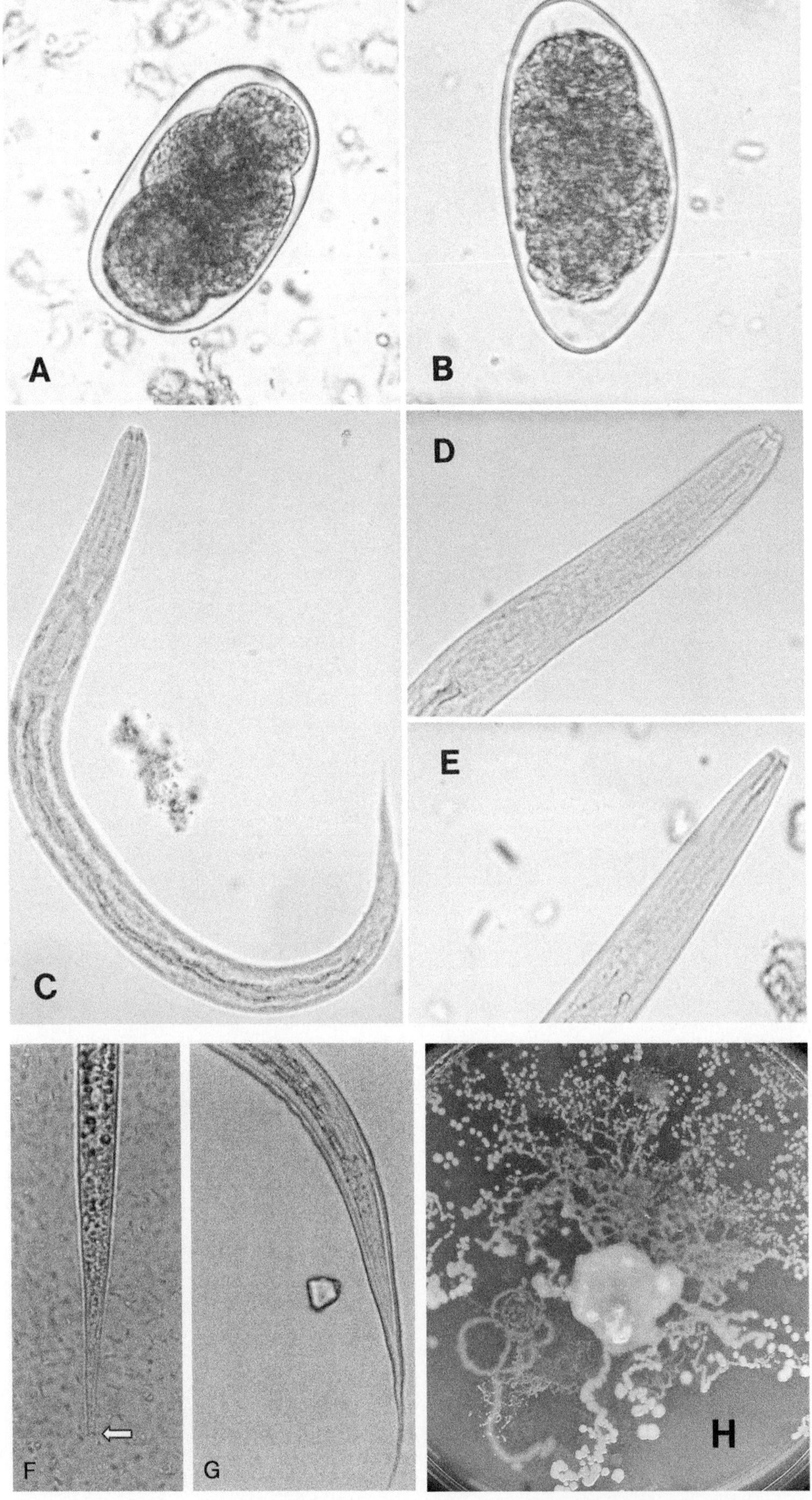
A
B
C
D
E
F
G
H

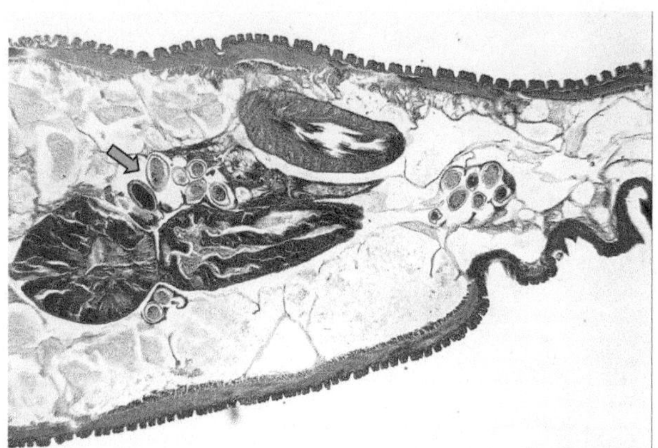

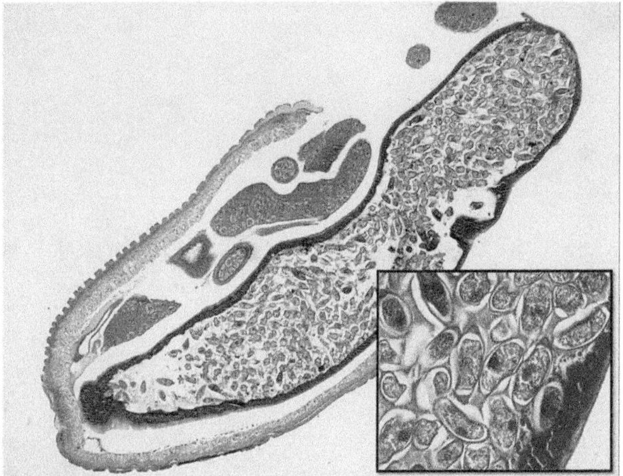

FIGURE 4 Sections of adult female worms taken at colonoscopy (hematoxylin and eosin stain). (A) *E. vermicularis* female showing characteristic eggs (arrow). Magnification, ×400. (B) *T. trichiura* female showing characteristic eggs. Magnification, ×100.

COLLECTION, TRANSPORT, AND STORAGE OF SPECIMENS

Specimens should be collected before antibiotics or antiparasitic drugs are given (for details, see chapter 136). It is important to transport and process fecal specimens for parasitic examination as soon as possible. Clinicians and collection staff should be encouraged to either send fresh specimens to the laboratory without delay or use commercially available preservative kits. If delay is inevitable, specimens should be refrigerated or transported in commercially available vials or kits with a preservative such as polyvinyl alcohol or sodium acetate-acetic acid-formalin. If these are not available at the point of collection, preservatives should be added as soon as the specimen is received in the laboratory. Excellent directions for proper collection are available with these kits. The choice of preservative depends on various considerations, such as whether permanent stained smears or immunoassays are required (for details, see reference 12). Two or three specimens collected over a period of 7 to 10 days is optimal. Specimens that are very small in volume or obviously dry should be rejected and a fresh specimen should be collected. Refrigeration and the use of preservatives should be avoided if agar plate culture (APC) or Baermann procedures for culture of *Strongyloides* larvae are required.

Worms retrieved at colonoscopy or submitted by the patient should be transported to the laboratory without delay. Worms can be preserved in 60% alcohol; the use of formalin should be avoided, as it causes contraction and hardening of tissues.

For sputum specimens, proper instructions should be given to patients emphasizing requirements, i.e., avoidance of saliva and avoiding use of a mouthwash before deep coughing (expectorating). Sputum and aspirates should be transported to the laboratory and processed immediately.

All specimens should be handled using standard precautions; e.g., latex gloves should be worn by anyone handling the specimens.

DIRECT EXAMINATION

The specimen should be handled in a work cabinet (biological safety cabinet), and gloves and gown should be worn. The specimen should be examined, and its consistency should be noted. Motile and nonmotile worms should be noted (Fig. 5A and B) or segments of worms. Areas that look watery, purulent, or bloody should be sampled. If feces are formed, several areas of the specimen should be sampled for the concentration technique.

Both the direct specimen and concentrate are examined as wet preps in saline and iodine. The whole coverslip area should be scanned at low-power magnification (×100). Most helminth eggs and larvae can be identified at this magnification and diagnosis confirmed at high power (×400) on the basis of their shape, size, and characteristic features (Fig. 1 to 3). Smears should be prepared from a centrifuged deposit (500 × *g* for 10 minutes) for permanent staining, but this technique is not the preferred method for identification of nematode eggs or larvae; it is primarily to diagnose mixed infections with protozoa.

ASCARIS LUMBRICOIDES (ROUNDWORM)

Taxonomy

The organisms in this group, in the modern classification of biological species, are in clade III (Chromadoria: Spururina) of the Nematoda, in the order Ascaridida and the family Ascarididae.

FIGURE 3 Eggs and larvae of intestinal nematodes (magnification, ×850). (A) Hookworm egg; (B) *Trichostrongylus* egg; (C) rhabditiform or first-stage larva of *S. stercoralis*; (D) anterior end of a rhabditiform larva of *S. stercoralis* showing the short buccal cavity; (E) anterior end of a rhabditiform hookworm larva showing long buccal cavity; (F) tail end of a filariform, or last-stage, larva of *S. stercoralis* with the notched tail (arrow); (G) tail end of a filariform, or last-stage, hookworm larva with a tapering tail; (H) APC showing tracks of bacterial colonies due to larval movement on the surface and inside the agar. The fecal specimen is placed in middle of the plate and sealed, as larvae are infectious.

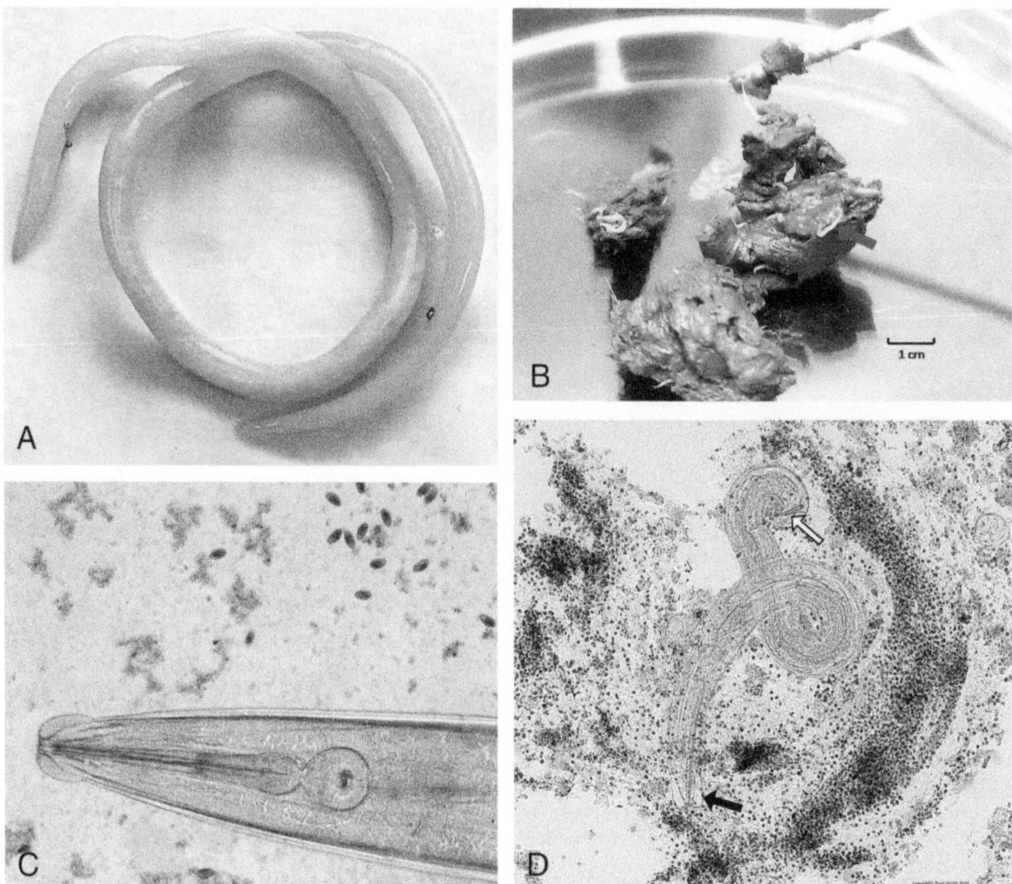

FIGURE 5 Various adult worms of intestinal nematodes. (A) *A. lumbricoides* adult worm with typical cylindrical body with tapering ends and thick cuticle. The *A. lumbricoides* adult worm is the largest of the human pathogenic nematodes, 15 to 35 cm in length. (B) Adult worms of *E. vermicularis* in feces (arrow). (C) Anterior end of an *E. vermicularis* adult female worm with the characteristic cervical alae ("lips"). Adult females are usually 8 to 13 by 0.3 to 0.5 mm. Typical eggs can also usually be seen in the field. (D) Anterior end of an *E. vermicularis* adult male worm with the characteristic cervical alae (arrow). These are only occasionally seen in feces. There is also a characteristic spicule at the posterior end (open arrow). Courtesy of Pam Smith, Royal Darwin Hospital.

Of the three genera of ascaridid nematodes regularly occurring as parasites of humans, only *Ascaris* is a true human parasite. The others (*Toxocara* and *Toxascaris*) are common parasites of cats and dogs and occasionally infect humans. Ascaridids are related to anisakids, with three distinct lips, but differ in that their life cycle is linked to terrestrial rather than aquatic conditions.

Ascaris suum was thought to be a separate species in pigs but has recently been found to be genetically similar to the human species *A. lumbricoides* (13).

Description of the Agent

Eggs

Eggs of *A. lumbricoides* (Fig. 2A to D) are usually seen in two forms: unfertilized and fertilized. The shell of a fertilized egg (45 to 75 by 35 to 50 μm) consists of an inner lipid layer responsible for selective permeability, a chitin-protein layer responsible for structural strength, and an outer vitelline layer. The inner layer contains a lipoprotein, ascaroside, which helps prevent formaldehyde, disinfectants, and other chemicals from contacting the embryo. The outer surface of the fertilized egg has an uneven deposit of mucopolysaccharide with adhesive properties. Eggs appear brown due to staining by bile. The unfertilized eggs have thinner walls and distorted mammillations. These eggs are usually more elongated, measure 85 to 95 by 43 to 47 μm, and may have either a pronounced mammillated coat or little or no mammillated layer. The presence of only unfertilized eggs suggests that only female worms are present in the intestine. Occasionally, a hatching larva may be seen (Fig. 2D). This could represent continuing development of the embryo despite the presence of fixative.

Larvae

During an incubation period of 2 to 3 weeks in soil, first-stage larvae develop inside the eggs and molt to form the second-stage larvae. Following ingestion of eggs, the larvae hatch in the jejunum; these second-stage larvae have a typical filariform appearance (measuring approximately 250 by 14 μm).They migrate across the intestinal wall and enter the circulation to reach the lungs, growing to approximately 560 by 28 μm. A further molt occurs in the lungs, and the larvae develop over 8 or 9 days to reach a size of 1.2 mm by 36 μm. They are carried to the throat and are swallowed. Growth is rapid after the fourth and final molt in the intestine.

Worms

Adult male and female *A. lumbricoides* worms (Fig. 5A) are light brown to pink when fresh, turning white with storage. Egg laying commences at 8 to 9 weeks, when females measure 15 to 20 cm, and they may reach 45 cm by 5 mm; males are generally smaller, at 15 to 31 cm by 3 mm. Males have a curved tail containing a cloaca, a pair of copulatory spicules, and caudal papillae. Adult worms live in the lumen of the small intestine and feed on digestion products.

Epidemiology and Prevention

A. lumbricoides infection is one of the most common human infections, with over a billion people estimated to be infected. It has a worldwide distribution and is most common in tropical and subtropical areas. It is particularly associated with crowding and poor sanitation. Contamination of soil by human excreta can result in a layer of eggs within silt that is easily disturbed, resulting in contamination of root and vegetable produce.

Preventive measures consist of health education about personal hygiene and sanitation, and drug therapy.

Transmission and Life Cycle (Fig. 6)

Eggs passed in feces (diagnostic stage) have an unsegmented ovum, which develops in the soil over 10 to 15 days to become an infective-stage larva (Table 1); eggs may survive in this form for years under favorable conditions of heat and humidity. Infection follows the ingestion of embryonated eggs (infective stage), which hatch in the small intestine. Larvae penetrate the intestinal mucosa, and the venous circulation carries them to the lungs. From here they migrate to the trachea and are swallowed. They then complete their

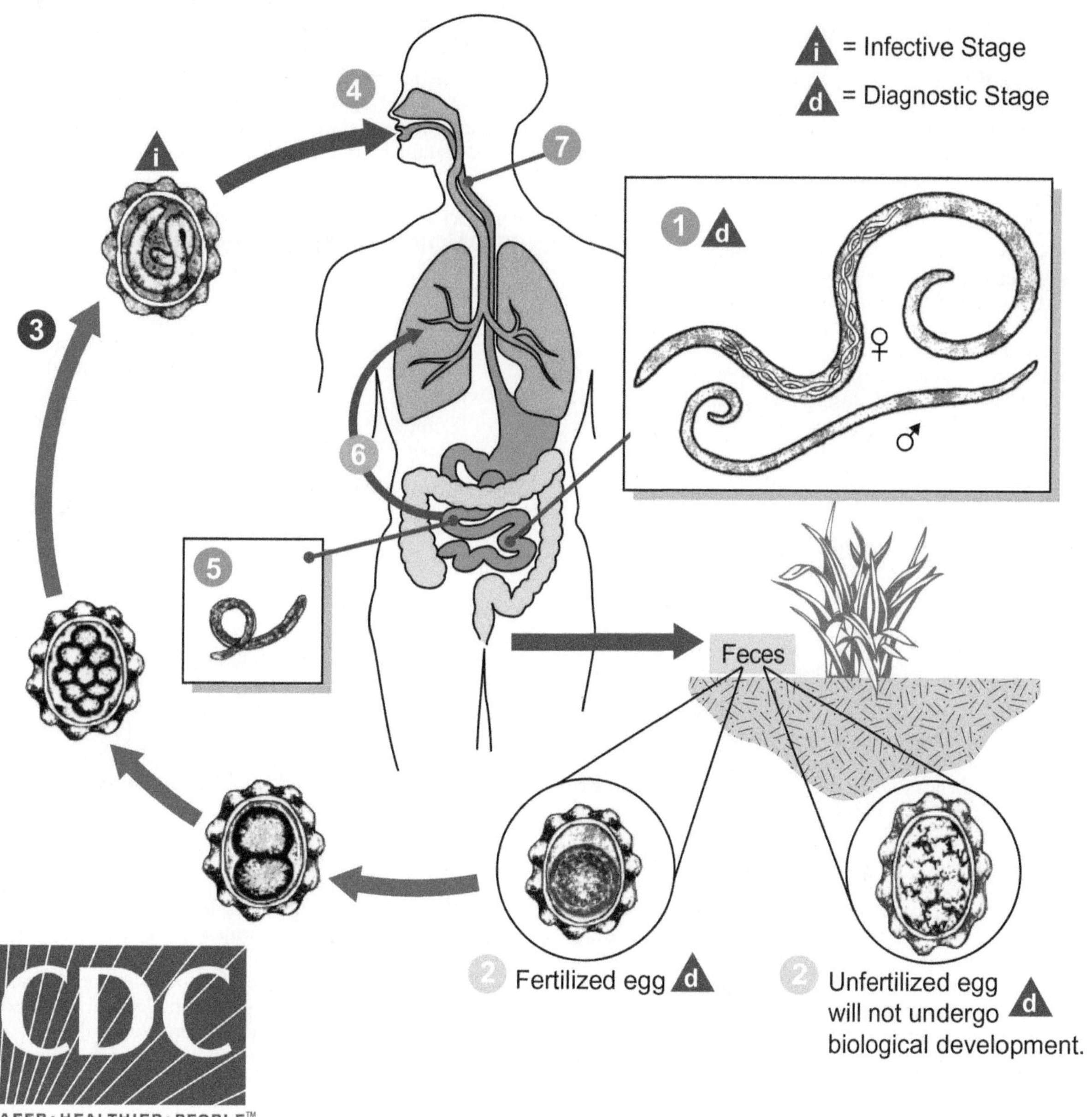

FIGURE 6 Life cycle of *A. lumbricoides*.

TABLE 1 Usual times for completion of life cycles under favorable conditions

Nematode	Time for life cycle completion	
	Within host	In external environment
A. lumbricoides	8 wk	10–15 days
E. vermicularis	4–7 wk	6 h
Hookworm	4–7 wk	5–6 days
S. stercoralis	4 wk	3–4 days (direct)
T. trichiura	10–12 wk	21 days

development into mature adult worms in the small intestine, with eggs being produced after 60 to 70 days. A minority of individuals develop heavy infections and act as an important source of transmission.

The prepatent period (from egg ingestion to egg production) is approximately 2 months.

Clinical Significance

Initial infection is usually asymptomatic. Migration of larvae through the lungs may result in an eosinophilic pneumonitis with cough, fever, and dyspnea. This may occur up to 2 weeks after infection and lasts approximately 3 weeks. Bronchospasm can be prominent and is occasionally fatal.

The clinical features of established infections relate to the worm burden. Most infections are light and asymptomatic, but nonspecific abdominal symptoms may occur. Heavy infections are associated with malnutrition and impaired growth in children. Intestinal obstruction is an uncommon complication in children with a very large worm burden and has a high mortality rate in some settings (3). Ectopic ascariasis occasionally occurs when adult worms attempt to escape the gut lumen. This may be a spontaneous event or occur in response to febrile illness, medication, or anesthesia. Worms may enter hepatobiliary and pancreatic ducts or the appendix and cause obstruction, resulting in biliary colic, cholecystitis, acute cholangitis, acute pancreatitis, appendicitis, or a hepatic abscess. It occurs more commonly in countries with high rates of infection where the parasite is endemic. (For more on the clinical manifestations of *A. lumbricoides*, see reference 14.)

Direct Examination

Microscopy

The primary diagnosis of infection is by demonstration of eggs in feces. The fertilized eggs are round or oval, bile stained, mammillated, and thick walled. Both fertilized and unfertilized eggs may be found in the same specimen. Multiple specimens taken on separate days may be required. Concentration methods such as formalin-ethyl acetate sedimentation should be used for optimal yield. The flotation technique is unsuitable, as unfertilized eggs have a high density. Decorticated fertile and infertile eggs may be difficult to recognize (Fig. 2A to C). Motile larvae may sometimes be seen in expectorated sputum but rarely in feces.

Macroscopic Examination

Occasionally, an adult worm (usually female) may be passed in feces or may spontaneously migrate out of the anus, mouth, or nares, particularly in children.

Identification is relatively straightforward, because no other human parasite is as large as *A. lumbricoides*. However, it should be noted that earthworms of comparable size can occasionally be retrieved from toilets and submitted for identification. The distinguishing features of *Ascaris* adult worms are that they have tapering ends (Fig. 5A), a lateral white line along the entire length of the body, three lips at the anterior end, and a tough cuticle.

Treatment

Albendazole and mebendazole are effective (see chapter 152) (1, 14). These benzimidazoles should not be used in first trimester of pregnancy or in children <12 months of age. The WHO recommends use in the second and third trimesters of pregnancy and in children >12 months of age.

For a summary of *A. lumbricoides*, see Table 2.

ENTEROBIUS VERMICULARIS (PINWORM OR THREADWORM)

Taxonomy

The organisms in this group, in the modern classification of biological species, are in clade III (Chromadoria: Spururina) of the Nematoda, in the order Oxyurida and the family Oxyuridae.

Only the genus *Enterobius* regularly occurs in humans and other primates.

Description of the Agent

Eggs

Pinworm eggs (Fig. 2E) are ovoid, 50 to 60 by 20 to 35 μm, and asymmetrically flattened on one side and appear colorless when recovered from the perianal skin. The outer layer of the eggshell is albuminous and sticky, enabling the egg to adhere readily. The egg contains an immature first-stage larva, but this develops rapidly to become infective.

Larvae

The larvae hatch in the small bowel and then migrate to the large bowel to complete molting and development.

Worms

Adult female worms (Fig. 5B and C) measure approximately 8 to 13 by 0.3 to 0.5 mm, with cervical alae or wing-like expansions at the mouth and a long, pointed tail (hence the name pinworm). Male worms are 2.5 by 0.2 mm but are rarely seen (Fig 5D).

Enterobius gregorii was thought to be a sister species of *E. vermicularis* and has a slightly smaller spicule (sexual organ). However, its existence is controversial, and some experts think that *E. gregorii* is a younger or immature stage of *E. vermicularis*, as no differences have been found on molecular analysis.

Epidemiology and Prevention

E. vermicularis infection has a worldwide distribution and is more common in children than in adults.

TABLE 2 Summary of common nematodes

Parasite	Major clinical presentations	Prepatent period	Laboratory findings	Treatment of choice
A. lumbricoides	Symptoms relate to worm burden; most infections are light and asymptomatic; migratory phase, eosinophilic pneumonitis. Symptoms of established infection include: • History of passing/vomiting worm • Mild gastrointestinal symptoms • Small-bowel obstruction in children with heavy worm burdens • Ectopic ascariasis involving appendix or hepatobiliary or pancreatic ducts • Malnutrition and growth retardation in children	2 mo	Demonstration of eggs in feces; identification of worm passed; eosinophilia low or absent	Albendazole or mebendazole
E. vermicularis	Many infections are asymptomatic; pruritus ani occurs mainly at night; excoriation from scratching and secondary infection are common; general symptoms include weight loss and loss of appetite; occasionally ectopic, involving appendix or female genital tract.	3–4 wk	Demonstration of eggs in sticky tape preparation; eosinophilia low or absent	Albendazole or mebendazole; prevent reinfection and treat contacts
Hookworms	Pruritic rash or "ground itch" on extremities at site of entry of larvae; migratory phase, cough and wheezing due to eosinophilic pneumonitis. Symptoms of established infection include: • Iron-deficiency anemia • Hypoproteinemia leading to chronic malnutrition and growth disorders in children • Enteropathy with gastrointestinal symptoms Light infections may be asymptomatic	4–8 wk	Demonstration of eggs or larvae in feces; culture (agar plate method or Harada-Mori technique); eosinophilia, usually moderate	Albendazole or mebendazole; iron therapy if anemia is present
S. stercoralis	Chronic infection occurs due to autoinfection; recurrent, migratory, linear rash when larvae enter perianal skin, or "larva currens"; urticarial rashes also occur; enteropathy causing intermittent or chronic diarrhea, sometimes with malabsorption; pulmonary symptoms and hypereosinophilia may occur during autoinfection; Loeffler-like syndrome; Gram-negative-bacterial septicemia or meningitis due to transfer of bowel flora by migrating larvae; hyperinfection syndrome(disseminated) in immunocompromised or debilitated individuals, leading to severe enteropathy and respiratory symptoms.	2–4 wk	Demonstration of larvae in feces; culture (agar plate method or Harada-Mori technique); demonstration of antibodies in serum; eosinophilia, variable but usually moderate; PCR, high specificity but variable sensitivity	Ivermectin
T. trichiura	Usually asymptomatic or mild gastrointestinal symptoms; epigastric pain, vomiting, distension, anorexia, and weight loss; *Trichuris* dysentery, sometimes with rectal prolapse, may occur in heavy infections; growth retardation in children due to chronic malnutrition and anemia	3 mo	Demonstration of eggs in feces; eosinophilia low or absent	Albendazole or mebendazole

Preventive measures consist of health education about personal hygiene and sanitation, and drug therapy.

Transmission and Life Cycle (Fig. 7)

Adult worms inhabit the cecum, appendix, and ascending colon. The female migrates down the colon when mature and deposits her eggs on perianal and perineal skin (diagnostic stage). More than 10,000 eggs may be deposited, become infective within 6 h, and remain viable for up to 5 days.

Transmission is either autoinfection, direct from the anal and perianal regions to the mouth, usually by fingernail contamination, or from exposure to a contaminated environment. When swallowed, the embryonated eggs (infective stage) hatch in the small bowel. Larvae migrate to the large bowel, where they mature into adult worms. Retroinfection, where larvae migrate from the anal skin back to the rectum, is thought to be possible.

The prepatent period (from egg ingestion to egg production) is 3 to 4 weeks.

Clinical Significance

Children are most commonly infected. Many patients are asymptomatic or present with pruritus ani and perineal pruritus, which may be severe and worse at night. Excoriation from scratching and secondary bacterial infection is often evident.

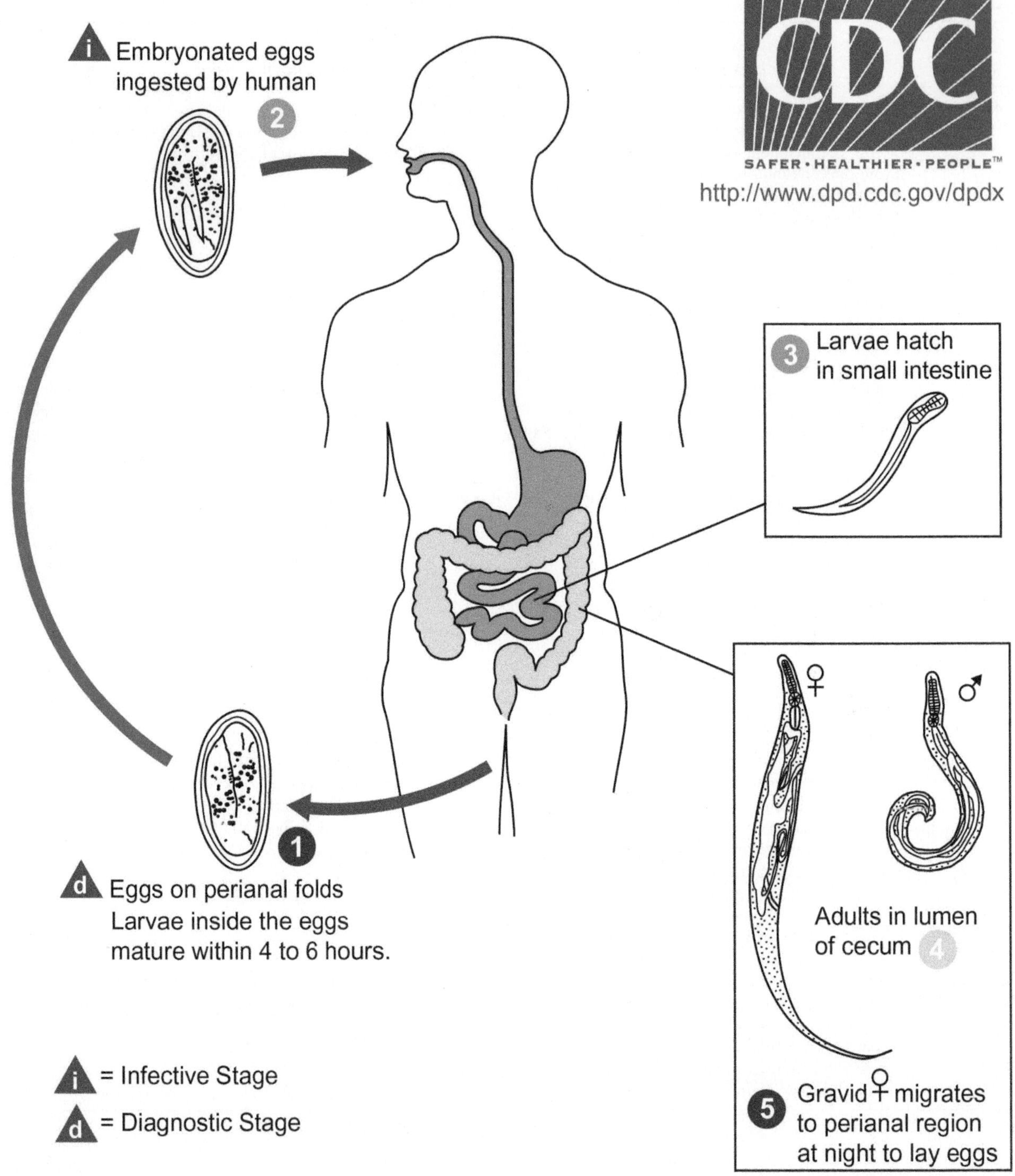

FIGURE 7 Life cycle of *E. vermicularis*.

With heavy worm burdens, poor concentration, enuresis, and emotional distress are features. General symptoms, including abdominal pain, weight loss, and loss of appetite, may occur. Occasionally, the presence of worms in the appendix contributes to inflammation and true appendicitis (15). Reinfection (autoinfection or retroinfection) is also possible.

The presence of ectopic worms and eggs in several sites, including the female genitourinary tract, the epididymis, and the peritoneum, has been reported. Some of these mimic tumor-like lesions (16) or endometriosis. They rarely cause serious complications. (For more on the clinical manifestations of *E. vermicularis*, see reference 14.)

Direct Examination

Microscopy

The primary diagnosis of infection is by demonstration of the presence of eggs on the skin in the perineal area by using the "sticky tape" method (eggs adhere to cellulose tape and can then be detected microscopically). Briefly, a strip of cellulose tape with adhesive side outwards on a microscopy slide is pressed firmly against the right and left perianal folds. The tape is then spread back over the slide with the adhesive side down and examined directly under the microscope. Visibility of eggs can be improved by lifting the tape from the slide, adding a drop of xylene or xylene substitute, and pressing the tape back down on the slide. This helps clear the preparation, and the eggs can be observed clearly (17, 18). If an opaque tape is submitted by mistake, a drop of immersion oil on the top of the tape will clear it enough for microscopy. Repeated preparations on two or three consecutive days may be required. Commercial collection kits (Evergreen Scientific, Los Angeles, CA, or Swube [Becton Dickinson], Sparks, MD) are available in some countries. Eggs are occasionally present in feces. Eggs are non-bile stained, ovoid, asymmetrical with a characteristic shape (concave on one side and flat on the other), smooth, and thick walled and may contain a partially or fully developed larva (Fig. 2E). Specimens should ideally be taken early in the morning prior to the child bathing or using the toilet.

Macroscopic Examination

Adult female worms may be seen in feces, observed around the anal opening, or detected at colonoscopy. They are white or cream-colored pinworms or threadlike worms. In rare instances, immature worms that lack the wing-like expansions at the mouth may be detected in feces. The mature, distended female contains copious eggs, and these may be extruded from the genital pore by applying pressure to the coverslip (Fig. 5C). A cross-section view of an adult female shows characteristic eggs in a histology section (Fig. 4A).

Treatment

Albendazole and mebendazole are the drugs of choice. These drugs should be avoided during pregnancy. Pyrantel and piperazine are also effective and can be used during pregnancy (see chapter 152) (1, 14).

It is important to treat other family members and close contacts and to decontaminate the environment by washing bed linen and clothes. Advice should be given on adequate hygiene and hand washing.

For a summary of *E. vermicularis*, see Table 2.

HOOKWORMS

Taxonomy

The organisms in this group, in the modern classification of biological species, are in clade V (Chromadoria: Rhabditina) of the Nematoda, in the order Rhabditida (Strongylida) and the family Ancylostomatidae.

Ancylostoma and *Necator* are the two genera of Ancylostomatidae that infect humans. Infective species include *Ancylostoma duodenale* (Old World hookworm), *Ancylostoma ceylanicum* (mainly described from Asia and the Pacific islands) (19), and *Necator americanus* (New World hookworm).

Description

Eggs

Eggs (Fig. 3A) of *A. duodenale*, *A. ceylanicum*, and *N. americanus* are indistinguishable; they are oval with a thin shell and measure approximately 56 to 75 by 36 to 40 μm. They have a clear space between the developing embryo and the thin eggshell. When passed, eggs are only at the four-cell stage; development of larvae occurs in moist, shady, warm soil, where larvae hatch within 1 to 2 days.

Larvae

First-stage rhabditoid larvae (Fig. 3E and G) from the hatched eggs measure about 200 μm in length. They feed on organic debris and undergo two further molts over a 5- to 8-day period. The infective, nonfeeding third-stage larvae measure from 500 to 700 μm, those of *Ancylostoma* being generally longer than those of *Necator*. These infective filariform larvae remain viable in the soil for several weeks. Variations in the morphology of the filariform larvae have been used to differentiate *A. duodenale* from *N. americanus*. However, *A. ceylanicum* filariform larvae share morphological features (prominent striations on the posterior sheath) with *N. americanus* and may have been be misidentified in previous studies (20).

Worms

For all three species, male worms (5 to 11 mm) are shorter than females (7 to 13 by 0.4 to 0.5 mm), and *A. duodenale* is generally longer and more sturdily built than *N. americanus*. These can also be differentiated on the basis of their anatomical differences in mouth parts and in caudal and buccal anatomy. Adult worms are rarely seen, since they remain firmly attached to the intestinal mucosa, feeding on blood obtained by puncturing the capillary network in the intestinal mucosa.

Epidemiology and Prevention

An estimated 740 million people are infected in poor regions of the tropics and subtropics, especially in Asia, Latin America, and the Caribbean and sub-Saharan Africa (3). *A. ceylanicum*, although previously considered to be largely a parasite of cats and dogs, is prevalent in humans in Southeast Asia, Australia, and the Pacific Islands, especially the Solomon Islands (20). Additionally, in a study conducted in Cambodia, sequencing of the cytochrome oxidase-1 gene identified two groups of *A. ceylanicum*, the first being restricted entirely to infections in humans and the second including isolates from humans and dogs, thus confirming that *A. ceylanicum* infection represents a true zoonosis (21). In addition to drug therapy, preventive measures consist of health education about personal hygiene, the need to wear shoes, and avoidance of soil contamination. A hookworm vaccine has completed phase 1 trials and will be advanced into clinical trials in children and eventual efficacy studies (22). The full sequencing of the genome of *N. americanus* also offers hope for new drug targets and recognition of immunomodulatory proteins (23).

Transmission and Life Cycle (Fig. 8)

Eggs are passed in the feces into the environment, where they hatch into rhabditiform larvae that mature into filariform larvae, with the potential to infect new hosts. Entry of third-stage or filariform larvae (infective stage) by direct penetration of the skin initiates human infection; within 10 days, this is followed by migration to the lungs. *A. duodenale* larvae can also infect if swallowed, to result in direct maturation to the adult stage in the anterior small intestine. In contrast, larvae of *N. americanus* require an obligatory lung migration to initiate infection. Larvae leave the lungs after 3 to 5 weeks, pass through the trachea and pharynx, enter the gastrointestinal tract, and attach to the intestinal

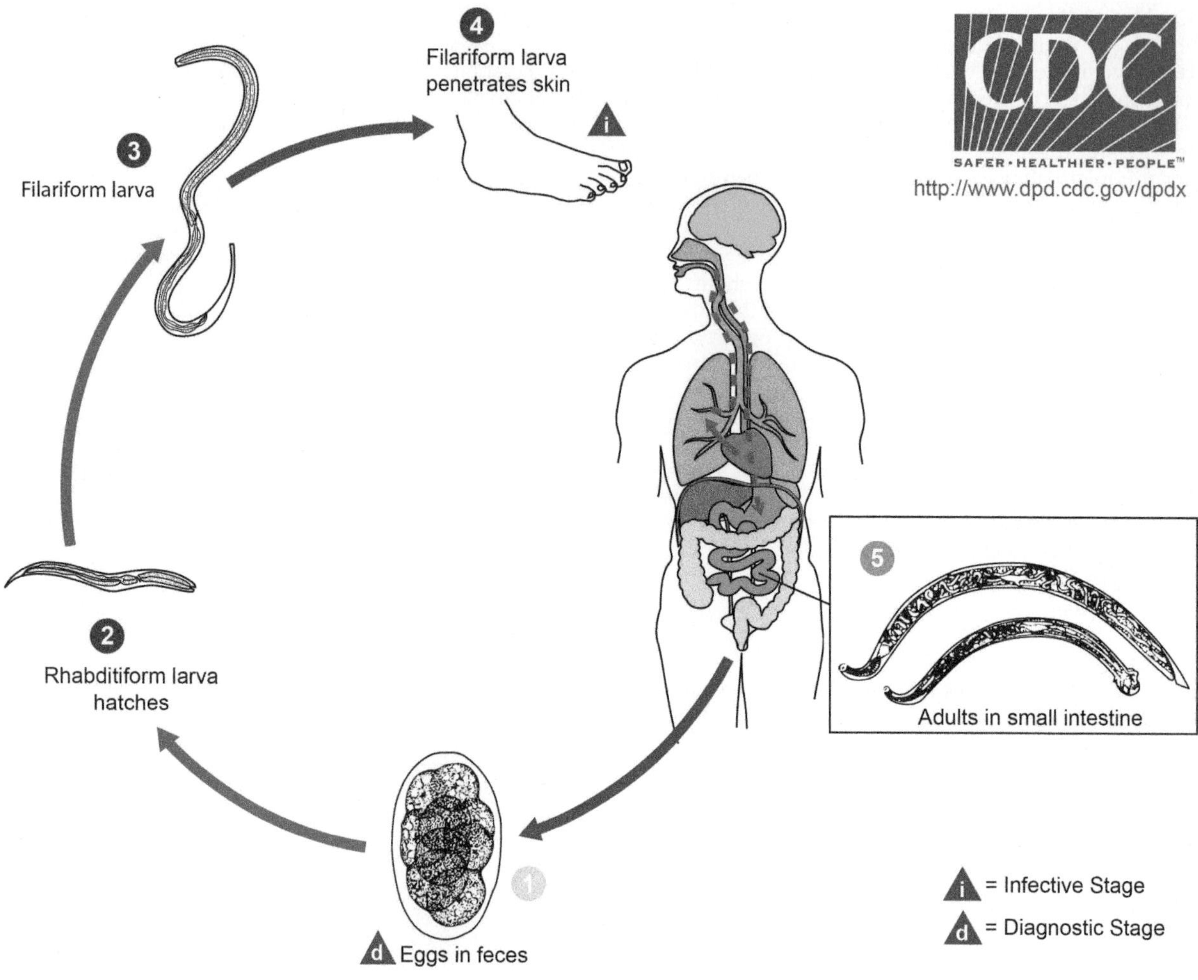

FIGURE 8 Life cycle of hookworms.

mucosa, where they mature into adults (Table 1). Attachment and the release of anticlotting factors result in blood loss, which, as indicated above, is greater with *A. duodenale*. Hookworms may survive in the host for several years. The prepatent period from larva penetration to egg production is 4 to 8 weeks.

Clinical Significance

The major clinical manifestation of hookworm infection is iron deficiency anemia due to intestinal blood loss and depletion of iron stores. The degree of iron deficiency induced by hookworms depends on the intensity and duration of infection, the species of hookworm, and the iron status of the host. It has been estimated that a single *A. duodenale* worm can withdraw as much as 0.2 ml of blood per day, whereas *N. americanus* withdraws approximately 0.05 ml. *A. ceylanicum* has also been recorded as causing a similar jejunal infection with associated anemia. In other cases, infection has been limited to the lower gastrointestinal tract, with symptoms more comparable to those seen with *Ancylostoma caninum* infection (19). Young children, women of reproductive age, and pregnant women are most at risk for iron deficiency anemia because of inadequate dietary iron and reduced iron reserves. Anemia during pregnancy is linked to maternal morbidity and mortality, impaired lactation, prematurity, and/or low-birth-weight infants. In children, iron deficiency anemia is associated with impaired neurocognitive development, reduced school performance, and exercise intolerance.

Patients with light worm burdens are usually asymptomatic. Moderate and heavy worm burdens cause epigastric pain and tenderness, nausea, weight loss, and diarrhea. This may lead to protein-losing enteropathy and hypoalbuminemia. In those who develop iron deficiency anemia, common symptoms are lethargy and fatigue, exertional dyspnea, and palpitations. In children, chronic malnutrition and developmental delay may occur.

A pruritic rash is often present at the site of penetration of larvae ("ground itch"). This must be differentiated from cercarial dermatitis and creeping eruptions from other causes. In some patients, mild cough and wheezing occur in response to larval migration through the lungs (For more on the clinical manifestations of hookworms, see reference 14.)

Direct Examination

Microscopy

The primary diagnosis of infection is by detection of eggs in feces. Multiple specimens taken on separate days may be required. For optimal yield, both direct and concentration methods such as formalin-ethyl acetate sedimentation should be used. Eggs are non-bile stained and usually have a 4- to 8-cell-stage embryo (Fig. 3A). Occasionally, a 16- to 32-cell-stage embryo or a developing larva may be seen, especially if there is delay in processing an unfixed fecal specimen. Hookworm eggs may be confused with *Trichostrongylus* eggs, but eggs of the latter species are more elongated and generally in an advanced stage of cleavage (Fig. 3B).

Culture

Culture for the detection of *Strongyloides stercoralis* larvae by the Harada-Mori technique or agar plate method may also show the presence of hookworm larvae (see "*Strongyloides stercoralis*" below for details) (Fig. 3C to G). Hookworm larvae can be differentiated from *S. stercoralis* larvae by their morphological features (Fig. 3C to G). Hookworm larvae are uncommon in adequately fixed fecal specimens, but motile larvae may be seen occasionally in expectorated sputum.

Macroscopic Examination

Usually, the worm is firmly attached to the small bowel mucosa and rarely passed in feces. However, worms may be detected during gastroscopy or colonoscopy, and a specimen may be recovered. The adult worm can be identified by the structure of the buccal capsule.

The diagnosis of hookworm infection should be considered for people who have resided in areas where the infection is endemic, especially if they have eosinophilia or iron deficiency anemia.

Treatment

The two most practical and effective drugs for treating hookworm infections are albendazole and mebendazole. These benzimidazoles should not be used in the first trimester of pregnancy and in children <12 months of age. The WHO recommends use in second and third trimester of pregnancy and in children >12 months of age. Pyrantel is also effective and can be used in pregnancy (see chapter 152) (1, 14).

Iron supplementation may be required for those who are iron deficient.

For a summary of hookworms, see Table 2.

STRONGYLOIDES STERCORALIS

Taxonomy

The organisms in this group, in the modern classification of biological species, are in clade V (Chromadoria: Rhabditina) of the Nematoda, in the order Rhabditida (Strongylida) and the family Strongylidae.

Members of the family Strongylidae exhibit an irregular alternation of generations, with a parasitic parthenogenetic female alternating with a free-living sexual generation. Only one genus, *Strongyloides*, occurs in humans.

Description, Transmission, and Life Cycle (Fig. 9)

Eggs

Eggs of the parasitic female are deposited within the mucosa of the small intestine and usually hatch within the crypts of Lieberkühn before reaching the lumen. As a result, they are rarely excreted in the feces (*Strongyloides fuelleborni*, seen in Zimbabwe and Zambia, and a similar species found in Papua New Guinea are the exceptions; see below). Eggs of the free-living adult female are partially embryonated and oval and measure approximately 50 to 70 μm in length.

Larvae

First-stage rhabditiform larvae (Fig. 3C, D, and F) measure approximately 180 to 380 by 14 to 20 μm and are characterized by a muscular esophagus comprising the anterior third of the body. A short buccal cavity (Fig 3D) and a prominent genital primordium located midbody (Fig. 3C) help to distinguish them from other nematodes, such as hookworms (Fig. 3E). In the soil, first-stage larvae follow a direct or indirect course of development. In the direct cycle, larvae develop rapidly into infective third-stage, filariform larvae; in the indirect cycle, first-stage larvae develop into a free-living generation of adult male and female worms. Third-stage, or filariform, larvae are 500 to 600 by 16 μm, and the ratio of esophageal to intestinal length is approximately 1:1. The tail of the larvae has a V-shaped notch, a feature that separates them from hookworm larvae, which have long pointed tails (Fig. 3F and G).

Worms

Parasitic male forms do not occur. Parasitic females are small and thin, measuring approximately 2 to 3 mm in length and 30 to 50 μm in width. The anterior portion is thicker than the posterior and contains the esophagus.

The free-living adult female is approximately half the size of its parasitic counterpart, although it is nearly twice as thick (approximately 80 μm). While the reproductive systems are morphologically similar, the uterus in the free-living adult female contains significantly more eggs. The free-living adult male is slightly smaller than the female, approximately 50 μm in width.

Transmission occurs when filariform (infective-stage) larvae penetrate the skin or mucous membranes, enter the venous circulation, and are carried to the lungs. Larvae penetrate alveolar walls, migrate through the tracheobronchial tree, are swallowed, and then embed within the mucosa of the upper small intestine. Here, they reach maturity and commence egg production by the process of parthenogenesis. The eggs hatch within the intestinal crypts to release rhabditiform larvae, most of which are excreted in feces (diagnostic stage). In the soil, they undergo several molts to become infective filariform larvae (Fig. 9).

Some rhabditiform larvae develop into infective filariform larvae in the bowel lumen and maintain a cycle of repeated migration by either penetration of the mucosa of the colon or small intestine or externally by crossing perianal skin, to repeat the cycle of maturation within the same host. This process of autoinfection results in chronic infections that may persist for 40 years or more. The prepatent period (from larva penetration to egg production) is 2 to 4 weeks.

Epidemiology and Prevention

Strongyloides worms live in warm, moist soil and are widely distributed in the tropics and subtropics, with distribution similar to that of hookworms. There are an estimated 30 to 100 million patients infected with *S. stercoralis* worldwide. Analysis of the limited prevalence data available identifies the geographical distribution and risk factors for *Strongyloides* infection. In particular, hot spots for infection have been identified, especially in Southeast Asia (24). However, the true prevalence is uncertain due to the low sensitivity of conventional methods typically used for the detection of other STH infections. More sensitive methods, such as the Baermann or APC method, are required to detect the variably low numbers of larvae typically excreted in chronic infection (2, 24). At-risk groups include those living in areas where the parasite is endemic,

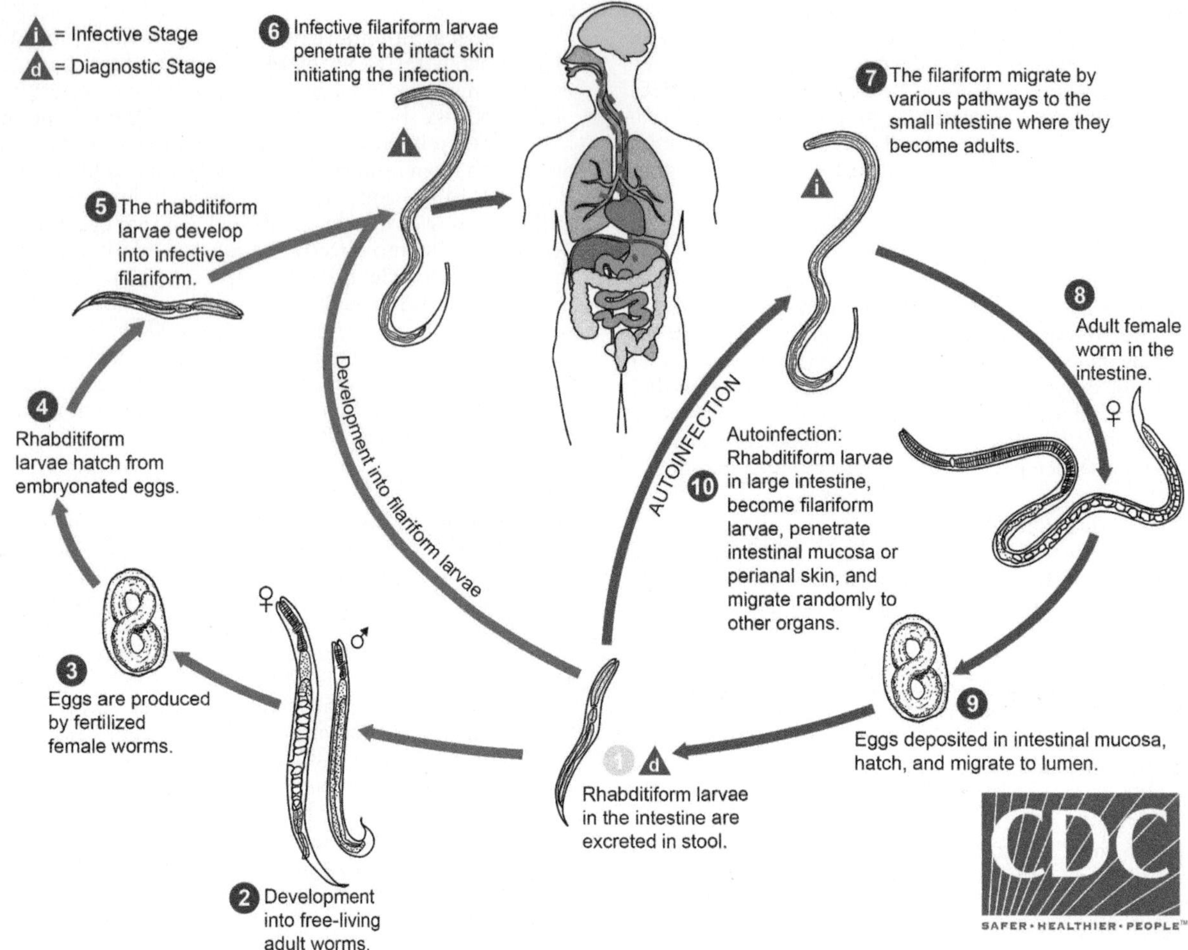

FIGURE 9 Life cycle of *S. stercoralis*.

as well as immigrants and refugees, indigenous peoples, and war veterans previously exposed in these regions. Screening and active treatment of patients undergoing immunosuppression should be considered for at-risk groups (8–10). Patients with hyperinfection syndrome also pose an infection risk for immediate family, laboratory workers, and those providing nursing care.

Preventive measures include good personal hygiene and wearing shoes in areas where transmission occurs. In a study conducted in northern Cambodia, populations of *S. stercoralis* isolated from dogs and humans were compared by whole-genome sequencing and nuclear and mitochondrial DNA sequence polymorphisms. This demonstrated that one population of *Strongyloides* spp. is found in dogs and humans, raising the possibility that dogs may represent a further, zoonotic source of infection (25).

Clinical Significance

S. stercoralis infections are often chronic, lasting for several decades. Most patients have low worm burdens and are asymptomatic or have intermittent cutaneous and/or gastrointestinal symptoms. Intermittent or chronic diarrhea, abdominal pain and bloating, nausea, and anorexia are the main gastrointestinal symptoms. Other manifestations (e.g., dermatological and pulmonary symptoms) are less common.

Recurrent pruritic, serpiginous, erythematous rashes may occur due to larval migration in the skin (larva currens). These are seen most commonly on the buttocks, groin, and trunk; movement under the skin may continue for 1 to 2 days. Other, less distinctive urticarial and papular rashes also occur. Although pulmonary symptoms are uncommon in uncomplicated strongyloidiasis, passage of larvae through the lung may be associated with a cough, wheezing, and dyspnea, as well as patchy infiltrates upon radiography (Loeffler-like syndrome).

It is thought that in chronic infection, there is a balance between immunity and the level of infection. However, this equilibrium may be lost when illness or drug therapy leads to immunosuppression. Exacerbation of symptoms can occur in as little as 6 days after commencement of treatment with corticosteroids. The resulting disseminated strongyloidiasis or hyperinfection syndrome has a very high fatality rate. Other conditions predisposing to these syndromes include chemotherapy, infection with human T-cell lymphotropic virus type 1, alcoholism, kidney disease, bone marrow transplantation, and hypogammaglobulinemia (9, 26).

In disseminated disease, migration of larvae extends to multiple organs, and this can be associated with bacteremia and even meningitis caused by Gram-negative bacilli carried from the gut during migration of the larvae. Hyperinfection results from proliferation of worms with no spreading beyond the normal pattern of migration. Large numbers of larvae (and occasionally embryonated eggs) in stool and sputum produce severe gastrointestinal and/or respiratory symptoms (27). Within the bowel, the range of symptoms includes generalized inflammation, colitis, proctitis, and mucosal ulceration. Most cases of strongyloidiasis associated with solid organ transplantation have been due to the reactivation of a latent infection in the recipient as a result of the immunosuppressive therapy; however, donor-derived infections are becoming increasingly frequent. Current practice guidelines need to be updated to incorporate immunological and molecular techniques for the rapid screening for strongyloidiasis prior to transplantation, and empirical treatment with ivermectin should be considered (28).

(For more on the clinical manifestations of *S. stercoralis*, see references 9 and 14.)

Direct Examination

The laboratory diagnosis of strongyloidiasis can be difficult (17, 18). It is based on demonstrating the presence of the larvae in feces, detecting DNA by real-time PCR (RT-PCR), or demonstrating antibodies to *S. stercoralis* in blood. The choice may be based on practicalities in different clinical settings (29, 30). Currently, serology is the best screening method, especially in settings where the disease is not endemic. APC and RT-PCR can be considered as confirmatory tests for selected cases (31).

Microscopy and Culture

Microscopy of feces may detect the first-stage (rhabditiform) larvae; eggs or adult worms are very rarely detected. In chronic infection, the sensitivity of microscopy is generally low, as larvae are shed sporadically and numbers depend on the stage and severity of the infection. For this reason, multiple specimens collected over several days should be examined. Coproculture is an alternative method of detection of larvae in freshly passed stool specimen. Ideally, this should be attempted for all suspected cases, especially with patients from areas where the infection is endemic. It is important that the specimen be sent directly to the laboratory, without refrigeration or addition of preservative. The critical factor in culture methods is that large quantities of stool can be processed. This improves the sensitivity over that of standard procedures, such as formalin ethyl acetate concentration or Kato-Katz smear. Care should be exercised in the handling of these cultures, as the larvae present are filariform, or infectious, and capable of crossing intact skin. The various methods available for culture are as follows (for details, see references 9, 12, and 32).

1. APC. A large amount (2 to 3 g) of feces is placed on the center of an agar plate, and the plate is sealed and incubated at room temperature. If larvae are present, they travel away from the initial inoculum carrying bacteria from the feces. Colonies of these bacteria appear on the surface as tracks (or occasionally inside the agar) with a characteristic sinusoidal pattern (Fig. 3H). The plates are examined by microscopy for confirmation of the presence of larvae. For safety, larvae should be recovered in a solution containing formaldehyde to allow confirmation of identity. This is the easiest culture method to perform and is now the recommended procedure.
2. Harada-Mori technique. The fecal specimen is smeared on the top of a strip of filter paper, dipping into 3 ml of water in a 15-ml sealed centrifuge tube. The tube is held at 25°C in the dark. After 7 to 10 days, the water can be tested by microscopy for the presence of larvae.
3. Petri dish methods. Either filter paper or a watch glass is used to hold the specimen. The larvae migrate to fresh water and light.
4. Baermann technique. This technique uses a modified funnel device to sample the water used to moisten the fecal specimen placed on a wire mesh covered with gauze. It relies on the principle that larvae will actively migrate out of the feces to fresh water and higher temperature.

Occasionally, hookworm larvae may hatch in feces that have been left at warm temperatures for long periods before processing. In contrast to *S. stercoralis*, hookworm larvae have a long buccal cavity and inconspicuous genital primordium (Fig. 3C to E). The presence of larvae of *Strongyloides* in expectorated sputum or duodenal aspirate obtained via enteroscopy may also be demonstrated. Filariform *Strongyloides* larvae may be seen in feces or sputum in cases of hyperinfection or in cases in which infection has been identified by the culture methods described above.

It is also noteworthy that a recent fatal case of infection in Australia with the free-living, neurotrophic parasite *Halicephalobus gingivalis* was detected as rhabditiform larvae in the central nervous system. The initial differential diagnosis included disseminated strongyloidiasis, but based on morphological assessment followed by molecular identification of the organism, strongyloidiasis was excluded (33).

Nucleic Acid Detection

Diagnosis by molecular techniques has been developed (7) and is now available in many reference laboratories but not available commercially at the time of writing. Various formats for detecting DNA in feces, such as RT-PCR, loop-mediated isothermal amplification, and nested PCR, have been shown to be useful (34–36). Overall, the specificity is very high but the sensitivity is variable due to low numbers and intermittent excretion of larvae in feces in different phases of the infection. Good reviews comparing different testing protocols are available (30, 32). Another possible approach is to detect parasite DNA in the urine (37). This may prove to be an advantage, especially in areas of endemicity where collection and transport of feces may be difficult. However, the utility, sensitivity, and specificity of this approach are yet to be proven.

Other Tests

Although peripheral blood eosinophilia is common especially during an initial acute infection, it does not reliably correlate with infection and may be intermittent in chronic infection. The concomitant use of steroids may significantly decrease eosinophilia in infected patients.

Serologic Tests

Demonstration of anti-*Strongyloides* antibodies in blood should be used as a screening test or as an adjunct for diagnosis. In most cases it is useful in monitoring treatment. Antibody levels decline after 6 to 12 months of effective treatment (38) and may be negative by 12 to 24 months (39). The sensitivity of one commercially available enzyme immunoassay (EIA) using *S. stercoralis* filariform antigens (Strongyloides IgG ELISA [EIA-4208]; DRG International, Inc., Springfield, NJ) is cited as being ~90% and is much higher than that of indirect hemagglutination assays and immunofluorescent assays. Higher sensitivity (~95%) has been reported for the U.S. Centers for Disease Control and Prevention *Strongyloides* EIA in patients with proven infection (38). Sensitivity may be lower in severely immunocompromised patients. The specificity of EIA is ~85%, as cross-reactions in patients with filarial and other nematode infections may occur. If antibodies are detected, efforts should be made to establish a parasitological diagnosis (microscopic and culture) and to exclude infection with other parasites that could result in cross-reacting antibodies. *Strongyloides* serology should be performed for all at-risk candidates for immunosuppressive therapy (e.g., prior to organ transplant or treatment for malignancies, etc.). Assessing the accuracy and sensitivity of serological methods is difficult because of the lack of sensitivity of a fecal-based reference standard (gold standard). However, in the past few years, tests based on a new recombinant antigen have been developed and are reported to have a higher specificity. One such assay, the SS-NIE-1 IgG_4 ELISA, uses the antigen NIE, a 31-kDa recombinant antigen derived from a *S. stercoralis* L3 cDNA library developed at the U.S. National Institutes of Health. This assay has a reported sensitivity and specificity of 93% and 95%, respectively (40), with fewer cross-reactions with other parasitic infections. A new assay, the luciferase immunoprecipitation system, is thought to perform better than the EIA format (41). This test has also been shown to work well on blood spots collected in remote areas where collection and transport of serum may be an issue (42). These new tests using the NIE antigen are not available commercially at the time of writing.

Treatment

S. stercoralis infection should always be treated because of the potential for developing severe complicated disease. Ivermectin is the drug of choice, but repeated cycles of treatment may be required in immunocompromised patients. Ivermectin should not be used during pregnancy or in children weighing <15 kg. Albendazole and mebendazole are less effective than ivermectin. Thiabendazole, although effective, is no longer used in many countries due to frequent severe side effects (see chapter 152) (1, 14). These benzimidazoles should not be used in the first trimester of pregnancy or in children <12 months of age. The WHO recommends use in the second and third trimesters of pregnancy and in children >12 months of age.

Monitoring (usually 6 to 12 months after treatment) with serology, stool microscopy (if positive), and eosinophil count is recommended until infection is eradicated. Guidelines are available for refugees and migrants from countries where the parasite is endemic (4).

For a summary of *S. stercoralis*, see Table 2.

STRONGYLOIDES FUELLEBORNI

S. fuelleborni is a parasite of non-human primates found in monkeys in Central and Eastern Africa. A similar species is found in Papua New Guinea, but no animal vector has been identified. Most human infections are asymptomatic in adults but may cause a severe protein loss enteropathy and abdominal distension (swollen belly syndrome) in infants. In contrast to *S. stercoralis*, ova of *S. fuelleborni* are found in feces in large numbers and resemble those of hookworms. The two *Strongyloides* species can be differentiated on the basis of adult worm morphology (43). Treatment is similar to that for *S. stercoralis*. The mortality rate associated with untreated infections is very high in infants.

TRICHURIS TRICHIURA (WHIPWORM)

Taxonomy

The organisms in this group, in the modern classification of biological species, are in clade I (Dorylaimia) of the Nematoda, in the order Trichocephalida and the family Trichuridae.

Description

Eggs

Eggs of *T. trichiura* (Fig. 2F) are lemon shaped with a mucous plug at both ends and an unsegmented nucleus. Eggs have a double shell, with the outer one bile stained; they measure 50 to 55 by 20 to 24 μm. Under favorable conditions in soil, the eggs become fully embryonated and infective in 2 to 4 weeks.

Larvae

Larvae emerge in the small intestine (the second-stage larvae measure about 260 by 15 μm in length). After a period of growth, they pass into the cecum, where they embed in the mucosa.

Worms

Adult worms have a highly characteristic shape from which the name whipworm is derived. The long, thin anterior end lies in a burrow in the mucosa, and the thicker end, which contains the reproductive tract, extends into the intestinal lumen. Worms are whitish; the males (30 to 45 mm) are shorter than the females (35 to 50 mm) and have a coiled posterior end. Adult females produce up to 20,000 eggs/day and live for approximately 3 years.

Epidemiology and Prevention

Trichuris has a worldwide distribution and is often associated with *Ascaris* and hookworm infections in children and pregnant women in tropical and subtropical areas.

Preventive measures include health education about personal hygiene, avoidance of soil contamination, and drug therapy programs in areas where infection is endemic.

Transmission and Life Cycle (Fig. 10)

Transmission is direct via oral ingestion of embryonated eggs (infective stage) from contaminated soil. Following ingestion, larvae are released and pass into the large bowel, where they mature into adults in mucosal crypts. The eggs passed in feces contain an unsegmented ovum (diagnostic stage), and once the eggs are in warm, moist conditions in soil, they become infective 2 to 4 weeks after passage (Table 1).

The prepatent period (from egg ingestion to egg production) is 3 months.

Clinical Significance

The clinical features are related to the intensity of infection; light infections are asymptomatic or present with mild gastrointestinal symptoms.

Epigastric pain, vomiting, distension, anorexia, and weight loss may occur with heavier infections, and *Trichuris* dysentery syndrome may be seen in extreme cases complicated by rectal prolapse. Children with severe infections may develop growth retardation due to chronic malnutrition and iron deficiency anemia. Iron deficiency anemia may also occur in pregnant women with a higher worm burden, especially when hookworm coinfection is present (44). The mechanisms by which *Trichuris* infection causes anemia

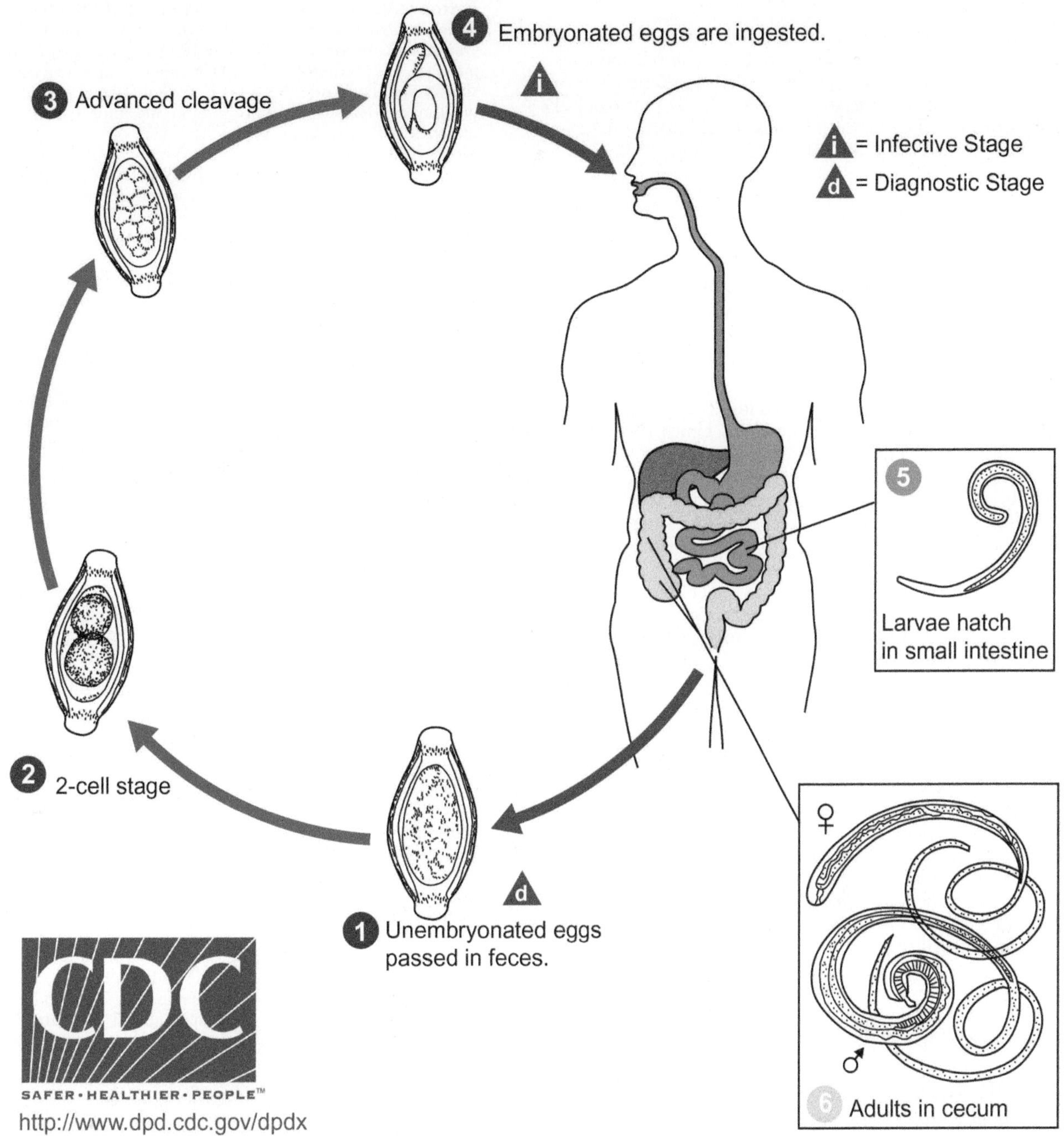

FIGURE 10 Life cycle of *T. trichiura*.

include blood loss from damage to the intestinal epithelium by adult worms and infection-attributable loss of appetite resulting in lower food (and iron) intake. The health impact from *T. trichiura* rises as the worm burden increases, resulting in chronic undernutrition. (For more on the clinical manifestations of *T. trichiura*, see reference 14.)

Direct Examination

Microscopy

The primary diagnosis of infection is by detection of eggs in feces. Multiple specimens collected on separate days may be required. Concentration methods such as formalin-ethyl acetate sedimentation should be used for optimal yield. The eggs are bile stained and double walled with mucoid plugs at both ends, giving them a characteristic "tea tray" appearance (Fig. 2F).

Macroscopic Examination

Adult worms are rarely passed in feces and are occasionally found on colonoscopy (45). They have a coiled, long, thin anterior region and a thicker tail, giving them the appearance of a whip (hence the name whipworm). The characteristic eggs can be seen in histology sections (Fig. 4B).

Treatment

Albendazole and mebendazole are the drugs of choice (see chapter 152) (1, 14). Failures are not uncommon, and multiple doses are required. Combination chemotherapies have showed the highest efficacy, e.g., albendazole plus oxantel pamoate (46). The benzimidazoles should not be used in the first trimester of pregnancy or in children <12 months of age. The WHO recommends use in the second and third trimesters of pregnancy and in children >12 months of age. For a summary of *T. trichiura*, see Table 2.

EVALUATION, INTERPRETATION, AND REPORTING OF RESULTS

The adequacy and quality of the specimen submitted should be noted. If it is inadequate, this should be mentioned in the report.

Any helminth eggs or larvae found in feces are significant, and treatment is recommended, even if the patient is asymptomatic. There is no need to quantitate helminth parasites, as this does not necessarily correlate with clinical illness. However, in rare instances, quantitation may be required for epidemiological studies or for clinical assessment of children.

The time of collection is also important, especially when *Enterobius* is suspected. If the specimen is inadequate, e.g., delayed, dry, or insufficient, a repeat specimen should be requested. A freshly collected specimen and/or use of preservative kits should be encouraged where possible.

Examples of interpretative comments used to ensure that adequate testing is performed are as follows.

1. Larvae of *S. stercoralis* not detected. A single negative result does not exclude the diagnosis of *Strongyloides*. Please send freshly collected feces and transport to laboratory without delay.
2. Eggs of *E. vermicularis* not detected on the sticky tape preparation. A single negative result does not exclude the diagnosis of pinworm infection. Please send properly collected repeat specimen, if clinically indicated. Contact the laboratory for instructions if required.
3. No parasites detected. Excretion of parasite forms may be variable or intermittent. Repeat testing is recommended if clinically indicated. Contact the laboratory for instructions if required.

REFERENCES

1. **World Health Organization.** 2017. Guideline: preventive chemotherapy to control soil-transmitted helminth infections in at-risk population groups. World Health Organization, Geneva, Switzerland. http://apps.who.int/iris/bitstream/10665/258983/1/9789241550116-eng.pdf
2. **Krolewiecki AJ, Lammie P, Jacobson J, Gabrielli A-F, Levecke B, Socias E, Arias LM, Sosa N, Abraham D, Cimino R, Echazú A, Crudo F, Vercruysse J, Albonico M.** 2013. A public health response against *Strongyloides stercoralis*: time to look at soil-transmitted helminthiasis in full. *PLoS Negl Trop Dis* **7:**e2165.
3. **Pullan RL, Smith JL, Jasrasaria R, Brooker SJ.** 2014. Global numbers of infection and disease burden of soil transmitted helminth infections in 2010. *Parasit Vectors* **7:**37.
4. **Chaves NJ, Paxton G, Biggs BA, Thambiran A, Smith M, Williams J, Gardiner J, Davis JS.** 2016. Recommendations for comprehensive post-arrival health assessment for people from refugee-like backgrounds. Australasian Society for Infectious Diseases, Surry Hills, New South Wales, Australia. https://www.asid.net.au/documents/item/1225.
5. **Easton AV, Oliveira RG, O'Connell EM, Kepha S, Mwandawiro CS, Njenga SM, Kihara JH, Mwatele C, Odiere MR, Brooker SJ, Webster JP, Anderson RM, Nutman TB.** 2016. Multi-parallel qPCR provides increased sensitivity and diagnostic breadth for gastrointestinal parasites of humans: field-based inferences on the impact of mass deworming. *Parasit Vectors* **9:**38–49.
6. **Mejia R, Vicuña Y, Broncano N, Sandoval C, Vaca M, Chico M, Cooper PJ, Nutman TB.** 2013. A novel, multi-parallel, real-time polymerase chain reaction approach for eight gastrointestinal parasites provides improved diagnostic capabilities to resource-limited at-risk populations. *Am J Trop Med Hyg* **88:**1041–1047.
7. **Verweij JJ, Canales M, Polman K, Ziem J, Brienen EA, Polderman AM, van Lieshout L.** 2009. Molecular diagnosis of *Strongyloides stercoralis* in faecal samples using real-time PCR. *Trans R Soc Trop Med Hyg* **103:**342–346.
8. **Puthiyakunnon S, Boddu S, Li Y, Zhou X, Wang C, Li J, Chen X.** 2014. Strongyloidiasis—an insight into its global prevalence and management. *PLoS Negl Trop Dis* **8:**e3018.
9. **Toledo R, Muñoz-Antoli C, Esteban JG.** 2015. Strongyloidiasis with emphasis on human infections and its different clinical forms. *Adv Parasitol* **88:**165–241.
10. **Davis JS, Currie BJ, Fisher DA, Huffam SE, Anstey NM, Price RN, Krause VL, Zweck N, Lawton PD, Snelling PL, Selva-Nayagam S.** 2003. Prevention of opportunistic infections in immunosuppressed patients in the tropical top end of the Northern Territory. *Commun Dis Intell Q Rep* **27:**526–532.
11. **Adl SM, Simpson AGB, Lane CE, Lukeš J, Bass D, Bowser SS, Brown MW, Burki F, Dunthorn M, Hampl V, Heiss A, Hoppenrath M, Lara E, Le Gall L, Lynn DH, McManus H, Mitchell EAD, Mozley-Stanridge SE, Parfrey LW, Pawlowski J, Rueckert S, Shadwick L, Schoch CL, Smirnov A, Spiegel FW.** 2012. The revised classification of eukaryotes. *J Eukaryot Microbiol* **59:**429–493. CORRECTION *J Eukaryot Microbiol* **60:**321.
12. **Shimizu RY, Garcia LS (section ed).** 2016. Parasitology, chapters 9.1–9.10. *In* Leber AL (ed), *Clinical Microbiology Procedures Handbook*, vol. 2, 4th ed. ASM Press, Washington, DC.
13. **Shao CC, Xu MJ, Alasaad S, Song HQ, Peng L, Tao JP, Zhu XQ.** 2014. Comparative analysis of microRNA profiles between adult *Ascaris lumbricoides* and *Ascaris suum*. *BMC Vet Res* **10:**99–104.
14. **Maguire JH.** 2015. Intestinal nematodes (roundworms), p 3199–3207. *In* Bennett JE, Dolin R, Blaser MJ (ed), *Mandell, Douglas, and Bennett's Principles and Practice of Infectious Diseases*, 8th ed. Elsevier, Saunders, Philadelphia, PA.
15. **Arca MJ, Gates RL, Groner JI, Hammond S, Caniano DA.** 2004. Clinical manifestations of appendiceal pinworms in children: an institutional experience and a review of the literature. *Pediatr Surg Int* **20:**372–375.
16. **Pampiglione S, Rivasi F.** 2009. Enterobiasis in ectopic locations mimicking tumor-like lesions. *Int J Microbiol* **2009:**642481.
17. **Ash LR, Orihel TC.** 2003. Intestinal helminths, p 2031–2046. *In* Murray PR, Baron EJ, Jorgensen JH, Pfaller MA, Yolken RH (ed), *Manual of Clinical Microbiology*, 8th ed. ASM Press, Washington, DC.
18. **Garcia LS.** 2016. Intestinal nematodes, p 299–335. *In* Garcia LS (ed), *Diagnostic Medical Parasitology*, 6th ed. ASM Press, Washington, DC.
19. **Traub RJ.** 2013. *Ancylostoma ceylanicum*, a re-emerging but neglected parasitic zoonosis. *Int J Parasitol* **43:**1009–1015.
20. **Bradbury RS, Hii SF, Harrington H, Speare R, Traub R.** 2017. *Ancylostoma ceylanicum* hookworm in the Solomon Islands. *Emerg Infect Dis* **23:**252–257.
21. **Inpankaew T, Schär F, Dalsgaard A, Khieu V, Chimnoi W, Chhoun C, Sok D, Marti H, Muth S, Odermatt P, Traub RJ.** 2014. High prevalence of *Ancylostoma ceylanicum* hookworm infections in humans, Cambodia, 2012. *Emerg Infect Dis* **20:**976–982.
22. **Brelsford JB, Plieskatt JL, Yakovleva A, Jariwala A, Keegan BP, Peng J, Xia P, Li G, Campbell D, Periago MV,**

Correa-Oliveira R, Bottazzi ME, Hotez PJ, Diemert D, Bethony JM. 2017. Advances in neglected tropical disease vaccines: developing relative potency and functional assays for the Na-GST-1/Alhydrogel hookworm vaccine. *PLoS Negl Trop Dis* **11:**e0005385.

23. **Tang YT, Gao X, Rosa BA, Abubucker S, Hallsworth-Pepin K, Martin J, Tyagi R, Heizer E, Zhang X, Bhonagiri-Palsikar V, Minx P, Warren WC, Wang Q, Zhan B, Hotez PJ, Sternberg PW, Dougall A, Gaze ST, Mulvenna J, Sotillo J, Ranganathan S, Rabelo EM, Wilson RW, Felgner PL, Bethony J, Hawdon JM, Gasser RB, Loukas A, Mitreva M.** 2014. Genome of the human hookworm *Necator americanus*. *Nat Genet* **46:**261–269.
24. **Schär F, Giardina F, Khieu V, Muth S, Vounatsou P, Marti H, Odermatt P.** 2016. Occurrence of and risk factors for *Strongyloides stercoralis* infection in South-East Asia. *Acta Trop* **159:**227–238.
25. **Jaleta TG, Zhou S, Bemm FM, Schär F, Khieu V, Muth S, Odermatt P, Lok JB, Streit A.** 2017. Different but overlapping populations of *Strongyloides stercoralis* in dogs and humans—dogs as a possible source for zoonotic strongyloidiasis. *PLoS Negl Trop Dis* **11:**e0005752.
26. **Fardet L, Généreau T, Poirot JL, Guidet B, Kettaneh A, Cabane J.** 2007. Severe strongyloidiasis in corticosteroid-treated patients: case series and literature review. *J Infect* **54:**18–27.
27. **Schroeder L, Banaei N.** 2013. *Strongyloides stercoralis* embryonated ova in the lung. *N Engl J Med* **368:**e15.
28. **Kim JH, Kim DS, Yoon YK, Sohn JW, Kim MJ.** 2016. Donor-derived strongyloidiasis infection in solid organ transplant recipients: a review and pooled analysis. *Transplant Proc* **48:**2442–2449.
29. **Levenhagen MA, Costa-Cruz JM.** 2014. Update on immunologic and molecular diagnosis of human strongyloidiasis. *Acta Trop* **135:**33–43.
30. **Buonfrate D, Formenti F, Perandin F, Bisoffi Z.** 2015. Novel approaches to the diagnosis of *Strongyloides stercoralis* infection. *Clin Microbiol Infect* **21:**543–552.
31. **Buonfrate D, Perandin F, Formenti F, Bisoffi Z.** 2017. A retrospective study comparing agar plate culture, indirect immunofluorescence and real-time PCR for the diagnosis of *Strongyloides stercoralis* infection. *Parasitology* **144:**812–816.
32. **Requena-Méndez A, Chiodini P, Bisoffi Z, Buonfrate D, Gotuzzo E, Muñoz J.** 2013. The laboratory diagnosis and follow up of strongyloidiasis: a systematic review. *PLoS Negl Trop Dis* **7:**e2002.
33. **Lim CK, Crawford A, Moore CV, Gasser RB, Nelson R, Koehler AV, Bradbury RS, Speare R, Dhatrak D, Weldhagen GF.** 2015. First human case of fatal *Halicephalobus gingivalis* meningoencephalitis in Australia. *J Clin Microbiol* **53:**1768–1774.
34. **Sultana Y, Jeoffreys N, Watts MR, Gilbert GL, Lee R.** 2013. Real-time polymerase chain reaction for detection of *Strongyloides stercoralis* in stool. *Am J Trop Med Hyg* **88:**1048–1051.
35. **Watts MR, James G, Sultana Y, Ginn AN, Outhred AC, Kong F, Verweij JJ, Iredell JR, Chen SC, Lee R.** 2014. A loop-mediated isothermal amplification (LAMP) assay for *Strongyloides stercoralis* in stool that uses a visual detection method with SYTO-82 fluorescent dye. *Am J Trop Med Hyg* **90:**306–311.
36. **Sharifdini M, Mirhendi H, Ashrafi K, Hosseini M, Mohebali M, Khodadadi H, Kia EB.** 2015. Comparison of nested polymerase chain reaction and real-time polymerase chain reaction with parasitological methods for detection of *Strongyloides stercoralis* in human fecal samples. *Am J Trop Med Hyg* **93:**1285–1291.
37. **Lodh N, Caro R, Sofer S, Scott A, Krolewiecki A, Shiff C.** 2016. Diagnosis of *Strongyloides stercoralis*: detection of parasite-derived DNA in urine. *Acta Trop* **163:**9–13.
38. **Loutfy MR, Wilson M, Keystone JS, Kain KC.** 2002. Serology and eosinophil count in the diagnosis and management of strongyloidiasis in a non-endemic area. *Am J Trop Med Hyg* **66:**749–752.
39. **Biggs BA, Caruana S, Mihrshahi S, Jolley D, Leydon J, Chea L, Nuon S.** 2009. Management of chronic strongyloidiasis in immigrants and refugees: is serologic testing useful? *Am J Trop Med Hyg* **80:**788–791.
40. **Rascoe LN, Price C, Shin SH, McAuliffe I, Priest JW, Handali S.** 2015. Development of Ss-NIE-1 recombinant antigen based assays for immunodiagnosis of strongyloidiasis. *PLoS Negl Trop Dis* **9:**e0003694.
41. **Bisoffi Z, Buonfrate D, Sequi M, Mejia R, Cimino RO, Krolewiecki AJ, Albonico M, Gobbo M, Bonafini S, Angheben A, Requena-Mendez A, Muñoz J, Nutman TB.** 2014. Diagnostic accuracy of five serologic tests for *Strongyloides stercoralis* infection. *PLoS Negl Trop Dis* **8:**e2640.
42. **Mounsey K, Kearns T, Rampton M, Llewellyn S, King M, Holt D, Currie BJ, Andrews R, Nutman T, McCarthy J.** 2014. Use of dried blood spots to define antibody response to the *Strongyloides stercoralis* recombinant antigen NIE. *Acta Trop* **138:**78–82.
43. **Brooker S, Bundy DAP.** 2014. Soil transmitted helminths (geohelminths), p 766–794. *In* Farrar J, Hotez PJ, Junghanss T, Kang G, Lalloo D, White N (ed), *Manson's Tropical Diseases*, 23rd ed. Elsevier Saunders, Philadelphia, PA.
44. **Gyorkos TW, Gilbert NL, Larocque R, Casapía M.** 2011. Trichuris and hookworm infections associated with anaemia during pregnancy. *Trop Med Int Health* **16:**531–537.
45. **Lorenzetti R, Campo SM, Stella F, Hassan C, Zullo A, Morini S.** 2003. An unusual endoscopic finding: *Trichuris trichiura*.. *Dig Liver Dis* **35:**811–813.
46. **Speich B, Ali SM, Ame SM, Bogoch II, Alles R, Huwyler J, Albonico M, Hattendorf J, Utzinger J, Keiser J.** 2015. Efficacy and safety of albendazole plus ivermectin, albendazole plus mebendazole, albendazole plus oxantel pamoate, and mebendazole alone against *Trichuris trichiura* and concomitant soil-transmitted helminth infections: a four-arm, randomised controlled trial. *Lancet Infect Dis* **15:**277–284.

Filarial Nematodes

CARMELLE T. NORICE-TRA AND THOMAS B. NUTMAN

147

Filarial worms are arthropod-transmitted nematodes or roundworms that dwell in the subcutaneous tissues and the lymphatics. Although eight filarial species infect humans, four are responsible for most of the pathology associated with these infections: *Wuchereria bancrofti*, *Brugia malayi*, *Onchocerca volvulus*, and *Loa loa*. The taxonomy of these parasites follows a newly adopted molecular approach (see chapter 135, Table 5) (1). In general, each of these parasites is transmitted by biting arthropods. Although these parasites are nonendemic in temperate or subtropical areas, they are often seen in individuals who have immigrated to, resided in, or traveled to filaria-endemic tropical areas. Infection is generally not established unless exposure to infective larvae is intense and prolonged. The distribution and vectors of all the filarial parasites of humans are given in Table 1.

All filariae go through a complex life cycle that includes an infective larval stage carried by the insects and an adult worm stage that resides in humans, either in the lymph nodes, in the adjacent lymphatics, or in the subcutaneous tissue. Development of the infective larva to the gravid, adult stage in the vertebrate host requires several months and in some cases a year or more. Adult female worms produce microfilariae that circulate in the blood or migrate through the skin. The microfilariae can then be ingested by the appropriate biting arthropod and develop into infective larvae that can initiate the life cycle once more. Certain species (*W. bancrofti*, *Brugia* spp., *L. loa*) circulate in the blood with a defined circadian rhythm or "periodicity," which can be nocturnal (typically the lymphatic filariae) or diurnal (*L. loa*). Other species lack periodicity and are found in the peripheral blood at all hours of the day and night. When absent from the peripheral blood, the microfilariae are found in the deeper visceral capillaries, particularly within the pulmonary vasculature. Because the adult worms are typically sequestered in subcutaneous or lymphatic tissues, the diagnosis of infection depends on the detection of microfilariae in either blood or skin, depending on the species. Adult worms may survive for decades (2), whereas the life spans of microfilariae range from 3 months to 3 years.

Microfilariae are relatively simple in their organization and structure (Fig. 1). They are vermiform and in stained preparations appear to be composed of a column of nuclei interrupted along its length by spaces and special cells that are the precursors of body organs or organelles. Some species of microfilariae are enveloped in a sheath, whereas others have no sheath (Table 1; Fig. 2).

There are significant differences in the clinical manifestations of filarial infections, or at least in the period over which the manifestations present, between patients native to the areas of endemicity and those who are travelers or recent arrivals in these same areas. Characteristically, the infection in previously unexposed individuals is more likely to be clinically symptomatic than the infection in natives of the region of endemicity (3, 4). Furthermore, symptoms tend to develop rather slowly.

LYMPHATIC FILARIAL PARASITES

Taxonomy

Wuchereria bancrofti, *Brugia malayi*, and *Brugia timori* belong to clade III (Chromadoria: Spirurina) of the Nematoda, in the superfamily Spiruromorpha, and the family Onchocercidae.

Description of the Agents

There are three lymphatic-dwelling filarial parasites of humans—*W. bancrofti*, *B. malayi*, and *B. timori*. The adult worms usually reside in either the afferent lymphatic channels or the lymph nodes. These adult parasites may remain viable in the human host for decades. The morphologic appearance and other characteristics of the parasite can be found in Table 1 and Fig. 1 and 2.

Epidemiology and Transmission

Wuchereria bancrofti

W. bancrofti is the most common and widespread species of filariae that infect humans. It has an extensive distribution throughout tropical and subtropical areas of the world, including Asia and the Pacific Islands, Africa, areas of South America, and the Caribbean Basin. Humans are the only definitive host for this parasite and are therefore the natural reservoir for infection. There are both periodic and subperiodic forms of the parasite. Nocturnally periodic forms have microfilariae present in the peripheral blood primarily at night (between 10 p.m. and 4 a.m.), whereas the subperiodic forms have microfilariae present in the blood at all times but with maximal levels in the afternoon.

TABLE 1 Filarial parasites of humans

Species	Distribution	Vector	Primary pathology	Location	Periodicity	Size	Tail	Sheath: Presence	Sheath: Staining properties
Wuchereria bancrofti	Tropics	Mosquito	Lymphatic, pulmonary	Blood, hydrocele fluid	Nocturnal, subperiodic	298 × 7.5–10 μm	Pointed tail devoid of nuclei	+	Does not stain
Brugia timori	Indonesia	Mosquito	Lymphatic	Blood	Nocturnal	300 × 5–6 μm	Nuclei in tail	+	Tends not to stain
Brugia malayi	South and Southeast Asia	Mosquito	Lymphatic, pulmonary	Blood	Nocturnal, subperiodic	270 × 5–6 μm	Nuclei in tail	+	Bright pink with Giemsa
Onchocerca volvulus	Africa and South America	Black fly	Dermal, ocular, lymphatic	Skin, eyes	None	309 × 5–9 μm	No nuclei in tail	–	
Mansonella streptocerca	Africa	Midge	Dermal	Skin	None	210 × 5–6 μm	"Crooked tail" in which column of nuclei extends	–	
Loa loa	Africa	Deerfly	Allergic	Blood	Diurnal	Up to 300 μm	Irregularly arranged nuclei extend to end of tail	+	Does not stain
Mansonella perstans	Africa, South America	Midge	Probably allergic	Blood	None	203 × 4–5 μm	Blunt tail contains nuclei	–	
Mansonella ozzardi	Central and South America	Midge, black fly	Ill defined	Blood	None	224 × 4–5 μm	Long tail with no nuclei in it	–	

Generally, the subperiodic form is found only in the Pacific Islands (including Cook and Ellis Islands, Fiji, New Caledonia, the Marquesas, Samoa, and the Society Islands). Elsewhere, *W. bancrofti* is nocturnally periodic. The natural vectors are *Culex fatigans* mosquitoes in urban settings and usually anopheline, aedean, or mansonian mosquitoes in rural areas.

Brugia malayi and *Brugia timori*

The distribution of brugian filariasis is limited primarily to China, India, Indonesia, Korea, Japan, Malaysia, and the Philippines. *B. timori* has been described only on two islands in Timor. Similar to the situation with *W. bancrofti*, there are both periodic and subperiodic forms of brugian filariasis. The nocturnal periodic form is more common and is transmitted in areas of coastal rice fields (by mansonian and anopheline mosquitoes), while the subperiodic form is found in the swamp forests (mansonian vector). Although humans are the common host, *B. malayi* also naturally infects cats.

Clinical Significance

Lymphatic filariasis (LF) is associated with a variety of clinical manifestations. The most common presentations are asymptomatic (or subclinical) microfilaremia, lymphedema, hydrocele, acute adenolymphangitis or dermatolymphangioadenitis, and elephantiasis. Less frequently, LF can present with chyluria or tropical eosinophilia (5–7). The range of clinical disease varies somewhat across geographic locations and according to the species of nematode causing the infection (8). Additionally, the disease in previously unexposed individuals is more acute and intense than that found in natives of the region of endemicity (3, 4). Patients with asymptomatic (or subclinical) microfilaremia rarely come to the attention of medical personnel except through the incidental finding of microfilariae in the peripheral blood. Although they may be clinically asymptomatic, virtually all persons with *W. bancrofti* or *B. malayi* microfilaremia have some degree of subclinical disease that includes dilated and tortuous lymphatics, which can be visualized by lymphoscintigraphy (9) and—in men with *W. bancrofti*—scrotal lymphangiectasia (detectable by ultrasound) (10). Despite these findings, the majority of individuals appear to remain clinically asymptomatic for years. Relatively few progress to either the acute or chronic stage of infection (11). Development of lymphedema may not occur until long after the initial infection. Lymphatic dysfunction develops as a primary event in response to adult filarial parasites and host immune responses in virtually all infected persons. This process has been shown to be progressive during infection and permanent once established (12). Lymphedema most commonly affects the lower extremities but can also affect arms, breasts in females, and the scrotum in males. Secondary effects such as thickening of the subcutaneous tissues, hyperkeratosis, fissuring of the skin, and hyperplastic skin changes can occur. Recurrent attacks of acute dermatolymphangioadenitis (ADLA)—characterized by edematous inflammatory plaques and systemic symptoms (fever, chills, myalgia, headache)—on the background of chronic skin changes and lymphatic dysfunction play a major role for lymphedema disease development and progression to elephantiasis (13, 14).

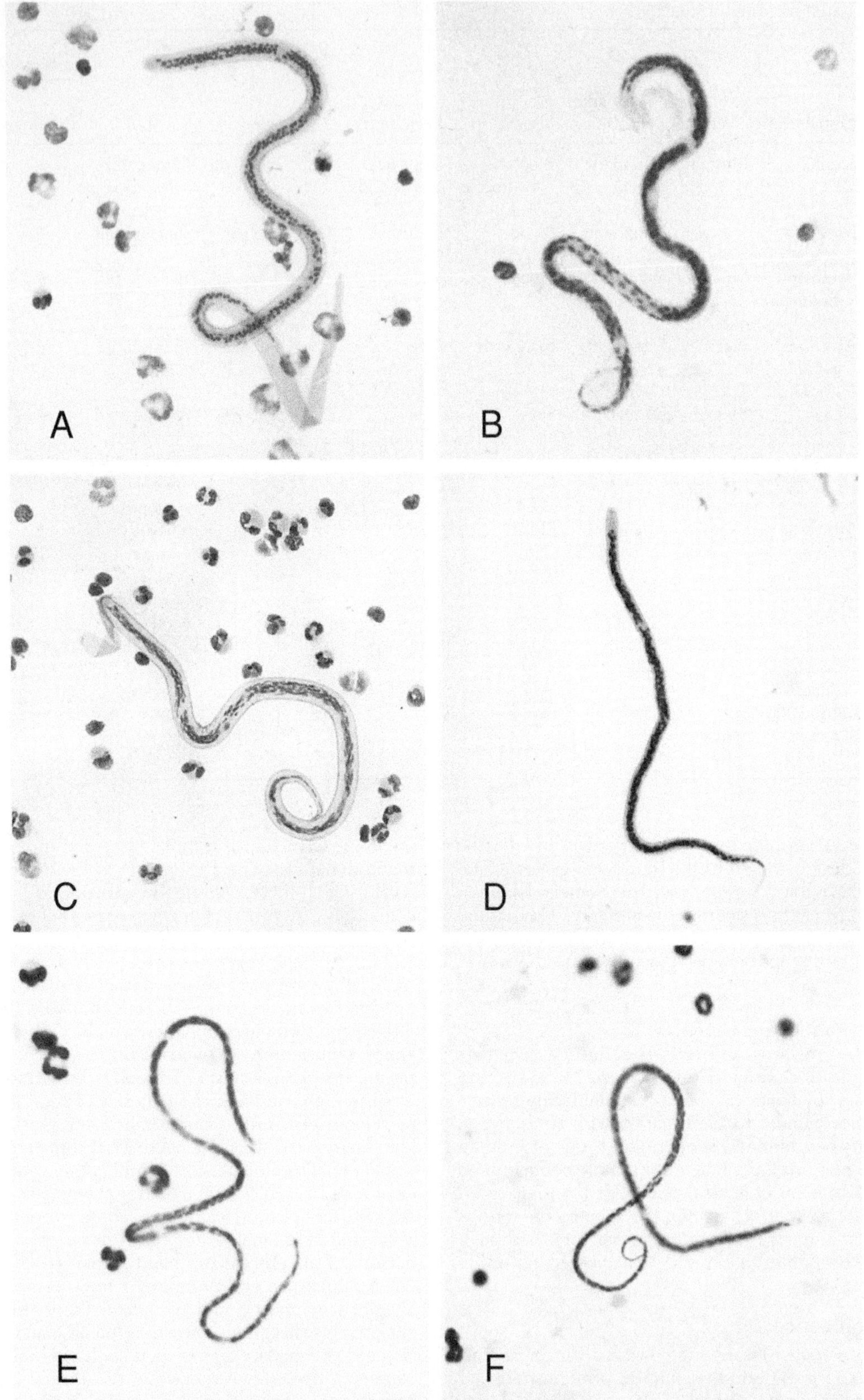

FIGURE 1 Common microfilariae found in humans. Hematoxylin stain. Magnification, ×325. (A) *W. bancrofti*; (B) *B. malayi*; (C) *L. loa*; (D) *O. volvulus*; (E) *M. perstans*; (F) *M. ozzardi*.

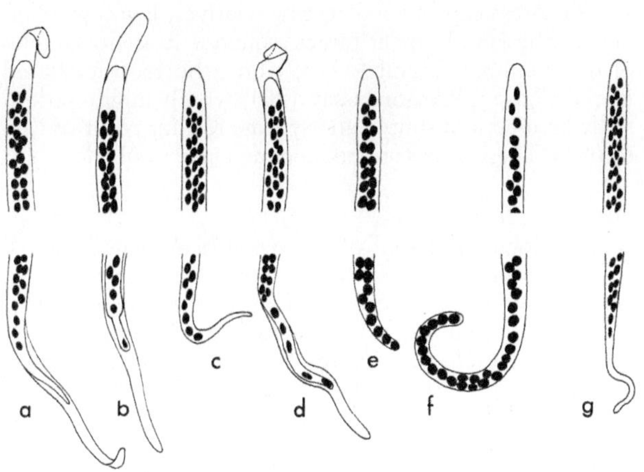

FIGURE 2 Diagrammatic representation of the anterior and posterior extremities of the common microfilariae found in humans. (A) *W. bancrofti*; (B) *B. malayi*; (C) *O. volvulus*; (D) *L. loa*; (E) *M. perstans*; (F) *M. streptocerca*; (G) *M. ozzardi*.

Acute attacks in LF cover a variety of clinical entities that present with inflammation. True filarial adenolymphangitis (ADL), felt to reflect the death of an adult worm, presents with inflammation, swelling, and retrograde lymphangitis extending peripherally from the draining node where the parasites presumably reside. Regional lymph nodes are often enlarged, and the entire lymphatic channel can become indurated and inflamed. The second type of acute attack is now labeled bacterial ADL or dermatoadenolymphangitis (DLA). Skin changes may result in entry lesions of the affected limb—particularly in the toe webs, which serve as portals of entry for skin biota (15, 16). For these reasons, limbs become susceptible to recurrent bacterial infections (17, 18). The clinical pattern of DLA is distinctly different from that of ADL (17). The lymphangitis develops in a reticular rather than in a linear pattern, and the local and systemic symptoms, including edema, pain, fever, and chills, are frequently more severe (19). These cause considerable acute morbidity and progression of lymphedema to elephantiasis (20). ADL and DLA occur in both the upper and lower extremities with both bancroftian and brugian filariasis, but involvement of the genital lymphatics occurs almost exclusively with *W. bancrofti* infection.

Hydrocele formation occurs in bancroftian filariasis when adult worms block retroperitoneal and subdiaphragmatic lymphatics. In males, this causes accumulation of straw-colored lymph either unilaterally or bilaterally between the visceral and parietal layers of the tunica vaginalis. The condition presents as a translucent mass obscuring palpation of the testis and differs from a congenital hydrocele or herniation in that the tunica is sealed at the top and peritoneal fluid is not communicating. If there is obstruction of the retroperitoneal lymphatics, renal lymphatic pressure can increase to the point at which they rupture into the renal pelvis or tubules so that chyluria is seen. The chyluria is characteristically intermittent and is often prominent in the morning just after the patient arises. In females, there have been reports of vulval lymphedema (also termed "vulval elephantiasis") as well (21, 22).

Tropical pulmonary eosinophilia (TPE) is a syndrome caused by immune hyperresponsiveness to microfilariae of LF species trapped in the lungs (5, 7, 23). This syndrome affects males more often than females, most commonly young adults, especially in the third decade of life. Most cases have been reported from India, Pakistan, Sri Lanka, Brazil, Guyana, and Southeast Asia, but it can occur in any area where filarial infections occur. The main features include a history of residence in filaria-endemic regions, paroxysmal cough and wheezing that are usually nocturnal, weight loss, low-grade fever, and adenopathy and pronounced blood eosinophilia (3,000 eosinophils/μl or more). Patients are rarely found to have microfilariae in the blood, and circulating filarial antigen may be undetectable. Chest radiographs generally show increased bronchoalveolar markings, diffuse interstitial lesions, and/or mottled opacities prominently in the lower lung fields, but may be normal in 20 to 30% of cases (24). Tests of pulmonary function show restrictive abnormalities in most cases and obstructive defects in half. Total serum IgE levels (10,000 to 100,000 ng/ml) and antifilarial antibody titers are characteristically elevated. Although there is no single clinical or laboratory criterion that aids in distinguishing TPE from other pulmonary diseases, residence in the tropics, the presence of high levels of antifilarial antibodies, and a rapid clinical response to diethylcarbamazine (DEC) favor the diagnosis of tropical eosinophilia (25).

Diagnosis

Diagnosis of bancroftian and brugian filarial infection can be made noninvasively in the right setting with clinical and historical information, by ultrasound, and/or by laboratory methods. Definitive identification of parasites can be achieved with appropriate samples of blood or tissue for microscopy of microfilariae, circulating antigen detection, or nucleic acid amplification test (NAAT) detection of filarial DNA. The timing of blood collection is critical and should be based on the periodicity of the microfilariae in the region of endemicity involved (Table 1). Recent developments in immunodiagnostic and molecular biology techniques give further options for diagnosis.

Ultrasound

Ultrasonography allows for visualization of adult worms in lymphatic channels or of lymphatics that have been dilated as a consequence of infection (26). In cases of suspected LF due to *W. bancrofti*, high-frequency ultrasound of the scrotum or female breast coupled with Doppler imaging may result in identification of motile adult worms ("filarial dance sign") within dilated lymphatics (27, 28). Adult worms may be visualized in the lymphatics of the spermatic cord in up to 80% of infected men with microfilaremia associated with *W. bancrofti* (11). In brugian filariasis, ultrasounds have been used successfully to localize the adult worms in the female breast, the inguinal lymph nodes, and the lymphatic vessels of the thigh and calf (29).

Direct Examination

Parasites can be identified by direct examination of blood or other fluids (such as chyle, urine, hydrocele fluid). Timing of the blood draw should take advantage of the periodicity of each organism; species identification is based on the characteristic morphologic appearance of the microfilariae (Table 1 and Fig. 2).

Microscopy

A small volume of fluid is spread on a clean slide. The slide is then air dried, stained with Giemsa, and examined microscopically. The microfilariae of *W. bancrofti* are sheathed, lie in smooth curves in stained smears, and are 298 μm × 7.5 to 10.0 μm. The column nuclei are dispersed; there is a short headspace, and the pointed tail is devoid of nuclei (Fig. 1A). The morphology of the *B. malayi* microfilariae is similar to that of the *W. bancrofti* microfilariae, being sheathed but somewhat smaller (279 μm × 5 to 6 μm), and can be differentiated from the *W. bancrofti* microfilariae by the presence of subterminal and terminal nuclei in the tail (Fig. 1, A and B). *B. timori* microfilariae are similar to those of *B. malayi* with conspicuous terminal and subterminal nuclei; however, *B. timori* microfilariae are larger (more than 300 μm long) than those of *B. malayi*. Additionally, the *B. malayi* sheath stains bright pink with Giemsa, whereas the *B. timori* sheath tends not to stain, and that of *W. bancrofti* never does.

Because microfilariae may be present in the blood in only small numbers, sensitive procedures such as Nuclepore filtration and Knott's concentration are also used routinely to detect infections.

Nuclepore Filtration

A known volume of anticoagulated blood is passed through a polycarbonate (Nuclepore) filter with a 3-μm pore. A large volume (50 ml) of distilled water is passed through (the water will lyse or break open the red blood cells, leaving the worms intact and more easily visible). The filter is then air dried, stained with Wright's or Giemsa stain, and examined by microscopy. For studies in the field, 1 ml of anticoagulated blood can be added to 9 ml of a solution of 2% formalin or 10% Teepol and stored for up to 9 months before performing filtration (30).

Knott's Concentration Technique

Anticoagulated blood (1 ml) is placed in 9 ml of 2% formalin. The tube is centrifuged at 1,500 rpm for 1 minute. The sediment is spread on a slide and dried thoroughly. The slide is then stained with Wright's or Giemsa stain and examined microscopically.

Antigen Detection

Assays for circulating antigens of *W. bancrofti* permit the diagnosis of microfilaremic and cryptic (amicrofilaremic) infection. Three tests are commercially available for testing of whole blood, plasma, or serum (although not in the United States): (i) Tropbio Filariasis Antigen II, an enzyme-linked immunosorbent assay (ELISA) available from Celllabs (Townsville, Queensland, Australia); (ii) BinaxNOW Filariasis, a rapid-format immunochromatographic card available from Alere International (Waltham, MA); and (iii) Alere Filariasis Test Strip, a new rapid-format immunochromatographic test also available from Alere International. The Alere Filariasis Test Strip detects a lower concentration of circulating filarial antigen than the BinaxNOW Filariasis test (31, 32). These assays have sensitivities that range from 96% to 100% and specificities that approach 98% (32, 33). All these tests can be used on blood drawn at any time of day or night, thus avoiding the need for specific bleeding times depending on the periodicity of microfilariae. None of the tests is FDA approved. There are currently no tests for circulating antigens in brugian filariasis.

Nucleic Acid Detection Techniques

In appropriate laboratories, NAAT can detect parasite DNA and is now the most sensitive technique for definitive diagnosis (34–36). For each of the lymphatic-dwelling parasites, primers and probes have been identified that are 100% specific and provide sensitivities that are up to 10-fold greater than parasite detection by direct examination. Recent diagnostic advances include highly sensitive real-time NAAT assays capable of detecting relatively low copy numbers of the *Hha* I repeat target sequence in small samples of dried human blood (37–39) and the loop-mediated isothermal application assay (40), which might potentially be used as a simple and specific test for point-of-care settings. These assays are not commercially available.

Serologic Tests

Immunologically based diagnosis with measured IgG or IgG4 responses against crude extracts of *Brugia* worms suffers from poor specificity. There is extensive cross-reactivity among filarial antigens and antigens of other helminths, including common intestinal roundworms. Furthermore, serologic tests are unable to distinguish between active and past infection. However, these tests still have a role in diagnosis, as a negative test effectively excludes past or present infection. These tests are available commercially and from the National Institutes of Health, from the U.S. Centers for Disease Control and Prevention, and at World Health Organization (WHO) Collaborating Centers for Lymphatic Filariasis worldwide.

For serologic detection specifically of *W. bancrofti* infections, an antigen termed Wb123 has been used, primarily in the context of epidemiologic studies. There are two commercial "research only" tests: a Filaria Detect IgG4 ELISA from InBios (Seattle, WA) and the SD Bioline Lymphatic Filariasis IgG4 rapid diagnostic test (RDT) from Standard Diagnostics (Seoul, South Korea) for the measurement of IgG4 to this antigen. These tests have sensitivities between 70% and 80% and specificities greater than 97% (41–43).

For brugian filariasis, the Brugia Rapid test for IgG4 immunoreactivity against the recombinant *B. malayi* antigen BmR1 may be employed (Reszon Diagnostics International, Subang Java, Selangor, Malaysia). A large multicenter evaluation of the performance of this test demonstrated 92.96% sensitivity and 100% specificity (44, 45).

Treatment and Prevention

The available chemotherapy for LF is DEC, ivermectin, and albendazole. DEC remains the treatment of choice for the individual with active LF (microfilaremia, antigen positivity, or adult worms on ultrasound), although albendazole has also been shown to have some macrofilaricidal efficacy. If the adult parasites survive, microfilaremia along with clinical symptoms can recur within months after conclusion of the therapy. Chronic low-dose DEC may also result in cure (e.g., in DEC salt). Evidence shows that these drugs are safe and more effective when used in combination (46–49). The current global elimination campaign uses these three drugs in various combinations for mass treatment of communities in areas of endemicity (50). Most pathogenic filarial nematodes apart from *L. loa* harbor bacterial endosymbionts. These *Wolbachia* are vital for parasite larval development and adult worm fertility and viability. Use of antibiotics (e.g., the tetracyclines) that target the *Wolbachia* has been shown to reduce microfilarial levels (51) and circulating filarial antigen (52).

Once lymphedema is established, antifilarial medication is not useful if the patient does not have active infection. Management of lymphedema should concentrate on exercise, elevation, and local skin care with appropriate treatment of entry lesions (51). There has, however, been some recent evidence that treatment with doxycycline may decrease the severity in early stages of lymphedema, independent of its antimicrobial effects (53). Antifilarial medication is also not indicated in management of bacterial ADLA, which is addressed with skin care and antibiotics, if indicated (15, 19). Hydroceles can be drained repeatedly or managed surgically (54–56).

Avoidance of mosquito bites is usually not feasible for residents of areas of endemicity, but visitors should make use of insect repellent and mosquito nets. Impregnated bed nets have been shown to have a salutary effect. Community-based intervention is the current approach to elimination of LF as a public health problem (57, 58). The underlying tenet of this approach is that mass annual distribution of anti-filarial drugs (albendazole with either DEC [for all areas except where onchocerciasis is coendemic] or ivermectin) will profoundly suppress microfilaremia. If the suppression is sustained, then transmission can be interrupted. Community education and clinical care for persons already suffering from the chronic sequelae of LF are important components of filariasis control and elimination programs (59). Vaccines are not currently available but may have a role in the future.

ONCHOCERCA VOLVULUS

Taxonomy

O. volvulus belongs to clade III (Chromadoria: Spirurina) of the Nematoda, in the superfamily Spiruromorpha, and the family Onchocercidae.

Description of the Agent

The adult worms of *O. volvulus* typically reside in nodules composed primarily of fibrous host tissue. These adult parasites may remain viable in the human host for decades. The morphologic appearance and other characteristics of microfilariae and adult worms can be found in Table 1 and Fig. 1 and 2.

Epidemiology and Transmission

Onchocerciasis, also known as "river blindness," is caused by infection with *O. volvulus*, a subcutaneous-dwelling filarial worm. Approximately 18 million people are infected, mostly in equatorial Africa, the Sahara, Yemen, and parts of Brazil and Venezuela. The infection is transmitted to humans through the bites of black flies of the genus *Simulium*, which breed along fast-flowing rivers in the above-mentioned tropical areas.

Clinical Significance

The major disease manifestations of onchocerciasis are localized to the skin, lymph nodes, and eyes. Onchocerciasis is a cumulative infection—intense infection leads to the most severe complications and is felt to reflect repeated inoculation with infective larvae.

Skin

Onchocercal skin disease may manifest as acute papular onchodermatitis, chronic papular onchodermatitis, lichenified onchodermatitis, skin atrophy, hanging groin, and depigmentation (60–62). Pruritus is the most frequent manifestation of onchocercal dermatitis and may be accompanied by the appearance of localized areas of edema and erythema. Typically, skin disease appears as a papular, pruritic dermatitis. If the infection is prolonged, lichenification and pigment changes (either hypo- or hyperpigmentation) can occur; these often lead to atrophy, "lizard skin," and mottling of the skin. Localized, hyperreactive onchodermatitis—a form of skin disease referred to as "sowda"—is a lichenified dermatitis characterized by intense pruritus and hyperpigmentation (63–67).

Onchocercomata

These subcutaneous nodules, which can be palpable and/or visible, contain the adult worm. In African patients, they are common over bony prominences; in Latin American patients, nodules tend to develop preferentially in the upper part of the body, particularly on the head. Nodules vary in size and characteristically are firm and nontender. It has been estimated that for every palpable nodule there are four deeper nonpalpable ones (68, 69).

Lymph Nodes

Lymphadenopathy is frequently found, particularly in the inguinal and femoral areas. The underlying pathology consists of scarring of the lymphoid areas (*O. volvulus* infection in Africa) or follicular hyperplasia (*O. volvulus* infection in Yemen). As the lymph nodes enlarge, they can come to lie within areas of loose skin (so-called "hanging groin") that predisposes to inguinal and femoral hernias.

Ocular Disease

Onchocercal ocular disease is usually seen in persons with moderate or heavy infections. Sparing no part of the eye, it may manifest as conjunctivitis, anterior uveitis, or iridocyclitis leading to secondary glaucoma, sclerosing keratitis, optic atrophy, and chorioretinal lesions (70, 71). Ultimately, the devastating consequences of severe vision loss or blindness are observed in a small percentage of patients with onchocerciasis.

Other Complications

Chronic infections are associated with low body weight and diffuse musculoskeletal pain. An acquired form of dwarfism called Nakalanga syndrome, which is characterized by growth retardation, endocrine dysfunction, mental impairment, and epilepsy, has been attributed to pituitary involvement in this disease (72, 73). An association with epilepsy has also been reported (72, 74, 75). Other conditions are reproductive abnormalities with secondary amenorrhea, spontaneous abortion, and infertility.

Diagnosis

Definitive diagnosis depends on finding an adult worm in an excised nodule or, more commonly, microfilariae in a skin snip. Microfilariae can occasionally be found in the blood and in urine, typically after treatment. Microfilariae may also be seen in the cornea and in the anterior chamber of the eye when viewed with a slit lamp.

For skin-snip evaluation, a small piece of skin is elevated by the tip of a needle or skin hook held parallel to the surface, and a scalpel blade is used to shave off the skin area stretched across the top surface of the needle. Alternatively, a sclerocorneal punch can be used to obtain a blood-free circular skin specimen. Skin snips are generally obtained from an area of affected skin or from the scapular, gluteal, and calf areas (in the African form) and from the scapular, deltoid, and gluteal areas (in the Central American form). Once obtained, the skin snips are incubated in a physiologic solution (such as normal saline). The emergent microfilariae can be seen under a microscope typically within 30 minutes in heavy infection or within 24 hours in light infections.

Direct Examination

Microscopy

Microfilariae lack a sheath and are approximately 309 μm long × 5 to 9 μm in diameter. The tail is tapered, usually bent or flexed, and without nuclei (Fig. 1D and 2C).

Nucleic Acid Detection Techniques

Assays using NAAT to detect onchocercal DNA by targeting O-150 repeat sequence in skin snips are now in use in research laboratories and are highly specific and sensitive, provided that organisms (or DNA) are present in the skin samples obtained (34, 76).

Serologic Tests

Because direct detection of parasites in the skin or eye is invasive and insensitive, immunodiagnostic assays may be preferable. IgG antifilarial antibody assays, while positive in individuals with onchocerciasis, suffer from the same lack of specificity and positive predictive value seen in the bloodborne filarial infections; however, the combined use of three groups of recombinant antigens in conventional ELISA provides sensitivity and specificities that approach 100% for the diagnosis of onchocerciasis (77). Another platform incorporates four recombinant antigens into a rapid, high-throughput luciferase immunoprecipitation system assay (LIPS) that is 100% sensitive and 80% to 90% specific in distinguishing onchocerciasis from related filarial infections (78).

For serologic detection of O. *volvulus* infections, an antigen termed OV-16 has been used as an early biomarker for infection. A commercially available RDT for OV-16 has been developed; this SD Bioline Onchocerciasis IgG4 RDT has a specificity that ranges from 95% to 99% and sensitivities of approximately 80% (79–82). Although used primarily as a surveillance tool for certifying elimination, it may be useful for confirming diagnosis in persons with suspected onchocerciasis.

Treatment

The major goals of therapy are to prevent irreversible lesions and to alleviate symptoms. Surgical excision of nodules is recommended when the nodules are located on the head because of the proximity of the microfilariae-producing adult worms to the eye, but chemotherapy is the mainstay of treatment. Ivermectin, a semisynthetic macrocyclic lactone, is now considered first-line therapy for onchocerciasis. It is characteristically given yearly or semiannually for the life of the adult worm (10 to 15 years). Most patients have limited to no reaction to treatment. Pruritus, cutaneous edema, and/or a maculopapular rash occur in approximately 1% to 10% of treated individuals. Significant ocular complications are extremely rare, as is hypotension.

Ivermectin is contraindicated for use in pregnant or breastfeeding women on the basis of toxicity and teratogenicity data from animal studies. Although ivermectin treatment results in a marked drop in skin microfilarial density, its effect can be short lived (less than 3 months in some cases). Thus, ivermectin can be given more frequently than each year for persistent symptoms (83).

In areas of Africa coendemic for O. *volvulus* and L. *loa*, however, ivermectin is contraindicated because of severe posttreatment encephalopathy seen in patients who are heavily microfilaremic with L. *loa* (84). However, a new mobile phone-based videomicroscopy platform called the LoaScope (85) has been used as a point-of-contact method of identifying those at risk (more than 20,000 microfilariae of L. *loa* per ml) for serious adverse events and excluding them from ivermectin-based MDA in a strategy termed "test and not treat" (86).

There is now a significant amount of evidence that a 6-week course of doxycycline-based therapy targeting *Wolbachia* endosymbiont macrofilaristatic, rendering the female adult worms sterile for long periods of time (87, 88).

Prevention

Prevention of infection is being achieved by mass-treatment programs using ivermectin (89, 90). Vector control has been beneficial in areas of high endemicity in which breeding sites are vulnerable to insecticide spraying, but most areas where onchocerciasis is endemic are not suited to this type of intervention. Community-based administration of ivermectin every 6 to 12 months is now being used to interrupt transmission in areas of endemicity. This measure has already helped eliminate the parasite in most of Latin America. No drug has proven useful for prophylaxis of O. *volvulus* infection, and no vaccine exists.

LOA LOA

Taxonomy

L. *loa* belongs to clade III (Chromadoria: Spirurina) of the Nematoda, in the superfamily Spiruromorpha, and the family Onchocercidae.

Description of the Agent

The adult parasite lives in the subcutaneous tissues in humans; microfilariae circulate in the bloodstream with a diurnal periodicity that peaks between 12:00 p.m. and 2:00 p.m. The morphologic appearance and other characteristics of adult worms and microfilariae can be found in Table 1 and Fig. 1 and 2.

Epidemiology and Transmission

The distribution of L. *loa* is limited to the rain forests of West and Central Africa (91). Tabanid flies (deer flies) of the genus *Chrysops* are the vectors.

Clinical Significance

L. *loa* infection may be associated with a clinically asymptomatic condition associated with microfilaremia, with the infection being recognized only after subconjunctival migration of an adult worm (the so-called eye worm). The classic clinical presentation is with episodic "Calabar swelling" (localized areas of transient angioedema) found predominantly on the extremities. If associated inflammation extends to the nearby joints or peripheral nerves, corresponding symptoms develop (e.g., entrapment neuropathy). Nephropathy (presumed to be immune complex mediated), encephalopathy, and cardiomyopathy may occur rarely.

There appear to be differences in the presentations of loiasis between those native to the area of endemicity and those who are visitors (92–94). The latter tend to have a greater predominance of allergic symptomatology. The episodes of Calabar swelling tend to be more frequent and debilitating, and such patients rarely have microfilaremia. In addition, those who are not native to the area of endemicity have extreme elevation of eosinophils in the blood as well as marked increases in antifilarial antibody titers.

Diagnosis

Definitive diagnosis is made parasitologically, either by finding microfilariae in the peripheral blood or by isolating the adult worm from the eye or subcutaneous biopsy material following treatment. The diagnosis must often be made on clinical grounds, however, particularly in travelers (usually amicrofilaremic) returning from stays in the region of *Loa* endemicity.

Direct Examination

Microscopy

The microfilariae are sheathed and are up to 300 μm long. Adult females are 50 to 70 mm long and 0.5 mm wide, whereas adult males are 25 to 35 mm long and 0.25 mm wide. In contrast to the LF, the nuclei extend to the end of the tail; however, they are somewhat irregularly arranged along the length of the tail (Fig. 1C and 2D). The sheath does not stain with Giemsa.

Nucleic Acid Detection Techniques

NAAT-based assays for the detection and quantitation of *L. loa* DNA in blood by targeting the *Loa* interspersed repeat sequence, LLMF72 and LLMF269, are now available in research laboratories and are highly sensitive and specific (34, 95).

Serologic Tests

Available methods using crude antigen extracts from *Brugia* or *Dirofilaria* species do not differentiate between *L. loa* and other filarial pathogens. The utility of such testing in endemic populations is limited by the presence of antifilarial antibodies in up to 95% of individuals in some regions. A *L. loa*-specific recombinant protein, LLSXP-1, has been tested and has good specificity but only limited (50%) sensitivity in conventional IgG4-based ELISA assays (96). Incorporation of LLSXP-1 into a LIPS assay increased sensitivity to near 100% while also allowing for rapid, high-throughput processing of samples (97). Most recently an RDT measuring IgG against LLSXP-1 has been developed and has shown to have a sensitivity greater than 90%, with specificity approaching 95% (98).

Antifilarial IgG and IgG4, while nonspecific, may be useful in confirming the diagnosis of loiasis in visitors to areas of endemicity with suggestive clinical symptoms or unexplained eosinophilia.

Treatment and Prevention

DEC is effective against both the adult and the microfilarial forms of *L. loa*, but multiple courses are frequently necessary before the disease resolves completely (99). It can be obtained from the U.S. Centers for Disease Control and Prevention under an Investigational New Drug. In cases of heavy microfilaremia, allergic or other inflammatory reactions can take place during treatment, including central nervous system involvement with coma and encephalitis (84, 100, 101). Heavy infections can be treated initially with apheresis to remove the microfilariae and with glucocorticoids followed by small doses of DEC. If antifilarial treatment has no adverse effects, the prednisone dose can be rapidly tapered, and the dose of DEC gradually increased. Albendazole or ivermectin (although not approved for this use by the FDA) has been shown to be effective in reducing microfilarial loads (102), but the use of ivermectin in heavily microfilaremic individuals is contraindicated (84, 100, 101). Weekly DEC can be used as an effective prophylactic regimen for loiasis in temporary residents of locations where *L. loa* is endemic (103).

MANSONELLA SPECIES

Taxonomy

Mansonella perstans, *Mansonella ozzardi*, and *Mansonella streptocerca* belong to clade III (Chromadoria: Spirurina) of the Nematoda, in the superfamily Spiruromorpha, and the family Onchocercidae.

Description of the Agents

The adult worms of *M. perstans* reside in the body cavities (pericardial, pleural, and peritoneal) as well as in the mesentery and the perirenal and retroperitoneal tissues, whereas the location of the adult worms of *M. ozzardi* is unknown. The microfilariae of both parasites circulate in the blood without periodicity. For *M. streptocerca*, the adult parasites reside in the skin. *M. streptocerca* microfilariae are found predominantly in the skin. The morphologic appearance and other characteristics of adult worms and microfilariae can be found in Table 1 and Fig. 1 and 2.

Epidemiology and Transmission

M. perstans is distributed across the center of Africa and in northeastern South America. The infection is transmitted to humans through the bites of midges (*Culicoides* species). *M. streptocerca* is largely found in the tropical forest belt of Africa from Ghana to Zaire. It is transmitted to the human host by biting midges (*Culicoides* species). The distribution of *M. ozzardi* is restricted to Central and South America as well as certain Caribbean islands. The parasite is transmitted to the human host by biting midges (*Culicoides furens*) and black flies (*Simulium amazonicum*).

Clinical Significance

Although most patients infected with *M. perstans* appear to be asymptomatic, clinical manifestations may include transient angioedematous swellings of the arms, face, or other body parts (similar to the Calabar swellings of *L. loa* infection); pruritus; fever; headache; arthralgias; neurologic or psychologic symptoms; and right-upper-quadrant pain. Occasionally, pericarditis and hepatitis occur (104).

The major clinical manifestations of *M. streptocerca* infections are related to the skin: pruritus, papular rashes, and pigmentation changes. These are thought to be secondary to inflammatory reactions around microfilariae. Most infected individuals also show inguinal lymphadenopathy. Lymph nodes of affected individuals may show chronic lymphadenitis with scarring; however, many patients are completely asymptomatic (105).

The clinical details of *M. ozzardi* infection are poorly characterized. Furthermore, many consider this organism to be nonpathogenic; however, headache, articular pain, fever, pulmonary symptoms, adenopathy, hepatomegaly, and pruritus have been ascribed to infection with this organism (106, 107). There have been reports of an association of *M. ozzardi* with keratitis (108).

Diagnosis

For *M. perstans* infections, diagnosis is made parasitologically by finding the microfilariae in the blood or in other body fluids (serosal effusions). Microfilariae are small (203 μm × 4 to 5 μm) and have a blunt tail filled with nuclei. Perstans filariasis is often associated with peripheral blood eosinophilia and antifilarial antibody elevations (104). The diagnosis of *M. ozzardi* infection is made by demonstrating the characteristic microfilariae in the peripheral blood. These are small (224 μm × 4 to 5 μm) and have long attenuated tails devoid of nuclei (Fig. 1F and 2G). NAAT-based assays of venous blood samples and dried blood spots for the ribosomal gene internal transcriber spacer target may provide increased sensitivity in submicroscopic infections (109). The diagnosis of streptocerciasis can be made by finding the characteristic microfilariae on skin-snip examination (see previous section on onchocerciasis diagnosis). In areas where both *O. volvulus* and *M. streptocerca* are endemic, care must be taken to correctly identify the microfilariae. M. *streptocerca* microfilariae have no sheath, are long and slender, and measure approximately 210 μm × 5 to 6 μm. The most characteristic feature of M. *streptocerca* is its crooked tail (Fig. 2F), which contains nuclei.

Treatment and Prevention

Mansonella perstans

A number of treatment regimens have been tried, but none has been shown to be particularly effective in M. *perstans* filariasis. However, consistent with the identification of a *Wolbachia* species in M. *perstans* (110), a randomized trial in Mali has demonstrated the utility of doxycycline (200 mg daily for 6 weeks) treatment for this infection (111).

Mansonella streptocerca

DEC is particularly effective in treating infection by both the microfilarial and the adult forms of the parasite. Following treatment, as in onchocerciasis, one can often see debilitating urticaria, arthralgias, myalgias, headaches, and abdominal discomfort. Nevertheless, because DEC is contraindicated in most of Africa because of concerns with posttreatment reactions in onchocerciasis, its use in this infection is limited. Consequently, ivermectin is currently the drug of choice for this infection (112).

Mansonella ozzardi

Ivermectin is the drug of choice for this infection (113, 114) but has been associated with significant posttreatment adverse events in some patients (115, 116). There currently are no good preventive measures for any of the *Mansonella* infections beyond personal protective equipment, clothing, and insect repellants such as DEET (*N*,*N*-diethyl-meta-toluamide) or permethrin.

REFERENCES

1. **Adl SM, Simpson AG, Lane CE, Lukeš J, Bass D, Bowser SS, Brown MW, Burki F, Dunthorn M, Hampl V, Heiss A, Hoppenrath M, Lara E, Le Gall L, Lynn DH, McManus H, Mitchell EA, Mozley-Stanridge SE, Parfrey LW, Pawlowski J, Rueckert S, Shadwick L, Schoch CL, Smirnov A, Spiegel FW.** 2012. The revised classification of eukaryotes. *J Eukaryot Microbiol* **59:**429–493.
2. **Antinori S, Schifanella L, Million M, Galimberti L, Ferraris L, Mandia L, Trabucchi G, Cacioppo V, Monaco G, Tosoni A, Brouqui P, Gismondo MR, Giuliani G, Corbellino M.** 2012. Imported *Loa loa* filariasis: three cases and a review of cases reported in non-endemic countries in the past 25 years. *Int J Infect Dis* **16:**e649–e662.
3. **Lipner EM, Law MA, Barnett E, Keystone JS, von Sonnenburg F, Loutan L, Prevots DR, Klion AD, Nutman TB, GeoSentinel Surveillance Network.** 2007. Filariasis in travelers presenting to the GeoSentinel Surveillance Network. *PLoS Negl Trop Dis* **1:**e88.
4. **Rajan TV.** 2000. *Lymphatic Filariasis: A Historical Perspective*, vol 1. Imperial College Press, London, United Kingdom.
5. **Ottesen EA, Nutman TB.** 1992. Tropical pulmonary eosinophilia. *Annu Rev Med* **43:**417–424.
6. **Dreyer G, Mattos D, Norões J.** 2007. [Chyluria]. *Rev Assoc Med Bras 1992* **53:**460–464.
7. **Vijayan VK.** 2007. Tropical pulmonary eosinophilia: pathogenesis, diagnosis and management. *Curr Opin Pulm Med* **13:**428–433.
8. **Sasa M.** 1976. *Human Filariasis. A Global Survey of Epidemiology and Control*, p 819. University Park Press, Baltimore, MD.
9. **Freedman DO, de Almeida Filho PJ, Besh S, Maia e Silva MC, Braga C, Maciel A.** 1994. Lymphoscintigraphic analysis of lymphatic abnormalities in symptomatic and asymptomatic human filariasis. *J Infect Dis* **170:**927–933.
10. **Norões J, Addiss D, Santos A, Medeiros Z, Coutinho A, Dreyer G.** 1996. Ultrasonographic evidence of abnormal lymphatic vessels in young men with adult *Wuchereria bancrofti* infection in the scrotal area. *J Urol* **156:**409–412.
11. **Dreyer G, Norões J, Figueredo-Silva J, Piessens WF.** 2000. Pathogenesis of lymphatic disease in bancroftian filariasis: a clinical perspective. *Parasitol Today* **16:**544–548.
12. **Dreyer G, Addiss D, Roberts J, Norões J.** 2002. Progression of lymphatic vessel dilatation in the presence of living adult *Wuchereria bancrofti*. *Trans R Soc Trop Med Hyg* **96:**157–161.
13. **Pani SP, Srividya A.** 1995. Clinical manifestations of bancroftian filariasis with special reference to lymphoedema grading. *Indian J Med Res* **102:**114–118.
14. **Olszewski WL, Jamal S, Manokaran G, Pani S, Kumaraswami V, Kubicka U, Lukomska B, Tripathi FM, Swoboda E, Meisel-Mikolajczyk F, Stelmach E, Zaleska M.** 1999. Bacteriological studies of blood, tissue fluid, lymph and lymph nodes in patients with acute dermatolymphangioadenitis (DLA) in course of 'filarial' lymphedema. *Acta Trop* **73:**217–224.
15. **Shenoy RK, Sandhya K, Suma TK, Kumaraswami V.** 1995. A preliminary study of filariasis related acute adenolymphangitis with special reference to precipitating factors and treatment modalities. *Southeast Asian J Trop Med Public Health* **26:**301–305.
16. **Ananthakrishnan S, Das LK.** 2004. Entry lesions in bancroftian filarial lymphoedema patients—a clinical observation. *Acta Trop* **90:**215–218.
17. **Dreyer G, Medeiros Z, Netto MJ, Leal NC, de Castro LG, Piessens WF.** 1999. Acute attacks in the extremities of persons living in an area endemic for bancroftian filariasis: differentiation of two syndromes. *Trans R Soc Trop Med Hyg* **93:**413–417.
18. **McPherson T, Persaud S, Singh S, Fay MP, Addiss D, Nutman TB, Hay R.** 2006. Interdigital lesions and frequency of acute dermatolymphangioadenitis in lymphoedema in a filariasis-endemic area. *Br J Dermatol* **154:**933–941.
19. **Shenoy RK, Kumaraswami V, Suma TK, Rajan K, Radhakuttyamma G.** 1999. A double-blind, placebo-controlled study of the efficacy of oral penicillin, diethylcarbamazine or local treatment of the affected limb in preventing acute adenolymphangitis in lymphoedema caused by brugian filariasis. *Ann Trop Med Parasitol* **93:**367–377.
20. **Pani SP, Yuvaraj J, Vanamail P, Dhanda V, Michael E, Grenfell BT, Bundy DA.** 1995. Episodic adenolymphangitis and lymphoedema in patients with bancroftian filariasis. *Trans R Soc Trop Med Hyg* **89:**72–74.
21. **Adesiyun AG, Samaila MO.** 2008. Huge filarial elephantiasis vulvae in a Nigerian woman with subfertility. *Arch Gynecol Obstet* **278:**597–600.
22. **Palanisamy AP, Kanakaram KK, Vadivel S, Kothandapany S.** 2015. Vulval elephantiasis. *Indian Dermatol Online J* **6:**371.
23. **Pinkston P, Vijayan VK, Nutman TB, Rom WN, O'Donnell KM, Cornelius MJ, Kumaraswami V, Ferrans VJ, Takemura T, Yenokida G.** 1987. Acute tropical pulmonary eosinophilia. Characterization of the lower respiratory tract inflammation and its response to therapy. *J Clin Invest* **80:**216–225.
24. **Udwadia F.** 1975. *Pulmonary Eosinophilia, Progress in Respiration Research*, vol 7. S. Karger, Basel, Switzerland.
25. **Udwadia FE.** 1993. Tropical eosinophilia: a review. *Respir Med* **87:**17–21.
26. **Amaral F, Dreyer G, Figueredo-Silva J, Noroes J, Cavalcanti A, Samico SC, Santos A, Coutinho A.** 1994. Live adult worms detected by ultrasonography in human Bancroftian filariasis. *Am J Trop Med Hyg* **50:**753–757.
27. **Mand S, Debrah A, Batsa L, Adjei O, Hoerauf A.** 2004. Reliable and frequent detection of adult *Wuchereria bancrofti* in Ghanaian women by ultrasonography. *Trop Med Int Health* **9:**1111–1114.
28. **Mand S, Supali T, Djuardi J, Kar S, Ravindran B, Hoerauf A.** 2006. Detection of adult *Brugia malayi* filariae by ultrasonography in humans in India and Indonesia. *Trop Med Int Health* **11:**1375–1381.

29. **Shenoy RK, Suma TK, Kumaraswami V, Padma S, Rahmah N, Abhilash G, Ramesh C.** 2007. Doppler ultrasonography reveals adult-worm nests in the lymph vessels of children with brugian filariasis. *Ann Trop Med Parasitol* **101:**173–180.
30. **Eberhard ML, Lammie PJ.** 1991. Laboratory diagnosis of filariasis. *Clin Lab Med* **11:**977–1010.
31. **Weil GJ, Curtis KC, Fakoli L, Fischer K, Gankpala L, Lammie PJ, Majewski AC, Pelletreau S, Won KY, Bolay FK, Fischer PU.** 2013. Laboratory and field evaluation of a new rapid test for detecting Wuchereria bancrofti antigen in human blood. *Am J Trop Med Hyg* **89:**11–15.
32. **Chesnais CB, Awaca-Uvon NP, Bolay FK, Boussinesq M, Fischer PU, Gankpala L, Meite A, Missamou F, Pion SD, Weil GJ.** 2017. A multi-center field study of two point-of-care tests for circulating *Wuchereria bancrofti* antigenemia in Africa. *PLoS Negl Trop Dis* **11:**e0005703.
33. **Tisch DJ, Bockarie MJ, Dimber Z, Kiniboro B, Tarongka N, Hazlett FE, Kastens W, Alpers MP, Kazura JW.** 2008. Mass drug administration trial to eliminate lymphatic filariasis in Papua New Guinea: changes in microfilaremia, filarial antigen, and Bm14 antibody after cessation. *Am J Trop Med Hyg* **78:**289–293.
34. **Fink DL, Fahle GA, Fischer S, Fedorko DF, Nutman TB.** 2011. Toward molecular parasitologic diagnosis: enhanced diagnostic sensitivity for filarial infections in mobile populations. *J Clin Microbiol* **49:**42–47.
35. **McCarthy JS, Zhong M, Gopinath R, Ottesen EA, Williams SA, Nutman TB.** 1996. Evaluation of a polymerase chain reaction-based assay for diagnosis of *Wuchereria bancrofti* infection. *J Infect Dis* **173:**1510–1514.
36. **Zhong M, McCarthy J, Bierwert L, Lizotte-Waniewski M, Chanteau S, Nutman TB, Ottesen EA, Williams SA.** 1996. A polymerase chain reaction assay for detection of the parasite *Wuchereria bancrofti* in human blood samples. *Am J Trop Med Hyg* **54:**357–363.
37. **Rao RU, Huang Y, Bockarie MJ, Susapu M, Laney SJ, Weil GJ.** 2009. A qPCR-based multiplex assay for the detection of *Wuchereria bancrofti, Plasmodium falciparum* and *Plasmodium vivax* DNA. *Trans R Soc Trop Med Hyg* **103:**365–370.
38. **Rao RU, Weil GJ, Fischer K, Supali T, Fischer P.** 2006. Detection of *Brugia* parasite DNA in human blood by real-time PCR. *J Clin Microbiol* **44:**3887–3893.
39. **Pilotte N, Torres M, Tomaino FR, Laney SJ, Williams SA.** 2013. A TaqMan-based multiplex real-time PCR assay for the simultaneous detection of *Wuchereria bancrofti* and *Brugia malayi*. *Mol Biochem Parasitol* **189:**33–37.
40. **Poole CB, Tanner NA, Zhang Y, Evans TC Jr, Carlow CK.** 2012. Diagnosis of brugian filariasis by loop-mediated isothermal amplification. *PLoS Negl Trop Dis* **6:**e1948.
41. **Kubofcik J, Fink DL, Nutman TB.** 2012. Identification of Wb123 as an early and specific marker of *Wuchereria bancrofti* infection. *PLoS Negl Trop Dis* **6:**e1930.
42. **Steel C, Golden A, Kubofcik J, LaRue N, de Los Santos T, Domingo GJ, Nutman TB.** 2013. Rapid *Wuchereria bancrofti*-specific antigen Wb123-based IgG4 immunoassays as tools for surveillance following mass drug administration programs on lymphatic filariasis. *Clin Vaccine Immunol* **20:**1155–1161.
43. **Steel C, Golden A, Stevens E, Yokobe L, Domingo GJ, de los Santos T, Nutman TB.** 2015. Rapid point-of-contact tool for mapping and integrated surveillance of *Wuchereria bancrofti* and *Onchocerca volvulus* infection. *Clin Vaccine Immunol* **22:**896–901.
44. **Noordin R, Shenoy RK, Rahman RA.** 2003. Comparison of two IgG4 assay formats (ELISA and rapid dipstick test) for detection of brugian filariasis. *Southeast Asian J Trop Med Public Health* **34:**768–770.
45. **Rahmah N, Shenoy RK, Nutman TB, Weiss N, Gilmour K, Maizels RM, Yazdanbakhsh M, Sartono E.** 2003. Multicentre laboratory evaluation of Brugia Rapid dipstick test for detection of brugian filariasis. *Trop Med Int Health* **8:**895–900.
46. **Fox LM, Furness BW, Haser JK, Desire D, Brissau JM, Milord MD, Lafontant J, Lammie PJ, Beach MJ.** 2005. Tolerance and efficacy of combined diethylcarbamazine and albendazole for treatment of *Wuchereria bancrofti* and intestinal helminth infections in Haitian children. *Am J Trop Med Hyg* **73:**115–121.
47. **Tisch DJ, Michael E, Kazura JW.** 2005. Mass chemotherapy options to control lymphatic filariasis: a systematic review. *Lancet Infect Dis* **5:**514–523.
48. **Dreyer G, Addiss D, Williamson J, Norões J.** 2006. Efficacy of co-administered diethylcarbamazine and albendazole against adult *Wuchereria bancrofti*. *Trans R Soc Trop Med Hyg* **100:**1118–1125.
49. **Thomsen EK, Sanuku N, Baea M, Satofan S, Maki E, Lombore B, Schmidt MS, Siba PM, Weil GJ, Kazura JW, Fleckenstein LL, King CL.** 2016. Efficacy, safety, and pharmacokinetics of coadministered diethylcarbamazine, albendazole, and ivermectin for treatment of bancroftian filariasis. *Clin Infect Dis* **62:**334–341.
50. **Ichimori K, King JD, Engels D, Yajima A, Mikhailov A, Lammie P, Ottesen EA.** 2014. Global programme to eliminate lymphatic filariasis: the processes underlying programme success. *PLoS Negl Trop Dis* **8:**e3328.
51. **Taylor MJ, Makunde WH, McGarry HF, Turner JD, Mand S, Hoerauf A.** 2005. Macrofilaricidal activity after doxycycline treatment of *Wuchereria bancrofti*: a double-blind, randomised placebo-controlled trial. *Lancet* **365:**2116–2121.
52. **Walker M, Specht S, Churcher TS, Hoerauf A, Taylor MJ, Basáñez MG.** 2015. Therapeutic efficacy and macrofilaricidal activity of doxycycline for the treatment of river blindness. *Clin Infect Dis* **60:**1199–1207.
53. **Mand S, Debrah AY, Klarmann U, Batsa L, Marfo-Debrekyei Y, Kwarteng A, Specht S, Belda-Domene A, Fimmers R, Taylor M, Adjei O, Hoerauf A.** 2012. Doxycycline improves filarial lymphedema independent of active filarial infection: a randomized controlled trial. *Clin Infect Dis* **55:**621–630.
54. **World Health Organization.** 1992. Lymphatic filariasis: the disease and its control. Fifth Report of the WHO Expert Committee on Filariasis. *World Health Organ Tech Rep Ser* **821:**1–71.
55. **Capuano GP, Capuano C.** 2012. Surgical management of morbidity due to lymphatic filariasis: the usefulness of a standardized international clinical classification of hydroceles. *Trop Biomed* **29:**24–38.
56. **Lim KH, Speare R, Thomas G, Graves P.** 2015. Surgical treatment of genital manifestations of lymphatic filariasis: a systematic review. *World J Surg* **39:**2885–2899.
57. **Ramaiah KD, Ottesen EA.** 2014. Progress and impact of 13 years of the global programme to eliminate lymphatic filariasis on reducing the burden of filarial disease. *PLoS Negl Trop Dis* **8:**e3319.
58. **Ottesen EA, Hooper PJ, Bradley M, Biswas G.** 2008. The global programme to eliminate lymphatic filariasis: health impact after 8 years. *PLoS Negl Trop Dis* **2:**e317.
59. **Seim AR, Dreyer G, Addiss DG.** 1999. Controlling morbidity and interrupting transmission: twin pillars of lymphatic filariasis elimination. *Rev Soc Bras Med Trop* **32:**325–328.
60. **Murdoch ME, Murdoch IE, Evans J, Yahaya H, Njepuome N, Cousens S, Jones BR, Abiose A.** 2017. Pre-control relationship of onchocercal skin disease with onchocercal infection in Guinea Savanna, Northern Nigeria. *PLoS Negl Trop Dis* **11:**e0005489.
61. **Murdoch ME, Asuzu MC, Hagan M, Makunde WH, Ngoumou P, Ogbuagu KF, Okello D, Ozoh G, Remme J.** 2002. Onchocerciasis: the clinical and epidemiological burden of skin disease in Africa. *Ann Trop Med Parasitol* **96:**283–296.
62. **Murdoch ME, Hay RJ, Mackenzie CD, Williams JF, Ghalib HW, Cousens S, Abiose A, Jones BR.** 1993. A clinical classification and grading system of the cutaneous changes in onchocerciasis. *Br J Dermatol* **129:**260–269.
63. **Abdul-Ghani R, Mahdy MAK, Beier JC.** 2016. Onchocerciasis in Yemen: time to take action against a neglected tropical parasitic disease. *Acta Trop* **162:**133–141.
64. **Baraka OZ, Mahmoud BM, Ali MM, Ali MH, el Sheikh EA, Homeida MM, Mackenzie CD, Williams JF.** 1995. Ivermectin treatment in severe asymmetric reactive onchodermatitis (sowda) in Sudan. *Trans R Soc Trop Med Hyg* **89:**312–315.

65. **Siddiqui MA, al-Khawajah MM.** 1991. The black disease of Arabia, Sowda-onchocerciasis. New findings. *Int J Dermatol* **30:**130–133.
66. **Connor DH, Gibson DW, Neafie RC, Merighi B, Buck AA.** 1983. Sowda—onchocerciasis in north Yemen: a clinicopathologic study of 18 patients. *Am J Trop Med Hyg* **32:**123–137.
67. **Anderson J, Fuglsang H, al-Zubaidy A.** 1973. Onchocerciasis in Yemen with special reference to sowda. *Trans R Soc Trop Med Hyg* **67:**30–31.
68. **Albiez EJ.** 1983. Studies on nodules and adult *Onchocerca volvulus* during a nodulectomy trial in hyperendemic villages in Liberia and Upper Volta. I. Palpable and impalpable onchocercomata. *Tropenmed Parasitol* **34:**54–60.
69. **Meyers WM, Neafie RC, Connor DH.** 1977. Onchocerciasis: invasion of deep organs by *Onchocerca volvulus*. *Am J Trop Med Hyg* **26:**650–657.
70. **Taylor HR.** 1985. Global priorities in the control of onchocerciasis. *Rev Infect Dis* **7:**844–846.
71. **Taylor HR.** 1990. Onchocerciasis. *Int Ophthalmol* **14:**189–194.
72. **Duke BO.** 1998. Onchocerciasis, epilepsy and hyposexual dwarfism. *Trans R Soc Trop Med Hyg* **92:**236.
73. **Föger K, Gora-Stahlberg G, Sejvar J, Ovuga E, Jilek-Aall L, Schmutzhard E, Kaiser C, Winkler AS.** 2017. Nakalanga syndrome: clinical characteristics, potential causes, and its relationship with recently described nodding syndrome. *PLoS Negl Trop Dis* **11:**e0005201.
74. **Pion SD, Boussinesq M.** 2012. Significant association between epilepsy and presence of onchocercal nodules: case-control study in Cameroon. *Am J Trop Med Hyg* **86:**557, author reply 558.
75. **Kaiser C, Pion SD, Boussinesq M.** 2013. Case-control studies on the relationship between onchocerciasis and epilepsy: systematic review and meta-analysis. *PLoS Negl Trop Dis* **7:**e2147.
76. **Zimmerman PA, Guderian RH, Aruajo E, Elson L, Phadke P, Kubofcik J, Nutman TB.** 1994. Polymerase chain reaction-based diagnosis of *Onchocerca volvulus* infection: improved detection of patients with onchocerciasis. *J Infect Dis* **169:**686–689.
77. **Ramachandran CP.** 1993. Improved immunodiagnostic tests to monitor onchocerciasis control programmes—a multicenter effort. *Parasitol Today* **9:**77–79.
78. **Burbelo PD, Leahy HP, Iadarola MJ, Nutman TB.** 2009. A four-antigen mixture for rapid assessment of *Onchocerca volvulus* infection. *PLoS Negl Trop Dis* **3:**e438.
79. **Weil GJ, Steel C, Liftis F, Li BW, Mearns G, Lobos E, Nutman TB.** 2000. A rapid-format antibody card test for diagnosis of onchocerciasis. *J Infect Dis* **182:**1796–1799.
80. **Lipner EM, Dembele N, Souleymane S, Alley WS, Prevots DR, Toe L, Boatin B, Weil GJ, Nutman TB.** 2006. Field applicability of a rapid-format anti-Ov-16 antibody test for the assessment of onchocerciasis control measures in regions of endemicity. *J Infect Dis* **194:**216–221.
81. **Golden A, Steel C, Yokobe L, Jackson E, Barney R, Kubofcik J, Peck R, Unnasch TR, Nutman TB, de los Santos T, Domingo GJ.** 2013. Extended result reading window in lateral flow tests detecting exposure to *Onchocerca volvulus*: a new technology to improve epidemiological surveillance tools. *PLoS One* **8:**e69231.
82. **Dieye Y, Storey HL, Barrett KL, Gerth-Guyette E, Di Giorgio L, Golden A, Faulx D, Kalnoky M, Ndiaye MKN, Sy N, Mané M, Faye B, Sarr M, Dioukhane EM, Peck RB, Guinot P, de Los Santos T.** 2017. Feasibility of utilizing the SD BIOLINE Onchocerciasis IgG4 rapid test in onchocerciasis surveillance in Senegal. *PLoS Negl Trop Dis* **11:**e0005884.
83. **Boatin BA, Richards FO Jr.** 2006. Control of onchocerciasis. *Adv Parasitol* **61:**349–394.
84. **Gardon J, Gardon-Wendel N, Demanga-Ngangue, Kamgno J, Chippaux JP, Boussinesq M.** 1997. Serious reactions after mass treatment of onchocerciasis with ivermectin in an area endemic for *Loa loa* infection. *Lancet* **350:**18–22.
85. **D'Ambrosio MV, Bakalar M, Bennuru S, Reber C, Skandarajah A, Nilsson L, Switz N, Kamgno J, Pion S, Boussinesq M, Nutman TB, Fletcher DA.** 2015. Point-of-care quantification of blood-borne filarial parasites with a mobile phone microscope. *Sci Transl Med* **7:**286re4.
86. **Kamgno J, Pion SD, Chesnais CB, Bakalar MH, D'Ambrosio MV, Mackenzie CD, Nana-Djeunga HC, Gounoue-Kamkumo R, Njitchouang GR, Nwane P, Tchatchueng-Mbouga JB, Wanji S, Stolk WA, Fletcher DA, Klion AD, Nutman TB, Boussinesq M.** 2017. A test-and-not-treat strategy for onchocerciasis in *Loa loa*-endemic areas. *N Engl J Med* **377:**2044–2052.
87. **Hoerauf A, Mand S, Adjei O, Fleischer B, Büttner DW.** 2001. Depletion of wolbachia endobacteria in *Onchocerca volvulus* by doxycycline and microfilaridermia after ivermectin treatment. *Lancet* **357:**1415–1416.
88. **Debrah AY, Specht S, Klarmann-Schulz U, Batsa L, Mand S, Marfo-Debrekyei Y, Fimmers R, Dubben B, Kwarteng A, Osei-Atweneboana M, Boakye D, Ricchiuto A, Büttner M, Adjei O, Mackenzie CD, Hoerauf A.** 2015. Doxycycline leads to sterility and enhanced killing of female *Onchocerca volvulus* worms in an area with persistent microfilaridermia after repeated ivermectin treatment: a randomized, placebo-controlled, double-blind trial. *Clin Infect Dis* **61:**517–526.
89. **Evans DS, Unnasch TR, Richards FO.** 2015. Onchocerciasis and lymphatic filariasis elimination in Africa: it's about time. *Lancet* **385:**2151–2152.
90. **Molyneux DH.** 2009. Filaria control and elimination: diagnostic, monitoring and surveillance needs. *Trans R Soc Trop Med Hyg* **103:**338–341.
91. **Zouré HG, Wanji S, Noma M, Amazigo UV, Diggle PJ, Tekle AH, Remme JH.** 2011. The geographic distribution of *Loa loa* in Africa: results of large-scale implementation of the Rapid Assessment Procedure for Loiasis (RAPLOA). *PLoS Negl Trop Dis* **5:**e1210.
92. **Nutman TB, Miller KD, Mulligan M, Ottesen EA.** 1986. *Loa loa* infection in temporary residents of endemic regions: recognition of a hyperresponsive syndrome with characteristic clinical manifestations. *J Infect Dis* **154:**10–18.
93. **Klion AD, Massougbodji A, Sadeler BC, Ottesen EA, Nutman TB.** 1991. Loiasis in endemic and nonendemic populations: immunologically mediated differences in clinical presentation. *J Infect Dis* **163:**1318–1325.
94. **Herrick JA, Legrand F, Gounoue R, Nchinda G, Montavon C, Bopda J, Tchana SM, Ondigui BE, Nguluwe K, Fay MP, Makiya M, Metenou S, Nutman TB, Kamgno J, Klion AD.** 2017. Posttreatment reactions after single-dose diethylcarbamazine or ivermectin in subjects with *Loa loa* infection. *Clin Infect Dis* **64:**1017–1025.
95. **Fink DL, Kamgno J, Nutman TB.** 2011. Rapid molecular assays for specific detection and quantitation of *Loa loa* microfilaremia. *PLoS Negl Trop Dis* **5:**e1299.
96. **Klion AD, Vijaykumar A, Oei T, Martin B, Nutman TB.** 2003. Serum immunoglobulin G4 antibodies to the recombinant antigen, Ll-SXP-1, are highly specific for *Loa loa* infection. *J Infect Dis* **187:**128–133.
97. **Burbelo PD, Ramanathan R, Klion AD, Iadarola MJ, Nutman TB.** 2008. Rapid, novel, specific, high-throughput assay for diagnosis of *Loa loa* infection. *J Clin Microbiol* **46:**2298–2304.
98. **Pedram B, Pasquetto V, Drame PM, Ji Y, Gonzalez-Moa MJ, Baldwin RK, Nutman TB, Biamonte MA.** 2017. A novel rapid test for detecting antibody responses to *Loa loa* infections. *PLoS Negl Trop Dis* **11:**e0005741.
99. **Klion AD, Ottesen EA, Nutman TB.** 1994. Effectiveness of diethylcarbamazine in treating loiasis acquired by expatriate visitors to endemic regions: long-term follow-up. *J Infect Dis* **169:**604–610.
100. **Boussinesq M, Gardon J, Gardon-Wendel N, Chippaux JP.** 2003. Clinical picture, epidemiology and outcome of *Loa*-associated serious adverse events related to mass ivermectin treatment of onchocerciasis in Cameroon. *Filaria J* **2**(Suppl 1)**:**S4.
101. **Duke BO.** 2003. Overview: report of a scientific working group on serious adverse events following Mectizan(R) treatment of onchocerciasis in *Loa loa* endemic areas. *Filaria J* **2**(Suppl 1)**:**S1.

102. **Klion AD, Massougbodji A, Horton J, Ekoué S, Lanmasso T, Ahouissou NL, Nutman TB.** 1993. Albendazole in human loiasis: results of a double-blind, placebo-controlled trial. *J Infect Dis* **168:**202–206.
103. **Nutman TB, Miller KD, Mulligan M, Reinhardt GN, Currie BJ, Steel C, Ottesen EA.** 1988. Diethylcarbamazine prophylaxis for human loiasis. Results of a double-blind study. *N Engl J Med* **319:**752–756.
104. **Adolph PE, Kagan IG, McQUAY RM.** 1962. Diagnosis and treatment of *Acanthocheilonema perstans* filariasis. *Am J Trop Med Hyg* **11:**76–88.
105. **Meyers WM, Connor DH, Harman LE, Fleshman K, Moris R, Neafie RC.** 1972. Human streptocerciasis. A clinico-pathologic study of 40 Africans (Zairians) including identification of the adult filaria. *Am J Trop Med Hyg* **21:**528–545.
106. **McNeeley DF, Raccurt CP, Boncy J, Lowrie RC Jr.** 1989. Clinical evaluation of *Mansonella ozzardi* in Haiti. *Trop Med Parasitol* **40:**107–110.
107. **Lima NF, Veggiani Aybar CA, Dantur Juri MJ, Ferreira MU.** 2016. *Mansonella ozzardi*: a neglected New World filarial nematode. *Pathog Glob Health* **110:**97–107.
108. **Vianna LM, Martins M, Cohen MJ, Cohen JM, Belfort R Jr.** 2012. Mansonella ozzardi corneal lesions in the Amazon: a cross-sectional study. *BMJ Open* **2:**e001266.
109. **Tang TH, López-Vélez R, Lanza M, Shelley AJ, Rubio JM, Luz SL.** 2010. Nested PCR to detect and distinguish the sympatric filarial species *Onchocerca volvulus*, *Mansonella ozzardi* and *Mansonella perstans* in the Amazon Region. *Mem Inst Oswaldo Cruz* **105:**823–828.
110. **Keiser PB, Coulibaly Y, Kubofcik J, Diallo AA, Klion AD, Traoré SF, Nutman TB.** 2008. Molecular identification of Wolbachia from the filarial nematode *Mansonella perstans*. *Mol Biochem Parasitol* **160:**123–128.
111. **Coulibaly YI, Dembele B, Diallo AA, Lipner EM, Doumbia SS, Coulibaly SY, Konate S, Diallo DA, Yalcouye D, Kubofcik J, Doumbo OK, Traore AK, Keita AD, Fay MP, Traore SF, Nutman TB, Klion AD.** 2009. A randomized trial of doxycycline for *Mansonella perstans* infection. *N Engl J Med* **361:**1448–1458.
112. **Fischer P, Tukesiga E, Büttner DW.** 1999. Long-term suppression of *Mansonella streptocerca* microfilariae after treatment with ivermectin. *J Infect Dis* **180:**1403–1405.
113. **Gonzalez AA, Chadee DD, Rawlins SC.** 1999. Ivermectin treatment of mansonellosis in Trinidad. *West Indian Med J* **48:**231–234.
114. **Nutman TB, Nash TE, Ottesen EA.** 1987. Ivermectin in the successful treatment of a patient with *Mansonella ozzardi* infection. *J Infect Dis* **156:**662–665.
115. **Gil-Setas A, Pérez Salazar M, Navascués A, Rodríguez Eleta F, Cebamanos JA, Rubio MT.** 2010. [*Loa loa* and *Mansonella perstans* coinfection in a patient from Guinea]. *An Sist Sanit Navar* **33:**227–231.
116. **Krolewiecki AJ, Cajal SP, Villalpando C, Gil JF.** 2011. Ivermectin-related adverse clinical events in patients treated for *Mansonella ozzardi* infections. *Rev Argent Microbiol* **43:**48–50.

Cestodes

HECTOR H. GARCIA, JUAN A. JIMENEZ, AND HERMES ESCALANTE

148

Cestodes have as their key characteristic a flattened body composed of the head, or scolex (bearing the fixation organs—suckers, hooks, and bothria), the neck (where the cellular reproduction occurs, to form the strobila), and the strobila, formed by numerous segments or proglottids. As new proglottids develop in the neck region, existing ones mature as they become more distal. The more distal proglottids are gravid, almost completely occupied by a uterus full of eggs, which are passed with the stools of the carrier, either inside complete proglottids or free after proglottid breakage. In some species, proglottids can actively migrate out of the anus.

Tapeworms live in the lumen of the small intestine with the head or scolex as the only fixation organ, attached to the mucosa. They absorb nutrients from the host's intestine both at the head and through their tegument. Accordingly, they have developed cephalic fixation organs such as hooks, suckers, or shallow grooves as longitudinal suction sulci (bothria) (Fig. 1), and a specialized tegument.

Four species of cestode tapeworms inhabit the human intestine with frequency: *Diphyllobothrium latum*, *Taenia saginata*, *Taenia solium*, and *Hymenolepis nana*. They differ widely in size, intermediate host, and other characteristics, from the 12-m *D. latum* to the 3-cm *H. nana* (Table 1). More rarely, *Dipylidium caninum* and *Hymenolepis diminuta* can also inhabit the human gut; these parasites are reviewed in chapter 150 of this *Manual*. In addition, a number of cestode larvae can produce human disease if infective tapeworm eggs are ingested, mainly cysticercosis (*T. solium*), cystic hydatid disease (*Echinococcus granulosus*), and alveolar hydatid disease (*Echinococcus multilocularis*). Rarer larval cestode infections affecting humans include coenurosis (*Taenia multiceps*), sparganosis (*Spirometra mansonoides*), and cysticercosis (*Taenia crassiceps*). Tapeworms, and especially tapeworm larval infections, still represent an important cause of morbidity and mortality, not only in most underdeveloped countries but also in industrialized countries, particularly in rural areas or among immigrants from areas of endemicity.

DIPHYLLOBOTHRIUM LATUM

Known as the fish tapeworm, *D. latum* is the longest intestinal parasite of humans. Also common in fish-eating mammals such as canids and felids (reservoir hosts), it differs from other adult tapeworms infecting humans in its morphology, biology, and epidemiology.

Taxonomy

D. latum is included in the phylum Platyhelminthes, subphylum Neodermata, class Cestoidea, subclass Eucestoda, order Pseudophyllidea, family Diphyllobothriidae, and genus *Diphyllobothrium*.

Description of the Agent

Adult Tapeworm

The adult parasite can grow to 15 m in length and can live for 20 years or longer in the small intestine. It is ivory in color and has a scolex which is provided with bothria on its dorsal and ventral aspects (1, 2). *Diphyllobothrium* proglottids are much wider than they are long (~8 by 4 mm) and are easy to recognize because their genital pore is located in the center of the proglottid rather than in the lateral edges as in all other tapeworms of humans. The coiled uterus in the center of the gravid proglottids looks yellow-brown in freshly passed specimens. The uterine pore is located in the center of the proglottid near the genital pore.

Eggs

Unembryonated, operculate eggs are passed in the feces. *D. latum* eggs are oval and resemble those of trematodes but are smaller (58 to 75 μm long by 44 to 50 μm wide) and have a better-defined wall. The abopercular end usually has a small knoblike protrusion. Eggs are usually numerous, and expulsion of proglottid chains is usual.

Larvae

After the eggs embryonate in a water environment for several weeks, ciliated six-hooked embryos (coracidia) hatch. Coracidia must be ingested by appropriate species of freshwater copepods (genus, *Cyclops*) for further development. In the copepod a solid-bodied larva, the procercoid, develops as a second larval stage and becomes infective for the second intermediate host (fish). In fish, the procercoid migrates to the flesh and develops in the third larval stage, the plerocercoid, or sparganum, which is the infective stage for human and animal (canids or felids) hosts.

Epidemiology, Transmission, and Prevention

The geographic distribution of *D. latum* includes lake areas in Scandinavia, other areas of northern Europe, the former Soviet Union, Finland, northern Japan, and North America,

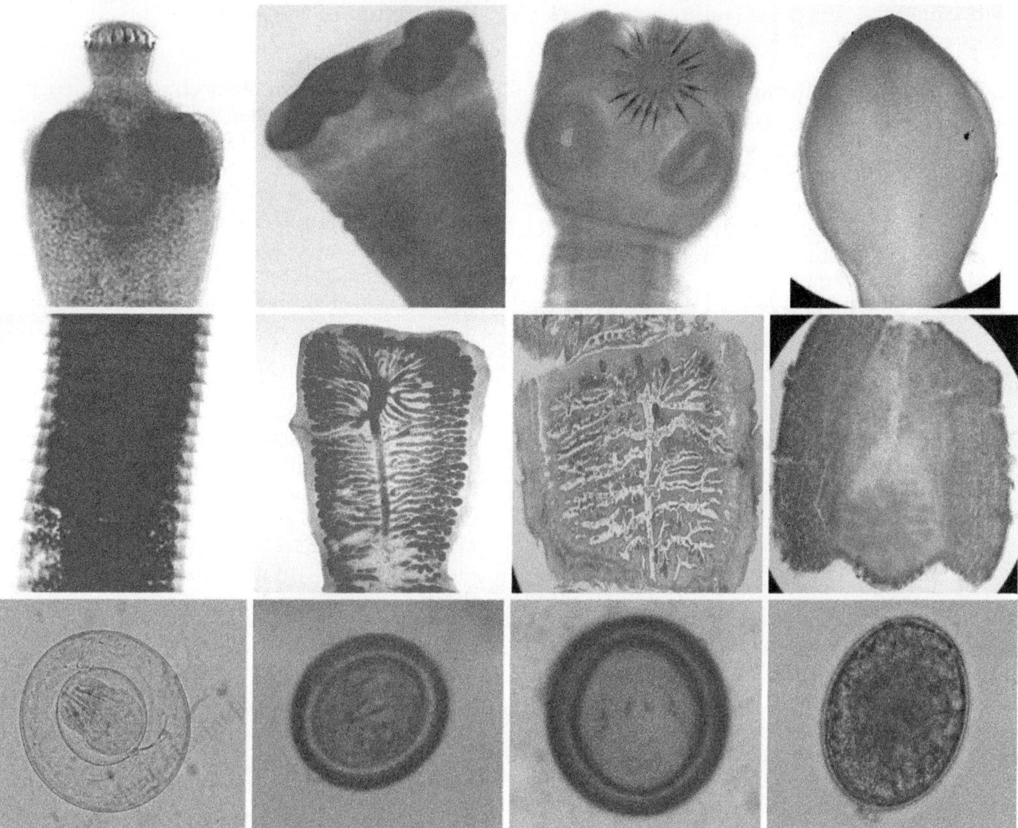

FIGURE 1 Scoleces (top panels), gravid proglottids (middle panels), and eggs (lower panels) of, from left to right, *H. nana*, *T. saginata*, *T. solium*, and *D. pacificum*. Note the coiled, central uterus in *D. pacificum*, the absence of hooks in the scolex of *T. saginata*, and the similar appearances of the eggs of *T. saginata* and *T. solium*. The morphological characteristics shown for *D. pacificum* are similar to those of *D. latum*.

principally the upper Midwest, Alaska, and Canada, and the southwestern coast of South America. Several other *Diphyllobothrium* species (*D. pacificum*, *D. cordatum*, *D. ursi*, *D. dendriticum*, *D. lanceolatum*, *D. dalliae*, and *D. yonagoensis*) have also been reported to infect humans but less frequently (2, 3). *D. pacificum*, identified by Nybellin in 1931, is a parasite of seawater found along the western coast of South America, specifically in Peru and Chile. *D. pacificum* is much smaller than *D. latum* and usually measures 50 to 200 cm long, although it can occasionally reach 3 to 4 m.

The most common sources of human *Diphyllobothrium* infection are the pike, burbot, perch, ruff, and turbot (2). Infected fish (undercooked, raw, or insufficiently treated flesh) transmit plerocercoids to humans or other fish-eating mammals. Infection with *Diphyllobothrium* is preventable by eating well-cooked fish or fish that has been deep-frozen (at least −10°C for 24 h).

Clinical Significance (Description of Clinical Presentation)

Infected individuals notice passing segment chains with their stools. The parasite may produce no clinical symptoms in some people, but when it reaches a large size it may cause mechanical bowel obstruction, diarrhea, abdominal pain, and particularly in northern European countries, pernicious anemia resulting from vitamin B_{12} deficiency because the tapeworm competes with the intestinal epithelium for the uptake of the vitamin. This condition is rare outside

TABLE 1 Some characteristics of main cestodes infecting humans

Organism	Length (cm)	Scolex	Gravid proglottids	Intermediate host(s)
D. latum	1,200	Spatulate, two bothria	Rosette-shaped central uterus	Copepods, fish
T. saginata	600	Squared, four suckers, no hooks	>15 main lateral uterine branches	Cattle
T. solium	300	Squared, four suckers, hooks (double crown)	<12 main lateral uterine branches	Pigs, humans
H. nana	3	Knoblike, four suckers, hooks (single crown)	Bag-shaped uterus	Insects, rodents, humans

Scandinavian countries, and some authors postulate a genetic predisposition.

Collection, Transport, and Storage of Specimens

For identification purposes, eggs are well preserved in 5 to 10% formalin solutions. For DNA recovery, 95% ethanol is a better option. Electron microscopy may require cacodylate buffer or other glutaraldehyde media. Adult tapeworm material is better defined if it is washed in saline, relaxed for better visualization of its internal structures by warming the saline at 55°C for a short period (5 min), and then placed between two glass slides and stored in a fixative solution. Fixatives could be 10% formalin, acetic acid-formaldehyde-alcohol, or sodium acetate-acetic acid-formaldehyde. Fixed pieces can be stained by injecting Semichon's carmine or India ink. The proglottids can also be sectioned and stained using hematoxylin and eosin; however, morphological characteristics can be more easily seen in whole mounts.

Direct Examination

Microscopy

Eggs can be easily seen by microscopical examination of stools. Either flotation or sedimentation techniques may be used. However, since the eggs are operculated, they generally do not float using the flotation concentration method; both the surface film and sediment need to be examined if this concentration method is used. For that reason, most laboratories routinely use the sedimentation concentration method. Low-magnification microscopy should easily permit identification of the characteristic scolex or proglottids when available (Fig. 1). Neither culture nor antigen detection is relevant for the detection and identification of *D. latum*.

Nucleic Acid Detection Techniques

Although several groups have described genus variation in *Diphyllobothrium* by using nucleic acid detection methods, the information has no clinical relevance in terms of routine tapeworm recovery and identification (4).

Serologic Tests

Serologic tests are not available.

Treatment

Both praziquantel and niclosamide are effective drugs. At recommended doses both are associated with only mild side effects, mostly gastrointestinal.

Evaluation, Interpretation, and Reporting of Results

Both stool microscopy and parasite identification are unambiguous. Eggs or tapeworm pieces should be reported as *D. latum* eggs (except in South America, where *D. pacificum* is more frequently found). Other human-infecting species are rarely found.

TAENIA SAGINATA

Known as the beef tapeworm, *T. saginata* is still endemic to most of the world. Humans are its only definitive host. While *T. saginata* infections do not carry major risks for the host, differential diagnosis with *T. solium* is important because the latter can cause neurocysticercosis.

Taxonomy

T. saginata is included in the phylum Platyhelminthes, subphylum Neodermata, class Cestoidea, subclass Eucestoda, order Cyclophyllidea, family Taeniidae, and genus *Taenia*.

Description of the Agent

Adult Tapeworm

The adult *T. saginata* tapeworm attains lengths of 4 to 8 m and has a scolex provided with four suckers and an unarmed (no hooks) rostellum. Gravid proglottids are longer than they are wide (18 to 20 mm by 5 to 7 mm). Each proglottid has a genital pore at the midlateral margin. In mature proglottids, the ovary has only two lobes and presents a vaginal sphincter. Gravid proglottids, which are highly muscular and active, break off from the strobila and actively migrate out of the anus (a pathognomic characteristic of this species).

Eggs

Eggs from *T. saginata* and *T. solium* are indistinguishable by morphological characteristics. They are spherical, measure 30 to 40 μm in diameter, and have a quite characteristic thick, yellow-brown, radiate shell (embryophore) composed of collagen subunits, which gets thicker as the eggs mature. Eggs are frequently surrounded by a thin layer of vitellum (Fig. 1). Within the egg is a six-hooked embryo, the oncosphere.

Larvae

The unarmed scolex is invaginated into a fluid-filled bladder, the cysticercus. Larval cysts are 4 to 6 mm long by 7 to 10 mm wide and have a pearl-like appearance in tissues.

Epidemiology, Transmission, and Prevention

T. saginata is distributed worldwide, although it is especially prevalent in some parts of Africa, Central and South America, eastern and western Asia, and some countries in Europe. Cattle serve as the intermediate host, and ingestion of eggs from contaminated pasturelands by grazing cattle results in development in cattle tissues of the infective cysticercus stage. After ingestion of the cysticercus in raw or inadequately cooked beef, it takes approximately 2 to 3 months for the infection to become patent in the human host.

In Southeast Asia there is a human tapeworm that is morphologically very similar to *T. saginata* (*T. saginata asiatica*, *Taenia asiatica*, or Taiwan taenia). In this tapeworm, the cysticercus stage occurs in the livers of pigs and, less frequently, in cattle. The adult tapeworm infects the human host, and its appearance is very similar to that of *T. saginata* (5, 6).

Clinical Significance (Description of Clinical Presentation)

Although patients may exhibit no symptoms with this infection, they usually notice passing proglottids or find them in their underwear. The mature worm can also cause abdominal discomfort, diarrhea, and occasionally intestinal obstruction as a result of its large size.

Collection, Transport, and Storage of Specimens

See instructions in "Collection, Transport, and Storage of Specimens" for *Diphyllobothrium*.

Direct Examination

Microscopy

Typical *Taenia* eggs can be found in feces. Sedimentation or the less frequently used Kato-Katz method is more sensitive for the detection of *Taenia* eggs in stools than other concentration techniques. Finding *Taenia* eggs does not allow a species-specific diagnosis of infection; it is usually made by identification of gravid proglottids that have been passed in feces or have actively migrated out of the anus. Identification of the proglottids is based on shape and size and mainly on the morphology of the uterus, which can be demonstrated after injection with India ink or staining with carmine or hematoxylin stains. In *T. saginata* there are 15 to 20 primary lateral branches on each side of the central uterine stem (Fig. 1).

Antigens in stools (coproantigen) have been detected by enzyme-linked immunosorbent assay (ELISA) since 1990, but this assay is used mainly in research settings because of scarce availability.

Nucleic Acid Detection Techniques

Species-specific PCR techniques have been described to detect parasite DNA and differentiate *T. saginata* from *T. solium*. Most of these assays require actual parasite material, although some are able to establish the difference with DNA from eggs in feces (7–10).

Serologic Tests

Serum antigen detection ELISAs for *T. saginata* cysticercosis in cattle have been developed using monoclonal antibodies to *T. saginata*. Although these assays can detect parasite burdens of <50 cysts per animal, they have not yet been routinely applied except in research settings (11–13).

Treatment

Both praziquantel and niclosamide are effective drugs. At recommended doses both are associated with only mild side effects, mostly gastrointestinal. In regions where *T. solium* is endemic, there is a possibility that latent neurocysticercosis may respond to praziquantel and cause severe headaches or seizures. Niclosamide is not absorbed from the gastrointestinal tract and thus does not carry this risk (14).

Evaluation, Interpretation, and Reporting of Results

Eggs should be reported as "*Taenia* sp." because direct observation does not confirm the species. The finding of *Taenia* sp. eggs should be communicated to the attending physician to ensure prompt treatment. The presence of the scolex in the expelled parasite material (spontaneously or posttreatment) should be reported both because it allows species diagnosis and because if it is not found, the chances of treatment failure increase.

TAENIA SOLIUM

Known as the pork tapeworm, *T. solium* has an extensive geographic distribution. This infection has a huge impact on human health because of its association with seizure disorders caused by infection of the human brain with its larval stage (neurocysticercosis) (15).

Taxonomy

T. solium is included in the phylum Platyhelminthes, subphylum Neodermata, class Cestoidea, subclass Eucestoda, order Cyclophyllidea, family Taeniidae, and genus *Taenia*.

Description of the Agent

Adult Tapeworm

The adult *T. solium* tapeworm measures 2 to 4 m and has a scolex provided with four suckers and a rostellum armed with two crowns of hooks. Gravid proglottids have similar length and width (approximately 1 cm). Each proglottid has a genital pore at the midlateral margin. In mature proglottids, the ovary has two main lobes and one accessory lobe (lacking in *T. saginata*), and a vaginal sphincter muscle is lacking (present in *T. saginata*). Gravid proglottids have few (<12) lateral branches on the central uterine stem (Fig. 1). Since the eggs of *T. solium* are infective to humans and can cause cysticercosis, extreme caution in the handling of these proglottids or infective stools is recommended.

Eggs

Eggs from *T. saginata* and *T. solium* are indistinguishable by morphological characteristics. They are spherical, measure 30 to 40 μm in diameter, and have a characteristic thick, yellow-brown, radiate shell (embryophore) composed of collagen subunits, which gets thicker as the eggs mature. Eggs are frequently surrounded by a thin layer of vitellum (Fig. 1). Within the egg is a six-hooked embryo, the oncosphere.

Larvae

The fluid-filled bladder (cysticercus) larvae are bigger than those of *T. saginata*, measuring approximately 8 to 10 mm in diameter. They lodge in the pig's tissues, mostly in muscle and brain.

Epidemiology, Transmission, and Prevention

T. solium taeniasis and cysticercosis are highly endemic to all parts of the developing world where pigs are raised as a food source, including Latin America, most of Asia, sub-Saharan Africa, and parts of Oceania. The infection is now also increasingly diagnosed in industrialized countries due to immigration of tapeworm carriers from zones of endemicity (6, 15).

As for *T. saginata*, humans are the only definitive host. Ingestion of contaminated pork containing *T. solium* cysticerci causes human taeniasis. Conversely, *T. solium* eggs cause cysticercosis in pigs (the usual intermediate host) and humans. Pigs acquire cysticercosis by eating stools contaminated with infective eggs in places where deficient sanitation exists. Humans are infected by fecal-oral contamination from a tapeworm carrier, commonly in the household or another close environment. A large field program in northern Peru demonstrated the feasibility of interrupting the transmission of *T. solium* using human deworming with niclosamide, pig treatment with oxfendazole, and pig vaccination (16), creating possibilities for its eventual elimination and eradication.

Clinical Significance (Description of Clinical Presentation)

Human *T. solium* taeniasis is acquired by ingestion of infective cysticerci in inadequately cooked pork or pork products. Taeniasis is mostly asymptomatic, and most patients do not even notice passing proglottids in stools. The clinical significance of *T. solium* infections relates to the risk of neurocysticercosis (see below), which is high for tapeworm carriers and their close contacts (15).

Collection, Transport, and Storage of Specimens

See instructions in "Collection, Transport, and Storage of Specimens" for *Diphyllobothrium*. Handling of *T. solium* proglottids or contaminated stools should be done with appropriate biosafety conditions (biosafety level 2 or higher) to avoid cysticercosis.

Direct Examination

Microscopy

Typical *Taenia* eggs can be found in feces. Sedimentation or the less frequently used Kato-Katz method is more sensitive for the detection of *Taenia* eggs in stools than other concentration techniques. Finding *Taenia* eggs does not allow a diagnosis of infection by the species, which is usually made by identification of gravid proglottids or, more rarely, the scolex passed in feces. Identification of the proglottids is based on shape and size and mainly on the morphology of the uterus, which can be demonstrated after injection with India ink or staining with carmine or hematoxylin stains. In *T. solium* there are few primary branches on each side of the central uterine stem (Fig. 1).

Antigens in stools (coproantigen) have been detected by ELISA since 1990. Coproantigen detection ELISA is much more sensitive than microscopy and thus is highly recommended for the diagnosis of human taeniasis (specifically in the case of *T. solium* because of the risks of cysticercosis transmission), as well as to monitor the effectiveness of treatment, but its availability is still limited (17).

Nucleic Acid Detection Techniques

Species-specific PCR techniques that differentiate *T. saginata* from *T. solium* have been described but are not yet commercially available. Most of these assays require actual parasite material, although some are able to establish the difference with DNA from eggs in feces (7–10).

Serologic Tests

Recently, stage-specific serologic assays directed to the adult tapeworm have been developed, with high sensitivity and specificity, although these are not yet commercially available. Mostly, serology is directed to the detection of *T. solium* antibodies in relation to the diagnosis of neurocysticercosis. Antibody detection by enzyme-linked immunoelectrotransfer blot assay is the method of choice, with a sensitivity of 98% in cases with more than one viable larval cyst and a specificity of 100% (18). *T. solium* antigen detection in serum or cerebrospinal fluid has been performed in cases of human cysticercosis, based on a known genus-specific cross-reaction in ELISAs for *T. saginata*. Although these assays can detect parasite burdens of <50 cysts in infected animals, they have not yet been routinely applied except in research settings. *T. solium* antigen detection is likely to be a helpful tool to monitor the evolution of patients with severe, subarachnoid neurocysticercosis, in which high antigen levels occur (19).

Treatment

Both praziquantel and niclosamide are effective drugs. At recommended doses both are associated with only mild side effects, mostly gastrointestinal. In regions where *T. solium* is endemic, there is a possibility that latent neurocysticercosis may respond to praziquantel and cause severe headaches or seizures. Niclosamide is not absorbed from the gastrointestinal tract and thus does not carry this risk (14).

Evaluation, Interpretation, and Reporting of Results

Eggs should be reported as "*Taenia* sp." because direct observation does not confirm the species. The finding of *Taenia* sp. eggs should be communicated to the attending physician to ensure prompt treatment and minimize the chances of cysticercosis in the patient or the patient's contacts. The presence of the scolex in the expelled parasite material (spontaneously or posttreatment) should be reported both because it allows species diagnosis and because if it is not found, the chances of treatment failure increase.

HYMENOLEPIS NANA

H. nana is the smallest of the intestinal tapeworms of humans and also the most common tapeworm infection throughout the world. It can be transmitted from person to person (an intermediate host is not necessarily required) (3).

Taxonomy

H. nana is included in the phylum Platyhelminthes, subphylum Neodermata, class Cestoidea, subclass Eucestoda, order Cyclophyllidea, family Hymenolepididae, and genus *Hymenolepis*.

Description of the Agent

Adult Tapeworm

The adult parasite measures 2 to 4 cm and lives for approximately 1 year. The scolex has four suckers and one crown of hooks.

Eggs

The eggs are 30 to 50 μm in diameter and thin shelled, and they contain a six-hooked oncosphere that lies in the center of the egg and is separated from the outer shell by considerable space. The oncosphere is surrounded by a membrane that has two polar thickenings from which arise four to eight filaments extending into the space between it and the outer shell (Fig. 1). These filaments are not seen in *H. diminuta*. Eggs may hatch inside the host's intestine, and the embryos (oncospheres) invade the mucosa to develop into larval stages.

Larvae

The cysticercoid larvae have an invaginated scolex but no fluid-filled bladder. They lodge in the intestinal mucosa and emerge in the intestinal lumen as young tapeworms after a few days.

Epidemiology, Transmission, and Prevention

H. nana is normally a parasite of mice, and its life cycle characteristically involves a beetle as an intermediate host. In humans, transmission is usually accomplished by direct ingestion of infective eggs containing oncospheres. When eggs are ingested, a solid-bodied larva, a cysticercoid, first develops in the wall of the small intestine. Subsequently, the larva migrates back into the intestinal lumen, where it reaches maturity as an adult tapeworm in 2 to 3 weeks. In beetles that ingest eggs of *H. nana*, the cysticercoids develop in the body cavity and have thick protective walls around them. Although humans may acquire the infection by accidental ingestion of infected beetles (often occurring in dry cereals), direct infection is far more common and is the primary reason why *H. nana* usually occurs in institutional and familial settings in which hygiene is substandard. A feature of human *H. nana* infection is the opportunity for internal autoinfection with the parasite, which may result in large worm burdens. Autoinfection occurs when eggs discharged by adult tapeworms in the lumen of the small intestine hatch rapidly and invade the wall of the intestine; here, cysticercoids are formed, and they subsequently reenter the intestine to mature as adult worms.

Clinical Significance (Description of Clinical Presentation)

Most infections cause no symptoms. However, hymenolepiasis can be associated with abdominal pain, diarrhea, headaches, or irritability, probably in infections with heavier worm burdens (20, 21). Invasion of lymph nodes and lungs by abnormal, proliferating, genetically altered tapeworm cells as in cancer metastasis has been demonstrated in an HIV-infected individual (22).

Collection, Transport, and Storage of Specimens

See instructions in "Collection, Transport, and Storage of Specimens" for *Diphyllobothrium*.

Direct Examination

Microscopy

Diagnosis of the infection rests on finding the spherical eggs in feces by microscopy. Either flotation or sedimentation techniques are helpful. Proglottids (Fig. 1) are rarely seen, since they disintegrate after breaking off from the main strobila. Neither culture, antigen detection, nor nucleic acid detection techniques are relevant for the detection and identification of *H. nana*.

Serologic Tests

Antibody detection ELISAs have been used in research settings but are of no clinical use (23).

Treatment

Both praziquantel and niclosamide are effective drugs. At recommended doses both are associated with only mild side effects, mostly gastrointestinal. A second dose of praziquantel after 10 to 15 days may decrease the likelihood of relapses. Niclosamide needs to be administered for 7 days because it is not absorbed and thus does not affect the cysticercoid larvae in the intestinal mucosa. Nitazoxanide has been reported to be useful as a therapeutic alternative (24).

Evaluation, Interpretation, and Reporting of Results

Eggs are characteristic and should be reported as *H. nana* eggs. The closest differential diagnosis is with *H. diminuta*, which rarely infects humans. The eggs of *H. diminuta* are bigger, lack polar filaments, and have a wider interior space and thus can be differentiated by microscopy.

LARVAL CESTODES INFECTING THE HUMAN HOST

The larval stages of *T. solium*, *E. granulosus*, *E. multilocularis*, and less frequently, *S. mansonoides*, *T. multiceps*, and *T. crassiceps* can invade the human tissues. These are briefly described below.

Cysticercosis (*T. solium*)

In the normal life cycle of *T. solium*, humans are the definitive host and pigs act as the intermediate host, hosting the larval stage, or cysticercus. Porcine cysticercosis is a serious economic problem for pig farmers. However, the most serious consequences are associated with human cysticercosis (15). Larval vesicles located in the human central nervous system (Fig. 2) cause seizures or other neurological

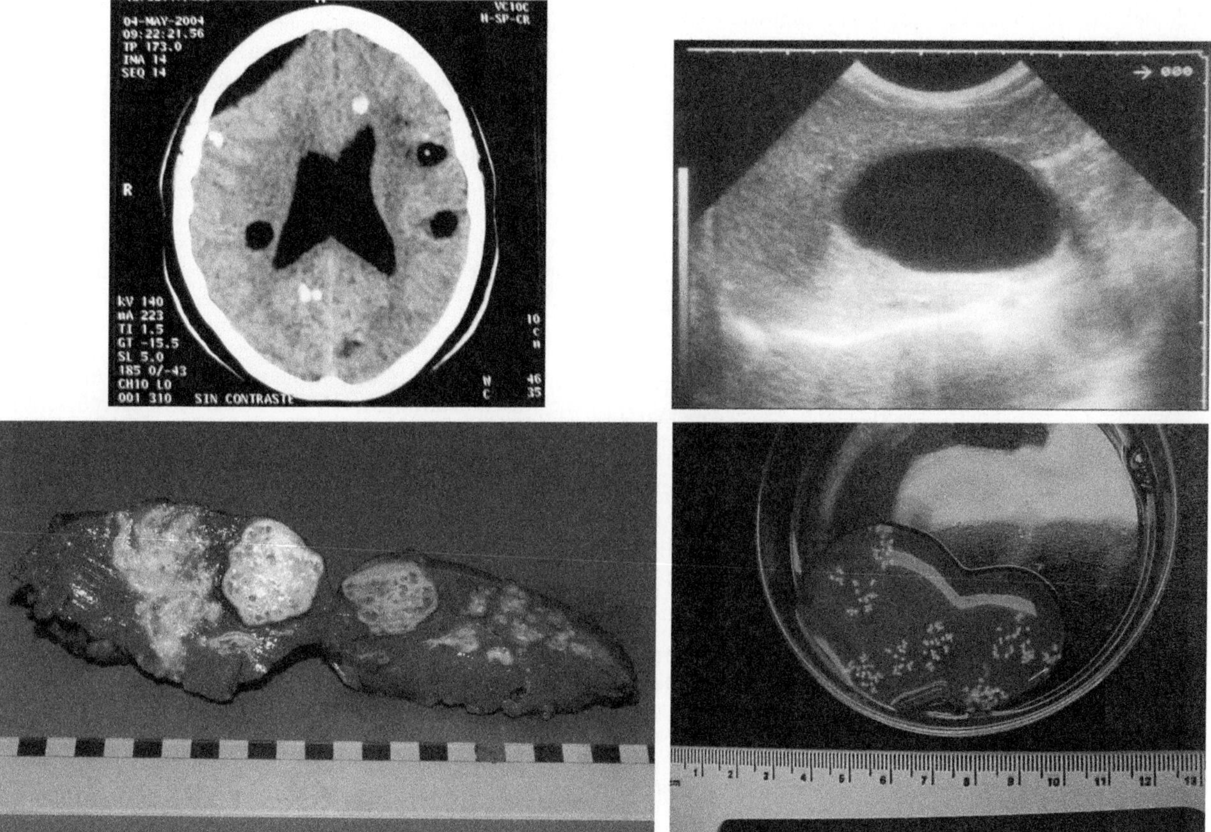

FIGURE 2 Larval cestodes infecting the human host. (Top left) *T. solium* cysticerci in the human brain (neurocysticercosis), shown in a noncontrasted CT scan of the brain; (top right) *E. granulosus* hydatid in the human liver (hydatid disease) as seen on liver ultrasound (kind contribution of Enrico Brunetti, Università di Pavia, Pavia, Italy); (bottom left) *Echinococcus multilocularis* alveolar hydatid disease in human liver (courtesy of K. Buttenschoen and P. Kern, University Hospital Ulm, Ulm, Germany); (bottom right) *T. multiceps* coenurus showing multiple scolices in the cystic wall.

symptoms. Indeed, neurocysticercosis is associated with a significant proportion of seizure cases in areas of endemicity (25, 26). Clinical manifestations of neurocysticercosis are related to individual differences in the number, size, and topography of lesions and in the severity of the host's immune response to the parasites. Symptoms and signs are varied and nonspecific. Parasites in the brain parenchyma usually cause seizures and headache, whereas those located in the cerebral ventricles or in the subarachnoid space ("racemose" cysticercosis) cause intracranial hypertension and hydrocephalus. Diagnosis is made using brain imaging, either computed tomography (CT) scan or magnetic resonance imaging (MRI), and confirmed by serology. CT has a lower cost (quite important for poor areas where the disease is endemic), is more widely available, and has better sensitivity for the detection of calcified parasites. Conversely, MRI has better sensitivity for small lesions, those located close to the skull, and intraventricular parasites. The serologic assay of choice is an immunoblot using seven purified glycoprotein larval antigens, which has 98% sensitivity and 100% specificity except in cases with a single lesion, for which sensitivity drops to approximately 70% (18, 19). Antigen detection assays have been described, but no controlled data on sensitivity and specificity are yet available. Treatment of neurocysticercosis uses antiparasitic agents (albendazole or praziquantel) for viable parasites, usually given with steroids to ameliorate the inflammation produced by the death of the cyst. Combined use of both agents increases their efficacy in individuals with multiple brain cysts (27). Surgery is limited to excision of single, big lesions or implantation of ventricle-peritoneal shunts. Antigen detection assays permit patient monitoring and follow-up of antiparasitic treatment (19, 28).

Cystic Hydatid Disease (*E. granulosus*)

In the normal life cycle of *E. granulosus*, the dog is the definitive host and herbivores (mainly sheep) act as the intermediate host. These become infected with the larval stage (cystic hydatid) by ingesting infective eggs dispersed from the feces of a tapeworm-infected dog. Human cystic hydatid disease is an important cause of human morbidity, requiring costly surgical and medical treatment. This cestodiasis is still endemic to most of the Old World, particularly Greece, Cyprus, Bulgaria, Lebanon, Turkey, some other European countries, South America, and Africa. Sporadic autochthonous transmission is currently recognized in Alaska and other states in the United States (29). The affected organs are most commonly the liver and lungs and, more rarely, the heart, brain, bones, and other locations. Diagnosis is made using ultrasound or CT scan for liver infection or chest X rays or CT for lung infections (Fig. 2). Antibody detection by serology is helpful, although sensitivity is lower than for other infections, reaching 80 to 85%. It is more sensitive for hepatic than for pulmonary cases. Treatment uses antiparasitic agents (albendazole or albendazole plus praziquantel) for small cysts or presurgery; PAIR (puncture, injection, aspiration, and reinjection), which is a technique of ultrasound- or CT-guided aspiration and sterilization of the cyst's contents; or either laparoscopic or open surgery (30, 31). Spillage of cyst contents could lead to acute anaphylactic reactions or dissemination of infection in the surrounding tissues. Cystic lesions may resolve without therapy in some patients (32).

Alveolar Hydatid Disease (*E. multilocularis*)

The adult stage of *E. multilocularis* lives in the small intestine of the definitive host, commonly wild predators in the Northern Hemisphere, occurring in parts of Europe, Asia, Japan, and North America, including Alaska (33, 34). The larval stages infect microtine rodents that usually serve as the common intermediate host. Human infections (causing alveolar hydatid disease) occur by accidental ingestion of the oncosphere by contamination with the feces of the definitive host. The manifestation of alveolar hydatid disease resembles a slowly developing "malignant tumor" of the liver, with subsequent invasion of the blood vessels and bile ducts and metastatic dissemination. The lesions vary in size and can produce minor foci up to large infiltrating structures in the host's tissue. Thus, alveolar hydatid disease differs greatly in the pathology and clinical course from cystic hydatid disease. This disease often affects people aged over 50 years and is characterized by a chronic course lasting for months or years. Clinical manifestations relate to the extent of tumor-like lesions of the cyst. Besides physical examination, diagnosis usually is based on imaging techniques, including ultrasound, CT, and MRI, supported by serology. Treatment is mainly surgical. Chemotherapy with benzimidazole agents is restricted to residual, postsurgical, or inoperable lesions (35).

Sparganosis (*S. mansonoides*)

Mainly found in Southeast Asian countries, the metacestode larvae of *Spirometra* species can invade the human tissues either by ingestion of contaminated crustaceans in drinking water, by ingestion of infected meat (frog or snake), or by direct contact via a poultice. The most commonly affected sites are subcutaneous tissues and the eye. The diagnosis rests on the pathological demonstration of the larvae after excision by biopsy (36).

Coenurosis (*T. multiceps* or *Taenia serialis*)

T. multiceps and *T. serialis* have canids as definitive hosts and sheep as their normal intermediate host, harboring the larva, or coenurus. The coenurus is a vesicle containing a transparent fluid, with a fine membrane in which multiple (500 to 700) scolices can be seen. Infected sheep lose their balance and rotate in circles continuously, become dizzy, and fall (screw disease). It infrequently causes coenuriasis in humans. Human infections have largely been confined to the African continent, but a few cases have been described from France, England, and North and South America. The space-occupying coenurus usually invades the brain, producing lethal lesions. Diagnosis is based on pathological demonstration of the typical larval membrane and multiple scolices (37, 38).

Cysticercosis (*T. crassiceps*)

T. crassiceps is a common tapeworm of the red fox. Larval forms are generally found in subcutaneous tissues and body cavities of rodents. Human cases are quite rare, mostly in immunocompromised patients (subcutaneous, muscular, or ocular infections) (39, 40).

REFERENCES

1. **Fuchizaki U, Ohta H, Sugimoto T.** 2003. Diphyllobothriasis. *Lancet Infect Dis* **3:**32.
2. **Scholz T, Garcia HH, Kuchta R, Wicht B.** 2009. Human broad tapeworm (genus *Diphyllobothrium*), including clinical relevance. *Clin Microbiol Rev* **22:**146–160.
3. **Raether W, Hänel H.** 2003. Epidemiology, clinical manifestations and diagnosis of zoonotic cestode infections: an update. *Parasitol Res* **91:**412–438.

4. **Logan FJ, Horák A, Stefka J, Aydogdu A, Scholz T.** 2004. The phylogeny of diphyllobothriid tapeworms (Cestoda: Pseudophyllidea) based on ITS-2 rDNA sequences. *Parasitol Res* **94:**10–15.
5. **Eom KS, Jeon HK, Kong Y, Hwang UW, Yang Y, Li X, Xu L, Feng Z, Pawlowski ZS, Rim HJ.** 2002. Identification of *Taenia asiatica* in China: molecular, morphological, and epidemiological analysis of a Luzhai isolate. *J Parasitol* **88:**758–764.
6. **Flisser A, Viniegra AE, Aguilar-Vega L, Garza-Rodriguez A, Maravilla P, Avila G.** 2004. Portrait of human tapeworms. *J Parasitol* **90:**914–916.
7. **González LM, Montero E, Harrison LJ, Parkhouse RM, Garate T.** 2000. Differential diagnosis of *Taenia saginata* and *Taenia solium* infection by PCR. *J Clin Microbiol* **38:**737–744.
8. **Mayta H, Gilman RH, Prendergast E, Castillo JP, Tinoco YO, Garcia HH, Gonzalez AE, Sterling CR, Cysticercosis Working Group in Peru.** 2008. Nested PCR for specific diagnosis of *Taenia solium* taeniasis. *J Clin Microbiol* **46:**286–289.
9. **Mayta H, Talley A, Gilman RH, Jimenez J, Verastegui M, Ruiz M, Garcia HH, Gonzalez AE.** 2000. Differentiating *Taenia solium* and *Taenia saginata* infections by simple hematoxylin-eosin staining and PCR-restriction enzyme analysis. *J Clin Microbiol* **38:**133–137.
10. **Yamasaki H, Allan JC, Sato MO, Nakao M, Sako Y, Nakaya K, Qiu D, Mamuti W, Craig PS, Ito A.** 2004. DNA differential diagnosis of taeniasis and cysticercosis by multiplex PCR. *J Clin Microbiol* **42:**548–553.
11. **Dorny P, Vercammen F, Brandt J, Vansteenkiste W, Berkvens D, Geerts S.** 2000. Sero-epidemiological study of *Taenia saginata* cysticercosis in Belgian cattle. *Vet Parasitol* **88:**43–49.
12. **Garcia HH, Parkhouse RM, Gilman RH, Montenegro T, Bernal T, Martinez SM, Gonzalez AE, Tsang VC, Harrison LJ, Cysticercosis Working Group in Peru.** 2000. Serum antigen detection in the diagnosis, treatment, and follow-up of neurocysticercosis patients. *Trans R Soc Trop Med Hyg* **94:**673–676.
13. **Onyango-Abuje JA, Hughes G, Opicha M, Nginyi KM, Rugutt MK, Wright SH, Harrison LJ.** 1996. Diagnosis of *Taenia saginata* cysticercosis in Kenyan cattle by antibody and antigen ELISA. *Vet Parasitol* **61:**221–230.
14. **Jeri C, Gilman RH, Lescano AG, Mayta H, Ramirez ME, Gonzalez AE, Nazerali R, Garcia HH.** 2004. Species identification after treatment for human taeniasis. *Lancet* **363:**949–950.
15. **García HH, Gonzalez AE, Evans CAW, Gilman RH, Cysticercosis Working Group in Peru.** 2003. *Taenia solium* cysticercosis. *Lancet* **362:**547–556.
16. **Garcia HH, Gonzalez AE, Tsang VC, O'Neal SE, Llanos-Zavalaga F, Gonzalvez G, Romero J, Rodriguez S, Moyano LM, Ayvar V, Diaz A, Hightower A, Craig PS, Lightowlers MW, Gauci CG, Leontsini E, Gilman RH, Cysticercosis Working Group in Peru.** 2016. Elimination of *Taenia solium* transmission in Northern Peru. *N Engl J Med* **374:**2335–2344.
17. **Bustos JA, Rodriguez S, Jimenez JA, Moyano LM, Castillo Y, Ayvar V, Allan JC, Craig PS, Gonzalez AE, Gilman RH, Tsang VC, Garcia HH, Cysticercosis Working Group in Peru.** 2012. Detection of *Taenia solium* taeniasis coproantigen is an early indicator of treatment failure for taeniasis. *Clin Vaccine Immunol* **19:**570–573.
18. **Tsang VC, Brand JA, Boyer AE.** 1989. An enzyme-linked immunoelectrotransfer blot assay and glycoprotein antigens for diagnosing human cysticercosis (*Taenia solium*). *J Infect Dis* **159:**50–59.
19. **Rodriguez S, Wilkins P, Dorny P.** 2012. Immunological and molecular diagnosis of cysticercosis. *Pathog Glob Health* **106:**286–298.
20. **Mirdha BR, Samantray JC.** 2002. *Hymenolepis nana*: a common cause of paediatric diarrhoea in urban slum dwellers in India. *J Trop Pediatr* **48:**331–334.
21. **Schantz PM.** 1996. Tapeworms (cestodiasis). *Gastroenterol Clin North Am* **25:**637–653.
22. **Muehlenbachs A, Bhatnagar J, Agudelo CA, Hidron A, Eberhard ML, Mathison BA, Frace MA, Ito A, Metcalfe MG, Rollin DC, Visvesvara GS, Pham CD, Jones TL, Greer PW, Vélez Hoyos A, Olson PD, Diazgranados LR, Zaki SR.** 2015. Malignant transformation of *Hymenolepis nana* in a human host. *N Engl J Med* **373:**1845–1852.
23. **Castillo RM, Grados P, Carcamo C, Miranda E, Montenegro T, Guevara A, Gilman RH.** 1991. Effect of treatment on serum antibody to *Hymenolepis nana* detected by enzyme-linked immunosorbent assay. *J Clin Microbiol* **29:**413–414.
24. **Rossignol JF, Maisonneuve H.** 1984. Nitazoxanide in the treatment of *Taenia saginata* and *Hymenolepis nana* infections. *Am J Trop Med Hyg* **33:**511–512.
25. **Medina MT, Durón RM, Martínez L, Osorio JR, Estrada AL, Zúniga C, Cartagena D, Collins JS, Holden KR.** 2005. Prevalence, incidence, and etiology of epilepsies in rural Honduras: the Salamá Study. *Epilepsia* **46:**124–131.
26. **Montano SM, Villaran MV, Ylquimiche L, Figueroa JJ, Rodriguez S, Bautista CT, Gonzalez AE, Tsang VC, Gilman RH, Garcia HH, Cysticercosis Working Group in Peru.** 2005. Neurocysticercosis: association between seizures, serology, and brain CT in rural Peru. *Neurology* **65:**229–233.
27. **Garcia HH, Gonzales I, Lescano AG, Bustos JA, Zimic M, Escalante D, Saavedra H, Gavidia M, Rodriguez L, Najar E, Umeres H, Pretell EJ, Cysticercosis Working Group in Peru.** 2014. Efficacy of combined antiparasitic therapy with praziquantel and albendazole for neurocysticercosis: a double-blind, randomised controlled trial. *Lancet Infect Dis* **14:**687–695.
28. **Garcia HH, Del Brutto OH, Cysticercosis Working Group in Peru.** 2005. Neurocysticercosis: updated concepts about an old disease. *Lancet Neurol* **4:**653–661.
29. **Eckert J, Deplazes P.** 2004. Biological, epidemiological, and clinical aspects of echinococcosis, a zoonosis of increasing concern. *Clin Microbiol Rev* **17:**107–135.
30. **Khuroo MS, Wani NA, Javid G, Khan BA, Yattoo GN, Shah AH, Jeelani SG.** 1997. Percutaneous drainage compared with surgery for hepatic hydatid cysts. *N Engl J Med* **337:**881–887.
31. **World Health Organization Informal Working Group in Echinococcosis.** 2001. *Puncture, Aspiration, Injection, Reaspiration. An Option for the Treatment of Cystic Echinococcosis.* World Health Organization, Geneva, Switzerland.
32. **Moro PL, Gilman RH, Verastegui M, Bern C, Silva B, Bonilla JJ.** 1999. Human hydatidosis in the central Andes of Peru: evolution of the disease over 3 years. *Clin Infect Dis* **29:**807–812.
33. **Craig PS, Rogan MT, Campos-Ponce M.** 2003. Echinococcosis: disease, detection and transmission. *Parasitology* **127**(Suppl)**:** S5–S20.
34. **Jiang CP, Don M, Jones M.** 2005. Liver alveolar echinococcosis in China: clinical aspect with relative basic research. *World J Gastroenterol* **11:**4611–4617.
35. **Kadry Z, Renner EC, Bachmann LM, Attigah N, Renner EL, Ammann RW, Clavien PA.** 2005. Evaluation of treatment and long-term follow-up in patients with hepatic alveolar echinococcosis. *Br J Surg* **92:**1110–1116.
36. **Wiwanitkit V.** 2005. A review of human sparganosis in Thailand. *Int J Infect Dis* **9:**312–316.
37. **Ing MB, Schantz PM, Turner JA.** 1998. Human coenurosis in North America: case reports and review. *Clin Infect Dis* **27:**519–523.
38. **Ozmen O, Sahinduran S, Haligur M, Sezer K.** 2005. Clinicopathologic observations on *Coenurus cerebralis* in naturally infected sheep. *Schweiz Arch Tierheilkd* **147:**129–134.
39. **François A, Favennec L, Cambon-Michot C, Gueit I, Biga N, Tron F, Brasseur P, Hemet J.** 1998. *Taenia crassiceps* invasive cysticercosis: a new human pathogen in acquired immunodeficiency syndrome? *Am J Surg Pathol* **22:**488–492.
40. **Maillard H, Marionneau J, Prophette B, Boyer E, Celerier P.** 1998. *Taenia crassiceps* cysticercosis and AIDS. *AIDS* **12:**1551–1552.

Trematodes

MALCOLM K. JONES, JENNIFER KEISER, AND DONALD P. McMANUS

149

This chapter focuses on members of the clade Digenea of the phylum Platyhelminthes (Neodermata: Trematoda: Digenea) (see chapter 135). At least 70 species of digenean trematode have been recorded as adult parasites in humans. These species are endoparasitic, occupying a variety of tissue sites (Tables 1 to 3). The prominent morphological features in most species are the two rounded suckers, an oral sucker that surrounds the mouth and a ventral sucker that lies approximately one-third of the way along the body and serves as a primary attachment organ (1). As endoparasites, adult specimens are rarely observed in clinical contexts, but they may be observed after anthelmintic purging or at autopsy. Their eggs are more commonly observed in excreta. With few exceptions (2, 3), the eggs have distinct morphology and their presence is pathognomonic of specific or at least familial infection. Despite the diverse range of body sites infected by these parasites, the eggs of most digeneans are voided with feces. Exceptions to this include *Schistosoma haematobium* and rarely other schistosomes, for which eggs are excreted with urine, and *Paragonimus* species, for which eggs can be observed in sputum as well as feces.

Detailed descriptions of the digenean life cycles are shown in Fig. 1 and 2. There are many subtle variations in life cycle patterns, but two predominant strategies exist for these trematodes (Fig. 1 and 2). The first strategy, exemplified by the schistosomes, is one in which humans are infected by direct invasion of the skin by cercariae. This form of life cycle strategy is termed waterborne transmission. The second strategy, apparent in the remainder of the human-infecting species, is foodborne transmission, and parasites that use this strategy can be termed collectively the foodborne digeneans (4). For these species, the human-infective stage, a metacercaria, is ingested with food (Fig. 2).

Two features of the digenean life cycle are noteworthy. First, digeneans often display high specificity in their choice of first intermediate host. So intimate are these host-parasite associations that the geographical distribution of a digenean will be determined largely by that of its snail host. For this reason, many digeneans display a focal distribution in countries where they are endemic. Second, most human parasites are zoonotic, requiring the co-occurrence of other mammalian or avian hosts in an area of endemicity to maintain human infection.

COLLECTION, TRANSPORT, AND STORAGE

As stated above, adult digeneans are rarely encountered in clinical settings. If they are observed, for example, after anthelmintic purging, they can be fixed for subsequent morphological, serological, or molecular investigations using standard procedures (5). Samples to be taken for diagnostic purposes include stool, urine, and sputum, depending on locality and other clinical signs. Detailed instructions on the collection, transport, and storage of digenean eggs in human fecal material are provided in chapter 136.

DIGENEANS OF THE CIRCULATORY SYSTEM: SCHISTOSOMES

Members of the genus *Schistosoma* (Strigeatida: Schistosomatidae) are blood flukes responsible for the important human disease schistosomiasis. Schistosomes responsible for human disease and their distribution, snail hosts, and treatment are shown in Table 1. Currently, an estimated 779 million people are at risk of infection, and 230 million people in 76 countries and territories have schistosomiasis, with 85% of cases occurring in sub-Saharan Africa (6). Of these, some 120 million people are symptomatic and 20 million have severe illness.

Description of the Agents

Adult schistosomes are intravascular parasites of humans, occupying either the veins of the mesenteries or the vesical plexus. Rarely among platyhelminths, the adults are dioecious and the slender female rests within a semiclosed gynecophoric canal, formed by the male wrapping its lateral margins ventrally. Morphological descriptions and primary taxonomic considerations of adult worms are summarized elsewhere (1). Five species commonly infect humans, of which three (*Schistosoma mansoni*, *S. japonicum*, and *S. haematobium*) contribute to most human cases (Table 1). Cross-hybridization between predominantly human- and animal-parasitic species is recognized as an increasing problem in Africa (7), and, alarmingly, recently in southern Europe (8, 9).

Clinical Significance

Cercarial dermatitis occurs in schistosomiasis but is more commonly reported after infection with avian schistosomes (Table 1) and *Schistosoma spindale*. The number of species

TABLE 1 Geographical distribution, intermediate hosts, and egg morphology of the major schistosomes infecting humans

Species	Disease and geographic area	Snail host(s)	Drug[a]	Egg
S. mansoni	Intestinal schistosomiasis, infecting humans and sometimes other mammals; Angola, Benin, Botswana, Burkina Faso, Burundi, Cameroon, Central African Republic, Chad, Congo, Côte D'Ivoire, Democratic Republic of the Congo, Equatorial Guinea, Eritrea, Ethiopia, Gabon, Gambia, Ghana, Guinea, Guinea-Bissau, Kenya, Liberia, Madagascar, Malawi, Mali, Mauritania, Mozambique, Namibia, Nigeria, Rwanda, Senegal, Sierra Leone, South Africa, Swaziland, Togo, Uganda, Tanzania, Zambia, Zimbabwe, Egypt, Libya, Oman, Saudi Arabia, Somalia, Sudan, Yemen, Antigua, Brazil, Dominican Republic, Guadeloupe, Martinique, Montserrat, Puerto Rico, St. Lucia, Suriname, Venezuela	*Biomphalaria* species; in Africa (Asia), many species in *B. alexandrina*, *B. choanomphala*, *B. pfeifferi*, *B. sudanica* species groups; in Americas, *B. glabrata* and 2 other species	Praziquantel, 20 mg/kg, 2 or 3 doses. Community programs usually give 40 mg/kg in a single dose.	Feces (rarely urinary); 140 × 61 μm
S. japonicum	Intestinal schistosomiasis, infecting humans and many other mammals; China, Indonesia, Philippines	*Oncomelania hupensis*, *O. nosophora*, *O. hupensis formasona*, *O. h. quadrasi*, and *O. lindoensis*	As above, but 60 mg/kg in a single dose in community programs	Feces; 85 × 60 μm
S. haematobium	Genitourinary schistosomiasis infecting humans; Algeria, Angola, Benin, Botswana, Burkina Faso, Burundi, Cameroon, Central African Republic, Chad, Congo, Côte d'Ivoire, Democratic Republic of the Congo, Egypt, Ethiopia, Gabon, Gambia, Ghana, Guinea, Guinea-Bissau, Iran, Iraq, Jordan, Kenya, Lebanon, Liberia, Libya, Madagascar, Malawi, Mali, Mauritania, Mauritius, Morocco, Mozambique, Namibia, Niger, Nigeria, Oman, Saudi Arabia, Senegal, Sierra Leone, Somalia, South Africa, Sudan, Swaziland, Syria, Togo, Tunisia, Uganda, Tanzania, Yemen, Zambia, Zimbabwe	Many species in the subgenera *Physopsis* and *Bulinus* of the genus *Bulinus*	As for *S. mansoni*	Urine (rarely feces); 150 × 62 μm
S. mekongi	Intestinal schistosomiasis infecting humans and other mammals; Cambodia, Laos, Thailand	*Neotricula aperta*	As for *S. japonicum*	Feces; 66 × 57 μm
S. intercalatum	Rectal schistosomiasis infecting humans; Cameroon, Central African Republic, Chad, Congo, Democratic Republic of the Congo (Zaire), Equatorial Guinea, Gabon, Mali, Nigeria, São Tomé and Principe	*Bulinus* (*Physopsis*) *africanus*, *Bulinus* (*B.*) *camerunensis*		Feces; 176 × 66 μm
S. bovis, *S. curassoni*, *S. guineensis*, *S. mattheei*, *S. margrebowiei*	African schistosomes infecting bovines and wildlife; rare human infections	*Bulinus* spp.		
S. sinensium, *S. malayensis*	Asian schistosomes infecting animals; rare human infections			
Species of *Austrobilharzia*, *Bilharziella*, *Gigantobilharzia*, *Macrobilharzia*, *Ornithobilharzia*, *Trichobilharzia*	Swimmers' itch, cercarial dermatitis; worldwide distribution	*Bulinus*, *Lymnaea*, *Nassarius*, *Physa*, *Planorbis*, *Stagnicola*		Eggs not observed in human excreta as the parasites do not reach sexual maturity in these hosts

TABLE 2 Geographical distribution, hosts, and life histories of lung and hepatic digeneans of humans[a]

Family	Species	Location(s) in human host	Disease and geographic area	Snail hosts	Source of metacercariae	Drug	Eggs
Fasciolidae	*Fasciola hepatica* and *F. gigantica*	Bile ducts	Fasciolosis; worldwide as disease of livestock; in humans in Australia, Bolivia, China, Cuba, Egypt, Ecuador, France, Iran, Peru, Portugal, Turkey, Vietnam	*Galba/Fossaria* group (*F. hepatica*), *Radix* spp. (*F. gigantica*)	Vegetation (wet grass, watercress, water mint, semiaquatic vegetables), contaminated water	T, 10 mg/kg (in severe cases for 2 days)	Feces; *F.h.*, 130–150 × 60–85 µm; *F.g.*, 160–190 × 70–90 µm
Opisthorchiidae	*Clonorchis sinensis*, *Opisthorchis viverrini* and *O. felineus*	Bile ducts	Opisthorchiasis/clonorchiasis; China, former Soviet Union, Cambodia, Korea, Laos, Taiwan, Thailand, Vietnam	*C.s.*, various freshwater snails (*Alocinma*, *Bulinus*, *Parafossarulus*); *O.v. and O.f.*, freshwater snails from genus *Bithynia* and related genera	Many species (>100) of freshwater fish	P, 25 mg/kg 3 times daily for 2 days	Feces; *C.s.*, 23–35 × 10–20 µm; *O.v.* and *O.f.*, 30 × 12 µm
Opisthorchiidae	*O. guayaquilensis*, *Metorchis albidus*, *M. comjunctus*, *Pseudamphistomum aethiopicum*, *P. truncatum*	Bile ducts	Opisthorchiasis; Asia	Not listed	Fish		
Opisthorchiidae	*Amphimerus*	Bile ducts	Opisthorchiasis; South America	Not listed	Fish		As for *Opisthorchis*, above
Troglotrematidae	*P. africanus*, *P calienssis*, *P. heterotremus*, *P. hueitungensis*, *P. kellicotti*, *P. mexicanus*, *P. miyazakii*, *P. skrjabini*, *P. uterobilateralis* *P. westermani*	Pulmonary cysts, also abdominal cavity, brain	Paragonimiasis: Cameroon, China, Colombia, Costa Rica, Cote d'Ivoire, Ecuador, Equatorial Guinea, Gabon, Guatemala, Honduras, India, Indonesia, Japan, Laos, Liberia, Malaysia, Mexico, Nepal, Nicaragua, Nigeria, North Korea, Panama, Papua New Guinea, Peru, Philippines, Poland(?), Southeast Siberia, Samoa, South Korea, Sri Lanka, Taiwan, Thailand, Venezuela, Vietnam, North America	Operculate snail: *Semisulcospira*, *Thiara*, *Oncomelania*	Freshwater crabs, crayfish	T, 20 mg/kg; P, 25 mg/kg 3 times daily for 2–3 days	Feces, sputum; size varies with species
Dicrocoeliidae	*Dicrocoelium* species	Bile ducts	Dicrocoeliasis; human cases in Czech Republic, Kenya, Nigeria, Russian Federation, Saudi Arabia, Somalia, Spain, U.S.	Land snails, order Stylommatophora	Insects (ants)	P?	Fecal, bile, 38–45 × 22–30 µm; brown, thick-walled, embryonated, operculate

[a]Abbreviations: P, praziquantel; T, triclabendazole; *C.s.*, *C. sinensis*; *F.h.*, *F. hepatica*; *O.f.*, *O. felineus*; *O.v.*, *O. viverrini*.

TABLE 3 Geographical distribution, intermediate hosts, and egg morphology of digeneans of the human gastrointestinal tract[a,b]

Family	Genera	Disease and geographic area	Snail host(s)	Source of metacercariae	Human infection	Drug	Egg
Echinostomatidae	*Acanthoparyphium*, *Artyfechinostomum*, *Echinochasmus*, *Echinoparyphium*, *Echinostoma*, *Episthmium*, *Euparpyhium*, *Himasthla*, *Hypoderaeum*, *Isthmiophora*, *Paryphostomum*	Echinostomiasis; China, Egypt, Hungary, India, Indonesia, Italy, Japan, Korea, Malaysia, North and South America, Philippines, Romania, Russian Federation, Siberia, Singapore, Taiwan, Thailand	Family Viviparidae, Planorbidae	Fish (loach), molluscs (snails, clams), amphibians (tadpoles, frogs)	Focal; prevalence, 5–44%	P (25 mg/kg)	Feces; 100 × 65–70 μm
Fasciolidae	*Fasciolopsis*	Fasciolopsiasis; Bangladesh, Cambodia, China, India, Indonesia, Korea, Laos, Pakistan, Taiwan, Thailand, Vietnam	Family Planorbidae	Water plants (water chestnut, caltrop, lotus roots, bamboo), other aquatic vegetation	Widespread but focal; prevalence, up to 60% in children	P, 15–40 mg/kg; MB, 100 mg/kg	Feces, 130–140 × 80–85 μm
Heterophyidae	*Appophalus*, *Centrocestus*, *Cryptocotyle*, *Diorchitrema*, *Haplorchis*, *Heterophyes*, *Heterophyopsis*, *Metagonimus*, *Phagicola*, *Procerovum*, *Pygidiopis*, *Stellantchasmus*, *Stichodora*	Metagonimiasis or heterophyiasis; Balkans, Brazil, China, Egypt, Greenland, Indonesia, Israel, Japan, Korea, Philippines, Russia, Spain, Sudan, Taiwan, Tunisia, Turkey, U.S.	Family Thiaridae, Littoriniidae	Fish (freshwater or brackish, carp, mullet, cyprinoids), crustaceans (shrimp)	Low prevalence, but common; cases with heavy infections of clinical significance	P, 10–20 mg/kg	Feces; 20–35 × 12–20 μm
Paramphistomidae	*Gastrodiscoides*, *Gastrodiscus*, *Watsonia*	Gastrodiscoidiasis; China, Guyana, India, Myanmar, Malaysia, Pakistan, Philippines, Russia, Thailand, Vietnam	*Helicorbus*	Squid, plants, crustaceans (crayfish), amphibians (frogs, tadpoles)	Rare, focal	NR	Feces; 127–169 × 62–75 μm
Troglotrematidae	*Nanophyetus salmincola and N. schikhobalowi*	Nanophyetiasis; Russia, U.S.	*Oxytrema silicula*	Fish (salmon, trout)	Rare	P	64–97 × 34–55 μm

[a]Modified from reference 79; used with permission.
[b]Abbreviations: NR, not recorded; MB, mebendazole; P, praziquantel.

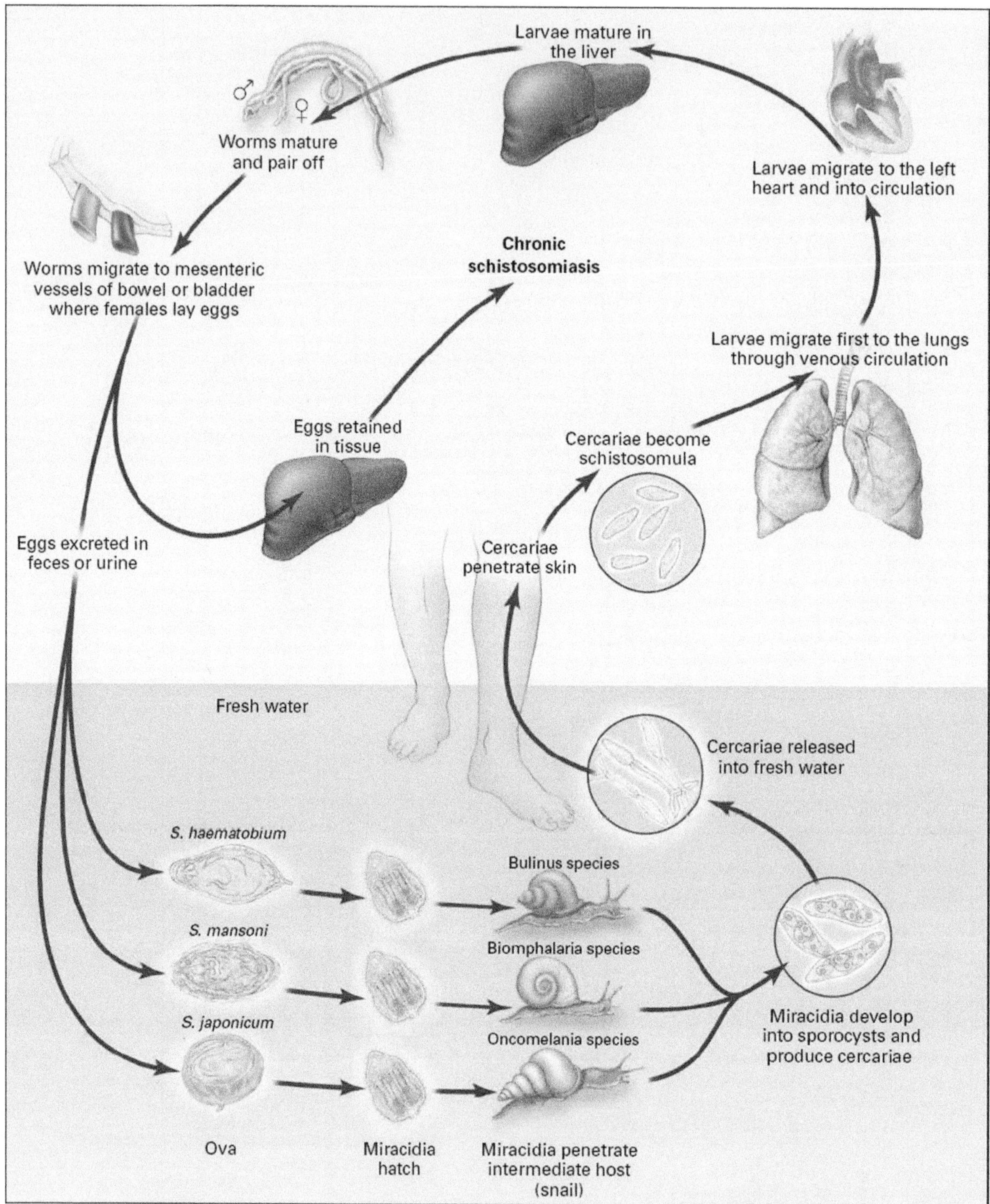

FIGURE 1 Five species of *Schistosoma* are known to infect humans. Infection with *S. mansoni*, *S. japonicum*, *S. mekongi*, or *S. intercalatum* adults occurs in mesenteric veins; *S. haematobium* adults infect the vesicle plexus. Humans are infected after cercarial penetration of the skin. After penetration, the cercariae shed their bifurcated tails, and the resulting schistosomula enter capillaries and lymphatic vessels en route to the lungs. After several days, the worms migrate to the portal venous system, where they mature and unite. Pairs of worms then migrate to the site of patent infection. Egg production commences 4 to 6 weeks after infection. Eggs pass from the lumen of blood vessels into adjacent tissues, and many then pass through the intestinal or bladder mucosa and are shed in the feces or urine (see the text). In freshwater, the eggs hatch, releasing miracidia that, in turn, infect specific freshwater snails (Table 1). Reprinted from the *New England Journal of Medicine* (41) with permission.

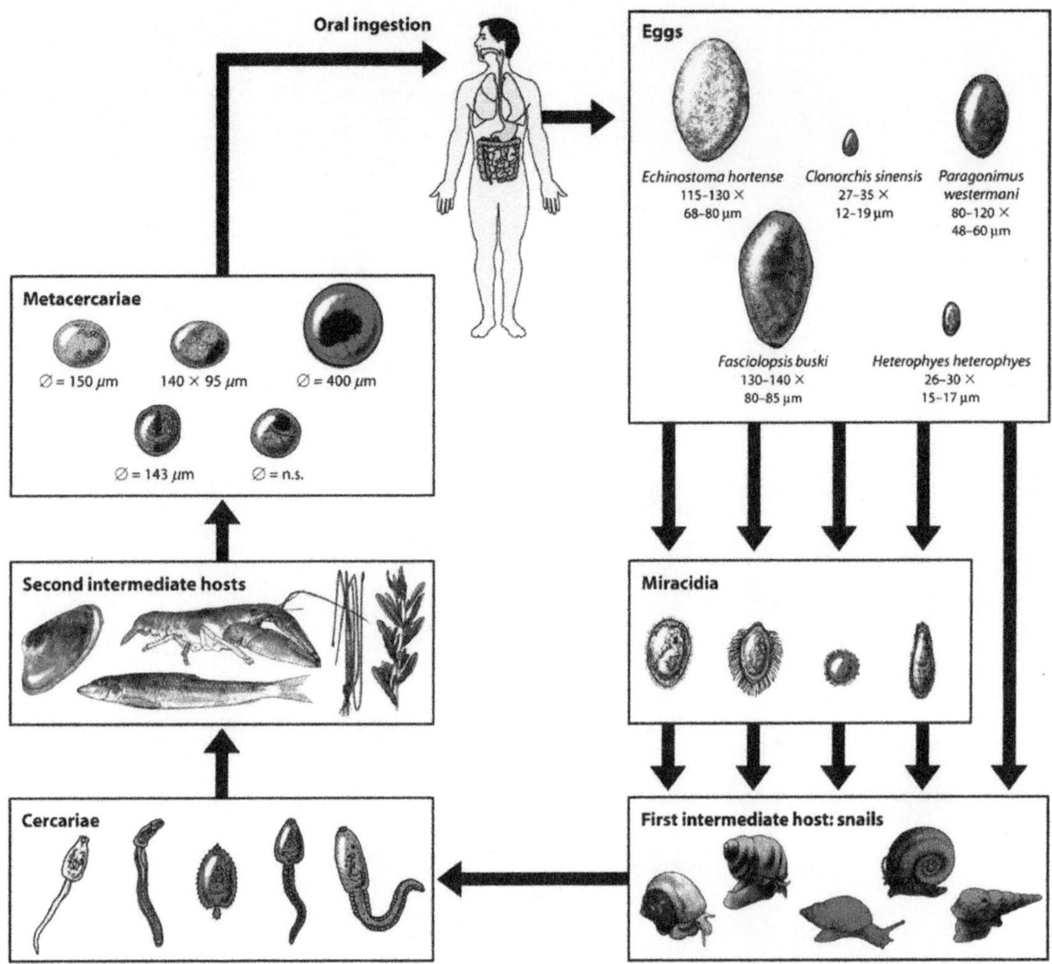

FIGURE 2 Life cycles of five foodborne trematodes, including intestinal flukes (*Echinostoma hortense*, *F. buski*, and *H. heterophyes*), a liver fluke (*C. sinensis*), and a lung fluke (*P. westermani*). Reprinted from *Clinical Microbiology Reviews* (50) with permission.

that may give rise to cercarial dermatitis in humans is likely underestimated, and a rich diversity of potential agents has been identified from the United States, South America, and Europe (10).

Acute toxemic schistosomiasis (Katayama fever) can occur with infection by any schistosome species but is more apparent in nonimmune individuals, resembling serum sickness in its manifestations (11).

Eggs (Fig. 3) are laid by female worms in the vasculature and must traverse endothelia and gut or bladder mucosa to escape the host. In schistosomes infecting the mesenteric veins, eggs pass through the wall of the intestine or rectum, while for *S. haematobium*, the eggs escape across the bladder wall. For all species, however, many eggs become entrapped in tissues. The chronic effects of schistosomiasis, therefore, relate to the site of adult infections and granulomatous and fibrotic responses to entrapped parasite eggs (12). Granulomas occur in many tissues in response to entrapped eggs; however, most accumulate in tissues drained by vasculature leading from the site of adult infection. Eggs retained in the gut wall induce inflammation, hyperplasia, and ulceration, and occult blood occurs in the feces. There is some evidence for a relationship between deposited eggs of intestinal schistosomes and colorectal cancer, but this requires further validation (13). Eggs entrapped in the liver lead to portal hypertension and splenic and hepatic enlargement, potentially giving rise to the formation of fragile esophageal varices. Ascites also is common.

In urinary schistosomiasis, the granulomatous inflammatory response to embolized eggs gives rise to dysuria, hematuria, proteinuria, calcifications in the bladder, obstruction of the ureter, renal colic, hydronephrosis, and renal failure. Secondary bacterial infection of the bladder and other affected tissues may occur. There is consistent association between *S. haematobium* infection and squamous-cell carcinoma of the bladder (14). Pathologic effects on the reproductive tract of males and females are common. *S. haematobium* infection causes genital disease in approximately one-third of infected women, leading to vulval and perineal disease and tubal infertility, and may lead to increased risk of infection with HIV (15).

Epidemiology, Transmission, and Prevention

The life cycle involves only two hosts (Fig. 1), a species of freshwater snail specific for each schistosome species and the human definitive host (or in the case of zoonotic species, species of domestic and wild mammals). Freshwater bodies containing the appropriate vector species of snail are essential for transmission.

All schistosomes of humans use a freshwater snail as the intermediate host. Humans are infected through exposure to water contaminated with infective larvae, the cercariae (Fig. 1), that enter the body by percutaneous penetration.

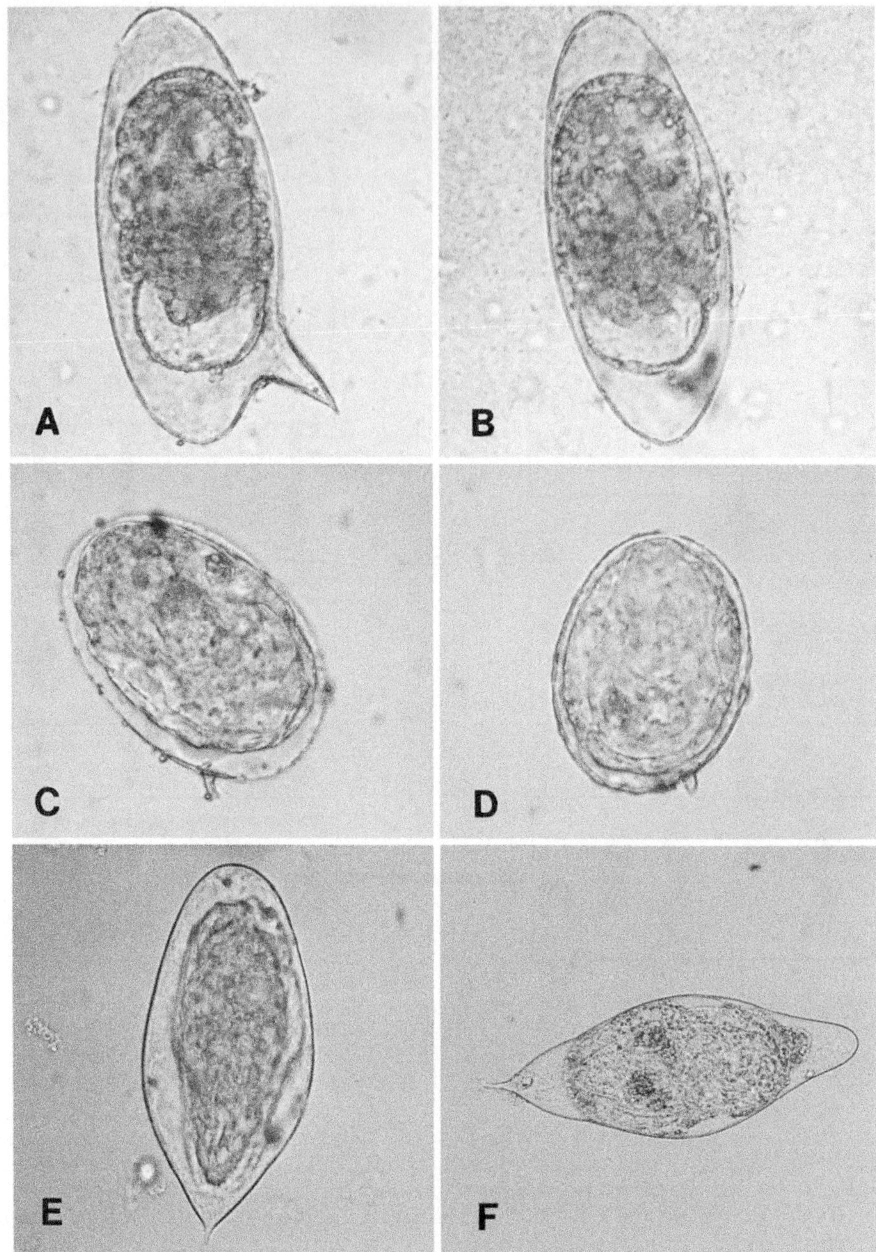

FIGURE 3 Eggs of schistosome species (magnification, ×600). (A) *S. mansoni*; (B) *S. mansoni* egg with typical lateral spine not in view; (C) *S. japonicum*; (D) *S. mekongi*; (E) *S. haematobium*; (F) *S. intercalatum*. Panels C through E are reprinted from reference 30 with permission.

Within regions of endemicity, factors contributing to schistosome transmission include the distribution biology and population dynamics of the snail hosts, the extent of contamination of freshwater with feces or urine, and the degree of exposure of humans to contaminated water. The recent development of large-scale dams in some countries where the parasite is endemic has led to changes in transmission dynamics (16). One interesting hypothesis is that dams alter the distribution of decapod crustaceans (prawns and shrimps) that would normally feed on vector hosts in calcium-depleted freshwater environments (17). The full impact of the Three Gorges Dam in China on transmission of *S. japonicum* remains uncertain (18), but there is evidence that it may be accelerating progress towards eliminating the transmission of schistosomiasis along the lower and middle reaches of the Yangtze River, although the ecological impact of the dam over the long term will require continued monitoring (19).

Hepatointestinal Schistosomiasis

The most extensively studied schistosome, *S. mansoni*, occurs throughout sub-Saharan Africa, Egypt, the Middle East, Madagascar, eastern countries of South America, and some islands of the Caribbean (Table 1). Large-scale control programs, facilitated by donated praziquantel, are ongoing in sub-Saharan Africa, supported by risk maps and geostatistical analysis depicting the geographical distribution of schistosomiasis (20). On the other hand, sparse data are available from the Latin American countries on the epidemiological status of schistosomiasis, and these data are crucial to tailor control and elimination programs (21). In many parts of Africa, the distribution of *S. mansoni* overlaps that of *S. haematobium*. *S. mansoni* was carried to South America with the slave trade, where it infected endemic species of *Biomphalaria*. In Brazil, species of rodent are known to carry this parasite.

S. japonicum is responsible for significant hepatointestinal disease in foci in Asia (22) (Table 1). Originally found in Japan, the parasite has been eliminated there and now exists in China, the Philippines, and a small focal region in Indonesia. Sustained control efforts in China have reduced the number of infected people from approximately 12 million in 1949 to under 200,000 in 2013 (23). While China has achieved success in disease control, the disease remains entrenched in the Philippines, where the parasite infects people in regions inaccessible to authorities due to conflict and geography. Schistosomiasis japonica is a zoonosis, and ruminants, particularly water buffalo, cattle, and goats, are of primary concern in perpetuating the life cycle (24).

Schistosoma mekongi has a highly focal distribution in the Mekong River basin, with foci of endemicity in Laos and Cambodia (25). Although originally regarded as a subspecies of *S. japonicum*, the species was recognized as distinct based on morphological and genetic characteristics, pathologic effects, and life cycle patterns. Sustained large-scale chemotherapy in provinces in Cambodia where the parasite is endemic has led to effective control of the disease in that country (26). The parasite remains an ongoing concern in the region, as a recent survey of humans living on Mekong River islands for *S. mekongi* found that 22% of the people were infected, with approximately 4% showing severe disease (27). Furthermore, the disease was highly represented among children less than 9 years of age. Companion animals represented a significant source of zoonotic infection.

Schistosoma intercalatum is responsible for rectal schistosomiasis in regions of Africa. The species occurs as two geographically isolated strains (now considered distinct species [28]), the Cameroon and the Democratic Republic of the Congo strains, which display highly focal distribution (22). This parasite belongs to the *S. haematobium* group of species, characterized by, among other features, eggs with a terminal spine (compare with Fig. 3).

Genitourinary Schistosomiasis

S. haematobium, the sole agent of urinary schistosomiasis, occurs in much of the African continent as well as Madagascar and the Middle East (1, 22) (Table 1). Adult worms live in the vesical plexus. Eggs escape the host across the bladder wall to be excreted with urine.

In recent years, many reports have indicated that the species is capable of cross-breeding with other schistosome species. Introgressions between *S. haematobium* and *Schistosoma bovis* and between *S. guineensis* and *S. intercalatum* have been confirmed or suggested. The capacity for formation of species hybrids and hybrids of distinct populations of *S. haematobium* that have distinct preferences with respect to their snail hosts remains an issue for ongoing control of these parasites, particularly with respect to their epidemiology (29).

Direct Examination by Microscopy

The presence of schistosome eggs (Fig. 3) (30) in feces or urine is diagnostic of schistosomiasis. Eggs of hepatosplenic schistosomes may be observed by light microscopy in stool specimens with or without suspension in saline. Recently, cameras of cell phones have been tested for rapid microscopic visualization of eggs from fecal and urine preparations (31). Formalin-based techniques for sedimentation and concentration are particularly useful, especially for patients releasing few eggs. Hatching tests, in which fecal matter is suspended in nonchlorinated water in darkened vessels with directed surface light, have been used to detect motile miracidia. In patients with chronic disease and with typical clinical presentation but negative urine and stool specimens, a biopsy of bladder or rectal mucosa may be helpful for diagnosis.

The Kato-Katz fecal smear method has long been used in field studies for diagnosis and quantification of schistosome egg burdens. The Kato-Katz test gives a theoretical sensitivity cutoff of 24 eggs per gram of feces (32), but large daily variations in egg shedding and the uneven distribution of eggs in feces may lead to inconsistent counts (33). New methods have been subjected to trials for direct observation of fecal eggs of agents of hepatointestinal schistosomiasis, among them the saline gradient method, the FLOTAC technique, and the Helmintex method (34, 35, 36). The Helmintex method exploits peculiar surface interaction between eggs and magnetic beads in a magnetic field to deliver high-sensitivity purification of eggs. While used in Brazil, Helmintex has not been approved by the U.S. Food and Drug Administration (FDA).

Sedimentation or concentration methods are most useful for diagnosis of *S. haematobium* from urine samples. In addition, the use of tests for blood, protein, and eosinophils in urine, while not specific, may be indicative of infection (37). Portable ultrasound is useful for assessment of pathologic damage to tissues. The use of questionnaires in populations where the disease is endemic is helpful in revealing infections for *S. japonicum* and *S. haematobium*, but for *S. mansoni*, it may lead to underestimation of prevalence (38).

Serologic Testing

A variety of serological tools have been developed for diagnosis of infections with the three major agents of schistosomiasis (39). The markers and methods are diverse, featuring cercarial, egg, and adult worm antigens for all three species. Serology can be most valuable for diagnosis of schistosomiasis in travelers returning from regions of endemicity or for patients living in areas from which schistosomiasis has been eliminated (36). Serological tests can have limitations with respect to sensitivity and specificity, in early stages of disease, and because of persistence of specific antibodies after worms have been controlled through drugs (36). If serology is used as the diagnostic test, it is recommended that two distinct tests be performed to improve sensitivity (39). In a recent advance, Cai and colleagues (40) showed that combining two recombinant *S. japonicum* proteins (the saposin SjSAP4, a lipid-binding protein secreted by the parasite gut epithelium, and Sj23-LHD, an extrinsic loop of a surface-exposed tetraspanin protein) in an antibody enzyme-linked immunosorbent assay (ELISA) has the potential to provide a diagnostic tool with high sensitivity and specificity, with the capability of identifying individuals with only a few worms, below the detection threshold of current fecal or circulating antigen tests.

Other indirect tests include assays for peripheral-blood eosinophilia, anemia, hypoalbuminemia, elevated urea and creatinine levels, and hypergammaglobulinemia (37, 41).

Direct Antigen Tests

Two antigens detected in urine of patients with schistosomiasis, the circulating anodic and cathodic antigens, have been targeted for point-of-care diagnosis of schistosomiasis, notably for detection of *S. mansoni* infection. A lateral flow kit for detection of circulating cathodic antigen is available commercially and has been widely utilized in studies in Africa and Brazil but does not have FDA approval. While significantly more sensitive than the Kato-Katz fecal smear procedure, the test has some limitations, notably in interpretation of trace or borderline results (42). Nevertheless, the rapid test is gaining wide acceptance in epidemiological surveys due to its rapidity and greater diagnostic accuracy. A flow assay targeting circulating anodic antigen remains under development but has been tested successfully for sensitive diagnosis of *S. japonicum* and *S. haematobium* in low-intensity and near-eradication settings (36).

Nucleic Acid Detection

Molecular detection methods have been used in many studies for high-sensitivity detection of schistosome infections in epidemiological surveys (36, 43), particularly since the advent of real-time PCR. A wide variety of target sequences are used, although mitochondrial sequences (*cox2* and *nad6* genes for *S. japonicum* and *S. mansoni*, *nad1* and *nad2* for *S. japonicum*, and *cox1* for *S. haematobium*) are commonly used (23, 43).

There has been interest in detection of cell-free schistosome DNA from plasma, blood, saliva, and urine samples (44, 45). A microfluidic chamber utilizing loop-mediated isothermal amplification (LAMP) of a highly repetitive 121-bp sequence was recently subjected to trials using blood from experimentally infected hosts (46). LAMP methods have also been developed for monitoring of schistosome-infected snails.

The molecular tests have proven highly sensitive and are suited to surveys in low-intensity settings, but relative costs of instrumentation and reagents remain an issue for point-of-care diagnosis with molecular tools.

Treatment

Praziquantel is the drug of choice for treatment of schistosomiasis. The drug has been used in mass treatment campaigns in many countries, a development facilitated in part by reductions in costs associated with manufacture of the drug. Despite this, the anthelmintic has some limitations, as it is effective against only adult stages (47) and does not protect against subsequent infection. Praziquantel disrupts calcium transport in cells and induces severe muscle contractions in treated parasites. Widespread resistance to praziquantel has not been observed clinically, but the application of the drug in mass treatment campaigns may result in the emergence of new resistant forms (48). Praziquantel is registered for children above the age of 5 years. However, in order to prevent morbidity in young children, efforts are ongoing to identify the correct dose for preschool-age children (49). Moreover, an oral dispersible tablet of praziquantel or its active enantiomer (L-praziquantel) for infants is currently in development.

A wide variety of compounds have been tested in *in vitro* and *in vivo* studies and in proof-of-concept studies, but no clinical alternatives to praziquantel are apparent. Several promising new agents have been identified in laboratory studies, but it would take another decade before they would reach the market (48).

FOODBORNE DIGENEANS

All other digeneans considered here represent a diverse assemblage of taxa which infect humans through ingestion of uncooked or undercooked food (Fig. 2; Tables 2 and 3). The impact of these foodborne trematodes on human health is large. Approximately one-seventh of the human population is at risk of infection, and over 56 million are infected (50). These species are zoonotic. The primary epidemiological features governing human infection include the distribution of suitable snail intermediate hosts, human food consumption behaviors, the presence of suitable zoonotic hosts, and the potential for water contamination with human or animal excreta (50).

Trematodes of the Respiratory System: *Paragonimus*

Paragonimiasis is caused by a number of species distributed throughout Asia, Africa, and the Americas (Table 2). The genus *Paragonimus*, of the clades Plagiorchiida and Troglotrematidae, is highly diverse, with most species occurring in Southeast Asia. Taxonomy of the group is complicated by genetic diversity with ongoing speciation (51). All species are zoonotic, infecting carnivores, pigs, and rodents. In North America, the zoonotic *Paragonimus kellicotti* primarily infects mammals that eat crustaceans (52). The most common species infecting humans is *Paragonimus westermani*, which occurs in China and other Southeast Asian nations.

Description of the Agents

Adult *Paragonimus* species inhabit the lungs, where they induce formation of encapsulating cysts. The flukes are large and fleshy, measuring 8 to 16 by 4 to 8 mm. Taxonomic information on these parasites is presented elsewhere (53).

Clinical Significance

Some 20.7 million people have paragonimiasis, and a further 293 million are at risk of infection (54). Signs of infection include fever with dry cough, sometimes blood-stained sputum containing eggs, chest pain, dyspnea, and bronchitis, and symptoms sometimes resemble those of pulmonary tuberculosis. Peripheral-blood eosinophilia is common. The flukes induce the formation of an epithelial cyst, measuring approximately 1 cm in diameter, which may calcify over time. Parasites may also occur in extrapulmonary locations, and serious complications occur when parasites are present in the brain (55).

In North America, *P. kellicotti* occurs in states of the north Midwest of the United States, particularly the state of Missouri, and in Canada (52). Although human infections are rare, they may be significant. Two recent cases presented with eosinophilic meningitis due to *P. kellicotti* infection (55), and paragonimiasis should be considered in cases of meningoencephalitis in regions where the organism is endemic.

Epidemiology, Transmission, and Prevention

The life cycle of *Paragonimus* is shown in Fig. 2 and Table 2. Of the approximately 30 species, 9 have been recorded as human parasites. Eggs are passed in the lungs and are transferred up the bronchial tree with sputum. Eggs may be expectorated with sputum or swallowed and passed with feces. The first intermediate hosts are freshwater snails. Human infection arises after ingestion of uncooked or marinated freshwater crabs or crayfish (56), but unwashed hands of food preparers and contaminated utensils may also be a source of human infection. Wild boar and deer can also act as paratenic hosts. After ingestion, the immature flukes penetrate the intestinal wall and migrate to the lungs through the body cavity.

Direct Examination by Microscopy

Diagnosis of paragonimiasis is largely dependent on observation of the eggs (30, 56) (Fig. 4) in sputum, feces,

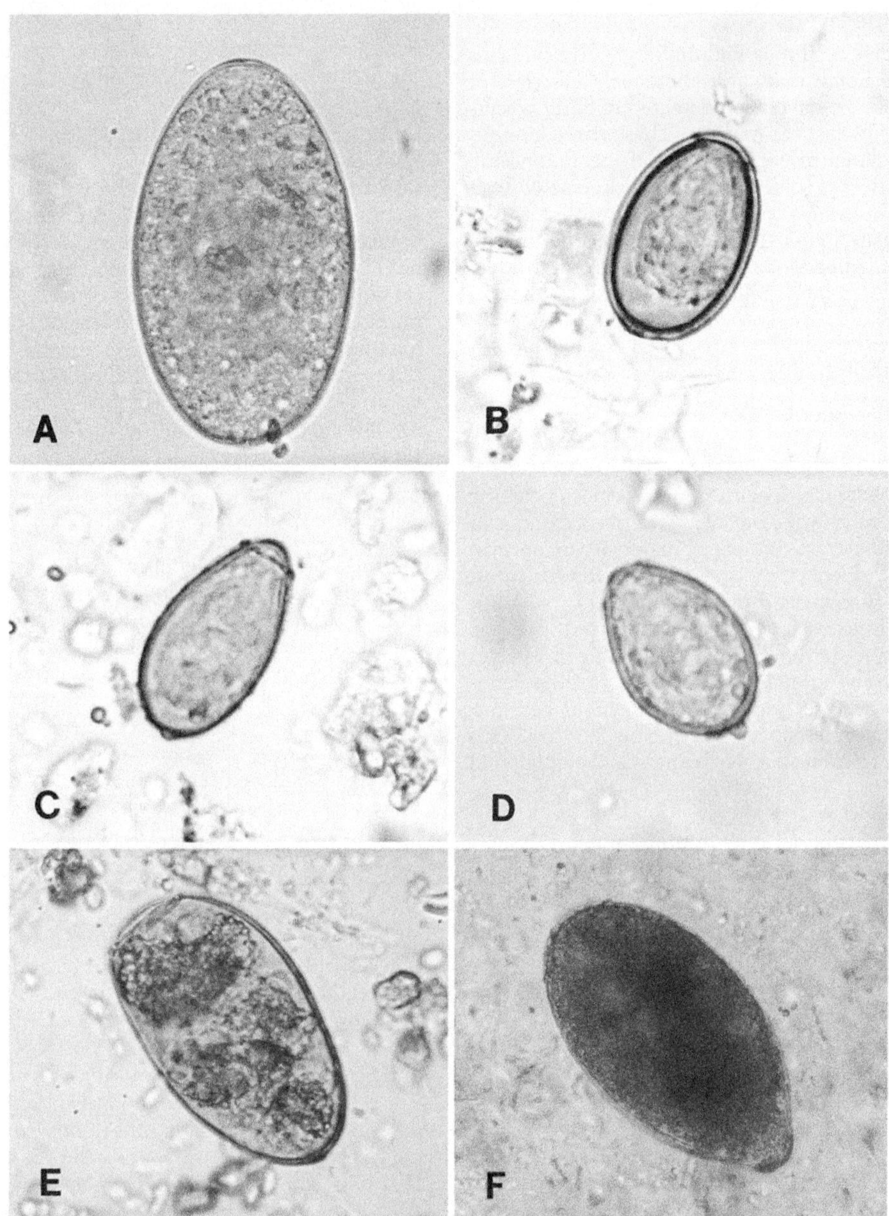

FIGURE 4 Eggs of trematode parasites. (A) *F. buski* (magnification, ×500); (B) *H. heterophyes* (magnification, ×1,500); (C) *C. sinensis* (magnification, ×1,500); (D) *O. viverrini* (magnification, ×1,500); (E) *P. westermani* (magnification, ×600); (F) *N. salmincola* (magnification, ×750). Panels B through D are reprinted from reference 30 with permission.

or pleural effusions. Demonstration of eggs can be difficult, however, as clinical symptoms may occur many weeks or months before eggs are observed in excreta (52). A cough with brown sputum is indicative of lung infection, and the sputum should be examined for eggs. The cysts formed around adult worms appear in X-rays as characteristic rings or nodules, but direct observation of eggs is required to differentiate the disease from pulmonary tuberculosis.

Serologic Testing and Nucleic Acid Detection

Serological tests include ELISAs using either 32- and 35-kDa antigens or parasite yolk ferritin as the antigen (37). For *P. kellicotti*, a Western blot assay using a parasite antigen has been developed (57). Pleurisy with eosinophilia and a dominant IgM antibody titer may be indicative of paragonimiasis (58).

A range of molecular methods for diagnosis of *Paragonimus* species, including conventional PCR, real-time PCR, and LAMP, have been tested (57). No systematic comparison of the methods has been made.

Treatment

The current WHO recommendation for treatment is administration of praziquantel, given at 25 mg/kg of body weight for 2 to 3 consecutive days. Triclabendazole at 10 mg/kg or 20 mg/kg in two divided doses holds promise as a therapeutic alternative (59).

Trematodes of the Liver

At least 13 species of flukes, belonging to the families Fasciolidae, Opisthorchiidae, and Dicrocoeliidae (lancet flukes) (60) (Table 2), have been detected as adult worms in the liver and bile ducts of humans. These three families are not closely related to each other, and the taxonomic differences are reflected somewhat in their diverse biology and life cycles. The groups of parasites responsible for liver fluke infection are discussed in separate sections below, beginning with members of the family Opisthorchiidae, then the family Fasciolidae, followed by a brief account of the Dicrocoeliidae.

■ Family Opisthorchiidae

Description of the Agents

Members of the first family of human liver fluke belong to the clades Opisthorchiida and Opisthorchiidae in the modern classification of biological species. Three species occurring in Asian regions, namely, *Opisthorchis viverrini*, *Opisthorchis felineus*, and *Clonorchis sinensis*, are of major significance in regions of Asia (Table 2). The three opisthorchiids infest the bile ducts of humans and other mammal hosts. Adult opisthorchiids of humans are elongate, lanceolate flukes, up to 20 mm in length and 2 to 4 mm wide. A fourth species from the same family, an undescribed member of the genus *Amphimerus*, has been recorded from indigenous communities in coastal rainforests of northern Ecuador (61). This species also lives in the bile ducts of humans and animals and produces characteristic opisthorchiid eggs (Table 2).

Epidemiology, Transmission, and Prevention

Life cycle information is presented in Fig. 2 and Table 2. Rarely among the trematodes, eggs of opisthorchiids of humans must be ingested by the snail host to hatch. In opisthorchiids, the metacercariae (Fig. 2) are found encysted in the muscles of cyprinid fish (60). Thus, humans are infected by eating raw or undercooked fish (3).

Clinical Significance

Disease severity varies among the different species (3) and with intensity of infection. *C. sinensis* infects approximately 15 million people in China, Hong Kong, India, North Korea, Siberia, Taiwan, and Vietnam (62). *O. viverrini* infects about 10 million people in Thailand, Laos, and Cambodia, and *O. felineus* is widespread throughout northern Europe and Asia, infecting about 1.5 million people (50). All three species live in the bile duct and are thought to feed on biliary epithelia. Light infections are usually asymptomatic, but heavy infections can induce disease. Symptoms most commonly observed are associated with an acute phase of infection and may include fever, abdominal pain, hepatitis-like symptoms, and eosinophilia. A number of asymptomatic hepatobiliary abnormalities are associated with infection (63). Severe infestations with these liver flukes, which are rare, might cause obstructive jaundice, cirrhosis, cholangitis, cholecystitis, bile peritonitis, biliary obstruction, intrahepatic stone formation, cholelithiasis, biliary and liver abscesses, pancreatitis, and hepatitis. The most serious complication of infections with *C. sinensis* and *O. viverrini* is cholangiocarcinoma, or malignant bile duct cancer. Recent evidence suggests an association between *O. felineus* infection and cholangiocarcinoma in the Russian Federation, indicating that all three species have carcinogenic potential (64).

Eggs of *Amphimerus* sp. from Ecuador were found in feces of indigenous people with a prevalence of 15 to 34%. Eggs were not observed in other people groups in the same region. This disparity in prevalence has been attributed to the diet of the native people, who eat smoked fish (61).

Direct Examination by Microscopy

Eggs of opisthorchiids (Fig. 4) are embryonated when laid and are oval, yellowish-brown, and operculate, with a shoulder or thickened region of shell surrounding the operculum. The shell surface may appear rough and may have a small knob at the abopercular pole (60). The eggs are smaller than those of many other digeneans of humans, ranging from 20 to 35 μm in length. Opisthorchiid eggs may be confused with those of other taxa, especially the heterophyids (see below). Differential diagnosis may be arrived at by patient history, by examination by the formalin-ether concentration technique, and by examination of purged worms in feces after anthelmintic treatment.

Serologic Testing and Nucleic Acid Detection

Many serologic tests for *O. viverrini* have entered trials, but most are plagued by cross-reactivity and persistence of antibodies after parasitological cure (65). A coproantigen ELISA has been developed using monoclonal antibodies raised against adult *O. viverrini* E/S antigen and has displayed high specificity and sensitivity, whereas ELISAs for circulating antibodies show high sensitivity but low specificity (37). An ELISA has been developed for *Amphimerus* from Ecuador (66).

PCR tests have been developed that detect and discriminate between fish-borne zoonoses caused by opisthorchiids and members of the related family Heterophyidae, based on mitochondrial (67) and ribosomal (68) sequences. More recently, a LAMP assay that targets eight sequences on the *cox1* mitochondrial gene was developed (69). This assay could detect egg burdens of approximately 10 eggs per gram of feces with high sensitivity and specificity. A LAMP assay has been devised for sensitive diagnosis of *Amphimerus* sp. based on internal transcribed spacer 2 sequences (70).

Treatment

Treatment for clonorchiasis or opisthorchiasis relies on oral administration of praziquantel (a dosage of 25 mg/kg three times per day for 2 consecutive days is commonly used in hospitals, while a single oral dose of 40 mg/kg is used for mass treatment programs). The Chinese anthelmintic tribendimidine possesses promising activities against *O. viverrini* and *C. sinensis*, as documented in proof-of-concept studies and phase 2a and b trials (71).

■ Family Fasciolidae

Description of the Agents

Fasciolids are large parasites of the clades Echinostomida and Fasciolidae. Fascioliasis, caused by flukes of the genus *Fasciola*, is primarily a disease of herbivorous mammals. Until recently, fascioliasis was considered a sporadic infection of humans, but it is now estimated that some 17 million people in 61 countries are infected, with 180 million at risk globally. The two causative species, *Fasciola hepatica* and *Fasciola gigantica*, have a worldwide distribution in domesticated animals, and human disease is focal, with recognized regions where human fascioliasis is endemic (1, 37, 72).

Epidemiology, Transmission, and Prevention

Fasciolid metacercariae encyst on semiaquatic or moistened vegetation, predominantly watercress, grass, water mint, or salad vegetables (Fig. 2; Table 2). The frequency of the parasites in domesticated animals does not necessarily correlate with human disease. Areas of low human endemicity include regions of France (<3.1 cases per 100,000 people in Basse-Normandie) and Chile; regions of high endemicity are in Peru (15.64 to 34.2% in regions of endemicity) and Bolivia (66.7% in the Bolivian Altiplano) (72). Most of the areas with high endemicity are regions where *F. hepatica* is present. While common zoonotic hosts are cattle and sheep, other hosts, such as pigs, equines, and rats, may serve as reservoir hosts for human infection. Children and young adults are more commonly infected than adults, suggestive of the presence of age-dependent acquired immunity (73).

Clinical Significance

Many infections with fasciolids remain asymptomatic. Acute disease arises because of extensive tissue damage as parasites migrate through the hepatic parenchyma to gain access to the bile ducts. Parasite activity in the bile ducts leads to proliferation of ductal epithelium, inflammation, and fibrosis. Heavy infections can lead to cholestasis and result in hepatic atrophy and periportal cirrhosis (37). Common symptoms in chronic infection include biliary colic and cholangitis. Eosinophilia is common in all stages of disease.

Diagnosis

The eggs of fasciolids are large compared with those of other digeneans (Table 2). *Fasciola* eggs cannot be distinguished from those of the related intestinal parasite *Fasciolopsis buski* (Fig. 4) and also resemble those of *Gastrodiscoides* (Table 3). Fasciolid eggs of individual species can also vary in morphology and size in different host species, complicating species identification in regions where more than one fasciolid is endemic (74). Liver fasciolids have a long (2-month) prepatent period, and because of this, fascioliasis is one disease where serological diagnosis is valuable. Immunological tests, particularly ELISAs, based on parasite excretory/secretory antigens, cysteine protease, or saposin-like antigens display high sensitivity and specificity (75). Detection of parasite antigen in stools is useful to distinguish between present and past infections (76). Molecular diagnosis, notably tests based on LAMP, for detection of parasite nucleic acid in feces offers promising alternatives.

Treatment

Fasciola species appear to be insensitive to praziquantel, and triclabendazole is the drug of choice (Table 2). There have been reports of triclabendazole-insensitive isolates in livestock (77).

■ Family Dicrocoeliidae

The lancet flukes belong to the clades Plagiorchiida and Dicrocoeliidae. Members parasitizing humans, *Dicrocoelium dendriticum* and *Dicrocoelium hospes*, are widespread in Europe, Asia, Africa, and North America, where they primarily infect ruminants and rabbits. The life cycle involves a terrestrial snail and ants as second intermediate hosts. Although it is rare, humans can become infected through ingestion of ants. Spurious infections are more common and are identified by the characteristic eggs in feces. Eggs are ovate, with an inconspicuous operculum, and have a dense shell. Such infections arise after ingestion of adult worms with undercooked livers of typical hosts. Brief information on human dicrocoeliasis is provided (Table 2), but the reader is referred to other reviews (1, 78) for more information on the lancet flukes.

Trematodes of the Intestine

Humans can serve as hosts to a wide variety of intestinal flukes. Summary information on some families of intestinal trematodes is presented in Table 3. The families Brachylaimidae, Diplostomidae, Gymnophallidae, Lecithodendriidae, Microphallidae, Paramphistomatidae, Plagiorchiidae, and Strigeidae are rarely encountered in humans and are not considered further in this chapter. For further information on intestinal trematodes not provided here, see the article by Fried et al. (79). Members of the clades Echinostomatidae, Heterophyidae, Fasciolidae, Opisthorchiidae, and Troglotrematidae are commonly encountered in some countries and are discussed below.

■ Echinostomatidae

Description of the Agents

Echinostomatid flukes, of the clade Echinostomida, are small, typically 3 to 10 mm in length and 1 to 3 mm in width, with a large ventral sucker and distinctive spinous head collar. At least 23 species are known to parasitize humans, mostly in Asia (Table 3) (80).

Epidemiology, Transmission, and Prevention

All human infections by echinostomatids are zoonotic and focal in distribution, and foci are often in the vicinity of freshwater or brackish-water habitats. Hosts of echinostomatids include planorbid, lymnaeid, and bulinid snails. Humans are infected by eating a range of raw or undercooked vertebrate and invertebrate foods, including fish, snails, and crustaceans (Table 3). Infection with echinostomes is thus related to life cycle preferences of species and human eating preferences in different geographic regions (80).

Clinical Significance

In most cases, infection is asymptomatic. Heavy infections can lead to a range of symptoms, including epigastric and abdominal pain, fatigue, diarrhea, and weight loss. Some heavy infections in children have been fatal.

Diagnosis

Eggs of echinostomatids are similar in shape to those of fasciolids but are smaller (Table 3). Interspecific variation in egg size occurs among the echinostomes, and species identification is not possible unless adult worms are obtained by purgation with anthelmintics. Evidence of wrinkles or thickening of the abopercular pole of the eggs may be used to assist in identification (80). Recently, a singleplex real-time fluorescence-activated PCR test with 28S ribosomal DNA as the target has been developed for discrimination of *Echinostoma malayanum* from *Paragonimus heterotremus* and *F. gigantica* infections (81). All three species have similar eggs, rendering specific diagnosis through microscopy methods difficult.

Treatment

A single dose of 25 mg/kg of praziquantel is recommended for treatment (77).

■ Fasciolidae

Description of the Agent

Another member of the clade Fasciolidae, *F. buski*, is the sole member of this family parasitizing the intestine of humans. This species is the largest fluke parasitic in humans, measuring 8 to 10 cm in length and 1 to 3 cm in width (82). Adult worms inhabit the duodenum and jejunum of humans and a small range of other hosts that includes pigs, horses, dogs, cattle, goats, and sheep. The species is distributed focally in many countries (Table 3).

Epidemiology, Transmission, and Prevention

The snail intermediate hosts of *F. buski* are shown in Table 3. Humans are infected by eating aquatic plants on which metacercariae are encysted or by drinking metacercariae that have encysted on the water surface (79).

Clinical Significance

Adults attach to and feed on the intestinal wall. Human disease relates to the severity of infection, and symptoms vary from intestinal disturbance and pain, associated with eosinophilia, to severe diarrhea, gastric pain, bowel obstruction, and nausea. Complications such as acute kidney injury and intestinal perforation have been reported, and heavy infection has resulted in death (83).

Diagnosis

Feces of infected patients are often profuse and yellow-green and may contain undigested food particles. The eggs of *F. buski* are large, operculate, nonembryonated, ellipsoidal, and yellow (Table 3; Fig. 4). The eggs are very similar to those of other fasciolids, and species may be distinguished by observation of purged adults. Attempts have been made towards development of a molecular diagnostic tool for discrimination of *F. buski* from other fasciolids using ribosomal sequences. With recent publication of the mitochondrial genome of the species (84), there is potential for an effective diagnostic molecular tool.

Treatment

The current drug of choice is praziquantel at a dose of 75 mg/kg, but albendazole and mebendazole have also been subjected to trials (77, 79).

■ Heterophyidae

Description of the Agents

Closely related to members of the trematode clade Opisthorchiidae (clade Opisthorchiida), heterophyids are mostly small trematodes, less than 0.5 mm in length. Commonly encountered heterophyids of humans are *Heterophyes heterophyes*, *Metagonimus yokogawai*, and *Haplorchis* species. *H. heterophyes* infection in humans has been reported from many countries in Asia, North Africa, and the Middle East (79). Other species are often encountered in rural Asia (85).

Epidemiology, Transmission, and Prevention

While many heterophyids of medical significance infect freshwater snails as first intermediate hosts, some species infect marine snails. Cercariae encyst in a range of fish, including mugilids, cyprinids, and gobiids. Humans are infected by consumption of raw, fresh-salted, or undercooked fish (Table 3). The adult flukes are intestinal inhabitants of a wide range of piscivorous birds and mammals. Eggs (Fig. 4) are embryonated when passed from the host but do not hatch until ingested by a snail intermediate host (1).

Clinical Significance

Disease symptoms in humans relate to infection intensity and arise because of parasite irritation of the intestinal mucosa. Eggs may on occasion pass into the bloodstream and lodge in tissues. These eggs have been known to cause fatal myocarditis in the Philippines (37).

Diagnosis

Diagnosis of heterophyids is facilitated by observation of eggs in feces (Table 3). Heterophyid eggs are similar in size to those of opisthorchiid liver flukes, and care must be taken to differentiate the infections. Often, this can be achieved only by examination of purged adult worms. The recommended treatment for heterophyid infection is a single dose of praziquantel (Table 3).

■ Troglotrematidae

Description of the Agents

Troglotrematidae is a member of the trematode clade Plagiorchiida. These trematodes are small oval flukes which parasitize mammals, including humans. Two species of the genus *Nanophyetus*, *Nanophyetus salmincola* and *Nanophyetus schikhobalowi*, are found along the North American and Asian coasts of the North Pacific Ocean, respectively. These so-called salmon fever flukes are small and rounded, approximately 2 to 4 mm long.

Epidemiology, Transmission, and Prevention

Both species cause human infections. The life cycle involves a cerithioidean snail as the primary host and a fish, usually a salmonid, as the secondary host. In North America, freshwater snails act as intermediate hosts. Humans can become infected by eating or handling undercooked fish. In regions where salmonid fish form a large part of the diet, such as in indigenous populations in the northeastern part of the Russian Federation, infection rates are as high as 95 to 98% (86). The species may be the most commonly encountered human trematode endemic to North America.

Clinical Significance

Infection with *Nanophyetus* species is associated with abdominal discomfort, nausea, vomiting, chronic diarrhea, eosinophilia, weight loss, and fatigue. A history of eating salmon flesh, either raw, undercooked, or smoked, is an important differential for infection in North America (87). Evidently, salmon roe may also be a source of infection. In North America, *N. salmincola* is a vector for the rickettsia *Neorickettsia helminthoeca*, the agent of salmon poisoning disease, a disease of dogs that is fatal if left untreated. The rickettsia has not been proven to be transmitted to humans.

Diagnosis

Diagnosis is made through detection of eggs in feces. The eggs of this species are ovoid, light brown, and operculate, measuring 87 to 97 μm in length. Adult worms produce very few eggs, and in light infections, stool examination may not reveal eggs. The use of trichrome staining of feces has been recommended to reveal eggs (88).

Treatment

Praziquantel (25 mg/kg) is recommended as being efficacious for nanophyetiasis.

Trematodes of the Eyes

Incidental ocular infections in humans have been recorded in a number of countries in Europe, Asia (including the Philippines), Africa, and North and South America. The avian eye fluke, *Philophthalmus* species (Echinostomida: Philophthalmidae), can develop to adult in the conjunctiva (89). Humans are presumably infected by ingesting encysted metacercariae that occur on aquatic vegetation. In India, species of *Procerovum* (Opisthorchiida: Heterophyidae) cause ocular infections, while trematodes of unknown identity are common causes of pediatric uveitis in the Nile River delta in Egypt (10).

REFERENCES

1. **Muller R (ed).** 2002. *Worms and Human Disease*, 2nd ed. CABI Publishing, Wallingford, United Kingdom.
2. **Jamornthanyawat N.** 2002. The diagnosis of human opisthorchiasis. *Southeast Asian J Trop Med Public Health* **33**(Suppl 3):86–91.
3. **Sithithaworn P, Haswell-Elkins M.** 2003. Epidemiology of *Opisthorchis viverrini*. *Acta Trop* **88:**187–194.
4. **Keiser J, Utzinger J.** 2005. Emerging foodborne trematodiasis. *Emerg Infect Dis* **11:**1507–1514.
5. **Cribb TH, Bray RA.** 2010. Gut wash, body soak, blender and heat-fixation: approaches to the effective collection, fixation and preservation of trematodes of fishes. *Syst Parasitol* **76:**1–7.
6. **Colley DG, Bustinduy AL, Secor WE, King CH.** 2014. Human schistosomiasis. *Lancet* **383:**2253–2264.
7. **Huyse T, Webster BL, Geldof S, Stothard JR, Diaw OT, Polman K, Rollinson D.** 2009. Bidirectional introgressive hybridization between a cattle and human schistosome species. *PLoS Pathog* **5:**e1000571.
8. **Boissier J, Moné H, Mitta G, Bargues MD, Molyneux D, Mas-Coma S.** 2015. Schistosomiasis reaches Europe. *Lancet Infect Dis* **15:**757–758.
9. **Kincaid-Smith J, Rey O, Toulza E, Berry A, Boissier J.** 2017. Emerging schistosomiasis in Europe: a need to quantify the risks. *Trends Parasitol* **33:**600–609.
10. **Pinto HA, Pulido-Murillo EA, de Melo AL, Brant SV.** 2017. Putative new genera and species of avian schistosomes potentially involved in human cercarial dermatitis in the Americas, Europe and Africa. *Acta Trop* **176:**415–420.
11. **Ross AG, Vickers D, Olds GR, Shah SM, McManus DP.** 2007. Katayama syndrome. *Lancet Infect Dis* **7:**218–224.
12. **deWalick S, Tielens AG, van Hellemond JJ.** 2012. *Schistosoma mansoni*: the egg, biosynthesis of the shell and interaction with the host. *Exp Parasitol* **132:**7–13.
13. **Nakatani K, Kato T, Okada S, Matsumoto R, Nishida K, Komuro H, Iida M, Tsujimoto S, Suganuma T.** 2016. Ascending colon cancer associated with deposited ova of *Schistosoma japonicum* in non-endemic area. *IDCases* **6:**52–54.
14. **Antoni S, Ferlay J, Soerjomataram I, Znaor A, Jemal A, Bray F.** 2017. Bladder cancer incidence and mortality: a global overview and recent trends. *Eur Urol* **71:**96–108.
15. **Brodish PH, Singh K.** 2016. Association between *Schistosoma haematobium* exposure and human immunodeficiency virus infection among females in Mozambique. *Am J Trop Med Hyg* **94:**1040–1044.
16. **Steinmann P, Keiser J, Bos R, Tanner M, Utzinger J.** 2006. Schistosomiasis and water resources development: systematic review, meta-analysis, and estimates of people at risk. *Lancet Infect Dis* **6:**411–425.
17. **Sokolow SH, Jones IJ, Jocque M, La D, Cords O, Knight A, Lund A, Wood CL, Lafferty KD, Hoover CM, Collender PA, Remais JV, Lopez-Carr D, Fisk J, Kuris AM, De Leo GA.** 2017. Nearly 400 million people are at higher risk of schistosomiasis because dams block the migration of snail-eating river prawns. *Philos Trans R Soc Lond B Biol Sci* **372:**20160127.
18. **McManus DP, Li Y, Gray DJ, Ross AG.** 2009. Conquering 'snail fever': schistosomiasis and its control in China. *Expert Rev Anti Infect Ther* **7:**473–485.
19. **Zhou YB, Liang S, Chen Y, Jiang QW.** 2016. The Three Gorges Dam: does it accelerate or delay the progress towards eliminating transmission of schistosomiasis in China? *Infect Dis Poverty* **5:**63.
20. **Lai YS, Biedermann P, Ekpo UF, Garba A, Mathieu E, Midzi N, Mwinzi P, N'Goran EK, Raso G, Assaré RK, Sacko M, Schur N, Talla I, Tchuenté LA, Touré S, Winkler MS, Utzinger J, Vounatsou P.** 2015. Spatial distribution of schistosomiasis and treatment needs in sub-Saharan Africa: a systematic review and geostatistical analysis. *Lancet Infect Dis* **15:**927–940.
21. **Zoni AC, Catalá L, Ault SK.** 2016. Schistosomiasis prevalence and intensity of infection in Latin America and the Caribbean countries, 1942–2014: a systematic review in the context of a regional elimination goal. *PLoS Negl Trop Dis* **10:**e0004493.
22. **Chitsulo L, Engels D, Montresor A, Savioli L.** 2000. The global status of schistosomiasis and its control. *Acta Trop* **77:**41–51.
23. **He P, Gordon CA, Williams GM, Li Y, Wang Y, Hu J, Gray DJ, Ross AP, Harn D, McManus DP.** 2017. Real-time PCR diagnosis of *Schistosoma japonicum* in low transmission areas of China. *Infect Dis Poverty* **7:**8.
24. **Van Dorssen CF, Gordon CA, Li Y, Williams GM, Wang Y, Luo Z, Gobert GN, You H, McManus DP, Gray DJ.** 2017. Rodents, goats and dogs—their potential roles in the transmission of schistosomiasis in China. *Parasitology* **144:**1633–1642.
25. **Attwood SW.** 2001. Schistosomiasis in the Mekong region: epidemiology and phylogeography. *Adv Parasitol* **50:**87–152.
26. **Sinuon M, Tsuyuoka R, Socheat D, Odermatt P, Ohmae H, Matsuda H, Montresor A, Palmer K.** 2007. Control of *Schistosoma mekongi* in Cambodia: results of eight years of control activities in the two endemic provinces. *Trans R Soc Trop Med Hyg* **101:**34–39.
27. **Vonghachack Y, Odermatt P, Taisayyavong K, Phounsavath S, Akkhavong K, Sayasone S.** 2017. Transmission of *Opisthorchis viverrini*, *Schistosoma mekongi* and soil-transmitted helminthes on the Mekong Islands, Southern Lao PDR. *Infect Dis Poverty* **6:**131.
28. **Kane RA, Southgate VR, Rollinson D, Littlewood DT, Lockyer AE, Pagès JR, Tchuem Tchuentè LA, Jourdane J.** 2003. A phylogeny based on three mitochondrial genes supports the division of *Schistosoma intercalatum* into two separate species. *Parasitology* **127:**131–137.
29. **Stauffer JR Jr, Madsen H, Rollinson D.** 2014. Introgression in Lake Malaŵi: increasing the threat of human urogenital schistosomiasis? *EcoHealth* **11:**251–254.
30. **Ash LR, Orihel TL.** 1997. *Atlas of Human Parasitology*, 4th ed. ASCP Press, Chicago, IL.
31. **Lo NC, Addiss DG, Hotez PJ, King CH, Stothard JR, Evans DS, Colley DG, Lin W, Coulibaly JT, Bustinduy AL, Raso G, Bendavid E, Bogoch II, Fenwick A, Savioli L, Molyneux D, Utzinger J, Andrews JR.** 2017. A call to strengthen the global strategy against schistosomiasis and soil-transmitted helminthiasis: the time is now. *Lancet Infect Dis* **17:**e64–e69.
32. **Doenhoff MJ, Chiodini PL, Hamilton JV.** 2004. Specific and sensitive diagnosis of schistosome infection: can it be done with antibodies? *Trends Parasitol* **20:**35–39.
33. **Kongs A, Marks G, Verlé P, Van der Stuyft P.** 2001. The unreliability of the Kato-Katz technique limits its usefulness for evaluating *S. mansoni* infections. *Trop Med Int Health* **6:**163–169.
34. **Fagundes Teixeira C, Neuhauss E, Ben R, Romanzini J, Graeff-Teixeira C.** 2007. Detection of *Schistosoma mansoni* eggs in feces through their interaction with paramagnetic beads in a magnetic field. *PLoS Negl Trop Dis* **1:**e73.
35. **Favero V, Frasca Candido RR, De Marco Verissimo C, Jones MK, St Pierre TG, Lindholz CG, Da Silva VD, Morassutti AL, Graeff-Teixeira C.** 2017. Optimization of the Helmintex method for schistosomiasis diagnosis. *Exp Parasitol* **177:**28–34.
36. **Utzinger J, Becker SL, van Lieshout L, van Dam GJ, Knopp S.** 2015. New diagnostic tools in schistosomiasis. *Clin Microbiol Infect* **21:**529–542.
37. **Acha PN, Szyfres B.**2003. *Zoonoses and Communicable Diseases Common to Man and Animals*, 3rd ed, vol 3. *Parasitoses*. Pan American Health Organization, Washington, DC.
38. **Utzinger J, N'Goran EK, Tanner M, Lengeler C.** 2000. Simple anamnestic questions and recalled water-contact patterns for self-diagnosis of *Schistosoma mansoni* infection among schoolchildren in western Côte d'Ivoire. *Am J Trop Med Hyg* **62:**649–655.
39. **Hinz R, Schwarz NG, Hahn A, Frickmann H.** 2017. Serological approaches for the diagnosis of schistosomiasis—a review. *Mol Cell Probes* **31:**2–21.

40. **Cai P, Weerakoon KG, Mu Y, Olveda DU, Piao X, Liu S, Olveda RM, Chen Q, Ross AG, McManus DP.** 2017. A parallel comparison of antigen candidates for development of an optimized serological diagnosis of schistosomiasis japonica in the Philippines. *EBioMedicine* **24:**237–246.
41. **Ross AG, Bartley PB, Sleigh AC, Olds GR, Li Y, Williams GM, McManus DP.** 2002. Schistosomiasis. *N Engl J Med* **346:**1212–1220.
42. **Ortu G, Ndayishimiye O, Clements M, Kayugi D, Campbell CH Jr, Lamine MS, Zivieri A, Magalhaes RS, Binder S, King CH, Fenwick A, Colley DG, Jourdan PM.** 2017. Countrywide reassessment of *Schistosoma mansoni* infection in Burundi using a urine-circulating cathodic antigen rapid test: informing the national control program. *Am J Trop Med Hyg* **96:**664–673.
43. **Weerakoon KG, Gobert GN, Cai P, McManus DP.** 2015. Advances in the diagnosis of human schistosomiasis. *Clin Microbiol Rev* **28:**939–967.
44. **Wichmann D, Panning M, Quack T, Kramme S, Burchard G-D, Grevelding C, Drosten C.** 2009. Diagnosing schistosomiasis by detection of cell-free parasite DNA in human plasma. *PLoS Negl Trop Dis* **3:**e422.
45. **Weerakoon KG, Gordon CA, Williams GM, Cai P, Gobert GN, Olveda RM, Ross AG, Olveda DU, McManus DP.** 2017. Droplet digital PCR diagnosis of human schistosomiasis: parasite cell-free DNA detection in diverse clinical samples. *J Infect Dis* **216:**1611–1622.
46. **Song J, Liu C, Bais S, Mauk MG, Bau HH, Greenberg RM.** 2015. Molecular detection of schistosome infections with a disposable microfluidic cassette. *PLoS Negl Trop Dis* **9:**e0004318.
47. **Greenberg RM.** 2005. Are Ca^{2+} channels targets of praziquantel action? *Int J Parasitol* **35:**1–9.
48. **Bergquist R, Utzinger J, Keiser J.** 2017. Controlling schistosomiasis with praziquantel: how much longer without a viable alternative? *Infect Dis Poverty* **6:**74.
49. **Coulibaly JT, Panic G, Silué KD, Kovač J, Hattendorf J, Keiser J.** 2017. Efficacy and safety of praziquantel in preschool-aged and school-aged children infected with *Schistosoma mansoni*: a randomised controlled, parallel-group, dose-ranging, phase 2 trial. *Lancet Glob Health* **5:**e688–e698.
50. **Keiser J, Utzinger J.** 2009. Food-borne trematodiases. *Clin Microbiol Rev* **22:**466–483.
51. **Blair D, Nawa Y, Mitreva M, Doanh PN.** 2016. Gene diversity and genetic variation in lung flukes (genus *Paragonimus*). *Trans R Soc Trop Med Hyg* **110:**6–12.
52. **Fischer PU, Weil GJ.** 2015. North American paragonimiasis: epidemiology and diagnostic strategies. *Expert Rev Anti Infect Ther* **13:**779–786.
53. **Blair D, Xu ZB, Agatsuma T.** 1999. Paragonimiasis and the genus *Paragonimus*. *Adv Parasitol* **42:**113–222.
54. **Fürst T, Keiser J, Utzinger J.** 2012. Global burden of human food-borne trematodiasis: a systematic review and meta-analysis. *Lancet Infect Dis* **12:**210–221.
55. **Bahr NC, Trotman RL, Samman H, Jung RS, Rosterman LR, Weil GJ, Hinthorn DR.** 2017. Eosinophilic meningitis due to infection with *Paragonimus kellicotti*. *Clin Infect Dis* **64:**1271–1274.
56. **Procop GW.** 2009. North American paragonimiasis (caused by *Paragonimus kellicotti*) in the context of global paragonimiasis. *Clin Microbiol Rev* **22:**415–446.
57. **Fischer PU, Curtis KC, Folk SM, Wilkins PP, Marcos LA, Weil GJ.** 2013. Serological diagnosis of North American paragonimiasis by Western blot using *Paragonimus kellicotti* adult worm antigen. *Am J Trop Med Hyg* **88:**1035–1040.
58. **Nakamura-Uchiyama F, Onah DN, Nawa Y.** 2001. Clinical features and parasite-specific IgM/IgG antibodies of paragonimiasis patients recently found in Japan. *Southeast Asian J Trop Med Public Health* **32**(Suppl 2)**:**55–58.
59. **Keiser J, Engels D, Büscher G, Utzinger J.** 2005. Triclabendazole for the treatment of fascioliasis and paragonimiasis. *Expert Opin Investig Drugs* **14:**1513–1526.
60. **Kaewkes S.** 2003. Taxonomy and biology of liver flukes. *Acta Trop* **88:**177–186.
61. **Calvopiña M, Cevallos W, Kumazawa H, Eisenberg J.** 2011. High prevalence of human liver infection by *Amphimerus* spp. flukes, Ecuador. *Emerg Infect Dis* **17:**2331–2334.
62. **Qian MB, Utzinger J, Keiser J, Zhou XN.** 2016. Clonorchiasis. *Lancet* **387:**800–810.
63. **Mairiang E, Mairiang P.** 2003. Clinical manifestation of opisthorchiasis and treatment. *Acta Trop* **88:**221–227.
64. **Fedorova OS, Kovshirina YV, Kovshirina AE, Fedotova MM, Deev IA, Petrovskiy FI, Filimonov AV, Dmitrieva AI, Kudyakov LA, Saltykova IV, Odermatt P, Ogorodova LM.** 2017. Opisthorchis felineus infection and cholangiocarcinoma in the Russian Federation: a review of medical statistics. *Parasitol Int* **66:**365–371.
65. **Wongratanacheewin S, Sermswan RW, Sirisinha S.** 2003. Immunology and molecular biology of *Opisthorchis viverrini* infection. *Acta Trop* **88:**195–207.
66. **Cevallos W, Calvopiña M, Nipáz V, Vicente-Santiago B, López-Albán J, Fernández-Soto P, Guevara Á, Muro A.** 2017. Enzyme-linked immunosorbent assay for diagnosis of *Amphimerus* spp. liver fluke infection in humans. *Mem Inst Oswaldo Cruz* **112:**364–369.
67. **Lovis L, Mak TK, Phongluxa K, Soukhathammavong P, Sayasone S, Akkhavong K, Odermatt P, Keiser J, Felger I.** 2009. PCR diagnosis of *Opisthorchis viverrini* and *Haplorchis taichui* infections in a Lao community in an area of endemicity and comparison of diagnostic methods for parasitological field surveys. *J Clin Microbiol* **47:**1517–1523.
68. **Traub RJ, Macaranas J, Mungthin M, Leelayoova S, Cribb T, Murrell KD, Thompson RCA.** 2009. A new PCR-based approach indicates the range of *Clonorchis sinensis* now extends to central Thailand. *PLoS Negl Trop Dis* **3:**e367.
69. **Rahman SMM, Song HB, Jin Y, Oh JK, Lim MK, Hong ST, Choi MH.** 2017. Application of a loop-mediated isothermal amplification (LAMP) assay targeting cox1 gene for the detection of *Clonorchis sinensis* in human fecal samples. *PLoS Negl Trop Dis* **11:**e0005995.
70. **Cevallos W, Fernández-Soto P, Calvopiña M, Fontecha-Cuenca C, Sugiyama H, Sato M, López Abán J, Vicente B, Muro A.** 2017. LAMPhimerus: a novel LAMP assay for detecting *Amphimerus* sp. DNA in human stool samples. *PLoS Negl Trop Dis* **11:**e0005672.
71. **Sayasone S, Odermatt P, Vonghachack Y, Xayavong S, Senggnam K, Duthaler U, Akkhavong K, Hattendorf J, Keiser J.** 2016. Efficacy and safety of tribendimidine against *Opisthorchis viverrini*: two randomised, parallel-group, single-blind, dose-ranging, phase 2 trials. *Lancet Infect Dis* **16:** 1145–1153.
72. **Mas-Coma MS, Esteban JG, Bargues MD.** 1999. Epidemiology of human fascioliasis: a review and proposed new classification. *Bull World Health Organ* **77:**340–346.
73. **Yilmaz H, Gödekmerdan A.** 2004. Human fasciolosis in Van province, Turkey. *Acta Trop* **92:**161–162.
74. **Valero MA, Perez-Crespo I, Periago MV, Khoubbane M, Mas-Coma S.** 2009. Fluke egg characteristics for the diagnosis of human and animal fascioliasis by *Fasciola hepatica* and *F. gigantica*. *Acta Trop* **111:**150–159.
75. **Córdova M, Reátegui L, Espinoza JR.** 1999. Immunodiagnosis of human fascioliasis with *Fasciola hepatica* cysteine proteinases. *Trans R Soc Trop Med Hyg* **93:**54–57.
76. **Cabada MM, White AC Jr.** 2012. New developments in epidemiology, diagnosis, and treatment of fascioliasis. *Curr Opin Infect Dis* **25:**518–522.
77. **Keiser J, Utzinger J.** 2004. Chemotherapy for major foodborne trematodes: a review. *Expert Opin Pharmacother* **5:** 1711–1726.
78. **Schweiger F, Kuhn M.** 2008. *Dicrocoelium dendriticum* infection in a patient with Crohn's disease. *Can J Gastroenterol* **22:**571–573.
79. **Fried B, Graczyk TK, Tamang L.** 2004. Food-borne intestinal trematodiases in humans. *Parasitol Res* **93:**159–170.
80. **Toledo R, Esteban JG.** 2016. An update on human echinostomiasis. *Trans R Soc Trop Med Hyg* **110:**37–45.
81. **Tantrawatpan C, Saijuntha W, Manochantr S, Kheolamai P, Thanchomnang T, Sadaow L, Intapan PM, Maleewong W.** 2016.

A singleplex real-time fluorescence resonance energy transfer PCR with melting curve analysis for the differential detection of *Paragonimus heterotremus*, *Echinostoma malayanum* and *Fasciola gigantica* eggs in faeces. *Trans R Soc Trop Med Hyg* **110:**74–83.
82. **Kuntz RE, Lo CT.** 1967. Preliminary studies on *Fasciolopsis buski* (Lankester, 1857) (giant Asian intestinal fluke) in the United States. *Trans Am Microsc Soc* **86:**163–166.
83. **Gupta A, Xess A, Sharma HP, Dayal VM, Prasad KM, Shahi SK.** 1999. Fasciolopsis buski (giant intestinal fluke)—a case report. *Indian J Pathol Microbiol* **42:**359–360.
84. **Biswal DK, Ghatani S, Shylla JA, Sahu R, Mullapudi N, Bhattacharya A, Tandon V.** 2013. An integrated pipeline for next generation sequencing and annotation of the complete mitochondrial genome of the giant intestinal fluke, *Fasciolopsis buski* (Lankester, 1857) Looss, 1899. *PeerJ* **1:**e207.
85. **Sayasone S, Vonghajack Y, Vanmany M, Rasphone O, Tesana S, Utzinger J, Akkhavong K, Odermatt P.** 2009. Diversity of human intestinal helminthiasis in Lao PDR. *Trans R Soc Trop Med Hyg* **103:**247–254.
86. **Dragomeretskaia AG, Zelia OP, Trotsenko OE, Ivanova IB.** 2014. [Social bases for the functioning of nanophyetiasis foci in the Amur region]. *Med Parazitol (Mosk)* **2014:**23–28. [In Russian.]
87. **Harrell LW, Deardorff TL.** 1990. Human nanophyetiasis: transmission by handling naturally infected coho salmon (*Oncorhynchus kisutch*). *J Infect Dis* **161:**146–148.
88. **Eastburn RL, Fritsche TR, Terhune CA Jr.** 1987. Human intestinal infection with *Nanophyetus salmincola* from salmonid fishes. *Am J Trop Med Hyg* **36:**586–591.
89. **Pinto RM, dos Santos LC, Tortelly R, Menezes RC, de Moraes W, Juvenal JC, Gomes DC.** 2005. Pathology and first report of natural infections of the eye trematode Philophthalmus lachrymosus Braun, 1902 (Digenea, Philophthalmidae) in a non-human mammalian host. *Mem Inst Oswaldo Cruz* **100:**579–583.

Less Common Helminths

GARY W. PROCOP AND RONALD C. NEAFIE

150

This chapter covers the less common causes of helminthic parasitic infections, particularly those caused by the less common nematodes and cestodes. The trematodes are discussed thoroughly in chapter 149 of this *Manual*. This chapter is not inclusive, given the wide variety of helminthic parasites that have been reported to cause human disease, but includes some of the most interesting and challenging parasitic diseases. Further information about these and other helminths of medical importance is available in *Pathology of Infectious Diseases*, volume 1, *Helminthiasis*, by the former Armed Forces Institute of Pathology (AFIP) (1); *Pathology of Infectious Diseases* (2); and at the Centers for Disease Control and Prevention's (CDC) parasitology diagnostic website (http://www.cdc.gov/dpdx).

COLLECTION, TRANSPORT, AND STORAGE OF SPECIMENS

Collection, transport, and storage of specimens are similar regardless of the type of helminth present, so guidelines are consolidated here to reduce duplication. Worms present in the lumen of the gastrointestinal tract, such as *Anisakis* and *Trichuris*, can be retrieved by endoscopy. Surgical resection specimens may contain a worm or larvae. The intact worm and surgical specimens may be preserved and transported in 60% ethanol or 10% neutral buffered formalin, with the former preferred because the latter hardens the tissues of the worm. Stool is an important diagnostic specimen for parasites that reproduce within the intestinal tract, such as *Ascaris lumbricoides* and *Capillaria philippinensis*, and should be collected and fixed in a standard manner (e.g., formalin and polyvinyl alcohol), as described in chapter 136 of this *Manual*. Blood for serology should be handled in a standard manner. Additional information about serologic tests for the diagnosis of parasites covered in this chapter is also available through the CDC at https://www.cdc.gov/dpdx/diagnosticprocedures/serum/tests.html.

LESS COMMON NEMATODES

Anisakis and Related Species

Taxonomy

The organisms in this group, in the modern classification of biological species, are in clade III (Chromadoria: Spururina) of the Nematoda, in the order Ascaridida, and in the family Anisakidae.

Description of the Agents

The organisms covered in this section include *Anisakis* species, for which *Anisakis simplex* is the type species, *Pseudoterranova decipiens*, and *Contracaecum* species.

Epidemiology, Transmission, and Prevention

The larvae of anisakids are present in many varieties of fish. Marine mammals are the definitive hosts; human infections occur when raw or poorly cooked infected fish is consumed (3). Fish that has been salted, pickled, smoked, or marinated in lime juice (e.g., ceviche) may still contain viable anisakid larvae. A single report claims possible transmission through the ingestion of clams (4). Disease may be prevented by consuming only thoroughly cooked fish.

Clinical Significance

The clinical features vary depending on the stage of disease and immunologic response of the host. Disease is caused by the physical presence of the worm and/or the human response to the helminth antigens. Most commonly, patients experience nonspecific, acute abdominal pain from the physical presence of the worm within 12 hours after eating infected fish; allergic reactions may occur within this same timeframe (5, 6). Infections vary from asymptomatic to dysentery (7, 8). The larvae are associated with the superficial aspects of the mucosa in the early stages of disease, and damage is caused by larval migration and the tissue reaction to helminth products. Larvae at this stage may migrate up the esophagus and cause coughing, potentially with expectoration of the worm; infestation of the palatine tonsil has also been described (9). Intraluminal transit of the worm may result in mid- to lower-abdominal pain, as the small intestine and colon are involved; *Anisakis* has been incidentally discovered in the colon of an asymptomatic individual (7). Severe symptoms manifest if the worm penetrates through the mucosa into the submucosal and deeper tissues (Fig. 1). This evokes leukocytosis and eosinophilia (10). Sudden, intense abdominal pain may be mistaken for appendicitis, acute gastritis, gastric ulcer disease, or chronic colitis (e.g., Crohn's disease) (11). Diarrhea and constipation may occur, and the stool may contain occult blood. Immunoglobulin E (IgE)–mediated hypersensitivity reactions to anisakids have been described and include acute urticaria and anaphylaxis (6, 12).

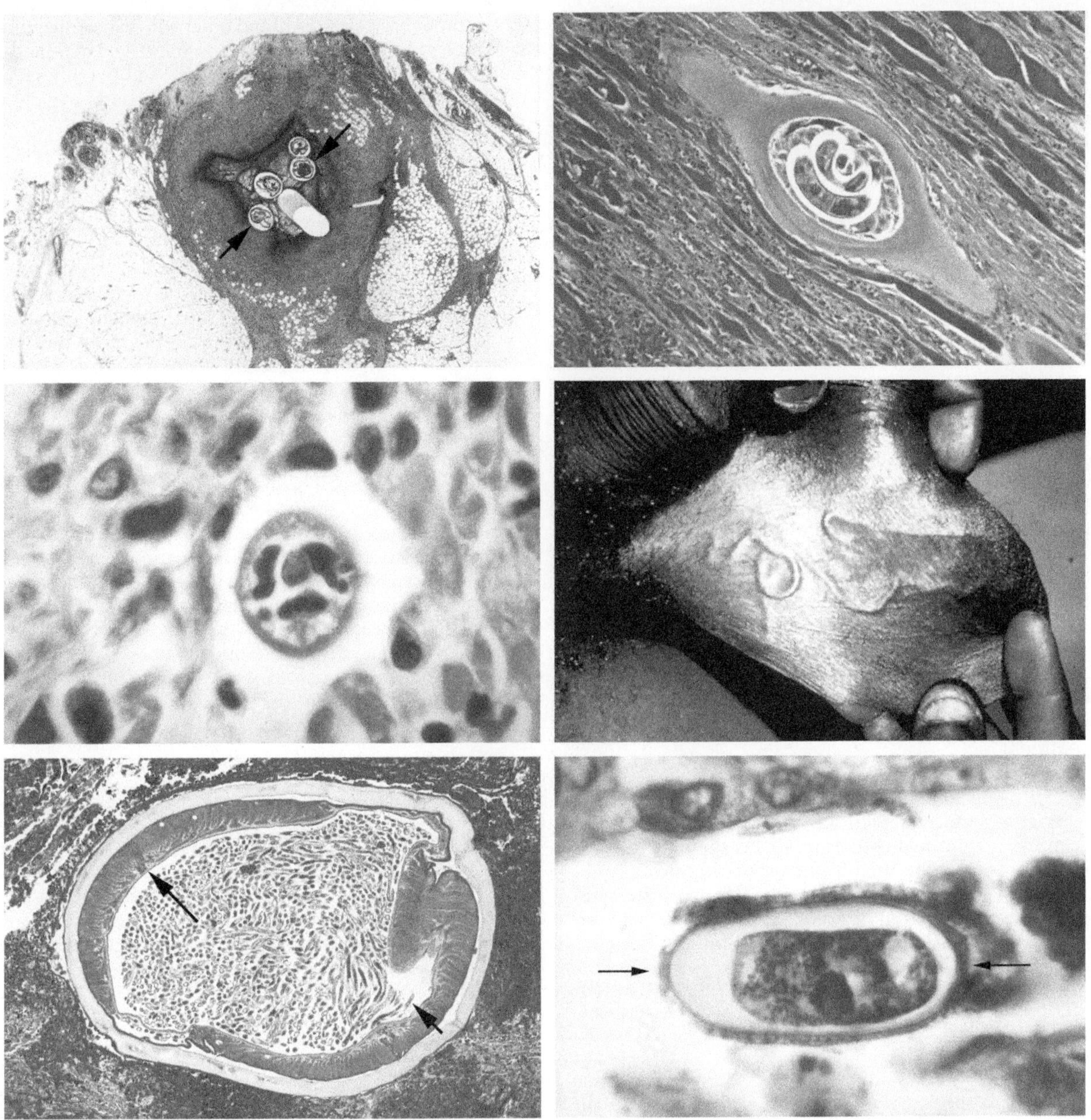

FIGURE 1 (Top row, left) This *Anisakis* species (arrows) has penetrated into the deep tissues of the abdomen. Multiple cross sections of the worm, which is 300 μm in diameter, are seen in the omentum. Movat stain; original magnification, ×2.5.

FIGURE 2 (Top row, right) This coiled first-stage *T. spiralis* larva is in a "nurse cell." Note the hyaline, amorphous appearance of the external aspect of the nurse cell and the surrounding chronic inflammatory infiltrate. The worm diameter is 35 μm. Hematoxylin and eosin stain; original magnification, ×30.

FIGURE 3 (Middle row, left) The minute lateral alae are useful in the identification of *Toxocara* species. The worm diameter is 18 μm. Hematoxylin and eosin stain; original magnification, ×500.

FIGURE 4 (Middle row, right) The serpiginous tract of a female *D. medinensis* worm is demonstrated in the scrotum of this patient.

FIGURE 5 (Bottom row, left) Rhabditiform larvae (short arrow) fill the body cavity of this gravid *D. medinensis* worm. Also note the presence of the two prominent bands of somatic muscle (long arrow). The worm diameter is 1.1 mm. Movat stain; original magnification, ×25.

FIGURE 6 (Bottom row, right) The bipolar plugs (arrows), pitted egg shell, and rectangular shape are characteristic of *Capillaria* species. This photomicrograph is from a human small intestine and demonstrates an egg that is 40 μm long. Hematoxylin and eosin stain; original magnification, ×490.

Direct Examination and Microscopy

The intact worms, best visualized with a dissecting microscope, are white to cream, nonsegmented larvae that measure 10 to 50 mm × 0.3 to 1.2 mm. One dorsal and two subventral reduced lips and a triangular boring tooth are useful for identification. The mucron or tail spine is another useful feature for the identification of *Anisakis* larvae. Histopathologic analysis of infected tissues often demonstrates cross sections of the worm and the host inflammatory response, which contains numerous eosinophils. Cross-sectional studies are useful for identifying the type of anisakid present, but the precise genus and species designation is not necessary for treatment. Molecular- and protein-based methods of detection and characterization have been described; these are most commonly used in the food industry and are usually unnecessary for the diagnosis of human infection (13).

Serologic Tests

Serologic tests to detect the immunologic response to *Anisakis* and related species are available at commercial reference laboratories in the United States. A variety of serologic assays have been developed, which vary in sensitivity and specificity. These identify 85 to 90% of infected individuals, with antibodies appearing from 10 to 35 days after infection. The specificity of these assays is limited predominantly because of cross-reactivity with other ascarids, which may limit the utility of these assays in certain populations (e.g., individuals with intestinal ascarids).

Treatment

Removal of the larva via endoscopy, while it is associated only with the superficial mucosa, is the most efficacious treatment. Surgical resection, however, may be needed for more deeply insinuated larvae. Anthelmintic drugs do not appear to be useful, but corticosteroids may be used to decrease the associated inflammation. Most recently, a combination of prednisolone and olopatadine hydrochloride has been successfully used to treat intestinal anisakiasis (14).

Trichinella Species

Taxonomy

The organisms in this group, in the modern classification of biological species, are in clade I (Dorylaimia) of the Nematoda in the order Trichocephalida and the family Trichinellidae. A full explanation of the modern classification system is provided in chapter 135 of this *Manual*.

Description of the Agents

Trichinella spiralis is the most important cause of human disease in this genus. *Trichinella nativa*, *T. pseudospiralis*, *T. nelson*, *T. britovi*, and other *Trichinella* species also cause trichinosis (15).

Epidemiology, Transmission, and Prevention

Trichinosis occurs worldwide (16). The life cycle of *T. spiralis* is different from that of other nematodes in that the infected mammal that serves as the definitive host also harbors infective larvae encysted within muscle (i.e., the intermediate host) (Fig. 2) (15). The domestic pig has historically been the most important host for the transmission of this roundworm to humans, wherein the parasitic cycle is propagated in the barnyard between pigs and rodents. Porcine transmission, however, has decreased significantly in areas with good animal husbandry practices. The meat of bears, walruses, and other wild game, including wild pigs and boars, may also contain infective larvae and is an important cause of human infection. Additionally, many other animals that are uncommon food sources, such as wolves, foxes, and raccoons, also harbor *Trichinella*. Disease may be prevented by eating only thoroughly cooked meat products of potential hosts and by attempting to control trichinosis in domesticated hosts through good animal husbandry practices.

Clinical Significance

Infections vary from mild, subclinical disease to severe illness, depending on the parasite load. The clinical manifestations vary with the stage of infection. Gastrointestinal symptoms, associated with adult worms, last only about a week and include nausea, vomiting, abdominal pain, and diarrhea. Fever, facial edema that is particularly predominant around the eyes, myalgia, splinter hemorrhages under the nails, and marked peripheral eosinophilia are cardinal features of trichinosis. The major clinical findings extracted from 5,377 well-documented patients with trichinosis were myalgia, diarrhea, fever, facial edema, and headaches (16). If larval migration involves the brain and meninges, then neurologic symptoms predominate, whereas involvement of the myocardium causes myocarditis and possibly arrhythmias or sudden cardiac death. Unlike skeletal muscle, the larvae do not encyst in these other tissues. Experimental animal models and paired serologic data from infants born to infected women support the possibility of vertical transmission during pregnancy (17, 18).

Direct Examination and Microscopy

The direct microscopic examination of a muscle biopsy, performed by simply compressing the fresh muscle fibers between glass slides and observing the specimen microscopically, may disclose larvae encysted within a nurse cell. *Trichinella pseudospiralis*, however, does not produce encystment. More commonly, larvae are detected by observing the infected tissues after histologic processing (i.e., in surgical pathology) (Fig. 2).

Nucleic Acid Detection Techniques

Although nucleic acid amplification assays have been developed for *Trichinella spiralis*, these are not used clinically. These assays, as well as enzyme immunoassays, rapid-cycle PCR, and, more recently, mass spectrometry, are methods used for assessing the presence of this parasite in animal products, and thereby the prevalence of infections in domestic pigs (19–21).

Serology

The antibody response begins 3 to 5 weeks after infection in 80 to 100% of patients and follows the acute phase of disease. Therefore, seroconversion during or immediately following an acute illness is evidence of disease. The tests are highly sensitive, and although they are less than 100% specific, with cross-reactivity usually occurring in patients with other helminth infections, they usually produce results in the equivocal range. These tests are available at the CDC and from several commercial laboratories.

Treatment

Therapy varies according to the stage of disease. Thiabendazole and albendazole are active against intestinal worms but not against the encysted larvae. There is no proven method to kill the encysted larvae; however, microcrystalized forms of therapeutics, which act during the intestinal phase, are being assessed for decreasing the parasitic muscle burden (22). Corticosteroids, salicylates, and antihistamines may lessen symptoms associated with inflammation.

Toxocara Species

Taxonomy

The organisms in this group, in the modern classification of biological species, are in clade III (Chromadoria: Spururina) of the Nematoda, in the order Ascaridida, and in the family Toxocaridae.

Description of the Agents

Toxocara canis is the intestinal ascarid of dogs and other canids, whereas *Toxocara cati* is the intestinal ascarid of cats. Although larvae of both species can cause toxocariasis in humans, most infections are caused by *T. canis* (23).

Epidemiology, Transmission, and Prevention

Toxocariasis has a worldwide distribution, but the prevalence of this zoonotic disease varies widely by geographic area. The seroprevalence of human disease reflects helminthic control in dogs and cats. The highest infection rates occur among the poor, and there is an association with dog and cat ownership (24). Large surveys in the Netherlands associated with the evaluation of fecal specimens from 960 household dogs and 670 cats confirmed that younger animals were more likely to be infected, as were animals that were allowed to roam; additionally, the knowledge of animal owners was found insufficient to rely on them to make sound decisions concerning deworming (25, 26).

The natural cycle of *Toxocara* begins with the passage of unembryonated eggs in the feces of the definitive host. An infected animal passes a large number of eggs per day; for instance, an infected puppy may pass more than 10,000 eggs per gram of feces (27). Therefore, one instance of stool contamination of the environment, such as in a sandbox, can cause significant contamination. The L2 (i.e., second-stage) larvae develop in the eggs after 10 to 20 days of incubation in the soil; the eggs at this stage are infective. If the eggs are ingested by a suitable definitive host, then the larvae penetrate the intestinal tract and migrate through the liver, bloodstream, and lungs. The larvae then migrate up the respiratory tract, are swallowed, and mature into adult worms in the intestinal tract. Paratenic hosts (e.g., rabbits) may also participate in the life cycle by harboring infective larvae after egg ingestion; ingestion of the paratenic host by the definitive host will allow the larvae to mature to adulthood. When the eggs are ingested by a nonpermissive host, such as a child, the resulting *Toxocara* larvae cannot complete their life cycle but rather wander aimlessly in the aberrant host, causing visceral larva migrans. Prevention is achieved foremost through zoonotic control by deworming dogs and cats. Deworming is most important for puppies, which are particularly permissive for infection and are often in close contact or proximity with children. Other preventive measures include avoidance of animal feces, thorough washing of fruits and vegetables, and thorough cooking of meats from potentially paratenic hosts (28).

Clinical Significance

Toxocara infections are common helminthic infections of humans. Fortunately, most infections are subclinical, producing only mild disease for which a definitive diagnosis is not sought. The most severe forms of disease occur with involvement of the eyes or significant involvement of the heart, liver, brain, or other vital organs (29, 30).

Direct Examination and Microscopy

Eggs are not produced in the human in toxocariasis, so a stool evaluation is not helpful for diagnosis. However, occasionally the eggs of another geohelminth, such as *Ascaris*, hookworm, or *Trichuris*, may be present because of common risk factors. The detection of the migrating larvae in surgically excised tissues by histopathologic evaluation provides the definitive morphological diagnosis, but larvae are not always present in biopsy specimens. When present, the single minute lateral ala and the cross-sectional diameter are useful criteria for identifying these parasites in histologic sections (Fig. 3) (31).

Serologic Tests

Serologic studies are important for the establishment of the diagnosis of toxocariasis; results of these should be used in conjunction with clinical findings as well as other laboratory findings, such as increased IgE and eosinophilia (32). Positive results in the absence of other corroborative findings could represent a previous, asymptomatic infection or cross-reactivity due to another helminth infection. The sensitivity and specificity of these assays are high but less than 100%. It is difficult to determine the precise parameters of serologic assays since there is not a better parasitological test (i.e., a gold standard) to confirm the presence of a true infection. These tests have also been used successfully in seroepidemiologic studies. Tests are available at the CDC and from commercial reference laboratories.

Treatment

There is no proven therapy. Anthelmintic therapy with albendazole or a similar therapeutic is often used, with claims of increased efficacy with long-term treatment (33). Corticosteroids may be necessary to control the inflammatory response in patients with a large parasite burden. Treatment for eye infections requires a combined medical and surgical approach (34).

Dracunculus medinensis

Taxonomy

Dracunculus medinensis, in the modern classification of biological species, is in clade III (Chromadoria: Spururina) of the Nematoda, in the order Camallanida, and in family Dracunculidae.

Description of the Agent

D. medinensis, also known as the Guinea worm, is not a filarial worm but rather is the only human parasite in the order Camallanida. Although other *Dracunculus* species exist, these infect a variety of other animals but do not cause human disease.

Epidemiology, Transmission, and Prevention

Dracunculiasis is found only in the rural parts of Africa. Infections occur more commonly in the dry season and affect men more commonly than women. Individuals of a wide age range (i.e., 10 to 60 years old) are affected, which adversely affects the productivity of communities in areas of endemicity. An ongoing and intensive effort by the World Health Organization, local governments, and numerous other humanitarian organizations has significantly decreased the annual incidence of disease (35). When eradication efforts began in 1986, an estimated 3.5 million people were infected with the Guinea worm (35). This number has been reduced to only 22 cases in 2015, a decrease of 83% compared with 2014 (35).

Although excellent progress has been made, efforts to completely eradicate this parasite have been difficult and new challenges have been recognized (36, 37). Updates and additional information are available from the WHO and CDC at the respective websites (i.e., http://www.who.int/topics/dracunculiasis/en/ and http://www.cdc.gov/parasites/guineaworm/).

Infection follows the consumption of freshwater copepods, usually in drinking water that harbors the infective larvae. After ingestion, the larvae migrate to the retroperitoneum, where they mature and mate. The female worm eventually migrates to a subcutaneous location, where a blister forms. The blister bursts on contact with water and releases numerous larvae. The larvae are ingested by a copepod, wherein they become infective. Preventive measures are centered on education and providing clean drinking water (38, 39).

Currently, ongoing transmission is present in four countries: Chad, Ethiopia, Mali, and South Sudan (35). Political unrest and war have hampered eradication efforts. Additionally, the recognition of canine infections and, more recently, transmission through the ingestion of meat from paratenic hosts (i.e., fish and frog) have significantly complicated eradication efforts (36, 37).

Clinical Significance

Patients are often asymptomatic during larval penetration of the gastrointestinal tract and retroperitoneal maturation and mating of the worms. Symptoms at this phase are secondary to inflammation and tissue damage caused by worm migration. Although lesions are most common in the lower extremities, they may occur anywhere in the body. The migrating worm produces a serpiginous tract under the skin (Fig. 4). The large blister that is formed may become secondarily infected. Dead worms may be absorbed, calcify, or produce symptoms secondary to location (e.g., arthritis due to involvement of a joint).

Direct Examination and Microscopy

The presence of the end of a worm protruding from a burst blister or ulcer in the appropriate setting is usually diagnostic. However, a cutaneous manifestation of sparganosis is in the differential diagnosis (40). The microscopic analysis of these worms in cross section demonstrates a 30- to 50-μm-thick cuticle, indistinct lateral cords, prominent dorsal and ventral bands of smooth muscle, and a large uterus filled with rhabditoid larvae that fills the body cavity (Fig. 5); these findings definitively differentiate *Dracunculus* from the agents of sparganosis.

Serologic Tests

Serologic tests are usually not necessary for diagnosis, given the obvious findings in people at risk for disease. However, seroprevalence studies are useful to identify infected individuals prior to the partial emergence of the adult worm.

Treatment

The oldest and traditional treatment, as depicted in an ancient Egyptian medical text, the *Papyrus Ebers*, consists of removing the gravid worm by wrapping the exposed end of the worm around a stick and applying gentle pressure each day for a number of days, until the worm is removed. Treatment with thiabendazole and metronidazole, although not lethal for the worm, facilitates removal by this process (38). Although it is often effective, risks include rupture or breaking of the worm prior to full removal. Currently, surgical excision is preferred (39). Anti-inflammatory agents and antihistamines are important for symptomatic relief. Antibiotics may be necessary to curtail secondary bacterial infections, and tetanus vaccination is important.

Capillaria philippinensis

Taxonomy

The organisms in this group, in the modern classification of biological species, are in clade I (Dorylaimia) of the Nematoda, in the order Trichocephalida, and in the family Capillariidae.

Description of the Agent

Capillaria philippinensis is a trichurid nematode responsible for intestinal capillariasis (41, 42). Other *Capillaria* species (*C. hepatica* and *C. aerophila*), which are less common causes of human disease, are not discussed further.

Epidemiology, Transmission, and Prevention

The natural parasitic cycle of *C. philippinensis* involves marine, fish-eating birds as the definitive hosts and fish as the intermediate hosts. Disease is endemic to the Philippines, Thailand, and other parts of Asia, with more recent concerns that this disease has spread to Upper Egypt (43). The means by which *C. philippinensis* has spread to Egypt is unknown, but the importation of infected live fish or the carriage of the parasite in infected migratory birds has been postulated (43). Humans become infected by ingesting raw or undercooked fish that harbor the infective larvae. Larvae at various stages of maturation may be found in the lumen of the intestine of the definitive host or the patient and may reinfect the intestinal mucosa, causing a hyperinfection. Thorough cooking of fish is protective.

Clinical Significance

Infections with *C. philippinensis* are relatively rare. Eighty-two patients with intestinal capillariasis were reported in Thailand from 1994 to 2006, whereas 24 infected patients from Buriram, Thailand, were reported in this same period (44). Rarely, because intraintestinal hyperinfection is possible, infections may be fatal (45, 46). Nonspecific gastrointestinal complaints predominate early in the course of disease; these include watery diarrhea, weight loss, abdominal pain, edema, and weakness (44). As the disease progresses and the number of worms increases, there is continued diarrhea, with malabsorption leading to cachexia (46). Endoscopy may be useful for establishing the diagnosis, but stool examination remains the diagnostic test of choice (47). Death occurs secondarily to malnutrition or because of secondary bacterial infections (e.g., septicemia).

Direct Examination and Microscopy

Microscopic examination of the stool may demonstrate a mixture of eggs, larvae, and adult parasites. The eggs of *C. philippinensis* (Fig. 6), which have bipolar plugs, are superficially reminiscent of the more commonly recognized trichurid worm, *Trichuris trichiura*. The plugs of *C. philippinensis*, however, are nonprotruding, the egg is more rectangular, and there is a distinctive pitting of the egg shell (48). The adults superficially resemble *Strongyloides stercoralis* but may be differentiated by the presence of stichocytes and three bacillary bands, with the latter being recognized most easily in cross section.

Serologic Tests

Serologic tests are not available from the CDC or from commercial reference laboratories in the United States.

An enzyme-linked immunosorbent assay for the screening of sera for antibodies directed against *C. philippinensis* has been developed and is reported to have high sensitivity and specificity (49). This assay is particularly useful in infected patients who are negative by conventional stool examination. Cross-reactivity may occur when other helminthic infections are present, which may affect the specificity of the assay.

Treatment

Albendazole, mebendazole, or thiabendazole may be used for therapy. Relapsing disease requires prolonged anthelmintic therapy. Aggressive electrolyte replacement and monitoring are critical, as are control of diarrhea and administration of nutrients.

Gnathostoma Species

Taxonomy

The organisms in this group, in the modern classification of biological species, are in clade III (Chromadoria: Spururina) of the Nematoda, in the order Spirurida, and in the family Gnathostomatidae.

Description of the Agents

Gnathostoma species are gastric spirurid nematode parasites for which the definitive hosts are a variety of mammals, not including humans (50). Infective L3 (i.e., third-stage) larvae predominantly cause disease in humans, but it is also thought that L2 (i.e., second-stage) larvae encountered in infected copepods in unclean drinking may also cause disease. *Gnathostoma* infections result in cutaneous and/or visceral larva migrans, the latter of which includes ocular and central nervous system manifestations. *Gnathostoma spinigerum* is the most common cause of human disease, but other species have also been reported to cause disease.

Epidemiology, Transmission, and Prevention

Gnathostoma spinigerum has essentially a worldwide distribution, with dogs and cats serving as the primary definitive hosts. *Gnathostoma hispidum* and *G. doloresi* infect wild and domestic pigs, whereas *G. nipponicum* is a parasite of weasels.

The adult male and female gnathostomes live in a tumor produced in the wall of the stomach of the definitive host, where they mate and produce eggs. The eggs are passed in the stool, and once in water, hatch and release first-stage larvae. These infect the copepod *Cyclops* and mature into second-stage larvae. When a variety of intermediate hosts, such as fish, snakes, eels, or frogs, eat the copepod, the larvae penetrate the gastric wall of the new host, wherein they develop into third-stage larvae (L3), migrate to the musculature, and encyst. When a definitive host eats the intermediate host, the L3 larvae excyst, penetrate the gastric wall, and subsequently migrate through the liver, muscles, and connective tissues, only to return to the stomach to mature into adults. Alternatively, paratenic hosts such as birds may eat the second intermediate host; the ingested L3 larvae remain viable within the paratenic host, which may be transmitted to either the definitive host or to humans.

The parasite is transmitted to humans through the ingestion of raw or undercooked meat from a secondary intermediate host or a paratenic host. Humans are accidental hosts in which the nematode larvae cannot mature to adulthood and continue to migrate aimlessly and aggressively (50). Disease can be prevented by thoroughly cooking potentially infected foods.

Clinical Significance

The clinical presentations of gnathostomiasis are protean because the wandering larvae may be present in any tissue or organ system (51–54). Although the infection is not commonly fatal, significant morbidity may result. The clinical manifestations depend on the tissues in which the larva is migrating. Panniculitis, creeping eruptions, and pseudofurunculosis are dermatologic manifestations of gnathostomiasis (52). Any visceral organ may be affected, including the eyes and central nervous system. (53, 54).

Direct Examination and Microscopy

The L3 larvae, rather than the mature (adult) gnathostomes, are present in humans. This form is morphologically similar to the adult form but smaller, measuring 3 to 4 mm in length by approximately 630 μm in diameter (*G. spinigerum*). The head bulb contains four rows of cephalic hooklets, with approximately 45 hooklets per row. The body of the larva, like that of the adult, is covered with transverse rows of sharply pointed spines that diminish toward the posterior end of the worm. An entire worm may be expelled spontaneously from the site of infection or may require surgical excision.

Serologic Tests

Serologic assays have been developed predominantly in areas of endemicity. These are not available in the United States, but the CDC can assist in identifying a source for testing, if necessary. The possibility of cross-reactivity should be considered with these tests and with other serologic assays for helminthic parasites.

Treatment

Surgical removal of the parasite is the most effective treatment, but it is difficult to achieve because of parasite migration; this may be aided by advanced imaging tools (55). Treatment usually involves some type of anthelmintic medication, such as albendazole or ivermectin. There remains controversy regarding the treatment of central nervous system gnathostomiasis, because there is a concern that anthelmintic therapy will kill the invading worms and increase the inflammatory reaction; treatment is supportive and may include corticosteroid use to control the inflammatory response (56).

Parastrongylus (*Angiostrongylus*) Species

Taxonomy

The organisms in this group, in the modern classification of biological species, are in clade V (Chromadoria: Rhabditina) of the Nematoda, in the order Rhabditida (Strongylida), and in the family Ancylostomatidae.

Description of the Agents

Parastrongylus cantonensis and *P. costaricensis* are filariform worms that are the most important causes of angiostrongyliasis (56).

Epidemiology, Transmission, and Prevention

Parastrongylus spp. are widely distributed throughout the world and represent an important public health threat, particularly in Southeast Asia, the Asian Pacific Islands, Africa, and the Caribbean. These parasites persist in a wide variety of rodents, which serve as the definitive host. The adult worms of *Parastrongylus cantonensis* reside in the pulmonary artery and the right side of the heart of the rodent, whereas the adults of *P. costaricensis* reside in arterioles in the ileum.

Eggs released from the adult worms lodge in capillaries, where they hatch and release larvae. The larvae subsequently migrate up the trachea, are swallowed, and are passed in the feces. These larvae infect mollusks, particularly snails and slugs, which are the intermediate host. Within the snail, they mature into the infective L3 larvae. A number of animals, including shrimp, crabs, fish, and frogs, that eat the infected mollusks serve as important paratenic hosts. Rodents that ingest either the infected mollusk or tissues from the paratenic host become infected. In the definitive host, the infective larvae penetrate the intestine, become bloodborne, and migrate to the central nervous system, where they molt twice. Thereafter, the worms reenter the systemic circulation and finally reside in either the right ventricle and pulmonary artery (*P. cantonensis*) or the ileum (*P. costaricensis*) to mature and complete the cycle.

Humans become infected through the ingestion of tissue from an infected mollusk, an infected paratenic host, and possibly through excretions from snails or slugs (i.e., slime) that contaminate other foodstuff (e.g., vegetables). Prevention of disease can be achieved through control of the local rat population, the thorough cooking of mollusks and meat from paratenic hosts, and the washing of vegetables that may be contaminated with snail or slug slime.

Clinical Significance

The clinical manifestations reflect the worm burden and the site of worm residence, the central nervous system for *P. cantonensis* and the ileocecal region for *P. costaricensis*. The worms of *P. cantonensis* remain juvenile, tend to remain associated with the brain and meninges in human infections (Fig. 7), and will usually die in this location. Conversely, *P. costaricensis* often reaches sexual maturity in the arterioles of the ileum and releases eggs into intestinal tissue. Patients with central nervous system disease demonstrate signs and symptoms typical of meningitis or meningoencephalitis, with headache, fever, possibly eosinophilia (10 to 60%), and a variety of neurologic disturbances, depending on the location of the worms. The cerebrospinal fluid (CSF) demonstrates pleocytosis, eosinophilia (26 to 75%), and elevated protein and occasionally will contain immature worms. Alternatively, patients may have infections of the eye, with retinal detachment and blindness. Less commonly, human infections may result in pulmonary disease. Infections with *P. costaricensis* result in eosinophilic enteritis with diarrhea and abdominal pain.

Direct Examination and Microscopy

Demonstration of the worms in histologic sections or intact in clinical specimens from the CSF, eye, or other infected tissue definitively establishes the diagnosis. Eosinophilia in the CSF may be the first indicator of a possible parasitic infection of the central nervous system. The differential diagnosis of the causes of CSF eosinophilia, however, is broad and includes other parasitic infections, e.g., with *Gnathostoma* or *Toxocara* spp., allergic reactions, and coccidioidomycosis. The gross appearance of an adult female worm is distinctive, with the spiral winding of the uteri and ovarian branches imparting a "barber pole" appearance. Cross section of the female demonstrates a large intestine and two uteri, whereas cross section of the male reveals a large intestine and a single reproductive tract. Eggs are not produced in human tissues by *P. cantonensis*, whereas they may be produced by *P. costaricensis*. The eggs of *P. costaricensis* remain embedded in tissue in the human host and do not appear in stool. The eggs are oval and thin-shelled, somewhat resemble a hookworm egg, and usually measure 60 to 65 by 40 to 45 μm.

Serologic Tests

Serologic assays are powerful tools for the diagnosis of parastrongyliasis, particularly since *P. cantonensis* is usually located in a difficult-to-access location, the central nervous system. The serologic assays that have been developed vary with respect to sensitivity and specificity, so it is important that the user understand the performance characteristics and the limitations of the assay under consideration (57). Although intrathecal antibody is not always produced during infection, when detected, the presence of intrathecal antibody synthesis provides strong evidence of infection. This assay is available from some commercial laboratories in the United States.

Treatment

An optimal treatment has not been established. Fortunately, the disease is often self-limited. Removal of CSF, to decrease intracranial pressure, and the administration of corticosteroids and nonsteroidal anti-inflammatory agents have been used to control pain and inflammation. A variety of anthelmintic medications have been used, with mebendazole being the current drug of choice and albendazole as an alternative. Careful monitoring of the patient is important

FIGURE 7 (Row 1, left) The immature *P. cantonensis* worm (arrows) in the meninges of this patient is eliciting a marked eosinophilic response. The worm is 200 μm in diameter. Hematoxylin and eosin stain; original magnification, ×50 (AFIP negative no. 73-6862).

FIGURE 8 (Row 1, right) The coiled remnants of an immature male *D. immitis* worm are present in this branch of the pulmonary artery. The maximum worm diameter is 250 μm. Movat stain; original magnification, ×15 (AFIP negative no. 71-11563).

FIGURE 9 (Row 2, left) The two uteri (arrows), muscle, trilaminar (arrowhead), and smooth cuticle are characteristic of an immature female *D. immitis* worm. The worm diameter is 250 μm. Movat stain; original magnification, ×80 (AFIP negative no. 72-2732).

FIGURE 10 (Row 2, right) The *Dirofilaria* species other than *D. immitis* have external longitudinal cuticular ridges, whereas the cuticle of *D. immitis* is smooth. *D. tenuis* is pictured here, in cross section; it is 270 μm in diameter and has obvious cuticular ridges (arrows). *Dirofilaria* species other than *D. immitis* are often found in a subcutaneous location rather than in the pulmonary arterial vasculature. Movat stain; original magnification, ×80 (AFIP negative no. 94-5122).

FIGURE 11 (Row 3, left) An egg packet of *D. caninum*, obtained from a crushed gravid proglottid, is 150 μm in diameter. The eggs within the packet are 40 μm in diameter. Unstained (AFIP negative no. 86-7369).

FIGURE 12 (Row 3, right) The thick inner membrane of the egg of *Hymenolepis diminuta* is surrounded by a gelatinous matrix and then by an outer striated shell. The eggs of *H. diminuta* are spherical, whereas those of *Hymenolepis nana* are ovoid. The egg pictured here is 80 μm in diameter. Unstained; original magnification, ×250 (AFIP negative no. 96-5119). See chapter 148, "Cestodes," for more detailed coverage of *Hymenolepis* spp.

FIGURE 13 (Row 4, left) A sparganum superficially resembles an adult tapeworm. Close inspection, however, clarifies its immature form, with a head with only a ventral groove or bothrium (arrow) and a lack of proglottids. The maximum width is 6 mm. Unstained; original magnification, ×0.5 (AFIP negative no. 70-15303).

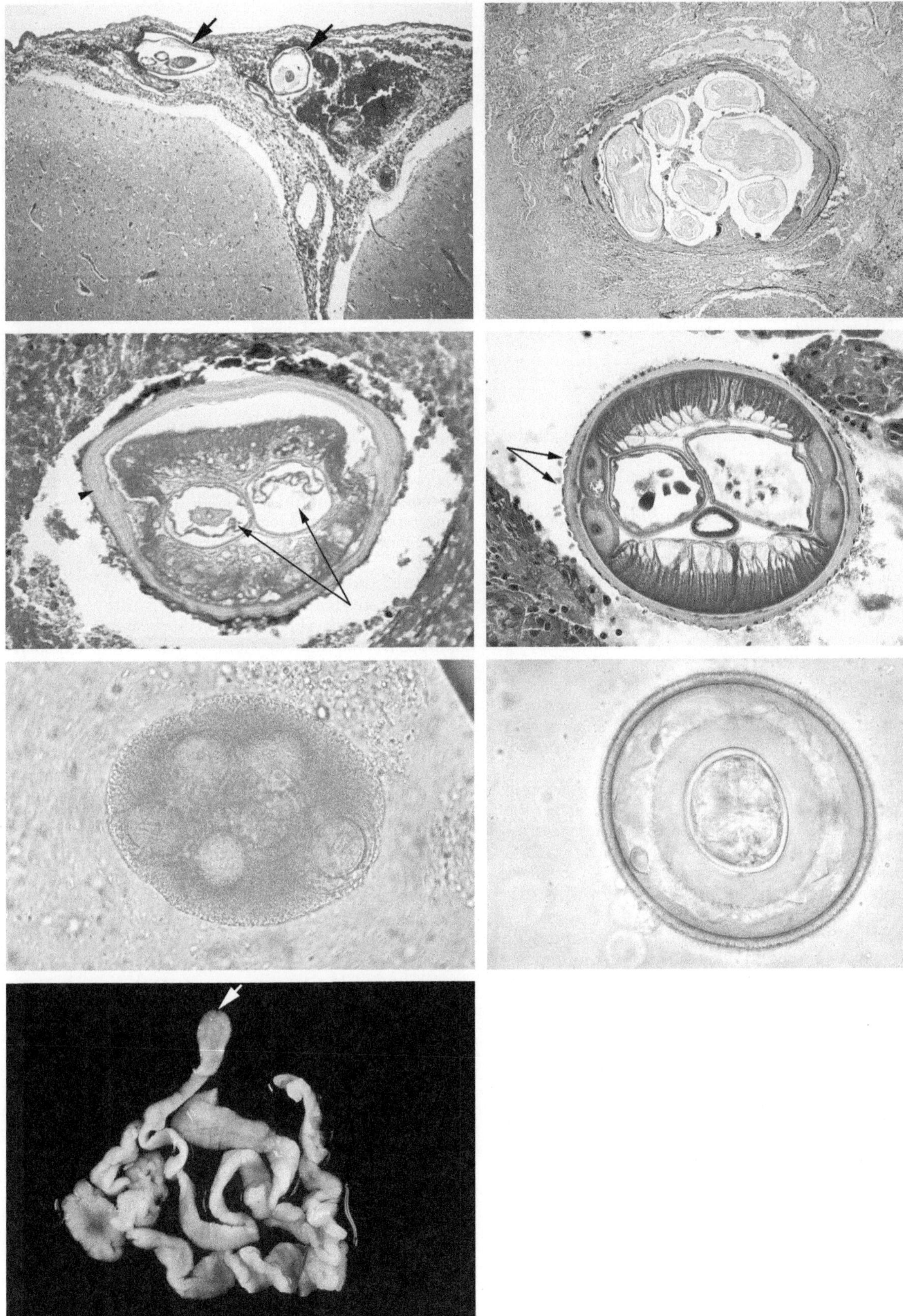

TABLE 1 Other less common nematodes

Organism	Definitive host	Intermediate host(s)/vectors	Disease(s) produced	Method of diagnosis
Zoonotic hookworms (e.g., *Ancylostoma ceylanicum*, *A. caninum*, *A. braziliense*, and *Uncinaria* (*stenocephala*)	Cats, dogs, and hamsters	Not applicable	Cutaneous larva migrans (creeping eruption)	Clinical findings or, rarely, detection of larvae in biopsy sample of skin
Gongylonema species	Various vertebrates	Various beetles	Larva migrans	Clinical findings; excision
Halicephalobus species	None; free living	None; free living	Meningoencephalitis	Biopsy
Dirofilaria species other than *D. immitis*, *D. tenuis*, *D. repens*, *D. ursi*, *D. subdermata*, and *D. striata*	Raccoons (*D. tenuis*), dogs and cats (*D. repens*), bears (*D. ursi*), porcupines (*D. subdermata*), wild cats (*D. striata*)	Mosquitoes, except for *D. ursi*, which is transmitted by black flies	Usually subcutaneous nodules that contain mature, immature, or degenerated worms	Morphological features of the worm in excised tissues (Fig. 10)

since anthelmintic therapy may sometimes exacerbate the symptoms (58). Corticosteroids may be used alone or in combination with anthelmintic therapy (58).

Dirofilaria immitis and Other *Dirofilaria* Species

Taxonomy

The organisms in this group, in the modern classification of biological species, are in clade III (Chromadoria: Spururina) of the Nematoda, in the order Spirurida, and in the family Onchocercidae.

Description of the Agents

The filarial dog heartworm, *Dirofilaria immitis*, has a worldwide distribution; when infections occur in humans, they cause pulmonary dirofilariasis (59). There are a variety of other *Dirofilaria* species that may also accidentally infect humans. *Dirofilaria tenuis* is a raccoon parasite common in the southeast United States; *D. ursi* infects bears in the northern United States and Canada, and *Dirofilaria repens* is a dog parasite restricted to the Old World (60, 61).

Epidemiology, Transmission, and Prevention

Although dogs are the most important host for *D. immitis*, other mammals, such as foxes and bears, are also suitable hosts. The blood of infected suitable hosts contains microfilariae that are released from the adult worm, which resides in the right ventricle of the heart. These are taken into the mosquito during a blood meal, wherein they mature into infective L3 larvae and are capable of transfer to another mammal during a blood meal. The larvae migrate through subcutaneous tissues and eventually enter the bloodstream and the right side of the heart, wherein they mature into adults in a permissive host. Humans, however, are unsuitable or nonpermissive hosts. The worm dies in human infections before it reaches maturity and is swept into the pulmonary arterial circulation. It subsequently becomes lodged in the subsegmental pulmonary arteries and arterioles and causes thrombosis, infarction, inflammation, and eventually a granulomatous reaction surrounded by a wall of fibrous tissue (Fig. 8).

The geographic distribution of disease reflects the prevalence of canine dirofilariasis. The areas of highest prevalence in the United States are in the South, particularly along the Gulf and Atlantic coasts and along the Mississippi River (61). *Dirofilaria immitis* is widely distributed, also occurring throughout South and Central America, Australia, and the South Pacific islands, as well as in parts of Europe, Russia, and Africa (59), Interestingly, dog ownership is not a risk factor for disease. Prevention is centered on the control of zoonotic disease. The use of mosquito repellents, particularly in areas of high endemicity, is also recommended to interrupt transmission.

Clinical Significance

Slightly more than half of the patients with dirofilariasis are asymptomatic. The findings in symptomatic patients are nonspecific symptoms, such as cough, chest pain, hemoptysis, low-grade fever, chills, and malaise (62). Peripheral eosinophilia is present in only 5 to 10% of patients. In addition to pulmonary manifestations, *D. immitis* has also rarely been identified in subcutaneous abscesses, the abdominal cavity, the eyes, and the testes. *Dirofilaria* species other than *D. immitis* are more likely to be found in a subcutaneous location (Table 1). Pampiglione et al. undertook a critical review of human pulmonary dirofilariasis in the Old World and suggested, on the basis of traditional morphologic findings, that the cause of pulmonary dirofilariasis in these geographic regions may more likely be because of a *Dirofilaria* species other than *D. immitis*, namely *D. repens* (63). The nodules caused by *D. immitis* are often discovered by a routine chest radiograph; they must be excised in most instances to exclude malignancy (61). These nodules are usually single, but occasionally two or three nodules may be present.

Direct Examination and Microscopy

The pulmonary nodules produced by *D. immitis* are characteristically small (0.8 to 4.5 cm; mean, 1.9 cm), subpleural, spherical, and well circumscribed. *D. immitis* has a smooth, thick cuticle (5 to 25 μm) with the three distinct layers characteristic of the genus *Dirofilaria*; other *Dirofilaria* species that infect humans have a similar cuticle but with external longitudinal ridges (Fig. 9 and 10). The thick, multilayered cuticle projects inwardly at the lateral chords, forming two prominent, opposing internal longitudinal ridges. The somatic musculature is typically prominent, but the lateral chords are usually poorly preserved. Transverse sections may reveal two large uteri and a much smaller intestine in female worms (Fig. 9); a single reproductive tract and an intestine are present in males. The definitive identification of the worm based on internal structures may be difficult or impossible, given the advanced stage of parasite degeneration in many of these specimens.

The presence of a parasitic worm in a pulmonary artery and in association with a pulmonary infarct, however, is usually sufficient for a diagnosis.

Serologic Tests

Serologic tests to detect antibody to *Dirofilaria* are commercially available from several reference laboratories. Although advances have been made to increase specificity without sacrificing sensitivity, cross-reactivity may occur in patients infected with other nematodes, particularly other filarial worms. As with many serologic assays, a positive test is useful, whereas a negative test does not exclude the possibility of infection.

Treatment

Excision of the nodule is curative. The organism is already dead, so antiparasitic therapy is not necessary.

Baylisascaris procyonis

Taxonomy

Baylisascaris species are in clade III (Chromadoria: Spururina) of the Nematoda, in the order Ascaridida, and in the family Ascarididae in the modern classification of biological species.

Description of the Agent

Baylisascaris procyonis is the roundworm of the raccoon (*Procyon lotor*) and the most important human pathogen of this genus. Although other *Baylisascaris* species exist, these have been only rarely associated with sporadic disease. The adults of *Baylisascaris* are large tan roundworms; the smaller males measure 9 to 11 cm in length, whereas the larger females measure 20 to 22 cm in length (64).

Epidemiology, Transmission, and Prevention

B. procyonis is as widespread as its definitive host, the North American raccoon. Although originally endemic only to North America, raccoons with this parasite have been exported worldwide as zoo animals, as fur-producing animals, or as pets, which is discouraged (64).

Young raccoons usually become infected through the direct ingestion of eggs, which are sometimes adherent to the fur of the mother raccoon. Mature raccoons are more commonly infected through the ingestion of infected animals, such as woodchucks, rabbits, and rodents, which are intermediate hosts that when infected develop larva migrans (65). Interestingly, if the paratenic host does not die of the larva migrans, the disease makes the animal more susceptible to opportunistic predation by raccoons. After ingestion, migration, and maturation, male and female worms develop in the small intestine of the raccoon and mate.

It has been estimated that the adult female produces between 115,000 and 179,000 eggs/worm/day (66). An infected raccoon passes 20,000 to 26,000 eggs per g of feces (EGF), with extremes of more than 250,000 EGF recorded (66). In addition to the high level of egg production, there is an enhanced risk of infection by *B. procyonis* compared with other *Baylisascaris* species because of the behavior of the raccoon host. Raccoons are known to defecate in large piles, which are known as raccoon latrines (66). This combination of large quantities of feces in a single location (i.e., a raccoon latrine), each of which contains high quantities of eggs, makes raccoon latrines a high-risk area for contracting infection.

Transmission occurs through the ingestion of material contaminated with egg-containing raccoon feces. The eggs of *Baylisascaris* are highly resistant to desiccation, remaining viable for years in the environment, long after the physical evidence of the presence of a raccoon latrine has been removed by environmental factors (e.g., rain) (65). Children, particularly male children for some reason, are most commonly infected (64, 65). The feces of raccoons may contain seeds and other objects of temptation for a young child, and pica is a common risk factor for infection (64, 65).

Although control of the local raccoon population is a preventive measure, this is often difficult to achieve, as these animals live and thrive near human habitats. Behaviors that encourage raccoons, such as feeding and uncovered trash bins, should be avoided. Awareness of the medical importance of raccoon latrines and their careful clearing, as well as keeping young children away from such areas, are important preventive measures.

Clinical Significance

B. procyonis readily infects humans and a variety of other animals, causing visceral, ocular, and neural larva migrans. Although less than 10% of the infecting larvae are thought to reach the brain, those that do produce severe disease because of their large size and aggressive migratory behavior (67). Six (40%) infections were fatal in a series of 15 reported patients; seven (47%) patients that survived were characterized as having severe neurologic deficits, and five were blind (65).

The history of a child entering and possibly eating material from a raccoon latrine is of paramount importance but may not be remembered, thought important, or even known by the parents. The presence of peripheral eosinophilia, eosinophilia of the CSF, and deep white matter changes on radiologic imaging are all clues to baylisascariasis in a child with unexplained meningoencephalomyelitis (65, 68, 69). Prompt antihelminthic and antiinflammatory therapy should be given prior to the establishment of a definitive diagnosis (see below), and serologic studies sent for confirmation.

In addition to the devastating presentations described, serologic studies suggest that low-level infections producing subclinical disease, likely from ingestion of a small inoculum, may be more common than is appreciated (64, 70).

Direct Examination and Microscopy

Direct examination and microscopy play a minor role in the prompt clinical diagnosis of baylisascariasis. Occasionally, if a biopsy is performed, then the migrating larvae may be seen. The migrating larvae of *Baylisascaris* are 60 to 80 μm in diameter and have a central intestine that is flanked on each side by a triangular lateral excretory column in midbody transverse section; a single lateral cuticular alae is located on each side of the larva (66). These features are sufficient to differentiate *Baylisascaris* from other causes of larva migrans. Unfortunately, not all biopsy specimens contain larvae, given the migratory nature of the larvae. The autopsy remains important to determine the cause of death for patients with fatal meningoencephalomyelitis of undetermined etiology.

Serologic Tests

Serologic studies are the most important laboratory tools to establish the diagnosis of baylisascariasis. These are available through the Centers for Disease Control and Prevention, as well as through the Department of Veterinary Pathobiology at Purdue University (64). Although these baylisascariasis infections are rare and large studies have not been performed, the serologic assays appear sufficiently sensitive to detect and confirm patients with infection. Importantly, these assays also appear highly specific, having been shown not to cross-react with specimens from patients with larva migrans caused by *Toxocara*.

Treatment

Mortality is high for patients with baylisascariasis, and significant long-term morbidity occurs in most patients who survive a serious clinical infection. Awareness of the possibility of this infection is critical for prompt therapy. Importantly, there is some evidence that treatment with albendazole in the very early stages of infection may reduce or eliminate the possibility of neural larva migrans (66, 71). This therapeutic opportunity, unfortunately, is often missed, and the possibility of this infection is not considered early in the patient evaluation.

The diagnosis, in most instances, is not considered until severe disease is established and other causes of encephalomyelitis have been excluded. Albendazole is recommended at the advanced stage of disease, but even with treatment prognosis is poor; it is often given in conjunction with corticosteroids (65). When ocular larva migrans is the predominant presentation, the direct photocoagulation of the larvae can be performed by an experienced ophthalmologist (65).

Other Less Common Nematodes

There are a number of less common nematodes other than those described here. Some of these and their important associated features are included in Table 1.

LESS COMMON CESTODES

The less common cestodes covered in detail below are *Dipylidium caninum*, commonly known as the dog tapeworm, and *Spirometra* species, the etiologic agent of sparganosis. Descriptions of a few of the other less common cestodes that may infect humans are given below in Table 2.

TABLE 2 Other less common cestodes[a]

Organism	Definitive host(s)	Intermediate host(s)	Disease produced	Diagnostic method
Hymenolepis diminuta, the rat tapeworm	Rats	Insects	Usually asymptomatic; heavy infections resemble heavy *H. nana* infections.	Eggs in the feces (Fig. 12); proglottids disintegrate before fecal passage.
Hymenolepis nana, the dwarf tapeworm[b]	Rats; human-to-human transmission possible	Fleas	This worm, the smallest adult tapeworm that infects humans, produces disease that is usually mild, and patients may be asymptomatic. Massive infections may produce abdominal pain, allergic reactions, anorexia, nausea, diarrhea or constipation, and flatulence.	Identification of characteristic eggs in the stool; proglottids disintegrate and release eggs before they are passed in the stool. The eggs are ovoid, in contrast to those of *H. diminuta*, which are spherical, and have an inner hyaline membrane, a thin egg shell, polar thickenings from which polar filaments arise, and a distinct oncosphere that contains six hooklets.
Less common *Taenia* species				
T. taeniaeformis	Cats	Rodents	Larval stage may infect liver, like cysticercosis.	Demonstration of strobilocercus in histologic sections.
T. multiceps, *T. serialis*	Canids	Sheep, rabbits	Coenurosis, an infection with the coenurus in the central nervous system, eyes, or subcutaneous tissues (like cysticercosis).	Demonstration of the coenurus in histologic sections.
Mesocestoides species	Foxes, dogs, cats, and other mammals	Unknown, possibly reptile or arthropod vectors	Asymptomatic or mild abdominal symptoms.	Detection of gravid proglottid with characteristic parauterine organ. Eggs are usually not present in the stool.
Bertiella species	Primates	Mites and possibly other insects	Asymptomatic or mild abdominal symptoms.	Motile proglottids in the stool, similar to *D. caninum* infection. Eggs within proglottids are not within packets.
Inermicapsifer madagascariensis		Raw sugar cane ingestion has been suggested	Asymptomatic to symptoms similar to *D. caninum* infections.	Motile proglottids in the stool, similar to *D. caninum* infection. Proglottid and egg morphology and number of eggs per packet are used for identification.
Raillietina species	Birds	Insects, slugs, snails	Asymptomatic or symptoms similar to *D. caninum* infections.	Motile proglottids in the stool, similar to *D. caninum* infection. Proglottid and egg morphology and number of eggs per packet are used for identification.

[a]Praziquantel is the treatment of choice for infections with adult tapeworms; it is also effective for treatment of coenurosis. Effective preventive measures are centered on controlling disease in the zoonotic host (e.g., cats or dogs) or controlling the zoonotic hosts themselves (e.g., rats). Controlling intermediate hosts is also effective but may prove more difficult.

[b]This parasite is covered in detail in chapter 148 of this *Manual*.

Dipylidium caninum

Taxonomy

The organisms in this group, in the modern classification of biological species, are in the Cestoda, in the order Cyclophyllidea, and in the family Dipylidiidae.

Description of the Agent

Dipylidium caninum, a common tapeworm of dogs and cats, also commonly infects children (72, 73).

Epidemiology, Transmission, and Prevention

Dipylidiasis occurs throughout the world. This disease, like hymenolepiasis, is transmitted primarily through the ingestion of an infected flea. In the natural cycle, the dog or cat contains the intestinal adult parasite, which releases gravid proglottids. The eggs are ingested by fleas or lice, which are the intermediate hosts. The eggs hatch within the intermediate host, releasing larvae that penetrate the body cavity, where they mature into infective cysticercoid larvae. When an infected intermediate host is ingested, the cysticercoid metacestode larva attaches to the small intestine and matures into an adult tapeworm, completing the cycle. Maturation to the adult tapeworm also occurs in humans when an infected intermediate host is ingested. Prevention is achieved by deworming animals and controlling fleas and lice.

Clinical Significance

Dipylidiasis is usually an innocuous infection. Larger worm burdens may cause weight loss, abdominal pain, failure to thrive, or the appearance of colic, but such severe disease is uncommon. Disease usually comes to the attention of parents and pediatricians when motile, gravid proglottids are seen in the stool. This observation has been mistaken for an *Enterobius* infection, which underscores the importance of laboratory-based parasite identification.

Direct Examination and Microscopy

The proglottids of *D. caninum* resemble a rice grain or cucumber seed on gross examination and may be motile. The presence of two genital pores (*dipylos* means two gates) differentiates this organism from most other cestodes. The genital pores are more readily appreciated with use of a dissecting microscope and compression of the proglottid between two glass slides. The identification may also be achieved by demonstrating the characteristic egg packets (Fig. 11) and/or characteristic eggs that have distinct morphological features (i.e., four envelopes). A fecal examination will likely be negative for eggs or egg packets because intact proglottids are usually passed in the stool. Microdissection or histologic examination of the proglottids will reveal the eggs and egg packets. In addition to the egg packets, the histologic examination of the proglottid will reveal other features common to cestodes, such as a tegument, smooth muscle, and calcareous corpuscles.

Serologic Tests

Serologic tests are not commonly performed because the disease is usually subclinical and unsuspected; the diagnosis is achieved when the proglottids are discovered and examined.

Treatment

Both praziquantel and niclosamide are effective against *D. caninum*. On discovery, examination and treatment of household pets should proceed, as should aggressive flea control.

Spirometra Species

Taxonomy

The organisms in this group, in the modern classification of biological species, are in the Cestoda, in the order Pseudophyllidea, and in the family Diphyllobothriidae.

Description of the Agents

Sparganosis is the infection of humans by L3 plerocercoid larvae of a pseudophyllidean tapeworm (74). The plerocercoid larva in a human host does not reach maturity and is known as a sparganum. The tapeworms that cause sparganosis are *Spirometra mansoni*, *Spirometra mansonoides*, *Spirometra ranarum*, and *Spirometra erinacei*. The precise taxonomic relationship of a cestode known as *Sparganum proliferum* is unclear, but this organism may simply represent a variant of *S. mansonoides* or *S. erinacei*. Additional information concerning this organism can also be found in chapter 148.

Epidemiology, Transmission, and Prevention

Adult *Spirometra* species are widely distributed tapeworms of animals, particularly dogs and cats. The parasitic cycle for these worms begins with the passage of eggs from an infected suitable host. The coracidium that emerges from the egg infects the first intermediate host, a copepod. The second intermediate host, which includes snakes, frogs, and fish, becomes infected by ingesting the infected copepod. The cycle is completed when a permissive (i.e., definitive) host ingests the second intermediate host. Humans are nonpermissive hosts and may become infected by ingesting raw or undercooked meat from a second intermediate host or by drinking contaminated water that contains the infected copepod *Cyclops*. Humans have also become infected by using infected animal flesh (e.g., frog flesh) as a poultice.

Clinical Significance

The results of ingesting a plerocercoid larva depend on both the species of the host and the species of the larva. For example, the ingestion of a plerocercoid larva of *Diphyllobothrium latum* by a human will result in the development of an adult tapeworm, whereas the ingestion of a plerocercoid larva of a *Spirometra* species will result only in the continued existence of the larva (i.e., the sparganum) in the new host (75). This is a situation wherein the human is behaving biologically like a second intermediate or paratenic host. The clinical features of disease are influenced by worm burden (most patients harbor only a single worm), worm location, and worm viability. Spargana migrate, but this migration usually does not cause symptoms. Migration to a subcutaneous location, however, may result in a nodule (40). This nodule may be excised to exclude the possibility of malignancy. Ocular sparganosis, particularly involving the conjunctiva, may result following the application of a folk-medicine poultice that contains raw snake or frog tissues. Inflammation and sometimes calcification ensue after death of the sparganum; when these symptoms occur in the brain, they may cause obstructive hydrocephalus (54). Subcutaneous spargana that become exposed through ulceration have been mistaken for *Dracunculus* in regions where this latter parasite is endemic (40).

Direct Examination and Microscopy

Spargana are flat, ribbon-like worms that superficially resemble adult tapeworms (Fig. 13). Closer inspection demonstrates an immature anterior end without hooklets; a cleft or ventral groove, termed a bothrium, is present (Fig. 13) (76).

Mature proglottids are not produced. Histopathologic examination of the sparganum demonstrates calcareous corpuscles characteristic of a cestode. Developed internal organs are not seen, but rather, irregularly scattered smooth muscle fibers and excretory ducts are seen in a loose stroma.

Serologic Tests

If the diagnosis is not suspected, it is usually made when a viable sparganum is unexpectedly discovered during surgery. The gross findings are largely diagnostic, but histopathologic examination can be used for confirmation. In such instances, serology is not useful. However, if this disease is clinically suspected, the diagnosis may be achieved through the combination of radiology and serology (77). Serologic tests for *Spirometra* are not commercially available, so sera should be sent to specialized centers.

Treatment

Medical therapy is currently deemed unsuitable for the treatment of sparganosis because the plerocercoid larva is resistant to praziquantel. Complete surgical excision is recommended. An incomplete excision, particularly if the anterior end of the larva remains in the tissue, may result in continued growth of the organism (1).

SUMMARY

There are a wide variety of less commonly encountered helminthic parasites, which may be nematodes, cestodes, or trematodes. The diseases caused by these parasites are interesting and demonstrate their highly evolved life cycles and the complex interactions with their hosts. Diseases produced range from subclinical, e.g., dipylidiasis, to possibly life threatening, e.g., baylisascariasis. In many instances, the disease occurs only in a particular geographic area, which is largely determined by the biological ranges of the definitive and intermediate hosts. Dietary and folk-medicine customs are also important in the prevalence of human disease, as many of these are associated with the ingestion or application of raw animal products. The treatment of these parasites varies depending on the infectious agent, but common preventive measures may significantly diminish the transmission of many of these parasitic diseases. These measures include the zoonotic control of parasitic disease in animal hosts and the vectors of transmission, washing of fruits and vegetables, access to clean drinking water, and thorough cooking of meats before consumption.

REFERENCES

1. **Armed Forces Institute of Pathology.** 2000. *Pathology of Infectious Diseases*, vol 1. Armed Forces Institute of Pathology, Washington, DC.
2. **Procop GW, Pritt BS (ed).** 2015. *Pathology of Infectious Diseases*. Elsevier Saunders, Philadelphia, PA.
3. **Pravettoni V, Primavesi L, Piantanida M.** 2012. *Anisakis simplex*: current knowledge. *Eur Ann Allergy Clin Immunol* **44:**150–156.
4. **Shweiki E, Rittenhouse DW, Ochoa JE, Punja VP, Zubair MH, Baliff JP.** 2014. Acute small-bowel obstruction from intestinal anisakiasis after the ingestion of raw clams; documenting a new method of marine-to-human parasitic transmission. *Open Forum Infect Dis*. **26:**ofu087.
5. **Bucci C, Gallotta S, Morra I, Fortunato A, Ciacci C, Iovino P.** 2013. *Anisakis*, just think about it in an emergency! *Int J Infect Dis* **17:**e1071–e1072.
6. **Moneo I, Carballeda-Sangiao N, González-Muñoz M.** 2017. New perspectives on the diagnosis of allergy to *Anisakis* spp. *Curr Allergy Asthma Rep* **17:**27.
7. **Tsukui M, Morimoto N, Kurata H, Sunada F.** 2016. Asymptomatic anisakiasis of the colon incidentally diagnosed and treated during colonoscopy by retroflexion in the ascending colon. *J Rural Med* **11:**73–75.
8. **Amir A, Ngui R, Ismail WH, Wong KT, Ong JS, Lim YA, Lau YL, Mahmud R.** 2016. Anisakiasis causing acute dysentery in Malaysia. *Am J Trop Med Hyg* **95:**410–412.
9. **Takano K, Okuni T, Murayama K, Himi T.** 2016. A case study of Anisakiasis in the palatine tonsils. *Adv Otorhinolaryngol* **77:**125–127.
10. **Daschner A, Pascual CY.** 2005. *Anisakis simplex*: sensitization and clinical allergy. *Curr Opin Allergy Clin Immunol* **5:**281–285.
11. **Madi L, Ali M, Legace-Wiens P, Duerksen DR.** 2013. Gastrointestinal manifestations and management of anisakiasis. *Can J Gastroenterol* **27:**126–127.
12. **Falcão H, Lunet N, Neves E, Iglésias I, Barros H.** 2008. *Anisakis simplex* as a risk factor for relapsing acute urticaria: a case-control study. *J Epidemiol Community Health* **62:**634–637.
13. **Chen Q, Yu HQ, Lun ZR, Chen XG, Song HQ, Lin RQ, Zhu XQ.** 2008. Specific PCR assays for the identification of common anisakid nematodes with zoonotic potential. *Parasitol Res* **104:**79–84.
14. **Toyoda H, Tanaka K.** 2016. Intestinal anisakiasis treated successfully with prednisolone and olopatadine hydrochloride. *Case Rep Gastroenterol* **10:**30–35.
15. **Knopp S, Steinmann P, Keiser J, Utzinger J.** 2012. Nematode infections: soil-transmitted helminths and trichinella. *Infect Dis Clin North Am* **26:**341–358.
16. **Murrell KD, Pozio E.** 2011. Worldwide occurrence and impact of human trichinellosis, 1986–2009. *Emerg Infect Dis* **17:**2194–2202.
17. **Riva E, Fiel C, Bernat G, Muchiut S, Steffan P.** 2017. Studies on vertical transmission of *Trichinella spiralis* in experimentally infected guinea pigs (*Cavia porcellus*). *Parasitol Res* **116:**2271–2276.
18. **Saracino MP, Calcagno MA, Beauche EB, Garnier A, Vila CC, Granchetti H, Taus MR, Venturiello SM.** 2016. *Trichinella spiralis* infection and transplacental passage in human pregnancy. *Vet Parasitol* **231:**2–7.
19. **Taher EE, Méabed EMH, El Akkad DMH, Kamel NO, Sabry MA.** 2017. Modified dot-ELISA for diagnosis of human trichinellosis. *Exp Parasitol* **177:**40–46.
20. **Cuttell L, Corley SW, Gray CP, Vanderlinde PB, Jackson LA, Traub RJ.** 2012. Real-time PCR as a surveillance tool for the detection of *Trichinella* infection in muscle samples from wildlife. *Vet Parasitol* **188:**285–293.
21. **Mayer-Scholl A, Murugaiyan J, Neumann J, Bahn P, Reckinger S, Nöckler K.** 2016. Rapid identification of the foodborne pathogen *Trichinella* spp. by matrix-assisted laser desorption/ionization mass spectrometry. *PLoS One* **11:**e0152062.
22. **García A, Barrera MG, Piccirilli G, Vasconi MD, Di Masso RJ, Leonardi D, Hinrichsen LI, Lamas MC.** 2013. Novel albendazole formulations given during the intestinal phase of *Trichinella spiralis* infection reduce effectively parasitic muscle burden in mice. *Parasitol Int* **62:**568–570.
23. **Rubinsky-Elefant G, Hirata CE, Yamamoto JH, Ferreira MU.** 2010. Human toxocariasis: diagnosis, worldwide seroprevalences and clinical expression of the systemic and ocular forms. *Ann Trop Med Parasitol* **104:**3–23.
24. **Won KY, Kruszon-Moran D, Schantz PM, Jones JL.** 2008. National seroprevalence and risk factors for zoonotic *Toxocara* spp. infection. *Am J Trop Med Hyg* **79:**552–557.
25. **Nijsse R, Ploeger HW, Wagenaar JA, Mughini-Gras L.** 2015. *Toxocara canis* in household dogs: prevalence, risk factors and owners' attitude towards deworming. *Parasitol Res* **114:**561–569.
26. **Nijsse R, Ploeger HW, Wagenaar JA, Mughini-Gras L.** 2016. Prevalence and risk factors for patent *Toxocara* infections in cats and cat owners' attitude towards deworming. *Parasitol Res* **115:**4519–4525.
27. **Jacobs DE, Fisher MA.** 1993. Recent developments in the chemotherapy of *Toxocara canis* infection in puppies and the prevention of toxocariasis, p 111–116. *In* Lewis JW, Maizels RM (ed), *Toxocara and Toxocariasis: Clinical, Epidemiological and Molecular Perspectives*. Institute of Biology, London, United Kingdom.

28. **Taira K, Saeed I, Permin A, Kapel CM.** 2004. Zoonotic risk of *Toxocara canis* infection through consumption of pig or poultry viscera. *Vet Parasitol* **121:**115–124.
29. **Shields JA.** 1984. Ocular toxocariasis. A review. *Surv Ophthalmol* **28:**361–381.
30. **Nicoletti A.** 2013. Toxocariasis. *Handb Clin Neurol* **114:**217–228.
31. **Nichols RL.** 1956. The etiology of visceral Larva migrans. II. Comparative larval morphology of *Ascaris lumbricoides, Necator americanus, Strongyloides stercoralis* and *Ancylostoma caninum*. *J Parasitol* **42**(4 Section 1):363–399.
32. **Cojocariu IE, Bahnea R, Luca C, Leca D, Luca M.** 2012. Clinical and biological features of toxocariasis. *Rev Med Chir Soc Med Nat Iasi* **116:**1162–1165.
33. **Hombu A, Yoshida A, Kikuchi T, Nagayasu E, Kuroki M, Maruyama H.** 2017. Treatment of larva migrans syndrome with long-term administration of albendazole. *J Microbiol Immunol Infect* **pii:**S1684-1182(17)30142-1.
34. **Good B, Holland CV, Taylor MR, Larragy J, Moriarty P, O'Regan M.** 2004. Ocular toxocariasis in schoolchildren. *Clin Infect Dis* **39:**173–178.
35. **Hopkins DR, Ruiz-Tiben E, Eberhard ML, Roy SL, Weiss AJ, Centers for Disease Control and Prevention.** 2016. Progress toward global eradication of dracunculiasis—January 2015–June 2016. *MMWR Morb Mortal Wkly Rep* **65:**1112–1116.
36. **Eberhard ML, Cleveland CA, Zirimwabagabo H, Yabsley MJ, Ouakou PT, Ruiz-Tiben E.** 2016. Guinea worm (*Dracunculus medinensis*) infection in a wild-caught frog, Chad. *Emerg Infect Dis* **22:**1961–1962.
37. **Eberhard ML, Yabsley MJ, Zirimwabagabo H, Bishop H, Cleveland CA, Maerz JC, Bringolf R, Ruiz-Tiben E.** 2016. Possible role of fish and frogs as paratenic hosts of *Dracunculus medinensis*, Chad. *Emerg Infect Dis* **22:**1428–1430.
38. **Chippaux JP.** 1991. Mebendazole treatment of dracunculiasis. *Trans R Soc Trop Med Hyg* **85:**280.
39. **Hesse AA, Nouri A, Hassan HS, Hashish AA.** 2012. Parasitic infestations requiring surgical interventions. *Semin Pediatr Surg* **21:**142–150.
40. **Eberhard ML, Thiele EA, Yembo GE, Yibi MS, Cama VA, Ruiz-Tiben E.** 2015. Thirty-seven human cases of sparganosis from Ethiopia and South Sudan caused by *Spirometra* spp. *Am J Trop Med Hyg* **93:**350–355.
41. **Moravec F.** 2001. Redescription and systematic status of *Capillaria philippinensis*, an intestinal parasite of human beings. *J Parasitol* **87:**161–164.
42. **Cross JH.** 1992. Intestinal capillariasis. *Clin Microbiol Rev* **5:**120–129.
43. **Attia RA, Tolba ME, Yones DA, Bakir HY, Eldeek HE, Kamel S.** 2012. *Capillaria philippinensis* in Upper Egypt: has it become endemic? *Am J Trop Med Hyg* **86:**126–133.
44. **Saichua P, Nithikathkul C, Kaewpitoon N.** 2008. Human intestinal capillariasis in Thailand. *World J Gastroenterol* **14:**506–510.
45. **Sadaow L, Sanpool O, Intapan PM, Sukeepaisarnjaroen W, Prasongdee TK, Maleewong W.** 2017. A hospital-based study of intestinal capillariasis in Thailand: clinical features, potential clues for diagnosis, and epidemiological characteristics of 85 patients. *Am J Trop Med Hyg* **98:**27–31.
46. **el-Karaksy H, el-Shabrawi M, Mohsen N, Kotb M, el-Koofy N, el-Deeb N.** 2004. *Capillaria philippinensis*: a cause of fatal diarrhea in one of two infected Egyptian sisters. *J Trop Pediatr* **50:**57–60.
47. **Wongsawasdi L, Ukarapol N, Lertprasertsuk N.** 2002. The endoscopic diagnosis of intestinal capillariasis in a child: a case report. *Southeast Asian J Trop Med Public Health* **33:**730–732.
48. **Canlas B, Cabrera B, Davis U.** 1967. Human intestinal capillariasis. 2. Pathological features. *Acta Med Philipp* **4:**84–91.
49. **Intapan PM, Maleewong W, Sukeepaisarnjaroen W, Morakote N.** 2010. An enzyme-linked immunosorbent assay as screening tool for human intestinal capillariasis. *Southeast Asian J Trop Med Public Health* **41:**298–305.
50. **Miyazaki I.** 1960. On the genus *Gnathostoma* and human gnathostomiasis, with special reference to Japan. *Exp Parasitol* **9:**338–370.
51. **Herman JS, Chiodini PL.** 2009. Gnathostomiasis, another emerging imported disease. *Clin Microbiol Rev* **22:**484–492.
52. **High WA, Bravo FG.** 2007. Emerging diseases in tropical dermatology. *Adv Dermatol* **23:**335–350.
53. **Pillai GS, Kumar A, Radhakrishnan N, Maniyelil J, Shafi T, Dinesh KR, Karim S.** 2012. Intraocular gnathostomiasis: report of a case and review of literature. *Am J Trop Med Hyg* **86:**620–623.
54. **Sawanyawisuth K, Chotmongkol V.** 2013. Eosinophilic meningitis. *Handb Clin Neurol* **114:**207–215.
55. **Bhende M, Biswas J, Gopal L.** 2005. Ultrasound biomicroscopy in the diagnosis and management of intraocular gnathostomiasis. *Am J Ophthalmol* **140:**140–142.
56. **Ramirez-Avila L, Slome S, Schuster FL, Gavali S, Schantz PM, Sejvar J, Glaser CA.** 2009. Eosinophilic meningitis due to *Angiostrongylus* and *Gnathostoma* species. *Clin Infect Dis* **48:**322–327.
57. **Eamsobhana P, Yong HS.** 2009. Immunological diagnosis of human angiostrongyliasis due to *Angiostrongylus cantonensis* (Nematoda: angiostrongylidae). *Int J Infect Dis* **13:**425–431.
58. **Hidelaratchi MD, Riffsy MT, Wijesekera JC.** 2005. A case of eosinophilic meningitis following monitor lizard meat consumption, exacerbated by anthelminthics. *Ceylon Med J* **50:**84–86.
59. **Simón F, Siles-Lucas M, Morchón R, González-Miguel J, Mellado I, Carretón E, Montoya-Alonso JA.** 2012. Human and animal dirofilariasis: the emergence of a zoonotic mosaic. *Clin Microbiol Rev* **25:**507–544.
60. **Canestri Trotti G, Pampiglione S, Rivasi F.** 1997. The species of the genus *Dirofilaria*, Railliet & Henry, 1911. *Parassitologia* **39:**369–374.
61. **Shah MK.** 1999. Human pulmonary dirofilariasis: review of the literature. *South Med J* **92:**276–279.
62. **Chitkara RK, Sarinas PS.** 1997. *Dirofilaria*, visceral larva migrans, and tropical pulmonary eosinophilia. *Semin Respir Infect* **12:**138–148.
63. **Pampiglione S, Rivasi F, Gustinelli A.** 2009. Dirofilarial human cases in the Old World, attributed to *Dirofilaria immitis*: a critical analysis. *Histopathology* **54:**192–204.
64. **Gavin PJ, Kazacos KR, Shulman ST.** 2005. Baylisascariasis. *Clin Microbiol Rev* **18:**703–718.
65. **Murray WJ, Kazacos KR.** 2004. Raccoon roundworm encephalitis. *Clin Infect Dis* **39:**1484–1492.
66. **Kazacos KR.** 2001. *Baylisascaris procyonis* and related species, p 301–341. *In* Samuels WM, Pybus MJ, Kocans AA (ed), *Parasitic Diseases of Wild Mammals*, 2nd ed. Iowa State University Press, Ames, IA.
67. **Kazacos KR, Boyce WM.** 1989. *Baylisascaris* larva migrans. *J Am Vet Med Assoc* **195:**894–903.
68. **Centers for Disease Control.** 2000. Raccoon roundworm encephalitis—Chicago, Illinois, and Los Angeles, California. *MMWR Morb Mortal Wkly Rep* **50:**1153–1155.
69. **Fox AS, Kazacos DR, Gould NS, Heydemann PT, Thomas C, Boyer KM.** 1985. Fatal eosinophilic meningoencephalitis and visceral larva migrans caused by the raccoon ascarid *Baylisascaris procyonis*. *N Engl J Med* **312:**1619–1623.
70. **Cunningham CK, Kazacos KR, McMillan JA, Lucas JA, McAuley JB, Wozniak EJ, Weiner LB.** 1994. Diagnosis and management of *Baylisascaris procyonis* infection in an infant with nonfatal meningoencephalitis. *Clin Infect Dis* **18:**868–872.
71. **Kazacos KR.** 2000. Protecting children from helminthic zoonoses. *Contemp Pediatr* **17**(Supple):1–24.
72. **Chappell CL, Enos JP, Penn HM.** 1990. *Dipylidium caninum*, an underrecognized infection in infants and children. *Pediatr Infect Dis J* **9:**745–747.
73. **Turner JA.** 1962. Human dipylidiasis (dog tapeworm infection) in the United States. *J Pediatr* **61:**763–768.
74. **Nakamura T, Hara M, Matsuoka M, Kawabata M, Tsuji M.** 1990. Human proliferative sparganosis. A new Japanese case. *Am J Clin Pathol* **94:**224–228.
75. **Dorny P, Praet N, Deckers N, Gabriel S.** 2009. Emerging food-borne parasites. *Vet Parasitol* **163:**196–206.
76. **Noya O, Alarcón de Noya B, Arrechedera H, Torres J, Argüello C.** 1992. *Sparganum proliferum*: an overview of its structure and ultrastructure. *Int J Parasitol* **22:**631–640.
77. **Rahman M, Lee EG, Bae YA.** 2011. Two-dimensional immunoblot analysis of antigenic proteins of *Spirometra plerocercoid* recognized by human patient sera. *Parasitol Int* **60:**139–143.

Arthropods of Medical Importance

SAM R. TELFORD III AND BLAINE A. MATHISON

151

Arthropods comprise a diverse group of invertebrate animals, united in a common body theme (bauplan) of a jointed, chitinous exoskeleton. Four major extant groupings contain those arthropods of medical importance: hexapods (insects), arachnids, crustaceans, and myriapods (e.g., millipedes and centipedes). All arthropod classes have existed for hundreds of millions of years, thereby providing ample opportunity for life history traits such as parasitism to independently evolve, and evolve multiple times, in each class.

Medically important arthropods have long been considered to mainly comprise ectoparasites, parasites that limit their activities to the skin. Parasitism, however, is only one of several associations that comprise the interaction of arthropods of medical importance with humans. Arthropods may actively defend themselves against predation (crushing or swatting) by biting, stinging, piercing, or secreting noxious chemicals. Such defenses would operate regardless of the attacker, be it human or other arthropod. Passive modes of defense may inadvertently affect humans, such as irritation after brushing the urticarial hairs of certain caterpillars. Arthropods may also be medically important due to indirect effects: fear of insects, delusion of parasitosis, or allergy due to dust mites. The various modes by which arthropods may affect human health thus reflect the diversity of these animals, but there are very few instances where it may be argued that natural selection favored the reproduction of those that focused on causing misery. Accordingly, arthropods should be viewed as a normal part of the environment that under individual circumstances may cause pathology. In addition, because of their ubiquity, spurious associations with pathology are common.

ARTHROPODS AS VECTORS

Arthropods are thought of by many in clinical settings with respect to their role as vectors, transmitters of infectious agents including viruses, bacteria, protozoa, and helminths. Infectious agents may have an obligate relationship with an arthropod (biological transmission) or may simply contaminate an arthropod (mechanical transmission). Malaria parasites undergo a complex developmental cycle within certain mosquitoes and could not perpetuate without them. In contrast, the agent of trachoma (*Chlamydia trachomatis*) is found on the external surfaces of eye gnats and flies (1) and may be transferred between hosts by the act of landing and crawling, but *C. trachomatis* more commonly perpetuates by direct contact of hosts. Mechanical transmission of an infectious agent is dependent on its stability and quantum of infection. HIV, for example, does not survive long outside of the body, and the femtoliter or so of material that may contaminate the mouthparts of a mosquito would not contain enough viable lymphocytes with HIV to initiate infection (2); thus, mosquitoes have never been epidemiologically linked with HIV transmission even though mosquitoes and other hematophagous arthropods obviously feed on viremic individuals.

There are five major groups of vectors: the Diptera (flies and mosquitoes), Hemiptera (kissing bugs), Siphonaptera (fleas), Psocodea (lice), and Acarines (ticks and mites). The general life history strategies for each group provide the basis for understanding vectorial capacity, which is the sum of physiological and ecological attributes that allow transmission. Specific vector-pathogen relationships are discussed in detail in other chapters in this *Manual* focusing on the respective agents but are succinctly summarized here in Table 1.

Diptera

The dipteran vectors are winged insects that include mosquitoes, sand flies, black flies, gnats, horse/deer flies, and tsetse flies. They range in size from minute (ceratopogonid midges less than 2 mm in length) to large (horse flies more than 2 cm in length). Unlike other winged insects, dipterans have only one functional pair of wings. Those that take blood meals as adult females may serve as vectors. Blood meals are used for nutrition to produce eggs (anautogeny); once those eggs are laid, another blood meal may be taken and more eggs produced. Thus, unless a mosquito inherits infection (transovarial or vertical transmission), the first blood meal infects it and the second allows the agent to be transmitted; under favorable environmental circumstances, a mosquito may survive for several weeks and take more than two blood meals. Both male and female flies and mosquitoes also require sugar meals (usually from plant nectar), but sugar meals can result in reproduction only in certain species (autogeny).

Eggs are laid in water or within detritus. Vermiform larvae emerge from the eggs, and develop through several stages (instars) in water or detritus, feeding on organic material or bacteria, culminating in pupae from which emerge new adults, thereby undergoing complete

TABLE 1 Summary of the major arthropod genera serving as vectors or scalars of infectious agents (not an exhaustive list)

Arthropod(s)	Etiologic agent(s)	Disease
Crustacea		
Decapods	*Paragonimus*	Paragonimiasis
Copepods	*Spirometra* sp.	Sparganosis
	Dracunculus medinensis	Guinea worm disease
	Gnathostoma spinigerum	Gnathostomiasis
Insecta		
Psocodea		
Pediculus	*Rickettsia prowazekii*	Epidemic typhus
	Bartonella quintana	Trench fever
	Borrelia recurrentis	Epidemic relapsing fever
Siphonaptera		
Xenopsylla, Nosopsyllus	*Yersinia pestis*	Plague
	Rickettsia typhi	Murine typhus
	Hymenolepis diminuta	Rat tapeworm
Pulex, Oropsylla	*Y. pestis*	Plague
Ctenocephalides	*Dipylidium caninum*	Dog tapeworm disease
Hemiptera		
Panstrongylus, Rhodnius, Triatoma	*Trypanosoma cruzi*	Chagas disease
Diptera		
Aedes	*Wuchereria, Brugia*	Filariasis
	Flaviviruses	Dengue, yellow fever
	Other arboviruses	Encephalitis
Anopheles	*Plasmodium*	Malaria
	Wuchereria, Brugia	Filariasis
	Arboviruses	Encephalitis
Culex	*Wuchereria*	Filariasis
	Arboviruses	Encephalitis
Culicoides	*Mansonella*	Filariasis
Glossina	*Trypanosoma brucei*	African sleeping sickness
Chrysops	*Loa loa*	Loiasis
	Francisella tularensis	Tularemia
Simulium	*Onchocerca volvulus*	Onchocerciasis
	Mansonella ozzardi	Filariasis
Phlebotomus, Lutzomyia	*Leishmania*	Leishmaniasis
	Bartonella bacilliformis	Bartonellosis
	Phlebovirus	Sandfly fever
Arachnida		
Acari (ticks)		
Ixodes	*Borrelia burgdorferi*	Lyme disease
	Anaplasma phagocytophilum	Human granulocytic ehrlichiosis
	Rickettsia conorii	Boutonneuse fever
	Babesia	Babesiosis
Dermacentor	*Rickettsia rickettsii*	Rocky Mountain spotted fever
	F. tularensis	Tularemia
	Coltivirus	Colorado tick fever
	Flavivirus	Omsk hemorrhagic fever
Amblyomma	*R. rickettsii*	Rocky Mountain spotted fever
	F. tularensis	Tularemia
	Ehrlichia chaffeensis	Human monocytic ehrlichiosis
Hyalomma	Nairovirus	Crimean-Congo hemorrhagic fever
Rhipicephalus	*Rickettsia conorii*	Boutonneuse fever
	R. rickettsii	Rocky Mountain spotted fever
Ornithodoros	*Borrelia*	Relapsing fever
Acari (mites)		
Leptotrombidium	*Orientia tsutsugamushi*	Scrub typhus
Liponyssoides	*Rickettsia akari*	Rickettsialpox

metamorphosis (holometabolous development). Depending on the species and ambient temperature, the duration of the dipteran life cycle may be as short as a week or so. Tsetse flies are an unusual exception to this pattern and produce only one advanced larva for each blood meal, with the larva nourished internally from milk gland analogs during a gestation of several weeks (3). This large maternal investment in offspring makes adulticiding (trapping, spraying) very effective in reducing tsetse populations and thereby reducing the transmission of the agents of sleeping sickness.

The Diptera are only transiently associated with a blood meal source. Host-seeking cues include body heat, carbon dioxide (exhaled by the host), mechanical vibrations, and lactic acid and other skin-associated compounds. The flies visually seek hosts with their compound eyes, mainly larger dark-colored objects with movement, but proximal odorant cues associated with a host seem to be required to initiate feeding. The widely used repellent DEET (diethyltoluamide) works by modulating the odor-gaited ion channel formed by the dipteran odorant receptor complex on the antennae (4). Once a host has been identified, feeding is initiated and completed within minutes. Sand flies, black flies, and mosquitoes have a diverse salivary armamentarium of pharmacologically active substances that promote finding and removing blood. During probing, antihemostatic and anti-inflammatory chemicals are secreted into the feeding channel created in the epidermis. Probing lacerates capillaries, and the ADP that is released from damaged endothelial cells promotes platelet activation, but by secreting an apyrase that cleaves ADP into a monophosphate, platelet aggregation is greatly reduced during blood feeding. In addition, local inflammatory processes are temporarily diminished due to secretion of chemicals such as prostaglandin E2 (5). Thus, the first few bites from a given species remain unnoticed by the host, although factors in the saliva of black flies may leave an egg-sized lump that is hot to the touch at the site of their bites. Such lumps may persist for several days and may be accompanied by low-grade fever. Such "black fly fever" should not be misinterpreted as infection; it resolves on its own without treatment.

The variety of proteins that are deposited within skin during vector feeding are the basis for hypersensitivity reactions, mainly itch, in hosts that are exposed to bites more than once over the course of weeks. Repeated exposure over months may lead to tolerance and a return to failing to react to bites. Although much work remains to be done, there appears to be some cross-reactivity between salivary products from different groups of vectors so that some individuals may equally react to the bites of mosquitoes, bugs, or ticks.

The blood-feeding flies have cruder salivary tools, reflecting their less elegant way of feeding, which usually involves scraping the skin with a roughened maxilla and feeding from the pooled blood or lymph. Accordingly, fly bites are more painful regardless of prior exposure, and few flies successfully engorge to repletion on humans.

Freshly blood-fed dipterans seek a resting place for diuresis and digestion, usually the nearest vertical surface. This behavior renders those species that bite within houses susceptible to control by indoor residual insecticide spraying.

The transient nature of infestation by blood-feeding dipterans means that few specimens are submitted to clinical laboratories. Other than analyses related to confirming the diagnosis of a vector-borne infection, dipterans come to the attention of laboratorians for issues related to hypersensitivity or for myiasis (see below).

Hemiptera

The only hemipterans that serve as vectors are the kissing, or reduviid, bugs, which belong to a diverse and speciose order of minute to large insects with compound eyes, antennae, sucking mouthparts, two pairs of wings (one delicate pair hidden under an outer pair of more robust ones), and a segmented abdomen. All are easily seen without magnification, adult bed bugs being roughly 1 cm in length, and adult triatomines ranging in size from 1 cm to more than 5 cm. Small numbers of eggs are produced by females, from which emerge miniature versions of the adults. These nymphs undergo an incomplete metamorphosis (hemimetabolous development), with development through 5 nymphal stages, each one requiring a blood meal to proceed. The full duration of the life cycle can be as short as 3 months or as long as 2 years. Reduviid bugs are cryptic, living within cracks of mud walls or other narrow, confined spaces. They serve as vectors of trypanosomes (*Trypanosoma cruzi*, the agent of Chagas disease, and *Trypanosoma rangeli*, an apparently nonpathogenic trypanosome that is often cotransmitted with *T. cruzi*) in the New World. *Triatoma rubrofasciata* transmits a trypanosome that infects monkeys in Southeast Asia, but to date there is no known bug-transmitted trypanosomiasis of humans in the Palearctic. Interestingly, there are good natural cycles of enzootic *T. cruzi* transmission within the United States from California through virtually all of the southern-central states, north to Maryland, but only rare human cases of autochthonous Chagas disease are reported. Two factors account for this paradox: people live in well-made houses that are less likely to have infestations of bugs, and more importantly, the main southern U.S. vector, *Triatoma sanguisuga*, does not defecate on the host while feeding (6). Transmission of *T. cruzi* to humans requires contamination of the site of the bite or mucosa by trypanosomes that are excreted in the bug feces, although recent outbreaks have been reported in Brazil which resulted from drinking sugar cane juice contaminated with reduviid excreta (7).

As with mosquitoes, salivary products from reduviids contain a variety of pharmacologically active compounds. Unlike those of mosquitoes, repeated reduviid feedings may cause a dangerous anaphylactoid reaction in residents of houses where the bugs are common. Scientists working with reduviid bugs often need to carry an epinephrine injector with them due to their propensity for feeding their colonies on themselves, thereby receiving large doses of salivary antigens.

Although it is possible that a true reduviid bug (Fig. 1) may be presented by a patient for identification in clinical settings outside of Latin America, it is more likely that such specimens are related heteropterans such as assassin bugs, which are insect predators, or the plant-feeding stink bugs, chinch bugs, harlequin bugs, or squash bugs. Assassin bugs may inflict extremely painful wounds by their piercing mouthparts, but these require only typical first aid measures and perhaps a booster of tetanus toxoid given the

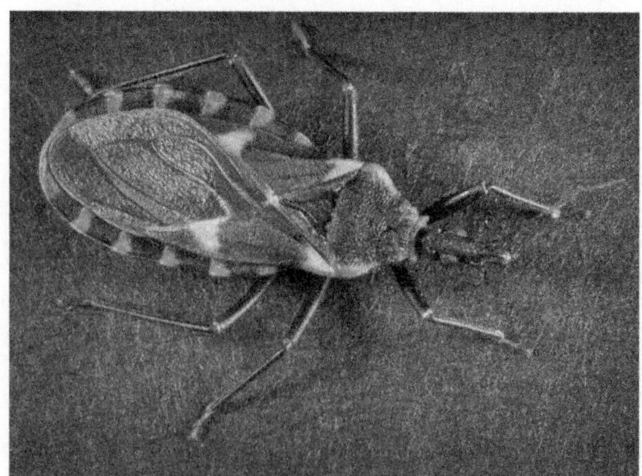

FIGURE 1 Reduviid bug (*Triatoma sanguisuga*). All reduviid bugs have a similar bauplan, with a dorsoventrally flattened body (often appearing crimped at the edge), folded wings, and "cone" nose. (Image courtesy of the CDC-DPDx.)

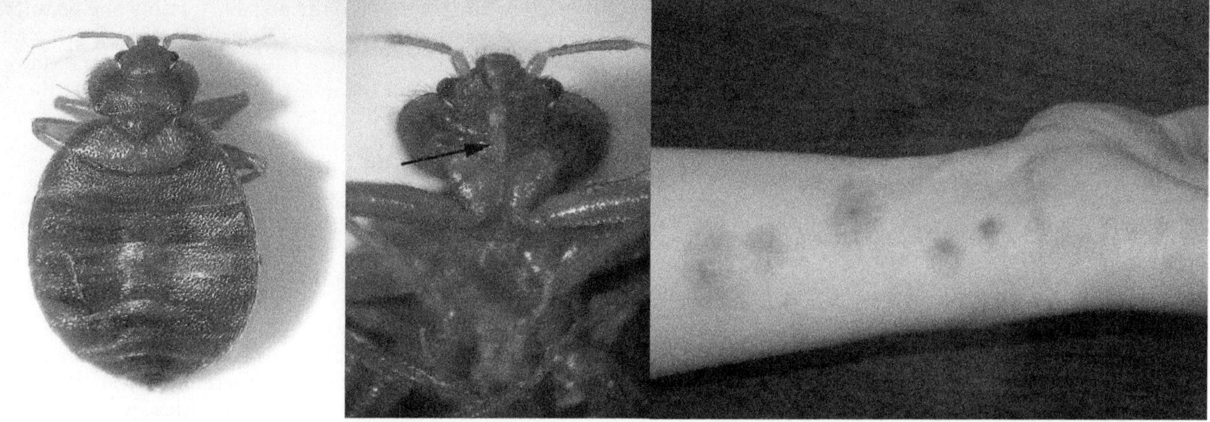

FIGURE 2 Bed bug, *Cimex lectularius*. Left panel, dorsal view; middle panel, ventral view showing piercing/sucking mouthparts (from reference 43, reproduced with permission). Right panel, arm with immediate-type hypersensitivity reaction to bed bug bites acquired in a four-star hotel in Dupont Circle, Washington, DC, December 2005.

depth of the puncture wound (probosces range in length from 3 to 8 mm). The plant feeders may issue noxious secretions, which may taste bad if accidentally ingested (from a bug that infested a fruit or vegetable that was eaten directly from the vine) but are otherwise not a cause for concern.

Bed bugs (*Cimex lectularius*, *Cimex hemipterus*) are hemipterans but are not known to serve as vectors for any pathogen. These bugs with short broad heads, oval bodies, and four-jointed antennae undergo incomplete metamorphosis with five nymphal stages, each requiring a blood meal to develop. The duration of the life cycle is roughly 6 to 8 weeks but may be as long as 11 months, depending on temperature and humidity; they may survive for months without feeding. They are small, 5 mm or less in length as adults (Fig. 2). They are cryptic and require hiding places such as cracks in walls, mattress foundations, or rattan furniture. At night, bed bugs emerge and infest sleeping people, taking 10 to 20 minutes for engorgement. Feeding is often interrupted by the movements of people during their sleep, so multiple bites may result from a single bed bug (Fig. 2). Blood meals may be taken every week or so, depending on the life cycle stage, with batches of 10 to 50 eggs laid; one female may lay 200 to 500 eggs in her life. Repeated exposure to bed bug bites may lead to anaphylactic reactions. Various laboratory studies have reported the survival of diverse agents such as HIV, hepatitis B virus, *Francisella tularensis*, and West Nile virus in artificially infected bed bugs. Epidemiologically, bed bugs have never been associated with any of these infections. Although it is not impossible, the likelihood that a bed bug has served as a vector is infinitesimally small, and a physician may want to question a patient more closely about known risky practices such as intravenous drug abuse. Bed bug infestations have emerged as a major complaint of urban dwellers (https://www.epa.gov/bedbugs), particularly those in multifamily homes in communities with great ethnic diversity. Bed bugs are easily transported in luggage or within discarded and repurposed furniture, particularly mattresses.

Bed bug control has become more challenging due to the development of insecticide resistance in many of their populations. A large proportion (>70%) of an infestation is associated with the bedding, the mattress and box spring, and the headboard and frame. The mattress and box spring should be encased in a bug-proof fabric bag. The headboard and frame need to be treated with an insecticide that penetrates all joints and cracks. All furniture in the home needs to be inspected and similarly treated, as do the baseboards of all walls and any other location where bugs and their eggs may be hiding; "bug bombs" are not appropriate for such treatments because their droplet size precludes deep penetration of such hiding places. Luggage may be treated prior to travel with the same insecticide, following the label instructions, to prevent the introduction of bed bugs to a home.

It is possible that bat- or bird-infesting species of cimicids (the family of bugs that includes bed bugs) may transiently infest people or be incidentally found. The life cycle of these blood-feeding bugs is not likely to be maintained on human blood alone, and thus careful examination of homes should reveal the existence of bird nests or bat roosts. Unlike bed bug infestations, bat or bird bugs may be easily eliminated by removing the nests or roosts that serve as their source. An entomologist might be consulted to identify a specimen that has been presented by a patient who insists that it is impossible for them to have acquired a bed bug infestation (e.g., an isolated rural home whose occupants do not travel and have not had visitors with luggage). Specific identification might remove the need for professional pest control services as opposed to simply using a broom.

Siphonaptera

Fleas are bilaterally compressed, heavily chitinized insects with greatly modified hind legs for their characteristic jumping mode of locomotion; they lack wings (Fig. 3). Fleas are generally small, no larger than 5 mm in length. Fleas undergo complete metamorphosis, starting from a worm-like larva feeding on organic debris and blood pellets expelled, often with remarkable force and over a long distance, from the anus of the adult flea. The larva develops through three molts (has three instars), then secretes a silk to form a cocoon, in which it pupates. The female flea requires blood for egg production; one bloodmeal may serve for the production of several dozen eggs, which are laid on the fur of the host. Eggs become detached from the host's fur, coming to rest within its nest. Most fleas are what are known as "nest parasites." Individual fleas usually live for a couple of months, laying eggs daily, but may rarely persist for as long as a year. As with most arthropods, the duration of the life cycle is affected by temperature and relative humidity, but on average most species take 30 to 75 days to develop from egg to adult.

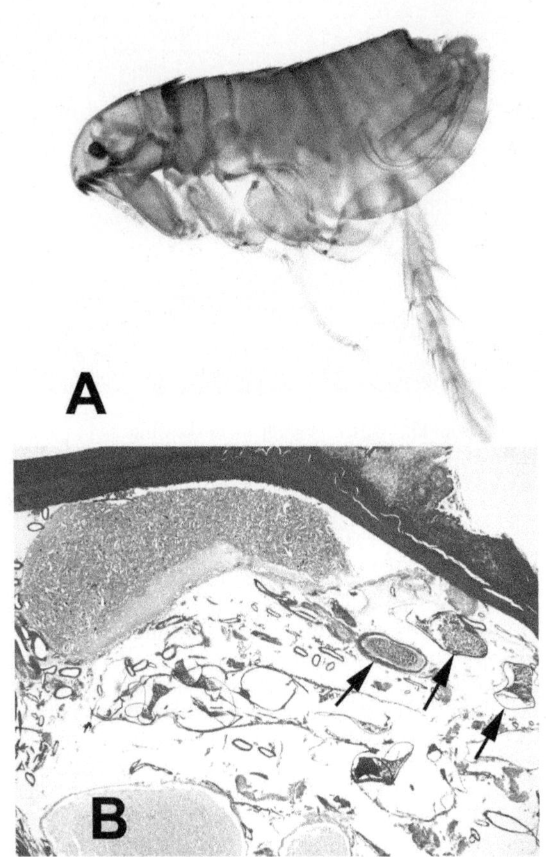

FIGURE 3 Fleas. (A) Cat flea (*Ctenocephalides felis*), showing typical flea morphologic features (from reference 43, reproduced with permission). (B) Histopathology section of the chigoe flea (*Tunga penetrans*) from a foot lesion, showing developing eggs (arrows).

Of the 2,000 or so flea species that have been described, the vast majority are from rodents and have varying degrees of host specificity. Because fleas are generally nest parasites, are relatively host specific, and cannot travel long distances (crawling or jumping on the order of a few meters, implying that humans must be directly associated with their habitat for infestation to occur), only a few species are of medical importance. These include the "human" flea (*Pulex irritans*), the dog and cat fleas (*Ctenocephalides canis* and *Ctenocephalides felis*), the main plague vector, the Oriental rat flea (*Xenopsylla cheopis*), and the sticktight flea (*Echidnophaga gallinacea*). Of these, *C. felis* fleas are the most notorious pests, feeding voraciously and rapidly developing dense infestations. Chronic infestations of homes are largely due to the presence of a cat or dog (despite its name, this flea feeds on either animal), the pet's bedding, wall-to-wall carpeting, and relatively high humidity within the home. (Cold climates rarely have self-sustaining infestations because winter heating tends to dry out the carpets and molding and other places where the larval fleas tend to be hidden.) Although bites sustained over several weeks usually induce a typical delayed-type hypersensitivity reaction, with an intensely itching red spot developing at the site of the bite (usually around the ankles), note that not all members of a household react in the same manner. Some people are more attractive to arthropods than others; others react differently to bites. It is quite possible for only one person to have itchy bites and others in the same house to have none, and thus a diagnosis of flea bite should not depend on the perception that if a household is infested, everyone should demonstrate similar lesions.

The human flea actually feeds on a variety of mammals, including domestic livestock. In tropical sites where homes have dirt floors and livestock share living accommodations, extremely dense infestations may develop. Although this flea is cosmopolitan in its distribution, the cat flea appears to have supplanted it as the major flea pest for humans in many countries.

An unusual flea, the chigoe or jigger (*Tunga penetrans*, *Tunga trimamillata*), attaches to a host and maintains a feeding site. Originally found in Latin America, the chigoe has been carried across to sub-Saharan Africa by humans and may be found anywhere there. This flea often penetrates under toenails or burrows into the skin between the toes or in the soles of the feet, an infestation known as tungiasis (Fig. 3). The female of *Tunga* spp. swells to 10 times its size, and the host's immune response causes skin to swell up and cover her, with only the end of the abdomen exposed. Through this opening, she deposits eggs and feces. When the flea dies, the lesion becomes secondarily infected, causing great irritation and pain. Tourists may become infested by walking barefoot in shady spots around beaches.

Perhaps the most famous flea is the plague vector, the Oriental rat flea, *X. cheopis*. Although it prefers rats (*Rattus rattus*, *Rattus norvegicus*) as hosts, in their absence (or when they die), *X. cheopis* feeds on humans and other animals. These fleas may be found on rats in virtually every tropical or warm temperate port city around the world, having been transported there with their hosts by trade ships. Plague is usually maintained in enzootic foci by wild rodents and their more specific fleas, but in Vietnam, Madagascar, and India rats and *X. cheopis* appear to be important for perpetuation. Although enzootic plague usually results in sporadic cases, the great fecundity of rats under the right circumstances means that explosive outbreaks of plague may occur in urban areas, with hundreds or thousands of cases. Human exposure in the western United States, where plague is enzootic, may be due to chance contact with ground squirrels or their fleas (often *Diamanus montanus*) in sheds, disused cabins, crawl spaces, or by digging around burrows. Domestic cats often serve as an intermediary, hunting moribund rodents and subsequently exposing their owners.

Psocodea

The order Psocodea includes bark lice, book lice, and parasitic lice. Infestation with lice is called pediculosis (head and body lice) or pthiriasis (pubic lice). The lice are wingless, flat (dorsoventrally), elongate, small (0.4 to 10 mm) insects that are generally characterized by strong host specificity. Classically, three orders were recognized: the Mallophaga (chewing lice), the Anoplura (the sucking lice), and the Psocoptera (bark lice and book lice); however, it is now believed that parasitism has evolved multiple times within the nonparasitic lice, and all three orders have been combined into the Psocodea, which contains about 4,000 species. Of these, the sucking lice are clinically relevant, although the chewing lice may be presented as spurious ectoparasites or associated with double-pored tapeworm (*Dipylidium caninum*) infection. Most chewing lice are commensals of birds, whereas the sucking lice feed mainly on mammals.

Lice undergo incomplete (hemimetabolous) development, with nymphal forms resembling adult lice and often found concurrently with the adults. Thus, size may appear to vary greatly within a single collection of specimens from one host. All lice are delicate and very sensitive to temperature and humidity requirements; all die within days without a host.

Chewing lice usually are found in the feathers of birds, feeding on skin fragments. Virtually all chewing lice lack piercing mouthparts and therefore do not feed on blood. The dog-biting louse (*Trichodectes canis*) may be presented as a specimen because it is a common commensal of dogs and may be spuriously associated with "bites." Dogs serve as definitive hosts for *D. caninum*, the eggs of which are shed in feces; the feces dry on the fur and the louse may then ingest the eggs. The tapeworm eggs hatch and a cysticercoid becomes localized in the hemocoel of the louse. Transmission is effected when the louse is accidentally ingested, usually when the dog is grooming; humans (usually children) are incidentally infected if their hands become contaminated and then touch food or drink or are placed in their mouths.

The nonparasitic Psocodea (booklice and barklice, formerly the Psocoptera) may resemble parasitic lice and live on molds infesting old books. They are frequently presented as specimens in diagnostic workups for itches of unknown etiology, but do not infest humans or any other animal.

The lice of greatest clinical importance (Fig. 4) are the head louse (*Pediculus humanus capitis*), the body louse (*P. humanus humanus*), and the pubic louse (*Pthirus pubis*). All of these sucking lice have prominent claws attached to each of their legs, morphologically adapted for grasping the hairs of their host. They feed at least daily and deposit 1 to 10 eggs from each blood meal, gluing one egg at a time onto the shafts of hairs (or in the case of the body louse, onto threads in clothing). The eggs, or nits, are almost cylindrical in shape and have an anterior operculum. Nits hatch within 4 to 15 days, and each of the three nymphal stages lasts 3 to 8 days. Lice are transferred between hosts by close physical contact or by sharing clothing in the case of body lice. Schools are excellent sites for the spread of a louse infestation, not only through the sharing of hats and scarves, but by children deliberately infesting others during play. It is possible that transient circumstances, such as a subway headrest recently used by an infested head, could serve as the means for transfer. Because body, head, and pubic lice do not survive long off the human host, it is not likely that an infestation may be acquired from an inanimate object. The presence of pubic lice on the eyebrows usually denotes a sexually transmitted infestation, and pubic louse infestation of a child is cause for an inquiry into the possibility of child abuse.

Body or pubic louse infestation may result in intense irritation for several days, with each bite generating a red papule. Chronically infested individuals may become desensitized or may develop a nonspecific febrile illness with lymphadenopathy, edema, and arthropathy (although such signs and symptoms should prompt a search for the agent of trench fever). A very few chronically infested individuals may develop "morbus errorum," or vagabond's disease (Fig. 4), with a thickening and dark pigmentation of the skin.

Although body louse or pubic louse infestation may be considered evidence of poor hygiene or poor judgment, infestation by head lice should not be a stigma, because it occurs in the best of families. Nor should head louse infestation be considered to be a public health menace or even a clinical problem. Very few infestations are dense enough to cause signs or symptoms, and head lice are not vectors. Nonetheless, draconian measures are taken by many school districts, banning an infested child until treatment is thorough enough to remove all nits. Many such schools fail to discriminate between live and dead nits, insisting that all traces of them be absent. Complete removal of all nit remnants can be very difficult, relying mainly on fine toothed combs, a tool that has been found in the tomb of an Egyptian pharaoh (8).

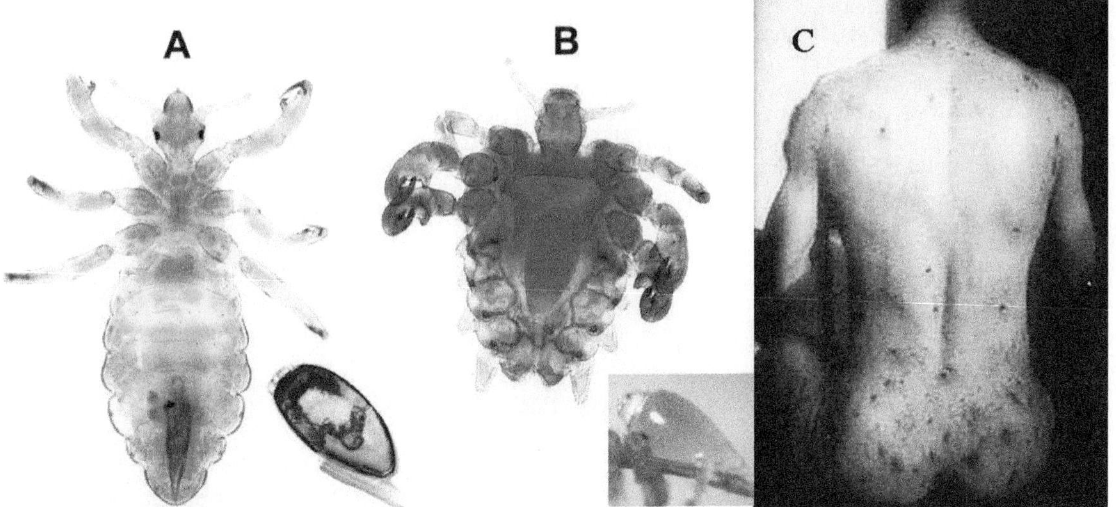

FIGURE 4 (A) Head-and-body louse (*Pediculus humanus*) (inset, nit). (B) Pubic louse (*Pthirus pubis*) (inset, nit). *P. humanus* is longer than it is wide, has a thorax narrower than the abdomen, and has claws that are the same size on each leg; the nit has a flattened operculum. *P. pubis* is nearly as wide as it is long, has a thorax wider than the abdomen, lateral protuberances on the abdominal segment, and claws on the middle and hind legs that are larger than those on the forelegs; the nit has a raised, conical operculum. (From reference 43, reproduced with permission.) (C) Vagabond's disease. The trunk of people chronically infested by body lice becomes hyperpigmented and hyperkeratotic due to scratching. (Courtesy of Department of Tropical Public Health, Harvard School of Public Health, Boston, MA.)

The sucking lice are important vectors as well as pests. Among the most notorious vectors in history are the body lice, which may serve as vectors for the agents of epidemic typhus, trench fever, and louse-borne relapsing fever. Napoleon's invasion of Russia in 1812 was probably thwarted by epidemic typhus decimating his troops. At the end of World War I, it is said that a typhus epidemic in Russia and Romania killed 800,000 people (9). Body lice are the product of poor hygiene, with clothes never or rarely being changed, such as in cold weather, by the homeless, or in refugee camps. Trench fever may be common in the homeless, and the most recent large outbreak of typhus was in Burundi, in Rwandan refugees. Oddly, even though the head louse is conspecific and appears vector competent in laboratory experiments, it has not been epidemiologically associated with any of these infections, nor has the pubic louse.

Body louse infestations are easily controlled by changing clothes frequently and bathing regularly. Clothes that have been removed from infested individuals should be destroyed, or at the very least, securely bagged in plastic and left for several weeks so that any lice that are present may starve. Clothing may also be washed in hot water and placed in a hot dryer for at least 30 minutes. Pubic lice may be treated by shaving the pubes and changing underwear regularly or by a topical pediculicide as for head lice. Although the increased prevalence of pubic grooming (e.g., Brazilian waxing) was suggested to have diminished the reported prevalence of pthiriasis, the evidence that was presented was a simple correlation analysis and not definitive. Pubic lice may survive on other kinds of hair. Head lice may be removed mechanically using specifically designed louse combs, but treatment using a pediculicide is more efficient. Although insecticide resistance is widespread, the common pediculicides containing permethrin or malathion should still be used as directed on the product label as the first line of therapy, along with environmental hygiene (laundering bedding and clothing, particularly hats; vacuuming cushions and mattresses) and screening of family members and close friends for infestation. Retreatment a week later is required because these topical pediculicides do not act efficiently on the developing louse within nits. If infestations persist after a retreatment complemented by environmental hygiene, the new generation of prescription pediculicides should be used. A single application of topical ivermectin (0.5%) or topical spinosad (0.9%) provides excellent efficacy in eliminating head louse infestations (10). Oral ivermectin (single dose 200 to 400 mg/kg with one retreatment for children >15 kg and nonpregnant females) is an effective off-label treatment for those who may have skin sensitivity to the topical formulations.

Acarina

The acarines are a subclass within the class Arachnida, which also contains the spiders. Acarina comprise the mites and ticks, tiny to small arthropods with eight legs as nymphs and adults (as opposed to six for insects) and with fused main body segments as opposed to three discrete ones for insects. Acarine baupläne are characterized by two functional body parts, the gnathosoma (or capitulum), which comprises the "head," and the idiosoma, which contains all the remaining functions (reproductive, motility, digestion). They undergo incomplete metamorphosis, passing through a larval and one to several nymphal stages before attaining sexual maturity. The mites are one of the most speciose groups of animals, with 45,000 recognized species. They are among the oldest terrestrial animals, dating in the fossil record to the Devonian (nearly 400 million years ago), and are found in every habitat on Earth. There are two major orders of the acarines, the Acariformes and the Parasitiformes. In the former, there are two main groups, the Sarcoptiformes (astigmata) and the Trombidiformes (prostigmata), both of which contain species of clinical significance (Fig. 5). The latter comprises three orders, the Holothyrida, the Ixodida, and the Mesostigmata. Of these, only the latter two are clinically significant; the holothyrids consist of about 20 species that are found only in Australasia and some neotropical forests and are unlikely to be encountered (although they are known to secrete a toxin that may incapacitate a human that has ingested such a mite). The Mesostigmata (also known as gamasida or dermanyssoida) include some mites that infest birds or rodents that under certain circumstances infest humans and cause itch. The Ixodida consist of the ticks, which are essentially very large mites.

Other than the ticks and some mesostigmatids, mites are generally not considered vectors of agents that infect humans. They are, however, important for their pest potential, causing itch, dermatitis, and allergy.

The house mouse mite (*Liponyssoides sanguineus*) is the vector for rickettsialpox due to infection by *Rickettsia akari*. The relatively mild disease, characterized by fever and exanthema, was first described after a garbage strike in Kew Gardens in the Bronx, New York, during the 1940s (11).

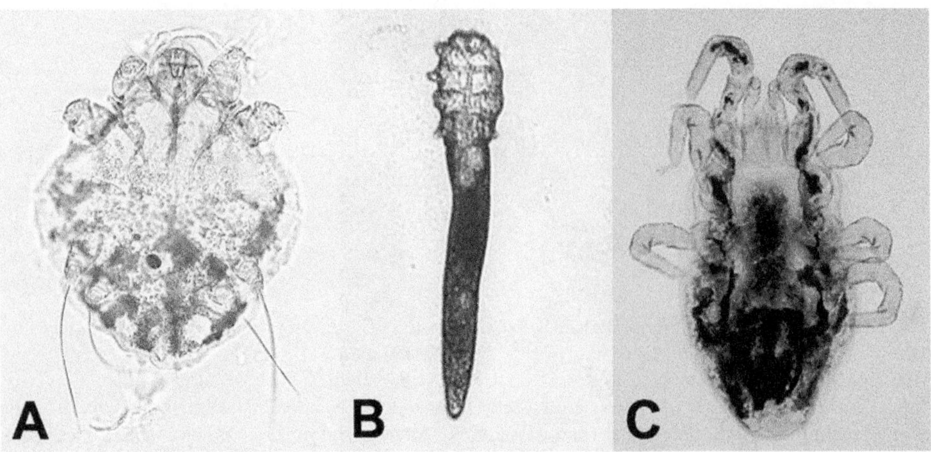

FIGURE 5 (A) Human itch mite, *Sarcoptes scabiei*. (B) Follicle mite, *Demodex folliculorum*. (C) Northern bird mite, *Ornithonyssus sylviarum*. (From reference 42.)

Garbage piled up, and house mice became dense. When the strike was resolved and the garbage was removed, the mice died or emigrated, leaving behind dense infestations of hungry mites. The prostigmatid trombiculid mites (chiggers) are the vectors for the agent of scrub typhus (*Orientia tsutsugamushi*), a rickettsiosis of Eurasia and northeastern Australia. A focus of scrub typhus has been described from an island off the coast of Chile, raising the possibility that the distribution of risk is not limited to the known focus regions of the Palearctic. More than 3 billion people live in countries where scrub typhus is endemic. Scrub typhus is acquired from infestation by tiny (0.2 mm) larval trombiculid mites such as *Leptotrombidium deliense* or *Leptotrombidium akamushi*; an eschar forms at the site of the chigger bite, with proximal lymphadenopathy, fever, headache, exanthema, and myalgia. Case fatality rates can range from 5 to 35%. Interestingly, the nymphal and adult stages of this mite feed on detritus or other arthropods and do not take vertebrate blood. Therefore, *O. tsutsugamushi* relies mainly on transovarial or vertical transmission (passage through the egg) for perpetuation, although rodent hosts that are infected may feed noninfected larvae and generate new matrilineages of infected mites. All other vector-borne agents have greater opportunities for horizontal transmission, that is, amplification by infecting a vertebrate host, and having multiple blood meals during development.

Mites are extremely difficult to identify, particularly given the likely confusion with dust mites or other ubiquitous free-living forms. All require clearing and mounting on a slide and examination under a compound microscope.

Ticks are prolific vectors, with more recognized transmitted agents than any arthropod other than mosquitoes. All of the nearly 900 known species of ticks require blood for their development and reproduction. Clinically relevant ticks (Fig. 6) belong to either the Ixodidae (the hard ticks) or the Argasidae (the soft ticks); a third family, the Nuttalliellidae, comprises a monotypic genus of soft ticks found in southern Africa, for which an association with a pathogenic agent has yet to be described. Hard ticks are so named because of the hardened sclerotized idiosomal shield or scutum. In female hard ticks, the scutum is on the anterior third of the idiosoma, with the remainder of the idiosoma consisting of pleated, leathery cuticle that allows for tremendous expansion during blood feeding. In male hard ticks, which may or may not feed at all, the scutum extends the length of the idiosoma. In contrast, soft ticks have no scutum; their entire idiosoma is leathery.

The "head," or capitulum, consists of the holdfast (hypostome), chelicerae (which are homologs of insect mandibles), and the palps, which cover the mouthparts (hypostome and chelicerae) and serve a sensory function. Chelicerae act as cutting organs, the two sides sliding past each other, with the cutting teeth at the end gaining a purchase in a host's skin. The hypostome is thereby inserted allows anchoring of the entire tick due to recurved, backward-facing teeth, or denticles (Fig. 7). Many hard ticks also secrete a cement around the hypostome. Often, when removing an attached dog tick (*Dermacentor variabilis*) from a host, a large piece of skin comes with the hypostome, mostly cement and surrounding epidermis. Thus, by virtue of the cement and denticles, tick hypostomes rarely emerge intact when a tick is removed. "Leaving the head in" is not critical, and usually the remnant is walled off as a foreign body or works itself out, perhaps by the act of scratching. Treatment therefore should simply be disinfection of the site of the bite and certainly not excavation of the epidermis looking for the "head." Soft ticks are transient feeders and are only rarely found attached.

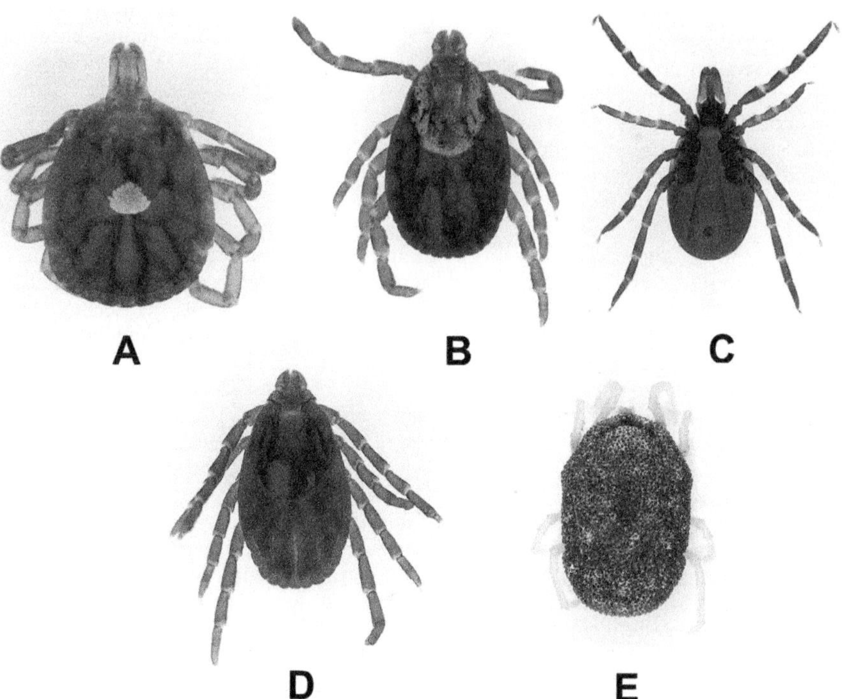

FIGURE 6 Medically important ticks of the United States. (A) Lone star tick, *Amblyomma americanum*. (B) American dog tick, *Dermacentor variabilis*. (C) Black-legged or deer tick, *Ixodes scapularis* or *I. dammini*. (D) Brown dog tick, *Rhipicephalus sanguineus*. (E) Soft tick, *Ornithodoros turicata*. (Images adapted from reference 43, reproduced with permission.)

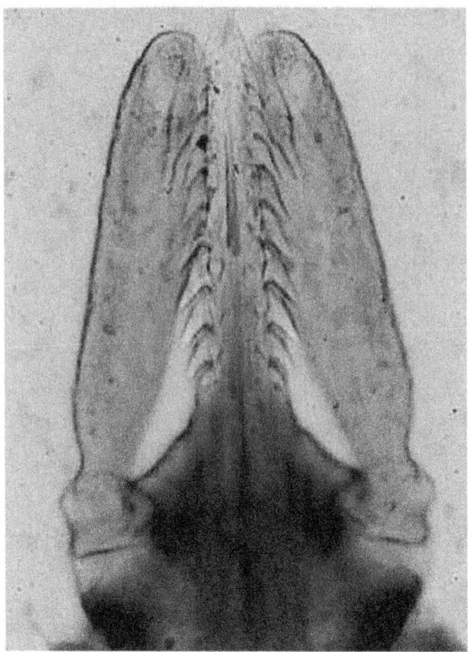

FIGURE 7 Tick hypostome ("holdfast"), showing recurved denticles that anchor the tick into the skin.

Hard ticks require several days to complete their blood meal; the number of days depends on the species and life cycle stage of the tick. The North American deer tick (*Ixodes dammini*, frequently referred to as *Ixodes scapularis*) (12) feeds 3 days as a larva, 4 days as a nymph, and 7 days as the female. The closely related European sheep or castor bean tick, *Ixodes ricinus*, feeds 2 days as a larva, 3 days as a nymph, and 7 days as the female. The duration of feeding depends also on host immune status (previous exposure may induce immediate-type hypersensitivity, which slows down the feeding process) and temperature (*I. dammini* and *I. ricinus* feed twice as long on cold reptiles as on ones that are held at 37°C). The extended duration of feeding is required for the cuticle to soften so that the idiosoma may accommodate 10 to 100 times its weight in blood, and the site of the bite is prepared so that a pool of lymph and blood is available for removal. During the first 70% of the feeding process, very little blood or lymph appears to be present within ticks, which remain dorsoventrally flat. Hemoglobin is excreted from the anus, lipids are retained, and water from the blood is recycled back into the host as saliva (13). In the last day, usually in the last 3 or 4 hours of the blood meal, the tick takes what has been termed "the big sip," removing a large volume of whole blood, then detaching and dropping from the host.

Because they must remain attached for days, hard ticks have evolved means of temporarily disabling a host's local inflammatory response, which might inhibit its feeding. Hard tick saliva is an extremely complex mixture of anticoagulant, anti-inflammatory, and antihemostatic agents (14) that act mainly at the site of the feeding lesion. Tick saliva also neutralizes Th2 responses systemically. Hosts that have never been exposed to ticks do not realize that a tick is attached. Indeed, most patients with Lyme disease or spotted fever never knew that they had been "bitten" (15, 16). The most dangerous tick is not necessarily the one that a patient finds and removes, aborting the transmission process, but the one that the patient never knew was there and which was able to complete its feeding.

In contrast, soft ticks are more like mosquitoes in their feeding, spending tens of minutes to no more than a few hours feeding, usually as their host is sleeping. Soft tick saliva does not need to be as biochemically complex, and some species have painful bites. The pajuello (pajaroello), *Ornithodoros coriaceous*, of California and Mexico is renowned for its "toxic bite," which causes local pain and burning.

Tick life cycles have an extended duration, usually months or years. Deer ticks, for example, take 2 years to go from egg to egg. For this reason, there is generally no risk associated with hard ticks engorging and dropping off of a companion animal in a patient's home. The engorged tick will not feed again and will take weeks to molt or lay eggs, and in the interim, usually the relative humidity in the house is too low for extended survival of the tick. On the other hand, cats as opposed to dogs appear to be a risk factor for acquiring Lyme disease, perhaps because deer ticks feed well on dogs but poorly on cats; ticks, particularly nymphs, detach in mid-feed and readily reattach to the cat's owner (17). The exceptions to the lack of risk associated with ticks engorging and detaching in the house is the brown dog tick (*Rhipicephalus sanguineus*), which is the vector of Marseille fever (Mediterranean spotted fever, boutonneuse fever), *Ehrlichia canis*, and has also recently been documented as a vector of Rocky Mountain spotted fever. These ticks hide behind wall molding to molt and are known for dense infestations covering the interior walls of dog kennels.

Ticks can be difficult to identify, depending on their state of engorgement and whether mouthparts are intact. The need for identification rests on whether a submitted specimen was associated with illness, in which case assigning it to a genus might contribute to a differential diagnosis. Although tick systematists have recently altered some of the generic epithets, in general the classic Centers for Disease Control and Prevention (CDC) diagrams of the mouthparts and idiosoma (Fig. 8) can be used to at least classify a tick to the genus. Often, simply knowing the country in which a tick may have been acquired significantly narrows down the list of possibilities (Table 2).

ARTHROPODS AS "SCALARS"

Vectors impart directionality to a pathogen. In contrast, there are arthropod-pathogen relationships that are not characterized by directionality, and analogous to mathematical terminology, arthropods that inadvertently serve as a source of infection are called scalars (18). Helminths may use an arthropod as an intermediate host, but that arthropod does not deliver the infectious stage of the helminth during an obligate behavior such as blood feeding. Drinking water with copepods (Crustacea) containing third-stage larvae of the filarial nematode *Dracunculus medinensis* initiates infection when the copepods are digested by stomach acids, thereby liberating the nematode larvae, but the copepods did not swim toward a vessel scooping water out for drinking. Accordingly, the patient's history needs to specifically address the possibility of exposure via drinking from natural bodies of water (copepods and *Dracunculus*); the presence of flour beetles, fleas, or roaches (hymenolepidid cestodes, *D. caninum*, *Gongylonema* spp., acanthocephalans); eating crabs or crayfish (*Paragonimus* spp.); or being in an environment with dense infestations of house flies (trachoma). With the exception of house flies and *C. trachomatis* (the causal agent of trachoma, which perpetuates in the absence of flies, spreading by direct contact with ocular exudates), all these are obligate relationships.

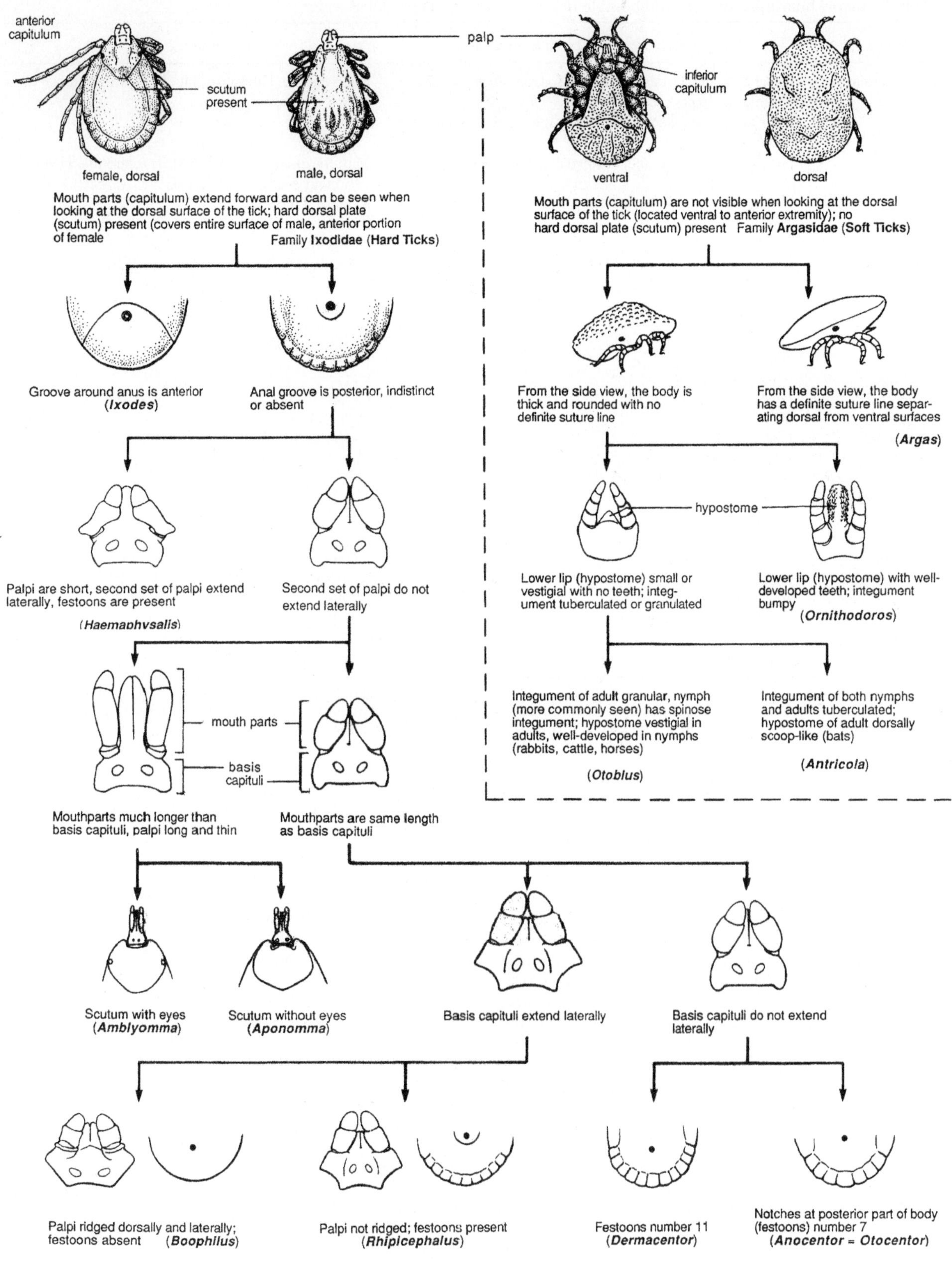

FIGURE 8 Pictorial key to major tick genera in the United States.

TABLE 2 Likely human-biting ticks and possible tick-borne infections by global region

Region	Likely tick(s) infesting humans	Possible zoonosis[a]
North America	*Ixodes dammini, Ixodes scapularis, Ixodes pacificus, Ixodes dentatus, Ixodes cookei*	Lyme disease, babesiosis, HGA, Powassan fever
	Dermacentor variabilis, Dermacentor andersoni, Dermacentor occidentalis	RMSF, CTF, tularemia
	Amblyomma americanum, Amblyomma maculatum	Masters' disease/STARI, RMSF, tularemia, HME, human ewingii ehrlichiosis
	Ornithodoros hermsi, Ornithodoros turicata	Relapsing fever
South America	*Amblyomma cajennense*	RMSF
	Ornithodoros spp.	Relapsing fever
Europe, Russia	*Ixodes ricinus, Ixodes persulcatus*	Lyme disease, babesiosis, HGA, TBE
	Dermacentor marginatus	TIBOLA
	Rhipicephalus sanguineus	Marseille fever, HME?
Japan, China, Korea	*Ixodes ovatus, I. persulcatus*	Lyme disease, babesiosis, HGA, TBE
	Dermacentor spp.	Tick typhus, JSF?
	Haemaphysalis spp.	JSF?
South Asia	*Haemaphysalis* spp.	KFD
	Hyalomma spp.	CCHF
	R. sanguineus	Tick typhus
Southeast Asia	*Ixodes granulatus*	Lyme disease?
	R. sanguineus	Tick typhus? HME?
Australia	*Ixodes holocyclus*	Tick typhus
North Africa	*Hyalomma* spp.	CCHF
	R. sanguineus	Marseille fever, HME?
	I. ricinus	Lyme disease
West Africa	*Hyalomma* spp.	CCHF
	Ornithodoros erraticus	Relapsing fever
	Amblyomma variegatum	ATBF
Sub-Saharan Africa	*A. variegatum, Amblyomma hebraeum, Haemaphysalis leachi*	ATBF
	Hyalomma spp.	CCHF
	Ornithodoros moubata	Relapsing fever

[a]HGA, human granulocytic anaplasmosis (*Anaplasma phagocytophilum*); HME, human monocytic ehrlichiosis (due to either *Ehrlichia chaffeensis* or *Ehrlichia canis*); RMSF, Rocky Mountain spotted fever; STARI, southern tick-associated rash illness (etiology unknown, possibly *Borrelia*); CTF, Colorado tick fever; TIBOLA, tick-borne lymphadenopathy (*Rickettsia slovaca*); JSF, Japanese spotted fever (*Rickettsia japonica*); TBE, tick-borne encephalitis; CCHF, Crimean-Congo hemorrhagic fever; KFD, Kyasanur Forest disease; ATBF, African tick bite fever (*Rickettsia africae*).

Muscoid Flies

The muscoid dipterans include the muscids (house flies, stable flies); the Calliphoridae (blow flies); and the Sarcophagidae (the flesh flies). Egg deposition and larval development occur in characteristic materials, *viz*., fecal material for house flies, decaying plant material for stable flies, live flesh for blow flies, and carrion for flesh flies. These flies can be remarkably prolific within short periods of time: a female house fly, for example, deposits 100 to 150 eggs in moist, decaying organic material, usually excrement, at one time, but may do so 20 or more times (19). Larvae emerge from the eggs within 12 hours. Three larval stages develop during a week, and a puparium is formed. The adult fly emerges from the pupa within 4 days, and copulation may occur within one day. Thus, a full life cycle may take as few as 12 days.

House flies have received much attention for their potential as scalars because of their association with poor hygiene. Flies are strong fliers and move readily from outdoors to indoors. A large fleshy structure at the apex of the proboscis provides a surface for contamination, as do the hairy body and legs of the fly. In addition, flies may regurgitate while feeding, and the vomitus may contain organisms that were acquired in a previous landing. House flies commonly feed on human excrement, and virtually every possible enteric pathogen (those causing amebiasis, cholera, typhoid, hepatitis A, poliomyelitis; even roundworms and *Helicobacter pylori*) has been detected within or upon them. With few exceptions, such findings are epidemiologically irrelevant inasmuch as all of the agents perpetuate in their absence. Polio virus, for example, was recovered in flies captured from sites where polio was actively being transmitted (20), but use of DDT failed to curtail the epidemic. In contrast, residual DDT treatment of army camps reduced the incidence of shigellosis (21). It is likely that individual cases of enteric disease may derive from fly contamination of food, but whether the risk of such an event merits worry by patients or their health care providers remains unclear. Dense infestations of flies should be reduced by source reduction (i.e., by preventing flies from getting access to garbage and excrement); a few flies in the house do not warrant setting off a bug bomb.

Cockroaches

Roaches are dorsoventrally flattened, smooth-bodied, winged insects with long antennae, biting-type mouthparts, and abdominal projections (cerci). The outer pair of wings is thick and leathery, and the inner pair is membranous. Roaches can fly but usually scuttle about on long spiny legs. They undergo incomplete metamorphosis, with the immature forms looking like miniature adults, although without wings. Eggs are laid within a hard capsule, the ootheca, which is deposited in a dark crevice. Development is slow, taking about 4 weeks between molts; many roaches only have one generation each year. Roaches can live for months without food, but water seems critical. They are omnivorous, feeding on the finest of foods to the vilest of waste, usually at night. Secretions deposited by scent glands (including trail and aggregation pheromones) give rise to a characteristic disagreeable odor that confirms an infestation even when live roaches cannot be found. Common roaches range in size from the small German cockroach (*Blatella germanica*), about half an inch in length, to the American cockroach, nearly 2 inches. Much work has been done attempting to incriminate roaches as scalars, even estimating nearly 14,000 CFU of bacteria (mainly *Staphylococcus* spp.) on the surface of the body of one German cockroach. Cholera-laden feces were fed to American cockroaches, with ingestion of as much as 200 μl of material and recovery of live vibrios 30 to 80 hours later from roach feces (22). A roundworm (*Gongylonema* sp.) normally infecting ungulates may encyst within roaches and be transmitted to humans when ingested, usually as a contaminant of food. People may similarly become infected by a zoonotic acanthocephalan worm (*Moniliformis moniliformis*) which uses cockroaches and other arthropods as intermediate hosts. As with flies, the presence of roaches suggests poor environmental hygiene, but only rare instances of enteric disease might be associated with them.

The main role of cockroaches in public health appears to be as a major cause of asthma, perhaps as commonly a cause as is the dust mite, as well as a cause of wheezing, rhinitis, and atopic dermatitis. Their feces (frass) contains the allergens Bla g 1 and Bla g 2, which cross-react with known allergens such as fungi, as well as tropomyosin, a panallergen found on dust mites, crustacea, and mollusks (23). Patients sensitized to cockroach allergens frequently (>70% of the time) have specific IgE reactivity to the 20- to 90-kDa Bla g 1 protein. Although sensitization is a main cause of frass-associated rhinitis, prior exposure is not required to trigger airway inflammation.

Dense infestations of cockroaches may develop quickly and promote respiratory illness. Hence, any detection of an active infestation should prompt control efforts. Control of roach infestations can be difficult. Boric acid, deposited along walls, behind moldings, and around other sites where they may hide, is effective in killing adults and nymphs by abrading the cuticle between abdominal segments, rendering the roach prone to desiccation. Removing standing water (wiping up and getting rid of clutter around sinks) can also reduce infestations by preventing access to water. Roach infestations are most common in apartment buildings serving transient student or immigrant populations, who bring the insects in with their household goods.

DIRECT INJURY DUE TO ARTHROPODS

Arthropods Typically Thought of as Vectors

Vectors such as lice, ticks, bugs, fleas, mosquitoes, and black flies may directly cause injury by their bites, either by hypersensitivity reactions or toxic effects of their salivary products. Hypersensitivity reactions mainly manifest as itch, with the concomitant potential for secondary infection due to scratching. Bed bug and flea bites may cause immediate-type hypersensitivity reactions with itchy erythema greater than 3 cm in diameter (Fig. 2). Ticks may induce a chronic local granulomatous lesion, persisting for months, perhaps due to remnants of the mouthparts (denticles) left within the epidermis. This phenomenon is particularly pronounced with "seed tick" infestation (stepping into a newly emerged batch of larval *Amblyomma* ticks, often thousands), where dozens or hundreds of ticks may attach at the belt line. Itch may be immediately relieved by calamine (or Caladryl with Benadryl) lotion or even by holding the affected part under very hot running water, which induces mast cells to degranulate. Over-the-counter hydrocortisone creams may help mild cases of itch, but severe cases may require prescription-strength steroid cream (e.g., betamethasone 0.05%). Daily application of hydrocortisone should promote a resolution of itch within a week. Tick granulomas may be treated with Retin A gel (0.05%), which may promote the turnover of epidermis and ejection of remaining antigenic material (S. Telford, personal observation).

As mentioned in the introduction to the section on Diptera, black fly bites may produce "black fly fever," usually as a dose-dependent reaction. Usually, the site of the bites becomes edematous, with a golf ball-sized lump and an oozing punctate lesion. Fever and myalgia manifest the night after the bite occurs and disappear within 24 hours. Such symptoms should not be construed as infection; few pathogens, if any, have such a short prepatent period. Treatment is symptomatic. Similarly, soft tick bites due to pajaroello or the African tampan (*Ornithodoros moubata*) may immediately cause pain, swelling, and irritation at the site of the bite, with raised hard wheals (24). The effects are said to last several days, with "irritability" of the affected part. Anecdotally, hunters in northern New England and the upper Great Lakes may complain of bites of *Dermacentor albipictus* larvae (a species that usually feeds only on ungulates such as deer or moose) during the early winter; apocrypha indicate that Native Americans called these larvae "bite all same as a piece of fire." The condition has not been studied.

An unusual toxicosis due to tick bite is tick paralysis. The presence of certain feeding ticks induces an acute ascending paralysis. First described for sheep and cattle in Australia in 1843, a similar disease was reported for a child in Oregon in 1912. The Australian *Ixodes holocyclus* attacks cattle, sheep, and dogs but rarely humans, and thus tick paralysis is not a common clinical condition there. However, in the western United States, bites of *Dermacentor andersoni* commonly produce cases of "staggers" in cattle or sheep, which may terminate fatally. Children are the usual victims of tick paralysis, with ticks attached at the nape of the neck. The illness is characterized by fatigue, irritability, distal paresthesias, leg weakness with reduced tendon reflexes, ataxia, and lethargy. Unless the tick is removed, quadriplegia and respiratory failure may result; the case fatality rate without treatment can be 10%. Removal of the tick induces a seemingly miraculous recovery within 48 hours. (Tick biologists unromantically suggest such an etiology for the tale of Snow White, who awakens after the prince bends over her and kisses her, probably removing a tick from behind her ear.) A 40- to 60-kDa toxin has been isolated from *I. holocyclus* and has been named holocyclotoxin (25); an antitoxin has been produced for veterinary use; other toxins with a much smaller molecular weight have also been isolated. The toxin has not been isolated from the American tick paralysis ticks. Other ticks (*Amblyomma americanum*, *Ixodes* spp.) have also been reported to induce tick paralysis.

An enigmatic red meat allergy has been associated with the bites of lone star ticks in the eastern United States. Similar associations have also been reported for Europe and Australia, with sheep ticks (*Ixodes ricinus*) and paralysis ticks (*I. holocyclus*), respectively, suspected as the culprits. A severe hypersensitivity reaction to treatment with cetuximab was found to be geographically limited and due to IgE reactivity with galactose-α-1,3-galactose (alpha-gal). Such IgE reactivity was also associated with a newly recognized red meat allergy, which manifested as urticaria or anaphylaxis 3 to 6 hours after ingesting beef, pork, or lamb.

The delayed onset of symptoms distinguishes this red meat allergy from other food allergies. Patients recalled recent multiple tick bites, and subsequently detailed studies of individual cases, epidemiological association between anti-alpha-gal IgE and lone star tick bites, and correlation of IgE to tick proteins and alpha-gal together have provided evidence for causality (26). The majority of patients have a blood type other than B, which is biologically consistent with the structural similarity of alpha-gal and the B blood group determinants. Alpha-gal is a major component of internal tick tissues, and hence the demonstrated associations are biologically plausible. Specific treatment has not been described other than avoidance of red meat and tick bites; apparently, the allergy resolves in the absence of additional tick bites. This unusual example of direct, delayed injury due to arthropods remains to be fully understood.

Endoparasitic Arthropods

Arthropods that invade a host's body and cause disease include mites (scabies), fleas (tungiasis), fly larvae (myiasis), and pentastomes (halzoun). Tungiasis is discussed in the flea section above. Pentastomes, or tongue worms, are primitive, elongate arthropods that live as adults in the lungs and air passages of hosts including fish, amphibians, reptiles, and some mammals. The body, like that of acarines, consists of a cephalothorax and indistinct abdomen, with no legs; often, the cuticle appears ringed or annulated. Chitinous hooks protrude from the head. Their size ranges from 1 to 10 cm. Although long thought to be in its own phylum, recent cladistic analyses based on morphologic and molecular characteristics place it within the Crustacea and most closely related to the branchiurid fish lice (27). Pentastomes undergo a complex life cycle with incomplete development, requiring intermediate hosts in which the nymphal stages may encyst.

Human infestation by *Linguatula serrata* may be due to ingestion of eggs (from contamination by nasal discharges from the dog intermediate host) or ingestion of encysted nymphs within the raw or poorly cooked liver, lungs, or mesentery of an intermediate host such as rabbits, cattle, or sheep (28). A nasopharyngeal syndrome results, known as halzoun in the Middle East and marrara in Sudan. Facial edema, nasal discharge, coughing, and sneezing are due to the migration of nymphal forms into the nasopharynx. Removal of the offending nymphs (by visual inspection and forceps) and symptomatic treatment with antihistamines to reduce edema may be helpful. *Armillifer armillatus* and *Porocephalus crotali* of snakes also cause infections in humans, probably as a result of drinking water contaminated with eggs from their feces and not because of ingestion of poorly cooked snake meat. Usually, human infection is noted only at autopsy or by the presence of calcified abdominal or lung objects in radiographs. Treatment is symptomatic.

The most common ectoparasite-caused direct injury is scabies, caused by infestation with the human scabies mite (*Sarcoptes scabiei*). A number of different populations of *S. scabiei* have been treated as full species based on their tropism for other animals (including dogs, pigs, sheep, cattle, and goats), but all are morphologically identical. Infestation may occur anywhere in the world. Canine sarcoptic mange is commonly associated with atypical scabies infestations in the owners of the dogs; mites derived from canines cannot perpetuate solely on human hosts, and they form papular lesions that may be the result of abortive infestation (29). In either animal or human scabies, transmission is by direct personal contact, and infestations often cluster among groups of people, particularly families. There is little evidence that environments become contaminated; fomites have not been identified.

The female scabies mite burrows beneath the stratum corneum (Fig. 9), leaving behind eggs and feces in a track-like trail. A few dozen eggs are deposited, and these hatch within a week. Larvae form new burrows but may also emerge from the skin and move freely about. Nymphs develop from fed larvae, and they in turn develop into the adult male and female. Normal infestations consist of a dozen or two dozen female mites. Nocturnal itching begins within a month of the first infestation but may begin

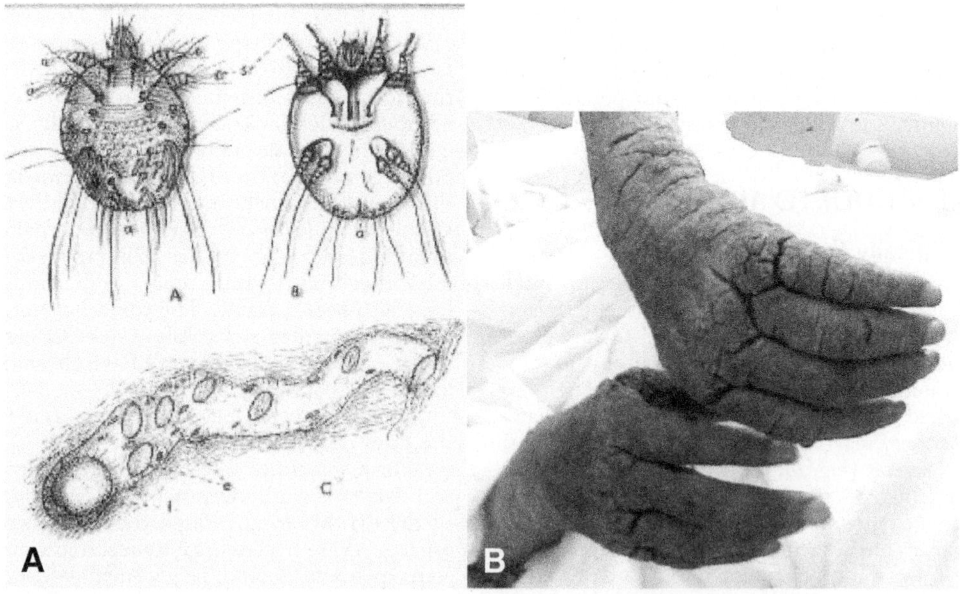

FIGURE 9 Scabies. (A) Diagram of feeding lesion and adult female mite. (B) Hands of a homeless individual with AIDS and severe scabies (crusted scabies) (courtesy of the Wikimedia Commons, Adam Cuerden; released into the public domain by author).

within a day in previously exposed individuals. Thus, newly exposed individuals, prior to their recognizing an infestation by the presence of itching, may contaminate other individuals. Erythematous papules and vesicles first appear on the webs of fingers, and spread to the arms, trunk, and buttocks. The burrows contain granular, highly antigenic feces (scybala), which cause both delayed- and immediate-type hypersensitivity reactions. Interestingly, in individuals who are immunocompromised, hundreds of female mites may be found, itching is minimal, but a hyperkeratosis is prominent. Such "crusted" or Norwegian scabies are highly infectious to other people.

Scabies infestations can be easily diagnosed by scraping a newly developed papule (not one that has been scratched) with a scalpel coated with mineral oil. The scrapings in the oil are transferred to a slide and examined at ×100 or ×400 brightfield for 300- to 400-micron-sized mites or the smaller black fecal granules. Scabies may be treated by topical 5% permethrin cream or 1% permethrin rinse (Nix, same as is used for head lice). Globally, 12.5% benzyl benzoate is the treatment of choice due to cost considerations but is not Food and Drug Administration (FDA) approved as a scabicide and hence is not used in the United States. Topical lindane (Kwell) is also effective, but the FDA now suggests the use of permethrin first and lindane only if that fails. Lindane can be neurotoxic to children and small adults. Although oral ivermectin has been suggested as being more effective, the FDA has not approved it as a scabies treatment, and at the moment, topical permethrin or benzyl benzoate is still considered to be the first-line treatment when correctly applied (24).

Demodex folliculorum and *Demodex brevis*, the follicle mites, infest virtually everybody. These elongate 500-micron-long mites (Fig. 5) may be found within follicles and sebaceous glands on the face, ear, and breast and are often brought to the attention of a physician because a tweezed eyelash may have a few mites at the base of the hair shaft. Although they appear to largely be nonpathogenic, they have been associated with several skin conditions, including rosacea and pityriasis folliculorum. However, it is thought that these associations are incidental. Related mites cause demodectic mange in dogs and cattle, but these species are not known to infest humans.

Dust mite allergies (one of many causes of asthma, rhinitis, and atopic dermatitis) are due to inhalation of feces excreted by *Dermatophagoides farinae* or related pyroglyphid mites, which are human commensals that feed on flakes of skin shed from a person. The mites themselves do not infest a person but remain in the environment (usually within bedding or carpets) to feed and develop. About a half gram of skin may be shed from a person each day; one female mite lays one egg a day for about 2 months; thus, large accumulations of mites may readily develop. The 300- to 400-micron-long mites may be presented by patients as suspects for other nonspecific lesions or sets of signs and symptoms because they may be found in virtually all houses and can be detected if dust is allowed to settle on standing water; the mites float and do move and can be seen at ×20 magnification. Humidity less than 60% greatly reduces dust mite infestations, as does periodic vacuuming and washing of bedding and carpets. A sublingual immunotherapy designed to tolerize patients to dust mite allergen has recently been approved by the FDA (Odactra; ALK, Inc.) and may be prescribed by an allergist.

Myiasis is the infestation of human or animal tissue by fly larvae, deposited as eggs or first-stage larvae; the larvae develop by feeding on the surrounding tissue, emerge as third-stage larvae, and pupate in the environment. Three kinds of myiasis have been classically recognized: obligate, facultative, and "accidental." Obligate myiasis reflects the need for larvae to feed well during development because adult flies do not feed or feed poorly. Bot flies are the main example of obligate myiasis. Most bot flies normally infest animals, and thus human bot fly infestation by these species is considered zoonotic. Two flies, *Dermatobia hominis* (human bot fly) and *Cordylobia anthropophaga* (tumbu fly), are more adapted to humans, as illustrated by their life cycles. The former fly lays its eggs on a transport (phoretic) host such as a mosquito, and when the mosquito feeds on a human, the eggs hatch during the course of the blood meal, and the larvae penetrate the skin at the site of the mosquito bite or burrow in on their own. The latter fly is attracted to sweat, urine, and feces and oviposits on clothing that has been spread out to dry on the ground or hung up to dry on areas of cloth that are redolent with such odors, which may remain when primitive clothes washing practices are used. The eggs hatch when placed close to the body, and the larvae burrow into the skin. Thus, any clothing washed in tropical countries without the aid of modern soap powders and dryers should be ironed before wearing. Other bot flies that can cause zoonotic infections include *Oestrus ovis* (the nasal bot fly of sheep, which can cause ophthalmomyiasis), *Hypoderma* spp. (the warble fly; causes cutaneous myiasis) and *Cuterebra* spp. (furuncular or respiratory myiasis).

Facultative myiasis is usually due to infestation by blowflies (*Phormia regina*), green bottle flies (*Lucilia sericata*) and related calliphorids, flesh flies (*Wohlfarhtia* spp.), or common house flies (*Musca domestica*). These flies normally deposit eggs into fecal or other rotting organic material but directly lay eggs in wounds or necrotic tissue, but the larvae may not confine themselves to such resources and may move into healthy tissue.

"Accidental myiasis," or pseudomyiasis, should not be considered myiasis, because it is almost always an incidental finding. Fly larvae, often house fly, may be found under wound dressings or in unusual sites such as the gastrointestinal tract. The rat-tailed maggot (*Eristalis tenax*) is actually a hoverfly (syrphid) that breeds in sewage or dirty water. Larvae may find their way into the lower gastrointestinal tract (30), although the means by which they do so (perhaps due to oviposition around the anus) have not been definitively demonstrated. Drinking unfiltered dirty water might cause temporary infestation of the gut, with larvae surviving into the lower intestine. More often, larvae are found in containers of stool samples that are intended for the clinical laboratory and are most likely due to oviposition after taking the sample. The relationship between the arthropod specimen and clinical signs and symptoms is almost always difficult to definitively demonstrate.

A variety of clinical presentations are evident depending on the site where the larvae are present. Bot flies cause furuncular lesions or migratory integumomyiasis (a serpiginous track may be produced in the skin). Wound myiasis comprises shallow or pocketlike initial lesions that become more deeply invasive. Maggots may invade the nose and accompanying structures, causing nasal or oral myiasis. Maggots may get into the ears, producing aural myiasis. Ophthalmomyiasis is due to external or internal infestation. Enteric, vaginal, or vesicomyiasis is due to invasion of the gut or genitalia, although in many instances the fly larva is an incidental finding or contamination. In all presentations, pathology may be due to tissue trauma or local destruction but is more often associated with secondary bacterial infection. On the other hand, many maggots do not promote bacterial infection but, rather, secrete bacteriolytic compounds and have been used as a surgical intervention to debride wounds (31). Indeed, sterile *L. sericata* maggots are available by prescription in the United States (www.monarchlabs.com) to help with wound debridement. Thus, the development of secondary bacterial infection in myiasis may suggest the death of the maggot.

In all cases, treatment is by removal of the maggots, laboriously picking them out using forceps. The maggots causing furuncular myiasis or migratory integumomyiasis have their posterior end visible within the lesion, exposing the spiracular plates that cover their tracheolar breathing apparatus. Although much lore exists on how to best remove such maggots, including "luring" the maggots with bacon or pork fat, the simplest method is to cover the lesion with petroleum jelly, thereby preventing the maggot from breathing. (Obstruction of the spiracles is probably the mode of action for bacon or pork rind, not a preference for tasty fat.) The maggot eventually moves out enough in an attempt to get air so that it may be grasped with forceps.

Identification of maggots can be difficult. The spiracular plates can be diagnostic (Fig. 10) and should be removed from the posterior end, mounted on slides in an appropriate mounting medium, and compared with pictorial keys. Often, a live maggot can be reared to pupation on raw meat, and the resulting adult fly identified. On the other hand, other than academic curiosity, most myiasis cases presenting in developed countries are the result of tourism, and not knowing the specific identity of the fly does not influence further preventive measures; treatment is sufficient. One important reason for accurately identifying a maggot is for forensic purposes: the developmental rates of the

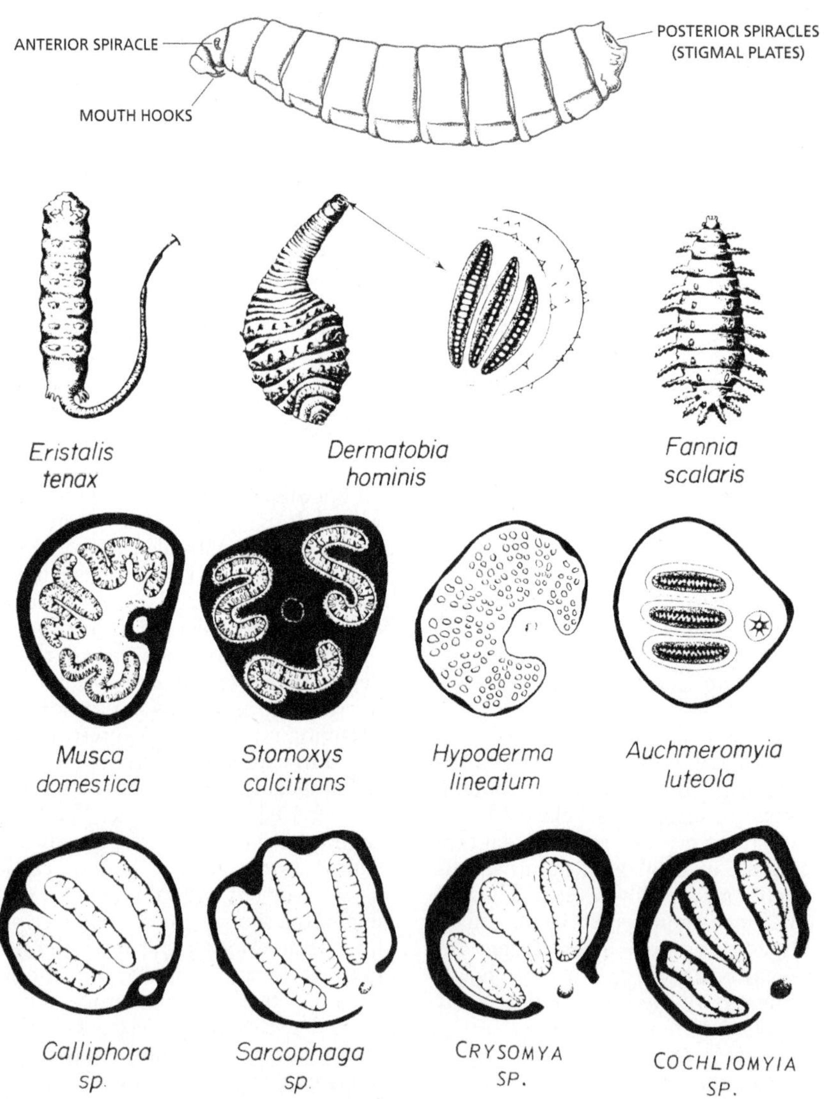

FIGURE 10 Myiasis. Pictorial key of characteristics of some myiasis-producing fly larvae. (Row 1) Mature larva of a muscoid fly (from R. Hegner et al., copyright 1938 by Appleton Century, Inc., New York, NY). (Row 2) Larva of *Eristalis tenax*, the rat-tailed maggot, *Dermatobia hominis*, the human bot fly (with an enlarged view of a posterior spiracle), and *Fannia scalaris*, the latrine fly. (Rows 3 and 4) Appearance of posterior spiracles of some species that produce accidental, facultative, or obligatory myiasis. (Centers for Disease Control and Prevention, Atlanta, GA.)

various obligate or facultative myiases have been described as a great aid in assigning time of death for cadavers. The American Board of Forensic Entomology (http://www.forensicentomologist.org) provides certification for experts in such tasks, and their membership may be consulted should a need for precise identification arise.

Stinging and Biting Resulting in Envenomation

Hymenoptera

Wasps, bees, and ants all belong to the order Hymenoptera, which contains well over 100,000 recognized species. Hymenoptera are minute to medium-sized insects with compound eyes, mandibles, and two pairs of transparent wings (although in the ants, wings may be seen on males or females only at certain times of the year). They undergo complete metamorphosis from a grub-like larva to a pupa. Those of clinical importance are within the Aculeata, particularly the Vespidae (social and solitary wasps), Apoidea (social and solitary bees), and Formicoidea (ants). Most of the Aculeata have a characteristic constriction between the first and second abdominal segments. These insects have complex social behavior, with males, females, and worker castes. Workers have a stinging organ, which is used for defending the colony or capturing prey.

Most stings by hymenopterans cause localized reactions, sometimes with extreme pain and resulting in a transient induration with hyperemia. By virtue of their living in large colonies, bees and ants may swarm an intruder, and dozens if not hundreds of stings may be sustained. Airway obstruction may result should multiple stings be received on the face or neck. Although the honey bee's agricultural value in pollinating plants greatly exceeds any slight risk due to their stings, African honey bees (*Apis mellifera adansoni*, a subspecies of the regular honey bee; also known as "killer bees"), which were imported into Brazil in the hopes that they would be better pollinators, can be dangerous because they are more aggressive than the typical honey bee. Bees differ from wasps and ants in that their stinging apparatus is forcibly torn out during the act of stinging, thereby ensuring the death of the individual bee as a result. Wasps and ants may sting multiple times; some fire ants may hang on by their mandibles and repeatedly insert their posteriorly located stinger.

Bee venom has been well characterized and consists of a large amount of a polypeptide (melittin), phospholipase A2, histamine, hyaluronidase, mast cell discharging peptide, and apamin. Histamine appears to be the cause of the acute pain of bee stings.

Bumble bees, paper wasps, yellowjackets, and hornets may all sting, usually as a result of intruding too near a nest. The most important clinical manifestation of bee or wasp stings is anaphylaxis. Chest tightness, nausea, vertigo, cyanosis, and urticaria may be seen even in individuals who apparently had never previously been exposed. Dozens of people die each year in the United States due to bee sting anaphylaxis.

Ants, on the other hand, rarely pose a risk for anaphylaxis but produce a reaction that may persist for a longer duration. An induration or wheal may be observed immediately after the sting, and a papule may develop that itches or remains irritated for several days. Secondary bacterial infection may ensue. Fire ants (*Solenopsis invicta*) may bite or sting, both modes accompanied by the injection of a venom, an ethyl ketone for the former and various 2,6 dialkypiperidines in the latter. Other ants (the Formicinae) have a venom that is mainly formic acid.

Urticating Caterpillars

Lepidoptera (moths and butterflies) undergo complete development, with the well-known caterpillar and cocoon stages. More than 100,000 species of these familiar insects have been described. Although certain adult moths (in four superfamilies) may imbibe blood or tears, no signs or symptoms are associated with what is evidently an independent evolution of hematophagy. About 12 families of Lepidoptera across the world, however, have caterpillars with urticating hairs, and some of the neotropical species can produce surprisingly severe reactions, including a hemorrhagic syndrome (*Lonomia achelous*, a saturniid moth of the Amazon) due to a fibrinolytic toxin exuding from poison spines. Caterpillar-associated disease is likely very underrecognized and underreported in even the most developed countries. The most common pathology comprises rashes caused by contact with hairs (erucism, or erucic rash). A common shade tree pest, the brown-tailed moth (*Nygmia phaeorrhoea*), in Europe and northeastern North America, liberates tiny barbed hairs when the caterpillar molts. Massive cyclical irruptions of the introduced gypsy moth (*Lymantria dispar*) in the New England states have recently caused increased visits by patients to dermatologists. The hairs of these caterpillars are blown about by the wind, and when skin is exposed, a severe dermatitis results. Dermatitis produced by urticating hairs typically comprises itchy, erythematous patches associated with small vesicles and edema. Prolonged contact (e.g., when detritus containing hairs or caterpillar "skins" contaminates sweaty skin under clothing) may result in ulceration, eschar formation, and scarring in some individuals (Fig. 11). Use of a masking tape-type lint roller can be very effective in removing urticating hairs, which may or may not be visible. Prompt showering after outdoor activities greatly reduces the likelihood of prolonged contact with the hairs.

Four other syndromes may be observed from contact with caterpillars (32). Lepidopterism, dendrolimiasis, ophthalmia nodosa, and a coagulopathy with fibrinolysis are less common but likely underrecognized. Lepidopterism is a systemic disease, suggesting aerogenic exposure to hairs, with generalized signs and symptoms such as headache, whole-body rash, pharyngitis, and respiratory distress. Conjunctivitis may also result. Dendrolimiasis is a subset of lepidopterism associated with Asian pine tree lappet moths (*Dendrolimus pini*). Exposure to moth cocoons or fluids from

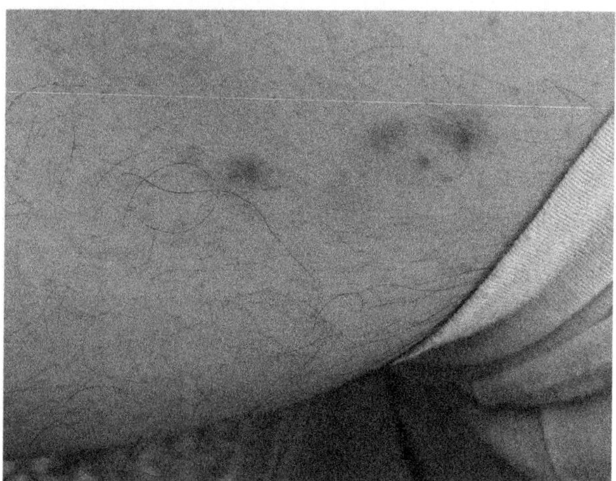

FIGURE 11 Caterpillar urticaria: chronic scarring 2 months after exposure to brown tail moth hairs, Massachusetts, 2017.

the caterpillars appears to trigger hypersensitivity reactions as well as chronic arthropathy. Ophthalmia nodosa is due to corneal penetration by caterpillar hairs (and also tarantula hairs) causing a chronic uveitis. Finally, *Lonomia* spp. caterpillars of South America can deliver a potent venom containing proteases and thrombolytics via a unique breakaway tip to their spiny "hairs." Penetration of the skin by the tips of these spines can cause immediate bleeding and ecchymoses, progressing to a frank hemorrhagic disease that may culminate in acute renal failure or intracerebral bleeds. Treatment comprises restoration of clotting factors and administration of antifibrinolytics. An experimental antivenin is being tested in Brazil, where a trend of increasing prevalence of *Lonomia* coagulopathy has been documented.

Scorpions

Scorpions are arachnids with a characteristic crablike appearance. The body consists of the cephalothorax and a segmented abdomen with a segmented tail, which terminates in a prominent stinging apparatus (aculeus). There are four pairs of legs that follow a pair of appendages (pedipalps) that terminate in well-defined characteristic pincers. Scorpions may range in size from 2 to 10 cm. Scorpions undergo incomplete development (immature stages look like miniature adults). Of the 1,000 or so species that are known, fewer than 50 have been reported to cause illness with their sting. Scorpions are problems mainly in the warmer climates. The bulbous end of the tail contains muscles that force venom through the stinger. All scorpions are predatory on other arthropods, immobilizing their prey with their venom. Humans are stung by walking barefoot at night, by not shaking their shoes out in the morning in an area of endemicity, by lifting rocks or logs, or in bedding that is on the floor. The stings cause local pain (probably due to the great biogenic amine content of the venom), edema, discoloration, and hypesthesia. Systemic signs can include shock, salivation, confusion or anxiety, nausea, tachycardia, and tetany. Venom characteristics differ depending on the genus of scorpion: some stimulate parasympathetic nerves and can lead to secondary stimulation of catecholamines, resulting in sympathetic stimulation, which in turn may contribute to respiratory failure (33). Others affect the central nervous system, are hemolytic, or cause local necrosis. Hypersensitivity and anaphylaxis may occur in individuals who are repeatedly exposed.

Treatment is usually symptomatic, although in areas with known dangerous species (Middle East: *Leiurus* spp., *Buthacus* spp., *Buthus* spp.; southern Africa: *Parabuthos* spp., *Buthos* spp., *Uroplectes* spp.; South and Central America: *Tityus* spp.; southern United States: *Centruroides* spp.), quickly getting a pressure bandage on over the sting and immobilizing the limb (if that is where the sting was) helps to prevent venom from traveling via the lymphatics. Lidocaine may be injected directly into the sting to reduce pain. Medical attention should be sought as soon as possible because antivenin, when administered promptly, reduces morbidity. However, antivenin is usually species specific, and without bringing the culprit in for identification, antivenin use would be on a presumptive basis.

Centipedes and Millipedes

The centipedes (class Chilopoda, 2,800 species) and millipedes (class Diplopoda, 8,000 species) are elongate, vermiform arthropods with dozens of segments, each of which bears a pair of legs. Both undergo incomplete development, with larvae looking like miniature adults. "Centipedes" would suggest having 100 segments (and pairs of legs) or fewer; "millipedes," more than 100 and up to 1,000. This simplification is not quite correct, but in general, many legs indicate a millipede, fewer legs (but more than insects or ticks) indicate a centipede. Other differences are apparent: millipedes are rounded in cross-section, but centipedes are dorsoventrally flattened; millipedes have mouthparts that are ventral and nonpiercing, whereas centipedes have mouthparts that protrude anteriorly and are clearly capable of piercing. Millipedes move slowly, reflecting their mode of life as feeders on detritus. Centipedes are very rapid predators of other arthropods.

The diversity of both millipedes and centipedes is greatest in the tropics, and virtually all those of medical importance are found in warm climates. Millipedes may squirt a noxious, corrosive fluid from pores on their segments. Such fluid may contain benzoquinone, aldehydes, and hydrocyanic acid and cause an immediate burning sensation followed by erythema and edema, even progressing to blistering (34). Most millipedes also have a repugnant smell; both the corrosive fluid and smell tend to protect them from predation. People become exposed when they step on or sleep on millipedes or provoke them (children playing with them are often victims). Treatment consists of washing the affected site as soon as possible to dilute and remove the corrosive fluids and is symptomatic for the skin lesions and pain. Millipedes can also serve as intermediate hosts of *Macracanthorhynchus ingens*, a zoonotic acanthocephalan. Centipedes have powerful biting mandibles and small fang-like structures (forcipules) situated between them and derived from the first pair of legs that may inject a venom. This venom is used to immobilize prey but is also used in defense. Centipede bites occur when people step on or sleep on them or play with them. Envenomation is manifested by local pain and swelling, with proximal lymphadenopathy. Headache, nausea, and anxiety are common. Skin lesions may ulcerate and become necrotic. Death due to centipede bite has only been confirmed for one case, a Filipino child who was bitten on the head by a large *Scolopendra* sp. The common house centipede, *Scutigera coleoptrata* of the eastern United States, is commonly found in bathtubs. This hairy-looking, small (5 to 8 cm long) centipede is actually beneficial, preying on roaches and other potential pests in houses. Its strong mandibles can, however, inflict a painful pinch, and it does have a mild venom that produces a bite similar in quality to a bee sting.

Spiders

The order Araneae comprises nearly 30,000 species, but only a fraction of them have any medical importance. Most are very small (0.5 cm or smaller in length), but a few are as large as a man's hand. Two major suborders are recognized, the Mygalomorphae, in which the fang-tipped chelicerae operate in parallel using an up-and-down strike, and the Aranaeomorphae, in which the chelicerae operate like insect mandibles, with a side-to-side motion. Spiders have an unsegmented cephalothorax, an abdomen, four pairs of legs, the prominent chelicerae, and spinnerets, specialized organs that secrete the silk for making webs. All spiders are predatory on other arthropods and use their venom to immobilize prey, which are stored live. Spiders rend their prey with their chelicerae and bathe them with a digestion fluid for hours prior to ingestion. Thus, although all spiders have stout chelicerae and can bite and all spiders have a venom with which to immobilize their prey, most are too small to be noticed by humans even if they were to be bitten. The spiders of main medical interest belong to four groups (35, 36): the funnel-web or trapdoor spiders of Australia (*Atrax* spp., *Hydronyche* spp.), New World and southern African recluse spiders (*Loxosceles* spp.), South American armed spiders (*Phoneutria* spp.), and the cosmopolitan widow spiders (*Latrodectus* spp.). The recluse and widows have been widely transported by humans.

The clinical manifestations and complications of envenomation differ among the four main spiders, and the syndromes caused by each have been given names that reflect the identity of the spider. With spider bites in general, there is local pain and erythema at the site of the bite, and this may be accompanied by fever, chills, nausea, and joint pains. In loxoscelism, the site of the bite ulcerates and becomes necrotic. Skin may slough, and there may be destruction of the adjacent tissues. Hemolysis, thrombocytopenia, and renal failure may ensue. With latrodectism, phoneutrism, and funnel-web neurotoxicity, the venoms have a strong neurotoxic action. Muscle rigidity and cramping (similar to acute abdomen) are seen with latrodectism; complications include electrocardiogram abnormalities and hypotension. With phoneutrism, visual disturbances, vertigo, and prostration may occur; complications include hypotension and respiratory paralysis. Funnel web spiders induce autonomic nervous system excitation, with muscular twitching, salivation and lachrymation, nausea and vomiting, and diarrhea; fatal respiratory arrest may result from apnea or laryngospasm (37).

Funnel web spider bites require prompt first aid, and the same recommendations could be used for latrodectism or phoneutrism. A compression bandage should be applied over the site of the bite, and the affected limb immobilized by splinting with a compression bandage if bitten on an extremity (standard procedures for snakebite). This may help prevent the venom from moving from the local lymphatics. The patient should seek medical attention as soon as possible for antivenin treatment. Otherwise, treatment is symptomatic with analgesics and antipyretics.

Tarantulas are popular pets and appear fearsome. Fortunately, most are docile, and most injuries associated with them are due to their urticating hairs, particularly with respect to conjunctivitis. They do, however, have robust mandibles and venom and should not be provoked; bites are similar in quality to a bee sting.

Necrotic dermal lesions are often classified as loxoscelism even if the appropriate spiders are not known to be present in the area: only 35 of 216 diagnoses of "brown recluse spider bites" proved to be supported by the minimum evidence for assigning such a specific etiology, *viz.*, the known presence of *Loxosceles reclusa* within the geographic area of exposure (38). In the eastern United States, some necrotic dermal lesions may actually be due to the bite of the yellow sac spider, *Cheiracanthium mildei*, or the related *Cheiracanthium inclusum*, causing a painful eschar that may last for weeks; however, a literature review failed to definitively incriminate these spiders as the cause (39). Severe reactions to tick bite, or even the erythema migrans of Lyme disease, may be confused with recluse or other spider bites (40).

Miscellaneous Injury Due to Arthropods

Beetles (Coleoptera) comprise 40% of all insect species, but even with this great diversity, very few may be harmful. Most injury is related to vesication by secretions containing cantharidin. Hemolymph (blood) of some of these beetles, generally called the blister beetles, also contains this irritant, and thus exposure may be by direct contact with live or dead (crushed) beetles. Cantharidin is the active ingredient of Spanish fly, the alleged aphrodisiac made from pulverized *Lytta vesicatoria* and other meloid beetles. Ingestion of Spanish fly irritates the ureter and urethra and causes painful priapism. Overdose or chronic use causes renal tubular necrosis. It is likely that Spanish fly is no longer in demand given the availability of nitric oxide inhibitors.

An unusual group of carabids, the bombardier beetles, spray a boiling hot (100°C) jet of benzoquinone as a defense (41), causing burns and blistering. Blistering is also produced by crushing the staphylinid beetle *Paederus fusca* of Southeast Asia, which contains a toxic alkaloid, pederin.

More commonly, carpet beetles (dermestids), which feed on wool rugs and other animal fur products, are associated with a papulovesicular eruption. In particular, larval dermestids and their hairs or shed skins (exuviae) cause a contact dermatitis.

Water bugs (colloquially known as water beetles but actually members of the Hemiptera), also known as toe-biters, can inflict strong pinches on unsuspecting toes wading through water.

OTHER INJURY

Delusion of Parasitosis

Illusory parasitosis is a condition in which a patient who has a real itch has the mistaken belief that the itch is due to active infestation by irrelevant arthropods. Often the itch is due to a drug reaction, sunburn, detergents, irritating dusts, poison ivy, or even *bona fide* arthropod bites (among many other potential sources of itch) that were sustained months in the past. Once a patient has been helped to identify the actual cause of the itch, he or she does not persist in blaming an arthropod. In contrast, in delusion of parasitosis (the terminology for the pathology that was known as delusory parasitosis continues to change, in an attempt to communicate with patients in a more neutral manner; another term is Ekbom syndrome) the patient cannot be dissuaded that the source of discomfort is probably not an arthropod. In some patients, there are no objective lesions but simply an insistence that the patient is infested. Many such cases are highly educated people who can describe their infestation with great detail. However, they rarely produce a specimen, and when they do, it is usually not an arthropod or part thereof. Delusion of parasitosis can be a serious illness which can be treated by experienced mental health professionals.

IDENTIFYING SUBMITTED SPECIMENS

For most purposes, identification to the species level ("This is *Eutrombicula alfreddugesi*.") may not provide any more clinically relevant information than identification to a higher taxonomic level ("This is a chigger."). In some cases, simply being able to say "This is definitely an arthropod part, perhaps beetle," may be all the information that is required (in this example, a beetle part may suggest dwarf tapeworm infection or be consistent with urticaria due to the hairs of dermestid beetle larvae or vesication due to the hot spray of the bombardier beetle). A whole arthropod may be compared with the bauplan diagram to place it within a general group. A classic pictorial key published by the CDC (available from http://www.dpd.cdc.gov/dpdx/HTML/CDProducts.htm) or simple tables or dichotomous keys (Table 3, Table 4) may be used to narrow the identification down to a known order or even genus of medically important arthropods (42, 43). Anything more specific usually requires consulting a taxonomic reference or finding

TABLE 3 Summary of the features of the major groups of arthropods of medical importance[a]

Group	Body regions	Legs	Antennae	Wings	Select medically important examples
Hexapoda (insects)	3 in adults (head, thorax, abdomen); larvae often lack defined regions	3 pairs in adults and some larvae; larvae may also contain pro-legs	Usually present in adults, 1 pair	Often present in adults, 1–2 pairs	Mosquitoes, lice, fleas, black flies, kissing bugs, bed bugs, stinging bees, wasps, ants
Arachnida (arachnids)	Usually 2 (cephalathorax and abdomen)	4 pairs in adults (mite, tick larvae have 3 pairs)	Always absent	Always absent	Ticks, itch and follicle mites, chiggers, venomous spiders and scorpions
Crustacea (crustaceans)	Variable, 1–2	Variable, usually 5–7 pairs in adults	Usually present, 2 pairs	Always absent	Tongue worms (pentastomes)
Chilopoda (centipedes)	2, head and body	≥15 pairs, 1 per body segment	Present, 1 pair	Always absent	Several venomous species
Diplopoda (millipedes)	2, head and body	>40 pairs, 2 per body segment	Present, 1 pair	Always absent	Some species produce poisonous secretions

[a]From reference 43. Reproduced with permission.

an entomologist who will help. Agricultural extension services, university entomology departments, local mosquito or pest control organizations, parasitologists, and local bug-collecting enthusiast clubs may all be of help in identifying a specimen and usually do not charge, out of professional courtesy. (Note that few such entities are CLIA certified, and thus fee for service is problematic.)

In some cases, a patient insists that an arthropod specimen be tested for the presence of an infectious agent. This is particularly common in areas that are endemic for Lyme disease. Numerous commercial laboratories test for the presence of Lyme disease spirochetes using a PCR assay, but given that the prevalence of infection in the vector may range from 15 to 70%, a positive test is likely. Some laboratories now offer a full range of PCR assays to include all of the deer tick microbial guild (44) (*Babesia microti, Borrelia miyamotoi, Anaplasma phagocytophilum*, deer tick virus). The value of such a practice is dubious, other than for psychologically satisfying the patient's demand. Physicians are often puzzled as to what to do with the information when confronted with the results of such a test by an otherwise healthy patient; most would not prescribe treatment based on a finding of infection in a tick. For Lyme disease, postexposure prophylaxis may be provided in the form of 1 or 2 doses of 100 mg doxycycline, which has been demonstrated by prospective randomized placebo-controlled clinical study to reduce the risk of infection after a recognized tick bite by 85%. The few epidemiological studies that have been performed suggest that about 70% of all Lyme disease or Rocky Mountain spotted fever patients never recall a tick bite preceding their acute disease (15, 16), and hence the tick that is found and submitted is usually by a healthy person.

The most important variable in determining the riskiness of a tick bite is how long the tick has fed (Fig. 12). If a deer tick is attached for no more than 24 hours, regardless of whether it is demonstrated to be infected with Lyme disease spirochetes, *Babesia microti*, or the agent of granulocytic ehrlichiosis, the likelihood of an infectious dose of organisms being transmitted is very small. The biological basis for this "grace period" is a phenomenon known as reactivation, wherein pathogens within ticks require a period of replication after emerging from a period of dormancy that they enter during the long interstadial period between blood meals (45). Reactivation was first described for the agent of Rocky Mountain spotted fever, which attains infectivity within tick salivary glands only after 12 to 18 hours of exposure to a host. Reactivation is probably a general phenomenon with most ixodid (hard) tick-transmitted agents, the only known exceptions being the viruses causing tick-borne encephalitis and the related Powassan fever, in which transmission is thought to be instantaneous with attachment.

Estimating the degree of engorgement may provide more of an index of individual risk than the actual presence or absence of infection. A simple measurement may be made with deer ticks and might be tried for other species of ticks. The scutal index (Fig. 12) is the ratio of the length of the tick from the tip of the mouthparts to the caudal edge of the tick to the width of the scutum, the dark shield on the dorsum of the tick. A scutal index of >2.5 suggests that a deer tick has been attached for more than 24 hours, and therefore transmission is likely (45). Such a finding might prompt a physician to provide prophylactic antibiotics, which would effectively abort Lyme disease or even human granulocytic anaplasmosis. Although such prophylaxis would not prevent babesiosis, note that of the agents transmitted by deer ticks, *B. microti* requires the greatest duration of attachment for infectivity, probably relating to the requirement for sporogony during attachment.

Much progress has been made in a universal barcoding system for identifying animals by means of DNA sequences. In particular, the 5′ end of the mitochondrial cytochrome C oxidase subunit I (COI), usually a 648-base pair portion, is used as a PCR target, and the nucleotide sequence that is obtained from the amplification product can be compared to a large online database (BOLD [46], http://ibol.org/). Most species of animals contain unique sequences in their COI gene and thus can be discriminated from other related species. Nearly 750,000 sequences have been accessioned in the BOLD database. For the phylum Arthropoda, barcode sequences exist for all 16 classes; for Insecta, all 30 orders are represented. Accordingly, virtually any putative arthropod sample may be identified to its order and possibly to family or genus by extracting its DNA, amplifying the COI gene, sequencing, and then submitting the data in FASTA format to the BOLD server. Assuming that the equipment

TABLE 4 Key to the common arthropod classes, subclasses, and orders of medical importance, adult stages only[a]

1. Three or four pairs of legs (2)
   Five or more pairs of legs (22)
2. Three pairs of legs with antennae **(insects: class Insecta)** (3)
   Four pairs of legs without antennae **(spiders, ticks, mites, scorpions: class Arachnida)** (20)
3. Wings present, well developed (4)
   Wings absent or rudimentary (12)
4. One pair of wings **(flies, mosquitoes, midges: order Diptera)** (5)
   Two pairs of wings (6)
5. Wings with scales **(mosquitoes: order Diptera)**
   Wings without scales **(other flies: order Diptera)**
6. Mouthparts adapted for sucking, with an elongate proboscis (7)
   Mouthparts adapted for chewing, without an elongate proboscis (8)
7. Wings densely covered with scales, proboscis coiled **(butterflies and moths: order Lepidoptera)**
   Wings not covered with scales, proboscis not coiled but directed backward **(bedbugs and kissing bugs: order Hemiptera)**
8. Both pairs of wings membranous, similar in structure, although size may vary (9)
   Front pair of wings leathery or shell-like, serving as covers for the second pair (10)
9. Both pairs of wings similar in size **(termites: order Isoptera)**
   Hind wings much smaller than front wings **(wasps, hornets, and bees: order Hymenoptera)**
10. Front wings horny or leathery, without distinct veins, meeting in a straight line down the middle (11)
    Front wings leathery or paperlike, with distinct veins, usually overlapping in the middle **(cockroaches: order Dictyoptera)**
11. Abdomen with prominent cerci or forceps; wings shorter than abdomen **(earwigs: order Dermaptera)**
    Abdomen without prominent cerci or forceps; wings covering abdomen **(beetles: order Coleoptera)**
12. Abdomen with three long terminal tails **(silverfish and firebrats: order Thysanura)**
    Abdomen without three long terminal tails (13)
13. Abdomen with narrow waist **(ants: order Hymenoptera)**
    Abdomen without narrow waist (14)
14. Abdomen with prominent pair of cerci or forceps **(earwigs: order Dermaptera)**
    Abdomen without cerci or forceps (15)
15. Body flattened laterally, antennae small, fitting into grooves in side of head **(fleas: order Siphonaptera)**
    Body flattened dorsoventrally, antennae projecting from side of head, not fitting into grooves (16)
16. Antennae with nine or more segments (17)
    Antennae with three to five segments (18)
17. Pronotum covering head **(cockroaches: order Dictyoptera)**
    Pronotum not covering head **(termites: order Isoptera)**
18. Mouthparts consisting of tubular joined beak; three- to five-segmented tarsi **(bedbugs: order Hemiptera)**
    Mouthparts retracted into head or of the chewing type; one- or two-segmented tarsi (19)
19. Mouthparts retracted into the head; adapted for sucking blood **(sucking lice: order Anopleura)**
    Mouthparts of the chewing type **(chewing lice: order Mallophaga)**
20. Body oval, consisting of a single saclike region **(ticks and mites: subclass Acari)**
    Body divided into two distinct regions, a cephalothorax and an abdomen (21)
21. Abdomen joined to the cephalothorax by a slender waist; abdomen with segmentation indistinct or absent; stinger absent **(spiders: subclass Araneae)**
    Abdomen broadly joined to the cephalothorax; abdomen distinctly segmented, ending with a stinger **(scorpions: subclass Scorpiones)**
22. Five to nine pairs of legs or swimmerets; one or two pairs of antennae; principally aquatic organisms **(copepods, crabs, and crayfish: class Crustacea)**
    Ten or more pairs of legs or swimmerets absent; one pair of antennae present; terrestrial organisms (23)
23. Body segments each with only one pair of legs **(centipedes: class Chilopoda)**
    Body segments each with two pairs of legs **(millipedes: class Diplopoda)**

[a]Data from references 49 and 50.

is available (thermal cycler, gel electrophoresis, pipettors and other materials common to molecular biology laboratories), such an identification might cost on the order of $150 to $200 (5 hours of technician time, PCR reagents, commercial rate for sequencing 300 base pairs) with a few days turnaround (usually 24 to 48 hours minimum from submission of the DNA to receipt of the sequencing chromatogram is required for DNA sequencing). A simple DNA extraction technique (HotSHOT, which uses hot sodium hydroxide and tris neutralization) may be used on most samples to prepare for PCR analysis (47). The assay conditions and PCR primers for amplifying an informative portion of the COI gene may be adopted from published analyses of preserved museum specimens, which often contain degraded DNA similar to many forensic or clinical samples (48). The advantage to the barcoding approach is that the method is not subjective and does not require the extensive training and expertise for morphological identification; anyone with general expertise in molecular biology may be engaged. Classically based methods, however,

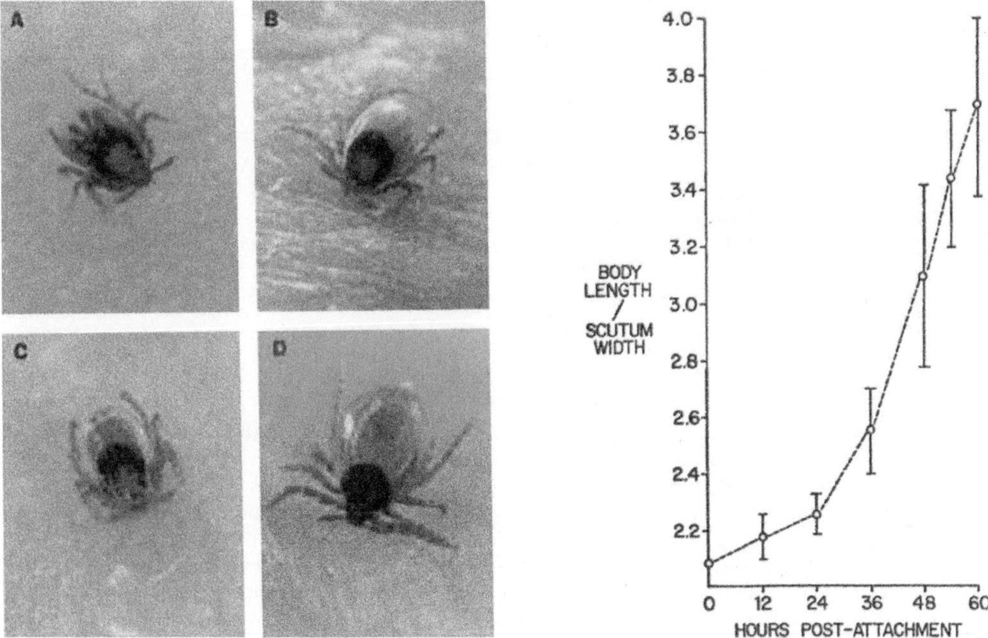

FIGURE 12 Gradual engorgement of feeding ixodid ticks. (Left panel) Four-day feeding sequence of nymphal *Ixodes ricinus* (reprinted from Matuschka FR, Spielman A, *Lancet* **342**:529, 1993, with permission from Elsevier). (Right panel) Scutal index of engorgement for *Ixodes dammini* (from reference 45, reprinted with permission of the American Society of Tropical Medicine and Hygiene).

require little more than a microscope, can be virtually instantaneous, and may be performed as a professional courtesy without a fee. Some commercial websites (e.g., www.identifyus.com) offer virtual morphologic identification in real time, with clients uploading a photograph of the offending arthropod to be identified quickly by an expert. Alternatively, amateur entomologist websites (e.g., www.bugguide.net) can be extremely helpful in identifying samples. "Dr. Google Images" may also be of great utility for both the pathology suspected of having an arthropod origin (e.g., for a query such as "skin blister burns after insect contact" yielding "blister beetle welt") or for a submitted specimen ("flat beetle from a bed" yielding pictures of bed bugs).

REFERENCES

1. **Jones BR.** 1975. The prevention of blindness from trachoma. *Trans Ophthalmol Soc U K* **95:**16–33.
2. **Jupp PG, Lyons SF.** 1987. Experimental assessment of bedbugs (*Cimex lectularius* and *Cimex hemipterus*) and mosquitoes (*Aedes aegypti formosus*) as vectors of human immunodeficiency virus. *AIDS* **1:**171–174.
3. **Buxton PA.** 1955. *The Natural History of Tsetse Flies*. H.K. Lewis, London, United Kingdom.
4. **Pellegrino M, Steinbach N, Stensmyr MC, Hansson BS, Vosshall LB.** 2011. A natural polymorphism alters odour and DEET sensitivity in an insect odorant receptor. *Nature* **478:**511–514.
5. **Ribeiro JMC.** 1995. Blood-feeding arthropods: live syringes or invertebrate pharmacologists? *Infect Agents Dis* **4:**143–152.
6. **Pung OJ, Banks CW, Jones DN, Krissinger MW.** 1995. *Trypanosoma cruzi* in wild raccoons, opossums, and triatomine bugs in southeast Georgia, U.S.A. *J Parasitol* **81:**324–326.
7. **Shikanai-Yasuda MA, Carvalho NB.** 2012. Oral transmission of Chagas disease. *Clin Infect Dis* **54:**845–852.
8. **Palma RL.** 1991. Ancient head lice found on wooden comb from Antinoe, Egypt. *J Egypt Archaeol* **77:**194.
9. **Zinsser H.** 1942. *Rats, Lice and History*, 4th ed. George Routledge, London, United Kingdom.
10. **Deeks LS, Naunton M, Currie MJ, Bowden FJ.** 2013. Topical ivermectin 0.5% lotion for treatment of head lice. *Ann Pharmacother* **47:**1161–1167.
11. **Huebner RJ, Stamps P, Armstrong C.** 1946. Rickettsialpox; a newly recognized rickettsial disease; isolation of the etiological agent. *Public Health Rep* **61:**1605–1614.
12. **Telford SR III.** 1998. The name *Ixodes dammini* epidemiologically justified. *Emerg Infect Dis* **4:**132–134.
13. **Balashov YS.** 1972. *Bloodsucking Ticks (Ixodoidea): Vectors of Diseases of Man and Animals. Misc Publ Entomol Soc Am*, vol. 8(5). Entomological Society of America, College Park, MD.
14. **Ribeiro JM, Makoul GT, Levine J, Robinson DR, Spielman A.** 1985. Antihemostatic, antiinflammatory, and immunosuppressive properties of the saliva of a tick, *Ixodes dammini*. *J Exp Med* **161:**332–344.
15. **Steere AC.** 1994. Lyme disease: a growing threat to urban populations. *Proc Natl Acad Sci U S A* **91:**2378–2383.
16. **Woodward TE, Cunha BA.** 2000. Rocky Mountain spotted fever, p 121–138. *In* Cunha BA (ed), *Tickborne Infectious Diseases: Diagnosis and Management*. Marcel Dekker, New York, NY.
17. **Curran KL, Fish D.** 1989. Increased risk of Lyme disease for cat owners. *N Engl J Med* **320:**183.
18. **Spielman A, Rossignol PA.** 1984. Insect vectors, 167–183. *In* Warren KS, Mahmoud AAF (ed), *Tropical and Geographical Medicine*. McGraw-Hill, New York, NY.
19. **Hewitt CG.** 1910. *The House Fly*. University Press, Manchester, United Kingdom.
20. **Ward R, Melnick JL, Horstmann DM.** 1945. Poliomyelitis virus in fly-contaminated food collected at an epidemic. *Science* **101:**491–493.
21. **Watt J, Lindsay DR.** 1948. Diarrheal disease control studies; effect of fly control in a high morbidity area. *Public Health Rep* **63:**1319–1333.
22. **Barber MA.** 1914. Cockroaches and ants as carriers of the vibrios of Asiatic cholera. *Philipp J Sci, Sect B* **9:**1.
23. **Portnoy J, Chew GL, Phipatanakul W, Williams PB, Grimes C, Kennedy K, Matsui EC, Miller JD, Bernstein D, Blessing-Moore J, Cox L, Khan D, Lang D, Nicklas R, Oppenheimer J, Randolph C, Schuller D, Spector S, Tilles SA, Wallace D, Seltzer J, Sublett J, Joint Task Force on

Practice Parameters. 2013. Environmental assessment and exposure reduction of cockroaches: a practice parameter. *J Allergy Clin Immunol* **132:**802–802.e5.

24. **Mounsey KE, McCarthy JS.** 2013. Treatment and control of scabies. *Curr Opin Infect Dis* **26:**133–139.
25. **Masina S, Broady KW.** 1999. Tick paralysis: development of a vaccine. *Int J Parasitol* **29:**535–541.
26. **Commins SP, James HR, Kelly LA, Pochan SL, Workman LJ, Perzanowski MS, Kocan KM, Fahy JV, Nganga LW, Ronmark E, Cooper PJ, Platts-Mills TA.** 2011. The relevance of tick bites to the production of IgE antibodies to the mammalian oligosaccharide galactose-α-1,3-galactose. *J Allergy Clin Immunol* **127:**1286–93.e6.
27. **Lavrov DV, Brown WM, Boore JL.** 2004. Phylogenetic position of the Pentastomida and (pan)crustacean relationships. *Proc Biol Sci* **271:**537–544.
28. **Riley J.** 1986. The biology of pentastomids. *Adv Parasitol* **25:**45–128.
29. **Aydıngöz IE, Mansur AT.** 2011. Canine scabies in humans: a case report and review of the literature. *Dermatology* **223:** 104–106.
30. **Raffray L, Malvy D.** 2014. Accidental intestinal myiasis caused by *Eristalis tenax* in France. *Travel Med Infect Dis* **12:**109e110
31. **Chernin E.** 1986. Surgical maggots. *South Med J* **79:** 1143–1145.
32. **Diaz JH.** 2005. The evolving global epidemiology, syndromic classification, management, and prevention of caterpillar envenoming. *Am J Trop Med Hyg* **72:**347–357.
33. **Amitai Y.** 1998. Clinical manifestations and management of scorpion envenomation. *Public Health Rev* **26:**257–263.
34. **Attygalle AB, Xu SC, Meinwald J, Eisner T.** 1993. Defensive secretion of the millipede *Floridobolus penneri*. *J Nat Prod* **56:**1700–1706.
35. **Bucherl W.** 1969. Biology and venoms of the most important South American spiders of the genera *Phoneutria, Loxosceles, Lycosa,* and *Latrodectus*. *Am Zool* **9:**157–159.
36. **Diaz JH.** 2004. The global epidemiology, syndromic classification, management, and prevention of spider bites. *Am J Trop Med Hyg* **71:**239–250.
37. **Miller MK, Whyte IM, White J, Keir PM.** 2000. Clinical features and management of *Hadronyche envenomation* in man. *Toxicon* **38:**409–427.
38. **Vetter RS, Cushing PE, Crawford RL, Royce LA.** 2003. Diagnoses of brown recluse spider bites (loxoscelism) greatly outnumber actual verifications of the spider in four western American states. *Toxicon* **42:**413–418.
39. **Vetter RS, Isbister GK, Bush SP, Boutin LJ.** 2006. Verified bites by yellow sac spiders (genus *Cheiracanthium*) in the United States and Australia: where is the necrosis? *Am J Trop Med Hyg* **74:**1043–1048.
40. **Masters EJ, King LE Jr.** 1994. Differentiating loxoscelism from Lyme disease. *Emerg Med* **26:**47–49.
41. **Dean J, Aneshansley DJ, Edgerton HE, Eisner T.** 1990. Defensive spray of the bombardier beetle: a biological pulse jet. *Science* **248:**1219–1221.
42. **Mathison BA, Pritt BS.** 2014. Laboratory identification of arthropod ectoparasites. *Clin Microbiol Rev* **27:**48–67.
43. **Mathison B, Pritt BS.** 2015. *Arthropod Benchtop Reference Guide*. College of American Pathologists, Chicago, IL.
44. **Katavolos P, Armstrong PM, Dawson JE, Telford SR III.** 1998. Duration of tick attachment required for transmission of granulocytic ehrlichiosis. *J Infect Dis* **177:**1422–1425.
45. **Piesman J, Spielman A.** 1980. Human babesiosis on Nantucket Island: prevalence of *Babesia microti* in ticks. *Am J Trop Med Hyg* **29:**742–746.
46. **Ratnasingham S, Hebert PDN.** 2007. BOLD: the Barcode of Life Data System. *Mol Ecol Notes.*
47. **Truett GE, Heeger P, Mynatt RL, Truett AA, Walker JA, Warman ML.** 2000. Preparation of PCR-quality mouse genomic DNA with hot sodium hydroxide and tris (HotSHOT). *Biotechniques* **29:**52–54, 54.
48. **Meusnier I, Singer GAC, Landry JF, Hickey DA, Hebert PDN, Hajibabaei M.** 2008. A universal DNA mini-barcode for biodiversity analysis. *BMC Genomics* **9:**214.
49. **Herms WB.** 1939. *Medical Entomology*, 3rd ed. Macmillan, New York, NY.
50. **Arnett RH.** 1985. *American Insects: A Handbook of the Insects of America North of Mexico*. Van Nostrand Reinhold Company, New York, NY.

ANTIPARASITIC AGENTS AND SUSCEPTIBILITY TEST METHODS

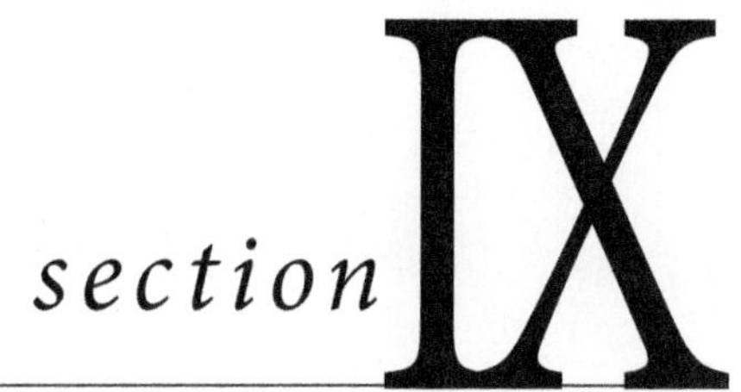

VOLUME EDITOR: DAVID W. WARNOCK
SECTION EDITOR: GARY W. PROCOP

Antiparasitic Agents

KARIN LEDER, SARAH L. McGUINNESS, AND PETER F. WELLER

152

A number of effective antiprotozoal and anthelmintic drugs are currently available. Antiparasitic agents are important both for therapy of infected individual patients and for control of parasitic infections at the community level. Large-scale chemotherapy is reducing transmission, morbidity, and mortality of certain infections, including lymphatic filariasis, onchocerciasis, schistosomiasis, and infections with intestinal nematodes. However, the lack of financial incentives to develop new agents is a major limitation to the future of antiparasitic chemotherapy. Emerging resistance among parasites, lack of effective antiparasitic vaccines, and the enormous burden of disease worldwide also pose challenges to the effective management of parasitic infections.

This chapter focuses on the mechanisms of action, pharmacology, clinical utility, and adverse effects of common first-line antiparasitic therapies and newer drug alternatives. Most helminth infections in humans can be treated with one of five drugs, namely, albendazole, mebendazole, praziquantel, ivermectin, and diethylcarbamazine (DEC), so these five drugs are reviewed in detail. Another agent, nitazoxanide, has both anthelmintic and antiprotozoal activity and is also discussed. Other major antiprotozoal drugs are also reviewed, including those used for malaria, infections with gastrointestinal protozoa, leishmaniasis, and trypanosomiasis, but an exhaustive list of all antiparasitic drugs is not included. Specifically, we exclude discussion of agents without a first-line indication or that are recommended only in special situations, such as furazolidone in children. Tribendimidine is a promising new agent for treatment of liver flukes (clonorchiasis and opisthorchiasis), but trials are still under way, and it has not yet been approved for use, so it is not discussed. Additionally, antibacterial and antifungal agents that can also be used for treatment of protozoal infections, such as the 5-nitroimidazoles, trimethoprim-sulfamethoxazole, azithromycin, and amphotericin, are not discussed in detail here, but their general indications for parasitic infections are shown in Tables 1 and 2. Resistance to antiparasitic agents and drug susceptibility testing are dealt with in separate chapters.

Throughout this chapter, we indicate which antiparasitic drugs are currently approved by the U.S. Food and Drug Administration (FDA). For those based in other countries, a table of national and regional drug regulatory authorities is provided at the end of the chapter.

ANTHELMINTIC AGENTS

Benzimidazoles

The benzimidazoles are antiparasitic agents with a broad spectrum of activity against many helminthic and certain protozoal infections. All members of the benzimidazole class have in common a bicyclic ring system into which benzene has been inserted. Mebendazole and albendazole, both of which are synthetic agents, are the most widely used drugs of this class. Mebendazole is 5-benzoyl-2-benzimidazole carbamic acid, and albendazole is methyl 5-(propylthio)-2-benzimidazole carbamate. The low cost, high efficacy, and ease of administration of these two agents have led to their widespread use for many human parasitic infections. Major indications for their use are shown in Tables 3 and 4. Although mebendazole has been approved for treatment of multiple nematode infections by the FDA, mebendazole is not currently available in the United States. Instead, albendazole is used preferentially as first-line treatment for many parasite infections but is nevertheless considered investigational and given as a "nonapproved indication" in all cases except when used as treatment for hydatid infections and neurocysticercosis (1).

Other members of this drug class include flubendazole, thiabendazole, and triclabendazole. Flubendazole, a parafluoro analogue of mebendazole, has the same mechanism of action as mebendazole and albendazole. It is licensed in Europe for the treatment of intestinal nematodes but is not licensed in the United States. It has shown good activity against adult filarial parasites in animal models if given parenterally (2). It also exhibits activity against protoscoleces of *Echinococcus granulosus*, but currently there are no data on its efficacy for treatment of hydatid disease in humans (3). Thiabendazole, 2-(4-thiazolyl)-1H-benzimidazole, has similar mechanisms of action as the other benzimidazoles, but it is frequently associated with side effects. It has now been replaced by other anthelmintic agents (4) but is sometimes still used topically for treatment of cutaneous larva migrans. Triclabendazole is a newer imidazole derivative that has been used as a veterinary agent for many years. It is thought to act on microtubules, causing decreased parasite motility. It is the drug of choice for fascioliasis and acts on both adult and immature worms (5), although resistance is emerging in animals and this may pose a threat to treatment of human patients (6–9). It is also an option for therapy of paragonimiasis (1, 10).

TABLE 1 Treatment of intestinal, blood and tissue (nonplasmodial), and urogenital protozoal infections[a]

Organism or disease	Primary agent used for treatment	Alternative agent(s)
Intestinal protozoa		
Entamoeba histolytica	Invasive trophozoites: metronidazole	Tinidazole
	Luminal agent: iodoquinol	Alternative luminal agents: diloxanide furoate, paromomycin
	Tetracycline	Metronidazole, iodoquinol
Neobalantidium coli	Nitazoxanide	
Cryptosporidium parvum	In patients with HIV/AIDS: restoration of immunity with antiretroviral therapy	Nitazoxanide[b]
Cyclospora cayetanensis	Trimethoprim-sulfamethoxazole	
Cystoisospora belli	Metronidazole	Iodoquinol, paromomycin
Dientamoeba fragilis	Metronidazole	Tinidazole, nitazoxanide, quinacrine, albendazole, furazolidone, paromomycin
Giardia duodenalis	Tinidazole	Metronidazole, nitazoxanide, albendazole, paromomycin, furazolidone, quinacrine
Blood and tissue protozoa		
Amebic meningoencephalitis	Amphotericin B	Miltefosine, variety of combinations; clindamycin plus quinine
Babesia species	Atovaquone plus azithromycin	Miltefosine, pentamidine, paromomycin
Leishmania species—visceral leishmaniasis[c]	Liposomal amphotericin B	Miltefosine, pentavalent antimonials, amphotericin B, pentamidine
Leishmania species—cutaneous or mucocutaneous leishmaniasis[c]	No treatment of choice; treatment should be individualized	
Toxoplasma gondii	Pyrimethamine plus sulfadiazine	
Trypanosoma brucei species (African trypanosomiasis)	Early: suramin (*T. b. rhodesiense*) or pentamidine (*T. b. gambiense*)	
	Late: melarsoprol (*T. b. rhodesiense*) or eflornithine plus nifurtimox (*T. b. gambiense*)	Benznidazole
Trypanosoma cruzi (American trypanosomiasis)	Nifurtimox	Benznidazole
Urogenital protozoa		
Trichomonas vaginalis	Metronidazole	Tinidazole

[a]Adapted from reference 1.
[b]See Table 8.
[c]Adapted from reference 167.

Triclabendazole is well tolerated, and few significant adverse effects have been described, but it is not recommended for use during pregnancy because of insufficient safety data. It is considered investigational by the FDA and may be obtained from the Centers for Disease Control and Prevention (CDC) in the United States for paragonimiasis, but it is not widely available. These three agents are not discussed further.

Mechanism of action. The antiparasitic activity of albendazole and mebendazole results mainly from their ability to bind to a cytoskeletal protein of parasites called β-tubulin, thereby inhibiting the polymerization of tubulin into microtubules (11). The disruption of microtubule synthesis within parasitic intestinal cells results in decreased absorptive function. In addition, mebendazole and albendazole directly inhibit glucose absorption by parasites, leading to a depletion of parasite glycogen stores, insufficient energy sources for formation of ATP, and an inability to reproduce or survive (12, 13). Although tubulin is also present in mammalian hosts, the benzimidazoles bind to parasite tubulin with an affinity that is hundreds of times greater than that with which they bind to mammalian tubulin, thereby causing minimal mammalian toxicity (4).

Pharmacokinetics. Benzimidazoles are poorly soluble in water and therefore are not well absorbed following oral administration. Although this limits their activity against tissue-dwelling parasites, it contributes to their minimal toxicity and to their efficacy in the treatment of many intestinal helminthic infections (14). Less than 20% of mebendazole is absorbed after oral administration, with peak plasma concentrations seen at 2 to 4 h. It is metabolized in the liver to inactive compounds, eliminated in the bile, and excreted predominantly in the feces. It is 95% protein bound in plasma, and its serum half-life is 2.5 to 5.5 h. Serum levels are markedly variable between individuals, but tissue and echinococcal cyst concentrations tend to be low (15).

The oral bioavailability of albendazole is also poor, with less than 10% absorption following an oral dose (16). Administration of albendazole with a fatty meal markedly improves bioavailability, up to 5-fold. It is rapidly metabolized in the liver, and concentrations of the parent drug in plasma are negligible. However, its primary metabolite, albendazole sulfoxide, also has anthelmintic activity (17). This results in a higher efficacy of albendazole than mebendazole for most indications. Albendazole sulfoxide is 70% protein bound and is widely distributed throughout the body. Peak plasma concentrations of albendazole sulfoxide are seen after 2 to 5 h but show great intersubject variability, ranging from 0.45 to 2.96 mg/liter following a single dose of 15 mg/kg of body weight (18). Albendazole induces enzymes of the cytochrome P450 system responsible

TABLE 2 Treatment of major helminthic infections[a]

Organism or disease[b]	Primary agent used for treatment	Alternative agent(s)
Nematodes		
Ancylostoma caninum (eosinophilic enterocolitis)	Albendazole	Mebendazole
Angiostrongylus cantonensis	Supportive	Albendazole plus steroids
Ascaris lumbricoides	Albendazole	Mebendazole, ivermectin
Capillaria species	Mebendazole	Albendazole
Cutaneous larva migrans	Albendazole	Ivermectin
Enterobius vermicularis	Albendazole	Mebendazole
Filariasis (*Wuchereria bancrofti*, *Brugia malayi*)	DEC with or without albendazole or ivermectin	
Gnathostoma species	Albendazole	Ivermectin, surgical removal
Hookworm	Albendazole	Mebendazole
Loa loa (only treat without high microfilaremia)	DEC with or without albendazole or ivermectin	
Onchocerca volvulus	Ivermectin	
Strongyloides stercoralis	Ivermectin	Albendazole
Toxocara species (visceral larva migrans)	Albendazole	Mebendazole
Trichinella spiralis	Albendazole plus steroids	Mebendazole
Trichostrongylus species	Albendazole	Mebendazole
Trichuris trichiura	Mebendazole	Albendazole, ivermectin
Cestodes		
Cysticercosis	Albendazole	Praziquantel
Diphyllobothrium latum	Praziquantel	
Dipylidium caninum	Praziquantel	
Echinococcus species	Albendazole	Praziquantel
Hymenolepis nana	Praziquantel	
Taenia saginata	Praziquantel	
Taenia solium	Praziquantel	
Trematodes		
Clonorchis sinensis	Praziquantel	Albendazole
Fasciola hepatica	Triclabendazole	
Intestinal flukes	Praziquantel	
Metorchis conjunctus	Praziquantel	
Opisthorchis viverrini	Praziquantel	
Paragonimus species	Triclabendazole	Praziquantel
Schistosoma species	Praziquantel	

[a]Adapted from reference 1.
[b]This is not an exhaustive list of all possible parasitic infections, but commonly encountered parasites are included.

TABLE 3 Major indications for albendazole[a]

Indication	Usual dose	Reported efficacy
Echinococcus granulosus	15 mg/kg/day (max, 800 mg) in 2 doses, usually a minimum of 1–6 mo	Clinical cure, as evidenced by cyst disappearance in one-third of recipients and improvement in radiological appearance in an additional 30–50%. Combined treatment with praziquantel can improve antiparasitic effectiveness.[b]
Cysticercosis	15 mg/kg/day (max, 800 mg) in 2 doses, usually for 8 days (8–30 days)	75–95% of parenchymal cysts destroyed and 40–70% of patients show resolution of all active cysts. Combined treatment with praziquantel improves cysticidal efficacy.[c]
Ascaris lumbricoides	Single 400-mg dose	Median cure rate of 95–98% and egg reduction rate of 99–100%
Cutaneous larva migrans	400 mg daily for 3 days	No large clinical trials; generally reserved for those with severe or disseminated infection
Enterobius vermicularis	400-mg dose, repeat in 2 wk	Cure rate close to 100%
Hookworm	Single 400-mg dose	Cure rate of 70–90% and egg reduction rate of 85–100%
Trichuris trichiura	400-mg dose for 3 days	Cure rate of 35–70% and egg reduction rate of 50–90%
Toxocariasis	400 mg twice daily for 5 days	No large clinical trials
Lymphatic filariasis	Single 400-mg dose	Microfilaremia reduced by 98–99% for prolonged periods when administered in combination with doxycycline, DEC, or ivermectin
Loa loa	Single 400-mg dose	No microfilaricidal effect, but partial macrofilaricidal effect with sterilization and/or death of adult worms
Giardia duodenalis	400 mg daily for 5 days	Cure rate of 80–97%
Gnathostoma spinigerum	400 mg twice daily for 21 days	No large clinical trials

[a]Adapted from reference 1.
[b]See reference 48.
[c]See reference 43.

TABLE 4 Major indications for mebendazole[a]

Indication	Usual dose	Reported efficacy
Ascaris lumbricoides	Single 500-mg dose or 100 mg twice daily for 3 days	Median cure rates of 95–98% and egg reduction rates of 99–100%
Enterobius vermicularis	Single 100-mg dose, repeated after 2–3 weeks	Mean cure rate of 95%
Hookworm	Single 500-mg dose or 100 mg twice daily for 3 days	Cure rates of 15–30% and egg reduction rates of 60–95% Approx 70% cure achieved with 3 days of mebendazole 500 mg daily
Trichuris trichiura	100 mg twice daily for 3 days	Cure rate of 70–90% and egg reduction rates of 90–95%
Toxocariasis	100–200 mg twice daily for 5 days	No large clinical trials

[a]Adapted from reference 1.

for its metabolism. Cimetidine and dexamethasone both raise drug levels and increase the area under the plasma concentration-time curve (19), and coadministration with praziquantel also increases the levels of albendazole (20–22). Albendazole sulfoxide has been detected in urine, bile, liver, cyst fluid, and cerebrospinal fluid (CSF). Levels in plasma have been reported to be 3- to 10-fold and 2- to 4-fold higher than in cyst fluid and CSF, respectively (23, 24), although the relationship between plasma levels and levels in other fluids shows individual variability (25). Albendazole sulfoxide has a half-life of ~9 h. It is oxidized further to inactive compounds such as albendazole sulfone and is excreted mainly in the urine.

Neither mebendazole nor albendazole is dialyzable. No dosage adjustment is required for individuals with renal impairment, but a reduction in dose should be considered if there is significant hepatic insufficiency. Benzimidazoles are not available as intravenous formulations.

Spectrum of activity. The benzimidazoles are effective against adult worms and developing helminthic embryos. Albendazole and mebendazole have similar and broad ranges of activity (Tables 3 and 4). Both drugs have good efficacy against many common intestinal nematode infections, including ascariasis, trichuriasis, enterobiasis, and hookworm infections. Three-day regimens of mebendazole and 1 to 3 days of albendazole are generally recommended for therapy of individual patients (with the longer duration being particularly preferable for trichuriasis therapy) (26, 27). A single dose of either drug is often used for mass or targeted community treatment of intestinal nematodes in areas where the parasites are endemic. Albendazole is preferred in most instances, but the efficacy of albendazole against very heavy infections with *Trichuris trichiura* is suboptimal, and mebendazole may be preferable in this circumstance. The reported curative efficacy of both drugs in different parasitic infections varies according to the baseline intensity of infection in the patient, geographical location, diagnostic tests employed, and duration of follow-up posttreatment (27).

Mebendazole and albendazole also have activity against other nematode infections, including angiostrongyliasis, trichostrongyliasis, capillariasis, trichinellosis, gnathostomiasis, toxocariasis, and cutaneous larva migrans. Additionally, albendazole is being increasingly being used, sometimes in combination with either DEC or ivermectin, for treatment of bancroftian or brugian filariasis and loiasis; it is particularly useful for these infections as part of a single-dose regimen for mass chemotherapy programs (28). Although albendazole displays some efficacy against *Strongyloides stercoralis*, ivermectin consistently yields higher cure rates and is the recommended treatment of choice.

Both mebendazole and albendazole also show activity in certain cestode infections. Albendazole is again preferred because of its more favorable pharmacokinetics, and it is now considered the drug of choice for medical management or adjunctive treatment of hydatid disease due to *E. granulosus*. Prolonged albendazole therapy (minimum of 10 years) can also be used in inoperable alveolar echinococcosis or as adjuvant therapy for patients with *Echinococcus multilocularis* infection. Additionally, albendazole is used for treatment of parenchymal neurocysticercosis. Although considered primarily an anthelmintic agent, albendazole is also an alternative agent for giardiasis (29).

Adverse effects. Adverse effects following short courses of the benzimidazoles mebendazole and albendazole are infrequent and generally mild. Transient abdominal pain, nausea, and diarrhea may develop. Headache, dizziness, insomnia, and allergic phenomena are also reported. With prolonged high-dose therapy, such as for echinococcosis, transient and reversible elevations of serum transaminases occur in 1 to 5% of recipients. Occasionally, alopecia (<1%) and reversible leukopenia (<1%) are seen. Discontinuation of therapy is infrequently needed, but a death related to albendazole-induced pancytopenia has been described (30). There are rare reports of albendazole therapy triggering seizures in people with undiagnosed neurocysticercosis (31, 32).

When mebendazole (pregnancy category C) has been used by pregnant women, the incidence of spontaneous abortions or fetal malformations has not been greater than the background population rate. There are also no reports of teratogenicity from albendazole (pregnancy category C), and women who have received it inadvertently during pregnancy have not experienced adverse fetal outcomes (33, 34). However, studies of benzimidazole drugs in animals suggest a possible teratogenic and embryotoxic effect. Since there are no good prospective safety data on either of these agents in humans, it is recommended that neither albendazole nor mebendazole be administered during pregnancy, particularly during the first trimester, unless the potential benefits justify the possible risk to the fetus. Albendazole and mebendazole are excreted in low concentrations in breast milk, and although they are unlikely to be harmful to the infant, these drugs should be used with caution in lactating women (35).

Praziquantel

Praziquantel is a synthetic heterocyclic isoquinoline-pyrazine derivative. Major indications for its use are shown in Table 5. It has been approved for use by the FDA (1). It has the unique characteristic of being active against almost all trematodes and cestodes, but it is not useful for treatment of nematode infections (4).

TABLE 5 Major indications for praziquantel[a]

Indication	Usual dose	Reported efficacy
Clonorchiasis	75 mg/kg/day in 3 doses for 2 days	Cure rate of 85–100%
Cysticercosis	50 mg/kg/day in 3 doses, usually for 15 days (1–30 days)	Combined treatment with albendazole improves cysticidal efficacy[b]
Opisthorchiasis	75 mg/kg/day in 3 doses for 2 days	Cure rate of >95%
Intestinal flukes	75 mg/kg/day in 3 doses for 1 day	No large clinical trials
Paragonimiasis	75 mg/kg/day in 3 doses for 2 days	>95% cure rate for pulmonary infections (may be lower in ectopic sites)
Schistosomiasis	40–60 mg/kg/day in 2 or 3 doses for 1 day	Cure rate of 75–100% and egg reduction rate of 90–95% in those not cured
Tapeworms (intestinal stage)	Single dose of 5–25 mg/kg	Cure rates of >95% for *Taenia*, *Diphyllobothrium*, and *Hymenolepis* species infections

[a]Adapted from reference 1.
[b]See reference 44.

Mechanism of action. Praziquantel induces ultrastructural changes in the teguments of parasites, resulting in increased permeability to calcium ions. Calcium ions accumulate in the parasite cytosol, leading to muscular contractions and ultimately to paralysis of adult worms. By damaging the tegument membrane, praziquantel also exposes parasite antigens to host immune responses (36–38). These effects lead to dislodgment of worms from their intestinal sites and subsequent expulsion by peristalsis.

Pharmacokinetics. Praziquantel is available for oral administration, with >80% of the drug being rapidly absorbed. Coadministration with a fatty or high-carbohydrate meal increases drug concentrations in serum (39, 40). Praziquantel is manufactured and administered as a racemic mixture of *S* and *R* stereoisomers: the anthelmintic properties of the drug are associated with (*R*)-praziquantel and the bitter taste lies predominantly with the inactive *S* isomer (38, 40). No parenteral formulation exists. The drug is biotransformed in the liver, and metabolites are excreted mainly in the urine. The cytochrome P450 hepatic metabolism of praziquantel is induced by corticosteroids, phenytoin, and phenobarbital. Serum levels of praziquantel are therefore lowered when any of these drugs are coadministered. Cimetidine, which inhibits P450-mediated metabolism, can be given concurrently to increase plasma praziquantel levels. Plasma levels peak after 1.5 to 2 h, and after a single 40-mg/kg dose, peak levels have been reported to be 1.007 to 1.625 mg/liter (41), with an area under the curve from 2,100 to 5,400 ng · h/ml (40, 42). Praziquantel crosses the blood-brain barrier, but levels in CSF are only approximately 20 to 25% of plasma levels (14, 39). It is 80% protein bound, and its half-life in serum is 1 to 3 h. It is not dialyzable, and no adjustment in dose is recommended in either renal or hepatic insufficiency.

Spectrum of activity. Praziquantel is active against the larval and adult stages of many trematodes. It is the drug of choice for schistosomiasis and is effective for all *Schistosoma* species that infect humans. It is used both for treatment of individuals and in mass community chemotherapy programs that lead to decreased transmission and prevalence of infection. Praziquantel is also used for treatment of opisthorchiasis, clonorchiasis, paragonimiasis, and intestinal fluke infections, including fasciolopsiasis, heterophyiasis, and metagonimiasis. In contrast to other human trematode infections, praziquantel has not proven to be effective in the treatment of *Fasciola hepatica*.

Many cestode infections can also be treated with praziquantel. Most tapeworm infections respond, including those caused by *Taenia*, *Diphyllobothrium*, and *Hymenolepis* species. Because praziquantel does not kill eggs, precautions should be taken to prevent autoinfection and laboratory-acquired infection, particularly for *Taenia solium*. Praziquantel is also used in the treatment of neurocysticercosis as an alternative or preferably as an adjunct to albendazole (43, 44).

Praziquantel has also been used in combination with albendazole for treatment of echinococcal infections. Praziquantel has high protoscolicidal activity *in vitro*, and reports have suggested superior efficacy of the combination compared to either drug alone (45–48).

Adverse effects. Adverse effects of praziquantel are generally mild, but many studies report that some side effects occur in over 30% of patients. Common reactions include dizziness, lethargy, headache, nausea, and abdominal pain. Hypersensitivity reactions occur rarely (49, 50). Severe adverse reactions are uncommon, although administration to individuals with neurocysticercosis can result in seizures and neurological sequelae related to precipitation of an inflammatory response (51).

Animal studies do not suggest a teratogenic effect of praziquantel (pregnancy category B), but an increased abortion rate has been seen in rats. There are minimal data on its safety in humans, but there is a very low potential for adverse effects on either the mother or her unborn child (52), and when praziquantel has been used during pregnancy, no increase in abortion rates, preterm deliveries, or congenital abnormalities has been noted (25, 53). Consequently, praziquantel can be given after the first trimester. No adverse effects of praziquantel administration during lactation have been reported, but it is excreted in human breast milk, and discontinuation of breast feeding on the day of therapy and for the following 72 h is sometimes suggested. However, owing to available data regarding its safety profile, in 2002 the World Health Organization recommended that it can be considered for use in pregnant and lactating women (54). It is FDA approved for children aged 4 years and over.

Ivermectin

Ivermectin is a semisynthetic macrocyclic lactone derivative of avermectins, which are natural substances derived from the actinomycete *Streptomyces avermitilis*. Major indications for its use are shown in Table 6. It was initially developed as an agent for veterinary use but is now used widely in humans. Ivermectin is a potent oral agent with a relatively broad spectrum of anthelmintic activity. It has been approved by the FDA as oral therapy for onchocerciasis and uncomplicated strongyloidiasis (1) and as a topical treatment for head lice.

TABLE 6 Major indications for ivermectin[a]

Indication	Usual dose	Reported efficacy
Ascaris lumbricoides	Single 150- to 200-μg/kg dose	Cure rates of 78–99%
Cutaneous larva migrans	200 μg/kg daily (usually 12 mg) for 1 or 2 days	Cure rates of 77–100%
Gnathostoma spinigerum	200 μg/kg daily for 2 days	Cure rates of 76–95%
Onchocerca volvulus	Single 150-μg/kg dose, repeat every 6–12 months until asymptomatic	Skin microfilarial counts reduced by 85–95%, and levels remain suppressed by >90% at 1 year
Strongyloides stercoralis	200 μg/kg daily for 2 doses (doses given either on consecutive days or 2 weeks apart)	Cure rates of 85–97% in uncomplicated infection (normal or immunocompromised hosts)
Trichuris trichiura	200 μg/kg daily for 3 days	Cure rates of 35–84%
Ectoparasites: scabies and lice	200-μg/kg dose, repeat after 2 weeks for scabies	Almost 100% efficacy

[a]Adapted from reference 1.

Mechanism of action. Ivermectin causes an influx of chloride ions across glutamate-gated chloride channels in nerve and muscle cell membranes, resulting in hyperpolarization of the affected cells and consequent paralysis and death of parasites (4, 55–59). It also acts as an antagonist of the neurotransmitter gamma-amino butyric acid (60). Although specific ivermectin binding sites have been identified in mammalian brain tissue, the affinity of ivermectin for sites within parasites is about 100 times greater than for mammalian tissue.

Pharmacokinetics. Ivermectin is available as an oral preparation. There is no parenteral preparation of ivermectin approved by the FDA, but it has been given via the rectal and subcutaneous routes to critically ill patients with disseminated strongyloidiasis who are unable to tolerate oral therapy (61–64). It is rapidly absorbed following oral administration. While recommendations are to administer the drug on an empty stomach with water to reduce side effects, bioavailability is thought to increase ~2.5-fold if the drug is taken with a high-fat meal (65). Ivermectin is metabolized in the liver and excreted almost entirely in the feces. Peak serum levels occur at 4 to 5 h, and levels of ~46 μg/liter have been reported after a single 12-mg dose (15). It is highly protein bound in plasma, and it has a half-life of 10 to 18 h. The drug accumulates in fat tissue and does not readily cross the blood-brain barrier (66).

Spectrum of activity. Ivermectin is the drug of choice for onchocerciasis and strongyloidiasis (1, 68). In onchocercal infections, ivermectin does not significantly affect the viability of adult worms, but it impairs release of microfilariae, is a potent microfilaricide, and leads to a sustained reduction in microfilaremia for many months (56). It can be used both for the treatment of individual patients and in mass chemotherapy programs in areas where onchocerciasis is endemic. The role of ivermectin combination therapy with doxycycline is being explored (69). In uncomplicated strongyloidiasis, ivermectin has excellent efficacy in immunocompetent patients (60). In disseminated strongyloidiasis, ivermectin is administered daily until stool and sputum exams are negative for larvae.

Ivermectin also has activity against microfilariae of *Wuchereria bancrofti*, *Brugia malayi*, and *Loa loa*. It does not have a significant effect on adult worm viability in these infections, so reduced microfilaremia is sustained only with repeated doses, and it has not replaced DEC as first-line therapy for these infections. Combination therapy with albendazole and/or DEC may increase efficacy (70). Ivermectin also has activity against *Mansonella ozzardi* and *M. streptocerca* microfilariae.

Ivermectin also has efficacy against many intestinal helminths, including *Ascaris lumbricoides*, *T. trichiura*, *Enterobius vermicularis*, and cutaneous larva migrans (57, 71–74). However, it is not generally used as first-line treatment for these indications due to the widespread availability and excellent efficacy of albendazole. It also can be used for treatment of gnathostomiasis (75, 76). It is not active against trematodes or cestodes. In addition to its anthelmintic activity, ivermectin is used for ectoparasitic infestations, including scabies and lice, for which it can be given either orally or topically.

In addition to its anthelmintic effects, ivermectin may reduce malaria transmission by killing mosquitoes that take blood meals from ivermectin-treated humans (77, 78). It has also been shown to impair development of malarial parasites inside hepatocytes, reducing the ensuing blood-stage parasitemia (79), so it may have a role as a tool to control malaria transmission.

Adverse effects. Ivermectin is generally well tolerated, with most adverse effects that occur following its administration being a result of the host's immune response to destruction of parasites rather than to toxic effects of the drug per se. Adverse effects include fever, rash, dizziness, pruritus, myalgia, arthralgia, and tender lymphadenopathy; the severity of these symptoms relates to the pretreatment intensity of infection rather than to ivermectin serum concentrations (80). Transaminitis is occasionally reported. Severe reactions occasionally occur, including a hypersensitivity response to dying microfilarial parasites known as the Mazzotti reaction. This anaphylactoid response is characterized by allergic manifestations, including pruritus, edema, fever, and systemic hypotension. However, these reactions are primarily restricted to individuals with high parasite loads. In patients infected with *L. loa* who have elevated levels of microfilaremia, ivermectin has been associated with the development of fatal encephalopathy (81) and so should be avoided.

Ivermectin (pregnancy category C) has been shown to be teratogenic in mice, rats, and rabbits when given in repeated doses of 0.2, 8.1, and 4.5 times the maximum recommended human dose, respectively. Teratogenicity was characterized in the three species tested by cleft palate; clubbed forepaws were additionally observed in rabbits. These developmental effects were found only at or near doses that were maternotoxic to the pregnant female (14, 56). There are insufficient data to recommend its use in pregnant women, although the risk of fetal damage in 203 pregnant women inadvertently treated with ivermectin was no greater than in controls, and it has been suggested that ivermectin can be given safely after the first trimester (82–84). It is excreted in breast milk in low concentrations and so should be avoided in lactating women when possible. It is not recommended for children weighing less than 15 kg.

Diethylcarbamazine

DEC is a piperazine derivative. Its main use is in filarial infections. Major indications for its use are shown in Table 7. DEC is not currently licensed for use in the United States, but it can be obtained from the CDC under the Investigational New Drug program.

Mechanism of action. The mode of action of DEC is uncertain. It is predominantly a microfilaricidal agent, and it is thought that its main effect is to inhibit arachidonic acid metabolism and alter the surface membrane of microfilariae, thereby enhancing destruction via host immune responses (12, 13). It also has some macrofilaricidal activity under certain conditions, likely via hyperpolarization and immobilization of adult worms (85).

Pharmacokinetics. DEC is available only in tablet form. It is freely soluble in water and is almost completely absorbed after oral administration. The drug is metabolized in the liver, although over 50% is excreted unchanged in the urine. There is negligible protein binding, and it is widely distributed in tissues. It readily crosses the blood-brain barrier. Peak plasma levels of 100 to 150 μg/liter at 1 to 2 h have been reported after a single 0.5-mg/kg dose (86). The half-life of DEC is 2 to 10 h. Renal excretion is reduced in the presence of an alkaline urinary pH, and dose reductions are required in patients with renal impairment.

Spectrum of activity. DEC is an effective microfilaricidal drug against *W. bancrofti*, *B. malayi*, *Brugia timori*, *Onchocerca volvulus*, *L. loa*, and *M. streptocerca*, but it has little or no effect on *Mansonella perstans* or *M. ozzardi* microfilariae (4). It has been the drug of choice for lymphatic filariasis for the last 50 years. It is used both for individual therapy for filarial infections and in mass community chemotherapy programs, either alone or in combination with ivermectin, albendazole, or doxycycline. It is predominantly a microfilaricidal agent, although it has some macrofilaricidal activity in *W. bancrofti*, *B. malayi*, *B. timori*, and *L. loa* infections (87–89). DEC has also been used in the treatment of toxocaral visceral larva migrans, but albendazole is now the preferred agent because of its better safety profile.

Adverse effects. The side effects of DEC include mild headache, dizziness, anorexia, nausea, and arthralgias. Administration of the drug to individuals with filarial infections can induce adverse results that are not due to the drug itself but instead are related to host responses, in part to release of *Wolbachia* endosymbionts from filariae, damage to adult worms (local reactions), and death of microfilariae (systemic reactions). These reactions tend to be relatively mild with lymphatic filariasis and infrequent with loiasis, but they can be severe with onchocerciasis or with heavy *L. loa* infections and result in intense pruritus, rash, fever, hypotension, and encephalopathy. The potentially fatal Mazzotti reaction and serious ophthalmic adverse effects can occur following treatment of *O. volvulus* with DEC, so DEC is contraindicated for onchocercal infections. For heavy *L. loa* infections, DEC is contraindicated to avoid potentially fatal encephalopathy. Animal studies have not shown DEC to be teratogenic, but it may increase the risk of abortion and so should be avoided in pregnancy when possible (14, 90). It is not excreted in breast milk and is safe during lactation.

Pyrantel Pamoate

Pyrantel, a tetrahydropyrimidine, is a relatively broad-spectrum agent against nematodes. It is associated with more side effects and lower efficacy than the benzimidazoles, so it has now largely been replaced. It is widely available without a prescription in the United States (1).

Mechanism of action. Pyrantel is a depolarizing neuromuscular blocking agent. It exerts its anthelmintic effect via release of acetylcholine and inhibition of helminthic acetylcholinesterase. This results in stimulation of ganglionic receptors and spastic paralysis of adult worms. The worms become dislodged from the intestinal wall and are expelled in the feces by normal peristalsis.

Pharmacokinetics. Pyrantel is administered orally but is almost insoluble in water and is therefore poorly absorbed from the gastrointestinal tract. Peak serum levels occur after 1 to 3 h. More than 50% is excreted unchanged in the feces. The absorbed drug is partially metabolized in the liver. There is no significant interaction with food.

Spectrum of activity. Pyrantel has excellent efficacy in the treatment of ascariasis and hookworm and pinworm infections (27). It also has some activity against *Trichostrongylus*. It is not active against *T. trichiura*; however, it is sometimes combined with its *m*-oxyphenol analogue, oxantel pamoate, to increase its efficacy (74, 91).

Adverse effects. Although pyrantel is generally well tolerated, it can lead to adverse reactions, including anorexia, nausea, vomiting, abdominal cramps, and diarrhea. It has also been associated with neurotoxic effects, including headache, dizziness, drowsiness, and insomnia. Transient increases in hepatic enzymes have also been reported, and one study reported nephrotic syndrome temporally related to it use (92). Animal studies have not shown adverse effects in the fetus, and it has been used during pregnancy in humans without harmful fetal effects (pregnancy category C) (93). It is not recommended for children <2 years of age.

TABLE 7 Major indications for DEC[a]

Indication	Usual dose	Reported efficacy
Loa loa	Up to 9 mg/kg/day in 3 doses for 12 days	Few large trials, but single course is curative in <50% of patients
Wuchereria bancrofti and *Brugia sp.* infections	Up to 6 mg/kg/day in 3 doses for 12 days (or repeated single doses)	>90–99% reduction in microfilaremia, but often need additional courses to eradicate adult worms

[a]Adapted from reference 1.

AN AGENT WITH ANTHELMINTIC AND ANTIPROTOZOAL ACTIVITIES: NITAZOXANIDE

Nitazoxanide is a 5-nitrothiazole derivative with broad-spectrum activity against numerous intestinal protozoa, helminths, and anaerobic bacteria. Major indications for its use are shown in Table 8. It was initially developed as a veterinary anthelmintic with activity against intestinal nematodes, cestodes, and liver trematodes (94). The FDA has approved it for use for the treatment of diarrhea caused by *Cryptosporidium* species and *Giardia duodenalis* in pediatric and adult patients (94, 95).

Mechanism of action. Nitazoxanide inhibits pyruvate ferredoxin oxidoreductase, an enzyme essential to anaerobic energy metabolism. This is its mechanism of action against anaerobic protozoa and bacteria (e.g., *Trichomonas vaginalis, Entamoeba histolytica*, and *Clostridium perfringens*), although for protozoa, additional mechanisms may also be involved (96). The exact mechanism of nitazoxanide's activity against helminths (e.g., *Hymenolepis nana*) has not yet been determined.

Pharmacokinetics. Nitazoxanide is given by the oral route and is available as a suspension or in tablet formulation. Bioavailability is nearly doubled by administration with food (97). It is absorbed from the gastrointestinal tract, with approximately one-third of the oral dose excreted in urine and two-thirds excreted in feces (98, 99). In blood, nitazoxanide is rapidly hydrolyzed to form an active metabolite, tizoxanide. The maximum concentration of tizoxanide in plasma following an oral dose of 500 mg of nitazoxanide is 2 mg/liter (6.5 μM), and its half-life in plasma is 1 to 2 h (100). Tizoxanide is extensively bound to plasma proteins (>99%), and its urinary elimination half-life is 7.3 h (101). Tizoxanide then undergoes glucuronidation to form tizoxanide glucuronide. Nitazoxanide is not detected in plasma, urine, bile, or feces, but tizoxanide is found in plasma, urine, bile, and feces, and tizoxanide glucuronide is found in plasma, bile, and urine (99). The pharmacokinetics of nitazoxanide in patients with impaired liver or renal function has not been studied, and the drug must be administered with caution to these patients (94).

Spectrum of activity. While nitazoxanide has been reported to have activity against a broad range of parasites (102, 103), it is FDA approved only for treatment of *Cryptosporidium* species and *G. duodenalis*, and its role in treating other infections is poorly defined.

Adverse effects. Nitazoxanide is well tolerated, with adverse effects similar to those of placebo. Mild and transient side effects have been seen in only 3 to 4% of patients, principally related to the gastrointestinal tract (abdominal pain, diarrhea, and nausea) (104). No significant adverse effects on electrocardiography, hematology, clinical chemistry, or urinalysis parameters in humans have been noted (96, 105). There are minimal data on the safety of nitazoxanide in pregnant (pregnancy category B) and lactating women (94).

ANTIMALARIALS

A number of agents are approved for use for treatment of malaria. The most commonly recommended agents are shown in Table 9.

Quinoline Derivatives

The quinoline derivatives can be divided into four groups: the 4-aminoquinolines, the cinchona alkaloids, synthetic compounds such as mefloquine and halofantrine, and the 8-aminoquinolines. A related drug, piperaquine, which is a bisquinoline, is now often used in combination with artemisinin derivatives for treatment of malaria. Although it used in Europe, it is not approved by the FDA.

4-Aminoquinolines

The 4-aminoquinolines include chloroquine, hydroxychloroquine, and amodiaquine. Chloroquine is the most widely used of these agents. It is an inexpensive, safe drug that has been used extensively for treatment and prophylaxis of all *Plasmodium* species that infect humans, although resistance to chloroquine in *Plasmodium falciparum* is prevalent globally in most malarious regions. Hydroxychloroquine is a related synthetic compound with an identical clinical spectrum, similar pharmacokinetics, and similar adverse effects. Amodiaquine is another related agent with the same mechanism of action and spectrum of activity. It is reported to be more effective than chloroquine for parasite clearance, but its use has been restricted due to uncommon serious side effects, as noted below. It is not approved by the FDA (1).

Mechanism of action. The main mechanism of action of the 4-aminoquinolines is thought to be via nonenzymatic inhibition of heme polymerization. Asexual intraerythrocytic malaria parasites actively concentrate quinoline ring compounds within hemoglobin-containing vesicles. In the absence of drug, plasmodia degrade host erythrocyte hemoglobin to provide amino acid nutrients essential for parasite growth. The degradation of hemoglobin produces free heme, which is stored as ferriprotoporphyrin IX within the red blood cell. Ferriprotoporphyrin IX is toxic to the parasite and is usually polymerized into nontoxic malaria pigment (hemozoin). In the presence of drug, there is inhibition of the conversion of heme into hemozoin, leading to the accu-

TABLE 8 Major indications for nitazoxanide

Indication	Usual dose[a]	Reported efficacy
Cryptosporidium parvum	Immunocompetent children 1–11 yr and adults: twice-daily treatment for 3 days[b]	Cure rates of 52–80%
	Immunocompromised: 1,000 mg twice daily for 2–8 weeks	Cure rates of 18–67% (efficacy varies with CD4$^+$-cell count in HIV-positive patients)
Giardia duodenalis	Twice-daily treatment for 3 days[c]	Cure rates of 71–94%

[a]Adapted from reference 94.

[b]The dosing schedule of nitazoxanide is as follows: for children 1 to 3 years of age, 100 mg twice daily for 3 days; for children 4 to 11 years of age, 200 mg twice daily for 3 days; and for adults, 500 mg twice daily for 3 days.

[c]Licensed for this use by the FDA.

TABLE 9 Treatment regimens for malaria[a]

Clinical presentation	Primary agent used for treatment	Alternative agents[b]
Severe malaria caused by any species (initial therapy)[c]	Intravenous or intramuscular artesunate	Intravenous quinine or quinidine
Uncomplicated *Plasmodium falciparum* malaria	ACT	Quinine sulfate plus clindamycin or doxycycline
Uncomplicated *P. vivax* and *P. ovale* malaria in areas with chloroquine-resistant infections	ACT, followed by primaquine	Quinine sulfate plus clindamycin or doxycycline, followed by primaquine
Uncomplicated *P. vivax* and *P. ovale* malaria in areas with chloroquine-susceptible infections	ACT or chloroquine, followed by primaquine	Quinine sulfate plus clindamycin or doxycycline, followed by primaquine
P. malariae or *P. knowlesi*	ACT or chloroquine	Quinine sulfate plus clindamycin or doxycycline

[a]Adapted from reference 111. ACT, artemisinin-based combination therapy.
[b]Atovaquone-proguanil may also be considered for the treatment of uncomplicated malaria in travelers outside areas where malaria is endemic provided that atovaquone-proguanil was not taken as malaria chemoprophylaxis.
[c]Parenteral therapy should be continued for at least 24 h. Once a patient has received at least 24 h of parenteral therapy and can tolerate oral therapy, treat as for uncomplicated malaria.

mulation of products toxic to the parasite and resulting in parasite death (106). These agents also inhibit protein synthesis by inhibiting incorporation of phosphate into DNA and RNA and by inhibiting DNA and RNA polymerases (13). Chloroquine also raises the pH of the vesicle (107).

Pharmacokinetics. The 4-aminoquinolines are extensively distributed in tissues and are characterized by a long elimination half-life. Despite similarities in their chemical structures, these drugs show differences in their biotransformation and routes of elimination (108).

Chloroquine is available in oral and parenteral forms. Many different formulations are manufactured worldwide. Oral administration is preferred, as excessively rapid administration via the parenteral route results in toxic peak plasma concentrations and a danger of fatal cardiovascular collapse (109). Chloroquine is rapidly absorbed from the gastrointestinal tract after oral administration and has oral bioavailability exceeding 75%. Food has variable effects on absorption. The drug is extensively distributed in body tissues and reaches high levels within the brain (110). Chloroquine binds to melanin-containing cells in the skin and eye and so can also reach high levels in these sites. There is marked variability in peak plasma concentrations between individuals, but within 3 h of initiating standard oral treatment doses (10 mg chloroquine base/kg at 0 and 24 h, followed by 5 mg/kg at 48 h) (111), blood concentrations remain above 1 mmol/liter for at least 4 days (112). Young children may require higher doses to achieve similar plasma concentrations (113, 114). It is ~60% protein bound and has a half-life of 3 to 6 days. Approximately 30 to 50% of the drug is metabolized in the liver to inactive compounds, and the remainder is excreted in the urine. Treatment reduction (usually 50% of the normal dose) is required in patients with severe renal or hepatic failure. It is not dialyzable.

In contrast, amodiaquine is a prodrug and is almost entirely metabolized to a biologically active metabolite, desethylamodiaquine, following oral administration. Otherwise, it has pharmacokinetic properties similar to those of chloroquine but has a smaller volume of distribution.

Spectrum of activity. The 4-aminoquinolines are efficient and rapidly acting blood schizonticides. They can be used both in the treatment and prophylaxis of susceptible malaria strains of all malaria species. They have no effect on tissue schizonts or exoerythrocytic stages. They are gametocytocidal for *Plasmodium vivax* and *Plasmodium malariae* but have minimal effect on *P. falciparum* gametocytes. Following infections with *P. vivax* or *Plasmodium ovale*, primaquine is also needed to eradicate liver hypnozoites and prevent relapses of infection.

Chloroquine is still a first-line option for therapy for some *P. vivax*, *Plasmodium knowlesi*, *P. malariae*, and *P. ovale* infections, but increasing resistance among *P. vivax* isolates globally, and especially among *P. vivax* infections acquired in Indonesia, East Timor, Papua New Guinea, and the Solomon Islands, is emerging. Chloroquine also remains the treatment of choice for susceptible *P. falciparum* strains, although *P. falciparum* strains from almost all areas of the world have developed resistance to it, so it is now rarely used for *P. falciparum*. It is also effective against *P. knowlesi* infections (115). Because of its potential toxicity, amodiaquine is not recommended for prophylaxis of malaria and is generally not used as first-line treatment. However, it results in faster parasite clearance and more rapid resolution of symptoms than chloroquine, and it may be effective in some cases of chloroquine-resistant malaria, so it is used as an alternative treatment regimen in some areas.

Chloroquine is also active against *E. histolytica* trophozoites but is rarely used for this indication, as the nitro-5-imidazoles are the drugs of choice.

Adverse effects. Chloroquine has a bitter taste. It is generally well tolerated at the doses required for malaria prevention or treatment, even when taken for prolonged periods. However, it can lead to nausea, abdominal discomfort, dizziness, retinal pigmentation, blurred vision, electrocardiographic changes, muscular weakness, and rarely transient psychiatric symptoms. It can also cause severe pruritus, particularly in African blacks. Irreversible neuroretinitis can result if it is taken at high doses for prolonged periods. If an overdose is taken, it can cause shock, arrhythmia, and death.

At the doses used for malaria treatment or prophylaxis, chloroquine has rarely been reported to cause adverse congenital effects (pregnancy category C) (116). However, affinity for melanin-containing tissues such as the retina, iris, and choroid of the eye has been reported, and definitive delineation of fetal risk remains undefined. It is commonly used for treatment and prophylaxis of malaria in pregnant women without evidence of teratogenicity, and it is generally agreed that the benefits of preventing and treating malaria in pregnant women outweigh the potential fetal risks. Chloroquine is excreted in breast milk in small amounts.

Amodiaquine is more palatable than chloroquine and seems to cause less itching. However, serious adverse events including agranulocytosis, aplastic anemia, and drug-induced hepatitis have been reported, predominantly following long-term amodiaquine use (mean, 7 to 8 weeks) for malaria prophylaxis (117). While short-term treatment regimens are thought to be safe (118), this drug is now uncommonly used.

Cinchona Alkaloids

The cinchona alkaloids, quinine and quinidine, contain a quinoline ring. Quinidine is the diastereoisomer of quinine. Quinine was originally extracted from the bark of the South American cinchona tree, but a synthetic form is now available, usually as a quinine sulfate salt. Quinidine is more active than quinine, but it is also more cardiotoxic.

Mechanism of action. The exact target of cinchona alkaloids is unknown. They are thought to act by forming complexes with ferriprotoporphyrin IX, thereby interfering with hemoglobin digestion and resulting in cell lysis and death of schizonts (119). They also interfere with the function of plasmodial DNA and inhibit the synthesis of parasite nucleic acids and proteins. Quinine also interacts with certain fatty acids present in parasitized erythrocytes, preventing lysis of red blood cells and interrupting schizont maturation (13). Additionally, it increases intracellular pH, resulting in lethal effects on the parasite.

Pharmacokinetics. Quinine is available for oral administration as a sulfate salt and for parenteral administration as quinine dihydrochloride. It is >80% absorbed from the gastrointestinal tract following oral doses. It is widely distributed in body tissues, but CSF concentrations are <10% of concurrent plasma levels. It is over 90% protein bound. Quinine is metabolized in the liver, and the native drug and its metabolites are excreted in the urine (110). It has a short half-life of 8 to 12 h, necessitating multiple daily doses. After a single dose of 650 mg of quinine sulfate, peak serum concentrations are ~3.2 mg/liter in healthy individuals but are higher (8.4 mg/liter) in patients with malaria. Intravenous quinine is used in many countries when oral therapy cannot be tolerated, but quinidine gluconate is considered the parenteral drug of choice in the United States (1). The two agents have similar pharmacokinetic properties.

The pharmacokinetic properties of the cinchona alkaloids are considerably altered in malaria, with a reduction in clearance that is proportional to the severity of disease. Consequently, doses should be decreased by 30 to 50% after the third day of treatment to avoid accumulation of drug in seriously ill patients (120). Drug levels may also be increased by administration with foods that alkalinize the urine, because increased tubular reabsorption results. Caution is recommended in patients with significant liver impairment, and dose reduction is required if there is renal impairment. Both agents are partially dialyzable.

Spectrum of activity. The cinchona alkaloids can be used in the treatment of all human *Plasmodium* infections. Their main indication is in chloroquine-resistant *P. falciparum*. Oral therapy is indicated in uncomplicated malaria, and parenteral formulations of quinine dihydrochloride or quinidine gluconate are used in severe infections.

Quinine and quinidine are blood schizonticides but have little effect on sporozoites or pre-erythrocytic forms of the parasite. Consequently, they do not eradicate *P. vivax* or *P. ovale* hypnozoites in the liver. They also are not gametocytocidal against *P. falciparum*. Although resistance to these agents has emerged in Southeast Asia and Africa, they remain useful drugs for the treatment of malaria worldwide, but in recent years they have been replaced by artemisinin derivatives for first-line malaria treatment.

Quinine is also used for the treatment of babesiosis. It is ineffective when used as a single agent but can be given with clindamycin or azithromycin (1).

Adverse effects. Quinine has an extremely bitter taste and can be associated with nausea, vomiting, and epigastric pain. It also often leads to the symptom complex of cinchonism (nausea, tinnitus, dysphoria, and reversible high-tone deafness). Quinine can also cause hyperinsulinemic hypoglycemia, especially in children and pregnant women with severe malaria, as it increases release of insulin from the pancreas. It has also been associated with massive hemolysis in patients with heavy *P. falciparum* infections. Additionally, agranulocytosis, thrombocytopenia, retinopathy, and tongue discoloration have been reported. Overdose of quinine can lead to ataxia, convulsions, and coma.

When used as treatment for severe malaria, intravenous quinidine is associated with cardiac arrhythmias. It prolongs the QT interval, widens the QRS complex, and prolongs the PR interval. It can therefore lead to hypotension and ventricular arrhythmias, including torsade de pointes. Consequently, it should be administered only in an intensive care setting with cardiac monitoring. As with quinine, administration can also result in blood dyscrasias and cinchonism.

Despite reports of congenital defects following administration of quinine during pregnancy, it can be administered during pregnancy when the benefits of maternal treatment outweigh the potential fetal risks (pregnancy category C) (121, 122). Quinidine has not been reported to be teratogenic, but published experience in pregnancy is limited (123). Quinine can have an abortifacient effect and lead to induction of labor. It is excreted in small amounts in breast milk but can be administered during breastfeeding when necessary.

Synthetic Quinoline Compounds

Mefloquine

Mefloquine is a synthetic 4-quinoline methanol compound structurally related to quinine.

Mechanism of action. Mefloquine interacts both with host cell phospholipids and with the ferriprotoporphyrin IX of the parasitized erythrocyte (13). Its action is thought to rely on interference with the digestion of hemoglobin during the blood stages of the malaria parasite's life cycle, likely via a similar mechanism to quinine (119). It does not inhibit protein synthesis.

Pharmacokinetics. Mefloquine is available for oral administration only. Food enhances bioavailability, and the drug should not be taken on an empty stomach. It is >85% absorbed following oral administration and is concentrated within red blood cells (124). It is >95% protein bound and has a half-life of 2 to 4 weeks. Because of its long half-life, mefloquine is frequently used for prophylaxis of malaria as a once-weekly dose. However, when mefloquine is administered weekly, it requires about 8 weeks before steady-state drug levels are reached, so a loading dose is often recommended. Peak plasma concentrations occur at 6 to 24 h, and following a single dose of 500 mg or 1,000 mg orally, they are 430 and 800 μg/liter, respectively. In healthy volunteers, a dose of 250 mg once weekly produces maximum steady-state plasma concentrations of 1,000 to 2,000 μg/liter, which are reached after 7 to 10 weeks. It is highly lipophilic and widely distributed throughout the body, and it can cross the blood-brain barrier. Mefloquine is metabolized in the liver and excreted through the bile and feces. There are no specific recommendations regarding the need for dosage adjustment in patients with renal or hepatic failure. It is not dialyzable.

Spectrum of activity. Mefloquine is active against the erythrocytic schizonts of all agents of human malaria, and it has been used for both chemoprophylaxis and therapy. Since weekly administration is sufficient for chemoprophylaxis, it is convenient for use in travelers to areas where malaria is endemic. Its main utility in malaria treatment results from its activity against most chloroquine-resistant *P. falciparum* strains, although resistance has been recognized, particularly in some areas of Southeast Asia. When used for therapy, it should be combined with another agent, usually an artemisinin derivative. Mefloquine does not kill tissue schizonts, so patients with *P. vivax* should be subsequently treated with an 8-aminoquinoline. It also has no effect on gametocytes.

Adverse effects. Adverse reactions to mefloquine include nausea and vomiting, agranulocytosis, and aplastic anemia, as well as central nervous system effects, such as dysphoria, dizziness, disturbed sleep, nightmares, and ataxia. Gastrointestinal side effects are dose dependent (125). Severe neuropsychiatric reactions including delirium and seizures have been reported occasionally and are thought to occur in approximately 1:200 to 1:1,300 patients treated for acute falciparum malaria (125–127). Mefloquine can also potentiate dysrhythmias in individuals on beta blockers. Mefloquine should be avoided in those with a history of a neuropsychiatric illness, including epilepsy (128). Mefloquine is teratogenic in high doses in animals, but reports in humans do not support teratogenic effects (pregnancy category B) (129, 130). A possible higher rate of spontaneous abortion has been suggested, so it is generally avoided in the first trimester of pregnancy if possible. However, limited data suggest that it is probably safe to use even during the first trimester, and it can be used in later stages of pregnancy if the benefits outweigh the potential risks (130, 131). It is excreted in low concentrations in breast milk but can be used in lactating women when necessary.

Halofantrine

Halofantrine is a synthetic phenanthrene-methanol compound. It is not approved by the FDA (1), and because of its potential cardiac side effects, it has limited indications for use.

Mechanism of action. Halofantrine has activity against the asexual erythrocytic stages of malaria parasites, although the exact mechanism of action is unclear.

Pharmacokinetics. Halofantrine is available only for oral administration but has variable bioavailability. Absorption is enhanced by administration with fatty food, but because high blood levels enhance toxicity, it is recommended for administration on an empty stomach. After three doses of 500 mg of halofantrine hydrochloride (at 0, 6, and 12 h), a maximum plasma concentration of 896 μg/liter has been reported (132). Halofantrine is metabolized in the liver to an active metabolite, *N*-desbutylhalofantrine. The half-lives of halofantrine and its metabolite are 6 to 10 days and 3 to 4 days, respectively. It is excreted mainly in the feces.

Spectrum of activity. Halofantrine is efficacious in the treatment of *P. vivax* and *P. falciparum* malaria, but data concerning *P. ovale* and *P. malariae* are limited (133). It is not recommended for prophylaxis of malaria because of toxicity. It is active against blood schizonts only and appears to have no effect against sporozoites, gametocytes, or tissue stages. Halofantrine is more active than mefloquine; however, cross-resistance between these drugs occurs. Its expense and potential toxicity also limit its use.

Adverse effects. Halofantrine leads to gastrointestinal adverse effects, including nausea, vomiting, diarrhea, and abdominal pain. It also has potential cardiovascular toxicity and causes concentration-dependent prolongation of the QT interval. It is therefore contraindicated in patients with long-QT syndrome, as it can lead to cardiac arrest (134). It can also lead to pruritus and hepatic enzyme elevations. Halofantrine is contraindicated in pregnancy. The degree of excretion in breast milk is unknown, and it is not advised for use in lactating women.

Lumefantrine

Lumefantrine is a drug with a similar structure to halofantrine. It is used as a long-acting partner drug to artemether in a widely used fixed-dose combination for malaria.

Mechanism of action. The exact mechanism by which lumefantrine exerts its antimalarial effect is unknown. However, it seems to inhibit the formation of β-hematin by forming a complex with hemin and inhibits nucleic acid and protein synthesis.

Pharmacokinetics. The oral bioavailability of lumefantrine is highly variable and increases up to 3- to 4-fold when taken with a high-fat meal. Peak plasma levels are seen after 6 to 8 h. Lumefantrine is 99.7% protein bound, and its half-life is 3 to 6 days. It is highly lipophilic and has an apparent large volume of distribution. Peak plasma levels vary considerably, but median plasma levels after six tablets containing 2,780 mg of 8 to 9 μg/ml are seen (135). Lumefantrine is extensively metabolized in the liver, and the major metabolite found in plasma is desbutyllumefantrine. It should be used with caution in patients with severe renal or hepatic failure.

Spectrum of activity. In its fixed-dose combination with artemether, lumefantrine has efficacy against all *Plasmodium* species.

Adverse effects. Lumefantrine is well tolerated, with rare mild adverse reactions, such as diarrhea, nausea, abdominal pain, and vomiting. There is no evidence of significant cardiotoxicity associated with lumefantrine use, but it is recommended that it be avoided in patients at risk for QT prolongation. Artemether-lumefantrine has been assigned to pregnancy category C by the FDA. There are no human data on the excretion of lumefantrine into breast milk, but animal data suggest some excretion. The effects in the nursing infant are unknown, and this drug should be used with caution in nursing women.

8-Aminoquinolines

The 8-aminoquinolines are primaquine and tafenoquine (WR-238605). Tafenoquine is not yet commercially available and has not been approved by the FDA (1).

Mechanism of action. The 8-aminoquinolines interfere with parasite mitochondrial enzymes involved in energy production. They also have an inhibitory action against DNA, although the exact mechanism by which this occurs in unclear (13). An active metabolite of the drug is thought to interrupt the mitochondrial transport system and pyrimidine synthesis in hypnozoites (136).

Pharmacokinetics. The 8-aminoquinolines are well absorbed after oral administration, with >90% bioavailability. Primaquine is rapidly metabolized in the liver, and its half-life is 4 to 9 h, so it needs to be administered daily. Following a single 45-mg oral dose, a mean peak serum level of 153.3 μg/liter was observed after 2 to 3 h (137). It is found at relatively low concentrations in most body sites. Tafenoquine has a longer half-life of 2 to 4 weeks. Weekly or possibly monthly doses seem to be sufficient when used for prophylaxis, thus making it better tolerated than primaquine (138). A single dose of tafenoquine may be sufficient for prevention of relapse following *P. vivax* infections (139). Optimal dose-finding studies are being performed.

Spectrum of activity. Primaquine is less active against blood-stage malarial parasites than most other antimalarial agents, but it is very active against pre-erythrocytic sporozoites and exoerythrocytic tissue schizonts of all malarial species. Its main use is to prevent relapse of *P. vivax* and *P. ovale* infections from latent hypnozoites following treatment with chloroquine. Additionally, it is gametocytocidal against *Plasmodium*, especially *P. falciparum*, and can interrupt transmission of malaria. It is also an effective causal prophylactic agent, but it has traditionally been used infrequently in this way for travelers. Tafenoquine is reported to be more active than primaquine and has higher schizonticidal activity (140).

Adverse effects. Mild gastrointestinal side effects, including nausea and abdominal pain, are common following 8-aminoquinoline administration. These drugs should not be used in people with glucose-6-phosphate dehydrogenase deficiency, as they can induce hemolysis. Patients with NADH methemoglobin reductase deficiency are at risk of developing methemoglobinemia. Primaquine also occasionally causes arrhythmias. Interference with visual accommodation has also been reported. These agents should also not be used during pregnancy or lactation because of the potential risk of hemolytic effects in the fetus.

Artemisinin (Qinghaosu) Derivatives

Artemisinin is an extract from the Chinese herbal plant *Artemisia annua*, also known as qinghaosu. It is a sesquiterpene lactone peroxide. Synthetic derivatives include artemether, dihydroartemisinin, arteether, and artesunate. Although not officially approved for use by the FDA, the intravenous formulation of artesunate is available via the CDC under the Investigational New Drug program for patients with severe malaria.

Mechanism of action. Artemisinin and its derivatives act mainly against the asexual erythrocytic stages of malaria. They have an antiparasitic effect, particularly on young, ring-form parasites, leading to their clearance and preventing development of more mature pathogenic forms. They bind to the parasite membrane and to ferriprotoporphyrin IX, so they are highly concentrated within parasites and reach concentrations in plasmodium-infected red cells that are 100 to 300 times higher than those in uninfected cells (141). By binding iron in the malarial pigment, they lead to production of toxic oxidative free radicals which damage parasite organelles and alkylate parasitic proteins, leading to inhibition of protein synthesis and ultimately to parasite death.

Pharmacokinetics. The derivatives of artemisinin have greater solubility and consequently have been developed for easier administration by a variety of routes. Artesunate is water soluble and can be given intravenously, intramuscularly, orally, or by suppository. Artemether and arteether are oil soluble and available in tablet, capsule, and intramuscular injection forms. Although artesunate is the most potent *in vitro*, there is no apparent clinical difference in efficacy between the formulations. The artemisinin derivatives have a short half-life of <1 to 2 h. They are usually administered once daily for a minimum of 3 days. All are metabolized to the active compound, dihydroartemisinin. Following a single oral dose of 2 mg of dihydroartemisinin/kg in healthy volunteers, median peak plasma values of 181 and 360 μg/liter, respectively, have been observed (142). Inhibitors of cytochrome P450, such as grapefruit juice, increase the plasma levels of artemether. Artemisinin is eliminated by glucuronidation to inactive metabolites (4, 143). The pharmacokinetics of artesunate may be altered by pregnancy and by acute malaria infection. Artemisinin derivatives should be used with caution in individuals with hepatic or renal impairment.

Spectrum of activity. The artemisinin derivatives are effective against *P. falciparum* and *P. vivax* and are the most potent and rapidly acting parasiticidal drugs. They act specifically against the erythrocytic stages of *Plasmodium*. They are effective against multidrug-resistant *P. falciparum* and are the drugs of choice against mefloquine- and/or quinine-resistant *P. falciparum* isolates and against chloroquine-resistant *P. vivax*. The artemisinin derivatives are also active against gametocytes, reducing gametocyte carriage by ~90% and interrupting transmission in areas where they are widely used (144–146). They are not effective against the intrahepatic hypnozoite stage of *P. vivax* or *P. ovale* infections. Late recrudescence is common unless these agents are combined with another drug, so they should be administered with a second agent, such as mefloquine or doxycycline, or in fixed combinations, such as artemether-lumefantrine, artesunate-amodiaquine, or dihydroartemisinin-piperaquine. The artemisinin derivatives are usually associated with quick clearance of parasitemia, and recent randomized trials comparing them with quinine have shown a benefit in terms of mortality in adults treated for severe *P. falciparum* malaria (147–149). However, artemisinin-resistant *P. falciparum* malaria is now also emerging, particularly along the Thai-Cambodian border, characterized clinically by a substantial delay in parasite clearance (150). Despite limited data, the oral artemisinin derivative combinations seem effective against *P. knowlesi* (151), *P. ovale*, and *P. malariae* infections. Intravenous artesunate is used for those affected by severe malaria due to *P. knowlesi* (152). The artemisinin derivatives also have antitrematode activity and have been studied in schistosomiasis. They are less effective than praziquantel but may have a role as part of combination therapy in the future (153–155).

Adverse effects. The artemisinin derivatives are very well tolerated, with no serious toxicity or subjective adverse effects, although hematopoietic suppression has been described. They have been associated with adverse neurological effects in animal models, but there is no evidence that this occurs in humans. Fetal deaths and congenital malformations, though seen in rodent studies, were not observed in clinical trials involving 1,837 pregnant women, including 176 patients in the first trimester exposed to an artemisinin agent or artemisinin-based combination therapy (156, 157). Although it is generally recommended that they be avoided in pregnancy because of insufficient safety data, they can be used, particularly after the first trimester, if the benefits outweigh the risks. The World Health Organization recommends the use of intravenous artesunate for severe malaria in pregnancy (111). The amount excreted in breast milk is unknown.

Antifolates

Pyrimethamine-sulfadoxine, also known as Fansidar, is still used for treatment of malaria in some countries despite widespread resistance. Pyrimethamine is a synthetic aminopyrimidine antimalarial agent, and sulfadoxine is a long-acting sulfonamide agent.

Mechanism of action. Pyrimethamine acts against the asexual erythrocytic stage of *Plasmodium* by inhibiting the plasmodial enzyme dihydrofolate reductase. Although it is active against *P. falciparum*, rapid development of resistance occurs and is a major factor limiting its use. Combining pyrimethamine with a sulfonamide or sulfone provides sequential, synergistic inhibition of the folate biosynthesis pathway. Malaria parasites are unable to utilize host-derived folic acid, so inhibition of folic acid biosynthesis prevents malarial DNA replication, ultimately leading to cell death.

Pharmacokinetics. Fansidar tablets are composed of 25 mg of pyrimethamine and 500 mg of sulfadoxine. Both drugs are well absorbed orally. After oral administration of a single tablet, peak plasma concentrations of pyrimethamine and sulfadoxine are 0.13 to 0.4 mg/liter and 51 to 76 mg/liter, respectively. The half-life of pyrimethamine is 80 to 95 h, and the half-life of sulfadoxine is 150 to 200 h (120). Both components are ~90% protein bound. Sulfadoxine is metabolized in the liver, and both agents are excreted mainly in the urine.

Spectrum of activity. Pyrimethamine-sulfadoxine is effective both for treatment and chemoprophylaxis of *P. falciparum* malaria. It is no longer recommended for routine prophylaxis because of the potential for severe adverse effects. It acts mainly against blood schizonts and does not have significant gametocytocidal activity. Pyrimethamine-sulfadoxine also has some efficacy in the treatment of *P. vivax*, but it has longer parasite and fever clearance times than chloroquine and higher failure rates (30 to 40%), so it is not recommended. The efficacy of pyrimethamine-sulfadoxine against *P. ovale* and *P. malariae* has not been adequately evaluated.

Pyrimethamine is also used in combination with sulfadiazine for the treatment of toxoplasmosis.

Adverse effects. Pyrimethamine-sulfadoxine can result in adverse effects, including rash, nausea, vomiting, headache, and peripheral neuritis. It can also be associated with more serious and occasionally fatal reactions, including the Stevens-Johnson syndrome and blood dyscrasias (particularly agranulocytosis and megaloblastic anemia) (117). Other reported adverse effects include hepatitis, toxic nephrosis, exfoliative dermatitis, and erythema multiforme. The long half-life of the sulfa component means that sensitivity reactions can be sustained for prolonged periods even after the drug is discontinued.

Pyrimethamine has been associated with teratogenic effects in animals. There are no controlled human studies; however, this drug has been used frequently during pregnancy and has been associated with good fetal outcome. The World Health Organization now recommends that women living in areas of Africa where malaria is endemic receive intermittent preventive treatment with pyrimethamine-sulfadoxine in the second and third trimesters of their first and second pregnancies (111). In other settings, it is officially recommended for use during pregnancy only when potential benefits outweigh the possible risks to the fetus. Fansidar can cause kernicterus in infants, so it should be used with caution in pregnant women late in the third trimester. Both pyrimethamine and sulfadoxine are excreted into breast milk and are preferably avoided during lactation.

Atovaquone-Proguanil (Malarone)

Malarone is a tablet combination of 250 mg of atovaquone and 100 mg of proguanil. Atovaquone is a hydroxynaphthoquinone, and proguanil is an antifolate. Malarone has been approved for use by the FDA for prophylaxis and treatment of malaria.

Mechanism of action. *Plasmodium* species are dependent on *de novo* pyrimidine biosynthesis, which is selectively coupled with electron transport. Atovaquone inhibits the electron transport system in the mitochondria of parasites, thereby blocking nucleic acid synthesis and inhibiting replication (158). When used as monotherapy, atovaquone is associated with high recrudescence rates. Proguanil also acts against the asexual erythrocytic stage of the parasite by selectively inhibiting plasmodial dihydrofolate reductase. However, in combination with atovaquone, it acts via a different mechanism and directly lowers the effective concentration at which atovaquone causes collapse of the mitochondrial membrane potential (159).

Pharmacokinetics. Atovaquone is a highly lipophilic compound with low aqueous solubility and poor and variable oral availability. Its absorption is increased if it is administered with fatty foods or a milky drink. It is not metabolized and is excreted almost exclusively in the feces. It is 99% plasma protein bound, and its half-life is 2 to 4 days. Atovaquone levels vary widely between individuals (160). Proguanil is rapidly and extensively absorbed after oral administration. It is metabolized by cytochrome P450 in the liver to the active cyclic triazine metabolite, cycloguanil. It is 75% protein bound and is excreted mainly in the urine. Its half-life is 12 to 21 h. After two Malarone tablets twice daily for 3 days, mean plasma levels of proguanil of 170 μg/liter have been reported. The pharmacokinetics of atovaquone-proguanil are altered during pregnancy. No dosing adjustments are required in the setting of mild to moderate hepatic or renal insufficiency. However, with severe renal impairment (creatinine clearance of <30 ml/min), use of atovaquone-proguanil is contraindicated for prophylaxis, but it can be used for treatment if the benefits outweigh the risks.

Spectrum of activity. Atovaquone-proguanil is effective against asexual and sexual forms of *P. falciparum* and is recommended for treatment and prophylaxis of falciparum malaria. It is used frequently for chemoprophylaxis in travelers to areas where malaria is endemic. Atovaquone-proguanil is also effective for treating *P. vivax* and *P. ovale*, but neither drug is effective against hypnozoites, so primaquine is additionally required to prevent relapses after drug discontinuation. Atovaquone-proguanil also shows good efficacy against *P. malariae* and *P. knowlesi* in limited studies (152, 161). Reports of clinical failures and resistance of *P. falciparum* isolates to atovaquone-proguanil resulting from single mutations to the cytochrome β gene are emerging.

Adverse effects. Atovaquone-proguanil is generally very well tolerated. Side effects are mild and include anorexia, nausea, vomiting, abdominal pain, diarrhea, pruritus, and headache. Between 5 and 10% of recipients develop transient asymptomatic elevations in transaminases and amylase. Because of inadequate safety data, it is not recommended for prophylaxis during pregnancy (pregnancy category C) or lactation. It is also not recommended for treatment during pregnancy but can be considered if warranted due to risks. There are insufficient safety data to recommend use in children weighing <5 kg.

OTHER ANTIPROTOZOAL AGENTS

Diloxanide Furoate

Diloxanide furoate, also known as Furamide, is a substituted acetanilide. Its main use is as a luminal amebicidal agent. It is not widely available in the United States and can be obtained only from specific pharmacies (1).

Mechanism of action. The mechanism of action of diloxanide furoate is unknown.

Pharmacokinetics. Diloxanide furoate is available in tablet form. The parent drug is poorly absorbed following oral administration, but it is hydrolyzed in the bowel lumen to an active compound, diloxanide. This is >90% absorbed and is glucuronidated in the liver, reaching peak serum levels within 1 to 2 h. Metabolites are excreted primarily in the urine.

Spectrum of activity. Diloxanide furoate acts primarily as a luminal agent and helps clear the bowel of *E. histolytica* cysts, thereby preventing relapse in cyst carriers (162, 163). It is not effective for amebae in the bowel wall or in other tissues, such as the liver, so it is generally given with a 5-nitroimidazole.

Adverse effects. Side effects are generally not severe but include rash, nausea, abdominal pain, diarrhea, and flatulence. It is not recommended in pregnancy or during lactation.

Iodoquinol

Iodoquinol is a halogenated 8-hydroxyquinoline derivative, diiodohydroxyquin.

Mechanism of action. Iodoquinol is thought to act by inactivating essential parasitic enzymes and inhibiting parasite multiplication (13).

Pharmacokinetics. Iodoquinol is available for oral administration but is very slowly absorbed, with <8% reaching the systemic circulation, so it is primarily excreted in the feces. Small amounts of absorbed drug are glucuronidated in the liver, and small quantities of glucuronic acid metabolites are excreted in the urine. It should not be used in individuals with renal or hepatic insufficiency, and it should be used with caution in patients with thyroid or neurologic disease.

Spectrum of activity. Iodoquinol is a potent amebicidal drug. It is effective against trophozoites and cysts of *E. histolytica* located within the lumen of the intestine and is used to eradicate amebic cysts to help prevent relapse of infection (162). Because it is poorly absorbed systemically, it is not effective for invasive intestinal or extraintestinal *E. histolytica* infections and is therefore frequently combined with a 5-nitroimidazole.

Iodoquinol also has activity against *Neobalantidium coli*, *Dientamoeba fragilis*, and *G. duodenalis*.

Adverse effects. The main side effects of iodoquinol include nausea, abdominal cramps, diarrhea, headache, pruritus, and rash. Skin and hair may be temporarily stained yellow-brown following exposure. At high doses or with prolonged use, it can cause optic neuritis, optic atrophy, peripheral neuropathy, ataxia, and seizures. It is also associated with nephrotoxicity. It should be avoided in individuals who are sensitive to iodine. The degree of safety associated with its use in pregnancy or lactation is uncertain, so it is recommended that it be avoided in pregnancy and during lactation.

Pentavalent Antimonial Compounds

The pentavalent antimony derivatives are used for treatment of leishmaniasis. They include sodium antimonylgluconate (or stibogluconate), also known as Pentostam, and *N*-methylglucamine antimoniate (or meglumine antimoniate), also known as Glucantime. Selection of one drug over the other is based primarily on cost and availability. Neither drug is licensed for use in the United States, but sodium stibogluconate is available from the CDC for individual patient use (1).

Mechanism of action. The precise mechanism of action of the pentavalent antimony derivatives remains unclear. They are thought to inhibit enzymes of glycolysis within parasites. Because glycolysis is the major source of parasitic ATP, the blockade of this source of energy is fatal to parasites (13).

Pharmacokinetics. The pentavalent antimonials are administered parenterally (intramuscularly or intravenously), or via intralesional injection. New formulations and drug delivery approaches are being investigated. They remain in plasma and are excreted predominantly by the kidneys. Small amounts are metabolized in the liver to trivalent antimony, which contributes to the toxicity associated with their use. Following intramuscular administration of an initial dose of 10 mg antimony per kg, mean peak antimony blood concentrations of 9 to 12 mg/liter have been reported at 2 h (164). There are no specific guidelines regarding dose adjustment in renal impairment.

Spectrum of activity. Antimony preparations are efficient in killing many protozoan and helminthic parasites, but they are no longer recommended for most parasitic infections because of their toxicity. They are still used for the treatment of visceral, mucocutaneous, and cutaneous leishmaniasis, as few effective alternatives exist, although drug resistance is increasing. Various treatment regimens are used, often involving 28 days of therapy, but the exact duration and efficacy vary depending on the type of leishmaniasis, the severity of the lesion, and the area of endemicity.

Adverse effects. Minor adverse effects from the pentavalent antimonials are common and include nausea, vomiting, headache, and malaise (165). More severe reactions, such as leukopenia, agranulocytosis, and electrocardiographic changes (prolongation of the QT interval and ventricular arrhythmias), can also occur. Renal insufficiency, proteinuria, and elevation of hepatic and pancreatic enzymes have also been described. Local hypersensitivity, erythema, and edema have been described with intralesional administration (166).

Miltefosine

Miltefosine is a phosphocholine analogue originally developed as an anticancer compound. It is the first effective oral agent for visceral leishmaniasis and is becoming increasingly important because of growing resistance of leishmania strains to pentavalent antimonials. In 2014, miltefosine was approved by the FDA as an oral treatment option for visceral leishmaniasis due to *Leishmania donovani*, cutaneous leishmaniasis due to *Leishmania braziliensis*, *Leishmania guyanensis*, and *Leishmania panamensis*, and mucosal leishmaniasis due to *L. braziliensis* in patients aged 12 years and over (167). Miltefosine has shown ameba-killing activity *in vitro* against the free-living ameba *Naegleria fowleri* and has been used successfully to treat patients with *Balamuthia* and disseminated *Acanthamoeba* infections.

Mechanism of action. The mechanism of action of miltefosine is not well understood. The drug interferes with cell-signaling pathways and appears to act on key enzymes involved in the metabolism of ether lipids present on the surface of parasites (168, 169). Miltefosine does not appear to have a direct immunostimulatory effect, but it does induce apoptosis (170, 171). It has been shown to be active against both the extracellular promastigote form and the intracellular amastigote form of *Leishmania* parasites both *in vitro* and *in vivo* (172).

Pharmacokinetics. Miltefosine is well absorbed after oral administration and is widely distributed. Minimal pharmacokinetic data for humans are available, but in rats, the drug is rapidly taken up and accumulates in the kidney, liver, lung, spleen, and adrenal glands (169). On oral administration of 30 mg of miltefosine/kg twice per day, concentrations of 155 to 189 nmol/g of tissue are achieved (168). Miltefosine has a long half-life of about 8 days and is slowly metabolized by phospholipase.

Spectrum of activity. Miltefosine has activity against *Leishmania* spp. and *Trypanosoma cruzi* both *in vitro* and *in vivo*, but clinical studies to date have been limited to leishmaniasis. *In vitro* activity of miltefosine against *Trypanosoma brucei* spp., *E. histolytica*, and *Acanthamoeba* spp. has also been demonstrated (173). In visceral leishmaniasis clinical trials, treatment with miltefosine has resulted in cure rates of >90% at 6 months in both adults and children (174, 175), although emerging resistance is reducing its efficacy. Different combination therapy strategies involving miltefosine are being used in various geographical regions. Recent studies have also examined its efficacy in New World cutaneous leishmaniasis and have generally found 70 to 90% efficacy for most species (176). It is also used for post-kala azar dermal leishmaniasis. There are also recent case reports of clinical success using miltefosine in combination with other agents for granulomatous amebic encephalitis (177, 178).

Adverse effects. In various clinical trials, toxic effects associated with miltefosine have usually been found to be tolerable and reversible, although the therapeutic window appears to be narrow (170). Mild to moderate gastrointestinal side effects, including nausea, vomiting, and diarrhea, occur in up to 60% of patients. Dose-related motion sickness is also reported in up 40% of patients (179). A mild increase in aspartate aminotransferase and creatinine and/or blood urea nitrogen level has been reported, with reversible hepatotoxicity and renal damage in a few cases (169, 174). One case of fatal acute pancreatitis secondary to miltefosine has been described (180). Miltefosine is abortifacient and teratogenic in animals and should not be used during pregnancy or breastfeeding (181). Contraception must be used in women of childbearing age during and for 3 to 5 months after treatment (167, 181).

Pentamidine

Pentamidine is an aromatic diamidine compound that is used as an antiprotozoal agent in the treatment of leishmaniasis and African trypanosomiasis. Its use has been approved by the FDA (1).

Mechanism of action. Pentamidine is chemically related to guanidine. Its mechanism of action has not been clearly defined and may not be uniform against different organisms. It is possible that it inhibits dihydrofolate reductase and interferes with aerobic glycolysis in protozoa. It may also interfere with amino acid transport, precipitate nucleotides and nucleotide-containing coenzymes, and inhibit DNA, RNA, and protein synthesis (182).

Pharmacokinetics. Pentamidine is currently available as an isethionate salt. It is poorly absorbed from the gastrointestinal tract. When used for protozoal infections, it is administered intramuscularly or intravenously, but it can be given via inhalation for prevention of *Pneumocystis jirovecii* pneumonia and via intralesional injection for cutaneous leishmaniasis (183). Following intravenous administration of a 4-mg/kg dose, plasma concentrations of 0.3 to 1.4 mg/liter have been reported (184). The highest concentrations of the drug are found in the kidney, liver, and spleen, and pentamidine penetrates poorly into the central nervous system. It has a short serum half-life of 6.5 to 9 h because it is rapidly and extensively taken up by tissues. Its extensive tissue binding results in prolonged excretion over a period of 6 to 8 weeks, and it is eliminated unchanged via the kidneys. Pentamidine should be used cautiously in the presence of renal or hepatic failure, but no dosage adjustment is recommended.

Spectrum of activity. The antiparasitic indications for pentamidine include leishmaniasis and African trypanosomiasis, but its main use is as an antifungal agent for treatment and prophylaxis of *P. jirovecii* pneumonia. Despite leishmanicidal activity, pentamidine's toxicity means that it is used predominantly in individuals intolerant of antimonial compounds, in disease that is refractory to other treatment, or in combination therapy. Pentamidine is also active against African trypanosomes, and it is first-line treatment in early disease, but its utility is restricted to trypanosomiasis without central nervous system involvement.

Since central nervous system involvement occurs early with *Trypanosoma brucei rhodesiense*, it is used more frequently for *T. b. gambiense* infections. Pentamidine is also sometimes used in combination therapy for granulomatous amebic encephalitis caused by *Acanthamoeba* and *Balamuthia* species.

Adverse effects. Over half of parenteral pentamidine recipients experience some adverse effect from therapy. Administration is associated with a variety of reactions that appear to be unrelated to drug concentrations in plasma (182). Immediate reactions include nausea, anorexia, dizziness, pruritus, and hypotension. Pentamidine can also produce local effects, including pain and necrosis at the site of injection. In addition, pentamidine administration is associated with hematologic effects, particularly leukopenia (up to 10% of recipients) and thrombocytopenia (~5% of recipients), as well as with electrolyte abnormalities, including hyperkalemia, hypomagnesemia, and hypocalcemia. Other severe adverse effects include ventricular arrhythmias, pancreatitis, hypo- or hyperglycemia, hepatotoxicity, and acute renal failure. Pentamidine has also been associated with Stevens-Johnson syndrome. Finally, occasional seizures and hallucinations have been reported. There are minimal available safety data regarding the use of pentamidine in pregnancy or lactation, and it is therefore not recommended.

Paromomycin

Paromomycin, which was initially named aminosidine, is an oral, poorly absorbed broad-spectrum aminoglycoside. It is active against Gram-negative and many Gram-positive bacteria as well as some protozoa and cestodes. It is approved by the FDA for use in noninvasive intestinal amebiasis and is sometimes used off-label for cryptosporidiosis, *D. fragilis* infection, and giardiasis. Paromomycin is used in parenteral intramuscular (visceral and cutaneous leishmaniasis), topical (Old World and New World cutaneous leishmaniasis [185]), and oral (protozoal infections) formulations.

Mechanism of action. Paromomycin is a protein synthesis inhibitor that exerts its function by binding to 16S rRNA, thus inhibiting protein synthesis. However, when used for treatment of leishmaniasis, it has additional mechanisms of action that are incompletely understood but seem to involve inhibition of parasite metabolism and mitochondrial respiration (186).

Pharmacokinetics. Paromomycin is not systemically absorbed after oral administration and is passed in feces without being metabolized. Following an intramuscular injection, peak plasma concentrations are achieved within 0.5 to 1.5 h, and the drug half-life is 2 to 3 h. Plasma protein binding is negligible. Mean plasma concentrations 1 h after a 12- to 15-mg/kg dose are 18.3 to 20.5 μg/ml. Paromomycin is widely distributed in the body after parenteral administration, with measurable concentrations achieved in bone, synovial fluid, and peritoneal fluid, but with negligible central nervous system penetration. It should be used with caution in patients with renal impairment.

Spectrum of activity. Oral paromomycin has activity against the intestinal protozoa *G. duodenalis*, *Cryptosporidium parvum*, and *D. fragilis*. It is the drug of choice for giardiasis in pregnancy because of its safety, and it is also used in cases that have not responded to other agents (187). In addition, it has activity as a luminal agent to clear intestinal infection with *E. histolytica*, but it is not effective in extraintestinal amebiasis. It has also been used for treatment of *Blastocystis hominis* (188), and it has activity against *T. vaginalis*. Paromomycin also is used parenterally or topically in visceral and cutaneous leishmaniasis, sometimes in combination with other agents. Although it has activity against most tapeworm infections, it is not used for this indication due to the availability of alternate agents (189, 190).

Adverse effects. The most common side effects of paromomycin are nausea, increased gastrointestinal motility, abdominal pain, and diarrhea. As with other aminoglycosides, systemic absorption of paromomycin following intramuscular injection may cause reversible ototoxicity and nephrotoxicity. It can also cause an increase in hepatic transaminases. With parenteral administration, ~50% of patients experience mild pain at the injection site.

Because oral paromomycin is not systemically absorbed, it does not adversely affect the fetus or infant, so it can be used during pregnancy and lactation. However, parenteral aminoglycosides cross the placenta and may accumulate in fetal plasma and amniotic fluid. No reproductive toxicity has been observed in animals, but data regarding the use of paromomycin in pregnant women are insufficient to recommend its use. All results to date indicate that parenteral paromomycin is safe during lactation provided that the mother and infant have normal renal function (186).

Suramin

Suramin is a polysulfonated naphthylamine derivative of urea. Its main indication is in the treatment of African trypanosomiasis. It is not licensed for use in the United States but is available from the CDC via a compassionate drug use protocol (1).

Mechanism of action. The mechanism of action of suramin is not fully understood, but it is thought to act via inhibition of enzymes associated with DNA metabolism and protein synthesis of the trypanosomal parasites (191).

Pharmacokinetics. Suramin is dispensed as a sodium salt and is soluble in water. It is not absorbed when given orally and is usually administered as a 10% solution by slow intravenous infusion. Following intravenous injection, it is rapidly distributed, and >99% becomes bound to plasma proteins. It does not cross the blood-brain barrier. It undergoes little or no metabolism and has a half-life of 41 to 78 days. It is excreted in the urine. It should not be used in the presence of renal failure or significant hepatic dysfunction.

Spectrum of activity. Suramin is an effective drug for early hemolymphatic stages of *T. b. gambiense* infections. It also has some effect in early *T. b. rhodesiense* infection, provided that there is no central nervous system involvement (192). Suramin was used to treat onchocerciasis prior to the development of ivermectin. An advantage of suramin is that it has macrofilaricidal activity, damaging the intestinal epithelium of adult *O. volvulus* worms and resulting in their death, but it is associated with frequent toxic effects at the required doses (193). Suramin also has activity against adult *W. bancrofti* worms but is not recommended for this indication (13).

Adverse effects. Potential side effects include an immediate reaction with nausea, vomiting, shock, and loss of consciousness following suramin injection. Other adverse effects include renal impairment, exfoliative dermatitis, and neurological toxicity. It has also been associated with pancytopenia. Suramin has been reported to be teratogenic in rodents (194). No case of infant malformation has been described in humans, but it is not recommended for use during pregnancy except in circumstances where there is no suitable alternative.

Melarsoprol

Melarsoprol is a trivalent arsenical compound. Its main use is in the treatment of African trypanosomiasis. It is not licensed for use in the United States but is available from the CDC via a compassionate drug use protocol (1).

Mechanism of action. Melarsoprol appears to act by binding to essential thiol groups of trypanosomes and has a particularly high affinity for the active site for pyruvate kinase. This results in interference with energy generation within parasites, thereby preventing trophozoite multiplication.

Pharmacokinetics. Melarsoprol is absorbed if given orally but is generally administered by the intravenous route. It is prepared as a solution in propylene glycol and is given by slow intravenous infusion. It is estimated that <1% penetrates the central nervous system, and CSF concentrations are up to 50-fold lower than serum concentrations (12, 195). However, it is an efficacious trypanocidal agent that can be used for late stages of trypanosomal disease, although resistance has been reported. Melarsoprol has a half-life of ~35 h. Its metabolism has not been well studied, but it is excreted predominantly in the urine.

Spectrum of activity. Melarsoprol is active in the treatment of all stages of African trypanosomiasis due to *T. b. gambiense* and *T. b. rhodesiense* and is the only available treatment for late-stage *T. b. rhodesiense* infection. Treatment courses have been reduced from 1 month to 10 days (196). However, because of its toxicity, it is generally reserved for use in late stages of disease involving the central nervous system (197).

Adverse effects. Melarsoprol is commonly associated with significant toxicity, including vomiting, abdominal pain, hepatotoxicity, peripheral neuropathy, hypersensitivity reactions, myocarditis, cardiac arrhythmias, and albuminuria. Administration can also lead to a reactive encephalopathy in up to 10% of patients, and this is associated with significant mortality. Hypersensitivity reactions are also relatively frequent. The injection is very irritating, and extravasation during intravenous administration should be avoided. There are minimal data available regarding potential teratogenic effects.

Eflornithine

The main indication for use of eflornithine (also known as difluoromethylornithine) is for treatment of African trypanosomiasis. Drug availability is limited, and it is not available in the United States for systemic use.

Mechanism of action. Eflornithine selectively and irreversibly inhibits ornithine decarboxylase, an enzyme required for the formation of polyamines needed for cellular proliferation and differentiation in parasites. It is trypanostatic rather than trypanocidal (197).

Pharmacokinetics. Eflornithine can be administered by mouth and has >50% oral bioavailability, but significant diarrhea frequently results, so it is usually given intravenously. No protein binding of the drug occurs following intravenous administration. It crosses the blood-brain barrier and produces CSF-to-blood ratios between 0.13 and 0.5 (198, 199). The half-life is 3 to 3.5 h, and ~80% of the dose is excreted unchanged by the kidneys. Dose reduction is required in patients with significant renal impairment.

Spectrum of activity. Eflornithine is used for treatment of *T. b. gambiense* when there is central nervous system involvement. Nifurtimox-eflornithine combination therapy is now standard first-line treatment for central nervous system-stage *T. b. gambiense* infection (196, 200). Eflornithine is ineffective as monotherapy in *T. b. rhodesiense* (201). It displays some activity against other parasites, including *Plasmodium* species, *C. parvum*, and *T. vaginalis*, but is not used for these indications because of toxicity.

Adverse effects. Side effects of eflornithine occur in up to 40% of patients. Common adverse reactions include vomiting, abdominal pain, diarrhea, dizziness, arthralgias, alopecia, and rash. Bone marrow toxicity resulting in anemia, thrombocytopenia, and leukopenia has also been described. Eflornithine has been shown to arrest embryonic development in animals (202). There are no good studies of its safety in pregnancy or lactation (pregnancy category C), so it should be used only when the potential maternal benefits outweigh the possible risks to the fetus.

Nifurtimox and Benznidazole

The two agents used for treatment of American trypanosomiasis are nifurtimox and benznidazole. Nifurtimox is a synthetic nitrofuran, and benznidazole is a 2-nitroimidazole derivative. Benznidazole was approved by the FDA in August 2017 for use in children aged 2 to 12 years with Chagas' disease. Nifurtimox can be obtained from the CDC under the Investigational New Drug program (203). As of May 2018, benznidazole is no longer available through the CDC Investigational New Drug program, and physician requests for benznidazole should now be directed to the drug company Exeltis (67).

Mechanism of action. Benznidazole has an inhibitory effect on protein and ribonucleic acid synthesis in *T. cruzi* cells (204). It is thought to cause increased phagocytosis, cytokine release, and production of reactive mitogen intermediates that result in destruction of intracellular parasites (205).

Nifurtimox is a prodrug that is activated by a parasite-encoded nitroreductase, generating cytotoxic nitrile metabolites that are toxic to trypanosomes (206). It may also cause direct inhibition of protein synthesis via damage to parasite DNA (207).

Pharmacokinetics. Benznidazole is available for oral administration and has a bioavailability of over 90%. It is ~40% protein bound. It has a half-life of ~12 h and has good tissue penetration (208, 209). Nifurtimox is administered orally but has poor oral bioavailability. It is metabolized in the liver and has a half-life of ~3 h. Dose reduction is advised for patients with significant hepatic or renal impairment, but no specific guidelines exist.

Spectrum of activity. Both benznidazole and nifurtimox are used for the treatment of acute *T. cruzi* infection (Chagas' disease). Neither agent has demonstrated efficacy in late stages of disease, and indications for treatment of chronic infection remain controversial but are expanding (210–212). No randomized trial has evaluated the comparative safety and efficacy of nifurtimox and benznidazole in adults (213). Nifurtimox is now also increasingly being used in combination with eflornithine for first-line treatment of *T. b. gambiense* infection. It also has been shown to have some activity in leishmaniasis but is not routinely used for this indication.

Adverse effects. Side effects are common with benznidazole and are seen in up to 40% of treated individuals, commonly including vomiting, abdominal pain, peripheral neuropathy, rash, and pruritus. Bone marrow suppression and neuropsychiatric reactions have also been reported. Nifurtimox has significant side effects that preclude the completion of therapy in many patients. Adverse effects include anorexia, nausea, rash, headache, sleep disturbance, peripheral neuropathy, and myalgias. Less frequent but more severe toxicity includes psychosis and convulsions. Benznidazole crosses the placenta, but there are minimal data regarding teratogenic effects for either agent in either animals or humans (214). Nifurtimox is detected in breast milk, so caution is recommended (215). Similarly, safety data for benznidazole and lactation are lacking, so withholding treatment while the patient is breastfeeding is again recommended.

APPENDIX

National and Regional Medicine Regulatory Authorities

The regulatory authorities listed here are members or associate members of the International Coalition of Medicines Regulatory Authorities (ICMRA). Individual websites can be accessed through links on the ICMRA website (http://www.icmra.info/drupal/participatingRegulatoryAuthorities).

Country or region	Regulatory body
Australia	Therapeutic Goods Administration (TGA)
Austria	Austrian Medicines and Medical Devices Agency (AGES MEA)
Brazil	National Health Surveillance Agency (ANVISA)
Canada	Health Products and Food Branch (HPFB), Health Canada
China	China Food and Drug Administration (CFDA)
Denmark	Danish Medicines Agency
Europe	European Commission—Directorate General for Health and Consumers (DG-SANCO) and European Medicines Agency (EMA)
France	French National Agency for Medicines and Health Products Safety (ANSM)
Germany	Paul-Ehrlich-Institut (PEI)
India	India Central Drugs Standard Control Organisation (CDSCO)
Ireland	Health Product Regulatory Authority (HPRA)
Italy	Italian Medicines Agency (AIFA)
Japan	Pharmaceuticals and Medical Devices Agency (PMDA), and the Ministry of Health, Labour and Welfare (MHLW)
Korea	Ministry of Food and Drug Safety (MFDS)
Mexico	Federal Commission for the Protection against Sanitary Risks (COFEPRIS)
Netherlands	Medicines Evaluation Board (MEB)
New Zealand	Medsafe, New Zealand Medicines and Medical Devices Safety
Nigeria	National Agency for Food Drug Administration and Control (NAFDAC)
Poland	The Office for Registration of Medicinal Products, Medical Devices and Biocidal Products (URPLWMiPB)
Russian Federation	Federal Service for Surveillance in Healthcare (Roszdravnadzor)
Singapore	Health Sciences Authority Singapore (HSA)
South Africa	Medicines Control Council (MCC), Department of Health
Spain	Spanish Agency of Medicines and Medical Devices (AEMPS)
Sweden	Sweden Medicinal Products Agency (MPA)
Switzerland	Swissmedic
United Kingdom	Medicines and Healthcare Products Regulatory Agency (MHRA)
United States	Food and Drug Administration (FDA)

REFERENCES

1. **The Medical Letter, Inc.** 2013. Drugs for parasitic infections. *Treat Guidel Med Lett* **11**(Suppl):e1–e31.
2. **Mackenzie CD, Geary TG.** 2011. Flubendazole: a candidate macrofilaricide for lymphatic filariasis and onchocerciasis field programs. *Expert Rev Anti Infect Ther* **9:**497–501.
3. **Ceballos L, Virkel G, Elissondo C, Canton C, Canevari J, Murno G, Denegri G, Lanusse C, Alvarez L.** 2013. A pharmacology-based comparison of the activity of albendazole and flubendazole against *Echinococcus granulosus* metacestode in sheep. *Acta Trop* **127:**216–225.
4. **van den Enden E.** 2009. Pharmacotherapy of helminth infection. *Expert Opin Pharmacother* **10:**435–451.
5. **Villegas F, Angles R, Barrientos R, Barrios G, Valero MA, Hamed K, Grueninger H, Ault SK, Montresor A, Engels D, Mas-Coma S, Gabrielli AF.** 2012. Administration of triclabendazole is safe and effective in controlling fascioliasis in an endemic community of the Bolivian Altiplano. *PLoS Negl Trop Dis* **6:**e1720.
6. **Cabada MM, White AC Jr.** 2012. New developments in epidemiology, diagnosis, and treatment of fascioliasis. *Curr Opin Infect Dis* **25:**518–522.
7. **Winkelhagen AJ, Mank T, de Vries PJ, Soetekouw R.** 2012. Apparent triclabendazole-resistant human *Fasciola hepatica* infection, the Netherlands. *Emerg Infect Dis* **18:**1028–1029.
8. **Fairweather I.** 2009. Triclabendazole progress report, 2005-2009: an advancement of learning? *J Helminthol* **83:**139–150.
9. **Cabada MM, Lopez M, Cruz M, Delgado JR, Hill V, White AC Jr.** 2016. Treatment failure after multiple courses of triclabendazole among patients with fascioliasis in Cusco, Peru: a case series. *PLoS Negl Trop Dis* **10:**e0004361.
10. **Keiser J, Engels D, Büscher G, Utzinger J.** 2005. Triclabendazole for the treatment of fascioliasis and paragonimiasis. *Expert Opin Investig Drugs* **14:**1513–1526.
11. **Lacey E.** 1990. Mode of action of benzimidazoles. *Parasitol Today* **6:**112–115.
12. **Gilman A, Rall TW, Nies AS (ed).** 1990. *Goodman and Gilman's the Pharmacological Basis of Therapeutics*, 8th ed. Pergamon Press, New York, NY.

13. **Frayha GJ, Smyth JD, Gobert JG, Savel J.** 1997. The mechanisms of action of antiprotozoal and anthelmintic drugs in man. *Gen Pharmacol* **28:**273–299.
14. **de Silva N, Guyatt H, Bundy D.** 1997. Anthelmintics. A comparative review of their clinical pharmacology. *Drugs* **53:**769–788.
15. **Edwards G, Breckenridge AM.** 1988. Clinical pharmacokinetics of anthelmintic drugs. *Clin Pharmacokinet* **15:**67–93.
16. **Marriner SE, Morris DL, Dickson B, Bogan JA.** 1986. Pharmacokinetics of albendazole in man. *Eur J Clin Pharmacol* **30:**705–708.
17. **Bogan JA, Marriner S.** 1980. Analysis of benzimidazoles in body fluids by high-performance liquid chromatography. *J Pharm Sci* **69:**422–423.
18. **Jung H, Hurtado M, Sanchez M, Medina MT, Sotelo J.** 1992. Clinical pharmacokinetics of albendazole in patients with brain cysticercosis. *J Clin Pharmacol* **32:**28–31.
19. **Jung H, Hurtado M, Medina MT, Sanchez M, Sotelo J.** 1990. Dexamethasone increases plasma levels of albendazole. *J Neurol* **237:**279–280.
20. **Garcia HH, Lescano AG, Lanchote VL, Pretell EJ, Gonzales I, Bustos JA, Takayanagui OM, Bonato PS, Horton J, Saavedra H, Gonzalez AE, Gilman RH, Cysticercosis Working Group in Peru.** 2011. Pharmacokinetics of combined treatment with praziquantel and albendazole in neurocysticercosis. *Br J Clin Pharmacol* **72:**77–84.
21. **Lima RM, Ferreira MA, de Jesus Ponte Carvalho TM, Dumêt Fernandes BJ, Takayanagui OM, Garcia HH, Coelho EB, Lanchote VL.** 2011. Albendazole-praziquantel interaction in healthy volunteers: kinetic disposition, metabolism and enantioselectivity. *Br J Clin Pharmacol* **71:**528–535.
22. **Pawluk SA, Roels CA, Wilby KJ, Ensom MHH.** 2015. A review of pharmacokinetic drug-drug interactions with the anthelmintic medications albendazole and mebendazole. *Clin Pharmacokinet* **54:**371–383.
23. **Morris DL, Chinnery JB, Georgiou G, Stamatakis G, Golematis B.** 1987. Penetration of albendazole sulphoxide into hydatid cysts. *Gut* **28:**75–80.
24. **Moskopp D, Lotterer E.** 1993. Concentrations of albendazole in serum, cerebrospinal fluid and hydatidous brain cyst. *Neurosurg Rev* **16:**35–37.
25. **Olveda RM, Acosta LP, Tallo V, Baltazar PI, Lesiguez JLS, Estanislao GG, Ayaso EB, Monterde DBS, Ida A, Watson N, McDonald EA, Wu HW, Kurtis JD, Friedman JF.** 2016. Efficacy and safety of praziquantel for the treatment of human schistosomiasis during pregnancy: a phase 2, randomised, double-blind, placebo-controlled trial. *Lancet Infect Dis* **16:** 199–208.
26. **Keiser J, Utzinger J.** 2008. Efficacy of current drugs against soil-transmitted helminth infections: systematic review and meta-analysis. *JAMA* **299:**1937–1948.
27. **Moser W, Schindler C, Keiser J.** 2017. Efficacy of recommended drugs against soil transmitted helminths: systematic review and network meta-analysis. *BMJ* **358:**j4307.
28. **Pion SDS, Chesnais CB, Weil GJ, Fischer PU, Missamou F, Boussinesq M.** 2017. Effect of 3 years of biannual mass drug administration with albendazole on lymphatic filariasis and soil-transmitted helminth infections: a community-based study in Republic of the Congo. *Lancet Infect Dis* **17:**763–769.
29. **Escobedo AA, Ballesteros J, González-Fraile E, Almirall P.** 2016. A meta-analysis of the efficacy of albendazole compared with tinidazole as treatments for *Giardia* infections in children. *Acta Trop* **153:**120–127.
30. **Opatrny L, Prichard R, Snell L, Maclean JD.** 2005. Death related to albendazole-induced pancytopenia: case report and review. *Am J Trop Med Hyg* **72:**291–294.
31. **Lillie P, McGann H.** 2010. Empiric albendazole therapy and new onset seizures—a cautionary note. *J Infect* **60:**403–404, author reply 404–405.
32. **Ramos-Zúñiga R, Pérez-Gómez HR, Jáuregui-Huerta F, del Sol López-Hernández M, Valera-Lizárraga JE, Paz-Vélez G, Becerra-Valdivia A.** 2013. Incidental consequences of antihelmintic treatment in the central nervous system. *World Neurosurg* **79:**149–153.
33. **Auer H, Kollaritsch H, Jüptner J, Aspöck H.** 1994. Albendazole and pregnancy. *Appl Parasitol* **35:**146–147.
34. **Torp-Pedersen A, Jimenez-Solem E, Cejvanovic V, Poulsen HE, Andersen JT.** 2016. Birth outcomes after exposure to mebendazole and pyrvinium during pregnancy—a Danish nationwide cohort study. *J Obstet Gynaecol* **36:** 1020–1025.
35. **Abdel-tawab AM, Bradley M, Ghazaly EA, Horton J, el-Setouhy M.** 2009. Albendazole and its metabolites in the breast milk of lactating women following a single oral dose of albendazole. *Br J Clin Pharmacol* **68:**737–742.
36. **Brindley PJ, Sher A.** 1990. Immunological involvement in the efficacy of praziquantel. *Exp Parasitol* **71:**245–248.
37. **Doenhoff MJ, Cioli D, Utzinger J.** 2008. Praziquantel: mechanisms of action, resistance and new derivatives for schistosomiasis. *Curr Opin Infect Dis* **21:**659–667.
38. **Cupit PM, Cunningham C.** 2015. What is the mechanism of action of praziquantel and how might resistance strike? *Future Med Chem* **7:**701–705.
39. **Sotelo J, Jung H.** 1998. Pharmacokinetic optimisation of the treatment of neurocysticercosis. *Clin Pharmacokinet* **34:** 503–515.
40. **Olliaro P, Delgado-Romero P, Keiser J.** 2014. The little we know about the pharmacokinetics and pharmacodynamics of praziquantel (racemate and R-enantiomer). *J Antimicrob Chemother* **69:**863–870.
41. **Kaojarern S, Nathakarnkikool S, Suvanakoot U.** 1989. Comparative bioavailability of praziquantel tablets. *DICP* **23:**29–32.
42. **Jung-Cook H.** 2012. Pharmacokinetic variability of anthelmintics: implications for the treatment of neurocysticercosis. *Expert Rev Clin Pharmacol* **5:**21–30.
43. **Garcia HH, Gonzales I, Lescano AG, Bustos JA, Zimic M, Escalante D, Saavedra H, Gavidia M, Rodriguez L, Najar E, Umeres H, Pretell EJ, Cysticercosis Working Group in Peru.** 2014. Efficacy of combined antiparasitic therapy with praziquantel and albendazole for neurocysticercosis: a double-blind, randomised controlled trial. *Lancet Infect Dis* **14:** 687–695.
44. **Garcia HH, Lescano AG, Gonzales I, Bustos JA, Pretell EJ, Horton J, Saavedra H, Gonzalez AE, Gilman RH, Cysticercosis Working Group in Peru.** 2016. Cysticidal efficacy of combined treatment with praziquantel and albendazole for parenchymal brain cysticercosis. *Clin Infect Dis* **62:** 1375–1379.
45. **Mohamed AE, Yasawy MI, Al Karawi MA.** 1998. Combined albendazole and praziquantel versus albendazole alone in the treatment of hydatid disease. *Hepatogastroenterology* **45:** 1690–1694.
46. **Cobo F, Yarnoz C, Sesma B, Fraile P, Aizcorbe M, Trujillo R, Diaz-de-Liaño A, Ciga MA.** 1998. Albendazole plus praziquantel versus albendazole alone as a pre-operative treatment in intra-abdominal hydatisosis caused by *Echinococcus granulosus*. *Trop Med Int Health* **3:**462–466.
47. **Bygott JM, Chiodini PL.** 2009. Praziquantel: neglected drug? Ineffective treatment? Or therapeutic choice in cystic hydatid disease? *Acta Trop* **111:**95–101.
48. **Alvela-Suárez L, Velasco-Tirado V, Belhassen-Garcia M, Novo-Veleiro I, Pardo-Lledías J, Romero-Alegría A, Pérez del Villar L, Valverde-Merino MP, Cordero-Sánchez M.** 2014. Safety of the combined use of praziquantel and albendazole in the treatment of human hydatid disease. *Am J Trop Med Hyg* **90:**819–822.
49. **Lee JM, Lim HS, Hong ST.** 2011. Hypersensitive reaction to praziquantel in a clonorchiasis patient. *Korean J Parasitol* **49:**273–275.
50. **Kyung SY, Cho YK, Kim YJ, Park JW, Jeong SH, Lee JI, Sung YM, Lee SP.** 2011. A paragonimiasis patient with allergic reaction to praziquantel and resistance to triclabendazole: successful treatment after desensitization to praziquantel. *Korean J Parasitol* **49:**73–77.
51. **Hewagama SS, Darby JD, Sheorey H, Daffy JR.** 2010. Seizures related to praziquantel therapy in neurocysticercosis. *Med J Aust* **193:**246–247.

52. **Olds GR.** 2003. Administration of praziquantel to pregnant and lactating women. *Acta Trop* **86:**185–195.
53. **Adam I, Elwasila T, Homeida M.** 2004. Is praziquantel therapy safe during pregnancy? *Trans R Soc Trop Med Hyg* **98:**540–543.
54. **Allen HE, Crompton DW, de Silva N, LoVerde PT, Olds GR.** 2002. New policies for using anthelmintics in high risk groups. *Trends Parasitol* **18:**381–382.
55. **Sutherland IH, Campbell WC.** 1990. Development, pharmacokinetics and mode of action of ivermectin. *Acta Leiden* **59:**161–168.
56. **Campbell WC.** 1993. Ivermectin, an antiparasitic agent. *Med Res Rev* **13:**61–79.
57. **Fox LM.** 2006. Ivermectin: uses and impact 20 years on. *Curr Opin Infect Dis* **19:**588–593.
58. **Geary TG, Moreno Y.** 2012. Macrocyclic lactone anthelmintics: spectrum of activity and mechanism of action. *Curr Pharm Biotechnol* **13:**866–872.
59. **Kircik LH, Del Rosso JQ, Layton AM, Schauber J.** 2016. Over 25 years of clinical experience with ivermectin: an overview of safety for an increasing number of indications. *J Drugs Dermatol* **15:**325–332.
60. **Ottesen EA, Campbell WC.** 1994. Ivermectin in human medicine. *J Antimicrob Chemother* **34:**195–203.
61. **Fusco DN, Downs JA, Satlin MJ, Pahuja M, Ramos L, Barie PS, Fleckenstein L, Murray HW.** 2010. Non-oral treatment with ivermectin for disseminated strongyloidiasis. *Am J Trop Med Hyg* **83:**879–883.
62. **Grein JD, Mathisen GE, Donovan S, Fleckenstein L.** 2010. Serum ivermectin levels after enteral and subcutaneous administration for *Strongyloides* hyperinfection: a case report. *Scand J Infect Dis* **42:**234–236.
63. **Bogoch II, Khan K, Abrams H, Nott C, Leung E, Fleckenstein L, Keystone JS.** 2015. Failure of ivermectin per rectum to achieve clinically meaningful serum levels in two cases of *Strongyloides* hyperinfection. *Am J Trop Med Hyg* **93:**94–96.
64. **Donadello K, Cristallini S, Taccone FS, Lorent S, Vincent JL, de Backer D, Jacobs F.** 2013. Strongyloides disseminated infection successfully treated with parenteral ivermectin: case report with drug concentration measurements and review of the literature. *Int J Antimicrob Agents* **42:**580–583.
65. **Miyajima A, Hirota T, Sugioka A, Fukuzawa M, Sekine M, Yamamoto Y, Yoshimasu T, Kigure A, Anata T, Noguchi W, Akagi K, Komoda M.** 2016. Effect of high-fat meal intake on the pharmacokinetic profile of ivermectin in Japanese patients with scabies. *J Dermatol* **43:**1030–1036.
66. **Baraka OZ, Mahmoud BM, Marschke CK, Geary TG, Homeida MM, Williams JF.** 1996. Ivermectin distribution in the plasma and tissues of patients infected with *Onchocerca volvulus*. *Eur J Clin Pharmacol* **50:**407–410.
67. **Herwaldt BL, Dougherty CP, Allen CK, Jolly JP, Brown MN, Yu P, Yu Y.** 2018. Characteristics of patients for whom benznidazole was released through the CDC-sponsored Investigational New Drug program for treatment of Chagas disease—United States, 2011–2018. *MMWR Morb Mortal Wkly Rep* **67:**803–805.
68. **Henriquez-Camacho C, Gotuzzo E, Echevarria J, White AC Jr, Terashima A, Samalvides F, Pérez-Molina JA, Plana MN.** 2016. Ivermectin versus albendazole or thiabendazole for *Strongyloides stercoralis* infection. *Cochrane Database Syst Rev* **2016**(1)**:**CD007745.
69. **Abegunde AT, Ahuja RM, Okafor NJ.** 2016. Doxycycline plus ivermectin versus ivermectin alone for treatment of patients with onchocerciasis. *Cochrane Database Syst Rev* **2016**(1)**:**CD011146.
70. **Thomsen EK, Sanuku N, Baea M, Satofan S, Maki E, Lombore B, Schmidt MS, Siba PM, Weil GJ, Kazura JW, Fleckenstein LL, King CL.** 2016. Efficacy, safety, and pharmacokinetics of coadministered diethylcarbamazine, albendazole, and ivermectin for treatment of bancroftian filariasis. *Clin Infect Dis* **62:**334–341.
71. **Naquira C, Jimenez G, Guerra JG, Bernal R, Nalin DR, Neu D, Aziz M.** 1989. Ivermectin for human strongyloidiasis and other intestinal helminths. *Am J Trop Med Hyg* **40:**304–309.
72. **Wen LY, Yan XL, Sun FH, Fang YY, Yang MJ, Lou LJ.** 2008. A randomized, double-blind, multicenter clinical trial on the efficacy of ivermectin against intestinal nematode infections in China. *Acta Trop* **106:**190–194.
73. **Knopp S, Mohammed KA, Speich B, Hattendorf J, Khamis IS, Khamis AN, Stothard JR, Rollinson D, Marti H, Utzinger J.** 2010. Albendazole and mebendazole administered alone or in combination with ivermectin against *Trichuris trichiura*: a randomized controlled trial. *Clin Infect Dis* **51:**1420–1428.
74. **Speich B, Ali SM, Ame SM, Bogoch II, Alles R, Huwyler J, Albonico M, Hattendorf J, Utzinger J, Keiser J.** 2015. Efficacy and safety of albendazole plus ivermectin, albendazole plus mebendazole, albendazole plus oxantel pamoate, and mebendazole alone against *Trichuris trichiura* and concomitant soil-transmitted helminth infections: a four-arm, randomised controlled trial. *Lancet Infect Dis* **15:**277–284.
75. **Kraivichian K, Nuchprayoon S, Sitichalernchai P, Chaicumpa W, Yentakam S.** 2004. Treatment of cutaneous gnathostomiasis with ivermectin. *Am J Trop Med Hyg* **71:**623–628.
76. **González P, González FA, Ueno K.** 2012. Ivermectin in human medicine, an overview of the current status of its clinical applications. *Curr Pharm Biotechnol* **13:**1103–1109.
77. **Ouédraogo AL, Bastiaens GJH, Tiono AB, Guelbéogo WM, Kobylinski KC, Ouédraogo A, Barry A, Bougouma EC, Nebie I, Ouattara MS, Lanke KHW, Fleckenstein L, Sauerwein RW, Slater HC, Churcher TS, Sirima SB, Drakeley C, Bousema T.** 2015. Efficacy and safety of the mosquitocidal drug ivermectin to prevent malaria transmission after treatment: a double-blind, randomized, clinical trial. *Clin Infect Dis* **60:**357–365.
78. **Alout H, Krajacich BJ, Meyers JI, Grubaugh ND, Brackney DE, Kobylinski KC, Diclaro JW II, Bolay FK, Fakoli LS, Diabaté A, Dabiré RK, Bougma RW, Foy BD.** 2014. Evaluation of ivermectin mass drug administration for malaria transmission control across different West African environments. *Malar J* **13:**417.
79. **Mendes AM, Albuquerque IS, Machado M, Pissarra J, Meireles P, Prudêncio M.** 2017. Inhibition of *Plasmodium* liver infection by ivermectin. *Antimicrob Agents Chemother* **61:**e02005-16.
80. **Njoo FL, Beek WM, Keukens HJ, van Wilgenburg H, Oosting J, Stilma JS, Kijlstra A.** 1995. Ivermectin detection in serum of onchocerciasis patients: relationship to adverse reactions. *Am J Trop Med Hyg* **52:**94–97.
81. **Twum-Danso NA.** 2003. Loa loa encephalopathy temporally related to ivermectin administration reported from onchocerciasis mass treatment programs from 1989 to 2001: implications for the future. *Filaria J* **2**(Suppl 1)**:**S7.
82. **Pacqué M, Muñoz B, Poetscke G, Foose J, Taylor HR, Greene BM.** 1990. Pregnancy outcome after inadvertent ivermectin treatment during community-based distribution. *Lancet* **336:**1486–1489.
83. **Goa KL, McTavish D, Clissold SP.** 1991. Ivermectin. A review of its antifilarial activity, pharmacokinetic properties and clinical efficacy in onchocerciasis. *Drugs* **42:**640–658.
84. **Gyapong JO, Chinbuah MA, Gyapong M.** 2003. Inadvertent exposure of pregnant women to ivermectin and albendazole during mass drug administration for lymphatic filariasis. *Trop Med Int Health* **8:**1093–1101.
85. **Klion AD, Ottesen EA, Nutman TB.** 1994. Effectiveness of diethylcarbamazine in treating loiasis acquired by expatriate visitors to endemic regions: long-term follow-up. *J Infect Dis* **169:**604–610.
86. **Edwards G, Awadzi K, Breckenridge AM, Gilles HM, Orme ML, Ward SA.** 1981. Diethylcarbamazine disposition in patients with onchocerciasis. *Clin Pharmacol Ther* **30:**551–557.
87. **Norões J, Dreyer G, Santos A, Mendes VG, Medeiros Z, Addiss D.** 1997. Assessment of the efficacy of diethylcarbamazine on adult *Wuchereria bancrofti* in vivo. *Trans R Soc Trop Med Hyg* **91:**78–81.
88. **Ottesen EA.** 1985. Efficacy of diethylcarbamazine in eradicating infection with lymphatic-dwelling filariae in humans. *Rev Infect Dis* **7:**341–356.
89. **Nicolas L, Plichart C, Nguyen LN, Moulia-Pelat JP.** 1997. Reduction of *Wuchereria bancrofti* adult worm circulating antigen after annual treatments of diethylcarbamazine combined with ivermectin in French Polynesia. *J Infect Dis* **175:** 489–492.

90. **Joseph CA, Dixon PA.** 1984. Possible prostaglandin-mediated effect of diethylcarbamazine on rat uterine contractility. *J Pharm Pharmacol* **36:**281–282.
91. **Speich B, Ame SM, Ali SM, Alles R, Huwyler J, Hattendorf J, Utzinger J, Albonico M, Keiser J.** 2014. Oxantel pamoate-albendazole for *Trichuris trichiura* infection. *N Engl J Med* **370:**610–620.
92. **Ferrara P, Bersani I, Bottaro G, Vitelli O, Liberatore P, Gatto A, del Bufalo F, Romano V, Stabile A.** 2011. Massive proteinuria: a possible side effect of pyrantel pamoate? *Ren Fail* **33:**534–536.
93. **Tietze PE, Jones JE.** 1991. Parasites during pregnancy. *Prim Care* **18:**75–99.
94. **Fox LM, Saravolatz LD.** 2005. Nitazoxanide: a new thiazolide antiparasitic agent. *Clin Infect Dis* **40:**1173–1180.
95. **Anonymous.** 2003. Nitazoxanide (Alinia)—a new anti-protozoal agent. *Med Lett Drugs Ther* **45:**29–31.
96. **Gilles HM, Hoffman PS.** 2002. Treatment of intestinal parasitic infections: a review of nitazoxanide. *Trends Parasitol* **18:** 95–97.
97. **Stockis A, Allemon AM, De Bruyn S, Gengler C.** 2002. Nitazoxanide pharmacokinetics and tolerability in man using single ascending oral doses. *Int J Clin Pharmacol Ther* **40:**213–220.
98. **Broekhuysen J, Stockis A, Lins RL, De Graeve J, Rossignol JF.** 2000. Nitazoxanide: pharmacokinetics and metabolism in man. *Int J Clin Pharmacol Ther* **38:**387–394.
99. **Ortiz JJ, Ayoub A, Gargala G, Chegne NL, Favennec L.** 2001. Randomized clinical study of nitazoxanide compared to metronidazole in the treatment of symptomatic giardiasis in children from northern Peru. *Aliment Pharmacol Ther* **15:**1409–1415.
100. **Adagu IS, Nolder D, Warhurst DC, Rossignol JF.** 2002. In vitro activity of nitazoxanide and related compounds against isolates of *Giardia intestinalis*, *Entamoeba histolytica* and *Trichomonas vaginalis*. *J Antimicrob Chemother* **49:**103–111.
101. **Stockis A, Deroubaix X, Lins R, Jeanbaptiste B, Calderon P, Rossignol JF.** 1996. Pharmacokinetics of nitazoxanide after single oral dose administration in 6 healthy volunteers. *Int J Clin Pharmacol Ther* **34:**349–351.
102. **Asai T, Còrdova Vidal C, Strauss W, Ikoma T, Endoh K, Yamamoto M.** 2016. Effect of mass stool examination and mass treatment for decreasing intestinal helminth and protozoan infection rates in Bolivian children: a cross-sectional study. *PLoS Negl Trop Dis* **10:**e0005147.
103. **Hotez PJ.** 2014. Could nitazoxanide be added to other essential medicines for integrated neglected tropical disease control and elimination? *PLoS Negl Trop Dis* **8:**e2758.
104. **Diaz E, Mondragon J, Ramirez E, Bernal R.** 2003. Epidemiology and control of intestinal parasites with nitazoxanide in children in Mexico. *Am J Trop Med Hyg* **68:**384–385.
105. **Olliaro P, Seiler J, Kuesel A, Horton J, Clark JN, Don R, Keiser J.** 2011. Potential drug development candidates for human soil-transmitted helminthiases. *PLoS Negl Trop Dis* **5:**e1138.
106. **Slater AF, Cerami A.** 1992. Inhibition by chloroquine of a novel haem polymerase enzyme activity in malaria trophozoites. *Nature* **355:**167–169.
107. **Krogstad DJ, Schlesinger PH, Gluzman IY.** 1989. Chloroquine and acid vesicle function. *Prog Clin Biol Res* **313:**53–59.
108. **Pussard E, Verdier F.** 1994. Antimalarial 4-aminoquinolines: mode of action and pharmacokinetics. *Fundam Clin Pharmacol* **8:**1–17.
109. **Abu-Aisha H, Abu-Sabaa HMA, Nur T.** 1979. Cardiac arrest after intravenous chloroquine injection. *J Trop Med Hyg* **82:**36–37.
110. **Krishna S, White NJ.** 1996. Pharmacokinetics of quinine, chloroquine and amodiaquine. Clinical implications. *Clin Pharmacokinet* **30:**263–299.
111. **WHO.** 2015. *Guidelines for the Treatment of Malaria*, 3rd ed. WHO Press, Geneva, Switzerland.
112. **Rombo L, Björkman A, Sego E, Ericsson O.** 1986. Whole blood concentrations of chloroquine and desethylchloroquine during and after treatment of adult patients infected with *Plasmodium vivax*, *P. ovale* or *P. malariae*. *Trans R Soc Trop Med Hyg* **80:**763–766.
113. **Añez A, Moscoso M, Garnica C, Ascaso C.** 2016. Evaluation of the paediatric dose of chloroquine in the treatment of *Plasmodium vivax* malaria. *Malar J* **15:**371.
114. **Ursing J, Eksborg S, Rombo L, Bergqvist Y, Blessborn D, Rodrigues A, Kofoed PE.** 2014. Chloroquine is grossly under dosed in young children with malaria: implications for drug resistance. *PLoS One* **9:**e86801.
115. **Daneshvar C, Davis TME, Cox-Singh J, Rafa'ee MZ, Zakaria SK, Divis PCS, Singh B.** 2010. Clinical and parasitological response to oral chloroquine and primaquine in uncomplicated human Plasmodium knowlesi infections. *Malar J* **9:**238.
116. **Levy M, Buskila D, Gladman DD, Urowitz MB, Koren G.** 1991. Pregnancy outcome following first trimester exposure to chloroquine. *Am J Perinatol* **8:**174–178.
117. **Phillips-Howard PA, West LJ.** 1990. Serious adverse drug reactions to pyrimethamine-sulphadoxine, pyrimethamine-dapsone and to amodiaquine in Britain. *J R Soc Med* **83:** 82–85.
118. **Olliaro P, Nevill C, LeBras J, Ringwald P, Mussano P, Garner P, Brasseur P.** 1996. Systematic review of amodiaquine treatment in uncomplicated malaria. *Lancet* **348:**1196–1201.
119. **Foley M, Tilley L.** 1997. Quinoline antimalarials: mechanisms of action and resistance. *Int J Parasitol* **27:**231–240.
120. **White NJ.** 1985. Clinical pharmacokinetics of antimalarial drugs. *Clin Pharmacokinet* **10:**187–215.
121. **Looareesuwan S, Phillips RE, White NJ, Kietinun S, Karbwang J, Rackow C, Turner RC, Warrell DA.** 1985. Quinine and severe falciparum malaria in late pregnancy. *Lancet* **ii:**4–8.
122. **Silver HM.** 1997. Malarial infection during pregnancy. *Infect Dis Clin North Am* **11:**99–107.
123. **Moore BR, Salman S, Davis TME.** 2016. Treatment regimens for pregnant women with falciparum malaria. *Expert Rev Anti Infect Ther* **14:**691–704.
124. **Karbwang J, White NJ.** 1990. Clinical pharmacokinetics of mefloquine. *Clin Pharmacokinet* **19:**264–279.
125. **Lee SJ, Ter Kuile FO, Price RN, Luxemburger C, Nosten F.** 2017. Adverse effects of mefloquine for the treatment of uncomplicated malaria in Thailand: a pooled analysis of 19, 850 individual patients. *PLoS One* **12:**e0168780.
126. **Hennequin C, Bourée P, Bazin N, Bisaro F, Feline A.** 1994. Severe psychiatric side effects observed during prophylaxis and treatment with mefloquine. *Arch Intern Med* **154:**2360–2362.
127. **van Riemsdijk MM, van der Klauw MM, van Heest JA, Reedeker FR, Ligthelm RJ, Herings RM, Stricker BH.** 1997. Neuro-psychiatric effects of antimalarials. *Eur J Clin Pharmacol* **52:**1–6.
128. **Grabias B, Kumar S.** 2016. Adverse neuropsychiatric effects of antimalarial drugs. *Expert Opin Drug Saf* **15:**903–910.
129. **Vanhauwere B, Maradit H, Kerr L.** 1998. Post-marketing surveillance of prophylactic mefloquine (Lariam) use in pregnancy. *Am J Trop Med Hyg* **58:**17–21.
130. **González R, Hellgren U, Greenwood B, Menéndez C.** 2014. Mefloquine safety and tolerability in pregnancy: a systematic literature review. *Malar J* **13:**75.
131. **Nosten F, Vincenti M, Simpson J, Yei P, Thwai KL, de Vries A, Chongsuphajaisiddhi T, White NJ.** 1999. The effects of mefloquine treatment in pregnancy. *Clin Infect Dis* **28:** 808–815.
132. **Veenendaal JR, Parkinson AD, Kere N, Rieckmann KH, Edstein MD.** 1991. Pharmacokinetics of halofantrine and n-desbutylhalofantrine in patients with falciparum malaria following a multiple dose regimen of halofantrine. *Eur J Clin Pharmacol* **41:**161–164.
133. **Bryson HM, Goa KL.** 1992. Halofantrine. A review of its antimalarial activity, pharmacokinetic properties and therapeutic potential. *Drugs* **43:**236–258.
134. **Bouchaud O, Imbert P, Touze JE, Dodoo AN, Danis M, Legros F.** 2009. Fatal cardiotoxicity related to halofantrine: a review based on a worldwide safety data base. *Malar J* **8:**289.
135. **Ezzet F, van Vugt M, Nosten F, Looareesuwan S, White NJ.** 2000. Pharmacokinetics and pharmacodynamics of lumefantrine (benflumetol) in acute falciparum malaria. *Antimicrob Agents Chemother* **44:**697–704.

136. **Warhurst DC.** 1984. Why are primaquine and other 8-aminoquinolines particularly effective against the mature gametocytes and the hypnozoites of malaria? *Ann Trop Med Parasitol* **78:**165.
137. **Mihaly GW, Ward SA, Edwards G, Orme ML, Breckenridge AM.** 1984. Pharmacokinetics of primaquine in man: identification of the carboxylic acid derivative as a major plasma metabolite. *Br J Clin Pharmacol* **17:**441–446.
138. **Nasveld PE, Edstein MD, Reid M, Brennan L, Harris IE, Kitchener SJ, Leggat PA, Pickford P, Kerr C, Ohrt C, Prescott W, Tafenoquine Study Team.** 2010. Randomized, double-blind study of the safety, tolerability, and efficacy of tafenoquine versus mefloquine for malaria prophylaxis in nonimmune subjects. *Antimicrob Agents Chemother* **54:**792–798.
139. **Walsh DS, Wilairatana P, Tang DB, Heppner DG Jr, Brewer TG, Krudsood S, Silachamroon U, Phumratanaprapin W, Siriyanonda D, Looareesuwan S.** 2004. Randomized trial of 3-dose regimens of tafenoquine (WR238605) versus low-dose primaquine for preventing *Plasmodium vivax* malaria relapse. *Clin Infect Dis* **39:**1095–1103.
140. **Brueckner RP, Coster T, Wesche DL, Shmuklarsky M, Schuster BG.** 1998. Prophylaxis of *Plasmodium falciparum* infection in a human challenge model with WR 238605, a new 8-aminoquinoline antimalarial. *Antimicrob Agents Chemother* **42:**1293–1294.
141. **Gu HM, Warhurst DC, Peters W.** 1984. Uptake of [3H] dihydroartemisinine by erythrocytes infected with *Plasmodium falciparum* in vitro. *Trans R Soc Trop Med Hyg* **78:** 265–270.
142. **Na-Bangchang K, Krudsood S, Silachamroon U, Molunto P, Tasanor O, Chalermrut K, Tangpukdee N, Matangkasombut O, Kano S, Looareesuwan S.** 2004. The pharmacokinetics of oral dihydroartemisinin and artesunate in healthy Thai volunteers. *Southeast Asian J Trop Med Public Health* **35:**575–582.
143. **Morris CA, Duparc S, Borghini-Fuhrer I, Jung D, Shin CS, Fleckenstein L.** 2011. Review of the clinical pharmacokinetics of artesunate and its active metabolite dihydroartemisinin following intravenous, intramuscular, oral or rectal administration. *Malar J* **10:**263.
144. **Price RN, Nosten F, Luxemburger C, ter Kuile FO, Paiphun L, Chongsuphajaisiddhi T, White NJ.** 1996. Effects of artemisinin derivatives on malaria transmissibility. *Lancet* **347:**1654–1658.
145. **Chen PQ, Li GQ, Guo XB, He KR, Fu YX, Fu LC, Song YZ.** 1994. The infectivity of gametocytes of *Plasmodium falciparum* from patients treated with artemisinin. *Chin Med J (Engl)* **107:**709–711.
146. **Ippolito MM, Johnson J, Mullin C, Mallow C, Morgan N, Wallender E, Li T, Rosenthal PJ.** 2017. The relative effects of artemether-lumefantrine and non-artemisinin antimalarials on gametocyte carriage and transmission of *Plasmodium falciparum*: a systematic review and meta-analysis. *Clin Infect Dis* **65:**486–494.
147. **South East Asian Quinine Artesunate Malaria Trial (SEAQUAMAT) Group.** 2005. Artesunate versus quinine for treatment of severe falciparum malaria: a randomised trial. *Lancet* **366:**717–725.
148. **Sinclair D, Donegan S, Isba R, Lalloo DG.** 2012. Artesunate versus quinine for treating severe malaria. *Cochrane Database Syst Rev* **2012:**CD005967.
149. **Dondorp AM, Fanello CI, Hendriksen IC, Gomes E, Seni A, Chhaganlal KD, Bojang K, Olaosebikan R, Anunobi N, Maitland K, Kivaya E, Agbenyega T, Nguah SB, Evans J, Gesase S, Kahabuka C, Mtove G, Nadjm B, Deen J, Mwanga-Amumpaire J, Nansumba M, Karema C, Umulisa N, Uwimana A, Mokuolu OA, Adedoyin OT, Johnson WB, Tshefu AK, Onyamboko MA, Sakulthaew T, Ngum WP, Silamut K, Stepniewska K, Woodrow CJ, Bethell D, Wills B, Oneko M, Peto TE, von Seidlein L, Day NP, White NJ, AQUAMAT group.** 2010. Artesunate versus quinine in the treatment of severe falciparum malaria in African children (AQUAMAT): an open-label, randomised trial. *Lancet* **376:**1647–1657.
150. **Talisuna AO, Karema C, Ogutu B, Juma E, Logedi J, Nyandigisi A, Mulenga M, Mbacham WF, Roper C, Guerin PJ, D'Alessandro U, Snow RW.** 2012. Mitigating the threat of artemisinin resistance in Africa: improvement of drug-resistance surveillance and response systems. *Lancet Infect Dis* **12:**888–896.
151. **Grigg MJ, William T, Barber BE, Rajahram GS, Menon J, Schimann E, Wilkes CS, Patel K, Chandna A, Price RN, Yeo TW, Anstey NM.** 2017. Artemether-lumefantrine versus chloroquine for the treatment of uncomplicated Plasmodium knowlesi malaria: an open-label randomized controlled trial CAN KNOW. *Clin Infect Dis* **66:**229–236.
152. **Antinori S, Galimberti L, Milazzo L, Corbellino M.** 2013. *Plasmodium knowlesi*: the emerging zoonotic malaria parasite. *Acta Trop* **125:**191–201.
153. **Utzinger J, Xiao SH, Tanner M, Keiser J.** 2007. Artemisinins for schistosomiasis and beyond. *Curr Opin Investig Drugs* **8:**105–116.
154. **Wikman-Jorgensen PE, Henríquez-Camacho CA, Serrano-Villar S, Pérez-Molina JA.** 2012. The role of artesunate for the treatment of urinary schistosomiasis in schoolchildren: a systematic review and meta-analysis. *Pathog Glob Health* **106:**397–404.
155. **Pérez del Villar L, Burguillo FJ, López-Abán J, Muro A.** 2012. Systematic review and meta-analysis of artemisinin based therapies for the treatment and prevention of schistosomiasis. *PLoS One* **7:**e45867.
156. **Nosten F, White NJ.** 2007. Artemisinin-based combination treatment of falciparum malaria. *Am J Trop Med Hyg* **77**(Suppl)**:**181–192.
157. **Li Q, Si Y, Xie L, Zhang J, Weina P.** 2009. Severe embryolethality of artesunate related to pharmacokinetics following intravenous and intramuscular doses in pregnant rats. *Birth Defects Res B Dev Reprod Toxicol* **86:**385–393.
158. **Looareesuwan S, Chulay JD, Canfield CJ, Hutchinson DB.** 1999. Malarone (atovaquone and proguanil hydrochloride): a review of its clinical development for treatment of malaria. Malarone Clinical Trials Study Group.. *Am J Trop Med Hyg* **60:**533–541.
159. **Srivastava IK, Vaidya AB.** 1999. A mechanism for the synergistic antimalarial action of atovaquone and proguanil. *Antimicrob Agents Chemother* **43:**1334–1339.
160. **Edstein MD, Looareesuwan S, Viravan C, Kyle DE.** 1996. Pharmacokinetics of proguanil in malaria patients treated with proguanil plus atovaquone. *Southeast Asian J Trop Med Public Health* **27:**216–220.
161. **Radloff PD, Philipps J, Hutchinson D, Kremsner PG.** 1996. Atovaquone plus proguanil is an effective treatment for *Plasmodium ovale* and *P. malariae* malaria. *Trans R Soc Trop Med Hyg* **90:**682.
162. **McAuley JB, Herwaldt BL, Stokes SL, Becher JA, Roberts JM, Michelson MK, Juranek DD.** 1992. Diloxanide furoate for treating asymptomatic *Entamoeba histolytica* cyst passers: 14 years' experience in the United States. *Clin Infect Dis* **15:**464–468.
163. **Marie C, Petri WA.** 2013. Amoebic dysentery. *BMJ Clin Evid* **2013:**0918.
164. **Chulay JD, Fleckenstein L, Smith DH.** 1988. Pharmacokinetics of antimony during treatment of visceral leishmaniasis with sodium stibogluconate or meglumine antimoniate. *Trans R Soc Trop Med Hyg* **82:**69–72.
165. **Oliveira LF, Schubach AO, Martins MM, Passos SL, Oliveira RV, Marzochi MC, Andrade CA.** 2011. Systematic review of the adverse effects of cutaneous leishmaniasis treatment in the New World. *Acta Trop* **118:**87–96.
166. **Brito NC, Rabello A, Cota GF.** 2017. Efficacy of pentavalent antimoniate intralesional infiltration therapy for cutaneous leishmaniasis: a systematic review. *PLoS One* **12:**e0184777.
167. **Aronson N, Herwaldt BL, Libman M, Pearson R, Lopez-Velez R, Weina P, Carvalho EM, Ephros M, Jeronimo S, Magill A.** 2016. Diagnosis and treatment of leishmaniasis: clinical practice guidelines by the Infectious Diseases Society of America (IDSA) and the American Society of Tropical Medicine and Hygiene (ASTMH). *Clin Infect Dis* **63:**e202–e264.

168. **Jha TK, Sundar S, Thakur CP, Bachmann P, Karbwang J, Fischer C, Voss A, Berman J.** 1999. Miltefosine, an oral agent, for the treatment of Indian visceral leishmaniasis. *N Engl J Med* **341:**1795–1800.
169. **More B, Bhatt H, Kukreja V, Ainapure SS.** 2003. Miltefosine: great expectations against visceral leishmaniasis. *J Postgrad Med* **49:**101–103.
170. **Prasad R, Kumar R, Jaiswal BP, Singh UK.** 2004. Miltefosine: an oral drug for visceral leishmaniasis. *Indian J Pediatr* **71:**143–144.
171. **Soto J, Soto P.** 2006. Miltefosine: oral treatment of leishmaniasis. *Expert Rev Anti Infect Ther* **4:**177–185.
172. **Sindermann H, Croft SL, Engel KR, Bommer W, Eibl HJ, Unger C, Engel J.** 2004. Miltefosine (Impavido): the first oral treatment against leishmaniasis. *Med Microbiol Immunol (Berl)* **193:**173–180.
173. **Croft SL, Seifert K, Duchêne M.** 2003. Antiprotozoal activities of phospholipid analogues. *Mol Biochem Parasitol* **126:**165–172.
174. **Bhattacharya SK, Jha TK, Sundar S, Thakur CP, Engel J, Sindermann H, Junge K, Karbwang J, Bryceson AD, Berman JD.** 2004. Efficacy and tolerability of miltefosine for childhood visceral leishmaniasis in India. *Clin Infect Dis* **38:**217–221.
175. **Sundar S, Jha TK, Thakur CP, Engel J, Sindermann H, Fischer C, Junge K, Bryceson A, Berman J.** 2002. Oral miltefosine for Indian visceral leishmaniasis. *N Engl J Med* **347:**1739–1746.
176. **Sundar S, Sinha P, Jha TK, Chakravarty J, Rai M, Kumar N, Pandey K, Narain MK, Verma N, Das VNR, Das P, Berman J, Arana B.** 2013. Oral miltefosine for Indian post-kala-azar dermal leishmaniasis: a randomised trial. *Trop Med Int Health* **18:**96–100.
177. **Webster D, Umar I, Kolyvas G, Bilbao J, Guiot MC, Duplisea K, Qvarnstrom Y, Visvesvara GS.** 2012. Treatment of granulomatous amoebic encephalitis with voriconazole and miltefosine in an immunocompetent soldier. *Am J Trop Med Hyg* **87:**715–718. *ERRATUM Am J Trop Med Hyg* **87:**1154.
178. **Martínez DY, Seas C, Bravo F, Legua P, Ramos C, Cabello AM, Gotuzzo E.** 2010. Successful treatment of *Balamuthia mandrillaris* amoebic infection with extensive neurological and cutaneous involvement. *Clin Infect Dis* **51:**e7–e11.
179. **Soto J, Toledo J, Gutierrez P, Nicholls RS, Padilla J, Engel J, Fischer C, Voss A, Berman J.** 2001. Treatment of American cutaneous leishmaniasis with miltefosine, an oral agent. *Clin Infect Dis* **33:**e57–e61.
180. **Pandey K, Singh D, Lal CS, Das VNR, Das P.** 2013. Fatal acute pancreatitis in a patient with visceral leishmaniasis during miltefosine treatment. *J Postgrad Med* **59:**306–308.
181. **Monge-Maillo B, López-Vélez R.** 2015. Miltefosine for visceral and cutaneous leishmaniasis: drug characteristics and evidence-based treatment recommendations. *Clin Infect Dis* **60:**1398–1404.
182. **Sands M, Kron MA, Brown RB.** 1985. Pentamidine: a review. *Rev Infect Dis* **7:**625–634.
183. **Soto J, Paz D, Rivero D, Soto P, Quispe J, Toledo J, Berman J.** 2016. Intralesional pentamidine: a novel therapy for single lesions of Bolivian cutaneous leishmaniasis. *Am J Trop Med Hyg* **94:**852–856.
184. **Waalkes TP, DeVita VT.** 1970. The determination of pentamidine (4,4′-diamidinophenoxypentane) in plasma, urine, and tissues. *J Lab Clin Med* **75:**871–878.
185. **Ben Salah A, Ben Messaoud N, Guedri E, Zaatour A, Ben Alaya N, Bettaieb J, Gharbi A, Belhadj Hamida N, Boukthir A, Chlif S, Abdelhamid K, El Ahmadi Z, Louzir H, Mokni M, Morizot G, Buffet P, Smith PL, Kopydlowski KM, Kreishman-Deitrick M, Smith KS, Nielsen CJ, Ullman DR, Norwood JA, Thorne GD, McCarthy WF, Adams RC, Rice RM, Tang D, Berman J, Ransom J, Magill AJ, Grogl M.** 2013. Topical paromomycin with or without gentamicin for cutaneous leishmaniasis. *N Engl J Med* **368:**524–532.
186. **Davidson RN, den Boer M, Ritmeijer K.** 2009. Paromomycin. *Trans R Soc Trop Med Hyg* **103:**653–660.
187. **Harris JC, Plummer S, Lloyd D.** 2001. Antigiardial drugs. *Appl Microbiol Biotechnol* **57:**614–619.
188. **van Hellemond JJ, Molhoek N, Wismans PJ, van Genderen PJJ, Koelewijn R.** 2013. Is paromomycin the drug of choice for eradication of *Blastocystis* in adults? *J Infect Chemother* **19:**545–548.
189. **Botero D.** 1970. Paromomycin as effective treatment of *Taenia* infections. *Am J Trop Med Hyg* **19:**234–237.
190. **Katz M.** 1977. Anthelmintics. *Drugs* **13:**124–136.
191. **Pépin J, Milord F.** 1994. The treatment of human African trypanosomiasis. *Adv Parasitol* **33:**1–47.
192. **Dumas M, Bouteille B.** 2000. Treatment of human African trypanosomiasis. *Bull World Health Organ* **78:**1474.
193. **Taylor HR.** 1984. Recent developments in the treatment of onchocerciasis. *Bull World Health Organ* **62:**509–515.
194. **Voogd TE, Vansterkenburg EL, Wilting J, Janssen LH.** 1993. Recent research on the biological activity of suramin. *Pharmacol Rev* **45:**177–203.
195. **Burri C, Baltz T, Giroud C, Doua F, Welker HA, Brun R.** 1993. Pharmacokinetic properties of the trypanocidal drug melarsoprol. *Chemotherapy* **39:**225–234.
196. **Lutje V, Seixas J, Kennedy A.** 2010. Chemotherapy for second-stage human African trypanosomiasis. *Cochrane Database Syst Rev* **2010:**CD006201.
197. **Eperon G, Balasegaram M, Potet J, Mowbray C, Valverde O, Chappuis F.** 2014. Treatment options for second-stage gambiense human African trypanosomiasis. *Expert Rev Anti Infect Ther* **12:**1407–1417.
198. **Huebert ND, Schwartz JJ, Haegele KD.** 1997. Analysis of 2-difluoromethyl-DL-ornithine in human plasma, cerebrospinal fluid and urine by cation-exchange high-performance liquid chromatography. *J Chromatogr A* **762:**293–298.
199. **Milord F, Loko L, Ethier L, Mpia B, Pépin J.** 1993. Eflornithine concentrations in serum and cerebrospinal fluid of 63 patients treated for *Trypanosoma brucei gambiense* sleeping sickness. *Trans R Soc Trop Med Hyg* **87:**473–477.
200. **Kennedy PGE.** 2013. Clinical features, diagnosis, and treatment of human African trypanosomiasis (sleeping sickness). *Lancet Neurol* **12:**186–194.
201. **Croft SL.** 1997. The current status of antiparasite chemotherapy. *Parasitology* **114**(Suppl):S3–S15.
202. **Fozard JR, Part ML, Prakash NJ, Grove J.** 1980. Inhibition of murine embryonic development by alpha-difluoromethylornithine, an irreversible inhibitor of ornithine decarboxylase. *Eur J Pharmacol* **65:**379–391.
203. **Bern C.** 2015. Chagas' disease. *N Engl J Med* **373:**456–466.
204. **Polak A, Richle R.** 1978. Mode of action of the 2-nitroimidazole derivative benznidazole. *Ann Trop Med Parasitol* **72:**45–54.
205. **Murta SM, Ropert C, Alves RO, Gazzinelli RT, Romanha AJ.** 1999. In-vivo treatment with benznidazole enhances phagocytosis, parasite destruction and cytokine release by macrophages during infection with a drug-susceptible but not with a derived drug-resistant *Trypansoma cruzi* population. *Parasite Immunol* **21:**535–544.
206. **Hall BS, Bot C, Wilkinson SR.** 2011. Nifurtimox activation by trypanosomal type I nitroreductases generates cytotoxic nitrile metabolites. *J Biol Chem* **286:**13088–13095.
207. **Gutteridge WE.** 1985. Existing chemotherapy and its limitations. *Br Med Bull* **41:**162–168.
208. **Workman P, White RA, Walton MI, Owen LN, Twentyman PR.** 1984. Preclinical pharmacokinetics of benznidazole. *Br J Cancer* **50:**291–303.
209. **Wiens MO, Kanters S, Mills E, Peregrina Lucano AA, Gold S, Ayers D, Ferrero L, Krolewiecki A.** 2016. Systematic review and meta-analysis of the pharmacokinetics of benznidazole in the treatment of Chagas disease. *Antimicrob Agents Chemother* **60:**7035–7042.
210. **Matta Guedes PM, Gutierrez FRS, Nascimento MSL, Do-Valle-Matta MA, Silva JS.** 2012. Antiparasitical chemotherapy in Chagas' disease cardiomyopathy: current evidence. *Trop Med Int Health* **17:**1057–1065.

211. **Bern C.** 2011. Antitrypanosomal therapy for chronic Chagas' disease. *N Engl J Med* **364:**2527–2534.
212. **Rassi A Jr, Rassi A, Marin-Neto JA.** 2010. Chagas disease. *Lancet* **375:**1388–1402.
213. **Jackson Y, Chatelain E, Mauris A, Holst M, Miao Q, Chappuis F, Ndao M.** 2013. Serological and parasitological response in chronic Chagas patients 3 years after nifurtimox treatment. *BMC Infect Dis* **13:**85.
214. **de Toranzo EG, Masana M, Castro JA.** 1984. Administration of benznidazole, a chemotherapeutic agent against Chagas disease, to pregnant rats. Covalent binding of reactive metabolites to fetal and maternal proteins. *Arch Int Pharmacodyn Ther* **272:**17–23.
215. **Garcia-Bournissen F, Altcheh J, Panchaud A, Ito S.** 2010. Is use of nifurtimox for the treatment of Chagas disease compatible with breast feeding? A population pharmacokinetics analysis. *Arch Dis Child* **95:**224–228.

Mechanisms of Resistance to Antiparasitic Agents

W. EVAN SECOR, JACQUES LE BRAS, AND JÉRÔME CLAIN

153

Parasitic diseases rank among the most prevalent and severe diseases worldwide. However, because no effective antiparasitic vaccines are available and implementation of other control measures often proves to be difficult in countries where parasitic diseases are endemic, control relies heavily on a single tool: the drugs used for chemotherapy or prophylaxis. The danger of depending on drugs alone is compounded by the relative paucity of the current armamentarium of antiparasitic products and the selection of drug-resistant parasites, a situation attributable largely to a lack of economic incentives for research and development. Furthermore, those drugs that are available are too often used incorrectly in communities and in control programs, a practice that encourages the selection of drug-resistant parasites.

The complex biologic interactions between parasites and their hosts (and at times vectors) significantly influence the emergence and expression of drug resistance. In many cases the observed resistance is true resistance, attributable to biologic characteristics of the parasites that enable them to survive drug concentrations that are lethal to susceptible members of the species. Mechanisms for such true resistance are varied; common mechanisms include decreases in drug accumulation within the parasite and modifications in parasite enzyme structure or metabolic pathways. However, various host factors modulate the clinical and parasitological responses to drug treatment, and observed responses do not necessarily reflect true parasite resistance or susceptibility. For example, in populations with high rates of parasitic infections, the resulting high rates of immunity might suffice to eliminate an infection even if parasites are resistant to drugs or are treated with a poorly effective drug. Conversely, treatment with a drug to which the parasite is biologically susceptible will not necessarily result in therapeutic success if the host takes an inadequate dose of the drug, absorbs it poorly, or lacks the immune response that might be needed for a successful antiparasitic synergism with the drug. Host factors may be especially important in the areas where most parasitic diseases prevail, where high rates of parasite transmission result in high rates of immunity in most of the population, or where, conversely, malnutrition and human immunodeficiency virus (HIV) infection compromise the patient's immune status.

Greater understanding of the epidemiology and mechanisms of drug resistance can provide valuable guidance for a better use of existing compounds and for the development of novel products. A selective review of drug resistance in five diseases will illustrate the existing problems and their potential solutions. A summary of the proposed mechanisms of resistance is provided in Table 1.

MALARIA

Overview

By 1955, the World Health Organization had established projects for malaria eradication based on use of indoor residual spraying of insecticides to limit contact between humans and the anopheline vector and mass administration of pyrimethamine and chloroquine to kill forms of the parasites that replicate in erythrocytes (1). As these programs faced infrastructure deficiencies and resistance to insecticides, vector control was often neglected, and the bulk of expenditure was devoted to treatment of febrile persons with presumed malaria, initially mainly with chloroquine and later with sulfadoxine-pyrimethamine. However, these programs were compromised as *Plasmodium falciparum*, the most virulent species, developed resistance to chloroquine and sulfadoxine-pyrimethamine, and further, to nearly all known drugs to various degrees. Sub-Saharan Africa alone contributes about 90% of the annual 212 million patients suffering worldwide from malaria, leading to an estimated 429,000 deaths worldwide (2). Severe malaria affects mainly those without adequate acquired clinical immunity, such as young children or particular groups, such as pregnant women. Since the beginning of the 21st century, expanded efforts to strengthen integrated malaria control have led to a reduction in malaria morbidity and mortality rates (2). Critical elements of these programs have included widespread use of long-lasting insecticidal nets (3) and the global establishment of diagnostic testing for malaria, followed by treatment with artemisinin-based combination therapies (ACTs). These therapies associate a curative drug that has a long elimination half-life with a rapidly active drug able to destroy a large parasite load in a few hours. Artemisinin, a substance extracted from sagebrush grown mainly in China, generates oxidative stress in the parasite. The combination of multiple drugs enhances clinical efficacy and may delay the acquisition of parasite resistance. Partner drugs combined with the artemisinin derivative currently

TABLE 1 Summary of proposed mechanisms of resistance to selected antiparasitic drugs

Disease	Drug(s)	Mechanism(s) of resistance
Malaria	Chloroquine	Decreased vacuolar accumulation of the drug by the parasite, resulting from altered transport properties of mutant PfCRT and PfPGH-1
	Mefloquine	Vacuolar sequestration of the drug by the parasite, resulting from overexpression of the vacuolar multidrug transporter PfPGH-1
	Pyrimethamine	Alteration in binding affinities between the drug and the parasite dihydrofolate reductase, resulting from mutations on the corresponding gene
	Sulfadoxine	Alteration in binding affinities between the drug and the parasite dihydropteroate synthase, resulting from mutations on the corresponding gene
	Atovaquone	Alteration in binding affinities between the drug and the parasite cytochrome *b*, resulting from mutations on the corresponding gene
	Artemisinins	Mutated kelch K13 protein; precise mechanism poorly understood
	Piperaquine	Increased expression of the vacuolar hemoglobinases plasmepsin 2 and 3 and altered vacuolar transport by mutant PfCRT
Trichomoniasis	Metronidazole, tinidazole	Reduced concentration of enzymes or coenzymes necessary to activate nitro group Reduced oxygen scavenging
Leishmaniasis	Pentavalent antimonials	Decreased active intracellular drug concentration through decreased uptake, increased efflux, or decreased conversion to active trivalent form
	Miltefosine	Replaced pentavalent antimonials as primary treatment in some areas, resistance by increased drug efflux or increases in strain infectivity
	Amphotericin B	Increased drug efflux, altered thiol metabolism
African trypanosomiasis	Pentamidine (1st stage)	Mutation or loss of P2 adenosine and/or aquaglyceroporin 2 transporters that uptake drug
	Suramin (1st stage)	Not useful in West Africa where *T. b. gambiense* is the primary infection because of severe allergic reactions in onchocerciasis patients
	Melarsoprol (2nd stage)	Mutation or loss of P2 adenosine and/or functional aquaglyceroporin 2 transporters that uptake drug
	Eflornithine or combination eflornithine and nifurtimox	*T. b. rhodesiense* naturally tolerant, thus only useful against *T. b. gambiense*
Schistosomiasis	Praziquantel	Widespread clinical resistance not currently recognized as an important public health problem Genetic bottlenecking observed in some treatment areas and resistance demonstrated in laboratory strains

include amodiaquine, lumefantrine, mefloquine, piperaquine, pyronaridine, or sulfadoxine-pyrimethamine. We need to consider the history of the emergence and spread of resistance to chloroquine and sulfadoxine-pyrimethamine as a warning of the risk of losing the effectiveness of ACTs if their use is not controlled. Indeed, resistance to ACTs has emerged and is spreading in Southeast Asia since the mid-2000s. Tri-therapies based on ACTs are currently in clinical testing in this region.

The 4-amino quinoline drug chloroquine, a cornerstone of antimalarial chemotherapy since the 1940s due to its low cost, safety, and rapid action, lost most of its usefulness as the frequency of chloroquine-resistant *P. falciparum* strains increased and peaked in the 1980s. From limited original foci in Southeast Asia, South America, and Papua New Guinea, resistance has spread inexorably and is now found in most areas of endemicity, including Africa, the continent with the heaviest malaria burden. Chloroquine no longer constitutes an appropriate option for prompt and effective treatment (or prophylaxis) in most countries where *P. falciparum* malaria is the dominant endemic species, although the level of resistance to chloroquine is decreasing in several areas since its use has officially ceased. With increased use of sulfadoxine-pyrimethamine, the second most affordable, relatively safe, and easily administered drug after chloroquine, parasite resistance to sulfadoxine-pyrimethamine has developed very quickly following the same routes as the spread of chloroquine resistance a few years before. Nevertheless, specific groups of people (e.g., pregnant women) in areas of endemicity still rely on sulfadoxine-pyrimethamine for presumptive treatment of fever or for intermittent preventive treatment as the most effective way to prevent severe consequences of malaria. Losing the two low-cost antimalarials is often seen by experts as a public health disaster. Reducing transmission intensity could slow the spread of resistance, but, paradoxically, below a critical level it may accelerate the selection of multigenic resistance (3). This critical situation has prompted international initiatives to help face the high cost of ACTs: to make affordable, rapid diagnostic tests available everywhere and to renew mosquito-control programs by an extensive distribution of insecticide-impregnated nets. Learning from the past that delay in detection and control of resistance to ACTs may ruin all programs without alternatives for some time, real-time drug-resistance surveillance and drug development must be reinforced.

Mechanisms of *P. falciparum* Resistance to Selected Antimalarials

Chloroquine concentrates from nanomolar levels outside the parasite to millimolar levels within the digestive vacuole of the intraerythrocytic trophozoite, where it inhibits hemoglobin degradation (4). Chloroquine forms complexes with hematin, a by-product of host-cell hemoglobin digestion by the parasite; this formation results in accumulation of ferriprotoporphyrin IX in large quantities that eventually kills the parasite. The resistant isolates share a defect in chloroquine accumulation in the digestive vacuole (5). Several mechanisms have been proposed to explain the altered chloroquine accumulation, such as changes in the pH gradient or altered membrane permeability leading to a decreased drug uptake or increased drug efflux (6). Chloroquine accumulation has high structural specificity, which suggests the involvement of either a specific transporter/permease or a molecule associated with hematin in the digestive vacuole (7). Following demonstration that chloroquine resistance is reversible by verapamil, earlier studies focused on the orthologue of the mammalian multidrug resistance (*mdr*) gene, whose products are overexpressed in cancer cells where they expel cytotoxic drugs (8). This strategy led to the identification of the *pfmdr1* gene product (protein PfPGH-1), a transporter located in the membrane of the parasite digestive vacuole (9). Chloroquine susceptibility is altered by PfPGH-1 mutated at specific amino acid residues and in specific parasite genetic backgrounds (10). However, current evidence indicates that *pfmdr1* does play a secondary role in chloroquine resistance, except in Madagascar where it plays a major role in chloroquine-treatment failures (11). More recently, by use of a genetic cross between chloroquine-sensitive and chloroquine-resistant parasites, inheritance data led to the key discovery of the *Plasmodium falciparum* chloroquine resistance transporter gene *pfcrt* (12, 13). The *pfcrt* gene encodes a transmembrane protein (PfCRT), as does PfPGH-1, located in the membrane of the digestive vacuole (13). A complex set of mutations (or haplotype) of this gene is found in most natural isolates from chloroquine-treatment failures and in isolates with an *in vitro* chloroquine-resistant phenotype (13–15). Finally, transfection of chloroquine-sensitive parasites with the mutant *pfcrt* genotypes found in resistant isolates suffices to confer chloroquine resistance (16). Mutant PfCRT has acquired the ability to excrete chloroquine out of the digestive vacuole (17) that is dependent on a positive charge loss at codon 76 (usually the K76T mutation) in the first transmembrane helix of the transporter (17, 18). The role of the other *pfcrt* mutations that systematically accompany K76T remains elusive (6). At least four independent mutant *pfcrt* haplotypes carrying the K76T mutation are seen, varying geographically: Asia-Africa, Papua, and twice in South America (15). A major event in chloroquine resistance was the emergence on the Thai-Cambodian border in the 1950s of the CVIET haplotype in codons 72 through 76 of the *pfcrt* gene under drug-pressure selection; this haplotype has now spread in the Asian and African regions (15, 19). Nonetheless, the wild-type *pfcrt* parasites have not been totally replaced, and their prevalence increases when drug pressure is removed (20). In French Guiana, reversal of chloroquine resistance occurred by acquisition of an additional mutation in the common South-American *pfcrt* mutant haplotype, likely driven by the concomitant acquisition of *pfcrt*-mediated piperaquine resistance (21). Besides the specific case of French Guiana, the *pfcrt* K76T mutation is now a valuable molecular marker used in epidemiological surveys of chloroquine resistance. Its estimated prevalence may offer a useful predictor of the clinical efficacy of chloroquine in a given area, provided that appropriate adjustments are made for host factors, particularly immunity, that may result in parasite clearance despite treatment with an ineffective drug (22).

Amodiaquine, piperaquine, and pyronaridine, which are in the first line of therapy as partners of artemisinins, share with chloroquine a quinoline scaffold, whereas mefloquine and lumefantrine, the other partners of ACTs, belong to amino-alcohols. Neither the mechanism of action of these drugs nor resistances to them are as clearly understood as for chloroquine. However, the *pfmdr1* gene appears to be involved in parasite response to diverse antimalarials as point mutations or amplification of the gene alter parasite susceptibility to desethyl amodiaquine, the active metabolite of amodiaquine, quinine, mefloquine, lumefantrine, and artemisinins (10, 23–26). Similarly, wild-type and various mutant *pfcrt* alleles associate with altered susceptibility to various antimalarials (lumefantrine, amodiaquine, piperaquine, artemisinin derivatives) in addition to chloroquine (6, 16, 27). Transporters other than PfCRT and PfPGH-1, such as PfMRP-1 and PfNHE-1, may be involved in resistance to mefloquine, lumefantrine, pyrimethamine (28, 29), and quinine, respectively. Gene amplification of *plasmepsin 2* and *3* encoding vacuolar proteases and specific *pfcrt* mutations associate with piperaquine resistance (30–33), suggesting a vacuolar target for piperaquine.

Resistance of *P. falciparum* to artemisinins initially emerged in the mid-2000s in Cambodia (34) and then spread in multiple Southeast-Asian locations. It manifests as a delayed parasite-clearance time following treatment initiation and as a higher failure rate of artemisinin-containing treatments (34–36). Extensive genetic studies pointed out specific regions of the parasite genome that are associated with the *in vivo* delayed parasite-clearance time (37, 38). Comparative genomics of laboratory-selected and Cambodian field-derived artemisinin-resistant parasites led to the identification of single amino acid changes in the kelch (or propeller) domain of the K13 protein as a genetic marker of artemisinin resistance (39). Gene editing of artemisinin-sensitive parasites demonstrated that introduction of *k13* mutations found in resistant isolates suffices to confer artemisinin resistance (40). Parasites carrying *k13* mutations exhibit a deceleration of cell development during the early intraerythrocytic stage and an altered proteostasis response (41, 42). At the biochemical level, the dominant *k13* C580Y mutation alters the binding of K13 with the parasite's phosphatidylinositol-3-kinase, and ubiquitin-mediated degradation is then decreased (43). The functional relationships between artemisinin resistance and the metabolic pathway(s) associated with phosphatidylinositol-3-kinase are currently unknown. Whereas multiple *k13* resistance mutations originated when artemisinin resistance was first detected, a single *k13* C580Y mutant parasite lineage is now spreading throughout the East Thailand-Cambodia-Lao PDR-Vietnam region, probably because of associated partner drug resistance and better fitness of the parasite (44, 45).

Regarding drugs that antagonize a single enzyme, such as antifolates or inhibitors of the mitochondrial respiratory chain, a single gene modification is often sufficient to generate high-grade resistance. Malaria parasites mostly rely on *de novo* synthesis for folate supply. Cycloguanil (produced by the prodrug proguanil) and its analogue, pyrimethamine, were the first satisfactory synthetic antifolate antimalarials to be on the market in the 1940s. Both inhibit the plasmodial dihydrofolate reductase (PfDHFR), a key enzyme in the folate synthesis pathway of the parasite. Unfortunately, resistance emerged almost instantaneously and independently from several areas where the drugs had been introduced, and these antimalarials were soon supplanted by chloroquine (46). Resurgence in the use of PfDHFR inhibitors took place with the demonstration in 1967 that potentiation with other antifolates from the sulfone/sulfonamide group (such as sulfadoxine or dapsone) bypassed resistance, and sulfadoxine-pyrimethamine became the new frontrunner to counter chloroquine resistance in Southeast Asia (46). However, resistance to sulfadoxine-pyrimethamine emerged soon after the increased use of sulfadoxine-pyrimethamine in Thailand. Resistance to PfDHFR inhibitors is conferred by mutant PfDHFR enzymes, to which antifolate drugs bind less efficiently than to the wild-type version (47, 48). Stepwise acquisition of pyrimethamine and then sulfadoxine-pyrimethamine resistance in *P. falciparum* is mirrored by the stepwise acquisitions of PfDHFR mutations: first the key S108N mutation, then the additive N51I and C59R mutations, and finally the additive I164L mutation (48, 49). Other additive mutations can be found in specific areas such as in South America (50). The quadruple-mutant N51I-C59R-S108N-I164L, which associates with the highest level of sulfadoxine-pyrimethamine resistance as well as with decreased sensitivity to chlorproguanil-dapsone (an attempt to develop a new antifolate combination similar to sulfadoxine-pyrimethamine), has been reported mostly in Southeast Asia. However, the triple mutant N51I-C59R-S108N, which is widespread in Africa, also associates with treatment failure to sulfadoxine-pyrimethamine (51). This triple mutant N51I-C59R-S108N *pfdhfr* gene emerged in Southeast Asia and then spread throughout Asia and Africa in the following years (52, 53).

Resistance to the sulfone/sulfonamide group (sulfadoxine being the major antimalarial compound) is conferred by mutant PfDHPS enzymes to which antifolate drugs bind less efficiently than to the wild-type version (54, 55). Resistance to sulfadoxine has been traced to a set of sequential mutations in the *pfdhps* gene. The likely initial event consisted of an A437G mutation, with subsequent additional mutations conferring increasing degrees of resistance (55). These resistance mutations have appeared independently multiple times and in multiple sites of endemicity (56). Altogether, resistance to the sulfadoxine-pyrimethamine combination appears to require three mutations in the *pfdhfr* gene (N51I-C59R-S108N), and the probability of sulfadoxine-pyrimethamine treatment failure increases with additional mutations in *pfdhps*. The clinical outcome of a sulfadoxine-pyrimethamine treatment is subject to additional host factors such as the level of folates and of acquired immunity, drug absorption, and metabolism (51, 57). Cross-resistance has been demonstrated between cycloguanil and pyrimethamine (47, 48, 58). Consequently, interest in other antifolates, such as chlorproguanil plus dapsone (LapDap), to treat parasites resistant to sulfadoxine-pyrimethamine has been limited.

The combination of atovaquone and proguanil was registered in 1996 in North America and Europe where, within 10 years, it became a popular antimalarial for prophylaxis and a first-line treatment of nonsevere *P. falciparum* malaria. It is now a second-line treatment after ACTs. Atovaquone is an ubiquinone analogue and binds to cytochrome *b* (PfCytB), a component of the complex III in the mitochondrial respiratory chain (59). In association with proguanil, the effective concentration at which it collapses the mitochondrial membrane potential is diminished (60). In addition, proguanil is partially metabolized to the antifolate cycloguanil by human P450 cytochromes. The contribution of the resulting low cycloguanil blood concentrations to the therapeutic efficacy of atovaquone-proguanil remains to be substantiated. As with the antifolates, atovaquone resistance emerged almost immediately (61). Resistance to atovaquone is conferred by mutant PfCytB, to which atovaquone binds less efficiently than to the wild-type version (62). The substitution of tyrosine for serine, cysteine, or asparagine in codon 268 of PfCytB is associated with treatment failures and confers a high level of atovaquone resistance (63) that proguanil could not thwart (64). Remarkably, the resistance mutation is extremely rarely detected in areas of endemicity, but it seems to evolve repeatedly during primary infections (65, 66). Because of the risk of rapid development of resistance and high cost of the drug, the deployment of atovaquone-proguanil in malaria-endemic regions has not yet been considered as a priority.

Drug resistance in *Plasmodium vivax*, the second most common malaria parasite, remains at much lower magnitude in many areas than in *P. falciparum*. Increasing attention has recently focused on tackling this threat, specifically with respect to chloroquine resistance that is now present throughout most countries where *P. vivax* is endemic (67). However, no validated molecular marker for chloroquine-resistant *P. vivax* is yet available. *P. vivax*, which relapses from dormant parasites in the liver, developed partial resistance to primaquine, the only drug active against liver forms (68). Primaquine's diminished efficacy against relapses from dormant *P. vivax* liver parasites is also associated with polymorphisms in the host cytochrome P450 2D6, resulting in altered concentrations of the active metabolites (69). Investigations on mechanisms of resistance in this species currently examine the potential role of *P. vivax* homologues of *pfcrt* (70), *pfmdr1* (71), *pfdhfr* (72), and *pfdhps* (73).

A recent, more comprehensive review on antimalarial drug resistance can be found in Blasco et al. (74).

TRICHOMONIASIS

Infection with *Trichomonas vaginalis* is one of the most common causes of human vaginitis as well as the most prevalent nonviral sexually transmitted disease (75). *T. vaginalis* infections damage the genital epithelium, cause malodorous vaginal discharge, and are associated with adverse outcomes of pregnancy such as preterm delivery, low birth weight, and long-term consequences for offspring. *T. vaginalis* infection is also associated with greater susceptibility to infection with HIV and increased shedding of virus in HIV-infected individuals (76–78). As a result, effective treatment of this infection has become an important public health goal (79, 80).

T. vaginalis is a facultative anaerobe, and trichomoniasis is most commonly treated with the 5-nitroimidazole class of drugs. Two members of this group, metronidazole and tinidazole, are the only drugs approved for treatment of trichomoniasis in the United States. Tinidazole is more active at equimolar concentrations than metronidazole and is recommended if treatment with metronidazole fails (81–83). However, strains clinically resistant to metronidazole can have cross-resistance to tinidazole. The molecular epidemiology of *T. vaginalis* suggests that clinically resistant isolates are genetically related and are concentrated within one of two major subpopulations (84–86). In a survey of women attending sexually transmitted disease clinics in six U.S. cities, 4.3% of isolates exhibited drug resistance (87), suggesting that almost 160,000 residents in the United States may be at risk for treatment failure (79, 80). As use of more sensitive nucleic acid amplification tests becomes more widespread, it is likely that additional asymptomatic infections will be identified that may not clear with nitroimidazole treatment. There is a need to determine how to manage asymptomatic trichomoniasis in general and how to manage treatment of nonresponsive infections with no apparent sequalae.

The 5-nitroimidazoles enter parasites in an inactive form by passive diffusion and are then reduced to the active nitro radical anion that is thought to cause parasite death by breaking or disrupting DNA. A number of electron donors in the hydrogenosome, which is the source of ATP generation in these amitochondriate parasites, have been suggested as important for drug activation, including ferredoxin, pyruvate-ferredoxin oxidoreductase (PFOR), and malic enzyme (88–90). Drug resistance occurs when transcription of one or more of these enzymes is decreased and there are lower levels of drug activation. Laboratory-generated resistant isolates have smaller hydrogenosomes; however, clinical resistance does not correlate with lower transcript levels of these enzymes or smaller hydrogenosome size (91, 92).

The nitroimidazole drugs are also reduced by the flavin enzyme thioredoxin reductase and nitroreductases (86, 93). An *in vitro*-induced nitroimidazole-resistant strain demonstrated reduced thioredoxin reductase activity, not as a result of decreased enzyme concentration but because of a deficiency in the necessary FAD cofactor. Furthermore, use of a flavin inhibitor rendered a normally susceptible isolate resistant to high concentrations of metronidazole (94). The role of nitroreductases was demonstrated by identification of single nucleotide polymorphisms (SNPs) that introduce premature stop codons in two nitroreductase genes and are associated with increased metronidazole resistance in clinical isolates (86). A third possible mechanism for nitroimidazole resistance is diminished intracellular oxygen scavenging in trichomonads, resulting in reoxidation, and therefore inactivation, of reduced nitroimidazoles. Flavin reductase 1 is important for oxygen scavenging in *T. vaginalis*, and some clinically resistant isolates express reduced levels of this enzyme (95). It remains unclear which, if any, of these mechanisms is responsible for the clinical nitroimidazole resistance observed in *T. vaginalis* infections, but sequencing of clinical isolates found associations of resistance with SNPs in genes for the enzymes described above as well as SNPs in as yet uncharacterized genes (96).

Treatment of patients who have metronidazole-resistant trichomoniasis often results in an immediate resolution of symptoms and a negative wet mount. However, within 3 to 4 weeks, in the absence of further exposure, symptoms may recur as the number of organisms rebounds. Thus, it is important to monitor efficacy of treatment for up to a month and to encourage patients to avoid unprotected intercourse during this time. When nitroimidazole resistance is encountered, patients are often successfully treated with increased doses of drug for a longer time (82, 83). However, many patients cannot tolerate high doses of metronidazole and stop treatment early, which may only exacerbate the development of drug resistance. In addition, some patients experience hypersensitivity reactions in response to metronidazole and tinidazole (97). Clearly, alternatives to the nitroimidazoles for treatment of *T. vaginalis* are needed, but the impetus for pharmaceutical companies to develop new drugs is low because metronidazole is now available as a very inexpensive generic drug and is effective for the vast majority of infections. Thus, repurposing existing drugs or using them in combination with a nitroimidazole may be an effective strategy (98). One promising drug is auranofin, which is used to treat rheumatoid arthritis. It functions by inhibiting thioredoxin reductase and shows activity against *T. vaginalis in vitro* and in animal models (99); however, efficacy for persons with trichomoniasis has not been evaluated. Intravaginal treatment with drugs such as furazolidone and paromomycin sulfate that are not absorbed well from the intestine or cannot be ingested has been successful to cure some patients but in general has limited efficacy (97, 100). Povidone-iodine, boric acid, and zinc sulfate have also shown efficacy for treating some patients, but additional clinical testing is needed (100–102).

LEISHMANIASIS

Leishmaniasis is transmitted to humans by phlebotomine sandfly vectors and manifests as a variety of syndromes. Depending in part on which of the possible 20 species of *Leishmania* that infect humans is present, pathology can range from a cutaneous lesion that is self-limiting to the more severe mucosal or visceral forms. The identification of leishmaniasis as an important opportunistic infection in patients with AIDS has presented new challenges for treatment of this disease, with increased treatment failures and drug toxicity in HIV-1-positive individuals (103, 104). Use of antileishmanial drugs is limited by their high cost, difficulty of administration (injection for several weeks), and/or associated toxicity. These factors are particularly consequential in developing countries where leishmaniasis is endemic as they can lead to premature self-termination of therapy, which in turn may promote increased levels of resistance. While true drug resistance has been described for isolates of some *Leishmania* spp., other species or isolates may just differ in their intrinsic sensitivity to certain compounds, with host factors also contributing to drug efficacy or failure (105–107). True resistance is more likely in anthroponotic forms of leishmaniasis, such as *Leishmania donovani* and *Leishmania tropica*, because the zoonotic species that primarily infect animals, with humans as an occasional host, rarely encounter drugs and serve as a reservoir for drug-sensitive parasites (108).

The frontline drugs for treating *Leishmania* infections regardless of species or clinical form have long been the pentavalent antimonial compounds such as sodium stibogluconate and meglumine antimoniate. These compounds are inexpensive compared to other antileishmanial drugs, but they are no longer effective in some areas of endemicity. For example, in the state of Bihar in India, rates of failure of treatment of visceral leishmaniasis (VL) caused by *L. donovani* are as high as 65% (109). Poor drug efficacy is likely multifactorial; causes may include lower intrinsic sensitivity of parasites that cause VL to antimonials and contamination of drinking water with arsenic (107, 110, 111). Evidence for true drug resistance in this setting comes from observations that isolates from clinically resistant patients require higher *in vitro* concentrations of drug to kill the parasites than do isolates from patients who respond to treatment (112). However, the correlation between clinical outcomes of treatment for leishmaniasis and the *in vitro* susceptibility of the causative isolate is not always clear (105, 108, 113).

Pentavalent antimonials are prodrugs that are reduced within the mammalian host cell or parasite to an active trivalent form that boosts the intracellular cytotoxic potential of macrophages and disrupts the parasite's redox metabolism. Many of the proposed mechanisms of resistance across the various *Leishmania* spp. involve a reduced intracellular concentration of active drug (114, 115). One mechanism by which this occurs is a decrease in aquaglyceroporin 1 (AQP1) on the parasite's surface, resulting in decreased uptake of drug (116, 117). Higher expression of AQP1 by the species that cause cutaneous leishmaniasis (CL) than by those that cause VL confers greater sensitivity of CL to antimonial treatment. Differences in AQP1 expression are a function of mRNA stability that is regulated by the 3′ untranslated region (110).

Resistance has also been associated with increased production of trypanothione or glutathione that binds with the trivalent antimonials and is sequestered in intracellular organelles by ATP-binding cassette (ABC) transporters (114, 118). Increased expression of the enzymes involved in thiol synthesis or of the ABC transporter promotes resistance to pentavalent antimonials, whereas inhibition of these pathways in resistant strains increases susceptibility to the drug (115, 116, 118–121). Adding to the difficulty of defining resistance mechanisms, more than one of these mechanisms may arise, even within closely related parasite strains (114, 117, 122, 123). Nevertheless, the pentavalent antimonials remain the preferred treatment for CL (124).

Because of a high level of pentavalent antimonial resistance in parts of India and Nepal, miltefosine became the primary treatment for VL (106, 125). However, relapse rates of 20% were reported within 1 year after the introduction of miltefosine (126). As with the antimonials, resistance to miltefosine is associated with mechanisms that decrease intracellular concentrations, and inhibitors of ABC transporters can restore drug susceptibility *in vitro* (127–129). However, recent studies suggest that these mechanisms do not explain all the clinical resistance to miltefosine; other mechanisms, such as infectivity of the parasite strain, may be involved (125, 126, 130, 131).

The drug now being used for primary treatment of VL on the Indian subcontinent is amphotericin B, which induces pore formation in the parasite plasma membranes (132). The use of amphotericin B has been limited in the past because of its high cost and toxicity; however, new lipid-associated formulations of amphotericin B have greatly reduced toxicities and retain good efficacy even when administered in lower doses (133, 134). Amphotericin B also seems to be superior to antimonials for treatment of leishmaniasis in HIV-infected individuals (103, 104). Lipid-associated formulations of amphotericin B are phagocytized by host monocytes and accumulate in the phagocytic lysosomes where *Leishmania* amastigotes reside. Interestingly, although the mode of action of amphotericin B is thought to differ greatly from that of the antimonials, field isolates with greater sodium antimony gluconate resistance also had greater *in vitro* resistance to amphotericin B (127). As with the other antileishmania drugs, amphotericin B resistance is associated with greater drug efflux and altered thiol metabolism (135). Amphotericin B-resistant strains also demonstrate upregulation of the tryparedoxin cascade, resulting in decreased intracellular concentration of toxic reactive oxygen species (132).

AFRICAN TRYPANOSOMIASIS

Trypanosoma brucei rhodesiense and *T. b. gambiense* are the etiologic agents of human African trypanosomiasis (HAT). The two subspecies are endemic in east and west central Africa, respectively, with *T. b. gambiense* causing the vast majority of infections (136, 137). Because these parasites possess antigenic switching mechanisms, host immune responses are ineffective and the prospects for the development of vaccines against these organisms are meager. *T. b. gambiense* infection generally only occurs in humans, and the key aspect of control is treatment of infected individuals detected through passive surveillance. Transmission of *T. b. rhodesiense* also involves domestic and wild animals; thus, control efforts include reduction of the tsetse fly vector and case detection and treatment (136, 138). Incidents of political unrest with subsequent loss of an effective public health infrastructure result in resurgence of disease. Nevertheless, HAT epidemics that occurred in the 1990s have now largely been controlled, with fewer than 3,000 cases reported in 2015 (136). There is now optimism for elimination of HAT as a public health problem by 2020, at least for *T. b. gambiense* infections (138).

HAT has two stages; the initial bloodstream stage is followed by invasion of the central nervous system in the second stage, which causes the meningoencephalitic symptoms associated with "sleeping sickness," the more familiar name for HAT. While both forms of HAT usually result in death in the absence of treatment, *T. b. rhodesiense* infections proceed more rapidly, with progression to second stage in a few weeks and death as quickly as 6 months. By contrast, death from untreated *T. b. gambiense* infections typically occurs 3 years after infection (136).

Pentamidine and suramin are the drugs used for treatment of first-stage disease. They are not used for second-stage disease because they are highly ionic and do not cross the blood-brain barrier. Furthermore, use of suramin is avoided for treatment of *T. b. gambiense* because of the risk of severe allergic reactions that it can cause in patients with onchocerciasis, which is often coendemic with HAT caused by *T. b. gambiense* (136, 137). While clinical resistance to these drugs does not seem to be a problem, failures can occur when infections are diagnosed and treated after disease has progressed past the hemolymphatic stage. Late-stage central nervous system disease is treated with melarsoprol for *T. b. rhodesiense* infections and eflornithine or nifurtimox-eflornithine combination therapy (NECT) for *T. b. gambiense* infections (136, 139). The drugs for HAT are difficult to administer, require a prolonged treatment regimen, and are relatively toxic; these issues can contribute to premature cessation of treatment, which can in turn contribute to the development of drug resistance.

Like treatment failures in leishmaniasis, HAT drug resistance is associated with decreased drug uptake. Pentamidine and melarsoprol share an amidinium-like moiety with amino purines that is recognized and actively taken up by nucleoside transporters in the trypanosome membrane (137). One of these receptors, the *T. brucei* P2 adenosine transporter, or TbAT1, has been extensively studied; resistance to pentamidine and melarsoprol is associated with loss of function mutations in *tbat1* expression, with resistant laboratory-induced and field isolates exhibiting the same set of point mutations (137, 140, 141). However, *tbat1* knockout parasites are only partially resistant, leading to the discovery of the role aquaglyceroporin 2 (AQP2) in HAT drug resistance. Mutations that cause loss of AQP2 or chimera formation between AQP2 and AQP3 confer a 3- to 5-fold decrease in sensitivity to melarsoprol resistance and a 40- to 50-fold decrease in sensitivity to pentamidine (141–143). Reintroduction of wild-type AQP2 into resistant clinical isolates restores drug susceptibility (144). However, not all treatment failures can be attributed to dysfunctional AQP2, suggesting that other mechanisms or even patient factors such as nutrition, immunologic status, or coinfections with other parasites may also contribute to treatment failures (145).

To date, clinical resistance to eflornithine and nifurtimox has not been documented. Nevertheless, resistance in laboratory strains has been readily induced for both drugs (146, 147). Eflornithine resistance is associated with the loss of a nonessential amino acid transporter that is responsible for drug uptake, raising the concern that field resistance could easily develop (146). The recent demonstration that treatment of *T. b. gambiense* infections with oral fexinidazole produced cure rates similar to NECT without an increase in treatment-related adverse events increases the optimism for achieving the 2020 HAT elimination goals (148).

SCHISTOSOMIASIS

Praziquantel is the only drug currently being used for treatment of schistosomiasis. It is effective against all schistosome species that infect humans and makes up the backbone of schistosomiasis control programs through mass drug administration (MDA). Typically, a single drug widely administered to large numbers of people is a recipe for driving development of drug resistance. However, although a few potential incidents of clinical praziquantel resistance have been described (149), there is as yet no widespread resistance in schistosomiasis, even in areas with high-intensity treatment pressure for a prolonged time (150–152). This fortuitous phenomenon may be aided by the fact that schistosomes do not asexually replicate within humans who receive treatment, although it does occur in the intermediate snail host. Thus, unlike protozoan parasites, selective drug pressure is absent during parasite multiplication, reducing the ease with which resistance could develop. Ironically, incomplete coverage of MDA in control programs leaves ample refugia of untreated worms that may also deter emergence of widespread resistance to praziquantel (153).

Nevertheless, eggs obtained from the feces of individuals who were not successfully cured have been used to establish infections in mice, confirming that a drug-resistance phenotype can develop (154–156). Laboratory and field studies have also shown decreased diversity of schistosomes following praziquantel treatment suggestive of a genetic bottleneck, a warning sign for development of drug resistance (157, 158). However, this observation has not been consistent in all field studies (159–161).

When considering treatment failures in schistosomiasis, it is important to distinguish characteristics leading to reduced drug efficacy from true drug resistance. For example, persons with very high levels of infection are less likely to cure with single-dose therapy than individuals with lower worm burdens (162). This result is in part related to the fact that praziquantel is only effective against the adult stage of the parasite and that even under the best conditions, a single dose does not demonstrate complete efficacy (153). Immature worms that may be present at the time of drug treatment, especially in areas of high transmission, are not susceptible to praziquantel and subsequently develop into patent infections that give the impression of treatment failure. As a result, two treatments spaced 4 to 6 weeks apart are more effective than a single treatment and should be attempted when drug resistance is suspected (163, 164). Rapid reinfection in areas of high transmission should also be considered as a possible explanation for suspected praziquantel treatment failure (165, 166).

The mechanism of action of praziquantel is not definitively understood, making it more difficult to identify occurrence and mechanisms of developed resistance. The unique beta subunit of the schistosome calcium ion channel is a molecular target for praziquantel, with treatment rapidly inducing a calcium-dependent sustained muscle contraction in the worm's tegument (167). The praziquantel-induced damage to the tegument of adult schistosomes renders the worms susceptible to attack and killing by the host's immune response. Resistant strains of parasites demonstrate less tegumental damage caused by praziquantel than do susceptible strains (168).

One potential mechanism of drug resistance may help explain the comparative susceptibility of juvenile and adult worms to praziquantel. There is increased expression of a P-glycoprotein ATP-dependent efflux pump homologue in parasite strains that have reduced susceptibility to praziquantel and in juvenile worms compared to adults (169–171). Pharmaceutical inhibitors of this pump, or suppression of its expression by RNA interference, increase susceptibility to praziquantel in both juvenile worms and otherwise resistant adults (172). Fortunately, the inhibitors are safe, inexpensive, and approved for human use, thus providing a potential strategy for combating praziquantel resistance should it arise.

As MDA programs are increasingly employed for schistosomiasis control, there is reasonable fear that reliance on a single drug may promote the emergence of resistance. This risk reiterates the need for ongoing monitoring for development of praziquantel resistance and efforts to discover new drugs or reposition existing compounds to treat schistosomiasis (153, 173, 174).

FUTURE PERSPECTIVES

Several factors contribute to the emergence of drug-resistant parasites. Those parasite species with short life cycles and high multiplication rates that occur in areas of intense transmission are most likely to develop resistant subpopulations. The selection of such populations is encouraged when the parasites are repeatedly exposed to suboptimal drug concentrations. This pattern can result from the use of drugs with long half-lives or, more typically, from the frequent, often unjustified, use of inadequate doses of drugs, a common occurrence in countries where parasite infections are endemic. Public health interventions to correct these factors have not always been successful and would benefit from a better understanding of the drug-resistance mechanisms used by parasites. These mechanisms are very diverse and have been difficult to study, but recent technological advances now provide long-awaited tools that will facilitate the task. The genome sequences for several *Plasmodium* species, *T. vaginalis*, *L. major*, *T. brucei*, *S. mansoni*, and *S. haematobium* have been compiled. When these data are used, for example, in combination with microarray technology or whole-genome sequencing, and the DNA of drug-resistant parasite strains is compared to drug-susceptible strains, identification of the genes that confer resistance should proceed even more rapidly than in the past few years. In addition, genomic, transcriptomic, and proteomic data may also be useful in the design of new chemotherapeutic agents as they help researchers identify metabolic processes of parasites that are sufficiently distinct from those of their human hosts to allow development of effective treatments.

The findings and conclusions in this report are those of the authors and do not necessarily represent the views of the CDC.

REFERENCES

1. **World Health Organization.** 1993. *A Global Strategy for Malaria Control.* World Health Organization, Geneva, Switzerland.
2. **World Health Organization.** 2016. *World Malaria Report 2016.* World Health Organization, Geneva, Switzerland.
3. **Bhatt S, Weiss DJ, Cameron E, Bisanzio D, Mappin B, Dalrymple U, Battle K, Moyes CL, Henry A, Eckhoff PA, Wenger EA, Briët O, Penny MA, Smith TA, Bennett A, Yukich J, Eisele TP, Griffin JT, Fergus CA, Lynch M, Lindgren F, Cohen JM, Murray CLJ, Smith DL, Hay SI, Cibulskis RE, Gething PW.** 2015. The effect of malaria control on *Plasmodium falciparum* in Africa between 2000 and 2015. *Nature* **526:**207–211.

4. **Fitch CD.** 1970. *Plasmodium falciparum* in owl monkeys: drug resistance and chloroquine binding capacity. *Science* **169:**289–290.
5. **Verdier F, Le Bras J, Clavier F, Hatin I, Blayo MC.** 1985. Chloroquine uptake by *Plasmodium falciparum*-infected human erythrocytes during *in vitro* culture and its relationship to chloroquine resistance. *Antimicrob Agents Chemother* **27:**561–564.
6. **Ecker A, Lehane AM, Clain J, Fidock DA.** 2012. PfCRT and its role in antimalarial drug resistance. *Trends Parasitol* **28:**504–514.
7. **Bray PG, Mungthin M, Ridley RG, Ward SA.** 1998. Access to hematin: the basis of chloroquine resistance. *Mol Pharmacol* **54:**170–179.
8. **Martin SK, Oduola AM, Milhous WK.** 1987. Reversal of chloroquine resistance in *Plasmodium falciparum* by verapamil. *Science* **235:**899–901.
9. **Foote SJ, Thompson JK, Cowman AF, Kemp DJ.** 1989. Amplification of the multidrug resistance gene in some chloroquine-resistant isolates of *P. falciparum*. *Cell* **57:**921–930.
10. **Reed MB, Saliba KJ, Caruana SR, Kirk K, Cowman AF.** 2000. Pgh1 modulates sensitivity and resistance to multiple antimalarials in *Plasmodium falciparum*. *Nature* **403:**906–909.
11. **Andriantsoanirina V, Ratsimbasoa A, Bouchier C, Tichit M, Jahevitra M, Rabearimanana S, Raherinjafy R, Mercereau-Puijalon O, Durand R, Ménard D.** 2010. Chloroquine clinical failures in *P. falciparum* malaria are associated with mutant *Pfmdr-1*, not *Pfcrt* in Madagascar. *PLoS One* **5:**e13281.
12. **Su X, Kirkman LA, Fujioka H, Wellems TE.** 1997. Complex polymorphisms in an approximately 330 kDa protein are linked to chloroquine-resistant *P. falciparum* in Southeast Asia and Africa. *Cell* **91:**593–603.
13. **Fidock DA, Nomura T, Talley AK, Cooper RA, Dzekunov SM, Ferdig MT, Ursos LM, Sidhu AB, Naudé B, Deitsch KW, Su XZ, Wootton JC, Roepe PD, Wellems TE.** 2000. Mutations in the *P. falciparum* digestive vacuole transmembrane protein PfCRT and evidence for their role in chloroquine resistance. *Mol Cell* **6:**861–871.
14. **Djimdé A, Doumbo OK, Cortese JF, Kayentao K, Doumbo S, Diourté Y, Coulibaly D, Dicko A, Su XZ, Nomura T, Fidock DA, Wellems TE, Plowe CV.** 2001. A molecular marker for chloroquine-resistant falciparum malaria. *N Engl J Med* **344:**257–263.
15. **Wootton JC, Feng X, Ferdig MT, Cooper RA, Mu J, Baruch DI, Magill AJ, Su XZ.** 2002. Genetic diversity and chloroquine selective sweeps in *Plasmodium falciparum*. *Nature* **418:**320–323.
16. **Sidhu AB, Verdier-Pinard D, Fidock DA.** 2002. Chloroquine resistance in *Plasmodium falciparum* malaria parasites conferred by *pfcrt* mutations. *Science* **298:**210–213.
17. **Martin RE, Marchetti RV, Cowan AI, Howitt SM, Bröer S, Kirk K.** 2009. Chloroquine transport via the malaria parasite's chloroquine resistance transporter. *Science* **325:** 1680–1682.
18. **Johnson DJ, Fidock DA, Mungthin M, Lakshmanan V, Sidhu AB, Bray PG, Ward SA.** 2004. Evidence for a central role for PfCRT in conferring *Plasmodium falciparum* resistance to diverse antimalarial agents. *Mol Cell* **15:**867–877.
19. **Ariey F, Fandeur T, Durand R, Randrianarivelojosia M, Jambou R, Legrand E, Ekala MT, Bouchier C, Cojean S, Duchemin JB, Robert V, Le Bras J, Mercereau-Puijalon O.** 2006. Invasion of Africa by a single *pfcrt* allele of South East Asian type. *Malar J* **5:**34.
20. **Kublin JG, Cortese JF, Njunju EM, Mukadam RA, Wirima JJ, Kazembe PN, Djimdé AA, Kouriba B, Taylor TE, Plowe CV.** 2003. Reemergence of chloroquine-sensitive *Plasmodium falciparum* malaria after cessation of chloroquine use in Malawi. *J Infect Dis* **187:**1870–1875.
21. **Pelleau S, Moss EL, Dhingra SK, Volney B, Casteras J, Gabryszewski SJ, Volkman SK, Wirth DF, Legrand E, Fidock DA, Neafsey DE, Musset L.** 2015. Adaptive evolution of malaria parasites in French Guiana: reversal of chloroquine resistance by acquisition of a mutation in *pfcrt*. *Proc Natl Acad Sci USA* **112:**11672–11677.
22. **Djimdé A, Doumbo OK, Steketee RW, Plowe CV.** 2001. Application of a molecular marker for surveillance of chloroquine-resistant falciparum malaria. *Lancet* **358:**890–891.
23. **Price RN, Uhlemann AC, Brockman A, McGready R, Ashley E, Phaipun L, Patel R, Laing K, Looareesuwan S, White NJ, Nosten F, Krishna S.** 2004. Mefloquine resistance in *Plasmodium falciparum* and increased *pfmdr1* gene copy number. *Lancet* **364:**438–447.
24. **Sidhu AB, Valderramos SG, Fidock DA.** 2005. *pfmdr1* mutations contribute to quinine resistance and enhance mefloquine and artemisinin sensitivity in *Plasmodium falciparum*. *Mol Microbiol* **57:**913–926.
25. **Veiga MI, Dhingra SK, Henrich PP, Straimer J, Gnädig N, Uhlemann AC, Martin RE, Lehane AM, Fidock DA.** 2016. Globally prevalent PfMDR1 mutations modulate *Plasmodium falciparum* susceptibility to artemisinin-based combination therapies. *Nat Commun* **7:**11553.
26. **Sidhu AB, Uhlemann AC, Valderramos SG, Valderramos JC, Krishna S, Fidock DA.** 2006. Decreasing *pfmdr1* copy number in *plasmodium falciparum* malaria heightens susceptibility to mefloquine, lumefantrine, halofantrine, quinine, and artemisinin. *J Infect Dis* **194:**528–535.
27. **Sisowath C, Petersen I, Veiga MI, Mårtensson A, Premji Z, Björkman A, Fidock DA, Gil JP.** 2009. In vivo selection of *Plasmodium falciparum* parasites carrying the chloroquine-susceptible *pfcrt* K76 allele after treatment with artemether-lumefantrine in Africa. *J Infect Dis* **199:**750–757.
28. **Dahlström S, Ferreira PE, Veiga MI, Sedighi N, Wiklund L, Mårtensson A, Färnert A, Sisowath C, Osório L, Darban H, Andersson B, Kaneko A, Conseil G, Björkman A, Gil JP.** 2009. *Plasmodium falciparum* multidrug resistance protein 1 and artemisinin-based combination therapy in Africa. *J Infect Dis* **200:**1456–1464.
29. **Dahlström S, Veiga MI, Mårtensson A, Björkman A, Gil JP.** 2009. Polymorphism in PfMRP1 (*Plasmodium falciparum* multidrug resistance protein 1) amino acid 1466 associated with resistance to sulfadoxine-pyrimethamine treatment. *Antimicrob Agents Chemother* **53:**2553–2556.
30. **Witkowski B, Duru V, Khim N, Ross LS, Saintpierre B, Beghain J, Chy S, Kim S, Ke S, Kloeung N, Eam R, Khean C, Ken M, Loch K, Bouillon A, Domergue A, Ma L, Bouchier C, Leang R, Huy R, Nuel G, Barale JC, Legrand E, Ringwald P, Fidock DA, Mercereau-Puijalon O, Ariey F, Ménard D.** 2017. A surrogate marker of piperaquine-resistant *Plasmodium falciparum* malaria: a phenotype-genotype association study. *Lancet Infect Dis* **17:**174–183
31. **Amato R, Lim P, Miotto O, Amaratunga C, Dek D, Pearson RD, Almagro-Garcia J, Neal AT, Sreng S, Suon S, Drury E, Jyothi D, Stalker J, Kwiatkowski DP, Fairhurst RM.** 2017. Genetic markers associated with dihydroartemisinin-piperaquine failure in *Plasmodium falciparum* malaria in Cambodia: a genotype-phenotype association study. *Lancet Infect Dis* **17:**164–173.
32. **Agrawal S, Moser KA, Morton L, Cummings MP, Parihar A, Dwivedi A, Shetty AC, Drabek EF, Jacob CG, Henrich PP, Parobek CM, Jongsakul K, Huy R, Spring MD, Lanteri CA, Chaorattanakawee S, Lon C, Fukuda MM, Saunders DL, Fidock DA, Lin JT, Juliano JJ, Plowe CV, Silva JC, Takala-Harrison S.** 2017. Association of a novel mutation in the *Plasmodium falciparum* chloroquine resistance transporter with decreased piperaquine sensitivity. *J Infect Dis* **216:** 468–476.
33. **Dhingra SK, Redhi D, Combrinck JM, Yeo T, Okombo J, Henrich PP, Cowell AN, Gupta P, Stegman ML, Hoke JM, Cooper RA, Winzeler E, Mok S, Egan TJ, Fidock DA.** 2017. A variant PfCRT isoform can contribute to *Plasmodium falciparum* resistance to the first-line partner drug piperaquine. *MBio* **8:**e00303-17.
34. **Dondorp AM, Nosten F, Yi P, Das D, Phyo AP, Tarning J, Lwin KM, Ariey F, Hanpithakpong W, Lee SJ, Ringwald P, Silamut K, Imwong M, Chotivanich K, Lim P, Herdman T, An SS, Yeung S, Singhasivanon P, Day NP, Lindegardh N, Socheat D, White NJ.** 2009. Artemisinin resistance in *Plasmodium falciparum* malaria. *N Engl J Med* **361:**455–467.

35. **Carrara VI, Lwin KM, Phyo AP, Ashley E, Wiladphaingern J, Sriprawat K, Rijken M, Boel M, McGready R, Proux S, Chu C, Singhasivanon P, White N, Nosten F.** 2013. Malaria burden and artemisinin resistance in the mobile and migrant population on the Thai-Myanmar border, 1999–2011: an observational study. *PLoS Med* **10:**e1001398.
36. **Phyo AP, Nkhoma S, Stepniewska K, Ashley EA, Nair S, McGready R, ler Moo C, Al-Saai S, Dondorp AM, Lwin KM, Singhasivanon P, Day NP, White NJ, Anderson TJ, Nosten F.** 2012. Emergence of artemisinin-resistant malaria on the western border of Thailand: a longitudinal study. *Lancet* **379:**1960–1966.
37. **Cheeseman IH, Miller BA, Nair S, Nkhoma S, Tan A, Tan JC, Al Saai S, Phyo AP, Moo CL, Lwin KM, McGready R, Ashley E, Imwong M, Stepniewska K, Yi P, Dondorp AM, Mayxay M, Newton PN, White NJ, Nosten F, Ferdig MT, Anderson TJ.** 2012. A major genome region underlying artemisinin resistance in malaria. *Science* **336:**79–82.
38. **Miotto O, et al.** 2013. Multiple populations of artemisinin-resistant *Plasmodium falciparum* in Cambodia. *Nat Genet* **45:**648–655.
39. **Ariey F, Witkowski B, Amaratunga C, Beghain J, Langlois AC, Khim N, Kim S, Duru V, Bouchier C, Ma L, Lim P, Leang R, Duong S, Sreng S, Suon S, Chuor CM, Bout DM, Ménard S, Rogers WO, Genton B, Fandeur T, Miotto O, Ringwald P, Le Bras J, Berry A, Barale JC, Fairhurst RM, Benoit-Vical F, Mercereau-Puijalon O, Ménard D.** 2014. A molecular marker of artemisinin-resistant *Plasmodium falciparum* malaria. *Nature* **505:**50–55.
40. **Straimer J, Gnädig NF, Witkowski B, Amaratunga C, Duru V, Ramadani AP, Dacheux M, Khim N, Zhang L, Lam S, Gregory PD, Urnov FD, Mercereau-Puijalon O, Benoit-Vical F, Fairhurst RM, Ménard D, Fidock DA.** 2015. Drug resistance. K13-propeller mutations confer artemisinin resistance in *Plasmodium falciparum* clinical isolates. *Science* **347:**428–431.
41. **Dogovski C, Xie SC, Burgio G, Bridgford J, Mok S, McCaw JM, Chotivanich K, Kenny S, Gnädig N, Straimer J, Bozdech Z, Fidock DA, Simpson JA, Dondorp AM, Foote S, Klonis N, Tilley L.** 2015. Targeting the cell stress response of *Plasmodium falciparum* to overcome artemisinin resistance. *PLoS Biol* **13:**e1002132.
42. **Mok S, Ashley EA, Ferreira PE, Zhu L, Lin Z, Yeo T, Chotivanich K, Imwong M, Pukrittayakamee S, Dhorda M, Nguon C, Lim P, Amaratunga C, Suon S, Hien TT, Htut Y, Faiz MA, Onyamboko MA, Mayxay M, Newton PN, Tripura R, Woodrow CJ, Miotto O, Kwiatkowski DP, Nosten F, Day NP, Preiser PR, White NJ, Dondorp AM, Fairhurst RM, Bozdech Z.** 2015. Drug resistance. Population transcriptomics of human malaria parasites reveals the mechanism of artemisinin resistance. *Science* **347:**431–435.
43. **Mbengue A, Bhattacharjee S, Pandharkar T, Liu H, Estiu G, Stahelin RV, Rizk SS, Njimoh DL, Ryan Y, Chotivanich K, Nguon C, Ghorbal M, Lopez-Rubio JJ, Pfrender M, Emrich S, Mohandas N, Dondorp AM, Wiest O, Haldar K.** 2015. A molecular mechanism of artemisinin resistance in *Plasmodium falciparum* malaria. *Nature* **520:**683–687.
44. **Anderson TJ, Nair S, McDew-White M, Cheeseman IH, Nkhoma S, Bilgic F, McGready R, Ashley E, Pyae Phyo A, White NJ, Nosten F.** 2017. Population parameters underlying an ongoing soft sweep in southeast Asian malaria parasites. *Mol Biol Evol* **34:**131–144.
45. **Imwong M, Hien TT, Thuy-Nhien NT, Dondorp AM, White NJ.** 2017. Spread of a single multidrug resistant malaria parasite lineage (PfPailin) to Vietnam. *Lancet Infect Dis* **17:**1022–1023.
46. **Gregson A, Plowe CV.** 2005. Mechanisms of resistance of malaria parasites to antifolates. *Pharmacol Rev* **57:**117–145.
47. **Peterson DS, Walliker D, Wellems TE.** 1988. Evidence that a point mutation in dihydrofolate reductase-thymidylate synthase confers resistance to pyrimethamine in falciparum malaria. *Proc Natl Acad Sci USA* **85:**9114–9118.
48. **Sirawaraporn W, Sathitkul T, Sirawaraporn R, Yuthavong Y, Santi DV.** 1997. Antifolate-resistant mutants of *Plasmodium falciparum* dihydrofolate reductase. *Proc Natl Acad Sci USA* **94:**1124–1129.
49. **Lozovsky ER, Chookajorn T, Brown KM, Imwong M, Shaw PJ, Kamchonwongpaisan S, Neafsey DE, Weinreich DM, Hartl DL.** 2009. Stepwise acquisition of pyrimethamine resistance in the malaria parasite. *Proc Natl Acad Sci USA* **106:**12025–12030.
50. **Cortese JF, Caraballo A, Contreras CE, Plowe CV.** 2002. Origin and dissemination of *Plasmodium falciparum* drug-resistance mutations in South America. *J Infect Dis* **186:**999–1006.
51. **Plowe CV, Cortese JF, Djimde A, Nwanyanwu OC, Watkins WM, Winstanley PA, Estrada-Franco JG, Mollinedo RE, Avila JC, Cespedes JL, Carter D, Doumbo OK.** 1997. Mutations in *Plasmodium falciparum* dihydrofolate reductase and dihydropteroate synthase and epidemiologic patterns of pyrimethamine-sulfadoxine use and resistance. *J Infect Dis* **176:**1590–1596.
52. **Roper C, Pearce R, Nair S, Sharp B, Nosten F, Anderson T.** 2004. Intercontinental spread of pyrimethamine-resistant malaria. *Science* **305:**1124.
53. **Maïga O, Djimdé AA, Hubert V, Renard E, Aubouy A, Kironde F, Nsimba B, Koram K, Doumbo OK, Le Bras J, Clain J.** 2007. A shared Asian origin of the triple-mutant *dhfr* allele in *Plasmodium falciparum* from sites across Africa. *J Infect Dis* **196:**165–172.
54. **Wang P, Read M, Sims PF, Hyde JE.** 1997. Sulfadoxine resistance in the human malaria parasite *Plasmodium falciparum* is determined by mutations in dihydropteroate synthetase and an additional factor associated with folate utilization. *Mol Microbiol* **23:**979–986.
55. **Triglia T, Wang P, Sims PF, Hyde JE, Cowman AF.** 1998. Allelic exchange at the endogenous genomic locus in *Plasmodium falciparum* proves the role of dihydropteroate synthase in sulfadoxine-resistant malaria. *EMBO J* **17:**3807–3815.
56. **Pearce RJ, Pota H, Evehe MS, Bâ H, Mombo-Ngoma G, Malisa AL, Ord R, Inojosa W, Matondo A, Diallo DA, Mbacham W, van den Broek IV, Swarthout TD, Getachew A, Dejene S, Grobusch MP, Njie F, Dunyo S, Kweku M, Owusu-Agyei S, Chandramohan D, Bonnet M, Guthmann JP, Clarke S, Barnes KI, Streat E, Katokele ST, Uusiku P, Agboghoroma CO, Elegba OY, Cissé B, A-Elbasit IE, Giha HA, Kachur SP, Lynch C, Rwakimari JB, Chanda P, Hawela M, Sharp B, Naidoo I, Roper C.** 2009. Multiple origins and regional dispersal of resistant *dhps* in African *Plasmodium falciparum* malaria. *PLoS Med* **6:**e1000055.
57. **Kublin JG, Dzinjalamala FK, Kamwendo DD, Malkin EM, Cortese JF, Martino LM, Mukadam RA, Rogerson SJ, Lescano AG, Molyneux ME, Winstanley PA, Chimpeni P, Taylor TE, Plowe CV.** 2002. Molecular markers for failure of sulfadoxine-pyrimethamine and chlorproguanil-dapsone treatment of *Plasmodium falciparum* malaria. *J Infect Dis* **185:**380–388.
58. **Basco LK, Ringwald P.** 2000. Molecular epidemiology of malaria in Yaounde, Cameroon. VI. Sequence variations in the *Plasmodium falciparum* dihydrofolate reductase-thymidylate synthase gene and in vitro resistance to pyrimethamine and cycloguanil. *Am J Trop Med Hyg* **62:**271–276.
59. **Srivastava IK, Morrisey JM, Darrouzet E, Daldal F, Vaidya AB.** 1999. Resistance mutations reveal the atovaquone-binding domain of cytochrome b in malaria parasites. *Mol Microbiol* **33:**704–711.
60. **Srivastava IK, Vaidya AB.** 1999. A mechanism for the synergistic antimalarial action of atovaquone and proguanil. *Antimicrob Agents Chemother* **43:**1334–1339.
61. **Looareesuwan S, Viravan C, Webster HK, Kyle DE, Hutchinson DB, Canfield CJ.** 1996. Clinical studies of atovaquone, alone or in combination with other antimalarial drugs, for treatment of acute uncomplicated malaria in Thailand. *Am J Trop Med Hyg* **54:**62–66.
62. **Kessl JJ, Ha KH, Merritt AK, Lange BB, Hill P, Meunier B, Meshnick SR, Trumpower BL.** 2005. Cytochrome b mutations that modify the ubiquinol-binding pocket of the cytochrome bc1 complex and confer anti-malarial drug resistance in *Saccharomyces cerevisiae*. *J Biol Chem* **280:**17142–17148.

63. **Musset L, Bouchaud O, Matheron S, Massias L, Le Bras J.** 2006. Clinical atovaquone-proguanil resistance of *Plasmodium falciparum* associated with cytochrome b codon 268 mutations. *Microbes Infect* **8:**2599–2604.
64. **Fivelman QL, Adagu IS, Warhurst DC.** 2004. Modified fixed-ratio isobologram method for studying in vitro interactions between atovaquone and proguanil or dihydroartemisinin against drug-resistant strains of *Plasmodium falciparum*. *Antimicrob Agents Chemother* **48:**4097–4102.
65. **Musset L, Le Bras J, Clain J.** 2007. Parallel evolution of adaptive mutations in *Plasmodium falciparum* mitochondrial DNA during atovaquone-proguanil treatment. *Mol Biol Evol* **24:**1582–1585.
66. **Cottrell G, Musset L, Hubert V, Le Bras J, Clain J, Atovaquone-Proguanil Treatment Failure Study Group.** 2014. Emergence of resistance to atovaquone-proguanil in malaria parasites: insights from computational modeling and clinical case reports. *Antimicrob Agents Chemother* **58:**4504–4514.
67. **Price RN, von Seidlein L, Valecha N, Nosten F, Baird JK, White NJ.** 2014. Global extent of chloroquine-resistant *Plasmodium vivax*: a systematic review and meta-analysis. *Lancet Infect Dis* **14:**982–991.
68. **Smoak BL, DeFraites RF, Magill AJ, Kain KC, Wellde BT.** 1997. *Plasmodium vivax* infections in U.S. Army troops: failure of primaquine to prevent relapse in studies from Somalia. *Am J Trop Med Hyg* **56:**231–234.
69. **Bennett JW, Pybus BS, Yadava A, Tosh D, Sousa JC, McCarthy WF, Deye G, Melendez V, Ockenhouse CF.** 2013. Primaquine failure and cytochrome P-450 2D6 in *Plasmodium vivax* malaria. *N Engl J Med* **369:**1381–1382.
70. **Nomura T, Carlton JM, Baird JK, del Portillo HA, Fryauff DJ, Rathore D, Fidock DA, Su X, Collins WE, McCutchan TF, Wootton JC, Wellems TE.** 2001. Evidence for different mechanisms of chloroquine resistance in 2 *Plasmodium* species that cause human malaria. *J Infect Dis* **183:**1653–1661.
71. **Brega S, Meslin B, de Monbrison F, Severini C, Gradoni L, Udomsangpetch R, Sutanto I, Peyron F, Picot S.** 2005. Identification of the *Plasmodium vivax mdr*-like gene (*pvmdr1*) and analysis of single-nucleotide polymorphisms among isolates from different areas of endemicity. *J Infect Dis* **191:**272–277.
72. **Hastings MD, Porter KM, Maguire JD, Susanti I, Kania W, Bangs MJ, Sibley CH, Baird JK.** 2004. Dihydrofolate reductase mutations in *Plasmodium vivax* from Indonesia and therapeutic response to sulfadoxine plus pyrimethamine. *J Infect Dis* **189:**744–750.
73. **Korsinczky M, Fischer K, Chen N, Baker J, Rieckmann K, Cheng Q.** 2004. Sulfadoxine resistance in *Plasmodium vivax* is associated with a specific amino acid in dihydropteroate synthase at the putative sulfadoxine-binding site. *Antimicrob Agents Chemother* **48:**2214–2222.
74. **Blasco B, Leroy D, Fidock DA.** 2017. Antimalarial drug resistance: linking *Plasmodium falciparum* parasite biology to the clinic. *Nat Med* **23:**917–928.
75. **World Health Organization.** 2012. Global incidence and prevalence of selected curable sexually transmitted infections—2008. http://apps.who.int/iris/bitstream/10665/75181/1/9789241503839_eng.pdf?ua=1 Accessed September 8, 2017.
76. **Silver BJ, Guy RJ, Kaldor JM, Jamil MS, Rumbold AR.** 2014. *Trichomonas vaginalis* as a cause of perinatal morbidity: a systematic review and meta-analysis. *Sex Transm Dis* **41:**369–376.
77. **Mann JR, McDermott S, Barnes TL, Hardin J, Bao H, Zhou L.** 2009. Trichomoniasis in pregnancy and mental retardation in children. *Ann Epidemiol* **19:**891–899.
78. **Kissinger P, Adamski A.** 2013. Trichomoniasis and HIV interactions: a review. *Sex Transm Infect* **89:**426–433.
79. **Secor WE, Meites E, Starr MC, Workowski KA.** 2014. Neglected parasitic infections in the United States: trichomoniasis. *Am J Trop Med Hyg* **90:**800–804.
80. **Meites E, Gaydos CA, Hobbs MM, Kissinger P, Nyirjesy P, Schwebke JR, Secor WE, Sobel JD, Workowski KA.** 2015. A review of evidence-based care of symptomatic trichomoniasis and asymptomatic *Trichomonas vaginalis* infections. *Clin Infect Dis* **61**(Suppl 8)**:**S837–S848.
81. **Crowell AL, Sanders-Lewis KA, Secor WE.** 2003. In vitro metronidazole and tinidazole activities against metronidazole-resistant strains of *Trichomonas vaginalis*. *Antimicrob Agents Chemother* **47:**1407–1409.
82. **Workowski KA, Bolan GA, Centers for Disease Control and Prevention.** 2015. Sexually transmitted diseases treatment guidelines, 2015. *MMWR Recomm Rep* **64**(RR-03)**:** 1–137.
83. **Bosserman EA, Helms DJ, Mosure DJ, Secor WE, Workowski KA.** 2011. Utility of antimicrobial susceptibility testing in *Trichomonas vaginalis*-infected women with clinical treatment failure. *Sex Transm Dis* **38:**983–987.
84. **Snipes LJ, Gamard PM, Narcisi EM, Beard CB, Lehmann T, Secor WE.** 2000. Molecular epidemiology of metronidazole resistance in a population of *Trichomonas vaginalis* clinical isolates. *J Clin Microbiol* **38:**3004–3009.
85. **Conrad MD, Gorman AW, Schillinger JA, Fiori PL, Arroyo R, Malla N, Dubey ML, Gonzalez J, Blank S, Secor WE, Carlton JM.** 2012. Extensive genetic diversity, unique population structure and evidence of genetic exchange in the sexually transmitted parasite *Trichomonas vaginalis*. *PLoS Negl Trop Dis* **6:**e1573.
86. **Paulish-Miller TE, Augostini P, Schuyler JA, Smith WL, Mordechai E, Adelson ME, Gygax SE, Secor WE, Hilbert DW.** 2014. *Trichomonas vaginalis* metronidazole resistance is associated with single nucleotide polymorphisms in the nitroreductase genes ntr4Tv and ntr6Tv. *Antimicrob Agents Chemother* **58:**2938–2943.
87. **Kirkcaldy RD, Augostini P, Asbel LE, Bernstein KT, Kerani RP, Mettenbrink CJ, Pathela P, Schwebke JR, Secor WE, Workowski KA, Davis D, Braxton J, Weinstock HS.** 2012. *Trichomonas vaginalis* antimicrobial drug resistance in 6 US cities, STD Surveillance Network, 2009–2010. *Emerg Infect Dis* **18:**939–943.
88. **Land KM, Delgadillo MG, Johnson PJ.** 2002. In vivo expression of ferredoxin in a drug resistant trichomonad increases metronidazole susceptibility. *Mol Biochem Parasitol* **121:** 153–157.
89. **Rasoloson D, Vanácová S, Tomková E, Rázga J, Hrdy I, Tachezý J, Kulda J.** 2002. Mechanisms of in vitro development of resistance to metronidazole in *Trichomonas vaginalis*. *Microbiology* **148:**2467–2477.
90. **Hrdý I, Cammack R, Stopka P, Kulda J, Tachezy J.** 2005. Alternative pathway of metronidazole activation in *Trichomonas vaginalis* hydrogenosomes. *Antimicrob Agents Chemother* **49:**5033–5036.
91. **Wright JM, Webb RI, O'Donoghue P, Upcroft P, Upcroft JA.** 2010. Hydrogenosomes of laboratory-induced metronidazole-resistant *Trichomonas vaginalis* lines are downsized while those from clinically metronidazole-resistant isolates are not. *J Eukaryot Microbiol* **57:**171–176.
92. **Mead JR, Fernadez M, Romagnoli PA, Secor WE.** 2006. Use of *Trichomonas vaginalis* clinical isolates to evaluate correlation of gene expression and metronidazole resistance. *J Parasitol* **92:**196–199.
93. **Leitsch D, Kolarich D, Binder M, Stadlmann J, Altmann F, Duchêne M.** 2009. *Trichomonas vaginalis*: metronidazole and other nitroimidazole drugs are reduced by the flavin enzyme thioredoxin reductase and disrupt the cellular redox system. Implications for nitroimidazole toxicity and resistance. *Mol Microbiol* **72:**518–536.
94. **Leitsch D, Kolarich D, Duchêne M.** 2010. The flavin inhibitor diphenyleneiodonium renders *Trichomonas vaginalis* resistant to metronidazole, inhibits thioredoxin reductase and flavin reductase, and shuts off hydrogenosomal enzymatic pathways. *Mol Biochem Parasitol* **171:**17–24.
95. **Leitsch D, Janssen BD, Kolarich D, Johnson PJ, Duchêne M.** 2014. *Trichomonas vaginalis* flavin reductase 1 and its role in metronidazole resistance. *Mol Microbiol* **91:**198–208.
96. **Bradic M, Warring SD, Tooley GE, Scheid P, Secor WE, Land KM, Huang PJ, Chen TW, Lee CC, Tang P, Sullivan SA, Carlton JM.** 2017. Genetic indicators of drug resistance in the highly repetitive genome of *Trichomonas vaginalis*. *Genome Biol Evol* **9:**1658–1672.

97. **Helms DJ, Mosure DJ, Secor WE, Workowski KA.** 2008. Management of *trichomonas vaginalis* in women with suspected metronidazole hypersensitivity. *Am J Obstet Gynecol* **198:**370.e1–370.e7.
98. **Goodhew EB, Secor WE.** 2013. Drug library screening against metronidazole-sensitive and metronidazole-resistant *Trichomonas vaginalis* isolates. *Sex Transm Infect* **89:**479–484.
99. **Hopper M, Yun JF, Zhou B, Le C, Kehoe K, Le R, Hill R, Jongeward G, Debnath A, Zhang L, Miyamoto Y, Eckmann L, Land KM, Wrischnik LA.** 2016. Auranofin inactivates *Trichomonas vaginalis* thioredoxin reductase and is effective against trichomonads in vitro and in vivo. *Int J Antimicrob Agents* **48:**690–694.
100. **Waters LJ, Dave SS, Deayton JR, French PD.** 2005. Recalcitrant *Trichomonas vaginalis* infection—a case series. *Int J STD AIDS* **16:**505–509.
101. **Muzny C, Barnes A, Mena L.** 2012. Symptomatic *Trichomonas vaginalis* infection in the setting of severe nitroimidazole allergy: successful treatment with boric acid. *Sex Health* **9:**389–391.
102. **Byun JM, Jeong DH, Kim YN, Lee KB, Sung MS, Kim KT.** 2015. Experience of successful treatment of patients with metronidazole-resistant *Trichomonas vaginalis* with zinc sulfate: a case series. *Taiwan J Obstet Gynecol* **54:**617–620.
103. **Jarvis JN, Lockwood DN.** 2013. Clinical aspects of visceral leishmaniasis in HIV infection. *Curr Opin Infect Dis* **26:**1–9.
104. **Cota GF, de Sousa MR, Fereguetti TO, Rabello A.** 2013. Efficacy of anti-leishmania therapy in visceral leishmaniasis among HIV infected patients: a systematic review with indirect comparison. *PLoS Negl Trop Dis* **7:**e2195.
105. **Torres DC, Ribeiro-Alves M, Romero GAS, Dávila AMR, Cupolillo E.** 2013. Assessment of drug resistance related genes as candidate markers for treatment outcome prediction of cutaneous leishmaniasis in Brazil. *Acta Trop* **126:**132–141.
106. **Berg M, Mannaert A, Vanaerschot M, Van Der Auwera G, Dujardin JC.** 2013. (Post-) Genomic approaches to tackle drug resistance in *Leishmania*. *Parasitology* **140:**1492–1505.
107. **Vanaerschot M, Dumetz F, Roy S, Ponte-Sucre A, Arevalo J, Dujardin JC.** 2014. Treatment failure in leishmaniasis: drug-resistance or another (epi-) phenotype? *Expert Rev Anti Infect Ther* **12:**937–946.
108. **Hendrickx S, Guerin PJ, Caljon G, Croft SL, Maes L.** 2016. Evaluating drug resistance in visceral leishmaniasis: the challenges. *Parasitology* **145:**453–463.
109. **Croft SL, Sundar S, Fairlamb AH.** 2006. Drug resistance in leishmaniasis. *Clin Microbiol Rev* **19:**111–126.
110. **Mandal G, Mandal S, Sharma M, Charret KS, Papadopoulou B, Bhattacharjee H, Mukhopadhyay R.** 2015. Species-specific antimonial sensitivity in *Leishmania* is driven by post-transcriptional regulation of AQP1. *PLoS Negl Trop Dis* **9:**e0003500.
111. **Perry M, Wyllie S, Prajapati V, Menten J, Raab A, Feldmann J, Chakraborti D, Sundar S, Boelaert M, Picado A, Fairlamb A.** 2015. Arsenic, antimony, and *Leishmania*: has arsenic contamination of drinking water in India led to treatment-resistant kala-azar? *Lancet* **385**(Suppl 1)**:**S80.
112. **Sundar S.** 2001. Drug resistance in Indian visceral leishmaniasis. *Trop Med Int Health* **6:**849–854.
113. **Adaui V, Maes I, Huyse T, Van den Broeck F, Talledo M, Kuhls K, De Doncker S, Maes L, Llanos-Cuentas A, Schönian G, Arevalo J, Dujardin JC.** 2011. Multilocus genotyping reveals a polyphyletic pattern among naturally antimony-resistant *Leishmania braziliensis* isolates from Peru. *Infect Genet Evol* **11:**1873–1880.
114. **Decuypere S, Vanaerschot M, Brunker K, Imamura H, Müller S, Khanal B, Rijal S, Dujardin JC, Coombs GH.** 2012. Molecular mechanisms of drug resistance in natural *Leishmania* populations vary with genetic background. *PLoS Negl Trop Dis* **6:**e1514.
115. **do Monte-Neto RL, Coelho AC, Raymond F, Légaré D, Corbeil J, Melo MN, Frézard F, Ouellette M.** 2011. Gene expression profiling and molecular characterization of antimony resistance in *Leishmania amazonensis*. *PLoS Negl Trop Dis* **5:**e1167.
116. **Rai S, Bhaskar, Goel SK, Nath Dwivedi U, Sundar S, Goyal N.** 2013. Role of efflux pumps and intracellular thiols in natural antimony resistant isolates of *Leishmania donovani*. *PLoS One* **8:**e74862.
117. **Mukherjee A, Boisvert S, Monte-Neto RL, Coelho AC, Raymond F, Mukhopadhyay R, Corbeil J, Ouellette M.** 2013. Telomeric gene deletion and intrachromosomal amplification in antimony-resistant *Leishmania*. *Mol Microbiol* **88:**189–202.
118. **Mukherjee A, Padmanabhan PK, Singh S, Roy G, Girard I, Chatterjee M, Ouellette M, Madhubala R.** 2007. Role of ABC transporter MRPA, γ-glutamylcysteine synthetase and ornithine decarboxylase in natural antimony-resistant isolates of *Leishmania donovani*. *J Antimicrob Chemother* **59:**204–211.
119. **Walker J, Gongora R, Vasquez JJ, Drummelsmith J, Burchmore R, Roy G, Ouellette M, Gomez MA, Saravia NG.** 2012. Discovery of factors linked to antimony resistance in *Leishmania panamensis* through differential proteome analysis. *Mol Biochem Parasitol* **183:**166–176.
120. **Mukhopadhyay R, Mukherjee S, Mukherjee B, Naskar K, Mondal D, Decuypere S, Ostyn B, Prajapati VK, Sundar S, Dujardin JC, Roy S.** 2011. Characterisation of antimony-resistant *Leishmania donovani* isolates: biochemical and biophysical studies and interaction with host cells. *Int J Parasitol* **41:**1311–1321.
121. **Manzano JI, García-Hernández R, Castanys S, Gamarro F.** 2013. A new ABC half-transporter in *Leishmania major* is involved in resistance to antimony. *Antimicrob Agents Chemother* **57:**3719–3730.
122. **Matrangolo FS, Liarte DB, Andrade LC, de Melo MF, Andrade JM, Ferreira RF, Santiago AS, Pirovani CP, Silva-Pereira RA, Murta SM.** 2013. Comparative proteomic analysis of antimony-resistant and -susceptible *Leishmania braziliensis* and *Leishmania infantum chagasi* lines. *Mol Biochem Parasitol* **190:**63–75.
123. **Berg M, Vanaerschot M, Jankevics A, Cuypers B, Maes I, Mukherjee S, Khanal B, Rijal S, Roy S, Opperdoes F, Breitling R, Dujardin JC.** 2013. Metabolic adaptations of *Leishmania donovani* in relation to differentiation, drug resistance, and drug pressure. *Mol Microbiol* **90:**428–442.
124. **Uliana SRB, Trinconi CT, Coelho AC.** 2017. Chemotherapy of leishmaniasis: present challenges. *Parasitology* **145:**464–480.
125. **Bhandari V, Kulshrestha A, Deep DK, Stark O, Prajapati VK, Ramesh V, Sundar S, Schonian G, Dujardin JC, Salotra P.** 2012. Drug susceptibility in *Leishmania* isolates following miltefosine treatment in cases of visceral leishmaniasis and post kala-azar dermal leishmaniasis. *PLoS Negl Trop Dis* **6:**e1657.
126. **Rijal S, Ostyn B, Uranw S, Rai K, Bhattarai NR, Dorlo TP, Beijnen JH, Vanaerschot M, Decuypere S, Dhakal SS, Das ML, Karki P, Singh R, Boelaert M, Dujardin JC.** 2013. Increasing failure of miltefosine in the treatment of Kala-azar in Nepal and the potential role of parasite drug resistance, reinfection, or noncompliance. *Clin Infect Dis* **56:**1530–1538.
127. **Kumar D, Kulshrestha A, Singh R, Salotra P.** 2009. In vitro susceptibility of field isolates of *Leishmania donovani* to Miltefosine and amphotericin B: correlation with sodium antimony gluconate susceptibility and implications for treatment in areas of endemicity. *Antimicrob Agents Chemother* **53:**835–838.
128. **Sánchez-Cañete MP, Carvalho L, Pérez-Victoria FJ, Gamarro F, Castanys S.** 2009. Low plasma membrane expression of the miltefosine transport complex renders *Leishmania braziliensis* refractory to the drug. *Antimicrob Agents Chemother* **53:**1305–1313.
129. **Pérez-Victoria JM, Bavchvarov BI, Torrecillas IR, Martínez-García M, López-Martín C, Campillo M, Castanys S, Gamarro F.** 2011. Sitamaquine overcomes ABC-mediated resistance to miltefosine and antimony in *Leishmania*. *Antimicrob Agents Chemother* **55:**3838–3844.

130. **Rai K, Cuypers B, Bhattarai NR, Uranw S, Berg M, Ostyn B, Dujardin JC, Rijal S, Vanaerschot M.** 2013. Relapse after treatment with miltefosine for visceral leishmaniasis is associated with increased infectivity of the infecting *Leishmania donovani* strain. *MBio* **4:**e00611–e00613.
131. **Hendrickx S, Eberhardt E, Mondelaers A, Rijal S, Bhattarai NR, Dujardin JC, Delputte P, Cos P, Maes L.** 2015. Lack of correlation between the promastigote back-transformation assay and miltefosine treatment outcome. *J Antimicrob Chemother* **70:**3023–3026.
132. **Cohen BE.** 2016. The role of signaling via aqueous pore formation in resistance responses to amphotericin B. *Antimicrob Agents Chemother* **60:**5122–5129.
133. **Sundar S, Chakravarty J.** 2013. Leishmaniasis: an update of current pharmacotherapy. *Expert Opin Pharmacother* **14:**53–63.
134. **Botero Aguirre JP, Restrepo Hamid AM.** 2015. Amphotericin B deoxycholate versus liposomal amphotericin B: effects on kidney function. *Cochrane Database Syst Rev* **23:**CD010481.
135. **Purkait B, Kumar A, Nandi N, Sardar AH, Das S, Kumar S, Pandey K, Ravidas V, Kumar M, De T, Singh D, Das P.** 2012. Mechanism of amphotericin B resistance in clinical isolates of *Leishmania donovani*. *Antimicrob Agents Chemother* **56:**1031–1041.
136. **Büscher P, Cecchi G, Jamonneau V, Priotto G.** 2017. Human African trypanosomiasis. *Lancet* **390:**2397–2409.
137. **Baker N, de Koning HP, Mäser P, Horn D.** 2013. Drug resistance in African trypanosomiasis: the melarsoprol and pentamidine story. *Trends Parasitol* **29:**110–118.
138. **Aksoy S, Buscher P, Lehane M, Solano P, Van Den Abbeele J.** 2017. Human African trypanosomiasis control: achievements and challenges. *PLoS Negl Trop Dis* **11:**e0005454.
139. **Barrett MP, Vincent IM, Burchmore RJ, Kazibwe AJ, Matovu E.** 2011. Drug resistance in human African trypanosomiasis. *Future Microbiol* **6:**1037–1047.
140. **Stewart ML, Burchmore RJ, Clucas C, Hertz-Fowler C, Brooks K, Tait A, Macleod A, Turner CM, De Koning HP, Wong PE, Barrett MP.** 2010. Multiple genetic mechanisms lead to loss of functional TbAT1 expression in drug-resistant trypanosomes. *Eukaryot Cell* **9:**336–343.
141. **Graf FE, Ludin P, Wenzler T, Kaiser M, Brun R, Pyana PP, Büscher P, de Koning HP, Horn D, Mäser P.** 2013. Aquaporin 2 mutations in *Trypanosoma brucei gambiense* field isolates correlate with decreased susceptibility to pentamidine and melarsoprol. *PLoS Negl Trop Dis* **7:**e2475.
142. **Baker N, Glover L, Munday JC, Aguinaga Andrés D, Barrett MP, de Koning HP, Horn D.** 2012. Aquaglyceroporin 2 controls susceptibility to melarsoprol and pentamidine in African trypanosomes. *Proc Natl Acad Sci USA* **109:**10996–11001.
143. **Munday JC, Eze AA, Baker N, Glover L, Clucas C, Aguinaga Andrés D, Natto MJ, Teka IA, McDonald J, Lee RS, Graf FE, Ludin P, Burchmore RJ, Turner CM, Tait A, MacLeod A, Mäser P, Barrett MP, Horn D, De Koning HP.** 2014. *Trypanosoma brucei* aquaglyceroporin 2 is a high-affinity transporter for pentamidine and melaminophenyl arsenic drugs and the main genetic determinant of resistance to these drugs. *J Antimicrob Chemother* **69:**651–663.
144. **Graf FE, Baker N, Munday JC, de Koning HP, Horn D, Mäser P.** 2015. Chimerization at the *AQP2-AQP3* locus is the genetic basis of melarsoprol-pentamidine cross-resistance in clinical *Trypanosoma brucei gambiense* isolates. *Int J Parasitol Drugs Drug Resist* **5:**65–68.
145. **Pyana PP, Sere M, Kaboré J, De Meeûs T, MacLeod A, Bucheton B, Van Reet N, Büscher P, Belem AMG, Jamonneau V.** 2015. Population genetics of *Trypanosoma brucei gambiense* in sleeping sickness patients with treatment failures in the focus of Mbuji-Mayi, Democratic Republic of the Congo. *Infect Genet Evol* **30:**128–133.
146. **Vincent IM, Creek D, Watson DG, Kamleh MA, Woods DJ, Wong PE, Burchmore RJ, Barrett MP.** 2010. A molecular mechanism for eflornithine resistance in African trypanosomes. *PLoS Pathog* **6:**e1001204.
147. **Sokolova AY, Wyllie S, Patterson S, Oza SL, Read KD, Fairlamb AH.** 2010. Cross-resistance to nitro drugs and implications for treatment of human African trypanosomiasis. *Antimicrob Agents Chemother* **54:**2893–2900.
148. **Mesu VKBK, Kalonji WM, Bardonneau C, Mordt OV, Blesson S, Simon F, Delhomme S, Bernhard S, Kuziena W, Lubaki JF, Vuvu SL, Ngima PN, Mbembo HM, Ilunga M, Bonama AK, Heradi JA, Solomo JLL, Mandula G, Badibabi LK, Dama FR, Lukula PK, Tete DN, Lumbala C, Scherrer B, Strub-Wourgaft N, Tarral A.** 2018. Oral fexinidazole for late-stage African *Trypanosoma brucei gambiense* trypanosomiasis: a pivotal multicentre, randomised, non-inferiority trial. *Lancet* **391:**144–154. 10.1016/S0140-6736(17)32758-7.
149. **Vale N, Gouveia MJ, Rinaldi G, Brindley PJ, Gärtner F, Correia da Costa JM.** 2017. Praziquantel for schistosomiasis: single-drug metabolism revisited, mode of action, and resistance. *Antimicrob Agents Chemother* **61:**e02582–e16.
150. **Black CL, Steinauer ML, Mwinzi PNM, Evan Secor W, Karanja DMS, Colley DG.** 2009. Impact of intense, longitudinal retreatment with praziquantel on cure rates of schistosomiasis mansoni in a cohort of occupationally exposed adults in western Kenya. *Trop Med Int Health* **14:**450–457.
151. **Guidi A, Andolina C, Makame Ame S, Albonico M, Cioli D, Juma Haji H.** 2010. Praziquantel efficacy and long-term appraisal of schistosomiasis control in Pemba Island. *Trop Med Int Health* **15:**614–618.
152. **Seto EY, Wong BK, Lu D, Zhong B.** 2011. Human schistosomiasis resistance to praziquantel in China: should we be worried? *Am J Trop Med Hyg* **85:**74–82.
153. **Cioli D, Pica-Mattoccia L, Basso A, Guidi A.** 2014. Schistosomiasis control: praziquantel forever? *Mol Biochem Parasitol* **195:**23–29.
154. **Melman SD, Steinauer ML, Cunningham C, Kubatko LS, Mwangi IN, Wynn NB, Mutuku MW, Karanja DM, Colley DG, Black CL, Secor WE, Mkoji GM, Loker ES.** 2009. Reduced susceptibility to praziquantel among naturally occurring Kenyan isolates of *Schistosoma mansoni*. *PLoS Negl Trop Dis* **3:**e504.
155. **Ismail M, Metwally A, Farghaly A, Bruce J, Tao LF, Bennett JL.** 1996. Characterization of isolates of *Schistosoma mansoni* from Egyptian villagers that tolerate high doses of praziquantel. *Am J Trop Med Hyg* **55:**214–218.
156. **Lamberton PHL, Hogan SC, Kabatereine NB, Fenwick A, Webster JP.** 2010. *In vitro* praziquantel test capable of detecting reduced in vivo efficacy in *Schistosoma mansoni* human infections. *Am J Trop Med Hyg* **83:**1340–1347.
157. **Coeli R, Baba EH, Araujo N, Coelho PM, Oliveira G.** 2013. Praziquantel treatment decreases *Schistosoma mansoni* genetic diversity in experimental infections. *PLoS Negl Trop Dis* **7:**e2596.
158. **Norton AJ, Gower CM, Lamberton PHL, Webster BL, Lwambo NJ, Blair L, Fenwick A, Webster JP.** 2010. Genetic consequences of mass human chemotherapy for *Schistosoma mansoni*: population structure pre- and post-praziquantel treatment in Tanzania. *Am J Trop Med Hyg* **83:**951–957.
159. **Blanton RE, Blank WA, Costa JM, Carmo TM, Reis EA, Silva LK, Barbosa LM, Test MR, Reis MG.** 2011. *Schistosoma mansoni* population structure and persistence after praziquantel treatment in two villages of Bahia, Brazil. *Int J Parasitol* **41:**1093–1099.
160. **Huyse T, Van den Broeck F, Jombart T, Webster BL, Diaw O, Volckaert FA, Balloux F, Rollinson D, Polman K.** 2013. Regular treatments of praziquantel do not impact on the genetic make-up of *Schistosoma mansoni* in Northern Senegal. *Infect Genet Evol* **18:**100–105.
161. **Lelo AE, Mburu DN, Magoma GN, Mungai BN, Kihara JH, Mwangi IN, Maina GM, Kinuthia JM, Mutuku MW, Loker ES, Mkoji GM, Steinauer ML.** 2014. No apparent reduction in schistosome burden or genetic diversity following four years of school-based mass drug administration in Mwea, central Kenya, a heavy transmission area. *PLoS Negl Trop Dis* **8:**e3221.

162. **Secor WE, Montgomery SP.** 2015. Something old, something new: is praziquantel enough for schistosomiasis control? *Future Med Chem* **7:**681–684.
163. **Tukahebwa EM, Vennervald BJ, Nuwaha F, Kabatereine NB, Magnussen P.** 2013. Comparative efficacy of one versus two doses of praziquantel on cure rate of *Schistosoma mansoni* infection and re-infection in Mayuge District, Uganda. *Trans R Soc Trop Med Hyg* **107:**397–404.
164. **King CH, Olbrych SK, Soon M, Singer ME, Carter J, Colley DG.** 2011. Utility of repeated praziquantel dosing in the treatment of schistosomiasis in high-risk communities in Africa: a systematic review. *PLoS Negl Trop Dis* **5:**e1321.
165. **Garba A, Lamine MS, Barkiré N, Djibo A, Sofo B, Gouvras AN, Labbo R, Sebangou H, Webster JP, Fenwick A, Utzinger J.** 2013. Efficacy and safety of two closely spaced doses of praziquantel against *Schistosoma haematobium* and *S. mansoni* and re-infection patterns in school-aged children in Niger. *Acta Trop* **128:**334–344.
166. **Webster BL, Diaw OT, Seye MM, Faye DS, Stothard JR, Sousa-Figueiredo JC, Rollinson D.** 2013. Praziquantel treatment of school children from single and mixed infection foci of intestinal and urogenital schistosomiasis along the Senegal River Basin: monitoring treatment success and re-infection patterns. *Acta Trop* **128:**292–302.
167. **Greenberg RM.** 2013. New approaches for understanding mechanisms of drug resistance in schistosomes. *Parasitology* **140:**1534–1546.
168. **Pinto-Almeida A, Mendes T, de Oliveira RN, Corrêa SA, Allegretti SM, Belo S, Tomás A, Anibal FF, Carrilho E, Afonso A.** 2016. Morphological characteristics of *Schistosoma mansoni* PZQ-resistant and -susceptible strains are different in presence of praziquantel. *Front Microbiol* **7:**594.
169. **Messerli SM, Kasinathan RS, Morgan W, Spranger S, Greenberg RM.** 2009. *Schistosoma mansoni* P-glycoprotein levels increase in response to praziquantel exposure and correlate with reduced praziquantel susceptibility. *Mol Biochem Parasitol* **167:**54–59.
170. **Greenberg RM.** 2013. ABC multidrug transporters in schistosomes and other parasitic flatworms. *Parasitol Int* **62:**647–653.
171. **Kasinathan RS, Morgan WM, Greenberg RM.** 2010. *Schistosoma mansoni* express higher levels of multidrug resistance-associated protein 1 (SmMRP1) in juvenile worms and in response to praziquantel. *Mol Biochem Parasitol* **173:**25–31.
172. **Kasinathan RS, Sharma LK, Cunningham C, Webb TR, Greenberg RM.** 2014. Inhibition or knockdown of ABC transporters enhances susceptibility of adult and juvenile schistosomes to Praziquantel. *PLoS Negl Trop Dis* **8:**e3265.
173. **Caffrey CR, Secor WE.** 2011. Schistosomiasis: from drug deployment to drug development. *Curr Opin Infect Dis* **24:**410–417.
174. **Bergquist R, Utzinger J, Keiser J.** 2017. Controlling schistosomiasis with praziquantel: how much longer without a viable alternative? *Infect Dis Poverty* **6:**74.

Susceptibility Test Methods: Parasites

JÉRÔME CLAIN, JACQUES LE BRAS, AND W. EVAN SECOR

154

Accurate methods for ascertaining responses of parasites to antiparasitic drugs can prove useful at several levels. They can assist in the clinical management of individual patients, yield epidemiologic information that may guide drug use policies and public health interventions, and offer crucial research tools for the development of new and better drugs. Drug susceptibility tests fall into four broad categories: *in vivo* tests, *in vitro* tests, tests with experimental animals, and molecular tests.

In vivo tests with patients directly assess the clinical efficacies of existing compounds. These tests are performed as part of epidemiologic investigations, and their modest technical requirements make them suitable for use under field conditions in developing countries. The interpretation of *in vivo* tests is limited by potential interference by factors related to the host (e.g., immunity or variations in drug intake or metabolism) or to the environment (e.g., reinfections). However, such tests have proven instrumental in guiding drug use policies, particularly for malaria.

In vitro tests circumvent these interferences by isolating the parasites from their hosts and investigating them in culture under controlled laboratory conditions, which provides opportunities for repeated assessments against multiple compounds, including experimental compounds. *In vitro* tests, however, are technically more demanding and therefore less amenable to performance under field conditions. They are most feasible for investigation of parasites that multiply rapidly in culture, a select group consisting mostly of protozoa. They are of limited use for assessing inactive drug precursors that must be activated by the host or drugs whose antiparasitic activities necessitate the synergistic effect of the host's immune defenses.

Tests with experimental animal models permit investigations of parasites that cannot be grown in culture or of drugs not yet approved for use in humans. This approach accommodates the advantages of human *in vivo* drug testing without the potential of exposing persons to toxic drugs that may be ineffective. However, its use is predicated on a suitable animal model for the infection and on the availability of appropriate facilities for maintaining the test animals. Furthermore, for animal models to be relevant, the pharmacokinetics of the drug under investigation should be similar in the particular model used and in humans.

Molecular tests detect genetic variations that are potentially linked with resistance. Such tests offer unique advantages. Nucleic acid amplification tests (NAATs) can be performed with minute amounts of nonviable parasite genetic material. They can be run in batches, allowing large-scale epidemiologic studies. Molecular analysis can circumvent potential ambiguities associated with the polyclonality of parasites infecting a single host, which are occasionally encountered in *in vivo* or *in vitro* tests, and allows the differentiation of such within-host parasite populations. Because of their short duration (hours), molecular diagnostic procedures can potentially be used to guide patient management. *In vivo* and *in vitro* tests usually require more time (days to weeks) and yield results that are used mainly for epidemiologic surveillance and experimental chemotherapy studies. Drawbacks of molecular tests reside in their technical requirements and in the need to be certain that the genes evaluated correlate with functional resistance. However, thanks to the development of more practical protocols and more robust automated equipment, as well as a better understanding of the genes that confer resistance, molecular techniques are being used in an increasing number of laboratories, including field facilities.

These different categories of tests provide complementary information. At one end of the spectrum, molecular tests analyze parasites at their most basic biologic level, without any outside interference. At the other end, *in vivo* tests in patients reflect complex interactions between host and parasite and are most relevant for clinicians and public health practitioners. While a good correlation based on various test methods is desirable, some degree of discrepancy should be expected to result from factors linked to the host or the culture conditions. Indeed, a judicious analysis of such discrepancies might provide valuable insights into the mechanisms of drug action and resistance.

These points are illustrated in the following discussion of test methods used for five parasitic diseases, selected for their particular chemotherapeutic challenges. A summary of these methods is provided in Table 1.

MALARIA

Most drug resistance tests in malaria focus on *Plasmodium falciparum*, the most prevalent and virulent species and the most prone to develop resistance. Initial recognition of drug-resistant malaria occurs most often in a clinical context, and confirmation is frequently sought by *in vivo* tests.

TABLE 1 Selected antiparasitic agents and susceptibility testing methods[a]

Disease and drugs	Testing method(s)	Remarks
Malaria[b] Chloroquine, amodiaquine, quinine, mefloquine, lumefantrine, piperaquine, pyronaridine, artemisinin, sulfadoxine-pyrimethamine, atovaquone-proguanil, primaquine, doxycycline, clindamycin, and others	*In vivo* tests in patients with *P. falciparum* or *P. vivax* malaria. Culture of erythrocytic stages of *P. falciparum*. Criteria for assessment are (i) microscopic examination (maturation from rings to schizonts; parasite multiplication and survival), (ii) metabolic activity (incorporation of [^{3}H]hypoxanthine; production of pLDH and HRP2), and (iii) DNA quantitation. PCR-based genetic analysis (mostly of *P. falciparum*) of mutations in and amplification of genes putatively involved in resistance to artemisinin derivatives (*k13*), piperaquine (*pfplasmepsin2*), chloroquine (*pfcrt, pfmdr1*), mefloquine (*pfmdr1*), antifolates (*dhfr* and *dhps* genes), atovaquone (cytochrome *b*), and others	Drug resistance is a major problem, especially in *P. falciparum*; it also occurs in *P. vivax*. Tests are used for epidemiologic assessment as well as for laboratory investigations. Short-term culture tests are also described for erythrocytic stages of *P. vivax*. On an experimental basis, there are *in vitro* tests to determine a drug's effect on liver stages and sexual stages (gametocytes).
Trichomoniasis[c] Metronidazole and tinidazole	Culture under aerobic and anaerobic conditions. The criterion for assessment is parasite mobility. PCR to detect mutation introducing stop codon into nitroreductase genes.	Resistance to metronidazole is relative; testing is performed over a wide range of concentrations. Results do not inform alternative treatment approaches.
Leishmaniasis[d] Sodium stibogluconate, meglumine antimoniate, pentamidine, amphotericin B, paromomycin, and miltefosine	Culture of promastigotes. Criteria for assessment are microscopic examination with parasite counting and metabolic activity (acid phosphatase activity; conversion of resazurin or tetrazolium salts). Culture of amastigotes in macrophage cell lines. Assessment by microscopic examination with counting of stained intracellular parasites or transformation of amastigotes back to promastigotes and counting by limiting dilution.	Problems with most drugs are their high cost, difficulty of administration, and toxicity. There is a high level of failure of pentavalent antimonials in some areas. The choices of promastigote or amastigote assay differ with the drug being tested. Tests using intracellular amastigotes show better correlation with clinical drug efficacy but are not absolute.
African trypanosomiasis[e] Pentamidine, suramin, melarsoprol, and eflornithine	Culture of trypomastigotes and assessment by microscopic examination with parasite counting or reduction of resazurin PCR and RFLP analysis	*In vitro* tests are used mainly for laboratory investigations. Detection of mutations in the aquaglyceroporin 2 transporter responsible for drug uptake may allow field-applicable tests.
Schistosomiasis[f] Praziquantel	Examination of damage to adult worms from experimental infections with suspected resistant strains by survival, motility, or metabolism Miracidial morphology when incubated with drug	*In vivo* animal tests are needed for confirmation due to the dependence of drug effect on the host immune response. Automated measurement of worm mobility or metabolism is more useful for new drug discovery than assessment of clinical resistance.

[a]See the text for details.
[b]Disease caused predominantly by *Plasmodium falciparum, Plasmodium vivax, Plasmodium ovale, Plasmodium malariae*, and *Plasmodium knowlesi*.
[c]Disease caused by *T. vaginalis*.
[d]Disease caused by one or several *Leishmania* species.
[e]Disease caused by *Trypanosoma brucei rhodesiense* and *T. brucei gambiense*.
[f]Disease caused predominantly by *Schistosoma mansoni, Schistosoma japonicum*, and *Schistosoma haematobium*.

In vitro tests aim to document the parasitological and clinical response of a malaria infection in a patient treated with a standard dose of the test drug and monitored under controlled conditions. Initially standardized by the WHO for the response of *P. falciparum* to chloroquine, *in vivo* tests have been modified several times for increased performance and assessments of other drugs (1). An increasing number of *in vivo* tests comparing drug schemes have been performed since 1996, as it was necessary to assess the response of *P. falciparum* to artemisinin-based combined therapy (2). With regard to the fast-acting artemisinin derivatives, measurement of parasite clearance times and determination of standard clinical outcomes have been introduced (3). Nevertheless, the diversity of study designs and analytical methods undermines the possibility of monitoring antimalarial drug efficacy over time from diverse regions of endemicity (4). Among key variables considered to determine the therapeutic response are *Plasmodium* species, outcome measured, level of immunity, and adjustment to discriminate recrudescence of the initial infection and recurrence (e.g., *Plasmodium vivax*) or reinfection. Incorporating consideration of pharmacokinetic parameters is of importance to identify true resistance to drugs partnered with artemisinins, because the partner drugs are frequently poorly absorbed or slowly eliminated drugs (5).

Experimental humanized mouse models containing human hepatocytes and erythrocytes are seeing early success and will permit preclinical investigations of human parasites and testing of drugs not yet approved for use in humans (6, 7).

The standard *in vitro* antimalarial drug susceptibility assay determines the *ex vivo* growth of intraerythrocytic parasites from the ring stage (the only asexual stage found in patient peripheral blood) to the schizont stage in 24 to 72 h in the presence of serial drug concentrations under conditions close to *in vivo* conditions. With regard to the standard assay, a well-suited 96-well microtiter plate format was designed using the Trager and Jensen cultivation parameters (hypoxia and buffered RPMI medium with human serum), which is the basis of the most-used tests (8, 9). The simplest test format has been adapted to field work and uses 100 μl of fingerstick capillary blood mixed with medium, a 24- to 30-h candle jar incubation, a microscopic count of multinucleated schizonts, and calculation of the 50% inhibitory concentration (IC_{50}) and IC_{90} or IC_{99} of the drug from a dose-response curve (10). Beyond this simplest format, for which standard reagents were prepared and commercialized through the WHO from 1980 to 1990, other *in vitro* tests that offer valuable advantages have been developed (11). All tests are applicable both to field-collected parasites and to the parasites growing asynchronously in long-term laboratory culture and can also be used for screening potential new antimalarials and for investigations on drug modes of action or resistance.

The activities of and resistance to some antimalarials, such as quinine and the artemisinins, respectively, address only a part of the asexual erythrocytic cycle. This implies that when long-term laboratory culture of patient isolates or reference clones is used, tight synchronization at the ring stage improves the reproducibility of susceptibility results. Parasite growth and inhibition can be assessed using different methods. A parasite count by microscopic examination of culture smears is cumbersome and often poorly reproducible. Measurement of uptake of [^{3}H]hypoxanthine offers a semiautomated, quantitative, high-output approach but necessitates the use of radioactive material and specialized equipment in authorized laboratories, leading to high costs because of the handling of nuclear waste (12). Measurement of highly produced *Plasmodium* proteins, such as parasite lactate dehydrogenase (13) or histidine-rich protein 2 (14), by double-site enzyme-linked immunosorbent assay demonstrates a higher sensitivity than the use of radioisotopes, although these tests are time-consuming and commercial kits are costly (15). Other tests measure the production of DNA during the maturation of parasites using SYBR green I fluorescent dye (16, 17).

The successful completion and interpretation of all *in vitro* tests depend on several factors that in turn depend on the characteristics of the samples, materials, culture, and statistical methods to generate inhibitory constants. Sample-related factors to be considered include recent intake of antimalarial drugs by the patient, which may decrease the test success rate; high parasite inocula, which can lead to an overestimation of resistance to some drugs (18); and the presence of folate and *para*-aminobenzoic acid in the culture medium, which antagonize the *in vitro* effect of antifolate drugs (19). Another sample factor is the short life of erythrocyte *P. falciparum* parasites outside the host; each day that passes at 4°C diminishes their capacity to survive and grow *in vitro* (20).

Critical aspects of the laboratory methods include the necessity of preparing and distributing dilutions of drugs in wells of plates, which results in particular difficulties for some drugs other than chloroquine, as most are poorly soluble or have limited shelf lives. Culture necessitates supplementation of RPMI medium with human serum or AlbuMAX, although this can affect IC_{50}s, as they interact with drugs differently (21). All these fundamental methodological issues undermine accurate comparisons of *in vitro* susceptibilities either between laboratories or within a single laboratory over time. Consensus exists on parameters of culture, and suggested improvements include measures of quality control of key parameters, such as predosed plates (titrated drug solutions) and reference of endpoints of isolate susceptibilities to those of reference clones with known susceptibilities (22). Finally, standardized mathematical analysis of concentration inhibition assays is possible through free Web-based tools (23, 24). Drug concentrations associated with the IC_{50} are determined by a modified sigmoid maximum-effect (E_{max}) model-fitting algorithm and display the precision of IC_{50} estimation. The standard *in vitro* antimalarial drug susceptibility assays described above, however, do not permit discrimination of parasites susceptible and resistant to the fast-acting artemisinin derivatives for which specific protocols have recently been developed (25–27). These new assays test the capacity of early-ring-stage parasites to survive a brief pulse exposure to high artemisinin concentrations (the so-called ring-stage survival assay), better mimicking the situation faced by parasites *in vivo*. In a study with Cambodian parasite isolates, the survival rate estimated with the ring-stage survival assay correlates with *in vivo* parasite clearance half-lives (26). Decreased susceptibility to piperaquine is also better explored using IC_{90} rather than IC_{50} estimation or a piperaquine survival assay (28, 29).

Tests exploring antimalarial efficacy at various stages of the *Plasmodium* life cycle have been designed but are more suitable for drug discovery purposes rather than routine laboratory use (30). However, the microtechnique has been adapted for testing of erythrocytic stages of *P. vivax* (31), and cultures of the liver and sexual blood stages of *Plasmodium* spp. and *P. falciparum* can also be used, although they are substantially more cumbersome (32, 33).

Genetic markers have been identified for several major antimalarials, making it possible to develop molecular tools to assess parasite drug resistance. Chloroquine resistance has been linked to a K76T change in the *P. falciparum* chloroquine resistance transporter, located in the membrane of *P. falciparum* digestive vacuole (34, 35). *P. falciparum* multidrug resistance gene 1 (*pfmdr1*) encodes a P-glycoprotein homologue of a human ABC transporter that transports toxic compounds across the digestive vacuole membrane. Point mutations and gene amplification of *pfmdr1* have been linked, to various extents, to altered susceptibilities to various antimalarials, including artemisinin-based combination therapies (chloroquine, amodiaquine, quinine, lumefantrine, mefloquine, and the active artemisinin metabolite dihydroartemisinin) (36–38). Gene amplification of *plasmepsin2*, encoding a vacuolar protease, has been linked to clinical piperaquine resistance (39, 40).

Regarding the artemisinins, several amino acid changes (chiefly C580Y) in a Kelch protein called K13 confer artemisinin resistance in *P. falciparum* parasites from Southeast Asia (41, 42). Resistance to antifolates, such as sulfadoxine-pyrimethamine, has been associated with combinations of S108N, C59R, and N51I changes in *P. falciparum* dihydrofolate reductase (43–45) or its homologues in *P. vivax* (46). High levels of resistance to antifolate drugs are associated with the additional *P. falciparum* dihydrofolate reductase change I164L (43, 47) or changes in the *P. falciparum* dihydropteroate synthase target of sulfa drugs (48). Resistance to atovaquone-proguanil has been linked to substitutions in codon Y268 of the *P. falciparum* mitochondrial cytochrome *b* gene, resulting in the amino acid change S, N, or C, leading to high-level resistance (49). Such genetic polymorphisms can be identified in individual parasite isolates by various standard techniques, which include mutation-specific nested PCR (50) or PCR followed by

Sanger sequencing (51), restriction fragment length polymorphism (RFLP) analysis (52), and single-nucleotide primer extension with detection of fluorescent products on a capillary sequencer (53), or by using a DNA microarray-based method (54). Next-generation sequencing techniques allow accurate, high-throughput detection of targeted drug resistance genotypes from either pooled or individual parasite isolates (55, 56). Genetic analysis and discovery of drug resistance are now accelerated using whole-genome sequencing (39, 41, 57). Possibilities for analyzing haplotypes in mixed parasite isolates may improve our ability to find the clinical relevance of combined mutations (58).

The judicious use of *in vivo*, *in vitro*, and molecular tests can yield valuable, complementary information that will enable adaptation of drug policies before extension of resistance brings about elevated morbidity consequences (59, 60).

TRICHOMONIASIS

Trichomonas vaginalis is the most common nonviral sexually transmitted infection in the United States and throughout the world; however, metronidazole and tinidazole are the only drugs currently approved by the U.S. Food and Drug Administration to treat trichomoniasis (61). With 4.3% of *T. vaginalis*-infected patients who attend sexually transmitted disease clinics in the United States demonstrating some degree of resistance to metronidazole, standard treatment regimens may not be effective for approximately 160,000 individuals (62, 63). Fortunately, drug susceptibility testing has proven useful to identify alternative treatment protocols that are usually successful to effect patient cure (64). *In vitro* testing for resistance to 5-nitroimidazoles is indicated following failure of standard treatments to cure the patient's infection (65).

Susceptibility testing for *T. vaginalis* uses a simple assay of parasite motility in the presence of drug (66). Axenic trichomonads are cultured in Diamond's Trypticase-yeast-maltose medium with serial dilutions (400 to 0.2 μg/ml) of metronidazole or tinidazole dissolved in dimethyl sulfoxide and the appropriate parallel concentrations of dimethyl sulfoxide in U-bottom microtiter plates. Plates are incubated at 37°C for 48 h and are then examined microscopically with an inverted phase-contrast microscope. The lowest concentration of drug in which no motile organisms are observed is defined as the minimum lethal concentration. Minimal lethal concentrations greater than 100 μg of metronidazole per ml have been associated with clinical resistance (67). This assay has been adapted to determine IC_{50}s and screen novel compounds for antitrichomonad activity by measuring incorporation of [^{3}H]thymidine (68, 69), acid phosphatase activity (70), or ATP-dependent luminescence (71). These modifications have not yet been adapted to monitor clinically resistant isolates, but theoretically, this could be accomplished rather easily.

One difficulty of the *in vitro* culture method for assessing the resistance of *T. vaginalis* isolates is the need to derive axenic cultures from clinical specimens. As individuals with trichomoniasis are often infected with other sexually transmitted disease organisms that also grow in Diamond's medium, this may require an extended time. Molecular detection of nitroimidazole resistance caused by reduced nitroreductase levels is possible through testing for a single nucleotide polymorphism (SNP) that results in a premature stop codon (72). Illumina sequencing of metronidazole-sensitive and -resistant *T. vaginalis* isolates suggests that additional genetic markers for nitroimidazole resistance could be identified (73). The prospect of a molecular marker for resistant *T. vaginalis* is exciting, as it may make possible a PCR-based assay for resistance and obviate the need for establishing axenic cultures, thus decreasing the amount of time needed to determine whether the parasite isolate is drug resistant. Identification of molecular resistance markers may also allow direct testing of specimens from patients who are suspected of harboring a resistant isolate or who have persistent, asymptomatic infections that are detected by NAATs but do not have sufficient parasites to culture and test using the traditional assay.

LEISHMANIASIS

Treatment failure in leishmaniasis may result from either true drug resistance, innate differences in the *Leishmania* sp. sensitivity to drugs, or patient factors, such as immunodeficiencies, that preclude effective chemotherapeutic action. Differentiation of these possible causes for treatment failure is important for both individual patient care and general public health (74). Drug susceptibility assays can either be performed using axenic cultures of promastigotes or intracellular cultures of amastigotes. Promastigote cultures are easier to perform, are more readily adapted from clinical isolates, and have higher throughput. However, they yield clinically reliable results only for drugs such as miltefosine and amphotericin B that do not require cellular mechanisms for activation (75, 76). In contrast, the more widely used pentavalent antimonials require reduction by host cells to the active trivalent form, and assays that test drug susceptibility of the intracellular amastigote form of leishmania parasites are recommended (77). Amastigote assays are also considered more clinically relevant (74). Unfortunately, intracellular assays are much more labor-intensive, are host cell dependent, and require much greater adaptation that could introduce differences from the clinical isolate. The lack of a standardized protocol for assessing drug resistance of *Leishmania* spp. makes test comparisons between laboratories and endemic settings challenging (74, 78).

Promastigote assays are performed by culturing parasites with drug in standard cell culture media (RPMI or M199) supplemented with bovine sera for 42 to 72 h at 26 to 37°C and assessing viability by absorbance at 600 nm (79), acid phosphatase activity (80), reduction of resazurin (76, 81), or conversion of tetrazolium salts [MTT: 3-(4,5-dimethylthiazol-2-yl)-2,5-diphenyltetrazolium bromide; XTT: 2,3-*bis*-(2-methoxy-4-nitro-5-sulfophenyl)-2*H*-tetrazolium-5-carboxanilide; or WST-8: 2-(2-methoxy-4-nitrophenyl)-3-(4-nitrophenyl)-5-(2,4-disulfophenyl)-2*H*-tetrazolium] (82–84). Each of these methods of detection has unique advantages and limitations. Acid phosphatase and conversion of tetrazolium salts are colorimetric assays that can be read with standard microplate readers, while resazurin assays require readers that can detect fluorescence. Resazurin (alamarBlue), MTT, and XTT are available as commercial products, facilitating their use. Direct comparison of the tetrazolium salts suggests that WST-8 has performance superior to that of MTT and XTT (84). Because resazurin and XTT do not require cell lysis (MTT does) or other manipulation of the parasites in order to read the assay, drug activities can be monitored at different time points after initiation of cultures for kinetic analysis.

Amastigote assays are performed by infecting macrophage cell lines (e.g., U-937, J774, and THP-1) with promastigotes isolated from clinical samples and incubating with different concentrations of the drug being tested at 34 to 37°C for 2 to 7 days (79, 80, 83, 85, 86). Following exposure of amastigote-infected macrophages to drug, cells are stained for microscopic counting of the proportion of infected macrophages and the number of amastigotes per 100 macrophages in drug-treated and control cultures. Typically, three or four replicates of each drug concentration are assessed. Alternatively, following incubation of infected cells with drug, controlled lysis of macrophages can be performed to release amastigotes that are then transformed back into promastigotes and enumerated by limiting dilution (83).

As molecular mechanisms of drug resistance in *Leishmania* spp. become better defined, it may be possible to utilize PCR and DNA sequencing of SNPs for epidemiologic studies of resistant isolates. Resistance-associated SNPs in genes for drug transporters, stress response, and thiol and redox metabolism have been identified from both visceral and cutaneous leishmania species (87, 88). These assays are of interest, as no manipulation beyond growing parasites is needed. However, it is likely that applicability will be species and drug restricted and would fail to detect novel mechanisms of resistance.

AFRICAN TRYPANOSOMIASIS

As in leishmania drug sensitivity testing, trypanosomes can be cultured *in vitro* with drug and monitored for viability by direct counting or incubation with resazurin for fluorescence detection (89–91). Parasites are cultured at 37°C for 24 to 72 h in 5% CO_2 in Iscove's or minimal essential medium supplemented with HEPES buffer, β-mercaptoethanol, and heat-inactivated bovine or horse serum. Resazurin is added for the last 4 hours of culture before the assays is read using 530-nm excitation and 590-nm emission wavelengths (89, 91). However, these assays are more useful for screening new compounds than for assessing drug resistance in clinical isolates, as adaptation to axenic culture may impose selective pressures on the parasites that could alter important characteristics (78).

Resistance of African trypanosomes to pentamidine and melarsoprol is primarily a function of mutations in the transporters required for their uptake, leading to decreased intracellular drug concentrations. PCR followed by RFLP analysis can be used to assess resistance in isolates obtained from persons who have relapsed after treatment (92). Using this approach, loss of functional aquaglyceroporin 2 (AQP2) was identified as more important for treatment failure than aminopurine transporter P2 (93–95). PCR-RFLP makes it easier to provide drug resistance information on samples obtained from patients, as no culture step is required. However, when analysis is focused on only one transporter, there is the potential to miss other possible drug resistance mechanisms. A case in point is the use of microsatellite markers and whole-genome sequencing of parasites from patients with relapsed infection, which suggested that mutation of AQP2 may not be solely responsible for clinically resistant human African trypanosomiasis phenotypes. There may be up to 23 additional genes affecting melarsoprol sensitivity, and nonparasite factors, such as host immunity and nutritional status, could also be important (96, 97). More clinical drug-resistant isolates will need to be evaluated to confirm the utility of this test, but it has potential for both management of individual patients' infections and tracking the spread of resistance in a population.

SCHISTOSOMIASIS

Drug resistance testing of schistosomes differs greatly from that of protozoan parasites in both purpose and methods. Adult worms do not replicate within the definitive host, thus circumventing one of the mechanisms associated with rapid development of drug resistance. As a result, widespread resistance to praziquantel, the drug of choice for schistosomiasis, has not emerged even under heavy drug pressure (98–100). Thus, the need to evaluate drug resistance for individual infections is rare. However, because reliance on a sole drug is risky and schistosomes have developed resistance to other drugs, techniques to monitor praziquantel resistance are needed. Here, the failure of adult worms to replicate makes drug susceptibility testing methods more challenging. Investigation of drug resistance has typically been performed by obtaining eggs from an unsuccessfully treated mammalian host, infecting the appropriate snail intermediate host, isolating cercariae from the infected snail, and infecting and treating experimental animals. A protocol to determine the 50% effective dose of antimicrobial compounds in mice has been developed and demonstrates good reproducibility among different laboratories (101). This approach has the drawbacks of being very time-consuming and technically challenging, especially in areas of endemicity that may not have well-developed experimental snail and rodent colonies.

Fifty-percent effective doses can also be estimated in an *in vitro* assay by assessing contraction or metabolism of worms following perfusion and incubation with praziquantel and correspond well with *in vivo* results (102–104). Although this approach is less complicated than infecting, treating, and perfusing additional mice, it still requires the availability of naïve snails and some mice to obtain the adult worms along with the time and expertise needed to perpetuate the life cycle. In addition, the parasites that successfully infect mice may not accurately represent diversity of the field isolate. An *in vitro* method that circumvents these problems has been adapted to field use (105, 106). Eggs from stools of infected individuals are isolated and hatched to release miracidia that are then exposed to praziquantel, and effects on morphology are monitored. When this technique was used, the miracidia from persons who cleared their infection following treatment were more affected by drug than miracidia from stools whose donors did not clear their infections. Evaluating changes in the parasite's population structure using miracidia obtained from eggs in patients' stools is another approach to monitor development of potential drug resistance. Changes in the genetic composition of schistosomes following treatment suggest praziquantel efficacy, while maintenance of the same microsatellite distribution may indicate treatment failure (107, 108). Ongoing surveillance for development of drug resistance will be an important component for schistosomiasis control programs that are dependent on mass drug administration.

FUTURE PERSPECTIVES

Most susceptibility tests for antiparasitic drugs are not routinely available in clinical diagnostic laboratories, because these procedures are not in frequent demand and present special technical requirements. Such tests are performed mainly in reference or research laboratories or during epidemiologic investigations in areas of endemicity. Thanks to recent advances in laboratory technology and genetic analysis of parasites, available tests are increasingly sophisticated and informative. The development of tests that are robust and simple to use will facilitate field studies that aim at optimizing the deployment of currently available drugs. These field tests usefully complement the more sophisticated procedures used in research laboratories whose main orientation is toward the development of novel antiparasitic compounds and deciphering drug resistance mechanisms.

The findings and conclusions in this report are those of the authors and do not necessarily represent the views of the CDC.

REFERENCES

1. **World Health Organization.** 2009. *Methods for Surveillance of Antimalarial Drug Efficacy*. World Health Organization, Geneva, Switzerland.
2. **World Health Organization.** 2005. Susceptibility of *P. falciparum* to antimalarial drugs: report on global monitoring: 1996–2004. WHO/HTM/MAL/2005.1103. World Health Organization, Geneva, Switzerland.
3. **Flegg JA, Guerin PJ, White NJ, Stepniewska K.** 2011. Standardizing the measurement of parasite clearance in falciparum malaria: the parasite clearance estimator. *Malar J* **10:**339.
4. **Price RN, Dorsey G, Ashley EA, Barnes KI, Baird JK, d'Alessandro U, Guerin PJ, Laufer MK, Naidoo I, Nosten F, Olliaro P, Plowe CV, Ringwald P, Sibley CH, Stepniewska K, White NJ.** 2007. World Antimalarial Resistance Network I: clinical efficacy of antimalarial drugs. *Malar J* **6:**119
5. **Barnes KI, Watkins WM, White NJ.** 2008. Antimalarial dosing regimens and drug resistance. *Trends Parasitol* **24:**127–134.
6. **Soulard V, Bosson-Vanga H, Lorthiois A, Roucher C, Franetich JF, Zanghi G, Bordessoulles M, Tefit M, Thellier M, Morosan S, Le Naour G, Capron F, Suemizu H, Snounou G, Moreno-Sabater A, Mazier D.** 2015. *Plasmodium falciparum* full life cycle and *Plasmodium ovale* liver stages in humanized mice. *Nat Commun* **6:**7690.
7. **Duffier Y, Lorthiois A, Cisteró P, Dupuy F, Jouvion G, Fiette L, Mazier D, Mayor A, Lavazec C, Moreno Sabater A.** 2016. A humanized mouse model for sequestration of *Plasmodium falciparum* sexual stages and in vivo evaluation of gametocytidal drugs. *Sci Rep* **6:**35025.
8. **Trager W, Jensen JB.** 1976. Human malaria parasites in continuous culture. *Science* **193:**673–675.
9. **Rieckmann KH, Campbell GH, Sax LJ, Ema JE.** 1978. Drug sensitivity of *Plasmodium falciparum*. An in-vitro microtechnique. *Lancet* **i:**22–23.
10. **World Health Organization.** 2001. In vitro micro-test (mark III) for the assessment of *P. falciparum* susceptibility to chloroquine, mefloquine, quinine, amodiaquine, sulfadoxine/pyrimethamine and artemisinin. CTD/MAL/9720 Rev 2. World Health Organization, Geneva, Switzerland.
11. **World Health Organization.** 2007. *Field Application of In Vitro Assays for the Sensitivity of Human Malaria Parasites to Antimalarial Drugs*. World Health Organization, Geneva, Switzerland.
12. **Desjardins RE, Canfield CJ, Haynes JD, Chulay JD.** 1979. Quantitative assessment of antimalarial activity in vitro by a semiautomated microdilution technique. *Antimicrob Agents Chemother* **16:**710–718.
13. **Moreno A, Brasseur P, Cuzin-Ouattara N, Blanc C, Druilhe P.** 2001. Evaluation under field conditions of the colourimetric DELI-microtest for the assessment of *Plasmodium falciparum* drug resistance. *Trans R Soc Trop Med Hyg* **95:**100–103.
14. **Noedl H, Attlmayr B, Wernsdorfer WH, Kollaritsch H, Miller RS.** 2004. A histidine-rich protein 2-based malaria drug sensitivity assay for field use. *Am J Trop Med Hyg* **71:**711–714.
15. **Kaddouri H, Nakache S, Houze S, Mentre F, Le Bras J.** 2006. Assessment of the drug susceptibility of *Plasmodium falciparum* clinical isolates from Africa by using a *Plasmodium* lactate dehydrogenase immunodetection assay and an inhibitory maximum effect model for precise measurement of the 50-percent inhibitory concentration. *Antimicrob Agents Chemother* **50:**3343–3349.
16. **Smilkstein M, Sriwilaijaroen N, Kelly JX, Wilairat P, Riscoe M.** 2004. Simple and inexpensive fluorescence-based technique for high-throughput antimalarial drug screening. *Antimicrob Agents Chemother* **48:**1803–1806.
17. **Rason MA, Randriantsoa T, Andrianantenaina H, Ratsimbasoa A, Ménard D.** 2008. Performance and reliability of the SYBR Green I based assay for the routine monitoring of susceptibility of *Plasmodium falciparum* clinical isolates. *Trans R Soc Trop Med Hyg* **102:**346–351.
18. **Duraisingh MT, Jones P, Sambou I, von Seidlein L, Pinder M, Warhurst DC.** 1999. Inoculum effect leads to overestimation of *in vitro* resistance for artemisinin derivatives and standard antimalarials: a Gambian field study. *Parasitology* **119:**435–440.
19. **Wang P, Sims PF, Hyde JE.** 1997. A modified *in vitro* sulfadoxine susceptibility assay for *Plasmodium falciparum* suitable for investigating Fansidar resistance. *Parasitology* **115:** 223–230.
20. **Basco LK.** 2004. Molecular epidemiology of malaria in Cameroon. XX. Experimental studies on various factors of in vitro drug sensitivity assays using fresh isolates of *Plasmodium falciparum*. *Am J Trop Med Hyg* **70:**474–480.
21. **Basco LK.** 2003. Molecular epidemiology of malaria in Cameroon. XV. Experimental studies on serum substitutes and supplements and alternative culture media for in vitro drug sensitivity assays using fresh isolates of *Plasmodium falciparum*. *Am J Trop Med Hyg* **69:**168–173.
22. **Bacon DJ, Jambou R, Fandeur T, Le Bras J, Wongsrichanalai C, Fukuda MM, Ringwald P, Sibley CH, Kyle DE.** 2007. World Antimalarial Resistance Network (WARN) II: in vitro antimalarial drug susceptibility. *Malar J* **6:**120–124.
23. **Le Nagard H, Vincent C, Mentré F, Le Bras J.** 2011. Online analysis of in vitro resistance to antimalarial drugs through nonlinear regression. *Comput Methods Programs Biomed* **104:**10–18.
24. **Woodrow CJ, Dahlström S, Cooksey R, Flegg JA, Le Nagard H, Mentré F, Murillo C, Ménard D, Nosten F, Sriprawat K, Musset L, Quashie NB, Lim P, Fairhurst RM, Nsobya SL, Sinou V, Noedl H, Pradines B, Johnson JD, Guerin PJ, Sibley CH, Le Bras J.** 2013. High-throughput analysis of antimalarial susceptibility data by the WorldWide Antimalarial Resistance Network (WWARN) *in vitro* analysis and reporting tool. *Antimicrob Agents Chemother* **57:**3121–3130.
25. **Klonis N, Xie SC, McCaw JM, Crespo-Ortiz MP, Zaloumis SG, Simpson JA, Tilley L.** 2013. Altered temporal response of malaria parasites determines differential sensitivity to artemisinin. *Proc Natl Acad Sci USA* **110:**5157–5162.
26. **Witkowski B, Amaratunga C, Khim N, Sreng S, Chim P, Kim S, Lim P, Mao S, Sopha C, Sam B, Anderson JM, Duong S, Chuor CM, Taylor WR, Suon S, Mercereau-Puijalon O, Fairhurst RM, Ménard D.** 2013. Novel phenotypic assays for the detection of artemisinin-resistant *Plasmodium falciparum* malaria in Cambodia: in-vitro and ex-vivo drug-response studies. *Lancet Infect Dis* **13:**1043–1049.
27. **Witkowski B, Khim N, Chim P, Kim S, Ke S, Kloeung N, Chy S, Duong S, Leang R, Ringwald P, Dondorp AM, Tripura R, Benoit-Vical F, Berry A, Gorgette O, Ariey F, Barale JC, Mercereau-Puijalon O, Ménard D.** 2013. Reduced artemisinin susceptibility of *Plasmodium falciparum* ring stages in western Cambodia. *Antimicrob Agents Chemother* **57:** 914–923.
28. **Agrawal S, Moser KA, Morton L, Cummings MP, Parihar A, Dwivedi A, Shetty AC, Drabek EF, Jacob CG, Henrich PP, Parobek CM, Jongsakul K, Huy R, Spring MD, Lanteri CA, Chaorattanakawee S, Lon C, Fukuda MM, Saunders DL, Fidock DA, Lin JT, Juliano JJ, Plowe CV, Silva JC, Takala-Harrison S.** 2017. Association of a novel mutation in the *Plasmodium falciparum* chloroquine resistance transporter with decreased piperaquine sensitivity. *J Infect Dis* **216:** 468–476.
29. **Duru V, Khim N, Leang R, Kim S, Domergue A, Kloeung N, Ke S, Chy S, Eam R, Khean C, Loch K, Ken M, Lek D, Beghain J, Ariey F, Guerin PJ, Huy R, Mercereau-Puijalon O, Witkowski B, Menard D.** 2015. *Plasmodium falciparum* dihydroartemisinin-piperaquine failures in Cambodia are associated with mutant K13 parasites presenting high survival rates in novel piperaquine in vitro assays: retrospective and prospective investigations. *BMC Med* **13:**305.

30. **Delves M, Plouffe D, Scheurer C, Meister S, Wittlin S, Winzeler EA, Sinden RE, Leroy D.** 2012. The activities of current antimalarial drugs on the life cycle stages of *Plasmodium*: a comparative study with human and rodent parasites. *PLoS Med* **9:**e1001169.
31. **Tasanor O, Noedl H, Na-Bangchang K, Congpuong K, Sirichaisinthop J, Wernsdorfer WH.** 2002. An in vitro system for assessing the sensitivity of *Plasmodium vivax* to chloroquine. *Acta Trop* **83:**49–61.
32. **Barata L, Houzé P, Boutbibe K, Zanghi G, Franetich JF, Mazier D, Clain J.** 2016. In vitro analysis of the interaction between atovaquone and proguanil against liver stage malaria parasites. *Antimicrob Agents Chemother* **60:**4333–4335.
33. **Vial H, Taramelli D, Boulton IC, Ward SA, Doerig C, Chibale K.** 2013. CRIMALDDI: platform technologies and novel anti-malarial drug targets. *Malar J* **12:**396.
34. **Fidock DA, Nomura T, Talley AK, Cooper RA, Dzekunov SM, Ferdig MT, Ursos LMB, Sidhu ABS, Naudé B, Deitsch KW, Su XZ, Wootton JC, Roepe PD, Wellems TE.** 2000. Mutations in the *P. falciparum* digestive vacuole transmembrane protein PfCRT and evidence for their role in chloroquine resistance. *Mol Cell* **6:**861–871.
35. **Ecker A, Lehane AM, Clain J, Fidock DA.** 2012. PfCRT and its role in antimalarial drug resistance. *Trends Parasitol* **28:**504–514.
36. **Pickard AL, Wongsrichanalai C, Purfield A, Kamwendo D, Emery K, Zalewski C, Kawamoto F, Miller RS, Meshnick SR.** 2003. Resistance to antimalarials in Southeast Asia and genetic polymorphisms in *pfmdr1*. *Antimicrob Agents Chemother* **47:**2418–2423.
37. **Price RN, Uhlemann AC, Brockman A, McGready R, Ashley E, Phaipun L, Patel R, Laing K, Looareesuwan S, White NJ, Nosten F, Krishna S.** 2004. Mefloquine resistance in *Plasmodium falciparum* and increased *pfmdr1* gene copy number. *Lancet* **364:**438–447.
38. **Veiga MI, Dhingra SK, Henrich PP, Straimer J, Gnädig N, Uhlemann AC, Martin RE, Lehane AM, Fidock DA.** 2016. Globally prevalent PfMDR1 mutations modulate *Plasmodium falciparum* susceptibility to artemisinin-based combination therapies. *Nat Commun* **7:**11553.
39. **Witkowski B, Duru V, Khim N, Ross LS, Saintpierre B, Beghain J, Chy S, Kim S, Ke S, Kloeung N, Eam R, Khean C, Ken M, Loch K, Bouillon A, Domergue A, Ma L, Bouchier C, Leang R, Huy R, Nuel G, Barale JC, Legrand E, Ringwald P, Fidock DA, Mercereau-Puijalon O, Ariey F, Ménard D.** 2017. A surrogate marker of piperaquine-resistant *Plasmodium falciparum* malaria: a phenotype-genotype association study. *Lancet Infect Dis* **17:**174–183.
40. **Amato R, Lim P, Miotto O, Amaratunga C, Dek D, Pearson RD, Almagro-Garcia J, Neal AT, Sreng S, Suon S, Drury E, Jyothi D, Stalker J, Kwiatkowski DP, Fairhurst RM.** 2017. Genetic markers associated with dihydroartemisinin-piperaquine failure in *Plasmodium falciparum* malaria in Cambodia: a genotype-phenotype association study. *Lancet Infect Dis* **17:**164–173.
41. **Ariey F, Witkowski B, Amaratunga C, Beghain J, Langlois AC, Khim N, Kim S, Duru V, Bouchier C, Ma L, Lim P, Leang R, Duong S, Sreng S, Suon S, Chuor CM, Bout DM, Ménard S, Rogers WO, Genton B, Fandeur T, Miotto O, Ringwald P, Le Bras J, Berry A, Barale JC, Fairhurst RM, Benoit-Vical F, Mercereau-Puijalon O, Ménard D.** 2014. A molecular marker of artemisinin-resistant *Plasmodium falciparum* malaria. *Nature* **505:**50–55.
42. **Straimer J, Gnädig NF, Witkowski B, Amaratunga C, Duru V, Ramadani AP, Dacheux M, Khim N, Zhang L, Lam S, Gregory PD, Urnov FD, Mercereau-Puijalon O, Benoit-Vical F, Fairhurst RM, Ménard D, Fidock DA.** 2015. K13-propeller mutations confer artemisinin resistance in *Plasmodium falciparum* clinical isolates. *Science* **347:** 428–431.
43. **Peterson DS, Walliker D, Wellems TE.** 1988. Evidence that a point mutation in dihydrofolate reductase-thymidylate synthase confers resistance to pyrimethamine in falciparum malaria. *Proc Natl Acad Sci USA* **85:**9114–9118.
44. **Cowman AF, Morry MJ, Biggs BA, Cross GA, Foote SJ.** 1988. Amino acid changes linked to pyrimethamine resistance in the dihydrofolate reductase-thymidylate synthase gene of *Plasmodium falciparum*. *Proc Natl Acad Sci USA* **85:**9109–9113.
45. **Müller IB, Hyde JE.** 2013. Folate metabolism in human malaria parasites—75 years on. *Mol Biochem Parasitol* **188:** 63–77.
46. **Hastings MD, Porter KM, Maguire JD, Susanti I, Kania W, Bangs MJ, Sibley CH, Baird JK.** 2004. Dihydrofolate reductase mutations in *Plasmodium vivax* from Indonesia and therapeutic response to sulfadoxine plus pyrimethamine. *J Infect Dis* **189:**744–750.
47. **Sirawaraporn W, Sathitkul T, Sirawaraporn R, Yuthavong Y, Santi DV.** 1997. Antifolate-resistant mutants of *Plasmodium falciparum* dihydrofolate reductase. *Proc Natl Acad Sci USA* **94:**1124–1129.
48. **Nzila AM, Mberu EK, Sulo J, Dayo H, Winstanley PA, Sibley CH, Watkins WM.** 2000. Towards an understanding of the mechanism of pyrimethamine-sulfadoxine resistance in *Plasmodium falciparum*: genotyping of dihydrofolate reductase and dihydropteroate synthase of Kenyan parasites. *Antimicrob Agents Chemother* **44:**991–996.
49. **Musset L, Bouchaud O, Matheron S, Massias L, Le Bras J.** 2006. Clinical atovaquone-proguanil resistance of *Plasmodium falciparum* associated with cytochrome b codon 268 mutations. *Microbes Infect* **8:**2599–2604.
50. **Djimdé A, Doumbo OK, Cortese JF, Kayentao K, Doumbo S, Diourté Y, Coulibaly D, Dicko A, Su XZ, Nomura T, Fidock DA, Wellems TE, Plowe CV.** 2001. A molecular marker for chloroquine-resistant falciparum malaria. *N Engl J Med* **344:**257–263.
51. **Basco LK, Ringwald P.** 2000. Molecular epidemiology of malaria in Yaounde, Cameroon. VI. Sequence variations in the *Plasmodium falciparum* dihydrofolate reductase-thymidylate synthase gene and *in vitro* resistance to pyrimethamine and cycloguanil. *Am J Trop Med Hyg* **62:**271–276.
52. **Syafruddin D, Asih PB, Casey GJ, Maguire J, Baird JK, Nagesha HS, Cowman AF, Reeder JC.** 2005. Molecular epidemiology of *Plasmodium falciparum* resistance to antimalarial drugs in Indonesia. *Am J Trop Med Hyg* **72:**174–181.
53. **Nair S, Brockman A, Paiphun L, Nosten F, Anderson TJ.** 2002. Rapid genotyping of loci involved in antifolate drug resistance in *Plasmodium falciparum* by primer extension. *Int J Parasitol* **32:**852–858.
54. **Crameri A, Marfurt J, Mugittu K, Maire N, Regös A, Coppee JY, Sismeiro O, Burki R, Huber E, Laubscher D, Puijalon O, Genton B, Felger I, Beck HP.** 2007. Rapid microarray-based method for monitoring of all currently known single-nucleotide polymorphisms associated with parasite resistance to antimalaria drugs. *J Clin Microbiol* **45:**3685–3691.
55. **Taylor SM, Parobek CM, Aragam N, Ngasala BE, Mårtensson A, Meshnick SR, Juliano JJ.** 2013. Pooled deep sequencing of *Plasmodium falciparum* isolates: an efficient and scalable tool to quantify prevailing malaria drug-resistance genotypes. *J Infect Dis* **208:**1998–2006.
56. **Nag S, Dalgaard MD, Kofoed PE, Ursing J, Crespo M, Andersen LO, Aarestrup FM, Lund O, Alifrangis M.** 2017. High throughput resistance profiling of *Plasmodium falciparum* infections based on custom dual indexing and Illumina next generation sequencing-technology. *Sci Rep* **7:**2398.
57. **MalariaGEN Plasmodium falciparum Community Project.** 2016. Genomic epidemiology of artemisinin resistant malaria. *eLife* **5:**e08714.
58. **Hastings IM, Smith TA.** 2008. MalHaploFreq: a computer programme for estimating malaria haplotype frequencies from blood samples. *Malar J* **7:**130.
59. **Sibley CH, Barnes KI, Plowe CV.** 2007. The rationale and plan for creating a World Antimalarial Resistance Network (WARN). *Malar J* **6:**118.
60. **Vestergaard LS, Ringwald P.** 2007. Responding to the challenge of antimalarial drug resistance by routine monitoring to update national malaria treatment policies. *Am J Trop Med Hyg* **77**(Suppl)**:**153–159.

61. **Meites E, Gaydos CA, Hobbs MM, Kissinger P, Nyirjesy P, Schwebke JR, Secor WE, Sobel JD, Workowski KA.** 2015. A review of evidence-based care of symptomatic trichomoniasis and asymptomatic *Trichomonas vaginalis* infections. *Clin Infect Dis* **61**(Suppl 8):S837–S848.
62. **Kirkcaldy RD, Augostini P, Asbel LE, Bernstein KT, Kerani RP, Mettenbrink CJ, Pathela P, Schwebke JR, Secor WE, Workowski KA, Davis D, Braxton J, Weinstock HS.** 2012. *Trichomonas vaginalis* antimicrobial drug resistance in 6 US cities, STD Surveillance Network, 2009-2010. *Emerg Infect Dis* **18:**939–943.
63. **Secor WE, Meites E, Starr MC, Workowski KA.** 2014. Neglected parasitic infections in the United States: trichomoniasis. *Am J Trop Med Hyg* **90:**800–804.
64. **Bosserman EA, Helms DJ, Mosure DJ, Secor WE, Workowski KA.** 2011. Utility of antimicrobial susceptibility testing in *Trichomonas vaginalis*-infected women with clinical treatment failure. *Sex Transm Dis* **38:**983–987.
65. **Workowski KA, Bolan GA, Centers for Disease Control and Prevention.** 2015. Sexually transmitted diseases treatment guidelines, 2015. *MMWR Recomm Rep* **64**(RR-03)**:**1–137.
66. **Meingassner JG, Thurner J.** 1979. Strain of *Trichomonas vaginalis* resistant to metronidazole and other 5-nitroimidazoles. *Antimicrob Agents Chemother* **15:**254–257.
67. **Müller M, Lossick JG, Gorrell TE.** 1988. In vitro susceptibility of *Trichomonas vaginalis* to metronidazole and treatment outcome in vaginal trichomoniasis. *Sex Transm Dis* **15:** 17–24.
68. **Crowell AL, Stephens CE, Kumar A, Boykin DE, Secor WE.** 2004. Activities of dicationic compounds against *Trichomonas vaginalis*. *Antimicrob Agents Chemother* **48:** 3602–3605.
69. **Goodhew EB, Secor WE.** 2013. Drug library screening against metronidazole-sensitive and metronidazole-resistant *Trichomonas vaginalis* isolates. *Sex Transm Infect* **89:** 479–484.
70. **Martínez-Grueiro MM, Montero-Pereira D, Giménez-Pardo C, Nogal-Ruiz JJ, Escario JA, Gómez-Barrio A.** 2003. *Trichomonas vaginalis:* determination of acid phosphatase activity as a pharmacological screening procedure. *J Parasitol* **89:**1076–1077.
71. **Hopper M, Yun JF, Zhou B, Le C, Kehoe K, Le R, Hill R, Jongeward G, Debnath A, Zhang L, Miyamoto Y, Eckmann L, Land KM, Wrischnik LA.** 2016. Auranofin inactivates *Trichomonas vaginalis* thioredoxin reductase and is effective against trichomonads in vitro and in vivo. *Int J Antimicrob Agents* **48:**690–694.
72. **Paulish-Miller TE, Augostini P, Schuyler JA, Smith WL, Mordechai E, Adelson ME, Gygax SE, Secor WE, Hilbert DW.** 2014. *Trichomonas vaginalis* metronidazole resistance is associated with single nucleotide polymorphisms in the nitroreductase genes $ntr4_{Tv}$ and $ntr6_{Tv}$. *Antimicrob Agents Chemother* **58:**2938–2943.
73. **Bradic M, Warring SD, Tooley GE, Scheid P, Secor WE, Land KM, Huang PJ, Chen TW, Lee CC, Tang P, Sullivan SA, Carlton JM.** 2017. Genetic indicators of drug resistance in the highly repetitive genome of *Trichomonas vaginalis*. *Genome Biol Evol* **9:**1658–1672.
74. **Hendrickx S, Guerin PJ, Caljon G, Croft SL, Maes L.** 2016. Evaluating drug resistance in visceral leishmaniasis: the challenges. *Parasitology* **145:**453–463.
75. **Vermeersch M, da Luz RI, Toté K, Timmermans J-P, Cos P, Maes L.** 2009. In vitro susceptibilities of *Leishmania donovani* promastigote and amastigote stages to antileishmanial reference drugs: practical relevance of stage-specific differences. *Antimicrob Agents Chemother* **53:**3855–3859.
76. **Kulshrestha A, Bhandari V, Mukhopadhyay R, Ramesh V, Sundar S, Maes L, Dujardin JC, Roy S, Salotra P.** 2013. Validation of a simple resazurin-based promastigote assay for the routine monitoring of miltefosine susceptibility in clinical isolates of *Leishmania donovani*. *Parasitol Res* **112:**825–828.
77. **Aït-Oudhia K, Gazanion E, Vergnes B, Oury B, Sereno D.** 2011. *Leishmania* antimony resistance: what we know what we can learn from the field. *Parasitol Res* **109:**1225–1232.
78. **Genetu Bayih A, Debnath A, Mitre E, Huston CD, Laleu B, Leroy D, Blasco B, Campo B, Wells TNC, Willis PA, Sjö P, Van Voorhis WC, Pillai DR.** 2017. Susceptibility testing of medically important parasites. *Clin Microbiol Rev* **30:**647–669.
79. **Mandal G, Mandal S, Sharma M, Charret KS, Papadopoulou B, Bhattacharjee H, Mukhopadhyay R.** 2015. Species-specific antimonial sensitivity in *Leishmania* is driven by post-transcriptional regulation of AQP1. *PLoS Negl Trop Dis* **9:**e0003500.
80. **Obonaga R, Fernández OL, Valderrama L, Rubiano LC, Castro MM, Barrera MC, Gomez MA, Gore Saravia N.** 2014. Treatment failure and miltefosine susceptibility in dermal leishmaniasis caused by *Leishmania* subgenus *Viannia* species. *Antimicrob Agents Chemother* **58:**144–152.
81. **Deep DK, Singh R, Bhandari V, Verma A, Sharma V, Wajid S, Sundar S, Ramesh V, Dujardin JC, Salotra P.** 2017. Increased miltefosine tolerance in clinical isolates of *Leishmania donovani* is associated with reduced drug accumulation, increased infectivity and resistance to oxidative stress. *PLoS Negl Trop Dis* **11:**e0005641.
82. **Zauli-Nascimento RC, Miguel DC, Yokoyama-Yasunaka JK, Pereira LI, Pelli de Oliveira MA, Ribeiro-Dias F, Dorta ML, Uliana SR.** 2010. In vitro sensitivity of *Leishmania (Viannia) braziliensis* and *Leishmania (Leishmania) amazonensis* Brazilian isolates to meglumine antimoniate and amphotericin B. *Trop Med Int Health* **15:**68–76.
83. **Varela-M RE, Villa-Pulgarin JA, Yepes E, Müller I, Modolell M, Muñoz DL, Robledo SM, Muskus CE, López-Abán J, Muro A, Vélez ID, Mollinedo F.** 2012. *In vitro* and *in vivo* efficacy of ether lipid edelfosine against *Leishmania spp*. and SbV-resistant parasites. *PLoS Negl Trop Dis* **6:**e1612.
84. **Ginouves M, Carme B, Couppie P, Prevot G.** 2014. Comparison of tetrazolium salt assays for evaluation of drug activity against *Leishmania spp*. *J Clin Microbiol* **52:**2131–2138.
85. **Fernández O, Diaz-Toro Y, Valderrama L, Ovalle C, Valderrama M, Castillo H, Perez M, Saravia NG.** 2012. Novel approach to in vitro drug susceptibility assessment of clinical strains of *Leishmania spp*. *J Clin Microbiol* **50:**2207–2211.
86. **Fernández OL, Diaz-Toro Y, Ovalle C, Valderrama L, Muvdi S, Rodríguez I, Gomez MA, Saravia NG.** 2014. Miltefosine and antimonial drug susceptibility of *Leishmania Viannia* species and populations in regions of high transmission in Colombia. *PLoS Negl Trop Dis* **8:**e2871. *CORRECTION PLoS Negl Trop Dis* **8:**e3026.
87. **Vanaerschot M, Decuypere S, Downing T, Imamura H, Stark O, De Doncker S, Roy S, Ostyn B, Maes L, Khanal B, Boelaert M, Schönian G, Berriman M, Chappuis F, Dujardin J-C, Sundar S, Rijal S.** 2012. Genetic markers for SSG resistance in *Leishmania donovani* and SSG treatment failure in visceral leishmaniasis patients of the Indian subcontinent. *J Infect Dis* **206:**752–755.
88. **Torres DC, Ribeiro-Alves M, Romero GAS, Dávila AMR, Cupolillo E.** 2013. Assessment of drug resistance related genes as candidate markers for treatment outcome prediction of cutaneous leishmaniasis in Brazil. *Acta Trop* **126:**132–141.
89. **Räz B, Iten M, Grether-Bühler Y, Kaminsky R, Brun R.** 1997. The Alamar Blue assay to determine drug sensitivity of African trypanosomes (T.b. rhodesiense and T.b. gambiense) in vitro. *Acta Trop* **68:**139–147.
90. **Kaminsky R, Zweygarth E.** 1989. Feeder layer-free in vitro assay for screening antitrypanosomal compounds against *Trypanosoma brucei brucei* and *T. b. evansi*. *Antimicrob Agents Chemother* **33:**881–885.
91. **Lim KT, Zahari Z, Amanah A, Zainuddin Z, Adenan MI.** 2016. Development of resazurin-based assay in 384-well format for high throughput whole cell screening of *Trypanosoma brucei rhodesiense* strain STIB 900 for the identification of potential anti-trypanosomal agents. *Exp Parasitol* **162:**49–56.
92. **Kazibwe AJ, Nerima B, de Koning HP, Mäser P, Barrett MP, Matovu E.** 2009. Genotypic status of the TbAT1/P2 adenosine transporter of *Trypanosoma brucei gambiense* isolates from Northwestern Uganda following melarsoprol withdrawal. *PLoS Negl Trop Dis* **3:**e523.

93. **Graf FE, Ludin P, Wenzler T, Kaiser M, Brun R, Pyana PP, Büscher P, de Koning HP, Horn D, Mäser P.** 2013. Aquaporin 2 mutations in *Trypanosoma brucei gambiense* field isolates correlate with decreased susceptibility to pentamidine and melarsoprol. *PLoS Negl Trop Dis* **7:**e2475.
94. **Pyana Pati P, Van Reet N, Mumba Ngoyi D, Ngay Lukusa I, Karhemere Bin Shamamba S, Büscher P.** 2014. Melarsoprol sensitivity profile of *Trypanosoma brucei gambiense* isolates from cured and relapsed sleeping sickness patients from the Democratic Republic of the Congo. *PLoS Negl Trop Dis* **8:**e3212.
95. **Munday JC, Settimo L, de Koning HP.** 2015. Transport proteins determine drug sensitivity and resistance in a protozoan parasite, *Trypanosoma brucei*. *Front Pharmacol* **6:**32.
96. **Pyana PP, Sere M, Kaboré J, De Meeûs T, MacLeod A, Bucheton B, Van Reet N, Büscher P, Belem AMG, Jamonneau V.** 2015. Population genetics of *Trypanosoma brucei gambiense* in sleeping sickness patients with treatment failures in the focus of Mbuji-Mayi, Democratic Republic of the Congo. *Infect Genet Evol* **30:**128–133.
97. **Richardson JB, Evans B, Pyana PP, Van Reet N, Sistrom M, Büscher P, Aksoy S, Caccone A.** 2016. Whole genome sequencing shows sleeping sickness relapse is due to parasite regrowth and not reinfection. *Evol Appl* **9:**381–393.
98. **Black CL, Steinauer ML, Mwinzi PNM, Evan Secor W, Karanja DMS, Colley DG.** 2009. Impact of intense, longitudinal retreatment with praziquantel on cure rates of *Schistosomiasis mansoni* in a cohort of occupationally exposed adults in western Kenya. *Trop Med Int Health* **14:**450–457.
99. **Guidi A, Andolina C, Makame Ame S, Albonico M, Cioli D, Juma Haji H.** 2010. Praziquantel efficacy and long-term appraisal of schistosomiasis control in Pemba Island. *Trop Med Int Health* **15:**614–618.
100. **Wang W, Dai J-R, Li H-J, Shen X-H, Liang Y-S.** 2010. Is there reduced susceptibility to praziquantel in *Schistosoma japonicum*? Evidence from China. *Parasitology* **137:** 1905–1912.
101. **Cioli D, Botros SS, Wheatcroft-Francklow K, Mbaye A, Southgate V, Tchuenté L-AT, Pica-Mattoccia L, Troiani AR, El-Din SHS, Sabra A-NA, Albin J, Engels D, Doenhoff MJ.** 2004. Determination of ED_{50} values for praziquantel in praziquantel-resistant and -susceptible *Schistosoma mansoni* isolates. *Int J Parasitol* **34:**979–987.
102. **Rinaldi G, Loukas A, Brindley PJ, Irelan JT, Smout MJ.** 2015. Viability of developmental stages of *Schistosoma mansoni* quantified with xCELLigence worm real-time motility assay (xWORM). *Int J Parasitol Drugs Drug Resist* **5:**141–148.
103. **Pica-Mattoccia L, Doenhoff MJ, Valle C, Basso A, Troiani A-R, Liberti P, Festucci A, Guidi A, Cioli D.** 2009. Genetic analysis of decreased praziquantel sensitivity in a laboratory strain of *Schistosoma mansoni*. *Acta Trop* **111:**82–85.
104. **Howe S, Zöphel D, Subbaraman H, Unger C, Held J, Engleitner T, Hoffmann WH, Kreidenweiss A.** 2015. Lactate as a novel quantitative measure of viability in *Schistosoma mansoni* drug sensitivity assays. *Antimicrob Agents Chemother* **59:**1193–1199.
105. **Liang YS, Coles GC, Doenhoff MJ, Southgate VR.** 2001. In vitro responses of praziquantel-resistant and -susceptible *Schistosoma mansoni* to praziquantel. *Int J Parasitol* **31:** 1227–1235.
106. **Lamberton PHL, Hogan SC, Kabatereine NB, Fenwick A, Webster JP.** 2010. *In vitro* praziquantel test capable of detecting reduced *in vivo* efficacy in *Schistosoma mansoni* human infections. *Am J Trop Med Hyg* **83:**1340–1347.
107. **Norton AJ, Gower CM, Lamberton PHL, Webster BL, Lwambo NJS, Blair L, Fenwick A, Webster JP.** 2010. Genetic consequences of mass human chemotherapy for *Schistosoma mansoni*: population structure pre- and post-praziquantel treatment in Tanzania. *Am J Trop Med Hyg* **83:**951–957.
108. **Huyse T, Van den Broeck F, Jombart T, Webster BL, Diaw O, Volckaert FAM, Balloux F, Rollinson D, Polman K.** 2013. Regular treatments of praziquantel do not impact on the genetic make-up of *Schistosoma mansoni* in northern Senegal. *Infect Genet Evol* **18:**100–105.

Author Index

Volume 1 comprises pages 1–1431; volume 2 comprises pages 1432–2690.

Subject Index

Volume 1 comprises pages 1–1431; volume 2 comprises pages 1432–2690.